16th Edition

HARRISON'S
PRINCIPLES OF
Internal
Medicine

16th Edition

HARRISON'S
PRINCIPLES OF
Internal
Medicine

Editors

DENNIS L. KASPER, MD

William Ellery Channing Professor of Medicine,
Professor of Microbiology and Molecular Genetics,
Harvard Medical School; Director, Channing
Laboratory, Department of Medicine, Brigham and
Women's Hospital, Boston

ANTHONY S. FAUCI, MD

Chief, Laboratory of Immunoregulation; Director,
National Institute of Allergy and Infectious Diseases,
National Institutes of Health, Bethesda

DAN L. LONGO, MD

Scientific Director, National Institute on Aging,
National Institutes of Health,
Bethesda and Baltimore

EUGENE BRAUNWALD, MD

Distinguished Hersey Professor of Medicine,
Harvard Medical School; Chairman, TIMI Study Group,
Brigham and Women's Hospital, Boston

STEPHEN L. HAUSER, MD

Robert A. Fishman Distinguished Professor and Chairman,
Department of Neurology,
University of California San Francisco, San Francisco

J. LARRY JAMESON, MD, PhD

Irving S. Cutter Professor and Chairman,
Department of Medicine,
Northwestern University Feinberg School of Medicine;
Physician-in-Chief, Northwestern
Memorial Hospital, Chicago

Volume II

McGraw-Hill
MEDICAL PUBLISHING DIVISION

New York   Chicago   San Francisco   Lisbon   London   Madrid
Mexico City   Milan   New Delhi   San Juan   Seoul   Singapore   Sydney   Toronto

Harrison's
PRINCIPLES OF INTERNAL MEDICINE
Sixteenth Edition

Copyright © 2005, 2001, 1998, 1994, 1991, 1987, 1983, 1980, 1977, 1974, 1970, 1966, 1962, 1958 by *The McGraw-Hill Companies, Inc.* All rights reserved. Printed in the United States of America. Except as permitted under the United States Copyright Act of 1976, no part of this publication may be reproduced or distributed in any form or by any means, or stored in a data base or retrieval system, without the prior written permission of the publisher.

234567890 DOWDOW 098765

ISBN 0-07-139140-1 (Set)
ISBN 0-07-139141-X (Vol. I)
ISBN 0-07-139142-8 (Vol. II)

ISBN 0-07-140235-7 (Combo)

FOREIGN LANGUAGE EDITIONS

Arabic (13e): McGraw-Hill Libri Italia srl (est. 1996)

Chinese Long Form (15e): McGraw-Hill International Enterprises, Inc., Taiwan

Chinese Short Form (15e): McGraw-Hill Education (Asia), Singapore

Croatian (13e): Placebo, Split, Croatia

French (15e): Medecine-Sciences Flammarion, Paris, France

German (15e): ABW Wissenschaftsverlagsgesellschaft mbH, Berlin, Germany

Greek (15e): Parissianos, S.A., Athens, Greece

Italian (15e): The McGraw-Hill Companies, Srl, Milan, Italy

Japanese (15e): MEDSI-Medical Sciences International Ltd, Tokyo, Japan

Korean (15e): McGraw-Hill Korea, Inc., Seoul, Korea

Polish (14e): Czelej Publishing Company, Lubin, Poland (est. 2000)

Portuguese (15e): McGraw-Hill Interamericana do Brazil, Rio de Janeiro, Brazil

Romanian (14e): Teora Publishers, Bucharest, Romania (est. 2000)

Serbian (15e): Publishing House Romanov, Bosnia & Herzegovina, Republic of Serbska

Spanish (15e): McGraw-Hill Interamericana de Espana S.A., Madrid, Spain

Turkish (15e): Nobel Tip Kitabevleri, Ltd., Istanbul, Turkey

Vietnamese (15e): McGraw-Hill Education (Asia), Singapore

This book was set in Times Roman by Progressive Information Technologies. The editors were Martin Wonsiewicz and Mariapaz Ramos Englis. The production director was Robert Laffler. The index was prepared by Barbara Littlewood. The text designer was Marsha Cohen/Parallelogram Graphics. Art director: Libby Pisacreta; cover design by Janice Bielawa. Medical illustrator: Jay McElroy, MAMS.

R. R. Donnelley and Sons, Inc., was the printer and binder.

Cover illustrations courtesy of Raymond J. Gibbons, MD; George V. Kelvin; Robert S. Hillman, MD; and Marilu Gorno-Tempini, MD.

Library of Congress Cataloging-in-Publication Data

Harrison's principles of internal medicine—16th ed./editors, Dennis L. Kasper . . . [et al.].   p. cm.
  Includes bibliographical references and index.
  ISBN 0-07-139140-1 (set)—ISBN 0-07-139141-X (v. 1)—ISBN 0-07-139142-8 (v. 2)—ISBN 0-07-140235-7 (combo)
    1. Internal medicine. I. Title: Principles of internal medicine. II. Kasper, Dennis L. III. Harrison, Tinsley Randolph, 1900– Principles of internal medicine.
  [DNLM: 1. Internal Medicine. WB 115 H322 2005]
  RC46.H333 2005
  616—dc21

2004044931

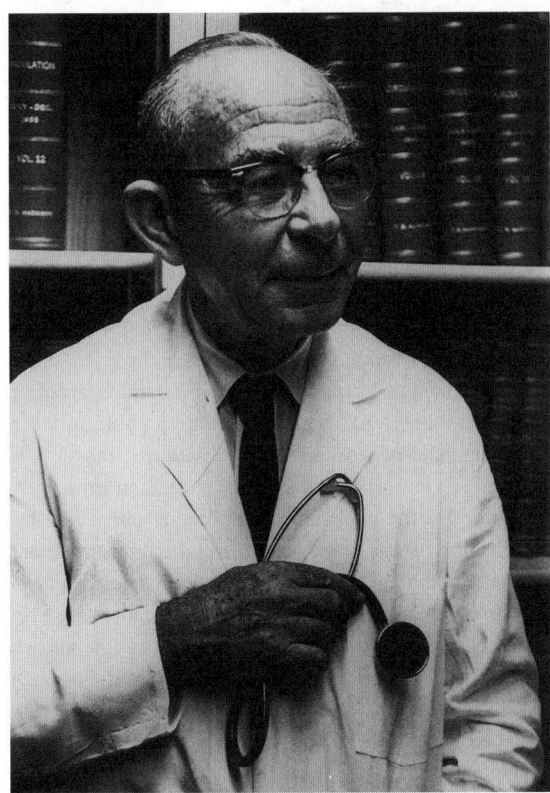

Tinsley R. Harrison

The 16th Edition of Harrison's Principles of Internal Medicine is dedicated to Tinsley R. Harrison, the founding editor and Editor-in-Chief for the first five editions.

From time to time a personality scintillates across the medical firmament who dazzles all beholders. Tinsley Harrison was such a person. A delightful, vivacious, passionate physician, he stimulated everyone with whom he came into contact, and he placed an indelible stamp on the medical events of his day.

Tinsley Randolph Harrison was born in Talladega, Alabama, on March 18, 1900. His father, Groce Harrison, was a sixth-generation physician, a student of William Osler who inculcated Osler's values into his son from an early age. Tinsley earned his undergraduate degree from the University of Michigan and his M.D. from Johns Hopkins School of Medicine. After a medical residency at the Peter Bent Brigham Hospital in Boston, where he developed his life-long interest in cardiovascular science and medicine, and additional training at Hopkins, Dr. Harrison served as chief medical resident and then joined the faculty of Vanderbilt University School of Medicine. His Chief of Medicine there, Canby Robinson, described him as "a human dynamo with unbounded energy." After a brief period of private practice, which Harrison later described as "perhaps the greatest educational experience of my entire life," he served successively as chair of medicine at Bowman-Gray School of Medicine, Winston-Salem, North Carolina; the Southwestern Medical School in Dallas, Texas; and the University of Alabama, Birmingham. He played a key role in organizing the Bowman-Gray and Southwestern medical schools. He also served as Dean of Southwestern and the University of Alabama and as Chief of Cardiology at the latter. Dr. Harrison died in Birmingham, on August 4, 1978.

For decades he was an active experimentalist, and his important contributions to the understanding of the pathophysiology of heart failure were all the more remarkable because they were obtained before the availability of measurements of intracardiac pressures, cardiac output, and regional blood flow. Harrison's research involved both basic studies in cardiovascular physiology as well as clinical research and were summarized in a classic text *Failure of the Circulation*. He was a founding member of the Council of the National Heart Institute and served as president of the American Society for Clinical Investigation and of the American Heart Association. Tinsley Harrison received the Gold Heart Award from the latter, the Kober Medal of the Association of American Physicians, and the Distinguished Teacher Award of the American College of Physicians. Few people of his generation surpassed him as a bedside teacher.

In 1945, stimulated by the publisher Blakiston, Harrison conceived of a new type of textbook of internal medicine, in which both of his interests—clinical medicine and the pathophysiologic mechanisms of disease—would be as closely interwoven as they were in his mind. He immediately recruited an editorial team; Harrison authored or co-authored almost the entire cardiovascular section. By 1950, the first edition of *Principles of Internal Medicine* was published.

Although Harrison was a distinguished investigator, teacher, academic leader, and editor, he was first and foremost a masterful physician who excelled in the care of the sick. The individual patient was always in the center of the stage. To put the disease first, to refer to the patient as "a case," would arouse Harrison's wrath. The words that he penned for the first edition of this book reflect the importance he attached to his role as a physician.

> *No greater opportunity or obligation can fall the lot of a human being than to be a physician. In the care of the suffering he needs technical skill, scientific knowledge, and human understanding. He who uses these with courage, humility, and wisdom will provide a unique service for his fellow man and will build an enduring edifice of character within himself. The physician should ask of his destiny no more than this, and he should be content with no less.*

These words express the philosophy of the original editors and of all those who have followed.

It is to the memory of this great physician, teacher, investigator, and editor, whose life and works have so inspired us, that this sixteenth edition of *Harrison's Principles of Internal Medicine* is dedicated.

THE EDITORS

CONTENTS

Part Fifteen
NEUROLOGIC DISORDERS

Part Sixteen
POISONING, DRUG OVERDOSE, AND ENVENOMATION

Numbers in brackets refer to chapters written or co-written by the contributor.

ELIAS ABRUTYN, MD
Professor of Medicine and Public Health, Associate Provost and Associate Dean for Faculty Affairs; Interim Chief, Infectious Diseases, Drexel University College of Medicine, Philadelphia [124,125]

JOHN C. ACHERMANN, MRCP, MRCPCH, MD
Wellcome Trust Clinician Scientist, Department of Medicine and Institute of Child Health, University College London, London, UK [328]

JOHN W. ADAMSON, MD
Executive Vice President for Research, Director, Blood Research Institute, Blood Center of Southeastern Wisconsin, Milwaukee [52, 90]

DAVID A. AHLQUIST, MD
Professor of Medicine, Mayo Clinic College of Medicine; Consultant in Gastroenterology, Division of Gastroenterology and Hepatology, Mayo Clinic, Rochester [35]

LEENA ALA-KOKKO, MD, PhD
Professor of Medicine, Center for Gene Therapy, Tulane University Health Sciences Center, New Orleans [342]

KENNETH C. ANDERSON, MD
Chief, Division of Hematologic Neoplasia; Director, Jerome Lipper Multiple Myeloma Center, Dana-Farber Cancer Institute; Kraft Family Professor of Medicine, Harvard Medical School, Boston [98, 99]

ELLIOTT M. ANTMAN, MD
Professor of Medicine, Harvard Medical School; Director, Samuel A. Levine Cardiac Unit, Brigham and Women's Hospital, Boston [228]

FREDERICK R. APPELBAUM, MD
Member and Director, Clinical Research Division, Fred Hutchinson Cancer Research Center; Professor and Head, Division of Medical Oncology, University of Washington School of Medicine, Seattle [100]

GORDON L. ARCHER, MD
Professor of Medicine and Microbiology/Immunology; Chair, Division of Infectious Diseases, Department of Medicine, Virginia Commonwealth University Medical Center, Richmond [118]

JAMES O. ARMITAGE, MD
Joe Shapiro Professor of Medicine, University of Nebraska, Omaha [97]

ARTHUR K. ASBURY, MD
Van Meter Professor of Neurology Emeritus, University of Pennsylvania School of Medicine, Philadelphia [22, 363, 365]

JOHN R. ASPLIN, MD
Assistant Professor of Medicine, Section of Nephrology, University of Chicago Pritzker School of Medicine, Chicago [265, 268]

JOHN C. ATHERTON, MD
Professor of Gastroenterology, Wolfson Digestive Diseases Centre and Institute of Infections, Immunity and Inflammation, University of Nottingham, Nottingham, England [135]

PAUL S. AUERBACH, MD, MS
Clinical Professor of Surgery, Department of Surgery, Division of Emergency Medicine, Stanford University School of Medicine, Los Altos [378]

K. FRANK AUSTEN, MD
AstraZeneca Professor of Respiratory and Inflammatory Diseases, Harvard Medical School; Director, Inflammation and Allergic Diseases Research Section, Division of Rheumatology, Immunology, and Allergy, Department of Medicine, Brigham and Women's Hospital, Boston [298]

BERNARD M. BABIOR, MD, PhD
Professor and Head, Division of Biochemistry, Department of Molecular and Experimental Medicine, The Scripps Research Institute, La Jolla [92]

LINDSEY R. BADEN, MD
Assistant Professor of Medicine, Harvard Medical School; Division of Infectious Diseases, Brigham and Women's Hospital, Boston [162]

KAMAL F. BADR, MD
Professor and Chair, Department of Internal Medicine, American University of Beirut (Lebanon); Attending Physician, American University of Beirut Medical Center, Beirut, Lebanon [267]

DONALD S. BAIM, MD
Professor of Medicine, Harvard Medical School; Director, Center for Integration of Medicine and Innovative Technology, Brigham and Women's Hospital, Boston [212, 229]

ROBERT L. BARBIERI, MD
Kate Macy Ladd Professor of Obstetrics, Gynecology, and Reproductive Biology, Harvard Medical School; Chairman, Obstetrics and Gynecology, Brigham and Women's Hospital, Boston [6]

TAMAR F. BARLAM, MD
Associate Professor of Medicine, Boston University School of Medicine, Boston [106, 131]

KENNETH J. BART, MD
Director, Graduate School of Public Health, Professor of Epidemiology and Biostatistics, San Diego State University, San Diego [107]

SHARI S. BASSUK, ScD
Epidemiologist, Division of Preventive Medicine, Brigham and Women's Hospital, Boston [327]

M. FLINT BEAL, MD
Anne Parrish Titzel Professor and Chair, Department of Neurology and Neuroscience, Weill Medical College of Cornell University; Neurologist-in-Chief, New York Presbyterian Hospital, New York [345, 355]

NICHOLAS J. BEECHING, FRCP, FRACP, DCH, DTM&H
Senior Lecturer in Infectious Diseases, Liverpool School of Tropical Medicine; Clinical Lead, Tropical and Infectious Disease Unit, Royal Liverpool University Hospital, Liverpool, United Kingdom [141]

ROBERT S. BENJAMIN, MD
Professor of Medicine, Chairman, Department of Sarcoma Medical Oncology, The University of Texas MD Anderson, Houston [84]

JOHN E. BENNETT, MD
Head, Clinical Mycology Section, Laboratory of Clinical Investigation, National Institute of Allergy and Infectious Diseases, National Institutes of Health, Potomac [182–190]

EDWARD J. BENZ, JR., MD
Richard and Susan Smith Professor of Medicine, Professor of Pediatrics, Professor of Pathology, Harvard Medical School; President and CEO, Dana-Farber Cancer Institute; Director, Dana-Farber/Harvard Cancer Center, Boston [91]

SHALENDAR BHASIN, MD
Professor of Medicine, University of California Los Angeles School of Medicine; Chief, Division of Endocrinology, Charles R. Drew University, Los Angeles [325]

DAVID R. BICKERS, MD
Carl Truman Nelson Professor and Chair, Department of Dermatology, College of Physicians and Surgeons, Columbia University Medical Center, New York [51]

HENRY J. BINDER, MD
Professor of Medicine, Professor of Cellular and Molecular Physiology, Yale University, New Haven [275]

THOMAS D. BIRD, MD
Professor of Neurology and Medicine, University of Washington; Veterans Affairs Puget Sound Medical Center, Seattle [350, 364]

NEIL R. BLACKLOW, MD
Chairman Emeritus, Department of Medicine, Professor of Medicine, University of Massachusetts Medical School, Worcester; Visiting Professor of Medicine, Harvard Medical School, Boston [168]

MARTIN J. BLASER, MD
Chairman, Department of Medicine, Frederick H. King Professor of Internal Medicine; Professor of Microbiology, New York University School of Medicine, New York [135, 139]

CLARA D. BLOOMFIELD, MD
William G. Pace III Professor of Cancer Research, Cancer Scholar and Senior Advisor, The Ohio State University Comprehensive Cancer and The Arthur G. James Cancer Hospital and Richard J. Solove Research Institute, Columbus [96]

RICHARD S. BLUMBERG, MD
Chief, Division of Gastroenterology, Hepatology, and Endoscopy, Brigham and Women's Hospital, Boston [276]

DAVID M. BODINE, PhD
Chief, Hematopoiesis Section, Genetics and Molecular Biology Branch, National Human Genome Research Institute, Bethesda [59]

JEAN L. BOLOGNIA, MD
Professor of Dermatology, Yale University School of Medicine, New Haven [48]

GEORGE J. BOSL, MD
Chairman, Department of Medicine, Memorial Sloan-Kettering Cancer Center; Professor of Medicine, Weill Medical College of Cornell University, New York [82]

RICHARD C. BOUCHER JR., MD
William Rand Kenan Professor of Medicine, University of North Carolina at Chapel Hill; Director, University of North Carolina Cystic Fibrosis Center, Chapel Hill [241]

KAREN D. BRADSHAW, MD
Professor of Obstetrics/Gynecology and Surgery, Helen J. and Robert S. Strauss and Diana K. and Richard C. Strauss Distinguished Professor in Women's Health, The University of Texas Southwestern Medical Center, Dallas [326]

HUGH R. BRADY, MD, PhD, FRCPI
Professor and Head, Department of Medicine and Therapeutics, University College Dublin, Dublin, Ireland [260, 264]

KENNETH D. BRANDT, MD
Professor of Medicine and Professor of Orthopaedic Surgery, Indiana University School of Medicine; Director, Indiana University Multipurpose Arthritis and Musculoskeletal Diseases Center, Indianapolis [312]

EUGENE BRAUNWALD, MD, MA(Hon), MD(Hon), ScD(Hon)
Distinguished Hersey Professor of Medicine, Harvard Medical School; Chairman, TIMI Study Group, Brigham and Women's Hospital, Boston [29, 31, 32, 208, 209, 215, 216, 219, 221, 222, 226–228]

IRWIN M. BRAVERMAN, MD
Professor of Dermatology, Yale University School of Medicine, New Haven [48]

OTIS W. BRAWLEY, MD
Professor of Hematology, Oncology, and Epidemiology, Emory University Medical School; Associate Director, Population Sciences and Cancer Control Program, Winship Cancer Institute, Atlanta [67]

JOEL G. BREMAN, MD, DTPH
Senior Scientific Advisor, Fogarty International Center, National Institutes of Health, Bethesda [195]

BARRY M. BRENNER, MD, DSc(Hon), DMSc(Hon)
Samuel A. Levine Professor of Medicine, Harvard Medical School; Director Emeritus, Renal Division, Brigham and Women's Hospital, Boston [40, 41, 259–262, 264, 266, 267, 270]

ROBERT M. BRENNER, MD
Associate Medical Director, Clinical Research, Amgen In., Thousand Oaks, California [259]

GEORGE J. BREWER, MD
Morton S. and Henrietta K. Sellner Active Emeritus Professor of Human Genetics, Active Emeritus Professor of Internal Medicine, University of Michigan Medical School, Ann Arbor [339]

F. RICHARD BRINGHURST, MD
Associate Professor of Medicine, Harvard Medical School, Boston [331]

CLAIRE V. BROOME, MD
Senior Advisor, Centers for Disease Control and Prevention, Atlanta [123]

ROBERT H. BROWN, JR., MD, DPHil
Associate Neurologist, Massachusetts General Hospital; Professor of Neurology, Harvard Medical School, Boston [353, 368]

GREGORY BULKLEY, MD
Mark M. Ravitch Professor of Surgery, The Johns Hopkins University School of Medicine, Baltimore [279]

H. FRANKLIN BUNN, MD
Professor of Medicine, Harvard Medical School, Boston [92, 93]

DAVID M. BURNS, MD
Professor of Family and Preventive Medicine, Professor of Medicine, University of California San Diego, San Diego [375]

MICHAEL J. BURNS, MD
Assistant Professor of Medicine, Harvard Medical School, Boston [377]

JOAN R. BUTTERTON, MD, DTM&H
Assistant Professor of Medicine, Harvard Medical School; Assistant in Medicine, Infectious Disease Division, Massachusetts General Hospital, Boston [113]

JOHN C. BYRD, MD
D. Warren Brown Professor of Leukemia Research, Associate Professor of Medicine and Medical Chemistry, The Ohio State University; Director of Hematologic Malignancies, Division of Hematology and Oncology, James Cancer Hospital and Solove Research Institute, Columbus [96]

STEPHEN B. CALDERWOOD, MD
Chief, Division of Infectious Diseases, Massachusetts General Hospital; Professor of Medicine (Microbiology and Molecular Genetics), Harvard Medical School, Boston [113]

MICHAEL V. CALLAHAN, MD, MSPH, DTM&H
Program Leader, Biological Threat Defense, Center for Integration of Medicine and Innovative Technologies, Massachusetts General Hospital, Boston [18]

MICHAEL CAMILLERI, MD
Atherton and Winifred W. Bean Professor, Professor of Medicine and Physiology, Mayo Clinic College of Medicine; Consultant in Gastroenterology, Mayo Clinic, Rochester [35]

G. DOUGLAS CAMPBELL, MD
Professor of Medicine, Director, Division of Pulmonary, Critical Care, and Sleep Medicine, University of Mississippi School of Medicine, Jackson [239]

GRANT L. CAMPBELL, MD, PhD
Chief, Epidemiology Activity, Arbovirus Diseases Branch, Division of Vector-Borne Infectious Diseases, National Center for Infectious Diseases, Centers for Disease Control and Prevention, Fort Collins [143]

CHRISTOPHER P. CANNON, MD
Associate Professor of Medicine, Harvard Medical School; Senior Investigator, TIMI Study Group, Cardiovascular Division, Brigham and Women's Hospital, Boston [227]

MARK D. CARLSON, MD
Professor of Medicine, Associate Vice President for Government Relations, Case Western Reserve University; Associate Dean, Case School of Medicine, Cleveland [20]

CHARLES B. CARPENTER, MD
Professor of Medicine, Harvard Medical School; Senior Physician, Brigham and Women's Hospital, Boston [263]

BRUCE R. CARR, MD
Professor and Director, Division of Reproductive Endocrinology and Infertility; Holder, Paul C. MacDonald Distinguished Chair in Obstetrics and Gynecology, The University of Texas Southwestern Medical Center, Dallas [326]

AGUSTIN CASTELLANOS, MD
Professor of Medicine; Director, Clinical Electrophysiology, University of Miami School of Medicine, Miami [256]

PHILIP F. CHANCE, MD
Professor of Pediatrics and Neurology, University of Washington School of Medicine; Chief, Division of Genetics and Development, Children's Hospital and Regional Medical Center, Seattle [364]

FENG-YEE CHANG, MD
Professor, Department of Medicine, National Defense Medical Center; Chief, Division of Infectious Diseases and Tropical Medicine, Department of Internal Medicine, Tri-Service General Hospital, Taipei, Taiwan [132]

YUAN-TSONG CHEN, MD, PhD
Professor and Chief, Division of Medical Genetics, Duke University Medical Center; Director, Institute of Biomedical Sciences, Durham [341]

JOHN S. CHILD, MD
Streisand Professor of Medicine/Cardiology; Co-Chief, Division of Cardiology, David Geffen School of Medicine at UCLA; Director, Ahmanson/UCLA Adult Congenital Heart Disease Center, UCLA Medical Center, Los Angeles [218]

KATARINA G. CHILLER, MD
Assistant Professor, Department of Dermatology, Emory University, Atlanta [73]

OLIVIER M. CHOSIDOW, MD, PhD
Department of Internal Medicine, Hôpital Pitié-Salpêtrière, Paris, France [50]

RAYMOND T. CHUNG, MD
Assistant Professor of Medicine, Harvard Medical School; Director, Hepatology Source, Medical Director, Lung Transplant Program, Associate Physician, Massachusetts General Hospital, Boston [289]

FREDRIC L. COE, MD
Professor of Medicine and Physiology, University of Chicago Pritzker School of Medicine, Chicago [265, 268]

ALAN S. COHEN, MD
Distinguished Professor of Medicine in Rheumatology, Emeritus, Boston University School of Medicine, Boston [310]

JEFFREY I. COHEN, MD
Head, Medical Virology Section, Laboratory of Infectious Diseases, National Institute of Allergy and Infectious Diseases, National Institutes of Health, Bethesda [165, 175]

FRANCIS S. COLLINS, MD, PhD
Director, National Human Genome Research Institute, National Institutes of Health, Bethesda [68]

WILSON S. COLUCCI, MD, FACC, FAHA
Thomas J. Ryan Professor of Medicine, Boston University School of Medicine; Chief, Cardiovascular Medicine, Boston University Medical Center, Boston [223]

JOEL D. COOPER, MD
Evarts A. Graham Professor of Surgery, Department of Surgery, Division of Cardiothoracic Surgery, Washington University School of Medicine, St. Louis [248]

MAX D. COOPER, MD
Professor of Medicine, Pediatrics, and Microbiology; Howard Hughes Medical Institute Investigator, University of Alabama at Birmingham, Birmingham [297]

MICHAEL J. CORBEL, PhD, DSc(Med), FIBiol, FRCPath
Head, Division of Bacteriology, National Institute for Biological Standards and Control, Potters Bar, United Kingdom [141]

LAWRENCE COREY, MD
Professor, Medicine and Laboratory Medicine; Head, Virology Division, University of Washington; Head, Program in Infectious Diseases, Fred Hutchinson Cancer Research Center, Seattle [163, 179]

FELICIA COSMAN, MD
Associate Professor of Clinical Medicine, Columbia University College of Physicians and Surgeons; Medical Director, Clinical Research Center, Helen Hayes Hospital, West Haverstraw, New York [333]

MARK A. CREAGER, MD
Professor of Medicine, Harvard Medical School; Physician, Brigham and Women's Hospital, Boston [231, 232]

PHILIP E. CRYER, MD
Irene E. and Michael M. Karl Professor of Endocrinology and Metabolism in Medicine, Washington University School of Medicine, St. Louis [324]

RONALD G. CRYSTAL, MD
Professor and Chair, Department of Genetic Medicine, Weill Medical College of Cornell University; Chief, Division of Pulmonary and Critical Care Medicine, New York Presbyterian Hospital-Weill Cornell Medical Center, New York [309]

JOHN J. CUSH, MD
Medical Director, Arthritis Center, Presbyterian Hospital of Dallas, Dallas [311]

CHARLES A. CZEISLER, MD, PhD
Professor of Medicine, Harvard Medical School; Chief, Division of Sleep Medicine; Director, Sleep Disorders and Circadian Medicine, Brigham and Women's Hospital, Boston [24]

MARINOS C. DALAKAS, MD
Professor of Neurology; Chief, Neuromuscular Diseases Section, National Institute of Neurological Disorders and Stroke, National Institutes of Health, Bethesda [369]

JOSEP DALMAU, MD, PhD
Associate Professor of Neurology, Department of Neurology, University of Pennsylvania, Philadelphia [87]

DANIEL F. DANZL, MD
Professor and Chair, Department of Emergency Medicine, University of Louisville School of Medicine, Louisville [19]

ROBERT B. DAROFF, MD
Professor of Neurology and Associate Dean, Case Western Reserve University School of Medicine, Cleveland [20]

CHARLES E. DAVIS, MD
Professor of Pathology and Medicine Emeritus, University of California San Diego School of Medicine; Director Emeritus, Microbiology Laboratory, University of California San Diego Medical Center, San Diego [192]

STEVEN R. DEITCHER, MD
Head, Section of Hematology and Coagulation Medicine, Department of Hematology-Medical Oncology, The Cleveland Clinic Foundation, Cleveland [103]

JOHN DEL VALLE, MD
Professor and Senior Associate Chair of Medicine, Graduate Medical Education, Department of Internal Medicine, University of Michigan Health System, Ann Arbor [274]

MAHLON R. DELONG, MD
Timmie Professor of Neurology; Director of Neuroscience, Emory University School of Medicine, Atlanta [351]

MARIE B. DEMAY, MD
Associate Professor of Medicine, Harvard Medical School, Boston [331]

BRADLEY M. DENKER, MD
Assistant Professor of Medicine, Harvard Medical School; Associate Physician, Brigham and Women's Hospital, Boston [40]

DAVID T. DENNIS, MD, MPH
Faculty Affiliate, Department of Microbiology, Colorado State University; Medical Epidemiologist, Division of Vector-Borne Infectious Diseases, Centers for Disease Control and Prevention, Fort Collins [143, 156]

ROBERT J. DESNICK, MD, PhD
Professor and Chair, Department of Human Genetics, Mount Sinai School of Medicine of New York University, New York [337]

BETTY DIAMOND, MD
Chief, Division of Rheumatology, Department of Microbiology and Immunology, Albert Einstein College of Medicine, New York [299]

JULES L. DIENSTAG, MD
Professor of Medicine, Harvard Medical School; Physician, Massachusetts General Hospital, Boston [78, 285–287, 291]

WILLIAM P. DILLON, MD
Professor of Radiology, Section Chief, Neuroradiology, Vice-Chair for Research Radiology, University of California San Francisco, San Francisco [347]

CHARLES A. DINARELLO, MD
Professor of Medicine, University of Colorado Health Sciences Center, Denver [16]

ROBERT G. DLUHY, MD
Professor of Medicine, Harvard Medical School, Brigham and Women's Hospital, Boston [321]

RAPHAEL DOLIN, MD
Maxwell Finland Professor of Medicine (Microbiology and Molecular Genetics); Dean for Academic and Clinical Programs, Harvard Medical School, Boston [162, 170, 171]

DAVID M. DOSA, MD, MPH
Assistant Professor of Medicine, Brown Medical School; Division of Geriatrics, Rhode Island Hospital, Providence [8]

DANIEL B. DRACHMAN, MD
Professor of Neurology and Neuroscience; WW Smith Charitable Foundation Professor of Neuroimmunology; Director, Neuromuscular Unit, The Johns Hopkins University School of Medicine, Baltimore [366]

JEFFREY M. DRAZEN, MD
Professor of Medicine, Harvard Medical School, Boston [233–235, 252]

THOMAS D. DUBOSE, JR., MD
Professor and Chair, Department of Internal Medicine, Professor, Department of Physiology and Pharmacology, Wake Forest University School of Medicine, Winston-Salem [42]

J. STEPHEN DUMLER, MD
Professor, Division of Medical Microbiology, Department of Pathology and the Program in Cellular and Molecular Medicine, The Johns Hopkins University School of Medicine; Department of Molecular Microbiology and Immunology, The Johns Hopkins University Bloomberg School of Public Health, Baltimore [158]

ANDREA E. DUNAIF, MD
Charles F. Kettering Professor of Medicine, Northwestern University Feinberg School of Medicine; Chief, Division of Endocrinology, Metabolism and Molecular Medicine, Northwestern University, Chicago [5]

SAMUEL C. DURSO, MD
Associate Professor of Medicine, Division of Geriatric Medicine and Gerontology, The Johns Hopkins University School of Medicine; Deputy Director of Education, Co-Director Fellowship Training Program, Director of Ambulatory Clinical Services, Baltimore [28]

JANICE P. DUTCHER, MD
Professor of Medicine, New York Medical College; Associate Director, Clinical Affairs, Our Lady of Mercy Cancer Center, Bronx [88]

JOHANNA T. DWYER, DSc
Professor of Medicine and Community Health, Tufts University School of Medicine and Friedman School of Nutrition; Director, Frances Stern Nutrition Center; Tufts-New England Medical Center Senior Scientist; Nutritional Epidemiology Program, Jean Mayer USDA Human Nutrition Center on Aging at Tufts, Boston [60]

VICTOR J. DZAU, MD
Hersey Professor of Medicine, Harvard Medical School; Chairman, Department of Medicine and Director of Research, Brigham and Women's Hospital, Boston [231, 232]

JEFFERY S. DZIECZKOWSKI, MD
Physician, New Britain General Hospital, New Britain [99]

J. DONALD EASTON, MD
Professor and Chair, Department of Clinical Neurosciences, Brown Medical School and Rhode Island Hospital, Providence [349]

DAVID A. EHRMANN, MD
Associate Professor, Section of Endocrinology, Department of Medicine, University of Chicago Pritzker School of Medicine, Chicago [44]

EZEKIEL J. EMANUEL, MD, PhD
Chief, Department of Clinical Bioethics, Warren G. Magnuson Clinical Center, National Institutes of Health, Bethesda [9]

LINDA L. EMANUEL, MD
Buehler Professor of Geriatric Medicine, Director, Buehler Center on Aging, Northwestern University School of Medicine, Chicago [9]

JOHN W. ENGSTROM, MD
Professor of Neurology; Vice Chairman, Residency Program Director, University of California San Francisco, San Francisco [15, 354]

ANTHONY S. FAUCI, MD
Chief, Laboratory of Immunoregulation; Director, National Institute of Allergy and Infectious Diseases, National Institutes of Health, Bethesda [172, 173, 205, 295, 306]

MURRAY J. FAVUS, MD
Professor of Medicine, University of Chicago Pritzker School of Medicine, Division of Biological Sciences, Chicago [268, 334]

ROBERT G. FENTON, MD, PhD
Associate Professor of Medicine, University of Maryland Greenebaum Cancer Center, Baltimore [69]

HOWARD L. FIELDS, MD, PhD
Professor of Neurology and Physiology, University of California San Francisco, San Francisco [11]

GREGORY A. FILICE, MD
Chief, Infectious Disease Section, Veterans Affairs Medical Center; Associate Professor, Department of Medicine, University of Minnesota, Minneapolis [146]

ROBERT W. FINBERG, MD
Professor and Chair, Department of Medicine, University of Massachusetts Medical School, Worcester [72, 117]

JOYCE D. FINGEROTH, MD
Assistant Professor of Medicine, Harvard Medical School; Division of Infectious Diseases, Beth Israel Deaconess Medical Center, Boston [117]

NAOMI D.L. FISHER, MD
Assistant Professor, Harvard Medical School; Director, Hypertension Service, Brigham and Women's Hospital, Boston [230]

JEFFREY S. FLIER, MD
Chief Academic Officer, Beth Israel Deaconess Medical Center; George C. Reisman Professor of Medicine, Harvard Medical School, Boston [64]

SONIA FRIEDMAN, MD
Instructor of Medicine, Harvard Medical School; Associate Physician, Brigham and Women's Hospital, Boston [276]

WILLIAM F. FRIEDMAN, MD
JH Nicholson Professor of Pediatrics (Cardiology); Senior Associate Dean for Academic Affairs, David Geffen School of Medicine at UCLA, Los Angeles [218]

ROBERT F. GAGEL, MD
Professor of Medicine and Head, Division of Internal Medicine, University of Texas MD Anderson Cancer Center, Houston [330]

JOHN I. GALLIN, MD
Director, NIH Warren Grant G. Magnuson Clinical Center; NIH Associate Director for Clinical Research; Chief Laboratory of Host Defenses, National Institute of Allergy and Infectious Diseases, National Institutes of Health, Bethesda [55]

SUSAN L. GEARHART, MD
Assistant Professor of Surgery, The Johns Hopkins University School of Medicine, Baltimore [279]

ROBERT H. GELBER, MD
Leonard Wood Memorial Scientific Director, American Leprosy Foundation; Clinical Professor of Medicine and Dermatology, University of California San Francisco, San Francisco [151]

JEFFREY A. GELFAND, MD
Visiting Professor of Medicine, Harvard Medical School; Professor of Medicine, Tufts University School of Medicine; Physician, Infectious Diseases Unit, Department of Medicine, Massachusetts General Hospital, Boston [16, 18]

DALE N. GERDING, MD
Chief, Medical Service, VA Chicago Health Care System—Lakeside Division; Professor and Associate Chairman, Department of Medicine, The Feinberg School of Medicine, Northwestern University, Chicago [114]

ANNE A. GERSHON, MD
Professor of Pediatrics; Director, Division of Pediatric Infectious Diseases, Columbia University Medical Center, New York [176–178]

MARC GHANY, MD
Medical Staff Fellow, Liver Diseases Section, Digestive Diseases Branch, National Institute of Diabetes and Digestive and Kidney Diseases, National Institutes of Health, Bethesda [282]

RAYMOND J. GIBBONS, MD
Arthur M. and Gladys D. Gray Professor of Medicine, Mayo Clinic College of Medicine, Rochester [211]

BRUCE C. GILLILAND, MD
Professor of Medicine and Laboratory Medicine, University of Washington School of Medicine, Seattle [303, 308, 315, 316]

ROGER I. GLASS, MD, PhD
Viral Gastroenteritis Section, Centers for Disease Control and Prevention, Atlanta [174]

ELI GLATSTEIN, MD
Morton M. Kligerman Professor and Vice Chairman, Clinical Director, Department of Radiation Oncology, University of Pennsylvania Medical Center, Philadelphia [71, 207]

ROBERT M. GLICKMAN, MD
Professor of Medicine and Dean, New York University School of Medicine; CEO New York University Hospitals Center, New York [39]

JAMES F. GLOCKNER, MD
Assistant Professor of Radiology, Mayo Clinic College of Medicine; Consultant, Department of Radiology, Mayo Clinic, Rochester [211]

ARY L. GOLDBERGER, MD
Associate Professor of Medicine, Harvard Medical School; Director, Margret and H.A. Rey Institute for Nonlinear Dynamics in Medicine, Beth Israel Deaconess Medical Center, Boston [210]

SAMUEL Z. GOLDHABER, MD
Associate Professor of Medicine, Harvard Medical School; Director, Venous Thromboembolism Research Group, Director, Anticoagulation Service and Staff Cardiologist, Brigham and Women's Hospital, Boston [244]

RALPH GONZALES, MD, MSPH
Associate Professor of Medicine, Epidemiology and Biostatistics, University of California San Francisco, San Francisco [27]

DOUGLAS S. GOODIN, MD
Professor of Neurology, University of California San Francisco, San Francisco [359]

RAJ K. GOYAL, MD
Mallinckrodt Professor of Medicine, Harvard Medical School, Boston [33, 273]

GREGORY A. GRABOWSKI, MD
Director, Division and Program in Human Genetics, Cincinnati Children's Hospital Research Foundation; Professor, Department of Pediatrics, and Molecular Genetics and Biochemistry, University of Cincinnati College of Medicine, Cincinnati [340]

JACOB GREEN, MD
Associate Professor of Medicine, Department of Nephrology, Technion Faculty of Medicine, Haifa, Israel [261]

NORTON J. GREENBERGER, MD
Professor of Medicine, Harvard Medical School; Senior Physician, Brigham and Women's Hospital, Boston [292–294]

DAVID E. GRIFFITH, MD
Director of Tuberculosis Services and Professor of Medicine, University of Texas Health Center, Tyler [149]

WILLIAM GROSSMAN, MD
Myer Friedman Distinguished Professor of Medicine, University of California San Francisco; Chief of Cardiology, University of California San Francisco Medical Center, San Francisco [212]

RASIM GUCALP, MD
Associate Professor of Medicine, Department of Oncology, Montefiore Medical Center, Albert Einstein College of Medicine, New York [88]

BEVRA HANNAHS HAHN, MD
Professor of Medicine, David Geffen School of Medicine at the University of California Los Angeles, Los Angeles [300]

STEPHEN M. HAHN, MD
Associate Professor, Department of Radiation Oncology, Division of Hematology Oncology, University of Pennsylvania, Philadelphia [71]

JANET E. HALL, MD
Associate Professor of Medicine, Harvard Medical School; Assistant Physician, Massachusetts General Hospital, Boston [45]

JESSE B. HALL, MD
Section Chief, Pulmonary and Critical Care Medicine; Professor of Medicine, Anesthesia and Critical Care, University of Chicago, Chicago [249]

SCOTT A. HALPERIN, MD
Professor of Pediatrics; Associate Professor of Microbiology and Immunology, Dalhousie University, Halifax, Nova Scotia, Canada [133]

CHARLES H. HALSTED, MD
Professor of Internal Medicine and Nutrition, University of California-Davis School of Medicine, Davis [62]

ROBERT I. HANDIN, MD
Professor of Medicine, Harvard Medical School, Boston [53, 101, 102]

CATHLEEN A. HANLON, VMD, PhD
Veterinary Medical Officer, Rabies Section, Centers for Disease Control and Prevention, Atlanta [179]

GAVIN HART, MD, MPH
Director, STD Services, Royal Adelaide Hospital; Clinical Associate Professor, School of Medicine, Flinders University, Adelaide, South Australia, Australia [145]

WILLIAM L. HASLER, MD
Associate Professor of Internal Medicine, Division of Gastroenterology, University of Michigan Medical Center, Ann Arbor [34, 271]

TERRY J. HASSOLD, PhD
Professor of Genetics, Case Western Reserve University School of Medicine, Cleveland [57]

STEPHEN L. HAUSER, MD
Robert A. Fishman Distinguished Professor and Chairman, Department of Neurology, University of California San Francisco, San Francisco [345, 346, 355, 356, 365]

EDWARD B. HAYES, MD
Medical Epidemiologist, Division of Vector-Borne Infectious Diseases, Centers for Disease Control and Prevention, Fort Collins [156]

BARTON F. HAYNES, MD
Frederic M. Hanes Professor of Medicine, Professor of Immunology, Duke University School of Medicine, Durham [295]

J. CLAUDE HEMPHILL III, MD
Assistant Professor of Neurology, University of California San Francisco; Director, Neurovascular and Neurocritical Care Program, San Francisco General Hospital, San Francisco [258]

PATRICK H. HENRY, MD
Principal Investigator, St. Louis-Cape Girardeau Community Clinical Oncology Program, St. Louis [54]

BARBARA L. HERWALDT, MD, MPH
Medical Epidemiologist, Division of Parasitic Diseases, Centers for Disease Control and Prevention, Atlanta [196]

MARTIN S. HIRSCH, MD
Professor of Medicine, Harvard Medical School; Professor of Immunology and Infectious Diseases, Harvard School of Public Health; Director of Clinical AIDS Research, Massachusetts General Hospital, Boston [166]

HELEN HASKELL HOBBS, MD
Investigator, Howard Hughes Medical Institute; Professor of Internal Medicine and Molecular Genetics, University of Texas Southwestern Medical Center, Dallas [335]

JUDITH S. HOCHMAN, MD, FACC
Harold Snyder Family Professor of Cardiology; Clinical Chief, Division of Cardiology; Director, Cardiovascular Clinical Research, New York University School of Medicine, New York [255]

STEVEN M. HOLLAND, MD
Senior Investigator and Head, Immunopathogenesis Unit, Clinical Pathophysiology Section, Laboratory of Host Defenses, National Institute of Allergy and Infectious Diseases, National Institute of Health, Bethesda [55]

KING K. HOLMES, MD, PhD
Professor of Medicine; Director, Center for AIDS and Sexually Transmitted Diseases, University of Washington, Seattle [115]

RANDALL K. HOLMES, MD, PhD
Professor and Chair, Department of Microbiology, University of Colorado Health Sciences Center, Denver [122]

JAY H. HOOFNAGLE, MD
Director, Liver Disease Research Branch, Division of Digestive Diseases and Nutrition, National Institute of Diabetes and Digestive and Kidney Diseases, National Institutes of Health, Bethesda [282]

ROBERT J. HOPKIN, MD
Assistant Professor of Clinical Pediatrics, The University of Cincinnati College of Medicine; Division and Program in Human Genetics, Cincinnati Children's Hospital Research Foundation, Cincinnati [340]

JONATHAN C. HORTON, MD, PhD
William F. Hoyt Professor of Neuro-Ophthalmology, Departments of Ophthalmology, Neurology, and Physiology, University of California San Francisco, San Francisco [25]

LYN HOWARD, MB, FRCP
Emeritus Professor of Medicine, Associate Professor of Pediatrics, Albany Medical College, Albany [63]

HOWARD HU, MD, MPH, ScD
Professor of Occupational and Environmental Medicine, Department of Environmental Health, Harvard School of Public Health; Associate Physician Channing Laboratory, Department of Medicine, Brigham and Women's Hospital; Associate Professor of Medicine, Harvard Medical School, Boston [376]

GARY W. HUNNINGHAKE, MD
Sterba Professor of Medicine, Director, Division of Pulmonary Critical Care and Occupational Medicine; Director, Graduate Program in Translational Biomedical Research, University of Iowa College of Medicine, Iowa City [237]

SHARON A. HUNT, MD
Professor, Division of Cardiovascular Medicine, Stanford University, Stanford [217]

CHARLES G. HURST, MD
Chief, Chemical Casualty Care Division, US Army Medical Research Institute of Chemical Defense, Maryland [206]

DAVID H. INGBAR, MD
Professor, Medicine Physiology and Pediatrics; Director, Pulmonary Allergy and Critical Care Division, University of Minnesota, Minneapolis [255]

EDWARD P. INGENITO, MD, PhD
Associate Physician, Brigham and Women's Hospital; Adjunct Assistant Professor, Harvard Medical School, Boston [250, 252]

ROLAND H. INGRAM, JR., MD
Martha West Looney Professor Emeritus, Emory University School of Medicine, Atlanta [29]

MARK A. ISRAEL, MD
Professor of Pediatrics and Genetics, Dartmouth Medical School; Director, Norris Cotton Cancer Center, Dartmouth–Hitchcock Medical Center, Lebanon [358]

KURT J. ISSELBACHER, MD
Distinguished Mallinckrodt Professor of Medicine, Harvard Medical School; Physician and Director, Massachusetts General Hospital Cancer Center, Boston [78, 285–287]

RICHARD F. JACOBS, MD
Horace C. Cabe Professor of Pediatrics, University of Arkansas for Medical Sciences College of Medicine; Chief, Pediatric Infectious Diseases, Arkansas Children's Hospital, Little Rock [142]

J. LARRY JAMESON, MD, PhD
Irving S. Cutter Professor and Chair, Department of Medicine, Northwestern University Feinberg School of Medicine; Physician-in-Chief, Northwestern Memorial Hospital, Chicago [56, 58, 59, 86, 317, 318, 320, 325, 328]

JAMES L. JANUZZI, JR., MD
Assistant Professor of Medicine, Harvard Medical School; Assistant Physician, Division of Cardiology and Department of Medicine, Massachusetts General Hospital, Boston [Appendices]

ROBERT T. JENSEN, MD
Chief, Digestive Diseases Branch, National Institute of Diabetes and Digestive and Kidney Diseases, National Institutes of Health, Bethesda [329]

BRUCE E. JOHNSON, MD
Associate Professor of Medicine, Brigham and Women's Hospital and Harvard Medical School; Program Director, Lowe Center for Thoracic Oncology, Dana-Farber Cancer Institute, Boston [86]

STUART JOHNSON, MD
Attending Physician, Hines VA Hospital; Associate Professor, Department of Medicine, Stritch School of Medicine, Loyola University, Maywood, IL [114]

S. CLAIBORNE JOHNSTON, MD, PhD
Associate Professor of Neurology and Epidemiology; Director, Stroke Service, University of California San Francisco, San Francisco [349]

MARK E. JOSEPHSON, MD
Professor of Medicine, Harvard Medical School; Chief, Cardiovascular Division, Beth Israel Deaconess Medical Center; Director, Harvard-Thorndike Electrophysiology Institute and Arrhythmia Service, Boston [213, 214]

JORGE L. JUNCOS, MD
Associate Professor of Neurology, Emory University School of Medicine; Director of Neurology, Wesley Woods Hospital, Atlanta [351]

EDWARD L. KAPLAN, MD
Professor of Pediatrics, University of Minnesota Medical School, Minneapolis [302]

MARSHALL M. KAPLAN, MD
Professor of Medicine, Tufts University School of Medicine, Boston [38, 283]

ADOLF W. KARCHMER, MD
Professor of Medicine, Harvard Medical School; Chief, Division of Infectious Diseases, Beth Israel Deaconess Medical Center, Boston [109]

DENNIS L. KASPER, MD, MA(Hon)
William Ellery Channing Professor of Medicine, Professor of Microbiology and Molecular Genetics, Harvard Medical School; Director, Channing Laboratory, Department of Medicine, Brigham and Women's Hospital, Boston [104, 106, 112, 126, 131, 148]

LLOYD H. KASPER, MD
Professor of Medicine (Neurology) and Microbiology/Immunology; Director, Multiple Sclerosis Center, Dartmouth Medical School, Lebanon [198]

DANIEL L. KASTNER, MD, PhD
Chief, Genetics and Genomics Branch, National Institute of Arthritis and Musculoskeletal and Skin Diseases, National Institutes of Health, Bethesda [278]

ELAINE T. KAYE, MD
Clinical Instructor in Dermatology, Harvard Medical School; Assistant in Medicine, Department of Medicine, Children's Hospital Medical Center, Boston [17]

KENNETH M. KAYE, MD
Assistant Professor of Medicine, Harvard Medical School; Associate Physician, Division of Infectious Diseases, Brigham and Women's Hospital, Boston [17]

GERALD T. KEUSCH, MD
Assistant Provost and Associate Dean for Global Health; Professor of Medicine and International Health, Boston University Medical Campus and School of Public Health, Boston [107, 138, 140]

JAY S. KEYSTONE, MD, MSC(CTM), FRCPC
Professor of Medicine, University of Toronto; Tropical Disease Unit, Division of Infectious Disease, Toronto General Hospital, University Health Network, Toronto, Ontario, Canada [108]

ELLIOTT KIEFF, MD, PhD
Harriet Ryan Albee Professor of Medicine and Microbiology and Molecular Genetics, Harvard Medical School; Senior Physician, Brigham and Women's Hospital, Boston [161]

TALMADGE E. KING, JR., MD
The Constance B. Wofsy Distinguished Professor and Vice Chairman, Department of Medicine, University of California San Francisco; Chief, Medical Services, San Francisco General Hospital, San Francisco [243]

LOUIS V. KIRCHHOFF, MD, MPH
Professor, Departments of Internal Medicine and Epidemiology, University of Iowa; Staff Physician, Department of Veterans Affairs Medical Center, Iowa City [197]

JOEL N. KLINE, MD, MS
Professor, Director, University of Iowa Adult Asthma Center, University of Iowa College of Medicine, Iowa City [237]

HOWARD K. KOH, MD, PhD
Professor and Associate Dean, Harvard School of Public Health, Boston [73]

DENNIS J. KOPECKO, PhD
Chief, Laboratory of Enteric and Sexually Transmitted Diseases, Center for Biologics Evaluation and Research, National Institutes of Health, Bethesda [138]

PETER KOPP, MD
Associate Professor, Division of Endocrinology, Metabolism, and Molecular Medicine, Northwestern University Feinberg School of Medicine, Chicago [56]

WALTER J. KOROSHETZ, MD
Vice Chair, Neurology Service, Massachusetts General Hospital, Associate Professor of Neurology, Harvard Medical School, Boston [361]

PHYLLIS E. KOZARSKY, MD
Professor of Medicine/Infectious Diseases, Emory University School of Medicine; Chief, Traveler's Health, Division of Global Migration and Quarantine, Centers for Disease Control and Prevention, Atlanta [108]

BARNETT S. KRAMER, MD, MPH
Associate Director for Disease Prevention, National Institutes of Health; Clinical Professor of Medicine, Uniformed Services University of the Health Sciences, Bethesda [67]

STEPHEN M. KRANE, MD
Persis, Cyrus, and Marlow B. Harrison Professor of Medicine, Harvard Medical School; Physician and Chief, Arthritis Unit, Massachusetts General Hospital, Boston [331]

ALEXANDER KRATZ, MD, PhD, MPH
Assistant Professor of Pathology, Harvard Medical School; Director, Clinical Hematology Laboratory, Massachusetts General Hospital [Appendices]

JOHN P. KRESS, MD
Assistant Professor of Medicine, University of Chicago Pritzker School of Medicine, Chicago [249]

HENRY M. KRONENBERG, MD
Professor of Medicine, Harvard Medical School; Chief, Endocrine Unit, Massachusetts General Hospital, Boston [331]

LOREN LAINE, MD
Professor of Medicine, Gastrointestinal Division, Department of Medicine, Keck School of Medicine, University of Southern California School of Medicine, Los Angeles [37]

ANIL K. LALWANI, MD
Mendik Foundation Professor and Chair, Department of Otolaryngology; Professor of Physiology and Neuroscience, New York University School of Medicine, New York [26]

LEWIS LANDSBERG, MD
Professor of Medicine, Dean and Vice President for Medical Affairs, Northwestern University Feinberg School of Medicine, Chicago [322]

H. CLIFFORD LANE, MD
Head, Clinical and Molecular Retrovirology Section, Laboratory of Immunoregulation; Clinical Director, National Institute of Allergy and Infectious Diseases, National Institutes of Health, Bethesda [173, 205]

CAROL A. LANGFORD, MD
Senior Investigator, Immunologic Diseases Section, NIAID, NIH, Bethesda [306]

THOMAS J. LAWLEY, MD
Dean, Emory University School of Medicine, Atlanta [46, 47, 49]

THOMAS H. LEE, MD
Associate Professor of Medicine, Harvard Medical School; Chief Executive Officer, Partners Community Health Care, Inc; Network President, Partners Health Care, Boston [12]

OFER LEHAVI, MD
Attending Physician, Department of Obstetrics and Gynecology, Tel-Aviv Medical Center, Israel [207]

CAMMIE F. LESSER, MD, PhD
Assistant Professor in Medicine, Harvard Medical School, Cambridge [137]

BRUCE D. LEVY, MD, FACP
Assistant Professor of Medicine, Harvard Medical School; Pulmonary and Critical Care Medicine, Brigham and Women's Hospital, Boston [251]

KENT B. LEWANDROWSKI, MD
Associate Chief of Pathology, Director, Core Laboratory, Massachusetts General Hospital; Associate Professor, Harvard Medical School, Boston [Appendices]

PETER LIBBY, MD
Mallinckrodt Professor of Medicine, Harvard Medical School; Chief, Cardiovascular Medicine, Brigham and Women's Hospital, Boston [224, 225]

RICHARD W. LIGHT, MD
Professor of Medicine, Vanderbilt University, Nashville [245]

CRAIG LILLY, MD
Associate Professor of Medicine, Harvard Medical School; Division of Pulmonary and Critical Care, Department of Medicine, Brigham and Women's Hospital, Boston [250]

CHRISTOPHER H. LINDEN, MD
Professor, Department of Emergency Medicine, Division of Medical Toxicology, University of Massachusetts Medical School, Worcester [377]

ROBERT LINDSAY, MD, PhD
Professor of Clinical Medicine, Columbia University College of Physicians and Surgeons; Chief, Internal Medicine, Helen Hayes Hospital, West Haverstraw, New York [333]

MARC E. LIPPMAN, MD
John G. Searle Professor and Chair, Department of Internal Medicine, University of Michigan Health System, Ann Arbor [76]

PETER E. LIPSKY, MD
Scientific Director, National Institute of Arthritis and Musculoskeletal and Skin Diseases, National Institutes of Health, Bethesda [299, 301, 311]

DAN L. LONGO, MD
Scientific Director, National Institute on Aging, National Institutes of Health, Bethesda and Baltimore [52, 54, 66, 69, 70, 89, 97, 98, 172]

NICOLA LONGO, MD, PhD
Professor of Pediatrics and Director, Metabolic Service, Division of Medical Genetics, Department of Pediatrics, University of Utah, Salt Lake City [343, 344]

DONALD E. LOW, MD
Chief, Department of Medicine, Toronto Medical Laboratories and Mount Sinai Hospital; Professor of Medicine and Microbiology, University of Toronto, Toronto, Ontario, Canada [239]

PHILLIP A. LOW, MD
Professor of Neurology, Mayo Medical School; Chairman, Division of Clinical Neurophysiology; Consultant in Neurology, Mayo Clinic, Rochester [354]

DANIEL H. LOWENSTEIN, MD
Professor of Neurology, Vice Chairman, Department of Neurology; Director, Physician-Scientist Education and Training Program; Director UCSF Epilepsy Center, University of California San Francisco, San Francisco [346, 348]

FRANKLIN D. LOWY, MD
Professor of Medicine and Physiology, Columbia University, New York [120]

SHEILA A. LUKEHART, PhD
Research Professor, University of Washington, Seattle [153,154]

LAWRENCE C. MADOFF, MD
Assistant Professor of Medicine, Harvard Medical School; Associate Physician, Brigham and Women's Hospital, Boston [104, 126, 314]

JAMES H. MAGUIRE, MD
Chief, Parasitic Diseases Branch, Centers for Disease Control and Prevention, Atlanta [111, 314, 379]

ADEL A. F. MAHMOUD, MD, PhD
President, Merck Vaccines, Merck & Co., Inc.; Adjunct Professor of Medicine, Case Western Reserve University, Whitehouse Station [203]

RONALD V. MAIER, MD
Professor and Vice Chair, Surgery, University of Washington; Surgeon-in-Chief, Harborview Medical Center, Seattle [253]

MARK E. MAILLIARD, MD
Associate Professor, Department of Internal Medicine, University of Nebraska College of Medicine; Chief, Section of Gastroenterology, Omaha Veterans Affairs Medical Center, Omaha [288]

JOANN E. MANSON, MD, DRPH
Professor of Medicine and the Elizabeth F. Brigham Professor of Women's Health, Harvard Medical School; Chief, Division of Preventive Medicine, Brigham and Women's Hospital, Boston [327]

ELEFTHERIA MARATOS-FLIER, MD
Associate Professor of Medicine, Harvard Medical School; Chief, Obesity Section, Joslin Diabetes Center, Boston [64]

DANIEL B. MARK, MD, MPH
Professor of Medicine, Duke University Medical Center; Director, Outcomes Research, Duke Clinical Research Institute, Durham [2]

THOMAS J. MARRIE, MD, FRCPC
Professor, Department of Medicine, Dean Faculty of Medicine and Dentistry, University of Alberta, Edmonton, Alberta, Canada [158, 239]

GARY J. MARTIN, MD
Raymond J. Lagenback, MD, Professor of Medicine, Vice Chairman, Department of Medicine, Northwestern University Feinberg School of Medicine, Chicago [4]

JOSEPH B. MARTIN, MD, PhD, MA(Hon)
Dean of the Faculty of Medicine; Caroline Shields Walker Professor of Neurobiology and Clinical Neuroscience, Harvard Medical School, Boston [11, 346]

ROBERT J. MAYER, MD
Vice Chair for Academic Affairs; Director, Center for Gastrointestinal Oncology, Dana-Farber Cancer Institute; Professor of Medicine, Harvard Medical School, Boston [77, 79]

CALVIN O. McCALL, MD
Assistant Professor of Dermatology, Department of Dermatology, Emory University School of Medicine, Atlanta [47]

WILLIAM M. McCORMACK, MD
Professor of Medicine; Chief, Infectious Diseases Division, State University of New York Downstate Medical Center, New York [159]

E. REGIS McFADDEN, JR., MD
Argyl J. Beams Professor of Medicine, MetroHealth Medical Center, Cleveland [236]

RONALD D.G. McKAY, PhD
Chief, Laboratory of Molecular Biology, National Institute of Neurologic Disorders and Stroke, NIH, Bethesda [59]

KEVIN T. McVARY, MD
Associate Professor of Urology, Northwestern University Feinberg School of Medicine, Chicago [43]

NANCY K. MELLO, PhD
Professor of Psychology, Harvard Medical School, Boston [374]

SHLOMO MELMED, MD
Professor and Associate Dean, David Geffen School of Medicine at University of California Los Angeles; Senior Vice President and Chief Academic Officer at Cedars-Sinai Medical Center, Los Angeles [318]

JERRY R. MENDELL, MD
Helen C. Kurtz Professor and Chairman of Neurology, Ohio State University, Columbus [367, 368]

JACK H. MENDELSON, MD
Professor of Psychiatry (Neuroscience), Harvard Medical School, Belmont [374]

M. -MARSEL MESULAM, MD
Ruth and Evelyn Dunbar Professor of Neurology and Psychiatry; Director, Center for Behavioral and Cognitive Neurology; Director, Alzheimer's Program, Northwestern University Feinberg School of Medicine, Chicago [23]

SUSAN MIESFELDT, MD
Maine Center for Cancer Medicine and Blood Disorders, Scarborough [58]

EDGAR L. MILFORD MD
Associate Professor of Medicine, Harvard Medical School; Brigham and Women's Hospital, Boston [263]

BRUCE L. MILLER, MD
AW and Mary Margaret Clausen Distinguished Chair, Professor of Neurology, University of California San Francisco, San Francisco [350, 362]

MARK MILLER, MD
Associate Director for Research; Director, Division of International Epidemiology and Population Studies, Fogarty International Center, National Institutes of Health, Bethesda [107]

SAMUEL I. MILLER, MD
Professor of Medicine, Microbiology, and Genome Sciences, University of Washington, Seattle [137]

JOHN D. MINNA, MD
Professor of Internal Medicine and Pharmacology; Director, Hamon Center for Therapeutic Oncology Research, University of Texas Southwestern Medical Center, Dallas [75]

THOMAS A. MOORE, MD, FACP
Clinical Associate Professor of Medicine, University of Kansas School of Medicine, Wichita [193]

PAT J. MORIN, PhD
Investigator, National Institute on Aging, National Institutes of Health; Assistant Professor, Department of Pathology, The Johns Hopkins School of Medicine, Baltimore [68]

ROBERT J. MOTZER, MD
Attending Physician, Memorial Sloan-Kettering Cancer Center; Professor of Medicine, Weill Medical College of Cornell University, New York [80, 82]

HARALAMPOS M. MOUTSOPOULOS, MD
Professor and Director, Department of Pathophysiology, National University School of Medicine; President of the National Organization for Medicines, Athens, Greece [304, 307]

ROBERT S. MUNFORD, MD
Jan and Henri Bromberg Professor of Internal Medicine, University of Texas Southwestern Medical Center, Dallas [127, 254]

TIMOTHY F. MURPHY, MD
Distinguished Professor of Medicine; Chief, Division of Infectious Diseases, State University of New York at Buffalo, Buffalo [130]

DANIEL M. MUSHER, MD
Chief, Infectious Diseases Section, Veterans Affairs Medical Center; Professor of Medicine, Professor of Molecular Virology and Immunology, Baylor College of Medicine, Houston [119, 129]

ROBERT J. MYERBURG, MD
Lemberg Professor of Medicine and Physiology, Director, Division of Cardiology, University of Miami School of Medicine; American Heart Association Chair in Cardiovascular Research, Miami [256]

GERALD T. NEPOM, MD, PhD
Director, Benaroya Research Institute at Virginia Mason; Professor (Affiliate), Department of Immunology, University of Washington School of Medicine, Seattle [296]

JONATHAN NEWMARK, MD
Chief, Operations, Chemical Casualty Care, US Army Medical Research Institute of Chemical Defense, Maryland [206]

RICHARD A. NISHIMURA, MD
Judd and Mary Morris Leighton Professor of Cardiovascular Diseases, Mayo Clinic College of Medicine, Rochester [211]

ROBERT L. NORRIS, MD
Associate Professor of Surgery, Department of Surgery, Division of Emergency Medicine, Stanford University School of Medicine, Stanford [378]

THOMAS B. NUTMAN, MD
Head, Helminth Immunology Section, and Head, Clinical Parasitology Unit, Laboratory of Parasitic Diseases, National Institute of Allergy and Infectious Diseases, National Institutes of Health, Bethesda [201, 202]

RICHARD J. O'BRIEN, MD
Head of Scientific Evaluation, Foundation for Innovative New Diagnostics, Geneva, Switzerland [150]

CHRISTOPHER A. OHL, MD
Associate Professor of Medicine, Section of Infectious Diseases, Wake Forest University School of Medicine; Director, Center for Antimicrobial Utilization, Stewardship, and Epidemiology, Baptist Medical Center, Winston-Salem [136]

RICHARD K. OLNEY, MD
Professor of Neurology, University of California San Francisco, San Francisco [21]

YVONNE M. O'MEARA, MD, FRCPI
Senior Lecturer in Medicine, University College Dublin; Consultant Nephrologist, Mater Misericordiae Hospital, Dublin, Ireland [264]

ROBERT A. O'ROURKE, MD
Charles Conrad Brown Distinguished Professor of Cardiovascular Science, University of Texas Health Science Center at San Antonio, San Antonio [209]

CHUNG OWYANG, MD
Professor of Internal Medicine, H. Marvin Pollard Collegiate Professor and Chief, Division of Gastroenterology, Department of Internal Medicine, University of Michigan Medical Center, Ann Arbor [271, 277]

UMESH D. PARASHAR, MBBS, MPH
Medical Epidemiologist, Respiratory and Enteric Viruses Branch, Centers for Disease Control and Prevention, Atlanta [174]

JEFFREY PARSONNET, MD
Associate Professor of Medicine and of Microbiology, Dartmouth Medical School; Staff Physician, Infectious Diseases Section, Dartmouth-Hitchcock Medical Center, Lebanon [111]

SHREYASKUMAR R. PATEL, MD
Associate Professor of Medicine, Deputy Chairman, Department of Sarcoma Medical Oncology, University of Texas, MD Anderson Cancer Center, Houston [84]

G. ALEXANDER PATTERSON, MD
Joseph C. Bancroft Professor of Surgery, Department of Surgery, Division of Cardiothoracic Surgery, Washington University School of Medicine, St. Louis [248]

GUSTAV PAUMGARTNER, MD
Professor of Medicine, Ludwig Maximiliam University of Munich, Durchwal, Germany [292]

MICHAEL C. PERRY, MD, FACP
Professor of Internal Medicine, Director, Division of Hematology/ Oncology, Nellie B. Smith Chair of Oncology, University of Missouri/ Ellis Fischer Cancer Center, Columbia [89]

CLARENCE J. PETERS, MD
John Sealy Distinguished University Chair in Tropical and Emerging Virology, Director for Biodefense, Center for Biodefense and Emerging Infectious Diseases, University of Texas Medical Branch in Galveston, Galveston [180, 181]

ELIOT A. PHILLIPSON, MD
Sir John and Lady Eaton Professor and Chair, Department of Medicine, University of Toronto, Toronto, Ontario, Canada [246, 247]

GERALD B. PIER, PhD
Professor of Medicine (Microbiology and Molecular Genetics), Harvard School of Medicine, Boston [105]

DANIEL K. PODOLSKY, MD
Mallinckrodt Professor of Medicine, Harvard Medical School; Chief, Gastroenterology, Massachusetts General Hospital, Boston [289, 290]

RONALD E. POLK, Pharm. D.
Professor of Pharmacy and Medicine, Chair, Department of Pharmacy, School of Pharmacy, Virginia Commonwealth University, Richmond [118]

MATTHEW POLLACK, MD
Professor of Medicine, Uniformed Services University; F. Edward Hébert School of Medicine; Attending Staff Physician, Internal Medicine and Infectious Diseases, National Naval Medical Center, Bethesda [136]

RICHARD J. POLLACK, PhD
Instructor of Tropical Public Health, Department of Immunology and Infectious Diseases, Harvard School of Public Health, Boston [379]

JOHN T. POTTS, JR., MD
Jackson Distinguished Professor of Clinical Medicine, Harvard Medical School, Boston [332]

LAWRIE W. POWELL, MD, PhD
Professor of Medicine, The University of Queensland and The Royal Brisbane and Women's Hospital, Brisbane, Queensland, Australia [336]

ALVIN C. POWERS, MD
Ruth K. Scoville Professor of Medicine, Division of Diabetes, Endocrinology, and Metabolism, Vanderbilt University Medical Center; Chief, Diabetes and Endocrinology Section, VA Tennessee Valley Healthcare System, Nashville [323]

DANIEL S. PRATT, MD
Assistant Professor of Medicine, Tufts University School of Medicine; Medical Director of Liver Transplantation, New England Medical Center, Boston [38, 283]

DANIEL T. PRICE, MD
Assistant Professor of Medicine, Boston University School of Medicine; Staff Physician, Boston Veterans Affairs Medical Center, West Roxbury [223]

DARWIN J. PROCKOP, MD, PhD
Director of Center for Gene Therapy and Professor of Biochemistry, Tulane Health Sciences Center, New Orleans [342]

STANLEY B. PRUSINER, MD
Director, Institute for Neurodegenerative Diseases; Professor, Departments of Neurology, Biochemistry and Biophysics, University of California San Francisco, San Francisco [362]

DANIEL J. RADER, MD
Associate Professor, Department of Medicine, University of Pennsylvania School of Medicine, Philadelphia [335]

SANJAY RAM, MD
Assistant Professor of Medicine, Section of Infectious Diseases, Boston University School of Medicine and Boston Medical Center, Boston [128]

DIDIER RAOULT, MD
Professor of Medicine, Unité des Rickettsies, School of Medicine, University of Aux-Marseille, Marseille, France [158]

NEIL H. RASKIN, MD
Professor of Neurology, University of California San Francisco, San Francisco [14]

MARIO C. RAVIGLIONE, MD
Director, Stop TB Department, World Health Organization, Geneva, Switzerland [150]

SHARON L. REED, MD
Professor of Pathology and Medicine, Director, Microbiology and Virology Laboratories, University of California Medical Center, San Diego [194]

ANTONIO J. REGINATO, MD
Professor of Medicine; Head, Division of Rheumatology, Cooper University Medical Center, Robert Wood Johnson Medical School at Camden, Camden [313]

RICHARD C. REICHMAN, MD
Professor of Medicine, Microbiology and Immunology; Head, Infectious Diseases Unit, Senior Associate Dean for Clinical Research, University of Rochester School of Medicine and Dentistry, Rochester [169]

CAROL M. REIFE, MD
Assistant Professor of Medicine, Jefferson Medical College of Thomas Jefferson University, Philadelphia [36]

JOHN J. REILLY, MD
Associate Professor of Medicine, Harvard Medical School; Clinical Director, Pulmonary and Critical Care Medicine, Brigham and Women's Hospital, Boston [242]

JOHN T. REPKE, MD, FACOG
Professor and Chair, Department of Obstetrics and Gynecology, Pennsylvania State University College of Medicine; Obstetrician-Gynecologist In-Chief, The Milton S. Hershey Medical Center, Hershey [6]

NEIL M. RESNICK, MD
Professor of Medicine, University of Pittsburgh School of Medicine; Chief, Division of Geriatric Medicine, University of Pittsburgh Institute on Aging, Pittsburgh [8]

VICTOR I. REUS, MD
Professor of Psychiatry, University of California San Francisco; Medical Director, Langley Porter Hospital, San Francisco [371]

C. FORDHAM VON REYN, MD
Professor of Medicine, Chief, Infectious Diseases and International Health, Dartmouth Medical School, Lebanon [152]

PETER A. RICE, MD
Professor of Medicine and Chief, Section of Infectious Diseases, Boston University Medical Center, Boston [128]

STUART RICH, MD
Professor of Medicine, Rush University Medical, Chicago [220]

GARY S. RICHARDSON, MD
Assistant Professor of Psychiatry, Case Western Reserve University, Cleveland; Senior Research Scientist, Sleep Disorders and Research Center, Henry Ford Hospital, Detroit [24]

GARY L. ROBERTSON, MD
Professor of Medicine and Neurology, Northwestern University Feinberg School of Medicine, Chicago [319]

DAN M. RODEN, MD
Professor of Medicine and Pharmacology; Chief, Division of Clinical Pharmacology, Vanderbilt University School of Medicine, Nashville [3]

JAMES A. ROMANO, JR., PhD
Commander, US Army Medical Research Institute of Chemical Defense, Maryland [206]

KAREN L. ROOS, MD
John and Nancy Nelson Professor of Neurology, Indiana University School of Medicine, Indianapolis [360]

ALLAN H. ROPPER, MD
Professor and Chairman of Neurology, Tufts University School of Medicine; Chief, Department of Neurology, St. Elizabeth's Medical Center, Boston [257, 356, 357]

ROGER N. ROSENBERG, MD
Zale Distinguished Chair and Professor of Neurology, University of Texas Southwestern Medical Center at Dallas; Attending Neurologist, Parkland Memorial Hospital and Zale-Lipsky University Hospital, Dallas [352]

MYRNA R. ROSENFELD, MD, PhD
Associate Professor of Neurology, Department of Neurology, University of Pennsylvania, Philadelphia [87]

WENDELL ROSSE, MD
Florence Reynaud McAlister Professor of Medicine and Medical Research, Department of Medicine, Duke University Medical School, Durham [93]

MICHAEL A. RUBIN, MD, PhD
Assistant Professor, Internal Medicine, Division of Infectious Diseases, Division of Clinical Epidemiology, Salt Lake City [27]

ROBERT M. RUSSELL, MD
Professor, Friedman School of Nutrition Science and Policy; Director and Scientist, Jean Mayer USDA Human Nutrition Center on Aging at Tufts, Boston [61]

THOMAS A. RUSSO, MD, CM
Assistant Professor of Medicine, Division of Infectious Diseases, Department of Medicine, State University of New York at Buffalo; Veterans Affairs Medical Center, Buffalo [134, 147]

STEPHEN M. SAGAR, MD
Professor of Neurology, Case Western Reserve School of Medicine; Director of Neuro-Oncology, Ireland Cancer Center, University Hospitals of Cleveland, Cleveland [358]

MERLE A. SANDE, MD
Professor of Medicine, University of Utah School of Medicine; President, Academic Alliance for AIDS Care and Prevention in Africa Foundation, Salt Lake City [27]

EDWARD A. SAUSVILLE, MD, PhD
Associate Director for Clinical Research, Greenebaum Cancer Center, University of Maryland, Baltimore [70]

MOHAMED H. SAYEGH, MD
Associate Professor of Medicine, Harvard Medical School; Director, Transplantation Research Center, Brigham and Women's Hospital and Children's Hospital, Boston [263]

HOWARD I. SCHER, MD
D. Wayne Calloway Chair in Urologic Oncology, Attending Physician and Chief, Genitourinary Oncology Service, Department of Medicine, Memorial Sloan-Kettering Cancer Center; Professor of Medicine, Weill Medical College of Cornell University, New York [80, 81]

HARRY W. SCHROEDER, JR., MD, PhD
Professor of Medicine and Microbiology, University of Alabama at Birmingham, Birmingham [297]

ANNE SCHUCHAT, MD
Chief, Respiratory Diseases Branch, National Center for Infectious Diseases, Centers for Disease Control and Prevention, Atlanta [123]

MARC A. SCHUCKIT, MD
Professor of Psychiatry, University of California, San Diego; Director, Alcohol Research Center; Director, Alcohol and Drug Treatment Program, Veterans Affairs San Diego Healthcare System, San Diego [372, 373]

STUART SCHWARTZ, PhD
Professor of Genetics and Oncology, Center for Human Genetics Laboratory, Cleveland [57]

DAVID S. SEGAL, PhD
Professor of Psychiatry, University of California San Diego, La Jolla [373]

JULIAN L. SEIFTER, MD
Associate Professor of Medicine, Harvard Medical School; Physician, Brigham and Women's Hospital, Boston [270]

ANDREW P. SELWYN, MD
Professor of Medicine, Harvard Medical School; Physician, Brigham and Women's Hospital, Boston [226]

STEVEN D. SHAPIRO, MD
Parker B. Francis Professor of Medicine, Harvard Medical School and Brigham and Women's Hospital, Boston [242, 250, 251]

STEVEN I. SHERMAN, MD
Associate Professor, University of Texas M.D. Anderson Cancer Center; Adjunct Associate Professor, Baylor College of Medicine, Houston [330]

WILLIAM SILEN, MD
Johnson and Johnson Distinguished Professor of Surgery, Emeritus, Harvard Medical School, Boston [13, 280, 281]

EDWIN K. SILVERMAN, MD, PhD
Assistant Professor of Medicine, Harvard Medical School; Brigham and Women's Hospital, Boston [242]

GARY G. SINGER, MD
Assistant Professor of Medicine, Washington University School of Medicine; Associate Director, Transplant Nephrology, Barnes Jewish Hospital, St. Louis [41]

AJAY K. SINGH, MD
Associate Professor of Medicine, Harvard Medical School; Director of Clinical Nephrology, Brigham and Women's Hospital, Boston [262]

JEAN DOW SIPE, PhD
Professor Emeritus, Boston University School of Medicine; Scientific Review Administrator, National Institutes of Health, Bethesda [310]

KARL SKORECKI, MD
Annie Chutick Professor of Medicine, Bruce Rappaport Faculty of Medicine, Technion-Israel Institute of Technology; Director, Department of Nephrology and Molecular Medicine, Rambam Medical Center, Haifa, Israel [261]

GERALD W. SMETANA, MD
Associate Professor of Medicine, Harvard Medical School; Division of General Medicine and Primary Care, Beth Israel Deaconess Medical Center, Boston [7]

PATRICK M. SLUSS, PhD
Director, Immunodiagnostics Laboratory, Department of Pathology, Massachusetts General Hospital; Assistant Professor, Harvard Medical School, Boston [Appendices]

WADE S. SMITH, MD
Associates Professor of Neurology; Director, Neurointensive Care Service, University of California San Francisco, San Francisco [349]

MICHAEL C. SNELLER, MD
Chief of Immunologic Diseases Section, NIAID, NIH, Bethesda [306]

JAMES B. SNOW, JR., MD
Professor Emeritus, Department of Otorhinolaryngology, University of Pennsylvania; former Director, National Institute on Deafness and Other Communication Disorders, National Institutes of Health, Bethesda [26]

ARTHUR J. SOBER, MD
Professor of Dermatology, Harvard Medical School; Associate Chief of Dermatology, Massachusetts General Hospital, Boston [73]

MICHAEL F. SORRELL, MD
Robert L. Grissom Professor of Medicine; Chief, Section of Gastroenterology and Hepatology, and Medical Director, Liver Transplantation, University of Nebraska Medical Center, Omaha [288]

PETER SPEELMAN, MD, PhD
Professor of Internal Medicine, Division of Infectious Diseases, Tropical Medicine and AIDS, Department of Internal Medicine, Academic Medical Center, University of Amsterdam, Amsterdam, The Netherlands [155]

FRANK E. SPEIZER, MD
Edward H. Kass Professor of Medicine, Harvard Medical School; Co-Director, Channing Laboratory, Brigham and Women's Hospital; Professor of Environmental Science, Harvard School of Public Health, Boston [238]

ANDREW SPIELMAN, ScD
Professor of Tropical Public Health, Harvard School of Public Health, Boston [379]

JERRY L. SPIVAK, MD
Professor of Medicine and Oncology, Johns Hopkins University School of Medicine, Baltimore [95]

WALTER E. STAMM, MD
Professor of Medicine and Head, Division of Allergy and Infectious Diseases, University of Washington School of Medicine, Seattle [160, 269]

ALLEN C. STEERE, MD
Professor of Medicine, Harvard Medical School; Director of Rheumatology, Massachusetts General Hospital, Boston [157]

DAVID S. STEPHENS, MD
Director, Division of Infectious Diseases, Emory University Hospital; Stephen W. Schwarzmann Professor and Executive Vice Chair, Department of Medicine, Emory University School of Medicine, Atlanta [127]

ROBERT S. STERN, MD
Carl J. Herzog Professor of Dermatology, Harvard Medical, Boston [50]

DENNIS L. STEVENS, MD, PhD
Professor of Medicine, University of Washington School of Medicine, Seattle; Chief, Infectious Diseases, VA Medical Center, Boise [110]

RICHARD M. STONE, MD
Clinical Director, Adult Leukemia Program, Dana-Farber Cancer Institute/Brigham and Women's Hospital; Associate Professor of Medicine, Harvard Medical School, Boston [85]

STEPHEN E. STRAUS, MD
Senior Investigator, Laboratory of Clinical Investigation, National Institute of Allergy and Infectious Diseases; Director, National Center for Complementary and Alternative Medicine, National Institutes of Health, Bethesda [10, 370]

MORTON N. SWARTZ, MD
Professor, Department of Medicine, Harvard Medical School; Chief Emeritus, Infectious Disease, Chief, James Jackson Firm Medical Services, Massachusetts General Hospital, Boston [361]

A. JAMIL TAJIK, MD
Thomas J. Watson, Jr., Professor; Professor of Medicine and Pediatrics, Mayo Clinic College of Medicine Chair (Emeritus); Division of Cardiovascular Diseases and Internal Medicine; Consultant, Section of Pediatric Cardiology, Mayo Clinic, Minnesota [211]

JOEL D. TAUROG, MD
Professor of Internal Medicine, and William M. and Gatha Burnett Professor for Arthritis Research, University of Texas Southwestern Medical Center, Dallas [296, 305]

SCOTT J. THALER, MD
Chief Medical Officer, AERAS Global TB Vaccine Foundation, Bethesda [314]

ZELIG A. TOCHNER, MD
Associate Professor, Department of Radiation Oncology, University of Pennsylvania Medical Center, Philadelphia [207]

LUCY STUART TOMPKINS, MD
Professor of Medicine (Infectious Diseases and Geographic Medicine), Professor of Microbiology, Immunology and Pathology, Stanford University School of Medicine, Stanford [144]

MARK TOPAZIAN, MD
Associate Professor of Medicine, Yale University School of Medicine; Assistant Director, Gastrointestinal Procedure Center, Yale New Haven Hospital, New Haven [272]

PHILLIP P. TOSKES, MD
Professor of Medicine and Director, Division of Gastroenterology, Hepatology and Nutrition; Associate Chairman for Clinical Affairs, Department of Medicine, University of Florida, Gainesville [293, 294]

JEFFREY M. TRENT, PhD
President and Scientific Director; Senior Investigator, Molecular Diagnostics and Target Validation Division, T-Gen, Phoenix [68]

ELBERT P. TRULOCK, MD
Rosemary and I. Jerome Flance Professor of Pulmonary Medicine, Washington University School of Medicine; Medical Director, Lung Transplantation Program, Barnes-Jewish Hospital, St. Louis [248]

KENNETH L. TYLER, MD
Reuler-Lewin Family Professor of Neurology; Professor of Medicine, Microbiology and Immunology, University of Colorado Health Sciences Center; Chief, Neurology Service, Denver VA Medical Center, Denver [360]

BERT VOGELSTEIN, MD
Professor of Oncology and Pathology, Howard Hughes Investigator, The Sidney Kimmel Comprehensive Cancer Center, The Johns Hopkins University School of Medicine, Baltimore [68]

EVERETT E. VOKES, MD
Director, Section of Hematology/Oncology; John E. Ultmann Professor of Medicine and Radiation Oncology, University of Chicago, Chicago [74]

TAMARA J. VOKES, MD
Assistant Professor of Clinical Medicine, University of Chicago Pritzker School of Medicine, Chicago [334]

MATTHEW K. WALDOR, MD, PhD
Associate Professor of Medicine and Microbiology, Tufts University School of Medicine, Boston [140]

DAVID H. WALKER, MD
Professor and Chairman, Department of Pathology; Director, WHO Collaborating Center for Tropical Diseases, University of Texas Medical Branch, Galveston [158, 239]

RICHARD J. WALLACE, JR., MD
Chairman, Department of Microbiology, John Chapman Professorship in Microbiology, Professor of Medicine, University of Texas Health Center, Tyler [149]

B. TIMOTHY WALSH, MD
Ruane Professor of Psychiatry, College of Physicians and Surgeons, Columbia University; Director, Eating Disorders Research Unit, New York State Psychiatric Institute, New York [65]

PETER D. WALZER, MD
Associate Chief of Staff for Research, Cincinnati VA Medical Center; Professor of Medicine, University of Cincinnati, Cincinnati [191]

FREDERICK C.S. WANG, MD
Associate Professor of Medicine, Harvard Medical School; Medical Director, Clinical Virology Laboratory, Brigham and Women's Hospital, Boston [161,167]

CARL V. WASHINGTON, JR., MD
Assistant Professor of Dermatology, Emory University School of Medicine; Director, Mohs Surgery Unit, The Emory Clinic, Atlanta [73]

ANTHONY P. WEETMAN, MD, DSc
Professor of Medicine and Dean, University of Sheffield Medical School; Consultant Physician, Northern General Hospital, Sheffield, UK [320]

STEVEN E. WEINBERGER, MD
Professor of Medicine, Harvard Medical School; Senior Vice President, Medical Knowledge and Education Division, American College of Physicians, Philadelphia [30, 233–235, 240]

ROBERT A. WEINSTEIN, MD
Professor of Medicine, Rush Medical College; Chair, Infectious Diseases, Cook County Hospital; Chief Operating Officer, The CORE Center, Chicago [116]

PETER F. WELLER, MD, FACP
Professor of Medicine, Harvard Medical School; Co-Chief, Infectious Diseases Division; Chief, Allergy and Inflammation Division; Senior Vice Chair of Research, Department of Medicine, Beth Israel Deaconess Medical Center, Boston [199–202, 204]

MICHAEL R. WESSELS, MD
Professor of Pediatrics and Medicine (Microbiology and Molecular Genetics), Harvard Medical School; Chief, Division of Infectious Diseases, Children's Hospital, Boston [121]

LEE M. WETZLER, MD
Associate Professor of Medicine and Microbiology, Boston University School of Medicine, Boston [127]

MEIR WETZLER, MD
Associate Professor of Medicine, Roswell Park Cancer Institute, Buffalo [96]

A. CLINTON WHITE, JR., MD
Professor, Infectious Diseases Section, Department of Medicine, Baylor College of Medicine, Houston [204]

NICHOLAS J. WHITE, MD, DSc
Professor of Tropical Medicine, Mahidol University, Bangkok, Thailand; and Oxford University, Oxford, UK [195]

RICHARD J. WHITLEY, MD
Loeb Eminent Scholar in Pediatrics; Professor of Pediatrics, Microbiology, Medicine, and Neurosurgery, University of Alabama at Birmingham, Birmingham [164]

GORDON H. WILLIAMS, MD
Professor of Medicine, Harvard Medical School; Chief, Cardiovascular Endocrinology Section, Brigham and Women's Hospital, Boston [230, 321]

JOHN W. WINKELMAN, MD, PhD
Assistant Professor of Psychiatry, Harvard Medical School; Medical Director, Sleep Health Center, Brigham and Women's Hospital, Boston [24]

BRUCE U. WINTROUB, MD
Professor and Chair of Dermatology, Associate Dean, School of Medicine, University of California San Francisco, San Francisco [50]

ALLAN W. WOLKOFF, MD
Professor of Medicine and Anatomy and Structural Biology, Albert Einstein College of Medicine, New York [284]

ROBERT L. WORTMANN, MD
Professor and Chair, Department of Internal Medicine, University of Oklahoma College of Medicine, Tulsa [338]

JOSHUA WYNNE, MD, MBA, MPH
Professor of Medicine, Wayne State University; Attending Physician, Detroit Medical Center, Detroit [221]

KIM B. YANCEY, MD
Professor and Chair, Department of Dermatology, Medical College of Wisconsin, Milwaukee [46, 49]

JAMES B. YOUNG, MD
Professor of Medicine, Executive Associate Dean for Faculty Affairs, Northwestern University Feinberg School of Medicine, Chicago [322]

NEAL S. YOUNG, MD
Chief, Hematology Branch, National Heart, Lung and Blood Institute, National Institutes of Health, Bethesda [94]

ROBERT C. YOUNG, MD
President, Fox Chase Cancer Center, Philadelphia [83]

ALAN S.L. YU, MD, BChir
Assistant Professor of Medicine, University of Southern California Keck School of Medicine, Los Angeles [266]

VICTOR L. YU, MD
Professor of Medicine, University of Pittsburgh; Chief, Infectious Disease Section, VA Medical Center, Pittsburgh [132]

DORI F. ZALEZNIK, MD
Associate Clinical Professor of Medicine, Harvard Medical School; Senior Physician, Beth Israel Deaconess Medical Center, Boston [112]

PETER J. ZIMETBAUM, MD
Assistant Professor of Medicine, Harvard Medical School; Beth Israel Deaconess Medical Center, Boston [213, 214]

The first edition of *Harrison's Principles of Internal Medicine* was published more than half a century ago. Over the decades, this textbook has evolved to reflect the continuing advances in the field of internal medicine and to meet the growing information base required of medical students and clinical practitioners. The users of this sixteenth edition of *Harrison's* will not even have to open the volume to see that it marks a transition point in the book's history. The new cover is only the most obvious indication of a new direction for *Harrison's*.

In shaping and revising this new version, the Editors have committed themselves to making the textbook as useful as possible to students and practitioners coping with the demands of modern medicine. The growth of evidence-based medicine, the prominence of managed care, and the explosion of information in fundamental areas such as the genetics of disease are only three of the many factors that make these demands different from those faced by physicians only a decade ago. Just as the cover retains key elements of the classic book, the content of the sixteenth edition retains the essential facts that remain clinically useful and important. However, through modifications in both its format and its content, the new *Harrison's* addresses the changing needs of its readers.

The sixteenth edition of *Harrison's* has a full-color format that facilitates quick reference and allows the inclusion of hundreds more high-quality illustrations than in previous editions. We expect that the reader's convenience will be well served by the placement of color illustrations within the chapters rather than in the separate color atlas used in earlier editions. While providing the basic-science information that is critical to an understanding of biology and pathophysiology, this edition focuses more directly and extensively than ever on crucial aspects of clinical practice. Areas of emphasis include the approach to the patient, differential diagnosis, state-of-the-art treatment options, and disease prevention. Key topics, such as the immune system and HIV infection/AIDS, are covered in chapters amounting to "mini-textbooks." New sections offer information on the formidable challenges posed by critical care medicine and by the threat of bioterrorism. New chapters provide coverage of highly relevant clinical topics such as disease screening, perimenopausal management and hormone replacement therapy, and end-of-life care. Virtually every chapter in this edition has been substantially rewritten, and 46 chapters either are entirely new or have new authors.

These are only highlights of the changes that the Editors hope will make the new *Harrison's* a helpful tool—not only for the student who needs an expert source of basic knowledge in internal medicine, but also for the pressured practitioner who needs a clear, concise, and balanced distillation of the best information on which to base daily clinical decisions.

Part One, "Introduction to Clinical Medicine," contains a new chapter that provides practical information about the screening approaches that every internist should consider for routine health maintenance. This chapter discusses the principles and guidelines used in screening for common conditions such as cancer, hypertension, lipid disorders, and osteoporosis. Another new chapter offers a pragmatic approach to the medical evaluation of patients who are about to undergo surgical procedures. In light of the growth of the hospice movement and the increased awareness of the sensitive issues—physical, mental, social, and existential—that surround end-of-life care, a new chapter on this complex topic provides insights, information, and guidance to practitioners dealing with dying patients and their families. The chapter on women's health has been entirely revised and offers a broad overview of the approach to disorders that affect women disproportionately.

Part Two, "Cardinal Manifestations and Presentation of Diseases,"

serves as a comprehensive introduction to clinical medicine as well as a practical guide to the care of patients with these manifestations. Each section focuses on a particular group of disorders, examining the concepts of pathophysiology and differential diagnosis that must be considered in caring for patients with these common clinical presentations. Major symptoms are reviewed and correlated with specific disease states, and clinical approaches to patients presenting with these symptoms are summarized. Every chapter has been updated, and three chapters have new authors. The chapter on sexual dysfunction now addresses disorders in both men and women.

Given the rapid advances in human genetics over the past several years, Part Three, "Genetics and Disease," has once again been completely updated. The material included in this edition is strongly geared toward clinical practice, in which genetic information increasingly comes into play. The new chapter on stem cell and gene transfer in clinical medicine addresses a timely and controversial topic, defining different types of stem cells and discussing their potential clinical applications.

Part Four, "Nutrition," covers nutritional considerations related to clinical medicine. Areas of focus include nutritional and dietary assessment, nutritional requirements, protein-energy malnutrition, eating disorders, obesity, and enteral and parenteral nutrition therapy.

The core of *Harrison's* continues to encompass the disorders of the organ systems and is contained in Parts Five through Sixteen. These sections include succinct accounts of the pathophysiology of diseases involving the major organ systems as well as infectious diseases, with an emphasis on clinical manifestations, diagnostic procedures, differential diagnosis, and treatment strategies and guidelines.

Part Five, "Oncology and Hematology," includes four chapters by new authors. An increasing proportion of patients who develop cancer are being cured. It is important to detect late consequences as early as possible in their natural history to optimize outcome. The chapter on the late consequences of cancer and its treatment helps physicians following such patients to know what to look for in addition to a recurrence of the cancer. Advances in the management of many cancers are highlighted—for example, the dramatic impact of imatinib mesylate (Gleevec) on chronic myeloid leukemia and gastrointestinal stromal cell tumors and the role of rituximab in the management of lymphoma and autoimmune diseases. The chapter delineating the principles of radiation therapy has been entirely rewritten by Eli Glatstein and is a companion piece to this author's chapter on radiation bioterrorism in Part Seven (see below). The hematology section features the World Health Organization's new classification of lymphoid and myeloid neoplasms. One of the most rapidly expanding areas of medicine is the development of novel agents to interfere with blood coagulation. With a new author who is an expert in this field, the chapter on anticoagulant, fibrinolytic, and antiplatelet therapy reviews all these new products and their indications.

Part Six, "Infectious Diseases," summarizes the latest information on pathology, genetics, and epidemiology while focusing sharply on the needs of clinicians who must accurately diagnose and treat infections under time pressure and cost constraints. In particular, the inclusion of dozens more illustrations in full color provides easily accessible information to assist clinicians with these challenges. Specific recommendations are provided for therapeutic regimens, including the drug of choice, dose, duration, and alternatives. Current trends in antimicrobial resistance are presented and considered in light of their impact on therapeutic choices. A new chapter offers key information on the management of the complex clinical issues raised by *Clostridium difficile*–associated disease, including pseudomembranous colitis. New authors cover the latest advances in the management of diseases caused by staphylococci and nontuberculous mycobacteria, viral gastroenteritis, and brucellosis. The superb chapter by Raphael Dolin on common viral respiratory infections has been expanded to include thorough coverage of severe acute respiratory syndrome (SARS). Now placed in a separate section with the overview of the human retroviruses, the chapter on HIV infection and AIDS by Anthony S. Fauci and H. Clifford Lane has been completely revised and updated, with an emphasis on therapeutic strategies. This chapter is widely considered to be a classic in the field; its clinically pragmatic focus in combination with its comprehensive and analytical approach to the pathogenesis of HIV disease has allowed its use as the sole complete reference on HIV/AIDS in medical schools.

In recent years, physicians have found themselves on the front line of response to bioterrorist attacks around the world. Since the attacks on the United States on September 11, 2001, and the subsequent anthrax attacks, the nation has been preparing for the further attacks that will inevitably come. Part Seven, "Bioterrorism and Clinical Medicine," consists of entirely new material written by authorities in three areas of bioterrorism: microbial, chemical, and radiation. Edited by *Harrison's* editor Anthony S. Fauci, these chapters are written succinctly and include easily readable charts, tables, and algorithms; their goal is to confer an understanding of the pathogenesis, diagnosis, treatment, and prognosis of the diseases in question.

Part Eight, "Disorders of the Cardiovascular System," is once again edited by the preeminent expert in the field, Eugene Braunwald. A new chapter covers the clinically important topics of unstable angina and non-ST-segment elevation myocardial infarction; three other chapters have new authors; and every chapter has been revised to reflect the latest trends and strategies for management. These include primary percutaneous coronary intervention for ST-segment elevation myocardial infarction as well as new drugs and devices for the treatment of heart failure.

Enormous strides have been made in the use of lung transplantation for selected patients with end-stage, irreversible, pulmonary parenchymal and vascular disease. Part Nine, "Disorders of the Respiratory System," includes a chapter by a new author that focuses on the selection of patients for this intervention. New authors have also taken on the broad topic of pneumonia and lung abscess, providing focus and a clinical perspective to help the reader grasp the central issues involved in the diagnosis and management of both community-acquired and nosocomial disease.

With advances in health care delivery and pressures aimed at cost containment, critical care units account for a growing percentage of hospital beds. Part Ten, "Critical Care Medicine," is a new section of *Harrison's* that is devoted to the provision of optimal care in this medical setting of growing importance. Incorporating both new chapters and refocused chapters on topics covered in previous editions, this part deals with three main areas: respiratory critical care, shock and cardiac arrest, and neurologic critical care. The approach to the patient and the central tenets underlying critical care are at the heart of this part of the sixteenth edition.

Part Eleven, "Disorders of the Kidney and Urinary Tract," includes contributions from several new authors and, as in previous editions, provides a thorough overview of the urinary-tract disorders encountered in internal medicine.

Part Twelve, "Disorders of the Gastrointestinal System," includes a new chapter on familial Mediterranean fever. The chapter on the approach to the patient with gastrointestinal disease has been completely reworked by a new author, as has the chapter on diverticular and vascular disease of the bowel. The chapters on the various categories of viral hepatitis have been extensively revised and updated to reflect breakthrough advances in treatment.

The first chapter in Part Thirteen, "Disorders of the Immune System, Connective Tissue, and Joints," provides an introduction to the immune system that has become a classic in its field and is often used as the textbook of immunology in postgraduate and medical school courses. This chapter combines an in-depth description and analysis of the principles of basic immunology with an easy flow into the application of these principles to clinical disease states. Its description of the relationship of innate to adaptive immunity is a model for understanding the intricacies of the human immune system. Once again, the authors have extensively revised this chapter to bring it up to date with regard to recent rapid advances in both basic and clinical immunology. In the section on disorders of immune-mediated injury, the spondyloarthropathies have been grouped together in one chapter that clearly and comprehensively discusses the similarities and dissimilarities among the various diseases in this category. The breakthrough advances in immunomodulatory therapy that have been realized in rheumatology over the past few years are captured in the spondyloarthropathy chapters and in the extensively revised chapters on rheumatoid arthritis and systemic lupus erythematosus. A new chapter covers fibromyalgia, arthritis associated with systemic disease, and other arthritides.

Part Fourteen, "Endocrinology and Metabolism," includes six chapters with new authors as well as a timely new chapter on the perimenopause transition and hormone replacement therapy. The writing of the latter chapter coincided with publication of results from the Women's Health Initiative that unexpectedly showed an increased risk of cardiovascular disease among women who received estrogen treatment. The author reviews the literature in this area and provides practical algorithms for the management of patients during this transition. The new authors of the chapter on disorders of sexual differentiation highlight novel insights derived from elucidation of the genetic basis of sex determination. The outstanding new review of bone and mineral metabolism lays a superb foundation for an understanding of the pathophysiology and treatment of various metabolic bone diseases. The newly authored version of the chapter on disorders of lipoprotein metabolism offers a much sharper focus on the classification, diagnosis, and treatment of disorders of cholesterol and triglyceride metabolism, emphasizing the use of statins for the reduction of cardiovascular risk. The new chapter on Wilson disease reports on the substantially modified treatment recommendations for this entity.

Part Fifteen, "Neurologic Disorders," has been extensively updated. A comprehensive new chapter on Alzheimer's disease and related dementias summarizes the recent explosion of knowledge on this topic, highlighting the new understanding of the genetics of these dementias and the molecules that trigger them as well as providing a clinical guide to diagnosis, differential diagnosis, and the latest treatments. The new chapter on Parkinson's disease reviews the recent genetic findings and provides an authoritative approach to therapy, including surgical options. The chapter on cerebrovascular diseases has been extensively rewritten, offering an evidence-based approach to the treatment and prevention of stroke, the third leading killer in the Western world. The updated chapter on multiple sclerosis presents the most recent advances in therapy and a practical approach to management of different stages of the disease. Finally, the recognition of bovine spongiform encephalopathy in many regions of the world has focused the global health care community on the biology and clinical manifestations of prion diseases; the sixteenth edition of *Harrison's* includes a comprehensive review of this subject by Nobel Laureate Stanley Prusiner.

Part Sixteen, "Poisoning, Drug Overdose, and Envenomation," has been thoroughly revised and streamlined to focus on the topics most relevant to internal medicine.

In view of the requirements for continuing education for licensure and relicensure as well as the emphasis on certification and recertification, a revision of the PreTest Self-Assessment and Review will again be published with this edition. This volume is in the capable hands of a new author, Dr. Charles Wiener from Johns Hopkins. It consists of several hundred questions based on the sixteenth edition of *Harrison's*, along with answers and explanations for the answers. The *Companion Handbook*, which was pioneered as a supplement to the eleventh edition of *Harrison's*, has been reworked as a concise quick-reference clinical manual; the *Manual of Medicine* will appear shortly after the publication of this edition, along with a PDA version, *Harrison's OnHand*. In 1998, *Harrison's* went online to provide a "living" textbook of internal medicine. In addition to permitting full search capabilities of the text, *Harrison's Online* offers frequent updates, reports of clinical trials, practice guidelines, online lectures, and concise reviews of timely topics as well as additional and updated references (with links to MEDLINE abstracts) and illustrations.

We wish to express our appreciation to our many associates and colleagues, who, as experts in their fields, have offered us constructive criticism and helpful suggestions. We acknowledge especially the contributions of the following individuals: Joseph Alpert, Michael Bray, Mark D. Carlson, Daniel H. Lowenstein, Lawrence C. Madoff, Thomas R. Martin, Chung Owyang, Alice Pau, and Mary Wright.

We thank in particular Kenneth and Elaine Kaye and Lindsey Baden, who gathered many high-quality illustrations of infectious disease manifestations. We also express our gratitude to Eileen J. Scott, who has applied her editorial expertise to the past six editions of *Harrison's*, and Marsha Cohen, who has been the text and cover designer for the past five editions.

This book could not have been edited without the dedicated help of our co-workers in the editorial offices of the individual editors. We are especially indebted to Patricia L. Duffey, Gregory K. Folkers, Sarah Matero, Julie B. McCoy, Jaylyn Olivo, Elizabeth Robbins, Leslie Runnels, Kathryn Saxon, Marie Scurti, and Sue Anne Tae.

Finally, we continue to be highly indebted to three outstanding members of the McGraw-Hill organization: Mariapaz Ramos Englis, Senior Managing Editor; Robert Laffler, Production Director; and Martin J. Wonsiewicz, Publisher. They are an effective team who have given the Editors constant encouragement and sage advice. They have been instrumental in guiding the many changes instituted with this edition of *Harrison's* and in bringing this volume to fruition in a timely manner.

THE EDITORS

16th Edition

HARRISON'S
PRINCIPLES OF
Internal
Medicine

208 APPROACH TO THE PATIENT WITH CARDIOVASCULAR DISEASE
Eugene Braunwald

THE MAGNITUDE OF THE PROBLEM

Cardiovascular diseases comprise the most prevalent serious disorders in the developed nations. The American Heart Association has reported that in 2002, 62 million Americans—32 million females and 30 million males (i.e., more than one in five persons)—had a cardiovascular disease (including hypertension). The prevalence rises progressively with age from 5% at age 20 to 75% at age >75 years.

Discharges from U.S. hospitals for cardiovascular disorders have been rising steadily and now exceed 6 million per year. Despite substantial progress in the primary and secondary prevention of coronary heart disease, approximately 6.5 million Americans suffer from angina pectoris and more than 1 million experience a myocardial infarction each year. About 4.8 million Americans have congestive heart failure and more than half a million new cases occur each year. Hospitalizations for heart failure have risen from 400,000 to 950,000 per year in the past 20 years. More than 1.4 million patients undergo cardiac catheterization each year, and approximately 1.2 million undergo revascularization (either percutaneous coronary intervention or coronary artery bypass grafting). There are approximately 1 million Americans with congenital heart disease now alive, and 40,000 babies with congenital heart disease are born each year. The annual total costs of cardiovascular diseases are estimated at $280 billion—$170 billion in direct costs and $110 billion in indirect costs in lost productivity.

Although age-adjusted death rates for coronary heart disease have declined by two-thirds from their peak in 1965, cardiovascular diseases remain the most common causes of death, responsible for 40% of all deaths, almost 1 million deaths each year. Approximately one-fourth of these deaths are sudden. Among developed nations, death rates from cardiovascular diseases are highest in the nations of the former Soviet Union, are intermediate in the United States and Western Europe, and lowest in Japan. The prevalence of cardiovascular disease, especially coronary artery disease, is rising alarmingly in China, India, Pakistan, and the Middle East, as nutritional and infectious causes of death decline in these regions. It has been projected that by 2020 cardiovascular diseases will be the leading causes of death worldwide.

CARDIAC SYMPTOMS

The symptoms caused by heart disease result most commonly from myocardial ischemia, from disturbance of the contraction and/or relaxation of the myocardium, from obstruction to blood flow, or from an abnormal cardiac rhythm or rate. Ischemia is manifest most frequently as chest discomfort, while reduction of the pumping ability of the heart commonly leads to fatigability and shortness of breath or, when severe, produces cyanosis, hypotension, syncope, and elevated intravascular pressure behind a failing ventricle. The latter results in abnormal fluid accumulation, which in turn leads to dyspnea, orthopnea, and systemic or pulmonary edema. Obstruction to blood flow, as in valvular stenosis, can cause symptoms resembling those resulting from congestive heart failure. Cardiac arrhythmias often develop suddenly, and the resulting signs and symptoms—palpitation, dyspnea, hypotension, presyncope, and syncope—generally occur abruptly and may disappear as rapidly as they develop. Ischemic heart disease, by far the most common form of heart disease in adults, may present with chest discomfort but also as heart failure, tachyarrhythmia, and sudden cardiac death.

Myocardial or coronary function that may be adequate at rest may be inadequate during exertion. Thus chest discomfort and/or dyspnea that appear only during activity are characteristic of heart disease, while the opposite pattern, i.e., the appearance of these symptoms at rest and their remission during exertion, is rarely observed in patients with organic heart disease.

Many patients with cardiocirculatory disease may also be asymptomatic, both at rest and during exertion, but may present an abnormal physical finding, such as a heart murmur, elevated arterial pressure, or an abnormality of the electrocardiogram (ECG) or of the cardiac silhouette on the chest roentgenogram. Patients may exhibit asymptomatic ischemia on an exercise stress test. In some asymptomatic patients the first clinical event may be catastrophic—sudden cardiac death, acute myocardial infarction, or stroke.

FEAR OF HEART DISEASE

Diseases of the heart and circulation are so common and the laity is so well acquainted with the major symptoms resulting from these disorders that patients, and occasionally physicians, erroneously attribute many noncardiac complaints to cardiovascular disease. The combination of the widespread fear of heart disease with the deep-seated emotional connotations concerning this organ's function results in the frequent development of symptoms that mimic those of organic disease in persons with normal cardiovascular systems. The unraveling of symptoms and signs due to organic heart disease from those not directly related is an important and challenging task in such patients.

Patients in whom heart disease has been confirmed, especially those who have experienced a major cardiovascular event such as a myocardial infarction or a serious arrhythmia, are often frightened and anxious about hospital discharge and resuming normal activity, including sexual relations. Attention to these matters is vital in the care of cardiac patients.

Dyspnea, one of the cardinal manifestations of heart failure, is not limited to patients with heart disease but is also observed in conditions as diverse as pulmonary disease, marked obesity, and anxiety (Chap. 29). Similarly, chest discomfort may result from a variety of causes other than myocardial ischemia (Chap. 12). Whether heart disease is responsible for these symptoms can frequently be determined by carrying out a careful clinical examination. Noninvasive testing using electrocardiography at rest and during exercise (Chap. 210), echocardiography (Chap. 211), roentgenography, and myocardial imaging usually provides important additional information to permit the correct interpretation of symptoms; more specialized invasive examinations (catheterization and angiography; Chap. 212) are occasionally necessary.

DIAGNOSIS

As outlined by the New York Heart Association, the elements of a complete cardiac diagnosis include consideration of the following:

1. *The underlying etiology.* Is the disease congenital, infectious, hypertensive, or ischemic in origin?

2. *The anatomic abnormalities.* Which chambers are involved? Are they hypertrophied, dilated, or both? Which valves are affected? Are they regurgitant and/or stenotic? Is there pericardial involvement? Has there been a myocardial infarction?

3. *The physiologic disturbances.* Is an arrhythmia present? Is there evidence of congestive heart failure or of myocardial ischemia?

4. *Functional disability.* How strenuous is the physical activity

required to elicit symptoms? The classification provided by the New York Heart Association has been found to be useful in describing functional disability (Table 208-1).

One example may serve to illustrate the importance of establishing a complete diagnosis. In a patient who presents with exertional chest pain, the identification of myocardial ischemia as the etiology is of great clinical importance. However, the simple recognition of ischemia is insufficient to formulate a therapeutic strategy or prognosis until the underlying anatomic abnormalities responsible for the myocardial ischemia, e.g., coronary atherosclerosis or aortic stenosis, are identified and a judgment made as to whether other physiologic disturbances that cause an imbalance between myocardial oxygen supply and demand, such as severe anemia, thyrotoxicosis, or supraventricular tachycardia, play a contributory role. Finally, the severity of the disability will govern the extent and tempo of the workup and strongly influence the therapeutic strategy that is selected.

The establishment of a correct and complete cardiac diagnosis often commences with the history and physical examination (Chap. 209). Indeed, the clinical examination remains the basis for the diagnosis of a wide variety of disorders (Table 208-2). The clinical examination may then be supplemented by four types of laboratory tests: (1) ECG (Chap. 210); (2) chest roentgenogram; (3) noninvasive graphic examinations (echocardiogram, radionuclide and imaging techniques; Chap. 211); and occasionally (4) specialized invasive examinations, i.e., cardiac catheterization, angiocardiography, and coronary angiography (Chap. 212).

THE DIAGNOSTIC PROCESS In the diagnostic process, the results obtained from each of these several modalities should be analyzed independently of one another as well as together. Only in this way can one avoid overlooking a subtle, though important, finding. For example, an ECG should be obtained in every patient suspected of heart disease. It may provide the critical clue in establishing the correct diagnosis, e.g., the finding of a mild atrioventricular conduction disturbance in a patient with unexplained syncope, even when all other methods of examination reveal no abnormal findings, can be the clue that advanced heart block and asystole might be the cause and can dictate electrophysiologic testing. On the other hand, when combined intelligently with the results of other methods of examination, the ECG may provide essential confirmatory data. Thus, the knowledge that a patient has an apical diastolic rumbling murmur may direct particular attention to the P waves, and the recognition of electrocardiographic left atrial enlargement supports the suggestion that the murmur is caused by mitral stenosis. The diagnosis can then be confirmed by echocardiography, a technique that can also determine the severity of the obstruction and its effects on pulmonary artery pressure and on right and left ventricular function.

FAMILY HISTORY In eliciting the history of a patient with known or suspected cardiovascular disease, particular attention should be directed to the family history. Familial clustering is common in many forms of heart disease. Mendelian transmission of single-gene defects may occur, as in hypertrophic cardiomyopathy (Chap. 221), the Marfan syndrome (Chap. 342), and sudden death associated with a pro-

TABLE 208-2 Conditions in Which Clinical Examination Is an Important Determinant of Diagnosis: Confirmation by Echocardiography Is Often Useful

Mitral valve prolapse	Tricuspid regurgitation
Congestive heart failure	Aortic stenosis
Cardiac tamponade	Acute pulmonary hypertension
Hypertension	Chronic pulmonary hypertension
Mitral stenosis	High-output states
Chronic mitral regurgitation	Atrial septal defect
Chronic aortic regurgitation	Anginal syndrome

longed QT syndrome (Chap. 214). Essential hypertension or coronary atherosclerosis are often polygenic disorders. While familial transmission may be less obvious than in the single-gene disorders, it is also helpful in assessing risk and prognosis. Familial clustering of cardiovascular diseases may occur not only on a genetic basis but may also be related to familial dietary or behavior patterns, such as excessive ingestion of salt or calories or cigarette smoking.

ASSESSMENT OF FUNCTIONAL IMPAIRMENT When an attempt is made to determine the severity of functional impairment in a patient with heart disease, it is helpful to ascertain with as much precision as possible the level of activity and the rate at which it is performed before symptoms develop. Thus, it is not sufficient to state that the patient complains of dyspnea. The breathlessness that occurs after running up two long flights of stairs denotes far less functional impairment than similar symptoms occurring after taking a few steps on the level. Also, the degree of customary physical activity at work and during recreation should be considered. The development of two-flight dyspnea in a well-conditioned marathon runner may be far more significant than the development of one-flight dyspnea in a previously sedentary person. Similarly, the history must include a detailed consideration of the patient's therapeutic regimen. For example, the persistence or development of edema, breathlessness, and other manifestations of heart failure in a patient whose diet is rigidly restricted in sodium content and who is receiving optimal doses of diuretics is far more grave than are similar manifestations in the absence of these measures. In an effort to determine the progression of symptoms, and thereby the severity of the underlying illness, it may be useful to ascertain what, if any, specific tasks the patient could carry out 1 year earlier that he or she cannot carry out at present.

THE PATIENT WITH A HEART MURMUR (Fig. 208-1) The cause of a heart murmur can often be readily elucidated from a systematic evaluation of its major attributes: timing, duration, intensity, quality, frequency, configuration, location, radiation, and response to maneuvers when considered in the light of the history, general physical examination, and other features of the cardiac examination, as described in Chap. 209.

The majority of heart murmurs are midsystolic and soft (grades I to II/VI). When such a murmur occurs in an asymptomatic child or young adult *without* other evidence of heart disease on clinical examination, it is usually benign and echocardiography is not generally required. On the other hand, two-dimensional and Doppler echocardiography (Chap. 211) are indicated in patients with loud systolic murmurs (grades ≥III/VI), especially those that are holosystolic or late systolic; in most patients with diastolic or continuous murmurs; and in patients with additional unexplained abnormal physical findings on cardiac examination.

ELECTROCARDIOGRAM (See also Chap. 210) Although an ECG should be recorded in every patient with known or suspected heart disease, with the exception of the identification of arrhythmias and of acute myocardial infarction, it rarely permits establishment of a specific diagnosis. The range of normal electrocardiographic findings is wide, and the tracing can be affected significantly by many noncardiac factors, such as age, body habitus, and serum electrolyte concentrations. In the absence of other abnormal findings, electrocardiographic changes must not be overinterpreted.

TABLE 208-1 New York Heart Association Functional Classification

Class I	Class III
No limitation of physical activity	Marked limitation of physical activity
No symptoms with ordinary exertion	Less than ordinary activity causes symptoms
Class II	Asymptomatic at rest
Slight limitation of physical activity	Class IV
Ordinary activity causes symptoms	Inability to carry out any physical activity without discomfort
	Symptoms at rest

Source: Modified from The Criteria Committee of the New York Heart Association.

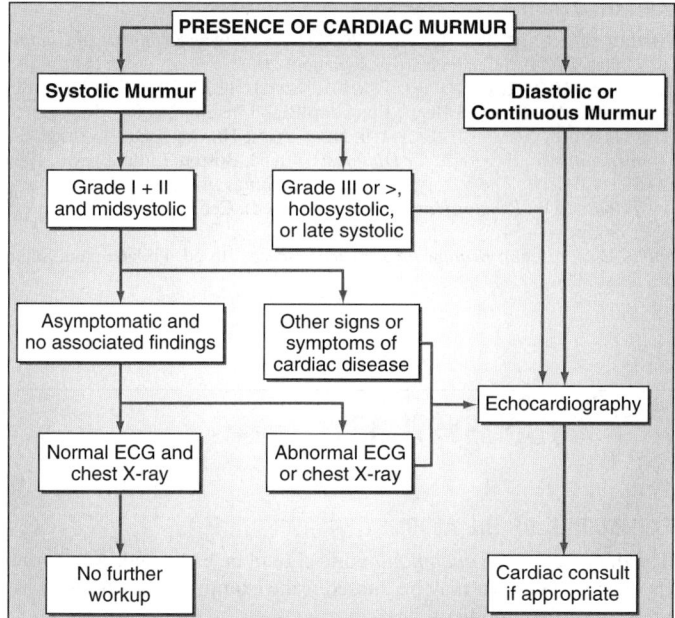

FIGURE 208-1   An alternative "echocardiography first" approach to the evaluation of a heart murmur that also uses the results of the electrocardiogram (ECG) and chest x-ray in asymptomatic patients with soft midsystolic murmurs and no other physical findings. This algorithm is useful to patients over age 40 years in whom the prevalence of coronary artery disease and aortic stenosis increases as the cause of systolic murmur. [From RA O'Rourke, in E Braunwald, L Goldman (eds): Primary Cardiology, 2d ed. Philadelphia, Saunders, 2003.]

NATURAL HISTORY   Cardiovascular disorders often present acutely, as in a previously asymptomatic patient with extensive coronary atherosclerosis who develops an acute myocardial infarction (Chap. 228) or the previously asymptomatic patient with hypertrophic cardiomyopathy (Chap. 221) whose first clinical manifestation is syncope or even sudden death. However, in both instances, the alert physician may recognize the patient at risk of these complications long before they occur and can often take measures to prevent their occurrence. For example, the patient with acute myocardial infarction may well have had risk factors for atherosclerosis for many years. Had these been recognized, their elimination or reduction might have delayed or even prevented the infarction. Similarly, the patient with hypertrophic cardiomyopathy may have had a heart murmur for years, and a positive family history might have led to an echocardiographic examination and the recognition of the condition and appropriate therapy long before the acute manifestations.

PITFALLS IN CARDIOVASCULAR MEDICINE

Increasing subspecialization in internal medicine and the perfection of advanced diagnostic techniques in cardiology can lead to several undesirable consequences. Examples include:

1.   Failure by the *noncardiologist* to recognize important cardiac manifestations of systemic illnesses. Examples of the latter are (a) stroke (secondary to atrial fibrillation or mitral stenosis); (b) skeletal muscular dystrophies (associated with cardiomyopathy); (c) hemochromatosis (associated with myocardial infiltration and restrictive cardiomyopathy); (d) congenital deafness (associated with prolonged QT interval and serious cardiac arrhythmias); (e) Raynaud's disease (associated with primary pulmonary hypertension and coronary vasospasm); (f) connective tissue disorders, e.g., the Marfan syndrome (aortic dilatation and aneurysm, prolapsed mitral valve); (g) hyperthyroidism (heart failure, atrial fibrillation); (h) hypothyroidism (pericardial effusion, coronary artery disease); (i) rheumatoid arthritis (pericarditis, aortic valve disease); (j) scleroderma (cor pulmonale, myocardial fibrosis, pericarditis); (k) systemic lupus erythematosus (valvulitis, myocarditis, pericarditis); and (l) sarcoidosis (arrhythmias, cardiomyopathy). In patients with these and other systemic disorders,

a cardiovascular examination should be carried out to identify and estimate the severity of cardiovascular involvement.

2.   Failure by the cardiologist to recognize underlying systemic disorders, such as those listed above, in patients with a cardiac disorder. Patients with heart disease should be assessed for the frequent *noncardiac* manifestations of systemic disorders with cardiovascular manifestations. For example, hyperthyroidism should be considered in an elderly patient with unexplained heart failure and atrial fibrillation. Similarly, Lyme disease should be considered in patients with unexplained fluctuating atrioventricular block. A cardiovascular abnormality may provide the clue critical to the recognition of some systemic disorders. For instance, unexplained atrial fibrillation may provide the first clue to the diagnosis of thyrotoxicosis.

3.   Overreliance on and overutilization of laboratory tests, particularly invasive techniques for the examination of the cardiovascular system. Cardiac catheterization and coronary arteriography (Chap. 212) provide precise diagnostic information under many circumstances. For example, they aid in establishing a specific anatomic diagnosis, which, in turn, may be critical to developing a therapeutic plan in patients with known or suspected ischemic heart disease. Although a great deal of attention has been lavished on these expensive examinations, it should be recognized that they serve to *supplement*, not *supplant*, a careful examination carried out by clinical and noninvasive techniques. A coronary arteriogram should not be carried out in lieu of a careful history in patients with chest pain suspected of having ischemic heart disease. Although coronary arteriography may establish whether the coronary arteries are obstructed, the results often do not provide a definite answer to the question of whether a patient's complaint of chest pain is attributable to coronary arteriosclerosis. Catheterization of the left side of the heart is all too frequently employed to assess patients with valvular heart disease when echocardiographic examination would actually provide more useful information.

Despite the enormous value of these invasive tests in certain circumstances, they entail some small risk to the patient, involve discomfort and substantial cost, and place a strain on medical facilities. Therefore, they should be carried out only if, after clinical examination and assessment by noninvasive tests, the results of the invasive examination can be expected to modify the patient's management.

MANAGEMENT

After a complete diagnosis has been established, a number of management options are usually available. Several examples may be used to demonstrate some of the principles of cardiovascular therapeutics:

1.   In the absence of evidence of heart disease, a clear, definitive statement to that effect should be made and the patient should *not* be asked to return at intervals for repeated examinations. If there is no evidence for disease, such continued attention may lead to the patient developing inappropriate anxiety and fixation on the heart.

2.   If there is no evidence of cardiovascular disease but the patient has one or more risk factors for the development of ischemic heart disease (Chap. 224), a plan for their reduction should be developed and the patient should be retested at intervals to assess that he or she is complying and that these risk factors are in fact being reduced.

3.   Asymptomatic or mildly symptomatic patients with valvular heart disease that is anatomically severe should be evaluated periodically, every 6 to 12 months, by clinical and noninvasive examinations. Early signs of deterioration of ventricular function can be detected in this manner and in appropriate patients may signify the need for surgical treatment before the development of disabling symptoms, irreversible myocardial damage, and excessive risk of surgical treatment (Chap. 219).

4.   It is critical to establish clear criteria for deciding on the form of treatment (medical, percutaneous coronary intervention, or surgical revascularization) in patients with ischemic heart disease (Chap. 226). Mechanical revascularization, i.e., the latter two modalities, is proba-

bly being employed too frequently in the United States; the mere presence of angina pectoris and/or the demonstration of critical coronary arterial narrowing at angiography should not reflexly evoke a decision to treat the patient by revascularization. Instead, this approach should be limited to those patients with ischemic heart disease whose angina has not responded adequately to medical treatment or in whom revascularization has been shown to improve the natural history (e.g., acute coronary syndrome, or multivessel coronary artery disease with left ventricular dysfunction).

FURTHER READING

AMERICAN HEART ASSOCIATION: *2004 Heart and Stroke Statistical Update.* Dallas, TX, American Heart Association, 2003

NATIONAL HEART, LUNG AND BLOOD INSTITUTE: *FY 2003 Fact Book.* Bethesda, MD, National Heart, Lung and Blood Institute, 2004

THE CRITERIA COMMITTEE OF THE NEW YORK HEART ASSOCIATION: *Nomenclature and Criteria for Diagnosis,* 9th ed. Boston, Little, Brown, 1994

VANDEN BELT J: The history, in *Classic Teachings in Clinical Cardiology: A Tribute to W. Proctor Harvey,* M Chizner (ed). Cedar Grove, NJ, Laennec, 1996, pp 41–54

ZIPES D et al (eds): *Braunwald's Heart Disease,* 7th ed. Philadelphia, Saunders, 2004

209 PHYSICAL EXAMINATION OF THE CARDIOVASCULAR SYSTEM
Robert A. O'Rourke, Eugene Braunwald

A meticulous physical examination is an often inadequately utilized low-cost method for assessing the cardiovascular system and frequently provides important information for the appropriate selection of additional tests. First, the general physical appearance should be evaluated. The patient may appear tired because of a chronic low cardiac output; the respiratory rate may be rapid in cases of pulmonary venous congestion. Central cyanosis, often associated with clubbing of the fingers and toes, indicates right-to-left cardiac or extracardiac shunting or inadequate oxygenation of blood by the lungs. Cyanosis in the distal extremities, cool skin, and increased sweating result from vasoconstriction in patients with severe heart failure (Chap. 31). Noncardiovascular details can be equally important. For example, infective endocarditis is the likely diagnosis in patients with petechiae, Osler's nodes, and Janeway lesions (Chap. 109).

The blood pressure should be taken in both arms and with the patient supine and upright; the heart rate should be timed for 30 s. Orthostatic hypotension and tachycardia may indicate a reduced blood volume, while resting tachycardia may be due to heart failure.

EXAMINATION OF THE RETINA

Inspection of the smaller vessels of the body is possible in the retina. The optic disc should be observed first, with a search for evidence of edema and blurred margins and for cupping with sharp contours. Neovascularization or the pallor of optic atrophy should be ruled out. Next, the examiner should scan along the superior temporal arcade, inspecting the arteries carefully for embolic plaques at each bifurcation and noting the arteriovenous crossing for evidence of obscuration of the vein and for pronounced nicking and banking of the vessels.

Early diabetic microaneurysms, a manifestation of diabetic microvascular disease, are found just temporal to the fovea, along the horizontal raphe, and cotton-wool infarcts are found circularly around the disc (see Fig. 323-9). Thus, the retina can be searched efficiently for evidence of cardiovascular disease.

Variations in the caliber of a single vessel are more important than determinations of arteriovenous ratios. These changes may take the form of focal narrowing, sometimes called *beading,* and are seen in hypercholesterolemia or spasm. In severe hypertension, hypertensive retinopathy with scattered flame-shaped hemorrhages, very constricted arterioles, and cotton-wool spots are evident (see Fig. 25-8).

Retinal emboli have particular cardiovascular significance. Of these, platelet emboli are both the most common and the most evanescent. Hollenhorst cholesterol plaques may be identified at the same bifurcations for months to years after the embolic shower. Platelet emboli, Hollenhorst plaques, and calcium emboli are usually seen along the course of a retinal artery, and their appearance indicates that a patient is shedding from the heart, aorta, great vessels, or carotid arteries (see Fig. 25-6). Roth spots and fat emboli may not appear to be intravascular and may not be associated with a vessel that is ophthalmoscopically visible.

EXAMINATION OF THE ABDOMEN

The diameter of the *abdominal* aorta should be estimated. An abdominal aortic aneurysm may be missed if the examiner fails to assess the area above the umbilicus.

Specific abnormalities of the abdomen may be secondary to heart disease. A large, tender liver is common in patients with heart failure or constrictive pericarditis. Systolic hepatic pulsations are frequent in patients with tricuspid regurgitation. A palpable spleen is a late sign in patients with severe heart failure and is also often present in patients with infective endocarditis.

Ascites may occur with heart failure alone, although it is less common with the use of diuretic therapy. Severe tricuspid regurgitation often results in an enlarged pulsating liver and ascites. Constrictive pericarditis should be considered when the ascites is out of proportion to peripheral edema. When there is an arteriovenous fistula, a continuous murmur may be heard over the abdomen. Fistulas due to trauma and surgery may occur.

A systolic bruit heard over the kidney areas may signify renal artery stenosis in patients with systemic hypertension.

EXAMINATION OF THE EXTREMITIES

Examination of the upper and lower extremities may provide important diagnostic information. Palpation of the peripheral arterial pulses in the upper and lower extremities is necessary to define the adequacy of systemic blood flow and to detect the presence of occlusive arterial lesions. Atherosclerosis of the peripheral arteries may produce intermittent claudication of the buttock, calf, thigh, or foot, with severe disease resulting in tissue damage of the toes. Peripheral atherosclerosis is an important risk factor for coincident ischemic heart disease.

Thrombophlebitis often causes pain (in the calf or thigh) or edema, and when present, pulmonary emboli should be considered as well. Edema is a late sign of heart failure; it frequently involves the right leg prior to the left. However, edema of the lower extremities may be secondary to local factors, such as varicose veins or thrombophlebitis, or to the removal of veins at coronary artery bypass surgery. Under such circumstances, the edema is often unilateral.

ARTERIAL PRESSURE PULSE

The normal central aortic pulse wave is characterized by a fairly rapid rise to a somewhat rounded peak (Fig. 209-1). The anacrotic shoulder, present on the ascending limb, occurs at the time of peak rate of aortic flow just before maximum pressure is reached. The less steep descending limb is interrupted by a sharp downward deflection, coincident with aortic valve closure, called the *incisura.* As the pulse wave is transmitted peripherally, the initial upstroke becomes steeper, the anacrotic shoulder becomes less apparent, and the incisura is replaced by the smoother dicrotic notch. Accordingly, palpation of a peripheral arterial pulse (e.g., the radial pulse) frequently gives less information than examination of a more central pulse (e.g., the carotid pulse) re-

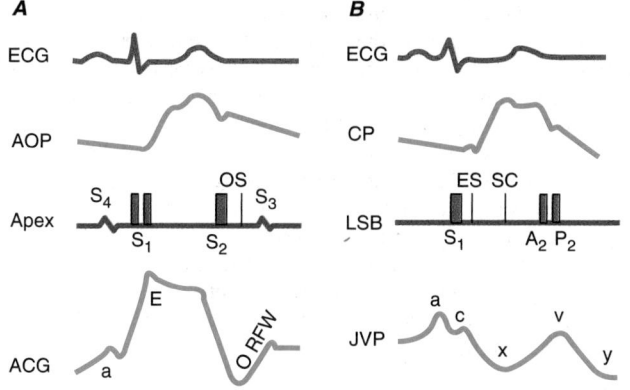

FIGURE 209-1 *A.* Schematic representation of electrocardiogram, aortic pressure pulse (AOP), phonocardiogram recorded at the apex, and apex cardiogram (ACG). On the phonocardiogram, S_1, S_2, S_3, and S_4 represent the first through fourth heart sounds; OS represents the opening snap of the mitral valve, which occurs coincident with the O point of the apex cardiogram. S_3 occurs coincident with the termination of the rapid-filling wave (RFW) of the ACG, while S_4 occurs coincident with the *a* wave of the ACG. *B.* Simultaneous recording of electrocardiogram, indirect carotid pulse (CP), phonocardiogram along the left sternal border (LSB), and indirect jugular venous pulse (JVP). ES, ejection sound; SC, systolic click.

garding alterations in left ventricular ejection or aortic valve function. However, certain findings, such as the bisferiens pulse of aortic regurgitation or pulsus alternans, are more evident in peripheral arteries (Fig. 209-2).

The carotid pulse is best examined with the sternocleidomastoid muscle relaxed and with the patient's head rotated slightly toward the examiner. In palpating the brachial arterial pulse, the examiner can support the patient's relaxed elbow with the right arm while compressing the brachial pulse with the thumb. The usual technique is to compress the artery with the thumb or forefinger until the maximum pulse is sensed. Varying degrees of pressure should then be applied while concentrating on the separate phases of the pulse wave. This method, known as *trisection*, is useful for assessing the sharpness of the upstroke, systolic peak, and diastolic slope of the arterial pulse. In most normal persons, a dicrotic wave is not palpable.

A small weak pulse, *pulsus parvus*, is common in conditions with a diminished left ventricular stroke volume, a narrow pulse pressure, and increased peripheral vascular resistance (Fig. 209-2). A *hypokinetic* pulse may be due to hypovolemia, to left ventricular failure, to restrictive pericardial disease, or to mitral valve stenosis. In aortic valve stenosis, the delayed systolic peak, *pulsus tardus*, results from obstruction to left ventricular ejection. In contrast, a large, bounding (*hyperkinetic*) pulse is usually associated with an increased left ventricular stroke volume, a wide pulse pressure, and a decrease in pe-

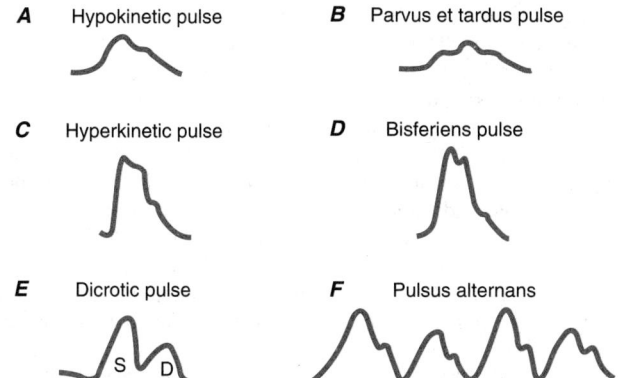

FIGURE 209-2 Schematic representation of arterial pulse waveforms that occur with alterations in cardiac hemodynamics, which may result from normal physiologic responses or may be due to cardiac disease. S, systole; D, diastole. [*Modified from RA O'Rourke, in Hurst's The Heart, 10th ed, V Fuster et al (eds). New York, McGraw-Hill, 2001, with permission.*]

ripheral vascular resistance. This pattern occurs characteristically in patients with an elevated stroke volume, as in complete heart block; with hyperkinetic circulation due to anxiety, anemia, exercise, or fever; or with a rapid runoff of blood from the arterial system (as caused by a patent ductus arteriosus or peripheral arteriovenous fistula). Patients with mitral regurgitation or a ventricular septal defect may also have a bounding pulse, since vigorous left ventricular ejection produces a rapid upstroke in the arterial pulse, even though the duration of systole and the forward stroke volume may be reduced. In aortic regurgitation, the rapidly rising, bounding arterial pulse results from an increased left ventricular stroke volume and an increased rate of ventricular ejection.

The *bisferiens pulse*, which has two systolic peaks, is characteristic of aortic regurgitation (with or without accompanying stenosis) and of hypertrophic cardiomyopathy (Chap. 221). In the latter condition, the pulse wave upstroke rises rapidly and forcefully, producing the first systolic peak ("percussion wave"). A brief decline in pressure follows because of the sudden midsystolic decrease in the rate of left ventricular ejection, when severe obstruction often develops. This pressure trough is followed by a smaller and more slowly rising positive pulse wave ("tidal wave") produced by continued ventricular ejection and by reflected waves from the periphery. The *dicrotic pulse* has two palpable waves, one in systole and one in diastole. It usually denotes a very low stroke volume, particularly in patients with dilated cardiomyopathy.

Pulsus alternans is a pattern in which there is regular alteration of the pressure pulse amplitude, despite a regular rhythm (Fig. 209-2). It is due to alternating left ventricular contractile force, usually indicates severe impairment of left ventricular function, and commonly occurs in patients who also have a loud third heart sound. Pulsus alternans may also occur during or following paroxysmal tachycardia or for several beats following a premature beat in patients without heart disease. In *pulsus bigeminus*, there is also a regular alteration of pressure pulse amplitude, but it is caused by a premature ventricular contraction that follows each regular beat. In *pulsus paradoxus*, the decrease in systolic arterial pressure that normally accompanies the reduction in arterial pulse amplitude during inspiration is accentuated. In patients with pericardial tamponade (Chap. 222), airway obstruction, or superior vena cava obstruction, the decrease in systolic arterial pressure frequently exceeds the normal decrease of 10 mmHg and the peripheral pulse may disappear completely during inspiration.

Simultaneous palpation of the radial and femoral arterial pulses, which normally are virtually coincident, is important to rule out aortic coarctation, in which the latter pulse is weakened and delayed (Chap. 218).

JUGULAR VENOUS PULSE (JVP)

The two main objectives of the examination of the neck veins are inspection of their waveform and estimation of the central venous pressure (CVP). In most patients, the right internal jugular vein is best for both purposes. Usually, the pulsation of the internal jugular vein is greatest when the trunk is inclined by less than 30°. In patients with elevated venous pressure, it may be necessary to elevate the trunk further, sometimes to as much as 90°. When the neck muscles are relaxed, shining a beam of light tangentially across the skin overlying the vein exposes the pulsations of the internal jugular vein. Simultaneous palpation of the left carotid artery aids the examiner in deciding which pulsations are venous and in relating the venous pulsations to their timing in the cardiac cycle.

The normal JVP reflects phasic pressure changes in the right atrium and consists of two or sometimes three positive waves and two negative troughs (Fig. 209-1). The positive presystolic *a* wave is produced by venous distention due to right atrial contraction and is the dominant wave in the JVP, particularly during inspiration. Large *a* waves indicate that the right atrium is contracting against an increased resistance (Fig. 209-3), such as occurs with tricuspid stenosis or more commonly

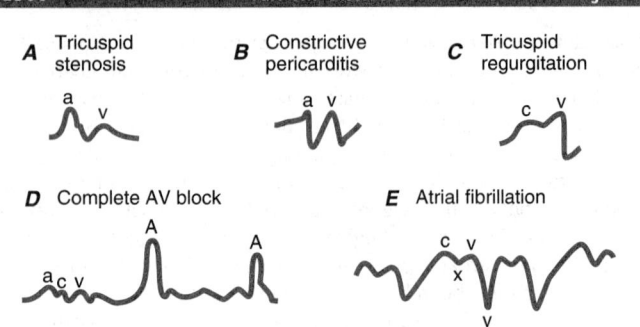

FIGURE 209-3 Abnormal jugular venous pulse waveforms commonly present in patients with cardiac disease and/or arrhythmias. See text. [*Modified from RA O'Rourke, in Hurst's The Heart, 10th ed, V Fuster et al (eds). New York, McGraw-Hill, 2001, with permission.*]

with increased resistance to right ventricular filling (pulmonary hypertension or pulmonic stenosis). Large *a* waves also occur during arrhythmias whenever the right atrium contracts while the tricuspid valve is closed by right ventricular systole. Such "cannon" *a* waves may occur regularly (as during junctional rhythm) or irregularly (as in atrioventricular dissociation with ventricular tachycardia or complete heart block). The *a* wave is absent in patients with atrial fibrillation, and there is an increased delay between the *a* wave and the carotid arterial pulse in patients with first-degree atrioventricular block.

The *c* wave, often observed in the JVP, is a positive wave produced by the bulging of the tricuspid valve into the right atrium during right ventricular isovolumetric systole and by the impact of the carotid artery adjacent to the jugular vein. The *x* descent is due both to atrial relaxation and to the downward displacement of the tricuspid valve during ventricular systole. The *x* descent wave during systole is often accentuated in patients with constrictive pericarditis (Fig. 209-3), but the nadir of this wave is reduced with right ventricular dilation and is often reversed in tricuspid regurgitation. The positive, late systolic *v* wave results from the increasing volume of blood in the right atrium during ventricular systole when the tricuspid valve is closed. Tricuspid regurgitation causes the *v* wave to be more prominent; when tricuspid regurgitation becomes severe, the combination of a prominent *v* wave and obliteration of the *x* descent results in a single large positive systolic wave. After the *v* wave peaks, the right atrial pressure falls because of the decreased bulging of the tricuspid valve into the right atrium as right ventricular pressure declines and the tricuspid valve opens (Fig. 209-3).

This negative descending limb—the *y* descent of the JVP—is produced mainly by the opening of the tricuspid valve and the subsequent rapid inflow of blood into the right ventricle. A rapid, deep *y* descent in early diastole occurs with severe tricuspid regurgitation. A venous pulse characterized by a sharp *y* descent, a deep *y* trough, and a rapid ascent to the baseline is seen in patients with constrictive pericarditis or with severe right-sided heart failure and a high venous pressure. A slow *y* descent in the JVP suggests an obstruction to right ventricular filling, as occurs with tricuspid stenosis or right atrial myxoma.

The right internal jugular is the best vein to use for accurate estimation of the CVP. The sternal angle is used as the reference point, because the center of the right atrium lies approximately 5 cm below the sternal angle in the average patient, regardless of body position. The patient is examined at the optimal degree of trunk elevation for visualization of venous pulsations. The vertical distance between the top of the oscillating venous column and the level of the sternal angle is determined; generally it is less than 3 cm (3 cm + 5 cm = 8 cm blood). The most common cause of a high venous pressure is an elevated right ventricular diastolic pressure.

In patients suspected of having right ventricular failure who have a normal CVP at rest, the *abdominojugular reflux test* may be helpful. The palm of the examiner's hand is placed over the abdomen, and firm pressure is applied for 10 s or more. In normal persons, this maneuver

does not alter the jugular venous pressure significantly, but when right heart function is impaired, the upper level of venous pulsation usually increases. A positive abdominojugular test is best defined as an increase in JVP during 10 s of firm midabdominal compression followed by a rapid drop in pressure of 4 cm blood on release of the compression. The most common cause of a positive test is right-sided heart failure secondary to elevated left heart filling pressures. Also, abdominal compression may elicit the JVP pattern typical of tricuspid regurgitation when the resting pulse wave is normal. *Kussmaul's sign*—an increase rather than the normal decrease in the CVP during inspiration—is most often caused by severe right-sided heart failure; it is a frequent finding in patients with constrictive pericarditis or right ventricular infarction.

PRECORDIAL PALPATION

The location, amplitude, duration, and direction of the cardiac impulse usually can be best appreciated with the fingertips. The normal left ventricular apex impulse is located at or medial to the left midclavicular line in the fourth or fifth intercostal space and is a tapping, early systolic outward thrust localized to a point usually less than 2.5 cm in diameter. It is due primarily to recoil of the heart as blood is ejected and should be evaluated with the patient supine and in the left lateral position. Left ventricular hypertrophy results in exaggeration of the amplitude, duration, and often size of the normal left ventricular thrust. The impulse may be displaced laterally and downward into the sixth or seventh intercostal space, particularly in patients with a left ventricular volume load such as occurs in cases of aortic regurgitation or dilated cardiomyopathy.

Additional abnormal features that are detectable at the left ventricular apex include (1) marked presystolic distention of the left ventricle, usually accompanied by a fourth heart sound in patients with an excessive left ventricular pressure load or myocardial ischemia/infarction; and (2) a prominent early diastolic rapid-filling wave, often accompanied by a third heart sound in patients with left ventricular failure or mitral valve regurgitation (Fig. 209-1). A double systolic apical impulse is palpable in many patients with hypertrophic cardiomyopathy.

Right ventricular hypertrophy often results in a sustained systolic lift at the lower left parasternal area, which starts in early systole and is synchronous with the left ventricular apical impulse.

Abnormal precordial pulsations occur during systole in patients with left ventricular dyssynergy due to ischemic heart disease or to diffuse myocardial disease from some other cause. These pulsations often occur in patients with a recent myocardial infarction and may be present in some patients only during episodes of angina. They are most commonly felt in the left midprecordium one or two interspaces above and/or 1 to 2 cm medial to the left ventricular apex. A systolic bulge occurring in the region of the apex is difficult to distinguish from the impulse of left ventricular hypertrophy.

A left parasternal lift is frequently present in patients with severe mitral regurgitation. This pulsation occurs distinctly later than the left ventricular apical impulse, is synchronous with the *v* wave in the left atrial pressure curve, and is due to anterior displacement of the right ventricle by an enlarged, expanding left atrium. A similar impulse occurs to the right of the sternum in some patients with severe tricuspid regurgitation and a giant right atrium. Pulsation of the right sternoclavicular joint may indicate a right-sided aortic arch or aneurysmal dilation of the ascending aorta. Pulmonary artery pulsation is often visible and palpable in the second left intercostal space. While it may be normal in children or thin young adults, this pulsation usually denotes pulmonary hypertension, increased pulmonary blood flow, or poststenotic pulmonary artery dilation.

Thrills are palpable, low-frequency vibrations associated with heart murmurs. The systolic murmur of mitral regurgitation may be palpated at the cardiac apex. When the palm of the hand is placed over the precordium, the thrill of aortic stenosis crosses the palm toward the right side of the neck, while the thrill of pulmonic stenosis radiates more often to the left side of the neck. The thrill due to a ventricular septal defect is usually located in the third and fourth intercostal spaces near the left sternal border.

Percussion should be performed in each patient to identify normal or abnormal position of the heart, stomach, and liver. However, in patients with a normal cardiac situs, percussion adds little to careful inspection and palpation in the recognition of cardiac enlargement.

CARDIAC AUSCULTATION

To obtain the most information from cardiac auscultation, the observer should keep in mind several principles: (1) Auscultation should be performed in a quiet room to avoid the distracting noises of normal activity. (2) For optimal auscultation, attention must be focused on the phase of the cardiac cycle during which the auscultatory event is expected to occur. (3) The timing of a heart sound or murmur can be determined accurately from its relation to other observable events in the cardiac cycle—the carotid arterial pulse, the apical impulse, or the JVP. (4) To define the significance of a cardiac sound or murmur, it is often necessary to observe alterations in its timing or intensity during various physiologic and/or pharmacologic interventions (Table 209-1).

HEART SOUNDS

The major components of heart sounds are vibrations associated with the abrupt acceleration or deceleration of blood in the cardiovascular system. Studies using simultaneous echocardiographic-phonocardiographic recordings indicate that the first and second heart sounds are produced primarily by the closure of the atrioventricular (AV) and semilunar valves and the events that accompany these closures. The intensity of the *first heart sound* (S_1) is influenced by (1) the position

---

TABLE 209-1 *Effects of Physiologic and Pharmacologic Interventions on the Intensity of Heart Murmurs and Sounds*

Respiration Systolic murmurs due to TR or pulmonic blood flow through a normal or stenotic valve and diastolic murmurs of TS or PR generally increase with inspiration, as do right-sided S_3 and S_4. Left-sided murmurs and sounds usually are louder during expiration.

Valsalva maneuver Most murmurs decrease in length and intensity. Two exceptions are the systolic murmur of HCM, which usually becomes much louder, and that of MVP, which becomes longer and often louder. Following release of the Valsalva maneuver, right-sided murmurs tend to return to control intensity earlier than left-sided murmurs.

After VPB or AF Murmurs originating at normal or stenotic semilunar valves increase in the cardiac cycle following a VPB or in the cycle after a long cycle length in AF. By contrast, systolic murmurs due to AV valve regurgitation either do not change, diminish (papillary muscle dysfunction), or become shorter (MVP).

Positional changes With *standing*, most murmurs diminish, two exceptions being the murmur of HCM, which becomes louder, and that of MVP, which lengthens and often is intensified. With *squatting*, most murmurs become louder, but those of HCM and MVP usually soften and may disappear. Passive leg raising usually produces the same results.

Exercise Murmurs due to blood flow across normal or obstructed valves (e.g., PS, MS) become louder with both isotonic and submaximal isometric (handgrip) exercise. Murmurs of MR, VSD, and AR also increase with handgrip exercise. However, the murmur of HCM often decreases with near maximum handgrip exercise. Left-sided S_4 and S_3 are often accentuated by exercise, particularly when due to ischemic heart disease.

Pharmacologic interventions During the initial relative hypotension following amyl nitrite inhalation, murmurs of MR, VSD, and AR decrease, while murmurs of aortic stenosis or sclerosis increase. During the later tachycardia phase, murmurs of MS and right-sided lesions also increase. The response in MVP often is biphasic (first softer and then louder than control). The arterial constrictor phenylephrine tends to produce the opposite effects.

Transient arterial occlusion Transient external compression of both arms by bilateral cuff inflation to 20 mmHg over peak systolic pressure augments the murmurs of MR, VSD, and AR, but not murmurs due to other causes.

Note: TR, tricuspid regurgitation; TS, tricuspid stenosis; PR, pulmonic regurgitation; HCM, hypertrophic cardiomyopathy; MVP, mitral valve prolapse; PS, pulmonic stenosis; MS, mitral stenosis; MR, mitral regurgitation; VSD, ventricular septal defect; AR, aortic regurgitation; VPB, ventricular premature beat; and AF, atrial fibrillation.

---

of the mitral leaflets at the onset of ventricular systole; (2) the rate of rise of the left ventricular pressure pulse; (3) the presence or absence of structural disease of the mitral valve; and (4) the amount of tissue, air, or fluid between the heart and the stethoscope. S_1 is louder if diastole is shortened because of tachycardia, if AV flow is increased because of high cardiac output or prolonged because of mitral stenosis, or if atrial contraction precedes ventricular contraction by an unusually short interval, reflected in a short PR interval. The loud S_1 in mitral stenosis usually signifies that the valve is pliable and that it remains open at the onset of isovolumetric contraction because of the elevated left atrial pressure. A soft S_1 may be due to poor conduction of sound through the chest wall, a slow rise of the left ventricular pressure pulse, a long PR interval, or imperfect closure due to reduced valve substance, as in mitral regurgitation. S_1 is also soft when the anterior mitral leaflet is immobile because of rigidity and calcification, even in the presence of predominant mitral stenosis.

Splitting of the two high-pitched components of S_1 by 10 to 30 ms is a normal phenomenon (Fig. 209-1). The first component of S_1 is usually attributed to mitral valve closure, and the second to tricuspid valve closure. Widening of the S_1 is due most often to complete right bundle branch block and the resulting delay in onset of the right ventricular pressure pulse. Reversed splitting of the S_1, in which the mitral component follows the tricuspid component, may be present in patients with severe mitral stenosis, left atrial myxoma, and left bundle branch block.

SPLITTING OF THE *SECOND HEART SOUND* This sound (S_2) normally splits into audibly distinct aortic (A_2) and pulmonic (P_2) components during inspiration, when the augmented inflow into the right ventricle increases its stroke volume and ejection period and thus delays closure of the pulmonic valve. P_2 is coincident with the incisura of the pulmonary artery pressure curve, which is separated from the right ventricular pressure tracing by an interval termed the *hangout time*. The absolute value of this interval reflects the resistance to pulmonary blood flow and the impedance characteristics of the pulmonary vascular bed. This interval is prolonged, and physiologic splitting of S_2 is accentuated, in conditions associated with right ventricular volume overload and a distensible pulmonary vascular bed. However, in patients with an increase in pulmonary vascular resistance, the hangout time is markedly reduced, and narrow splitting of S_2 is present. Splitting that persists with expiration (heard best at the pulmonic area or left sternal border) is usually abnormal when the patient is in the upright position. Such splitting may be due to many causes: delayed activation of the right ventricle (right bundle branch block); left ventricular ectopic beats; a left ventricular pacemaker; prolongation of right ventricular contraction with an increased right ventricular pressure load (pulmonary embolism or pulmonic stenosis); or delayed pulmonic valve closure because of right ventricular volume overload associated with right ventricular failure or diminished impedance of the pulmonary vascular bed and a prolonged hangout time (atrial septal defect).

In pulmonary hypertension, P_2 is loud, and splitting of the second heart sound may be diminished, normal, or accentuated, depending on the cause of the pulmonary hypertension, the pulmonary vascular resistance, and the presence or absence of right ventricular decompensation. Early aortic valve closure, occurring with mitral regurgitation or a ventricular septal defect, may also produce splitting that persists during expiration. It may also occur with constrictive pericarditis. In patients with an atrial septal defect, the proportion of right atrial filling contributed by the left atrium and the venae cavae varies reciprocally during the respiratory cycle, so that right atrial inflow remains relatively constant. Therefore, the volume and duration of right ventricular ejection are not significantly increased by inspiration, and there is little inspiratory exaggeration of the splitting of S_2. This phenomenon, termed *fixed splitting* of the second heart sound, is of considerable diagnostic value.

A delay in aortic valve closure causing P_2 to precede A_2 results in so-called reversed (paradoxic) splitting of S_2. Splitting is then maximal in expiration and decreases during inspiration with the normal delay of pulmonic valve closure. The most common causes of reversed splitting of S_2 are left bundle branch block and delayed excitation of the left ventricle from a right ventricular ectopic beat. Mechanical prolongation of left ventricular systole, resulting in reversed splitting of S_2, may also be caused by severe aortic outflow obstruction, a large aorta-to-pulmonary artery shunt, systolic hypertension, and ischemic heart disease or cardiomyopathy with left ventricular failure. P_2 is normally softer than A_2 in the second left intercostal space; a P_2 that is greater than A_2 in this area suggests pulmonary hypertension, except in patients with atrial septal defect.

SYSTOLIC SOUNDS   The *ejection sound* is a sharp, high-pitched event occurring in early systole and closely following the first heart sound. Ejection sounds occur in the presence of semilunar valve stenosis and in conditions associated with dilation of the aorta or pulmonary artery. The aortic ejection sound is usually heard best at the left ventricular apex and the second right intercostal space; the pulmonary ejection sound is loudest at the upper left sternal border. The latter, unlike most other right-sided acoustical events, is heard better during expiration.

Nonejection clicks, or *midsystolic clicks*, occurring with or without a late systolic murmur, often denote prolapse of one or both leaflets of the mitral valve (Chap. 219). They also may be caused by tricuspid valve prolapse. They probably result from chordae tendineae that are functionally unequal in length on either or both AV valves and are heard best along the lower left sternal border and at the left ventricular apex. Systolic clicks may be single or multiple, and they may occur at any time in systole but are usually later than the systolic ejection sound.

DIASTOLIC SOUNDS   The *opening snap* (OS) is a brief, high-pitched, early diastolic sound, which is usually due to stenosis of an AV valve, most often the mitral valve. It is generally heard best at the lower left sternal border and radiates well to the base of the heart. The A_2-OS interval is inversely related to the height of the mean left atrial pressure and ranges from 0.04 to 0.12 s. In the second intercostal space, an OS is often confused with P_2. However, careful auscultation will reveal both components of S_2, followed by the OS. The OS of tricuspid stenosis occurs later in diastole than the mitral OS and is often overlooked in patients with more prominent mitral valve disease.

The *third heart sound* (S_3) is a low-pitched sound produced in the ventricle 0.14 to 0.16 s after A_2, at the termination of rapid filling. This sound is frequent in normal children and in patients with high cardiac output. However, in patients over 40 years old, an S_3 usually indicates impairment of ventricular function, AV valve regurgitation, or other conditions that increase the rate or volume of ventricular filling. The left-sided S_3 is best heard with the bell piece of the stethoscope at the left ventricular apex during expiration and with the patient in the left lateral position. The right-sided S_3 is best heard at the left sternal border or just beneath the xiphoid and is usually louder with inspiration. Often it is accompanied by the systolic murmur of functional tricuspid regurgitation. Third heart sounds often disappear with treatment of heart failure.

An S_3 that is earlier (0.10 to 0.12 s after A_2) and higher-pitched than normal (a pericardial knock) often occurs in patients with constrictive pericarditis (Chap. 222); its presence depends on the restrictive effect of the adherent pericardium, which abruptly halts diastolic filling.

The *fourth heart sound* (S_4) is a low-pitched, presystolic sound produced in the ventricle during ventricular filling; it is associated with an effective atrial contraction and is best heard with the bell piece of the stethoscope. The sound is absent in patients with atrial fibrillation. The S_4 occurs when diminished ventricular compliance increases the resistance to ventricular filling, and it is frequently present in patients with systemic hypertension, aortic stenosis, hypertrophic cardiomyopathy, ischemic heart disease, and acute mitral regurgitation. Most patients with an acute myocardial infarction and sinus rhythm have an audible S_4. The fourth heart sound is frequently accompanied by visible and palpable presystolic distention of the left ventricle. It is loudest at the left ventricular apex when the patient is in the left lateral position and is accentuated by mild isotonic or isometric exercise in the supine position. The right-sided S_4 is present in patients with right ventricular hypertrophy secondary to either pulmonic stenosis or pulmonary hypertension and frequently accompanies a prominent presystolic *a* wave in the JVP.

An S_4 frequently accompanies delayed AV conduction even in the absence of clinically detectable heart disease. The incidence of an audible S_4 increases with increasing age. Whether an audible S_4 in adults without other evidence of cardiac disease is abnormal remains controversial. Both left-sided S_3 and S_4 sounds increase with isometric exercise and both may radiate to the subclavian and carotid arteries.

HEART MURMURS

Cardiac murmurs result from vibrations set up in the bloodstream and the surrounding heart and great vessels as a result of turbulent blood flow, the formation of eddies, and cavitation (bubble formation as a result of sudden decrease in pressure).

The evaluation of the patient with a heart murmur may vary greatly depending on many of the considerations discussed below. These include the intensity of the cardiac murmur, its timing in the cardiac cycle, its location and radiation, and its response to various physiologic maneuvers. Also of importance are the presence or absence of cardiac and noncardiac symptoms and whether other cardiac or noncardiac physical findings suggest that the cardiac murmur is clinically significant. The skill and confidence of the cardiac auscultator, the relative costs of various diagnostic approaches, and the accuracy and reliability of additional tests in the laboratory where they are performed are also important factors.

The intensity (loudness) of murmurs may be graded from I to VI. A grade I murmur is so faint that it can be heard only with special effort; a grade IV murmur is commonly accompanied by a thrill; and a grade VI murmur is audible with the stethoscope removed from contact with the chest. The configuration of a murmur may be crescendo, decrescendo, crescendo-decrescendo (diamond-shaped), or plateau (Fig. 209-4). The precise time of onset and time of cessation of a murmur depend on the instant in the cardiac cycle at which an adequate pressure difference between two chambers arises and disappears (Fig. 209-5).

The location on the chest wall where the murmur is best heard and the areas to which it radiates can aid in identifying the cardiac structure from which the murmur originates. For example, the murmur of aortic valve stenosis is usually loudest in the second right intercostal space and radiates to the carotid arteries. By contrast, the murmur of mitral regurgitation is most often loudest at the cardiac apex. It may radiate to the left sternal border and base of the heart when the posterior mitral leaflet is predominantly involved or to the axilla and back when the anterior leaflet is more severely affected. In the latter case, the regurgitant blood is directed toward the posterior left atrial wall.

EFFECTS OF PHYSIOLOGIC INTERVENTIONS   It is often difficult to classify a cardiac murmur with certainty on the basis of its timing, configuration, location, radiation, pitch, or intensity. However, by noting changes in the characteristics of the murmur during maneuvers that alter cardiac hemodynamics, the auscultator can often identify its correct origin and significance (Table 209-1).

Accentuation of a murmur during inspiration (a maneuver that augments systemic venous return) implies that it originates on the right side of the circulation; expiratory exaggeration has less significance. Prolonged expiratory pressure against a closed glottis (i.e., the Valsalva maneuver) reduces the intensity of most murmurs by diminishing both right and left ventricular filling (i.e., ventricular preload). The systolic murmur associated with *hypertrophic cardiomyopathy* and the late systolic murmur due to *mitral valve prolapse* are exceptions and may be paradoxically accentuated during the Valsalva maneuver. Mur-

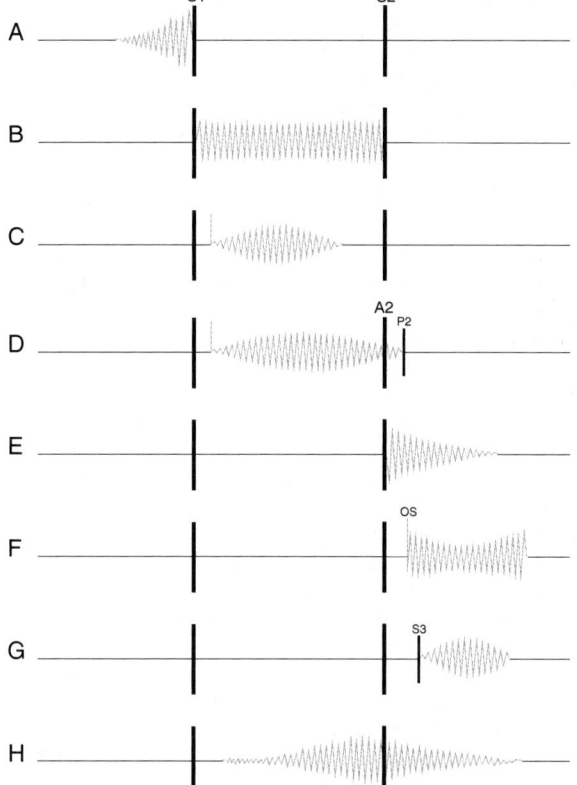

FIGURE 209-4 Diagram depicting principal heart murmurs. *A.* Presystolic murmur of mitral or tricuspid stenosis. *B.* Holosystolic (pansystolic) murmur of mitral or tricuspid regurgitation or of ventricular septal defect. *C.* Aortic ejection murmur beginning with an ejection click and fading before the second heart sound. *D.* Systolic murmur in pulmonic stenosis spilling through the aortic second sound, pulmonic valve closure being delayed. *E.* Aortic or pulmonary diastolic murmur. *F.* Long diastolic murmur of mitral stenosis following the opening snap. *G.* Short middiastolic inflow murmur following a third heart sound. *H.* Continuous murmur of patent ductus arteriosus *(Adapted by P O'Gara from P Wood, Diseases of the Heart and Circulation. Philadelphia, Lippincott, 1968, with permission.)*

murs due to flow across a normal or obstructed semilunar valve increase in intensity in the cycle following a premature ventricular beat or a long RR interval in atrial fibrillation. In contrast, murmurs due to AV valve regurgitation or a ventricular septal defect do not change appreciably during the beat following a prolonged diastole. Standing, which decreases left ventricular volume, accentuates the murmur of hypertrophic cardiomyopathy and occasionally the murmur due to mitral valve prolapse. Squatting, which increases both venous return and systemic arterial resistance and thus ventricular afterload, increases most murmurs, except those due to hypertrophic cardiomyopathy and mitral regurgitation due to a prolapsed mitral valve, which often decrease. In the patient who cannot squat, jackknifing the legs will produce the same response. Sustained handgrip exercise, which increases systemic arterial pressure and heart rate, often accentuates the murmurs of mitral regurgitation, aortic regurgitation, and mitral stenosis but usually diminishes those due to aortic stenosis or hypertrophic cardiomyopathy.

SYSTOLIC MURMURS ■ Holosystolic (Pansystolic) Murmurs These are generated when there is flow between two chambers that have widely different pressures throughout systole, such as the left ventricle and either the left atrium or the right ventricle (Fig. 209-5). The pressure gradient occurs early in contraction and lasts until relaxation is almost complete. Therefore, holosystolic murmurs begin before aortic ejection, and at the area of maximal intensity they begin with S_1 and end after S_2 (Fig. 209-4*B*). Holosystolic murmurs accompany mitral or tricuspid regurgitation, ventricular septal defect, and, under certain circumstances, aortopulmonary shunts. Although the typical high-pitched murmur of mitral regurgitation usually continues throughout systole,

the shape of the murmur may vary considerably. The holosystolic murmurs of mitral regurgitation and ventricular septal defect are augmented by transient exercise.

The murmur of tricuspid regurgitation associated with pulmonary hypertension is holosystolic and frequently increases during inspiration. Not all patients with mitral or tricuspid regurgitation or ventricular septal defect have holosystolic murmurs. Often, a mild valvular regurgitant jet, detected by color flow Doppler techniques (Chap. 211), is not associated with an audible murmur despite optimal auscultation. Such regurgitant jets usually do not indicate clinical heart disease. Trivial mitral regurgitation can be detected by Doppler in up to 45% of normal individuals; tricuspid regurgitation in up to 70%; and pulmonic regurgitation in up to 88%. Aortic regurgitation is encountered much less frequently in normal persons, and its incidence increases with advancing age. An overinterpretation of the significance of mild regurgitation by echocardiographers often results in a misdiagnosis of "echocardiographic heart disease," resulting in unnecessary patient anxiety and infective endocarditis prophylaxis.

Midsystolic Murmurs These also called *systolic ejection murmurs*, which are often crescendo-decrescendo in shape, and occur when blood is ejected across the aortic or pulmonic outflow tracts (Figs. 209-4*C* and 209-5). The murmur starts shortly after S_1, when the ventricular pressure becomes high enough to open the semilunar valve. As the velocity of ejection increases, the murmur gets louder; as ejection declines, it diminishes. The murmur ends before the ventricular pressure falls enough to permit closure of the aortic or pulmonic leaflets. When the semilunar valves are normal, an increased flow rate (as occurs in states of elevated cardiac output), ejection into a dilated vessel beyond the valve, or increased transmission of sound through a thin chest wall may be responsible for this murmur. Most benign, functional murmurs are midsystolic and originate from the pulmonary outflow tract. Valvular or subvalvular obstruction of either ventricle may also cause such a midsystolic murmur, the intensity being related to the flow rate.

The murmur of aortic stenosis is the prototype of the left-sided midsystolic murmur. The location and radiation of this murmur are influenced by the direction of the high-velocity jet within the aortic

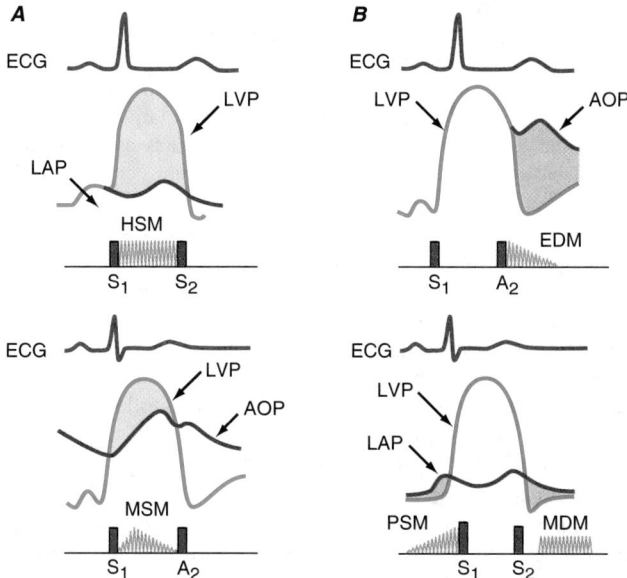

FIGURE 209-5 *A.* Schematic representation of ECG, aortic pressure (AOP), left ventricular pressure (LVP), and left atrial pressure (LAP). The shaded areas indicate a transvalvular pressure difference during systole. HSM, holosystolic murmur; MSM, midsystolic murmur. *B.* Graphic representation of ECG, aortic pressure (AOP), left ventricular pressure (LVP), and left atrial pressure (LAP) with shaded areas indicating transvalvular diastolic pressure difference. EDM, early diastolic murmur; PSM, presystolic murmur; MDM, middiastolic murmur.

root. In *valvular aortic stenosis*, the murmur is usually maximal in the second right intercostal space, with radiation into the neck. In *supravalvular aortic stenosis*, the murmur is occasionally loudest even higher, with disproportionate radiation into the right carotid artery. In hypertrophic cardiomyopathy, the midsystolic murmur originates in the left ventricular cavity and is usually maximal at the lower left sternal edge and apex, with relatively little radiation to the carotids. When the aortic valve is immobile (calcified), the aortic closure sound (A_2) may be soft and inaudible so that the length and configuration of the murmur are difficult to determine. Midsystolic murmurs also occur in patients with mitral regurgitation or, less frequently, tricuspid regurgitation resulting from papillary muscle dysfunction. Such murmurs due to mitral regurgitation are often confused with those originating in the aorta, particularly in elderly patients.

The patient's age and the area of maximal intensity aid in determining the significance of midsystolic murmurs. Thus, in a young adult with a thin chest and a high velocity of blood flow, a faint or moderate midsystolic murmur heard only in the pulmonic area is usually without clinical significance, while a somewhat louder murmur in the aortic area may indicate congenital aortic stenosis. In elderly patients, pulmonic flow murmurs are rare, while aortic systolic murmurs are common and may be due to aortic dilation, to a significant degree of valvular aortic stenosis, or to nonstenotic thickening of the aortic valve leaflets. Midsystolic aortic and pulmonic murmurs are intensified after amyl nitrite inhalation and during the cardiac cycle following a premature ventricular beat, while those due to mitral regurgitation are unchanged or softer. Aortic systolic murmurs are diminished by interventions that increase aortic impedance, such as transient arterial occlusion. Echocardiography or cardiac catheterization may be necessary to separate a prominent and exaggerated functional murmur from one due to congenital or acquired semilunar valve stenosis.

Early Systolic Murmurs   These murmurs begin with the first heart sound and end in midsystole. In *large ventricular septal defects with pulmonary hypertension*, the shunting at the end of systole may be small or absent, resulting in an early systolic murmur. A similar murmur may occur with very small *muscular ventricular septal defects*, the shunt being interrupted in late systole. An early systolic murmur is a feature of *tricuspid regurgitation occurring in the absence of pulmonary hypertension*. This lesion is common in narcotics abusers with infective endocarditis, in whom a tall regurgitant right atrial *v* wave reaches the level of the normal right ventricular pressure in late systole, confining the murmur to early systole. Patients with acute mitral regurgitation into a noncompliant left atrium and a large *v* wave often have a loud early systolic murmur that diminishes as the pressure gradient between the left ventricle and left atrium decreases in late systole (Chap. 219).

Late Systolic Murmurs   These murmurs are faint or moderately loud, high-pitched apical murmurs that start well after ejection and do not mask either heart sound. They are probably related to papillary muscle dysfunction caused by infarction or ischemia of these muscles or to their distortion by left ventricular dilation. They may appear only during angina but are common in patients with myocardial infarction or diffuse myocardial disease. Late systolic murmurs following midsystolic clicks are due to late systolic mitral regurgitation caused by prolapse of the mitral valve into the left atrium (Chap. 219).

DIASTOLIC MURMURS ■ **Early Diastolic Murmurs** (Figs. 209-4*E*, 209-5) These murmurs begin with or shortly after S_2, as soon as the corresponding ventricular pressure falls enough below that in the aorta or pulmonary artery. The high-pitched murmurs of aortic regurgitation or of pulmonic regurgitation due to pulmonary hypertension are generally decrescendo, since there is a progressive decline in the volume or rate of regurgitation during diastole. Faint, high-pitched murmurs of aortic regurgitation are difficult to hear unless they are specifically sought by applying firm pressure with the diaphragm over the left midsternal border while the patient sits leaning forward and holds a

breath in full expiration. The diastolic murmur of aortic regurgitation is enhanced by an acute elevation of the arterial pressure, such as occurs with handgrip exercise; it diminishes with a decrease in arterial pressure, as with amyl nitrite inhalation. The diastolic murmur of congenital pulmonic regurgitation without pulmonary hypertension is low- to medium-pitched. The onset of this murmur is delayed because the regurgitant flow is minimal at the onset of pulmonic valve closure when the reverse pressure gradient responsible for the regurgitation is negligible.

Middiastolic Murmurs   These usually arise from the mitral or tricuspid valves, occur during early ventricular filling, and are due to disproportion between valve orifice size and flow rate. Such murmurs may be quite loud (grade III), despite only slight AV valve stenosis, when there is normal or increased blood flow. Conversely, the murmurs may be soft or even absent despite severe obstruction if the cardiac output is markedly reduced. When stenosis is marked, the diastolic murmur is prolonged, and the duration of the murmur is more reliable than its intensity as an index of the severity of valve obstruction.

The low-pitched, middiastolic murmur of mitral stenosis characteristically follows the OS (Fig. 209-4*F*). It should be specifically sought by placing the bell of the stethoscope at the site of the left ventricular impulse, which is best localized with the patient on the left side. Frequently, the murmur of mitral stenosis is present only at the left ventricular apex, and it may be increased in intensity by mild supine exercise or by inhalation of amyl nitrite. In tricuspid stenosis, the middiastolic murmur is localized to a relatively limited area along the left sternal edge and may be louder during inspiration.

Middiastolic murmurs may be generated across the mitral valve in cases of mitral regurgitation, patent ductus arteriosus, or ventricular septal defect, and across the tricuspid valve in cases of tricuspid regurgitation or atrial septal defect. These murmurs are related to the very rapid flow across an AV valve, usually follow an S_3 (Fig. 209-4*G*), and tend to occur with large left-to-right shunts or severe AV valve regurgitation. A soft middiastolic murmur may sometimes be heard in patients with acute rheumatic fever (Carey-Coombs murmur). It has been attributed to inflammation of the mitral valve cusps or excessive left atrial blood flow as a consequence of mitral regurgitation.

In acute, severe aortic regurgitation, the left ventricular diastolic pressure may exceed the left atrial pressure, resulting in a middiastolic murmur due to "diastolic mitral regurgitation." In severe, chronic aortic regurgitation, a murmur is frequently present that may be either middiastolic or presystolic (Austin-Flint murmur). This murmur appears to originate at the anterior mitral valve leaflet when blood enters the left ventricle simultaneously from both the aortic root and the left atrium.

Presystolic Murmurs (Fig. 209-4*A*)   These murmurs begin during the period of ventricular filling that follows atrial contraction and therefore occur in sinus rhythm. They are usually due to AV valve stenosis and have the same quality as the middiastolic filling rumble, but they are usually crescendo, reaching peak intensity at the time of a loud S_1. The presystolic murmur corresponds to the AV valve gradient, which may be minimal until the moment of right or left atrial contraction. It is the presystolic murmur that is most characteristic of tricuspid stenosis and sinus rhythm. A right or left *atrial myxoma* may occasionally cause either middiastolic or presystolic murmurs that resemble the murmurs of mitral or tricuspid stenosis.

CONTINUOUS MURMURS   These begin in systole, peak near S_2, and continue into all or part of diastole (Fig. 209-4*H*). These murmurs result from continuous flow due to a communication between high- and low-pressure areas that persists through the end of systole and the beginning of diastole. A *patent ductus arteriosus* causes a continuous murmur as long as the pressure in the pulmonary artery is much below that in the aorta. The murmur is intensified by elevation of the systemic arterial pressure. When pulmonary hypertension is present, the diastolic portion may disappear, leaving the murmur confined to systole. A continuous murmur is uncommon in cases of aortopulmonary septal defect, which usually is associated with severe pulmonary hypertension. Surgically produced connections and the subclavian–pulmonary artery anastomosis result in murmurs similar to that of a patent ductus.

Continuous murmurs may result from congenital or acquired *systemic arteriovenous fistula*, *coronary arteriovenous fistula*, anomalous origin of the left coronary artery from the pulmonary artery, and *communications between the sinus of Valsalva and the right side of the heart*. Continuous murmurs may also occur in patients with a small atrial septal defect with a high left atrial pressure. Murmurs associated with *pulmonary arteriovenous fistulas* may be continuous but are usually only systolic. Continuous murmurs may also be due to disturbances of flow pattern in constricted systemic (e.g., renal) or pulmonary arteries when marked pressure differences between the two sides of the narrow segment persist; a continuous murmur in the back may be present in *coarctation of the aorta*; *pulmonary embolism* may cause continuous murmurs in partially occluded vessels.

In nonconstricted arteries, continuous murmurs may be due to rapid flow through a tortuous bed. Such murmurs typically occur within the bronchial arterial collateral circulation in cyanotic patients with severe pulmonary outflow obstruction. The "mammary souffle," an innocent murmur heard over the breasts during late pregnancy and in the early postpartum period, may be systolic or continuous. The innocent cervical venous hum is a continuous murmur usually audible over the medial aspect of the right supraclavicular fossa with the patient upright. The hum is usually louder during diastole and can be abolished instantaneously by digital compression of the ipsilateral internal jugular vein. Transmission of a loud venous hum to the area below the clavicles may result in a mistaken diagnosis of patent ductus arteriosus.

PERICARDIAL FRICTION RUB These adventitious sounds may have presystolic, systolic, and early diastolic scratchy components and may be confused with a murmur or extracardiac sound when heard only in systole. A pericardial friction rub is best appreciated with the patient upright and leaning forward and may be accentuated during inspiration.

FURTHER READING

ABRAMS J: *Synopsis of Cardiac Physical Diagnosis*, 2d ed. Boston, Butterworth, 2001

BRAUNWALD E: The clinical examination, in *Primary Cardiology*, 2d ed, E Braunwald, L Goldman (eds). Philadelphia, Saunders, 2003

CHISNER MA: The diagnosis of heart disease by clinical assessment alone. Curr Probl Cardiol 26:285, 2001

CHOONG CY et al: Prevalence of valvular regurgitation by Doppler echocardiography in patients with structurally normal hearts by 2-dimensional echocardiography. Am Heart J 117:636, 1989

CLEMENT DL, COHN JN: Salvaging the history, physical examination and doctor-patient relationship in a technological cardiology environment. J Am Coll Cardiol 33:892, 1999

O'ROURKE RA: Approach to a patient with a heart murmur, in *Primary Cardiology*, 2d ed, E Braunwald, L Goldman (eds). Philadelphia, Saunders, 2003

PERLOFF JK (ed): *Physical Examination of the Heart and Circulation*, 3d ed. Philadelphia, Saunders, 2000

VLACHOPOULOUS C, O'ROURKE RA: Genesis of the normal and abnormal arterial pulse. Curr Probl Cardiol 25:297, 2000

210 ELECTROCARDIOGRAPHY
Ary L. Goldberger

The electrocardiogram (ECG or EKG) is a graphic recording of electric potentials generated by the heart. The signals are detected by means of metal electrodes attached to the extremities and chest wall and are then amplified and recorded by the electrocardiograph. ECG *leads* actually display the instantaneous *differences* in potential between these electrodes.

The clinical utility of the ECG derives from its immediate availability as a noninvasive, inexpensive, and highly versatile test. In addition to its use in detecting arrhythmias, conduction disturbances, and myocardial ischemia, electrocardiography may reveal other findings related to life-threatening metabolic disturbances (e.g., hyperkalemia) or increased susceptibility to sudden cardiac death (e.g., QT prolongation syndromes). The advent of coronary thrombolysis or angioplasty in the early therapy of acute myocardial infarction (Chap. 228) has refocused particular attention on the sensitivity and specificity of ECG signs of myocardial ischemia.

ELECTROPHYSIOLOGY (See also Chaps. 213 and 214)

Depolarization of the heart is the initiating event for cardiac contraction. The electric currents that spread through the heart are produced by three components: cardiac pacemaker cells, specialized conduction tissue, and the heart muscle itself. The ECG, however, records only the depolarization (stimulation) and repolarization (recovery) potentials generated by the atrial and ventricular myocardium.

The depolarization stimulus for the normal heartbeat originates in the *sinoatrial (SA) node* (Fig. 210-1), or *sinus node*, a collection of *pacemaker cells*. These cells fire spontaneously; that is, they exhibit *automaticity*. The first phase of cardiac electrical activation is the spread of the depolarization wave through the right and left atria, followed by atrial contraction. Next, the impulse stimulates pacemaker and specialized conduction tissues in the atrioventricular (AV) nodal and His-bundle areas; together, these two regions constitute the AV junction. The bundle of His bifurcates into two main branches, the right and left bundles, which rapidly transmit depolarization wavefronts to the right and left ventricular myocardium by way of Purkinje fibers. The main left bundle bifurcates into two primary subdivisions, a left anterior fascicle and a left posterior fascicle. The depolarization wavefronts then spread through the ventricular wall, from endocardium to epicardium, triggering ventricular contraction.

Since the cardiac depolarization and repolarization waves have direction and magnitude, they can be represented by vectors. *Vectorcardiograms* that measure and display these instantaneous potentials are no longer used much in clinical practice. However, the general principles of vector analysis remain fundamental to understanding the genesis of normal and pathologic ECG waveforms. Vector analysis illustrates a central concept of electrocardiography—that the ECG re-

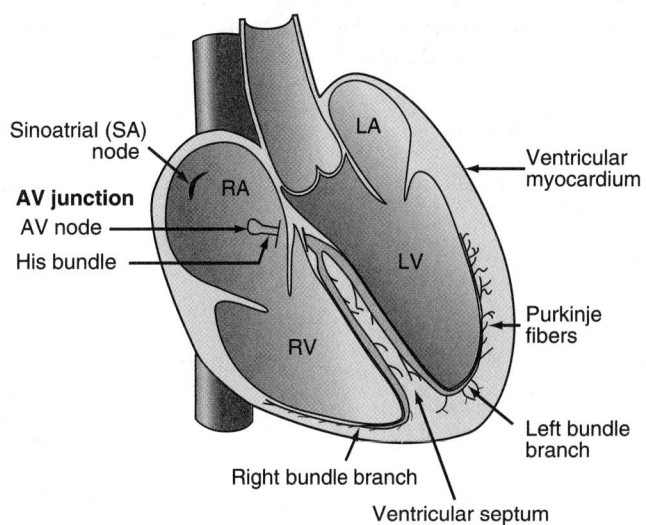

FIGURE 210-1 Schematic of the cardiac conduction system.

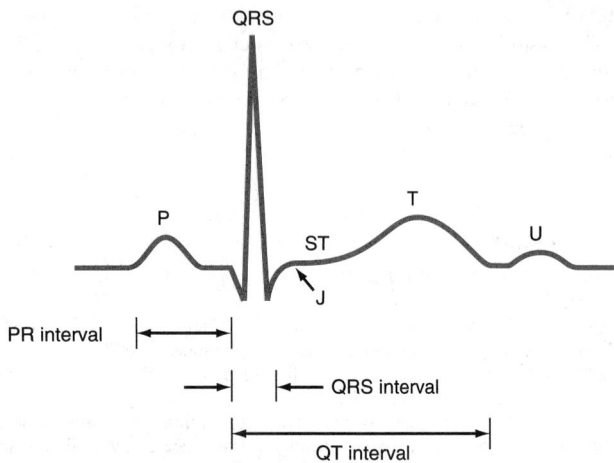

FIGURE 210-2 Basic ECG waveforms and intervals. Not shown is the R-R interval, the time between consecutive QRS complexes.

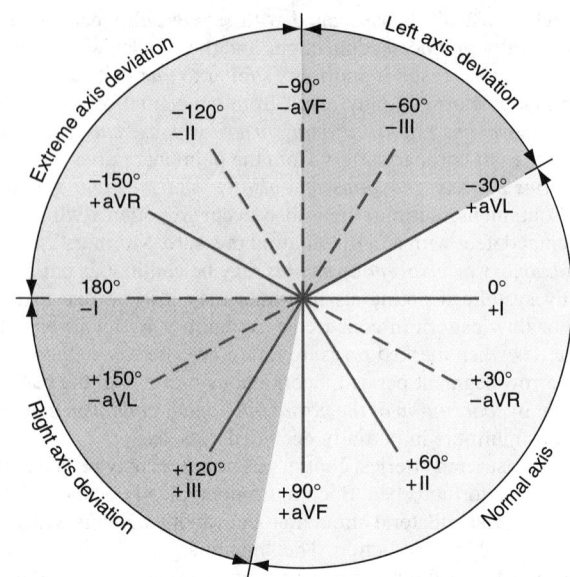

FIGURE 210-4 The frontal plane (extremity or limb) leads are represented on a hexaxial diagram. Each ECG lead has a specific spatial orientation and polarity. The positive pole of each lead axis (*solid line*) and negative pole (*hatched line*) are designated by their angular position relative to the positive pole of lead I (0°). The mean electrical axis of the QRS complex is measured with respect to this display.

cords the complex spatial and temporal summation of electrical potentials from multiple myocardial fibers conducted to the surface of the body. This principle accounts for inherent limitations in both ECG *sensitivity* (activity from certain cardiac regions may be canceled out or may be too weak to be recorded) and *specificity* (the same vectorial sum can result from either a selective gain or a loss of forces in opposite directions).

ECG WAVEFORMS AND INTERVALS

The ECG waveforms are labeled alphabetically, beginning with the P wave, which represents atrial depolarization (Fig. 210-2). The QRS complex represents ventricular depolarization, and the ST-T-U complex (ST segment, T wave, and U wave) represents ventricular repolarization. The J point is the junction between the end of the QRS complex and the beginning of the ST segment. Atrial repolarization is usually too low in amplitude to be detected, but it may become apparent in such conditions as acute pericarditis or atrial infarction.

The QRS-T waveforms of the surface ECG correspond in a general way with the different phases of simultaneously obtained ventricular *action potentials*, the intracellular recordings from single myocardial fibers (see Fig. 213-2). The rapid upstroke (phase 0) of the action potential corresponds to the onset of QRS. The plateau (phase 2) corresponds to the isoelectric ST segment, and active repolarization (phase 3) to the inscription of the T wave. Factors that decrease the slope of phase 0 by impairing the influx of Na^+ (e.g., drugs such as flecainide or procainamide, or hyperkalemia) tend to increase QRS duration. Conditions that prolong phase 2 (use of amiodarone, hypocalcemia) increase the QT interval. In contrast, shortening of ventric-

ular repolarization (phase 2), as by digitalis administration or hypercalcemia, abbreviates the ST segment.

The electrocardiogram is ordinarily recorded on special graph paper which is divided into 1-mm² gridlike boxes. Since the ECG paper speed is generally 25 mm/s, the smallest (1 mm) horizontal divisions correspond to 0.04 s (40 ms), with heavier lines at intervals of 0.20 s (200 ms). Vertically, the ECG graph measures the amplitude of a given wave or deflection (1 mV = 10 mm with standard calibration; the voltage criteria for hypertrophy mentioned below are given in millimeters). There are four major ECG intervals: R-R, PR, QRS, and QT (Fig. 210-2). The heart rate (beats per minute) can be readily computed from the interbeat (R-R) interval by dividing the number of large (0.20 s) time units between consecutive R waves into 300 or the number of small (0.04 s) units into 1500. The PR interval measures the time (normally 120 to 200 ms) between atrial and ventricular depolarization, which includes the physiologic delay imposed by stimulation of cells in the AV junction area. The QRS interval (normally 100 ms or less) reflects the duration of ventricular depolarization. The QT interval includes both ventricular depolarization and repolarization times and varies inversely with the heart rate. A rate-related ("corrected") QT interval, QT_c, can be calculated as $QT/\sqrt{R\text{-}R}$ and normally is ≤0.44 s.

The QRS complex is subdivided into specific deflections or waves. If the initial QRS deflection in a given lead is negative, it is termed a *Q wave*; the first positive deflection is termed an *R wave*. A negative deflection after an R wave is an *S wave*. Subsequent positive or negative waves are labeled R′ and S′, respectively. Lowercase letters (qrs) are used for waves of relatively small amplitude. An entirely negative QRS complex is termed a *QS wave*.

ECG LEADS

The 12 conventional ECG leads record the difference in potential between electrodes placed on the surface of the body. These leads are divided into two groups: six extremity (limb) leads and six chest (precordial) leads. The extremity leads record potentials transmitted onto the *frontal plane* (Fig. 210-3A), and the chest leads record potentials transmitted onto the *horizontal plane* (Fig. 210-3B). The six extremity leads are further subdivided into three *bipolar leads* (I, II, and III) and three *unipolar*

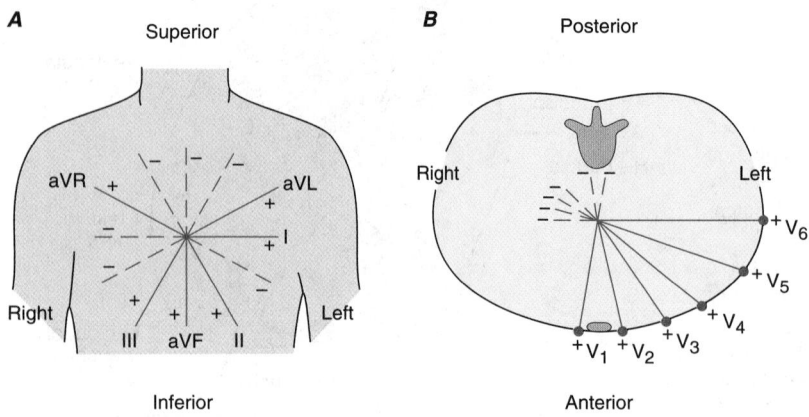

FIGURE 210-3 The six frontal plane (*A*) and six horizontal plane (*B*) leads provide a three-dimensional representation of cardiac electrical activity.

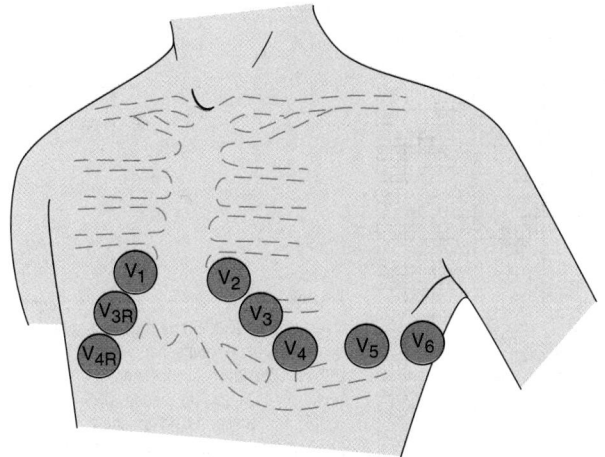

FIGURE 210-5 The horizontal plane (chest or precordial) leads are obtained with electrodes in the locations shown.

leads (aVR, aVL, and aVF). Each bipolar lead measures the difference in potential between electrodes at two extremities: lead I = left arm − right arm voltages, lead II = left leg − right arm, and lead III = left leg − left arm. The unipolar leads measure the voltage (V) at one locus relative to an electrode (called the *central terminal* or *indifferent electrode*) that has approximately zero potential. Thus, aVR = right arm, aVL = left arm, and aVF = left leg (foot). The lowercase *a* indicates that these unipolar potentials are electrically augmented by 50%. The right leg electrode functions as a ground. The spatial orientation and polarity of the six frontal plane leads is represented on the hexaxial diagram (Fig. 210-4).

The six chest leads (Fig. 210-5) are unipolar recordings obtained by electrodes in the following positions: lead V_1, fourth intercostal space, just to the right of the sternum; lead V_2, fourth intercostal space, just to the left of the sternum; lead V_3, midway between V_2 and V_4; lead V_4, midclavicular line, fifth intercostal space; lead V_5, anterior axillary line, same level as V_4; and lead V_6, midaxillary line, same level as V_4 and V_5.

Together, the frontal and horizontal plane electrodes provide a three-dimensional representation of cardiac electrical activity. Each lead can be likened to a different camera angle "looking" at the same events—atrial and ventricular depolarization and repolarization—from different spatial orientations. The conventional 12-lead ECG can be supplemented with additional leads under special circumstances. For example, right precordial leads V_3R, V_4R, etc. are useful in detecting evidence of acute right ventricular ischemia. Bedside monitors and ambulatory ECG (Holter) recordings usually employ only one or two modified leads. →*Intracardiac electrocardiography and electrophysiologic testing are discussed in Chaps. 213 and 214.*

The ECG leads are configured so that a positive (upright) deflection is recorded in a lead if a wave of depolarization spreads toward the positive pole of that lead, and a negative deflection if the wave spreads toward the negative pole. If the mean orientation of the depolarization vector is at right angles to a given lead axis, a biphasic (equally positive and negative) deflection will be recorded.

GENESIS OF THE NORMAL ECG

P WAVE

The normal atrial depolarization vector is oriented downward and toward the subject's left, reflecting the spread of depolarization from the sinus node to the right and then the left atrial myocardium. Since this vector points toward the positive pole of lead II and toward the negative pole of lead aVR, the normal P wave will be positive in lead II and negative in lead aVR. By contrast, activation of the atria from an ectopic pacemaker in the lower part of either atrium or in the AV junction region may produce retrograde P waves (negative in lead II, positive in lead aVR).

QRS COMPLEX

Normal ventricular depolarization proceeds as a rapid, continuous spread of activation wavefronts. This complex process can be divided into two major, sequential phases, and each phase can be represented by a mean vector (Fig. 210-6). The first phase is depolarization of the interventricular septum from the left to the right and anteriorly (vector 1). The second results from the simultaneous depolarization of the right and left ventricles; it is normally dominated by the more massive left ventricle, so that vector 2 points leftward and posteriorly. Therefore, a right precordial lead (V_1) will record this biphasic depolarization process with a small positive deflection (septal r wave) followed by a larger negative deflection (S wave). A left precordial lead, e.g., V_6, will record the same sequence with a small negative deflection (septal q wave) followed by a relatively tall positive deflection (R wave). Intermediate leads show a relative increase in R-wave amplitude (normal R-wave progression) and a decrease in S-wave amplitude progressing across the chest from the right to left. The precordial lead where the R and S waves are of approximately equal amplitude is referred to as the *transition zone* (usually V_3 or V_4) (Fig. 210-7).

The QRS pattern in the extremity leads may vary considerably from one normal subject to another depending on the *electrical axis* of the QRS, which describes the mean orientation of the QRS vector with reference to the six frontal plane leads. Normally, the QRS axis ranges from −30° to +100° (Fig. 210-4). An axis more negative than −30° is referred to as *left axis deviation*, while an axis more positive than +100° is referred to as *right axis deviation*. Left axis deviation may

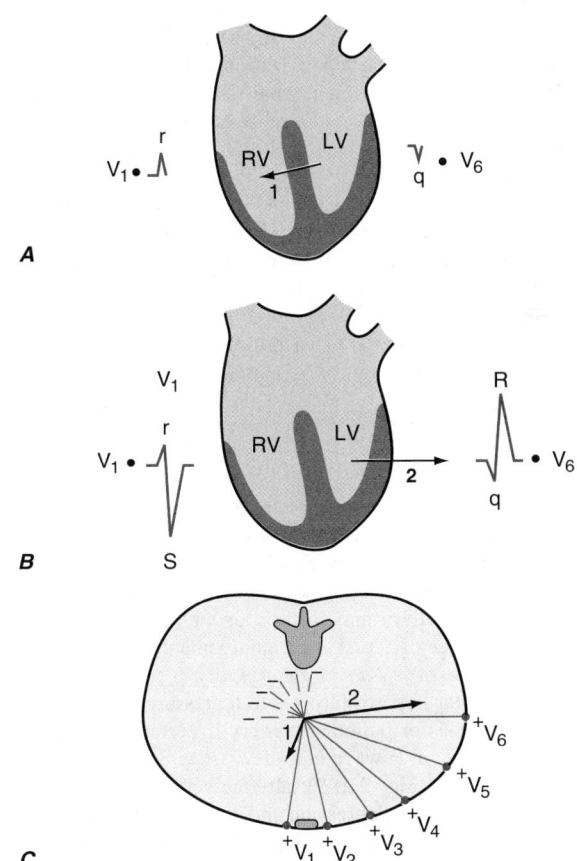

FIGURE 210-6 Ventricular depolarization can be divided into two major phases, each represented by a vector. *A.* The first phase (*arrow 1*) denotes depolarization of the ventricular septum, beginning on the left side and spreading to the right. This process is represented by a small "septal" r wave in lead V_1 and a small septal q wave in lead V_6. *B.* Simultaneous depolarization of the left and right ventricles (LV and RV) constitutes the second phase. Vector 2 is oriented to the left and posteriorly, reflecting the electrical predominance of the LV. *C.* Vectors (*arrows*) representing these two phases are shown in reference to the horizontal plane leads. (*After Goldberger, 1999.*)

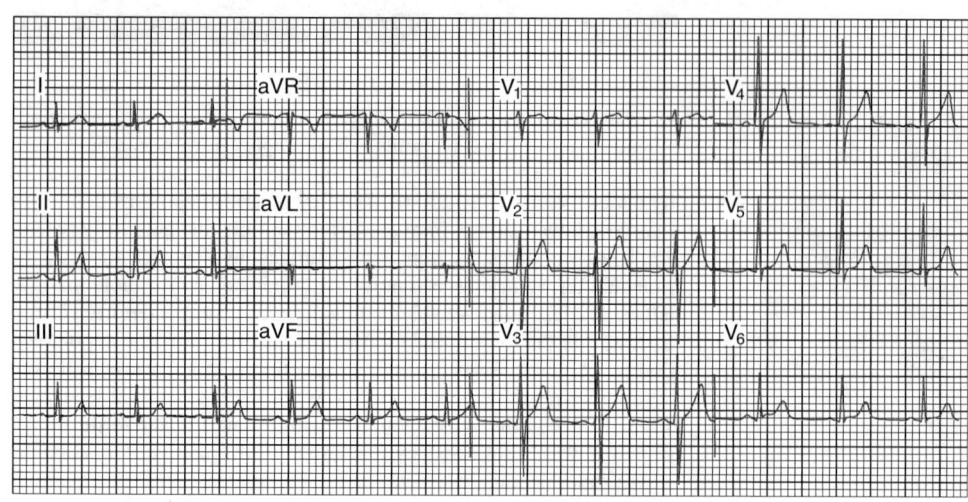

FIGURE 210-7 Normal electrocardiogram from a healthy subject. Sinus rhythm is present with a heart rate of 75 beats per minute. PR interval is 0.16 s; QRS interval (duration) is 0.08 s; QT interval is 0.36 s; the mean QRS axis is about +70°. The precordial leads show normal R-wave progression with the transition zone (R wave = S wave) in lead V_3.

occur as a normal variant but is more commonly associated with left ventricular hypertrophy, a block in the anterior fascicle of the left bundle system (left anterior fascicular block or hemiblock), or inferior myocardial infarction. Right axis deviation may also occur as a normal variant (particularly in children and young adults); as a spurious finding due to reversal of the left and right arm electrodes; or in conditions such as right ventricular overload (acute or chronic), infarction of the lateral wall of the left ventricle, dextrocardia, left pneumothorax, or left posterior fascicular block.

T WAVE AND U WAVE

Normally, the mean T-wave vector is oriented roughly concordant with the mean QRS vector. Since depolarization and repolarization are electrically opposite processes, this normal QRS–T-wave vector concordance indicates that repolarization must normally proceed in the reverse direction from depolarization (i.e., from ventricular epicardium to endocardium). The normal U wave is a small, rounded deflection (≤1 mm) that follows the T wave and usually has the same polarity as the T wave. An abnormal increase in U-wave amplitude is most commonly due to drugs (e.g., quinidine, procainamide, disopyramide) or hypokalemia. Very prominent U waves are a marker of increased susceptibility to the *torsades de pointes* type of ventricular tachycardia (Chap. 214). Inversion of the U wave in the precordial leads is abnormal and may be a subtle sign of ischemia.

MAJOR ECG ABNORMALITIES

CARDIAC ENLARGEMENT AND HYPERTROPHY

Right atrial overload (acute or chronic) may lead to an increase in P-wave amplitude (≥2.5 mm) (Fig. 210-8). Left atrial overload typically produces a biphasic P wave in V_1 with a broad negative component or a broad (≥120 ms), often notched P wave in one or more limb leads (Fig. 210-8). This pattern may also occur with left atrial conduction delays in the absence of actual atrial enlargement, leading to the more general designation of *left atrial abnormality*.

Right ventricular hypertrophy due to a pressure load (as from pulmonic valve stenosis or pulmonary artery hypertension) is characterized by a relatively tall R wave in lead V_1 (R ≥ S wave), usually with right axis deviation (Fig. 210-9); alternatively, there may be a qR pattern in V_1 or V_3R. ST depression and T-wave inversion in the right to midprecordial leads are also often present. This so-called ventricular strain pattern is attributed to repolarization abnormalities in hypertrophied muscle. Right ventricular hypertrophy due to ostium secundum–type atrial septal defects, with the accompanying right ventricular volume overload, is commonly associated with an incomplete or complete right bundle branch block pattern with a rightward QRS axis.

Acute cor pulmonale due to pulmonary embolism (Chap. 244), for example, may be associated with a normal ECG or a variety of abnormalities. Sinus tachycardia is the most common arrhythmia, al-

though other tachyarrhythmias, such as atrial fibrillation or flutter, may occur. The QRS axis may shift to the right, sometimes in concert with the so-called $S_1Q_3T_3$ pattern (prominence of the S wave in lead I, Q wave in lead III, with T-wave inversion in lead III). Acute right ventricular dilation may also be associated with poor R-wave progression and T-wave inversions in V_1 to V_4 (right ventricular "strain") simulating acute anterior infarction. A right ventricular conduction disturbance may appear.

Chronic cor pulmonale due to obstructive lung disease (Chap. 220) usually does not produce the classic ECG patterns of right ventricular hypertrophy noted above. Instead of tall right precordial R waves, chronic lung disease more typically is associated with small R waves in right to midprecordial leads (poor R-wave progression) due in part to downward displacement of the diaphragm and the heart. Low-voltage complexes are commonly present, owing to hyperaeration of the lungs.

A number of different voltage criteria for *left ventricular hypertrophy* (Fig. 210-9) have been proposed on the basis of the presence of tall left precordial R waves and deep right precordial S waves [e.g., $SV_1 + (RV_5 \text{ or } RV_6) \geq 35$ mm; or $(RV_5 \text{ or } RV_6) \geq 25$ mm]. Repolarization abnormalities (ST depression with T-wave inversions) may

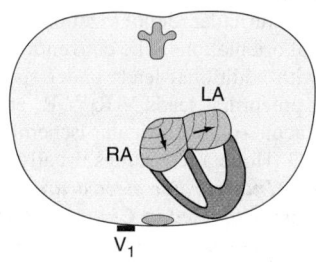

	Normal	Right	Left
II	RA → ← LA	RA ↑ ← LA	RA ← → LA
V_1	RA / LA	RA ↑ / LA	RA / LA ↓

FIGURE 210-8 Right atrial (RA) overload may cause tall, peaked P waves in the limb or precordial leads. Left atrial (LA) abnormality may cause broad, often notched P waves in the limb leads and a biphasic P wave in lead V_1 with a prominent negative component representing delayed depolarization of the LA. (*After MK Park, WG Guntheroth: How to Read Pediatric ECGs, 3d ed. St. Louis, Mosby–Year Book, 1992.*)

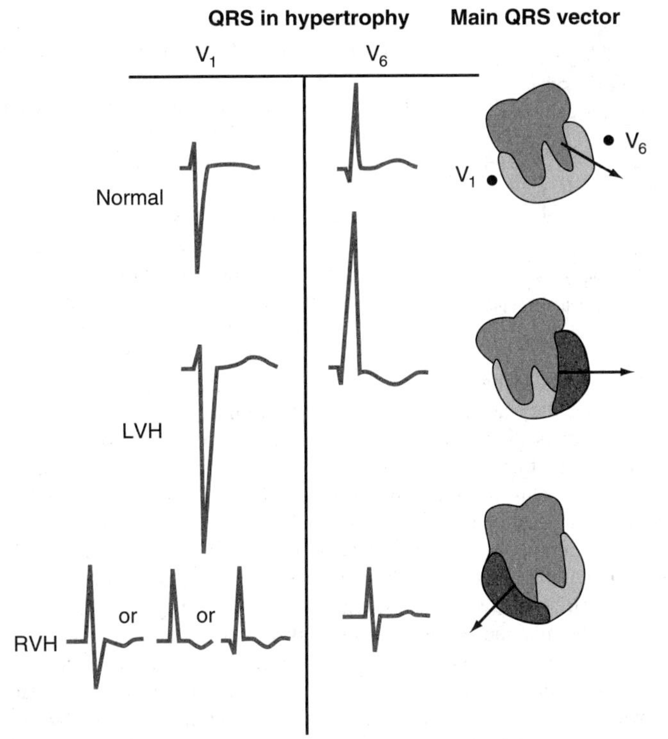

QRS in hypertrophy   Main QRS vector

V₁   V₆

Normal

LVH

RVH   or   or

FIGURE 210-9   Left ventricular hypertrophy (LVH) increases the amplitude of electrical forces directed to the left and posteriorly. In addition, repolarization abnormalities may cause ST-segment depression and T-wave inversion in leads with a prominent R wave ("strain" pattern). Right ventricular hypertrophy (RVH) may shift the QRS vector to the right; this effect usually is associated with an R, RS, or qR complex in lead V₁. T-wave inversions may be present in right precordial leads ("strain" pattern).

also appear (left ventricular "strain" pattern) in leads with prominent R waves. However, prominent precordial voltages may occur as a normal variant, especially in athletic or young individuals. Left ventricular hypertrophy may increase limb lead voltage (e.g., RaVL ≥ 11 to 13 mm, RaVF ≥ 20 mm; $R_1 + S_{III} \geq 25$ mm) with or without increased precordial voltage. The presence of left atrial abnormality increases the likelihood of underlying left ventricular hypertrophy in cases with borderline voltage criteria. Left ventricular hypertrophy often progresses to incomplete or complete left bundle branch block. The sensitivity of conventional voltage criteria for left ventricular hypertrophy is decreased in obese persons and in smokers. ECG evidence for left ventricular hypertrophy is a major noninvasive marker of increased risk of cardiovascular morbidity and mortality, including sudden cardiac death. However, because of false-positive and false-negative diagnoses, the ECG is of limited utility in diagnosing atrial or ventricular enlargement. More definitive information is provided by echocardiography (Chap. 211).

BUNDLE BRANCH BLOCKS

Intrinsic impairment of conduction in either the right or left bundle system (intraventricular conduction disturbances) leads to prolongation of the QRS interval. With complete bundle branch blocks the QRS interval is ≥120 ms in duration; with incomplete blocks the QRS interval is between 100 and 120 ms. The QRS vector is usually oriented in the direction of the myocardial region where depolarization is delayed (Fig. 210-10). Thus, with right bundle branch block, the terminal QRS vector is oriented anteriorly and to the right (rSR′ in V₁ and qRS in V₆, typically). Left bundle branch block alters both early and later phases of ventricular depolarization. The major QRS vector is directed to the left and posteriorly. In addition, the normal early left-to-right pattern of septal activation is disrupted such that septal depolarization proceeds from right to left as well. As a result, left bundle branch block generates wide, predominantly negative (QS) complexes in lead V₁ and entirely positive (R) complexes in lead V₆. A pattern identical to that of left bundle branch block, preceded by a sharp spike,

is seen in most cases of electronic right ventricular pacing because of the relative delay in left ventricular activation.

Bundle branch block may occur in a variety of conditions. In subjects without structural heart disease, right bundle branch block is seen more commonly than left bundle branch block. Right bundle branch block also occurs with heart disease, both congenital (e.g., atrial septal defect) and acquired (e.g., valvular, ischemic). Left bundle branch block is often a marker of one of four underlying conditions: coronary heart disease (often with impaired left ventricular function), hypertensive heart disease, aortic valve disease, and cardiomyopathy. Bundle branch blocks may be chronic or intermittent. A bundle branch block may be rate-related; for example, it often occurs when the heart rate exceeds some critical value.

Bundle branch blocks and depolarization abnormalities secondary to artificial pacemakers not only affect ventricular depolarization (QRS) but are also characteristically associated with *secondary repolarization* (ST-T) abnormalities. With bundle branch blocks, the T wave is typically opposite in polarity to the last deflection of the QRS (Fig. 210-10). This discordance of the QRS–T-wave vectors is caused by the altered sequence of repolarization that occurs secondary to altered depolarization. In contrast, *primary repolarization* abnormalities are independent of QRS changes and are related instead to actual alterations in the electrical properties of the myocardial fibers themselves (e.g., in the resting membrane potential or action potential duration), not just to changes in the sequence of repolarization. Ischemia, electrolyte imbalance, and drugs such as digitalis all cause such primary ST–T-wave changes. Primary and secondary T-wave changes may coexist. For example, T-wave inversions in the right precordial leads with left bundle branch block or in the left precordial leads with right bundle branch block may be important markers of underlying ischemia or other abnormalities.

Partial blocks ("hemiblocks") in the left bundle system (left anterior or posterior fascicular blocks) generally do not prolong the QRS duration substantially but instead are associated with shifts in the frontal plane QRS axis (leftward or rightward, respectively). More complex combinations of fascicular and bundle branch blocks may occur involving the left and right bundle system. Examples of *bifascicular*

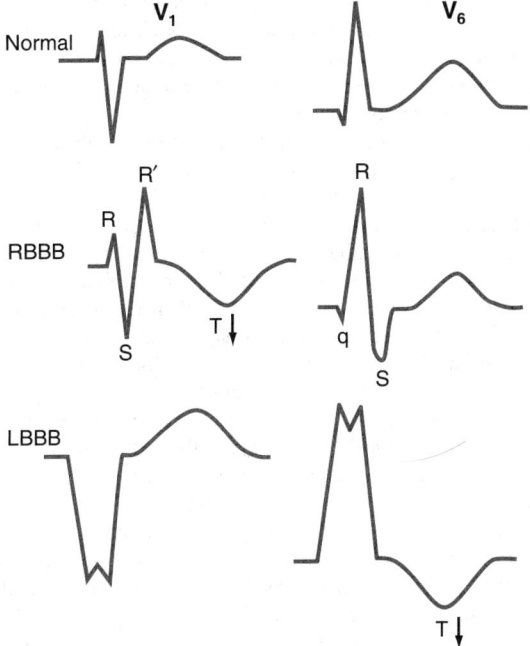

FIGURE 210-10   Comparison of typical QRS-T patterns in right bundle branch block (RBBB) and left bundle branch block (LBBB) with the normal pattern in leads V₁ and V₆. Note the secondary T-wave inversions (*arrows*) in leads with an rSR′ complex with RBBB and in leads with a wide R wave with LBBB.

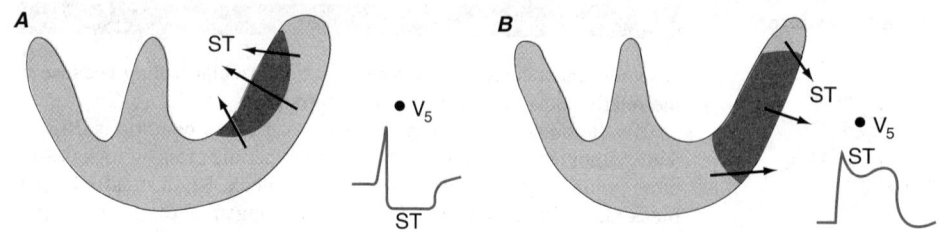

FIGURE 210-11 Acute ischemia causes a current of injury. With predominant subendocardial ischemia (A), the resultant ST vector will be directed toward the inner layer of the affected ventricle and the ventricular cavity. Overlying leads therefore will record ST depression. With ischemia involving the outer ventricular layer (B) (transmural or epicardial injury), the ST vector will be directed outward. Overlying leads will record ST elevation.

block include right bundle branch block and left posterior fascicular block, right bundle branch block with left anterior fascicular block, and complete left bundle branch block. Chronic bifascicular block in an asymptomatic individual is associated with a relatively low risk of progression to high-degree AV heart block. In contrast, new bifascicular block with acute anterior myocardial infarction carries a much greater risk of complete heart block. Alternation of right and left bundle branch block is a sign of *trifascicular disease.* However, the presence of a prolonged PR interval and bifascicular block does not necessarily indicate trifascicular involvement, since this combination may arise with AV node disease and bifascicular block. Intraventricular conduction delays can also be caused by extrinsic (toxic) factors that slow ventricular conduction, particularly hyperkalemia or drugs (class 1 antiarrhythmic agents, tricyclic antidepressants, phenothiazines).

Prolongation of QRS duration does not necessarily indicate a conduction delay but may be due to *preexcitation* of the ventricles via a bypass tract, as in the Wolff-Parkinson-White (WPW) syndrome (Chap. 214) and related variants. The diagnostic triad of WPW consists of a wide QRS complex associated with a relatively short PR interval and slurring of the initial part of the QRS (delta wave), the latter effect due to aberrant activation of ventricular myocardium. The presence of a bypass tract predisposes to reentrant supraventricular tachyarrhythmias.

MYOCARDIAL ISCHEMIA AND INFARCTION (See also Chap. 228)

The ECG is a cornerstone in the diagnosis of acute and chronic ischemic heart disease. The findings depend on several key factors: the nature of the process [reversible (i.e., ischemia) versus irreversible (i.e., infarction)], the duration (acute versus chronic), extent (transmural versus subendocardial), and localization (anterior versus inferoposterior), as well as the presence of other underlying abnormalities (ventricular hypertrophy, conduction defects).

Ischemia exerts complex time-dependent effects on the electrical properties of myocardial cells. Severe, acute ischemia lowers the resting membrane potential and shortens the duration of the action potential. Such changes cause a voltage gradient between normal and ischemic zones. As a consequence, current flows between these regions. These currents of injury are represented on the surface ECG by deviation of the ST segment (Fig. 210-11). When the acute ischemia is *transmural,* the ST vector is usually shifted in the direction of the outer (epicardial) layers, producing ST elevations and sometimes, in the earliest stages of ischemia, tall, positive so-called hyperacute T waves over the ischemic zone. With ischemia confined primarily to the *subendocardium,* the ST vector typically shifts toward the subendocardium and ventricular cavity, so that overlying (e.g., anterior precordial) leads show ST-segment depression (with ST elevation in lead aVR). Multiple factors affect the amplitude of acute ischemic ST deviations. Profound ST elevation or depression in multiple leads usually indicates very severe ischemia. From a clinical viewpoint, the division of acute myocardial infarction into ST segment elevation and non-ST elevation types is useful since the efficacy of acute reperfusion therapy is limited to the former group.

The ECG leads are more helpful in localizing regions of ST elevation than non-ST elevation ischemia. For example, acute transmural anterior (including apical and lateral) wall ischemia is reflected by ST

elevations or increased T-wave positivity (Fig. 210-12) in one or more of the precordial leads (V_1 to V_6) and leads I and aVL. Inferior wall ischemia produces changes in leads II, III, and aVF. Posterior wall ischemia may be indirectly recognized by *reciprocal* ST depressions in leads V_1 to V_3. Prominent reciprocal ST depressions in these leads also occur with certain inferior wall infarcts, particularly those with posterior or lateral wall extension. Right ventricular ischemia usually produces ST elevations in right-sided chest leads (Fig. 210-5). When ischemic ST elevations occur as the earliest sign of acute infarction, they are typically followed within a period ranging from hours to days by evolving T-wave inversions and often by Q waves occurring in the same lead distribution. (T-wave inversions due to evolving or chronic ischemia correlate with prolongation of repolarization and are often associated with QT lengthening.) Reversible transmural ischemia, for example, due to coronary vasospasm (Prinzmetal's variant angina), may cause transient ST-segment elevations without development of Q waves. Depending on the severity and duration of such ischemia, the ST elevations may either resolve completely in minutes or be followed by T-wave inversions that persist for hours or even days. Patients with ischemic chest pain who present with deep T-wave inversions in multiple precordial leads (e.g., V_1 to V_4) with or without cardiac enzyme elevations typically have severe obstruction in the left anterior descending coronary artery system (Fig. 210-13). In contrast, patients whose baseline ECG already shows abnormal T-wave inversions may develop T-wave normalization (pseudonormalization) during episodes of acute transmural ischemia.

With infarction, depolarization (QRS) changes often accompany repolarization (ST-T) abnormalities. Necrosis of sufficient myocardial tissue may lead to decreased R-wave amplitude or abnormal Q waves in the anterior or inferior leads (Fig. 210-14). Previously, abnormal Q waves were considered to be markers of transmural myocardial in-

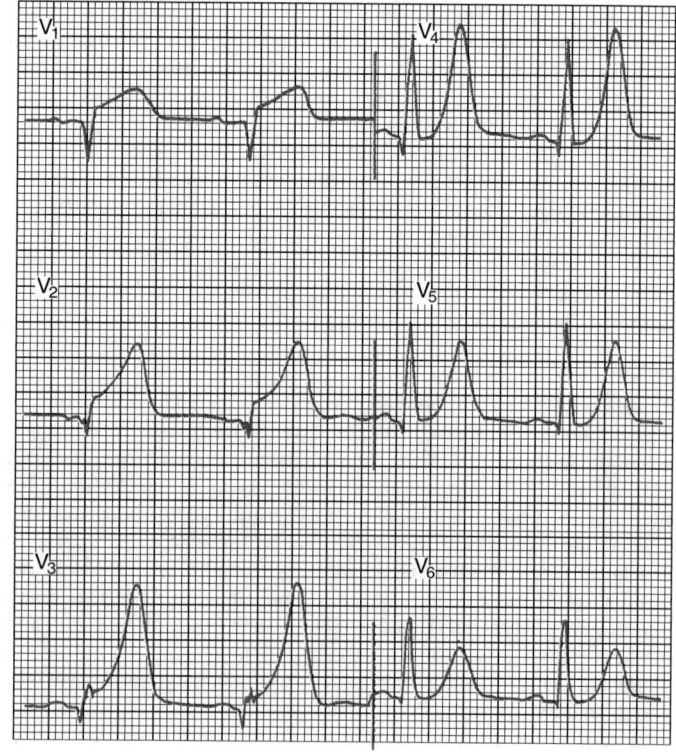

FIGURE 210-12 Hyperacute phase of anteroseptal myocardial infarction (MI). Note the tall positive T waves (V_2 to V_3) along with ST-segment elevations and Q waves (V_1 to V_3).

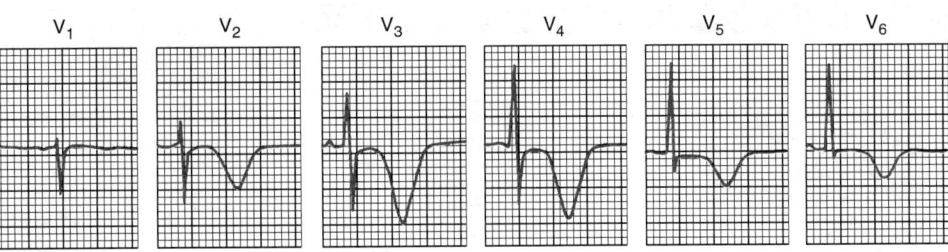

FIGURE 210-13 Severe anterior wall ischemia (with or without infarction) may cause prominent T-wave inversions in the precordial leads. This pattern is usually associated with a high-grade stenosis of the left anterior descending coronary artery.

farction, while subendocardial infarcts were thought not to produce Q waves. However, careful ECG-pathology correlative studies have indicated that transmural infarcts may occur without Q waves and that subendocardial (nontransmural) infarcts may sometimes be associated with Q waves. Therefore, infarcts are more appropriately classified as "Q-wave" or "non-Q-wave." The major acute ECG changes in syndromes of ischemic heart disease are schematically summarized in Fig. 210-15. Loss of depolarization forces due to posterior or lateral infarction may cause reciprocal increases in R-wave amplitude in leads V_1 and V_2 without diagnostic Q waves in any of the conventional leads. Atrial infarction may be associated with PR-segment deviations due to an atrial current of injury, changes in P-wave morphology, or atrial arrhythmias. In the weeks and months following infarction, these ECG changes may persist or begin to resolve. Complete normalization of the ECG following Q-wave infarction is uncommon but may occur, particularly with smaller infarcts. In contrast, ST-segment elevations that persist for several weeks or more after a Q-wave infarct usually correlate with a severe underlying wall motion disorder (akinetic or dyskinetic zone), although not necessarily a frank ventricular aneurysm.

ECG changes due to ischemia may occur spontaneously or may be provoked by various exercise protocols (stress electrocardiography) (Chap. 226). In patients with severe ischemic heart disease, exercise testing is most likely to elicit signs of subendocardial ischemia (horizontal or downsloping ST depression in multiple leads). ST-segment elevation during exercise is most often observed after a Q-wave infarct. This repolarization change does not necessarily indicate active ischemia but correlates strongly with the presence of an underlying ventricular wall motion abnormality. However, in patients *without* prior

infarction, transient ST-segment elevation with exercise is a reliable sign of transmural ischemia.

The ECG has important limitations in both sensitivity and specificity in the diagnosis of ischemic heart disease. Although a single normal ECG does not exclude ischemia or even acute infarction, a normal ECG *throughout* the course of an acute infarct is distinctly uncommon. Prolonged chest pain without diagnostic ECG changes, therefore, should always prompt a careful search for other noncoronary causes of chest pain (Chap. 12). Furthermore, the diagnostic changes of acute or evolving ischemia are often masked by the presence of left bundle branch block, electronic ventricular pacemaker patterns, and WPW preexcitation. On the other hand, clinicians may overdiagnose ischemia or infarction based on the presence of ST-segment elevations or depressions, T-wave inversions, tall positive T waves, or Q waves *not* related to ischemic heart disease (pseudoinfarct patterns). For example, ST-segment elevations simulating ischemia may occur with acute pericarditis (Fig. 210-16) or myocarditis, as a normal variant ("early repolarization" pattern), or in a variety of other conditions (Table 210-1). Similarly, tall, positive T waves do not invariably represent hyperacute ischemic changes but may also be caused by normal variants, hyperkalemia, cerebrovascular injury, and left ventricular volume overload due to mitral or aortic regurgitation, among other causes. ST-segment elevations and tall, positive T waves are common findings in leads V_1 and V_2 in left bundle branch block or left ventricular hypertrophy in the absence of ischemia. The differential diagnosis of Q waves (Table 210-2) includes physiologic or positional variants, ventricular hypertrophy, acute or chronic noncoronary myocardial injury, hypertrophic cardiomyopathy, and ventricular conduction disorders. Digitalis, ventricular hypertrophy, hypokalemia, and a variety of other

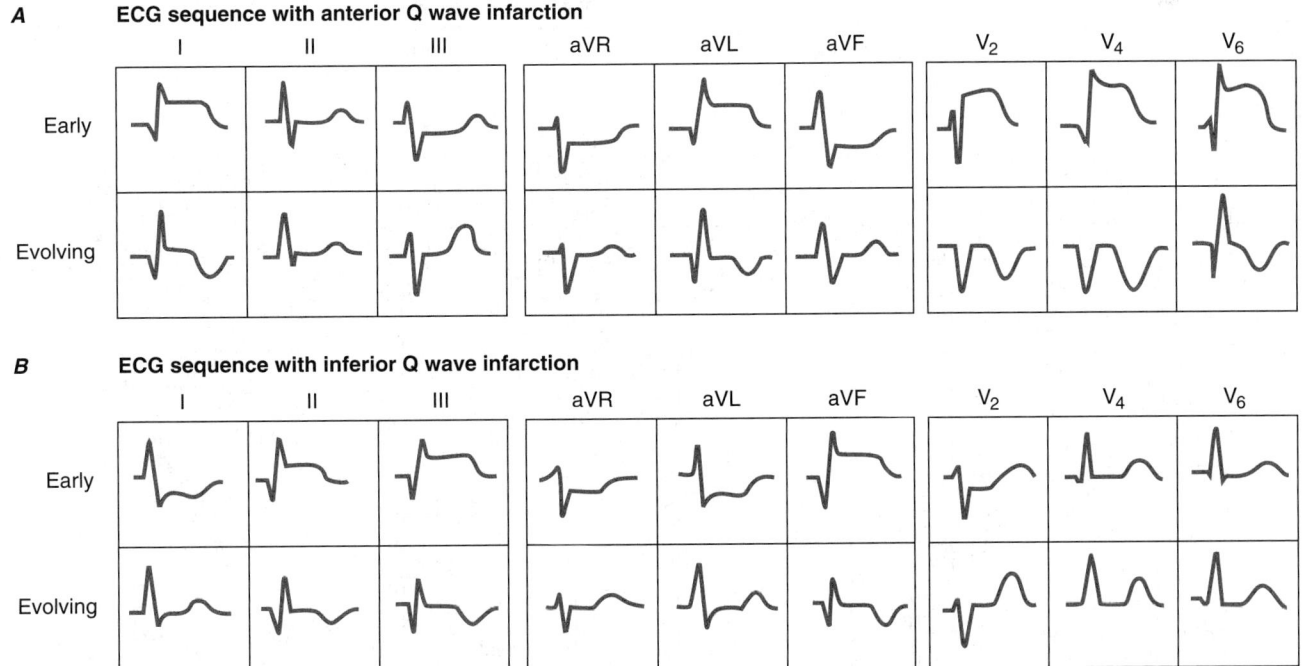

A **ECG sequence with anterior Q wave infarction**

B **ECG sequence with inferior Q wave infarction**

FIGURE 210-14 Sequence of depolarization and repolarization changes with (*A*) acute anterior and (*B*) acute inferior wall Q-wave infarctions. With anterior infarcts, ST elevation in leads I, aVL, and the precordial leads may be accompanied by reciprocal ST depressions in leads II, III, and aVF. Conversely, acute inferior (or posterior) infarcts may be associated with reciprocal ST depressions in leads V_1 to V_3. (*After Goldberger, 1999.*)

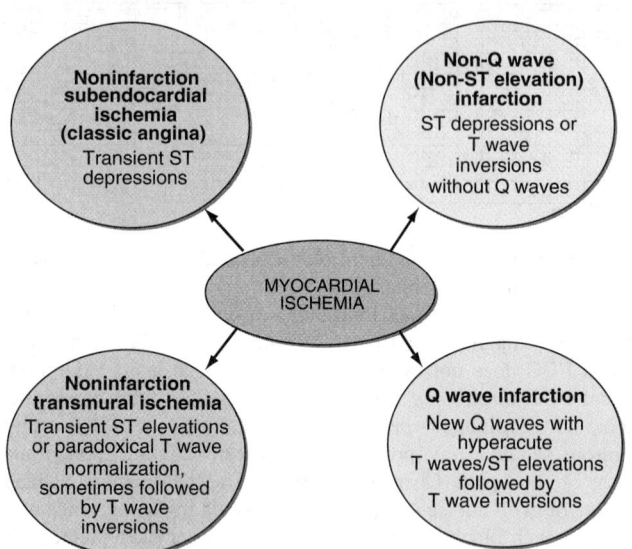

FIGURE 210-15 Variability of ECG patterns with acute myocardial ischemia. The ECG also may be normal or nonspecifically abnormal. Furthermore, these categorizations are not mutually exclusive. For example, a non-ST elevation infarct may evolve into a Q-wave infarct; ST elevations may be followed by a non-Q-wave infarct; or ST depressions and T-wave inversions may be followed by a Q-wave infarct. (*After Goldberger, 1991.*)

factors may cause ST-segment depression mimicking subendocardial ischemia. Prominent T-wave inversion may occur with ventricular hypertrophy, cardiomyopathy, myocarditis, and cerebrovascular injury (particularly intracranial bleeds; Fig. 210-17), among many other conditions.

METABOLIC FACTORS AND DRUG EFFECTS

A variety of metabolic and pharmacologic agents alter the ECG and, in particular, cause changes in repolarization (ST-T-U) and sometimes QRS prolongation. Certain life-threatening electrolyte disturbances may be diagnosed initially and monitored from the ECG. *Hyperkalemia* produces a sequence of changes usually beginning with narrowing and peaking (tenting) of the T waves. Further elevation of extracellular K^+ leads to AV conduction disturbances, diminution in P-wave amplitude, and widening of the QRS interval. Severe hyperkalemia eventually causes cardiac arrest with a slow sinusoidal type of mechanism ("sine-wave" pattern) followed by asystole. *Hypokalemia* (Fig. 210-17) prolongs ventricular repolarization, often with prominent U waves.

TABLE 210-1   Differential Diagnosis of ST Segment Elevations

Ischemia/myocardial infarction
    Noninfarction, transmural ischemia (Prinzmetal's angina pattern)
    Acute myocardial infarction
    Postmyocardial infarction (ventricular aneurysm pattern)
Acute pericarditis
Normal variant ("early repolarization" pattern)
Left ventricular hypertrophy/left bundle branch block[a]
Other (rarer)
    Brugada syndrome (right bundle branch block-like pattern with ST
       elevations in right precordial leads)[a]
    Class 1C antiarrhythmic drugs[a]
    DC cardioversion
    Hypercalcemia[a]
    Hyperkalemia[a]
    Hypothermia (J wave/Osborn wave)
    Myocardial injury
       Myocarditis
       Tumor invading left ventricle
       Trauma to ventricles

[a] Usually localized to V_1-V_2 or V_3
Source: Modified from Goldberger, 1999.

TABLE 210-2   Differential Diagnosis of Q Waves (with Selected Examples)

Physiologic or positional factors
1. Normal variant "septal" q waves
2. Normal variant Q waves in V_1 to V_2, aVL, III, and aVF
3. Left pneumothorax or dextrocardia: loss of lateral R-wave progression
Myocardial injury or infiltration
1. Acute processes: myocardial ischemia or infarction, myocarditis, hyperkalemia
2. Chronic processes: myocardial infarction, idiopathic cardiomyopathy, myocarditis, amyloid, tumor, sarcoid, scleroderma, Chagas' disease, echinococcus cyst
Ventricular hypertrophy/enlargement
1. Left ventricular (poor R-wave progression[a])
2. Right ventricular (reversed R-wave progression[b] or poor R-wave progression[a], particularly with chronic obstructive lung disease)
3. Hypertrophic cardiomyopathy (may simulate anterior, inferior, posterior, or lateral infarcts)
Conduction abnormalities
1. Left bundle branch block (poor R-wave progression[a])
2. Wolff-Parkinson-White patterns

[a] Small or absent R waves in the right to midprecordial leads.
[b] Progressive decrease in R-wave amplitude from V_1 to the mid- or lateral precordial leads.
Source: After Goldberger, 1991.

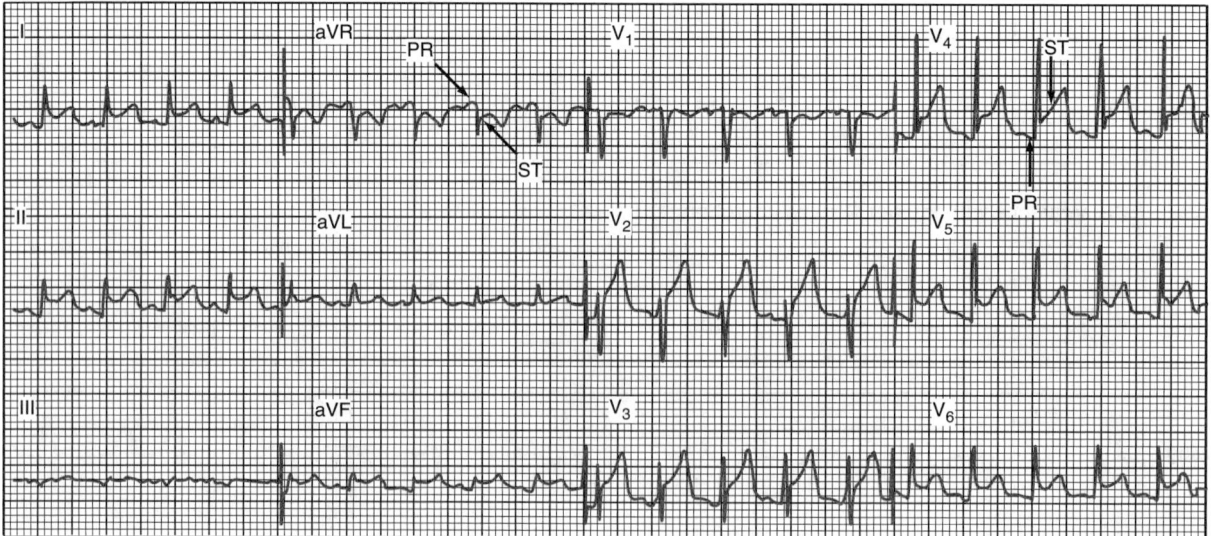

FIGURE 210-16 Acute pericarditis often produces diffuse ST-segment elevations (in this case in leads I, II, aVF, and V_2 to V_6) due to a ventricular current of injury. Note also the characteristic PR-segment deviation (opposite in polarity to the ST segment) due to a concomitant atrial injury current.

Prolongation of the QT interval (Fig. 210-17) is also seen with drugs that increase the duration of the ventricular action potential—class 1A antiarrhythmic agents and related drugs (e.g., quinidine, disopyramide, procainamide, tricyclic antidepressants, phenothiazines) and class III agents (amiodarone, sotalol, ibutilide). Marked QT prolongation, sometimes with deep, wide T-wave inversions, may occur with intracranial bleeds, particularly subarachnoid hemorrhage ("CVA T-wave" pattern) (Fig. 210-17). Systemic *hypothermia* (Fig. 210-17) also prolongs repolarization, usually with a distinctive convex elevation of the J point (Osborn wave). *Hypocalcemia* typically prolongs the QT interval (ST portion), while *hypercalcemia* shortens it (Fig. 210-18). Digitalis glycosides also shorten the QT interval, often with a characteristic "scooping" of the ST–T-wave complex (*digitalis effect*).

Many other factors are associated with ECG changes, particularly alterations in ventricular repolarization. T-wave flattening, minimal T-wave inversions, or slight ST-segment depression ("nonspecific ST–T-wave changes") may occur with a variety of electrolyte and acid-base disturbances, a variety of infectious processes, central nervous system disorders, endocrine abnormalities, many drugs, ischemia, hypoxia, and virtually any type of cardiopulmonary abnormality. While subtle ST–T-wave changes may be markers of ischemia, transient nonspecific repolarization changes may also occur following a meal or with postural (orthostatic) change, hyperventilation, or exercise in healthy individuals.

ELECTRICAL ALTERNANS

Electrical alternans—a beat-to-beat alternation in one or more components of the ECG signal—is a common type of nonlinear cardiovascular response to a variety of hemodynamic and electrophysiologic perturbations. Total electrical alternans (P-QRS-T) with sinus tachycardia is a relatively specific sign of pericardial effusion, usually with cardiac tamponade. The mechanism relates to a periodic swinging motion of the heart in the effusion at a frequency exactly one-half the heart rate. Repolarization (ST-T) alternans is a sign of electrical instability and may precede ventricular tachyarrhythmias.

CLINICAL INTERPRETATION OF THE ECG

Accurate analysis of ECGs requires thoroughness and care. The patient's age, gender, and clinical status should always be taken into account. For example, T-wave inversions in leads V_1 to V_3 are more

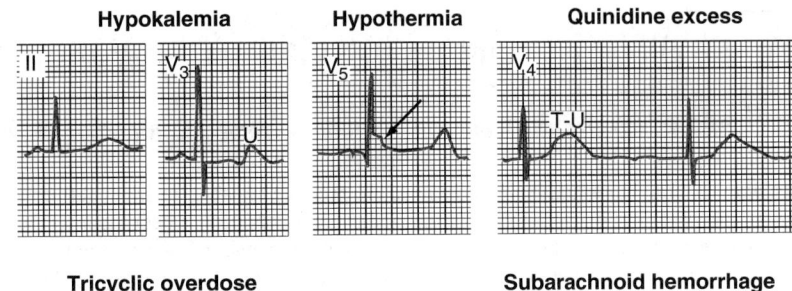
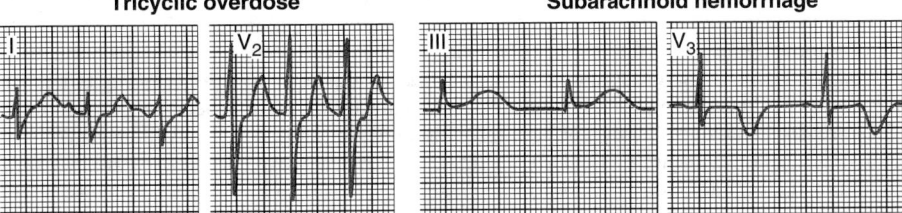

FIGURE 210-17 A variety of metabolic derangements, drug effects, and other factors may prolong ventricular repolarization with QT prolongation or prominent U waves. Repolarization prolongation, particularly if due to hypokalemia or pharmacologic agents, indicates increased susceptibility to *torsades de pointes* type ventricular tachycardia. Hypothermia is associated with a distinctive convex "hump" at the J point (Osborn wave, *arrow*). Note QRS and QT prolongation along with sinus tachycardia in the case of tricyclic antidepressant overdose.

likely to represent a normal variant in a healthy young adult woman ("persistent juvenile T-wave pattern") than in an elderly man with chest discomfort. Similarly, the likelihood that ST-segment depression during exercise testing represents ischemia depends partly on the prior probability of coronary artery disease.

Many mistakes in ECG interpretation are errors of omission. Therefore, a systematic approach is desirable. The following 14 points should be analyzed carefully in every ECG: (1) standardization (calibration) and technical features (including lead placement and artifacts); (2) heart rate; (3) rhythm; (4) PR interval; (5) QRS interval; (6) QT interval; (7) mean QRS electrical axis; (8) P waves; (9) QRS voltages; (10) precordial R-wave progression; (11) abnormal Q waves; (12) ST segments; (13) T waves; (14) U waves.

Only after analyzing all these points should the interpretation be formulated. Where appropriate, important clinical correlates or inferences should be mentioned. For example, the combination of left atrial abnormality (enlargement) and signs of right ventricular hypertrophy suggests mitral stenosis. Low voltage with sinus tachycardia raises the possibility of pericardial tamponade or chronic obstructive lung disease. Sinus tachycardia with QRS and QT (U) prolongation suggests tricyclic antidepressant overdose (Fig. 210-17). Comparison with previous ECGs is essential. →*The diagnosis and management of specific cardiac arrhythmias and conduction disturbances are discussed in Chaps. 213 and 214.*

COMPUTERIZED ELECTROCARDIOGRAPHY

Computerized ECG systems are widely used. Digital systems provide for convenient storage and immediate retrieval of thousands of ECG records. Despite advances, computer interpretation of ECGs has important limitations. Incomplete or inaccurate readings are most likely with arrhythmias and complex abnormalities. Therefore, computerized interpretation (including measurements of basic ECG intervals) should not be accepted without careful physician review.

FURTHER READING

ASHLEY EA et al: An evidence-based review of the resting electrocardiogram as a screening technique for heart disease. Prog Cardiovasc Dis 44:55, 2001

GOLDBERGER AL: *Clinical Electrocardiography: A Simplified Approach*, 6th ed. St. Louis, Mosby, 1999

——— AL: *Myocardial Infarction: Electrocardiographic Differential Diagnosis*, 4th ed. St. Louis, Mosby–Year Book, 1991

SURAWICZ B, KNILANS TK: *Chou's Electrocardiography in Clinical Practice*, 5th ed. Philadelphia, Saunders, 2001

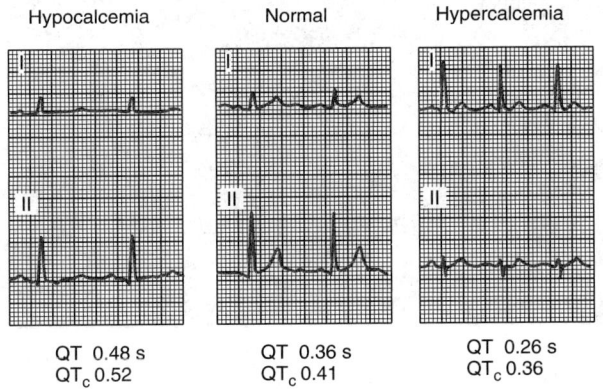

FIGURE 210-18 Prolongation of the Q-T interval (ST-segment portion) is typical of hypocalcemia. Hypercalcemia may cause abbreviation of the ST segment and shortening of the QT interval.

Cardiovascular imaging has significantly enhanced the practice of cardiology over the past few decades. Two-dimensional (2D) echocardiography is able to visualize the heart directly in real time using ultrasound, providing instantaneous assessment of the myocardium, cardiac chambers, valves, pericardium, and great vessels. Doppler echocardiography measures the velocity of moving red blood cells and has become a noninvasive alternative to cardiac catheterization for assessment of hemodynamics. Transesophageal echocardiography (TEE) provides a unique window for high-resolution imaging of posterior structures of the heart, particularly the left atrium, mitral valve, and aorta. Nuclear cardiology uses isotopes to assess myocardial perfusion and function and has contributed greatly to the evaluation of patients with ischemic heart disease. Cardiac magnetic resonance imaging (MRI) and computed tomography (CT) can delineate cardiac structure and function with high resolution. They are particularly useful in the examination of cardiac masses, the pericardium, and the great vessels and there is growing interest in their utility in patients with suspected coronary artery disease (CAD). This chapter provides an overview of the basic concepts of these cardiac imaging modalities, as well as the clinical indications for each procedure.

ECHOCARDIOGRAPHY

TWO-DIMENSIONAL ECHOCARDIOGRAPHY ■ Basic Principles 2D echocardiography uses the principle of ultrasound reflection off cardiac structures to produce images of the heart (Table 211-1). The imaging is performed from multiple acoustic windows with different transducer rotations so that the entire heart and great vessels can be displayed in real time and in various 2D planes. Most information from a study is obtained from a visual analysis of the 2D images, although objective measurements of cardiac dimensions can be obtained. For a transthoracic echocardiogram (TTE), the imaging is performed with a handheld transducer placed directly on the chest wall. In selected patients, a TEE may be performed, in which an ultrasound transducer is mounted on the tip of an endoscope placed in the esophagus and directed toward the cardiac structures, so that high-resolution images of the posterior structures are obtained.

Current echocardiographic machines are portable; they can be wheeled directly to the patient's bedside. Thus, a major advantage of echocardiography over other imaging modalities is the ability to obtain instantaneous images of the cardiac structures for immediate interpretation, even in emergency or trauma units or in critical care settings.

"Handheld" echocardiographic units weighing less than 6 lb have now become available, further enhancing the ease and portability of echocardiography. These units can easily be carried to the bedside of the patient. Although prototype instruments had only 2D echocardiographic capabilities, there are now units that can also perform pulsed Doppler, continuous-wave Doppler, and color-flow Doppler imaging. As these units become smaller and more functional, they may soon become an essential part of the physical examination.

A limitation of a 2D echocardiogram performed via a transthoracic approach is the inability to obtain high-quality images in all patients, especially those with a thick chest wall or severe lung disease. Ultrasound waves are poorly transmitted through lung parenchyma. The diagnostic accuracy of an echocardiogram is highly dependent on both the operator of the echocardiographic equipment and the interpreter of the study.

Chamber Size and Function 2D echocardiography is an ideal imaging modality for assessing left ventricular (LV) size and function (Fig. 211-1). A qualitative assessment of the cavity size of the ventricle and systolic function can be made directly from the 2D image by experienced observers (Fig. 211-2). Quantitative assessment of LV size and function can be made by electronic calipers (measuring systolic and diastolic dimensions of the short axis of the LV) or quantitative 2D echocardiography. With quantitative 2D echocardiography, endocardial outlines of the LV cavity are traced in systole and diastole and the LV cavity areas are then fitted to computer models of the LV to obtain systolic and diastolic volumes. The presence or absence of regional wall motion abnormalities can be visually assessed by examining endocardial motion as well as wall thickening. 2D echocardiography is useful in the diagnosis of LV hypertrophy, seen as an

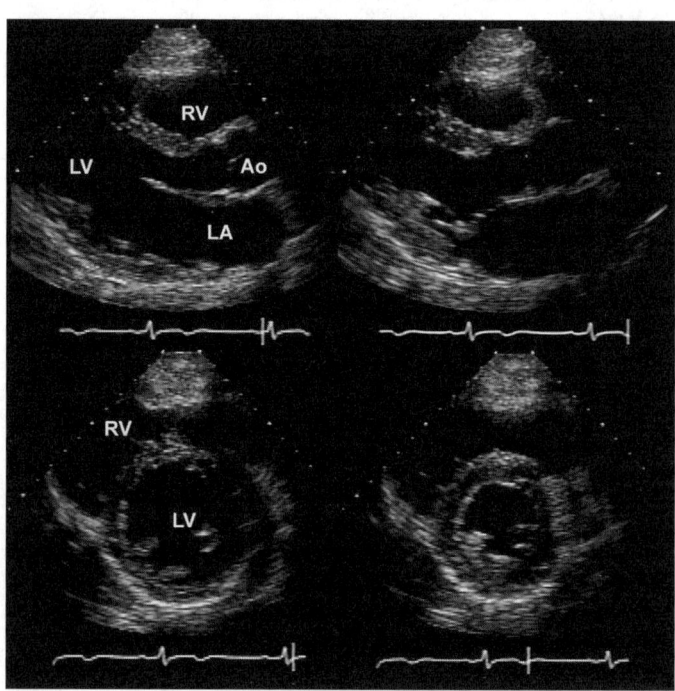

FIGURE 211-1 Two-dimensional echocardiographic still-frame images from a normal patient with a normal heart. *Upper:* Parasternal long axis view during systole and diastole (*left*) and systole (*right*). During systole, there is thickening of the myocardium and reduction in the size of the left ventricle (LV). The valve leaflets are thin and open widely. *Lower:* Parasternal short axis view during diastole (*left*) and systole (*right*) demonstrating a decrease in the left ventricular cavity size during systole as well as an increase in wall thickening. LA, left atrium; RV, right ventricle; Ao, aorta.

TABLE 211-1 Clinical Uses of Echocardiography

Two-Dimensional Echocardiography	Doppler Echocardiography
Cardiac chambers	Valve stenosis
Chamber size	Gradient
Left ventricular	Valve area
Hypertrophy	Valve regurgitation
Regional wall motion abnormalities	Semiquantitation
Valve	Intracardiac pressures
Morphology and motion	Volumetric flow
Pericardium	Diastolic filling
Effusion	Intracardiac shunts
Tamponade	**Transesophageal Echocardiography**
Masses	Inadequate transthoracic images
Great vessels	Aortic disease
Stress Echocardiography	Infective endocarditis
Two-dimensional	Source of embolism
Myocardial ischemia	Valve prosthesis
Viable myocardium	Intraoperative
Doppler	
Valve disease	

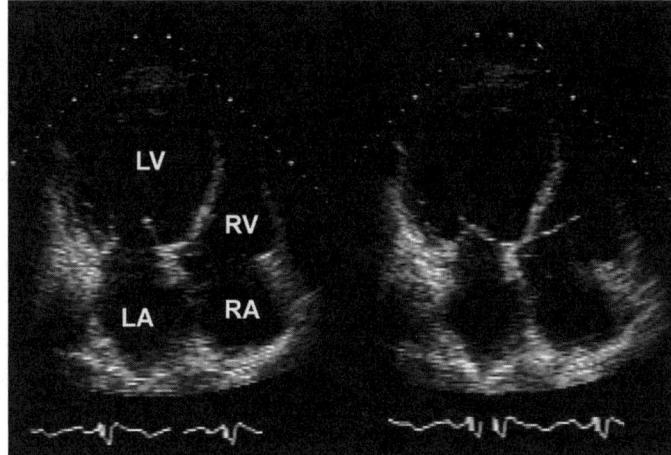

FIGURE 211-2 Apical four-chamber view from a patient with a dilated cardiomyopathy. The left ventricle (LV) is dilated, and there is little change in the LV cavity size from diastole (*left*) to systole (*right*). RV, right ventricle; RA, right atrium; LA, left atrium.

increase in wall thickness. Other chamber sizes are assessed by visual analysis, including the left atrium and right-sided chambers. There is no method for quantitative analysis of right ventricular size and function by 2D echocardiography, due to the complex geometry of the right ventricle.

Valve Abnormalities (See also Chap. 219)   2D echocardiography is the gold standard for imaging valve morphology and motion (Fig. 211-1). Leaflet thickness and mobility, valve calcification, and the appearance of subvalvular and supravalvular structures can be assessed. Valve stenosis is reliably diagnosed by the thickening and decreased mobility of the valve. 2D echocardiography is the gold standard for the diagnosis of mitral stenosis, which produces typical tethering and diastolic doming. The severity of the stenosis can be obtained from a direct planimeter measurement of the mitral valve orifice from the short axis view. The presence and etiology of stenosis of the semilunar valves can be made by 2D echocardiography. Estimating the severity of the stenosis by 2D echocardiography alone is less reliable and requires Doppler echocardiography. The diagnosis of valvular regurgitation must be made by Doppler echocardiography, but 2D echocardiography is valuable for determining the etiology of the regurgitation. Annular dilatation, prolapse, flail leaflets, vegetation, and rheumatic involvement can be diagnosed and the LV response to volume overload can be assessed by 2D echocardiography.

Pericardial Effusion (See also Chap. 222)   2D echocardiography is the imaging modality of choice for the detection of pericardial effusion, which is easily visualized as a black echolucent ovoid structure surrounding the heart. In the hemodynamically unstable patient with pericardial tamponade, typical echo findings of right ventricular collapse, right atrial collapse, and a dilated inferior vena cava are seen (see Fig. 222-2). In patients with subclinical tamponade, these 2D echocardiographic features may not be present, but the diagnosis of elevated pericardial pressure can be made by Doppler findings of variations of inflow velocities with respiration (see Fig. 222-3). Echocardiographically guided pericardiocentesis has now become a standard of care. A 2D echocardiogram can directly visualize the location of the pericardial fluid in relationship to the entry point, and this technique has led to a low complication rate. Increased thickness of the pericardium is difficult to assess by 2D echocardiography. Subtle clues to pericardial constriction can be seen on

2D echocardiography from enhanced ventricular interaction, but Doppler imaging is required for confirmation of this diagnosis.

Intracardiac Masses (See also Chap. 223)   Intracardiac masses can be visualized on 2D echocardiography, provided that image quality is adequate. Solid masses appear as echo-dense structures, which can be located inside the cardiac chambers or infiltrating into the myocardium or pericardium (see Fig. 223-1). Although an echocardiographic examination cannot provide pathologic confirmation of the etiology of a mass, there are several instances in which the diagnosis of the mass can be suspected from its appearance, mobility, attachments, and the concomitant abnormalities seen. *LV* thrombus appears as an echo-dense structure, usually in the apical region associated with regional wall motion abnormalities. The appearance and mobility of the thrombus are predictive of embolic events. *Atrial myxoma* can be diagnosed by the appearance of a well-circumscribed mobile mass with attachments to the atrial septum. Prominent benign structures, such as *lipomatous infiltration of the atrial septum* and a *calcified mitral annulus*, may appear as cardiac masses. The high-resolution images provided by TEE may be required for further delineation of myocardial masses.

Aortic Disease (See also Chap. 231)   2D echocardiography can provide extremely useful information on diseases of the aorta. The proximal ascending aorta, the arch, and the distal descending aorta can usually be visualized via the transthoracic approach. For patients in whom a dilated aorta is well visualized, 2D echocardiography can be used for serial follow-up. Aortic dissection can be diagnosed when an intimal flap is visualized on a TTE. However, the definitive diagnosis of an aortic dissection usually requires a TEE.

DOPPLER ECHOCARDIOGRAPHY ■ Basic Principles   Doppler echocardiography uses ultrasound reflecting off moving red blood cells to measure the velocity of blood flow across valves, within cardiac chambers, and through the great vessels. Normal and abnormal blood flow patterns can be assessed noninvasively. Color-flow Doppler imaging (Fig. 211-3) displays the blood velocities in real time superimposed upon a 2D echocardiographic image. The different colors indicate the direction of blood flow (blue toward and red away from the transducer), with green superimposed when there is turbulent flow. Thus regurgitant lesions and shunts may be assessed by color-flow Doppler. Pulsed-wave Doppler measures the blood flow velocity in a specific location on the 2D echocardiographic image and displays the velocities in a spectral pattern using time as the *x*-axis. Continuous-wave Doppler

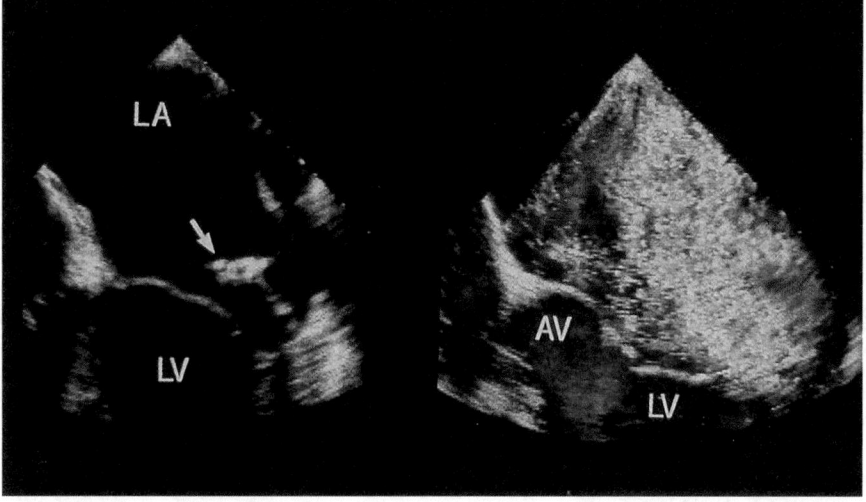

FIGURE 211-3   *Left:* Transesophageal echocardiographic view of a patient with severe mitral regurgitation due to a flail posterior leaflet. The arrow points to the portion of the posterior leaflet that is unsupported and moves into the left atrium during systole. *Right:* Color-flow imaging demonstrating a large mosaic jet of mitral regurgitation during systole. LA, left atrium; LV, left ventricle; AV, aortic valve.

echocardiography can measure high velocities of blood flow directed along the line of the Doppler beam, such as occur in the presence of valve stenosis, valve regurgitation, or intracardiac shunts. These high velocities can be used to determine intracardiac pressure gradients by a modified Bernoulli equation:

$$\text{Pressure change} = 4 \times (\text{velocity})^2$$

The derived pressure gradient can be used to determine intracardiac pressures and stenosis severity.

Tissue Doppler echocardiography measures the velocity of the myocardium. The velocity of myocardium is several magnitudes lower than the velocity of moving red blood cells. Analysis of specific myocardial motion allows for quantification of regional myocardial contraction and relaxation.

Valve Gradients (See also Chap. 219)   In the presence of valvular stenosis, there is an increase in the velocity of blood flow across the stenotic valve. A continuous-wave Doppler beam can be placed into this jet of blood, and the measured velocity used to determine an instantaneous gradient across the valve by applying the modified Bernoulli equation. Integration of this velocity over time provides an accurate measurement of the mean gradient across the valve. Since the valve gradient is dependent upon transvalvular flow, a calculated "valve area" is of clinical benefit and can be derived noninvasively.

Valvular Regurgitation (See also Chap. 219)   Valvular regurgitation is diagnosed by Doppler echocardiography when there is an abnormal retrograde flow across the valve. Color-flow imaging is the Doppler method used most frequently to detect valve regurgitation by visualization of a high-velocity turbulent jet in the chamber proximal to the regurgitant valve. The sensitivity of Doppler echocardiography for the detection of regurgitant lesions is high, and even trivial or mild regurgitation in the absence of clinical auscultatory evidence of a regurgitant murmur may be detected. The size and extent of the color-flow jet into the receiving cardiac chamber provide a semiqualitative estimate of the severity of regurgitation, but there are many limitations to using color jet size alone.

Intracardiac Pressures   These can be calculated from the peak continuous-wave Doppler signal of a regurgitant lesion. The Bernoulli equation is applied to the peak velocity to obtain the pressure gradient between two cardiac chambers. This is commonly applied to a tricuspid regurgitant jet, from which the systolic pressure gradient between the right atrium and right ventricle can be calculated. Adding an assumed right atrial pressure to this gradient will give a derived right ventricular systolic pressure, which provides the pulmonary artery systolic pressure in the absence of right ventricular outflow tract obstruction. Change in pressure over time during isovolumic contraction can be derived from a mitral regurgitation signal. This measurement provides an index of systolic contractility.

Cardiac Output   Volume flow rates can be reliably measured noninvasively from Doppler echocardiography. Using the hydrodynamic principle of flow through a rigid tube, the volume of flow can be calculated from the area of an orifice through which blood flows multiplied by the time of the velocity. The most accurate site for this measurement is through the LV outflow tract. The product of the outflow area and velocity provides a beat-to-beat measurement of stroke volume, which, when multiplied by heart rate, provides a measurement of cardiac output.

Diastolic Filling (See also Chap. 215)   Doppler echocardiography allows noninvasive evaluation of ventricular diastolic filling. The transmitral velocity curves reflect the relative pressure gradients between the left atrium and LV throughout the diastolic filling period. They are influenced by the rate of ventricular relaxation, the driving force across the valve, and the compliance of the LV. There is a progression of diastolic dysfunction in disease states, which can be assessed by Doppler flow velocity curves (Fig. 211-4). In the early phase of diastolic

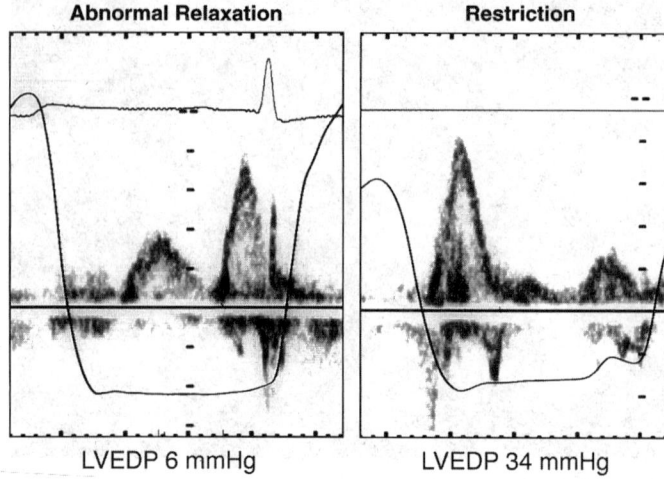

Abnormal Relaxation   **Restriction**

LVEDP 6 mmHg   LVEDP 34 mmHg

FIGURE 211-4   High-fidelity left ventricular pressure curve superimposed on a mitral inflow velocity curve obtained by Doppler echocardiography. The ratio of early and late diastolic flows is termed an *E:A ratio*. *Left*: In early stages of diastolic dysfunction, there is an abnormality of relaxation. There is a decrease in the early diastolic filling and an increase with filling at atrial contraction, resulting in a low E:A ratio of 0.5, with deceleration time (DT) of 280 ms. In this instance, the left ventricular end-diastolic pressure (LVEDP) is low at 6 mmHg. *Right*: As diastolic dysfunction progresses, there is a restriction to filling, in which there is a high early diastolic velocity and low velocity at atrial contraction resulting in a high E:A ratio of 3.0, with DT of 120 ms. In this instance, the LVEDP is markedly elevated to 34 mmHg. The DT reflects the rate of decline of the early velocity and is a measure of the effective operative compliance of the left ventricle. (See text for explanation.)

dysfunction there is primarily an abnormality of relaxation, with decreased early transmitral flow and a compensatory increase in flow during atrial contraction. As disease progresses, there is a higher left atrial pressure and reduced compliance of the LV, resulting in a higher early transmitral velocity and shortening of the deceleration of flow in early diastole, termed *restriction to filling*. These transmitral flow curves can be used to estimate ventricular filling pressures and to determine prognosis in certain disease entities. The addition of Doppler interrogation of pulmonary venous flow, analysis of Doppler tissue velocities of annular motion, and right-sided chamber flow velocities provides further information concerning the diastolic properties. Grading of the severity of diastolic dysfunction is now possible based on the Doppler velocities (Grades I–IV).

Congenital Heart Disease (See also Chap. 218)   Doppler echocardiography has been useful in the evaluation of patients with congenital heart disease. Congenital stenotic or regurgitant valve lesions can be assessed. The detection and semiquantitation of intracardiac shunts is possible by Doppler echocardiography. Patency of surgical shunts and conduits can be determined.

STRESS ECHOCARDIOGRAPHY (See also Chap. 226)   2D and Doppler echocardiography are usually performed in the resting state. Further information can be obtained by reimaging during either exercise or pharmacologic stress. The primary indications for stress echocardiography are to confirm the suspicion of CAD and estimate its severity. Stress echocardiography using both 2D echocardiography and Doppler echocardiography provides additional information for the patient with valvular heart disease.

The response of the myocardium to ischemia consists of a cascade of events. A decrease in systolic contraction of the ischemic area, termed a *regional wall motion abnormality*, occurs before symptoms or electrocardiographic changes. During a stress echocardiogram, 2D echocardiographic images at rest and during stress are digitized and displayed in a side-by-side format so that induced regional wall motion abnormalities may be detected. Changes in overall systolic function as well as end-systolic volume are also assessed. New regional wall motion abnormalities, a decline in ejection fraction, and an increase in end-systolic volume with stress are all indicators of myocardial ischemia (Fig. 211-5).

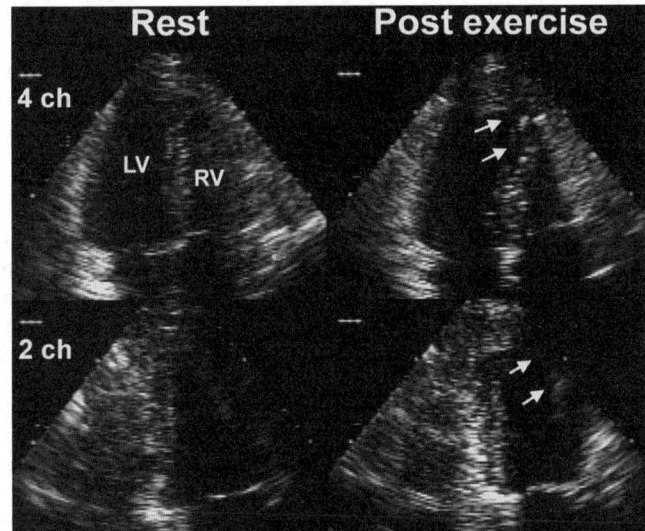

FIGURE 211-5 Stress echocardiographic images in a patient with known coronary artery disease. *Left*: The systolic views from a patient in the resting state is shown. The upper frame is taken from a four-chamber view and the lower frame is taken from a two-chamber view. *Right*: The systolic views are shown immediately after exercise. The arrows point to the appearance of a regional wall motion abnormality in the anterior and apical segments. LV, left ventricle; RV, right ventricle. *(From JK Oh et al, The Echo Manual, 2d ed. Philadelphia, Lippincott, Williams & Wilkins, 1999; with permission.)*

Exercise stress testing is usually done with exercise protocols using either upright treadmill or bicycle exercise. The echocardiographic imaging is done at baseline and then immediately after exercise. In patients who are not able to exercise, pharmacologic testing can be performed by infusion of dobutamine to increase myocardial oxygen demand. Dobutamine echocardiography has also been used to assess myocardial viability in patients with poor systolic function and concomitant CAD. In this type of study, dobutamine is started at a low dose of 5 to 10 μg/kg per min and then incrementally increased every few minutes. In the presence of viable myocardium, an increase in the systolic contraction of the myocardium is evident at low doses of dobutamine, and is followed by an ischemic response at higher doses.

It is important that the images be obtained as soon as possible after exercise is stopped since regional wall motion abnormalities may dissipate rapidly with time. Interpretation of the images is highly operator-dependent, and thus this technique requires an experienced echocardiographer.

Doppler echocardiography can be used at rest and during exercise in patients with valvular heart disease to determine the hemodynamic response to stress. Gradients across stenotic valves can be measured at rest and immediately after exercise; this provides information previously obtained by right heart catheterization during exercise. Pulmonary pressures can be obtained from the tricuspid regurgitation velocities at rest and during exercise.

TRANSESOPHAGEAL ECHOCARDIOGRAPHY This technique has provided an additional window to the heart (see Fig. 211-3). Because of the close proximity of the esophagus to the heart, high-resolution images of posterior structures are consistently obtained. TEE should be performed when further information is required after comprehensive 2D and Doppler transthoracic echocardiograms. Diseases of the aorta, such as aortic dissection, can be readily diagnosed and quantitated by TEE (Fig. 211-6; Chap. 231). Defining the source of embolism is a common indication for TEE, as abnormalities such as atrial thrombi, patent foramen ovale, and aortic debris can be detected. Other masses, particularly those in the atria, can be visualized. The presence of vegetations for the diagnosis of infective endocarditis and its compli-

cations can be assessed by TEE (Chap. 109). The evaluation of suspected abnormalities of a mitral prosthesis is an indication for TEE, as the posterior imaging window will avoid the problems of acoustic reflection caused by the prosthetic valve seen with TTE. TEE can be used during cardiac surgery to guide various operations, such as mitral valve repair and septal myectomy. When limited information is obtained from a TTE due to poor imaging windows, TEE can be useful.

Patients presenting with atrial fibrillation of indeterminate duration pose a difficult therapeutic challenge. Cardioversion may be the preferred treatment modality for these patients but if the time of onset of the atrial fibrillation is either greater than 48 h or unclear, there may be a higher risk of an embolic event at the time of cardioversion. In this situation, TEE has been used before cardioversion to look for a thrombus in the left atrium or left atrial appendage. If no thrombus is present, cardioversion can be safely performed emergently, as long as there is full dose anticoagulation before, during, and after the procedure.

EMERGENCY ECHOCARDIOGRAPHY A major advantage of echocardiography is the ability to obtain instantaneous images of the cardiac structures for immediate interpretation at the patient's bedside. Thus, echocardiography has become an ideal imaging modality for cardiac emergencies.

Unstable Hemodynamics For the patient with unstable hemodynamics, echocardiography can determine left ventricular size and function, right ventricular size and function, and the presence of acute valvular regurgitation and pericardial tamponade. Echocardiography is especially useful in the hemodynamically unstable patient following myocardial infarction, where acute mechanical complications (e.g., papillary muscle rupture, ventricular septal defect, myocardial perforation with tamponade, and right ventricular infarction) can be diagnosed and need to be differentiated from severe left ventricular systolic dysfunction. An enlarged right ventricle in a hemodynamically unstable patient can indicate the presence of acute right ventricular pressure overload, which is seen in acute pulmonary embolism. Echocardiography is the imaging modality of choice for the diagnosis of pericardial tamponade. 2D echocardiography can also be used to guide emergency pericardiocentesis.

Chest Pain Syndromes (See also Chap. 12) Echocardiography can be useful in selected patients with chest pain syndromes. For those patients who have an equivocal electrocardiogram, the presence of regional wall motion abnormalities on an echocardiogram can lead to the diagnosis of myocardial ischemia as an etiology for the pain. Other

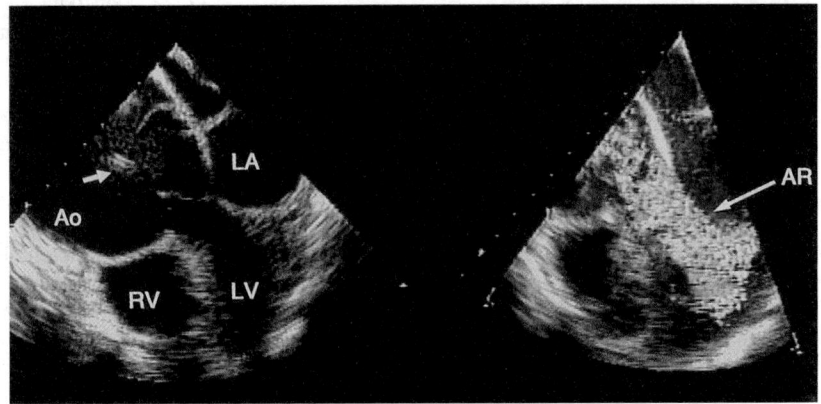

FIGURE 211-6 Transesophageal echocardiographic view of a patient with a dilated aorta, aortic dissection, and severe aortic regurgitation. The arrow points to the intimal flap that is seen in the dilated ascending aorta. *Left*: The long axis apex down view of the black and white two-dimensional image in diastole. *Right*: Color-flow imaging that demonstrates a large mosaic jet of aortic regurgitation. Ao, aorta; RV, right ventricle; AR, aortic regurgitation.

etiologies of chest pain, such as acute dissection or pericarditis with effusion, can also be diagnosed by echocardiography.

NUCLEAR CARDIOLOGY

BASIC PRINCIPLES OF NUCLEAR CARDIOLOGY All nuclear cardiology studies depend on the injection into the patient of an isotope that emits photons, generally gamma rays generated during radioactive decay when the nucleus of an isotope changes from one energy level to a lower one. Radionuclide imaging uses a special camera that images these photons. A common problem with all nuclear studies is that photons are emitted in all directions from the point of origin, and scattering, attenuation, and absorption of the photons can occur. The higher the energy of the isotope, the less chance for scatter or absorption. The two most commonly used isotopes are technetium 99m (^{99m}Tc) and thallium 201 (^{201}Tl).

ASSESSMENT OF VENTRICULAR FUNCTION Equilibrium radionuclide angiography, also known as *multiple-gated blood pool imaging*, is useful for the noninvasive assessment of ventricular function. It involves the imaging of ^{99m}Tc-labeled albumin or red cells that are uniformly distributed throughout the blood volume. Resting images of the blood pool of isotopes within the cardiac chambers are obtained by electrocardiographic gating through multiple cycles, so that sufficient counts can be detected to obtain an image. This requires that the heart rate be reasonably constant without significant arrhythmia. It provides an accurate, reproducible method for assessment of LV function. Other clinical variables that can be obtained include size and function of the right ventricle, size of atrial chambers and great vessels, diastolic filling parameters, and the severity of valvular regurgitation.

First-pass radionuclide angiography is an alternative method for the noninvasive assessment of ventricular function that involves the recording of the movement of a bolus of radionuclide during its "first pass" through the central circulation. This does not require labeling of red blood cells. ^{99m}Tc is utilized because of its low cost and short half-life. During this testing, the passage of the radioisotope through the right atrium, right ventricle, pulmonary circulation, left atrium, left ventricle, and aorta is recorded with a high-count (usually multicrystal) camera. The high count rates allow temporal definition of the passage of the bolus. The disadvantage of first-pass radionuclide angiography compared to equilibrium testing is its poorer resolution of ventricular wall motion.

Gated single-photon emission computed tomography (SPECT) can also be used to assess ejection fraction and regional wall motion (usually poststress) by gating the acquisition of SPECT myocardial perfusion images (see below). Although this can potentially be done using ^{201}Tl, ^{99m}Tc- labeled compounds are preferable because of their higher count rates. An automated technique determines the endocardial borders of the LV cavity and a geometric model is used to calculate the ejection fraction. As for equilibrium radionuclide angiography, the heart rhythm should be regular without significant arrhythmia.

ASSESSMENT OF MYOCARDIAL PERFUSION Myocardial perfusion imaging by nuclear techniques is now widely applied for the evaluation of ischemic heart disease (Chap. 226). Injection of radioisotopes at rest and during stress is performed to produce images of myocardial regional uptake proportional to regional blood flow. With maximal exercise, myocardial blood flow is increased up to fivefold above the resting condition. In the presence of a fixed coronary stenosis, there is an inability to increase myocardial perfusion in the territory supplied by the stenosis, creating a flow differential and inhomogeneous distribution of the isotope. In patients who are unable to exercise, pharmacologic agents are used to increase blood flow and create similar inhomogeneities. The preferred pharmacologic agents are adenosine or dipyridamole, which increase blood flow to a similar degree as exercise. In patients with bronchospastic lung disease, which is a contraindication to the use of adenosine or dipyridamole, dobutamine may

be used as an alternative, although it does not increase blood flow to the same extent.

^{201}Tl is a potassium analogue and is avidly taken up by viable myocardial cells. The degree of uptake is related directly to the coronary blood flow. An initial injection is usually performed at peak exercise, and hypoperfused myocardium will have less thallium uptake than a region of normal perfusion. Over the next several hours, a complex process occurs that is known as "redistribution." There is a continuous input of thallium into the myocardium from a large reservoir of thallium in the blood pool. At the same time, thallium continuously washes out of portions of the myocardium at a rate that is dependent on local myocardial perfusion. The final result is that a region of ischemia that initially appears as an area of reduced uptake becomes apparently normal over time; this redistribution is seen on delayed imaging. In regions of fibrosis (infarction), there will be no redistribution on delayed imaging. A "reinjection" of additional thallium before acquisition of the delayed images enhances the detection of ischemia. The presence of redistribution in areas of hypokinesia has been associated with recovery of LV function after revascularization.

Other findings on thallium imaging may be of considerable clinical importance. Increased lung uptake of thallium may be seen immediately after stress and assessed either quantitatively or qualitatively. This finding reflects increased pulmonary capillary wedge pressure during stress. It occurs in the presence of severe CAD and/or LV dysfunction. It provides important adverse prognostic information that is incremental to other clinical, stress, and coronary angiographic variables. Thallium images may also show evidence of transient poststress LV dilatation. This finding is also associated with severe CAD and/or LV dysfunction as well as with an adverse prognosis.

^{99m}Tc-labeled compounds have a higher photon energy and shorter half-life than ^{201}Tl, permitting the injection of larger doses (Fig. 211-7). As a result, these compounds generally provide higher quality scans with fewer artifacts. Three technetium-labeled agents have been approved for general use: teboroxime, tetrofosmin, and sestamibi. The last is the best studied of these agents and is currently used most frequently. Like thallium, sestamibi distributes to the myocardium in relation to blood flow, and its uptake requires a viable myocardial cell and an intact cell membrane. It is transported through the cytoplasm and bound to the mitochondria in a nearly irreversible fashion. Compared to thallium, there is far less redistribution. As a result, the agent must generally be injected twice—once at rest and once during stress.

COMPARISON OF THALLIUM AND TECHNETIUM Both ^{201}Tl- and ^{99m}Tc-labeled compounds provide clinically useful myocardial perfusion images in the majority of patients. The choice between the two is often dictated by local experience and economics. However, in selected patients, there may be factors that suggest a clear advantage for one or the other. The relative advantages of both agents are listed in Table 211-2.

POSITRON EMISSION TOMOGRAPHY The underlying physics of positron emission tomography (PET) scanning is quite different from that involved in the standard radionuclide techniques described above. The annihilation of the positron leads to the simultaneous emission of two very high energy (511 keV) photons in opposite directions. These can then be imaged by a series of detectors placed in a ring around the patient. The very high energy of the photons results in far less scatter and attenuation than with conventional nuclear cardiology techniques. PET cameras are considerably more expensive than conventional nuclear cardiology cameras. The radiopharmaceuticals involved require a cyclotron for production and generally have half-lives that are so short that transportation beyond the immediate local region is not feasible. Although the initial availability of PET was limited, the increasing role of PET imaging in oncology has increased its availability for cardiac imaging.

Positron emitters can be employed to study both myocardial blood flow and myocardial metabolism. Nitrogen-13 ammonia, oxygen-15 water, and rubidium-82 have all been employed to assess myocardial blood flow. They permit measurement of absolute regional blood flows, in contrast to the relative blood flows that are assessed with

FIGURE 211-7 *A.* Exercise sestamibi study on a 71-year-old, white female with atypical angina. *Left:* Stress images; *right:* rest images. The images are normal. There is even sestamibi update throughout the myocardium at rest and during stress. *B.* Exercise sestamibi study on a 75-year-old male with a history of typical angina. *Left:* Stress images; *right:* rest images. The stress images show a large defect involving the apex, lateral, and inferior walls (thick arrows), which improves at rest (thin arrows). Subsequent coronary angiography demonstrates severe three-vessel coronary artery disease. SA, short axis; Mid, middle of the left ventricle; VLA, vertical long axis; HLA, horizontal long axis.

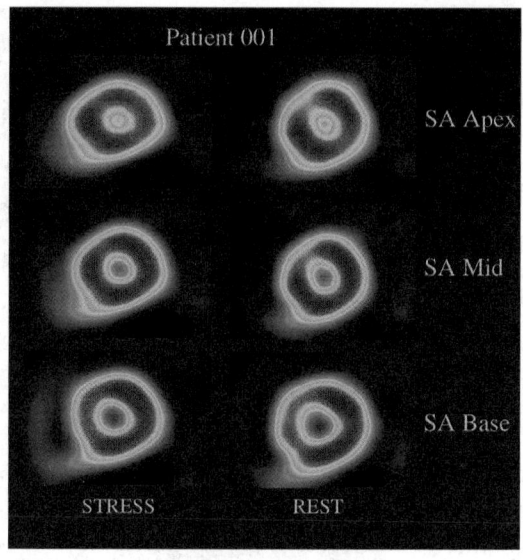

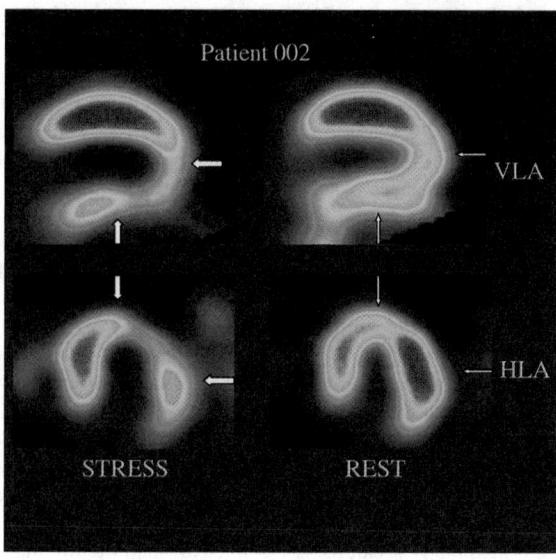

^{201}Tl- or ^{99m}Tc-labeled compounds. This advantage has been utilized for research purposes but has not yet been exploited clinically. Myocardial metabolism is most often assessed using fluorine-18 deoxyglucose. This agent permits the detection and quantification of exogenous glucose utilization in areas of hypoperfused myocardium.

The clinical application of PET scanning that has been most well studied is the assessment of myocardial viability. The pattern of enhanced fluorodeoxyglucose uptake in regions of decreased perfusion (termed *glucose/blood flow "mismatch"*) indicates the presence of ischemic myocardium that has preferentially shifted its metabolic substrate toward glucose rather than fatty acid or lactate. This pattern identifies regions of ischemic or hibernating myocardium that are likely to improve in function after revascularization (Chap. 226).

Careful studies have consistently shown the ability of PET to identify ischemic or hibernating myocardium in 10 to 20% of regions that would be classified as fibrotic (infarcted) by ^{201}Tl- or ^{99m}Tc-labeled compounds. For that reason, this technique is generally regarded as the gold standard for the assessment of myocardial viability. When large fixed defects (infarcts) are detected by ^{201}Tl- or ^{99m}Tc-labeled-compounds in patients who are candidates for coronary revascularization, PET imaging can suggest if the risk of revascularization is justified by the potential benefit.

Within the past few years, specially modified conventional gamma cameras have been employed to image fluorodeoxyglucose in an attempt to avoid the expense related to cameras dedicated to PET. The limited evidence available suggests that this approach is inferior to standard PET.

TABLE 211-2 *Relative Advantages of Thallium 201 and Technetium 99m Sestamibi*
THALLIUM
Lower radiopharmaceutical cost
Measurement of increased pulmonary uptake
Detection of resting ischemia (hibernating myocardium)
SESTAMIBI
Better image quality (particularly in obese patients or female patients with breast attenuation)
Ventricular function assessment (first-pass or gated SPECT)
Shorter imaging times (lower cost)
Shorter imaging protocols (patient/scheduling convenience)
Acute imaging in myocardial infarction (myocardium at risk) and unstable angina (chest pain triage)
Superior quantification, particularly of resting perfusion defect (infarct size)

Note: SPECT, single-photon emission computed tomography.

OVERVIEW OF STRESS TESTING

CHOOSING THE APPROPRIATE INITIAL STRESS TEST The choice of an initial stress testing modality should be based on the evaluation of the patient's resting electrocardiogram, the physical ability to perform exercise, and the local expertise and technology available in an institution. For the standard risk assessment of CAD, the exercise electrocardiographic test (Chap. 226) should be the initial mode of stress testing in patients with a normal electrocardiogram who are not taking digoxin and who are able to exercise. If there are resting electrocardiographic abnormalities (ST depression >1 mm, LV hypertrophy, bundle branch block, paced rhythm, pre-excitation) or the patient is taking digoxin or has had a prior coronary revascularization, an imaging modality (either nuclear imaging or echocardiography) should be used for initial evaluation. Pharmacologic stress testing with imaging should be used in patients who are unable to exercise.

When an imaging modality is appropriate, the decision as to whether to use an echocardiographic or a nuclear test is dependent not only on the patient's situation but also on the local expertise and technology available in the institution. Both echocardiography and nuclear imaging require expertise in the performance and interpretation of the tests and the best information is obtained from the imaging modality in which there is most expertise and experience. There are, however, certain situations in which one imaging modality has an advantage over the other.

Echocardiography provides additional structural information. Therefore, if there is a question of concomitant valve disease, pericardial disease, or aortic disease, echocardiography is able to provide information regarding these issues. The major limitation of echocardiography is the inability to obtain diagnostic images in all patients, especially those with chronic obstructive pulmonary disease or severe obesity. Tissue harmonic imaging and contrast injection may help in further delineating endocardial motion in these patients. However, if there is inadequate definition of endocardial motion on the resting echocardiogram, stress echocardiography should not be performed. If the patient has had a previous infarction and one needs to determine whether a specific area of the myocardium is ischemic, nuclear imaging is the preferred modality. Nuclear imaging using ^{99m}Tc-labeled compounds is preferred in obese patients and those with severe lung disease. Nuclear imaging is more sensitive and less specific than echocardiography for the detection of myocardial ischemia.

There are certain instances in which there are false-positives with imaging stress testing. In patients with left bundle branch block, exercise may provoke abnormalities in regional perfusion and regional ventricular function in the absence of CAD. Therefore, the modality of choice in these patients is pharmacologic perfusion imaging.

STRESS TESTING FOR PROGNOSIS Exercise electrocardiography, stress nuclear imaging, and stress echocardiography can all provide important information regarding diagnosis and the patient's subsequent risk for cardiac death. The results are often pivotal in defining the need for coronary angiography and coronary revascularization. For the exercise electrocardiogram, the Duke treadmill score is a well-validated index that is useful for both diagnosis and prognosis. Patients who exercise for > 5 min on the treadmill using a Bruce protocol without angina or ST segment changes have a low risk of subsequent cardiac death (< 1% annual mortality). In contrast, patients with markedly abnormal stress tests are at high risk for subsequent death (> 3% annual mortality); coronary angiography and possible revascularization are appropriate. For the exercise electrocardiogram, a high-risk Duke score consists of a low exercise workload with angina and early ST segment changes.

The imaging tests can add further prognostic information, especially when the results of an exercise electrocardiogram fall into an intermediate risk category. For nuclear imaging, normal stress (exercise) or pharmacologic myocardial perfusion scans (p. 1325) are highly predictive of the absence of significant coronary disease and a low risk of subsequent cardiac death. For stress (exercise or dobutamine) echocardiography, an increase in ejection fraction and a decrease in end-systolic volume at a high workload predict the absence of significant coronary disease and a low risk of subsequent cardiac death. For nuclear imaging, large stress-induced defects, multiple stress-induced defects of moderate size, or a large fixed defect with LV dilatation or increased ^{201}Tl lung uptake are high-risk findings. For stress echocardiography, patients with a drop in ejection fraction, the appearance of multiple regional wall motion abnormalities, and an increase in end-systolic volume are at high risk.

MRI AND CT IMAGING

MRI MRI is a technique based on the magnetic properties of hydrogen nuclei. In the presence of a large magnetic field, nuclear spin transitions from the ground state to excited states can be induced, and as the nuclei relax and return to their ground state, they release energy in the form of electromagnetic radiation that is detected and processed into an image. Contrast agents are frequently employed in MRI to provide magnetic resonance angiograms (MRAs). These provide enhanced soft-tissue contrast as well as the opportunity to obtain rapid angiographic images during the first pass of contrast through the vascular system. Cardiac MRI is particularly challenging because of the rapid physiologic motion of the heart and coronary arteries. Both static and cine images can be obtained using electrocardiographic triggering, often within a short breath-hold of 10 to 15 s (Fig. 211-8). Cine images can be acquired in any plane with excellent blood-myocardial contrast, and these images can be used to quantify ejection fraction, end-systolic and end-diastolic volumes, and cardiac mass with high accuracy and reliability.

Clinical Utility The multiplanar capabilities of MRI, coupled with excellent contrast and spatial resolution, are often valuable in defining anatomic relationships in patients with complex congenital heart disease. Cardiac masses can be characterized and their relationship to normal anatomic structures defined. Likewise, MRI is often the examination of choice to determine whether a mediastinal or pulmonary mass has invaded the pericardium or heart. The entire pericardium can be visualized in multiple planes, and MRI has proved useful in characterization of pericardial effusions, pericardial thickening, and constrictive pericarditis in patients with indeterminate results on echocardiography. MRI is an important technique for evaluation of patients with suspected arrhythmogenic right ventricular dysplasia, where fatty infiltration of the right ventricular free wall can be identified, as can right ventricular dilatation and dyskinesis.

MRA is a standard technique for imaging the aorta and large vessels of the chest and abdomen, with results essentially identical to

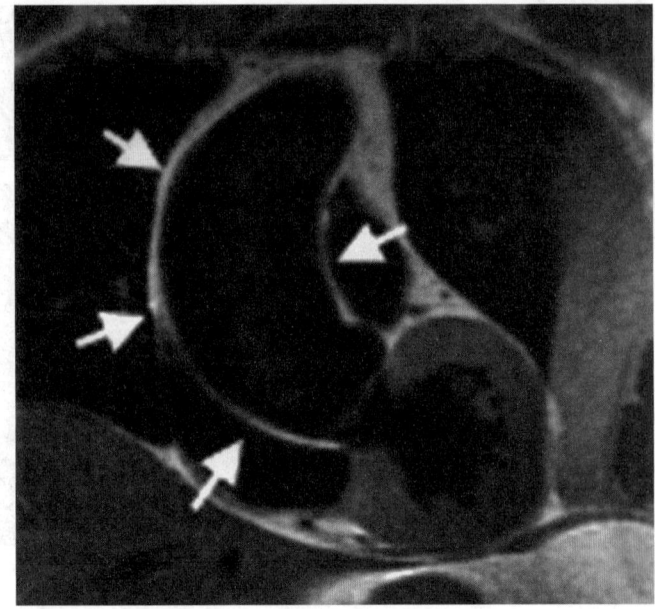

FIGURE 211-8 Axial dark-blood MRI from a patient with aortic stenosis and dilatation of the ascending aorta (arrows). Image was acquired in approximately 10 s during suspended respiration.

conventional catheter-based angiography. MRA of the coronary arteries is a much more difficult challenge, both because of the small size of these vessels and because of their rapid and complex motion during the cardiac cycle. Although promising results have been achieved, coronary MRA is not yet an accurate and reliable clinical technique.

MRI is a promising technology for the evaluation of myocardial perfusion. Myocardial perfusion is evaluated by injecting a bolus of contrast and then continuously scanning the heart as the contrast passes through the cardiac chambers and into the myocardium. Relative perfusion deficits are reflected as regions of low signal intensity within the myocardium. Myocardial viability may be determined by imaging the heart 10 to 20 min after contrast injection, as infarcted tissue retains contrast by virtue of its larger extracellular volume. Specialized pulse sequences have been designed to measure the velocity of blood in each pixel of the image, so that flow across valves and within blood vessels may be accurately determined. These techniques may allow characterization of the severity of valvular disease as well as quantification of shunt volumes.

Cardiac MRI has several limitations. Absolute contraindications include the presence of pacemakers, internal defibrillators, or cerebral aneurysm clips. A small percentage of patients are claustrophobic and unable to tolerate the examination within the relatively confined quarters of the magnet bore. Examination of clinically unstable patients is problematic, since close monitoring is difficult.

CT IMAGING CT is fast, simple, and noninvasive, and it provides images with excellent spatial resolution and good soft-tissue contrast. Imaging the heart is a more difficult problem, however, because image acquisition times for conventional CT have until recently been on the order of 1 s, far too long to freeze cardiac motion.

Electron-beam CT employs a fixed detector array and radiation source. The x-rays are generated by an electron beam sweeping continuously across the target anode ring. This is accomplished very rapidly, on the order of 50 to 100 ms. The electron beam can be triggered by the electrocardiogram trace, and single static images or cine images are generated with excellent temporal resolution.

Clinical Applications Cardiac CT has several clinical applications. Pericardial calcification is an important sign of constrictive pericarditis and is easily detected by CT. CT is useful in characterizing cardiac masses, particularly those containing fat or calcium. The ability to detect small amounts of fat with high spatial resolution makes CT an

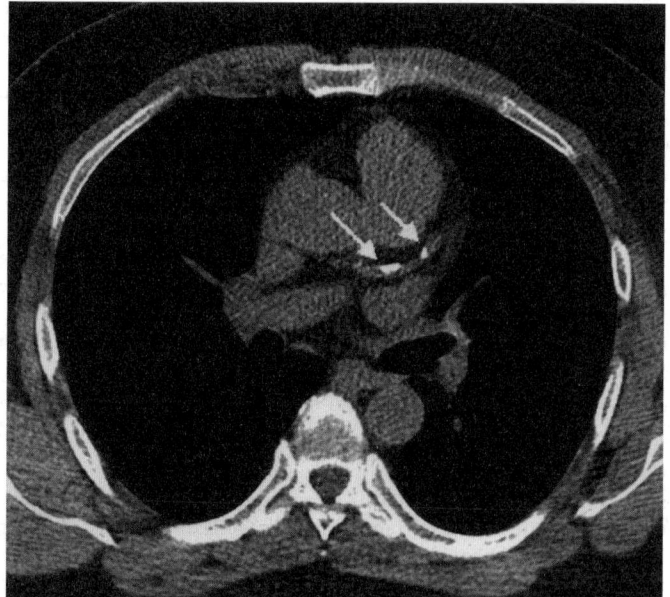

FIGURE 211-9 Noncontrast image from electron-beam CT revealing small foci of calcification in the left anterior descending coronary artery (arrow).

attractive technique for imaging patients with suspected arrhythmogenic right ventricular dysplasia. Cine images can be used to evaluate wall motion and determine ejection fraction, end-diastolic and end-systolic volumes, and cardiac mass.

CT angiography (CTA) has demonstrated accuracy similar to MRA in imaging the aorta and great vessels, and CTA is rapidly becoming the examination of choice in the evaluation of patients with suspected pulmonary embolus. Coronary CTA with multidetector spiral CT is in the developmental stage. Both CT and MRI are valuable in delineating the presence and course of anomalous coronary vessels; however, the clinical utility of either technique in detecting and grading coronary artery stenoses has not been widely demonstrated.

Coronary Calcification Calcium in the coronary arteries occurs in atherosclerosis and is absent in the normal coronary artery. CT is very sensitive for the detection of coronary artery calcification and is being promoted as a noninvasive modality for the screening and diagnosis of CAD (Fig. 211-9). The amount of coronary calcification (coronary

calcium score) is related to the severity of coronary disease. However, although CT has a very high sensitivity for the detection of CAD, it has a low specificity. The overall predictive accuracy for angiographic obstructive coronary disease in a typical CAD patient population is similar to other imaging modalities, such as SPECT. Due to its low specificity, CT should not be used for the diagnosis of obstructive coronary disease. However, in asymptomatic patients, more severe coronary atherosclerosis (and thus a higher calcium score) is associated with a higher risk of future cardiac events. Nonetheless, there are no data to show that the information from CT is additive to standard clinical assessment of the risk of CAD and coronary events. The results of properly designed outcomes research studies are required for determination of the ultimate clinical role of CT scanning in patients with known or suspected CAD.

Limitations of CT Limitations of CT include ionizing radiation and the need for iodinated contrast, which is problematic in patients with renal insufficiency or contrast allergy. Radiation doses tend to increase as the spatial and temporal resolution improve; however, the dose for cardiac CT is almost always significantly lower than the dose delivered during cardiac catheterization.

FURTHER READING

DUTKA DP et al: The contribution of positron emission tomography to the study of ischemic heart failure. Prog Cardiovasc Dis 43:399, 2001

GIBBONS RJ et al: ACC/AHA guideline update for exercise testing: A report of the American College of Cardiology/American Heart Association Task Force on Practice Guidelines Circulation 106:1883, 2002

GIBBONS RJ: Myocardial perfusion imaging. Heart 83:355, 2000

HABERL R et al: Correlation of coronary calcification and angiographically documented stenoses in patients with suspected coronary artery disease: Results of 1,764 patients. J Am Coll Cardiol 37:451, 2001

KIMURA BJ et al: Screening cardiac ultrasonographic examination in patients with suspected cardiac disease in the emergency department. Am Heart J 142:324, 2001

MAZUR W: Myocardial viability: Recent developments in detection and clinical significance. Curr Opin Cardiol 16:277, 2001

MULVAGH SL et al: Contrast echocardiography: Current and future applications. J Am Soc Echocardiogr 13:331, 2000

TRAMBAIOLO P et al: New insights into regional systolic and diastolic left ventricular function with tissue Doppler echocardiography: From qualitative analysis to a quantitative approach. J Am Soc Echocardiogr 14:85, 2001

212 DIAGNOSTIC CARDIAC CATHETERIZATION AND ANGIOGRAPHY
Donald S. Baim, William Grossman

Despite progressive improvements in noninvasive techniques, cardiac catheterization remains a key clinical tool for assessing the anatomy and physiology of the heart and its associated vasculature. It involves the insertion of small (diameter, 2 to 3 mm), hollow plastic tubes or catheters into a peripheral artery or vein under local anesthesia, and passage of their tips into the heart for pressure measurement or for the injection of a liquid radiographic contrast agent. The findings of diagnostic cardiac catheterization characterize the extent and severity of cardiac disease and thereby help in deciding on the most appropriate plan for medical, surgical, or catheter-based treatment. While the majority of patients with coronary artery disease (CAD) or valvular disease can be managed using only clinical and noninvasive data, more than 2 million cardiac catheterization and angiographic procedures are performed each year for diagnostic or interventional purposes, or both. This chapter focuses on the uses of cardiac catheterization as a diagnostic tool. →*For further discussion of catheter-based interventions, see Chap. 229.*

INDICATIONS, CONTRAINDICATIONS, AND COMPLICATIONS

INDICATIONS Given the expense and small, but real, risks of cardiac catheterization, its performance is not routine whenever cardiac disease is diagnosed or suspected. Instead, cardiac catheterization is recommended only when there is a need to confirm the presence of a clinically suspected condition, define its anatomic and physiologic severity, and determine whether important associated conditions are present. This need most commonly arises when a patient is experiencing limiting or escalating symptoms of cardiac dysfunction (Chap. 216) or myocardial ischemia (Chap. 226) or when objective measures (such as exercise testing or echocardiography) suggest that the patient has a high risk of progressing to rapid functional deterioration, myocardial infarction, or other adverse events. Under these circumstances, catheterization may serve as a checkpoint prior to treatment by cardiac surgery or a catheter-based intervention. While cardiac catheterization was previously considered mandatory in *all* patients being considered for cardiac surgery, currently many patients with congenital or valvular

TABLE 212-1 *Relative Contraindications to Cardiac Catheterization and Angiography*

Uncontrolled ventricular irritability: increased risk of ventricular tachycardia and fibrillation during catheterization if ventricular irritability is uncontrolled

Uncorrected hypokalemia or digitalis toxicity

Uncorrected hypertension: predisposes to myocardial ischemia and/or heart failure during angiography

Intercurrent febrile illness

Decompensated heart failure: especially acute pulmonary edema, unless catheterization can be done with patient sitting up

Anticoagulated state: prothrombin time >18 s

Severe allergy to radiographic contrast agent

Severe renal insufficiency and/or anuria: unless dialysis is planned to remove fluid and radiographic contrast load

heart disease undergo surgical correction based solely on clinical and noninvasive test data. Cardiac catheterization and coronary arteriography still remain, however, the only way to define *coronary anatomy* with sufficient precision to inform decisions regarding coronary surgery or catheter-based interventions in patients with CAD. In patients with other forms of heart disease (e.g., dilated cardiomyopathy, valvular heart disease), cardiac catheterization can provide hemodynamic characterization essential for the design of an appropriate medical regimen, or to assess prognosis.

CONTRAINDICATIONS When there is a clinical "need to know," there are very few absolute contraindications to diagnostic cardiac catheterization in a patient who understands and accepts the associated risks. Some relative contraindications to cardiac catheterization, however, are listed in Table 212-1. Most center on factors that increase the risk of the procedure above the baseline mortality risk of roughly 1 in 1000 for clinically stable patients. For example, risk is increased more than tenfold in patients with severe symptoms, certain types of coronary anatomy, valve disease, left ventricular dysfunction, or severe noncardiac disease, as outlined in Table 212-2.

COMPLICATIONS Beyond the mortality risk, cardiac catheterization carries a 1 in 1000 risk of stroke or myocardial infarction. Other problems, such as transient tachy- or bradyarrhythmias or bruising or bleeding at the catheter insertion site, occur in fewer than 1% of patients and respond to drug therapy, countershock, or vascular surgical repair, without long-term sequelae. Although serious, problems such as cardiac perforation or arterial dissection are very rare in the modern era of cardiac catheterization.

Some patients, however, are intolerant of the iodinated contrast agents used for angiography, which may produce transient deterioration in renal function (particularly in patients with baseline renal dys-

TABLE 212-2 *Patient Characteristics Associated with Increased Mortality from Cardiac Catheterization*

Age Infants (<1 month old) and the elderly (>85 years old) are at increased risk of death during cardiac catheterization. Elderly women appear to be at higher risk than elderly men.

Functional class Mortality in class IV patients is more than 10 times greater than in class I–II patients.

Severity of coronary obstruction Mortality for patients with left main coronary artery disease is more than 10 times greater than in patients with one- or two-vessel disease.

Valvular heart disease Especially when severe and combined with coronary disease, is associated with a higher risk of death at cardiac catheterization than coronary artery disease alone.

Left ventricular dysfunction Mortality in patients with a left ventricular ejection fraction <30% is more than 10 times greater than in patients with an ejection fraction ≥50%.

Severe noncardiac disease Patients with renal insufficiency, insulin-requiring diabetes, advanced cerebrovascular and/or peripheral vascular disease, or severe pulmonary insufficiency have an increased incidence of death and other major complications from cardiac catheterization.

function or proteinuria who are not adequately prehydrated) or *allergic reactions* ranging from urticaria to frank anaphylaxis in sensitive patients. These allergic reactions can be suppressed by pretreatment with glucocorticoids (prednisone, 20 to 40 mg every 6 h), conventional antihistamines (e.g., diphenhydramine, 25 mg every 6 h), and H_2 antagonists (cimetidine, 300 mg every 6 h), starting 18 to 24 h prior to the procedure. Despite these precautions, anaphylactic reactions during radiographic contrast angiography may require emergency treatment with intravenous epinephrine. In contemporary practice, however, use of newer nonionic contrast agents has almost eliminated these severe allergic reactions. Compared to the original high-osmolar agents, the newer contrast agents also have a lesser myocardial depressant effect and produce fewer side effects (hypotension, nausea, bradycardia, or a sensation of marked warmth following injection).

TECHNIQUES

Cardiac catheterization is performed with the patient in the fasting state and awake but lightly sedated. Typical preprocedure sedatives include diazepam (Valium, 5 to 10 mg orally) or midazolam (Versed, 1 mg intravenously). Although cardiac catheterization was previously performed exclusively as an inpatient procedure, current practice is to perform most elective procedures on an *outpatient* basis, with the patient discharged 2 to 4 h after the procedure is completed. Since cardiac catheterization is a sterile procedure, prophylactic antibiotics are not necessary. To minimize the risks of bleeding at the local catheter insertion site, patients who have been anticoagulated chronically with warfarin should have this agent discontinued at least 48 h prior to the procedure, so that the INR falls below 2. Oral aspirin (325 mg per day) is recommended in patients undergoing diagnostic catheterization for suspected coronary disease, since aspirin pretreatment is required if a coronary intervention is to be performed.

Most (>95%) cardiac catheterizations are performed by the percutaneous femoral technique, in which a needle puncture is performed in the femoral artery (for left heart catheterization) and the femoral vein (for right heart catheterization). A flexible guidewire is inserted through this needle, over which a vascular access sheath is placed, through which the desired catheters can be advanced. This percutaneous technique has been modified for other sites, including the brachial and radial artery. The brachial or radial approach has an advantage in the patient with peripheral vascular disease involving the abdominal aorta and iliac or femoral arteries or in whom immediate postprocedure ambulation is desired, but it involves some limitations in the range of devices that can be used if the diagnostic procedure evolves into a catheter-based intervention. With these alternatives, the original cut-down, or Sones, technique of cardiac catheterization by direct exposure of the brachial artery and vein in the antecubital fossa is rarely used.

Cardiac catheterization may include a variety of different measurements of pressure and flow (hemodynamics) as well as a variety of different contrast injections recorded as x-ray movies (angiography). The exact types of testing performed in any given procedure depend on the nature of the clinical problem being evaluated. In patients with CAD, the procedure may include only left ventriculography and coronary angiography, while in patients with valvular heart disease, full left and right heart hemodynamic studies may be performed.

RIGHT HEART CATHETERIZATION

Measurement of the pressures in the right side of the heart was once a routine part of each cardiac catheterization, but it is now used in fewer than 25% of procedures since it adds little to the evaluation of the patient with CAD. It is still useful, however, when significant left and/or right ventricular dysfunction, valve disease, myopericardial disease, or intracardiac shunting is suspected. The right heart catheterization procedure is similar to the placement of a Swan-Ganz catheter at the bedside in the intensive care unit, except that it is performed under fluoroscopic guidance. A balloon flotation catheter is advanced from a suitable vein (femoral, brachial, subclavian, or internal jugular) into the superior vena cava, where blood is sampled for oximetry. The catheter is then positioned in the right atrium, where pressure is measured. The balloon is inflated with air (or carbon dioxide, if intracardiac shunting is suspected) and advanced sequentially into the right ventricle, pulmonary artery, and pulmonary artery wedge position. Pressure is recorded at each of these locations, with normal values for pressures measured during cardiac catheterization summarized in Table 212-3. After recording the pulmonary wedge pressure (which approximates left atrial pressure), the balloon is deflated so that pulmonary artery pressure can be monitored and blood samples obtained for oximetry. Comparison of oxygen saturations in the superior and inferior vena cava, the chambers of the right heart, and pulmonary artery permits assessment of the presence of a left-to-right shunt at the atrial, ventricular, or pulmonary artery level, which will be manifested as an increase ("step-up") in oxygen saturation of blood as it traverses these vessels and chambers.

MEASUREMENT OF CARDIAC OUTPUT   Measurements of the pulmonary artery and aortic oxygen content and oxygen consumption allow calculation of the cardiac output by the Fick principle, which states that

$$Q \text{ (L/min)} = \frac{O_2 \text{ consumption (mL/min)}}{\text{arteriovenous } O_2 \text{ difference (mL/L)}}$$

In order to compare individuals of different body weights and sizes, cardiac output (Q) is commonly divided by body surface area to yield the cardiac index (CI). Normal values for O_2 consumption and cardiac output are given in Table 212-3. It should be noted, however, that dividing the O_2 consumption by the arteriovenous O_2 difference across the lungs (estimated pulmonary venous–pulmonary arterial O_2 content) actually measures the *pulmonary* blood flow (Q_p). In patients with an intracardiac left-to-right shunt at the atrial, ventricular, or pulmonary artery levels, this calculated pulmonary blood flow overestimates systemic blood flow by the amount flowing through the shunt. In such cases, calculation of systemic blood flow (Q_s) requires dividing O_2 consumption by the *systemic* arteriovenous O_2 difference, estimated as the systemic arterial blood O_2 content minus the mixed venous blood O_2 content derived from the chamber immediately proximal to the level of the shunt. The Fick method is most dependable when the cardiac output is low and a large arteriovenous oxygen difference can be measured.

Another approach to the measurement of cardiac output during right heart catheterization is the thermodilution technique, in which a thermistor is mounted on the tip of a balloon flotation catheter and positioned in the pulmonary artery. An aliquot (10 mL) of room temperature or chilled intravenous solution is then injected into the vena cava or right atrium via a proximal port on the catheter. The resulting change in temperature at the thermistor is monitored, and the integral of temperature drop at the thermistor is calculated electronically. By conservation of heat, this temperature integral is inversely proportional to the volume flow rate past the thermistor, allowing calculation of the

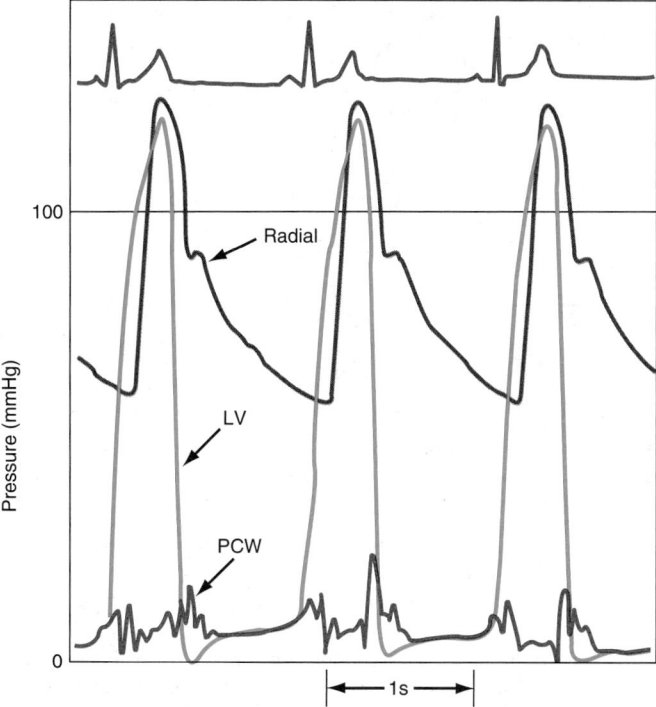

FIGURE 212-1   Left ventricular (LV), radial artery, and pulmonary capillary wedge (PCW) pressures in a patient with normal cardiovascular function. Note the absence of a pressure gradient between the LV and radial artery in systole and between the LV and PCW in diastole.

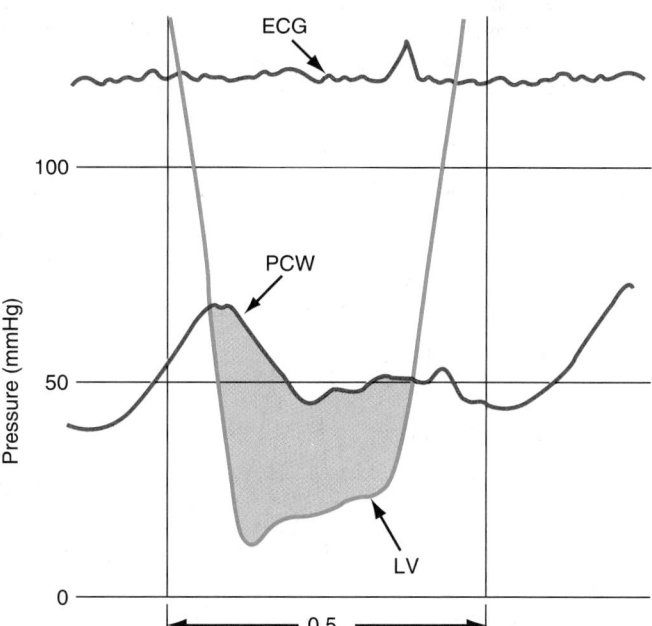

FIGURE 212-2   Pulmonary capillary wedge (PCW) and left ventricular (LV) pressure tracings in a 40-year-old woman with mitral stenosis. This patient also had systemic hypertension and significant elevation of her LV diastolic pressure. [*From BA Carabello, W Grossman, in Grossman's Cardiac Catheterization, Angiography, and Intervention, 6th ed, DS Baim, W Grossman (eds). Baltimore, Lippincott Williams & Wilkins, 2000.*]

TABLE 212-3 *Normal Values for Hemodynamic Parameters*	
Pressures (mmHg)	
Systemic arterial	
Peak systolic/end-diastolic	100–140/60–90
Mean	70–105
Left ventricle	
Peak systolic/end-diastolic	100–140/3–12
Left atrium (or pulmonary capillary wedge)	
Mean	2–10
a wave	3–15
v wave	3–15
Pulmonary artery	
Peak systolic/end-diastolic	15–30/4–12
Mean	9–18
Right ventricle	
Peak systolic/end-diastolic	15–30/2–8
Right atrium	
Mean	2–8
a wave	2–10
v wave	2–10
Resistances [(dyn·s)/cm⁵]	
Systemic vascular resistance	700–1600
Pulmonary vascular resistance	20–130
Cardiac index [(L/min)/m²]	2.6–4.2
Oxygen consumption index [(L/min)/m²]	110–150
Arteriovenous oxygen difference (mL/L)	30–50

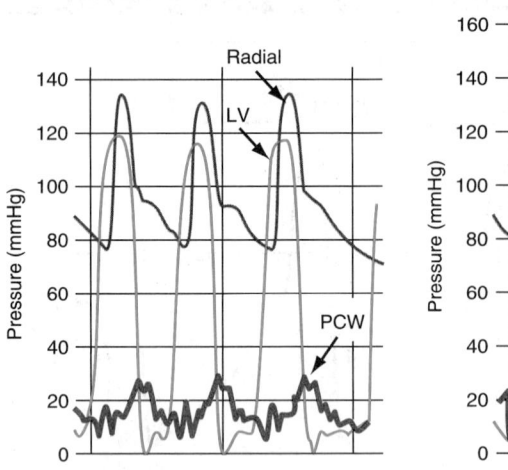
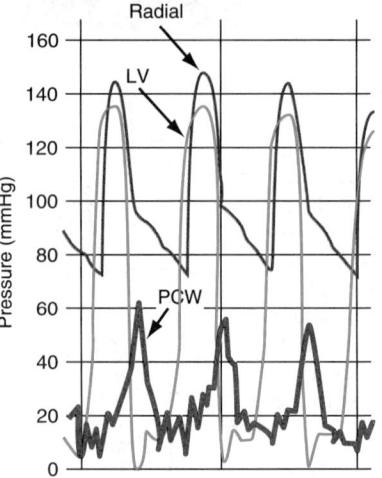

FIGURE 212-3   Hemodynamic findings at rest and during exercise in a patient with mitral regurgitation. Left ventricular (LV), pulmonary capillary wedge (PCW), and radial artery pressure tracings are shown before (*left*) and during (*right*) the sixth minute of supine bicycle exercise. PCW mean pressure and *v* wave increase substantially with exercise. [*From BH Lorell, W Grossman, in Grossman's Cardiac Catheterization, Angiography, and Intervention, 6th ed, DS Baim, W Grossman (eds). Baltimore, Lippincott Williams & Wilkins, 2000.*]

corresponding pulmonary blood flow. In contrast to the Fick method, the indicator-dilution method is least reliable when the cardiac output is low and transit of the cold bolus through the right heart is delayed.

LEFT HEART CATHETERIZATION

Whether performed using the femoral, brachial, or radial approach, the left heart catheter is advanced under fluoroscopic guidance into the central aorta, where pressure is measured and recorded. Next, the catheter is advanced in retrograde fashion across the aortic valve into the left ventricle, where pressure is measured. If a right heart catheter is in place, this is an appropriate time for simultaneous measurement and recording of left heart, right heart, and peripheral arterial pressures together with a determination of cardiac output by either thermodilution or the Fick method. This hemodynamic "snap-shot" allows assessment of possible pressure gradients across the mitral and aortic valves and calculation of systemic and pulmonary vascular resistances. The resistance to blood flow through the systemic vascular bed is

$$SVR = 80(MAP - RA)/SBF$$

where SVR is systemic vascular resistance [(dyn·s)/cm^5], MAP and RA

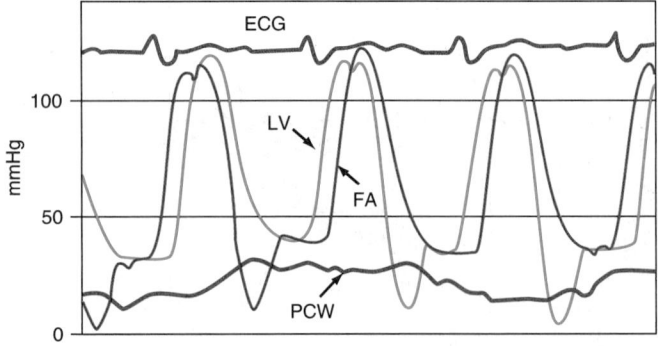

FIGURE 212-4   Severe aortic regurgitation. There is equilibration between the left ventricular (LV) and aortic or femoral artery (FA) pressures in diastole. Also, LV diastolic pressure exceeds pulmonary capillary wedge (PCW) pressure early in diastole, indicating premature closure of the mitral valve (a characteristic feature of severe aortic regurgitation). [*From W Grossman, in Grossman's Cardiac Catheterization, Angiography, and Intervention, 6th ed, DS Baim, W Grossman (eds). Baltimore, Lippincott Williams & Wilkins, 2000.*]

are mean aortic and right atrial pressures (mmHg), 80 a constant for converting to metric units, and SBF is systemic blood flow (L/min). Resistance to blood flow through the pulmonary vascular bed is

$$PVR = 80(PA - PCW \text{ or } LA)/PBF$$

where PVR is pulmonary vascular resistance [(dyn·s)/cm^5]; PA, PCW, and LA are pulmonary artery, pulmonary capillary wedge, and left atrial mean pressures, respectively (mmHg); and PBF is pulmonary blood flow (L/min). Normal values for pulmonary and systemic vascular resistances are given in Table 212-3.

When valvular stenosis is present, the measurements of the upstream and downstream pressures and flow allow calculation of the valve orifice using the Gorlin formula

$$A = flow/K\sqrt{\Delta P}$$

where A is the valve orifice area (cm^2), *flow* is the blood flow (mL/s) across the stenotic valve; ΔP is the mean pressure gradient (mmHg) during the period of blood flow; and K is a constant (44.3 for the aortic valve and 37.7 for the mitral valve).

In the normal heart, left ventricular and aortic pressures should be essentially equal during systole, while left atrial (pulmonary capillary wedge) and left ventricular pressures should be equal during diastole, as seen in Fig. 212-1. The presence of a systolic pressure gradient between the left ventricle and aorta indicates obstruction at the level of the aortic valve (e.g., calcific *aortic stenosis*) or at subaortic level (e.g., *hypertrophic obstructive cardiomyopathy*). Similarly, the presence of a diastolic pressure gradient between the left atrium (or pulmonary capillary wedge pressure) and the left ventricle generally indicates *mitral stenosis*, although it may also be seen in rare conditions such as cor triatriatum and left atrial myxoma. An example of a large diastolic pressure gradient in a patient with mitral stenosis is seen in Fig. 212-2. As seen in Fig. 212-3, patients with significant mitral regurgitation may have a prominent *v* wave in the pulmonary capillary wedge pressure, which often increases substantially during modest exercise. Severe *aortic regurgitation* produces a widening of the aortic pulse pressure, with equilibration of aortic and left ventricular pressures in diastole (Fig. 212-4). In the presence of valvular heart disease affecting the tricuspid or pulmonic valves, right-sided pressures exhibit characteristic deformities. In patients with severe *tricuspid regurgitation*, the right atrial pressure resembles the right ventricular pressure closely in appearance. Mean right atrial pressure and right ventricular end-diastolic pressure are both elevated in tricuspid regurgitation. In *tricuspid stenosis*, there is a pressure gradient between the right atrium and ventricle during diastole.

In *cardiac tamponade* or *pericardial constriction* (Chap. 222), there is equalization of left and right ventricular diastolic pressures. In pericardial tamponade, diastolic pressures continue to increase gradually throughout diastole, but in constrictive pericarditis ventricular filling ceases shortly after mitral and tricuspid valve opening. This produces an abrupt rise in ventricular diastolic pressure with a mid- and late-ventricular pressure plateau, giving the so-called square root sign (Fig. 212-5).

Congestive heart failure due to myocardial contractile dysfunction is associated with characteristic alterations in the ventricular pressure waveforms seen at cardiac catheterization. Neither the rise nor the decline in isovolumic pressure is as steep as in the normal heart. The reduced slopes of pressure rise and decline are associated with an abbreviated ejection period, giving the left ventricular pressure tracing a triangular appearance (Fig. 212-6). Also, the pressure decline does not continue to zero, so the minimal left ventricular pressure may be elevated. This hemodynamic finding correlates with an increased ventricular end-systolic volume, which is a sign of depressed contractile function of the left ventricular myocardium.

CARDIAC ANGIOGRAPHY

LEFT VENTRICULOGRAPHY

Following the measurement of cardiac pressures, the angiographic portion of the cardiac catheterization usually begins with left ventriculography—the injection of radiographic contrast material directly into the left ventricular cavity. A power injector is used to inject 30 to 45 mL of radiographic contrast material into the left ventricular chamber at a rate of 10 to 12 mL/s. The resulting radiographic images are recorded, and the left ventricular silhouette is defined at end-diastole and end-systole. This permits calculation of the left ventricular chamber volumes and ejection fraction, as well as qualitative assessment of regional wall motion abnormalities. The normal left ventricle ejects 50 to 80% of its end-diastolic volume with each beat; i.e., its *ejection fraction* is 0.50 to 0.80. In adults, normal values for left ventricular volumes are, for end-diastolic volume, 72 ± 15 mL/m^2 (mean $\pm$ standard deviation) and, for end-systolic volume, 20 ± 8 mL/m^2. Regional abnormalities of wall motion are illustrated in Fig. 212-7 and include diminished inward motion of a myocardial segment (*hypokinesis*), absence of inward movement of a myocardial segment (*akinesis*), and paradoxical systolic expansion of a regional myocardial segment (*dyskinesis*).

Performing left ventriculography in the right anterior oblique projection allows assessment of the mitral and aortic valves. Mitral regurgitation is easily visualized as the leakage of radiographic contrast material back into the left atrium during left ventricular systole. Its severity can be estimated qualitatively using a grading system of 1+ (mild; radiographic contrast material clears with each beat and never opacifies the entire left atrium) to 4+ (severe; opacification of the

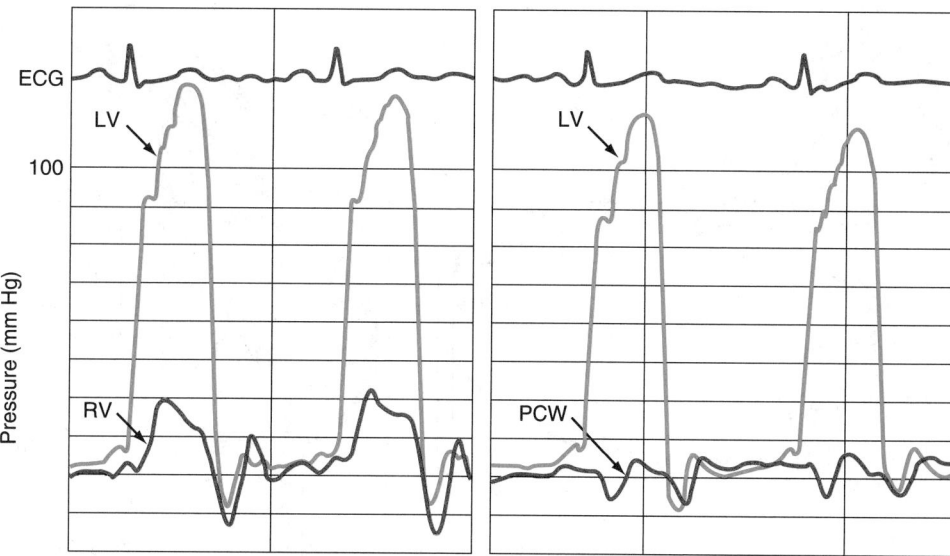

FIGURE 212-5 Left ventricular (LV), right ventricular (RV), and pulmonary capillary wedge (PCW) pressure tracings in a patient with severe constrictive pericarditis. Note the diastolic dip and plateau ("square root sign") pattern for left and right ventricular diastolic pressures (*left*). The wedge pressure (*right*) shows early systolic and early diastolic dips.

entire left atrium occurs within one beat, and contrast material can be seen refluxing into the pulmonary veins).

On occasion, left ventriculography may also be performed in the *left* anterior oblique projection to evaluate contraction of the septal or lateral walls or to detect abnormal communications such as ventricular septal defect (Chap. 218). In the most common form of hypertrophic cardiomyopathy (idiopathic hypertrophic subaortic stenosis; Chap. 221), left ventriculography in this projection shows anterior motion of the anterior leaflet of the mitral valve during systole and bulging of the interventricular septum into the left ventricular cavity, especially in the subaortic region. Mural thrombi within the left ventricular chamber may be well visualized during left ventriculography; they occur most commonly in the left ventricular apex.

It should be pointed out, however, that many of these findings could

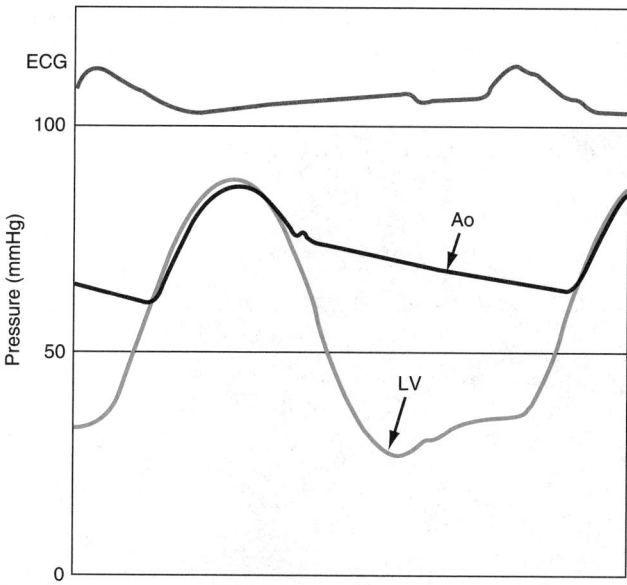

FIGURE 212-6 Left ventricular (LV) and aortic (Ao) pressures in a patient with advanced dilated cardiomyopathy. Marked slowing of the rates of LV pressure rise and fall (impairment of contractility and relaxation) give the LV pressure pulse a triangular appearance. Also, the minimal value for LV diastolic pressure is markedly elevated, suggesting an increased end-systolic volume and a reduced LV ejection fraction. *[From W Grossman, in Grossman's Cardiac Catheterization, Angiography, and Intervention, 6th ed, DS Baim, W Grossman (eds). Baltimore, Lippincott Williams & Wilkins, 2000.]*

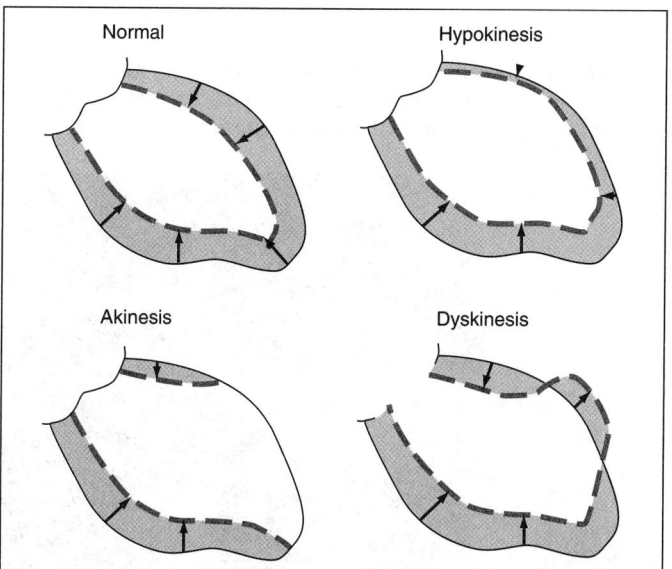

FIGURE 212-7 Diagrammatic representation of end-diastolic (*solid line*) and end-systolic (*dashed line*) silhouettes of left ventricular cineangiograms in various forms of localized wall motion disorder in patients with coronary heart disease. Normal wall motion is symmetric; a patient with *hypokinesis* exhibits reduced contraction, seen here over the anterior and apical surfaces; a patient with *akinesis* exhibits absent wall motion, seen here over the anteroapical surface; a patient with *dyskinesis* exhibits paradoxic bulging of a small portion of the anterior wall with systole.

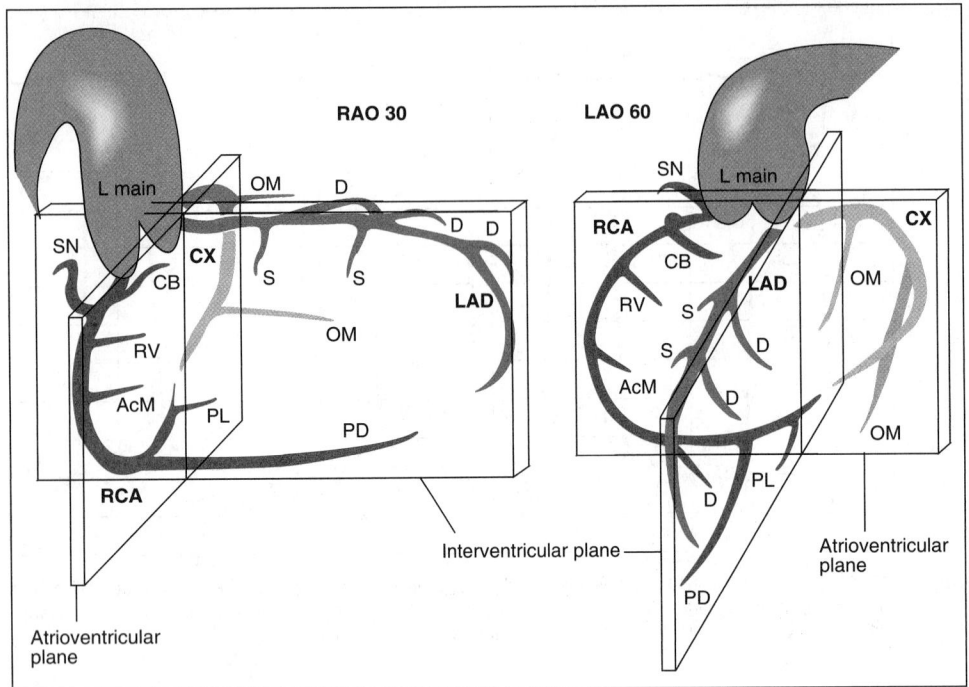

FIGURE 212-8 Representation of coronary anatomy relative to the interventricular and atrioventricular valve planes. Coronary branches are indicated as L Main (left main), LAD (left anterior descending), D (diagonal), S (septal), CX (circumflex), OM (obtuse marginal), RCA (right coronary artery), CB (conus branch), SN (sinus node), AcM (acute marginal), PD (posterior descending), PL (posterolateral left ventricular). RAO, right anterior oblique, LAO, left anterior oblique. *[From DS Baim, W Grossman, in Grossman's Cardiac Catheterization, Angiography, and Intervention, 6th ed, DS Baim, W Grossman (eds). Baltimore, Lippincott Williams & Wilkins, 2000.]*

also be evaluated using either cardiac echo or cardiac magnetic resonance imaging. This allows avoidance of left ventriculography in patients where a reduction in total contrast load is desired.

AORTOGRAPHY

Rapid injection of radiographic contrast material into the ascending aorta allows detection of abnormalities that involve the aorta and aortic valve. When suspected clinically, aortography permits detection and qualitative assessment of the severity of abnormalities such as aortic regurgitation, which is graded using a 1+ to 4+ scale, as for mitral regurgitation. Abnormal communications between the aorta and right side of the heart, such as a patent ductus arteriosus or ruptured aneurysm of a sinus of Valsalva, may be visualized. Aortography can permit identification of aortic aneurysm and of aortic dissection (Chap. 231) by visualizing an intimal flap within the aortic lumen.

CORONARY ANGIOGRAPHY

This common procedure involves the selective injection of a radiographic contrast agent into the coronary arteries. Placement of the catheter tip into the right and left coronary arteries is carried out under fluoroscopic guidance, and contrast agent is injected by hand during recording of the radiographic image. Each coronary artery is usually viewed in several projections to permit assessment of the severity of stenosis and to minimize the overlap of adjacent vessels. In addition to the detection of coronary artery stenoses, coronary angiography evaluates the rapidity of coronary flow, the blush of capillary filling in the myocardium, the presence of congenital abnormalities of the coronary circulation, and patency of any coronary artery bypass grafts. Examples of normal and abnormal coronary anatomy are shown in Figs. 212-8 and 212-9. The location, severity, and morphology of the stenotic lesions can be analyzed in great detail, and the resulting information is essential to planning either bypass surgery or catheter-based intervention (Fig. 212-10). This is usually done by visual estimation of percent diameter stenosis of each lesion relative to the "uninvolved" adjacent reference segment, with stenosis > 50% taken as being hemodynamically significant (that is capable of interfering with maximal increases in perfusion of the subserved myocardial territory during stress).

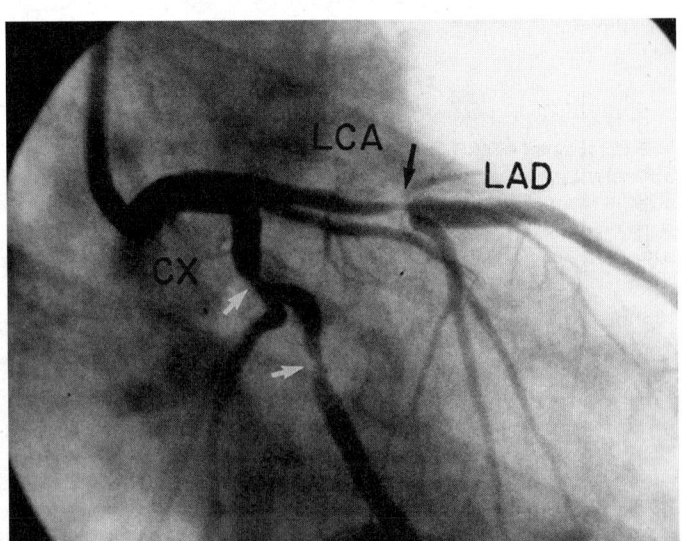

FIGURE 212-9 Coronary angiogram showing a right coronary artery (RCA) with a severe (95%) stenosis at its midpoint (*arrow*).

FIGURE 212-10 Coronary angiogram of a left coronary artery (LCA) with a tight stenosis in the proximal left anterior descending (LAD) artery (*black arrow*) immediately prior to the origin of a large septal branch. The circumflex artery (CX) has two moderately severe stenoses (*white arrows*).

POSTPROCEDURE CARE

The average diagnostic cardiac catheterization procedure takes roughly 30 min. Intravenous heparin (2000 to 3000 IU) may be given at the time of catheter insertion and reversed with intravenous protamine at the conclusion, but increasingly diagnostic catheterization is being performed without anticoagulant administration. The vascular sheaths are removed at the end of the procedure, and hemostasis is achieved by applying local pressure over the puncture site for 10 to 15 min, followed by a 2- to 4-h period of bed rest before ambulation and discharge. Alternatively, a variety of devices are now available for sealing the arterial puncture site, to allow a shorter period of bed rest and earlier ambulation. Most patients with suitable anatomy, however, now undergo a catheter-based intervention during the same procedure as the diagnostic cardiac catheterization, entailing an overnight hospital stay (Chap. 229).

FURTHER READING

BAIM DS, GROSSMAN W (eds): *Grossman's Cardiac Catheterization, Angiography, and Intervention*, 6th ed. Baltimore, Lippincott Williams & Wilkins, 2000

DAVIDSON CJ et al: Cardiac catheterization, in *Braunwald's Heart Disease*, 7th ed, D Zipes et al (eds). Philadelphia, Saunders, 2004

KERN MJ et al: Interpretation of cardiac pathophysiology from pressure waveform analysis: Simultaneous left and right ventricular pressure measurements. Cathet Cardiovasc Diagn 28:51, 1993

RYAN TJ: The coronary angiogram and its seminal contributions to cardiovascular medicine over five decades. Circulation 106:752, 2002

SCANLON PJ et al: AHA/ACC guidelines for coronary angiography—executive summary and recommendations. Circulation 99:2345, 1999

Section 2   Disorders of Rhythm

213 THE BRADYARRHYTHMIAS: DISORDERS OF SINUS NODE FUNCTION AND AV CONDUCTION DISTURBANCES
Mark E. Josephson, Peter Zimetbaum

ANATOMY OF THE CONDUCTING SYSTEM Under normal conditions, the pacemaker function of the heart resides in the sinoatrial (SA) node, which lies at the junction of the right atrium and superior vena cava. The SA node is approximately 1.5 cm long and 2 to 3 mm wide and is supplied by the sinus node artery, which arises from either the right coronary artery (60%) or the left circumflex coronary artery (40%). Once the impulse exits the sinus node and perinodal tissue, it traverses the atrium until it reaches the atrioventricular (AV) node. The blood supply of the AV node is derived from the posterior descending coronary artery (90%). The AV node lies at the base of the interatrial septum just above the tricuspid annulus and anterior to the coronary sinus. The electrophysiologic properties of the AV node result in slow conduction, which is responsible for the normal delay in AV conduction, i.e., the PR interval.

The bundle of His emerges from the AV node, enters the fibrous skeleton of the heart, and courses anteriorly across the membranous interventricular septum. It has a dual blood supply from the AV nodal artery and a branch of the anterior descending coronary artery. The branching (distal) portion of the bundle of His gives rise to a broad sheet of fibers that course over the left side of the interventricular septum to form the left bundle branch and a narrow cable-like structure on the right side that forms the right bundle branch. The arborization of both the right and left bundle branches gives rise to the distal His-Purkinje system, which ultimately extends throughout the endocardium of the right and left ventricles.

The SA node, atrium, and AV node are significantly influenced by autonomic tone. Vagal influences depress automaticity of the SA node, depress conduction, and prolong refractoriness in the tissue surrounding the SA node; inhomogeneously decrease atrial refractoriness and slow atrial conduction; and prolong AV nodal conduction and refractoriness. Sympathetic influences exert the opposite effect.

ELECTROPHYSIOLOGIC PRINCIPLES

In the resting state, the interior of most cardiac cells, with the exception of the SA and AV nodes, is approximately −80 to −90 mV, negative with respect to a reference extracellular electrode. The resting membrane potential is determined primarily by the concentration gradient of potassium across the cell membrane. Activation of cardiac cells results from movement of ions across the cell membrane, causing a transient depolarization known as the *action potential*. The ionic species responsible for the action potential varies among the cardiac tissues, and the configuration of the action potential is therefore unique to each tissue (Fig. 213-1).

The action potential of the His-Purkinje system has five phases (Fig. 213-2). The rapid depolarizing current (phase 0) is mainly determined by an influx of sodium into myocardial cells followed by a secondary (slower) influx of calcium, which produces a slow inward current. The repolarization phases of the action potential (phases 1 to 3) are primarily related to outward flux of potassium. The resting membrane potential is phase 4. Recent studies have demonstrated hetero-

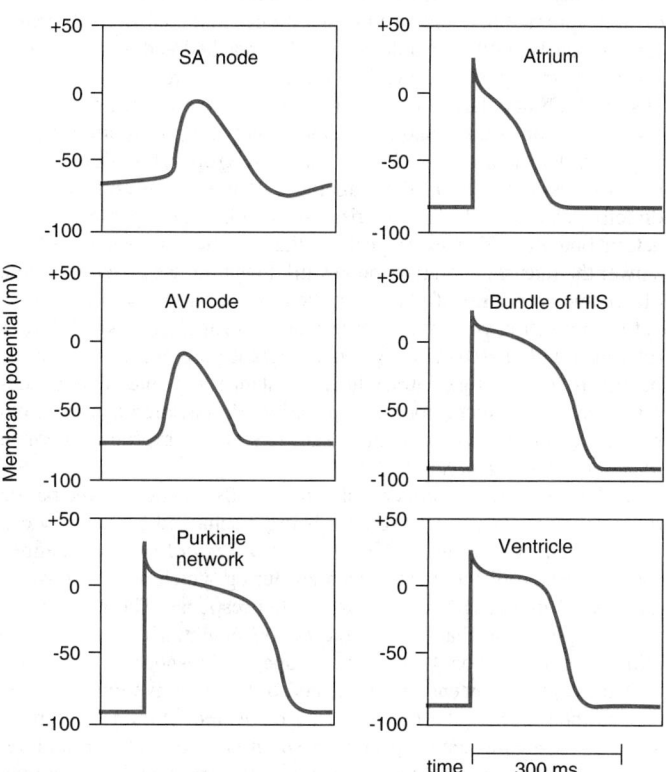

FIGURE 213-1 Action potential configurations in different regions of the mammalian heart. *(From AM Katz, Physiology of the Heart, 2d ed. New York, Raven, 1992, with permission.)*

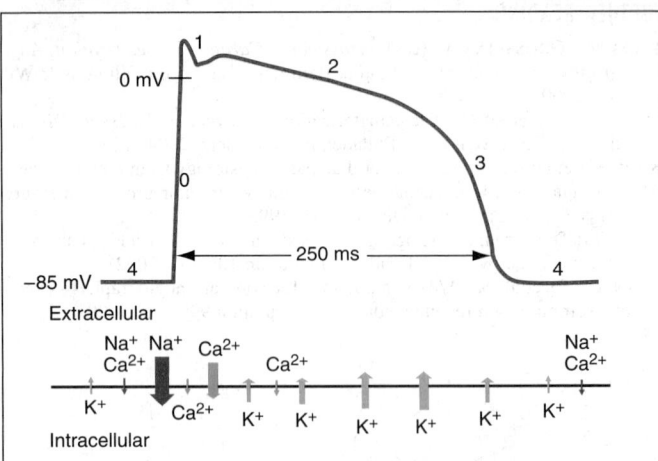

FIGURE 213-2 Schematic representation of the action potential in normal ventricle depicting the direction, strength, and period of flow of the ionic currents underlying the action potential. The arrow's direction and size indicate whether current is inward- or outward-directed and the approximate current strength of the ion identified at the arrow's base. The horizontal position of the arrow corresponds to the same moment in the time course of action potential (see text). The five phases of the action potential are indicated by the numerals placed along the waveform. *(From Ten Eick et al, Prog Cardiovasc Dis 24:157, 1981, with permission.)*

geneity of action potentials in the epicardium, mid-myocardium, and endocardium as well as between right and left ventricles. These differences are due to different ion currents in different layers.

The bradyarrhythmias result from abnormalities either of impulse formation, i.e., automaticity, or of conduction. *Automaticity*, which is normally observed in the sinus node, the specialized fibers of the His-Purkinje system, and some specialized atrial fibers, is the property of a cardiac cell that causes it to depolarize spontaneously during phase 4 of the action potential, leading to the generation of an impulse. To exhibit automaticity, the resting membrane potential must decrease spontaneously until threshold potential is reached and an all-or-none regenerative response occurs. The ionic currents producing spontaneous diastolic depolarization appear to involve the inward currents of sodium and/or calcium and a decreasing outward potassium current.

The velocity of *conduction*, i.e., impulse propagation through cardiac tissues, depends on the magnitude of inward current, which is directly related to the rate of rise and amplitude of phase 0 of the action potential. The more positive the threshold potential and the slower the rate of depolarization toward threshold, the lower is the rate of rise and amplitude of phase 0 of the action potential and the slower is the conduction velocity. Disease states or drugs may result in lower rates of rise of phase 0 at any given membrane potential. Passive membrane properties (e.g., intracellular resistance and intercellular coupling) can also affect impulse propagation. Propagation is more rapid parallel to fiber orientation than transverse to it, a property termed *anisotropic conduction*.

Refractoriness is a property of cardiac cells that defines the period of recovery that cells require after being discharged before they can be reexcited by a stimulus. The *absolute refractory period* is defined by that portion of the action potential during which no stimulus, regardless of its strength, can evoke another response. The *effective refractory period* is that part of the action potential during which a stimulus can evoke only a local, nonpropagated response. The *relative refractory period* extends from the end of the effective refractory period to the time that the tissue is fully recovered. During this time, a stimulus of greater than threshold strength is required to evoke a response, which is propagated more slowly than normal. In the normal His-Purkinje system or ventricular myocytes, excitability is recovered following completion of the action potential, and evoked responses

have characteristics similar to the spontaneous normal response. In the AV node, recovery of excitability occurs well after completion of the action potential.

INTRACARDIAC RECORDINGS OF THE SPECIALIZED CONDUCTING SYSTEM Electrode catheters allow the recording of activation of portions of the specialized conducting system, including the bundle of His. To obtain a recording from the bundle of His, the electrode catheter is positioned across the tricuspid valve (Fig. 213-3). The interval from local atrial depolarization in the His bundle recording to the onset of depolarization of the His bundle deflection is called the *AH interval* (normal = 60 to 125 ms) and represents an indirect method of assessing AV nodal conduction time. The interval from the beginning of the His bundle deflection to the earliest onset of ventricular activation, as measured from any of multiple-surface electrocardiogram (ECG) leads or the intracardiac ventricular electrogram, is called the *HV interval* (normal = 35 to 55 ms) and represents conduction time through the His-Purkinje system. Electrode catheters can be positioned in the area of the sinus node to record high right atrial activity. Left atrial activity may be recorded directly via a catheter placed across a patent foramen ovale or indirectly using a catheter inserted into the coronary sinus. The atrial activation sequence may be "mapped," and sites of intra- and interatrial conduction abnormalities may be ascertained.

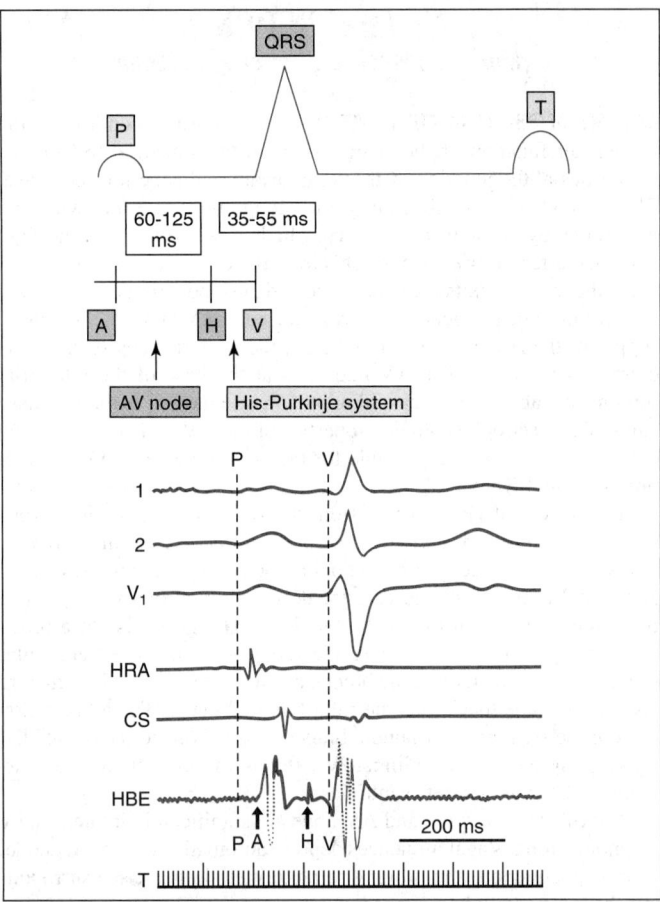

FIGURE 213-3 *(Top)* Schema relating the surface electrocardiogram with intracardiac conduction. The normal AV nodal conduction time (AH interval) is 60–125 ms and normal His-Purkinje conduction time (HV interval) is 35–55 ms. Surface ECG leads I, II, and V_1 are displayed with intracardiac ECGs from the high right atrium (HRA), left atrium from the coronary sinus (CS), and AV junction to obtain a His bundle electrogram (HBE). T, time lines; A, atrial activation; H, His bundle activation; V, ventricular activation. Atrial activation begins in the HRA and spreads inferiorly to the low atrial septum, as recorded in the HBE, and the left atrium, as recorded in the CS. The AH and HV intervals represent AV nodal and His-Purkinje conduction times, respectively. *(Bottom)* Normal intracardiac recording. Normal atrioventricular conduction. Vertical lines at bottom = 0.10 s. *(From ME Josephson, Clinical Cardiac Electrophysiology: Techniques and Interpretations, 3d ed. Philadelphia, Lippincott Williams & Wilkins 2002, with permission.)*

SINUS NODE DYSFUNCTION

The SA node is normally the dominant cardiac pacemaker because its intrinsic discharge rate is the highest of all potential cardiac pacemakers. Its responsiveness to alterations in autonomic nervous system tone is responsible for the normal acceleration of heart rate during exercise and the slowing that occurs during rest and sleep. Increases in sinus rate normally result from an increase in parasympathetic tone acting

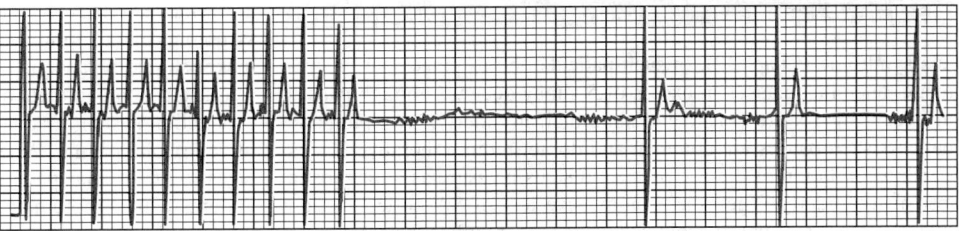

FIGURE 213-4 Tachycardia-bradycardia syndrome. Rhythm strip of ECG lead II showing spontaneous cessation of supraventricular tachycardia followed by a 6-s pause prior to resumption of sinus activity. The patient was asymptomatic during supraventricular tachycardia, but the sinus pause caused severe light-headedness.

via muscarinic receptors and/or an increase in sympathetic tone acting via β-adrenergic receptors. Slowing of the heart rate is normally due to opposite alterations. In adults, the normal sinus rate under basal conditions is 60 to 100 beats/min. *Sinus bradycardia* is said to exist when the sinus rate is <60 beats/min, and *sinus tachycardia* when it is >100 beats/min. However, there is wide variation among individuals, and rates <60 beats/min do not necessarily indicate pathologic states. For example, trained athletes often exhibit resting rates <50 beats/min due to increases in vagal tone. Normal elderly individuals may also show marked sinus bradycardia at rest.

ETIOLOGY SA node dysfunction is most often found in the elderly as an isolated phenomenon. Although interruption of the blood supply to the SA node may produce dysfunction, the correlation between obstruction of the sinus node artery and clinical evidence of SA node dysfunction is poor. Specific disease states associated with SA node dysfunction include senile amyloidosis and other conditions associated with infiltration of the atrial myocardium. Sinus bradycardia is associated with hypothyroidism, advanced liver disease, hypothermia, typhoid fever, and brucellosis; it occurs during episodes of hypervagotonia (vasovagal syncope), severe hypoxia, hypercapnia, acidemia, and acute hypertension. However, most cases of SA node dysfunction are due to idiopathic degeneration or are secondary to pharmacologic agents.

MANIFESTATIONS Although marked and/or inappropriate (≤50 beats/min) sinus bradycardia may cause fatigue and other symptoms due to inadequate cardiac output, more commonly sinus node dysfunction is manifest as paroxysmal dizziness, presyncope, or syncope. These symptoms usually result from abrupt, prolonged sinus pauses caused by failure of sinus impulse formation (sinus arrest) or block of conduction of sinus impulses to the surrounding atrial tissue (sinus exit block). In either case, the ECG manifestation is a prolonged period (3 s) of atrial asystole. In some patients, SA node dysfunction is accompanied by abnormalities in AV conduction. In addition to the absence of atrial activity, lower pacemakers fail to emerge during the sinus pauses, resulting in periods of ventricular asystole and syncope. Occasionally, SA node dysfunction is manifested by an inadequate acceleration in sinus rate in response to a stress such as exercise or fever. In some patients, SA node dysfunction may become manifest only in the presence of certain cardioactive drugs: cardiac glycosides, β-adrenergic blocking drugs, calcium channel blockers, amiodarone, and other antiarrhythmic agents. These agents, which do not usually cause sinus node dysfunction in normal individuals, may unmask evidence of sinus node dysfunction in susceptible individuals.

The *sick sinus syndrome* refers to a combination of symptoms (dizziness, confusion, fatigue, syncope, and congestive heart failure) caused by SA node dysfunction and manifested by marked sinus bradycardia, sinoatrial block, or sinus arrest. Because these symptoms are nonspecific, and because ECG manifestations of sinus node dysfunction are often intermittent, it may be difficult to prove that such symptoms are actually caused by SA node dysfunction.

Atrial tachyarrhythmias such as atrial fibrillation, atrial flutter, or atrial tachycardia may be accompanied by SA node dysfunction. The *bradycardia-tachycardia syndrome* refers to paroxysmal atrial arrhythmia that upon termination is followed by prolonged sinus pauses

(Fig. 213-4) or in which there are alternating periods of tachyarrhythmia and bradyarrhythmia. Syncope or presyncope may result from failure of the sinus node to recover function following suppression of automaticity by atrial tachyarrhythmia.

DIAGNOSIS *First-degree sinoatrial exit block* denotes a prolonged conduction time from the SA node to the surrounding atrial tissue. It cannot be recognized on a standard (surface) ECG but requires invasive intracardiac recordings, which can detect this condition indirectly, by measuring the sinus response to atrial premature beats, or directly, by recording SA node electrograms. *Second-degree sinoatrial exit block* denotes the intermittent failure of conduction of sinus impulses to the surrounding atrial tissue; it is manifested as the intermittent absence of P waves (Fig. 213-5). *Third-degree*, or *complete, sinoatrial block* is characterized by a lack of atrial activity or by the presence of an ectopic subsidiary atrial pacemaker. On the standard ECG it cannot be distinguished from sinus arrest, but direct intracardiac recordings of SA node activity permit this distinction. The bradycardia-tachycardia syndrome is manifested on the standard ECG as tachyarrhythmias (Fig. 213-4). Most often these are atrial flutter or fibrillation, although any tachycardia during which the atria are activated may cause overdrive suppression of the sinus node, resulting in clinical appearance of this syndrome.

The most important step in the diagnosis of sick sinus syndrome is to correlate symptoms with ECG evidence of SA node dysfunction. While ambulatory ECG (Holter) monitoring remains a mainstay in evaluating sinus node function, most episodes of syncope are paroxysmal and unpredictable. Single and even multiple 24-h Holter monitor recordings may fail to include a symptomatic episode. Caution must be taken in interpreting the Holter monitor results. For instance, a pause during sleep is often a normal finding associated with heightened vagal tone. This should not be interpreted as sinus node dysfunction requiring pacemaker implantation. Continuous-loop event records represent a more specific diagnostic tool. These devices may be worn for prolonged periods of time and allow close correlation between electrocardiographic findings and symptoms. They do require the patient's ability to activate the monitor at the time of symptoms. More recently, an implantable event recorder, which can be interrogated like a pacemaker, has been developed for patients with rare events.

The response to carotid sinus pressure and pharmacologic autonomic "denervation" of the heart may be helpful. Carotid sinus pressure can be particularly useful in patients in whom paroxysmal dizziness or syncope is compatible with the hypersensitive carotid si-

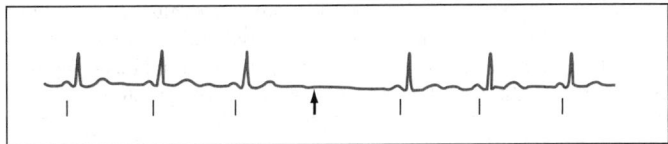

FIGURE 213-5 Second-degree sinoatrial exit block. Surface ECG denoting abrupt absence of P wave during sinus rhythm. Prior to the pause, the sinus rate is regular. The interval of the pause is exactly twice the basal sinus cycle length. The arrow marks the appropriate location for the absent P wave. SA exit block can be 2:1 as above or longer, as shown in Fig. 213-6.

nus syndrome (Chap. 20). In such patients, the response can be dramatic, and sinus pauses in excess of 5 s may occur. Although pauses in excess of 3 s are considered abnormal, in elderly, asymptomatic patients such pauses are common and do not require therapy. This is a major limitation of the use of carotid sinus pressure as a diagnostic test in the elderly. The other noninvasive test of SA node function involves the use of pharmacologic agents to manipulate the autonomic nervous system and assess the balance of parasympathetic and sympathetic activity on the sinus node. Physiologic or pharmacologic maneuvers that are vagomimetic (Valsalva maneuver or phenylephrine-induced hypertension), vagolytic (atropine), sympathomimetic (isoproterenol or hypotension by nitroprusside), or sympatholytic (β-adrenergic blocking agents) can be utilized, singly and in combination. These studies are designed to test the response of the sinus node to autonomic stimulation and inhibition and thereby characterize the status of autonomic regulation of the sinus node. Abnormalities of the autonomic control of sinus function are particularly common in patients in whom asymptomatic sinus bradycardia is documented.

Intrinsic Heart Rate This is a manifestation of the primary activity of the SA node, and its determination requires chemical autonomic blockade of the heart with a combination of atropine and a beta blocker. Normal values of intrinsic heart rate (in beats per minute) are calculated by the formula $118.1 - (0.57 \times \text{age})$. The use of autonomic blockade can separate patients with asymptomatic sinus bradycardia into a group with primary sinus node dysfunction (slow intrinsic heart rate) and a group with autonomic imbalance (normal intrinsic heart rate). Autonomic blockade is particularly useful when combined with invasive assessment of sinus node function. Autonomic blockade may depress conduction in patients with intrinsic disease of the conduction system and should be carried out only in a setting where arrhythmias can be monitored and treated rapidly.

EVALUATION The invasive electrophysiologic investigation of SA node dysfunction should be undertaken in patients who have had symptoms compatible with SA node dysfunction and in whom no documentation of the arrhythmia responsible for these symptoms has been obtained by prolonged monitoring. Asymptomatic patients with sinus bradycardia need not be tested, since no therapy is indicated. Similarly, symptomatic patients with ECG documentation of asystole, sinoatrial block or arrest, or the bradycardia-tachycardia syndrome do not require electrophysiologic tests for diagnosis. However, in symptomatic patients without documentation of an arrhythmia, electrophysiologic assessment of SA node function can yield information that may be used to guide appropriate therapy. The tools most commonly employed are the sinus node recovery time (a response to overdrive atrial pacing) and sinoatrial conduction time calculated indirectly by response to atrial premature complexes or recorded directly by a sinus node electrogram.

The results of electrophysiologic tests of sinus node function must be interpreted with caution. SA node dysfunction coexists frequently with other disorders such as AV conduction disturbances, which may cause symptoms such as syncope. Electrophysiologic evaluation of patients with symptoms such as undiagnosed syncope must not stop with the demonstration of abnormalities of SA node dysfunction or carotid sinus hypersensitivity. Instead, complete evaluation, including His bundle recordings and programmed atrial and ventricular stimulation (Chap. 214), is necessary to search for additional electrophysiologic abnormalities that could be responsible for symptoms.

℞ TREATMENT

Permanent pacemakers (p. 1339) are the mainstay of therapy for patients with symptomatic SA node dysfunction. Patients with intermittent paroxysms of bradycardia or sinus arrest and with the cardioinhibitory form of the hypersensitive carotid sinus syndrome are usually adequately treated by demand ventricular pacemakers. These devices

are reliable, relatively inexpensive, and suffice to prevent episodic symptoms due to abrupt bradycardia. Although an atrial demand pacemaker should be adequate for patients with SA node dysfunction, the frequent accompaniment of dysfunction in other portions of the cardiac conduction system mandates placement of a pacemaker also capable of ventricular pacing. Whether dual-chamber pacing offers any advantages to ventricular pacing in such circumstances remains uncertain. Patients with symptomatic chronic sinus bradycardia or frequent prolonged episodes of sinus node dysfunction do better with dual-chamber pacemakers that preserve the normal AV activation sequence. Recent studies suggest that AV sequential pacing may also be useful in preventing atrial fibrillation, an important component of the bradycardia-tachycardia syndrome, and stroke, a known complication of atrial fibrillation.

AV CONDUCTION DISTURBANCES

The specialized cardiac conducting system normally ensures synchronous conduction of each sinus impulse from the atria to the ventricles. Abnormalities of conduction of the sinus impulse to the ventricles may portend the development of heart block, which can ultimately lead to syncope or cardiac arrest. In order to evaluate the clinical significance of conduction abnormalities, the physician must assess (1) the site of conduction disturbance, (2) the risk of progression to complete block, and (3) the probability that a subsidiary escape rhythm arising distal to the site of block will be electrophysiologically and hemodynamically stable. This latter point is perhaps the most important, since the rate and stability of the escape pacemaker determine what symptoms result from heart block. The escape pacemaker following AV nodal block is usually in the His bundle, which generally has a stable rate of 40 to 60 beats/min and is associated with a QRS complex of normal duration (in the absence of a preexisting intraventricular conduction defect). This contrasts with escape rhythms arising in the distal His-Purkinje system, which have lower intrinsic rates (25 to 45 beats/min), manifest wide QRS complexes with prolonged duration, and are unstable. Thus, the most important issue is to assess the risk of infra- or intra-His block (which always mandates a pacemaker) or AV nodal block in which the frequency of the escape pacemaker is not sufficient to meet hemodynamic requirements (Table 213-1). Although prolonged QRS complexes are invariable when the distal His-Purkinje pacemakers form the escape mechanism, wide QRS complexes can also coexist with AV nodal block and a His bundle rhythm. Therefore, QRS morphology alone may not be adequate to identify the site of block.

ETIOLOGY The AV node is supplied by the parasympathetic and sympathetic nervous systems and is sensitive to variations in autonomic tone. Chronic slowing of AV nodal conduction may be seen in highly trained athletes who have hypervagotonia at rest. A variety of diseases and drugs can also influence AV nodal conduction. These include acute processes such as myocardial infarction (particularly inferior); coronary spasm (usually of the right coronary artery); digitalis intoxication; excesses of beta and/or calcium blockers; acute infections such as viral myocarditis, acute rheumatic fever, infectious mononucleosis; and miscellaneous disorders such as Lyme disease, sarcoidosis, amyloidosis, and neoplasms, particularly cardiac mesotheliomas. AV nodal block may also be congenital.

TABLE 213-1 *Atrioventricular Conduction Evaluation*

1. Atrial activation times: Measurement of intraatrial conduction times. Prolonged activation times may be associated with atrial flutter or fibrillation.
2. Measurement of AH and HV intervals: Prolongation of AH interval (>125 ms) or prolongation of the HV interval (>55 ms) may help localize the site of delay.
3. Incremental atrial pacing: To determine the cycle length at which block occurs in the AV node and/or His-Purkinje system. Block below the His bundle at rates of <150 beats per minute portends the development of infra-His block.

Two degenerative diseases are commonly responsible for damage to the specialized conducting system and produce AV block usually associated with bundle branch block (Chap. 210). In *Lev's disease,* there are calcification and sclerosis of the fibrous cardiac skeleton, which frequently involve the aortic and mitral valves, the central fibrous body, and the summit of the ventricular septum. *Lenegre's disease* appears to be a primary sclerodegenerative disease of the conducting system with no involvement of the myocardium or the fibrous skeleton of the heart. These two diseases are probably the most common causes of isolated chronic heart block in adults. Hypertension and aortic and/or mitral stenosis are specific disorders that either accelerate the degeneration of the conducting system or have a direct effect by calcification and fibrosis involving the conducting system.

First-degree AV block, more properly termed *prolonged AV conduction,* is classically characterized by a PR interval >0.20 s, but use of this value may be misleading in terms of clinical significance. Since the PR interval is determined by atrial, AV nodal, and His-Purkinje activation, delay in any one or more of these structures can contribute to a prolonged PR interval. In the presence of a QRS complex of normal duration, a PR interval >0.24 s almost invariably is due to a delay within the AV node. If the QRS is prolonged, delays may be present at any of the levels mentioned above. Delay within the His-Purkinje system is always accompanied by a prolonged QRS duration but can occur with a relatively normal PR interval (Fig. 213-6). However, as indicated below, it is only with intracardiac recordings that the exact site of delay can be determined.

Second-degree heart block (intermittent AV block) is present when some atrial impulses fail to conduct to the ventricles. Mobitz type I second-degree AV block (AV Wenckebach block) is characterized by progressive PR interval prolongation prior to block of an atrial impulse (Fig. 213-7A). The pause that follows is less than fully compensatory (i.e., is less than two normal sinus intervals), and the PR interval of the first conducted impulse is shorter than the last conducted atrial impulse prior to the blocked P wave. Usually the difference between the longest and shortest PR intervals exceeds 100 ms. This type of block is almost always localized to the AV node and associated with a normal QRS duration, although bundle branch block may be present. It is seen most often as a transient abnormality with inferior wall infarction or with drug intoxication, particularly digitalis, beta blockers, and occasionally calcium channel antagonists. This type of block can

also be observed in normal individuals with heightened vagal tone. Although Mobitz type I block can progress to complete heart block, this is uncommon, except in the setting of acute inferior wall myocardial infarction. Even when it does, however, the heart block is usually well tolerated because the escape pacemaker usually arises in the proximal His bundle and provides a stable rhythm. As a result, the presence of Mobitz type I second-degree AV block rarely mandates aggressive therapy. Therapeutic decisions depend on the ventricular response and the symptoms of the patient. If the ventricular rate is adequate and the patient is asymptomatic, observation is sufficient.

In Mobitz type II second-degree AV block, conduction fails suddenly and unexpectedly without a preceding change in PR intervals (Fig. 213-7B). It is generally due to disease of the His-Purkinje system and is most often associated with a prolonged QRS duration. When Mobitz type II block occurs with a normal QRS duration, an intra-His site of block should be expected. It is important to recognize this type of block because it has a high incidence of progression to complete heart block with an unstable, slow, lower escape pacemaker. Therefore, pacemaker implantation is necessary in this condition. Mobitz type II block may occur in the setting of anteroseptal infarction or in the primary or secondary sclerodegenerative or calcific disorders of the fibrous skeleton of the heart. In so-called high-degree AV block there are periods of two or more consecutively blocked P waves, but intermittent conduction can be demonstrated. Block is usually in the His-Purkinje system, but simultaneous block in the AV node may also be present. Regardless of the site of origin of the escape rhythm, if it is slow and the patient is symptomatic, a cardiac pacemaker is mandatory.

Third-degree AV block is present when no atrial impulse propagates to the ventricles. If the QRS complex of the escape rhythm is of normal duration, occurs at a rate of 40 to 55 beats/min, and increases with atropine or exercise, AV nodal block is probable. Congenital complete AV block is usually localized to the AV node. If the block is within the His bundle, the escape pacemaker is usually less responsive to these perturbations. If the escape rhythm of the QRS is wide and associated with rates ≤40 beats/min, block is usually localized in, or distal to, the His bundle and mandates a pacemaker, since the escape rhythm in this setting is unreliable (Fig. 213-8). Some patients with infra-His bundle block are capable of retrograde conduction. In such patients, a "pacemaker syndrome" (see below) may develop if a simple ventricular pacemaker is used. Dual-chamber pacemakers eliminate this potential problem.

AV DISSOCIATION AV dissociation exists whenever the atria and ventricles are under the control of two separate pacemakers and, while present in complete AV block, can occur in the absence of a primary conduction disturbance. AV dissociation unrelated to heart block may occur under two circumstances: First, it may develop with an AV junctional rhythm in response to severe sinus bradycardia. When the sinus rate and the escape rate are similar and the P waves occur just before, in, or following the QRS complex, isorhythmic AV dissociation is said to be present. Treatment usually consists of removal of the offending cause of sinus bradycardia (i.e., discontinuation of digitalis, beta blockers, or calcium antagonists), accelerating the sinus node by vagolytic agents, or insertion of a pacemaker if the escape rhythm is slow and results in symptoms. Second, AV dissociation can be caused by an enhanced lower (junctional or ventricular) pacemaker that competes with normal sinus rhythm and frequently exceeds it. This has been called *interference AV dissociation* because the rapid lower pacemaker results in bombardment of the AV node in a retrograde fashion, rendering it refractory to the normal sinus impulses. Thus failure of antegrade conduction is a physiologic response in this circumstance. Interference dissociation commonly occurs during ventricular tachycardia, accelerated junctional or ventricular rhythms seen with digitalis intoxication, myocardial ischemia and/or infarction, or local irritation following cardiac surgery. The accelerated rhythm should be treated

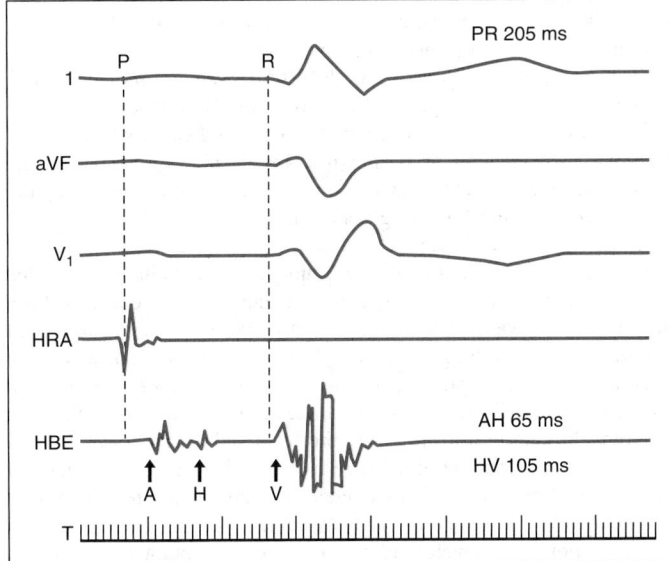

FIGURE 213-6 Example of marked His-Purkinje system disease with a relatively normal PR interval. Surface leads I, aVF, and V₁ are shown with electrograms from the high right atrium (HRA), His bundle electrogram (HBE), and time lines (T). The QRS shows right bundle branch block and left anterior hemiblock; the PR interval is minimally elevated at 205 ms, but the HV interval exceeds 100 ms. Such a prolonged HV interval mandates a pacemaker.

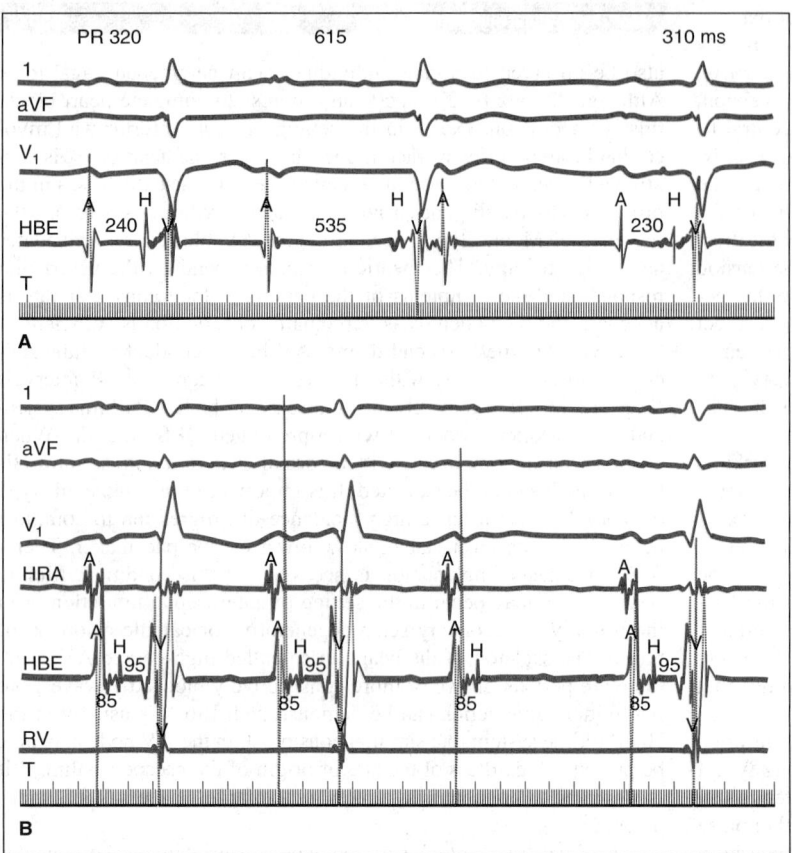

FIGURE 213-7 A. Mobitz type I second-degree AV block. Intracardiac recordings demonstrate that the PR prolongation (320, 615 ms) is localized to the AV node (AH 240, 535 ms, respectively). HBE, His bundle electrogram; A, atrium; H, His; V, ventricle. Time lines (T) = 100 ms. B. Mobitz type II second-degree AV block. Intracardiac recordings document block below the His bundle. During sinus rhythm right bundle branch block is present. AV nodal conduction is normal (AH, 85 ms), but His-Purkinje conduction is markedly prolonged (HV, 95 ms). The third sinus P wave suddenly blocks below the recorded His deflection without any preceeding change in AV conduction. (From ME Josephson, Clinical Cardiac Electrophysiology: Techniques and Interpretations, 3d ed. Philadelphia, Lippincott Williams & Wilkins 2002, with permission.)

with either antiarrhythmic drugs (Chap. 214), removal of an offending drug, or correction of the metabolic abnormality or ischemia.

INTRACARDIAC ELECTROCARDIOGRAPHIC RECORDINGS IN DIAGNOSIS AND MANAGEMENT The main therapeutic decision in patients with AV conduction disturbance is whether or not a permanent pacemaker is required, and a number of circumstances exist in which His bundle electrocardiography can be a useful diagnostic tool upon which to base

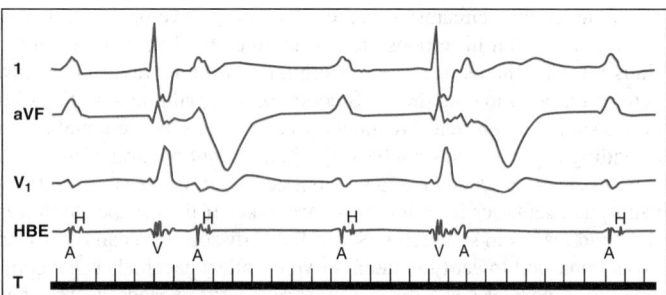

FIGURE 213-8 Third-degree AV block. The figure shows surface leads 1, aVF, V₁, and an intracardiac His bundle recording (HBE). Complete heart block is evident on the surface leads. The intracardiac recording demonstrates an absence of QRS deflection (V) after a His bundle (H) spike. This indicates block below the His bundle. Note that following the second QRS complex (V), there is an atrial (A) deflection indicating retrograde conduction. Retrograde conduction is often present when block is in the His-Purkinje system but is virtually never present when block is in the AV node. (From ME Josephson, Clinical Cardiac Electrophysiology: Techniques and Interpretations, 3d ed. Philadelphia, Lippincott Williams & Wilkins, 2002, with permission.)

this decision. It is unquestionable that patients with symptomatic second- or third-degree AV block should be paced, and therefore these patients do not require electrophysiologic study. However, intracardiac ECG recordings can be useful in at least the following four groups of patients:

1. *Patients with syncope and bundle branch or bifascicular block without documentation of AV block.* In such patients, the demonstration of marked infra-His bundle conduction disturbances, i.e., a prolonged HV interval (>100 ms), may usually be taken as an indication of the need for the insertion of the permanent pacemaker. Complete electrophysiologic evaluation, including atrial and ventricular programmed stimulation, is indicated to help identify other possible cardiac etiologies for the syncope. Since the incidence of significant advanced AV block is low in asymptomatic patients who have bifascicular block, electrophysiologic evaluation or permanent pacemakers are not cost-effective. In this group, observation appears most reasonable.

2. *Patients with 2:1 AV conduction.* Intracardiac recordings are necessary to ascertain the site of the conduction disturbance because the typical ECG features of Mobitz type I or Mobitz type II block cannot be discerned during a 2:1 pattern of AV conduction on the surface ECG. Intracardiac recordings may demonstrate that AV nodal block, intra-His bundle block, infra-His bundle block, or combinations of block may be responsible (Figs. 213-7 and 213-8). A surface ECG finding that suggests an infra-His bundle lesion is the presence of alternating bundle branch block associated with changing PR intervals. Intracardiac recordings in such patients confirm that the block is almost always in the His-Purkinje system. Increasing block with exercise or following atropine suggests intra- or infra-His block (Table 213-2). The finding of infra- or intra-His bundle block in patients with asymptomatic second-degree AV block mandates pacemaker therapy because of the high likelihood of the development of symptomatic high-grade AV block and syncope.

3. *Patients with Wenckebach block in the presence of bundle branch block.* This situation, particularly when the maximal change in PR interval is 50 ms, can suggest intra- or infra-His Wenckebach block, in which case a pacemaker is mandated. Intracardiac recordings are necessary to make this diagnosis.

4. *Asymptomatic patients with third-degree AV block.* In such patients, electrophysiologic studies may be useful in assessing the stability of the junctional pacemaker. Pacing is indicated when the His bundle escape pacemaker is shown to be unstable by an inadequate response to exercise, atropine, or isoproterenol or by a prolonged junctional recovery time following ventricular pacing.

GENETIC CONSIDERATIONS A number of congenital and familial syndromes involving the cardiac conduction system have been described. An example of a congenital condition that is transmitted but not genetic is congenital complete heart block associated with maternal systemic lupus erythematosus. This disorder is associated with maternal IgG autoantibodies to several ribonucleoproteins that are transplacentally transmitted to the fetus and damage the fetal AV node. The fetal conduction disease is generally clinically evident by the second trimester and is associated with significant fetal mortality and neonatal requirement of cardiac pacing.

The embryonic development of the cardiac septa and conduction system occur together, and clinical disorders have been described, including the *Holt-Oram syndrome*, an autosomal dominant disorder including upper limb dysplasia and atrial septal defect, often with conduction disturbances in the AV node. Studies of families with a high incidence of congenital heart disease, including ostium secundum atrial septal defect and conduction disorders in the AV node, have

TABLE 213-2 *Site of 2:1 Atrioventricular Block*

Characteristic	Observation—Site of Block
1. QRS width	BBB—anywhere
	Normal QRS—in AV node or His bundle
2. PR interval of conducted P wave	>0.30 s—in AV node
	≤0.16 s—in HPS or His bundle[a]
3. Atropine or exercise	Improve conduction—in AV node
	Worsen conduction—in HPS or His bundle[a]
4. CSP	Worsen conduction—in AV node
	Improve conduction—in HPS or His bundle[a]
5. Retrograde conduction	Present—in HPS or His bundle[a]
	Absent—may be anywhere

[a] Use of a pacemaker is indicated.
Note: BBB, bundle branch block; HPS, His-Purkinje system; CSP, carotid sinus pressure.

identified the gene NKX2-5 on chromosome 5q35 as important in the regulation of septation and in the development and function of the AV node. A familial syndrome of progressive complete heart block has also long been recognized. The gene for this disorder has been mapped to a region on chromosome 19q13. Familial disorders of SA node function have also been described, but specific details of abnormal genetic sites are not available.

Rx TREATMENT

Pharmacologic Therapy Pharmacologic therapy is usually reserved for acute situations. Atropine (0.5 to 2.0 mg intravenously) and isoproterenol (1 to 4 μg/min intravenously) are useful in increasing heart rate and decreasing symptoms in patients with sinus bradycardia or AV block localized to the AV node. They have an insignificant effect on lower pacemakers. In patients with neurocardiac syncope, beta blockers and disopyramide have been suggested as methods to depress left ventricular function and decrease mechanoreceptor-related reflexes. Mineralocorticoids, midodrine, ephedrine, and theophylline have also been reported to be of benefit to occasional patients. Unfortunately, no controlled study has shown that any of these pharmacologic modalities works in a predictable fashion in all patients. Recently, serotonin-reuptake inhibitors have been shown to benefit some patients. Further work on delineating different mechanisms in different patient groups may allow us to apply pharmacologic agents more appropriately. Long-term therapy of bradyarrhythmias is best accomplished by pacemakers.

Pacemakers External energy sources can be used to stimulate the heart when disorders in impulse formation and/or transmission lead to symptomatic bradyarrhythmias. Pacer stimuli can be applied to the atria and/or ventricles. Indications for pacemaker insertion are listed in the guidelines summarized on p. 1340.

TEMPORARY PACING This is usually instituted to provide immediate stabilization prior to permanent pacemaker placement or to provide pacemaker support when a bradycardia is precipitated by what is presumed to be a transient event such as ischemia or drug toxicity. Temporary pacing is usually achieved by the transvenous insertion of an electrode catheter with the catheter positioned in the right ventricular apex and attached to an external generator. This procedure is associated with a small risk of cardiac perforation, infection at the insertion site, and thromboembolism; the risk of the latter two complications increases markedly if the pacing wire is left in place for >48 h. The development of an entirely external transthoracic cardiac pacing system may preclude the need for transvenous pacing in selected patients. However, occasional failure of ventricular capture and significant discomfort related to the large current required for effective transthoracic ventricular stimulation preclude the uniform use of this approach.

PERMANENT PACING This mode of pacing is instituted for persistent or intermittent symptomatic bradycardia not related to a self-limiting pre-

cipitating factor or for documented infranodal second- or third-degree AV block. Permanent pacing leads are usually inserted transvenously through the subclavian or cephalic vein with the leads positioned in the right atrial appendage for atrial pacing and the right ventricular apex for ventricular pacing. The leads are then attached to the pulse generator, which is inserted into a subcutaneous pocket below the clavicle. Epicardial lead placement is used when (1) transvenous access cannot be obtained; (2) the chest is already open, i.e., in the course of a cardiac operation; and (3) adequate endocardial lead placement cannot be achieved. Most pacemaker generators are powered by lithium batteries. The life expectancy of the generator is related to (1) voltage output required for capture, (2) requirement for incessant or intermittent pacing, and (3) number of cardiac chambers paced. Life expectancy of the simple ventricular demand pacemaker can exceed 10 years.

PACING CODE A code consisting of three to five letters has been developed for describing pacemaker type and function (Table 213-3). The first letter indicates the chamber(s) paced and is designated V for ventricular pacing, A for atrial pacing, or D for dual-chamber (both atrial and ventricular) pacing. The second letter indicates the chamber in which electrical activity is sensed and is also indicated by A, V, or D. An additional designation, O, has been used when pacemaker discharge is not dependent on a sensed electrical activity. The third letter refers to the response to a sensed electric signal. The letter O represents no response to an underlying electric signal, usually related to the absence of associated sensing function; I represents inhibition of pacing function; T represents triggering of pacing function; and D indicates a dual response, i.e., spontaneous atrial and ventricular activity inhibiting atrial and ventricular pacing and atrial activity triggering a ventricular response. Additional fourth and fifth letters of the pacing code have been recommended to indicate whether the pacemaker is programmable and has rate modulation (fourth) and whether special antitachycardia functions are available (i.e., antitachycardia pacing, T, and delivery of high- or low-energy shocks). In the fourth category, M represents multiprogrammability and R represents rate response ("physiologic") pacing.

It follows from the described code that the standard VVIR (ventricular demand pacemaker) paces the ventricle, senses the ventricle, is inhibited by sensed spontaneous ventricular activity, and has rate modulation, while the DDDR pulse generator is capable of sensing and pacing both the atria and ventricles and has a dual response to the sensed atrial and ventricular activity as described above (Fig. 213-9). Both pacemakers have rate modulation (R). "Physiologic" pacemakers use sensors (muscular activity, respiratory rate, temperature, O_2 saturation, QT interval, etc.) as methods to allow the pacemaker to increase the heart rate in response to physiologic demands, i.e., exercise. These pacemakers are essential when chronotropic incompetence is present and an increase in heart rate is required to enhance physiologic performance. Studies have shown that such "physiologic" pacemakers improve exercise tolerance and relieve symptoms to a greater degree than fixed-rate pacemakers.

Selection of the appropriate pacemaker and pacing mode depends on the clinical condition and the type of bradyarrhythmia being treated. The two most common pacing mode selections are DDD and VVI. DDD provides AV sequential pacing, which is ideally suited for the relatively young and active patient who has intact sinus node function or intermittent dysfunction and high-grade persistent or intermittent AV block. The DDD mode will allow for physiologic atrial sensed and ventricular paced rates and improve exercise tolerance. AV synchrony and dual-chamber pacing may also be desirable in patients with borderline hemodynamic reserve who are dependent on atrial contribution to cardiac output and in those patients who develop the pacemaker syndrome (see below) in response to ventricular demand pacing.

Rate-responsive DDD (i.e., DDDR) pacing is indicated when chronotropic incompetence is present in a patient who requires AV synchrony. The DDD pacing mode is contraindicated in chronic atrial

Acquired AV Block in Adults

Class I

1. Third-degree and advanced second-degree AV block, associated with any one of the following:
   a. Symptomatic bradycardia
   b. Arrhythmias and other conditions that require drugs that result in symptomatic bradycardia
   c. Documented periods of asystole ≥ 3.0 s or any escape rate less than 40 beats/min
   d. After catheter ablation of the AV junction
   e. Postoperative AV block that is not expected to resolve
   f. Neuromuscular diseases

Class IIa

1. Asymptomatic third-degree block with average awake ventricular rates of ≥ 40 beats/min
2. Asymptomatic type II second-degree AV block with a narrow QRS
3. Asymptomatic type I second-degree AV block at intra- or infra-His levels
4. First- or second-degree AV block with symptoms similar to those of pacemaker syndrome

Class IIb

1. Marked first-degree AV block (> 0.3 s) in patients with LV dysfunction in whom a shorter AV interval results in hemodynamic improvement, presumably by decreasing left atrial filling pressure

Class III

1. Intermittent third-degree AV block
2. Asymptomatic type I second-degree AV block at the AV node
3. AV block expected to resolve

Chronic Bifascicular and Trifascicular Block

Class I

1. Intermittent third-degree AV block
2. Type II second-degree AV block
3. Alternating bundle-branch block

Class IIa

1. Syncope when other likely causes have been excluded
2. Incidental finding at EP study of HV interval ≥ 100 ms
3. Incidental finding at EP study

Class IIb

1. Neuromuscular diseases

Class III

1. Fascicular block without AV block or symptoms
2. Fascicular block with first-degree AV block without symptoms

After Acute Myocardial Infarction

Class I

1. Persistent second-degree AV block in the His-Purkinje system with bilateral bundle branch block or third-degree AV block
2. Transient advanced (second- or third-degree) infranodal AV block and associated bundle branch block
3. Persistent and symptomatic second- or third-degree AV block

Class IIb

1. Persistent second- or third-degree AV nodal block

Class III

1. Transient AV block in the absence of intraventricular conduction defects
2. Transient AV block in the presence of isolated left anterior fascicular block
3. Acquired left anterior fascicular block in absence of AV block
4. Persistent first-degree AV block in the presence of old bundle branch block

Sinus Node Dysfunction

Class I

1. With documented symptomatic bradycardia
2. Symptomatic chronotropic incompetence

Class IIa

1. With heart rate < 40 beats/min not associated with symptoms
2. With syncope of unexplained origin

Class IIb

1. With minimal symptoms

Class III

1. Asymptomatic patients
2. In patients with symptoms documented as not associated with a slow heart rate
3. With symptomatic bradycardia due to nonessential drug therapy

Pacemakers That Automatically Detect and Pace to Terminate Tachycardias

Class I

1. Symptomatic recurrent supraventricular tachycardia that is reducibly terminated by pacing after drugs and catheter ablation failure
2. Symptomatic recurrent sustained VT as part of an automatic defibrillator system

Pacing Recommendations to Prevent Tachycardia

Class I

1. Sustained pause-dependent VT

Class IIa

1. High-risk patients with congenital long-QT syndrome

Class IIb

1. AV reentrant or AV node reentrant supraventricular tachycardia not responsive to therapy
2. Prevention of symptomatic, drug-refractory, recurrent atrial fibrillation

Hypersensitive Carotid Sinus Syndrome and Neurocardiogenic Syncope

Class I

1. Recurrent syncope caused by carotid sinus stimulation
2. Minimal carotid sinus pressure induces ventricular asystole of >3 s duration in the absence of any medication that depresses the sinus node or AV conduction

Class IIa

1. Recurrent syncope without clear, provocative events and with a hypersensitive cardioinhibitory response
2. Syncope of unexplained origin when major abnormalities of sinus node function or AV conduction are discovered or provoked in EP studies
3. Significantly symptomatic and recurrent neurocardiogenic syncope associated with bradycardia documented spontaneously or at the time of tilt-table testing

Class IIb

1. Neurally mediated syncope with significant bradycardia reproduced by a head-up tilt

Class III

1. Hyperactive cardioinhibitory response to carotid sinus stimulation in the absence of symptoms
2. Recurrent syncope, lightheadedness, or dizziness in the absence of a hyperactive cardioinhibitory response

Note: Class I: Evidence that procedure/treatment is indicated; Class IIa: Conflicting evidence but weight of evidence in favor; Class IIb: Efficacy less well established; Class III: Evidence that procedure/treatment is not effective; EP: electrophysiologic.

Source: Adapted from the American College of Cardiology/American Heart Association: J Am Coll Cardiol 31:1175, 1998, and incorporating new recommendations from G Gregoratas: Circulation 106:2145, 2002.

fibrillation or flutter, because rapid and irregular ventricular pacing will occur to the upper rate limit. In some cases this will produce a more rapid ventricular rate than the patient's own rate in the absence of a pacemaker. DDD pacemakers must either automatically switch (i.e., mode-switching function) or be reprogrammed to the VVI mode. Almost all such pacemakers are now combined with some form of rate responsiveness so that when the device functions in the VVI mode, it also will respond to physiologic demands (VVIR).

Chronotropic insufficiency (i.e., the inability of the sinus rate to accelerate) is a contraindication for a DDD pacemaker, since such a pacemaker will act as a "fixed-rate" pacemaker at the programmed lower rate. In these situations, a rate-adaptive or "physiologic" pace-maker is indicated (VVIR or DDDR). In patients with impaired sinus node function or chronic atrial fibrillation, a sensor-driven, rate-adaptive pacemaker must be implanted. As mentioned earlier, these pacemakers automatically adjust ventricular pacing rates to a sensed indicator of exertion. The DDD pacing mode may also be contraindicated in patients with intermittent or persistent ventriculoatrial conduction, who may develop pacemaker-mediated tachycardia (see below).

Specific pacemaker programming is often effective for the management of vasovagal syncope. These algorithms result in rapid pacing (≥ 100 beats/min) following the detection of an abrupt and significant drop in sinus rates. Biventricular pacing is a new therapy for class 3

TABLE 213-3 *The NASPE/BPEG Generic Pacemaker Code*

Position Category	I Chamber(s) Paced	II Chamber(s) Sensed	III Response to Sensing	IV Programmability, Rate Modulation	V Antitachyarrhythmia Function(s)
	O, None	O, None	O, None	O, None	O, None
	A, Atrium	A, Atrium	T, Triggered	P, Simple programmable	P, Pacing (antitachyarrhythmia)
	V, Ventricle	V, Ventricle	I, Inhibited	M, Multiprogrammable	S, Shock
	D, Dual (A + V)	D, Dual (A + V)	D, Dual (T + I)	C, Communicating	D, Dual (P + S)
				R, Rate modulation	
Manufacturer's designation	S, Single (A or V)	S, (A or V)			

Source: From DP Zipes, in *Braunwald's Heart Disease: A Textbook of Cardiovascular Medicine,* 7th ed. Philadelphia, Saunders, 2005.

and 4 heart failure with QRS prolongation (Chap. 216). This technique involves the addition of a lead placed in the coronary sinus to pace the posterolateral aspect of the left ventricle. The synchronized activation of the lateral (coronary sinus lead) and septal (right ventricular lead) aspects of the left ventricle results in improved hemodynamic function in some patients.

PROGRAMMABILITY OF PACEMAKERS This allows for modification of pacing function after implantation and for adaptation to changes in clinical needs. Pacemaker programming is accomplished by activation of the programming head positioned over the implanted pulse generator after making the desired changes in programmable parameters (Table 213-3). A radio frequency system is routinely used to communicate the program to the pacemaker. A high degree of sophistication is required to recognize the presence and causes of pacemaker malfunction and their treatment.

COMPLICATIONS Adverse effects of permanent pacing are usually associated with failure or malfunction of the pacing system. These problems are usually secondary to over- or undersensing, output failure, and/or lead fracture or displacement. Two other problems may occur. The *pacemaker syndrome* consists of fatigue, dizziness, syncope, and distressing pulsations in the neck and chest and can be associated with adverse hemodynamic effects. The pathophysiologic contributors to

the pacemaker syndrome include (1) loss of atrial contribution to ventricular systole; (2) vasodepressor reflex initiated by cannon *a* waves, which are caused by atrial contractions against a closed tricuspid valve and observed in the jugular venous pulse (Chap. 209); and (3) systemic and pulmonary venous regurgitation due to atrial contraction against a closed AV valve. The symptoms associated with the pacemaker syndrome can be prevented by maintaining AV synchrony by dual-chamber pacing or, in the case of a ventricular demand pacemaker, by programming an escape rate 15 to 20 beats/min below that of the paced rate (i.e., hysteresis). As a result of this programming, sinus activity and thus atrial contraction will be less likely to occur at the same time as ventricular pacing and ventricular contraction. The second major problem peculiar to dual-chamber pacemakers is the development of *pacemaker-mediated tachycardia.* In this instance, retrograde depolarization of the atria, resulting from a premature ventricular depolarization or a paced ventricular complex, is sensed and leads to subsequent triggering of ventricular pacing. This, in turn, can result in repetition of the phenomenon of ventriculoatrial conduction with the development of an endless-loop, pacemaker-mediated tachycardia. It may be corrected by reprogramming the atrial refractory period.

FURTHER READING

ABRAHAM WT et al: Cardiac resynchronization in chronic heart failure. N Engl J Med 346:1845, 2002

BRINK P et al: Gene for progressive familial heart block type 1 maps to chromosome 19q13. Circulation 91:1633, 1995

BUYON J et al: Autoimmune associated congenital heart block: Demographics, mortality, morbidity and recurrence rates obtained from a national neonatal lupus registry. J Am Coll Cardiol 31:1685, 1998

ELLENBOGEN KA et al: New insights into pacemaker syndrome gained from hemodynamic, humoral and vascular responses during ventriculo-atrial pacing. Am J Cardiol 65:53, 1990

GREGORATAS G: ACC/AHA/NASPE 2002 Guideline for implantation of cardiac pacemakers and antiarrhythmia devices: Summary article. Circulation 106:2145, 2002

HAYES DL, ZIPES DP: Cardiac pacemakers, in *Braunwald's Heart Disease: A Textbook of Cardiovascular Medicine,* 7th ed, D Zipes et al (eds). Philadelphia, Saunders, 2005

HUANG SK et al: Carotid sinus hypersensitivity in patients with unexplained syncope: Clinical, electrophysiologic and long-term follow-up observations. Am Heart J 116:989, 1988

JOSEPHSON ME: *Clinical Cardiac Electrophysiology: Techniques and Interpretations,* 3d ed. Philadelphia, Lippincott Williams & Wilkins, 2002, Chaps 3,4,5,11

MENDES LA, DAVIDOFF R: Cardiogenic seizure with bradyarrhythmia: Documentation of the mechanism during asystole. Am Heart J 125:1786, 1993

SCHOTT J et al: Congenital heart disease caused by mutations in the transcription factor NKX2-5. Science, 1998; 281:108–111

WALLER BF et al: Anatomy, histology and pathology of the cardiac conduction system: Part II. Clin Cardiol 16:347, 1993

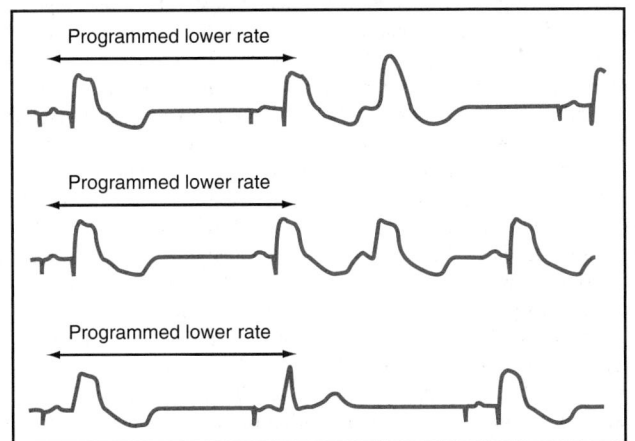

FIGURE 213-9 Normally functioning DDD pacemaker. All three panels show a lead II rhythm strip at 50 mm/s. The programmed lower rate is approximately 55 beats/min. (*Top*) AV sequential pacing with a paced AV interval of 160 ms is shown for the first two complexes. A ventricular premature complex occurs and is sensed, resetting the cycle. (*Middle*) The first beat is AV paced, but spontaneous sinus P waves and atrial premature complex trigger a ventricular paced complex with a sensed P to QRS of 120 ms. (*Bottom*) After the first AV paced complex, a paced atrial complex conducts to the ventricle with a PR of 120 ms, inhibiting the ventricular pacemaker.

MECHANISMS OF TACHYARRHYTHMIAS

Tachyarrhythmias may be divided into disorders of impulse propagation and disorders of impulse formation.

REENTRY Disorders of impulse propagation (reentry) are generally considered to be the most common mechanism of sustained paroxysmal tachyarrhythmia. The requirements for initiating reentry include (1) electrophysiologic inhomogeneity (i.e., differences in conduction and/or refractoriness) in two or more regions of the heart connected with each other to form a potentially closed loop; (2) unidirectional block in one pathway; (3) slow conduction over an alternative pathway, allowing time for the initially blocked pathway to recover excitability; and (4) reexcitation of the initially blocked pathway to complete a loop of activation (Fig. 214-1). Repetitive circulation of the impulse over this loop can produce a sustained tachyarrhythmia. While anatomic obstacles may underlie reentry and provide an inexcitable center around which the impulse can circulate, they are not essential. Reentrant arrhythmias can be reproducibly initiated and terminated by premature complexes and rapid stimulation. The response of these arrhythmias to stimulation can help distinguish them from arrhythmias caused by triggered activity.

ENHANCED AUTOMATICITY Disorders of impulse formation can be subdivided into tachyarrhythmias caused by enhanced automaticity and those caused by triggered activity. In addition to the sinus node, automatic pacemaker activity can be observed in specialized atrial fibers, fibers of the atrioventricular (AV) junction, and Purkinje fibers (Chap. 213). Myocardial cells do not normally possess pacemaker activity. Enhancement of normal automaticity in latent pacemaker fibers or the development of abnormal automaticity due to partial depolarization of the resting membrane occurs as a consequence of a variety of pathophysiologic states, which include (1) increased endogenous or exogenous catecholamines, (2) electrolyte disturbances (e.g., hypokalemia), (3) hypoxia or ischemia, (4) mechanical effects (e.g., stretch), and (5) drugs (e.g., digitalis). Tachycardia caused by automaticity cannot be started or stopped by pacing.

TRIGGERED ACTIVITY Rhythms due to triggered activity are events that do not occur spontaneously but require a change in cardiac electrical frequency as a trigger. Triggered activity may be caused by early afterdepolarizations, which occur during phases 2 and 3 of the action potential, or delayed afterdepolarizations, which occur following completion of phase 3 of the action potential (Fig. 213-2). Triggered activity has been observed in atrial, ventricular, and His-Purkinje tissue under conditions such as increased local catecholamine concentration, hypercalcemia, and digitalis intoxication (delayed afterdepolariza-

tions) or during bradycardia, hypokalemia, or other situations prolonging action potential duration (early afterdepolarizations). All of these conditions produce an accumulation of intracellular calcium. With increasing amplitude of the afterdepolarizations, threshold can be reached and repetitive activity produced. The exact role of triggered activity in spontaneous clinical arrhythmias is unknown, but tachyarrhythmias associated with digitalis intoxication, accelerated idioventricular rhythm in acute infarction and/or reperfusion, and exercise-induced ventricular tachycardia (VT) are believed to be caused by triggered activity due to delayed afterdepolarizations. *Torsades de pointes* ("twisting of the points"; polymorphic VT associated with long QT intervals) may be caused by triggered activity due to early afterdepolarizations, although reentry may also be operative.

The use of electrophysiologic studies, i.e., intracardiac recordings and programmed stimulation, has greatly expanded the understanding of the mechanisms of tachyarrhythmias. In addition to helping diagnose arrhythmias, these techniques may be of value in determining the most appropriate types of therapy because they allow the physician to observe the hemodynamic and symptomatic consequences of the arrhythmia in the presence or absence of therapy. Electrophysiologic studies of tachycardias require the positioning of multiple electrode catheters at critical areas within the heart. These electrodes must be capable of both stimulating and recording from multiple sites in the atria and/or ventricles.

PREMATURE COMPLEXES

ATRIAL PREMATURE COMPLEXES (APCs) APCs can be found on 24-h Holter monitoring in over 60% of normal adults. APCs are usually asymptomatic and benign, although at times they may be associated with palpitations. In susceptible patients, they can initiate paroxysmal supraventricular tachycardias (PSVTs). APCs may originate from any location in either atrium, and they are recognized on the electrocardiogram (ECG) as early P waves with a morphology that differs from the sinus P wave (Fig. 214-2). While APCs usually conduct to the ventricles when they occur late in the cardiac cycle, early APCs may reach the AV conduction system while it is still in its relative refractory period, resulting in a conduction delay manifested by a prolonged PR interval following the premature P wave (Fig. 214-2). Very early APCs may even be blocked in the AV node if this structure is encountered during its effective refractory period. APCs, whether conducted or not, are usually followed by a pause before a return to sinus activity. Most commonly, an APC enters and resets the sinus node, so the sum of the pre- and postextrasystolic PP intervals is less than the sum of two sinus PP intervals (Fig. 214-2). In this case, the pause is said to be less than fully compensatory. The QRS complex following most APCs is normal, although early APCs may be followed by aberrantly conducted QRS complexes due to the premature complex falling within the relative refractory period of the His-Purkinje system.

Since most APCs are asymptomatic, treatment is not required. When they cause palpitations or trigger PSVTs (see below), treatment may be useful. Factors that precipitate APCs, such as alcohol, tobacco, or adrenergic stimulants, should be identified and eliminated; in their absence, mild sedation or the use of a beta blocker may be tried.

AV JUNCTIONAL COMPLEXES The site of origin of these complexes is thought to be in the bundle of His, since the normal AV node in vivo possesses no automaticity. AV junctional complexes are less common than either atrial or ventricular premature complexes and are more often associated with cardiac disease or digitalis intoxication. Junctional premature impulses can conduct both antegradely to the ventricles and retrogradely to the atrium and, on rare occasions, may fail to conduct in either direction. Premature AV junctional complexes can be recognized by normal-appearing QRS complexes that are not preceded by a P wave. Retrograde P waves (inverted in leads II, III, and aVF) may be observed after the QRS complex.

While often asymptomatic, junctional premature complexes may be associated with palpitations and cause cannon *a* waves, which may

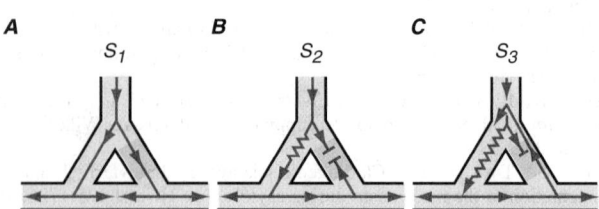

FIGURE 214-1 Schema of reentry. Y branching of the Purkinje system to ventricular muscle is shown in panels *A* through *C*. The right limb (*blue*) of the Purkinje system has a longer refractory period than the left. *A*. During a slow stimulated rate (S₁), conduction proceeds normally over both Purkinje fibers, resulting in collision in the ventricular muscle. *B*. An early premature stimulus (S₂) results in block in the Purkinje fiber on the right and slow conduction down the left. The impulse conducts through the ventricle and attempts to reenter the initial site of block but fails because this site has not fully recovered excitability. *C*. An earlier stimulus (S₃) again results in block on the left. The resulting slower propagation down the left fiber provides enough time for the initial site of block to recur and allows the impulse to conduct through it to produce a reentrant circuit.

result in distressing pulsations in the neck. When symptomatic, they should be treated like APCs.

VENTRICULAR PREMATURE COMPLEXES (VPCs)

These are among the most common arrhythmias and occur in patients with and without heart disease. Of adult males, ≥60% will exhibit VPCs during a 24-h Holter monitoring. In patients without heart disease, VPCs have not been shown to be associated with any increased incidence in mortality or morbidity. VPCs may occur in up to 80% of patients with previous myocardial infarction, and in this setting, if frequent (>10 per hour) and/or complex (occurring in couplets), they have been associated with increased mortality. However, cardiac mortality in such patients usually occurs in association with significantly impaired ventricular function. While frequent and complex ventricular ectopy is an independent risk factor, it is not as strong a risk factor as is impaired ventricular function. Moreover, even though VT and/or ventricular fibrillation (VF) may be the basis for the sudden death in these patients, this does not a priori establish a cause-and-effect relation between spontaneous ectopy and life-threatening VT or VF. Very early cycle (R-on-T) VPCs have been stated by some to increase the risk of sudden death. Although this has been observed during acute ischemia and in the setting of QT prolongation, frequently, VT or VF is precipitated by VPCs that occur after the T wave of the prior beat.

VPCs are recognized by wide (usually >0.14 s), bizarre QRS complexes that are not preceded by P waves (Fig. 214-3A). However, when they arise in the specialized conduction system (e.g., fascicles) they may be <0.12 s in duration. They may bear a relatively fixed relationship to the preceding sinus complex (i.e., fixed coupled VPCs). When fixed coupling is not present and the interval between VPCs has a common denominator, *ventricular parasystole* is said to be present (Fig. 214-4). Under these circumstances, the VPCs are a manifestation of abnormal automaticity of a protected ventricular focus. Because this focus is not penetrated by sinus impulses, it is not reset by them, and the interectopic intervals remain relatively fixed (≤120 ms variation of mean RR cycle length).

VPCs may occur singly; in patterns of bigeminy, in which every sinus beat is followed by a VPC; in trigeminy, in which two sinus beats are followed by a VPC; in quadrigeminy, etc. Two successive VPCs are termed *pairs* or *couplets*, while three or more consecutive VPCs are termed *ventricular tachycardia* when the rate exceeds 100 beats/min (Fig. 214-3B). VPCs may have similar morphologies (monomorphic, or uniform) or different morphologies (polymorphic, or multiformed).

Most commonly, VPCs are not conducted retrogradely to the atrium to reset the sinoatrial node. Thus they result in a fully compensatory pause, i.e., the interval between conducted sinus beats that bracket the VPC equals two basic RR intervals. Ventricular impulses may also manifest retrograde conduction to the atrium and cause inverted P waves in leads II, III, and aVF. This retrograde atrial activation can reset the sinus node, and the pause that results may therefore be less than compensatory. In many instances, the VPC will not be associated with retrograde ventriculoatrial (VA) conduction but may block retrogradely

in the AV node. This renders the AV node refractory to the subsequent sinus beat and causes slowed conduction (i.e., prolonged PR interval) or block of the next sinus P wave. This prolonged PR interval is said to be a manifestation of concealed retrograde conduction of the ventricular impulse into the AV node. A VPC that does not produce any manifestation of retrograde concealed conduction and fails to influence the oncoming sinus impulse is termed an *interpolated VPC*.

VPCs can cause palpitations or neck pulsations secondary to either the occurrence of cannon *a* waves or the increased force of contraction due to postextrasystolic potentiation of ventricular contractility. Patients with frequent VPCs or bigeminy may rarely develop syncope or lightheadedness because the VPCs do not result in an adequate stroke volume and the cardiac output is reduced by the "halving" of the heart rate.

℞ TREATMENT

In the absence of cardiac disease, isolated asymptomatic VPCs, regardless of configuration and frequency, need no treatment. When arrhythmias are symptomatic, the symptoms should first be addressed by either allaying the patient's anxiety or, if this is not successful, reducing the frequency of the VPCs with antiarrhythmic agents. β-Adrenergic blockers may be successful in managing VPCs that occur primarily in the daytime or under stressful situations and in specific settings such as mitral valve prolapse and thyrotoxicosis. While other antiarrhythmic agents may be tried should this be unsuccessful, their risk may outweigh any benefits. In patients with cardiac disease, fre-

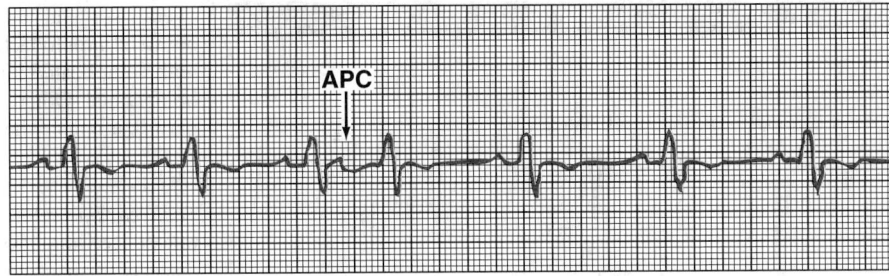

FIGURE 214-2 ECG lead II. Sinus rhythm with one atrial premature complex (*arrow*). Note the difference in P-wave configuration between sinus and the premature atrial complexes. In addition, note that the PR interval of the premature complex is prolonged, due to slowed conduction of the premature impulse through the AV conduction system.

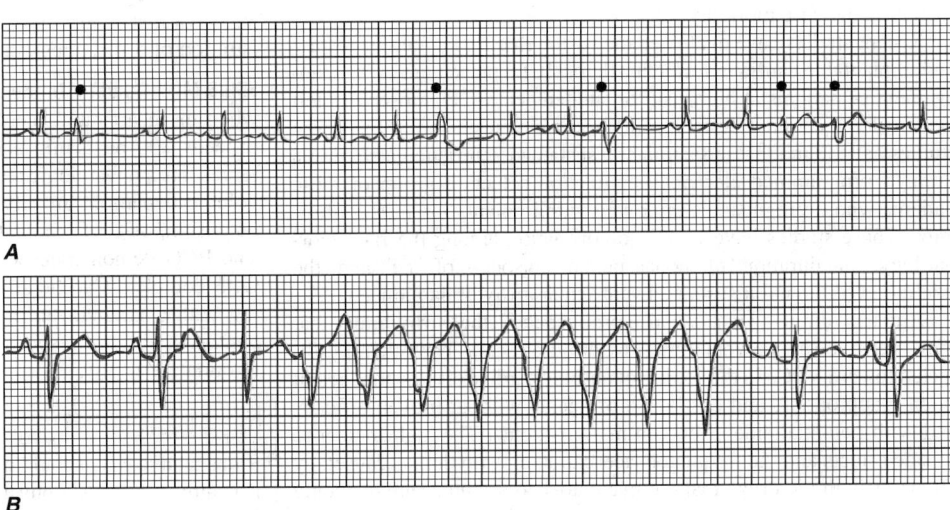

FIGURE 214-3 *A.* Single ventricular ectopy. During sinus rhythm, five premature ventricular complexes (*filled circles*) occur. Note that the QRS configuration is bizarre and different from that during sinus rhythm. The premature ventricular complexes are not preceded by P waves. The QRS widths of the premature complexes are 120–160 ms and multiple morphologies are present. The pause following the premature complexes is fully compensatory, the sinus beat after the premature complex occurring on time. *B.* Nonsustained ventricular tachycardia (VT). Following two sinus beats, an atrial premature contraction with long PR interval initiates an 8-beat run of wide complex tachycardia. Atrial activity can be seen following the fourth and seventh beats. The greater number of QRS complexes compared with P waves confirms the diagnosis of VT.

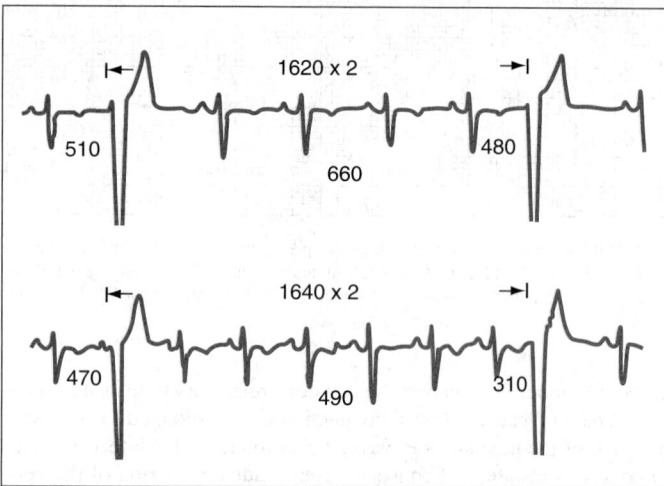

FIGURE 214-4 Ventricular parasystole. At varying sinus cycle lengths during exercise, interectopic intervals remain constant at 1620 to 1640 ms. However, the coupling intervals between sinus and ectopic complexes vary between 510 and 310 ms.

quent VPCs are associated with an increased risk of sudden and non-sudden cardiac death, and many physicians have attempted to eliminate or reduce the frequency of these VPCs in an attempt to reduce this risk. However, the cause-and-effect relationship of the VPCs to fatal events has never been established.

The ability of pharmacologic antiarrhythmic therapy guided by continuous ECG monitoring to reduce the risk of sudden death in postmyocardial infarction patients with frequent (≥ 6 per minute) VPCs was tested by the Cardiac Arrhythmia Suppression Trial (CAST). This study compared mortality in patients whose ectopy was suppressed by one of three agents (encainide, flecainide, or moricizine) and then randomized to treatment with either the "effective" drug or placebo. After a mean follow-up of 2 years, the study was discontinued because both the sudden death and overall mortality rate were significantly increased in patients receiving antiarrhythmic agents (encainide, flecainide). This study has shown that in patients having the characteristics of the study population, abolition of ventricular ectopy by pharmacologic therapy cannot be used as a marker to define reduction of the risk of sudden death after myocardial infarction and, in fact, may increase mortality.

Recent studies have evaluated the use of electrophysiologic testing and implantable cardioverter/defibrillator (ICD) placement in the management of patients at high risk for sudden death (i.e., those with left ventricular ejection fractions <40% and nonsustained VT). These studies have found that induction of a sustained ventricular arrhythmia through programmed electrical stimulation selects a group of these patients whose prognosis is improved with implantation of a defibrillator. These studies have found no correlation among the rate, morphology, or duration of nonsustained episodes of VT and the likelihood of having a sustained ventricular arrhythmia induced.

Antiarrhythmic agents can also produce the lethal arrhythmias that they are given to prevent (proarrhythmic effects). Thus therapy directed toward VPCs in the setting of chronic cardiac disease may result in an inappropriate and costly use of agents without proven efficacy and with potential side effects in many patients. The high incidence of side effects and the frequent exacerbation of arrhythmias caused by all antiarrhythmic drugs make it mandatory to monitor patients being treated with such agents. Congestive heart failure (CHF) is the most important risk factor for proarrhythmia.

In acute myocardial infarction, the greatest incidence of primary VF occurs within the first 24 h (Chap. 228). Temporary prophylactic antiarrhythmic therapy with lidocaine or procainamide was formerly recommended for all patients with acute infarction, regardless of the presence or degree of spontaneous ectopy. However, failure to improve overall survival and drug toxicity have led most physicians to recommend prophylactic antiarrhythmic therapy only to young patients with complicated infarctions, where a favorable risk-benefit ratio may be obtained. Other studies have shown that intravenous beta blockers may also reduce the incidence of primary VF.

TACHYCARDIAS

Tachycardias refer to arrhythmias with three or more complexes at rates exceeding 100 beats/min; they occur more often in structurally diseased than in normal hearts. Those paroxysmal tachycardias that are initiated by APCs or VPCs are considered to be due to reentry, except some of the digitalis-induced tachyarrhythmias, which are probably due to triggered activity (see below).

If the patient is hemodynamically stable, an attempt should be made to determine the mechanism and origin of the tachycardia, since this will usually lead to an appropriate therapeutic decision. Information to be obtained from the ECG includes (1) the presence, frequency, morphology, and regularity of P waves and QRS complexes; (2) the relationship between atrial and ventricular activity; (3) a comparison of the QRS morphology during sinus rhythm and during the tachycardia; and (4) the response to carotid sinus massage or other vagal maneuvers. It is useful first to compare a 12-lead ECG during the tachycardia with one recorded during sinus rhythm. One can also utilize the electrodes situated at the end of a flexible pacing catheter inserted into the esophagus behind the left atrium to record atrial activity.

Observation of the jugular venous pulse can provide clues to the presence of atrial activity and its relationship to ventricular ectopy. Intermittent cannon *a* waves suggest AV dissociation, while persistent cannon *a* waves suggest 1:1 VA conduction. Flutter waves may be seen or no atrial activity may be apparent, as in the presence of atrial flutter and atrial fibrillation (AF), respectively. The arterial pulse may also manifest AV dissociation or AF by demonstrating variations in amplitude. A first heart sound of variable intensity during a regular rhythm also suggests AV dissociation or AF.

Carotid sinus pressure should be applied only while the patient is electrocardiographically monitored with resuscitative equipment available to manage the rare episode of asystole and/or VF associated with this procedure. Carotid sinus massage should not be performed in patients with carotid arterial bruits. The patient should be positioned flat with the neck extended. Massage of one carotid bulb at a time should be performed by applying firm pressure just underneath the angle of the jaw for up to 5 s. Alternative vagomimetic maneuvers include the Valsalva maneuver, immersion of the face in cold water, and administration of 5 to 10 mg edrophonium.

SINUS TACHYCARDIA   In the adult, sinus tachycardia is said to be present when the heart rate exceeds 100 beats/min. Sinus tachycardia rarely exceeds 200 beats/min and is not a primary arrhythmia; instead, it represents a physiologic response to a variety of stresses, such as fever, volume depletion, anxiety, exercise, thyrotoxicosis, hypoxemia, hypotension, or CHF. Sinus tachycardia has a gradual onset and offset. The ECG demonstrates P waves with sinus contour preceding each QRS complex. Carotid sinus pressure usually produces modest slowing with a gradual return to the previous rate upon cessation. This contrasts with the response of PSVTs, which may slow slightly and terminate abruptly.

℞ TREATMENT

Sinus tachycardia should not be treated as a primary arrhythmia, since it is almost always a physiologic response to a demand placed on the heart. As such, therapy should be directed to the primary disorder. However, in the setting of CHF, enhanced sympathetic activity has detrimental effects on myocardial function and merits treatment. Use of beta blockers in this situation decreases the effects of neurohormonal activation that leads to worsening CHF. Angiotensin-converting enzyme (ACE) inhibitors and angiotensin receptor blockers are additional drugs affecting neurohormonal activation in heart failure whose use improves outcomes. The other situations in which sinus tachycardia is a consequence (listed above) can all be readily treated.

ATRIAL FIBRILLATION AF is a common arrhythmia that may occur in paroxysmal and persistent forms. It may be seen in normal individuals, particularly during emotional stress or following surgery, exercise, acute alcoholic intoxication, or a prominent surge of vagal tone (i.e., vasovagal response). It may also occur in patients with heart or lung disease who develop acute hypoxia, hypercapnia, or metabolic or hemodynamic derangements. Persistent AF usually occurs in patients with cardiovascular disease, most commonly rheumatic heart disease, nonrheumatic mitral valve disease, hypertensive cardiovascular disease, chronic lung disease, atrial septal defect, and a variety of miscellaneous cardiac abnormalities. AF may be the presenting finding in thyrotoxicosis. So-called lone AF, which occurs in patients without underlying heart disease, often represents the tachycardia phase of the tachycardia-bradycardia syndrome.

The morbidity associated with AF is related to (1) excessive ventricular rate, which in turn may lead to hypotension, pulmonary congestion, or angina pectoris in susceptible individuals, and in some patients can produce a tachycardia-mediated cardiomyopathy; (2) the pause following cessation of AF, which can cause syncope; (3) systemic embolization, which occurs most commonly in patients with rheumatic heart disease (Table 214-1); (4) loss of the contribution of atrial contraction to cardiac output, which may cause fatigue; and (5) anxiety secondary to palpitations. In patients with severe cardiac dysfunction, particularly those with hypertrophied, noncompliant ventricles, the combination of the loss of the atrial contribution to ventricular filling and the abbreviated filling period due to the rapid ventricular rate in AF can produce marked hemodynamic instability, resulting in hypotension, syncope, or heart failure. In patients with mitral stenosis, in whom ventricular filling time is critical, development of AF with a rapid ventricular rate may precipitate pulmonary edema (Chap. 219). AF may also cause a cardiomyopathy related to persistent rapid rates (so-called tachycardia-induced cardiomyopathy).

AF is characterized by disorganized atrial activity without discrete P waves on the surface ECG (Fig. 214-5A). Atrial activation is manifested by an undulating baseline or by more sharply inscribed atrial deflections of varying amplitude and frequency ranging from 350 to 600 beats/min. The ventricular response is irregularly irregular. This results from the large number of atrial impulses that penetrate the AV node, making it partially refractory to subsequent impulses. This effect of nonconducted atrial impulses to influence the response to subsequent atrial impulses is termed *concealed conduction*. As a result, the ventricular response is relatively slow, considering the actual atrial rate. AF may convert to atrial flutter, especially in response to antiarrhythmic drugs such as quinidine or flecainide. If AF converts to atrial flutter, which has a slower atrial rate, the effect of concealed conduction may be diminished, and a paradoxical increase in the ventricular response may occur. The main factor determining the rate of the ventricular response is the functional refractory period of the AV node or the most rapid paced rate at which 1:1 conduction through the AV node can be observed.

If, in the presence of AF, the ventricular rhythm becomes regular and slow (e.g., 30 to 60 beats/min), complete heart block is suggested,

TABLE 214-1 *Factors Associated with High Risk of Stroke in Patients with Atrial Fibrillation*

1. Age >65
2. Hypertension
3. Rheumatic heart disease
4. Prior stroke or transient ischemic attack
5. Diabetes mellitus
6. Congestive heart failure
7. Transesophageal echocardiographic characteristics
   Spontaneous echo contrast in left atrium
   Left atrial appendage velocity <20 cm/s
   Complex aortic atheroma

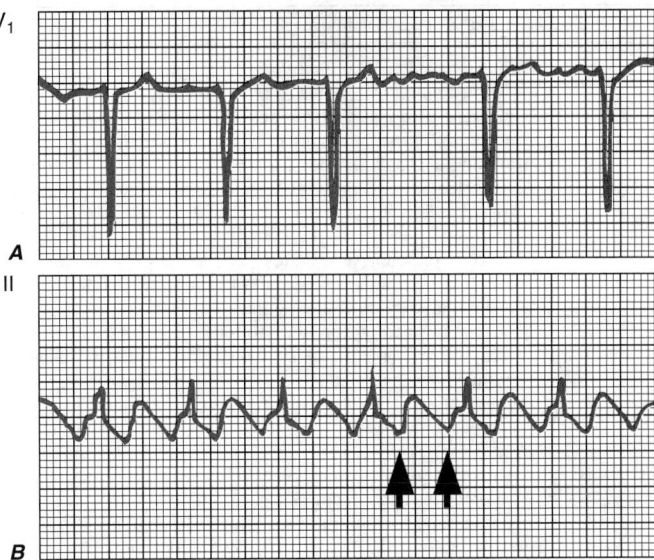

FIGURE 214-5 Atrial fibrillation and atrial flutter. *A.* Lead V_1 demonstrating an irregular ventricular rhythm associated with poorly defined irregular atrial activity consistent with atrial fibrillation. *B.* Lead II demonstrates atrial flutter, identified by the regular "sawtooth-like" activity (*arrows*) at an atrial rate of 300 beats/min with 2:1 ventricular response.

and if the ventricular rhythm is regular and rapid (e.g., ≥100 beats/min), a tachycardia arising in the AV junction or ventricle should be suspected. Digitalis intoxication is a common cause of both phenomena.

Patients with AF exhibit a loss of *a* waves in the jugular venous pulse and variable pulse pressures in the carotid arterial pulse. The first heart sound usually varies in intensity. On echocardiography, the left atrium is frequently enlarged, and in patients in whom the left atrial diameter >4.5 cm, it may be difficult to convert AF to sinus rhythm and/or maintain the latter, despite therapy.

TREATMENT

In acute AF, a precipitating factor such as fever, pneumonia, alcoholic intoxication, thyrotoxicosis, pulmonary emboli, CHF, or pericarditis should be sought. When such a factor is present, therapy should be directed toward the primary abnormality. If the patient's clinical status is severely compromised, electrical cardioversion is the treatment of choice. In the absence of severe cardiovascular compromise, slowing of the ventricular rate becomes the initial therapeutic goal. This may be most rapidly accomplished with β-adrenergic blockers and/or calcium channel antagonists. Both prolong the refractory period of the AV node and slow conduction within it. When catecholamine levels or sympathetic nervous system tone are likely to be elevated, beta blockers may be favored. Digitalis preparations are less effective, take longer to act, and are associated with more toxicity. Conversion to sinus rhythm may then be attempted. Prior to cardioversion, precautions must be taken to reduce the risk of systemic embolization. Patients should be anticoagulated to an INR of at least 1.8 for the prior 3 consecutive weeks or have had AF for <48 h. Alternatively, for those patients with AF for >48 h who are not anticoagulated, a transesophageal echocardiogram can exclude the presence of left atrial thrombus and allow safe cardioversion. Following cardioversion, anticoagulation must be maintained for at least 4 weeks until atrial mechanical function returns to normal.

Antiarrhythmic medications in either oral or intravenous form may be employed but are only modestly effective in restoring sinus rhythm. When antiarrhythmic agents such as the quinidine-like drugs (class IA) or the flecainide-like agents (class IC) are used (Table 214-2), it is important to increase AV node refractoriness prior to administering

TABLE 214-2 *Classification of Antiarrhythmic Drugs*

Class I	Drugs that reduce maximal velocity of phase of depolarization (V_{max}) due to block of inward Na^+ current in tissue with fast response action potentials
IA	$\downarrow V_{max}$ at all heart rates and $\uparrow$ action potential duration, e.g., quinidine, procainamide, disopyramide
IB	Little effect at slow rates on V_{max} in normal tissue; $\downarrow V_{max}$ in partially depolarized cells with fast response action potentials Effects increased at faster rates No change or $\downarrow$ in action potential duration, e.g., lidocaine, phenytoin, tocainide, mexiletine
IC	$\downarrow V_{max}$ at normal rates in normal tissue Minimal effect on action potential duration, e.g., flecainide, propafenone, moricizine
Class II	Antisympathetic agents, e.g., propranolol and other β-adrenergic blockers: $\downarrow$ SA nodal automaticity, $\uparrow$ AV nodal refractoriness, and $\downarrow$ AV nodal conduction velocity
Class III	Agents that prolong action potential duration in tissue with fast-response action potentials, e.g., bretylium, amiodarone, sotalol, ibutilide, dofetilide
Class IV	Calcium (slow) channel blocking agents: $\downarrow$ conduction velocity and $\uparrow$ refractoriness in tissue with slow-response action potentials, e.g., verapamil, diltiazem
Drugs that cannot be classified by this schema: Digitalis, Adenosine	

Note: SA, sinoatrial; AV, atrioventricular.

such drugs because their vagolytic effect and/or their ability to convert AF to atrial flutter may reduce the concealed conduction in the AV node and lead to an excessively rapid ventricular response. β-Adrenergic blockers are especially useful in this regard. Intravenous ibutilide, a class III agent, is reasonably effective in converting new-onset AF to sinus rhythm.

Direct-current (DC) electrical cardioversion is a highly effective method to restore sinus rhythm, either as a primary method of therapy or following the failure of antiarrhythmic medications. DC cardioversion is accomplished through the delivery of at least 200 W·s of energy between electrodes placed to the right of the sternum and the cardiac apex or to the left of the scapula. New methods of cardioversion using biphasic waveforms have increased the efficacy of transthoracic cardioversion to >90%. If external cardioversion is unsuccessful, internal cardioversion with energy delivered between two catheters inside the heart or one inside and a patch outside the heart may prove effective. Recent studies suggest pretreatment with ibutilide can facilitate cardioversion.

It is unlikely that patients with chronic AF will convert to and remain in sinus rhythm in the presence of long-standing rheumatic heart disease and/or when the atria are markedly enlarged. The goal of therapy in patients in whom AF cannot be converted to sinus rhythm is control of the ventricular response. This can usually be accomplished by beta blockers, calcium channel blockers, or digitalis, singly or in combination. In occasional patients, the ventricular response cannot be controlled by pharmacologic therapy alone. In such patients, the creation of complete heart block by radiofrequency catheter ablation of the AV junction followed by permanent pacemaker implantation is appropriate.

If sinus rhythm is restored electrically or pharmacologically, quinidine or related agents as well as the class IC agents (e.g., flecainide or propafenone), sotalol, dofetilide, or amiodarone may be used to prevent recurrence. In patients in whom cardioversion is unsuccessful or in whom AF has recurred or is likely to recur despite antiarrhythmic therapy, it is probably wisest to allow the patient to remain in AF and to control the ventricular response with calcium antagonists, β-adrenergic blockers, or digitalis glycosides. Since such patients are always at risk of systemic embolization, particularly in the presence of organic heart disease, chronic anticoagulation must be considered (Table 214-3). Chronic anticoagulation is particularly important in the elderly, where the attributable risk of AF for stroke approaches 30%. Several

TABLE 214-3 *Recommendations for Long-Term Anticoagulation in Patients with Chronic Atrial Fibrillation*

Age, years	Risk Factors[a]	Recommendations
<65	Absent	Aspirin
	Present	Warfarin [target INR 2.5 (range 2.0–3.0)]
65–75	Absent	Aspirin or warfarin
	Present	Warfarin [target INR 2.5 (range 2.0–3.0)]
>75	All patients	Warfarin [target INR 2.5 (range 2.5–3.0)]

[a] Risk factors are prior transient ischemic attack, systemic embolus or stroke, hypertension, poor left ventricular function, rheumatic mitral valve disease, prosthetic heart valve, congestive heart failure.
Source: From ACC/AHA/ESC.

studies have now demonstrated conclusively that the incidence of embolization in patients with AF not associated with valvular heart disease is reduced by chronic anticoagulation with warfarin-like agents. Recommendation for chronic anticoagulation should be instituted based on clinical risk factors for stroke regardless of whether or not an antiarrhythmic medication is utilized. Studies have demonstrated that antiarrhythmic drugs are not associated with stroke reduction perhaps because of asymptomatic (unrecognized) recurrences. Aspirin also may be effective for this purpose in patients who are not at high risk for stroke. Although anticoagulation may be associated with hemorrhagic complications, the risk is largely associated with INRs above the recommended range of 2.0 to 3.0. Recommendations for the selection of antiarrhythmic medications to prevent the recurrence of AF are shown in Fig. 214-6.

Ablation therapy for cure of AF is an active area of investigation. This therapy is generally employed for patients with paroxysmal AF. This type of AF is often triggered by automatic foci located in the pulmonary veins. Ablation around the pulmonary veins to prevent electrical transit of impulses from the pulmonary veins to and from the left atrium may be curative. While ablation or isolation of these foci is possible, the procedure can result in pulmonary vein stenosis, pulmonary hypertension, and stroke. The MAZE procedure is a surgical approach to cure AF through the creation of multiple scars in the right and left atria to compartmentalize the electrical conduction in these chambers and disallow the propagation of fibrillatory waves. The

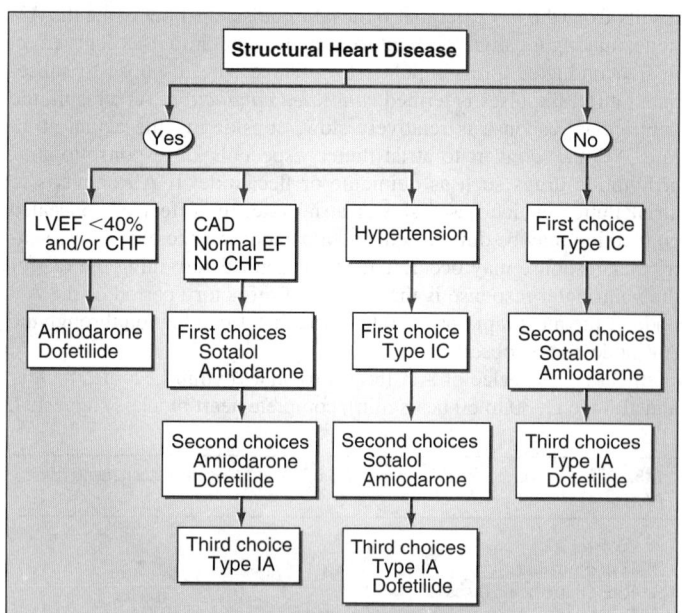

FIGURE 214-6 Recommendations for the selection of antiarrhythmic medications to prevent the recurrence of atrial fibrillation. See Tables 214-2 and 214-4 for definition of class IA and IC drugs. An atrioventricular nodal blocking agent (i.e., beta blocker, calcium channel blocker, or digoxin) should be added to all class IC and IA agents as well as to dofetilide. LVEF, left ventricular ejection fraction; CHF, congestive heart failure; CAD, coronary artery disease; EF, ejection fraction.

morbidity, mortality, and success rate of such catheter-based procedures render them experimental at this time.

ATRIAL FLUTTER This arrhythmia occurs most often in patients with organic heart disease. Flutter may be paroxysmal, in which case there is usually a precipitating factor, such as pericarditis or acute respiratory failure, or it may be persistent. Atrial flutter (as well as AF) is very common during the first week following open-heart surgery. Atrial flutter is usually less long-lived than is AF, although on occasion it may persist for months to years. Often, if it lasts for more than a week, atrial flutter will convert to AF. Systemic embolization is less common in atrial flutter than in AF.

Atrial flutter is characterized by an atrial rate between 250 and 350 beats/min. Typically, the ventricular rate is half the atrial rate, i.e., ~150 beats/min because of 2:1 block in the AV node. If the atrial rate is slowed to <220 beats/min by antiarrhythmic agents such as quinidine, which also possess vagolytic properties, the ventricular rate may rise suddenly because of the development of 1:1 AV conduction. Classically, flutter waves are seen as regular sawtooth-like atrial activity, most prominent in the inferior leads (Fig. 214-5B). When the ventricular response is regular and not a simple fraction of the atrial rate, complete AV block is present, which may be a manifestation of digitalis toxicity. Activation mapping suggests that atrial flutter is a form of atrial reentry localized to the right atrium.

℞ TREATMENT

The most effective treatment of atrial flutter is DC cardioversion, which can be accomplished at low energy (25 to 50 W·s) under mild sedation. Higher energies (100 to 200 W·s) are often used because they are less likely to cause AF, which not infrequently occurs following lower energy delivery. Although atrial flutter is associated with a slightly lower risk of embolization than AF, the same precautions should be followed in regard to anticoagulation as are used with AF. The reason for the increased risk of emboli in atrial flutter is uncertain, but the coexistence of AF is common. In patients who develop atrial flutter following open-heart surgery or recurrent flutter in the setting of acute myocardial infarction, particularly if they are being treated with digitalis, atrial pacing (using temporary pacing wires implanted at the time of operation or a pacing lead inserted into the atrium pervenously) at rates of 115 to 130% of the atrial flutter rate can usually convert the atrial flutter to sinus rhythm. Atrial pacing may also result in the conversion of atrial flutter to AF, which allows for easier control of the ventricular response.

If immediate conversion of atrial flutter is not mandated by the patient's clinical status, the ventricular response should first be slowed by blocking the AV node with a beta blocker, calcium antagonist, or digitalis. Digitalis is the least effective and occasionally converts atrial flutter into AF. Once AV nodal conduction is slowed with any of these drugs, an attempt to convert flutter to sinus rhythm using a class I (A or C) agent or amiodarone should be made. Increasing doses of the drug selected are administered until the rhythm converts or side effects occur. Ibutilide is a new antiarrhythmic agent that is administered intravenously and appears to be particularly effective for conversion of atrial flutter to sinus rhythm.

Quinidine, other class IA drugs, flecainide, propafenone, sotalol, dofetilide, and amiodarone (Table 214-4) may be useful in preventing recurrences of atrial flutter. Radiofrequency ablation is a highly effective treatment for patients with the most typical forms of atrial flutter, which are due to reentry around the tricuspid valve in a counterclockwise or clockwise fashion. The coronary sinus and inferior vena cava cause the wavefront of activation to pass between them and the tricuspid valve. Ablation of the narrowed isthmus using radiofrequency energy can cure flutter in >85% of cases. This is far more successful than the response to drugs. As such, ablation is considered by many to be the therapy of choice for recurrent atrial flutter.

PAROXYSMAL SUPRAVENTRICULAR TACHYCARDIAS (Fig. 214-7) In most cases, functional differences in conduction and refractoriness in the

AV node or the presence of an AV bypass tract provide the substrate for the development of PSVT (previously termed *paroxysmal atrial tachycardia*). Electrophysiologic studies have demonstrated that reentry is responsible for the vast majority of cases of PSVT. Reentry has been localized to the sinus node, atrium, AV node, or a macroreentrant circuit involving conduction in the antegrade direction through the AV node and retrograde through an AV bypass tract (Fig. 214-8). Such a bypass tract may also conduct antegradely, in which case the Wolff-Parkinson-White (WPW) syndrome is said to be present. When the bypass tract manifests only retrograde conduction, it is termed a *concealed bypass tract* (Fig. 214-7B). In these cases, the QRS complex during sinus rhythm is normal. In the absence of the WPW syndrome, reentry through the AV node or through a concealed bypass tract makes up nearly 90% of all PSVTs. Atrial tachycardias due to automaticity are not paroxysmal and often present as an incessant arrhythmia.

AV NODAL REENTRANT TACHYCARDIA There is no age or disease predisposition for the development of AV nodal reentrant tachycardia, the most common cause of supraventricular tachycardia. It is, however, more commonly observed in women. It usually presents as a regular narrow QRS complex tachycardia at rates of 120 to 250 beats/min. APCs that initiate the arrhythmia are almost always associated with a prolonged PR interval. Retrograde P waves may be absent, buried in the QRS complex, or appear as distortions at the terminal parts of the QRS complex (Fig. 214-7A).

AV nodal reentrant PSVT (Fig. 214-7A) can be reproducibly initiated and terminated by appropriately timed atrial premature stimuli. The onset of the tachycardia is almost always associated with prolongation of the PR interval due to marked AV nodal conduction delay (prolonged AH interval) following the APC that is critical for the genesis of the arrhythmia. The sudden prolongation of the AH interval is consistent with the concept of dual AV nodal pathways: a *fast pathway*, which exhibits rapid conduction and a long refractory period, and a *slow pathway*, which has a short refractory period but conducts slowly. During sinus rhythm, only conduction over the fast pathway is manifest, resulting in a normal PR interval (Fig. 214-8). Atrial extrastimuli at a critical coupling interval are blocked in the fast pathway because of its longer refractory period and are conducted slowly through the slow pathway. If conduction down the slow pathway is slow enough to allow the previously refractory fast pathway time to recover excitability, a single atrial (echo) reentrant beat or sustained tachycardia ensues. A critical balance between conduction velocity and refractoriness within the node is required to sustain AV nodal reentry. Retrograde atrial and antegrade ventricular activation occur simultaneously, explaining why P waves may not be apparent on the surface ECG.

Clinical Features AV nodal reentry may produce palpitations, syncope, and heart failure depending on the rate and duration of the arrhythmia and the presence and severity of any underlying heart disease. Hypotension and syncope may occur due to both the sudden loss of the atrial contribution to ventricular filling and a reflex baroreceptor response to simultaneous atrial and ventricular contraction, which produce high atrial pressures. This situation can also result in acute pulmonary edema.

℞ TREATMENT

In patients without hypotension, vagal maneuvers, particularly carotid sinus massage, can terminate the arrhythmia in 80% of cases. If these maneuvers are unsuccessful, adenosine (12 mg intravenously) is the agent of choice. Beta blockers may also be used to slow or terminate the tachycardia but are agents of second choice. Digitalis glycosides have a slower onset of action and should *not* be used for acute therapy. When these drugs fail to terminate the tachycardia, or when the tachycardia is recurrent, atrial or ventricular pacing via a temporary pacemaker inserted pervenously may be used to terminate the arrhythmia.

TABLE 214-4 *Drugs Used to Treat Cardiac Tachyarrhythmias*

Drug	Mode of Administration	$t_{1/2}$ (oral), h	Route of Metabolism	Clinical Effects and/or Indications for Use
Digoxin	IV, 0.25–1.5 mg Oral, 0.75–1.5 mg loading dose over 12–24 h Maintenance, 0.23–0.50 mg/kg	36	Renal	Slowing of ventricular rate during AF, flutter, and other atrial tachycardias in the absence of preexcitation; slowing, termination, and/or prevention of SVT due to AV nodal reentry and AV reentry utilizing bypass tracts; may terminate or prevent intraatrial reentrant tachycardias; ineffective in prevention of automatic atrial tachycardias
Adenosine	IV bolus, 6–12 mg	<10s		Acute termination of regular reentrant SVT involving the AV node
Quinidine (class IA)	Oral, 200–400 mg q6h	8–9	Hepatic, 80% Renal, 20%	Atrial and ventricular tachyarrhythmias; all types of SVT; control of ventricular rate in patients with preexcitation and AF and flutter
Procainamide (class IA)	IV, 40–50 mg/min to total of 10–20 mg/kg Oral, 500–1000 mg q6h (sustained-release forms)	3–5	Hepatic, 50% Renal, 50%	Same as quinidine
Disopyramide (class IA)	Oral, 100–300 mg q6h	8–9	Hepatic, 50% Renal, 50%	Same as quinidine
Lidocaine (class IB)	IV, 20–50 mg/min to total of 5 mg/kg loading dose, followed by 1–4 mg/kg	1–2	Hepatic	VT and VF, especially during acute ischemia and myocardial infarction
Phenytoin (class IB)	IV, 20 mg/kg to total dose of 1000 mg Oral, 1000-mg loading dose over 24 h Maintenance, 100–400 mg/d	18–36	Hepatic	Tachyarrhythmias induced by digitalis; occasionally effective for ventricular tachyarrhythmias not induced by digitalis alone or in combination with other antiarrhythmic agents; polymorphic VT associated with increased QT interval
Mexiletine (class IB)	Oral, 100–300 mg q6–8h	9–12	Hepatic	Ventricular tachyarrhythmias; secondary agent in combination with other class I medication
Flecainide (class IC)	Oral, begin at 50–100 mg bid, increase by ≤50 mg in 4-day intervals to a maximum of mg daily	7–23	Hepatic, 75% Renal, 25%	Supraventricular tachyarrhythmias including atrial fibrillation and flutter; also ventricular arrhythmias refractory to other medications or radiofrequency ablation
Propafenone (class IC)	Oral, 150–300 mg q8h	5–8	Hepatic	Same as flecainide
Moricizine (class IC)	Oral, 200–400 mg q8h	2–6	Hepatic	Same as flecainide
Beta blockers (class II) e.g., metoprolol	IV, load with 5–10 mg q5min for 3 doses, then 3 mg q6h Oral, 25–100 mg bid	3–4	Hepatic	Slowing of ventricular rate during AF, atrial flutter, and other atrial tachyarrhythmias in the absence of preexcitation; SVT due to AV nodal reentry; reentry utilizing bypass tracts; arrhythmias (e.g., VT) induced by exercise or occurring in the presence of hyperthyroidism; polymorphic VT associated with congenital long QT syndrome
Bretylium (class III)	IV, 1–2 mg/kg per min to total load, 5–10 mg/kg Maintenance, 0.5–2 mg/kg	8–14	Renal	Refractory VT and VF, especially due to acute ischemia
Amiodarone (class III)	IV, 5–10 mg/kg load over 20 min, then 1 g/24 h Oral, load 800–1600 mg/d for 1 week, then 400–600 mg/d for 3 weeks, then 200–400 mg/d thereafter	13–103	Hepatic	Sustained VT and VF AF and atrial flutter, other types of SVT, VT, VF
Sotalol (class III)	Oral, 80–320 mg q12h	10–20	Renal, 90% Hepatic, 10%	Atrial and ventricular tachyarrhythmias
Ibutilide (class III)	IV, <60 kg: 0.01 mg/kg over 10 min IV, ≥60 kg: 1 mg over 10 min, repeat after 10 min if no effect	2–6	Hepatic	AF, atrial flutter, and other SVTs including preexcitation tachycardias
Dofetilide	125–250 mg PO bid	8–12	Renal	AF, atrial flutter, and other SVTs
Calcium channel blockers (class IV) e.g., verapamil	IV, 2.5–10 mg over 1–2 min to total of 0.15 mg/kg Oral, 240–480 qd	6–24	Hepatic	Slowing of ventricular rate during AF and flutter, and other SVTs in the absence of preexcitation; idiopathic VT
Diltiazem	IV, load with 0.25 mg/kg over 2 min; if needed, repeat after 15 min with 0.35 mg over 2 min Maintenance, 10–15 mg/h		Hepatic	Same as verapamil

Note: AF, atrial fibrillation; AV, atrioventricular; SVT, supraventricular tachycardia; VF, ventricular fibrillation; VT, ventricular tachycardia.

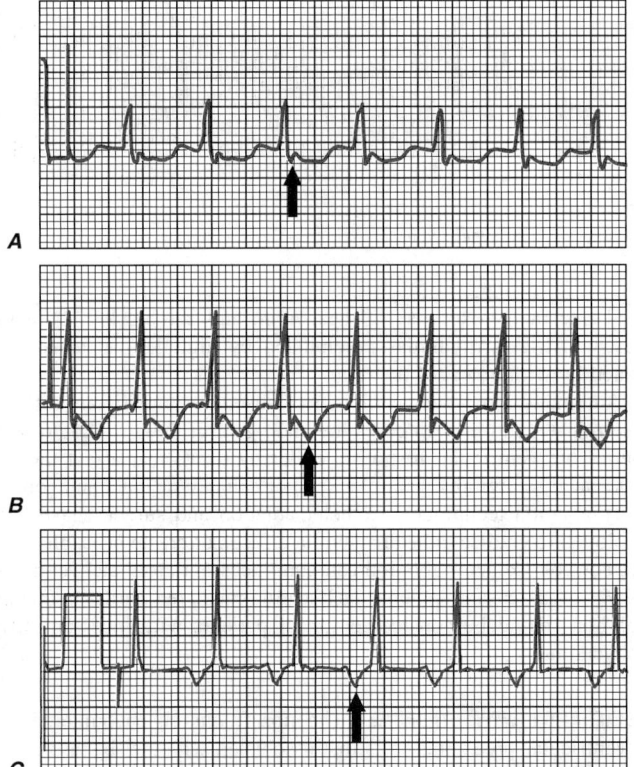

FIGURE 214-7 Examples of supraventricular tachycardia (SVT). Arrows indicate P waves. *A.* AV nodal reentry. Upright P waves are visible at the end of the QRS complex. *B.* AV reentry using a concealed bypass tract. Inverted retrograde P waves are superimposed on the T waves. *C.* Automatic atrial tachycardia. Inverted P waves follow the T waves and precede the QRS complex.

However, if severe ischemia and/or hypotension is caused by the tachycardia, (DC) cardioversion should be considered.

AV nodal reentry can usually be prevented by the use of drugs that act primarily on the antegrade slow pathway (such as digitalis, beta blockers, or calcium channel antagonists) or on the fast pathway (class IA or IC; Table 214-4). We favor initial therapy with beta blockers, calcium channel antagonists, or digoxin because the risk-benefit ratio associated with treatment with these agents is more favorable than that of IA or IC agents. Drugs most likely to avert recurrences prevent induction of the arrhythmias by programmed stimulation. This technique utilizes temporary pacemaker catheters connected to a physiologic stimulator capable of variable rate pacing and stimulation with one or more precisely timed premature impulses. In the past decade it has been recognized that in symptomatic patients who require chronic therapy, radiofrequency catheter modification of the AV node should be considered the treatment of choice. This technique can cure AV nodal reentry in >95% of cases and has been proven to be safe, although a 1 to 2% risk of AV block requiring a permanent pacemaker exists.

AV REENTRANT TACHYCARDIA PSVT due to AV reentry incorporates a concealed AV bypass tract as part of the tachycardia circuit. Thus the impulse passes antegradely from the atria through the AV node and His-Purkinje system to the ventricles and then retrogradely through the (concealed) bypass tract back to

the atrium. Patients with this disorder manifest the same type of PSVT as do patients with the WPW syndrome (see below), but the bypass tract cannot conduct in an antegrade direction during sinus rhythm or other atrial tachyarrhythmias.

AV reentrant tachycardia can be initiated and terminated by either APCs or VPCs. Initiation of PSVT by a VPC is virtually diagnostic of AV reentry. Alternation of the QRS complexes occurs in approximately one-third of such tachycardias. Since atrial activation must follow ventricular activation during AV reentry, the P wave usually occurs after the QRS complex (Fig. 214-7*B*).

Atrial activation mapping is of major value in evaluating the origin of these tachycardias. Most concealed bypass tracts are left-sided. Thus, during PSVT or during ventricular pacing, the earliest activation sequence is recorded in the left atrium, usually via a catheter in the coronary sinus. This eccentric atrial activation is quite distinct from the normal retrograde activation sequence in which the earliest activation of the atria is in the area of the AV junction. The ability of a ventricular stimulus to conduct to the atrium at a time when the bundle of His is refractory or more specifically terminate the tachycardia without depolarizing the atria is diagnostic of retrograde conduction over a concealed bypass tract.

℞ TREATMENT

This is similar to the treatment for AV nodal reentry tachycardia. Although pharmacologic agents may be used, patients who require chronic therapy should be considered candidates for radiofrequency catheter ablation of the bypass tract. This requires detailed electrophysiologic study to exclude other arrhythmias that may be responsible for patients' symptoms and to determine the location of the bypass tract(s). The efficacy of this procedure exceeds 90%, with minimal risks. In the remaining small number of patients failing catheter ablation, surgical ablation or pharmacologic therapy can be used.

SINUS NODE REENTRY AND OTHER ATRIAL TACHYCARDIAS Reentry in the region of the sinus node or within the atria is invariably initiated by APCs. These arrhythmias are less common than AV nodal or AV

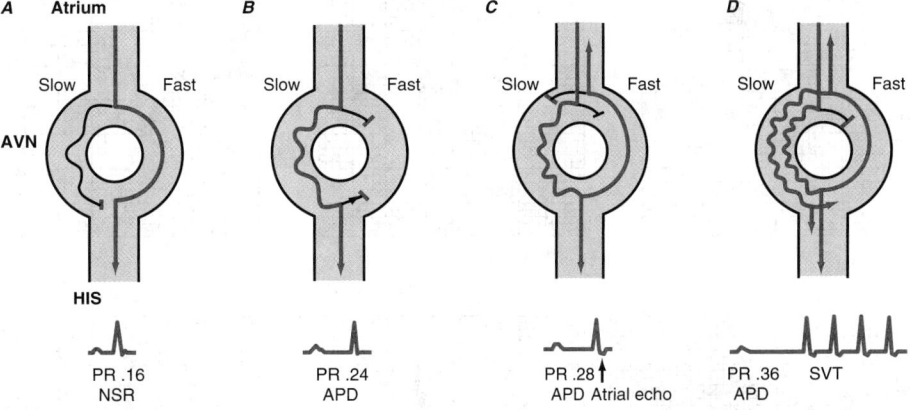

FIGURE 214-8 Mechanism of AV nodal reentry: The atrium, AV node (AVN), and His bundle are shown schematically. The AV node is longitudinally dissociated into two pathways, slow and fast, with different functional properties (see text). In each panel of this diagram, red lines denote excitation in the AV node, which is manifest on the surface electrocardiogram (ECG), while black lines denote conduction that is concealed and not apparent on the surface electrocardiogram. *A.* During sinus rhythm (NSR) the impulse from the atrium conducts down both pathways. However, only conduction over the fast pathway is manifest on the surface ECG, producing a normal PR interval of 0.16 s. *B.* An atrial premature depolarization (APD) blocks in the fast pathway. The impulse conducts over the slow pathway to the His bundle and ventricles, producing a PR interval of 0.24 s. Because the impulse is premature, conduction over the slow pathway occurs more slowly than it would during sinus rhythm. *C.* A more premature atrial impulse blocks in the fast pathway, conducting with increased delay in the slow pathway, producing a PR interval of 0.28 s. The impulse conducts retrogradely up the fast pathway producing a single atrial echo. Sustained reentry is prevented by subsequent block in the slow pathway. *D.* A still more premature atrial impulse blocks initially in the fast pathway, conducting over the slow pathway with increasing delay, producing a PR interval of 0.36 s. Retrograde conduction occurs over the fast pathway and reentry occurs, producing a sustained tachycardia (SVT). *(After ME Josephson: Clinical Cardiac Electrophysiology, 2d ed. Philadelphia, Lea & Febiger, 2002; with permission.)*

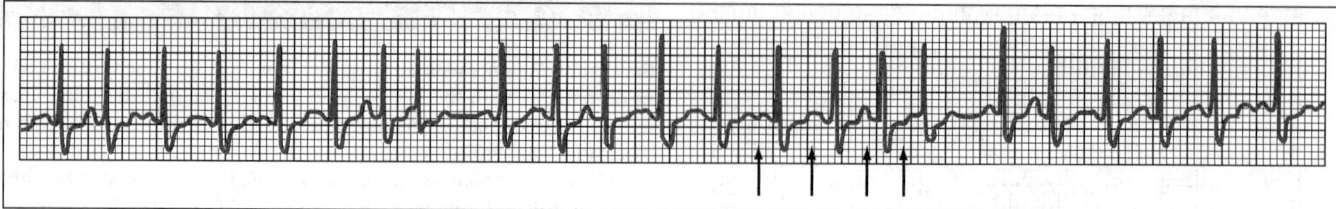

FIGURE 214-9 Multifocal atrial tachycardia. A lead I rhythm strip demonstrates a multifocal atrial tachycardia defined by ≥3 consecutive P waves of variable morphology and rate >100 beats/min (*arrows*).

reentry and are more often associated with underlying cardiac disease. During sinus node reentry, the P-wave morphology is identical to that occurring in sinus rhythm, but the PR interval is prolonged. This is in contrast to sinus tachycardia, in which the PR interval tends to shorten. With intraatrial reentry, the P-wave configuration differs from that during sinus rhythm, and the PR interval is prolonged.

℞ TREATMENT

Sinus node and atrial reentrant arrhythmias are managed like other reentrant PSVTs, except that catheter ablation is less successful because multiple foci may be present.

NONREENTRANT ATRIAL TACHYCARDIAS   These may be a manifestation of digitalis intoxication or may be associated with severe pulmonary or cardiac disease, with hypokalemia, or with the administration of theophylline or adrenergic drugs. Multifocal atrial tachycardia (MAT) (Fig. 214-9) is particularly common following theophylline administration. By definition, MAT requires three or more consecutive P waves of different morphologies at rates greater than 100 beats/min. MAT usually has an irregular ventricular rate because of varying AV conduction. There is a high incidence of AF (50 to 70%) in patients with MAT.

℞ TREATMENT

Treatment should be directed at the underlying disorder. The digitalis-induced arrhythmias are caused by triggered activity. In such atrial tachycardias with AV block secondary to digitalis intoxication, the atrial rate rarely exceeds 180 beats/min, and 2:1 block is typically present. Atrial arrhythmias precipitated by digitalis can usually be treated by withdrawal of the drug.

Automatic atrial tachycardias not caused by digitalis are difficult to terminate, and in such cases the main goal of therapy should be to control the ventricular response, either by drugs that affect the AV node, such as digitalis, beta blockers, or calcium channel antagonists, or by ablation techniques. Catheter ablation and surgery have been employed to eradicate the arrhythmia's focus or create heart block for rate control. Catheter ablation can cure incessant atrial tachycardia in <75% of cases and reverse tachycardia-mediated cardiomyopathy. Ablation should be considered for all patients with incessant atrial tachycardia.

PREEXCITATION (WPW) SYNDROME   The most frequently encountered type of ventricular preexcitation is that associated with AV bypass tracts. These connections are composed of strands of atrial-like muscle, which may occur almost anywhere around the AV rings. The term *Wolff-Parkinson-White syndrome* is applied to patients with both preexcitation on the ECG and paroxysmal tachycardias. AV bypass tracts can be associated with certain congenital abnormalities, the most important of which is Ebstein's anomaly.

AV bypass tracts that conduct in an antegrade direction produce a typical ECG pattern of a short PR interval (<0.12 s), a slurred upstroke of the QRS complex (delta wave), and a wide QRS complex. This pattern results from a fusion of activation of the ventricles over both the bypass tract and the AV nodal His-Purkinje system (Fig. 214-10). The relative contribution of activation over each system determines the amount of preexcitation.

During PSVT in WPW, the impulse is usually conducted antegradely over the normal AV system and retrogradely through the bypass tract. The characteristics are identical to those described on p. 1347. Rarely (~5%), tachycardias occurring in patients with WPW will exhibit a reverse pattern with antegrade conduction through the bypass tract and retrograde conduction through the normal AV system. This produces a tachycardia with a wide QRS complex in which the ventricles are totally activated by the bypass tract. Atrial flutter and AF also occur commonly in patients with WPW syndrome. Since the bypass tract does not have the same decremental conducting properties as the AV node, the ventricular responses during atrial flutter or fibrillation may be unusually rapid and may cause VF.

The goals of electrophysiologic evaluation in patients suspected of having the WPW syndrome are (1) to confirm the diagnosis, (2) to localize the bypass tract and determine how many

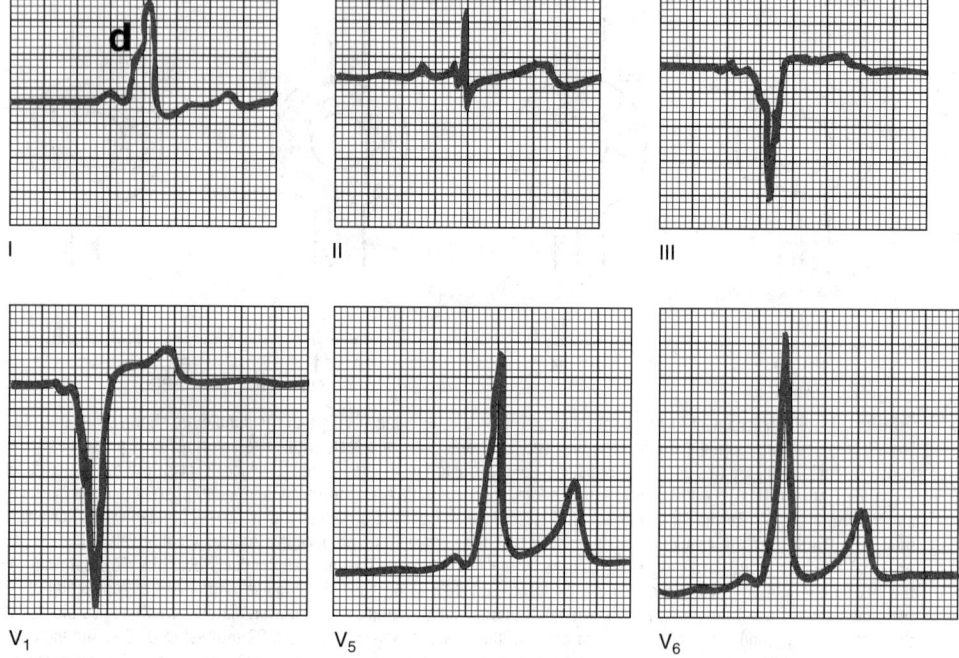

FIGURE 214-10   ECG in Wolff-Parkinson-White syndrome. There is a short PR interval (0.11 s), a wide QRS complex (0.12 s), and slurring on the upstroke of the QRS produced by early ventricular activation over the bypass tract (delta wave, d in lead I). The negative delta waves in V_1 are diagnostic of a right-sided bypass tract. Note the Q wave (negative delta wave) in lead III, mimicking myocardial infarction.

bypass tracts are present, (3) to demonstrate the role of the bypass tract in the genesis of the arrhythmias, (4) to determine the potential for the development of possibly life-threatening rates during atrial flutter or fibrillation, and (5) to evaluate therapeutic options.

℞ TREATMENT

Pharmacologic therapy is aimed at altering the electrophysiologic properties (i.e., refractoriness or conduction velocity) of one or more components of the reentrant circuit. This is most often accomplished by agents such as beta blockers or calcium channel blockers that slow conduction and increase refractoriness of the AV node or by agents such as quinidine or flecainide that slow conduction and increase refractoriness primarily in the bypass tract. Some drugs may affect multiple sites.

Acute management of episodes of PSVT in patients with WPW syndrome is similar to that of PSVT in patients with concealed bypass tracts.

In patients with the WPW syndrome and AF, DC cardioversion should be carried out if there is a life-threatening, rapid ventricular response. In non-life-threatening situations, lidocaine (3 to 5 mg/kg) or procainamide (15 mg/kg) administered intravenously over 15 to 20 min will usually slow the ventricular response. More recently, ibutilide has become available as an alternative therapy for preexcitation tachycardia. Caution should be employed when using digitalis or intravenous verapamil in patients with the WPW syndrome and AF, since these drugs can shorten the refractory period of the accessory pathway and can increase the ventricular rate, thereby placing the patient at increased risk for VF. Chronic oral therapy with verapamil is not associated with this risk. In addition to these drugs, beta-blocking agents are of no utility in controlling the ventricular response during AF when conduction proceeds over the bypass tract. Although atrial or ventricular pacing can almost always terminate PSVT in patients with the WPW syndrome, they can induce AF. As such, chronic pacemaker therapy is to be discouraged.

While surgical ablation of bypass tracts offers a permanent cure of supraventricular tachycardia (SVT) and most AFs associated with SVT, the advent of radiofrequency catheter ablation has virtually eliminated the need for surgery. Catheter ablation of bypass tracts is possible in >90% of patients and is the treatment of choice in patients with symptomatic arrhythmias. It is safer, more cost-effective, and just as successful as surgery. Nevertheless, surgical ablation may be required in the occasional patient in whom catheter ablation fails.

NONPAROXYSMAL JUNCTIONAL TACHYCARDIA This rhythm usually results from conditions that produce enhanced automaticity or triggered activity in the AV junction and is most commonly due to digitalis intoxication, inferior wall myocardial infarction, myocarditis, endogenous or exogenous catecholamine excess, acute rheumatic fever, or valve surgery.

The onset of nonparoxysmal junctional tachycardia is usually gradual, with a "warm-up" period prior to stabilization of the rate, which can range from 70 to 150 beats/min, faster rates usually being associated with digitalis intoxication. Nonparoxysmal junctional tachycardia is recognized by a QRS complex identical to that of sinus rhythm. The rate can be influenced by autonomic tone and can be increased by catecholamines, vagolytic agents, or exercise and slowed somewhat by carotid sinus pressure. When this rhythm is due to digitalis intoxication, it usually is associated with AV block and/or dissociation. Soon after cardiac surgery, retrograde conduction is more likely to be present because of the heightened sympathetic state.

℞ TREATMENT

This is directed toward elimination of the underlying etiologic factors. Since digitalis is the most common cause of this rhythm, discontinuation of this drug is indicated. If the rhythm is associated with other serious manifestations of digitalis intoxication, such as ventricular or atrial irritability, active intervention with lidocaine or a beta blocker

may be useful, and in some instances use of digitalis antibodies (Fab fragments) should be considered. Cardioversion of this rhythm should not be attempted, particularly in the setting of digitalis intoxication. When AV conduction is intact, atrial pacing can capture and override the junctional focus and provide the AV synchrony necessary to maximize cardiac output. Nonparoxysmal junctional tachycardia is usually not a chronic, recurrent problem, and attention to the acute precipitating events can often resolve the tachycardia.

VENTRICULAR TACHYCARDIA *Sustained ventricular tachycardia* is defined as VT that persists for >30 s or requires termination because of hemodynamic collapse. VT generally accompanies some form of structural heart disease, most commonly chronic ischemic heart disease associated with a prior myocardial infarction. Sustained VT may also be associated with nonischemic cardiomyopathies, metabolic disorders, drug toxicity, or prolonged QT syndrome, and it occurs occasionally in the absence of heart disease or other predisposing factors. Nonsustained VT (three beats to 30 s) is also associated with cardiac disease but occurs in its absence more often than the sustained arrhythmia. While nonsustained VT usually does not produce symptoms, sustained VT is almost always symptomatic and is often associated with marked hemodynamic compromise and/or the development of myocardial ischemia. A fixed anatomic substrate, not acute ischemia, is responsible for most recurrent episodes of sustained uniform VT. Acute ischemia appears to have little role in the genesis of sustained uniform VT associated with chronic infarction but may play a role in the degeneration of stable VT into VF or initiation of polymorphic VT. Most episodes of VF begin with VT.

The ECG diagnosis of VT is suggested by a wide-complex QRS tachycardia at a rate exceeding 100 beats/min. The QRS configuration during any episode of VT may be uniform (monomorphic) or it may vary from beat to beat (polymorphic). *Bidirectional tachycardia* refers to VT that shows an alternation in QRS axis. Typically this appears as a QRS with a right bundle branch block pattern with alternating superior (leftward) and inferior axes (rightward). While the rhythm is usually quite regular, slight irregularity may exist. Atrial activity may be dissociated from ventricular activity, or the atria may be depolarized retrogradely. The onset of the tachycardia is generally abrupt, but in nonparoxysmal tachycardias it can be gradual. Paroxysmal VT is usually initiated by a VPC.

It is important to distinguish SVT with aberration of intraventricular conduction from VT because the clinical implications and management of these two arrhythmias are totally different. The most important clinical predictor of VT is the presence of structural heart disease. The observation of intermittent cannon *a* waves and varying first heart sounds suggests AV dissociation and is diagnostic of VT. In a majority of cases, the diagnosis can and should be made by close examination of the 12-lead ECG. Pharmacologic maneuvers, such as administration of intravenous verapamil or adenosine, can be hazardous and should be avoided. It is always useful to have a 12-lead ECG recorded during sinus rhythm for comparison with that during tachycardia. When the tracing obtained during sinus rhythm demonstrates the same morphologic features as those during the tachycardia, the diagnosis of PSVT with aberration is favored. An infarction pattern on the sinus rhythm tracing suggests the potential presence of the anatomic substrate necessary for VT.

Characteristics of the 12-lead ECG during the tachycardia that suggest a ventricular origin for the arrhythmia are (1) a QRS complex >0.14 s in the absence of antiarrhythmic therapy, (2) AV dissociation (with or without fusion or captured beats) or variable retrograde conduction (Fig. 214-11), (3) a superior QRS axis in the presence of a right bundle branch block pattern, (4) concordance of the QRS pattern in all precordial leads (i.e., all positive or all negative deflections), and (5) other QRS patterns (morphology) with prolonged duration that are inconsistent with typical right or left bundle branch block patterns (Table 214-5). A wide, complex, bizarre tachycardia that is very ir-

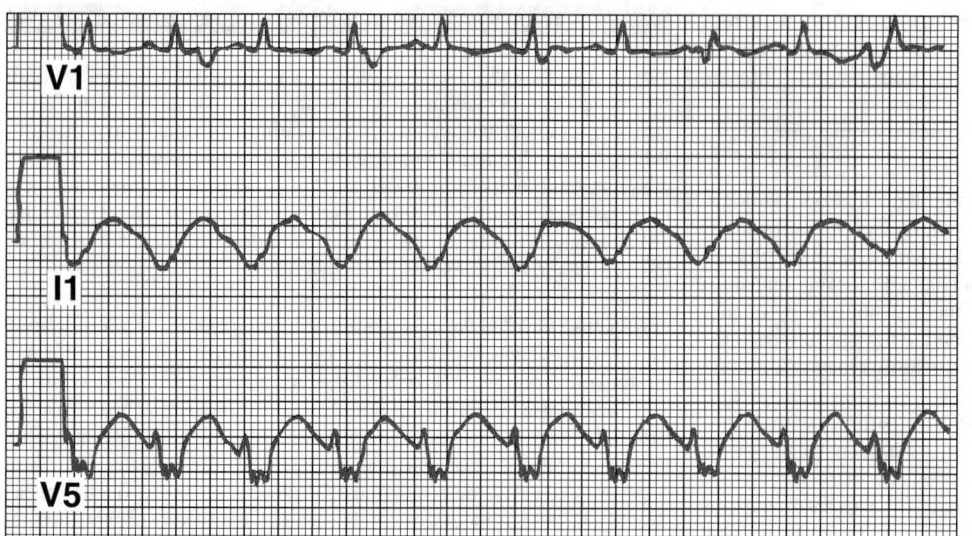

FIGURE 214-11 Ventricular tachycardia with AV dissociation. P waves are dissociated from the underlying wide complex rhythm (best seen on lead V₁).

regular suggests AF with conduction over an AV bypass tract. Similarly, a QRS complex in excess of 0.20 s is uncommon during VT in the absence of drug therapy and is more common with preexcitation. Intravenous verapamil will stop most recalcitrant SVTs involving the AV junction, but it is rarely effective for VT. Because of this property, verapamil has been utilized to attempt to differentiate SVT with aberrant conduction from VT. However, this is extremely hazardous, since intravenous verapamil can precipitate cardiac arrest in patients with VT. A similar caveat can be made for use of adenosine. This agent can produce a coronary stent in patients with multivessel disease and produce a cardiac arrest.

It has been possible to replicate sustained uniform VT in >95% of patients with this arrhythmia using programmed electrical stimulation. In most patients the tachycardia is initiated with ventricular premature stimuli. A sustained monomorphic VT with a morphology identical to that of the spontaneous arrhythmia is the rule. The clinical significance of polymorphic VT initiated by programmed stimulation is not clear, since more aggressive stimulation (i.e., the use of three or four extrastimuli) can induce polymorphic VT and even VF in some normal subjects and in patients who have never had a clinical arrhythmia.

Sustained uniform VT can be terminated by programmed stimulation or rapid pacing in at least 75% of patients; the remainder require cardioversion. The ability to reproducibly initiate and terminate a sustained, uniform VT permits assessment of pharmacologic and electrical therapy of these arrhythmias.

The reproducible termination of VT by programmed stimulation permits evaluation of the effectiveness of antitachycardia pacemakers for long-term therapy of paroxysmal episodes of arrhythmia. Unfortunately, rapid pacing, the most effective form of therapy, can accelerate the tachycardia and/or produce VF. Therefore, antitachycardia pacing is a viable form of therapy only when the pacing device includes backup defibrillation capabilities.

Clinical Features Symptoms resulting from VT depend on the ventricular rate, duration of the tachycardia, and presence and extent of underlying cardiac disease. When the tachycardia is rapid and associated with severe myocardial dysfunction and cerebrovascular disease, hypotension and syncope are common. However, the presence of hemodynamic stability does not preclude a diagnosis of VT. The rate, loss of the atrial contribution to ventricular filling, and abnormal sequence of ventricular activation are important factors producing a decreased cardiac output during VT.

The *prognosis* of VT depends on the underlying disease state. If sustained VT develops within the first 6 weeks following acute myocardial infarction, the prognosis is poor, with a 75% mortality rate at 1 year. Patients with nonsustained VT following myocardial infarction

have a threefold greater risk of death than a comparable group of patients without this arrhythmia. However, a cause-and-effect relationship between the nonsustained tachycardia and subsequent sudden death has not been established. Patients without heart disease who have uniform VT have a good prognosis and an extremely low risk of sudden death.

℞ TREATMENT

The risk-benefit ratio of treating each specific type of VT should be considered before beginning therapy. This is important because antiarrhythmic agents can produce or exacerbate the very arrhythmias that they are given to prevent. In general, patients with VT but without organic heart disease have a benign course; such patients with asymptomatic, nonsustained VT need not be treated because their prognosis will not be affected. An exception is the patient with congenital long QT syndrome. Such patients have recurrent polymorphic VT and a high mortality from sudden death if untreated. Patients with sustained VT in the absence of heart disease usually require therapy because the arrhythmia causes symptoms. These tachycardias may respond to beta blockers; verapamil; class IA, IC, or III agents; or amiodarone.

In patients with VT and organic heart disease, if marked hemodynamic compromise is present or if there is evidence of ischemia, CHF, or central nervous system hypoperfusion, the rhythm should be promptly terminated by (DC) cardioversion (see below). If the patient with organic heart disease tolerates the VT well, pharmacologic therapy may be tried. Procainamide is probably the most effective agent

TABLE 214-5 *Wide Complex Tachycardia*
ECG CRITERIA THAT FAVOR VENTRICULAR TACHYCARDIA

1. AV dissociation
2. QRS width: >0.14 s with RBBB configuration
   >0.16 s with LBBB configuration
3. QRS axis: Left axis deviation with RBBB morphology
   Extreme left axis deviation (northwest axis) with LBBB morphology
4. Concordance of QRS in precordial leads
5. Morphologic patterns of the QRS complex
   RBBB: Mono- or biphasic complex in V₁
   RS (*only with left axis deviation*) or QS in V₆

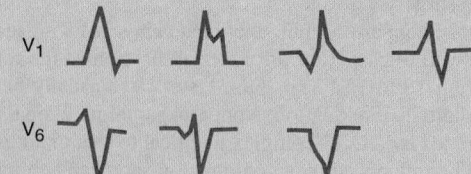

   LBBB: Broad R wave in V₁ or V₂ ≥0.04 s
   Onset of QRS to nadir of S wave in V₁ or V₂ of ≥0.07 s
   Notched downslope of S wave in V₁ or V₂
   Q wave in V₆

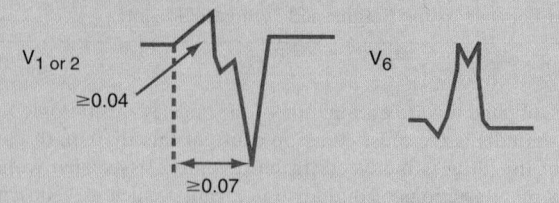

Note: AV, atrioventricular; BBB, bundle branch block.

for acute therapy. It may or may not terminate the tachycardia but almost always slows the rate. In stable patients in whom these drugs do not terminate the arrhythmia, a pacing catheter can be inserted pervenously into the right ventricular apex, and the tachycardia can be terminated by overdrive pacing.

Although programmed stimulation has been used to select the appropriate antiarrhythmic agent to prevent recurrent, sustained VT, recent data suggest ICD implantation is more effective. As such, drugs are used in patients in whom ICDs are contraindicated or according to patient preference. These drugs may also be used as adjunctive therapy with ICDs to suppress recurrent ventricular or coexisting supraventricular arrhythmias.

Antitachycardia pacing has been used as a means to terminate tachycardias that have been reproducibly terminated by pacing in the electrophysiology laboratory. Automatic antitachycardia pacing devices are not used alone because pacing during VT may accelerate tachycardia, converting a stable arrhythmia into an unstable one and resulting in severe hemodynamic compromise. However, devices combining antitachycardia pacing with an ICD (see below) afford a "backup" means of terminating unstable arrhythmias.

The advent of endocardial catheter and intraoperative mapping led to the development of surgical techniques for the management of VT. Even though most patients with VT and ischemic heart disease have markedly impaired left ventricular function and multivessel coronary artery disease, the operative mortality rate has ranged between 8 and 15%. Following operation, >90% of survivors are controlled either off (two-thirds of patients) or on (one-third) antiarrhythmic agents that were previously ineffective in controlling these rhythms. With the development of radiofrequency ablation and refinement of mapping criteria to locate the critical sites of the VT circuit precisely, catheter ablation can be performed as a curative procedure in selected patients. In experienced centers, cure of VT in these *selected* patients approaches 75%.

Specific Types of VT *Torsades de pointes* (Fig. 214-12) refers to VT characterized by polymorphic QRS complexes that change in amplitude and cycle length, giving the appearance of oscillations around the baseline. This rhythm is, by definition, associated with QT prolongation. The latter may result from electrolyte disturbances (particularly hypokalemia and hypomagnesemia), use of a variety of antiarrhythmic drugs (especially quinidine), phenothiazines and tricyclic antidepressants, liquid protein diets, intracranial events, and bradyarrhythmias, particularly third-degree AV block. It may also occur as a congenital anomaly that most often presents with torsades de pointes (syncope or sudden death) at a young age.

The electrocardiographic hallmark is polymorphic VT preceded by marked QT prolongation, often in excess of 0.60 s. These patients often have multiple episodes of nonsustained polymorphic VT associated with recurrent syncope, but they may also develop VF and sudden cardiac death.

℞ TREATMENT

This should be directed at removing the precipitating factors, i.e., correcting metabolic abnormalities and removing drugs that have induced the prolonged QT interval. In the setting of drug-induced torsades de pointes, atrial or ventricular overdrive pacing and the administration of magnesium have also been useful in terminating and preventing the arrhythmia. For patients with the congenital prolonged QT interval syndrome, β-adrenergic blocking agents have been the mainstay of therapy; agents that shorten the QT interval may also be useful (e.g., phenytoin). Cervicothoracic sympathectomy has been proposed as a form of therapy for congenital prolonged QT syndrome, but it is not often effective as the sole therapy. Pacing in combination with beta blockers and sympathectomy has been used by some investigators when beta blockers fail, but it is not uniformly successful and results in a Horner's syndrome. ICDs with dual-chambered pacing capability and beta blockers have become the treatment of choice for patients with recurrent episodes despite beta blockers.

Polymorphic tachycardias associated with normal QT intervals in patients with ischemic heart disease that are initiated by "R-on-T" VPCs are probably caused by reentry, and their treatment is totally different. They should not be considered torsades de pointes. In such cases, class I or III agents may be the most effective form of therapy and should be administered in full antiarrhythmic doses. However, these arrhythmias may also result from acute, severe ischemia and will only respond to abolition of the ischemia, usually by revascularization. Another group of patients has recently been defined who have polymorphic VT initiated by short coupled VPCs during exercise or other catecholamine states due to triggered activity associated with release of Ca^{2+} from the sarcoplasmic reticulum. This is a lethal syndrome requiring an implantable defibrillator.

Accelerated idioventricular rhythm, also termed *slow VT*, with a rate that ranges from 60 to 120 beats/min, usually occurs in acute myocardial infarction, often during reperfusion. It may also be seen following cardiac operations; in patients with cardiomyopathy, rheumatic fever, or digitalis intoxication; and in patients with no evidence of heart disease. The rhythm is usually transient and rarely causes significant hemodynamic compromise or symptoms. Treatment is rarely necessary and should usually be considered only if symptoms arise due to impaired hemodynamics, most commonly due to AV dissociation. In most cases, atropine can accelerate the sinus rate to overdrive the ventricular rhythm.

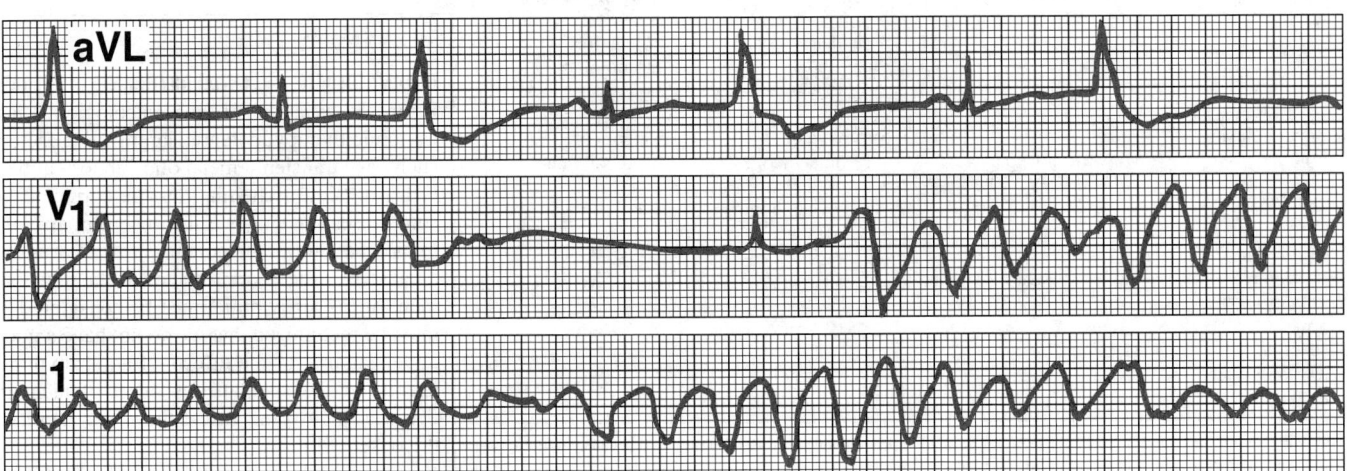

FIGURE 214-12 Rhythm strips of patients with drug (disopyramide)-induced torsades de pointes. The polymorphic ventricular tachycardia is associated with very long QT intervals.

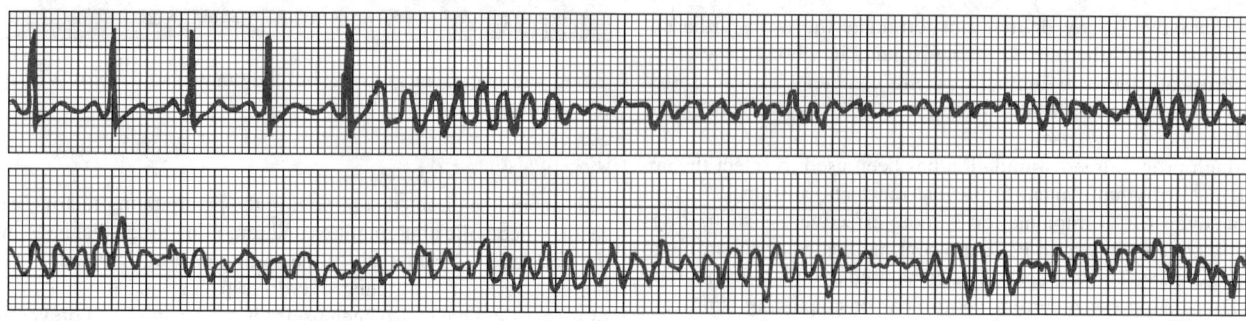

FIGURE 214-13 Ventricular fibrillation. In a patient with coronary disease, ventricular fibrillation is initiated by an early ventricular premature complex that produces a rapid polymorphic ventricular tachycardia, which rapidly degenerates to ventricular fibrillation (note the undulating baseline with indistinguishable systole and diastole).

VENTRICULAR FLUTTER AND VENTRICULAR FIBRILLATION (Fig. 214-13; see also Chap. 256) These arrhythmias occur most often in patients with ischemic heart disease. They also occur following administration of antiarrhythmic drugs, particularly those that induce prolonged QT intervals and torsades de pointes (see above), in patients with severe hypoxia or ischemia, and in those with WPW syndrome who develop AF with an extremely rapid ventricular response (p. 1345). Electrical accidents frequently cause cardiac arrest due to the development of VF. The onset of these arrhythmias is rapidly followed by loss of consciousness and, if untreated, death. Episodes of cardiac arrest recorded during Holter monitoring reveal that approximately three-fourths of the sudden deaths are due to VT or VF.

In patients with nonischemic VF, the onset usually begins with a short run of rapid VT, which is initiated by a relatively late coupled VPC. In patients with acute myocardial infarction or ischemia, however, VF is usually precipitated by a single early ventricular complex beat falling on the T wave (the vulnerable period), which produces a rapid VT that degenerates into VF (Fig. 214-13).

The clinical setting in which VF occurs is important. Most patients who have primary VF within the first 48 h of the onset of acute infarction have a good long-term prognosis, with a very low rate of recurrence or sudden cardiac death. Their short-term mortality may, however, be slightly increased. In contrast, patients who experience VF unassociated with the development of acute myocardial infarction have a recurrence rate of 20 to 30% in the year following the event (Chap. 256).

Ventricular flutter usually appears as a sine wave with a rate between 150 and 300 beats/min. These oscillations make it impossible to assign a specific morphology to the arrhythmia and in some cases to distinguish it from rapid VT. VF is recognized by grossly irregular undulations of varying amplitudes, contours, and rates (Fig. 214-13). Electrophysiologic studies have demonstrated that regardless of the apparent gross irregularity on the surface ECG, VF usually starts out with a rapid repetitive sequence of VT that ultimately breaks down into multiple wavelets of reentry.

Electrophysiologic studies have been useful in patients who have been resuscitated from cardiac arrest. In approximately 70% of patients with prior infarction, programmed stimulation can reproducibly initiate a sustained VT. Ablation may be possible in some of these patients, particularly if the VT can be slowed so that it can be mapped. Several recent secondary prevention trials have demonstrated superior survival (3 years) in patients treated with ICDs versus amiodarone (Table 214-6). However, in patients with ejection fractions >35% or <20%, survival was comparable.

GENETIC CONSIDERATIONS Many advances have been made in the identification of genes responsible for syndromes associated with VTs and sudden cardiac death. Specific examples include the congenital long QT syndrome (LQTS), hypertrophic obstructive cardiomyopathy (Chap. 221), arrhythmogenic right ventricular dysplasia, catecholamine-related VT/VF, and the *Brugada syndrome* (Table 214-7). The latter is a recently described disorder characterized by the electrocardiographic profile of a pseudo right bundle branch block pattern with ST elevation and terminal T-wave inversion in leads V_1-V_3 (Fig. 214-14). The clinical presentation is VF in patients with structurally normal hearts. A mutation in the cardiac sodium channel, SCN 5A, is believed to be responsible. While the same gene is responsible for the LQTS, the mutation is different in the two syndromes.

℞ TREATMENT

PHARMACOLOGIC ANTIARRHYTHMIC THERAPY Prior to initiation of pharmacologic antiarrhythmic therapy, potential aggravating factors such as transient metabolic abnormalities, CHF, or acute ischemia must be corrected; in some cases this may suffice to control arrhythmias. In addition, the potential role of drugs as a cause or exacerbating factor in the development of the arrhythmia must be considered. It must be recognized that we do not have a good understanding of the effects of antiarrhythmic agents on the spontaneous onset of tachyarrhythmias. In some cases, they may facilitate the onset.

Antiarrhythmic drugs are used in three principal situations: (1) to terminate an acute arrhythmia, (2) to prevent recurrence of an

TABLE 214-6 *Trials of ICD Therapy for Secondary Prevention in VT/VF Patients*

	AVID			CIDS	CASH
Protocol	ICD vs. empiric amiodarone or sotolol (mainly amiodarone)			ICD vs. empiric amiodarone	ICD vs. empiric amiodarone, metoprolol, and propafenone[a]
Sample size	$n = 1016$ AAD = 509 ICD = 507			$n = 659$ Amiodarone = 331 ICD = 328	$n = 346$ Amiodarone = 92 Metoprolol = 97 Propafenone[a] = 58 ICD = 99
Patient inclusion criteria	Survivors of VF VT with syncope VT with EF ≤ 40%			Survivors of VF VT with syncope VT with EF ≤ 35% and cycle length ≤ 400 ms	Survivors of VF (no EF requirement)
Mortality in "drug" or "control" arm	17.7% 1 year	25.3% 2 years	35.9% 3 years	30% 3 years	19.6% 2 years
Mortality in ICD arm	10.7% 1 year	18.4% 2 years	24.6% 3 years	25% 3 years	12.1% 2 years
Reduction in mortality with ICD	39% 1 year	27% 2 years	31% 3 years	20% 3 years	37% 2 years

[a] Following an interim analysis in March, 1992, enrollment in propafenone arm was discontinued because mortality was increased significantly over mortality in the ICD arm.

Note: EF, ejection fraction; ICD, implanted cardioverter/defibrillator; VF, ventricular fibrillation; VT, ventricular tachycardia.

Sources: AVID Investigators: N Engl J Med 337(22):1576, 1997; K Kuck, S Connolly: ACC NewsOnline, 1998.

arrhythmia, and (3) to prevent a life-threatening arrhythmia for which the patient is perceived to be at risk but which has never occurred.

Most currently available antiarrhythmic agents (Table 214-4) have a relatively low toxic/therapeutic ratio; all can exert proarrhythmic effects (Table 214-8) and therefore may exacerbate underlying arrhythmias. Serum levels can be determined for most currently available antiarrhythmic agents. Standards for therapeutic and toxic levels can serve only as a rough guide for selecting the appropriate dose in any individual patient. In the final analysis, the therapeutic level in

TABLE 214-7 *Genetically Determined Arrhythmia Syndromes*

Disease	Inheritance	Involved Gene	Protein
LQT	Autosomal dominant	KVLQT 1	I_{KS} K channel
		HERG	I_{Kr} K channel
		SCN5A	I_{Na} Na channel
		LQT 4	Unknown
		minK	I_{KS} K channel
		MiRP1	I_{Kr} K channel
	Autosomal recessive (with neural deafness)	KVLQT 1	I_{KS} K channel
		MinK	I_{KS} K channel
	Drug-induced	HERG	I_{Kr} K channel
		MiRP1	I_{Kr} K channel
Brugada syndrome	Autosomal dominant	SNC5A	I_{Na} Na channel
Catecholamine VT	Autosomal dominant	RyR2	Ryanodine receptor
	Autosomal recessive	CASQ2	Calsequestran receptor
Arrhythmogenic RV dysplasia	Autosomal dominant	Unknown genes	
Hypertrophic cardiomyopathy	Autosomal dominant	Multiple cardiac sarcomeric genes (troponin T, troponin I, myosin heavy chain, myosin binding protein C, α tropomyosin)	

a given patient is the concentration that achieves the desired antiarrhythmic effect, and the toxic level for each patient is the concentration at which undesirable side effects occur. Since many adverse effects are directly related to drug concentrations, the lowest serum level that achieves an effective antiarrhythmic response should be chosen.

In order to determine the therapeutic level for a patient, one must have a standard to judge drug efficacy. For a patient with an incessant arrhythmia, antiarrhythmic drugs may be administered empirically until the arrhythmia is suppressed. If a reproducible precipitating factor such as exercise can be identified, serial drug testing during such a provocative maneuver may be performed. Unfortunately, most arrhythmias are sporadic and occur unpredictably without identifiable precipitating factors. In these cases, if one waits to observe spontaneous recurrences on each antiarrhythmic drug, assessment of drug efficacy may require months. This type of assessment of efficacy may be adequate for arrhythmias that are not life-threatening such as AF or SVT. In the current era, most patients with ventricular arrhythmia have ICDs, and recurrence can be monitored through ICD arrhythmic logs. However, this mode of assessment is inadequate for arrhythmias that compromise hemodynamic stability, result in syncope, or cause cardiac arrest.

CLASSIFICATION OF ANTIARRHYTHMIC DRUGS A number of classifications of antiarrhythmic drugs have been proposed; the most frequently used is a modification of one proposed by Vaughan-Williams (Table 214-2). This classification is based in part on the ability of antiarrhythmic drugs to modify the cardiac cellular (1) excitatory currents (Na^+ or Ca^{2+}), (2) action potential duration, and (3) automaticity (phase 4 depolarization). These effects of the drugs on isolated cardiac cells are thought to account for some of the antiarrhythmic properties of the drugs. Thus depression of excitatory currents by class I and class IV antiarrhythmics results in slowing of conduction velocity and may interrupt arrhythmias by blocking conduction in areas of marginal excitability, where conduction velocity is already slow. Class III antiarrhythmics allegedly exert their action by increasing refractoriness through prolongation of the action potential duration. However, this classification has a number of limitations. The electrophysiologic effects of these drugs in vivo may differ from their effects on isolated cells. Also, the effects of heart rate and fiber geometry are not considered. Not all drugs (e.g., adenosine) fit into the classifications. Finally, some drugs (e.g., amiodarone) exhibit properties consistent with multiple classes. The uses, actions, and toxic actions of currently available antiarrhythmic drugs are summarized in Tables 214-4 and 214-7.

ELECTRICAL THERAPY OF TACHYARRHYTHMIAS ■ Pacemakers Cardiac pacing can be used to terminate and, in selected cases, prevent recurrent supraventricular and ventricular arrhythmias. Because many tachyarrhythmias appear to be due to a reentrant mechanism with the impulse

traveling in a circuit, a properly timed paced impulse can penetrate and prematurely depolarize part of the circuit, rendering it refractory to the next circulating wavefront and thereby interrupting the circus movement. Pacing therapy for arrhythmias is generally reserved for patients whose arrhythmias are refractory to drug therapy and who remain hemodynamically stable during the tachycardia. All forms of pacing therapy require repeated demonstration of their effectiveness and reliability in terminating the arrhythmias during electrophysiologic testing prior to implantation of the pacing device.

The type of pacing device and modality selected for arrhythmia termination depend on (1) the rate of the tachycardia (rates >160 beats/min are rarely terminated by a single premature stimulus), (2) the type of arrhythmia (atrial flutter and VT are rarely terminated by single extrastimuli), and (3) concomitant drug therapy.

Because many tachycardias cannot be terminated by single premature stimuli, pacemakers have been developed that allow for multiple extrastimuli (burst pacing) to be introduced. In the current era, antitachycardia pacing is used almost exclusively for ventricular arrhythmias because of the success of radiofrequency ablative therapy for supraventricular arrhythmias.

Cardiac pacing has also been used to prevent ventricular tachyarrhythmias. Polymorphic VT associated with a long QT interval and bradycardia (torsades de pointes, p. 1351) is most likely to respond. Pacing the atrium and/or ventricle at rates between 90 and 120 beats/min appears to increase the homogeneity of electrical recovery and markedly reduces the propensity for a recurrence of arrhythmias.

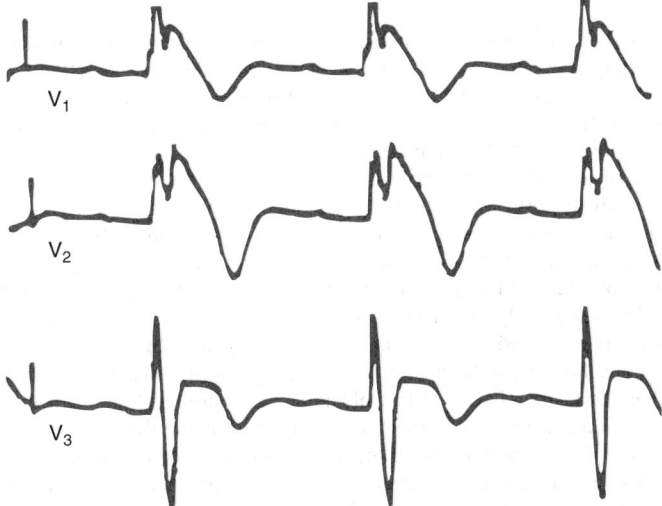

FIGURE 214-14 Brugada syndrome. Note ST elevation with terminal T wave inversion in leads V_1–V_3 mimicking right bundle branch block.

TABLE 214-8 *Toxicity of Most Frequently Used Antiarrhythmic Agents*

Drug	Nonarrhythmic Toxicity	Proarrhythmic Toxicity			
		TDP[a]	A Flutter 1:1	VT/VF	Bradycardia
Digoxin	Anorexia, nausea, vomiting, visual changes	Atrial tachycardia, VT, AV nodal block, accelerated junctional rhythms, atrial and ventricular premature depolarizations; acceleration of ventricular rate during atrial fibrillation or flutter in the presence of preexcitation			
Quinidine[b]	Anorexia, nausea, vomiting, diarrhea, cinchonism, tinnitus, hearing and visual changes, thrombocytopenia, hemolytic anemia, rash, potentiation of digoxin levels	2%	++	++	+
Procainamide[b]	Lupus erythematosus–like syndrome, anorexia, nausea	2%	+	++	+
Disopyramide[b]	Anticholinergic actions: dry mouth, urinary retention, visual disturbances (avoid in narrow-angle glaucoma) constipation, congestive heart failure	2%	+	++	+
Lidocaine	Dizziness, confusion, delirium, seizures, coma; side effects potentiated by liver and heart failure	—	—	—	+[b]
Mexiletine	Ataxia, tremor, gait disturbances, rash, vomiting	—	—	—	—
Flecainide	Dizziness, nausea	Rare	+++	++	++
Propafenone[c]	Taste disturbance, bronchospasm	Rare	+++	++	++
Amiodarone	Pulmonary infiltrates and fibrosis, hepatitis, hypo- and hyperthyroidism, photosensitivity, peripheral neuropathy, tremor	Rare	+++	+++	+++
Sotalol	Bronchospasm	+++	+	+	+++

[a] TDP (torsades de pointes) occurs most often in the setting of slow heart rates, QT prolongation, and hypokalemia or hypomagnesemia and at the time of conversion from atrial fibrillation to sinus rhythm. QT prolongation and torsades de pointes are not dose-related phenomena. QRS prolongation is a dose-related phenomenon also and will occur at toxic concentrations. QT and WRS intervals should be monitored and dose reductions made for interval prolongations.

[b] May suppress sinus node function in patients with underlying sinus node dysfunction. May suppress escape foci in patients with complete heart block.

[c] Avoid in patients with prior myocardial infarction and depressed left ventricular function. Use in combination with AV nodal blocking agent to limit risk of atrial flutter with 1:1 conduction.

Note: A flutter 1:1, atrial flutter with 1:1 atrioventricular (AV) conduction; VT/VF, ventricular tachycardia/ventricular fibrillation.

Pacemakers may be self-contained or energized by an external radiofrequency source. The self-contained pacemaker may function automatically [i.e., it incorporates an arrhythmia-recognition program (circuit)], or it may be activated by an external magnet. The major advantage of a fully automatic system is that there is no need for the patient to recognize the arrhythmia in order for termination to occur. The advantages of the externally activated system (rarely used today) include (1) the decreased risk of unnecessary treatment because of faulty sensing, and (2) the opportunity to initiate monitoring at the time of attempted termination of arrhythmia. This type of monitoring is frequently helpful if pacing techniques are employed to terminate VT, given the risk of acceleration of the arrhythmia by pacing.

The limitations of pacing therapy are primarily related to (1) the changes in the characteristics of the arrhythmia over time such that programmed pacing parameters no longer terminate the tachycardia; (2) the risk of acceleration of the tachycardia with the development of AF when stimulating the atrium and the development of rapid VT and VF when stimulating the ventricles; and (3) inappropriate recognition of supraventricular tachyarrhythmias as VTs, leading to delivery of therapy unnecessarily, which can initiate VT or VF. Future pacing generators that can perform cardioversion and defibrillation will increase the applicability of pacing therapy for the treatment of arrhythmias (see below).

Cardioversion and Defibrillation Electrical cardioversion and defibrillation remain the most reliable methods for terminating arrhythmias. By depolarizing all or at least a large portion of excitable myocardium in a near homogeneous fashion, the electrical shock can interrupt reentrant arrhythmias. External cardioversion is routinely performed by placing two paddles 12 cm in diameter in firm contact with the chest wall, with one paddle usually located to the right of the sternum at the level of the second rib and the other in the left anterior axillary line in the fifth intercostal space. If the patient is conscious, a short-acting anesthetic or an amnesic drug should be administered to prevent patient discomfort. A person skilled in maintaining an airway should be present.

Energy is delivered synchronously with the QRS complex for all arrhythmias except ventricular flutter and VF, since asynchronous shocks can produce VF. The amount of energy used will vary with the type of tachycardia being treated. With the exception of AF, SVTs can frequently be terminated with energy levels in the range of 25 to 50 W·s, while AF usually requires ≥100 W·s for termination. For terminating VT, energy levels ≥100 W·s should probably be employed. While energies as low as 25 W·s may be used successfully, they also have a higher incidence of producing VF or AF. At least 200 W·s of energy should be used for initial attempts at terminating VF. If the initial shock fails, all repeated attempts at defibrillation should be with the maximum energy that the defibrillator is capable of delivering (320 to 400 W·s). As noted earlier, biphasic cardioversion has proven more effective with lower energy requirements than monophasic cardioversion.

Indications for cardioversion depend on the clinical setting and the patient's general condition. Any tachycardia (except sinus tachycardia) that produces hypotension, myocardial ischemia, or heart failure warrants consideration of prompt termination using external cardioversion. Arrhythmias that fail to terminate with pharmacologic therapy may also be terminated by electrical cardioversion. Transient bradycardias and supraventricular and ventricular irritability following cardioversion are common and usually do not warrant antiarrhythmic intervention.

Implanted Cardioverter/Defibrillator ICD devices have been developed that will promptly recognize and terminate life-threatening ventricular arrhythmias. These devices can deliver <1 to 40 W·s, the amount of which can be programmed. Current devices have antitachycardia pacing capabilities such that VT can be sensed and terminated without resorting to a painful shock. In such devices, high-energy shocks are reserved for hypotensive VT, acceleration of VT, or failure to terminate VT after a programmed duration (Fig. 214-15). ICDs are generally implanted transvenously, in a manner similar to pacemakers. Clinical trials testing the function of these devices in patients with drug-refractory ventricular arrhythmias have demonstrated survival from sudden death at 1 year ranging between 92 and 100%. Currently, ICDs

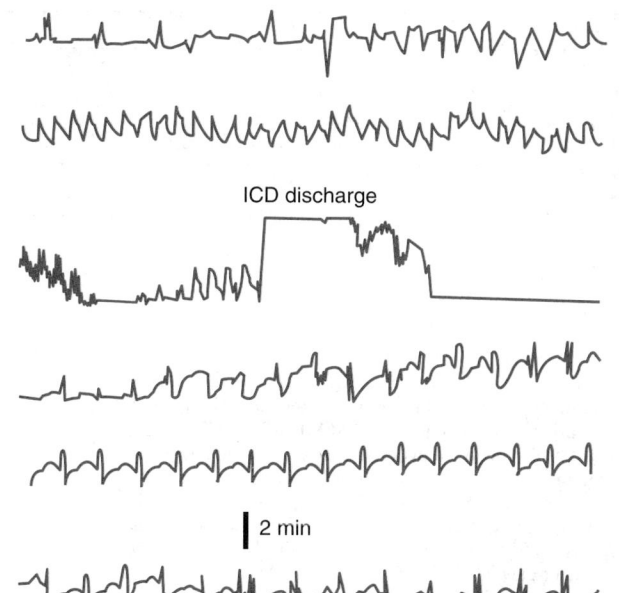

ICD discharge

| 2 min

FIGURE 214-15 Normally functioning implantable defibrillators. A continuous Holter monitoring tracing is shown. On the top strip, a rapid polymorphic tachycardia is initiated which beats more uniformly. The automatic implantable cardioverter/defibrillator (ICD) senses the rhythm and delivers a shock which restores sinus rhythm.

should be considered for patients with VT that is not hemodynamically tolerated. As mentioned earlier, recent randomized trials suggest that ICDs confer improved mortality over amiodarone in patients with hemodynamically untolerated VT and a cardiac arrest not due to reversible causes (Table 214-9). Finally, they are indicated for patients with depressed left ventricular function, prior myocardial infarction, and nonsustained and sustained VT at electrophysiologic study (Table 214-9). A more recent study has defined a mortality benefit conferred by ICDs in patients with coronary artery disease and severely depressed ventricular function, regardless of the presence of nonsustained VT in electrophysiologic study results. Guidelines for their use are given in Table 214-10.

The most frequent problem with the ICD has been its inappropriate discharge in the absence of sustained ventricular arrhythmias. Additional potential problems include an increase in defibrillation threshold and decrease in tachycardia rates below the rate cut-off of the device in response to many antiarrhythmic drugs. Permanently implanted ventricular pacemakers may interfere with the device's ability to sense VF. This can be avoided by using committed bipolar pacing systems that are better able to sense local ventricular activity. Diagnostic fea-

tures of newer, all-in-one devices are able to identify the probable cause of an inappropriate ICD discharge (e.g., AF, SVT, fractured lead) and to adjust pharmacologic therapy or reprogram the device to avoid such inappropriate shocks. These newer devices have the capability to take a "second look" prior to shock delivery and thus may abort delivery for self-terminating arrhythmias. In addition, the range of candidates suitable for implantation will be expanded because the newer devices have the capability of shock therapy for patients whose arrhythmias do not cause loss of consciousness.

Newer generations of ICDs are smaller and frequently allow placement of a second lead in the right atrium. This lead senses atrial activity and provides enhanced discrimination of atrial from ventricular electrical activity. This enhanced discrimination of SVT from VT prevents inappropriate shocks for SVT that may be misinterpreted as VT and allows the device to switch from a dual-chamber to a single-chamber device should an SVT-like AF develop. These dual-chamber devices also allow AV sequential pacing.

DEVICES FOR HEART FAILURE MANAGEMENT (See also Chap. 216) The addition of a lead in the coronary sinus to pace the left ventricle at the same time that the right ventricle is being paced is called *cardiac resynchronization*. This technique has proven complementary to standard pharmacologic management of CHF. Resynchronization with biventricular pacing can be instituted with a pacemaker or ICD.

Ablative Therapy for Arrhythmias Catheter-based mapping techniques have provided a nonoperative approach to the identification and cure of a variety of arrhythmias. In fact, catheter ablation techniques are now the procedures of choice for symptomatic patients with (1) concealed or manifest (WPW) bypass tracts; (2) AV nodal reentrant SVT; (3) typical atrial flutter; and (4) poorly controlled ventricular responses to atrial arrhythmias, most commonly AF. Successful ablation of bypass tracts and modifications of the AV node by radiofrequency energy are extremely successful and cost-effective and are the procedure of choice for patients with recurrent episodes. The creation of AV block with implantation of a pacemaker is the method of choice in managing patients with AF and poorly controlled ventricular response. Idiopathic VTs and some VTs that are associated with coronary artery disease are also amenable to ablation, but the result is less successful than for ablation of SVTs.

Surgical therapy is now relegated to cases of sustained VT associated with coronary artery disease when operative intervention is needed for coronary bypass surgery and/or aneurysmectomy or VT associated with specific structural abnormalities [e.g., idiopathic left ventricle aneurysm, status post (s/p) surgery for tetralogy of Fallot]. It may also be undertaken for the unusual instances of failed catheter ablation for SVTs associated with bypass tracts and for AF.

TABLE 214-9 *Trials of ICD Therapy for Primary Prevention of Sudden Cardiac Death*

	MADIT	MUSTT	MADIT II
Protocol	ICD vs conventional (AAD, primary empirical amiodarone)	EP-guided Rx (AAD, ICD) vs. control	ICD vs. conventional drug therapy (beta blockers), ACD inhibitor
Sample size	$n = 196$ Conventional = 101 ICD = 95	$n = 704$ EP-guided Rx = 351 Control = 353	$n = 1232$ ICD = 742 Conventional drug therapy = 490
Patient inclusion	S/P MI, EF ≤ 35% NSVT, inducible sustained VT not suppressible by procainamide	CAD, EF ≤ 40%, NSVT, inducible sustained VT	S/P MI, LVEF ≤ 30%
Total mortality	Conventional = 39% ICD = 16% (27 months)	Control = 48% EP-guided Rx = 42% AAD = 55% ICD = 24% (60 months)	Conventional = 19.6% ICD = 14.2% (23 months)

Note: AAD, antiarrhythmic drug; CAD, coronary artery disease; EF, ejection fraction; EP, electrophysiology; ICD, implantable cardioverter/defibrillator; MADIT, Multicenter Automatic Defibrillator Trial; MUSTT, Multicenter Unsustained Tachycardia Trial; NSVT, nonsustained ventricular tachycardia; Rx, therapy; S/P MI, status post–myocardial infarction; VT, ventricular tachycardia.
Source: From Buxton et al; Moss et al.

TABLE 214-10 *Guidelines for ICD Implantation*

CLASS 1[a]

1. Cardiac arrest due to VF or VT not due to a transient or reversible cause.
2. Spontaneous sustained VT in association with structural heart disease.
3. Syncope of undetermined origin with clinically relevant, hemodynamically significantly sustained VT or VF induced at EP study when drug therapy is ineffective, not tolerated, or not preferred.
4. Nonsustained VT in patients with coronary disease, prior myocardial infarction, LV dysfunction, and inducible VT or sustained VT at electrophysiological study that is not suppressible by a class I antiarrhythmic drug.
5. Spontaneous sustained VT in patients who do not have structured heart disease that is not amenable to other treatments.

CLASS 2[a]

1. Patients with LV ejection fraction ≤30%, at least 1 month post-MI and 3 months post-coronary artery revascularization.*

CLASS 2[b]

1. Cardiac arrest presumed to be due to VF when EP testing is precluded by other medical conditions.
2. Severe symptoms (e.g., syncope) attributable to ventricular tachyarrhythmia in patients awaiting cardiac transplantation.
3. Familial or inherited conditions with a high risk for life-threatening ventricular tachyarrhythmias such as long QT syndrome or hypertrophic cardiomyopathy.
4. Nonsustained VT with coronary artery disease, prior MI, and LV dysfunction, and inducible sustained VT or VF at EP study.
5. Recurrent syncope of undetermined etiology in the presence of ventricular dysfunction and inducible ventricular arrhythmias at EP study, when other causes of syncope have been excluded.
6. Syncope of unexplained etiology or family history of unexplained death in association with typical or atypical right bundle branch block and ST-segment elevations (Brugada syndrome).

CLASS 3[c]

1. Syncope of undetermined cause in a patient without inducible ventricular tachyarrhythmias and without structural heart disease.
2. Incessant VT or VF.
3. VF or VT resulting from arrhythmias amenable to surgical or catheter ablation; e.g., atrial arrhythmias associated with the Wolff-Parkinson-White syndrome, right ventricular outflow tract VT, idiopathic LV tachycardia, or fascicular VT.
4. Ventricular tachyarrhythmias due to a transient or reversible disorder when correction of the disorder is considered feasible and likely to substantially reduce the risk of recurrent arrhythmia.

[a] Evidence and/or agreement that procedure is indicated.
[b] Divergence in evidence opinion that procedure is indicated.
[c] Evidence/agreement that procedure is not indicated or is harmful.
Note: EP, electrophysiology; ICD, implantable cardioverter/defibrillator; LV, left ventricular; MI, myocardial infarction; VF, ventricular fibrillation, VT, ventricular tachycardia.

Sources: Adapted from American College of Cardiology/American Heart Association: J Am Coll Cardiol 31:1175, 1998, and incorporating new recommendations from G Gregoratas: Circulation 106:2145, 2002, with permission.
*The benefit of an ICD is greatest in this subgroup when the QRS duration is greater than 0.12 seconds.

FURTHER READING

ACC/AHA/ESC: Guidelines for the management of patients with atrial fibrillation. Executive Summary. J Am Coll Cardiol 38:1231, 2001

BUXTON AE et al: A randomized study of the prevention of sudden death in patients with coronary artery disease. N Engl J Med 341:1882, 1999

CLANCY CE, RUDY Y: Na$^{(+)}$ channel mutation that causes both Brugada and long QT syndrome phenotypes: A simulation study of mechanism. Circulation 105:1208, 2002

JOSEPHSON ME: *Clinical Cardiac Electrophysiology: Techniques and Interpretations*, 3d ed. Philadelphia, Lippincott Williams & Wilkins, 2002

KEATING MJ, SANGUINETTI MC: Molecular and cellular mechanisms of cardiac arrhythmia. Cell 104:569, 2001

MOSS AJ et al. Prophylactic implantation of a defibrillator in patients with myocardial infarction and reduced ejection fraction. N Engl J Med 346: 877, 2002

OZCAN C et al: Long-term survival after ablation of the atrioventricular node and implantation of a permanent pacemaker in patients with atrial fibrillation. N Engl J Med 377:1043, 2001

TANG W et al: A comparision of biphasic and monophasic waveform defibrillation after prolonged ventricular fibrillation. Chest 120:948, 2001

THE ATRIAL FIBRILLATION FOLLOW-UP INVESTIGATION OF RHYTHM MANAGEMENT (AFFIRM) Investigators: A comparison of rate control and rhythm control in patients with atrial fibrillation. N Engl J Med 347:1825, 2002

ZIPES DP: Specific arrhythmias: Diagnosis and treatment, in *Braunwald's Heart Disease: A Textbook of Cardiovascular Medicine,* 7th ed, DP Zipes et al (eds). Philadelphia, Saunders, 2005

Section 3   Disorders of the Heart

215 | NORMAL AND ABNORMAL MYOCARDIAL FUNCTION
Eugene Braunwald

CELLULAR BASIS OF CARDIAC CONTRACTION

THE CARDIAC ULTRASTRUCTURE

About three-fourths of the ventricular *myocardium* is composed of individual striated muscle cells (myocytes), normally 60 to 140 μm in length and 17 to 25 μm in diameter (Fig. 215-1*A*). Each fiber contains multiple, rodlike cross-banded strands (myofibrils) that run the length of the fiber and are, in turn, composed of serially repeating structures, the sarcomeres. The cytoplasm between the myofibrils contains other cell constituents (Fig. 215-1*B*), such as the single centrally-located nucleus, numerous mitochondria, and the intracellular membrane system, the sarcoplasmic reticulum.

The *sarcomere*, the structural and functional unit of contraction, is delimited by two adjacent dark lines, the Z lines (Fig. 215-1*C*). The distance between Z lines varies with the degree of contraction or stretch of the muscle and ranges between 1.6 and 2.2 μm. Within the confines of the sarcomere are alternating light and dark bands, giving the myocardial fibers their striated appearance under the light microscope. At the center of the sarcomere is a dark band of constant length (1.5 μm), the A band, which is flanked by two lighter bands, the I bands, which are of variable length. The sarcomere of heart muscle, like that of skeletal muscle, is made up of two sets of interdigitating myofilaments (Fig. 215-1D). Thicker filaments, composed principally of the protein myosin, traverse the A band. They are about 10 nm (100 Å) in diameter, with tapered ends, and measure 1.5 to 1.6 μm in length. Thinner filaments, composed primarily of actin, course from the Z line through the I band into the A band. They are approximately 5 nm (50 Å) in diameter and 1.0 μm in length. Thus there is overlapping of thick and thin filaments only within the A band, while the I band contains only thin filaments (Fig. 215-1C). On electron-microscopic (EM) examination, bridges may be seen to extend between the thick and thin filaments within the A band.

THE CONTRACTILE PROCESS

The sliding model for muscle contraction rests on the fundamental observation that the thick and thin filaments are constant in overall length during both contraction and relaxation. With activation, the actin filaments are propelled further into the A band. In the process, the A band remains constant in length, whereas the I band shortens and the Z lines move toward one another.

The *myosin* molecule is a complex, asymmetric fibrous protein with a molecular weight of about 500,000; it has a rodlike portion that is about 150 nm (1500 Å) in length with a globular portion at its end (Fig. 215-1D). This globular portion of the myosin forms the bridges between the myosin and actin and is the site of ATPase activity. In forming the thick myofilament, which is composed of ~300 longitudinally stacked myosin molecules, the rodlike segments of the myosin molecules are laid down in an orderly, polarized manner, leaving the globular portions projecting outward so that they can interact with actin to generate force and shortening (Fig. 215-2).

Actin has a molecular weight of about 47,000. The thin filament is composed of a double helix of two chains of actin molecules wound about each other on a larger molecule, tropomyosin, which serves as a "backbone" to the thin filament. A group of these regulatory proteins, troponins C, I, and T, are spaced at regular intervals on this filament (Fig. 215-3). In contrast to myosin, actin has no intrinsic enzymatic activity, but it has the ability to combine reversibly with myosin in the presence of ATP and Ca^{2+}. The latter activates the myosin ATPase, which in turn breaks down ATP, the energy source for contraction. In relaxed muscle this interaction is inhibited by tropomyosin. *Titin* (Fig. 215-1D) is a large, flexible, myofibrillar protein that connects myosin to the Z line. Its stretching is believed to contribute to the elasticity of the heart.

During activation of the myocyte, Ca^{2+} becomes attached to troponin C, which results in a conformational change in the regulatory protein tropomyosin; the latter in turn exposes the actin cross-bridge interaction sites. Repetitive interaction between myosin heads and actin filaments is termed *cross-bridge cycling*, which results in sliding of the actin along the myosin filaments, ultimately causing muscle shortening and/or the development of tension. The splitting of ATP, which is synthesized in the mitochondria, then dissociates the myosin cross-bridge from the actin. In the presence of ATP (Fig. 215-2), linkages between actin and myosin filaments are made and broken cyclically as long as sufficient Ca^{2+} is present; these linkages cease when $[Ca^{2+}]$ falls below a critical level, and the troponin-tropomyosin complex once more prevents interactions between the myosin cross-bridges and the actin filaments. Intracytoplasmic Ca^{2+} is a principal mediator of the inotropic state of the heart. The fundamental action of most positive inotropic drugs, including the digitalis glycosides, β-

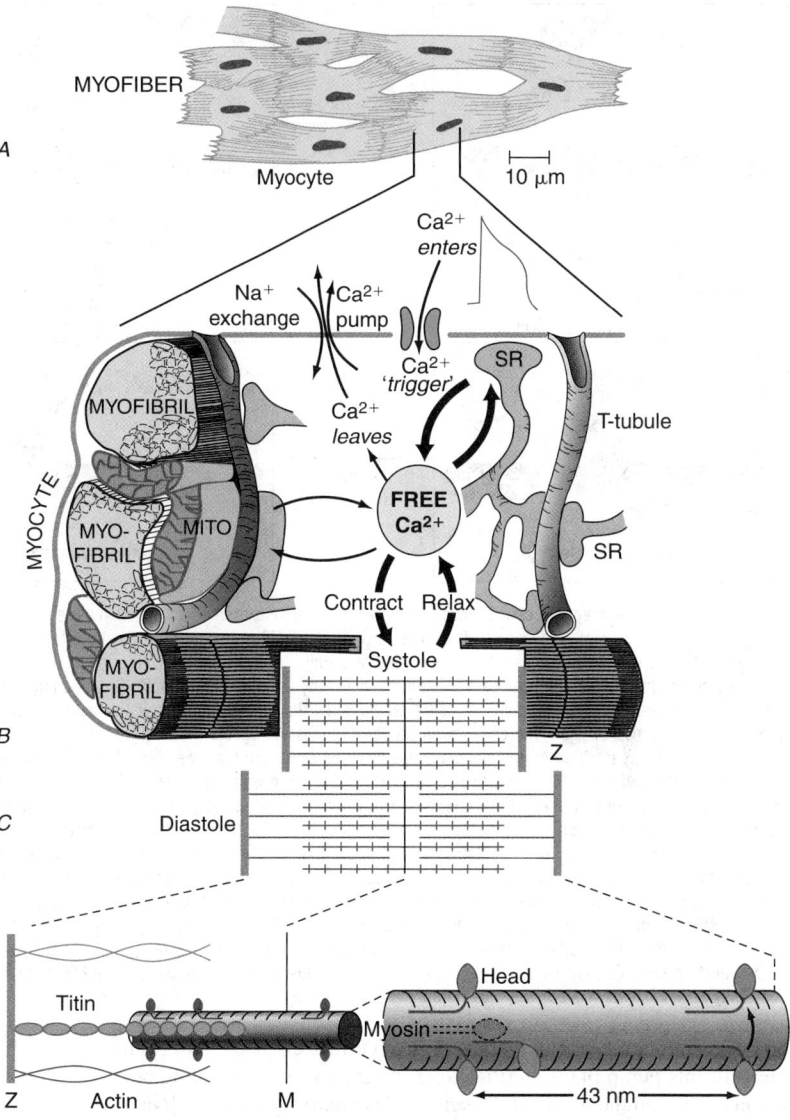

FIGURE 215-1 *A.* Microscopic evidence of heart muscle. *B.* Cardiac contraction and relaxation result from changing concentrations of Ca^{2+} ions in the myocardial cytosol. Ca^{2+} ions are shown schematically as entering via the calcium channel, which opens in response to the wave of depolarization that travels along the sarcolemma. These Ca^{2+} ions "trigger" the release of more calcium from the sarcoplasmic reticulum (SR) and thereby initiate a contraction-relaxation cycle. Eventually, the small amount of calcium that has entered the cell leaves, predominantly by a Na^+-Ca^{2+} exchanger with a lesser role for the sarcolemmal calcium pump. *C.* The varying actin-myosin overlap is shown for systole and diastole. *D.* The myosin heads, attached to the thick filaments, interact with the thin actin filaments. *(Copyright 2001 LH Opie. Reprinted with permission.)*

adrenergic agonists, and phosphodiesterase inhibitors, is to raise the $[Ca^{2+}]$ in the vicinity of the myofilaments.

The *sarcoplasmic reticulum* (SR) (Fig. 215-1B) is a complex network of anastomosing intracellular channels that invests the myofibrils. Its longitudinally disposed membrane-lined tubules are closely applied to the surfaces of individual sarcomeres but have no direct continuity with the outside of the cell. However, closely related to the SR, both structurally and functionally, are the transverse tubules, or T system, formed by tubelike invaginations of the sarcolemma that extend into the myocardial fiber along the Z lines, i.e., the ends of the sarcomeres.

CARDIAC ACTIVATION

In the inactive state, the cardiac cell is polarized, i.e., the interior has a negative charge relative to the outside of the cell, with a transmembrane potential of −80 to −100 mV (Chap. 213). The sarcolemma, which in the resting state is largely impermeable to Na^+, has a Na^+-

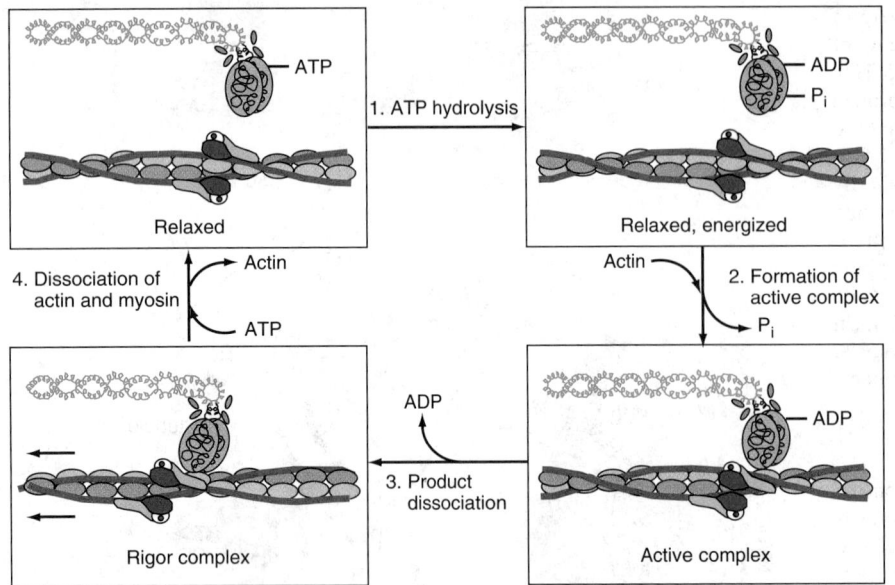

FIGURE 215-2 Four steps in cardiac muscle contraction and relaxation. In relaxed muscle (*upper left*), ATP bound to the myosin cross-bridge dissociates the thick and thin filaments. *Step 1:* Hydrolysis of myosin-bound ATP by the ATPase site on the myosin head transfers the chemical energy of the nucleotide to the activated cross-bridge (*upper right*). When cytosolic Ca^{2+} concentration is low, as in relaxed muscle, the reaction cannot proceed because tropomyosin and the troponin complex on the thin filament do not allow the active sites on actin to interact with the cross-bridges. Therefore, even though the cross-bridges are energized, they cannot interact with actin. *Step 2:* When Ca^{2+} binding to troponin C has exposed active sites on the thin filament, actin interacts with the myosin cross-bridges to form an active complex (lower right) in which the energy derived from ATP is retained in the actin-bound cross-bridge, whose orientation has not yet shifted. *Step 3:* The muscle contracts when ADP dissociates from the cross-bridge; this step leads to the formation of the low-energy rigor complex (lower left), in which the chemical energy derived from ATP hydrolysis has been expended to perform mechanical work (the "rowing" motion of the cross-bridge). *Step 4:* The muscle returns to its resting state, and the cycle ends when a new molecule of ATP binds to the rigor complex and dissociates the cross-bridge from the thin filament. This cycle continues until calcium is dissociated from troponin C in the thin filament, which causes the contractile proteins to return to the resting state with the cross-bridge in the energized state. [*From AM Katz, in WS Colucci (ed): Heart Failure: Cardiac Function and Dysfunction, in Atlas of Heart Diseases, 3d ed, E Braunwald (series ed). Philadelphia, Current Medicine, 2002. Reprinted with permission.*]

The ATP formed from substrate oxidation is the principal source of energy for almost all of the mechanical work of contraction performed by the myocardial cell. The high-energy phosphate stores in ATP are in equilibrium with those in creatine phosphate. The activity of myosin ATPase determines the rate of forming and breaking of the actin-myosin cross-bridges and ultimately the velocity of muscle contraction.

THE ROLE OF MUSCLE LENGTH

In cardiac muscle, indeed in all striated muscle, the force of contraction depends on initial muscle length. The sarcomere length associated with the most forceful contraction is approximately 2.2 μm. At this length the two sets of myofilaments of the sarcomere are configured so as to provide the greatest area for their interaction (Fig. 215-1). The length of the sarcomere also regulates the extent of activation of the contractile system, i.e., its sensitivity to Ca^{2+}. According to this concept, termed *length-dependent activation*, at the optimal sarcomere length of 2.2 μm, the myofilament sensitivity to Ca^{2+} is also maximal.

The relation between the initial length of the muscle fibers and the developed force is of prime importance for the function of heart muscle. This forms the basis of the Frank-Starling relation (Starling's law of the heart), which states that, within limits, the force of ventricular contraction is a function of the end-diastolic length of the cardiac muscle; in the intact heart the latter is closely related to the ventricular end-diastolic volume.

and K^+-stimulating pump energized by ATP that extrudes Na^+ from the cell; this pump plays a critical role in establishing the resting potential. Thus, on the inside of the cell $[K^+]$ is relatively high and $[Na^+]$ is far lower, while in the extracellular milieu $[Na^+]$ is high and $[K^+]$ is low. At the same time, in the resting state, the extracellular $[Ca^{2+}]$ greatly exceeds the free intracellular $[Ca^{2+}]$. →*The four phases of the action potential are discussed and illustrated in Chapter 213.*

During the plateau of the action potential (phase 2) there is a slow inward current through L-type Ca^{2+} channels in the sarcolemma (Fig. 215-4). The absolute quantity of Ca^{2+} that crosses the surface membrane is relatively small and itself appears to be insufficient to bring about full activation of the contractile apparatus. The depolarizing current not only extends across the surface of the cell but penetrates deeply into the cell by way of the ramifying T system; this Ca^{2+} current triggers the release of much larger quantities of Ca^{2+} from the SR, a process termed *Ca^{2+}-induced Ca^{2+} release.*

The Ca^{2+} released from the SR then diffuses toward the myofibrils, where, as already described, it combines with troponin C. By repressing this inhibitor of contraction, Ca^{2+} activates the myofilaments to shorten. During repolarization the activity of the Ca^{2+} pump in the SR reaccumulates Ca^{2+} against a concentration gradient, and the Ca^{2+} is stored by its attachment to a protein *calsequestrin*. This is an energy-requiring process that lowers the $[Ca^{2+}]$ in the vicinity of the myofibrils to a level that inhibits the actin-myosin interaction responsible for contraction and in this manner leads to relaxation. Also, there is an exchange of Ca^{2+} for Na^+ at the sarcolemma, reducing the cytoplasmic $[Ca^{2+}]$. Thus, the combination of the cell membrane, transverse tubules, and SR, with their ability to transmit the action potential, to release, and then to reaccumulate Ca^{2+}, appears to play a fundamental role in the rhythmic contraction and relaxation of heart muscle.

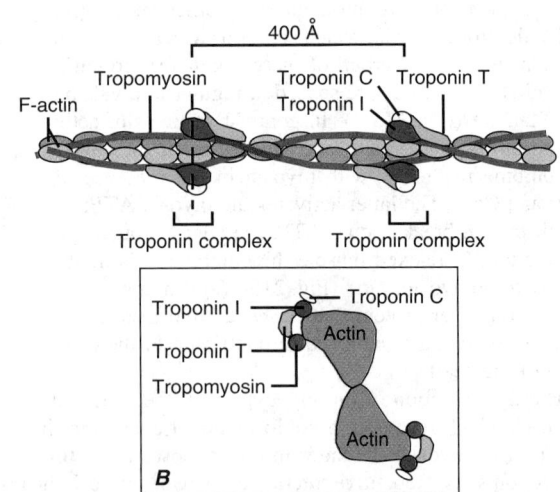

FIGURE 215-3 Structure of the thin filament. *A.* The "backbone" of the thin filament, seen in a longitudinal view, is F-actin, which contains two strands of actin monomers (blue and white). Troponin complexes, made up of one molecule each of troponin C, troponin I, and troponin T, are distributed at approximately 40 nm (400 Å) intervals along the thin filament. Elongated tropomyosin molecules (solid line in the grooves between the two actin strands). *B.* A cross-section of the thin filament at the level where the troponin complexes are located shows probable relationships between actin, tropomyosin, and the three components of the troponin complex. The strength of the bond linking troponin I and actin varies, depending on whether Ca^{2+} is bound to troponin C. [*Adapted from AM Katz, Molecular and cellular basis of contraction, in WS Colucci (ed): Heart Failure: Cardiac Function and Dysfunction, in Atlas of Heart Diseases, 3d ed, E Braunwald (series ed). Philadelphia, Current Medicine, 2002. Reprinted with permission.*]

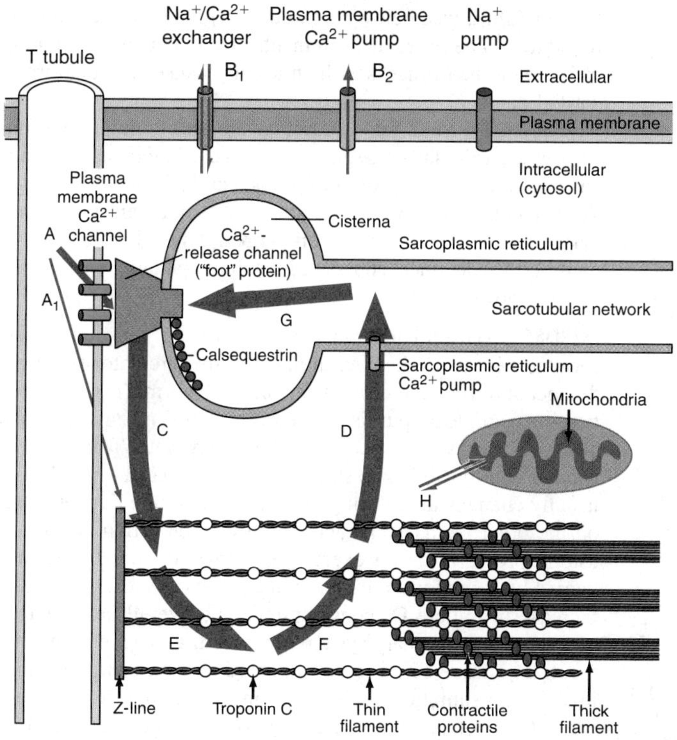

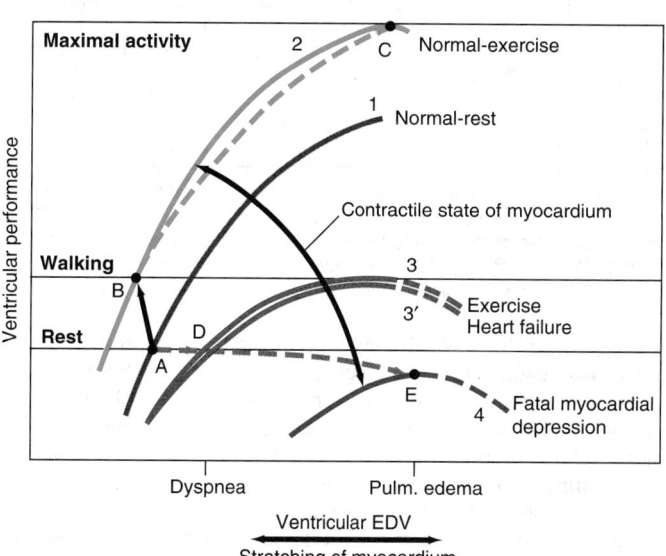

FIGURE 215-4

FIGURE 215-4 The Ca²⁺ fluxes and key structures involved in cardiac excitation-contraction coupling. The *arrows* denote the direction of Ca²⁺ fluxes. The thickness of each arrow indicates the magnitude of the calcium flux. Two Ca²⁺ cycles regulate excitation-contraction coupling and relaxation. The larger cycle is entirely intracellular and involves Ca²⁺ fluxes into and out of the sarcoplasmic reticulum, and Ca²⁺ binding to and release from troponin C. The smaller extracellular Ca²⁺ cycle occurs when this cation moves into and out of the cell. The action potential opens plasma membrane Ca²⁺ channels to allow passive entry of Ca²⁺ into the cell from the extracellular fluid (*arrow A*). Only a small portion of the Ca²⁺ that enters the cell directly activates the contractile proteins (*arrow A₁*). The extracellular cycle is completed when Ca²⁺ is actively transported back out to the extracellular fluid by way of two plasma membrane fluxes mediated by the sodium-calcium exchanger (*arrow B₁*) and the plasma membrane calcium pump (*arrow B₂*). In the intracellular Ca²⁺ cycle, passive Ca²⁺ release occurs through channels in the cisternae (*arrow C*) and initiates contraction, and active Ca²⁺ uptake by the Ca²⁺ pump of the sarcotubular network (*arrow D*) relaxes the heart. Diffusion of Ca²⁺ within the sarcoplasmic reticulum (*arrow G*) returns this activator cation to the cisternae, where it is stored in a complex with calsequestrin and other calcium-binding proteins. Ca²⁺ released from the sarcoplasmic reticulum initiates systole when it binds to troponin C (*arrow E*). Lowering of cytosolic [Ca²⁺] by the SR cause this ion to dissociate from troponin (*arrow F*) and relaxes the heart. Ca²⁺ may also move between mitochondria and cytoplasm (H). (*Adapted from Katz, with permission.*)

MYOCARDIAL MECHANICS AND CARDIAC FUNCTION

THE FORCE-VELOCITY CURVE

The mechanical activity of cardiac muscle may be expressed externally in two ways: shortening and tension development. In both skeletal and cardiac muscle the velocity of shortening is inversely related to the development of tension, an expression of the so-called force-velocity relation. Expressed simply, the greater the load the muscle is called upon to lift, the lower its velocity (and extent) of shortening, and vice versa. However, the contractile activity of cardiac muscle is readily altered under physiologic conditions by changes in resting fiber length and by changes in the contractility, both of which shift the myocardial force-velocity curve.

VENTRICULAR EJECTION

Analysis of the heart as a pump has classically centered on the relation between the end-diastolic volume of the ventricle (which is related to the length of the muscle fibers) and its stroke volume (the Frank-Starling relation). The end-diastolic or "filling" pressure of the ventricle is sometimes used as a surrogate for the end-diastolic volume. In the heart-lung preparation the stroke volume varies directly with the

diastolic fiber length (preload) and inversely with the arterial resistance (afterload), and as the heart fails it delivers a progressively smaller stroke volume from a normal or even elevated end-diastolic volume. The relation between the ventricular end-diastolic pressure and the stroke work of the ventricle (the ventricular function curve) provides a useful definition of the level of *contractility* of the intact heart. An increase in ventricular contractility is accompanied by a shift of the ventricular function curve upward and to the left [greater stroke work at any level of ventricular end-diastolic pressure (or volume), or lower end-diastolic pressure at any level of stroke work], while depression of contractility is characterized by a shift downward and to the right (Fig. 215-5).

Increased impulse traffic in the cardiac adrenergic nerves stimulates ventricular function as a consequence of the release of norepinephrine from adrenergic nerve endings in the heart. Norepinephrine activates myocardial β receptors and through the Gs-stimulated guanine nucleotide binding protein activates the enzyme adenylate cyclase, which leads to the formation of the intracellular second messenger cyclic AMP from ATP (Fig. 215-6). Cyclic AMP, in turn, activates protein kinase, which causes a more rapid, forceful contraction by phosphorylating the Ca²⁺ channel in the myocardial sarcolemma, thereby enhancing the influx of Ca²⁺ into the myocyte. Ca²⁺ acts on the contractile apparatus, as described on p. 1359. Cyclic AMP also phosphorylates the SR protein phospholamban, which increases the uptake of Ca²⁺ by the SR, increasing the rate of relaxation and providing larger quantities of Ca²⁺ in the SR to be released by subsequent depolarization and thereby further stimulating contraction. Adrenergic activation is evidenced by tachycardia, increased rates of ejection and filling, and a reduction in cardiac dimensions.

ASSESSMENT OF CARDIAC FUNCTION

Several techniques are available for defining impaired cardiac function. The cardiac output and stroke volume may be depressed in the presence of heart failure (HF), but not uncommonly these variables are within normal limits. A more sensitive index is the ejection fraction, i.e., the ratio of stroke volume to end-diastolic volume (normal

FIGURE 215-5 Diagram showing the interrelations among influences on ventricular end-diastolic volume (EDV) through stretching of the myocardium and the contractile state of the myocardium. Levels of ventricular EDV associated with filling pressures that result in dyspnea and pulmonary edema are shown on the abscissa. Levels of ventricular performance required when the subject is at rest, while walking, and during maximal activity are designated on the ordinate. The broken lines are the descending limbs of the ventricular-performance curves, which are rarely seen during life but which show the level of ventricular performance if end-diastolic volume could be elevated to very high levels. For further explanation see text. (*Modified from E Braunwald et al: Mechanisms of Contraction of the Normal and Failing Heart. Boston, Little, Brown, 1976.*)

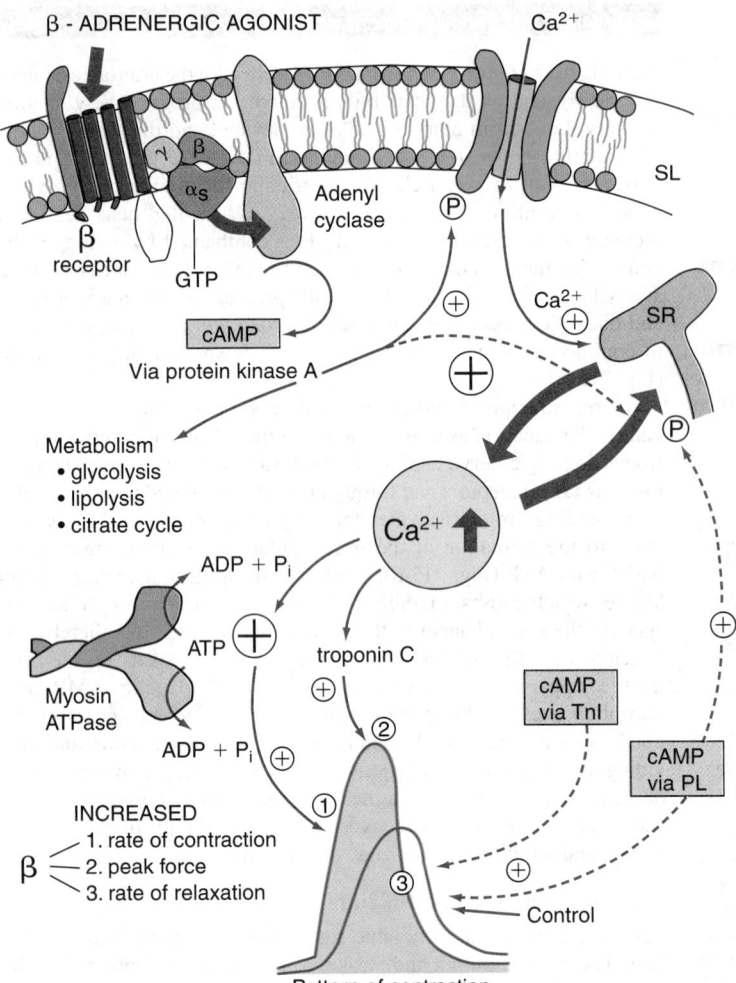

β - ADRENERGIC AGONIST

β receptor

GTP

α_s β γ

Adenyl cyclase

cAMP

Via protein kinase A

Metabolism
• glycolysis
• lipolysis
• citrate cycle

ADP + P_i

ATP ⊕

Myosin ATPase

ADP + P_i ⊕

INCREASED

β ⎰ 1. rate of contraction
   ⎱ 2. peak force
     3. rate of relaxation

Ca^{2+}

troponin C ⊕

② ⊕
①

③

Pattern of contraction

Control

Ca^{2+}

SL

P

Ca^{2+} ⊕

SR

⊕

P

⊕

cAMP via TnI

cAMP via PL

⊕

FIGURE 215-6 Signal systems involved in positive intropic and lusitropic (enhanced relaxation) effects of β-adrenergic stimulation. When the β-adrenergic agonist interacts with the β receptor, a series of G protein-mediated changes leads to activation of adenylate cyclase and formation of cyclic AMP (cAMP). The latter acts via protein kinase A to stimulate metabolism (left) and to phosphorylate the Ca^{2+} channel protein (right). The result is an enhanced opening probability of the Ca^{2+} channel, thereby increasing the inward movement of Ca^{2+} ions through the sarcolemma (SL) of the T tubule. These Ca^{2+} ions release more calcium from the sarcoplasmic reticulum (SR) to increase cytosolic Ca^{2+} and to activate troponin C. Ca^{2+} ions also increase the rate of breakdown of ATP to ADP and inorganic phosphate (P_i). Enhanced myosin ATPase activity explains the increased rate of contraction, with increased activation of troponin C explaining increased peak force development. An increased rate of relaxation is explained because cyclic AMP also activates the protein phospholamban, situated on the membrane of the SR, that controls the rate of uptake of calcium into the SR. The latter effect explains enhanced relaxation (lusitropic effect). P, phosphorylation; PL, phospholamban; SL, sarcolemma; SR, sarcoplasmic reticulum; TnI, troponin I. *(Copyright 2001, L Opie. Reprinted with permission.)*

tricular filling (see below), as well as regional contraction and relaxation. The latter measurements are particularly important in ischemic heart disease which usually causes regional myocardial damage.

The end-systolic left ventricular pressure-volume relationship is a particularly useful index of ventricular performance since it is independent of both preload and afterload (Fig. 215-7). At any level of myocardial contractility, left ventricular end-systolic volume varies inversely with end-systolic pressure; as contractility declines, end-systolic volume (at any level of end-systolic pressure) rises.

EXERCISE A useful technique for evaluating ventricular performance involves the measurement of the circulatory changes that occur during exercise. In persons with normal cardiac function, the cardiac output rises by more than 500 mL/min for each 100 mL increase in O_2 consumption per minute. The left ventricular end-diastolic pressure at rest is less than 12 mmHg and usually changes little during exercise. The failing left ventricle, on the other hand, is characterized by an elevation of end-diastolic pressure during exercise to above 12 mmHg, accompanied by a subnormal increase in cardiac output related to the increase in minute O_2 consumption. The overall performance of the cardiopulmonary system in delivering oxygen to the metabolizing tissue can also be estimated by measuring the maximal O_2 consumption achieved during escalating treadmill exercise ($\dot{V}_{maxO_2}$). Normal values exceed 20 mL/min per kg, while values under 10 mL/min per kg represent severe impairment of function, usually seen in patients with severe heart failure and a poor prognosis.

The potential value of stressing the left ventricle to assess its performance is emphasized by the fact that the normal ranges of left ventricular end-diastolic pressure, cardiac index, and ventricular stroke work in the resting state are wide, with values that frequently overlap those seen in patients with ventricular dysfunction.

DIASTOLIC FUNCTION (Fig. 215-8)

This important variable is best assessed by continuously measuring the flow velocity across the mitral valve using Doppler echocardiography. Normally, the velocity of inflow is more rapid in early diastole than during atrial systole; with impaired relaxation the rate of early diastolic filling declines, while the rate of presystolic filling rises. With severe impairment of filling the pattern is "pseudo-normalized" and early ventricular filling becomes more rapid as left atrial pressure upstream to the stiff left ventricle rises (Fig. 211-4).

CONTROL OF CARDIAC PERFORMANCE AND OUTPUT

The extent of shortening of heart muscle and, therefore, the stroke volume of the intact ventricle are determined by three major influences: (1) the length of the muscle at the onset of contraction, i.e., the preload; (2) the contractility of the muscle, i.e., the position of its force-velocity-length relation; and (3) the tension that the muscle is called upon to develop during contraction, i.e., the afterload. Ventricular filling is influenced by the extent and speed of myocardial relaxation, which in turn is determined by the rate of uptake of Ca^{2+} by the SR; the latter may be enhanced by adrenergic activation and reduced by ischemia. Filling may also be impeded by the stiffness of the ventricular wall, which may be increased by ventricular hypertrophy and conditions that infiltrate the ventricle, such as amyloid, or by an extrinsic constraint (e.g., pericardial compression) (Fig. 215-8).

VENTRICULAR END-DIASTOLIC VOLUME (PRELOAD)

At any level of contractility, the performance of the myocardium is influenced profoundly by ventricular end-diastolic fiber length and therefore by diastolic ventricular volume, i.e., by operation of the

value = $67 \pm 8\%$), which may be estimated by radiocontrast or radionuclide angiography or echocardiography, and it is frequently depressed in systolic heart failure even when the stroke volume itself is normal. Alternatively, the abnormally elevated ventricular end-diastolic volume (normal value = 75 ± 20 mL/m²) or end-systolic volume (normal value = 25 ± 7 mL/m²) signify impairment of left ventricular systolic function. A limitation of measuring cardiac output, ejection fraction, and ventricular volumes is that these variables are influenced strongly by ventricular loading conditions. Thus, a depressed ejection fraction and lowered cardiac output may be observed in patients with normal ventricular function but reduced preload, as occurs in hypovolemia, or with increased afterload, as occurs in acutely elevated arterial pressure.

Noninvasive techniques, particularly echocardiography and radionuclide angiography (Chap. 211), are of great value in the clinical assessment of myocardial function. They provide measurements of end-diastolic and end-systolic volumes, global ejection fraction, and systolic shortening rate and they allow assessment of ven-

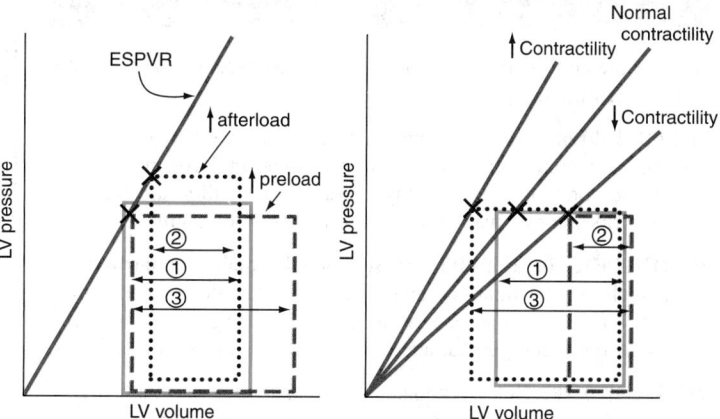

FIGURE 215-7 *The responses of the left ventricle to increased afterload, increased preload, and increased and reduced contractility are shown in the pressure-volume plane. ESPVR, end-systolic pressure-volume relation; E_{ES}, the slope of the end-systolic pressure-volume relation. Left. Effects of increases in preload and afterload on the pressure-volume loop. Since there has been no change in contractility, ESPVR is unchanged. With an increase in afterload, stroke volume falls (1 → 2); with an increase in preload, stroke volume rises (1 → 3). Right. With increased myocardial contractility, the normal ESPVR moves to the left of the normal line (lower end-systolic volume at any end-systolic pressure) and stroke volume rises (1 → 3). With reduced myocardial contractility, the ESPVR moves to the right; end-systolic volume is increased and stroke volume falls (1 → 2).*

Frank-Starling mechanism (Fig. 215-5). The following are the major determinants of ventricular preload in the intact organism:

TOTAL BLOOD VOLUME When blood volume is depleted, as in hemorrhage or dehydration (Chap. 253), venous return to the heart declines and ventricular end-diastolic volume (preload) falls, as does ventricular performance, as reflected in stroke volume, cardiac output, and ventricular work.

DISTRIBUTION OF BLOOD VOLUME The ventricular end-diastolic volume is influenced by the distribution of blood volume between the intra- and extrathoracic compartments. This distribution in turn is influenced by the following:

1. *Body position.* Gravitational forces pool blood in dependent portions of the body; upright posture augments extrathoracic at the expense of intrathoracic blood volume and reduces ventricular work.

2. *Intrathoracic pressure.* Normally, mean intrathoracic pressure is negative, which increases thoracic blood volume and enhances the return of blood to the heart, particularly when this pressure becomes more negative during inspiration. Elevation of intrathoracic pressure, as occurs during the Valsalva maneuver, prolonged bouts of coughing, or positive-pressure ventilation, has the opposite effect.

3. *Intrapericardial pressure.* When this pressure is elevated, as in pericardial tamponade (Chap. 222), there is interference with cardiac

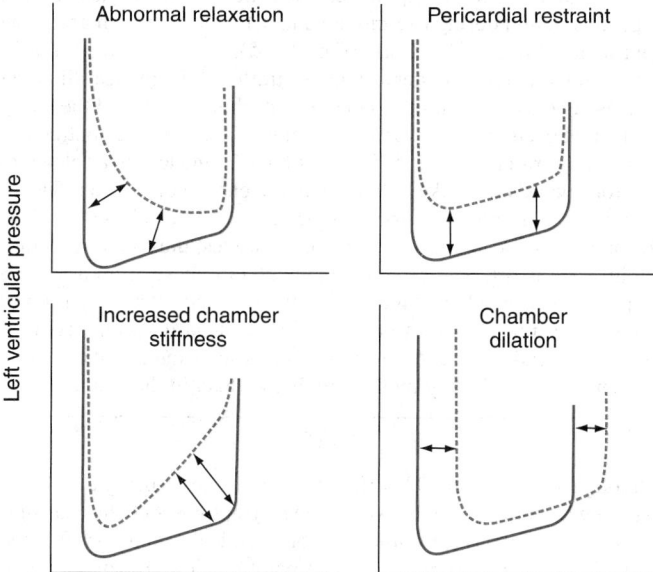

FIGURE 215-8 *Mechanisms that cause diastolic dysfunction reflected in the pressure-volume relation. The bottom half of the pressure-volume loop is depicted. Solid lines represent normal subjects; dashed lines represent patients with diastolic dysfunction. (From MR Zile: Diastolic dysfunction: detection, consequences, and treatment: II. Diagnosis and treatment of diastolic function. Mod Concepts Cardiovasc Dis 59:1, 1990. Reprinted with permission.)*

filling, and the resultant reduction in ventricular diastolic volume reduces stroke volume and ventricular work.

4. *Venous tone.* The venous system is not a simple system of passive conduits between the systemic capillary bed and the right atrium. Instead, the smooth muscle in the walls of the venules and veins responds to a variety of neural and humoral stimuli. Venoconstriction occurs during muscular exercise, deep respiration, fright, or hypovolemic shock, enhancing venous return to the heart and thereby effecting ventricular performance.

5. *The pumping action of skeletal muscle.* During muscular exercise the contracting skeletal muscles squeeze blood out of the venous bed and, with the aid of the venous valves, displace it centrally, thereby increasing intrathoracic blood volume, ventricular end-diastolic volume, and ventricular work.

ATRIAL CONTRACTION Vigorous, appropriately-timed atrial contraction augments ventricular filling and end-diastolic volume. The atrial contribution to ventricular filling, the so-called "atrial kick," is of particular importance in patients with concentric ventricular hypertrophy. In such patients, the loss of atrial systole (as occurs with the development of atrial fibrillation) reduces ventricular end-diastolic pressure and volume, ultimately lowering myocardial performance.

MYOCARDIAL CONTRACTILITY

A number of factors determine the level of ventricular performance at any given ventricular end-diastolic volume, i.e., the position of the ventricular function curve (Fig. 215-5) as well as the position of the left ventricular end-systolic pressure-volume relation (Fig. 215-7). These influences may be considered to operate by modifying myocardial force-velocity relations. In the final analysis, most of these influences act by altering the $[Ca^{2+}]$ in the vicinity of the myofilaments, which in turn trigger cross-bridge cycling (p. 1359).

ADRENERGIC NERVE ACTIVITY The quantity of norepinephrine released by adrenergic nerve endings in the heart is determined by the adrenergic nerve impulse traffic; norepinephrine acts on the β-adrenergic receptors in the myocardium. This mechanism is the most important one that acutely modifies myocardial contractility under physiologic conditions.

CIRCULATING CATECHOLAMINES When it is stimulated by adrenergic nerve impulses, the adrenal medulla releases catecholamines, which augment both heart rate and myocardial contractility when they reach the heart.

FORCE-FREQUENCY RELATION Myocardial contractility is also influenced by the rate and rhythm of cardiac contraction. The contractility of the normal (but to a lesser extent the failing) heart is augmented by an increase in frequency of contraction, and ventricular extrasystoles result in post-extrasystolic potentiation, presumably by increasing the quantity of Ca^{2+} that enters the cardiac cell.

EXOGENOUSLY ADMINISTERED INOTROPIC AGENTS Isoproterenol, dopamine, dobutamine, and other sympathomimetic agents, cardiac glycosides, Ca^{2+}, and the phosphodiesterase inhibitors amrinone and milrinone all improve the contractility and therefore may be used to stimulate ventricular performance.

PHYSIOLOGIC DEPRESSANTS   Included among these are severe myocardial hypoxia, ischemia, and acidosis. Acting either singly or in combination, these conditions depress myocardial contractility and left ventricular work at any given ventricular end-diastolic volume.

PHARMACOLOGIC DEPRESSANTS   These include many antiarrhythmic drugs such as procainamide and disopyramide; calcium antagonists such as verapamil; β-adrenergic blockers; and large doses of barbiturates, alcohol, and general anesthetics as well as many other drugs.

MYOCARDIAL DEPRESSION   Although the fundamental mechanisms responsible for depression of myocardial contractility in most cases of chronic congestive heart failure secondary to prolonged ventricular overload or cardiomyopathy remain to be elucidated it is now apparent that in this condition the inotropic state of individual myocytes is depressed, and as a consequence the ventricular performance at any ventricular preload and afterload is lowered.

VENTRICULAR AFTERLOAD

The stroke volume is ultimately a function of the extent of ventricular fiber shortening. In the intact heart, as in isolated cardiac muscle, the extent (and velocity) of shortening of ventricular muscle fibers at any level of preload and of myocardial contractility are inversely related to the afterload, i.e., the load that opposes shortening. In the intact heart the afterload may be defined as the tension or stress developed in the ventricular wall during ejection. It is determined by the aortic pressure as well as by the volume and thickness of the ventricular cavity. Laplace's law indicates that the tension of the myocardial fiber is a function of the product of the intracavitary ventricular pressure and ventricular radius divided by the wall thickness. Therefore, at any given level of aortic pressure, the afterload on a dilated left ventricle of normal thickness is higher than that on a normal-sized ventricle. Conversely, at the same aortic pressure and ventricular diastolic volume, the afterload of a hypertrophied ventricle is lower than of a normal chamber. The aortic pressure, in turn, is determined by the peripheral vascular resistance, the physical characteristics of the arterial tree, and the volume of blood it contains at the onset of ejection.

The critical role played by the ventricular afterload in cardiovascular regulation is shown in Fig. 215-9. As already noted, elevations of both preload and contractility increase myocardial fiber shortening, while increases in afterload reduce it. The extent of myocardial fiber shortening and left ventricular size are the determinants of stroke volume. Arterial pressure, in turn, is related to the product of cardiac output and systemic vascular resistance, while afterload is a function of left ventricular volume, wall thickness, and arterial pressure. An increase in arterial pressure induced by vasoconstriction, for example, augments afterload, which opposes myocardial fiber shortening, reducing stroke volume. This in turn tends to limit the increase in pressure.

When myocardial contractility becomes impaired and the ventricle dilates, afterload rises and limits cardiac output. Increased afterload may result from neural and humoral stimuli that occur in response to a fall in cardiac output. This increased afterload may reduce cardiac output further while increasing myocardial O_2 requirements, and can initiate a vicious circle in patients with ischemic heart disease and limited myocardial O_2 supply. Treatment with vasodilators has the opposite effect; by reducing afterload, cardiac output rises (Chap. 216).

Under normal circumstances, the various influences acting on cardiac performance enumerated above interact in a complex fashion to maintain cardiac output at a level appropriate to the requirements of the metabolizing tissues; interference with a single mechanism may not influence the cardiac output. For example, a moderate reduction of blood volume or the loss of the atrial contribution to ventricular contraction can ordinarily be sustained without a reduction in the car-

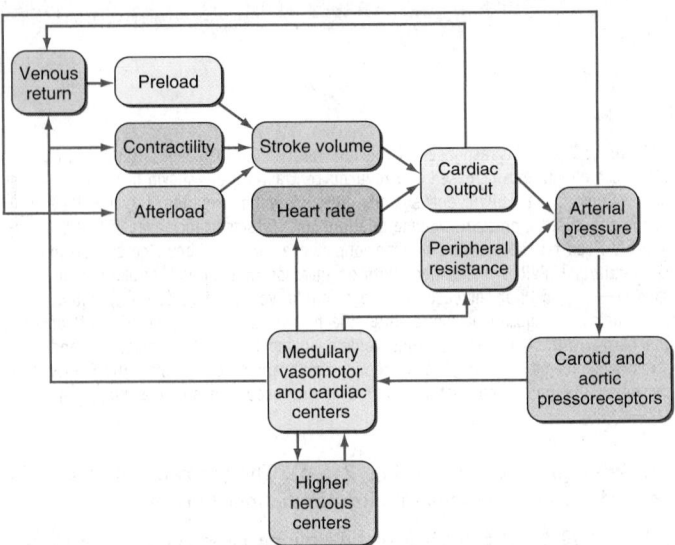

FIGURE 215-9   Interactions in the intact circulation of preload, contractility and afterload in producing stroke volume. Stroke volume combined with heart rate determines cardiac output, which, in turn, when combined with peripheral vascular resistance, determines arterial pressure for tissue perfusion. The characteristics of the arterial system also contribute to afterload, an increase of which reduces stroke volume. The interaction of these components with carotid and aortic baroreceptors provides a feedback mechanism to higher medullary and vasomotor cardiac centers and to higher levels in the central nervous system to affect a modulating influence on heart rate, peripheral vascular resistance, venous return, and contractility. [From MR Starling: Physiology of myocardial contraction, in WS Colucci and E Braunwald (eds). Atlas of Heart Failure: Cardiac Function and Dysfunction, 3d ed, Philadelphia: Current Medicine, 2002, pp 19–35. Adapted from FR Badke and RA O'Rourke: Cardiovascular physiology, in JH Stein (ed): Internal Medicine, ed 1. Boston: Little, Brown and Co. 1983:407–423.]

diac output at rest. Under these circumstances, other factors, such as increases in the frequency of adrenergic nerve impulses to the heart, in heart rate, and in venous tone will, in a normal individual, serve as compensatory mechanisms and sustain cardiac output.

EXERCISE

Hyperventilation, the pumping action of the exercising muscles, and venoconstriction during exercise all augment venous return and hence ventricular filling and preload (Fig. 215-5). Simultaneously, the increase in the adrenergic nerve impulse traffic to the myocardium, the increased concentration of circulating catecholamines, and the tachycardia that occur during exercise combine to augment the contractility of the myocardium (Fig. 215-5, curves 1 and 2) and lead to an elevation of stroke work and stroke volume, without change or even a reduction of end-diastolic pressure and volume (Fig. 215-5, points A and B). Vasodilatation occurs in the exercising muscles, thus tending to limit the increase in arterial pressure that would otherwise occur as cardiac output rises to levels as high as five times greater than basal during maximal exercise. This vasodilatation ultimately allows the achievement of a greatly elevated cardiac output during exercise, at an arterial pressure (afterload) only moderately higher than in the resting state.

THE FAILING HEART

Although heart failure (HF) may be readily described as a clinical syndrome, characterized by well-known symptoms and physical signs (Chap. 216), a precise physiologic or biochemical definition is far more difficult. However, from the clinical point of view, HF may be considered to be the condition in which *an abnormality of cardiac structure or function is responsible for the inability of the heart to fill with or eject blood at a rate commensurate with the requirements of the metabolizing tissues.*

Abnormalities during systole and/or diastole may be present in HF. In so-called *systolic heart failure* (p. 1369), an impairment of myocardial contractility causes weakened systolic contraction, which leads,

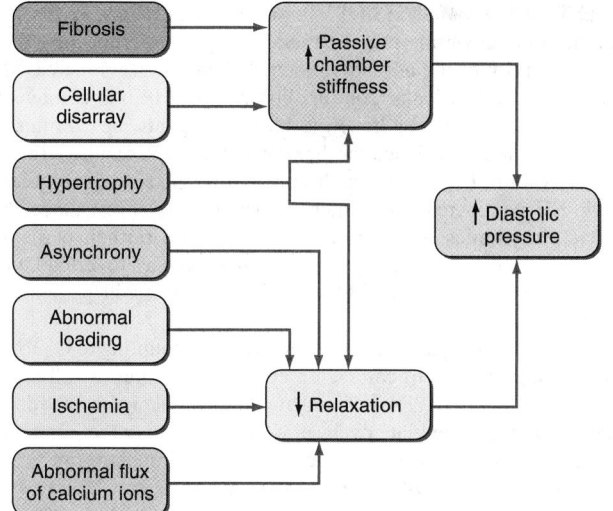

FIGURE 215-10 Mechanisms responsible for diastolic dysfunction in hypertrophic and ischemic heart disease. These factors, alone or in combination, contribute to the increased left ventricular chamber stiffness and impaired myocardial relaxation. As a result, left ventricular diastolic pressures are increased and filling is impaired. *[From WH Gaasch, EC Schick: Heart failure with normal left ventricular ejection fraction: A manifestation of diastolic dysfunction, in MH Crawford et al (eds). Cardiology. London, Mosby, 2001, pp 6.1–6.8. Reprinted with permission.]*

ultimately, to a reduction in stroke volume and cardiac output, inadequate ventricular emptying, cardiac dilatation, and often elevation of ventricular diastolic pressure. Idiopathic dilated cardiomyopathy (Chap. 221) and cardiogenic shock secondary to acute myocardial infarction (Chap. 255) are the prototypes of chronic and acute systolic HF, respectively.

In *diastolic heart failure* (p. 1369), the principal abnormality is impaired relaxation and filling of the ventricle, which leads to an elevation of ventricular diastolic pressure at any given diastolic volume (Fig. 215-8). Failure of relaxation can be functional and transient, as during ischemia, which reduces the ATP required for the SR pump to lower cytoplasmic [Ca^{2+}]. Chronically impaired ventricular filling can be caused by a stiffened, thickened ventricle and a number of conditions illustrated in Fig. 215-10. Typical conditions in which diastolic HF occurs are restrictive cardiomyopathy secondary to infiltrative conditions, such as amyloidosis or hemochromatosis, and hypertrophic cardiomyopathy (Chap. 221). The concentric hypertrophy associated with chronic hypertension can also impair ventricular filling. In many patients with cardiac hypertrophy and dilatation, systolic and diastolic HF coexist; the left ventricle both empties and fills abnormally.

MECHANISMS OF HEART FAILURE

ADAPTIVE AND MALADAPTIVE MECHANISMS
A number of mechanisms aid the heart faced with an increased hemodynamic burden (such as pressure or volume overload) or one that has sustained loss of myocardium or contractility. On a short-term basis many of these responses are adaptive (beneficial). However, on a long-term basis these responses are often maladaptive (deleterious) (Table 215-1).

1. The *Frank-Starling mechanism* operates through an increase in preload (p. 1361). As outlined above, an increase in the end-diastolic volume of the ventricle is associated with stretching of the sarcomeres, which increases the interaction between actin and myosin filaments and their sensitivity to Ca^{2+},

thereby enhancing contraction. However, ventricular dilatation may become maladaptive when it becomes excessive, as may occur in severe valvular regurgitation, dilatation increases wall stress through the operation of Laplace's law and thereby reduces shortening.

2. *Compensatory hypertrophy* occurs in hemodynamic overload, which in turn restores elevated ventricular wall stress to normal (Fig. 216-1). If the hypertrophy is insufficient to restore wall stress to normal, the ventricle dilates and this increases wall stress further, leading to a vicious circle. Also, severe ventricular hypertrophy may impair ventricular filling and cause myocardial ischemia.

3. In *ventricular remodeling* there are changes in the size, mass, and configuration of the ventricle as a consequence of hemodynamic changes following mechanical overload, hypertension, cardiomyopathy, and myocardial infarction. Remodeling is triggered by myocyte growth, interstitial fibrosis and apoptosis (Table 215-2), ischemia, vasoactive peptides, and fibrosis. A change to a more spherical shape, which decreases the effectiveness of ejection, is common in the remodeled ventricle.

4. *Redistribution of a subnormal cardiac output* away from the skin, skeletal muscle, and kidneys with maintenance of blood flow to the most vital organs, i.e., the brain and the heart, occurs. The vasoconstriction, however, may increase afterload, thereby reducing cardiac output further.

REDUCTION IN CARDIAC EFFICIENCY The common forms of low-output systolic HF, secondary to coronary atherosclerosis, hypertension, cardiomyopathy, and certain valvular and congenital lesions, are characterized by a reduction in the external work performed by the heart, while myocardial oxygen consumption remains normal or nearly so. Therefore, the external efficiency, i.e., the ratio of external work performed to energy consumed, is often depressed.

ALTERATIONS IN ENERGY METABOLISM When HF occurs in the presence of acute or chronic ischemia, it can be attributed to reduced supply of oxygen with a resultant reduction of ATP generation. Severe ventricular hypertrophy and/or dilatation from any etiology can contribute to ischemia, especially in the subendocardium, and this can impair both ventricular contraction and filling. In some forms of HF without ischemia, myocardial energy stores in the form of creatine phosphate are decreased, as is the activity of the enzyme creatine kinase required for the shuttling of high-energy phosphate between creatine phosphate and ADP, suggesting that reductions in myocardial energy reserves may play a role in nonischemic conditions as well.

ALTERATIONS IN SARCOMERIC PROTEINS Hemodynamic overload, neurohormonal and/or cytokine stimulation and gene mutations in familial cardiomyopathies may all reinduce the expression of fetal sarcomeric

TABLE 215-1 *Short-Term and Long-Term Responses to Impaired Cardiac Performance*

Response	Short-term Effects (mainly adaptive; hemorrhage, acute heart failure)	Long-term Effects (mainly deleterious; chronic heart failure)
Salt and water retention	Augments preload	Pulmonary congestion, anasarca
Vasoconstriction	Maintains pressure for perfusion of vital organs (brain, heart)	Exacerbates pump dysfunction, increases cardiac energy expenditure
Sympathetic stimulation	Increases heart rate and ejection	Increases energy expenditure
Cytokine activation	Vasodilatation	Skeletal muscle catabolism, deterioration of endothelial function, impaired contraction, LV remodeling.
Hypertrophy	Unloads individual muscle fibers	Deterioration and death of cardiac cells: cardiomyopathy of overload
Increased collagen	May reduce dilatation	Impairs relaxation

LV, left ventricle.
Source: From H Drexler, G Hasenfuss: Physiology of the normal and failing heart, in MH Crawford and JP DeMarco et al (eds): *Cardiology*. London, Mosby, 2001, pp 1.1–1.16, Modified from AM Katz: Cardiomyopathy of overload. A major determinant of prognosis in congestive heart failure. N Engl J Med 322:100, 1990

TABLE 215-2 *Factors that Lead to the Progressive Remodeling of the Left Ventricle*

Mechanism of Progressive Remodeling and Heart Failure			
Cell Growth	Fibrosis	Apoptosis	Counter-regulatory Factors
Angiotensin II	Angiotensin II	TNF-α	ANP
Catecholamines	Endothelin	*Fas* ligand	Bradykinin
Endothelin	Aldosterone		Nitric oxide
TNF-α	TGF-β		BNP
Growth hormone			
IGF			
Cardiotrophin-1			
Mechanical stretch			

Growth of cardiac myocytes is a primary feature and is due to a number of growth factors, including neurohormones and cytokines as well as mechanical stretch. Fibrosis is promoted by activation of the renin-angiotensin-aldosterone axis and through activation of endothelin and TGF-β. Apoptosis regulation is altered via changes in the expression of *p53*, *Bcl-2*, and *Bax* genes, perhaps as a consequence of increases in TNF-α acting to stimulate the *Fas* ligand. Programmed cell death is enhanced, producing cell drop-out. Counter-regulatory forces, including atrial natriuretic peptide (ANP) and brain natriuretic peptide (BNP) are activated. Nitric oxide, driven by bradykinin and ANP, may have antigrowth properties and hold uncontrolled growth in check to some extent; however, on balance, cardiac myocytes elongate, which contributes to left ventricular remodeling. IGF, insulin-like growth factor.
Source: G. Francis: Changing the remodeling process in heart failure: basic mechanisms and laboratory results. Curr Opin Cardiol 13:156, 1998

proteins whose contractility is depressed. It has been postulated that these alterations in sarcomeric proteins cause systolic HF. A reduction of myosin ATPase activity, which may be caused by an alteration in the expression of troponin T and/or of myosin light chain kinase 2, may also lower the rate of interaction between myosin and actin myofilaments and impair muscle shortening.

MYOCARDIAL CELL DEATH When a sufficiently large portion of ventricular myocardium becomes nonfunctional or necrotic, as occurs transiently during ischemia (Chap. 226) and permanently in myocardial infarction (Chap. 228), total ventricular performance at any given level of end-diastolic volume becomes depressed. Apoptosis of myocytes, like the reinduction of fetal sarcomeric proteins, can be caused by hemodynamic overload, excessive neurohormone and/or cytokine stimulation, as well as by severe ischemia. As a consequence of cell death, whatever the mechanism, the load on surviving myocytes is increased, setting the stage for a vicious circle of repeated cell death.

ABNORMALITIES OF EXCITATION-CONTRACTION COUPLING Substantial evidence supports the view that in many forms of heart failure the delivery of Ca^{2+} to the contractile sites is disturbed, thereby impairing cardiac performance. However, the molecular basis of this abnormality—indeed of the subcellular structures involved, i.e., the sarcolemma, T tubules, and/or SR—has yet to be defined. There is, however, evidence for a reduction in the activity of the Ca^{2+} release (ryanodine) channel in the SR and of messenger RNAs of the proteins regulating Ca^{2+} movements. The latter include the sarcolemmal Na^+-Ca^{2+} channels, and the activity of the SR Ca^{2+} uptake pump (SERCa-2a), which play critical roles in the movement of Ca^{2+} between the SR and the cytoplasm. Impaired expression of the genes encoding these proteins can impair both myocardial contraction and relaxation and thereby contribute to the development of HF.

NEUROHUMORAL AND CYTOKINE ADJUSTMENTS

A reduction in cardiac performance evokes a series of neurohumoral adjustments, which may at different times be adaptive or maladaptive (Table 215-1). These adjustments are adaptive when they maintain arterial perfusion pressure in the face of a sudden reduction of cardiac output. However, they are maladaptive when they increase the hemodynamic burden and oxygen requirements of the failing ventricle and when they exacerbate myocardial injury (Fig. 215-11).

THE ADRENERGIC NERVOUS SYSTEM In patients with HF the levels of circulating norepinephrine may be markedly elevated, reflecting the increased activity of the adrenergic nervous system. This increased activity supports ventricular contractility in acute HF that is intensified when large doses of β-adrenergic blocking agents are administered acutely, providing evidence for the protective action of adrenergic nervous activation. However, the chronic adrenergic stimulation that occurs in HF may increase afterload by raising vascular resistance, cause cardiac arrhythmias, and may damage myocytes further, perhaps by increasing myocardial energy expenditures and Ca^{2+} overload. Gradually increasing doses of β blockers are of benefit in patients with chronic HF (Chap. 216).

The density of β_1 adrenergic receptors, their coupling to G proteins, and the concentration of cardiac norepinephrine stores are all reduced in chronic, severe HF. These changes are accompanied by a reduction in the activity of adenylate cyclase, which may lower the intracellular concentration of cyclic AMP (Fig. 215-6). The reduction in turn depresses the activation of protein kinase, the phosphorylation of Ca^{2+} channels and transarcolemmal Ca^{2+} entry. It also reduces the phosphorylation of phospholamban, a protein in the SR, which in its unphosphorylated state inhibits the reuptake of Ca^{2+} by the SR. Changes in the G proteins, which couple the β receptor to adenylate cyclase (which is responsible for the production of cyclic AMP), may also occur in HF, with increased activity of the inhibitory subunit of the proteins.

THE RENIN-ANGIOTENSIN-ALDOSTERONE SYSTEM When cardiac output declines, the renin-angiotensin-aldosterone system (Chap. 321) is activated. Concentrations of both circulating angiotensin II and aldosterone are increased, the former contributing to excess vasoconstriction and the latter to the retention of salt and water and perhaps to cardiac fibrosis (Table 215-1). The local (tissue) renin-angiotensin system is also activated in HF and angiotensin II exerts a local cardiotoxic effect by stimulating G_q proteins that activate phospholipase C, which in turn activates protein kinase C. The latter stimulates cardiac hypertrophy and causes ventricular remodeling. Patients with HF are usually improved by blocking this system with angiotensin-converting enzyme (ACE) inhibitors, angiotensin II receptor blockers, and aldosterone antagonists (Chap. 216).

ENDOTHELIN AND TUMOR NECROSIS FACTOR α The concentration of circulating endothelin, a polypeptide that is a very powerful vasoconstrictor, is increased in HF and it contributes to the excessive afterload. The overexpression of a number of cytokines also appears to play a

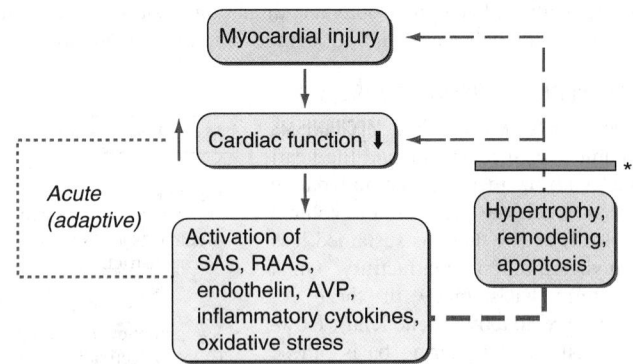

FIGURE 215-11 Interplay between cardiac function and neurohumoral and cytokine systems. Myocardial injury, of many etiologies, can depress cardiac function, which in turn causes activation of the sympathoadrenal system (SAS) and the renin-angiotensin-aldosterone system (RAAS) and the elaboration of endothelin, arginine vasopressin (AVP), and cytokines such as tumor necrosis factor (TNF) α. In acute heart failure (*left*), these are adaptive and tend to maintain arterial pressure and cardiac function. In chronic heart failure (*right*) they cause maladaptive hypertrophic remodeling and apoptosis, which cause further myocardial injury and impairment of cardiac function. The horizontal line on the right (*) shows that chronic maladaptive influences can be inhibited by angiotensin converting enzyme inhibitors, β-adrenergic blockers, angiotensin type I receptor blockers, and aldosterone antagonists.

prominent role in the pathogenesis of HF. It has now been well established that patients with HF exhibit elevated levels of TNF-α, both in the circulation and in cardiac muscle; the pathophysiologic significance of this finding is just unfolding. Transgenic mice with overexpressed cardiac TNF-α exhibit systolic dysfunction, myocarditis, ventricular dilatation, HF, and shortened survival. The infusion of TNF-α impairs ventricular function. However, thus far, blockade of endothelin and TNF-α have not been shown to improve the outcome of patients with HF.

VASODILATOR PEPTIDES   A number of vasodilator peptides are released by the dilated heart. Best known are the natriuretic peptides atrial natriuretic peptide (ANP) and brain natriuretic peptide (BNP). When stretch receptors in the atria (site of ANP and BNP stores) and ventricles (site of BNP stores) are stimulated, these hormones (or their prohormones) are released and act on specific natriuretic peptide receptors, which increase the concentrations of cyclic GMP in the kidney, adrenal glomerulosa, vascular smooth muscle, and platelets. Urine volume and sodium excretion are augmented, vascular resistance is reduced, and the release of renin and the secretion of aldosterone are reduced. These effects, while beneficial, are not sufficiently powerful to neutralize the sodium-retaining and vasoconstrictor influences of the aforementioned neurohumoral systems activated in HF. Elevated circulating concentrations of ANP and particularly BNP correlate with a poor prognosis in HF. The direct administration of recombinant BNP in acute pulmonary edema is promising.

Figure 215-11 illustrates current concepts of neurohumoral-cytokine activation in HF. The activation of the adrenergic nervous system and the renin-angiotensin-aldosterone system and the enhanced elaboration of endothelin and arginine vasopressin appear to be adaptive in *acute*, severe HF. However, they all appear to exert a maladaptive response in chronic HF. Inflammatory cytokines and oxidative stress are emerging as potent noxious stimuli as well. Together they result in a vicious circle, causing myocyte hypertrophy, remodeling, and cell death, the latter often due to myocardial apoptosis (see below), all resulting in further impairment of cardiac function and myocardial injury. Agents that interfere with the adverse effects of these stimuli on cardiac function, especially β-adrenergic blockers, ACE inhibitors, angiotensin receptor blockers, aldosterone receptor blockers, and perhaps arginine vasopressin blockers appear to be capable of blocking this vicious circle.

ABNORMALITIES OF THE INTERNAL AND EXTERNAL SKELETONS   Both hemodynamic overload and mutations of genes encoding cytoskeletal proteins interfere with the regulation of myocyte architecture and thereby interfere with contraction and relaxation. Proliferation of the *extracellular matrix* occurs in myocardial infarction, longstanding hypertension, and a variety of cardiomyopathic disorders. Since this matrix forms the extracellular "skeleton" of the heart, its excessive proliferation can interfere with both systolic shortening and diastolic lengthening. Thus abnormalities of both the internal and external skeleton can contribute to the progression of HF.

HEART FAILURE—A DISTURBANCE OF THE MYOCARDIAL PUMP
(See also Chap. 216)

In the final analysis, in systolic HF the basic problem is depression of the myocardial force-velocity relationship and of the length–active tension curve, reflecting reductions in myocardial contractility (Fig. 215-5, curves 1 to 3, Fig. 215-7, right). In diastolic HF there is upward displacement of the diastolic pressure–volume relation (Fig. 215-8). In many instances, cardiac output and external ventricular performance at rest are within normal limits but are maintained at these levels only by an increased end-diastolic fiber length and an elevated ventricular end-diastolic volume, i.e., through the operation of the Frank-Starling mechanism (Fig. 215-5, points A to D). The elevation of left ventricular preload is associated with increases in the pulmonary capillary pressure, contributing to the dyspnea experienced by patients with HF, while elevation of right ventricular preload raises systemic venous pressure and contributes to the development of edema. The improvement of contractility that normally accompanies augmented adrenergic activity during exercise is attenuated or even prevented by norepinephrine depletion and downregulation of myocardial β receptors, which occur in severe HF (Fig. 215-5, curves 3 and 3′).

The factors that augment ventricular filling during exercise in the normal individual push the failing myocardium along its flattened length–active tension curve. Although the function of left ventricle may be improved at this higher diastolic volume, through the operation of the Frank-Starling mechanism, this improvement occurs only as a consequence of an inordinate elevation of ventricular end-diastolic volume and pressure and, therefore, of the pulmonary capillary pressure. The latter intensifies dyspnea and limits the intensity of exercise that the patient can perform. Left ventricular failure becomes fatal when the myocardial length–active tension curve is depressed (Fig. 215-5, curve 4) to the point at which cardiac performance fails to satisfy the requirements of the peripheral tissues even at rest, and/or the left ventricular end-diastolic and pulmonary capillary pressures are elevated to levels that result in pulmonary edema (Fig. 215-5, point E).

FURTHER READING

ALPERT NR et al: The failing human heart. Cardiovasc Res 54:1, 2002

ANVERSA P et al: Myocyte death in heart failure. Curr Opin Cardiol 11:245, 1996

BRAUNWALD E: Congestive heart failure: A half century perspective. The Denolin lecture. Eur Heart J 22:825, 2001

COLUCCI WS (ed): Heart failure: Cardiac function and dysfunction, in *Atlas of Heart Diseases*, 3d ed, E Braunwald (series ed). Philadelphia, Current Medicine, 2002

KATZ AM: *Heart Failure*, New York, Raven, 2000, pp 381

CARROLL J, HESS O: Assessment of cardiac function, in *Braunwald's Heart Disease*, 7th ed, D Zipes et al (eds). Philadelphia, Saunders, 2005

OPIE LH: Mechanisms of cardiac contraction and relaxation, in *Heart Disease*, 6th ed, E Braunwald et al (ed). Philadelphia, Saunders, 2001

SCHWARTZ K, MERCADIER J-J: Molecular and cellular biology of heart failure. Curr Opin Cardiol 11:227, 1996

216 | HEART FAILURE AND COR PULMONALE
Eugene Braunwald

HEART FAILURE

Heart failure (HF) is a clinical syndrome in which an abnormality of cardiac structure or function is responsible for the inability of the heart to eject or fill with blood at a rate commensurate with the requirements of the metabolizing tissues. HF results in a constellation of clinical manifestations, including, in various combinations, circulatory congestion, dyspnea, fatigue, and weakness. The severity of the clinical manifestations are commonly described according to criteria developed by the New York Heart Association.

HF is a major public health problem in industrialized nations. It appears to be the only common cardiovascular condition that is increasing in prevalence and incidence in North America and Europe. In the United States, HF is responsible for almost 1 million hospital admissions and 50,000 deaths annually. Since HF is more common in the elderly, its prevalence is likely to continue to increase as the population ages.

HF is frequently, but not always, caused by a defect in myocardial contraction, and then the term *myocardial failure* is appropriate. The latter may result from a primary abnormality in heart muscle, as occurs in the cardiomyopathies, or in viral myocarditis (Chap. 221). HF also results commonly from coronary atherosclerosis, which interferes with cardiac contraction by causing myocardial infarction and ischemia. HF may also occur in congenital, valvular, and hypertensive heart disease in which the myocardium is damaged by the long-standing hemodynamic overload. In other patients with HF, however, a similar clinical syndrome is present but without any detectable abnormality of *myocardial* function. In some cases the normal heart is suddenly presented with a mechanical load that exceeds its capacity, such as an acute hypertensive crisis, rupture of an aortic valve leaflet, in endocarditis or with a massive pulmonary embolism. HF in the presence of normal systolic function also occurs in chronic conditions in which there is impaired filling of the ventricles due to a mechanical abnormality such as tricuspid and/or mitral stenosis without myocardial involvement, endocardial fibrosis, and some forms of hypertrophic cardiomyopathy (see Fig. 215-8).

CAUSES OF HEART FAILURE

UNDERLYING CAUSES　Although HF may occur as a consequence of most forms of heart disease, in the United States and Western Europe, ischemic heart disease is responsible for about three-quarters of all cases. Cardiomyopathies are second in frequency, while congenital, valvular, and hypertensive heart disease are less common causes. It is important to identify potentially treatable underlying causes of HF, such as the latter three groups of disorders.

PRECIPITATING CAUSES　In evaluating patients with HF, it is important to identify not only the *underlying* but also the *precipitating cause*. Frequently, clinical manifestations of HF are seen for the first time in the course of an acute disturbance that places an additional load on a myocardium that is chronically excessively burdened. Such a heart may be adequately compensated under normal circumstances but have little additional reserve, the additional load imposed by a precipitating cause results in further deterioration of cardiac function. The ten most common precipitating causes are described below.

1. *Infection.* Patients with pulmonary vascular congestion due to left ventricular failure are more susceptible to pulmonary infection than are normal persons; however, any infection may precipitate HF. The resulting fever, tachycardia, hypoxemia, and the increased metabolic demands may place a further burden on an overloaded, but compensated, myocardium of a patient with chronic heart disease.

2. *Arrhythmias.* These are among the most frequent precipitating causes of HF. They exert a deleterious effect on cardiac function through a variety of mechanisms: (a) Tachyarrhythmias reduce the time available for ventricular filling, contributing especially to diastolic HF; they may also cause ischemic myocardial dysfunction in patients with ischemic heart disease. (b) The dissociation between atrial and ventricular contractions characteristic of many brady- and tachyarrhythmias results in the loss of the atrial booster pump mechanism, i.e., the "atrial kick," thereby raising atrial pressures. (c) Cardiac performance may become further impaired because of the loss of normally synchronized ventricular contraction in any arrhythmia associated with abnormal intraventricular conduction (see resynchronization therapy below). (d) Slowing of the heart rate associated with complete atrioventricular block or other severe bradyarrhythmias reduces cardiac output unless stroke volume rises reciprocally; this compensatory response is limited in myocardial dysfunction, even in the absence of overt HF.

3. *Physical, Dietary, Fluid, Environmental, and Emotional Excesses.* The sudden augmentation of sodium intake as with a large holiday meal, the inappropriate discontinuation of drugs or other therapy for HF, blood transfusions, physical overexertion, excessive environmental heat or humidity, and emotional crises all may precipitate HF in patients who were previously compensated.

4. *Myocardial Infarction.* In patients with chronic but compen-

sated ischemic heart disease, a new infarct, sometimes otherwise silent clinically, may further impair ventricular function and precipitate HF (Chap. 228).

5. *Pulmonary Embolism.* Physically inactive patients with low cardiac output are at increased risk of developing thrombi in the veins of the lower extremities or the pelvis. Pulmonary emboli may result in further elevation of pulmonary arterial pressure, which in turn may produce or intensify ventricular failure. In the presence of pulmonary vascular congestion, such emboli also may cause pulmonary infarction (Chap. 244).

6. *Anemia.* In the presence of anemia, the oxygen needs of the metabolizing tissues can be met only by an increase in the cardiac output (Chap. 52). Such an increase may be sustained by a normal heart. However, a diseased, overloaded, but otherwise compensated heart may be unable to augment sufficiently the volume of blood that it delivers to the periphery. In this manner, the combination of anemia and previously compensated heart disease can precipitate HF and lead to inadequate delivery of oxygen to the periphery.

7. *Thyrotoxicosis and Pregnancy.* Similar to anemia and fever, thyrotoxicosis and pregnancy are also high cardiac output states. The development or intensification of HF in a patient with previously compensated heart disease may actually be one of the first clinical manifestations of hyperthyroidism (Chap. 320). Similarly, HF may occur for the first time during pregnancy in women with rheumatic valvular disease, in whom cardiac compensation may return following delivery (Chap. 6).

8. *Aggravation of Hypertension.* Rapid elevation of arterial pressure, as may occur in some instances of renal hypertension or upon abrupt discontinuation of antihypertensive medication in patients with essential hypertension, may result in cardiac decompensation.

9. *Rheumatic, Viral, and Other Forms of Myocarditis.* Acute rheumatic fever and a variety of other inflammatory or infectious processes affecting the myocardium may precipitate HF in patients with or without preexisting heart disease (Chaps. 221 and 302).

10. *Infective Endocarditis.* The additional valvular damage, anemia, fever, and myocarditis that often occur as a consequence of infective endocarditis may, singly or in combination, precipitate HF (Chap. 109).

A systematic search for these precipitating causes should be made in every patient with the new development or recent intensification of HF. If properly recognized, the precipitating cause of HF usually can be treated effectively. Therefore, the prognosis in patients with HF in whom a precipitating cause can be identified, treated, and eliminated is more favorable than in patients in whom the underlying disease process has progressed to the point of producing HF without a detectable precipitating cause.

HF resembles but should be distinguished from (1) conditions in which there is circulatory congestion secondary to abnormal salt and water retention but in which there is no disturbance of cardiac function *per se*, as occurs in renal failure; and (2) noncardiac causes of inadequate cardiac output, such as hypovolemic shock (Chap. 253).

The ventricles respond to chronic hemodynamic overload with the development of hypertrophy (Fig. 216-1). When the ventricle is called on to deliver an elevated cardiac output for prolonged periods, as in valvular regurgitation, it develops *eccentric hypertrophy*, i.e., cavity dilatation, with an increase in muscle mass so that the ratio between wall thickness and ventricular cavity diameter remains relatively constant early in the process. With chronic pressure overload, as in valvular aortic stenosis or untreated hypertension, *concentric ventricular hypertrophy* develops; in this condition the ratio between wall thickness and ventricular cavity size increases. In both eccentric and concentric hypertrophy, wall tension is initially maintained at a normal level and cardiac function may remain stable for many years. However, myocardial function may ultimately deteriorate, leading to HF. Often at this time, the ventricle dilates and the ratio between wall thickness and cavity size declines, leading to increased stress on each unit of myocardium, further dilatation, and a vicious cycle is initiated. Remodeling of the ventricle occurs with a change to a more spherical

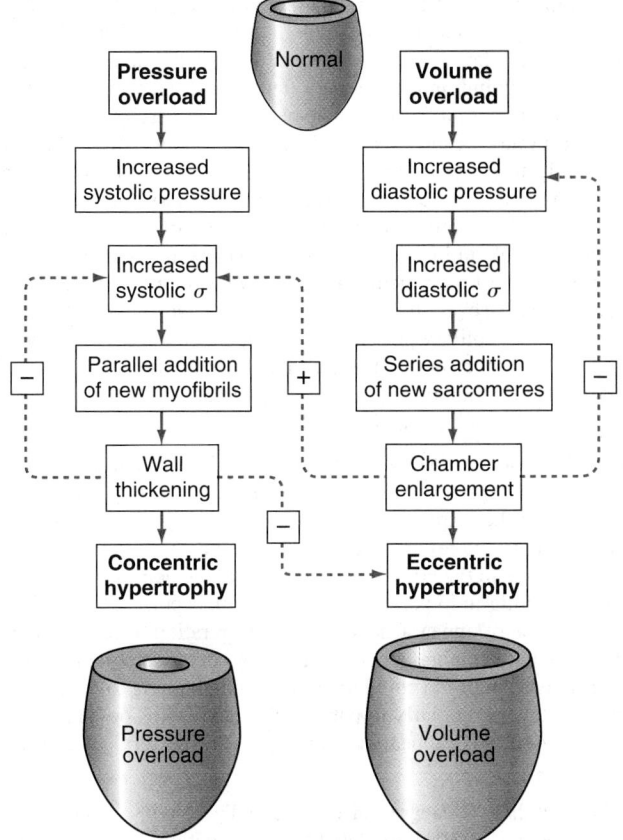

FIGURE 216-1 Patterns of ventricular hypertrophy. Specific patterns of ventricular remodeling occur in response to the imposed augmentation in work load. A pattern of hypertrophic growth characterized as concentric, in which increased mass is out of proportion to chamber volume, is particularly effective in reducing systolic wall stress (σ) under conditions of heightened pressure load. In contrast, in volume overload conditions, in which the major stimulus is diastolic loading, a predominant finding is a great increase in the cavity size or volume. Although there can be extensive increases in mass, the relationship between mass and volume is either preserved or, in severe cases, reduced. The fundamental response is generated by cellular hypertrophy. However, the configuration of the new contractile tissue is specific and offsets the mechanical stimulus. *[Modified from W Grossman et al in NR Alpert (ed): Perspectives in Cardiovascular Research. Myocardial Hypertrophy and Failure, vol 7. New York, Raven Press, 1993, with permission.]*

shape, which increases the hemodynamic stresses on the wall and may cause or intensify mitral regurgitation. Activation of endogenous neurohormonal systems and cytokines (Chap. 215) appears to be involved in ventricular remodeling and thereby the progression of HF. Remodeling is particularly prominent in patients with transmural myocardial infarction, in whom the infarcted area stretches and the remaining viable portion of the ventricle dilates.

FORMS OF HEART FAILURE

HF may be described as *systolic* or *diastolic*, *high-output* or *low-output*, *acute* or *chronic*, *right-sided* or *left-sided*, and *forward* or *backward*. These descriptors are often useful in a clinical setting, particularly early in the patient's course, but the differences often become blurred late in the course of chronic HF.

SYSTOLIC VERSUS DIASTOLIC FAILURE The distinction between these two forms of HF relates to whether the principal abnormality is the inability of the ventricle to contract normally and expel sufficient blood (systolic failure) or to relax and fill normally (diastolic failure). The manifestations of systolic failure relate to an inadequate cardiac output with weakness, fatigue, reduced exercise tolerance, and other symptoms of hypoperfusion, while in diastolic HF the manifestations relate principally to the elevation of filling pressures in the left and/or right ventricles. Diastolic HF is usually defined as HF in patients with an ejection fraction >50%.

Diastolic HF (see Fig. 215-8) may be caused by increased resistance to ventricular inflow and reduced ventricular diastolic capacity (constrictive pericarditis and restrictive, hypertensive, and hypertrophic cardiomyopathy), impaired ventricular relaxation (acute myocardial ischemia), and myocardial fibrosis and infiltration (restrictive cardiomyopathy). Diastolic HF occurs more frequently in women than men, especially elderly women with hypertension. In most patients with HF, abnormalities both of contraction and relaxation coexist.

LOW-OUTPUT VERSUS HIGH-OUTPUT HEART FAILURE *Low-output HF* occurs secondary to ischemic heart disease, hypertension, dilated cardiomyopathy, and valvular and pericardial disease, while *high-output HF* occurs in patients with reduced systemic vascular resistance, i.e., hyperthyroidism, anemia, pregnancy, arteriovenous fistulas, beriberi, and Paget's disease. In clinical practice, however, low-output and high-output HF cannot always be readily distinguished. The normal range of cardiac output is wide (2.2 to 3.5 L/min per m²); in many patients with low-output HF, the cardiac output may actually be just above the lower limit of normal range at rest (although lower than it had been previously), but fails to rise normally during exertion. On the other hand, in patients with so-called high-output HF, the output may not exceed the upper limits of normal (although it would have been abnormally elevated had it been measured before HF supervened); instead, it may have fallen to within normal limits with HF.

The hemodynamic burden placed on the myocardium by many forms of high-output heart failure resembles that produced by chronic aortic regurgitation. In addition, thyrotoxicosis and beriberi may also impair myocardial metabolism directly, while very severe anemia may interfere with myocardial function by producing myocardial anoxia, especially in the subendocardium and in the presence of underlying obstructive coronary artery disease.

ACUTE VERSUS CHRONIC HEART FAILURE An example of causes of *acute HF* are the sudden rupture of a cardiac valve leaflet secondary to trauma or infective endocarditis or a massive myocardial infarction in a patient who previously had no cardiac dysfunction. In acute HF the sudden reduction in cardiac output often results in systemic hypotension without peripheral edema. *Chronic HF* is typically observed in patients with dilated cardiomyopathy or multivalvular heart disease and develops or progresses slowly. Vascular congestion is common in chronic HF, but arterial pressure is ordinarily well maintained until very late.

RIGHT-SIDED VERSUS LEFT-SIDED HEART FAILURE Many of the clinical manifestations of HF result from the accumulation of fluid upstream to (behind) the ventricles that is initially affected. For example, patients in whom the left ventricle is hemodynamically overloaded (e.g., aortic regurgitation) or weakened due to myocyte loss (e.g., postmyocardial infarction) develop dyspnea and orthopnea as a result of pulmonary congestion, a condition referred to as *left-sided HF*. When the underlying abnormality affects the right ventricle primarily (e.g., primary pulmonary hypertension secondary to chronic pulmonary thromboembolism), symptoms resulting from pulmonary congestion are uncommon, and edema, congestive hepatomegaly, and systemic venous distention, i.e., clinical manifestations of *right-sided HF*, are prominent. The muscle bundles composing both ventricles are continuous, and both ventricles share a common wall, the interventricular septum. The biochemical changes that occur in the myocardium in HF (Chap. 215) usually occur in the myocardium of *both* ventricles. Therefore, when HF has existed for months or years, localization of excess fluid behind one ventricle may no longer exist.

BACKWARD VERSUS FORWARD HEART FAILURE A controversy has revolved around the mechanism of the clinical manifestations resulting from HF. The concept of *backward HF* contends that in HF, one or the other ventricle fails to discharge its contents or fails to fill normally. As a consequence, the pressures in the atrium and venous system behind (upstream to) the failing ventricle rise, and retention of sodium and water occurs as a consequence of the elevation of systemic venous and capillary pressures and the resultant transudation of fluid into the pulmonary or systemic interstitial space. On the other hand, proponents of the *forward HF* hypothesis maintain that the clinical manifestations of HF result directly from an inadequate discharge of blood into the arterial system. According to this concept, salt and water retention is a consequence of diminished renal perfusion and excessive proximal and distal tubular reabsorption of sodium, the latter through activation of the renin-angiotensin-aldosterone system (RAAS) (Chap. 32).

The rate of onset of HF often influences the clinical manifestations. For example, when a large portion of the left ventricle is suddenly destroyed, as in myocardial infarction, the patient may succumb to acute pulmonary edema, a manifestation of *backward failure*. If the patient survives the acute insult, clinical manifestations resulting from a chronically depressed cardiac output, including the abnormal retention of fluid within the systemic vascular bed, may develop, which is a manifestation of *forward failure*.

SALT AND WATER RETENTION (See also Chap. 32)   When the volume of blood pumped by the left ventricle into the systemic vascular bed is reduced, a complex sequence of adjustments occurs that ultimately results in the abnormal accumulation of fluid. This may be considered a two-edged sword. Many of the troubling clinical manifestations of HF, such as pulmonary congestion and edema, are secondary to this excessive retention of fluid (see Fig. 32-1). However, this abnormal fluid accumulation and the expansion of blood volume that accompanies it also constitute an important compensatory mechanism that tends to maintain cardiac output and therefore perfusion of the vital organs. Except in the terminal stages of HF, the ventricle operates on an ascending, albeit depressed and flattened, function curve (see Fig. 215-5), and the augmented ventricular end-diastolic volume characteristic of HF must be regarded as helping to maintain the reduced cardiac output, despite causing pulmonary and/or systemic venous congestion.

CLINICAL MANIFESTATIONS OF HEART FAILURE

RESPIRATORY DISTURBANCES ■ Dyspnea (Chap. 29)   In early HF, dyspnea is observed only during exertion, when it may simply represent an aggravation of the breathlessness that occurs normally. As HF advances, dyspnea occurs with progressively less strenuous activity and ultimately it is present even at rest. The principal difference between exertional dyspnea in normal persons and in patients with HF is the degree of exertion necessary to induce this symptom. Cardiac dyspnea is observed most frequently in patients with elevations of pulmonary venous and capillary pressures who have engorged pulmonary vessels and interstitial accumulation of interstitial fluid. The activation of receptors in the lungs results in the rapid, shallow breathing characteristic of cardiac dyspnea. The oxygen cost of breathing is increased by the excessive work of the respiratory muscles required to move air into and out of the congested lungs. This is coupled with the diminished delivery of oxygen to these muscles, a consequence of a reduced cardiac output. This imbalance may contribute to fatigue of the respiratory muscles and the sensation of shortness of breath.

Orthopnea   This symptom, i.e., dyspnea in the recumbent position, is usually a later manifestation of HF than exertional dyspnea. Orthopnea results from the redistribution of fluid from the abdomen and lower extremities into the chest during recumbency, which increases the pulmonary capillary pressure, combined with elevation of the diaphragm. Patients with orthopnea must elevate their head on several pillows at night and frequently awaken short of breath and/or coughing if their head slips off the pillows. Orthopnea is usually relieved by sitting upright, and some patients report that they find relief from sitting in front of an open window. In advanced HF, patients cannot lie down at all and must spend the entire night in a sitting position.

Paroxysmal (Nocturnal) Dyspnea   This term refers to attacks of severe shortness of breath and coughing that generally occur at night, usually

awaken the patient from sleep, and may be quite frightening. Though simple orthopnea may be relieved by sitting upright at the side of the bed with legs dependent, in the patient with paroxysmal nocturnal dyspnea, coughing and wheezing often persist even in this position. Paroxysmal nocturnal dyspnea may be caused in part by the depression of the respiratory center during sleep, which may reduce ventilation sufficiently to lower arterial oxygen tension, particularly in patients with interstitial lung edema and reduced pulmonary compliance. *Cardiac asthma* is closely related to paroxysmal nocturnal dyspnea and nocturnal cough and is characterized by wheezing secondary to bronchospasm—most prominent at night. *Acute pulmonary edema* (Chaps. 29 and 255) is a severe form of cardiac asthma due to marked elevation of pulmonary capillary pressure leading to alveolar edema, associated with extreme shortness of breath, rales over the lung fields, and the expectoration of blood-tinged fluid. If not treated promptly, acute pulmonary edema may be fatal.

Cheyne-Stokes Respiration   Also known as *periodic respiration* or *cyclic respiration*, Cheyne-Stokes respiration is characterized by diminished sensitivity of the respiratory center to arterial P_{CO_2}. There is an apneic phase, during which the arterial P_{O_2} falls and the arterial P_{CO_2} rises. These changes in the arterial blood stimulate the depressed respiratory center, resulting in hyperventilation and hypocapnia, followed in turn by recurrence of apnea. Cheyne-Stokes respiration occurs most often in patients with cerebral atherosclerosis and other cerebral lesions, but the prolongation of the circulation time from the lung to the brain that occurs in HF, particularly in patients with hypertension and coronary artery disease, also appears to contribute to this form of disordered breathing.

OTHER SYMPTOMS ■ Fatigue and Weakness   These nonspecific but common symptoms of HF are related to the reduction of skeletal muscle perfusion. Exercise capacity is reduced by the limited ability of the failing heart to increase its output and deliver oxygen to the exercising muscles.

Abdominal Symptoms   Anorexia and nausea associated with abdominal pain and fullness are frequent complaints and may be related to the congested liver and portal venous system.

Cerebral Symptoms   Patients with severe HF, particularly elderly patients with cerebral arteriosclerosis, reduced cerebral perfusion, and arterial hypoxemia, may develop alterations in the mental state characterized by confusion, difficulty in concentration, impairment of memory, headache, insomnia, and anxiety. *Nocturia* is common in HF and may contribute to insomnia.

PHYSICAL FINDINGS (See Chap. 209)   In mild or moderately severe HF, the patient appears in no distress at rest except feeling uncomfortable when lying flat for more than a few minutes. In severe HF, the pulse pressure may be diminished, reflecting a reduction in stroke volume, and the diastolic arterial pressure may be elevated as a consequence of generalized vasoconstriction. In severe acute HF, systolic hypotension may be present, with cool, diaphoretic extremities, and Cheyne-Stokes respiration. There may be cyanosis of the lips and nail beds (Chap. 31) and sinus tachycardia. *Systemic venous pressure* is often abnormally elevated, and this may be reflected in distention of the jugular veins. In the early stages of HF, the venous pressure may be normal at rest but may become abnormally elevated, with sustained pressure on the abdomen (positive abdominojugular reflux).

Third and fourth heart sounds are often audible but are not specific for HF, and *pulsus alternans*, i.e., a regular rhythm with alternation of strong and weak cardiac contractions and therefore alternation in the strength of the peripheral pulses, may be present. This sign of severe HF may be detected by sphygmomanometry and in more severe cases even by palpation; it frequently follows an extrasystole and is observed most commonly in patients with cardiomyopathy, hypertensive, or ischemic heart disease.

Pulmonary Rales   Moist, inspiratory, crepitant rales and dullness to percussion over the lung bases are common in patients with HF and elevated pulmonary venous and capillary pressures. In patients with pulmonary edema, rales may be heard widely over both lung fields; they are frequently coarse and sibilant and may be accompanied by expiratory wheezing. Rales may, however, be caused by many conditions other than left ventricular failure. Some patients with longstanding HF and elevated pulmonary vascular pressures have no rales because of increased lymphatic drainage of alveolar fluid.

Cardiac Edema (See Chap. 32)   This is usually symmetric and dependent in HF, occurring in the legs, particularly in the ankles and pretibial region in ambulatory patients, in whom it is most prominent in the evening. In patients who are bedridden, cardiac edema occurs in the sacral region.

Hydrothorax and Ascites   Pleural effusion in HF (hydrothorax) results from the elevation of pleural capillary pressure and the resultant transudation of fluid into the pleural cavities. Since the pleural veins drain into *both* the systemic and pulmonary veins, hydrothorax occurs most commonly with marked elevation of pressure in both venous systems but may also be seen with marked elevation of pressure in either venous bed. It occurs more frequently in the right pleural cavity than in the left. *Ascites* also occurs as a consequence of transudation and results from increased pressure in the hepatic veins and the veins draining the peritoneum (Chap. 39). Among patients with HF, ascites occurs most frequently in those with constrictive pericarditis and those with tricuspid valve disease.

Congestive Hepatomegaly   Like edema, an enlarged, tender, pulsating liver also accompanies systemic venous hypertension. With prolonged, severe hepatomegaly, as in patients with tricuspid valve disease or chronic constrictive pericarditis, enlargement of the spleen, i.e., congestive splenomegaly, may also occur.

Jaundice   This is a late finding in HF and is associated with elevations of both direct and indirect bilirubin. It results from impairment of hepatic function secondary to hepatic congestion and the hepatocellular hypoxia associated with central lobular atrophy. Hepatic enzymes are frequently elevated. If hepatic congestion occurs acutely, the jaundice may be severe and the enzymes strikingly elevated.

Cardiac Cachexia   With severe chronic HF there may be marked weight loss and cachexia because of: (1) elevation of the metabolic rate, which results in part from the extra work performed by the respiratory muscles, the increased O_2 needs of the hypertrophied heart, and/or the discomfort associated with severe HF; (2) anorexia, nausea, and vomiting due to congestive hepatomegaly and abdominal fullness and/or digitalis intoxication (see below); (3) impairment of intestinal absorption due to congestion of the intestinal veins; (4) elevation of circulating concentrations of cytokines such as tumor necrosis factor; and (5) rarely, due to protein-losing enteropathy in patients with particularly severe failure of the right side of the heart.

Other Manifestations   With reduction of blood flow, the skin, especially in the extremities, may be cold, pale, and diaphoretic. Urine flow is depressed, contains albumin, has a high specific gravity, and a low concentration of sodium. In addition, prerenal azotemia may be present. In patients with long-standing severe HF, depression and sexual dysfunction are common.

DIFFERENTIAL DIAGNOSIS   The diagnosis of congestive HF may be established by observing some combination of the clinical manifestations of HF described above, together with the findings characteristic of one of the underlying forms of heart disease. Table 216-1 shows the Framingham criteria, which are useful in the diagnosis of HF. Since chronic HF is often associated with cardiac enlargement, the diagnosis should be questioned, but is by no means excluded, when all chambers are normal in size. HF is sometimes difficult to distinguish from *pulmonary disease*, and the differential diagnosis is discussed in Chap. 29. *Pulmonary embolism* also presents many of the manifestations of HF, but hemoptysis, pleuritic chest pain, a right ventricular lift, and the characteristic mismatch between ventilation and perfusion on lung scan should point to this diagnosis (Chap. 244).

TABLE 216-1   *Framingham Criteria for Diagnosis of Congestive Heart Failure[a]*

MAJOR CRITERIA

Paroxysmal nocturnal dyspnea
Neck vein distention
Rales
Cardiomegaly
Acute pulmonary edema
S_3 gallop
Increased venous pressure (>16 cmH$_2$O)
Positive hepatojugular reflux

MINOR CRITERIA

Extremity edema
Night cough
Dyspnea on exertion
Hepatomegaly
Pleural effusion
Vital capacity reduced by one-third from normal
Tachycardia (≥120 bpm)

MAJOR OR MINOR

Weight loss ≥4.5 kg over 5 days' treatment

[a] To establish a clinical diagnosis of congestive heart failure by these criteria, at least one major and two minor criteria are required.
Source: KKL Ho et al, Circulation 88:107, 1993.

Ankle edema may be due to varicose veins, cyclic edema, or gravitational effects (Chap. 32), but in patients with these conditions, there is no jugular venous hypertension at rest or with pressure over the abdomen. Edema secondary to *renal disease* can usually be recognized by appropriate renal function tests and urinalysis and it is rarely associated with elevation of venous pressure. Enlargement of the liver and ascites occur in patients with *hepatic cirrhosis* and also may be distinguished from HF by normal jugular venous pressure and the absence of a positive abdominojugular reflux.

BRAIN NATRIURETIC PEPTIDE (BNP)   Pre pro-BNP is formed in the ventricles and, with myocyte stretch, is broken down to N-terminal-pro-BNP (NT-pro-BNP) and BNP. These hormones are highly accurate for identifying or excluding HF with high sensitivity and specificity and add significant independent predictive power when added to the chemical features. BNP is particularly valuable in differentiating cardiac from pulmonary causes of dyspnea. The availability of a bedside assay makes BNP useful in evaluating patients in the Emergency Department.

APPROACH TO THE PATIENT

In addition to a detailed clinical examination, a two-dimensional echocardiogram with Doppler flow studies is of critical importance in determining the underlying causes of HF and in assessing the severity of ventricular systolic and/or diastolic dysfunction, as well as valvular dysfunction. Such ultrasound studies are part of the workup of all patients in whom the diagnosis of HF is considered. The electrocardiogram is rarely normal in systolic HF. The chest roentgenogram is helpful in detecting cardiomegaly and pulmonary congestion. BNP is extremely useful in diagnosis, prognosis, and monitoring therapy.

℞ TREATMENT

A simple rule for the treatment of all patients with HF cannot be formulated because of its varied etiologies, hemodynamic features, clinical manifestations, and severity. The treatment of HF may be divided into five components: (1) general measures; (2) correction of the underlying cause; (3) removal of the precipitating cause; (4) prevention of deterioration of cardiac function; and (5) control of the congestive HF state. An example of correction of the underlying course is the surgical repair or replacement of a deformed valve. An example of removal of a precipitating cause is the restoration of sinus rhythm in a patient with atrial fibrillation and a rapid ventricular rate. An approach that applies to many patients is shown in Table 216-2 and Fig. 216-2.

GENERAL MEASURES Every effort should be made to prevent HF, not only by treating hypertension and other coronary risk factors (Chap. 225) but also by the administration of angiotensin-converting enzyme (ACE) inhibitors (or, in patients who are intolerant of them, angiotensin receptor blockers, ARBs), even in asymptomatic patients with a history of atherosclerotic vascular disease, diabetes mellitus, or hypertension.

General measures in patients with HF include moderate dietary Na$^+$ restriction (see below), daily measurement of weight to aid in the adjustment of diuretic dosage, as well as immunization with influenza and pneumococcal vaccines to prevent respiratory infection. Education of the patient and family about the condition and the critical importance of close attention to compliance with the medical regimen and supervision of outpatient care by a specially trained nurse or physician assistant have all been found to be helpful. Excessive alcohol, temperature extremes, and tiring trips should be avoided.

Activity In acute, severe HF, meals should be small in quantity, but more frequent, and every effort should be made to diminish anxiety; sometimes drugs such as diazepam (2 to 5 mg tid) for several days are useful. Physical and emotional rest tends to lower arterial pressure and reduce the load on the myocardium by diminishing the requirements for cardiac output. Reduced physical exertion should be continued for several days after the patient's condition has stabilized. The hazards of phlebothrombosis and pulmonary embolism which occur with bed rest may be reduced with anticoagulants, leg exercises, and elastic stockings. *Absolute* bed rest is rarely required or advisable, and even the patient with severe HF should ordinarily be encouraged to sit in a chair. In ambulatory patients with chronic, moderately severe HF, additional periods of rest on weekends frequently allow continuation of gainful employment. A scheduled nap or rest following lunch and the avoidance of particularly strenuous exertion are often helpful.

Once the patient has become compensated, regular isotonic exercise such as walking or riding a stationary-bicycle ergometer as tolerated should be strongly encouraged. Some trials of exercise training have led to encouraging results with reduced symptoms, increased exercise capacity, and improved quality of life. Weight reduction by restriction of caloric intake in obese patients with HF also diminishes cardiac work load and is an essential component of the therapeutic program.

CONTROL OF EXCESSIVE FLUID Many of the clinical manifestations of HF result from expansion of the extracellular fluid volume. A negative Na$^+$ balance can be achieved in such patients by reducing the dietary intake and increasing the urinary excretion of this ion with the aid of diuretics. Rarely, in severe HF, mechanical removal of extracellular fluid by means of thoracentesis and paracentesis may be necessary.

Diet In patients with mild HF, symptomatic improvement may result simply from reducing the sodium intake. The normal diet contains approximately 6 to 10 g NaCl per day; this intake can be reduced in half simply by excluding salt-rich foods and salt added at the table. Further reduction of the ordinary dietary intake of NaCl to approximately one-fourth of normal may be achieved if, in addition, NaCl is omitted from cooking. In patients with severe HF who have fluid accumulation despite vigorous diuretic therapy (see below), the dietary intake of NaCl should be reduced to 1 g/d. In order to achieve this, milk, cheese, bread, cereals, canned vegetables and soups, some salted cuts of meat, and some fresh vegetables (including spinach, celery, and beets) must be eliminated. A variety of fresh fruit, green vegeta-

---

TABLE 216-2 *Stages in the Evolution of Heart Failure/Recommended Therapy by Stage*

Stage A ⟶		Stage B ⟶		Stage C ⟶		Stage D
At high risk for heart failure but without structural heart disease or symptoms of HF		Structural heart disease but without symptoms of HF		Structural heart disease with prior or current symptoms of HF		Refractory HF requiring specialized interventions
Patients with hypertension coronary artery disease diabetes mellitus *or* Patients using cardiotoxins with FHx CM	Structural heart disease	Patients with previous MI LV systolic dysfunction asymptomatic valvular disease	Symptoms of HF develop	Patients with known structural heart disease shortness of breath and fatigue, reduced exercise tolerance	Refractory symptoms of HF at rest	Patients who have marked symptoms at rest despite maximal medical therapy (e.g., those who are recurrently hospitalized or cannot be safely discharged from the hospital without specialized interventions)

THERAPY

Stage A		Stage B		Stage C		Stage D
Treat hypertension Encourage smoking cessation Treat lipid disorders Encourage regular exercise Discourage alcohol intake, illicit drug use ACE inhibition		All measures under stage A ACE inhibitors in appropriate patients Beta-blockers		All measures under stage A Drugs for routine use: Diuretics ACE inhibitors Beta-blockers Digitalis Dietary Salt restriction		All measures under stages A, B, and C Mechanical assist devices Heart transplantation Continuous (not intermittent) IV inotropic infusions for palliation Hospice care

Abbreviations: HF, heart failure, FHxCM, family history of cardiomyopathy; ACE, angiotensin-converting enzyme; MI, myocardial infarction; LV, left ventricular; IV, intravenous.

Source: Modified from S Hunt: J Am Coll Cardiology, 38:2101, 2001, with permission.

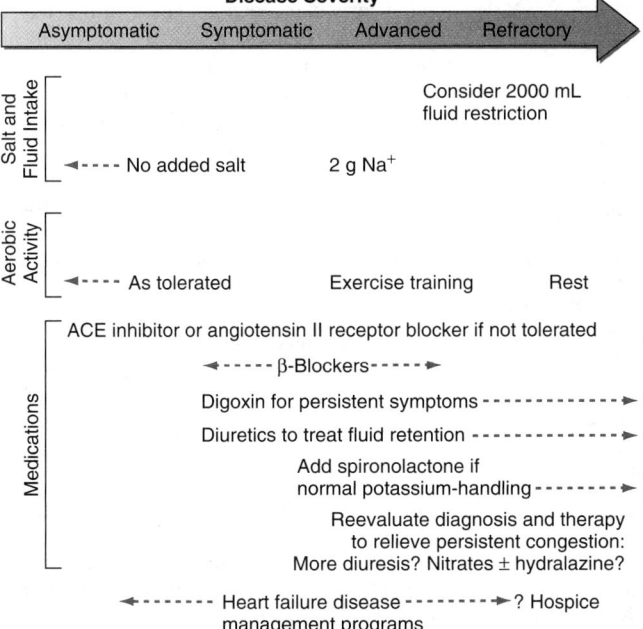

Stepped Therapy for Heart Failure

Disease Severity

Asymptomatic   Symptomatic   Advanced   Refractory

Salt and Fluid Intake

Consider 2000 mL fluid restriction

◀---- No added salt   2 g Na$^+$

Aerobic Activity

◀---- As tolerated   Exercise training   Rest

Medications

ACE inhibitor or angiotensin II receptor blocker if not tolerated

◀----- β-Blockers ----- ▶

Digoxin for persistent symptoms ------------- ▶

Diuretics to treat fluid retention ------------- ▶

Add spironolactone if normal potassium-handling -------- ▶

Reevaluate diagnosis and therapy to relieve persistent congestion: More diuresis? Nitrates ± hydralazine?

◀-------- Heart failure disease --------▶ ? Hospice management programs

Transplantation/mechanical assist devices

FIGURE 216-2 The step diagram demonstrates addition of therapies in relation to the clinical severity of heart failure with reduced left ventricular ejection fraction. Angiotensin-converting enzyme (ACE) inhibitors are prescribed at every level of disease severity. Angiotensin receptor-blocking agents (ARBs) are a reasonable alternative for patients who cannot tolerate ACE inhibitors due to angioedema or severe cough. β-Adrenergic blocking agents are prescribed for patient with mild to moderate symptoms of heart failure, but they are not initiated in patients with severe symptoms of heart failure unresponsive to stabilization with other therapies. Diuretics are prescribed to maintain fluid balance, with spironolactone added in patients with severely symptomatic disease when renal function and potassium handling are preserved. When severe symptoms persist, patients may benefit from addition of nitrates with or without hydralazine. Transplantation and mechanical assist devices are relevant to only a very small population with advanced heart failure. Restriction of sodium and fluid intake is increasingly required as heart failure becomes more severe. Heart failure management programs are most cost-effective in patients at high risk for repeated heart failure hospitalization. *(From A Nohria et al, 2002, with permission.)*

bles, specially processed breads and milk, and NaCl substitutes are permissible. Late in the course of HF, dilutional hyponatremia may develop in patients who are unable to excrete an H_2O load, sometimes because of excessive secretion of antidiuretic hormone. In such cases, both H_2O and NaCl must be restricted.

Diuretics (See also Chap. 230) These agents should be given to achieve euvolemia and reduce or prevent edema and jugular venous distention. A variety of diuretics is available (Tables 216-3 and 230-8), and almost all are effective in patients with mild HF. However, in the more severe forms of HF, the selection of diuretics is more difficult, and abnormalities in serum electrolytes must be watched for. On the other hand, overtreatment with diuretics must be avoided, since the resultant hypovolemia may reduce cardiac output, interfere with renal function, and produce profound weakness and lethargy.

THIAZIDE DIURETICS These agents are useful by themselves in patients with mild HF and in combination with other diuretics in patients with severe HF. In patients with chronic mild HF, the continued administration of a thiazide diuretic abolishes or diminishes the need for *rigid* dietary Na$^+$ restriction, although salty foods and table salt still should be avoided. Thiazide diuretics reduce the reabsorption of Na$^+$ and Cl$^-$ in the first half of the distal convoluted tubule and a portion of the cortical ascending limb of the loop of Henle, and H_2O follows the unreabsorbed salt. However, thiazides can cause excretion of a hypertonic urine and contribute to dilutional hyponatremia. As a con-

sequence of increased delivery of Na$^+$ to the distal nephron, Na$^+$-K$^+$ exchange is enhanced, and kaliuresis results.

K$^+$ depletion and metabolic alkalosis (the latter due to increased H$^+$ secretion as a substitute for the depleted intracellular stores of K$^+$) are the chief adverse metabolic effects following prolonged administration of the thiazides, and also of metolazone, and of the loop diuretics. Hypokalemia may seriously enhance the dangers of digitalis intoxication (see below), and induce fatigue and lethargy; it may be prevented by oral supplementation with KCl or preferably by the addition of a K$^+$-retaining diuretic. Other side effects of thiazides include reduction of the excretion of uric acid, which may lead to hyperuricemia, and impaired glucose tolerance. Skin rashes, thrombocytopenia, and granulocytopenia have also been reported.

Thiazide diuretics are effective and useful in the treatment of HF as long as the glomerular filtration rate exceeds approximately one half of normal. Chlorothiazide (25 to 50 mg/d) is especially useful since it may be administered once daily.

METOLAZONE This quinethazone derivative has a site of action and potency similar to the thiazides but is effective in the presence of moderate renal failure. Both metolazone and thiazides potentiate the diuretic efficacy of intravenous loop diuretics.

FUROSEMIDE, BUMETANIDE, AND TORSEMIDE These "loop" diuretics are similar physiologically but differ chemically from one another. They reversibly inhibit the reabsorption of Na$^+$, K$^+$, and Cl$^-$ in the thick ascending limb of Henle's loop, apparently by blocking a cotransport system in the luminal membrane. They may induce renal cortical vasodilatation and can produce rates of urine formation that may be as high as one-fourth of the glomerular filtration rate. Metabolic alkalosis may be caused by a large increase in the urinary excretion of Cl$^-$, H$^+$, and K$^+$. Hypokalemia, hyperuricemia, and hyperglycemia are observed occasionally, as with thiazide diuretics. The reabsorption of free H_2O is decreased. These three drugs are usually effective both intravenously and by mouth, and are excreted in the bile and urine. Weakness, nausea, and dizziness may complicate the administration of all loop diuretics.

These powerful diuretics are useful in all forms of HF, particularly in patients with otherwise refractory HF and pulmonary edema. They have been shown to be effective in patients with hypoalbuminemia, hyponatremia, hypochloremia, and with reductions in glomerular filtration rate, and to produce a diuresis in patients in whom thiazide diuretics and potassium-sparing diuretics, alone and in combination, are ineffective. In patients with refractory HF, the action of loop diuretics may be potentiated by intravenous administration and by the addition of other diuretics, i.e., thiazides, metozalone, and the potassium-sparing diuretics.

POTASSIUM-SPARING DIURETICS These agents act on the distal tubule and cortical collecting ducts, are relatively weak, and therefore are rarely indicated as sole agents. Spironolactone resemble aldosterone structurally and acts by competitive inhibition of aldosterone, thereby blocking the exchange between Na$^+$ and both K$^+$ and H$^+$ in the distal tubules and collecting ducts. Amiloride and triamterene have a similar effect but act directly on the distal tubule/collecting duct. These agents produce a Na$^+$ diuresis, and in contrast to the thiazides, metolazone and the thiazides result in K$^+$ *retention*.

Potassium-sparing diuretics are most effective when administered in combination with loop and/or thiazide diuretics. The opposing action of these drugs on urine and serum potassium makes possible a sodium diuresis without either hyper- or hypokalemia when spironolactone and one of these other agents are administered in combination. Also, since potassium-sparing diuretics act on the distal tubule, they are particularly effective when used in combination with one of the other diuretics that act more proximally. Spironolactone, triamterene, and amiloride should *not* be administered to patients with serum K$^+$ > 5 mmol/L, renal failure, or hyponatremia. Reported complications include nausea, epigastric distress, mental confusion, drowsiness,

TABLE 216-3   *Common Medications for Heart Failure*

Medication	Initial Dose	Maximum Dose
Loop diuretics		
Furosemide	20–40 mg 1–2 times daily PO; 20 mg IV	400 mg/d; 80 mg IV
Bumetanide	0.5–1.0 mg 1–2 times daily PO; 0.5 mg IV	10 mg/d; 2 mg IV
Torsemide	10 mg 1–2 times daily PO; 5 mg IV	200 mg/d; 20 mg IV
Supplemental thiazides		
Metolazone	2.5 mg 1–2 times daily	10 mg/d
Hydrochlorathiazide	25 mg/d	100 mg/d
Chlorthalidone	50 mg/d	100 mg/d
Spironolactone (only with loop diuretics)	25 mg/d or every other day	25 mg twice daily, occasionally higher for refractory hypokalemia
Angiotensin-converting enzyme inhibitors		
Captopril	6.25 mg/d or every other day	50–100 mg 4 times daily
Enalapril maleate	2.5 mg twice daily	10–20 mg twice daily
Fosinopril sodium	5–10 mg/d	40 mg/d
Lisinopril	2.5–5.0 mg/d	20–40 mg/d
Quinapril hydrochloride	10 mg twice daily	40 mg twice daily
Ramipril	1.25–2.5 mg/d	10 mg/d
β-Blockers		
Bisoprolol	1.25 mg/d	10 mg/d
Carvedilol	3.125 mg twice daily	25–50 mg twice daily
Metoprolol tartrate	6.25 mg twice daily	75 mg twice daily
Metoprolol CR/XL*	12.5–25 mg/d	200 mg/d
Digoxin	0.125 mg every other day to 0.25 mg/d	0.50 mg/d to avoid toxic effects
Other vasodilators		
Isosorbide dinitrate	10 mg 3 times daily	80 mg 3 times daily
Sublingual isosorbide	2.5 mg as occasion requires or prior to exercise to decrease dyspnea	
Hydralazine	25 mg 3 times daily	150 mg 4 times daily

* CR/XL indicates controlled-release extended release metoprolol succinate
Source: Modified from Nohria A et al, 2002; data adapted from Hunt et al: ACC/AHA Guidelines for the Evaluation and Management of Chronic Heart Failure in the Adult. *J Am Coll Cardiol.* 38:2101, 2001

gynecomastia, and erythematous eruptions. As mentioned below, a lower dose of spironolactone (25 mg/d), which exerts little if any diuretic effect, has been shown to prolong life in patients with advanced HF (Table 216-3).

Triamterene and *amiloride* exert renal effects similar to those of spironolactone. However, their action does not depend on the presence of aldosterone. The effective dose of triamterene is 100 to 200 mg/d, and that of amiloride is 5 to 10 mg/d. Side effects include nausea, vomiting, diarrhea, headache, granulocytopenia, eosinophilia, and skin rash. Combination therapy, e.g., spironolactone and hydrochlorothiazide in a single tablet (e.g. Aldactazide) have proved popular.

When *choosing a diuretic*, an orally administered loop diuretic, thiazide or metolazone are the agents of choice in the treatment of chronic cardiac edema of mild to moderate degree in patients without hyperglycemia, hyperuricemia, or hypokalemia. Spironolactone, triamterene, and amiloride potentiate the thiazide and loop diuretics. In severe HF, the combination of a loop diuretic, a thiazide, and a potassium-sparing diuretic is required. In acute HF, especially pulmonary edema, intravenous loop diuretics are often effective.

PREVENTION OF DETERIORATION OF MYOCARDIAL INFARCTION   *Chronic* activation of the renin-angiotensin-aldosterone system (RAAS) and of the adrenergic nervous systems in HF cause ventricular remodeling, further deterioration of cardiac function and/or potentially fatal arrhythmias (Chap. 215). Drugs that block these two systems have been found to be useful in the management of HF (Tables 216-2 and 216-3).

Angiotensin-Converting Enzyme (ACE) Inhibitors   ACE inhibitors play a central role in the prevention and treatment of HF at almost all stages.

In addition to slowing maladaptive remodeling of the injured or abnormally burdened ventricle, ACE inhibitors reduce the impedance to left ventricular ejection. These drugs may be particularly helpful in (but are by no means limited to) patients with systolic HF due to myocardial infarction, hypertension, and valvular regurgitation. In patients with systolic HF who are treated with ACE inhibitors, cardiac output rises, the pulmonary wedge pressure falls, the signs and symptoms of HF are relieved, and a new steady state is achieved in which cardiac output is higher and afterload lower with no or only mild reduction of arterial pressure.

The administration of ACE inhibitors has been shown to prevent or retard the development of HF in patients with left ventricular dysfunction without HF, to reduce symptoms, enhance exercise performance, and to reduce long-term mortality and the need for rehospitalization in patients with HF, in patients shortly after acute myocardial infarction as well as in patients with vascular disease who are at high risk for recurrent events. These beneficial effects are related only in part to the salutary hemodynamic effects, i.e., the reduction of preload and afterload. The major effect of ACE inhibitors appears to be on inhibition of local (tissue) renin-angiotensin systems. Once begun and an optimal dose has been reached (Table 216-3) an ACE inhibitor should be maintained indefinitely. However, ACE inhibition should *not* be used in hypotensive patients.

Angiotensin Receptor Blockers   In patients who cannot tolerate ACE inhibitors because of cough, angioneurotic edema, leukopenia, an angiotensin II receptor blocker (type AT1) antagonist may be used instead and appears to be equally effective.

Aldosterone Antagonist   The activation of the RAAS in HF increases not only the circulating and tissue angiotensin II but also aldosterone. The latter, in addition to causing Na+ retention and worsening edema (Chaps. 32 and 321), causes sympathetic activation, myocardial, vascular, and perivascular fibrosis, and reduces arterial compliance. In one large multicenter trial in patients with HF with recent or current class IV symptoms and reduced ejection fraction who were receiving ACE inhibitors, diuretics and digoxin, the addition of spironolactone, 25 mg/d reduced total mortality, as well as sudden death and death from pump failure. Since spironolactone is also a useful, albeit weak, diuretic (see above), its widespread use in severe systolic HF should be considered.

Beta-Adrenoceptor Blockers   While the abrupt administration of large doses of beta-adrenergic receptor blockers can intensify HF, especially acute HF, the administration of gradually escalating doses has been reported to improve the symptoms of HF, and to reduce all-cause death, cardiovascular death, sudden death, rehospitalization for HF, and pump failure death in patients with chronic heart failure already receiving ACE inhibitors (Table 216-3). These drugs are indicated in patients with moderately severe HF (classes II and III), but are not indicated with unstable HF, in hypotensive patients (systolic pressure < 90 mmHg), in patients with severe fluid overload, in patients who have required recent treatment with an intravenous inotropic agent, and in patients with sinus bradycardia, atrioventricular block, or a bronchospastic disorder.

Three beta-adrenergic blockers (metoprolol, bisoprolol and carvedilol) have been shown to improve survival in patients with HF. The first two are selective and block only β_1 receptors, while the third blocks both β_1 and β_2 receptors as well as α receptors, thereby causing mild vasodilation. Carvedilol also appears to exert antioxidant activity.

Before commencing beta-blocker therapy, patients should be stabilized on an ACE inhibitor, diuretics and possibly digoxin. They should be begun in very low doses, e.g., carvedilol 3.125 mg bid or metoprolol XL 12.5 mg qd and titrated upward slowly every 2 to 4 weeks. During titration, the patients should be observed closely for hypertension, bradycardia, and worsening HF. Approximately 15% of patients cannot tolerate beta blockade, and an equal number cannot tolerate target doses (carvedilol 25 mg bid and metoprolol XL 200 mg). In the latter, low-dose beta-blocker therapy is preferred to no therapy.

Once a maintenance dose has been achieved, administration of the beta blocker should be continued indefinitely. If treatment of a patient on a beta blocker with a positive inotropic agent is required, a phosphodiesterase III inhibitor (see below) should be used.

ENHANCEMENT OF MYOCARDIAL CONTRACTILITY ■ Digitalis
The improvement of myocardial contractility by means of cardiac glycosides is useful in the control of HF. Cardiac glycosides inhibit the monovalent cation transport enzyme–coupled Na^+, K^+-ATPase and increase intracellular $[Na^+]$; the latter, in turn, increases intracellular $[Ca^{2+}]$ through a Na^+-Ca^{2+} exchange carrier mechanism. The increased myocardial $[Ca^{2+}]$ augments Ca^{2+} released to the myofilaments during excitation and, therefore, invokes a positive inotropic response (Chap. 215). Cardiac glycosides causes increased automaticity and ectopic impulse activity. They also prolong the effective refractory period of the atrioventricular node and thereby slow ventricular rate in atrial flutter and fibrillation.

Digitalis is effective in patients with systolic HF complicated by atrial flutter and fibrillation and a rapid ventricular rate, who benefit both from slowing of the ventricular rate and from the positive inotropic effect. Although digitalis does not improve survival in patients with systolic HF and sinus rhythm, it reduces symptoms of HF and the need for hospitalization. Digitalis is of *little* or *no* value in patients with HF, sinus rhythm, and the following conditions: hypertrophic cardiomyopathy, myocarditis, mitral stenosis, chronic constrictive pericarditis, and any form of diastolic HF.

Digoxin, which has a half-life of 1.6 days, is filtered in the glomeruli and secreted by the renal tubules. Significant reductions of the glomerular filtration rate reduce the elimination of digoxin and, therefore, may prolong digoxin's effect, allowing it to accumulate to toxic levels, unless the dose is reduced.

DIGITALIS INTOXICATION This is a serious and potentially fatal complication. Advanced age, hypokalemia, hypomagnesemia, hypoxemia, renal insufficiency, hypercalcemia, and acute myocardial infarction all may reduce tolerance to digitalis. Chronic digitalis intoxication may be insidious in onset and is characterized by anorexia, nausea, and vomiting, exacerbations of HF, weight loss, cachexia, neuralgias, gynecomastia, yellow vision, and delirium.

The most frequent disturbances of cardiac rhythm are ventricular premature beats, bigeminy, ventricular tachycardia, and, rarely, ventricular fibrillation. Atrioventricular block and nonparoxysmal atrial tachycardia with variable atrioventricular block are characteristic of digitalis intoxication; withdrawal of the drug and treatment with β-adrenoceptor blocker or lidocaine are indicated. If hypokalemia is present, potassium should be administered cautiously by the oral route. Fab fragments of purified, intact digitalis antibodies are a potentially lifesaving approach to the treatment of severe intoxication.

The administration of quinidine, verapamil, amiodarone, and propafenone to patients receiving digoxin raises the serum concentration of the latter, increasing the propensity to digitalis intoxication. The dose of digitalis should be reduced by half in patients receiving these drugs.

Sympathomimetic Amines Two sympathomimetic amines that act largely on β-adrenergic receptors—dopamine and dobutamine—improve myocardial contractility and are effective in the management of severe,

acute HF. They must be administered by constant intravenous infusion and can be given for several days to patients with intractable, severe HF, particularly those with a reversible component, such as exists in patients who have undergone cardiac surgery, as well as to patients with acute myocardial infarction and shock or pulmonary edema (Chap. 255), and they may be used in patients with refractory HF as a "bridge" to cardiac transplantation. The administration of sympathomimetic amines should be accompanied by careful and continuous monitoring of the electrocardiogram, arterial pressure, and, if possible, pulmonary artery wedge pressure.

Dopamine is a naturally occurring, immediate precursor of norepinephrine and has a combination of actions that makes it particularly useful in the treatment of a variety of hypotensive states and HF. At very low doses (i.e., 1 to 2 μg/kg per min), it dilates renal and mesenteric blood vessels through stimulation of specific dopaminergic receptors, thereby augmenting renal and mesenteric blood flow and sodium excretion. In the range of 2 to 10 μg/kg per min, dopamine stimulates myocardial β_1 receptors but induces relatively little tachycardia, while at higher doses it also stimulates α-adrenergic receptors and elevates arterial pressure.

Dobutamine is a synthetic sympathomimetic agent that acts on β_1, β_2, and α_1 receptors. It exerts a potent inotropic action, has only a modest cardio accelerating effect, and lowers peripheral vascular resistance. Since it simultaneously raises cardiac output, it may not lower systemic arterial pressure in patients with severe HF. Dobutamine, given in continuous infusions of 2.5 to 10 μg/kg per min, is useful in the treatment of acute HF without hypotension.

A major problem with all sympathomimetics is the loss of responsiveness, apparently due to "downregulation" of adrenergic receptors, which becomes evident within 8 h of continuous administration. This problem may be managed by intermittent therapy.

Phosphodiesterase Inhibitors These bipyridines, amrinone and milrinone, are noncatecholamine, nonglycoside agents that exert both *positive* inotropic and vasodilator actions by inhibiting phosphodiesterase III, an enzyme that breaks down intracytoplasmic cyclic AMP, the second messenger which is critical to adrenergic stimulation. These agents are administered intravenously; by simultaneously stimulating cardiac contractility and dilating the systemic vascular bed they reverse the major hemodynamic abnormalities associated with HF. Amrinone and milrinone may be administered for the same conditions in which dopamine or dobutamine are useful; they may be employed together with and potentiate the sympathomimetics.

VASODILATORS Direct vasodilators may be useful in patients with severe, acute HF who demonstrate systemic vasoconstriction despite ACE inhibitor therapy. The ideal vasodilator for the treatment of *acute* HF should have a rapid onset and brief duration of action when administered by intravenous infusion; sodium nitroprusside (0.1 to 3.0 μg/kg per min) qualifies as such a drug, but its use requires careful monitoring of the arterial pressure and, if possible, of the pulmonary artery wedge pressure. Intravenous nitroglycerin (beginning at 20 μg/min and titrated upwards to achieve the desired result or a maximum of 400 μg/min) and nesiritide (recombinant BNP, I.V. bolus = 2 μg/kg followed by 0.01 μg/kg per min) are effective vasodilators. The combination of hydralazine (up to 100 mg tid orally) and isosorbide dinitrate (up to 60 mg tid orally) may be useful for chronic oral administration.

VENTRICULAR RESYNCHRONIZATION Intraventricular conduction is depressed in about one-fourth of patients with chronic HF. This depression is manifest in prolongation of the QRS complex to more than 120 ms, leading to dyssynchrony of cardiac contraction, which further impairs cardiac contraction and thereby aggravates HF. "Resynchronization" with a device that has three pacing leads (right atrium, right ventricle, and cardiac vein, which provides left ventricular stimulation) has been shown to improve performance in patients with HF. This device, which has been approved by the FDA, has been demonstrated to increase ejection fraction as well as the distance walked in 6 min, improved functional New York Heart Association class, and the quality of life. Hospitalization for worsening HF and/or requiring use of intravenous medication were reduced in half. Device placement was not possible or complications occurred in 8% of patients. Devices that incorporate the ability to achieve resynchronization and internal cardioversion-defibrillation are now also available and may simultaneously improve contraction and prevent sudden death due to ventricular fibrillation in patients with HF (see below).

MANAGEMENT OF ARRHYTHMIAS   Premature ventricular contractions and episodes of asymptomatic ventricular tachycardia are common in advanced HF. Sudden death, presumably due to ventricular fibrillation, is responsible for about one-half of all deaths in this condition. The remainder are due to failure of the cardiac pump. The management of arrhythmias should commence with correction of electrolyte and acid-base disturbances (Chaps. 41 and 42), especially diuretic-induced hypokalemia, as well as digitalis intoxication (see above). Treatment with class I antiarrhythmics such as quinidine, procainamide, or flecainide (Chap. 214) is *contraindicated* because these drugs are proarrhythmic in patients with HF. Amiodarone, a class III antiarrhythmic, on the other hand, is well tolerated and is the drug of choice for patients with HF and atrial fibrillation.

Patients who have been resuscitated from sudden death, those with syncope or presyncope due to ventricular arrhythmias, and those with asymptomatic ventricular tachyarrhythmias in whom ventricular tachycardia can be induced during electrophysiologic testing should be strongly considered for the implantable automatic defibrillator (ICD). The MADIT II trial showed a 30% reduction in all-cause mortality in patients with a prior myocardial infarction and a left ventricular ejection fraction ≤30% in whom an ICD had been implanted. Although the societal costs of treating the majority of all such patients with a prophylactic ICD will be immense, this may soon become the treatment of choice in patients with severe systolic HF. The addition to the device of the capacity for "back-up pacing" may prevent sudden death due to bradyarrhythmias. (See also Chap. 214.)

Anticoagulants   Patients with severe HF are at increased risk of pulmonary emboli secondary to venous thrombosis and of systemic emboli secondary to intracardiac thrombi and should be treated with warfarin. Patients with HF and atrial fibrillation, previous venous thrombosis, and pulmonary or systemic emboli are at especially high risk and should receive heparin followed by warfarin.

DIASTOLIC HEART FAILURE   The major goal in the treatment of this condition is to eliminate or reduce the causes of diastolic dysfunction, such as ventricular hypertrophy, fibrosis, or ischemia. The second goal is to reduce pulmonary and/or systemic venous congestion, a major consequence of diastolic dysfunction. Dietary Na^+ restriction and diuretics are useful for this purpose. Slowing of heart rate with beta blockers or nondihydropyridine calcium antagonists is also important since it provides more time for ventricular filling.

REFRACTORY HEART FAILURE   When the response to ordinary treatment as described above is inadequate, HF is considered to be refractory. Before assuming that this condition simply reflects terminal myocardial depression, careful consideration must be given to several possibilities: (1) an underlying or precipitating cause that may be amenable to specific surgical or medical therapy, such as infective endocarditis, thyrotoxicosis, or silent aortic or mitral stenosis has been overlooked; and (2) complications of overly vigorous therapy, such as digitalis intoxication, hypovolemia, or electrolyte imbalance. Recognition and proper treatment of the aforementioned problems, if they exist, are likely to restore responsiveness to therapy.

Patients with refractory HF ordinarily require hospital management (Table 216-4). The combination of an intravenously administered vasodilator such as nitroglycerin, niseritide, *or.* of a phosphodiesterase inhibitor (amrinone or milrinone), together with a sympathomimetic

TABLE 216-4   *Therapeutic Options for Patients with Refractory Heart Failure*

Combination diuretics	Left ventricular or biventricular pacing
Additional vasodilators	Novel cardiac surgery
Positive inotropic agents	Ventricular remodeling surgery
Mechanical circulatory support	Dynamic cardiomyoplasty
Cardiac transplantation	Mitral valve repair

Source: From MM Givertz, JN Cohn in EM Antman (ed): *Cardiovascular Therapeutics*, 2d ed. Philadelphia, Saunders, 2002, with permission.

amine (dopamine or dobutamine) often results in additive effects, raising cardiac output and lowering filling pressure further.

In hospitalized patients with refractory HF, therapy guided by hemodynamic measurements provided by a balloon flotation (Swan-Ganz) catheter may be helpful. The goal of manipulating diuretics, inotropic agents, and vasodilators is to achieve a pulmonary capillary wedge pressure of 15 to 18 mmHg, a right atrial pressure of 5 to 8 mmHg, a cardiac index >2.2 L/min per m², and a systemic vascular resistance of 800 to 1200 dyne · s/cm⁵. Once these values are achieved, an attempt should be made to convert the patient from intravenous to oral vasodilator therapy.

ASSISTED CIRCULATION/CARDIAC TRANSPLANTATION   When patients with HF become unresponsive to a combination of all the aforementioned therapeutic measures, are in New York Heart Association class IV, and are deemed unlikely to survive one year, they should be considered for assisted circulation and/or cardiac transplantation (see Chap. 217). Prolonged left ventricular assistance may be used as a "bridge to transplantation." In a small (~10%) of patients receiving this therapy, there is sufficient improvement in cardiac function after two or three months to allow recovery after withdrawal of the device.

Treatment of Acute Pulmonary Edema   →*Cardiogenic pulmonary edema is described in Chap. 29. Its management is described in Chap. 255.*

PROGNOSIS

The prognosis in patients with HF depends primarily on the nature of the underlying heart disease and on the presence or absence of a precipitating factor that can be treated. When one of the latter can be identified and removed, the outlook for immediate survival is far better than if HF occurs without any obvious precipitating cause. The long-term prognosis is more favorable when the underlying forms of heart disease, e.g., valvular heart disease, can be treated effectively. When this is not possible, the prognosis can be estimated by observing the response to treatment. When patients can be rendered free of congestion, survival may be 80% at two years. Survival may be as low as 50% at six months in patients with refractory symptoms (Fig. 216-3).

Other factors that have been shown to be associated with a poor

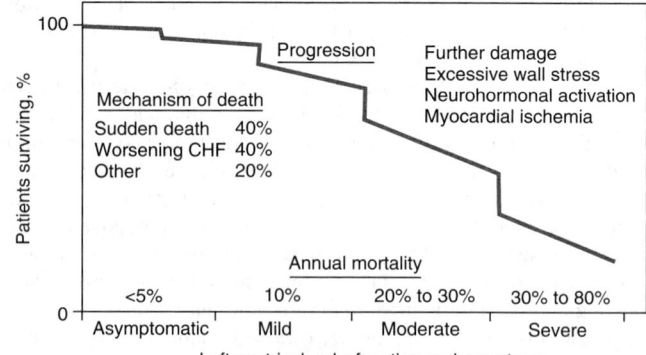

FIGURE 216-3   The natural history of congestive heart failure (CHF). Once left ventricular systolic dysfunction is present, it usually progresses, albeit not predictably. As left ventricular dysfunction progresses and symptoms increase, mortality rate increases and the process becomes inexorable. Myocyte loss and fibrosis become irreversible. An effective preventive measure must be introduced before onset or early in the course of progressive left ventricular dysfunction. (*From BM Massie, NH Shah: Curr Opin Cardiol 11:221, 1996; with permission.*)

prognosis include a severely depressed ejection fraction (<15%), a reduced maximal O_2 uptake (<10 mL/kg per min), the inability to walk on a level and at a normal pace for more than 3 min, reduced serum Na^+ concentration (<133 mEq/L), reduced serum K^+ (<3 meq/L), a markedly elevated (>500 pg/mL) BNP, as well as frequent ventricular extrasystoles. If sudden cardiac death is prevented by implantation of an ICD, patients may later go on to develop and succumb to pump failure and the number of such patients is likely to grow. When all available therapeutic measures have been exhausted, comfort care, sometimes in a hospice, with continued infusions of inotropic agents, diuretics, and the administration of anxiolytics and analgesics should be considered.

COR PULMONALE

Cor pulmonale is defined as enlargement of the right ventricle (RV) secondary to abnormalities of the lungs, thorax, pulmonary ventilation, or circulation. It sometimes leads to RV failure, with an elevation of transmural RV end-diastolic pressure.

NORMAL FUNCTION OF THE PULMONARY CIRCULATION

PATHOPHYSIOLOGY The stroke volume of the RV, as of the left, is regulated by its preload, contractility, and afterload (Chap. 215). Since the RV is a relatively thin, compliant reservoir, acute changes in venous return (e.g., an increase with inhalation and decline with exhalation) can occur with little change in transmural RV pressure. However, the ability of the RV to increase its systolic pressure is limited. Normally, the RV afterload, which is closely related to the pulmonary artery pressure, is low. The pulmonary artery pressure normally rises slightly when blood is displaced into the chest at the start of exercise; on assuming recumbency; or with cold, anxiety, or pain. A driving pressure of only about 5 cmH_2O between the pulmonary artery (15 cmH_2O) and the left atrium (10 cmH_2O) normally propels the entire cardiac output of approximately 5 L/min at rest through the lungs, and only a modest increase in pressure is necessary to drive a flow of up to 25 L/min through the pulmonary capillary bed during maximal exercise.

The severity of RV enlargement in cor pulmonale is a function of the increase in afterload. When the pulmonary vascular resistance is elevated and relatively fixed, as in pulmonary vascular or severe parenchymal lung disease, an elevation in cardiac output, as occurs with physical exertion, can elevate pulmonary artery pressure markedly. RV afterload may be augmented when the lungs are hyperinflated, as in chronic obstructive lung disease (COLD), due to the compression of the alveolar capillaries and the lengthening of the pulmonary vessels (Chap. 242). RV afterload can also increase when lung volume is reduced following extensive pulmonary resection, as well as in restrictive lung diseases in which pulmonary vessels are compressed and distorted. RV afterload rises with hypoxic pulmonary vasoconstriction caused by hypoxia or acidosis, which are important causes of pulmonary hypertension (Chap. 220).

The elevation of RV afterload responsible for cor pulmonale is caused principally by pulmonary vascular or parenchymal disease.

PULMONARY VASCULAR DISEASES In these conditions the RV afterload is elevated as a consequence of restriction to pulmonary blood flow. In cor pulmonale secondary to pulmonary vascular disease, pulmonary hypertension is usually more severe than in pulmonary parenchymal disease. Chronic cor pulmonale secondary to pulmonary vascular disease may result from repeated pulmonary emboli, pulmonary vasculitis, pulmonary vasoconstriction secondary to high altitude, congenital heart disease with left-to-right shunting (e.g., atrial or ventricular septal defect, patent ductus arteriosus; Chap. 218), as well as pulmonary venoocclusive disease. When the cause of elevated pulmonary vascular resistance responsible for cor pulmonale cannot be defined, the condition is referred to as *primary pulmonary hypertension* (Chap. 220).

COR PULMONALE DUE TO PULMONARY EMBOLI This condition is associated with two distinct syndromes.

Acute Cor Pulmonale It has been estimated that in the United States about 50,000 people die each year from pulmonary thromboembolism

(Chap. 244). Probably half die within the first hour from acute right heart failure due to massive or multiple emboli. A sudden, large embolic burden causes a low-output state resulting from the RV's inability to generate the pressure necessary to drive blood through the acutely compromised pulmonary vascular bed. Depression of cardiac output can also occur with a moderate-sized embolism if the pulmonary circulation has been critically compromised by previous pulmonary vascular or parenchymal disease. The RV begins to fail when systolic pressure is forced to double acutely, i.e., to exceed approximately 50 mmHg. Acute RV failure secondary to pulmonary embolism is suggested by the history of the sudden onset of severe dyspnea and cardiovascular collapse in a patient with, or predisposed to, venous thrombosis.

Clinical Manifestations Acute RV failure causes pallor, sweating, hypotension, and a rapid pulse of small amplitude. The neck veins are distended and often exhibit prominent *v* waves secondary to tricuspid regurgitation. The liver may be pulsatile, distended, and tender. A systolic murmur of tricuspid regurgitation along the left sternal border may be accompanied by a presystolic (S_4) gallop sound. Arterial blood gas frequently shows reduced Pa_{O_2} due to ventilation/perfusion mismatching and a low Pa_{CO_2} due to hyperventilation.

℞ TREATMENT

The treatment of pulmonary embolism is described in Chap. 244. In acute cor pulmonale [and in RV failure due to acute RV infarction (Chap. 228)], an increase in RV preload can be achieved by a cautious expansion of blood volume, which helps to maintain cardiac output. When hypoxic pulmonary vasoconstriction contributes to pulmonary hypertension, inhalation of 100% O_2 reduces RV afterload.

CHRONIC COR PULMONALE SECONDARY TO PULMONARY VASCULAR DISEASE In contrast to acute, massive thromboembolism, when the elevation in pulmonary vascular resistance and the RV hypertrophy develop gradually, higher pulmonary vascular pressures, sometimes even approaching systemic arterial levels, may be generated. Chronic cor pulmonale can be caused by recurrent, medium-sized emboli that fail to lyse, but organize, resulting in chronic thromboembolic pulmonary hypertension. Particles from intravenous drug abuse, parasites, or tumor tissue that embolizes into the pulmonary vascular bed may also cause persistent pulmonary hypertension. Chronic cor pulmonale can also be caused by *primary pulmonary hypertension* (Chap. 220) or any chronic widespread vasculitis, such as occurs in association with collagen vascular disorders and that may affect the pulmonary vascular bed, particularly the CREST syndrome (Chap. 303).

Clinical Manifestations Dyspnea and tachypnea are characteristic features of pulmonary hypertension secondary to pulmonary vascular disease. They may be distressing during mild exertion or even at rest and are *not* relieved by sitting upright. An unproductive cough is another frequent complaint. Anterior chest pain, due to acute dilation of the root of the pulmonary artery or RV ischemia, can occur. The elevation in systemic venous pressure can cause hepatomegaly and ankle edema.

Occasionally there is cyanosis due to arterial hypoxemia and low cardiac output. An RV heave may be palpable along the left sternal border or in the epigastrium, and a high-pitched pulmonary ejection click may be audible to the left of the upper sternum. The second (pulmonary) component of the second heart sound is intensified and may be palpable; fixed, narrow splitting of the second heart sound and a right ventricular protodiastolic gallop (S_3) that may increase during inspiration can be present. A systolic murmur of tricuspid regurgitation, which is augmented by inspiration, is often audible; occasionally, a diastolic murmur of pulmonary regurgitation is also heard. Prominent *a* (and sometimes also *v*) waves in the jugular venous pulse are evident. The onset of RV failure is reflected by an increase of venous pressure, the development of larger *v* waves associated with increasing tricuspid regurgitation, a positive hepatojugular reflux, and a gallop rhythm with both third and fourth heart sounds. These physical findings of RV failure can disappear rapidly when pulmonary artery pressure is reduced by relief of hypoxemia.

Laboratory Examination On *radiologic examination* the pulmonary trunk and hilar vessels are enlarged, as is the descending right pulmonary artery. Ventilation and perfusion lung scans and systemic venography showing deep vein thrombosis in the lower extremities are helpful in confirming the diagnosis of embolic pulmonary vascular disease. In the presence of severe pulmonary hypertension, the *electrocardiogram* (ECG) shows P pulmonale, right axis deviation, and RV hypertrophy (Chap. 210).

Echocardiography allows measurement of the thickness of the RV wall and may show enlargement of the RV cavity in relation to the left. The interventricular septum may be displaced leftward and may move paradoxically during the cardiac cycle. Pulmonary artery and RV systolic pressure can be estimated from measurement of the peak tricuspid regurgitant flow and pulmonic regurgitant flow with Doppler echocardiography.

Magnetic resonance imaging is useful for measuring RV mass, wall thickness, cavity volume, and ejection fraction.

Cardiac catheterization provides precise measurement of pulmonary vascular pressures, calculation of pulmonary vascular resistance, and their responses to oxygen and vasodilators. Catheterization is sometimes helpful in patients with cor pulmonale to exclude congenital and left heart diseases, and it allows pulmonary angiography to be carried out to confirm the nature of the pulmonary vascular obstruction. Measurements of pulmonary vascular pressure and flow during exercise may reveal abnormal pressure increments of pulmonary artery systolic and diastolic and RV diastolic pressures and an inadequate response to cardiac output.

Lung biopsy can be useful in demonstrating vasculitis in some types of pulmonary vascular disease such as the collagen vascular diseases, rheumatoid arthritis, and Wegener's granulomatosis.

PARENCHYMAL PULMONARY DISEASES Cor pulmonale may be caused by both obstructive and restrictive lung diseases, more frequently the former. In these conditions there are usually only modest elevations of pulmonary artery pressure. The development of cor pulmonale confers a poor prognosis on patients with respiratory disease, not because RV failure cannot be treated, but because it reflects the seriousness of the underlying pulmonary disease.

℞ **TREATMENT** (See Chap. 242)

Acute respiratory infection, often the precipitant of RV failure, must be treated promptly and vigorously. Alveolar hypoxia at rest and during exertion and sleep should be corrected by improving alveolar ventilation through relieving the airflow obstruction and by judiciously increasing the inspired O_2 concentration. Long-term O_2 therapy is helpful in patients with severe COLD and reduces pulmonary artery pressure and pulmonary vascular resistance. Bronchodilators and antibiotics lessen airflow obstruction, and diuretics relieve the edema. Loop diuretics must be used with care since they may cause a metabolic alkalosis and thereby blunt the respiratory drive. Digitalis should be used cautiously in the presence of overt RV failure, and small phlebotomies should be considered when the hematocrit exceeds 55 to 60%. Inhalation of nitric oxide and infusion of prostacyclin are undergoing evaluation as agents to reduce pulmonary hypertension.

FURTHER READING

ABRAHAM WT et al: Cardiac resynchronization in chronic heart failure. N Engl J Med 346:1845, 2002

ACC/AHA Guidelines for the Evaluation and Management of Chronic Heart Failure in the Adult—Executive Summary. J Am Coll Cardiol 38:2101, 2001. Full report found at www.acc.org/clinical/guidelines/failure/hf_index.htm; www.americanheart.org/presenter

ASHER CR, KLEIN AL: Diastolic heart failure: Restrictive cardiomyopathy, constrictive pericarditis and cardiac tamponade: Clinical and echocardiographic evaluation. Card Review 10:218, 2002

BRAUNWALD E, BRISTOW MR: Congestive heart failure: Fifty years of progress. Circulation 102:IV-14, 2000

GARG R, YUSUF S: Overview of randomized trials of angiotensin-converting enzyme inhibitors on mortality and morbidity in patients with heart failure. Collaborative Group on ACE Inhibitor Trials. JAMA 274:462, 1995

KITZMAN DW et al: Pathophysiological characterization of isolated diastolic heart failure in comparison to systolic heart failure. JAMA 288:2144, 2002

MAISEL AS et al: Rapid measurement of B-type natriuretic peptide in the emergency diagnosis of heart failure. N Engl J Med 347:161, 2002

MCCULLOUGH PA et al: Uncovering heart failure in patients with a history of pulmonary disease: Rationale for the early use of B-type natriuretic peptide in the emergency department. Acad Emerg Med 10:275, 2003

MOSS AJ et al: Prophylactic implantation of a defibrillator in patients with myocardial infarction and reduced ejection fraction. N Engl J Med 346:877, 2002

NOHRIA A et al: Medical management of advanced heart failure. JAMA 287:628, 2002

PITT B et al: The effect of spironolactone on morbidity and mortality in patients with severe heart failure. N Engl J Med 341:709, 1999

PUBLICATION COMMITTEE FOR THE VMAC INVESTIGATORS: Intravenous nesiritide vs. nitroglycerin for treatment of decompensated congestive heart failure: A randomized controlled trial. JAMA 287:1531, 2002

RAPAPORT E: Cor pulmonale, in *Textbooks of Respiratory Medicine*, JF Murray, JA Nadel (eds). Philadelphia, Saunders, 2000

RICH S: Pulmonary hypertension and cor pulmonale, in *Braunwald's Heart Disease*, 7th ed, D Zipes et al (eds). Philadelphia, Saunders, 2005

WEITZENBLUM E: Chronic cor pulmonale. Heart 89:225, 2003

WILCOX CS: Diuretics, in *The Kidney*, 7th ed, BM Brenner (ed). Philadelphia, Saunders, 2004

---

217 | CARDIAC TRANSPLANTATION AND PROLONGED ASSISTED CIRCULATION
Sharon A. Hunt

Advanced or end-stage heart failure is an increasingly frequent sequela as progressively more effective palliation for the earlier stages of heart disease and prevention of sudden death associated with heart disease become more widely recognized and employed (Chap. 216). When patients with end-stage or refractory heart failure are identified, the physician is faced with the decision of advising compassionate end-of-life care or choosing to recommend extraordinary life-extending measures. For the occasional patient who is relatively young and without serious comorbidities, the latter may represent a reasonable option. Current therapeutic options are limited to cardiac transplantation (with the option of mechanical cardiac assistance as a "bridge" to transplantation), but the option of permanent mechanical assistance of the circulation is not far off.

CARDIAC TRANSPLANTATION

Surgical techniques for orthotopic transplantation of the heart were devised in the 1960s and taken into the clinical arena in 1967. The procedure did not gain widespread clinical acceptance until the introduction of "modern" and more effective immunosuppression in the early 1980s. By the 1990s the demand for transplantable hearts met, and then exceeded, the available donor supply and peaked at 4400 annually worldwide in the early 1990s and declined to about 3000 in 2002.

SURGICAL TECHNIQUE Donor and recipient hearts are excised in virtually identical operations with incisions made across the atria and atrial septa at the midatrial level (leaving the posterior of the atria in place)

and across the great vessels just above the semilunar valves. The donor heart is generally "harvested" in an anatomically identical manner by a separate surgical team and transported from the donor hospital in a bag of iced saline solution and then is reanastomosed into the waiting recipient in the orthotopic or normal anatomical position. The only change in surgical technique since this method was first described has been a movement in recent years to move the right atrial anastamosis back to the level of the superior and inferior vena cavae in order to better preserve right atrial geometry and prevent atrial arrhythmias. This method of implantation leaves the recipient with a surgically denervated heart that does not respond to any direct sympathetic or parasympathetic stimuli but does respond to circulating catecholamines. The physiologic responses of the denervated heart to the demands of exercise are atypical but quite adequate to carry on normal physical activity.

DONOR ALLOCATION SYSTEM In the United States the allocation of donor organs is accomplished under the supervision of the United Network for Organ Sharing (UNOS), a private organization under contract to the federal government. The United States is divided geographically into eleven regions for donor heart allocation. Allocation of donor hearts within a region is decided according to a system of priority that takes into account (1) the severity of illness, (2) geographic distance from the donor, and (3) patient time on the waiting list. A physiologic limit of approximately 3 h of "ischemic" (out of body) time for hearts precludes a national sharing of hearts. This allocation system design is reissued annually and is responsive to input from a variety of constituencies, including donor families and transplant professionals.

At the current time, higher priority according to severity of illness is assigned only to patients requiring hospitalization for intravenous inotropic support either with a pulmonary artery catheter in place for hemodynamic monitoring or without hemodynamic monitoring. All other patients have priority according to their time on the waiting list, and matching is achieved only according to ABO blood group compatibility and gross body size compatibility.

INDICATIONS/CONTRAINDICATIONS Heart failure is an increasingly common cause of death, particularly in the elderly. Most patients who reach what has recently been categorized as stage D, or refractory end-stage heart failure, are appropriately treated with compassionate end-of-life care. A subset of such patients who are younger and without significant comorbidities can be considered as candidates for heart transplantation. Exact criteria vary in different centers but generally take into consideration the patient's physiologic age and the existence of comorbidities such as peripheral or cerebrovascular disease, obesity, diabetes, cancer, or chronic infection.

RESULTS A registry organized by the International Society for Heart and Heart-Lung Transplantation has tracked worldwide and U.S. survival rates after heart transplantation since 1982. The most recent update reveals 83% and 76% survival 1 and 3 years posttransplant or a posttransplant "half-life" of 9.3 years (Fig. 217-1). The quality of life in these patients is generally excellent, with well over 90% of patients in the registry returning to normal and unrestricted function following transplantation.

IMMUNOSUPPRESSION Medical regimens employed to provide suppression of the normal immune response to a solid organ allograft vary from center to center and are in a constant state of evolution as more effective agents with improved side-effect profiles and less toxicity are introduced. All currently used regimens are nonspecific, providing general hyporeactivity to foreign antigens rather than donor-specific hyporeactivity and the attendant, and unwanted, susceptibility to infections and malignancy. Most cardiac transplant programs currently use a three-drug regimen including a calcineurin inhibitor (cyclosporine or tacrolimus), an inhibitor of T cell proliferation or differentiation (azathioprine, mycophenolate mofetil, or sirolimus), and at least a short initial course of glucocorticoids. Many programs also include an initial "induction" course of polyclonal or monoclonal anti-T cell antibodies in the perioperative period to decrease the frequency or severity of early posttransplant rejection. Most recently introduced have been monoclonal antibodies (daclizumab and basiliximab), which

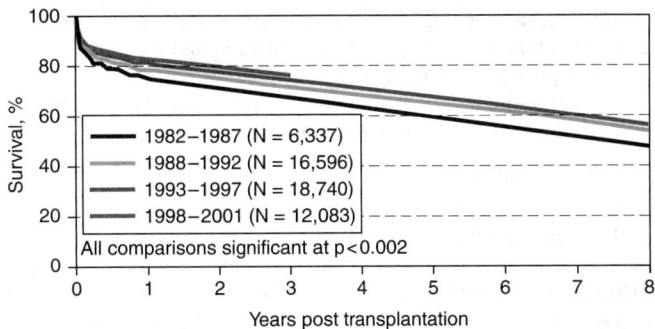

FIGURE 217-1 Actuarial survival for heart transplants performed between 1982 and 2001 by era of transplantation. (*Data by permission from United Network for Organ Sharing/International Society for Heart and Heart-Lung Transplantation Registry.*)

block the interleukin 2 receptor and may provide prevention of allograft rejection without additional global immunosuppression.

Diagnosis of cardiac allograft rejection is usually made with the use of endomyocardial biopsy, either done on a surveillance basis or in response to clinical deterioration. Therapy consists of augmentation of immunosuppression, the intensity and duration of which is dictated by the severity of the rejection.

LATE POSTTRANSPLANT MANAGEMENT ISSUES Increasing numbers of heart transplant patients are surviving for years following transplantation and constitute a population of patients with long-term management issues.

Allograft Coronary Artery Disease Despite having young donor hearts, cardiac allograft recipients are prone to develop coronary artery disease (CAD). This CAD is generally a diffuse, concentric, and longitudinal process that is quite different from "ordinary" atherosclerotic CAD, which is more focal and often eccentric. The underlying etiology is most likely primarily immunologic injury of the vascular endothelium, but a variety of risk factors influence its existence and progression. It is hoped that newer and improved immunosuppressive modalities will reduce the incidence and impact of these devastating complications, which currently account for the majority of late posttransplant deaths. Palliation of the disease with percutaneous interventions is probably safe and effective in the short term. Because of the denervated status of the organ, patients rarely experience angina pectoris, even with advanced stages of the disease.

Retransplantation is the only definitive form of therapy for advanced allograft CAD, but inferior survival rates after retransplantation and the scarcity of donor hearts make the decision to pursue retransplantation a difficult one in an individual patient, as well as a difficult ethical issue.

Malignancy The occurrence of an increased incidence of malignancy is a well-recognized sequela of any program of chronic immunosuppression, and organ transplantation is no exception. Lymphoproliferative disorders are among the most frequent posttransplant complications and, in most cases, seem to be driven by the Epstein-Barr virus. Effective therapy includes reduction of immunosuppression (a clear "double-edged sword" in the setting of a life-sustaining organ), antiviral agents, and traditional chemo- and radiotherapy. Most recently, specific antilymphocyte (CD20) therapy has shown great promise. Cutaneous malignancies (both basal cell and squamous cell carcinomas) also occur with increased frequency in transplant recipients and can pursue very aggressive courses. The role of decreasing immunosuppression for treatment of these cancers is much less clear.

Infections The use of currently available nonspecific immunosuppressive modalities to prevent allograft rejection naturally results in an increased susceptibility to infectious complications in transplant recipients. Although their incidence has decreased since the introduction of cyclosporine, infections with unusual and opportunistic organisms remain the major cause of death during the first postoperative year and remain a threat to the chronically immunosuppressed patient throughout life. Effective therapy depends on careful surveillance for early signs and symptoms of opportunistic infection and an extremely aggressive approach to obtaining a specific diagnosis as well as expertise in recognizing the more common clinical presentations of cytomegalovirus, *Aspergillus*, and other opportunistic infectious agents.

PROLONGED ASSISTED CIRCULATON

The modern era of mechanical circulatory support can be traced back to 1953 when cardiopulmonary bypass was first used in a clinical setting and ushered in the possibility of brief periods of circulatory support to permit open heart surgery. There have subsequently been developed a variety of extracorporeal pumps to provide circulatory support for brief periods of time. The use of a mechanical device to support the circulation for more than a few hours got off to a slow start in the 1980s when the first artificial hearts were introduced with much publicity but failed to produce the hoped-for treatment of end-stage heart disease. Subsequently, technology evolved to provide mechanical assistance to (rather than replacement of) the failing ventricle, although newer versions of the total artificial heart are now once again in preliminary clinical trials.

Although conceived of initially as alternatives to biologic replacement of the heart, left ventricular assist devices (LVADs) were introduced as, and are still employed primarily as, temporary "bridges" to heart transplantation in candidates who begin to fail medical therapy before a donor heart becomes available. Several devices are approved by the U.S. Food and Drug Administration (FDA) and are currently in widespread use. Those that are implantable within the body are compatible with hospital discharge and offer the patient chance for life at home while waiting for a donor heart. However successful such "bridging" is for the individual patient, it does nothing to alleviate the scarcity of donor hearts, and the ultimate goal in the field remains that of providing a reasonable alternative to biologic replacement of the heart—one that is widely and easily available and cost effective.

AVAILABLE DEVICES   In the United States there are currently three FDA-approved devices that are used as bridges to transplantation. None as yet are totally implantable, and, because of this need for transcutaneous connections, all share a common problem with infectious complications. Likewise, all share some tendency to thromboembolic complications as well as the expected possibility of mechanical device failure common to any man-made machine.

The Thoratec LVAD (Thoratec Corp., Pleasanton, CA) is an extracorporeal pump that takes blood from a large cannula placed in the left ventricular apex and propels it forward through an outflow cannula inserted into the ascending aorta. The pump itself sits in the paracorporeal position on the abdomen and is attached to a device console cart with wheels, allowing for limited ambulation. The extracorporeal nature of this pump allows it to be used for small adults for whom the intracorporeal pumps would be too large.

The Novacor LVAD (WorldHeart Inc., Oakland, CA) also takes blood from the left ventricular apex through a cannula and propels it into the ascending aorta through a second cannula. With this device the pump itself is placed in a surgically created pocket in the preperitoneal fascia in the abdomen. A drive line that connects to the power source is tunneled subcutaneously and usually exits in the right upper quadrant of the abdomen.

The HeartMate LVAD (Thoratec Corp., Pleasanton, CA) uses a configuration identical to that of the Novacor device (Fig. 217-2). Differences between the two have to do with the materials used and the tendency for thromboembolic complications. Both commonly lead to hospital discharge and an outpatient wait for a donor heart.

RESULTS   The use of these devices in the United States is limited mainly to patients with postcardiac surgery shock and those who are "bridged" to transplantation. Approximately 6000 patients per year receive support devices after cardiac surgery, with hospital survival

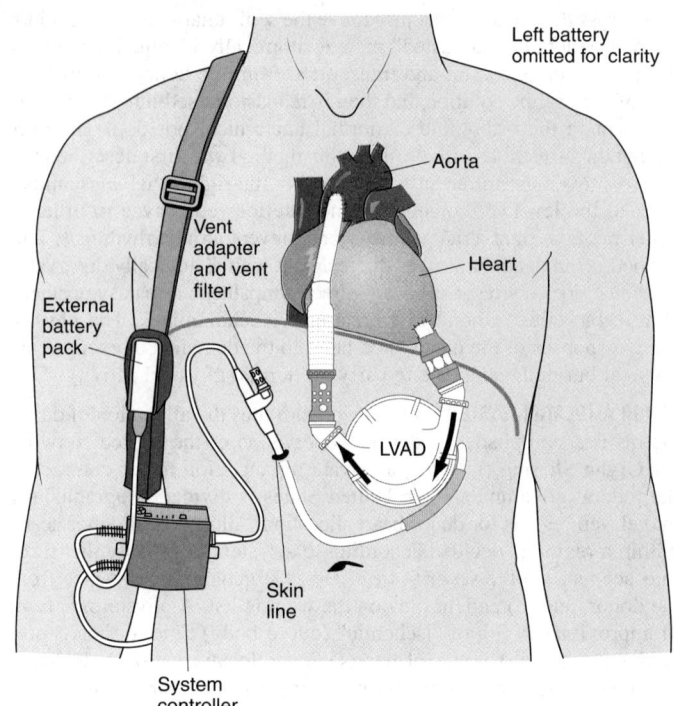

FIGURE 217-2   Diagram of HeartMate left ventricular assist device. (*Reprinted with permission from Thoratec Corp., Pleasanton, CA.*)

rates between 20 and 40%. Approximately 300 to 400 patients per year have devices placed as bridges to transplantation, with an overall discharge rate of 50 to 70% from implantation through transplantation.

GOALS   Future developments in this field can be expected in two directions. First, newer generations of the pumps will likely be smaller and simpler mechanically and, most important, totally implantable. Several much smaller devices, which use a mechanical propeller to provide axial, or non-pulsatile, flow of blood, are already in clinical trials. Second, use of the pumps as "permanent" (destination) therapy in patients with end-stage heart failure who are not considered eligible for transplantation will likely happen in the near future. In a randomized trial of long-term circulatory support with the HeartMate device in such patients, survival with the device was superior to continued medical management. FDA approval of the HeartMate device as permanent circulatory support for patients not eligible for transplantation was granted in 2002. Eventually it is hoped that improved assist devices will be accepted as valid alternatives to biologic replacement of the heart even in transplant-eligible patients and help to modify the supply/demand mismatch for cardiac replacement therapy.

FURTHER READING

BENIAMINOVITZ A et al: Prevention of rejection in cardiac transplantation by blockade of the interleukin-2 receptor with a monoclonal antibody. N Engl J Med 342:613, 2000

GARNIER JL et al: Treatment of post-transplant lymphomas with anti-B-cell monoclonal antibodies. Recent Results Cancer Res 159:113, 2002

HERTZ MI et al: The registry of the International Society for Heart and Lung Transplantation: Nineteenth official report—2002. J Heart Lung Transplant 21:950, 2002

HUNT SA et al: ACC/AHA Practice Guidelines: ACC/AHA Guidelines for the Evaluation and Management of Chronic Heart Failure in the Adult: A report of the American College of Cardiology/American Heart Association Task Force on Practice Guidelines. J Am Coll Cardiol 38:2101, 2001

ROSE EA et al: Long-term use of a left ventricular assist device for end-stage heart failure. N Engl J Med 345:1435, 2001

SCHNETZLER B et al: The role of percutaneous transluminal coronary angioplasty in heart transplant recipients. J Heart Lung Transplant 19:557, 2000

STEVENSON LW, KORMOS RL: Mechanical cardiac support 2000: Current applications and future trial design. Circulation 103:337, 2001

Congenital heart disease complicates ~1% of all live births. It occurs in about 4% of offspring of women with congenital heart disease. Substantial numbers of affected infants reach adulthood because of successful medical and/or surgical management, or because the alteration caused in cardiovascular physiology is well tolerated.

ETIOLOGY Congenital cardiovascular malformations are generally the result of aberrant embryonic development of a normal structure, or failure of such a structure to progress beyond an early stage of embryonic or fetal development. Malformations are due to complex multifactorial genetic and environmental causes. Recognized chromosomal aberrations and mutations of single genes account for <10% of all cardiac malformations (Table 218-1).

The presence of a cardiac malformation as one component of the multiple system involvement in Down's, Turner's, and the trisomy 13-15(D1) and 17-18 (E) syndromes may be anticipated in occasional pregnancies by detection of abnormal chromosomes in fetal cells obtained from amniotic fluid or chorionic villus biopsy. Identification in such cells of the enzyme disorders characteristic of Hurler's syndrome, homocystinuria, or type II glycogen storage disease may also allow one to predict cardiac disease.

PATHOPHYSIOLOGY The anatomic and physiologic changes in the heart and circulation due to any specific congenital cardiocirculatory lesion are not static but rather progress from prenatal life to adulthood. Thus, malformations that are benign or escape detection in childhood may become clinically significant in the adult. For example, the functionally normal, congenitally bicuspid aortic valve may thicken and calcify with time, resulting in significant aortic stenosis; or the well-tolerated left-to-right shunt of an atrial septal defect may not result in cardiac decompensation, with or without pulmonary hypertension, until the fourth or fifth decade.

Pulmonary Hypertension This is a common companion of many congenital cardiac lesions, and the status of the pulmonary vascular bed is often the principal determinant of the clinical manifestations, the course, and the feasibility of surgical repair. Increases in pulmonary arterial pressure result from elevation of pulmonary blood flow and/or resistance, the latter due sometimes to an increase in vascular tone but usually the result of obstructive, obliterative structural changes within the pulmonary vascular bed. Because pulmonary vascular obstructive disease can be the determining factor in assessing the advisability of operation, it is important to quantitate and compare pulmonary to systemic flows and resistances in patients with severe pulmonary hypertension. The causes of pulmonary vascular obstructive disease are unknown, although increased pulmonary blood flow, increased pulmonary arterial blood pressure, elevated pulmonary venous pressure, erythrocytosis, systemic hypoxemia, acidosis, and the bronchial circulation have been implicated. The designation *Eisenmenger syndrome* is applied to patients with a large communication between the two circulations at the aortopulmonary, ventricular, or atrial levels and bidirectional or predominantly right-to-left shunts because of high-resistance and obstructive pulmonary hypertension. No specific treatment has proved beneficial for obstructive pulmonary vascular disease, although newer pulmonary vasodilators and both single lung transplantation with intracardiac defect repair and total heart-lung transplantation are under investigation (Chaps. 217 and 248).

Erythrocytosis The chronic hypoxemia in cyanotic congenital heart disease results in *erythrocytosis* due to increased erythropoietin production (Chap. 31). The commonly used term *polycythemia* is a misnomer because white cell counts are normal and platelet counts are normal to decreased. Cyanotic patients with erythrocytosis may have compensated or decompensated hematocrits. Compensated erythrocytosis with iron-replete equilibrium hematocrits rarely result in symptoms of hyperviscosity at hematocrits <65% and occasionally not even with hematocrits ≥70%. Therapeutic phlebotomy is rarely required in compensated erythrocytosis. In contrast, patients with decompensated erythrocytosis fail to establish equilibrium with unstable, rising hematocrits and recurrent hyperviscosity symptoms. Therapeutic phlebotomy, a two-edged sword, allows temporary relief of symptoms but begets instability of the hematocrit and compounds the problem by iron depletion. Iron-deficiency symptoms are usually indistinguishable from those of hyperviscosity; progressive symptoms after recurrent phlebotomy are usually due to iron depletion with hypochromic microcytosis. Iron depletion results in a larger number of smaller (microcytic) hypochromic red cells that are less capable of carrying oxygen and less deformable in the microcirculation. Because these microcytes are less deformable in the microcirculation and there are more of them relative to the plasma volume, the viscosity is greater than for an equivalent hematocrit with fewer, larger, iron-replete, deformable cells. As such, iron-depleted erythrocytosis results in increasing symptoms due to decreased oxygen delivery to the tissues.

Hemostasis is abnormal in cyanotic congenital heart disease, due in part to the increased blood volume and engorged capillaries, abnormalities in platelet function and sensitivity to aspirin or nonsteroidal anti-inflammatory agents, and abnormalities of the extrinsic and intrinsic coagulation system. Oral contraceptives are contraindicated for cyanotic women because of the enhanced risk of vascular thrombosis.

The risk of stroke is greatest in children <4 years with cyanotic heart disease and iron deficiency, often with dehydration as an aggravating cause. In contrast, adults with cyanotic congenital heart disease do not appear to be at increased risk for stroke, unless there are excessive injudicious phlebotomies, inappropriate use of aspirin or anticoagulants, or the presence of atrial arrhythmias or infective endocarditis.

Symptoms of hyperviscosity can be produced in any cyanotic patient with erythrocytosis if dehydration causes a reduction of plasma volume. Phlebotomy, when required for symptoms of hyperviscosity not due to dehydration or iron deficiency, is a simple outpatient removal of 500 mL of blood over 45 min with isovolumetric replacement with isotonic saline (5% dextrose if congestive heart failure exists). Acute phlebotomy without volume replacement is contraindicated. Iron repletion in decompensated iron-depleted erythrocytosis ameliorates iron-deficiency symptoms but must be done gradually to avoid a sudden excessive rise in hematocrit and resultant hyperviscosity.

Pregnancy The physiologic alterations during normal gestation (Chap. 6) can create symptoms and physical findings that may be attributed erroneously to heart disease. Dyspnea due to the hormonal influence of progesterone and elevation of the diaphragm in association with peripheral edema and fatigability may be attributed inappropriately to heart failure. The jugular venous pulsations normally become more apparent after the twentieth week. Elevation of the diaphragm can cause basal rales (which disappear with deep breathing). Both ventricles are more easily palpated due to the normal increase in ventricular volumes and elevation of the diaphragm. Third heart sounds, already relatively frequent in normal nongravid young women, increase in frequency and intensity with pregnancy because of increased heart rate and volume of flow across the mitral and tricuspid valves. Midsystolic murmurs across the pulmonary outflow tract and supraclavicular systolic murmurs are caused by increased cardiac output. Venous hums and mammary souffles are usual during pregnancy.

These normal circulatory changes may impinge upon the woman's cardiac reserve. The mother is most at risk if she has a cardiovascular lesion associated with pulmonary vascular disease and pulmonary hypertension (e.g., Eisenmenger's physiology or mitral stenosis) or left

TABLE 218-1 *Syndromes with Associated Cardiovascular Involvement*

Syndrome (Genetic Locus)	Major Cardiovascular Manifestations	Major Noncardiac Abnormalities
HERITABLE AND POSSIBLY HERITABLE		
Ellis–van Creveld	Single atrium or atrial septal defect	Chondrodystrophic dwarfism, nail dysplasia, polydactyly
TAR (thrombocytopenia-absent radius)	Atrial septal defect, tetralogy of Fallot	Radial aplasia or hypoplasia, thrombocytopenia
Holt-Oram (12q21–q3)	Atrial septal defect (other defects common)	Skeletal upper limb defect, hypoplasia of clavicles
Kartagener	Dextrocardia	Situs inversus, sinusitis, bronchiectasis
Laurence-Moon-Biedl-Bardet	Variable defects	Retinal pigmentation, obesity, polydactyly
Noonan (12q24)	Pulmonic valve dysplasia, cardiomyopathy (usually hypertrophic)	Webbed neck, pectus excavatum, cryptorchidism
Tuberous sclerosis (type 1—4q); type 2—16p)	Rhabdomyoma, cardiomyopathy	Phakomatosis, bone lesions, hamartomatous skin lesions
Multiple lentigines (LEOPARD) syndrome	Pulmonic stenosis	Basal cell nevi, broad facies, rib anomalies, deafness
Rubenstein-Taybi (16p13.3)	Patent ductus arteriosus (others)	Broad thumbs and toes, hypoplastic maxilla, slanted palpebral fissures
Familial deafness	Arrhythmias, sudden death	Sensorineural deafness
Weber-Osler-Rendu (9q33)	Arteriovenous fistulas (lung, liver, mucous membranes)	Multiple telangiectasias
Apert (10q26)	Ventricular septal defect	Craniosynostosis, midfacial hypoplasia, syndactyly
Crouzon (10q26, 4p16.3)	Patent ductus arteriosus, aortic coarctation	Ptosis with shallow orbits, craniosynostosis, maxillary hypoplasia
Hypertrophic cardiomyopathy (locus heterogeneity, 14q11.2–12, 1q32, 15q22, 11p11.2, etc.)	Asymmetric septal hypertrophy	Family history of sudden death
Incontinentia pigmenti	Patent ductus arteriosus	Irregular pigmented skin lesions, patchy alopecia, hypodontia
Alagille (arteriohepatic dysplasia) (20p12)	Peripheral pulmonic stenosis, pulmonic stenosis	Biliary hypoplasia, vertebral anomalies, prominent forehead, deep-set eyes
Catch-22 (DiGeorge) (22q11)	Interrupted aortic arch, tetralogy of Fallot, truncus arteriosus	Thymic hypoplasia or aplasia, parathyroid aplasia or hypoplasia, abnormal facies
Shprintzen (velocardiofacial) (22q11.2)	Ventricular septal defect, tetralogy of Fallot, right aortic arch	Cleft palate, prominent nose, slender hands, learning disability
Williams (7q11.23)	Supravalvular aortic stenosis, peripheral pulmonic stenosis	Mental deficiency, elfin facies, loquacious personality, hoarse voice
Long QT (Jervell and Lange-Nielsen, Romano-Ward) (11p15.5, 7q35, 3p21, 21q22)	Long QT interval, ventricular arrhythmias	Family history of sudden death, congenital deafness (not in Romano-Ward)
Friedreich's ataxia (9q)	Hypertrophic or dilated cardiomyopathy; conduction defects	Ataxia, speech defect, degeneration of spinal cord dorsal columns
Muscular dystrophy	Cardiomyopathy	Pseudohypertrophy of calf muscles, weakness of trunk and proximal limb muscles
Cystic fibrosis (7q)	Cor pulmonale	Pancreatic insufficiency, malabsorption, chronic lung disease
Sickle cell anemia	Cardiomyopathy, mitral regurgitation	Hemoglobin SS
Conradi-Hunermann	Ventricular septal defect, patent ductus arteriosus	Asymmetrical limb shortness, early punctate mineralization, large skin pores
Cockayne	Accelerated atherosclerosis	Cachectic dwarfism, retinal pigment abnormalities, photosensitivity dermatitis
Progeria	Accelerated atherosclerosis	Premature aging, alopecia, atrophy of subcutaneous fat, skeletal hypoplasia
CONNECTIVE TISSUE DISORDERS		
Cutis laxa	Peripheral pulmonic stenosis	Generalized disruption of elastic fibers, diminished skin resilience, hernias
Ehlers-Danlos (2q31)	Arterial dilatation and rupture, mitral regurgitation	Hyperextensible joints, hyperelastic and friable
Marfan (15q21.1)	Aortic dilatation, aortic and mitral incompetence	Gracile habitus, arachnodactyly with hyperextensibility, lens subluxation
Osteogenesis imperfecta (4.17)	Aortic incompetence	Fragile bones, blue sclerae
Pseudoxanthoma elasticum	Peripheral and coronary arterial disease	Degeneration of elastic fibers in skin, retinal angioid streaks
INBORN ERRORS OF METABOLISM		
Pompe disease	Glycogen storage disease of heart	Acid maltase deficiency, muscular weakness
Homocystinuria	Aortic and pulmonary arterial dilatation, intravascular thrombosis	Cystathionine synthetase deficiency, lens subluxation, osteoporosis
Mucopolysaccharidoses: Hurler; Hunter	Multivalvular and coronary and great artery disease, cardiomyopathy	Hurler: Deficiency of α-L-iduronidase, corneal clouding, coarse features, growth and mental retardation
		Hunter: Deficiency of L-iduranosulfate sulfatase, coarse facies, clear cornea, growth and mental retardation

(continued)

TABLE 218-1—(Continued)

Syndrome (Genetic Locus)	Major Cardiovascular Manifestations	Major Noncardiac Abnormalities
Morquio; Scheie; Maroteaux-Lamy	Aortic regurgitation	Morquio: Deficiency of *N*-acetylhexosamine sulfate sulfatase, cloudy cornea, severe bone changes involving vertebrae and epiphyses Scheie: Deficiency of α-L-iduronidase, cloudy cornea, normal intelligence, peculiar facies Maroteaux-Lamy: Deficiency of arylsulfatase B, cloudy cornea, osseous changes
CHROMOSOMAL ABNORMALITIES		
Trisomy 21 (Down syndrome)	Endocardial cushion defect, atrial or ventricular septal defect, tetralogy of Fallot	Hypotonia, hyperextensible joints, mongoloid facies, mental retardation
Trisomy 13 (D)	Ventricular septal defect, patent ductus arteriosus, double-outlet right ventricle	Single midline intracerebral ventricle with midfacial defects, polydactyly, nail changes, mental retardation
Trisomy 18 (E)	Congenital polyvalvular dysplasia, ventricular septal defect, patent ductus	Clenched hand, short sternum, low arch dermal ridge pattern on fingertips, mental retardation
Cri du chat (short-arm deletion-5)	Ventricular septal defect	Cat cry, microcephaly, antimongoloid slant of palpebral fissures, mental retardation
XO (Turner)	Coarctation of aorta, bicuspid aortic valve, aortic dilatation	Short female, broad chest, lymphedema, webbed neck
XXXY and XXXXX	Patent ductus arteriosus	XXXY: Hypogenitalism, mental retardation, radial-ulnar synostosis XXXXX: Small hands, incurving of fifth fingers, mental retardation
SPORADIC DISORDERS		
VATER association	Ventricular septal defect	Vertebral anomalies, anal atresia, tracheo-esophageal fistula, radial and renal anomalies
CHARGE association	Tetralogy of Fallot (other defects common)	Colobomas, choanal atresia, mental and growth deficiency, genital and ear anomalies
Cornelia de Lange	Ventricular septal defect	Micromelia, synophrys, mental and growth deficiency
TERATOGENIC DISORDERS		
Rubella	Patent ductus arteriosus, pulmonic valvular and/or arterial stenosis, atrial septal defect	Cataracts, deafness, microcephaly
Alcohol	Ventricular septal defect (other defects)	Microcephaly, growth and mental deficiency, short palpebral fissures, smooth philtrum, thin upper lip
Dilantin	Pulmonic stenosis, aortic stenosis, coarctation, patent ductus arteriosus	Hypertelorism, growth and mental deficiency, short phalanges, bowed upper lip
Thalidomide	Variable	Phocomelia
Lithium	Ebstein's anomaly, tricuspid atresia	None

Source: Modified from WF Friedman and N Silverman: Congenital heart disease in infancy and childhood, in E Braunwald et al (eds), *Heart Disease*, 6th ed. Philadelphia, Saunders, 1998; with permission.

ventricular (LV) outflow tract obstruction (e.g., aortic stenosis) but also risks death with any malformation that may cause heart failure or a hemodynamically important arrhythmia (Table 218-2). The fetus is most at risk in the presence of maternal cyanosis, heart failure, or pulmonary hypertension. Women with aortic coarctation or Marfan's syndrome are at risk for aortic dissection. Patients with cyanotic heart disease, pulmonary hypertension, or Marfan's syndrome should not become pregnant; those with correctable lesions should be counseled about the risks of pregnancy with an uncorrected malformation versus repair and later pregnancy. The effect of pregnancy in postoperative patients depends on the outcome of the repair including the presence and severity of residua, sequelae, or complications. Contraception is an important topic with such patients. Tubal ligation should be considered in those in whom pregnancy is strictly contraindicated.

INFECTIVE ENDOCARDITIS (See also Chap. 109) Routine antimicrobial prophylaxis is recommended for most patients with congenital heart disease whether operated on or not. Antibiotic prophylaxis is not uniformly effective. Nonetheless, it is recommended for all dental procedures, gastrointestinal and genitourinary surgery, and diagnostic procedures such as proctosigmoidoscopy and cystoscopy. The clinical and bacteriologic profile of infective endocarditis in patients with congenital heart disease has changed with the advent of intracardiac surgery and of prosthetic devices. Two major predisposing causes of infective endocarditis are a susceptible cardiovascular substrate and a

source of bacteremia. Prophylaxis includes both chemotherapeutic (antimicrobial) and nonchemotherapeutic (hygienic) measures. Meticulous dental and skin care is required.

TABLE 218-2 *Tolerance of Pregnancy by Patients with Various Congenital Cardiac Malformations*

Well Tolerated	Intermediate Effect	Poorly Tolerated
NYHA class I	NYHA class II–III	NHYA class IV
Left-right shunts without PHTN	Repaired transposition of the great arteries	Right-left shunt, unrepaired cyanotic heart disease
Aortic or mitral valvular regurgitation (mild-moderate)	Fontan repairs	PHTN and/or pulmonary vascular disease (e.g., Eisenmenger's, "primary PHTN")
Pulmonic or tricuspid regurgitation (if low pressure, even severe)	Aortic or mitral stenosis (moderate)	Aortic or mitral stenosis (severe)
Pulmonic stenosis (mild-moderate)	Ebstain's anomaly	Pulmonic stenosis (severe)
Well-repaired tetralogy of Fallot		Marfan's or aortic coarctation

Note: NYHA, New York Heart Association; PHTN, pulmonary hypertension.

EXERCISE   Advice on athletics and exercise is governed by the nature of the exercise and by the type and severity of the congenital cardiovascular lesion. Patients with lesions characterized by LV outflow tract obstruction, if more than mild to moderate, or pulmonary vascular disease, risk syncope or even sudden death. In Fallot's tetralogy, isotonic exercise–induced decrease in systemic vascular resistance relative to the right ventricular (RV) outflow obstruction augments the right-to-left shunt, increases hypoxemia, and causes an increase in subjective breathlessness due to the response of the respiratory center to the changes in blood gases and pH.

INSURABILITY AND EMPLOYABILITY   Most patients with congenital heart disease must pay significantly more than standard life insurance rates, assuming their anomaly places them in a category that companies have determined is eligible for insurance. A paucity of actuarial survival data beyond adolescence for persons with most congenital cardiac lesions that have undergone operative repair has made it difficult to convince insurance companies to offer reasonable cost insurance even to individual patients whose long-term prognosis is quite good.

Employment is affected by the patient's physical capacity relative to the type of job sought. Job discrimination exists, often because the employer is reluctant to accept health insurance responsibilities. Eligibility for some occupations is governed by public safety regulations, e.g., airline pilots, bus drivers.

SPECIFIC CARDIAC DEFECTS

Table 218-3 provides a classification of cardiac anomalies that recognizes the general categories of clinical presentation, functional consequences, and site of origin of congenital defects.

Categorizing the defect(s) in an individual patient requires an answer to a number of basic questions. Is the patient acyanotic or cyanotic? Is pulmonary arterial blood flow increased or not? Does the malformation originate in the left or right side of the heart? Which is the dominant ventricle? Is pulmonary hypertension present or not? With the above information as a foundation, the use of more refined

---

TABLE 218-3   *Classification of Congenital Heart Disease*

ACYANOTIC WITH LEFT-TO-RIGHT SHUNT

I. Atrial level shunt
  A. Atrial septal defect
    1. Ostium primum
    2. Ostium secundum
    3. Sinus venosus
  B. Atrial septal defect with mitral stenosis (Lutembacher's syndrome)
  C. Partial anomalous pulmonary venous connection
II. Ventricular level shunt
  A. Ventricular septal defect
    1. Inlet septum
    2. Muscular septum
    3. Perimembranous septum
    4. Infundibular septum
  B. Ventricular septal defect with aortic regurgitation
  C. Ventricular septal defect with left ventricular to right atrial shunt

III. Aortic root to right heart shunt
  A. Ruptured sinus of Valsalva aneurysm
  B. Coronary arteriovenous fistula
  C. Anomalous origin of the left coronary artery from the pulmonary trunk
IV. Aortopulmonary level shunt
  A. Aortopulmonary window
  B. Patent ductus arteriosus
V. Multiple level shunts
  A. Complete common atrioventricular canal
  B. Ventricular septal defect with atrial septal defect
  C. Ventricular septal defect with patent ductus arteriosus

ACYANOTIC WITHOUT A SHUNT

I. Left heart malformations
  A. Congenital obstruction to left atrial inflow
    1. Pulmonary vein stenosis
    2. Mitral stenosis
    3. Cor triatriatum
  B. Mitral regurgitation
    1. Atrioventricular septal (endocardial cushion)
    2. Congenitally corrected transposition of the great arteries
    3. Anomalous origin of the left coronary artery from the pulmonary trunk
    4. Miscellaneous (double-orifice mitral valve, congenital perforations, accessory commissures with anomalous chordal insertion, congenitally short or absent chordae, cleft posterior leaflet, parachute mitral valve, etc.)
  C. Primary dilated endocardial fibroelastosis

  D. Aortic stenosis
    1. Discrete subvalvular
    2. Valvular
    3. Supravalvular
  E. Aortic valve regurgitation
  F. Coarctation of the aorta
II. Right heart malformations
  A. Acyanotic Ebstein's anomaly of the tricuspid valve
  B. Pulmonic stenosis
    1. Subinfundibular
    2. Infundibular
    3. Valvular
    4. Supravalvular (stenosis of pulmonary artery and its branches)
  C. Congenital pulmonary valve regurgitation
  D. Idiopathic dilatation of the pulmonary trunk

CYANOTIC

I. Increased pulmonary blood flow
  A. Complete transposition of the great arteries
  B. Double-outlet right ventricle of the Taussig-Bing type
  C. Truncus arteriosus
  D. Total anomalous pulmonary venous connection
  E. Single ventricle without pulmonic stenosis
  F. Common atrium
  G. Tetralogy of Fallot with pulmonary atresia and increased collateral arterial flow
  H. Tricuspid atresia with large ventricular septal defect and no pulmonic stenosis
  I. Hypoplastic left heart (aortic atresia, mitral atresia)

II. Normal or decreased pulmonary blood flow
  A. Tricuspid atresia
  B. Ebstein's anomaly with right-to-left atrial shunt
  C. Pulmonary atresia with intact ventricular septum
  D. Pulmonic stenosis or atresia with ventricular septal defect (tetralogy of Fallot)
  E. Pulmonic stenosis with right-to-left atrial shunt
  F. Complete transposition of the great arteries with pulmonic stenosis
  G. Double-outlet right ventricle with pulmonic stenosis
  H. Single ventricle with pulmonic stenosis
  I. Pulmonary arteriovenous fistula
  J. Vena caval to left atrial communication

OTHER

I. Congenitally corrected transposition of the great arteries
II. The cardiac malpositions

III. Congenital complete heart block

Source: Modified from JK Perloff, *The Clinical Recognition of Congenital Heart Disease*, Philadelphia, Saunders, 1991.

diagnostic techniques such as transthoracic (precordial) and transesophageal echocardiography and Doppler imaging, magnetic resonance imaging, and/or hemodynamic study and angiocardiography leads to a precise anatomic and functional assessment.

ACYANOTIC CONGENITAL HEART DISEASE WITH A LEFT-TO-RIGHT SHUNT

ATRIAL SEPTAL DEFECT This common cardiac anomaly in adults occurs more frequently in females. The *sinus venosus* type occurs high in the atrial septum near the entry of the superior vena cava and is associated frequently with anomalous connection of pulmonary veins from the right lung to the junction of the superior vena cava and right atrium. *Ostium primum* anomalies are a form of atrioventricular septal defect that lie immediately adjacent to the atrioventricular valves, either of which may be deformed and incompetent. Ostium primum defects occur commonly in patients with Down's syndrome, although the more complex atrioventricular septal defects with a common atrioventricular valve and a posterior defect of the basal portion of the interventricular septum are more characteristic of this chromosomal defect. The most common atrial septal defect involves the fossa ovalis, is midseptal in location, and is of the *ostium secundum type*. This type of defect should not be confused with a *patent foramen ovale*. Anatomic obliteration of the foramen ovale ordinarily follows its functional closure soon after birth, but residual "probe patency" is a normal variant; atrial septal defect denotes a true deficiency of the atrial septum and implies functional and anatomic patency.

The magnitude of the left-to-right shunt through an atrial septal defect depends on the defect size, the diastolic properties of both ventricles, and the relative impedance in the pulmonary and systemic circulations. The left-to-right shunt causes diastolic overloading of the right ventricle and increased pulmonary blood flow.

Patients with atrial septal defect are usually asymptomatic in early life, although there may be some physical underdevelopment and an increased tendency for respiratory infections; cardiorespiratory symptoms occur in many older patients. Beyond the fourth decade, a significant number of patients develop atrial arrhythmias, pulmonary arterial hypertension, bidirectional and then right-to-left shunting of blood, and cardiac failure. Patients exposed to the chronic environmental hypoxia of high altitude tend to develop pulmonary hypertension at younger ages. In some older patients, left-to-right shunting across the defect increases as progressive systemic hypertension and/or coronary artery disease result in reduced compliance of the left ventricle.

Physical Examination Examination usually reveals a prominent right ventricular impulse and palpable pulmonary artery pulsation. The first heart sound is normal or split, with accentuation of the tricuspid valve closure sound. Increased flow across the pulmonic valve is responsible for a midsystolic pulmonary outflow murmur. The second heart sound is widely split and is relatively fixed in relation to respiration. A mid-diastolic rumbling murmur, loudest at the fourth intercostal space and along the left sternal border, reflects increased flow across the tricuspid valve. In patients with ostium primum defects, an apical thrill and holosystolic murmur indicate associated mitral or tricuspid incompetence or a ventricular septal defect.

The physical findings are altered when an increase in the pulmonary vascular resistance results in diminution of the left-to-right shunt. Both the pulmonary and tricuspid murmurs decrease in intensity, the pulmonic component of the second heart sound and a systolic ejection sound are accentuated, the two components of the second heart sound may fuse, and a diastolic murmur of pulmonic regurgitation appears. Cyanosis and clubbing accompany the development of a right-to-left shunt.

In adults with an atrial septal defect and atrial fibrillation, the physical findings may be confused with the findings of mitral stenosis with pulmonary hypertension because the tricuspid flow murmur and widely split second heart sound may be mistakenly thought to represent the diastolic murmur of mitral stenosis and the mitral "opening snap," respectively.

Electrocardiogram In patients with an ostium secundum defect, the electrocardiogram (ECG) usually shows right axis deviation and an rSr' pattern in the right precordial leads representing delayed posterobasal activation of the ventricular septum and enlargement of the RV outflow tract. An ectopic atrial pacemaker or first-degree heart block occurs occasionally in patients with defects of the sinus venous type. In patients with an ostium primum defect, the RV conduction defect is characteristically accompanied by left axis deviation and by superior orientation and counterclockwise rotation of the QRS loop in the frontal plane. Varying degrees of RV and right atrial (RA) hypertrophy may occur with each type of defect, depending on the height of the pulmonary artery pressure. *Chest roentgenograms* reveal enlargement of the right atrium and right ventricle, dilatation of the pulmonary artery and its branches, and increased pulmonary vascular markings.

Echocardiogram This test shows pulmonary arterial and RV dilatation, and anterior systolic (paradoxical) or flat interventricular septal motion if a significant RV volume overload is present. The defect may be visualized directly from subcostal, right parasternal, or apical echocardiographic windows. In most institutions, two-dimensional echocardiography, supplemented by conventional or color Doppler flow examination, has supplanted cardiac catheterization as the confirmatory test for atrial septal defect. Transesophageal echocardiography is indicated if the transthoracic echocardiogram is ambiguous, which is often the case with sinus venosus defects. Cardiac catheterization is then performed if inconsistencies exist in the clinical data, if significant pulmonary hypertension or associated malformations are suspected, or if coronary artery disease is a possibility.

℞ TREATMENT

Operative repair, usually with a patch of pericardium or of prosthetic material, or percutaneous transcatheter device closure, ideally in children ages 3 to 6, should be advised for all patients with uncomplicated secundum atrial septal defects in whom there is significant left-to-right shunting, i.e., pulmonary-to-systemic flow ratios ~2.0:1.0. Excellent results may be anticipated, at low risk, even in patients >40 years, in the absence of pulmonary hypertension. Patients with ostium primum defects, cleft, deformed, and incompetent valves require repair in addition to patch closure of the atrial defect. Intraoperative transesophageal echocardiography is used to monitor the surgical results of atrioventricular valve repair. Closure should not be carried out in patients with small defects and trivial left-to-right shunts or in those with severe pulmonary vascular disease without a significant left-to-right shunt.

Patients with atrial septal defect of the sinus venosus or ostium secundum types rarely die before the fifth decade. During the fifth and sixth decades the incidence of progressive symptoms, often leading to severe disability, increases substantially. Medical management should include prompt treatment of respiratory tract infections, antiarrhythmic medications for atrial fibrillation or supraventricular tachycardia, and the usual measures for hypertension, coronary disease, or heart failure (Chap. 216), if these complications occur. The risk of infective endocarditis is quite low unless the defect is complicated by valvular regurgitation or has recently been repaired with a patch (Chap. 109).

VENTRICULAR SEPTAL DEFECT Defects of the ventricular septum are common as isolated defects and as one component of a combination of anomalies. The opening is usually single and situated in the membranous portion of the septum. The functional disturbance is dependent primarily on its size and on the status of the pulmonary vascular bed, rather than on the location of the defect. Only small or moderate-size defects are usually seen initially in adulthood as most patients with isolated large defects come to medical and, often, surgical attention very early in life.

A wide spectrum exists in the natural history of ventricular septal defect, ranging from spontaneous closure to congestive cardiac failure and death in early infancy. Within this spectrum is the possible development of pulmonary vascular obstruction, RV outflow tract obstruction, aortic regurgitation, and infective endocarditis. Spontaneous closure is more common in patients born with a small ventricular septal defect and occurs in early childhood in most patients.

Patients with large ventricular septal defects and pulmonary hypertension are those at greatest risk for developing pulmonary vascular obstruction. Thus, large defects should be corrected surgically early in life when pulmonary vascular disease is still reversible or not yet developed. In patients with severe pulmonary vascular obstruction (Eisenmenger syndrome), symptoms in adult life consist of exertional dyspnea, chest pain, syncope, and hemoptysis. The right-to-left shunt leads to cyanosis, clubbing, and erythrocytosis. In all patients, the degree to which pulmonary vascular resistance is elevated before operation is a critical factor determining prognosis. If the pulmonary vascular resistance is one-third or less of the systemic value, progression of pulmonary vascular disease after operation is unusual. However, if a moderate to severe increase in pulmonary vascular resistance exists preoperatively, either no change or a progression of pulmonary vascular disease is common postoperatively.

RV outflow tract obstruction develops in ~5 to 10% of patients who present in infancy with a moderate to large left-to-right shunt. With time, as subvalvular RV outflow tract obstruction progresses, the findings in these patients begin to resemble more closely those of the cyanotic tetralogy of Fallot.

In ~5% of patients, incompetence of the aortic valve results from insufficient cusp tissue or prolapse of the cusp through the interventricular defect; the aortic regurgitation then complicates and usually dominates the clinical course.

Two-dimensional *echocardiography* with conventional or color Doppler examination can usually define the number and location of defects in the ventricular septum and detect associated anomalies. Hemodynamic and angiographic study may be employed to assess the status of the pulmonary vascular bed and clarify details of the altered anatomy.

Rx TREATMENT

Surgery is not recommended for patients with normal pulmonary arterial pressures with small shunts (pulmonary-to-systemic flow ratios of <1.5 to 2.0:1.0). Operative correction is indicated when there is a moderate to large left-to-right shunt with a pulmonary-to-systemic flow ratio >1.5:1.0 or 2.0:1.0, in the absence of prohibitively high levels of pulmonary vascular resistance.

PATENT DUCTUS ARTERIOSUS　The ductus arteriosus is a vessel leading from the bifurcation of the pulmonary artery to the aorta just distal to the left subclavian artery. Normally, the vascular channel is open in the fetus but closes immediately after birth. The flow across the ductus is determined by the pressure and resistance relationships between the systemic and pulmonary circulations and by the cross-sectional area and length of the ductus. In most adults with this anomaly, pulmonary pressures are normal and a gradient and shunt from aorta to pulmonary artery persist throughout the cardiac cycle, resulting in a characteristic thrill and a continuous "machinery" murmur with a late systolic accentuation at the upper left sternal edge. In adults who were born with a large left-to-right shunt through the ductus arteriosus, pulmonary vascular obstruction (Eisenmenger syndrome) with pulmonary hypertension, right-to-left shunting, and cyanosis have usually developed. Severe pulmonary vascular disease results in reversal of flow through the ductus; unoxygenated blood is shunted to the descending aorta; and the toes, but not the fingers, become cyanotic and clubbed, a finding termed *differential cyanosis*. The leading causes of death in adults with patent ductus are cardiac failure and infective endocarditis; occasionally severe pulmonary vascular obstruction may cause aneurysmal dilatation, calcification, and rupture of the ductus.

Rx TREATMENT

In the absence of severe pulmonary vascular disease and predominant left-to-right shunting of blood, the patent ductus should be surgically ligated or divided. Transcatheter closure using coils, buttons, plugs, and umbrellas has become commonplace for appropriately shaped defects. Thoracoscopic surgical approaches are considered experimental. Operation should be deferred for several months in patients treated successfully for infective endocarditis, because the ductus may remain somewhat edematous and friable.

AORTIC ROOT TO RIGHT HEART SHUNTS　The three most common causes of aortic root to right heart shunts are congenital aneurysm of an aortic sinus of Valsalva with fistula, coronary arteriovenous fistula, and anomalous origin of the left coronary artery from the pulmonary trunk. *Aneurysm of an aortic sinus of Valsalva* consists of a separation or lack of fusion between the media of the aorta and the annulus of the aortic valve. Rupture usually occurs in the third or fourth decade of life; most often the aorticocardiac fistula is between the right coronary cusp and the right ventricle, but occasionally, when the noncoronary cusp is involved, the fistula drains into the right atrium. Abrupt rupture causes chest pain, bounding pulses, a continuous murmur accentuated in diastole, and volume overload of the heart. Diagnosis is confirmed by two-dimensional and Doppler echocardiographic studies; cardiac catheterization quantitates the left-to-right shunt, and thoracic aortography visualizes the fistula. Medical management is directed at cardiac failure, arrhythmias, or endocarditis. At operation, the aneurysm is closed and amputated, and the aortic wall is reunited with the heart, either by direct suture or with a prosthesis.

Coronary arteriovenous fistula, an unusual anomaly, consists of a communication between a coronary artery and another cardiac chamber, usually the coronary sinus, right atrium, or right ventricle. The shunt is usually of small magnitude, and myocardial blood flow is not usually compromised. Potential complications include infective endocarditis, thrombus formation with occlusion or distal embolization, rupture of an aneurysmal fistula, and rarely, pulmonary hypertension and congestive failure. A loud, superficial, continuous murmur at the lower or midsternal border usually prompts a further evaluation of asymptomatic patients. Doppler echocardiography demonstrates the site of drainage; if the site of origin is proximal, it may be detectable by two-dimensional echocardiography. Retrograde thoracic aortography or coronary arteriography permits identification of the size and anatomic features of the fistulous tract, which may be closed by suture or transcatheter obliteration.

The third anomaly causing a shunt from the aortic root to the right heart is *anomalous origin of the left coronary artery from the pulmonary artery*. Myocardial infarction and fibrosis commonly lead to death within the first year, though up to 20% of patients survive to adolescence and beyond without surgical correction. The diagnosis is supported by the ECG findings of an anterolateral myocardial infarction. Operative management of adults consists of coronary artery bypass with an internal mammary artery graft or saphenous vein–coronary artery graft.

ACYANOTIC CONGENITAL HEART DISEASE WITHOUT A SHUNT

CONGENITAL AORTIC STENOSIS　Malformations that cause obstruction to LV outflow include congenital valvular aortic stenosis, discrete subaortic stenosis, supravalvular aortic stenosis, and hypertrophic obstructive cardiomyopathy (Chap. 221).

Valvular Aortic Stenosis　This malformation occurs three to four times more often in males than in females. The congenital bicuspid aortic valve, which is not necessarily stenotic, is one of the most common congenital malformations of the heart, although it may go undetected in early life. Because bicuspid valves may become stenotic with time or be the site of the infective endocarditis, the lesion may be difficult to distinguish in adults from acquired rheumatic or degenerative calcific aortic stenosis.

The dynamics of blood flow associated with a congenitally deformed, rigid aortic valve commonly lead to thickening of the cusps and, in later life, to calcification. Hemodynamically significant obstruction causes concentric hypertrophy of the LV wall. The ascending aorta is often dilated, misnamed "poststenotic" dilatation; this is due to histologic abnormalities similar to those in Marfan syndrome, and may result in aortic dissection. →*The clinical manifestations and hemodynamic abnormalities are discussed in Chap. 219.*

℞ TREATMENT

The medical management of congenital valvular aortic stenosis includes prophylaxis against infective endocarditis and, in patients with diminished cardiac reserve, the administration of digitalis and diuretics and sodium restriction while awaiting operation. A dilated aortic root may require beta blockers. If severe aortic stenosis is present, strenuous physical activity should be avoided even when the patient is asymptomatic, and participation in competitive sports should probably be restricted in patients with milder degrees of obstruction. Aortic valve replacement is indicated in adults with critical obstruction, i.e., with an aortic valve area <0.5 cm^2/m^2, with symptoms secondary to LV dysfunction or myocardial ischemia, or with hemodynamic evidence of LV dysfunction. In asymptomatic children or adolescents or young adults with critical aortic stenosis without valvular calcification or these features, aortic balloon valvuloplasty is often useful (Chap. 229). If surgery is contraindicated in older patients because of a complicating medical problem such as malignancy or renal or hepatic failure, balloon valvuloplasty may provide short-term improvement. It may serve as a bridge to aortic valve replacement in patients with severe heart failure.

Subaortic Stenosis The most common form of subaortic stenosis is the *idiopathic hypertrophic* variety, also termed *hypertrophic cardiomyopathy*, which is present at birth in about one-third of the patients and is discussed in Chap. 221. In contrast, both clinically and physiologically, the *discrete* form of subaortic stenosis resembles valvular aortic stenosis. The lesion usually consists of a membranous diaphragm or fibrous ring encircling the LV outflow tract just beneath the base of the aortic valve. Echocardiography demonstrates the subaortic obstruction; Doppler studies show turbulence proximal to the aortic valve and also detect and quantitate the pressure gradient and severity of aortic regurgitation. Treatment consists of excision of the membrane or fibrous ridge.

Supravalvular Aortic Stenosis This anomaly consists of a localized or diffuse narrowing of the ascending aorta originating just above the level of the coronary arteries at the superior margin of the sinuses of Valsalva. In contrast to other forms of aortic stenosis, the coronary arteries are subjected to elevated systolic pressures from the left ventricle, are often dilated and tortuous, and are susceptible to premature atherosclerosis. In most patients a genetic defect for the anomaly is located in the same chromosomal subunit as elastin on chromosome 7.

COARCTATION OF THE AORTA Narrowing or constriction of the lumen of the aorta may occur anywhere along its length but is most common distal to the origin of the left subclavian artery near the insertion of the ligamentum arteriosum. Coarctation occurs in ~7% of patients with congenital heart disease, is twice as common in males as in females, and is most frequent in patients with gonadal dysgenesis. Clinical manifestations depend on the site and extent of obstruction and the presence of associated cardiac anomalies, most commonly a bicuspid aortic valve. Aneurysmal arterial dilatation of the circle of Willis produces a high risk of sudden rupture and death.

Most children and young adults with isolated, discrete coarctation are asymptomatic. Headache, epistaxis, cold extremities, and claudication with exercise may occur, and attention is usually directed to the cardiovascular system when a heart murmur or hypertension in the upper extremities and absence, marked diminution, or delayed pulsations in the femoral arteries are detected on physical examination.

Enlarged and pulsatile collateral vessels may be palpated in the intercostal spaces anteriorly, in the axillae, or posteriorly in the interscapular area. The upper extremities and thorax may be more developed than the lower extremities. A midsystolic murmur over the anterior part of the chest, back, and spinous processes may become continuous if the lumen is narrowed sufficiently to result in a high-velocity jet across the lesion throughout the cardiac cycle. Additional systolic and continuous murmurs over the lateral thoracic wall may reflect increased flow through dilated and tortuous collateral vessels. The ECG usually reveals LV hypertrophy. Roentgenograms may show a dilated left subclavian artery high on the left mediastinal border and a dilated ascending aorta. Indentation of the aorta at the site of coarctation and pre- and poststenotic dilatation (the "3" sign) along the left paramediastinal shadow are almost pathognomonic. Notching of the ribs, an important radiographic sign, is due to erosion by dilated collateral vessels. Two-dimensional echocardiography from para- or suprasternal windows identifies the site and length of coarctation, while Doppler studies record and quantitate the pressure gradient. Transesophageal echocardiography and magnetic resonance imaging or three-dimensional computed tomography allow visualization of the length and severity of the obstruction and the associated collateral arteries. In adults, cardiac catheterization is indicated primarily to evaluate the coronary arteries.

The chief hazards result from severe hypertension and include the development of cerebral aneurysms and hemorrhage, dissection and/or rupture of the aorta, premature coronary arteriosclerosis, LV failure, and infective endocarditis.

℞ TREATMENT

Treatment is usually surgical; resection and end-to-end anastomosis or subclavian flap angioplasty are used commonly, although it may be necessary to use a tubular graft, patch, or bypass conduit if the narrowed segment is long. Systemic hypertension postoperatively, in the absence of residual coarctation, appears to be related to the duration of preoperative hypertension. Percutaneous balloon dilatation is controversial in native unoperated aortic coarctation but commonly successful for postsurgical recoarctation, often with deployment of a stent.

PULMONARY STENOSIS WITH INTACT VENTRICULAR SEPTUM Obstruction to RV outflow may be localized to the supravalvular, valvular, or subvalvular levels or occur at a combination of these sites. Multiple sites of narrowing of the peripheral pulmonary arteries are a feature of *rubella embryopathy* and may occur with both the familial and sporadic forms of supravalvular aortic stenosis. Valvular pulmonic stenosis is the most common form of isolated RV obstruction.

The severity of the obstructing lesion, rather than the site of narrowing, is the most important determinant of the clinical course. In the presence of a normal cardiac output, a peak systolic transvalvular pressure gradient between 50 and 80 mmHg is considered to be moderate stenosis; levels below and above that range are classified as mild and severe, respectively. Patients with mild pulmonic stenosis are generally asymptomatic and demonstrate little or no progression in the severity of obstruction with age. In patients with more significant stenosis, the severity may increase with time. Symptoms vary with the degree of obstruction. Fatigue, dyspnea, RV failure, and syncope may limit the activity of older patients, in whom moderate or severe obstruction may prevent an augmentation of cardiac output with exercise. In patients with severe obstruction, the systolic pressure in the right ventricle may exceed that in the left ventricle, since the ventricular septum is intact. RV ejection is prolonged with moderate or severe stenosis, and the sound of pulmonary valve closure is delayed and soft. RV hypertrophy reduces the compliance of that chamber, and a forceful RA contraction is necessary to augment RV filling.

A fourth heart sound, prominent *a* waves in the jugular venous pulse, and, occasionally, presystolic pulsations of the liver reflect vigorous atrial contraction. The clinical diagnosis is supported by a left parasternal lift and harsh systolic crescendo-decrescendo murmur and thrill at the upper left sternal border, typically preceded by a systolic ejection sound, if the obstruction is valvular. The holosystolic decrescendo murmur of tricuspid regurgitation may accompany severe pulmonic stenosis, especially in the presence of congestive heart failure. Cyanosis usually reflects right-to-left shunting through a patent foramen ovale or atrial septal defect. In patients with supravalvular or peripheral pulmonary arterial stenosis, the murmur is systolic or continuous and is best heard over the area of narrowing, with radiation to the peripheral lung fields.

The ECG may be helpful in assessing the degree of RV obstruction. In mild cases, the ECG is often normal, whereas moderate and severe stenoses are associated with right axis deviation and RV hypertrophy. A ventricular strain pattern, as well as high-amplitude P waves in leads II and V_1, indicating RA enlargement, are associated with severe stenosis. The chest roentgenogram with mild or moderate pulmonic stenosis often shows a heart of normal size and normal vascularity of the lungs. In the presence of valvular stenosis, dilatation of the main and left pulmonary arteries may be evident, in part poststenotic and in part due to intrinsic tissue weakness. With severe obstruction and resultant RV failure, RA and RV enlargement are generally evident. The pulmonary vascularity may be reduced with severe stenosis, RV failure, and/or a right-to-left shunt at the atrial level. Two-dimensional echocardiography visualizes pulmonary valve morphology; the outflow tract pressure gradient can be estimated by Doppler ultrasonography.

℞ TREATMENT

The cardiac catheter technique of balloon valvuloplasty (Chap. 212) is usually effective. Direct surgical relief of moderate and severe obstruction may be accomplished at a low risk. Multiple stenoses of the peripheral pulmonary arteries are usually inoperable, but narrowing of a single branch or at the bifurcation of the main pulmonary trunk may be surgically corrected or undergo balloon dilatation and stenting.

CYANOTIC CONGENITAL HEART DISEASE WITH INCREASED PULMONARY BLOOD FLOW

COMPLETE TRANSPOSITION OF THE GREAT ARTERIES   In this condition the aorta arises from the right ventricle to the right of and anterior to the pulmonary artery, which emerges from the left ventricle (Fig. 218-1, *left panel*). This results in two separate and parallel circulations, and some communication between them must exist after birth to sustain life. Most patients have an interatrial communication, two-thirds have a patent ductus arteriosus, and about one-third have an associated ven-

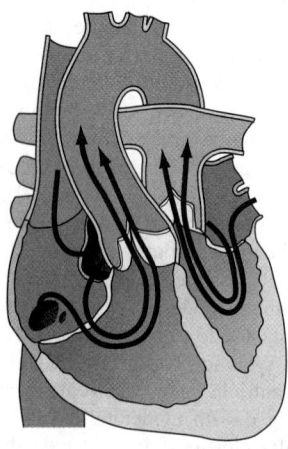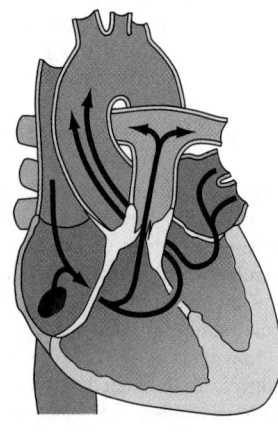

FIGURE 218-1   Complete transposition of the great arteries is depicted in the left panel. The aorta arises from the right ventricle and the pulmonary artery from the left ventricle. The only mixing between the two circulations occurs across a patent foramen ovale. In the right panel, the tetralogy of Fallot drawing illustrates the two most important anatomic findings, a large ventricular septal defect and RV outflow tract obstruction. A right-to-left shunt is shown across the ventricular septum.

tricular septal defect. Transposition is more common in males and accounts for ~10% of cyanotic heart disease.

The course is determined by the degree of tissue hypoxia, the ability of each ventricle to sustain an increased work load in the presence of reduced coronary arterial oxygenation, the nature of the associated cardiovascular anomalies, and the status of the pulmonary vascular bed. Pulmonary vascular obstruction develops by 1 to 2 years of age in patients with an associated large ventricular septal defect or large patent ductus arteriosus in the absence of obstruction to LV outflow.

℞ TREATMENT

The balloon or blade catheter or surgical creation or enlargement of an interatrial communication in the neonate is the simplest procedure for providing increased intracardiac mixing of systemic and pulmonary venous blood. Systemic–pulmonary artery anastomosis may be indicated in the patient with severe obstruction to LV outflow and diminished pulmonary blood flow. Intracardiac repair may be accomplished by rearranging the venous returns (intraatrial switch, i.e., Mustard or Senning operation) so that the systemic venous blood is directed to the mitral valve and thence to the left ventricle and pulmonary artery, while the pulmonary venous blood is diverted through the tricuspid valve and right ventricle to the aorta. The late survival after these repairs is good, but late sudden death is the most worrisome feature. Preferably, this malformation is corrected in infancy by transposing both coronary arteries to the posterior artery and transecting, contraposing, and anastomosing the aorta and pulmonary arteries (arterial switch operation). For those patients with a ventricular septal defect in whom it is necessary to bypass a severely obstructed LV outflow tract, corrective operation employs an intracardiac ventricular baffle and extracardiac prosthetic conduit to replace the pulmonary artery (Rastelli procedure).

SINGLE VENTRICLE   This is a family of complex lesions with both atrioventricular valves or a common atrioventricular valve opening to a single ventricular chamber. Associated anomalies include abnormal great artery positional relationships, pulmonic valvular or subvalvular stenosis, and subaortic stenosis.

Survival to adulthood depends on a relatively normal pulmonary blood flow, yet normal pulmonary resistance, and good ventricular function. Modifications of the Fontan approach are generally applied to carefully selected patients with creation of a pathway(s) from the systemic veins to the pulmonary arteries.

CYANOTIC CONGENITAL HEART DISEASE WITH DECREASED PULMONARY BLOOD FLOW

TRICUSPID ATRESIA   This malformation is characterized by atresia of the tricuspid valve, an interatrial communication, and, frequently, hypoplasia of the right ventricle and pulmonary artery. The clinical picture is usually dominated by severe cyanosis due to obligatory admixture of systemic and pulmonary venous blood in the left ventricle. The ECG characteristically shows RA enlargement, left axis deviation, and LV hypertrophy.

Atrial septostomy and palliative operations to increase pulmonary blood flow, often by anastomosis of a systemic artery or vein to a pulmonary artery, may allow survival to the second or third decade. A Fontan atriopulmonary or total cavopulmonary connection may then allow functional correction in those patients with normal or low pulmonary arterial resistance pressure and good LV function.

EBSTEIN'S ANOMALY   Characterized by a downward displacement of the tricuspid valve into the right ventricle, due to anomalous attachment of the tricuspid leaflets, the Ebstein tricuspid valve tissue is dysplastic and results in tricuspid regurgitation. The abnormally situated tricuspid orifice produces an "atrialized" portion of the right ventricle lying between the atrioventricular ring and the origin of the valve, which is continuous with the RA chamber. Often the right ventricle is hypoplastic. Although the clinical manifestations are variable, some patients come to initial attention because of progressive cyanosis from right-to-left atrial shunting, or symptoms due to tricuspid regurgitation and RV dysfunction, or paroxysmal atrial tachyarrhythmias with or without atrioventricular bypass tracts ("WPW" syndrome). Diagnostic findings by two-dimensional echocardiography include the abnormal positional relation between the tricuspid and mitral valves with apical displacement of the septal tricuspid leaflet. Tricuspid regurgitation is quantitated by Doppler examination. Surgical approaches include prosthetic replacement of the tricuspid valve when the leaflets are tethered or repair of the native valve.

TETRALOGY OF FALLOT   The four components of the tetralogy of Fallot are malaligned ventricular septal defect, obstruction to RV outflow, aortic override of the ventricular septal defect, and RV hypertrophy (Fig. 218-1, *right panel*).

The severity of RV outflow obstruction determines the clinical presentation. The severity of hypoplasia of the RV outflow tract varies from mild to complete (pulmonary atresia). Pulmonary valve stenosis and supravalvular and peripheral pulmonary arterial obstruction may coexist; rarely there is unilateral absence of a pulmonary artery (usually the left). A right-sided aortic arch and descending aorta occur in ~25% of patients with tetralogy.

The relationship between the resistance of blood flow from the ventricles into the aorta and into the pulmonary vessels plays a major role in determining the hemodynamic and clinical picture. Thus, the severity of obstruction to RV outflow is of fundamental significance. When the obstruction is severe, the pulmonary blood flow is reduced markedly, and a large volume of desaturated systemic venous blood is shunted from right to left across the ventricular septal defect. Severe cyanosis and erythrocytosis occur, and symptoms and sequelae of systemic hypoxemia are prominent. In many infants and children the obstruction is mild but progressive.

The ECG ordinarily shows RV and, less often, RA hypertrophy. Radiologic examination characteristically reveals a normal-sized, boot-shaped heart (*coeur en sabot*) with prominence of the right ventricle and a concavity in the region of the pulmonary conus. The pulmonary vascular markings are typically diminished, and the aortic arch and knob may be on the right side. Two-dimensional echocardiography from the parasternal or subcostal windows demonstrates the malalignment of the ventricular septal defect and the subpulmonary stenosis. Selective angiocardiography with RV injection provides architectural details of the RV outflow tract, pulmonary valve and annulus, and caliber of the main branches of the pulmonary artery; coronary arteriography identifies the anatomy and course of the coronary arteries.

℞ TREATMENT

Factors that may complicate the treatment of patients with tetralogy of Fallot include infective endocarditis, paradoxic embolism, excessive erythrocytosis, coagulation defects, and cerebral infarction or abscess. Corrective operation is advisable at some point for almost all patients with this anomaly. Successful correction avoids progressive infundibular obstruction, delayed growth, and complications due to hypoxemia and excessive erythrocytosis. The size of the pulmonary arteries rather than the age or size of the infant or child is the most important determinant in establishing candidacy for primary repair. Pronounced hypoplasia of the pulmonary arteries is a relative contraindication for an early corrective surgical procedure. When this problem is present, a palliative operation, such as creation of a systemic arterial–pulmonary arterial shunt, is carried out and is usually followed by complete correction, which can be carried out at a lower risk later in childhood.

OTHER FORMS OF CONGENITAL HEART DISEASES

CONGENITALLY CORRECTED TRANSPOSITION   The two fundamental anatomic abnormalities in this malformation are transposition of the ascending aorta and pulmonary trunk and inversion of the ventricles. This arrangement results in desaturated systemic venous blood passing from the right atrium through the mitral valve to the left ventricle and into

the pulmonary trunk, whereas oxygenated pulmonary venous blood flows from the left atrium through the tricuspid valve to the right ventricle and into the aorta. Thus, the circulation is corrected functionally. The clinical presentation, course, and prognosis of patients with congenitally corrected transposition vary depending on the nature and severity of any complicating intracardiac anomalies and of development of dysfunction of the systemic subaortic RV. Ebstein-type anomalies of the left-side tricuspid atrioventricular valve, with progressive regurgitation, ventricular septal defect, obstruction to outflow from the venous ventricle, and congenital heart block are often associated with corrected transposition. The diagnosis of the malformation and associated lesions can be established by two-dimensional echocardiography and Doppler examination.

MALPOSITIONS OF THE HEART   Positional anomalies refer to conditions in which the cardiac apex is in the right side of the chest (*dextrocardia*), or at the midline (*mesocardia*), or in which there is a normal location of the heart in the left side of the chest but abnormal position of the viscera (*isolated levocardia*). Knowledge of the position of the abdominal organs and of the branching pattern of the main stem bronchi is important in categorizing these malpositions. When dextrocardia occurs without situs inversus, when the visceral situs is indeterminate, or if isolated levocardia is present, associated, often complex, multiple cardiac anomalies are usually present. In contrast, mirror-image dextrocardia is usually observed with complete situs inversus, which occurs most frequently in individuals whose hearts are otherwise normal.

SURGICALLY MODIFIED CONGENITAL HEART DISEASE

Because of the enormous strides in cardiovascular surgical techniques that have occurred in the past 20 years, a large number of long-term survivors of corrective operations in infancy and childhood have reached adulthood. These patients are often challenging because of the diversity of anatomic, hemodynamic, and electrophysiologic residua and sequelae of cardiac operations.

The proper care of the survivor of operation for congenital heart disease requires that the clinician understand the details of the malformation before operation; pay meticulous attention to the details of the operative procedure; and recognize the postoperative residua (conditions left totally or partially uncorrected), the sequelae (conditions caused by surgery), and the complications that may have resulted from the operation. With the exception of ligation and division of an uncomplicated patent ductus arteriosus, almost every other surgical repair of an anomaly leaves behind or causes some abnormality of the heart and circulation that may range from trivial to serious. Intraoperative transesophageal echocardiography assists in detecting unsuspected lesions, in monitoring the repair, and in verifying a satisfactory result or directing further repair. Thus, even with results that are considered clinically to be good to excellent, continued long-term postoperative follow-up is advisable.

Table 218-4 lists the categories of common late postoperative problems. Cardiac operations importantly involving the atria, such as closure of atrial septal defect, repair of total or partial anomalous pulmonary venous return, or venous switch corrections of complete transposition of the great arteries (the Mustard or Senning operations), may be followed years later by sinus node or atrioventricular node dysfunction or by atrial arrhythmias. Intraventricular surgery may also result in electrophysiologic consequences, including complete heart block necessitating pacemaker insertion to avoid sudden death. In ad-

TABLE 218-4   *Potential Late Postoperative Problems*

Residual shunts	Arrhythmias and conduction defects
Residual ventricular outflow obstruction	Myocardial dysfunction
Residual valvular anomalies	Prosthetic valve malfunction
Systemic arterial hypertension	Prosthetic conduit obstruction
Pulmonary vascular obstruction	Infective endocarditis

dition, valvular problems may arise late after initial cardiac operation. An example is the progressive stenosis of an initially nonobstructive bicuspid aortic valve in the patient who underwent aortic coarctation repair. Such aortic valves may also be the site of infective endocarditis. After repair of the ostium primum atrial septal defect, the cleft mitral valve may become progressively incompetent. Tricuspid regurgitation may also be progressive in the postoperative patient with tetralogy of Fallot if RV outflow tract obstruction was not relieved adequately at initial surgery. In many patients with surgically modified congenital heart disease, inadequate relief of an obstructive lesion, or a residual regurgitant lesion, or a residual shunt will cause or hasten the onset of clinical signs and symptoms of myocardial dysfunction. Despite a good hemodynamic repair, many patients with a subaortic right ventricle develop RV decompensation and signs of "left heart failure." In many patients, particularly those who were cyanotic for many years before operation, a preexisting compromise in ventricular performance is due to the original underlying malformation.

A final category of postoperative problems involves the use of prosthetic valves, patches, or conduits in the operative repair. The special risks include infective endocarditis, thrombus formation, and prema-

ture degeneration and calcification of the prosthetic materials. There are many patients in whom extracardiac conduits are required to correct the circulation functionally and often to carry blood to the lungs from the right atrium or right ventricle. These conduits may develop intraluminal obstruction, and, if they include a prosthetic valve, it may show progressive calcification and thickening.

FURTHER READING

BRICKNER ME et al: Congenital heart disease in adults (2 parts). N Engl J Med 342:256, and 334, 2000

GERSONY WM, ROSENBAUM MS: *Congenital Heart Disease in the Adult.* New York, McGraw-Hill, 2002

PERLOFF JK: *Clinical Recognition of Congenital Heart Disease*, 5th ed. Philadelphia, Saunders, 2003

———, WARNES CA: Challenges posed by adults with repaired congenital heart disease. Circulation 103:2637, 2001

SIU SC et al: Prospective multicenter study of pregnancy outcomes in women with heart disease. Circulation 104:515, 2001

WEBB G, REDINGTON A: Congenital heart disease in children and adults, in *Braunwald's Heart Disease*, 7th ed, DP Zipes et al (eds). Philadelphia, Saunders, 2005

ZHONG-DONG D et al: Comparison between transcatheter and surgical closure of secundum atrial septal defect in children and adults. Results of a multicenter nonrandomized trial. J Am Coll Cardiol 39:1836, 2002

219 VALVULAR HEART DISEASE
Eugene Braunwald

The role of physical examination in the evaluation of patients with valvular disease is also considered in Chap. 209; of electrocardiography (ECG) in Chap. 210; of echocardiography in Chap. 211; and of cardiac catheterization and angiography in Chap. 212.

MITRAL STENOSIS

ETIOLOGY AND PATHOLOGY Two-thirds of all patients with mitral stenosis (MS) are female. MS and mixed MS and mitral regurgitation (MR) are generally rheumatic in origin; very rarely, MS is congenital. Pure or predominant MS occurs in approximately 40% of all patients with rheumatic heart disease. In other patients with rheumatic heart disease, lesser degrees of MS may accompany MR and aortic valve lesions. With reductions in the incidence of acute rheumatic fever, particularly in temperate climates and developed nations, the incidence of MS is declining. However, it remains a major problem in developing nations, especially in tropical and semitropical climates.

In rheumatic stenosis the valve leaflets are diffusely thickened by fibrous tissue and/or calcific deposits. The mitral commissures fuse, the chordae tendineae fuse and shorten, the valvular cusps become rigid, and these changes, in turn, lead to narrowing at the apex of the funnel-shaped ("fish-mouth") valve. Although the initial insult to the mitral valve is rheumatic, the later changes may be a nonspecific process resulting from trauma to the valve caused by altered flow patterns due to the initial deformity. Calcification of the stenotic mitral valve immobilizes the leaflets and narrows the orifice further. Thrombus formation and arterial embolization may arise from the calcific valve itself, but more frequently arise from the dilated left atrium (LA) in patients with atrial fibrillation (AF).

PATHOPHYSIOLOGY In normal adults the mitral valve orifice is 4 to 6 cm². In the presence of significant obstruction, i.e., when the orifice is less than approximately 2 cm², blood can flow from the LA to the left ventricle (LV) only if propelled by an abnormally elevated left atrioventricular pressure gradient (see Fig. 212-2), the hemodynamic hallmark of MS. When the mitral valve opening is reduced to 1 cm², often referred to as "critical" MS, a LA pressure of approximately 25 mmHg is required to maintain a normal cardiac output (CO). The elevated pulmonary venous and pulmonary arterial (PA) wedge pressures re-

duce pulmonary compliance, contributing to exertional dyspnea. The first bouts of dyspnea are usually precipitated by clinical events that increase the rate of blood flow across the mitral orifice, resulting in further elevation of the LA pressure (see below). To assess the severity of obstruction, both the transvalvular pressure gradient and the flow rate must be measured (Chap. 212). The latter depends not only on the CO but on the heart rate as well. An increase in heart rate shortens diastole proportionately more than systole and diminishes the time available for flow across the mitral valve. Therefore, at any given level of CO, tachycardia including that resulting from atrial fibrillation augments the transvalvular gradient and elevates further the LA pressure. Similar considerations apply to the tricuspid stenosis.

The LV diastolic pressure and ejection fraction (EF) are normal in isolated MS. In MS and sinus rhythm, the elevated LA and PA wedge pressures exhibit a prominent atrial contraction (*a* wave) and a gradual pressure decline after mitral valve opening (*y* descent) (see Fig. 212-2). In severe MS and whenever pulmonary vascular resistance is significantly increased, the pulmonary arterial pressure (PAP) is elevated at rest and rises further during exercise, often causing secondary elevations of right ventricle (RV) end-diastolic pressure and volume.

Cardiac Output In patients with moderately severe MS (mitral valve orifice 1.2 cm² to 1.7 cm²), the CO is normal or almost so at rest but rises subnormally during exertion. In patients with critical MS, particularly those in whom pulmonary vascular resistance is strikingly elevated, the CO is subnormal at rest and may fail to rise or may even decline during activity.

Pulmonary Hypertension The clinical and hemodynamic features of MS are influenced importantly by the level of the PAP. Pulmonary hypertension results from (1) passive backward transmission of the elevated LA pressure; (2) pulmonary arteriolar constriction, which presumably is triggered by LA and pulmonary venous hypertension (reactive pulmonary hypertension); (3) interstitial edema in the walls of the small pulmonary vessels; and (4) organic obliterative changes in the pulmonary vascular bed. Severe pulmonary hypertension results in tricuspid regurgitation (TR) and pulmonary incompetence as well as right-sided heart failure.

SYMPTOMS In temperate climates the latent period between the initial attack of rheumatic carditis (in the increasingly rare circumstances in which a history of one can be elicited) and the development of symptoms due to MS is generally about two decades; most patients begin to experience disability in the fourth decade of life. Studies carried out before the development of mitral valvotomy revealed that once a patient with MS became seriously symptomatic, the disease progressed continuously to death within 2 to 5 years. In economically deprived areas, in tropical and subtropical climates, particularly on the Indian subcontinent, in Central America, and in the Middle East, MS tends to progress more rapidly and frequently causes serious symptoms in patients less than 20 years of age. In contrast, slowly progressive MS in the elderly is being recognized with increasing frequency in the United States and Western Europe.

When valvular obstruction is mild, the physical signs of MS may be present without symptoms. However, even in patients whose mitral orifices are large enough to accommodate a normal blood flow with only mild elevations of LA pressure, marked elevations of this pressure leading to dyspnea and cough may be precipitated by severe exertion, excitement, fever, severe anemia, paroxysmal atrial fibrillation and other tachycardias, sexual intercourse, pregnancy, and thyrotoxicosis. As MS progresses, lesser stresses precipitate dyspnea, and the patient becomes limited in daily activities. The redistribution of blood from the dependent portions of the body to the lungs, which occurs when the recumbent position is assumed, leads to orthopnea and paroxysmal nocturnal dyspnea. *Pulmonary edema* develops when there is a sudden surge in flow across a markedly narrowed mitral orifice. When moderately severe MS has existed for several years, *atrial arrhythmias* occur with increasing frequency. The development of permanent AF often marks a turning point in the patient's course and is generally associated with acceleration of the rate at which symptoms progress.

Hemoptysis (Chap. 30) results from rupture of pulmonary-bronchial venous connections secondary to pulmonary venous hypertension. It occurs most frequently in patients who have elevated LA pressures without markedly elevated pulmonary vascular resistances and is almost never fatal. *Recurrent pulmonary emboli* (Chap. 244), sometimes with infarction, are an important cause of morbidity and mortality late in the course of MS. *Pulmonary infections*, i.e., bronchitis, bronchopneumonia, and lobar pneumonia, commonly complicate untreated MS. *Infective endocarditis* (Chap. 109) is rare in isolated MS.

Pulmonary Changes   In addition to the aforementioned changes in the pulmonary vascular bed, fibrous thickening of the walls of the alveoli and pulmonary capillaries occurs commonly in MS. The vital capacity, total lung capacity, maximal breathing capacity, and oxygen uptake per unit of ventilation are reduced (Chap. 234), and the latter fails to rise normally during exertion. Pulmonary compliance falls further as pulmonary capillary pressure rises during exercise. In some patients, airway resistance is abnormally increased and the diffusing capacity may be reduced. These changes in the lungs are due, in part, to increased transudation of fluid from the pulmonary capillaries into the interstitial and alveolar spaces. However, the increased capacity of the pulmonary lymphatic system to drain excess fluid retards the development of alveolar edema.

Thrombi and Emboli   *Thrombi* may form in the left atria, particularly in the enlarged atrial appendages of patients with MS. Embolization occurs much more frequently in patients with AF, in older patients, and in those with a reduced cardiac output (CO). However, systemic embolization may be the presenting complaint in otherwise asymptomatic patients with mild MS. Rarely, a large pedunculated or a freefloating thrombus may suddenly obstruct the stenotic mitral orifice and cause syncope, angina, and changing auscultatory signs with alterations in position.

PHYSICAL FINDINGS (See also Chap. 209) ■ **Inspection and Palpation**   In patients with severe MS, there may be a malar flush with pinched and blue facies. In patients with sinus rhythm and severe pulmonary hypertension or associated tricuspid stenosis (TS), the jugular venous pulse reveals prominent *a* waves due to vigorous right atrial systole. The systemic arterial pressure is usually normal or slightly low. An RV tap along the left sternal border signifies an enlarged RV. A dia-

stolic thrill is frequently present at the cardiac apex, with the patient in the left lateral recumbent position.

Auscultation   The first heart sound (S_1) is generally accentuated and snapping, and slightly delayed. The pulmonary component of the second heart sound (P_2) is often accentuated, and the two components of the second heart sound (S_2) are closely split or fixed. A pulmonary systolic ejection click may be heard in patients with severe pulmonary hypertension. The opening snap (OS) of the mitral valve is most readily audible in expiration at, or just medial to the cardiac apex. This sound generally follows the sound of aortic valve closure (A_2) by 0.05 to 0.12 s. The time interval between A_2 and OS varies inversely with the severity of the MS. The OS is followed by a low-pitched, rumbling, diastolic murmur, heard best at the apex with the patient in the left lateral recumbent position (see Fig. 209-5*B*). It is accentuated by mild exercise (e.g., a few rapid situps) carried out just before auscultation. In general, the duration of this murmur correlates with the severity of the stenosis. In patients with sinus rhythm, the murmur often reappears or becomes reaccentuated during atrial systole. Soft grade I or II/VI systolic murmurs are commonly heard at the apex or along the left sternal border in patients with pure MS and do not necessarily signify the presence of MR. Hepatomegaly, ankle edema, ascites, and pleural effusion, particularly in the right pleural cavity, may occur in patients with MS and RV failure.

Associated Lesions   With severe pulmonary hypertension, a pansystolic murmur produced by functional TR may be audible along the left sternal border. Characteristically, this murmur is accentuated by inspiration and diminishes during forced expiration (Carvallo's sign); it should not be confused with the apical pansystolic murmur of MR. When the S_1 and/or the OS are soft or absent in a patient with mitral valve disease who also has an apical systolic murmur, it is likely that significant MR and/or serious calcification of the deformed mitral valve leaflets are present. When the CO is markedly reduced in MS, the typical auscultatory findings, including the diastolic rumbling murmur, may not be detectable (silent MS), but they may reappear as compensation is restored. The *Graham Steell murmur* of pulmonary regurgitation (PR), a high-pitched, diastolic, decrescendo blowing murmur along the left sternal border, results from dilatation of the pulmonary valve ring and occurs in patients with mitral valve disease and severe pulmonary hypertension. This murmur may be indistinguishable from the more common murmur produced by aortic regurgitation (AR).

LABORATORY EXAMINATION ■ EKG   In MS and sinus rhythm, the P wave usually suggests LA enlargement (see Fig. 210-8). It may become tall and peaked in lead II and upright in lead V_1 when severe pulmonary hypertension or TS complicates MS and right atrial (RA) enlargement occurs. The QRS complex is usually normal. However, with severe pulmonary hypertension, right axis deviation and RV hypertrophy are often present.

Echocardiogram   (See also Chap. 211)   This is the most sensitive and specific noninvasive method for diagnosing MS. Transthoracic two-dimensional color flow Doppler echocardiographic imaging and Doppler ultrasound provide critical information, including an estimate of the transvalvular gradient and of mitral orifice size, the presence and severity of accompanying MR, the extent of restriction of valve leaflets, their thickness, the degree of distortion of the subvalvular apparatus, and the anatomic suitability for balloon mitral valvotomy (see below). In addition, echocardiography provides an assessment of the size of the cardiac chambers, an estimation of the LV function, an estimation of the PAP, and an indication of the presence and severity of associated valvular lesions. Transesophageal echocardiography provides superior images and should be employed when transthoracic imaging is inadequate for guiding therapy.

Lesion	Symptom Control	Secondary Prevention and Natural History
Mitral stenosis	Diuretics for heart failure; Digoxin, β blockers, and rate-limiting calcium antagonists for rate control in atrial fibrillation	Penicillin prophylaxis against recurrent episodes of rheumatic fever; Anticoagulants to prevent systemic thromboembolism.
Mitral regurgitation	Diuretics and vasodilators (usually ACE inhibitors) for heart failure	No proven treatment
Aortic stenosis	Diuretics for heart failure; nitrates and β blockers for angina	No proven treatment but lipid lowering therapy may slow progression of calcific aortic stenosis
Aortic regurgitation	Diuretics and vasodilators (usually ACE inhibitors) for heart failure	Vasodilators (nifedipine or ACE inhibitors) to protect the left ventricular myocardium and delay the need for surgery

Source: NA Boon, P Bloomfield: The medical management of valvular heart disease. Heart 87:395, 2002, with permission

Roentgenogram The earliest changes are straightening of the left border of the cardiac silhouette, prominence of the main pulmonary arteries, dilatation of the upper lobe pulmonary veins, and backward displacement of the esophagus by an enlarged LA. In severe MS, however, all chambers and vessels upstream to the narrowed valve are prominent. Kerley B lines are fine, dense, opaque, horizontal lines that are most prominent in the lower and midlung fields and that result from distention of interlobular septa and lymphatics with edema when the resting mean LA pressure exceeds approximately 20 mmHg.

DIFFERENTIAL DIAGNOSIS Like MS, significant MR may also be associated with a prominent diastolic murmur at the apex, but in MR this diastolic murmur commences slightly later than in patients with MS, and there is often clear-cut evidence of LV enlargement. An apical pansystolic murmur of at least grade III/VI intensity as well as an S_3 suggests significant associated MR. Similarly, the apical middiastolic murmur associated with AR (*Austin Flint murmur*) may be mistaken for MS. TS, which occurs rarely in the absence of MS, may mask many of the clinical features of MS.

Atrial septal defect (Chap. 218) may be mistaken for MS; in both conditions there is often clinical, EKG, and roentgenographic evidence of RV enlargement and accentuation of the pulmonary vascularity. The widely split S_2 of atrial septal defect may be confused with the mitral OS, and the diastolic flow murmur across the tricuspid valve may be mistaken for the mitral diastolic murmur. However, the absence of LA enlargement and of Kerley B lines and the demonstration of fixed splitting of S_2 all favor atrial septal defect over MS.

Left atrial myxoma (Chap. 223) may obstruct LA emptying, causing dyspnea, a diastolic murmur, and hemodynamic changes resembling those of MS. However, patients with an LA myxoma often have features suggestive of a systemic disease, such as weight loss, fever, anemia, systemic emboli, and elevated serum IgG concentrations. The auscultatory findings may change markedly with body position. The diagnosis can be established by the demonstration of a characteristic echo-producing mass in the LA with two-dimensional echocardiography.

CARDIAC CATHETERIZATION AND ANGIOCARDIOGRAPHY

Left heart catheterization is useful when there is a discrepancy between clinical and echocardiographic findings. It is helpful in assessing associated lesions such as aortic stenosis (AS) and aortic regurgitation (AR). Catheterization and coronary arteriography are not usually necessary to aid in the decision about surgery in younger patients with typical findings of severe obstruction on clinical examination and echocardiography. In males over 45 years of age, females over 55 years of age, and younger patients with coronary risk factors, especially those with positive noninvasive stress tests for myocardial ischemia, coronary angiography is usually advisable preoperatively to detect patients with critical coronary obstructions that should be bypassed at the time of operation. Catheterization and LV angiography are also indicated in most patients who have undergone balloon mitral valvot-

omy or previous mitral valve operations and who have redeveloped serious symptoms.

℞ TREATMENT

Penicillin prophylaxis of β-hemolytic streptococcal infections (Chap. 302) to prevent rheumatic fever and prophylaxis for infective endocarditis (Chap. 109) are important for all patients (Table 219-1). In symptomatic patients, some improvement usually occurs with restriction of sodium intake and maintenance doses of oral diuretics. Digitalis glycosides usually do not benefit patients with MS and sinus rhythm but are helpful in slowing the ventricular rate of patients with AF. Beta blockers or nondihydropyridine calcium antagonists (e.g., verapamil or diltiazem) are useful in this regard. Warfarin to an INR of 2-3:1 should be administered for at least 1 year to patients with MS who have suffered systemic and/or pulmonary embolization and permanently to those with AF.

If AF is of relatively recent origin in a patient whose MS is not severe enough to warrant balloon mitral valvotomy or surgical valvotomy, reversion to sinus rhythm pharmacologically or by means of electrical countershock is indicated. Usually this reversion should be undertaken after the patient has had 3 weeks of anticoagulant treatment. Conversion to sinus rhythm is rarely helpful in patients with severe MS, particularly those in whom the LA is especially enlarged or in whom AF has been present for more than 1 year, since sinus rhythm is rarely sustained in such patients.

Mitral Valvotomy Unless there is a contraindication, mitral valvotomy is indicated in symptomatic patients with isolated MS whose effective orifice is less than approximately 1.0 cm²/m² body surface area, or <1.7 cm² in normal-sized adults. Mitral valvotomy can be carried out by two techniques: percutaneous balloon mitral valvotomy and surgical valvotomy. In balloon mitral valvotomy (Figs. 219-1 and 219-2), a catheter is directed into the LA after transseptal puncture and a single or double balloon (Inoue balloon) is directed across the valve and inflated in the valvular orifice. Ideal patients have relatively mobile, thin leaflets with no or little calcium, without extensive subvalvular thickening and with no or mild MR. The short- and long-term results of this procedure in appropriate patients are similar to those of surgical valvotomy, but with less morbidity and a lower mortality rate. Therefore, balloon valvotomy has become the procedure of choice for such patients. Transthoracic echocardiography is helpful in identifying patients for the percutaneous procedure (Fig. 219-3).

In patients in whom percutaneous valvotomy is not possible, unsuccessful, or in those with restenosis, an "open" valvotomy using cardiopulmonary bypass is necessary. In addition to opening the valve

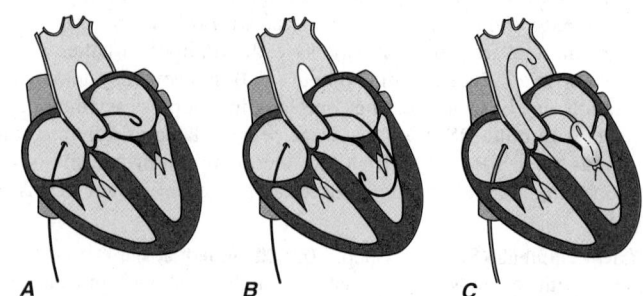

A   **B**   **C**

FIGURE 219-1 Technique of double balloon mitral valvuloplasty. *A.* The position of the guidewire in the left atrium after left atrial puncture using the Brockenbrough needle. *B.* The position of the guidewire as it is advanced into the left ventricle across the stenotic mitral valve. *C.* Partial inflation of a balloon catheter across the stenotic mitral valve. [*From JP Srebro, TA Ports, Catheter-balloon valvuloplasty, in K Chatterjee et al (eds): Cardiology: An Illustrated Text. Philadelphia, Lippincott, 1991.*]

PREDILATATION

ECG

MEAN MITRAL GRADIENT 15 mmHg
Cardiac output 3.0 L/min
Mitral valve area 0.6 cm²

POSTDILATATION

ECG

Mean mitral gradient 3 mmHg
Cardiac output 3.8 L/min
Mitral valve area 1.8 cm²

FIGURE 219-2 Simultaneous left atrial (LA) and left ventricular (LV) pressure before and after balloon mitral valvuloplasty in a patient with severe mitral stenosis. *(Courtesy of Raymond G. McKay, MD).*

commissures, it is important to loosen any subvalvular fusion of papillary muscles and chordae tendineae and to remove large deposits of calcium, thereby improving valvular function, as well as to remove atrial thrombi. The mortality rate is approximately 2%.

Successful valvotomy, whether balloon or surgical, usually results in striking symptomatic and hemodynamic improvement and prolongs survival. However, there is no evidence that the procedure improves the prognosis of patients with slight or no functional impairment. Therefore, unless recurrent systemic embolization or severe pulmonary hypertension has occurred, valvotomy is *not* recommended for patients who are entirely asymptomatic. When there is little symptomatic improvement after valvotomy, it is likely that the procedure was ineffective, that it induced MR, or that associated valvular or myocardial disease was present. About half of all patients undergoing mitral valvotomy require reoperation by 10 years. In the pregnant patient with MS, valvotomy should be carried out if pulmonary congestion occurs despite intensive medical treatment.

Mitral valve replacement (MVR) is necessary in patients with MS and significant associated MR, those in whom the valve has been severely distorted by previous transcatheter or operative manipulation, or those in whom the surgeon does not find it possible to improve

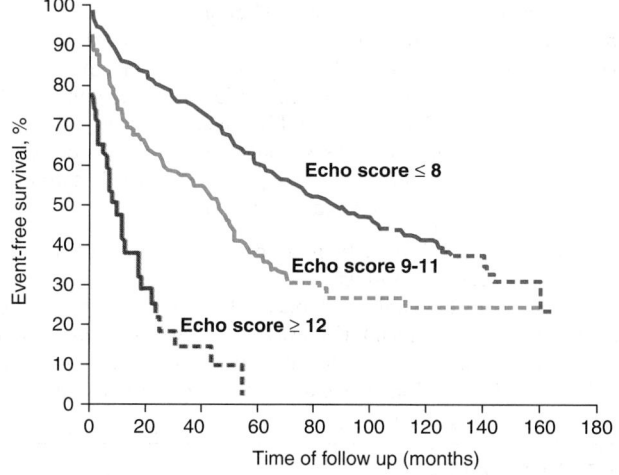

FIGURE 219-3 Event-free survival following percutaneous balloon mitral valvuloplasty. The echo score is derived from examining leaflet rigidity, thickening, calcification and the extent of subvalvular disease and grading each from 1 (not detectable) to 4 (very severe) and calculating the total. The minimum score is 4 and the maximum is 16. Event-free survival is survival without mitral valve replacement or repeat balloon valvuloplasty. *(From Palacios et al 2002.)*

TABLE 219-2 *Mortality Rates After Valve Replacement and Repair*

Operative Category	Number	Operative Mortality (%)
AVR (isolated)	26,317	4.3
MVR (isolated)	13,936	6.4
Multiple valve replacement	3,840	9.6
AVR + CAB	22,713	8.0
MVR + CAB	8,788	15.3
Multiple valve replacement + CAB	1,424	18.8
AVR + any valve repair	938	7.4
MVR + any valve repair	1,266	12.5
Aortic valve repair	597	5.9
Mitral valve repair	4,167	3.0
Tricuspid valve repair	144	13.9

Note: AVR, aortic valve replacement; CAB, coronary artery bypass; MVR, mitral valve replacement.
Source: Modified from Jamieson et al.

valve function significantly. Since the operative mortality rate of isolated MVR is still approximately 6% (Table 219-2), and since there are long-term complications of valve replacement, patients in whom preoperative evaluation suggests the possibility that MVR may be required should be operated on only if they have critical MS, i.e., an orifice ≤1 cm² area and are in New York Heart Association class III, i.e., symptomatic with ordinary activity despite optimal medical therapy. The overall 10-year survival of surgical survivors is approximately 70%. Long-term prognosis is worse in older patients and those with marked disability and striking depression of the cardiac index preoperatively.

MITRAL REGURGITATION

ETIOLOGY Chronic rheumatic heart disease is the cause of severe MR in only about one-third of cases and occurs more frequently in males. The rheumatic process produces rigidity, deformity, and retraction of the valve cusps and commissural fusion, as well as shortening, contraction, and fusion of the chordae tendineae. MR may occur as a congenital anomaly (Chap. 218), most commonly as a defect of the endocardial cushions (atrioventricular cushion defects). MR is frequently secondary to ischemia. Thus, it may occur as a consequence of ventricular remodeling or with fibrosis of a papillary muscle in patients with healed myocardial infarction. It may develop acutely in patients with acute infarction involving the base of a papillary muscle. Transient MR also may occur during periods of ischemia involving a papillary muscle or the adjacent myocardium and may accompany bouts of angina pectoris. MR may occur with marked LV enlargement of any cause in which dilatation of the mitral annulus and lateral displacement of the papillary muscles interfere with coaptation of the valve leaflets, most commonly ischemia. In hypertrophic cardiomyopathy, the anterior leaflet of the mitral valve is displaced anteriorly during systole, causing MR (Chap. 221). Calcification of the mitral annulus of unknown cause, presumably degenerative, which occurs most commonly in elderly women, also can be responsible for significant MR. Acute MR may occur secondary to infective endocarditis involving the valve leaflets or chordae tendineae, or as a consequence of trauma. Mitral valve prolapse (MVP), an important cause of MR, is considered in the next section.

Irrespective of cause, severe MR is often progressive, since enlargement of the LA places tension on the posterior mitral leaflet, pulling it away from the mitral orifice and thereby aggravating the valvular dysfunction. Similarly, LV dilatation increases the regurgitation, which in turn enlarges the LA and LV further, causing chordal rupture and resulting in a vicious circle; hence the aphorism, "mitral regurgitation begets mitral regurgitation."

PATHOPHYSIOLOGY The resistance to LV emptying is reduced in patients with MR. As a consequence, the LV is decompressed into the LA during ejection, and with the reduction in LV size during systole, there is a rapid decline in LV tension. The initial compensation to acute MR is more complete LV emptying. However, LV volume increases progressively as the severity of the regurgitation increases and as LV function deteriorates. This increase in LV volume is often accompanied by a reduced forward CO. The regurgitant volume varies directly with the LV systolic pressure and the size of the regurgitant orifice; as mentioned above, the latter, in turn, is influenced profoundly by the extent of LV dilatation. Since ejection fraction (EF) rises in severe MR in the presence of normal LV function, even a modest reduction in this parameter (<60%) reflects significant dysfunction.

The v wave in the LA pressure pulse is usually prominent (see Fig. 212-3). During early diastole, as the distended LA empties, there is a particularly rapid y descent (as long as there is no associated MS). In chronic MR, there is often an increase in LV compliance, so that LV volume rises with little elevation in LV diastolic pressure. The effective (forward) CO is usually reduced in seriously symptomatic patients. A brief, early diastolic atrioventricular pressure gradient (often accompanying a murmur) may occur in patients with pure MR as a result of the very rapid flow of blood across a normal-sized mitral orifice.

The prompt appearance of contrast material in the LA after its injection into the LV signifies the presence of MR. The regurgitant volume can be measured by determining the difference between the total LV stroke volume, estimated angiocardiographically, and the effective forward stroke volume determined by the Fick method (Chap. 212). In severe cases, as much as 50% of the total LV stroke volume regurgitates with each beat. Qualitative, but clinically useful, estimates of the severity of regurgitation may be made by observation on cineangiograms of the degree of LA opacification after the injection of contrast material into the LV. Color flow Doppler imaging is most commonly used for this purpose (see below).

Left ventricular contractility becomes reduced, sometimes irreversibly, with longstanding MR. The compliance, i.e., the pressure-volume relationship of the LA and pulmonary venous bed affects the clinical picture. Patients with acute MR usually have *normal or reduced LA compliance*, with little enlargement of the LA, but marked elevation of the LA pressure, particularly of the v wave. Severe pulmonary congestion and pulmonary edema are common in this group. Patients with a *marked increase in LA compliance* are at the opposite end of the spectrum, having longstanding, severe MR, marked enlargement of the LA, and normal or only slightly elevated LA and PA pressures. These patients usually complain of severe fatigue and exhaustion secondary to a low CO, while symptoms resulting from pulmonary congestion are less prominent; AF is almost invariably present. Most common are patients whose clinical and hemodynamic features are intermediate between those in the two aforementioned groups.

SYMPTOMS Fatigue, exertional dyspnea, and orthopnea are the most prominent complaints in patients with chronic, severe MR. Systemic embolism occurs less frequently than in MS. Right-sided heart failure, with painful hepatic congestion, ankle edema, distended neck veins, ascites, and TR, occur in patients with MR who have associated pulmonary vascular disease and marked pulmonary hypertension. In patients with acute, severe MR, LV failure with acute pulmonary edema is common.

PHYSICAL FINDINGS The arterial pressure is usually normal, and in patients with severe MR the arterial pulse may show a sharp upstroke. The jugular venous pulse shows abnormally prominent a waves in patients with sinus rhythm and marked pulmonary hypertension and prominent v waves in those with accompanying severe TR. A systolic thrill is often palpable at the cardiac apex, the LV is hyperdynamic with a brisk systolic impulse and a palpable rapid-filling wave, and the apex beat is often displaced laterally. An RV tap and the shock of pulmonary valve closure may be palpable in patients with marked pulmonary hypertension.

Auscultation The S_1 is generally absent, soft, or buried in the systolic murmur. In patients with severe MR, the aortic valve may close prematurely, resulting in wide splitting of the S_2. An OS indicates associated MS but does not exclude predominant regurgitation. A low-pitched S_3 occurring 0.12 to 0.17 s after the aortic valve closure sound, i.e., at the completion of the rapid-filling phase of the LV, is believed to be caused by the sudden tensing of the papillary muscles, chordae tendineae, and valve leaflets and is an important auscultatory feature of severe MR. The S_3 may be followed by a short, rumbling, diastolic murmur, even in the absence of MS. A fourth heart sound is often audible in patients with acute, severe MR of recent onset who are in sinus rhythm. A presystolic murmur is not ordinarily heard with isolated MR but is present in patients with sinus rhythm and associated MS.

A systolic murmur of at least grade III/VI intensity, is the most characteristic auscultatory finding in severe MR. It is usually holosystolic (see Figs. 209-4 and 209-5A), but it may be decrescendo and cease in late systole in patients with acute, severe MR. In MR due to papillary muscle dysfunction or MVP, the systolic murmur commences in midsystole (see below). The systolic murmur is usually most prominent at the apex and radiates to the axilla. However, in patients with ruptured chordae tendineae or primary involvement of the posterior mitral leaflet, the regurgitant jet strikes the LA wall adjacent to the aortic root. In this situation, the systolic murmur is transmitted to the base of the heart and therefore may be confused with the murmur of AS. In patients with ruptured chordae tendineae the systolic murmur may have a cooing or "sea gull" quality, while a flail leaflet may cause a murmur with a musical quality. The systolic murmur of MR is intensified by isometric strain but is reduced during the Valsalva maneuver.

LABORATORY EXAMINATION ■ Electrocardiogram In patients with sinus rhythm there is evidence of LA enlargement, but RA enlargement also may be present when pulmonary hypertension is severe. Chronic, severe MR is generally associated with AF. In many patients there is no clear-cut electrocardiographic evidence of enlargement of either ventricle. In others, the signs of LV hypertrophy are present.

Echocardiogram Color flow Doppler imaging is the most accurate noninvasive technique for the detection and estimation of MR. Two-dimensional echocardiography is useful for assessing the cause of MR and for estimating LV function from end-systolic and end-diastolic volumes and EF. The LA is usually enlarged and/or exhibits increased pulsation while the LV may be hyperdynamic. Findings that help to determine the etiology of MR, such as mitral annular calcification and LV dyskinesis in ischemic MR, can often be identified by two-dimensional echocardiography. With ruptured chordae tendineae or a flail leaflet, coarse, erratic motion of the involved leaflets may be noted. Vegetations associated with infective endocarditis, incomplete coaptation of the anterior and posterior mitral leaflets, and annular calcification, as well as MR secondary to LV dilatation, aneurysm, or dyskinesis may be recognized. Transesophageal imaging provides greater detail than transthoracic imaging (see Fig. 211-3). The echocardiogram in patients with MVP is described in the next section.

Roentgenogram The LA and LV are the dominant chambers; late in the course of the disease, the former may be massively enlarged and forms the right border of the cardiac silhouette. Pulmonary venous congestion, interstitial edema, and Kerley B lines are sometimes noted. Marked calcification of the mitral leaflets occurs commonly in patients with longstanding combined MR and MS. Calcification of the mitral annulus may be visualized.

℞ TREATMENT

MEDICAL (Table 219-1) The nonsurgical management of patients with severe MR begins with restricting those physical activities that regularly produce dyspnea and excessive fatigue, reducing sodium intake, and enhancing sodium excretion with the appropriate use of diuretics (Chap. 216). Vasodilators and digitalis glycosides increase the forward output of the failing LV. Intravenous nitroprusside or nitroglycerin reduce afterload and thereby the volume of regurgitant flow and are useful in stabilizing patients with acute and/or severe MR. Angiotensin-converting enzyme (ACE) inhibitors are useful in the treatment of chronic MR. The same considerations as in patients with MS apply to the reversion of AF to sinus rhythm. In the late stages of heart failure anticoagulants and leg binders are used to diminish the likelihood of venous thrombi and pulmonary emboli. Endocarditis prophylaxis is important. In patients with severe MR secondary to dilated cardiomyopathy, intensive medial therapy can reduce the severity of MR.

SURGICAL In the selection of patients with severe MR for surgical treatment, the chronic, often slowly progressive nature of the condition must be balanced against the immediate and long-term risks associated with the operation. Patients with MR who are asymptomatic or who are limited only during strenuous exertion and whose LV functions are normal are not considered to be candidates for surgical treatment, since their condition may remain stable for years. By contrast, unless there are contraindications, surgical treatment should be offered to patients with severe MR whose limitations do not allow fulltime employment or the performance of normal household activities despite optimal medical management. Surgical treatment of severe MR should be considered even in asymptomatic patients or those with mild symptoms when LV dysfunction is progressive, with LV EF declining below 60% and/or end-systolic cavity dimension on echocardiography rising above 45 mm. In patients with impaired LV function, the risk of surgery rises, the recovery of LV performance is incomplete, and the long-term survival is reduced (Fig. 219-4). However, conservative management has little to offer these patients, so operative treatment may be indicated and occasionally, the clinical and hemodynamic improvement that follows surgical treatment of patients with advanced disease is dramatic. However, unless chordal continuity can be preserved, operation is contraindicated in patients whose LV ejection fraction has declined to below 30%. Though most patients who survive surgery appear to be greatly improved, some degree of myocardial dysfunction often persists.

When surgical treatment is contemplated, left-sided heart catheterization and angiocardiography may be helpful in confirming the presence of severe MR in patients in whom there is a discrepancy between the clinical picture and the echocardiographic findings; these procedures may also aid in detecting and assessing the severity of associated valve lesions. Importantly, coronary arteriography identifies patients who require concomitant coronary revascularization.

Surgical treatment of MR, especially that caused by valves that are markedly deformed, with shrunken, calcified leaflets secondary to rheumatic fever, requires MVR with a prosthesis. However, in an increasing number of patients, particularly those with severe annular dilatation, flail leaflets, MVP, ruptured chordae, or infective endocarditis, reconstruction of the mitral valve apparatus (mitral valvuloplasty) and/or mitral annuloplasty with an annuloplasty ring may be successful. Valve reconstruction should be carried out whenever fea-

sible since the operative risk is about half (~3%) of that associated with MVR (Table 219-1). Also, reconstruction spares the patient the long-term adverse consequences of valve replacement, i.e., thromboembolic and hemorrhagic complications in the case of mechanical prostheses and late valve failure necessitating repeat valve replacement in the case of bioprostheses. In addition, by preserving the integrity of the papillary muscles, subvalvular apparatus and chordae tendinae, mitral repair and valvuloplasty maintains LV function. In asymptomatic patients with preserved left ventricular function, surgical treatment can be considered as long as mitral repair seems feasible and pulmonary hypertension or recent atrial fibrillation are present.

MITRAL VALVE PROLAPSE

MVP, also variously termed the *systolic click-murmur syndrome, Barlow's syndrome, floppy-valve syndrome,* and *billowing mitral leaflet syndrome,* is a relatively common, but highly variable clinical syndrome resulting from diverse pathogenic mechanisms of the mitral valve apparatus. Among these are excessive or redundant mitral leaflet tissue, which is commonly associated with myxomatous degeneration and greatly increased concentrations of acid mucopolysaccharide. MVP is a frequent finding in patients with heritable disorders of connective tissue, including the Marfan syndrome (Chap. 342), osteogenesis imperfecta, and the Ehler-Danlos syndrome. In most patients with MVP, however, myxomatous degeneration is confined to the mitral (or less commonly the tricuspid or aortic) valves without other clinical or pathologic manifestations of disease. The posterior leaflet is usually more affected than the anterior, and the mitral valve annulus is often greatly dilated. In many patients, elongated redundant chordae tendineae cause or contribute to the regurgitation.

In most patients with MVP, the cause is unknown, but in some it appears to be a genetically determined collagen tissue disorder. A reduction in the production of type III collagen has been incriminated, and electron microscopy has revealed fragmentation of collagen fibrils. MVP may be associated with thoracic skeletal deformities similar to but not as severe as those in the Marfan syndrome, including a high-arched palate and alterations of the chest and thoracic spine, including the so-called straight back syndrome. MVP also may occur as a sequel of acute rheumatic fever, in ischemic heart disease, and in cardiomyopathies, as well as in 20% of patients with ostium secundum atrial septal defect.

MVP may lead to excessive stress on the papillary muscles, which in turn leads to dysfunction and ischemia of the papillary muscles and the subjacent ventricular myocardium. Rupture of chordae tendineae and progressive annular dilatation and calcification also contribute to valvular regurgitation, which then places more stress on the diseased mitral valve apparatus, thereby creating a vicious circle. The electrocardiographic changes (see below) and ventricular arrhythmias appear to result from regional ventricular dysfunction related to increased stress placed on the papillary muscles.

CLINICAL FEATURES MVP is more common in females. It affects individuals in a wide age range but most commonly those between the ages of 14 and 30 years. The clinical course is often benign. MVP may also be observed in older (>50 years) patients, often males, and in them MR is more often severe and requires surgical treatment. There is an increased familial incidence for some patients, suggesting an autosomal dominant form of inheritance. MVP encompasses a broad spectrum of severities, ranging from only a systolic click and murmur and mild prolapse of the posterior leaflet of the mitral valve to severe MR due to chordal rupture and massive prolapse of both leaflets. In many patients, this condition progresses over years or decades.

Most patients are asymptomatic and remain so for their entire lives. However, MVP is now the most common cause of isolated severe MR requiring surgical treatment in North America. Arrhythmias, most commonly ventricular premature contractions and paroxysmal supraventricular and ventricular tachycardia, have been reported and may

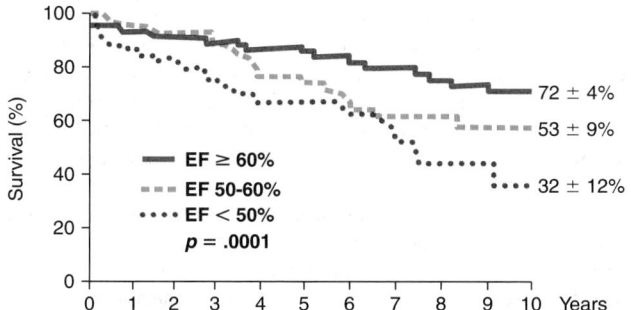

FIGURE 219-4 Late survival rates of patients surviving surgical correction of MR according to preoperative echocardiographic ejection fraction (EF). *(From M Enriquez-Sarano et al: Echocardiographic prediction of survival after surgical correction of organic mitral regurgitation. Circulation 90:833, 1994, with permission.)*

cause palpitations, light-headedness, and syncope. Sudden death is a very rare complication. Many patients have chest pain that is difficult to evaluate. It is often substernal, prolonged, poorly related to exertion, and rarely resembles angina pectoris. Transient cerebral ischemic attacks secondary to emboli from the mitral valve due to endothelial disruption have been reported. Infective endocarditis may occur in patients with MR associated with MVP.

Auscultation   The most important finding is the mid- or late (nonejection) systolic click, which occurs 0.14 s or more after the S_1 and is thought to be generated by the sudden tensing of slack, elongated chordae tendineae or by the prolapsing mitral leaflet when it reaches its maximum excursion. Systolic clicks may be multiple and may be followed by a high-pitched, late systolic crescendo-decrescendo murmur, which occasionally is "whooping" or "honking," and is heard best at the apex. The click and murmur occur earlier with standing, during the strain of the Valsalva maneuver, and with any intervention that decreases LV volume, exaggerating the propensity of mitral leaflet prolapse. Conversely, squatting and isometric exercise, which increase LV volume, diminish MVP, and the click-murmur complex is delayed and may even disappear. Some patients have a midsystolic click without the murmur; others have the murmur without a click. Still others have both sounds at different times.

LABORATORY EXAMINATION   The ECG most commonly is normal but may show biphasic or inverted T waves in leads II, III, and aVF, and occasionally supraventricular or ventricular premature contractions. *Two-dimensional echocardiography* is particularly effective in identifying the abnormal position and prolapse of the mitral valve leaflets. A useful echocardiographic definition of MVP is systolic displacement (in the parasternal view) of the mitral valve leaflets by at least 2 mm into the LA superior to the plane of the mitral annulus. Thickening of the mitral valve leaflets identifies a subgroup of patients at higher risk of infective endocarditis and the development of severe MR. Prolapse of the tricuspid and/or aortic valve may be found. *Color-imaging* and *Doppler studies* are helpful in revealing and evaluating accompanying MR. *Angiocardiography* generally shows prolapse of the posterior and sometimes of both mitral valve leaflets.

℞ TREATMENT

The management of patients with MVP consists of the asymptomatic patient without severe MR or arrhythmias and the prevention of infective endocarditis with antibiotic prophylaxis in patients with a systolic murmur and/or thickening of mitral valve leaflets on endocardiography. Beta blockers sometimes relieve chest pain. If symptomatic tachyarrhythmias have occurred, antiarrhythmic agents as dictated by electrophysiologic studies should be administered. If the patient is symptomatic from severe MR, mitral valve repair (or rarely, replacement) is indicated. Antiplatelet aggregation agents such as aspirin should be given to patients with transient ischemic attacks, and if these are not effective, anticoagulants should be used.

AORTIC STENOSIS

AS occurs in about one-fourth of all patients with chronic valvular heart disease; approximately 80% of adult patients with symptomatic valvular AS are male.

ETIOLOGY   AS in adults may be due to degenerative calcification of the aortic cusps. It may be congenital in origin or it may be secondary to rheumatic inflammation. *Age-related degenerative calcific AS* (also known as senile or sclerocalcific AS) is now the most common cause of AS in adults in North America and Western Europe. About 30% of persons >65 years exhibit aortic valve sclerosis, many of whom have a systolic murmur of AS but without obstruction, while an additional 2% exhibit frank stenosis. On histologic examination these valves frequently exhibit inflammatory changes similar to those seen in athero-

sclerotic vessels. Interestingly, risk factors for atherosclerosis, such as age, male sex, smoking, diabetes mellitus, hypertension, increased LDL, reduced HDL cholesterol, and elevated C-reactive protein are all risk factors for aortic valve calcification.

The *congenitally affected valve* may be stenotic at birth (Chap. 218) and may become progressively more fibrotic, calcified, and stenotic. In other cases the valve may be congenitally deformed, usually bicuspid, without serious narrowing of the aortic orifice during childhood; its abnormal architecture makes its leaflets susceptible to otherwise ordinary hemodynamic stresses, which ultimately lead to valvular thickening, calcification, increased rigidity, and narrowing of the aortic orifice.

Rheumatic endocarditis of the aortic leaflets produces commissural fusion, sometimes resulting in a bicuspid valve. This condition in turn, makes the leaflets more susceptible to trauma and ultimately leads to fibrosis, calcification, and further narrowing. By the time the obstruction to LV outflow causes serious clinical disability, the valve is usually a rigid calcified mass, and careful examination may make it difficult or even impossible to determine the etiology of the underlying process. Rheumatic AS is almost always associated with involvement of the mitral valve and by associated severe AR.

OTHER FORMS OF OBSTRUCTION TO LEFT VENTRICULAR OUTFLOW   Besides valvular AS, three other lesions may be responsible for obstruction to LV outflow.

1. *Hypertrophic cardiomyopathy* (Chap. 221). This condition is characterized by marked hypertrophy of the LV and involves in particular the interventricular septum; it may cause subaortic obstruction.

2. *Discrete congenital subvalvular AS* (Chap. 218). This congenital anomaly is produced by either a membranous diaphragm or a fibrous ridge just below the aortic valve.

3. *Supravalvular AS* (Chap. 218). This uncommon congenital anomaly is produced by narrowing of the ascending aorta or by a fibrous diaphragm with a small opening just above the aortic valve.

PATHOPHYSIOLOGY   The obstruction to LV outflow produces a systolic pressure gradient between the LV and aorta. When severe obstruction is suddenly produced experimentally, the LV responds by dilatation and reduction of stroke volume. However, in patients the obstruction may be present at birth and/or increase gradually over the course of many years, and LV output is maintained by the presence of concentric LV hypertrophy. This serves as a useful compensatory mechanism because it reduces toward normal the systolic stress developed by the myocardium. A large transaortic valvular pressure gradient may exist for many years without a reduction of CO or LV dilatation; ultimately, however, these changes occur.

A peak systolic pressure gradient >50 mmHg in the face of a normal cardiac output or an effective aortic orifice less than approximately 1.0 cm^2 or <0.6 cm^2/m^2 body surface area, i.e., less than approximately one-third of the normal orifice, is generally considered to represent severe obstruction to LV outflow. The elevated LV end-diastolic pressure observed in many patients with severe AS signifies the presence of LV dilatation and/or diminished compliance of the hypertrophied LV wall. A large *a* wave in the LA pressure pulse is usually present. Although the CO at rest is within normal limits in most patients with severe AS, it usually fails to rise normally during exercise. Loss of an appropriately timed, vigorous atrial contraction, as occurs in AF or atrioventricular dissociation, may cause a rapid progression of symptoms. Late in the course the CO and LV–aortic pressure gradient decline, and the mean LA, PA, and RV pressures rise.

The hypertrophied LV muscle mass elevates myocardial oxygen requirements. In addition, even in the absence of obstructive coronary artery disease, there may be interference with coronary blood flow. This is because the pressure compressing the coronary arteries exceeds the coronary perfusion pressure, often causing ischemia, especially in the subendocardium, and during tachycardia, both in the presence and in the absence of coronary arterial narrowing.

SYMPTOMS AS is rarely of clinical importance until the valve orifice has narrowed to approximately 0.5 cm^2/m^2 body surface area in adults. Even severe AS may exist for many years without producing any symptoms because of the ability of the hypertrophied LV to generate the elevated intraventricular pressures required for a normal stroke volume.

Most patients with pure or predominant AS have gradually increasing obstruction for years but do not become symptomatic until the sixth to eighth decades. Exertional dyspnea, angina pectoris, and syncope are the three cardinal symptoms. Often there is a history of insidious progression of fatigue and dyspnea associated with gradual curtailment of activities. *Dyspnea* results primarily from elevation of the pulmonary capillary pressure caused by elevations of LV diastolic pressures secondary to reduced compliance. *Angina pectoris* usually develops somewhat later and reflects an imbalance between the augmented myocardial oxygen requirements and reduced oxygen availability; the former results from the increased myocardial mass and intraventricular pressure, while the latter may result from accompanying coronary artery disease, which is not uncommon in patients with AS, as well as from compression of the coronary vessels by the hypertrophied myocardium. Therefore, angina may occur in severe AS even without obstructive epicardial coronary artery disease. *Exertional syncope* may result from a decline in arterial pressure caused by vasodilatation in the exercising muscles and inadequate vasoconstriction in nonexercising muscles in the face of a fixed CO, or from a sudden fall in CO produced by an arrhythmia.

Since the CO at rest is usually well maintained until late in the course, marked fatigability, weakness, peripheral cyanosis, and other clinical manifestations of a low CO are usually not prominent until this stage is reached. Orthopnea, paroxysmal nocturnal dyspnea, and pulmonary edema, i.e., symptoms of LV failure, also occur only in the advanced stages of the disease. Severe pulmonary hypertension leading to RV failure and systemic venous hypertension, hepatomegaly, AF, and TR are usually late findings in patients with isolated, severe AS.

When AS and MS coexist, the reduction of cardiac output induced by MS lowers the pressure gradient across the aortic valve and thereby masks many of the clinical findings produced by AS. Left heart catheterization is helpful in defining the relative importance of each valvular abnormality.

PHYSICAL FINDINGS The rhythm is generally regular until very late in the course; at other times, AF should suggest the possibility of associated mitral valve disease. The systemic arterial pressure is usually within normal limits. In the late stages, however, when stroke volume declines, the systolic pressure may fall and the pulse pressure narrow. Systemic hypertension is unusual in patients with severe AS. The peripheral arterial pulse, as palpated in the carotid or brachial arteries, rises slowly to a delayed sustained peak (pulsus parvus et tardus) (see Fig. 209-2). In the elderly, the stiffening of the arterial wall may mask this important physical sign. A palpable double systolic arterial pulse, the so-called bisferiens pulse, excludes pure or predominant AS and signifies dominant AR. In the late stages of AS, when the pulse pressure is reduced, the pulse amplitude may be so small that the anacrotic nature of the pulse and the delay in its upstroke may become difficult to appreciate. In many patients the *a* wave in the jugular venous pulse is accentuated. This results from the diminished distensibility of the RV cavity caused by the bulging, hypertrophied intraventricular septum.

The LV impulse is usually active and displaced laterally, reflecting the presence of LV hypertrophy. A double apical impulse may be recognized, particularly with the patient in the left lateral recumbent position. A systolic thrill is generally present at the base of the heart, in the jugular notch, and along the carotid arteries. In patients who do not have marked pulmonary emphysema, a thick chest wall, thoracic deformity, or heart failure, the absence of a systolic thrill suggests that the AS is relatively mild.

Auscultation An early systolic ejection sound, actually the OS of the aortic valve, is frequently audible in children and adolescents with congenital noncalcific valvular AS. This sound usually disappears when the valve becomes calcified and rigid. As AS increases in severity, LV systole may become prolonged so that the aortic valve closure sound no longer precedes the pulmonic valve closure sound, and the two components may become synchronous, or aortic valve closure may even follow pulmonic valve closure, causing paradoxic splitting of the S$_2$ (Chap. 209). The sound of aortic valve closure can be heard most frequently in patients with AS who have pliable valves, and calcification diminishes the intensity of this sound. Frequently, an S$_4$ is audible at the apex and reflects the presence of LV hypertrophy and an elevated LV end-diastolic pressure; an S$_3$ generally occurs when the LV dilates.

The murmur of AS is characteristically an ejection (mid) systolic murmur that commences shortly after the S$_1$, increases in intensity to reach a peak toward the middle of ejection, and ends just before aortic valve closure (see Figs. 209-4 and 209-5A). It is characteristically low-pitched, rough and rasping in character, and loudest at the base of the heart, most commonly in the second right intercostal space. It is transmitted upward along the carotid arteries. Occasionally, it is transmitted downward and to the apex where it may be confused with the systolic murmur of MR. In almost all patients with severe obstruction, the murmur is at least grade III/VI. In patients with mild degrees of obstruction or in those with severe stenosis with heart failure in whom the stroke volume and therefore the transvalvular flow rate are reduced, the murmur may be relatively soft and brief.

LABORATORY EXAMINATION ■ **Electrocardiogram** In most patients with severe AS there is LV hypertrophy (see Fig. 210-9). In advanced cases, ST-segment depression and T-wave inversion (LV "strain") in standard leads I and aVL and in the left precordial leads are evident. However, there is no close correlation between the ECG and the hemodynamic severity of obstruction, and the absence of ECG signs of LV hypertrophy does not exclude severe obstruction.

The key findings are LV hypertrophy and, in patients with valvular calcification (i.e., most adult patients with symptomatic AS), multiple, bright, thick, echoes from within the aortic root. Eccentricity of the aortic valve cusps is characteristic of congenitally bicuspid valves. Transesophageal imaging usually displays the obstructed orifice extremely well. The transaortic valvular gradient can be estimated by Doppler echocardiography. LV dilatation and reduced systolic shortening reflect impairment of LV function. Echocardiography is also useful for identifying valvular abnormalities such as MS and AR, which sometimes accompany AS, and for differentiating valvular AS from obstructive hypertrophic cardiomyopathy.

Roentgenogram The chest roentgenogram may show no or little overall cardiac enlargement for many years, since the development of concentric LV hypertrophy is the initial response to obstruction to LV outflow. Hypertrophy without dilatation may produce some rounding of the cardiac apex in the frontal projection and slight backward displacement in the lateral view; critical AS is often associated with poststenotic dilatation of the ascending aorta (Fig. 211-5). Aortic calcification is usually readily apparent on fluoroscopic examination or by echocardiography; the absence of valvular calcification in an adult suggests that severe valvular AS is not present. In later stages of the disease as the LV dilates, there is increasing roentgenographic evidence of LV enlargement; pulmonary congestion; and enlargement of the LA, PA, and right side of the heart.

Catheterization Catheterization of the left side of the heart and coronary arteriography should generally be carried out in patients suspected of having severe AS who are being considered for operative treatment. These investigations are especially indicated in the following:

1. *Patients with clinical signs of AS and symptoms of myocardial ischemia,* in whom associated coronary artery disease is suspected. An

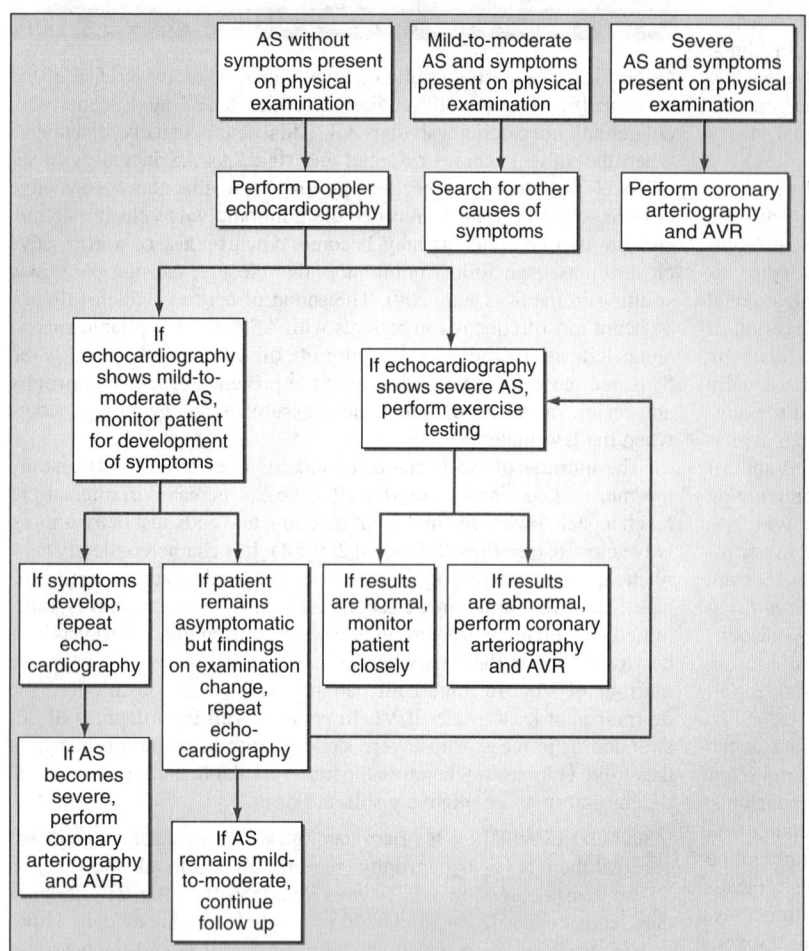

FIGURE 219-5 Algorithm for the management of aortic stenosis. AS, aortic stenosis; AVR, aortic valve replacement. *(From Carabello, 2002.)*

effort should be made to determine whether AS or coronary atherosclerosis is primarily responsible for the symptoms. Coronary arteriography should be carried out to identify patients who require coronary bypass grafting at the time of aortic valve surgery.

2. *Patients with multivalvular disease*, in whom the role played by each valvular deformity should be defined to aid in the planning of definitive operative treatment.

3. *Young, asymptomatic patients with noncalcific congenital AS*, to define with precision the severity of obstruction to LV outflow, since operation [which does not usually require aortic valve replacement (AVR)] or balloon valvotomy may be indicated if severe AS is present, even in the absence of symptoms. Balloon valvotomy may follow left heart catheterization immediately.

4. *Patients in whom it is suspected that the obstruction to LV outflow may not be at the aortic valve* but rather in the sub- or supravalvular regions.

NATURAL HISTORY Death in patients with severe AS occurs most commonly in the seventh and eighth decades. Based on data obtained at postmortem examination in patients before surgical treatment became widely available, the average time to death after the onset of various symptoms was as follows: angina pectoris, 3 years; syncope, 3 years; dyspnea, 2 years; and congestive heart failure, 1.5 to 2 years. Moreover, in >80% of patients who died with AS, symptoms had existed for <4 years. Congestive heart failure was considered to be the cause of death in one-half to two-thirds of patients. Among adults dying with valvular AS, sudden death, which presumably resulted from an arrhythmia, occurred in 10 to 20% and at an average age of 60 years. However, most sudden deaths occur in patients who had previously been symptomatic; thus sudden death is very uncommon (3 per 1000 patient years) in asymptomatic patients with severe AS. Obstructive

calcific AS is a progressive disease, with an annual reduction in valve area of approximately 0.1 mm²/year.

℞ TREATMENT

Medical Treatment (Fig. 219-5, Table 219-1) In patients with severe AS (<0.5 cm²/m²), strenuous physical activity should be avoided, even in the asymptomatic stage. Sodium restriction, the cautious administration of diuretics and digitalis glycosides are indicated in the treatment of congestive heart failure, but care must be taken to avoid volume depletion since this may cause a marked reduction of CO. Nitroglycerin is helpful in relieving angina pectoris. Retrospective studies have shown that patients with degenerative calcific AS who receive HMG-CoA reductase inhibitors ("statins") exhibit slower progression of leaflet calcification and aortic valve area reduction than those who do not. Treatment with these relatively safe agents should be considered while the results of clinical trials are awaited.

Surgical Treatment The most critical decision in the management of AS concerns the advisability of surgical treatment which, in most adults with calcific AS and severe obstruction consists of AVR. However, these patients should be followed carefully for the development of symptoms and by serial echocardiograms for evidence of deteriorating LV function. Operation is generally indicated in patients with severe AS (valve area <1.0 cm² or 0.6 cm²/m² body surface area) who are symptomatic, those who exhibit LV dysfunction, as well as those with an expanding poststenotic aortic root, even if they are asymptomatic. In patients without heart failure, the operative risk of AVR is approximately 4% (Table 219-2). In most instances, it is prudent to postpone operation in patients with severe calcific AS who are asymptomatic and who exhibit normal LV function, i.e., EF >50%, since they may continue to do well for many years. The risk of surgical mortality exceeds that of sudden death in asymptomatic patients. However, AVR can be carried out in asymptomatic patients with severe stenosis who undergo coronary artery bypass grafting.

Operation should, if possible, be carried out before frank LV failure develops; at this late stage, the aortic valve pressure gradient declines as the stroke volume and ejection fraction decline. In such patients, the operative risk is high (15 to 20%), and evidence of myocardial disease may persist even when the operation is technically successful. Furthermore, long-term postoperative survival also correlates inversely with preoperative LV dysfunction. Nonetheless, in view of the even worse prognosis of such patients when they are treated medically, there is usually little choice but to advise surgical treatment, especially in patients in whom contractile reserve can be demonstrated by dobutamine echocardiography. In patients in whom severe AS and coronary artery disease coexist, relief of the AS and revascularization of the myocardium by means of aortocoronary bypass grafting may result in striking clinical and hemodynamic improvement.

Because many patients with calcific AS are elderly, particular attention must be directed to the adequacy of hepatic, renal, and pulmonary function before AVR is recommended. The mortality rate depends to a substantial extent on the patient's preoperative clinical and hemodynamic state. The 10-year survival rate of patients with AVR is approximately 60%. Approximately 30% of bioprosthetic valves evidence primary valve failure in 10 years, requiring rereplacement, and an approximately equal percentage of patients with mechanical prostheses develop significant hemorrhagic complications as a consequence of treatment with anticoagulants.

Percutaneous Balloon Aortic Valvuloplasty This procedure is preferable to operation in children and young adults with congenital, noncalcific AS. It is not commonly used in adults with severe calcific AS because of a high restenosis rate, but has on occasion been used successfully in patients as a "bridge to operation" in patients with severe LV dysfunction who are too ill to tolerate surgery.

AORTIC REGURGITATION

ETIOLOGY AR may be caused by primary valve disease or by primary aortic root disease.

Primary Valve Disease Approximately three-fourths of patients with pure or predominant valvular AR are males; females predominate among patients with primary valvular AR who have associated mitral valve disease. In approximately two-thirds of patients with AR the disease is rheumatic in origin, resulting in thickening, deformity, and shortening of the individual aortic valve cusps, changes that prevent their proper opening during systole and closure during diastole. A rheumatic origin is less common in patients with isolated AR. Patients with congenital membranous subaortic stenosis often develop thickening of the aortic valve leaflets, which makes the valves particularly susceptible to endocarditis. AR also may occur in patients with rheumatoid spondylitis and in patients with congenital bicuspid aortic valves. Prolapse of an aortic cusp, resulting in progressive chronic AR, occurs in approximately 15% of patients with ventricular septal defect (Chap. 218). Congenital fenestrations of the aortic valve occasionally produce mild AR.

Acute AR may result from infective endocarditis, which can develop on a valve previously affected by rheumatic disease, a congenitally deformed valve, or, rarely, on a normal aortic valve, and perforate or erode one or more of the leaflets. Although traumatic rupture of the aortic valve is an uncommon cause of acute AR, it does represent the most frequent serious lesion in patients surviving nonpenetrating cardiac injuries. The coexistence of hemodynamically significant AS with AR usually excludes all the rarer forms of AR because it occurs almost exclusively in patients with rheumatic or congenital AR. In patients with AR due to primary valvular disease, dilatation of the aortic annulus may occur secondarily and intensify the regurgitation.

Primary Aortic Root Disease AR, both acute and chronic, also may be due entirely to marked aortic dilatation, i.e., aortic root disease, without primary involvement of the valve leaflets; widening of the aortic annulus and separation of the aortic leaflets are responsible for the AR (Chap. 231). Cystic medial necrosis of the ascending aorta, which may or may not be associated with other manifestations of the Marfan syndrome, idiopathic dilatation of the aorta, osteogenesis imperfecta, and severe hypertension all may widen the aortic annulus and lead to progressive AR. Occasionally, AR is caused by retrograde dissection of the aorta involving the aortic annulus. Syphilis and rheumatoid ankylosing spondylitis may be associated with cellular infiltration and scarring of the media of the thoracic aorta, leading to aortic dilatation, aneurysm formation, and severe regurgitation. In syphilis of the aorta, now a very rare condition (Chap. 153), the involvement of the intima may narrow the coronary ostia, which in turn may be responsible for myocardial ischemia.

PATHOPHYSIOLOGY The total stroke volume ejected by the LV (i.e., the sum of the effective forward stroke volume and the volume of blood that regurgitates back into the LV) is increased in patients with AR. In patients with wide-open (free) AR, the volume of regurgitant flow may equal the effective forward stroke volume. In contrast to MR, in which a fraction of the LV stroke volume is delivered into the low-pressure LA, in AR the entire LV stroke volume is ejected into a high-pressure zone, the aorta. An increase in the LV end-diastolic volume (increased preload) constitutes the major hemodynamic compensation for AR. The dilatation and eccentric hypertrophy of the LV allows this chamber to eject a larger stroke volume without requiring any increase in the relative shortening of each myofibril. Therefore, severe AR may occur with a normal effective forward stroke volume and a normal left ventricular EF [total (forward plus regurgitant) stroke volume/end-diastolic volume], together with an elevated LV end-diastolic pressure and volume. However, through the operation of Laplace's law (which

holds that myocardial wall tension is the product of intracavitary pressure and LV radius), LV dilatation increases the LV systolic tension required to develop any given level of systolic pressure. Ultimately, these adaptive measures fail. As LV function deteriorates, the end-diastolic volume rises further and the forward stroke volume and EF decline. Deterioration of LV function often precedes the development of symptoms. Considerable thickening of the LV wall also occurs with chronic AR, and at autopsy the hearts of these patients may be among the largest encountered, sometimes weighing >1000 g.

The reverse pressure gradient from aorta to LV, which drives the AR flow, falls progressively during diastole (see Fig. 212-4), accounting for the decrescendo nature of the diastolic murmur. Equilibration between aortic and LV pressures may occur toward the end of diastole in patients with severe AR, particularly when the heart rate is slow, and the LV end-diastolic pressure may be elevated, occasionally to extremely high levels (>40 mmHg). Rarely, in acute, severe AR, the LV pressure exceeds the LA pressure toward the end of diastole, and this reversed pressure gradient closes the mitral valve prematurely or causes diastolic MR.

In patients with severe AR, the effective forward CO usually is normal or only slightly reduced at rest, but often it fails to rise normally during exertion. Early signs of LV dysfunction include reduction in the EF, determined by echocardiography or radionuclide angiography. In advanced stages there may be considerable elevation of the LA, PA wedge, PA, and RV pressures and lowering of the forward CO at rest.

Myocardial ischemia may occur in patients with AR because myocardial oxygen requirements are elevated by both LV dilatation and elevated LV systolic tension. However, a large fraction of coronary blood flow occurs during diastole, when arterial pressure is subnormal, thereby reducing coronary perfusion pressure. This combination of increased oxygen demand and reduced supply may cause myocardial ischemia, particularly of the subendocardium, even in the absence of concomitant coronary artery disease.

HISTORY A family history may frequently be elicited from patients with AR associated with the Marfan syndrome. A history compatible with infective endocarditis may sometimes be elicited from patients with rheumatic or congenital involvement of the aortic valve, and the infection often precipitates or seriously aggravates preexisting symptoms. Ankylosing spondylitis is usually self evident.

In patients with *acute, severe AR*, as may occur in infective endocarditis or trauma, the LV cannot dilate sufficiently to maintain stroke volume, and LV diastolic pressure rises rapidly with associated elevations of LA and PA wedge pressures. Pulmonary edema and/or cardiogenic shock may develop rapidly.

Chronic, severe AR may have a long latent period, and patients may remain relatively asymptomatic for as long as 10 to 15 years. However, uncomfortable awareness of the heartbeat, especially on lying down, may be an early complaint. Sinus tachycardia during exertion or with emotion, or premature ventricular contractions may produce particularly uncomfortable palpitations, as well as head pounding. These complaints may persist for many years before the development of exertional dyspnea, usually the first symptom of diminished cardiac reserve. The dyspnea is followed by orthopnea, paroxysmal nocturnal dyspnea, and excessive diaphoresis. Anginal chest pain occurs frequently in patients with severe AR, even in younger patients, and it is not necessary to invoke the presence of coronary artery disease to explain this symptom in patients with severe AR. Anginal pain may develop at rest as well as during exertion. Nocturnal angina may be a particularly troublesome symptom, and it may be accompanied by marked diaphoresis. The anginal episodes can be prolonged and often do not respond satisfactorily to sublingual nitroglycerin. Systemic fluid accumulation, including congestive hepatomegaly and ankle edema, may develop late in the course of the disease.

PHYSICAL FINDINGS In severe AR, the jarring of the entire body and the bobbing motion of the head with each systole can be appreciated, and

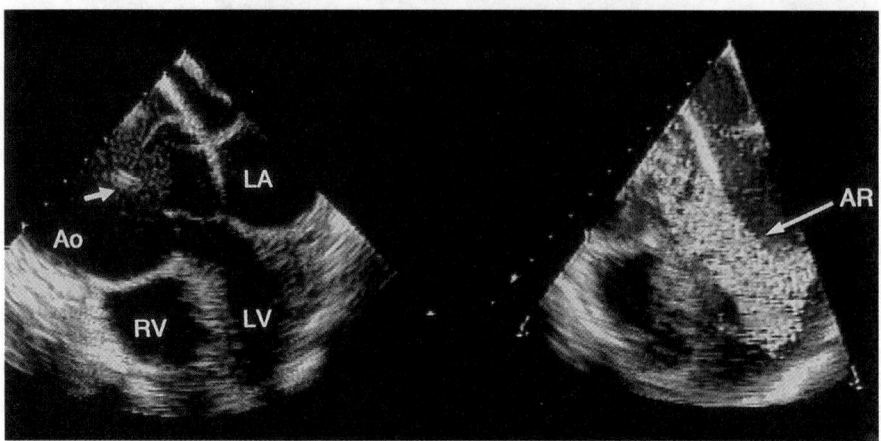

FIGURE 219-6 Transesophageal echocardiographic view of a patient with a dilated aorta, aortic dissection, and severe aortic regurgitation. The *arrow* points to the intimal flap that is seen in the dilated ascending aorta. *Left:* the long axis apex down view of the black and white two-dimensional image in diastole. *Right:* color flow imaging that demonstrates a large mosaic jet of aortic regurgitation. AO, aorta; RV, right ventricle; AR, aortic regurgitation.

the abrupt distention and collapse of the larger arteries are easily visible. The examination should be directed toward the detection of conditions predisposing to AR, such as the Marfan syndrome, rheumatoid ankylosing spondylitis, and ventricular septal defect.

Arterial Pulse   A rapidly rising "water-hammer" pulse, which collapses suddenly as arterial pressure falls rapidly during late systole and diastole (Corrigan's pulse), and capillary pulsations, an alternate flushing and paling of the skin at the root of the nail while pressure is applied to the tip of the nail (Quincke's pulse), are characteristic of free AR. A booming, "pistol-shot" sound can be heard over the femoral arteries (Traube's sign), and a to-and-fro murmur (Duroziez's sign) is audible if the femoral artery is lightly compressed with a stethoscope.

The arterial pulse pressure is widened, with an elevation of the systolic pressure, sometimes to as high as 300 mmHg, and a depression of the diastolic pressure. The measurement of arterial diastolic pressure with a sphygmomanometer may be complicated by the fact that systolic sounds are frequently heard with the cuff completely deflated. However, the level of cuff pressure at the time of muffling of the Korotkoff sounds (Phase IV) generally corresponds fairly closely to the true intraarterial diastolic pressure. The severity of AR does not always correlate directly with the arterial pulse pressure, and severe regurgitation may exist in patients with arterial pressures in the range of 140/60 mmHg. As the disease progresses and the LV end-diastolic pressure rises markedly, the arterial diastolic pressure may actually rise also, since the aortic diastolic pressure cannot fall below the LV end-diastolic pressure. For the same reason, *severe, acute* AR may also be accompanied by only light widening of the pulse pressure.

Palpation   The LV impulse is heaving and displaced laterally and inferiorly. The systolic expansion and diastolic retraction of the apex are prominent and contrast with the sustained systolic thrust characteristic of severe AS. A diastolic thrill is often palpable along the left sternal border, and a prominent systolic thrill may be palpable in the jugular notch and transmitted upward along the carotid arteries. This systolic thrill and the accompanying murmur are due to the markedly increased blood flow across the aortic orifice and do not necessarily signify the coexistence of AS. In many patients with pure AR or with combined AS and AR, the carotid arterial pulse is bisferiens, i.e., with two systolic waves separated by a trough.

Auscultation   In patients with severe AR, the aortic valve closure sound (A_2) is usually absent. An S_3 and systolic ejection sound are frequently audible, and occasionally, an S_4 also may be heard. The murmur of chronic AR is typically a high-pitched, blowing, decrescendo diastolic murmur, heard best in the third intercostal space along the left sternal border (see Fig. 209-5*B*). In patients with mild AR, this murmur is

brief, but as the severity increases, generally becomes louder and longer, indeed holodiastolic. When the murmur is soft, it can be heard best with the diaphragm of the stethoscope and with the patient sitting up, leaning forward, and with the breath held in forced expiration. In patients in whom the AR is caused by primary valvular disease, the diastolic murmur is usually louder along the left than the right sternal border. However, when the murmur is heard best along the right sternal border, it suggests that the AR is caused by aneurysmal dilatation of the aortic root. "Cooing" or musical diastolic murmurs suggest eversion of an aortic cusp vibrating in the regurgitant stream.

A midsystolic ejection murmur is frequently audible in AR. It is generally heard best at the base of the heart and is transmitted along the carotid vessels. This murmur may be quite loud without signifying aortic obstruction; it is often higher pitched, shorter, and less rasping in quality than the ejection systolic murmur heard in patients with predominant AS. A third murmur frequently heard in patients with severe AR is the *Austin Flint murmur*, a soft, low-pitched, rumbling middiastolic bruit. It is probably produced by the diastolic displacement of the anterior leaflet of the mitral valve by the AR stream but does not appear to be associated with hemodynamically significant mitral obstruction and, in contrast to the diastolic murmur of MS, it is not accompanied by an OS or loud S_1. The auscultatory features of AR are intensified by isometric exercise such as strenuous handgrip, which augments systemic resistance, and reduced by inhalation of amyl nitrite.

In *severe, acute* AR, the elevation of LV end-diastolic pressure may lead to early closure of the mitral valve, an associated middiastolic sound, a soft or absent S_1, a pulse pressure that is not particularly wide, and a soft, short diastolic murmur of AR.

LABORATORY EXAMINATION ■ EKG   In patients with severe, chronic AR, the EKG signs of LV hypertrophy become manifest (Chap. 210). In addition, these patients frequently exhibit ST-segment depression and T-wave inversion in leads I, aVL, V_5, and V_6 ("LV strain"). Left axis deviation and/or QRS prolongation denote diffuse myocardial disease, generally associated with patchy fibrosis, and usually signify a poor prognosis.

Echocardiogram   The extent and velocity of wall motion are normal or even supernormal, until myocardial contractility declines. A rapid, high-frequency fluttering of the anterior mitral leaflet produced by the impact of the regurgitant jet is a characteristic finding. The echocardiogram is also useful in determining the cause of AR, by detecting dilatation of the aortic annulus (Fig. 219-6). Thickening and failure of coaptation of the leaflets also may be noted. Color flow Doppler echocardiographic imaging is very sensitive in the detection of AR, and Doppler echocardiography is helpful in assessing its severity. Serial two-dimensional echocardiography is valuable in assessing LV performance and in detecting progressive myocardial dysfunction.

Roentgenogram   In severe chronic AR, the apex is displaced downward and to the left in the frontal projection, and frequently the cardiac shadow extends below the left diaphragm. LV enlargement also may be apparent in the left anterior oblique and lateral projections, in which the LV is displaced posteriorly and encroaches on the spine. In patients in whom primary valvular disease is responsible for the AR, the ascending aorta and aortic knob may be moderately dilated. When AR is caused by primary disease of the aortic wall, aneurysmal dilatation of the aorta may be noted, and the aorta may fill the retrosternal space in the lateral view.

Cardiac Catheterization and Angiography   In addition to providing an accurate confirmation of the magnitude of regurgitation and the status of

LV function, the condition of the coronary arterial bed should ordinarily be evaluated preoperatively.

Rx TREATMENT

Medical Treatment (Table 219-1) Although operation constitutes the definitive treatment of AR and should be carried out before the development of heart failure, the latter usually responds briefly to treatment with digitalis glycosides, salt restriction, diuretics, and vasodilators, especially ACE inhibitors. Digitalis also may be indicated in patients with severe regurgitation and dilated left ventricles without frank LV failure. Cardiac arrhythmias and infections are poorly tolerated in patients with severe AR and must be treated promptly and vigorously. Although nitroglycerin and long-acting nitrates are not as helpful in relieving anginal pain as they are in patients with ischemic heart disease, they are worth a trial. Long-acting nifedipine has been found to delay the need for operation. Patients with syphilitic aortitis should receive a full course of penicillin therapy (Chap. 153).

Surgical Treatment In deciding on the advisability and proper timing of surgical treatment, two points should be kept in mind: (1) patients with chronic AR usually do not become symptomatic until *after* the development of myocardial dysfunction, and (2) when delayed too long, surgical treatment often does not restore normal LV function. Therefore, in patients with severe AR, careful clinical follow-up and noninvasive testing with echocardiography at approximately 6-month intervals are necessary if operation is to be undertaken at the optimal time, i.e., *after* the onset of LV dysfunction but *prior* to the development of severe symptoms. Operation can be deferred as long as the patient both remains asymptomatic and retains normal LV function. In general, operation should be carried out even in asymptomatic patients with progressive LV dysfunction and a left ventricular ejection fraction (LVEF) <55% or a LV end-systolic volume >55 mL/m². These parameters have been referred to as the "55/55 rule."

AVR with a suitable mechanical or tissue prosthesis is generally necessary in patients with rheumatic AR and in many patients with other forms of regurgitation. Rarely, when a leaflet has been perforated during infective endocarditis or torn from its attachments to the aortic annulus by thoracic trauma, surgical repair may be possible. When AR is due to aneurysmal dilatation of the annulus and ascending aorta rather than to primary valvular involvement, it may be possible to reduce the regurgitation by narrowing the annulus or by excising a portion of the aortic root without replacing the valve. More frequently, however, regurgitation can be eliminated only by replacing the aortic valve, excising the dilated or aneurysmal ascending aorta responsible for the regurgitation, and replacing it with a graft. This formidable procedure entails a higher risk than isolated AVR.

As in patients with other valvular abnormalities, both the operative risk and the late mortality are largely dependent on the stage of the disease and on myocardial function at the time of operation. The overall operative mortality for isolated AVR is 4.3% (Table 219-2). However, patients with marked cardiac enlargement and prolonged LV dysfunction experience an operative mortality rate of approximately 10% and a late mortality rate of approximately 5% per year due to LV failure despite a technically satisfactory operation. Nonetheless, because of the very poor prognosis with medical management, even patients with LV failure should be considered for operation.

Patients with acute, severe AR require prompt surgical treatment, which may be lifesaving.

TRICUSPID STENOSIS

TS, a relatively uncommon valvular lesion in North America and Western Europe, is more common in tropical and subtropical climates, especially in southern Asia and in Latin America. It is generally rheumatic in origin and is more common in females than in males. It does not occur as an isolated lesion and is usually associated with MS. Hemodynamically significant TS occurs in 5 to 10% of patients with severe MS; rheumatic TS is commonly associated with some degree of TR.

PATHOPHYSIOLOGY A diastolic pressure gradient between the RA and RV can be recorded with a double-lumen cardiac catheter. It is augmented when the transvalvular blood flow increases during inspiration and declines during expiration. A mean diastolic pressure gradient of 4 mmHg is usually sufficient to elevate the mean RA pressure to levels that result in systemic venous congestion. Unless sodium intake has been restricted and diuretics administered, this venous congestion is associated with ascites and edema, sometimes severe. In patients with sinus rhythm, the RA *a* wave may be extremely tall and may even approach the level of the RV systolic pressure. The CO at rest is usually depressed and it fails to rise during exercise. The low CO is responsible for the normal or only slightly elevated LA, PA, and RV systolic pressures despite the presence of MS. Thus, the presence of TS can mask the hemodynamic and clinical features of the MS which usually accompanies it.

SYMPTOMS Since the development of MS generally precedes that of TS, many patients initially have symptoms of pulmonary congestion. Amelioration of these symptoms should raise the possibility that TS may be developing. Characteristically, patients complain of relatively little dyspnea for the degree of hepatomegaly, ascites, and edema that they have. However, fatigue secondary to a low CO and discomfort due to refractory edema, ascites, and marked hepatomegaly are common in patients with TS and/or TR. In some patients, TS may be suspected for the first time when symptoms of RV failure persist after an adequate mitral valvotomy.

PHYSICAL FINDINGS

Since TS usually occurs in the presence of other obvious valvular disease, the diagnosis may be missed unless it is specifically searched for. Severe TS is associated with marked hepatic congestion, often resulting in cirrhosis, jaundice, serious malnutrition, anasarca, and ascites. Congestive hepatomegaly and, in cases of severe tricuspid valve disease, splenomegaly are present. The jugular veins are distended, and in patients with sinus rhythm there may be giant *a* waves. The *v* waves are less conspicuous, and since tricuspid obstruction impedes RA emptying during diastole, there is a slow *y* descent. In patients with sinus rhythm there may be prominent presystolic pulsations of the enlarged liver as well.

On auscultation, the pulmonic valve closure sound is not accentuated, and occasionally, an OS of the tricuspid valve may be heard approximately 0.06 s after pulmonic valve closure. The diastolic murmur of TS has many of the qualities of the diastolic murmur of MS, and since TS almost always occurs in the presence of MS, the less common valvular lesion may be missed. However, the tricuspid murmur is generally heard best along the left lower sternal margin and over the xiphoid process and is most prominent during presystole in patients with sinus rhythm. The diastolic murmur is reduced in amplitude as the stethoscope is inched laterally, only to intensify or reappear as the mitral murmur at the apex. The murmur of TS is augmented during inspiration, and it is reduced during expiration and particularly during the strain of Valsalva maneuver, when tricuspid blood flow is reduced.

LABORATORY EXAMINATION The ECG features of RA enlargement (Chap. 210) include tall, peaked P waves in lead II, as well as prominent, upright P waves in lead V_1. The *absence* of ECG evidence of right ventricular hypertrophy (RVH) in a patient with right-sided heart failure who is believed to have MS should suggest associated tricuspid valve disease. The chest roentgenogram in patients with combined TS and MS shows particular prominence of the RA and superior vena cava without much enlargement of the PA and with less evidence of pulmonary vascular congestion than occurs in patients with isolated MS. On echocardiographic examination, the tricuspid valve is usually thickened; the transvalvular gradient can be estimated by Doppler echocardiography.

℞ TREATMENT

Patients with TS generally exhibit marked systemic venous congestion; intensive salt restriction and diuretic therapy are required during the preoperative period. Such a preparatory period may diminish hepatic congestion and thereby improve hepatic function sufficiently so that the risks of operation are diminished. Surgical relief of the TS should be carried out, preferably at the time of surgical mitral valvotomy or MVR, in patients with moderate or severe TS who have mean diastolic pressure gradients exceeding approximately 4 mmHg and tricuspid orifices less than 1.5 to 2.0 cm². TS is almost always accompanied by significant TR. Open-heart repair may permit substantial improvement of tricuspid valve function. If this cannot be accomplished, the tricuspid valve may have to be replaced with a prosthesis, preferably a large bioprosthetic valve.

TRICUSPID REGURGITATION

Most commonly, TR is functional and secondary to marked dilatation of the tricuspid annulus. Functional TR may complicate RV enlargement of any cause, including inferior wall infarcts that involve the RV. It is commonly seen in the late stages of heart failure due to rheumatic or congenital heart disease with severe pulmonary hypertension, as well as in ischemic heart disease, cardiomyopathy, and cor pulmonale. It is in part reversible if pulmonary hypertension is relieved. Rheumatic fever may produce organic TR, often associated with TS. Infarction of RV papillary muscles, tricuspid valve prolapse, carcinoid heart disease, endomyocardial fibrosis, infective endocarditis, and trauma all may produce TR. Less commonly, TR results from congenitally deformed tricuspid valves, and it occurs with defects of the atrioventricular canal as well as with Ebstein's malformation of the tricuspid valve (Chap. 218).

As is the case for TS, the clinical features of TR result primarily from systemic venous congestion and reduction of CO. With the onset of TR in patients with pulmonary hypertension, symptoms of pulmonary congestion diminish, but the clinical manifestations of right-sided heart failure become intensified. The neck veins are distended with prominent v waves; and marked hepatomegaly, ascites, pleural effusions, edema, systolic pulsations of the liver, and a positive hepatojugular reflux are common. A prominent RV pulsation along the left parasternal region and a blowing holosystolic murmur along the lower left sternal margin, which may be intensified during inspiration and reduced during expiration or the strain of the Valsalva maneuver, are characteristic findings; AF is usually present.

The ECG usually shows changes characteristic of the lesion responsible for the enlargement of the RV that leads to TR, e.g., inferior wall myocardial infarction or severe RVH. Echocardiography may be helpful by demonstrating RV dilatation and prolapsing or flail tricuspid leaflets; the diagnosis of TR can be made by color flow Doppler echocardiography, and the severity estimated by Doppler examination. The latter is also useful in estimating PA pressure. Roentgenographic examination usually reveals enlargement of both the RA and RV.

In patients with severe TR, the CO is usually markedly reduced, and the RA pressure pulse may exhibit no x descent during early systole but a prominent c-v wave with a rapid y descent. The mean RA and the RV end-diastolic pressures are often elevated.

℞ TREATMENT

Isolated TR, in the absence of pulmonary hypertension, such as that occurring as a consequence of infective endocarditis or trauma, is usually well tolerated and does not require operation. Indeed, even total excision of an infected tricuspid valve may be well tolerated for several years if the PA pressure is normal. Treatment of the underlying cause of heart failure usually reduces the severity of functional TR by reducing the size of the tricuspid annulus. In patients with mitral valve disease and TR secondary to pulmonary hypertension and massive RV enlargement, effective surgical correction of the mitral valvular abnormality results in lowering of the PA pressures and gradual reduction or disappearance of the TR without direct treatment of the tricuspid valve. However, recovery may be much more rapid in patients with severe secondary TR if, at the time of mitral valve surgery, tricuspid annuloplasty (generally with the insertion of a plastic ring), open tricuspid valve repair, or, in the rare instance of severe organic tricuspid valve disease, tricuspid valve replacement is performed. Surgical treatment of the TR also should be carried out in patients with severe regurgitation secondary to deformity of the tricuspid valve due to rheumatic fever, particularly those *without* severe pulmonary hypertension.

PULMONIC VALVE DISEASE

The pulmonic valve is affected by rheumatic fever far less frequently than are the other valves, and it is uncommonly the seat of infective endocarditis. The most common *acquired* abnormality affecting the pulmonic valve is regurgitation secondary to dilatation of the pulmonic valve ring as a consequence of severe pulmonary hypertension. This produces the *Graham Steell murmur*, a high-pitched, decrescendo, diastolic blowing murmur along the left sternal border, which is difficult to differentiate from the far more common murmur produced by AR. It is usually of little hemodynamic significance; indeed, surgical removal or destruction of the pulmonic valve by infective endocarditis does not produce heart failure unless serious pulmonary hypertension is also present. The *carcinoid syndrome* may cause pulmonic stenosis and/or regurgitation. →*Congenital pulmonic stenosis is discussed in Chap. 218.*

VALVE REPLACEMENT

The results of replacement of any valve are dependent primarily on (1) the patient's myocardial function and general medical condition at the time of operation; (2) the technical abilities of the operative team and the quality of the postoperative care; and (3) the durability, hemodynamic characteristics, and thrombogenicity of the prosthesis. Increased operative mortality is associated with advanced age, comorbidity (e.g., pulmonary or renal disease, the need for nonvalvular cardiovascular surgery, diabetes mellitus) as well as with higher levels of preoperative functional disability and pulmonary hypertension. Late complications of valve replacement include paravalvular leakage, thromboemboli, bleeding due to anticoagulants, mechanical dysfunction of the prosthesis, and infective endocarditis.

The considerations involved in the choice between a bioprosthetic (tissue) and artificial mechanical valve are similar in the mitral and aortic sites and in the treatment of stenotic, regurgitant, or mixed lesions. All patients who have undergone replacement of any valve with a mechanical prosthesis are at risk of thromboembolic complications and must be maintained permanently on anticoagulants, a treatment that imposes a hazard of hemorrhage. The primary advantage of bioprostheses over mechanical prostheses is the virtual absence of thromboembolic complications 3 months after implantation, and except for patients with chronic AF, few such instances have been associated with their use. The major disadvantage of bioprosthetic valves is their mechanical deterioration, the incidence of which is inversely proportional to the patient's age. This results in the need to replace the prosthesis in 30% of patients by 10 years and in 50% by 15 years. Because this complication is age-related, bioprostheses are ordinarily not used in patients under 65 years but are particularly useful in the elderly (>70 years), in whom there is more concern about chronic anticoagulation than about long-term (>20 years) valve durability. Patients between 65 and 70 years should be evaluated on a case-by-case basis as to the use of a bioprosthetic or mechanical valve. Bioprosthetic valves are also indicated in women who expect to become pregnant, as well as others in whom anticoagulation may be contraindicated. Alternative bioprostheses are xenografts [i.e., porcine aortic valves; cryopreserved, mounted bovine pericardium; homograft (allograft) aortic valves obtained from cadavers as well as pulmonary autografts transplanted into the aortic position.]

In patients without contraindications to anticoagulants, particularly those under 65 years, a mechanical prosthesis may be preferable. Many surgeons now select the St. Jude prosthesis, a double-disk tilting prosthesis, for replacement of both aortic and mitral valves because of favorable hemodynamic characteristics and possible association with lower thrombogenicity.

FURTHER READING

BONOW RO et al: ACC/AHA Guidelines for the management of patients with valvular heart disease. J Am Coll Cardiol 32:1486, 1998

BONOW RD, BRAUNWALD E: Valvular heart disease, in D Zipes et al (eds): *Braunwald's Heart Disease*, 7th ed. Philadelphia, Saunders, 2005

CANNEGIETER SC et al: Oral anticoagulant treatment in patients with mechanical heart valves: How to reduce the risk of thromboembolic and bleeding complications. J Intern Med 245:369, 1999

CARABELLO BA: Aortic stenosis. N Engl J Med 346:677, 2002

ENRIQUEZ-SARANO M: Timing of mitral valve surgery. Heart 87:79, 2002

FANN JI, BURDON TA: Are the indications for tissue valves different in 2001 and how do we communicate these changes to our cardiology colleagues? Curr Opin Cardiol 16:126, 2001

HA JW et al: Tricuspid stenosis and regurgitation: Doppler and color flow echocardiography and cardiac catheterization findings. Clin Cardiol 23:51, 2000

HUNG L, RAHIMTOOLA SH: Prosthetic heart valves and pregnancy. Circulation 107:1240, 2003

JAMIESON WRE et al: Risk stratification for cardiac valve replacement. National Cardiac Surgery Database. Ann Thorac Surg 67:943, 1999

NOVARO GM et al: Effect of hydroxymethylglutaryl coenzyme A reductase inhibitors on the progression of calcific aortic stenosis. Circulation 104:2205, 2001

PALACIOS IF et al: Which patients benefit from percutaneous mitral balloon valvuloplasty? Prevalvuloplasty and postvalvuloplasty variables that predict long-term outcome. Circulation 105:1465, 2002

PEREIRA JJ et al: Survival after aortic valve replacement for severe aortic stenosis with low transvalvular gradients and severe left ventricular dysfunction. J Am Coll Cardiol 39:1356, 2002

220 PULMONARY HYPERTENSION
Stuart Rich

Pulmonary hypertension, an abnormal elevation in pulmonary artery pressure, may reflect an increase in left heart filling pressure in the presence of normal pulmonary vascular resistance, pulmonary vascular or parenchymal disease with an elevation in pulmonary vascular resistance, or a combination of these initiating factors. Whether the pulmonary hypertension arises from cardiac, pulmonary, or intrinsic vascular disease, it generally is a feature of advanced disease. Because the causes of pulmonary hypertension are so diverse, it is essential that the etiology underlying the pulmonary hypertension be clearly determined before embarking on treatment. Recent data suggest that mild increases in pulmonary artery pressure also occur with age as the pulmonary circulation becomes less compliant.

Cor pulmonale (Chap. 216) is a term used to indicate right ventricular (RV) enlargement secondary to any underlying cardiac or pulmonary disease. Pulmonary hypertension is the most common cause of cor pulmonale. Advanced cor pulmonale is associated with the development of RV failure.

PATHOPHYSIOLOGY The right ventricle responds to an increase in resistance within the pulmonary circulation by increasing RV systolic pressure as necessary to preserve cardiac output. The increase in pulmonary vascular resistance may be attributed to excessive production of vascular growth factors, mechanical obstruction of the pulmonary arteries, hypoxia, or other stimuli. Over time, chronic changes occur in the pulmonary circulation resulting in remodeling of the vasculature, which can sustain or promote pulmonary hypertension even if the initiating factor is removed.

On occasion a patient may have marked elevations in pulmonary artery pressure in association with obstructive or interstitial lung disease, essential hypertension, ischemic heart disease, or valvular heart disease. Although it may appear that the pulmonary hypertension is out of proportion to the underlying associated condition, it likely represents a pulmonary vasoconstrictor response to the associated condition, which serves as a trigger of the pulmonary arteriopathy. The distinction is important because the treatment of pulmonary hypertension should include treating the underlying associated cause whenever possible.

The ability of the right ventricle to adapt to increased vascular resistance is influenced by several factors including age and the rapidity of the development of pulmonary hypertension. For example, a large acute pulmonary thromboembolism can result in RV failure and shock, whereas chronic thromboembolic disease of equal severity may result in only mild exercise intolerance. Coexisting hypoxemia from

lung disease or myocardial ischemia from coronary artery disease can impair the ability of the ventricle to compensate. The onset of clinical RV failure, usually manifest by peripheral edema, is associated with a poor outcome.

DIAGNOSIS A thorough diagnostic evaluation of all potential causes of pulmonary hypertension should be undertaken (Fig. 220-1). The most

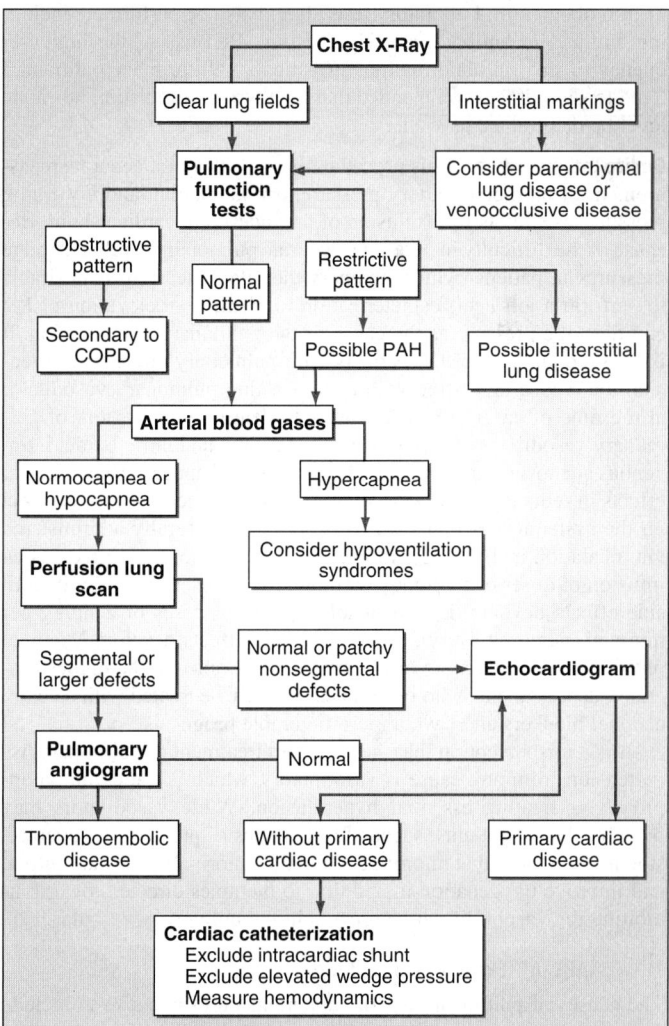

FIGURE 220-1 An algorithm for the workup of a patient with unexplained pulmonary hypertension. (*Adapted with permission from Rich.*)

common symptom attributable to pulmonary hypertension is exertional dyspnea. Other common symptoms are fatigue, angina pectoris that may represent RV ischemia, syncope, near syncope, and peripheral edema.

The physical examination typically reveals increased jugular venous pressure, a reduced carotid pulse, and a palpable RV lift. Most patients have an increased pulmonic component of the second heart sound and a right-sided fourth heart sound (Chap. 209). Tricuspid regurgitation is a clinical feature of RV failure. Peripheral cyanosis and/or edema tend to occur in later stages of the disease. The presence of clubbing can be a clinical clue that the patient has underlying congenital heart disease or hypoxemic lung disease.

Laboratory Findings The chest x-ray generally shows enlarged central pulmonary arteries. The lung fields may or may not reveal other pathology. The electrocardiogram usually reveals right axis deviation and RV hypertrophy. The echocardiogram commonly demonstrates RV and right atrial enlargement, a reduction in left ventricular (LV) cavity size, and a tricuspid regurgitant jet that can be used to estimate RV systolic pressure. Pulmonary function tests are helpful in documenting underlying obstructive airways disease or severe restrictive lung disease. Hypoxemia and an abnormal diffusing capacity for carbon monoxide are common findings of pulmonary hypertension of most causes. A perfusion lung scan is almost always abnormal in patients with thromboembolic pulmonary hypertension (Chap. 244). However, diffuse patchy filling defects of a nonsegmental nature can often be seen in longstanding pulmonary hypertension in the absence of thromboemboli. Laboratory tests should also be performed, including antinuclear antibody and HIV testing. Because of the high frequency of thyroid abnormalities in patients with primary pulmonary hypertension, it is recommended that the thyroid-stimulating hormone level be determined as well.

Cardiac Catheterization This procedure is mandatory for accurate measurement of pulmonary artery pressure, cardiac output, and LV filling pressure, as well as for exclusion of an underlying cardiac shunt. Because of the difficulty in obtaining accurate pulmonary capillary wedge pressures in patients with pulmonary vascular disease, it is desirable to perform a left heart catheterization to identify an elevation of LV end-diastolic pressure as the cause of the pulmonary hypertension. It is also recommended that patients with pulmonary arterial hypertension undergo drug testing with a short-acting pulmonary vasodilator at the time of cardiac catheterization to determine the extent of pulmonary vasodilator reactivity (Fig. 220-2). Inhaled nitric oxide, intravenous adenosine, and intravenous epoprostenol appear to have similar effects in reducing pulmonary artery pressure acutely with little effect on the systemic vascular bed. Nitric oxide is generally administered via inhalation in 10 to 20 parts per million. Adenosine is given as an infusion of doses of 50 μg/kg per min and increased every 2 min until side effects develop. Epoprostenol is given in doses of 2 ng/kg per min and increased every 30 min until side effects develop. Maximal physiologic effectiveness of the drug is determined at the highest tolerated dose. Patients who respond can usually be treated with calcium channel blockers and have a more favorable prognosis.

It is a misperception that the preferred treatment of pulmonary hypertension from any cause is vasodilators, which is the common approach to treating essential hypertension. While vasodilators may benefit selected patients, successful therapies of pulmonary hypertension include those that improve RV function, normalize cardiac output, and improve oxygenation in addition to therapies directed toward inhibiting the vasoproliferative process in the pulmonary vascular bed.

PULMONARY ARTERIAL HYPERTENSION

The causes of pulmonary arterial hypertension (Table 220-1) include primary pulmonary hypertension, pulmonary hypertension associated with the collagen vascular diseases, congenital systemic to pulmonary shunts, portal hypertension, HIV infection, anorexigen use, and per-

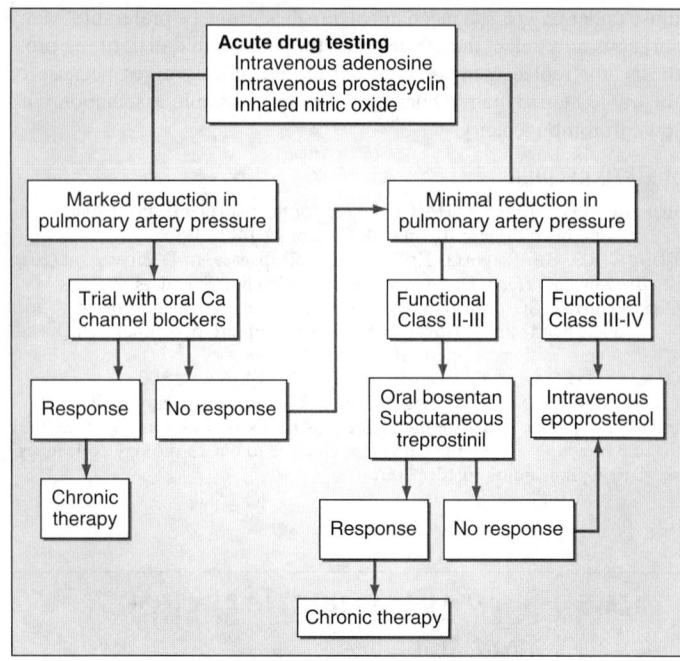

FIGURE 220-2 An algorithm for the selection of optimal drug treatment of a patient with pulmonary arterial hypertension. (*Adapted with permission from Rich.*)

sistent pulmonary hypertension of the newborn. These patients share a common histopathology that includes pulmonary vascular abnormalities involving the endothelium, smooth-muscle cells, and extracellular matrix. The most common features are medial hypertrophy, eccentric and concentric intimal fibrosis, recanalized thrombi appearing as fibrous webs, and plexiform lesions.

Pathobiology There are likely several pathobiologic processes that result in pulmonary arterial hypertension as a final common pathway. These include inhibition of the voltage-regulated potassium channel producing vasoconstriction of the pulmonary artery smooth-muscle cells, reduced expression of nitric oxide synthase in the endothelium of the pulmonary arterial bed, increased expression of endothelin and basic fibroblast growth factor, and thrombin deposition related to a procoagulant state. The types of abnormalities that occur are likely influenced by the patient's genotype and exposure to risk factors that serve to trigger these processes.

TABLE 220-1 *Additional Diagnostic Tests to Evaluate the Suspected Cause of Pulmonary Hypertension*

Cause	Diagnostic Test
Collagen vascular disease	Serologic and immunogenetic studies
Congenital heart disease	Transesophageal echocardiography with contrast
Portal hypertension	Ultrasonography, computed tomography (CT)
Human immunodeficiency virus	HIV serologic test
Left ventricular diastolic dysfunction	Left ventricular end-diastolic pressure or left atrial pressure measurement
Mitral valve disease	Echocardiography with Doppler
Mediastinal fibrosis	CT, magnetic resonance imaging
Chronic obstructive lung disease	Pulmonary function tests
Obstructive sleep apnea	Sleep apnea study
Pulmonary fibrosis	High-resolution chest CT
Interstitial pneumonitis	Transbronchial or open-lung biopsy
Pulmonary thromboembolic disease	Perfusion lung scan, contrast-enhanced Spiral CT, pulmonary angiography
Sarcoidosis	Lung or lymph node biopsy

PRIMARY PULMONARY HYPERTENSION

Primary pulmonary hypertension (PPH) is uncommon, with an estimated incidence of 2 cases per million. There is a strong female predominance, with most patients presenting in the fourth and fifth decades, although the age range is from infancy to >60 years.

GENETIC CONSIDERATIONS Familial PPH accounts for 12 to 20% of cases of PPH and is characterized by autosomal dominant inheritance, variable age of onset, and incomplete penetrance. The clinical and pathologic features of familial and sporadic PPH are identical. Heterozygous germline mutations that involve the gene coding the type II bone morphogenetic protein receptor (BMPR II), a member of the transforming growth factor β superfamily, have been found to underlie many cases of familial PPH. This gene, which is located on chromosome 2q31, has been designated as the PPH I gene. An interruption in the BMP-mediated signaling pathway predisposes the cells within the small pulmonary arteries to proliferation rather than apoptosis. These observations support the concept that PPH is a result of abnormal proliferation of pulmonary vascular endothelial and smooth-muscle cells.

NATURAL HISTORY The natural history of PPH is uncertain because initially the disease can be asymptomatic. Because the predominant symptom is dyspnea, which can have an insidious onset, the disease is typically diagnosed late in its course. Prior to current therapies, a mean survival of 2 to 3 years from the time of diagnosis was reported. It appears that the survival of patients with pulmonary hypertension secondary to congenital heart disease is longer than for patients with PPH, while the survival of patients with pulmonary hypertension secondary to scleroderma is shorter. Functional class remains a strong predictor of survival, with patients who are in New York Heart Association (NYHA) functional class IV having a mean survival of <6 months. The cause of death is usually RV failure, which is manifest by progressive hypoxemia, tachycardia, hypotension, and edema.

℞ TREATMENT

Because the pulmonary artery pressure in PPH increases dramatically with exercise, patients should be cautioned against participating in activities that demand increased physical stress. Digoxin may increase cardiac output and lower circulating levels of norepinephrine. Diuretic therapy relieves peripheral edema and may be useful in reducing RV volume overload in the presence of tricuspid regurgitation. Resting and exercise pulse oximetry should be obtained, as oxygen supplementation helps to alleviate dyspnea and RV ischemia in patients whose arterial oxygen saturation is reduced. Anticoagulant therapy is advocated for all patients with PPH since thrombin deposition occurs in the pulmonary circulation; thrombin can serve as a growth factor to promote the disease process. One retrospective study and one prospective study demonstrated that the anticoagulant warfarin increases survival of patients with PPH. The dose of warfarin is generally titrated to achieve an INR of two to three times control.

Calcium Channel Blockers Patients who have substantial reductions in pulmonary arterial pressure in response to short-acting vasodilators at the time of cardiac catheterization may be candidates for oral calcium channel blockers. Typically, patients require high doses (e.g., nifedipine, 240 mg/d, or amlodipine, 20 mg/d[1]). Patients who respond favorably usually have dramatic reductions in pulmonary artery pressure and pulmonary vascular resistance associated with improved symptoms, regression of RV hypertrophy, and improved survival with chronic therapy. However, <20% of patients respond to calcium channel blockers in the long term. These drugs can be particularly hazardous when given to patients who are unresponsive, as they can result in hypotension, hypoxemia, tachycardia, and worsening right heart failure.

---

[1]These agents have not been approved for the treatment of primary pulmonary hypertension by the U.S. Food and Drug Administration.

Prostacyclins *Epoprostenol* is the best characterized approved treatment of pulmonary arterial hypertension for patients who are NYHA functional class III or IV and unresponsive to other therapies. Clinical trials have demonstrated an improvement in symptoms, exercise tolerance, and survival even if no acute hemodynamic response to drug challenge occurs. Recent reports have documented sustained benefits for >10 years in some patients. The drug can only be administered intravenously and requires placement of a permanent central venous catheter and infusion through an ambulatory infusion pump system. It generally takes several months to titrate the dose gradually upwards to optimal clinical efficacy, which is usually between 25 and 50 ng/kg per min. Side effects include flushing, jaw pain, and diarrhea, which are generally tolerated by most patients. The major problem with this therapy is infection related to the venous catheter, which requires close monitoring and diligence on behalf of the patient.

Recently, *treprostinil* has been approved for patients with PPH who are NYHA functional classes II to IV and who are unresponsive to conventional therapy, defined as anticoagulation, diuretics, and calcium blockers. An analogue of epoprostenol, treprostinil has a longer half-life and is stable at room temperature, allowing it to be administered subcutaneously through a small infusion pump that was originally developed for insulin. Short-term clinical trials have demonstrated an increase in exercise capacity and a reduction of dyspnea. The major problem with this treatment has been local pain at the infusion site, which has caused patients to discontinue therapy.

Endothelin Receptor Antagonists The nonselective endothelin receptor antagonist *bosentan* was recently approved as an oral treatment of PPH for patients who are NYHA functional classes III and IV and who are unresponsive to conventional therapy. In randomized clinical trials, bosentan was shown to improve exercise tolerance as measured by an increase in 6-min walk distance, improve functional class, and extend time until clinical worsening versus placebo. Therapy is initiated at 62.5 mg bid for the first month and then increased to 125 mg bid thereafter. Because of the high frequency of abnormal hepatic function tests associated with drug use, primarily an increase in transaminases, it is recommended that liver function be monitored monthly throughout the duration of use. Bosentan is also contraindicated in patients who are currently on cyclosporine or glyburide. There are no data to support the use of bosentan for other forms of pulmonary hypertension.

Sildenafil There have been several case reports on the use of sildenafil (Viagra), an oral phosphodiesterase-5 inhibitor, in the treatment of pulmonary hypertension. Phosphodiesterase-5 is responsible for the hydrolysis of cyclic GMP in pulmonary vascular smooth muscles, the mediator through which nitric oxide lowers pulmonary artery pressure and inhibits pulmonary vascular growth. These reports suggest that oral sildenafil has a similar efficacy to inhaled nitric oxide. Large randomized clinical trials using sildenafil as a treatment of pulmonary hypertension are under consideration.

Lung Transplantation (See also Chap. 248) Lung transplantation is considered for patients who, while on epoprostenol, continue to manifest right heart failure. Acceptable results have been achieved with heart-lung, bilateral lung, and single lung transplant. The availability of donor organs often influences the choice of procedure. The recurrence of PPH has never been reported in a patient who has undergone lung transplantation.

CONDITIONS ASSOCIATED WITH PULMONARY HYPERTENSION

COLLAGEN VASCULAR DISEASE All of the collagen vascular diseases may be associated with pulmonary arterial hypertension. This complication occurs commonly with the CREST syndrome (calcinosis, Raynaud's phenomenon, esophageal involvement, sclerodactyly, and telangiectasia) and in scleroderma (Chap. 303), and less frequently in systemic lupus erythematosus (Chap. 300), Sjögrens syndrome (Chap. 304), dermatomyositis, polymyositis (Chap. 306), and rheumatoid arthritis (Chap. 301). It is usual for these patients to have some element of coexistent interstitial pulmonary fibrosis even though it may not be apparent on chest x-ray, computed tomography, or pulmonary function tests. Consequently, these patients tend to have hypoxemia as an important clinical feature, along with the other classic findings of pulmonary hypertension.

Treatment for these patients is identical to that for patients with PPH (see above) but is less effective. It is rare for these patients to respond to calcium channel blockers. Bosentan, treprostinil, and epoprostenol have been effective in clinical trials. The treatment of the pulmonary hypertension, however, does not affect the natural history of the underlying collagen vascular disease.

CONGENITAL SYSTEMIC TO PULMONARY SHUNTS It is common for large post-tricuspid cardiac shunts (e.g., ventricular septal defect, patent ductus arteriosus) to produce severe pulmonary hypertension (Chap. 218), which, although less common, may also occur in pre-tricuspid shunts (e.g., atrial septal defect, anomalous pulmonary venous drainage). In patients with uncorrected shunts, the clinical features include those associated with right-to-left shunting such as hypoxemia and peripheral cyanosis, which worsen dramatically with exertion (Chap. 31). Pulmonary arterial hypertension may occur years or even decades after surgical correction of these lesions, in which case there will be no associated right-to-left shunting. These patients present similarly to patients with PPH but tend to have better long-term survival. This has been attributed to the more slowly progressive nature of the underlying vascular disease. The treatments are similar to those for PPH.

PORTAL HYPERTENSION Portal hypertension is associated with pulmonary arterial hypertension, but the mechanism remains unknown. The risk is not related to the severity of underlying liver disease. Patients with advanced cirrhosis can have the combined features of a high-output cardiac state in association with the features of pulmonary hypertension and RV failure. Thus, a normal cardiac output may actually reflect a marked impairment of RV function. The etiology of ascites and edema can be confusing in these patients since it can have both cardiac and hepatic causes. Venous congestion from right heart failure, however, is poorly tolerated by cirrhotic livers. Patients with mild pulmonary hypertension who have a favorable response to epoprostenol have undergone successful liver transplantation with improvement of the pulmonary vascular disease.

HIV INFECTION The mechanism by which HIV infection produces pulmonary hypertension remains unknown (Chap. 173). The evaluation and treatment are identical to those for PPH. Treatment of the HIV infection does not appear to affect the severity or natural history of the underlying pulmonary hypertension.

ANOREXIGENS A causal relationship has been established between exposure to several anorexigens, including aminorex and the fenfluramines, and the development of pulmonary arterial hypertension. Although the fenfluramines were removed from the world markets in 1997, there are still patients who were exposed prior to that time who are now developing pulmonary hypertension. While the clinical features are identical to those of PPH, the patients appear to be less responsive to medical treatments and have a poorer prognosis.

PULMONARY VENOOCCLUSIVE DISEASE Pulmonary venoocclusive disease is a rare and distinct pathologic entity found in <10% of patients who present with the diagnosis of unexplained pulmonary hypertension. Histologically it is manifest by widespread intimal proliferation and fibrosis of the intrapulmonary veins and venules, occasionally extending to the arteriolar bed. The pulmonary venous obstruction explains the increase in pulmonary capillary wedge pressure observed in patients with advanced disease. These patients may develop orthopnea that can mimic LV failure. The therapy of this condition is not established.

PULMONARY CAPILLARY HEMANGIOMATOSIS Pulmonary capillary hemangiomatosis is a very rare form of pulmonary hypertension. Histologically it is characterized by the presence of infiltrating thin-walled blood vessels throughout the pulmonary interstitium and walls of the pulmonary arteries and veins. The presenting symptoms are usually those of PPH but often with hemoptysis as a clinical feature. The diagnosis can be made with pulmonary angiography. The clinical course is usually one of progressive deterioration leading to severe pulmonary hypertension, right-sided heart failure, and death. There is no established therapy.

PULMONARY VENOUS HYPERTENSION

Pulmonary hypertension occurs as a result of increased resistance to pulmonary venous drainage. It is often associated with diastolic dysfunction of the left ventricle; diseases affecting the pericardium or mitral or aortic valves; or rare entities such as cor triatriatum, left atrial myxoma, extrinsic compression of the central pulmonary veins from fibrosing mediastinitis, and pulmonary venoocclusive disease. Pulmonary venous hypertension affects the pulmonary veins and venules, producing arterialization of the external elastic lamina, medial hypertrophy, and focal eccentric intimal fibrosis. Microcirculatory lesions include capillary congestion, focal alveolar edema, and dilatation of the interstitial lymphatics. Although these lesions are potentially reversible, regression may take years after the underlying cause is removed. In some patients pulmonary venous hypertension triggers reactive vasoconstriction in the pulmonary arterial bed and results in proliferative changes of the intima and media that can produce severe elevations in pulmonary artery pressure. Clinically it may be confusing and appear as if two separate disease processes are occurring simultaneously.

LEFT VENTRICULAR DIASTOLIC DYSFUNCTION Pulmonary hypertension as a result of LV diastolic failure is common but often unrecognized (Chap. 216). It can occur with or without LV systolic failure. The most common causes are hypertensive heart disease; coronary artery disease; or impaired LV compliance related to age, diabetes, and hypoxemia. Symptoms of orthopnea and paroxysmal nocturnal dyspnea are prominent. Many patients improve considerably if LV end-diastolic pressure is lowered.

MITRAL VALVE DISEASE Mitral stenosis and mitral regurgitation represent important causes of pulmonary hypertension (Chap. 219). These patients often have superimposed pulmonary vasoconstriction resulting in marked elevations in pulmonary artery pressures. An echocardiogram usually shows abnormalities such as thickened mitral valve leaflets with reduced mobility or severe mitral regurgitation documented by Doppler echocardiography (Chap. 211). At cardiac catheterization a pressure gradient between the pulmonary capillary wedge pressure and LV end-diastolic pressure is diagnostic of mitral stenosis.

In patients with mitral stenosis corrective surgery of the mitral valve or mitral balloon valvuloplasty predictably results in a reduction in pulmonary artery pressure and pulmonary vascular resistance. Patients with mitral regurgitation, however, may not have as dramatic a response from surgery due to persistent elevations in LV end-diastolic pressure.

PULMONARY HYPERTENSION ASSOCIATED WITH LUNG DISEASE AND HYPOXEMIA

The mechanism of hypoxic pulmonary vasoconstriction involves the inhibition of potassium currents and membrane depolarization of pulmonary vascular smooth muscle as a result of the change in membrane sulfhydryl redox status. Increased calcium entry into the vascular smooth-muscle cells mediates hypoxic pulmonary vasoconstriction. Pulmonary vascular remodeling in response to chronic hypoxia is also mediated by a reduction in nitric oxide production; an increase in endothelin 1; and increased expression of platelet-derived growth factors, vascular endothelial growth factor, and angiotensin II. Chronic hypoxia results in muscularization of the arterioles with minimal effects on the intima. When it occurs as an isolated entity, the changes produced are potentially reversible.

Although chronic hypoxia is an established cause of pulmonary hypertension, it rarely leads to an increase in the mean pulmonary artery pressure >40 mmHg. Polycythemia in response to the hypoxemia is a characteristic finding. Hypoxia may also occur in conjunction with other causes of pulmonary hypertension associated with more extensive vascular changes. Clinically, the hypoxia will tend to have an added adverse affect. Patients with chronic hypoxia who have a marked elevation in pulmonary pressure should be evaluated for other causes of the pulmonary hypertension.

CHRONIC OBSTRUCTIVE LUNG DISEASE Chronic obstructive lung disease (COLD) is a common cause of pulmonary hypertension in the advanced stages (Chap. 242). Pulmonary hypertension has been attributed to multiple factors, including hypoxic pulmonary vasoconstriction, acidemia, hypercapnia, the mechanical effects of high lung volume on pulmonary vessels, the loss of small vessels in the vascular bed, and regions of emphysematous lung destruction.

Although the elevation of pulmonary artery pressure associated with COLD tends to be mild, the presence of pulmonary hypertension confers a worse outcome. The only effective therapy is supplemental oxygen. Several large clinical trials have documented that continuous oxygen therapy relieves some of the pulmonary vasoconstriction, relieves chronic ischemia throughout the systemic and pulmonary vascular beds, and improves survival. Long-term oxygen therapy is indicated if the resting arterial P_{O_2} remains <55 mmHg.

INTERSTITIAL LUNG DISEASE Pulmonary hypertension from interstitial lung disease is often associated with obliteration of the pulmonary vascular bed by lung destruction and fibrosis (Chap. 243). In addition, hypoxemia and pulmonary vasculopathy can be contributory factors. A large number of patients have pulmonary fibrosis of unknown etiology. Interstitial lung disease is often associated with the collagen vascular diseases. Patients are commonly older than 50 years and report an insidious onset of progressive dyspnea and cough for months to years. A definitive diagnosis requires an open-lung biopsy to rule out other diseases such as bronchiolitis obliterans, nonspecific interstitial pneumonia, and hypersensitivity pneumonitis. Management of these disorders is discussed in Chap. 243. None of the medical treatments developed for pulmonary arterial hypertension have been shown to be effective in these patients.

SLEEP-DISORDERED BREATHING *Sleep apnea*, defined as repeated episodes of obstructive apnea and hypopnea during sleep together with daytime somnolence and altered cardiopulmonary function, is a common condition (Chap. 247). The incidence of pulmonary hypertension in the setting of obstructive sleep apnea appears to be <20% and is generally mild. Therapeutic strategies for patients with sleep apnea should be directed towards establishing normal nocturnal oxygenation and ventilation, abolishing snoring, eliminating disruption of sleep due to upper airway closure, and avoiding factors that tend to aggravate the condition such as alcohol, sedatives, and hypnotic agents. The most important advance in medical treatment has been positive airway pressure delivered through a face mask during sleep.

When mild pulmonary hypertension is associated with sleep apnea, the treatments directed towards the sleep apnea are often effective in reducing pulmonary arterial pressure. Some patients, however, will present with severe pulmonary hypertension in conjunction with sleep apnea, which may or may not be related. In these cases it is recommended that the patients be treated for sleep apnea for a minimum of 3 months before treating the pulmonary arterial hypertension as a separate entity.

ALVEOLAR HYPOVENTILATION Pulmonary hypertension can occur in patients with chronic hypoventilation and hypoxia secondary to thoracovertebral deformities. Symptoms are slowly progressive and related to hypoxemia (Chap. 246). In patients with advanced disease, intermittent positive-pressure breathing and supplemental oxygen have been used successfully.

Pulmonary hypertension secondary to hypoxemia has been reported in patients with neuromuscular disease as a result of generalized weakness of the respiratory muscles and in patients with diaphragmatic paralysis. Diaphragmatic paralysis is generally a result of trauma to the phrenic nerve. Patients with nontraumatic bilateral diaphragmatic paralysis may go unrecognized until they present with either respiratory failure or pulmonary hypertension.

PULMONARY HYPERTENSION DUE TO THROMBOEMBOLIC DISEASE
ACUTE PULMONARY THROMBOEMBOLISM See Chap. 244

CHRONIC THROMBOEMBOLIC PULMONARY HYPERTENSION Patients appropriately treated for acute pulmonary thromboembolism with intravenous heparin and chronic oral warfarin therapy rarely develop chronic pulmonary hypertension. However, there is a subset of patients with impaired fibrinolytic resolution of the thromboembolism, which leads to organization and incomplete recanalization and chronic obstruction of the pulmonary vascular bed. The entity of chronic thromboembolic pulmonary hypertension has been well characterized and often mimics PPH. In many patients, the initial pulmonary thromboembolism was undetected or untreated.

Diagnosis The physical examination is typical of pulmonary hypertension but may include bruits heard over areas of the lung, representing blood flow through vessels with partial occlusion. A perfusion lung scan or contrast-enhanced spiral computed tomography scan usually reveals underlying thromboemboli. However, pulmonary angiography is necessary to determine the precise location and proximal extent of the thromboemboli, and hence the potential for operability.

℞ TREATMENT

Pulmonary thromboendarterectomy is an established surgical treatment in patients whose thrombi are accessible to surgical removal. The operative mortality is fairly high, at ~12% in experienced centers. Postoperative survivors who have a good result can expect to realize an improvement in functional class and exercise tolerance. Life-long anticoagulation using warfarin is mandatory. Thrombolytic therapy is rarely of help in patients with chronic thromboembolic pulmonary hypertension and may expose these patients to the increased risk of bleeding without potential benefit. Patients who are not surgical candidates have a poor outcome.

SICKLE CELL DISEASE Cardiovascular system abnormalities are prominent in the clinical spectrum of sickle cell disease, and pulmonary hypertension has been reported to occur in 20% of patients (Chap. 91). The pulmonary hypertension can usually be attributed to LV diastolic dysfunction. Although patients with sickle cell disease have an increased risk of thromboembolism, sickle cell disease rarely produces pulmonary arterial hypertension.

OTHER DISORDERS DIRECTLY AFFECTING PULMONARY VASCULATURE
SARCOIDOSIS Sarcoidosis can produce severe pulmonary hypertension as a result of chronic severe fibrocystic lung involvement (Chap. 309). In addition, direct cardiovascular involvement can coexist. Consequently, patients with sarcoidosis who present with progressive dyspnea and clinical features of pulmonary hypertension need a thorough evaluation. There is a subset of patients with sarcoidosis who present with severe pulmonary hypertension believed to be due to direct pulmonary vascular involvement. Many of these patients exhibit a favorable response to intravenous epoprostenol therapy.

SCHISTOSOMIASIS Although extremely rare in North America, schistosomiasis is the most common cause of pulmonary hypertension worldwide (Chap. 203). The development of pulmonary hypertension almost always occurs in the setting of hepatosplenic disease and portal hypertension. Schistosome ova can embolize from the liver to the lungs, where they result in an inflammatory pulmonary vascular reaction and chronic changes. The diagnosis is confirmed by finding the parasite ova in the urine or stools of patients with symptoms, which can be difficult. The efficacy of therapies directed towards pulmonary hypertension in these patients is unknown.

FURTHER READING

ARCHER S, RICH S: Primary pulmonary hypertension: A vascular biology and translational research "Work in Progress." Circulation 102:2781, 2000

HUMBERT M, TREMBATH RC: Genetics of pulmonary hypertension: From bench to bedside. Eur Respir J 20:741, 2002

MCLAUGHLIN WV, SHILLINGTON A et al: Survival in primary pulmonary hypertension: The impact of epoprostenol therapy. Circulation 106:1477, 2002

MICHELAKIS E et al: Oral sildenafil is an effective and specific pulmonary vasodilator in patients with pulmonary arterial hypertension. Circulation 105:2398, 2002

RICH S: Primary pulmonary hypertension, in *World Symposium—Primary Pulmonary Hypertension*, S Rich (ed). 1998. Also available from the World Health Organization via the Internet (*http://www.who.int/ncd/cvd/pph.html*)

RUBIN L et al: Bosentan therapy for pulmonary arterial hypertension. N Engl J Med 346:896, 2002

SIMONNEAU G et al: Continuous subcutaneous infusion of treprostinil, a prostacyclin analogue, in patients with pulmonary arterial hypertension: A double-blind, randomized, placebo-controlled trial. Am J Respir Crit Care Med 165:800, 2002

---

221 CARDIOMYOPATHY AND MYOCARDITIS
Joshua Wynne, Eugene Braunwald

The cardiomyopathies are a group of diseases that affect the heart muscle itself and are not the result of hypertension or congenital or acquired valvular, coronary, or pericardial abnormalities. The diffuse myocardial fibrosis that accompanies multiple myocardial scars produced by extensive coronary artery disease can impair left ventricular function and is frequently referred to as *ischemic cardiomyopathy*. This colloquial use of the term should be avoided; the term *cardiomyopathy* should be restricted to a condition *primarily* involving the myocardium. When the cardiomyopathies are classified on an etiologic basis, two fundamental forms are recognized: (1) a primary type, consisting of heart muscle disease of unknown cause; and (2) a secondary type, consisting of myocardial disease of known cause or associated with a disease involving other organ systems (Table 221-1). (In the World Health Organization classification, the term *specific cardiomyopathy* is used to describe heart muscle diseases associated with certain systemic or cardiac disorders; examples include hypertensive and metabolic cardiomyopathy.) In many cases, however, it is not possible to arrive at a specific etiologic diagnosis, and thus it is often more desirable to classify the cardiomyopathies into one of three types

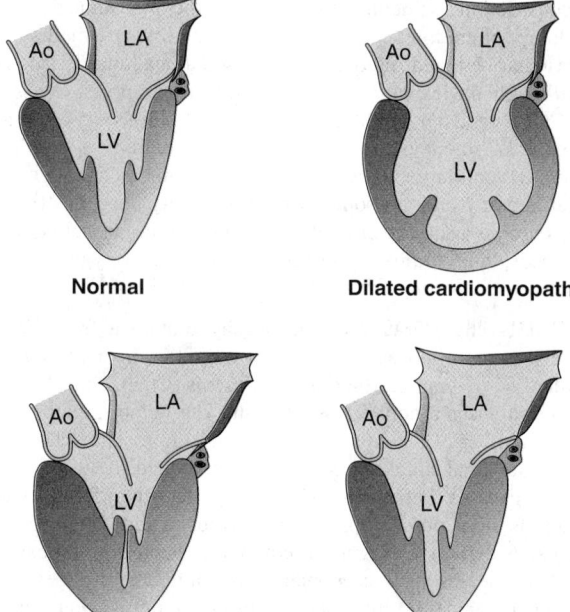

FIGURE 221-1 Drawing comparing the three broad classes of cardiomyopathies. Ao, aorta; LA, left atrium; LV, left ventricle. (*From BF Waller: J Am Soc Echocardiogr 1:4, 1988.*)

(dilated, restrictive, hypertrophic) on the basis of differences in their pathophysiology and clinical presentation (Fig. 221-1; Tables 221-2 and 221-3).

DILATED CARDIOMYOPATHY

About one in three cases of congestive heart failure (CHF) is due to dilated cardiomyopathy, with the remainder the consequence of coronary artery disease. Left and/or right ventricular systolic pump function is impaired, leading to progressive cardiac enlargement and hypertrophy, a process called *remodeling*. Symptoms of CHF typically appear only after remodeling has been ongoing for some time (months or even years). There is, however, no close correlation between the degree of contractile dysfunction and the severity of symptoms.

Although no cause is apparent in many cases, dilated cardiomyopathy is probably the end result of myocardial damage produced by

---

TABLE 221-1 *Etiologic Classification of Cardiomyopathies*

PRIMARY MYOCARDIAL INVOLVEMENT

Idiopathic (D,R,H)
Familial (D,R,H)
Eosinophilic endomyocardial disease (R)
Endomyocardial fibrosis (R)

SECONDARY MYOCARDIAL INVOLVEMENT

Infective (D)	Connective tissue disorders (D)
Viral myocarditis	Systemic lupus erythematosus
Bacterial myocarditis	Polyarteritis nodosa
Fungal myocarditis	Rheumatoid arthritis
Protozoal myocarditis	Progressive systemic sclerosis
Metazoal myocarditis	Dermatomyositis
Spirochetal	Infiltrations and granulomas (R,D)
Rickettsial	Amyloidosis
Metabolic (D)	Sarcoidosis
Familial storage disease (D,R)	Malignancy
Glycogen storage disease	Neuromuscular (D)
Mucopolysaccharidoses	Muscular dystrophy
Hemochromatosis	Myotonic dystrophy
Fabry's disease	Friedreich's ataxia (H,D)
Deficiency (D)	Sensitivity and toxic reactions (D)
Electrolytes	Alcohol
Nutritional	Radiation
	Drugs
	Peripartum heart disease (D)

Note: The principal clinical manifestation(s) of each etiologic grouping is denoted by D (dilated), R (restrictive), or H (hypertrophic) cardiomyopathy.
Source: Adapted from the WHO/ISFC task force report on the definition and classification of cardiomyopathies, 1980.

TABLE 221-2 *Clinical Classification of Cardiomyopathies*

1. Dilated: Left and/or right ventricular enlargement, impaired systolic function, congestive heart failure, arrhythmias, emboli
2. Restrictive: Endomyocardial scarring or myocardial infiltration resulting in restriction to left and/or right ventricular filling
3. Hypertrophic: Disproportionate left ventricular hypertrophy, typically involving septum more than free wall, with or without an intraventricular systolic pressure gradient; usually of a nondilated left ventricular cavity

a variety of toxic, metabolic, or infectious agents. Dilated cardiomyopathy may be the late sequel of acute viral myocarditis, possibly mediated through an immunologic mechanism. Although it may occur in any patient population, it is most commonly a disease of middle-aged men and is more common in African Americans than in whites. The prevalence of this condition is increasing. A reversible form of dilated cardiomyopathy may be found with alcohol abuse, pregnancy, thyroid disease, cocaine use, and chronic uncontrolled tachycardia. Obesity increases the risk of developing heart failure, as does sleep apnea. At least 20% (and perhaps as many as 40%) of patients have familial forms of the disease, with mutations of genes encoding cytoskeletal (such as the dystrophin and desmin genes), contractile, nuclear membrane (such as the lamin A/C gene), and other proteins. The disease is genetically heterogeneous but most commonly autosomal dominant in transmission; autosomal recessive, mitochondrial (especially in children), and X-linked inheritance is found as well.

Right ventricular dysplasia is a unique familial cardiomyopathy marked by progressive replacement of the right ventricular wall with adipose tissue. Often associated with ventricular arrhythmias, the clinical course is variable, but sudden death is a constant threat. Catheter ablation of arrhythmia sites and insertion of an implantable cardioverter-defibrillator are often employed.

CLINICAL MANIFESTATIONS Symptoms of left- and right-sided congestive failure develop gradually in most patients (Chap. 216). Some patients have left ventricular dilatation for months or even years before becoming symptomatic. Although vague chest pain may be present, typical angina pectoris is unusual and suggests the presence of concomitant ischemic heart disease. Syncope due to arrhythmias and systemic embolism (often emanating from a ventricular thrombus) may occur.

PHYSICAL EXAMINATION Variable degrees of cardiac enlargement and findings of CHF are noted. In patients with advanced disease, the pulse pressure is narrow and the jugular venous pressure is elevated. Third and fourth heart sounds are common, and mitral or tricuspid regurgitation may occur.

LABORATORY EXAMINATIONS The chest roentgenogram demonstrates enlargement of the cardiac silhouette due to left ventricular dilatation, although generalized cardiomegaly is often seen. The lung fields may demonstrate evidence of pulmonary venous hypertension and interstitial or alveolar edema. The electrocardiogram often shows sinus tachycardia or atrial fibrillation, ventricular arrhythmias, left atrial abnormality, diffuse nonspecific ST-T-wave abnormalities and sometimes intraventricular conduction defects and low voltage. Echocardiography and radionuclide ventriculography show left ventricular dilatation, with normal, minimally thickened, or thinned walls, and systolic dysfunction (reduced ejection fraction). The detection of elevated circulating levels of brain natriuretic peptide (Chaps. 32 and 216) may help clarify which patients with dyspnea of uncertain etiology actually have heart failure rather than pulmonary disease as the cause of their symptoms, and indentifies patients at increased risk of sudden death.

Cardiac catheterization and coronary angiography are often performed to exclude ischemic heart disease, and bedside hemodynamic monitoring may be helpful in the management of the acutely decompensated patient. Angiography reveals a dilated, diffusely hypokinetic left ventricle, often with some degree of mitral regurgitation. Transvenous endomyocardial biopsy is usually not necessary in idiopathic

TABLE 221-3 *Laboratory Evaluation of the Cardiomyopathies*

	Dilated	Restrictive	Hypertrophic
Chest roentgenogram	Moderate to marked cardiac silhouette enlargement Pulmonary venous hypertension	Mild cardiac silhouette enlargement	Mild to moderate cardiac silhouette enlargement
Electrocardiogram	ST-segment and T-wave abnormalities	Low voltage, conduction defects	ST-segment and T-wave abnormalities Left ventricular hypertrophy Abnormal Q waves
Echocardiogram	Left ventricular dilatation and dysfunction	Increased left ventricular wall thickness Normal or mildly reduced systolic function	Asymmetric septal hypertrophy (ASH) Systolic anterior motion (SAM) of the mitral valve
Radionuclide studies	Left ventricular dilatation and dysfunction (RVG)	Normal or mildly reduced systolic function (RVG)	Vigorous systolic function (RVG) Perfusion defect (^{201}Tl)
Cardiac catheterization	Left ventricular dilatation and dysfunction Elevated left- and often right-sided filling pressures Diminished cardiac output	Normal or mildly reduced systolic function Elevated left- and right-sided filling pressures	Vigorous systolic function Dynamic left ventricular outflow obstruction Elevated left- and right-sided filling pressures

Note: RVG, radionuclide ventriculogram; ^{201}Tl, thallium 201.

or familial dilated cardiomyopathy. However, it may be helpful in the recognition of secondary cardiomyopathies, such as amyloidosis and acute myocarditis.

 TREATMENT

Most patients pursue an inexorably downhill course, and the majority, particularly those >55 years, die within 3 years of the onset of symptoms. African Americans are more likely to suffer progressive heart failure and death than Caucasians. Spontaneous improvement or stabilization occurs in about a quarter of patients. Death is due to either CHF or ventricular tachy- or bradyarrhythmia; sudden death is a constant threat. Systemic embolization is a concern, and patients should be considered for chronic anticoagulation. Standard therapy of heart failure with salt restriction, angiotensin-converting enzyme (ACE) inhibitors, diuretics, and digitalis produces symptomatic improvement (Chap. 216). An angiotensin II receptor blocker may be substituted in ACE-intolerant patients. Most patients should be treated with a β-adrenergic blocker. Spironolactone should be added for most patients with recent or current advanced heart failure. Some patients with dilated cardiomyopathy who have biopsy evidence of myocardial inflammation have been treated with immunosuppressive therapy, but long-term evidence of efficacy is lacking. Alcohol should be avoided because of its cardiac toxic effects, as should calcium channel blockers and nonsteroidal anti-inflammatory drugs. Antiarrhythmic agents are best avoided for fear of proarrhythmia, unless they are needed to treat symptomatic or serious arrhythmias. For the one in three patients with an intraventricular conduction delay (such as right or left bundle branch block), biventricular pacing (termed *resynchronization therapy*) improves symptoms, reduces hospitalizations, and perhaps reduces mortality. Insertion of an implantable cardioverter-defibrillator is useful in patients with symptomatic ventricular arrhythmias, and its use in other patients is evolving. In patients with advanced disease who are refractory to medical therapy, cardiac transplantation should be considered (Chap. 217).

ALCOHOLIC CARDIOMYOPATHY Individuals who consume large quantities of alcohol over many years may develop a clinical picture identical to idiopathic dilated cardiomyopathy. The risk of developing cardiomyopathy is partially genetically determined. Reducing or ceasing alcohol consumption before severe heart failure has developed may halt the progression or even reverse the course of this disease. Alcoholic patients with advanced heart failure have a poor prognosis, particularly if they continue to drink; fewer than one-quarter survive 3 years.

A second presentation of alcoholic cardiotoxicity may be found in individuals without overt heart failure and consists of recurrent supraventricular or ventricular tachyarrhythmias. Termed the *holiday heart syndrome*, it typically appears after a drinking binge; atrial fibrillation is seen most frequently, followed by atrial flutter and ventricular premature depolarizations.

PERIPARTUM CARDIOMYOPATHY (See also Chap. 6)   Cardiac dilatation and CHF of unexplained cause may develop during the last trimester of pregnancy or within 6 months after delivery; most women develop symptoms in the month before or immediately after delivery. The patient who develops peripartum cardiomyopathy typically is multiparous, African American, and over the age of 30, although the disease may be found in a wide spectrum of patients. The symptoms, signs, and treatment are similar to those in patients with idiopathic dilated cardiomyopathy. The mortality rate is around 10 to 20%. The prognosis in these patients appears to be related to whether the heart size returns to normal after the first episode of CHF. If it does, subsequent pregnancies may sometimes be tolerated, albeit with an increased risk of recurrent heart failure; if the heart remains enlarged, however, further pregnancies frequently produce additional myocardial damage, ultimately leading to refractory CHF and death. Those who recover should be encouraged to avoid further pregnancies, particularly if cardiomegaly persists.

NEUROMUSCULAR DISEASE (See also Chap. 367)   Cardiac involvement is common in many of the muscular dystrophies. In *Duchenne's progressive muscular dystrophy*, mutations in a gene that encodes a cardiac structural protein (*dystrophin*) lead to myocyte death. Myocardial involvement is most frequently indicated by a distinctive and unique electrocardiographic pattern consisting of tall R waves in right precordial leads with an R/S ratio >1.0, often associated with deep Q waves in the limb and lateral precordial leads. A variety of supraventricular and ventricular arrhythmias are frequently found. Rapidly progressive CHF may develop despite extended periods of apparent circulatory stability during which the only detectable abnormalities are in the electrocardiogram. *Myotonic dystrophy* is characterized by a variety of electrocardiographic abnormalities, especially disorders of impulse formation and conduction, but other overt clinical evidence of heart disease is uncommon. Because of these abnormalities, syncope and sudden death are major hazards; in appropriate patients, insertion of a permanent pacemaker may be effective. Involvement of the heart is very common in *Friedreich's ataxia* (manifested by abnormal electrocardiographic or echocardiographic findings), with as many as half the patients developing cardiac symptoms. The electrocardiogram most commonly demonstrates ST-segment and T-wave abnormalities. The echocardiogram may demonstrate left ventricular hypertrophy, with either symmetric or asymmetric hypertrophy of the left ventricular septum compared with the free wall. Although morphologically similar to some cases of hypertrophic cardiomyopathy, cellular disarray is lacking.

DRUGS   A variety of pharmacologic agents may damage the myocardium acutely, producing a pattern of inflammation (myocarditis), or they may lead to chronic damage of the type seen with idiopathic dilated cardiomyopathy. Certain drugs produce only electrocardiographic abnormalities, while others may precipitate fulminant CHF and death.

The anthracycline derivatives, particularly doxorubicin (Adriamycin), are powerful antineoplastic agents that, when given in high doses (>550 mg/m² for doxorubicin), may produce fatal heart failure. The incidence of heart failure is related not only to the dose of the drug but also to the presence or absence of several risk factors (cardiac irradiation, age >70 years, underlying heart disease, hypertension, treatment with cyclophosphamide); at any dose of doxorubicin, patients with these risk factors have an eight- to tenfold greater frequency

of developing heart failure than do patients lacking them. Radionuclide ventriculography and echocardiography, usually combined with exercise stress, may document preclinical deterioration of left ventricular function and allow appropriate dose adjustments. By monitoring left ventricular function, it is often possible to continue doxorubicin even in patients at high risk for developing heart failure. Efforts to modify the dose schedule by giving the drug more slowly, along with the selective use of potentially cardioprotective agents such as the iron-chelator dexrazoxone, have further reduced the risk of cardiotoxicity. Some patients with CHF, even those with severe depression of left ventricular function, have demonstrated recovery of cardiac function with aggressive management with ACE inhibitors and diuretics. In others, late asymptomatic contractile dysfunction may occur, even in those without initial cardiotoxicity.

High-dose *cyclophosphamide* may produce CHF acutely or within 2 weeks of administration; a characteristic histopathologic feature is myocardial edema and hemorrhagic necrosis. Electrocardiographic changes and arrhythmias may result from treatment with tricyclic antidepressants, the phenothiazines, emetine, lithium, and various aerosol propellants. *Cocaine abuse* is associated with a variety of life-threatening cardiac complications, including sudden death, myocarditis, dilated cardiomyopathy, and acute myocardial infarction (resulting from coronary spasm and/or thrombosis with or without underlying coronary artery stenosis). Nitrates, calcium channel blockers, and benzodiazepines have been used to treat cocaine-induced cardiotoxicities; β-adrenergic blockers should be avoided.

HYPERTROPHIC CARDIOMYOPATHY

Hypertrophic cardiomyopathy (HCM) is characterized by left ventricular hypertrophy, typically of a nondilated chamber, without obvious cause such as hypertension or aortic stenosis. It is found in about 1 in 500 of the general population. Two features of HCM have attracted the greatest attention: (1) asymmetric left ventricular hypertrophy, often with preferential hypertrophy of the interventricular septum; and (2) a dynamic left ventricular outflow tract pressure gradient, related to a narrowing of the subaortic area as a consequence of the midsystolic apposition of the anterior mitral valve leaflet against the hypertrophied septum, i.e., systolic anterior motion (SAM) of the mitral valve. Initial studies of this disease emphasized the dynamic "obstructive" features, and it has been termed *idiopathic hypertrophic subaortic stenosis* and *hypertrophic obstructive cardiomyopathy*. It has become clear, however, that only about one-quarter of patients with HCM demonstrate an outflow tract pressure gradient. The ubiquitous pathophysiologic abnormality is not systolic but rather *diastolic* dysfunction (Chap. 215), characterized by increased stiffness of the hypertrophied muscle. This results in elevated diastolic filling pressures and is present despite a hyperdynamic left ventricle.

The pattern of hypertrophy is distinctive in HCM and differs from that seen in secondary hypertrophy (as in hypertension). Most patients have striking regional variations in the extent of hypertrophy in different portions of the left ventricle, and the majority demonstrate a ventricular septum whose thickness is disproportionately increased when compared with the free wall. Other patients may demonstrate disproportionate involvement of the apex or left ventricular free wall; 10% or more of patients have concentric involvement of the ventricle. A bizarre and disorganized arrangement of cardiac muscle cells in the septum occurs, with disorganization of the myofibrillar architecture, along with a variable degree of myocardial fibrosis and thickening of the small intramural coronary arteries. In some children, systolic compression of an intramyocardial segment of a coronary artery may lead to ischemia and death.

GENETIC CONSIDERATIONS   About half of all patients with HCM have a positive family history compatible with autosomal-dominant transmission. More than 150 different mutations of 10 different genes that encode sarcomeric proteins have been identified. About 40% of these are associated with mutations of the cardiac β-myosin heavy chain gene on chromosome 14, with certain mutations associated with more malignant prognoses. About 15% have a mutation of the cardiac troponin T gene on chromosome 1, 20% a mutation of myosin-binding protein C (chromosome 11), and ~5% a mutation of the α-tropomyosin gene. The remainder of familial cases are due to mutations of other genes such as the gene for troponin I. Echocardiographic studies have confirmed that about one-third of the first-degree relatives of patients with familial HCM have evidence of the disease, although in many of these patients the extent of hypertrophy is mild, no outflow tract pressure gradient is present, and symptoms are not prominent. Since the hypertrophic characteristics may not be apparent in childhood and often appear first in adolescence, a single normal echocardiogram in a child does not exclude the presence of the disease. Many sporadic cases of HCM probably represent spontaneous mutations.

CLINICAL FEATURES The clinical course of HCM is highly variable. Many patients are asymptomatic or mildly symptomatic and may be relatives of patients with known disease. Unfortunately, the first clinical manifestation of the disease may be sudden death, frequently occurring in children and young adults, often during or after physical exertion. In symptomatic patients, the most common complaint is dyspnea, largely due to increased stiffness of the left ventricular walls, which impairs ventricular filling and leads to elevated left ventricular diastolic and left atrial pressures. Other symptoms include angina pectoris, fatigue, and syncope. Symptoms are not closely related to the presence or severity of an outflow pressure gradient. Most patients with gradients demonstrate a double or triple apical precordial impulse, a rapidly rising carotid arterial pulse, and a fourth heart sound. The hallmark of obstructive HCM is a systolic murmur, which is typically harsh, diamond-shaped, and usually begins well after the first heart sound, since ejection is unimpeded early in systole. The murmur is best heard at the lower left sternal border as well as at the apex, where it is often more holosystolic and blowing in quality, no doubt due to the mitral regurgitation that usually accompanies obstructive HCM.

HEMODYNAMICS In contrast to the obstruction produced by a fixed narrowed orifice, such as valvular aortic stenosis, the pressure gradient in HCM, when present, is dynamic and may change between examinations and even from beat to beat. Obstruction appears to result from further narrowing of an already small left ventricular outflow tract by SAM of the mitral valve against the hypertrophied septum. While SAM is occasionally found in a variety of conditions besides HCM, it is *always* found when obstruction is present in HCM. Three basic mechanisms are involved in the production and intensification of the dynamic pressure gradient: (1) increased left ventricular contractility, (2) decreased ventricular volume (preload), and (3) decreased aortic impedance and pressure (afterload). Interventions that increase myocardial contractility, such as exercise, sympathomimetic amines, and digitalis glycosides, and those that reduce ventricular volume, such as the Valsalva maneuver, sudden standing, nitroglycerin, amyl nitrite, or tachycardia, may all cause an increase in the gradient and the murmur. Conversely, elevation of arterial pressure by phenylephrine, squatting, sustained handgrip, augmentation of venous return by passive leg raising, and expansion of the blood volume all increase ventricular volume and ameliorate the gradient and murmur.

LABORATORY EVALUATION The *electrocardiogram* commonly shows left ventricular hypertrophy and widespread, deep, broad Q waves that suggest an old myocardial infarction. Many patients demonstrate arrhythmias, both atrial (supraventricular tachycardia or atrial fibrillation) and ventricular (ventricular tachycardia), during ambulatory (Holter) monitoring. *Chest roentgenography* may be normal, although a mild to moderate increase in the cardiac silhouette is common. The mainstay of the diagnosis of HCM is the *echocardiogram*, which demonstrates left ventricular hypertrophy, often with the septum 1.3 or more times the thickness of the high posterior left ventricular free wall. The septum may demonstrate an unusual "ground-glass" appearance, probably related to its abnormal cellular architecture and myocardial fibrosis. SAM of the mitral valve is found in patients with pressure

gradients. The left ventricular cavity typically is small in HCM, with vigorous posterior wall motion but reduced septal excursion. A rare form of HCM, characterized by apical hypertrophy, is often associated with giant negative T waves on the electrocardiogram and a "spade-shaped" left ventricular cavity on angiography; it usually has a benign clinical course. *Radionuclide scintigraphy* with thallium 201 frequently reveals evidence of myocardial perfusion defects even in asymptomatic patients.

Although cardiac catheterization is not required to diagnose HCM, the two typical *hemodynamic* features are an elevated left ventricular diastolic pressure due to diminished left ventricular compliance and, when obstruction is present, a systolic pressure gradient between the body of the left ventricle and the subaortic region. When a gradient is not present, it can be induced in some patients by provocative maneuvers such as infusion of isoproterenol, inhalation of amyl nitrite, or the Valsalva maneuver.

℞ TREATMENT

Since sudden death often occurs during or just after physical exertion, competitive sports and probably strenuous activity should be proscribed. Dehydration should be avoided, and diuretics should be used with caution. β-Adrenergic blockers are often used and ameliorate angina pectoris and syncope in one-third to one-half of patients. Resting intraventricular pressure gradients are usually unchanged, although these drugs may limit the increase in the gradient that occurs during exercise. It does not appear that β-adrenergic blockers offer any protection against sudden death. Amiodarone appears to be effective in reducing the frequency of supraventricular as well as life-threatening ventricular arrhythmias, and anecdotal data suggest that it may reduce the risk of sudden death. Verapamil and diltiazem may reduce the stiffness of the ventricle, reduce the elevated diastolic pressures, increase exercise tolerance, and, in some instances, reduce the severity of outflow tract pressure gradients, although adverse side effects occur in about one-quarter of patients. Nifedipine should be avoided. Disopyramide has been used in some patients to reduce left ventricular contractility and the outflow pressure gradient.

If atrial fibrillation occurs, a strenuous effort should be made to restore and then maintain sinus rhythm. Dual-chamber permanent pacing with a short PR interval has been reported to improve symptoms and reduce the outflow gradient in some patients with severe symptoms, presumably by altering the pattern of ventricular depolarization and contraction, although much of the putative benefit has been attributed to a placebo effect. Infarction of the interventricular septum induced by ethanol injections into the septal artery has also been reported to reduce obstruction. A surgical myotomy/myectomy of the hypertrophied septum may result in lasting symptomatic improvement in about three-quarters of severely symptomatic patients with large pressure gradients who are unresponsive to medical management. Digitalis, diuretics, nitrates, vasodilators, and β-adrenergic agonists are best avoided if possible, particularly in patients with known left ventricular outflow tract pressure gradients. Even social alcohol ingestion may produce sufficient vasodilatation to exacerbate an outflow pressure gradient. First-degree relatives of patients with HCM should be screened by echocardiography. The insertion of an implantable cardioverter defibrillator should be considered in patients (Chap. 214) with a high-risk profile for sudden cardiac death (see below).

PROGNOSIS The natural history of HCM is variable, although many patients never exhibit any clinical manifestations. Atrial fibrillation is common late in the course of the disease; its onset often leads to an increase in symptoms in two out of three patients, due to loss of the atrial contribution to filling of the thickened ventricle. Infective endocarditis occurs in <10% of patients, but endocarditis prophylaxis is indicated, particularly in patients with resting obstruction and mitral regurgitation. Progression of HCM to left ventricular dilatation and dysfunction with wall thinning without an outflow pressure gradient occurs in about 5 to 10% of patients. The major cause of mortality in HCM is sudden death, which may occur in asymptomatic patients or interrupt an otherwise stable course in symptomatic ones. The annual risk of dying from HCM is about 1% per year, similar to the normal adult population. Patients at higher risk of sudden death include those with a history of resuscitation from sudden cardiac death, ventricular tachycardia on ambulatory monitoring or at electrophysiologic testing, marked ventricular hypertrophy, (ventricular septal thickness >30 mm), syncope (especially in children), genetic mutations associated with an increased risk, an abnormal blood pressure response to exercise, and a family history of sudden death. There is no correlation between the risk of sudden death and the severity of symptoms, but there is an increased risk of death in patients with outflow gradients.

RESTRICTIVE CARDIOMYOPATHY

The hallmark of the restrictive cardiomyopathies is abnormal diastolic function (Chap. 215); the ventricular walls are excessively rigid and impede ventricular filling. Myocardial fibrosis, hypertrophy, or infiltration due to a variety of causes is usually responsible. The infiltrative diseases, which represent important causes for secondary restrictive cardiomyopathy, may also show some impairment of systolic function. Myocardial involvement with *amyloid* is a common cause of secondary restrictive cardiomyopathy, although restriction is also seen in hemochromatosis, glycogen deposition, endomyocardial fibrosis, sarcoidosis, Fabry's disease, the eosinophilias, and scleroderma; in the transplanted heart and following mediastinal irradiation; and in neoplastic infiltration and myocardial fibrosis of diverse causes. In many of these conditions, particularly those with substantial concomitant endocardial involvement, partial obliteration of the ventricular cavity by fibrous tissue and thrombus contributes to the abnormally increased resistance to ventricular filling. Thromboembolic complications ensue in about a third of patients.

The inability of the ventricle to fill limits cardiac output and raises filling pressure. Therefore, exercise intolerance and dyspnea are usually the most prominent symptoms. As a result of persistently elevated venous pressure, these patients commonly have dependent edema, ascites, and an enlarged, tender, and often pulsatile liver. The jugular venous pressure is elevated and does not fall normally, or it may rise with inspiration (Kussmaul's sign). The heart sounds may be distant, and third and fourth heart sounds are common. In contrast to constrictive pericarditis, which the restrictive cardiomyopathies resemble in many respects, the apex impulse is usually easily palpable, and mitral regurgitation is more common. The electrocardiogram often shows low-voltage, nonspecific ST-T-wave changes and various arrhythmias. Pericardial calcification on x-ray, which occurs in constrictive pericarditis, is absent. Echocardiography typically reveals symmetrically thickened left ventricular walls and normal or slightly reduced ventricular volumes and systolic function. Cardiac catheterization shows a decreased cardiac output, elevation of the right and left ventricular end-diastolic pressures, and a dip-and-plateau configuration of the diastolic portion of the ventricular pressure pulse resembling that seen in constrictive pericarditis.

Differentiation from constrictive pericarditis may be challenging (Chap. 222). This distinction is of importance because the latter condition is potentially curable by operation. Helpful in the differentiation of these two diseases are right ventricular transvenous endomyocardial biopsy (by revealing myocardial infiltration or fibrosis in restrictive cardiomyopathy) and computed tomography or magnetic resonance imaging (by demonstrating a thickened pericardium in constrictive pericarditis). Treatment is usually disappointing, except for hemochromatosis (where deferoxamine has been helpful in reducing myocardial iron content), and Fabry's disease (where infusion of galactose stimulates the activity of the deficient enzyme with attendant improvement in cardiac function). Chronic anticoagulation is often recommended to reduce the risk of embolization from the heart.

ENDOMYOCARDIAL FIBROSIS   This is a progressive disease of unknown cause that occurs most commonly in children and young adults residing in tropical and subtropical Africa, particularly Uganda and Nigeria. Endomyocardial fibrosis is a frequent cause of heart failure in Africa, accounting for up to one-quarter of deaths due to heart disease. The condition is characterized by fibrous endocardial lesions of the inflow portion of the right or left ventricle (or both) and often involves the atrioventricular valves, producing valvular regurgitation. The apex of the ventricles may be obliterated by a mass of thrombus and fibrous tissue. In some ways this disease resembles eosinophilic endomyocardial disease (see below), although they occur in quite different geographic areas and age groups and generally are felt to be different diseases.

The clinical picture depends on which ventricle and atrioventricular valve show predominant involvement; left-sided involvement results in symptoms of pulmonary congestion, while predominant right-sided disease presents features of a restrictive cardiomyopathy. Medical treatment is often disappointing, and surgical excision of the fibrotic endocardium and replacement of the involved atrioventricular valve have led to substantial symptomatic improvement in some patients.

EOSINOPHILIC ENDOMYOCARDIAL DISEASE   Also called *Loeffler's endocarditis* and *fibroplastic endocarditis*, this disease appears to be a subcategory of the hypereosinophilic syndrome in which the heart is predominantly involved, with cardiac damage the apparent result of the toxic effects of eosinophilic proteins. Typically, the endocardium of either or both ventricles thickens markedly, with involvement of the underlying myocardium. Large mural thrombi may develop in either ventricle, thereby compromising the size of the ventricular cavity and serving as a source of pulmonary and systemic emboli. Hepatosplenomegaly and localized eosinophilic infiltration of other organs are usually present. Management usually includes diuretics, afterload-reducing agents, and anticoagulation. The use of glucocorticoids and cytotoxic drugs (hydroxyurea in particular) appears to have improved survival substantially. Surgical treatment, as for endomyocardial fibrosis, may be helpful in selected patients.

DIFFERENTIAL DIAGNOSIS   Involvement of the heart is the most frequent cause of death in *primary amyloidosis* (Chap. 310), while clinically significant cardiac involvement is uncommon in the secondary form. Focal deposits of amyloid in elderly patients (*senile cardiac amyloidosis*) are common and usually clinically insignificant. Aspiration of abdominal fat or biopsy of the myocardium or other organs permits the diagnosis to be made before death in over three-quarters of cases. The heart is firm, rubbery, and noncompliant, and four clinical presentations (alone or in combination) are seen: (1) diastolic dysfunction (restrictive cardiomyopathy), (2) systolic dysfunction, (3) arrhythmias and conduction disturbances, and (4) orthostatic hypotension. The two-dimensional echocardiogram may be helpful in making the diagnosis of amyloidosis and may show a thickened myocardial wall with a distinctive "speckled" appearance. Chemotherapy, often with alkylating agents, appears to have improved survival in specific cases, and heart transplantion (often combined with bone marrow transplantation, or liver or kidney transplantation for hereditary amyloidosis) may help selected patients, but the overall prognosis is poor, especially in the primary form with advanced cardiac involvement.

Hemochromatosis (Chap. 336) is often the result of multiple transfusions or a hemoglobinopathy; the familial (autosomal recessive) form should be suspected if cardiomyopathy occurs in the setting of diabetes mellitus, hepatic cirrhosis, and increased skin pigmentation. The diagnosis may be confirmed by endomyocardial biopsy. Phlebotomy may be of some benefit if employed early in the course of the disease. Continuous subcutaneous administration of deferoxamine may reduce body iron stores and result in clinical improvement.

Myocardial *sarcoidosis* (Chap. 309) is generally associated with other manifestations of systemic disease and may cause restrictive as well as congestive features, since cardiac infiltration by sarcoid granulomas results not only in increased stiffness of the myocardium but also in diminished systolic contractile function. A variety of arrhythmias, including high-grade atrioventricular block, have been noted. A common cardiac manifestation of systemic sarcoidosis is right heart overload due to pulmonary artery hypertension as a result of parenchymal pulmonary involvement. Many patients are treated empirically with glucocorticoids. The *carcinoid syndrome* results in endocardial fibrosis and stenosis and/or regurgitation of the tricuspid and/or pulmonary valve (Chap. 219); morphologically similar lesions have been seen with the use of the anorexic agents fenfluramine and phentermine.

MYOCARDITIS

Myocarditis, i.e., cardiac inflammation, is most commonly the result of an infectious process. Myocarditis may also result from a hypersensitivity to drugs or may be caused by radiation, chemicals, or physical agents. In an unknown number of cases, acute myocarditis progresses to chronic dilated cardiomyopathy. While almost every infectious agent is capable of producing myocarditis (Table 221-1), clinically significant acute myocarditis in the United States is caused most commonly by viruses, especially coxsackievirus B. The clinical manifestations range from an asymptomatic state, with the presence of myocarditis inferred only by the finding of transient electrocardiographic ST-T-wave abnormalities, to a fulminant condition with arrhythmias, heart failure, and death. In some patients, myocarditis simulates acute myocardial infarction, with chest pain, electrocardiographic changes, and elevated serum levels of myocardial enzymes. Patients with myocarditis and pulmonary hypertension are at a particularly high risk of death.

The physical examination is often normal, although more severe cases may show a muffled first heart sound, along with a third heart sound and a murmur of mitral regurgitation. A pericardial friction rub may be audible in patients with associated pericarditis.

Though viral myocarditis is most often self-limited and without sequelae, severe involvement may recur, and it is likely that acute viral myocarditis occasionally progresses to a chronic form and to dilated cardiomyopathy. Patients with viral myocarditis often give a history of a preceding upper respiratory febrile illness or a flulike syndrome, and viral nasopharyngitis or tonsillitis may be evident clinically. The isolation of virus from the stool, pharyngeal washings, or other body fluids and changes in specific antibody titers are helpful clinically. Endomyocardial biopsy, carried out early in the illness, may show round-cell infiltration and necrosis of adjacent myocytes.

Exercise may be deleterious in patients with viral myocarditis, and strenuous activity should be proscribed until the electrocardiogram has returned to normal. Patients who develop CHF respond to the usual measures (ACE inhibitors, diuretics, and salt restriction), but they appear to be unusually sensitive to digitalis. Arrhythmias are common and are occasionally difficult to manage. Deaths attributed to heart failure, tachyarrhythmias, and heart block have been reported, and it seems prudent to monitor the electrocardiogram of patients with arrhythmias, especially during the acute illness. Patients with fulminant myocarditis may require mechanical cardiopulmonary support or cardiac transplantation, but the majority survive and many demonstrate substantial recovery of ventricular function.

HIV MYOCARDITIS (See also Chap. 173) Many HIV-infected patients have subclinical cardiac involvement, including pericardial effusion, right-sided chamber enlargement, and neoplastic involvement. Overt clinical involvement is seen in 10% of HIV patients, and the most common finding is left ventricular dysfunction that in some cases appears to be due to infiltration of the myocardium by the virus itself. In other patients, the heart is affected by any of the various opportunistic infections common in AIDS, such as toxoplasmosis, as well as by cardiac metastases in Kaposi's sarcoma. The clinical manifestations of cardiac involvement may be incorrectly attributed to concurrent noncardiac problems such as pneumonia. This is unfortunate, since the dilated cardiomyopathy of HIV infection may respond at least transiently to standard therapy with digitalis, diuretics, and ACE inhibitors.

BACTERIAL MYOCARDITIS Bacterial involvement of the heart is uncommon, but when it does occur, it is usually as a complication of endocarditis. Myocardial abscess formation may involve the valve rings and interventricular septum. *Diphtheritic myocarditis* develops in over one-quarter of the patients with diphtheria, is one of the most serious complications, and is the most common cause of death (Chap. 122). Cardiac damage is due to the liberation of a toxin that inhibits protein synthesis and leads to a dilated, flabby, hypocontractile heart; the conduction system is frequently involved as well. Cardiomegaly and severe CHF typically appear after the first week of illness. Prompt therapy with antitoxin is crucial; antibiotic therapy is also indicated but is of less urgency.

CHAGAS DISEASE Chagas disease, caused by the protozoan *Trypanosoma cruzi* and transmitted by an insect vector (Chap. 197), produces an extensive myocarditis that typically becomes evident years after the initial infection. It is one of the most common causes of heart disease encountered in Central and South America; in rural endemic areas 20 to 75% of the population may be affected. An increasing number of cases are found in the United States as patients migrate from endemic areas; in rare cases, it has been transmitted by transfusion and organ donation. Although only about 1% of infected individuals have an acute illness, which may include acute myocarditis, upwards of one-third develop chronic myocardial damage many years later. The chronic form is characterized by dilatation of several cardiac chambers, fibrosis and thinning of the ventricular wall, aneurysm formation (especially at the left ventricular apex), and mural thrombi. Chronic progressive heart failure is the rule and is associated with poor survival. The electrocardiogram is abnormal in most patients with cardiac involvement and typically shows right bundle branch block and left anterior hemiblock, which may progress to complete atrioventricular block. The *echocardiogram* may reveal a unique pattern of hypokinesis of the posterior left ventricular wall and relatively preserved septal motion. Ventricular arrhythmias are common and are seen especially during and after exertion; oral amiodarone appears to be particularly effective in treating ventricular tachyarrhythmias. The cause of death is either intractable CHF or an arrhythmia, with a minority of patients dying from embolic phenomena.

℞ TREATMENT

Therapy is directed toward amelioration of the CHF and arrhythmias; progressive conduction system disease and heart block may require implantation of a pacemaker. Anticoagulation (if feasible) may reduce the risk of thromboembolism. Medical therapy is often unsatisfactory or unavailable (especially in poor rural areas), however, and a more promising tactic in endemic areas has been the use of insecticides to eliminate the vector.

GIANT CELL MYOCARDITIS This rare myocarditis of unknown cause is characterized by rapidly fatal CHF and arrhythmia in young to middle-aged adults. At necropsy, the distinctive features include cardiac enlargement, ventricular thrombi, grossly visible serpiginous areas of myocardial necrosis in both ventricles, and microscopic evidence of giant cells within an extensive inflammatory infiltrate. The cause of giant cell myocarditis remains obscure, although it occurs in association with thymoma, systemic lupus erythematosus, and thyrotoxicosis. While treatment with immunosuppressive therapy may help some patients, cardiac transplantation is the treatment of choice.

LYME CARDITIS (See also Chap. 157) Lyme disease is caused by a tick-borne spirochete and is most common in the Northeast, upper Midwest, and Pacific Coastal regions of the United States during the summer months. About 10% of patients develop symptomatic cardiac involvement during the acute phase of the disease. Conduction abnormalities are the most common manifestations of involvement and may lead to syncope. Concomitant myopericarditis is not uncommon, and mild asymptomatic left ventricular dysfunction may occur. Intravenous ceftriaxone or penicillin is used in all but the mildest forms of Lyme carditis, in which case oral amoxicillin or doxycycline is employed. Hospitalization with electrocardiographic monitoring is indicated in patients with second- or third-degree atrioventricular block. A temporary pacemaker may be needed for symptomatic heart block, but permanent pacing is rarely required. The utility of glucocorticoids in reversing heart block is uncertain, but they are often employed. Long-term cardiac manifestations of Lyme disease are uncommon.

FURTHER READING

BANSCH D et al: Primary prevention of sudden cardiac death in idiopathic dilated cardiomyopathy: The Cardiomyopathy Trial (CAT). Circulation 105:1453, 2002

ELKAYAM U et al: Maternal and fetal outcomes of subsequent pregnancies in women with peripartum cardiomyopathy. N Engl J Med 344:1567, 2001

LANGE RA, HILLIS LD: Cardiovascular complications of cocaine use. N Engl J Med 345:351, 2001

LOWES BD et al: Myocardial gene expression in dilated cardiomyopathy treated with beta-blocking agents. N Engl J Med 346:1357, 2002

MARON MS et al: Effect of left ventricular outflow tract obstruction on clinical outcome in hypertrophic cardiomyopathy. N Engl J Med 348:295, 2003

MCCARTHY RE 3rd et al: Long-term outcome of fulminant myocarditis as compared with acute (nonfulminant) myocarditis. N Engl J Med 342:690, 2000

NICOLAS JM et al: The effect of controlled drinking in alcoholic cardiomyopathy. Ann Intern Med 136:192, 2002

WYNNE J: Stirred, not shaken. Ann Intern Med 136:247, 2002

———, BRAUNWALD E: The cardiomyopathies, in *Braunwald's Heart Disease*, 7th ed, D Zipes et al (eds). Philadelphia, Saunders, 2005

YAZAKI Y et al: Prognostic determinants of long-term survival in Japanese patients with cardiac sarcoidosis treated with prednisone. Am J Cardiol 88:1006, 2001

222   PERICARDIAL DISEASE
Eugene Braunwald

NORMAL FUNCTIONS OF THE PERICARDIUM   The visceral pericardium is a serous membrane that is separated by a small quantity (15 to 50 mL) of fluid, an ultrafiltrate of plasma from a fibrous sac, the parietal pericardium. The pericardium normally prevents sudden dilatation of the cardiac chambers during exercise and with hypervolemia. The pericardium also restricts the anatomic position of the heart, minimizes friction between the heart and surrounding structures, prevents displacement of the heart and kinking of the great vessels, and probably retards the spread of infections from the lungs and pleural cavities to the heart. Notwithstanding the foregoing, total absence of the pericardium does not produce obvious clinical disease. In partial left pericardial defects, the main pulmonary artery and left atrium may bulge through the defect; very rarely, herniation and subsequent strangulation of the left atrium may cause sudden death.

ACUTE PERICARDITIS

Acute pericarditis, by far the most common pathologic process involving the pericardium, may be classified both clinically and etiologically (Table 222-1). Pain, a pericardial friction rub, electrocardiographic changes, and pericardial effusion with cardiac tamponade and paradoxical pulse are cardinal manifestations of many forms of acute pericarditis.

Chest pain is an important but not invariable symptom in various forms of acute pericarditis (Chap. 12); it is usually present in the acute infectious types and in many of the forms presumed to be related to hypersensitivity or autoimmunity. Pain is often absent in a slowly developing tuberculous, postirradiation, neoplastic, or uremic pericarditis. The pain of pericarditis is often severe, retrosternal and left precordial, and referred to the back and the left trapezius ridge. Often the pain is pleuritic consequent to accompanying pleural inflammation, i.e., sharp and aggravated by inspiration, coughing, and changes in body position, but sometimes it is a steady, constricting pain that radiates into either arm or both arms and resembles that of myocardial ischemia; therefore, confusion with acute myocardial infarction (AMI) is common. Characteristically, however, pericardial pain may be relieved by sitting up and leaning forward and is intensified by lying supine. The differentiation of AMI from acute pericarditis becomes perplexing when, with acute pericarditis, serum biomarkers of myocardial damage such as creatine kinase and troponin rise, presumably because of concomitant involvement of the epicardium. However, these elevations, if they occur, are quite modest, given the extensive electrocardiographic ST-segment elevation in pericarditis.

The *pericardial friction rub,* the most important physical sign of acute pericarditis, may have up to three components per cardiac cycle and is high-pitched, scratching, and grating, as described in Chap. 209; it can sometimes be elicited only when firm pressure with the diaphragm of the stethoscope is applied to the chest wall at the left lower sternal border. It is heard most frequently during expiration with the patient in the sitting position. The rub is often inconstant, and the loud to-and-fro leathery sound may disappear within a few hours, possibly to reappear the following day.

The *electrocardiogram* (ECG) in acute pericarditis without massive effusion usually displays changes secondary to acute subepicardial inflammation (see Fig. 210-16). There is widespread elevation of the ST segments, often with upward concavity, involving two or three standard limb leads and V_2 to V_6, with reciprocal depressions only in aVR and sometimes V_1. Usually there are no significant changes in QRS complexes, except for some reduction in voltage in patients with large pericardial effusions. After several days, the ST segments return to normal, and only then do the T waves become inverted. In contrast, in AMI, ST elevations are convex, and reciprocal depression is usually more prominent; QRS changes occur, particularly the development of Q waves, as well as notching and loss of R-wave amplitude; and T-wave inversions are usually seen within hours *before* the ST segments have become isoelectric. Sequential ECGs are useful in distinguishing acute pericarditis from AMI. In the latter, elevated ST segments return to normal within hours. Early repolarization is a normal variant and may also cause widespread ST-segment elevation, most prominent in left precordial leads. However, in this condition the T waves are usually tall and the ST/T ratio is <0.25, but this ratio is higher in acute pericarditis. Depression of the PR segment (below the TP segment) is also common and reflects atrial involvement.

PERICARDIAL EFFUSION   In acute pericarditis, effusion is usually associated with pain and/or the above-mentioned ECG changes characteristic of pericarditis and an enlargement of the cardiac silhouette. Pericardial effusion is especially important clinically when it develops within a relatively short time, since it may lead to cardiac tamponade (see below). Differentiation from cardiac enlargement may be difficult on physical examination, but heart sounds tend to become faint with pericardial effusion; the friction rub may disappear, and the apex impulse may vanish, but sometimes it remains palpable, albeit medial to the left border of cardiac dullness. The base of the left lung may be compressed by pericardial fluid, producing Ewart's sign, a patch of dullness beneath the angle of the left scapula. The chest roentgenogram may show a "water bottle" configuration of the cardiac silhouette (Fig. 222-1) but may also be normal or almost so. Lucent pericardial fat lines may be seen deep within the cardiopericardial silhouette. Fluoroscopic examination may show the ventricular pulsations to be diminished.

Diagnosis   *Echocardiography* (Chap. 211) is the most effective imaging technique available, since it is sensitive, specific, simple, non-

TABLE 222-1 *Classification of Pericarditis*

CLINICAL CLASSIFICATION

I. Acute pericarditis (<6 weeks)
   A. Fibrinous
   B. Effusive (serous or sanguineous)
II. Subacute pericarditis (6 weeks to 6 months)
   A. Effusive-constrictive
   B. Constrictive
III. Chronic pericarditis (<6 months)
   A. Constrictive
   B. Effusive
   C. Adhesive (nonconstrictive)

ETIOLOGIC CLASSIFICATION

I. Infectious pericarditis
   A. Viral (coxsackievirus A and B, echovirus, mumps, adenovirus, hepatitis, HIV)
   B. Pyogenic (pneumococcus, streptococcus, staphylococcus, *Neisseria, Legionella*)
   C. Tuberculous
   D. Fungal (histoplasmosis, coccidioidomycosis, *Candida,* blastomycosis)
   E. Other infections (syphilitic, protozoal, parasitic)
II. Noninfectious pericarditis
   A. Acute myocardial infarction
   B. Uremia
   C. Neoplasia
     1. Primary tumors (benign or malignant, mesothelioma)
     2. Tumors metastatic to pericardium (lung and breast cancer, lymphoma, leukemia)
   D. Myxedema
   E. Cholesterol
   F. Chylopericardium
   G. Trauma
     1. Penetrating chest wall
     2. Nonpenetrating
   H. Aortic dissection (with leakage into pericardial sac)
   I. Postirradiation
   J. Familial Mediterranean fever
   K. Familial pericarditis
     1. Mulibrey nanism[a]
   L. Acute idiopathic
   M. Whipple's disease
   N. Sarcoidosis
III. Pericarditis presumably related to hypersensitivity or autoimmunity
   A. Rheumatic fever
   B. Collagen vascular disease (SLE, rheumatoid arthritis, ankylosing spondylitis, scleroderma, acute rheumatic fever, Wegener's granulomatosis)
   C. Drug-induced (e.g., procainamide, hydralazine, phenytoin, isoniazide, minoxidil, anticoagulants, methysergide)
   D. Postcardiac injury
     1. Postmyocardial infarction (Dressler's syndrome)
     2. Postpericardiotomy
     3. Posttraumatic

[a] An autosomal recessive syndrome, characterized by growth failure, muscle hypotonia, hepatomegaly, ocular changes, enlarged cerebral ventricles, mental retardation, and chronic constrictive pericarditis.

invasive, may be performed at the bedside, and can identify accompanying cardiac tamponade (see below) (Fig. 222-2). The presence of pericardial fluid is recorded by two-dimensional transthoracic echocardiography as a relatively echo-free space between the posterior pericardium and left ventricular epicardium in patients with small effusions and as a space between the anterior right ventricle and the parietal pericardium just beneath the anterior chest wall in those with larger effusions. In the latter the heart may swing freely within the pericardial sac; when severe, the extent of this motion alternates and may be associated with electrical alternans. Echocardiography allows localization and estimation of the quantity of pericardial fluid. The diagnosis of pericardial fluid or thickening may be confirmed by computed tomography (CT) or magnetic resonance imaging (MRI); these techniques may be superior to echocardiography in detecting loculated pericardial effusions and pericardial thickening.

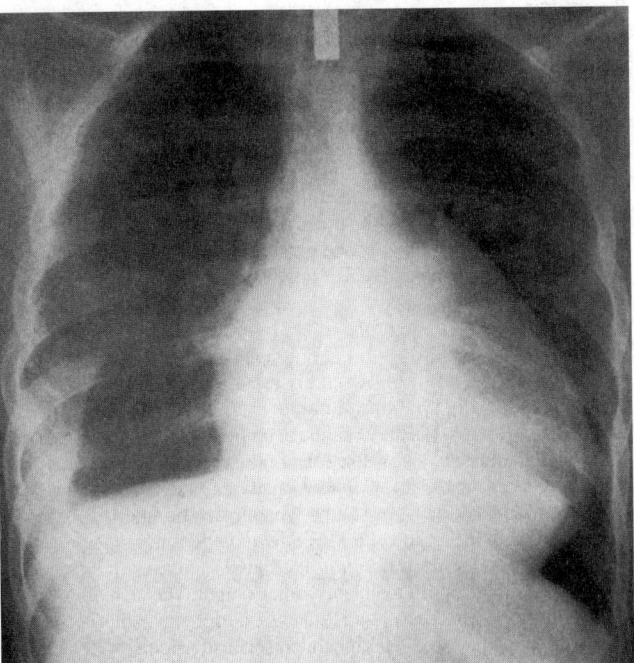

FIGURE 222-1 Chest radiogram from a patient with a pericardial effusion showing typical "water bottle" heart. There is also a right pleural effusion. *[From SS Kabbani, M LeWinter, in MH Crawford et al (eds): Cardiology. London, Mosby, 2001.]*

Pericardiocentesis When pericardial fluid is removed for diagnostic and/or therapeutic purposes, a needle attached to a properly grounded ECG lead is inserted into the pericardial space, usually through a subxiphoid approach, and, if possible, using echocardiographic control. Intrapericardial pressure should be measured before fluid is withdrawn. Pericardial effusion nearly always has the physical characteristics of an exudate. Bloody fluid is commonly due to tuberculosis or neoplasm but may also be found in the effusion of rheumatic fever, post-cardiac injury, and post-myocardial infarction (MI) and in uremic pericarditis. Transudative pericardial effusions may occur in heart failure.

CARDIAC TAMPONADE The accumulation of fluid in the pericardium in a quantity sufficient to cause serious obstruction to the inflow of blood

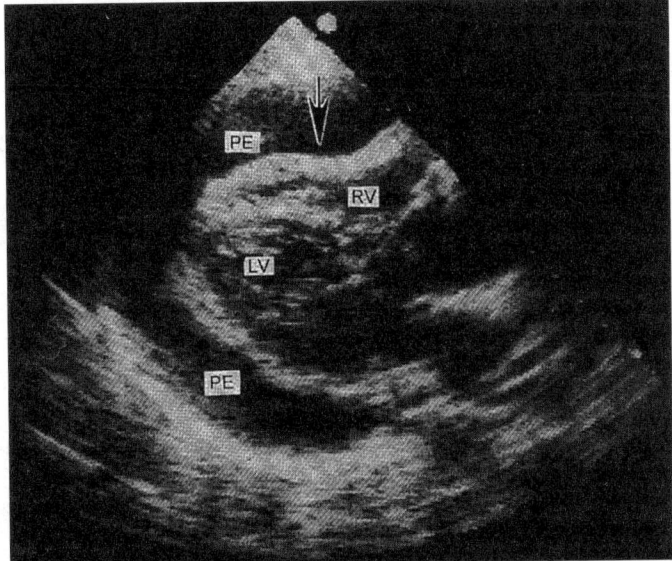

FIGURE 222-2 Large pericardial effusion (PE) with tamponade. Arrow indicates right ventricular (RV) collapse. LV, left ventricle. *(From LeWinter, with permission.)*

TABLE 222-2 *Features That Distinguish Cardiac Tamponade from Constrictive Pericarditis and Similar Clinical Disorders*

Characteristic	Tamponade	Constrictive Pericarditis	Restrictive Cardiomyopathy	RVMI
Clinical				
Pulsus paradoxus	Common	Usually absent	Rare	Rare
Jugular veins				
Prominent *y* descent	Absent	Usually present	Rare	Rare
Prominent *x* descent	Present	Usually present	Present	Rare
Kussmaul's sign	Absent	Present	Absent	Absent
Third heart sound	Absent	Absent	Rare	May be present
Pericardial knock	Absent	Often present	Absent	Absent
Electrocardiogram				
Low ECG voltage	May be present	May be present	May be present	Absent
Electrical alternans	May be present	Absent	Absent	Absent
Echocardiography				
Thickened pericardium	Absent	Present	Absent	Absent
Pericardial calcification	Absent	Often present	Absent	Absent
Pericardial effusion	Present	Absent	Absent	Absent
RV size	Usually small	Usually normal	Usually normal	Enlarged
Myocardial thickness	Normal	Normal	Usually increased	Normal
Right atrial collapse and RVDC	Present	Absent	Absent	Absent
Increased early filling, ↑ mitral flow velocity	Absent	Present	Present	May be present
Exaggerated respiratory variation in flow velocity	Present	Present	Absent	Absent
CT/MRI				
Thickened/calcific pericardium	Absent	Present	Absent	Absent
Cardiac catheterization				
Equalization of diastolic pressures	Usually present	Usually present	Usually absent	Absent or present
Cardiac biopsy helpful?	No	No	Sometimes	No

Abbreviations: RV, right ventricle; RVMI, right ventricular myocardial infarction; RVDC, right ventricular diastolic collapse; ECG, electrocardiograph.
Source: From GM Brockington et al, Cardiol Clin 8:645, 1990, with permission.

to the ventricles results in cardiac tamponade. This complication may be fatal if it is not recognized and treated promptly. The three most common causes of tamponade are neoplastic disease, idiopathic pericarditis, and uremia. Tamponade may also result from bleeding into the pericardial space either following cardiac operations and trauma (including cardiac perforation during cardiac catheterization or insertion of pacemaker wires) or from tuberculosis and hemopericardium. The latter may occur when a patient with any form of acute pericarditis is treated with anticoagulants.

The three principal features of tamponade are elevation of intracardiac pressures, limitation of ventricular filling, and reduction of cardiac output. The quantity of fluid necessary to produce this critical state may be as small as 200 mL when the fluid develops rapidly or >2000 mL in slowly developing effusions when the pericardium has had the opportunity to stretch and adapt to an increasing volume. The volume of fluid required to produce tamponade also varies directly with the thickness of the ventricular myocardium and inversely with the thickness of the parietal pericardium.

Table 222-2 lists the features that distinguish cardiac tamponade from constrictive pericarditis. The classic findings of falling arterial pressure, rising venous pressure, and faint heart sounds usually occur only with severe, acute tamponade, as occurs with cardiac trauma or rupture. Tamponade may also develop more slowly, and under these circumstances the clinical manifestations may resemble those of heart failure, including dyspnea, orthopnea, hepatic engorgement, and jugular venous hypertension. A high index of suspicion for cardiac tamponade is required, since, in many instances, no obvious cause for pericardial disease is apparent. Tamponade should be considered in

any patient with hypotension and elevation of jugular venous pressure with a prominent *x* descent and a diminutive or absent *y* descent. In contrast, in constrictive pericarditis, the *y* descent is prominent (Chap. 209). A positive Kussmaul sign (see below) is rare in cardiac tamponade, as is a pericardial knock. Their presence suggests that an organizing process and epicardial constriction are present in addition to effusion. A widening of the area of flatness to percussion across the anterior aspect of the chest wall, a paradoxical pulse (see below), hypotension, relatively clear lung fields, diminished pulsations of the cardiac silhouette on fluoroscopy, enlargement of the cardiac silhouette (especially in subacute or chronic tamponade), reduction in amplitude of the QRS complexes, and *electrical alternans* of the P, QRS, and T waves should raise the suspicion of cardiac tamponade.

Paradoxical Pulse This important clue to the presence of cardiac tamponade consists of *a greater than normal (10 mmHg) inspiratory decline in systolic arterial pressure.* When severe, it may be detected by palpating weakness or disappearance of the arterial pulse during inspiration, but usually sphygmomanometric measurement of systolic pressure during slow respiration is required.

Since both ventricles share a tight incompressible covering, i.e., the pericardial sac, the inspiratory enlargement of the right ventricle in cardiac tamponade compresses and reduces left ventricular volume; leftward bulging of the interventricular septum further reduces the left ventricular cavity as the right ventricle enlarges during inspiration. Thus, in cardiac tamponade the normal inspiratory augmentation of right ventricular volume causes an exaggerated reciprocal reduction in left ventricular volume. Also, respiratory distress increases the fluctuations in intrathoracic pressure, which exaggerates the mechanism just described. Right ventricular infarction (Chap. 228) may resemble cardiac tamponade with hypotension, elevated jugular venous pressure, an absent *y* descent in the jugular venous pulse, and occasionally pulsus paradoxus. The differences between these two conditions are shown in Table 222-2.

Paradoxical pulse occurs not only in cardiac tamponade but also in approximately one-third of patients with constrictive pericarditis. This physical finding is not pathognomonic of pericardial disease because it may be observed in some cases of hypovolemic shock, acute and chronic obstructive airways disease, and pulmonary embolus.

Low-pressure tamponade refers to mild tamponade in which the intrapericardial pressure is increased from its slightly subatmospheric levels to +5 to +10 mmHg; in some instances hypovolemia coexists. As a consequence, the central venous pressure is normal or only slightly elevated, while arterial pressure is unaffected and there is no paradoxical pulse. The patients are asymptomatic or complain of mild weakness and dyspnea. The diagnosis is aided by echocardiography, and both hemodynamic and clinical manifestations improve following pericardiocentesis.

Diagnosis Since immediate treatment of cardiac tamponade may be lifesaving, prompt measures to establish the diagnosis by echocardiography should be undertaken (Fig. 222-2). When pericardial effusion causes tamponade, Doppler ultrasound shows that tricuspid and pulmonic valve flow velocities increase markedly during inspiration, while pulmonic vein, mitral, and aortic flow velocities diminish (Fig. 222-3). Often the right ventricular cavity is reduced in diameter, and there is late diastolic inward motion (collapse) of the right ventricular free wall and of the right atrium. Transesophageal echocardiography may be necessary to diagnose a loculated effusion or hemorrhage responsible for cardiac tamponade.

℞ TREATMENT

Patients with acute pericarditis should be observed frequently for the development of an effusion; if a large effusion is present, the patient should be hospitalized and watched closely for signs of tamponade. In the presence of an effusion, arterial and venous pressures and heart rate should be monitored or followed carefully and serial echocardiograms obtained. If manifestations of tamponade appear, pericardiocentesis must be carried out at once, since relief of the intrapericardial pressure may be lifesaving. Intravenous saline may be administered as the patient is being readied. It is helpful, though not essential, to carry this out in the catheterization laboratory with hemodynamic and fluoroscopic monitoring. A small, multiholed catheter advanced over the needle inserted into the pericardial cavity may be left in place to allow draining of the pericardial space if fluid reaccumulates. When a *diagnostic* pericardiocentesis of a large effusion is carried out, an attempt should be made to remove as much fluid as possible. Surgical drainage through a limited (subxiphoid) thoracotomy may be required in recurrent tamponade, when it is necessary to remove loculated effusions, and/or when it is necessary to obtain tissue for diagnosis.

VIRAL OR IDIOPATHIC FORM OF ACUTE PERICARDITIS In some cases of this common disorder, an A or B coxsackievirus or the virus of influenza, echovirus, mumps, herpes simplex, chickenpox, adenovirus, or Epstein-Barr has been isolated from pericardial fluid and/or appropriate elevations in viral antibody titers have been noted. In many instances, acute pericarditis occurs in association with illnesses of known viral origin and, presumably, are caused by the same agent. Commonly, there is an antecedent infection of the respiratory tract, but in many patients such an association is not evident and viral isolation and serologic studies are negative. Most frequently, a viral causation cannot be established; the term *acute idiopathic pericarditis* is then appropriate. Pericardial effusion is the most common cardiac manifestation of HIV; it is usually secondary to infection (often mycobacterial) or neoplasm—most frequently lymphoma or Kaposi's sarcoma. Approx-

imately 80% are asymptomatic, while dyspnea or chest pain occur in the remainder. Pericardial effusion in full-blown AIDS is associated with a shortened survival (Chap. 173).

Acute pericarditis occurs at all ages but is more frequent in young adults and is often associated with pleural effusions and pneumonitis. The almost simultaneous development of fever and precordial pain, often 10 to 12 days after a presumed viral illness, constitutes an important feature in the differentiation of acute pericarditis from AMI, in which pain precedes fever. The constitutional symptoms are usually mild to moderate, and a pericardial friction rub is often audible. The disease ordinarily runs its course in a few days to 4 weeks, but one or more recurrences occur in about one-fourth of patients. Although accumulation of some pericardial fluid is common, tamponade is unusual, and constrictive pericarditis is a possible complication. The ST-segment alterations in the ECG usually disappear after 1 or more weeks, but the abnormal T waves may persist for several years and be a source of confusion in persons without a clear history of pericarditis. Pleuritis and pneumonitis frequently accompany pericarditis. Granulocytosis followed by lymphocytosis is common.

℞ TREATMENT

There is no specific therapy, but bed rest and anti-inflammatory treatment with aspirin may be given. If this is ineffective, one of the nonsteroidal anti-inflammatory agents, such as indomethacin (25 to 75 mg qid), or a glucocorticoid (e.g., prednisone, 40 to 80 mg daily) usually suppresses the clinical manifestations of the acute illness and may be useful in patients in whom the purulent and tuberculous forms of pericarditis have been excluded. Anticoagulants should be avoided. After the patient has been asymptomatic and afebrile for about a week, the dose of the anti-inflammatory agent is gradually tapered. Colchicine may prevent recurrences, but when recurrences are multiple, frequent, disabling, and continue beyond 2 years, pericardiectomy may be effective in terminating the illness.

POST-CARDIAC INJURY SYNDROME Acute pericarditis may appear under a variety of circumstances that have one common feature: previous injury to the myocardium, with blood in the pericardial cavity. The syndrome may develop after a cardiac operation (postpericardiotomy syndrome); after cardiac trauma (Chap. 223), e.g., a stab wound, contusions after a nonpenetrating blow to the chest; or after perforation of the heart with a catheter. Rarely, it follows AMI.

The clinical picture mimics acute viral or idiopathic pericarditis. The principal symptom is the pain of acute pericarditis, which usually develops 1 to 4 weeks following the cardiac injury but sometimes appears only after an interval of months. Recurrences are common and may occur up to 2 years or more after the injury. Fever with temperature up to 40°C, pericarditis, pleuritis, and pneumonitis are the outstanding features, and the bout of illness usually subsides in 1 or 2 weeks. The pericarditis may be of the fibrinous variety or it may be a pericardial effusion, which is often serosanguineous, and may be accompanied by arthralgias, but rarely causes tamponade. Leukocytosis, an increased sedimentation rate, and electrocardiographic changes typical of acute pericarditis may also occur.

The mechanisms responsible for this syndrome have not been identified, but they are probably the result of a hypersensitivity reaction in which the antigen originates from injured myocardial tissue and/or pericardium; the suggested designation of *post-cardiac injury syndrome* for this group of disorders implies that they may have a common pathogenetic mechanism. Circulating autoantibodies to myocardium occur frequently, but their precise role has not been defined. Viral infection may also play an etiologic role, since antiviral antibodies are often elevated in patients who develop this syndrome following cardiac surgery.

Often no treatment is necessary aside from aspirin and analgesics. The management of pericardial effusion and tamponade has already been discussed. When the illness is followed by a series of disabling

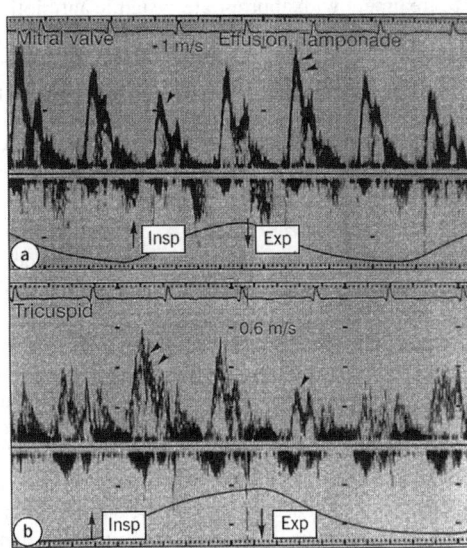

FIGURE 222-3 Doppler tracing of (*A*) mitral and (*B*) tricuspid inflow velocities in a patient with cardiac tamponade. Note the marked respiratory variation from inspiration (Insp) to (exp) expiration. (*From JJ Schultzman et al. Am J Cardiol 70:1353, 1992; with permission.*)

recurrences, therapy with a nonsteroidal anti-inflammatory agent or a glucocorticoid is usually effective.

DIFFERENTIAL DIAGNOSIS Since there is no specific test for *acute idiopathic pericarditis*, the diagnosis is one of exclusion. Consequently, all other disorders that may be associated with acute fibrinous pericarditis must be considered. A common diagnostic error is mistaking acute viral or idiopathic pericarditis for AMI and vice versa. When acute fibrinous pericarditis is associated with AMI, it may be confused with acute viral or idiopathic pericarditis; this complication of infarction, described in Chap. 228, is characterized by fever, pain, and a friction rub in the first 4 days following the development of the infarct. ECG abnormalities (such as the appearance of Q waves, brief ST-segment elevations with reciprocal changes, and earlier T-wave changes in MI) and the extent of the elevations of myocardial enzymes are helpful in differentiating pericarditis from AMI.

Pericarditis secondary to post-cardiac injury is differentiated from acute idiopathic pericarditis chiefly by timing. If it occurs within a few weeks of an MI or a chest blow, it may be justified to conclude that the two are probably related. If the infarct has been silent or the chest blow forgotten, the relationship to the pericarditis may not be recognized.

It is important to distinguish *pericarditis due to collagen vascular disease* from acute idiopathic pericarditis. Most important in the differential diagnosis is the pericarditis due to systemic lupus erythematosus (SLE; Chap. 300) or drug-induced (procainamide or hydralazine) lupus. Pain is often present in pericarditis due to collagen vascular disease. Sometimes in SLE the pericarditis appears as an asymptomatic effusion and, rarely, tamponade develops. When pericarditis occurs in the absence of any obvious underlying disorder, the diagnosis may be made on discovery of LE cells or a rise in the titer of antinuclear antibodies. Acute pericarditis may complicate the viral, pyogenic, mycobacterial, and fungal infections that occur in AIDS. Acute pericarditis is an occasional complication of *rheumatoid arthritis*, *scleroderma*, and *polyarteritis nodosa*, and other evidence of these diseases is usually obvious. Asymptomatic pericardial effusion is also frequent in these disorders. It is important to question every patient with acute pericarditis about the ingestion of procainamide, hydralazine, isoniazid, cromolyn, and minoxidil, since these drugs can cause this syndrome.

The pericarditis of *acute rheumatic fever* is generally associated with evidence of severe pancarditis and with cardiac murmurs (Chap. 302). *Pyogenic (purulent) pericarditis* is usually secondary to cardiothoracic operations, immunosuppressive therapy, rupture of the esophagus into the pericardial sac, or rupture of a ring abscess in a patient with infective endocarditis and with septicemia complicating aseptic pericarditis. It is accompanied by fever, chills, septicemia, and evidence of infection elsewhere.

Uremic pericarditis (Chap. 261) occurs in up to one-third of patients with chronic uremia and is seen most frequently in patients undergoing chronic hemodialysis. It may be fibrinous and is generally associated with an effusion that may be sanguineous. A friction rub is common, but pain is usually absent. Treatment with an anti-inflammatory agent and intensification of hemodialysis is usually adequate. Pericardial instillation of glucocorticoids may be helpful. Occasionally, tamponade occurs and pericardiocentesis is required. When uremic pericarditis is recurrent or persistent, pericardiectomy may be necessary. Pericarditis due to *neoplastic diseases* results from extension or invasion of metastatic tumors (most commonly carcinoma of the lung and breast, malignant melanoma, lymphoma, and leukemia) to the pericardium; pain, atrial arrhythmias, and tamponade are complications that occur occasionally. *Mediastinal irradiation* for neoplasm may cause acute pericarditis and/or chronic constrictive pericarditis after eradication of the tumor. Unusual causes of acute pericarditis include syphilis, fungal infection (histoplasmosis, blastomycosis, aspergillosis, and candidiasis), and parasitic infestation (amebiasis, toxoplasmosis, echinococcosis, trichinosis).

CHRONIC PERICARDIAL EFFUSIONS Chronic pericardial effusions are sometimes encountered in patients without an antecedent history of acute pericarditis. They may cause few symptoms per se, and their presence may be detected by finding an enlarged cardiac silhouette on chest roentgenogram.

Tuberculosis This is a common cause of chronic pericardial effusion, although less so in the United States than in other parts of the world (Chap. 150). The clinical picture is that of a chronic, systemic illness in a patient with pericardial effusion. It is important to consider this condition in a middle-aged or elderly person with fever and enlargement of the cardiac silhouette of undetermined origin, with or without elevation of venous pressure. Weight loss, fever, and fatigability are sometimes observed. Inasmuch as treatment is quite effective, overlooking a tuberculous pericardial effusion may have serious consequences. If the etiology of chronic pericardial effusion remains obscure, a pericardial biopsy, preferably by a limited thoracotomy, should be performed. If definitive evidence is then still lacking but the specimen shows caseation necrosis, antituberculous chemotherapy is indicated. If the biopsy specimen shows a thickened pericardium, pericardiectomy should be carried out in order to prevent the development of constriction.

Other Causes *Myxedema* may be responsible for a pericardial effusion that is sometimes massive but rarely, if ever, causes cardiac tamponade. The cardiac silhouette is markedly enlarged, and an echocardiogram is necessary to distinguish cardiomegaly from pericardial effusion. The diagnosis of myxedema is frequently overlooked. It is important, therefore, to carry out appropriate tests for thyroid function (Chap. 320) as well as echocardiography in patients with an enlarged cardiac outline of undetermined origin. Myxedematous pericardial effusion responds to thyroid hormone replacement. *Cholesterol pericardial disease* is sometimes associated with myxedema. It is characterized by large pericardial effusions with a high cholesterol content, which may induce an inflammatory response and constrictive pericarditis.

Neoplasms, SLE, rheumatoid arthritis, mycotic infections, radiation therapy, pyogenic infections, severe chronic anemia, and chylopericardium may also cause chronic pericardial effusion and should be considered and specifically looked for in such patients.

Aspiration and analysis of the pericardial fluid are often helpful in diagnosis, especially in patients with chronic large effusions that are nonresponsive to nonsteroidal anti-inflammatory drugs. Fluid should be sent for hematocrit, cell count, protein, culture, and cytology. In infections the organism can often be identified by smear or culture and should lead to treatment with appropriate systemic antibiotics. Grossly sanguineous pericardial fluid results most commonly from a neoplasm, tuberculosis, uremia, or slow leakage from an aortic aneurysm. Pericardiocentesis may resolve large effusions, but pericardiectomy may be required with recurrence. Intrapericardial instillation of sclerosing agents or anti-neoplastc agents (e.g., bleomycin) may be used to prevent reaccumulation of fluid.

CHRONIC CONSTRICTIVE PERICARDITIS

This disorder results when the healing of an acute fibrinous or serofibrinous pericarditis or a chronic pericardial effusion is followed by obliteration of the pericardial cavity with the formation of granulation tissue. The latter gradually contracts and forms a firm scar, encasing the heart and interfering with filling of the ventricles. In some reports, a high percentage of cases has been of tuberculous origin, but in North America, tuberculosis is now an infrequent cause. Chronic constrictive pericarditis may also follow trauma, cardiac operation of any type, mediastinal irradiation, purulent infection, histoplasmosis, neoplastic disease (especially breast cancer, lung cancer, and lymphoma), acute viral or idiopathic pericarditis, rheumatoid arthritis, SLE, and chronic renal failure with uremia treated by chronic dialysis. In many patients the cause of the pericardial disease is undetermined, and in them an asymptomatic or forgotten bout of viral pericarditis, acute or idiopathic, may have been the inciting event. The heart may also be constricted and compressed by malignant tumors or organized blood clot in the pericardial cavity.

The basic physiologic abnormality in symptomatic patients with chronic constrictive pericarditis, as in those with cardiac tamponade, is the inability of the ventricles to fill because of the limitations imposed by the rigid, thickened pericardium or the tense pericardial fluid. In constrictive pericarditis, ventricular filling is unimpeded during early diastole but is reduced abruptly when the elastic limit of the pericardium is reached, while in cardiac tamponade, ventricular filling is impeded throughout diastole. In chronic constrictive pericarditis, ventricular end-diastolic and stroke volumes are reduced and the end-diastolic pressures in both ventricles and the mean pressures in the atria, pulmonary veins, and systemic veins are all elevated to similar levels, i.e., within 5 mmHg of one another. The fibrotic process may extend into the myocardium and cause myocardial scarring, and venous congestion may then be due to the combined effects of the myocardial and pericardial lesions. Despite these hemodynamic changes, myocardial function may be normal or only slightly impaired.

In constrictive pericarditis, the central venous and right and left atrial pressure pulses display an M-shaped contour, with prominent *x* and *y* descents; the *y* descent, which is absent or diminished in cardiac tamponade, is the most prominent deflection in constrictive pericarditis and is interrupted by a rapid rise in pressure during early diastole, when ventricular filling is impeded by the constricting pericardium. These characteristic changes are transmitted to the jugular veins, where they may be recognized by inspection. In constrictive pericarditis, the ventricular pressure pulses in both ventricles exhibit characteristic "square root" signs during diastole (Fig. 222-4). These hemodynamic changes, although characteristic, are not pathognomonic of constrictive pericarditis but may also be observed in cardiomyopathies characterized by restriction of ventricular filling (Chap. 221).

CLINICAL AND LABORATORY FINDINGS (Table 222-2) Weakness, fatigue, weight gain, increased abdominal girth, abdominal discomfort, and edema are common. The patient often appears chronically ill with decreased skeletal muscle mass and a protuberant abdomen. Exertional dyspnea is common, and orthopnea may occur, although it is usually not severe. Acute left ventricular failure (acute pulmonary edema) is very uncommon. The cervical veins are distended and may remain so even after intensive diuretic treatment, and venous pressure may fail to decline during inspiration (Kussmaul's sign). The latter is frequent in chronic pericarditis but may also occur in tricuspid stenosis, right ventricular infarction, and restrictive cardiomyopathy. The pulse pressure is normal or reduced. In about one-third of the cases a paradoxical pulse can be detected. Congestive hepatomegaly is pronounced and may impair hepatic function; ascites is common and is usually more prominent than dependent edema. In about half of patients the heart is normal in size. The apical pulse is reduced and retracts in systole.

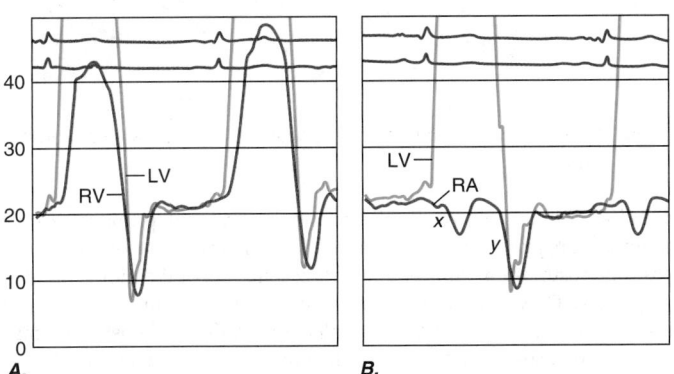

FIGURE 222-4 Pressure recording in a patient with constrictive pericarditis. *A.* Simultaneous right ventricular (RV) and left ventricular (LV) pressure tracings with equalization of diastolic pressure as well as "dip and plateau" morphology. *B.* Simultaneous right atrial (RA) and LV pressure with equalization of RA and LV diastolic pressure. Note the prominent *y* descent. *(From P Vaitkus et al: Circulation 93:834, 1996; with permission.)*

The heart sounds may be distant; an early third heart sound, i.e., a pericardial knock, occurring 0.09 to 0.12 s after aortic valve closure is often conspicuous. Protein-losing enteropathy is a rare complication.

The *ECG* frequently displays low voltage of the QRS complex and diffuse flattening or inversion of the T waves. Atrial fibrillation is present in about one-third of patients. The *chest roentgenogram* shows a normal or slightly enlarged heart, sometimes with pericardial calcification.

Inasmuch as the usual physical signs of cardiac disease (murmurs, cardiac enlargement) may be inconspicuous or absent in chronic constrictive pericarditis, hepatic enlargement and dysfunction associated with intractable ascites may lead to a mistaken diagnosis of cirrhosis of the liver. This error can be avoided if the neck veins are inspected carefully in patients with ascites and hepatomegaly. *Given a clinical picture resembling hepatic cirrhosis, but with the added feature of distended neck veins, careful search for calcification of the pericardium by chest roentgenography and CT or MRI should be carried out and may disclose this curable or remediable form of heart disease.*

The echocardiogram typically shows pericardial thickening, atrial enlargement, dilatation of the inferior vena cava and hepatic veins, and a sharp halt in ventricular filling in early diastole, with normal ventricular systolic function and flattening of the left ventricular posterior wall endocardium. There is a distinctive pattern of transvalvular flow velocity on Doppler echocardiography, with an exaggerated reduction in blood flow velocity in the pulmonary veins and across the mitral valve during inspiration, and the opposite occurring during expiration. Diastolic flow velocity in the vena cavae into the right atrium and across the tricuspid valve increases in an exaggerated manner during inspiration and declines during expiration. However, echocardiography cannot definitively exclude the diagnosis. MRI and CT scanning, especially the latter, are more accurate than echocardiography in establishing or excluding the presence of a thickened pericardium. Pericardial thickening and even pericardial calcification, however, are not synonymous with constrictive pericarditis since they may occur without seriously impairing ventricular filling.

DIFFERENTIAL DIAGNOSIS Like cor pulmonale (Chap. 216), chronic constrictive pericarditis may be associated with severe systemic venous hypertension but little pulmonary congestion; the heart is usually not enlarged, and a paradoxical pulse may be present. However, in cor pulmonale advanced parenchymal pulmonary disease is usually obvious and venous pressure *falls* during inspiration, i.e., Kussmaul's sign is negative. *Tricuspid stenosis* (Chap. 219) may also simulate chronic constrictive pericarditis; congestive hepatomegaly, splenomegaly, ascites, and venous distention may be equally prominent, and the manifestations of left-sided heart failure may be inconspicuous. However, in tricuspid stenosis, a characteristic murmur as well as mitral stenosis are usually present. In tricuspid stenosis, a paradoxical pulse and a steep, deep *y* descent in the jugular venous pulse do not occur, serving to differentiate it from chronic constrictive pericarditis.

Because constrictive pericarditis can be corrected surgically, it is important, though often difficult, to distinguish chronic constrictive pericarditis from restrictive cardiomyopathy (Chap. 221), which has a similar physiologic abnormality, i.e., restriction of ventricular filling. In many of these patients the ventricular wall is thickened on echocardiographic examination (Table 222-2). The features favoring the diagnosis of restrictive cardiomyopathy over chronic constrictive pericarditis include a well-defined apex beat, cardiac enlargement, and pronounced orthopnea with attacks of acute left ventricular failure, left ventricular hypertrophy, gallop sounds (in place of a pericardial knock), bundle branch block, and in some cases abnormal Q waves on the ECG. The echocardiogram in chronic constrictive pericarditis characteristically shows pericardial thickening, i.e., a distinct echo posterior to the left ventricular wall, and paradoxical septal motion.

The left ventricular wall moves sharply outward in early diastole on Doppler myocardial imaging. Marked respiratory variations in atrio-ventricular flow velocities on Doppler echocardiography are also characteristic of constrictive pericarditis but not restrictive cardiomyopathy (Fig. 222-4). The definitive diagnosis of restrictive cardiomyopathy, when it is due to an infiltrative disease such as amyloidosis, can often be established by endomyocardial biopsy. CT scanning and MRI are very useful in distinguishing between restrictive cardiomyopathy and chronic constrictive pericarditis. In the former, the ventricular walls are hypertrophied, while in the latter the pericardium is thickened and sometimes calcified.

When a patient has progressive, disabling, and unresponsive congestive failure and displays any of the features of constrictive heart disease, the most careful and detailed clinical and laboratory studies must be carried out in order to detect or exclude constrictive pericarditis, since the latter is usually curable.

℞ TREATMENT

Pericardial resection is the only definitive treatment of constrictive pericarditis, but dietary sodium restriction and diuretics are useful during preoperative preparation. The benefits derived from cardiac decortication are often striking, and the improvement, though slight at first, is usually progressive over a period of months. The risk of this operation depends on the extent of penetration of the myocardium by the calcific process, by the severity of myocardial atrophy, by the extent of secondary impairment of hepatic and/or renal function, and by the patient's general condition. Operative mortality is in the range of 5 to 15%; the patients with the most severe and/or advanced disease are at highest risk. Therefore, surgical treatment should be carried out relatively early in the course.

Many cases of constrictive pericarditis are of tuberculous origin. Antituberculous therapy during the phase of effusion may prevent the development of constriction, and such therapy should be carried out before and after operation if a tuberculous origin can be diagnosed or suspected (Chap. 150).

Subacute Effusive-Constrictive Pericarditis   This form of pericardial disease is characterized by the combination of a tense effusion in the pericardial space and constriction of the heart by thickened pericardium. It shares a number of features both with chronic pericardial effusion producing cardiac compression and with pericardial constriction. It may be caused by tuberculosis, multiple attacks of acute idiopathic pericarditis, radiation, traumatic pericarditis, uremia, and scleroderma. The heart is generally enlarged, and a paradoxical pulse and a prominent x descent (without a prominent y descent) are present in the atrial and jugular venous pressure pulses. Following pericardiocentesis, the physiologic findings may change from those of cardiac tamponade to those of pericardial constriction, with a "square root" sign in the ventricular pressure pulse and a prominent y descent in the atrial and jugular venous pressure pulses. Furthermore, the intrapericardial pressure and the central venous pressure may decline, but not to normal. In many patients the condition progresses to the chronic constrictive form of the disease. Wide excision of both the visceral and parietal pericardium is usually effective.

OTHER DISORDERS OF THE PERICARDIUM

Pericardial cysts appear as rounded or lobulated deformities of the cardiac silhouette, most commonly at the right cardiophrenic angle. They do not cause symptoms, and their major clinical significance lies in the possibility of confusion with a tumor, ventricular aneurysm, or massive cardiomegaly. *Tumors* involving the pericardium are most commonly secondary to malignant neoplasms originating in or invading the mediastinum, including carcinoma of the bronchus and breast, lymphoma, and melanoma. The most common *primary* malignant tumor is the mesothelioma. The usual clinical picture of malignant pericardial tumor is an insidiously developing, often bloody, pericardial effusion. Surgical exploration is required to establish a definitive diagnosis and to carry out definitive or, more commonly, palliative treatment.

FURTHER READING

Hoit BD: Management of effusive and constrictive pericardial heart disease. Circulation 105:2939, 2002

LeWinter M: Pericardial diseases, in D Zipes et al (eds): *Braunwald's Heart Disease*, 7th ed. Philadelphia, Saunders, 2005

Ling LH et al: Constrictive pericarditis in the modern era: Evolving clinical spectrum and impact on outcome after pericardiectomy. Circulation 100:1380, 1999

Oh JK et al: Diagnostic role of Doppler echocardiography in constrictive pericarditis. J Am Coll Cardiol 23:154, 1994

Rajagopalan N et al: Comparison of new Doppler echocardiographic methods to differentiate constrictive pericardial heart disease and restrictive cardiomyopathy. Am J Cardiol 87:86, 2001

Sagrista A et al: Long-term follow-up of idiopathic chronic pericardial effusions. N Engl J Med 341:2054, 1999

223 CARDIAC TUMORS, CARDIAC MANIFESTATIONS OF SYSTEMIC DISEASES, AND TRAUMATIC CARDIAC INJURY
Wilson S. Colucci, Daniel T. Price

TUMORS OF THE HEART

PRIMARY TUMORS

Primary tumors of the heart are rare. Approximately three-quarters are histologically benign, and the remainder, which in almost all cases are sarcomas, are malignant (Table 223-1). Because all cardiac tumors have the potential to cause life-threatening complications, and many are now curable by surgery, it is important that the diagnosis be made whenever possible.

CLINICAL PRESENTATION   Cardiac tumors may present with a wide array of cardiac and noncardiac manifestations. The location and the size of the tumor are the major determinants of the specific signs and symptoms, many of which are present in more common forms of heart disease, such as chest pain, syncope, heart failure, murmurs, arrhyth-mias, conduction disturbances, and pericardial effusion with or without tamponade.

MYXOMA   Myxomas are the most common type of primary cardiac tumor in all age groups, accounting for one-third to one-half of all cases at postmortem and for about three-quarters of the tumors treated surgically. They occur at all ages, most commonly in the third through sixth decades, with a female predilection. Although most myxomas are sporadic, some are familial with autosomal dominant transmission or are part of a syndrome that involves a complex of abnormalities including lentigines or pigmented nevi, primary nodular adrenal cortical disease with or without Cushing's syndrome, myxomatous mammary fibroadenomas, testicular tumors, and/or pituitary adenomas with gigantism or acromegaly. Patients with Carney complex have spotty skin pigmentation, myxomas, endocrine overactivity, and schwanno-

TABLE 223-1	Relative Incidence of Primary Tumors of the Heart	
Type	Number	Percent
Benign	199	58.0
Myxoma	114	33.2
Rhabdomyoma	20	5.8
Fibroma	20	5.8
Hemangioma	17	5.0
Atrioventricular nodal	10	2.9
Granular cell	4	1.2
Lipoma	2	0.6
Paraganglioma	2	0.6
Myocytic hamartoma	2	0.6
Histiocytoid cardiomyopathy	2	0.6
Inflammatory psuedotumor	2	0.6
Other benign tumors	4	1.2
Malignant	144	42.0
Sarcoma	137	39.9
Lymphoma	7	2.1

Source: Modified from A Burke; R Virmani: *Atlas of Tumor Pathology. Tumors of the Heart and Great Vessels.* Washington, DC, Armed Forces Institute of Pathology 1996, p 231; with permission.

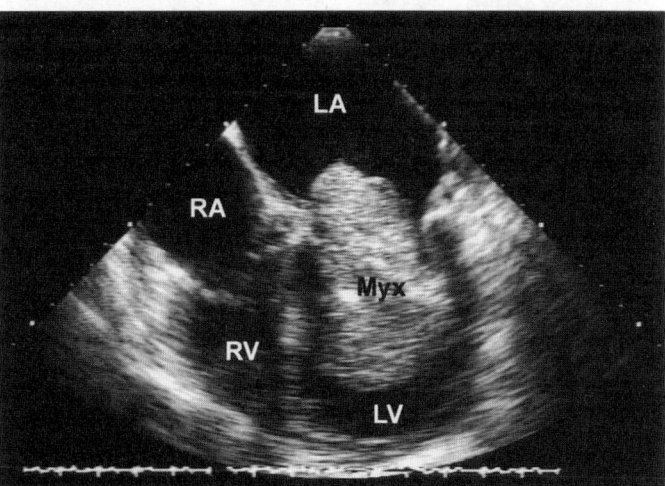

FIGURE 223-1 Transthoracic echocardiogram during diastole demonstrating a large myocardial mass, which is an atrial myxoma (Myx) that prolapses into the left ventricle (LV). LA, left atrium; RA, right atrium; RV, right ventricle. (*Courtesy of Dr. Rick Nishimura.*)

mas that are due to mutations of the gene encoding the protein kinase A type I-α regulatory subunit. Certain constellations of findings have been referred to as the *NAME* syndrome (nevi, atrial myxoma, myxoid neurofibroma, and ephelides) or the *LAMB* syndrome (lentigines, atrial myxoma, and blue nevi). Approximately 7% of cardiac myxomas are familial or part of the myxoma syndrome with the complex of abnormalities described above.

Pathologically, myxomas are gelatinous structures consisting of myxoma cells imbedded in a stroma rich in glycosaminoglycans. Most are pedunculated on a fibrovascular stalk and average 4 to 8 cm in diameter. Most are solitary and located in the atria, particularly the left, where they arise from the interatrial septum in the vicinity of the fossa ovalis. In contrast to sporadic tumors, familial or myxoma syndrome tumors tend to occur in younger individuals, be multiple or ventricular in location, and have more postoperative recurrences, probably reflecting their multicentric nature.

Myxomas commonly present with obstructive, embolic, or constitutional signs and symptoms. The most common clinical presentation mimics that of mitral valve disease—either stenosis due to tumor prolapse into the mitral orifice, or regurgitation due to tumor-induced valvular trauma. Ventricular myxomas may cause outflow obstruction similar to that caused by subaortic or subpulmonic stenosis. The symptoms and signs of myxoma may be of sudden onset or positional in nature, reflecting changes in tumor position due to gravity. An auscultatory finding, termed a "tumor plop," is a characteristic low-pitched sound that may be audible during early or mid-diastole and is thought to result from the tumor abruptly stopping as it strikes the ventricular wall. Myxomas may also present with peripheral or pulmonary emboli, or constitutional signs and symptoms including fever, weight loss, cachexia, malaise, arthralgias, rash, clubbing, Raynaud's phenomenon, hypergammaglobulinemia, anemia, polycythemia, leukocytosis, elevated erythrocyte sedimentation rate, thrombocytopenia, or thrombocytosis. Not surprisingly, myxomas are frequently misdiagnosed as endocarditis, collagen vascular disease, or noncardiac tumor.

Two-dimensional transthoracic or transesophageal echocardiography is useful in the diagnosis of cardiac myxoma and allows determination of the site of tumor attachment and tumor size, which are important considerations in the planning of surgical excision (Fig. 223-1). Computed tomography (CT) and particularly magnetic resonance imaging (MRI) may provide important information regarding size, shape, composition, and surface characteristics of the tumor. Because myxomas may be familial, echocardiographic screening of first-degree relatives is appropriate, particularly if the patient is young and has multiple tumors or evidence of myxoma syndrome. Although cardiac catheterization and angiography have previously been performed rou-

tinely before surgery, catheterization of the chamber from which the tumor arises carries the risk of tumor emboli. Catheterization is no longer considered mandatory when adequate noninvasive information is available and other cardiac diseases (e.g., coronary artery disease) are not considered likely.

℞ TREATMENT

Surgical excision utilizing cardiopulmonary bypass is indicated and is generally curative. Myxomas recur in approximately 12 to 22% of familial cases and in about 1 to 2% of sporadic cases. Tumor recurrence is most likely due to multifocal lesions in the former and inadequate resection in the latter.

OTHER BENIGN TUMORS Cardiac *lipomas*, although relatively common, are usually incidental findings at postmortem examination. However, they may grow as large as 15 cm and may present with symptoms due to mechanical interference with cardiac function, arrhythmias, or conduction disturbances, or as an abnormality of the cardiac silhouette on chest x-ray. *Papillary fibroelastomas*, similarly, are relatively common findings on cardiac valves or the adjacent endothelium at postmortem, but seldom result in clinical symptoms. Occasionally, these growths may cause mechanical interference with valve function. *Rhabdomyomas* and *fibromas*, the most frequent tumors in infants and children, most commonly occur in the ventricles and therefore produce signs and symptoms by mechanical obstruction that may mimic valvular stenosis, congestive heart failure, restrictive or hypertrophic cardiomyopathy, and pericardial constriction. Rhabdomyomas are probably hamartomatous growths; are multiple in 90% of cases; and may be associated with tuberous sclerosis, adenoma sebaceum, and benign kidney tumors in approximately 30% of patients. Calcification of a cardiac tumor strongly suggests that it is a fibroma, although myxomas and sarcomas also may be calcified. *Hemangiomas* and *mesotheliomas* are generally small tumors, most often intramyocardial in location, and may cause atrioventricular (AV) conduction disturbances and even sudden death as a result of their predilection for the region of the AV node. Other benign tumors arising from the heart include *teratoma*, *chemodectoma*, *neurilemoma*, *granular cell myoblastoma*, and *bronchogenic cysts*.

SARCOMA Almost all primary cardiac malignancies are sarcomas, which may be of several histologic types. In general, these tumors are characterized by a rapidly downhill course leading to the patient's death in weeks to months from the time of presentation as a result of hemodynamic compromise, local invasion, or distant metastases. Sarcomas commonly involve the right side of the heart, and because of their rapid growth, invasion of the pericardial space and obstruction of the cardiac chambers or vena cavae are common. Sarcomas can also occur on the left side of the heart and may be mistaken for myxomas.

℞ TREATMENT

At the time of presentation these tumors have often spread too extensively for surgical excision. Although scattered reports exist of palliation with surgery, radiotherapy, and/or chemotherapy, the overall experience with cardiac sarcomas is poor. The one exception appears to be cardiac lymphosarcomas, which may respond to a combination of chemo- and radiotherapy.

TUMORS METASTATIC TO THE HEART

Tumors metastatic to the heart are much more common than primary tumors, and their incidence is likely to increase as the life expectancy of patients with various forms of malignant neoplasms is extended by more effective therapy. Although cardiac metastases occur in 1 to 20% of all tumor types, the relative incidence is especially high in malignant melanoma and, to a somewhat lesser extent, in leukemia and lymphoma. In absolute numbers, the most common primary originating sites of cardiac metastases are carcinoma of the breast and lung, reflecting the high incidence of these cancers. Cardiac metastases almost always occur in the setting of widespread primary disease, and most often either primary or metastatic disease exists elsewhere in the thoracic cavity. Nevertheless, a cardiac metastasis may occasionally be the initial presentation of a tumor elsewhere in the body.

Cardiac metastases reach the heart from the blood stream, the lymphatics, or by direct invasion. They generally are small, firm nodules. Diffuse infiltration may also occur, especially with sarcomas or hematologic neoplasms. The pericardium is most often involved, followed by myocardial involvement of any chamber, and, rarely, by involvement of the endocardium or cardiac valves.

Cardiac metastases result in clinical manifestations only about 10% of the time and rarely are the cause of death. In most instances the metastases are not the cause of the presenting clinical features but occur in the setting of a previously recognized malignant neoplasm. Although cardiac metastases may present with a large number of nonspecific signs and symptoms, the most common are dyspnea, signs of acute pericarditis, cardiac tamponade, a rapid increase in the cardiac silhouette on chest x-ray, new onset of ectopic tachyarrhythmia or AV block, and congestive heart failure. As with primary cardiac tumors, the clinical presentation is more closely related to the location and size of the tumor than to histologic type. Many of these signs and symptoms also occur with myocarditis, pericarditis, or cardiomyopathy resulting from radiotherapy or chemotherapy.

Electrocardiographic (ECG) findings are nonspecific. On chest x-ray the cardiac silhouette is most often normal but may reveal a pericardial effusion or bizarre contour. Echocardiography is useful for the diagnosis of pericardial effusion and the visualization of larger metastases. Computed tomography (CT), MRI, and radionuclide imaging with gallium or thallium may provide useful anatomic information. Angiography may delineate discrete lesions, and pericardiocentesis can allow a specific cytologic diagnosis.

℞ TREATMENT

Because most patients with cardiac metastases have widespread disease, therapy generally consists of treatment of the primary tumor. Symptomatic malignant effusions are treated by removal of fluid by pericardiocentesis, with or without concomitant instillation of a sclerosing agent (e.g., tetracycline), or placement of a pericardial window for drainage to the pleural space, to palliate symptoms, and to delay or prevent reaccumulation of the effusion.

CARDIAC EFFECTS OF CANCER THERAPY See Chap. 221

CARDIOVASCULAR MANIFESTATIONS OF SYSTEMIC DISEASES

DIABETES MELLITUS (See also Chap. 323)

There is an increased incidence of large-vessel atherosclerosis and myocardial infarction in patients with both insulin- and noninsulin-dependent diabetes mellitus. Coronary artery disease is the most common cause of death in adults with diabetes mellitus. Diabetes mellitus is an independent risk factor for coronary artery disease (Chap. 224), and the incidence of coronary artery disease is related to the duration of diabetes. In patients with diabetes mellitus, myocardial infarctions are not only more frequent but also tend to be larger in size and more likely to result in complications such as heart failure, shock, and death. Patients with diabetes mellitus are more likely to have an abnormal or absent pain response to myocardial ischemia, probably as a result of generalized autonomic nervous system dysfunction. Ambulatory ECG monitoring has shown that up to 90% of episodes of ischemia are silent in diabetic patients with coronary artery disease; the presentation of their ischemia may be exertional or episodic dyspnea, flash pulmonary edema, arrhythmias, heart block, or syncope. Since coronary artery disease is more common in patients with diabetes mellitus and often is not associated with typical anginal symptoms, the threshold for the diagnosis should be low, particularly when the duration of disease is long and concomitant risk factors for coronary artery disease (e.g., hypertension, smoking, hyperlipidemia) are present.

Patients with diabetes mellitus may also have myocardial dysfunction characteristic of a restrictive cardiomyopathy in the absence of large-vessel (epicardial) coronary artery disease, with abnormal relaxation of the myocardium, and evidenced clinically by elevated left ventricular filling pressures. Histologically, these patients have interstitial fibrosis with increased amounts of collagen, glycoprotein, triglycerides, and cholesterol in the myocardial interstitium. In some cases intimal thickening, hyaline deposition, and inflammatory changes have been observed in small intramural arteries. Patients with diabetes mellitus have an increased risk of developing clinical heart failure, even after correction for the presence of coronary artery disease, hypertension, and obesity, and it is likely that diabetic cardiomyopathy contributes to excessive cardiovascular morbidity and mortality in these patients. There is some evidence that insulin therapy results in an amelioration of the myocardial dysfunction.

MALNUTRITION AND VITAMIN DEFICIENCY MALNUTRITION
(See also Chap. 62)

In patients whose intake of protein, calories, or both is severely deficient, the heart may become thin, pale, and flabby with myofibrillar atrophy and interstitial edema. The systolic pressure and cardiac output are low, and the pulse pressure is narrow. Generalized edema is common and is due to a combination of factors, including reduced serum oncotic pressure and myocardial dysfunction. Such profound states of malnutrition, termed *marasmus* in the case of caloric deficiency and *kwashiorkor* in the case of relative protein deficiency, are most common in underdeveloped countries. However, significant nutritional heart disease may also occur in developed nations, particularly in patients with chronic diseases such as AIDS, in patients with anorexia nervosa, and in patients with severe cardiac failure in whom gastrointestinal hypoperfusion and venous congestion may lead to anorexia and malabsorption. Open-heart surgery poses increased risk in malnourished patients, and they may benefit from preoperative hyperalimentation.

THIAMINE DEFICIENCY (BERIBERI) (See also Chap. 61)   In many cases, malnutrition is accompanied by thiamine deficiency, although this hypovitaminosis may also occur in the presence of an adequate protein and caloric intake, particularly in the Far East, where polished rice deficient in thiamine may be a major dietary component. In Western nations, the widespread use of thiamine-enriched flour limits the presence of deficiency primarily to alcoholics and food faddists. The measurement of the thiamine-pyrophosphate effect (TPPE) can biochemically quantitate thiamine stores. An elevated TPPE, indicative of thiamine deficiency, has been found in 20 to 90% of patients with chronic heart failure. The deficiency appears to result from both reduced dietary intake and a diuretic-induced increase in the urinary excretion of thiamine. The acute administration of thiamine to these patients increases the left ventricular ejection fraction and the excretion of salt and water.

Clinically, there is usually evidence of generalized malnutrition, peripheral neuropathy, glossitis, and anemia. The characteristic cardiovascular syndrome is heart failure with increased cardiac output, tachycardia, and often elevated filling pressures in the left and right sides of the heart. The major cause of the high-output cardiac state is vasomotor depression, the precise mechanism of which is not understood but which leads to a reduced systemic vascular resistance. The cardiac examination reveals a wide pulse pressure, tachycardia, a third heart sound, and, frequently, an apical systolic murmur. The ECG may show decreased voltage, a prolonged QT interval, and T-wave abnormalities. The chest x-ray generally shows a large heart with signs of congestive heart failure. The response to thiamine is often dramatic, with an increase in systemic vascular resistance, decrease in cardiac output, clearing of pulmonary congestion, and a reduction in heart size often occurring in 12 to 48 h. Although the response to digitalis and diuretics may be poor before thiamine therapy, these agents may be important *after* thiamine is given, since the left ventricle may not be capable of dealing with the increased work load presented by the return of vascular tone.

VITAMIN B₆, B₁₂, AND FOLATE DEFICIENCY (See also Chap. 61) These vitamin cofactors in the metabolism of homocysteine probably contribute to the majority of cases of hyperhomocysteinemia in the general population. Hyperhomocysteinemia is associated with increased risk of atherosclerosis. Supplementation of these vitamins has reduced the incidence of hyperhomocysteinemia in the United States. The clinical benefit of normalizing elevated homocysteine levels, however, remains unproven.

OBESITY (See also Chap. 64)

Severe obesity, particularly when it occurs in an upper-body distribution, is associated with an increase in cardiovascular morbidity and mortality. Although obesity itself is not considered a disease, there is clearly an increased prevalence of hypertension, glucose intolerance, and atherosclerotic coronary artery disease in obese patients. In addition, these patients have a distinct abnormality of the cardiovascular system characterized by increases in total and central blood volumes, cardiac output, and left ventricular filling pressure. The elevated cardiac output appears to be required to support the metabolic needs of the excessive adipose tissue. Left ventricular filling pressure is often at the upper limits of normal and rises excessively with exercise. As a result of chronic volume overload, eccentric cardiac hypertrophy with cardiac dilatation and abnormal ventricular function may develop. Pathologically, there are left and, in some cases, right ventricular hypertrophy and generalized cardiac dilatation, which is not due simply to fatty infiltration of the myocardium. Although these patients may develop pulmonary congestion, peripheral edema, and exercise intolerance, the recognition of these findings may be difficult in massively obese patients.

Weight reduction is the most effective therapy and results in reduction in blood volume and in the return of cardiac output toward normal. However, rapid weight reduction may be dangerous, as cardiac arrhythmias and sudden death due to electrolyte imbalance have been described. Digitalis, sodium restriction, and diuretics may also be useful. This form of heart disease should be distinguished from the Pickwickian syndrome (Chap. 246), which may share several of the cardiovascular features of heart disease secondary to severe obesity but, in addition, frequently has components of central apnea, hypoxemia, pulmonary hypertension, and cor pulmonale.

THYROID DISEASE (See also Chap. 320)

Thyroid hormone exerts a major influence on the cardiovascular system by a number of direct and indirect mechanisms, and not surprisingly, cardiovascular effects are prominent in both hypo- and hyperthyroidism. Thyroid hormone causes increases in total-body metabolism and oxygen consumption that indirectly place an increased work load on the heart. In addition, although the exact mechanism has not been defined, thyroid hormone exerts direct inotropic, chronotropic, and dromotropic effects that are similar to those seen with adrenergic stimulation (e.g., tachycardia, increased cardiac output). Thyroid hormone increases the synthesis of myosin and of Na^+,K^+-ATPase, as well as the density of myocardial β-adrenergic receptors.

HYPERTHYROIDISM Cardiovascular presentations of hyperthyroidism include palpitations, systolic hypertension, fatigue, or, in patients with underlying heart disease, angina or heart failure. Sinus tachycardia is found in about 40% of patients and atrial fibrillation in about 15%. Other findings include a hyperdynamic precordium, a widened pulse pressure, an increase in the intensity of the first heart sound and the pulmonic component of the second heart sound, and a third heart sound. An increased incidence of mitral valve prolapse has been associated with hyperthyroidism, and in some cases there may be a midsystolic murmur heard best at the left sternal border with or without a systolic ejection click. A *Means-Lerman scratch* is a systolic scratchy sound, heard at the left second intercostal space during expiration; it is thought to result from the rubbing of the hyperdynamic pericardium against the pleura.

Elderly patients with hyperthyroidism, so-called apathetic hyperthyroidism, may present with only the cardiovascular manifestations of thyrotoxicosis, such as atrial fibrillation, which may be resistant to therapy until the hyperthyroidism is controlled. Angina pectoris and congestive heart failure are unusual unless there is coexistent underlying heart disease, and in many cases symptoms resolve with treatment of the hyperthyroidism.

HYPOTHYROIDISM Cardiac manifestations of hypothyroidism include a reduction in cardiac output, stroke volume, heart rate, blood pressure, and pulse pressure. In about one-third of patients there is a pericardial effusion which only rarely results in tamponade. Increased capillary permeability results in pleural and pericardial effusions. Other clinical signs include cardiomegaly, bradycardia, weak arterial pulses, and distant heart sounds. Although the signs and symptoms of myxedema may suggest the diagnosis of congestive heart failure, in the absence of other cardiac disease, myocardial failure is uncommon. The ECG generally shows sinus bradycardia and low voltage and may show prolongation of the QT interval, decreased P-wave voltage, prolonged AV conduction time, intraventricular conduction disturbances, and nonspecific ST-T wave abnormalities. Chest x-ray may show cardiomegaly, often with a "water bottle" configuration, pleural effusions, and, in some cases, evidence of congestive heart failure. Pathologically, the heart is pale, dilated, and flabby, often with myofibrillar swelling, loss of striations, and interstitial fibrosis.

Patients with hypothyroidism frequently have elevations of cholesterol and triglycerides, and severe atherosclerotic coronary artery disease. Before treatment with thyroid hormone, patients with hypothyroidism frequently do not have angina pectoris, presumably because of the low metabolic demands caused by their condition. However, angina and myocardial infarction may be precipitated during initiation of thyroid hormone replacement, especially in elderly patients with underlying heart disease. Therefore, replacement should be done with care, starting with low doses that are increased gradually.

MALIGNANT CARCINOID (See also Chap. 329)

These tumors elaborate a variety of vasoactive amines (e.g., serotonin), kinins, indoles, and other substances believed to be responsible for the diarrhea, flushing, and labile blood pressure in these patients. The cardiac lesions due to gastrointestinal carcinoids are almost exclusively in the right side of the heart and occur only when there are hepatic metastases, suggesting that the substance responsible for the cardiac lesions is inactivated by passage through the liver and lungs. Similar lesions occur in the left side of the heart when there exists a right-to-left shunt or when the tumor is located in the lungs. These lesions are fibrous plaques on the endothelium of the cardiac chambers, valves, and great vessels. These plaques, which result in distortion of the cardiac valves, consist of smooth-muscle cells embedded in a stroma of acid mucopolysaccharide and collagen and presumably result from healing of endothelial injury.

The clinical syndrome is most often that of tricuspid regurgitation, pulmonic stenosis, or both. In some cases a high-output cardiac state may occur, presumably as a result of a decrease in systemic vascular resistance due to a vasoactive substance released by the tumor. Progression of the cardiac lesions does not appear to be affected by treatment with serotonin antagonists, and, in some severely symptomatic patients, valve replacement is indicated. Coronary artery spasm, presumably due to a circulating vasoactive substance, may occur in patients with carcinoid syndrome.

PHEOCHROMOCYTOMA (See also Chap. 322)

In addition to causing labile or sustained hypertension, the high circulating levels of catecholamines as a result of the pheochromocytoma may also cause direct myocardial injury. Focal myocardial necrosis and inflammatory cell infiltration are present in about 50% of patients who die with pheochromocytoma and may contribute to clinically significant left ventricular failure and pulmonary edema. In addition, hypertension results in left ventricular hypertrophy. Left ventricular function and congestive heart failure may resolve after removal of the tumor.

ACROMEGALY (See also Chap. 318)

The effect of excessive growth hormone on cardiac function results in congestive heart failure that may be due to high cardiac output, diastolic dysfunction due to ventricular hypertrophy (with increased left ventricular chamber size or wall thickness), or global systolic dysfunction. Hypertension occurs in up to one-third of patients and is characterized by suppression of the renin-aldosterone axis and increases in total body sodium and plasma volume. Cardiac disease occurs in about one-third of patients with acromegaly, and is associated with a doubling in the risk of death from heart disease.

RHEUMATOID ARTHRITIS AND THE COLLAGEN VASCULAR DISEASES

RHEUMATOID ARTHRITIS (See also Chap. 301)   There may be inflammation of any or all anatomical parts of the heart in patients with rheumatoid arthritis. Pericarditis is the most common cause of clinically apparent disease and may be found by echocardiography in 10 to 50% of all patients with rheumatoid arthritis, particularly those with subcutaneous nodules. However, only a small fraction of these patients have clinical evidence of pericarditis, which usually follows a benign course but occasionally may progress to cardiac tamponade or constrictive pericarditis. The pericardial fluid is generally an exudate, with decreased concentrations of complement and glucose, and elevated cholesterol. Coronary arteritis with intimal inflammation and edema is present in about 20% of cases but only rarely results in angina pectoris or myocardial infarction. The cardiac valves, most often the mitral and aortic, may be involved by inflammation and granuloma formation that in some cases may cause clinically significant regurgitation due to valve deformity. Myocarditis rarely results in cardiac dysfunction.

Treatment is directed at the underlying rheumatoid arthritis and may include glucocorticoids. Pericardiectomy is usually required in cases of tamponade or persistent effusion.

SERONEGATIVE ARTHROPATHIES (See also Chap. 305)   The seronegative arthropathies, ankylosing spondylitis, Reiter's syndrome, psoriatic ar-

thritis, and the arthritides associated with ulcerative colitis and regional enteritis all may be accompanied by a pancarditis and proximal aortitis; the latter may result in aortic regurgitation and may extend into the anterior mitral valve ring and/or AV node. Conduction disturbances are common, occurring in up to one-third of patients; they are more common in patients with aortic valve disease and appear to be associated with the presence of the HLA-B27 antigen. Both aortic regurgitation and AV block are more common in patients with peripheral joint involvement and longstanding disease; treatment with aortic valve replacement and permanent pacemaker placement may be required. Up to one-fifth of patients with peripheral joint involvement and disease for more than 30 years have significant aortic regurgitation. Occasionally, aortic regurgitation precedes the onset of arthritis, and, therefore, the diagnosis of a seronegative arthritis should be considered in young males with isolated aortic regurgitation.

SYSTEMIC LUPUS ERYTHEMATOSUS (SLE) (See also Chap. 300)   Pericarditis is common, occurring in about two-thirds of patients, and generally follows a benign course, although rarely tamponade or constriction may result. The characteristic *endocardial lesions* of SLE, described by Libman and Sacks, consist of wartlike lesions most often located at the angles of the AV valves or on the ventricular surface of the mitral valve. Hemodynamically important valvular regurgitation is rare. Patients with the antiphospholipid syndrome have a higher incidence of cardiovascular abnormalities, including valvular disease (particularly regurgitant lesions), a variety of thrombotic disorders (venous and arterial thrombosis, thrombocytopenia, premature stroke), myocardial infarction, pulmonary hypertension, and cardiomyopathy. Myocarditis generally parallels the activity of the disease and, although common histologically, seldom results in clinical heart failure unless associated with hypertension. Although arteritis of large coronary arteries may rarely result in myocardial ischemia, there is also an increased frequency of coronary atherosclerosis that may be related to hypertension or glucocorticoid therapy.

TRAUMATIC CARDIAC INJURY

Traumatic cardiac damage may be due to either penetrating or nonpenetrating injuries. The most frequent cause of a *nonpenetrating injury* is the impact of the chest against the steering wheel of an automobile. The absence of external signs of thoracic trauma does not exclude serious injury of the heart. Although the most common injury is myocardial contusion, any structure of the heart may be affected by the trauma.

Myocardial contusions are often not immediately recognized in trauma patients due to focus on more obvious injuries. Myocardial contusion may cause arrhythmias, bundle branch block, or ECG abnormalities resembling those of infarction or pericarditis; hence, it is important to consider trauma as a cause of otherwise unexplained ECG changes. Serum creatine kinase (CK-MB) isoenzyme levels are increased in about 20% of patients, but false-positive elevations of MB may occur in the presence of massive injuries associated with large increases in total CK. Cardiac troponin levels may have a greater diagnostic value than CK-MB levels. Echocardiography can detect abnormal wall motion and the presence of pericardial effusion, in addition to aiding in diagnosis of other forms of cardiac trauma. Myocardial contusion may produce positive radionuclide scans and regional impairment of ventricular function, as occurs in myocardial infarction (Chap. 228). Pericardial effusion may occur weeks or even months after the accident. In these cases, the pericardial effusion is a manifestation of the postcardiac injury syndrome, which resembles the post-pericardiotomy syndrome (Chap. 222).

Rupture of the heart valves or the supporting structures leads to acute valvular incompetence. The presence of a loud heart murmur followed by the development of rapidly progressive heart failure after trauma heralds this diagnosis, which can be made by either transthoracic or transesophageal echocardiography.

The most serious consequence of nonpenetrating injury is myocardial rupture, leading to tamponade or intracardiac shunting. Although it is generally immediately fatal, up to 40% of patients with cardiac rupture have been reported to survive long enough to reach a specialized trauma center. Hemopericardium may also follow tearing of a pericardial vessel or coronary artery.

Rupture of the aorta is a common consequence of nonpenetrating chest trauma. Indeed, rupture of the aorta at the isthmus or just above the aortic valve is the most common vascular deceleration injury. The clinical presentation is similar to that of aortic dissection (Chap. 231). The arterial pressure and pulse amplitude may be increased in the upper extremities and decreased in the lower extremities, and on chest x-ray there may be widening of the mediastinum. Occasionally, aortic rupture is limited by the aortic adventitia and results in a silent false aneurysm that may be discovered months or years after the injury.

Penetrating injuries of the heart, produced by bullets or stab wounds, usually result in immediate or very rapid death because of hemopericardium or massive hemorrhage. However, up to half of such patients may survive if they are resuscitated and/or survive long enough to reach a specialized trauma center. Perforation complicating the placement of an intravenous intracardiac catheter or pacemaker lead is another common cause of penetrating injuries to the heart and great vessels.

When great vessel rupture is due to a penetrating injury, there is usually a hemothorax and, less often, a hemopericardium. Hematoma formation may compress major vessels, and AV fistulae may form, sometimes resulting in high-output congestive heart failure.

Patients who suffer penetrating injuries of the heart should be carefully examined several weeks after the event to rule out a ventricular septal defect or mitral regurgitation that may have gone undetected at the time of emergency surgery. Sometimes the patient survives the acute incident and presents with a cardiac murmur and congestive heart failure. A left-to-right shunt due to traumatic ventricular septal defect, aortopulmonary artery fistula, or coronary AV fistula may be suspected and confirmed by cardiac catheterization and angiocardiography.

℞ TREATMENT

The treatment of an uncomplicated myocardial contusion, with or without myocardial infarction, is similar to that for a myocardial infarction, except that anticoagulation is contraindicated, and should include monitoring for the development of complications such as arrhythmia and cardiac rupture (Chap. 228). Acute myocardial failure resulting from the rupture of a valve usually requires operative correction. Immediate thoracotomy should be carried out for most cases of penetrating injury, or if there is evidence of cardiac tamponade and/or shock regardless of the type of trauma. Pericardiocentesis may be helpful in patients with tamponade, but usually only as a temporizing maneuver on the way to the operating room. Pericardial hemorrhage often leads to constriction, which must be treated by decortication.

FURTHER READING

KENCHAIAH S et al: Obesity and the risk of heart failure. N Engl J Med 347: 305, 2002

KLEIN I, OJAMAA K: Thyroid hormone and the cardiovascular system. N Engl J Med 344:501, 2001

KLUKE MH, MAYER RJ: Carcinoid tumors. N Engl J Med 340:858, 1999

MATTOX KL: Traumatic heart disease, in *Braunwald's Heart Disease*, 7th ed, DP Zipes et al (eds). Philadelphia, Saunders, 2005

REYMAN K: Cardiac myxomas. N Engl J Med 333:1610, 1995

RHEE PM et al: Penetrating cardiac injuries: A population-based study. J Trauma 45:366, 1998

SABATINE M, SCHOEN F: Primary tumors of the heart, in *Braunwald's Heart Disease*, 7th ed, DP Zipes et al (eds). Philadelphia, Saunders, 2005

SOWERS JR: Diabetes mellitus and cardiovascular disease in women. Arch Intern Med 158:617, 1998

VAUGHAN CJ et al: Tumors and the heart: Molecular genetic advances. Curr Opin Cardiol 16:195, 2001

Section 4   Vascular Disease

224 THE PATHOGENESIS OF ATHEROSCLEROSIS
Peter Libby

Atherosclerosis is the leading cause of death and disability in the developed world. Despite our familiarity with this disease, some of its fundamental characteristics remain poorly recognized and understood. Although many generalized or systemic risk factors predispose to its development, atherosclerosis affects various regions of the circulation preferentially and yields distinct clinical manifestations depending on the particular circulatory bed affected. Atherosclerosis of the coronary arteries commonly causes myocardial infarction (Chap. 228) and angina pectoris (Chap. 226). Atherosclerosis of the arteries supplying the central nervous system frequently provokes strokes and transient cerebral ischemia (Chap. 349). In the peripheral circulation, atherosclerosis causes intermittent claudication and gangrene and can jeopardize limb viability. Involvement of the splanchnic circulation can cause mesenteric ischemia. Atherosclerosis can affect the kidneys either directly (e.g., renal artery stenosis) or as a frequent site of atheroembolic disease (Chap. 231).

Even within a given arterial bed, atherosclerosis tends to occur focally, typically in certain predisposed regions. In the coronary circulation, for example, the proximal left anterior descending coronary artery exhibits a particular predilection for developing atherosclerotic occlusive disease. Likewise, atherosclerosis preferentially affects the proximal portions of the renal arteries and, in the extracranial circulation to the brain, the carotid bifurcation. Indeed, atherosclerotic lesions often form at branching points of arteries, regions of disturbed blood flow. Not all manifestations of atherosclerosis result from stenotic, occlusive disease. Ectasia and development of aneurysmal disease, for example, frequently occur in the aorta (Chap. 231). The mechanisms that underlie this discontinuous anatomic distribution of atherosclerosis remain uncertain.

Atherosclerosis manifests itself focally not only in space, as just described, but in time as well. Atherogenesis in humans typically occurs over a period of many years, usually many decades. Growth of atherosclerotic plaques probably does not occur in a smooth linear fashion, but rather discontinuously, with periods of relative quiescence punctuated by periods of rapid evolution. After a generally prolonged "silent" period, atherosclerosis may become clinically manifest. The clinical expressions of atherosclerosis may be *chronic*, as in the development of stable, effort-induced angina pectoris or of predictable and reproducible intermittent claudication. Alternatively, a much more dramatic *acute* clinical event such as myocardial infarction, a cerebrovascular accident, or sudden cardiac death may first herald the presence of atherosclerosis. Other individuals may never experience clinical manifestations of arterial disease despite the presence of widespread atherosclerosis demonstrated post mortem.

INITIATION OF ATHEROSCLEROSIS

FATTY STREAK FORMATION An integrated view of experimental results in animals and study of human atherosclerosis suggests that the "fatty streak" represents the initial lesion of atherosclerosis. The formation of these early lesions of atherosclerosis most often seems to arise from focal increases in the content of lipoproteins within regions of the intima. This accumulation of lipoprotein particles may not result simply from an increased permeability, or "leakiness," of the overlying endothelium (Fig. 224-1). Rather, these lipoproteins may collect in the intima of arteries because they bind to constituents of the extracellular matrix, increasing the residence time of the lipid-rich particles within the arterial wall. Lipoproteins that accumulate in the extracellular space of the intima of arteries often associate with proteoglycan molecules of the arterial extracellular matrix, an interaction that may promote the retention of lipoprotein particles by binding them and slowing their egress from the intima.

Lipoprotein particles in the extracellular space of the intima, particularly those bound to matrix macromolecules, may undergo chemical modifications. Accumulating evidence supports a pathogenic role for such modifications of lipoproteins in atherogenesis. Two types of such alterations in lipoproteins bear particular interest in the context of understanding how risk factors actually promote atherogenesis: oxidation and nonenzymatic glycation.

Lipoprotein Oxidation   Lipoproteins sequestered from plasma antioxidants in the extracellular space of the intima become susceptible to oxidative modification. Oxidatively modified low-density lipoprotein (LDL), rather than being a defined homogenous entity, actually comprises a variable and incompletely defined mixture. Both the lipid and protein moieties of these particles can participate in oxidative modification. Modifications of the lipids may include formation of hydroperoxides, lysophospholipids, oxysterols, and aldehydic breakdown products of fatty acids. Modifications of the apoprotein moieties may include breaks in the peptide backbone as well as derivatization of certain amino acid residues. A more recently recognized modification may result from local hypochlorous acid production by inflammatory cells within the plaque, giving rise to chlorinated species such as chlorotyrosyl moieties. Considerable evidence supports the presence of such oxidation products in atherosclerotic lesions.

Nonenzymatic Glycation   In diabetic patients with sustained hyperglycemia, nonenzymatic glycation of apolipoproteins and other arterial proteins likely occurs that may alter their function and propensity to accelerate atherogenesis. A good deal of experimental work suggests that both oxidatively modified and glycated lipoproteins or their constituents can contribute to many of the subsequent cellular events of lesion development.

LEUKOCYTE RECRUITMENT   After the accumulation of extracellular lipid, recruitment of leukocytes occurs as a second step in the formation of the fatty streak (Fig. 224-1). The white blood cell types typically found in the evolving atheroma include primarily cells of the mononuclear lineage: monocytes and lymphocytes. A number of adhesion molecules or receptors for leukocytes expressed on the surface of the arterial endothelial cell likely participate in the recruitment of leukocytes to the nascent fatty streak. Constituents of oxidatively modified LDL can augment expression of leukocyte adhesion molecules. This example illustrates how the accumulation of lipoproteins in the arterial intima may link mechanistically with leukocyte recruitment and subsequent events in lesion formation.

Laminar shear forces, such as those encountered in most regions of normal arteries, can also suppress the expression of leukocyte adhesion molecules. Sites of predilection for forming atherosclerotic lesions (e.g., branch points) often have disturbed laminar flow. Ordered laminar shear of normal blood flow augments the production of nitric oxide by endothelial cells. This molecule, in addition to its vasodilator properties, can act at the low levels constitutively produced by arterial endothelium as a local anti-inflammatory autacoid, for example, limiting local adhesion molecule expression. These examples indicate how hemodynamic forces may influence the cellular events that underlie atherosclerotic lesion initiation and provide a potential explanation for the focal distribution of atherosclerotic lesions at certain sites predetermined by altered flow patterns.

Once adherent to the surface of the arterial endothelial cell via interaction with adhesion receptors, the monocytes and lymphocytes penetrate the endothelial layer and take up residence in the intima. In addition to products of modified lipoproteins, cytokines (a class of protein mediators of inflammation) can regulate the expression of adhesion molecules involved in leukocyte recruitment. For example, the cytokines interleukin 1 (IL-1) or tumor necrosis factor α (TNF-α) induce or augment the expression of leukocyte adhesion molecules on endothelial cells. Because modified lipoproteins can induce cytokine release from vascular wall cells, this pathway may provide an additional link between accumulation and modification of lipoproteins and leukocyte recruitment. The directed migration of leukocytes into the arterial wall may also result from the actions of modified lipoprotein. For example, oxidized LDL may promote the chemotaxis of leukocytes. Also, oxidatively modified lipoproteins can elicit the production

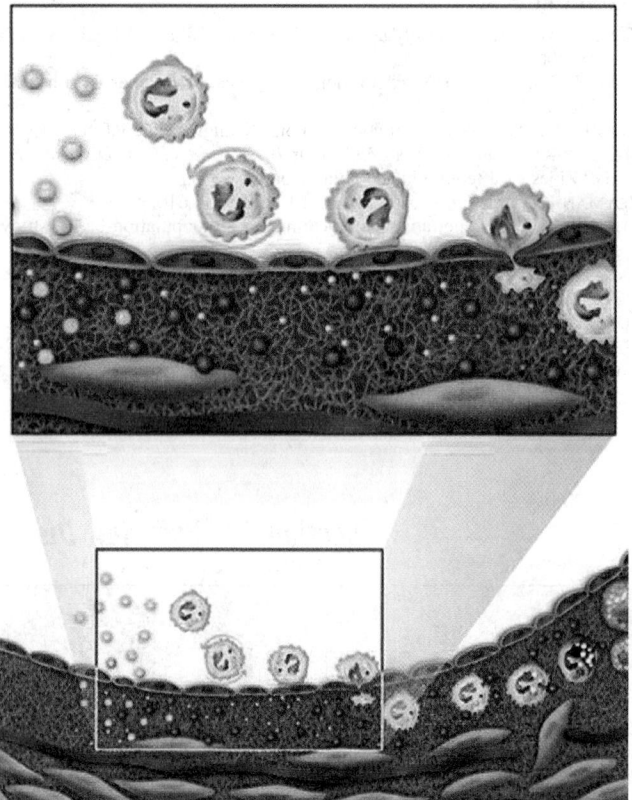

FIGURE 224-1   Cross-sectional view of an artery depicting steps in development of an atheroma, from left to right. The *upper panel* shows a detail of the boxed area below. The endothelial monolayer overlying the intima contacts blood. Hypercholesterolemia promotes accumulation of LDL particles (light spheres) in the intima. The lipoprotein particles often associate with constituents of the extracellular matrix, notably proteoglycans. Sequestration within the intima separates lipoproteins from some plasma antioxidants and favors oxidative modification. Such modified lipoprotein particles (darker spheres) may trigger a local inflammatory response responsible for signaling subsequent steps in lesion formation. The augmented expression of various adhesion molecules for leukocytes recruits monocytes to the site of a nascent arterial lesion.

Once adherent, some white blood cells will migrate into the intima. The directed migration of leukocytes probably depends on chemoattractant factors including modified lipoprotein particles themselves and chemoattractant cytokines depicted by the smaller spheres, such as the chemokine macrophage chemoattractant protein 1 produced by vascular wall cells in response to modified lipoproteins. Leukocytes in the evolving fatty streak can divide and exhibit augmented expression of receptors for modified lipoproteins (scavenger receptors). These mononuclear phagocytes ingest lipids and become foam cells, represented by a cytoplasm filled with lipid droplets. As the fatty streak evolves into a more complicated atherosclerotic lesion, smooth-muscle cells migrate from the media (*bottom of lower panel*), through the internal elastic membrane (*solid wavy line*), and accumulate within the expanding intima where they lay down extracellular matrix that forms the bulk of the advanced lesion (*bottom panel, right-hand side*).

by vascular wall cells of chemoattractant cytokines such as monocyte chemoattractant protein 1.

FOAM CELL FORMATION Once resident within the intima, the mononuclear phagocytes differentiate into macrophages and transform into lipid-laden foam cells. The conversion of mononuclear phagocytes into foam cells requires the uptake of lipoprotein particles by receptor-mediated endocytosis. One might suppose that the well-recognized "classical" receptor for LDL mediates this lipid uptake. Patients or animals lacking effective LDL receptors due to genetic alterations (e.g., familial hypercholesterolemia), however, have abundant arterial lesions and extraarterial xanthomata rich in macrophage-derived foam cells. Also, the exogenous cholesterol suppresses expression of the LDL receptor, such that under hypercholesterolemic conditions the level of this cell-surface receptor for LDL decreases. Candidates for alternative receptors that can mediate lipid-loading of foam cells include a growing number of macrophage "scavenger" receptors, which preferentially endocytose modified lipoproteins, and other receptors for oxidized LDL or β-VLDL (very low density lipoprotein), a type of lipoprotein commonly encountered in certain hypercholesterolemic states (Chap. 335). By ingesting lipids from the extracellular space, the mononuclear phagocytes bearing such scavenger receptors may remove lipoproteins from the developing lesion. Some lipid-loaded macrophages may leave the artery wall, functioning to clear lipid from the artery. Lipid accumulation, and hence propensity to form atheroma, ensues if the amount of lipid entering the artery wall exceeds that exported by mononuclear phagocytes or other pathways. Macrophages may thus play a vital role in the dynamic economy of lipid accumulation in the arterial wall during atherogenesis. Some lipid-laden foam cells within the expanding intimal lesion perish. Some foam cells may die as a result of programmed cell death known as *apoptosis*. This death of mononuclear phagocytes results in formation of the lipid-rich center, often called the *necrotic core*, of more complicated atherosclerotic plaques.

Macrophages taking up modified lipoproteins, much like intrinsic vascular wall cells, may elaborate cytokines and growth factors that can further signal some of the cellular events in lesion complication. A number of growth factors or cytokines elaborated by mononuclear phagocytes can stimulate smooth-muscle cell proliferation and production of extracellular matrix, which accumulates in atherosclerotic plaques. Cytokines found in the plaque, including IL-1 or TNF-α, can induce local production of growth factors such as forms of platelet-derived growth factor (PDGF), fibroblast growth factor, and others that may contribute to plaque evolution and complication. Other cytokines, notably interferon γ (IFN-γ) derived from activated T cells within lesions, can inhibit smooth-muscle proliferation and synthesis of interstitial forms of collagen. These examples illustrate how atherogenesis likely depends on a complex balance between mediators that can promote lesion formation and other pathways that can mitigate the atherogenic process.

FACTORS THAT MODULATE INHIBITION OF ATHEROMA

Elaboration of small molecules by activated mononuclear phagocytes and vascular wall cells in the evolving lesion may also modulate atherogenesis. Notably, reactive oxygen species can modulate growth of smooth-muscle cells, activate inflammatory gene expression via the nuclear factor kappa B (NFκB) transcriptional control system, and annihilate NO radicals, decreasing the effect of this endogenous vasodilator. However, the macrophage in the lesion may be activated to express the inducible form of the enzyme that can synthesize NO, known as inducible NO synthase. This high-capacity form of the enzyme can produce relatively large, potentially cytotoxic amounts of NO radicals. While at the low concentrations of NO produced by the constitutive NO synthase in endothelial cells, this radical may produce beneficial effects; when overproduced by activated phagocytes, however, it may prove deleterious.

Export by phagocytes may constitute one response to local lipid overload in the evolving lesion. Another mechanism, reverse cholesterol transport mediated by high-density lipoproteins (HDL), may provide an independent pathway for lipid removal from atheroma. This transfer of cholesterol from the cell to the HDL particle involves specialized cell surface molecules such as the ATP binding cassette transporter (ABCA1) (the gene mutated in Tangier disease, a condition characterized by very low HDL levels) and a family of scavenger receptors (the "B" family). Such "reverse cholesterol transport" explains part of HDL's antiatherogenic action.

Although clear evidence supports lipoprotein disorders as predisposing factors for atheroma formation, other etiologies may contribute to or modulate atherogenesis (see Table 225-1). For example, hypertension constitutes an independent risk factor for coronary events. Male gender and the postmenopausal state also augment the risk of developing coronary artery disease. Premenopausal women have increased HDL levels compared to age-matched men. However, a favorable lipoprotein pattern only partially accounts for the protection against atherosclerosis conferred by the premenopausal state. Although laboratory studies suggest that estrogens have direct beneficial effects on the arterial wall, clinical trials have not shown that estrogen replacement therapy prevents recurrent myocardial infarction in postmenopausal women. Indeed, treatment with a combination of estrogen and progesterone appears to augment cardiovascular events in women with or without prior myocardial infarction.

Diabetes mellitus aggravates atherogenesis. In addition to the well-known microvascular complications of diabetes (Chap. 323), macrovascular disease such as atherosclerosis causes a great deal of excess mortality in the diabetic population. Diabetes-associated dyslipidemias strongly promote atherogenesis. In particular, the constellation of insulin resistance, high triglycerides, and low HDL, often in association with the central adiposity and hypertension frequently seen in type 2 diabetic patients, seems to accelerate atherogenesis potently. As noted above, hyperglycemia may promote the nonenzymatic glycation of LDL. LDL modified in this manner, like oxidatively modified LDL, may signal many of the initial events in atherogenesis. Triglyceride-rich lipoprotein particles, often elevated in poorly controlled diabetic patients, also accentuate atherogenesis.

Lp(a) (often pronounced "lipoprotein little a" to distinguish it from apolipoprotein AI and others found in HDL) provides a potential link between hemostasis and blood lipids. The Lp(a) particle consists of an apoprotein (a) molecule bound by a sulfhydryl link to the apolipoprotein B moiety of an LDL particle. Apoprotein (a) has homology with plasminogen and may inhibit fibrinolysis by competing with plasminogen. Other risk factors for atherosclerosis related to blood clotting include elevated levels of fibrinogen or of the inhibitor of fibrinolysis, plasminogen-activator inhibitor 1 (PAI-1). Another nonlipid risk factor for coronary events, elevated levels of *homocysteine*, may act by promoting thrombosis, although the pathophysiology of this association is uncertain at present. Although individuals with marked elevations of Lp(a) or homocysteine do appear to have heightened risk of coronary thrombosis, in the population at large these factors show a much weaker correlation with vascular events than LDL, HDL, or the global inflammatory marker C-reactive protein (CRP).

The relationship between *tobacco use* and atherosclerosis also remains poorly understood. The rapid reduction in risk for cardiac events after cessation of cigarette smoking implies that tobacco may promote thrombosis or some other determinant of plaque stability as well as contribute to the evolution of the atherosclerotic lesion itself. For example, tobacco smokers have elevated fibrinogen levels, a variable associated with increased atherosclerosis and acute cardiovascular events.

INFLAMMATION In other situations, antecedent inflammatory states may predispose toward atherosclerosis. For example, *Kawasaki disease* in childhood may promote development of vascular lesions in the arteries of adults. Infectious agents continue to be proposed as instigators or potentiators of atherogenesis. However, in humans, an atherogenic role for viral or microbial pathogens (e.g., Herpesviridiae, including cytomegalovirus, or *Chlamydia*) remains speculative. In some patients, immune or autoimmune reactions may contribute to atherogenesis. In the particular example of the accelerated form of coronary arteriopathy that plagues heart transplant recipients, immunologic factors may contribute importantly to the pathogenesis.

Known monogenic defects in lipoprotein metabolism account for only a fraction of the familial risk for coronary artery disease. Thus, other as yet undefined and perhaps multiple genetic factors may contribute to coronary risk. Mechanisms of disease susceptibility involving the arterial wall might account for some of the genetic predisposition to atherosclerosis unexplained by lipoprotein disorders. Application of molecular genetic techniques may identify new polymorphisms linked to coronary risk and may eventually shed light on new pathophysiologic mechanisms. For example, some data suggest a link between certain alleles of the genes encoding angiotensin-converting enzyme, the cytokine lymphotoxin, or PAI-1 with increased risk of myocardial infarction. Application of genomic technologies may aid identification of "modifier" genes that modulate individual responses to established risk factors. Large studies currently in progress should clarify these and other potential genetic factors that influence atherosclerosis.

ATHEROMA EVOLUTION AND COMPLICATIONS

INVOLVEMENT OF ARTERIAL SMOOTH-MUSCLE CELLS Although the fatty streak commonly precedes the development of a more advanced atherosclerotic plaque, not all fatty streaks progress to form complex atheromas. Why do some fatty streaks progress to fibrous lesions while others do not? By what mechanisms do fatty streaks evolve into more complex lesions? While accumulation of lipid-laden macrophages is the hallmark of the fatty streaks, accumulation of fibrous tissue typifies the more advanced atherosclerotic lesion. The smooth-muscle cell synthesizes the bulk of the extracellular matrix of the complex atherosclerotic lesion. Hence, arrival of smooth-muscle cells and their elaboration of extracellular matrix probably provides a critical transition, yielding a fibrofatty lesion in place of a simple accumulation of macrophage-derived foam cells.

Recent research has provided insight into the mechanisms that may trigger migration and proliferation of smooth-muscle cells into and within the evolving intimal lesion and signal the accumulation of extracellular matrix. Cytokines and growth factors elicited by modified lipoproteins or other agents from both vascular wall cells and infiltrating leukocytes can modulate functions of the smooth-muscle cell (Fig. 224-1). For example, PDGF elaborated by activated endothelial cells can stimulate the migration of smooth-muscle cells. In this manner, smooth-muscle cells resident in the tunica media may migrate into the intima. Various growth factors produced locally can stimulate the proliferation of both resident smooth-muscle cells in the intima and those that have migrated from the media. Transforming growth factor β (TGF-β), among other mediators, potently stimulates interstitial collagen production by smooth-muscle cells. These mediators may arise not only from neighboring vascular cells or leukocytes (a "paracrine" pathway) but also, in some instances, from the same cell that responds to the factor (an "autocrine" pathway). Together, these alterations in smooth-muscle cells, signaled by these mediators acting at short distances, can hasten transformation of the fatty streak into a more fibrous smooth-muscle cell and extracellular matrix-rich lesion.

BLOOD COAGULATION In addition to locally produced mediators, atherogenic risk factor signals related to blood coagulation and thrombosis likely contribute to atheroma evolution and complication. Current evidence suggests that fatty streak formation begins underneath a morphologically intact endothelium. In advanced fatty streaks, however, microscopic breaches in endothelial integrity may occur. Microthrombi rich in platelets can form at such sites of limited endothelial denudation, due to exposure of the highly thrombogenic extracellular

matrix of underlying basement membrane. Activated platelets release numerous factors that can promote the fibrotic response. In addition to PDGF and TGF-β, low-molecular-weight mediators such as serotonin can also alter smooth-muscle function. Most of these microthrombi probably resolve without clinical manifestation by a process of local fibrinolysis, resorption, and endothelial repair.

MICROVESSELS As atherosclerotic lesions advance, abundant plexi of microvessels develop in connection with the artery's vasa vasorum. These newly developing microvascular networks may contribute to lesion complication in several ways. These blood vessels provide an abundant surface area for leukocyte trafficking and may serve as the portal of entry and exit of white blood cells from the established atheroma. The plaques' microvessels may also furnish foci for intraplaque hemorrhage. Like the neovessels in the diabetic retina, microvessels of the plaque may be friable and prone to rupture and produce focal hemorrhage. Such a vascular leak leads to thrombosis in situ and thrombin generation from prothrombin. In addition to its role in blood coagulation, thrombin can modulate many aspects of vascular cell function including stimulation of proliferation and cytokine release from smooth-muscle cells and production of growth factors such as PDGF from endothelial cells. Atherosclerotic plaques often contain fibrin and hemosiderin, indicating episodes of intraplaque hemorrhage as an element in plaque complication.

As they advance, atherosclerotic plaques also accumulate *calcium*. Proteins that are usually associated with bone also occur in atherosclerotic lesions. For example, osteocalcin, osteopontin, and bone morphogenetic proteins localize in atherosclerotic plaques. In fact, mineralization of the atherosclerotic plaque recapitulates many aspects of bone formation.

PLAQUE EVOLUTION Traditionally, atherosclerosis research has focused much attention on proliferation of smooth-muscle cells, yet these cells actually replicate rather slowly in complicated atherosclerotic lesions. Estimates of the rate of smooth-muscle cell division in such lesions at a given time show a replicative rate below 1%. Such observations do not exclude bursts of proliferative activity at certain junctures in the history of an atheroma, perhaps in association with local thrombin generation due to microvascular hemorrhage or formation of a microthrombus at a site of localized endothelial denudation, as discussed above. On the other hand, cell death has been recognized as a component of atherogenesis since the time of Virchow in the mid-nineteenth century. Indeed, complex atheroma often have a primarily fibrous character lacking the hypercellular appearance of less advanced lesions and actually exhibiting a paucity of smooth-muscle cells. This relative lack of smooth-muscle cells in advanced atheroma may result from the ultimate predominance of cytostatic mediators such as TGF-β or IFN-γ, which can inhibit smooth-muscle cell proliferation. Also, smooth-muscle cells as well as macrophages in advanced atherosclerotic lesions can undergo programmed cell death, or apoptosis. Some of the same cytokines that activate atherogenic functions of vascular wall cells can also trigger apoptosis in these cells.

Thus, during the evolution of the atherosclerotic plaque, a complex balance between entry and egress of lipoproteins and leukocytes, cell proliferation and cell death, extracellular matrix production and remodeling, as well as calcification and neovascularization contribute to lesion formation. Multiple and often competing signals trigger these various cellular events. Increasingly, we appreciate links between atherogenic risk factors and the altered behavior of intrinsic vascular wall cells and infiltrating leukocytes that underlie the complex pathogenesis of these lesions.

CLINICAL SYNDROMES OF ATHEROSCLEROSIS

Atherosclerotic lesions occur ubiquitously in Western societies. Most atheroma produce no symptoms, and many never cause clinical manifestations. Numerous patients with diffuse atherosclerosis may succumb to unrelated illnesses without ever having experienced a clinically significant manifestation of atherosclerosis. What accounts for this variability in the clinical expression of atherosclerotic disease?

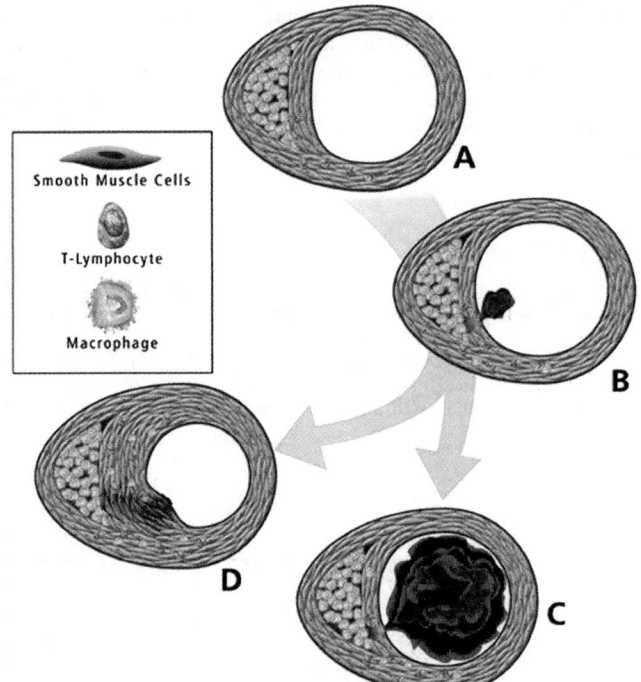

FIGURE 224-2   Plaque rupture, thrombosis, and healing. *A.* Arterial remodeling during atherogenesis. During the initial part of the life history of an atheroma, growth is often outward, preserving the caliber of lumen. This phenomenon of "compensatory enlargement" accounts in part for the tendency of coronary arteriography to underestimate the degree of atherosclerosis. *B.* Rupture of the plaque's fibrous cap causes thrombosis. Physical disruption of the atherosclerotic plaque commonly causes arterial thrombosis by allowing blood coagulant factors to contact thrombogenic collagen found in the arterial extracellular matrix and tissue factor produced by macrophage-derived foam cells in the lipid core of lesions. In this manner, sites of plaque rupture form the nidus for thrombi. The normal artery wall possesses several fibrinolytic or antithrombotic mechanisms that tend to resist thrombosis and lyse clots that begin to form in situ. Such antithrombotic or thrombolytic molecules include thrombomodulin, tissue and urokinase-type plasminogen activators, heparan sulfate proteoglycans, prostacyclin, and nitric oxide. *C.* When the clot overwhelms the endogenous fibrinolytic mechanisms, it may propagate and lead to arterial occlusion. The consequences of this occlusion depend on the degree of existing collateral vessels. In a patient with chronic multivessel, occlusive coronary artery disease, collateral channels have often formed. In such circumstances, even a total arterial occlusion may not lead to myocardial infarction, or it may produce an unexpectedly modest or a non-ST segment elevation infarct because of collateral flow. In the patient with less advanced disease and without substantial stenotic lesions to provide a stimulus to collateral vessel formation, sudden plaque rupture and arterial occlusion commonly produces ST-segment elevation infarction. These are the types of patients who may present with myocardial infarction or sudden death as a first manifestation of coronary atherosclerosis. In some cases, the thrombus may lyse or organize into a mural thrombus without occluding the vessel. Such instances may be clinically silent. *D.* The subsequent thrombin-induced fibrosis and healing causes a fibroproliferative response that can lead to a more fibrous lesion, one that can produce an eccentric plaque that causes a hemodynamically significant stenosis. In this way, a nonocclusive mural thrombus, even if clinically silent or causing unstable angina rather than infarction, can provoke a healing response that can promote lesion fibrosis and luminal encroachment. Such a sequence of events may convert a "vulnerable" atheroma with a thin fibrous cap prone to rupture into a more "stable" fibrous plaque with a reinforced cap. Angioplasty of unstable coronary lesions may "stabilize" the lesions by a similar mechanism, producing a wound followed by healing.

Arterial remodeling during atheroma formation (Fig. 224-2*A*) represents a frequently overlooked but clinically important feature of lesion evolution. During the initial phases of atheroma development, the plaque usually grows outward, in an abluminal direction. Vessels affected by atherogenesis tend to increase in diameter, a phenomenon known as *compensatory enlargement*, a type of vascular remodeling. The growing atheroma does not encroach upon the arterial lumen until the burden of atherosclerotic plaque exceeds approximately 40% of the area encompassed by the internal elastic lamina. Thus, during much of its life history, an atheroma will not cause stenosis that can limit tissue perfusion.

Flow-limiting stenoses commonly form later in the history of the plaque. Many such plaques cause stable syndromes such as demand-induced angina pectoris or intermittent claudication in the extremities. In the coronary and other circulations, even occlusion due to atheroma does not invariably lead to infarction. The hypoxic stimulus of repeated bouts of ischemia characteristically induces formation of collateral vessels in the myocardium, mitigating the consequences of an acute occlusion of an epicardial coronary artery. On the other hand, we now appreciate that many lesions that cause acute or unstable atherosclerotic syndromes, particularly in the coronary circulation, may arise from atherosclerotic plaques that do not produce a flow-limiting stenosis. Such lesions may produce only minimal luminal irregularities on traditional angiograms and often do not meet the traditional criteria for "significance" by arteriography. Instability of such nonocclusive stenoses may explain the frequency of myocardial infarction as an initial manifestation of coronary artery disease (in at least a third of cases) in patients who report no prior history of angina pectoris, a syndrome usually caused by flow-limiting stenoses.

PLAQUE INSTABILITY AND RUPTURE   Pathologic studies afford considerable insight into the microanatomic substrate underlying the "instability" of plaques that are not critically stenotic. A superficial erosion of the endothelium or a frank plaque rupture or fissure usually produces the thrombus that causes episodes of unstable angina pectoris or the occlusive and relatively persistent thrombus that causes acute myocardial infarction (Fig. 224-2*B*). In the case of carotid atheroma, a deeper ulceration that provides a nidus for formation of platelet thrombi may underlie the unstable syndromes that cause transient ischemic attacks.

Rupture of the plaque's fibrous cap (Fig. 224-2*C*) permits contact between coagulation factors in the blood with highly thrombogenic tissue factor expressed by macrophage foam cells in the plaque's lipid-rich core. If the ensuing thrombus is nonocclusive or transient, the episode of plaque disruption may not cause symptoms or may result in ischemic symptoms such as rest angina. Occlusive thrombi that endure will often cause acute myocardial infarction, particularly in the absence of a well-developed collateral circulation supplying the affected territory. Repetitive episodes of plaque disruption and healing provide one likely mechanism of transition of the fatty streak to a more complex fibrous lesion (Fig. 224-2*D*). The healing process in arteries, as in skin wounds, involves the laying down of new extracellular matrix and fibrosis.

Not all atheroma exhibit the same propensity to rupture. Pathologic studies of culprit lesions that have caused acute myocardial infarction reveal several characteristic features. Plaques that have proved vulnerable tend to have thin fibrous caps, relatively large lipid cores, and a high content of macrophages. Morphometric studies of such culprit lesions show that macrophages and T lymphocytes predominate at the site of plaque rupture. On the other hand, sites of plaque rupture contain relatively few smooth-muscle cells. The cells that concentrate at sites of plaque rupture bear markers of inflammatory activation. The presence of the transplantation, or histocompatibility, antigen HLA-DR provides one convenient gauge of the degree of inflammation in cells in atheroma. Resting cells in normal arteries seldom express this transplantation antigen. However, macrophages and smooth-muscle cells at sites of human coronary artery plaque disruption do bear this inducible cell-surface marker. Therefore, the presence of HLA-DR-positive macrophages and T cells indicates an ongoing inflammatory response at sites of plaque rupture.

Inflammatory mediators may actually regulate processes that govern the integrity of the plaque's fibrous cap and hence its propensity to rupture. For example, the T cell–derived cytokine IFN-γ, found in atherosclerotic plaques and required to induce the HLA-DR present at sites of rupture, can inhibit growth and collagen synthesis of smooth-muscle cells. Cytokines derived from activated macrophages such as TNF-α or IL-1 in addition to T cell–derived IFN-γ can elicit the expression of genes that encode proteolytic enzymes that can degrade the extracellular matrix of the plaque's fibrous cap. Thus, inflammatory mediators can impair collagen synthesis required for maintenance and repair of the fibrous cap and trigger degradation of extracellular matrix macromolecules, processes that weaken the plaque's fibrous cap and enhance its vulnerability to rupture. In contrast to vulnerable plaques, those with a dense extracellular matrix and relatively thick fibrous cap without substantial tissue factor-rich lipid cores seem generally resistant to rupture and unlikely to provoke thrombosis.

CONCLUSION

We now appreciate that features of the biology of the atheromatous plaque in addition to its degree of luminal encroachment influence the clinical manifestations of this disease. This enhanced understanding

of plaque biology provides insight into the diverse ways in which atherosclerosis can present clinically and why the disease may remain silent or stable for prolonged periods, punctuated by acute complications at certain times. Increased understanding of atherogenesis provides new insight into the ways in which current therapies may improve outcomes and also suggests new targets for future intervention.

FURTHER READING

GLASS CK, WITZTUM JL: Atherosclerosis. The road ahead. Cell 104:503, 2001
LIBBY P: Current concepts of the pathogenesis of the acute coronary syndromes. Circulation 104:365, 2001
——— et al: Inflammation and atherosclerosis. Circulation 105:1135, 2002
LUSIS AJ: Atherosclerosis. Nature 407:233, 2000
VIRMANI R et al: Pathology of the unstable plaque. Prog Cardiovasc Dis 44: 349, 2002

225 PREVENTION AND TREATMENT OF ATHEROSCLEROSIS
Peter Libby

Atherosclerosis remains the major cause of death and premature disability in developed societies. Moreover, current predictions estimate that by the year 2020 cardiovascular diseases, notably atherosclerosis, will become the leading global cause of total disease burden, defined as the years subtracted from healthy life by disability or premature death. Substantial success has been achieved in recent years in reducing morbidity and mortality due to acute coronary events. However, the treatment of the underlying disease process, atherosclerosis, and preventing its acute complications presents an enormous challenge and opportunity simultaneously.

THE CONCEPT OF ATHEROSCLEROTIC RISK FACTORS

During the first half of the twentieth century, animal experiments and clinical observation linked certain variables, such as hypercholesterolemia, to the risk of atherosclerotic events. The systematic study of risk factors in humans, however, began approximately mid-century. The prospective, community-based Framingham Heart Study provided rigorous support for the concept that hypercholesterolemia, hypertension, and other factors correlated with cardiovascular risk. Similar observational studies performed in the United States and abroad provided independent support for the concept of "risk factors" for cardiovascular disease. Numerous data suggested a link between dietary habits and cardiovascular risk based upon population surveys.

From a practical viewpoint, the cardiovascular risk factors that have emerged from such studies fall into two categories: those modifiable by lifestyle and/or pharmacotherapy and those that are essentially unmodifiable. The weight of evidence supporting various risk factors differs. For example, hypercholesterolemia and hypertension certainly predict coronary risk, but other so-called nontraditional risk factors, such as levels of homocysteine, lipoprotein (a) [Lp(a)], or infection, remain controversial. One must further distinguish factors that actually participate in atherogenesis from those that may merely serve as markers of risk without direct involvement in pathogenesis. Table 225-1 lists the risk factors recognized by the current National Cholesterol Education Project Adult Treatment Panel III (ATP III). The sections below will consider some of these risk factors and approaches to their modification.

LIPID DISORDERS Abnormalities in plasma lipoproteins and derangements in lipid metabolism rank as the most firmly established and best understood risk factors for atherosclerosis. Chap. 335 describes the lipoprotein classes and provides a detailed discussion of lipoprotein metabolism. Chap. 224 considers the mechanisms by which lipopro-

TABLE 225-1 *Major Risk Factors (Exclusive of LDL Cholesterol) That Modify LDL Goals*

Cigarette smoking
Hypertension (BP $\geq$ 140/90 mmHg or on antihypertensive medication)
Low HDL cholesterol[a] [<1.0 mmol/L (<40 mg/dL)]
Diabetes mellitus
Family history of premature CHD
    CHD in male first-degree relative <55 years
    CHD in female first-degree relative <65 years
Age (men $\geq$45 years; women $\geq$55 years)
Lifestyle risk factors
    Obesity (BMI $\geq$ 30 kg/m^2)
    Physical inactivity
    Atherogenic diet
Emerging risk factors
    Lipoprotein(a)
    Homocysteine
    Prothrombotic factors
    Proinflammatory factors
    Impaired fasting glucose
    Subclinical atherogenesis

[a] HDL cholesterol $\geq$1.6 mmol/L ($\geq$60 mg/dL) counts as a "negative" risk factor; its presence removes one risk factor from the total count.
Note: LDL, low-density lipoprotein; BP, blood pressure; HDL, high-density lipoprotein; CHD, coronary heart disease; BMI, body-mass index.
Source: Modified from Expert Panel on Detection, Evaluation, and Treatment of High Blood Cholesterol in Adults (Adult Treatment Panel III). JAMA 285:2486, 2001.

teins may influence atherogenesis. Therefore, this section will focus on preventive aspects of the treatment of lipid disorders.

Current ATP III guidelines recommend cholesterol screening in all adults >20 years. The screen should include a fasting lipid profile [total cholesterol, triglycerides, low-density lipoprotein (LDL) cholesterol, and high-density lipoprotein (HDL) cholesterol] repeated every 5 years. The ATP III guidelines strive to match the intensity of treatment to an individual's risk. A quantitative estimate of risk places individuals in one of three treatment strata (Table 225-2). The first step in applying these guidelines is to count an individual's risk factors (Table 225-1). Individuals with fewer than two risk factors fall into the lowest treatment intensity stratum [LDL goal <4.1 mmol/L (< 160 mg/dL)]. In those with two or more of these risk factors, the next step involves a simple calculation of an estimate of the 10-year risk of developing coronary heart disease (CHD) (Table 225-1); (see also *http://www.nhlbi.nih.gov/guidelines/cholesterol/* for the algorithm and a downloadable risk calculator). Those with a 10-year risk $\leq$ 20% fall into the intermediate stratum [LDL goal <3.4 mmol/L (< 130 mg/

dL)]. Those with a calculated 10-year CHD risk of > 20%, any evidence of established atherosclerosis, or diabetes (now considered a CHD risk-equivalent) fall into the most intensive treatment group [LDL goal <2.6 mmol/L (< 100 mg/dL)]. The first maneuver to achieve the LDL goal involves therapeutic lifestyle changes (TLC), including specific diet and exercise recommendations established by the guidelines. According to ATP III criteria, those with LDL levels exceeding goal for their risk group by >0.8 mmol/L (> 30 mg/dL) merit consideration for drug therapy. In patients with triglycerides >2.6 mmol/L (>200 mg/dL), ATP III guidelines specify a secondary goal for therapy, "non-HDL cholesterol" (simply the HDL cholesterol level subtracted from the total cholesterol). Cutpoints for therapeutic decision for non-HDL cholesterol are 0.8 mmol/L (30 mg/dL) more than those for LDL. A robust body of clinical trial evidence now supports the effectiveness of aggressive management of dyslipidemia. Addition of drug therapy to dietary and other nonpharmacologic measures reduces cardiovascular risk in patients with established coronary atherosclerosis and in individuals who have not previously suffered CHD events as well (Fig. 225-1). As guidelines inevitably lag the emerging clinical trial evidence base, the practitioner may elect to exercise clinical judgement in making therapeutic decisions in individual patients.

Lipid-lowering therapies do not appear to exert their beneficial effect on cardiovascular events by causing a marked "regression" of obstructive coronary lesions. Angiographically monitored studies of lipid lowering have shown at best a modest reduction in coronary artery stenoses over the duration of study. Yet these same studies consistently show substantial decreases in coronary events. These results suggest that the beneficial mechanism of lipid lowering does not require a substantial reduction in the fixed stenoses. Rather, the benefit may derive from "stabilization" of atherosclerotic lesions without decreased stenosis. Such stabilization of atherosclerotic lesions and the attendant decrease in coronary events may result from the egress of lipids or by favorably influencing aspects of the biology of atherogenesis discussed in Chap. 224. In addition, as sizeable lesions may protrude abluminally rather than into the lumen, shrinkage of such plaques might not be apparent on angiograms.

The benefit of LDL lowering by HMG-CoA reductase inhibitor (statin) therapy on cardiovascular events seems to require 6 to 24 months of treatment. Improvement of vasomotor responses to endothelial-dependent vasodilators occurs much more rapidly, requiring ≤6 months. Thus, HMG-CoA reductase inhibitors may act by two or more mechanisms on the arteries of hypercholesterolemic individuals. The relatively rapid improvement in endothelial-dependent vasomotion may reflect enhanced production or reduced destruction of the endogenous vasodilator nitric oxide at the level of the arterial endothelium. Reduction in the thrombotic complications of atherosclerosis, such as myocardial infarction or unstable angina, probably requires more prolonged treatment to effect removal of lipid from deeper within the atheroma, yielding improvements in the biology underlying plaque destabilization described in Chap. 224. In addition to their potent beneficial effects on the lipid profile, statins may have direct actions on the biology of the atheroma independent of lipid lowering.

In addition to statins, clinical trials have shown reductions in CHD events in certain populations with drugs that affect the lipoprotein profile, including fibric acid derivatives and nicotinic acid. New classes of lipid-lowering medications, including cholesterol absorption inhibitors, may prove useful adjuncts to current therapies; however, clinical trial evidence demonstrating benefits for CHD outcomes are not yet available.

Current understanding of the mechanism by which elevated LDL levels promote atherogenesis relates to oxidative modification of these particles within the artery wall, promoting formation of macrophage-derived foam cells and providing a stimulus for inflammation (Chap. 224). These concepts stimulated interest in the possibility that anti-

Risk Category	LDL Goal, mmol/L (mg/dL)	LDL Level at which to Initiate TLC, mmol/L (mg/dL)	LDL Level at which to Consider Drug Therapy, mmol/L (mg/dL)
CHD or CHD risk equivalents[a] (10-year risk >20%)	<2.6 (<100)	≥2.6 (≥100)	≥3.4 (≥130) [drug optional between 2.6 and 3.3 (100 and 129)]
2+ Risk factors (10-year risk ≤20%)	<3.4 (<130)	≥3.4 (≥130)	10-Year risk 10–20%: ≥3.4 (≥130) 10-Year risk 10%: ≥4.1 (≥160)
0–2 Risk factors	<4.1 (<160)	≥4.1 (≥160)	≥4.9 (≥190) [drug optional between 4.1 and 4.9 (160 and 189)]

TABLE 225-2 LDL Cholesterol Goals and Cutpoints for Therapeutic Lifestyle Changes (TLC) and Drug Therapy in Different Risk Categories

[a] Diabetes mellitus is a CHD risk equivalent.
Note: LDL, low-density lipoprotein; CHD, coronary heart disease.

oxidants, either dietary or pharmacologic, might reduce CHD events. Both experimental and observational clinical studies supported this notion. However, rigorous and well-controlled clinical trials have consistently shown that antioxidant vitamin therapy does *not* improve CHD outcomes. Therefore, the current evidence base does *not* support the use of antioxidant vitamins for this indication.

HYPERTENSION (See also Chap. 230)   A wealth of epidemiologic data support a relationship between hypertension and atherosclerotic risk, and extensive clinical trial evidence has established that pharmacologic treatment of hypertension can reduce the risk of stroke and heart failure. More recent studies also show a reduction in CHD risk by antihypertensive therapy, particularly interruption of the renin-angiotensin system.

DIABETES MELLITUS, INSULIN RESISTANCE, AND THE METABOLIC SYNDROME (See also Chap. 323)   Diabetes mellitus is a CHD risk equivalent; most patients with diabetes mellitus die of atherosclerosis and its complications. Aging and rampant obesity in the U.S. population underlie a current epidemic of type 2 (non-insulin-dependent) diabetes mellitus. The abnormal lipoprotein profile associated with insulin resistance, known as *diabetic dyslipidemia*, accounts for part of the elevated cardiovascular risk in patients with type 2 diabetes. While diabetic patients often have LDL cholesterol levels near average, the LDL particles tend to be smaller and denser and thus more atherogenic (Chap. 335). Other features of diabetic dyslipidemia include low HDL and elevated triglyceride levels. Hypertension also frequently accompanies

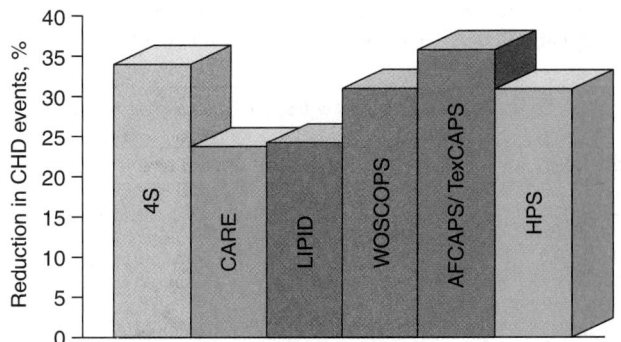

FIGURE 225-1 Lipid lowering reduces coronary events, as reflected on this graph showing the reduction percentages for onset of the acute coronary syndromes achieved by participants in six major clinical studies. 4S, Scandinavian Simvastatin Survival Study (patients with coronary heart disease and elevated cholesterol); CARE, Cholesterol and Recurrent Events (patients with coronary heart disease and average cholesterol); LIPID, Long-Term Intervention with Pravastatin in Ischemic Disease (patients with coronary heart disease and average cholesterol); WOSCOPS, West of Scotland Coronary Prevention Study (normal patients with elevated cholesterol); AFCAPS/TexCAPS, Air Force Coronary Atherosclerosis Prevention Study/Texas Coronary Atherosclerosis Prevention Study (normal patients with average cholesterol); HPS, Heart Protection Study (patients with coronary heart disease, or at high risk, with a wide range of cholesterol).

obesity, insulin resistance, and dyslipidemia. Indeed, the ATP III guidelines now recognize this cluster of risk factors and provide criteria for diagnosis of the "metabolic syndrome" (Table 225-3).

Therapeutic objectives for intervention in these patients include addressing the underlying causes, including obesity and low physical activity, by initiating TLC. The ATP III guidelines provide an explicit step-by-step plan for implementing TLC. Treatment of the component risk factors should accompany TLC. Establishing that strict glycemic control reduces the risk of macrovascular complications of diabetes has proved much more elusive than the established beneficial effects on microvascular complications such as retinopathy or renal disease. In the absence of clear-cut evidence that tight glycemic control reduces coronary risk in diabetic patients, attention to other aspects of risk in this patient population assumes even greater importance. In this regard, multiple clinical trials have demonstrated unequivocal benefit of HMG-CoA reductase inhibitor therapy in diabetic patients over all ranges of LDL cholesterol levels. The Veterans Affairs HDL Intervention Trial showed that gemfibrozil, a fibric acid derivative, reduced CHD and stroke in a population of men, many of whom had features of the metabolic syndrome. Diabetic populations appear to derive particular benefit from antihypertensive strategies that block the action of angiotensin II. Thus, the antihypertensive regimen for patients with the metabolic syndrome should include angiotensin-converting enzyme inhibitors or angiotensin receptor blockers when possible. Most of these individuals will require more than one antihypertensive agent to achieve the current American Diabetes Association blood pressure goal of 130/85 mmHg.

MALE GENDER/POSTMENOPAUSAL STATE Decades of observational studies have verified excess coronary risk in men compared with premenopausal women. After menopause, however, coronary risk accelerates in women. At least part of the apparent protection against CHD in premenopausal women derives from their relatively higher HDL levels compared with those of men. After menopause, HDL values fall in concert with increased coronary risk. Estrogen therapy lowers LDL cholesterol and raises HDL cholesterol, changes that should decrease coronary risk.

Multiple observational and experimental studies suggested that estrogen therapy (ET) might reduce coronary risk. However, several recent clinical trials have failed to demonstrate a net benefit of estrogen when combined with progestin on CHD outcomes. In the Heart and Estrogen/Progestin Replacement Study, postmenopausal female survivors of acute myocardial infarction were randomized to an estrogen/progestin combination or to placebo. This study showed no overall reduction in recurrent coronary events in the active treatment arm. Indeed, early in the 5-year course of this trial, there was a trend toward

an actual increase in vascular events in the treated women. Extended follow-up of this cohort did not disclose an accrual of benefit in the treatment group. The Women's Health Initiative (WHI) study arm using a similar ET plus progesterone regimen was halted because of a small but significant hazard of cardiovascular events, stroke, and breast cancer. The excess cardiovascular events may result from an increase in thromboembolism (Chap. 327).

These clinical trials do not exclude a potential CHD benefit of estrogen alone or selective estrogen receptor modulator regimens; the estrogen *without progestin* arm of the WHI continues and should prove informative in this regard. Physicians should work with women to provide information and help weigh the small but evident CHD risk of estrogen/progestin vs. the benefits on postmenopausal symptoms and osteoporosis, taking personal preferences into account. The current disappointment surrounding estrogen/progestin therapy as a means of reducing cardiovascular risk highlights the need for redoubled attention to known modifiable risk factors in women. In the recent clinical trials with HMG-CoA reductase inhibitors, women, when included, have derived benefits at least commensurate with those seen in men.

DYSREGULATED COAGULATION OR FIBRINOLYSIS Thrombosis ultimately causes the gravest complications of atherosclerosis. The propensity to form thrombi and/or to lyse clots once they form clearly influences the manifestations of atherosclerosis. Thrombosis provoked by atheroma rupture and subsequent healing may promote plaque growth (Chap. 224). Certain individual characteristics can influence thrombosis or fibrinolysis and have received attention as potential coronary risk factors. For example, fibrinogen levels correlate with coronary risk and provide information regarding coronary risk independent of the lipoprotein profile. Elevated fibrinogen levels might promote a thrombotic diathesis. Alternatively, fibrinogen, an acute-phase reactant, may serve as a marker of inflammation rather than directly participating in the pathogenesis of coronary events.

The stability of an arterial thrombus depends on the balance between fibrinolytic factors, such as plasmin, and inhibitors of the fibrinolytic system, such as plasminogen activator inhibitor (PAI) 1. However, the levels of tissue plasminogen activator and PAI-1 in plasma have not proven to add information beyond the lipid profile to assessment of cardiovascular risk. Lp(a) (Chap. 335) may modulate fibrinolysis, and although individuals with elevated Lp(a) levels have increased CHD risk, Lp(a) levels do not potently predict risk in the population at large.

Aspirin reduces CHD events in several contexts. Chap. 226 discusses aspirin therapy in stable ischemic heart disease, Chap. 227 reviews recommendations for aspirin treatment in acute coronary syndromes, and Chap. 349 describes aspirin's role in preventing recurrent ischemic stroke. In primary prevention, pooled trial data show that low-dose aspirin treatment (81 mg qd to 325 mg qod) can reduce risk of first myocardial infarction in men. Individuals with CHD risk factors, and especially men > 45 years old, should take aspirin in the absence of contraindications.

HOMOCYSTEINE A large body of literature suggests a relationship between hyperhomocysteinemia and coronary events. Several mutations in the enzymes involved in homocysteine accumulation correlate with thrombosis and, in some studies, coronary risk. Prospective studies have not shown a robust utility of hyperhomocysteinemia in CHD risk stratification, and there are no clinical trial data showing that intervention to lower homocysteine levels reduces CHD events. Fortification of the U.S. diet with folic acid to reduce neural tube defects has lowered homocysteine levels in the population at large. Measurement of homocysteine levels should be reserved for individuals with atherosclerosis at a young age or out of proportion to established risk factors. Physicians who advise consumption of supplements containing folic acid should consider that this treatment might mask pernicious anemia.

INFLAMMATION/INFECTION An accumulation of clinical evidence shows that markers of inflammation correlate with coronary risk. For example, variations of plasma levels of C-reactive protein (CRP), as mea-

TABLE 225-3 *Clinical Identification of the Metabolic Syndrome—Any Three Risk Factors*

Risk Factor	Defining Level
Abdominal obesity[a]	
Men (waist circumference)[b]	>102 cm (>40 in.)
Women	>88 cm (>35 in.)
Triglycerides	>1.7 mmol/L (>150 mg/dL)
HDL cholesterol	
Men	<1.0 mmol/L (<40 mg/dL)
Women	<1.3 mmol/L (<50 mg/dL)
Blood pressure	≥130/≥85 mmHg
Fasting glucose	>6.1 mmol/L (>110 mg/dL)

[a] Overweight and obesity are associated with insulin resistance and the metabolic syndrome. However, the presence of abdominal obesity is more highly correlated with the metabolic risk factors than is an elevated body-mass index (BMI). Therefore, the simple measure of waist circumference is recommended to identify the BMI component of the metabolic syndrome.

[b] Some male patients can develop multiple metabolic risk factors when the waist circumference is only marginally increased, e.g., 94–102 cm (37–39 in.). Such patients may have a strong genetic contribution to insulin resistance. They should benefit from lifestyle changes, similarly to men with categorical increases in waist circumference.

sured by a high-sensitivity assay, can prospectively predict risk of myocardial infarction. CRP levels also correlate with outcome of patients with acute coronary syndromes. In contrast to several other novel risk factors, CRP adds predictive information to that derived from established risk factors such as cholesterol (Fig. 225-2). Elevated levels of the acute-phase reactant CRP may merely reflect ongoing inflammation rather than a direct etiologic role for CRP in coronary artery disease. Elevations in acute-phase reactants such as fibrinogen or CRP could reflect overall atherosclerotic burden and/or extravascular inflammation that could potentiate atherosclerosis or its complications. In all likelihood, both factors contribute to elevation of inflammatory markers in patients at risk for coronary events. Indeed, lipid-lowering therapy may reduce coronary events in part by reducing the inflammatory aspects of the pathogenesis of atherosclerosis.

One source of inflammatory stimulus could arise from infectious agents. Interest has resurged in the possibility that infections may cause or contribute to atherosclerosis. A spate of recent publications has furnished evidence that supports a role of *Chlamydia pneumoniae*, cytomegalovirus, or other infectious agents in atherosclerosis and restenosis following coronary intervention. Some microorganisms exist in human atherosclerotic plaques. However, prospective and well-controlled seroepidemiologic studies show little or no association between infection with various agents and atherosclerosis. At present no sufficiently powered clinical trial supports the use of antibiotics to reduce CHD risk.

LIFESTYLE MODIFICATION The prevention of atherosclerosis presents a long-term challenge to all health care professionals and for public health policy as well. Both individual practitioners and organizations providing health care should strive to help patients optimize their risk factor profile long before atherosclerotic disease becomes manifest. The care plan for all patients seen by internists should include measures to assess and minimize cardiovascular risk. Physicians must counsel patients regarding the health risks of tobacco use and provide guidance regarding smoking cessation. Likewise, physicians should advise all patients about prudent dietary and exercise habits for maintaining ideal body weight. The recent National Institutes of Health Consensus Panel on Physical Activity and Cardiovascular Health established a goal of accumulating at least 30 min of moderate-intensity physical activity on a daily basis. Obesity, particularly the male pattern of centripetal or visceral fat accumulation, can contribute to the elements of the metabolic syndrome (Table 225-3). Physicians should encourage their patients to take responsibility for behavior related to modifiable risk factors for development of premature atherosclerotic disease. Conscientious counseling and patient education may forestall the need for pharmacologic measures intended to reduce coronary risk.

ISSUES IN RISK ASSESSMENT A growing panel of markers of coronary risk presents a perplexing array to the practitioner. Markers measured in peripheral blood include size fractions of LDL particles and concentrations of homocysteine, Lp(a), fibrinogen, CRP, and PAI-1

among others. In general, such specialized tests add little to the information available from a careful history and physical examination combined with measurement of a plasma lipoprotein profile and fasting blood sugar. The high-sensitivity CRP measurement may well prove an exception in view of its robustness in risk prediction, its ease of reproducible and standardized measurement, its relative stability in individuals over time, and, most importantly, its ability to add to the risk information disclosed by standard measurements such as the lipid profile. Given the utility of high-sensitivity CRP measurement in predicting a gamut of important cardiovascular outcomes, this simple blood test may prove useful in the future in guiding therapy, particularly in primary prevention. Current guidelines, however, recommend the use of this test only in individuals with intermediate risk of a CHD event (10–20%, 10-year risk).

Similar concerns pertain to the use of specialized radiographic estimations of coronary artery calcification. Accumulating information indicates that the amount of calcium determined by such techniques as electron beam computed tomography correlates with coronary risk. However, the utility of using such estimates of coronary artery calcium content as a guide to therapy remains unproven, particularly in asymptomatic individuals. Inappropriate use of such imaging modalities might promote excessive invasive diagnostic and therapeutic procedures. Widespread application of such modalities for screening should await proof that clinical benefit derives from their application.

THE CHALLENGE OF IMPLEMENTATION: CHANGING PHYSICIAN AND PATIENT BEHAVIOR

Despite declining age-adjusted rates of coronary death, cardiovascular mortality is on the rise due to the aging of the population overall. There is a powerful global trend toward increased atherosclerotic disease. Enormous challenges remain regarding translation of the current evidence base into practice. We must learn how to help individuals adopt a healthy lifestyle and learn to deploy our increasingly powerful pharmacologic tools most economically and effectively. The obstacles to implementation of current evidence-based prevention and treatment of atherosclerosis include economics, education, physician awareness, and patient adherence to recommended regimens. Future goals in the field of treatment of atherosclerosis should include application of the current knowledge regarding risk-factor management and, when appropriate, drug therapy.

FURTHER READING

BECKMAN JA et al: Diabetes and atherosclerosis: Epidemiology, pathophysiology, and management. JAMA 287:2570, 2002

GAZIANO JM et al: Primary and secondary prevention of coronary heart disease, in *Braunwald's Heart Disease: A Textbook of Cardiovascular Medicine*. 7th ed, D Zipes et al (eds). Philadelphia, Saunders, 2005

GRADY D et al: Cardiovascular disease outcomes during 6.8 years of hormone therapy: Heart and Estrogen/Progestin Replacement Study follow-up (HERS II). JAMA 288:49, 2002

MRC/BHF HEART PROTECTION STUDY OF ANTIOXIDANT VITAMIN SUPPLEMENTATION IN 20,536 HIGH-RISK INDIVIDUALS: A randomised placebo-controlled trial. Lancet 360:23, 2002

THE NATIONAL CHOLESTEROL EDUCATION PROGRAM: Executive summary of the third report of the NCEP expert panel on detection, evaluation, and treatment of high blood cholesterol in adults (Adult Treatment Panel). JAMA 285:2486, 2001

PEARSON TA et al: Markers of inflammation and cardiovascular disease: Application to clinical and public health practice. A statement for healthcare professionals from the Centers for Disease Control and Prevention and The American Heart Association. Circulation 107:499, 2003

RIDKER PM: Role of inflammatory biomarkers in prediction of coronary heart disease. Lancet 358:946, 2001

WOMEN'S HEALTH INITIATIVE RANDOMIZED CONTROLLED TRIAL: Principal results on the risks and benefits of estrogen plus progestin in healthy postmenopausal women. JAMA 288:321, 2002

YUSUF S et al: Effects of an angiotensin-converting-enzyme inhibitor, ramipril, on cardiovascular events in high-risk patients. The Heart Outcomes Prevention Evaluation Study Investigators. N Engl J Med 342:145, 2000

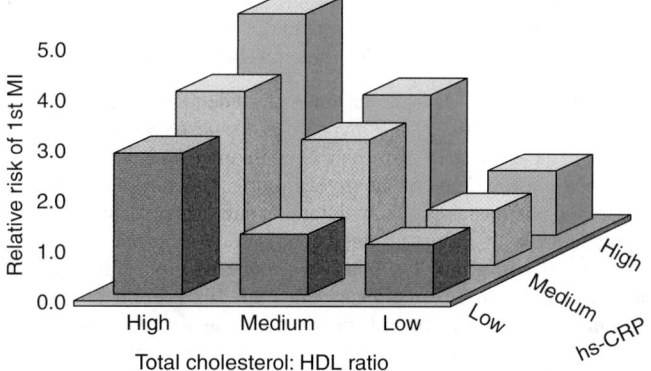

FIGURE 225-2 Measurement of C-reactive protein (CRP) level adds predictive value to TC:HDL ratio in determining risk of first MI among apparently healthy men. TC, total cholesterol; HDL, high-density lipoprotein; MI, myocardial infarction; hs-CRP, high-sensitivity measurement of CRP. (*Adapted from PM Ridker et al: Circulation 97:2007, 1998*).

Ischemia refers to a lack of oxygen due to inadequate perfusion of the myocardium, which causes an imbalance between oxygen supply and demand. The most common cause of myocardial ischemia is obstructive atherosclerotic disease of epicardial coronary arteries.

EPIDEMIOLOGY Ischemic heart disease (IHD) causes more deaths and disability and incurs greater economic costs than any other illness in the developed world. IHD is the most common, serious, chronic, life-threatening illness in the United States, where >12 million persons have IHD, >6 million have angina pectoris, and >7 million have sustained a myocardial infarction. A high-fat and energy-rich diet, smoking, and a sedentary life-style are associated with the emergence of IHD (Chap. 225). In the United States and western Europe, it is growing amongst the poor rather than the rich (who are adopting more healthful life-styles), while primary prevention has delayed the disease to later in life in all socioeconomic groups. Obesity, insulin resistance, and type 2 diabetes mellitus are increasing and are powerful risk factors for IHD. With urbanization in the developing world, the prevalence of risk factors for IHD is increasing rapidly in these regions. Large increases in IHD throughout the world are projected, and IHD is likely to become the most common cause of death worldwide by 2020.

PATHOPHYSIOLOGY Although the large epicardial coronary arteries are capable of constriction and relaxation, in healthy persons they serve as conduits and are referred to as *conductance vessels*, while the intramyocardial arterioles normally exhibit changes in tone and are therefore referred to as *resistance vessels*. Abnormal constriction of the conductance vessels can cause severe ischemia in Prinzmetal's angina (Chap. 227). Abnormal constriction or failure of normal dilation of the coronary resistance vessels can also cause ischemia. When it causes angina this condition is referred to as *microvascular angina*.

The normal coronary circulation is dominated and controlled by the heart's requirements for oxygen. This need is met by the ability of the coronary vascular bed to vary its resistance (and therefore blood flow) considerably while the myocardium extracts a high and relatively fixed percentage of oxygen. Normally, intramyocardial resistance vessels demonstrate an immense capacity for dilation. For example, the changing oxygen needs of the heart with exercise and emotional stress affect coronary vascular resistance and in this manner regulate the supply of oxygen and substrate to the myocardium (*metabolic regulation*). The coronary resistance vessels also adapt to physiologic alterations in blood pressure in order to maintain coronary blood flow at levels appropriate to myocardial needs (*autoregulation*).

By reducing the lumen of the coronary arteries, atherosclerosis limits appropriate increases in perfusion when the demand for flow is augmented, as occurs during exertion or excitement. When the luminal reduction is severe, myocardial perfusion in the basal state is reduced. Coronary blood flow can also be limited by spasm, arterial thrombi, and, rarely, coronary emboli as well as by ostial narrowing due to luetic aortitis. Congenital abnormalities, such as origin of the left anterior descending coronary artery from the pulmonary artery, may cause myocardial ischemia and infarction in infancy, but this cause is very rare in adults. Myocardial ischemia can also occur if myocardial oxygen demands are markedly increased, and when coronary blood flow may be limited, as occurs in severe left ventricular hypertrophy due to aortic stenosis. The latter can present with angina that is indistinguishable from that caused by coronary atherosclerosis (Chap. 219). A reduction in the oxygen-carrying capacity of the blood, as in extremely severe anemia or in the presence of carboxyhemoglobin, rarely causes myocardial ischemia by itself but it may lower the threshold for ischemia in patients with moderate coronary obstruction. Not infrequently, two or more causes of ischemia coexist, such as an increase in oxygen demand due to left ventricular hypertrophy secondary to

hypertension and a reduction in oxygen supply secondary to coronary atherosclerosis and anemia.

CORONARY ATHEROSCLEROSIS Epicardial coronary arteries are the major site of atherosclerotic disease. The major risk factors for atherosclerosis [high plasma low-density lipoprotein (LDL), low plasma high-density lipoprotein (HDL), cigarette smoking, hypertension, and diabetes mellitus (Chaps. 224 and 225)] disturb the normal functions of the vascular endothelium. These functions include local control of vascular tone, maintenance of an anticoagulant surface, and defense against inflammatory cells. The loss of these defenses leads to inappropriate constriction, luminal clot formation, and abnormal interactions with blood monocytes and platelets. The latter results in the subintimal collections of fat, smooth-muscle cells, fibroblasts, and intercellular matrix (i.e., atherosclerotic plaques), which develop at irregular rates in different segments of the epicardial coronary tree and lead eventually to segmental reductions in cross-sectional area. When a stenosis reduces the cross-sectional area by ~75%, a full range of increases in flow to meet increased myocardial demand is not possible. When the luminal area is reduced by ≥80%, blood flow at rest may be reduced, and further minor decreases in the stenotic orifice can reduce coronary flow dramatically and cause myocardial ischemia.

Segmental atherosclerotic narrowing of epicardial coronary arteries is caused most commonly by the formation of a plaque, which is subject to fissuring, erosion, hemorrhage, and thrombosis. Any of these events can temporarily worsen the obstruction, reduce coronary blood flow, and cause clinical manifestations of myocardial ischemia, as described below. The location of the obstruction influences the quantity of myocardium rendered ischemic and determines the severity of the clinical manifestations. Thus, critical obstructions in vessels such as the left main coronary artery or the proximal left anterior descending coronary artery are particularly hazardous. Severe coronary narrowing and myocardial ischemia are frequently accompanied by the development of collateral vessels, especially when the narrowing develops gradually. When well developed, such vessels can, by themselves, provide sufficient blood flow to sustain the viability of the myocardium at rest but not during conditions of increased demand.

Once stenosis of a proximal epicardial artery has reduced the cross-sectional area by ≥70%, the distal resistance vessels (when they function normally) dilate to reduce vascular resistance and maintain coronary blood flow. A pressure gradient develops across the proximal stenosis, and poststenotic pressure falls. When the resistance vessels are maximally dilated, myocardial blood flow becomes dependent on the pressure in the coronary artery distal to the obstruction. In these circumstances ischemia, manifest clinically by angina or electrocardiographically by ST-segment depression, can be precipitated by increases in myocardial oxygen demands caused by physical activity, emotional stress, and/or tachycardia. Changes in the caliber of the stenosed coronary artery due to physiologic vasomotion, loss of endothelial control of dilation, pathologic spasm (Prinzmetal's angina), or small platelet plugs can also upset the critical balance between oxygen supply and demand and thus precipitate myocardial ischemia.

EFFECTS OF ISCHEMIA During episodes of inadequate perfusion caused by coronary atherosclerosis, myocardial tissue oxygen tension falls and may cause transient disturbances of the mechanical, biochemical, and electrical functions of the myocardium. The abrupt development of severe ischemia, as occurs with total or subtotal coronary occlusion, is associated with almost instantaneous failure of normal muscle contraction and relaxation. The relatively poor perfusion of the subendocardium causes more intense ischemia of this portion of the wall. Ischemia of large portions of the ventricle causes transient left ventricular failure, and if the papillary muscles are involved, mitral regurgitation can complicate this event. When ischemia is transient, it may be associated with angina pectoris; when it is prolonged, it can lead to myocardial necrosis and scarring with or without the clinical picture of acute myocardial infarction (Chap. 228). Coronary atherosclerosis is a focal process that usually causes nonuniform ischemia.

Regional disturbances of ventricular contractility cause segmental akinesis or, in severe cases, bulging (dyskinesia), which can greatly reduce myocardial pump function.

A wide range of abnormalities in cell metabolism, function, and structure underlie these mechanical disturbances during ischemia. The normal myocardium metabolizes fatty acids and glucose to carbon dioxide and water. With severe oxygen deprivation, fatty acids cannot be oxidized, and glucose is broken down to lactate; intracellular pH is reduced, as are the myocardial stores of high-energy phosphates, i.e., ATP and creatine phosphate. Impaired cell membrane function leads to the leakage of potassium and the uptake of sodium by myocytes. The severity and duration of the imbalance between myocardial oxygen supply and demand determine whether the damage is reversible (≤ 20 min for total occlusion in the absence of collaterals) or whether it is permanent, with subsequent myocardial necrosis (>20 min).

Ischemia also causes characteristic changes in the electrocardiogram (ECG) such as repolarization abnormalities, as evidenced by inversion of T waves and, when more severe, by displacement of ST segments (Chap. 210). Transient ST-segment depression often reflects subendocardial ischemia, while ST-segment elevation is thought to be caused by more severe transmural ischemia. Another important consequence of myocardial ischemia is electrical instability, which may lead to ventricular tachycardia or ventricular fibrillation (Chap. 214). Most patients who die suddenly from IHD do so as a result of ischemia-induced ventricular tachyarrhythmias (Chap. 256).

ASYMPTOMATIC VERSUS SYMPTOMATIC IHD Postmortem studies on accident victims and military casualties in western countries have shown that coronary atherosclerosis often begins to develop prior to age 20 and is widespread even among adults who were asymptomatic during life. Exercise stress tests in asymptomatic persons may show evidence of silent myocardial ischemia, i.e., exercise-induced ECG changes not accompanied by angina pectoris; coronary angiographic studies of such persons may reveal coronary artery obstruction (Chap. 212)]. Postmortem examination of patients with such obstruction without a history of clinical manifestations of myocardial ischemia often shows macroscopic scars secondary to myocardial infarction in regions supplied by diseased coronary arteries. According to population studies, ~25% of patients who survive acute myocardial infarction may not reach medical attention, and these patients carry the same adverse prognosis as those who present with the classic clinical syndrome (Chap. 228). Sudden death may be unheralded and is a common presenting manifestation of IHD (Chap. 256). Patients with IHD can also present with cardiomegaly and heart failure secondary to ischemic damage of the left ventricular myocardium that may have caused no symptoms prior to the development of heart failure; this condition is referred to as *ischemic cardiomyopathy*. In contrast to the asymptomatic phase of IHD, the symptomatic phase is characterized by chest discomfort due to either angina pectoris or acute myocardial infarction (Chap. 228). Having entered the symptomatic phase, the patient may exhibit a stable or progressive course, revert to the asymptomatic stage, or suddenly die.

STABLE ANGINA PECTORIS

This episodic clinical syndrome is due to transient myocardial ischemia. Various diseases that cause myocardial ischemia as well as the numerous forms of discomfort with which it may be confused are discussed in Chap. 12. Males constitute ~70% of all patients with angina pectoris and an even greater fraction of those <50 years.

HISTORY The typical patient with angina is a man >50 years or a woman >60 years who complains of chest discomfort, usually described as heaviness, pressure, squeezing, smothering, or choking and only rarely as frank pain. When the patient is asked to localize the sensation, he or she will typically press on the sternum, sometimes with a clenched fist, to indicate a squeezing, central, substernal discomfort (Levine's sign). Angina is usually crescendo-decrescendo in nature, typically lasts 2 to 5 min, and can radiate to the left shoulder and to both arms, especially to the ulnar surfaces of the forearm and

hand. It can also arise in or radiate to the back, interscapular region, root of the neck, jaw, teeth, and epigastrium. Angina is rarely localized below the umbilicus or above the mandible.

Although episodes of angina are typically caused by exertion (e.g., exercise, hurrying, or sexual activity) or emotion (e.g., stress, anger, fright, or frustration) and are relieved by rest, they may also occur at rest [see "Unstable Angina Pectoris," (Chap. 227)] and at night while the patient is recumbent (angina decubitus). The patient may be awakened at night distressed by typical chest discomfort and dyspnea. Nocturnal angina may be due to episodic tachycardia or to the expansion of the intrathoracic blood volume that occurs with recumbency; the latter causes an increase in cardiac size and myocardial oxygen demand that lead to ischemia and transient left ventricular failure.

The threshold for the development of angina pectoris may vary by time of day and emotional state. Many patients report a fixed threshold for angina, which occurs predictably at a certain level of activity, such as climbing two flights of stairs at a normal pace. In these patients coronary stenosis and myocardial oxygen supply are fixed and ischemia is precipitated by an increase in myocardial oxygen demand. In other patients the threshold for angina may vary considerably within any given day and from day to day. In such patients variations in myocardial oxygen supply, most likely due to changes in coronary vascular tone, may play an important role. A patient may report symptoms upon minor exertion in the morning (a short walk or shaving) yet by midday may be capable of much greater effort without symptoms. Angina may also be precipitated by unfamiliar tasks, a heavy meal, exposure to cold, or a combination. Exertional angina is typically relieved by rest in 1 to 5 min and even more rapidly by rest and sublingual nitroglycerin (see below). Indeed, the diagnosis of angina should be suspect if it does not respond to the combination of these two measures. The severity of angina can be expressed by the Canadian Cardiac Society functional classification (Table 226-1).

Sharp, fleeting chest pain or prolonged, dull aches localized to the left submammary area are rarely due to myocardial ischemia. However, angina pectoris may be atypical in location and not strictly related to provoking factors. In addition, this symptom may exacerbate and remit over days, weeks, or months. Its occurrence can be seasonal, being more frequent in the winter in temperate climates. Anginal "equivalents" are symptoms of myocardial ischemia other than angina. These include dyspnea, fatigue, and faintness and are more common in the elderly and in diabetic patients.

TABLE 226-1 *Grading of Angina Pectoris According to CCS Classification*

Class	Description of Stage
I	"Ordinary physical activity does not cause . . . angina," such as walking or climbing stairs. Angina occurs with strenuous, rapid, or prolonged exertion at work or recreation.
II	"Slight limitation of ordinary activity." Angina occurs on walking or climbing stairs rapidly; walking uphill; walking or stair climbing after meals; in cold, in wind, or under emotional stress; or only during the few hours after awakening. Angina occurs on walking >2 blocks on the level and climbing >1 flight of ordinary stairs at a normal pace and under normal conditions.
III	"Marked limitations of ordinary physical activity." Angina occurs on walking 1 to 2 blocks on the level and climbing 1 flight of stairs under normal conditions and at a normal pace.
IV	"Inability to carry on any physical activity without discomfort—anginal symptoms may be present at rest."

Note: CCS, Canadian Cardiovascular Society.
Source: Braunwald E et al. ACC/AHA guidelines for the management of patients with unstable angina-non-ST segment elevation myocardial infarction: A report of the American College of Cardiology/American Heart Association Task Force on Practice Guidelines (Committee on the Management of Patients with Unstable Angina). J Am Coll Cardiol 36: 970, 2000. Adapted with permission from L Campeau: Grading of angina pectoris (letter). Circulation 54:522, 1976, with permission, American Heart Association, Inc.

Systematic questioning of the patient with suspected IHD is important to uncover the features of an unstable syndrome associated with increased risk, such as angina occurring at rest or awakening the patient from sleep. Since coronary atherosclerosis is often accompanied by similar diseases in other arteries, the patient with angina should be questioned and examined for peripheral arterial disease (intermittent claudication, Chap. 232), stroke, or transient ischemic attacks (Chap. 349). It is also important to uncover a family history of premature IHD (<45 years in first-degree male relatives and <55 in female relatives) and the presence of diabetes mellitus, hyperlipidemia, hypertension, cigarette smoking, and other risk factors for coronary atherosclerosis (Chap. 224). The history of typical angina pectoris establishes the diagnosis of IHD until proven otherwise. In patients with atypical angina (Chap. 12), the coexistence of advanced age, male gender, the postmenopausal state, and risk factors for atherosclerosis increase the likelihood of important coronary disease.

PHYSICAL EXAMINATION This is often normal in patients with stable angina, but it may reveal evidence of atherosclerotic disease at other sites, such as an abdominal aortic aneurysm, carotid arterial bruits, and diminished arterial pulse in the lower extremities, or of risk factors for atherosclerosis, such as xanthelasma and xanthomas (Chap. 224). Examination of the fundi may reveal increased light reflexes and arteriovenous nicking as evidence of hypertension. There may also be signs of anemia, thyroid disease, and nicotine stains on the fingertips from cigarette smoking. Palpation may reveal cardiac enlargement and abnormal contraction of the cardiac impulse (left ventricular akinesia or dyskinesia). Auscultation can uncover arterial bruits, a third and/or fourth heart sound, and, if acute ischemia or previous infarction has impaired papillary muscle function, an apical systolic murmur due to mitral regurgitation. These auscultatory signs are best appreciated with the patient in the left decubitus position. Aortic stenosis, aortic regurgitation (Chap. 219), pulmonary hypertension (Chap. 220), and hypertrophic cardiomyopathy (Chap. 221) must be excluded, since these disorders may cause angina in the absence of coronary atherosclerosis. Examination during an anginal attack is useful, since ischemia can cause transient left ventricular failure with the appearance of a third and/or fourth heart sound, a dyskinetic cardiac apex, mitral regurgitation, and even pulmonary edema. Tenderness of the chest wall or reproduction of the pain with palpation of the chest discomfort makes it unlikely that it is caused by angina.

LABORATORY EXAMINATION Although the diagnosis of IHD can be made with confidence from the clinical examination, a number of simple laboratory tests can be helpful. The urine should be examined for evidence of diabetes mellitus and renal disease (including microalbuminuria) since these conditions accelerate atherosclerosis. Similarly, examination of the blood should include measurements of lipids (cholesterol—total, LDL, HDL—and triglycerides), glucose, creatinine, hematocrit, and, if indicated based on the physical examination, thyroid function. A chest x-ray is important, since it may show the consequences of IHD, i.e., cardiac enlargement, ventricular aneurysm, or signs of heart failure. These signs can support the diagnosis of IHD and are important in assessing the degree of cardiac damage.

ELECTROCARDIOGRAM A 12-lead ECG recorded at rest is normal in about half the patients with typical angina pectoris, but there may be signs of an old myocardial infarction (Chap. 210). Although repolarization abnormalities, i.e., ST-segment and T-wave changes as well as left ventricular hypertrophy and intraventricular conduction disturbances, are suggestive of IHD, they are nonspecific, since they can also occur in pericardial, myocardial, and valvular heart disease or, in the case of the former, transiently with anxiety, changes in posture, drugs, or esophageal disease. Typical ST-segment and T-wave changes that accompany episodes of angina pectoris and disappear thereafter are more specific.

STRESS TESTING ■ Electrocardiographic The most widely used test for both the diagnosis of IHD and estimating the prognosis involves recording the 12-lead ECG before, during, and after exercise, usually on a treadmill. The test consists of a standardized incremental increase in external workload while the symptoms, ECG, and arm blood pressure are monitored. Performance is usually symptom-limited, and the test is discontinued upon evidence of chest discomfort, severe shortness of breath, dizziness, severe fatigue, ST-segment depression > 0.2 mV (2 mm), a fall in systolic blood pressure >10 mmHg, or the development of a ventricular tachyarrhythmia. This test seeks to discover any limitation in exercise performance, to detect typical ECG signs of myocardial ischemia, and to establish their relationship to chest discomfort. The ischemic ST-segment response is generally defined as flat depression of the ST segment >0.1 mV below baseline (i.e., the PR segment) and lasting longer than 0.08 s (Fig. 226-1). Upsloping or junctional ST-segment changes are not considered characteristic of ischemia and do not constitute a positive test. Although T-wave abnormalities, conduction disturbances, and ventricular arrhythmias that develop during exercise should be noted, they are also not diagnostic. Negative exercise tests in which the target heart rate (85% of maximal heart rate for age and sex) is not achieved are considered to be nondiagnostic.

When interpreting ECG stress tests, the probability that coronary artery disease (CAD) exists in the patient or population under study (i.e., pretest probability) should be considered (Fig. 2-2). Overall, false-positive or false-negative results occur in one-third of cases. However, a positive result on exercise indicates that the likelihood of CAD is 98% in males >50 years with a history of typical angina pectoris and who develop chest discomfort during the test. The likelihood decreases if the patient has atypical or no chest pain by history and/or during the test. The incidence of false-positive tests is significantly increased in patients with low probabilities of IHD, such as asymptomatic men under the age of 40 or in premenopausal women with no risk factors for premature atherosclerosis. It is also increased in patients taking cardioactive drugs, such as digitalis and quinidine, or in those with intraventricular conduction disturbances, resting ST-segment and T-wave abnormalities, ventricular hypertrophy, or abnormal serum potassium levels. Obstructive disease limited to the circumflex coronary artery may result in a false-negative stress test since the posterior portion of the heart which this vessel supplies is not well represented on the surface 12-lead ECG. Since the overall sensitivity of exercise stress electrocardiography is only ~75%, a negative result does not exclude CAD, although it makes the likelihood of three-vessel or left main CAD extremely unlikely.

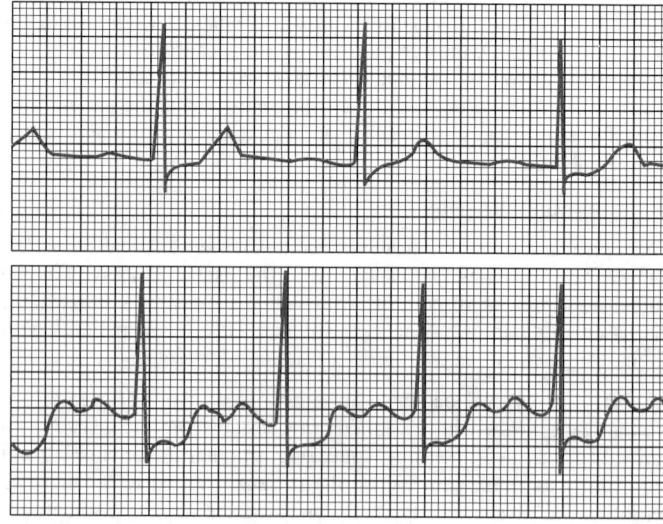

FIGURE 226-1 Lead V_4 at rest (*top*) and after 4½ min of exercise (*bottom*). There is 3 mm (0.3 mV) of horizontal ST-segment depression, indicating a positive test for ischemia. [*Modified from BR Chaitman, in E Braunwald et al (eds): Heart Disease, 6th ed, Philadelphia, Saunders, 2001.*]

The physician should be present throughout the exercise test, and it is important to measure total duration of exercise, the times to the onset of ischemic ST-segment change and chest discomfort, the external work performed (generally expressed as the stage of exercise), and the internal cardiac work performed, i.e., by the heart rate–blood pressure product. The depth of the ST-segment depression and the time needed for recovery of these ECG changes are also important. Because the risks of exercise testing are small but real—estimated at one fatality and two nonfatal complications per 10,000 tests—equipment for resuscitation should be available. Modified (heart rate–limited rather than symptom-limited) exercise tests can be performed safely in patients as early as 6 days after uncomplicated myocardial infarction. Contraindications to exercise stress testing include rest angina within 48 h, unstable rhythm, severe aortic stenosis, acute myocarditis, uncontrolled heart failure, and active infective endocarditis.

The normal response to graded exercise includes progressive increases in heart rate and blood pressure. Failure of the blood pressure to increase or an actual decrease with signs of ischemia during the test is an important adverse prognostic sign, since it may reflect ischemia-induced global left ventricular dysfunction. The development of angina and/or severe (>0.2 mV) ST-segment depression at a low workload, i.e., before completion of stage II of the Bruce protocol, and/or ST-segment depression that persists for >5 min after the termination of exercise increases the specificity of the test and suggests severe IHD and a high risk of future adverse events.

Cardiac Imaging (See also Chap. 211)   When the resting ECG is abnormal (e.g., Wolff-Parkinson-White syndrome, >1 mm of resting ST-segment depression, left bundle branch block, paced ventricular rhythm), information gained from an exercise test can be enhanced by stress myocardial perfusion imaging after the intravenous administration of thallium 201 or technetium 99m sestamibi during exercise (or a pharmacologic) stress; the imaging is carried out both immediately after cessation of exercise to detect regional ischemia and 4 h later to confirm reversible ischemia and regions of persistent absent uptake that signify infarction.

A sizable fraction of patients who need noninvasive stress testing to identify myocardial ischemia and increased risk of coronary events cannot exercise because of peripheral vascular or musculoskeletal disease, exertional dyspnea, or deconditioning. In these circumstances intravenous dipyridamole or adenosine can be used in place of exercise. The development of a transient perfusion defect with a tracer such as radioactive thallium or technetium 99m sestamibi is used to detect myocardial ischemia. Ambulatory monitoring of the ECG can assess myocardial ischemia as episodes of ST-segment depression. These techniques are sensitive and capable of identifying patients with ischemia who are at increased risk of coronary events.

Two-dimensional echocardiography can assess both global and regional wall motion abnormalities of the left ventricle due to myocardial infarction or persistent ischemia. Stress (exercise or dobutamine) echocardiography may cause the emergence of regions of akinesis or dyskinesis not present at rest. Stress echocardiography, like stress myocardial perfusion imaging, is more sensitive than exercise electrocardiography in the diagnosis of IHD. The relative advantages of stress echocardiography and stress radionuclide perfusion imaging in the diagnosis of IHD are shown in Table 226-2.

Echocardiography or radionuclide angiography should be carried out to assess left ventricular function in patients with chronic stable angina and in patients with a history of a prior myocardial infarction, pathologic Q waves, or clinical evidence of heart failure.

CORONARY ARTERIOGRAPHY (See also Chap. 212)   This diagnostic method outlines the lumina of the coronary arteries and can be used to detect or exclude serious coronary obstruction. However, coronary arteriography provides no information regarding the arterial wall, and severe atherosclerosis that does not encroach on the lumen may go undetected.

Indications   Coronary arteriography is indicated in (1) patients with chronic stable angina pectoris who are severely symptomatic despite

---

TABLE 226-2 *Comparative Advantages of Stress Echocardiography and Stress Radionuclide Perfusion Imaging in Diagnosis of CAD*

Advantages of stress echocardiography
1. Higher specificity
2. Versatility—more extensive evaluation of cardiac anatomy and function
3. Greater convenience/efficacy/availability
4. Lower cost

Advantages of stress perfusion imaging
1. Higher technical success rate
2. Higher sensitivity—especially for single vessel coronary disease involving the left circumflex
3. Better accuracy in evaluating possible ischemia when multiple resting LV wall motion abnormalities are present
4. More extensive published data base—especially in evaluation of prognosis

Note: CAD, coronary artery disease; LV, left ventricular.
Source: From Gibbons RJ et al, 1999, with permission.

---

medical therapy and who are being considered for revascularization, i.e., a percutaneous coronary intervention (PCI) or coronary artery bypass grafting (CABG); (2) patients with troublesome symptoms that present diagnostic difficulties in whom there is need to confirm or rule out the diagnosis of IHD; (3) patients with known or possible angina pectoris who have survived cardiac arrest; (4) patients with angina or evidence of ischemia on noninvasive testing with clinical or laboratory evidence of ventricular dysfunction; and (5) patients judged to be at high risk of sustaining coronary events based on signs of severe ischemia on noninvasive testing, regardless of the presence or severity of symptoms (see below).

Examples of other indications include:

1. Patients with chest discomfort suggestive of angina pectoris but a negative or nondiagnostic stress test who require a definitive diagnosis for guiding medical management, alleviating psychological stress, career or family planning, or insurance purposes.
2. Patients who have been admitted repeatedly to the hospital for suspected acute coronary syndromes (acute myocardial infarction or unstable angina) but in whom this diagnosis has not been established and in whom the presence or absence of CAD should be determined.
3. Patients with careers that involve the safety of others (e.g., pilots, fire fighters, police) who have questionable symptoms, suspicious or positive noninvasive tests, and in whom there are reasonable doubts about the state of the coronary arteries.
4. Patients with aortic stenosis or hypertrophic cardiomyopathy and angina in whom the chest pain could be due to IHD.
5. Male patients >45 and females >55 years who are to undergo a cardiac operation, such as valve replacement or repair, and who may or may not have clinical evidence of myocardial ischemia.
6. Patients who are at high risk after myocardial infarction because of the recurrence of angina or the presence of heart failure, frequent ventricular premature contractions, or signs of ischemia on the stress test.
7. Patients with angina pectoris, regardless of severity, in whom noninvasive testing indicates a high risk of coronary events.
8. Patients in whom coronary spasm or another nonatherosclerotic cause of myocardial ischemia (e.g., coronary artery anomaly, Kawasaki's disease) is suspected.

PROGNOSIS   The principal prognostic indicators in patients known to have IHD are age, the functional state of the left ventricle, the location(s) and severity of coronary artery narrowing, and the severity or activity of myocardial ischemia. Angina pectoris of recent onset, unstable angina (Chap. 227), early post-myocardial infarction angina, angina that is unresponsive or poorly responsive to medical therapy or is accompanied by symptoms of congestive heart failure all indicate an increased risk for adverse coronary events. The same is true for the physical signs of heart failure, episodes of pulmonary edema, transient third heart sounds, or mitral regurgitation, and for echocardiographic or radioisotopic (or roentgenographic) evidence of cardiac enlargement and reduced (<0.40) ejection fraction. Most importantly, any of the following signs during noninvasive testing indicate a high risk for coronary events: inability to exercise for 6 minutes, i.e., stage II (Bruce protocol) of the exercise test; a strongly positive exercise test showing onset of myocardial ischemia at low workloads (≥ 0.1 mV ST-segment depression before completion of stage II; ≥ 0.2 mV ST depression at any stage; ST depression for >5 min following the cessation of exercise; a decline in systolic pressure >10 mmHg during exercise; the development of ventricular tachyarrhythmias during exercise); the development of large or multiple perfusion defects or increased lung uptake during stress radioisotope perfusion imaging; and a decrease in left ventricular ejection fraction during exercise on radionuclide ventriculography or during stress echocardiography. Conversely, patients who can complete stage III of the Bruce exercise protocol and have a normal stress perfusion scan or negative stress echocardiographic evaluation are at very low risk of future coronary events.

On cardiac catheterization, elevations of left ventricular end-diastolic pressure and ventricular volume and reduced ejection fraction are the most important signs of left ventricular dysfunction and are associated with a poor prognosis. Patients with chest discomfort but normal left ventricular function and normal coronary arteries have an excellent prognosis. In patients with normal left ventricular function and mild angina but with critical stenoses ($\geq 70\%$ luminal diameter) of one, two, or three epicardial coronary arteries, the 5-year mortality rates are approximately 2, 8, and 11%, respectively. Obstructive lesions of the left anterior descending coronary artery proximal to the origin of the first septal artery are associated with a greater risk than are lesions of the right or left circumflex coronary artery, since the former vessel usually perfuses a greater quantity of myocardium. Stenosis (>50% luminal diameter) of the left main coronary artery is associated with a mortality rate of about 15% per year. The segmental atherosclerotic plaques in epicardial arteries with fissuring or filling defects indicates increased risk. These lesions go through phases of inflammatory cellular activity, degeneration, endothelial instability, abnormal vasomotion, platelet aggregation, and fissuring or hemorrhage. These factors can temporarily worsen the stenosis and cause abnormal reactivity of the vessel wall, thus exacerbating the manifestations of ischemia. The recent onset of symptoms, the development of severe ischemia during stress testing (see above), and unstable angina pectoris (Chap. 227) all reflect episodes of rapid progression in coronary lesions.

With any degree of obstructive CAD, mortality is greatly increased when left ventricular function is impaired; conversely, at any level of left ventricular function, the prognosis is influenced importantly by the quantity of myocardium perfused by critically obstructed vessels. Therefore, it is useful to collect all the evidence substantiating past myocardial damage (evidence of myocardial infarction on ECG, echocardiography, radioisotope imagine, or left ventriculography), residual left ventricular function (ejection fraction and wall motion), and risk of future damage from coronary events (extent of coronary disease and severity of ischemia defined by noninvasive stress testing). The larger the quantity of established myocardial necrosis, the less the heart is able to withstand additional damage and the poorer the prognosis. All the above signs of past damage plus the risk of future damage should be considered indicators of risk.

The plasma level of C-reactive protein is an indicator of inflammation and risk of future adverse coronary events in populations with atherosclerosis (Chap. 225). Similarly, electron beam computed tomography to measure coronary calcification and ultrasound measures of carotid intimal thickening can be used for the same purpose. The presence of other risk factors for coronary atherosclerosis [advanced age (>75 years), diabetes, morbid obesity, accompanying peripheral and/or cerebrovascular disease, previous myocardial infarction] worsen the prognosis of angina.

℞ TREATMENT

Each patient must be evaluated individually with respect to his or her expectations and goals, control of symptoms, and prevention of adverse clinical outcomes such as myocardial infarction and premature death. The degree of disability as well as the physical and emotional stress that precipitate angina must be carefully recorded in order to set treatment goals. The management plan should include the following components: (1) explanation and reassurance, (2) identification and treatment of aggravating conditions, (3) adaptation of activity, (4) treatment of risk factors that will decrease the occurrence of adverse coronary outcomes, (5) drug therapy for angina, and (6) consideration of mechanical revascularization (Table 226-3).

Explanation and Reassurance   Patients with IHD need to understand their condition as best they can and to realize that a long and useful life is possible even though they suffer from angina pectoris or have experienced and recovered from an acute myocardial infarction. Offering case histories of persons in public life who have lived with coronary disease as well as results of national studies showing improved outcomes can be of great value when encouraging patients to resume or maintain activity and return to their occupation. A planned program of rehabilitation can encourage patients to lose weight, improve exercise tolerance, and control risk factors with more confidence.

Identification and Treatment of Aggravating Conditions   A number of conditions may either increase oxygen demand or decrease oxygen supply to the myocardium and may precipitate or exacerbate angina in patients with IHD. Aortic valve disease and hypertrophic cardiomyopathy may cause or contribute to angina and should be excluded or treated. Obesity, hypertension, and hyperthyroidism should be treated aggressively in order to reduce the frequency and severity of anginal episodes. Decreased myocardial oxygen supply may be due to reduced oxygenation of the arterial blood (e.g., in pulmonary disease or, when carboxyhemoglobin is present, due to cigarette or cigar smoking) or decreased oxygen-carrying capacity (e.g., in anemia). Correction of these abnormalities, if present, may reduce or even eliminate angina pectoris.

Adaptation of Activity   Myocardial ischemia is caused by a discrepancy between the demand of the heart muscle for oxygen and the ability of the coronary circulation to meet this demand. Most patients can be helped to understand this concept and utilize it in the rational programming of activity. Many tasks that ordinarily evoke angina may be accomplished without symptoms simply by reducing the speed at which they are performed. Patients must appreciate the diurnal variation in their tolerance of certain activities and should reduce their energy requirements in the morning, immediately after meals, and in cold or inclement weather.

It may be necessary to recommend a change in employment or residence to avoid physical stress. However, with the exception of manual laborers, most patients with IHD can continue to function merely by allowing more time to complete each task. In some patients, anger and frustration may be the most important factors precipitating myocardial ischemia. If these cannot be avoided, training in stress management may be useful. A treadmill exercise test to determine the approximate heart rate at which ischemic ECG changes or symptoms develop may be helpful in the development of a specific exercise program.

Physical conditioning usually improves the exercise tolerance of patients with angina and exerts substantial psychological benefits. It may also improve the chances of surviving a myocardial infarction. A regular program of isotonic exercise within the limits of each patient's threshold for the development of angina pectoris and that does not exceed 80% of the heart rate associated with ischemia on exercise testing should be strongly encouraged.

TABLE 226-3 *Guidelines for the Treatment of Chronic Stable Angina*

Treatment of Symptoms
Class I[a]
1. Aspirin
2. β-blockers—particularly with a prior history of MI
3. Calcium antagonists as initial therapy
   a. If β-blockers are contraindicated
   b. With β-blockers to control symptom
   c. When β-blockers are stopped due to side effects
4. Sublingual nitroglycerin (tablets or spray) for relief of symptoms
5. Lipid lowering; LDL <2.6 mmol/L (100 mg/dL)
6. Health-promoting behaviors including smoking cessation, treatment of obesity, low-fat diet, supervised exercise program
Class IIa[b]
1. Clopidogrel when aspirin is contraindicated
2. Long-acting nondihydropyridine calcium antagonists (not short-acting) instead of β-blockers as initial therapy
3. Add long-acting nitrates and β-blockers or calcium antagonists for symptoms as needed
Class III[d]
1. Dypiridamole
2. Chelation therapy

Treatment of Risk Factors to Improve Outcomes
Class I
1. Smoking cessation
2. Treatment of dyslipidemia; LDL ≤2.6 mmol/L (100 mg/dL)
3. Angiotensin-converting enzyme inhibitor
4. Treatment of hypertension
5. Ideal weight and supervised exercise program
6. Low-fat diet
7. Treatment of diabetes using ADA National Guidelines
Class IIb[c]
1. Folate therapy for elevated homocysteine
2. Interventions directed at psychosocial stress
Class III
1. Hormone replacement therapy in postmenopausal women
2. Vitamins E and C
3. Treatment of depression
4. Chelation therapy
5. Herbal remedies and acupuncture

Treatment Using Revascularization
Class I
1. Coronary artery bypass surgery (CABG) for significant left main disease
2. CABG for 3-vessel coronary disease and reduced (≤50%) left ventricular function
3. CABG for 2-vessel CAD including LAD disease and reduced LV function
4. CABG for 3-vessel CAD plus high risk for percutaneous coronary intervention (PCI), abnormal (high risk) stress test, or diabetes
5. CABG in patients with prior CABG or PCI, recurrent restenosis, and high risk on noninvasive testing
6. PCI for 1- to 3-vessel CAD, normal LV function, no diabetes, lesions suitable (low risk) for PCI
7. PCI or CABG for failed medical therapy and acceptable risk with either modality

Class IIa
1. Repeat CABG for multiple vein graft stenoses, particularly including the LAD
2. PCI for simple focal vein graft stenosis
3. PCI or CABG for 1- or 2-vessel disease and moderate ischemia on noninvasive testing, including disease of the LAD
Class IIb
1. PCI instead of CABG in 2- or 3-vessel CAD (including the LAD) with controlled diabetes and lesions suitable (low risk) for PCI
2. PCI for technically suitable left main disease when CABG is not possible
3. PCI instead of CABG in 1- to 3-vessel CAD when each lesion is suitable (low risk) but the patient exhibits reduced LV function, treated diabetes, history of malignant arrhythmia, survived sudden death
Class III
1. PCI in left main disease or 3-vessel CAD with diabetes or poor LV function in patients who are candidates for CABG surgery
2. PCI or CABG in patients with mild symptoms, no evidence of ischemia in noninvasive testing, and not yet given an adequate trial of medical therapy
3. Baseline coronary stenoses (≤ 60%) and no signs of ischemia on noninvasive testing

Follow-up—Monitoring Disease, Testing, and Therapies
Class I
1. Chest x-ray with new evidence of congestive heart failure (CHF)
2. LV function testing for new evidence of CHF or MI
3. Echocardiogram for worsening of valvular disease
4. Treadmill testing for any change in clinical state
5. Stress imaging for any change in clinical state if the ECG cannot be interpreted or patient cannot exercise
6. Stress imaging for patients with prior revascularization and any change in clinical state
7. Coronary angiography in patients with obvious change in clinical state and limitations in daily activity despite medical therapy
Class IIb
1. Repeat annual treadmill exercise testing in patients with no change in clinical state, who can exercise, have no ECG abnormalities at rest, with an estimated morality of ≤ 1% per year
Class III
1. Echo or nuclear stress imaging for LV function and ischemia with no change in symptoms, normal ECG, no MI, and no CHF
2. Repeat treadmill stress test in ≤ 3 years in stable patients with estimated annual mortality ≤1% on an initial evaluation shown by:
   a. Low-risk Duke treadmill score
   b. Negative imaging study
   c. Normal LV function and no obstructive CAD
3. Stress imaging if stable, can exercise, normal resting ECG
4. Repeat coronary arteriogram with no change in clinical state, exercise testing, or stress imaging or insignificant CAD on initial examination

[a] Class I, therapies supported by evidence of efficacy.
[b] Class IIa, weight of evidence in favor of a therapy.
[c] Class IIb, evidence of efficacy less well established.
[d] Class III, therapies that are not useful and can be harmful.

Note: MI, myocardial infarction; LDL, low-density lipoprotein; ADA, American Diabetes Association; CAD, coronary artery disease; LAD, left anterior descending (coronary artery); LV, left ventricular; ECG, electrocardiogram.
Source: Adapted from Gibbons et al., 1999.

Treatment of Risk Factors A *family history* of premature IHD is an important indicator of increased risk and should trigger a search for treatable risk factors such as hyperlipidemia, hypertension, and diabetes. *Obesity* impairs the treatment of other risk factors and increases the risk of adverse coronary events. In addition, obesity is often accompanied by three other risk factors—diabetes mellitus, hypertension, and hyperlipidemia. The treatment of obesity and these accompanying risk factors is an important component of any management plan. A diet low in saturated fatty acids and a caloric intake to achieve optimal body weight is a cornerstone in the management of chronic IHD. Small controlled trials have shown that the combination of a 10% fat vegetarian diet, aerobic exercise, stress management training, smoking cessation, and psychosocial support can reduce the progression of coronary obstructive lesions, reduce angina, and result in fewer coronary events.

Cigarette smoking accelerates coronary atherosclerosis in both sexes and at all ages and increases the risk of thrombosis, plaque instability, myocardial infarction, and death (Chap. 225). Also, by increasing myocardial oxygen needs and reducing oxygen supply, it aggravates angina. Smoking cessation studies have demonstrated important benefits with a significant decline in the occurrence of these adverse outcomes. The physician's message must be clear and strong and supported by programs that achieve and monitor abstinence (Chap. 375). *Hypertension* (Chap. 230) is associated with increased risk of adverse clinical events from coronary atherosclerosis as well as stroke. In addition, the left ventricular hypertrophy that results from sustained

TABLE 226-4 Drugs Commonly Used for Angina Pectoris

Drug	Usual Dose	Side Effects	Contraindications
NITRATES			
Sublingual NTG	0.3–0.6 mg	Flushing, headache	Intolerance of side effects
Isosorbide dinitrate SR			
Oral	10–60 mg q8h	Flushing, headache,	As above, worsening
Sublingual	2.5–10 mgq4–6h	tolerance after 24 h	ischemia on withdrawal
Transdermal NTG patch	0.4–1.2 mg/h for 12–14 h	Flushing, headache, tolerance after 24 h	As above, worsening ischemia on withdrawal
Isosorbide-5-monitrate			
Oral	20–30 mg bid	Flushing, headache,	As above, worsening is-
Oral SR	60–240 mg once daily	tolerance after 24 h	chemia on withdrawal
BETA BLOCKERS			
Propranolol	20–80 mg qid	Depression, constipation, impotence, bronchospasm, heart failure, bradycardia	Asthma, AV conduction block, heart failure
Metoprolol	25–200 mg bid	As above	As above
Atenolol	50–150 mg once daily	As above	As above
CALCIUM CHANNEL BLOCKING DRUGS			
Nifedipine XL	30–90 mg daily	Hypotension, flushing, edema, worsening angina	Hypotension, intolerance of side effects
Diltiazem SR	60–120 mg bid	Constipation, AV conduction block, worsening heart failure	AV conduction block, impaired LV function, bradycardia
Verapamil SR	180–240 mg daily	Constipation, AV conduction block, worsening heart failure	AV conduction delay, impaired LV function, bradycardia
Amlodipine	5–10 mg daily	Edema	Intolerance of side effects

Note: NTG, nitroglycerin; SR, slow release; XL, slow release preparation.

hypertension aggravates ischemia. There is evidence that long-term, effective treatment of hypertension can decrease the occurrence of adverse coronary events. *Diabetes mellitus* (Chap. 323) accelerates coronary and peripheral atherosclerosis and is frequently associated with dyslipidemias and increases in the risk of angina, myocardial infarction, and sudden coronary death. Strict control of the dyslipidemia and hypertension that are frequently found in diabetic patients is essential, as described below.

Dyslipidemia The treatment of dyslipidemia is central when aiming for long-term relief from angina, reduced need for revascularization, and reduction in myocardial infarction and death. Epidemiologic observations, angiographic trials, and controlled trials have shown that (1) men >45 years and women >55 years with two risk factors (family history of premature IHD, cigarette smoking, hypertension), diabetes mellitus, or evidence of atherosclerotic disease should have a total cholesterol ≤ 5.17 mmol/L (≤200 mg/dL), LDL ≤ 2.58 mmol/L (≤100 mg/dL), and HDL ≥ 1.03 mmol/L (≥40 mg/dL). The control of lipids can be achieved by the combination of a diet low in saturated fatty acids, exercise, and weight loss. Frequently, HMG-CoA reductase inhibitors (statins) are required and can lower LDL cholesterol (25 to 50%), raise HDL cholesterol (5 to 9%), and lower triglycerides (5 to 30%). Niacin or fibrates can be used to raise HDL cholesterol and lower triglycerides (Chaps. 225 and 335). Controlled trials with lipid-regulating regimens have shown equal proportional benefit for men, women, the elderly, diabetics, and even smokers.

Risk Reduction in Women with IHD The incidence of clinical IHD in premenopausal women is very low. However, following the menopause, the atherogenic risk factors increase (e.g., increased LDL, reduced HDL) and the rate of clinical coronary events accelerates to the levels observed in men. Women have not given up cigarette smoking as effectively as have men. Diabetes mellitus, which is more common in women, greatly increases the occurrence of clinical IHD and amplifies the deleterious effects of hypertension, hyperlipidemia, and

smoking. Cardiac catheterization and coronary revascularization are often applied more sparingly in women and at a later, and more severe, stage of the disease than in men. When cholesterol lowering, beta blockers after myocardial infarction, and coronary artery bypass grafting (CABG) are applied in the appropriate patient groups, women enjoy the same benefits of improved outcome as do men.

Compliance with regard to the health-promoting behaviors listed above is generally very poor, and the conscientious physician must not underestimate the major effort required to meet this challenge. Fewer than one-half of patients in the United States discharged from the hospital with proven coronary disease receive treatment for dyslipidemia. Given the proof that treating dyslipidemia brings major benefits, physicians need to secure treatment pathways, monitor compliance, and follow up.

Drug Therapy The commonly used drugs for the treatment of angina pectoris are summarized in Table 226-4.

NITRATES This valuable class of drugs in the management of angina pectoris acts by causing systemic venodilation, thereby reducing myocardial wall tension and oxygen requirements, and by dilating the epicardial coronary vessels and increasing blood flow in collateral vessels. The nitrates likely bind to guanylate cyclase in vascular smooth-muscle cells, oxidize sulfhydryl groups, and are converted to *S*-nitrosothiols. This leads to an increase in cyclic guanosine monophosphate, which causes relaxation of vascular smooth muscle. The absorption of these agents is most rapid and complete through the mucous membranes. For this reason, nitroglycerin is most commonly administered sublingually in tablets of 0.4 or 0.6 mg. Patients with angina should be instructed to take the medication both to relieve angina and also approximately 5 min before stress that is likely to induce an episode. The value of this prophylactic use of the drug cannot be overemphasized.

A pulsating feeling in the head or headache is the most common side effect of nitroglycerin and fortunately is only rarely disturbing at the doses usually required to relieve or prevent angina. Postural dizziness has also been reported. Nitroglycerin deteriorates with exposure to air, moisture, and sunlight, so that if the drug neither relieves discomfort nor produces a slight sensation of burning at the sublingual site of absorption, the preparation may be inactive and a fresh supply should be obtained. If relief is not achieved by rest and within 2 or 3 min after nitroglycerin, a second or third dose may be given at 5-min intervals. If discomfort continues despite treatment, the patient should consult a physician or report promptly to a hospital emergency room for evaluation of possible unstable angina or acute myocardial infarction (Chap. 228).

Nitrates improve exercise tolerance in patients with chronic angina and relieve ischemia in patients with unstable angina as well as in patients with Prinzmetal's variant angina (Chap. 227). A diary of angina and nitroglycerin use may be valuable for detecting changes in the frequency, severity, or threshold for discomfort that may signify the development of unstable angina pectoris and/or herald an impending myocardial infarction.

Long-Acting Nitrates None of the long-acting nitrates is as effective as sublingual nitroglycerin for the acute relief of angina. These preparations can be swallowed, chewed, or administered as a patch or paste by the transdermal route. They can provide effective plasma levels for up to 24 h, but the therapeutic response is highly variable. Different preparations and/or administration during the daytime should be tried only to prevent discomfort while avoiding side effects such as headache and dizziness. Individual dose titration is important in order to prevent side effects. Useful preparations include isosorbide dinitrate (10 to 60 mg orally bid or tid), nitroglycerin ointment (0.5 to 2.0 in. qid), or sustained-release transdermal patches (5 to 25 mg/d). Tolerance with loss of efficacy develops with 12 to 24 h of continuous exposure to all of the long-acting nitrates due to depletion of sulfhydryl groups, decreased benefit through increased generation of oxygen free radicals, and to counterregulatory alterations in intravascular fluid balance with fluid retention. In order to minimize the effects of tolerance, the minimum effective dose should be used and a minimum of 8 h each day kept free of the drug so as to restore any useful response(s).

β-ADRENERGIC BLOCKERS These drugs represent an important component of the pharmacologic treatment of angina pectoris. They reduce myocardial oxygen demand by inhibiting the increases in heart rate, arterial pressure, and myocardial contractility caused by adrenergic activation. Beta blockade reduces these variables most strikingly during exercise while causing only small reductions at rest. Long-acting beta-blocking drugs (e.g., atenolol, 50 to 100 mg/d, or nadolol, 40 to 80 mg/d) offer the advantage of once-a-day dosage (Table 226-4). The therapeutic aims include relief of angina and ischemia. These drugs can also reduce mortality and reinfarction in patients after myocardial infarction and are moderately effective antihypertensive agents. Relative contraindications include asthma and reversible airway obstruction in patients with chronic lung disease, atrioventricular conduction disturbances, severe bradycardia, Raynaud's phenomenon, and a history of mental depression. Side effects include fatigue, reduced exercise tolerance, nightmares, impotence, cold extremities, intermittent claudication, bradycardia (sometimes severe), impaired atrioventricular conduction, left ventricular failure, bronchial asthma, worsening claudication, and intensification of the hypoglycemia produced by oral hypoglycemic agents and insulin. Reducing the dose or even discontinuation may be necessary if these side effects develop and persist. Since sudden discontinuation can intensify ischemia, the doses should be tapered over 2 weeks.

Beta blockers with relative β_1-receptor specificity, such as metoprolol and atenolol, may be preferable in patients with mild bronchial obstruction, insulin-requiring diabetes mellitus, or intermittent claudication.

CALCIUM ANTAGONISTS Slow-release nifedipine (30 to 90 mg once daily), verapamil (80 to 120 mg tid), diltiazem (30 to 90 mg qid), amlodipine (2.5 to 10 mg daily), and other calcium antagonists are coronary vasodilators that produce variable and dose-dependent reductions in myocardial oxygen demand, contractility, and arterial pressure. These combined pharmacologic effects are advantageous and make these agents as effective as beta blockers in the treatment of angina pectoris. They are indicated when beta blockers are contraindicated, poorly tolerated, or ineffective. Verapamil and diltiazem may produce symptomatic disturbances in cardiac conduction and bradyarrhythmias.They also exert negative inotropic actions and are more likely to aggravate left ventricular failure, particularly when used in patients with left ventricular dysfunction, especially if they are also receiving beta blockers. Although useful effects are usually achieved when calcium antagonists are combined with beta blockers and nitrates, careful individual titrations of the doses are essential with these combinations. Variant (Prinzmetal's) angina responds particularly well to calcium antagonists, supplemented when necessary by nitrates (Chap. 227). Nifedipine as well as other calcium antagonists are formulated as long-acting preparations, including diltiazem (60 to 120 mg twice daily) and verapamil (180 to 240 mg once daily).

Verapamil should not ordinarily be combined with beta blockers because of the combined effects on heart rate and contractility. Diltiazem can be combined with beta blockers with caution in patients with

normal ventricular function and no conduction disturbances. Amlodipine and beta blockers have complementary actions on coronary blood supply and myocardial oxygen demands. While the former decreases blood pressure and dilates coronary arteries, the latter slows heart rate and decreases contractility. Amlodipine and the other second-generation dihydropyridine calcium antagonists (nicardipine, isradipine, long-acting nifedipine, and felodipine) are potent vasodilators and useful in the simultaneous treatment of angina and hypertension. Short-acting dihydropyridines should be avoided because of the risk of precipitating infarction, particularly in the absence of beta blockers.

CHOICE BETWEEN BETA BLOCKERS AND CALCIUM ANTAGONISTS FOR INITIAL THERAPY Since beta blockers have been shown to improve life expectancy following acute myocardial infarction (Chap. 228) while calcium antagonists have not, the former may also be preferable in patients with chronic IHD. However, calcium antagonists are indicated in patients with the following: (1) inadequate responsiveness to the combination of beta blockers and nitrates; many such patients do well with a combination of a beta blocker and a dihydropyridine calcium antagonist; (2) adverse reactions to beta blockers such as depression, sexual disturbances, and fatigue; (3) angina and a history of asthma or chronic obstructive pulmonary disease; (4) sick-sinus syndrome or significant atrioventricular conduction disturbances; (5) Prinzmetal's angina; or (6) symptomatic peripheral arterial disease.

ANTIPLATELET DRUGS Aspirin is an irreversible inhibitor of platelet cyclooxygenase activity and thereby interferes with platelet activation. Chronic administration of 75 to 325 mg orally per day has been shown to reduce coronary events in asymptomatic adult men, patients with chronic stable angina, and patients with or who have survived unstable angina and myocardial infarction. Administration of this drug should be considered in all patients with IHD in the absence of gastrointestinal bleeding, allergy, or dyspepsia. Clopidogrel (300 mg loading and 75 mg/d) is an oral agent that blocks ADP receptor–mediated platelet aggregation. It provides the same benefits as aspirin, if not better, particularly if aspirin causes the side effects listed above. Clopidogrel with aspirin can improve coronary outcomes when given to patients for 1 year after an episode of unstable angina but with some increase in the risk of bleeding (Chap. 227). This increased risk is improved when the dose of aspirin is reduced.

Other Therapies The angiotensin-converting enzyme inhibitors have become widely used in the treatment of survivors of myocardial infarction, patients with hypertension or chronic IHD including angina pectoris, and those at high risk of vascular disease, such as diabetes. A large clinical trial (the Heart Outcomes Prevention Evaluation Study) has shown that up to 10 mg/d of ramipril can result in the reduction of major adverse events (death, myocardial infarction, and stroke), angina, and the need for revascularization in a group of high-risk patients with atherosclerotic cardiovascular disease (including chronic IHD) and normal left ventricular function. →*The dosing and side effects of these agents are discussed in Chaps. 216, 228, and 230.*

Enhanced external counterpulsation utilizes pneumatic cuffs on the lower extremities to provide diastolic augmentation and systolic unloading of blood pressure in order to decrease cardiac work and oxygen consumption while enhancing coronary blood flow. Recent trials have shown that regular application improves angina, exercise capacity, and regional myocardial perfusion.

In summary, a regimen of diet, exercise, smoking cessation, together with treatment of hypertension and dyslipidemia and use of aspirin and beta blockers form a treatment plan that reduces angina, the need for revascularization, myocardial infarction, and coronary death. ACE inhibitors should be used in patients with angina, particularly those with hypertension and/or diabetes.

ANGINA AND HEART FAILURE   Transient left ventricular failure with angina can be controlled by the use of nitrates. For patients with established congestive heart failure the increased left ventricular wall tension raises myocardial oxygen demand. Treatment of congestive heart failure with an angiotensin-converting enzyme inhibitor, diuretic, and digitalis (Chap. 216) reduces heart size, wall tension, and myocardial oxygen demand, which, in turn, helps to control angina and ischemia. If the symptoms and signs of heart failure are controlled, every effort should be made to cautiously use beta blockers not only for angina but because trials in heart failure have shown significant improvement in survival. Nocturnal angina can often be relieved by the treatment of heart failure. Nitrates are useful and can simultaneously improve the disturbed hemodynamics of congestive heart failure by vasodilatation, thereby reducing preload, and relieve angina by preventing or reversing myocardial ischemia. The combination of congestive heart failure and angina in patients with IHD usually indicates a poor prognosis and warrants serious consideration of cardiac catheterization and coronary revascularization.

CORONARY REVASCULARIZATION

While the basic management of patients with IHD is medical, as described above, many patients are improved by coronary revascularization procedures. These interventions should be employed in conjunction with but do not replace the continuing need to modify risk factors and medical therapy.

PERCUTANEOUS CORONARY INTERVENTION (See also Chap. 229 and Table 226-5)   PCI, most commonly percutaneous transluminal coronary angioplasty with stenting, is widely used to achieve revascularization of the myocardium in patients with symptomatic IHD and suitable stenoses of epicardial coronary arteries. Whereas patients with stenosis of the left main coronary artery and those with three-vessel IHD (especially with diabetes and/or impaired left ventricular function) who require revascularization are best treated with CABG, PCI is widely employed in patients with symptoms and evidence of ischemia due to stenoses of one or two vessels, and even in selected patients with three-vessel disease, and may offer many advantages over surgery.

Indications and Patient Selection   The most common clinical indication for PCI is angina pectoris, despite medical therapy, accompanied by

evidence of ischemia during a stress test. PCI is more effective than medical therapy for the relief of angina. Whereas PCI improves outcomes in patients with unstable angina and myocardial infarction, the value of this procedure in reducing the occurrence of coronary death and myocardial infarction in patients with chronic stable angina has not been established. PCI can be used to treat stenoses in native coronary arteries as well as in bypass grafts in patients who have recurrent angina following CABG. This is an important indication when the technical difficulties and the increased mortality that accompanies reoperation are considered. PCI has also been carried out in patients with recent total occlusion (within 3 months) of a coronary artery and angina; in this group the primary success rate is slightly decreased.

Risks   When coronary stenoses are discrete and symmetric, two and even three vessels can be dilated in sequence. However, case selection is essential in order to avoid a prohibitive risk of complications, which are usually due to dissection or thrombosis with vessel occlusion, uncontrolled ischemia, and ventricular failure. Oral aspirin, clopidogrel, and intravenous heparin are given to reduce coronary thrombus formation. In unstable angina and when intracoronary thrombus is seen, the use of specific platelet glycoprotein receptor (GpIIb/IIIa) antagonists further reduces thrombotic complications and increases success. In experienced hands, the overall mortality rate is <0.5%, the need for emergency coronary surgery <1%, and the occurrence of clinical myocardial infarction <2%. Minor complications occur in 5 to 10% of patients and include occlusion of a branch of a coronary artery, myocardial infarction manifest only by release of CK-MB into the circulation, and complications of arterial catheterization. Left main coronary artery stenosis is generally regarded as a contraindication to PCI; such patients should be treated with CABG.

Efficacy   Primary success, i.e., adequate dilation (an increase in luminal diameter >20% to a residual diameter obstruction <50%) with relief of angina, is achieved in >95% of cases. Recurrent stenosis of the dilated vessels occurs in ~20% of cases within 6 months of PCI with base metal stents, and angina will recur within 6 months in 10% of cases. Restenosis is more common in patients with diabetes mellitus, arteries with small caliber, incomplete dilation of the stenosis, occluded vessels, obstructed vein grafts, dilation of the left anterior descending coronary artery, and stenoses containing thrombi. It is usual clinical practice to administer aspirin for months after the procedure. Although aspirin and the antiplatelet drug clopidogrel may help prevent acute coronary thrombosis during and shortly following PCI with stenting, there is no evidence that these medications reduce the incidence of restenosis. Controlled trials have shown that the catheter-based local delivery of beta irradiation can significantly reduce the recurrence of in-stent restenosis. In diseased vein grafts procedural success has been improved by the use of capture devices or filters that prevent embolization, ischemia, and infarction. Moreover, the use of stents that locally deliver antiproliferative drugs such as rapamycin can reduce restenosis to near zero within the stent and 3 to 7% at the edges. These significant advances are extending the use of PCI.

Successful PCI produces effective relief of angina in >95% of cases and has been shown to be more effective than medical therapy for up to 2 years. More than one-half of patients with symptomatic IHD who require revascularization can be treated initially by PCI. Successful PCI is less invasive and expensive than CABG, usually requires only 1 to 2 days in the hospital, and permits considerable savings in the initial cost of care. Successful PCI also allows earlier return to work and the resumption of an active life. However, this economic benefit is reduced over time because of the greater need for follow-up and for repeat procedures. Clinical trials in patients after PCI have shown improvements in outcome with statin treatment.

CORONARY ARTERY BYPASS GRAFTING (See Table 226-5)   Anastomosis of one or both of the internal mammary arteries or a radial artery to the coronary artery distal to the obstructive lesion is carried out. For additional obstructions that cannot be bypassed by an artery, a section of a vein (usually the saphenous) is used to form a connection between the aorta and the coronary artery distal to the obstructive lesion.

TABLE 226-5 *Comparison of Revascularization Procedures in Multivessel Disease*

Procedure	Advantages	Disadvantages
Percutaneous coronary intervention (PCI)	Less invasive Shorter hospital stay Lower initial cost Easily repeated Effective in relieving symptoms	Restenosis High incidence of incomplete revascularization Unknown effect on outcomes in patients with severe left ventricular dysfunction Limited to specific anatomic subsets Poor outcome in diabetics with 2- or 3-vessel coronary disease
Coronary artery bypass grafting (CABG)	Effective in relieving symptoms Improved survival in certain subsets Ability to achieve complete revascularization	Cost Increased risk of a repeat procedure due to late graft closure Morbidity and mortality of major surgery

Source: Modified from DP Faxon, in GA Beller (ed), *Chronic Ischemic Heart Disease,* in E Braunwald (series ed), *Atlas of Heart Diseases,* Philadelphia, Current Medicine, 1995.

Although some indications for CABG are controversial, certain areas of agreement exist:

1. The operation is relatively safe, with mortality rates <1% in patients without serious comorbid disease and normal left ventricular function, and when the procedure is performed by an experienced surgical team.
2. Intraoperative and postoperative mortality increase with the severity of ventricular dysfunction, comorbidities, age >80 years, and lack of surgical experience. The effectiveness and risk of CABG vary widely depending on case selection and the skill and experience of the surgical team.
3. Occlusion of *venous* grafts is observed in 10 to 20% of patients during the first postoperative year and in approximately 2% per year during 5- to 7-year follow-up and 4% per year thereafter. Long-term patency rates are considerably higher for internal mammary and radial artery implantations than saphenous vein grafts. In patients with left anterior descending coronary artery obstruction, survival is better when coronary bypass involves the internal mammary artery rather than a saphenous vein. Graft patency and outcomes are improved by meticulous treatment of risk factors, particularly dyslipidemia.
4. Angina is abolished or greatly reduced in ~90% of patients following complete revascularization. Although this is usually associated with graft patency and restoration of blood flow, the pain may also have been alleviated as a result of infarction of the ischemic segment or a placebo effect. Within 3 years, angina recurs in about one-fourth of patients but is rarely severe.
5. Survival may be improved by operation in patients with stenosis of the left main coronary artery as well as in patients with three- or two-vessel disease with significant obstruction of the proximal left anterior descending coronary artery. The survival benefit is greater in patients with abnormal left ventricular function (ejection fraction < 50%). Survival *may* also be improved in the following patients: (1) with obstructive CAD who have survived sudden cardiac death or sustained ventricular tachycardia; (2) who have undergone previous CABG and who have multiple saphenous vein graft stenoses, especially of a graft supplying the left anterior descending coronary artery; and (3) with recurrent stenosis following PCI, and high-risk criteria on noninvasive testing.
6. Minimally invasive CABG through a small thoracotomy and/or off-pump surgery can reduce morbidity and shorten convalescence in suitable patients.

Indications for CABG are usually based on the severity of symptoms, coronary anatomy, and ventricular function. The ideal candidate is male, <80 years of age, has no other complicating disease, has troublesome or disabling angina that is not adequately controlled by medical therapy or does not tolerate medical therapy and wishes to lead a more active life, and has severe stenoses of two or three epicardial coronary arteries with objective evidence of myocardial ischemia as a cause of the chest discomfort. Great symptomatic benefit can be anticipated in such patients. Congestive heart failure and/or left ventricular dysfunction, advanced age (>80 years), reoperation, urgent need for surgery, and the presence of diabetes mellitus are all associated with a higher perioperative mortality.

Left ventricular dysfunction can be due to noncontractile segments that are viable (hibernating myocardium). These can be detected by using radionuclide scans of myocardial perfusion and metabolism, positron emission tomography, or delayed scanning with thallium-201 or by improvement of regional functional impairment, provoked by low-dose dobutamine. In such patients, revascularization can return function and improve survival.

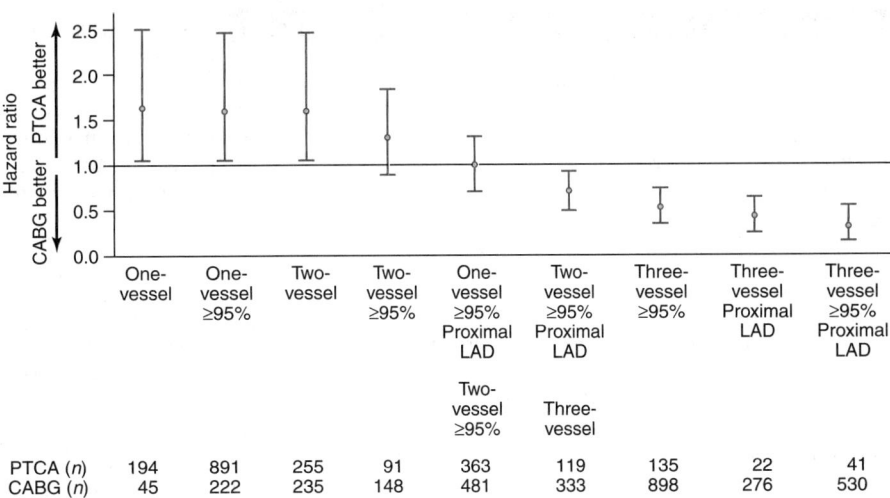

	One-vessel	One-vessel ≥95%	Two-vessel	Two-vessel ≥95%	One-vessel ≥95% Proximal LAD / Two-vessel ≥95%	Two-vessel ≥95% Proximal LAD / Three-vessel	Three-vessel ≥95%	Three-vessel Proximal LAD	Three-vessel ≥95% Proximal LAD
PTCA (n)	194	891	255	91	363	119	135	22	41
CABG (n)	45	222	235	148	481	333	898	276	530

FIGURE 226-2 Results from the Duke database comparing percutaneous transluminal coronary angioplasty (PTCA) and coronary artery bypass grafting (CABG). The preferred method of therapy depends on the extent and severity of coronary disease. PTCA seems to be superior in patients with less extensive disease, whereas CABG is more advantageous for patients with more extensive coronary disease. LAD, left anterior descending [*Modified from RH Jones et al. J Thorac Cardiovasc Surg III: 1013, 1996; with permission.*]

The Choice between PCI and CABG (Table 226-5; Fig. 226-2) A number of randomized clinical trials have compared PCI and CABG in patients with multivessel CAD who were suitable technically for both procedures. The redevelopment of angina requiring repeat coronary angiography and repeat revascularization due to restenosis was higher in the PCI groups. (This disadvantage of PCI may be abolished by the use of drug-eluting stents.) However, the occurrence of death or myocardial infarction has been found to be similar between both groups for up to 5 years. In patients with diabetes mellitus as well as obstruction of two or more coronary arteries, CABG results in significantly better outcomes and survival and should be the revascularization technique of choice.

Based on these trials and observational studies, it is now recommended that patients with an unacceptable level of angina despite optimal medical management be considered for coronary revascularization. Patients with single- or two-vessel disease with normal left ventricular function and anatomically suitable lesions are ordinarily advised to undergo PCI (Chap. 229). Patients with three-vessel disease (or two-vessel disease that includes the proximal left desending coronary artery) and impaired global left ventricular function (left ventricular ejection fraction < 50%) or diabetes mellitus or those with left main coronary artery disease or other lesions unsuitable for catheter-based procedures should be considered for CABG as the initial method of revascularization (Table 226-3, Table 226-5, and Fig. 226-2).

ASYMPTOMATIC (SILENT) ISCHEMIA

Obstructive CAD, acute myocardial infarction, and transient myocardial ischemia are frequently asymptomatic. During continuous ambulatory ECG monitoring, the majority of ambulatory patients with typical chronic stable angina are found to have objective evidence of myocardial ischemia (ST-segment depression) during episodes of chest discomfort while they are active outside the hospital, but many of these patients have more frequent episodes of asymptomatic ischemia. In addition, there is a large (but as yet unknown) number of totally asymptomatic persons with severe coronary atherosclerosis who exhibit ST-segment changes during activity. Some of these patients exhibit higher thresholds to electrically induced pain, others show higher endorphin levels, and still others may be diabetics with autonomic dysfunction.

Frequent episodes of ischemia (symptomatic and asymptomatic) during daily life appear to be associated with an increased likelihood of adverse coronary events (death and myocardial infarction). In addition, patients with asymptomatic ischemia after suffering a myocardial infarction are at greater risk for a second coronary event. The widespread use of exercise ECG during routine examinations has also identified some of these heretofore unrecognized patients with asymptomatic CAD. Longitudinal studies have demonstrated an increased incidence of coronary events in asymptomatic patients with positive exercise tests.

℞ TREATMENT

The management of patients with asymptomatic ischemia must be individualized. Thus, the physician should consider the following: (1) the degree of positivity of the stress test, particularly the stage of exercise at which ECG signs of ischemia appear, the magnitude and number of the perfusion defect(s) on thallium scintigraphy, and the change in left ventricular ejection fraction which occurs on radionuclide ventriculography or echocardiography during ischemia and/or during exercise; (2) the ECG leads showing a positive response, with changes in the anterior precordial leads indicating a less favorable prognosis than changes in the inferior leads; and (3) the patient's age, occupation, and general medical condition. Most would agree that an asymptomatic 45-year-old commercial airline pilot with 0.4-mV ST-segment depression in leads V_1 to V_4 during mild exercise should undergo coronary arteriography, whereas the asymptomatic, sedentary 75-year-old retiree with 0.1-mV ST-segment depression in leads II and III during maximal activity need not. However, there is no consensus about the appropriate procedure in the large majority of patients for whom the situation is less extreme. Asymptomatic patients with silent ischemia, three-vessel CAD, and impaired left ventricular function may be considered appropriate candidates for CABG.

The treatment of risk factors, particularly lipid lowering as described above, and the use of aspirin and beta blockers have been shown to reduce events and improve outcomes in asymptomatic as well as symptomatic patients with ischemia and proven CAD. While the incidence of asymptomatic ischemia can be reduced by treatment with beta blockers, calcium channel antagonists, and long-acting nitrates, it is not clear whether this is necessary or desirable in patients who have not suffered a myocardial infarction. However, there is evidence that β-adrenoceptor blockade begun 7 to 35 days after acute myocardial infarction improves survival (Chap. 228).

FURTHER READING

BLUMENTHAL RS et al: Medical therapy versus coronary angioplasty in stable coronary artery disease: A critical review of the literature. J Am Coll Cardiol 36:668, 2000

CLEEMAN JI et al: Executive summary of the Third Report of the National Cholesterol Education Program (NCEP) Expert Panel on Detection, Evaluation, and Treatment of High Blood Cholesterol in Adults (Adult Treatment Panel III). JAMA 285:2486, 2001

DEFEYTER PJ et al: Bypass surgery versus stenting for the treatment of multivessel disease in patients with unstable angina compared with stable angina. Circulation 105:2367, 2002

GIBBONS RJ et al: ACC/AHA/ACP-ASIM Guidelines for the Management of Patients with Chronic Stable Angina: Executive summary and recommendations. A report of the American College of Cardiology/American Heart Association Task Force on Practice Guidelines (Committee on Management of Patients with Chronic Stable Angina). Circulation 99:2829, 1999

KIM MC et al: Refractory angina pectoris. Mechanism and therapeutic options. J Am Coll Cardiol 39:923, 2002

LEE TH et al: Noninvasive tests in patients with stable coronary artery disease. N Engl J Med 344:1840, 2001

MORROW D et al: Chronic ischemic heart disease, in Braunwald's Heart Disease, 7th ed, D Zipes et al (eds). Philadelphia, Saunders, 2005

VAN DEN BRAND MJBM et al: The effect of completeness of revascularization on event-free survival at one year in the ARTS trial. J Am Coll Cardiol 39:559, 2002

YUSUF S et al: Effects of an angiotensin-converting enzyme inhibitor, ramipril, on cardiovascular events in high-risk patients. The Heart Outcomes Prevention Evaluation Study Investigators. N Engl J Med 342:145, 2000

227 UNSTABLE ANGINA AND NON–ST-ELEVATION MYOCARDIAL INFARCTION
Christopher P. Cannon, Eugene Braunwald

Patients with ischemic heart disease fall into two large groups: patients with stable angina secondary to chronic coronary artery disease (Chap. 226) and patients with acute coronary syndromes (ACS). The latter group, in turn, is composed of patients with acute myocardial infarction (MI) with ST-segment elevation on their presenting electrocardiogram (STEMI; Chap. 228) and those with unstable angina (UA) and non-ST-segment elevation MI (UA/NSTEMI; Fig. 228-1). Every year in the United States, ~1.4 million patients are admitted to hospitals with UA/NSTEMI as compared with 400,000 patients with acute STEMI.

DEFINITION The diagnosis of UA is based largely on the clinical presentation. *Stable* angina pectoris is characterized by chest or arm discomfort that is rarely described as pain, but that is reproducibly associated with physical exertion or stress and is relieved within 5 to 10 min by rest and/or sublingual nitroglycerin (Chaps. 12 and 226). UA is defined as angina pectoris or equivalent ischemic discomfort with at least one of three features: (1) it occurs at rest (or with minimal exertion) usually lasting > 10 min, (2) it is severe and of new onset (i.e., within the prior 4 to 6 weeks), and/or (3) it occurs with a crescendo pattern (i.e., distinctly more severe, prolonged, or frequent than previously). The diagnosis of NSTEMI is established if a patient with the clinical features of UA develops evidence of myocardial necrosis, as reflected in elevated cardiac biomarkers.

PATHOPHYSIOLOGY UA/NSTEMI can be caused by a reduction in oxygen supply and/or by an increase in myocardial oxygen demand (e.g., by tachycardia or severe anemia) superimposed on a coronary obstruction. Four pathophysiologic processes that may contribute to the development of UA have been identified: (1) plaque rupture or erosion with superimposed nonocclusive thrombus, believed to be the most common cause; (2) dynamic obstruction [e.g., coronary spasm, as in Prinzmetal's variant angina (p. 1448)]; (3) progressive mechanical obstruction [e.g., rapidly advancing coronary atherosclerosis or restenosis following percutaneous coronary intervention (PCI)]; and (4) secondary UA related to increased myocardial oxygen demand and/or decreased supply (e.g., anemia). More than one of these processes may be involved in many patients.

Among patients with UA/NSTEMI studied at angiography, ~5% have left main stenosis, 15% have three-vessel coronary artery disease, 30% have two-vessel disease, 40% have single-vessel disease, and 10% have no critical coronary stenosis; some of the latter have Prinzmetal's variant angina (see below). The "culprit lesion" on angiography may show an eccentric stenosis with scalloped or overhanging edges and a narrow neck. Angioscopy may reveal "white" (platelet-rich) thrombi, as opposed to "red" thrombi, more often seen in patients with acute STEMI.

CLINICAL PRESENTATION ■ History and Physical Examination The clinical hallmark of UA/NSTEMI is chest pain, typically located in the substernal region or sometimes in the epigastrium, that frequently radiates to the neck, left shoulder, and left arm (Chap. 12). This discomfort is usually severe enough to be considered painful. Anginal "equivalents" such as dyspnea and epigastric discomfort may also occur. The examination resembles that in patients with stable angina (Chap. 226) and may be unremarkable. If the patient has a large area of myocardial ischemia or a large NSTEMI, the physical findings can include diaphoresis, pale cool skin, sinus tachycardia, a third and/or fourth heart sound, basilar rales, and sometimes hypotension, resembling the findings of large STEMI.

Electrocardiogram In UA, ST-segment depression, transient ST-segment elevation, and/or T-wave inversion occur in 30 to 50% of patients, depending on the severity of the clinical presentation. In patients with the clinical features of UA, the presence of new ST-segment deviation, even of only 0.05 mV, is an important predictor of adverse outcome. T-wave changes are sensitive for ischemia but are less specific, unless they are new, deep T-wave inversions ($\geq$0.3 mV).

Cardiac Biomarkers Patients with UA who have elevated biomarkers of necrosis, such as CK-MB and troponin (a much more specific marker of myocardial necrosis), are at increased risk for death or recurrent MI. Elevated levels of these markers distinguish patients with NSTEMI from those with UA. There is a direct relationship between the degree of troponin elevation and mortality. However, in patients *without* a clear clinical history of myocardial ischemia, minor troponin elevations have been reported and can be caused by congestive heart failure, myocarditis, or pulmonary embolism or may be false-positive readings. Thus, in patients with an *unclear* history, small troponin elevations may not be diagnostic of an ACS.

DIAGNOSTIC EVALUATION (See also Chap. 12) Approximately 6 to 7 million persons per year in the United States present to hospital emergency departments (EDs) with a complaint of chest pain or other symptoms suggestive of ACS. A diagnosis of an ACS is established in 20 to 25% of such patients. The first step in evaluating patients with possible UA/NSTEMI is to determine the *likelihood* that coronary artery disease is the cause of the presenting symptoms. The 2002 American College of Cardiology/American Heart Association (ACC/AHA) Guidelines include, among the factors associated with a high likelihood of ACS, a clinical history typical of ischemic discomfort, a history of established coronary artery disease by angiography, prior MI, congestive heart failure, new electrocardiographic (ECG) changes, or elevated cardiac biomarkers. Factors associated with an intermediate likelihood of ACS in patients with the clinical features of this condition are: age >70 years, male gender, diabetes mellitus, known peripheral arterial or cerebrovascular disease, and old ECG abnormalities.

Diagnostic Pathways There are four major diagnostic tools used in the diagnosis of UA/NSTEMI in the ED—the clinical history, the ECG, cardiac markers, and stress testing. The goals are to: (1) recognize or exclude MI (using cardiac markers), (2) evaluate for rest ischemia (chest pain at rest, serial or continuous ECGs), and (3) evaluate for significant coronary artery disease (using provocative stress testing). Typical pathways begin with assessment of the likelihood that the presenting symptoms are due to ischemia. Patients with a low likelihood of ischemia are usually managed with an ED-based critical pathway (which in some institutions is carried out in a "chest pain unit" (Fig. 227-1). Evaluation of such patients includes clinical monitoring for recurrent ischemic discomfort, serial ECGs, and cardiac markers, typically performed at baseline and at 4 to 6 h and 12 h after presentation. If new elevations in cardiac markers (currently CK-MB and troponin) or ECG changes are noted, the patient is admitted to the hospital. If the patient remains pain free and the markers are negative, the patient may go on to stress testing. This may be performed as early as 6 h after presentation in the ED or chest pain center, or on an outpatient basis within 72 h. For most patients, standard treadmill ECG stress testing is used, but for patients with fixed abnormalities on the ECG (e.g., left bundle branch block), perfusion or echocardiographic imaging is used. For patients who cannot walk, pharmacologic stress is used. By demonstrating normal myocardial perfusion, sestamibi or thallium imaging (Chap. 211) can reduce unnecessary hospitalizations by excluding acute ischemia.

RISK STRATIFICATION AND PROGNOSIS Patients with documented UA/NSTEMI exhibit a wide spectrum of early (30 day) risk, ranging from ~2 to 10%, and of new or recurrent infarction of 3 to 10%. Assessment of "global risk" can be accomplished by clinical risk scoring systems

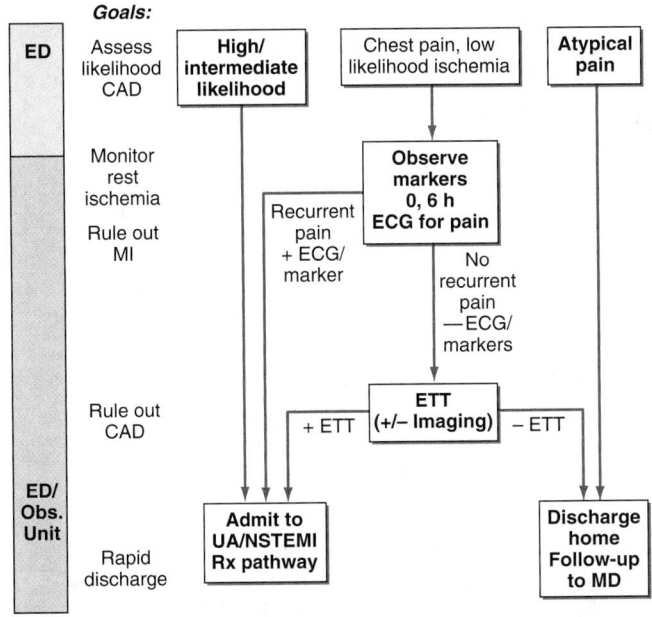

Critical Pathway for ED Evaluation of Chest Pain/ "Rule Out MI"

FIGURE 227-1 Diagnostic evaluation of patients presenting with suspected UA/NSTEMI. The first step is to assess the likelihood of coronary artery disease. Patients at high or intermediate likelihood are admitted to the hospital. Those with clearly atypical chest pain are discharged home. Patients with a *low* likelihood of ischemia enter the pathway and are observed in a monitored bed in the emergency department (ED) or observation unit over a period of 6 h and 12-lead electrocardiograms are performed if the patient has recurrent chest discomfort. A panel of cardiac markers (e.g., troponin and CK-MB) are drawn at baseline and 6 h later. If the patient develops recurrent pain, has ST-segment or T-wave changes, or had positive cardiac markers, he/she is admitted to the hospital and treated for UA/NSTEMI. If the patient has negative markers and no recurrence of pain, he/she is sent for exercise treadmill testing, with imaging reserved for patients with abnormal baseline electrocardiograms (e.g., left bundle branch block or left ventricular hypertrophy). If positive, the patient is admitted; if negative, the patient is discharged home with follow-up to his/her primary physician. (CAD, coronary artery disease; ECG, electrocardiogram; E.D., emergency department; ETT, exercise tolerance test; MI, myocardial infarction; OBS, observation unit.) [*Adapted from CP Cannon, E Braunwald, in E Braunwald et al (eds): Heart Disease: A Textbook of Cardiovascular Medicine, 6th ed. Philadelphia, Saunders, 2001.*]

such as that used in the Thrombolysis in Myocardial Ischemia Trial (TIMI), which includes seven independent risk factors: age $\geq$ 65 years, three or more risk factors for coronary artery disease, documented coronary artery disease at catheterization, development of UA/NSTEMI while on aspirin, more than two episodes of angina within the preceeding 24 h, ST deviation $\geq$ 0.5 mm, and an elevated cardiac marker (Fig. 227-2).

Early risk assessment (especially using troponin, ST-segment changes, and/or a global risk scoring system) is useful both in predicting the risk of recurrent cardiac events and in identifying those patients who would derive the greatest benefit from the newer and more potent antithrombotic therapies, such as low-molecular-weight heparin (LMWH) and glycoprotein (GP)IIb/IIIa inhibitors, and from an early invasive strategy. For example, in the TACTICS-TIMI 18 Trial, an early invasive strategy conferred a 40% reduction in recurrent cardiac events in patients with a positive troponin level, whereas no benefit was observed in those with a negative troponin level.

Among other cardiac biomarkers under intensive investigation are C-reactive protein, B-type natriuretic peptide, and CD-40 ligand, all of which correlate independently with increased mortality and recurrent cardiac events in patients presenting with UA/NSTEMI. Multimarker strategies are now gaining favor both to define the pathophysiologic mechanisms underlying a given patient's presentation more fully and to stratify the patient's risk further.

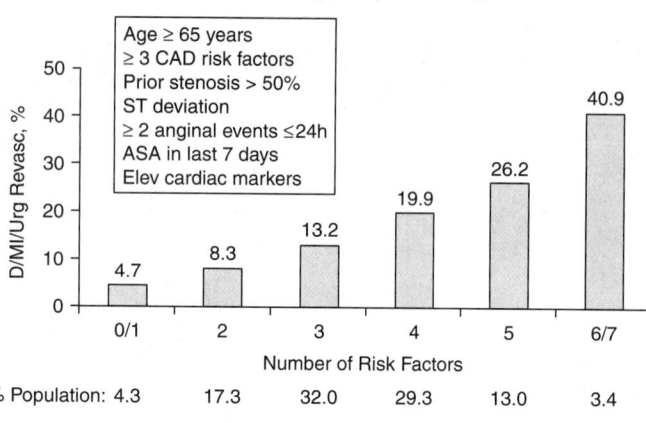

Age ≥ 65 years
≥ 3 CAD risk factors
Prior stenosis > 50%
ST deviation
≥ 2 anginal events ≤24h
ASA in last 7 days
Elev cardiac markers

% Population: 4.3   17.3   32.0   29.3   13.0   3.4

FIGURE 227-2 The TIMI Risk Score for UA/NSTEMI, a simple but comprehensive clinical risk stratification score to identify increasing risk of death, myocardial infarction, or urgent revascularization to day 14. (*Adapted from Antman et al.*)

℞ TREATMENT

Medical Treatment   Patients with UA/NSTEMI should be placed at bed rest with continuous ECG monitoring for ST-segment deviation and cardiac rhythm. Ambulation is permitted if the patient shows no recurrence of ischemia (discomfort or ECG changes) and does not develop a biomarker of necrosis for 12 to 24 h. Medical therapy involves simultaneous anti-ischemic treatment and antithrombotic treatment.

Anti-Ischemic Treatment (Table 227-1)   In order to provide relief and prevention of recurrence of chest pain, initial treatment should include nitrates and beta blockers.

NITRATES   Nitrates should first be given sublingually or by buccal spray (0.3 to 0.6 mg) if the patient is experiencing ischemic pain. If pain persists after three doses given 5 min apart, intravenous nitroglycerin (5 to 10 μg/min using nonabsorbing tubing) is recommended. The rate of the infusion may be increased by 10 μg/min every 3 to 5 min until symptoms are relieved or systolic arterial pressure falls to <100 mmHg. Topical or oral nitrates (Chap. 226) can be used once the pain has resolved, or they may replace intravenous nitroglycerin when the

TABLE 227-1   *Drugs Commonly Used in Intensive Medical Management of Patients with Unstable Angina and Non-ST Elevation MI*

Drug Category	Clinical Condition	When to Avoid[a]	Dosage
Nitrates	Symptoms are not fully relieved with three sublingual nitroglycerin tablets and initiation of beta-blocker therapy	Hypotension	5–10 μg/min by continuous infusion Titrated up to 75–100 μg/min until relief of symptoms or limiting side effects (headache or hypotension with a systolic blood pressure <90 mmHg or more than 30% below starting mean arterial pressure levels if significant hypertension is present) Topical, oral, or buccal nitrates are acceptable alternatives for patients without ongoing or refractory symptoms
Beta blockers[b]	Unstable angina	PR interval (ECG) >0.24 s 2° or 3° atrioventricular block Heart rate <60 beats/min Blood pressure <90 mmHg Shock Left ventricular failure with congestive heart failure Severe reactive airway disease	Metoprolol[c] 5-mg increments by slow (over 1–2 min IV administration Repeated every 5 min for a total initial dose of 15 mg Followed in 1–2 h by 25–50 mg by mouth every 6 h If a very conservative regimen is desired, initial doses can be reduced to 1–2 mg Esmolol[c] Starting maintenance dose of 0.1 mg/kg per min IV Titration in increments of 0.05 mg/kg per min every 10–15 min as tolerated by blood pressure until the desired therapeutic response has been obtained, limiting symptoms develop, or a dose of 0.20 mg/kg per min is reached Optional loading dose of 0.5 mg/kg may be given by slow IV administration (2–5 min) for more rapid onset of action
Calcium channel blockers	Patients whose symptoms are not relieved by adequate doses of nitrates and beta blockers or in patients unable to tolerate adequate doses of one or both of these agents or in patients with variant angina	Pulmonary edema Evidence of left ventricular dysfunction (for diltiazem or verapamil)	Dependent on specific agent
Morphine sulfate	Patients whose symptoms are not relieved after three serial sublingual nitroglycerin tablets or whose symptoms recur with adequate anti-ischemic therapy	Hypotension Respiratory depression Confusion Obtundation	2–5 mg IV dose May be repeated every 5–30 min as needed to relieve symptoms and maintain patient comfort

[a] Allergy or prior intolerance is a contraindication for all categories of drugs listed in this chart.
[b] Choice of the specific agent is not as important as ensuring that appropriate candidates receive this therapy. If there are concerns about patient intolerance owing to existing pulmonary disease, especially asthma, left ventricular dysfunction, or risk of hypotension or severe bradycardia, initial selection should favor a short-acting agent, such as propranolol or metoprolol or the ultra-short-acting agent esmolol. Mild wheezing or a history of chronic obstructive pulmonary disease should prompt a trial of a short-acting agent at a reduced dose (e.g., 2.5 mg IV metoprolol, 12.5 mg oral metoprolol, or 25 μg/kg per min esmolol as initial doses) rather than complete avoidance of beta-blocker therapy.

[c] Metoprolol and esmolol are two of several beta blockers that may be employed.
Note: Some of the recommendations in this guide suggest the use of agents for purposes or in doses other than those specified by the U.S. Food and Drug Administration. Such recommendations are made after consideration of concerns regarding nonapproved indications. Where made such recommendations are based on more recent clinical trials or expert consensus.
IV, intravenous; aPTT, activated partial thromboplastin time; ECG, electrocardiogram; 2°, second-degree; 3°, third-degree.
Source: Modified from E Braunwald et al: Circulation 1994;90:613–622.

patient has been pain free for 12 to 24 h. The only absolute contraindications to the use of nitrates are hypotension or the use of sildenafil (Viagra) or other drugs in that class within the previous 24 h.

β-ADRENERGIC BLOCKADE These agents are the other mainstay of antiischemic treatment. Intravenous beta blockade followed by oral beta blockade targeted to a heart rate of 50 to 60 beats/min is recommended. Heart rate–slowing calcium channel blockers, e.g., verapamil or diltiazem, are recommended in patients who have persistent or recurrent symptoms after treatment with full-dose nitrates and beta blockers and in patients with contraindications to beta blockade. Additional medical therapy includes angiotensin-converting enzyme (ACE) inhibition and HMG-CoA reductase inhibitors (statins) for long-term secondary prevention.

If pain persists despite intravenous nitroglycerin and beta blockade, morphine sulfate, 1 to 5 mg intravenously, can be administered every 5 to 30 min as needed.

Antithrombotic Therapy (Table 227-2) This is the other main component of treatment for UA/NSTEMI. Initial treatment should begin with the platelet cyclooxygenase inhibitor aspirin (Fig. 227-3). The thienopyridine clopidogrel, which blocks the platelet adenosine receptor (in combination with aspirin), was shown in the CURE trial to confer a 20% relative reduction in cardiovascular death, MI, or stroke compared with aspirin alone in both low- and high-risk patients with UA/NSTEMI, but to be associated with a moderate (absolute 1%) increase in serious bleeding, which is more marked in patients who undergo coronary artery bypass grafting. Pretreatment with clopidogrel has also been shown to reduce adverse outcomes associated with and following PCI (Chap. 229). Continued benefit of long-term (~1 year) treatment with the combination of clopidogrel and aspirin has been observed both in patients treated conservatively and in those who underwent a PCI. This combination is recommended for all patients with UA/NSTEMI who are not at excessive risk for bleeding.

Unfractionated heparin (UFH) or LMWH should be added to aspirin and clopidogrel. Based on several randomized trials showing the superiority of the LMWH enoxaparin to UFH in reducing recurrent cardiac events, the 2002 ACC/AHA UA/NSTEMI guidelines favor enoxaparin as the preferred antithrombin. Direct thrombin inhibitors and factor Xa inhibitors are being studied as replacements for heparin.

Intravenous GP IIb/IIIa inhibitors have also been shown to be beneficial in treating UA/NSTEMI (Fig. 227-3). For "upstream" management of high-risk patients in whom an invasive management is intended (i.e., initiating therapy when the patient first presents to the hospital), the small molecule inhibitors eptifibatide and tirofiban show benefit, while the monoclonal antibody abciximab appears not to be effective in patients treated conservatively, (i.e., in those not undergoing coronary angiography or PCI). However, abciximab has been shown to be beneficial in patients with UA/NSTEMI undergoing PCI. As with all antithrombotic agents, bleeding is the most important adverse effect of these drugs. Thus, patients with a history of bleeding must be screened carefully and given fewer antithrombotic agents.

INVASIVE VERSUS CONSERVATIVE STRATEGY Multiple clinical trials have shown the benefit of an early invasive strategy in high-risk patients, i.e., patients with multiple clinical risk factors, ST-segment deviation, and/or positive biomarkers (Table 227-3). In this strategy, following treatment with anti-ischemic and antithrombotic agents, coronary arteriography is carried out within ~48 h of admission, followed by coronary revascularization (PCI or coronary artery bypass grafting), depending on the coronary anatomy.

Such a strategy is quite cost-effective in high-risk patients. In low-risk patients, the outcomes from an invasive strategy are similar to those obtained from a conservative strategy, which consists of anti-

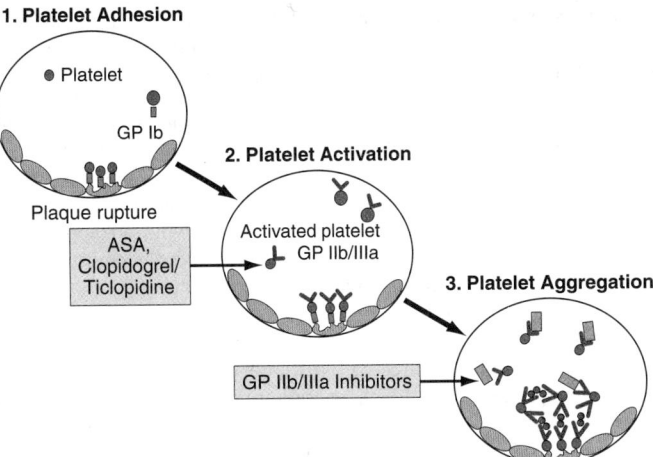

FIGURE 227-3 Platelets initiate thrombosis at the site of a ruptured plaque: *platelet adhesion* occurs via: (1) the GP 1b receptor in conjunction with von Willebrand factor. This is followed by *platelet activation* (2), which leads to a shape change in the platelet, degranulation of the alpha and dense granules, and expression of glycoprotein IIb/IIIa receptors on the platelet surface with activation of the receptor, such that it can bind fibrinogen. The final step is *platelet aggregation* (3), in which fibrinogen (or von Willebrand factor) binds to the activated GP IIb/IIIa receptors. Aspirin (ASA) and clopidogrel act to decrease platelet activation, whereas the glycoprotein IIb/IIIa inhibitors inhibit the final step of platelet aggregation. [*From CP Cannon, E Braunwald, in E Braunwald et al (eds): Heart Disease: A Textbook of Cardiovascular Medicine, 6th ed. Philadelphia, Saunders, 2001.*]

TABLE 227-2   *Clinical Use of Antithrombotic Therapy*

ORAL ANTIPLATELET THERAPY

Aspirin	Initial dose of 162–325 mg nonenteric formulation followed by 75–160 mg/d of an enteric or a nonenteric formulation
Clopidogrel (Plavix)	Loading dose of 300 mg followed by 75 mg/d

HEPARINS[a]

Dalteparin (Fragmin)	120 IU/kg SC every 12 h (maximum 10,000 IU twice daily)
Enoxaparin (Lovenox)	1 mg/kg SC every 12 h; the first dose may be preceded by a 30-mg IV bolus
Heparin (UFH)	Bolus 60–70 U/kg (maximum 5000 U) IV followed by infusion of 12–15 U/kg per h (initial maximum 1000 U/h) titrated to a PTT 1.5–2.5 times control

INTRAVENOUS ANTIPLATELET THERAPY

Abciximab (ReoPro)	0.25 mg/kg bolus followed by infusion of 0.125 µg/kg per min (maximum 10 µg/min) for 12 to 24 h
Eptifibatide (Integrilin)	180 µg/kg bolus followed by infusion of 2.0 µg/kg per min for 72 to 96 h
Tirofiban (Aggrastat)	0.4 µg/kg per min for 30 min followed by infusion of 0.1 µg/kg per min for 48 to 96 h

[a] Other LMWH exist beyond those listed.
Note: IV, intravenous; SC, subcutaneously; UFH, unfractionated heparin.
Source: Modified from E Braunwald et al: J Am Coll Cardiol 2000;36:970–1056.

TABLE 227-3   *Class I Recommendations for Use of an Early Invasive Strategy*[a]

Class I (level of evidence: A) indications
  Recurrent angina at rest/low-level activity despite Rx
  Elevated TnT or TnI
  New ST-segment depression
  Rec. angina/ischemia with CHF symptoms, rales, MR
  Positive stress test
  EF < 0.40
  Decreased BP
  Sustained VT
  PCI < 6 mos, prior CABG

[a] Any one of the high-risk indicators.
Abbreviations: TnT, troponin T; TnI, troponin I; CHF, congestive heart failure; MR, mitral regurgitation; EF, ejection fraction; BP, blood pressure; VT, ventricular tachycardia; PCI, percutaneous coronary intervention; CABG, coronary artery bypass grafting.
Source: From E Braunwald et al: Circulation 106:1893, 2002.

ischemic and antithrombotic therapy followed by "watchful waiting," in which coronary arteriography is carried out only if rest pain or ST-segment changes recur or there is evidence of ischemia on a stress test.

LONG-TERM MANAGEMENT   The time of hospital discharge is a "teachable moment" for the patient, when the physician can review and optimize the medical regimen. Risk factor modification is key, and the physician should discuss with the patient the importance of smoking cessation, achieving optimal weight, daily exercise, following an appropriate diet, blood pressure control, tight control of hyperglycemia (for diabetic patients), and lipid management, as recommended for patients with chronic stable angina (Chap. 225).

There is evidence of benefit with long-term therapy with five classes of drugs that are directed at different components of the atherothrombotic process. Beta blockers are appropriate anti-ischemic therapy and may help decrease triggers for MI. Statins and ACE inhibitors are recommended for long-term plaque stabilization. Antiplatelet therapy, now recommended to be the combination of aspirin and clopidogrel for at least 9 to 12 months, with aspirin continued thereafter, prevents or reduces the severity of any thrombosis that would occur if a plaque does rupture. Thus, a multifactorial approach to long-term medical therapy is directed at preventing the various components of atherothrombosis.

PRINZMETAL'S VARIANT ANGINA

In 1959, Prinzmetal et al. described a syndrome of ischemic pain that occurs at rest but not usually with exertion and is associated with transient ST-segment elevation. This syndrome is due to focal spasm of an epicardial coronary artery, leading to severe myocardial ischemia. Although it is frequently thought that the spasm occurs in arteries without stenosis, many Prinzmetal patients have spasm adjacent to atheromatous plaques. The exact cause of the spasm is not well defined, but it may be related to hypercontractility of vascular smooth muscle due to vasoconstrictor mitogens, leukotrienes, or serotonin. In some patients it is a manifestation of a vasospastic disorder and is associated with migraine, Raynaud's phenomenon, or aspirin-induced asthma.

CLINICAL AND ANGIOGRAPHIC MANIFESTATIONS   Patients with variant angina are younger and have fewer coronary risk factors (with the exception of cigarette smoking) than patients with UA secondary to coronary atherosclerosis. The anginal discomfort is often extremely severe and has usually not progressed from a period of chronic stable angina. Cardiac examination is usually normal in the absence of ischemia.

The clinical diagnosis of variant angina is made with the detection of transient ST-segment *elevation* with rest pain. Many patients also exhibit multiple episodes of asymptomatic ST-segment elevation (*silent ischemia*). Small elevations of CK-MB may occur in patients with prolonged attacks of variant angina. Exercise testing in patients with variant angina is of limited value because the patients can demonstrate ST elevation, depression, or no ST changes.

Coronary angiography demonstrates transient coronary spasm as the diagnostic hallmark of Prinzmetal's angina. Significant proximal coronary stenosis of at least one major vessel occurs in the majority of patients, and in them spasm usually occurs within 1 cm of the

obstruction. Focal spasm is most common in the right coronary artery, and it may occur at one or more sites in one artery or in multiple arteries simultaneously. Ergonovine, acetylcholine, other vasoconstrictor medications, and hyperventilation have been used to provoke and demonstrate focal coronary stenosis to establish the diagnosis. Hyperventilation has also been used to provoke rest angina, ST-segment elevation, and spasm on coronary arteriography.

℞ TREATMENT

Nitrates and calcium channel blockers are the main treatments for patients with variant angina. Sublingual or intravenous nitroglycerin often abolishes episodes of variant angina promptly, and long-acting nitrates are useful in preventing recurrences. Calcium antagonists are extremely effective in preventing the coronary artery spasm of variant angina, and they should be prescribed in maximally tolerated doses. Similar efficacy rates have been noted among the various types of calcium antagonists. Prazosin, a selective α-adrenoreceptor blocker, has also been found to be of value in some patients, while aspirin may actually increase the severity of ischemic episodes. The response to beta blockers is variable. Coronary revascularization may be helpful in patients with variant angina who also have discrete, proximal fixed obstructive lesions.

PROGNOSIS   Many patients with Prinzmetal's angina pass through an acute, active phase, with frequent episodes of angina and cardiac events during the first 6 months after presentation. Long-term survival at 5 years is excellent (~90 to 95%). Patients with no or mild fixed coronary obstruction tend to experience a more benign course than do patients with associated severe obstructive lesions. Nonfatal MI occurs in up to 20% of patients by 5 years. Patients with variant angina who develop serious arrhythmias during spontaneous episodes of pain are at a higher risk for sudden death. In most patients who survive an infarction or the initial 3- to 6-month period of frequent episodes, the condition stabilizes and there is a tendency for symptoms and cardiac events to diminish with time.

FURTHER READING

ANTMAN EM et al: The TIMI risk score for unstable angina/non-ST elevation MI: A method for prognostication and therapeutic decision making. JAMA 284:835, 2000

BOERSMA E et al: Platelet glycoprotein IIb/IIIa inhibitors in acute coronary syndromes: A meta-analysis of all major randomised clinical trials. Lancet 359:189, 2002

BRAUNWALD E: Unstable angina: A classification. Circulation 80:410, 1989
——— et al: ACC/AHA guideline update for the management of patients with unstable angina and non-ST segment elevation myocardial infarction: A report of the American College of Cardiology/American Heart Association Task Force on Practice Guidelines (Committee on the Management of Unstable Angina). www.acc.org 2002; accessed 3/15/2002

CANNON CP, BRAUNWALD E: Unstable angina, in *Braunwald's Heart Disease*, 7th ed, DP Zipes et al (eds). Philadelphia, Saunders, 2005
——— et al: Comparison of early invasive and conservative strategies in patients with unstable coronary syndromes treated with the glycoprotein IIb/IIIa inhibitor tirofiban. N Engl J Med 344:1879, 2001

CLOPIDOGREL IN UNSTABLE ANGINA TO PREVENT RECURRENT EVENTS TRIAL INVESTIGATORS: Effects of clopidogrel in addition to aspirin in patients with acute coronary syndromes without ST-segment elevation. N Engl J Med 345:494, 2001

228 ST-SEGMENT ELEVATION MYOCARDIAL INFARCTION
Elliott M. Antman, Eugene Braunwald

Acute myocardial infarction (AMI) is one of the most common diagnoses in hospitalized patients in industrialized countries. In the United States, approximately 650,000 patients experience a new AMI and 450,000 experience a recurrent AMI each year. The early (30-day) mortality rate from AMI is ~30%, with more than half of these deaths occurring before the stricken individual reaches the hospital. Although the mortality rate after admission for AMI has declined by ~30% over the past two decades, approximately 1 of every 25 patients who survives the initial hospitalization dies in the first year after AMI. Survival is markedly reduced in elderly patients (over age 75).

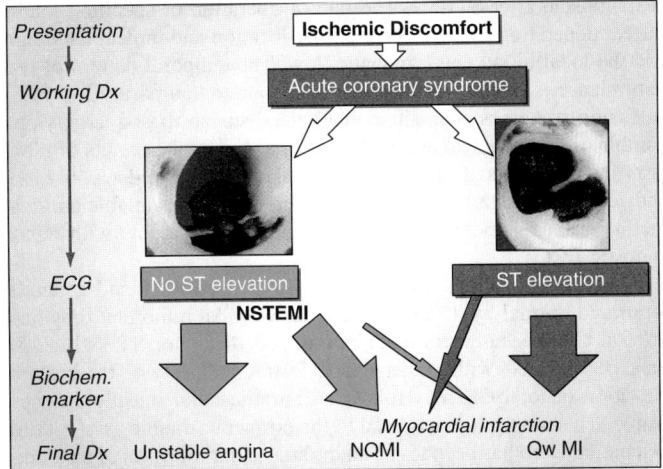

FIGURE 228-1 Acute coronary syndromes. Following disruption of a vulnerable plaque, patients experience ischemic discomfort resulting from a reduction of flow through the affected epicardial coronary artery. The flow reduction may be caused by a completely occlusive thrombus (right) or subtotally occlusive thrombus (left). Patients with ischemic discomfort may present with or without ST-segment elevation. Of patients with ST-segment elevation, the majority (*large red arrow*) ultimately develop a Q-wave MI (QwMI), while a minority (*small red arrow*) develop a non-Q-wave MI (NQMI). Patients who present without ST-segment elevation are suffering from either unstable angina or a non-ST-segment elevation MI (NSTEMI) (*large green arrows*), a distinction that is ultimately made on the presence or absence of a serum cardiac marker such as CKMB or a cardiac troponin detected in the blood. The majority presenting with NSTEMI ultimately develop a NQMI on the ECG; a minority develop a QwMI (*small green arrow*). (*Adapted from CW Hamm et al: Lancet 358:1533, 2001, and MJ Davies: Heart 83:361, 2000; with permission from the BMJ Publishing Group.*)

When patients with acute ischemic discomfort are first seen, the working diagnosis is that they are suffering from an acute coronary syndrome (Fig. 228-1). The 12-lead electrocardiogram (ECG) is at the center of the decision pathway for management since it permits distinction of those patients presenting with ST-segment elevation from those presenting without ST-segment elevation. Serum cardiac biomarkers are obtained to distinguish unstable angina from non-ST-segment MI (NSTEMI) (Chap. 227) and to assess the magnitude of an ST-segment elevation MI (STEMI).

PATHOPHYSIOLOGY: ROLE OF ACUTE PLAQUE RUPTURE

STEMI generally occurs when coronary blood flow decreases abruptly after a thrombotic occlusion of a coronary artery previously affected by atherosclerosis. Slowly developing, high-grade coronary artery stenoses do not usually precipitate STEMI because of the development of a rich collateral network over time. Instead, STEMI occurs when a coronary artery thrombus develops rapidly at a site of vascular injury. This injury is produced or facilitated by factors such as cigarette smoking, hypertension, and lipid accumulation. In most cases, infarction occurs when an atherosclerotic plaque fissures, ruptures, or ulcerates and when conditions (local or systemic) favor thrombogenesis, so that a mural thrombus forms at the site of rupture and leads to coronary artery occlusion. Histologic studies indicate that the coronary plaques prone to rupture are those with a rich lipid core and a thin fibrous cap (Chap. 224). After an initial platelet monolayer forms at the site of the ruptured plaque, various agonists (collagen, ADP, epinephrine, serotonin) promote platelet activation. After agonist stimulation of platelets, there are production and release of thromboxane A$_2$ (a potent local vasoconstrictor), further platelet activation, and potential resistance to thrombolysis.

In addition to the generation of thromboxane A$_2$, activation of platelets by agonists promotes a conformational change in the glycoprotein IIb/IIIa receptor (Chap. 101). Once converted to its functional state, this receptor develops a high affinity for amino acid sequences on soluble adhesive proteins (i.e., integrins) such as von Willebrand factor (vWF) and fibrinogen. Since vWF and fibrinogen are multiva-

lent molecules, they can bind to two different platelets simultaneously, resulting in platelet cross-linking and aggregation.

The coagulation cascade is activated on exposure of tissue factor in damaged endothelial cells at the site of the ruptured plaque. Factors VII and X are activated, ultimately leading to the conversion of prothrombin to thrombin, which then converts fibrinogen to fibrin (Chap. 102). Fluid-phase and clot-bound thrombin participate in an autoamplification reaction that leads to further activation of the coagulation cascade. The culprit coronary artery eventually becomes occluded by a thrombus containing platelet aggregates and fibrin strands.

In rare cases, STEMI may be due to coronary artery occlusion caused by coronary emboli, congenital abnormalities, coronary spasm, and a wide variety of systemic—particularly inflammatory—diseases. The amount of myocardial damage caused by coronary occlusion depends on (1) the territory supplied by the affected vessel, (2) whether or not the vessel becomes totally occluded, (3) the duration of coronary occlusion, (4) the quantity of blood supplied by collateral vessels to the affected tissue, (5) the demand for oxygen of the myocardium whose blood supply has been suddenly limited, (6) native factors that can produce early spontaneous lysis of the occlusive thrombus, and (7) the adequacy of myocardial perfusion in the infarct zone when flow is restored in the occluded epicardial coronary artery.

Patients at increased risk of developing STEMI include those with multiple coronary risk factors (Chap. 224) and those with unstable angina or Prinzmetal's variant angina (Chap. 227). Less common underlying medical conditions predisposing patients to STEMI include hypercoagulability, collagen vascular disease, cocaine abuse, and intracardiac thrombi or masses that can produce coronary emboli.

CLINICAL PRESENTATION

In up to one-half of cases, a precipitating factor appears to be present before STEMI, such as vigorous physical exercise, emotional stress, or a medical or surgical illness. Although STEMI may commence at any time of the day or night, circadian variations have been reported such that clusters are seen in the morning within a few hours of awakening.

Pain is the most common presenting complaint in patients with STEMI. The pain is deep and visceral; adjectives commonly used to describe it are *heavy*, *squeezing*, and *crushing*, although occasionally it is described as stabbing or burning (Chap. 12). It is similar in character to the discomfort of angina pectoris (Chap. 226) but is usually more severe and lasts longer. Typically the pain involves the central portion of the chest and/or the epigastrium, and on occasion it radiates to the arms. Less common sites of radiation include the abdomen, back, lower jaw, and neck. The frequent location of the pain beneath the xiphoid and patients' denial that they may be suffering a heart attack are chiefly responsible for the common mistaken impression of indigestion. The pain of STEMI may radiate as high as the occipital area but not below the umbilicus. It is often accompanied by weakness, sweating, nausea, vomiting, anxiety, and a sense of impending doom. The pain may commence when the patient is at rest, but when it begins during a period of exertion, it does not usually subside with cessation of activity, in contrast to angina pectoris.

The pain of STEMI can simulate pain from acute pericarditis (Chap. 222), pulmonary embolism (Chap. 244), acute aortic dissection (Chap. 231), costochondritis, and gastrointestinal disorders. These conditions should therefore be considered in the differential diagnosis. Radiation of discomfort to the trapezius is not seen in patients with STEMI and may be a useful distinguishing feature that suggests pericarditis is the correct diagnosis. However, *pain is not uniformly present in patients with STEMI.* The proportion of painless STEMIs is greater in patients with diabetes mellitus, and it increases with age. In the elderly, STEMI may present as sudden-onset breathlessness, which may progress to pulmonary edema. Other less common presentations, with or without pain, include sudden loss of consciousness, a confusional state, a sensation of profound weakness, the appearance of an arrhythmia, evidence of peripheral embolism, or merely an unexplained drop in arterial pressure.

PHYSICAL FINDINGS   Most patients are anxious and restless, attempting unsuccessfully to relieve the pain by moving about in bed, altering their position, and stretching. Pallor associated with perspiration and coolness of the extremities occurs commonly. The combination of substernal chest pain persisting for >30 min and diaphoresis strongly suggests STEMI. Although many patients have a normal pulse rate and blood pressure within the first hour of STEMI, about one-fourth of patients with anterior infarction have manifestations of sympathetic nervous system hyperactivity (tachycardia and/or hypertension), and up to one-half with inferior infarction show evidence of parasympathetic hyperactivity (bradycardia and/or hypotension).

The precordium is usually quiet, and the apical impulse may be difficult to palpate. In patients with anterior wall infarction, an abnormal systolic pulsation caused by dyskinetic bulging of infarcted myocardium may develop in the periapical area within the first days of the illness and then may resolve. Other physical signs of ventricular dysfunction include fourth (S_4) and third (S_3) heart sounds, decreased intensity of the first heart sound, and paradoxical splitting of the second heart sound (Chap. 209). A transient midsystolic or late systolic apical systolic murmur due to dysfunction of the mitral valve apparatus may be present. A pericardial friction rub is heard in many patients with transmural STEMI at some time in the course of the disease, if they are examined frequently. The carotid pulse is often decreased in volume, reflecting reduced stroke volume. Temperature elevations up to 38°C may be observed during the first week after STEMI. The arterial pressure is variable; in most patients with transmural infarction, systolic pressure declines by approximately 10 to 15 mmHg from the preinfarction state.

LABORATORY FINDINGS

Myocardial infarction (MI) progresses through the following temporal stages: (1) acute (first few hours to 7 days), (2) healing (7 to 28 days), and (3) healed (≥29 days). When evaluating the results of diagnostic tests for STEMI, the temporal phase of the infarction process must be considered. The laboratory tests of value in confirming the diagnosis may be divided into four groups: (1) ECG, (2) serum cardiac biomarkers, (3) cardiac imaging, and (4) nonspecific indexes of tissue necrosis and inflammation.

ELECTROCARDIOGRAM   The electrocardiographic manifestations of STEMI are described in Chap. 210. During the initial stage of the acute phase of MI, total occlusion of an epicardial artery produces ST-segment elevation. Most patients initially presenting with ST-segment elevation evolve Q waves on the ECG and are ultimately diagnosed as having sustained a Q-wave MI (Fig. 228-1). A small proportion may sustain only a non-Q-wave MI. When the obstructing thrombus is not totally occlusive, obstruction is transient, or if a rich collateral network is present, no ST-segment elevation is seen. Such patients are initially considered to be experiencing either unstable angina or NSTEMI (Chap. 227). Among patients presenting *without* ST-segment elevation, if a serum cardiac biomarker of necrosis (see below) is detected and no Q wave develops, the diagnosis of non-Q-wave MI is ultimately made (Fig. 228-1). A minority of patients who present initially without ST-segment elevation may develop a Q-wave MI. Previously it was believed that transmural MI is present if the ECG demonstrates Q waves or loss of R waves, and nontransmural MI may be present if the ECG shows only transient ST-segment and T-wave changes. However, electrocardiographic-pathologic correlations are far from perfect; therefore a more rational nomenclature for designating electrocardiographic infarction is now commonly in use, with the terms *Q-wave MI* and *non-Q-wave MI* replacing the terms *transmural MI* and *nontransmural MI*, respectively (Fig. 228-1).

SERUM CARDIAC BIOMARKERS   Certain proteins, called serum cardiac markers, are released into the blood in large quantities from necrotic

heart muscle after STEMI. The rate of liberation of specific proteins differs depending on their intracellular location and molecular weight and the local blood and lymphatic flow. The temporal pattern of protein release is of diagnostic importance, but contemporary urgent reperfusion strategies necessitate making a decision (based largely on a combination of clinical and ECG findings) before the results of blood tests have returned from the central laboratory. Rapid whole-blood bedside assays for serum cardiac markers are now available and may facilitate management decisions, particularly in patients with nondiagnostic ECGs.

Creatine phosphokinase (CK) rises within 4 to 8 h and generally returns to normal by 48 to 72 h (Fig. 228-2). An important drawback of total CK measurement is its lack of specificity for STEMI, as CK may be elevated with skeletal muscle trauma. A two- to threefold elevation of total CK may follow an intramuscular injection, for example. This ambiguity may lead to the erroneous diagnosis of STEMI in a patient who has been given an intramuscular injection of a narcotic for chest pain of noncardiac origin. Other potential sources of total CK elevation are (1) skeletal muscular diseases, including muscular dystrophy, myopathies, and polymyositis; (2) electrical cardioversion; (3) hypothyroidism; (4) stroke; (5) surgery; and (6) skeletal muscle damage secondary to trauma, convulsions, and prolonged immobilization.

The MB isoenzyme of CK has the advantage over total CK that it is not present in significant concentrations in extracardiac tissue and therefore is considerably more specific. However, cardiac surgery, myocarditis, and electrical cardioversion often result in elevated serum levels of the MB isoenzyme. A ratio (relative index) of CKMB mass: CK activity ≥2.5 suggests but is not diagnostic of a myocardial rather than a skeletal muscle source for the CKMB elevation. This ratio is less useful when levels of total CK are high owing to skeletal muscle injury or when the total CK level is within the normal range but CKMB is elevated.

Cardiac-specific troponin T (cTnT) and *cardiac-specific troponin I* (cTnI) have amino acid sequences different from those of the skeletal muscle forms of these proteins. These differences permitted the development of quantitative assays for cTnT and cTnI with highly specific monoclonal antibodies. Since cTnT and cTnI are not normally detectable in the blood of healthy individuals but may increase after

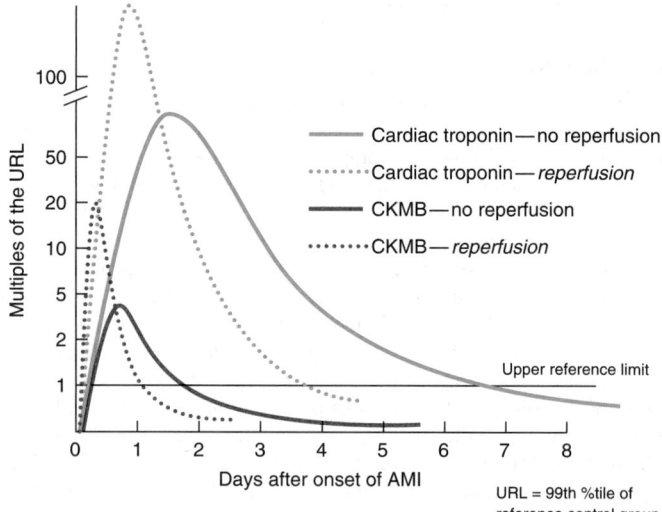

FIGURE 228-2   Typical cardiac biomarkers that are used to evaluate patients with STEMI include the MB isoenzyme of CK (CKMB) and cardiac-specific troponins. The white horizontal line depicts the upper reference limit (URL) for the cardiac biomarker in the clinical chemistry laboratory. The kinetics of release of CKMB and cardiac troponin in patients who do not undergo reperfusion are shown in the solid green and red curves as multiples of the URL. When patients with STEMI undergo reperfusion, as depicted in the dashed green and red curves, the cardiac biomarkers are detected sooner, rise to a higher peak value, but decline more rapidly, resulting in a smaller area under the curve and limitation of infarct size. (*Adapted from JS Alpert et al: J Am Coll Cardiol 36:959, 2000, and AH Wu et al: Clin Chem 45:1104, 1999.*)

STEMI to levels >20 times higher than the upper reference limit, the noise level of the assay), the measurement of cTnT or cTnI is of considerable diagnostic usefulness, and they are now the preferred biochemical markers for MI (Fig. 228-2). The cardiac troponins are particularly valuable when there is clinical suspicion of either skeletal muscle injury or a small MI that may be below the detection limit for CK and CKMB measurements. Levels of cTnI and cTnT may remain elevated for 7 to 10 days after STEMI.

Myoglobin is released into the blood within only a few hours of the onset of STEMI. Although myoglobin is one of the first serum cardiac markers that rises above the normal range after STEMI, it lacks cardiac specificity, and it is rapidly excreted in the urine, so that blood levels return to the normal range within 24 h of the onset of infarction.

Many hospitals are using cTnT or cTnI rather than CKMB as the routine serum cardiac marker for diagnosis of STEMI, although any of these analytes remains clinically acceptable. It is *not* cost-effective to measure both a cardiac-specific troponin and CKMB at all time points in every patient. However, in view of the prolonged elevation of cardiac-specific troponins (>1 week), episodes of recurrent ischemic discomfort and suspected recurrent MI are more readily diagnosed with a serum cardiac marker that remains elevated in the blood more briefly, such as CKMB or myoglobin.

While it has long been recognized that the total quantity of protein released correlates with the size of the infarct, the peak protein concentration correlates only weakly with infarct size. Recanalization of a coronary artery occlusion (either spontaneously or by mechanical or pharmacologic means) in the early hours of STEMI causes earlier and higher peaking (at about 8 to 12 h after reperfusion) of serum cardiac markers (Fig. 228-2).

For the purposes of confirming the diagnosis of MI, serum cardiac markers should be measured on admission, 6 to 9 h after admission, and 12 to 24 h after admission if the diagnosis remains uncertain.

The *nonspecific reaction* to myocardial injury is associated with polymorphonuclear leukocytosis, which appears within a few hours after the onset of pain and persists for 3 to 7 days; the white blood cell count often reaches levels of 12,000 to 15,000/μL. The erythrocyte sedimentation rate rises more slowly than the white blood cell count, peaking during the first week and sometimes remaining elevated for 1 or 2 weeks.

CARDIAC IMAGING Abnormalities of wall motion on *two-dimensional echocardiography* (Chap. 211) are almost universally present. Although acute STEMI cannot be distinguished from an old myocardial scar or from acute severe ischemia by echocardiography, the ease and safety of the procedure make its use appealing as a screening tool. In the emergency department setting, early detection of the presence or absence of wall motion abnormalities by echocardiography can aid in management decisions, such as whether the patient should receive reperfusion therapy [e.g., fibrinolysis or a percutaneous coronary intervention (PCI)]. Echocardiographic estimation of left ventricular (LV) function is useful prognostically; detection of reduced function serves as an indication for therapy with an angiotensin-converting enzyme (ACE) inhibitor (see "Angiotensin-Converting Enzyme Inhibitors," below). Echocardiography may also identify the presence of right ventricular (RV) infarction, ventricular aneurysm, pericardial effusion, and LV thrombus. In addition, Doppler echocardiography is useful in the detection and quantitation of a ventricular septal defect and mitral regurgitation, two serious complications of STEMI (see below).

Several *radionuclide imaging techniques* (Chap. 211) are available for evaluating patients with suspected STEMI. However, these imag-

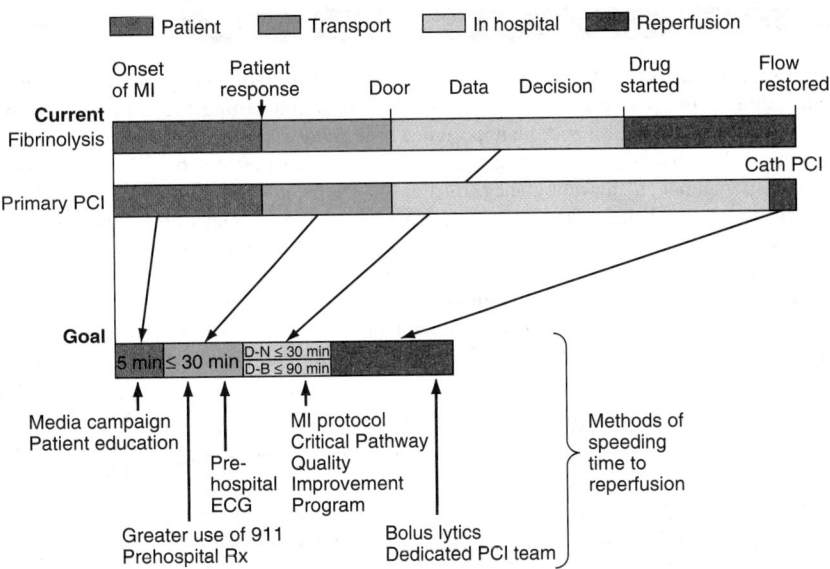

FIGURE 228-3 Major components of time delay between onset of symptoms from STEMI and restoration of flow in the infarct-related artery. Plotted sequentially from left to right are shown the times for patients to recognize symptoms and seek medical attention, transportation to the hospital, in-hospital decision-making, implementation of reperfusion strategy, and restoration of flow once the reperfusion strategy has been initiated. The time to initiate fibrinolytic therapy is the "door-to-needle" (D-N) time; this is followed by the period of time required for pharmacologic restoration of flow. More time is required to move the patient to the catheterization laboratory for a percutaneous coronary interventional (PCI) procedure, referred to as the "door-to-balloon" (D-B) time, but restoration of flow in the epicardial infarct-related artery occurs promptly after PCI. At the bottom are shown a variety of methods for speeding the time to reperfusion along with the goals for the time intervals for the various components of the time delay. (*Adapted from CP Cannon et al: J Thromb Thrombol 1:27, 1994.*)

ing modalities are used less often than echocardiography because they are more cumbersome and lack sensitivity and specificity in many clinical circumstances. Myocardial perfusion imaging with ^{201}Tl or ^{99m}Tc-sestamibi, which are distributed in proportion to myocardial blood flow and concentrated by viable myocardium (Chap. 226), reveal a defect ("cold spot") in most patients during the first few hours after development of a transmural infarct. However, although perfusion scanning is extremely sensitive, it cannot distinguish acute infarcts from chronic scars and thus is not specific for the diagnosis of *acute* MI. Radionuclide ventriculography, carried out with ^{99m}Tc-labeled red blood cells, frequently demonstrates wall motion disorders and reduction in the ventricular ejection fraction in patients with STEMI. While of value in assessing the hemodynamic consequences of infarction and in aiding in the diagnosis of RV infarction when the RV ejection fraction is depressed, this technique is nonspecific, as many cardiac abnormalities other than MI alter the radionuclide ventriculogram.

INITIAL MANAGEMENT

PREHOSPITAL CARE The prognosis in STEMI is largely related to the occurrence of two general classes of complications: (1) electrical complications (arrhythmias) and (2) mechanical complications ("pump failure"). Most out-of-hospital deaths from STEMI are due to the sudden development of ventricular fibrillation. The vast majority of deaths due to ventricular fibrillation occur within the first 24 h of the onset of symptoms, and, of these, over half occur in the first hour. Therefore, the major elements of prehospital care of patients with suspected STEMI include (1) recognition of symptoms by the patient and prompt seeking of medical attention; (2) rapid deployment of an emergency medical team capable of performing resuscitative maneuvers, including defibrillation; (3) expeditious transportation of the patient to a hospital facility that is continuously staffed by physicians and nurses skilled in managing arrhythmias and providing advanced cardiac life support; and (4) expeditious implementation of reperfusion therapy (Fig. 228-3). The biggest delay usually occurs not during transportation to the hospital but rather between the onset of pain and the patient's decision to call for help. This delay can best be reduced by education of the public by health care professionals concerning the significance of chest pain and the importance of seeking early medical attention. Increasingly, monitoring and treatment are carried out by trained personnel in the ambulance, further shortening the time between the onset of the infarction and appropriate treatment. General guidelines for initiation of fibrinolysis in the prehospital setting include the ability to transmit 12-lead ECGs to confirm the diagnosis, the presence of paramedics in the ambulance, training of paramedics in the interpretation of ECGs and management of STEMI, and online medical command and control that can authorize the initiation of treatment in the field.

MANAGEMENT IN THE EMERGENCY DEPARTMENT   In the emergency department, the goals for the management of patients with suspected STEMI include control of cardiac pain, rapid identification of patients who are candidates for urgent reperfusion therapy, triage of lower-risk patients to the appropriate location in the hospital, and avoidance of inappropriate discharge of patients with STEMI. Many aspects of the treatment of STEMI are initiated in the emergency department and then continued during the in-hospital phase of management.

Aspirin is essential in the management of patients with suspected STEMI and is effective across the entire spectrum of acute coronary syndromes (Fig. 228-1). Rapid inhibition of cyclooxygenase in platelets followed by a reduction of thromboxane A_2 levels is achieved by buccal absorption of a chewed 160- to 325-mg tablet in the emergency department. This measure should be followed by daily oral administration of aspirin in a dose of 75 to 162 mg.

In patients whose arterial oxygen saturation is normal as estimated by pulse oximetry or measured by an arterial blood gas specimen, supplemental oxygen is of limited if any clinical benefit and therefore is not cost-effective. However, when hypoxemia is present, oxygen should be administered by nasal prongs or face mask (2 to 4 L/min) for the first 6 to 12 h after infarction; the patient should then be reassessed to determine if there is a continued need for such treatment.

Control of Pain   Sublingual *nitroglycerin* can be given safely to most patients with STEMI. Up to three doses of 0.4 mg should be administered at about 5-min intervals. In addition to diminishing or abolishing chest discomfort, nitroglycerin may be capable of both decreasing myocardial oxygen demand (by lowering preload) and increasing myocardial oxygen supply (by dilating infarct-related coronary vessels or collateral vessels). In patients whose initially favorable response to sublingual nitroglycerin is followed by the return of chest pain, particularly if accompanied by other evidence of ongoing ischemia such as further ST-segment or T-wave shifts, the use of intravenous nitroglycerin should be considered. Therapy with nitrates should be avoided in patients who present with low systolic arterial pressure (<90 mmHg) or in whom there is clinical suspicion of RV infarction (inferior infarction on ECG, elevated jugular venous pressure, clear lungs, and hypotension). Nitrates should not be administered to patients who have taken the phosphodiesterase-5 inhibitor sildenafil for erectile dysfunction within the preceding 24 h since it may potentiate the hypotensive effects of nitrates. An idiosyncratic reaction to nitrates, consisting of sudden marked hypotension, sometimes occurs but can usually be reversed promptly by the rapid administration of intravenous atropine.

Morphine is a very effective analgesic for the pain associated with STEMI. However, it may reduce sympathetically mediated arteriolar and venous constriction, and the resulting venous pooling may reduce cardiac output and arterial pressure. These hemodynamic disturbances usually respond promptly to elevation of the legs, but in some patients volume expansion with intravenous saline is required. The patient may experience diaphoresis and nausea, but these events usually pass and are replaced by a feeling of well-being associated with the relief of pain. Morphine also has a vagotonic effect and may cause bradycardia or advanced degrees of heart block, particularly in patients with pos-

teroinferior infarction. These side effects usually respond to atropine (0.5 mg intravenously). Morphine is routinely administered by repetitive (every 5 min) intravenous injection of small doses (2 to 4 mg) rather than by the subcutaneous administration of a larger quantity, because absorption may be unpredictable by the latter route.

Intravenous *beta blockers* are also useful in the control of the pain of STEMI. These drugs control pain effectively in some patients, presumably by diminishing myocardial oxygen demand and hence ischemia. More important, there is evidence that intravenous beta blockers reduce in-hospital mortality, particularly in high-risk patients (see "Beta-Adrenoceptor Blockers," below). A commonly employed regimen is metoprolol, 5 mg every 2 to 5 min for a total of three doses, provided the patient has a heart rate > 60 beats per minute (bpm), systolic pressure > 100 mmHg, a PR interval < 0.24 s, and rales that are no higher than 10 cm up from the diaphragm. Fifteen minutes after the last intravenous dose, an oral regimen is initiated of 50 mg every 6 h for 48 h, followed by 100 mg every 12 h.

Unlike beta blockers, calcium antagonists are of little value in the acute setting, and there is evidence that short-acting dihydropyridines may be associated with an increased mortality risk.

Management Strategies   The primary tool for screening patients and making triage decisions is the initial 12-lead ECG. When ST-segment elevation of at least 2 mm in two contiguous precordial leads and 1 mm in two limb leads is present, a patient should be considered a candidate for *reperfusion therapy* (Fig. 228-4). The process of selecting patients for fibrinolysis versus primary PCI (angioplasty, or stenting; Chap. 229) is discussed below. In the absence of ST-segment elevation, fibrinolysis is not helpful, and evidence exists suggesting that it may be harmful.

Limitation of Infarct Size   The quantity of myocardium that becomes necrotic as a consequence of a coronary artery occlusion is determined by factors other than just the site of occlusion. While the central zone of the infarct contains necrotic tissue that is irretrievably lost, the fate of the surrounding ischemic myocardium may be improved by timely restoration of coronary perfusion, reduction of myocardial oxygen demands, prevention of the accumulation of noxious metabolites, and blunting of the impact of mediators of reperfusion injury (e.g., calcium overload and oxygen-derived free radicals). Up to one-third of patients with STEMI may achieve *spontaneous* reperfusion of the infarct-related coronary artery within 24 h and experience improved healing of infarcted tissue. Reperfusion either pharmacologically (by fibrinolysis)

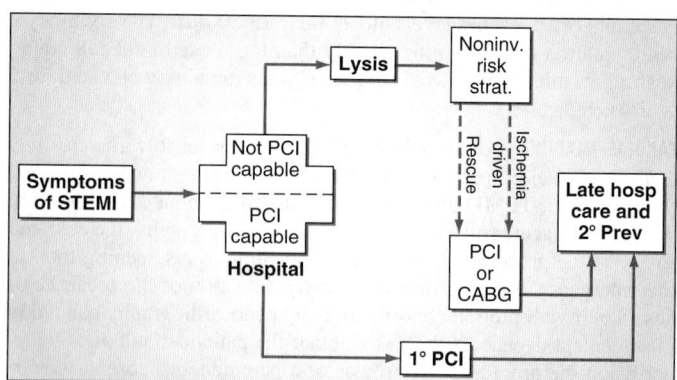

FIGURE 228-4   Reperfusion strategies for STEMI. Following the onset of symptoms of STEMI, the patient is transported to the hospital where reperfusion options are assessed. If the hospital is not capable of performing percutaneous coronary intervention (PCI), the patient is treated with fibrinolytic therapy; if the hospital is capable of performing PCI, reperfusion is implemented in the form of primary PCI. Patients who receive fibrinolytic therapy should undergo noninvasive risk stratification (Noninv. Risk Strat.). Patients with continued chest pain or failure to resolve ST-segment elevation by about 90 min should be referred for rescue PCI; if spontaneous recurrent ischemia or provoked ischemia is detected on noninvasive testing later in the hospital, patients should be referred for PCI or coronary artery bypass graft (CABG) surgery. All patients should receive therapies for secondary prevention of STEMI. (*Adapted from PW Armstrong, D Collen, EM Antman: Circulation 107:2533, 2003, with permission.*)

or by PCI accelerates the occluded infarct-related artery in those patients in whom spontaneous thrombolysis ultimately would have occurred and also greatly increases the number of patients in whom restoration of flow in the infarct-related artery is accomplished. Timely restoration of flow in the epicardial infarct–related artery combined with improved perfusion of the downstream zone of infarcted myocardium results in a limitation of infarct size. Protection of the ischemic myocardium by the maintenance of an optimal balance between myocardial oxygen supply and demand through pain control, treatment of congestive heart failure (CHF), and minimization of tachycardia and hypertension extends the "window" of time for the salvage of myocardium by reperfusion strategies.

Glucocorticoids and nonsteroidal anti-inflammatory agents, with the exception of aspirin, should be avoided in the setting of STEMI. They can impair infarct healing and increase the risk of myocardial rupture, and their use may result in a larger infarct scar. In addition, they can increase coronary vascular resistance, thereby potentially reducing flow to ischemic myocardium.

Primary Percutaneous Coronary Intervention (See also Chap. 229) PCI, usually angioplasty and/or stenting without preceding fibrinolysis, referred to as *primary PCI*, is effective in restoring perfusion in STEMI when carried out on an emergency basis in the first few hours of MI. It has the advantage of being applicable to patients who have contraindications to fibrinolytic therapy but otherwise are considered appropriate candidates for reperfusion. It appears to be more effective than fibrinolysis in opening occluded coronary arteries and, *when performed by experienced operators [≥75 PCI cases (not necessarily primary) per year] in dedicated medical centers (≥36 primary PCI cases per year)*, is associated with better short-term and long-term clinical outcomes. Compared with fibrinolysis, primary PCI is generally preferred when the diagnosis is in doubt, cardiogenic shock is present (especially in patients <75 years), bleeding risk is increased, or symptoms have been present for at least 2 to 3 h when the clot is more mature and less easily lysed by fibrinolytic drugs. However, PCI is expensive in terms of personnel and facilities, and its applicability is limited by its availability, around the clock, in only a minority of hospitals.

Fibrinolysis If no contraindications are present (see below), fibrinolytic therapy should ideally be initiated within 30 min of presentation (i.e., door-to-needle time ≤30 min). The principal goal of fibrinolysis is prompt restoration of full coronary arterial patency. The fibrinolytic agents tissue plasminogen activator (tPA), streptokinase, tenecteplase (TNK), and reteplase (rPA) have been approved by the U.S. Food and Drug Administration for intravenous use in the setting of STEMI. These drugs all act by promoting the conversion of plasminogen to plasmin, which subsequently lyses fibrin thrombi. Although considerable emphasis was first placed on a distinction between more fibrin-specific agents, such as tPA, and non-fibrin-specific agents, such as streptokinase, it is now recognized that these differences are only relative, as some degree of systemic fibrinolysis occurs with tPA. TNK and rPA are referred to as *bolus fibrinolytics* since their administration does not require a prolonged intravenous infusion.

When assessed angiographically, flow in the culprit coronary artery is described by a simple qualitative scale called the *thrombolysis in myocardial infarction (TIMI) grading system*: grade 0 indicates complete occlusion of the infarct-related artery; grade 1 indicates some penetration of the contrast material beyond the point of obstruction but without perfusion of the distal coronary bed; grade 2 indicates perfusion of the entire infarct vessel into the distal bed but with flow that is delayed compared with that of a normal artery; and grade 3 indicates full perfusion of the infarct vessel with normal flow. Early reports frequently lumped TIMI grades 2 and 3 under the general category of *patency*, but it is now recognized that grade 3 flow is the goal of reperfusion therapy, because full perfusion of the infarct-related coronary artery yields far better results in terms of limiting infarct size, maintenance of LV function, and reduction of both short- and long-term mortality rates. Relatively new methods of angiographic assessment of the efficacy of fibrinolysis include counting the number of

frames on the cine film required for dye to flow from the origin of the infarct-related artery to a landmark in the distal vascular bed (*TIMI frame count*) and determining the rate of entry and exit of contrast dye from the microvasculature in the myocardial infarct zone (*TIMI myocardial perfusion grade*).

Fibrinolytic therapy can reduce the relative risk of in-hospital death by up to 50% when administered within the first hour of the onset of symptoms of STEMI, and much of this benefit is maintained for at least 10 years. Appropriately used fibrinolytic therapy appears to reduce infarct size, limit LV dysfunction, and reduce the incidence of serious complications such as septal rupture, cardiogenic shock, and malignant ventricular arrhythmias. Since myocardium can be salvaged only before it has been irreversibly injured, the timing of reperfusion therapy, by fibrinolysis or a catheter-based approach, is of extreme importance in achieving maximum benefit. While the upper time limit depends on specific factors in individual patients, it is clear that "every minute counts" and that patients treated within 1 to 3 h of the onset of symptoms generally benefit most. Although reduction of the mortality rate is more modest, the therapy remains of benefit for many patients seen 3 to 6 h after the onset of infarction, and some benefit appears to be possible up to 12 h, especially if chest discomfort is still present and ST segments remain elevated in ECG leads that do not yet demonstrate new Q waves. Compared with PCI for STEMI (primary PCI), fibrinolysis is generally the preferred reperfusion strategy for patients presenting in the first hour of symptoms, if there are logistical concerns about transportation of the patient to a suitable PCI center (experienced operator and team with a track record for a "door-to-balloon" time of < 2 h), or there is an anticipated delay of at least 1 h between the time that fibrinolysis could be started versus implementation of PCI. Although patients <75 years achieve a greater relative reduction in the mortality rate with fibrinolytic therapy than do older patients, the higher *absolute* mortality rate (15 to 25%) in the latter results in similar absolute reductions in the mortality rates for both age groups.

tPA and the other relatively fibrin-specific plasminogen activators rPA and TNK are more effective than streptokinase at restoring full perfusion—i.e., TIMI grade 3 coronary flow—and have a small edge in improving survival as well. The current recommended regimen of tPA consists of a 15-mg bolus followed by 50 mg intravenously over the first 30 min, followed by 35 mg over the next 60 min. Streptokinase is administered as 1.5 million units (MU) intravenously over 1 h. rPA is administered in a double-bolus regimen consisting of a 10-MU bolus given over 2 to 3 min followed by a second 10-MU bolus 30 min later. TNK is given as a single weight-based intravenous bolus of 0.53 mg/kg over 10 s. In addition to the fibrinolytic agents discussed above, pharmacologic reperfusion typically involves adjunctive antiplatelet and antithrombotic drugs, as discussed subsequently.

Alternative pharmacologic regimens for reperfusion combine an intravenous glycoprotein IIb/IIIa inhibitor with a reduced dose of a fibrinolytic agent. Compared with fibrinolytic agents that involve a prolonged infusion (e.g., tPA) such combination reperfusion regimens facilitate the rate and extent of fibrinolysis by inhibiting platelet aggregation, weakening the clot structure, and allowing penetration of the thrombolytic agent deeper into the clot. However, combination reperfusion regimens have similar efficacy as compared with bolus fibrinolytics (e.g., rPA) and are associated with an increased risk of bleeding, especially in patients >75 years. Therefore, combination reperfusion regimens have not been approved for use but remain under active investigation to determine if they are helpful for preparing patients who are referred promptly for PCI—an experimental strategy called *facilitated PCI*.

CONTRAINDICATIONS AND COMPLICATIONS Clear contraindications to the use of fibrinolytic agents include a history of cerebrovascular hemorrhage at any time, a nonhemorrhagic stroke or other cerebrovascular event within the past year, marked hypertension (a reliably determined systolic arterial pressure > 180 mmHg and/or a diastolic pressure > 110 mmHg) at any time during the acute presentation, suspicion of aortic dissection, and active internal bleeding (excluding menses). While advanced age is associated with an increase in hemorrhagic complications, the benefit of fibrinolytic therapy in the elderly appears to justify its use if no other contraindications are present and the amount of myocardium in jeopardy appears to be substantial.

Relative contraindications to fibrinolytic therapy, which require assessment of the risk:benefit ratio, include current use of anticoagulants (international normalized ratio ≥2), a recent (<2 weeks) invasive or surgical procedure or prolonged (>10 min) cardiopulmonary resuscitation, known bleeding diathesis, pregnancy, a hemorrhagic ophthalmic condition (e.g., hemorrhagic diabetic retinopathy), active peptic ulcer disease, and a history of severe hypertension that is currently adequately controlled. Because of the risk of an allergic reaction, patients should not receive streptokinase if that agent had been received within the preceding 5 days to 2 years.

Allergic reactions to streptokinase occur in ~2% of patients who receive it. While a minor degree of hypotension occurs in 4 to 10% of patients given this agent, marked hypotension occurs, although rarely, in association with severe allergic reactions.

Hemorrhage is the most frequent and potentially the most serious complication. Because bleeding episodes that require transfusion are more common when patients require invasive procedures, unnecessary venous or arterial interventions should be avoided in patients receiving thrombolytic agents. Hemorrhagic stroke is the most serious complication and occurs in ~0.5 to 0.9% of patients being treated with these agents. This rate increases with advancing age, with patients >70 years experiencing roughly twice the rate of intracranial hemorrhage as those <65 years. Large-scale intervention trials have suggested that the rate of intracranial hemorrhage with tPA or rPA is slightly higher than with streptokinase.

Cardiac catheterization and coronary angiography should be carried out after fibrinolytic therapy if there is evidence of either (1) failure of reperfusion (persistent chest pain and ST-segment elevation >90 min), in which case a *rescue PCI* should be considered; or (2) coronary artery reocclusion (reelevation of ST segments and/or recurrent chest pain) or the development of recurrent ischemia (such as recurrent angina in the early hospital course or a positive exercise stress test before discharge), in which case an *elective PCI* should be considered. The potential benefits of routine angiography after PCI even in asymptomatic patients following administration of fibrinolytic therapy are controversial, but such an approach may have merit given the numerous technological advances that have occurred in the catheterization laboratory and the increasing number of skilled interventionalists. Coronary artery bypass surgery should be reserved for patients whose coronary anatomy is unsuited to angioplasty but in whom revascularization appears to be advisable because of extensive jeopardized myocardium or recurrent ischemia.

HOSPITAL PHASE MANAGEMENT

CORONARY CARE UNITS These units are routinely equipped with a system that permits continuous monitoring of the cardiac rhythm of each patient and hemodynamic monitoring in selected patients. Defibrillators, respirators, noninvasive transthoracic pacemakers, and facilities for introducing pacing catheters and flow-directed balloon-tipped catheters are also usually available. Equally important is the organization of a highly trained team of nurses who can recognize arrhythmias; adjust the dosage of antiarrhythmic, vasoactive, and anticoagulant drugs; and perform cardiac resuscitation, including electroshock, when necessary.

Patients should be admitted to a coronary care unit early in their illness when it is expected that they will derive benefit from the sophisticated and expensive care provided. The availability of electrocardiographic monitoring and trained personnel outside the coronary care unit has made it possible to admit lower-risk patients (e.g., those not hemodynamically compromised and without active arrhythmias) to "intermediate care units."

The duration of stay in the coronary care unit is dictated by the ongoing need for intensive care. If STEMI has been ruled out (ideally within 8 to 12 h) and symptoms are controlled with oral therapy, patients may be transferred out of the coronary care unit. Also, patients who have a confirmed STEMI but who are considered to be at low risk (no prior infarction and no persistent chest discomfort, CHF, hypotension, or cardiac arrhythmias) may be safely transferred out of the coronary care unit within 24 h.

Activity Factors that increase the work of the heart during the initial hours of infarction may increase the size of the infarct. Therefore, patients with STEMI should be kept at bed rest for the first 12 h. However, in the absence of complications, patients should be encouraged, under supervision, to resume an upright posture by dangling their feet over the side of the bed and sitting in a chair within the first 24 h. This practice is psychologically beneficial and usually results in a reduction in the pulmonary capillary wedge pressure. In the absence of hypotension and other complications, by the second or third day patients typically are ambulating in their room with increasing duration and frequency, and they may shower or stand at the sink to bathe. By day 3 after infarction, patients should be increasing their ambulation progressively to a goal of 185 m (600 ft) at least three times a day.

Diet Because of the risk of emesis and aspiration soon after MI, patients should receive either nothing or only clear liquids by mouth for the first 4 to 12 h. The typical coronary care unit diet should provide ≤30% of total calories as fat and have a cholesterol content of ≤300 mg/d. Complex carbohydrates should make up 50 to 55% of total calories. Portions should not be unusually large, and the menu should be enriched with foods that are high in potassium, magnesium, and fiber but low in sodium. Diabetes mellitus and hypertriglyceridemia are managed by restriction of concentrated sweets in the diet.

Bowels Bed rest and the effect of the narcotics used for the relief of pain often lead to constipation. A bedside commode rather than a bedpan, a diet rich in bulk, and the routine use of a stool softener such as dioctyl sodium sulfosuccinate (200 mg/d) are recommended. If the patient remains constipated despite these measures, a laxative can be prescribed. Contrary to prior belief, it is safe to perform a gentle rectal examination on patients with STEMI.

Sedation Many patients require sedation during hospitalization to withstand the period of enforced inactivity with tranquillity. Diazepam (5 mg), oxazepam (15 to 30 mg), or lorazepam (0.5 to 2 mg), given three or four times daily, is usually effective. An additional dose of any of the above medications may be given at night to ensure adequate sleep. Attention to this problem is especially important during the first few days in the coronary care unit, where the atmosphere of 24-h vigilance may interfere with the patient's sleep. However, sedation is no substitute for reassuring, quiet surroundings. Many drugs used in the coronary care unit, such as atropine, H_2 blockers, and narcotics, can produce delirium, particularly in the elderly. This effect should not be confused with agitation, and it is wise to conduct a thorough review of the patient's medications before arbitrarily prescribing additional doses of anxiolytics.

PHARMACOTHERAPY

ANTITHROMBOTIC AGENTS The use of antiplatelet and antithrombin therapy during the initial phase of STEMI is based on extensive laboratory and clinical evidence that thrombosis plays an important role in the pathogenesis of this condition. The primary goal of treatment with antiplatelet and antithrombin agents is to establish and maintain patency of the infarct-related artery. A secondary goal is to reduce the patient's tendency to thrombosis and thus the likelihood of mural thrombus formation or deep venous thrombosis, either of which could result in pulmonary embolization. The degree to which antiplatelet and antithrombin therapy achieves these goals partly determines how effectively it reduces the risk of mortality from STEMI.

As noted previously (see "Management in the Emergency Department," above), aspirin is the standard antiplatelet agent for patients with STEMI. The most compelling evidence for the benefits of anti-platelet therapy (mainly with aspirin) in STEMI is found in the comprehensive overview by the Antiplatelet Trialists' Collaboration. Data from nearly 20,000 patients with MI enrolled in 15 randomized trials were pooled and revealed a relative reduction of 27% in the mortality rate, from 14.2% in control patients to 10.4% in patients receiving antiplatelet agents.

The glycoprotein IIb/IIIa receptor is the focus of intense investigation (Chaps. 101 and 103). Glycoprotein inhibitors appear useful for preventing thrombotic complications in patients with STEMI undergoing PCI.

The standard antithrombin agent used in clinical practice is unfractionated heparin (UFH). Despite numerous clinical trials, the precise role of heparin in patients treated with fibrinolytic agents remains uncertain. The available data fail to show any convincing benefit of UFH with respect to either coronary arterial patency or mortality rate when UFH is added to a regimen of aspirin and a non-fibrin-specific thrombolytic agent such as streptokinase. Although not conclusively proven, it appears that the immediate administration of intravenous UFH, in addition to a regimen of aspirin and relatively fibrin-specific fibrinolytic agents (tPA, rPA, or TNK), helps to facilitate thrombolysis and to establish and maintain patency of the infarct-related artery. This effect is achieved at the cost of a small increased risk of bleeding. The recommended dose of UFH is an initial bolus of 60 U/kg (maximum 4000 U) followed by an initial infusion of 12 U/kg per hour (maximum 1000 U/h). The activated partial thromboplastin time during maintenance therapy should be 1.5 to 2 times the control value.

An alternative to UFH for anticoagulation of patients with STEMI that is being used with increased frequency in patients with unstable angina/NSTEMI (Chap. 227) are the low-molecular-weight heparin (LMWH) preparations, which are formed by enzymatic or chemical depolymerization to produce saccharide chains of varying length but with a mean molecular weight of about 5000 Da. The risks and benefits of LMWHs for management of patients with STEMI are under investigation.

Patients with an anterior location of the infarction, severe LV dysfunction, CHF, a history of embolism, two-dimensional echocardiographic evidence of mural thrombus, or atrial fibrillation are at increased risk of systemic or pulmonary thromboembolism. Such individuals should receive full therapeutic levels of antithrombin therapy (UFH or LMWHs) while hospitalized, followed by at least 3 months of warfarin therapy.

BETA-ADRENOCEPTOR BLOCKERS The benefits of beta blockers in patients with STEMI can be divided into those that occur immediately when the drug is given acutely and those that accrue over the long term when the drug is given for secondary prevention after an infarction. Acute intravenous beta blockade improves the myocardial oxygen supply-demand relationship, decreases pain, reduces infarct size, and decreases the incidence of serious ventricular arrhythmias. An overview of the data from 27,000 patients enrolled in nine randomized trials in the prethrombolytic era indicates that intravenous followed by oral beta blockade is associated with a 15% relative reduction in mortality, nonfatal reinfarction, and nonfatal cardiac arrest. In patients who undergo fibrinolysis soon after the onset of chest pain, no incremental reduction in mortality rate is seen with beta blockers, but recurrent ischemia and reinfarction are reduced.

Thus, beta blocker therapy after STEMI is useful for most patients (including those treated with an ACE inhibitor) except those in whom it is specifically contraindicated (patients with heart failure or severely compromised LV function, heart block, orthostatic hypotension, or a history of asthma) and perhaps those whose excellent long-term prognosis (defined as an expected mortality rate of <1% per year) markedly diminishes any potential benefit (patients <55 years with normal ventricular function, no complex ventricular ectopy, and no angina).

ANGIOTENSIN-CONVERTING ENZYME INHIBITORS ACE inhibitors reduce the mortality rate after STEMI, and the mortality benefits are additive to those achieved with aspirin and beta blockers. The maximum benefit is seen in high-risk patients (those who are elderly or who have an anterior infarction, a prior infarction, and/or globally depressed LV

function), but evidence suggests that a short-term benefit occurs when ACE inhibitors are prescribed unselectively to all hemodynamically stable patients with STEMI (i.e., those with a systolic pressure > 100 mmHg). The mechanism involves a reduction in ventricular remodeling after infarction (see "Ventricular Dysfunction," below) with a subsequent reduction in the risk of CHF. The rate of recurrent infarction may also be lower in patients treated chronically with ACE inhibitors after infarction.

ACE inhibitors should be prescribed within 24 h to all patients with STEMI. Before hospital discharge, LV function should be assessed with an imaging study. ACE inhibitors should be continued indefinitely in patients who have clinically evident CHF, in patients in whom an imaging study shows a reduction in global LV function or a large regional wall motion abnormality, or in those who are hypertensive. The use of angiotensin receptor blockers (ARBs) has not been as thoroughly explored as ACE inhibitors in STEMI patients. However, clinical experience in the management of patients with heart failure as well as data from clinical trials in STEMI patients suggest that ARBs may be useful in patients with depressed LV function or with clinical heart failure who are intolerant of an ACE inhibitor.

OTHER AGENTS Although the actual impact on the mortality rate is slight (three to four lives saved per 1000 patients treated), *nitrates* (intravenous or oral) may be useful in the relief of pain associated with STEMI. Favorable effects on the ischemic process and ventricular remodeling (see below) previously led many physicians to routinely use *intravenous nitroglycerin* (5 to 10 μg/min initial dose and up to 200 μg/min as long as hemodynamic stability is maintained) for the first 24 to 48 h after the onset of infarction. However, the benefits of routine use of intravenous nitroglycerin are less in the contemporary era where beta-adrenoceptor blockers and ACE inhibitors are routinely prescribed for patients with STEMI.

Results of multiple trials of different calcium antagonists have failed to establish a role for these agents in the treatment of most patients with STEMI, in contrast to the more consistent data that exist for other drugs (e.g., beta blockers, aspirin, fibrinolytic agents). The routine use of calcium antagonists cannot be recommended. Strict control of blood glucose in diabetic patients with STEMI has been shown to reduce the mortality rate. Serum magnesium should be measured in all patients on admission, and any demonstrated deficits should be corrected to minimize the risk of arrhythmias.

COMPLICATIONS AND THEIR MANAGEMENT

VENTRICULAR DYSFUNCTION After STEMI, the left ventricle undergoes a series of changes in shape, size, and thickness in both the infarcted and noninfarcted segments. This process is referred to as *ventricular remodeling* and generally precedes the development of clinically evident CHF in the months to years after infarction. Soon after STEMI, the left ventricle begins to dilate. Acutely, this results from expansion of the infarct, i.e., slippage of muscle bundles, disruption of normal myocardial cells, and tissue loss within the necrotic zone, resulting in disproportionate thinning and elongation of the infarct zone. Later, lengthening of the noninfarcted segments occurs as well. The overall chamber enlargement that occurs is related to the size and location of the infarct, with greater dilation following infarction of the apex of the left ventricle and causing more marked hemodynamic impairment, more frequent heart failure, and a poorer prognosis. Progressive dilation and its clinical consequences may be ameliorated by therapy with ACE inhibitors and other vasodilators (e.g., nitrates). In patients with an ejection fraction <40%, regardless of whether or not heart failure is present, ACE inhibitors should be prescribed.

HEMODYNAMIC ASSESSMENT Pump failure is now the primary cause of in-hospital death from STEMI. The extent of ischemic necrosis correlates well with the degree of pump failure and with mortality, both early (within 10 days of infarction) and later. The most common clinical signs are pulmonary rales and S_3 and S_4 gallop sounds. Pulmonary congestion is also frequently seen on the chest roentgenogram. Elevated LV filling pressure and elevated pulmonary artery pressure are the characteristic hemodynamic findings, but these findings may result from a reduction of ventricular compliance (diastolic failure) and/or a reduction of stroke volume with secondary cardiac dilation (systolic failure) (Chap. 215).

A classification originally proposed by Killip divides patients into four groups: class I, no signs of pulmonary or venous congestion; class II, moderate heart failure as evidenced by rales at the lung bases, S_3 gallop, tachypnea, or signs of failure of the right side of the heart, including venous and hepatic congestion; class III, severe heart failure, pulmonary edema; and class IV, shock with systolic pressure < 90 mmHg and evidence of peripheral vasoconstriction, peripheral cyanosis, mental confusion, and oliguria. When this classification was established in 1967, the expected hospital mortality rate of patients in these classes was as follows: class I, 0 to 5%; class II, 10 to 20%; class III, 35 to 45%; and class IV, 85 to 95%. With advances in management, the mortality rate in each class has fallen, perhaps by as much as one-third to one-half.

Hemodynamic evidence of abnormal LV function appears when contraction is seriously impaired in 20 to 25% of the left ventricle. Infarction of ≥40% of the left ventricle usually results in cardiogenic shock (Chap. 255). Positioning of a balloon flotation catheter in the pulmonary artery permits monitoring of LV filling pressure; this technique is useful in patients who exhibit hypotension and/or clinical evidence of CHF. Cardiac output can also be determined with a pulmonary artery catheter. With the addition of intraarterial pressure monitoring, systemic vascular resistance can be calculated as a guide to adjusting vasopressor and vasodilator therapy. Some patients with STEMI have markedly elevated LV filling pressures (>22 mmHg) and normal cardiac indexes [>2.6 and >3.6 L/(min/m²)], while others have relatively low LV filling pressures (<15 mmHg) and reduced cardiac indexes. The former patients usually benefit from diuresis, while the latter may respond to volume expansion by means of intravenous administration of colloid-containing solutions.

Hypovolemia   This is an easily corrected condition that may contribute to the hypotension and vascular collapse associated with STEMI in some patients. It may be secondary to previous diuretic use, to reduced fluid intake during the early stages of the illness, and/or to vomiting associated with pain or medications. Consequently, hypovolemia should be identified and corrected in patients with STEMI and hypotension before more vigorous forms of therapy are begun. Central venous pressure reflects RV rather than LV filling pressure and is an inadequate guide for adjustment of blood volume, since LV function is almost always affected much more adversely than RV function in patients with STEMI. The optimal LV filling or pulmonary artery wedge pressure may vary considerably among patients. Each patient's ideal level (generally ~20 mmHg) is reached by cautious fluid administration during careful monitoring of oxygenation and cardiac output. Eventually, the cardiac output level plateaus, and further increases in LV filling pressure only increase congestive symptoms and decrease systemic oxygenation without raising arterial pressure.

R𝗑 TREATMENT

The management of CHF in association with STEMI is similar to that of acute heart failure secondary to other forms of heart disease (avoidance of hypoxemia, diuresis, afterload reduction, inotropic support) (Chap. 216), except that the benefits of digitalis administration to patients with STEMI are unimpressive. By contrast, diuretic agents are extremely effective, as they diminish pulmonary congestion in the presence of systolic and/or diastolic heart failure (Chap. 255). LV filling pressure falls and orthopnea and dyspnea improve after the intravenous administration of furosemide or other loop diuretics. These drugs should be used with caution, however, as they can result in a massive diuresis with associated decreases in plasma volume, cardiac output, systemic blood pressure, and hence coronary perfusion. Nitrates in various forms may be used to decrease preload and congestive

symptoms. Oral isosorbide dinitrate, topical nitroglycerin ointment, or intravenous nitroglycerin all have the advantage over a diuretic of lowering preload through venodilation without decreasing the total plasma volume. In addition, nitrates may improve ventricular compliance if ischemia is present, as ischemia causes an elevation of LV filling pressure. Vasodilators must be used with caution to prevent serious hypotension. As noted earlier, ACE inhibitors are an ideal class of drugs for management of ventricular dysfunction after STEMI, especially for the long term.

CARDIOGENIC SHOCK   Efforts to reduce infarct size and prompt treatment of ongoing ischemia and other complications of MI appear to have reduced the incidence of cardiogenic shock from 20% to about 7%. Only 10% of patients with this condition present with it on admission, while 90% develop it during hospitalization. Typically, patients who develop cardiogenic shock have severe multivessel coronary artery disease with evidence of "piecemeal" necrosis extending outward from the original infarct zone. →*The evaluation and management of cardiogenic shock and severe power failure after STEMI are discussed in detail in Chap. 255.*

RIGHT VENTRICULAR INFARCTION   Approximately one-third of patients with inferoposterior infarction demonstrate at least a minor degree of RV necrosis. An occasional patient with inferoposterior LV infarction also has extensive RV infarction, and rare patients present with infarction limited primarily to the right ventricle. Clinically significant RV infarction causes signs of severe RV failure [jugular venous distention, Kussmaul's sign (Chap. 209), hepatomegaly] with or without hypotension. ST-segment elevations of right-sided precordial ECG leads, particularly lead V_4R, are frequently present in the first 24 h in patients with RV infarction. Two-dimensional echocardiography is helpful in determining the degree of RV dysfunction. Catheterization of the right side of the heart often reveals a distinctive hemodynamic pattern resembling cardiac tamponade or constrictive pericarditis (steep right atrial "y" descent and an early diastolic dip and plateau in RV waveforms) (Chap. 222). Therapy consists of volume expansion to maintain adequate RV preload and efforts to improve LV performance with attendant reduction in pulmonary capillary wedge and pulmonary arterial pressures.

ARRHYTHMIAS   (See also Chaps. 213 and 214)   The incidence of arrhythmias after STEMI is higher in patients seen early after the onset of symptoms. The mechanisms responsible for infarction-related arrhythmias include autonomic nervous system imbalance, electrolyte disturbances, ischemia, and slowed conduction in zones of ischemic myocardium. An arrhythmia can usually be managed successfully if trained personnel and appropriate equipment are available when it develops. Since most deaths from arrhythmia occur during the first few hours after infarction, the effectiveness of treatment relates directly to the speed with which patients come under medical observation. The prompt management of arrhythmias constitutes a significant advance in the treatment of STEMI.

Ventricular Premature Beats   Infrequent, sporadic ventricular premature depolarizations occur in almost all patients with STEMI and do not require therapy. Whereas in the past, frequent, multifocal, or early diastolic ventricular extrasystoles (so-called warning arrhythmias) were routinely treated with antiarrhythmic drugs to reduce the risk of development of ventricular tachycardia and ventricular fibrillation, pharmacologic therapy is now reserved for patients with sustained ventricular arrhythmias. Prophylactic antiarrhythmic therapy (either intravenous lidocaine early or oral agents later) is contraindicated for ventricular premature beats in the absence of clinically important ventricular tachyarrhythmias, as such therapy may actually increase the mortality rate. Beta-adrenoceptor blocking agents are effective in abolishing ventricular ectopic activity in patients with STEMI and in the prevention of ventricular fibrillation. As described above (see "Beta-Adrenoceptor Blockers"), they should be used routinely in patients without contraindications. In addition, hypokalemia and hypomagnesemia are risk factors for ventricular fibrillation in patients with

STEMI; the serum potassium concentration should be adjusted to approximately 4.5 mmol/L and magnesium to about 2.0 mmol/L.

Ventricular Tachycardia and Fibrillation Within the first 24 h of STEMI, ventricular tachycardia and fibrillation can occur without prior warning arrhythmias. The occurrence of ventricular fibrillation can be reduced by prophylactic administration of intravenous lidocaine. However, prophylactic use of lidocaine has not been shown to reduce overall mortality from STEMI. In fact, in addition to causing possible non-cardiac complications, lidocaine may predispose to an excess risk of bradycardia and asystole. For these reasons, and with earlier treatment of active ischemia, more frequent use of beta-blocking agents, and the nearly universal success of electrical cardioversion or defibrillation, routine prophylactic antiarrhythmic drug therapy *is no longer recommended*. It should be reserved for patients who cannot reach a hospital or for those treated in hospitals that lack the constant presence in the coronary care unit of a physician or nurse trained in the recognition and treatment of ventricular fibrillation.

Sustained ventricular tachycardia that is well tolerated hemodynamically should be treated with an intravenous regimen of amiodarone (bolus of 150 mg over 10 min, followed by infusion of 1.0 mg/min for 6 h and then 0.5 mg/min); or procainamide (bolus of 15 mg/kg over 20 to 30 min; infusion of 1 to 4 mg/min); if it does not stop promptly, electroversion should be used (Chap. 214). An unsynchronized discharge of 200 to 300 J (defibrillation) is used immediately in patients with ventricular fibrillation or when ventricular tachycardia causes hemodynamic deterioration. Ventricular tachycardia or fibrillation that is refractory to electroshock may be more responsive after the patient is treated with epinephrine (1 mg intravenously or 10 mL of a 1:10,000 solution via the intracardiac route), bretylium (a 5-mg/kg bolus), or amiodarone (a 75- to 150-mg bolus).

Ventricular arrhythmias, including the unusual form of ventricular tachycardia known as *torsades de pointes* (Chap. 214), may occur in patients with STEMI as a consequence of other concurrent problems (such as hypoxia, hypokalemia, or other electrolyte disturbances) or of the toxic effects of an agent being administered to the patient (such as digoxin or quinidine). A search for such secondary causes should always be undertaken.

Although the in-hospital mortality rate is increased, the long-term survival is good in patients who survive to hospital discharge after *primary* ventricular fibrillation, i.e., ventricular fibrillation that is a primary response to acute ischemia and is not associated with predisposing factors such as CHF, shock, bundle branch block, or ventricular aneurysm. This result is in sharp contrast to the poor prognosis for patients who develop ventricular fibrillation *secondary* to severe pump failure. For patients who develop ventricular tachycardia or ventricular fibrillation late in their hospital course (i.e., after the first 48 h), the mortality rate is increased both in-hospital and during long-term follow-up. Such patients should be considered for electrophysiologic study and implantation of a cardioverter/defibrillator (Fig. 228-5) (Chap. 214).

Accelerated Idioventricular Rhythm Accelerated idioventricular rhythm (AIVR, "slow ventricular tachycardia"), a ventricular rhythm with a rate of 60 to 100 bpm, occurs in 25% of patients with STEMI. It often occurs transiently during fibrinolytic therapy at the time of reperfusion. The rate of AIVR is usually similar to that of the sinus rhythm that precedes and follows it, and this similarity of rate plus the relatively minor hemodynamic effects make this rhythm more difficult to detect except by electrocardiographic monitoring. For the most part, AIVR is benign and does not presage the development of classic ventricular tachycardia. Most episodes of AIVR do not require treatment if the patient is monitored carefully, as degeneration into a more serious arrhythmia is rare, and, if it occurs, AIVR can generally be treated readily with a drug that increases the sinus rate (atropine).

Supraventricular Arrhythmias Sinus tachycardia is the most common supraventricular arrhythmia. If it occurs secondary to another cause (such as anemia, fever, heart failure, or a metabolic derangement), the primary problem should be treated first. However, if it appears to be due

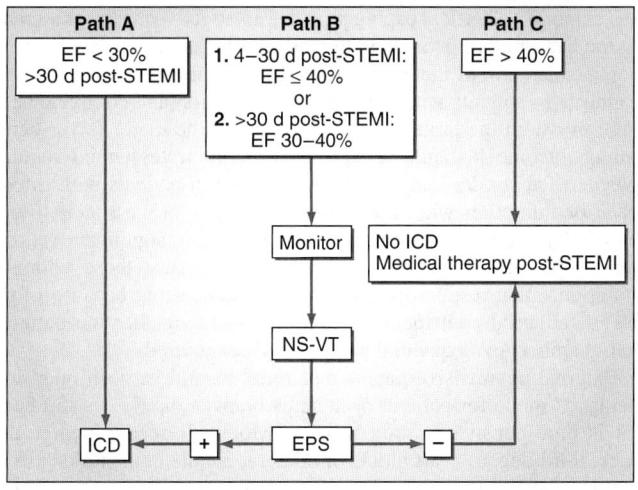

FIGURE 228-5 Algorithm for assessment of need for electrophysiologic study and implantation of a cardioverter/defibrillator. The appropriate management path is selected based upon the timing of and measurement of left ventricular ejection fraction (table at top of figure). In path A, patients with markedly depressed left ventricular function at least 1 month post-STEMI are referred for insertion of an implantable cardioverter/defibrillator (ICD). Path B illustrates the management of patients in an intermediate-risk category who require further evaluation with an electrophysiology study (EPS). If the EPS reveals inducible ventricular tachycardia/ventricular fibrillation, an ICD is implanted; if the EPS is negative, no ICD is implanted and the patient receives medical therapy post-STEMI. Path C illustrates the management of patients with preserved left ventricular function who do not receive an ICD and are treated with medical therapy post-STEMI. (*Adapted from EM Antman et al: ACC/AHA guidelines for the management of patients with ST elevation myocardial infarction. Circulation and JACC, 2004, in press; with permission.*)

to sympathetic overstimulation (e.g., as part of a hyperdynamic state), then treatment with a beta blocker is indicated. Other common arrhythmias in this group are atrial flutter and atrial fibrillation, which are often secondary to LV failure. Digoxin is usually the treatment of choice for supraventricular arrhythmias if heart failure is present. If heart failure is absent, beta blockers, verapamil, or diltiazem are suitable alternatives for controlling the ventricular rate, as they may also help to control ischemia. If the abnormal rhythm persists for >2 h with a ventricular rate >120 bpm or if tachycardia induces heart failure, shock, or ischemia (as manifested by recurrent pain or ECG changes), a synchronized electroshock (100 to 200 J) should be used.

Accelerated junctional rhythms have diverse causes but may occur in patients with inferoposterior infarction. Digitalis excess must be ruled out. In some patients with severely compromised LV function, the loss of appropriately timed atrial systole results in a marked decrease in cardiac output. Right atrial or coronary sinus pacing is indicated in such instances.

Sinus Bradycardia Treatment of sinus bradycardia is indicated if hemodynamic compromise results from the slow heart rate. Atropine is the most useful drug for increasing heart rate and should be given intravenously in doses of 0.5 mg initially. If the rate remains <50 to 60 bpm, additional doses of 0.2 mg, up to a total of 2.0 mg, may be given. Persistent bradycardia (<40 bpm) despite atropine may be treated with electrical pacing. Isoproterenol should be avoided.

Atrioventricular and Intraventricular Conduction Disturbances (See also Chap. 213) Both the in-hospital mortality rate and the post-discharge mortality rate of patients who have complete atrioventricular (AV) block in association with anterior infarction are markedly higher than those of patients who develop AV block with inferior infarction. This difference is related to the fact that heart block in inferior infarction is commonly a result of increased vagal tone and/or the release of adenosine and therefore is transient. In anterior wall infarction, heart block is usually related to ischemic malfunction of the conduction system, which is commonly associated with extensive myocardial necrosis.

Temporary electrical pacing provides an effective means of increasing the heart rate of patients with bradycardia due to AV block. However, acceleration of the heart rate may have only a limited impact on prognosis in patients with anterior wall infarction and complete heart block in whom the large size of the infarct is the major factor determining outcome. It should be carried out if it improves hemodynamics, however. Pacing does appear to be beneficial in patients with infero-posterior infarction who have complete heart block associated with heart failure, hypotension, marked bradycardia, or significant ventricular ectopic activity. A subgroup of these patients, those with RV infarction, often respond poorly to ventricular pacing because of the loss of the atrial contribution to ventricular filling. In such patients, dual-chamber AV sequential pacing may be required.

External noninvasive pacing electrodes should be positioned in a "demand" mode for patients with sinus bradycardia (rate < 50 bpm) that is unresponsive to drug therapy, Mobitz II second-degree AV block, third-degree heart block, or bilateral bundle branch block (e.g., right bundle branch block plus left anterior fascicular block). Retrospective studies suggest that permanent pacing may reduce the long-term risk of sudden death due to bradyarrhythmias in the rare patient who develops combined persistent bifascicular and transient third-degree heart block during the acute phase of MI.

OTHER COMPLICATIONS ▪ Recurrent Chest Discomfort Recurrent angina develops in ~25% of patients hospitalized for STEMI. This percentage is even higher in patients who undergo successful thrombolysis. Since recurrent or persistent ischemia often heralds extension of the original infarct or reinfarction in a new myocardial zone and is associated with a doubling of risk after STEMI, patients with these symptoms should be referred for prompt coronary arteriography and mechanical revascularization. Repeat administration of a fibrinolytic agent is an alternative to early mechanical revascularization.

Pericarditis (See also Chap. 222) Pericardial friction rubs and/or pericardial pain are frequently encountered in patients with transmural STEMI. This complication can usually be managed with aspirin (650 mg qid). It is important to diagnose the chest pain of pericarditis accurately, since failure to recognize it may lead to the erroneous diagnosis of recurrent ischemic pain and/or infarct extension, with resulting inappropriate use of anticoagulants, nitrates, beta blockers, or coronary arteriography. When it occurs, complaints of pain radiating to either trapezius muscle is helpful since such a pattern of discomfort is typical of pericarditis but rarely occurs with ischemic discomfort. Anticoagulants potentially could cause tamponade in the presence of acute pericarditis (as manifested by either pain or persistent rub) and therefore should not be used unless there is a compelling indication.

Thromboembolism Clinically apparent thromboembolism complicates STEMI in ~10% of cases, but embolic lesions are found in 20% of patients in necropsy series, suggesting that thromboembolism is often clinically silent. Thromboembolism is considered to be an important contributing cause of death in 25% of patients with STEMI who die after admission to the hospital. Arterial emboli originate from LV mural thrombi, while most pulmonary emboli arise in the leg veins.

Thromboembolism typically occurs in association with large infarcts (especially anterior), CHF, and a LV thrombus detected by echocardiography. The incidence of arterial embolism from a clot originating in the ventricle at the site of an infarction is small but real. Two-dimensional echocardiography reveals LV thrombi in about one-third of patients with anterior wall infarction but in few patients with inferior or posterior infarction. Arterial embolism often presents as a major complication, such as hemiparesis when the cerebral circulation is involved or hypertension if the renal circulation is compromised. When a thrombus has been clearly demonstrated by echocardiographic or other techniques or when a large area of regional wall motion abnormality is seen even in the absence of a detectable mural thrombus, systemic anticoagulation should be undertaken (in the absence of contraindications), as the incidence of embolic complications appears to

be markedly lowered by such therapy. The appropriate duration of therapy is unknown, but 3 to 6 months is probably prudent.

Left Ventricular Aneurysm The term *ventricular aneurysm* is usually used to describe *dyskinesis* or local expansile paradoxical wall motion. Normally functioning myocardial fibers must shorten more if stroke volume and cardiac output are to be maintained in patients with ventricular aneurysm; if they cannot, overall ventricular function is impaired. True aneurysms are composed of scar tissue and neither predispose to nor are associated with cardiac rupture.

The complications of LV aneurysm do not usually occur for weeks to months after STEMI; they include CHF, arterial embolism, and ventricular arrhythmias. Apical aneurysms are the most common and the most easily detected by clinical examination. The physical finding of greatest value is a double, diffuse, or displaced apical impulse. Ventricular aneurysms are readily detected by two-dimensional echocardiography, which may also reveal a mural thrombus in an aneurysm.

Rarely, myocardial rupture may be contained by a local area of pericardium, along with organizing thrombus and hematoma. Over time, this *pseudoaneurysm* enlarges, maintaining communication with the LV cavity through a narrow neck. Because a pseudoaneurysm often ruptures spontaneously, it should be surgically repaired if recognized.

POSTINFARCTION RISK STRATIFICATION AND MANAGEMENT

Many clinical factors have been identified that are associated with an increase in cardiovascular risk after initial recovery from STEMI. Some of the most important factors include persistent ischemia (spontaneous or provoked), depressed LV ejection fraction (<40%), rales above the lung bases on physical examination or congestion on chest radiograph, and symptomatic ventricular arrhythmias. Other features associated with increased risk include a history of previous MI, age >75, diabetes mellitus, prolonged sinus tachycardia, hypotension, ST-segment changes at rest without angina ("silent ischemia"), an abnormal signal-averaged ECG, nonpatency of the infarct-related coronary artery (if angiography is undertaken), and persistent advanced heart block or a new intraventricular conduction abnormality on the ECG. Therapy must be individualized on the basis of the relative importance of the risk(s) present.

The goal of preventing reinfarction and death after recovery from STEMI has led to strategies to evaluate risk after infarction. In stable patients, submaximal exercise stress testing may be carried out before hospital discharge to detect residual ischemia and ventricular ectopy and to provide the patient with a guideline for exercise in the early recovery period. Alternatively, or in addition, a maximal (symptom-limited) exercise stress test may be carried out 4 to 6 weeks after infarction. Evaluation of LV function is usually warranted as well. Recognition of a depressed LV ejection fraction by echocardiography or radionuclide ventriculography identifies patients who should receive ACE inhibitors (see "Angiotensin-Converting Enzyme Inhibitors," above). Patients in whom angina is induced at relatively low workloads, those who have a large reversible defect on perfusion imaging or a depressed ejection fraction, those with demonstrable ischemia, and those in whom exercise provokes symptomatic ventricular arrhythmias should be considered at high risk for recurrent MI or death from arrhythmia (Fig. 228-5). Cardiac catheterization with coronary angiography and/or invasive electrophysiologic evaluation is advised.

Exercise tests also aid in formulating an individualized exercise prescription, which can be much more vigorous in patients who tolerate exercise without any of the above-mentioned adverse signs. Additionally, predischarge stress testing may provide an important psychological benefit, building the patient's confidence by demonstrating a reasonable exercise tolerance. Furthermore, particularly when no arrhythmias or signs of ischemia are identified, the patient benefits by the physician's reassurance that objective evidence suggests no immediate jeopardy.

In many hospitals a cardiac rehabilitation program with progressive exercise is initiated in the hospital and continued after discharge. Ideally, such programs should include an educational component that informs patients about their disease and its risk factors.

The usual duration of hospitalization for an uncomplicated STEMI is about 5 days. The remainder of the convalescent phase may be accomplished at home. During the first 1 to 2 weeks, the patient should be encouraged to increase activity by walking about the house and outdoors in good weather. Normal sexual activity may be resumed during this period. After 2 weeks, the physician must regulate the patient's activity on the basis of exercise tolerance. Most patients will be able to return to work within 2 to 4 weeks.

SECONDARY PREVENTION

Various secondary preventive measures are at least partly responsible for the improvement in the long-term mortality and morbidity rates after STEMI. Long-term treatment with an antiplatelet agent (usually aspirin) after STEMI is associated with a 25% reduction in the risk of recurrent infarction, stroke, or cardiovascular mortality (36 fewer events for every 1000 patients treated). In addition, in patients taking aspirin chronically, STEMIs tend to be smaller and are more likely to be non-Q-wave in nature. An alternative antiplatelet agent that may be used for secondary prevention in patients intolerant of aspirin is the ADP receptor antagonist clopidogrel (75 mg orally daily). ACE inhibitors should be used indefinitely by patients with clinically evident heart failure, a moderate decrease in global ejection fraction, or a large regional wall motion abnormality to prevent late ventricular remodeling and recurrent ischemic events.

The chronic routine use of oral beta-adrenoceptor blockers for at least 2 years after STEMI is supported by well-conducted, placebo-controlled trials that have convincingly demonstrated reductions in the rates of total mortality, sudden death, and, in some instances, reinfarction. In contrast, calcium antagonists are not recommended for routine secondary prevention.

Evidence suggests that warfarin lowers the risk of late mortality and the incidence of reinfarction after STEMI. Most physicians prescribe aspirin routinely for all patients without contraindications and add warfarin for patients at increased risk of embolism (see "Thromboembolism," above). Several studies suggest that in patients <75 years a low dose of aspirin (75 to 81 mg/d) in combination with warfarin administered to achieve an INR > 2.0 is more effective than aspirin alone for preventing recurrent MI and embolic cerebrovascular accident. However, there is an increased risk of bleeding and a high rate of discontinuation of warfarin that has limited clinical acceptance of combination antithrombotic therapy. Combination antiplatelet therapy with aspirin and clopidogrel has been established as an important treatment strategy for reducing the risk of death and recurrent ischemic events in the year following presentation with unstable angina/NSTEMI. Trials are underway to assess whether such combined antiplatelet therapy is also effective and safe in patients recovering from STEMI.

Finally, risk factors for *atherosclerosis* (Chap. 224) should be discussed with the patient, and, when possible, favorably modified. In particular, efforts should be made to ensure the cessation of smoking and the control of hypertension and hyperlipidemia [the target low-density lipoprotein level is <2.6 mmol/L (<100 mg/dL)]. In addition, regular physical exercise and reduction of emotional stress should be encouraged. Hormone replacement therapy prevention of coronary events should not be given de novo to postmenopausal women after STEMI. Postmenopausal women already taking estrogen plus progestin at the time of STEMI may continue that therapy.

FURTHER READING

AMERICAN HEART ASSOCIATION: *Heart and Stroke Facts: 2002 Statistical Supplement.* Dallas, American Heart Association, 2003
ANTMAN EM, BRAUNWALD E: Acute myocardial infarction, in *Braunwald's Heart Disease*, 7th ed, DP Zipes et al. (eds). Philadelphia, Saunders, 2005
——— et al: ACC/AHA guidelines for the management of patients with ST elevation myocardial infarction. Circulation and JACC, 2004, in press; www.acc.org/clinical/guidelines/stemi/index.htm
BOERSMA E et al: Acute myocardial infarction. Lancet 361:847, 2003
FALK E et al: Coronary plaque disruption. Circulation 92:657, 1995
FIBRINOLYTIC THERAPY TRIALISTS (FTT) COLLABORATIVE GROUP: Indications for fibrinolytic therapy in suspected acute myocardial infarction: Collaborative overview of early mortality and major morbidity results from all randomised trials of more than 1000 patients. Lancet 343:311, 1994
GOTTLIEB SS et al: Effect of beta-blockade on mortality among high-risk and low-risk patients after myocardial infarction. N Engl J Med 339:489, 1998
MICHAELS AD, GOLDSCHLAGER N: Risk stratification after acute myocardial infarction in the reperfusion era. Prog Cardiovasc Dis 42:273, 2000
MONTALESCOT G et al: Platelet glycoprotein IIb/IIIa inhibition with coronary stenting for acute myocardial infarction. N Engl J Med 344:1895, 2001
TOPOL EJ: Acute myocardial infarction: Thrombolysis. Heart 83:122, 2000

229 PERCUTANEOUS CORONARY REVASCULARIZATION
Donald S. Baim

While bypass surgery was once the only means of coronary revascularization, in 1977 Andreas Gruntzig introduced a form of catheter-based coronary revascularization that he termed *percutaneous transluminal coronary angioplasty (PTCA)*. Given the limitations of his early equipment, fewer than 1000 PTCA procedures were performed worldwide each year. By the mid-1980s, progressive improvements in the balloon angioplasty equipment led to improved results, expanded indications for use, and explosive growth in the numbers of PTCA procedures; the annual number of PTCA procedures (~300,000) then roughly matched the number of surgical bypass operations. During the 1990s, a number of newer devices (including stents and atherectomy devices) were introduced that further improved the acute success, safety, and long-term durability and allowed the number of percutaneous coronary revascularizations (PCRs), or percutaneous coronary interventions (PCIs), to grow further (from 800,000 to 1 million procedures annually), more than double the annual number of coronary bypass operations (~400,000). This dominant role of catheter-based intervention in the treatment of coronary artery disease has led to creation of a separate area within the field of cardiovascular diseases known as *interventional cardiology*, with incremental fellowship requirements and Board certification based on training, ongoing experience (75 procedures per year), and a written examination.

All catheter-based coronary interventions are derivatives of diagnostic cardiac catheterization (Chap. 212), in which catheters are introduced into the arterial circulation by needle puncture, advanced into the heart under fluoroscopic guidance, and used for pressure measurements or injections of radiopaque liquid contrast agents. Interventional procedures differ in that the catheter placed into the ostium of the narrowed coronary artery has a slightly larger lumen diameter to allow passage of a flexible, steerable guidewire (diameter <0.5 mm) down the coronary artery lumen, through the narrowing, and into the vessel beyond. This guidewire then serves as the rail over which angioplasty balloons or other therapeutic devices are advanced and used to enlarge the narrowed segment of coronary artery (Fig. 229-1). Because PCR is performed with local anesthesia and requires only a short (1-day) hospitalization, its use in suitable patients can greatly decrease recovery time and expense compared to coronary bypass surgery. While not all types of coronary narrowing are well suited to catheter-based intervention, PCR is the treatment of choice for roughly 70% of patients with symptomatic single-vessel disease and roughly 20% of patients with symptomatic three-vessel disease. Selection of suitable cases for PCR versus bypass surgery takes into account the anatomic restrictions of PCR (in dealing with diffuse disease, bifurcation lesions, etc.). Both patient and physician need to be aware that while catheter-based in-

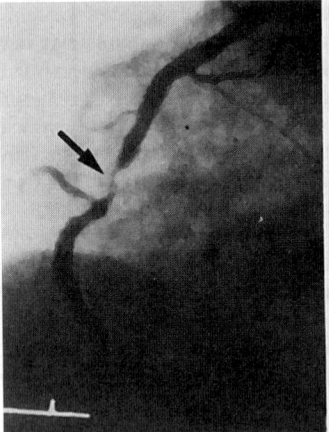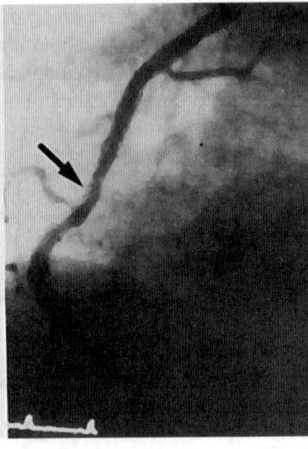

FIGURE 229-1 Focal discrete stenosis of the mid-right coronary angioplasty in a patient with unstable angina, shown before (*left panel*) and after (*right panel*) inflation of the PTCA balloon catheter. The lesion is typical of the straightforward lesion anatomy treated by early (pre-1985) coronary angioplasty.

tervention is done under anesthesia and has a lower elective mortality rate than bypass surgery (0.4 to 1.0%, compared to a rate of 1 to 3%), it is still an invasive procedure whose risks and benefits need to be weighed carefully for each individual patient. To decide which patients should undergo revascularization (rather than continued medical management), and to select which patients should undergo catheter-based rather than surgical revascularization, a detailed understanding of both clinical and coronary angiographic factors, as well as the applicability of various interventional techniques, is required.

INDICATIONS

The fundamental indication for PCR is the presence of one or more coronary stenoses that are approachable by catheter-based techniques and are thought to be responsible for a clinical syndrome that warrants revascularization. Moreover, the risks and benefits of revascularization by PCR for the individual patient should compare favorably with those of surgery. In patients with significant narrowing of a single coronary artery, the main benefit of revascularization lies in relief of anginal symptoms rather than in increasing their already good prognosis with medical therapy. By contrast, for the patient with significant left main stenosis or multivessel disease, revascularization may both relieve angina *and* improve long-term survival. For most patients with multivessel coronary disease, the current choice is surgical rather than catheter-based revascularization, particularly when one or more vessels supplying significant areas of viable myocardium are not well suited to PCR due to unfavorable anatomic features. In patients for whom either PCR or bypass surgery is a possible treatment for multivessel coronary artery disease, randomized trials have suggested that the two procedures are essentially equivalent in terms of in-hospital and 3- to 5-year mortality rates, except for patients with diabetes mellitus and multivessel coronary artery disease where surgical treatment appears to offer improved 5- to 7-year survival compared to PCR. However, patients who undergo PCR are more likely to need a second revascularization procedure (generally repeat PCR to treat restenosis) to maintain an equivalent level of symptom relief at 5 years. Repeat procedures will thus be needed in 50% of patients undergoing PTCA and in 20% of patients undergoing stenting, compared to 7 to 10% for patients undergoing bypass surgery, for multivessel disease.

The current clinical indications for PCR cover the spectrum of ischemic heart disease, from patients with unstable angina or acute infarction to patients with silent ischemia, as summarized in the recent ACC/AHA guidelines. One clear indication is *moderately severe, chronic, stable angina,* which persists despite medical antianginal therapy (Chap. 226). Occasionally, PCR is offered to patients with objective evidence of ischemia on noninvasive testing (i.e., an abnormal exercise test) and suitable coronary lesions, even though they have comparatively mild anginal symptoms. At the other extreme, many patients undergo PCR for more pressing indications, including unstable angina or acute myocardial infarction (MI) (with or without prior thrombolytic therapy). An aggressive approach to the treatment of unstable angina is now favored. It involves initial stabilization with beta blockers, nitrates, heparin, and antiplatelet agents (aspirin and frequently a platelet glycoprotein IIb/IIIa receptor blocker), followed by prompt diagnostic catheterization and same-procedure PCR of the culprit blockage. This approach offers the patient a more rapid return to work, fewer readmissions and late revascularizations, and potentially a reduction in late events compared to more prolonged initial trials of medical stabilization before proceeding with invasive evaluation and treatment.

In the early 1980s the introduction of intravenous fibrinolytic agents to reopen the occluded infarct-related vessel represented a major advance in the treatment of acute MI (Chap. 228). While use of immediate PCR would be expected to improve the results of fibrinolytic therapy further (by treating the underlying atherosclerotic stenosis), randomized trials showed that routine PCR after thrombolytic administration had no benefit compared to "watchful waiting," reserving PCR for patients who exhibited spontaneous or exercise-induced ischemia. In contrast, there is now strong evidence that *primary* or direct PCR (that is, PCR used instead of fibrinolytic therapy) can reduce the in-hospital mortality rate (from roughly 7 to 4%) when performed promptly by a skilled operator (Fig. 229-2). Another advantage of PCR is that it can be performed even in acute MI patients who have relative contraindications to fibrinolytic therapy (advanced age, hypertension, prior stroke, recent surgery, etc.).

As the clinical indications for PCR have broadened, so have its anatomic capabilities. Largely through the introduction of newer interventional devices

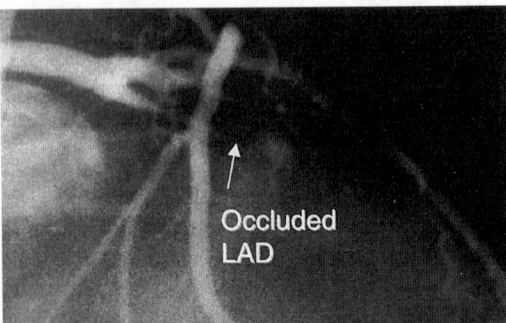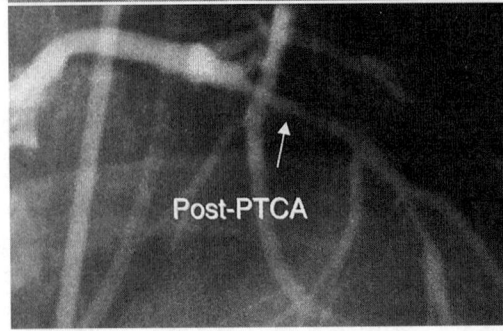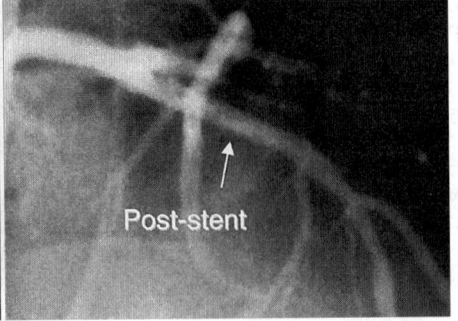

FIGURE 229-2 Left coronary angiogram in a patient with acute anterior myocardial infarction and cardiogenic shock shows occlusion of the proximal left anterior descending coronary artery (*top panel, arrow*) with only faint filling beyond the obstructing thrombus. After initial PTCA (*lower left panel*), there is restored antegrade flow with residual stenosis. After stent placement (*lower right panel*), there is no residual stenosis and brisk flow. This improvement was associated with reversal of shock hemodynamics, including normalization of severe lactic acidosis.

such as stents, PCR has advanced well beyond the treatment of proximal, discrete, subtotal, concentric, noncalcified lesions. Calcified, complex, or diffuse disease lesions respond well to coronary stent placement, sometimes after pretreatment with rotational atherectomy. Even totally occluded coronary arteries (particularly ones that have been occluded for <6 months) can be crossed and dilated effectively, although the success rate remains lower than for subtotal lesions (60% versus 90% for subtotal stenotic lesions). In addition to lesions in the native coronary tree, obstructions in the saphenous vein (Fig. 229-3) or internal mammary artery bypass grafts can also be dilated successfully to treat postbypass angina. If multiple lesions are responsible for the clinical syndrome, they generally can be dilated during a single procedure. When the severity of some individual lesions is unclear based on prior stress testing and angiography, special guidewires can be used to measure their physiologic severity during maximal coronary flow induced by adenosine infusion.

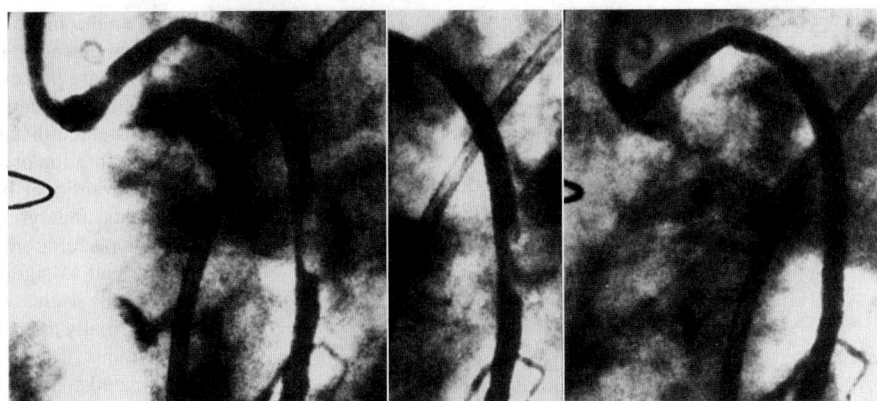

FIGURE 229-3   Stent placement in a diseased saphenous vein graft. *Left*: Severe eccentric stenosis in an 8-year-old saphenous vein graft to the left anterior descending coronary artery. *Middle*: After balloon angioplasty, the lumen remains stenotic due to elastic recoil of the vessel wall and disruption (dissection) of the plaque. *Right*: After placement of a coronary stent, both recoil and dissection have been overcome, providing a large smooth lumen.

NONBALLOON TECHNIQUES

While conventional balloon angioplasty (PTCA) offered anatomic versatility and acceptable short- and long-term results, it was limited when used to approach certain anatomic lesion types (e.g., calcified eccentric, ostial, thrombus-containing, or bifurcation lesions). It was also plagued by the problems of intimal dissection (which led to abrupt closure of the dilated segment in 3% of cases, requiring emergency bypass surgery) and restenosis of 30 to 40% of the dilated segments within 6 months of initially successful treatment. These problems motivated the development of a number of newer, nonballoon techniques that entered routine clinical practice during the early 1990s. These include atherectomy and stent placement, the latter of which now dominates current PCR (see below). In parallel, improvements in adjunctive pharmacotherapy (especially thienopyridines and platelet glycoprotein IIb/IIIa receptor blockers) has helped produce significant improvements in the success, safety, and long-term results. While most newer PCR procedures have higher in-hospital cost than conventional balloon angioplasty, much of this incremental cost can be recouped by the reduction in acute complications and the treatment of subsequent restenosis.

STENTS   These are metallic scaffolds that are inserted into a diseased vessel segment in their collapsed form and are then deployed by balloon inflation or self-expansion (after removal of an external constraining membrane) (Fig. 229-4). They overcome two of the principal limitations of balloon dilatation—local dissection of the plaque and the tendency for elastic recoil of the vessel wall—allowing stents consistently to establish a normal-appearing vessel lumen. Since 1994, when the first two balloon-expandable stent designs were approved by the U.S. Food and Drug Administration (FDA), a number of second- and third-generation stent designs have been developed that offer easier delivery of a wider variety of sizes and lengths, into tortuous or distal lesions. Other refinements in stent design include optional membranous coverings (to seal aneurysms or perforations) and drug-eluting coatings (to suppress stent thrombosis and in-stent proliferation).

In the early experience, metallic stents proved prone to thrombotic occlusion, either acute (<24 h) or subacute (1 to 14 days with a peak at 6 days), requiring an aggressive anticoagulation regimen (aspirin, dipyridamole, and warfarin) to reduce such thromboses to ~3%. This aggressive anticoagulant regimen prolonged hospitalization and increased the incidence of local vascular complications at the femoral arterial entry site. Many of these thrombotic complications were the result of incomplete stent expansion, and greater attention to full initial deployment allowed even more favorable thrombosis rates (<1%), with only antiplatelet drugs (aspirin plus the platelet ADP-receptor blockers, ticlopidine or clopidogrel). This rapid evolution in devices, concomitant medications, and indications has led to the dominance of stent placement in catheter-based coronary revascularization, with placement of one or more stents in 85% of all procedures.

In addition to controlling complications related to abrupt vessel closure, the fact that stenting provides a large acute luminal area compared to PTCA alone has reduced the incidence of subsequent restenosis (e.g., angiographic restenosis rates of 20% versus 33%, and clinical restenosis rates of 10% versus 16 to 20%). When in-stent restenosis does occur, it is the consequence of excessive neointimal hyperplasia within the stent (Fig. 229-5). This can be treated by balloon dilatation, followed by catheter-delivered local β or γ radiation to suppress subsequent neointimal regrowth. Since such radiation treatment also inhibits endothelialization, placement of new stents at the time of radiation should be avoided or they should be protected by prolonging antiplatelet therapy to 9 to 12 months. More recent research has demonstrated that stents can be coated to elute antiproliferative agents such as rapamycin or taxol that inhibit excessive proliferation. Local release of these agents has further decreased angiographic restenosis rates (to <10%) and clinical restenosis rates (to roughly 5%)—benefits that have broadened the use of stents and PCR following their release in early 2003.

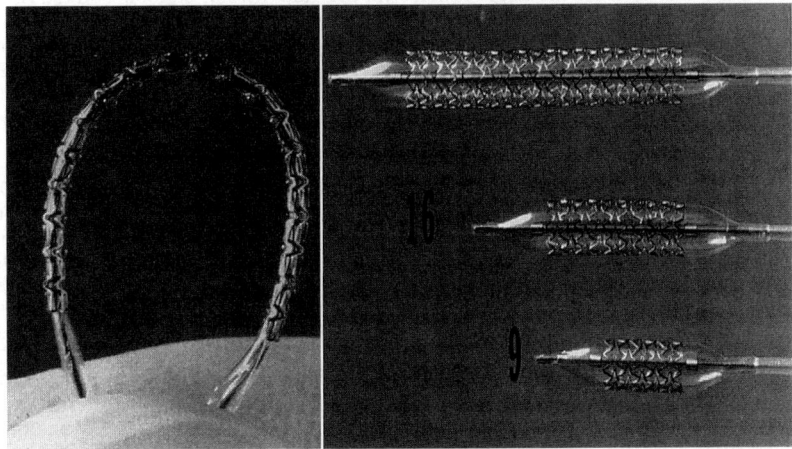

FIGURE 229-4   Second-generation stent. *Left*: The flexibility typical of second-generation stents is shown in bending the collapsed stent on its delivery balloon. *Right*: The same stent design is shown in its balloon-expanded configuration, in some of the available lengths [32 mm (*top*), 16 mm, and 9 mm]. The availability of a variety of second-generation stents since 1997 has helped make stent placement a part of more than 85% of all PCRs.

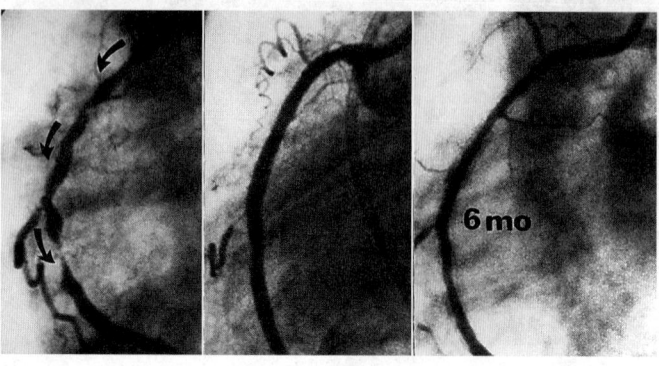

FIGURE 229-5 Short- and long-term results in a long lesion in the right coronary artery. *Left:* A long (~50 mm) area of disease (*arrows*) is present in the right coronary artery. *Middle:* Contrast injection after placement of two long second-generation stents (25 and 35 mm long) shows excellent patency throughout the proximal- and mid-portions of the vessel. *Right:* Follow-up angiogram 6 months after stent placement shows mild lumen reduction throughout the stented segment due to neointimal hyperplasia within the stent (note the separation between the stent shadows and the contrast-filled lumen). Mild degrees of proliferative narrowing are benign and common within stents (particularly long stents such as this one). Had the degree of lumen reduction been greater and associated with recurrent symptoms or an abnormal exercise test, however, re-intervention would have been performed, possibly followed by local radiation delivery (brachytherapy) to inhibit excessive subsequent tissue regrowth. Use of a drug-eluting stent would have virtually eliminated this in-stent neointimal hyperplasia.

ATHERECTOMY Whereas both balloon angioplasty and stent placement enlarge the coronary lumen by displacing plaque, atherectomy catheters enlarge the lumen by removing plaque mass from the treated lesion. Several mechanical atherectomy devices were developed in the 1990s, including directional, rotational, extraction, and laser atherectomy. Although each has certain applications, the greater technical difficulty and procedural complication profile of atherectomy compared to stenting has relegated these devices to niche roles in current PCR. Suction thrombectomy devices may be useful when large intracoronary thrombi are present (e.g., acute MI), and embolic protection devices (distal filters or occlusion/aspiration devices) may be useful adjuncts during the treatment of saphenous vein graft or other lesions prone to the liberation of debris that may compromise the distal myocardial microcirculation.

RESULTS

The success rate for PCR—defined as leaving a residual diameter stenosis <50% (<30% when a stent has been used), without producing an associated complication—now exceeds 97%. Failures may result from inability to cross the target lesion with the guidewire or balloon catheter, particularly when that target lesion is a chronic total occlusion, or failure to dilate a rigid calcified stenosis (now treated by rotational atherectomy). Before the advent of stents, some local dissection was present in virtually all successful balloon dilatation procedures, and more extensive dissection led to abrupt closure of the dilated segment soon after withdrawal of the balloon catheter, necessitating emergency bypass surgery in approximately 3% of cases. In the stent era, however, the incidence of emergency bypass surgery is now <0.3%. The main remaining hazards of PCR are thrombosis and vessel perforation, each of which is well below 1%.

Since PCR causes local endothelial injury and leaves metallic foreign bodies (stents) in the vessel lumen, platelet activation and thrombosis are expected potential complications. All PCRs are thus performed under systemic anticoagulation (heparin, 7000 to 10,000 units, or a direct-acting thrombin inhibitor), to maintain an activated clotting time of 250 to 300, and antiplatelet therapy (aspirin, 325 mg/d starting at least 24 h before PCR and continued for at least 3 to 6 months after the procedure). If a coronary stent has been placed, aspirin is supplemented by a blocker of the platelet ADP receptor, clopidogrel, to reduce the likelihood of stent thrombosis. Intravenous antiplatelet agents (blockers of the platelet glycoprotein IIb/IIIa receptors) may reduce

further the incidence of ischemic complications (especially postprocedural elevation of cardiac enzymes). They are used prophylactically in what are perceived to be high-risk interventions or provisionally in interventions that have left behind an imperfect mechanical result (e.g., a nonstented distal dissection).

Perforation of a coronary artery was an extremely rare complication of conventional balloon angioplasty but may occur in up to 1% of patients undergoing more aggressive atherectomy procedures. Even small perforations of the distal vessel by the angioplasty guidewire may lead to significant hemopericardium requiring urgent pericardiocentesis in the setting of intense anticoagulant and antiplatelet therapy. Finally, catheter-based interventions are subject to all of the complications of diagnostic catheterization, including adverse reactions to iodinated contrast agents and groin hematoma. For most patients, however, catheter-based coronary revascularization offers a safe and effective alternative to surgical revascularization.

FOLLOW-UP

After successful PCR of all "culprit" lesions, marked improvement or complete resolution of the presenting ischemic syndrome should be evident. In approximately 20% of patients, however, evidence of recurrent ischemia develops within 6 months, reflecting restenosis of the dilated segment in response to the local injury of PCR. When recurrent ischemia develops later than 6 months after PCR, it tends to reflect progression of disease at another site, rather than restenosis of a previous treatment site. Whether due to restenosis or disease progression, most post-PCR ischemia can be treated by repeat PCR, so that only about 10% of patients require bypass surgery during the 5 years after a successful procedure. Since all post-PCR patients have provided evidence of severe obstructive coronary atherosclerosis requiring revascularization, an aggressive program to reduce atherosclerotic risk factors and thereby slow the pace of development of new lesions should be part of any post-PCR regimen. This should include control of hypertension, hyperlipidemia, and smoking cessation (Chap. 226).

SUMMARY

Over the past 25 years, the development of new techniques (such as stent placement), new drug regimens, and refinements in practice driven by "evidence-based" medicine, catheter-based revascularization (PCR) has developed from a procedural curiosity to what is now the dominant form of coronary revascularization. As short- and long-term results have improved and the number of procedures has continued to grow, the pace of development continues to accelerate.

FURTHER READING

BAIM DS: Coronary angioplasty, in *Cardiac Catheterization, Angiography and Intervention*, 6th ed, D Baim, W Grossman (eds). Philadelphia, Lippincott Williams & Wilkins, 2000

BERGER PB et al: Survival following coronary angioplasty versus coronary artery bypass in anatomic subsets in which coronary artery bypass improves survival compared with medical therapy—results from the Bypass Angioplasty Revascularization Investigation (BARI). J Am Coll Cardiol 38:1440, 2001

BROWN DL et al: Meta-analysis of effectiveness and safety of abciximab versus eptifibatide or tirofiban in percutaneous coronary intervention. Am J Cardiol 87:537, 2001

CUTLIP DE et al: Stent thrombosis in the modern era—a pooled analysis of multicenter stent clinical trials. Circulation 103:1967, 2001

DE FEYTER PJ et al: Bypass surgery versus stenting for the treatment of multivessel disease in patients with unstable angina compared with stable angina. Circulation 105:2367, 2002

LEON MD et al: Localized intracoronary gamma radiation therapy to inhibit the recurrence of restenosis after stenting. N Engl J Med 344:250, 2001

MORRICE MC et al: A randomized comparison of a sirolimus-eluting stent with a standard stent for coronary revascularization. N Engl J Med 346: 1773, 2002

SMITH SC et al: ACC/AHA guidelines of percutaneous coronary interventions. J Am Coll Cardiol 37:2215, 2001

VAN DE WERF F et al: Reperfusion for ST-elevation myocardial infarction—an overview of current treatment options. Circulation 105:2813, 2002

An elevated arterial pressure is probably the most important public health problem in developed countries. It is common, asymptomatic, readily detectable, usually easily treatable, and often leads to lethal complications if left untreated. As a result of extensive educational programs in the late 1960s and 1970s by both private and government agencies, the number of undiagnosed and/or untreated patients was reduced significantly by the late 1980s to a level of ~25%, with a concomitant decline in cardiovascular mortality. Unfortunately, by the mid-1990s, this beneficial trend began to wane. The number of undiagnosed patients with hypertension increased to nearly 33%, the decline in cardiovascular mortality flattened, and the number of individuals with chronic diseases with untreated or poorly treated hypertension increased. For example, the prevalence of end-stage renal disease per million population increased from <100 in 1982 to >250 in 1995, and the prevalence of congestive heart failure from ages 55 to 75 more than doubled between 1976 to 1980 and 1988 to 1991. Thus, although our understanding of the pathophysiology of elevated arterial pressure has increased, in 90 to 95% of cases the etiology (and thus potentially the means of prevention or cure) is still largely unknown. As a consequence, in most cases the hypertension is treated nonspecifically, resulting in a large number of minor side effects and a relatively high (50 to 60%) noncompliance rate.

PREVALENCE The prevalence of hypertension depends on both the racial composition of the population studied and the criteria used to define the condition. In a white suburban population like that in the Framingham Study, nearly one-fifth of individuals have blood pressures >160/95 mmHg, while almost one-half have pressures >140/90 mmHg. An even higher prevalence has been documented in the nonwhite population. In females the prevalence is closely related to age, with a substantial increase occurring after age 50. This increase is presumably related to the hormonal changes of menopause, although the mechanism is unclear. Thus, the ratio of hypertension frequency in women versus men increases from 0.6 to 0.7 at age 30 to 1.1 to 1.2 at age 65.

The prevalence of various forms of secondary hypertension depends on the nature of the population studied and on how extensive the evaluation is. There are no available data to define the frequency of secondary hypertension in the general population, although in middle-aged males it has been reported to be 6%. On the other hand, in referral centers where patients undergo an extensive evaluation, it has been reported to be as high as 35%. The various forms of hypertension are outlined in Table 230-1, and their relative frequencies are given in Table 230-2.

ESSENTIAL HYPERTENSION

Patients with arterial pressure and no definable cause are said to have *primary*, *essential*, or *idiopathic hypertension*. Undoubtedly, the primary difficulty in uncovering the responsible mechanisms in these patients is attributable to the variety of systems that are involved in the regulation of arterial pressure: peripheral and/or central adrenergic, renal, hormonal, and vascular. In addition, these systems are interrelated in a complex fashion, with input from multiple genes (see below). Several abnormalities have been described in patients with essential hypertension, often with a claim that one or more of them are primarily responsible for the hypertension. While it is still uncertain whether these individual abnormalities are primary or secondary, varying expressions of a single disease process, or reflective of separate disease entities, the accumulating data increasingly support the latter hypothesis. Therefore, just as pneumonia is caused by a variety of infectious agents, even though the clinical picture observed may be similar, so essential hypertension likely has a number of distinct causes. Thus, the distinction between primary and secondary hypertension has become blurred, and the approach to both the diagnosis and therapy of

hypertensive patients has been modified. For example, when a group of patients with essential hypertension is separated into a distinct subset (e.g., low-renin essential hypertension), the patients have not been reclassified as having a form of secondary hypertension but rather remain in the essential hypertensive group. In this chapter, individuals in whom a specific structural organ or gene defect is responsible for hypertension are defined as having a *secondary* form of hypertension. In contrast, individuals in whom generalized or functional abnormalities may be the cause of hypertension, even if the abnormalities are discrete, are defined as having *essential* hypertension.

ENVIRONMENT A number of environmental factors have been implicated in the development of hypertension, including salt intake, obesity, occupation, alcohol intake, family size, and crowding. These factors have all been assumed to be important in the increase in blood pressure with age in more affluent societies, in contrast to the decline in blood pressure with age in less affluent groups.

SALT SENSITIVITY The environmental factor that has received the greatest attention is salt intake. Even this factor illustrates the heterogeneous nature of the essential hypertensive population, in that the blood pressure is particularly responsive to the level of sodium intake in only ~60% of hypertensives. The cause of this special sensitivity to salt

---

TABLE 230-1 *Classification of Arterial Hypertension*

SYSTOLIC HYPERTENSION WITH WIDE PULSE PRESSURE

  I. Decreased compliance of aorta (arteriosclerosis)
 II. Increased stroke volume
    A. Aortic regurgitation
    B. Thyrotoxicosis
    C. Hyperkinetic heart syndrome
    D. Fever
    E. Arteriovenous fistula
    F. Patent ductus arteriosus

SYSTOLIC AND DIASTOLIC HYPERTENSION (INCREASED PERIPHERAL VASCULAR RESISTANCE)

  I. Renal
    A. Chronic pyelonephritis
    B. Acute and chronic glomerulonephritis
    C. Polycystic renal disease
    D. Renovascular stenosis or renal infarction
    E. Most other severe renal diseases (arteriolar nephrosclerosis, diabetic nephropathy, etc.)
    F. Renin-producing tumors
 II. Endocrine
    A. Oral contraceptives
    B. Adrenocortical hyperfunction
       1. Cushing's disease and syndrome
       2. Primary hyperaldosteronism
       3. Congenital or hereditary adrenogenital syndromes (17α-hydroxylase and 11β-hydroxylase defects)
    C. Pheochromocytoma
    D. Myxedema
    E. Acromegaly
III. Neurogenic
    A. Psychogenic
    B. Diencephalic syndrome
    C. Familial dysautonomia (Riley-Day)
    D. Polyneuritis (acute porphyria, lead poisoning)
    E. Increased intracranial pressure (acute)
    F. Spinal cord section (acute)
IV. Miscellaneous
    A. Coarctation of aorta
    B. Increased intravascular volume (excessive transfusion, polycythemia vera)
    C. Polyarteritis nodosa
    D. Hypercalcemia
    E. Medications, e.g., glucocorticoids, cyclosporine
  V. Unknown etiology
    A. Essential hypertension (>90% of all cases of hypertension)
    B. Toxemia of pregnancy
    C. Acute intermittent porphyria

TABLE 230-2 *Prevalence of Various Forms of Hypertension in the General Population and in Specialized Referral Clinics[a]*

Diagnosis	General Population, %	Specialty Clinic, %
Essential hypertension	92–94	65–85
Renal hypertension:		
Parenchymal	2–3	4–5
Renovascular	1–2	4–16
Endocrine hypertension:		
Primary aldosteronism	0.3	0.5–12
Cushing's syndrome	<0.1	0.2
Pheochromocytoma	<0.1	0.2
Oral contraceptive–induced	0.5–1	1–2
Miscellaneous	0.2	1

[a] Estimates based on a number of reports in the literature.

varies, with primary aldosteronism, bilateral renal artery stenosis, renal parenchymal disease, and low-renin essential hypertension accounting for about half the patients. In the remainder, the pathophysiology is still uncertain, but postulated contributing factors include chloride intake, calcium intake, a generalized cellular membrane defect, insulin resistance, and "nonmodulation" (see below).

ROLE OF RENIN Renin is an enzyme secreted by the juxtaglomerular cells of the kidney and linked with aldosterone in a negative feedback loop (Chap. 321). While a variety of factors can modify its rate of secretion, the primary determinant is the volume status of the individual, particularly as related to changes in dietary sodium intake. The end product of the action of renin on its substrate is the generation of the peptide angiotensin II. The response of target tissues to this peptide is uniquely determined by the prior dietary electrolyte intake. For example, sodium intake normally modulates adrenal and renal vascular responses to angiotensin II. With sodium restriction, adrenal responses are enhanced and the renal vascular responses reduced. Sodium loading has the opposite effect. The range of plasma renin activities observed in hypertensive subjects is broader than in normotensive individuals. In consequence, some hypertensive patients have been defined as having *low-renin* and others as having *high-renin* essential hypertension.

Low-Renin Essential Hypertension Approximately 20% of patients who by all other criteria have essential hypertension have suppressed plasma renin activity. Low-renin essential hypertension describes a widely recognized classification validated by clinical features, including salt-sensitivity of blood pressure and diuretic responsiveness. This situation is more common in individuals of African descent than in white patients, and in diabetics and the elderly. Though these patients are not hypokalemic, they have been reported to have expanded extracellular fluid volumes, and one unproven suggestion is that they have sodium retention and renin suppression due to excessive production of an unidentified mineralocorticoid. There are data to suggest that the low-renin state confers a beneficial natural history compared to that in patients with normal- or high-renin hypertension.

Nonmodulating Essential Hypertension Another subset of hypertensive patients who are also salt-sensitive has a reduced adrenal response to sodium restriction. In these individuals, sodium intake does not modulate either adrenal or renal vascular responses to angiotensin II. Hypertensives in this subset have been termed *nonmodulators* because of the absence of the sodium-mediated modulation of target tissue responses to angiotensin II. These individuals make up 25 to 30% of the hypertensive population, have plasma renin activity levels that are normal to high if measured when the patient is on a low-salt diet, and have hypertension that is salt-sensitive because of a defect in the kidney's ability to excrete sodium appropriately. They also are more insulin-resistant than other hypertensive patients, and the pathophysiologic characteristics can be corrected by the administration of an angiotensin-converting enzyme (ACE) inhibitor. Nonmodulation is much more frequent among males and postmenopausal females. Furthermore, the nonmodulation characteristic appears to be genetically determined (associated with a certain allele of the angiotensinogen gene). Thus, nonmodulators are probably the most completely characterized intermediate phenotype in the hypertensive population.

High-Renin Essential Hypertension Approximately 15% of patients with essential hypertension have plasma renin activity levels above the normal range. It has been suggested that plasma renin plays an important role in the pathogenesis of the elevated arterial pressure in these patients. However, most studies have found that saralasin (a substance that, like losartan, acts as a competitive antagonist of angiotensin II) significantly reduces blood pressure in fewer than half of these patients. This finding has led some investigators to postulate that the elevated renin levels and blood pressure may both be secondary to an increase in adrenergic system activity. It has been proposed that in patients with angiotensin-dependent high-renin hypertension whose arterial pressures are lowered by an angiotensin II antagonist, the mechanism responsible for the increase in renin and, therefore, for the hypertension is the nonmodulating defect.

SODIUM ION VERSUS CHLORIDE OR CALCIUM Most studies assessing the role of salt in the hypertensive process have assumed that it is the sodium ion that is important. However, some investigators have suggested that the chloride ion may be equally important. This suggestion is based on the observation that feeding chloride-free sodium salts to salt-sensitive hypertensive animals fails to increase arterial pressure. Calcium has also been implicated in the pathogenesis of some forms of essential hypertension. A low-calcium intake has been associated with an increase in blood pressure in epidemiologic studies; an increase in leukocyte cytosolic calcium levels has been reported in some hypertensives. Finally, calcium entry blockers are effective antihypertensive agents. Several studies have reported a potential link between the salt-sensitive forms of hypertension and calcium. It has been postulated that salt loading in combination with a defect in the kidney's ability to excrete salt may lead to a secondary increase in circulating natriuretic factors. One of these factors, the so-called digitalis-like natriuretic factor, inhibits ouabain-sensitive Na^+,K^+-ATPase and thereby leads to intracellular calcium accumulation and a hyperreactive vascular smooth muscle.

CELL MEMBRANE DEFECT Another postulated explanation for salt-sensitive hypertension is a generalized cell membrane defect. This hypothesis derives most of its data from studies on circulating blood elements, particularly red blood cells, in which abnormalities in the transport of sodium across the cell membrane have been documented. Since both increases and decreases in the activity of different transport systems have been reported, it is likely that some abnormalities are primary and some are secondary. It has been assumed that an abnormality in sodium transport reflects an undefined alteration in the cell membrane and that this defect occurs in many, perhaps all, cells of the body, particularly the vascular smooth-muscle cells. The defect leads to an abnormal accumulation of calcium in vascular smooth muscle, resulting in a heightened vascular responsiveness to vasoconstrictor agents. This defect has been proposed to be present in 35 to 50% of essential hypertensive persons on the basis of studies using red cells. Other studies suggest that the abnormality in red cell sodium transport is not fixed but can be modified by environmental factors.

The common final pathway in all these hypotheses is an increase in cytosolic calcium resulting in increased vascular reactivity. However, as described above, several mechanisms might produce this calcium accumulation.

INSULIN RESISTANCE Insulin resistance and/or hyperinsulinemia have been suggested as being responsible for the increased arterial pressure in some patients with hypertension. This feature is now widely recognized as part of syndrome X, or the metabolic syndrome (Chap. 225), marked also by central obesity, dyslipidemia (especially elevated triglycerides), and high blood pressure. While it is clear that a substantial fraction of the hypertensive population has insulin resistance and hyperinsulinemia, it is less certain that this is more than an association. Insulin resistance is common in patients with diabetes mellitus type 2 and in obesity; both of these conditions are more common in hypertensive than in normotensive subjects. However, several studies have found that hyperinsulinemia and insulin resistance are present even in lean hypertensive patients without type 2 diabetes, suggesting that this relationship is more than a coincidence. As noted earlier, these individuals seem to be concentrated in the nonmodulation phenotype.

Hyperinsulinemia can increase arterial pressure by one or more of four mechanisms. An underlying assumption in each case is that some, but not all, of the target tissues of insulin are resistant to its effects. Specifically, tissues involved in glucose homeostasis are resistant (thereby producing the hyperinsulinemia), while tissues involved in the hypertensive process are not. First, hyperinsulinemia produces renal sodium retention (at least acutely) and increases sympathetic activity. Either or both of these effects could lead to an increase in arterial pressure. Another mechanism is vascular smooth-muscle hypertrophy secondary to the mitogenic action of insulin. Third, insulin also modifies ion transport across the cell membrane, thereby potentially increasing the cytosolic calcium levels of insulin-sensitive vascular or renal tissues. This mechanism would increase arterial pressure for reasons similar to those described above for the membrane-defect hypothesis. Finally, insulin resistance may be a marker for another pathologic process, e.g., nonmodulation, which could be the primary mechanism increasing blood pressure. It is important to point out, however, that the role of insulin in controlling arterial pressure is only vaguely understood, and, therefore, its potential as a pathogenic factor in hypertension remains unclear.

Few of the features of hypertension discussed above remain constant in a given patient. Some may be a reflection of the current metabolic and hormonal status of the patient rather than a permanent feature of the disease process. For example, at one point a patient might have insulin resistance secondary to obesity, which could lead to sodium retention, intravascular volume expansion, and renin suppression. This patient would be labeled as having "low-renin essential hypertension." If the patient lost weight, however, the salt-retaining tendency would be reversed. If the blood pressure did not normalize, the patient might then have "normal- or high-renin essential hypertension." Thus, the features reviewed above should not be considered mutually exclusive or permanent characteristics in a given patient with hypertension.

GENETIC CONSIDERATIONS Hypertension is one of the most common complex genetic disorders, with genetic heritability averaging ~30%. Data supporting this view emerge from animal studies as well as in population studies in humans. One approach has been to assess the correlation of blood pressure in families (familial aggregation). From these studies, the minimum size of the genetic factor can be expressed by a correlation coefficient of ~0.2. However, the variation in the size of the genetic factor in different studies reemphasizes the probably heterogeneous nature of the essential hypertensive population. In addition, most studies support the concept that the inheritance is probably multifactorial or that a number of different genetic defects each have an elevated blood pressure as one of their phenotypic expressions.

However, genes responsible for three distinct but rare monogenic hypertensive syndromes have been identified, two of which are inherited in a dominant fashion. Patients with *glucocorticoid-remediable hypertension* (GRA) have characteristically early-onset hypertension with increased frequency of strokes and evidence of hyperaldosteronism. Plasma aldosterone concentrates are high, plasma renin activity is low, and hypokalemia is frequent. A chimeric gene containing the promoter of the 11β-hydroxylase gene and the coding sequence for the aldosterone synthase gene has been identified in these patients, resulting in the ectopic production of aldosterone, which is corticotropin-dependent. The second dominant form is also a rare familial syndrome in which patients also *appear* to have elevated aldosterone

activity, with suppressed plasma renin activity and hypokalemia. In these patients, however, plasma aldosterone is normal. Mutations in the epithelial amiloride-sensitive sodium channel located in the collecting cortical tubule are responsible. The third monogenic syndrome is also a low-renin state, termed the *syndrome of apparent mineralocorticoid excess* (AME), caused by a defect in renal 11β-hydroxysteroid dehydrogenase. In these patients, the protective conversion of cortisol to the inactive cortisone does not occur, and local cortisol binds to the renal mineralocorticoid receptor.

In addition to these monogenic syndromes, susceptibility genes have now been reported which have as one of their consequences an increased arterial pressure (see below and Chap. 321). The most promising of these is the gene for renin substrate, angiotensinogen, in which a substitution of threonine for methionine at codon 235 has been associated with hypertension. Also, in patients with low-renin essential hypertension, an association with the G460W polymorphism of the α-adducin gene has been demonstrated. One of the hints of the genetic heritability of the low-renin state has emerged from studies revealing the familial aggregation of low-renin hypertension.

More than 50 genes have been examined in association studies with hypertension, and the number is constantly growing. As can be seen in Table 230-3, most studies of likely genes have failed to document linkage or consistent association with hypertension. However, uncertainty exists as to the validity of these negative conclusions. A positive relationship between hypertension and a gene could be obscured by the high probability of a false-negative result because of the heterogeneity of the hypertensive population. Thus, intermediate phenotypes in the hypertensive population need to be identified to differentiate patients into more homogeneous subgroups; the role of a specific candidate gene can then be more readily assessed. Such an approach is illustrated in Table 230-4.

TABLE 230-3 Genesis Hypothesized to be Involved in Essential Hypertension

Gene	Linkage +/−	Association +/−
Renin-angiotensin-aldosterone system/sodium-volume		
Angiotensin-converting enzyme	0/1	12/14
Angiotensinogen	3/4	12/9
Aldosterone synthase	1/1	5/7
α-Adducin	0/1	5/3
AT1 receptor		4/6
Atrial natriuretic peptide		2/5
Human natriuretic peptide receptor (A)		1/1
Human natriuretic peptide receptor (B)		1/2
Renin	3/2	2/2
Adrenergic		
β_2-Adrenergic receptor		3/4
β_3-Adrenergic receptor		3/1
Dopamine D$_2$ receptor		2/0
α_2-Adrenergic receptor		1/1
Vascular		
Endothelin-1		3/1
Nitric oxide synthase, endothelial (NOS3)	0/2	5/10
Nitric oxide synthase, inducible (NOS2A)		1/1
Metabolic		
Glycogen synthase		1/1
Insulin receptor	0/1	3/0
Lipoprotein lipase		1/2
Apolipoprotein C-III		1/1
Miscellaneous		
G protein β_3 subunit		3/5

[a] Number of pertinent positive (+) and negative (−) published studies in humans.

TABLE 230-4 *Role of Intermediate Phenotypes in Genetic Analysis*

Gene	Phenotype	
	Intermediate	*Distant*
Converting enzyme ⎫	Angiotensin II effect	Increases BP
Angiotensinogen ⎭	on kidney	Increases BP
Aldo synthase	Increases 18-OH cortisol	Increases BP
Kallikrein	Decreases urine kallikrein	Increases BP
Na^+/H^+ exchanger	Increases Na/Li CTT	Increases BP
α-adducin	Low-renin hypertension	Increases BP
11 HSD_2	↑Cortisol/cortisone	Increases BP
ENaC	↓Renin, ↓aldosterone, ↓K^+	Increases BP

Note: BP, blood pressure; OH, hydroxy; CTT, countertransport; HSD, hydroxy steroid-dehydrogenase; eNac, epithelial sodium channel.

FACTORS THAT MODIFY THE COURSE OF ESSENTIAL HYPERTENSION Age, race, sex, smoking, alcohol intake, serum cholesterol, glucose intolerance, and weight all may alter the prognosis of this disease. The younger the patient when hypertension is first noted, the greater is the reduction in life expectancy if the hypertension is left untreated. In the United States, urban blacks have about twice the prevalence of hypertension as whites and more than four times the hypertension-induced morbidity rate. At all ages and in both white and nonwhite populations, females with hypertension fare better than males up to the age of 65, and the prevalence of hypertension in premenopausal females is substantially less than that in age-matched males or postmenopausal women. Yet, compared with their normotensive counterparts, females with hypertension run the same relative risk of a morbid cardiovascular event as do males. Accelerated atherosclerosis is an invariable companion of hypertension. Thus, it is not surprising that independent risk factors associated with the development of atherosclerosis, such as an elevated serum cholesterol, glucose intolerance, and/or cigarette smoking, significantly enhance the effect of hypertension on mortality rate regardless of age, sex, or race (Chap. 224). There is also no question that a positive correlation exists between obesity and arterial pressure. A gain in weight is associated with an increased frequency of hypertension in persons with previously normal blood pressure, and weight loss in obese persons with hypertension lowers their arterial pressure and, if they are being treated for hypertension, the intensity of therapy required to keep them normotensive. Whether these changes are mediated by changes in insulin resistance is unknown.

NATURAL HISTORY Because essential hypertension is a heterogeneous disorder, variables other than the arterial pressure modify its course. Thus, the probability of developing a morbid cardiovascular event with a given arterial pressure may vary as much as 20-fold depending on whether associated risk factors are present (Table 230-5). Although exceptions have been reported, most untreated adults with hypertension will develop further increases in arterial pressure with time. Furthermore, it has been demonstrated from both actuarial data and experience in the era prior to effective therapy that untreated hypertension is associated with a shortening of life by 10 to 20 years, usually related to an acceleration of the atherosclerotic process, with the rate of acceleration in part related to the severity of the hypertension. Even individuals who have relatively mild disease—i.e., without evidence of end-organ damage—that is left untreated for 7 to 10 years have a high risk of developing significant complications. Nearly 30% will exhibit atherosclerotic complications, and >50% will have end-organ damage related to the hypertension itself, such as cardiomegaly, congestive heart failure, retinopathy, a cerebrovascular accident, and/or renal insufficiency. Thus, even in its mild forms, hypertension is a progressive and lethal disease if left untreated.

SECONDARY HYPERTENSION

As noted earlier, in only a small minority of patients with elevated arterial pressure can a specific cause be identified. Yet these patients should not be ignored for at least two reasons: (1) correction of the

TABLE 230-5 *Risk Factors for An Adverse Prognosis in Hypertension*

Black race
Youth
Male sex
Persistent diastolic pressure >115 mmHg
Smoking
Diabetes mellitus
Hypercholesterolemia
Obesity
Excess alcohol intake
Evidence of end organ damage
1. Cardiac
   a. Cardiac enlargement
   b. Electrocardiographic signs of ischemia or left ventricular strain
   c. Myocardial infarction
   d. Congestive heart failure
2. Eyes
   a. Retinal exudates and hemorrhages
   b. Papilledema
3. Renal: impaired renal function
4. Nervous system: cerebrovascular accident

cause may cure their hypertension, and (2) these secondary forms of the disease may provide insight into the etiology of essential hypertension. Nearly all the secondary forms of hypertension are related to an alteration in hormone secretion and/or renal function and are discussed in detail in other chapters.

RENAL HYPERTENSION (See also Chap. 267) Hypertension produced by renal disease is the result of either (1) an alteration in renal secretion of vasoactive materials resulting in a systemic or local change in arteriolar tone, or (2) a derangement in the renal handling of sodium and fluids leading to volume expansion. The main subdivisions of renal hypertension are renovascular hypertension, including preeclampsia and eclampsia, and renal parenchymal hypertension. A simple explanation for *renal vascular hypertension* is that decreased perfusion of renal tissue due to stenosis of a main or branch renal artery activates the renin-angiotensin system, described in Chap. 321. Circulating angiotensin II elevates arterial pressure by directly causing vasoconstriction, by stimulating aldosterone secretion with resulting sodium retention, and/or by stimulating the adrenergic nervous system. In practice, only about one-half of patients with renovascular hypertension have an absolute elevation in renin activity in peripheral plasma, although when renin measurements are referenced against an index of sodium balance, a much higher fraction have inappropriately high values.

Activation of the renin-angiotensin system has also been offered as an explanation for the hypertension in both acute and chronic *renal parenchymal disease*. In this formulation, the only difference between renovascular and renal parenchymal hypertension is that the decreased perfusion of renal tissue in the latter case results from inflammatory and fibrotic changes involving multiple small intrarenal vessels. There are enough differences between the two conditions, however, to suggest that other mechanisms are active in renal parenchymal disease. Specifically, (1) peripheral plasma renin activity is elevated far less frequently in renal parenchymal than in renovascular hypertension; (2) cardiac output is said to be normal in renal parenchymal hypertension (unless uremia and anemia are present) but slightly elevated in renovascular hypertension; (3) circulatory responses to tilting and to the Valsalva maneuver are exaggerated in the latter condition; and (4) blood volume tends to be high in patients with severe renal parenchymal disease and low in patients with severe unilateral renovascular hypertension. Alternative explanations for the hypertension in renal parenchymal disease include the possibilities that the damaged kidneys (1) produce an unidentified vasopressor substance other than renin, (2) fail to produce a necessary humoral vasodilator substance (perhaps prostaglandin or bradykinin), (3) fail to inactivate circulating vasopressor substances, and/or (4) are ineffective in disposing of sodium. In the last case, the retained sodium would be responsible for the hypertension as outlined earlier.

Although all of these explanations, including participation of the renin-angiotensin system, probably have some validity in individual patients, the hypothesis involving sodium retention is particularly attractive. It is supported by the observation that those patients with chronic pyelonephritis or polycystic renal disease who are salt wasters do not develop hypertension and by the observation that removal of salt and water by dialysis or diuretics is effective in controlling arterial pressure in most patients with renal parenchymal disease.

A rare form of renal hypertension results from the excess secretion of renin by juxtaglomerular cell tumors or nephroblastomas. The initial presentation is similar to that of hyperaldosteronism, with hypertension, hypokalemia, and overproduction of aldosterone. However, in contrast to primary aldosteronism, peripheral renin activity is *elevated instead of subnormal*. This disease can be distinguished from other forms of secondary aldosteronism by the presence of normal renal function and unilateral increases in renal vein renin concentration without a renal artery lesion.

ENDOCRINE HYPERTENSION ■ **Adrenal Hypertension** Hypertension is a feature of a variety of adrenal cortical abnormalities. In *primary aldosteronism* (Chap. 321), there is a clear relationship between the aldosterone-induced sodium retention and the hypertension. Normal individuals given aldosterone develop hypertension only if they also ingest sodium. Since aldosterone causes sodium retention by stimulating renal tubular exchange of sodium for potassium, hypokalemia is a prominent feature in most patients with primary aldosteronism, and, therefore, the measurement of serum potassium provides a simple screening test. The effect of sodium retention and volume expansion in chronically suppressing plasma renin activity is critical for the definitive diagnosis. In most clinical situations, plasma renin activity and plasma or urinary aldosterone levels parallel each other, but in patients with primary aldosteronism, aldosterone levels are high and relatively fixed because of autonomous aldosterone secretion, whereas plasma renin activity levels are suppressed and respond sluggishly to sodium depletion. Primary aldosteronism may be secondary to either a tumor or bilateral adrenal hyperplasia. It is important to distinguish between these two conditions preoperatively, since the hypertension in the latter case is usually not modified by operation.

The sodium-retaining effect of large amounts of glucocorticoids (perhaps resulting in part from saturation of the 11β-hydroxysteroid hydrogenase enzyme system in the kidney by the increased concentration of cortisol) also offers an explanation for the hypertension in severe cases of Cushing's syndrome (Chap. 321). Moreover, increased production of mineralocorticoids has also been documented in some patients with Cushing's syndrome. However, the hypertension in many cases of Cushing's syndrome does not seem volume-dependent, leading investigators to speculate that it may be secondary to glucocorticoid-induced production of renin substrate (angiotensin-mediated hypertension). In the forms of the adrenogenital syndrome due to C-11 or C-17 hydroxylase deficiency (Chap. 321), deoxycorticosterone accounts for the sodium retention and the resulting hypertension, which is accompanied by suppression of plasma renin activity.

In patients with pheochromocytoma (Chap. 322), increased secretion of epinephrine and norepinephrine by a tumor (most often located in the adrenal medulla) causes excessive stimulation of adrenergic receptors, which results in peripheral vasoconstriction and cardiac stimulation. This diagnosis is confirmed by demonstrating increased urinary excretion of epinephrine and norepinephrine and/or their metabolites.

Acromegaly (See also Chap. 318) Hypertension, coronary atherosclerosis, and cardiac hypertrophy are frequent complications of this condition.

Hypercalcemia (See also Chap. 331) The hypertension that occurs in up to one-third of patients with hyperparathyroidism ordinarily can be attributed to renal parenchymal damage due to nephrolithiasis and nephrocalcinosis. However, increased calcium levels can also have a direct vasoconstrictive effect. In some cases, the hypertension disappears when the hypercalcemia is corrected. Thus, paradoxically, the increased serum calcium level in hyperparathyroidism raises blood pressure, while epidemiologic studies suggest that a high calcium intake lowers blood pressure. To confuse the issue further, calcium entry-blocking agents are effective antihypertensive agents. Additional studies are needed to resolve these seemingly conflicting observations.

COARCTATION OF THE AORTA (See also Chap. 218) The hypertension associated with coarctation may be caused by the constriction itself or perhaps by the changes in the renal circulation, which result in an unusual form of renal arterial hypertension. The diagnosis of coarctation is usually evident from physical examination and routine x-ray findings.

EFFECTS OF HYPERTENSION

Patients with hypertension die prematurely; the most common cause of death is heart disease, with stroke and renal failure also frequent, particularly in patients with significant retinopathy.

EFFECTS ON THE HEART Cardiac compensation for the excessive workload imposed by increased systemic pressure is at first sustained by concentric left ventricular hypertrophy, characterized by an increase in wall thickness. Ultimately, the function of this chamber deteriorates, the cavity dilates, and the symptoms and signs of heart failure appear (Chap. 215). Angina pectoris may also occur because of the combination of accelerated coronary arterial disease and increased myocardial oxygen requirements as a consequence of the increased myocardial mass (Chap. 226). On physical examination, the heart is enlarged and has a prominent left ventricular impulse. The sound of aortic closure is accentuated, and there may be a faint murmur of aortic regurgitation. Presystolic (atrial, fourth) heart sounds appear frequently in hypertensive heart disease, and a protodiastolic (ventricular, third) heart sound or summation gallop rhythm may be present. Electrocardiographic changes of left ventricular hypertrophy (Chap. 210) may occur, but the electrocardiogram substantially underestimates the frequency of cardiac hypertrophy compared with that observed with the echocardiogram. Evidence of ischemia or infarction may be observed late in the disease. Most deaths due to hypertension result from myocardial infarction or congestive heart failure. Recent data suggest that some of the myocardial damage may be mediated by aldosterone in the presence of a normal/high salt intake rather than just the increased blood pressure or an increase in angiotensin II levels per se.

NEUROLOGIC EFFECTS The neurologic effects of long-standing hypertension may be divided into retinal and central nervous system changes. Because the retina is the only tissue in which the arteries and arterioles can be examined directly, repeated ophthalmoscopic examination provides the opportunity to observe the progress of the vascular effects of hypertension. The Keith-Wagener-Barker classification of the *retinal changes* in hypertension has provided a simple and excellent means for serial evaluation of hypertensive patients (see Fig. 25-1).

Central nervous system dysfunction also occurs frequently in patients with hypertension. Occipital headaches, most often occurring in the morning, are among the most prominent early symptoms of hypertension. Dizziness, light-headedness, vertigo, tinnitus, and dimmed vision or syncope may also be observed, but the more serious manifestations are due to vascular occlusion, hemorrhage, or encephalopathy (Chap. 349). The pathogeneses of the former two disorders are quite different. *Cerebral infarction* is secondary to the increased atherosclerosis observed in hypertensive patients, whereas *cerebral hemorrhage* is the result of both the elevated arterial pressure and the development of cerebral vascular microaneurysms (Charcot-Bouchard aneurysms). Only age and arterial pressure are known to influence the development of the microaneurysms. Thus, it is not surprising that arterial pressure shows a better association with cerebral hemorrhage than with either cerebral or myocardial infarction.

Hypertensive encephalopathy (see p. 1480) consists of the following symptom complex: severe hypertension, disordered consciousness, increased intracranial pressure, retinopathy with papilledema, and seizures. The pathogenesis is uncertain but is probably not related to arteriolar spasm or cerebral edema. Focal neurologic signs are infrequent and, if present, suggest that infarction, hemorrhage, or transient ischemic attacks are more likely diagnoses. Although some investigators have suggested that prompt lowering of arterial pressure in these patients may adversely affect cerebral blood flow, most studies indicate that this is not the case.

EFFECTS ON THE KIDNEY (See also Chap. 267) Arteriosclerotic lesions of the afferent and efferent arterioles and the glomerular capillary tufts are the most common renal vascular lesions in hypertension and result in a decreased glomerular filtration rate and tubular dysfunction. Proteinuria and microscopic hematuria occur because of glomerular lesions, and ~10% of the deaths caused by hypertension result from renal failure. Blood loss in hypertension occurs not only from renal lesions; epistaxis, hemoptysis, and metrorrhagia also occur frequently in these patients.

APPROACH TO THE PATIENT

DEFINITION Since there is no dividing line between normal and high blood pressure, arbitrary levels have been established to define persons who have an increased risk of developing a morbid cardiovascular event and/or will benefit from medical therapy. These should be based upon not only the level of diastolic pressure but also systolic pressure, age, sex, race, and concomitant diseases. For example, patients with a diastolic pressure >90 mmHg have a significant reduction in morbidity and mortality rate if they receive adequate therapy. These, then, are patients who have hypertension and who should be considered for treatment.

The level of *systolic* pressure is very important in assessing the influence of arterial pressure on cardiovascular morbidity. Data increasingly suggest that it may be more important than diastolic pressure, especially in those over the age of 50. For example, males with normal diastolic pressures (<82 mmHg) but elevated systolic pressures (>158 mmHg) have a cardiovascular mortality rate 2.5 times higher than individuals who have similar diastolic pressures but whose systolic pressures clearly are normal (<130 mmHg). A reduction in mortality and morbidity with treatment, specifically in the elderly, has been documented in these patients. This beneficial effect results mainly from a reduction in strokes and occurs in women as well. Other significant demographic factors that modify the influence of blood pressure on the frequency of morbid cardiovascular events are age, race, and sex, with young black males being most adversely affected by hypertension.

When hypertension is suspected, blood pressure should be measured at least twice during two separate examinations after the initial screening. In adults, a *diastolic* pressure <85 mmHg is considered to be normal; one between 85 and 89 mmHg is high normal; one of 90 to 99 mmHg represents stage 1 or mild hypertension; one of 100 to 109 mmHg represents stage 2 or moderate hypertension; and one of ≥110 mmHg represents stage 3 or severe hypertension. A systolic pressure <130 mmHg indicates normal blood pressure; one between 130 and 139 mmHg indicates high normal; one between 140 and 159 mmHg indicates stage 1 or mild hypertension; one between 160 and 179 mmHg indicates stage 2 or moderate hypertension; and one ≥180 mmHg indicates stage 3 or severe hypertension. Isolated systolic hypertension, common among the elderly, is defined by systolic pressure <140 mmHg together with a normal diastolic pressure. *White coat hypertension* describes a significant percentage of individuals whose blood pressure, measured in the office by a professional, is persistently higher than when measured at home or under casual circumstances. Current estimates are that 10 to 20% of patients declared hypertensive in their doctors' offices are normotensive outside it; this diagnosis is relatively more common among the elderly and pregnant women.

Increasing use of ambulatory blood pressure monitoring (ABPM) may provide additional useful information in patients who are difficult to classify. These devices measure blood pressure over a 12- or 24-h period as patients perform normal activities and during sleep. However, normal values for this procedure and its usefulness in relation to therapeutic outcomes are not currently known. A useful classification of hypertension derived from the 2003 European Society of Hypertension Guidelines is shown in Table 230-6. Of note, the Seventh US Joint National Committee on Prevention, Detection, Evaluation, and Treatment of High Blood Pressure (JNC 7) published a new classification in 2003 which limited normal blood pressure to <120 mmHg systolic and <80 mmHg diastolic, and added a new category of "prehypertension" defined by systolic pressure between 120 and 139 or diastolic blood pressure between 80 and 89 mm. Prevention strategies are recommended for this population.

Arterial pressure fluctuates in most persons, whether they are normotensive or hypertensive. Patients who are classified as having *labile hypertension* are those who sometimes, but not always, have arterial pressures in the hypertensive range. These patients are often considered to have borderline hypertension. Sustained hypertension can become accelerated or enter a malignant phase (p. 1480), although that is unusual in treated patients. *Accelerated hypertension* is defined as a significant recent increase over previous hypertensive levels associated with evidence of vascular damage on funduscopic examination but without papilledema.

PATIENT EVALUATION In evaluating patients with hypertension, the initial history, physical examination, and laboratory tests should be directed at (1) uncovering correctable secondary forms of hypertension (see below), (2) establishing a pretreatment baseline, (3) assessing factors that may influence the type of therapy or be changed adversely by therapy, (4) determining if target organ damage is present, and (5) determining whether other risk factors for the development of arteriosclerotic cardiovascular disease are present (Table 230-5).

Symptoms and Signs Most patients with hypertension have no specific symptoms referable to their blood pressure elevation and are identified only in the course of a physical examination. When symptoms do bring the patient to the physician, they fall into three categories. They are related to (1) the elevated pressure itself, (2) the hypertensive vascular disease, and (3) the underlying disease, in the case of secondary hypertension. Though popularly considered a symptom of elevated arterial pressure, headache is characteristic of only severe hypertension; most commonly such headaches are localized to the occipital region and are present when the patient awakens in the morning but subside spontaneously after several hours. Other complaints that may be related to elevated blood pressure include dizziness, palpitations, easy fatigability, and

---

TABLE 230-6 *Classification of Blood Pressure for Adults ≥18 Years Old*

Category	Systolic Pressure, mmHg	Diastolic Pressure, mmHg
Optimal	<120	<80
Normal	<130	<85
High normal	130–139	85–89
Hypertension[a]		
Stage 1 (mild)	140–159	90–99
Stage 2 (moderate)	160–179	100–109
Stage 3 (severe)	≥180	≥110
Isolated systolic hypertension	≥140	<90

[a] Based on the average of ≥2 readings taken at each of two or more visits after an initial screening.

Note: Classification of blood pressure for adults aged 18 years and older not taking antihypertensive drugs and not acutely ill. When systolic and diastolic pressures fall into different categories, the higher category should be selected to classify the individual's blood pressure status.

Source: 2003 European Society of Hypertension—European Society of Cardiology guidelines for the management of arterial hypertension.

impotence. Complaints referable to vascular disease include epistaxis, hematuria, blurring of vision owing to retinal changes, episodes of weakness or dizziness due to transient cerebral ischemia, angina pectoris, and dyspnea due to cardiac failure. Pain due to dissection of the aorta or to a leaking aneurysm is a rare presenting symptom.

Examples of symptoms related to the underlying disease in secondary hypertension are polyuria, polydipsia, and muscle weakness secondary to hypokalemia in patients with primary aldosteronism or weight gain, and emotional lability in patients with Cushing's syndrome. The patient with a pheochromocytoma may present with episodic headaches, palpitations, diaphoresis, and postural dizziness.

History A strong family history of hypertension, along with the reported finding of intermittent pressure elevation in the past, favors the diagnosis of essential hypertension. Secondary hypertension often develops before the age of 35 years or after 55. A history of repeated urinary tract infections suggests chronic pyelonephritis, although this condition may occur in the absence of symptoms. A history of weight gain is compatible with Cushing's syndrome, and one of weight loss is compatible with pheochromocytoma. A number of aspects of the history aid in determining whether vascular disease has progressed to a dangerous stage. These include angina pectoris and symptoms of cerebrovascular insufficiency, congestive heart failure, and/or peripheral vascular insufficiency. Other risk factors that should be asked about include cigarette smoking, diabetes mellitus, lipid disorders, and a family history of early deaths due to cardiovascular disease. Finally, aspects of the patient's lifestyle that could contribute to the hypertension or affect its treatment should be assessed, including diet, physical activity, family status, work, and educational level.

Physical Examination The physical examination starts with the patient's general appearance. For instance, are the round face and truncal obesity of Cushing's syndrome present? Is muscular development in the upper extremities out of proportion to that in the lower extremities, suggesting coarctation of the aorta? The next step is to compare the blood pressures and pulses in the two upper extremities and in the supine and standing positions (for at least 2 min). A rise in diastolic pressure when the patient goes from the supine to the standing position is most compatible with essential hypertension; a fall, in the absence of antihypertensive medications, suggests secondary forms of hypertension. Funduscopic findings provide one of the best indications of the duration of hypertension and of prognosis. A useful guide is the Keith-Wagener-Barker classification of funduscopic changes, in which classification from normal through grade IV retinopathy is based upon the presence of arteriolar light reflex, arteriovenous crossing defects, hemmorhages and exudates; the specific changes in each fundus should be recorded and a grade assigned (see Fig. 25-8). Palpation and auscultation of the carotid arteries for evidence of stenosis or occlusion should be carried out. In examination of the heart and lungs, evidence of left ventricular hypertrophy and cardiac decompensation should be sought. Is there a left ventricular lift? Are third and fourth heart sounds present? Are there pulmonary rales? A third heart sound and pulmonary rales are unusual in uncomplicated hypertension. Their presence suggests ventricular dysfunction. Chest examination also includes a search for extracardiac murmurs and palpable collateral vessels that may result from coarctation of the aorta.

The most important part of the abdominal examination is auscultation for bruits originating in stenotic renal arteries. Bruits due to renal arterial narrowing nearly always have a diastolic component or may be continuous and are best heard just to the right or left of the midline above the umbilicus or in the flanks. The abdomen should also be palpated for an abdominal aneurysm and for the enlarged kidneys of polycystic renal disease. The femoral pulses should be felt, and, if they are decreased and/or delayed in comparison with the radial pulse, the blood pressure in the lower extremities must be measured. Even if the femoral pulse is normal to palpation, arterial pressure in the lower extremities should be recorded at least once in patients in whom hypertension is discovered before the age of 30 years.

Laboratory Investigation The *basic* laboratory studies that should be performed in all patients are described in Table 230-7. Renal status is evaluated by assessing the presence of protein, blood, and glucose in the urine and measuring serum creatinine and/or blood urea nitrogen. Microscopic examination of the urine is also helpful. The serum potassium level should be measured both as a screen for mineralocorticoid-induced hypertension and to provide a baseline before diuretic therapy is begun. A blood glucose determination is helpful both because diabetes mellitus may be associated with accelerated arteriosclerosis, renal vascular disease, and diabetic nephropathy in patients with hypertension and because primary aldosteronism, Cushing's syndrome, and pheochromocytoma may all be associated with hyperglycemia. The possibility of hypercalcemia may also be investigated. Serum cholesterol, high-density lipoprotein cholesterol, and triglyceride levels identify other factors that predispose to the development of arteriosclerosis.

An electrocardiogram should be obtained in all cases. The echocardiogram is more sensitive than either the electrocardiogram or physical examination in determining whether cardiac hypertrophy is present and may be a useful addition to the *baseline* evaluation of a hypertensive patient, particularly as left ventricular hypertrophy is an independent cardiovascular risk factor and its presence indicates the need for vigorous antihypertensive therapy. Because of the cost of an echocardiogram and the uncertainty as to whether the resultant information would modify therapy, it is unclear that routine *follow-up* echocardiograms during therapy are justified. The chest roentgenogram may also be helpful by providing the opportunity to identify aortic dilation or elongation and the rib notching that occurs in coarctation of the aorta.

Most patients do not require ABPM, but readings are useful in diagnosing white coat hypertension and also in evaluating refractory hypertension, circadian patterns of blood pressure, and relation

---

TABLE 230-7 *Laboratory Tests for Evlution of Hypertension*

BASIC TESTS FOR INITIAL EVALUATION

1. Always included
   a. Urine for protein, blood, and glucose
   b. Microscopic urinalysis
   c. Hematocrit
   d. Serum potassium
   e. Serum creatinine and/or blood urea nitrogen
   f. Fasting glucose
   g. Total cholesterol
   h. Electrocardiogram
2. Usually included, depending on cost and other factors
   a. Thyroid-stimulating hormone
   b. White blood cell count
   c. HDL and LDL cholesterol and triglycerides
   d. Serum calcium and phosphate
   e. Chest x-ray; limited echocardiogram

SPECIAL STUDIES TO SCREEN FOR SECONDARY HYPERTENSION

1. Renovascular disease: angiotensin-converting enzyme inhibitor radionuclide renal scan, renal duplex Doppler flow studies, and MRI angiography
2. Pheochromocytoma: 24-h urine assay for creatinine, metanephrines, and catecholamines
3. Cushing's syndrome: overnight dexamethasone suppression test or 24-h urine cortisol and creatinine
4. Primary aldosteronism: plasma aldosterone: renin activity ratio

Note: HDL, high-density lipoprotein; LDL, low-density lipoprotein; MRI, magnetic resonance imaging.

of blood pressure to symptoms like dizziness and visual changes. ABPM readings are good predictors of future cardiovascular events. Mean 24-h systolic pressure ≥135 mmHg has been associated with a nearly double cardiovascular risk. When the normal nocturnal decline in blood pressure ("dipping") is absent, readings correlate well with the prevalence and extent of target organ damage in hypertensive individuals.

DIAGNOSIS OF SECONDARY HYPERTENSION   The abrupt onset of severe hypertension and/or the onset of hypertension of any severity in a patient under the age of 35 or over the age of 55 should lead to laboratory tests to exclude renovascular hypertension and pheochromocytoma, and the finding on physical examination of bilateral upper abdominal masses consistent with polycystic renal disease should lead to the performance of an abdominal ultrasound. An elevated creatinine or blood urea nitrogen level, associated with proteinuria and hematuria, should prompt a detailed workup for renal insufficiency (Chap. 259). A familial history of hypertension, particularly with early age of onset, should spark consideration of a genetic form. Special studies for secondary hypertension are also indicated if there is therapeutic failure with the initial drug program. The specific diagnostic measures depend on the most likely causes of secondary hypertension.

Pheochromocytoma (See also Chap. 322)   A history of headaches, palpitations, anxiety attacks, unusual sweating, hyperglycemia, and weight loss should also lead to tests to exclude pheochromocytoma. The easiest and best screening procedure for pheochromocytoma is the measurement of catecholamines and their metabolites in a 24-h urine sample collected while the patient is hypertensive. Measurement of plasma catecholamine levels may also be useful, while the assay of plasma-free metanephrines holds promise for heightened sensitivity. These tests may be indicated even in patients who do not have episodic hypertension, since over half the patients with pheochromocytoma have fixed hypertension. Provocative tests are seldom, if ever, indicated, although occasionally a suppressive test may be useful.

Cushing's Syndrome (See also Chap. 321)   A 24-h urine test for cortisol and creatinine or the administration of 1 mg of dexamethasone at bedtime, followed by the measurement of plasma cortisol at 7 to 10 A.M., is the best test to screen for the presence of Cushing's syndrome. A urine cortisol level of <2750 nmol (100 μg) or suppression of the plasma cortisol level to <140 nmol/L (5 μg/dL) effectively rules out Cushing's syndrome.

Renovascular Hypertension (See also Chap. 267)   The presence of an abdominal bruit should lead to a workup for renovascular hypertension. Suspicion for this form of hypertension should also be especially high in patients with deterioration of renal function after institution of ACE inhibitor therapy or in older patients with atherosclerotic disease. Over the past decades the standard approach to screen for renovascular hypertension has progressed from the rapid-sequence intravenous pyelogram to one of three noninvasive techniques: the captopril-enhanced radionuclide renal scan (the preferred choice), a duplex Doppler flow study, or magnetic resonance (MR) angiography with gadolinium enhancements. Perhaps the most sensitive and specific screening test, the spiral computed tomography (CT) scan, which gives a three-dimensional view, also requires giving an intravenous contrast agent.

The definitive test for surgically correctable renal disease is the combination of a renal angiogram and renal vein renin determinations. The renal arteriogram both establishes the presence of a renal arterial lesion and aids in the determination of whether the lesion is due to atherosclerosis or to one of the fibrous or fibromuscular dysplasias. It does not, however, prove that the lesion is responsible for the hypertension, nor does it permit prediction of the chances of surgical cure. It must be noted that (1) renal artery stenosis is a frequent finding by angiography and at postmortem in normotensive individuals, and (2) essential hypertension is a common condition and may occur in combination with renal arterial stenosis that is not responsible for the hypertension. Bilateral renal vein catheterization for measurement of plasma renin activity is therefore used to assess the functional significance of any lesion noted on arteriography. When one kidney is ischemic and the other is normal, all the renin released comes from the involved kidney. In the most straightforward situation, the ischemic kidney has a significantly higher venous plasma renin activity than the normal kidney, by a factor of ≥1.5. Moreover, the renal venous blood draining the uninvolved kidney exhibits levels similar to those in the inferior vena cava below the entrance of the renal veins.

Significant benefit from operative correction may be anticipated in at least 80% of patients with the findings described above if care is taken to prepare the patient properly before renal vein blood sampling, i.e., by discontinuing renin-suppressing drugs, such as beta blockers, for at least 10 days; restricting the patient to a low-sodium intake for 4 days; and/or giving a converting-enzyme inhibitor for 24 h. When obstructing lesions in the *branches* of the renal arteries are demonstrated by arteriography, an attempt to obtain blood samples from the *main branches* of the renal vein should be made in an effort to identify a localized intrarenal arterial lesion responsible for the hypertension.

Primary Aldosteronism (See also Chap. 321)   These patients usually exhibit hypokalemia. Diuretic therapy often complicates the picture when the hypokalemia is first observed and needs to be assessed. Given the presence of hypokalemia, the relation between plasma renin activity and the aldosterone level becomes the key to the diagnosis of primary aldosteronism. The aldosterone concentration or excretion rate is high and plasma renin activity is low in primary aldosteronism, and these levels are relatively unaffected by changes in sodium balance. Thus, the aldosterone:renin ratio is high. A critical part of the evaluation after primary aldosteronism has been established is to determine whether disease is unilateral or bilateral, because surgical removal of the lesion usually reduces arterial pressure only in patients with unilateral disease.

℞ TREATMENT

INDICATIONS FOR THERAPY   Patients with a diastolic pressure repeatedly >90 mmHg or systolic pressure >140 mmHg should be treated unless specific contraindications exist. Patients with isolated *systolic* hypertension (levels >160 mmHg with diastolic pressure <89 mmHg) should also be treated if they are over age 65 (Fig. 230-1). Patients with labile hypertension or isolated systolic hypertension who are not treated should have regular follow-up examinations at 6-month intervals because of the frequent development of progressive and/or sustained hypertension. Finally, patients with atherosclerotic vascular disease or diabetes mellitus and diastolic blood pressures between 85 and 90 mmHg should also receive antihypertensive therapy (Fig. 230-2).

Appropriate therapy for patients with white coat hypertension is debated, largely because the ultimate risk of cardiovascular events in these patients is still unknown. Some believe that subjects whose blood pressure is susceptible to apprehension and anxiety in the doctor's office are likely to have elevations during other periods of stress in their lives. Others hold white coat hypertension to be a tightly circumscribed phenomenon. In either case, these individuals would clearly benefit from life-style modifications to reduce progression to sustained hypertension. At present, there are insufficient data to warrant treatment with antihypertensive therapy unless other risk factors are present.

What should the blood pressure goal be? Previously it was assumed that 140/90 mmHg was the desired level. This still seems reasonable for nondiabetic patients since the Hypertension Optimal Treatment (HOT) study did not detect a significant difference in cardiovascular risk between nondiabetic patients treated to goal diastolic blood pressures of 90 versus 80 mmHg. However, in patients with

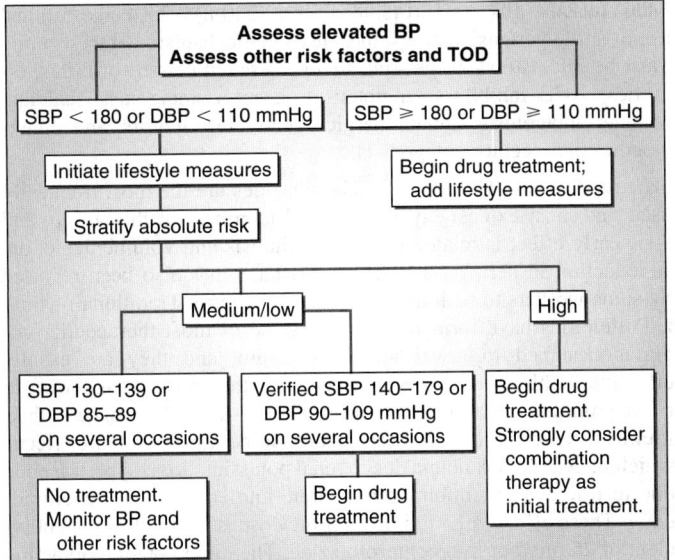

FIGURE 230-1 Initiation of treatment in patients with hypertension. See Table 230-11 for listing of classes of agents to use initially. In the initial evaluation, patients are stratified for cardiovascular risk using: level of blood pressure; the presence of risk factors—smoking, obesity, male gender, etc.—which vary from 0 factors (low risk) to three or more factors (high risk equivalent to having diabetes mellitus), target organ damage (TOD, i.e., clinical cardiovascular or renal disease) or diabetes (both high risk if present regardless of other risk factors). SBP, systolic blood pressure; DBP, diastolic blood pressure

diabetes this is not the case. In the U.K. Prospective Diabetes Study (UKPDS), patients reaching a blood pressure of 144/82 mmHg had a substantially lower risk compared to those with a blood pressure of 154/87 mmHg. The HOT study investigators documented a similar finding in their diabetic subset. Importantly, these studies have failed to document the existence of a "J" or "U" curve, indicating no increased risk of excessive blood pressure reduction. Thus, it is reasonable to target a blood pressure well within the normal range for diabetic patients, at most 130/85 mmHg. Newer studies may force this recommended goal even lower (see "Diabetes Mellitus," below). While not definitively proven, it seems prudent to use the same goal in patients with target organ damage, and in young and middle-aged patients, depending on what other cardiovascular risk factors are present. For elderly individuals, a goal of 140/90 mmHg is appropriate. Importantly, how aggressive one should be in achieving these blood pressure goals depends on the number and severity of other risk factors present.

Probably fewer than one-third of hypertensive patients in the United States are being treated effectively. Only a small number of these failures are related to drug unresponsiveness. Most are related to (1) failure to detect hypertension, (2) failure to institute effective treatment of an asymptomatic hypertensive patient, and (3) failure of the asymptomatic hypertensive patient to adhere to therapy. To help with the latter problem, patients must be educated to continue treatment once an effective regimen has been identified. Side effects and inconveniences of treatment must be minimized or counteracted in order to obtain the patient's continued cooperation.

The identification of an operable form of secondary hypertension does not automatically mean that surgical treatment is indicated. The decision depends on the age and general health of the patient, the natural history of the lesion, and the response of the arterial pressure to drug therapy. In patients with renovascular hypertension, the feasibility of renal angioplasty, the advantages of surgical repair versus nephrectomy, and the degree of overall renal functional impairment must be considered. Age and general health are important in patients with renovascular hypertension due to arteriosclerosis, because there is no evidence that repair of the stenosis increases life expectancy in the elderly patient with other evidence of vascular disease. Knowledge of the natural history of the disease is especially important when making a decision in the case of a young patient with renal artery stenosis due to fibrous dysplasia. If the arteriographic appearance suggests that the stenosis is due to intimal or subadventitial fibroplasia, the lesion may be expected to progress, and operation or angioplasty is required. Medial fibroplasia, on the other hand, often remains stable, and operation or angioplasty may not be necessary if pressure can be controlled by drug therapy.

The decision regarding operation should also be considered carefully in patients with primary aldosteronism when neither abdominal CT nor bilateral adrenal venous sampling for aldosterone demonstrates a tumor, because such patients may prove to have multinodular hyperplasia. In that case, bilateral adrenalectomy would be required to eliminate the aldosterone excess, and, even then, hypertension would usually persist. If hypokalemia can be controlled by an aldosterone receptor antagonist, e.g., spironolactone, or other drug therapy and arterial pressure lowered with antihypertensive agents, then it is reasonable to withhold operative treatment.

GENERAL MEASURES Nondrug therapeutic intervention is probably indicated in all patients with sustained hypertension and probably in most with labile hypertension. The general measures employed include (1) relief of stress, (2) dietary management, (3) regular aerobic exercise, (4) weight reduction (if needed), and (5) control of other risk factors contributing to the development of arteriosclerosis. Though it

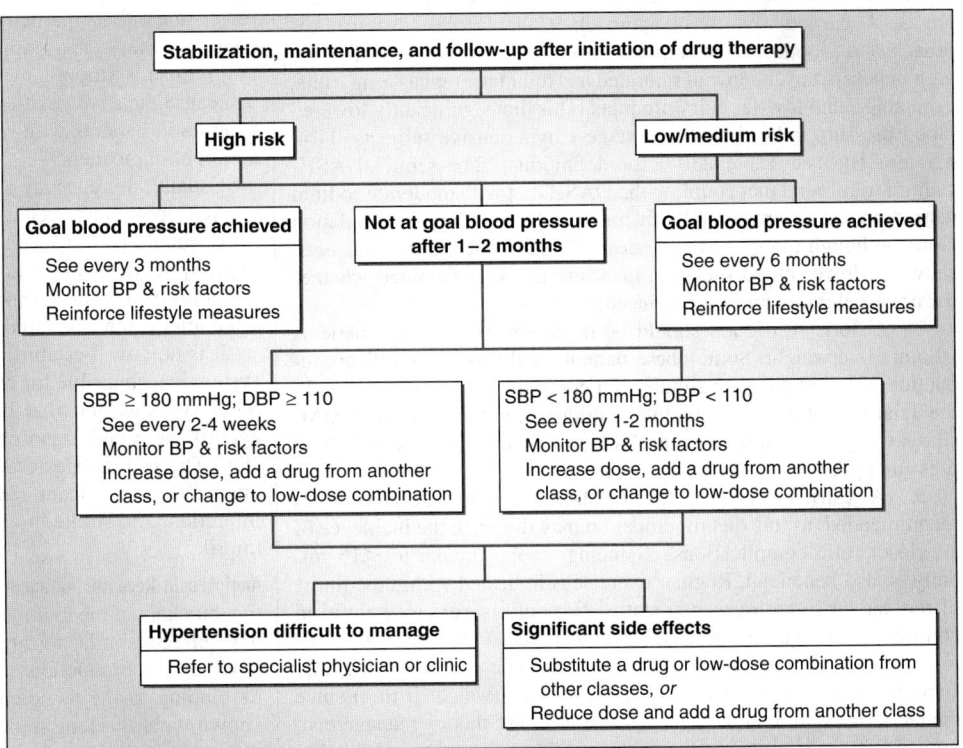

FIGURE 230-2 Approach to the hypertensive patient after initiating antihypertensive drug treatment. See Fig. 230-1 for initial steps and definition of risk and Table 230-11 for initial choice of agents.

is usually impossible to extricate the hypertensive patient from all internal and external stresses, he or she should be advised to avoid unnecessary tensions. In rare instances, it may be appropriate to recommend a change of job or of life-style. It has been suggested that relaxation techniques may also lower arterial pressure.

Dietary management has three aspects:

1. Because of the documented efficacy of sodium restriction and volume contraction in lowering blood pressure, patients previously were instructed to curtail sodium intake drastically. Some investigators have suggested that this is not necessary. They base their conclusion on two observations: (1) In many patients the blood pressure is not sensitive to the level of sodium intake, and (2) diuretics provide another method of decreasing body sodium stores in individuals whose blood pressure is sodium-sensitive. However, meta-analyses of previous diet studies have documented a 5-mmHg reduction in systolic pressure and a 2.6-mmHg reduction in diastolic pressure when sodium intake is reduced by ~75 meq/d. In addition, several reports have documented that, while mild sodium restriction has little if any direct action on blood pressure, it significantly potentiates the efficacy of nearly all antihypertensive agents. Thus, by making it possible to control blood pressure with lower doses of drugs, sodium restriction leads to a reduction in side effects. In addition, it is quite clear that some hypertensive patients are salt-sensitive (p. 1463), and the level of sodium intake does influence the blood pressure. Thus, since there is no apparent risk to mild sodium restriction, the most practical approach is to advise mild dietary sodium restriction (up to 5 g NaCl per day), which can be achieved by eliminating all additions of salt to food that is prepared normally. Some studies have also reported a lowering of arterial pressure related to an *increase* in potassium and/or calcium intake. For example, in one meta-analysis, dietary potassium supplements of 50 to 120 meq/d reduced blood pressure by about the same amount as salt restriction (by 6 mmHg systolic and 3.4 mmHg diastolic). While the advisability of these forms of dietary alteration is still controversial, the fact that a moderately high calcium intake (1.5 g elemental calcium daily) probably also reduces the extent of age-related osteoporosis, combined with the results of the potassium supplementation studies, indicate that they are probably useful adjuncts. A particularly useful approach is the DASH (Dietary Approaches to Stop Hypertension) diet, which uses natural foods that are high in potassium and low in saturated and total fat, emphasizing fruits, vegetables, and low-fat dairy products. This diet significantly lowered blood pressure in borderline and stage 1 hypertensive subjects (11.4/5.5 mm Hg)(see Table 230-6 for definitions). The sequel DASH-sodium trial found that coupling the DASH diet with moderate sodium restriction led to greater falls in pressure than dietary manipulation alone, although the gain was modest. While salt restriction has been shown to lower blood pressure, no study has yet examined whether cardiovascular outcomes are reduced.

2. Caloric restriction should be urged for hypertensive patients who are overweight. Some obese patients will show a significant reduction in blood pressure simply as a consequence of weight loss. In the Trial of Antihypertensive Interventions and Management (TAIM) study, weight reduction (average 4.4 kg over 6 months) lowered blood pressure by 2.5 mmHg.

3. A restriction in the intake of cholesterol and saturated fats is recommended, as this diet modification may diminish the incidence of arteriosclerotic complications. Reducing alcohol intake to <15 mL daily is also beneficial. Regular exercise is indicated within the limits of the patient's cardiovascular status. Not only is exercise helpful in controlling weight, but there is also evidence that physical conditioning itself may lower arterial pressure. Isotonic exercises (jogging, swimming) are better than isometric exercises (weight lifting) since the latter, if anything, raises arterial pressure. The dietary management outlined above is aimed at the control of other risk factors. Probably the most significant additional step that could be taken in this area would be to convince the smoker to give up cigarettes.

DRUG THERAPY FOR HYPERTENSION (Table 230-8) To make rational use of antihypertensive drugs, the sites and mechanisms of their action must be understood. In general, there are seven classes of drugs: diuretics, ACE inhibitors, angiotensin receptor antagonists, calcium channel antagonists; antiadrenergic agents, vasodilators, and mineralocorticoid receptor antagonists.

Diuretics (See also Chap. 216) The thiazides are the most frequently used and most extensively investigated members of this group, and their early effect is related to sodium diuresis and volume depletion. A reduction in peripheral vascular resistance has also been reported by some workers to be important in the long term. Traditionally, thiazide diuretics have formed the cornerstone of most therapeutic programs designed to lower arterial pressure, and they are usually effective within 3 to 4 days. Furthermore, they have been shown to reduce mortality and morbidity in long-term trials. Resistance to their routine use arose primarily because of their adverse metabolic effects, which include hypokalemia due to renal potassium loss, hyperuricemia due to uric acid retention, carbohydrate intolerance, and hyperlipidemia. These effects are minimized if the dose is kept below the equivalent of 25 mg/d of hydrochlorothiazide. The more potent loop-acting diuretics furosemide and bumetanide have also been shown to be antihypertensive but have been used less extensively for this indication, primarily because of their shorter duration of action. Triamterene and amiloride also impede sodium reabsorption, although triamterene has little intrinsic antihypertensive effect. Their major disadvantage is that they can produce hyperkalemia, particularly in patients with impaired renal function. Any of the potassium-sparing diuretics can also be given along with thiazide diuretics to minimize renal potassium loss.

ACE Inhibitors Drugs in this group inhibit the enzyme converting angiotensin I into angiotensin II—ACE. These agents are an increasingly popular choice for initial therapy. They are useful because they not only inhibit the generation of a potent vasoconstrictor (angiotensin II) but also retard the degradation of a potent vasodilator (bradykinin), alter prostaglandin production, and can modify the activity of the adrenergic nervous system. They are especially useful in renal or renovascular hypertension and in diabetic patients, as well as in accelerated and malignant hypertension. They are also as effective in mild, uncomplicated hypertension as beta blockers and thiazides—and have fewer side effects, particularly ones that adversely affect the patient's quality of life, such as fatigue, impotence, and forgetfulness. Ten ACE inhibitors are currently available in the United States. As a group they can cause the adverse effects of cough in 5 to 10% of patients, hyperkalemia in patients with renal insufficiency, and the idiosyncratic reaction of angioedema.

Usually, diuretics are stopped 2 to 3 days before administration of an ACE inhibitor is begun and are added back later if needed. These drugs should be used with caution when the renin system is activated (e.g., by severe heart failure, prior diuretic therapy, or substantial salt restriction) to avoid profound hypotension. In patients with bilateral renal artery stenosis, rapid deterioration of renal function may occur.

It is now well-established than activation of the renin-angiotensin system is responsible for detrimental effects on the cardiovascular and renal systems, and that blockade with ACE inhibitors is effective against these end-organ changes, even in patients without hypertension. The HOPE (Heart Outcomes Prevention Evaluation) trial demonstrated a significant reduction in the rates of death, myocardial infarction, and stroke in a broad range of high-risk patients given ramipril.

Angiotensin Receptor Antagonists (ARBs) These drugs are the most selective blockers of the renin-angiotensin system currently available. They have effects similar to those of ACE inhibitors. However, instead of blocking the production of angiotensin II, they competitively inhibit its binding to the angiotensin II AT$_1$ receptor subtype. It is not yet known what the long-term effects, in any, will be from exposure of the angiotensin II receptors to chronic increased circulating concentrations of angiotensin II. The utility, efficacy, and tolerability of ARBs are similar to those of the ACE inhibitors, but they appear to cause

Site of Action	Drug	Dosage	Indications	Contraindications/Cautions	Frequent or Peculiar Side Effects
DIURETICS					
Renal tubule	Thiazides: e.g., hydrochloro-thiazide	Depends on specific drug Oral: 12.5–25 mg daily	Mild hypertension; as adjunct in treatment of moderate to severe hypertension	Diabetes mellitus, hyperuricemia, primary aldosteronism	Potassium depletion, hyperglycemia, hyperuricemia, hypercholesterolemia, dermatitis, purpura, depression, hypercalcemia
	Loop-acting: e.g., furosemide	Oral: 20–80 mg 2 or 3 times a day	Mild hypertension; as adjunct in severe or malignant hypertension, particularly with renal failure	Hyperuricemia, primary aldosteronism	Potassium depletion, hyperuricemia, hyperglycemia, hypocalcemia, blood dyscrasias, rash, nausea, vomiting, diarrhea
	Potassium-sparing: Spironolactone	Oral: 25 mg 2 to 4 times daily	Hypertension due to hypermineralocorticoidism; as adjunct to thiazide therapy	Renal failure	Hyperkalemia, diarrhea, gynecomastia, menstrual irregularities
	Triamterene	Oral: 25–100 mg daily			Hyperkalemia, nausea, vomiting, leg cramps, nephrolithiasis, GI disturbances
	Amiloride	Oral: 5–10 mg daily			
ANTIADRENERGIC AGENTS					
Central	Clonidine	Oral: 0.05–0.6 mg twice daily	Mild to moderate hypertension, renal disease with hypertension		Postural hypotension, drowsiness, dry mouth, rebound hypertension after abrupt withdrawal, insomnia
	Guanabenz	Oral: 4–16 mg twice daily			
	Guanfacine	Oral: 1–3 mg daily			
	Methyldopa (also acts by blocking sympathetic nerves)	Oral: 250–1000 mg twice daily IV: 250–1000 mg every 4–6 h (tolerance may develop)	Mild to moderate hypertension (oral), malignant hypertension (IV)	Pheochromocytoma, active hepatic disease (IV), during MAO inhibitor administration	Postural hypotension, sedation, fatigue, diarrhea, impaired ejaculation, fever, gynecomastia, lactation, positive Coombs' tests (occasionally associated with hemolysis), chronic hepatitis, acute ulcerative colitis, lupus-like syndrome
Autonomic ganglia	Trimethaphan	IV: 1–6 mg/min	Severe or malignant hypertension	Severe coronary artery disease, cerebrovascular insufficiency, diabetes mellitus (on hypoglycemic therapy), glaucoma, prostatism	Postural hypotension, visual symptoms, dry mouth, constipation, urinary retention, impotence
Nerve endings	Guanethidine	Oral: 10–150 mg daily	Moderate to severe hypertension	Pheochromocytoma, severe coronary artery disease, cerebrovascular insufficiency, during MAO inhibitor administration	Postural hypotension, bradycardia, dry mouth, diarrhea, impaired ejaculation, fluid retention, asthma
	Guanadrel	Oral: 5–50 mg twice daily			
α Receptors	Phentolamine	IV: 1–5 mg bolus	Suspected or proved pheochromocytoma	Severe coronary artery disease	Tachycardia, weakness, dizziness, flushing
	Phenoxybenza-mine	Oral: 10–50 mg once or twice daily (tolerance may develop)	Proved pheochromocytoma		Postural hypotension, tachycardia, miosis, nasal congestion, dry mouth
	Prazosin	Oral: 1–10 mg twice daily	Mild to moderate hypertension	Use with caution in the elderly	Sudden syncope, headache, sedation, dizziness, tachycardia, anticholinergic effect, fluid retention
	Terazosin	Oral: 1–20 mg daily			
	Doxazosin	Oral: 1–16 mg daily			
β Receptors	Propranolol	Oral: 10–120 mg 2 to 4 times daily	Mild to moderate hypertension (especially with evidence of hyperdynamic circulation); as adjunct to hydralazine therapy	Congestive heart failure, asthma, diabetes mellitus (on hypoglycemic therapy), during MAO inhibitor administration, COPD, sick sinus syndrome, 2d or 3d degree heart block	Dizziness, depression, bronchospasm, nausea, vomiting, diarrhea, constipation, heart failure, fatigue, Raynaud's phenomenon, hallucinations, hypertriglyceridemia, hypercholesterolemia, psoriasis; sudden withdrawal may precipitate angina or myocardial injury in patients with heart disease
	Metoprolol	Oral: 25–150 mg twice daily			
	Nadolol	Oral: 20–120 mg daily			
	Atenolol	Oral: 25–100 mg daily			
	Timolol	Oral: 5–15 mg twice daily			

(continued)

Site of Action	Drug	Dosage	Indications	Contraindications/Cautions	Frequent or Peculiar Side Effects
α/β Receptors	Betaxolol	Oral: 10–20 mg daily			
	Carteolol	Oral: 2.5–10 mg daily			
	Pindolol	Oral: 5–30 mg twice daily			Less resting bradycardia than other beta blockers
	Acebutolol	Oral: 200–600 mg twice daily			
	Labetalol	Oral: 100–600 mg twice daily IV: 2 mg/min			Similar to beta blockers with more postural effects
	Carvediol	Oral: 12.5–50 mg daily or in divided doses			

VASODILATORS

Site of Action	Drug	Dosage	Indications	Contraindications/Cautions	Frequent or Peculiar Side Effects
Vascular smooth muscle	Hydralazine	Oral: 10–75 mg 4 times daily IV or IM: 10–50 mg every 6 h (tolerance may develop)	As adjunct in treatment of moderate to severe hypertension (oral), malignant hypertension (IV or IM), renal disease with hypertension	Lupus erythematosus, severe coronary artery disease	Headache, tachycardia, angina pectoris, anorexia, nausea, vomiting, diarrhea, lupus-like syndrome, rash, fluid retention
	Minoxidil	Oral: 2.5–40 mg twice daily	Severe hypertension	Severe coronary artery disease	Tachycardia, aggravates angina, marked fluid retention, hair growth on face and body, coarsening of facial features, possible pericardial effusions
	Diazoxide	IV: 1–3 mg/kg up to 150 mg rapidly	Severe or malignant hypertension	Diabetes mellitus, hyperuricemia, congestive heart failure	Hyperglycemia, hyperuricemia, sodium retention
	Nitroprusside	IV: 0.5–8 (μg/kg)/min	Malignant hypertension		Apprehension, weakness, diaphoresis, nausea, vomiting, muscle twitching, cyanide toxicity

ANGIOTENSIN-CONVERTING ENZYME INHIBITORS

Site of Action	Drug	Dosage	Indications	Contraindications/Cautions	Frequent or Peculiar Side Effects
Converting enzyme	Captopril	Oral: 12.5–75 mg twice daily	Mild to severe hypertension, renal artery stenosis	Renal failure (reduction of dose), bilateral renal artery stenosis, pregnancy	Leukopenia, pancytopenia, hypotension, cough, angioedema, urticarial rash, fever, loss of taste, acute renal failure in bilateral renal artery stenosis, hyperkalemia
	Benazepril	Oral: 5–40 mg daily			Same as captopril, but little evidence for leukopenia, but perhaps increased frequency of cough and angioedema. All can be given once daily, but side effects are reduced if one-half dose is given twice daily. Fosinopril is excreted more in bile than the others.
	Enalapril	Oral: 2.5–40 mg daily			
	Enalaprilat	IV: 0.625–1.25 mg over 5 min every 6–8 h			
	Fosinopril	Oral: 10–40 mg daily			
	Lisinopril	Oral: 5–40 mg daily			
	Quinapril	Oral: 5–80 mg daily			
	Ramipril	Oral: 1.25–20 mg daily			
	Trandolapril	Oral: 1–4 mg daily			

ANGIOTENSIN RECEPTOR ANTAGONISTS

Site of Action	Drug	Dosage	Indications	Contraindications/Cautions	Frequent or Peculiar Side Effects
	Losartan	Oral: 25–50 mg once or twice daily	Mild to severe hypertension, renal artery stenosis	Pregnancy, bilateral renal artery stenosis	Hypotension, acute renal failure in bilateral renal artery stenosis, hyperkalemia
	Valsartan	Oral: 80–320 mg			
	Irbesartan	Oral: 150–300 mg daily			

(continued)

TABLE 230-8—(Continued)

Site of Action	Drug	Dosage	Indications	Contraindications/Cautions	Frequent or Peculiar Side Effects
CALCIUM CHANNEL ANTAGONISTS					
Vascular smooth muscle	Dihydropyridines: Nifedipine XL Amlodipine	Oral: 30–90 mg daily Oral: 2.5–10 mg daily	Mild to moderate hypertension	Heart failure, 2d or 3d degree heart block	Tachycardia, flushing, gastrointestinal disturbances, hyperkalemia, edema, headache
	Felodipine XL Isradipine	Oral: 5–10 mg daily Oral: 2.5–10 mg daily			
	Nicardipine	Oral: 20–40 mg 3 times daily			
	Benzothiazepines: Diltiazem	Oral: 30–90 mg 4 times daily or as CD form 180–300 mg daily	Mild to moderate hypertension	Heart failure, 2d or 3d degree heart block	Same as amlodipine, except no tachycardia or edema, but can cause heart block, constipation, and liver dysfunction
	Phenylalkylamine: Verapamil	Oral: 30–120 mg 4 times daily or as SR form 120–480 mg daily	Mild to moderate hypertension	Heart failure, 2d or 3d degree heart block	
MINERALOCORTICOID RECEPTOR ANTAGONISTS					
Renal tubule	Spironolactone	Oral: 25–50 mg 2 to 4 times daily	Hypertension due to hypermineralo-corticoidism; as adjunct to thiazide therapy	Renal failure	Hyperkalemia, diarrhea, menstrual irregularities, gynecomastia
	Eplerenone	50–100 mg daily	Hypertension due to hypermineralo-corticoidism; as adjunct to thiazide therapy	Renal failure, diabetic nephropathy	Hyperkalemia, no anti-androgenic or progesterone side effects

Note: MAO, monoamine oxidase; COPD, chronic obstructive pulmonary disease; XL, CD, SR are long-acting or sustained-release formulations.

fewer side effects. Specifically, they do not cause excessive cough or angioedema. There appears to be variation within the class in terms of antihypertensive efficacy. No studies are available to allow comparison of efficacy between ACE inhibitors and ARBs, and their joint use, while already in clinical practice, awaits more substantiating data.

A number of large-scale prospective studies are under way to investigate the effects of ARBs on mortality and morbidity in patients with cardiovascular disease. The Losartan Intervention for Endpoint Reduction in Hypertension (LIFE) study has shown that losartan-based antihypertensive treatment was superior to atenolol in reducing cardiovascular mortality and morbidity, especially stroke and regression of left ventricular hypertrophy (Table 230-9). Three studies have demonstrated that irbesartan and losartan significantly reduce the progression on diabetic nephropathy in patients with type 2 diabetes mellitus.

Calcium Channel Antagonists There are three subclasses of calcium channel antagonists: the phenylalkylamine derivatives (e.g., verapamil), the benzothiazepines (e.g., diltiazem), and the dihydropyridines (e.g., amlodipine). To date, there is only one therapeutic agent in each of the first two classes but a number of agents in the third class. All three subclasses modify calcium entry into cells by interacting with specific binding sites on the α_1 subunit of the L-type voltage-dependent calcium channel. Thus, since there are other calcium channels (e.g., the T and N types), the actions of these drugs only partially modify total calcium transport into cells. The relative specificity of each agent stems from the fact that each class has a unique binding site on the α_1 subunit, and these sites are variably expressed in different tissues. Thus, while agents from all three subclasses cause vasodilation, usually only the dihydropyridines produce reflex tachycardia. Diltiazem and verapamil can both slow atrioventricular conduction—a feature not observed with the dihydropyridines. While calcium channel antagonists are also useful in angina pectoris (Chap. 226), because of their negative inotropic actions, they should be used with caution in hypertensive patients with heart failure.

Considerable controversy has surrounded the use of calcium channel antagonists in the treatment of hypertension. In part the controversy was secondary to the inadequacy of the data and the confusion between the use of short-acting agents (e.g., nifedipine) and long-acting agents. Several facts have helped partially to resolve this controversy. First has been the general recognition that despite its previously frequent use as an antihypertensive agent, short-acting nifedipine rarely, if ever, should be used to treat hypertension, since it has been reported to increase the incidence of acute coronary events. Second, the results of the SYST-EUR (Systolic Hypertension in Europe) trial documented, in patients over the age of 60 with isolated systolic hypertension, that a long-acting dihydropyridine calcium channel antagonist reduced cardiovascular morbidity and mortality to an extent equivalent to that previously reported for diuretics and beta blockers. The effect was greater among diabetics. Thus, long-acting calcium channel antagonists are often used as first-line hypertension therapy.

Antiadrenergic Agents ■ *β-ADRENERGIC RECEPTOR BLOCKERS* (See also Chap. 226) A number of effective β-adrenergic receptor blocking agents are available that block sympathetic effects on the heart and are most effective in reducing cardiac output and in lowering arterial pressure when there is increased cardiac sympathetic nerve activity. These agents are also often used as first-line therapy. In addition, they block the adrenergic nerve–mediated release of renin from the renal juxtaglomerular cells. This action may be an important component of their blood pressure–lowering action. β-Adrenergic blockers are particularly useful when employed in conjunction with vasodilators, which tend to evoke a reflex increase in heart rate, and with diuretics, the administration of which often results in an elevation of circulating renin activity. In practice, beta blockers appear to be effective even when there is no evidence of increased sympathetic tone, with about one-half or more of all hypertensive patients showing a fall in pressure. Furthermore, like diuretics, they have been shown to reduce morbidity and mortality in long-term clinical trials. However, these agents can precipitate congestive heart failure and asthma in susceptible individuals, and they must be used with caution in diabetic patients receiving

TABLE 230-9 *Randomized Clinical Trials in Hypertension*

Trial Reference	Patient Number and Characteristics	Trial Arms	Endpoints	Results	Conclusion
SYST-EUR, JA Staessen et al, Lancet 350: 757, 1997	4695, >60 years old 2 years' follow-up	Nitrendipine/ enalapril or HTZ Placebo	Primary: Death, all cardiovascular events, strokes	Active treatment reduced total stroke rate 42% ($p = .003$); nonfatal stroke decreased 44% ($p = .007$). All fatal and nonfatal cardiac endpoints declined 26% ($p = .03$). Cardiovascular mortality decreased 27% ($p = .07$).	Among elderly patients with isolated systolic hypertension, nitrendipine reduced cardiovascular complications; treatment of 1000 patients for 5 years with this regimen may prevent 29 strokes and/or 53 major cardiovascular endpoints
SYST-EUR, J Tuomilehto et al, N Engl J Med 341:372, 1999	4695 (diabetic = 492) >60 years old 2 years' follow-up	Nitrendipine/enalapril or HTZ Placebo	Primary: Death, all cardiovascular events, strokes	In diabetics total mortality reduced 55%; mortality from cardiovascular disease by 76%; all cardiovascular events combined by 69%; nonfatal stroke by 73% Reductions in mortality and all cardiovascular events were significantly larger among diabetic than nondiabetic patients ($p = .04$ to $.01$).	Calcium channel antagonist significantly reduces cardiovascular morbidity and mortality in elder hypertensive patients; the effect is greater in diabetic than nondiabetic subjects
CAPPP Trial, L Hansson et al, Lancet 353: 611, 1999	10,985, age 25–66, diastolic BP $\geq$ 100 mmHg 2–3 years' follow-up	Captopril Diuretics/beta blocker	Primary: Composite of fatal and nonfatal myocardial infarction, stroke, and other cardiovascular deaths	Primary endpoint relative risk 1.05, $p = .52$; Cardiovascular mortality was lower with captopril, relative risk (RR) 0.77, $p = .092$ Fatal and nonfatal stroke was more common with captopril, RR 1.25, $p = .044$	Captopril and conventional treatment did not differ in preventing cardiovascular morbidity and mortality
HOT Study, Hansson et al, Lancet 351: 1755, 1998	18,790, 50–80 years with diastolic BP 100–115 mmHg 3–4 years' follow-up	Felodipine plus four other agents to reduce diastolic BP to 90 mmHg or 85 mmHg or 80 mmHg	Major cardiovascular events	Lowest cardiovascular mortality occurred at 86.5 mmHg; further reduction below these BPs was safe but no further reduction in risk; in patients with diabetes, a 51% reduction in cardiovascular events in target group = 80 mmHg compared with target group = 90 mmHg (p for trend = .006)	Intensive lowering of BP was associated with a low rate of cardiovascular events down to a diastolic BP of 82.6 mmHg
DASH Trial, LJ Appel et al, N Engl J Med 336:1117, 1997	459 with diastolic blood pressure 80–95 mmHg; 8 wks. Sodium intake and body weight were maintained constant.	Diet rich in fruits and vegetables Diet rich in fruits, vegetables, and low-fat dairy products Control (average U.S. diet)	Blood pressure	Combination diet reduced systolic and diastolic BP by 5.5 and 3.0 mmHg more than the control diet ($p < .001$); the fruit and vegetable diet had an intermediate effect	A diet rich in fruits, vegetables, and low-fat dairy food can substantially lower BP
FG Messerli et al, JAMA 279: 1903, 1998	Meta-analysis of efficacy of beta blockers vs. diuretics as first-line therapy for elderly patients (>60 years) with hypertension Approximate mean of 5 years' follow-up	Diuretics, 8 trials Beta blockers, 2 trials	Cerebrovascular events, coronary heart disease, stroke mortality, cardiovascular mortality, all-cause mortality	Diuretics significantly reduced cerebrovascular events odds ratio (0.61), coronary heart disease odds ratio (0.74), stroke mortality odds ratio (0.67), cardiovascular mortality odds ratio (0.75), and all-cause mortality odds ratio (0.86); beta blockers significantly reduced only cerebrovascular events odds ratio (0.74)	In elderly patients with hypertension, first-line diuretics reduced morbidity and mortality better than beta blockers

(continued)

TABLE 230-9— (Continued)

Trial Reference	Patient Number and Characteristics	Trial Arms	Endpoints	Results	Conclusion
HOPE, S Yusuf et al, 2000	9297 high-risk patients (≥55 years old) with vascular disease or diabetes plus one other cardiovascular risk factor	Ramipril vs. placebo for a mean of 5 years	Primary: Composite of myocardial infarction, stroke, or death from cardiovascular causes	Ramipril significantly reduced the rates of death from cardiovascular causes (RR 0.74), MI (RR 0.80), stroke (RR 0.68), cardiac arrest (RR 0.62), heart failure (RR 0.77), and complications related to diabetes (RR 0.84).	Ramipril significantly reduced the rates of death, MI, and stroke in high-risk patients not known to have a low ejection fraction or heart failure.
LIFE, B Dahlof et al, Lancet 359: 995, 2002	9193, age 55–80, with essential hypertension and LVH by ECG	Once daily losartan-based or atenolol-based antihypertensive treatment for at least 4 years and until 1040 patients had primary cardiovascular event	Primary cardiovascular event (death, MI, or stroke)	BP fell by 30.2/16.6 (SD 18.5/10.1) and 29.1/16.8 mmHg (19.2/10.1) in the losartan vs. atenolol groups. The primary composite endpoint occurred in 508 losartan and 588 atenolol patients (RR 0.87). New-onset diabetes was less frequent with losartan	Losartan prevented more cardiovascular morbidity and death than atenolol for similar reduction in BP
ALLHAT, ALLHAT Collaborative Research Group, 2002	42,419 high-risk hypertensives ≥ 55 years	Chlorthalidone vs. lisinopril vs. amlodipine vs. doxazosin	Fatal coronary heart disease and nonfatal MI	Doxazosin arm stopped after 3 years because of increased rate of heart failure	No difference in primary endpoints or in all-cause mortality between ACE inhibition, calcium channel blockade, and diuretics

Note: HTZ, hydrochlorothiazine; BP, blood pressure; MI, myocardial infarction; LVH, left ventricular hypertrophy; ECG, electrocardiogram.

hypoglycemic therapy because they inhibit the usual sympathetic responses to hypoglycemia.

Cardioselective beta-blocking agents (so-called beta$_1$ blockers, e.g., metoprolol, atenolol) have been developed and may be superior to nonselective beta blockers such as propranolol and timolol in patients with bronchospasm. Nadolol, a nonselective beta blocker, unlike other drugs of this class, is excreted unchanged in the urine and has a half-life of 14 to 20 h; only one dose a day is required. Atenolol also usually needs to be given only once a day. Pindolol and acebutolol are nonselective beta blockers that have partial agonist activity and, therefore, produce less bradycardia. Labetalol exerts both α- and β-adrenergic blocking actions. Thus, it lowers arterial pressure not only by the same complex actions as do beta blockers but also directly by reducing systemic vascular resistance. Usually it has a more rapid onset of action but produces more postural symptoms and sexual dysfunction than the other beta blockers. It is usually not used as first-line therapy as there is no mortality study in which it has been tested.

Centrally acting agents include clonidine and methyldopa. These drugs and their metabolites stimulate α_2 receptors in the vasomotor centers of the brain, thereby reducing sympathetic outflow and arterial pressure. Usually a fall in cardiac output and heart rate also occurs. Since the baroreceptor reflex is intact, postural symptoms are absent. However, rebound hypertension may occur rarely when clonidine is stopped. This effect is probably secondary to an increase in norepinephrine release, which is inhibited by these agents owing to their agonist effect on presynaptic α receptors. They are usually not used as first-line therapy.

α-ADRENERGIC RECEPTOR BLOCKERS These agents are also not usually used as first-line therapy. Phentolamine and phenoxybenzamine block the action of norepinephrine at α-adrenergic receptor sites. These two compounds block both presynaptic (α_2) and postsynaptic (α_1) α receptors, and the former action accounts for the tolerance that develops. Prazosin, terazosin, and doxazosin are more effective because they selectively block only *postsynaptic* α receptors, i.e., α_1 receptors. Thus, presynaptic α activity remains, suppressing norepinephrine release, and tolerance occurs only infrequently. Accordingly, these three agents can produce substantial hypotension following the first dose. Their use has decreased with a report of their association with an increase in cardiovascular events. The doxazosin arm of the Antihypertensive and Lipid Lowering Treatment to Prevent Heart Attack Trial (ALLHAT) was terminated prematurely because of a significant increase in the risk of congestive heart failure.

Vasodilators These agents are usually not used for initial therapy. Hydralazine is the most versatile of the drugs that cause direct relaxation of vascular smooth muscle; it acts mainly on arterial resistance. Unfortunately, the effect of hydralazine on peripheral resistance is partly negated by a reflex increase in sympathetic discharge that raises heart rate and cardiac output, limiting the usefulness of hydralazine, especially in patients with severe coronary artery disease. Minoxidil is even more potent than hydralazine but unfortunately produces significant hypertrichosis and fluid retention and, therefore, is mainly limited to patients with severe hypertension and renal insufficiency.

Diazoxide is restricted in its application to acute situations. It begins to act immediately to lower blood pressure, and its effects may last for several hours. Nitroprusside given intravenously also acts as a direct vasodilator, with onset and offset of actions that are almost immediate. Nitroglycerin is a third direct-acting vasodilator useful as an intravenous agent. These latter three drugs are useful only for the treatment of hypertensive emergencies (Table 230-10).

Mineralocorticoid Receptor Antagonists In addition to its classic hormonal effects on the kidney causing sodium retention and potassium excretion, aldosterone is now recognized as a paracrine hormone that can act locally not only in the kidneys but also in the heart and blood vessels, contributing to fibrosis and hypertrophy. Aldosterone antagonists are emerging as agents that may counter these detrimental ef-

TABLE 230-10 *Therapeutic Agents Used to Treat Malignant Hypertension*

Drug	Route	Starting Dose	Time Course of Action			Oral Preparation Available
			Onset	Peak	Duration	
IMMEDIATE ONSET						
Nitroprusside	Continuous IV	0.25 μg/kg per min	<1 min	1–2 min	2–5 min	No
Nitroglycerin	Continuous IV	5 μg/min	1–5 min	2–6 min	3–10 min	No
Diazoxide	IV bolus	50 mg q5–10min up to 600 mg	1–5 min	2–4 min	4–12 h	No
Fenoldopan	Continuous IV	0.1–0.3 μg/kg per min	<5 min	5–10 min	30 min	No
Esmolol	Continuous IV	250–500 μg/min $\times$ 1 min; then 50–100 μg/kg per min $\times$ 4 min	1–2 min	2–3 min	10–20 min	No
DELAYED ONSET						
Enalaprilat	IV	1.25 mg q6h	10–15 min	3–4 h	6–24 h	Yes
Hydralazine	IV, IM	5–10 mg q20min $\times$ 3	10–20 min	20–40 min	4–12 h	Yes
Labetalol	IV	20–80 mg q10min up to 300 mg	5 min	20–30 min	3–6 h	Yes
Nicardipine	IV	5–15 mg/h	5–10 min	20–40 min	1–4 h	Yes

fects of aldosterone, including but not limited to hypertension. Spironolactone causes renal sodium loss by blocking the effect of mineralocorticoids, and it was initially employed as more effective management in hypertensive patients whose mineralocorticoid levels are excessive, such as patients with primary or secondary aldosteronism. However, the Randomized Aldactone Evaluation Study (RALES) clinical trial in heart failure using low doses of spironolactone achieved a 30% reduction in mortality, suggesting that an aldosterone receptor antagonist may be beneficial even when aldosterone levels are relatively normal (Chap. 216). Eplerenone is a new, selective mineralocorticoid receptor antagonist without clinically significant androgen receptor blocking or progesterone receptor stimulating activities, which translates into absence of gynecomastia and impotence in men and of menstrual irregularity in women. Both agents, like ACE inhibitors and angiotensin II receptor antagonists, can increase potassium levels significantly in patients with renal insufficiency. Initial close monitoring of serum potassium levels in patients with compromised renal function is, therefore, advised.

APPROACH TO DRUG THERAPY The aim of drug therapy is to use the agents described, alone or in combination, to return arterial pressure to normal levels with minimal side effects. Ideally, one would choose a therapeutic program that specifically corrects the underlying defect resulting in the elevated blood pressure, e.g., treatment with spironolactone or eplerenone for patients with primary aldosteronism. As our knowledge of the mechanisms underlying the hypertension in individual patients increases, more specific drug programs will become available. Such programs presumably will result in normalization of blood pressure with fewer side effects. In the absence of this information, an empirical approach is used, which takes into consideration efficacy, safety, impact on the quality of life, compliance, ease of administration, and cost. When used in combination, drugs are chosen for their different sites of action. Three major trials of anti-hypertensive agents have been reported recently. The mammoth ALLHAT trial resulted in no difference in either combined fatal coronary heart disease or nonfatal myocardial infarction between patients started on treatment with an ACE inhibitor, diuretic, or calcium channel blocker. In an Australian randomized trial of >6000 elderly hypertensives, in contrast, treatment with ACE inhibitors resulted in fewer cardiovascular events than treatment with diuretic agents, despite similar reductions of blood pressure. Guidelines for the initiation of antihypertensive therapy should be based upon two criteria: level of systolic and diastolic blood pressure and the total level of cardiovascular risk.

Since many effective antihypertensive agents are available, a number of useful therapeutic regimens have been developed. There are two major authoritative groups that have published treatment guidelines in 2003: The US Joint National Committee (JNC) and the European Society of Hypertension (ESH) and the European Society of Cardiology (ESC). In the absence of specific therapy, their approaches are similar in many respects, relying heavily on the results of randomized clinical trials (Table 230-9), except for which drugs should be used to initiate therapy. JNC7 recommends starting with diuretics because mortality trials have demonstrated a positive effect of treatment with these agents. The ESH/ESC guidelines recommend initiating therapy with any of five classes of agents (Table 230-11), or with a combination; recent study results from ALLHAT have made it advisable to remove alpha blockade from this list (see below). The different rec-

TABLE 230-11 *Guidelines for Selecting Initial Drug Treatment of Hypertension*

Class of Drug	Compelling Indications	Possible Indications	Compelling Contraindications	Possible Contraindications
Diuretics	Heart failure Elderly patients Systolic hypertension	Diabetes	Gout	Dyslipidemia Sexually active males
β-Blockers	Angina After myocardial infarct Tachyarrhythmias	Heart failure Pregnancy Diabetes	Asthma and COPD Heart block[a]	Dyslipidemia Athletes and physically active patients Peripheral vascular disease
ACE inhibitors	Heart failure Left ventricular dysfunction After myocardial infarct Diabetic nephropathy		Pregnancy Hyperkalemia Bilateral renal artery stenosis	
Calcium antagonists	Angina Elderly patients Systolic hypertension	Peripheral vascular disease	Heart block[b]	Congestive heart failure[c]
Angiotensin II antagonists	ACE inhibitor cough	Heart failure	Pregnancy Bilateral renal artery stenosis Hyperkalemia	

[a] Grade 2 or 3 atrioventricular block.
[b] Grade 2 or 3 atrioventricular block with verapamil or diltiazem.
[c] Verapamil or diltiazem.

Note: COPD, chronic obstructive pulmonary disease; ACE, angiotensin-converting enzyme.
Source: Adapted with permission from 1999 WHO.

ommendations, in part, reflect the fact that European committees reviewed more recent data from mortality clinical trials that, in one case, documented reductions in morbidity and mortality with a long-acting calcium channel antagonist versus placebo similar to previous reports for diuretics and beta blockers; in another case, ACE inhibitors were shown to be as effective as beta blockers and diuretics in reducing mortality. Practically, it has become less important which agent is chosen as "initial therapy" since the majority of hypertensive patients will require more than one agent to reach goal blood pressure.

There are several critical caveats common to both the JNC 7 and ESH/ESC approaches:

1. Start with an agent that may also treat and/or not harm a coexisting condition.
2. Start with an agent that the patient is likely to tolerate best; long-term compliance is related to tolerability and efficacy of the first agent used.
3. For low- or medium-risk patients, start with a low dose of an agent and, if blood pressure is not controlled, increase only moderately.
4. Add an additional agent from a different, complementary class if blood pressure is not controlled with a moderate dose of the first agent.
5. Use a diuretic when two agents are used, in nearly all cases.
6. Use thiazide diuretics only at low doses, i.e., ≤25 mg/d of hydrochlorothiazide or its equivalent, unless some pressing reason exists.
7. For medium- to high-risk patients, strongly consider low-dose combination therapy as initial therapy:
   a. A diuretic with a beta blocker, ACE inhibitor, or angiotensin II antagonist;
   b. A calcium channel blocker with an ACE inhibitor or a beta blocker.

If therapy with low doses of two drugs does not achieve blood pressure control, the primary agent should be increased to full dose, e.g., 20 mg of enalapril or 360 mg of diltiazem. If the blood pressure is still not controlled, then a detailed search for a secondary cause of hypertension, as outlined above, is indicated, with lower levels of suspicion in diabetics and the elderly. If none is found, then a dietary assessment will often reveal a high sodium intake. With reduction in salt intake to ≤5 g/d, blood pressure is often controlled. If the blood pressure is still not controlled, a third agent should be added. Caution should be used with the addition of an ACE inhibitor, as administration of such an agent to a patient who is already taking a diuretic occasionally may lead to profound hypotension.

If the blood pressure is controlled, then a stepwise reduction in the dose and/or withdrawal of some of the agents should be carried out to determine the minimal therapeutic program that will maintain the blood pressure at ≤140/90 mmHg. Fewer than 5% of patients will still be hypertensive at this point. For these, one first should consider the reasons for therapeutic failure, as shown in Table 230-12. If none can be identified, then one of the other agents listed in Table 230-11 should be added. If blood pressure is still not controlled, then consideration should be given to an alternate class as listed in Table 230-8. If blood

TABLE 230-12 *Reasons for Poor Therapeutic Response in Patients with Hypertension*

Inadequate patient compliance
Volume expansion
  Caused by excessive sodium intake
  Caused by nondiuretic antihypertensive agent
  Caused by renal damage
Excessive weight gain
Inadequate doses
Drug antagonism
Cold remedies
Sympathomimetics
Oral contraceptives (estrogens)
Adrenal steroids
Secondary forms of hypertension

pressure is controlled, previous drugs are withdrawn sequentially to determine the minimal therapeutic program that will maintain a normal blood pressure.

While the recommendations outlined above are satisfactory for a large majority of patients, it is important to use a flexible approach, because individual patients may respond differently to individual drugs and drug combinations. For those patients requiring multiple drugs, once the appropriate combination has been found, the use of a single formulation with the appropriate combination of drugs may simplify the regimen and thereby increase compliance. Every effort should be made to reduce the number of times each day the patients must interrupt their schedules for the medication. Pharmacologic treatment of essential hypertension is usually lifelong, and since most patients are asymptomatic, compliance with a complex regimen may be a serious problem, particularly if the therapeutic regimen has a negative impact on the quality of the patient's life. Finally, it is uncertain what level of arterial pressure should be accepted as representing adequate control. It is clear that reducing diastolic blood pressure to <90 mmHg is appropriate and reduces morbidity and/or mortality.

SPECIAL CONSIDERATIONS Five groups of patients with hypertension require special consideration because of associated conditions: those with renal disease, coronary artery disease, or diabetes mellitus; women of reproductive age; and the elderly. These groups are considered in the following sections.

Renal Disease Reduction of arterial pressure in hypertensive patients with impaired renal function is often accompanied initially by an increase in serum creatinine. This change does not represent further structural renal damage and should not deter the physician from continuing the therapy, since achievement of blood pressure control may eventually reduce the value toward normal. However, if serum creatinine increases in a patient treated with an ACE inhibitor, care needs to be exercised, because these patients may have bilateral renal artery disease. Their renal function will continue to deteriorate as long as the ACE inhibitor is given. Thus, ACE inhibitors should be used cautiously in patients with impaired renal function, and renal function should be assessed frequently (every 4 to 5 days) for the first 3 weeks. While these drugs are contraindicated in patients with bilateral renal artery stenosis, together with angiotensin receptor blockers they are the drugs of choice in patients with unilateral renal artery stenosis and a normally functioning contralateral kidney and probably also in patients with chronic renal failure with or without diabetes mellitus.

Coronary Artery Disease Beta blockers, important in reducing mortality after myocardial infarction and in the treatment of angina, are useful antihypertensive agents in patients with coronary artery disease. ACE inhibitors are useful in these patients as well, especially those with hypertension and left ventricular dysfunction.

Diabetes Mellitus The diabetic patient with hypertension is particularly challenging to treat because multiple agents are usually needed to achieve goal blood pressure and because many of the agents used to lower blood pressure can affect glucose metabolism adversely. ACE inhibitors or angiotensin receptor blockers should be first-line therapy in hypertensive individuals with type 2 diabetes. They have no known adverse effects on glucose or lipid metabolism and minimize the development of diabetic nephropathy by reducing renal vascular resistance and renal perfusion pressure—the primary factor underlying renal deterioration in these patients (Chap. 323). Meta-analyses of clinical studies have demonstrated that setting a lower blood pressure goal in diabetic patients is ideal to prevent progression of end-organ disease, with current recommendations shifting from 130/85 mmHg downward to 130/80. The average hypertensive diabetic patient will require at least three medications to achieve appropriate control.

Women of Reproductive Age ■ *ORAL CONTRACEPTIVES* Several years ago, a common cause of endocrine hypertension was the use of estrogen-containing oral contraceptives. However, more recent studies have suggested that this is no longer true, probably owing to the lower estrogen content of modern oral contraceptives. In patients receiving these agents who do become hypertensive, the mechanism is likely to be activation of the renin-angiotensin-aldosterone system. The estrogen component of oral contraceptive agents stimulates the hepatic synthesis of the renin substrate angiotensinogen, which in turn favors the increased production of angiotensin II and secondary aldosteronism. However, only a small number of women taking oral contraceptives actually have an increase in arterial pressure to a level >140/90mmHg, and in about half of these, the hypertension will remit within 6 months of stopping the drug. Why some women taking oral contraceptives develop hypertension and others do not is unclear but may be related to (1) increased vascular sensitivity to angiotensin II, (2) the presence of mild renal disease, (3) familial factors (>50% have a positive family history for hypertension), (4) age (hypertension is significantly more prevalent in women over age 35), (5) the estrogen content of the contraceptive, and/or (6) obesity. Indeed, some investigators have suggested that oral contraceptives simply unmask women with essential hypertension.

PREGNANCY (See also Chap. 6)   The patient who is pregnant and hypertensive or who develops hypertension during pregnancy (pregnancy-induced hypertension, preeclampsia, eclampsia) is particularly difficult to treat. Because it is uncertain whether autoregulation of uterine blood flow occurs, lowering blood pressure in the pregnant hypertensive patient may result in reduced placental and fetal perfusion. Thus, a conservative approach to lowering blood pressure is usually indicated. In the second and third trimesters, antihypertensive agents are often not indicated unless the diastolic pressure exceeds 95 mmHg. In general, severe salt restriction and/or diuretics are not used because of the associated increase in fetal wastage. Beta blockers need to be used cautiously for similar reasons. Methyldopa and hydralazine, and to a lesser extent calcium channel antagonists, are the antihypertensive agents used most often, because they have no known adverse effects on the fetus. Little is known about the safety of other antihypertensive agents in pregnancy, except that nitroprusside, ACE inhibitors, and angiotensin receptor blockers may cause adverse effects on the fetus and are contraindicated.

Elderly Patients   Hypertensive patients who are over age 65, and particularly those over age 75, offer substantial challenges to the physician. Several studies have reported that healthy elderly patients, whether male or female, who are treated with relatively modest doses of antihypertensive agents show a substantial reduction in strokes and stroke-related deaths. This is true whether the patient has systolic and diastolic hypertension or isolated systolic hypertension. What is not clear from these studies is how broadly the results can be extrapolated, since the studies were performed in healthy elderly patients, while many such patients have other diseases. Thus, in the elderly hypertensive patient, individualization of therapy is warranted.

MALIGNANT HYPERTENSION

In addition to marked blood pressure elevation (usually diastolic blood pressure > 130 mmHg) in association with papilledema and retinal hemorrhages and exudates, the full-blown medical emergency of malignant hypertension may include manifestations of hypertensive encephalopathy, such as severe headache, vomiting, visual disturbances (including transient blindness), transient paralyses, convulsions, stupor, and coma. These manifestations have been attributed to spasm of cerebral vessels and to cerebral edema. In some patients who have died, multiple small thrombi have been found in the cerebral vessels. Cardiac decompensation and rapidly declining renal function are other critical features of malignant hypertension. Oliguria may, in fact, be the presenting feature. The vascular lesion characteristic of malignant hypertension is fibrinoid necrosis of the walls of small arteries and arterioles, and this development can be reversed by effective antihypertensive therapy.

The pathogenesis of malignant hypertension is unknown. However, at least two independent processes—dilation of cerebral arteries and generalized arteriolar fibrinoid necrosis—contribute to the associated signs and symptoms. The cerebral arteries dilate because the normal autoregulation of cerebral blood flow decompensates as a result of the markedly elevated arterial pressure. Cerebral blood flow therefore is excessive, producing the encephalopathy associated with malignant hypertension. Many patients also show evidence of a microangiopathic hemolytic anemia; this secondary phenomenon could contribute to the deterioration of renal function. Most patients also have elevated levels of peripheral plasma renin activity and increased aldosterone production, and these effects may be involved in causing vascular damage.

Perhaps <1% of hypertensive patients develop the malignant phase, which can occur in the course of both essential and secondary hypertension. Rarely, it is the first recognized manifestation of hypertension, and it is unusual for it to occur in patients under treatment. The average age at diagnosis is 40, and men are affected more often than women. Prior to the availability of effective therapy, the life expectancy after diagnosis of malignant hypertension was <2 years, with most deaths being due to renal failure, cerebral hemorrhage, or congestive heart failure. With the advent of effective antihypertensive therapy, at least half the patients survive for >5 years.

℞ TREATMENT

Malignant hypertension is a medical emergency that requires immediate therapy. However, it needs to be distinguished from severe hypertension, in which overly aggressive therapy could result in a potentially hazardous reduction in myocardial and cerebral perfusion. The initial aims of therapy should be (1) correction of medical complications, and (2) reduction of diastolic pressure by one-third, but not to a level <95 mmHg. The drugs available for treatment of malignant hypertension can be divided into two groups on the basis of time of onset of action (Table 230-9). If the patient has hypertensive encephalopathy or pulmonary edema, and if arterial pressure must be reduced rapidly, then one from the immediate-acting group should be used, but they are not satisfactory for long-term management.

Furosemide is an important adjunct to the therapy just discussed. Given either orally or intravenously, it serves to maintain sodium diuresis in the face of a falling arterial pressure and thus will speed recovery from encephalopathy and congestive heart failure as well as maintain the sensitivity to the primary antihypertensive drug. Digitalis (Chap. 216) may also be indicated if there is evidence of cardiac decompensation.

In patients with malignant hypertension in whom the existence of pheochromocytoma is suspected, urine should be collected for measurement of the products of catecholamine metabolism, and drugs that might release additional catecholamines, such as methyldopa, reserpine, and guanethidine, must be avoided. The parenteral drug of choice in these patients is phentolamine, administered with care to avoid a precipitous reduction in arterial pressure.

FURTHER READING

ALLHAT COLLABORATIVE RESEARCH GROUP: The Antihypertensive and Lipid Lowering Treatment to Prevent Heart Attack Trial (ALLHAT). Major outcomes in high-risk hypertensive patients randomized to angiotensin converting enzyme inhibitor or calcium channel blocker vs. diuretic. JAMA 288:2981, 2002

CHOBANIAN AV et al: The Seventh Report of the Joint National Committee on Prevention Detection, Evaluation, and Treatment of High Blood Pressure: The JNC 7 report. JAMA 289:2560, 2003

CLEMENT DL et al: Prognostic value of ambulatory blood-pressure recordings in patients with treated hypertension. N Engl J Med 348:2407, 2003

DOMINICZAK AF et al: Genes and hypertension: From gene mapping in experimental models to vascular gene transfer strategies. Hypertension 35:164, 2000

GUIDELINES COMMITTEE. 2003 European Society of Hypertension—European Society of Cardiology guidelines for the management of arterial hypertension. J Hypertens 21:1011, 2003

KAPLAN N: Systemic hypertension: Mechanisms and diagnosis, in *Braunwald's Heart Disease*, 7th ed, D Zipes et al (eds). Philadelphia, Saunders, 2005

MORTENSEN RM, WILLIAMS GH: Aldosterone action (physiology), in *Endocrinology*, 4th ed, LJ DeGroot et al (eds). Philadelphia, Saunders, 2000

O'BRIEN E et al: Use and interpretation of ambulatory blood pressure monitoring: Recommendations of the British Hypertension Society. BMJ 320:1128, 2000

PRISANT LM, MOSER M: Hypertension in the elderly: Can we improve results of therapy? Arch Intern Med 160:283, 2000

REEVES RA: Does this patient have hypertension? How to measure blood pressure. JAMA 273:1211, 1995

SACKS FM et al: Effects on blood pressure of reduced dietary sodium and the Dietary Approaches to Stop Hypertension (DASH) diet. N Engl J Med 344:3, 2001

WING LM et al: SA comparison of outcomes with angiotensin-converting enzyme inhibitors and diuretics for hypertension in the elderly. N Engl J Med 13:583, 2003

1999 WORLD HEALTH ORGANIZATION–INTERNATIONAL SOCIETY OF HYPERTENSION GUIDELINES FOR THE MANAGEMENT OF HYPERTENSION. J Hypertens 17:151, 1999

YUSUF S et al: Effects of an angiotensin-converting-enzyme inhibitor, ramipril, on cardiovascular events in high-risk patients. The Heart Outcomes Prevention Evaluation Study Investigators. N Engl J Med 342:145, 2000

231 DISEASES OF THE AORTA
Victor J. Dzau, Mark A. Creager

The aorta is the conduit through which the blood ejected from the left ventricle is delivered to the systemic arterial bed. In adults, its diameter is approximately 3 cm at the origin, 2.5 cm in the descending portion in the thorax, and 1.8 to 2 cm in the abdomen. The aortic wall consists of a thin intima composed of endothelium, subendothelial connective tissue, and an internal elastic lamina; a thick tunica media composed of smooth-muscle cells and extracellular matrix; and an adventitia composed primarily of connective tissue enclosing the vasa vasorum and nervi vascularis. In addition to its conduit function, the viscoelastic and compliant properties of the aorta also subserve a buffering function. The aorta is distended during systole to enable a portion of the stroke volume to be stored, and it recoils during diastole so that blood continues to flow to the periphery. Because of its continuous exposure to high pulsatile pressure and shear stress, the aorta is particularly prone to injury and disease resulting from mechanical trauma (Table 231-1). The aorta is also more prone to rupture than any other vessel, especially with the development of aneurysmal dilatation, since its wall tension, as governed by Laplace's law (i.e., proportional to the product of pressure and radius), would be increased.

AORTIC ANEURYSM

An *aneurysm* is defined as a pathologic dilatation of a segment of a blood vessel. A *true aneurysm* involves all three layers of the vessel wall and is distinguished from a *pseudoaneurysm*, in which the intimal and medial layers are disrupted and the dilatation is lined by adventitia only and sometimes by perivascular clot. Aneurysms may also be classified according to their gross appearance. A *fusiform aneurysm* affects the entire circumference of a segment of the vessel, resulting in a diffusely dilated lesion. In contrast, a *saccular aneurysm* involves only a portion of the circumference, resulting in an outpouching of the vessel wall. Aortic aneurysms are also classified according to location, i.e., abdominal versus thoracic. Aneurysms of the descending thoracic aorta are usually contiguous with infradiaphragmatic aneurysms and are referred to as *thoracoabdominal aortic aneurysms*.

TABLE 231-1 *Diseases of the Aorta: Etiology and Associated Factors*

Aortic aneurysm	Aortic occlusion
Atherosclerosis	Atherosclerosis
Cystic medial necrosis	Thromboembolism
Tuberculosis	Aortitis
Syphilitic infection	Syphilitic aortitis
Mycotic infection	Rheumatic aortitis
Rheumatic aortitis	Takayasu's arteritis
Trauma	Giant cell arteritis
Aortic dissection	
Cystic medial necrosis	
Systemic hypertension	
Atherosclerosis	
Takayasu's arteritis	
Giant cell arteritis	

ETIOLOGY The most common pathologic condition associated with aortic aneurysm is *atherosclerosis*. It is controversial whether atherosclerosis itself actually causes aortic aneurysms or whether atherosclerosis develops as a secondary event in the dilated aorta. Causality is implied by studies that have shown that many patients with aortic aneurysms have coexisting risk factors for atherosclerosis (Chap. 224), particularly cigarette smoking, as well as atherosclerosis in other blood vessels. Seventy-five percent of atherosclerotic aneurysms are located in the distal abdominal aorta, below the renal arteries.

Cystic medial necrosis is the term used to describe the degeneration of collagen and elastic fibers in the tunica media of the aorta, as well as the loss of medial cells that are replaced by multiple clefts of mucoid material. Cystic medial necrosis characteristically affects the proximal aorta, results in circumferential weakness and dilatation, and leads to development of fusiform aneurysms involving the ascending aorta and the sinuses of Valsalva. This condition is particularly prevalent in patients with Marfan syndrome and Ehlers-Danlos syndrome type IV (Chap. 342) but also occurs in pregnant women, in patients with hypertension, and in those with valvular heart disease. Sometimes it appears as an isolated condition in patients without any other apparent disease. Familial clusterings of aortic aneurysms occur in 20% of patients, suggesting a hereditary basis of the disease. Mutations of the genes encoding fibrillin-1 and type III procollagen have been implicated in some cases. Linkage analysis has identified loci on chromosomes 5q13-14 and 11q23.3-q24 in several families, although the specific culprit genes have not been described. *Syphilis* (Chap. 153) is a relatively uncommon cause of aortic aneurysm. Syphilitic periaortitis and mesoaortitis damage elastic fibers, resulting in thickening and weakening of the aortic wall. Approximately 90% of syphilitic aneurysms are located in the ascending aorta or aortic arch. *Tuberculous aneurysms* (Chap. 150) typically affect the thoracic aorta and result from direct extension of infection from hilar lymph nodes or contiguous abscesses or from bacterial seeding. Loss of aortic wall elasticity results from granulomatous destruction of the medial layer. A *mycotic aneurysm* is a rare condition that develops as a result of staphylococcal, streptococcal, or salmonella infections of the aorta, usually at an atherosclerotic plaque. These aneurysms are usually saccular. Blood cultures are often positive and reveal the nature of the infecting agent.

Vasculitides associated with aortic aneurysm include Takayasu's arteritis and giant cell arteritis, which may cause aneurysms of the aortic arch and descending thoracic aorta. Spondyloarthropathies such as ankylosing spondylitis, rheumatoid arthritis, psoriatic arthritis, relapsing polychondritis and Reiter's syndrome are associated with dilatation of the ascending aorta. Behçet's disease (Chap. 307) causes thoracic and abdominal aortic aneurysms. *Traumatic aneurysms* may develop after penetrating or nonpenetrating chest trauma and most commonly affect the descending thoracic aorta just beyond the site of insertion of the ligamentum arteriosum. *Congenital aortic aneurysms* may be primary or associated with anomalies such as a bicuspid aortic valve or aortic coarctation.

THORACIC AORTIC ANEURYSMS The clinical manifestations and natural history of thoracic aortic aneurysms depend on their location. Cystic medial necrosis is the most common cause of ascending aortic aneurysms, whereas atherosclerosis is the condition most frequently associated with aneurysms of the aortic arch and descending thoracic aorta. The average growth rate of thoracic aneurysms is 0.1 to 0.4 cm per year. The risk of rupture is related to the size of the aneurysm and the presence of symptoms; it increases substantially for ascending aortic aneurysms >6 cm and descending thoracic aneurysms >7 cm. Most thoracic aortic aneurysms are asymptomatic. However, compression or erosion of adjacent tissue by aneurysms may cause symptoms such as chest pain, shortness of breath, cough, hoarseness, or dysphagia. Aneurysmal dilatation of the ascending aorta may cause congestive heart failure as a consequence of aortic regurgitation; and compression of the superior vena cava may produce congestion of the head, neck, and upper extremities.

A chest x-ray may be the first test to suggest the diagnosis of a thoracic aortic aneurysm (Fig. 231-1). Findings include widening of the mediastinal shadow and displacement or compression of the trachea or left mainstem bronchus. Two-dimensional echocardiography, and particularly transesophageal echocardiography, can be used to assess the proximal ascending aorta and descending thoracic aorta. Both contrast-enhanced computed tomography (CT) and magnetic resonance imaging (MRI) are sensitive and specific tests for assessment of aneurysms of the thoracic aorta. In asymptomatic patients whose aneurysms are too small to justify surgery, noninvasive testing with either contrast-enhanced CT or MRI should be performed at least every 6 to 12 months to monitor expansion. Contrast aortography is frequently required preoperatively to assess the length of the aneurysm and involvement of branch vessels (Fig. 231-2).

Patients with thoracic aortic aneurysms, and particularly patients with Marfan syndrome who have evidence of aortic root dilatation, should receive long-term beta-blocker therapy. Additional medical therapy should be given, as necessary, to control hypertension. Operative repair with placement of a prosthetic graft is indicated in patients with symptomatic thoracic aortic aneurysms, and in those in whom the aortic diameter is >6 cm or has increased by >1 cm per year. In patients with Marfan syndrome, thoracic aortic aneurysms >5 cm should be considered for surgery.

ABDOMINAL AORTIC ANEURYSMS Abdominal aortic aneurysms occur more frequently in males than in females, and the incidence increases with age. Abdominal aortic aneurysms may affect 1 to 2% of men older than 50 years. At least 90% of all abdominal aortic aneurysms >4.0 cm are affected by atherosclerosis, and most of these aneurysms are below the level of the renal arteries. Prognosis is related to both the size of the aneurysm and the severity of coexisting coronary artery and cerebrovascular disease. The risk of rupture increases with the size of the aneurysm. The 5-year risk of rupture for aneurysms <5 cm is 1 to 2%, whereas it is 20 to 40% for aneurysms >5 cm in diameter. The formation of mural thrombi within the aneurysm may predispose to peripheral embolization.

An abdominal aortic aneurysm commonly produces no symptoms. It is usually detected on routine examination as a palpable, pulsatile, and nontender mass, or it is an incidental finding during an abdominal x-ray or ultrasound performed for other reasons. However, as abdominal aortic aneurysms expand, they may become painful. Some patients complain of strong pulsations in the abdomen; others experience pain in the chest, lower back, or scrotum. Aneurysmal pain is usually a harbinger of rupture and represents a medical emergency. More often, acute rupture occurs without any prior warning, and this complication is always life-threatening. Rarely, there is leakage of the aneurysm with severe pain and tenderness. Acute pain and hypotension occur with rupture of the aneurysm, which requires emergency operation.

Abdominal radiography may demonstrate the calcified outline of the aneurysm. However, about 25% of aneurysms are not calcified and cannot be visualized by plain x-ray. An abdominal ultrasound can delineate the transverse and longitudinal dimensions of an abdominal aortic aneurysm and may detect mural thrombus. Abdominal ultra-

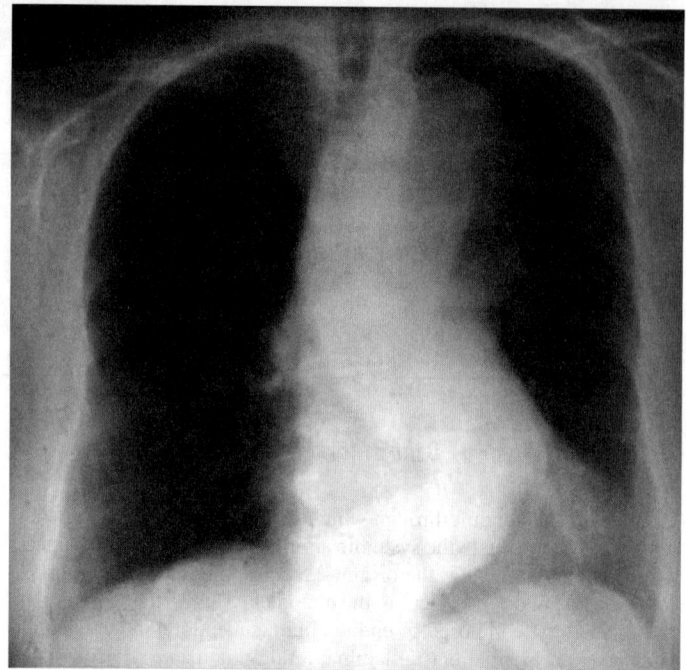

FIGURE 231-1   A chest x-ray of a patient with a thoracic aortic aneurysm.

sound is useful for serial documentation of aneurysm size and can be used to screen patients at risk for developing aortic aneurysm, such as those with affected siblings, peripheral atherosclerosis, or peripheral artery aneurysms. In one larger study, ultrasound screening of men aged 65 to 74 years was associated with a risk reduction in aneurysm-related death by 42%. CT with contrast and MRI are accurate, noninvasive tests to determine the location and size of abdominal aortic aneurysms (Fig. 231-3). Contrast aortography is used for the evaluation of patients with aneurysms before surgery, but the procedure carries a small risk of complications, such as bleeding, allergic reactions, and atheroembolism. This technique is useful in documenting the length of the aneurysm, especially its upper and lower limits, and the extent of associated atherosclerotic vascular disease. However, since the presence of mural clots may reduce the luminal size, aortography may underestimate the diameter of an aneurysm.

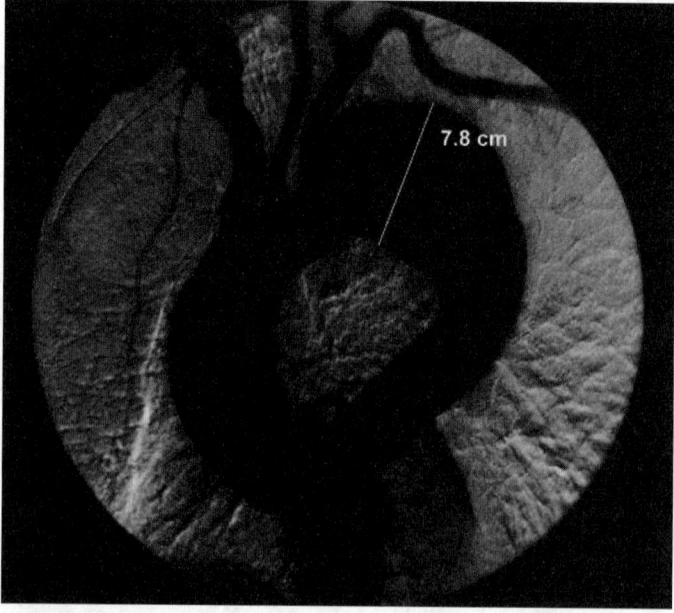

FIGURE 231-2   An aortogram demonstrating a large fusiform aneurysm of the descending thoracic aorta.

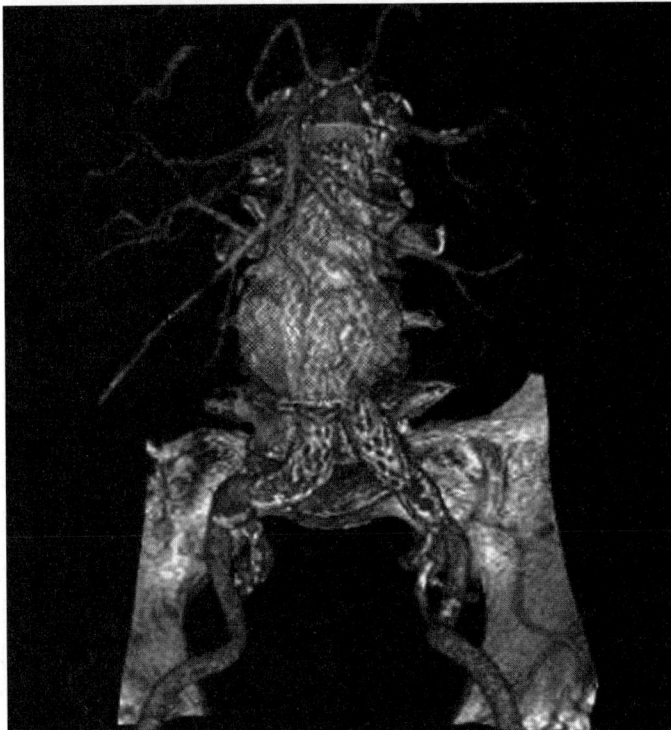

FIGURE 231-3 A computed tomographic angiogram (CTA) depicting a fusiform abdominal aortic aneurysm that has been treated with a bifurcated stent graft.

℞ TREATMENT

Operative repair of the aneurysm and insertion of a prosthetic graft is indicated for abdominal aortic aneurysms of any size that are expanding rapidly or are associated with symptoms. For asymptomatic aneurysms, operation is indicated if the diameter is >5.5 cm. Operation may be recommended in patients with aneurysm diameters of 4 to 5 cm, except for patients with exceptionally high operative risk. However, in recent randomized trials of patients with abdominal aortic aneurysms <5.5 cm, there was no difference in the long-term (5- to 8-year) mortality rate between those followed with ultrasound surveillance and those undergoing elective aneurysm repair. Thus, serial noninvasive follow-up of smaller aneurysms (<5 cm) is an alternative to immediate surgery. Percutaneous placement of endovascular stent grafts (Fig. 231-3) for treatment of infrarenal abdominal aortic aneurysms is currently available for selected patients, and initial reports have been favorable.

In surgical candidates, careful preoperative cardiac and general medical evaluations (followed by appropriate therapy of complicating conditions) are essential. Preexisting coronary artery disease, congestive heart failure, pulmonary disease, diabetes, and advanced age add to the risk of surgery. Perioperative management should include the placement of a Swan-Ganz catheter and arterial line to monitor and optimize left ventricular filling pressure, cardiac output, and arterial pressure, especially during clamping and unclamping of the aorta, as well as during the immediate postoperative period. With careful preoperative cardiac evaluation and postoperative care, the operative mortality rate approximates 1 to 2%. After acute rupture, the mortality rate of emergent operation generally exceeds 50%.

AORTIC DISSECTION

Aortic dissection is caused by a circumferential or, less frequently, transverse tear of the intima. It often occurs along the right lateral wall of the ascending aorta where the hydraulic shear stress is high. Another common site is the descending thoracic aorta just below the ligamentum arteriosum. The initiating event is either a primary intimal tear with secondary dissection into the media or a medial hemorrhage that dissects into and disrupts the intima. The pulsatile aortic flow then dissects along the elastic lamellar plates of the aorta and creates a false lumen. The dissection usually propagates distally down the descending aorta and into its major branches, but it may also propagate proximally. In some cases, a secondary distal intimal disruption occurs, resulting in the reentry of blood from the false to the true lumen.

There are at least two important pathologic and radiologic variants: intramural hematoma without an intimal flap and penetrating atherosclerotic ulcer. The clinical picture and therapeutic management of intramural hematoma are similar to those for classic aortic dissection. By contrast, penetrating ulcers are usually localized and are not associated with extensive propagation. They are primarily found in the mid and distal portions of the descending thoracic aorta and are associated with extensive atherosclerotic disease. The ulcer can erode beyond the intimal border, leading to medial hematoma, and may progress to false aneurysm formation or rupture.

DeBakey and coworkers initially classified aortic dissections as type I, in which an intimal tear occurs in the ascending aorta but which involves the descending aorta as well; type II, in which the dissection is limited to the ascending aorta; and type III, in which the intimal tear is located in the descending area with distal propagation of the dissection (Fig. 231-4). Another classification (Stanford) is that of type A, in which the dissection involves the ascending aorta (proximal dissection), and type B, in which it is limited to the descending aorta (distal dissection). From a management standpoint, classification into type A or B is more practical and useful, since DeBakey types I and II are managed in a similar manner.

The factors that predispose to aortic dissection include systemic hypertension, a coexisting condition in 70% of patients, and cystic medial necrosis. Aortic dissection is the major cause of morbidity and mortality in patients with Marfan syndrome (Chap. 342) and similarly may affect patients with Ehlers-Danlos syndrome. The incidence is

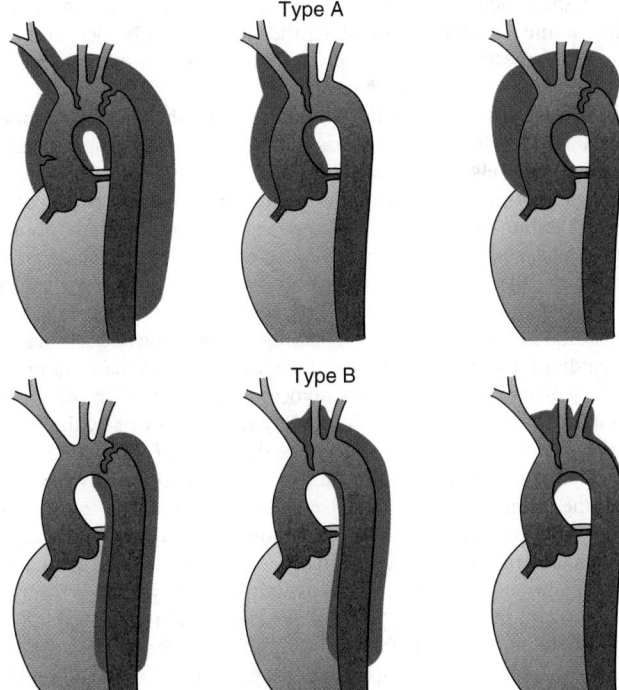

FIGURE 231-4 Classification of aortic dissections. Stanford classification: Type A dissections (*top panels*) involve the ascending aorta independent of site of tear and distal extension; type B dissections (*bottom panels*) involve transverse and/or descending aorta without involvement of the ascending aorta. DeBakey classification: Type I dissection involves ascending to descending aorta (*top left*); type II dissection is limited to ascending or transverse aorta, without descending aorta (*top center + top right*); type III dissection involves descending aorta only (*bottom left*). [From DC Miller, in RM Doroghazi, EE Slater (eds): *Aortic Dissection*. New York, McGraw-Hill, 1983, with permission.]

also increased in patients with inflammatory aortitis (i.e., Takayasu's arteritis, giant cell arteritis), congenital aortic valve anomalies (e.g., bicuspid valve), in those with coarctation of the aorta, and in otherwise normal women during the third trimester of pregnancy.

CLINICAL MANIFESTATIONS   The peak incidence is in the sixth and seventh decades. Men are more affected than women by a ratio of 2:1. The presentations of aortic dissection and its variants are the consequences of intimal tear, dissecting hematoma, occlusion of involved arteries, and compression of adjacent tissues. Acute aortic dissection presents with the sudden onset of pain (Chap. 12), which is often described as very severe and tearing and is associated with diaphoresis. The pain may be localized to the front or back of the chest, often the interscapular region, and typically migrates with propagation of the dissection. Other symptoms include syncope, dyspnea, and weakness. Physical findings may include hypertension or hypotension, loss of pulses, aortic regurgitation, pulmonary edema, and neurologic findings due to carotid artery obstruction (hemiplegia, hemianesthesia) or spinal cord ischemia (paraplegia). Bowel ischemia, hematuria, and myocardial ischemia have all been observed. These clinical manifestations reflect complications resulting from the dissection occluding the major arteries. Furthermore, clinical manifestations may result from the compression of adjacent structures (e.g., superior cervical ganglia, superior vena cava, bronchus, esophagus) by the expanding dissection causing aneurysmal dilatation, and include Horner's syndrome, superior vena caval syndrome, hoarseness, dysphagia, and airway compromise. Hemopericardium and cardiac tamponade may complicate a type A lesion with retrograde dissection. Acute aortic regurgitation is an important and common (>50%) complication of proximal dissection. It is the outcome of either a circumferential tear that widens the aortic root or a disruption of the annulus by dissecting hematoma that tears a leaflet(s) or displaces it below the line of closure. Signs of aortic regurgitation include bounding pulses, a wide pulse pressure, a diastolic murmur often radiating along the right sternal border, and evidence of congestive heart failure. The clinical manifestation depends on the severity of the regurgitation.

In dissections involving the ascending aorta, the chest x-ray often reveals a widened superior mediastinum. A pleural effusion (usually left-sided) may also be present. This effusion is typically serosanguineous and not indicative of rupture unless accompanied by hypotension and falling hematocrit. In dissections of the descending thoracic aorta, a widened mediastinum may also be observed on chest x-ray. In addition, the descending aorta may appear to be wider than the ascending portion. An electrocardiogram that shows no evidence of myocardial ischemia is helpful in distinguishing aortic dissection from myocardial infarction. Rarely, the dissection involves the right or left coronary ostium and causes acute myocardial infarction. The diagnosis of aortic dissection can be established by aortography or by the use of noninvasive techniques such as echocardiography, CT, or MRI. Aortography may be used to document the diagnosis; to identify the entry point, the intimal flap, and the false and true lumina; and to establish the extent of dissection into the major arteries. Coronary angiography may be performed concomitantly in high-risk patients in the evaluation and preparation for surgery. The sensitivity of aortography is 70% for visualizing an intimal flap, 56% for the site of intimal tear, and 87% for false lumen. It is unable to recognize intramural hemorrhage. Transthoracic echocardiography can be performed simply and rapidly and has an overall sensitivity of 60 to 85%. For diagnosing proximal ascending aortic dissections, its sensitivity exceeds 80%; it is less useful for detecting dissection of the arch and descending thoracic aorta. Transesophageal echocardiography requires greater skill and patient cooperation but is very accurate in identifying dissections of the ascending and descending thoracic aorta, but not the arch, achieving 98% sensitivity and approximately 90% specificity. Echocardiography also provides important information regarding the presence and severity of aortic regurgitation and pericardial effusion. CT and MRI are both highly accurate in identifying the intimal flap and the extent of the dissection; each has a sensitivity and specificity >90%. They are useful in recognizing intramural hemorrhage and penetrating ulcers. MRI can also detect blood flow, which may be useful in characterizing antegrade versus retrograde dissection. Transesophageal echocardiography, CT, and MRI are the diagnostic procedures of choice over contrast aortography. Their relative utility depends on the availability and expertise in individual institutions as well as on the hemodynamic stability of the patient, with CT and MRI obviously less suitable for unstable patients.

℞ TREATMENT

Medical therapy should be initiated as soon as the diagnosis is considered. The patient should be admitted to an intensive care unit for monitoring hemodynamics and urine output. Unless hypotension is present, therapy should be aimed at reducing cardiac contractility and systemic arterial pressure, and thereby shear stress. For acute dissection, unless contraindicated, β-adrenergic blockers should be administered parenterally, using intravenous propranolol, metoprolol, or the short-acting esmolol to achieve a heart rate of approximately 60 beats/min. This should be accompanied by sodium nitroprusside infusion to lower systolic blood pressure to ≤ 120 mmHg. Labetalol (Chap. 230), a drug with both β- and α-adrenergic blocking properties, is also used as a parenteral agent in the acute therapy of dissection.

The calcium channel antagonists, verapamil and diltiazem, may be used intravenously if nitroprusside or labetalol cannot be employed. The addition of a parenteral angiotensin-converting enzyme (ACE) inhibitor, such as enalaprilat, to a β-adrenergic blocker may also be considered. Isolated use of direct vasodilators, such as diazoxide and hydralazine, is contraindicated because these agents can increase hydraulic shear and may propagate dissection.

Emergent or urgent surgical correction is the preferred treatment for ascending aortic dissections (type A) and complicated type B dissections including those characterized by propagation, compromise of major aortic branches, impending rupture, or continued pain. Surgery involves excision of the intimal flap, obliteration of the false lumen, and placement of an interposition graft. A composite valve-graft conduit is used if the aortic valve is disrupted. The overall in-hospital mortality rate after surgical treatment of patients with aortic dissection is reported to be 15 to 25%. The major causes of perioperative mortality and morbidity include myocardial infarction, paraplegia, renal failure, tamponade, hemorrhage, and sepsis. Reports of the use of endoluminal stent grafts in selected patients with type B dissection are encouraging. Other transcatheter techniques, such as fenestration of the intimal flaps and stenting of narrowed branch vessels to increase flow to compromised organs, are also under investigation. For uncomplicated and stable distal dissection (type B), medical therapy is the preferred treatment. The in-hospital mortality rate of medically treated patients with type B dissection is 10 to 20%. Long-term therapy for patients with aortic dissection (with or without surgery) consists of the control of hypertension and reduction of cardiac contractility with the use of beta blockers plus other antihypertensive agents such as ACE inhibitors or calcium antagonists. Patients with chronic type B dissection should be followed on an outpatient basis every 6 to 12 months by contrast-enhanced CT or MRI to detect propagation or expansion. Patients with Marfan syndrome are at high risk for postdissection complications. The long-term prognosis for patients with treated dissections is generally good with careful follow-up; the 10-year survival rate is approximately 60%.

AORTIC OCCLUSION

CHRONIC ATHEROSCLEROTIC OCCLUSIVE DISEASE   Atherosclerosis may affect the thoracic and abdominal aorta. Occlusive aortic disease caused by atherosclerosis is usually confined to the distal abdominal aorta below the renal arteries. Frequently the disease extends to the iliac arteries (Chap. 232). Claudication characteristically involves the lower back, buttocks, and thighs and may be associated with impotence in males

(Leriche syndrome). The severity of the symptoms depends on the adequacy of collaterals. With sufficient collateral blood flow, a complete occlusion of the abdominal aorta may occur without the development of ischemic symptoms. The physical findings include absence of femoral and other distal pulses bilaterally and the detection of an audible bruit over the abdomen (usually at or below the umbilicus) and the common femoral arteries. Atrophic skin, loss of hair, and coolness of the lower extremities are usually observed. In advanced ischemia, rubor on dependency and pallor on elevation can be seen.

The diagnosis is usually established by the physical examination and noninvasive testing, including leg pressure measurements, Doppler velocity analysis, pulse volume recordings, and duplex ultrasonography. The anatomy may be defined by MRI, CT or conventional aortography before revascularization. Operative treatment is indicated in patients with debilitating symptoms and/or with the development of leg ischemia.

ACUTE OCCLUSION Acute occlusion in the distal abdominal aorta represents a medical emergency because it threatens the viability of the lower extremities. It usually results from an occlusive embolus that almost always originates from the heart. Rarely, acute occlusion may occur as the result of in situ thrombosis in a preexisting severely narrowed segment of the aorta or plaque rupture and hemorrhage into such an area.

The clinical picture is one of acute ischemia of the lower extremities. Severe rest pain, coolness, and pallor of the lower extremities and the absence of distal pulses bilaterally are the usual manifestations. Diagnosis should be established rapidly by aortography. Emergency thrombectomy or revascularization is indicated.

AORTITIS

Aortitis frequently affects the thoracic aorta and may result in aneurysmal dilatation and aortic regurgitation; it occasionally obstructs branch vessels of the aorta.

SYPHILITIC AORTITIS This late manifestation of luetic infection (Chap. 153) usually affects the proximal ascending aorta, particularly the aortic root, resulting in aortic dilatation and aneurysm formation. Syphilitic aortitis may occasionally involve the aortic arch or the descending aorta. The aneurysms may be saccular or fusiform and are usually asymptomatic, but compression of and erosion into adjacent structures may result in symptoms; rupture may also occur.

The initial lesion is an obliterative endarteritis of the vasa vasorum, especially in the adventitia. This is an inflammatory response to the invasion of the adventitia by the spirochetes. Destruction of the aortic media occurs as the spirochetes spread into this layer, usually via the lymphatics accompanying the vasa vasorum. Destruction of collagen and elastic tissues leads to dilation of the aorta, scar formation, and calcification. These changes account for the characteristic radiographic appearance of a calcified ascending aortic aneurysm.

The disease typically presents as an incidental chest radiographic finding 15 to 30 years after initial infection. Symptoms may result from aortic regurgitation, narrowing of coronary ostia due to syphilitic aortitis, compression of adjacent structures (e.g., esophagus), or rupture. Diagnosis is established by a positive serologic test, i.e., rapid plasmin reagin (RPR) or fluorescent treponemal antibody. Treatment includes penicillin and surgical excision and repair.

RHEUMATIC AORTITIS Rheumatoid arthritis (Chap. 301), ankylosing spondylitis (Chap. 305), psoriatic arthritis (Chap. 305), Reiter's syndrome (Chap. 305), relapsing polychondritis, and inflammatory bowel disorders may all be associated with aortitis involving the ascending aorta. The inflammatory lesions usually involve the ascending aorta and may extend to the sinuses of Valsalva, the mitral valve leaflets, and adjacent myocardium. The clinical manifestations are aneurysm, aortic regurgitation, and involvement of the cardiac conduction system.

TAKAYASU'S ARTERITIS This inflammatory disease often affects the ascending aorta and aortic arch causing obstruction of the aorta and its major arteries. Takayasu's arteritis is also termed *pulseless disease* because of the frequent occlusion of the large arteries originating from the aorta. It may also involve the descending thoracic and abdominal aorta and occlude large branches such as the renal arteries. Aortic aneurysms may also occur. The pathology is a panarteritis, characterized by mononuclear cells and occasionally giant cells, with marked intimal hyperplasia, medial and adventitial thickening, and, in chronic form, fibrotic occlusion. The disease is most prevalent in young females of Asian descent but does occur in women of other geographic and ethnic origins and also in young men. During the acute stage, fever, malaise, weight loss, and other systemic symptoms may be evident. An elevation of the erythrocyte sedimentation rate is common. The chronic stages of the disease present with symptoms related to large artery occlusion, such as upper extremity claudication, cerebral ischemia, and syncope. The chronic disease is intermittently active. Since the process is progressive and there is no definitive therapy, the prognosis is usually poor. Glucocorticoids and immunosuppressive agents have been reported to be effective in some patients during the acute phase. Occasionally, anticoagulation prevents thrombosis and complete occlusion of a large artery. Surgical bypass or endovascular intervention of a critically stenotic artery may be necessary.

GIANT CELL ARTERITIS (See also Chap. 306) This vasculitis occurs in older individuals and affects women more often than men. Primarily large and medium-sized arteries are affected. The pathology is that of focal granulomatous lesions involving the entire arterial wall. It may be associated with polymyalgia rheumatica. Obstruction of medium-sized arteries (e.g., temporal and ophthalmic arteries) and of major branches of the aorta and the development of aortitis and aortic regurgitation are some of the complications of the disease. High-dose glucocorticoid therapy may be effective when given early.

FURTHER READING

THE ANEURYSM DETECTION AND MANAGEMENT VETERANS AFFAIRS COOPERATIVE STUDY GROUP: Immediate repair compared with surveillance of small abdominal aortic aneurysms. N Engl J Med 346:1437, 2002

GANAHA F et al: Prognosis of aortic intramural hematoma with and without penetrating atherosclerotic ulcer. A clinical and radiological analysis. Circulation 106:342, 2002

GUO D et al: Familial thoracic aortic aneurysms and dissections: Genetic heterogeneity with a major locus mapping to 5q13-14. Circulation 103:2461, 2001

HAGAN PG et al: The International Registry of Acute Aortic Dissection (IRAD): New insights into an old disease. JAMA 283:897, 2000

HASHIMOTO H: Takayasu's arteritis and giant cell (temporal or cranial) arteritis. Intern Med 39:4, 2000

ISSELBACHER EM et al: Diseases of the aorta, in *Braunwald's Heart Disease: A Textbook of Cardiovascular Medicine,* 7th ed, DP Zipes et al (eds). Philadelphia, Saunders, 2005

THE MULTICENTRE ANEURYSM SCREENING STUDY GROUP: The Multicentre Aneurysm Screening Study (MASS) into the effect of abdominal aortic aneurysm screening on mortality in men: A randomized controlled trial. Lancet 360:1531, 2002

PARODI JC et al: Endovascular treatment of aneurysmal disease. Cardiol Clin 20:579, 2002

THE UK SMALL ANEURYSM TRIAL PARTICIPANTS: Long-term outcomes of immediate repair compared with surveillance of small abdominal aortic aneurysms. N Engl J Med 346:1445, 2002

VAUGHAN CJ et al: Identification of a chromosome 11q23.2-q24 locus for familial aortic aneurysm disease, a genetically heterogeneous disorder. Circulation 103:2469, 2001

ARTERIAL DISORDERS

PERIPHERAL ARTERIAL DISEASE Atherosclerosis is the leading cause of occlusive arterial disease of the extremities in patients over 40 years old; the highest incidence occurs in the sixth and seventh decades of life. As in patients with atherosclerosis of the coronary and cerebral vasculature, there is an increased prevalence of peripheral atherosclerotic disease in individuals with diabetes mellitus, hypercholesterolemia, hypertension, or hyperhomocysteinemia and in cigarette smokers.

Pathology (See also Chap. 224)   Segmental lesions causing stenosis or occlusion are usually localized in large and medium-sized vessels. The pathology of the lesions includes atherosclerotic plaques with calcium deposition, thinning of the media, patchy destruction of muscle and elastic fibers, fragmentation of the internal elastic lamina, and thrombi composed of platelets and fibrin. The primary sites of involvement are the abdominal aorta and iliac arteries (30% of symptomatic patients), the femoral and popliteal arteries (80 to 90% of patients), and the more distal vessels, including the tibial and peroneal arteries (40 to 50% of patients). Atherosclerotic lesions occur preferentially at arterial branch points, sites of increased turbulence, altered shear stress, and intimal injury. Involvement of the distal vasculature is most common in elderly individuals and patients with diabetes mellitus.

Clinical Evaluation   Fewer than 50% of patients with peripheral arterial disease (PAD) are symptomatic, though many have a slow or impaired gait. The most common *symptom* is intermittent claudication, which is defined as a pain, ache, cramp, numbness, or a sense of fatigue in the muscles; it occurs during exercise and is relieved by rest. The site of claudication is distal to the location of the occlusive lesion. For example, buttock, hip, and thigh discomfort occur in patients with aortoiliac disease (Leriche syndrome), whereas calf claudication develops in patients with femoral-popliteal disease. Symptoms are far more common in the lower than in the upper extremities because of the higher incidence of obstructive lesions in the former region. In patients with severe arterial occlusive disease, critical limb ischemia may develop. Patients will complain of rest pain or a feeling of cold or numbness in the foot and toes. Frequently, these symptoms occur at night when the legs are horizontal and improve when the legs are in a dependent position. With severe ischemia, rest pain may be persistent.

Important *physical findings* of PAD include decreased or absent pulses distal to the obstruction, the presence of bruits over the narrowed artery, and muscle atrophy. With more severe disease, hair loss, thickened nails, smooth and shiny skin, reduced skin temperature, and pallor or cyanosis are frequent physical signs. In addition, ulcers or gangrene may occur. Elevation of the legs and repeated flexing of the calf muscles produce pallor of the soles of the feet, whereas rubor, secondary to reactive hyperemia, may develop when the legs are dependent. The time required for rubor to develop or for the veins in the foot to fill when the patient's legs are transferred from an elevated to a dependent position is related to the severity of the ischemia and the presence of collateral vessels. Patients with severe ischemia may develop peripheral edema because they keep their legs in a dependent position much of the time. Ischemic neuritis can result in numbness and hyporeflexia.

Noninvasive Testing   The history and physical examination are usually sufficient to establish the diagnosis of PAD. An objective assessment of the severity of disease is obtained by noninvasive techniques. These include digital pulse volume recordings, Doppler flow velocity waveform analysis, duplex ultrasonography (which combines B-mode imaging and pulse-wave Doppler examination), segmental pressure measurements, transcutaneous oximetry, stress testing (usually using a treadmill), and tests of reactive hyperemia. In the presence of significant PAD, the volume displacement in the leg is decreased with each pulse, and the Doppler velocity contour becomes progressively flatter. Duplex ultrasonography is often useful in detecting stenotic lesions in native arteries and bypass grafts.

Arterial pressure can be recorded noninvasively along the legs by serial placement of sphygmomanometric cuffs and use of a Doppler device to auscultate or record blood flow. Normally, systolic blood pressure in the legs and arms is similar. Indeed, ankle pressure may be slightly higher than arm pressure due to pulse-wave reflection. In the presence of hemodynamically significant stenoses, the systolic blood pressure in the leg is decreased. Thus, if one were to obtain a ratio of the ankle and brachial artery pressures (termed the *ankle:brachial index*, or ABI), it would be ≥ 1.0 in normal individuals and <1.0 in patients with peripheral arterial disease. A ratio of <0.5 is consistent with severe ischemia.

Treadmill testing allows the physician to assess functional limitations objectively. Decline of the ankle-brachial systolic pressure ratio immediately after exercise may provide further support for the diagnosis of PAD in patients with equivocal symptoms and findings on examination. Exercise testing also allows simultaneous evaluation for the presence of coronary artery disease.

Magnetic resonance angiography and conventional contrast angiography should not be used for routine diagnostic testing but are performed prior to potential revascularization. Either test is useful in defining the anatomy to assist operative planning and is also indicated if nonsurgical interventions are being considered, such as percutaneous transluminal angioplasty (PTA) or thrombolysis. Studies have suggested that magnetic resonance angiography has diagnostic accuracy comparable to that of contrast angiography.

Prognosis   The natural history of patients with PAD is influenced primarily by the extent of coexisting coronary artery and cerebral vascular disease. Studies using coronary angiography have estimated that approximately one-half of patients with symptomatic PAD also have significant coronary artery disease. Life-table analysis has indicated that patients with claudication have a 70% 5-year and a 50% 10-year survival rate. Most deaths are either sudden or secondary to myocardial infarction. The likelihood of symptomatic progression of PAD appears less than the chance of succumbing to coronary artery disease. Approximately 75% of nondiabetic patients who present with mild to moderate claudication remain symptomatically stable or improve. Deterioration is likely to occur in the remainder, with approximately 5% of the group ultimately undergoing amputation. The prognosis is worse in patients who continue to smoke cigarettes or who have diabetes mellitus.

℞ TREATMENT

Therapeutic options include supportive measures, pharmacologic treatment, nonoperative interventions, and surgery. Supportive measures include meticulous care of the feet, which should be kept clean and protected against excessive drying with moisturizing creams. Well-fitting and protective shoes are advised to reduce trauma. Sandals and shoes made of synthetic materials that do not "breathe" should be avoided. Elastic support hose should be avoided, as they reduce blood flow to the skin. In patients with ischemia at rest, shock blocks under the head of the bed together with a canopy over the feet may improve perfusion pressure and ameliorate some of the rest pain.

Treatment of associated factors that contribute to the development of atherosclerosis should be initiated. The importance of discontinuing cigarette smoking cannot be overemphasized. The physician must assume a major role in this life-style modification. It is important to control blood pressure in hypertensive patients but to avoid hypotensive levels. Treatment of hypercholesterolemia is advocated, although reduction in cholesterol levels has not been shown unequivocally to reverse peripheral atherosclerotic lesions. However, it has been shown to prevent or to slow progression of the disease and to improve survival in patients with atherosclerosis. Patients with claudication should also be encouraged to exercise regularly and at progressively more strenuous levels. Supervised exercise training programs may improve muscle efficiency and prolong walking distance. Patients also should be advised to walk for 30 to 45 min daily, stopping at the onset of claudication and resting until the symptoms resolve before resuming ambulation.

Pharmacologic Management This form of treatment of patients with PAD has not been as successful as the medical treatment of coronary artery disease (Chap. 226). In particular, vasodilators as a class have not proved to be beneficial. During exercise, peripheral vasodilation occurs distal to sites of significant arterial stenoses. As a result, perfusion pressure falls, often to levels less than that generated in the interstitial tissue by the exercising muscle. Drugs such as α-adrenergic blocking agents, calcium channel antagonists, papaverine, and other vasodilators have not been shown to be effective in patients with PAD. Pentoxifylline, a substituted xanthine derivative, has been reported to decrease blood viscosity and to increase red cell flexibility, thereby increasing blood flow to the microcirculation and enhancing tissue oxygenation. Several placebo-controlled studies have found that pentoxifylline increased the duration of exercise in patients with claudication, but its efficacy has not been confirmed in all clinical trials.

Cilostazol, a phosphodiesterase inhibitor with vasodilator and antiplatelet properties, has been reported to increase claudication distance in multiple trials. Several studies have suggested that long-term parenteral administration of vasodilator prostaglandins decreases pain and facilitates healing of ulcers in patients with severe limb ischemia. Clinical trials with angiogenic growth factors such as vascular endothelial growth factor (VEGF) and basic fibroblast growth factor (bFGF) are proceeding. One placebo-controlled trial reported that intraarterial administration of recombinant bFGF modestly increased walking time in patients with claudication. Intramuscular gene transfer of DNA encoding VEGF or bFGF may promote collateral blood vessel growth in patients with critical limb ischemia, but evidence documenting clinical efficacy is not available and awaits the outcome of ongoing trials.

Platelet inhibitors, particularly aspirin, reduce the risk of adverse cardiovascular events in patients with peripheral atherosclerosis. Clopidogrel, a drug that inhibits platelet aggregation via its effect on ADP-dependent platelet-fibrinogen binding, appears to be more effective than aspirin in reducing cardiovascular morbidity and mortality in patients with PAD. The anticoagulants heparin and warfarin have not been shown to be effective in patients with chronic PAD but may be useful in acute arterial obstruction secondary to thrombosis or systemic embolism. Similarly, thrombolytic intervention using drugs such as streptokinase, urokinase, or recombinant tissue plasminogen activator (tPA) (alteplase) may have a role in the treatment of acute thrombotic arterial occlusion but is not effective in patients with chronic arterial occlusion secondary to atherosclerosis.

Revascularization Revascularization procedures, including nonoperative as well as operative interventions, are usually reserved for patients with progressive, severe, or disabling symptoms and ischemia at rest, as well as for individuals who must be symptom-free because of their occupation. Angiography should be performed mainly in patients who are being considered for a revascularization procedure. Nonoperative interventions include PTA, stent placement, and atherectomy (Chap. 229). PTA of the iliac artery is associated with a higher success rate than PTA of the femoral and popliteal arteries. Approximately 90 to 95% of iliac PTAs are initially successful, and the 3-year patency rate is >75%. Patency rates may be higher if a stent is placed in the iliac artery. The initial success rate for femoral-popliteal PTA is approximately 80%, with a 60% 3-year patency rate. Patency rates are influenced by the severity of pretreatment stenoses; the prognosis of

total occlusive lesions is worse than that of nonocclusive stenotic lesions.

Several operative procedures are available for treating patients with aortoiliac and femoral-popliteal artery disease. The preferred operative procedure depends on the location and extent of the obstruction(s) and general medical condition of the patient. Operative procedures for aortoiliac disease include aortobifemoral bypass, axillofemoral bypass, femoral-femoral bypass, and aortoiliac endarterectomy. The most frequently used procedure is the aortobifemoral bypass using knitted Dacron grafts. Immediate graft patency approaches 99%, and 5- and 10-year graft patency in survivors is >90 and 80%, respectively. Operative complications include myocardial infarction and stroke, infection of the graft, peripheral embolization, and sexual dysfunction from interruption of autonomic nerves in the pelvis. Operative mortality ranges from 1 to 3%, mostly due to ischemic heart disease.

Operative therapy for femoral-popliteal artery disease includes in situ and reverse autogenous saphenous vein bypass grafts, placement of polytetrafluoroethylene (PTFE) or other synthetic grafts, and thromboendarterectomy. Operative mortality ranges from 1 to 3%. The long-term patency rate depends on the type of graft used, the location of the distal anastomosis, and the patency of runoff vessels beyond the anastomosis. Patency rates of femoral-popliteal saphenous vein bypass grafts at 1 year approach 90% and at 5 years, 70 to 80%. Five-year patency rates of infrapopliteal saphenous vein bypass grafts are 60 to 70%. In contrast, 5-year patency rates of infrapopliteal PTFE grafts are <30%. Lumbar sympathectomy alone or as an adjunct to aorto-femoral reconstruction has fallen into disfavor.

Preoperative cardiac risk assessment may identify individuals especially likely to experience an adverse cardiac event during the perioperative period. Patients with angina, prior myocardial infarction, ventricular ectopy, heart failure, or diabetes are among those at increased risk. Noninvasive tests, such as treadmill testing (if feasible), dipyridamole or adenosine radionuclide myocardial perfusion imaging, dobutamine echocardiography, and ambulatory ischemia monitoring permit further stratification of patient risk (Chap. 229). Patients with abnormal test results require close supervision and adjunctive management with anti-ischemic medications. β-Adrenergic blockers reduce the risk of postoperative cardiovascular complications. It is not known whether coronary angiography and coronary arterial revascularization reduce overall perioperative mortality in high-risk patients undergoing peripheral vascular surgery, but cardiac catheterization should be considered in patients suspected of having left main or three-vessel coronary artery disease.

FIBROMUSCULAR DYSPLASIA This is a hyperplastic disorder affecting medium-sized and small arteries. It occurs predominantly in females and usually involves renal and carotid arteries but can affect extremity vessels such as the iliac and subclavian arteries. The histologic classification includes intimal, medial, and periadventitial dysplasia. Medial dysplasia is the most common type and is characterized by hyperplasia of the media with or without fibrosis of the elastic membrane. It is identified angiographically by a "string of beads" appearance caused by thickened fibromuscular ridges contiguous with thin, less involved portions of the arterial wall. When limb vessels are involved, clinical manifestations are similar to those for atherosclerosis, including claudication and rest pain. PTA and surgical reconstruction have been beneficial in patients with debilitating symptoms or threatened limbs.

THROMBOANGIITIS OBLITERANS Thromboangiitis obliterans (Buerger's disease) is an inflammatory occlusive vascular disorder involving small and medium-sized arteries and veins in the distal upper and lower extremities. Cerebral, visceral, and coronary vessels may also be affected. This disorder develops most frequently in men under age 40. The prevalence is higher in Asians and individuals of eastern European descent. While the cause of thromboangiitis obliterans is not known, there is a definite relationship to cigarette smoking in patients with this disorder.

In the initial stages of thromboangiitis obliterans, polymorphonuclear leukocytes infiltrate the walls of the small and medium-sized arteries and veins. The internal elastic lamina is preserved, and thrombus may develop in the vascular lumen. As the disease progresses, mononuclear cells, fibroblasts, and giant cells replace the neutrophils. Later stages are characterized by perivascular fibrosis and recanalization.

The clinical features of thromboangiitis obliterans often include a triad of claudication of the affected extremity, Raynaud's phenomenon (p. 1489), and migratory superficial vein thrombophlebitis. Claudication is usually confined to the calves and feet or the forearms and hands, because this disorder primarily affects distal vessels. In the presence of severe digital ischemia, trophic nail changes, painful ulcerations, and gangrene may develop at the tips of the fingers or toes. The physical examination shows normal brachial and popliteal pulses but reduced or absent radial, ulnar, and/or tibial pulses. Arteriography is helpful in making the diagnosis. Smooth, tapering segmental lesions in the distal vessels are characteristic, as are collateral vessels at sites of vascular occlusion. Proximal atherosclerotic disease is usually absent. The diagnosis can be confirmed by excisional biopsy and pathologic examination of an involved vessel.

There is no specific treatment except abstention from tobacco. The prognosis is worse in individuals who continue to smoke, but results are discouraging even in those who do stop smoking. Arterial bypass of the larger vessels may be used in selected instances, as well as local debridement, depending on the symptoms and severity of ischemia. Antibiotics may be useful; anticoagulants and glucocorticoids are not helpful. If these measures fail, amputation may be required.

VASCULITIS   Other vasculitides may affect the arteries supplying the upper and lower extremities. →*Takayasu's arteritis and giant cell (temporal) arteritis are discussed in Chap. 306.*

ACUTE ARTERIAL OCCLUSION   This results in the sudden cessation of blood flow to an extremity. The severity of ischemia and the viability of the extremity depend on the location and extent of the occlusion and the presence and subsequent development of collateral blood vessels. There are two principal causes of acute arterial occlusion: embolism and thrombus in situ.

The most common sources of arterial emboli are the heart, aorta, and large arteries. Cardiac disorders that cause thromboembolism include atrial fibrillation, both chronic and paroxysmal; acute myocardial infarction; ventricular aneurysm; cardiomyopathy; infectious and marantic endocarditis; prosthetic heart valves; and atrial myxoma. Emboli to the distal vessels may also originate from proximal sites of atherosclerosis and aneurysms of the aorta and large vessels. Less frequently, an arterial occlusion results paradoxically from a venous thrombus that has entered the systemic circulation via a patent foramen ovale or other septal defect. Arterial emboli tend to lodge at vessel bifurcations because the vessel caliber decreases at these sites; in the lower extremities, emboli lodge most frequently in the femoral artery, followed by the iliac artery, aorta, and popliteal and tibioperoneal arteries.

Acute arterial thrombosis in situ occurs most frequently in atherosclerotic vessels at the site of an atherosclerotic plaque or aneurysm and in arterial bypass grafts. Trauma to an artery may also result in the formation of an acute arterial thrombus. Arterial occlusion may complicate arterial punctures and placement of catheters. Less frequent causes include the thoracic outlet compression syndrome, which causes subclavian artery occlusion, and entrapment of the popliteal artery by abnormal placement of the medial head of the gastrocnemius muscle. Polycythemia and hypercoagulable disorders (Chaps. 95 and 103) are also associated with acute arterial thrombosis.

Clinical Features   The symptoms of an acute arterial occlusion depend on the location, duration, and severity of the obstruction. Often, severe pain, paresthesia, numbness, and coldness develop in the involved extremity within 1 h. Paralysis may occur with severe and persistent ischemia. Physical findings include loss of pulses distal to the occlusion, cyanosis or pallor, mottling, decreased skin temperature, muscle stiffening, loss of sensation, weakness, and/or absent deep tendon reflexes. If acute arterial occlusion occurs in the presence of an adequate collateral circulation, as is often the case in acute graft occlusion, the symptoms and findings may be less impressive. In this situation, the patient complains about an abrupt decrease in the distance walked before claudication occurs or of modest pain and paresthesia. Pallor and coolness are evident, but sensory and motor functions are generally preserved. The diagnosis of acute arterial occlusion is usually apparent from the clinical presentation. Arteriography is useful for confirming the diagnosis and demonstrating the location and extent of occlusion.

℞ TREATMENT

Once the diagnosis is made, the patient should be anticoagulated with intravenous heparin to prevent propagation of the clot. In cases of severe ischemia of recent onset, and particularly when limb viability is jeopardized, immediate intervention to ensure reperfusion is indicated. Endovascular or surgical thromboembolectomy or arterial bypass procedures are used to restore blood flow to the ischemic extremity promptly, particularly when a large proximal vessel is occluded.

Intraarterial thrombolytic therapy is effective when acute arterial occlusion is caused by a thrombus in an atherosclerotic vessel or arterial bypass graft. Thrombolytic therapy may also be indicated when the patient's overall condition contraindicates surgical intervention or when smaller distal vessels are occluded, thus preventing surgical access. One approach for administering intraarterial urokinase is to give 240,000 IU/h for 4 h, followed by 120,000 IU/h for a maximum of 48 h. Intraarterial recombinant tPA may be administered at infusion rates of 1 mg/h or 0.05 mg/kg per hour. Meticulous observation for hemorrhagic complications is required during intraarterial thrombolytic therapy.

If the limb is not in jeopardy, a more conservative approach that includes observation and administration of anticoagulants may be taken. Anticoagulation prevents recurrent embolism and reduces the likelihood of thrombus propagation. It can be initiated with intravenous heparin and followed by oral warfarin. Recommended dosages are the same as those used for deep vein thrombosis (see below). Emboli resulting from infectious endocarditis, the presence of prosthetic heart valves, or atrial myxoma often require surgical intervention to remove the cause.

ATHEROEMBOLISM   Atheroembolism constitutes a subset of acute arterial occlusion. In this condition, multiple small deposits of fibrin, platelet, and cholesterol debris embolize from proximal atherosclerotic lesions or aneurysmal sites. Large protruding aortic atheromas are a source of emboli that may lead to stroke and renal insufficiency as well as limb ischemia. Atheroembolism may occur after intraarterial procedures. Since the emboli tend to lodge in the small vessels of the muscle and skin and may not occlude the large vessels, distal pulses usually remain palpable. Patients complain of acute pain and tenderness at the site of embolization. Digital vascular occlusion may result in ischemia and the "blue toe" syndrome; digital necrosis and gangrene may develop (Fig. 232-1). Localized areas of tenderness, pallor, and livedo reticularis (see below) occur at sites of emboli. Skin or muscle biopsy may demonstrate cholesterol crystals.

Ischemia resulting from atheroemboli is notoriously difficult to treat. Usually neither surgical revascularization procedures nor thrombolytic therapy is helpful because of the multiplicity, composition, and distal location of the emboli. Some evidence suggests that platelet inhibitors prevent atheroembolism. Surgical intervention to remove or bypass the atherosclerotic vessel or aneurysm that causes the recurrent atheroemboli may be necessary.

THORACIC OUTLET COMPRESSION SYNDROME   This is a symptom complex resulting from compression of the neurovascular bundle (artery, vein,

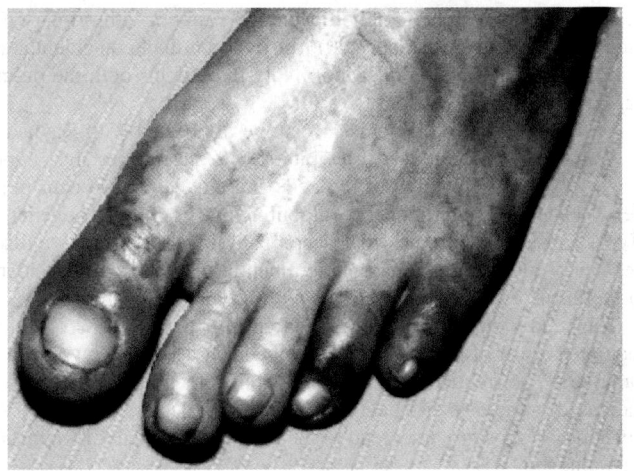

FIGURE 232-1 Atheroembolism causing cyanotic discoloration and impending necrosis of the toes (blue toe syndrome).

or nerves) at the thoracic outlet as it courses through the neck and shoulder. Cervical ribs, abnormalities of the scalenus anticus muscle, proximity of the clavicle to the first rib, or abnormal insertion of the pectoralis minor muscle may compress the subclavian artery and brachial plexus as these structures pass from the thorax to the arm. Patients may develop shoulder and arm pain, weakness, paresthesia, claudication, Raynaud's phenomenon, and even ischemic tissue loss and gangrene. Examination is often normal unless provocative maneuvers are performed. Occasionally, distal pulses are decreased or absent and digital cyanosis and ischemia may be evident. Tenderness may be present in the supraclavicular fossa. Abducting the affected arm by 90° and externally rotating the shoulder may precipitate symptoms. Several additional maneuvers are used to confirm the diagnosis of vascular compression and to suggest the location of the abnormality. These include the scalene maneuver (extension of the neck and rotation of the head to the side of the symptoms), the costoclavicular maneuver (posterior rotation of shoulders), and the hyperabduction maneuver (raising the arm 180°), which may cause subclavian bruits and loss of pulses in the arm. A chest x-ray will indicate the presence of cervical ribs. The electromyogram will be abnormal if the brachial plexus is involved.

℞ TREATMENT

Most patients can be managed conservatively. They should be advised to avoid the positions that cause symptoms. Many patients benefit from shoulder girdle exercises. Surgical procedures such as removal of the first rib or resection of the scalenus anticus muscle are necessary occasionally for relief of symptoms or treatment of ischemia.

ARTERIOVENOUS FISTULA Abnormal communications between an artery and a vein, bypassing the capillary bed, may be congenital or acquired. Congenital arteriovenous fistulas are the result of persistent embryonic vessels that fail to differentiate into arteries and veins; they may be associated with birthmarks, can be located in almost any organ of the body, and frequently occur in the extremities. Acquired arteriovenous fistulas are either created to provide vascular access for hemodialysis or occur as a result of a penetrating injury such as a gunshot or knife wound or as complications of arterial catheterization or surgical dissection. An infrequent cause of arteriovenous fistula is rupture of an arterial aneurysm into a vein.

The clinical features depend on the location and size of the fistula. Frequently, a pulsatile mass is palpable, and a thrill and bruit lasting throughout systole and diastole are present over the fistula. With long-standing fistulas, clinical manifestations of chronic venous insufficiency, including peripheral edema, large, tortuous varicose veins, and stasis pigmentation become apparent because of the high venous pressure. Evidence of ischemia may occur in the distal portion of the extremity. Skin temperature is higher over the arteriovenous fistula.

Large arteriovenous fistulas may result in an increased cardiac output with consequent cardiomegaly and high-output heart failure (Chap. 216).

Diagnosis The diagnosis is often evident from the physical examination. Compression of a large arteriovenous fistula may cause reflex slowing of the heart rate (Nicoladoni-Branham sign). Arteriography can confirm the diagnosis and is useful in demonstrating the site and size of the arteriovenous fistula.

℞ TREATMENT

Management of arteriovenous fistulas may involve surgery, radiotherapy, or embolization. Congenital arteriovenous fistulas are often difficult to treat because the communications may be numerous and extensive, and new ones frequently develop after ligation of the most obvious ones. Many of these lesions are best treated conservatively using elastic support hose to reduce the consequences of venous hypertension. Occasionally, embolization with autologous material, such as fat or muscle, or with hemostatic agents, such as gelatin sponges or silicon spheres, is used to obliterate the fistula. Acquired arteriovenous fistulas are usually amenable to surgical treatment that involves division or excision of the fistula. Occasionally, autogenous or synthetic grafting is necessary to reestablish continuity of the artery and vein.

RAYNAUD'S PHENOMENON Raynaud's phenomenon is characterized by episodic digital ischemia, manifested clinically by the sequential development of digital blanching, cyanosis, and rubor of the fingers or toes following cold exposure and subsequent rewarming. Emotional stress may also precipitate Raynaud's phenomenon. The color changes are usually well demarcated and are confined to the fingers or toes. Typically, one or more digits will appear white when the patient is exposed to a cold environment or touches a cold object. The blanching, or pallor, represents the ischemic phase of the phenomenon and results from vasospasm of digital arteries. During the ischemic phase, capillaries and venules dilate, and cyanosis results from the deoxygenated blood that is present in these vessels. A sensation of cold or numbness or paresthesia of the digits often accompanies the phases of pallor and cyanosis.

With rewarming, the digital vasospasm resolves, and blood flow into the dilated arterioles and capillaries increases dramatically. This "reactive hyperemia" imparts a bright red color to the digits. In addition to rubor and warmth, patients often experience a throbbing, painful sensation during the hyperemic phase. Although the triphasic color response is typical of Raynaud's phenomenon, some patients may develop only pallor and cyanosis; others may experience only cyanosis.

Pathophysiology Raynaud originally proposed that cold-induced episodic digital ischemia was secondary to exaggerated reflex sympathetic vasoconstriction. This theory is supported by the fact that α-adrenergic blocking drugs as well as sympathectomy decrease the frequency and severity of Raynaud's phenomenon in some patients. An alternative hypothesis is that the digital vascular responsiveness to cold or to normal sympathetic stimuli is enhanced. It is also possible that normal reflex sympathetic vasoconstriction is superimposed on local digital vascular disease or that there is enhanced adrenergic neuroeffector activity.

Raynaud's phenomenon is broadly separated into two categories: the idiopathic variety, termed *Raynaud's disease*, and the secondary variety, which is associated with other disease states or known causes of vasospasm (Table 232-1).

Raynaud's Disease This appellation is applied when the secondary causes of Raynaud's phenomenon have been excluded. Over 50% of patients with Raynaud's phenomenon have Raynaud's disease. Women are affected about five times more often than men, and the age of presentation is usually between 20 and 40 years. The fingers

TABLE 232-1   Classification of Raynaud's Phenomenon

Primary or idiopathic Raynaud's phenomenon: Raynaud's disease
Secondary Raynaud's phenomenon
  Collagen vascular diseases: scleroderma, systemic lupus
    erythematosus, rheumatoid arthritis, dermatomyositis, polymyositis
  Arterial occlusive diseases: atherosclerosis of the extremities,
    thromboangiitis obliterans, acute arterial occlusion, thoracic outlet
    syndrome
  Pulmonary hypertension
  Neurologic disorders: intervertebral disk disease, syringomyelia, spinal
    cord tumors, stroke, poliomyelitis, carpal tunnel syndrome
  Blood dyscrasias: cold agglutinins, cryoglobulinemia,
    cryofibrinogenemia, myeloproliferative disorders, Waldenström's
    macroglobulinemia
  Trauma: vibration injury, hammer hand syndrome, electric shock, cold
    injury, typing, piano playing
  Drugs: ergot derivatives, methysergide, β-adrenergic receptor
    blockers, bleomycin, vinblastine, cisplatin

are involved more frequently than the toes. Initial episodes may involve only one or two fingertips, but subsequent attacks may involve the entire finger and may include all the fingers. The toes are affected in 40% of patients. Although vasospasm of the toes usually occurs in patients with symptoms in the fingers, it may happen alone. Rarely, the earlobes and the tip of the nose are involved. Raynaud's phenomenon occurs frequently in patients who also have migraine headaches or variant angina. These associations suggest that there may be a common predisposing cause for the vasospasm.

Results of physical examination are often entirely normal; the radial, ulnar, and pedal pulses are normal. The fingers and toes may be cool between attacks and may perspire excessively. Thickening and tightening of the digital subcutaneous tissue (*sclerodactyly*) develop in 10% of patients. Angiography of the digits for diagnostic purposes is not indicated.

In general, patients with Raynaud's disease appear to have the milder forms of Raynaud's phenomenon. Fewer than 1% of these patients lose a part of a digit. After the diagnosis is made, the disease improves spontaneously in approximately 15% of patients and progresses in about 30%.

Secondary Causes of Raynaud's Phenomenon   Raynaud's phenomenon occurs in 80 to 90% of patients with systemic sclerosis (scleroderma) and is the presenting symptom in 30% (Chap. 303). It may be the only symptom of scleroderma for many years. Abnormalities of the digital vessels may contribute to the development of Raynaud's phenomenon in this disorder. Ischemic fingertip ulcers may develop and progress to gangrene and autoamputation. About 20% of patients with systemic lupus erythematosus (SLE) have Raynaud's phenomenon (Chap. 300). Occasionally, persistent digital ischemia develops and may result in ulcers or gangrene. In most severe cases, the small vessels are occluded by a proliferative endarteritis. Raynaud's phenomenon occurs in about 30% of patients with dermatomyositis or polymyositis (Chap. 369). It frequently develops in patients with rheumatoid arthritis and may be related to the intimal proliferation that occurs in the digital arteries.

Atherosclerosis of the extremities is a frequent cause of Raynaud's phenomenon in men over age 50. Thromboangiitis obliterans is an uncommon cause of Raynaud's phenomenon but should be considered in young men, particularly in those who are cigarette smokers. The development of cold-induced pallor in these disorders may be confined to one or two digits of the involved extremity. Occasionally, Raynaud's phenomenon may follow acute occlusion of large and medium-sized arteries by a thrombus or embolus. Embolization of atheroembolic debris may cause digital ischemia. The latter situation often involves one or two digits and should not be confused with Raynaud's phenomenon. In patients with the thoracic outlet syndrome, Raynaud's phenomenon may result from diminished intravascular pressure, stimulation of sympathetic fibers in the brachial plexus, or a combination

of both. Raynaud's phenomenon occurs in patients with primary pulmonary hypertension (Chap. 220); this is more than coincidental and may reflect a neurohumoral abnormality that affects both the pulmonary and digital circulations.

A variety of blood dyscrasias may be associated with Raynaud's phenomenon. Cold-induced precipitation of plasma proteins, hyperviscosity, and aggregation of red cells and platelets may occur in patients with cold agglutinins, cryoglobulinemia, or cryofibrinogenemia. Hyperviscosity syndromes that accompany myeloproliferative disorders and Waldenström's macroglobulinemia should also be considered in the initial evaluation of patients with Raynaud's phenomenon.

Raynaud's phenomenon occurs often in patients whose vocations require the use of vibrating hand tools, such as chain saws or jackhammers. The frequency of Raynaud's phenomenon also seems to be increased in pianists and keyboard operators. Electric shock injury to the hands or frostbite may lead to the later development of Raynaud's phenomenon.

Several drugs have been causally implicated in Raynaud's phenomenon. These include ergot preparations; methysergide; β-adrenergic receptor antagonists; and the chemotherapeutic agents bleomycin, vinblastine, and cisplatin.

Rx TREATMENT

Most patients with Raynaud's phenomenon experience only mild and infrequent episodes. These patients need reassurance and should be instructed to dress warmly and avoid unnecessary cold exposure. In addition to gloves and mittens, patients should protect the trunk, head, and feet with warm clothing to prevent cold-induced reflex vasoconstriction. Tobacco use is contraindicated.

Drug treatment should be reserved for the severe cases. The calcium channel antagonists, especially nifedipine and diltiazem, decrease the frequency and severity of Raynaud's phenomenon. Adrenergic blocking agents, such as reserpine, have been shown to increase nutritional blood flow to the fingers. The postsynaptic α_1-adrenergic antagonist prazosin has been used with favorable responses. Doxazosin and terazosin may also be effective. Other sympatholytic agents, such as methyldopa, guanethidine, and phenoxybenzamine, may be useful in some patients. Surgical sympathectomy is helpful in some patients who are unresponsive to medical therapy, but benefit is often transient.

ACROCYANOSIS   In this condition, there is arterial vasoconstriction and secondary dilation of the capillaries and venules with resulting persistent cyanosis of the hands and, less frequently, the feet. Cyanosis may be intensified by exposure to a cold environment. Women are affected much more frequently than men, and the age of onset is usually <30 years. Generally, patients are asymptomatic but seek medical attention because of the discoloration. Examination reveals normal pulses, peripheral cyanosis, and moist palms. Trophic skin changes and ulcerations do *not* occur. The disorder can be distinguished from Raynaud's phenomenon because it is persistent and not episodic, the discoloration extends proximally from the digits, and blanching does not occur. Ischemia secondary to arterial occlusive disease can usually be excluded by the presence of normal pulses. Central cyanosis and decreased arterial oxygen saturation are not present. Patients should be reassured and advised to dress warmly and avoid cold exposure. Pharmacologic intervention is not indicated.

LIVEDO RETICULARIS   In this condition, localized areas of the extremities develop a mottled or netlike appearance of reddish to blue discoloration. The mottled appearance may be more prominent following cold exposure. The idiopathic form of this disorder occurs equally in men and women, and the most common age of onset is in the third decade. Patients with the idiopathic form are usually asymptomatic and seek attention for cosmetic reasons. Livedo reticularis can also occur following atheroembolism (see above). Rarely, skin ulcerations develop. Patients should be reassured and advised to avoid cold environments. No drug treatment is indicated.

PERNIO (CHILBLAINS)   This is a vasculitic disorder associated with exposure to cold; acute forms have been described. Raised erythematous lesions develop on the lower part of the legs and feet in cold weather. These are associated with pruritus and a burning sensation, and they may blister and ulcerate. Pathologic examination demonstrates angiitis characterized by intimal proliferation and perivascular infiltration of mononuclear and polymorphonuclear leukocytes. Giant cells may be present in the subcutaneous tissue. Patients should avoid exposure to cold, and ulcers should be kept clean and protected with sterile dressings. Sympatholytic drugs may be effective in some patients.

ERYTHROMELALGIA (ERYTHERMALGIA)   This disorder is characterized by burning pain and erythema of the extremities. The feet are involved more frequently than the hands, and males are affected more frequently than females. Erythromelalgia may occur at any age but is most common in middle age. It may be primary or secondary to myeloproliferative disorders such as polycythemia vera and essential thrombocytosis, or it may occur as an adverse effect of drugs such as nifedipine or bromocriptine. Patients complain of burning in the extremities that is precipitated by exposure to a warm environment and aggravated by a dependent position. The symptoms are relieved by exposing the affected area to cool air or water or by elevation. Erythromelalgia can be distinguished from ischemia secondary to peripheral arterial disorders and peripheral neuropathy because the peripheral pulses are present and the neurologic examination is normal. There is no specific treatment; aspirin may produce relief in patients with erythromelalgia secondary to myeloproliferative disease. Treatment of associated disorders in secondary erythromelalgia may be helpful.

FROSTBITE   In this condition, tissue damage results from severe environmental cold exposure or from direct contact with a very cold object. Tissue injury results from both freezing and vasoconstriction. Frostbite usually affects the distal aspects of the extremities or exposed parts of the face, such as the ears, nose, chin, and cheeks. Superficial frostbite involves the skin and subcutaneous tissue. Patients experience pain or paresthesia, and the skin appears white and waxy. After rewarming, there is cyanosis and erythema, wheal-and-flare formation, edema, and superficial blisters. Deep frostbite involves muscle, nerves, and deeper blood vessels. It may result in edema of the hand or foot, vesicles and bullae, tissue necrosis, and gangrene.

Initial treatment is rewarming, performed in an environment where reexposure to freezing conditions will not occur. Rewarming is accomplished by immersion of the affected part in a water bath at temperatures of 40 to 44°C (104 to 111°F). Massage, application of ice water, and extreme heat are contraindicated. The injured area should be cleansed with soap or antiseptic and sterile dressings applied. Analgesics are often required during rewarming. Antibiotics are used if there is evidence of infection. The efficacy of sympathetic blocking drugs is not established. Following recovery, the affected extremity may exhibit increased sensitivity to cold.

DISORDERS OF THE VEINS AND LYMPHATICS
VENOUS DISORDERS

Veins in the extremities can be broadly classified as either superficial or deep. In the lower extremity, the superficial venous system includes the greater and lesser saphenous veins and their tributaries. The deep veins of the leg accompany the major arteries. Perforating veins connect the superficial and deep systems at multiple locations. Bicuspid valves are present throughout the venous system to direct the flow of venous blood centrally.

VENOUS THROMBOSIS   The presence of thrombus within a superficial or deep vein and the accompanying inflammatory response in the vessel wall is termed *venous thrombosis* or *thrombophlebitis*. Initially, the thrombus is composed principally of platelets and fibrin. Red cells become interspersed with fibrin, and the thrombus tends to propagate in the direction of blood flow. The inflammatory response in the vessel wall may be minimal or characterized by granulocyte infiltration, loss of endothelium, and edema.

TABLE 232-2 *Conditions Associated with an Increased Risk for Development of Venous Thrombosis*

Surgery
   Orthopedic, thoracic, abdominal, and genitourinary procedures
Neoplasms
   Pancreas, lung, ovary, testes, urinary tract, breast, stomach
Trauma
   Fractures of spine, pelvis, femur, or tibia; spinal cord injuries
Immobilization
   Acute myocardial infarction, congestive heart failure, stroke, postoperative convalescence
Pregnancy
Estrogen use (for replacement or contraception)
Hypercoagulable states
   Resistance to activated protein C; deficiencies of antithrombin III, protein C, or protein S; antiphospholipid antibodies; myeloproliferative diseases; dysfibrinogenemia; disseminated intravascular coagulation
Venulitis
   Thromboangiitis obliterans, Behçet's disease, homocysteinuria
Previous deep vein thrombosis

The factors that predispose to venous thrombosis were initially described by Virchow in 1856 and include stasis, vascular damage, and hypercoagulability. Accordingly, a variety of clinical situations are associated with increased risk of venous thrombosis (Table 232-2). Venous thrombosis may occur in >50% of patients having orthopedic surgical procedures, particularly those involving the hip or knee, and in 10 to 40% of patients who undergo abdominal or thoracic operations. The prevalence of venous thrombosis is particularly high in patients with cancer of the pancreas, lungs, genitourinary tract, stomach, and breast. Approximately 10 to 20% of patients with idiopathic deep vein thrombosis have or develop clinically overt cancer; there is no consensus on whether these individuals should be subjected to intensive diagnostic workup to search for occult malignancy.

The risk of thrombosis is increased following trauma, such as fractures of the spine, pelvis, femur, and tibia. Immobilization, regardless of the underlying disease, is a major predisposing cause of venous thrombosis. This fact may account for the relatively high incidence in patients with acute myocardial infarction or congestive heart failure. The incidence of venous thrombosis is increased during pregnancy, particularly in the third trimester and in the first month postpartum, and in individuals who use oral contraceptives or receive postmenopausal hormone replacement therapy. A variety of clinical disorders that produce systemic hypercoagulability, including resistance to activated protein C (factor V Leiden); prothrombin G20210A gene mutation; antithrombin III, protein C, and protein S deficiencies; antiphospholipid syndrome; hyperhomocysteinemia; SLE; myeloproliferative diseases; dysfibrinogenemia; and disseminated intravascular coagulation, are associated with venous thrombosis. Venulitis occurring in thromboangiitis obliterans, Behçet's disease, and homocysteinuria may also cause venous thrombosis.

DEEP VENOUS THROMBOSIS (DVT)   The most important consequences of this disorder are pulmonary embolism (Chap. 244) and the syndrome of chronic venous insufficiency. DVT of the iliac, femoral, or popliteal veins is suggested by unilateral leg swelling, warmth, and erythema. Tenderness may be present along the course of the involved veins, and a cord may be palpable. There may be increased tissue turgor, distention of superficial veins, and the appearance of prominent venous collaterals. In some patients, deoxygenated hemoglobin in stagnant veins imparts a cyanotic hue to the limb, a condition called *phlegmasia cerulea dolens*. In markedly edematous legs, the interstitial tissue pressure may exceed the capillary perfusion pressure, causing pallor, a condition designated *phlegmasia alba dolens*.

The diagnosis of DVT of the calf is often difficult to make at the bedside. This is so because only one of multiple veins may be involved, allowing adequate venous return through the remaining patent vessels. The most common complaint is calf pain. Examination may reveal posterior calf tenderness, warmth, increased tissue turgor or modest swelling, and, rarely, a cord. Increased resistance or pain during dorsiflexion of the foot (Homans' sign) is an unreliable diagnostic sign.

DVT occurs less frequently in the upper extremity than in the lower extremity, but the incidence is increasing because of greater utilization of indwelling central venous catheters. The clinical features and complications are similar to those described for the leg.

Diagnosis D-Dimer, a degradation product of cross-linked fibrin, is often elevated in patients with venous thrombosis. It is a sensitive, but not specific, test for venous thrombosis. The noninvasive test used most often to diagnose DVT is duplex venous ultrasonography (B-mode, i.e., two-dimensional, imaging, and pulse-wave Doppler interrogation). By imaging the deep veins, thrombus can be detected either by direct visualization or by inference when the vein does not collapse on compressive maneuvers. The Doppler ultrasound measures the velocity of blood flow in veins. This velocity is normally affected by respiration and by manual compression of the foot or calf. Flow abnormalities occur when deep venous obstruction is present. The sensitivity of duplex venous ultrasonography approaches 95% for proximal DVT and 75% for symptomatic calf vein thrombosis.

Magnetic resonance imaging (MRI) is another noninvasive means to detect DVT. Its diagnostic accuracy for assessing proximal DVT is similar to that of duplex ultrasonography. It is useful in patients with suspected thrombosis of the superior and inferior venae cavae or pelvic veins.

DVT can also be diagnosed by venography. Contrast medium is injected into a superficial vein of the foot and directed to the deep system by the application of tourniquets. The presence of a filling defect or absence of filling of the deep veins is required to make the diagnosis.

DVT must be differentiated from a variety of disorders that cause unilateral leg pain or swelling, including muscle rupture, trauma, or hemorrhage; a ruptured popliteal cyst; and lymphedema. It may be difficult to distinguish swelling caused by the postphlebitic syndrome from that due to acute recurrent DVT. Leg pain may also result from nerve compression, arthritis, tendinitis, fractures, and arterial occlusive disorders. A careful history and physical examination can usually determine the cause of these symptoms.

Rx TREATMENT

Anticoagulants (See also Chap. 244)   Prevention of pulmonary embolism is the most important reason for treating patients with DVT, since in the early stages the thrombus may be loose and poorly adherent to the vessel wall. Patients should be placed in bed, and the affected extremity should be elevated above the level of the heart until the edema and tenderness subside. Anticoagulants prevent thrombus propagation and allow the endogenous lytic system to operate. Initial therapy should include either unfractionated heparin or low-molecular-weight heparin. Unfractionated heparin should be administered intravenously as an initial bolus of 7500 to 10,000 IU, followed by a continuous infusion of 1000 to 1500 IU/h. The rate of the heparin infusion should be adjusted so that the activated partial thromboplastin time (aPTT) is approximately twice the control value. Subcutaneous injection of heparin has been used as an alternative form of therapy. In <5% of patients, heparin therapy may cause thrombocytopenia (heparin-induced thrombocytopenia, HIT). Infrequently, these patients develop arterial thrombosis and ischemia.

Low-molecular-weight (4000 to 6000 Da) heparins are as effective as or better than conventional, unfractionated heparin in preventing extension or recurrence of venous thrombosis. Depending on the specific preparation, low-molecular-weight heparin is administered subcutaneously, in fixed doses, once or twice daily; for example, the dose of enoxaparin is 1 mg/kg subcutaneously bid. The incidence of throm-

bocytopenia is less with low-molecular-weight heparin than with conventional preparations. A direct thrombin inhibitor, such as lepirudin or argatroban, may be used as initial anticoagulant therapy for patients in whom heparin is contraindicated because of HIT. Warfarin is administered during the first week of treatment with heparin and may be started as early as the first day of heparin treatment if the aPTT is therapeutic. It is important to overlap heparin treatment with oral anticoagulant therapy for at least 4 to 5 days because the full anticoagulant effect of warfarin is delayed. The dose of warfarin should be adjusted to maintain the prothrombin time at an international normalized ratio (INR) of 2.0 to 3.0.

Anticoagulant treatment is indicated for patients with proximal DVT, since pulmonary embolism may occur in ~50% of untreated individuals. The use of anticoagulants for isolated DVT of the calf is controversial. However, approximately 20 to 30% of calf thrombi propagate to the thigh, thereby increasing the risk of pulmonary embolism. The overall incidence of pulmonary embolism in patients presenting initially with deep calf vein thrombosis is 5 to 20%. Also, isolated calf vein thrombosis has been identified as a cause of embolic stroke via a patent foramen ovale.

Therefore, patients with calf vein thrombosis should either receive anticoagulants or be followed with serial noninvasive tests to determine whether proximal propagation has occurred. Anticoagulant treatment should be continued for at least 3 to 6 months for patients with acute idiopathic DVT and for those with a temporary risk factor for venous thrombosis to decrease the chance of recurrence. In a recent study of patients with idiopathic venous thromboembolism, long-term management with low-intensity warfarin using a targeted INR of 1.5 to 2.0, following at least 3 months of therapy with full-dose anticoagulation, reduced the risk of recurrent DVT and pulmonary embolism. The duration of treatment is indefinite for patients with recurrent DVT and for those in whom associated causes, such as malignancy or hypercoagulability, have not been eliminated. If treatment with anticoagulants is contraindicated because of a bleeding diathesis or risk of hemorrhage, protection from pulmonary embolism can be achieved by mechanically interrupting the flow of blood through the inferior vena cava. Inferior vena cava plication generally has been replaced by percutaneous insertion of a filter.

Thrombolytics   Thrombolytic drugs such as streptokinase, urokinase, and tPA may also be used, but there is no evidence that thrombolytic therapy is more effective than anticoagulants in preventing pulmonary embolism. However, early administration of thrombolytic drugs may accelerate clot lysis, preserve venous valves, and decrease the potential for developing postphlebitic syndrome.

Prophylaxis   Prophylaxis should be considered in clinical situations where the risk of DVT is high. Low-dose unfractionated heparin (5000 units 2 h prior to surgery and then 5000 units every 8 to 12 h postoperatively), warfarin, and external pneumatic compression are all useful. Low-dose heparin reduces the risk of DVT associated with thoracic and abdominal surgery and with prolonged bed rest. Low-molecular-weight heparins have been shown to prevent DVT in patients undergoing general or orthopedic surgery and in acutely ill medical patients. They are said to be more effective than conventional heparin and to cause an equal or lower incidence of bleeding. Danaparoid, a low-molecular-weight heparinoid, may be used for prophylaxis in patients undergoing hip surgery. Fondaparinux, a synthetic pentasaccharide capable of catalysing antithrombin-mediated inhibition of factor Xa, may be used for prophylaxis in patients undergoing major orthopedic surgery. Warfarin in a dose that yields a prothrombin time equivalent to an INR of 2.0 to 3.0 is effective in preventing DVT associated with bone fractures and orthopedic surgery. Warfarin is started the night before surgery and continued throughout the convalescent period. External pneumatic compression devices applied to the legs are used to prevent DVT when even low doses of heparin or warfarin might cause serious bleeding, as during neurosurgery or transurethral resection of the prostate.

SUPERFICIAL VEIN THROMBOSIS Thrombosis of the greater or lesser saphenous veins or their tributaries—i.e., superficial vein thrombosis—does not result in pulmonary embolism. It is associated with intravenous catheters and infusions, occurs in varicose veins, and may develop in association with DVT. Migrating superficial vein thrombosis is often a marker for a carcinoma and may also occur in patients with vasculitides, such as thromboangiitis obliterans. The clinical features of superficial vein thrombosis are easily distinguished from those of DVT. Patients complain of pain localized to the site of the thrombus. Examination reveals a reddened, warm, and tender cord extending along a superficial vein. The surrounding area may be red and edematous.

℞ TREATMENT

Treatment is primarily supportive. Initially, patients can be placed at bed rest with leg elevation and application of warm compresses. Nonsteroidal anti-inflammatory drugs may provide analgesia but may also obscure clinical evidence of thrombus propagation. If a thrombosis of the greater saphenous vein develops in the thigh and extends toward the saphenofemoral vein junction, it is reasonable to consider anticoagulant therapy to prevent extension of the thrombus into the deep system and a possible pulmonary embolism.

VARICOSE VEINS Varicose veins are dilated, tortuous superficial veins that result from defective structure and function of the valves of the saphenous veins, from intrinsic weakness of the vein wall, from high intraluminal pressure, or, rarely, from arteriovenous fistulas. Varicose veins can be categorized as primary or secondary. Primary varicose veins originate in the superficial system and occur two to three times as frequently in women as in men. Approximately half of patients have a family history of varicose veins. Secondary varicose veins result from deep venous insufficiency and incompetent perforating veins or from deep venous occlusion causing enlargement of superficial veins that are serving as collaterals.

Patients with venous varicosities are often concerned about the cosmetic appearance of their legs. Symptoms consist of a dull ache or pressure sensation in the legs after prolonged standing; it is relieved with leg elevation. The legs feel heavy, and mild ankle edema develops occasionally. Extensive venous varicosities may cause skin ulcerations near the ankle. Superficial venous thrombosis may be a recurring problem, and, rarely, a varicosity ruptures and bleeds. Visual inspection of the legs in the dependent position usually confirms the presence of varicose veins.

Varicose veins can usually be treated with conservative measures. Symptoms often decrease when the legs are elevated periodically, when prolonged standing is avoided, and when elastic support hose are worn. External compression stockings provide a counterbalance to the hydrostatic pressure in the veins. Small symptomatic varicose veins can be treated with sclerotherapy, in which a sclerosing solution is injected into the involved varicose vein and a compression bandage is applied. Surgical therapy usually involves extensive ligation and stripping of the greater and lesser saphenous veins and should be reserved for patients who are very symptomatic, suffer recurrent superficial vein thrombosis, and/or develop skin ulceration. Surgical therapy may also be indicated for cosmetic reasons.

CHRONIC VENOUS INSUFFICIENCY Chronic venous insufficiency may result from DVT and/or valvular incompetence. Following DVT, the delicate valve leaflets become thickened and contracted so that they cannot prevent retrograde flow of blood; the vein becomes rigid and thick-walled. Although most veins recanalize after an episode of thrombosis, the large proximal veins may remain occluded. Secondary incompetence develops in distal valves because high pressures distend the vein and separate the leaflets. Primary deep venous valvular dysfunction may also occur without previous thrombosis. Patients with venous insufficiency often complain of a dull ache in the leg that worsens with prolonged standing and resolves with leg elevation. Examination demonstrates increased leg circumference, edema, and su-

perficial varicose veins. Erythema, dermatitis, and hyperpigmentation develop along the distal aspect of the leg, and skin ulceration may occur near the medial and lateral malleoli. Cellulitis may be a recurring problem. Patients should be advised to avoid prolonged standing or sitting; frequent leg elevation is helpful. Graduated compression stockings should be worn during the day. These efforts should be intensified if skin ulcers develop. Ulcers should be treated with applications of wet to dry dressings and, occasionally, dilute topical antibiotic solutions. Commercially available dressings comprising antiseptic solutions and compressive bandages may be applied and should be changed weekly until healing occurs. Recurrent ulceration and severe edema may be treated by surgical interruption of incompetent communicating veins. Rarely, surgical valvuloplasty and bypass of venous occlusions are employed.

LYMPHATIC DISORDERS

Lymphatic capillaries are blind-ended tubes formed by a single layer of endothelial cells. The absent or widely fenestrated basement membrane of lymphatic capillaries allows access to interstitial proteins and particles. Lymphatic capillaries merge to form larger vessels that contain smooth muscle and are capable of vasomotion. Small and medium-sized lymphatic vessels empty into progressively larger channels, most of which drain into the thoracic duct. The lymphatic circulation is involved in the absorption of interstitial fluid and in the response to infection.

LYMPHEDEMA Lymphedema may be categorized as primary or secondary (Table 232-3). The prevalence of primary lymphedema is approximately 1 per 10,000 individuals. Primary lymphedema may be secondary to agenesis, hypoplasia, or obstruction of the lymphatic vessels. It may be associated with Turner syndrome, Klinefelter syndrome, Noonan syndrome, the yellow nail syndrome, the intestinal lymphangiectasia syndrome, and lymphangiomyomatosis. Women are affected more frequently than men. There are three clinical subtypes: congenital lymphedema, which appears shortly after birth; lymphedema praecox, which has its onset at the time of puberty; and lymphedema tarda, which usually begins after age 35. Familial forms of congenital lymphedema (Milroy's disease) and lymphedema praecox (Meige's disease) may be inherited in an autosomal dominant manner with variable penetrance; autosomal or sex-linked recessive forms are less common.

Secondary lymphedema is an acquired condition resulting from damage to or obstruction of previously normal lymphatic channels (Table 232-3). Recurrent episodes of bacterial lymphangitis, usually caused by streptococci, are a very common cause of lymphedema. The most common cause of secondary lymphedema worldwide is filariasis (Chap. 202). Tumors, such as prostate cancer and lymphoma, can also obstruct lymphatic vessels. Both surgery and radiation therapy for breast carcinoma may cause lymphedema of the upper extremity. Less common causes include tuberculosis, contact dermatitis, lymphogranuloma venereum, rheumatoid arthritis, pregnancy, and self-induced or factitious lymphedema following application of tourniquets.

Lymphedema is generally a painless condition, but patients may experience a chronic dull, heavy sensation in the leg, and most often

---

TABLE 232-3   Causes of Lymphedema

Primary
   Congenital (includes Milroy's disease)
   Lymphedema praecox (includes Meige's disease)
   Lymphedema tarda
Secondary
   Recurrent lymphangitis
   Filariasis
   Tuberculosis
   Neoplasm
   Surgery
   Radiation therapy

they are concerned about the appearance of the leg. Lymphedema of the lower extremity, initially involving the foot, gradually progresses up the leg so that the entire limb becomes edematous. In the early stages, the edema is soft and pits easily with pressure. In the chronic stages, the limb has a woody texture, and the tissues become indurated and fibrotic. At this point the edema may no longer be pitting. The limb loses its normal contour, and the toes appear square. Lymphedema should be distinguished from other disorders that cause unilateral leg swelling, such as DVT and chronic venous insufficiency. In the latter condition, the edema is softer, and there is often evidence of a stasis dermatitis, hyperpigmentation, and superficial venous varicosities.

The evaluation of patients with lymphedema should include diagnostic studies to clarify the cause. Abdominal and pelvic ultrasound and computed tomography can be used to detect obstructing lesions such as neoplasms. MRI may reveal edema in the epifascial compartment and identify lymph nodes and enlarged lymphatic channels. Lymphoscintigraphy and lymphangiography are rarely indicated, but either can be used to confirm the diagnosis or to differentiate primary from secondary lymphedema. Lymphoscintigraphy involves the injection of radioactively labeled technetium-containing colloid into the distal subcutaneous tissue of the affected extremity. In lymphangiography, contrast material is injected into a distal lymphatic vessel that has been isolated and cannulated. In primary lymphedema, lymphatic channels are absent, hypoplastic, or ectatic. In secondary lymphedema, lymphatic channels are usually dilated, and it may be possible to determine the level of obstruction.

℞ TREATMENT

Patients with lymphedema of the lower extremities must be instructed to take meticulous care of their feet to prevent recurrent lymphangitis. Skin hygiene is important, and emollients can be used to prevent drying. Prophylactic antibiotics are often helpful, and fungal infection should be treated aggressively. Patients should be encouraged to participate in physical activity; frequent leg elevation can reduce the amount of edema. Physical therapy, including massage to facilitate lymphatic drainage, may be helpful. Patients can be fitted with graduated compression hose to reduce the amount of lymphedema that develops with upright posture. Occasionally, intermittent pneumatic compression devices can be applied at home to facilitate reduction of the edema. Diuretics are contraindicated and may cause depletion of intravascular volume and metabolic abnormalities. Microsurgical lymphatico-venous anastomotic procedures have been performed to rechannel lymph flow from obstructed lymphatic vessels into the venous system.

FURTHER READING

AGNELLI G: Three months versus one year of oral anticoagulant therapy for idiopathic deep venous thrombosis. Warfarin Optimal Duration Italian Trial Investigators. N Engl J Med 345:165, 2001

BOUNAMEAUX H, PERNEGER T: Fondaparinux: A new synthetic pentasaccharide for thrombosis prevention. Lancet 359:1710, 2002

HIATT WR: Medical treatment of peripheral arterial disease and claudication. N Engl J Med 344:1608, 2001

KEARON C et al: Management of suspected deep venous thrombosis in outpatients by using clinical assessment and D-dimer testing. Ann Intern Med 135:108, 2001

McDERMOTT MM et al: The ankle brachial index is associated with leg function and physical activity: The Walking and Leg Circulation Study. Ann Intern Med 136:873, 2002

MILLER J et al: Postmenopausal estrogen replacement and risk for venous thromboembolism: A systematic review and meta-analysis for the U.S. Preventive Services Task Force. Ann Intern Med 136:680, 2002

OLIN JW: Thromboangiitis obliterans (Buerger's disease). N Engl J Med 343:864, 2000

RIDKER PM et al, on behalf of the Prevention of Recurrent Venous Thromboembolism (PREVENT) Investigators: Long-term, low-intensity warfarin therapy for the prevention of recurrent venous thromboembolism: A randomized, double-blind, placebo-controlled trial. N Engl J Med 348:1425, 2003

WIGLEY FM: Clinical practice. Raynaud's phenomenon. N Engl J Med 347:1001, 2002

233 | APPROACH TO THE PATIENT WITH DISEASE OF THE RESPIRATORY SYSTEM
Jeffrey M. Drazen, Steven E. Weinberger

Patients with disease of the respiratory system generally present because of symptoms, an abnormality on a chest radiograph, or both. These findings often lead to a set of diagnostic possibilities; the differential diagnosis is then refined on the basis of additional information gleaned from physical examination, pulmonary function testing, additional imaging studies, and bronchoscopic examination. This chapter will consider the approach to the patient based on the major patterns of presentation, focusing on the history, the physical examination, and the chest radiograph. →*For further discussion of pulmonary function testing, see Chap. 234, and of other diagnostic studies, see Chap. 235.*

CLINICAL PRESENTATION

HISTORY   Dyspnea (shortness of breath) and cough are common presenting symptoms for patients with respiratory system disease. Less common symptoms include hemoptysis (the coughing up of blood) and chest pain, often with a pleuritic quality.

Dyspnea (See also Chap. 29)   When evaluating a patient with shortness of breath, one should first determine the time course over which the symptom has become manifest. Patients who were well previously and developed *acute* shortness of breath (over a period of hours to days) can have acute disease affecting the airways (an acute attack of asthma), the pulmonary parenchyma (acute pulmonary edema or an acute infectious process such as a bacterial pneumonia), the pleural space (a pneumothorax), or the pulmonary vasculature (a pulmonary embolus). A *subacute* presentation (over days to weeks) can suggest an exacerbation of preexisting airways disease (asthma or chronic bronchitis), an indolent parenchymal infection (*Pneumocystis carinii* pneumonia in a patient with AIDS, mycobacterial or fungal pneumonia), a noninfectious inflammatory process that proceeds at a relatively slow pace (Wegener's granulomatosis, eosinophilic pneumonia, bronchiolitis obliterans with organizing pneumonia, and many others), neuromuscular disease (Guillain-Barré syndrome, myasthenia gravis), pleural disease (pleural effusion from a variety of possible causes), or chronic cardiac disease (congestive heart failure). A *chronic* presentation (over months to years) often indicates chronic obstructive lung disease, chronic interstitial lung disease, or chronic cardiac disease. Chronic diseases of airways (not only chronic obstructive lung disease but also asthma) are characterized by exacerbations and remissions. Patients often have periods when they are severely limited by shortness of breath, but these may be interspersed with periods in which symptoms are minimal or absent. In contrast, many of the diseases of pulmonary parenchyma are characterized by a slow but inexorable progression.

Other Respiratory Symptoms   *Cough* (Chap. 30) may indicate the presence of lung disease, but cough per se is not useful for the differential diagnosis. The presence of sputum accompanying the cough often suggests airway disease and may be seen in asthma, chronic bronchitis, or bronchiectasis.

Hemoptysis (Chap. 30) can originate from disease of the airways, the pulmonary parenchyma, or the vasculature. Diseases of the airways can be inflammatory (acute or chronic bronchitis, bronchiectasis, or cystic fibrosis) or neoplastic (bronchogenic carcinoma or bronchial carcinoid tumors). Parenchymal diseases causing hemoptysis may be either localized (pneumonia, lung abscess, tuberculosis, or infection with *Aspergillus*) or diffuse (Goodpasture's syndrome, idiopathic pul-

monary hemosiderosis). Vascular diseases potentially associated with hemoptysis include pulmonary thromboembolic disease and pulmonary arteriovenous malformations.

Chest pain (Chap. 12) caused by diseases of the respiratory system usually originates from involvement of the parietal pleura. As a result, the pain is accentuated by respiratory motion and is often referred to as *pleuritic*. Common examples include primary pleural disorders, such as neoplasm or inflammatory disorders involving the pleura, or pulmonary parenchymal disorders that extend to the pleural surface, such as pneumonia or pulmonary infarction.

Additional Historic Information   Information about risk factors for lung disease should be explicitly explored to assure a complete basis of historic data. A history of current and past smoking, especially of cigarettes, should be sought from all patients. The smoking history should include the number of years of smoking, the intensity (i.e., number of packs per day), and, if the patient no longer smokes, the interval since smoking cessation. The risk of lung cancer falls progressively in the decade following discontinuation of smoking, and loss of lung function above the expected age-related decline ceases with the discontinuation of smoking. Even though chronic obstructive lung disease and neoplasia are the two most important respiratory complications of smoking, other respiratory disorders (e.g., spontaneous pneumothorax, respiratory bronchiolitis–interstitial lung disease, eosinophilic granuloma of the lung, and pulmonary hemorrhage with Goodpasture's syndrome) are also associated with smoking. A history of significant secondhand (passive) exposure to smoke, whether in the home or at the workplace, should also be sought as it may be a risk factor for neoplasia or an exacerbating factor for airways disease.

The patient may have been exposed to other inhaled agents associated with lung disease, which act either via direct toxicity or through immune mechanisms (Chaps. 237 and 238). Such exposures can be either occupational or avocational, indicating the importance of detailed occupational and personal histories, the latter stressing exposures related to hobbies or the home environment. Important agents include the inorganic dusts associated with pneumoconiosis (especially asbestos and silica dusts) and organic antigens associated with hypersensitivity pneumonitis (especially antigens from molds and animal proteins). Asthma, which is more common in women than men, is often exacerbated by exposure to environmental allergens (dust mites, pet dander, or cockroach allergens in the home or allergens in the outdoor environment such as pollen and ragweed) or may be caused by occupational exposures (diisocyanates). Exposure to particular infectious agents can be suggested by contacts with individuals with known respiratory infections (especially tuberculosis) or by residence in an area with endemic pathogens (histoplasmosis, coccidioidomycosis, blastomycosis).

A history of coexisting nonrespiratory disease or of risk factors for or previous treatment of such diseases should be sought, as they may predispose a patient to both infectious and noninfectious respiratory system complications. Common examples include systemic rheumatic diseases that are associated with pleural or parenchymal lung disease (Chap. 301), metastatic neoplastic disease in the lung, or impaired host defense mechanisms and secondary infection, which occur in the case of hematologic and lymph node malignancies. Risk factors for AIDS should be sought, as the lungs are not only the most common site of AIDS-defining infection but can also be involved by noninfectious complications of AIDS (Chap. 173). Treatment of nonrespiratory dis-

TABLE 233-1 *Typical Chest Examination Findings in Selected Clinical Conditions*

Condition	Percussion	Fremitus	Breath Sounds	Voice Transmission	Adventitious Sounds
Normal	Resonant	Normal	Vesicular (at lung bases)	Normal	Absent
Consolidation or atelectasis (with patent airway)	Dull	Increased	Bronchial	Bronchophony, whispered pectoriloquy, egophony	Crackles
Consolidation or atelectasis (with blocked airway)	Dull	Decreased	Decreased	Decreased	Absent
Asthma	Resonant	Normal	Vesicular	Normal	Wheezing
Interstitial lung disease	Resonant	Normal	Vesicular	Normal	Crackles
Emphysema	Hyperresonant	Decreased	Decreased	Decreased	Absent or wheezing
Pneumothorax	Hyperresonant	Decreased	Decreased	Decreased	Absent
Pleural effusion	Dull	Decreased	Decreased[a]	Decreased[a]	Absent or pleural friction rub

[a] May be altered by collapse of underlying lung, which will increase transmission of sound.
Source: Adapted from Weinberger.

ease can be associated with respiratory complications, either because of effects on host defense mechanisms (immunosuppressive agents, cancer chemotherapy) with resulting infection or because of direct effects on the pulmonary parenchyma (cancer chemotherapy, radiation therapy, or treatment with other agents, such as amiodarone) or on the airways (β-blocking agents causing airflow obstruction, angiotensin-converting enzyme inhibitors causing cough) (Chap. 237).

Family history is important for evaluating diseases that have a genetic component. These include disorders such as cystic fibrosis, α_1-antitrypsin deficiency, pulmonary hypertension, pulmonary fibrosis, and asthma.

PHYSICAL EXAMINATION The general principles of inspection, palpation, percussion, and auscultation apply to the examination of the respiratory system. However, the physical examination should be directed not only toward ascertaining abnormalities of the lungs and thorax but also toward recognizing other findings that may reflect underlying lung disease.

On *inspection*, the rate and pattern of breathing as well as the depth and symmetry of lung expansion are observed. Breathing that is unusually rapid, labored, or associated with the use of accessory muscles of respiration generally indicates either augmented respiratory demands or an increased work of breathing. Asymmetric expansion of the chest is usually due to an asymmetric process affecting the lungs, such as endobronchial obstruction of a large airway, unilateral parenchymal or pleural disease, or unilateral phrenic nerve paralysis. Visible abnormalities of the thoracic cage include kyphoscoliosis and ankylosing spondylitis, either of which can alter compliance of the thorax, increase the work of breathing, and cause dyspnea.

On *palpation*, the symmetry of lung expansion can be assessed, generally confirming the findings observed by inspection. Vibration produced by spoken sounds is transmitted to the chest wall and is assessed by the presence or absence and symmetry of tactile fremitus. Transmission of vibration is decreased or absent if pleural liquid is interposed between the lung and the chest wall or if an endobronchial obstruction alters sound transmission. In contrast, transmitted vibration may increase over an area of underlying pulmonary consolidation. Palpation may also reveal focal tenderness, as seen with costochondritis or rib fracture.

The relative resonance or dullness of the tissue underlying the chest wall is assessed by *percussion*. The normal sound of underlying air-containing lung is resonant. In contrast, consolidated lung or a pleural effusion sounds dull, while emphysema or air in the pleural space results in a hyperresonant percussion note.

On *auscultation* of the lungs, the examiner listens for both the quality and intensity of the breath sounds and for the presence of extra, or adventitious, sounds. Normal breath sounds heard through the stethoscope at the periphery of the lung are described as *vesicular breath sounds*, in which inspiration is louder and longer than expiration. If sound transmission is impaired by endobronchial obstruction or by air or liquid in the pleural space, breath sounds are diminished in intensity or absent. When sound transmission is improved through consolidated lung, the resulting *bronchial breath sounds* have a more tubular quality and a more pronounced expiratory phase. Sound transmission can also be assessed by listening to spoken or whispered sounds; when these are transmitted through consolidated lung, *bronchophony* and *whispered pectoriloquy*, respectively, are present. The sound of a spoken E becomes more like an A, though with a nasal or bleating quality, a finding that is termed *egophony*.

The primary adventitious (abnormal) sounds that can be heard include crackles (rales), wheezes, and rhonchi. *Crackles* are the discontinuous, typically inspiratory, sound created when alveoli and small airways open and close with respiration. They are often associated with interstitial lung disease, microatelectasis, or filling of alveoli by liquid. *Wheezes*, which are generally more prominent during expiration than inspiration, reflect the oscillation of airway walls that occurs when there is airflow limitation, as may be produced by bronchospasm, airway edema or collapse, or intraluminal obstruction by neoplasm or secretions. *Rhonchi* is the term applied to the sounds created when there is free liquid in the airway lumen; the viscous interaction between the free liquid and the moving air creates a low-pitched vibratory sound. Other adventitious sounds include pleural friction rubs and stridor. The gritty sound of a *pleural friction rub* indicates inflamed pleural surfaces rubbing against each other, often during both inspiratory and expiratory phases of the respiratory cycle. *Stridor*, which occurs primarily during inspiration, represents flow through a narrowed upper airway, as occurs in an infant with croup.

A summary of the patterns of physical findings on pulmonary examination in common types of respiratory system disease is shown in Table 233-1.

A meticulous *general physical examination* is mandatory in patients with disorders of the respiratory system. Enlarged lymph nodes in the cervical and supraclavicular regions should be sought. Disturbances of mentation or even coma can occur in patients with acute carbon dioxide retention and hypoxemia. Telltale stains on the fingers point to heavy cigarette smoking; infected teeth and gums may occur in patients with aspiration pneumonitis and lung abscess.

Clubbing of the digits can be found in lung cancer, interstitial lung disease, and chronic infections in the thorax, such as bronchiectasis, lung abscess, and empyema. Clubbing can also be seen with congenital heart disease associated with right-to-left shunting and with a variety of chronic inflammatory or infectious diseases, such as inflammatory bowel disease and endocarditis. A number of systemic diseases, such as systemic lupus erythematosus, scleroderma, and rheumatoid arthritis, may be associated with pulmonary complications, even though their primary clinical manifestations and physical findings are not primarily related to the lungs. Conversely, other diseases that most commonly affect the respiratory system, such as sarcoidosis, can have findings on physical examination not related to the respiratory system, including ocular findings (uveitis, conjunctival granulomas) and skin findings (erythema nodosum, cutaneous granulomas).

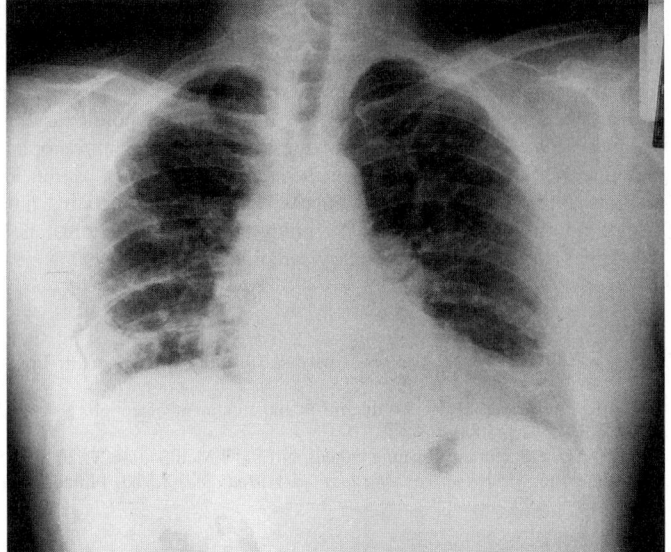

FIGURE 233-1   Posteroanterior (PA) chest radiograph of a patient with diffuse interstitial lung disease due to idiopathic pulmonary fibrosis. (*From Weinberger, with permission.*)

CHEST RADIOGRAPHY

Chest radiography is often the initial diagnostic study performed to evaluate patients with respiratory symptoms, but it can also provide the initial evidence of disease in patients who are free of symptoms. Perhaps the most common example of the latter situation is the finding of one or more nodules or masses when the radiograph is performed for a reason other than evaluation of respiratory symptoms.

A number of diagnostic possibilities are often suggested by the radiographic pattern (Figs. 233-1 and 233-2). A localized region of opacification involving the pulmonary parenchyma can be described as a nodule (usually <3 cm in diameter), a mass (usually ≥3 cm in diameter), or an infiltrate. Diffuse disease with increased opacification is usually characterized as having an alveolar, an interstitial, or a nodular pattern. In contrast, increased radiolucency can be localized, as seen with a cyst or bulla, or generalized, as occurs with emphysema. The chest radiograph is also particularly useful for the detection of pleural disease, especially if manifested by the presence of air or liquid in the pleural space. An abnormal appearance of the hila and/or the mediastinum can suggest a mass or enlargement of lymph nodes.

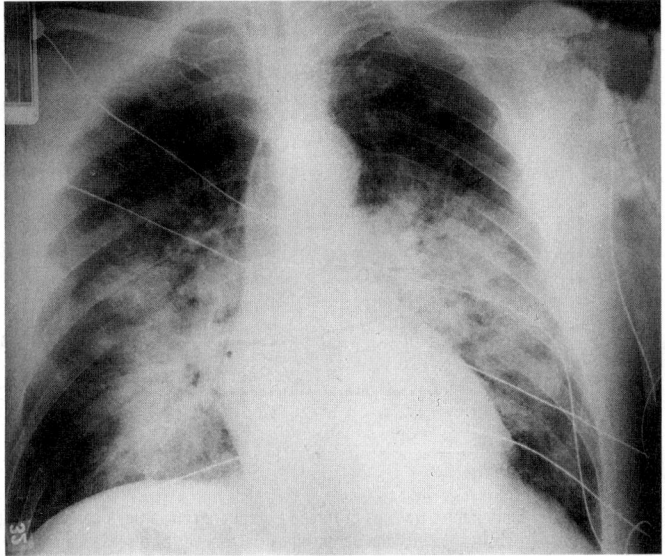

FIGURE 233-2   Anteroposterior (AP) chest radiograph demonstrating a diffuse alveolar filling pattern due to the acute respiratory distress syndrome (ARDS).

A summary of representative diagnoses suggested by these common radiographic patterns is presented in Table 233-2.

ADDITIONAL DIAGNOSTIC EVALUATION   Further information for clarification of radiographic abnormalities is frequently obtained with computed tomographic scanning of the chest (see Figs. 235-1, -2; 243-1, -2; 251-3). This technique is more sensitive than plain radiography in detecting subtle abnormalities and can suggest specific diagnoses based on the pattern of abnormality. →*For further discussion of the use of other imaging studies, including magnetic resonance imaging, scintigraphic studies, ultrasound, and angiography, see Chap. 235.*

Alteration in the function of the lungs as a result of respiratory system disease is assessed objectively by pulmonary function tests, and effects on gas exchange are evaluated by measurement of arterial blood gases or by oximetry (Chap. 234). As part of pulmonary function testing, quantitation of forced expiratory flow assesses the presence of obstructive physiology, which is consistent with diseases affecting the structure or function of the airways, such as asthma and chronic obstructive lung disease. Measurement of lung volumes assesses the presence of restrictive disorders, seen with diseases of the pulmonary parenchyma or respiratory pump and with space-occupying processes within the pleura.

Bronchoscopy is useful in some settings for visualizing abnormalities of the airways and for obtaining a variety of samples from either the airway or the pulmonary parenchyma (Chap. 235).

INTEGRATION OF THE PRESENTING CLINICAL PATTERN AND DIAGNOSTIC STUDIES

Patients with respiratory symptoms but a normal chest radiograph most commonly have diseases affecting the airways, such as asthma or chronic obstructive pulmonary disease. However, the latter diagnosis

TABLE 233-2   *Major Respiratory Diagnoses with Common Chest Radiographic Patterns*

Solitary circumscribed density—nodule (<3 cm) or mass (≥3 cm)
  Primary or metastatic neoplasm
  Localized infection (bacterial abscess, mycobacterial or fungal infection)
  Wegener's granulomatosis (one or several nodules)
  Rheumatoid nodule (one or several nodules)
  Vascular malformation
  Bronchogenic cyst

Localized opacification (infiltrate)
  Pneumonia (bacterial, atypical, mycobacterial, or fungal infection)
  Neoplasm
  Radiation pneumonitis
  Bronchiolitis obliterans with organizing pneumonia
  Bronchocentric granulomatosis
  Pulmonary infarction

Diffuse interstitial disease
  Idiopathic pulmonary fibrosis
  Pulmonary fibrosis with systemic rheumatic disease
  Sarcoidosis
  Drug-induced lung disease
  Pneumoconiosis
  Hypersensitivity pneumonitis
  Infection (*Pneumocystis*, viral pneumonia)
  Eosinophilic granuloma

Diffuse alveolar disease
  Cardiogenic pulmonary edema
  Acute respiratory distress syndrome
  Diffuse alveolar hemorrhage
  Infection (*Pneumocystis*, viral or bacterial pneumonia)
  Sarcoidosis

Diffuse nodular disease
  Metastatic neoplasm
  Hematogenous spread of infection (bacterial, mycobacterial, fungal)
  Pneumoconiosis
  Eosinophilic granuloma

is also commonly associated with radiographic abnormalities, such as diaphragmatic flattening and attenuation of vascular markings. Other disorders of the respiratory system for which the chest radiograph is normal include disorders of the respiratory pump (either the chest wall or the neuromuscular apparatus controlling the chest wall) or pulmonary circulation and occasionally interstitial lung disease. Chest examination and pulmonary function tests are generally helpful in sorting out these diagnostic possibilities. Obstructive diseases associated with a normal or relatively normal chest radiograph are often characterized by findings on physical examination and pulmonary function testing that are typical for these conditions. Similarly, diseases of the respiratory pump or interstitial diseases may also be suggested by findings on physical examination or by particular patterns of restrictive disease seen on pulmonary function testing.

When respiratory symptoms are accompanied by radiographic abnormalities, diseases of the pulmonary parenchyma or the pleura are usually present. Either diffuse or localized parenchymal lung disease is generally visualized well on the radiograph, and both air and liquid in the pleural space (pneumothorax and pleural effusion, respectively) are usually readily detected by radiography.

Radiographic findings in the absence of respiratory symptoms often indicate localized disease affecting the airways or the pulmonary parenchyma. One or more nodules or masses can suggest intrathoracic malignancy, but they can also be the manifestation of a current or previous infectious process. Patients with diffuse parenchymal lung disease on radiographic examination may be free of symptoms, as is sometimes the case with pulmonary sarcoidosis.

FURTHER READING

ALBERT RK et al (eds): *Comprehensive Respiratory Medicine*. St. Louis, Mosby, 1999

IRWIN RS, MADISON JM: The diagnosis and treatment of cough. N Engl J Med 343:1715, 2000

PATZ EF et al: Screening for lung cancer. N Engl J Med 343:1627, 2000

WEINBERGER SE: *Principles of Pulmonary Medicine*, 3d ed. Philadelphia, Saunders, 1998

234   DISTURBANCES OF RESPIRATORY FUNCTION
Steven E. Weinberger, Jeffrey M. Drazen

The respiratory system includes the lungs, the central nervous system (CNS), the chest wall (with the diaphragm and intercostal muscles), and the pulmonary circulation. The CNS controls the activity of the muscles of the chest wall, which constitute the pump of the respiratory system. Because these components of the respiratory system act in concert to achieve gas exchange, malfunction of an individual component or alteration of the relationships among components can lead to disturbances in function. In this chapter we consider three major aspects of disturbed respiratory function: (1) disturbances in ventilatory function, (2) disturbances in the pulmonary circulation, and (3) disturbances in gas exchange. →*For further discussion of disorders relating to CNS control of ventilation, see Chap. 246.*

DISTURBANCES IN VENTILATORY FUNCTION

Ventilation is the process whereby the lungs replenish the gas in the alveoli. Measurements of ventilatory function in common diagnostic use consist of quantification of the gas volume contained in the lungs under certain circumstances and the rate at which gas can be expelled from the lungs. The two measurements of lung volume commonly used for respiratory diagnosis are (1) total lung capacity (TLC), the volume of gas contained in the lungs after a maximal inspiration; and (2) residual volume (RV), the volume of gas remaining in the lungs at the end of a maximal expiration. The volume of gas that is exhaled from the lungs in going from TLC to RV is the *vital capacity* (VC) (Fig. 234-1).

Common clinical measurements of airflow are obtained from maneuvers in which the subject inspires to TLC and then forcibly exhales to RV. Three measurements are commonly made from a recording of forced exhaled volume versus time—i.e., a *spirogram*: (1) the volume of gas exhaled during the first second of expiration [forced expiratory volume (FEV) in 1 s, or FEV_1], (2) the total volume exhaled [forced vital capacity (FVC)], and (3) the average expiratory flow rate during the middle 50% of the VC [forced expiratory flow (FEF) between 25 and 75% of the VC, or $FEF_{25-75\%}$, also called the maximal midexpiratory flow rate (MMFR)] (Fig. 234-2).

PHYSIOLOGIC FEATURES

The lungs are elastic structures, containing collagen and elastic fibers that resist expansion. For normal lungs to contain air, they must be distended either by a positive internal pressure—i.e., by a pressure in

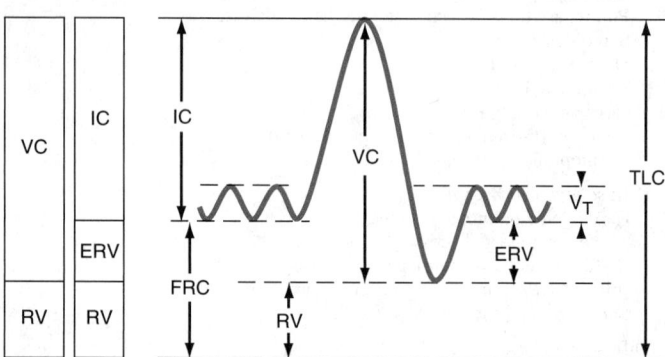

FIGURE 234-1   Lung volumes, shown by block diagrams *(left)* and by a spirographic tracing *(right)*. TLC, total lung capacity; VC, vital capacity; RV, residual volume; IC, inspiratory capacity; ERV, expiratory reserve volume; FRC, functional residual capacity; V_T, tidal volume. *(From Weinberger, with permission.)*

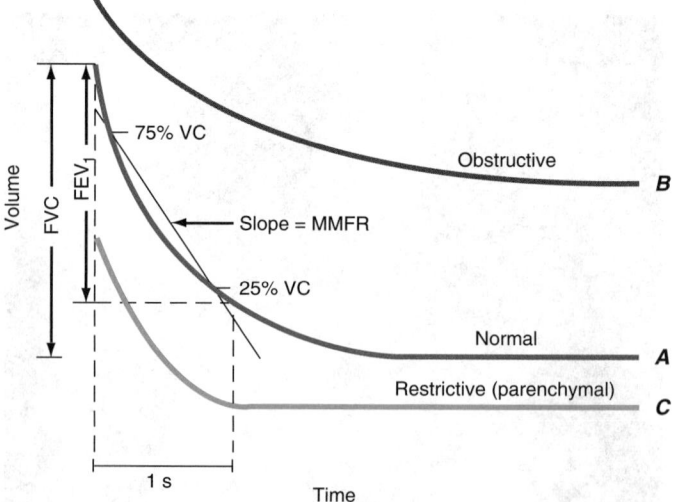

FIGURE 234-2   Spirographic tracings of forced expiration, comparing a normal tracing *(A)* and tracings in obstructive *(B)* and parenchymal restrictive *(C)* disease. Calculations of FVC, FEV_1, and $FEF_{25-75\%}$ are shown only for the normal tracing. Since there is no measure of absolute starting volume with spirometry, the curves are artificially positioned to show the relative starting lung volumes in the different conditions.

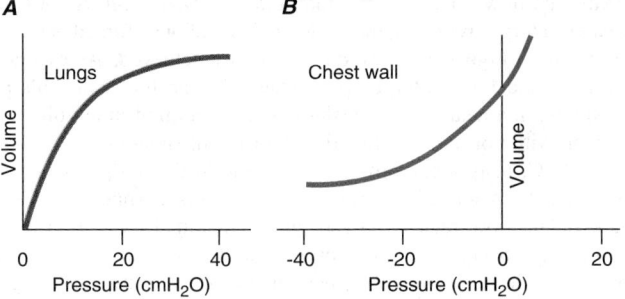

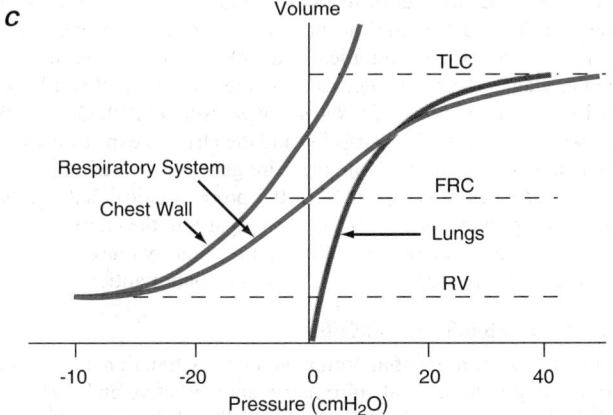

FIGURE 234-3 *A.* Pressure-volume curve of the lungs. *B.* Pressure-volume curve of the chest wall. *C.* Pressure-volume curve of the respiratory system, showing the superimposed component curves of the lungs and the chest wall. RV, residual volume; FRC, functional residual capacity; TLC, total lung capacity. *(From Weinberger, with permission.)*

the airways and alveolar spaces—or by a negative external pressure—i.e., by a pressure outside the lung. The relationship between the volume of gas contained in the lungs and the distending pressure (the *transpulmonary pressure*, or P_{TP}, defined as alveolar pressure minus pleural pressure) is described by the pressure-volume curve of the lungs (Fig. 234-3*A*).

The chest wall is also an elastic structure, with properties similar to those of an expandable and compressible spring. The relationship between the volume enclosed by the chest wall and the distending pressure for the chest wall is described by the pressure-volume curve of the chest wall (Fig. 234-3*B*). For the chest wall to assume a volume different from its resting volume, the internal or external pressures acting on it must be altered.

At functional residual capacity (FRC), defined as the volume of gas in the lungs at the end of a normal exhalation, the lungs are partially inflated, so their elastic recoil exerts a force tending to empty the lungs. At the same time, chest wall volume is such that its elastic recoil promotes outward expansion. FRC occurs at the lung volume at which the tendency of the lungs to contract is opposed by the equal and opposite tendency of the chest wall to expand (Fig. 234-3*C*).

For the lungs and the chest wall to achieve a volume other than the resting volume (FRC), either the pressures acting on them must be changed passively—e.g., by a mechanical ventilator that delivers positive pressure to the airways and alveoli—or the respiratory muscles must actively oppose the tendency of the lungs and the chest wall to return to FRC. During inhalation to volumes above FRC, the inspiratory muscles actively overcome the tendency of the respiratory system to decrease volume back to FRC. During active exhalation to volumes below FRC, expiratory muscle activity must overcome the tendency of the respiratory system to increase volume back to FRC.

At TLC, the maximal force applied by the inspiratory muscles to expand the lungs is opposed mainly by the inward recoil of the lungs. As a consequence, the major determinants of TLC are the stiffness of the lungs and inspiratory muscle strength. If the lungs become stiffer—

i.e., less compliant—TLC is decreased. If the lungs become less stiff (more compliant), TLC is increased. If the inspiratory muscles are significantly weakened, they are less able to overcome the inward elastic recoil of the lungs, and TLC is lowered.

At RV, the force exerted by the expiratory muscles to decrease lung volume further is balanced by the outward recoil of the chest wall, which becomes extremely stiff at low lung volumes. Two factors influence the volume of gas contained in the lungs at RV. The first is the ability of the subject to exert a prolonged expiratory effort, which is related to muscle strength and the ability to overcome sensory stimuli from the chest wall. The second is the ability of the lungs to empty to a small volume. In normal lungs, as P_{TP} is lowered, lung volume decreases. In lungs with diseased airways, as P_{TP} is lowered, flow limitation or airway closure may limit the amount of gas that can be expired. Consequently, either weak expiratory muscles or intrinsic airways disease can result in an elevation in measured RV.

Dynamic measurements of ventilatory function are made by having the subject inhale to TLC and then perform a forced expiration to RV. If a subject performs a series of such expiratory maneuvers using increasing muscular intensity, expiratory flow rates will increase until a certain level of effort is reached. Beyond this level, additional effort at any given lung volume will not increase the forced expiratory flow rate; this phenomenon is known as the *effort independence* of forced expiratory flow. The physiologic mechanisms determining the flow rates during this effort-independent phase of forced expiratory flow have been shown to be the elastic recoil of the lung, the airflow resistance of the airways between the alveolar zone and the physical site of flow limitation, and the airway wall compliance up to the site of flow limitation. Physical processes that decrease elastic recoil, increase airflow resistance, or increase airway wall compliance decrease the flow rate that can be achieved at any given lung volume. Conversely, processes that increase elastic recoil, decrease resistance, or stiffen airway walls increase the flow rate that can be achieved at any given lung volume.

MEASUREMENT OF VENTILATORY FUNCTION

Ventilatory function is measured under static conditions for determination of lung volumes and under dynamic conditions for determination of forced expiratory flow rates. VC, expiratory reserve volume (ERV), and inspiratory capacity (IC) (Fig. 234-1) are measured by having the patient breathe into and out of a spirometer, a device capable of measuring expired or inspired gas volume while plotting volume as a function of time. Other volumes—specifically, RV, FRC, and TLC —cannot be measured in this way because they include the volume of gas present in the lungs even after a maximal expiration. Two techniques are commonly used to measure these volumes: helium dilution and body plethysmography. In the helium dilution method, the subject repeatedly breathes in and out from a reservoir with a known volume of gas containing a trace amount of helium. The helium is diluted by the gas previously present in the lungs and very little is absorbed into the pulmonary circulation. From knowledge of the reservoir volume and the initial and final helium concentrations, the volume of gas present in the lungs can be calculated. The helium dilution method may underestimate the volume of gas in the lungs if there are slowly communicating airspaces, such as bullae. In this situation, lung volumes can be measured more accurately with a body plethysmograph, a sealed box in which the patient sits while panting against a closed mouthpiece. Because there is no airflow into or out of the plethysmograph, the pressure changes in the thorax during panting cause compression and rarefaction of gas in the lungs and simultaneous rarefaction and compression of gas in the plethysmograph. By measuring the pressure changes in the plethysmograph and at the mouthpiece, the volume of gas in the thorax can be calculated using Boyle's law.

Lung volumes and measurements made during forced expiration are interpreted by comparing the values measured with the values expected given the age, height, sex, and weight of the patient (Appendix

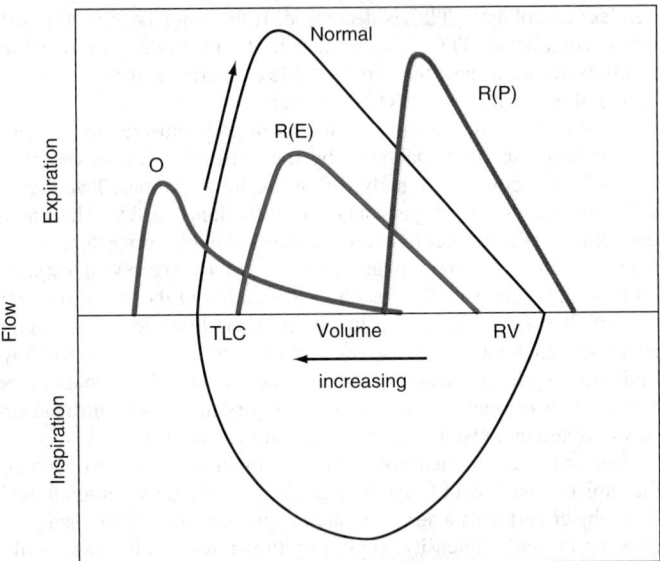

FIGURE 234-4 Flow-volume curves in different conditions: O, obstructive disease; R(P), parenchymal restrictive disease; R(E), extraparenchymal restrictive disease with limitation in inspiration and expiration. Forced expiration is plotted in all conditions; forced inspiration is shown only for the normal curve. TLC, total lung capacity; RV, residual volume. By convention, lung volume increases to the left on the abscissa. The arrow alongside the normal curve indicates the direction of expiration from TLC to RV.

Table C-4). Regression curves have been constructed on the basis of data obtained from large numbers of normal, nonsmoking individuals without evidence of lung disease. Predicted values for a given patient can then be obtained by using the patient's age and height in the appropriate regression equation; different equations are used depending on the patient's race and sex. Because there is some variability among normal individuals, values between 80 and 120% of the predicted value have traditionally been considered normal. Increasingly, calculated percentiles are used in determining normality. Specifically, values of individual measurements falling below the fifth percentile are considered to be below normal.

The normal value for the ratio FEV_1/FVC is approximately 0.75 to 0.80, although this value does fall somewhat with advancing age. The $FEF_{25-75\%}$ is often considered a more sensitive measurement of early airflow obstruction, particularly in small airways. However, this measurement must be interpreted cautiously in patients with abnormally small lungs (low TLC and VC). These patients exhale less air during forced expiration, and the $FEF_{25-75\%}$ may appear abnormal relative to the usual predicted value, even though it is normal relative to the size of the patient's lungs.

It is also a common practice to plot expiratory flow rates against lung volume (rather than against time); the close linkage of flow rates to lung volumes produces a typical *flow-volume curve* (Fig. 234-4). In addition, the spirometric values mentioned above can be calculated from the flow-volume curve. Commonly, flow rates during a maximal inspiratory effort performed as rapidly as possible are plotted as well,

making the flow-volume curve into a *flow-volume loop*. At TLC, before expiratory flow starts, the flow rate is zero; once forced expiration has begun, a high peak flow rate is rapidly achieved. As expiration continues and lung volume approaches RV, the flow rate falls progressively, in a nearly linear fashion as a function of lung volume for a person with normal lung function. During maximal inspiration from RV to TLC, inspiratory flow is most rapid at the midpoint of inspiration, so the inspiratory portion of the loop is U-shaped or saddle-shaped. The flow rates achieved during maximal expiration can be analyzed quantitatively by comparing the flow rates at specified lung volumes with the predicted values, or qualitatively by analyzing the shape of the descending limb of the expiratory curve.

Assessing the strength of respiratory muscles is an additional part of the overall evaluation of some patients with respiratory dysfunction. When a patient exhales completely to RV and then tries to inspire maximally against an occluded airway, the pressure that can be generated is called the *maximal inspiratory pressure* (MIP). On the other hand, when a patient inhales to TLC and then tries to expire maximally against an occluded airway, the pressure generated is called the *maximal expiratory pressure* (MEP). In the proper clinical setting, these studies may provide useful information regarding the cause of abnormal lung volumes and the possibility that respiratory muscle weakness may be causally related to the lung volume abnormalities.

PATTERNS OF ABNORMAL FUNCTION

The two major patterns of abnormal ventilatory function, as measured by static lung volumes and spirometry, are restrictive and obstructive patterns. In the *obstructive pattern*, the hallmark is a decrease in expiratory flow rates. With fully established disease, the ratio FEV_1/FVC is decreased, as is the $FEF_{25-75\%}$ (Fig. 234-2, line *B*). The expiratory portion of the flow-volume loop demonstrates decreased flow rates for any given lung volume. Nonuniform emptying of airways is reflected by a coved (scooped) configuration of the descending part of the expiratory curve (Fig. 234-4). With early obstructive disease, which originates in the small airways, FEV_1/FVC may be normal; the only abnormalities noted on routine testing of pulmonary function may be a depression in $FEF_{25-75\%}$ and an abnormal, i.e., coved, configuration in the terminal portion of the forced expiratory flow-volume curve.

In *obstructive* disease, the TLC is normal or increased. When helium equilibration tests are used to measure lung volumes, the measured volume may be less than the actual volume if helium was not well distributed to all regions of the lung. Residual volume is elevated as a result of airway closure during expiration, and the ratio RV/TLC is increased. VC is frequently decreased in obstructive disease because of the striking elevations in RV with only minor changes in TLC.

The hallmark of a *restrictive pattern* is a decrease in lung volumes, primarily TLC and VC. Disorders resulting in a restrictive pattern can be broadly divided into two subgroups, depending on the location of the pathology: pulmonary parenchymal and extraparenchymal. In pulmonary parenchymal disease, RV is also generally decreased, and forced expiratory flow rates are preserved. In fact, when FEV_1 is considered as a percentage of the FVC, the flow rates are often supranormal, i.e., disproportionately high relative to the size of the lungs (Fig. 234-2, line *C*). The flow-volume curve may graphically demonstrate this disproportionate relationship between flow rates and lung volumes, since the expiratory portion of the curve appears relatively tall (preserved flow rates) but narrow (decreased lung volumes), as shown in Fig. 234-4.

With extraparenchymal disease, dysfunction can be predominantly in inspiration or in both inspiration and expiration (Table 234-1). In the extraparenchymal pattern characterized by *inspiratory dysfunction*, caused by either inspiratory muscle weakness or a stiff chest wall, inadequate distending forces are exerted on an otherwise nor-

TABLE 234-1 *Alterations in Ventilatory Function*

	TLC	RV	VC	FEV_1/FVC	MIP	MEP
Obstructive	N to ↑	↑	↓	↓[a]	N	N
Restrictive						
Pulmonary parenchymal	↓	↓	↓	N to ↑	N	N
Extraparenchymal—inspiratory	↓	N to ↓	↓	N	↓/N[b]	N
Extraparenchymal—inspiratory + expiratory	↓	↑	↓	Variable	↓/N[b]	↓/N[b]

[a] Mild obstructive (small airways) disease may have decreased $FEF_{25-75\%}$ with normal (N) FEV_1/FVC.
[b] Reduced if due to respiratory muscle weakness; normal if due to chest wall stiffness.
Note: N, normal; for other abbreviations, see text.

TABLE 234-2 *Common Respiratory Diseases by Diagnostic Categories*

Obstructive
Asthma
Chronic obstructive lung disease (chronic bronchitis, emphysema)
Bronchiectasis
Cystic fibrosis
Bronchiolitis
Restrictive—Parenchymal
Sarcoidosis
Idiopathic pulmonary fibrosis
Pneumoconiosis
Drug- or radiation-induced interstitial lung disease
Restrictive—Extraparenchymal

Neuromuscular	Chest wall
Diaphragmatic weakness/paralysis	Kyphoscoliosis
Myasthenia gravis[a]	Obesity
Guillain-Barré syndrome[a]	Ankylosing spondylitis[a]
Muscular dystrophies[a]	
Cervical spine injury[a]	

[a] Can have inspiratory and expiratory limitation (see text).

mal lung. As a result, TLC values are less than predicted, RV is often not significantly affected, and expiratory flow rates are preserved. If inspiratory muscle weakness is the cause of this pattern, then MIP is decreased. In the extraparenchymal pattern characterized by *inspiratory and expiratory dysfunction*, the ability to expire to a normal RV is also limited, because of either expiratory muscle weakness or a deformed chest wall that is abnormally rigid at volumes below FRC. Consequently, RV is often elevated, unlike the pattern observed in the other restrictive subcategories. The ratio FEV_1/FVC is variable and depends on expiratory muscle strength. If expiratory muscle strength is significantly decreased, then MEP is decreased, the ability to expire rapidly is impaired, and FEV_1/FVC may be decreased even though there is no airflow obstruction. If expiratory muscle strength is normal but the chest wall is abnormally stiff below FRC, then FEV_1/FVC is normal or increased.

CLINICAL CORRELATIONS

Table 234-1 summarizes the typical patterns of altered ventilatory function as indicated by pulmonary function testing. This information can then be useful in diagnosis, as outlined in Table 234-2.

DISTURBANCES IN THE PULMONARY CIRCULATION

PHYSIOLOGIC FEATURES

The pulmonary vasculature must handle the entire output of the right ventricle, approximately 5 L/min in a normal adult at rest. The comparatively thin-walled vessels of the pulmonary arterial system provide relatively little resistance to flow and are capable of handling this large volume of blood at perfusion pressures that are low compared with those of the systemic circulation. The normal mean pulmonary artery pressure is 15 mmHg, as compared to approximately 95 mmHg for the normal mean aortic pressure. Regional blood flow in the lung is dependent on vascular geometry and on hydrostatic forces. In an upright person, perfusion is least at the apex of the lung and greatest at the base. When cardiac output increases, as occurs during exercise, the pulmonary vasculature is capable of recruiting previously unperfused vessels and distending underperfused vessels, thus responding to the increase in flow with a decrease in pulmonary vascular resistance. In consequence, the increase in mean pulmonary arterial pressure (PAP), even with a three- to fourfold increase in cardiac output, is small.

METHODS OF MEASUREMENT

Assessment of circulatory function in the pulmonary vasculature depends on measuring pulmonary vascular pressures and cardiac output. Clinically, these measurements are commonly made in intensive care units capable of invasive monitoring and in cardiac catheterization laboratories. With a flow-directed pulmonary arterial (Swan-Ganz) catheter, PAP and pulmonary capillary wedge pressure can be mea-

sured directly, and cardiac output can be obtained by the thermodilution method. Pulmonary vascular resistance (PVR) can then be calculated according to the equation

$$PVR = 80(PAP - PCW)/CO$$

where PVR = pulmonary vascular resistance ($dyn \cdot s/cm^5$); PAP = mean pulmonary arterial pressure (mmHg); PCW = pulmonary capillary wedge pressure (mmHg); and CO = cardiac output (L/min).

The normal value for pulmonary vascular resistance is approximately 50 to 150 $dyn \cdot s/cm^5$.

MECHANISMS OF ABNORMAL FUNCTION (See also Chap. 220)

PVR may increase by a variety of mechanisms. Pulmonary arterial and arteriolar vasoconstriction is a prominent response to alveolar hypoxia. PVR also increases if intraluminal thrombi or proliferation of smooth muscle in vessel walls diminishes the luminal cross-sectional area. If small pulmonary vessels are destroyed, either by scarring or by loss of alveolar walls, the total cross-sectional area of the pulmonary vascular bed diminishes, and PVR increases. When PVR is elevated, either PAP rises to maintain normal cardiac output or cardiac output falls if PAP does not increase.

CLINICAL CORRELATIONS

Disturbances in the function of the pulmonary vasculature as a result of primary cardiac disease, either congenital heart disease or conditions that elevate left atrial pressure, such as mitral stenosis, are beyond the scope of this chapter and are discussed in Chaps. 218 and 219, respectively. Instead, the focus will be on the pulmonary vasculature as its function is affected by diseases primarily involving the respiratory system, including the pulmonary vessels themselves.

All diseases of the respiratory system causing hypoxemia are potentially capable of increasing PVR, since alveolar hypoxia is a very potent stimulus for pulmonary vasoconstriction. The more prolonged and intense the hypoxic stimulus, the more likely it is that a significant increase in PVR producing pulmonary hypertension will result. In practice, patients with hypoxemia caused by chronic obstructive lung disease, interstitial lung disease, chest wall disease, and the obesity hypoventilation–sleep apnea syndrome are particularly prone to developing pulmonary hypertension. If there are additional structural changes in the pulmonary vasculature secondary to the underlying process, these will increase the likelihood of developing pulmonary hypertension.

With diseases directly affecting the pulmonary vessels, a decrease in the cross-sectional area of the pulmonary vascular bed is primarily responsible for increased PVR, while hypoxemia generally plays a lesser role. In the case of recurrent pulmonary emboli, parts of the pulmonary arterial system are occluded by intraluminal thrombi originating in the systemic venous system. With primary pulmonary hypertension (Chap. 220) or with pulmonary vascular disease secondary to scleroderma, the small pulmonary arteries and arterioles are affected by a generalized obliterative process that narrows and occludes these vessels. PVR increases, and significant pulmonary hypertension often results.

DISTURBANCES IN GAS EXCHANGE

PHYSIOLOGIC FEATURES

The primary functions of the respiratory system are to remove the appropriate amount of CO_2 from blood entering the pulmonary circulation and to provide adequate O_2 to blood leaving the pulmonary circulation. For these functions to be carried out properly, there must be adequate provision of fresh air to the alveoli for delivery of O_2 and removal of CO_2 (ventilation), adequate circulation of blood through the pulmonary vasculature (perfusion), adequate movement of gas between alveoli and pulmonary capillaries (diffusion), and appropriate contact between alveolar gas and pulmonary capillary blood (ventilation-perfusion matching).

A normal individual at rest inspires approximately 12 to 16 times per minute, each breath having a tidal volume of approximately 500 mL. A portion (approximately 30%) of the fresh air inspired with each breath does not reach the alveoli but remains in the conducting airways of the lung. This component of each breath, which is not generally available for gas exchange, is called the *anatomic dead space component*. The remaining 70% reaches the alveolar zone, mixes rapidly with the gas already there, and can participate in gas exchange. In this example, the total ventilation each minute is approximately 7 L, composed of 2 L/min of dead space ventilation and 5 L/min of alveolar ventilation. In certain diseases, some alveoli are ventilated but not perfused, so that some ventilation in addition to the anatomic dead space component is wasted. If total dead space ventilation is increased but total minute ventilation is unchanged, then alveolar ventilation must fall correspondingly.

Gas exchange is dependent on alveolar ventilation rather than total minute ventilation, as outlined below. The partial pressure of CO_2 in arterial blood (Pa_{CO_2}) is directly proportional to the amount of CO_2 produced per minute ($\dot{V}_{CO_2}$) and inversely proportional to alveolar ventilation ($\dot{V}_A$), according to the relationship

$$Pa_{CO_2} = 0.863 \times \dot{V}_{CO_2}/\dot{V}_A$$

where $\dot{V}_{CO_2}$ is expressed in mL/min, $\dot{V}_A$ in L/min, and Pa_{CO_2} in mmHg. At fixed $\dot{V}_{CO_2}$, when alveolar ventilation increases, Pa_{CO_2} falls, and when alveolar ventilation decreases, Pa_{CO_2} rises. Maintaining a normal level of O_2 in the alveoli (and consequently in arterial blood) also depends on provision of adequate alveolar ventilation to replenish alveolar O_2. This principle will become more apparent from consideration of the alveolar gas equation below.

DIFFUSION OF O_2 AND CO_2 Both O_2 and CO_2 diffuse readily down their respective concentration gradients through the alveolar wall and pulmonary capillary endothelium. Under normal circumstances, this process is rapid, and equilibration of both gases is complete within one-third of the transit time of erythrocytes through the pulmonary capillary bed. Even in disease states in which diffusion of gases is impaired, the impairment is unlikely to be severe enough to prevent equilibration of CO_2 and O_2. Consequently, a diffusion abnormality rarely results in arterial hypoxemia at rest. If erythrocyte transit time in the pulmonary circulation is shortened, as occurs with exercise, and diffusion is impaired, then diffusion limitation may contribute to hypoxemia. Exercise testing can often demonstrate such physiologically significant abnormalities due to impaired diffusion. Even though diffusion limitation rarely makes a clinically significant contribution to resting hypoxemia, clinical measurements of what is known as *diffusing capacity* (see below) can be a useful measure of the integrity of the alveolar-capillary membrane.

VENTILATION-PERFUSION MATCHING In addition to the absolute levels of alveolar ventilation and perfusion, gas exchange depends critically on the proper matching of ventilation and perfusion. The spectrum of possible ventilation-perfusion ($\dot{V}/\dot{Q}$) ratios in an alveolar-capillary unit ranges from zero, in which ventilation is totally absent and the unit behaves as a shunt, to infinity, in which perfusion is totally absent and the unit behaves as dead space. The P_{O_2} and P_{CO_2} of blood leaving each alveolar-capillary unit depend on the gas tension (of blood and air) entering that unit and on the particular $\dot{V}/\dot{Q}$ ratio of the unit. At one extreme, when an alveolar-capillary unit has a $\dot{V}/\dot{Q}$ ratio of 0 and behaves as a shunt, blood leaving the unit has the composition of mixed venous blood entering the pulmonary capillaries, i.e., $P\bar{v}_{O_2} \approx 40$ mmHg and $P\bar{v}_{CO_2} \approx 46$ mmHg. At the other extreme, when an alveolar-capillary unit has a high $\dot{V}/\dot{Q}$ ratio, it behaves almost like dead space, and the small amount of blood leaving the unit has partial pressures of O_2 and CO_2 ($P_{O_2} \approx 150$ mmHg, $P_{CO_2} \approx 0$ mmHg while breathing room air) approaching the composition of inspired gas.

In the ideal situation, all alveolar-capillary units have equal matching of ventilation and perfusion, i.e., a ratio of approximately 1 when each is expressed in L/min. However, even in the normal individual, some $\dot{V}/\dot{Q}$ mismatching is present, since there is normally a gradient of blood flow from the apices to the bases of the lungs. There is a similar gradient of ventilation from the apices to the bases, but it is less marked than the perfusion gradient. As a result, ventilation-perfusion ratios are higher at the lung apices than at the lung bases. Therefore, blood coming from the apices has a higher P_{O_2} and lower P_{CO_2} than blood coming from the bases. The net P_{O_2} and P_{CO_2} of the blood mixture coming from all areas of the lung is a flow-weighted average of the individual components, which reflects both the relative amount of blood from each unit and the O_2 and CO_2 *content* of the blood coming from each unit. Because of the sigmoid shape of the oxyhemoglobin dissociation curve (see Fig. 91-2), it is important to distinguish between the partial pressure and the content of O_2 in blood. Hemoglobin is almost fully (~90%) saturated at a P_{O_2} of 60 mmHg, and little additional O_2 is carried by hemoglobin even with a substantial elevation of P_{O_2} above 60 mmHg. On the other hand, significant O_2 desaturation of hemoglobin occurs once P_{O_2} falls below 60 mmHg and onto the steep descending limb of the curve. As a result, blood coming from regions of the lung with a high $\dot{V}/\dot{Q}$ ratio and a high P_{O_2} has only a small elevation in O_2 content and cannot compensate for blood coming from regions with a low $\dot{V}/\dot{Q}$ ratio and a low P_{O_2}, which has a significantly decreased O_2 content. Although $\dot{V}/\dot{Q}$ mismatching can influence P_{CO_2}, this effect is less marked and is often overcome by an increase in overall minute ventilation.

MEASUREMENT OF GAS EXCHANGE

ARTERIAL BLOOD GASES The most commonly used measures of gas exchange are the partial pressures of O_2 and CO_2 in arterial blood, i.e., Pa_{O_2} and Pa_{CO_2}, respectively. These partial pressures do not measure directly the quantity of O_2 and CO_2 in blood but rather the driving pressure for the gas in blood. The actual quantity or content of a gas in blood also depends on the solubility of the gas in plasma and the ability of any component of blood to react with or bind the gas of interest. Since hemoglobin is capable of binding large amounts of O_2, oxygenated hemoglobin is the primary form in which O_2 is transported in blood. The actual content of O_2 in blood therefore depends both on the hemoglobin concentration and on the Pa_{O_2}. The Pa_{O_2} determines what percentage of hemoglobin is saturated with O_2, based on the position on the oxyhemoglobin dissociation curve. Oxygen content in normal blood (at 37°C, pH 7.4) can be determined by adding the amount of O_2 dissolved in plasma to the amount bound to hemoglobin, according to the equation

$$O_2 \text{ content} = 1.34 \times [\text{hemoglobin}] \times \text{saturation} + 0.0031 \times P_{O_2}$$

since each gram of hemoglobin is capable of carrying 1.34 mL O_2 when fully saturated, and the amount of O_2 that can be dissolved in plasma is proportional to the P_{O_2}, with 0.0031 mL O_2 dissolved per deciliter of blood per mmHg P_{O_2}. In arterial blood, the amount of O_2 transported dissolved in plasma (approximately 0.3 mL O_2 per deciliter of blood) is trivial compared with the amount bound to hemoglobin (approximately 20 mL O_2 per deciliter of blood).

Most commonly, P_{O_2} is the measurement used to assess the effect of respiratory disease on the oxygenation of arterial blood. Direct measurement of O_2 saturation in arterial blood by oximetry is also important in selected clinical conditions. For example, in patients with carbon monoxide intoxication, carbon monoxide preferentially displaces O_2 from hemoglobin, essentially making a portion of hemoglobin unavailable for binding to O_2. In this circumstance, carbon monoxide saturation is high and O_2 saturation is low, even though the driving pressure for O_2 to bind to hemoglobin, reflected by P_{O_2}, is normal. Measurement of O_2 saturation is also important for the determination of O_2 content when mixed venous blood is sampled from a pulmonary arterial catheter to calculate cardiac output by the Fick technique. In mixed venous blood, the P_{O_2} is normally about 40 mmHg, but small changes in P_{O_2} may reflect relatively large changes in O_2 saturation.

A useful calculation in the assessment of oxygenation is the alveolar-arterial O_2 difference ($PA_{O_2} - Pa_{O_2}$), commonly called the *alveolar-arterial O_2 gradient* (or A − a gradient). This calculation takes into account the fact that alveolar and, hence, arterial P_{O_2} can be expected to change depending on the level of alveolar ventilation, reflected by the arterial P_{CO_2}. When a patient hyperventilates and has a low P_{CO_2} in arterial blood and alveolar gas, alveolar and arterial P_{O_2} will rise; conversely, hypoventilation and a high P_{CO_2} are accompanied by a decrease in alveolar and arterial P_{O_2}. These changes in arterial P_{O_2} are independent of abnormalities in O_2 transfer at the alveolar-capillary level and reflect only the dependence of alveolar P_{O_2} on the level of alveolar ventilation.

In order to determine the alveolar-arterial O_2 difference, the alveolar P_{O_2} (PA_{O_2}) must first be calculated. The equation most commonly used for this purpose, a simplified form of the alveolar gas equation, is

$$PA_{O_2} = FI_{O_2} \times (P_B - P_{H_2O}) - Pa_{CO_2}/R$$

where FI_{O_2} = fractional concentration of inspired O_2 (≈ 0.21 when breathing room air); P_B = barometric pressure (approximately 760 mmHg at sea level); P_{H_2O} = water vapor pressure (47 mmHg when air is fully saturated at 37°C); and R = respiratory quotient (the ratio of CO_2 production to O_2 consumption, usually assumed to be 0.8). If the preceding values are substituted into the equation for the patient breathing air at sea level, the equation becomes

$$PA_{O_2} = 150 - 1.25 \times Pa_{CO_2}$$

The alveolar-arterial O_2 difference can then be calculated by subtracting measured Pa_{O_2} from calculated PA_{O_2}. In a healthy young person breathing room air, the $PA_{O_2} - Pa_{O_2}$ is normally less than 15 mmHg; this value increases with age and may be as high as 30 mmHg in elderly patients.

The adequacy of CO_2 elimination is measured by the partial pressure of CO_2 in arterial blood, i.e., Pa_{CO_2}. A more complete understanding of the mechanisms and chronicity of abnormal levels of P_{CO_2} also requires measurement of pH and/or bicarbonate (HCO_3^-), since P_{CO_2} and the patient's acid-base status are so closely intertwined (Chap. 42).

PULSE OXIMETRY Because measurement of Pa_{O_2} requires arterial puncture, it is not ideal either for office use or for routine or frequent measurement in the inpatient setting. Additionally, because it provides intermittent rather than continuous data about the patient's oxygenation, it is not ideal for close monitoring of unstable patients. Pulse oximetry, an alternative method for assessing oxygenation, is readily available in many clinical settings. Using a probe usually clipped over a patient's finger, the pulse oximeter calculates oxygen saturation (rather than Pa_{O_2}) based on measurements of absorption of two wavelengths of light by hemoglobin in pulsatile, cutaneous arterial blood. Because of differential absorption of the two wavelengths of light by oxygenated and nonoxygenated hemoglobin, the percentage of hemoglobin that is saturated with oxygen, i.e., the Sa_{O_2}, can be calculated and displayed instantaneously.

Although the pulse oximeter has been a major advance in the noninvasive, continuous monitoring of oxygenation, there are several issues and potential problems concerning its use. First, the clinician must be aware of the relationship between oxygen saturation and tension as shown by the oxyhemoglobin dissociation curve (see Fig. 91-2). Because the curve becomes relatively flat above an arterial P_{O_2} of 60 mmHg (corresponding to Sa_{O_2} = 90%), the oximeter is relatively insensitive to changes in Pa_{O_2} above this level. In addition, the position of the curve and therefore the specific relationship between Pa_{O_2} and Sa_{O_2} may change depending on factors such as temperature, pH, and the erythrocyte concentration of 2,3-diphosphoglycerate. Second, when cutaneous perfusion is decreased, e.g., owing to low cardiac output or the use of vasoconstrictors, the signal from the oximeter may be less reliable or even unobtainable. Third, other forms of hemoglobin, such as carboxyhemoglobin and methemoglobin, are not distinguishable from oxyhemoglobin when only two wavelengths of light are used. The Sa_{O_2} values reported by the pulse oximeter are not reliable in the presence of significant amounts of either of these forms of hemoglobin. In contrast, the device used to measure oxygen saturation in samples of arterial blood, called the CO-oximeter, uses at least four wavelengths of light and is capable of distinguishing oxyhemoglobin, deoxygenated hemoglobin, carboxyhemoglobin, and methemoglobin. Finally, the clinician must remember that the often-used goal of $Sa_{O_2} \geq 90\%$ does not indicate anything about CO_2 elimination and therefore does not ensure a clinically acceptable P_{CO_2}.

DIFFUSING CAPACITY The ability of gas to diffuse across the alveolar-capillary membrane is ordinarily assessed by the diffusing capacity of the lung for carbon monoxide (DL_{CO}). In this test, a small concentration of carbon monoxide (0.3%) is inhaled, usually in a single breath that is held for approximately 10 s. The carbon monoxide is diluted by the gas already present in the alveoli and is also taken up by hemoglobin as the erythrocytes course through the pulmonary capillary system. The concentration of carbon monoxide in exhaled gas is measured, and DL_{CO} is calculated as the quantity of carbon monoxide absorbed per minute per mmHg pressure gradient from the alveoli to the pulmonary capillaries. The value obtained for DL_{CO} depends on the alveolar-capillary surface area available for gas exchange and on the pulmonary capillary blood volume. In addition, the thickness of the alveolar-capillary membrane, the degree of $\dot{V}/\dot{Q}$ mismatching, and the patient's hemoglobin level will affect the measurement. Because of this effect of hemoglobin levels on DL_{CO}, the measured DL_{CO} is frequently corrected to take the patient's hemoglobin level into account. The value for DL_{CO}, ideally corrected for hemoglobin, can then be compared with a predicted value, based either on age, height, and gender or on the alveolar volume (VA) at which the value was obtained. Alternatively, the DL_{CO} can be divided by VA and the resulting value for DL_{CO}/VA compared with a predicted value.

APPROACH TO THE PATIENT

ARTERIAL BLOOD GASES Hypoxemia is a common manifestation of a variety of diseases affecting the lungs or other parts of the respiratory system. The broad clinical problem of hypoxemia is often best characterized according to the underlying mechanism. The four basic, and not mutually exclusive, mechanisms of hypoxemia are (1) a decrease in inspired P_{O_2}, (2) hypoventilation, (3) shunting, and (4) $\dot{V}/\dot{Q}$ mismatching. Hypoxemia due to decreased diffusion occurs only under selected clinical circumstances and is not usually included among the general categories of hypoxemia. Determining the underlying mechanism for hypoxemia depends on measurement of the Pa_{CO_2}, calculation of $PA_{O_2} - Pa_{O_2}$, and knowledge of the response to supplemental O_2. A flowchart summarizing the approach to the hypoxemic patient is given in Fig. 234-5. →*See also Chap. 31.*

A decrease in the inspired P_{O_2} and hypoventilation both cause hypoxemia by lowering PA_{O_2} and therefore Pa_{O_2}. In each case, gas exchange at the alveolar-capillary level occurs normally, and $PA_{O_2} - Pa_{O_2}$ is not elevated. Hypoxemia due to decreased inspired P_{O_2} can be diagnosed from knowledge of the clinical situation. Inspired P_{O_2} is lowered either because the patient is at a high altitude, where barometric pressure is low, or, much less commonly, because the patient is breathing a gas mixture containing less than 21% O_2. The hallmark of hypoventilation as a cause of hypoxemia is an elevation in Pa_{CO_2}. This is associated with an increase in PA_{CO_2} and a fall in PA_{O_2}. When hypoxemia is due purely to a low inspired P_{O_2} or to alveolar hypoventilation, $PA_{O_2} - Pa_{O_2}$ is normal. If $PA_{O_2} - Pa_{O_2}$ and Pa_{CO_2} are both elevated, then an additional mechanism, such as $\dot{V}/\dot{Q}$ mismatching or shunting, is contributing to hypoxemia.

Shunting is a cause of hypoxemia when desaturated blood effectively bypasses oxygenation at the alveolar-capillary level. This situation occurs either because a structural problem allows desaturated blood to bypass the normal site of gas exchange or because

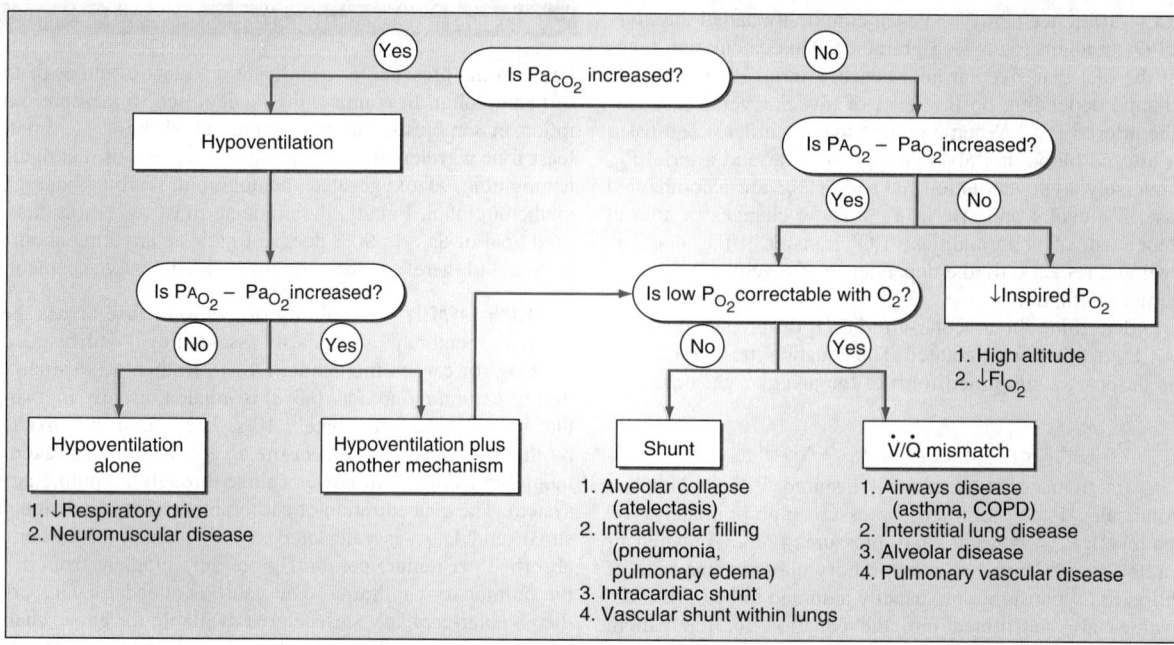

FIGURE 234-5 Flow diagram outlining the diagnostic approach to the patient with hypoxemia ($Pa_{O_2} < 80$ mmHg). $PA_{O_2} - Pa_{O_2}$ is usually < 15 mmHg for subjects ≤ 30 years old and increases by ~ 3 mmHg per decade after age 30. COPD, chronic obstructive pulmonary disease.

perfused alveoli are not ventilated. Shunting is associated with an elevation in the $PA_{O_2} - Pa_{O_2}$ value. When shunting is an important contributing factor to hypoxemia, the lowered Pa_{O_2} is relatively refractory to improvement by supplemental O_2.

Finally, the largest clinical category of hypoxemia is $\dot{V}/\dot{Q}$ mismatching. With $\dot{V}/\dot{Q}$ mismatching, regions with low $\dot{V}/\dot{Q}$ ratios contribute blood with a low P_{O_2} and a low O_2 content. Corresponding regions with high $\dot{V}/\dot{Q}$ ratios contribute blood with a high P_{O_2}. However, because blood is already almost fully saturated at a normal P_{O_2}, elevation of the P_{O_2} to a high value does not significantly increase O_2 saturation or content and therefore cannot compensate for the reduction of O_2 saturation and content in blood coming from regions with a low $\dot{V}/\dot{Q}$ ratio. When $\dot{V}/\dot{Q}$ mismatch is the primary cause of hypoxemia, $PA_{O_2} - Pa_{O_2}$ is elevated, and P_{CO_2} generally is normal. Supplemental O_2 corrects the hypoxemia by raising the P_{O_2} in blood coming from regions with a low $\dot{V}/\dot{Q}$ ratio; this response distinguishes hypoxemia due to $\dot{V}/\dot{Q}$ mismatching from that due to true shunt.

The essential mechanism underlying all cases of hypercapnia is alveolar ventilation that is inadequate for the amount of CO_2 produced. It is conceptually useful to characterize CO_2 retention further, based on a more detailed examination of the potential contributing factors. These include (1) increased CO_2 production; (2) decreased ventilatory drive ("won't breathe"); (3) malfunction of the respiratory pump or increased airways resistance, which makes it more difficult to sustain adequate ventilation ("can't breathe"); and (4) inefficiency of gas exchange (increased dead space or $\dot{V}/\dot{Q}$ mismatch) necessitating a compensatory increase in overall minute ventilation. In practice, more than one of these mechanisms is commonly responsible for hypercapnia, since increased minute ventilation is capable of compensating for increased CO_2 production and for inefficiencies of gas exchange.

DIFFUSING CAPACITY Although abnormalities in diffusion are rarely responsible for hypoxemia, clinical measurement of diffusing capacity is frequently used to assess the functional integrity of the alveolar-capillary membrane, which includes the pulmonary capillary bed. Diseases that affect solely the airways generally do not lower DL_{CO}, whereas diseases that affect the alveolar walls or the pulmonary capillary bed will have an effect on DL_{CO}. Even though DL_{CO} is a useful marker for assessing whether disease affecting the alveolar-capillary bed is present, an abnormal DL_{CO} does not necessarily imply that diffusion limitation is responsible for hypoxemia in a particular patient.

CLINICAL CORRELATIONS

Useful clinical correlations can be made with the mechanisms underlying hypoxemia (Fig. 234-5). A lowered inspired P_{O_2} contributes to hypoxemia if either the patient is at high altitude or the concentration of inspired O_2 is less than 21%. The latter problem occurs if a patient receiving anesthesia or ventilatory support is inadvertently given a gas mixture to breathe containing less than 21% O_2 or if O_2 is consumed from the ambient gas, as can occur during smoke inhalation from a fire. The primary feature of hypoventilation as a cause of hypoxemia is an elevation in arterial P_{CO_2}. →*For further discussion of the clinical correlations with hypoventilation, see Chap. 246.*

Shunting as a cause of hypoxemia can reflect transfer of blood from the right to the left side of the heart without passage through the pulmonary circulation, as occurs with an intracardiac shunt. This problem is most common in the setting of cyanotic congenital heart disease, when an interatrial or interventricular septal defect is associated with pulmonary hypertension so that shunting is in the right-to-left rather than the left-to-right direction. Shunting of blood through the pulmonary parenchyma is most frequently due to disease causing absence of ventilation to perfused alveoli. This can occur if the alveoli are atelectatic or if they are filled with fluid, as in pulmonary edema (both cardiogenic and noncardiogenic), or with extensive intraalveolar exudation of fluid due to pneumonia. Less commonly, vascular anomalies with arteriovenous shunting in the lung can cause hypoxemia. These anomalies can be hereditary, as found with hereditary hemorrhagic telangiectasia (Osler-Rendu-Weber syndrome), or acquired, as in pulmonary vascular malformations secondary to hepatic cirrhosis, which are similar to the commonly recognized cutaneous vascular malformations ("spider hemangiomas").

Ventilation-perfusion mismatch is the most common cause of hypoxemia clinically. Most of the processes affecting either the airways or the pulmonary parenchyma are distributed unevenly throughout the lungs and do not necessarily affect ventilation and perfusion equally. Some areas of lung may have good perfusion and poor ventilation, whereas others may have poor perfusion and relatively good ventilation. Important examples of airways diseases in which $\dot{V}/\dot{Q}$ mismatch causes hypoxemia are asthma and chronic obstructive lung disease.

Parenchymal lung diseases causing $\dot{V}/\dot{Q}$ mismatch and hypoxemia include interstitial lung disease and pneumonia.

Clinically important alterations in CO_2 elimination range from excessive ventilation and hypocapnia to inadequate CO_2 elimination and hypercapnia. →*For further discussion of these clinical problems, see Chap. 246.*

DIFFUSING CAPACITY Measurement of DL_{CO} may be useful for assessing disease affecting the alveolar-capillary bed or the pulmonary vasculature. In practice, three main categories of disease are associated with lowered DL_{CO}: interstitial lung disease, emphysema, and pulmonary vascular disease. With interstitial lung disease, scarring of alveolar-capillary units diminishes the area of the alveolar-capillary bed as well as pulmonary blood volume. With emphysema, alveolar walls are destroyed, so the surface area of the alveolar-capillary bed is again diminished. In patients with disease causing a decrease in the cross-sectional area and volume of the pulmonary vascular bed, such as recurrent pulmonary emboli or primary pulmonary hypertension, DL_{CO} is commonly diminished.

Diffusing capacity may be elevated if pulmonary blood volume is increased, as may be seen in congestive heart failure. However, once interstitial and alveolar edema ensue, the net DL_{CO} depends on the opposing influences of increased pulmonary capillary blood volume elevating DL_{CO} and pulmonary edema decreasing it. Finding an elevated DL_{CO} may be useful in the diagnosis of alveolar hemorrhage, as in Goodpasture's syndrome. Hemoglobin contained in erythrocytes in the alveolar lumen is capable of binding carbon monoxide, so the exhaled carbon monoxide concentration is diminished and the measured DL_{CO} is increased.

FURTHER READING

AMERICAN THORACIC SOCIETY: Lung function testing: Selection of reference values and interpretative strategies. Am Rev Respir Dis 144:1202, 1991

CELLI BR: The importance of spirometry in COPD and asthma: Effect on approach to management. Chest 117:15S, 2000

CHUPP GL (ed): Pulmonary function testing. Clin Chest Med 22:599, 2001

LAFFEY JG, KAVANAGH BP: Hypocapnia. N Engl J Med 347:43, 2002

LEVITZKY MG: *Pulmonary Physiology,* 5th ed. New York, McGraw-Hill, 1999

WEINBERGER SE: *Principles of Pulmonary Medicine,* 3d ed. Philadelphia, Saunders, 1998

235 DIAGNOSTIC PROCEDURES IN RESPIRATORY DISEASE
Steven E. Weinberger, Jeffrey M. Drazen

The diagnostic modalities available for assessing the patient with suspected or known respiratory system disease include imaging studies and techniques for acquiring biologic specimens, some of which involve direct visualization of part of the respiratory system. →*Methods used to characterize the functional changes developing as a result of disease, including pulmonary function tests and measurements of gas exchange, are discussed in Chap. 234.*

IMAGING STUDIES

ROUTINE RADIOGRAPHY Routine chest radiography, which generally includes both posteroanterior and lateral views, is an integral part of the diagnostic evaluation of diseases involving the pulmonary parenchyma, the pleura, and, to a lesser extent, the airways and the mediastinum (see Figs. 233-1 and 233-2). Lateral decubitus views are often useful for determining whether pleural abnormalities represent freely flowing fluid, whereas apical lordotic views can often visualize disease at the lung apices better than the standard posteroanterior view. Portable equipment, which is often used for acutely ill patients who either cannot be transported to a radiology suite or cannot stand up for posteroanterior and lateral views, generally yields just a single radiograph taken in the anteroposterior direction. →*Common radiographic patterns and their clinical correlates are reviewed in Chap. 233.*

COMPUTED TOMOGRAPHY Computed tomography (CT) offers several advantages over routine chest radiography (Figs. 235-1, -2; 243-1, -2; 251-3). First, the use of cross-sectional images often makes it possible to distinguish between densities that would be superimposed on plain radiographs. Second, CT is far better than routine radiographic studies at characterizing tissue density, distinguishing subtle differences in density between adjacent structures, and providing accurate size assessment of lesions. As a result, CT is particularly valuable in assessing hilar and mediastinal disease (which is often poorly characterized by plain radiography), in identifying and characterizing disease adjacent to the chest wall or spine (including pleural disease), and in identifying areas of fat density or calcification in pulmonary nodules (Fig. 235-1). Its utility in the assessment of mediastinal disease has made CT an important tool in the staging of lung cancer (Chap. 75), as an assessment of tumor involvement of mediastinal lymph nodes is critical to proper staging. With the additional use of contrast material, CT also makes it possible to distinguish vascular from nonvascular structures, which is particularly important in distinguishing lymph nodes and masses from vascular structures.

Helical CT scanning allows the collection of continuous data over a larger volume of lung during a single breath-holding maneuver than is possible with conventional CT. With CT angiography, in which intravenous contrast is administered and images are acquired rapidly by helical scanning, pulmonary emboli can be detected in segmental and larger pulmonary arteries. With high-resolution CT (HRCT), the thickness of individual cross-sectional images is approximately 1 to 2 mm, rather than the usual 7 to 10 mm, and the images are reconstructed using high-spatial-resolution algorithms. The detail that can be seen on HRCT scans allows better recognition of subtle parenchymal and airway disease, such as bronchiectasis, emphysema, and diffuse parenchymal disease (Fig. 235-2). Certain nearly pathognomonic patterns have now been recognized for many of the interstitial lung diseases, such as lymphangitic carcinoma, idiopathic pulmonary fibrosis, sarcoidosis, and eosinophilic granuloma; however, it is not yet

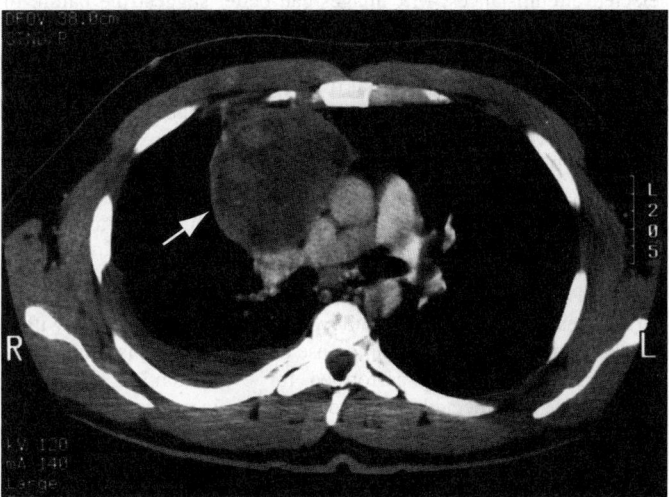

FIGURE 235-1 CT scan demonstrating a mediastinal mass of heterogeneous density (*arrow*). CT is superior to plain radiography for the detection of abnormal mediastinal densities and the distinction of masses from adjacent vascular structures.

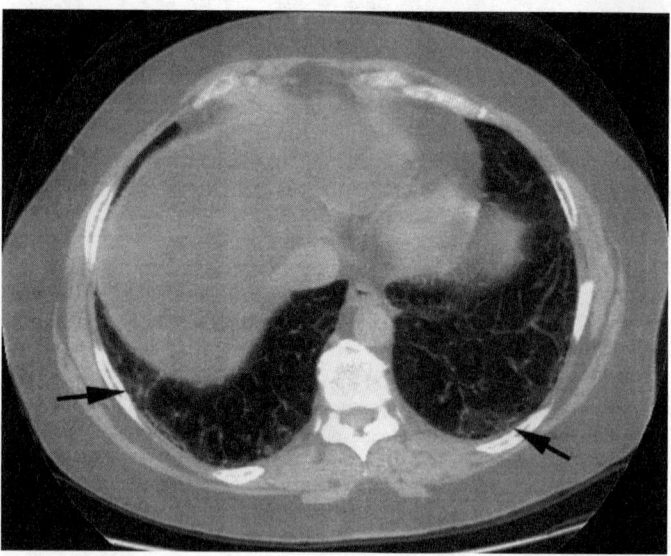

FIGURE 235-2 High-resolution CT scan from a patient with idiopathic pulmonary fibrosis. There are scattered reticular densities (arrows point to examples) that are especially prominent at the periphery of the lungs. This particular cross-section is from the base of the lungs, where the findings in idiopathic pulmonary fibrosis tend to be most marked.

clear in what settings these patterns obviate the need for obtaining lung tissue.

Recent advances in computer processing of the data acquired by helical scanning have allowed images to be presented in novel ways. For example, images may be displayed in views and planes other than the traditional cross-sectional view, and sophisticated three-dimensional reconstructions produce images (called *virtual bronchoscopy*) that mimic those seen by direct visualization through a bronchoscope.

MAGNETIC RESONANCE IMAGING The role of magnetic resonance (MR) imaging in the evaluation of respiratory system disease is less well defined than that of CT. Because MR generally provides a less detailed view of the pulmonary parenchyma as well as poorer spatial resolution, its usefulness in the evaluation of parenchymal lung disease is limited at present. However, MR images can be reconstructed in sagittal and coronal as well as transverse planes, so that the technique is well suited for imaging abnormalities near the lung apex, the spine, and the thoracoabdominal junction. MR images are dependent on tissue characteristics other than tissue density, unlike CT scanning. Therefore, in selected circumstances, MR images can better suggest the nature of abnormal tissue than can density-determined CT images. Finally, MR can be used to evaluate cardiac and vascular pathology within the thorax and to distinguish vascular from nonvascular structures without the need for contrast. Flowing blood does not produce a signal on MR imaging, so vessels appear as hollow tubular structures. This feature can be useful in determining whether abnormal hilar or mediastinal densities are vascular in origin and in defining aortic lesions such as aneurysms or dissection. In addition, gadolinium can be used as an intravascular contrast agent for MR angiography.

SCINTIGRAPHIC IMAGING Radioactive isotopes, administered by either intravenous or inhaled routes, allow the lungs to be imaged with a gamma camera. The most common use of such imaging is ventilation-perfusion lung scanning performed for evaluation of pulmonary embolism. When injected intravenously, albumin macroaggregates labeled with technetium 99m become lodged in pulmonary capillaries; therefore, the distribution of the trapped radioisotope follows the distribution of blood flow. When inhaled, radiolabeled xenon gas can be used to demonstrate the distribution of ventilation. For example, pulmonary thromboembolism usually produces one or more regions of ventilation-perfusion mismatch—that is, regions in which there is a

defect in perfusion that follows the distribution of a vessel and that is not accompanied by a corresponding defect in ventilation (Chap. 244). Another common use of such radioisotope scans is in a patient with impaired lung function who is being considered for lung resection. The distribution of the isotope(s) can be used to assess the regional distribution of blood flow and ventilation, allowing the physician to estimate the level of postoperative lung function.

POSITRON EMISSION TOMOGRAPHIC SCANNING Positron emission tomographic (PET) scanning is increasingly being used to identify malignant lesions in the lung based on their increased uptake and metabolism of glucose. The technique involves injection of a radiolabeled glucose analogue, ^{18}F-fluoro-2-deoxyglucose (FDG), which is taken up by metabolically active malignant cells. However, FDG is trapped within the cell following phosphorylation, and the unstable fluorine 18 decays by emission of positrons, which can be detected by a specialized PET camera or by a gamma camera that has been adapted for imaging of positron-emitting radionuclides. This technique has been used in the evaluation of solitary pulmonary nodules and as an aid to staging lung cancer, through identification of mediastinal lymph node involvement by malignancy.

PULMONARY ANGIOGRAPHY The pulmonary arterial system can be visualized by pulmonary angiography, in which radiopaque contrast medium is injected through a catheter previously threaded into the pulmonary artery. When performed in cases of pulmonary embolism, pulmonary angiography demonstrates the consequences of an intravascular clot—either a defect in the lumen of a vessel (a "filling defect") or an abrupt termination ("cutoff") of the vessel. Other, less common indications for pulmonary angiography include visualization of a suspected pulmonary arteriovenous malformation and assessment of pulmonary arterial invasion by a neoplasm. However, with advances in CT scanning, traditional pulmonary angiography is increasingly being replaced by CT angiography. The latter allows rapid acquisition of images with a less invasive procedure, since the radiocontrast material is injected intravenously rather than into a pulmonary artery.

ULTRASOUND Because ultrasound energy is rapidly dissipated in air, ultrasound imaging is not useful for evaluation of the pulmonary parenchyma. However, it is helpful in the detection and localization of pleural abnormalities and is often used as a guide to placement of a needle for sampling of pleural liquid (i.e., for thoracentesis).

TECHNIQUES FOR OBTAINING BIOLOGIC SPECIMENS
COLLECTION OF SPUTUM Sputum can be collected either by spontaneous expectoration or after inhalation of an irritating aerosol, such as hypertonic saline. The latter method, called *sputum induction*, is commonly used to obtain sputum for diagnostic studies, either because sputum is not spontaneously being produced or because of an expected higher yield of certain types of findings. Knowledge of the appearance and quality of the sputum specimen obtained is especially important when one is interested in Gram's staining and culture. Because sputum consists mainly of secretions from the tracheobronchial tree rather than the upper airway, the finding of alveolar macrophages and other inflammatory cells is consistent with a lower respiratory tract origin of the sample, whereas the presence of squamous epithelial cells in a "sputum" sample indicates contamination by secretions from the upper airways.

Besides processing for routine bacterial pathogens by Gram's staining and culture, sputum can be processed for a variety of other pathogens, including staining and culture for mycobacteria or fungi, culture for viruses, and staining for *Pneumocystis carinii*. In the specific case of sputum obtained for evaluation of *P. carinii* pneumonia in a patient infected with HIV, for example, sputum should be collected by induction, rather than spontaneous expectoration, and an immunofluorescent stain should be used to detect the organisms. Cytologic staining of sputum for malignant cells, using the traditional Papanicolaou method, allows noninvasive evaluation for suspected lung cancer. Traditional stains and cultures are now also being supplemented in some cases by immunologic techniques and by molecular biologic methods, including the use of polymerase chain reaction amplification and DNA probes.

PERCUTANEOUS NEEDLE ASPIRATION A needle can be inserted through the chest wall into a pulmonary lesion for the purpose of aspirating material for analysis by cytologic or microbiologic techniques. The procedure is usually carried out under CT guidance, which assists in the positioning of the needle and assures that it is localized in the lesion. Although the potential risks of this procedure include intrapulmonary bleeding and creation of a pneumothorax with collapse of the underlying lung, the low risk of complication in experienced hands is usually worth the information obtained. However, a limitation of the technique is sampling error due to the small amount of material obtained. Thus, findings other than a specific cytologic or microbiologic diagnosis are of limited clinical value.

THORACENTESIS Sampling of pleural liquid by thoracentesis is commonly performed for diagnostic purposes or, in the case of a large effusion, for palliation of dyspnea. Diagnostic sampling, either by blind needle aspiration or after localization by ultrasound, allows the collection of liquid for microbiologic and cytologic studies. Analysis of the fluid obtained for its cellular composition and chemical constituents, including glucose, protein, and lactate dehydrogenase, allows the effusion to be classified as either exudative or transudative (Chap. 245).

BRONCHOSCOPY Bronchoscopy is the process of direct visualization of the tracheobronchial tree. Although bronchoscopy is now performed almost exclusively with flexible fiberoptic instruments, rigid bronchoscopy, generally performed in an operating room on a patient under general anesthesia, still has a role in selected circumstances, primarily because of a larger suction channel and the fact that the patient can be ventilated through the bronchoscope channel. These situations include the retrieval of a foreign body and the suctioning of a massive hemorrhage, for which the small suction channel of the bronchoscope may be insufficient.

Flexible Fiberoptic Bronchoscopy This is an outpatient procedure that is usually performed in an awake but sedated patient. The bronchoscope is passed through either the mouth or the nose, between the vocal cords, and into the trachea. The ability to flex the scope makes it possible to visualize virtually all airways to the level of subsegmental bronchi. The bronchoscopist is able to identify endobronchial pathology, including tumors, granulomas, bronchitis, foreign bodies, and sites of bleeding. Samples from airway lesions can be taken by several methods, including washing, brushing, and biopsy. Washing involves instillation of sterile saline through a channel of the bronchoscope and onto the surface of a lesion. A portion of the liquid is collected by suctioning through the bronchoscope, and the recovered material can be analyzed for cells (cytology) or organisms (by standard stains and cultures). Brushing or biopsy of the surface of the lesion, using a small brush or biopsy forceps at the end of a long cable inserted through a channel of the bronchoscope, allows recovery of cellular material or tissue for analysis by standard cytologic and histopathologic methods.

The bronchoscope can be used to sample material not only from the regions that can be directly visualized (i.e., the airways) but also from the more distal pulmonary parenchyma. With the bronchoscope wedged into a subsegmental airway, aliquots of sterile saline can be instilled through the scope, allowing sampling of cells and organisms even from alveolar spaces. This procedure, called *bronchoalveolar lavage*, has been particularly useful for the recovery of organisms such as *P. carinii* in patients with HIV infection.

Brushing and biopsy of the distal lung parenchyma can also be performed with the same instruments that are used for endobronchial sampling. These instruments can be passed through the scope into small airways, where they penetrate the airway wall, allowing biopsy of peribronchial alveolar tissue. This procedure, called *transbronchial biopsy*, is used when there is either relatively diffuse disease or a localized lesion of adequate size. With the aid of fluoroscopic imaging,

the bronchoscopist is able to determine not only whether and when the instrument is in the area of abnormality, but also the proximity of the instrument to the pleural surface. If the forceps are too close to the pleural surface, there is a risk of violating the visceral pleura and creating a pneumothorax; the other potential complication of transbronchial biopsy is pulmonary hemorrhage. The incidence of these complications is less than several percent.

Another procedure involves use of a hollow-bore needle passed through the bronchoscope for sampling of tissue adjacent to the trachea or a large bronchus. The needle is passed through the airway wall, and cellular material can be aspirated from mass lesions or enlarged lymph nodes, generally in a search for malignant cells. This procedure can facilitate the staging of lung cancer by identifying mediastinal lymph node involvement and in some cases obviates the need for a more invasive procedure. Other new techniques that are not yet widely available include fluorescence bronchoscopy (to detect early endobronchial malignancy) and endobronchial ultrasound (to identify and localize mediastinal pathology).

The bronchoscope may provide the opportunity for treatment as well as diagnosis. For example, an aspirated foreign body may be retrieved with an instrument passed through the scope, and bleeding may be controlled with a balloon catheter similarly introduced. Newer interventional techniques performed through a bronchoscope include methods for achieving and maintaining patency of airways that are partially or completely occluded, especially by tumors. These techniques include laser therapy, cryotherapy, electrocautery, and stent placement.

VIDEO-ASSISTED THORACIC SURGERY Recent advances in video technology have allowed the development of thoracoscopy, or video-assisted thoracic surgery (VATS), for the diagnosis and management of pleural as well as parenchymal lung disease. This procedure involves the passage of a rigid scope with a distal lens through a trocar inserted into the pleura. A high-quality image is shown on a monitor screen, allowing the operator to manipulate instruments passed into the pleural space through separate small intercostal incisions. With these instruments, the operator can biopsy lesions of the pleura under direct vision. In addition, this procedure is now used commonly to biopsy peripheral lung tissue or to remove peripheral nodules, for both diagnostic and therapeutic purposes. Because this procedure is much less invasive than the traditional thoracotomy performed for lung biopsy, it has largely supplanted "open lung biopsy."

THORACOTOMY Although frequently replaced by VATS, thoracotomy remains an option for the diagnostic sampling of lung tissue. It provides the largest amount of material, and it can be used to biopsy and/or excise lesions that are too deep or too close to vital structures for removal by VATS. The choice between VATS and thoracotomy needs to be made on a case-by-case basis, and the relative indications for each are still evolving as more experience is being gained with VATS.

MEDIASTINOSCOPY AND MEDIASTINOTOMY Tissue biopsy is often critical for the diagnosis of mediastinal masses or enlarged mediastinal lymph nodes. Although CT and PET scanning are useful for determining the size and nature of mediastinal lymph nodes as part of the staging of lung cancer, confirmation that enlarged lymph nodes are actually involved with tumor generally requires biopsy and histopathologic examination. The two major procedures used to obtain specimens from masses or nodes in the mediastinum are mediastinoscopy (via a suprasternal approach) and mediastinotomy (via a parasternal approach). Both procedures are performed under general anesthesia by a qualified surgeon. In the case of suprasternal mediastinoscopy, a rigid mediastinoscope is inserted at the suprasternal notch and passed into the mediastinum along a pathway just anterior to the trachea. Tissue can be obtained with biopsy forceps passed through the scope, sampling masses or nodes that are in a paratracheal or pretracheal position. Left paratracheal and aortopulmonary lymph nodes are not accessible by this route and thus are commonly sampled by parasternal mediastinotomy (the Chamberlain procedure). This approach involves either a right or left parasternal incision and dissection directly down to a mass or node that requires biopsy.

FURTHER READING

BOLLIGER CT, MATHUR PN: ERS/ATS statement on interventional pulmonology. Eur Respir J 19:356, 2002

GOULD MK et al: Accuracy of positron emission tomography for diagnosis of pulmonary nodules and mass lesions. A meta-analysis. JAMA 285:914, 2001

MEHTA AC (ed): Flexible bronchoscopy update. Clin Chest Med 22:225, 2001

MÜLLER NL: Computed tomography and magnetic resonance imaging: Past, present and future. Eur Respir J 19(suppl 35):3s, 2002

RYU JH et al: Diagnosis of pulmonary embolism with use of computed tomographic angiography. Mayo Clin Proc 76:59, 2001

SEIJO LM, STERMAN DH: Interventional pulmonology. N Engl J Med 344: 740, 2001

WEINBERGER SE: Principles of Pulmonary Medicine, 3d ed. Philadelphia, Saunders, 1998

Section 2   Diseases of the Respiratory System

236   ASTHMA
E. R. McFadden, Jr.

Asthma is defined as a chronic inflammatory disease of airways that is characterized by increased responsiveness of the tracheobronchial tree to a multiplicity of stimuli. It is manifested physiologically by a widespread narrowing of the air passages, which may be relieved spontaneously or as a result of therapy, and clinically by paroxysms of dyspnea, cough, and wheezing. Asthma is an episodic disease, with acute exacerbations interspersed with symptom-free periods. Typically, most attacks are short-lived, lasting minutes to hours, and clinically the patient seems to recover completely after an attack. However, there can be a phase in which the patient experiences some degree of airway obstruction daily. This phase can be mild, with or without superimposed severe episodes, or much more serious, with severe obstruction persisting for days or weeks; the latter condition is known as *status asthmaticus*. In unusual circumstances, acute episodes can cause death.

PREVALENCE AND ETIOLOGY   Asthma is a very common disease with immense social impact. The prevalence of asthma is rising in many parts of the world, but it is unclear whether this is due to an actual increase in incidence or merely to the fact that the size of the overall population is growing. It is estimated that 4 to 5% of the population of the United States is affected. Data from the Centers for Disease Control and Prevention suggest that 10 to 11 million persons had acute attacks in 1998, which resulted in 13.9 million outpatient visits, 2 million requests for urgent care, and 423,000 hospitalizations, with a total cost >$6 billion. The impact of the disease appears to fall more heavily on minorities and inner-city African-American and Hispanic persons.

Bronchial asthma occurs at all ages but predominantly in early life. About one-half of cases develop before age 10, and another third occur before age 40. In childhood, there is a 2:1 male/female preponderance, but the sex ratio equalizes by age 30. From an etiologic standpoint, asthma is a heterogeneous disease and genetic (atopic) and environmental factors, such as viruses, occupational exposures, and allergens, contribute to its initiation and continuance.

Atopy is the single largest risk factor for the development of asthma. *Allergic asthma* is often associated with a personal and/or family history of allergic diseases such as rhinitis, urticaria, and eczema; with positive wheal-and-flare skin reactions to intradermal injection of extracts of airborne antigens; with increased levels of IgE in the serum; and/or with a positive response to provocation tests involving the inhalation of specific antigen.

A significant fraction of patients with asthma present with no personal or family history of allergy, with negative skin tests, and with normal serum levels of IgE, and therefore have disease that cannot be classified on the basis of currently defined immunologic mechanisms. These patients are said to have *idiosyncratic asthma* or *nonatopic asthma*. Many patients have disease that does not fit clearly into either of the preceding categories but instead falls into a mixed group with features of each. In general, asthma that has its onset in early life tends to have a strong allergic component, whereas asthma that develops late tends to be nonallergic or to have a mixed etiology.

PATHOGENESIS (See also Chap. 298)   Asthma results from a state of persistent subacute inflammation of the airways. Even in asymptomatic patients, the airways can be edematous and infiltrated with eosinophils, neutrophils, and lymphocytes, with or without an increase in the collagen content of the epithelial basement membrane. Overall, there is a generalized increase in cellularity associated with an elevated capillary density. There may also be glandular hypertrophy and denudation of the epithelium. These changes may persist despite treatment and often do not relate to the severity of the disease.

The physiologic and clinical features of asthma derive from an interaction among the resident and infiltrating inflammatory cells in the airway surface epithelium, inflammatory mediators, and cytokines. The cells thought to play important parts in the inflammatory response are mast cells, eosinophils, lymphocytes, and airway epithelial cells. The roles of neutrophils, macrophages, and other cellular constituents of the airways are less well defined. Each of the major cell types can contribute mediators and cytokines to initiate and amplify both acute inflammation and the long-term pathologic changes described (Fig. 236-1). The mediators released produce an intense, immediate inflammatory reaction involving bronchoconstriction, vascular congestion, edema formation, increased mucus production, and impaired mucociliary transport. This intense local event can then be followed by a more chronic one. Other elaborated chemotactic factors (eosinophil and neutrophil chemotactic factors of anaphylaxis and leukotriene B_4) also bring eosinophils, platelets, and polymorphonuclear leukocytes to the site of the reaction. The airway epithelium is both the target of, and a contributor to, the inflammatory cascade. This tissue both amplifies bronchoconstriction and promotes vasodilatation through the release of the compounds shown in Fig. 236-2.

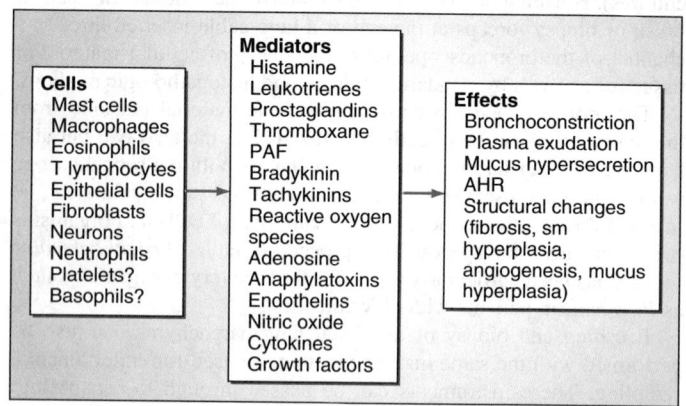

Cells	Mediators	Effects
Mast cells Macrophages Eosinophils T lymphocytes Epithelial cells Fibroblasts Neurons Neutrophils Platelets? Basophils?	Histamine Leukotrienes Prostaglandins Thromboxane PAF Bradykinin Tachykinins Reactive oxygen species Adenosine Anaphylatoxins Endothelins Nitric oxide Cytokines Growth factors	Bronchoconstriction Plasma exudation Mucus hypersecretion AHR Structural changes (fibrosis, sm hyperplasia, angiogenesis, mucus hyperplasia)

FIGURE 236-1   Cellular sources of inflammatory mediators and their physiologic effects. PAF, platelet-activating factor; AHR, antihyaluronidase reaction. [*From PJ Barnes, in E Middleton et al (eds): Allergy Principles and Practice, 5th ed. St. Louis, Mosby, 1998, with permission.*]

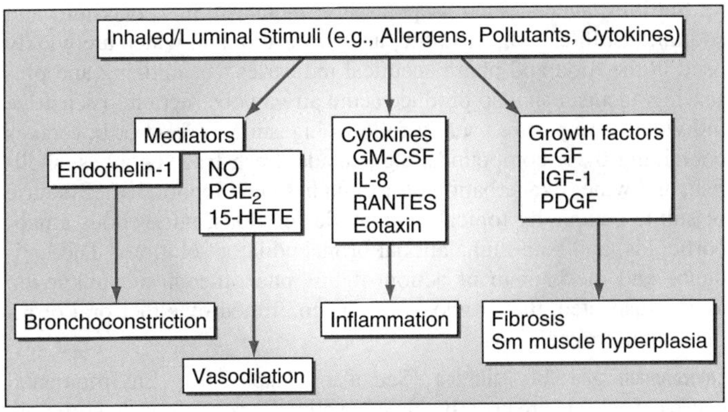

Inhaled/Luminal Stimuli (e.g., Allergens, Pollutants, Cytokines)

Mediators
Endothelin-1 | NO
PGE₂
15-HETE

Cytokines
GM-CSF
IL-8
RANTES
Eotaxin

Growth factors
EGF
IGF-1
PDGF

Bronchoconstriction

Inflammation

Fibrosis
Sm muscle hyperplasia

Vasodilation

FIGURE 236-2 Inflammatory mediators derived from epithelial sources. NO, nitrous oxide; PGE₂, prostaglandin E₂; GM-CSF, granulocyte-macrophage colony-stimulating factor; IL, interleukin; RANTES, regulated on activation, T cell expressed and secreted; EGF, epidermal growth factor; IGF, insulin-like growth factor; PDGF, platelet-derived growth factor. [*From PJ Barnes, in E Middleton et al (eds): Allergy Principles and Practice, 5th ed. St. Louis, Mosby, 1998, with permission.*]

The eosinophil appears to play an important part in the infiltrative component. Interleukin (IL) 5 stimulates the release of these cells into the circulation and extends their survival. Once activated, these cells are a rich source of leukotrienes, and the granular proteins released (major basic protein and eosinophilic cationic protein) and oxygen-derived free radicals are capable of destroying the airway epithelium, which then is sloughed into the bronchial lumen in the form of Creola bodies. Besides resulting in a loss of barrier and secretory function, such damage elicits the production of chemotactic cytokines, leading to further inflammation. In theory, it can also expose sensory nerve endings, thus initiating neurogenic inflammatory pathways. That, in turn, could convert a primary local event into a generalized reaction via a reflex mechanism. Although an important element in inflammation, the role that the eosinophil plays in establishing and maintaining airway hyperresponsiveness is undergoing reevaluation. Studies using antibodies against IL-5 show a disassociation between the inflammatory and physiologic events following an antigen challenge and blood and sputum eosinophilia. The cytokine network possibly involved in asthma is shown in Fig. 236-3.

T lymphocytes also appear to be important in the inflammatory response. Activated T_H2 cells are present in increased numbers in asthmatic airways and produce cytokines such as IL-4 that initiate humoral (IgE) immune responses. They also elaborate IL-5 with its effect on eosinophils. Data are accumulating that asthma may be related to an imbalance between T_H1 and T_H2 immune responses, but firm conclusions are not yet available.

GENETIC CONSIDERATIONS Although there is little doubt that asthma has a strong familial component, the identification of the genetic mechanisms underlying the illness has proven difficult for such fundamental reasons as a lack of uniform agreement on the definition of the disease, the inability to define a single phenotype, non-Mendelian modes of inheritance, and an incomplete understanding of how environmental factors modify genetic expression. Screening families for candidate genes has identified multiple chromosomal regions that relate to atopy, elevated IgE levels, and airway hyperresponsiveness. Evidence for genetic linkage of high total serum IgE levels and atopy has been observed on chromosomes 5q, 11q, and 12q in a number of populations scattered throughout the world. Regions of the genome demonstrating evidence for linkage to bronchial hyperreactivity also typically show evidence for linkage to elevated total serum IgE levels. Excellent candidate genes exist for specific abnormalities in asthma within the regions that were identified in the linkage studies. For example, chromosome 5q contains cytokine clusters including IL-4, IL-5, IL-9, and IL-13. Other regions on chromosome 5q also contain the β-adrenergic receptors and the glucocorticoid receptors. Chromosome 6p contains regions that are important in antigen presentation and me-

diation of the inflammatory response. Chromosome 12q contains two genes that could influence atopy and airway hyperresponsiveness, including nitric oxide synthase.

STIMULI THAT INCITE ASTHMA The stimuli that incite acute episodes of asthma can be grouped into seven major categories: allergenic, pharmacologic, environmental, occupational, infectious, exercise-related, and emotional.

Allergens Allergic asthma is dependent on an IgE response controlled by T and B lymphocytes and activated by the interaction of antigen with mast cell–bound IgE molecules. The airway epithelium and submucosa contain dendritic cells that capture and process antigen. After taking up an immunogen, these cells migrate to the local lymph nodes where they present the material to T cell receptors. In the appropriate genetic setting, the interaction of antigen with a naïve T cell T_H0 in the presence of IL-4 leads to the differentiation of the cell to a T_H2 subset. This process not only helps facilitate the inflammation of asthma but also causes B lymphocytes to switch their antibody production from IgG and IgM to IgE.

Once synthesized and released by B cells, IgE circulates in the blood until it attaches to high-affinity receptors on mast cells and low-affinity receptors on basophils. Most of the allergens that provoke asthma are airborne, and to induce a state of sensitivity they must be reasonably abundant for considerable periods of time. Once sensitization has occurred, however, the patient can exhibit exquisite responsivity, so that minute amounts of the offending agent can produce significant exacerbations of the disease. Immune mechanisms appear to be causally related to the development of asthma in 25 to 35% of all cases and to be contributory in perhaps another third. Higher prev-

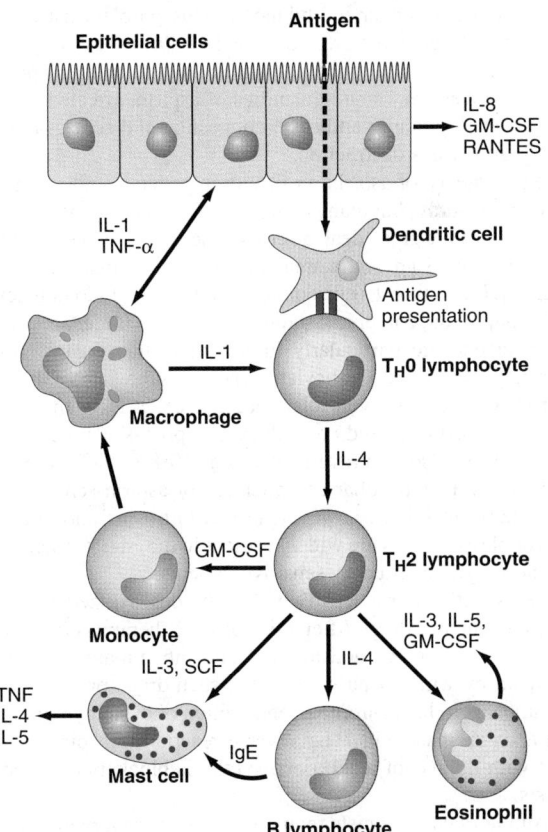

FIGURE 236-3 Cytokine network in allergic asthma. IL, interleukin; GM-CSF, granulocyte-macrophage colony-stimulating factor; RANTES, regulated on activation, T cell expressed and secreted; TNF, tumor necrosis factor; SCS, stem cell factor. [*From PJ Barnes, in E Middleton et al (eds): Allergy Principles and Practice, 5th ed. St. Louis, Mosby, 1998, with permission.*]

alences have been suggested, but it is difficult to know how to interpret the data because of confounding factors. Allergic asthma is frequently seasonal, and it is most often observed in children and young adults. A nonseasonal form may result from allergy to feathers, animal danders, dust mites, molds, and other environmental antigens that are present continuously. Exposure to antigen typically produces an immediate response in which airway obstruction develops in minutes and then resolves. In 30 to 50% of patients, a second wave of bronchoconstriction, the so-called late reaction, develops 6 to 10 h later. In a minority, only a late reaction occurs. It was formerly thought that the late reaction was essential to the development of the increase in airway reactivity that follows antigen exposure. This is now known not to be the case.

The mechanism by which an inhaled allergen provokes an acute episode of asthma depends in part on antigen-antibody interactions on the surface of pulmonary mast cells, with the subsequent generation and release of the mediators of immediate hypersensitivity. Current hypotheses hold that very small antigenic particles penetrate the lung's defenses and come in contact with mast cells that interdigitate with the epithelium at the luminal surface of the central airways. The subsequent elaboration of mediators and cytokines then produces the sequence outlined above.

Pharmacologic Stimuli   The drugs most commonly associated with the induction of acute episodes of asthma are aspirin, coloring agents such as tartrazine, β-adrenergic antagonists, and sulfiting agents. It is important to recognize drug-induced bronchial narrowing because its presence is often associated with great morbidity. Furthermore, death sometimes has followed the ingestion of aspirin (or other nonsteroidal anti-inflammatory agents) or β-adrenergic antagonists. The typical aspirin-sensitive respiratory syndrome primarily affects adults, although the condition may occur in childhood. This problem usually begins with perennial vasomotor rhinitis that is followed by a hyperplastic rhinosinusitis with nasal polyps. Progressive asthma then appears. On exposure to even very small quantities of aspirin, affected individuals typically develop ocular and nasal congestion and acute, often severe episodes of airways obstruction.

The prevalence of aspirin sensitivity in patients with asthma varies from study to study, but many authorities feel that 10% is a reasonable figure. There is a great deal of cross-reactivity between aspirin and other nonsteroidal anti-inflammatory compounds that inhibit prostaglandin G/H synthase 1 (cyclooxygenase type 1). Indomethacin, fenoprofen, naproxen, zomepirac sodium, ibuprofen, mefenamic acid, and phenylbutazone are particularly important in this regard. However, acetaminophen, sodium salicylate, choline salicylate, salicylamide, and propoxyphene are well tolerated. The exact frequency of cross-reactivity to tartrazine and other dyes in aspirin-sensitive individuals with asthma is also controversial; again, 10% is the commonly accepted figure. This peculiar complication of aspirin-sensitive asthma is particularly insidious, however, in that tartrazine and other potentially troublesome dyes are widely present in the environment and may be unknowingly ingested by sensitive patients.

Patients with aspirin sensitivity can be desensitized by daily administration of the drug. After this form of therapy, cross-tolerance also develops to other nonsteroidal anti-inflammatory agents. The mechanism by which aspirin and other such drugs produce bronchospasm appears to be a chronic overexcretion of cysteinyl leukotrienes, which activate mast cells. The adverse reaction to aspirin can be inhibited with the use of leukotriene synthesis blockers or receptor antagonists.

β-Adrenergic antagonists regularly obstruct the airways in individuals with asthma as well as in others with heightened airway reactivity and should be avoided by such individuals. Even the selective beta$_1$ agents have this propensity, particularly at higher doses. In fact, the local use of beta$_1$ blockers in the eye for the treatment of glaucoma has been associated with worsening asthma.

Sulfiting agents, such as potassium metabisulfite, potassium and sodium bisulfite, sodium sulfite, and sulfur dioxide, which are widely used in the food and pharmaceutical industries as sanitizing and preserving agents, can also produce acute airway obstruction in sensitive individuals. Exposure usually follows ingestion of food or beverages containing these compounds, e.g., salads, fresh fruit, potatoes, shellfish, and wine. Exacerbation of asthma has been reported after the use of sulfite-containing topical ophthalmic solutions, intravenous glucocorticoids, and some inhalational bronchodilator solutions. The incidence and mechanism of action of this phenomenon are unknown. When suspected, the diagnosis can be confirmed by either oral or inhalational provocations.

Environment and Air Pollution   (See also Chap. 238)   Environmental causes of asthma are usually related to climatic conditions that promote the concentration of atmospheric pollutants and antigens. These conditions tend to develop in heavily industrial or densely populated urban areas and are frequently associated with thermal inversions or other situations creating stagnant air masses. In these circumstances, although the general population can develop respiratory symptoms, patients with asthma and other respiratory diseases tend to be more severely affected. The air pollutants known to have this effect are ozone, nitrogen dioxide, and sulfur dioxide. All produce greater effects during periods of high ventilation. In some regions of North America, seasonal concentrations of airborne antigens such as pollen can rise high enough to result in epidemics of asthma admissions to hospitals and an increase in the death rate. These events may be ameliorated by treating patients prophylactically with anti-inflammatory drugs before the allergy season begins.

Occupational Factors   (See also Chap. 238)   Occupation-related asthma is a significant health problem, and acute and chronic airway obstruction have been reported to follow exposure to a large number of compounds used in many types of industrial processes. In general, the agents can be classified into high-molecular-weight compounds, which are believed to induce asthma through immunologic mechanisms, and low-molecular-weight agents, which serve as haptines or can release bronchoconstrictor substances. High-molecular-weight compounds of importance are *wood and vegetable dusts* (e.g., those of oak, grain, flour, castor bean, green coffee bean, mako, gum acacia, karay, gum, and tragacanth), *pharmaceutical agents* (e.g., antibiotics, piperazine, and cimetidine), *biologic enzymes* (e.g., laundry detergents, pancreatic enzymes, and *Bacillus subtilis*), and *animal and insect dusts, serums, and secretions* (e.g., laboratory animals, chickens, crabs, prawns, oysters, flys, bees, and moths). Troublesome low-molecular-weight compounds are *metal salts* (e.g., platinum, chrome, vanadium, and nickel) and *industrial chemicals and plastics* (e.g., toluene diisocyanate, phthalic acid anhydride, trimellitic anhydride, persulfates, ethylenediamine, *p*-phenylenediamine, western red cedar, azidrocarbonamide, and various dyes). Formaldehyde and urea formaldehyde also fall into this group. It is important to recognize that exposure to sensitizing chemicals, particularly those used in paints, solvents, and plastics, can also occur during leisure or non-work-related activities.

If the occupational agent causes an immediate or dual immunologic reaction, the history is similar to that which occurs with exposure to other antigens. Often, however, patients will give a characteristic cyclic history. They are well when they arrive at work, and symptoms develop toward the end of the shift, progress after the work site is left, and then regress. Absence from work during weekends or vacations brings about remission. Frequently, there are similar symptoms in fellow employees.

Infections   Respiratory infections are the most common of the stimuli that evoke acute exacerbations of asthma. Respiratory viruses and not bacteria or allergy to microorganisms are the major etiologic factors. In young children, the most important infectious agents are respiratory syncytial virus and parainfluenza virus. In older children and adults, rhinovirus and influenza virus predominate as pathogens. Simple colonization of the tracheobronchial tree is insufficient to evoke acute episodes of bronchospasm, and attacks of asthma occur only when symptoms of an ongoing respiratory tract infection are, or have been, present. Viral infections can actively and chronically destabilize asthma, and they are perhaps the only stimuli that can produce constant symptoms for weeks. The mechanism by which viruses induce exacerbations of asthma may be related to the production of T cell–derived cytokines that potentiate the infiltration of inflammatory cells into already susceptible airways.

Exercise Exercise is a very common precipitant of acute episodes of asthma. This stimulus differs from other naturally occurring provocations, such as antigens, viral infections, and air pollutants, in that it does not evoke any long-term sequelae, nor does it increase airway reactivity. Typically the attacks follow exertion and do not occur during it. The critical variables that determine the severity of the postexertional airway obstruction are the levels of ventilation achieved and the temperature and humidity of the inspired air. The higher the ventilation and the lower the heat content of the air, the greater the response. For the same inspired air conditions, running produces a more severe attack of asthma than walking because of its greater ventilatory cost. Conversely, for a given task, the inhalation of cold air markedly enhances the response, while warm, humid air blunts or abolishes it. Consequently, activities such as ice hockey, cross-country skiing, and ice skating (high ventilations of cold air) are more provocative than is swimming in an indoor, heated pool (relatively low ventilation of humid air). The mechanism by which exercise produces obstruction may be related to a thermally produced hyperemia and capillary leakage in the airway wall.

Emotional Stress Psychological factors can worsen or ameliorate asthma. Changes in airway caliber seem to be mediated through modification of vagal efferent activity, but endorphins may also play a role. The extent to which psychological factors participate in the induction and/or continuation of any given acute exacerbation is not established but probably varies from patient to patient and in the same patient from episode to episode.

PATHOLOGY In a patient who has died of acute asthma, the most striking feature of the lungs at necropsy is their gross overdistention and failure to collapse when the pleural cavities are opened. When the lungs are cut, numerous gelatinous plugs of exudate are found in most of the bronchial branches down to the terminal bronchioles. Histologic examination shows hypertrophy of the bronchial smooth muscle, hyperplasia of mucosal and submucosal vessels, mucosal edema, denudation of the surface epithelium, pronounced thickening of the basement membrane, and eosinophilic infiltrates in the bronchial wall. There is an absence of any of the well-recognized forms of destructive emphysema.

PATHOPHYSIOLOGY The pathophysiologic hallmark of asthma is a reduction in airway diameter brought about by contraction of smooth muscle, vascular congestion, edema of the bronchial wall, and thick, tenacious secretions. The net result is an increase in airway resistance, a decrease in forced expiratory volumes and flow rates, hyperinflation of the lungs and thorax, increased work of breathing, alterations in respiratory muscle function, changes in elastic recoil, abnormal distribution of both ventilation and pulmonary blood flow with mismatched ratios, and altered arterial blood gas concentrations. Thus, although asthma is considered to be primarily a disease of airways, virtually all aspects of pulmonary function are compromised during an acute attack. In addition, in very symptomatic patients there frequently is electrocardiographic evidence of right ventricular hypertrophy and pulmonary hypertension. When a patient presents for therapy, the 1-s forced expiratory volume (FEV_1) or peak expiratory flow rate (PEFR) is typically <40% of predicted. In keeping with the alterations in mechanics, the associated air trapping is substantial. In acutely ill patients, residual volume frequently approaches 400% of normal, while functional residual capacity doubles.

Hypoxia is a universal finding during acute exacerbations, but frank ventilatory failure is relatively uncommon, being observed in 10 to 15% of patients presenting for therapy. Most individuals with asthma have hypocapnia and a respiratory alkalosis. In acutely ill patients, the finding of a normal arterial carbon dioxide tension tends to be associated with quite severe levels of obstruction. Consequently, when found in a symptomatic individual, it should be viewed as representing impending respiratory failure, and the patient should be treated accordingly. Equally, the presence of metabolic acidosis in the setting of acute asthma signifies severe obstruction. Cyanosis is a very late sign. Trying to judge the state of an acutely ill patient's ventilatory status on clinical grounds alone can be extremely hazardous, and clinical indicators should not be relied on with any confidence. Therefore, in patients with suspected alveolar hypoventilation, arterial blood gas tensions must be measured.

CLINICAL FEATURES The symptoms of asthma consist of a triad of dyspnea, cough, and wheezing, the last often being regarded as the sine qua non. In its most typical form, all three symptoms coexist. At the onset of an attack, patients experience a sense of constriction in the chest, often with a nonproductive cough. Respiration becomes audibly harsh; wheezing in both phases of respiration becomes prominent; expiration becomes prolonged; and patients frequently have tachypnea, tachycardia, and mild systolic hypertension. The lungs rapidly become overinflated, and the anteroposterior diameter of the thorax increases. If the attack is severe or prolonged, there may be a loss of adventitial breath sounds, and wheezing becomes very high pitched. Furthermore, the accessory muscles become visibly active, and a paradoxical pulse often develops. These two signs are extremely valuable in indicating the severity of the obstruction. In the presence of either, pulmonary function tends to be significantly more impaired than in their absence. It is important to note that the development of a paradoxical pulse depends on the generation of large negative intrathoracic pressures. Thus, if the patient's breathing is shallow, this sign and/or the use of accessory muscles could be absent even though obstruction is quite severe. The other signs and symptoms of asthma only imperfectly reflect the physiologic alterations that are present. Indeed, if the disappearance of subjective complaints or even of wheezing is used as the end point at which therapy for an acute attack is terminated, an enormous reservoir of residual disease will be missed.

The end of an episode is frequently marked by a cough that produces thick, stringy mucus, which often takes the form of casts of the distal airways (Curschmann's spirals) and, when examined microscopically, often shows eosinophils and Charcot-Leyden crystals. In extreme situations, wheezing may lessen markedly or even disappear, cough may become extremely ineffective, and the patient may begin a gasping type of respiratory pattern. These findings imply extensive mucus plugging and impending suffocation. Ventilatory assistance by mechanical means may be required. Atelectasis due to inspissated secretions occasionally occurs with asthmatic attacks. Spontaneous pneumothorax and/or pneumomediastinum occur but are rare.

Less typically, a patient with asthma may complain of intermittent episodes of nonproductive cough or exertional dyspnea. Unlike other individuals with asthma, when these patients are examined during symptomatic periods, they tend to have normal breath sounds but may wheeze after repeated forced exhalations and/or may show ventilatory impairments when tested in the laboratory. In the absence of both these signs, a bronchoprovocation test may be required to make the diagnosis.

DIFFERENTIAL DIAGNOSIS The differentiation of asthma from other diseases associated with dyspnea and wheezing is usually not difficult, particularly if the patient is seen during an acute episode. The physical findings and symptoms listed above and the history of periodic attacks are quite characteristic. A personal or family history of allergic diseases such as eczema, rhinitis, or urticaria is valuable contributory evidence. An extremely common feature of asthma is nocturnal awakening with dyspnea and/or wheezing. In fact, this phenomenon is so prevalent that its absence raises doubt about the diagnosis.

Upper airway obstruction by tumor or *laryngeal edema* can occa-

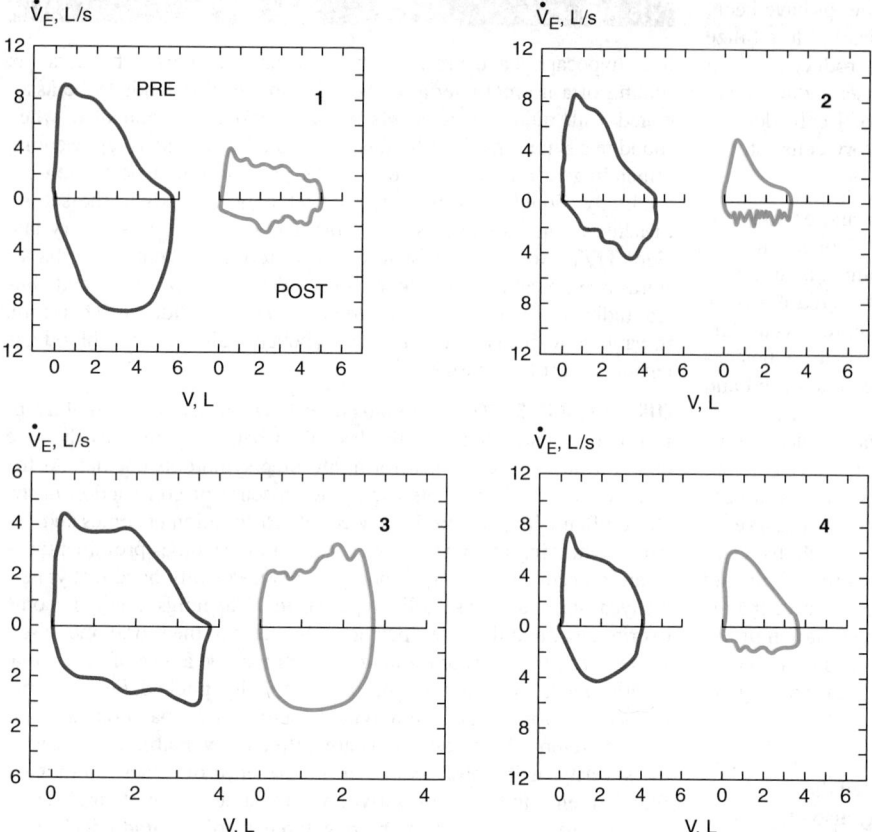

FIGURE 236-4 Representative examples of glottic dysfunction in four patients. The left-hand panels show normal flow-volume curves (red). The right-hand panels (green) represent the development of glottic dysfunction after exercise challenges (green). Note the variable waveforms that can exist. When the patients' attacks ended, the post provocation flow-volume curves returned to normal. $\dot{V}_E$, ventilation; L/s, liters/second; V, L, lung volume in liters.

sionally be confused with asthma. Typically, a patient with such a condition will present with stridor, and the harsh respiratory sounds can be localized to the area of the trachea. Representative flow–volume curves are shown in Fig. 236-4. Diffuse wheezing throughout both lung fields is usually absent. However, differentiation can sometimes be difficult, and indirect laryngoscopy or bronchoscopy may be required. Asthma-like symptoms have been described in patients with glottic dysfunction. These individuals narrow their glottis during inspiration and expiration, producing episodic attacks of severe airway obstruction. Occasionally, carbon dioxide retention develops. However, unlike in asthma, the arterial oxygen tension is well preserved, and the alveolar-arterial gradient for oxygen narrows during the episode, instead of widening as with lower airway obstruction. To establish the diagnosis of glottic dysfunction, the glottis should be examined when the patient is symptomatic. Normal findings at such a time exclude the diagnosis; normal findings during asymptomatic periods do not.

Persistent wheezing localized to one area of the chest in association with paroxysms of coughing indicates *endobronchial disease* such as foreign-body aspiration, a neoplasm, or bronchial stenosis.

The signs and symptoms of *acute left ventricular failure* occasionally mimic asthma, but the findings of moist basilar rales, gallop rhythms, blood-tinged sputum, and other signs of heart failure (Chap. 216) allow the appropriate diagnosis to be reached.

Recurrent episodes of bronchospasm can occur with *carcinoid tumors* (Chap. 329), *recurrent pulmonary emboli* (Chap. 244), and *chronic bronchitis* (Chap. 242). In chronic bronchitis there are no true symptom-free periods, and one can usually obtain a history of chronic cough and sputum production as a background on which acute attacks of wheezing are superimposed. Recurrent emboli can be very difficult to separate from asthma. Frequently, patients with this condition present with episodes of breathlessness, particularly on exertion, and

they sometimes wheeze. Lung scans may not be diagnostic because of the ventilation-perfusion abnormalities characteristic of asthma, and pulmonary angiography may be necessary to establish the correct diagnosis.

Eosinophilic pneumonias (Chap. 237) are often associated with asthmatic symptoms, as are various chemical pneumonias and exposures to insecticides and cholinergic drugs. Bronchospasm is occasionally a manifestation of *systemic vasculitis* with pulmonary involvement.

DIAGNOSIS The diagnosis of asthma is established by demonstrating reversible airway obstruction. *Reversibility* is traditionally defined as a $\geq 15\%$ increase in FEV_1 after two puffs of a β-adrenergic agonist. When the spirometry results are normal at presentation, the diagnosis can be made by showing heightened airway responsiveness to challenges with histamine, methacholine, or isocapnic hyperventilation of cold air. Once the diagnosis is confirmed, the course of the illness and the effectiveness of therapy can be followed by measuring PEFRs at home and/or the FEV_1 in the office or laboratory. Positive wheal-and-flare reactions to skin tests can be demonstrated to various allergens, but such findings do not necessarily correlate with the intrapulmonary events. Sputum and blood eosinophilia and measurement of serum IgE levels are also helpful but are not specific for asthma. Chest roentgenograms showing hyperinflation are also nondiagnostic.

Rx TREATMENT

Elimination of the causative agent(s) from the environment of an allergic individual with asthma is the most successful means available for treating this condition (for details on avoidance, see Chap. 298). Desensitization or immunotherapy with extracts of the suspected allergens has enjoyed widespread favor, but controlled studies are limited and have not proved to be highly effective.

DRUG TREATMENT The available agents for treating asthma can be divided into two general categories: drugs that inhibit smooth-muscle contraction, i.e., the so-called "quick relief medications" (β-adrenergic agonists, methylxanthines, and anticholinergics) and agents that prevent and/or reverse inflammation, i.e., the "long-term control medications" (glucocorticoids, long-acting β_2-agonists, combined medications, mast cell–stabilizing agents, leukotriene modifiers, and methylxanthines (Table 236-1).

Quick Relief Medications ■ *ADRENERGIC STIMULANTS* The drugs in this category consist of the catecholamines, resorcinols, and saligenins. These agents produce airway dilation through stimulation of β-adrenergic receptors and activation of G proteins with the resultant formation of cyclic adenosine monophosphate (AMP). They also decrease release of mediators and improve mucociliary transport. The catecholamines (epinephrine, isoproterenol, and isoetharine) are short-acting (30 to 90 min) and are effective only when administered by inhalational or parenteral routes. Their use has been superceded by the longer acting selective β_2-agonists terbutaline, fenoterol (a resorsinol), and albuterol (a saligenin). The resorcinols and saligenins are highly selective for the respiratory tract and are virtually devoid of significant cardiac effects except at high doses.

Their major side effect is tremor. They are active by all routes of administration and are relatively long-lasting (4 to 6 h). Inhalation is the preferred route because it allows maximal bronchodilation with fewer side effects. In treating episodes of severe asthma, intravenous administration offers no advantages over the inhaled route.

Very long lasting compounds (salmeterol and formoterol) are available and provide sustained effects for 9 to 12 h (Table 236-1). They are particularly helpful for conditions such as nocturnal and exercise-induced asthma. Salmeterol is not recommended for the treatment of acute episodes because of its relatively slow onset of action (~30 min), nor is it intended as a rescue drug for breakthrough symptoms. In addition, its long half-life means that administration of extra doses can cause cumulative side effects. The limits to the use of formoterol are not yet fully established. These compounds are now thought of as long-term controller medications by some, presumably because of their anti-inflammatory activities. The clinical significance of this aspect of their pharmacology has yet to be completely elucidated.

METHYLXANTHINES Theophylline and its various salts are medium-potency bronchodilators with questionable anti-inflammatory properties. The therapeutic plasma concentrations of theophylline lie between 5 and 15 μg/mL. The dose required to achieve the desired level varies widely from patient to patient owing to differences in the metabolism of the drug. Clearance falls with age and the concurrent use of erythromycin and other macrolide antibiotics, the quinolone antibiotics, and troleandomycin, allopurinol, cimetidine, and propranolol. It rises with use of cigarettes, marijuana, phenobarbital, phenytoin, or any other drug that is capable of inducing hepatic microsomal enzymes.

For maintenance therapy, long-acting theophylline compounds are available and are usually given once or twice daily. The dose is adjusted on the basis of the clinical response with the aid of serum theophylline measurements. Single-dose administration in the evening reduces nocturnal symptoms and helps keep the patient complaint-free during the day. However, the methylxanthines can disrupt sleep architecture. They are now considered second-line therapy, and as such they are rarely used in acute situations and infrequently in chronic ones. There is minimal evidence for additional benefit when used with optimal doses of β-adrenergics. There are some data that the methylxanthines can decrease inflammation, but as with the long-acting β_2-agonists, the effect is not large and its clinical impact is undefined. Nonetheless, some authorities now place these compounds in the "controller" class (Fig. 236-1). The most common side effects are nervousness, nausea, vomiting, anorexia, and headache. At plasma levels >30 μg/mL there is a risk of seizures and cardiac arrhythmias.

ANTICHOLINERGICS Anticholinergic drugs such as ipratropium bromide have been found to be both effective and free of untoward effects. They may be of particular benefit for patients with coexistent heart disease, in whom the use of methylxanthines and β-adrenergic stimulants may be dangerous. The major disadvantages of the anticholinergics are that they are slow to act (60 to 90 min may be required before peak bronchodilation is achieved) and they are of only modest potency.

Long-Term Controller Medications (Table 236-1) ■ *GLUCOCORTICOIDS* Glucocorticoids are the most potent and most effective anti-inflammatory medications available. Systemic or oral steroids are most beneficial in acute illness, when severe airway obstruction is not resolving or is worsening despite intense optimal bronchodilator therapy, and in chronic disease, when there has been failure of a previously optimal regimen with frequent recurrences of symptoms of increasing severity. Inhaled glucocorticoids are used in the long-term control of asthma.

Glucocorticoids are not bronchodilators, and the correct dose to use in acute situations is a matter of debate. In the United States, the recommended starting dose is 120 to 180 mg of methylprednisolone intravenously every 6 h. Since intravenous and oral administration produce the same effects, prednisone, 60 mg every 6 h, can be substituted. Clinical impressions suggest that smaller quantities may work as effectively, but there are no confirmatory data. In the United Kingdom and elsewhere, acute asthma both in and out of hospital is frequently treated with doses of prednisolone ranging from 30 to 40 mg given once daily. It should be emphasized that the effects of steroids in acute asthma are not immediate and may not be seen for ≥6 h after the initial administration. Consequently, it is mandatory to continue vigorous bronchodilator therapy during this interval.

Some believe that glucocorticoids should be given to all acutely ill patients upon presentation because of their long delay to peak effect. While there is some merit to this argument, glucocorticoids are often not necessary; the symptoms of ~80% of patients seen in emergency departments resolve rapidly with only inhaled β-agonists. Those who need steroids can be rapidly identified by monitoring their PEFR. Irrespective of the regimen chosen, it is important to appreciate that rapid tapering of glucocorticoids frequently results in recurrent obstruction. Most authorities recommend reducing the dose by one-half every third to fifth day, over 10 to 12 days, after an acute episode. Beyond this point, the drug can be abruptly stopped. In situations in which it appears that continued steroid therapy is needed, an alternate-day schedule should be instituted to minimize side effects. This is particularly important in children, since continuous glucocorticoid administration interrupts growth. Long-acting preparations such as dexamethasone should not be used in this approach, for they defeat the purpose of alternate-day schedules by causing prolonged suppression of the pituitary-adrenal axis. The availability of inhaled agents has all but eliminated the need for this form of therapy. The usual doses of

TABLE 236-1 *Usual Dosages for Long-Term-Control Medications*

Medication	Dosage Form	Adult Dose
Inhaled glucocorticoids	*(See Table 236-2)*	
Systemic glucocorticoids	*(Applies to all three formulations)*	
Methylprednisolone	2-, 4-, 8-, 16-, 32-mg tablets	7.5–60 mg daily in a single dose in A.M. or qod as needed for control
Prednisolone	5-mg tablets, 5 mg/5 mL, 15 mg/5 mL	Short-course "burst" to achieve control: 40–60 mg/d as single or 2 divided doses for 3–10 days
Prednisone	1, 2.5, 5, 10, 20, 50 mg tablets; 5 mg/mL, 5 mg/5 mL	
Long-acting inhaled β_2-agonists *(Should not be used for symptom relief or for exacerbations. Use with inhaled glucocorticoids.)*		
Salmeterol	MDI 21 μg/puff	2 puffs q 12 h
	DPI 50 μg/blister	1 blister q 12 h
Formoterol	DPI 12 μg/single-use capsule	1 capsule q 12 h
Combined medication		
Fluticasone/salmeterol	DPI 100, 250, or 500 μg/50 μg	1 inhalation bid; dose depends on severity of asthma
Cromolyn and Nedocromil		
Cromolyn	MDI 1 mg/puff	2–4 puffs tid-qid
	Nebulizer 20 mg/ampule	1 ampule tid-qid
Nedocromil	MDI 1.75 mg/puff	2–4 puffs bid-qid
Leukotriene modifiers		
Montelukast	4- or 5-mg chewable tablet, 10-mg tablet	10 mg qhs
Zafirlukast	10- or 20-mg tablet	40 mg daily (20-mg tablet bid)
Zileuton	300- or 600-mg tablet	2400 mg daily (given tablets qid)
Methylxanthines *[Serum monitoring is important (serum concentration of 5–15 μg/mL at steady state)].*		
Theophylline	Liquids, sustained-release tablets, and capsules	Starting dose 10 mg/kg per day up to 300 mg max; usual max, 800 mg/d

Note: MDI, metered-dose inhaler; DPI, daily permissible intake.

TABLE 236-2 *Comparative Daily Doses for Inhaled Steroids*

Drug	How Supplied	Dose Range		
		Low	Medium	High
Beclomethasone		168–540 μg	504–840 μg	>840 μg
	42 μg/puff	4–12 puffs	10–12 puffs	>20 puffs
	84 μg/puff	2–6 puffs	6–10 puffs	>10 puffs
Budesonide		200–400 μg	400–600 μg	>600 μg
	200 μg/dose	1–2 inhalations	2–3 inhalations	>3 inhalations
Flunisolide		500–1000 μg	1000–2000 μg	>2000 μg
	250 μg/dose	2–4 puffs	4–8 puffs	>8 puffs
Fluticasone		88–264 μg	264–660 μg	>660 μg
	MDI: 44,110, 220 μg/puff	2–6 puffs (44 μg) 2 puffs (110 μg)	2–6 puffs (110 μg)	>6 puffs (110 μg)
	DPI: 50,100, 250 μg/puff	2–6 inhalations (50 μg)	3–6 inhalations (100 μg)	>6 inhalations (100 μg)
Triamcinolone		400–1000 μg	1000–2000 μg	>2000 μg
	100 μg/puff	4–10 puffs	10–20 puffs	>20 puffs

Note: MDI, metered-dose inhaler; DPI, daily permissible intake.

oral glucocorticoids for nonemergent episodes of asthma are summarized in Table 236-1.

Inhaled Glucocorticoids These drugs are indicated in patients with persistent symptoms. The agents currently available in the United States and their comparative doses are presented in Table 236-2. These drugs share the ability to control inflammation, facilitate the long-term prevention of symptoms, reduce the need for oral glucocorticoids, minimize acute occurrences, and prevent hospitalizations.

There is no fixed dose of inhaled steroid that works for all patients. Requirements are dictated by the response of the individual and wax and wane in concert with progression of the disease. Generally, the worse the patient's condition, the more inhaled steroid is needed to gain control. Once achieved, however, remission can often be maintained with quantities as low as one or two puffs/day. Inhaled steroids can take up to a week or more to produce improvements; consequently, in rapidly deteriorating situations, it is best to prescribe oral preparations and initiate inhaled drugs as the dose of the former is reduced. In less emergent circumstances, the quantity of inhaled drug can be increased up to 2 to 2.5 times the recommended starting doses. The side effects increase in proportion to the dose-time product. In addition to thrush and dysphonia, the increased systemic absorption that accompanies larger doses of inhaled steroids has been reported to produce adrenal suppression, cataract formation, decreased growth in children, interference with bone metabolism, and purpura. As is the case with oral agents, suppression of inflammation, per se, cannot be relied upon to provide optimal results. It is essential to continue adrenergic or methylxanthine bronchodilators if the patient's disease is unstable. The combination of a long acting β-agonist and inhaled steroid seems particularly efficacious in patients with mild to moderate disease.

COMBINED MEDICATIONS The combination of an inhaled steroid and a long-acting β_2 agonist is gaining popularity. The only such combination available in the United States at present is fluticasone and salmeterol. Other combinations are being tested but are not yet available. There is little question that combinations of agents add a significant degree of convenience in the care of chronic asthma. They tend to work best in patients with milder disease. It has been suggested that the combination provides better pharmacologic activity than the individual drugs given alone.

MAST CELL–STABILIZING AGENTS Cromolyn sodium and nedocromil sodium do not influence airway tone. Their major therapeutic effect is to inhibit the degranulation of mast cells, thereby preventing the release of the chemical mediators of anaphylaxis.

Cromolyn sodium and nedocromil sodium, like the inhaled steroids, improve lung function, reduce symptoms, and lower airway reactivity in persons with asthma. They are most effective in atopic patients who have either seasonal disease or perennial airway stimulation. A therapeutic trial of two puffs four times daily for 4 to 6 weeks is frequently necessary before the beneficial effects of the drug appear. Unlike steroids, nedocromil and cromolyn sodium, when given prophylactically, block the acute obstructive effects of exposure to antigen, industrial chemicals, exercise, or cold air. With antigen, the late response is also abolished. Therefore, a patient who has intermittent exposure to either antigenic or nonantigenic stimuli that provoke acute episodes of asthma need not use these drugs continuously but instead can obtain protection by taking the drug only 15 to 20 min before contact with the precipitant.

LEUKOTRIENE MODIFIERS As mentioned earlier, the cysteinyl leukotrienes (LTC$_4$, LTD$_4$, and LTE$_4$) produce many of the critical elements of asthma, and drugs have been developed that either reduce the synthesis of all of the leukotrienes by inhibiting 5-lipoxygenase (5-LO), the enzyme involved in their production, or competitively antagonize the principal moiety (LTD$_4$). Zileuton is the only 5-LO synthesis inhibitor that is available in the United States. It is a modest bronchodilator that reduces asthma morbidity, provides protection against exercise-induced asthma, and diminishes nocturnal symptoms, but it has limited effectiveness against allergens. Hepatic enzyme levels can be elevated after its use, and there are significant interactions with other drugs metabolized in the liver. The LTD$_4$ receptor antagonists (zafirlukast and montelukast) have therapeutic and toxicologic profiles similar to that of zileuton but are long acting and permit twice- to once-daily dose schedules.

This class of drugs does not appear to be uniformly effective in all patients with asthma. Although precise figures are lacking, most authorities put the number of positive responders at <50%. As yet, there is no way of determining prospectively who will benefit, so clinical trials are required. Typically, if there is no improvement after 1 month, treatment can be discontinued. The leukotriene blockers have been associated with uncovering of Churg-Strauss syndrome (Chap. 306).

Miscellaneous Agents It has been suggested that steroid-dependent patients might benefit from the use of immunosuppressant agents such as methotrexate, gold salts, or colchicine. The effects of these agents on steroid dosage and disease activity are minor, and side effects can be considerable. Opiates, sedatives, and tranquilizers should be absolutely avoided in the acutely ill patient with asthma because the risk of depressing alveolar ventilation is great, and respiratory arrest has been reported to occur shortly after their use. Admittedly, most individuals are anxious and frightened, but experience has shown that they can be calmed equally well by the physician's presence and reassurances. β-Adrenergic blockers and parasympathetic agonists are contraindicated because they can cause marked deterioration in lung function.

Expectorants and mucolytic agents have enjoyed great vogue in the past, but they do not add significantly to the treatment of the acute or chronic phases of this disease. The use of intravenous fluids in the treatment of acute asthma has also been advocated. There is little evidence that this adjunct hastens recovery. Nonstandard bronchodilators, such as intravenous magnesium sulfate, for the treatment of acute asthma attacks are not yet warranted in clinical practice because of the controversy surrounding their efficacy.

Special Instructions The treatment of patients with asthma who have coexisting conditions such as heart disease or pregnancy does not differ materially from that outlined above. Therapy with inhaled β_2-selective and anti-inflammatory agents is the mainstay. The lowest doses of adrenergics that produce the desired effects should be used.

Framework for Management ■ *EMERGENCY SITUATIONS* The most effective treatment for acute episodes of asthma requires a systematic approach based on the aggressive use of sympathomimetic agents and serial objective monitoring of key indices of improvement. Reliance on empiricism and subjective assessment is no longer acceptable. Multiple inhalations of a short-acting sympathomimetic, such as albuterol, are the cornerstone of most regimens. These drugs provide three to four times more relief than does intravenous aminophylline. Anticholinergic drugs are not first-line therapy because of their long lag time to onset (~30 to 40 min) and their relatively modest bronchodilator properties. In emergency situations, β_2-agonists can be given every 20 min by handheld nebulizer for 2 to 3 doses. The optimum cumulative dose of albuterol appears to lie between 5 and 10 mg. It does not matter how the adrenergic agonists are inhaled. Treatment with albuterol administered by jet nebulizer, metered dose inhaler, or dry powder inhaler all provide equal resolution in acute situations when the doses are matched. Continuous nebulization of β_2-agonists has also been employed, but it is unclear if it is materially better than the other forms of treatment. Ipratropium can be added to the regimen in an attempt to speed resolution. The benefits on lung function are small, but the need for admission has decreased in some studies. There are no hard and fast rules as to who should be admitted.

Acute episodes of bronchial asthma are one of the most common respiratory emergencies, and it is essential that the physician recognize which episodes of airway obstruction are life-threatening and which patients demand what level of care. These distinctions can be made readily by assessing selected clinical parameters in combination with measures of expiratory flow and gas exchange. The presence of a paradoxical pulse, use of accessory muscles, and marked hyperinflation of the thorax signify severe airways obstruction, and failure of these signs to remit promptly after aggressive therapy mandates objective monitoring of the patient with measurements of arterial blood gases and PEFR or FEV_1. Although pulse and respiratory rates are commonly recorded, there is no relationship between these variables and the severity of the obstruction or the outcome of treatment.

Patients with the most impairment typically require the most extensive therapy for resolution. If the PEFR or FEV_1 is ≤20% of predicted on presentation and does not double within an hour of receiving the preceding therapy, the patient is likely to require extensive treatment, including glucocorticoids, before the obstruction dissipates. This group represents ~20% of all the patients who present for acute care. They generally require inpatient treatment before becoming asymptomatic. In such patients, if the clinical signs of a paradoxical pulse and accessory muscle use are diminishing and/or the PEFR is increasing, there is no need to change medications or doses, but the patient needs to be followed closely. However, if the PEFR falls by >20% of its previous value or if the magnitude of the pulsus paradoxicus is increasing, serial measures of arterial blood gases are required, as well as a reconsideration of the therapeutic modalities being employed. If the patient has hypocarbia, one can afford to continue the current approaches a while longer. On the other hand, if the Pa_{CO_2} is within the normal range or is elevated, the patient should be monitored in an intensive care setting, and therapy should be intensified to reverse or arrest the patient's respiratory failure.

Treatment with 70 to 80% helium (balance oxygen) may be beneficial in patients with severe airway obstruction. This gas mixture reduces airway resistance and improves the effect of aerosolized bronchodilators. This form of treatment should be considered in patients whose airway obstruction and gas exchange are worsening despite aggressive therapy. However, there are no large-scale clinical trials comparing this approach with other forms of treatment. The criteria for intubation and ventilatory support have not been standardized. The decision to use this therapy should be made by physicians with the most experience in caring for severely ill asthmatic patients.

Chronic Treatment The goal of chronic therapy is to achieve a stable, asymptomatic state with the best pulmonary function possible using the least amount of medication. The specific recommmendations from consensus guidelines are to promote a state of health encompassing the following: (1) minimal or absent daytime or nocturnal chronic symptoms, (2) minimal or absent exacerbations, (3) no limitation on activities, (4) no absences from school or work, (5) maintenance of normal or near-normal pulmonary functions, (6) the minimal use of short-acting β_2-agonists (< once per day, <1 canister/month), (7) and minimal or absent adverse effects from medications. A primary step is to educate patients to function as partners in their management. The severity of the illness needs to be assessed and monitored with objective measures of lung function. Asthma triggers should be avoided or controlled, and plans should be made for both chronic management and treatment of exacerbations. Regular follow-up care is mandatory.

A stepwise pharmacologic approach recommended by the National Asthma Education and Prevention Program is presented in Table 236-3. The purpose of this schema is to assist and not replace the clinical decision-making required to meet individual patient needs. In general, the simplest approach works best. Infrequent symptoms (step 1) require only the use of an inhaled sympathomimetic on an "as-needed" basis. When the disease worsens to a persistent state (step 2), as manifested by nocturnal awakenings and daytime symptoms, inhaled steroids, mast cell–stabilizing agents, and/or leukotriene modifiers should be added. Methylxanthines can also be employed. If symptoms do not abate (step 3), the dose of inhaled steroids can be increased. An upper limit has not yet been established, but side effects of glucocorticoid excess begin to appear more frequently when the dose exceeds 2.0 mg/kg per d. Persistent asthma complaints can be treated with low- to medium-dose inhaled glucocorticoids and long-acting inhaled β_2-agonists. Alternative treatments include leukotriene modifiers or sustained-release theophylline. In patients with recurrent or perennial symptoms and unstable lung function (step 4), the preferred treatment is high-dose inhaled glucocorticoids and long-acting inhaled β_2-agonists. If needed, oral glucocorticoids in a single daily dose are added to the regimen. Acute symptoms are treated with short-acting rescue medications such as albuterol alone or in combination with a parasympatholytic.

Once control is reached and sustained for several weeks, a stepdown reduction in therapy should be undertaken, beginning with the most toxic drug, to find the minimum amount of medication required to keep the patient well. During this process, the PEFR should be monitored and medication adjustments should be based on objective changes in lung function as well as on the patient's symptoms. The recommendations in the step-down mode are that treatment be reviewed every 1 to 6 months. In many instances, shorter periods can be employed. We have found that 2 to 4 weeks are a reasonable period. When a patient's asthma is destabilizing, frequent assessments are required. It is important to gain control as quickly as possible and then step down to the least medication necessary to maintain control. If there are difficulties in achieving this goal, then referral to an asthma specialist should be considered. Prior to increasing treatment, an important component is to review patients' inhaler technique, their adherence to therapeutic recommendations, and environment control.

PROGNOSIS AND CLINICAL COURSE The mortality rate from asthma is small. The most recent figures for the United States indicate fewer than 6000 deaths per year out of a population of ~10 million patients at risk. Death rates, however, appear to be rising in inner-city areas where there is limited availability of health care. Even so, only 0.09 to 0.25% of admissions to hospital are at risk of an untoward event.

Information on the clinical course of asthma suggests a good prognosis, particularly for those whose disease is mild and develops in childhood. The number of children who still have asthma 7 to 10 years after the initial diagnosis varies from 26 to 78%, averaging 46%; how-

TABLE 236-3 *Stepwise Approach for Managing Asthma in Adults*

Classify Severity: Clinical Features Before Treatment or Adequate Control

	Symptoms		PEFR or FEV₁	
	Day	Night	(PEFR Variability)	Daily Medications to Maintain Long-Term Control
Step 1: Mild intermittent	≤2 days/week	≤ 2 nights/month	≥80% (< 20%)	No daily medication needed. Severe exacerbations may occur, separated by long periods of normal lung function and no symptoms. A course of systemic glucocorticoids is recommended.
Step 2: Mild persistent	> 2 days/week but <1 per day	>2 nights/months	≥ 80% (20–30%)	Low-dose inhaled glucocorticoids Alternative treatment (listed alphabetically): cromolyn, leukotriene modifier, nedocromil, *or* sustained-release theophylline to serum concentration of 5–15 μg/mL.
Step 3: Moderate persistent	Daily	> 1 night/week	> 60%–< 80% (>30%)	Low- to medium-dose inhaled glucocorticoids and long-acting inhaled β_2-agonists. Alternative treatment: leukotriene modifier or theophylline instead of β_2 agents
Step 4: Severe persistent	Continual	Frequent	≤60% (> 30%)	High-dose inhaled glucocorticoids *and* Long-acting inhaled β_2-agonists *and*, if needed, Glucocorticoid tablets or syrup long term (2mg/kg per day, generally do not exceed 60 mg/d). (Make repeat attempts to reduce systemic glucocorticoids and maintain control with high-dose inhaled glucocorticoids.)
Quick relief for all patients	Short-acting bronchodilator: 2–4 puffs short-acting inhaled β_2-agonists as needed for symptoms. Intensity of treatment will depend on severity of exacerbation; up to 3 treatments at 20-min intervals or a single nebulizer treatment as needed. Course of systemic glucocorticoids may be needed. Use of short-acting β_2-agonists >2 times a week in intermittent asthma (daily, or increasing use in persistent asthma) may indicate the need to initiate (increase) long-term control therapy.			

Note: PEFR, peak expiratory flow rate; FEV₁, forced expiratory volume in 1 s.

Source: Modified from National Asthma Education and Prevention Program.

ever, the percentage who continue to have severe disease is relatively low (6 to 19%).

Although there are reports of patients with asthma developing irreversible changes in lung function, these individuals frequently have comorbid stimuli such as cigarette smoking that could account for these findings. Even when untreated, individuals with asthma do not continuously move from mild to severe disease with time. Rather, their clinical course is characterized by exacerbations and remissions. Some studies suggest that spontaneous remissions occur in approximately 20% of those who develop the disease as adults, and that ~40% can be expected to experience improvement, with less frequent and severe attacks, as they grow older.

FURTHER READING

BEASLEY DM et al: Prevalence and etiology of asthma. J Allergy Clin Immunol 105:S466, 2000

BUSSE WW: Anti-immunoglobulin E (omalizumab) therapy in allergic asthma. Am J Respir Crit Care Med 164:S12, 2001

————, LEMANSKE RF: Asthma. N Engl J Med 344:350, 2001

FITZGERALD M: Acute asthma. BMJ 323:841, 2001

HALL JB: Concise review: Contemporary management of status asthmaticus. New York: McGraw-Hill, www.harrisonsonline.com

ISRAEL E et al: The effect of polymorphisms of the beta2-adrenergic receptor on the response to regular use of albuterol in asthma. Am J Respir Crit Care Med 162:75, 2000

LAZARUS SC et al: Long-acting β_2-agonist monotherapy vs continued therapy with inhaled corticosteroids in patients with persistent asthma: A randomized controlled trial. JAMA 285:2583, 2001

MARTIN RJ et al: Systemic effect comparisons of six inhaled corticosteroid preparations. Am J Respir Crit Care Med 165:1377, 2002

THE NAEPP EXPERT PANEL REPORT: *Guidelines for the Diagnosis and Management of Asthma—Update on Selected Topics, 2002.* NIH publication no. 02-5075

O'BYRNE PM et al: Low dose inhaled budesonide and formoterol in mild persistent asthma: The OPTIMA randomized trial. Am J Respir Crit Care Med 164:1392, 2001

SZCZEKLIK A, STEVENSON DD: Aspirin-induced asthma: Advances in pathogenesis, diagnosis, and management. J Allergy Clin Immunol 111:913, 2003

TOGIAS A: Rhinitis and asthma: evidence for respiratory system integration. J Allergy Clin Immunol 111:1171, 2003

237 HYPERSENSITIVITY PNEUMONITIS AND PULMONARY INFILTRATES WITH EOSINOPHILIA
Joel N. Kline, Gary W. Hunninghake

HYPERSENSITIVITY PNEUMONITIS

First described in 1874, hypersensitivity pneumonitis (HP), or extrinsic allergic alveolitis, is an inflammatory disorder of the lung, involving alveolar walls and terminal airways, that is induced by repeated inhalation of a variety of organic agents by a susceptible host. Factors responsible for the expression of HP include both those related to the host (susceptibility) and the inciting agent. Causes of HP are typically designated with colorful names denoting the occupational or avocational risk associated with the disease; "farmer's lung" is the term most commonly used for HP due to inhalation of antigens present in moldy hay, such as thermophilic actinomyces, *Micropolyspora faeni*, and As-

pergillus species. The frequency of HP is unknown but varies with the environmental exposure and the specific antigen involved. The prevalence of farmer's lung among Wisconsin dairy farmers has been reported as 4.2 per 1000 and a Finnish cohort study demonstrated an annual incidence of 5 per 10,000 farmers. The diagnosis of HP requires a constellation of clinical, radiographic, physiologic, pathologic, and immunologic criteria, each of which is rarely pathognomonic alone, and the preferred treatment is avoidance of the causative antigen.

ETIOLOGY Agents implicated as causes of HP are diverse and include those listed in Table 237-1. Many cases of HP occurring in various occupations involve exposure to similar agents, particularly the thermophilic actinomycetes. In the United States, the most common types of HP are farmer's lung, bird fancier's lung, and chemical worker's lung. In *farmer's lung*, inhalation of proteins such as thermophilic bacteria and fungal spores that are present in moldy bedding and feed are most commonly responsible for the development of HP. These antigens are probably also responsible for the etiology of *mushroom worker's disease* (moldy composted growth medium is the source of the proteins) and *bagassosis* (moldy sugar cane is the source). *Bird fancier's lung* (and the related disorders of duck fever, turkey handler's lung, and dove pillow's lung) is a response to inhalation of proteins from feathers and droppings. *Chemical worker's lung* is an example of how simple chemicals, such as isocyanates, may also cause immune-mediated diseases. In this case, antihapten antibodies may be responsible for the development of HP. Although HP requires an immunulogic response to the inciting agent, such a response alone does not ensure the development of disease. Environmental factors such as ambient humidity and temperature play an important role in the development of disease, as do the concentration, frequency, and duration of exposure as well as the nature and size of the antigen particles. In some cases, the responsible exposure environment (for example, metalworking fluid) may be identified without implicating a specific antigen. Finally, personal habits may alter the apperance and course of disease: smokers appear more likely to present with chronic rather than acute HP, suggesting that smoking may inhibit antibody production.

PATHOGENESIS The finding that precipitating antibodies against extracts of moldy hay were demonstrable in most patients with farmer's lung led to the early conclusion that HP was an immune complex–mediated reaction. Subsequent investigations of HP in human beings and animal models provided evidence for the importance of cell-mediated hypersensitivity. The very early (acute) reaction is characterized by an increase in polymorphonuclear leukocytes in the alveoli and small airways. This early lesion is followed by an influx of mononuclear cells into the lung and the formation of granulomas that appear to be the result of a classic delayed (T cell mediated) hypersensitivity reaction to repeated inhalation of antigen and adjuvant-active materials. Studies in animal models suggest that the disease is a T_H1-mediated immune response to antigen, with both interferon-α and interleukin (IL) 12 contributing to disease expression. Most likely, multiple cytokines [including also IL-1β, transforming growth factor (TGF) β, tumor necrosis factor (TNF) α and others] interact to promote HP; their source includes both alveolar macrophages and T lymphocytes in the lung. Observations support a genetic predisposition to the development of HP; certain polymorphisms of the TNF-α promoter region reportedly confer an enhanced susceptibility to pigeon breeder's disease.

The attraction and accumulation of inflammatory cells in the lung

may be due to one or more of the following mechanisms: induction of the adhesion molecules L-selectin and E-selectin; elaboration by dendritic cells of CC chemokine 1 [dendritic cell–derived chemokine-1 (DC-CK-1)/cysteine-cysteine chemokine 18 (CCL18)]; and increased levels of Fas protein and FasL in the lung. Bronchoalveolar lavage (BAL) in patients with HP consistently demonstrates an increase in T lymphocytes in lavage fluid (a finding that is also observed in patients with other granulomatous lung disorders). Patients with recent or continual exposure to antigen may have an increase in polymorphonuclear leukocytes in lavage fluid; this has been associated with lung fibrosis. A role for oxidant injury has been proposed in HP, which is supported by the finding that BAL levels of the antioxidant glutathione are reduced following airway challenge in patients with HP, whereas they are increased in asymptomatic controls. In most patients examined during recovery from acute disease, the T lymphocytes in lavage fluid are predominantly the CD8+ T cell subset. In patients with very recent exposure to antigen, however, the numbers of CD4+ T cells may increase in lavage fluid. These observations and

TABLE 237-1 Selected Examples of Hypersensitivity Pneumonitis (HP)

Disease	Antigen	Source of Antigen
Bagassosis	Thermophilic actinomycetes[a]	"Moldy" bagasse (sugar cane)
Bird fancier's, breeder's, or handler's lung[b]	Parakeet, pigeon, chicken, turkey proteins	Avian droppings or feathers
Cephalosporium HP	Contaminated basement (sewage)	*Cephalosporium*
Cheese washer's lung	*Penicillium casei*	Moldy cheese
Chemical worker's lung[a]	Isocyanates	Polyurethane foam, varnishes, lacquer
Coffee worker's lung	Coffee bean dust	Coffee beans
Compost lung	*Aspergillus*	Compost
Detergent worker's disease	*Bacillus subtilis* enzymes (subtilisins)	Detergent
Familial HP	*Bacillus subtilis*	Contaminated wood dust in walls
Farmer's lung[a]	Thermophilic actinomycetes[b]	"Moldy" hay, grain, silage
Fish food lung	Unknown	Fish food
Fish meal worker's lung	Fish meal dust	Fish meal
Furrier's lung	Animal fur dust	Animal pelts
Hot tub lung	*Cladosporium* sp.	Mold on ceiling
Humidifier or air-conditioner lung (ventilation pneumonitis)	*Aureobasidium pullulans, Candida albicans*, other microorganisms	Contaminated water in humidification or forced-air air-conditioning systems
Japanese summer-type HP	*Trichosporon cutaneum, asahii,* and *mucoides*	House dust? Bird droppings
Laboratory worker's HP	Male rat urine	Laboratory rat
Lycoperdonosis	*Lycoperdon* puffballs	Puffball spores
Malt worker's lung	*Aspergillus fumigatus* or *A. clavatus*	Moldy barley
Maple bark disease	*Cryptostroma corticale*	Maple bark
Miller's lung	*Sitophilus granarius* (wheat weevil)	Infested wheat flour
Miscellaneous medication	Amiodarone, bleomycin, efavrienz, hydralazine, hydroxyurea, iosoniazid, methotrexate, paclitaxel, penicillin, procarbazine, propanolol, sulfasalazine	Medication
Mushroom worker's lung	Thermophilic actinomycetes,[b] *Hypsizigus marmoreus*, others	Mushroom compost
Pituitary snuff taker's lung	Animal proteins	Heterologous pituitary snuff
Potato riddler's lung	Thermophilic actinomycetes,[a] *Aspergillus*	"Moldy" hay around potatoes
Sauna taker's lung	*Aureobasidium* sp., other	Contaminated sauna water
Sausage worker's lung	*Penicillium nalgiovense*	Dry sausage mold
Sequoiosis	*Aureobasidium, Graphium* sp.	Redwood sawdust
Streptomyces albus HP	*Streptomyces albus*	Contaminated fertilizer
Suberosis	Cork dust mold	Cork dust
Tap water lung	Unknown	Contaminated tap water
Thatched roof disease	*Saccharomonospora viridis*	Dried grasses and leaves
Tobacco worker's disease	*Aspergillus* sp.	Mold on tobacco
Winegrower's lung	*Botrytis cinerea*	Mold on grapes
Wood trimmer's disease	*Rhizopus* sp., *Mucor* sp.	Contaminated wood trimmings
Woodman's disease	*Penicillium* sp.	Oak and maple trees
Woodworker's lung	Wood dust, *Alternaria*	Oak, cedar, pine, and mahogany dusts

[a] Thermophilic actinomycetes species include *Micropolyspora faeni, Thermoactinomyces vulgaris, T. saccharrii, T. viridis,* and *T. candidus.*
[b] Most common causes of hypersensitivity pneumonitis in the United States.

others in animal models suggest that there is an active modulation of granuloma formation in the lung by immunoregulatory T cells and associated cytokines in this disorder.

CLINICAL PRESENTATION The clinical picture is that of an interstitial pneumonitis, which varies from patient to patient and seems related to the frequency and intensity of exposure to the causative antigen and perhaps other host factors. The presentation can be *acute, subacute,* or *chronic*. In the *acute form,* symptoms such as cough, fever, chills, malaise, and dyspnea may occur 6 to 8 h after exposure to the antigen and usually clear within a few days if there is no further exposure to antigen. The *subacute form* often appears insidiously over a period of weeks marked by cough and dyspnea and may progress to cyanosis and severe dyspnea requiring hospitalization. In some patients, a subacute form of the disease may persist after an acute presentation of the disorder, especially if there is continued exposure to antigen. In most patients with the acute or subacute form of HP, the symptoms, signs, and other manifestations of HP disappear within days, weeks, or months if the causative agent is no longer inhaled. Transformation to a chronic form of the disease may occur in patients with continued antigen exposure, but the frequency of such progression is uncertain. The *chronic form* of HP may be clinically indistinguishable from pulmonary fibrosis due to a wide variety of causes. Physical examination may reveal clubbing. This stage may progressively worsen, resulting in dependence on supplemental oxygen, pulmonary hypertension, and death from respiratory failure. An indolent, gradually progressive form of the disease can be associated with cough and exertional dyspnea without a prior history consistent with acute or subacute manifestations. Such a gradual onset frequently occurs with low-dose exposure to the antigen.

As strict definitions of acute, subacute, and chronic stages of hypersensitivity pneumonitis have not been generally agreed on, interpretation of epidemiologic and clinical studies can be difficult. Because of this, it has been proposed that hypersensitivity pneumonitis be described as recently diagnosed, recurrent or progressive, or residual disease. For these categories, required diagnostic criteria include the history of symptoms following an exposure to a putative HP agent and symptoms associated with re-exposure; compatible radiologic findings; if performed, lymphocytic alveolitis on BAL; and, if performed, compatible histopathology on biopsy. Supportive criteria include bibasilar crackles, diminished carbon monoxide diffusion capacity, and hypoxemia.

DIAGNOSIS Following acute exposure to antigen, neutrophilia and lymphopenia are frequently present. Eosinophilia is not a feature. All forms of the disease may be associated with elevations in erythrocyte sedimentation rate, C-reactive protein, rheumatoid factor, and serum immunoglobulins. Antinuclear antibodies are rarely present and appear to have no pathogenic role. Examination for *serum precipitins* against suspected antigens, such as those listed in Table 237-1, is an important part of the diagnostic workup and should be performed on any patient with interstitial lung disease, especially if a suggestive exposure history is elicited. If found, precipitins indicate sufficient exposure to the causative agent for generation of an immunologic response. The diagnosis of HP is not established solely by the presence of precipitins, however, as precipitins are found in sera of many individuals exposed to appropriate antigens who demonstrate no other evidence of HP. False-negative results may occur because of poor-quality antigens or an inappropriate choice of antigens. Extraction of antigens from the suspected source may at times be helpful.

Chest x-ray shows no specific or distinctive changes in HP. It can be normal even in symptomatic patients. The acute or subacute phase may be associated with poorly defined, patchy, or diffuse infiltrates or with discrete, nodular infiltrates. In the chronic phase, the chest x-ray usually shows a diffuse reticulonodular infiltrate. Honeycombing may eventually develop as the condition progresses. Apical sparing is common, suggesting that disease severity correlates with inhaled antigen

load, but no particular distribution or pattern is classic for HP. Abnormalities rarely seen in HP include pleural effusion or thickening, and hilar adenopathy. High-resolution chest computed tomography (CT) has become the procedure of choice for imaging of HP, and a consensus is developing as to the typical appearance of the disease. Although pathognomonic features have not been identified, ground grass changes predominate in the lower lobes, especially in acute disease; this pattern is more common in workers whose exposure to antigen continues rather than those in whom removal from antigen exposure has occurred. Centrilobular nodules are also commonly seen. In chronic HP, patchy emphysema is seen more often than interstitial fibrosis, although neither predominates in the lower lobes; CT is far more sensitive than plain films at detecting these changes. Hilar or mediastinal adenopathy is not associated with HP, but its presence has no diagnostic significance (Fig. 237-1). Although not currently clinically used, *radionuclide studies* may have a role in the future diagnosis of HP: several case reports have inadvertently demonstrated rapid pulmonary uptake of radionuclides associated with a lymphocytic alveolitis in acute HP.

Pulmonary function studies in all forms of HP may show a restrictive or obstructive pattern with loss of lung volumes, impaired diffusion capacity, decreased compliance, and an exercise-induced hypoxemia. A resting hypoxemia may also be found. Bronchospasm and bronchial hyperreactivity are sometimes found in acute hypersensitivity pneumonitis. With antigen avoidance, the pulmonary function abnormalities are usually reversible, but they may gradually increase in severity or may occur rapidly following acute or subacute exposure to antigen.

Bronchoalveolar lavage is used in some centers to aid in diagnostic evaluation. A marked lymphocytic alveolitis on (BAL) is almost universal, although not pathognomonic. Lymphocytes typically have a decreased helper/suppressor ratio, and are activated. Alveolar neutrophilia is also prominent acutely, but tends to fade in the absence of recurrent exposure. Bronchoalveolar mastocytosis may correlate with disease activity. *Lung biopsy,* obtained through flexible bronchoscopy, open-lung procedures, or thoracoscopy, may be diagnostic. Although the histopathology is distinctive, it may not be pathognomonic of HP (Fig. 237-2). When the biopsy is taken during the active phase of disease, typical findings include an interstitial alveolar infiltrate consisting of plasma cells, lymphocytes, and occasional eosinophils and neutrophils, usually with accompanying loose, noncaseating peribronchial granulomas. Interstitial fibrosis may be present but most often is mild in earlier stages of the disease. Some degree of bronchiolitis is found in about half the cases, whereas vasculitis is not a feature of the

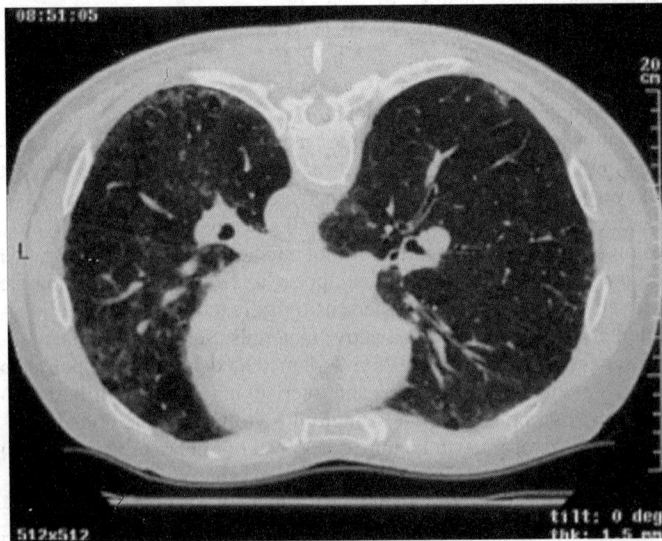

FIGURE 237-1 Chest CT scan of a case of acute hypersensitivity pneumonitis in which scattered regions of ground glass and nodular infiltrates are seen bilaterally. *(Courtesy of JS Wilson.)*

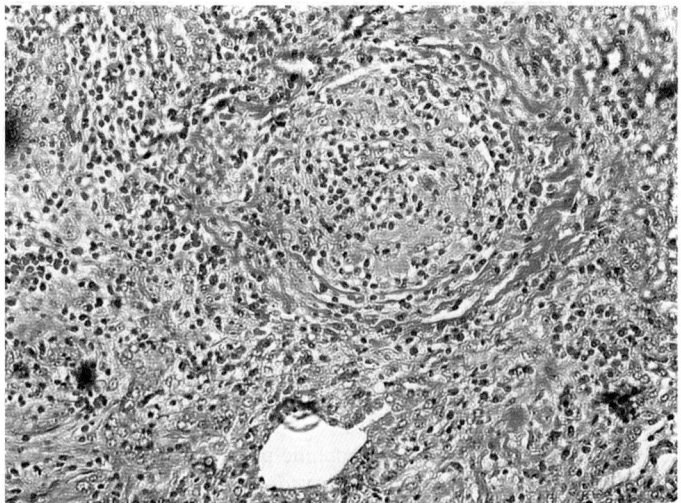

FIGURE 237-2 Open lung biopsy of a case of acute hypersensitivity pneumonitis demonstrating loose, nonnecrotizing granulomas and thickened interstitium with an associated interstitial inflammatory response. *(Courtesy of B DeYoung.)*

disorder. Rarely, bronchiolitis obliterans with organizing pneumonia (BOOP) can be seen. The triad of mononuclear bronchiolitis; interstitial infiltrates of lymphocytes and plasma cells; and single, nonnecrotizing, and randomly scattered parenchymal granulomas without mural vascular involvement is consistent with but not specific for HP.

Inhalation challenge studies have been described as useful to differentiate between HP and other interstitial lung diseases; a positive response to inhaled antigen may include fever, chills, dyspnea, diminished oxygen saturation, transient airflow obstruction, and peripheral and bronchoalveolar leukocytosis. These tests should be performed in a center that specializes in provocation testing for reasons of both safety and accuracy. Moreover, as the antigens used for provocation testing are not standardized, interpretation of these tests is difficult. In general, these tests may be used to support a diagnosis of HP, but they are not sufficiently accepted to either confirm or deny the diagnosis. The lack of standardized, nonirritating antigens and of proven controlled protocols makes *skin testing* useful only for research purposes. Similarly, in vitro tests of cell-mediated (delayed) hypersensitivity have not consistently been shown to correlate with clinical HP and have no place in the routine diagnostic workup.

In summary, the diagnosis in most cases is established by (1) consistent history, physical findings, pulmonary function tests, and chest x-ray; (2) exposure to a recognized antigen; and (3) finding an antibody to that antigen. In a few circumstances, (BAL) and/or lung biopsy may be needed. Provocation tests may be useful but are not essential. The most important tool in diagnosing HP may, in fact, be a high index of suspicion.

DIFFERENTIAL DIAGNOSIS Chronic HP may often be difficult to distinguish from a number of other interstitial lung disorders such as idiopathic pulmonary fibrosis, sarcoidosis, interstitial lung disease associated with a collagen vascular disorder, and drug-induced lung diseases. A negative history for use of relevant drugs and no evidence of a systemic disorder usually exclude the presence of drug-induced lung disease or a collagen vascular disorder. BAL often shows predominance of neutrophils in idiopathic pulmonary fibrosis and a predominance of CD4+ lymphocytes in sarcoidosis. Hilar/paratracheal lymphadenopathy or evidence of multisystem involvement also favors the diagnosis of sarcoidosis. In some patients, a lung biopsy may be required to differentiate chronic HP from other interstitial diseases. The lung disease associated with acute or subacute HP may clinically resemble other disorders that present with systemic symptoms and recurrent pulmonary infiltrates, including the allergic bronchopulmonary mycoses and other eosinophilic pneumonias.

Eosinophilic pneumonia is often associated with asthma and is typified by peripheral eosinophilia; neither of these is a feature of HP.

Allergic bronchopulmonary aspergillosis (ABPA) is the most common example of the allergic bronchopulmonary mycoses and is sometimes confused with HP because of the presence of precipitating antibodies to *Aspergillus fumigatus*. ABPA is associated with allergic (atopic) asthma. Acute HP may be confused with *organic dust toxic syndrome* (ODTS), a condition that is more common than HP. ODTS follows heavy exposure to organic dusts and is characterized by transient fever and muscle aches, with or without dyspnea and cough. Serum precipitins are absent and the chest x-ray is usually normal. Studies have shown no immunologic basis for ODTS, and endotoxin is suspected to be involved in its pathogenesis. This distinction is important, as ODTS is a self-limited disorder without significant long-term sequelae, whereas continued antigen exposure in HP can result in permanent disability. Massive exposure to moldy silage may result in a syndrome termed *pulmonary mycotoxicosis*, with fever, chills, and cough and the presence of pulmonary infiltrates within a few hours of exposure. No previous sensitization is required, and precipitins are absent to *Aspergillus*, the suspected causative agent.

℞ TREATMENT

Because effective treatment depends largely on avoiding the antigen, identification of the causative agent and its source is essential. This is usually possible if the physician takes a careful environmental and occupational history or, if necessary, visits the patient's environment. The simplest way to avoid the incriminated agent is to remove the patient from the environment or the source of the agent from the patient's environment. This recommendation cannot be taken lightly when it completely changes the lifestyle or livelihood of the patient. In many cases, however, the source of exposure (birds, humidifiers) can easily be removed. If occupational exposure is involved, an initial attempt can be made at antigen avoidance maneuvers least disruptive to the patient's livelihood, which usually means avoiding areas associated with heavy exposure and wearing an appropriate mask. This will not suffice for small-molecular-weight agents such as isocyanates, which require more elaborate respiratory systems. Pollen masks, personal dust respirators, airstream helmets, and ventilated helmets with a supply of fresh air are increasingly efficient means of purifying inhaled air. If symptoms recur or physiologic abnormalities progress in spite of these measures, then more effective measures to avoid antigen exposure must be pursued. Compromises with environmental control pertain primarily to the acute, recurrent, transient clinical form of HP and must be accompanied by careful follow-up. Subacute forms are ordinarily the result of a heavy, sustained exposure. The chronic form typically results from low-grade or recurrent exposure over many months to years, and the lung disease may already be partially or completely irreversible. These patients are usually advised to avoid all possible contact with the offending agent, although follow-up studies of farmer's lung and bird fancier's lung have found resolution of the disease despite continued exposure in some patients.

Patients with the *acute*, recurrent form of HP usually recover without need for glucocorticoids. *Subacute* HP may be associated with severe symptoms and marked physiologic impairment and may continue to progress for several days despite hospitalization. Urgent establishment of the diagnosis and prompt institution of glucocorticoid treatment are indicated in such patients. Such therapy may also hasten recovery in patients with lesser involvement. Prednisone at a dosage of 1 mg/kg per day or its equivalent is continued for 7 to 14 days and then tapered over the ensuing 2 to 6 weeks at a rate that depends on the patient's clinical status. Patients with *chronic* HP may gradually recover without therapy following environmental control. In many patients, however, a trial of prednisone may be useful to obtain maximal reversibility of the lung disease. Following initial prednisone therapy (1 mg/kg per day for 2 to 4 weeks), the drug is tapered to the lowest dosage that will maintain the functional status of the patient. Many patients will not require or benefit from long-term therapy if there is no further exposure to antigen. Available studies report no effect of glucocorticoid therapy on long-term prognosis of farmer's lung.

PULMONARY INFILTRATES WITH EOSINOPHILIA

Pulmonary infiltrates with eosinophilia (PIE, eosinophilic pneumonias) include distinct individual syndromes characterized by eosinophilic pulmonary infiltrates and, commonly, peripheral blood eosinophilia. Since Loeffler's initial description of a transient, benign syndrome of migratory pulmonary infiltrates and peripheral blood eosinophilia of unknown cause, this group of disorders has been enlarged to include several diseases of both known and unknown etiology (Table 237-2). These diseases may be considered as immunologically mediated lung diseases, but are not to be confused with HP, in which eosinophilia is not a feature. When an eosinophilic pneumonia is associated with bronchial asthma, it is important to determine if the patient has atopic asthma and has wheal-and-flare skin reactivity to *Aspergillus* or other relevant fungal antigens. If so, other criteria should be sought for diagnosis of ABPA (Table 237-3) or other, rarer examples of allergic bronchopulmonary mycosis such as those caused by *Penicillium, Candida, Curvularia,* or *Helminthosporium* spp. *A. fumigatus* is the most common cause of ABPA, although other *Aspergillus* species have also been implicated. ABPA has been reported to complicate cystic fibrosis. The chest roentgenogram in ABPA may show transient, recurrent infiltrates or may suggest the presence of proximal bronchiectasis. High-resolution chest CT is a sensitive, noninvasive technique for the recognition of proximal bronchiectasis. The bronchial asthma of ABPA likely involves an IgE-mediated hypersensitivity, whereas the bronchiectasis associated with this disorder is thought to result from a deposition of immune complexes in proximal airways. Adequate treatment usually requires the long-term use of systemic glucocorticoids.

Tropical eosinophilia is usually caused by filarial infection; however, eosinophilic pneumonias also occur with other parasites such as *Ascaris, Ancyclostoma* sp., *Toxocara* sp., and *Strongyloides stercoralis.* Tropical eosinophilia due to *Wuchereria bancrofti* or *W. malayi* occurs most commonly in southern Asia, Africa, and South America, and is treated successfully with diethylcarbamazine.

Drug-induced eosinophilic pneumonias are exemplified by acute reactions to nitrofurantoin, which may begin 2 h to 10 days after nitrofurantoin is started, with symptoms of dry cough, fever, chills, and dyspnea; an eosinophilic pleural effusion accompanying patchy or diffuse pulmonary infiltrates may also occur. Other drugs associated with eosinophilic pneumonias include sulfonamides, penicillin, chlorpropamide, thiazides, tricyclic antidepressants, hydralazine, mephenesin, mecamylamine, nickel carbonyl vapor, gold salts, isoniazid, para-amnosalicylic acid, indomethacin, and others. One recent report has identified anti-TNF-α monoclonal antibody therapy as a cause of eosinophilic pneumonitis. Treatment consists of withdrawal of the incriminated drugs and the use of glucocorticoids, if necessary. The eosinophilia-myalgia syndrome, caused by dietary supplements of impure L-tryptophan, is occasionally associated with pulmonary infiltrates.

TABLE 237-2 *Pulmonary Infiltrates with Eosinophilia*

ETIOLOGY KNOWN
Allergic bronchopulmonary mycoses
Parasitic infestations
Drug reactions
Eosinophilia-myalgia syndrome

IDIOPATHIC
Loeffler's syndrome
Acute eosinophilic pneumonia
Chronic eosinophilic pneumonia
Allergic granulomatosis of Churg and Strauss
Hypereosinophilic syndrome

TABLE 237-3 *Diagnostic Features of Allergic Bronchopulmonary Aspergillosis (ABPA)*

MAIN DIAGNOSTIC CRITERIA
Bronchial asthma
Pulmonary infiltrates
Peripheral eosinophilia ($>1000/\mu$L)
Immediate wheal-and-flare response to *A. fumigatus*
Serum precipitins to *A. fumigatus*
Elevated serum IgE
Central bronchiectasis

OTHER DIAGNOSTIC FEATURES
History of brownish plugs in sputum
Culture of *A. fumigatus* from sputum
Elevated IgE (and IgG) class antibodies specific for *A. fumigatus*

The group of idiopathic eosinophilic pneumonias consists of diseases of varying severity. *Loeffler's syndrome* was originally reported as a benign, acute eosinophilic pneumonia of unknown cause characterized by migrating pulmonary infiltrates and minimal clinical manifestations. In some patients, these clinical characteristics may prove to be secondary to parasites or drugs. *Acute eosinophilic pneumonia* has been described as an idiopathic acute febrile illness of less than 7 days' duration with severe hypoxemia, pulmonary infiltrates, and no history of asthma. *Chronic eosinophilic pneumonia* presents with significant systemic symptoms including fever, chills, night sweats, cough, anorexia, and weight loss of several weeks' to months' duration. The chest x-ray classically shows peripheral infiltrates resembling a photographic negative of pulmonary edema. Some patients also have bronchial asthma of the intrinsic or nonallergic type. Dramatic clearing of symptoms and chest x-rays is often noted within 48 h after initiation of glucocorticoid therapy.

Allergic angiitis and granulomatosis of Churg and Strauss is a multisystem vasculitic disorder that frequently involves the skin, kidney, and nervous system in addition to the lung. The disorder may occur at any age and is almost invariably found in patients with a history of bronchial asthma. The asthma often is progressive until the onset of fever and exaggerated eosinophilia, at which time the symptoms of asthma may ease. The illness may be fulminating and the prognosis grave unless treated aggressively with glucocorticoids and, at times, immunosuppressive therapy. The use of leukotriene-modifying agents (zafirlukast, zyleuton, and montelukast) has been associated with Churg-Strauss syndrome, but it remains uncertain whether the drugs cause the disease or rather unmask previously undiagnosed vasculitis, perhaps suppressed by the use of inhaled or systemic glucocorticoids.

The *hypereosinophilic syndrome* is characterized by the presence of over 1500 eosinophils per microliter of peripheral blood for 6 months or longer; lack of evidence for parasitic, allergic, or other known causes of eosinophilia; and signs or symptoms of multisystem organ dysfunction. Consistent features are blood and bone marrow eosinophilia with tissue infiltration by relatively mature eosinophils. The heart may be involved with tricuspid valve abnormalities or endomyocardial fibrosis and a restrictive, biventricular cardiomyopathy. Other organs affected typically include the lungs, liver, spleen, skin, and nervous system. Therapy of the disorder consists of glucocorticoids and/or hydroxyurea, plus therapy as needed for cardiac dysfunction, which is frequently responsible for much of the morbidity and mortality in this syndrome. Pulmonary eosinophilia has also been associated with T cell lymphoma, and has been reported following lung and bone marrow transplantation.

FURTHER READING

CORMIER Y et al: High-resolution computed tomographic characteristics in acute farmer's lung and in its follow-up. Eur Respir J 16:56, 2000

GLAZER CS et al: Acute eosinophilic pneumonia in AIDS. Chest 120:1732, 2001

JOHKOH T et al: Eosinophilic lung diseases: Diagnostic accuracy of thin-section CT in 111 patients. Radiology 216:773, 2000

KATZENSTEIN AL: Diagnostic features and differential diagnosis of Churg-Strauss syndrome in the lung. A review. Am J Clin Pathol 114:767, 2000

KAZUYOSHI K et al: Expression of FasL and Fas protein and their soluble form in patients with hypersensitivity pneumonitis. Int Arch Allergy Immunol 122:209, 2000

NAVARRO C et al: Up-regulation of L-selectin and E-selectin in hypersensitivity pneumonitis. Chest 121:354, 2002

OHTANI Y et al: Inhalation provocation tests in chronic bird fancier's lung. Chest 118:1382, 2000

PARDO A et al: Increase of lung neutrophils in hypersensitivity pneumonitis is associated with lung fibrosis. Am J Respir Crit Care Med 161:1698, 2000

PATEL AM et al: Hypersensitivity pneumonitis: Current concepts and future questions. J Allergy Clin Immunol 108:661, 2001

ROSENOW EC III et al: Drug-induced pulmonary disease. An update. Chest 102:239, 1992

ZACHARISEN MC et al: The long-term outcome in acute, subacute, and chronic forms of pigeon breeder's disease hypersensitivity pneumonitis. Ann Allergy Asthma Immunol 88:175, 2002

238 ENVIRONMENTAL LUNG DISEASES
Frank E. Speizer

This chapter provides perspectives on ways to assess pulmonary diseases for which environmental or occupational causes are suspected. This assessment is important because removal of the patient from harmful exposure is often the only intervention that might prevent further significant deterioration or lead to improvement in a patient's condition. Furthermore, the identification of an environment-associated disease in a single patient may lead to primary preventive strategies affecting other similarly exposed people who have not yet developed disease.

The exact magnitude of the problem is unknown, but there is no question that large numbers of individuals are at risk for developing serious respiratory disease as a result of occupational or environmental exposures. For example, recent estimates suggest that approximately 2.4 million workers in the United States have been exposed to crystalline silica or asbestos dust in mining and nonmining industries. Even if only 5% of these workers (a conservative estimate) are to suffer from respiratory disease as a result of their exposure, this figure represents more than 100,000 individuals.

HISTORY AND PHYSICAL EXAMINATION

The patient's history is of paramount importance in assessing any potential occupational or environmental exposure. Inquiry into specific work practices should include questions about specific contaminants involved, the availability and use of personal respiratory protection devices, the size and ventilation of workspaces, and whether coworkers have similar complaints. The temporal association of exposure at work and symptoms may provide clues to occupation-related disease. In addition, the patient must be questioned about alternative sources for potentially toxic exposures, including hobbies or other environmental exposures at home. Short-term exposures to potential toxic agents in the distant past must also be considered (Chap. 376).

Many people are aware of the potential hazards in their workplaces, and many states require that employees be informed about potentially hazardous exposures. These requirements include the provision of specific educational materials (including Material Safety Data Sheets), personal protective equipment and instructions in its use, and information on environmental control procedures. Reminders posted in the workplace may warn workers about hazardous substances. Protective clothing, lockers, and shower facilities may be considered necessary parts of the job. However, even in these more progressive industries, the introduction of new processes, particularly when related to the use of new chemical compounds, may change exposure significantly, and often only the employee on the production line is aware of the change. For the physician who regularly sees patients from a particular industry, a visit to the work site can be very instructive. Alternatively, physicians can request inspections by appropriate federal and/or state authorities.

The physical examination of patients with environment-related lung diseases may help to determine the nature and severity of the pulmonary condition. Unfortunately, the pulmonary response to most injurious agents is the development of a limited number of nonspecific physical signs. These findings do not point to the specific causative agent, and other types of information must be used to arrive at an etiologic diagnosis.

PULMONARY FUNCTION TESTS AND CHEST RADIOGRAPHY

Many mineral dusts produce characteristic alterations in the mechanics of breathing and lung volumes that clearly indicate a restrictive pattern (Chaps. 234 and 243). Exposures to a number of organic dusts or chemical agents capable of producing occupational asthma result in pronounced obstructive patterns of pulmonary dysfunction that may be reversible (Chap. 236). Measurement of change in forced expiratory volume (FEV_1) before and after a working shift can be used to detect an acute inflammatory or bronchoconstrictive response. An acute decrement of FEV_1 over the first work shift of the week is a characteristic feature of cotton textile workers with byssinosis.

The chest radiograph is useful in detecting and monitoring the pulmonary response to mineral dusts. The International Labour Organisation (ILO) International Classification of Radiographs of Pneumoconioses classifies chest radiographs according to the nature and size of opacities seen and the extent of involvement of the parenchyma. In general, opacities may be round or irregular, small (<10 mm in diameter) or large. They may be few in number, with visible normal lung markings, partially obscure normal markings, or totally obscure normal markings. Although useful for screening large numbers of workers, the ILO system lacks specificity and may over- or underestimate the functional impact of pneumoconiosis. With dusts causing rounded, regular opacities like those evident in coal worker's pneumoconiosis, the degree of involvement on the chest radiograph may be extensive, while pulmonary function may be only minimally impaired. In contrast, in pneumoconiosis causing linear, irregular opacities like those seen in asbestosis, the radiograph may lead to underestimation of the severity of the impairment until relatively late in the disease. For the individual patient with a history of exposure, conventional computed tomography (CT) and high-resolution computed tomography (HRCT) have improved the sensitivity of identifying diffuse parenchymal abnormalities of the lung. The procedures have been shown to provide earlier detection of silicosis and asbestosis.

Other diagnostic procedures of use in identifying environment-induced lung disease include evaluation of heavy metal concentrations in urine (arsenic in smelter workers, cadmium in battery plant workers); bacteriologic studies (tuberculosis in medical care personnel, anthrax in wool sorters); fungal studies (coccidioidomycosis in southwestern farm workers, histoplasmosis in poultry or pigeon handlers); and serologic studies (psittacosis in pet shop workers or owners of sick birds, Q fever in tanners or slaughterhouse workers). Ultimately, a lung biopsy may be required both for morphologic diagnosis of the underlying pulmonary disease and for attempted identification of the specific etiologic agent.

MEASUREMENT OF EXPOSURE

If reliable environmental sampling data are available, this information should be used in assessing a patient's exposure. Since many of the chronic diseases result from exposure over many years, current environmental measurements should be combined with work histories to arrive at estimates of past exposure.

In situations where individual exposure to specific agents—either in a work setting or via ambient air pollutants—has been determined, transport of these agents through the airways may be an important factor affecting dose. Highly soluble gases such as sulfur dioxide are absorbed in the upper airway and presumably produce their effects by reflex response of sensitive neural fibrils in the trachea or larger airways. In contrast, nitrogen dioxide, which is less soluble, may reach the bronchioles and alveoli in sufficient quantities to result in an acute life-threatening disease in farmers exposed even briefly to the gas evolved from moldy hay in silos (silo-filler's disease).

Particle size and chemistry of air contaminants must also be considered. Particles above 10 to 15 μm in diameter, because of their settling velocities in air, do not penetrate beyond the upper airways. These larger particles are often referred to as "fugitive dusts" and include pollens, other windblown dusts, and dusts resulting from mechanical industrial processes. They have little or no role in chronic respiratory disease except perhaps as related to cancer (see below).

Particles below 10 μm in size are created by the burning of fossil fuels or high-temperature industrial processes resulting in condensation products from gases, fumes, or vapors. These particles are divided into three size fractions on the basis of their size characteristics and sources. Particles of approximately 2.5 to 10 μm (coarse-mode fraction) contain crustal elements, such as silica, aluminum, and iron. These particles mostly deposit relatively high in the tracheobronchial tree. Although the total mass of an ambient sample is dominated by these larger respirable particles, the number of particles, and therefore the surface area on which potential toxic agents can deposit and be carried to the lower airways, is dominated by particles smaller than 2.5 μm (fine-mode fraction or accumulation mode). The smallest particles, those less than 0.1 μm in size, represent the ultrafine fraction and make up the largest number of particles, which tend to remain in the airstream and deposit in the lung only on a random basis as they come into contact with the alveolar walls.

Besides the size characteristics of particles and the solubility of gases, the actual chemical composition, mechanical properties, and immunogenicity or infectivity of inhaled material determine in large part the nature of the diseases found among exposed persons.

OCCUPATIONAL EXPOSURES AND PULMONARY DISEASE

Table 238-1 provides broad categories of exposure in the workplace and diseases associated with chronic exposure in these industries.

ASBESTOSIS

Except in localized regions with single industrial exposures, such as coal-mining or granite-quarrying regions, the most frequent inorganic dust-related chronic pulmonary diseases are associated with industries using *asbestiform fibers*. *Asbestos* is a generic term for several different mineral silicates, including chrysolite, amosite, anthophyllite, and crocidolite. Besides workers involved in the mining, milling, and manufacturing of asbestos products, workers in the building trades, including pipe fitters and boilermakers, were exposed to asbestos, which was widely used in construction because of its exceptional thermal and electric insulation properties. In addition, asbestos was used in the manufacture of fire-smothering blankets and safety garments, as filler for plastic materials, in cement and floor tiles, and in friction materials, such as brake and clutch linings.

Exposure to asbestos is not limited to persons who directly handle the material. Cases of asbestos-related diseases have been encountered in individuals with only moderate exposure, such as the painter or electrician who works alongside the insulation worker in a shipyard or the housewife who does no more than shake out and wash her husband's work clothes. Community exposure has probably resulted from the use of asbestos-containing material sprayed on steel girders in many large buildings as a safety feature to prevent buckling in case of fire.

Asbestos was first used extensively in the 1940s. Starting in 1975 it was mostly replaced with synthetic mineral fibers, such as fiberglass or slag wool, but it continues to be used increasingly in the developing world. Despite current regulations mandating adequate training for any worker potentially exposed to asbestos, exposure probably continues among inexperienced demolition workers. The major health effects from exposure to asbestos are pulmonary fibrosis (asbestosis) and cancers of the respiratory tract, the pleura, and (in rare cases) the peritoneum.

Asbestosis is a diffuse interstitial fibrosing disease of the lung that is directly related to the intensity and duration of exposure. Except for its association with a history of exposure to asbestos (generally in a work setting), asbestosis resembles the other forms of diffuse interstitial fibrosis (Chap. 243). Usually, moderate to severe exposure has taken place for at least 10 years before the disease becomes manifest.

Physiologic studies reveal a restrictive pattern with a decrease in lung volumes. Flow rates are commonly reduced less than would be predicted on the basis of the volume reduction. An early sign of severe disease may be a reduction in diffusing capacity.

Pulmonary fibrosis may occur following sufficient exposure to any of the asbestiform fiber types. The fibrotic lesions result from proinflammatory effects of reactive oxygen species released from phagocytes reacting with transition metals on the surface of the fibers. The clinical manifestations are typical of those physical findings in any patient with pulmonary fibrosis (Chap. 243).

DIAGNOSIS The chest radiograph can be used to detect a number of manifestations of asbestos exposure as well as to identify specific lesions. Past exposure is specifically indicated by pleural plaques, which are characterized by either thickening or calcification along the parietal pleura, particularly along the lower lung fields, the diaphragm, and the cardiac border. Without additional manifestations, pleural plaques imply only exposure, not pulmonary impairment. Benign pleural effusions may occur, particularly in patients with asbestosis, but are not necessarily restricted to those with overt disease. The fluid is sterile but may be a serous or blood-stained exudate and may occur bilaterally. The effusion may be slowly progressive or may resolve spontaneously.

The radiographic diagnosis of asbestosis depends on the presence of irregular or linear opacities, usually first noted in the lower lung fields and spreading into the middle and upper lung fields as the disease progresses. An indistinct heart border or a "ground glass" appearance in the lung fields is seen in some cases. In cases in which the x-ray changes are less obvious, HRCT may show distinct changes of subpleural curvilinear lines 5 to 10 cm in length that appear to be parallel to the pleural surface.

In general, newly diagnosed cases will have resulted from exposure levels that were present many years before and, in spite of the patients' having left the industry, are attributable to that former exposure. Since the patient may be eligible for compensation within a specific time frame after the diagnosis of an asbestos-related disease is made, the physician making the diagnosis should be certain to inform the patient promptly. On occasion, the physician may have reason to suspect ongoing exposure from a patient's current job description or actual monitoring data. In such cases, federal or state health authorities may need to be notified.

Casual, nonoccupational exposure to undisturbed sources of asbestos-containing materials—e.g., in walls of schools or other buildings—represents little if any hazard to people who inhabit or work in such buildings. Because the association of smoking and asbestos exposure increases the risk of developing lung cancer (see below), it is extremely important to advise patients with a history of exposure to asbestos to stop smoking. No specific therapy is available in the management of patients with asbestosis. The supportive care is the same as that given to any patient with diffuse interstitial fibrosis from any cause.

Lung cancer (Chap. 75), either squamous cell carcinoma or adenocarcinoma, is the most frequent cancer associated with asbestos ex-

TABLE 238-1 *Categories of Occupational Exposures and Number of Workers at Risk for Respiratory Diseases*

Occupational Exposures	Estimated Number of Workers Exposed	Nature of Respiratory Responses
Inorganic dusts		
Asbestos: mining	~250,000	Fibrosis (asbestosis), COPD, cancer,
Processing, nonagricultural	4.20×10^6	mesothelioma
Silica: mining, stone cutting, construction, quarrying	2.3×10^6	Fibrosis (silicosis), PMF, silicotuberculosis
Coal dust: mining	200,000	Fibrosis, pneumoconiosis
Beryllium: processing alloys for high tech industries	800,000	Acute pneumonitis, chronic granulomatous disease
Other metals: aluminum, chromium, cobalt, nickel, titanium, tungsten	~500,000	Wide variety of conditions from acute pneumonitis to lung cancer and asthma
Organic dusts		
Cotton dust: milling, processing	>800,000	Chronic bronchitis, reduced pulmonary function, byssinosis
Grain dust: elevator agents, dock workers, milling, bakers	>500,000	Asthma, chronic phlegm production, obstructive airways disease
Other agricultural dusts: fungal spores, vegetable product, insect fragments, animal dander, bird and rodent feces, endotoxins, microorganisms, pollens	~5×10^6	Hypersensitivity pneumonitis (farmers' lung), asthma, chronic bronchitis
Toxic chemicals: wide variety of industries—see Table 238-3	>9×10^6 (does not include firefighters)	See Table 238-2
Other respiratory environmental carcinogens: (proven or highly suspect): uranium and radon daughters, environmental tobacco smoke, nickel compounds, chromium salts, polycyclic hydrocarbons, mustard gas, diesel exhaust, welding fumes, woods or wood finishing products	Essentially unknowable, but a major fraction of U.S. population is exposed to low environmental levels of one or more of these agents	Estimates vary from ~3% to <10% of all lung cancers

Note: COPD, chronic obstructive pulmonary disease; PMF, progressive massive fibrosis.

posure. The excess frequency of lung cancer in asbestos workers is associated with a minimum lapse of 15 to 19 years between first exposure and development of the disease. Persons with more exposure are at greater risk of disease. In addition, there appears to be a significant multiplicative effect that leads to a far greater risk of lung cancer in persons who are cigarette smokers and have asbestos exposure than would be expected from the additive risk of each factor. To date, efforts to consider these high-risk individuals for special surveillance studies, including sputum cytologic examinations and repeated chest x-rays as frequently as every 4 to 6 months, have resulted in neither significant early detection nor prolonged survival once the lung cancer is found. The use of HRCT in such at-risk subjects is currently under investigation.

Mesotheliomas (Chap. 245), both pleural and peritoneal, are also associated with asbestos exposure. In contrast to lung cancers, these tumors do not appear to be associated with smoking. Relatively short-term asbestos exposures of 1 to 2 years or less occurring some 20 to 25 years in the past have been associated with the development of mesotheliomas (an observation that emphasizes the importance of obtaining a complete environmental exposure history). The risk for this type of tumor peaks 30 to 35 years after initial exposure. Since maximum exposure took place in the United States between 1930 and 1960, peak incidence of disease in men occurred in 1997, with a total of 2300 cases. Incidence is expected to decline over the next 30+ years to about 500 cases per year.

Although approximately 50% of mesotheliomas metastasize, the tumor generally is locally invasive, and death usually results from local extension. Most patients present with effusions that may obscure the underlying pleural tumor. In contrast to the findings in effusion due to other causes, because of the restriction placed on the chest wall, no shift of mediastinal structures toward the opposite side of the chest will be seen. The major diagnostic problem is differentiation from peripherally spreading pulmonary adenocarcinoma or from adenocarcinoma metastasized to pleura from an extrathoracic primary site. Although a needle biopsy may be diagnostic, an open biopsy is often necessary, and even the latter procedure may not provide a definitive diagnosis of the origin of the tumor.

Since epidemiologic studies have shown that more than 80% of mesotheliomas may be associated with asbestos exposure, documented mesothelioma in a worker with occupational exposure to asbestos may be compensable in many parts of the United States.

SILICOSIS

In spite of the technical adequacy of existing protective equipment, *free silica* (SiO_2), or crystalline quartz, is still a major occupational hazard. In the United States, estimates of potential numbers of exposed workers range between 1.2 and 3 million persons. The major occupational exposures include: mining; stonecutting; employment in abrasive industries, such as stone, clay, glass, and cement manufacturing; foundry work; packing of silica flour; and quarrying, particularly of granite. Most often, progressive pulmonary fibrosis (silicosis) occurs in a dose-response fashion after many years of exposure.

Workers exposed through sandblasting in confined spaces, tunneling through rock with high quartz content (15 to 25%), or the manufacture of abrasive soaps may develop acute silicosis with as little as 10 months' exposure. The disease may be rapidly fatal in less than 2 years, despite the discontinuation of exposure. A radiographic picture of profuse miliary infiltration or consolidation is characteristic of acute silicosis.

In long-term, less intense exposure, small rounded opacities in the upper lobes, with retraction and hilar adenopathy, classically appear on the radiograph after 15 to 20 years. Calcification of hilar nodes may occur in as many as 20% of cases and produces the characteristic "eggshell" pattern. These changes may be preceded by or associated with a reticular pattern of irregular densities that are uniformly present throughout the upper lung zones.

The nodular fibrosis may be progressive in the absence of further exposure, with coalescence and formation of nonsegmental conglomerates of irregular masses in excess of 1 cm in diameter. These masses become quite large and are characteristic of progressive massive fibrosis (PMF). Significant functional impairment with both restrictive and obstructive components may be associated with this form of silicosis. In the late stages of the disease, ventilatory failure may develop. In more subtle cases, CT may be helpful both in identifying nodules, which are preferentially located in the posterior aspect of the upper lobes, as well as in identifying larger opacities and more coalescence than might be noted on regular chest x-rays. Patients with silicosis are at greater risk of acquiring *Mycobacterium tuberculosis* infections (silicotuberculosis) and atypical mycobacterial infections. Because the frequency with which tuberculosis has been found at autopsy in patients with PMF exceeds considerably the frequency of premorbid diagnosis, treatment for tuberculosis is indicated in any patient with silicosis and a positive tuberculin test.

Other less hazardous silicates include Fuller's earth, kaolin, mica, diatomaceous earths, silica gel, soapstone, carbonate dusts, and cement dusts. The production of fibrosis in workers exposed to these agents is believed to be related either to the free silica content of these dusts or, for substances that contain no free silica, to the potentially large dust loads to which these workers may be exposed.

Other silicates, including *talc dusts*, may be contaminated with asbestos and/or free silica. Accidental exposure to significant quantities of talc may result in an acute syndrome with cough, cyanosis, and labored breathing (acute talcosis). Severe progressive fibrosis with respiratory failure may ensue within a few years. Fibrosis and/or pleural or lung cancer have been associated with chronic exposure to commercial talc. Pure talc does not produce fibrosis; thus, it is difficult to sort out whether the effects are due to the contamination of commercial talc by asbestos or by free silica.

COAL WORKER'S PNEUMOCONIOSIS (CWP)

Coal dust is associated with CWP, which has enormous social, economic, and medical significance in every nation in which coal mining is an important industry. Simple radiographically identified CWP is seen in 12% of all miners and in as many as 50% of anthracite miners with more than 20 years' work on the coal face. The prevalence of disease is lower in workers in bituminous coal mines. Since much western U.S. coal is bituminous, CWP is less prevalent in that region.

Much of the symptomatology associated with simple CWP appears to be similar and additive to the effects of cigarette smoking on the development of chronic bronchitis and obstructive lung disease (Chap. 242). In the early stages of simple CWP, radiographic abnormalities consist of small, irregular opacities (reticular pattern). With prolonged exposure, one sees small, rounded, regular opacities, 1 to 5 mm in diameter (nodular pattern). Calcification is generally not seen, although approximately 10% of older anthracite miners have calcified nodules.

Complicated CWP is manifested by the appearance on the chest radiograph of nodules ranging from 1 cm in diameter to the size of an entire lobe, generally confined to the upper half of the lungs. This condition, considered a form of PMF, is accompanied by a significant reduction in diffusing capacity and is associated with premature mortality.

Caplan's syndrome (Chap. 301), first described in coal miners but subsequently found in patients with a variety of pneumoconioses, includes seropositive rheumatoid arthritis with characteristic PMF. The syndrome suggests an immunopathologic mechanism. Over the past decade, the mechanisms by which the chronic inhalation of mineral dusts produce an increase in inflammatory cells (including macrophages and neutrophils), which in turn causes PMF, have been explored. All of these inorganic dusts can: (1) be directly cytotoxic; (2) stimulate reactive oxygen species; (3) activate macrophages to produce cytokines and enhance production of (anti)fibrogenic factors such as tumor necrosis factor-α; (4) increase protease activity; and (5) increase inactivation of α_1-antitrypsin and leukocyte elastase activity. The final pathologic pathway may be fibrosis resulting from the interactions of a variety of these mechanisms.

BERYLLIOSIS

Beryllium may produce an acute pneumonitis or, far more commonly, a chronic granulomatous disease. Unless one inquires specifically about occupational exposures to beryllium in the manufacture of alloys, ceramics, high-technology electronics, and (before the 1950s) the production of fluorescent lights, one may miss entirely the etiologic relationship to an occupational exposure. Nonspecific pulmonary function tests may be normal or may indicate evidence of restrictive disease. Between 2 and 15 years of exposure, depending on its intensity, are required for the disease to become manifest. On open lung biopsy, granulomatous formation similar to that seen in sarcoidosis (Chap. 309) may make differentiation impossible unless tissue levels of be-

ryllium are measured. Recent studies have identified T cell clones in the lungs of affected patients that suggest a gene-by-environment interaction that is necessary for the disease to become manifest.

Other hard metals, including aluminum powders, chromium, cobalt, titanium dioxide, and tungsten, may produce an interstitial pneumonitis, but this is rare.

OTHER INORGANIC DUSTS

Other dusts are considered *nuisance dusts* because their major environmental and health effects seem to be reduction in visibility and irritation of eyes, ears, nasal passages, and other mucous membranes, respectively. If they penetrate to the lower airways, these dusts do not affect the architecture of the terminal bronchioles or acinar spaces nor do they destroy collagen. Generally, clinical effects are reversible. Pulmonary function tests are usually normal unless another disease process coexists. If the dusts are radiodense, macular collections may produce striking radiographic pictures that are so characteristic that patients with a history of significant exposure are easily diagnosed as having the condition that bears the name reflecting the nature of the dust. Examples of radiodense dusts include iron and iron oxides from welding or silver finishing (*siderosis*); tin oxide used in metallurgy, color stabilization, printing, and the manufacture of porcelain, glass, and fabric (*stannosis*); and barium sulfate used as a catalyst for organic reactions, drilling mud components, and electroplating (*baritosis*). Other metal dusts producing similar radiodense pictures include *cerium dioxide* and *antimony salts*.

Most of the inorganic dusts discussed thus far are associated with the production of either dust macules or interstitial fibrotic changes in the lung. Another set of dusts (Table 238-2), along with some of the dusts previously discussed, is associated with chronic mucous hypersecretion (chronic bronchitis), with or without reduction of expiratory flow rates. These conditions are caused by cigarette smoking, and any effort to attribute some component of the disease to occupational and environmental exposures must take cigarette smoking into account. Most studies suggest an additive effect of dust exposure and smoking. The pattern of the effect is similar to that of cigarette smoking, suggesting that small airway inflammation may be the initial site of pathologic response in those cases associated with the development of obstructive lung disease. Cigarette smoke is usually the more noxious agent, and dust effects may be discernible only in nonsmokers.

ORGANIC DUSTS

Some of the specific diseases associated with organic dusts are discussed in detail in the chapters on asthma (Chap. 236) and hypersensitivity pneumonitis (Chap. 237). Many of these diseases are named for the specific setting in which they are found, e.g., farmer's lung, malt worker's disease, or mushroom worker's disease. Often the temporal relation of symptoms to exposure furnishes the best evidence for the diagnosis. Three occupational groups are singled out for discussion because they represent the largest proportion of people affected by the diseases resulting from organic dusts.

COTTON DUST (BYSSINOSIS)   Estimates of the number of exposed persons in the United States vary, but probably over 800,000 persons are exposed occupationally to cotton, flax, or hemp in the production of yarns for cotton, linen, and rope making. Although this discussion focuses on cotton, the same syndrome—albeit somewhat less severe—has been reported in association with exposure to flax, hemp, and jute.

Exposure occurs throughout the manufacturing process but is most pronounced in those portions of the factory involved with the treatment of the cotton prior to spinning—i.e., blowing, mixing, and carding (straightening of fibers). Attempts to control dust levels by use of exhaust hoods, general increases in ventilation, and wetting procedures in some settings have been highly successful. However, respiratory protective equipment appears to be required during certain operations to prevent workers from being exposed to levels of dust that exceed the current U.S. cotton dust standard.

TABLE 238-2 *Selected Occupational Dusts Believed to Be Associated with Mucous Hypersecretion and/or Obstructive Airway Disease and Other Respiratory Diseases*[a]

Agent (Exposure)	Mucous Hypersecretion	Obstruction	Other Conditions[b]
INORGANIC DUSTS			
Antimony (storage batteries, solder, ceramics, glass, plastics)	X		P
Arsenic (manufacture of pesticides, pigments, glass, alloys)	X		C
Barium and compounds including BaO, BaSO$_4$, BaCO$_3$ (catalysts, drilling mud, electroplating)	X		P
Cadmium dust (electroplating, battery manufacture, welding, smelting, aluminum soldering)	X	X	P
Cement dust (construction trades, manufacture of cement blocks)	X	X	
Chromium and CrO$_3$, CrF$_2$ (corrosion inhibitor pigment, metallurgy, electroplating)	X		C
Coal dust (mining)	X		P
Coke oven emissions (retort house, coke ovens)	X	X	P, C
Graphite (steelmaking, lubricants, pencils, paints, stove polish)	X	X	P
Iron dust (steel and nonferrous foundry workers, welding)	X		P
Mica (insulation, roofing shingles, oil refining, rubber manufacturing)	X		P
Phosphorus, elemental chlorides, sulfides (manufacture of fireworks, agricultural chemicals, insecticides, pesticides)	X	X	
Rock dusts (miners, tunnelers, quarry workers)	X		P
Vanadium pentoxide (welding electrodes, additive to steel, by-product in ash from oil burning)	X	X	
ORGANIC DUSTS (SEE CHAP. 237)			
Cotton dust, flax, hemp (manufacture of yarns for linen, rope, cotton; ginning, cottonseed crushing; waste fiber processing)	X	X	
Grain dusts (farmers, workers in grain elevators, barge and grain ship crew members)	X	X	
Moldy hay (farmers, other animal attendants)	X		HP

[a] The table excludes agents associated with asthma as the primary disease (see Chap. 236).
[b] Other conditions include hypersensitivity pneumonitis (HP), pneumoconiosis (P), and cancers (C).
Note: X indicates that mucous hypersecretion or obstruction is associated with exposure.

Byssinosis is characterized clinically as occasional (early stage) and then regular (late stage) chest tightness toward the end of the first day of the workweek ("Monday chest tightness"). In epidemiologic studies, depending on the level of exposure via the carding room air, up to 80% of employees may show a significant drop in their FEV$_1$ over the course of a Monday shift.

Initially the symptoms do not recur on subsequent days of the week. However, in 10 to 25% of workers, the disease may be progressive, with chest tightness recurring or persisting throughout the workweek. After more than 10 years of exposure, workers with recurrent symptoms are more likely to have an obstructive pattern on pulmonary function testing. There is an additive effect of cotton dust exposure plus cigarette smoking. The highest grades of impairment are generally seen in smokers.

Treatment in the early stages of the disease is directed toward reversing the bronchospasm with bronchodilators; however, the chest tightness appears to relate, at least in part, to histamine release, and antihistamines have been shown to lessen the anticipated fall in FEV$_1$ the first day of the week. Clearly, reduction of dust exposure is of primary importance. All workers with persistent symptoms or significantly reduced levels of pulmonary function should be moved to areas of lower risk of exposure. Regular surveillance of pulmonary function in the industry has made it easier to identify affected persons. Persons with reduced pulmonary function, a personal history of respiratory allergy, and a history of continued cigarette smoking should be considered at increased risk of developing byssinosis in association with work in the cotton industry.

GRAIN DUST Although the exact number of workers at risk in the United States is not known, at least 500,000 people work in grain elevators, and over 2 million farmers are potentially exposed to grain dust. The presentation of disease in grain elevator employees or in workers in flour or feed mills is virtually identical to the characteristic findings in cigarette smokers, i.e., persistent cough, mucous hypersecretion, wheeze and dyspnea on exertion, and reduced FEV$_1$ and FEV$_1$/FVC ratio (Chap. 234).

Dust concentrations in grain elevators vary greatly but appear to be in excess of 10,000 μg/m^3; approximately one-third of the particles, by weight, are in the respirable range. The effect of grain dust exposure is additive to that of cigarette smoking, with approximately 50% of workers who smoke having symptoms. Among nonsmoking grain elevator operators, approximately one-quarter have mucous hypersecretion, about five times the number that would be expected in unexposed nonsmokers. However, evidence of obstruction on pulmonary function studies is observed only in workers who smoke.

FARMER'S LUNG This condition results from exposure to moldy hay containing spores of thermophilic actinomycetes that produce a hypersensitivity pneumonitis (Chap. 237). There are few good population-based estimates of the frequency of occurrence of this condition in the United States. However, among farmers in Great Britain, the rate of disease ranges from approximately 10 to 50 per 1000. The prevalence of disease varies in association with rainfall, which determines the amount of fungal growth, and with differences in agricultural practices related to turning and stacking hay.

The patient with acute farmer's lung presents 4 to 8 h after exposure with fever, chills, malaise, cough, and dyspnea without wheezing. The history of exposure is obviously essential to distinguish this disease from influenza or pneumonia with similar symptoms. In the chronic form of the disease, the history of repeated attacks after similar exposure is important in differentiating this syndrome from other causes of patchy fibrosis (e.g., sarcoidosis).

A wide variety of other organic dusts are associated with the occurrence of hypersensitivity pneumonitis (Chap. 237). For those patients who present with hypersensitivity pneumonitis, specific and careful inquiry about occupations, hobbies, or other home environmental exposures will, in most cases, reveal the source of the etiologic agent.

TOXIC CHEMICALS

Exposure to toxic chemicals affecting the lung generally involves gases and vapors. A common accident is one in which the victim is trapped in a confined space where the chemicals have accumulated to toxic levels. In addition to the specific toxic effects of the chemical, the victim will often sustain considerable anoxia, which can play a dominant role in determining whether the individual survives.

Table 238-3 lists a variety of toxic agents that can produce acute and sometimes life-threatening reactions in the lung. All these agents in sufficient concentrations have been demonstrated, at least in animal studies, to affect the lower airways and disrupt alveolar architecture, either acutely or as a result of chronic exposure. Some of these agents may be generated acutely in the environment. For example, when plastics burn, a number of compounds, including hydrogen cyanide and hydrochloric acid, may be formed and released.

Firefighters and fire victims are at risk of *smoke inhalation*, a numerically important cause of acute cardiorespiratory failure. Smoke inhalation kills more fire victims than does thermal injury. Carbon monoxide poisoning with resulting significant hypoxemia can be life-threatening (Chap. 377). The use of synthetic materials (plastic, polyurethanes), which, when burned, may release a variety of other toxic agents (such as cyanide or hydrochloric acid), must be considered when evaluating smoke inhalation victims. Exposed victims may suffer some degree of lower respiratory tract inflammation and/or pulmonary edema.

Firefighters and victims may also be exposed to large quantities of particulate smoke. Significant long-term effects are not clearly associated with this particulate exposure except as related to the production of irritating effects on the upper airways; however, increased airway responsiveness in firefighters with repeated episodes of smoke inhalation has been demonstrated.

Some agents used in the manufacture of synthetic materials have resulted in some workers' being sensitized to extremely low levels of *isocyanates*, *aromatic amines*, or *aldehydes*. Repeated exposure to these agents causes some workers to develop chronic cough and sputum production, asthma, or episodes of low-grade fever and malaise.

Fluoropolymers, which at normal temperatures produce no reaction, upon heating become volatilized. The inhaled agents cause a characteristic syndrome of fever, chills, malaise, and occasionally mild wheezing leading to the diagnosis of *polymer fume fever* or, in the

TABLE 238-3 *Selected Common Toxic Chemical Agents Affecting the Lung*

Agent(s)	Selected Exposures	Acute Effects from High or Accidental Exposure	Chronic Effects from Relatively Low Exposure
Acid fumes: H_2SO_4, HNO_3	Manufacture of fertilizers, chlorinated organic compounds, dyes, explosives, rubber products, metal etching, plastics	Mucous membrane irritation, followed by chemical pneumonitis 2–3 days later	Bronchitis and suggestion of mildly reduced pulmonary function in children with lifelong residential exposure to high levels; clinical significance unknown
Ammonia	Refrigeration; petroleum refining; manufacture of fertilizers, explosives, plastics, and other chemicals	Same as for acid fumes	Chronic bronchitis
Cyanides	Electroplating; extraction of gold or silver; manufacture of mirrors, fumigants, photo supplies	Increase in respiratory rate followed by respiratory arrest, lactic acidosis, pulmonary edema, death	No data
Diazomethane	Methylating agent for acid compounds; laboratory workers	Violent coughing, dyspnea, wheezing, pulmonary edema	No data
Formaldehyde	Manufacture of resins, leathers, rubber, metals, and woods; laboratory workers, embalmers; emission from urethane foam insulation	Same as for acid fumes	Cancers in one species; no data on humans
Halides (Cl, Br, F)	Bleaching in pulp, paper, textile industry; manufacture of chemical compounds; synthetic rubber, plastics, disinfectant, rocket fuel, gasoline	Mucous membrane irritation, pulmonary edema; possible reduced FVC 1–2 yrs after exposure	Dryness of mucous membrane, epistaxis, dental fluorosis, tracheobronchitis
Hydrogen sulfide	By-product of many industrial processes, oil, other petroleum processes and storage	Respiratory paralysis similar to cyanides	Conjunctival irritation, chronic bronchitis, recurrent pneumonitis
Isocyanates (TDI, HDI, MDI)	Production of polyurethane foams, plastics, adhesives, surface coatings	Mucous membrane irritation, dyspnea, cough, wheeze, pulmonary edema	Upper respiratory tract irritation, cough, asthma, allergic alveolitis
Nitrogen dioxide	Silage, metal etching, explosives, rocket fuels, welding, by-product of burning fossil fuels	Cough, dyspnea, pulmonary edema may be delayed 4–12 h; possible result from acute exposure: bronchiolitis obliterans in 2–6 wks	Emphysema in animals, ?chronic bronchitis, associated with reduced lung function in children with lifelong residential exposure, clinical significance unknown
Ozone	Arc welding, flour bleaching, deodorizing, emissions from copying equipment, photochemical air pollutant	Mucous membrane irritant, pulmonary hemorrhage and edema, reduced pulmonary function transiently in children and adults exposed to summer haze	Chronic eye irritation
Phosgene	Organic compound, metallurgy, volatilization of chlorine-containing compounds	Delayed onset of bronchiolitis and pulmonary edema	Chronic bronchitis
Phthalic anhydride	Manufacture of resin esters, polyester resins, thermoactivated adhesives	Nasal irritation, cough	Asthma, chronic bronchitis
Sulfur dioxide	Manufacture of sulfuric acid, bleaches, coating of nonferrous metals, food processing, refrigerant, burning of fossil fuels, wood pulp industry	Mucous membrane irritant, epistaxis	?Chronic bronchitis

meat industry, *meat wrappers' asthma*. A similar self-limited, influenza-like syndrome—*metal fume fever*—results from acute exposure to fumes or smoke of zinc, copper, magnesium, and other volatilized metals. The syndrome may begin several hours after work and resolves within 24 h, only to return on repeated exposure. A proper occupational history should make the diagnosis evident.

ENVIRONMENTAL RESPIRATORY CARCINOGENS

Historically, it has been the astute clinician who has recognized a higher incidence of malignant tumors associated with certain environmental exposures. When these observations are linked to an occupational setting, they must be pursued by epidemiologic studies of relatively large groups of both current and former workers. Often the concentration and/or exact nature of the substances involved in the putative exposures cannot be determined. Rarely, the possibility that a substance can play an etiologic role in cancer is supported by observing that a few cases of a very rare tumor in a particular group represent "an epidemic." Examples are nasal sinus and lung cancer in nickel workers, angiosarcomas of the liver in vinyl chloride workers, and adenocarcinomas of the nose in woodworkers.

In addition to asbestos exposures, other occupational exposures associated with either proven or suspected respiratory carcinogens include those to acrylonitrile, arsenic compounds, beryllium (animal studies only), bis(chloromethyl) ether, chromium, polycyclic hydrocarbons (through coke oven emissions), iron oxide, isopropyl oil (nasal sinuses), mustard gas, the various ores used to produce pure nickel, talc (possible asbestos contamination in both mining and milling), vinyl chloride, welding materials, wood used in woodworking (nasal cancer only), and uranium. The occurrence of excess cancers in uranium miners raises the possibility that a large number of workers are at risk by virtue of exposure to similar radiation hazards. This number includes not only workers involved in processing uranium but also workers exposed in underground mining operations where radon daughters may be emitted from rock formations.

ASSESSMENT OF DISABILITY

Most commonly the need for disability assessment comes about because of the patient's complaint of shortness of breath. Pathophysiologically, dyspnea most often results from cardiac, respiratory, or neuromuscular diseases. With regard to respiratory diseases, the complaint most often relates to asthma. It is the physician's task to assess both the degree to which the symptoms are related to work or other environmental exposures and the severity of the symptoms, which result in the disability that may prevent the individual from performing his or her normal work tasks. Evaluating relation to work exposure requires a detailed work history, as previously discussed in this chapter. Objective assessment of severity of symptoms can generally be measured with pulmonary function tests including simple spirometry, lung volume measures, and diffusing capacity. In cases where these tests are normal, repeated measures of spirometry, airways hyperactivity, or degree of oxygen desaturation after modest exercise may be sufficient to demonstrate impairment. Occasionally, challenge to the putative work environment with repeated pulmonary function measures may be required.

With these data the physician should be able to make a judgment about the degree of impairment and its relation to exposure. How this information is formally used is often beyond the physician's control. Administrative panels, legal authorities, and sometimes confrontational employer/employee relations, as in a worker's compensation case, may have alternative reasons for collecting and using such data. Different authorities may have different guidelines and rules for setting levels of disability. What the physician may consider significant impairment may not be considered a disability for a worker with a sedentary job. Nevertheless, the treating physician is often asked for an opinion and must respond as objectively as possible. When this is being done for the physician's own patient, he or she needs to indicate to the patient what his or her specific role is and that most often the physician is not in the position of making the adjudicating decision.

If the physician is operating as an independent medical examiner, he or she should make clear to the agency that hires him or her that, from a medical-ethical perspective, the patient will be informed of all findings.

GENERAL ENVIRONMENTAL EXPOSURES

AIR POLLUTION

Dramatic and disastrous episodes of air pollution inversion have been documented in many industrialized centers in the world. Each of these episodes has been associated with excess acute mortality in the very old, the very young, and those with chronic cardiopulmonary diseases. The most dramatic event was the London fog of 1952, in which approximately 4000 excess deaths occurred over a 2-week period following 5 days of severe cold and dense fog. Similar episodes in the United States, although less dramatic in terms of total deaths, occurred in Donora, Pennsylvania, in 1948 and in New York City in the 1960s. In these episodes, which were generally associated with cold temperature and air stagnation, patients with underlying cardiopulmonary disease were most severely affected.

In addition to significant excess mortality during these episodes, a large number of people required medical care for cardiorespiratory complaints. Subsequent follow-up studies failed to implicate these episodic disasters in the etiology of chronic respiratory disease in adults. On the other hand, many epidemiologic studies of both international and regional differences in the prevalences of chronic respiratory disease suggest that long-term exposures in polluted areas in the early to middle part of the twentieth century were associated with excess chronic respiratory disease.

In 1970, the U.S. government established air quality standards for several pollutants believed to be responsible for excess cardiorespiratory diseases. Primary standards regulated by the Environmental Protection Agency (EPA) designed to protect the public health with an adequate margin of safety exist for sulfur dioxide, particulates <10 μm in size, nitrogen dioxide, ozone, lead, and carbon monoxide. Standards for each of these pollutants are updated regularly through an extensive review process conducted by the EPA. In 1997, a new standard was added for particles less than 2.5 μm; however, up through 2002 that new standard has not been implemented.

Pollutants are generated from both stationary sources (power plants and industrial complexes) and mobile sources (automobiles), and none of the pollutants occurs in isolation. Thus, except for the change in carboxyhemoglobin from carbon monoxide exposure, it becomes extremely difficult to relate any specific health effect to any single pollutant. Furthermore, pollutants may be changed by chemical reactions after being emitted. For example, reducing agents, such as sulfur dioxide and particulate matter from a power plant stack, may react in air to produce acid sulfates and aerosols, which can be transported long distances in the atmosphere. Oxidizing substances, such as oxides of nitrogen and oxidants from automobile exhaust, may react with sunlight to produce ozone. Although originally a problem confined to the southwestern part of the United States, in recent years, at least during the summertime, elevated ozone and acid aerosol levels have been documented throughout the United States. Both acute and chronic effects of these exposures have also been documented.

The symptoms and diseases associated with air pollution are the same as the nononcogenic conditions commonly associated with cigarette smoking. In addition, respiratory illness in early childhood has been associated with chronic exposure to only modestly elevated levels of traffic-related gases and respirable particles. Recent population-based studies comparing cities that have relatively high levels of particulate exposures with less polluted communities suggest excess morbidity and mortality from cardiorespiratory conditions in long-term residents of the former communities. This finding, in part, has led to greater emphasis on publicizing pollution alert levels. One can only advise individuals with significant cardiopulmonary impairment to stay indoors during periods when pollution exceeds current standards.

INDOOR EXPOSURE

Over the past 15 years, greater attention has been given to the effects of *passive cigarette smoking* (Chap. 375). Several studies have shown that the respirable particulate load in any household is directly proportional to the number of cigarette smokers living in the home. Increases in prevalence of respiratory illnesses and reduced levels of pulmonary function measured with simple spirometry have been found in children of smoking parents in a number of studies.

Evidence from numerous case-control and cohort studies shows modest excess disease associations for cardiopulmonary diseases and lung cancer. Because most of these excess relative risks appear to be below 50%, it is virtually impossible for any one of the studies to be considered definitive. Thus, the techniques of meta-analysis have been used effectively to combine data from the best of these studies. The most recent meta-analyses for lung cancer, cardiac disease, and respiratory disease in terms of excess mortality suggest an approximately 25% increase for each condition, even after adjustment for major potential confounders. According to measures of plasma cotinine, a metabolite of nicotine, a nonsmoker living with a smoker is exposed to approximately 1% of the level of tobacco smoke to which a smoker of 20 cigarettes a day is exposed. In spite of some prominent detractors, these combined relative risks appear to be consistent with the estimated exposure levels and suggest a consensus that the associations are causal.

Radon gas is believed to be a risk factor for lung cancer. The main radon product (radon 222) is a gas that results from the decay series of uranium 238, with the immediate precursor being radium 226. The amount of radium in earth materials determines how much radon gas will be emitted. Outdoors, the concentrations are trivial. Indoors, levels are dependent on the ventilation rate and the size of the space into which the gas is emitted. Levels associated with excess lung cancer risk may be present in as many as 10% of the houses in the United States. When smokers reside in the household, the problem is potentially greater, since the molecular size of radon particles allows them to readily attach to smoke particles that are inhaled. Fortunately, technology is available for assessing and reducing the level of exposure.

Other indoor exposures associated with an increased risk of atopy and asthma include those to such specific recognized putative biologic agents as cockroach antigen, dust mites, and pet danders. Other indoor chemical agents include formaldehyde, perfumes, and latex particles. Nonspecific responses associated with "tight-building syndrome," in which no particular agent has been implicated, have included a wide variety of complaints, among them respiratory symptoms, that are relieved only by avoiding exposure in the building in question. The degree to which "smells" or other sensory stimuli are involved in the triggering of potentially incapacitating psychological or physical responses has yet to be determined, and the long-term consequences of such environmental exposures are as yet unknown.

PORTAL OF ENTRY

The lung is a primary point of entry into the body for a number of toxic agents that affect other organ systems. For example, the lung is a route of entry for benzene (bone marrow), carbon disulfide (cardiovascular and nervous systems), cadmium (kidney), and metallic mercury (kidney, central nervous system). Thus, in any disease state of obscure origin, it is important to consider the possibility of inhaled environmental agents. Such consideration can sometimes furnish the clue needed to identify a specific external cause for a disorder that might otherwise be labeled "idiopathic."

FURTHER READING

BLANC PD: Acute pulmonary responses to toxic exposures, in *Textbook of Respiratory Medicine*, 3d ed, JF Murray, JA Nadel (eds). Philadelphia, Saunders, 2000, pp 1903–1914

CASTRANOVA V, VALLYATHAN V: Silicosis and coal workers' pneumoconiosis. Environ Health Perspect 108 (Suppl 4):675, 2000

CHAN-YEUNG M, MALO J-L: Occupational asthma. N Engl J Med 333: 107, 1995

CHEN R et al: Environmental tobacco smoke and lung function in employees who never smoked: The Scottish MONICA Study. Occup Environ Med 58: 563, 2001

MAIER LA et al: Angiotensin-1 converting enzyme polymorphisms in chronic beryllium disease. Am J Respir Crit Care Med 159:1342, 1999

MANNING CV et al: Diseases caused by asbestos: Mechanisms of injury and disease development. Int Immunopharmacol 2:191, 2002

PARKES WR: *Occupational Lung Disorders*, 3d ed. Oxford, Butterworth-Heinemann, 1994

SCHINS RP, BORM PJ: Mechanisms and mediators in coal dust–induced toxicity: A review. Ann Occup Hyg 43:7, 1999

YCESOY B et al: Association of tumor necrosis factor-α and interleukin-1 gene polymorphism with silicosis. Toxicol Appl Pharmacol 172:75, 2001

239 PNEUMONIA
Thomas J. Marrie, G. Douglas Campbell, David H. Walker, Donald E. Low

To the pathologist, pneumonia is an infection of the alveoli, distal airways, and interstitium of the lung that is manifested by increased weight of the lungs, replacement of the normal lung's sponginess by consolidation, and alveoli filled with white blood cells, red blood cells, and fibrin. To the clinician, pneumonia is a constellation of symptoms and signs (fever, chills, cough, pleuritic chest pain, sputum production, hyper- or hypothermia, increased respiratory rate, dullness to percussion, bronchial breathing, egophony, crackles, wheezes, pleural friction rub) in combination with at least one opacity on chest radiography. There is often a degree of uncertainty about the clinical diagnosis of pneumonia, since a number of noninfectious disorders may mimic this entity.

Pneumonia can be broadly categorized as community-acquired or hospital-acquired (nosocomial). When pneumonia occurs in residents of long-term-care facilities (LTCFs), it is treated as community-acquired by some physicians and as nosocomial by others. It is also useful to subdivide cases of community-acquired pneumonia (CAP) into those that can be treated in an ambulatory setting and those that are severe enough to require admission to the hospital. Similarly, nosocomial pneumonia can be categorized as ventilator-associated or non-ventilator-associated. These categories provide a rough guide as to likely pathogens and disease severity.

HOST DEFENSES PROTECTING THE LUNGS   With a surface area of ~70 m^2 that is exposed to the external environment, the lungs are protected by an elegant defense system aimed at preventing potential pathogens from reaching this site and at containing and eliminating the organisms that do gain entry. The pulmonary host defenses can be classified as innate (nonspecific) and acquired (specific).

Anatomical features of the upper airway constitute the first line of innate defense. The nasal turbinates and the sharp angular turn from the naso- and anterior oropharynx into the posterior pharynx act as baffles where inhaled particulate matter can impact. The mucociliary transport system includes ciliated cells of the trachea, bronchi, and terminal bronchioles as well as the overlying mucus layer. The ciliated cells move a mucus layer (produced by goblet cells and submucosal glands), which "floats" on a solute layer to the back of the throat and is swallowed. Mucus consists of complex glycoproteins called *mucins* that trap microorganisms. To prevent pathogens from attaching to and colonizing upper respiratory tract surfaces, binding is inhibited by a decreased mucosal pH, the presence of naturally occurring bacterial and epithelial cell binding analogues, secretory IgA, and the constant desquamation of epithelial cells. In addition, the naso-oropharynx is colonized with nonpathogenic bacteria that can interfere with attachment of pathogens to host cells by a variety of mechanisms.

The entry to the lower respiratory tract is protected by the glottis. If secretions do enter the lower respiratory tract, they can be cleared readily by coughing. In the lower respiratory tract, nonspecific defenses include macrophages, fibronectin, lysozymes, lactoferrin, IgG, defensins, cathelicidins, collectins (including surfactant proteins A and D), and complement. Surfactant is bactericidal to certain pathogens and, along with IgG and fibronectin, can opsonize bacteria. Alveolar macrophages (present at a density of one per alveolus) play a role in both innate and acquired immunity. Their long life span (20 to 80 days) and their ability to phagocytose multiple times are characteristics that particularly suit their role as primary lung phagocytes in innate immunity. As components of acquired immunity, alveolar macrophages present antigens to T cells and produce many regulatory cytokines and mediators. If, however, the concentration of organisms is great (e.g., with gross aspiration) or if especially virulent pathogens are present, the macrophages recruit polymorphonuclear leukocytes (PMNs), and a more intense inflammatory process ensues.

The epithelial cells act as a barrier to dissemination of microorganisms and serve an important immune function. Throughout the lower respiratory tract, these cells produce antimicrobial molecules and participate in the upregulation of inflammation by recruiting phagocytic cells and by producing certain chemokines, including interleukin (IL) 8, macrophage-inflammatory protein 2, granulocyte-macrophage colony-stimulating factor, and by-products of the arachidonic acid cascade. In addition, epithelial cells regulate the expression of endothelial adhesion molecules, thereby targeting the recruitment of PMNs to the lung.

The advantages of the specific host defenses, which require T cell activation, are that they specifically target the offending pathogen, further upregulate the inflammatory response, and result in lifelong immunity to the offending antigen. Lymphocytes and mononuclear phagocytes are present throughout the respiratory tract, from the submucosa of the nasopharynx to the interstitial and alveolar spaces of the pulmonary parenchyma; their presence ensures a fast response of immunoreactive cells to events in the respiratory tract. →*Specific host defenses are discussed in detail in Chap. 295.*

FACTORS IN PATHOGENESIS ■ Routes of Infection For pneumonia to occur, a potential pathogen must reach the lower respiratory tract in sufficient numbers or with sufficient virulence to overwhelm host defenses. Possible routes include gross aspiration, microaspiration, aerosolization, hematogenous spread from a distant infected site, and direct spread from a contiguous infected site. By far the most common route for bacterial pneumonia is microaspiration of oropharyngeal secretions colonized with pathogenic microorganisms. Oropharyngeal colonization by *Streptococcus pneumoniae* and by *Haemophilus influenzae* may occur among healthy individuals (with persistence for weeks) but is more likely with significant comorbidities, antibiotic therapy, or physiologic stress (e.g., due to surgery). Gross aspiration can occur postoperatively and in patients with central nervous system disorders that affect swallowing (seizures, strokes); common pathogens include anaerobic organisms and gram-negative bacilli. Hematogenous spread can take place in the setting of endocarditis, intravenous catheter infections, or infections at other sites, such as the urinary tract. *Staphylococcus aureus* (including methicillin-resistant *S. aureus*, or MRSA) frequently infects the lungs in association with intravascular catheter-related infections, in endocarditis, and with a decreased level of consciousness following head trauma. *Escherichia coli* commonly originates from urinary tract infections. Aerosolization is the route by which *Mycobacterium tuberculosis*, endemic fungi (*Coccidioides immitis, Blastomyces dermatitidis, Histoplasma capsulatum*), *Legionella* spp., *Coxiella burnetii*, and many respiratory viruses (especially influenza viruses A and B) reach the lungs.

Microbial Factors Pathogenic microorganisms have developed a variety of mechanisms to counteract host defenses. *Chlamydia pneumoniae* produces a ciliostatic factor; *Mycoplasma pneumoniae* can shear off cilia; influenza virus infection markedly reduces tracheal mucus velocity within hours of onset and for up to 12 weeks afterward. *S. pneumoniae* and *Neisseria meningitidis* produce proteases that can split secretory IgA. *Mycobacterium, Nocardia,* and *Legionella* spp. are resistant to the microbicidal activity of phagocytes. The pneumococcal capsule inhibits phagocytosis. Another virulence factor produced by all pneumococci is the 53-kDa polypeptide pneumolysin, a thiol-activated cytolysin that interacts with any cell whose membrane contains cholesterol. Pneumococci also produce neuraminidase, hyaluronidase, and IgA1 protease.

Host Factors Pneumonia is more common when host defense is impaired, as it is in severe underlying illness. Hypogammaglobulinemia, defects in phagocytosis or ciliary function, neutropenia, functional or anatomical asplenia, or a reduction in CD4+ T lymphocyte counts are all host defense deficits that can result in increased frequency or severity of pneumonia. Viral infection of alveolar macrophages may explain in part the very high rate of pneumococcal disease in the HIV-infected population. Anatomical defects such as obstructed bronchus, bronchiectasis, or sequestration of a pulmonary segment all lead to recurrent pneumonia or the failure of pneumonia to resolve.

A number of polymorphisms in or near the tumor necrosis factor α (TNF-α) gene are associated with variability in TNF-α production and with outcomes in pneumonia. In patients with CAP, the TNF-α 238 GA genotype is an independent risk factor for a fatal outcome, the lymphotoxin-α (LT-α) +250 AA genotype is a risk factor for septic shock, and the TNF-α 308:LT-α +250 GC haplotype is protective against septic shock. Patients with the DRB1*1501/DQB1*0602 haplotype have been found to mount significantly reduced responses to invasive group A streptococcal pulmonary infection and to be less likely to develop severe disease. In one study, 50% of patients with bacteremic pneumococcal pneumonia—but only 29% of uninfected controls—were homozygous for FcγRIIa-R31, which binds weakly to IgG2; this difference suggested that genetic factors may also be important risk factors for bacteremic pneumococcal pneumonia.

Functional or anatomical asplenia is an important risk factor for pneumonia presenting as overwhelming infection, with 80% of cases due to *S. pneumoniae*. Such overwhelming infection has a mortality rate of ~45%.

PATHOPHYSIOLOGY Vital capacity, lung compliance, functional residual capacity, and total lung capacity are below normal in patients with pneumonia. Ventilation-perfusion mismatch and intrapulmonary shunting are responsible for the hypoxemia that occurs in many patients with pneumonia.

PATHOLOGY The pathology of pneumonia manifests as four general patterns: lobar pneumonia, bronchopneumonia, interstitial pneumonia, and miliary pneumonia.

Lobar Pneumonia *Lobar pneumonia* classically involves an entire lung lobe relatively homogeneously, although in some patients a small portion of the lobe may be unaffected or at an earlier stage of involvement. Four stages of lobar pneumonia may exist simultaneously in the same lung, as the tendency of the progression to be synchronous is not absolute.

The first stage—*congestion*—occurs during the first 24 h and is characterized grossly by redness and a doughy consistency and microscopically by vascular congestion and alveolar edema. At this stage, many bacteria are present and are swept by the rapid expansion of edema fluid throughout the lobe via the pores of Kohn. Only a few neutrophils are seen at this stage. The second stage—termed *red hepatization* because of the color of the lung and the similarity of its airless, noncrepitant firmness to the consistency of liver—is characterized microscopically by the presence of many erythrocytes, neutrophils, desquamated epithelial cells, and fibrin in the alveolar spaces. In the third stage—*gray hepatization*—the lung is dry, friable, and gray-brown to yellow as a consequence of a persistent fibrinopurulent exudate, a progressive disintegration of red blood cells, and the variable presence of hemosiderin. The exudate contains macrophages as well as neutrophils, but bacteria are seldom visible. The second and third stages last for 2 to 3 days each, with a 2- to 6-day duration of maximal consolidation. The final stage—*resolution*—is characterized by enzymatic digestion of the alveolar exudate; resorption, phagocytosis, or coughing up of the residual debris; and restoration of the pulmonary architecture. Fibrinous inflammation may extend to and across the pleural space, causing a rub heard by auscultation, and may lead to resolution or to organization and pleural adhesions.

Bronchopneumonia *Bronchopneumonia*, a patchy consolidation involving one or several lobes, usually involves the dependent lower and posterior portions of the lung—a pattern attributable to the distribution of aspirated oropharyngeal contents by gravity. The consolidated areas are usually poorly demarcated, although in some cases there is an abrupt delimitation of the pneumonia at interlobular septa. The neutrophilic exudate is centered in bronchi and bronchioles, with centrifugal spread to the adjacent alveoli and diminishing cellular exudate; often there is only edema in the periphery of the lesion.

Interstitial Pneumonia *Interstitial pneumonia* is defined by histopathologic identification of an inflammatory process predominantly involving the interstitium, including the alveolar walls and the connective tissue around the bronchovascular tree. The inflammation may be patchy or diffuse. The alveolar septa contain an infiltration of lymphocytes, macrophages, and plasma cells. The alveoli do not contain a significant exudate, but protein-rich hyaline membranes similar to those found in adult respiratory distress syndrome (ARDS) may line the alveolar spaces. Some viruses with tropism for epithelial cells of the airways and alveoli may cause necrosis of the epithelium. In some instances, there may be a significant inflammatory exudate, with extensive degradation of inflammatory cells. Bacterial superinfection of viral pneumonia can also produce a mixed pattern of interstitial and alveolar airspace inflammation.

Miliary Pneumonia The original description of miliary pneumonia was based on the resemblance of the diffusely distributed 2- to 3-mm lesions of hematogenous tuberculosis to millet seeds. The current concept of *miliary pneumonia* is based on its numerous discrete lesions resulting from the spread of the pathogen to the lungs via the bloodstream. The varying degrees of immunocompromise in miliary tuberculosis, histoplasmosis, and coccidioidomycosis manifest as variations in the tissue reaction (from granulomas with caseous necrosis to foci of necrosis); the fibrinous exudate; and the weak, poorly formed cellular reaction. Miliary herpesvirus, cytomegalovirus, or varicella-zoster virus infection in severely immunocompromised patients results in numerous acute necrotizing hemorrhagic lesions.

PULMONARY COMPLICATIONS OF PNEUMONIA Uncontrolled infection by particular agents may lead to necrotizing pneumonia, formation of abscesses, vascular invasion with infarction, cavitation, and extension to the pleura with empyema or bronchopleural fistula. Complications of mechanical ventilation and supplemental oxygen administration include interstitial emphysema, pneumothorax, and ARDS. In patients with severe damage, tissue repair may lead to fibrosis with various anatomical distributions, such as organizing pneumonia, bronchiolitis obliterans, and pleural adhesions.

COMMUNITY-ACQUIRED PNEUMONIA

EPIDEMIOLOGY With an annual cost of $9.7 billion, CAP affects 4 million adults per year in the United States, ~20% of whom are admitted to a hospital for treatment. The overall rate of pneumonia ranges from 8 to 15 per 1000 persons per year, with the highest rates at the extremes of age and during the winter months. Rates of pneumonia are higher for men than for women and for black than for white persons.

Independent risk factors for CAP include alcoholism [RR (relative risk) 9], asthma (RR 4.2), immunosuppression (RR 1.9), and an age of >70 years (RR 1.5 vs. an age of 60 to 69 years). Dementia, seizures, congestive heart failure, cerebrovascular disease, tobacco smoking, alcoholism, and chronic obstructive pulmonary disease (COPD) are risk factors for pneumococcal pneumonia. Independent risk factors for invasive pneumococcal disease include male gender, black race, chronic illness, current tobacco smoking, and passive exposure to tobacco smoke. Cigarette smoking is the strongest independent predictor of invasive pneumococcal disease among immunocompetent young adults. The rate of pneumococcal pneumonia is up to 40 times higher among HIV-infected patients than among age-matched patients not infected with HIV. Risk factors for Legionnaires' disease include male gender, current tobacco smoking, diabetes, hematologic malignancy, cancer, end-stage renal disease, and HIV infection. Probable aspiration, previous hospital admission, previous antimicrobial treatment, and bronchiectasis are predictive of pneumonia due to gram-negative bacteria, including *Pseudomonas aeruginosa*. Heavy drinkers (i.e., those consuming >100 g of ethanol per day for the preceding 2 years) have a higher incidence of gram-negative bacterial pneumonia, experience worse clinical symptoms, and require longer courses of intravenous antibiotic therapy than do nondrinkers. More prolonged fever, slower resolution, and a higher rate of empyema have been noted in pneumococcal pneumonia patients with chronic alcoholism than in their nondrinking counterparts. The clinical entity designated ALPS—alcoholism, leukopenia, and pneumococcal sepsis—is associated with a mortality rate of 80%. In addition, excessive alcohol use is an independent risk factor for the development of ARDS.

ETIOLOGY The organism causing pneumonia may be identified from cultures of blood, sputum, pleural fluid, pulmonary tissue, or endobronchial secretions obtained with a bronchial brush or via lavage. Other methods for determining the etiology of pneumonia include the detection of an IgM response or a fourfold rise in the titer of antibody to an antigen of a particular microorganism and the detection of an antigen in urine, serum, or pleural fluid. In some instances, amplification of DNA or RNA of a respiratory pathogen from one of the above specimens or from material collected with a nasopharyngeal swab can be used for this purpose.

Identification of an etiologic agent in a case of pneumonia should be categorized as definite, probable, or possible, depending on the source of the microorganism or the test used to detect it (Table 239-1). Such diagnostic categorization is useful not only in comparative studies of pneumonia etiology but also in the approach to the patient with pneumonia.

The past 30 years have seen the identification of new etiologic agents of CAP, often during the detailed investigation of dramatic outbreaks. Thus *Legionella pneumophila* was isolated during the investigation of an outbreak of pneumonia at a convention of the American Legion in Philadelphia in 1976. Other etiologic agents identified during this period include *C. pneumoniae*, hantavirus, Nipah virus, Hendra virus, and metapneumovirus. Investigations of an outbreak of severe acute respiratory syndrome (SARS) originating in China and Hong Kong during the winter of 2003 and subsequently found to be caused by a novel coronavirus are ongoing.

The >100 documented microbial causes of CAP include bacteria, fungi, viruses, and parasites. Fortunately, most cases of pneumonia are caused by a few common respiratory pathogens, including *S. pneumoniae*, *H. influenzae*, *S. aureus*, *M. pneumoniae*, *C. pneumoniae*, *Moraxella catarrhalis*, *Legionella* spp., aerobic gram-negative bacteria, influenza viruses, adenoviruses, and respiratory syncytial virus. The relative frequency of these pathogens differs with the age of the patient and the severity of the pneumonia (Table 239-2). Overall, *S. pneumoniae* accounts for ~50% of all cases of CAP requiring admission to the hospital, although in everyday practice the etiology of CAP is unknown in up to 70% of patients.

Determination of the etiology of pneumonia starts with the gathering of clues from the history and physical examination (Table 239-3)

TABLE 239-1 *Categories Reflecting the Certainty of an Etiologic Diagnosis of Pneumonia*

Category	Definition
Definite	Pathogen recovered from blood, pleural fluid, or lung tissue Isolation of *Legionella* spp. or *Mycobacterium tuberculosis* from sputum Positive urinary antigen test for *Legionella*
Probable	Isolation from a purulent sputum specimen of any of the following microorganisms, with a morphologically compatible organism seen in moderate or large numbers on Gram's staining: *Staphylococcus aureus, Streptococcus pneumoniae, Haemophilus influenzae, Moraxella catarrhalis, Pseudomonas aeruginosa* Fourfold or greater rise in titer of antibody to a respiratory pathogen between acute- and convalescent-phase serum samples Positive urinary antigen test for *S. pneumoniae* in adults[a]
Possible	1. Gram's stain of an acceptable sputum specimen[b] showing a predominance of gram-positive diplococci (*S. pneumoniae*), gram-positive cocci in clusters (*S. aureus*), or gram-negative coccobacilli (*H. influenzae*) 2. Isolation of a pathogen from a purulent sputum specimen in the absence of a compatible Gram's stain 3. High single or static titer of antibody to *Legionella pneumophila* ($\geq$1:1024) or *Mycoplasma pneumoniae* ($\geq$1:64)

[a] Nasopharyngeal carriage of *S. pneumoniae* may be associated with a positive test in children.
[b] An acceptable sputum specimen is one with >25 white blood cells and <10 squamous epithelial cells per low-power field.

and proceeds to a diagnostic workup tailored to the severity of the pneumonia or to other circumstances, such as the setting of an outbreak. All patients with pneumonia who are admitted to the hospital should have blood cultured, and sputum should be cultured when the patient has a productive cough. This basic workup should be supplemented with more aggressive diagnostic methods (such as bronchoscopy with bronchoalveolar lavage or bronchial brush specimens) for patients admitted to intensive care units (ICUs).

TABLE 239-2 *Frequency of Most Common Pathogens Causing Community-Acquired Pneumonia, According to Severity of Illness*

Severity of Pneumonia	Rank Order of Pathogens
Ambulatory	1. *Streptococcus pneumoniae* 2. *Mycoplasma pneumoniae* 3. *Chlamydia pneumoniae* 4. *Haemophilus influenzae* 5. Influenza viruses 6. *Pneumocystis*
Treated on hospital ward	1. *S. pneumoniae* 2. Mixed etiology 3. Viruses 4. *H. influenzae* 5. *C. pneumoniae* 6. *Legionella* spp. 7. *M. pneumoniae* 8. *Staphylococcus aureus* 9. *Moraxella catarrhalis* 10. Aerobic gram-negative bacilli 11. *Mycobacterium tuberculosis* 12. *Pneumocystis*
Treated in intensive care unit	1. *S. pneumoniae* 2. *S. aureus* 3. Viruses 4. Mixed etiology 5. Aerobic gram-negative bacilli 6. *Legionella* spp. 7. *M. pneumoniae* 8. *Pneumocystis* 9. *H. influenzae*

TABLE 239-3 *Clues to the Etiology of Pneumonia from History and Physical Examination*

Factor	Possible Agent(s)
OCCUPATIONAL HISTORY	
Health care worker	*Mycobacterium tuberculosis*
Veterinarian, farmer, abattoir worker	*Coxiella burnetii*
Cooling tower maintenance worker	*Legionella* spp.
HOST FACTOR	
Diabetic ketoacidosis	*Streptococcus pneumoniae, Staphylococcus aureus*
Alcoholism	*S. pneumoniae, Klebsiella pneumoniae, S. aureus*, oral anaerobes, *Acinetobacter* spp.
Chronic obstructive pulmonary disease	*S. pneumoniae, Haemophilus influenzae, Moraxella catarrhalis*
Solid organ transplantation	*S. pneumoniae, H. influenzae, Legionella* spp., *Pneumocystis*, cytomegalovirus, *Strongyloides stercoralis*
Sickle cell disease	*S. pneumoniae*
HIV infection and CD4+ lymphocyte count of <200/μL	*S. pneumoniae, Pneumocystis, H. influenzae, Cryptococcus neoformans, M. tuberculosis, Rhodococcus equi*
Dementia, stroke, altered level of consciousness	Agents of aspiration pneumonitis (see text)
Structural lung disease (bronchiectasis)	*Pseudomonas aeruginosa*
TRAVEL AND OTHER ENVIRONMENTAL FACTORS	
Travel to Southeast Asia	*Burkholderia pseudomallei,[a] M. tuberculosis*
Travel to China, Taiwan, Toronto (Canada)[b]	Coronavirus causing severe acute respiratory syndrome (SARS)
Travel to many countries	*M. tuberculosis*
Travel to Arizona, parts of California	*Coccidioides immitis*
Travel to Ohio and St. Lawrence river valleys	*Histoplasma capsulatum*
Exposure to contaminated air-conditioning cooling towers, hot tub, grocery store mist machine; recent stay in a hotel; visit to or recent stay in a hospital with Legionellaceae-contaminated drinking water	*Legionella pneumophila*, other Legionellaceae
Exposure to mouse droppings in an endemic area	Hantavirus
Exposure to windstorm in an endemic area	*C. immitis, C. burnetii*
Pneumonia outbreak in shelter for homeless men or in jail	*S. pneumoniae, M. tuberculosis*
Pneumonia outbreak in military training camp	*S. pneumoniae, Chlamydia pneumoniae*, adenovirus
Pneumonia outbreak in nursing home	*C. pneumoniae, S. pneumoniae*, respiratory syncytial virus, influenza A virus, *M. tuberculosis*
Lawn mowing in an endemic area	*Francisella tularensis*
Exposure to bats, excavation or residence in an endemic area[c]	*H. capsulatum*
Exposure to parturient cats in an endemic area	*C. burnetii*
Sleeping in a rose garden	*Sporothrix schenckii*
Camping, cutting down trees in an endemic area	*Blastomyces dermatitidis*
Exposure to Vancouver Island (camping, residence)	*C. neoformans* var. *gattii*

[a] Agent of melioidosis.
[b] In 2003.
[c] Ohio and Mississippi river valleys.

TABLE 239-4 *British Thoracic Society Rule for Definition of Severe Community-Acquired Pneumonia (Acronym: CURB)*

Confusion
Urea[a]: >7 mmol/L
Respiratory rate: >30/min
Blood pressure: diastolic <60 mmHg or systolic <90 mmHg

[a] Blood urea nitrogen (BUN).

CLINICAL MANIFESTATIONS Pneumonia can range in severity from mild to fulminant and fatal, with serious disease developing even in previously healthy persons. The onset may be sudden and dramatic or insidious. Fever, cough (nonproductive or productive of purulent or rust-colored sputum), pleuritic chest pain, chills or rigors, and shortness of breath are typical—albeit nonspecific—manifestations of pneumonia. Symptoms reported with some frequency include headache, nausea, vomiting, diarrhea, myalgia, arthralgia, and/or fatigue. Falls and new-onset or worsening confusion may be important manifestations in an elderly person. The physical signs associated with pneumonia are tachypnea, dullness to percussion, increased tactile and vocal fremitus, egophony, whispering pectoriloquy, crackles, and pleural friction rub. In two studies, patients with a respiratory rate of >25/min had a pneumonia likelihood ratio of 1.5 to 3.4. In another study, patients with a heart rate of ≤100/min, a temperature of ≤37.8°C, and a respiratory rate of ≤20/min were five times less likely to have pneumonia than patients who had all of these abnormal parameters. A diagnosis of pneumonia based on physical examination has a sensitivity of 47 to 69% and a specificity of 58 to 75%; thus a clinical diagnosis of pneumonia should be confirmed by chest radiography. For patients who have pneumonia clinically diagnosed in an office setting, the physician must decide whether or not to obtain a chest radiograph. Even if the clinical assessment suggests mild disease, all patients with pneumonia who have an oral temperature of >38.5°C or who have pleuritic chest pain should have a chest radiograph. Pulmonary embolus is always a consideration with pleuritic chest pain, and further investigations are warranted if the chest radiograph is normal in this setting. If pneumonia is extensive in a patient with this degree of fever, further evaluation and perhaps hospitalization are necessary.

The single most useful clinical sign of the severity of pneumonia is a respiratory rate of >30/min in a person without underlying lung disease. Of the several measures of pneumonia severity, the simplest is the British Thoracic Society rule, which relies on three clinical findings and one laboratory finding (Table 239-4). If none of these features is present, the mortality rate is 2.4%; with one feature, the mortality rate is 8%; with two, 23%; with three, 33%; and with all four, 83%. The American Thoracic Society criteria for severe pneumonia are given in Table 239-5. To derive a scoring system for classifying pneumonia cases across the spectrum from mild to severe, the Pneumonia Patient Outcomes Research Team (PORT) assigned points to each of 20 items associated with mortality (Table 239-6). The resulting PORT score allowed categorization of patients with pneumonia into five risk groups (Table 239-7). Although this system was developed as a mortality prediction tool and is no substitute for clinical judgment, it is often used in making site-of-treatment decisions (see "Treatment," below).

Certain causes of pneumonia and organisms within a species are

TABLE 239-5 *American Thoracic Society Definition of Severe Pneumonia*

Category	Criteria
Major	Need for mechanical ventilation
	Requirement for vasopressors: >4 h
Minor	Systolic blood pressure: <90 mmHg
	Pa$_{O_2}$/Fi$_{O_2}$: <250
	Multilobar involvement

TABLE 239-6 *Severity-of-Illness Scoring System Based on Pneumonia Patient Outcomes Research Team (PORT) Cohort Study Data*

Patient Characteristic	No. of Points
Age	
Men	Age, years
Women	Age, years −10
Nursing home residents	Age, years +10
Coexisting illnesses	
Neoplastic disease[a]	30
Liver disease[b]	20
Congestive heart failure[c]	10
Cerebrovascular disease[d]	10
Renal disease[e]	10
Physical examination findings	
Altered mental status[f]	20
Respiratory rate >30/min	20
Systolic blood pressure <90 mmHg	20
Temperature <35°C (<95°F) or >40°C (>104°F)	15
Pulse rate >125/min	10
Laboratory and radiographic findings	
Arterial pH < 7.35	30
Blood urea nitrogen >30 mg/dL (>11 mmol/L)	20
Sodium <130 mmol/L	20
Glucose >250 mg/dL (>14 mmol/L)	10
Hematocrit <30%	10
Partial pressure of arterial oxygen <60 mmHg	10
Pleural effusion	10

[a] Any cancer (except basal or squamous cell carcinoma of the skin) active at presentation or within 1 year of presentation with community-acquired pneumonia.
[b] Clinical or histologic cirrhosis or chronic active hepatitis.
[c] Diagnosis documented by history or by findings on physical examination, chest radiography, echocardiography, multiple gated acquisition scan, or left ventriculography.
[d] Clinical diagnosis of stroke or transient ischemic attack; stroke documented by magnetic resonance imaging or computed tomography.
[e] History of chronic renal disease or abnormal blood urea nitrogen and creatinine concentrations documented in medical record.
[f] Disorientation as to person, place, or time that is not known to be chronic; stupor or coma.

associated with a high mortality rate. The mortality rate is highest (>50%) for pneumonia due to *P. aeruginosa*, followed by the rates for *Klebsiella* spp., *E. coli*, *S. aureus*, and *Acinetobacter* spp. (all 30 to 35%). The capsular serotype 3 pneumococcus is associated with a much higher mortality rate than serotype 1, as are M serotypes 1 and 3 of group A *Streptococcus* (compared with other serotypes).

Young, otherwise healthy adults who develop pneumonia and who are treated as outpatients usually feel well enough to return to work in 4 or 5 days, and almost all will have recovered in 2 weeks. However, those with relatively severe symptoms may require longer to recover. About 2 to 4% of those who are treated as outpatients experience a progression of symptoms and require admission to the hospital. In general, those admitted during the first week after the initial visit are admitted because pneumonia has worsened, while those admitted later are often admitted because of worsening of comorbid illnesses (e.g., diabetes mellitus, congestive heart failure, asthma, or ischemic heart disease). Currently, up to 25% of persons treated for pneumonia as outpatients are >65 years old, and the natural history of ambulatory

TABLE 239-7 *Mortality Rate at 30 Days among Patients with Community-Acquired Pneumonia, According to PORT Risk Class[a]*

Risk Class	Criteria	% Mortality Outpatient	% Mortality Inpatient
I	Age <50 years No existing illnesses or vital-sign abnormalities	0	0.5
II	70 points	0.4	0.9
III	71−90 points	0	1.25
IV	91−130 points	12.5	9.0
V	131 points	NA	27.1
Mean		0.6	8.0

[a] PORT, Pneumonia Patient Outcomes Research Team.

pneumonia in this group is probably different from that in younger patients.

Among patients admitted to the hospital for the treatment of pneumonia, clinical stability is usually attained in 3 to 7 days, depending on the definition used. In one study, a median of 2 days was required to achieve a heart rate of ≤100/min and 3 days to achieve a respiratory rate of ≤24/min, an oxygen saturation of ≥90%, and a temperature of ≤37.2°C. Once stability is attained, clinical deterioration is uncommon.

Since most patients admitted to the hospital with pneumonia are elderly and have multiple comorbid conditions, it is not uncommon for complications to occur during the hospital stay. The most common complications are respiratory failure, congestive heart failure, shock, atrial dysrhythmias, myocardial infarction, gastrointestinal bleeding, and renal insufficiency. Indeed, only ~30% of patients hospitalized for the treatment of pneumonia have no complications.

The in-hospital mortality rate from pneumonia is ~8%. The most common immediate causes of death among patients with pneumonia are respiratory failure, heart disease, and infections. About half of deaths are related to pneumonia, and the other half are due to comorbid illnesses. Pneumonia-related deaths are much more likely to occur during the first week of hospitalization. Factors independently associated with pneumonia-unrelated mortality include dementia, immunosuppression, active cancer, systolic hypotension, male gender, and multilobar pulmonary infiltrates. Increasing age and evidence of aspiration independently predict both pneumonia-related and comorbidity-related mortality.

DIAGNOSIS The usual standard for the diagnosis of pneumonia is chest radiography, which, however, is not 100% sensitive. High-resolution computed tomography (CT) occasionally detects pulmonary opacities in patients with symptoms and signs suggestive of pneumonia in whom chest radiographs are reported as not showing pneumonia. CT is also more likely than chest radiography to show bilateral involvement. If pneumonia is strongly suspected on clinical grounds and no opacity is seen on the initial chest radiograph, it is useful to repeat the radiograph in 24 to 48 h or to perform CT. It is important to remember that an opacity visible on chest radiograph may not be due to pneumonia; many other disease processes can result in opacities. Furthermore, there is variability among radiologists in the interpretation of chest radiographs; most commonly, subsegmental lower-lobe opacities in patients with suboptimal chest radiographs may be reported as atelectasis by one radiologist and as pneumonia by another. Occasionally, an etiologic diagnosis is suggested by the findings on chest radiography. For example, a cavitating upper-lobe lesion raises the likelihood of tuberculosis, and pneumatoceles suggest *S. aureus* pneumonia. An air-fluid level suggests a pulmonary abscess, which is often polymicrobial. In the immunocompromised host, a crescent (meniscus) sign suggests aspergillosis. In most instances, however, no etiologic inference can be made from radiographic findings.

Concomitant diseases (such as congestive heart failure or pulmonary fibrosis) may make both the clinical and the radiologic diagnosis of pneumonia difficult. However, serial clinical and radiographic observations usually allow the clinician to determine whether there are two diseases or just one and to identify which one is causing the clinical and radiographic findings.

Etiologic Diagnosis ■ *BLOOD CULTURE* Blood should be obtained for culture from patients to be treated on an ambulatory basis if they have been receiving antibiotic therapy and have presented because of any of the following: hyperthermia (temperature >38.5°C), hypothermia (temperature <36°C), homelessness, or alcohol abuse. All patients who are admitted to the hospital for CAP should have two sets of blood cultures done before initiation of antibiotic therapy (positivity rate: 6 to 20%). The most common isolates, in descending order, are *S. pneumoniae* (~60%), *S. aureus*, and *E. coli*.

SPUTUM STAINS AND CULTURE Gram's stain is used to screen a sputum sample for suitability for culture and to make a presumptive etiologic

diagnosis. A sputum sample with >25 white blood cells and <10 squamous epithelial cells per low-power field is suitable for culture. There is a great deal of interobserver variability in the interpretation of gram-stained sputum smears. The presence of any gram-positive diplococci has a sensitivity of 100% but a specificity of 0 for a diagnosis of pneumococcal infection. The presence of >10 gram-positive diplococci per oil-immersion field has a sensitivity of 55% and a specificity of 85% for this diagnosis. Culture results should always be correlated with those of Gram's staining. If an organism is isolated from sputum and its morphologic correlate is not seen on Gram's staining, the isolate may be colonizing the upper airway. Certain microorganisms, if isolated from sputum, should always be considered pathogens. These include *M. tuberculosis*, *Legionella* spp., *B. dermatitidis*, *H. capsulatum*, and *C. immitis*. In practice, only about one-third of elderly patients admitted with CAP produce sputum suitable for culture, and one-third of these specimens fail to yield a pathogen.

Other types of sputum staining are also useful for determining the etiology of CAP. A variety of stains for acid-fast bacilli are used to diagnose tuberculosis; *Pneumocystis* pneumonia can be diagnosed with monoclonal antibody staining; and special stains for fungi are useful in selected patients, as are cytologic stains.

DETECTION OF ANTIGENS OF PULMONARY PATHOGENS IN URINE *L. pneumophila* serogroup 1 antigen can be detected in the urine of patients with Legionnaires' disease due to this organism by means of an enzyme-linked immunosorbent assay (ELISA). The sensitivity of this assay is 69 to 72% on average, 88 to 100% in severe disease, and 40 to 53% in mild disease. The assay's sensitivity is low in nosocomial Legionnaires' disease. The results may be negative early in the illness, and antigen excretion can be prolonged. The test should be used in patients in whom Legionnaires' disease is strongly suspected, including those with rapidly progressive pneumonia. The urine antigen test is now the most frequently used diagnostic method for Legionnaires' disease. A critical point, however, is that infection with *Legionella* spp. other than *L. pneumophila* serogroup 1 gives a negative test result.

S. pneumoniae urinary antigen detection by ELISA has a sensitivity of 80% and a specificity of 97 to 100% in patients with bacteremic pneumococcal pneumonia. The antigen may be detected for up to 1 month after the onset of pneumonia, and the results can be available in 15 min. In children, nasopharyngeal carriage of *S. pneumoniae* can result in a positive urinary antigen test.

SEROLOGY The detection of IgM antibody or the demonstration of a fourfold rise in the titer of antibody to a particular agent between acute and convalescent-phase serum samples is generally considered good evidence that this agent is the cause of the pneumonia. The following etiologic agents are often diagnosed serologically: *M. pneumoniae*, *C. pneumoniae*, *Chlamydia psittaci*, *Legionella* spp., *C. burnetii*, adenovirus, parainfluenza viruses, and influenza virus A. The various serologic tests include complement fixation, indirect immunofluorescence, and ELISA. Separate IgM and IgG antibody detection tests can be performed with the latter two assays. One difficulty in relying on serology is that a polyclonal antibody response to one agent may result in a fourfold rise in antibody titer to others; thus the results may be nonspecific. Serologic testing is not recommended for routine use; however, if agents such as *C. burnetii* are suspected, such testing is necessary. Serology is also a useful part of the workup of outbreaks of pneumonia associated with negative blood and sputum cultures.

POLYMERASE CHAIN REACTION Amplification of the DNA or RNA of microorganisms that are not part of the pharyngeal flora (from microbial cells collected by throat swab) has been used to infer that the implicated microorganism is the cause of pneumonia. A multiplex polymerase chain reaction allows detection of DNA of *Legionella* spp., *M. pneumoniae*, and *C. pneumoniae*. This test is expensive and is not routinely available.

℞ TREATMENT

Successful treatment of CAP involves all the elements listed in Tables 239-8, 239-9, and 239-10.

Site of Care   As described above, the PORT score (based on a pneumonia-specific severity-of-illness scoring system; Tables 239-6 and 239-7) has been advocated as a tool to guide the decision regarding the site of care (home vs. hospital). Because of the low mortality rates in risk classes I and II, it is recommended that these patients be treated at home, while patients in risk classes IV and V require hospital admission. Patients in class III may benefit from a period of observation in the emergency room before a decision is made regarding the site of care. Reliance on this or any other such system as the sole criterion for this decision has several limitations: (1) These systems are mortality prediction tools only and do not take into account psychosocial reasons for admission. (2) Although illness is dynamic, scoring systems capture events at a single point in time. (3) A physician's judgment is often the most critical element in decision-making and should override any scoring system. For example, some patients in classes I to III may have a complicated hospital course and may even require admission to an ICU, although the scoring system would dictate that they should be sent home. In practice, a physician should use a number of approaches in deciding on the site of care—intuition, specific assessment of the severity of illness, and the parameters given in Table 239-10. When a patient with pneumonia is sent home from the emergency room or the physician's office, it is advisable to follow up with a telephone call within 48 h. In our experience, most patients have begun to feel better by this time, ~10% are unchanged, and ~5% are worse; this last group of patients should be reassessed by a physician. Patients who are treated on an ambulatory basis should be given written information about the warning signs of pneumonia exacerbation, such as shortness of breath while walking on level ground (for those who have no underlying lung disease), a temperature of >38.5°C after 72 h of antibiotic therapy, or a new onset of confusion or pleuritic chest pain. In addition, patients should be advised to report hemoptysis to their physicians.

TABLE 239-8   *Approach to the Patient with Community-Acquired Pneumonia*

1. Assess pneumonia severity. Pay attention to vital signs, including oxygen saturation. Always count the respiratory rate yourself for 1 min.
2. Ensure adequate oxygenation and support of circulation.
3. Perform etiologic workup (dictated by pneumonia severity).
4. Determine site of treatment: home, hospital (ward or intensive care unit), or long-term-care facility.
5. Institute empirical antibiotic therapy.
6. Rule out empyema in all patients with a pleural effusion of >1 cm on lateral decubitus chest radiography.
7. Never forget tuberculosis and *Pneumocystis* infection as possible etiologies. Check your hospital policy regarding the isolation of patients with CAP. In some centers where tuberculosis is common, all patients with CAP are isolated until sputum smears are found to be negative for acid-fast bacilli.
8. Consider pulmonary embolus in all patients with pleuritic chest pain.
9. Consider end-of-life decision-making.
10. Monitor and treat comorbid illnesses.
11. Monitor for achievement of stability of selected physiologic parameters.
12. Assess ability to perform activities of daily living.
13. Assess mental status.
14. Consider preventive measures:
    a. Smoking cessation counseling (if appropriate)
    b. Assessment of pneumococcal and influenza vaccination status, with vaccine administration as necessary
    c. Assessment of risk of aspiration and institution of preventive measures
15. Follow up to ensure radiographic clearance of pneumonia. All patients >40 years old and all tobacco smokers should have a follow-up chest radiograph to document pneumonia resolution.

Antibiotic Therapy ■ *EMPIRICAL TREATMENT AND DRUG RESISTANCE*   Since the etiology of pneumonia is frequently unknown, initial antibiotic therapy is often empirical. There are currently three sets of North American guidelines for empirical antibiotic treatment of CAP: those developed under the auspices of the Infectious Diseases Society of America, the American Thoracic Society, and the Canadian Infectious Diseases and Canadian Thoracic Societies. Table 239-9 combines various elements of these guidelines with the opinions of the authors.

There are no data from randomized clinical trials to indicate that one antibiotic or combination of antibiotics is better than another for the empirical treatment of CAP. A retrospective review of 12,945 Medicare patients (all >65 years old) indicated that treatment with a macrolide plus a second-generation or nonpseudomonal third-generation cephalosporin was associated with a significantly lower mortality rate than treatment with a second- or third-generation cephalosporin alone. Use of a fluoroquinolone alone was likewise associated with a significantly lower mortality rate, while the combination of an aminoglycoside and any other antibiotic resulted in a significantly higher mortality rate. Data from the Medicare study also indicated that timely administration is important: Patients who received antibiotics within 8 h after arrival at the emergency room had a lower mortality rate than those who received the first dose >8 h afterward. Data from a retrospective review of bacteremic pneumococcal pneumonia indicated that therapy with a single antimicrobial agent was not as effective as therapy with two or more agents effective against *S. pneumoniae*; data from randomized clinical trials must confirm or refute this observation.

In the selection of empirical antibiotic therapy, risk factors for drug-resistant *S. pneumoniae* must be considered (Table 239-9). Before 1980, strains of *S. pneumoniae* were almost universally susceptible to penicillin and other antimicrobial drugs. [The current National Committee for Clinical Laboratory Standards interpretive breakpoints for the minimal inhibitory concentration (MIC) of penicillin are ≤0.06 μg/mL (susceptible), 0.12 to 1.0 μg/mL (intermediate), and ≥2.0 μg/mL (resistant). Isolates classified as either intermediately resistant or resistant are considered nonsusceptible. Isolates resistant to three or more classes of drugs are termed multidrug-resistant.] In the late 1980s, the prevalence of penicillin-nonsusceptible *S. pneumoniae* in the United States was 4.0%; less than a decade later, it was 35%. In the United States, a multicenter national surveillance study conducted from November 1999 through April 2000 found that 35% of pneumococci were nonsusceptible to penicillin, with 60% of these isolates resistant. Resistance to non-β-lactam antibiotics also emerged among North American *S. pneumoniae* strains during the 1990s. In 1999 to 2000, the rate of resistance among U.S. isolates of *S. pneumoniae* was 25.9% for macrolides, 8.8% for clindamycin, 16.4% for tetracyclines, 8.4% for chloramphenicol, and 30.3% for trimethoprim-sulfamethoxazole. Furthermore, 22.5% of clinical isolates of *S. pneumoniae* were multidrug-resistant. The dominant factor in the emergence of drug-resistant *S. pneumoniae* in North America has been human-to-human spread of relatively few clonal groups that harbor resistance determinants to multiple classes of antibiotics. Serotypes 6A, 6B, 9V, 14, 19F, and 23F accounted for 92.3% of penicillin-resistant pneumococcal isolates in one study.

Emergence of pneumococcal resistance to quinolones has been described in Canada, Spain, Hong Kong, Eastern and Central Europe, and (to a lesser extent) the United States. In Canada, the prevalence of ciprofloxacin-resistant pneumococci (MIC ≥ 4 μg/mL) increased from 0 in 1993 to 1.7% in 1997 to 1998 (p = .01); the figures for adults were 0 in 1993 and 3.7% in 1998. The Active Bacterial Core Surveillance program carried out by the U.S. Centers for Disease Control and Prevention during 1995 to 1999 reported levofloxacin nonsusceptibility rates of 0.2%. The emergence of quinolone resistance has been documented in two pandemic multidrug-resistant pneumococcal clones, Spain 23F-1 and Spain 9V-3. Strains of the Spain 23F-1 clone have been found to be resistant to quinolones in the United States, Europe, and Hong Kong.

The rapid increase in drug resistance has not been accompanied by clear evidence of therapy failure among patients with pneumococcal

CAP. There have been only a few controlled studies on the impact of pneumococcal resistance to penicillin on CAP outcomes. Overall, the results from these studies suggest that mortality is not higher among patients with penicillin-nonsusceptible pneumococcal isolates than among patients with susceptible isolates, particularly when an isolate's MIC is ≤2 μg/mL. Two case-control studies have reported adverse outcomes among patients with CAP due to penicillin-nonsusceptible pneumococci. In one study, after the exclusion of deaths occurring during the first 4 days of hospitalization, there was a significant risk of death among patients whose pneumococcal isolates had a penicillin MIC of at least 4 μg/mL or a cefotaxime MIC of at least 2 μg/mL. While the risk of death was not elevated among patients with penicillin-nonsusceptible pneumococcal pneumonia, the risk of suppurative complications was greater than that among patients with penicillin-susceptible infections.

Given their excellent activity against *S. pneumoniae* as well as against the so-called atypical pathogens *M. pneumoniae*, *C. pneumoniae*, and *Legionella* spp., macrolide antibiotics (either alone or combined with β-lactams) have been widely used to treat CAP. Despite the rapid escalation of macrolide resistance in *S. pneumoniae*, there is little evidence of therapy failures, especially among nonbacteremic patients treated in the community. However, there is now evidence of breakthrough bacteremia during macrolide or azalide treatment of patients infected with erythromycin-resistant *S. pneumoniae*. Doxycycline, which is active against penicillin-susceptible *S. pneumoniae* and against the atypical pathogens, is underused for the treatment of CAP in an ambulatory setting.

Although anecdotal, a number of reports have described failures of quinolone therapy for CAP due to *S. pneumoniae* resistant to the specific agent used. Among the risk factors that identify patients likely to be colonized or infected with quinolone-resistant pneumococci are an age of >64 years and a history of COPD and/or quinolone exposure. Indeed, patients with pneumonia who have been treated with a quinolone in the past 3 months should receive treatment with another class of antibiotics.

If there is clinical evidence of meningitis in a patient with CAP, vancomycin and ceftriaxone should be used (Table 239-9) to ensure that potentially drug-resistant *S. pneumoniae* is adequately treated.

SWITCH FROM INTRAVENOUS TO ORAL ANTIBIOTIC THERAPY Switching from intravenous to oral antibiotics can be done safely when (1) the white blood cell count is returning toward normal, (2) there are two normal temperature readings (<37.5°C) 16 h apart, and (3) there is improvement in cough and shortness of breath. Some antibiotics, such as amoxicillin and respiratory quinolones (moxifloxacin, gatifloxacin, and levofloxacin), are so well absorbed from the gastrointestinal tract that intravenous therapy is necessary only when the patient is hypotensive, is nauseated, and/or is vomiting.

TABLE 239-9 *Initial Empirical Antibiotic Therapy for Community-Acquired Pneumonia*

Treatment Setting; Patient's Condition	Regimen[a]
Outpatient; no cardiopulmonary disease, no risk factors for DRSP infection[b]	Macrolide (e.g., clarithromycin 500 mg bid PO × 10 days; or azithromycin 500 mg PO once, then 250 mg/d × 4 days) *or* Doxycycline 100 mg bid PO × 10 days
Outpatient; cardiopulmonary disease and/or (1) risk factors for DRSP infection or (2) high DRSP prevalence in community	Quinolone with enhanced activity against *Streptococcus pneumoniae*—e.g., levofloxacin 500 mg/d PO (or, with C_{cr} <50 mL/min, 250 mg/d), moxifloxacin 400 mg/d PO, or gatifloxacin 400 mg/d PO *or* β-Lactam (cefpodoxime 200 mg bid, cefuroxime axetil 750 mg tid, or amoxicillin 1000 mg tid, PO; amoxicillin/clavulanic acid 875/175 mg tid) plus macrolide or doxycycline *or* Telithromycin 800 mg q24h × 10 days
Hospital ward	Cefuroxime 750 mg q8h IV or ceftriaxone 1 g/d IV or cefotaxime 2 g q6h IV or ampicillin/sulbactam 1.5–3 g q6h IV *plus* Azithromycin 1 g/d IV followed by 500 mg/d IV *or* Quinolone with enhanced activity against *S. pneumoniae* (see above)[c]
Intensive care unit; no risk factors for *Pseudomonas aeruginosa* infection	Azithromycin 1 g IV, then start 500 mg IV 24 h later *plus* Ceftriaxone 1 g q12h IV *or* Cefotaxime 2 g q6h IV *or* Quinolone IV
Intensive care unit; risk factors for *P. aeruginosa*[b]	Imipenem (or meropenem) 500 mg q6h IV *or* Piperacillin/tazobactam 3.375 g q6h IV *plus* Ciprofloxacin 750 mg q8h IV
Nursing home[d]	Amoxicillin/clavulanic acid 875/125 mg tid PO *plus* Macrolide PO (see above) *or* Quinolone PO with enhanced activity against *S. pneumoniae* (see above) *or* Ceftriaxone 500–1000 mg/d IM or cefotaxime 500 mg IM q12h *plus* Macrolide (see above)
Aspiration pneumonitis (presumed to be due to effects of gastric acid or other irritants)	Wait 24 h; if symptoms persist, give antibiotic therapy delineated below for aspiration pneumonia.
Aspiration pneumonia; poor dental hygiene or putrid sputum, alcoholism (anaerobic infection suspected)	Metronidazole 500 mg q12h PO[e] *or* Piperacillin/tazobactam 3.375 g q6h IV *or* Imipenem 500 mg q6h IV *plus* One of the following: levofloxacin 500 mg/d IV or PO, moxifloxacin 400 mg/d PO, gatifloxacin 400 mg/d IV or PO, ceftriaxone, or cefotaxime
Aspiration pneumonia; community-acquired	Levofloxacin, moxifloxacin, gatifloxacin, ceftriaxone, or cefotaxime (see above)
Concomitant meningitis (suspected pneumococcal)	Vancomycin 1 g q12h IV *plus* Ceftriaxone 2 g q12h IV

[a] The optimal duration of therapy for CAP is unknown. With the exception of azithromycin (which has a long half-life), a 7- to 10-day course is usually recommended. Pneumonia due to *Legionella* spp., *P. aeruginosa*, or Enterobacteriaceae usually requires therapy of longer duration (often up to 21 days).

[b] Risk factors: (1) For penicillin-resistant *S. pneumoniae*: Previous use (within 3 months) of β-lactam antibiotics, alcoholism, age <5 years or >65 years, and (in some areas) residence in a nursing home. (2) For macrolide-resistant *S. pneumoniae*: Age <5 years or nosocomial acquisition of infection. (3) For quinolone-resistant *S. pneumoniae*: Older age, nursing home residence, chronic obstructive pulmonary disease, previous exposure to quinolones (especially ciprofloxacin in patients with chronic obstructive pulmonary disease) in the past 3 months, multiple hospitalizations, and β-lactam use. (4) For *P. aeruginosa*: Bronchiectasis, malnutrition, treatment with >10 mg of prednisone/d, previously undiagnosed HIV infection, and broad-spectrum antibiotic therapy for >7 days in the past month.

[c] Some authorities suggest that a β-lactam be added if a quinolone is chosen as empirical therapy until it is clear that quinolone-resistant pneumococci are not involved.

[d] For nursing home residents transferred to the hospital for treatment, see appropriate hospital/intensive care unit recommendations.

[e] Clindamycin could be used, but, because of the increased rate of *Clostridium difficile*–associated diarrhea associated with this drug, metronidazole is preferred.

Note: DRSP, drug-resistant *S. pneumoniae*.

DURATION OF ANTIBIOTIC THERAPY The standard duration of treatment for most patients with CAP is 10 to 14 days. However, no data from randomized clinical trials indicate the optimal duration. Patients treated on an ambulatory basis with an antibiotic with a long half-life

1. Respiratory rate >28/min
2. Systolic blood pressure <90 mmHg or 30 mmHg below baseline
3. New-onset confusion or impaired level of consciousness
4. Hypoxemia: P_{O_2} <60 mmHg while breathing room air or oxygen saturation <90%
5. Unstable comorbid illness (e.g., decompensated congestive heart failure, uncontrolled diabetes mellitus, alcoholism, immunosuppression)
6. Multilobar pneumonia, if hypoxemia is present
7. Pleural effusion that is >1 cm on lateral decubitus chest radiography and has the characteristics of a complicated parapneumonic effusion on pleural fluid analysis

[a] Patient should be admitted if any of the above criteria applies. Social factors such as homelessness must also be considered in the admission decision.

(e.g., azithromycin) require only 5 days of treatment. Patients with severe Legionnaires' disease require 21 days of therapy, as do those with pneumonia due to *P. aeruginosa* or other aerobic gram-negative bacilli.

Discharge from the Hospital   The decision about when to discharge a patient with pneumonia is often a complicated matter. Once physiologic stability is achieved (defined as an oral temperature of <37.5°C for 24 h, a heart rate of <100/min, a respiratory rate of <24/min, a systolic blood pressure of >90 mmHg, an oxygen saturation of >90% while breathing room air, and the ability to eat and drink well enough to maintain hydration), clinical deterioration requiring admission to a critical-care unit or telemetry monitoring has occurred in <1% of patients. Since most patients hospitalized with CAP are elderly, it is necessary to assess functional and mental status before discharge. Comorbid illnesses should be stable, and any complications that have occurred during the hospital stay should have been addressed. Instability at the time of discharge is associated with higher rates of mortality and readmission than have been documented among patients stable at discharge.

In one study, patients with HIV infection and *Pneumocystis* pneumonia who were treated by an experienced medical team had a lower mortality rate than those who were treated by a team that managed such patients infrequently. Patients with pneumonia who were treated by subspecialists working outside their specialty had an 18% longer hospital stay and a slightly higher mortality rate than patients with pneumonia who were treated by general internists. High patient-to-nurse ratios are associated with increased mortality rates on surgical floors, and this association is likely to hold true and to be linked with suboptimal outcomes among patients hospitalized with pneumonia as well.

Failure to Improve   When a patient with pneumonia fails to improve despite therapy, an organized approach that considers all the factors listed in Table 239-11 is useful. Many noninfectious conditions may mimic pneumonia, including lung cancer, pulmonary thromboembolic disease with infarction, collagen vascular diseases involving the lungs, and hypersensitivity pneumonitis due to drugs and a variety of antigens. A careful physical examination, with a search for metastatic foci of infection or physical signs suggestive of other diseases (e.g., subconjunctival petechiae, a new cardiac murmur suggestive of endocarditis), should be conducted and should be followed by blood, urine, and sputum cultures and repeat chest radiography. Depending on the results of chest radiography, high-resolution CT of the chest may be the next step. Indeed, CT of the chest in patients who fail to respond to therapy results in new findings not seen on chest radiographs 50% of the time, and these findings frequently lead to a change in therapy. If these investigations are unrewarding and pulmonary infection is still thought to be the most likely diagnosis, bronchoscopy with bronchoalveolar lavage is indicated. The respiratory secretions obtained should be cultured both aerobically and anaerobically as well as for *M. tuberculosis*, atypical mycobacteria, respiratory viruses, and fungi. Monoclonal antibody staining for *Pneumocystis* should be done. The secretions should also be examined cytologically; although this type of examination is usually undertaken to detect malignant cells, the investigator is occasionally surprised by the finding of *Strongyloides stercoralis* larvae in immunosuppressed patients with hyperinfection syndrome.

FOLLOW-UP   Up to 2% of patients hospitalized with CAP are found to have cancer of the lung (with pneumonia distal to an obstructed bronchus). In 50% of these patients, the cancer is evident on the initial chest radiograph; however, in the remaining 50%, the cancer manifests as failure of the pneumonia to resolve radiographically and is evident only when bronchoscopy is performed to determine the reason for delayed pneumonia resolution. The rate of radiographic resolution of pneumonia is influenced by the age of the patient and the underlying lung disease. Thus patients with bacteremic pneumococcal pneumonia who are >60 years old and have COPD require up to 12 weeks for pneumonia resolution. The question, then, is the optimal timing of the follow-up chest radiograph among patients who are clinically well. In elderly patients with COPD, it is reasonable to wait 8 to 12 weeks. Nonsmoking patients <50 years of age who have no underlying lung disease should experience complete resolution of pneumonia within 6 weeks.

PREVENTION   All patients with pneumonia who are tobacco smokers should be encouraged to join smoking cessation programs. Influenza and pneumococcal vaccination status should be ascertained and vaccines offered when appropriate. When a patient is prone to aspiration, preventive measures should be taken.

SELECTED COMPLICATIONS OF CAP ■ Complicated Pleural Effusion   About 40% of patients hospitalized with CAP have a pleural effusion that can be documented by special techniques, such as CT of the chest. All patients with a pleural effusion should have a lateral decubitus chest radiograph with the affected side down. If the size of the effusion is >1 cm, the fluid should be aspirated. If the fluid has a pH of <7, a glucose level of <2.2 mmol/L, and a lactate dehydrogenase content of >1000 units and is positive on Gram's staining or culture, it should be drained. If frank pus is aspirated, insertion of a chest tube and treatment with intrapleural lytic agents are recommended. Thoracotomy and decortication may be necessary. All patients with a complicated pleural effusion, as defined above, should have a consultation with a thoracic surgeon.

Lung Abscess   A lung abscess is a localized area of suppuration within lung tissue that leads to parenchymal destruction and is manifest radiographically as a cavity with an air-fluid level. Lung abscesses are currently uncommon, with an incidence of 4 to 5 cases per 10,000 hospital admissions. Risk factors for lung abscess include conditions associated with impaired cough reflex and/or aspiration, such as al-

TABLE 239-11   *Possibilities to Consider When a Patient with Community-Acquired Pneumonia Fails to Improve Despite Treatment*

1. Reconsider the diagnosis. Is this another illness presenting as pneumonia? Collagen vascular diseases involving the lung are frequently diagnosed at first as pneumonia.
2. Are you treating the wrong pathogen? For example, if you are treating conventional bacterial causes of pneumonia, is this case actually due to *Mycobacterium tuberculosis*, *Pneumocystis*, or another fungus?
3. Are you treating the right pathogen with the wrong drug? For example, if you are using nafcillin or cloxacillin to treat *Staphylococcus aureus* and your patient is infected with methicillin-resistant *S. aureus*, you should be using vancomycin or linezolid.
4. Is there a mechanical reason for the patient's failure to improve (e.g., obstructed bronchus due to carcinoma or sequestration of a segment of lung)?
5. Have you overlooked an undrained or metastatic pyogenic focus (e.g., empyema, brain abscess, endocarditis, splenic abscess, osteomyelitis)?
6. Does the patient have drug-associated fever?

coholism, anesthesia, drug abuse, epilepsy, and stroke. Dental caries, bronchiectasis, bronchial carcinoma, and pulmonary infarction are also risk factors. Most aspiration-associated lung abscesses are due to a combination of aerobic and anaerobic bacteria, with an average of six or seven bacterial species identified in an individual case. The implicated anaerobic bacteria include the *Bacteroides fragilis* group, *Bacteroides gracilis*, *Prevotella intermedia*, *Prevotella denticola*, *Prevotella melaninogenicus*, *Prevotella oralis*, *Fusobacterium nucleatum*, *Peptostreptococcus micros*, *Peptostreptococcus anaerobius*, and *Peptostreptococcus magnus*. *Streptococcus milleri* is one of the principal aerobic pathogens; *S. aureus*, *S. pneumoniae*, *H. influenzae*, *P. aeruginosa*, *E. coli*, and *Klebsiella pneumoniae* are also isolated frequently. Rarely, *S. pneumoniae* alone (usually capsular type 3) can cause a lung abscess. In HIV-infected patients, lung abscesses can be due to *Pneumocystis*, *Rhodococcus equi*, and *Cryptococcus neoformans* as well as the bacteria noted above.

The clinical presentation is usually indolent, with weight loss, malaise, night sweats, fever, and productive cough. Patients with anaerobic lung abscess have foul-smelling, often foul-tasting sputum. Clubbing of the fingers occurs in ~10% of patients, usually in those who have been symptomatic for >3 weeks.

Spontaneous drainage occurs via bronchial communication and is accompanied by the production of copious amounts of purulent sputum. Percutaneous catheter drainage can be both diagnostic and therapeutic. Antibiotic therapy should be directed at the organisms isolated and should be continued until the abscess has resolved radiographically. The treatment of a lung abscess requires a prolonged duration of therapy (usually 6 to 8 weeks, depending on clinical response). Medical management is unsuccessful in ~10% of cases. When medical management fails or the lung abscess is large, percutaneous drainage or lobectomy should be considered. When empyema is present, closed thoracostomy or open surgical drainage with or without decortication should be performed.

Not all pulmonary cavities are lung abscesses. Cavitating carcinoma, Wegener's granulomatosis, rheumatoid nodules, pulmonary infarcts, tuberculosis, and fungal infections are included in the differential diagnosis.

Recurrent Pneumonia Of patients admitted to the hospital for the treatment of CAP, 10 to 15% have another episode within 2 years. If the recurrence affects the same anatomical location as the previous episode, the most likely cause is an obstructed bronchus due to either a tumor or a foreign body. COPD and repeated macroaspiration are the most common causes of recurrent pneumonia. Persons without COPD, with pneumonia in a different location from the previous episode, and with no risk factors for aspiration should undergo evaluation for immunodeficiency, including HIV testing, immunoglobulin determination, protein electrophoresis, and enumeration of T and B cells. CT of the chest often detects pulmonary anatomical defects such as bronchiectasis that might be the cause of the recurrent pneumonia.

CAP IN LONG-TERM-CARE FACILITIES

EPIDEMIOLOGY About 4% of persons >65 years of age and 15% of those >85 years of age reside in LTCFs. LTCF residents range from healthy, self-sufficient individuals to frail persons who may be bedridden. Pneumonia is the leading cause of infection requiring transfer of nursing home residents to the hospital, accounting for 10 to 18% of all pneumonia admissions in North America. Profound disability (Karnofsky score of <10), bedridden state, urinary incontinence, male gender, difficulty swallowing, and inability to take oral medications are risk factors for pneumonia among LTCF residents, whereas receipt of influenza vaccine is protective. Malnutrition, tube feedings, hyperextended neck, contractures, and use of benzodiazepine and anticholinergic medications are risk factors for aspiration pneumonia in this population.

ETIOLOGY The most common etiologic agents associated with LTCF-acquired pneumonia are *S. aureus* (including MRSA), aerobic gram-negative bacilli, *S. pneumoniae*, *M. tuberculosis* (~2% of cases), and

the agents of aspiration pneumonitis/pneumonia (about one-third of cases).

CLINICAL PRESENTATION In the frail or functionally impaired LTCF resident, pneumonia may present as an insidious or nonspecific deterioration in general health and/or activity level (e.g., confusion, falls, or sudden exacerbation of—or slow recovery from—an existing primary disease). An increase in respiratory rate to ≥28/min may be the first manifestation of pneumonia and often develops 24 to 48 h before clinical diagnosis. The in-hospital mortality rate can be as high as 30%, and the 1-year mortality rate is >50%.

℞ TREATMENT

Site of Care Nursing homes vary greatly in terms of the facilities and nursing staff available to provide care to very ill patients. Thus decisions about treatment site must be made with knowledge of the available resources as well as the wishes of patients and their families. Criteria helpful in deciding who should be transferred from an LTCF to the hospital for treatment of pneumonia are listed in Table 239-12.

Antibiotic Therapy Suggested regimens for the treatment of pneumonia in LTCF residents—either at the facility or in the hospital—are provided in Table 239-9.

PREVENTION Minimizing the risk of aspiration is a key factor in prevention of LTCF-associated pneumonia. Swallowing should be assessed in at-risk patients. Patients should be positioned upright for meals and during tube feeding. Use of sedatives/hypnotics should be minimized. Attention should be given to oral hygiene and dental care.

All residents should have a two-step Mantoux test at admission to the LTCF, and those with a positive result should be evaluated for evidence of active tuberculosis, with isoniazid treatment or prophylaxis given as needed. Humidifiers should be avoided or used only with sterile water. All LTCF workers should receive influenza vaccine annually.

SEVERE CAP

Severe CAP is generally defined as pneumonia requiring admission to the ICU. The criteria for severe CAP given in Table 239-4 are 100% sensitive and 72.8% specific and have a positive predictive value of 26.4%. Clinical judgment clearly remains paramount in this management decision.

EPIDEMIOLOGY The most common causes of severe CAP are listed in Table 239-2.

VENTILATORY SUPPORT While mechanical ventilation is commonly used to treat the hypoxemia associated with severe CAP, other therapies are also employed. Continuous positive airway pressure is widely used in hypoxemic patients with *Pneumocystis* pneumonia, and early studies suggest that it has the potential to hasten recovery. Hypoxemia is the result of intrapulmonary shunting and ventilation-perfusion mismatch, affecting up to 50% of cardiac output in patients with severe CAP. In patients with unilateral pneumonia, simply positioning the unaffected lung downward may result in improved ventilation-perfusion matching and an increase in Pa$_{O_2}$ of 10 to 15 mmHg. More experimental ap-

TABLE 239-12 *Criteria for Treatment of Pneumonia in a Nursing Home*

1. Respiratory rate <30/min
2. Oxygen saturation ≥92% while breathing room air
3. Pulse rate <90/min
4. Temperature 36.5°C to 38.1°C
5. Systolic and diastolic blood pressure within 10 mmHg of usual readings
6. No feeding tube present
7. Patient conscious
8. Availability of medical and nursing care
9. Wishes of patient and family

proaches include the use of cyclooxygenase inhibitors (e.g., aspirin and indomethacin) to help partially reverse hypoxic pulmonary artery vasoconstriction and the aerosolization of prostacycline (PGI_2) or nitric oxide to reduce intrapulmonary shunting and pulmonary hypertension.

ASPIRATION PNEUMONITIS/PNEUMONIA

Aspiration syndromes refer to the clinical and pathophysiologic effects resulting from the introduction of foreign objects or substances into the lower respiratory tract. The most commonly involved areas—those that are most dependent in the supine position—are the posterior segments of the upper lobes and the superior segments of the lower lobes.

ETIOLOGY   The usual causes of aspiration pneumonia in the elderly are Enterobacteriaceae, *S. aureus*, *S. pneumoniae*, and *H. influenzae*.

EPIDEMIOLOGY   Aspiration syndromes include two distinct clinical entities. In aspiration pneumonitis, gastric contents (sterile as long as gastric acid is present) are aspirated into the lungs, with a consequent inflammatory response. Pneumonia results from the aspiration of oropharyngeal flora into the lungs, with consequent bacterial infection. The risk factors for aspiration include altered level of consciousness, incompetent gastroesophageal junction, elevated intragastric pressure or volume, and neuromuscular diseases that interfere with glottic closure.

The number of cases of aspiration pneumonia diagnosed in Medicare patients increased by 93.5% between 1991 and 1998. The mortality rate among patients with aspiration pneumonia was 23.1%, compared with 7.6% among those with pneumococcal pneumonia.

CLINICAL FEATURES   The manifestations of aspiration pneumonia vary with the volume and nature of the material aspirated. Gastric acid aspiration results in a chemical pneumonitis that can be very severe, requiring assisted ventilation. A pH of <2.5 and a gastric aspirate volume of >0.3 mL/kg (20 to 25 mL in adults) are required for the development of aspiration pneumonitis. There is an acute onset of dyspnea, tachypnea, bronchospasm, and cyanosis, with a chest radiograph often showing diffuse opacities.

Many elderly patients are achlorhydric and so may not fit the typical presentation described above. Indeed, in many of these patients, aspiration pneumonitis is often indistinguishable from pneumonia. A history or a witnessed account of an aspiration event (one or more instances of vomiting, coughing while eating, displacement of a feeding tube, or vomitus or tube feeding on bedclothes or on the patient within 24 h of the diagnosis of pneumonia) is documented in only 40% of definite aspiration events among LTCF residents. Thus the diagnosis of aspiration pneumonitis/pneumonia requires a high index of suspicion. The location of the pneumonia depends on the position of the patient when aspiration occurred. An opacity involving the posterior segment of the upper lobes (especially the right upper lobe) is found in persons who have aspirated in the recumbent position, while aspiration in the upright or semirecumbent position results in involvement of the posterior basal segments of the lower lobes.

In the setting of aspiration of oropharyngeal contents and poor dental hygiene, anaerobic bacteria may be present, and lung abscess is not an uncommon complication. Particulate matter may be aspirated, with consequent mechanical obstruction of the airway.

℞ TREATMENT

Treatment for aspiration occurring in a community setting is outlined in Table 239-9.

PREVENTION   Good oral hygiene reduces the risk of aspiration pneumonia among patients with cerebrovascular disease and swallowing impairment. Patients at high risk for aspiration (e.g., those who have had a stroke) should be assessed for aspiration. This evaluation is easily done by having an alert patient sit up and take increasing amounts of water, starting with one spoonful. Water leaking out of the corners of the mouth, coughing, and shortness of breath are all suggestive of aspiration and indicate the need for further evaluation.

CAP IN THE IMMUNOCOMPROMISED HOST

HIV-INFECTED PERSONS   See Chap. 173.

TRANSPLANT RECIPIENTS (See also Chap. 117)   Organ transplant recipients who develop pneumonia need a comprehensive diagnostic workup (diagnostic yield, 80%) and careful follow-up. Almost all of these patients require admission to the hospital. Newer immunosuppressive regimens and suppressive therapy for cytomegalovirus infection are changing the types and times of onset of opportunistic infections in this population.

An acute onset of symptoms, with presentation to the physician within 24 h, suggests bacterial pneumonia, pulmonary emboli with infarction, or pulmonary hemorrhage. A subacute onset over a few days to a week suggests viral, *Mycoplasma*, or *Pneumocystis* infection. A more chronic course over ≥1 week suggests fungal, nocardial, or tuberculous infection. Bacterial pneumonia is the most common infection in lung transplant recipients, accounting for almost half of the infections in this population. The incidence of pneumonia among these patients peaks in the first 4 to 8 weeks after transplantation and declines by the fourth month.

Nocardia spp., *R. equi*, and *Legionella* spp. are the major opportunistic bacterial pathogens in the lungs of organ transplant recipients; cytomegalovirus, varicella-zoster virus, influenza A and B viruses, respiratory syncytial virus, and adenovirus are the principal viral pathogens; and *Pneumocystis*, *C. neoformans*, *Aspergillus* spp., and Mucoraceae are the major fungal pathogens. *Aspergillus* spp., often in combination with aerobic gram-negative bacilli, is the most common cause of CAP among hematopoietic stem cell transplant recipients with graft-versus-host disease. CT of the chest is particularly useful if aspergillosis is suspected, in that it reveals pulmonary nodules, cavities, and halo or air-crescent signs.

HOSPITAL-ACQUIRED (NOSOCOMIAL) PNEUMONIA

EPIDEMIOLOGY   Hospital-acquired pneumonia (HAP) is defined as pneumonia occurring at least 48 h after hospital admission and not incubating at the time of admission (Chap. 116). The incidence of HAP is estimated at 5 to 10 cases per 1000 hospital discharges, with ~300,000 cases annually. HAP is uncommon on obstetrical and psychiatric wards but reportedly develops in 5 to 10% of all hospital discharges on medical and surgical wards. HAP is the second most common nosocomial infection, accounting for up to 30% of all nosocomial infections; it carries the highest morbidity and mortality; it lengthens hospital stay by an average of 7 to 9 days per affected patient; and it increases costs by $2 billion annually. The incidence of HAP is highest among patients in the ICU who are undergoing mechanical ventilation. About 10% of general surgical postoperative patients, 20% of intubated patients, and up to 70% of patients with ARDS develop HAP during their stay in the ICU. A subset of HAP—ventilator-acquired pneumonia (VAP)—has been defined as pneumonia occurring after at least 48 h of mechanical ventilation and not incubating at the time of intubation. Because most patients undergo mechanical ventilation for only a short period, half of all cases of VAP occur within the first 4 days of intubation. The rate of VAP development is 3% for days 1 through 5, 2% for days 6 through 10, and 1% for days 11 through 15 after intubation. Among nonventilated patients, HAP is reported to occur at a median rate of 3.2 cases per 1000 ICU days; the corresponding figure for mechanically ventilated patients is 34.4 cases per 1000 ICU days. The incidence of pneumonia is reported to be 6 to 20 times higher among mechanically ventilated patients than among other hospitalized patients.

Crude mortality rates for HAP range from 30 to 70% and are highest among bacteremic patients, patients infected with high-risk pathogens (e.g., *P. aeruginosa*), and ICU patients. In the ICU setting, risk factors for death include shock, coma, ultimately or rapidly fatal underlying disease, systemic inflammatory response syndrome, a high APACHE score, bilateral pulmonary infiltrates on chest radiography, ARDS, and respiratory failure. Despite high crude mortality rates, not all deaths are due to pneumonia; some patients with HAP die of their underlying illness. The attributable mortality due to HAP (i.e., the percentage of deaths among patients with HAP that would not have occurred in the absence of pneumonia) has been studied and remains controversial, but several studies suggest that one-third to one-half of all HAP deaths are due to infection.

About 1.5% of patients develop pneumonia postoperatively. The mortality rate at 1 month is tenfold higher (21% vs. 2%) among these patients than among those who do not develop postoperative pneumonia. An age of >80 years, poor functional status, recent weight loss, and alcohol use are predictors of postoperative pneumonia. Abdominal aortic aneurysm repair, thoracic surgery, and emergency surgery carry the highest risk for postoperative pneumonia, and general anesthesia carries a higher risk than other types of anesthesia.

PATHOGENESIS In addition to the factors that are important in the pathogenesis of CAP overall, other factors play an important role in the pathogenesis of HAP. Moreover, certain risk factors increase the likelihood of infection by specific pathogens (see below).

The patient's host defense system can be adversely affected by a number of risk factors. Factors that affect upper-respiratory host defenses (nasogastric or endotracheal intubation/reintubation, enteral feedings) increase the risk of both gross aspiration and microaspiration. Endotracheal intubation increases the risk of pneumonia in several ways. The tube serves as a direct conduit for bacterial introduction into the lower respiratory tract, prevents effective coughing to clear lower respiratory secretions, damages the tracheal epithelium, and allows the accumulation of oropharyngeal secretions (which are frequently colonized with bacteria) just above the cuff. Colonization of the endotracheal tube with pathogenic organisms can cause the formation of a biofilm that can be dislodged into the lower respiratory tract during suctioning. Poor infection-control measures and prolonged use of inappropriate antimicrobial agents increase the risk of spread of antimicrobial-resistant and/or especially virulent pathogens.

The presence of nasotracheal or nasogastric tubes increases the risk of nosocomial sinusitis, which occurs in more than half of all patients intubated for >7 days and which is also a risk factor for VAP. In one study, the same organism was isolated by transnasal culture and by protected specimen brushing in 20% of all patients with radiographic evidence of sinusitis. Moreover, the mortality rate was significantly lower when nosocomial sinusitis was identified and aggressively treated with antibiotics and nasal lavage every 8 h.

The role of the stomach as a reservoir for organisms that cause HAP remains controversial. It is accepted that elevation in gastric pH by antacids, H$_2$ antagonists, or enteral gastric feedings often leads to gastric bacterial overgrowth, which could be aspirated into the lower respiratory tract. Patients in the ICU are at high risk of aspiration because of reflux in the supine position, stomach placement of the enteral feeding tube, and large gastric volume.

In mechanically ventilated patients, tracheobronchitis frequently precedes the development of VAP by several days. Tracheobronchitis does not inevitably result in VAP, but bacterial concentrations in the bronchi may reach levels of at least 10^3 colony-forming units (CFU) per milliliter. In addition to fever and purulent sputum, tracheobronchitis may cause a false-positive culture result when lower respiratory tract secretions are sampled with a protected specimen brush (PSB).

ETIOLOGY In a national survey in the United States, 64% of all microorganisms isolated from the lungs of patients with nosocomial pneumonia were gram-negative bacilli, including *P. aeruginosa* (21%), *Acinetobacter* spp. (6%), and traditional enteric pathogens such as *Enterobacter* spp. (9%) and *K. pneumoniae* (8%).

S. aureus is the most common cause of nosocomial pneumonia in the United States. The increasing prevalence of MRSA among nosocomial isolates of *S. aureus* (from 2% in 1974 to as high as 64% in recent surveys) is of great concern in this context. In a comparative

study of pneumonia due to MRSA and that due to methicillin-susceptible *S. aureus* (MSSA) in patients in an ICU, MRSA pneumonia resulted in a significantly greater frequency of bacteremia (36.4% vs. 10.5%; RR 3.4) and septic shock (27.3% vs. 7.9%; RR 3.4) and a significantly higher infection-associated mortality rate (54.5% vs. 2.6%; RR 20.7). Mortality rates among patients with MRSA and MSSA pneumonia who are treated with vancomycin are very high, possibly because of the low levels of vancomycin in the lungs 24 h after the initiation of treatment. In some in vitro studies, the bactericidal action of vancomycin against *S. aureus* has been weaker and slower than that of other antimicrobial agents, such as cloxacillin.

The Enterobacteriaceae account for ~30% of cases of ICU-acquired pneumonia. More than one-third of *Enterobacter* strains acquired in this setting are resistant to third-generation cephalosporins. The predominant mechanism of cephalosporin resistance in the Enterobacteriaceae is the production of β-lactamases, of which >300 have been described. The emergence of plasmid-mediated extended-spectrum β-lactamases (ESBLs) in members of the family Enterobacteriaceae has become a worldwide problem. ESBL molecular class A possesses an extended hydrolysis spectrum toward oxyimino-β-lactams and aztreonam but remains susceptible to cefoxitin and β-lactamase inhibitors.

The cephamycins (cefoxitin, cefotetan, and cefmetazole) are structurally different from the true cephalosporins and display enhanced stability in the presence of ESBLs. More than 90% of ESBL-producing organisms are susceptible to cephamycins.

Of major concern is the discovery of plasmid-mediated carbapenemases in Enterobacteriaceae. These enzymes inactivate all carbapenems, cephalosporins, and antipseudomonal penicillins.

Among patients on hospital wards who have no risk factors associated with specific pathogens, the pathogens most frequently causing nosocomial pneumonia include *S. pneumoniae*, *H. influenzae*, *S. aureus*, and enteric gram-negative bacilli (i.e., *E. coli*, *Klebsiella* spp., *Proteus* spp., and *Serratia marcescens*). These organisms have been designated "core pathogens" in the American Thoracic Society's guidelines for the treatment of nosocomial pneumonia.

The spectrum of potential pathogens is increased among patients with mild to moderate HAP if risk factors for specific pathogens are present. If the patient has had recent abdominal surgery or if an aspiration has been witnessed, the involvement of anaerobes should be considered. *S. aureus* (including MRSA) is more common among patients in a coma or with head trauma, diabetes mellitus, or renal failure. In the setting of potable-water contamination by *Legionella* spp., the use of high-dose glucocorticoids increases the risk of infection with this organism.

Among previously healthy patients with severe HAP requiring ICU care, length of stay before the onset of HAP affects the spectrum of pathogens. The most common pathogens among these patients with early-onset HAP or VAP (<5 days after admission) are the core pathogens (see above).

The most important risk factors for HAP due to resistant microorganisms are late onset of infection (>5 days after admission) and recent antibiotic therapy. The most common resistant organisms are MRSA, *Acinetobacter calcoaceticus-baumannii*, *Stenotrophomonas maltophilia*, and ESBL-producing Enterobacteriaceae. In addition, there are risk factors for specific resistant microorganisms. Glucocorticoid therapy, malnutrition, structural lung disease, mechanical ventilation, and underlying fatal medical conditions are risk factors for *P. aeruginosa*. Neurosurgery, head trauma, ARDS, and aspiration are risk factors for *Acinetobacter*. *S. maltophilia* is associated with increased ICU stay, tracheostomy, treatment with cefepime, and severe trauma with lung contusion. Isolation of MRSA has been associated with prior antibiotic therapy (especially with quinolones and macrolides), previous hospitalization, enteral feeding, surgery, and late-onset VAP. ESBL-producing Enterobacteriaceae have been associated with intubation, previous antibiotic therapy, and central venous catheterization. The latter organisms may also be community-acquired and are now a problem in chronic-care facilities.

CLINICAL MANIFESTATIONS The definition of HAP includes the presence of a new or progressive infiltrate on chest radiography plus at least two of the following: fever [>37.8°C (>100°F)], leukocytosis (>10,000 white blood cells/μL), and the production of purulent sputum. Other findings, such as dyspnea, hypoxemia, and pleuritic chest pain, should prompt investigations for nosocomial pneumonia. It is important to exclude noninfectious causes of pulmonary infiltrates when evaluating a patient who presents with possible HAP.

DIAGNOSIS One of the most controversial areas in the management of HAP is how best to ascertain whether pneumonia is present and to determine the most appropriate therapy. Diagnostic accuracy is particularly important in mechanically ventilated patients, in whom VAP is frequently overdiagnosed. Invasive diagnostic testing is generally performed on intubated patients with VAP. The sampling methods used include endotracheal aspiration, PSB or bronchoalveolar lavage (BAL)

sampling via a fiberoptic bronchoscope (FOB), or blinded invasive methods [blinded bronchial sampling (BBS), mini-BAL, and blinded PSB (BPSB)].

Endotracheal aspiration is most sensitive when patients have not received antimicrobial therapy. However, its specificity is low, and the sensitivity and specificity of cultures of endotracheal aspirates vary widely. If the patient has recently received any antibiotics, sensitivity and specificity are further decreased. The reported sensitivity and specificity of quantitative endotracheal aspiration range from 38 to 100% and from 14 to 100%, respectively. Visualization of elastin fibrils on Gram's staining and antibody coating of bacteria are unreliable indicators of infection.

Use of FOB-directed PSB and/or BAL has been advocated by many authorities; when performed at the same time, these studies are generally considered complementary. PSB is considered positive when at least 10^3 CFU of bacteria per brush are obtained, and BAL is considered positive when the recovered lavage fluid contains at least 10^4 CFU of bacteria per milliliter. The sensitivity of PSB ranges from 33 to 100% (median, 67%), and the specificity ranges from 50 to 100% (median, 95%). The sensitivity of BAL ranges from 42 to 93% (median, 73%), while the specificity ranges from 45 to 100% (median,

TABLE 239-13 *Empirical Antibiotic Therapy for Hospital-Acquired Pneumonia (HAP)*

Treatment Setting; Patient's Condition	Risk Factor/Usual Pathogen(s)	Regimen
Hospital ward; mild to moderate HAP, no risk factors for specific pathogens	—	Second-generation cephalosporin (cefuroxime 750 mg q8h IV) *or* Nonpseudomonal third-generation cephalosporin (ceftriaxone 1 g/d IV) *or* β-Lactam/β-lactamase inhibitor combination (piperacillin/tazobactam 3.375 g q6h IV) Penicillin allergy: Respiratory quinolone (levofloxacin 500 mg/d IV, moxifloxacin 400 mg/d IV, or gatifloxacin 400 mg/d IV) *or* Clindamycin plus aztreonam
Hospital ward; mild to moderate HAP with specific risk factors	—	Treat for usual pathogens (enteric gram-negative bacilli, *Staphylococcus aureus*, *Streptococcus pneumoniae*, *Haemophilus influenzae*) with cefuroxime, ceftriaxone, or piperacillin/tazobactam (see above) *plus* Treat for other pathogens related to risk factors (see below)
	Witnessed aspiration, recent abdominal surgery/ anaerobes	Standard treatment (see above) *plus* Clindamycin 450–900 mg q8h IV *or* β-Lactam/β-lactamase inhibitor combination (piperacillin/tazobactam 3.375 g q6h IV)
	Coma, head trauma, diabetes mellitus, renal failure/*S. aureus*, risk for MRSA	Standard treatment (see above) *plus* Vancomycin 1 g q12h IV
	High-dose glucocorticoids/*Legionella*	Standard treatment (see above) *plus* Macrolide (azithromycin 500 mg/d IV) *or* Respiratory quinolone (see above)
Intensive care unit; severe HAP, early onset, no specific risk factors	—	Second-generation cephalosporin, nonpseudomonal third-generation cephalosporin, or β-lactam/β-lactamase inhibitor combination (see above) Penicillin allergy: Respiratory quinolone (see above)
Intensive care unit; severe HAP, late onset or specific risk factors	—	Treat for usual pathogens (enteric gram-negative bacilli, *S. aureus*, *S. pneumoniae*, *H. influenzae*) with cefuroxime, ceftriaxone, or piperacillin/tazobactam (see above) *plus* Treat for other pathogens related to risk factors (see below)
	Malnutrition, structural lung disease, glucocorticoid therapy/*Pseudomonas aeruginosa*; neurosurgery, head trauma, ARDS, aspiration/*Acinetobacter* spp.	Standard treatment (see above) *plus* Aminoglycoside or ciprofloxacin 500 mg q12h IV plus one of the following: antipseudomonal penicillin (piperacillin 4 g q6h IV or piperacillin/tazobactam 4.5 g q6h IV) or cefepime 1–2 g q12h IV or imipenem (or meropenem) 500 mg q8h IV
	Prior antibiotic therapy (especially with quinolones or macrolides), previous hospitalization, enteral feeding/MRSA	Standard treatment (see above) *plus* Vancomycin 1 g q12h IV

Note: ARDS, adult respiratory distress syndrome; MRSA, methicillin-resistant *S. aureus*.

82%). Both procedures require a well-trained, experienced operator and rapid transportation of samples to the laboratory. Because results are not available for at least 18 h, a portion of the BAL fluid should be centrifuged, the pellet stained with Giemsa or Gram's stain, and the stained preparation examined to determine the percentage of white blood cells with intracellular bacteria. Both 1% and 5% of cells containing intracellular bacteria have been used as significant breakpoints for diagnosing pneumonia. The effect of antibiotic therapy on the sensitivity and specificity of PSB and BAL is uncertain.

Blind mini-BAL and BBS have been introduced relatively recently. These tests are easier to perform and are less expensive than FOB-directed BAL. The sensitivity and specificity are 74 to 97% and 74 to 100%, respectively, for BPSB; 63 to 100% and 66 to 96% for mini-BAL; and 58 to 86% and 71 to 100% for blind mini-BAL and BBS. Risks from these procedures appear to be minimal.

℞ TREATMENT

Most initial therapy for HAP is empirical (Table 239-13). The selection of drugs should be guided by an understanding of local patterns of antimicrobial resistance. If MRSA is highly prevalent in the institution and the patient is at risk for MRSA infection, empirical therapy should include vancomycin. Quinupristin-dalfopristin and linezolid can also be used to treat MRSA.

Evaluation of a patient whose condition is not improving or is actually deteriorating despite treatment involves the same considerations in HAP as in CAP (Table 239-11). Broadening the spectrum of antimicrobial therapy should be considered, with administration continued at least until the results of additional tests become available. Lower respiratory tract secretions should be sampled immediately by endotracheal aspiration, FOB-directed PSB or BAL, or a blinded sampling procedure.

PREVENTION A number of measures can reduce the risk of HAP. Health care providers must adhere strictly to hand-washing protocols. Surveillance of pneumonia rates should be routinely performed and reported. In patients undergoing mechanical ventilation, a concerted effort should be made to extubate rapidly, to minimize ventilator circuit changes, and to ensure careful periodic drainage of tubing condensate. Use of endotracheal tubes with a separate posterior lumen that allows continuous suctioning of subglottic secretions has been reported to decrease the incidence of early-onset VAP; heat-moisture exchanges reportedly reduce the risk of late-onset VAP. When the patient is receiving enteral feedings, a small-bore feeding tube should be placed distal to the pylorus, and large gastric residuals should be avoided. Elevation of the head of the bed by at least 30° lessens the risk of pneumonia, as does the use of kinetic beds. Earlier studies did not support the use of selective decontamination of the digestive tract as a method for preventing HAP. A recent study showed a significant reduction in mortality and colonization with resistant gram-negative aerobic bacteria among critically ill patients admitted to an ICU who underwent selective decontamination.

FURTHER READING

Bartlett JG et al: Practice guidelines for the management of community-acquired pneumonia in adults. Clin Infect Dis 31:347, 2000
de Jonge E et al: Effects of selective decontamination of digestive tract in mortality and acquisition of resistant bacteria in intensive care: A randomised controlled trial. Lancet 362:1011, 2003
File TM: Community-acquired pneumonia. Lancet 36:1991, 2003
Garau J: Treatment of drug-resistant pneumococcal pneumonia. Lancet Infect Dis 2:404, 2002
Halm EA et al: Instability on hospital discharge and the risk of adverse outcomes in patients with pneumonia. Arch Intern Med 162:1278, 2002
Mandell LA et al: Canadian guidelines for the initial management of community-acquired pneumonia: An evidence-based update by the Canadian Infectious Diseases Society and the Canadian Thoracic Society. Clin Infect Dis 31:383, 2000
——— et al: Update of practice guidelines for the management of community-acquired pneumonia in immunocompetent adults. Clin Infect Dis 37:1405, 2003
Medina-Walpole AM, Katz PR: Nursing home–acquired pneumonia. J Am Geriatr Soc 47:1005, 1999
Metlay JP, Fine MJ: Testing strategies in the initial management of patients with community-acquired pneumonia. Ann Intern Med 138:109, 2003
Minogue MF et al: Patients hospitalized after initial outpatient treatment for community-acquired pneumonia. Ann Emerg Med 31:376, 1998
Neiderman MS et al: Guidelines for the management of adults with community-acquired pneumonia. Diagnosis, assessment of severity, antimicrobial therapy and prevention. Am J Respir Crit Care Med 163:1730, 2001
Whitney CG et al: Increasing prevalence of multidrug-resistant Streptococcus pneumoniae in the United States. N Engl J Med 343:1917, 2000

240 BRONCHIECTASIS
Steven E. Weinberger

DEFINITION Bronchiectasis is an abnormal and permanent dilatation of bronchi. It may be either focal, involving airways supplying a limited region of pulmonary parenchyma, or diffuse, involving airways in a more widespread distribution. Although this definition is based on pathologic changes in the bronchi, diagnosis is often suggested by the clinical consequences of chronic or recurrent infection in the dilated airways and the associated secretions that pool within these airways.

PATHOLOGY The bronchial dilatation of bronchiectasis is associated with destructive and inflammatory changes in the walls of medium-sized airways, often at the level of segmental or subsegmental bronchi. The normal structural components of the wall, including cartilage, muscle, and elastic tissue, are destroyed and may be replaced by fibrous tissue. The dilated airways frequently contain pools of thick, purulent material, while more peripheral airways are often occluded by secretions or obliterated and replaced by fibrous tissue. Additional microscopic features include bronchial and peribronchial inflammation and fibrosis, ulceration of the bronchial wall, squamous metaplasia, and mucous gland hyperplasia. The parenchyma normally supplied by the affected airways is abnormal, containing varying combinations of fibrosis, emphysema, bronchopneumonia, and atelectasis. As a result of the inflammation, vascularity of the bronchial wall increases, with associated enlargement of the bronchial arteries and anastomoses between the bronchial and pulmonary arterial circulations.

Three different patterns of bronchiectasis were described by Reid in 1950. In *cylindrical bronchiectasis* the bronchi appear as uniformly dilated tubes that end abruptly at the point that smaller airways are obstructed by secretions. In *varicose bronchiectasis* the affected bronchi have an irregular or beaded pattern of dilatation resembling varicose veins. In *saccular (cystic) bronchiectasis* the bronchi have a ballooned appearance at the periphery, ending in blind sacs without recognizable bronchial structures distal to the sacs.

ETIOLOGY AND PATHOGENESIS Bronchiectasis is a consequence of inflammation and destruction of the structural components of the bronchial wall. Infection is the usual cause of the inflammation; microorganisms such as *Pseudomonas aeruginosa* and *Haemophilus influenzae* produce pigments, proteases, and other toxins that injure the respiratory epithelium and impair mucociliary clearance. The host inflammatory response induces epithelial injury, largely as a result of mediators released from neutrophils. As protection against infection is compromised, the dilated airways become more susceptible to colonization and growth of bacteria. Thus, a reinforcing cycle can result, with inflammation producing airway damage, impaired clearance of microorganisms, and further infection, which then completes the cycle by inciting more inflammation.

Infectious Causes   Adenovirus and influenza virus are the main viruses that cause bronchiectasis in association with lower respiratory tract involvement. Virulent bacterial infections, especially with potentially necrotizing organisms such as *Staphylococcus aureus*, *Klebsiella*, and anaerobes, remain important causes of bronchiectasis when antibiotic treatment of a pneumonia is not given or is significantly delayed. Bronchiectasis has been reported in patients with HIV infection, perhaps at least partly due to recurrent bacterial infection. Tuberculosis can produce bronchiectasis by a necrotizing effect on pulmonary parenchyma and airways and indirectly as a consequence of airway obstruction from bronchostenosis or extrinsic compression by lymph nodes. Nontuberculous mycobacteria are frequently cultured from patients with bronchiectasis, often as secondary infections or colonizing organisms. However, it has now also been recognized that these organisms, especially those of the *Mycobacterium avium* complex, can serve as primary pathogens associated with the development and/or progression of bronchiectasis. Mycoplasmal and necrotizing fungal infections are rare causes of bronchiectasis.

Impaired host defense mechanisms are often involved in the predisposition to recurrent infections. The major cause of localized impairment of host defenses is endobronchial obstruction. Bacteria and secretions cannot be cleared adequately from the obstructed airway, which develops recurrent or chronic infection. Slowly growing endobronchial neoplasms such as carcinoid tumors may be associated with bronchiectasis. Foreign-body aspiration is another important cause of endobronchial obstruction, particularly in children. Airway obstruction can also result from bronchostenosis, from impacted secretions, or from extrinsic compression by enlarged lymph nodes.

Generalized impairment of pulmonary defense mechanisms occurs with immunoglobulin deficiency, primary ciliary disorders, or cystic fibrosis. Infections and bronchiectasis are therefore often more diffuse. With panhypogammaglobulinemia, the best described of the immunoglobulin disorders associated with recurrent infection and bronchiectasis, patients often also have a history of sinus or skin infections. Selective deficiency of an IgG subclass, especially IgG2, has also been described in a small number of patients with bronchiectasis.

The primary disorders associated with ciliary dysfunction, termed *primary ciliary dyskinesia*, are responsible for 5 to 10% of cases of bronchiectasis. Numerous defects are encompassed under this category, including structural abnormalities of the dynein arms, radial spokes, and microtubules. The cilia become dyskinetic; their coordinated, propulsive action is diminished, and bacterial clearance is impaired. The clinical effects include recurrent upper and lower respiratory tract infections, such as sinusitis, otitis media, and bronchiectasis. Because normal sperm motility also depends on proper ciliary function, males are generally infertile (Chap. 325). Approximately half of patients with primary ciliary dyskinesia fall into the subgroup of *Kartagener's syndrome*, in which situs inversus accompanies bronchiectasis and sinusitis.

In cystic fibrosis (Chap. 241), the tenacious secretions in the bronchi are associated with impaired bacterial clearance, resulting in colonization and recurrent infection with a variety of organisms, particularly mucoid strains of *P. aeruginosa* but also *S. aureus*, *H. influenzae*, *Escherichia coli*, and *Burkholderia cepacia*.

Noninfectious Causes   Some cases of bronchiectasis are associated with exposure to a toxic substance that incites a severe inflammatory response. Examples include inhalation of a toxic gas such as ammonia or aspiration of acidic gastric contents, though the latter problem is often also complicated by aspiration of bacteria. An immune response in the airway may also trigger inflammation, destructive changes, and bronchial dilatation. This mechanism is presumably important for bronchiectasis with allergic bronchopulmonary aspergillosis (ABPA), which is due at least in part to an immune response to *Aspergillus* organisms that have colonized the airway (Chap. 237). Bronchiectasis accompanying ABPA often involves proximal airways and is associated with mucoid impaction. Bronchiectasis also occurs rarely in ulcerative colitis, rheumatoid arthritis, and Sjögren's syndrome, but it is not known whether an immune response triggers airway inflammation in these patients.

In α_1-antitrypsin deficiency, the usual respiratory complication is the early development of panacinar emphysema, but affected individuals may occasionally have bronchiectasis. In the *yellow nail syndrome*, which is due to hypoplastic lymphatics, the triad of lymphedema, pleural effusion, and yellow discoloration of the nails is accompanied by bronchiectasis in approximately 40% of patients.

CLINICAL MANIFESTATIONS   Patients typically present with persistent or recurrent cough and purulent sputum production. Hemoptysis occurs in 50 to 70% of cases and can be due to bleeding from friable, inflamed airway mucosa. More significant, even massive bleeding is often a consequence of bleeding from hypertrophied bronchial arteries.

When a specific infectious episode initiates bronchiectasis, patients may describe a severe pneumonia followed by chronic cough and sputum production. Alternatively, patients without a dramatic initiating event often describe the insidious onset of symptoms. In some cases, patients are either asymptomatic or have a nonproductive cough, often associated with "dry" bronchiectasis in an upper lobe. Dyspnea or wheezing generally reflects either widespread bronchiectasis or underlying chronic obstructive pulmonary disease. With exacerbations of infection, the amount of sputum increases, it becomes more purulent and often more bloody, and patients may become febrile. Such episodes may be due solely to exacerbations of the airway infection, but associated parenchymal infiltrates sometimes reflect an adjacent pneumonia.

Physical examination of the chest overlying an area of bronchiectasis is quite variable. Any combination of crackles, rhonchi, and wheezes may be heard, all of which reflect the damaged airways containing significant secretions. As with other types of chronic intrathoracic infection, clubbing may be present. Patients with severe, diffuse disease, particularly those with chronic hypoxemia, may have associated cor pulmonale and right ventricular failure. Amyloidosis can result from chronic infection and inflammation but is now seldom seen.

RADIOGRAPHIC AND LABORATORY FINDINGS   Though the chest radiograph is important in the evaluation of suspected bronchiectasis, the findings are often nonspecific. At one extreme, the radiograph may be normal with mild disease. Alternatively, patients with saccular bronchiectasis may have prominent cystic spaces, either with or without air-liquid levels, corresponding to the dilated airways. These may be difficult to distinguish from enlarged airspaces due to bullous emphysema or from regions of honeycombing in patients with severe interstitial lung disease. Other findings are due to dilated airways with thickened walls, which result from peribronchial inflammation. Because of decreased aeration and atelectasis of the associated pulmonary parenchyma, these dilated airways are often crowded together in parallel. When seen longitudinally, the airways appear as "tram tracks"; when seen in cross-section, they produce "ring shadows." Because the dilated airways may be filled with secretions, the lumen may appear dense rather than radiolucent, producing an opaque tubular or branched tubular structure.

Bronchography, which involves coating the airways with a radiopaque, iodinated lipid dye instilled through a catheter or bronchoscope, can provide excellent visualization of bronchiectatic airways. However, this technique has now been replaced by computed tomography (CT), which also provides an excellent view of dilated airways as seen in cross-sectional images (Fig. 240-1). With the advent of high-resolution CT scanning, in which the images are 1.0 to 1.5 mm thick, the sensitivity for detecting bronchiectasis has improved even further. Other features on high-resolution CT scanning can suggest a specific etiology of the bronchiectasis. For example, bronchiectasis of relatively proximal airways suggests ABPA, whereas the presence of multiple small pulmonary nodules (nodular bronchiectasis) suggests infection with *M. avium* complex.

Examination of sputum often reveals an abundance of neutrophils

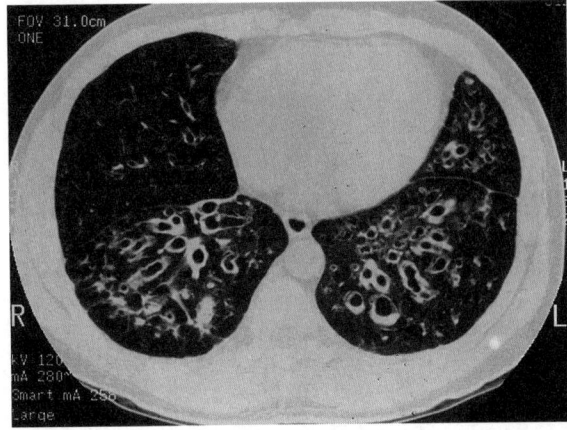

FIGURE 240-1 High-resolution CT scan of bronchiectasis showing dilated airways in both lower lobes and in the lingula. When seen in cross-section, the dilated airways have a ringlike appearance. (*From SE Weinberger: Principles of Pulmonary Medicine, 3d ed. Philadelphia, Saunders, 1998; with permission*).

and colonization or infection with a variety of possible organisms. Appropriate staining and culturing of sputum often provide a guide to antibiotic therapy.

Additional evaluation is aimed at diagnosing the cause for the bronchiectasis. When bronchiectasis is focal, fiberoptic bronchoscopy may reveal an underlying endobronchial obstruction. In other cases, upper lobe involvement may be suggestive of either tuberculosis or ABPA. With more widespread disease, measurement of sweat chloride levels for cystic fibrosis, structural or functional assessment of nasal or bronchial cilia or sperm for primary ciliary dyskinesia, and quantitative assessment of immunoglobulins may explain recurrent airway infection. In an asthmatic person with proximal bronchiectasis or other historical features to suggest ABPA, skin testing, serology, and sputum culture for *Aspergillus* are helpful in confirming the diagnosis.

Pulmonary function tests may demonstrate airflow obstruction as a consequence of diffuse bronchiectasis or associated chronic obstructive lung disease. Bronchial hyperreactivity, e.g., to methacholine challenge, and some reversibility of the airflow obstruction with inhaled bronchodilators are relatively common.

℞ TREATMENT

Therapy has four major goals: (1) elimination of an identifiable underlying problem; (2) improved clearance of tracheobronchial secretions; (3) control of infection, particularly during acute exacerbations; and (4) reversal of airflow obstruction. Appropriate treatment should be instituted when a treatable cause is found, for example, treatment of hypogammaglobulinemia with immunoglobulin replacement, tuberculosis with antituberculous agents, and ABPA with glucocorticoids.

Secretions are typically copious and thick and contribute to the symptoms. A variety of mechanical methods and devices accompanied by appropriate positioning can facilitate drainage in patients with copious secretions. Mucolytic agents to thin secretions and allow better clearance are controversial. Aerosolized recombinant DNase, which decreases viscosity of sputum by breaking down DNA released from neutrophils, has been shown to improve pulmonary function in cystic fibrosis, but similar benefits have not been found with bronchiectasis due to other etiologies.

Antibiotics have an important role in management. For patients with infrequent exacerbations characterized by an increase in quantity and purulence of the sputum, antibiotics are commonly used only during acute episodes. Although choice of an antibiotic may be guided by Gram's stain and culture of sputum, empiric coverage (e.g., with ampicillin, amoxicillin, trimethoprim-sulfamethoxazole, or cefaclor) is often given initially. When *P. aeruginosa* is present, oral therapy with a quinolone or parenteral therapy with an aminoglycoside or third-generation cephalosporin may be appropriate. In patients with chronic purulent sputum despite short courses of antibiotics, more prolonged courses, e.g., with an oral antibiotic or inhaled aminoglycosides, or intermittent but regular courses of single or rotating antibiotics have been used.

Bronchodilators to improve obstruction and aid clearance of secretions are particularly useful in patients with airway hyperreactivity and reversible airflow obstruction. Although surgical therapy was common in the past, more effective antibiotic and supportive therapy has largely replaced surgery. However, when bronchiectasis is localized and the morbidity is substantial despite adequate medical therapy, surgical resection of the involved region of lung should be considered.

When massive hemoptysis, often originating from the hypertrophied bronchial circulation, does not resolve with conservative therapy, including rest and antibiotics, therapeutic options are either surgical resection or bronchial arterial embolization (Chap. 30). Although resection may be successful if disease is localized, embolization is preferable with widespread disease. In patients with extensive disease, chronic hypoxemia and cor pulmonale may indicate the need for long-term supplemental oxygen. For selected patients who are disabled despite maximal therapy, lung transplantation is a therapeutic option.

FURTHER READING

ANGRILL J et al: Bacterial colonisation in patients with bronchiectasis: microbiologic pattern and risk factors. Thorax 57:15, 2002

BARKER AF: Bronchiectasis. N Engl J Med 346:1383, 2002

KUMAR NA et al: Bronchiectasis: Current clinical and imaging concepts. Semin Roentgenol 36:41, 2001

LILLINGTON GA: Dyskinetic cilia and Kartagener's syndrome. Bronchiectasis with a twist. Clin Rev Allergy Immunol 21:65, 2001

241 CYSTIC FIBROSIS
Richard C. Boucher

Cystic fibrosis (CF) is a monogenic disorder that presents as a multisystem disease. The first signs and symptoms typically occur in childhood, but about 7% of patients in the United States are diagnosed as adults. Due to improvements in therapy, >38% of patients are now adults (18 years of age) and 13% are past the age of 30. The median survival is >32 years for males and 29 years for females with CF. Thus, CF is no longer only a pediatric disease, and internists must be prepared to recognize and treat its many complications. This disease is characterized by chronic airways infection that ultimately leads to bronchiectasis and bronchiolectasis, exocrine pancreatic insufficiency and intestinal dysfunction, abnormal sweat gland function, and urogenital dysfunction.

PATHOGENESIS

GENETIC CONSIDERATIONS CF is an autosomal recessive disease resulting from mutations in a gene located on chromosome 7. The prevalence of CF varies with the ethnic origin of a population. CF is detected in approximately 1 in 3000 live births in the Caucasian population of North America and northern Europe, 1 in 17,000 live births of African Americans, and 1 in 90,000 live births of the Asian population of Hawaii. The most common mutation in the CF gene (~70% of CF chromosomes) is a 3-bp deletion that results in an absence of phenylalanine at amino acid position 508 (ΔF_{508}) of the CF gene protein product, known as the CF transmembrane conductance regulator (CFTR). The large number (>1000) of relatively uncommon (<2%) mutations identified in the CF gene makes it difficult to use DNA diagnostic technologies for identifying heterozygotes in populations at large, and no simple physiologic measurements allow heterozygote detection.

CFTR PROTEIN   The CFTR protein is a single polypeptide chain, containing 1480 amino acids, that appears to function both as a cyclic AMP–regulated Cl⁻ channel and, as its name implies, a regulator of other ion channels. The fully processed form of CFTR is found in the plasma membrane in normal epithelia (Fig. 241-1). Biochemical studies indicate that the ΔF_{508} mutation leads to improper processing and intracellular degradation of the CFTR protein. Thus, absence of CFTR at appropriate cellular sites is often part of the pathophysiology of CF. However, other mutations in the CF gene produce CFTR proteins that are fully processed but are nonfunctional or only partially functional at the appropriate cellular sites.

EPITHELIAL DYSFUNCTION   The epithelia affected by CF exhibit different functions in their native state, i.e., some are volume-absorbing (airways and distal intestinal epithelia), some are salt-absorbing but not volume-absorbing (sweat duct), whereas others are volume-secretory (proximal intestine and pancreas). Given this diverse array of native activities, it should not be surprising that CF produces very different effects on patterns of electrolyte and water transport. However, the unifying concept is that all affected tissues express abnormal ion transport function.

ORGAN-SPECIFIC PATHOPHYSIOLOGY ■ **Lung**   The diagnostic biophysical hallmark of CF is the raised transepithelial electric potential difference detected in airway epithelia. The transepithelial potential difference reflects components of both the rate of active ion transport and the resistance to ion flow of the superficial epithelium. CF airway epithelia exhibit both raised Na⁺ transport rates and decreased Cl⁻ secretion (Fig. 241-2). The Cl⁻ secretory defect reflects the absence of cyclic AMP–dependent kinase and protein kinase C–regulated Cl⁻ transport that is mediated by the Cl⁻ channel function of CFTR. An important observation is that there is an "alternative" Ca²⁺-regulated Cl⁻ channel expressed in airway epithelia. This Cl⁻ channel is different from CFTR and is regulated by intracellular Ca²⁺ levels. This channel can substitute for CFTR with regard to net Cl⁻ transport and may be a potential therapeutic target.

Raised Na⁺ absorption is a feature of CF airway epithelia. Na⁺ transport abnormalities in CF are not a widespread feature of the CF epithelial phenotype and appear confined to volume-absorbing epithelia. Recent studies demonstrate that the increased Na⁺ absorption re-

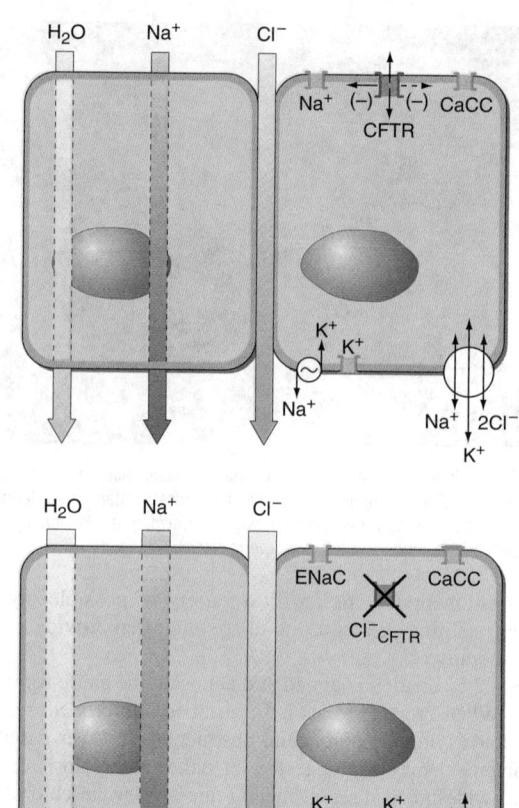

FIGURE 241-2 Comparison of ion transport properties of normal *(top)* and CF *(bottom)* airway epithelia. The vectors describe routes and magnitudes of Na⁺ and Cl⁻ transport that is accompanied by osmotically driven water flow. The normal basal pattern for ion transport is absorption of Na⁺ from the lumen via an amiloride-sensitive Na⁺ channel. This process is accelerated in CF. The capacity to initiate cyclic AMP–mediated Cl⁻ secretion is diminished in CF airway epithelia due to absence/dysfunction of the CFTR Cl⁻ channel. The accelerated Na⁺ absorption in CF reflects the absence of CFTR inhibitory effects on Na⁺ channels.

flects a second function of CFTR: it acts as a tonic inhibitor of the epithelial Na⁺ channel. The molecular mechanism mediating this action of CFTR is still unknown.

Mucus clearance appears to be a primary innate defense mechanism for the airways against infection by inhaled bacteria. Normal airways can vary the rates of active Na⁺ absorption and Cl⁻ secretion to adjust the volume of liquid (water) on airway surfaces for efficient mucus clearance. The central hypothesis of CF airways pathophysiology is that an abnormally high rate of Na⁺ absorption and low rate of Cl⁻ secretion reduce the salt and water content of mucus and deplete the volume of the periciliary liquid. Both the thickening of mucus and the depletion of the periciliary liquid lead to adhesion of mucus to the airway surface. Mucus adhesion leads to a failure to clear mucus normally from the airways by either ciliary or airflow-dependent (cough) mechanisms. Recent data from both human cell culture models and CF mice in vivo support this hypothesis.

The infection that characterizes CF airways involves the mucus layer rather than epithelial or airway wall invasion. The unique predisposition of CF airways to chronic infection by *Staphylococcus aureus* and *Pseudomonas aeruginosa* is consistent with failure to clear mucus, but it has also suggested that as yet undefined abnormalities in airway surface liquid may also contribute to selection of these organisms. Recently, it has been demonstrated that reduced O₂ tension in CF mucus before, and particularly after, infection may in part select for these bacteria and be responsible for their phenotype. Thus, both mucus stasis and mucus hypoxia may contribute to the propensity for *Pseudomonas* to grow in biofilm colonies within mucus plaques adherent to CF airway surfaces.

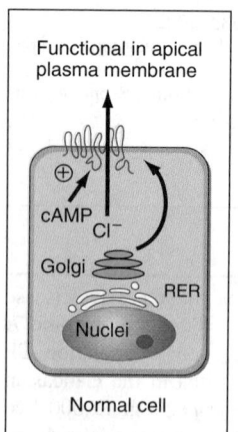
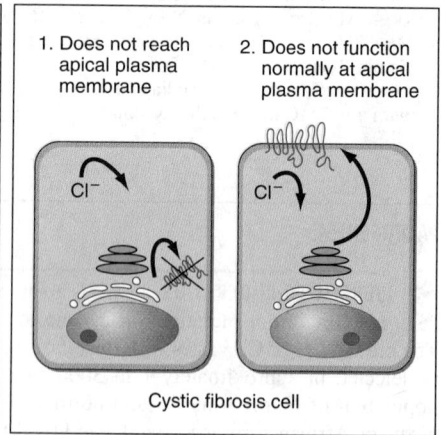

FIGURE 241-1 Cellular metabolism of the cystic fibrosis transmembrane regulator (CFTR) protein conductance (red). In a normal cell *(left)*, CFTR is synthesized in the rough endoplasmic reticulum (RER), is glycosylated in the Golgi apparatus, and functions as a Cl⁻ channel and regulator of other ion channels when located in the plasma membrane. Two possible outcomes of mutations in the CF gene are shown *(right)*. (1) If a mutation disturbs protein folding, e.g., the ΔF_{508} mutation, CFTR is degraded intracellularly so that no protein is transported to the plasma membrane. (2) With other mutations, the abnormal protein is processed and traffics to the plasma membrane but functions abnormally at that site.

Gastrointestinal Tract The gastrointestinal effects of CF are diverse. In the exocrine pancreas, the absence of the CFTR Cl^- channel in the apical membrane of pancreatic ductal epithelia limits the function of an apical membrane Cl^--HCO_3^- exchanger to secrete bicarbonate and Na^+ (by a passive process) into the duct. The failure to secrete Na^+ HCO_3^- and water leads to retention of enzymes in the pancreas and ultimately destruction of virtually all pancreatic tissue. The CF intestinal epithelium, because of the lack of Cl^- and water secretion, fails to flush secreted mucins and other macromolecules from intestinal crypts. The diminished CFTR-mediated secretion of liquid may be exacerbated by excessive absorption of liquid, reflecting abnormalities of CFTR-mediated regulation of Na^+ absorption (both mediated by Na^+ channels and possibly other Na^+ transporters, e.g., Na^+-H^+ exchangers). Both dysfunctions lead to dessicated intraluminal contents and obstruction of both the small and large intestine. In the hepatobiliary system, defective hepatic ductal salt (Cl^-) and water secretion causes retention of biliary secretion, focal biliary cirrhosis, and bile duct proliferation in approximately 25 to 30% of patients with CF. The inability of the CF gallbladder epithelium to secrete salt and water can lead to both chronic cholecystitis and cholelithiasis.

Sweat Gland CF patients secrete nearly normal volumes of sweat in the sweat acinus. However, CF patients are not able to absorb NaCl from sweat as it moves through the sweat duct due to the inability to absorb Cl^- across the ductal epithelial cells.

CLINICAL FEATURES

Most patients with CF present with signs and symptoms of the disease in childhood. Approximately 18% of patients present within the first 24 h of life with gastrointestinal obstruction, termed *meconium ileus.* Other common presentations within the first year or two of life include respiratory tract symptoms, most prominently cough and/or recurrent pulmonary infiltrates, and failure to thrive. A significant proportion of patients (~7%), however, are diagnosed after age 18.

RESPIRATORY TRACT Upper respiratory tract disease is almost universal in patients with CF. Chronic sinusitis is common in childhood and leads to nasal obstruction and rhinorrhea. The occurrence of nasal polyps approaches 25% and often requires surgery.

In the lower respiratory tract, the first symptom of CF is cough. With time, the cough becomes persistent and produces viscous, purulent, often greenish-colored sputum. Inevitably, periods of clinical stability are interrupted by "exacerbations," defined by increased cough, weight loss, increased sputum volume, and decrements in pulmonary function. These exacerbations require aggressive therapy, including frequent postural drainage and oral antibiotics, and often intravenous antibiotics (see below), with the goal being recovery of lung function. Over the course of years, the exacerbations become more frequent and the recovery of lost lung function incomplete, leading to respiratory failure.

CF patients exhibit a characteristic sputum microbiology. *Haemophilus influenzae* and *S. aureus* are often the first organisms recovered from samples of lung secretions in newly diagnosed patients with CF. *P. aeruginosa* is typically cultured from lower respiratory tract secretions thereafter. After repetitive antibiotic exposure, *P. aeruginosa*, often in a mucoid form, is usually the predominant organism recovered from sputum and may be present as several strains with different antibiotic sensitivities. *Burkholderia* (formerly *Pseudomonas*) *cepacia* has been recovered from CF sputum and is also pathogenic. Patient-to-patient spread of certain strains of this organism indicates that strict infection control in the hospital should be practiced. Other gram-negative rods recovered from CF sputum include *Xanthomonas xylosoxidans* and *B. gladioli*, and occasionally mucoid forms of *Proteus, Escherichia coli,* and *Klebsiella.* Up to 50% of CF patients have *Aspergillus fumigatus* in their sputum, and up to 10% of these patients exhibit the syndrome of allergic bronchopulmonary aspergillosis. *Mycobacterium tuberculosis* is rare in patients with CF. However, 10 to 20% of adult patients with CF have sputum cultures positive for nontuberculous mycobacteria, and in some patients these microorganisms are associated with disease.

The first lung function abnormalities observed in CF children, increased ratios of residual volume to total lung capacity, suggest that small airways disease is the first functional lung abnormality in CF. As the disease progresses, both reversible and irreversible changes in forced vital capacity and forced expiratory volume in 1 s are noted. The reversible component reflects the accumulation of intraluminal secretions and/or airway reactivity, which occurs in 40 to 60% of patients with CF. The irreversible component reflects chronic destruction of the airway wall and bronchiolitis.

The earliest chest x-ray change in CF lungs is hyperinflation, reflecting small airways obstruction. Later, signs of luminal mucus impaction, bronchial cuffing, and finally bronchiectasis, e.g., ring shadows, are noted. For reasons that are still unknown, the right upper lobe displays the earliest and most severe changes.

CF pulmonary disease is associated with many intermittent complications. Pneumothorax is common (>10% of patients). The production of small amounts of blood in sputum is common in CF patients with advanced pulmonary disease and appears to be associated with lung infection. Massive hemoptysis is life-threatening and difficult to localize bronchoscopically. With advanced lung disease, digital clubbing becomes evident in virtually all patients with CF. As late events, respiratory failure and cor pulmonale are prominent features of CF.

GASTROINTESTINAL TRACT The syndrome of meconium ileus in infants presents with abdominal distention, failure to pass stool, and emesis. The abdominal flat plate can be diagnostic, with small-intestinal airfluid levels, a granular appearance representing meconium, and a small colon. In children and young adults, a syndrome termed *meconium ileus equivalent* or *distal intestinal obstruction syndrome* occurs. The syndrome presents with right lower quadrant pain, loss of appetite, occasionally emesis, and often a palpable mass. The syndrome can be confused with appendicitis, which occurs frequently in CF patients. The characteristic intestinal abnormalities are complicated by exocrine pancreatic insufficiency in >90% of patients with CF. Insufficient pancreatic enzyme release yields the typical pattern of protein and fat malabsorption, with frequent, bulky, foul-smelling stools. Signs and symptoms of malabsorption of fat-soluble vitamins, including vitamins E and K, are also noted. Pancreatic beta cells are typically spared, but function decreases with age, causing hyperglycemia and increasing requirements for insulin in older patients with CF.

GENITOURINARY SYSTEM Late onset of puberty is common in both males and females with CF. The delayed maturational pattern is likely secondary to the effects of chronic lung disease and inadequate nutrition on reproductive endocrine function. More than 95% of male patients with CF are azoospermic, reflecting obliteration of the vas deferens that is probably a result of defective liquid secretion. Some 20% of CF women are infertile due to effects of chronic lung disease on the menstrual cycle; thick, tenacious cervical mucus that blocks sperm migration; and possibly fallopian tube/uterine wall abnormalities in liquid transport. More than 90% of completed pregnancies produce viable infants, and women with CF are generally able to breast-feed infants normally.

DIAGNOSIS

Because of the large number of CF mutations, DNA analysis is not used for primary diagnosis. The diagnosis of CF rests on a combination of clinical criteria and analyses of sweat Cl^- values. The values for the Na^+ and Cl^- concentration in sweat vary with age, but typically in adults a Cl^- concentration of >70 meq/L discriminates between patients with CF and patients with other lung diseases.

DNA analyses are being performed increasingly in patients with CF. Comprehensive genotype-phenotype relationships have not yet been established sufficiently for prognosis. A relationship between ΔF_{508} homozygosity and pancreatic insufficiency has been established, but no predictive relationship holds for ΔF_{508} homozygosity and lung disease.

Between 1 and 2% of patients with the clinical syndrome of CF have normal sweat Cl^- values. In most of these patients, the nasal transepithelial potential difference is raised into the diagnostic range for CF, and sweat acini do not secrete in response to injected β-adrenergic agonists. A single mutation of the CFTR gene, 3849 + 10 kb $C \rightarrow T$, is associated with approximately 50% of CF patients with normal sweat Cl^- values.

℞ TREATMENT

The major objectives of therapy for CF are to promote clearance of secretions and control infection in the lung, provide adequate nutrition, and prevent intestinal obstruction. Ultimately, gene therapy or therapies that restore the processing of misfolded CFTR may be the treatments of choice.

Lung Disease The principal techniques for clearing pulmonary secretions are breathing exercises, flutter valves, and chest percussion. Regular use of these maneuvers is effective in preserving lung function. There is increasing interest in the use of hypertonic saline (3 to 7%) aerosols to augment the clearance of secretions.

More than 95% of CF patients die of complications resulting from lung infection. Antibiotics are the principal agents available for treating lung infection, and their use should be guided by sputum culture results. Early intervention with antibiotics is useful, and long courses of treatment are the rule. Because of increased total-body clearance and volume of distribution of antibiotics in CF patients, the required doses are higher for patients with CF than for patients with similar chest infections who do not have CF.

Increased cough and mucus production are treated with antibiotics given orally. Typical oral agents used to treat *Staphylococcus* include a semisynthetic penicillin or a cephalosporin. Oral ciprofloxacin may reduce pseudomonal bacterial counts and control symptoms. However, its clinical usefulness may be limited by rapid emergence of resistant organisms, and, accordingly, courses should be intermittent (2 to 3 weeks) and not chronic. More severe exacerbations, or exacerbations associated with bacteria resistant to oral antibiotics, require intravenous antibiotics. Traditionally, intravenous therapy has been given in the hospital, but outpatient intravenous antibiotic administration has gained widespread acceptance. Usually, two drugs with different mechanisms of action (e.g., a cephalosporin and an aminoglycoside) are used to treat *P. aeruginosa* to hinder emergence of resistant organisms. Drug dosage should be monitored so that levels for gentamicin or tobramycin peak at ranges of $\sim 10 \, \mu g/mL$ and exhibit troughs of $<2 \, \mu g/mL$. Cephalosporins (e.g., ceftazidime) and penicillin derivatives also require higher doses. Antibiotics directed at *Staphylococcus* and/or *H. influenzae* are added, depending on the results of the culture. Aerosolized antibiotics also have an important role in treating CF lung infection. Large doses of aminoglycosides, e.g., 300 mg tobramycin twice daily, via aerosol are effective at delaying exacerbations. Aerosol administration also permits other drugs, e.g., colistin, to be utilized that are relatively ineffective by the intravenous route.

A number of pharmacologic agents for increasing mucus clearance are in use. *N*-acetylcysteine, which solubilizes mucous glycoproteins, has not been shown to have clinically significant effects on mucus clearance and/or lung function. Recombinant human DNAse, however, degrades the concentrated DNA in CF sputum, decreases sputum viscosity, and increases airflow during short-term administration. Long-term (6 months) DNAse treatment increases the time between pulmonary exacerbations. Most patients receive a therapeutic trial of DNAse to test for efficacy, and a sizeable minority demonstrate persistent objective benefits. Clinical trials of experimental drugs aimed at restoring salt and water content of secretions are underway. However, these drugs are not yet available clinically.

Inhaled β-adrenergic agonists can be useful to control airways constriction. They achieve a short-term increase in airflow, but long-term benefit has not been shown. Inhaled anticholinergics provide an alternative. Oral glucocorticoids may reduce airways inflammation, but their long-term use has been limited by adverse side effects; however, they may be useful for treating allergic bronchopulmonary aspergillosis.

The chronic damage to airway walls reflects to some extent the destructive activities of inflammatory enzymes generated in part by inflammatory cells. To date, specific therapies with antiproteases have not been successfully developed. However, a subset of adolescents with CF appear to benefit from long-term, high dose nonsteroidal (ibuprofen) therapy.

A number of pulmonary complications require acute interventions. Atelectasis is best treated with chest physiotherapy and antibiotic therapy. Pneumothoraces involving ≤10% of the lung can be observed without intervention. The use of chest tubes to expand collapsed, diseased lung often requires long periods of time, and sclerosing agents should be used with caution because of possible limitations for subsequent lung transplantation. Small-volume hemoptysis requires no specific therapy other than treatment of lung infection and assessment of coagulation and vitamin K status. If massive hemoptysis occurs, bronchial artery embolization can be successful. The most ominous complications of CF are respiratory failure and cor pulmonale. The most effective conventional therapy for these conditions is vigorous medical management of the lung disease and O_2 supplementation. Ultimately, the only effective treatment for respiratory failure in CF is lung transplantation (Chap. 248). The 2-year survival for lung transplantation exceeds 60%, and deaths in transplant patients result principally from graft rejection, often involving obliterative bronchiolitis. The transplanted lungs do not develop a CF-specific phenotype.

Gastrointestinal Disease Maintenance of adequate nutrition is critical for the health of the patient with CF. Most (>90%) of CF patients benefit from pancreatic enzyme replacement. Capsules generally contain between 4000 and 20,000 units of lipase. The dose of enzymes (typically no more than 2500 units/kg per meal) should be adjusted on the basis of weight gain, abdominal symptomatology, and character of stools. Replacement of fat-soluble vitamins, particularly vitamins E and K, is usually required. Hyperglycemia most often becomes manifest in the adult and typically requires insulin treatment.

For treatment of acute obstruction due to distal intestinal obstruction syndrome, megalodiatrizoate or other hypertonic radiocontrast materials delivered by enema to the terminal ileum are utilized. For control of symptoms, adjustment of pancreatic enzymes and the supplementation of intake by salt solutions containing osmotically active agents, e.g., propyleneglycol, are utilized. Persistent symptoms may indicate a diagnosis of gastrointestinal malignancy, which is increased in incidence in patients with CF. Hepatic and gallbladder complications are treated as for patients without CF. End-stage liver disease can be treated by transplantation, which has a 2-year survival rate >50%.

Psychosocial Factors CF imposes a tremendous burden on patients. Health insurance, career options, family planning, and life expectancy become major issues. Thus, assisting patients with the psychosocial adjustments required by CF is critical.

FURTHER READING

BRENNAN AL, GEDDES DM: Cystic fibrosis. Curr Opin Infect Dis 15:175, 2002

GELLER DE et al: Pharmacokinetics and bioavailability of aerosolized tobramycin in cystic fibrosis. Chest 122:219, 2002

GRIESENBACH U et al: Gene therapy progress and prospects: Cystic fibrosis. Gene Ther 9:1344, 2002

HENNEMAN L et al: Evaluation of cystic fibrosis carrier screening programs according to genetic screening criteria. Genet Med 4:241, 2002

MATSUI H et al: Evidence for periciliary liquid layer depletion, not abnormal ion composition, in the pathogenesis of cystic fibrosis airways disease. Cell 95:1005, 1998

PRINCE AS: Biofilms, antimicrobial resistance, and airway infection. N Engl J Med 347:1110, 2002

WORLITSCH D et al: Effects of reduced mucus oxygen concentration in airway pseudomonas infections of cystic fibrosis patients. J Clin Invest 109:317, 2002

Chronic obstructive pulmonary disease (COPD) has been defined by the Global Initiative for Chronic Obstructive Lung Disease (GOLD) as a disease state characterized by airflow limitation that is not fully reversible (http://www.goldcopd.com/). COPD includes *emphysema*, an anatomically defined condition characterized by destruction and enlargement of the lung alveoli; *chronic bronchitis*, a clinically defined condition with chronic cough and phlegm; and *small airways disease*, a condition in which small bronchioles are narrowed. COPD is present only if chronic airflow obstruction occurs; chronic bronchitis *without* chronic airflow obstruction is *not* included within COPD.

COPD is the fourth leading cause of death and affects >16 million persons in the United States. COPD is also a disease of increasing public health importance around the world. GOLD estimates suggest that COPD will rise from the sixth to the third most common cause of death worldwide by 2020.

RISK FACTORS ■ **Cigarette Smoking** By 1964, the Advisory Committee to the Surgeon General of the United States concluded that cigarette smoking was a major risk factor for mortality from chronic bronchitis and emphysema. Subsequent longitudinal studies have shown accelerated decline in the volume of air exhaled within the first second of the forced expiratory maneuver (FEV_1) in a dose-response relationship to the intensity of cigarette smoking, which is typically expressed as pack-years (average number of packs of cigarettes smoked per day multiplied by the total number of years of smoking). This dose-response relationship between reduced pulmonary function and cigarette smoking intensity accounts for the higher prevalence rates for COPD with increasing age. The historically higher rate of smoking among males is the likely explanation for the higher prevalence of COPD among males; however, the prevalence of COPD among females is increasing as the gender gap in smoking rates has diminished in the past 50 years.

Although the causal relationship between cigarette smoking and the development of COPD has been absolutely proven, there is considerable variability in the response to smoking. Although pack-years of cigarette smoking is the most highly significant predictor of FEV_1 (Fig. 242-1), only 15% of the variability in FEV_1 is explained by pack-years. This finding suggests that additional environmental and/or genetic factors contribute to the impact of smoking on the development of airflow obstruction.

Although cigar and pipe smoking may also be associated with the development of COPD, the evidence supporting such associations is less compelling, likely related to the lower dose of inhaled tobacco byproducts during cigar and pipe smoking.

Airway Responsiveness and COPD A tendency for increased bronchoconstriction in response to a variety of exogenous stimuli, including methacholine and histamine, is one of the defining features of asthma (Chap. 236). However, many patients with COPD also share this feature of airway hyperresponsiveness. The considerable overlap between persons with asthma and those with COPD on airway responsiveness, airflow obstruction, and pulmonary symptoms led to the formulation of the Dutch hypothesis. This suggests that asthma, chronic bronchitis, and emphysema are variations of the same basic disease, which is modulated by environmental and genetic factors to produce these pathologically distinct entities. The alternative British hypothesis contends that asthma and COPD are fundamentally different diseases: Asthma is viewed as largely an allergic phenomenon, while COPD results from smoking-related inflammation and damage. Determination of the validity of the Dutch hypothesis vs. the British hypothesis awaits identification of the genetic predisposing factors for asthma and/or COPD, as well as the interactions between these postulated genetic factors and environmental risk factors.

Longitudinal studies that compared airway responsiveness at the

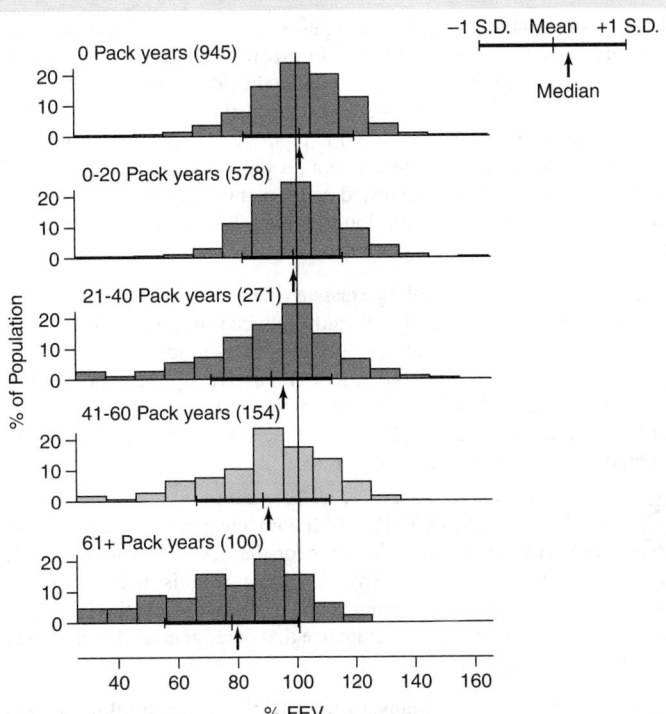

FIGURE 242-1 Distributions of forced expiratory volume in 1 s (FEV_1) values in a general population sample, stratified by pack-years of smoking. Means, medians, and ± 1 standard deviation of percent predicted FEV_1 are shown for each smoking group. Although a dose-response relationship between smoking intensity and FEV_1 was found, marked variability in pulmonary function was observed among subjects with similar smoking histories. (*From Burrows et al, with permission.*)

beginning of the study to subsequent decline in pulmonary function have demonstrated that increased airway responsiveness is clearly a significant predictor of subsequent decline in pulmonary function. Thus, airways hyperresponsiveness is a risk factor for COPD.

Respiratory Infections These have been studied as potential risk factors for the development and progression of COPD in adults; childhood respiratory infections have also been assessed as potential predisposing factors for the eventual development of COPD. The impact of adult respiratory infections on decline in pulmonary function is controversial, but significant long-term reductions in pulmonary function are not typically seen following an episode of bronchitis or pneumonia. The impact of the effects of childhood respiratory illnesses on the subsequent development of COPD has been difficult to assess due to a lack of adequate longitudinal data. Thus, although respiratory infections are important causes of exacerbations of COPD, the association of both adult and childhood respiratory infections to the development and progression of COPD remains to be proven.

Occupational Exposures Increased respiratory symptoms and airflow obstruction have been suggested as resulting from general exposure to dust at work. Several specific occupational exposures, including coal mining, gold mining, and cotton textile dust, have been suggested as risk factors for chronic airflow obstruction. However, although nonsmokers in these occupations developed some reductions in FEV_1, the importance of dust exposure as a risk factor for COPD, independent of cigarette smoking, is not certain. Among workers exposed to cadmium (a specific chemical fume), FEV_1, FEV_1/FVC, and DL_{CO} were significantly reduced (FVC, forced vital capacity; DL_{CO}, carbon monoxide diffusing capacity of the lung; Chap. 234), consistent with airflow obstruction and emphysema. Although several specific occupational dusts and fumes are likely risk factors for COPD, the magnitude of these effects appears to be substantially less important than the effect of cigarette smoking.

Ambient Air Pollution Some investigators have reported increased respiratory symptoms in those living in urban compared to rural areas, which may relate to increased pollution in the urban settings. However, the relationship of air pollution to chronic airflow obstruction remains unproven. With high rates of COPD reported in nonsmoking women in many developing countries, indoor air pollution, usually associated with cooking, has been suggested as a potential contributor. In most populations, ambient air pollution is a much less important risk factor for COPD than cigarette smoking.

Passive, or Second-Hand, Smoking Exposure Exposure of children to maternal smoking results in significantly reduced lung growth. In utero tobacco smoke exposure also contributes to significant reductions in postnatal pulmonary function. Although passive smoke exposure has been associated with reductions in pulmonary function, the importance of this risk factor in the development of the severe pulmonary function reductions in COPD remains uncertain.

GENETIC CONSIDERATIONS Although cigarette smoking is the major environmental risk factor for the development of COPD, the development of airflow obstruction in smokers is highly variable. Severe α_1 antitrypsin (α_1AT) deficiency is a proven genetic risk factor for COPD; there is increasing evidence that other genetic determinants also exist.

α_1 ANTITRYPSIN DEFICIENCY Many variants of the protease inhibitor (PI) locus that encodes α_1AT have been described. The common M allele is associated with normal α_1AT levels. The S allele, associated with slightly reduced α_1AT levels, and the Z allele, associated with markedly reduced α_1AT levels, also occur with frequencies >1% in most Caucasian populations. Rare individuals inherit null alleles, which lead to the absence of any α_1AT production through a heterogeneous collection of mutations. Individuals with two Z alleles or one Z and one null allele are referred to as Pi^Z, which is the most common form of severe α_1AT deficiency.

Although only 1 to 2% of COPD patients inherit severe α_1AT deficiency, these patients demonstrate that genetic factors can have a profound influence on the susceptibility for developing COPD. Pi^Z individuals often develop early-onset COPD, but the ascertainment bias in the published series of Pi^Z individuals—which have usually included many Pi^Z subjects who were tested for α_1AT deficiency because they had COPD—means that the fraction of Pi^Z individuals who will develop COPD and the age-of-onset distribution for the development of COPD in Pi^Z subjects remain unknown. Approximately 1 in 3000 individuals in the United States inherits severe α_1AT deficiency, but only a small minority of these individuals have been recognized.

A significant percentage of the variability in pulmonary function among Pi^Z individuals is explained by cigarette smoking; cigarette smokers with severe α_1AT deficiency are more likely to develop COPD at early ages. However, the development of COPD in Pi^Z subjects, even among current or ex-smokers, is not absolute. Among Pi^Z nonsmokers, impressive variability has been noted in the development of airflow obstruction. Other genetic and/or environmental factors likely contribute to this variability.

The clinical laboratory test used most frequently to screen for α_1AT deficiency is measurement of the immunologic level of α_1AT in serum (see "Laboratory Findings," below). Specific treatment in the form of α_1AT augmentation therapy is available for severe α_1AT deficiency as a weekly intravenous infusion (see "Treatment" below).

The risk of lung disease in heterozygous Pi^{MZ} individuals, who have intermediate serum levels of α_1AT (~60% of Pi^{MM} levels), is controversial. Although previous general population surveys have not typically shown increased rates of airflow obstruction in Pi^{MZ} com-

pared to Pi^{MM} individuals, case-control studies that compared COPD patients to control subjects have usually found an excess of Pi^{MZ} genotypes in the COPD patient group. Several recent large population studies have suggested that Pi^{MZ} subjects are at slightly increased risk for the development of airflow obstruction, but it remains unclear if all Pi^{MZ} subjects are at slightly increased risk for COPD or if a subset of Pi^{MZ} subjects are at substantially increased risk for COPD due to other genetic or environmental factors.

OTHER GENETIC RISK FACTORS Studies of pulmonary function measurements performed in general population samples have suggested that genetic factors other than PI type influence variation in pulmonary function. Familial aggregation of airflow obstruction within families of COPD patients has also been demonstrated.

Association studies have compared the distribution of variants in genes hypothesized to be involved in the development of COPD in COPD patients and control subjects. However, the results have been quite inconsistent, and no genetic determinants of COPD other than severe α_1AT deficiency have been definitively proven. Recent genome scan linkage analyses of early-onset COPD families have found evidence for linkage of spirometric phenotypes to several chromosomal regions, but the specific genetic determinants in those regions have yet to be identified.

NATURAL HISTORY The effects of cigarette smoking on pulmonary function appear to depend on the intensity of smoking exposure, the timing of smoking exposure during growth, and the baseline lung function of the individual; other environmental factors may have similar effects. Although rare individuals may demonstrate precipitous declines in pulmonary function, most individuals follow a steady trajectory of increasing pulmonary function with growth during childhood and adolescence, followed by a gradual decline with aging. Individuals appear to track in their quartile of pulmonary function based upon environmental and genetic factors that put them on different tracks. The risk of eventual mortality from COPD is closely associated with reduced levels of FEV$_1$. A graphic depiction of the natural history of COPD is shown as a function of the influences on tracking curves of FEV$_1$ in Fig. 242-2. Death or disability from COPD can result from a normal rate of decline after a reduced growth phase (curve B), an early initiation of pulmonary function decline after normal growth (curve C), or an accelerated decline after normal growth (curve D). The rate of decline in pulmonary function can be modified by changing environmental exposures (i.e., quitting smoking), with smoking cessation at an earlier age providing a more beneficial effect than smoking cessation after marked reductions in pulmonary function have already

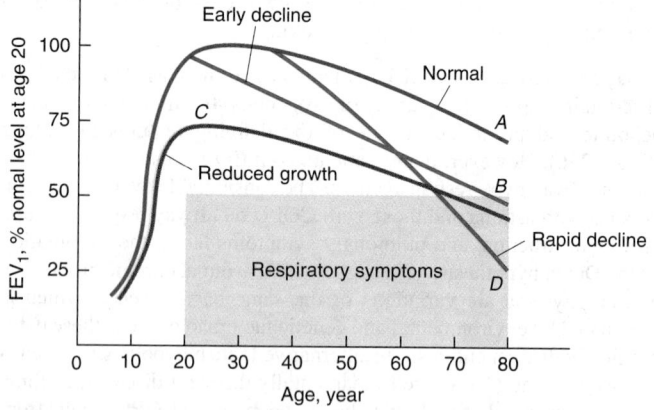

FIGURE 242-2 Hypothetical tracking curves of FEV$_1$ for individuals throughout their lifespans. The normal pattern of growth and decline with age is shown by curve A. Significantly reduced FEV$_1$ (<65% of predicted value at age 20) can develop from a normal rate of decline after a reduced pulmonary function growth phase (curve B), early initiation of pulmonary function decline after normal growth (curve C), or accelerated decline after normal growth (curve D). (From B Rijcken: Doctoral dissertation, p 133, University of Groningen, 1991; with permission.)

developed. Genetic factors likely contribute to the level of pulmonary function achieved during growth and to the rate of decline in response to smoking and potentially to other environmental factors as well.

PATHOPHYSIOLOGY Persistent reduction in forced expiratory flow rates is the most typical finding in COPD. Increases in the residual volume and the residual volume/total lung capacity ratio, nonuniform distribution of ventilation, and ventilation-perfusion mismatching also occur.

Airflow Obstruction Airflow limitation, also known as airflow obstruction, is typically determined by spirometry, which involves forced expiratory maneuvers after the subject has inhaled to total lung capacity (Fig. 234-4). Key phenotypes obtained from spirometry include FEV_1 and the total volume of air exhaled during the entire spirometric maneuver (FVC). Patients with airflow obstruction related to COPD have a chronically reduced ratio of FEV_1/FVC. In contrast to asthma, the reduced FEV_1 in COPD seldom shows large responses to inhaled bronchodilators, although improvements up to 15% are common. Asthma patients can also develop chronic (not fully reversible) airflow obstruction. Maximal inspiratory flow can be relatively well preserved in the presence of a markedly reduced FEV_1. Airflow during forced exhalation is the result of the balance between the elastic recoil of the lungs promoting flow and the resistance of the airways limiting flow. In normal lungs, as well as in lungs affected by COPD, maximal expiratory flow diminishes as the lungs empty because the lung parenchyma provides progressively less elastic recoil and because the cross-sectional area of the airways falls, raising the resistance to airflow. The decrease in flow coincident with decreased lung volume is readily apparent on the expiratory limb of a flow-volume curve. In the early stages of COPD, the abnormality in airflow is only evident at lung volumes at or below the functional residual capacity (closer to residual volume), appearing as a scooped-out lower part of the descending limb of the flow-volume curve. In more advanced disease the entire curve has decreased expiratory flow compared to normal.

Hyperinflation Lung volumes are also routinely assessed in pulmonary function testing. In COPD there is often "air trapping" (increased residual volume and increased ratio of residual volume to total lung capacity) and progressive hyperinflation (increased total lung capacity) late in the disease. Hyperinflation of the thorax during tidal breathing preserves maximum expiratory airflow, because as lung volume increases, elastic recoil pressure increases and airways enlarge so that airway resistance decreases. Consequently, hyperinflation helps to compensate for airway obstruction. However, hyperinflation can push the diaphragm into a flattened position with a number of adverse effects. First, by decreasing the zone of apposition between the diaphragm and the abdominal wall, positive abdominal pressure during inspiration is not applied as effectively to the chest wall, hindering rib cage movement and impairing inspiration. Second, because the muscle fibers of the flattened diaphragm are shorter than those of a more normally curved diaphragm they are less capable of generating inspiratory pressures than normal. Third, the flattened diaphragm (with increased radius of curvature, r) must generate greater tension (t) to develop the transpulmonary pressure (p) required to produce tidal breathing. This follows from Laplace's law, $p = 2t/r$. Also, because the thoracic cage is distended beyond its normal resting volume, during tidal breathing the inspiratory muscles must do work to overcome the resistance of the thoracic cage to further inflation instead of gaining the normal assistance from the chest wall recoiling outward towards its resting volume.

Gas Exchange Although there is considerable variability in the relationships between the FEV_1 and other physiologic abnormalities in COPD, certain generalizations may be made. The Pa_{O_2} usually remains near normal until the FEV_1 is decreased to ~50% of predicted, and even much lower FEV_1's can be associated with a normal Pa_{O_2}, at least at rest. An elevation of Pa_{CO_2} is not expected until the FEV_1 is ≤25% of predicted, and even then may not occur. Pulmonary hypertension severe enough to cause cor pulmonale and right ventricular failure due

to COPD occurs only in those individuals who have marked decreases in FEV_1 (<25% of predicted) together with chronic hypoxemia (Pa_{O_2} < 55 mmHg), although earlier in the course some elevation of pulmonary artery pressure, particularly with exercise, may occur (Chap. 220).

Nonuniform ventilation and ventilation-perfusion mismatching are characteristic of COPD, reflecting the heterogeneous nature of the disease process within the airways and lung parenchyma. Nitrogen wash-out while breathing 100% oxygen is delayed due to regions that are poorly ventilated, and the profile of the nitrogen wash-out curve is consistent with multiple parenchymal compartments having different wash-out rates due to regional differences in compliance and airway resistance. Ventilation/perfusion mismatching accounts for essentially all of the reduction in Pa_{O_2} that occurs in COPD; shunting is minimal. This finding explains the effectiveness of modest elevations of inspired oxygen in treating hypoxemia due to COPD and therefore the need to consider problems other than COPD when hypoxemia is difficult to correct with modest levels of supplemental oxygen in the patient with COPD.

PATHOLOGY Cigarette smoke exposure may affect the large airways, small airways (<2 mm diameter), and alveolar space. Changes in large airways cause cough and sputum, while changes in small airways and alveoli are responsible for physiologic alterations. Emphysema and small airway pathology are both present in most persons with COPD, and their relative contributions to obstruction vary from one person to another. Small airway obstruction likely contributes more to initial obstruction, with emphysema predominating later in the course.

Large Airway Cigarette smoking often results in mucous gland enlargement and goblet cell hyperplasia. These changes are proportional to cough and mucus production that define chronic bronchitis, but these abnormalities are not related to airflow limitation. Goblet cells not only increase in number but in extent through the bronchial tree. Bronchi also undergo squamous metaplasia, which not only predisposes to carcinogenesis but also disrupts mucociliary clearance. Although not as prominent as in asthma, patients may have smooth-muscle hypertrophy and bronchial hyperreactivity leading to airflow limitation. Neutrophil influx has been associated with purulent sputum of upper respiratory tract infections that hamper patients with COPD. Independent of its proteolytic activity, neutrophil elastase is among the most potent secretagogues identified.

Small Airways The major site of increased resistance in most individuals with COPD is in airways ≤2 mm diameter. Characteristic cellular changes include goblet cell metaplasia and replacement of surfactant-secreting Clara cells with mucus-secreting and infiltrating mononuclear inflammatory cells. Smooth-muscle hypertrophy may also be present. These abnormalities may cause luminal narrowing by excess mucus, edema, and cellular infiltration. Reduced surfactant may increase surface tension at the air-tissue interface, predisposing to airway narrowing or collapse. Fibrosis in the wall may cause airway narrowing directly or, as in asthma, predispose to hyperreactivity. Respiratory bronchiolitis with mononuclear inflammatory cells collecting in distal airway tissues may cause proteolytic destruction of elastic fibers in the respiratory bronchioles and alveolar ducts where the fibers are concentrated as rings around alveolar entrances. The resulting distortion and narrowing of these structures could be involved in the early airflow obstruction in COPD related to cigarette smoking.

Because small airway patency is maintained by the surrounding lung parenchyma that provides radial traction on bronchioles at points of attachment to alveolar septa, loss of bronchiolar attachments as a result of extracellular matrix destruction may cause airway distortion and narrowing in COPD. Although the significance of alveolar attachments is not resolved, the concept of decreased alveolar attachments leading to small airway obstruction is appealing because it underscores the mechanistic relationship between loss of elastic recoil and increased resistance to airflow in small airways.

Lung Parenchyma Emphysema is characterized by destruction of gas-exchanging airspaces, i.e., the respiratory bronchioles, alveolar ducts, and alveoli. Their walls become perforated and later obliterated with coalescence of small distinct airspaces into abnormal and much larger airspaces. Macrophages accumulate in respiratory bronchioles of young smokers. Bronchoalveolar lavage fluid from such individuals contains roughly five times as many macrophages as lavage from non-smokers. In smokers' lavage fluid, macrophages comprise >95% of the total cell count and neutrophils, nearly absent in nonsmokers' lavage, account for 1 to 2% of the cells. T lymphocytes, particularly CD8+ cells, are also increased in the alveolar space of smokers.

Emphysema is classified into distinct pathologic types, the most important types being centriacinar and panacinar. *Centriacinar emphysema*, the type most frequently associated with cigarette smoking, is characterized by enlarged airspaces found (initially) in association with respiratory bronchioles. Centriacinar emphysema is most prominent in the upper lobes and superior segments of lower lobes and is often quite focal. *Panacinar emphysema* refers to abnormally large airspaces evenly distributed within and across acinar units. Panacinar emphysema is usually observed in patients with $\alpha_1 AT$ deficiency, which has a predilection for the lower lobes. Distinctions between centriacinar and panacinar emphysema are interesting and may ultimately be shown to have different mechanisms of pathogenesis. However, garden-variety, smoking-related emphysema is usually mixed, particularly in advanced cases, and these pathologic classifications are not helpful in the care of patients with COPD.

PATHOGENESIS Airflow limitation, the major physiologic change in COPD, can result from both small airway obstruction and emphysema, as discussed above. Pathologic findings that can contribute to small airway obstruction are described above, but their relative importance is unknown. Fibrosis surrounding the small airways appears to be a significant contributor. Mechanisms leading to collagen accumulation around the airways in the face of increased collagenase activity remain an enigma. Although seemingly counterintuitive, there are several potential mechanisms whereby a proteinase can predispose to fibrosis including proteolytic activation of transforming growth factor β, and insulin-like growth factor (IGF) binding protein degradation releasing profibrotic IGF. Largely due to availability of suitable animal models, we know much more about the mechanisms involved in emphysema than in small airway obstruction.

The pathogenesis of emphysema can be dissected into three interrelated events (Fig. 242-3): (1) Chronic exposure to cigarette smoke may lead to inflammatory cell recruitment within the terminal airspaces of the lung, (2) these inflammatory cells release elastolytic proteinases that damage the extracellular matrix of the lung, and (3) ineffective repair of elastin and perhaps other extracellular matrix components results in pulmonary emphysema.

Inflammation Synthesis of existing data regarding inflammatory cell responses in human lungs following cigarette smoke exposure suggests the following sequence of events: (1) Macrophages patrol the lower airspace under normal conditions, and (2) cigarette smoke comes into contact with and activates lung epithelial cells and alveolar macrophages, leading to cytokine/chemokine release followed by acute neutrophil recruitment and subacute accumulation of macrophages in the respiratory bronchioles and alveolar spaces. T cells (CD8+ > CD4+) and perhaps other inflammatory and immune cells are also recruited. Concomitant cigarette smoke–induced loss of cilia in the airway epithelium predisposes to bacterial infection with neutrophilia. Surprisingly, in end-stage lung disease, long after smoking cessation, there remains an exuberant inflammatory response, suggesting that mechanisms of cigarette smoke–induced inflammation that initiate the disease differ from mechanisms that sustain inflammation after smoking cessation. Thus, multiple interacting inflammatory cell types are present and contribute to disease pathogenesis.

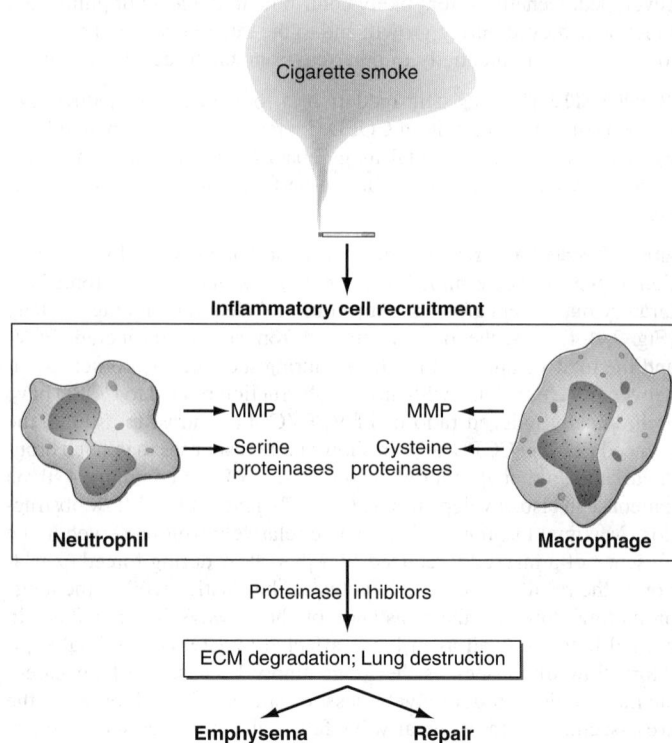

FIGURE 242-3 Pathogenesis of emphysema. Upon long-term exposure to cigarette smoke, inflammatory cells are recruited to the lung; they release proteinases in excess of inhibitors, and, if repair is abnormal, this leads to airspace destruction and enlargement or emphysema.

Extracellular Matrix Proteolysis Elastin, the principal component of elastic fibers, is a highly stable component of the extracellular matrix that is critical to the integrity of both the small airways and the lung parenchyma. The elastase:antielastase hypothesis proposed in the mid-1960s states that the balance of elastin-degrading enzymes and their inhibitors determines the susceptibility of the lung to destruction that results in airspace enlargement. Neutrophil elastase is a potent serine proteinase that clearly plays a major role in emphysema with associated $\alpha_1 AT$ deficiency and also contributes to the usual forms of emphysema. The neutrophil also possesses serine proteinase 3 and cathepsin G as well as matrix metalloproteinases (MMPs), neutrophil collagenase (MMP-8), and gelatinase B (MMP-9). The macrophage is becoming recognized as a critical cell, producing several elastolytic MMPs including matrilysin (MMP-7), MMP-9, and macrophage elastase (MMP-12). Macrophages also produce potent cysteine proteinases (cathepsins S, L, and K). Animal models, including gene-targeted mice, suggest that macrophage elastases contribute to cigarette smoke–induced emphysema. Collagen degradation is more complex in that, while there is clearly collagen turnover in COPD, there is a net increase in collagen deposition, particularly around the small airways.

Cell Death Airspace enlargement with loss of alveolar units obviously requires disappearance of both extracellular matrix and cells. Traditional theories suggest that inflammatory cell proteinases degrade lung extracellular matrix as the primary event, with subsequent loss of cell anchoring leading to apoptosis. Recent studies suggest that endothelial and epithelial cell death could be primary events (presumably with secretion of proteinases to dissolve the matrix). Whether these mechanisms play a role in human COPD is unknown; however, it has been shown that there is increased septal cell death associated with reduced lung expression of vascular endothelial growth factor (VEGF) and its receptor VEGFR-2 (KDR/Flk-1) in human emphysematous lungs.

Ineffective Repair The ability of the adult lung to repair damaged alveoli appears limited. Whether the process of septation that is responsible for alveogenesis during lung development can be reinitiated is not clear. In animal models, treatment with all-*trans* retinoic acid results in some repair. Also, lung resection results in compensatory lung growth in the remaining lung in animal models. In addition to restoring cellularity following injury, it appears difficult for an adult to restore completely an appropriate extracellular matrix, particularly functional elastic fibers.

CLINICAL PRESENTATION ■ History

The three most common symptoms in COPD are cough, sputum production, and exertional dyspnea. Many patients have such symptoms for months or years before seeking medical attention. Although the development of airflow obstruction is a gradual process, many patients date the onset of their disease to an acute illness or exacerbation. A careful history, however, usually reveals the presence of symptoms prior to the acute exacerbation. The development of exertional dyspnea, often described as increased effort to breathe, heaviness, air hunger, or gasping, can be insidious. It is best elicited by a careful history focused on typical physical activities and how the patient's ability to perform them has changed. Activities involving significant arm work, particularly at or above shoulder level, are particularly difficult for patients with COPD. Conversely, activities that allow the patient to brace the arms and use accessory muscles of respiration are better tolerated. Examples of such activities include pushing a shopping cart, walking on a treadmill, or pushing a wheelchair. As COPD advances, the principal feature is worsening dyspnea on exertion with increasing intrusion on the ability to perform vocational or avocational activities. In the most advanced stages, patients are breathless doing simple activities of daily living.

Accompanying worsening airflow obstruction is an increased frequency of exacerbations (described below). Patients may also develop resting hypoxemia and require institution of supplemental oxygen.

Physical Findings In the early stages of COPD, patients may have an entirely normal physical examination. Current smokers may have signs of active smoking, including an odor of smoke or nicotine staining of fingernails. In patients with more severe disease, the physical examination is notable for a prolonged expiratory phase and expiratory wheezing. In addition, signs of hyperinflation include a barrel chest and enlarged lung volumes with poor diaphragmatic excursion as assessed by percussion. Patients with severe airflow obstruction may also exhibit use of accessory muscles of respiration, sitting in the characteristic "tripod" position to facilitate the actions of the sternocleidomastoid, scalene, and intercostal muscles. Patients may develop cyanosis, visible in the lips and nail beds. Patients with predominant emphysema are classically referred to as "pink puffers," a reference to the lack of cyanosis, the use of accessory muscles, and pursed-lip breathing. Such patients also have a dramatic decrease in breath sounds throughout the chest. Patients with a clinical syndrome of chronic bronchitis are classically labeled "blue bloaters," a reference to fluid retention and more marked cyanosis. Typically patients have elements of each and cannot be simply classified. Advanced disease may be accompanied by systemic wasting, with significant weight loss, bitemporal wasting, and diffuse loss of subcutaneous adipose tissue. This syndrome has been associated with both inadequate oral intake and elevated levels of inflammatory cytokines (TNF-α). Such wasting is an independent poor prognostic factor in COPD. Some patients with advanced disease have paradoxical inward movement of the rib cage with inspiration (Hoover's sign), the result of alteration of the vector of diaphragmatic contraction on the rib cage as a result of chronic hyperinflation.

TABLE 242-1 GOLD Criteria for COPD Severity

GOLD Stage	Severity	Symptoms	Spirometry
0	At Risk	Chronic cough, sputum production	Normal
I	Mild	With or without chronic cough or sputum production	$FEV_1/FVC < 0.7$ and $FEV_1 \geq 80\%$ predicted
IIA	Moderate	With or without chronic cough or sputum production	$FEV_1/FVC < 0.7$ and $50\% \leq FEV_1 < 80\%$ predicted
III	Severe	With or without chronic cough or sputum production	$FEV_1/FVC < 0.7$ and $30\% \leq FEV_1 < 50\%$ predicted
IV	Very Severe	With or without chronic cough or sputum production	$FEV_1/FVC < 0.7$ and $FEV_1 < 30\%$ predicted *or* $FEV_1 < 50\%$ predicted with respiratory failure or signs of right heart failure

Note: GOLD, Global Initiative for Chronic Obstructive Pulmonary Disease (COPD).
Source: From Pauwels et al.

Signs of overt right heart failure, termed *cor pulmonale*, are relatively infrequent since the advent of supplemental oxygen therapy. Prior to the availability of such therapy, patients with advanced disease would develop elevated jugular venous pressures, a right ventricular heave or third heart sound, hepatic congestion, ascites, and peripheral edema as the right ventricle decompensated as a result of chronic pulmonary hypertension.

Clubbing of the digits is not a sign of COPD, and its presence should alert the clinician to initiate an investigation for causes of clubbing. In this population, the development of lung cancer is the most likely explanation for newly developed clubbing.

Laboratory Findings The hallmark of COPD is airflow obstruction (discussed above). Pulmonary function testing shows airflow obstruction with a reduction in FEV_1 and FEV_1/FVC (Chap. 234). With worsening disease severity, lung volumes may increase, resulting in an increase in total lung capacity, functional residual capacity, and residual volume. In patients with emphysema, the diffusing capacity may be reduced, reflecting the parenchymal destruction characteristic of the disease. The degree of airflow obstruction is an important prognostic factor in COPD and is the basis for the GOLD disease classification (Table 242-1).

While arterial blood gases and oximetry are not sensitive (discussed above), they may demonstrate resting or exertional hypoxemia. Arterial blood gases provide additional information about alveolar ventilation and acid-base status by measuring arterial P_{CO_2} and pH. The change in pH with P_{CO_2} is 0.08 units/10 mmHg acutely and 0.03 units/ 10 mmHg in the chronic state. Knowledge of the arterial pH therefore allows the classification of ventilatory failure, defined as $P_{CO_2} > 45$ mmHg, into acute or chronic conditions (Chap. 250). The arterial blood gas is an important component of the evaluation of patients presenting with symptoms of an exacerbation. An elevated hematocrit suggests the presence of chronic hypoxemia, as does the presence of signs of right ventricular hypertrophy on electrocardiography.

Radiographic studies may assist in the classification of the type of COPD. Obvious bullae, paucity of parenchymal markings, or hyperlucency suggest the presence of emphysema. Increased lung volumes and flattening of the diaphragm suggest hyperinflation, but do not provide information about chronicity of the changes. Computed tomography (CT) scan is the current definitive test for establishing the presence or absence of emphysema. From a practical perspective, the CT scan does little to influence therapy of COPD except in those individuals considering surgical therapy for their disease (described below).

In patients presenting at ≤ 50 years, those with a strong family history, those with predominant basilar disease or those with a minimal smoking history, the serum level of (α_1AT) should be measured. The definitive diagnosis of α_1AT deficiency requires PI type determination. This is typically performed by isoelectric focusing of serum, which reflects the genotype at the PI locus for the common alleles and many of the rare PI alleles as well. Molecular genotyping can be performed for the common PI alleles (M, S, and Z).

Rx TREATMENT

Stable Phase COPD   Only two interventions, smoking cessation and oxygen therapy in chronically hypoxemic patients, have been demonstrated to influence the natural history of patients with COPD. All other current therapies are directed at improving symptoms and decreasing the frequency and severity of exacerbations. The institution of these therapies should involve an assessment of symptoms, potential risks, costs, and benefits of therapy. This should be followed by an assessment of response to therapy, and a decision should be made whether or not to continue treatment.

Pharmacotherapy ■ *SMOKING CESSATION* (See also Chap. 375) It has been shown that middle-aged smokers who were able to successfully stop smoking experienced a significant improvement in the rate of decline in pulmonary function, returning to annual changes similar to that of nonsmoking patients. Thus, all patients with COPD should be strongly urged to quit and educated about the benefits of quitting. An emerging body of evidence demonstrates that combining pharmacotherapy with traditional supportive approaches considerably enhances the chances of successful smoking cessation. There are two principal pharmacologic approaches to the problem: bupropion, originally developed as an antidepressant medication, and nicotine replacement therapy. The latter is available as gum, transdermal patches, inhaler, and nasal spray. Current recommendations from the U.S. Surgeon General are that all smokers considering quitting be offered pharmacotherapy, in the absence of any contraindication to treatment.

BRONCHODILATORS   In general, bronchodilators are used for symptomatic benefit in patients with COPD. The inhaled route is preferred for medication delivery as the incidence of side effects is lower than that seen with the use of parenteral medication delivery.

ANTICHOLINERGIC AGENTS   While regular use of ipratropium bromide does not appear to influence the rate of decline of lung function, it has been reported to improve symptoms and produce acute improvement in FEV_1. Side effects are minor, and a trial of inhaled anticholinergics is recommended in symptomatic patients with COPD.

BETA AGONISTS   These provide symptomatic benefit. The main side effects are tremor and tachycardia. Long-acting inhaled β agonists, such as salmeterol, have benefits comparable to ipratropium bromide. Their use is more convenient than short-acting agents. The addition of a β agonist to inhaled anticholinergic therapy has been demonstrated to provide incremental benefit.

INHALED GLUCOCORTICOIDS   Several recent trials have *failed* to find a beneficial effect for the regular use of inhaled glucocorticoids on the rate of decline of lung function, as assessed by FEV_1. Patients studied included those with mild to severe airflow obstruction and current and ex-smokers. Patients with significant acute response to inhaled β agonists were excluded from these trials. Inhaled glucocorticoids were demonstrated to reduce the frequency of exacerbations by 25 to 30%, but their use has been associated with increased rates of oropharyngeal candidiasis and an increased rate of loss of bone density. A trial of inhaled glucocorticoids should be considered in patients with frequent exacerbations, defined as two or more per year, and in patients who demonstrate a significant amount of acute reversibility in response to inhaled bronchodilators.

PARENTERAL CORTICOSTEROIDS   The chronic use of oral glucocorticoids for treatment of COPD is not recommended because of an unfavorable benefit/risk ratio. The chronic use of oral glucocorticoids is associated with significant side effects, including osteoporosis, weight gain, cataracts, glucose intolerance, and increased risk of infection. A recent study demonstrated that patients tapered off chronic low-dose prednisone ($\sim$10 mg/d) did not experience any adverse effect on the frequency of exacerbations, health-related quality of life, or lung function. On average, patients lost $\sim$4.5 kg ($\sim$10 lb) when steroids were withdrawn.

THEOPHYLLINE   Theophylline produces modest improvements in expiratory flow rates and vital capacity and a slight improvement in arterial oxygen and carbon dioxide levels in patients with moderate to severe COPD. Nausea is a common side effect; tachycardia and tremor have also been reported.

OXYGEN   Supplemental O_2 is the only therapy demonstrated to decrease mortality in patients with COPD. For patients with resting hypoxemia (resting O_2 saturation <88% or <90% with signs of pulmonary hypertension or right heart failure), the use of O_2 has been demonstrated to have a significant impact on mortality. The Medical Research Council Trial demonstrated that 12 h per day was superior to no O_2 supplementation. The Nocturnal Oxygen Therapy Trial demonstrated that O_2 use 19 h per day was superior to 12 h per day. Various delivery systems are available, including portable systems that patients may carry to allow mobility outside the home.

Supplemental O_2 is commonly prescribed for patients with exertional hypoxemia or nocturnal hypoxemia. Although the rationale for supplemental O_2 in these settings is physiologically sound, the benefits of such therapy are not well substantiated.

OTHER AGENTS   *N*-acetyl cysteine has been used in patients with COPD for both its mucolytic and antioxidant properties. The latter aspect of its use is the subject of ongoing clinical trials. Specific treatment in the form of intravenous $\alpha_1 AT$ augmentation therapy is available for individuals with severe $\alpha_1 AT$ deficiency. Despite heat treatment of this product and the absence of reported cases of viral infection from therapy, hepatitis B vaccination is recommended prior to starting augmentation therapy. Although biochemical efficacy of $\alpha_1 AT$ augmentation therapy has been shown, a randomized controlled trial of $\alpha_1 AT$ augmentation therapy has never proven the efficacy of augmentation therapy in reducing decline of pulmonary function. Eligibility for $\alpha_1 AT$ augmentation therapy requires a serum $\alpha_1 AT$ level <11 μ M. Typically, Pi^z individuals will qualify, although other rare types associated with severe deficiency (e.g., null-null) are also eligible. Since only a fraction of individuals with severe $\alpha_1 AT$ deficiency will develop COPD, $\alpha_1 AT$ augmentation therapy is *not* recommended for severely $\alpha_1 AT$-deficient persons with normal pulmonary function and a normal chest CT scan.

Nonpharmacologic Therapies ■ *GENERAL MEDICAL CARE* Patients with COPD should receive the influenza vaccine annually. Polyvalent pneumococcal vaccine is also recommended, although proof of efficacy in this patient population is not definitive.

PULMONARY REHABILITATION   This refers to a treatment program that incorporates education and cardiovascular conditioning. In COPD, pulmonary rehabilitation has been demonstrated to improve health-related quality of life, dyspnea, and exercise capacity. It has also been shown to reduce rates of hospitalization over a 6- to 12-month period.

LUNG VOLUME REDUCTION SURGERY (LVRS)   Surgery to reduce the volume of lung in patients with emphysema was first introduced with minimal success in the 1950s and was reintroduced in the 1990s. It has been reported to produce symptomatic and functional benefit in selected patients, particularly those with emphysema, which is predominant in the upper lobes. The operation may be performed via either a median sternotomy or a thoracoscopic approach. Patients are excluded if they have significant pleural disease (a pulmonary artery systolic pressure > 45 mmHg), extreme deconditioning, congestive heart failure, or other severe comorbid conditions. Recent data demonstrate that patients with an FEV_1 < 20% of predicted and either diffusely distributed emphysema on CT scan or DL_{CO} < 20% of predicted have an increased mortality after the procedure and thus are not candidates for LVRS.

The National Emphysema Treatment trial demonstrated that LVRS offers both a mortality benefit and a symptomatic benefit in certain patients with emphysema. The anatomic distribution of emphysema and postrehabilitation exercise capacity are important prognostic characteristics. Patients with upper lobe–predominant emphysema and a low postrehabilitation exercise capacity are most likely to benefit from LVRS.

LUNG TRANSPLANTATION (See also Chap. 248) COPD is the single leading indication for lung transplantation. Current recommendations are that candidates for lung transplantation should be ≤65 years; have severe disability despite maximal medical therapy; and be free of comorbid conditions such as liver, renal, or cardiac disease. In contrast to LVRS, the anatomic distribution of emphysema and the presence of pulmonary hypertension are not contraindications to lung transplantation. Unresolved issues concerning lung transplantation and COPD include whether single- or double-lung transplant is the preferred procedure.

Exacerbations of COPD Exacerbations are a prominent feature of the natural history of COPD. Exacerbations are commonly considered to be episodes of increased dyspnea and cough and change in the amount and character of sputum. They may or may not be accompanied by other signs of illness, including fever, myalgias, and sore throat. Self-reported health-related quality of life correlates with frequency of exacerbations more closely than it does with the degree of airflow obstruction. Economic analyses have shown that >70% of COPD-related health care expenditures go to emergency department visits and hospital care; this translates to >$10 billion annually in the United States. The frequency of exacerbations increases as airflow obstruction increases; patients with moderate to severe airflow obstruction [GOLD stages III,IV (Table 242-1)] have one to three episodes per year.

The approach to the patient experiencing an exacerbation includes an assessment of the severity of the patient's illness, both acute and chronic components; an attempt to identify the precipitant of the exacerbation; and the institution of therapy.

PRECIPITATING CAUSES AND STRATEGIES TO REDUCE FREQUENCY OF EXACERBATIONS
A variety of stimuli may result in the final common pathway of airway inflammation and increased symptoms that are characteristic of COPD exacerbations. Bacterial infections play a role in many, but by no means all, episodes. Viral respiratory infections are present in approximately one-third of COPD exacerbations. In a significant minority of instances (20 to 35%), no specific precipitant can be identified.

Despite the frequent implication of bacterial infection, chronic suppressive or "rotating" antibiotics are not beneficial in patients with COPD. This is in contrast to their apparent efficacy in patients with significant bronchiectasis. In patients with bronchiectasis due to cystic fibrosis, suppressive antibiotics have been shown to reduce frequency of hospital admissions.

The role of anti-inflammatory therapy in reducing exacerbation frequency is less well studied. Chronic oral glucocorticoids are not recommended for this purpose. Inhaled glucocorticoids did reduce the frequency of exacerbations by 25 to 30% in large clinical trials. It is important to realize that patients with significant pulmonary function reversibility to inhaled bronchodilators were excluded from these trials. Thus, the use of inhaled glucocorticoids should be considered in patients with frequent exacerbations or those who have an asthmatic component, i.e., significant reversibility on pulmonary function testing or marked symptomatic improvement after inhaled bronchodilators.

PATIENT ASSESSMENT The practitioner should attempt to establish the severity of the exacerbation as well as the severity of preexisting COPD. The more severe either of these two components, the more likely that the patient will require hospital admission. The history should include quantification of the degree of dyspnea by asking about breathlessness during activities of daily living and typical activities for the patient. The patient should be asked about fever; change in character of sputum; any ill contacts; and associated symptoms such as nausea, vomiting, diarrhea, myalgias, and chills. Inquiring about the frequency and severity of prior exacerbations can provide important information. The physical examination should incorporate an assessment of the degree

of distress of the patient. Specific attention should be focused on tachycardia, tachypnea, use of accessory muscles, signs of perioral or peripheral cyanosis, the ability to speak in complete sentences, and the patient's mental status. The chest examination should establish the presence or absence of focal findings, degree of air movement, presence or absence of wheezing, asymmetry in the chest examination (suggesting large airway obstruction or pneumothorax mimicking an exacerbation), and the presence or absence of paradoxical motion of the abdominal wall.

Patients with severe underlying COPD who are in moderate or severe distress or those with focal findings should have a chest x-ray. Approximately 25% of x-rays in this clinical situation will be abnormal, with the most frequent findings being pneumonia and congestive heart failure. Patients with advanced COPD, those with a history of hypercarbia, those with mental status changes (confusion, sleepiness), or those in significant distress should have an arterial blood gas measurement. The presence of hypercarbia, defined as a $P_{CO_2} > 45$ mmHg, has important implications for treatment (discussed below). In contrast to its utility in the management of exacerbations of asthma, measurement of pulmonary function has not been demonstrated to be helpful in the diagnosis or management of exacerbations of COPD.

There are no definitive guidelines concerning the need for inpatient treatment of exacerbations. Patients with respiratory acidosis and hypercarbia, significant hypoxemia, or severe underlying disease or those whose living situation is not conducive to careful observation and the delivery of prescribed treatment should be admitted to the hospital.

Acute Exacerbations ■ *BRONCHODILATORS* Typically, patients are treated with an inhaled β agonist, often with the addition of an anticholinergic agent. These may be administered separately or together, and the frequency of administration depends on the severity of the exacerbation. Patients are often treated initially with nebulized therapy, as such treatment is often easier to administer in older patients or to those in respiratory distress. It has been shown, however, that conversion to metered-dose inhalers is effective when accompanied by education and training of patients and staff. This approach has significant economic benefits and also allows an easier transition to outpatient care. The addition of methylxanthines (such as theophylline) to this regimen can be considered, although convincing proof of its efficacy is lacking. If added, serum levels should be monitored in an attempt to minimize toxicity.

ANTIBIOTICS Patients with COPD are frequently colonized with potential respiratory pathogens and it is often difficult to identify conclusively a specific species of bacteria responsible for a particular clinical event. Bacteria frequently implicated in COPD exacerbations include *Streptococcus pneumoniae*, *Haemophilus influenzae*, and *Moraxella catarrhalis*. In addition, *Mycoplasma pneumoniae* or *Chlamydia pneumoniae* are found in 5 to 10% of exacerbations. The choice of antibiotic should be based on local patterns of antibiotic susceptibility of the above pathogens, as well as the patient's clinical condition. Most practitioners treat patients with moderate or severe exacerbations with antibiotics, even in the absence of data implicating a specific pathogen.

GLUCOCORTICOIDS Among patients admitted to hospital, the use of glucocorticoids has been demonstrated to reduce the length of stay, hasten recovery, and reduce the chance of subsequent exacerbation or relapse for a period of up to 6 months. A recent study demonstrated that 2 weeks of glucocorticoid therapy produced benefit indistinguishable from 8 weeks of therapy. The GOLD guidelines recommend 30 to 40 mg of oral prednisolone or its equivalent for a period of 10 to 14 days. Hyperglycemia, particularly in patients with preexisting diagnosis of diabetes, is the most frequently reported acute complication of glucocorticoid treatment.

OXYGEN Supplemental O_2 should be supplied to keep arterial saturations ≥90%. Hypoxic respiratory drive plays a small role in patients with COPD. Studies have demonstrated that in patients with both acute and chronic hypercarbia, the administration of supplemental O_2 does not reduce minute ventilation. It does, in some patients, result in modest increases in arterial P_{CO_2}, chiefly by altering ventilation-perfusion relationships within the lung. This should not deter practitioners from providing the oxygen needed to correct hypoxemia.

MECHANICAL VENTILATORY SUPPORT   Recent studies have demonstrated that the initiation of noninvasive positive pressure ventilation (NIPPV) in patients with respiratory failure, defined as $P_{CO_2} > 45$ mmHg, results in a significant reduction in mortality, need for intubation, complications of therapy, and hospital length of stay. Contraindications to NIPPV include cardiovascular instability, impaired mental status or inability to cooperate, copious secretions or the inability to clear secretions, craniofacial abnormalities or trauma precluding effective fitting of mask, extreme obesity, or significant burns.

Invasive (conventional) mechanical ventilation via an endotracheal tube is indicated for patients with severe respiratory distress despite initial therapy, life-threatening hypoxemia, severe hypercapnia and/or acidosis, markedly impaired mental status, respiratory arrest, hemodynamic instability, or other complications. The goal of mechanical ventilation is to correct the aforementioned conditions. Factors to consider during mechanical ventilatory support include the need to provide sufficient expiratory time in patients with severe airflow

obstruction and the presence of auto-PEEP (positive end-expiratory pressure) which can result in patients having to generate significant respiratory effort to trigger a breath during a demand mode of ventilation. The mortality of patients requiring mechanical ventilatory support is 17 to 30% for that particular hospitalization. For patients aged ≥ 65 admitted to the intensive care unit for treatment, the mortality doubles over the next year to 60%, regardless of whether mechanical ventilation was required.

FURTHER READING

BURROWS B et al: Quantitative relationships between cigarette smoking and ventilatory function. Am Rev Respir Dis 115:195, 1977

CELLI BR et al: Standards for the diagnosis and care of patients with chronic obstructive pulmonary disease. Official Statement of the American Thoracic Society. Am J Respir Crit Care Med. 152:S77, 1995

FIORE MC et al: *Treating Tobacco Use and Dependence*, Clinical Practice Guideline. Rockville, MD: U.S. Department of Health and Human Services. Public Health Service, June, 2000

KASAHARA Y et al: Inhibition of VEGF receptors causes lung cell apoptosis and emphysema. J Clin Invest 106:1311, 2000

PAUWELS RA et al: Global strategy for the diagnosis, management, and prevention of chronic obstructive pulmonary disease. NHLBI/WHO Global Initiative for Chronic Obstructive Lung Disease (GOLD) Workshop summary. Am J Respir Crit Care Med 163:1256, 2001

SENIOR RM, SHAPIRO SD: Chronic obstructive pulmonary disease: Epidemiology, pathophysiology, and pathogenesis, in *Fishman's Pulmonary Diseases and Disorders*, 3d ed, AD Fishman et al (eds). New York, McGraw-Hill, 1998, pp 659–681

243 INTERSTITIAL LUNG DISEASES
Talmadge E. King, Jr.

The interstitial lung diseases (ILDs) represent a large number of conditions that involve the parenchyma of the lung—the alveoli, the alveolar epithelium, the capillary endothelium, and the spaces between these structures, as well as the perivascular and lymphatic tissues. This heterogeneous group of disorders is classified together because of similar clinical, roentgenographic, physiologic, or pathologic manifestations. These disorders are often associated with considerable morbidity and mortality, and there is little consensus regarding the best management of most of them.

ILDs have been difficult to classify because more than 200 known individual diseases are characterized by diffuse parenchymal lung involvement, either as the primary condition or as a significant part of a multiorgan process, as may occur in the connective tissue diseases (CTDs). One useful approach to classification is to separate the ILDs into two groups based on the major underlying histopathology: (1) those associated with predominant inflammation and fibrosis, and (2) those with a predominantly granulomatous reaction in interstitial or vascular areas (Table 243-1). Each of these groups can be further subdivided according to whether the cause is known or unknown. For each ILD there may be an acute phase, and there is usually a chronic one as well. Rarely, some are recurrent, with intervals of subclinical disease.

Sarcoidosis (Chap. 309), idiopathic pulmonary fibrosis (IPF), and pulmonary fibrosis associated with CTDs (Chaps. 300 to 306) are the most common ILDs of unknown etiology. Among the ILDs of known cause, the largest group comprises occupational and environmental exposures, especially the inhalation of inorganic dusts, organic dusts, and various fumes or gases (Chaps. 237 and 238). A clinical diagnosis is possible for many forms of ILD, especially if an occupational and environmental history is aggressively pursued. For other forms, tissue examination, usually obtained by thoracoscopic or open-lung biopsy, is critical to confirmation of the diagnosis. High-resolution computed tomography (HRCT) scanning promises to improve diagnostic accuracy further as histologic-image correlation is perfected.

PATHOGENESIS

The ILDs are nonmalignant disorders and are not caused by identified infectious agents. The precise pathway(s) leading from injury to fibrosis is not known. Although there are multiple initiating agent(s) of injury, the immunopathogenic responses of lung tissue are limited, and the mechanisms of repair have common features. As mentioned above, the two major histopathologic patterns are a granulomatous pattern and a pattern in which inflammation and fibrosis predominate.

GRANULOMATOUS LUNG DISEASE   This process is characterized by an accumulation of T lymphocytes, macrophages, and epithelioid cells organized into discrete structures (granulomas) in the lung parenchyma. The granulomatous lesions can progress to fibrosis. Many patients with granulomatous lung disease remain free of severe impairment of lung function, or, when symptomatic, they improve after treatment. The main differential diagnosis is between sarcoidosis (Chap. 309) and hypersensitivity pneumonitis (Chap. 237).

INFLAMMATION AND FIBROSIS   The initial insult is an injury to the epithelial surface causing inflammation in the air spaces and alveolar walls. If the disease becomes chronic, inflammation spreads to adjacent portions of the interstitium and vasculature and eventually causes interstitial fibrosis. Important histopathologic patterns found in the ILDs include: usual interstitial pneumonia (UIP), nonspecific interstitial pneumonia, respiratory bronchiolitis, organizing pneumonia [bronchiolitis obliterans with organizing pneumonia (BOOP) pattern], diffuse alveolar damage (acute or organizing), desquamative interstitial pneumonia, and lymphocytic interstitial pneumonia. The development of irreversible scarring (fibrosis) of alveolar walls, airways, or vasculature is the most feared outcome in all of these conditions because it is often progressive and leads to significant derangement of ventilatory function and gas exchange.

INITIAL EVALUATION

Patients with ILDs come to medical attention mainly because of the onset of progressive exertional dyspnea or a persistent, nonproductive cough. Hemoptysis, wheezing, and chest pain may be present. Often, the identification of interstitial opacities on chest x-ray focuses the diagnostic approach toward one of the ILDs.

TABLE 243-1 *Major Categories of Alveolar and Interstitial Inflammatory Lung Disease*

Lung Response: Alveolitis, Interstitial Inflammation, and Fibrosis

KNOWN CAUSE

Asbestos	Radiation
Fumes, gases	Aspiration pneumonia
Drugs (antibiotics, amiodarone, gold) and chemotherapy drugs	Residual of adult respiratory distress syndrome

UNKNOWN CAUSE

Idiopathic interstitial pneumonias	Pulmonary alveolar proteinosis
Idiopathic pulmonary fibrosis (usual interstitial pneumonia)	Lymphocytic infiltrative disorders (lymphocytic interstitial pneumonitis associated with connective tissue disease)
Desquamative interstitial pneumonia	
Respiratory bronchiolitis-associated interstitial lung disease	Eosinophilic pneumonias
	Lymphangioleiomyomatosis
Acute interstitial pneumonia (diffuse alveolar damage)	Amyloidosis
	Inherited diseases
Cryptogenic organizing pneumonia (bronchiolitis obliterans with organizing pneumonia)	Tuberous sclerosis, neurofibromatosis, Niemann-Pick disease, Gaucher's disease, Hermansky-Pudlak syndrome
Nonspecific interstitial pneumonia	
Connective tissue diseases	
Systemic lupus erythematosus, rheumatoid arthritis, ankylosing spondylitis, systemic sclerosis, Sjögren's syndrome, polymyositis-dermatomyositis	Gastrointestinal or liver diseases (Crohn's disease, primary biliary cirrhosis, chronic active hepatitis, ulcerative colitis)
Pulmonary hemorrhage syndromes	Graft-vs.-host disease (bone marrow transplantation; solid organ transplantation)
Goodpasture's syndrome, idiopathic pulmonary hemosiderosis, isolated pulmonary capillaritis	

Lung Response: Granulomatous

KNOWN CAUSE

Hypersensitivity pneumonitis (organic dusts)	Inorganic dusts: beryllium silica

UNKNOWN CAUSE

Sarcoidosis	Bronchocentric granulomatosis
Langerhans cell granulomatosis (eosinophilic granuloma of the lung)	Lymphomatoid granulomatosis
Granulomatous vasculitides	
Wegener's granulomatosis, allergic granulomatosis of Churg-Strauss	

HISTORY ■ **Duration of Illness** *Acute presentation* (days to weeks), while unusual, occurs with allergy (drugs, fungi, helminths), acute idiopathic interstitial pneumonia, eosinophilic pneumonia, and hypersensitivity pneumonitis. These conditions may be confused with atypical pneumonias because of diffuse alveolar opacities on chest x-ray. *Subacute presentation* (weeks to months) may occur in all ILDs but is seen especially in sarcoidosis, drug-induced ILDs, the alveolar hemorrhage syndromes, cryptogenic organizing pneumonia (COP), and the acute immunologic pneumonia that complicates systemic lupus erythematosus (SLE) or polymyositis. In most ILDs the symptoms and signs form a *chronic presentation* (months to years). Examples include IPF, sarcoidosis, pulmonary Langerhans cell histiocytosis (PLCH) (also known as Langerhans cell granulomatosis, eosinophilic granuloma, or histiocytosis X), pneumoconioses, and CTDs. *Episodic presentations* are unusual and include eosinophilic pneumonia, hypersensitivity pneumonitis, COP, vasculitides, pulmonary hemorrhage, and Churg-Strauss syndrome.

Age Most patients with sarcoidosis, ILD associated with CTD, lymphangioleiomyomatosis (LAM), PLCH, and inherited forms of ILD

(familial IPF, Gaucher's disease, Hermansky-Pudlak syndrome) present between the ages of 20 and 40 years. Most patients with IPF are older than 50 years.

Gender LAM and pulmonary involvement in tuberous sclerosis occur exclusively in premenopausal women. Also, ILD in Hermansky-Pudlak syndrome and in the CTDs is more common in women; an exception is ILD in rheumatoid arthritis (RA), which is more common in men. Because of occupational exposures, pneumoconioses also occur more frequently in men.

Family History Family associations (with an autosomal dominant pattern) have been identified in tuberous sclerosis and neurofibromatosis. An autosomal recessive pattern of inheritance occurs in Niemann-Pick disease, Gaucher's disease, and the Hermansky-Pudlak syndrome. Familial clustering has been increasingly identified in sarcoidosis. Familial lung fibrosis has been associated with mutations in the surfactant protein C gene and is characterized by several patterns of interstitial pneumonia, including nonspecific interstitial pneumonia, desquamative interstitial pneumonia, and UIP.

Smoking History Patients with PLCH, desquamative interstitial pneumonia (DIP), Goodpasture's syndrome, respiratory bronchiolitis, and pulmonary alveolar proteinosis are almost always current or former smokers. Two-thirds to 75% of patients with IPF have a history of smoking.

Occupation and Environmental History A strict chronologic listing of the patient's lifelong employment must be sought, including specific duties and known exposures. In hypersensitivity pneumonitis (see Fig. 237-1), respiratory symptoms, fever, chills, and an abnormal chest roentgenogram are often temporally related to a hobby (pigeon breeder's disease) or to the workplace (farmer's lung) (Chap. 237). Symptoms may diminish or disappear after the patient leaves the site of exposure for several days; similarly, symptoms may reappear on returning to the exposure site.

Other Important Past History Parasitic infections may cause pulmonary eosinophilia, and therefore a travel history should be taken in patients with known or suspected ILD. History of risk factors for HIV infection should be elicited from all patients with ILD because several processes may occur at the time of initial presentation or during the clinical course, e.g., HIV infection, BOOP, acute interstitial pneumonia (AIP), lymphocytic interstitial pneumonitis, or diffuse alveolar hemorrhage.

RESPIRATORY SYMPTOMS AND SIGNS Dyspnea is a common and prominent complaint in patients with ILD, especially the idiopathic interstitial pneumonias, hypersensitivity pneumonitis, COP, sarcoidosis, eosinophilic pneumonias, and PLCH. Some patients, especially patients with sarcoidosis, silicosis, PLCH, hypersensitivity pneumonitis, lipoid pneumonia, or lymphangitis carcinomatosis, may have extensive parenchymal lung disease on chest x-ray without significant dyspnea, especially early in the course of the illness. Wheezing is an uncommon manifestation of ILD but has been described in patients with chronic eosinophilic pneumonia, Churg-Strauss syndrome, respiratory bronchiolitis, and sarcoidosis. Clinically significant chest pain is uncommon in most ILDs. However, substernal discomfort is common in sarcoidosis. Sudden worsening of dyspnea, especially if associated with acute chest pain, may indicate a spontaneous pneumothorax, which occurs in PLCH, tuberous sclerosis, LAM, and neurofibromatosis. Frank hemoptysis and blood-streaked sputum are rarely presenting manifestations of ILD but can be seen in the diffuse alveolar hemorrhage (DAH) syndromes, LAM, tuberous sclerosis, and the granulomatous vasculitides. Fatigue and weight loss are common in all ILDs.

PHYSICAL EXAMINATION The findings are usually not specific. Most commonly, physical examination reveals tachypnea and bibasilar end-inspiratory dry crackles, which are common in most forms of ILD associated with inflammation but are less likely to be heard in the granulomatous lung diseases. Crackles may be present in the absence of radiographic abnormalities on the chest radiograph. Scattered late inspiratory high-pitched rhonchi—so-called inspiratory squeaks—are heard in patients with bronchiolitis. The cardiac examination is usually normal except in the mid or late stages of the disease, when findings of pulmonary hypertension and cor pulmonale may become evident (Chap. 220). Cyanosis and clubbing of the digits occur in some patients with advanced disease.

LABORATORY   Antinuclear antibodies, anti-immunoglobulin antibodies (rheumatoid factors), and circulating immune complexes are identified in some patients, even in the absence of a defined CTD. A raised LDH is a nonspecific finding common to ILDs. Elevation of the serum angiotensin-converting enzyme level is common in sarcoidosis. Serum precipitins confirm exposure when hypersensitivity pneumonitis is suspected, although they are not diagnostic of the process. Antineutrophil cytoplasmic or anti-basement membrane antibodies are useful if vasculitis is suspected. The electrocardiogram is usually normal unless pulmonary hypertension is present; then it demonstrates right-axis deviation, right ventricular hypertrophy, or right atrial enlargement or hypertrophy. Echocardiography also reveals right ventricular dilatation and/or hypertrophy in the presence of pulmonary hypertension.

CHEST IMAGING STUDIES ■ Chest X-ray   ILD may be first suspected on the basis of an abnormal chest radiograph, which most commonly reveals a bibasilar reticular pattern. A nodular or mixed pattern of alveolar filling and increased reticular markings may also be present (see Fig. 233-1). A subgroup of ILDs exhibit nodular opacities with a predilection for the upper lung zones [sarcoidosis, PLCH, chronic hypersensitivity pneumonitis, silicosis, berylliosis, RA (necrobiotic nodular form), ankylosing spondylitis]. The chest x-ray correlates poorly with the clinical or histopathologic stage of the disease. The radiographic finding of honeycombing correlates with pathologic findings of small cystic spaces and progressive fibrosis; when present, it portends a poor prognosis. In most cases, the chest radiograph is nonspecific and usually does not allow a specific diagnosis.

Computed Tomography   HRCT is superior to the plain chest x-ray for early detection and confirmation of suspected ILD (Fig. 243-1). Also, HRCT allows better assessment of the extent and distribution of disease, and it is especially useful in the investigation of patients with a normal chest radiograph. Coexisting disease is often best recognized on HRCT scanning, e.g., mediastinal adenopathy, carcinoma, or emphysema. In the appropriate clinical setting HRCT may be sufficiently characteristic to preclude the need for lung biopsy in IPF, sarcoidosis,

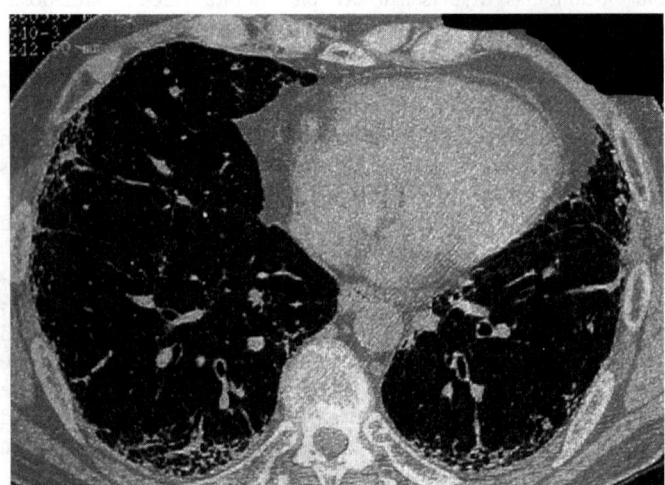

FIGURE 243-1 Idiopathic pulmonary fibrosis. High-resolution computed tomographic image shows bibasal, peripheral predominant reticular abnormality with traction bronchiectasis and honeycombing. The lung biopsy showed the typical features of usual interstitial pneumonia.

hypersensitivity pneumonitis, asbestosis, lymphangitic carcinoma, and PLCH. When a lung biopsy is required, HRCT scanning is useful for determining the most appropriate area from which biopsy samples should be taken.

Radionuclide Scanning   Gallium-67 or ^{99m}Tc-diethylenetriamene pentaacetate (DTPA) scanning have limited roles in evaluating the inflammatory component of ILD.

PULMONARY FUNCTION TESTING ■ Spirometry and Lung Volumes   Measurement of lung function is important in assessing the extent of pulmonary involvement in patients with ILD. Most forms of ILD produce a restrictive defect with reduced total lung capacity (TLC), functional residual capacity, and residual volume (Chap. 234). Forced expiratory volume in one second (FEV_1) and forced vital capacity (FVC) are reduced, but these changes are related to the decreased TLC. The FEV_1/FVC ratio is usually normal or increased. Lung volumes decrease as lung stiffness worsens with disease progression. A few disorders produce interstitial opacities on chest x-ray and obstructive airflow limitation on lung function testing (uncommon in sarcoidosis and hypersensitivity pneumonitis, while common in tuberous sclerosis and LAM).

Diffusing Capacity   A reduction in the diffusing capacity of the lung for carbon monoxide (DL_{CO}) is a common but nonspecific finding in most ILDs. This decrease is due, in part, to effacement of the alveolar capillary units but, more importantly, to mismatching of ventilation and perfusion ($\dot{V}/\dot{Q}$). Lung regions with reduced compliance due to either fibrosis or cellular infiltration may be poorly ventilated but may still maintain adequate blood flow and the ventilation-perfusion mismatch in these regions acts like true venous admixture. The severity of the reduction in DL_{CO} does not correlate with disease stage.

Arterial Blood Gas   The resting arterial blood gas may be normal or reveal hypoxemia (secondary to a mismatching of ventilation to perfusion) and respiratory alkalosis. A normal arterial O_2 tension (or saturation by oximetry) at rest does not rule out significant hypoxemia during exercise or sleep. CO_2 retention is rare and is usually a manifestation of end-stage disease.

CARDIOPULMONARY EXERCISE TESTING   Because hypoxemia at rest is not always present and because severe exercise-induced hypoxemia may go undetected, it is useful to perform exercise testing with measurement of arterial blood gases to detect abnormalities of gas exchange. Arterial oxygen desaturation, a failure to decrease dead space appropriately with exercise [i.e., a high VD/VT ratio (Chap. 234)], and an excessive increase in respiratory rate with a lower-than-expected recruitment of tidal volume provide useful information about physiologic abnormalities and extent of disease. Serial assessment of resting and exercise gas exchange is an excellent method for following disease activity and responsiveness to treatment, especially in patients with IPF.

FIBEROPTIC BRONCHOSCOPY AND BRONCHOALVEOLAR LAVAGE (BAL)   In selected diseases (e.g., sarcoidosis, hypersensitivity pneumonitis, DAH syndrome, cancer, pulmonary alveolar proteinosis), cellular analysis of BAL fluid may be useful in narrowing the differential diagnostic possibilities among various types of ILD. The role for BAL in defining the stage of disease and assessment of disease progression or response to therapy remains poorly understood, and the usefulness of BAL in the clinical assessment and management remains to be established.

TISSUE AND CELLULAR EXAMINATION   Lung biopsy is the most effective method for confirming the diagnosis and assessing disease activity. The findings may identify a more treatable process than originally suspected, particularly chronic hypersensitivity pneumonitis, COP, respiratory bronchiolitis–associated ILD, or sarcoidosis. Biopsy should be obtained before initiation of treatment. A definitive diagnosis avoids confusion and anxiety later in the clinical course if the patient does not respond to therapy or suffers serious side effects from it.

Fiberoptic bronchoscopy with multiple transbronchial lung biopsies (four to eight biopsy samples) is often the initial procedure of choice, especially when sarcoidosis, lymphangitic carcinomatosis, eosinophilic pneumonia, Goodpasture's syndrome, or infection are suspected. If a specific diagnosis is not made by transbronchial biopsy, then surgical lung biopsy by video-assisted thoracic surgery or open thoracotomy is indicated. Adequate-sized biopsies from multiple sites, usually from two lobes, should be obtained. Relative contraindications to lung biopsy include serious cardiovascular disease, honeycombing and other roentgenographic evidence of diffuse end-stage disease, severe pulmonary dysfunction, or other major operative risks, especially in the elderly.

with traction bronchiectasis and honeycombing (Fig. 243-1). Atypical findings that should suggest an alternative diagnosis include: extensive ground-glass abnormality, nodular opacities, upper or mid-zone predominance, and prominent hilar or mediastinal lymphadenopathy. Pulmonary function tests often reveal a restrictive pattern, a reduced DL_{CO}, and arterial hypoxemia that is exaggerated or elicited by exercise.

Histologic Findings Confirmation of the presence of the UIP pattern on histologic examination is essential to confirm this diagnosis. Transbronchial biopsies are not helpful in making the diagnosis of UIP, and surgical biopsy is usually required. The histologic hallmark and chief diagnostic criterion of UIP is a heterogeneous appearance at low magnification with alternating areas of normal lung, interstitial inflammation, foci of proliferating fibroblasts, dense collagen fibrosis, and honeycomb changes. These histologic changes affect the peripheral, subpleural parenchyma most severely. The interstitial inflammation is usually patchy and consists of a lymphoplasmacytic infiltrate in the alveolar septa, associated with hyperplasia of type 2 pneumocytes. The fibrotic zones are composed mainly of dense collagen, although scattered foci of proliferating fibroblasts are a consistent finding. The extent of fibroblastic proliferation is predictive of disease progression. Areas of honeycomb change are composed of cystic fibrotic air spaces that are frequently lined by bronchiolar epithelium and filled with mucin. Smooth-muscle hyperplasia is commonly seen in areas of fibrosis and honeycomb change. Histopathologic examinations during this accelerated phase show a combination of UIP and diffuse alveolar damage. A UIP-like pattern can also be seen with CTDs, pneumoconioses (e.g., asbestosis), radiation injury, certain drug-induced lung diseases (e.g., nitrofurantoin), and chronic aspiration. Also, a fibrotic pattern may be found in the chronic stage of several specific disorders such as sarcoidosis, chronic hypersensitivity pneumonitis, organized chronic eosinophilic pneumonia, and PLCH. Since other histopathologic features are frequently present in these syndromes, the term UIP is used for those patients in whom the lesion is idiopathic and not associated with another condition.

℞ TREATMENT

Although the course of ILD is variable, progression is common and often insidious. All treatable possibilities should be carefully considered. Since therapy does not reverse fibrosis, the major goals of treatment are permanent removal of the offending agent, when known, and early identification and aggressive suppression of the acute and chronic inflammatory process, thereby reducing further lung damage.

Hypoxemia (Pa_{O_2} < 55 mmHg) at rest and/or with exercise should be managed by supplemental oxygen. If cor pulmonale develops, diuretic therapy and phlebotomy may occasionally be required (Chap. 220).

DRUG THERAPY Glucocorticoids are the mainstay of therapy for suppression of the alveolitis present in ILD, but the success rate is low. There have been no placebo-controlled trials of glucocorticoids in ILD, so there is no direct evidence that steroids improve survival in many of the diseases for which they are commonly used. Glucocorticoid therapy is recommended for symptomatic ILD patients with idiopathic interstitial pneumonias, eosinophilic pneumonias, COP, CTD, sarcoidosis, acute inorganic dust exposures, acute radiation pneumonitis, DAH, and drug-induced ILD. In organic dust disease, glucocorticoids are recommended for both the acute and chronic stages.

The optimal dose and proper length of therapy with glucocorticoids in the treatment of most ILDs are not known. A common starting dose is prednisone, 0.5 to 1 mg/kg in a once-daily oral dose (based on the patient's lean body weight). This dose is continued for 4 to 12 weeks, at which time the patient is reevaluated. If the patient is stable or improved, the dose is tapered to 0.25 to 0.5 mg/kg and is maintained at this level for an additional 4 to 12 weeks depending on the course. Rapid tapering or a shortened course of glucocorticoid treatment can result in recurrence. If the patient's condition continues to decline while on glucocorticoids, a second agent (see below) is often added and the prednisone dose is lowered to or maintained at 0.25 mg/kg per day.

Cyclophosphamide and azathioprine (1 to 2 mg/kg lean body weight per day), with or without glucocorticoids, have been tried with variable success in IPF, vasculitis, and other ILDs. An objective response usually requires at least 8 to 12 weeks to occur. In situations in which these drugs have failed or could not be tolerated, other agents, including methotrexate, colchicine, penicillamine, and cyclosporine, have been tried. However, their role in the treatment of ILDs remains to be determined.

Many cases of ILD are chronic and irreversible despite the therapy discussed above, and lung transplantation may then be considered (Chap. 248).

INDIVIDUAL FORMS OF ILD

IDIOPATHIC PULMONARY FIBROSIS IPF is the most common form of idiopathic interstitial pneumonia. Separating IPF from other forms of lung fibrosis is an important step in the evaluation of all patients presenting with ILD. IPF has a distinctly poor response to therapy and prognosis.

Clinical Manifestations Exertional dyspnea, a nonproductive cough, and inspiratory crackles with or without digital clubbing may be present on physical examination. The HRCT lung scans typically show patchy, predominantly basilar, subpleural reticular opacities, often associated

℞ TREATMENT

The clinical course is variable, with a 5-year survival rate of 20 to 40% after diagnosis. Treatment options include glucocorticoids, cytotoxic agents (e.g., azathioprine, cyclophosphamide), and antifibrotic agents (e.g., colchicine, pirfenidone, or interferon gamma-1b), alone or in combination with glucocorticoids. However, there is no firm evidence that any of these treatment approaches improves survival or the quality of life. Because of the poor prognosis in untreated patients, a therapeutic trial may be tried. If therapy is recommended, it should be started at the first identification of clinical or physiologic evidence of impairment of lung function. Lung transplantation should be considered for those patients who experience progressive deterioration despite optimal medical management and who meet the established criteria (Chap. 248).

DESQUAMATIVE INTERSTITIAL PNEUMONIA DIP is a rare but distinct clinical and pathologic entity found exclusively in cigarette smokers. The histologic hallmark is the extensive accumulation of macrophages in intraalveolar spaces with minimal interstitial fibrosis. The peak incidence is in the fourth and fifth decades. Most patients present with dyspnea. Lung function testing shows a restrictive pattern with reduced DL_{CO} and arterial hypoxemia. The chest x-ray and HRCT scans usually shows diffuse hazy opacities. Clinical recognition of DIP is important because the process is associated with a better prognosis (10-year survival rate is ~70%) and a better response to smoking cessation and systemic glucocorticoids than the more common IPF. Respiratory bronchiolitis–associated ILD is considered to be a subset of DIP and is characterized by the accumulation of macrophages in peribronchial alveoli.

ACUTE INTERSTITIAL PNEUMONIA (HAMMAN-RICH SYNDROME)   AIP is a rare, fulminant form of lung injury characterized histologically by diffuse alveolar damage on lung biopsy. Most patients are older than 40 years. AIP is similar in presentation to the acute respiratory distress syndrome (ARDS) (Chap. 251) and probably corresponds to the subset of cases of idiopathic ARDS. The onset is usually abrupt in a previously healthy individual. A prodromal illness, usually lasting 7 to 14 days before presentation, is common. Fever, cough, and dyspnea are frequent manifestations at presentation. Diffuse, bilateral, air-space opacification is present on chest radiograph. HRCT scans show bilateral, patchy, symmetric areas of ground-glass attenuation. Bilateral areas of air-space consolidation may also be present. A predominantly subpleural distribution may be seen. The diagnosis of AIP requires the presence of a clinical syndrome of idiopathic ARDS and pathologic confirmation of organizing diffuse alveolar damage. Therefore, lung biopsy is required to confirm the diagnosis. Most patients have moderate to severe hypoxemia and develop respiratory failure. Mechanical ventilation is often required. The mortality rate is high (>60%), with most patients dying within 6 months of presentation. Recurrences have been reported. However, those who recover often have substantial improvement in lung function. The main treatment is supportive. It is not clear that glucocorticoid therapy is effective.

NONSPECIFIC INTERSTITIAL PNEUMONIA (NSIP)   This condition defines a subgroup of the idiopathic interstitial pneumonias that can be distinguished clinically and pathologically from UIP, DIP, AIP, and idiopathic BOOP. NSIP is a subacute restrictive process with a presentation similar to IPF but usually at a younger age. It is often associated with a febrile illness and there is a relative lack of clubbing. HRCT shows bilateral, subpleural ground-glass opacities, often associated with lower lobe volume loss (Fig. 243-2). Patchy areas of airspace consolidation and reticular abnormalities may be present, but honeycombing is unusual. Unlike patients with IPF (UIP), the majority of patients with NSIP have a good prognosis with most showing improvement after treatment with glucocorticoids.

ILD ASSOCIATED WITH CONNECTIVE TISSUE DISORDERS   Clinical findings suggestive of a CTD (musculoskeletal pain, weakness, fatigue, fever, joint pains or swelling, photosensitivity, Raynaud's phenomenon, pleuritis, dry eyes, dry mouth) should be sought in any patient with ILD. The CTDs may be difficult to rule out since the pulmonary manifestations occasionally precede the more typical systemic manifesta-

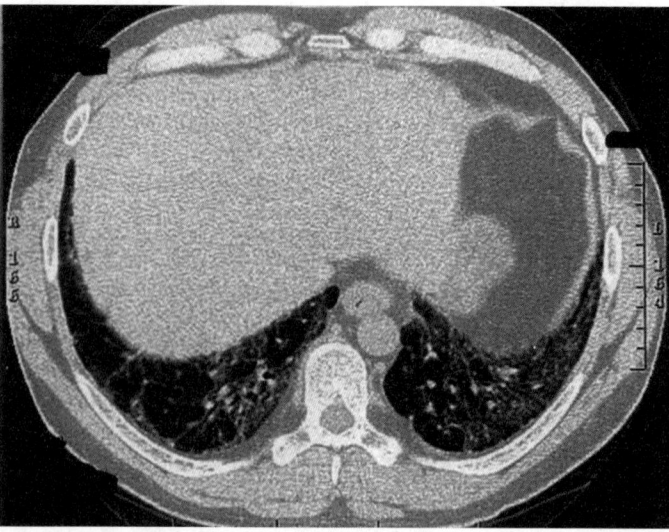

FIGURE 243-2   Nonspecific interstitial pneumonia. High-resolution computed tomography through the lower lung shows volume loss with extensive ground-glass abnormality, reticular abnormality and traction bronchiectasis. There is sparing on the lung immediately adjacent to the pleura. Histology showed a combination of inflammation and mild fibrosis.

tions by months or years. The most common form of pulmonary involvement is a chronic interstitial pattern similar to that in patients with IPF. However, determining the precise nature of lung involvement in most of the CTDs is difficult due to the high incidence of lung involvement caused by disease-associated complications of esophageal dysfunction (predisposing to aspiration and secondary infections), respiratory muscle weakness (atelectasis and secondary infections), complications of therapy (opportunistic infections), and associated malignancies.

Progressive Systemic Sclerosis (PSS) (See also Chap. 303)   Clinical evidence of ILD is present in about one-half of patients with PSS, and pathologic evidence in three-quarters. Pulmonary function tests show a restrictive pattern and impaired diffusing capacity, often before any clinical or radiographic evidence of lung disease appears. Pulmonary vascular disease alone or in association with pulmonary fibrosis, pleuritis, or recurrent aspiration pneumonitis is strikingly resistant to current modes of therapy.

Rheumatoid Arthritis (See also Chap. 301)   ILD associated with RA is more common in men. Pulmonary manifestations of RA include pleurisy with or without effusion, ILD in up to 20% of cases, necrobiotic nodules (nonpneumoconiotic intrapulmonary rheumatoid nodules) with or without cavities, Caplan's syndrome (rheumatoid pneumoconiosis), pulmonary hypertension secondary to rheumatoid pulmonary vasculitis, BOOP, and upper airway obstruction due to arytenoid arthritis.

Systemic Lupus Erythematosus (See also Chap. 300)   Lung disease is a common complication in SLE. Pleuritis with or without effusion is the most common pulmonary manifestation. Other lung manifestations include the following: atelectasis, diaphragmatic dysfunction with loss of lung volumes, pulmonary vascular disease, pulmonary hemorrhage, uremic pulmonary edema, infectious pneumonia, and BOOP. Acute lupus pneumonitis characterized by pulmonary capillaritis leading to alveolar hemorrhage is uncommon. Chronic, progressive ILD is uncommon. It is important to exclude pulmonary infection. Although pleuropulmonary involvement may not be evident clinically, pulmonary function testing, particularly DL_{CO}, reveals abnormalities in many patients with SLE.

Polymyositis and Dermatomyositis (PM/DM) (See also Chap. 369)   ILD occurs in ~10% of patients with PM/DM, and the clinical features are similar to those of IPF. Diffuse reticular or nodular opacities with or without an alveolar component occur radiographically, with a predilection for the lung bases. ILD occurs more commonly in the subgroup of patients with an anti-Jo-1 antibody that is directed to histidyl tRNA synthetase. Weakness of respiratory muscles contributing to aspiration pneumonia may be present. A rapidly progressive illness characterized by diffuse alveolar damage may cause respiratory failure.

Sjögren's Syndrome (See also Chap. 304)   General dryness and lack of airways secretion cause the major problems of hoarseness, cough, and bronchitis. Lymphocytic interstitial pneumonitis, lymphoma, pseudolymphoma, bronchiolitis, and bronchiolitis obliterans are associated with this condition. Lung biopsy is frequently required to establish a precise pulmonary diagnosis. Glucocorticoids have been used in the management of ILD associated with Sjögren's syndrome with some degree of clinical success.

DRUG-INDUCED ILD   Many classes of drugs have the potential to induce diffuse ILD, which is manifest most commonly as exertional dyspnea and nonproductive cough. A detailed history of the medications taken by the patient is needed to identify drug-induced disease, including over-the-counter medications, oily nose drops, or petroleum products (mineral oil). In most cases, the pathogenesis is unknown, although a combination of direct toxic effects of the drug (or its metabolite) and indirect inflammatory and immunologic events is likely. The onset of the illness may be abrupt and fulminant, or it may be insidious, extending over weeks to months. The drug may have been taken for several years before a reaction develops (e.g., amiodarone), or the lung disease may occur weeks to years after the drug has been discontinued (e.g., carmustine). The extent and severity of disease are usually dose related. Treatment consists of discontinuation of any possible offending drug and supportive care.

CRYPTOGENIC ORGANIZING PNEUMONIA   Also known as idiopathic BOOP, COP is a clinicopathologic syndrome of unknown etiology. The onset is usually in the fifth and sixth decades. The presentation may be of a flulike illness with cough, fever, malaise, fatigue, and weight loss. Inspiratory crackles are frequently present on examination. Pulmonary function is usually impaired, with a restrictive defect and arterial hypoxemia being most common. The roentgenographic manifestations are distinctive, revealing bilateral, patchy, or diffuse alveolar opacities in the presence of normal lung volume. Recurrent and migratory pulmonary opacities are common. HRCT shows areas of air-space consolidation, ground-glass opacities, small nodular opacities, and bronchial wall thickening and dilation. These changes occur more frequently in the periphery of the lung and in the lower lung zone. Lung biopsy shows granulation tissue within small airways, alveolar ducts, and airspaces, with chronic inflammation in the surrounding alveoli. Glucocorticoid therapy induces clinical recovery in two-thirds of patients. A few patients have rapidly progressive courses with fatal outcomes despite glucocorticoids.

Foci of organizing pneumonia (i.e., a "BOOP pattern") is a nonspecific reaction to lung injury found adjacent to other pathologic processes or as a component of other primary pulmonary disorders (e.g., cryptococcosis, Wegener's granulomatosis, lymphoma, hypersensitivity pneumonitis, and eosinophilic pneumonia). Consequently, the clinician must carefully reevaluate any patient found to have this histopathologic lesion to rule out these possibilities.

EOSINOPHILIC PNEUMONIA See Chap. 237

PULMONARY ALVEOLAR PROTEINOSIS   Although not strictly an ILD, pulmonary alveolar proteinosis (PAP) resembles and is therefore considered with these conditions. It has been proposed that a defect in macrophage function, more specifically an impaired ability to process surfactant, may play a role in the pathogenesis of PAP. This diffuse disease is characterized by the accumulation of an amorphous, periodic acid–Schiff–positive lipoproteinaceous material in the distal air spaces. There is little or no lung inflammation, and the underlying lung architecture is preserved. Mutant mice lacking the gene for granulocyte-macrophage colony-stimulating factor (GM-CSF) have a similar accumulation of surfactant and surfactant apoprotein in the alveolar spaces. Moreover, reconstitution of the respiratory epithelium of GM-CSF knockout mice with the GM-CSF gene completely corrects the alveolar proteinosis. Data from BAL studies in patients suggest that PAP is an autoimmune disease with neutralizing antibody of immunoglobulin G isotype against GM-CSF. These findings suggest that neutralization of GM-CSF bioactivity by the antibody causes dysfunction of alveolar macrophages, which results in reduced surfactant clearance. There are three distinct classes of PAP: acquired (>90% of all cases), congenital, and secondary. Congenital PAP is transmitted in an autosomal recessive manner and is caused by homozygosity for a frame shift mutation (121ins2) in the SP-B gene, which leads to an unstable SP-B mRNA, reduced protein levels, and secondary disturbances of SP-C processing. Secondary PAP is rare among adults and is caused by lysinuric protein intolerance, acute silicosis and other inhalational syndromes, immunodeficiency disorders, and malignancies (almost exclusively of hematopoietic origin) and hematopoietic disorders.

The typical age of presentation is 30 to 50 years, and males predominate. The clinical presentation is usually insidious and manifested by progressive exertional dyspnea, fatigue, weight loss, and low-grade fever. A nonproductive cough is common, but occasionally expectoration of "chunky" gelatinous material may occur. Polycythemia, hypergammaglobulinemia, and increased LDH levels are frequent. Markedly elevated serum levels of lung surfactant proteins A and D have been found in PAP. Radiographically, bilateral symmetric alve-

olar opacities located centrally in mid and lower lung zones result in a "bat-wing" distribution. HRCT shows a ground-glass opacification and thickened intralobular structures and interlobular septa. Whole lung lavage(s) through a double-lumen endotracheal tube provides relief to many patients with dyspnea or progressive hypoxemia and also may provide long-term benefit.

PULMONARY LYMPHANGIOLEIOMYOMATOSIS   Pulmonary LAM is a rare condition that afflicts premenopausal women and should be suspected in young women with emphysema, recurrent pneumothorax, or chylous pleural effusion. It is often misdiagnosed as asthma or chronic obstructive pulmonary disease. Pathologically, LAM is characterized by the proliferation of atypical pulmonary interstitial smooth muscle and cyst formation. The immature-appearing smooth-muscle cells react with monoclonal antibody HMB45, which recognizes a 100-kDa glycoprotein (gp100) originally found in human melanoma cells. Caucasians are affected much more commonly than members of other racial groups. The disease accelerates during pregnancy and abates after oopherectomy. Common complaints at presentation are dyspnea, cough, and chest pain. Hemoptysis may be life threatening. Spontaneous pneumothorax occurs in 50% of patients; it may be bilateral and necessitate pleurodesis. Meningioma and renal angiomyolipomas (hamartomas), characteristic findings in the genetic disorder tuberous sclerosis, are also common in patients with LAM. Chylothorax, chyloperitonium (chylous ascites), chyluria, and chylopericardium are other complications. Pulmonary function testing usually reveals an obstructive or mixed obstructive-restrictive pattern, and gas exchange is often abnormal. HRCT shows thin-walled cysts surrounded by normal lung without zonal predominance. Progression is common, with a median survival of 8 to 10 years from diagnosis. Oophorectomy, progesterone (10 mg/d), and, more recently, tamoxifen and luteinizing hormone–releasing hormone analogues have been used. Lung transplantation offers the only hope for cure despite reports of recurrent disease in the transplanted lung.

SYNDROMES OF ILD WITH DIFFUSE ALVEOLAR HEMORRHAGE   Injury to arterioles, venules, and the alveolar septal (alveolar wall or interstitial) capillaries can result in hemoptysis secondary to disruption of the alveolar-capillary basement membrane. This results in bleeding into the alveolar spaces, which characterizes DAH. Pulmonary capillaritis, characterized by a neutrophilic infiltration of the alveolar septae, may lead to necrosis of these structures, loss of capillary structural integrity, and the pouring of red blood cells into the alveolar space. Fibrinoid necrosis of the interstitium and red blood cells within the interstitial space are sometimes seen. Bland pulmonary hemorrhage (i.e., DAH without inflammation of the alveolar structures) may also occur.

The clinical onset is often abrupt, with cough, fever, and dyspnea. Severe respiratory distress requiring ventilatory support may be evident at initial presentation. Although hemoptysis is expected, it can be absent at the time of presentation in one-third of the cases. For patients without hemoptysis, new alveolar opacities, a falling hemoglobin level, and hemorrhagic BAL fluid point to the diagnosis. The chest radiograph is nonspecific and most commonly shows new patchy or diffuse alveolar opacities. Recurrent episodes of DAH may lead to pulmonary fibrosis, resulting in interstitial opacities on the chest radiograph. An elevated white blood cell count and falling hematocrit are frequent. Evidence for impaired renal function caused by focal segmental necrotizing glomerulonephritis, usually with crescent formation, may also be present.

Varying degrees of hypoxemia may occur and are often severe enough to require ventilatory support. The DL_{CO} may be increased, resulting from the increased hemoglobin within the alveoli compartment. Evaluation of either lung or renal tissue by immunofluorescent techniques indicates an absence of immune complexes (pauci-immune) in Wegener's granulomatosis, microscopic polyangiitis pauci-immune glomerulonephritis, and isolated pulmonary capillaritis. A granular pattern is found in the CTDs, particularly SLE, and a characteristic linear deposition is found in Goodpasture's syndrome. Granular deposition of IgA-containing immune complexes is present in Henoch-Schönlein purpura.

The mainstay of therapy for the DAH associated with systemic vasculitis, CTD, Goodpasture's syndrome, and isolated pulmonary capillaritis is intravenous methylprednisolone, 0.5 to 2.0 g daily in divided doses for up to 5 days, followed by a gradual tapering, and then maintenance on an oral preparation. Prompt initiation of therapy is important, particularly in the face of renal insufficiency, since early initiation of therapy has the best chance of preserving renal function. The decision to start other immunosuppressive therapy (cyclophosphamide or azathioprine) acutely depends on the severity of illness.

Goodpasture's Syndrome   Pulmonary hemorrhage and glomerulonephritis are features in most patients with this disease. Autoantibodies to renal glomerular and lung alveolar basement membranes are present. This syndrome can present and recur as DAH without an associated glomerulonephritis. In such case, circulating anti-basement membrane antibody is often absent, and the only way to establish the diagnosis is by demonstrating linear immunofluorescence in lung tissue. The underlying histology may be bland hemorrhage or DAH associated with capillaritis. Plasmapheresis has been recommended as adjunctive treatment.

INHERITED DISORDERS ASSOCIATED WITH ILD   Pulmonary opacities and respiratory symptoms typical of ILD can develop in related family members and in several inherited diseases. These include the phakomatoses, tuberous sclerosis and neurofibromatosis (Chap. 358), and the lysosomal storage diseases, Niemann-Pick disease and Gaucher's disease (Chap. 340). The Hermansky-Pudlak syndrome (Chap. 101) is an autosomal recessive disorder in which granulomatous colitis and ILD may occur. It is characterized by oculocutaneous albinism, bleeding diathesis secondary to platelet dysfunction, and the accumulation of a chromolipid, lipofuscin material in cells of the reticuloendothelial system. A UIP-like pattern is found on lung biopsy, but the alveolar macrophages may contain cytoplasmic ceroid-like inclusions.

ILD WITH A GRANULOMATOUS RESPONSE IN LUNG TISSUE OR VASCULAR STRUCTURES   Inhalation of organic dusts, which cause hypersensitivity pneumonitis, or of inorganic dust, such as silica, which elicits a granulomatous inflammatory reaction leading to ILD, produces diseases of known etiology (Table 243-1) that are discussed in Chaps. 237 and 238. Sarcoidosis (Chap. 309) is prominent among granulomatous diseases of unknown cause in which ILD is an important feature.

Pulmonary Langerhans Cell Histiocytosis   PLCH is a rare, smoking-related, diffuse lung disease that primarily affects men between the ages of 20 and 40 years. The clinical presentation varies from an asymptomatic state to a rapidly progressive condition. The most common clinical manifestations at presentation are cough, dyspnea, chest pain, weight loss, and fever. Pneumothorax occurs in about 25% of patients. Hemoptysis and diabetes insipidus are rare manifestations. The radiographic features vary with the stage of the disease. The combination of ill-defined or stellate nodules (2 to 10 mm in diameter), reticular or nodular opacities, bizarre-shaped upper zone cysts, preservation of lung volume, and sparing of the costophrenic angles are characteristics of PLCH. HRCT that reveals a combination of nodules and thin-walled cysts is virtually diagnostic of PLCH. The most frequent pulmonary function abnormality is a markedly reduced DL_{CO}, although varying degrees of restrictive disease, airflow limitation, and diminished exercise capacity may occur. Discontinuance of smoking is the key treatment, resulting in clinical improvement in one-third of patients. Most patients with PLCH suffer persistent or progressive disease. Death due to respiratory failure occurs in ~10% of patients.

Granulomatous Vasculitides   (See also Chap. 306)   The granulomatous vasculitides are characterized by pulmonary angiitis (i.e., inflammation and necrosis of blood vessels) with associated granuloma formation (i.e., infiltrates of lymphocytes, plasma cells, epithelioid cells, or his-

tiocytes, with or without the presence of multinucleated giant cells, sometimes with tissue necrosis). The lungs are almost always involved, although any organ system may be affected. Wegener's granulomatosis and allergic angiitis and granulomatosis (Churg-Strauss syndrome) primarily affect the lung but are associated with a systemic vasculitis as well. The granulomatous vasculitides generally limited to the lung include necrotizing sarcoid granulomatosis and benign lymphocytic angiitis and granulomatosis. Granulomatous infection and pulmonary angiitis due to irritating embolic material (e.g., talc) are important known causes of pulmonary vasculitis.

LYMPHOCYTIC INFILTRATIVE DISORDERS   This group of disorders features lymphocyte and plasma cell infiltration of the lung parenchyma. The disorders either are benign or can behave as low-grade lymphomas. Included are angioimmunoblastic lymphadenopathy with dysproteinemia, a rare lymphoproliferative disorder characterized by diffuse lymphadenopathy, fever, hepatosplenomegaly, and hemolytic anemia, with ILD in some cases.

Lymphocytic Interstitial Pneumonitis   This rare form of ILD occurs in adults, some of whom have an autoimmune disease or dysproteinemia. It has been reported in patients with Sjögren's syndrome and HIV infection.

Lymphomatoid Granulomatosis   This multisystem disorder of unknown etiology is an angiocentric malignant (T cell) lymphoma characterized by a polymorphic lymphoid infiltrate, an angiitis, and granulomatosis. Although it may affect virtually any organ, it is most frequently characterized by pulmonary, skin, and central nervous system involvement.

BRONCHOCENTRIC GRANULOMATOSIS   Rather than a specific clinical entity, bronchocentric granulomatosis (BG) is a descriptive histologic term that describes an uncommon and nonspecific pathologic response to a variety of airway injuries. There is evidence that BG is caused by a hypersensitivity reaction to *Aspergillus* or other fungi in patients with asthma. About half of the patients described have chronic asthma with severe wheezing and peripheral blood eosinophilia. In patients with asthma, BG probably represents one pathologic manifestation of allergic bronchopulmonary aspergillosis or another allergic mycosis. In patients without asthma, BG has been associated with RA and a variety of infections, including tuberculosis, echinococcosis, histoplasmosis, coccidioidomycosis, and nocardiosis. The chest roentgenogram reveals irregularly shaped nodular or mass lesions with ill-defined margins, which are usually unilateral and solitary, with an upper-lobe predominance. Glucocorticoids are the treatment of choice, often with excellent outcome, although recurrences may occur as therapy is tapered or stopped.

FURTHER READING

AMERICAN THORACIC SOCIETY/EUROPEAN RESPIRATORY SOCIETY: Idiopathic pulmonary fibrosis: Diagnosis and treatment. International consensus statement. Am J Respir Crit Care Med 161:646, 2000

————: International multidisciplinary consensus classification of the idiopathic interstitial pneumonias. Am J Respir Crit Care Med 165:277, 2002

FREEMER M, KING TE JR: Connective tissue disease, in MI Schwarz, TE King, Jr (eds): *Interstitial Lung Diseases*, 4th ed. Hamilton, Ontario, BC Decker, 2003, pp 535–598

KING TE Jr: Idiopathic interstitial pneumonias, in MI Schwarz, TE King, Jr (eds): *Interstitial Lung Diseases,* 4th ed. Hamilton, Ontario, BC Decker, 2003, pp 701–786

SELMAN M et al: Idiopathic pulmonary fibrosis: Prevailing and evolving hypotheses about its pathogenesis and implications for therapy. Ann Intern Med 134:136, 2001

SEYMOUR JF, PRESNEILL JJ: Pulmonary alveolar proteinosis: Progress in the first 44 years. Am J Respir Crit Care Med 166:215, 2002

SULLIVAN EJ: Lymphangioleiomyomatosis: A review. Chest 114:1689, 1998

THOMAS AQ et al: Heterozygosity for a surfactant protein C gene mutation associated with usual interstitial pneumonitis and cellular nonspecific interstitial pneumonitis in one kindred. Am J Respir Crit Care Med 165:1322, 2002

VASSALLO R et al: Clinical outcomes of pulmonary Langerhans'-cell histiocytosis in adults. N Engl J Med 346:484, 2002

PREDISPOSITION TO PULMONARY THROMBOEMBOLISM

Acquired and genetic factors contribute to the likelihood of venous thromboembolism. Acquired predispositions include long-haul air travel, obesity, cigarette smoking, oral contraceptives, pregnancy, postmenopausal hormone replacement, surgery, trauma, and medical conditions such as antiphospholipid antibody syndrome, cancer, systemic arterial hypertension, and chronic obstructive pulmonary disease. Thrombophilia contributes greatly to the risk of venous thrombosis, often due to an inherited risk factor in combination with an acquired predisposition. The two most common autosomal dominant genetic mutations are the factor V Leiden and the prothrombin gene mutations (Chap. 56). Only a minority of patients with venous thromboembolism has identifiable predisposing genetic factors. Some patients with predisposing genetic factors will never develop clinical evidence of clotting.

PATHOPHYSIOLOGY

EMBOLIZATION When venous thrombi dislodge from their site of formation, they embolize to the pulmonary arterial circulation or, paradoxically, to the arterial circulation through a patent foramen ovale or atrial septal defect. About half of patients with pelvic vein thrombosis or proximal leg deep venous thrombosis (DVT) have pulmonary thromboembolism (PE), which is usually asymptomatic. Isolated calf vein thrombi pose a lower risk of PE, but they are the most common source of paradoxical embolism. With increased use of chronic indwelling central venous catheters for hyperalimentation and chemotherapy, as well as more frequent insertion of permanent pacemakers and internal cardiac defibrillators, upper extremity venous thrombosis is becoming a more common problem. These thrombi may also embolize and cause PE.

PHYSIOLOGY Pulmonary embolism can have the following effects:

1. *Increased pulmonary vascular resistance* due to vascular obstruction or platelet secretion of neurohumoral agents including serotonin
2. *Impaired gas exchange* due to increased alveolar dead space from vascular obstruction, hypoxemia from alveolar hypoventilation relative to perfusion in the nonobstructed lung, right-to-left shunting, and impaired carbon monoxide transfer due to loss of gas exchange surface
3. *Alveolar hyperventilation* due to reflex stimulation of irritant receptors
4. *Increased airway resistance* due to constriction of airways distal to the bronchi
5. *Decreased pulmonary compliance* due to lung edema, lung hemorrhage, or loss of surfactant

Right Ventricular Dysfunction Progressive right heart failure is the usual cause of death from PE. In the International Cooperative Pulmonary Embolism Registry (ICOPER), the presence of right ventricular dysfunction on baseline echocardiography of PE patients was associated with a doubling of the 3-month mortality rate. As pulmonary vascular resistance increases, right ventricular wall tension rises and perpetuates further right ventricular dilatation and dysfunction. Consequently, the interventricular septum bulges into and compresses an intrinsically normal left ventricle. Increased right ventricular wall tension also compresses the right coronary artery and may precipitate myocardial ischemia and right ventricular infarction. Underfilling of the left ventricle may lead to a fall in left ventricular output and systemic arterial pressure, thereby provoking myocardial ischemia due to compromised coronary artery perfusion. Eventually, circulatory collapse and death may ensue.

DIAGNOSIS

The clinical setting, including risk factors such as family history or personal prior history of venous thromboembolism, can help suggest the diagnosis of PE. Semi-quantitative clinical scoring systems such as the Wells Diagnostic Scoring System are beginning to replace "gestalt" estimates of clinical likelihood (Table 244-1).

CLINICAL SYNDROMES Patients with *massive PE* present with systemic arterial hypotension and usually have anatomically widespread thromboembolism. Primary therapy with thrombolysis or embolectomy offers the greatest chance of survival. Those with *moderate to large PE* have right ventricular hypokinesis on echocardiography but normal systemic arterial pressure. Optimal management is controversial; such patients may benefit from thrombolysis or embolectomy rather than anticoagulation alone. Patients with *small to moderate PE* have both normal right heart function and normal systemic arterial pressure. They have a good prognosis with either adequate anticoagulation. The presence of *pulmonary infarction* usually indicates a small PE, but one that is exquisitely painful, because it lodges peripherally, near the innervation of pleural nerves. However, larger, more central PEs can occur concomitantly with peripheral pulmonary infarction.

Nonthrombotic pulmonary embolism may be easily overlooked. Possible etiologies include fat embolism after blunt trauma and long bone fractures, tumor embolism, or air embolism. Intravenous drug users may inject themselves with a wide array of substances, such as hair, talc, or cotton. *Amniotic fluid embolism* occurs when fetal membranes leak or tear at the placental margin. The pulmonary edema seen in this syndrome is probably due primarily to alveolar capillary leakage.

SYMPTOMS AND SIGNS Dyspnea is the most frequent symptom of PE, and tachypnea is its most frequent sign. Whereas dyspnea, syncope, hypotension, or cyanosis indicates a massive PE, pleuritic pain, cough, or hemoptysis often suggests a small embolism located distally near the pleura. On physical examination, young and previously healthy individuals may simply appear anxious but otherwise seem deceptively well, even with an anatomically large PE. They may only have dyspnea with moderate exertion. They often lack "classic" signs such as tachycardia, low-grade fever, neck vein distention, or an accentuated pulmonic component of the second heart sound. Sometimes, a paradoxical bradycardia occurs.

In older patients who complain of vague chest discomfort, the diagnosis of PE may not be apparent unless signs of right heart failure are present. Unfortunately, because acute coronary ischemic syndromes are so common, one may overlook the possibility of life-threatening PE and may inadvertently discharge these patients from the hospital after the exclusion of myocardial infarction with serial blood tests to detect cardiac injury and serial electrocardiograms.

DIFFERENTIAL DIAGNOSIS The differential diagnosis of PE is broad (Table 244-2). Although PE is known as "the great masquerader," quite often other illnesses simulate PE. For example, when the proposed diagnosis of PE is supposedly confirmed with a combination of dysp-

TABLE 244-1 *Wells Diagnostic Scoring System^a for Suspected PE*	
	Points
• Clinical signs and symptoms of DVT (minimum of leg swelling and pain with palpation of the deep veins)	3.0
• An alternative diagnosis is less likely than PE	3.0
• Heart rate >100 beats/min	1.5
• Immobilization or surgery in the previous 4 weeks	1.5
• Previous DVT/PE	1.5
• Hemoptysis	1.0
• Malignancy (on treatment, treated in the past 6 months, or palliative)	1.0

^{a} The Wells Scoring System has a maximum of 12.5 points. If the score is ≤ 4 points, the likelihood of PE is only 8%.
Note: DVT, deep vein thrombosis; PE, pulmonary thromboembolism.
Source: Adapted with permission from PS Wells et al: Thromb Haemost 83:416, 2000.

TABLE 244-2 *Differential Diagnosis of Pulmonary Thromboembolism*

Acute coronary syndrome, including unstable angina and acute myocardial infarction

Pneumonia, bronchitis, exacerbation of asthma or chronic obstructive pulmonary disease

Congestive heart failure

Pericarditis

Pleurisy, including "viral syndrome," costochondritis, other musculoskeletal discomfort

Rib fracture, pneumothorax

Primary pulmonary hypertension

Anxiety

nea, chest pain, and an abnormal lung scan, the correct diagnosis of pneumonia might become apparent 12 h later when an infiltrate blossoms on chest x-ray, purulent sputum is first produced, and high fever and shaking chills develop.

Some patients have PE and a coexisting illness such as pneumonia or heart failure. In such circumstances, clinical improvement will often fail to occur despite standard medical treatment of the concomitant illness. This situation can serve as a clinical clue to the possible coexistence of PE.

NONIMAGING DIAGNOSTIC MODALITIES   These are generally less expensive but also less specific than diagnostic modalities that employ imaging.

Blood Tests   The quantitative *plasma D-dimer enzyme-linked immunosorbent assay (ELISA)* level is elevated (>500 ng/mL) in more than 90% of patients with PE, reflecting plasmin's breakdown of fibrin and indicating endogenous (though clinically ineffective) thrombolysis. However, the D-dimer assay is not specific and therefore has no useful role among patients who are already hospitalized. Levels increase in patients with myocardial infarction, sepsis, or almost any systemic illness. The plasma D-dimer ELISA has a high negative predictive value and can be used to help exclude PE. In a prospective 1-year evaluation, the Emergency Department at Brigham and Women's Hospital mandated obtaining a D-dimer ELISA in all 1106 patients suspected of PE. It served as an excellent screening test, with a sensitivity of 96.4% and negative predictive value of 99.6%.

Data from the Prospective Investigation of Pulmonary Embolism Diagnosis (PIOPED) indicate that, contrary to classic teaching, *arterial blood gases* lack diagnostic utility for PE, even though the P_{O_2} and P_{CO_2} will often both decrease. Among patients suspected of PE, neither the room air arterial P_{O_2} nor calculation of the alveolar-arterial oxygen gradient can reliably differentiate or triage patients who actually have PE at angiography.

Electrocardiogram   Classic abnormalities include sinus tachycardia; new-onset atrial fibrillation or flutter; and an S wave in lead I, a Q wave in lead III, and an inverted T wave in lead III (Chap. 210). Often, the QRS axis is greater than 90°. T-wave inversion in leads V_1 to V_4, perhaps the most frequent but least publicized change, reflects right ventricular strain.

NONINVASIVE IMAGING MODALITIES ■ Chest Roentgenography   A normal or near-normal chest x-ray in a dyspneic patient suggests PE. Well-established abnormalities include focal oligemia (Westermark's sign), a peripheral wedged-shaped density above the diaphragm (Hampton's hump), or an enlarged right descending pulmonary artery (Palla's sign).

Venous Ultrasonography   Confirmed DVT is usually an adequate surrogate for PE. Ultrasonography of the deep venous system relies upon loss of vein compressibility as the primary criterion for DVT. About one-half of patients with PE have no imaging evidence of DVT, probably because the clot has already embolized to the lung or is in the pelvic veins, where ultrasonography is usually inadequate. Therefore, the workup for PE should continue if there is high clinical suspicion, despite a normal ultrasound examination.

Chest CT   Computed tomography (CT) of the chest with intravenous contrast (ordinarily, 100 mL administered at 3 to 4 mL/s via an antecubital vein) is superseding lung scanning (see below) as the principal imaging test for the diagnosis of PE. Chest CT effectively diagnoses large, central PE (Fig. 244-1). New generation multislice scanners image the entire thorax with 1-mm thin sections during a single 12- to 15-s breath-hold and can detect peripherally located thrombi in fifth order branches. In patients without PE, the lung parenchymal images may establish alternative diagnoses not apparent on chest x-ray that explain the presenting symptoms and signs, such as pneumonia, emphysema, pulmonary fibrosis, pulmonary mass, or aortic pathology.

Lung Scanning (See also Chap. 235)   Small particulate aggregates of albumin labeled with a gamma-emitting radionuclide are injected intravenously and are trapped in the pulmonary capillary bed. The perfusion scan defect indicates absent or decreased blood flow, possibly due to PE. Ventilation scans, obtained with radiolabeled inhaled gases such as xenon or krypton, improve the specificity of the perfusion scan. Abnormal ventilation scans indicate abnormal nonventilated lung, thereby providing possible explanations for perfusion defects other than acute PE. A high probability scan for PE is defined as having two or more segmental perfusion defects in the presence of normal ventilation (Fig. 244-2).

The diagnosis of PE is very unlikely in patients with normal and near-normal scans but is about 90% certain in patients with high-probability scans. Unfortunately, most patients have nondiagnostic scans, and fewer than half of patients with angiographically confirmed PE have a high-probability scan. Importantly, as many as 40% of patients with high clinical suspicion for PE and "low-probability" scans do, in fact, have PE at angiography.

Magnetic Resonance (MR) (Contrast-Enhanced)   MR pulmonary angiography utilizes gadolinium contrast agent, which unlike iodinated contrast agents used in CT angiography, is not nephrotoxic. The risk of a contrast reaction with gadolinium is very low, and no ionizing radiation is used. When compared with first-generation chest CT scanning, results are similar. MR also assesses right ventricular function, thus making it a promising single test for both diagnosis of PE and assessment of hemodynamic effect.

Echocardiography   More than half of patients with PE will have normal echocardiograms Nevertheless, this imaging test helps with the rapid triage of extremely ill patients who may have PE. Bedside echocardiography can usually reliably differentiate among illnesses that have radically different treatment, including acute myocardial infarction, pericardial tamponade, dissection of the aorta, and PE complicated by right heart failure. McConnell's sign, i.e., right ventricular free wall hypokinesis with normal right ventricular apical motion, appears to be specific for PE. Detection of right ventricular dysfunction due to PE

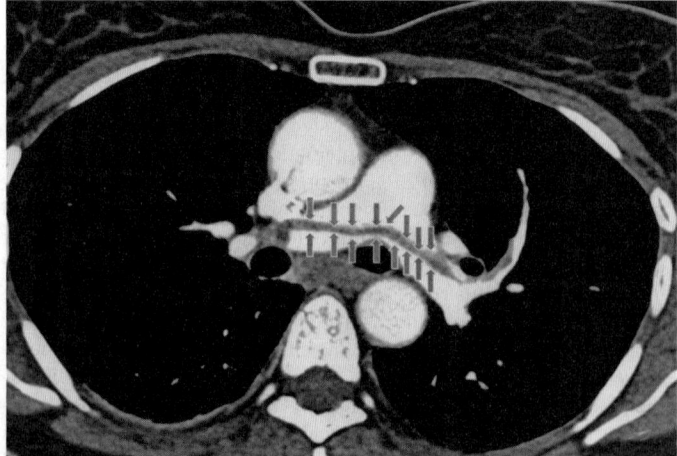

FIGURE 244-1   Bilateral "saddle" pulmonary thromboembolism computed tomography scan of the chest. The arrows outline the "saddle" (*Courtesy of Philip Costello, MD.*)

helps to stratify the risk, delineate the prognosis, and plan optimal management.

INVASIVE DIAGNOSTIC MODALITIES ■ Pulmonary Angiography Selective pulmonary angiography is the most specific examination available for establishing the definitive diagnosis of PE and can detect emboli as small as 1 to 2 mm. A definitive diagnosis of PE depends upon visualization of an intraluminal filling defect in more than one projection. Secondary signs of PE include abrupt occlusion ("cut-off") of vessels; segmental oligemia or avascularity; a prolonged arterial phase with slow filling; or tortuous, tapering peripheral vessels. Chest CT scanning is replacing diagnostic pulmonary angiography, because it is less invasive. In the current era of chest CT with contrast, pulmonary angiography is reserved for (1) patients with technically inadequate CT scans, (2) scans performed on older machines that cannot image fourth- and fifth-order pulmonary arteries, and (3) patients who will undergo interventions such as catheter embolectomy or catheter-directed thrombolysis.

Contrast Phlebography Venous ultrasonography has virtually replaced contrast phlebography, which is costly, uncomfortable, and occasionally results in contrast allergy or contrast-induced phlebitis.

INTEGRATED DIAGNOSTIC APPROACH We advocate an integrated diagnostic approach to streamline the workup of PE (Fig. 244-3). This strategy combines the clinical likelihood of PE with the results of noninvasive testing, especially D-dimer ELISA, venous ultrasonography, and chest CT or lung scanning to determine whether pulmonary angiography is warranted.

Rx TREATMENT

Primary Therapy versus Secondary Prevention *Primary therapy* consists of clot dissolution with thrombolysis or removal of PE by embolectomy. Anticoagulation with heparin and warfarin or placement of an inferior vena caval filter constitutes *secondary prevention* of recurrent PE rather than primary therapy.

Risk Stratification Risk stratification is crucial in determining treatment strategy. The presence of hemodynamic instability, right ventricular dysfunction, or elevation of the troponin level due to right ventricular microinfarction can identify high-risk patients.

Primary therapy should be reserved for patients at high risk of an adverse clinical outcome. When right ventricular function remains normal in a hemodynamically stable patient, a good clinical outcome is highly likely with anticoagulation alone (Fig. 244-4).

Adjunctive Therapy Important adjunctive measures include pain relief (especially with nonsteroidal anti-inflammatory agents), supplemental oxygenation, and psychological support. Dobutamine—a β-adrenergic agonist with positive inotropic and pulmonary vasodilating actions—may be effective in the treatment of right heart failure and cardiogenic shock. Volume loading should be undertaken cautiously because increased right ventricular dilatation can lead to even further reductions in left ventricular forward output.

Heparin Heparin binds to and accelerates the activity of antithrombin III, an enzyme that inhibits the coagulation factors thrombin (factor IIa), Xa, IXa, XIa, and XIIa. Heparin thus prevents additional thrombus formation and permits endogenous fibrinolytic mechanisms to lyse clot that has already formed. After 5 to 7 days of heparin, residual thrombus begins to stabilize in the endothelium of the vein or pulmonary artery. However, heparin does *not* directly dissolve thrombus that already exists.

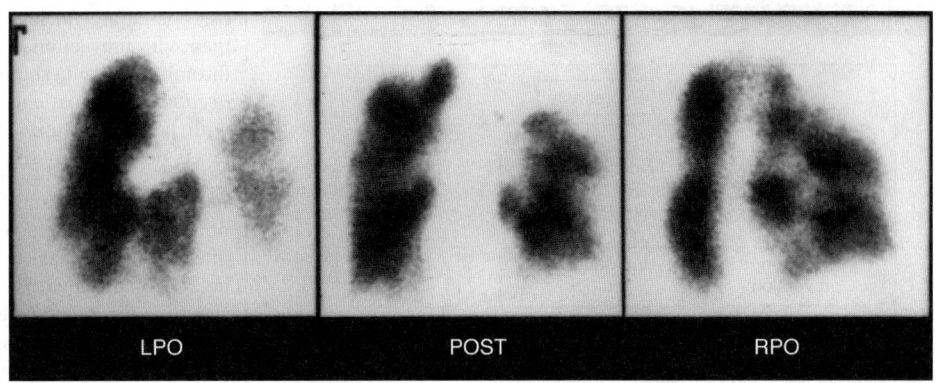

FIGURE 244-2 Three views of the pulmonary perfusion scan illustrating multiple segmental perfusion defects in both lung fields. The ventilation scan, which is normal, is not shown. The marked mismatch between normal ventilation and abnormal perfusion makes this lung scan *high probability* for pulmonary thromboembolism. LPO, left posterior oblique; POST, posterior; RPO, right posterior oblique.

MODIFIED CONSENSUS GUIDELINES FOR THE TREATMENT OF PULMONARY EMBOLISM FROM THE AMERICAN COLLEGE OF CHEST PHYSICIANS

1. Treat DVT or PE with therapeutic levels of unfractionated intravenous heparin, adjusted subcutaneous heparin, or low-molecular-weight heparin for at least 5 days, and overlap with oral anticoagulation for at least 4 to 5 days. Consider a longer course of heparin, approximately 10 days, for massive PE or severe iliofemoral DVT.

2. For most patients, heparin and oral anticoagulation can be started

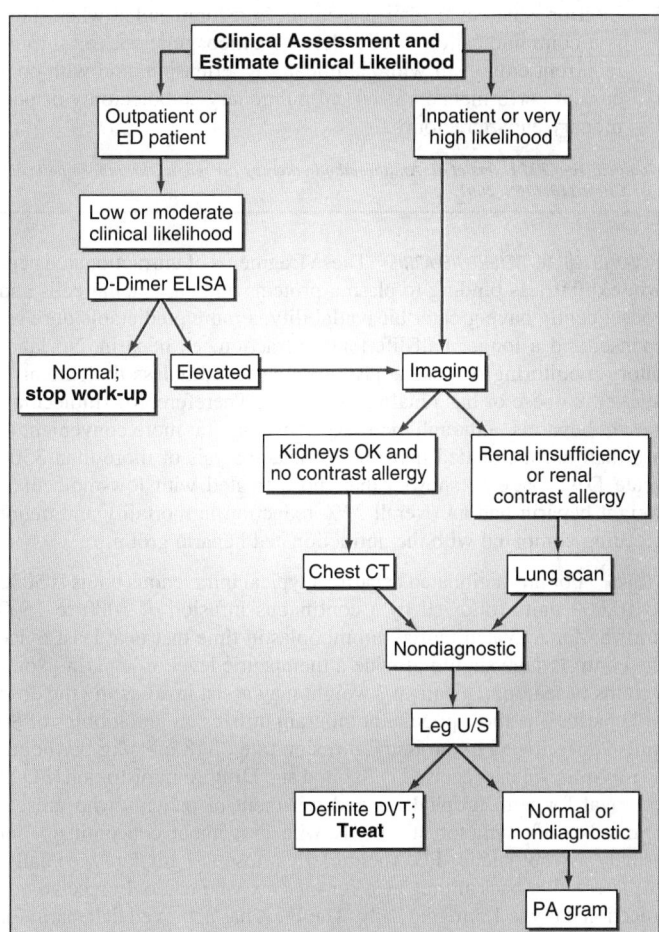

FIGURE 244-3 Diagnosis strategy for pulmonary thromboembolism: An integrated diagnostic approach. ED, emergency department; ELISA, enzyme-linked immunosorbent assay; CT, computed tomography; U/S, ultrasound; DVT, deep vein thrombosis; PA gram, pulmonary arteriogram.

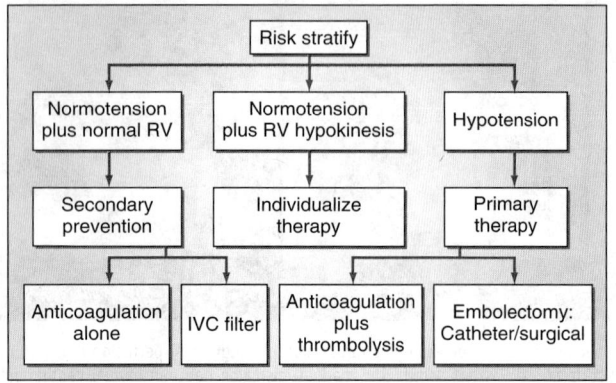

FIGURE 244-4 Acute management of pulmonary thromboembolism: RV, right ventricular; IVC, inferior vena cava.

together and heparin discontinued on day 5 or 6 if the INR has been therapeutic for two consecutive days.

3. Treat patients with reversible or time-limited risk factors for at least 3 months. Patients with a first episode of idiopathic DVT should be treated indefinitely. A proven regimen is warfarin, target INR of 2.0 to 3.0 for 6 months, followed by low-intensity warfarin, target INR of 1.5 to 2.0.

4. The use of thrombolytic agents continues to be highly individualized, and clinicians should have some latitude in using these agents. Patients with hemodynamically unstable PE or massive iliofemoral thrombosis are the best candidates.

5. Inferior vena caval filter placement is recommended when there is a contraindication to or failure of anticoagulation, for chronic recurrent embolism with pulmonary hypertension, and with concurrent performance of surgical pulmonary embolectomy or pulmonary endarterectomy.

Modified from TM Hyers et al: Antithrombotic therapy for venous thromboembolic disease Chest 119:176S, 2001.

LOW-MOLECULAR-WEIGHT HEPARINS These fragments of unfractionated heparin exhibit less binding to plasma proteins and endothelial cells and consequently have greater bioavailability, a more predictable dose response, and a longer half-life than unfractionated heparin. No laboratory monitoring or dose adjustment is needed unless the patient is markedly obese or has renal insufficiency. Therefore, low-molecular-weight heparins, although more expensive, are far more convenient to use than unfractionated heparin. A meta-analysis of more than 3500 acute DVT patients showed that those treated with low-molecular-weight heparin had an overall 29% reduction in mortality and major bleeding compared with the unfractionated heparin group.

DOSING For unfractionated heparin, a typical intravenous bolus is 5000 to 10,000 units followed by a continuous infusion of 1000 to 1500 units/h. An activated partial thromboplastin time that is at least twice the control value should provide a therapeutic level of heparin. Nomograms based upon a patient's weight may assist in adjusting the dose of heparin. The most popular nomogram utilizes an initial bolus of 80 units/kg, followed by an initial infusion rate of 18 units/kg per hour.

Enoxaparin has received U.S. Food and Drug Administration (FDA) approval for both prophylaxis and treatment of patients who present primarily with symptomatic DVT, with or without concomitant (but usually asymptomatic) PE. The preferred dose is 1 mg/kg twice daily. An alternative back-up regimen for patients who can only receive one injection daily is 1.5 mg/kg daily. The FDA has approved dalteparin for prophylaxis but not for treatment of venous thromboembolism.

COMPLICATIONS The most important adverse effect of heparin is hemorrhage. For life-threatening or intracranial hemorrhage, protamine sulfate can be administered. Heparin-induced thrombocytopenia and

osteopenia are far less common with low-molecular-weight heparins than with unfractionated heparin. Thrombosis due to heparin-induced thrombocytopenia should be managed with a direct thrombin inhibitor: *argatroban* for patients with renal insufficiency or *hirudin* for patients with hepatic failure. Heparin-associated elevations in transaminase levels occur commonly but are rarely associated with clinical toxicity.

Warfarin This vitamin K antagonist prevents γ carboxylation activation of coagulation factors II, VII, IX, and X. The full effect of warfarin often requires 5 days, even if the prothrombin time, used for monitoring, becomes elevated more rapidly. When warfarin is initiated during an active thrombotic state, the levels of protein C and S decline, thus creating a paradoxical thrombogenic potential. By overlapping either unfractionated or low-molecular-weight heparin and warfarin for 5 days, the early procoagulant effect of unopposed warfarin can be counteracted. Thus, heparin acts as a "bridge" until the full anticoagulant effect of warfarin is obtained.

DOSING In an average-sized adult, warfarin is usually initiated in a dose of 5 mg. Doses of 7.5 or 10 mg can be used in obese or large-framed young patients who are otherwise healthy. Patients who are malnourished or who have received prolonged courses of antibiotics are probably deficient in vitamin K and should receive smaller initial doses of warfarin, such as 2.5 mg. An uncommon genetic mutation delays the metabolism of warfarin, resulting in a very low dose requirement, 1 to 2 mg daily, to achieve a therapeutic affect. The prothrombin time is standardized with the INR, which assesses the anticoagulant effect of warfarin (Chap. 103). The target INR is usually 2.5, with a range of 2.0 to 3.0.

COMPLICATIONS As with heparin, bleeding is the most important and common complication associated with warfarin administration. Life-threatening bleeding can be treated with cryoprecipitate or fresh-frozen plasma (usually 2 units) to achieve immediate hemostasis. Recombinant factor VIIa is an effective, novel therapy for life-threatening bleeding in the setting of excessive warfarin. For less serious bleeding, or an excessively high INR in the absence of bleeding, vitamin K may be administered. Reversing excessive INRs by withholding warfarin and prescribing a low dose of oral vitamin K, such as 2.5 mg, will facilitate reestablishing a stable dose of warfarin.

Warfarin-induced skin necrosis is a rare complication that may be related to warfarin-induced reduction of protein C. It is usually associated with administration of a high initial dose of warfarin during an acute thrombotic state in which heparin is withheld.

During pregnancy, warfarin should be avoided if possible because of warfarin embryopathy, which is most common with exposure during the sixth through twelfth weeks of gestation. However, women can take warfarin postpartum and breast feed safely. Warfarin can also be administered safely during the second trimester.

DURATION OF ANTICOAGULATION Patients with PE following surgery or trauma ordinarily have a low rate of recurrence after 6 months of anticoagulation. In contrast, among patients with "idiopathic" PE, the recurrence rate is surprisingly high after cessation of anticoagulation. The PREVENT Trial establishes intensive anticoagulation with warfarin for 6 months, target INR of 2.0 to 3.0 followed by an indefinite duration of anticoagulation with low-intensity warfarin, target INR of 1.5 to 2.0.

Inferior Vena Caval Filters The two principal indications for insertion of an inferior vena caval filter are: (1) active bleeding that precludes anticoagulation, and (2) recurrent venous thrombosis despite intensive anticoagulation. Prevention of recurrent PE in patients with right heart failure who are not candidates for thrombolysis or prophylaxis of extremely high-risk patients are "softer" indications that are being utilized less frequently. The filter itself may fail by permitting the passage of small to medium-sized clots or because large thrombi embolize to the pulmonary arteries via collateral veins that develop. A more common complication is caval thrombosis with marked bilateral leg swelling. Paradoxically, by providing a nidus for clot formation, filters double the DVT rate over the ensuing 2 years following placement.

Thrombolysis Successful thrombolytic therapy rapidly reverses right heart failure and leads to a lower rate of death and recurrent PE. Thrombolysis usually: (1) dissolves much of the anatomically obstructing pulmonary arterial thrombus; (2) prevents the continued release of serotonin and other neurohumoral factors that exacerbate pulmonary hypertension; and (3) dissolves much of the source of the thrombus in the pelvic or deep leg veins, thereby decreasing the likelihood of recurrent PE.

The preferred thrombolytic regimen is 100 mg of recombinant tissue plasminogen activator (tPA) administered as a continuous peripheral intravenous infusion over 2 h. Patients appear to respond to thrombolysis for up to 14 days after the PE has occurred. MAPPET-3 (Management Strategy and Prognosis of Pulmonary Embolism Trial) is the largest randomized trial of thrombolysis (using 100 mg of tPA plus anticoagulation versus anticoagulation alone); 247 patients were enrolled with hemodynamically stable PE. Escalation of therapy (including use of pressors or intubation) was necessary in 24% of those receiving anticoagulation alone compared with 12% of those receiving tPA.

Contraindications to thrombolysis include intracranial disease, recent surgery, or trauma. There is a 1 to 2% risk of intracranial hemorrhage. Careful screening of patients for contraindications to thrombolysis is the best way to minimize bleeding risk.

Embolectomy The risk of intracranial hemorrhage with thrombolysis has prompted reevaluation of surgical embolectomy for acute PE. At Brigham and Women's Hospital, 29 patients with massive PE were operated on in 25 months, with an 89% survival rate. This high survival rate may be attributed to improved surgical technique, rapid diagnosis and triage, and careful patient selection. A possible alternative to open surgical embolectomy is catheter embolectomy.

Pulmonary Thromboendarterectomy Patients who develop chronic pulmonary hypertension due to prior PE may become severely dyspneic at rest or with minimal exertion. They should be considered for pulmonary thromboendarterectomy which, if successful, can markedly reduce and at times even cure pulmonary hypertension (Chap. 220).

PREVENTION

Prophylaxis against PE is of paramount importance because venous thromboembolism is difficult to detect and poses an excessive medical and economic burden. Mechanical and pharmacologic measures often succeed in preventing this complication (Table 244-3). Patients at high risk can receive a combination of mechanical and pharmacologic modalities. Graduated compression stockings and pneumatic compression devices may complement mini-dose unfractionated heparin (5000 units subcutaneously twice or preferably three times daily), low-molecular-weight heparin, a pentasaccharide or warfarin administration. Computerized reminder systems can increase the use of preventive care among these patients. Patients who have undergone total hip replacement, total knee replacement, or cancer surgery will benefit from extended pharmacologic prophylaxis for a total of 4 to 6 weeks, especially with low-molecular-weight heparin.

TABLE 244-3 *Prevention of Pulmonary Thromboembolism*

Condition	Prophylaxis Strategy
High-risk general surgery	Mini-UFH + GCS *or* LMWH + GCS
Thoracic surgery	Mini-UFH + IPC
Cancer surgery, including gynecologic cancer surgery	LMWH, consider 1 month of prophylaxis
Total hip replacement, total knee replacement, hip fracture surgery	LMWH, fondaparinux (a pentasaccharide) 2.5 mg sc, once daily *or* (except for total knee replacement) warfarin (target INR 2.5)
Neurosurgery	GCS + IPC
Neurosurgery for brain tumor	Mini-UFH *or* LMWH, + IPC, + predischarge venous ultrasonography
Benign gynecologic surgery	Mini-UFH + GCS
Medically ill patients	Mini-UFH *or* LMWH
Anticoagulation contraindicated	GCS + IPC
Long-haul air travel	Consider LMWH for very high risk patients

Note: Mini-UFH, minidose unfractionated heparin, 5000 units subcutaneously twice (less effective) or three times daily (more effective); GCS, graduated compression stockings, usually 10–18 mm Hg; LMWH, low-molecular-weight heparin, typically in the United States, enoxaparin, 40 mg once daily, or dalteparin, 2500 or 5000 units once daily; IPC, intermittent pneumatic compression devices.

FURTHER READING

AKLOG L et al: Acute pulmonary embolectomy: A contemporary approach. Circulation 105:1416, 2002

DECOUSUS H et al: A clinical trial of vena caval filters in the prevention of pulmonary embolism in patients with proximal deep-vein thrombosis. N Engl J Med 338:409, 1998

DUNN KL et al: Normal D-dimer levels in emergency department patients suspected of acute pulmonary embolism. J Am Coll Cardiol 40:1475, 2002

GOLDHABER SZ: Echocardiography in the management of pulmonary embolism. Ann Intern Med 136:691, 2002

———— et al: Acute pulmonary embolism: Clinical outcomes in the International Cooperative Pulmonary Embolism Registry (ICOPER). Lancet 353:1386, 1999

———— et al: New onset of venous thromboembolism among hospitalized patients at Brigham and Women's Hospital is caused more often by prophylaxis failure than by withholding treatment. Chest 118:1680, 2000

HIGASHI MK et al: Association between CYP2C9 genetic variants and anticoagulation-related outcomes during warfarin therapy. JAMA 287:1690, 2002

KONSTANTINIDES S et al: Heparin plus alteplase compared with heparin alone in patients with submassive pulmonary embolism. N Engl J Med 347:1143, 2002

LAPOSTOLLE F et al: Severe pulmonary embolism associated with air travel. N Engl J Med 345:779, 2001

RIDKER P et al: Long-term, low-intensity warfarin therapy for the prevention of recurrent venous thromboembolism. N Engl J Med 348:1425, 2003

245 DISORDERS OF THE PLEURA, MEDIASTINUM, DIAPHRAGM, AND CHEST WALL
Richard W. Light

DISORDERS OF THE PLEURA

PLEURAL EFFUSION The pleural space lies between the lung and chest wall and normally contains a very thin layer of fluid, which serves as a coupling system. A pleural effusion is present when there is an excess quantity of fluid in the pleural space.

Etiology Pleural fluid accumulates when pleural fluid formation exceeds pleural fluid absorption. Normally, fluid enters the pleural space from the capillaries in the parietal pleura and is removed via the lymphatics situated in the parietal pleura. Fluid can also enter the pleural space from the interstitial spaces of the lung via the visceral pleura or from the peritoneal cavity via small holes in the diaphragm. The lymphatics have the capacity to absorb 20 times more fluid than is normally formed. Accordingly, a pleural effusion may develop when there is excess pleural fluid formation (from the interstitial spaces of the lung, the parietal pleura, or the peritoneal cavity) or when there is decreased fluid removal by the lymphatics.

Diagnostic Approach When a patient is found to have a pleural effusion, an effort should be made to determine the cause (Fig. 245-1). The first step is to determine whether the effusion is a transudate or an exudate. A *transudative pleural effusion* occurs when *systemic factors* that in-

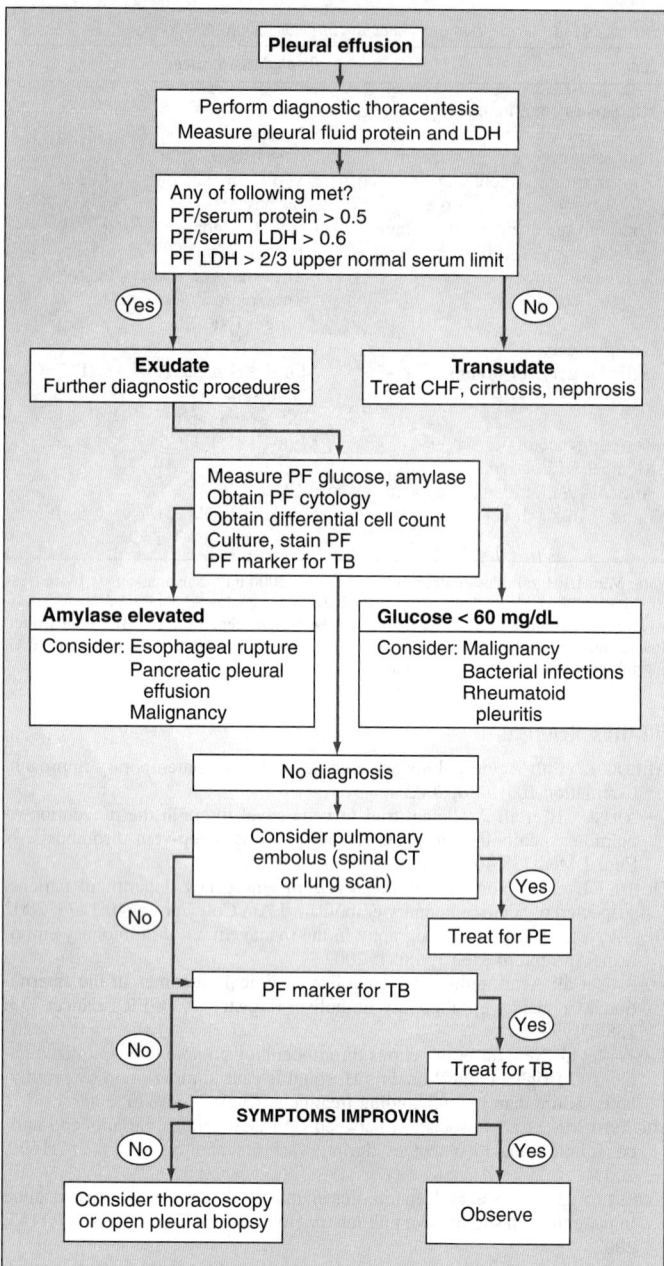

FIGURE 245-1   Approach to the diagnosis of pleural effusions. CHF, congestive heart failure; CT, computed tomography; LDH, lactate dehydrogenase; PE, pulmonary embolism; TB, tuberculosis; PF, pleural fluid.

fluence the formation and absorption of pleural fluid are altered. The leading causes of transudative pleural effusions in the United States are left ventricular failure, pulmonary embolism, and cirrhosis. An *exudative pleural effusion* occurs when *local factors* that influence the formation and absorption of pleural fluid are altered. The leading causes of exudative pleural effusions are bacterial pneumonia, malignancy, viral infection, and pulmonary embolism. The primary reason to make this differentiation is that additional diagnostic procedures are indicated with exudative effusions to define the cause of the local disease.

Transudative and exudative pleural effusions are distinguished by measuring the lactate dehydrogenase (LDH) and protein levels in the pleural fluid. Exudative pleural effusions meet at least one of the following criteria, whereas transudative pleural effusions meet none:

1. pleural fluid protein/serum protein >0.5
2. pleural fluid LDH/serum LDH >0.6

3. pleural fluid LDH more than two-thirds normal upper limit for serum

The above criteria misidentify approximately 25% of transudates as exudates. If one or more of the exudative criteria are met and the patient is clinically thought to have a condition producing a transudative effusion, the difference between the albumin levels in the serum and the pleural fluid should be measured. If this gradient is greater than 12 g/L (1.2 g/dL), the exudative categorization by the above criteria can be ignored because almost all such patients have a transudative pleural effusion.

If a patient has an exudative pleural effusion, the following tests on the pleural fluid should be obtained: description of the fluid, glucose level, differential cell count, microbiologic studies, and cytology.

Effusion due to Heart Failure   The most common cause of pleural effusion is left ventricular failure. The effusion occurs because the increased amounts of fluid in the lung interstitial spaces exit in part across the visceral pleura. This overwhelms the capacity of the lymphatics in the parietal pleura to remove fluid. A diagnostic thoracentesis should be performed if the effusions are not bilateral and comparable in size, if the patient is febrile, or if the patient has pleuritic chest pain to verify that the patient has a transudative effusion. Otherwise the patient is best treated with diuretics. If the effusion persists despite diuretic therapy, a diagnostic thoracentesis should be performed.

Hepatic Hydrothorax   Pleural effusions occur in approximately 5% of patients with cirrhosis and ascites. The predominant mechanism is the direct movement of peritoneal fluid through small holes in the diaphragm into the pleural space. The effusion is usually right-sided and frequently is large enough to produce severe dyspnea. If medical management does not control the ascites and the effusion, the best treatment is a liver transplant. If the patient is not a candidate for this, the best alternative is insertion of a transjugular intrahepatic portal systemic shunt.

Parapneumonic Effusion   Parapneumonic effusions are associated with bacterial pneumonia, lung abscess, or bronchiectasis and are probably the most common exudative pleural effusion in the United States. *Empyema* refers to a grossly purulent effusion.

Patients with aerobic bacterial pneumonia and pleural effusion present with an acute febrile illness consisting of chest pain, sputum production, and leukocytosis. Patients with anaerobic infections present with a subacute illness with weight loss, a brisk leukocytosis, mild anemia, and a history of some factor that predisposes them to aspiration.

The possibility of a parapneumonic effusion should be considered whenever a patient with a bacterial pneumonia is initially evaluated. The presence of free pleural fluid can be demonstrated with a lateral decubitus radiograph, computed tomography (CT) of the chest, or ultrasound. If the free fluid separates the lung from the chest wall by more than 10 mm on one of these examinations, a therapeutic thoracentesis should be performed. Factors indicating the likely need for a procedure more invasive than a thoracentesis (in increasing order of importance) include:

1. loculated pleural fluid
2. pleural fluid pH < 7.20
3. pleural fluid glucose <3.3 mmol/L (<60 mg/dL)
4. positive Gram stain or culture of the pleural fluid
5. the presence of gross pus in the pleural space

If the fluid recurs after the initial therapeutic thoracentesis, a repeat thoracentesis should be performed if any of the above characteristics are present. If the fluid recurs a second time, tube thoracostomy should be performed if any of the poor prognostic factors are present. If the fluid cannot be completely removed with the therapeutic thoracentesis, consideration should be given to inserting a chest tube and instilling a thrombolytic (streptokinase, 250,000 units) or performing thoracoscopy with the breakdown of adhesions. Decortication should be considered when the above are ineffective.

Effusion Secondary to Malignancy   Malignant pleural effusions secondary to metastatic disease are the second most common type of exudative pleural effusion. The three tumors that cause approximately 75% of all malignant pleural effusions are lung carcinoma, breast carcinoma, and lymphoma. Most patients complain of dyspnea, which is frequently out of proportion to the size of the effusion. The pleural fluid is an exudate, and its glucose level may be reduced if the tumor burden in the pleural space is high.

The diagnosis is usually made via cytology of the pleural fluid. If the initial cytologic examination is negative, then thoracoscopy is the best next procedure if malignancy is strongly suspected. At the time of thoracoscopy, a procedure such as pleural abrasion should be performed to effect a pleurodesis. If thoracoscopy is unavailable, then needle biopsy of the pleura should be performed.

Patients with a malignant pleural effusion are treated symptomatically for the most part, since the presence of the effusion indicates disseminated disease and most malignancies associated with pleural effusion are not curable with chemotherapy. The only symptom that can be attributed to the effusion itself is dyspnea. If the patient's lifestyle is compromised by dyspnea, and if the dyspnea is relieved with a therapeutic thoracentesis, then one of the following procedures should be considered: (1) tube thoracostomy with the instillation of a sclerosing agent such as doxycycline, 500 mg; or (2) outpatient insertion of a small indwelling catheter.

Mesothelioma Malignant mesotheliomas are primary tumors that arise from the mesothelial cells that line the pleural cavities. Most are related to asbestos exposure. Patients with mesothelioma present with chest pain and shortness of breath. The chest radiograph reveals a pleural effusion, generalized pleural thickening, and a shrunken hemithorax. Thoracoscopy or open pleural biopsy is usually necessary to establish the diagnosis. Various treatment modalities, including radical surgery, chemotherapy, and radiation therapy, have been tried, but none has been proven to be more effective than symptomatic therapy. It is recommended that chest pain be treated with opiates and that shortness of breath be treated with oxygen and/or opiates.

Effusion Secondary to Pulmonary Embolization The diagnosis most commonly overlooked in the differential diagnosis of a patient with an undiagnosed pleural effusion is pulmonary embolism. Dyspnea is the most common symptom. The pleural fluid is usually exudative but can be transudative. The diagnosis is established by spiral CT scan or pulmonary arteriography (Chap. 244). Treatment of the patient with a pleural effusion secondary to pulmonary embolism is the same as for any patient with pulmonary emboli. If the pleural effusion increases in size after anticoagulation, the patient probably has recurrent emboli or another complication such as a hemothorax or a pleural infection.

Tuberculous Pleuritis (See also Chap. 150) In many parts of the world, the most common cause of an exudative pleural effusion is tuberculosis (TB), but this is relatively uncommon in the United States. Tuberculous pleural effusions are thought to be due primarily to a hypersensitivity reaction to tuberculous protein in the pleural space. Patients with tuberculous pleuritis present with fever, weight loss, dyspnea, and/or pleuritic chest pain. The pleural fluid is an exudate with predominantly small lymphocytes. The diagnosis is established by demonstrating high levels of TB markers in the pleural fluid (adenosine deaminase $>$ 45 IU/L, interferon γ > 140 pg/mL, or positive polymerase chain reaction (PCR) for tuberculous DNA). Alternatively, the diagnosis can be established by culture of the pleural fluid, needle biopsy of the pleura, or thoracoscopy. The recommended treatment of pleural and pulmonary tuberculosis is identical (Chap. 150).

Effusion Secondary to Viral Infection Viral infections are probably responsible for a sizable percentage of undiagnosed exudative pleural effusions. In many series, no diagnosis is established for approximately 20% of exudative effusions, and these effusions resolve spontaneously with no long-term residua. The importance of these effusions is that one should not be too aggressive in trying to establish a diagnosis for the undiagnosed effusion, particularly if the patient is improving clinically.

AIDS Pleural effusions are uncommon in such patients. The most common cause is Kaposi's sarcoma, followed by parapneumonic ef-

fusion. Other common causes are TB, cryptococcosis, and primary effusion lymphoma. Pleural effusions are very uncommon with *Pneumocystis carinii* infection.

Chylothorax A chylothorax occurs when the thoracic duct is disrupted and chyle accumulates in the pleural space. The most common cause of chylothorax is trauma, but it also may result from tumors in the mediastinum. Patients with chylothorax present with dyspnea, and a large pleural effusion is present on the chest radiograph. Thoracentesis reveals milky fluid, and biochemical analysis reveals a triglyceride level that exceeds 1.2 mmol/L (110 mg/dL). Patients with chylothorax and no obvious trauma should have a lymphangiogram and a mediastinal CT scan to assess the mediastinum for lymph nodes. The treatment of choice for most chylothoraces is implantation of a pleuroperitoneal shunt. Patients with chylothoraces should not undergo prolonged tube thoracostomy with chest tube drainage because this will lead to malnutrition and immunologic incompetence.

Hemothorax When a diagnostic thoracentesis reveals bloody pleural fluid, a hematocrit should be obtained on the pleural fluid. If the hematocrit is >50% that of the peripheral blood, the patient has a hemothorax. Most hemothoraces are the result of trauma; other causes include rupture of a blood vessel or tumor. Most patients with hemothorax should be treated with tube thoracostomy, which allows continuous quantification of bleeding. If the bleeding emanates from a laceration of the pleura, apposition of the two pleural surfaces is likely to stop the bleeding. If the pleural hemorrhage exceeds 200 mL/h, consideration should be given to thoracotomy.

Miscellaneous Causes of Pleural Effusion There are many other causes of pleural effusion (Table 245-1). Key features of some of these conditions are as follows: If the pleural fluid amylase level is elevated, the diagnosis of esophageal rupture or pancreatic disease is likely. If the

---

TABLE 245-1 *Differential Diagnoses of Pleural Effusions*

TRANSUDATIVE PLEURAL EFFUSIONS

1. Congestive heart failure	5. Peritoneal dialysis
2. Cirrhosis	6. Superior vena cava obstruction
3. Pulmonary embolization	7. Myxedema
4. Nephrotic syndrome	8. Urinothorax

EXUDATIVE PLEURAL EFFUSIONS

1. Neoplastic diseases	6. Post-coronary artery bypass
a. Metastatic disease	surgery
b. Mesothelioma	7. Asbestos exposure
2. Infectious diseases	8. Sarcoidosis
a. Bacterial infections	9. Uremia
b. Tuberculosis	10. Meigs' syndrome
c. Fungal infections	11. Yellow nail syndrome
d. Viral infections	12. Drug-induced pleural disease
e. Parasitic infections	a. Nitrofurantoin
3. Pulmonary embolization	b. Dantrolene
4. Gastrointestinal disease	c. Methysergide
a. Esophageal perforation	d. Bromocriptine
b. Pancreatic disease	e. Procarbazine
c. Intraabdominal abscesses	f. Amiodarone
d. Diaphragmatic hernia	13. Trapped lung
e. After abdominal surgery	14. Radiation therapy
f. Endoscopic variceal	15. Post-cardiac injury syndrome
sclerotherapy	16. Hemothorax
g. After liver transplant	17. Iatrogenic injury
5. Collagen-vascular diseases	18. Ovarian hyperstimulation
a. Rheumatoid pleuritis	syndrome
b. Systemic lupus	19. Pericardial disease
erythematosus	20. Chylothorax
c. Drug-induced lupus	
d. Immunoblastic lympha-	
denopathy	
e. Sjögren's syndrome	
f. Wegener's granulomatosis	
g. Churg-Strauss syndrome	

patient is febrile, has predominantly polymorphonuclear cells in the pleural fluid, and has no pulmonary parenchymal abnormalities, an intraabdominal abscess should be considered. The diagnosis of an asbestos pleural effusion is one of exclusion. Benign ovarian tumors can produce ascites and a pleural effusion (Meigs' syndrome), as can the ovarian hyperstimulation syndrome. Several drugs can cause pleural effusion; the associated fluid is usually eosinophilic. Pleural effusions commonly occur following coronary artery bypass surgery. Effusions occurring within the first weeks are typically left-sided and bloody, with large numbers of eosinophils, and respond to one or two therapeutic thoracenteses. Effusions occurring after the first few weeks are typically left-sided and clear yellow, with predominantly small lymphocytes, and tend to recur. Other medical manipulations that induce pleural effusions include abdominal surgery, endoscopic variceal sclerotherapy, radiation therapy, liver or lung transplantation, or the intravascular insertion of central lines.

PNEUMOTHORAX Pneumothorax is the presence of gas in the pleural space. A *spontaneous pneumothorax* is one that occurs without antecedent trauma to the thorax. A *primary spontaneous pneumothorax* occurs in the absence of underlying lung disease, while a *secondary spontaneous pneumothorax* occurs in its presence. A *traumatic pneumothorax* results from penetrating or nonpenetrating chest injuries. A *tension pneumothorax* is a pneumothorax in which the pressure in the pleural space is positive throughout the respiratory cycle.

Primary Spontaneous Pneumothorax Primary spontaneous pneumothoraces are usually due to rupture of apical pleural blebs, small cystic spaces that lie within or immediately under the visceral pleura. Primary spontaneous pneumothoraces occur almost exclusively in smokers, which suggests that these patients have subclinical lung disease. Approximately one-half of patients with an initial primary spontaneous pneumothorax will have a recurrence. The initial recommended treatment for primary spontaneous pneumothorax is simple aspiration. If the lung does not expand with aspiration, or if the patient has a recurrent pneumothorax, thoracoscopy with stapling of blebs and pleural abrasion is indicated. Thoracoscopy or thoracotomy with pleural abrasion is almost 100% successful in preventing recurrences.

Secondary Spontaneous Pneumothorax Most secondary spontaneous pneumothoraces are due to chronic obstructive pulmonary disease, but pneumothoraces have been reported with virtually every lung disease. Pneumothorax in patients with lung disease is more life-threatening than it is in normal individuals because of the lack of pulmonary reserve in these patients. Nearly all patients with secondary spontaneous pneumothorax should be treated with tube thoracostomy and the instillation of a sclerosing agent such as doxycycline. Patients with secondary spontaneous pneumothoraces who have a persistent air leak, an unexpanded lung after 3 days of tube thoracostomy, or a recurrent pneumothorax should be subjected to thoracoscopy with bleb resection and pleural abrasion.

Traumatic Pneumothorax Traumatic pneumothoraces can result from both penetrating and nonpenetrating chest trauma. Traumatic pneumothoraces should be treated with tube thoracostomy unless they are very small. If a hemopneumothorax is present, one chest tube should be placed in the superior part of the hemithorax to evacuate the air, and another should be placed in the inferior part of the hemithorax to remove the blood. Iatrogenic pneumothorax is a type of traumatic pneumothorax that is becoming more common. The leading causes are transthoracic needle aspiration, thoracentesis, and the insertion of central intravenous catheters. The treatment differs according to the degree of distress and can be observation, supplemental oxygen, aspiration, or tube thoracostomy.

Tension Pneumothorax This condition usually occurs during mechanical ventilation or resuscitative efforts. The positive pleural pressure is life-threatening both because ventilation is severely compromised and because the positive pressure is transmitted to the mediastinum, which

results in decreased venous return to the heart and reduced cardiac output.

Difficulty in ventilation during resuscitation or high peak inspiratory pressures during mechanical ventilation strongly suggests the diagnosis. The diagnosis is made by the finding of an enlarged hemithorax with no breath sounds and shift of the mediastinum to the contralateral side. Tension pneumothorax must be treated as a medical emergency. If the tension in the pleural space is not relieved, the patient is likely to die from inadequate cardiac output or marked hypoxemia. A large-bore needle should be inserted into the pleural space through the second anterior intercostal space. If large amounts of gas escape from the needle after insertion, the diagnosis is confirmed. The needle should be left in place until a thoracostomy tube can be inserted.

DISORDERS OF THE MEDIASTINUM

The mediastinum is the region between the pleural sacs. It is separated into three compartments. The *anterior mediastinum* extends from the sternum anteriorly to the pericardium and brachiocephalic vessels posteriorly. It contains the thymus gland, the anterior mediastinal lymph nodes, and the internal mammary arteries and veins. The *middle mediastinum* lies between the anterior and posterior mediastina and contains the heart; the ascending and transverse arches of the aorta; the venae cavae; the brachiocephalic arteries and veins; the phrenic nerves; the trachea, main bronchi, and their contiguous lymph nodes; and the pulmonary arteries and veins. The *posterior mediastinum* is bounded by the pericardium and trachea anteriorly and the vertebral column posteriorly. It contains the descending thoracic aorta, esophagus, thoracic duct, azygos and hemiazygos veins, and the posterior group of mediastinal lymph nodes.

MEDIASTINAL MASSES The first step in evaluating a mediastinal mass is to place it in one of the three mediastinal compartments, since each has different characteristic lesions. The most common lesions in the anterior mediastinum are thymomas, lymphomas, teratomatous neoplasms, and thyroid masses. The most common masses in the middle mediastinum are vascular masses, lymph node enlargement from metastases or granulomatous disease, and pleuropericardial and bronchogenic cysts. In the posterior mediastinum, neurogenic tumors, meningoceles, meningomyeloceles, gastroenteric cysts, and esophageal diverticula are commonly found.

CT scanning is the most valuable imaging technique for evaluating mediastinal masses and is the only imaging technique that should be done in most instances. Barium studies of the gastrointestinal tract are indicated in many patients with posterior mediastinal lesions, since hernias, diverticula, and achalasia are readily diagnosed in this manner. An ^{131}I nuclear medicine scan can efficiently establish the diagnosis of intrathoracic goiter.

A definite diagnosis can be obtained with mediastinoscopy or anterior mediastinotomy in many patients with masses in the anterior or middle mediastinal compartments. A diagnosis can be established without thoracotomy via percutaneous fine-needle aspiration biopsy or endoscopic ultrasound-guided biopsy of mediastinal masses. In many cases the diagnosis can be established and the mediastinal mass removed with video-assisted thoracoscopy.

ACUTE MEDIASTINITIS Most cases of acute mediastinitis either are due to esophageal perforation or occur after median sternotomy for cardiac surgery. Patients with esophageal rupture are acutely ill with chest pain and dyspnea due to the mediastinal infection. The esophageal rupture can occur spontaneously or as a complication of esophagoscopy or the insertion of a Blakemore tube. Appropriate treatment is exploration of the mediastinum with primary repair of the esophageal tear and drainage of the pleural space and the mediastinum.

The incidence of mediastinitis following median sternotomy is 0.4 to 5.0%. Patients most commonly present with wound drainage. Other presentations include sepsis or a widened mediastinum. The diagnosis is usually established with mediastinal needle aspiration. Treatment includes immediate drainage, debridement, and parenteral antibiotic therapy, but the mortality still exceeds 20%.

CHRONIC MEDIASTINITIS The spectrum of chronic mediastinitis ranges from granulomatous inflammation of the lymph nodes in the mediastinum to fibrosing mediastinitis. Most cases are due to TB or histoplasmosis, but sarcoidosis, silicosis, and other fungal diseases are at times causative. Patients with granulomatous mediastinitis are usually asymptomatic. Those with fibrosing mediastinitis usually have signs of compression of some mediastinal structure such as the superior vena cava or large airways, phrenic or recurrent laryngeal nerve paralysis, or obstruction of the pulmonary artery or proximal pulmonary veins. Other than antituberculous therapy for tuberculous mediastinitis, no medical or surgical therapy has been demonstrated to be effective for mediastinal fibrosis.

PNEUMOMEDIASTINUM In this condition, there is gas in the interstices of the mediastinum. The three main causes are: (1) alveolar rupture with dissection of air into the mediastinum; (2) perforation or rupture of the esophagus, trachea, or main bronchi; and (3) dissection of air from the neck or the abdomen into the mediastinum. Typically, there is severe substernal chest pain with or without radiation into the neck and arms. The physical examination usually reveals subcutaneous emphysema in the suprasternal notch and *Hamman's sign*, which is a crunching or clicking noise synchronous with the heartbeat and best heard in the left lateral decubitus position. The diagnosis is confirmed with the chest radiograph. Usually no treatment is required, but the mediastinal air will be absorbed faster if the patient inspires high concentrations of oxygen. If mediastinal structures are compressed, the compression can be relieved with needle aspiration.

DISORDERS OF THE DIAPHRAGM

DIAPHRAGMATIC PARALYSIS The presence of bilateral diaphragmatic paralysis almost always causes severe morbidity in adults. The most common causes include high spinal cord injury, thoracic trauma (including cardiac surgery), multiple sclerosis, anterior horn disease, and muscular dystrophy. Most patients with severe diaphragmatic weakness present with hypercapnic respiratory failure, frequently complicated by cor pulmonale and right ventricular failure, atelectasis, and pneumonia.

The degree of diaphragmatic weakness is best quantitated by measuring transdiaphragmatic pressures. The treatment of choice is assisted ventilation for all or part of each day. This is best accomplished without tracheostomy using nasal intermittent positive airway pressure. If the nerve to the diaphragm is intact, diaphragmatic pacing may be a viable alternative. If the paralysis occurs during open heart surgery, recovery frequently occurs, but it may take 6 months or more.

Unilateral paralysis of the diaphragm is much more common than is bilateral paralysis. The most common cause is nerve invasion from malignancy, usually a bronchogenic carcinoma. If the patient does not have malignancy, then usually no cause for the paralysis is found. The diagnosis is suggested by finding an elevated hemidiaphragm on the chest roentgenogram. Confirmation is best established with the "sniff test." When a patient is observed with fluoroscopy while sniffing, the paralyzed diaphragm will move paradoxically upward due to the negative intrathoracic pressure. Patients with a unilateral paralyzed diaphragm are usually asymptomatic. Their vital capacity and total lung capacity are each reduced about 25%. If a patient has a mediastinal mass in conjunction with the diaphragmatic paralysis, further workup should be done. However, if the patient is asymptomatic with a normal chest radiograph, no invasive procedures are warranted.

DISORDERS OF THE CHEST WALL

KYPHOSCOLIOSIS Kyphoscoliosis is a combination of excessive anteroposterior and lateral curvature of the thoracic spine. Abnormalities of the spinal curvature are common, occurring in about 3% of the population. However, deformity of a sufficient degree to lead to symptoms and signs referable to the heart or lungs is rare, occurring in fewer than 3% of those with abnormal curvature. The major pathophysiologic effects of severe kyphoscoliosis are restrictive lung disease and ventilation-perfusion imbalances that result in chronic alveolar hypoventilation, hypoxic vasoconstriction, and eventually pulmonary arterial hypertension and cor pulmonale.

The severity of the cardiopulmonary disease correlates roughly with the degree of scoliosis. If the angle of curvature is <60°, ventilatory impairment is rare, while if it is >90°, marked ventilatory abnormalities develop commonly.

Although much effort has been devoted to restoring the normal curvature by either internal fixation or an external device, these efforts result in more improvement in the cosmetic appearance than in pulmonary function. However, the earlier that corrective actions are undertaken, the better the results. Once cardiorespiratory failure has developed, there is a high mortality from operative intervention. Patients with kyphoscoliosis and recurrent episodes of respiratory failure benefit from chronic nocturnal mechanical ventilation or nasal continuous positive airway pressure.

PECTUS EXCAVATUM (FUNNEL CHEST) In this congenital condition, the lower portion of the sternum is displaced posteriorly and the anterior ribs are markedly bowed, which results in a depressed panel in the anterior chest. Respiratory symptoms are uncommon, and pulmonary function tests are nearly normal. Surgical correction is seldom indicated and then only to treat psychological upset resulting from the cosmetic deformity.

PECTUS CARINATUM (PIGEON BREAST) This condition is the reverse of pectus excavatum with the sternum protruding anteriorly. This deformity is associated with congenital atrial or ventricular septal defects and severe prolonged childhood asthma. The deformity itself does not cause symptoms, and surgery is for cosmetic purposes only.

FURTHER READING

BAUMANN MH et al: Management of spontaneous pneumothorax: An American College of Chest Physicians Delphi Consensus Statement. Chest 119: 590, 2001

LARSEN SS et al: Endoscopic ultrasound guided biopsy of mediastinal lesions has a major impact on patient management. Thorax 57:98, 2002

LIGHT RW: *Pleural Diseases*, 4th ed. Philadelphia, Lippincott Williams & Wilkins, 2001

———: Pleural effusion. N Engl J Med 346:1971, 2002

MCCOOL FD, ROCHESTER DF: The lungs and chest wall diseases, in *Textbook of Respiratory Medicine*, JF Murray, JA Nabel (eds). Philadelphia, Saunders, 2000, pp 2357–2376

ZWISCHENBERGER JB et al: Mediastinal transthoracic needle and core lymph node biopsy. Should it replace mediastinoscopy? Chest 121:1165, 2002

246 DISORDERS OF VENTILATION
Eliot A. Phillipson

HYPOVENTILATION

DEFINITION AND ETIOLOGY Alveolar hypoventilation exists by definition when arterial P_{CO_2} (Pa_{CO_2}) increases above the normal range of 37 to 43 mmHg, but in clinically important hypoventilation syndromes Pa_{CO_2} is generally in the range of 50 to 80 mmHg. Hypoventilation disorders can be acute or chronic. The acute disorders, which represent life-threatening emergencies, are discussed in Chap. 251; this chapter deals with chronic hypoventilation syndromes.

Chronic hypoventilation can result from numerous disease entities (Table 246-1), but in all cases the underlying mechanism involves a defect in either the metabolic respiratory control system, the respiratory neuromuscular system, or the ventilatory apparatus. Disorders associated with impaired respiratory drive, defects in the respiratory neuromuscular system, some chest wall disorders such as obesity, and

TABLE 246-1   *Chronic Hypoventilation Syndromes*

Mechanism	Site of Defect	Disorder
Impaired respiratory drive	Peripheral and central chemoreceptors	Carotid body dysfunction, trauma Prolonged hypoxia Metabolic alkalosis
	Brainstem respiratory neurons	Bulbar poliomyelitis, encephalitis Brainstem infarction, hemorrhage, trauma Brainstem demyelination, degeneration Chronic drug administration Primary alveolar hypoventilation syndrome
Defective respiratory neuromuscular system	Spinal cord and peripheral nerves	High cervical trauma Poliomyelitis Motor neuron disease Peripheral neuropathy
	Respiratory muscles	Myasthenia gravis Muscular dystrophy Chronic myopathy
Impaired ventilatory apparatus	Chest wall	Kyphoscoliosis Fibrothorax Thoracoplasty Ankylosing spondylitis Obesity hypoventilation
	Airways and lungs	Laryngeal and tracheal stenosis Obstructive sleep apnea Cystic fibrosis Chronic obstructive pulmonary disease

Source: From Phillipson and Slutsky, with permission.

upper airway obstruction produce an increase in Pa_{CO_2}, despite normal lungs, because of a reduction in overall minute volume of ventilation and hence in alveolar ventilation. In contrast, most disorders of the chest wall and disorders of the lower airways and lungs may produce an increase in Pa_{CO_2}, despite a normal or even increased minute volume of ventilation, because of severe ventilation-perfusion mismatching that results in net alveolar hypoventilation.

Several hypoventilation syndromes involve combined disturbances in two elements of the respiratory system. For example, patients with chronic obstructive pulmonary disease may hypoventilate not simply because of impaired ventilatory mechanics but also because of a reduced central respiratory drive, which can be inherent or secondary to a co-existing metabolic alkalosis (related to diuretic and steroid therapy).

PHYSIOLOGIC AND CLINICAL FEATURES   Regardless of cause, the hallmark of all alveolar hypoventilation syndromes is an increase in alveolar P_{CO_2} (PA_{CO_2}) and therefore in Pa_{CO_2} (Fig. 246-1). The resulting respiratory acidosis eventually leads to a compensatory increase in plasma HCO_3^- concentration and a decrease in Cl^- concentration. The increase in PA_{CO_2} produces an obligatory decrease in PA_{O_2}, resulting in hypoxemia. If severe, the hypoxemia manifests clinically as cyanosis and can stimulate erythropoiesis and induce secondary polycythemia. The combination of chronic hypoxemia and hypercapnia may also induce pulmonary vasoconstriction, leading eventually to pulmonary hypertension, right ventricular hypertrophy, and congestive heart failure. The disturbances in arterial blood gases are typically magnified during sleep because of a further reduction in central respiratory drive. The resulting increased nocturnal hypercapnia may cause cerebral vasodilation leading to morning headache; sleep quality may also be severely impaired, resulting in morning fatigue, daytime somnolence, mental confusion, and intellectual impairment. Other clinical features associated with hypoventilation syndromes are related to the specific underlying disease (Table 246-1).

DIAGNOSIS   Investigation of the patient with chronic hypoventilation involves several laboratory tests that will usually localize the disorder

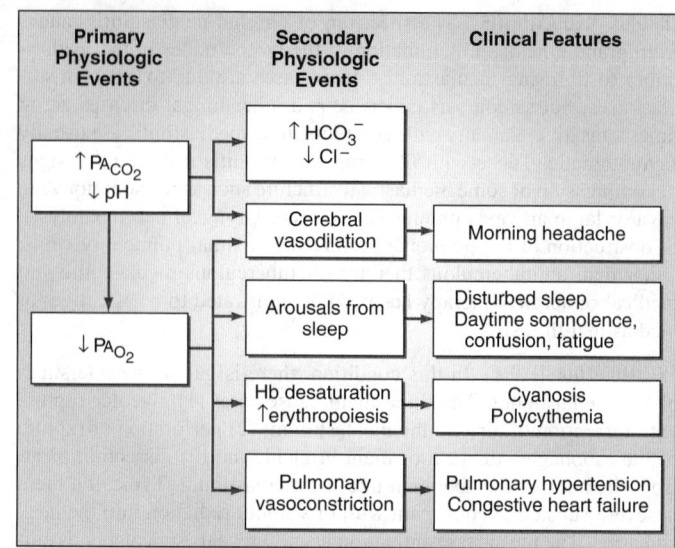

FIGURE 246-1   Physiologic and clinical features of alveolar hypoventilation. Hb, hemoglobin; PA_{CO_2}, alveolar P_{CO_2}; PA_{O_2}, alveolar P_{O_2}. *(After Phillipson and Slutsky.)*

to either the metabolic respiratory control system, the neuromuscular system, or the ventilatory apparatus (Fig. 246-2). Defects in the control system impair responses to chemical stimuli, including ventilatory, occlusion pressure, and diaphragmatic electromyographic (EMG) responses. During sleep, hypoventilation is usually more marked, and central apneas and hypopneas are common. However, because the behavioral respiratory control system (which is anatomically distinct from the metabolic control system), the neuromuscular system, and the ventilatory apparatus are intact, such patients can usually hyperventilate voluntarily, generate normal inspiratory and expiratory muscle pressures (PI_{max}, PE_{max}, respectively) against an occluded airway, generate normal lung volumes and flow rates on routine spirometry, and have normal respiratory system resistance and compliance and a normal alveolar-arterial $P_{O_2}[(A - a)P_{O_2}]$ difference. Patients with defects in the respiratory neuromuscular system also have impaired responses to chemical stimuli but in addition are unable to hyperventilate voluntarily or to generate normal static respiratory muscle pressures, lung volumes, and flow rates. However, at least in the early stages of the disease, the resistance and compliance of the respiratory system and the alveolar-arterial oxygen difference are normal.

In contrast to patients with disorders of the respiratory control or neuromuscular systems, patients with disorders of the chest wall, lungs, and airways typically demonstrate abnormalities of respiratory system resistance and compliance and have a widened $(A - a)P_{O_2}$. Because of the impaired mechanics of breathing, routine spirometric tests are abnormal, as is the ventilatory response to chemical stimuli. However, because the neuromuscular system is intact, tests that are independent of resistance and compliance are usually normal, including tests of respiratory muscle strength and of respiratory control that do not involve airflow.

℞ TREATMENT

The management of chronic hypoventilation must be individualized to the patient's particular disorder, circumstances, and needs and should include measures directed toward the underlying disease. Coexistent metabolic alkalosis should be corrected, including elevations of HCO_3^- that are inappropriately high for the degree of chronic hypercapnia. Administration of supplemental oxygen is effective in attenuating hypoxemia, polycythemia, and pulmonary hypertension but can aggravate CO_2 retention and the associated neurologic symptoms. For this reason, supplemental oxygen must be prescribed judiciously and the results monitored carefully. Pharmacologic agents that stimulate respiration (particularly progesterone) are of benefit in some patients, but generally, results are disappointing.

Site of defect	Responses to CO$_2$, hypoxia			Sleep studies	Voluntary hyperventil.	PI$_{max}$ PE$_{max}$	Volume flow rates	Resistance, compliance	(A − a) Po$_2$
	Ventil.	P.1	EMGdi						
Metabolic control system (chemoreceptors, brainstem integrating neurons) ↓	↓	↓	↓	↑ Hypoventil, central apneas	N	N	N	N	N
Respiratory neuromuscular system (brainstem motoneurons, spinal cord, respiratory nerves, and muscles) ↓	↓	↓	↓	↑ Hypoventil, central apneas	↓	↓	↓	N	N
Ventilatory apparatus (chest wall, lungs, airways)	↓	N	N	Variable	↓	N	Abnormal	Abnormal	↑

FIGURE 246-2   Pattern of laboratory test results in alveolar hypoventilation syndromes, based on the site of defect. Ventil, ventilation; P.1, mouth pressure generated after 0.1 s of inspiration against an occluded airway; EMGdi, diaphragmatic EMG; PI$_{max}$, PE$_{max}$, maximum inspiratory or expiratory pressure that can be generated against an occluded airway; (A − a)P$_{O_2}$, alveolar-arterial P$_{O_2}$ difference; N, normal. Defects in the metabolic control system impair central respiratory drive in response to chemical stimuli (CO$_2$ or hypoxia); therefore responses of EMGdi, P.1, and minute volume of ventilation are reduced and hypoventilation during sleep is aggravated. In contrast, tests of voluntary respiratory control, muscle strength, lung mechanics, and gas exchange [(A − a)P$_{O_2}$] are normal. Defects in the respiratory neuromuscular system impair muscle strength; therefore all tests dependent on muscular activity (voluntary or in response to metabolic stimuli) are abnormal, but lung resistance, lung compliance, and gas exchange are normal. Defects in the ventilatory apparatus usually impair gas exchange. Because resistance and compliance are also impaired, all tests dependent on ventilation (whether voluntary or in response to chemical stimuli) are abnormal; in contrast, tests of muscle activity or strength that do not involve airflow (i.e., P.1, EMGdi, PI$_{max}$, PE$_{max}$) are normal. (After Phillipson and Slutsky.)

Most patients with chronic hypoventilation related to impairment of respiratory drive or neuromuscular disease eventually require mechanical ventilatory assistance for effective management. When hypoventilation is severe, treatment may be required on a 24-h basis, but in most patients ventilatory assistance only during sleep produces dramatic improvement in clinical features and daytime arterial blood gases. In patients with reduced respiratory drive but intact respiratory lower motor neurons, phrenic nerves, and respiratory muscles, diaphragmatic pacing through an implanted phrenic electrode can be very effective. However, for patients with defects in the respiratory nerves and muscles, electrophrenic pacing is contraindicated. Such patients can usually be managed effectively with either intermittent negative-pressure ventilation in a cuirass or intermittent positive-pressure ventilation delivered through a tracheostomy or nose mask. For patients who require ventilatory assistance only during sleep, positive-pressure ventilation through a nose mask is the preferred method because it obviates a tracheostomy and avoids the problem of upper airway occlusion that can arise in a negative-pressure ventilator. Hypoventilation related to restrictive disorders of the chest wall (Table 246-1) can also be managed effectively with nocturnal intermittent positive-pressure ventilation through a nose mask or tracheostomy.

HYPOVENTILATION SYNDROMES

PRIMARY ALVEOLAR HYPOVENTILATION   Primary alveolar hypoventilation (PAH) is a disorder of unknown cause characterized by chronic hypercapnia and hypoxemia in the absence of identifiable neuromuscular disease or mechanical ventilatory impairment. The disorder is thought to arise from a defect in the metabolic respiratory control system, but few neuropathologic studies have been reported in such patients. Studies in animals suggest an important role for genetic factors in the pathogenesis of hypoventilation, and familial cases in humans have been described. Isolated PAH is relatively rare, and although it occurs in all age groups, the majority of reported cases in adults have been in males aged 20 to 50 years. The disorder typically develops insidiously and often first comes to attention when severe respiratory depression follows administration of standard doses of sedatives or anesthetics. As the degree of hypoventilation increases, patients typically develop lethargy, fatigue, daytime somnolence, disturbed sleep, and morning headaches; eventually cyanosis, polycythemia, pulmonary hypertension, and congestive heart failure occur (Fig. 246-1). Despite severe arterial blood gas derangements, dyspnea is uncommon, presumably because of impaired chemoreception and ventilatory drive. If left untreated, PAH is usually progressive over a period of months to years and ultimately fatal.

The key diagnostic finding in PAH is a chronic respiratory acidosis in the absence of respiratory muscle weakness or impaired ventilatory mechanics (Fig. 246-2). Because patients can hyperventilate voluntarily and reduce Pa$_{CO_2}$ to normal or even hypocapnic levels, hypercapnia may not be demonstrable in a single arterial blood sample, but the presence of an elevated plasma HCO$_3$$^-$ level should draw attention to the underlying chronic disturbance. Despite normal ventilatory mechanics and respiratory muscle strength, ventilatory responses to chemical stimuli are reduced or absent (Fig. 246-2), and breath-holding time may be markedly prolonged without any sensation of dyspnea.

Patients with PAH maintain rhythmic respiration when awake, although the level of ventilation is below normal. However, during sleep, when breathing is critically dependent on the metabolic control system, there is typically a further deterioration in ventilation with frequent episodes of central hypopnea or apnea.

PAH must be distinguished from other central hypoventilation syndromes that are secondary to underlying neurologic disease of the brainstem or chemoreceptors (Table 246-1). This distinction requires a careful neurologic investigation for evidence of brainstem or autonomic disturbances. Unrecognized respiratory neuromuscular disorders, particularly those that produce diaphragmatic weakness, are often misdiagnosed as PAH. However, such disorders can usually be suspected on clinical grounds (see below) and can be confirmed by the finding of reduced voluntary hyperventilation, as well as PI$_{max}$ and PE$_{max}$.

Some patients with PAH respond favorably to respiratory stimulant medications and to supplemental oxygen. However, the majority eventually require mechanical ventilatory assistance. Excellent long-term benefits can be achieved with diaphragmatic pacing by electrophrenic stimulation or with negative- or positive-pressure mechanical ventilation. The administration of such treatment only during sleep is sufficient in most patients.

RESPIRATORY NEUROMUSCULAR DISORDERS   Several primary disorders of the spinal cord, peripheral respiratory nerves, and respiratory muscles produce a chronic hypoventilation syndrome (Table 246-1). Hypoventilation usually develops gradually over a period of months to years and often first comes to attention when a relatively trivial increase in mechanical ventilatory load (such as mild airways obstruction) produces severe respiratory failure. In some of the disorders (such as motor neuron disease, myasthenia gravis, and muscular dystrophy), involvement of the respiratory nerves or muscles is usually a later feature of a more widespread disease. In other disorders, respiratory involvement can be an early or even isolated feature, and hence the underlying problem is often not suspected. Included in this category are the postpolio syndrome (a form of chronic respiratory insufficiency that develops 20 to 30 years following recovery from poliomyelitis), the myopathy associated with adult acid maltase deficiency, and idiopathic diaphragmatic paralysis.

Generally, respiratory neuromuscular disorders do not result in chronic hypoventilation unless there is significant weakness of the diaphragm. Distinguishing features of bilateral diaphragmatic weakness include orthopnea, paradoxical movement of the abdomen in the supine posture, and paradoxical diaphragmatic movement under fluoroscopy. However, the absence of these features does not exclude diaphragmatic weakness. Important laboratory features are a rapid deterioration of ventilation during a maximum voluntary ventilation maneuver and reduced PI_{max} and PE_{max} (Fig. 246-2). More sophisticated investigations reveal reduced or absent transdiaphragmatic pressures, calculated from simultaneous measurement of esophageal and gastric pressures; reduced diaphragmatic EMG responses (recorded from an esophageal electrode) to transcutaneous phrenic nerve stimulation; and marked hypopnea and arterial oxygen desaturation during rapid eye movement sleep, when there is normally a physiologic inhibition of all nondiaphragmatic respiratory muscles and breathing becomes critically dependent on diaphragmatic activity.

The management of chronic alveolar hypoventilation due to respiratory neuromuscular disease involves treatment of the underlying disorder, where feasible, and mechanical ventilatory assistance as described for the PAH syndrome. However, electrophrenic diaphragmatic pacing is contraindicated in these disorders, except for high cervical spinal cord lesions in which the phrenic lower motor neurons and nerves are intact.

OBESITY-HYPOVENTILATION SYNDROME   Massive obesity represents a mechanical load to the respiratory system because the added weight on the rib cage and abdomen serves to reduce the compliance of the chest wall. As a result, the functional residual capacity (i.e., end-expiratory lung volume) is reduced, particularly in the recumbent posture. An important consequence of breathing at a low lung volume is that some airways, particularly those in the lung bases, may be closed throughout part or even all of each tidal breath, resulting in underventilation of the lung bases and widening of the $(A - a)P_{O_2}$. Nevertheless, in the majority of obese individuals, central respiratory drive is increased sufficiently to maintain a normal Pa_{CO_2}. However, a small proportion of obese patients develop chronic hypercapnia, hypoxemia, and eventually polycythemia, pulmonary hypertension, and right-sided heart failure. Studies in mice demonstrate that genetically obese mice lacking circulating leptin also develop chronic hypoventilation that can be reversed by leptin infusions. In humans with obesity-hypoventilation syndrome, serum leptin levels are elevated, suggesting that leptin resistance may play a role in the pathogenesis of the disorder. In many patients, obstructive sleep apnea is a prominent feature, and even in those patients without sleep apnea, sleep-induced hypoventilation is an important element of the disorder and contributes to its progression. Most patients demonstrate a decrease in central respiratory drive, which may be inherent or acquired, and many have mild to moderate degrees of airflow obstruction, usually related to smoking. Based on these considerations, several therapeutic measures can be of considerable benefit, including weight loss, cessation of smoking, elimination of obstructive sleep apnea, and enhancement of respiratory drive by medications such as progesterone.

HYPERVENTILATION AND ITS SYNDROMES

DEFINITION AND ETIOLOGY   Alveolar hyperventilation exists when Pa_{CO_2} decreases below the normal range of 37 to 43 mmHg. *Hyperventilation* is not synonymous with *hyperpnea*, which refers to an increased minute volume of ventilation without reference to Pa_{CO_2}. Although hyperventilation is frequently associated with dyspnea, patients who are

TABLE 246-2   Hyperventilation Syndromes

1. Hypoxemia
   a. High altitude
   b. Pulmonary disease
   c. Cardiac shunts
2. Pulmonary disorders
   a. Pneumonia
   b. Interstitial pneumonitis, fibrosis, edema
   c. Pulmonary emboli, vascular disease
   d. Bronchial asthma
   e. Pneumothorax
   f. Chest wall disorders
3. Cardiovascular disorders
   a. Congestive heart failure
   b. Hypotension
4. Metabolic disorders
   a. Acidosis (diabetic, renal, lactic)
   b. Hepatic failure
5. Neurologic and psychogenic disorders
   a. Psychogenic or anxiety hyperventilation
   b. Central nervous system infection, tumors
6. Drug-induced
   a. Salicylates
   b. Methylxanthine derivatives
   c. β-Adrenergic agonists
   d. Progesterone
7. Miscellaneous
   a. Fever, sepsis
   b. Pain
   c. Pregnancy

hyperventilating do not necessarily complain of shortness of breath; and conversely, patients with dyspnea need not be hyperventilating.

Numerous disease entities can be associated with alveolar hyperventilation (Table 246-2), but in all cases the underlying mechanism involves an increase in respiratory drive that is mediated through either the behavioral or the metabolic respiratory control systems (Fig. 246-3). Thus hypoxemia drives ventilation by stimulating the peripheral chemoreceptors, and several pulmonary disorders and congestive heart failure drive ventilation by stimulating afferent vagal receptors in the lungs and airways. Low cardiac output and hypotension stimulate the peripheral chemoreceptors and inhibit the baroreceptors, both of which increase ventilation. Metabolic acidosis, a potent respiratory stimulant, excites both the peripheral and central chemoreceptors and increases the sensitivity of the peripheral chemoreceptors to coexistent hypoxemia. Hepatic failure can also produce hyperventilation, presumably as a result of metabolic stimuli acting on the peripheral and central chemoreceptors.

Several neurologic and psychological disorders are thought to drive ventilation through the behavioral respiratory control system. Included in this category are psychogenic or anxiety hyperventilation and severe cerebrovascular insufficiency, which may interfere with the inhibitory influence normally exerted by cortical structures on the brainstem respiratory neurons. Rarely, disorders of the midbrain and hypothalamus induce hyperventilation, and it is conceivable that fever and sepsis also cause hyperventilation through effects on these structures. Several drugs cause hyperventilation by stimulating the central or peripheral chemoreceptors or by direct action on the brainstem respiratory neurons. Chronic hyperventilation is a normal feature of pregnancy and

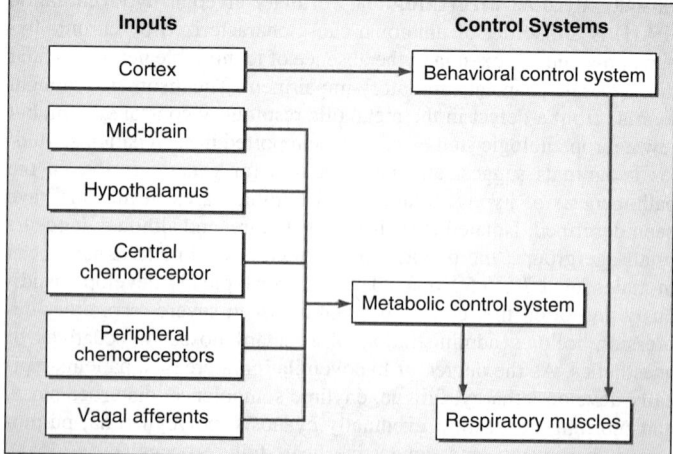

FIGURE 246-3   Schematic diagram of the mechanisms involved in alveolar hyperventilation. (*From Slutsky and Phillipson.*)

results from the effects of progesterone and other hormones acting on the respiratory neurons.

PHYSIOLOGIC AND CLINICAL FEATURES Because hyperventilation is associated with increased respiratory drive, muscle effort, and minute volume of ventilation, the most frequent symptom associated with hyperventilation is dyspnea. However, there is considerable discrepancy between the degree of hyperventilation, as measured by Pa_{CO_2}, and the degree of associated dyspnea. From a physiologic standpoint, hyperventilation is beneficial in patients who are hypoxemic, because the alveolar hypocapnia is associated with an increase in alveolar and arterial P_{O_2}. Conversely, hyperventilation can also be detrimental. In particular, the alkalemia associated with hypocapnia may produce neurologic symptoms, including dizziness, visual impairment, syncope, and seizure activity (secondary to cerebral vasoconstriction); paresthesia, carpopedal spasm, and tetany (secondary to decreased free serum calcium); and muscle weakness (secondary to hypophosphatemia); and may be associated with panic attacks. Severe alkalemia can also induce cardiac arrhythmias and evidence of myocardial ischemia. Patients with a primary respiratory alkalosis are also prone to periodic breathing and central sleep apnea (Chap. 247).

DIAGNOSIS In most patients with a hyperventilation syndrome, the cause is readily apparent on the basis of history, physical examination, and knowledge of coexisting medical disorders (Table 246-2). In patients in whom the cause is not clinically apparent, investigation begins with arterial blood gas analysis, which establishes the presence of alveolar hyperventilation (decreased Pa_{CO_2}) and its severity. Equally important is the arterial pH, which generally allows the disorder to be classified as either a primary respiratory alkalosis (elevated pH) or a primary metabolic acidosis (decreased pH). Also of importance is the Pa_{O_2} and calculation of the $(A - a)P_{O_2}$, since a widened alveolar-arterial oxygen difference suggests a pulmonary disorder as the underlying cause. The finding of a reduced plasma HCO_3^- level establishes the chronic nature of the disorder and points toward an organic cause. Measurements of ventilation and arterial or transcutaneous P_{CO_2} during sleep are very useful in suspected psychogenic hyperventilation, since such patients do not maintain the hyperventilation during sleep.

The disorders that most frequently give rise to unexplained hyperventilation are pulmonary vascular disease (particularly chronic or recurrent thromboembolism) and psychogenic or anxiety hyperventilation. Hyperventilation due to pulmonary vascular disease is associated with exertional dyspnea, a widened $(A - a)P_{O_2}$ and maintenance of hyperventilation during exercise. In contrast, patients with psychogenic hyperventilation typically complain of dyspnea at rest and not during mild exercise and of the need to sigh frequently. They are also more likely to complain of dizziness, sweating, palpitations, and paresthesia. During mild to moderate exercise, their hyperventilation tends to disappear and $(A - a)P_{O_2}$ is normal, but heart rate and cardiac output may be increased relative to metabolic rate.

℞ TREATMENT

Mild alveolar hyperventilation is usually of relatively minor clinical consequence and therefore is generally managed by appropriate treatment of the underlying cause. In the few patients in whom alkalemia is thought to be inducing significant cerebral vasoconstriction, paresthesia, tetany, or cardiac disturbances, acute inhalation of a low concentration of CO_2 can be very beneficial. For patients with disabling psychogenic hyperventilation, careful explanation of the basis of their symptoms can be reassuring and is often sufficient. Others have benefited from β-adrenergic antagonists or an exercise program. Specific treatment for anxiety may also be indicated.

FURTHER READING

LAFFEY JG, KAVANAGH BP: Hypocapnia. N Engl J Med 347:43, 2002

O'DONNELL CP et al: Leptin prevents respiratory depression in obesity. Am J Respir Crit Care Med 159:1477, 1999

PHILLIPSON EA, SLUTSKY AS: Hypoventilation and hyperventilation syndromes, in *Textbook of Respiratory Medicine*, 3d ed, JF Murray, JA Nadel (eds). Philadelphia, Saunders, 2000, pp 2139–2152

PHIPPS PR: Association of serum leptin with hypoventilation in human obesity. Thorax 57:75, 2002

247 SLEEP APNEA
Eliot A. Phillipson

Sleep apnea is defined as an intermittent cessation of airflow at the nose and mouth during sleep. By convention, apneas of at least 10 s duration have been considered important, but in most patients the apneas are 20 to 30 s in duration and may be as long as 2 to 3 min. *Sleep apnea syndrome* refers to a clinical disorder that arises from recurrent apneas during sleep. The clinical importance of sleep apnea arises from the fact that it is one of the leading causes of excessive daytime sleepiness and contributes to important cardiovascular disorders. Indeed, epidemiologic studies have established a prevalence of clinically important sleep apnea of at least 2% in middle-aged women and 4% in middle-aged men.

Sleep apneas can be central or obstructive in type. In central sleep apnea (CSA) the neural drive to all the respiratory muscles is transiently abolished. In contrast, in obstructive sleep apnea (OSA) airflow ceases despite continuing respiratory drive because of occlusion of the oropharyngeal airway.

OBSTRUCTIVE SLEEP APNEA

PATHOGENESIS The definitive event in OSA is occlusion of the upper airway usually at the level of the oropharynx. The resulting apnea leads to progressive asphyxia until there is a brief arousal from sleep, whereupon airway patency is restored and airflow resumes. The patient then returns to sleep, and the sequence of events is repeated, often up to 400 to 500 times per night, resulting in marked fragmentation of sleep.

The immediate factor leading to collapse of the upper airway in OSA is the generation of a critical subatmospheric pressure during inspiration that exceeds the ability of the airway dilator and abductor muscles to maintain airway stability. During wakefulness, upper airway muscle activity is greater than normal in patients with OSA, presumably to compensate for airway narrowing (see below) and a high upper airway resistance. Sleep plays a permissive but crucial role by reducing the activity of the muscles and their protective reflex response to subatmospheric airway pressures. Alcohol is frequently an important cofactor because of its depressant influence on the upper airway muscles and on the arousal response that terminates each apnea. In most patients the patency of the airway is also compromised structurally and is therefore predisposed to occlusion. In a minority of patients the structural compromise is due to obvious anatomic disturbances, such as adenotonsillar hypertrophy, retrognathia, and macroglossia. However, in the majority of patients the structural defect is simply a subtle reduction in airway size that can often be appreciated clinically as "pharyngeal crowding" and that can usually be demonstrated by imaging techniques. Obesity frequently contributes to the reduction in size of the upper airways, either by increasing fat deposition in the soft tissues of the pharynx or by compressing the pharynx by superficial fat masses in the neck. More sophisticated studies also demonstrate a high airway compliance—i.e., the airway is "floppy" and therefore prone to collapse.

PATHOPHYSIOLOGIC AND CLINICAL FEATURES The narrowing of the upper airways during sleep, which predisposes to OSA, inevitably results in snoring. In most patients, snoring usually antedates the development of obstructive events by several years. However, the majority of snor-

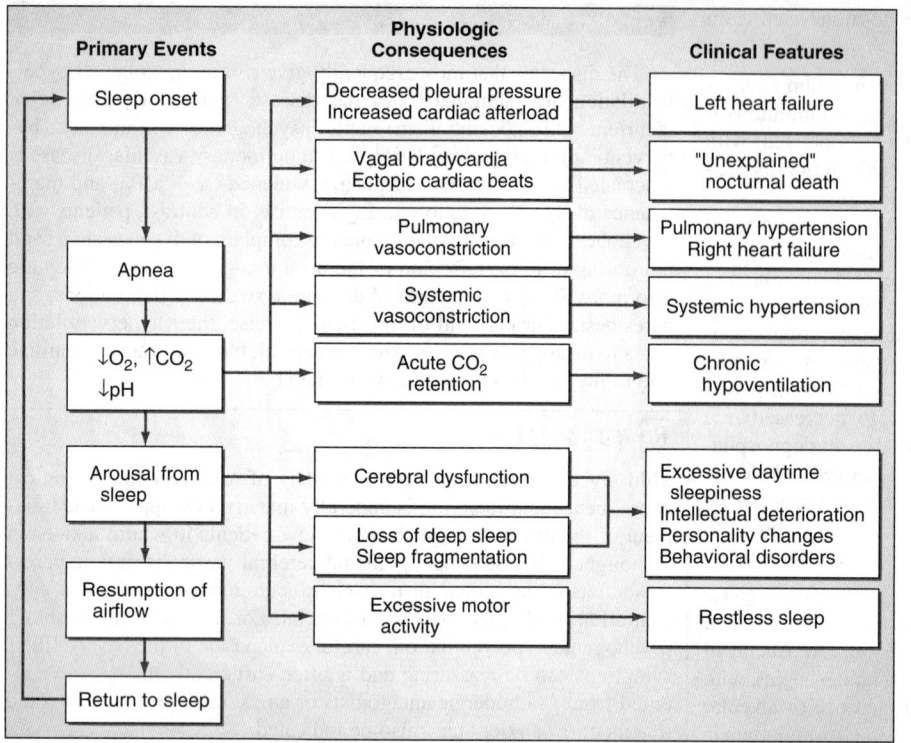

Primary Events	Physiologic Consequences	Clinical Features
Sleep onset	Decreased pleural pressure Increased cardiac afterload	Left heart failure
	Vagal bradycardia Ectopic cardiac beats	"Unexplained" nocturnal death
Apnea	Pulmonary vasoconstriction	Pulmonary hypertension Right heart failure
$\downarrow O_2$, $\uparrow CO_2$ $\downarrow pH$	Systemic vasoconstriction	Systemic hypertension
	Acute CO_2 retention	Chronic hypoventilation
Arousal from sleep	Cerebral dysfunction	Excessive daytime sleepiness Intellectual deterioration Personality changes Behavioral disorders
	Loss of deep sleep Sleep fragmentation	
Resumption of airflow	Excessive motor activity	Restless sleep
Return to sleep		

FIGURE 247-1 The primary sequence of events, physiologic responses, and clinical features of obstructive sleep apnea.

ing individuals do not have an OSA disorder, nor is there definitive evidence that snoring per se is associated with long-term health risks. Hence, in the absence of other symptoms, snoring alone does not warrant an investigation for OSA but does call for preventive counselling, particularly with regard to weight gain and alcohol consumption, and, when habitual, warrants conservative treatment similar to that for mild OSA (see below).

The recurrent episodes of nocturnal asphyxia and of arousal from sleep that characterize OSA lead to a series of secondary physiologic events, which in turn give rise in some patients to the clinical complications of the syndrome (Fig. 247-1). The most common manifestations are cognitive and behavioral disturbances that are thought to arise from the fragmentation of sleep and loss of slow-wave sleep induced by the recurrent arousal responses, and from nocturnal cerebral hypoxia. The most pervasive manifestation is excessive daytime sleepiness. Initially, daytime sleepiness manifests under passive conditions, such as reading or watching television; but as the disorder progresses, sleepiness encroaches into all daily activities and can become disabling and dangerous. Several studies have demonstrated two to seven times more motor vehicle accidents in patients with OSA compared with other drivers. Other related symptoms include intellectual impairment, memory loss, and personality disturbances.

The other major manifestations of OSA are cardiorespiratory in nature and are thought to arise from the recurrent episodes of nocturnal asphyxia and of negative intrathoracic pressure, which increases left ventricular afterload (Fig. 247-1). Many patients demonstrate a cyclical slowing of the heart during the apneas to 30 to 50 beats per minute, followed by a tachycardia of 90 to 120 beats per minute during the ventilatory phase. A small number of patients develop severe bradycardia or dangerous tachyarrhythmias, leading to the notion that OSA may result in sudden death during sleep, but corroborative data are lacking. Unlike in healthy subjects, in patients with OSA systemic blood pressure fails to decrease during sleep. In fact, blood pressure typically rises abruptly at the termination of each obstructive event as a result of sympathetic nervous activation and reflex vasoconstriction. Furthermore, over 50% of patients with OSA have systemic hypertension. Several epidemiologic studies have implicated OSA as a risk factor for the development of systemic hypertension, and studies in an

animal model demonstrate directly that OSA can cause sustained increases in daytime blood pressure. Emerging data also suggest that OSA can precipitate myocardial ischemia in patients with coronary artery disease and can adversely affect left ventricular function, both acutely and chronically, in patients with congestive heart failure. This complication is probably due to the combined effects of increased left ventricular afterload during each obstructive event, secondary to increased negative intrathoracic pressure (Fig. 247-1), recurrent nocturnal hypoxemia, and chronically elevated sympathoadrenal activity. Treatment of OSA in such patients often results in dramatic improvement in left ventricular function and in clinical cardiac status.

DIAGNOSIS Although OSA occurs at any age, and is considerably more prevalent in women than was previously thought, the typical patient is a male aged 30 to 60 years who presents with a history of snoring, excessive daytime sleepiness, nocturnal choking or gasping, witnessed apneas during sleep, moderate obesity and large neck circumference, and often mild to moderate hypertension. In women with OSA, who are typically postmenopausal, the complaint of snoring is less frequent than in men, and daytime fatigue may be more common than outright sleepiness.

The definitive investigation for suspected OSA is polysomnography, a detailed overnight sleep study that includes recording of (1) electrographic variables (electroencephalogram, electrooculogram, and submental electromyogram) that permit the identification of sleep and its various stages, (2) ventilatory variables that permit the identification of apneas and their classification as central or obstructive, (3) arterial O_2 saturation by ear or finger oximetry, and (4) heart rate. Continuous measurement of transcutaneous P_{CO_2} (which reflects arterial P_{CO_2}) can also be very useful, particularly in patients with CSA. The key diagnostic finding in OSA is episodes of airflow cessation or reduction at the nose and mouth despite evidence of continuing respiratory effort. By the time most patients come to clinical attention they have at least 10 to 15 obstructive events per hour of sleep. Although controversial, recent data suggest that a high upper airway resistance during sleep (manifested by snoring) that is accompanied by recurrent arousals from sleep, even in the absence of apneas and hypopneas, can result in a clinically important sleep-related syndrome. Therefore, the absence of outright apneas and hypopneas in a symptomatic patient may not definitely exclude a sleep-related respiratory disorder.

Because polysomnography is a time-consuming and expensive test, there is considerable interest in the role of screening tests and of unattended home sleep-monitoring for the investigation of OSA. However, the predictive value of most screening tests is too low to be clinically definitive, and the role of unattended, simplified sleep studies in routine practice has yet to be established. Nevertheless, in patients with a high probability of OSA (based on a history of habitual snoring, nocturnal choking or gasping, witnessed apneas during sleep, and daytime sleepiness or fatigue), overnight recording of arterial O_2 saturation by oximetry can be used to *confirm* the diagnosis and obviate the need for full polysomnography by demonstrating recurrent episodes of desaturation (at a rate of at least 10 to 15 events per hour). Negative results in such a patient do not exclude the diagnosis and mandate that the patient proceeds to polysomnography. In contrast, when the probability of OSA is low (only occasional snoring, no witnessed apneas, and no daytime sleepiness, fatigue, or other symptoms), the absence of nocturnal desaturation can be used to *exclude* OSA and obviate the need for full polysomnography. Based on these scenarios, it has been

TABLE 247-1 *Management of Obstructive Sleep Apnea (OSA)*

Mechanism	Mild to Moderate OSA	Moderate to Severe OSA
↑ Upper airway muscle tone	Avoidance of alcohol, sedatives	—
↑ Upper airway lumen size	Weight reduction	Uvulopalatopharyngo-plasty
	Avoidance of supine posture	
	Oral prosthesis	
↓ Upper airway subatmospheric pressure	Improved nasal patency	Nasal continuous positive airway pressure
Bypass occlusion		Tracheostomy

Source: From Phillipson, with permission.

estimated that overnight oximetry can obviate the need for polysomnography in about one-third of clinic patients referred for consideration of OSA.

℞ TREATMENT

Several approaches to treatment of OSA have been advocated, based on an understanding of the mechanisms involved ((Table 247-1). In establishing a treatment strategy, defining the severity of the disorder is essential, as indicated by the degree of clinical symptoms (particularly daytime sleepiness and fatigue) and the objective level of nocturnal respiratory and sleep disturbance. In severe OSA (significant daytime sleepiness or >30 obstructive events and arousals per hour of sleep), nasal continuous positive airway pressure (CPAP) is the treatment of choice. Nasal CPAP prevents upper airway occlusion by splinting the pharyngeal airway with a positive pressure delivered through a nasal mask. It is well tolerated and effective in >80% of patients, provided that they have received proper training. The established beneficial effects of CPAP include improvements in sleep quality, reduced daytime sleepiness and driving accidents, and decreased nocturnal hypertension. In patients with ischemic heart disease or congestive heart failure who also have OSA, nasal CPAP is the preferred treatment and the only one demonstrated to have a beneficial effect on cardiac status.

In patients with severe OSA who cannot tolerate nasal CPAP, upper airway surgery can be considered, with uvulopalatopharyngoplasty being the most commonly performed procedure. This operation is designed to increase the pharyngeal lumen by resecting redundant soft tissue. When applied to unselected patients with OSA, the response rate is <50%, but more discriminating selection of patients yields a higher rate of success. Other surgical approaches, including maxillofacial surgery, have variable results, but can be particularly effective in patients with craniofacial skeletal abnormalities.

In patients with mild to moderate OSA, nasal CPAP is superior to more conservative therapy but is often less well tolerated. Such patients can sometimes be managed effectively by modest weight reduction, avoidance of alcohol, improvement of nasal patency, cessation of smoking, and avoidance of sleeping in the supine posture. In addition, intraoral appliances, designed to modify the position of the mandible and tongue, can be effective and often better tolerated than nasal CPAP. Medications are generally ineffective in the management of OSA, except in patients with predominantly rapid eye movement (REM) sleep–related events in whom protriptyline or fluoxetine may be beneficial.

CENTRAL SLEEP APNEA

PATHOGENESIS The definitive event in CSA is transient abolition of central drive to the ventilatory muscles. Several underlying mechanisms can result in CSA (Table 247-2). First are defects in the metabolic respiratory control system and respiratory neuromuscular apparatus. Such defects usually produce a chronic alveolar hypoventilation syndrome (in addition to CSA) that becomes more severe during sleep when the stimulatory effect of wakefulness on breathing is abolished.

TABLE 247-2 *Mechanisms Underlying Central Sleep Apnea*

Underlying Mechanism	Clinical Example
Defects in metabolic control system or respiratory muscles	Primary and secondary central alveolar hypoventilation syndromes
	Respiratory muscle weakness
Transient instabilities in central respiratory drive	Sleep onset
	Hyperventilation-induced hypocapnia
	Idiopathic
	Hypoxia (high altitude, pulmonary disease)
	Cardiovascular disease, pulmonary congestion
	Central nervous system disease
	Prolonged circulation time

Source: From Phillipson, with permission.

In contrast are CSA disorders that arise from transient instabilities in an otherwise intact respiratory control system. Common to all these disorders is a P_{CO_2} level during sleep that falls transiently below the critical P_{CO_2} required for respiratory rhythm generation. This type of instability is frequent at sleep onset, because the P_{CO_2} level of wakefulness is generally lower than that required for rhythm generation in sleep; hence with loss of the stimulatory effect of wakefulness on breathing (referred to as the *waking neural drive*), an apnea develops at sleep onset until P_{CO_2} rises to the critical level (Fig. 247-2). However, if the central nervous system state fluctuates at sleep onset between "asleep" and "awake," a pattern of periodic breathing with central apneas or hypopneas develops as respiration follows the changes in state.

In most patients with CSA, the tendency to develop periodic breathing and central apneas during sleep is enhanced by some degree of chronic hyperventilation during wakefulness that drives the P_{CO_2} level below the threshold required for rhythm generation during sleep.

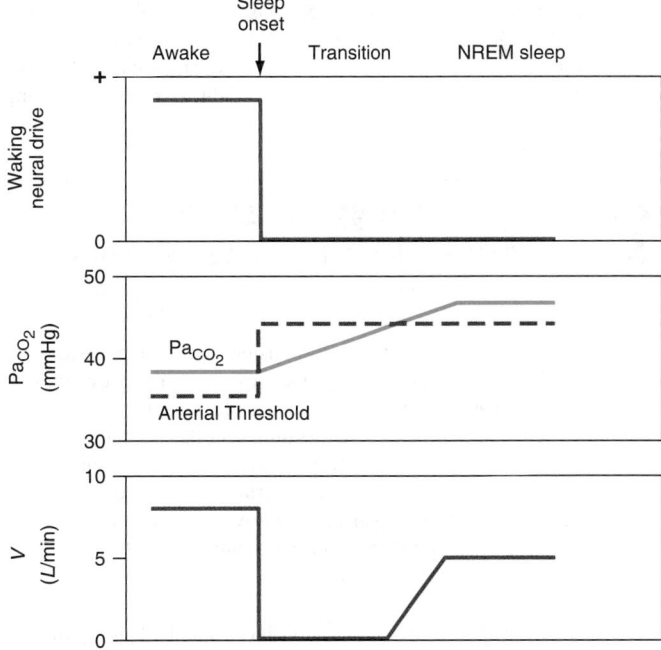

FIGURE 247-2 Schematic diagram of the mechanisms underlying central sleep apnea at sleep onset. With loss of the waking neural drive to breathing, the arterial threshold P_{CO_2} for rhythm generation increases above the Pa_{CO_2} present during wakefulness; ventilation (V) falls to zero and apnea ensues until Pa_{CO_2} rises above the threshold for rhythm generation during sleep. NREM, nonrapid eye movement. (*From TD Bradley, EA Phillipson, Clin Chest Med 13:439, 1992.*)

Such hyperventilation is frequently idiopathic in nature. Hypoxia, whether due to high altitude or to underlying cardiorespiratory disease, enhances the tendency to periodic breathing and CSA by a similar mechanism. Periodic breathing and CSA are also common in patients with congestive heart failure, in whom the periodic breathing is characterized by a classic crescendo-decrescendo pattern (Cheyne-Stokes respiration). Patients with heart failure and CSA have a higher left ventricular end-diastolic volume and filling pressure than do heart failure patients without CSA, suggesting that their hyperventilation results, at least in part, from pulmonary congestion and stimulation of pulmonary vagal receptors.

PATHOPHYSIOLOGIC AND CLINICAL FEATURES   In those patients whose CSA is a component of a chronic alveolar hypoventilation syndrome, daytime hypercapnia and hypoxemia are usually evident, and the clinical picture is dominated by a history of recurrent respiratory failure, polycythemia, pulmonary hypertension, and right-sided heart failure. Complaints of sleeping poorly, morning headache, and daytime fatigue and sleepiness are also prominent. In contrast, in patients whose CSA results from an instability in respiratory drive, the clinical picture is dominated by features related to sleep disturbance, including recurrent nocturnal awakenings, morning fatigue, and daytime sleepiness. In patients with congestive heart failure, CSA can be an important (and frequently overlooked) cause of daytime sleepiness and fatigue. In addition, studies indicate a higher mortality rate and higher rate of cardiac transplantation in congestive heart failure patients with CSA than in those without CSA, even when matched for functional class and left ventricular ejection fraction. This outcome probably relates to the fact that CSA can trigger sympathetic nervous activation in patients with heart failure and thereby exert a secondary deleterious effect on the underlying cardiac disorder.

DIAGNOSIS   Initially, many patients with CSA, particularly of the idiopathic type, are suspected clinically of having OSA because of a history of snoring, sleep disturbance, and daytime sleepiness. However, obesity and hypertension are less prominent in CSA than in OSA. Definitive diagnosis of CSA requires a polysomnographic study, with the *key observation being recurrent apneas that are not accompanied by respiratory effort*. Measurements of transcutaneous P_{CO_2} are particularly useful in CSA. Those patients with a defect in respiratory control or neuromuscular function typically demonstrate an elevated P_{CO_2} that tends to increase progressively during the night, particularly during REM sleep. In contrast, patients with instabilities in the respiratory control system typically demonstrate a mild degree of hypocapnia, which is an integral pathogenetic feature of their disorder (see above).

℞ TREATMENT

The management of patients whose CSA is a component of an alveolar hypoventilation syndrome is essentially the same as management of the underlying hypoventilation disorder (Chap. 246). Management of patients whose CSA arises from an instability of respiratory drive is more problematic. Patients with hypoxemia usually respond favorably to nocturnal supplemental oxygen. For those with idiopathic CSA, respiratory stimulation with acetazolamide or central nervous system sedation with triazolam have been advocated, but results are variable and efficacy has not been established. Nasal CPAP (as for OSA) can be effective in idiopathic CSA, although definitive long-term trials are lacking and the treatment is less well tolerated than in patients with OSA. The mechanism by which CPAP abolishes central apneas may involve a small increase in Pa_{CO_2} as a result of the added expiratory mechanical load. In patients whose CSA is secondary to congestive heart failure, CPAP is particularly effective in improving sleep quality and daytime cardiac function. In fact, short-term randomized trials have demonstrated that CPAP has a beneficial effect on several surrogate markers of mortality in patients with congestive heart failure, including left ventricular ejection fraction, functional mitral regurgitation, and norepinephrine concentrations. Small, 5-year follow-up studies in such patients demonstrate that CPAP results in a decreased mortality rate. Larger randomized trials are currently in progress.

FURTHER READING

JAVAHERI S et al: Sleep apnea in 81 ambulatory male patients with stable heart failure. Circulation 97:2154, 1998

KANEKO Y et al: Cardiovascular effects of continuous positive airway pressure in patients with heart failure and obstructive sleep apnea. N Engl J Med 348:1233, 2003

MCNICHOLAS WT, PHILLIPSON EA (eds): *Breathing Disorders in Sleep*. London, Saunders, 2002

PHILLIPS BG, SOMERS VK: Neural and humeral mechanisms mediating cardiovascular responses to obstructive sleep apnea. Resp Physiol 119:181, 2000

PHILLIPSON EA: Sleep disorders, in *Textbook of Respiratory Medicine*, 3d ed, JF Murray, JA Nadel (eds). Philadelphia, Saunders, 2000, pp 2153–2170

YOUNG T et al: Population-based study of sleep-disordered breathing as a risk factor for hypertension. Arch Intern Med 157:1746, 1997

---

248   LUNG TRANSPLANTATION
Elbert P. Trulock, G. Alexander Patterson, Joel D. Cooper

Lung transplantation is a therapeutic consideration for patients with most nonmalignant end-stage lung diseases. Activity grew rapidly through the mid-1990s and then reached a plateau of 1400 to 1500 transplants per year worldwide. Unfortunately, the demand exceeds the supply of donor organs, and deaths while awaiting transplantation are not unusual. Nonetheless, in appropriately selected recipients, transplantation prolongs survival and improves quality of life, but it is also associated with significant morbidity and mortality.

INDICATIONS

The indications for lung transplantation have spanned the gamut of lung diseases. The distribution reflects the prevalence and natural history of the various diseases, and the most common indications are shown in Table 248-1. "Other indications" in this table comprise many less prevalent lung diseases. During the past decade the proportion of recipients with primary pulmonary hypertension (PPH) steadily declined from 13% in 1990 to 4% in 2001 as medical therapy improved, and the fraction of recipients with chronic obstructive lung disease (COPD) or α_1-antitrypsin deficiency emphysema increased from 21 to 42%. During the same era, there was a trend toward more bilateral lung transplants, and since 1995 the annual numbers of single and bilateral procedures have been nearly equal.

RECIPIENT SELECTION

Transplantation should be considered when other therapeutic options have been expended and when the patient's prognosis will be improved by the procedure. Survival rates after transplantation can be compared with predictive indices for the underlying disease, but each patient's clinical course must be integrated into the assessment, too. Quality of life is the primary motive for transplantation for many patients, and the prospect of an improved quality-adjusted survival is often attractive to them, even if the survival advantage itself seems marginal.

Disease-specific guidelines for referring patients for transplantation are summarized in Table 248-2. These criteria are derived from prognostic information about the diseases and from clinical experience, and they are intended to identify patients who may benefit from transplantation. Although no randomized trial of transplantation has been carried out, relative risk analyses have demonstrated that transplantation

TABLE 248-1 *Indications for Adult Lung Transplantation (1995–2001)*

Diagnosis	Single Lung Transplantation (n = 4663)		Bilateral Lung Transplantation (n = 4118)		Total (n = 8781)	
Chronic obstructive pulmonary disease	2536	54.4%	926	22.5%	3462	39.4%
Idiopathic pulmonary fibrosis	1110	23.8%	376	9.1%	1486	16.9%
Cystic fibrosis	52	1.1%	1360	33.0%	1412	16.1%
α_1-Antitrypsin deficiency emphysema	408	8.7%	407	9.9%	815	9.3%
Primary pulmonary hypertension	61	1.3%	340	8.3%	401	4.6%
Sarcoidosis	126	2.7%	106	2.6%	232	2.6%
Bronchiectasis	14	0.3%	176	4.3%	190	2.2%
Eisenmenger's syndrome	8	0.2%	95	2.3%	103	1.2%
Lymphoangioleiomyomatosis	42	0.9%	53	1.3%	95	1.1%
Retransplantation	77	1.6%	79	1.9%	156	1.8%
Other indications	229	4.9%	200	4.9%	429	4.9%

Source: Adapted from Hertz et al.

confers a survival advantage in patients with COPD, idiopathic pulmonary fibrosis (IPF), cystic fibrosis (CF), and PPH.

Candidates for lung transplantation are thoroughly screened for any comorbidity that might adversely affect the outcome, and consensus guidelines for selecting potential recipients have been published. In general, suitable candidates should have clinically and physiologically severe lung disease (Table 248-2), but otherwise they must be in reasonably good health. The typical upper age limit is approximately 65 years at most centers. Absolute exclusions include HIV infection, chronic hepatitis B antigenemia or chronic active hepatitis C infection, uncured malignancy, active cigarette smoking, drug or alcohol dependency or abuse, uncontrolled or untreatable pulmonary or extrapulmonary infection, irreversible physical deconditioning, chronic noncompliance with medical care, and significant dysfunction of any vital organ other than the lungs.

Other problems that either increase the risk of complications or will be aggravated by the posttransplantation medical regimen consti-

tute relative contraindications. Some typical issues are ventilator-dependent respiratory failure, previous thoracic surgical procedures, osteoporosis, systemic hypertension, diabetes mellitus, severe obesity or cachexia, and psychosocial problems. Chronic infection poses a unique concern in patients with bronchiectasis. Infection with antibiotic-resistant *Pseudomonas* species is not unusual after years of treatment, and infection with *Burkholderia* species complicates the course of some patients with CF. In addition, infection with *Aspergillus* species or nontuberculous mycobacteria occurs in some cases. Pretransplantation *Burkholderia* infection has been associated with persistent posttransplantation infection and poor outcomes; however, pretransplantation infection with *Pseudomonas* species that are not panresistant to antibiotics, with *Aspergillus* that is not invasive, and with mycobacteria has not compromised the results of transplantation. The potential impact of these and many other factors have to be judged in their clinical context to determine an individual candidate's suitability for transplantation.

WAITING LIST AND ORGAN ALLOCATION

Suitable candidates for transplantation are placed on a waiting list, but there is a critical shortage of cadaveric donor organs. Organ allocation policies are influenced by ethical, medical, geographic, and political factors, and systems vary from country to country. Under the present lung allocation algorithm in the United States, after matching for body size and blood group compatibility between the donor and patients on the waiting list, donor lungs are assigned to recipients by their seniority on the waiting list. At this time, there is no priority for medical urgency, but the allocation scheme is being reviewed, and modifications may be proposed.

In the United States the median time to transplantation was 1064 days for patients who initially registered on the national waiting list in 1998. Because of the long waiting time, approximately 10% of patients who were at risk have died each year before an organ became available. However, the death rate while waiting has been much higher for patients with IPF, PPH, and CF than for those with COPD or α_1-antitrypsin deficiency emphysema.

TRANSPLANT PROCEDURE

Bilateral transplantation is mandatory for bronchiectasis because the risk of spillover infection from a remaining native lung precludes single lung transplantation. Heart-lung transplantation is obligatory for Eisenmenger's syndrome with complex anomalies that are not readily amenable to surgical repair and for concomitant end-stage lung disease and cardiac disease. However, cardiac replacement is *not* necessary for cor pulmonale because right ventricular function will recover when pulmonary vascular afterload is normalized by lung transplantation.

Either bilateral or single lung transplantation is an acceptable alternative for other diseases unless there are special considerations. However, bilateral transplantation provides more reserve lung function as a buffer against complications, and in recipients with COPD and α_1-antitrypsin deficiency emphysema, survival has been significantly

TABLE 248-2 *Disease-Specific Guidelines for Selecting Candidates for Lung Transplantation*

COPD and α_1-antitrypsin deficiency emphysema
  $FEV_1 < 25\%$ of predicted normal value (post-bronchodilator)
  $Pa_{CO_2} > 55$ mmHg
  Pulmonary arterial hypertension (mean pulmonary artery pressure > 25 mmHg)
Cystic fibrosis/bronchiectasis
  $FEV_1 < 30\%$ of predicted normal value
  $Pa_{CO_2} > 50$ mmHg
  $Pa_{O_2} > 50$ mmHg (on room air)
  Pulmonary arterial hypertension
  Adverse clinical course in spite of optimal medical management
    Increasing hospitalizations
    Recurrent, massive hemoptysis
    Rapidly declining FEV_1
    Cachexia
Idiopathic pulmonary fibrosis
  VC or TLC < 60–70% of predicted normal value
  $DL_{CO} < 50$–60% of predicted normal value
  Pulmonary arterial hypertension
  Hypoxemia ($Pa_{O_2} < 60$ mmHg or $SpO_2 < 90\%$) at rest or with activity (on room air)
  Progressive disease in spite of drug therapy
Primary pulmonary hypertension
  New York Heart Association functional class III or IV in spite of optimal drug therapy
  Unfavorable hemodynamic profile
    Right atrial pressure > 15 mmHg
    Mean pulmonary artery pressure > 55 mmHg
    Cardiac index < 2 (L/min)/m^2

Abbreviations: VC, vital capacity; TLC, total lung capacity; FEV_1, forced expiratory volume in 1 s; DL_{CO}, diffusing capacity for carbon monoxide; Pa_{O_2} and Pa_{CO_2}, partial pressure of oxygen and carbon dioxide, respectively, in arterial blood; SpO_2, oxygen saturation by pulse oximetry.
Source: Modified from International Guidelines for the Selection of Lung Transplant Candidates. Am J Respir Crit Care Med 158:335, 1998; with permission.

TABLE 248-3 *Recipient Survival, by Pretransplantation Diagnosis (1990–2000)*

		Survival Rate, %			
Diagnosis	n	3 Months	1 Year	3 Years	5 Years
Chronic obstructive pulmonary disease	4643	89	79	61	45
α_1-Antitrypsin deficiency emphysema	1288	85	74	59	50
Cystic fibrosis	1809	87	79	62	52
Idiopathic pulmonary fibrosis	1981	79	66	50	38
Primary pulmonary hypertension	714	81	68	53	48

Source: Data from Hertz et al.

better after bilateral transplantation. Nevertheless, single lung transplantation has been the preponderant procedure for COPD and IPF (Table 248-1). Bilateral transplantation has become the preferable operation for pulmonary vascular disease.

Living donor lobar transplantation has played a limited role in adult lung transplantation. It has been performed predominantly in teenagers or young adults with CF. A right lower lobe is obtained from one living donor and a left lower lobe from another, and these lobes are implanted to replace the right and left lungs, respectively, in the recipient. Since a lobe must replace a whole lung, donor-recipient size considerations are crucial, and the procedure is feasible only in recipients of relatively small stature. The results have been comparable to those with transplantation from cadaveric donors. The usual morbidities associated with a lobectomy have been encountered among the donors, but no deaths have yet been reported. Because of ethical concerns, this approach has been restricted to patients who were unlikely to survive the wait for a cadaveric donor.

POSTTRANSPLANTATION MANAGEMENT

Most recipients are managed with a three-drug maintenance immunosuppressive regimen that includes a calcineurin inhibitor (cyclosporine or tacrolimus), a purine synthesis antagonist (azathioprine or mycophenolate mofetil) and prednisone. Prophylaxis for *Pneumocystis carinii* pneumonia is standard, and prophylaxis against cytomegalovirus (CMV) infection is prescribed in many protocols. The dose of cyclosporine or tacrolimus is adjusted by blood-level monitoring. Both are metabolized by the hepatic cytochrome P450 system, and interactions with other medications that affect the pertinent cytochrome P450 pathways can profoundly alter the clearance and blood levels of these key immunosuppressants.

Routine management is designed to prevent complications or to detect them as soon as possible. The techniques include periodic contact with a transplant nurse coordinator, appointments with a physician, chest radiographs, blood tests, spirometry, and bronchoscopy. Lung function rapidly improves and then stabilizes by 3 to 6 months after transplantation. Subsequently, the coefficient of variation in spirometric measurements is small, and a sustained decline of 10 to 15% or more signals a potentially significant problem.

OUTCOMES

RESULTS Survival results are published regularly from large registries (Table 248-3) and can be accessed via the Internet (www.ishlt.org; www.ustransplant.org).

The main sources of perioperative mortality include technical complications of the operation, primary graft failure that is usually caused by ischemia-reperfusion lung injury, and infections. Although acute rejection and CMV infection are common problems in the first year, they have rarely been fatal. Beyond the first year, chronic rejection and non-CMV infections have caused the majority of deaths.

OUTCOMES Regardless of the pretransplantation diagnosis, successful transplantation has impressively restored cardiopulmonary function. Both overall and health-related quality of life have been enhanced after lung transplantation. With multidimensional profiles, improvements have extended across most domains and have been sustained longitudinally unless a complication such as chronic rejection has developed. However, fewer than one-half of recipients have reported either full- or part-time employment in 1-, 3-, and 5-year posttransplantation surveys.

COST The cost-effectiveness of lung transplantation has not been thoroughly analyzed. In the 1990s transplant hospitalization costs in the range of $160,000 were reported from two centers, but the charge would certainly be higher now. At these centers, the cost per quality-adjusted life-year gained through transplantation was estimated at approximately $155,000 to $175,000. Obviously, as recipients survive longer, the cost per quality-adjusted life-year will decrease, and the cost per quality-adjusted life-year for a 5-year survivor was appraised at $31,494 at one of the centers.

COMPLICATIONS

GRAFT DYSFUNCTION Graft dysfunction is not unusual in the first week after transplantation, and it has been referred to as *reperfusion edema*, *reimplantation response*, and *ischemia-reperfusion injury*. It is a form of acute lung injury with increased vascular permeability, but the severity is variable. Pulmonary venous obstruction and hyperacute rejection can produce a similar clinical picture in the first few days. The treatment is the conventional, supportive paradigm for acute lung injury, but inhaled nitric oxide and extracorporeal membrane oxygenation have been used successfully in severe cases. Most recipients recover, but graft failure is a leading cause of early death.

AIRWAY COMPLICATIONS The bronchial blood supply to the donor lung is disrupted. Consequently, when the lung is implanted in the recipient, the bronchus is dependent on retrograde bronchial blood flow through the pulmonary circulation and is vulnerable to ischemia.

The prevalence of major airway complications—dehiscence, stenosis, and bronchomalacia—has ranged from 4 to 20%, but the associated mortality has been very low. Management depends on the specific features. Laser therapy is effective for removing granulation tissue or fibrous webs. Sometimes, a stricture or stenosis can be managed by dilatation, but stent placement is often necessary for strictures and for bronchomalacia.

ACUTE REJECTION This is an immunologic response to direct or indirect alloantigen recognition, and it is characterized by arteriolar and bronchiolar lymphocytic inflammation. With current immunosuppressive regimens, 50% or more of recipients have at least one episode of acute rejection in the first year. Symptoms and signs can include cough, low-grade fever, dyspnea, hypoxemia, inspiratory crackles, interstitial infiltrates, and declining lung function. The signs and symptoms are nonspecific and overlap with infections like CMV pneumonia, hence the diagnosis should be confirmed by transbronchial biopsy. Treatment usually includes a short course of high-dose steroid therapy and adjustment of the maintenance immunosuppressive regimen.

CHRONIC REJECTION This complication is the main impediment to better medium-term survival rates, and it is the source of substantial morbidity because of its impact on lung function and quality of life. Both alloimmune inflammatory and non-alloimmune fibroproliferative mechanisms are probably important in the pathogenesis.

Clinically, chronic rejection is a form of graft dysfunction that is synonymous with bronchiolitis obliterans syndrome (BOS) (Chap. 243). BOS is characterized primarily by airflow limitation, and a formal diagnosis of BOS requires either a sustained decrement of 20% or more in the FEV_1 or biopsy proof of bronchiolitis obliterans. Clinically, the most useful is the $FEF_{25-75\%}$, which will usually decline before the FEV_1 and may presage BOS.

The prevalence of BOS approaches 50% by 3 years after transplantation. Both antecedent acute rejection and lymphocytic bronchiolitis are risk factors for subsequent BOS, and CMV pneumonitis has been implicated inconsistently. BOS is usually treated with augmented immunosuppression. While immunosuppressive therapy may stabilize lung function, the overall results of treatment have been disappointing, probably because the fibroproliferative process is already well established.

INFECTION The lung allograft is especially susceptible to infection, and infection has been one of the leading causes of death. In addition to a blunted immune response from the immunosuppressive drugs, other normal defenses are breached; the cough reflex is diminished, and mucociliary clearance is impaired in the transplanted lung. The spectrum of infections includes both opportunistic and nonopportunistic pathogens.

Bacterial bronchitis and pneumonia can occur at any time but are almost universal in the early postoperative period. Later, episodes of bronchitis are quite common, especially in recipients with BOS, and *P. aeruginosa* is often the culprit.

CMV is the most frequent viral infection after lung transplantation. Although gastroenteritis, colitis, and hepatitis can occur, CMV viremia and CMV pneumonia are the main illnesses. Most episodes occur in the first 6 months, and treatment with ganciclovir is effective unless resistance develops with repeated exposure. *Aspergillus* species have been the most problematic fungal infection.

OTHER COMPLICATIONS Other potential complications of the transplant operation are phrenic nerve injury with diaphragmatic dysfunction and vagal nerve injury with gastroparesis. Side effects and toxicities of the immunosuppressive drugs can cause new medical problems or aggravate preexisting conditions.

FURTHER READING

ARCASOY SM, KOTLOFF RM: Medical progress: Lung transplantation. N Engl J Med 340:1081, 1999

DeMEESTER J et al: Listing for lung transplantation: Life expectancy and transplant effect, stratified by type of end-stage lung disease, the Eurotransplant experience. J Heart Lung Transplant 20:518, 2001

ESTENNE M et al: Bronchiolitis obliterans syndrome 2001: An update of the diagnostic criteria. J Heart Lung Transplant 21:297, 2002

HERTZ MI et al: The Registry of the International Society for Heart and Lung Transplantation. Nineteenth official report—2002. J Heart Lung Transplant 21:950, 2002

249 PRINCIPLES OF CRITICAL CARE MEDICINE
John P. Kress, Jesse B. Hall

The care of critically ill patients requires a thorough understanding of pathophysiology and is centered initially around resuscitation of patients at extremes of physiologic deterioration. This resuscitation is often fast-paced and may have to be begun without a detailed awareness of the patient's chronic medical problems. While physiologic stabilization is taking place, intensivists attempt to gather important background medical information to supplement the real-time assessment of the patient's current physiologic conditions. Numerous tools are available to assist intensivists in the accurate assessment of pathophysiology and to support incipient organ failures, thus offering a window of opportunity for diagnosing and treating underlying disease(s) in a stabilized patient. Indeed, the use of invasive interventions such as mechanical ventilation and renal replacement therapy as well as diagnostic tools such as central venous and pulmonary artery catheters are commonplace in the intensive care unit (ICU).

ASSESSMENT OF SEVERITY OF ILLNESS Categorization of a patient's illness into grades of severity occurs frequently in the ICU. There are numerous severity-of-illness scoring systems that have been developed and validated over the past two decades. While these scoring systems have been validated as tools to assess populations of critically ill patients accurately, their utility in predicting individual patient outcomes is not clear.

Severity-of-illness scoring systems are important for defining populations of critically ill patients. This allows effective comparison of groups of patients enrolled in clinical trials. To be assured that a purported benefit of a therapy is real, investigators must be assured that different groups involved in a clinical trial have similar illness severities. These scores are also useful in guiding hospital administrative policies. Allocation of resources, such as nursing and ancillary care, can be directed by such scoring systems. Severity-of-illness scoring systems can also assist in the assessment of quality of ICU care over time.

Currently, the most commonly utilized scoring systems are the APACHE (acute physiology and chronic health evaluation) system, the MPM (mortality probability model), and the SAPS (simplified acute physiology score) system. These were all designed to predict outcomes in critical illness. All of these severity-of-illness scoring systems have common variables. These common threads include age; vital signs; assessments of respiratory, renal, and neurologic function; and an evaluation of chronic medical illnesses.

APACHE II Scoring System (Table 249-1) APACHE II is the most commonly used severity-of-illness scoring system in North America. Age, type of ICU admission (after elective surgery vs. nonsurgical or after emergency surgery), a chronic health problem score, and 12 physiologic variables (the most severely abnormal of each in the first 24 h of ICU admission) are used to derive a score. The predicted hospital mortality is derived from a formula that takes into account the APACHE II score; the need for emergency surgery; and a weighted, disease-specific diagnostic category (Fig. 249-1). The validation of this score is based upon 5815 ICU admissions from 13 different hospitals. Importantly, several studies have reported limitations of scoring systems such as APACHE II in predicting outcomes in specific subgroups of patients, such as postoperative coronary artery bypass graft patients. This is presumably related to the "controlled" temporary physiologic derangements that can occur in such patients (e.g., hypothermia, hypotension). More recently, the APACHE III scoring system has been

released. This scoring system is similar to APACHE II, in that it is based upon age, physiologic abnormalities, and chronic medical comorbidities. Although the APACHE III score can be calculated, conversion of the score to a mortality probability is only available as a proprietary commercial product.

The SAPS II score, used more frequently in Europe, is not disease-specific but rather incorporates three underlying disease variables (AIDS, metastatic cancer, and hematologic malignancy). The MPM can be used to calculate a direct probability of death in patients admitted to the ICU. It has been validated in 19,124 ICU admissions in 12 countries.

Severity-of-illness scoring systems suffer from the problem of inability to predict survival in individual patients. Accordingly, the use of these scoring systems to direct therapy and clinical decision-making cannot be recommended at present. Rather, these tools should be used as important data to complement clinical bedside decision-making. While they can provide valuable statistical probabilities for outcomes in similar groups of patients, they cannot reliably forecast outcomes in individual cases.

SHOCK (See also Chap. 253)

INITIAL EVALUATION Shock is a common condition necessitating admission to the ICU or occurring in the course of critical care. Shock is defined by the presence of multisystem end-organ hypoperfusion. Clinical indicators include reduced mean arterial pressure, tachycardia, tachypnea, cool skin and extremities, acute altered mental status, and oliguria. Hypotension is usually, though not always, present. The end result of multiorgan hypoperfusion is tissue hypoxia, often clinically manifested by lactic acidosis. Since the mean arterial pressure is the product of the cardiac output (CO) and the systemic vascular resistance (SVR), reductions in blood pressure can be categorized by decreased CO and/or decreased SVR. Accordingly, the initial evaluation of a hypotensive patient should evaluate the adequacy of the CO. This should be part of the earliest assessment of the patient by the clinician at the bedside once shock is considered (Fig. 249-2). Clinical evidence of diminished CO includes a narrow pulse pressure (the difference between systolic and diastolic blood pressure—a marker that correlates well with stroke volume) and cool extremities with delayed capillary refill. Signs of increased CO include a widened pulse pressure (particularly with a reduced diastolic pressure), warm extremities with bounding pulses, and rapid capillary refill. If a hypotensive patient has clinical signs of increased CO, it can be inferred that the reduced blood pressure is a result of decreased SVR.

In hypotensive patients with clinical evidence of reduced CO, an assessment of intravascular and cardiac volume status is appropriate. A hypotensive patient with decreased intravascular and cardiac volume status may have a history suggesting hemorrhage or other volume losses (e.g., vomiting, diarrhea, polyuria). The jugular venous pressure is often reduced in such a patient, while the change in pulse pressure as a function of respiration is increased. A hypotensive patient with an increased intravascular and cardiac volume status may have S_3 and/or S_4 gallop sounds on cardiac examination, increased jugular venous pressure, extremity edema, and rales on lung auscultation. The chest x-ray may show cardiomegaly, widening of the vascular pedicle, Kerley B lines, and pulmonary edema. Chest pain and electrocardiographic changes consistent with ischemia may also be noted.

In hypotensive patients with clinical evidence of *increased* CO, a

ACUTE PHYSIOLOGY SCORE

Score	4	3	2	1	0	1	2	3	4
Rectal temperature, °C	≥41	39.0–40.9		38.5–38.9	36.0–38.4	34.0–35.9	32.0–33.9	30.0–31.9	≤29.9
Mean blood pressure, mmHg	≥160	130–159	110–129		70–109		50–69		≤49
Heart rate	≥180	140–179	110–139		70–109		55–69	40–54	≤39
Respiratory rate	≥50	35–49		25–34	12–24	10–11	6–9		≤5
Arterial pH	≥7.70	7.60–7.69		7.50–7.59	7.33–7.49		7.25–7.32	7.15–7.24	<7.15
Oxygenation									
If $FI_{O_2} > 0.5$, use $(A - a) D_{O_2}$	≥500	350–499	200–349		<200				
If $FI_{O_2} \leq 0.5$, use Pa_{O_2}					>70	61–70		55–60	<55
Serum sodium, mEq/L	≥180	160–179	155–159	150–154	130–149		120–129	111–119	≤110
Serum potassium, meq/L	≥7.0	6.0–6.9		5.5–5.9	3.5–5.4	3.0–3.4	2.5–2.9		<2.5
Serum creatinine, mg/dL	≥3.5	2.0–3.4	1.5–1.9		0.6–1.4		<0.6		
Hematocrit	≥60		50–59.9	46–49.9	30–45.9		20–29.9		<20
WBC count, 10^3/mL	≥40		20–39.9	15–19.9	3–14.9		1–2.9		<1

GLASGOW COMA SCORE[b,c]

Eye Opening	Verbal (Nonintubated)	Verbal (Intubated)	Motor Activity
4—Spontaneous	5—Oriented and talks	5—Seems able to talk	6—Verbal command
3—Verbal stimuli	4—Disoriented and talks	3—Questionable ability to talk	5—Localizes to pain
2—Painful stimuli	3—Inappropriate words	1—Generally unresponsive	4—Withdraws to pain
1—No response	2—Incomprehensible sounds		3—Decorticate
	1—No response		2—Decerebrate
			1—No response

POINTS ASSIGNED TO AGE AND CHRONIC DISEASE AS PART OF THE APACHE II SCORE

Age, Years	Score
<45	0
45–54	2
55–64	3
65–74	5
≥75	6

Chronic Health (History of Chronic Conditions)[d]	Score
None	0
If patient is admitted after elective surgery	2
If patient is admitted after emergency surgery or for reason other than after elective surgery	5

[a] APACHE II score is the sum of the acute physiology score (vital signs, oxygenation, laboratory values) Glasgow coma score, age, and chronic health points. Worst values during first 24 h in the ICU should be used.

[b] Glasgow coma score (GCS) = eye-opening score + verbal (intubated or nonintubated) score + motor score.

[c] For GCS component of acute physiology score, subtract GCS from 15 to obtain points assigned.

[d] Chronic health conditions: liver, cirrhosis with portal hypertension or encephalopathy; cardiovascular, class IV angina (at rest or with minimal self-care activities); pulmonary, chronic hypoxemia or hypercapnia, polycythemia, ventilator dependent; kidney, chronic peritoneal or hemodialysis; immune, immunocompromised host.

Note: $(A - a) D_{O_2}$, alveolar-arterial oxygen difference; WBC, white blood (cell) count.

search for causes of decreased SVR is appropriate. The most common cause of high CO hypotension is sepsis (Chap. 254). Other causes include liver failure, severe pancreatitis, burns and other trauma that elicit the systemic inflammatory response syndrome (SIRS), anaphylaxis, thyrotoxicosis, and peripheral arteriovenous shunts. In summary, the three most common categories of shock (Table 253-1, p. 1600) are cardiogenic, hypovolemic, and high CO with decreased SVR (high-output hypotension). These categories may overlap and occur simultaneously (e.g., hypovolemic and septic shock, septic and cardiogenic shock).

The initial assessment of a patient in shock as outlined above should take only a few minutes. It is important that aggressive, early resuscitation be instituted based on the initial assessment, particularly since there are recent data suggesting that early resuscitation of septic and cardiogenic shock may improve survival. If the initial bedside assessment yields equivocal or confounding data, more objective assessments such as echocardiography and/or central venous or pulmonary artery catheterization may be useful. The goal of early resuscitation is to reestablish adequate tissue perfusion to prevent or minimize end-organ injury.

MECHANICAL VENTILATORY SUPPORT (See also Chap. 252)   During the initial resuscitation of patients in shock, principles of advanced cardiac life support should be followed. Since patients in shock may be obtunded and unable to protect the airway, an early assessment of the patient's airway is mandatory during resuscitation from shock. Early intubation and mechanical ventilation are often required. Reasons for institution of endotracheal intubation and mechanical ventilation include acute hypoxemic respiratory failure and ventilatory failure, which frequently accompany shock. Acute hypoxemic respiratory failure (Chap. 250) may occur in cardiogenic shock (high-pressure pulmonary edema, Chap. 255) and in septic shock (Chap. 254). Ventilatory failure often occurs as a result of an increased load on the respiratory system, which may present in the form of acute metabolic acidosis (often lactic acidosis) or decreased compliance of the lungs ("stiff" lungs) as a result of pulmonary edema. Inadequate perfusion of respiratory muscles in the setting of shock may be another reason for early intubation and mechanical ventilation. Normally, the respiratory muscles receive a very small percentage of the CO. However, in patients who are in shock with respiratory distress for the reasons listed above, the percentage of CO dedicated to respiratory muscles may increase tenfold or more. Lactic acid production from inefficient respiratory muscle activity presents an additional ventilatory load.

Mechanical ventilation may relieve the patient of the work of breathing and allow redistribution of a limited CO to other vital organs,

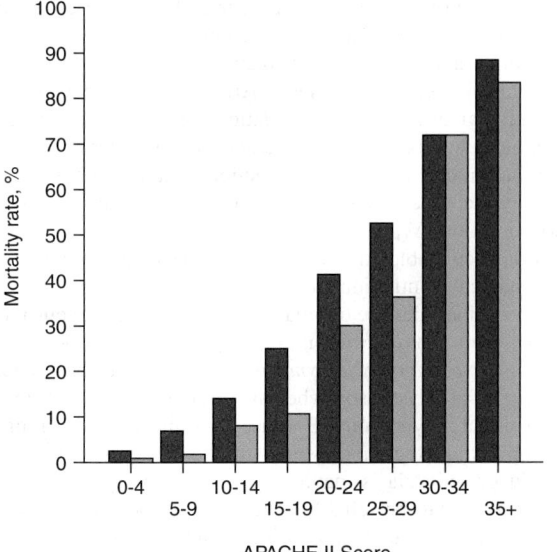

FIGURE 249-1   APACHE II mortality curve. Blue ■, nonoperative; green, postoperative.

often with an improvement in lactic acidosis. Patients demonstrate signs of respiratory muscle fatigue with a number of clinical signs including inability to speak full sentences, use of accessory respiratory muscles, paradoxical abdominal muscle activity, extreme tachypnea (>40 breaths/min), and decreasing respiratory rate despite an increasing drive to breathe. When patients with shock are treated with mechanical ventilation, a major goal of ventilator settings is to assume all or the majority of the work of breathing, facilitating a state of minimal respiratory muscle work. With the institution of mechanical

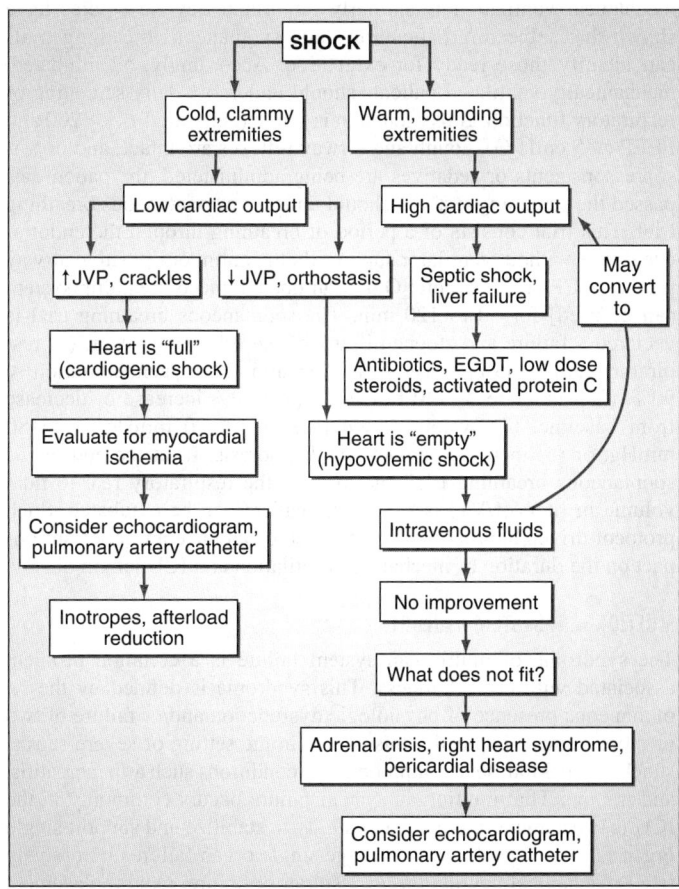

FIGURE 249-2   Approach to the patient in shock. JVP, jugular venous pulse; EGDT, early goal-directed therapy.

ventilation for shock, further worsening of blood pressure is frequently seen. The reasons for this include impedance of venous return with positive-pressure ventilation, reduced endogenous catecholamine secretion once the stress associated with respiratory failure is abated, and drugs used to facilitate endotracheal intubation (e.g., barbiturates, benzodiazepines, opiates), all of which may result in hypotension. Accordingly, hypotension after endotracheal intubation and positive-pressure ventilation should be anticipated. Many of these patients have a component of hypovolemia, which may respond to intravenous volume administration. →*For further discussion of individual forms of shock, see Chap. 253, Chap. 254, and Chap. 255.*

RESPIRATORY FAILURE (See also Chap. 250)

Respiratory failure is one of the most common reasons patients are admitted to the ICU. In some ICU settings, ≥75% of patients require mechanical ventilation during their ICU stay. Respiratory failure can be categorized mechanically, based on pathophysiologic derangements in respiratory function. Accordingly, four different types of respiratory failure can be described, based upon these pathophysiologic derangements.

TYPE I OR ACUTE HYPOXEMIC RESPIRATORY FAILURE   This form of respiratory failure occurs when alveolar flooding and subsequent intrapulmonary shunt physiology occur. Alveolar flooding may be a consequence of pulmonary edema, pneumonia, or alveolar hemorrhage. Pulmonary edema can be further categorized as occurring due to elevated intravascular pressures seen in heart failure and intravascular volume overload or to acute lung injury ("low-pressure pulmonary edema") (Chaps. 29 and 255). The acute respiratory distress syndrome (ARDS) describes an extreme degree of lung injury. This syndrome is defined by diffuse bilateral airspace edema seen by chest radiography (Figs. 233-2 and 251-2), the absence of evidence of left atrial hypertension (pulmonary capillary occlusion pressure <18 mmHg), profound shunt physiology with a ratio of Pa_{O_2} to fraction of inspired oxygen (Pa_{O_2}/Fi_{O_2}) of <200 (a Pa_{O_2}/Fi_{O_2} < 300 is described as *acute lung injury*), and a clinical setting where this syndrome is known to occur. Common clinical settings associated with acute lung injury and ARDS include sepsis, gastric aspiration, pneumonia, near-drowning, multiple blood transfusions, and pancreatitis.

The mortality rate of patients with ARDS was traditionally very high (50 to 70%), but recent changes in ventilator management strategy have led to reports of mortality in the low 30% range (see below). For many years, physicians have suspected that mechanical ventilation of patients with acute lung injury and ARDS may propagate lung injury. Cyclical collapse and reopening of alveoli may be partly responsible for this. As shown in Fig. 249-3, the pressure-volume relationship of the lung in ARDS is not linear. Alveoli may collapse at very low lung volumes. Animal studies have suggested that stretching and overdistention of injured alveoli during mechanical ventilation can further injure the lung.

Concern over this alveolar overdistention, termed *ventilator-induced "volutrauma,"* led to a multicenter, randomized, prospective trial to compare traditional ventilator strategies for acute lung injury and ARDS (large tidal volume—12 mL/kg ideal body weight) to a low tidal volume (6 mL/kg ideal body weight). This study showed a dramatic reduction in mortality in the low tidal volume group (large tidal volume—39.8% mortality—versus low tidal volume—31% mortality) and confirmed that ventilator management could impact outcomes in these patients.

TYPE II RESPIRATORY FAILURE   This ventilatory failure occurs as a result of alveolar hypoventilation and results in the inability to effectively eliminate carbon dioxide. Mechanisms by which this occurs are categorized as: (1) impaired central nervous system (CNS) drive to breathe, (2) impaired strength with failure of neuromuscular function in the respiratory system, (3) and increased load(s) on the respiratory system. Reasons for diminished CNS drive to breathe include drug overdose,

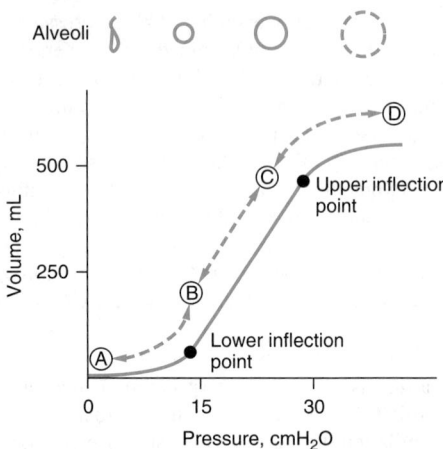

FIGURE 249-3   Pressure-volume relationship of the lungs of a patient with acute respiratory distress syndrome. At the lower inflection point, collapsed alveoli begin to open and the lung compliance changes. At the upper inflection point, alveoli become overdistended. The shape and size of alveoli are illustrated at the top.

brainstem injury, sleep-disordered breathing, and hypothyroidism. Reduced strength can be due to impaired neuromuscular transmission (e.g., myasthenia gravis, Guillain-Barré syndrome, amyotrophic lateral sclerosis, phrenic nerve injury) or respiratory muscle weakness (e.g., myopathy, electrolyte derangements, fatigue).

The overall load on the respiratory system can be classified into: resistive loads (e.g., bronchospasm), loads due to reduced lung compliance [e.g., alveolar edema, atelectasis, intrinsic positive end-expiratory pressure (autoPEEP)—see below], loads due to reduced chest wall compliance (e.g., pneumothorax, pleural effusion, abdominal distention), and loads due to increased minute ventilation requirements (e.g., pulmonary embolus with increased dead space fraction, sepsis).

The mainstays of therapy for type II respiratory failure are treatments directed at reversing the underlying cause(s) of ventilatory failure. Noninvasive positive-pressure ventilation using a mechanical ventilator with a tight-fitting face or nasal mask that avoids endotracheal intubation can often be used to stabilize these patients. This approach has clearly been shown to be beneficial in treating patients with exacerbations of chronic obstructive pulmonary disease. Noninvasive ventilation has been tested less extensively in other types of ventilatory failure but may be attempted nonetheless, in the absence of contraindications (hemodynamic instability, inability to protect airway, respiratory arrest).

TYPE III RESPIRATORY FAILURE   This form occurs as a result of lung atelectasis. Because atelectasis occurs so commonly in the perioperative period, this is also called *perioperative respiratory failure*. After general anesthesia, decreases in functional residual capacity lead to collapse of dependent lung units. Such atelectasis can be treated by frequent changes in position, chest physiotherapy, upright positioning, and aggressive control of incisional and/or abdominal pain. Noninvasive positive-pressure ventilation may also be used to reverse regional atelectasis.

TYPE IV RESPIRATORY FAILURE   This form occurs because of hypoperfusion of respiratory muscles in patients in shock. Normally, respiratory muscles consume <5% of the total CO and oxygen delivery. Patients in shock often suffer respiratory distress due to pulmonary edema, lactic acidosis, and anemia. In this setting, up to 40% of the CO may be distributed to the respiratory muscles. Intubation and mechanical ventilation can allow redistribution of the CO away from the respiratory muscles and back to vital organs while the shock is treated.

CARE OF THE MECHANICALLY VENTILATED PATIENT   Mechanically ventilated patients frequently require sedatives and analgesics. Most patients undergoing mechanical ventilation experience pain, which can be elicited

by the presence of the endotracheal tube and endotracheal suctioning. Accordingly, early and aggressive attention to pain control is extremely important. Opiates are the mainstay of therapy for pain control in mechanically ventilated patients. After assuring adequate pain control, additional indications for sedation for mechanically ventilated patients include: anxiolysis; treatment of subjective dyspnea; psychosis; facilitation of nursing care; reduction of autonomic hyperactivity, which may precipitate myocardial ischemia; and reducing global oxygen consumption (V_{O_2}).

Neuromuscular blocking agents are occasionally needed to facilitate mechanical ventilation in patients with profound dyssynchrony with the ventilator despite optimal sedation. The use of neuromuscular blocking agents may result in prolonged weakness—a myopathy known as the *postparalytic syndrome*. As a result, these agents are typically used as a last resort when aggressive sedation fails to achieve patient-ventilator synchrony. Because neuromuscular blocking agents result in pharmacologic paralysis without altering mental status, sedative-induced amnesia is mandatory when such agents are administered. Amnesia can be reliably achieved with benzodiazepines, such as lorazepam or midazolam, or with the intravenous anesthetic agent propofol. Outside of the setting of pharmacologic paralysis, there are few data supporting the idea that amnesia is mandatory in all patients who require intubation and mechanical ventilation. Sedatives and opiates may accumulate in critically ill patients when they are given for prolonged periods of time, since many of these patients have impaired hepatic and renal function. A protocol-driven approach to sedation of mechanically ventilated patients with daily interruption of sedative infusions has been shown to prevent excessive drug accumulation and shorten the duration of mechanical ventilation and length of stay in the ICU.

Weaning from Ventilation   While a thorough understanding of the pathophysiology of respiratory failure is essential in order to optimize patient care, recognition of a patient's readiness to be liberated from mechanical ventilation is similarly important. Several studies have shown that subjecting patients to daily spontaneous breathing trials can identify those ready for extubation. Accordingly, all intubated, mechanically ventilated patients should undergo a daily screening of respiratory function. If oxygenation is stable (i.e., $Pa_{O_2}/FI_{O_2} > 200$ and PEEP ≤ 5 cmH$_2$O), cough and airway reflexes are intact, and no vasopressor agents or sedatives are being administered, the patient has passed the screening test and should undergo a spontaneous breathing trial. This trial consists of a period of breathing through the endotracheal tube without ventilator support [both continuous positive airway pressure (CPAP) of 5 cmH$_2$O and an open T-piece breathing system can be used] for 30 to 120 min. The spontaneous breathing trial is declared a failure and stopped if any of the following occur: (1) respiratory rate > 35 breaths/min for >5 min (2) oxygen saturation < 90%, (3) heart rate > 140 beats/min or a 20% increase or decrease from baseline, (4) systolic blood pressure < 90 mmHg or >180 mmHg, or (5) increased anxiety or diaphoresis. If, at the end of the spontaneous breathing trial, the ratio of the respiratory rate to tidal volume in liters (f/V_T) is <105, the patient can be extubated. Such protocol-driven approaches to patient care can have an important impact on the duration of mechanical ventilation and ICU length of stay.

MULTIORGAN SYSTEM FAILURE

The syndrome of multiorgan system failure is a common problem associated with critical illness. This syndrome is defined by the simultaneous presence of physiologic dysfunction and/or failure of two or more organs. Typically, this occurs in the setting of severe sepsis, shock of any kind, severe inflammatory conditions such as pancreatitis, and trauma. That multiorgan system failure occurs commonly in the ICU is a testament to our current ability to stabilize and support single organ failure. The ability to manage single organ failure aggressively (e.g., mechanical ventilation for respiratory failure, renal replacement therapy for acute renal failure) has greatly reduced early mortality in critical illness. As such, it is uncommon for critically ill patients to die in the initial stages of resuscitation. Instead, many patients succumb to critical illness later in the ICU stay, after the initial presenting problem has been stabilized.

While there is debate regarding specific definitions of organ failure, several general principles governing the syndrome of multiorgan system failure apply. First, organ failure, no matter how defined, must persist beyond 24 h. Second, mortality risk increases as patients accrue additional organ failures. Third, prognosis is worsened by increased duration of organ failure. These observations remain true across various critical care settings (e.g., both medical and surgical). SIRS is a common basis for multiorgan system failure. Although infection is a common cause of SIRS, "sterile" triggers such as pancreatitis, trauma, and burns often are responsible for multiorgan system failure.

Gastrointestinal Tract Considerable attention has been directed to the liver and gastrointestinal tract as contributors to the syndrome of multiorgan system failure. Kupffer cells and macrophages in the liver play an important role in the uptake and clearance of endotoxin, cytokines, leukotrienes, and bacteria migrating from the lumen of the bowel to regional lymph nodes and then to the circulation (a process called *translocation*). Since the liver is positioned downstream from the venous drainage of the gastrointestinal tract, it plays a vital role in first-pass clearance of translocated bacteria, endotoxin, and cytokines. Mesenteric hypoperfusion plays a pivotal role in endotoxemia and bacterial translocation from the lumen of the gastrointestinal tract. It appears that mesenteric hypoperfusion leads to loss of integrity of the intestinal mucosa, with subsequent leakage of intact bacteria and endotoxin into mesenteric lymph nodes, mesenteric venous drainage, and the portal venous system. An imbalance favoring a pro-inflammatory state ensues, with overexpression of tumor necrosis factor-α and interleukins (IL), such as IL-1, IL-6, and IL-10. Leukocyte (particularly neutrophil) adherence to endothelial cells and subsequent diapedesis follows, propagating SIRS, which may progress in an unregulated manner.

Lungs While the gastrointestinal tract has received much attention with regard to its role as a nidus for the propagation of multiorgan system failure, other organs may also release inflammatory mediators in an unregulated manner and contribute to the propagation of SIRS and subsequent multiorgan system failure. Recent data suggest that the lungs may be a source of inflammatory cytokines, particularly when patients suffer from acute lung injury or ARDS (Chap. 251). It has been proposed that mechanical ventilation may propagate lung injury and the release of inflammatory cytokines from the lung itself.

MONITORING IN THE ICU

Because respiratory and circulatory failure occur commonly in critically ill patients, monitoring of the respiratory and cardiovascular systems is undertaken frequently in the ICU. Evaluation of respiratory gas exchange is routine in critical illness. The "gold standard" remains arterial blood-gas analysis, where pH, partial pressures of oxygen and carbon dioxide, and oxygen saturation are measured directly. With arterial blood-gas analysis, the two main functions of the lung—oxygenation of arterial blood and elimination of CO_2—can be assessed directly. Importantly, the blood pH, which has a profound effect on the drive to breathe, can only be assessed by sampling of arterial blood. Though sampling of arterial blood is generally safe, it may be painful and cannot provide continuous information for clinicians routinely. Given these limitations, noninvasive monitoring of respiratory function is often employed in the critical care setting.

PULSE OXIMETRY This is the most commonly utilized noninvasive monitor of respiratory function. The technique takes advantage of differences in the absorptive properties of oxygenated and deoxygenated hemoglobin. At wavelengths of 660 nm, oxyhemoglobin reflects light more effectively than does deoxyhemoglobin, whereas the reverse is true in the infrared spectrum (940 nm). A pulse oximeter passes both wavelengths of light through a perfused digit such as a finger, and the relative intensity of light transmission at these two wavelengths is

recorded. This allows the derivation of the relative percent of oxyhemoglobin. Since arterial pulsations produce phasic changes in the intensity of transmitted light, the pulse oximeter is designed to detect only light of alternating intensity. This allows distinction of arterial and venous blood saturation.

RESPIRATORY SYSTEM MECHANICS These can be measured during mechanical ventilation (Chap. 252). When volume-controlled modes of mechanical ventilation are used, accompanying airway pressures can be easily measured. The peak airway pressure is determined by two variables—the airways resistance and respiratory system compliance. At the end of inspiration, inspiratory flow can be stopped transiently. This end-inspiratory pause (*plateau pressure*) is a static measurement, impacted only by respiratory system compliance, not airways resistance. The difference between the peak (airways resistance + respiratory system compliance) and plateau (respiratory system compliance only) airway pressure provides a quantitative assessment of airways resistance. Accordingly, during volume-controlled ventilation, patients with increases in airways resistance (e.g., in asthma) typically have increased peak airway pressures as well as an abnormally high gradient between peak and plateau airway pressures (typically >15 cmH$_2$O). In such patients, the use of bronchodilators and/or glucocorticoids may be beneficial.

The plateau airway pressure is a static measurement, determined by the compliance of the respiratory system. Pathophysiologic processes such as pleural effusions, pneumothorax, increased abdominal girth from ascites or obesity all reduce chest wall compliance. Lung compliance may be reduced by pneumonia, pulmonary edema from any cause, or autoPEEP, which occurs when there is insufficient time for emptying of alveoli prior to the next inspiratory cycle. Since the alveoli have not decompressed completely, alveolar pressure remains positive at end-exhalation (functional residual capacity). This phenomenon is caused most commonly by critical narrowing of distal airways in disease processes such as asthma and chronic obstructive pulmonary disease. Modern mechanical ventilators allow breath-to-breath display of pressure and flow, which may allow detection of problems such as patient-ventilator dyssynchrony, airflow obstruction, and autoPEEP.

CIRCULATORY STATUS Monitors to characterize the circulatory status of critically ill patients are used commonly in the ICU. One of the most frequently used is the pulmonary artery catheter, also known as the right heart catheter or Swan-Ganz catheter. This catheter was originally designed as a tool to guide therapy in acute myocardial infarction but is currently used in the ICU for evaluation and treatment of a variety of other conditions such as ARDS, septic shock, congestive heart failure, and acute renal failure. This device has never been validated as a tool associated with reduction in morbidity and mortality.

Pulmonary Artery Catheter (See also Chap. 212) This is inserted via a central vein (jugular, subclavian, femoral) and is sequentially directed to the right atrium, right ventricle, and pulmonary artery after a balloon is inflated to facilitate its flow-directed placement. Waveform pressures in the right atrium, right ventricle, and pulmonary artery can be measured. When the balloon at the end of the pulmonary artery catheter is inflated, the catheter advances into a distal pulmonary artery until it "wedges" into place. Once the catheter is wedged, the measured pressure is transmitted from the "downstream" pulmonary veins and left atrium. Accordingly, the pulmonary capillary occlusion, or wedge, pressure is equal to the left atrial pressure under most circumstances. With a pulmonary artery catheter, the cardiac output can be measured directly using the thermodilution technique. When cool saline is injected into the proximal port of the catheter, the temperature change at the distal port can be measured. The measured temperature change is related to the volume of saline injected (which is known) and the CO. Blood from the pulmonary artery can be obtained from this catheter to measure oxygen saturation. This "mixed" venous saturation allows assessment of the adequacy of whole-body oxygen delivery.

Oxygen delivery is a function of CO and the content of O_2 in the arterial blood. The vast majority of O_2 delivered to tissues is bound to hemoglobin, and the dissolved O_2 contributes very little to O_2 content in arterial blood or O_2 delivery. The normal tissue extraction ratio for O_2 is ~25%. A pulmonary artery catheter allows measurements of O_2 delivery and oxygen extraction ratio.

The mixed venous O_2 saturation allows assessment of global tissue perfusion. A reduced mixed venous O_2 saturation may be caused by inadequate cardiac output, reduced hemoglobin concentration, and/or reduced arterial O_2 saturation. An abnormally high O_2 consumption, which may be caused by a multitude of problems such as fever, agitation, shivering, or thyrotoxicosis, may also lead to a reduced mixed venous O_2 saturation if O_2 delivery is not concomitantly increased.

Pulmonary artery catheters are invasive monitors and may be associated with a number of complications. Since the catheter is inserted via a central vein, all of the complications associated with central venous catheterization are present. These include central venous catheter–related infections, pneumothorax, arterial puncture with or without cannulation, bleeding, air embolism, venous thrombosis, and catheter embolism. The insertion of the pulmonary artery catheter also carries a number of risks, including dysrrhythmias, heart block, cardiac perforation, and balloon fragmentation. After the catheter is placed, pulmonary infarction, pulmonary artery rupture, and pulmonic valve insufficiency may occur. Fortunately, most of these complications are quite rare.

Misinterpretation of data derived from the pulmonary artery catheter may be the most common "complication" seen with these monitors. Pressure measurements in various cardiac chambers require careful zeroing of the pressure transducer relative to atmospheric pressure and placement at the proper adjustment, generally 5 cm inferior to the sternal angle in a supine patient. Another potential source of error is the variation in arterial pressure measurements as a function of the respiratory cycle. The atrial chambers are subjected to pleural pressure; therefore, atrial pressure typically falls during inspiration in a spontaneously breathing patient. Conversely, atrial pressure often rises during inspiration in a patient undergoing positive-pressure ventilation. As such, atrial pressure measurements should be made at end-expiration when there is no movement of air in or out of the thorax, often difficult to recognize in patients on mechanical ventilation.

PREVENTION OF COMPLICATIONS OF CRITICAL ILLNESS

SEPSIS IN THE CRITICAL CARE UNIT (See also Chap. 254)   Sepsis is a significant problem in the care of critically ill patients. It is the leading cause of death in noncoronary ICUs in the United States. Current estimates suggest that >750,000 patients are affected each year, and these numbers are expected to increase as the population continues to age and a greater percentage of persons vulnerable to infection will likely seek medical care.

Many therapeutic interventions in the ICU are invasive and predispose patients to infectious complications. These interventions include endotracheal intubation, indwelling vascular catheters, nasally placed enteral feeding tubes, transurethral bladder catheters, and other catheters placed into sterile body cavities (e.g., tube thoracostomy, percutaneous intraabdominal drainage catheters). The longer such devices remain in place, the more prone to these infections patients become. For example, ventilator-associated pneumonia correlates strongly with the duration of intubation and mechanical ventilation. Therefore, an important aspect of preventive care is the timely removal of invasive devices as soon as they are no longer needed. Multidrug resistant organisms are commonplace in the ICU.

An important aspect of critical care is infection control in the ICU. Simple measures such as frequent handwashing are effective but underutilized strategies. Protective isolation of patients with colonization or infection by drug-resistant organisms is another frequently used strategy in the critical care setting. Antibiotic-coated vascular catheters or endotracheal tubes with specialized suction ports above the cuff to decrease pooling and aspiration of oral secretions are other strategies

that may be used, with varying degrees of effectiveness reported. Surveillance programs monitoring adherence to infection control practices such as those described here may reduce the incidence of nosocomial infections.

DEEP VENOUS THROMBOSES   All ICU patients are at high risk for this complication, given their predilection toward immobility. Therefore, all ICU patients should receive some form of prophylaxis against deep venous thrombosis (DVT). Traditional forms of prophylaxis are subcutaneous low-dose heparin or low-molecular-weight heparin injections and sequential compression devices for the lower extremities. Recently, an observational study reported an alarming incidence of the occurrence of DVTs despite the use of these standard prophylactic regimens. Heparin prophylaxis may result in heparin-induced thrombocytopenia—another relatively common nosocomial complication in critically ill patients. Low-molecular-weight heparins such as enoxaparin are more effective than unfractionated heparin for DVT prophylaxis in high-risk patients, such as those undergoing orthopedic surgery, and they have a lower incidence of heparin-induced thrombocytopenia. Fondaparinux, a selective factor Xa inhibitor, is even more effective than enoxaparin in high-risk orthopedic patients.

STRESS ULCERS   Prophylaxis against stress ulcers is frequently administered in most ICUs. Typically, histamine-2 antagonists are administered. Currently available data suggest that high-risk patients, such as those with shock or respiratory failure requiring mechanical ventilation, benefit from such prophylactic treatment. Proton pump inhibitors are also used as agents for prophylaxis against stress ulcers, though outcomes data supporting the benefits of these drugs are largely lacking.

ANEMIA (See also Chap. 52)   This is a common problem in critically ill patients. Most suffer from anemia of chronic inflammation. Recent studies have demonstrated that erythropoietin levels are inappropriately reduced in most ICU patients and that exogenous erythropoietin administration may reduce transfusion requirements in the ICU. Phlebotomy contributes significantly to anemia in ICU patients. The hemoglobin level that merits transfusion in critically ill patients has been a long standing area of controversy. A large, multicenter study involving patients in many different ICU settings challenged a conventional notion that a hemoglobin level of 100 g/L (10 g/dL) is needed in critically ill patients. Patients prospectively randomized to red blood cell transfusions only when the hemoglobin level was ≤70 g/L (7 g/dL) had no difference in mortality than those liberally transfused to a target hemoglobin of 100 g/L (10 g/dL). It is noteworthy that even those with risk factors for coronary artery disease did not show increased morbidity or mortality with a restrictive transfusion strategy. Red blood cell transfusion is associated with impairment of immune function, increased risk of infections, acute lung injury, and volume overload—all of which may explain the findings in this study. Accordingly, a conservative transfusion strategy should be the rule in managing critically ill patients who are not actively hemorrhaging.

ACUTE RENAL FAILURE (See also Chap. 260)   This complication occurs in a significant percentage of critically ill patients. The most common underlying etiology is acute tubular necrosis, usually precipitated by hypoperfusion and/or nephrotoxic agents. Currently, there are no pharmacologic agents available for prevention of renal injury in critical illness. A recent study showed convincingly that low-dose dopamine is *not* effective in protecting the kidneys from acute injury. Other drugs, such as fenoldapam and vasopressin, have the potential to prove useful as agents for renal protection; however, more data are needed before firm conclusions can be drawn.

MALNUTRITION   This is a common problem in the critically ill patient; it may exacerbate respiratory failure, impair wound healing, and debilitate effective immune response. Nutritional support in the management of these patients is of the greatest importance. Early enteral feeding is reasonable, though no data are available to suggest that this improves patient outcome per se. Certainly, enteral feeding, if possible, is preferred over parenteral nutrition, which is associated with numerous complications including hyperglycemia, fatty liver, cholestasis, and sepsis. In addition, enteral feeding may prevent bacterial translocation across the gut mucosa (see "Multiorgan system failure", above). The catabolic state induced by critical illness mandates aggressive nutritional support; these patients often have higher caloric needs than normal patients, and nutrition support teams can play an important role in their management. Another recent study showed a significant mortality benefit when glucose levels were aggressively normalized in a large group of ICU patients, most of whom had recently undergone operations.

NEUROLOGIC DYSFUNCTION IN CRITICALLY ILL PATIENTS

Neurologic dysfunction is common in critically ill patients and a frequent cause of admission to the ICU.

DELIRIUM (See also Chap. 257) This state is defined by (1) an acute onset of changes or fluctuations in the course of mental status, (2) inattention, (3) disorganized thinking, and (4) an altered level of consciousness (i.e., other than alert). A recent study reported delirium in >80% of patients admitted to the ICU. A rapid test—the Confusion Assessment Method—to assess critically ill patients for delirium is available and has recently been validated. This assessment asks patients to answer simple questions and perform simple tasks and can be completed by the bedside nurse in about 2 min. The differential diagnosis of delirium in the ICU patient is broad and includes infectious etiologies (including sepsis), medications (particularly sedatives and analgesics), drug withdrawal, metabolic/electrolyte derangements, intracranial pathology (e.g., stroke, intracranial hemorrhage), seizures, hypoxia, hypertensive crisis, shock, and vitamin deficiencies (particularly thiamine).

ANOXIC CEREBRAL INJURY (See also Chap. 258) This condition is common following cardiac arrest and often results in severe and permanent brain injury in patients whose cardiac arrest is resuscitated. Active cooling of patients after cardiac arrest has been shown to improve neurologic outcomes. As such, all patients who present to the ICU after circulatory arrest from ventricular fibrillation or pulseless ventricular tachycardia should be actively cooled with cooling blankets and ice packs if necessary to achieve a core body temperature of 32 to 34°C.

STROKE (See also Chap. 349) This is a common cause of critical neurologic illness. Hypertension must be managed carefully, since abrupt reductions in blood pressure may be associated with further brain ischemia and injury. Acute ischemic stroke treated with tissue plasminogen activator (tPA) shows improved neurologic outcome when treatment is given within 3 h of onset of symptoms. However, mortality is not improved when tPA is compared to placebo, despite improved neurologic outcome, and cerebral hemorrhage is significantly higher in patients given tPA. A treatment benefit is *not* seen when tPA is given beyond 3 h. Heparin has not been shown to demonstrate improved outcomes convincingly in patients with acute ischemic stroke.

SUBARACHNOID HEMORRHAGE (See also Chap. 349) This may occur secondary to aneurysm rupture and is often complicated by cerebral vasospasm, rebleeding, and hydrocephalus. Vasospasm can be detected by either transcranial Doppler assessment or cerebral angiography; it is typically treated with the calcium channel blocker nimodipine; aggressive intravenous fluid administration; and therapy aimed at increasing the blood pressure, typically with vasoactive drugs such as phenylephrine. The intravenous fluids and vasoactive drugs (hypertensive hypervolemic therapy) are used to overcome the cerebral vasospasm. Early surgical clipping of aneurysms is advocated to prevent complications related to rebleeding. Hydrocephalus, typically heralded by a decreased level of consciousness, may require ventriculostomy drainage.

STATUS EPILEPTICUS (See also Chap. 348) Recurrent or relentless seizure activity is a medical emergency. Cessation of seizure activity is required to prevent irreversible neurologic injury. Lorazepam is the most effective benzodiazepine for treating status epilepticus and is the treatment of choice for controlling seizures acutely. Phenytoin or fosphenytoin should be given concomitantly since lorazepam has a short half-life. Other drugs such as gabapentin, carbamazepine, and phenobarbital should be reserved for patients with contraindications to phenytoin (e.g., allergy or pregnancy) or ongoing seizures despite phenytoin.

BRAIN DEATH (See also Chap. 258) Although critically ill patients usually die from irreversible cessation of circulatory and respiratory function, a diagnosis of death may also be established by irreversible cessation of all functions of the entire brain, including the brainstem, even if circulatory and respiratory functions remain intact as a result of artificial life support. Patients must demonstrate absence of cerebral function (unresponsive to all external stimuli) and brainstem functions [e.g., unreactive pupils, absent ocular movement to head turning or ice water irrigation of ear canals, positive apnea test (no drive to breathe)]. Absence of brain function must have an established cause and be permanent without possibility of recovery (e.g., must confirm the absence of sedative effect, hypothermia, hypoxemia, neuromuscular paralysis, or severe hypotension). If there is uncertainty about the cause of coma, studies of cerebral blood flow and electroencephalography should be performed.

WITHHOLDING AND WITHDRAWING CARE (See also Chap. 9)

The withholding and withdrawing of care occurs commonly in the ICU setting. Concerns about the provision of care deemed futile are occasionally raised during the care of critically ill patients. The Task Force on Ethics of the Society of Critical Care Medicine reported in a consensus statement that it is ethically sound to withhold or withdraw care if a patient or surrogate makes such a request or if the goals of therapy are not achievable according to the physician. Since all medical treatments are justified by their expected benefits, the loss of such an expectation justifies the act of withdrawing or withholding such a treatment. As such, the act of withdrawing care is fundamentally similar to the act of withholding care. An underlying stipulation derived from this task force report is that the informed patient should have his or her wishes respected with regard to life-sustaining therapy. Implicit in this stipulation is the need to ensure that patients are thoroughly and accurately informed regarding the plausibility and expected results of various therapies. The act of informing patients and/or surrogate decision makers is the responsibility of the physician and other health care providers. In the event a patient or surrogate desires therapy deemed futile by the treating physician, the physician is not ethically obligated to provide such treatment. Rather, arrangements may be made to transfer the patient's care to another care provider.

Decisions to withhold or withdraw care should occur only after extensive discussions with the patient (if this is possible), surrogate(s), and other health-care providers, usually in the form of one or more multiple formal meetings. In addition, most institutions have ethics committees to assist in the withholding and withdrawal of care. Though not required routinely, such committees are available to safeguard against patients or surrogates making capricious requests to withhold or withdraw care. In addition, such consultation may be considered in the event that a patient or surrogate does not agree with the physician's impression that care should be withheld or withdrawn.

It is noteworthy that decisions to withhold and withdraw life support from the critically ill are increasing, with recent reports of up to 90% of patients dying in the ICU after care was withheld or withdrawn. Critical care providers should meet regularly with patients and/or surrogates to discuss prognosis when the withholding or withdrawal of care is being considered. After a consensus amongst caregivers has been reached regarding withholding or withdrawal of care, this should be relayed to the patient and/or surrogate decision maker. If a decision to withhold or withdraw life-sustaining care for a patient has been reached, aggressive attention to analgesia and anxiolysis is needed. Opiates and benzodiazepines are typically used to achieve these goals.

Patients may have their death hastened by the aggressive administration of analgesic and anxiolytic drugs; however, if the intent of this therapy is to alleviate suffering and not to hasten death, this "double effect" is ethically acceptable.

FURTHER READING

ELY EW et al: Delirium in mechanically ventilated patients: Validity and reliability of the confusion assessment method for the intensive care unit (CAM-ICU). JAMA 286:2703, 2001

KNAUS WA et al: APACHE II: A severity of disease classification system. Crit Care Med 13:818, 1985

KRESS JP et al: Daily interruption of sedative infusions in critically ill patients undergoing mechanical ventilation. N Engl J Med 342:1471, 2000

RIVERS E et al: Early goal directed therapy in the treatment of severe sepsis and septic shock. N Engl J Med 346:305, 2002

SCHIFFL H et al: Daily hemodialysis and the outcome of acute renal failure. N Engl J Med 346:305, 2002

TASK FORCE ON ETHICS OF THE SOCIETY OF CRITICAL CARE MEDICINE: Consensus report on the ethics of foregoing life-sustaining treatments in the critically ill. Crit Care Med 18:1424, 1990

THE ACUTE RESPIRATORY DISTRESS SYNDROME NETWORK: Ventilation with lower tidal volumes as compared with traditional tidal volumes for acute lung injury and the acute respiratory distress syndrome. N Engl J Med 342:1301, 2000

THE HYPOTHERMIA AFTER CARDIAC ARREST STUDY GROUP: Mild therapeutic hypothermia to improve the neurologic outcome after cardiac arrest. N Engl J Med 346:549, 2002

VAN DEN BERGHE G et al: Intensive insulin therapy in the surgical intensive care unit. N Engl J Med 345:1359, 2001

250 RESPIRATORY FAILURE
Craig Lilly, Edward P. Ingenito, Steven D. Shapiro

DEFINITION AND CLASSIFICATION Respiratory failure is defined as a failure of gas exchange due to inadequate function of one or more essential components of the respiratory system. Clinically, respiratory failure can be manifest either as hypoxemia ($P_{O_2} < 60$ mmHg at sea level), i.e., inadequate blood oxygenation; hypercarbia ($P_{CO_2} > 45$ mmHg), i.e., excess of circulating carbon dioxide; or frequently, a combination of both types of gas exchange abnormalities. Respiratory failure is classified as hypoxemic, hypercarbic, or combined.

Respiratory failure is also commonly described in terms of its acuity, since it may develop either acutely or chronically. In *acute respiratory failure*, a sudden, catastrophic event leads to life-threatening respiratory insufficiency. In *chronic respiratory failure*, gradual worsening of respiratory function leads to progressive impairment of gas exchange, the metabolic effects of which are partially compensated by adaptations in other systems. In patients with long-standing respiratory disease, compensated *chronic respiratory insufficiency* may exist for many years, resulting in a state in which patients do not have true respiratory failure but have little or no functional respiratory reserve. In such cases, even a mild insult to the respiratory system can precipitate *acute on chronic respiratory failure*.

Independent of cause, as respiratory demand exceeds the functional capacity of the respiratory system, respiratory failure evolves and immediate medical intervention is required.

EPIDEMIOLOGY Respiratory failure is a common diagnosis among patients in medical intensive care units (ICUs) and is associated with a poor prognosis. The incidence of respiratory failure is 137 cases per 100,000 population, or 360,000 cases per year in the United States, with 36% of these individuals failing to survive the hospitalization. Both the incidence of and mortality from respiratory failure increase exponentially with age and in the presence of other comorbid conditions. Therapeutic advances in both mechanical ventilation and airway management have improved the prognosis for patients with respiratory failure over the past several decades. Even patients with irreversible chronic respiratory failure can now be provided with ventilator support systems that allow an acceptable quality of life and can be managed at home. Lung transplantation is also an option for selected patients with chronic respiratory failure (Chap. 248), although the widespread use of transplantation is limited by both the availability of organ donors and the number of qualified transplant centers.

PHYSIOLOGY Describing respiratory failure as either hypoxemic or hypercarbic provides some information about the physiologic deficit. However, a better understanding of the underlying pathophysiology and potential treatment strategies can be gained by considering the individual components of the respiratory system that are required for effective function under physiologic conditions. Normal respiration requires the integrated function of five separate components.

1. *Nervous system*. This is the control system, and it comprises the dorsal and ventral nuclei of the medullary respiratory control group and their associated afferent and efferent neural pathways. These act in concert with the cerebral cortex to determine respiratory rate and breathing effort. Respiratory failure due to diseases that cause dysfunction of the central control system can be thought of as *controller dysfunction*, or central apnea.

2. *Musculature* (the pump). The inspiratory muscles of breathing consist primarily of the diaphragm, but accessory muscles also contribute, including the internal intercostals, suprasternal, and sternocleidomastoid, as do supporting structures of the chest wall, which lower the pressure in the pleural space between the chest wall and lung during inspiration, establishing a pressure gradient between the airway opening and alveolar compartment that causes gas to flow into the lung. Respiratory failure due to diseases that cause ineffective function of the respiratory pump can be thought of as *pump dysfunction*. Under normal conditions, only elastic recoil is required for expiration, but during respiratory failure accessory muscles of expiration are required.

3. *Airways* (a complex conduit system for bulk delivery of gases). These consist of the upper airways, cartilaginous bronchi, and small airways distal to the terminal bronchioles capable of conducting gas quickly and evenly into and out of the alveolar compartment where gas exchange can occur. Respiratory failure involving diseases that cause marked obstruction or dysfunction of the air passages can be thought of as *airway system dysfunction*.

4. *Alveolar units* (an efficient, distensible, compact membrane system). This system consists of the respiratory bronchioles, alveolar ducts, and alveoli; these provide sufficient surface area to allow for rapid exchange of gases and sufficient elasticity so that following expansion, the membrane can generate adequate recoil pressure to empty the lung passively during exhalation. Respiratory failure as a result of diseases that cause collapse, flooding, or injury to the alveolar network can be thought of as *alveolar compartment dysfunction*.

5. *Vasculature* (a network of conduits capable of transporting dissolved gases to and from the functioning organs throughout the body). This consists of the pulmonary capillary network, intimately associated with the membrane system, but distinct both in structure and with respect to the types of diseases that can alter its normal function. Respiratory failure as a result of disease involving the pulmonary vasculature can be thought of as *pulmonary vascular dysfunction*.

Failure of any *one* of these essential components or significant dysfunction of more than one essential component can lead to *failure of the integrated system* and produce clinical respiratory failure.

Many diseases cause dysfunction of several of the essential components of the respiratory system, and ultimately this leads to abnormalities in gas exchange. Understanding which components of the respiratory system have failed in a given case provides valuable insight into the underlying disease process that cannot be gained from a simple analysis of the gas exchange abnormalities. For example, a patient with severe asthma, a patient with a large pulmonary embolus, and a patient with pulmonary edema may all present with hypoxemic respiratory failure. In each case, however, the cause and treatment of the respiratory failure are distinct. Developing a clinical approach for evaluating the five different functional components of the respiratory system is essential for identifying the cause of respiratory failure and quickly developing an effective management plan.

CLINICAL EVALUATION ■ Initial Assessment and Stabilization of Respiratory Failure Initial evaluation of the respiratory system includes an immediate determination of upper airway patency and an examination for central and peripheral cyanosis, followed by measurement of the respiratory rate and observation of the depth and pattern of respiration. One should simultaneously note the presence or absence of signs of respiratory distress including flaring of nostrils, pursed-lip breathing, and use of accessory muscles of respiration. Next, one should assess the configuration of the chest wall and its movement during the respiratory cycle. This is followed by palpation and auscultation over each hemithorax. These observations allow an initial assessment of respiratory drive, pump function, and delivery of gas to the lungs. This examination is supplemented by an estimation of the oxygen and carbon dioxide content of arterial blood determined by arterial blood-gas measurement. Oximetry provides a rapid way to determine blood oxygen content but does not provide information regarding alveolar ventilation and P_{CO_2} levels; an arterial blood-gas measurement is required to assess these parameters.

In contrast to many clinical conditions, the emergent nature of acute respiratory failure and the potential for rapid progression to a life-threatening situation require that initial therapy be implemented before the specific etiology of the respiratory failure is diagnosed and treated. Adequate airway protection, oxygenation, and ventilation should be assured prior to further diagnostic testing. Thus, in concert with the initial assessment one must stabilize the patient with respiratory failure quickly since hypoxemia and hypercarbia can rapidly lead to circulatory failure and death (see "Initial Management," below). Cardiovascular stability must also be rapidly assessed and achieved (see Chap. 253). From the standpoint of respiratory failure, the first priority is to establish adequate oxygenation and ventilation. Administration of supplemental oxygen might be all that is initially required, but if the patient is in distress, artificial ventilation is needed. Initially, ventilation is often administered manually using a bag-valve-mask device followed by use of a mechanical ventilator (Chap. 252). Once an endotracheal tube has been placed and secured, and its position verified, ventilator support can be initiated to help normalize oxygenation and CO_2 elimination. Following stabilization of the patient, a systematic

and thorough evaluation of the cause of respiratory failure can safely be carried out.

Clinical Evaluation of Respiratory Failure Based on Physiologic Principles Simple bedside techniques can be used to assess which of the five components of the respiratory system are no longer functioning normally in a patient with respiratory failure (Table 250-1). This assessment can provide great insight into the clinical cause of respiratory failure and assist with management planning.

CONTROLLER DYSFUNCTION This is perhaps the least common primary cause of respiratory failure, and it can be difficult to assess in the intubated ICU patient because many medications used to ensure comfort also affect the level of consciousness and limit respiratory drive. Nevertheless, useful information can frequently be obtained about respiratory drive by simple observation and history. The most frequent cause of controller dysfunction is the presence of medications that impair respiratory drive, many of which also impair the level of consciousness. A history of the use of respiratory depressants or an impaired level of consciousness prior to the administration of medications to facilitate intubation suggests the possibility of controller dysfunction. The awake, minimally sedated patient with either significant hypercarbia or hypoxemia who demonstrates no elevation in respiratory rate (i.e., <12 breaths/min) and no use of accessory muscles is likely to have a defect in regulating respiratory drive. In respiratory failure due solely to controller dysfunction, such as an opiate overdose, the degree of hypoxemia is in direct proportion to the degree of hypercarbia, i.e., the patient will have a normal alveolar-arterial gradient (Chap. 234). This can be calculated with the information obtained from an arterial blood-gas measurement. More formal tests of respiratory drive, including determining if the respiratory rate increases to at least 25 breaths/min when the patient inhales a mixture of 5% CO_2 and 15% O_2 (the CO_2 challenge test) and measuring the pressure generated 0.1 s after the start of inhalation (the $P_{0.1}$ test), have been described for outpatient investigation of respiratory controller problems, but they are not used in the ICU setting.

PUMP DYSFUNCTION This is a common cause of respiratory failure in ICU patients with respiratory failure and is usually multifactorial. Various medications, prolonged periods of mechanical ventilator support, and polyradiculopathy associated with critical illness can all adversely affect the respiratory muscles. In the patient who is not intubated, one must assess degree of respiratory distress as described above. In addition, abdominal paradoxus indicates diaphragmatic fatigue, a hallmark of pump failure. For patients who are mechanically ventilated, a

TABLE 250-1 *Methods for Assessing Controller, Pump, Airway, Alveolar Compartment, and Pulmonary Vascular Dysfunction at the Bedside*

Type of Dysfunction	Test	Method of Determination	Findings Consistent with Dysfunction
Controller	Respiratory rate	Clinical observation in spontaneously breathing patient	< 12/min in presence of hypoxia or hypercarbia and acidemia
Pump	Vital capacity, inspiratory force	Bedside measurement in awake patient	Presence of paradoxical respiratory motions. VC < 10 mL/kg IF < −20 cmH₂O RSBI > 105
Airway	Wheezing or ronchi on auscultation	Physical examination	Presence of wheezing
	Airway resistance measurement	Bedside measurement in cooperative or sedated patient	Raw > 10 cmH₂O/L per second
	Clinical evidence of auto-PEEP	Auscultation or bedside measurement in sedated patient	Presence of autoPEEP
Alveolar	Arterial blood gas	Arterial blood sample	Exam suggestive of consolidation
	Respiratory system compliance	Bedside measurement in sedated patient	Abnormal Pa_{O_2}/Fi_{O_2} ratio or elevated Pa_{CO_2}; Crs > 30 mL/cmH₂O
	Chest radiograph	Bedside x-ray	Alveolar infiltrates
Pulmonary vascular	Assessment of right heart function	JVP−central venous pressure	Elevation
		ECG	Right heart strain or RBBB

Note: VC, vital capacity; IF, inspiratory force; RSBI, rapid-shallow-breathing index; raw, raw airway resistance; auto-PEEP, intrinsic positive end-expiratory pressure; Crs, respiratory system compliance; JVP, jugular venous pressure; ECG, electrocardiogram; RBBB, right bundle branch block.

variety of simple bedside tests have been used to assess respiratory muscle function. Measurement of vital capacity and inspiratory force are the most frequently used; they provide an assessment of both the volume the respiratory muscles can generate against the impedance of the respiratory system and the isovolumetric pressure the respiratory muscles can generate during a maximal effort. Vital capacity < 10 mL/kg and inspiratory force measurements that fail to achieve a negative pressure of at least −20 cmH₂0 indicate a component of respiratory muscle insufficiency. The rapid-shallow-breathing index (respiratory rate/tidal volume) is an integrative index of respiratory performance that predicts success of liberation from mechanical ventilation when it is <105. More sophisticated measurements of respiratory muscle function, including transdiaphragmatic pressure measurements using esophageal balloons and bedside electromyography and nerve conduction studies, can be used in special circumstances to obtain detailed information about respiratory muscle dysfunction when warranted.

AIRWAY DYSFUNCTION   This can also be readily assessed at the bedside in the patient with respiratory failure using simple bedside measurements and clinical assessment. Stridor suggests the presence of large airway or laryngeal obstruction. Bronchospasm can be diagnosed by auscultation and detection of wheezing and/or rhonchi. Coarse breath sounds or rhonchi present during the inspiratory phase of respiration usually indicate obstruction of the large airways, frequently from retained secretions. High-pitched wheezing during expiration indicates obstruction of the small airways and is commonly associated with bronchospasm. In cases of severe airflow obstruction, wheezing may be reduced because airflow is minimal. In these cases, the obstruction may be manifest as dynamic hyperinflation or intrinsic positive end-expiratory pressure (autoPEEP), and detected by persistent, faint wheezing that continues throughout expiration to the point of initiation of the subsequent inspiration.

Simple bedside measurements can also be used to detect airflow obstruction, although they require that the patient be synchronous with the ventilator and not tachypneic. Therefore these tests are best performed in the sedated patient. By programming the ventilator to impose a brief pause (0.5 to 1 s in duration) at the end of inspiration, the driving pressure to overcome airway resistance during inspiration, equal to the peak inspiratory pressure minus the airway pressure measured at the end of the pause (i.e., plateau pressure), can be determined. Dividing this pressure difference by the end-inspiratory flow rate gives an estimate of airway resistance. Normal values in the intubated patient range from 3 to 8 cmH₂O/L per second, depending upon the size of the endotracheal tube. Values significantly greater than this indicate airflow obstruction. More detailed information about lung impedance, including airway resistance and dynamic compliance, can be obtained by measuring transpulmonary pressures, volumes, and flows using an esophageal balloon and bedside pneumotachograph system. However, such detailed measurements are usually made only for research purposes.

ALVEOLAR COMPARTMENT DYSFUNCTION   This can be assessed using several distinct and complementary bedside techniques, in addition to simple gas exchange measurements. Findings on physical examination that are suggestive of consolidation, such as tubular breath sounds, dullness to percussion, and egophony, establish alveolar compartment dysfunction. Lung stiffness, as reflected in static respiratory system compliance, can be assessed by measuring the distending pressure required to inflate the lung once inspiratory flow has ceased. This is calculated by measuring the end-inspiratory plateau pressure and dividing the inspiratory volume by end-inspiratory plateau pressure minus whatever level of PEEP is being applied. A normal value of static respiratory system compliance measured using this approach is 35 to 50 mL/cmH₂O. Values <30 during conventional tidal volume inflation (7 to 12 mL/kg tidal volumes) indicate increased stiffness of the lung, chest wall, or both.

The chest radiograph is also a useful tool for assessing the pathology of the alveolar compartment. Radiographic densities consistent with air-space disease point to alveolar infection, injury, or flooding and, together with a reduced lung compliance and reduced arterial oxygen level, favor a diagnosis of alveolar compartment dysfunction.

PULMONARY VASCULAR DYSFUNCTION   This cannot be directly assessed at the bedside but may be reflected by signs of right heart dysfunction, such as elevated jugular venous pressures, a pronounced or delayed pulmonic component of the second heart sound, a right-sided heave, a right-sided third heart sound, or a murmur of tricuspid regurgitation. In the absence of these signs it can be suggested by exclusion in cases where abnormal gas exchange exists in the apparent absence of controller, pump, airway, or alveolar compartment dysfunction. Pulmonary vascular disease can cause abnormalities in routine clinical tests including the electrocardiogram (ECG) and chest radiograph. It can cause right heart strain or right bundle branch block which will show on the electrocardiogram, and pulmonary artery enlargement can be seen on radiographic studies. More definitive testing including echocardiography, right heart catheterization, or contrast-enhanced computed tomography of the chest is often required to identify the presence of pulmonary vascular disease.

Making a Definitive Diagnosis   Approaching respiratory failure from a physiologic perspective can provide important clues about its specific etiology, which in turn can lead to the formulation of a more effective diagnostic approach and a definitive therapeutic plan. Once a patient has been stabilized by establishing a stable airway and providing mechanical ventilatory support (if indicated), a thorough evaluation of the cause of respiratory failure can be safely undertaken. Table 250-2 summarizes common disease states representative of each type of respiratory system dysfunction listed above. The associated blood-gas findings and additional confirmatory tests that may be useful in further evaluating each of these conditions are also presented.

INITIAL MANAGEMENT   Treatment for many of the specific disorders identified in Table 250-2 is addressed in subsequent chapters; in this chapter the focus is on the initial management that is common to all patients with respiratory failure. As discussed above, one must first focus on physiologic stabilization. The first priority is to establish adequate oxygenation through the administration of supplemental oxygen in patients with hypoxemia. For patients with hypercarbic respiratory failure leading to significant acidemia or hypoxemia inadequately corrected by supplemental oxygen, the mainstay of supportive care for respiratory failure is mechanical ventilation (Chap. 252). Although mechanical ventilation can sometimes be provided without placement of an artificial airway (i.e., mask ventilation), in the majority of cases the first step in stabilizing the patient with respiratory failure involves placement of an endotracheal tube. This can be achieved via either the orotracheal or nasotracheal route, usually using a combination of parenteral and local anesthesia to ensure patient comfort. Following placement, the tube must be secured and its position verified so as to provide 100% O₂ and adequate ventilation immediately.

Obstruction of the upper airway is a medical emergency. In an unconscious patient this is often due to occlusion by the tongue or soft tissues of the pharynx. The airway is immediately opened with the head tilt–chin lift maneuver and the patient assessed for spontaneous respirations. When a spontaneously breathing patient is unable to dislodge a foreign object, a forceful subdiaphragmatic thrust can facilitate removal of the object. Removal may require laryngoscopy and removal with forceps. Liquids such as vomitus or blood are removed by suctioning under direct vision. In some cases of respiratory failure the airway is secure without instrumentation, but in most a stable airway is achieved by passing an endotracheal tube. When the airway cannot be secured using these techniques a tracheostomy or cricothyrotomy should be performed.

One of the most effective ways to improve the O₂ content of blood is to increase its concentration in alveolar gas by administering O₂, initally with an FI$_{O_2}$ of 100%. Oxygen delivery to the alveoli can also

TABLE 250-2 *Clinical Syndromes Associated with Dysfunction of the Components of the Respiratory System*

Type of Dysfunction	Specific Representative Conditions	Predominant Gas Exchange Abnormality	Additional Testing/Evaluation
Controller	Sedative medications	Hypercarbia	Review of medications
	Chronic obstructive or interstitial lung disease	Hypoxemia + hypercarbia	History of daytime somnulence, lung function
	Toxic overdoses	Hypoxemia + hypercarbia	Toxicology screen
	Hypothermia post operatively	Hypercarbia	Measurement of core body temperature
	Brainstem stroke	Hypercarbia	Head CT/MRI scans
Pump	Medications/toxins	Hypercarbia	Review of medical history
	Paralytics		
	Aminoglycosides		
	Steroids		
	Botulism		
	Myopathy	Hypercarbia	Strength testing, EMG/NCV studies
	Myositis	Hypercarbia	Clinical exam, serum CK and aldolase
	Metabolic abnormalities	Hypercarbia	TSH, serum phosphate
	Hypothyroidism		
	Hypophosphatemia		
	Myasthenia gravis	Hypercarbia	EMG/NVC studies, Tensilon test
	Guillain-Barré syndrome	Hypercarbia	Clinical evaluation, EMG/NCV studies
	Paraneoplastic syndromes	Hypercarbia	Clinical evaluation, EMG/NCV studies
	Polyradiculopathy of critical illness	Hypercarbia	Clinical evaluation, EMG/NCV studies
	Postoperative or postradiation therapy phrenic nerve dysfunction	Hypercarbia	Diaphragmatic ultrasound, fluoroscopy of diaphragm
	Postoperative pain/splitting	Hypoxemia + hypercarbia	Clinical assessment
Airway	Asthma	Mild: hypoxemia + hypocarbia	Pulmonary function testing
		Severe: hypoxemia + hypercarbia	Functional response to bronchodilators
	Emphysema/chronic bronchitis	Hypoxemia + hypercarbia	Pulmonary function testing, chest x-ray
	Bronchiolitis	Hypoxemia + hypercarbia	Pulmonary function testing, chest CT, lung biopsy
	Endobronchial tumor, mass, or stricture	Variable	Pulmonary function testing, CT imaging, bronchoscopy
Alveolar	Pneumonia	Hypoxemia + hypercarbia	Smear and culture of secretions
	Pulmonary edema	Hypoxemia + hypercarbia	Examination of the heart Chest x-ray
	Pulmonary hemorrhage	Hypoxemia + hypercarbia	Chest x-ray, bronchoscopy
	ARDS	Hypoxemia + hypercarbia	Chest x-ray, arterial blood gas
	Drug reaction	Hypoxemia + hypercarbia	Drug exposure, toxicology screen, lung biopsy
	Pulmonary contusion	Hypoxemia + hypercarbia	Chest wall pain, chest x-ray
Pulmonary vascular	Acute pulmonary embolus	New-onset hypoxemia with or without hypercarbia	Ventilation-perfusion scanning, CT pulmonary embolism study
	Pulmonary hypertension	Exertional hypoxemia	Echocardiogram, right heart catheterization
	AVM or intracardiac shunt	Hypoxemia that is refractory to oxygen therapy	Echocardiogram with bubble study, high-resolution CT scan

Note: CT, computed tomography; MRI, magnetic resonance imaging; CK, creatine kinase; TSH, thyroid stimulating hormone; EMG, electromyography; NCV, nerve conduction velocity study; ARDS, adult respiratory distress syndrome; AVM, arteriovenous malformation.

be improved by applying PEEP in patients receiving mechanical ventilatory support. Increasing alveolar ventilation with a mechanical ventilator eliminates CO_2 and corrects acidemia. In the setting of acute respiratory failure, it is important to document that adequate oxygenation and elimination of CO_2 have been achieved before adjustment of the O_2 content and other ventilator settings.

The effective management of respiratory failure depends on identifying and optimally managing all of the treatable factors that impair the respiratory system. This includes removing excess secretion by suctioning, treating infections with effective antimicrobials, suppressing inflammation with anti-inflammatory or immunosuppressive drugs, treating obstruction with bronchodilators, avoiding the harmful effects of excess oxygen or mechanical forces from the mechanical ventilator, dissolving blood clots with anticoagulants or thrombolytics, providing pulmonary vasodilatation, and removing transudated fluid with diuretics. Some forms of chronic respiratory system failure, such as sleep apnea syndrome and post-polio syndrome, are ultimately re-

sponsive to nocturnal mechanical ventilation or continuous positive airway pressure (Chap. 252). Finally, selected patients with isolated severe chronic respiratory failure may have the quality of their lives improved by lung transplantation.

FURTHER READING

BEHRENDT CF: Acute respiratory failure in the United States: Incidence and 31-day survival. Chest 118:1100, 2000

HERTZ MI et al: The registry of the international society for heart and lung transplantation: Nineteenth official report: 2002. J Heart Lung Transplant 21:950, 2002

TOBIN MJ: *Principles and Practice of Mechanical Ventilation*. New York, McGraw-Hill, 1994

——: Advances in mechanical ventilation. N Engl J Med 344:1986, 2001

VINCENT JL et al: The epidemiology of acute respiratory failure in critically ill patients. Chest 121:1602, 2002

YANG KI, TOBIN MJ: A prospective study of indexes predicting the outcome of trials of weaning from mechanical ventilation. N Engl J Med 324:1445, 1991

Acute respiratory distress syndrome (ARDS) is a clinical syndrome of severe dyspnea of rapid onset, hypoxemia, and diffuse pulmonary infiltrates leading to respiratory failure. ARDS is caused by diffuse lung injury from many underlying medical and surgical disorders. The lung injury may be direct, as occurs in toxic inhalation, or indirect, as occurs in sepsis (Table 251-1). The clinical features of ARDS are listed in Table 251-2. Acute lung injury (ALI) is a less severe disorder but has the potential to evolve into ARDS (Table 251-2). The arterial (a) P_{O_2} (in mmHg)/ FI_{O_2} (inspiratory O_2 fraction) <200 mmHg is characteristic of ARDS, while a Pa_{O_2}/FI_{O_2} between 200 and 300 identifies patients with ALI who are likely to benefit from aggressive therapy.

The annual incidences of ALI and ARDS are estimated to be 30/100,000 and 10/100,000, respectively. Approximately 10% of all intensive care unit (ICU) admissions suffer from acute respiratory failure (Chap. 250), with ~20% of these patients meeting criteria for ALI or ARDS.

ETIOLOGY While many medical and surgical illnesses have been associated with the development of ALI and ARDS, most cases (>80%) are caused by a relatively small number of clinical disorders, namely, severe sepsis syndrome and/or bacterial pneumonia (~40 to 50%), trauma, multiple transfusions, aspiration of gastric contents, and drug overdose. Among patients with trauma, pulmonary contusion, multiple bone fractures, and chest wall trauma/flail chest are the most frequently reported surgical conditions in ARDS, whereas head trauma, near-drowning, toxic inhalation, and burns are rare causes. The risks of developing ARDS are increased in patients suffering from more than one predisposing medical or surgical condition; e.g., the risk for ARDS increases from 25% in patients with severe trauma to 56% in patients with trauma and sepsis.

Several other clinical variables have been associated with the development of ARDS. These include older age, chronic alcohol abuse, metabolic acidosis, and severity of critical illness. Trauma patients with an acute physiology and chronic health evaluation (APACHE) II score $\geq$ 16 (Chap. 249) have a 2.5-fold increase in the risk of developing ARDS, and those with a score > 20 have an incidence of ARDS that is more threefold greater than those with APACHE II scores $\leq$ 9.

CLINICAL COURSE AND PATHOPHYSIOLOGY The natural history of ARDS is marked by three phases—exudative, proliferative, and fibrotic—each with characteristic clinical and pathologic features (Fig. 251-1).

Exudative Phase In this phase, alveolar capillary endothelial cells and type I pneumocytes (alveolar epithelial cells) are injured, leading to the loss of the normally tight alveolar barrier to fluid and macromolecules. Edema fluid that is rich in protein accumulates in the interstitial and alveolar spaces. Significant concentrations of cytokines (e.g., interleukin 1, interleukin 8, and tumor necrosis factor α) and lipid mediators (e.g., leukotriene B_4) are present in the lung in this early phase. In response to proinflammatory mediators, leukocytes (especially neutrophils) traffick into the pulmonary interstitium and alveoli. In addi-

tion, condensed plasma proteins aggregate in the air spaces with cellular debris and dysfunctional pulmonary surfactant to form hyaline membrane whorls. Pulmonary vascular injury also occurs early in ARDS, with vascular obliteration by microthrombi and fibrocellular proliferation.

Alveolar edema predominantly involves *dependent* portions of the lung, leading to diminished aeration and atelectasis. Collapse of large sections of dependent lung markedly decreases lung compliance. Consequently, intrapulmonary shunting and hypoxemia develop and the work of breathing rises, leading to dyspnea. The pathophysiologic alterations in alveolar spaces are exacerbated by microvascular occlusion, which leads to reductions in pulmonary arterial blood flow to ventilated portions of the lung, increasing the dead space, and pulmonary hypertension. Thus, in addition to severe hypoxemia, hypercapnia secondary to an increase in pulmonary dead space is also prominent in early ARDS.

The exudative phase encompasses the first 7 days of illness after exposure to a precipitating ARDS risk factor, with the patient experiencing the onset of respiratory symptoms. Although usually present within 12 to 36 h after the initial insult, symptoms can be delayed by 5 to 7 days. Dyspnea develops with a sensation of rapid shallow breathing and an inability to get enough air. Tachypnea and increased work of breathing frequently result in respiratory fatigue and ultimately in respiratory failure. Laboratory values are generally nonspecific and primarily indicative of underlying clinical disorders. The chest radiograph usually reveals alveolar and interstitial opacities involving at least three-quarters of the lung fields (Fig. 251-2). While characteristic for ARDS or ALI, these radiographic findings are not specific and can be indistinguishable from cardiogenic pulmonary edema (Chaps. 29 and 255). Unlike the latter, however, the chest x-ray in ARDS rarely shows cardiomegaly, pleural effusions or pulmonary vascular redistribution. Chest computed tomography (CT) scanning in ARDS reveals extensive heterogeneity of lung involvement (Fig. 251-3).

Because the early features of ARDS and ALI are nonspecific, alternative diagnoses must be considered. In the differential diagnosis of ARDS, the most common disorders are cardiogenic pulmonary edema, diffuse pneumonia, and alveolar hemorrhage. Less frequent diagnoses to consider include acute interstitial lung diseases [e.g., acute interstitial pneumonitis (Chap. 243)], acute immunologic injury [e.g, hypersensitivity pneumonitis (Chap. 237)], toxin injury (e.g., radiation pneumonitis), and neurogenic pulmonary edema (Chap. 29).

Proliferative Phase This phase of ARDS usually lasts from day 7 to day 21. Most patients recover rapidly and are liberated from mechanical ventilation during this phase. Despite this improvement, many still experience dyspnea, tachypnea, and hypoxemia. Some patients develop progressive lung injury and early changes of pulmonary fibrosis during the proliferative phase. Histologically, the first signs of resolution are often evident in this phase with the initiation of lung repair,

TABLE 251-1 *Clinical Disorders Commonly Associated with ARDS*

Direct Lung Injury	Indirect Lung Injury
Pneumonia	Sepsis
Aspiration of gastric contents	Severe trauma
Pulmonary contusion	Multiple bone fractures
Near-drowning	Flail chest
Toxic inhalation injury	Head trauma
	Burns
	Multiple transfusions
	Drug overdose
	Pancreatitis
	Post-cardiopulmonary bypass

TABLE 251-2 *Diagnostic Criteria for ALI and ARDS*

Oxygenation	Onset	Chest Radiograph	Absence of Left Atrial Hypertension
ALI: $Pa_{O_2}/FI_{O_2} \leq$ 300 mmHg ARDS: $Pa_{O_2}/FI_{O_2} \leq$ 200 mmHg	Acute	Bilateral alveolar or interstitial infiltrates	PCWP $\leq$ 18 mmHg *or* no clinical evidence of increased left atrial pressure

Note: ALI, acute lung injury; ARDS, acute respiratory distress syndrome; Pa_{O_2} = arterial partial pressure of O_2; FI_{O_2}, inspired O_2 percentage; PCWP, pulmonary capillary wedge pressure.

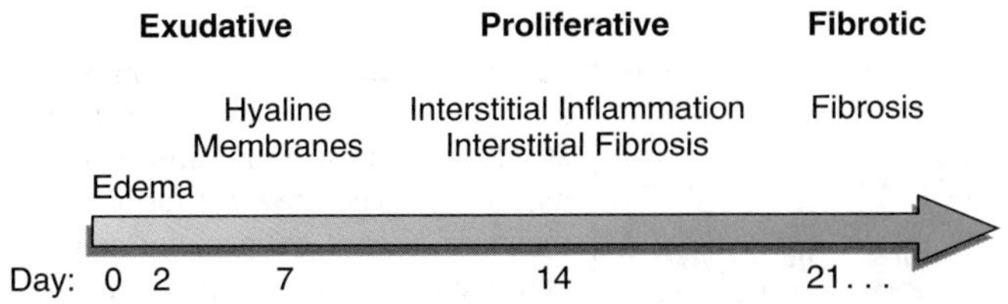

Exudative   Proliferative   Fibrotic

Hyaline   Interstitial Inflammation   Fibrosis
Membranes   Interstitial Fibrosis
Edema

Day: 0 2   7   14   21...

FIGURE 251-1   Diagram illustrating the time course for the development and resolution of ARDS. The exudative phase is notable for early alveolar edema and neutrophil-rich leukocytic infiltration of the lungs with subsequent formation of hyaline membranes from diffuse alveolar damage. Within 7 days, a proliferative phase ensues with prominent interstitial inflammation and early fibrotic changes. Approximately 3 weeks after the initial pulmonary injury, some patients enter the fibrotic phase, with substantial fibrosis and bullae formation.

organization of alveolar exudates, and a shift from a neutrophil to a lymphocyte-predominant pulmonary infiltrate. As part of the reparative process, there is a proliferation of type II pneumocytes along alveolar basement membranes. These specialized epithelial cells synthesize new pulmonary surfactant and differentiate into type I pneumocytes. The presence of alveolar type III procollagen peptide, a marker of pulmonary fibrosis, is associated with a protracted clinical course and increased mortality from ARDS.

Fibrotic Phase   While many patients with ARDS recover lung function 3 to 4 weeks after the initial pulmonary injury, some will enter a fibrotic phase that may require long-term support on mechanical ventilators and/or supplemental oxygen. Histologically, the alveolar edema and inflammatory exudates of earlier phases are now converted to extensive ductal and interstitial fibrosis. Acinar architecture is markedly disrupted, leading to emphysema-like changes with large bullae. Intimal fibroproliferation in the pulmonary microcirculation leads to progressive vascular occlusion and pulmonary hypertension. The physiologic consequences include an increased risk of pneumothorax, reductions in lung compliance, and increased pulmonary dead space. Patients in this late phase experience a substantial burden of excess morbidity. Lung biopsy evidence for pulmonary fibrosis in any phase of ARDS is associated with increased mortality.

℞ TREATMENT

General Principles   Recent reductions in ARDS/ALI mortality are largely the result of general advances in the care of critically ill patients (Chap. 249). Thus, caring for these patients requires close attention to: (1) the recognition and treatment of the underlying medical and surgical disorders (e.g., sepsis, aspiration, trauma); (2) minimizing procedures and their complications; (3) prophylaxis against venous thromboembolism, gastrointestinal bleeding, and central venous catheter infections; (4) the prompt recognition of nosocomial infections; and (5) provision of adequate nutrition.

Management of Mechanical Ventilation (See also Chap. 252) ■ *VENTILATOR-INDUCED LUNG INJURY*   Despite its life-saving potential, mechanical ventilation can aggravate lung injury. Experimental models have demonstrated that ventilator-induced lung injury appears to require two processes: repeated alveolar overdistention and recurrent alveolar collapse. Clearly evident by chest CT (Fig. 251-3), ARDS is a heterogeneous disorder, principally involving dependent portions of the lung with relative sparing of other regions. Because of their differing compliance, attempts to fully inflate the consolidated lung may lead to overdistention and injury to the more "normal" areas of lung. Ventilator-induced injury can be demonstrated in experimental models of ALI, with high tidal volume ventilation resulting in additional, synergistic alveolar damage. These findings led to the hypothesis that ventilating patients suffering from ALI or ARDS with lower tidal volumes would protect against ventilator-induced lung injury and improve clinical outcomes.

A large-scale, randomized controlled trial sponsored by the National Institutes of Health and conducted by the ARDS Network compared low tidal volume (6 mL/kg predicted body weight) ventilation to conventional tidal volume (12 mL/kg predicted body weight) ventilation. Mortality was significantly lower in the low tidal volume patients (31%) compared to the conventional tidal volume patients (40%). This improvement in survival represents the most substantial benefit in ARDS mortality demonstrated for *any* therapeutic intervention in ARDS to date.

PREVENTION OF ALVEOLAR COLLAPSE   In ARDS, the presence of alveolar and interstitial fluid and the loss of surfactant can lead to a marked reduction of lung compliance. Without an increase in end-expiratory pressure, significant alveolar collapse can occur at end-expiration, impairing oxygenation. In most clinical settings, positive end-expiratory pressure (PEEP) is empirically set to minimize FI_{O_2} and maximize Pa_{O_2}. On most modern mechanical ventilators, it is possible to construct a static pressure–volume curve for the respiratory system. The lower inflection point on the curve represents alveolar opening (or "recruitment"). The pressure at this point, usually 12 to 15 mmHg in ARDS, is a theoretical "optimal PEEP" for alveolar recruitment. Titration of the PEEP to the lower inflection point on the static pressure–volume curve has been hypothesized to keep the lung open, improving oxygenation and protecting against lung injury. The ARDS Network investigators are currently studying the effect of PEEP on clinical out-

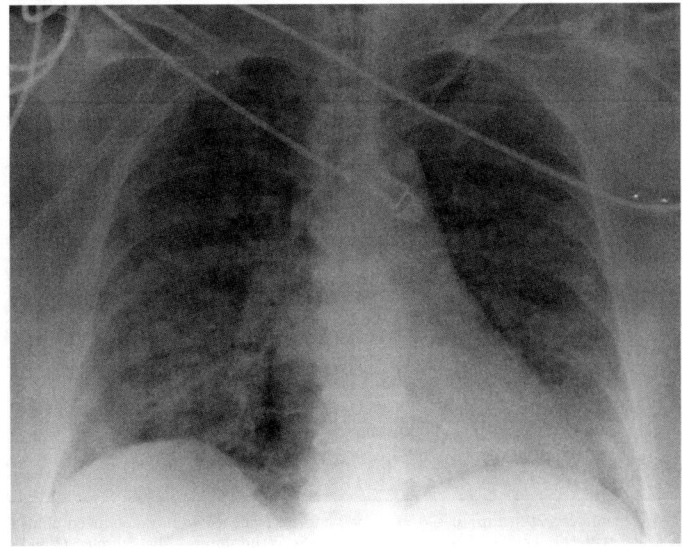

FIGURE 251-2   A representative anteroposterior (AP) chest x-ray in the exudative phase of ARDS that shows diffuse interstitial and alveolar infiltrates, which can be difficult to distinguish from left ventricular failure.

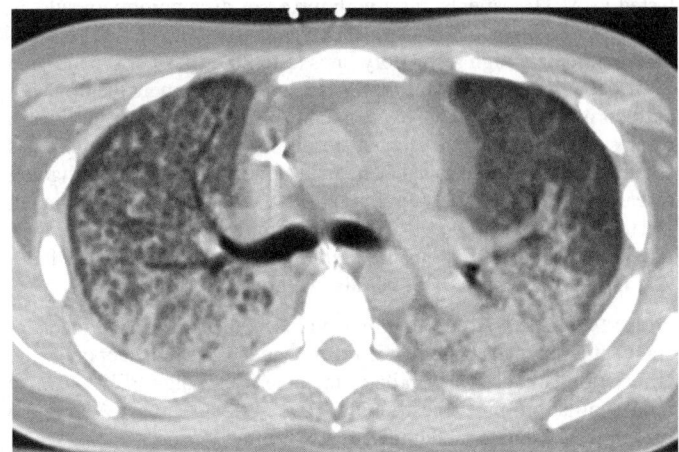

FIGURE 251-3   A representative computed tomographic scan of the chest during the exudative phase of ARDS in which *dependent* alveolar edema and atelectasis predominate.

TABLE 251-3 A Stepwise Approach to Mechanical Ventilation in ARDS

1. Calculate predicted body weight (PBW) in kilogram	Men = 50 + 5.42[height (cm) − 60] Women = 45.5 + 5.42[height (cm) − 60]
2. Ventilator mode	Volume cycle, assist control
3. Tidal volume (V_T)	Initial V_T 8 mL/kg PBW Reduce to 6 mL/kg over 2–4 h if ventilation adequate Goal inspiratory plateau pressures < 30 cmH$_2$O; reduce V_T to as low as 4 mL/kg as needed (and permitted by ventilation) to achieve this goal
4. Oxygenation	Pa$_{O_2}$ goal = 55 – 80 mmHg or pulse oximetry oxygen saturation 88–95% Use the minimal amount of PEEP to keep Fi$_{O_2}$ ≤ 0.6 and meet Pa$_{O_2}$ goal
5. Respiratory rate and acidosis management	Goal arterial pH = 7.30–7.40 If pH < 7.30, increase respiratory rate up to 35 breaths/min If pH < 7.30 and respiratory rate = 35, consider starting intravenous bicarbonate (or equivalent buffer)

If the above strategy fails and the patient is suffering from persistent hypoxemic respiratory failure, *consider* the following:
1. Neuromuscular blocking agents (if not already in use)
2. Prone position ventilation
3. Recruitment maneuvers
4. Inverse ratio ventilation, nitric oxide, high-frequency ventilation, extracorporeal membrane oxygenation, or partial liquid ventilation as part of a clinical research trial.

Note: PEEP, positive end-expiratory pressure.

comes in ARDS; until the results of these studies are available, it is advisable to set PEEP to minimize Fi$_{O_2}$ and optimize Pa$_{O_2}$ using parameters similar to those used by the ARDS Network (Table 251-3).

Oxygenation can also be improved by increasing mean airway pressure with "inverse ratio ventilation." In this technique, the inspiratory (*I*) time is lengthened so that it is longer than the expiratory (*E*) time (*I:E* >1:1). With diminished time to exhale, dynamic hyperinflation leads to increased end-expiratory pressure, similar to ventilator-prescribed PEEP. This mode of ventilation has the advantage of improving oxygenation with lower peak pressures than conventional ventilation. Although inverse ratio ventilation can improve oxygenation and help reduce Fi$_{O_2}$ to ≤ 0.60 to avoid possible oxygen toxicity, no mortality benefit in ARDS has been demonstrated.

Mechanical ventilation in the prone position improves arterial oxygenation, but its effect on important clinical outcomes remains uncertain. Moreover, unless the critical care team is experienced in "proning," repositioning critically ill patients can be hazardous, leading to accidental endotracheal extubation, loss of central venous catheters, and orthopedic injury. Until further studies validate its efficacy, prone position ventilation should be reserved for only the most critically ill ARDS patients.

OTHER STRATEGIES IN MECHANICAL VENTILATION Several additional mechanical ventilation strategies that utilize specialized equipment have been tested in ARDS patients, most with mixed or disappointing results in adults. These include high-frequency ventilation (HFV), i.e., ventilating at extremely high respiratory rates (5 to 20 cycles per second) and low tidal volumes (1 to 2 mL/kg). Also, lung replacement therapy with extracorporeal membrane oxygenation (ECMO), which provides a clear survival benefit in neonatal respiratory distress syndrome, has yet to have proven survival benefit in adults with ARDS. Ongoing research on partial liquid ventilation (PLV) with perfluorocarbon, an inert, high-density liquid that easily solubilizes oxygen and carbon dioxide, has revealed promising preliminary data on pulmonary function in patients with ARDS, but also without survival benefit.

RECOMMENDATIONS Based on current evidence, the approach to mechanical ventilation in Table 251-3 is recommended. Data in support of the efficacy of "adjunctive" ventilator therapies (e.g., high PEEP, inverse ratio ventilation, prone positioning, HFV, ECMO, and PLV) remain incomplete, so these modalities are not routinely used.

Fluid Management Increased pulmonary vascular permeability leading to interstitial and alveolar edema rich in protein is a central feature of ARDS. In addition, impaired vascular integrity augments the normal increase in extravascular lung water that occurs with increasing left atrial pressure. Maintaining a normal or low left atrial filling pressure minimizes pulmonary edema and prevents further decrements in arterial oxygenation and lung compliance, improves pulmonary mechanics, shortens ICU stay and the duration of mechanical ventilation, and is associated with a lower mortality. Thus, aggressive attempts to reduce left atrial filling pressures with fluid restriction and diuretics should be an important aspect of ARDS management, limited only by hypotension and hypoperfusion of critical organs, such as the kidneys.

Glucocorticoids Inflammatory mediators and leukocytes are abundant in the lungs of patients with ARDS. Many attempts have been made to treat both early and late ARDS with glucocorticoids to reduce this potentially deleterious pulmonary inflammation. Few studies have shown any benefit. The ARDS Network is currently conducting a large-scale study of glucocorticoids in ALI and ARDS. Current evidence does *not* support their use in the care of early ARDS patients. On the other hand, if patients fail to improve after 1 week of supportive therapy and have no contraindications to glucocorticoid therapy, providers may wish to consider an *empirical* trial of them in an attempt to speed ARDS resolution.

Other Therapies Clinical trials of surfactant replacement therapy have proven disappointing. Similarly, although several randomized clinical trials of inhaled nitric oxide (NO) in ARDS have demonstrated improved oxygenation, no significant improvement in survival or decrements in time on mechanical ventilation has been observed. Therefore, the use of NO is *not* currently recommended in ARDS.

Recommendations Many clinical trials have been undertaken to improve the outcome of patients with ARDS; most have been unsuccessful in modifying the natural history. The large number and uncertain clinical efficacy of ARDS therapies can make it difficult for clinicians to select a rational treatment plan, and these patients' critical illness can tempt physicians to try unproven and potentially harmful therapies. While results of large clinical trials must be judiciously administered to *individual* patients, an evidenced-based recommendation for ARDS management is summarized in Table 251-4.

PROGNOSIS ■ Mortality Recent mortality estimates for ARDS range from 41 to 65%. There is substantial variability, but a trend towards improved ARDS outcomes appears evident. Of interest, mortality in ARDS

TABLE 251-4 Evidence-Based Recommendations for ARDS Therapies

Treatment	Recommendation[a]
Mechanical ventilation:	
Low tidal volume	A
High-PEEP or "open-lung"	C
Prone position	C
High-frequency ventilation and ECMO	D
Minimize left atrial filling pressures	B
Glucocorticoids	C
Surfactant replacement, inhaled nitric oxide, and other anti-inflammatory therapy (e.g., ketoconazole, PGE$_1$, NSAIDs)	D

[a] A, recommended therapy based on strong clinical evidence from randomized clinical trials; B, recommended therapy based on supportive but limited clinical data; C, indeterminate evidence: recommended only as alternative therapy; D, not recommended based on clinical evidence against efficacy of therapy.
Note: PEEP, positive end-expiratory pressure; ECMO, extracorporeal membrane oxygenation; PGE$_1$, prostaglandin E$_1$; NSAIDs, nonsteroidal anti-inflammatory drugs.

is largely attributable to nonpulmonary causes, with sepsis and nonpulmonary organ failure accounting for >80% of deaths. Thus, improvement in survival is likely secondary to advances in the care of septic/infected patients and those with multiple organ failure (Chap. 249).

Several risk factors for mortality to help estimate prognosis have been identified. Similar to the risk factors for developing ARDS, the major risk factors for ARDS mortality are also nonpulmonary. Advanced age is an important risk factor. Patients >75 years have a substantially increased mortality (~60%) compared to those <45 (~20%). Also, patients >60 years with ARDS and sepsis have a threefold higher mortality compared to those <60. Preexisting organ dysfunction from chronic medical illness is an important additional risk factor for increased mortality. In particular, chronic liver disease, cirrhosis, chronic alcohol abuse, chronic immunosuppression, sepsis, chronic renal disease, any nonpulmonary organ failure, and increased APACHE II scores (Chap. 249) have also been linked to increased ARDS mortality. Several factors related to the presenting clinical disorders also increase risk for ARDS mortality. Patients with ARDS from direct lung injury (including pneumonia, pulmonary contusion, and aspiration; Table 251-1) have nearly twice the mortality of those with indirect causes of lung injury, while surgical and trauma patients with ARDS, especially those without direct lung injury, have a better survival rate than other ARDS patients.

Surprisingly, there is little value in predicting ARDS mortality from the extent of hypoxemia and any of the following measures of the severity of lung injury: the level of PEEP used in mechanical ventilation, the respiratory compliance, the extent of alveolar infiltrates on chest radiography, and the lung injury score (a composite of all these variables). However, recent data indicate that an early (within 24 h of presentation) elevation in dead space may predict increased mortality from ARDS.

Functional Recovery in ARDS Survivors While it is common for patients with ARDS to experience prolonged respiratory failure and remain dependent on mechanical ventilation for survival, it is a testament to the resolving powers of the lung that the majority of patients recover nearly normal lung function. Patients usually recover their maximum lung function within 6 months. One year after endotracheal extubation, over a third of ARDS survivors have normal spirometry values and diffusion capacity. Most of the remaining patients have only mild abnormalities in their pulmonary function. Unlike the risk for mortality, recovery of lung function is strongly associated with the extent of lung injury in early ARDS. Low static respiratory compliance, high levels of required PEEP, longer durations of mechanical ventilation, and high lung injury scores are all associated with worse recovery of pulmonary function. When caring for ARDS survivors it is important to be aware of the potential for a substantial burden of emotional and respiratory symptoms. There are significant rates of depression and posttraumatic stress disorder in ARDS survivors.

FURTHER READING

BERNSTEN AD et al: Incidence and mortality of acute lung injury and the acute respiratory distress syndrome in three Australian states. Am J Respir Crit Care Med 165:443, 2002

GATTINONI L et al: Lung structure and function in different stages of severe adult respiratory distress syndrome. JAMA, 271:1772, 1994

HERRIDGE MS et al: One-year outcomes in survivors of the acute respiratory distress syndrome. N Engl J Med 348:683, 2003

MILBERG JA et al: Improved survival of patients with acute respiratory distress syndrome (ARDS): 1983–1993. JAMA 273:306, 1995

THE ACUTE RESPIRATORY DISTRESS SYNDROME NETWORK: Ventilation with lower tidal volumes as compared with traditional tidal volumes for acute lung injury and the acute respiratory distress syndrome. N Engl J Med 342:1301, 2000

WARE LB and MATTHAY MA, The acute respiratory distress syndrome. N Engl J Med 342:1334, 2000

252 MECHANICAL VENTILATORY SUPPORT
Edward P. Ingenito, Jeffrey M. Drazen

Ventilators are specially designed pumps that can support the ventilatory function of the respiratory system and improve oxygenation through application of high oxygen content gas and positive pressure. They are a mainstay of physiologic supportive care (see also Chap. 249).

INDICATIONS FOR MECHANICAL VENTILATION

There are two basic types of respiratory failure, the primary indication for initiation of mechanical ventilation (see also Chap. 250).

1. *Hypoxemic respiratory failure* most commonly results from pulmonary conditions such as severe pneumonia, pulmonary edema, pulmonary hemorrhage, and respiratory distress syndrome causing ventilation-perfusion ($\dot{V}/\dot{Q}$) mismatch and shunt. Hypoxemic respiratory failure is present when arterial O_2 saturation (Sa_{O_2}) < 90% is observed despite an inspired O_2 fraction (FI_{O_2}) > 0.6. The goal of ventilator treatment in this setting is to provide adequate Sa_{O_2} through a combination of supplemental O_2 and specific patterns of ventilation that enhance oxygenation by improving $\dot{V}/\dot{Q}$ matching and reducing intrapulmonary shunt.

2. *Hypercarbic respiratory failure* results from disease states causing either a decrease in minute ventilation or an increase in physiologic dead space such that, despite adequate total minute ventilation, alveolar ventilation is inadequate to meet metabolic demands. Common clinical conditions associated with hypercarbic respiratory failure include neuromuscular diseases, such as myasthenia gravis, ascending polyradiculopathy, and myopathies, and diseases that cause respiratory muscle fatigue due to increased workload, such as asthma, chronic obstructive pulmonary disease, and restrictive lung disease. *Acute* hypercarbic respiratory failure is characterized by arterial P_{CO_2} values >50 mmHg and an arterial pH <7.30.

Mechanical ventilation generally should be instituted in acute hypercarbic respiratory failure. In contrast, the decision to institute ventilator support when components of both acute and chronic hypercarbic respiratory failure are present depends on blood gas parameters and clinical evaluation. In particular, if a patient is not in respiratory distress and is not mentally impaired by CO_2 accumulation, it is not mandatory to initiate mechanical ventilation while other forms of treatment are being administered. The goal of ventilator treatment in hypercarbic respiratory failure is to normalize arterial pH through changes in CO_2 tensions. In patients with severe obstructive or restrictive lung disease, potentially injurious elevation in airway pressures may limit tidal volumes to the extent that normalization of pH is not possible, a situation known as *permissive hypercapnia*.

Accepted therapeutic applications of mechanical ventilation include controlled hyperventilation to reduce cerebral blood flow in patients with increased intracranial pressure (ICP) or to improve pulmonary hemodynamics in patients with postoperative pulmonary hypertension. Mechanical ventilation has also been used to reduce the work of breathing in patients with congestive heart failure, especially in the presence of myocardial ischemia. Ventilator support is also frequently used in conjunction with endotracheal intubation to prevent aspiration of gastric contents in otherwise unstable patients during gastric lavage for suspected drug overdose or during upper gastrointestinal endoscopy. In the critically ill patient, intubation and mechanical ventilation are indicated before essential diagnostic or therapeutic studies if it appears that respiratory failure may occur during these maneuvers.

PHYSIOLOGIC ASPECTS OF MECHANICAL VENTILATION

Mechanical ventilators provide warmed and humidified gas to the airway opening in conformance with various specific volume, pressure, and time patterns. The ventilator serves as the energy source for inspiration, replacing the muscles of the diaphragm and chest wall. Expiration is passive, driven by the recoil of the lungs and chest wall; at the completion of inspiration, internal ventilator circuitry vents the airway to atmospheric pressure or a specified level of positive end-expiratory pressure (PEEP).

PEEP helps maintain patency of alveoli and small airways in the presence of destabilizing factors and therefore reverses hypoxemia and atelectasis by improving matching of ventilation and perfusion. PEEP levels between 0 and 10 cmH$_2$O are generally safe and effective; higher levels are recommended only in the management of significant refractory hypoxemia unresponsive to increments in F$_{IO_2}$ up to 0.6.

ESTABLISHING AND MAINTAINING AN AIRWAY A cuffed endotracheal tube is often inserted to allow positive-pressure ventilators to deliver conditioned gas, at pressures above atmospheric pressure, to the lungs in a controlled fashion. If neuromuscular paralysis is to be induced during intubation, the use of agents whose mechanism of action includes depolarization at the neuromuscular junction, such as succinylcholine chloride, should be avoided in patients with renal failure, tumor lysis syndrome, crush injuries, medical conditions associated with elevated serum potassium levels, and muscular dystrophy syndromes. Opiates and benzodiazepines can have a deleterious effect on hemodynamics in patients with depressed cardiac function or low systemic vascular resistance and should be used cautiously in this setting. Morphine can promote histamine release from tissue mast cells and may worsen bronchospasm in patients with asthma; fentanyl, sufentanil, and alfentanil are acceptable alternatives to morphine. Ketamine may increase systemic arterial pressure as well as ICP and has been associated with dramatic hallucinatory responses; it should be used with caution in patients with hypertensive crisis, increased ICP, or a history of psychiatric disorders. Newer agents such as etomidate and propofol have also been used for both induction and maintenance of anesthesia in patients receiving mechanical ventilator support. They are shorter acting and have fewer adverse hemodynamic effects, but are significantly more expensive than older agents.

Patients who require ventilator support for extended periods of time may be candidates for tracheostomy. Although definitive guidelines for performing a tracheostomy in the ventilated patient have not been established, in current clinical practice patients who are anticipated to require ventilator therapy for more than 3 weeks should be considered for this procedure. While it does not clearly reduce the incidence of laryngeal injury or tracheal stenosis, tracheostomy has been associated with improved patient comfort and enhanced ability to partake in rehabilitation-oriented activities.

VENTILATOR MODES *Mode* refers to the manner in which ventilator breaths are triggered, cycled, and limited; commonly used modes of mechanical ventilation are given in Table 252-1. The *trigger*, either an inspiratory effort or a time-based signal, defines what the ventilator senses to initiate an assisted breath. *Cycle* refers to the factors that determine the end of inspiration. For example, in volume-cycled ventilation, inspiration ends when a specific tidal volume is delivered to the patient. Other types of cycling include pressure cycling, time cycling, and flow cycling. *Limiting factors* are operator-specified values, such as airway pressure, that are monitored by transducers internal to the ventilator circuit throughout the respiratory cycle; if the specified

TABLE 252-1 *Clinical Characteristics of Commonly Used Modes of Mechanical Ventilation*

Ventilator Mode	Independent Variables (Set by User)	Dependent Variables (Monitored by User)	Trigger/Cycle Limit	Advantages	Disadvantages	Initial Settings
ACMV[a]	F$_{IO_2}$ Tidal volume Ventilator rate Level of PEEP Inspiratory flow pattern Peak inspiratory flow Pressure limit	Peak airway pressure, Pa$_{O_2}$, Pa$_{CO_2}$ Mean airway pressure I/E ratio	Patient/timer Pressure limit	Timer backup Patient-vent synchrony Patient controls minute ventilation	Not useful for weaning Potential for dangerous respiratory alkalosis	F$_{IO_2}$ = 1.0[b] V$_t$ = 10–15 mL/kg[a] f = 12–15/min PEEP = 0–5 cmH$_2$O Inspiratory flow = 60 L/min
SIMV[a]	Same as for ACMV	Same as for ACMV	Same as for ACMV	Timer backup useful for weaning	Potential dysynchrony	Same as for ACMV[a]
CPAP	F$_{IO_2}$ Level of CPAP	Tidal volume Rate, flow pattern Airway pressure Pa$_{O_2}$, Pa$_{CO_2}$, I/E ratio	No trigger Pressure limit	Allows assessment of spontaneous function Helps prevent atelectasis	No backup	F$_{IO_2}$ = 0.5–1.0[b] CPAP = 5–15 cmH$_2$O
PCV[a]	F$_{IO_2}$ Inspiratory pressure level Ventilator rate Level of PEEP Pressure limit I/E ratio	Tidal volume Flow rate, pattern Minute ventilation Pa$_{O_2}$, Pa$_{CO_2}$	Timer/patient Timer/pressure limit	System pressures regulated Useful for barotrauma treatment Timer backup	Requires heavy sedation Not useful for weaning	F$_{IO_2}$ = 1.0[b] PC = 20–40 cmH$_2$O[a] PEEP = 5–10 cmH$_2$O f = 12–15/min I/E = 0.7/1–4/1
PSV	F$_{IO_2}$ Inspiratory pressure level PEEP Pressure limit	Same as for PCV + I/E ratio	Inspiratory flow Pressure limit	Assures synchrony Good for weaning	No timer backup	F$_{IO_2}$ = 0.5–1.0[b] PS = 10–30 cmH$_2$O 5 cmH$_2$O usually the level used PEEP = 0–5 cmH$_2$O

[a] Open lung ventilation (OLV) involves the use of any of these specific modes with tidal volumes (or applied pressures) to achieve 5–6 mL/kg, and positive end expiratory pressures achieve maximal alveolar recruitment.

[b] F$_{IO_2}$ is usually set to 1.0 initially, unless there is a specific clinical indication to minimize F$_{IO_2}$, such as history of chemotherapy with bleomycin. Once adequate oxygenation is documented by blood gas analysis, F$_{IO_2}$ should be decreased in decrements of 0.1–0.2 as tolerated, until the lowest F$_{IO_2}$ required for an Sa$_{O_2}$ >90% is achieved.

Abbreviations: f, frequency; I/E, inspiration/expiration; F$_{IO_2}$, inspired O$_2$; PEEP, positive end-expiratory pressure; for ventilator modes, see text; V$_t$, tidal ventilation.

values are exceeded, inspiratory flow is immediately stopped, and the ventilator circuit is vented to atmospheric pressure or the specified PEEP.

Assist Control Mode Ventilation (ACMV) An inspiratory cycle is initiated either by the patient's inspiratory effort or, if no patient effort is detected within a specified time window, by a timer signal within the ventilator. Every breath delivered, whether patient or timer triggered, consists of the operator-specified tidal volume. Ventilatory rate is determined either by the patient or by the operator-specified backup rate, whichever is of higher frequency (Fig. 252-1A). ACMV is commonly used for initiation of mechanical ventilation because it ensures a backup minute ventilation in the absence of an intact respiratory drive

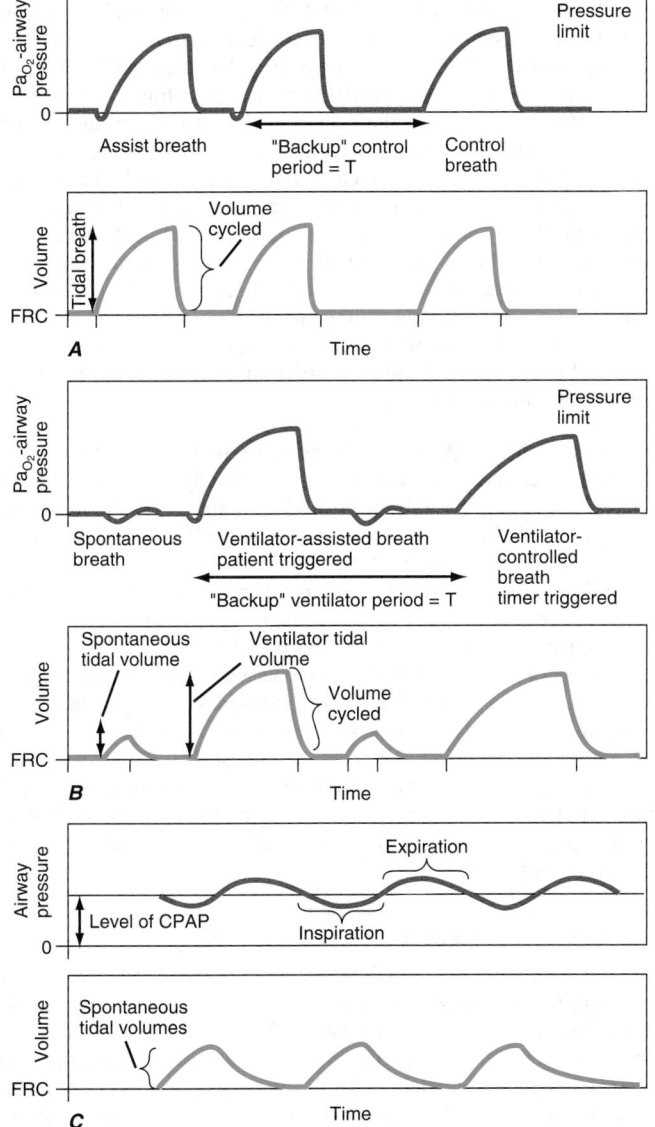

A. Airway pressure and lung volume versus time profile during assist control mode ventilation (ACMV). Assisted breaths are triggered by the patient's effort. Controlled breaths are triggered by the ventilator timer. Every breath, whether triggered by the patient or by the timer, is a complete volume-cycled breath, with airway pressure as a dependent variable. The pressure limit is set above the peak inspiratory pressure. **B.** Airway pressure and lung volume versus time profiles during synchronized intermittent mandatory ventilation (SIMV). Spontaneous breaths occur between patient-triggered assisted breaths and timer-triggered breaths. The tidal volume of the spontaneous breaths is determined by the patient's effort and lung impedance. Assisted and controlled breaths are volume cycled. **C.** Airway pressure and lung volume versus time profiles during continuous positive airway pressure (CPAP). Breathing is spontaneous, and no ventilator assist is provided. The spontaneous profile is superimposed on an elevated mean airway pressure that the user specifies. FRC, functional residual capacity.

FIGURE 252-1

and allows for synchronization of the ventilator cycle with the patient's inspiratory effort.

Problems can arise when ACMV is used in patients with tachypnea due to nonrespiratory or nonmetabolic factors such as anxiety, pain, or airway irritation. Respiratory alkalemia may develop and trigger myoclonus or seizures. Dynamic hyperinflation (so-called auto-PEEP) may occur if the patient's respiratory mechanics are such that inadequate time is available for complete exhalation between inspiratory cycles. Auto-PEEP can limit venous return, decrease cardiac output, and increase airway pressures, predisposing to barotrauma. ACMV is not effective for weaning patients from mechanical ventilation because it provides full ventilator assistance on each patient-initiated breath.

Synchronized Intermittent Mandatory Ventilation (SIMV) The major difference between SIMV and ACMV is that in the former the patient is allowed to breathe spontaneously, i.e., without ventilator assist, between delivered ventilator breaths. However, mandatory breaths are delivered in synchrony with the patient's inspiratory efforts at a frequency determined by the operator. If the patient fails to initiate a breath, the ventilator delivers a fixed-tidal-volume breath and resets the internal timer for the next inspiratory cycle (Fig. 252-1B). SIMV differs from ACMV in that only the preset number of breaths is ventilator-assisted.

SIMV allows patients with an intact respiratory drive to exercise inspiratory muscles between assisted breaths, making it useful for both supporting and weaning intubated patients. SIMV may be difficult to use in patients with tachypnea because they may attempt to exhale during the ventilator-programmed inspiratory cycle. When this occurs, the airway pressure may exceed the inspiratory pressure limit, the ventilator-assisted breath will be aborted, and minute volume may drop below that programmed by the operator. In this setting, if the tachypnea is in response to respiratory or metabolic acidosis, a change to ACMV will increase minute ventilation and help normalize the pH while the underlying process is further evaluated.

Continuous Positive Airway Pressure (CPAP) This is not a true support-mode of ventilation, inasmuch as all ventilation occurs through the patient's spontaneous efforts. The ventilator provides fresh gas to the breathing circuit with each inspiration and charges the circuit to a constant, operator-specified pressure that can range from 0 to 20 cmH$_2$O (Fig. 252-1C). CPAP is used to assess extubation potential in patients who have been effectively weaned and are requiring little ventilator support and in patients with intact respiratory system function who require an endotracheal tube for airway protection.

Pressure-Control Ventilation (PCV) This form of ventilation is time triggered, time cycled, and pressure limited. During the inspiratory phase, a given pressure is imposed at the airway opening, and the pressure remains at this user-specified level throughout inspiration (Fig. 252-2A). Since inspiratory airway pressure is specified by the operator, tidal volume and inspiratory flow rate are *dependent* rather than *independent* variables and are not user specified. PCV is the preferred mode of ventilation for patients with documented barotrauma, because airway pressures can be limited, and for postoperative thoracic surgical patients, in whom the shear forces across a fresh suture line should be limited. When PCV is used, minute ventilation and tidal volume must be monitored; minute ventilation is altered through changes in rate or in the pressure-control value.

PCV with the use of a prolonged inspiratory time is frequently applied to patients with severe hypoxemic respiratory failure. This approach, called inverse inspiratory-to-expiratory ratio ventilation (IRV), increases mean distending pressures without increasing peak airway pressures. It is thought to work in conjunction with PEEP to open collapsed alveoli and improve oxygenation. IRV may be associated with fewer deleterious effects than conventional volume-cycled ventilation, which requires higher peak airway pressures to achieve an equivalent reduction in shunt fraction, but there are no convincing data to show that IRV improves outcomes.

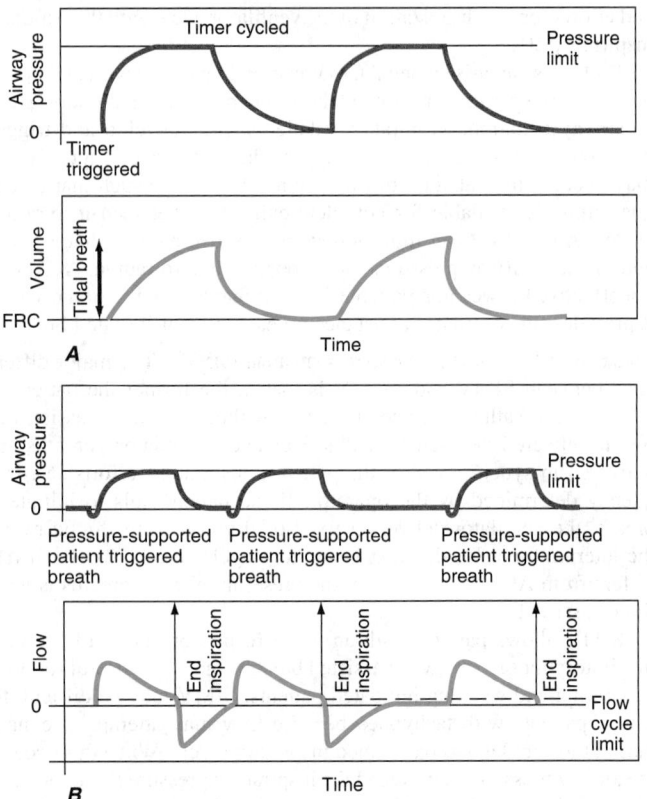

FIGURE 252-2 *A.* Airway pressure and lung volume versus time profiles during pressure-control ventilation (PCV). All breaths are timer triggered, timer cycled, and pressure limited. Peak airway pressure is set by the operator, and tidal volume is a dependent variable. The profiles shown here display the pressure limit as slightly higher than pressure-control level. This need not be the case, but it is appropriate to set the pressure limit only slightly above the pressure-control level when using this mode of ventilation for management of the patient with barotrauma. *B.* Airway pressure and airway flow versus time profiles during pressure-support ventilation (PSV). All breaths are patient triggered and flow cycled. Inspiration is cycled off when the inspiratory flow drops below a predetermined threshold internally set in the ventilator circuit. In the example shown, the pressure limit is slightly greater than the pressure-support level. Since each can be set independently, this need not be the case. FRC, functional residual capacity.

Pressure-Support Ventilation (PSV) This form of ventilation is patient triggered, flow cycled, and pressure limited; it is specifically designed for use in the weaning process. During PSV, the inspiratory phase is terminated when inspiratory airflow falls below a certain level; in most ventilators this flow rate cannot be adjusted by the operator. When PSV is used, patients receive ventilator assist only when the ventilator detects an inspiratory effort (Fig. 252-2B). PSV can also be used in combination with SIMV to ensure volume-cycled backup for patients whose respiratory drive is depressed.

PSV is well tolerated by most patients who are being weaned; PSV parameters can be set to provide fully or nearly fully ventilatory support and can be withdrawn slowly over a period of days in a systematic fashion to gradually load the respiratory muscles.

Open Lung Ventilation (OLV) OLV is not a distinct mode of ventilation, but rather a strategy for applying either volume-cycled or pressure-control ventilation to patients with severe respiratory failure. In OLV, the primary objectives of ventilator support are maintenance of adequate oxygenation and avoidance of cyclic opening and closing of alveolar units by selecting a level of PEEP that allows the majority of units to remain inflated during tidal ventilation. Achievement of eucapnia and normal blood pH through adjustments in ventilator tidal volume and breathing frequency are of lower priority. Clinical and experimental observations indicate that high airway pressures and repeated opening and closing of alveoli can cause microstructural lung

damage, propagation of lung injury through generation of inflammatory cytokines, and direct barotrauma. Current data suggest that a small tidal volume (i.e., 6 mL/kg) provides adequate ventilatory support with a lower incidence of adverse effects than more conventional tidal volumes of 10 to 15 mL/kg. Hypercapnia and consequent respiratory acidosis tend to be well tolerated physiologically, except in patients with significant hemodynamic compromise, ventricular dysfunction, cardiac dysrrhythmias, or increased ICP. Furthermore, there are recent data to suggest that hypercapnia may have direct beneficial anti-inflammatory effects. OLV has been used most extensively in the management of patients with hypoxemic respiratory failure due to acute lung injury. Although few randomized clinical trials of OLV have been performed, available data suggest that this strategy reduces the mortality rate and improves gas exhange in patients with acute lung injury.

Prone Positioning during Mechanical Ventilation Patients with acute respiratory distress syndrome (ARDS) experience hypoxemia as a result of intrapulmonary shunt due to regional atelectasis (see Chap. 251). Recent studies in patients with ARDS have demonstrated that collapse occurs most extensively in the dependent regions of the lung. Prone positioning increases transdiaphragmatic pressures in these atelectatic, dorsal lung zones by altering their position relative to the hydrostatic pressures generated by abdominal contents. Thus, distending pressures in these areas are increased through positioning without the need to apply additional airway pressures that can overdistend less damaged areas of lung and potentially cause additional damage. While conceptually appealing and simple to implement, a recently completed randomized trial in patients with acute lung injury failed to demonstrate a survival advantage with prone positioning despite demonstration of transient physiologic benefit.

Noninvasive Ventilation (NIV) Noninvasive ventilator support through a tight-fitting facemask or nasal mask, traditionally used for treatment of sleep apnea, has recently been used as primary ventilator support in patients with impending respiratory failure. Facemask and nasal devices for administering NIV therapy are most frequently combined with PSV or bi-level positive airway pressure ventilation, inasmuch as both of these modes are well tolerated by the conscious patient and optimize patient-ventilator synchrony. NIV has met with varying degrees of success when applied to patients with acute or chronic respiratory failure. The major limitation to its widespread application has been patient intolerance, because the tight-fitting mask required for NIV can cause both physical and emotional discomfort in patients with dyspnea. Aggressive medical therapy directed at the cause of impending respiratory failure, together with an experienced respiratory therapy and physician team, appear to be the keys to successful use of NIV in intensive care units.

GUIDELINES FOR MANAGING THE VENTILATED PATIENT

Most patients who are started on ventilator support receive ACMV or SIMV, because these modes ensure user-specified backup minute ventilation in the event that the patient fails to initiate respiratory efforts. Once the intubated patient has been stabilized with respect to oxygenation, definitive therapy for the underlying process responsible for respiratory failure is formulated and initiated. Subsequent modifications in ventilator therapy must be provided in parallel with changes in the patient's clinical status. As improvement in respiratory function is noted, the first priorities are to reduce PEEP and supplemental O_2. Once a patient can achieve adequate arterial saturation with an $FI_{O_2} \leq$ 0.5 and 5 cmH$_2$O PEEP, attempts should be made to reduce the level of mechanical ventilatory support. Patients previously on full ventilator support should be switched to a ventilator mode that allows for weaning, such as SIMV, PSV, or SIMV combined with PSV. Ventilator therapy can then be gradually removed, as outlined in the section on weaning. Patients whose condition continues to deteriorate after ventilator support is initiated may require increased O_2, PEEP, and alternative modes of ventilation such as IRV or OLV.

Patients who are started on mechanical ventilation usually require some form of sedation and analgesia to maintain an acceptable level of comfort. Often, this regimen consists of a combination of a benzodiazepine and opiate administered intravenously. Medications commonly used for this purpose include lorazepam, midazolam, diazepam, morphine, and fentanyl.

Immobilized patients in the intensive care unit on mechanical ventilator support are at increased risk for deep venous thrombosis; accepted practice consists of administering prophylaxis in the form of subcutaneous heparin and/or pneumatic compression boots. Fractionated low-molecular-weight heparin has also been used for this purpose; it appears to be equally effective and is associated with a decreased incidence of heparin-associated thrombocytopenia.

Prophylaxis against diffuse gastrointestinal mucosal injury is indicated for patients who have suffered a neurologic insult or those with severe respiratory failure in association with ARDS. Histamine receptor antagonists (H_2-receptor antagonists), antacids, and cytoprotective agents such as carafate have all been used for this purpose and appear to be effective. Recent data suggest that carafate use is associated with a reduction in the incidence of nosocomial pneumonias, since it does not cause changes in stomach pH and is less likely to permit colonization of the gastrointestinal tract by nosocomial organisms at neutral pH.

Nutrition support by enteral feeding through either a nasogastric or an orogastric tube should be maintained in all intubated patients whenever possible. In those patients with a normal baseline nutritional state, support should be initiated within 7 days. In malnourished patients, nutrition support should be initiated within 72 h. Delayed gastric emptying is common in critically ill patients on sedative medications but often responds to promotility agents such as metoclopramide. Parenteral nutrition is an alternative to enteral nutrition in patients with severe gastrointestinal pathology.

COMPLICATIONS OF MECHANICAL VENTILATION

Endotracheal intubation and positive-pressure mechanical ventilation have direct and indirect effects on several organ systems, including the lung and upper airways, the cardiovascular system, and the gastrointestinal system. Pulmonary complications include barotrauma, nosocomial pneumonia, oxygen toxicity, tracheal stenosis, and deconditioning of respiratory muscles. *Barotrauma*, which occurs when high pressures (i.e., > 50 cmH_2O) overdistend and disrupt lung tissue, is clinically manifest by interstitial emphysema, pneumomediastinum, subcutaneous emphysema, or pneumothorax. Although the first three conditions may resolve simply through the reduction of airway pressures, clinically significant pneumothorax, as indicated by hypoxemia, decreased lung compliance, and hemodynamic compromise, requires tube thoracostomy.

Patients intubated for longer than 72 h are at high risk for ventilator associated pneumonia as a result of aspiration from the upper airways through small leaks around the endotracheal tube cuff; the most common organisms responsible for this condition are enteric gram-negative rods, *Staphylococcus aureus*, and anaerobic bacteria. Because the endotracheal tube and upper airways of patients on mechanical ventilation are commonly colonized with bacteria, the diagnosis of nosocomial pneumonia requires "protected brush" bronchoscopic sampling of airway secretions coupled with quantitative microbiologic techniques to differentiate colonization from infection.

Hypotension resulting from elevated intrathoracic pressures with decreased venous return is almost always responsive to intravascular volume repletion. In patients judged to have hypotension or respiratory failure on the basis of alveolar edema, hemodynamic monitoring with a pulmonary arterial catheter may be of value in optimizing O_2 delivery via manipulation of intravascular volume and $F_{I_{O_2}}$ and PEEP levels.

Gastrointestinal effects of positive-pressure ventilation include *stress ulceration* and *mild to moderate cholestasis*. It is common practice to provide prophylaxis with H_2-receptor antagonists or sucralfate for stress-related ulcers. Mild cholestasis [i.e., total bilirubin values ≤68 μmol/L (≤4.0 mg/dL)] attributable to the effects of increased intrathoracic pressures on portal vein pressures is common and generally self-limited. Cholestasis of a more severe degree should not be attributed to a positive-pressure ventilation response and is more likely due to a primary hepatic process.

WEANING FROM MECHANICAL VENTILATION

Removal of mechanical ventilator support requires that a number of criteria be met. Upper airway function must be intact for a patient to remain extubated but is difficult to assess in the intubated patient. Therefore, if a patient can breathe on his or her own through an endotracheal tube but develops stridor or recurrent aspiration once the tube is removed, upper airway dysfunction or an abnormal swallowing mechanism should be suspected and plans for achieving a stable airway developed. An intact cough during suctioning is a good indicator of a patient's ability to mobilize secretions. Respiratory drive and chest wall function are assessed by observation of respiratory rate, tidal volume, inspiratory pressure, and vital capacity. The weaning index, defined as the ratio of breathing frequency to tidal volume (breaths per minute per liter), is both sensitive and specific for predicting the likelihood of successful extubation. When this ratio is less than 105 with the patient breathing without mechanical assistance through an endotracheal tube, successful extubation is likely. An inspiratory pressure of more than −30 cmH_2O and a vital capacity of greater than 10 mL/kg are considered indicators of acceptable chest wall and diaphragm function. Alveolar ventilation is generally adequate when elimination of CO_2 is sufficient to maintain arterial pH in the range of 7.35 to 7.40, and an Sa_{O_2} > 90% can be achieved with an $F_{I_{O_2}}$ < 0.5 and a PEEP ≤ 5 cmH_2O. Although many patients may not meet all criteria for weaning, the likelihood that a patient will tolerate extubation without difficulty increases as more criteria are met.

Many approaches to weaning patients from ventilator support have been advocated. T-piece and CPAP weaning are best tolerated by patients who have undergone mechanical ventilation for brief periods and require little respiratory muscle reconditioning, whereas SIMV and PSV are best for patients who have been intubated for extended periods and require gradual respiratory-muscle reconditioning.

T-piece weaning involves brief spontaneous breathing trials with supplemental O_2. These trials are usually initiated for 5 min/h followed by a 1-h interval of rest. T-piece trials are increased in 5- to 10-min increments until the patient can remain ventilator independent for periods of several hours. Extubation can then be attempted. CPAP weaning is similar to T-piece weaning except that trials of spontaneous breathing are conducted on the ventilator in CPAP mode.

Weaning by means of SIMV involves gradually tapering the mandatory backup rate in increments of 2 to 4 breaths per minute while monitoring blood gas parameters and respiratory rates. Rates of greater than 25 breaths per minute on withdrawal of mandatory ventilator breaths generally indicate respiratory muscle fatigue and the need to combine periods of exercise with periods of rest. Exercise periods are gradually increased until a patient remains stable on SIMV at 4 breaths per minute or less without needing rest at higher SIMV rates. A CPAP or T-piece trial can then be attempted before planned extubation.

PSV, as described in detail above, is used primarily for weaning from mechanical ventilation. PSV is usually initiated at a level adequate for full ventilator support (PSV_{max}); i.e., PSV is set slightly below the peak inspiratory pressures required by the patient during volume-cycled ventilation. The level of pressure support is then gradually withdrawn in increments of 5 cmH_2O until a level is reached at which the respiratory rate increases to 25 breaths per minute. At this point, intermittent periods of higher-pressure support are alternated with periods of lower-pressure support to provide muscle reconditioning without causing diaphragmatic fatigue. Gradual withdrawal of PSV continues until the level of support is just adequate to overcome the resistance of the endotracheal tube (approximately 5 to 10 cmH_2O). Support can be discontinued and the patient extubated.

FURTHER READING

AMATO MBP et al: Effect of a protective-ventilation strategy on mortality in the acute respiratory distress syndrome. N Engl J Med 338:347, 1998
BOZEMAN YP et al: Etomidate as a sole agent for endotracheal intubation in the prehospital air medical setting. Air Med J 21:32, 2002

ESTEBAN A et al: A comparison of four methods of weaning patients from mechanical ventilation. N Engl J Med 332:345, 1995
GATTINONI L et al: Effect of prone positioning on the survival of patients with acute respiratory failure. N Engl J Med 345:568, 2001
INGENITO EP, DRAZEN JM: Mechanical ventilators, in *Principles of Critical Care*, 2d ed, JB Hall, GA Schmidt, LDH Wood (eds). New York, McGraw-Hill, 1997, pp 142–154
TOBIN MJ: Advances in mechanical ventilation. N Engl J Med 344:1986, 2001

Section 2   Shock and Cardiac Arrest

253   APPROACH TO THE PATIENT WITH SHOCK
Ronald V. Maier

Shock is the clinical syndrome that results from inadequate tissue perfusion. Irrespective of cause, the hypoperfusion-induced imbalance between the delivery of and requirements for oxygen and substrate leads to cellular dysfunction. The cellular injury created by the inadequate delivery of oxygen and substrates also induces the production and release of inflammatory mediators that further compromise perfusion through functional and structural changes within the microvasculature. This leads to a vicious cycle in which impaired perfusion is responsible for cellular injury which causes maldistribution of blood flow, further compromising cellular perfusion; the latter causes multiple organ failure and, if the process is not interrupted, leads to the death of the patient. The clinical manifestations of shock are the result, in part, of sympathetic neuroendocrine responses to hypoperfusion as well as the breakdown in organ function induced by severe cellular dysfunction.

When very severe and/or persistent, inadequate oxygen delivery leads to irreversible cell injury; thus, only rapid restoration of oxygen delivery can reverse the progression of the shock state. The fundamental approach to management, therefore, is to recognize overt and impending shock in a timely fashion and to intervene emergently to restore perfusion. This requires the expansion or reexpansion of blood volume. Control of any inciting pathologic process, e.g., continued hemorrhage, impairment of cardiac function, or infection, must occur simultaneously.

Clinical shock is usually accompanied by hypotension, i.e., a mean arterial pressure <60 mmHg in previously normotensive persons. Multiple classification schemes have been developed in an attempt to synthesize the seemingly dissimilar processes leading to shock. Strict adherence to a classification scheme may be difficult from a clinical standpoint because of the frequent combination of two or more causes of shock in any individual patient, but the classification shown in Table 253-1 provides a useful reference point from which to discuss and further delineate the underlying processes.

PATHOGENESIS AND ORGAN RESPONSE

MICROCIRCULATION Normally when cardiac output falls, systemic vascular resistance rises to maintain a level of systemic pressure that is adequate for perfusion of the heart and brain at the expense of other tissues such as muscle, skin, and especially the gastrointestinal tract. Systemic vascular resistance is determined primarily by the luminal diameter of arterioles. The metabolic rates of the heart and brain are high, and their stores of energy substrate are low. These organs are critically dependent on a continuous supply of oxygen and nutrients, and neither tolerates severe ischemia for more than brief periods. Au-

TABLE 253-1 *Classification of Shock*	
Hypovolemic	Septic
Traumatic	Hyperdynamic
Cardiogenic	Hypodynamic
Intrinsic	Neurogenic
Compressive	Hypoadrenal

toregulation, i.e., the maintenance of blood flow over a wide range of perfusion pressures, is critical in sustaining cerebral and coronary perfusion despite significant hypotension. However, when mean arterial pressure drops to ≤60 mmHg, flow to these organs falls and their function deteriorates.

Arteriolar vascular smooth muscle has both α- and β-adrenergic receptors. The α_1 receptors mediate vasoconstriction, while the β_2 receptors mediate vasodilation. Efferent sympathetic fibers release norepinephrine, which acts primarily on α_1 receptors in one of the most fundamental compensatory responses to reduced perfusion pressure. Other constrictor substances that are increased in most forms of shock include angiotensin II, vasopressin, endothelin-1, and thromboxane A_2. Both norepinephrine and epinephrine are released by the adrenal medulla, and the concentrations of these catecholamines in the bloodstream rise. Circulating vasodilators in shock include prostacyclin [prostaglandin $(PG)I_2$], nitric oxide (NO), and, importantly, products of local metabolism such as adenosine that match flow to the metabolic needs of the tissue. The balance between these various vasoconstrictor and vasodilator influences acting upon the microcirculation determines local perfusion.

Transport to cells depends on microcirculatory flow; capillary permeability; the diffusion of oxygen, carbon dioxide, nutrients, and products of metabolism through the interstitium; and the exchange of these products across cell membranes. Impairment of the microcirculation, which is central to the pathophysiologic responses in the late stages of all forms of shock, results in the derangement of cellular metabolism, which is ultimately responsible for organ failure.

The endogenous response to mild or moderate hypovolemia is an attempt at restitution of intravascular volume through alterations in hydrostatic pressure and osmolarity. Constriction of arterioles leads to reductions in both the capillary hydrostatic pressure and the number of capillary beds perfused, thereby limiting the capillary surface area across which filtration occurs. When filtration is reduced while intravascular oncotic pressure remains constant or rises, there is net reabsorption of fluid into the vascular bed, in accord with Starling's law of capillary-interstitial liquid exchange (Chap. 29). Metabolic changes (including hyperglycemia and elevations in the products of glycolysis, lipolysis, and proteolysis) raise extracellular osmolarity, leading to an osmotic gradient between cells and interstitium that increases interstitial and intravascular volume at the expense of intracellular volume.

CELLULAR RESPONSES Interstitial transport of nutrients is impaired, leading to a decline of intracellular high-energy phosphate stores. Mitochondrial dysfunction and uncoupling of oxidative phosphorylation are the most likely causes for decreased amounts of ATP. As a consequence, there is an accumulation of hydrogen ions, lactate, and other products of anaerobic metabolism. As shock progresses, these vasodilator metabolites override vasomotor tone, causing further hypotension and hypoperfusion. Dysfunction of cell membranes is thought to represent a common end-stage pathophysiologic pathway in the various forms of shock. Normal cellular transmembrane potential falls, and there is an associated increase in intracellular sodium and water, leading to cell swelling, which interferes further with microvascular perfusion.

NEUROENDOCRINE RESPONSE Hypovolemia, hypotension, and hypoxia are sensed by baroreceptors and chemoreceptors, which contribute to an autonomic response that attempts to restore blood volume, maintain central perfusion, and mobilize metabolic substrates. Hypotension disinhibits the vasomotor center, resulting in increased adrenergic output and reduced vagal activity. Release of norepinephrine induces peripheral and splanchnic vasoconstriction, a major contributor to the maintenance of central organ perfusion, while reduced vagal activity increases the heart rate and cardiac output. The effects of circulating epinephrine released by the adrenal medulla in shock are largely metabolic, causing increased glycogenolysis and gluconeogenesis and reduced pancreatic insulin release. Epinephrine also inhibits production and release of inflammatory mediators through stimulation of β-adrenergic receptors on innate immune cells.

Severe pain and other severe stress cause the hypothalamic release of adrenocorticotropic hormone (ACTH). This stimulates cortisol secretion, which contributes to decreased peripheral uptake of glucose and amino acids, enhances lipolysis, and increases gluconeogenesis. Increased pancreatic secretion of glucagon during stress accelerates hepatic gluconeogenesis and further elevates blood glucose concentration. These hormonal actions act synergistically in the maintenance of blood volume. Many critically ill patients exhibit low plasma cortisol levels and an impaired response to ACTH stimulation. The importance of the cortisol response to stress is illustrated by the profound circulatory collapse that occurs in hypoadrenal patients (see below).

Renin release is increased in response to adrenergic discharge and reduced perfusion of the juxtaglomerular apparatus in the kidney. Renin induces the formation of angiotensin I, which is then converted to angiotensin II, an extremely potent vasoconstrictor and stimulator of aldosterone release by the adrenal cortex and of vasopressin by the posterior pituitary. Aldosterone contributes to the maintainance of intravascular volume by enhancing renal tubular reabsorption of sodium, resulting in the excretion of a low-volume, concentrated, sodium-free urine. Vasopressin has a direct action on vascular smooth muscle, contributing to vasoconstriction, and acts on the distal renal tubules to enhance water reabsorption.

CARDIOVASCULAR RESPONSE Three variables—ventricular filling (preload), the resistance to ventricular ejection (afterload), and myocardial contractility—are paramount in controlling stroke volume (Chap. 215). Cardiac output, the major determinant of tissue perfusion, is the product of stroke volume and heart rate. Hypovolemia leads to decreased ventricular preload, which in turn reduces the stroke volume. An increase in heart rate is a useful but limited compensatory mechanism to maintain cardiac output. A shock-induced reduction in myocardial compliance is frequent, reducing ventricular end-diastolic volume and hence stroke volume at any given ventricular filling pressure. Restoration of intravascular volume returns stroke volume to normal but only at elevated filling pressures. In addition, sepsis, ischemia, myocardial infarction, severe tissue trauma, hypothermia, general anesthesia, prolonged hypotension, and acidemia may all impair myocardial contractility and also reduce the stroke volume at any given ventricular end-diastolic volume. The resistance to ventricular ejection is significantly influenced by the systemic vascular resistance, which is elevated in most forms of shock. However, resistance is depressed in the early hyperdynamic stage of septic shock (see below), thereby allowing the cardiac output to be maintained or elevated.

The venous system contains nearly two-thirds of the total circulating blood volume, most in the small veins, and serves as a dynamic reservoir for autoinfusion of blood. Active venoconstriction as a consequence of α-adrenergic activity is an important compensatory mechanism for the maintenance of venous return and therefore of ventricular filling during shock. On the other hand, venous dilatation, as occurs in neurogenic shock, reduces ventricular filling and hence stroke volume and cardiac output (see below).

PULMONARY RESPONSE The response of the pulmonary vascular bed to shock parallels that of the systemic vascular bed, and the relative increase in pulmonary vascular resistance, particularly in septic shock, may exceed that of the systemic vascular resistance. Shock-induced tachypnea reduces tidal volume and increases both dead space and minute ventilation. Relative hypoxia and the subsequent tachypnea induce a respiratory alkalosis. Recumbency and involuntary restriction of ventilation secondary to pain reduce functional residual capacity and may lead to atelectasis. Shock is recognized as a major cause of acute lung injury and subsequent acute respiratory distress syndrome (ARDS; Chap. 251). These disorders are characterized by noncardiogenic pulmonary edema secondary to diffuse pulmonary capillary endothelial and alveolar epithelial injury, hypoxemia, and bilateral diffuse pulmonary infiltrates. Hypoxemia results from perfusion of underventilated and nonventilated alveoli. Loss of surfactant and lung volume in combination with increased interstitial and alveolar edema reduce lung compliance. The work of breathing and the oxygen requirements of respiratory muscles increase.

RENAL RESPONSE Acute renal failure (Chap. 260), a serious complication of shock and hypoperfusion, occurs less frequently than heretofore because of early aggressive volume repletion. Acute tubular necrosis is now more frequently seen as a result of the interactions of shock, sepsis, the administration of nephrotoxic agents (such as aminoglycosides and angiographic contrast media), and rhabdomyolysis; the latter may be particularly severe in skeletal muscle trauma. The physiologic response of the kidney to hypoperfusion is to conserve salt and water. In addition to decreased renal blood flow, increased afferent arteriolar resistance accounts for diminished glomerular filtration rate, which together with increased aldosterone and vasopressin is responsible for reduced urine formation. Toxic injury causes necrosis of tubular epithelium and tubular obstruction by cellular debris with back-leak of filtrate. The depletion of renal ATP stores that occurs with prolonged renal hypoperfusion contributes to subsequent impairment of renal function. There is no convincing evidence that low-dose dopamine protects against acute renal failure.

METABOLIC DERANGEMENTS During shock, there is disruption of the normal cycles of carbohydrate, lipid, and protein metabolism. Through the citric acid cycle, alanine in conjunction with lactate (which is converted from pyruvate in the periphery in the presence of oxygen deprivation) enhances the hepatic production of glucose. With reduced availability of oxygen, the breakdown of glucose to pyruvate and ultimately lactate represents an inefficient cycling of substrate with minimal net energy production. An elevated plasma lactate/pyruvate ratio is consistent with anaerobic metabolism and reflects inadequate tissue perfusion. Decreased clearance of exogenous triglycerides coupled with increased hepatic lipogenesis causes a significant rise in serum triglyceride concentrations. There is increased protein catabolism, a negative nitrogen balance, and, if the process is prolonged, severe muscle wasting.

INFLAMMATORY RESPONSES Activation of an extensive network of proinflammatory mediator systems plays a significant role in the progression of shock and contributes importantly to the development of organ injury and failure.

Multiple humoral mediators are activated during shock and tissue injury. The complement cascade, activated through both the classic and alternate pathways, generates the anaphylatoxins C3a and C5a. Direct complement fixation to injured tissues can progress to the C5-C9 attack complex, causing further cell damage. Activation of the coagulation cascade causes microvascular thrombosis, with subsequent lysis leading to repeated episodes of ischemia and reperfusion. Components of the coagulation system, such as thrombin, are potent proinflammatory mediators that cause expression of adhesion molecules on endothelial cells and activation of neutrophils, leading to microvascular injury. Coagulation also activates the kallekrein-kininogen cascade, contributing to hypotension.

TABLE 253-2 Normal Hemodynamic Parameters

Parameter	Calculation	Normal Values
Cardiac output (CO)	$SV \times HR$	4–8 L/min
Cardiac index (CI)	CO/BSA	2.6–4.2 (L/min)/m²
Stroke volume (SV)	CO/HR	50–100 mL/beat
Systemic vascular resistance (SVR)	$[(MAP - RAP)/CO] \times 80$	700–1600 dynes · s/cm⁵
Pulmonary vascular resistance (PVR)	$[(PAP_m - PCWP)/CO] \times 80$	20–130 dynes · s/cm⁵
Left ventricular stroke work (LVSW)	$SV(MAP - PCWP) \times 0.0136$	60–80 g-m/beat
Right ventricular stroke work (RVSW)	$SV(PAP_m - RAP)$	10–15 g-m/beat

Note: HR, heart rate; BSA, body surface area; MAP, mean arterial pressure; RAP, right atrial pressure; PAP_m, pulmonary artery pressure—mean; PCWP, pulmonary capillary wedge pressure.

Eicosanoids are vasoactive and immunomodulatory products of arachidonic acid metabolism that include cyclooxygenase-derived prostaglandins and thromboxane A_2 as well as lipoxygenase-derived leukotrienes and lipoxins. Thromboxane A_2 is a potent vasoconstrictor that contributes to the pulmonary hypertension and acute tubular necrosis of shock. PGI_2 and PGE_2 are potent vasodilators that enhance capillary permeability and edema formation. The cysteinyl leukotrienes LTC_4 and LTD_4 are pivotal mediators of the vascular sequelae of anaphylaxis, as well as of shock states resulting from sepsis or tissue injury. LTB_4 is a potent neutrophil chemoattractant and secretagogue that stimulates the formation of reactive oxygen species. Platelet-activating factor, an ether-linked, arachidonyl-containing phospholipid mediator, causes pulmonary vasoconstriction, bronchoconstriction, systemic vasodilation, increased capillary permeability, and the priming of macrophages and neutrophils to produce enhanced levels of inflammatory mediators.

Tumor necrosis factor (TNF) α, produced by activated macrophages, reproduces many components of the shock state including hypotension, lactic acidosis, and respiratory failure. Interleukin (IL) 1, produced by tissue-fixed macrophages, is critical to the inflammatory response. Chemokines such as IL-8 are potent neutrophil chemoattractants and activators that upregulate adhesion molecules on the neutrophil to enhance aggregation, adherence, and damage to the vascular endothelium. While the endothelium normally produces nitric oxide (NO), the inflammatory response stimulates the inducible isoform of NO synthase (iNOS), which is overexpressed and produces toxic NO and oxygen-derived free radicals which contribute to the hyperdynamic cardiovascular response in sepsis.

Multiple inflammatory cells, including neutrophils, macrophages, and platelets, are a major contributor to inflammation-induced injury. Margination of activated neutrophils in the microcirculation is a common pathologic finding in shock, causing secondary injury due to the release of toxic oxygen radicals and proteases. Tissue-fixed macrophages produce virtually all major components of the inflammatory response and orchestrate the progression and duration of the inflammatory response.

Monitoring Patients in shock require care in an intensive care unit. Careful and continuous assessment of the physiologic status is necessary. Arterial pressure through an indwelling line, pulse, and respiratory rate should be monitored continuously; a Foley catheter should be inserted to follow urine flow; and mental status assessed frequently.

Although there is ongoing debate as to the indications for using the flow-directed pulmonary artery catheter (PAC, Swan-Ganz catheter), most intensivists believe that the ability to predict the hemodynamic profiles of patients in shock accurately without a PAC is poor. The PAC is placed percutaneously via the subclavian or jugular vein through the central venous circulation and right heart into the pulmonary artery. There are ports both proximal in the right atrium and distal in the pulmonary artery to provide access for infusions and for cardiac output measurements. Right atrial and pulmonary artery pressures are measured, and the pulmonary capillary wedge pressure (PCWP) serves as an approximation of the left atrial pressure. Normal hemodynamic parameters are shown in Table 212-3 and Table 253-2.

Cardiac output is determined by the thermodilution technique, and high-resolution thermistors can also be used to determine right ventricular end-diastolic volume to monitor further the response of the right heart to fluid resuscitation. A PAC with an oximeter port offers the additional advantage of on-line monitoring of the mixed venous oxygen saturation, an important index of tissue perfusion. Systemic and pulmonary vascular resistances are calculated as the ratio of the pressure drop across these vascular beds to the cardiac output (Chap. 212). Determinations of oxygen content in arterial and venous blood, together with cardiac output and hemoglobin concentration, allow calculation of oxygen delivery, oxygen consumption, and oxygen-extraction ratio (Table 253-3). The hemodynamic patterns associated with the various forms of shock are shown in Table 253-4.

In resuscitation from shock, it is critical to restore tissue perfusion and optimize oxygen delivery, hemodynamics, and cardiac function rapidly. A reasonable goal of therapy is to achieve normal mixed venous oxygen saturation and arteriovenous oxygen-extraction ratio. To enhance oxygen delivery, red cell mass, arterial oxygen saturation, and cardiac output may be augmented singly or simultaneously. An increase in oxygen delivery not accompanied by an increase in oxygen consumption implies that oxygen availability is adequate and that oxygen consumption is not flow-dependent. Conversely, an elevation of oxygen consumption with increased cardiac output implies that the oxygen supply was inadequate. A reduction in systemic vascular resistance accompanying an increase in cardiac output indicates that compensatory vasoconstriction is reversing due to improved tissue perfusion. The determination of stepwise expansion of blood volume on cardiac performance allows identification of the optimum preload (Starling's law). An algorithm for the resuscitation of the patient in shock is shown in Fig. 253-1.

SPECIFIC FORMS OF SHOCK

HYPOVOLEMIC SHOCK This most common form of shock results either from the loss of red blood cell mass and plasma from hemorrhage or from the loss of plasma volume alone arising

TABLE 253-3 Oxygen Transport Calculations

Parameter	Calculation	Normal Values
Oxygen-carrying capacity of hemoglobin		1.39 mL/g
Plasma O_2 concentration		$P_{O_2} \times 0.0031$
Arterial O_2 concentration (Ca_{O_2})	$1.39\ Sa_{O_2} + 0.0031\ Pa_{O_2}$	20 vol%
Venous O_2 concentration (Cv_{O_2})	$1.39\ Sv_{O_2} + 0.0031\ Pv_{O_2}$	15.5 vol%
Arteriovenous O_2 difference ($Ca_{O_2} - Cv_{O_2}$)	$1.39\ (Sa_{O_2} - Sv_{O_2}) + 0.0031\ (Pa_{O_2} - Pv_{O_2})$	3.5 vol%
Oxygen delivery (D_{O_2})	$Ca_{O_2} \times CO\ (L/min) \times 10\ (dL/L)$ $1.39\ Sa_{O_2} \times CO \times 10$	800–1600 mL/min
Oxygen uptake (V_{O_2})	$(Ca_{O_2} - Cv_{O_2}) \times CO \times 10$ $1.39\ (Sa_{O_2} - Sv_{O_2}) \times CO \times 10$	150–400 mL/min
Oxygen delivery index ($D_{O_2}I$)	D_{O_2}/BSA	520–720 (mL/min)/m²
Oxygen uptake index ($V_{O_2}I$)	V_{O_2}/BSA	115–165 (mL/min)/m²
Oxygen extraction ratio (O_2ER)	$[1 - (\dot{V}_{O_2}/\dot{D}_{O_2})] \times 100$	22–32%

Note: P_{O_2}, partial pressure of oxygen; Sa_{O_2}, saturation of hemoglobin with O_2 in arterial blood; Pa_{O_2}, partial pressure of O_2 in arterial blood; Sv_{O_2}, saturation of hemoglobin with O_2 in venous blood; Pv_{O_2}, partial pressure of O_2 in venous blood; CO, cardiac output; BSA, body surface area.

TABLE 253-4 *Physiologic Characteristics of the Various Forms of Shock*

Type of Shock	CVP and PCWP	Cardiac Output	Systemic Vascular Resistance	Venous O_2 Saturation
Hypovolemic	↓	↓	↑	↓
Cardiogenic	↑	↓	↑	↓
Septic				
Hyperdynamic	↓↑	↑	↓	↑↓
Hypodynamic	↓↑	↓	↓	↑↓
Traumatic	↓	↓↑	↑↓	↓
Neurogenic	↓	↓	↓	↓
Hypoadrenal	↓↑	↓	=↓	↓

Note: CVP, central venous pressure; PCWP, pulmonary capillary wedge pressure.

from extravascular fluid sequestration or gastrointestinal, urinary, and insensible losses. The signs and symptoms of nonhemorrhagic hypovolemic shock are the same as those of hemorrhagic shock, although they may have a more insidious onset. The normal physiologic response to hypovolemia is to maintain perfusion of the brain and heart while restoring an effective circulating blood volume. There is an increase in sympathetic activity, hyperventilation, collapse of venous capacitance vessels, release of stress hormones, and expansion of intravascular volume through the recruitment of interstitial and intracellular fluid and reduction of urine output.

Mild hypovolemia (≤20% of the blood volume) generates mild tachycardia but relatively few external signs, especially in a supine resting young patient (Table 253-5). With moderate hypovolemia (~20 to 40% of the blood volume) the patient becomes increasingly anxious and tachycardic; although normal blood pressure may be maintained in the supine position, there may be significant postural hypotension and tachycardia. If hypovolemia is severe (≥~40% of the blood volume), the classic signs of shock appear; the blood pressure declines and becomes unstable even in the supine position, and the patient develops marked tachycardia, oliguria, and agitation or confusion. Perfusion of the central nervous system is well maintained until shock becomes severe. Hence, mental obtundation is an ominous clinical sign. The transition from mild to severe hypovolemic shock can be insidious or extremely rapid. If severe shock is not reversed rapidly, especially in elderly patients and those with comorbid illnesses, death is imminent. A very narrow time frame separates the derangements found in severe shock that can be reversed with aggressive resuscitation from those of progressive decompensation and irreversible cell injury.

Diagnosis Hypovolemic shock is readily diagnosed when there are signs of hemodynamic instability and the source of volume loss is obvious. The diagnosis is more difficult when the source of blood loss is occult, as into the gastrointestinal tract, or when plasma volume alone is depleted. After acute hemorrhage, hemoglobin and hematocrit values do not change until compensatory fluid shifts have occurred or exogenous fluid is administered. Thus, an initial normal hematocrit does not disprove

the presence of significant blood loss. Plasma losses cause hemoconcentration, and free water loss leads to hypernatremia. These findings should suggest the presence of hypovolemia.

It is essential to distinguish between hypovolemic and cardiogenic shock (see below) because definitive therapy differs significantly. Both forms are associated with a reduced cardiac output and a compensatory sympathetic mediated response characterized by tachycardia and elevated systemic vascular resistance. However, the findings in cardiogenic shock of jugular venous distention, rales, and an S_3 gallop distinguish it from hypovolemic shock and signify that ongoing volume expansion is undesirable.

℞ TREATMENT

Initial resuscitation requires rapid reexpansion of the circulating blood volume along with interventions to control ongoing losses. In accordance with Starling's law (Chap. 215), stroke volume and cardiac output rise with the increase in preload. After resuscitation, the compliance of the ventricles may remain reduced due to increased interstitial fluid in the myocardium. Therefore, elevated filling pressures are required to maintain adequate ventricular performance.

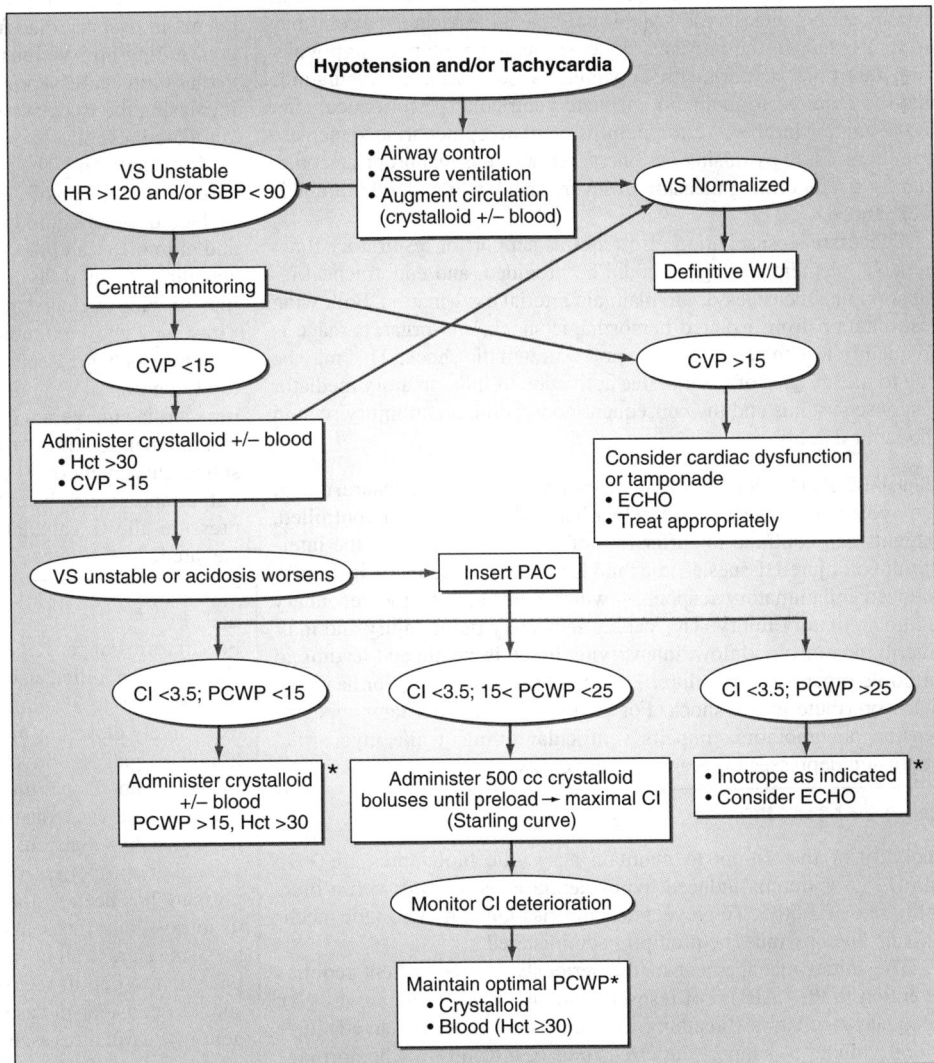

FIGURE 253-1   An algorithm for the resuscitation of the patient in shock. VS, vital signs; HR, heart rate; SBP, systolic blood pressure; W/U, work up; CVP, central venous pressure; Hct, hematocrit; ECHO, echocardiogram; PAC, pulmonary artery catheter; CI, cardiac index in (L/min)/m²; PCWP, pulmonary capillary wedge pressure in mmHg.
   *Monitor SV$_{O_2}$, SVRI, and RVEDVI as additional markers of correction for perfusion and hypovolemia. Consider age-adjusted CI. SV$_{O_2}$, saturation of hemoglobin with O_2 in venous blood; SVRI, systemic vascular resistance index; RVEDVI, right-ventricular end-diastolic volume index.

TABLE 253-5 *Hypovolemic Shock*

Mild (<20% Blood Volume)	Moderate (20–40% Blood Volume)	Severe (>40% Blood Volume)
Cool extremities Increased capillary refill time Diaphoresis Collapsed veins Anxiety	Same, plus: Tachycardia Tachypnea Oliguria Postural changes	Same, plus: Hemodynamic instability Marked tachycardia Hypotension Mental status deterioration (coma)

Volume resuscitation is initiated with the rapid infusion of isotonic saline (although care must be taken to avoid hyperchloremic acidosis) or a balanced salt solution such as Ringer's lactate through large-bore intravenous lines. No distinct benefit from the use of colloid has been demonstrated and, in trauma patients, it is associated with a higher mortality. The infusion of 2 to 3 L over 20 to 30 min should restore normal hemodynamic parameters. Continued hemodynamic instability implies that shock has not been reversed and/or that there are significant ongoing blood or volume losses. Continuing blood loss, with hemoglobin concentrations declining to ≤100 g/L (10 g/dL), should initiate blood transfusion, preferably as fully cross-matched blood. In extreme emergencies, type-specific or O-negative packed red cells may be transfused. In the presence of severe and/or prolonged hypovolemia, inotropic support with dopamine, vasopressin, or dobutamine may be required to maintain adequate ventricular performance, after blood volume has been restored. Infusion of norepinephrine to increase arterial pressure by raising peripheral resistance is inappropriate, other than as a temporizing measure in severe shock while blood volume is reexpanded.

Successful resuscitation also requires support of respiratory function. Supplemental oxygen should be provided, and endotracheal intubation may be necessary to maintain arterial oxygenation. Following resuscitation from isolated hemorrhagic shock, end-organ damage is frequently less than following septic or traumatic shock. This may be due to the absence of the massive activation of inflammatory mediator response systems and the consequent nonspecific organ injury seen in the latter conditions.

TRAUMATIC SHOCK   Shock following trauma is, in large measure, due to hypovolemia. However, even when hemorrhage has been controlled, patients can continue to suffer loss of plasma volume into the interstitium of injured tissues. These fluid losses are compounded by injury-induced inflammatory responses, which contribute to the secondary microcirculatory injury. This causes secondary tissue injury and maldistribution of blood flow, intensifying tissue ischemia and leading to multiple organ system failure. Trauma to the heart, chest, or head can also contribute to the shock. For example, pericardial tamponade or tension pneumothorax impairs ventricular filling, while myocardial contusion depresses myocardial contractility.

℞ TREATMENT

Inability of the patient to maintain a systolic blood pressure ≥90 mmHg after trauma-induced hypovolemia is associated with a mortality rate of ~50%. To prevent decompensation of homeostatic mechanisms, therapy must be promptly administered.

The initial management of the seriously injured patient requires attention to the "ABCs" of resuscitation: assurance of an airway (A), adequate ventilation (breathing, B), and establishment of an adequate blood volume to support the circulation (C). Control of hemorrhage requires immediate attention. Early stabilization of fractures, debridement of devitalized or contaminated tissues, and evacuation of hematomata all reduce the subsequent inflammatory response to the initial insult and minimize subsequent organ injury. Supplementation of depleted endogenous antioxidants also reduces subsequent organ failure and mortality.

INTRINSIC CARDIOGENIC SHOCK   This form of shock is caused by failure, often sudden, of the heart as an effective pump. It occurs most commonly as a complication of acute myocardial infarction (AMI; Chaps. 228 and 255), but it may also be seen in patients with severe brady- or tachyarrhythmias, valvular heart disease, significant cardiac contusion, or in the terminal stage of chronic heart failure of any cause, including ischemic heart disease and dilated cardiomyopathy. Cardiogenic shock is characterized by a low cardiac output, diminished peripheral perfusion, pulmonary congestion, and elevation of systemic vascular resistance and pulmonary vascular pressures. Acute right heart failure can arise as the result of right ventricular infarction or may complicate ARDS and severe pulmonary hypertension of any etiology. As a consequence of right ventricular failure, left ventricular preload falls, and this, in turn, reduces systemic perfusion. In contrast to other forms of shock, absolute or relative hypovolemia is usually not present in cardiogenic shock.

The ineffective contractile activity of either the right or left side of the heart leads to the accumulation of blood in the venous circulation upstream to the failing ventricle. Cardiogenic shock with left-sided heart failure increases fluid in the lungs that can overwhelm the capacity of the pulmonary lymphatics and causes interstitial and eventually alveolar edema. Interstitial lung edema usually occurs at pulmonary capillary pressures >18 mmHg, and overt pulmonary alveolar edema develops at pressures >24 mmHg (Chap. 29). Pulmonary edema impacts cardiac function further by impairing diffusion of oxygen, setting up a vicious cycle. The increase in interstitial and intraalveolar fluid causes a progressive reduction in lung compliance, thereby increasing the work of ventilation while increasing perfusion of poorly ventilated alveoli.

In establishing the diagnosis of cardiogenic shock, a history of cardiac disease or of AMI is of value. Associated physical findings include those of hemodynamic instability, peripheral vasoconstriction, and pulmonary and/or systemic venous congestion, as well as findings specific to the underlying cardiac abnormalities. An electrocardiogram may provide evidence of AMI or preexisting cardiac disease. The chest x-ray may show pulmonary edema and cardiomegaly. Transthoracic or transesophageal echocardiograms assist in the diagnosis of structural abnormalities and/or functional impairment of contractility. Serum cardiac markers will support the diagnosis of acute cardiac injury. Hemodynamic monitoring is usually necessary in the presence of shock. Placement of a PAC is helpful and will show a reduced cardiac output and an elevated PCWP, and direct measurement of right atrial pressure allows calculation of systemic vascular resistance which is elevated.

℞ TREATMENT

For all forms of cardiogenic shock, preload, afterload, and contractility should be modified using the information provided by the PAC. A PCWP of 15 to 20 mmHg should be the initial goal. If the PCWP is excessively elevated, inotropic agents may provide significant reduction. The goal is to increase contractility without significant increases in heart rate. Dopamine, norepinephrine, or vasopressin exert both inotropic and vasoconstrictor actions that are useful in the presence of persistent hypotension. Dobutamine, a positive inotropic agent with vasodilator properties, or vasodilators may be substituted when arterial pressure has been restored. Pulmonary congestion may be responsive to intravenous furosemide. Patients with an inadequate response to these measures can be supported by using intraaortic balloon counterpulsation to permit recovery of myocardial function. Additional measures to consider in cases of refractory cardiogenic shock include urgent myocardial revascularization in patients with AMI, correction of anatomic cardiac defects such as rupture of the papillary muscles of the interventricular septum, the placement of ventricular assist devices, and even urgent cardiac transplantation.

COMPRESSIVE CARDIOGENIC SHOCK   With compression, the heart and surrounding structures are less compliant and, thus, normal filling pressures generate inadequate diastolic filling. Blood or fluid within the poorly distensible pericardial sac may cause tamponade (Chap. 222). Any cause of increased intrathoracic pressure, such as tension pneumothorax, herniation of abdominal viscera through a diaphragmatic hernia, or excessive positive pressure ventilation to support pulmonary function, can also cause compressive cardiogenic shock while simultaneously impeding venous return. Acute right heart failure with a sudden decline in cardiac output can be caused by pulmonary embolism obstructing right ventricular outflow and impairing left ventricular filling. Although initially responsive to increased filling pressures produced by volume expansion, as compression increases, cardiogenic shock recurs.

The diagnosis of compressive cardiogenic shock is most frequently based on clinical findings, the chest radiograph, and an echocardiogram. The diagnosis of compressive cardiac shock may be more difficult to establish in the setting of trauma when hypovolemia and cardiac compression are present simultaneously. The classic findings of pericardial tamponade include the triad of hypotension, neck vein distention, and muffled heart sounds (Chap. 222). Pulsus paradoxus, i.e., an inspiratory reduction in systolic pressure >10 mmHg, may also be noted. The diagnosis is confirmed by echocardiography, and treatment consists of immediate pericardiocentesis. A tension pneumothorax produces ipsilateral decreased breath sounds, tracheal deviation away from the affected thorax, and jugular venous distention. Radiographic findings include increased intrathoracic volume, depression of the diaphragm of the affected hemithorax, and shifting of the mediastinum to the contralateral side. Chest decompression must be carried out immediately. Release of air and restoration of normal cardiovascular dynamics are both diagnostic and therapeutic.

SEPTIC SHOCK (See also Chap. 254) This form of shock is caused by the systemic response to a severe infection. It occurs most frequently in elderly or immunocompromised patients and in those who have undergone an invasive procedure in which bacterial contamination has occurred. Infections of the lung, abdomen, or urinary tract are most common, and approximately half of the patients have bacteremia. Gram-positive and -negative bacteria, viruses, fungi, rickettsiae, and protozoa have all been reported to produce the clinical picture of septic shock, and the overall response is generally independent of the specific type of invading organism. The clinical findings in septic shock are a consequence of the combination of metabolic and circulatory derangements driven by the systemic infection and the release of toxic components of the infectious organisms, e.g., the endotoxin of gram-negative bacteria or the exotoxins and enterotoxins of gram-positive bacteria. Organism toxins lead to the release of cytokines, including IL-1 and TNF-α, from tissue macrophages. Tissue factor expression and fibrin deposition are increased, and disseminated intravascular coagulation may develop. The inducible form of NO synthase is stimulated, and NO, a powerful vasodilator, is released. Hemodynamic changes in septic shock occur in two characteristic patterns: early, or hyperdynamic, and late, or hypodynamic, septic shock.

Hyperdynamic Response In hyperdynamic septic shock, tachycardia is present, the cardiac output is normal or elevated, and the systemic vascular resistance is reduced while the pulmonary vascular resistance is elevated. The extremities are usually warm. However, splanchnic vasoconstriction with decreased visceral flow is present. The venous capacitance is increased, which decreases venous return. With volume expansion cardiac output becomes supranormal. Myocardial contractility is depressed in septic shock by mediators including NO, IL-1, and/or TNF-α. Inflammatory mediator–induced processes include increased capillary permeability and continued loss of intravascular volume.

In septic shock, in contrast to other types of shock, total oxygen delivery may be increased while oxygen extraction is reduced due to maldistribution of microcirculatory perfusion and impaired mitochondrial utilization. In this setting the presence of a normal mixed venous oxygen saturation is not indicative of adequate peripheral perfusion, and even though the cardiac output may be elevated, it is still inadequate to meet the total metabolic needs. The toxicity of the infectious agents and their byproducts and the subsequent metabolic dysfunction drive the progressive deterioration of cellular and organ function. ARDS, thrombocytopenia, and neutropenia are common complications.

Hypodynamic Response As sepsis progresses, vasoconstriction occurs and the cardiac output declines. The patient usually becomes markedly tachypneic, febrile, diaphoretic, and obtunded, with cool, mottled, and often cyanotic extremities. Oliguria, renal failure, and hypothermia develop; there may be striking increases in serum lactate.

 TREATMENT

Aggressive volume expansion with a crystalloid solution to a PCWP of ~15 mmHg and the restoration of arterial oxygenation with inspired oxygen and frequently with mechanical ventilation are the highest priorities. In the presence of sepsis, augmentation of cardiac output may require inotropic support with dopamine, norepinephrine, or vasopressin in the presence of hypotension or with dobutamine if arterial pressure is normal. High-dose, *a*ctivated *p*rotein *C* (APC) provides a survival benefit in patients with severe sepsis and septic shock. Antibiotics should be administered, either appropriate for the results of cultures or empirical therapy based on the likely source of infection. Surgical debridement or drainage may also be necessary to control the infection.

NEUROGENIC SHOCK Interruption of sympathetic vasomotor input after a high cervical spinal cord injury, inadvertent cephalad migration of spinal anesthesia, or severe head injury may result in neurogenic shock. In addition to arteriolar dilatation, venodilation causes pooling in the venous system, which decreases venous return and cardiac output. The extremities are often warm, in contrast to the usual vasoconstriction-induced coolness in hypovolemic or cardiogenic shock. Treatment involves a simultaneous approach to the relative hypovolemia and to the loss of vasomotor tone. Excessive volumes of fluid may be required to restore normal hemodynamics. Once hemorrhage has been ruled out, norepinephrine may be necessary to augment vascular resistance.

HYPOADRENAL SHOCK (See also Chap. 321) The normal host response to the stress of illness, operation, or trauma requires that the adrenal glands hypersecrete cortisol in excess of that normally required. Hypoadrenal shock occurs in settings in which unrecognized adrenal insufficiency complicates the host response to the stress induced by acute illness or major surgery. Adrenocortical insufficiency may occur as a consequence of the chronic administration of high doses of exogenous glucocorticoids. Recent studies have shown that critical illness, including trauma and sepsis, may also induce a relative hypoadrenal state. Other, less common causes include adrenal insufficiency secondary to idiopathic atrophy, tuberculosis, metastatic disease, bilateral hemorrhage, and amyloidosis. The shock produced by adrenal insufficiency is characterized by reductions in systemic vascular resistance, hypovolemia, and reduced cardiac output. The diagnosis of adrenal insufficiency may be established by means of an ACTH stimulation test.

 TREATMENT

In the hemodynamically unstable patient, dexamethasone sodium phosphate, 4 mg, should be given intravenously. This agent is preferred because unlike hydrocortisone it does not interfere with the ACTH stimulation test. If the diagnosis of absolute or relative adrenal insufficiency has been established as shown by non-response to corticotropin stimulation, the patient has a reduced risk of death if treated with hydrocortisone, 100 mg every 6 to 8 h, and tapered as the patient achieves hemodynamic stability. Simultaneous volume resuscitation and pressor support are required.

ADJUNCTIVE THERAPIES

As described above, the sympathomimetic amines dobutamine, dopamine, and norepinephrine are widely used in the treatment of all forms of shock. Arginine-vasopressin (antidiuretic hormone) is also being used increasingly and may better protect vital organ blood flow and prevent pathologic vasodilation.

POSITIONING   Positioning of the patient may be a valuable adjunct in the initial treatment of hypovolemic shock. Elevating the foot of the bed (i.e., placing it on "shock blocks") and assumption of the Trendelenburg position without flexion at the knees are effective but may increase work of breathing and risk for aspiration. Simply elevating both legs may be the optimal approach.

PNEUMATIC ANTISHOCK GARMENT (PASG)   The PASG and the military antishock trousers (MAST) are inflatable external compression devices that can be wrapped around the legs and abdomen and have been widely used in the prehospital setting as a means of providing temporary support of central hemodynamics in shock. They cause an increase in systemic vascular resistance and blood pressure by arterial compression, without causing a significant change in cardiac output. The most appropriate use appears to be as a means to tamponade bleeding and augment hemostasis. Inflation of the suit provides splinting of fractures of the pelvis and lower extremities and arrests hemorrhage.

REWARMING   Hypothermia is a potential adverse consequence of massive volume resuscitation. The infusion of large volumes of refrigerated blood products and room-temperature crystalloid solutions can rapidly drop core temperatures if fluid is not run through warming devices. Hypothermia may depress cardiac contractility and thereby further impair cardiac output and oxygen delivery. Hypothermia, particularly temperatures $<35°$ C, directly impairs the coagulation pathway, sometimes causing a significant coagulopathy. Rapid rewarming to $>35°$ C significantly decreases the requirement for blood products and produces an improvement in cardiac function. The most effective method for rewarming is extracorporeal countercurrent warmers through femoral artery and vein cannulation. This process does not require a pump and can rewarm from 30° to 35°C in <30 min.

FURTHER READING

ANNANE D et al: Effect of treatment with low doses of hydrocortisone and fludrocortisone on mortality in patients with septic shock. JAMA 288:862, 2002

BERNARD GR et al: Pulmonary artery catheterization and clinical outcomes: National Heart, Lung, and Blood Institute and Food and Drug Administration Workshop Report Consensus Statement. JAMA 283:2568, 2000

CHEN P: Vasopressin: New uses in critical care. Am J Med Sci 324:146, 2002

CHOI PT et al: Crystalloids vs. colloids in fluid resuscitation: A systematic review. Crit Care Med 27:200, 1999

MCGEE S et al: The rational clinical examination. Is this patient hypovolemic? JAMA 281:1022, 1999

RIVERS E et al: Early goal-directed therapy in the treatment of severe sepsis and septic shock. N Engl J Med 345:1368, 2001

254   SEVERE SEPSIS AND SEPTIC SHOCK
Robert S. Munford

DEFINITIONS (See Table 254-1)   Animals mount both local and systemic responses to microbes that traverse epithelial barriers and invade underlying tissues. Fever or hypothermia, leukocytosis or leukopenia, tachypnea, and tachycardia are the cardinal signs of the systemic response often called the *systemic inflammatory response syndrome* (SIRS). SIRS may have an infectious or a noninfectious etiology. If infection is suspected or proven, a patient with SIRS is said to have *sepsis*. When sepsis is associated with dysfunction of organs distant from the site of infection, the patient has *severe sepsis*. Severe sepsis may be accompanied by hypotension or evidence of hypoperfusion. When hypotension cannot be corrected by infusing fluids, the diagnosis is *septic shock*. These definitions were proposed by a consensus conference committee in 1992 and are now widely used; there is evidence that the different stages form a continuum. As sepsis progresses to septic shock, the risk of dying increases substantially. Sepsis is usually reversible, whereas patients with septic shock often succumb despite aggressive therapy.

ETIOLOGY   Severe sepsis can be a response to any class of microorganism. Microbial invasion of the bloodstream is not essential for the development of severe sepsis, since local inflammation can also elicit distant organ dysfunction and hypotension. In fact, blood cultures yield bacteria or fungi in only ~20 to 40% of cases of severe sepsis and 40 to 70% of cases of septic shock. Individual gram-negative or gram-positive bacteria account for ~70% of these isolates; the remainder are fungi or a mixture of microorganisms (Table 254-2). In patients whose blood cultures are negative, the etiologic agent is often established by culture or microscopic examination of infected material from a local site. In some case series, a majority of patients with a clinical picture of severe sepsis or septic shock have had negative microbiologic data. Factors that predispose to infections with positive blood cultures are listed in (Table 254-3). Among patients who have positive blood cultures, the risk of developing severe sepsis is greater in persons >50 years old and in those with a primary pulmonary, abdominal, or neuromeningeal site of infection.

EPIDEMIOLOGY   The septic response is a contributing factor in $>200,000$ deaths per year in the United States. The incidence of severe sepsis and septic shock has increased over the past 20 years, and the annual number of cases is now $>300,000$. Approximately two-thirds of cases occur in patients hospitalized for other illnesses. The increasing incidence of severe sepsis in the United States is attributable to the aging of the population, the increasing longevity of patients with chronic diseases, and the relatively high frequency with which sepsis develops in patients with AIDS. The widespread use of antimicrobial agents, glucocorticoids, indwelling catheters and mechanical devices, and mechanical ventilation also plays a role.

PATHOPHYSIOLOGY   Most cases of severe sepsis are triggered by bacteria or fungi that do not ordinarily cause systemic disease in immunocompetent hosts (Table 254-2). These microbes probably exploit deficiencies in innate host defenses (e.g., phagocytes, complement, and natural antibodies) to survive within the body. Microbial pathogens, in contrast, are able to circumvent innate defenses by elaborating toxins or other virulence factors. In both cases, the body can fail to kill the invaders despite mounting a vigorous inflammatory reaction that can progress to severe sepsis. The septic response may also be induced by microbial exotoxins that act as superantigens (e.g., toxic shock syndrome toxin 1; Chap. 120).

Host Mechanisms for Sensing Microbes   Animals have exquisitely sensitive mechanisms for recognizing and responding to conserved microbial molecules. The lipid A moiety of lipopolysaccharide (LPS, also called *endotoxin*; Chap. 105) is the best-studied example. Lipid A is the bioactive center of the LPS of all gram-negative bacteria found in nature. A host protein (LPS-binding protein, or LBP) binds lipid A and transfers LPS to CD14 on the surfaces of monocytes, macrophages, and neutrophils. LPS and CD14 then interact with toll-like receptor (TLR) 4 and MD-2 to form a molecular complex that transduces the LPS signal to the interior of the cell. This signal rapidly triggers the production and release of mediators, such as tumor necrosis factor (TNF) α (see below), that amplify the LPS signal and transmit it to other cells and tissues. Bacterial peptidoglycan, lipoteichoic acids, DNA, certain polysaccharides, and fimbriae elicit responses in animals that are similar to those induced by LPS; whereas some of

TABLE 254-1 *Definitions Used to Describe the Condition of Septic Patients*

Bacteremia	Presence of bacteria in blood, as evidenced by positive blood cultures
Septicemia	Presence of microbes or their toxins in blood
Systemic inflammatory response syndrome (SIRS)	Two or more of the following conditions: (1) fever (oral temperature >38°C) or hypothermia (<36°C); (2) tachypnea (>24 breaths/min); (3) tachycardia (heart rate > 90 beats/min); (4) leukocytosis (>12,000/μL), leukopenia (<4,000/μL), or >10% bands; may have a noninfectious etiology
Sepsis	SIRS that has a proven or suspected microbial etiology
Severe sepsis (similar to "sepsis syndrome")	Sepsis with one or more signs of organ dysfunction—for example: 1. *Cardiovascular:* Arterial systolic blood pressure ≤90 mmHg or mean arterial pressure ≤ 70 mmHg that responds to administration of intravenous fluid 2. *Renal:* Urine output < 0.5 mL/kg per hour for 1 h despite adequate fluid resuscitation 3. *Respiratory:* Pa_{O_2}/FI_{O_2} ≤ 250 or, if the lung is the only dysfunctional organ, ≤200 4. *Hematologic:* Platelet count < 80,000/μL or 50% decrease in platelet count from highest value recorded over previous 3 days 5. *Unexplained metabolic acidosis:* A pH ≤ 7.30 or a base deficit ≥ 5.0 mEq/L and a plasma lactate level > 1.5 times upper limit of normal for reporting lab 6. *Adequate fluid resuscitation:* Pulmonary artery wedge pressure ≥ 12 mmHg or central venous pressure ≥ 8 mmHg
Septic shock	Sepsis with hypotension (arterial blood pressure <90 mmHg systolic, or 40 mmHg less than patient's normal blood pressure) for at least 1 h despite adequate fluid resuscitation; *or* Need for vasopressors to maintain systolic blood pressure ≥ 90 mmHg *or* mean arterial pressure ≥ 70 mmHg
Refractory septic shock	Septic shock that lasts for >1 h and does not respond to fluid or pressor administration
Multiple-organ dysfunction syndrome (MODS)	Dysfunction of more than one organ, requiring intervention to maintain homeostasis

Source: Adapted from the American College of Chest Physicians/Society of Critical Care Medicine Consensus Conference Committee and Bernard et al.

these molecules also bind CD14, they interact with several different TLRs. CD14 thus attracts numerous non-self molecules to the surfaces of cells, greatly increasing the sensitivity with which these molecules can be recognized by the host. Having numerous TLR-based receptor complexes (10 different TLRs have been identified so far) allows cells to recognize many conserved microbial molecules. The ability of some

TABLE 254-2 *Microorganisms Involved in Episodes of Severe Sepsis at Eight Academic Medical Centers*

Microorganisms	Episodes with Blood-stream Infection, % (n = 436)	Episodes with Documented Infection but No Bloodstream Infection, % (n = 430)	Total Episodes, % (n = 866)
Gram-negative bacteria[a]	35	44	40
Gram-positive bacteria[b]	40	24	31
Fungi	7	5	6
Polymicrobial	11	21	16
Classic pathogens[c]	<5	<5	<5

[a] Enterobacteriaceae, pseudomonads, *Haemophilus* spp., other gram-negative bacteria.
[b] *Staphylococcus aureus*, coagulase-negative staphylococci, enterococci, *Streptococcus pneumoniae*, other streptococci, other gram-positive bacteria.
[c] Such as *Neisseria meningitidis*, *S. pneumoniae*, *H. influenzae*, and *Streptococcus pyogenes*.
Source: Adapted from Sands et al.

TABLE 254-3 *Conditions That May Predispose to Infections with Positive Blood Cultures*

Microbial Isolate	Condition
Gram-negative bacilli	Diabetes mellitus Lymphoproliferative diseases Cirrhosis of the liver Burns Invasive procedures or devices Neutropenia Indwelling urinary catheter Diverticulitis, perforated viscus
Gram-positive bacteria	Intravascular catheters Indwelling mechanical devices Burns Neutropenia Intravenous drug use Infection with superantigen-producing *Streptococcus pyogenes*
Fungi	Neutropenia Broad-spectrum antimicrobial therapy

of the TLRs to serve as receptors for host ligands (e.g., hyaluronans) raises the possibility that they play a role in producing noninfectious sepsis-like states. Other molecular pattern-recognition proteins that are important for sensing microbial invasion include complement (principally the alternative pathway), mannose-binding lectin, bactericidal permeability-increasing protein, and C-reactive protein.

Local and Systemic Host Responses to Invading Microbes Recognition of microbial molecules by tissue phagocytes triggers the production and/or release of numerous host molecules (cytokines, chemokines, prostanoids, leukotrienes, and others) that increase blood flow to the infected tissue, enhance the permeability of local blood vessels, recruit neutrophils to the site of infection, and elicit pain. These phenomena are familiar elements of local inflammation, the body's major innate immune mechanism for eliminating microbial invaders. Systemic responses may be activated by neural and/or humoral communication with the hypothalamus and brainstem; these responses may enhance local defenses by increasing blood flow to the infected area, augmenting the number of circulating neutrophils, and elevating blood levels of numerous molecules (such as the microbial recognition proteins discussed above) that have anti-infective functions.

CYTOKINES AND OTHER MEDIATORS Cytokines can exert endocrine, paracrine, and autocrine effects (Chap. 295). TNF-α stimulates leukocytes and vascular endothelial cells to release other cytokines (as well as additional TNF-α), to express cell-surface molecules that enhance neutrophil-endothelial adhesion at sites of infection, and to increase prostaglandin and leukotriene production. Animals that are unable to produce or respond to TNF-α are abnormally susceptible to infection. Whereas blood levels of TNF-α are not elevated in individuals with localized infections, they increase in most patients with severe sepsis or septic shock. Moreover, intravenous infusion of TNF-α can elicit many of the characteristic abnormalities of sepsis, including fever, tachycardia, tachypnea, leukocytosis, myalgias, and somnolence. In animals, larger doses of TNF-α induce shock, disseminated intravascular coagulation (DIC), and death.

Although TNF-α is a central mediator, it is only one of many proinflammatory molecules that contribute to innate host defense. Chemokines, most prominently interleukin (IL) 8, attract circulating neutrophils to the infection site. IL-1β exhibits many of the same activities as TNF-α. TNF-α, IL-1β, interferon γ, IL-12, and other cytokines probably interact synergistically with one another and with additional mediators. Recent evidence suggests that proinflammatory cytokines that circulate in blood often originate in an inflamed local site.

COAGULATION FACTORS Intravascular thrombosis, a hallmark of the local inflammatory response, may help wall off invading microbes and prevent infection and inflammation from spreading to other tissues. Intravascular fibrin deposition, thrombosis, and DIC can also be important features of the systemic response. IL-6 and other mediators promote intravascular coagulation initially by inducing blood monocytes and vascular endothelial cells to express tissue factor (Chap. 53). When tissue factor is expressed on cell surfaces, it binds to factor VIIa to form an active complex that can convert factors X and IX to enzymatically active forms. The result is activation of both extrinsic and intrinsic clotting pathways, culminating in the generation of fibrin. Clotting is also favored by impaired function of the protein C–protein S inhibitory pathway and depletion of antithrombin and protein C, while fibrinolysis is prevented by increased plasma levels of plasminogen activator inhibitor 1. Thus, there may be a striking propensity to intravascular fibrin deposition, thrombosis, and bleeding (Chap. 127). Contact-system activation occurs during sepsis but contributes more to the development of hypotension than to DIC.

CONTROL MECHANISMS   Elaborate control mechanisms operate within both local sites of inflammation and the systemic circulation. The available evidence suggests that the body's systemic responses to injury and infection normally prevent inflammation within organs distant from a site of infection.

The signaling apparatus that links microbial recognition to cellular responses is greatly diminished in the blood. Whereas LBP plays a role in recognizing the presence of LPS, for example, in plasma it also prevents LPS signaling by transferring LPS molecules into plasma lipoprotein particles, which sequester the lipid A moiety so that it cannot interact with cells. At concentrations found in blood, LBP also inhibits monocyte responses to LPS, and the soluble (circulating) form of CD14 strips off LPS that has bound to monocyte cell surfaces. The blood concentrations of both LBP and soluble CD14 increase during the response to infection, enhancing the body's ability to prevent activation of blood cells by LPS.

Systemic responses to infection also diminish cellular responses to microbial molecules. Circulating levels of anti-inflammatory cytokines (e.g., IL-6 and IL-10) increase even in patients with mild infections. Glucocorticoids inhibit cytokine synthesis by monocytes in vitro; the increase in blood cortisol levels early in the systemic response presumably plays a similar inhibitory role. Epinephrine inhibits the TNF-α response to endotoxin infusion in humans while augmenting and accelerating the release of IL-10; prostaglandin E_2 has a similar "reprogramming" effect on the responses of circulating monocytes to LPS and other bacterial agonists. Cortisol, epinephrine, IL-10, and C-reactive protein reduce the ability of neutrophils to attach to vascular endothelium, favoring their demargination and thus contributing to leukocytosis while preventing neutrophil-endothelial adhesion in uninflamed organs.

The acute-phase response increases the blood concentrations of numerous molecules that have anti-inflammatory actions. Blood levels of IL-1 receptor antagonist (IL-1Ra) often greatly exceed those of circulating IL-1β, for example, and this excess may result in inhibition of the binding of IL-1β to its receptors. High levels of soluble TNF receptors neutralize TNF-α that enters the circulation. Other acute-phase proteins are protease inhibitors; these may neutralize proteases released from neutrophils and other inflammatory cells.

Organ Dysfunction and Shock   As the body's responses to infection intensify, the mixture of circulating cytokines and other molecules becomes very complex: elevated blood levels of more than 50 molecules have been found in patients with septic shock. Although high concentrations of both pro- and anti-inflammatory molecules are found, the net mediator balance in the plasma of these extremely sick patients may actually be anti-inflammatory. In addition, blood leukocytes from patients with severe sepsis are often hyporesponsive to agonists such as LPS. In patients with severe sepsis, persistence of leukocyte hyporesponsiveness has been associated with an increased risk of dying. How the body's pro- and anti-inflammatory forces contribute to hy-

potension and the dysfunction of organs distant from a site of infection is not known.

ENDOTHELIAL INJURY   Most investigators have favored widespread vascular endothelial injury as the major mechanism for multiorgan dysfunction. In keeping with this idea, one study found high numbers of vascular endothelial cells in the peripheral blood of septic patients. Leukocyte-derived mediators and platelet-leukocyte-fibrin thrombi may contribute to vascular injury, but the vascular endothelium also seems to play an active role. Stimuli such as TNF-α induce vascular endothelial cells to produce and release cytokines, procoagulant molecules, platelet-activating factor (PAF), nitric oxide, and other mediators. In addition, regulated cell-adhesion molecules promote the adherence of neutrophils to endothelial cells. While these responses can attract phagocytes to infected sites and activate their antimicrobial arsenals, endothelial cell activation can also promote increased vascular permeability, microvascular thrombosis, DIC, and hypotension.

Tissue oxygenation may be diminished as the number of functional capillaries is reduced by luminal obstruction due to swollen endothelial cells, decreased deformability of circulating erythrocytes, leukocyte-platelet-fibrin thrombi, or compression by edema fluid. One study using orthogonal polarization spectral imaging of the microcirculation in the tongue found that sepsis-associated derangements in capillary flow could be reversed by applying acetylcholine to the surface of the tongue; this observation suggested a neuroendocrine basis for the loss of capillary filling. Cellular ATP and antioxidant stores may become depleted as the production of lactate increases. Programmed cell death may ensue.

SEPTIC SHOCK   The hallmark of septic shock is a decrease in peripheral vascular resistance that occurs despite increased levels of vasopressor catecholamines. Cardiac output increases, as does blood flow to peripheral tissues. Oxygen utilization by these tissues may be greatly impaired by maldistribution of blood flow as well as by microcirculatory dysfunction (see above).

Prominent hypotensive molecules include nitric oxide, β-endorphin, bradykinin, PAF, and prostacyclin. Agents that inhibit the synthesis or action of each of these mediators can prevent or reverse endotoxic shock in animals. However, in clinical trials, neither a PAF receptor antagonist nor a bradykinin antagonist improved the survival rate of patients with septic shock, and a nitric oxide synthetase inhibitor, L-N^G-methylarginine HCl, actually increased the mortality rate.

Patients with septic shock often show diminished vasoconstrictor responses to catecholamines. This loss of sensitivity has been attributed to downregulation of adrenergic receptors and to elevated levels of nitric oxide. In patients with septic shock, plasma vasopressin levels do not increase to augment vasoconstriction; in several small series of patients with septic shock, infusion of vasopressin has increased blood pressure and reduced the requirement for catecholamine infusion. Administering hydrocortisone may also improve vascular sensitivity to catecholamines in many patients with septic shock.

Severe Sepsis: A Single Pathogenesis?   In some cases, circulating bacteria and their products almost certainly elicit multiorgan dysfunction and hypotension by directly stimulating inflammatory responses within the vasculature. In patients with fulminant meningococcemia, for example, mortality has correlated well with blood endotoxin levels and with the occurrence of DIC (Chap. 127). In most patients with nosocomial infections, in contrast, circulating bacteria or bacterial molecules may reflect uncontrolled infection at a local tissue site and have little or no direct impact on distant organs; in these patients, inflammatory mediators arising from the local site seem to be the key triggers for severe sepsis and septic shock. Support for this concept comes from a study in which *Pseudomonas aeruginosa* bacteremia was induced in rabbits either by constant intravenous infusion of bacteria or by intratracheal inoculation to produce pneumonia. Only the animals with pneumonia developed septic shock. Hypotension occurred only when TNF could move from the lungs into the blood. Shock could be prevented by use of a *P. aeruginosa* strain that did not disrupt alveolar epithelial permeability or by administration of an anti-TNF antibody prior to the onset of pneumonia. Clinical observations also suggest that uncontrolled local inflammation may drive the septic reaction. In a large series of patients with positive blood cultures, the risk of developing severe sepsis was strongly related to the site of primary infection: bacteremia arising from a pulmonary or abdominal source was eightfold more likely to be associated with severe sepsis than was bacteremic urinary tract infection, even after controlling for age, the kind of bacteria isolated from the blood, and other factors. A third pathogenesis may be represented by severe sepsis due to superantigen-producing *Staphylococcus aureus* or *Streptococcus pyogenes*, since the T cell activation induced by these toxins produces a cytokine profile that differs substantially from that elicited by gram-negative bacterial infection.

In summary, the pathogenesis of severe sepsis may differ according to the infecting microbe, the site of the primary infection, the presence or absence of immune defects, and the prior physiologic status of the host. Genetic factors may also be important. In patients who have sustained major trauma, for example, studies in different ethnic groups have identified associations between allelic polymorphisms in TNF-α and interferon-γ genes and risk of developing severe sepsis. Further studies in this area are needed.

CLINICAL MANIFESTATIONS

The manifestations of the septic response are usually superimposed on the symptoms and signs of the patient's underlying illness and primary infection. The rate at which signs and symptoms develop may differ from patient to patient, and there are striking individual variations in presentation. For example, some patients with sepsis are normo- or hypothermic; the absence of fever is most common in neonates, in elderly patients, and in persons with uremia or alcoholism.

Hyperventilation is often an early sign. Disorientation, confusion, and other manifestations of encephalopathy may also develop early in the septic response, particularly in the elderly and in individuals with preexisting neurologic impairment. Focal neurologic signs are uncommon, although preexisting focal deficits may become more prominent.

Hypotension and DIC predispose to acrocyanosis and ischemic necrosis of peripheral tissues, most commonly the digits. Cellulitis, pustules, bullae, or hemorrhagic lesions may develop when hematogenous bacteria or fungi seed the skin or underlying soft tissue. Bacterial toxins may also be distributed hematogenously and elicit diffuse cutaneous reactions. On occasion, skin lesions may suggest specific pathogens. When sepsis is accompanied by cutaneous petechiae or purpura, infection with *Neisseria meningitidis* (or, less commonly, *Haemophilus influenzae*) should be suspected (Fig. 127-1); in a patient who has been bitten by a tick while in an endemic area, petechial lesions also suggest Rocky Mountain spotted fever (Fig. 158-1). A cutaneous lesion seen almost exclusively in neutropenic patients is ecthyma gangrenosum, usually caused by *P. aeruginosa*. It is a bullous lesion, surrounded by edema, that undergoes central hemorrhage and necrosis (see Fig. 136-1). Histopathologic examination shows bacteria in and around the wall of a small vessel, with little or no neutrophilic response. Hemorrhagic or bullous lesions in a septic patient who has recently eaten raw oysters suggest *Vibrio vulnificus* bacteremia, while such lesions in a patient who has recently suffered a dog bite may indicate bloodstream infection due to *Capnocytophaga canimorsus* or *C. cynodegmi*. Generalized erythroderma in a septic patient suggests the toxic shock syndrome due to *S. aureus* or *S. pyogenes*.

Gastrointestinal manifestations such as nausea, vomiting, diarrhea, and ileus may suggest acute gastroenteritis. Stress ulceration can lead to upper gastrointestinal bleeding. Cholestatic jaundice, with elevated levels of serum bilirubin (mostly conjugated) and alkaline phosphatase, may precede other signs of sepsis. Hepatocellular or canalicular dysfunction appears to underlie most cases, and the results of hepatic function tests return to normal with resolution of the infection. Prolonged or severe hypotension may induce acute hepatic injury or ischemic bowel necrosis.

Many tissues may be unable to extract oxygen normally from the blood, so that anaerobic metabolism occurs despite near-normal mixed

venous oxygen saturation. Blood lactate levels rise early, in part because of increased glycolysis with impaired clearance of the resulting lactate and pyruvate by the liver and kidneys. As hypoperfusion develops, tissue hypoxia generates more lactic acid, contributing to metabolic acidosis. The blood glucose concentration often increases, particularly in patients with diabetes, although impaired gluconeogenesis and excessive insulin release on occasion produce hypoglycemia. The cytokine-driven acute-phase response inhibits the synthesis of transthyretin while enhancing the production of C-reactive protein, fibrinogen, and complement components. Protein catabolism is often markedly accelerated.

MAJOR COMPLICATIONS ■ Cardiopulmonary Complications
Ventilation-perfusion mismatching produces a fall in arterial P_{O_2} early in the course. Increasing alveolar capillary permeability results in an increased pulmonary water content, which decreases pulmonary compliance and interferes with oxygen exchange. Progressive diffuse pulmonary infiltrates and arterial hypoxemia (Pa_{O_2}/FI_{O_2}, < 200) indicate the development of the acute respiratory distress syndrome (ARDS). ARDS develops in ~50% of patients with severe sepsis or septic shock. The failure of the respiratory muscles can exacerbate hypoxemia and hypercapnia. An elevated pulmonary capillary wedge pressure (>18 mmHg) suggests fluid volume overload or cardiac failure rather than ARDS. Pneumonia caused by viruses or by *Pneumocystis* may be clinically indistinguishable from ARDS.

Sepsis-induced hypotension (see "Septic Shock," above) usually results from a generalized maldistribution of blood flow and blood volume and from hypovolemia that is due, at least in part, to diffuse capillary leakage of intravascular fluid. Other factors that may decrease effective intravascular volume include dehydration from antecedent disease or insensible fluid losses, vomiting or diarrhea, and polyuria. During early septic shock, systemic vascular resistance is usually elevated and cardiac output may be low. After fluid repletion, in contrast, cardiac output typically increases and systemic vascular resistance falls. Indeed, normal or increased cardiac output and decreased systemic vascular resistance distinguish septic shock from cardiogenic, extracardiac obstructive, and hypovolemic shock; other processes that can produce this combination include anaphylaxis, beriberi, cirrhosis, and overdoses of nitroprusside or narcotics.

Depression of myocardial function, manifested as increased end-diastolic and systolic ventricular volumes with a decreased ejection fraction, develops within 24 h in most patients with severe sepsis. Cardiac output is maintained despite the low ejection fraction because ventricular dilatation permits a normal stroke volume. In survivors, myocardial function returns to normal over several days. Although myocardial dysfunction may contribute to hypotension, refractory hypotension is usually due to a low systemic vascular resistance, and death results from refractory shock or the failure of multiple organs rather than from cardiac dysfunction per se.

Renal Complications
Oliguria, azotemia, proteinuria, and nonspecific urinary casts are frequently found. Many patients are inappropriately polyuric; hyperglycemia may exacerbate this tendency. Most renal failure is due to acute tubular necrosis induced by hypotension or capillary injury, although some patients also have glomerulonephritis, renal cortical necrosis, or interstitial nephritis. Drug-induced renal damage may complicate therapy, particularly when hypotensive patients are given aminoglycoside antibiotics.

Coagulation
Although thrombocytopenia occurs in 10 to 30% of patients, the underlying mechanisms are not understood. Platelet counts are usually very low ($<50,000/\mu L$) in patients with DIC; these low counts may reflect diffuse endothelial injury or microvascular thrombosis.

Neurologic Complications
When the septic illness lasts for weeks to months, "critical-illness" polyneuropathy may prevent weaning from ventilatory support and produce distal motor weakness. Electrophys-

iologic studies are diagnostic. Guillain-Barré syndrome, metabolic disturbances, and toxin activity must be ruled out.

LABORATORY FINDINGS   Abnormalities that occur early in the septic response may include leukocytosis with a left shift, thrombocytopenia, hyperbilirubinemia, and proteinuria. Leukopenia may develop. The neutrophils may contain toxic granulations, Döhle bodies, or cytoplasmic vacuoles. As the septic response becomes more severe, thrombocytopenia worsens (often with prolongation of the thrombin time, decreased fibrinogen, and the presence of D-dimers, suggesting DIC), azotemia and hyperbilirubinemia become more prominent, and levels of aminotransferases rise. Active hemolysis suggests clostridial bacteremia, malaria, a drug reaction, or DIC; in the case of DIC, microangiopathic changes may be seen on a blood smear.

During early sepsis, hyperventilation induces respiratory alkalosis. With respiratory muscle fatigue and the accumulation of lactate, metabolic acidosis (with increased anion gap) typically supervenes. Evaluation of arterial blood gases reveals hypoxemia, which is initially correctable with supplemental oxygen but whose later refractoriness to 100% oxygen inhalation indicates right-to-left shunting. The chest radiograph may be normal or may show evidence of underlying pneumonia, volume overload, or the diffuse infiltrates of ARDS. The electrocardiogram may show only sinus tachycardia or nonspecific ST–T-wave abnormalities.

Most diabetic patients with sepsis develop hyperglycemia. Severe infection may precipitate diabetic ketoacidosis, which may exacerbate hypotension (Chap. 323). Hypoglycemia occurs rarely. The serum albumin level, initially within the normal range, declines as sepsis continues. Serum lipid concentrations are often elevated. Hypocalcemia is rare.

DIAGNOSIS   There is no specific diagnostic test for the septic response. Diagnostically sensitive findings in a patient with suspected or proven infection include fever or hypothermia, tachypnea, tachycardia, and leukocytosis or leukopenia (Table 254-1); acutely altered mental status, thrombocytopenia, or hypotension also suggests the diagnosis. The septic response can be quite variable, however. In one study, 36% of patients with severe sepsis had a normal temperature, 40% had a normal respiratory rate, 10% had a normal pulse rate, and 33% had normal white blood cell counts. Moreover, the systemic responses of uninfected patients with other conditions may be similar to those characteristic of sepsis. Noninfectious etiologies of SIRS (Table 254-1) include pancreatitis, burns, trauma, adrenal insufficiency, pulmonary embolism, dissecting or ruptured aortic aneurysm, myocardial infarction, occult hemorrhage, cardiac tamponade, post-cardiopulmonary bypass syndrome, anaphylaxis, and drug overdose.

Definitive etiologic diagnosis requires isolation of the microorganism from blood or a local site of infection. At least two blood samples (10 mL each) should be obtained (from different venipuncture sites) for culture. Because gram-negative bacteremia is typically low-grade (<10 organisms per milliliter of blood), multiple blood cultures or prolonged incubation of cultures may be necessary; *S. aureus* grows more readily and is detectable in blood cultures within 48 h in most instances. In many cases, blood cultures are negative; this result can reflect prior antibiotic administration, the presence of slow-growing or fastidious organisms, or the absence of microbial invasion of the bloodstream. In these cases, Gram's staining and culture of material from the primary site of infection or of infected cutaneous lesions may help establish the microbial etiology. The skin and mucosae should be examined carefully and repeatedly for lesions that might yield diagnostic information. With overwhelming bacteremia (e.g., pneumococcal sepsis in splenectomized individuals or fulminant meningococcemia), microorganisms are sometimes visible on buffy coat smears of peripheral blood.

Detection of endotoxin in blood by the limulus lysate test may portend a poor outcome, but this assay is not useful for diagnosing gram-negative bacterial infections, including gram-negative bactere-mia. Although blood levels of IL-6 may also correlate with prognosis, cytokine assays are poorly standardized and currently have limited clinical value.

℞ TREATMENT

Patients in whom sepsis is suspected must be managed expeditiously. This task is best accomplished by personnel who are experienced in the care of the critically ill. Successful management requires urgent measures to treat the local site of infection, to provide hemodynamic and respiratory support, and to eliminate the offending microorganism. The outcome is also influenced by the patient's underlying disease, which should be managed aggressively.

ANTIMICROBIAL AGENTS   Antimicrobial chemotherapy should be initiated as soon as samples of blood and other relevant sites have been cultured. The choice of initial therapy is based on knowledge of the likely pathogens at specific sites of local infection. Available information about patterns of antimicrobial susceptibility among bacterial isolates from the community, the hospital, and the patient also should be taken into account. It is important, pending culture results, to initiate empirical antimicrobial therapy that is effective against both gram-positive and gram-negative bacteria (Table 254-4). Maximal recommended doses of antimicrobial drugs should be given intravenously, with adjustment for impaired renal function when necessary. When culture results become available, the regimen can often be simplified, as a single antimicrobial agent is frequently adequate for the treatment of a known pathogen. Most patients require antimicrobial therapy for at least 1 week; the duration of treatment is typically influenced by factors such as the site of tissue infection, the adequacy of surgical drainage, the patient's underlying disease, and the antimicrobial susceptibility of the bacterial isolate(s).

REMOVAL OF THE SOURCE OF INFECTION   Removal or drainage of a focal source of infection is essential. Sites of occult infection should be sought carefully. Indwelling intravenous catheters should be removed, the tip rolled over a blood agar plate for quantitative culture, and a new catheter inserted at a different site. Foley and drainage catheters should be replaced. The possibility of paranasal sinusitis (often caused by gram-negative bacteria) should be considered if the patient has undergone nasal intubation. In patients with extensive abnormalities on chest radiographs, computed tomography (CT) of the chest may identify unsuspected parenchymal, mediastinal, or pleural disease. In the neutropenic patient, cutaneous sites of tenderness and erythema, particularly in the perianal region, must be carefully sought. In patients with sacral or ischial decubitus ulcers, it is important to exclude pelvic or other soft tissue pus collections (by CT or magnetic resonance imaging, if necessary). In patients with severe sepsis arising from the urinary tract, sonography or CT should be used to rule out ureteral obstruction, perinephric abscess, and renal abscess. These studies are not so urgent in patients with less severe urosepsis, provided that a clinical response is evident within 48 to 72 h.

HEMODYNAMIC, RESPIRATORY, AND METABOLIC SUPPORT   The primary goal is to restore adequate oxygen and substrate delivery to the tissues. Adequate organ perfusion is essential. Effective intravascular volume depletion is common in patients with sepsis, and initial management of hypotension should include the administration of intravenous fluids, typically 1 to 2 L of normal saline over 1 to 2 h. To avoid pulmonary edema, the pulmonary capillary wedge pressure should be maintained between 12 and 16 mmHg or the central venous pressure between 8 and 12 cmH$_2$O. The urine output rate should be kept at >0.5 mL/kg per hour by continuing fluid administration; a diuretic such as furosemide may be used if needed. In about one-third of patients, hypotension and organ hypoperfusion respond to fluid resuscitation; a reasonable goal is to maintain a mean arterial blood pressure of >65 mmHg (systolic pressure, >90 mmHg) and a cardiac index of ≥4 L/min per m². If these guidelines cannot be met by volume infusion, inotropic and vasopressor therapy is indicated. Circulatory adequacy is also assessed by clinical parameters (mentation, urine output, skin perfusion) and, when possible, by measurements of oxygen delivery and consumption. A recent study found that prompt resuscitative measures, including maintenance of central venous oxygen saturation at >70% (by administration of dobutamine, if needed), were associated with significantly improved survival in patients who were admitted to the emergency department with severe sepsis.

Adrenal insufficiency should be considered in septic patients with refractory hypotension, fulminant *N. meningitidis* bacteremia, prior glucocorticoid use, disseminated tuberculosis, or AIDS. The cosyntropin ($\alpha^{1\text{-}24}$-ACTH) stimulation test (Chap. 321) may suggest absolute or partial adrenal insufficiency. Supplemental hydrocortisone (50 mg intravenously every 6 h) may be given while the results of the cosyntropin test are awaited (see "Antimediator Agents," below).

Plasma vasopressin levels do not increase in patients with septic shock. Recent studies have found that vasopressin infusion can reverse septic shock in some patients, reducing or eliminating the need for catecholamine pressors. An adequately powered and randomized trial of vasopressin infusion has not been performed, however, and its impact on end-organ function and survival is not known.

Ventilator therapy is indicated for progressive hypoxemia, hypercapnia, neurologic deterioration, or respiratory muscle failure. Sustained tachypnea (respiratory rate, >30 breaths/min) is frequently a harbinger of impending respiratory collapse; mechanical ventilation is often initiated to ensure adequate oxygenation, divert blood from the muscles of respiration, prevent aspiration of oropharyngeal contents, and reduce the cardiac afterload. Erythrocyte transfusion is indicated if oxygen delivery is compromised by a low hemoglobin concentration (<7 g/dL).

Bicarbonate is sometimes administered for severe metabolic acidosis (arterial pH <7.2). DIC, if complicated by major bleeding, should be treated with transfusion of fresh-frozen plasma and platelets. Successful treatment of the underlying infection is essential to reverse both acidosis and DIC.

GENERAL SUPPORT In patients with prolonged severe sepsis (i.e., that lasting more than 2 or 3 days), nutritional supplementation may reduce the impact of protein hypercatabolism; available evidence favors the enteral delivery route. Recovery is also assisted by preventing skin breakdown, deep venous thrombosis, nosocomial infections, and stress ulcers.

OTHER MEASURES Despite aggressive management, many patients with severe sepsis or septic shock die. Three kinds of agents that may help prevent these deaths are being investigated: (1) drugs that neutralize bacterial endotoxin, thereby potentially benefiting the fraction (approximately half) of septic patients who have gram-negative bacterial infection; (2) anti-inflammatory drugs that interfere with one or more mediators of the inflammatory response; and (3) anticoagulant drugs intended to prevent or reverse microthrombosis.

Antiendotoxin Agents Despite much effort to develop drugs that neutralize endotoxin in vivo, the potential of endotoxin as a target for therapeutic intervention remains controversial. In placebo-controlled clinical trials, two monoclonal antibodies to endotoxin did not prevent the

TABLE 254-4 *Initial Antimicrobial Therapy for Severe Sepsis with No Obvious Source in Adults with Normal Renal Function*

Clinical Condition	Antimicrobial Regimens (Intravenous Therapy)
Immunocompetent adult	The many acceptable regimens include (1) ceftriaxone (2 g q24h) *or* ticarcillin-clavulanate (3.1 g q4–6h) *or* piperacillin-tazobactam (3.375 g q4–6h); (2) imipenem-cilastatin (0.5 g q6h) *or* meropenem (1 g q8h) *or* cefepime (2 g q12h). Gentamicin *or* tobramycin (5–7 mg/kg q24h) may be *added* to either regimen. If the patient is allergic to β-lactam agents, use ciprofloxacin (400 mg q12h) *or* levofloxacin (500–750 mg q12h) *plus* clindamycin (600 mg q8h). If the institution has a high incidence of MRSA infections, add vancomycin (15 mg/kg q12h) to each of the above regimens.
Neutropenia[a] (<500 neutrophils/μL)	Regimens include (1) imipenem-cilastatin (0.5 g q6h) *or* meropenem (1 g q8h) *or* cefepime (2 g q8h); (2) ticarcillin-clavulanate (3.1 g q4h) *or* piperacillin-tazobactam (3.375 g q4h) *plus* tobramycin (5–7 mg/kg q24h). Vancomycin (15 mg/kg q12h) and cefepime should be used if the patient has an infected vascular catheter, if staphylococci are suspected, if the patient has received quinolone prophylaxis, if the patient has received intensive chemotherapy that produces mucosal damage, or if the institution has a high incidence of MRSA infections.
Splenectomy	Cefotaxime (2 g q6–8h) *or* ceftriaxone (2 g q12h) should be used. If the local prevalence of cephalosporin-resistant pneumococci is high, *add* vancomycin. If the patient is allergic to β-lactam drugs, vancomycin (15 mg/kg q12h) *plus* ciprofloxacin (400 mg q12h) *or* levofloxacin (750 mg q12h) *or* aztreonam (2 g q8h) should be used.
IV drug user	Nafcillin or oxacillin (2 g q8h) plus gentamicin (5–7 mg/kg q24h). If the local prevalence of MRSA is high or if the patient is allergic to β-lactam drugs, vancomycin (15 mg/kg q12h) with gentamicin should be used.
AIDS	Cefepime (2 g q8h), ticarcillin-clavulanate (3.1 g q4h), *or* piperacillin-tazobactam (3.375 g q4h) *plus* tobramycin (5–7 mg/kg q24h) should be used. If the patient is allergic to β-lactam drugs, ciprofloxacin (400 mg q12h) *or* levofloxacin (750 mg q12h) *plus* vancomycin (15 mg/kg q12h) *plus* tobramycin should be used.

[a] Adapted in part from WT Hughes et al: Clin Infect Dis 25:551, 1997.
Note: MRSA, methicillin-resistant *Staphylococcus aureus.*

death of patients with severe gram-negative bacterial sepsis. These antibodies did not bind to LPS with high affinity, and one was later reported to be a polyreactive autoantibody. A theoretically more promising agent is bactericidal permeability-increasing (BPI) protein, a human neutrophil protein that neutralizes lipid A and may be lethal for many gram-negative bacteria. In one clinical trial, infusion of BPI protein decreased the incidence of severe thrombotic events among children with fulminant meningococcemia. Other investigational drugs include nontoxic lipid A analogues that reduce host responses to endotoxins by competing with lipid A for interaction with the TLR4 signaling complex.

Antimediator Agents Other adjunctive therapies are intended to control the inflammatory response, regardless of the microbial stimulus. However, numerous agents that directly or indirectly interfere with the actions of inflammatory mediators have not prevented the death of patients with severe sepsis or septic shock. Many factors have probably contributed to the unsuccessful outcomes of these trials, including problems with study design (inappropriate end points, inadequate sample size, population heterogeneity, multiple covariates) and drug administration (wrong dose, time, or duration of administration). Anti-inflammatory drugs tested in clinical trials include methylprednisolone, dexamethasone, ibuprofen, PAF antagonists, recombinant IL-1Ra, genetically engineered soluble receptors for TNF-α, and monoclonal antibodies to TNF-α.

Whereas large doses of glucocorticoids have not improved survival, recent evidence suggests that many septic patients have inadequate adrenal reserve and that these individuals may benefit from low doses of glucocorticoid and mineralocorticoid. A recent study measured each patient's plasma cortisol response to a bolus infusion of 250 μg of synthetic ACTH. In the study population of severely septic patients, an increment of ≤9 μg/dL correlated with partial adrenal insufficiency and identified a group of patients who benefited from the administration of hydrocortisone (50 mg intravenously every 6 h) and 9-α-fludrocortisone (50 μg/d via nasogastric tube) for 7 days. The 28-day mortality was 53% among adrenal-deficient (nonresponder) patients who received combined steroid therapy and 63% in the placebo group (*p* < .02). Patients who had normal adrenal reserve did not benefit from steroid administration. Although these results have not been confirmed in a second clinical trial, the strategy has a strong physiologic rationale.

Anticoagulant Agents   Recombinant activated protein C (aPC) recently became the first drug to be approved by the U.S. Food and Drug Administration (FDA) for the treatment of patients with severe sepsis or septic shock. In a randomized controlled trial in which drug or placebo was given within 24 h of the patient's first sepsis-related organ dysfunction, 28-day mortality was significantly lower among recipients of aPC than among patients who received placebo (24.7% vs. 30.8%; *p* < .005). In addition, aPC recipients were more likely than placebo recipients to have severe bleeding (3% vs. 2%). Survival improved only for patients who had an APACHE II score of ≥25 during the 24 h before initiation of aPC infusion. Specifically, the FDA has approved aPC for use in adults (>18 years of age) who meet the APACHE II criterion and have a low risk of hemorrhage-related side effects. The drug is administered as a constant intravenous infusion of 24 μg/kg per hour for 96 h. Each patient's clotting parameters must be monitored carefully. Intracranial hemorrhage, the most serious complication noted to date, has occurred infrequently but seems to be more common among patients with platelet counts of <30,000/μL or meningitis at the time of infusion.

The long-term impact of aPC treatment is uncertain. In the pivotal clinical trial, the treatment and placebo groups did not differ significantly in the percentage of patients who had been discharged from the hospital by treatment day 28. Long-term survival data have not been released by the sponsor. Although the theoretical rationale for treating septic patients with anticoagulants is strong, two other human anticoagulant proteins (antithrombin III and tissue factor pathway inhibitor) did not improve patient survival in recent clinical trials, and the apparent efficacy of aPC did not correlate with preinfusion blood levels of protein C or other clotting parameters. In vitro studies suggest that aPC has anti-inflammatory activities that could contribute to its therapeutic effect.

Studies are needed to determine the relative benefits of hydrocortisone and mineralocorticoid treatment (in patients with adrenal insufficiency), vasopressin, and aPC and to learn how these agents should best be used—singly, together, or in combination with other agents.

PROGNOSIS   Approximately 20 to 35% of patients with severe sepsis and 40 to 60% of patients with septic shock die within 30 days. Others die within the ensuing 6 months. Late deaths often result from poorly controlled infection, complications of intensive care, failure of multiple organs, or the patient's underlying disease.

Prognostic stratification systems such as APACHE II indicate that factoring in the patient's age, underlying condition, and various physiologic variables can yield estimates of the risk of dying of severe sepsis. Of the individual covariates, the severity of underlying disease most strongly influences the risk of dying. Septic shock is also a strong predictor of short- and long-term mortality. Case-fatality rates are similar for culture-positive and culture-negative severe sepsis.

PREVENTION   Prevention offers the best opportunity to reduce morbidity and mortality. In developed countries, most episodes of severe sepsis and septic shock are complications of nosocomial infections. These cases might be prevented by reducing the number of invasive procedures undertaken, by limiting the use (and duration of use) of indwelling vascular and bladder catheters, by reducing the incidence and duration of profound neutropenia (<500 neutrophils/μL), and by more aggressively treating localized nosocomial infections. Indiscriminate use of antimicrobial agents and glucocorticoids should be avoided, and optimal infection-control measures (Chap. 116) should be used. Several studies point to associations between allelic polymorphisms in cytokine genes and risk of developing severe sepsis; if these associations prove to be broadly applicable, such polymorphisms can be used prospectively to identify high-risk patients and to target preventive and/or therapeutic measures to them. Studies indicate that 50 to 70% of patients who develop nosocomial severe sepsis or septic shock have experienced a less severe stage of the septic response (e.g., SIRS, sepsis) on at least one previous day in the hospital. Research is needed to develop adjunctive agents that can damp the septic response before organ dysfunction or hypotension occurs.

FURTHER READING

ANNANE D et al: Effect of treatment with low doses of hydrocortisone and fludrocortisone on mortality in patients with septic shock. JAMA 288:862, 2002

BERNARD GR et al: Efficacy and safety of recombinant human activated protein C for severe sepsis. N Engl J Med 344:699, 2001

DE BACKER D et al: Microvascular blood flow is altered in patients with sepsis. Am J Respir Crit Care Med 166:98, 2002

HOLMES CL et al: Physiology of vasopressin relevant to management of septic shock. Chest 120:989, 2001

HOTCHKISS RS, KARL IE: The pathophysiology and treatment of sepsis. N Engl J Med 348:138, 2003

MUNFORD RS, PUGIN J: Normal responses to injury prevent systemic inflammation and can be immunosuppressive. Am J Respir Crit Care Med 163:316, 2001

RIVERS E et al: Early goal-directed therapy in the treatment of severe sepsis and septic shock. N Engl J Med 345:1368, 2001

SANDS KE et al: Epidemiology of sepsis syndrome in 8 academic medical centers. JAMA 278:234, 1997

255   CARDIOGENIC SHOCK AND PULMONARY EDEMA
Judith S. Hochman, David Ingbar

Cardiogenic shock and pulmonary edema are life-threatening conditions that should be treated as medical emergencies. The most common etiology for both is severe left ventricular (LV) dysfunction, leading to pulmonary congestion and/or systemic hypoperfusion (Fig. 255-1). →*The pathophysiology of pulmonary edema and shock are discussed in Chaps. 29 and 253, respectively.*

CARDIOGENIC SHOCK

Cardiogenic shock (CS) is characterized by systemic hypoperfusion due to severe depression of the cardiac index [<2.2 (L/min)/m²] and sustained systolic arterial hypotension (<90 mmHg), despite an elevated filling pressure [pulmonary capillary wedge pressure (PCWP) > 18 mmHg]. It is associated with in-hospital mortality rates >50%. The major causes of CS are listed in Table 255-1. Circulatory failure based on cardiac dysfunction may be caused by primary myocardial failure, most commonly secondary to acute myocardial infarction (MI) (Chap. 228), and less frequently by cardiomyopathy or myocarditis (Chap. 221) or cardiac tamponade (Chap. 222).

INCIDENCE   CS is the leading cause of death of patients hospitalized with MI. Early reperfusion therapy for acute MI decreases the incidence of CS. The rate of CS complicating acute MI fell from 20% in the 1960s but has plateaued at ~8% for over 20 years. Shock is typically associated with ST elevation MI and is less common with non-ST elevation MI (Chap. 228).

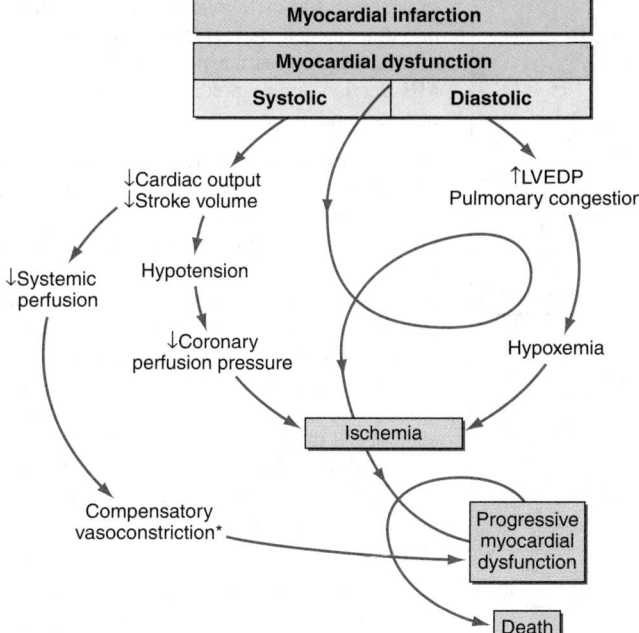

FIGURE 255-1 Pathophysiology of cardiogenic shock. Systolic and diastolic myocardial dysfunction result in a reduction in cardiac output and often pulmonary congestion. Systemic and coronary hypoperfusion occur, resulting in progressive ischemia. Although a number of compensatory mechanisms are activated in an attempt to support the circulation, these compensatory mechanisms may become maladaptive and produce a worsening of hemodynamics. *Release of inflammatory cytokines after myocardial infarction may lead to inducible nitrous oxide expression, excess NO, and inappropriate vasodilation. This causes further reduction in systemic and coronary perfusion. A vicious spiral of progressive myocardial dysfunction occurs that ultimately results in death if it is not interrupted. LVEDP, left ventricular end-diastolic pressure. (*From SM Hollenberg et al: Ann Intern Med 131:47, 1999.*)

LV failure accounts for ~80% of the cases of CS complicating acute MI. Acute severe mitral regurgitation (MR), ventricular septal rupture (VSR), predominant right ventricular (RV) failure, and free wall rupture or tamponade account for the remainder.

PATHOPHYSIOLOGY CS is characterized by a vicious circle in which depression of myocardial contractility, usually due to ischemia, results in reduced cardiac output and arterial pressure, which result in hypoperfusion of the myocardium and further ischemia and depression of the cardiac output (Fig. 255-1). Systolic myocardial dysfunction reduces stroke volume and, together with diastolic dysfunction, leads to elevated LV end-diastolic pressure and PCWP as well as to pulmonary congestion. Reduced coronary perfusion leads to worsening ischemia and progressive myocardial dysfunction and a rapid downward spiral, which, if uninterrupted, is often fatal. A systemic inflammatory response syndrome may accompany large infarctions and shock. Inflammatory cytokines, inducible nitric oxide synthase, and excess nitric oxide and peroxynitrite may contribute to the genesis of CS as they do to other forms of shock (Chap. 253). Hypoxemia and lactic acidosis develop as a result of pump failure and then contribute to the vicious circle by worsening myocardial ischemia and hypotension. Severe acidosis (pH <7.25) reduces the efficacy of endogenous and exogenously administered catecholamines. Refractory sustained ventricular or atrial tachyarrhythmias can cause or exacerbate CS.

Autopsy specimens often reflect the stuttering course and piecemeal necrosis of the left ventricle, often showing varying stages of infarction. Reinfarction is apparent as new areas of necrosis contiguous with or remote from a slightly older infarct. Typically, at least 40% of the LV myocardium is damaged by a combination of old scar and new infarcts. Infarctions that extend through the full myocardial thickness and result in rupture of the interventricular septum, papillary muscle, or ventricular free wall may result in shock (Chap. 228 and p. 1616).

PATIENT PROFILE In patients with acute MI, older age, female sex, prior MI, diabetes, and anterior MI location are all associated with increased risk of CS. Shock associated with a first inferior MI should prompt a search for a mechanical cause. In patients with non-ST elevation acute coronary syndrome (ACS), prior heart failure (HF), coronary artery bypass graft (CABG) surgery, and peripheral vascular disease are additional important risk factors. Reinfarction soon after MI increases the risk of CS. Severe and extensive coronary artery atherosclerotic lesions are typically present in MI patients who develop shock. Two-thirds of patients with CS have flow-limiting stenoses in all three major coronary arteries, and 20% have left main coronary artery stenosis.

TIMING Shock is present on admission in only 10 to 15% of patients who develop CS complicating MI; one-half develop it rapidly thereafter, within 6 h of MI onset. Another quarter develop shock later on the first day. Subsequent onset of CS may be due to reinfarction, marked infarct expansion, or a mechanical complication.

DIAGNOSIS Due to the unstable condition of these patients, supportive therapy must be initiated simultaneously with diagnostic evaluation (Fig. 255-2). A focused history and physical examination should be performed, blood specimens sent to the laboratory, and an electrocardiogram and chest x-ray obtained. A two-dimensional echocardiogram with color flow Doppler is an invaluable diagnostic tool in patients suspected of CS.

Clinical Findings Most patients have continuing chest pain and dyspnea and appear pale, apprehensive, cyanotic, and diaphoretic. Mentation may be altered, with varying degrees of somnolence, confusion, and

TABLE 255-1   *Etiologies of Cardiogenic Shock (CS)[a] and Cardiogenic Pulmonary Edema[b]*

ETIOLOGIES OF CARDIOGENIC SHOCK OR PULMONARY EDEMA

Acute myocardial infarction/ischemia
    LV failure
    VSR
    Papillary muscle/chordal rupture—severe MR
    Ventricular free wall rupture with subacute tamponade
    Other conditions complicating large MIs
        Hemorrhage
        Infection
        Excess negative inotropic or vasodilator medications
        Prior valvular heart disease
        Hyperglycemia/ketoacidosis
Post-cardiac arrest
Post-cardiotomy
Refractory sustained tachyarrhythmias
Acute fulminant myocarditis
End-stage cardiomyopathy
Hypertrophic cardiomyopathy with severe outflow obstruction
Aortic dissection with aortic insufficiency or tamponade
Pulmonary embolus
Severe valvular heart disease
    Critical aortic or mitral stenosis
    Acute severe aortic or MR
Toxic-metabolic
    Beta-blocker or calcium channel antagonist overdose

OTHER ETIOLOGIES OF CARDIOGENIC SHOCK[c]

RV failure due to:
    Acute myocardial infarction
    Acute coronary pulmonale
Refractory sustained bradyarrhythmias
Pericardial tamponade
Toxic/metabolic
    Severe acidosis, severe hypoxemia

[a] The etiologies of CS are listed. Most of these can cause pulmonary edema instead of shock or pulmonary edema with CS.
[b] Etiologies of noncardiogenic pulmonary edema are in Chap. 29.
[c] These cause CS but not pulmonary edema.

Note: LV, left ventricular; VSR, ventricular septal rupture; MR, mitral regurgitation; RV, right ventricular.

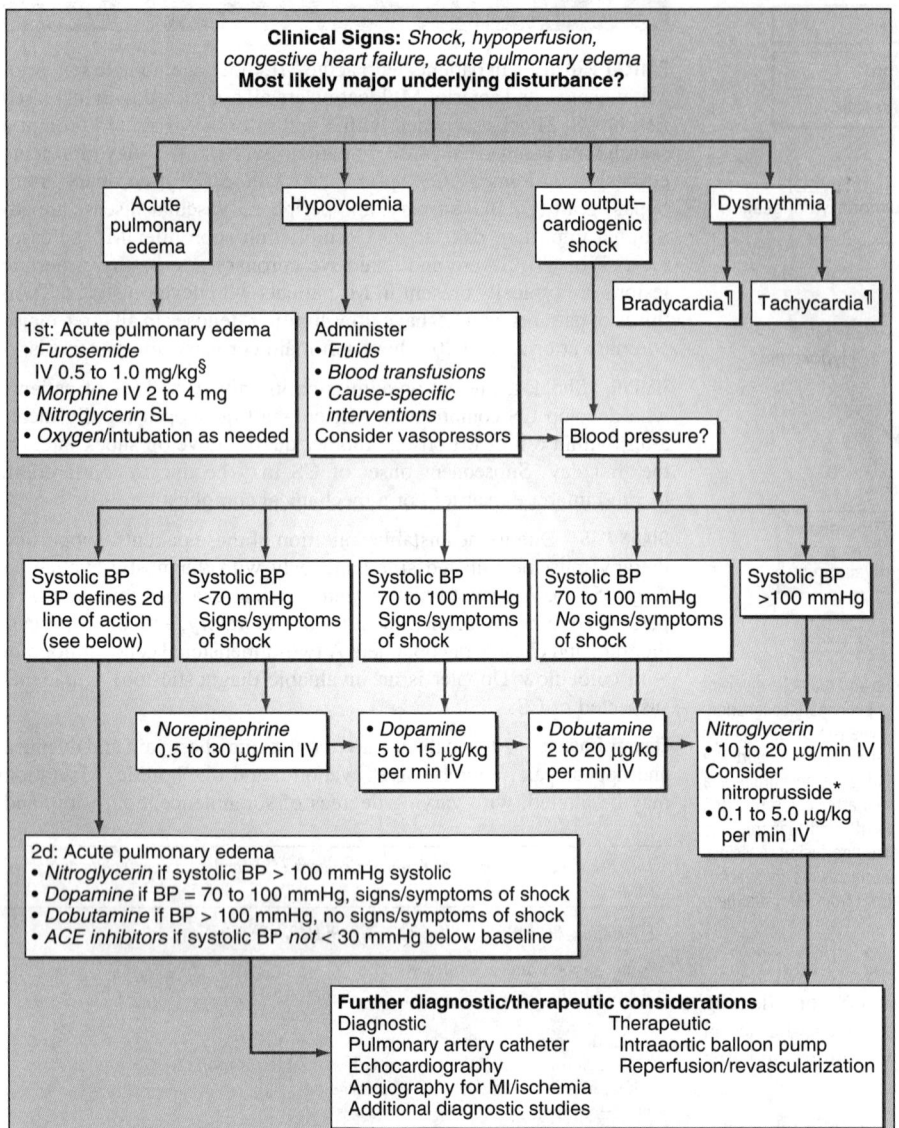

Clinical Signs: *Shock, hypoperfusion, congestive heart failure, acute pulmonary edema*
Most likely major underlying disturbance?

Acute pulmonary edema | Hypovolemia | Low output–cardiogenic shock | Dysrhythmia

Bradycardia¶ | Tachycardia¶

1st: Acute pulmonary edema
• *Furosemide* IV 0.5 to 1.0 mg/kg§
• *Morphine* IV 2 to 4 mg
• *Nitroglycerin* SL
• *Oxygen*/intubation as needed

Administer
• *Fluids*
• *Blood transfusions*
• *Cause-specific interventions*
Consider vasopressors

Blood pressure?

Systolic BP BP defines 2d line of action (see below) | Systolic BP <70 mmHg Signs/symptoms of shock | Systolic BP 70 to 100 mmHg Signs/symptoms of shock | Systolic BP 70 to 100 mmHg *No* signs/symptoms of shock | Systolic BP >100 mmHg

• *Norepinephrine* 0.5 to 30 µg/min IV | • *Dopamine* 5 to 15 µg/kg per min IV | • *Dobutamine* 2 to 20 µg/kg per min IV | *Nitroglycerin* • 10 to 20 µg/min IV Consider nitroprusside* • 0.1 to 5.0 µg/kg per min IV

2d: Acute pulmonary edema
• *Nitroglycerin* if systolic BP > 100 mmHg systolic
• *Dopamine* if BP = 70 to 100 mmHg, signs/symptoms of shock
• *Dobutamine* if BP > 100 mmHg, no signs/symptoms of shock
• *ACE inhibitors* if systolic BP *not* < 30 mmHg below baseline

Further diagnostic/therapeutic considerations
Diagnostic
Pulmonary artery catheter
Echocardiography
Angiography for MI/ischemia
Additional diagnostic studies

Therapeutic
Intraaortic balloon pump
Reperfusion/revascularization

FIGURE 255-2 The emergency management of patients with cardiogenic shock, acute pulmonary edema, or both is outlined. *Nitroprusside is contraindicated in states of reduced coronary artery perfusion. §Furosemide: <0.5 mg/kg for new-onset acute pulmonary edema without hypervolemia; 1 mg/kg for acute on chronic volume overload, renal insufficiency. ¶For management of bradycardia and tachycardia, see Chaps. 213 and 214. ACE, angiotensin-converting enzyme; BP, blood pressure; MI, myocardial infarction. *[Modified from Guidelines 2000 for Cardiopulmonary Resuscitation and Emergency Cardiovascular Care Part 7: The Era of Reperfusion. Section 1: Acute Coronary Syndromes (Acute Myocardial Infarction). Circulation 102 (suppl I): I-172, 2000. Reprinted with permission from Circulation].*

agitation. The pulse is typically weak and rapid, often in the range of 90 to 110 beats/min, or severe bradycardia due to high-grade heart block may be present. Systolic arterial pressure is reduced (<90 mmHg) with a narrow pulse pressure (<30 mmHg), but occasionally arterial pressure may be maintained by very high systemic vascular resistance. Tachypnea, Cheyne-Stokes respirations, and jugular venous distention may be present. The precordium is typically quiet, with a weak apical pulse. S1 is usually soft, and an S3 gallop may be audible. Acute, severe MR and VSR are usually associated with characteristic systolic murmurs (Chap. 228). Rales are audible in most patients with LV failure causing CS. Oliguria (urine output < 30 mL/h) is common.

Laboratory Findings The white blood cell count is typically elevated with a left shift. In the absence of prior renal insufficiency, renal function is initially normal, but blood urea nitrogen and creatinine rise progressively. Hepatic transaminases may be markedly elevated due to liver hypoperfusion. Lactic acid levels are elevated in severe shock, and electrolytes may reflect anion-gap acidosis. Prior to ventilatory support with supplemental O_2, arterial blood gases usually demonstrate

hypoxemia and metabolic acidosis, which may be compensated by respiratory alkalosis. Cardiac markers, creatine phosphokinase and its MB fraction, are markedly elevated, as are troponins I and T.

Electrocardiogram In CS due to acute MI with LV failure, Q waves and/or >2-mm ST elevation in multiple leads or left bundle branch block are usually present. More than one-half of all infarcts associated with shock are anterior. Global ischemia due to severe left main stenosis is usually accompanied by severe (e.g., >3 mm) ST depressions in multiple leads.

The chest x-ray typically shows pulmonary vascular congestion and often pulmonary edema, but these findings may be absent in up to a third of patients. The heart size is usually normal when CS results from a first MI but is enlarged when it occurs in a patient with a previous MI.

Echocardiogram A two-dimensional echocardiogram with color flow Doppler (Chap. 211) should be obtained promptly in patients with suspected CS to help define its etiology. Doppler mapping demonstrates a left-to-right shunt in patients with VSR and the severity of MR when the latter is present. Proximal aortic dissection with aortic regurgitation or tamponade may be visualized or evidence for pulmonary embolism obtained (Chap. 244).

Pulmonary Artery Catheterization There is controversy regarding the use of pulmonary artery balloon flotation (Swan-Ganz) catheters in patients with established or suspected CS (Chaps. 212 and 249). However, given the ominous prognosis, their use is generally recommended for measurement of filling pressures and cardiac output to confirm the diagnosis and help optimize use of intravenous fluids, inotropic agents, and vasopressors (Table 255-2). Blood samples for O_2 saturation measurement should be obtained from the right atrium, right ventricle, and pulmonary artery to rule out a left-to-right shunt. Mixed venous O_2 saturations are low and arterial-venous O_2 differences are elevated, reflecting increased O_2 extraction and low cardiac index, and the PCWP is elevated. However, these measurements, as well as systemic arterial pressure, may have returned toward normal in the presence of sympathomimetic amines. Systemic vascular resistance may be normal or elevated in CS. Equalization of right- and left-sided filling pressures (right atrial and PCWP) suggests cardiac tamponade as the cause of CS (Chap. 222).

Left Heart Catheterization and Coronary Angiography Measurement of LV pressure, definition of the coronary anatomy, and left ventriculography provide useful information and are indicated in most patients with CS complicating MI. Because of the procedural risk in this critically ill population, cardiac catheterization should be performed when there is a plan and capability for immediate coronary intervention (see below) or when a definitive diagnosis has not been made by other tests.

R̶x TREATMENT (Fig. 255-2)

General Measures In addition to the usual treatment of acute MI (Chap. 228), initial therapy is aimed at maintaining systemic and coronary perfusion by raising systolic blood pressure to ~90 mmHg with vaso-

TABLE 255-2 *Hemodynamic Patterns*[a]

	RA, mmHg	RVS, mmHg	RVD, mmHg	PAS, mmHg	PAD, mmHg	PCW, mmHg	CI, (L/min)/m²	SVR, (dyn · s)/cm⁵
Normal values	< 6	< 25	0–12	< 25	0–12	< 6–12	≥2.5	(800–1600)
MI without pulmonary edema[b]	—	—	—	—	—	~13 (5–18)	~2.7 (2.2–4.3)	—
Pulmonary edema	↔↑	↔↑	↔↑	↑	↑	↑	↔↓	↑
Cardiogenic shock								
LV failure	↔↑	↔↑	↔↑	↔↑	↑	↑	↓	↔↑
RV failure[c]	↑	↓↔↑[d]	↑	↓↔↑[d]	↔↓↑[d]	↓↔↑[d]	↓	↔↑
Cardiac tamponade	↑	↔↑	↑	↑	↑	↔↑	↓	↑
Acute mitral regurgitation	↔↑	↔↑	↔↑	↑	↑	↔↑	↔↓	↔↑
Ventricular septal rupture	↑	↔↑	↑	↔↑	↔↑	↔↑	↑ PBF ↓ SBF	↔↑
Hypovolemic shock	↓	↔↓	↔↓	↓	↓	↓	↓	↑
Septic shock	↓	↔↓	↔↓	↓	↓	↓	↑	↓

[a] There is significant patient-to-patient variation. Pressure may be normalized if cardiac output is low.

[b] Forrester et al classified non-reperfused MI patients into four hemodynamic subsets. (From Forrester JS et al: N Engl J Med 295:1356, 1976.) PCWP and CI in clinically stable subset 1 patients are shown. Values in parentheses represent range.

[c] "Isolated" or predominant RV failure.

[d] PCW and PA pressures may rise in RV failure after volume loading due to RV dilation, right to left shift of the interventricular septum, resulting in impaired LV filling. When biventricular failure is present, the patterns are similar to those shown for LV failure.

Note: RA, right atrium; RVS/D, right ventricular systolic/diastolic; PAS/D, pulmonary artery systolic/diastolic; PCW, pulmonary capillary wedge; CI, cardiac index; SVR, systemic vascular resistance; MI, myocardial infarction; P/SBF, pulmonary/systemic blood flow.

Source: Table prepared with the assistance of Krishnan Ramanathan, MD.

pressors and adjusting volume status to a level that ensures optimum LV filling pressure (PCWP ~ 20 mmHg). Hypoxemia and acidosis must be corrected; most patients require endotracheal intubation to correct these abnormalities and reduce the work of breathing (see "Pulmonary Edema," below). Negative inotropic agents should be discontinued and the doses of renally cleared medications adjusted. Hyperglycemia should be corrected with continuous infusion of insulin. Bradyarrhythmias may require transvenous pacing. Recurrent ventricular tachycardia or rapid atrial fibrillation may require immediate treatment (Chap. 214).

Vasopressors Various intravenous drugs may be used to augment blood pressure and cardiac output in patients with CS. All have important disadvantages, and none has been shown to change the outcome in patients with established shock. *Norepinephrine* is a potent vasoconstrictor and inotropic stimulant that increases myocardial O₂ consumption; it should be reserved for patients with CS and refractory hypotension without elevated systemic vascular resistance. It should be started at a dosage of 2 to 4 μg/min and titrated upward as necessary. If systolic pressure cannot be maintained at 90 mmHg with a dosage of 15 μg/min, it is unlikely that a further increase will be beneficial.

Dopamine is useful in many patients; at low doses (≤2 μg/kg per min), it dilates the renal vascular bed; at moderate doses (2 to 10 μg/kg per min), it has positive chronotropic and inotropic effects as a consequence of β-receptor stimulation. At higher doses, a vasoconstrictor effect results from α-receptor stimulation. It is started at an infusion rate of 2 to 5 μg/kg per min, and the dosage is increased every 2 to 5 min to a maximum of 20 to 50 μg/kg per min. Systolic blood pressure should be maintained at ~90 mmHg. *Dobutamine* is a synthetic sympathomimetic amine with positive inotropic action and minimal positive chronotropic activity at low doses (2.5 μg/kg per min) but moderate chronotropic activity at higher doses. Although the usual dosage is up to 10 μg/kg per min, its vasodilating activity precludes its use when a vasoconstrictor effect is required.

Aortic Counterpulsation In CS, mechanical assistance with an intraaortic balloon pumping (IABP) system capable of augmenting both arterial diastolic pressure and cardiac output is helpful in rapidly stabilizing patients. A sausage-shaped balloon at the end of a catheter is introduced into the aorta percutaneously via the femoral artery, and the balloon is automatically inflated during early diastole, augmenting coronary blood flow. The balloon collapses in early systole, reducing the afterload against which the left ventricle ejects. IABP improves hemodynamic status at least temporarily in the majority of patients. In contrast to vasopressors and inotropic agents, myocardial O₂ consumption is reduced, leading to amelioration of ischemia. In the absence of early revascularization, however, long-term survival after this mode of therapy in patients with CS is disappointing. IABP is useful as a stabilizing measure in patients with CS prior to and during cardiac catheterization and percutaneous coronary intervention (PCI) or prior to urgent surgery. IABP is contraindicated if aortic regurgitation is present or aortic dissection is suspected. Ventricular assist devices may be considered for eligible young patients with refractory shock as a bridge to cardiac transplantation.

Reperfusion-Revascularization The rapid establishment of blood flow in the infarct-related artery is essential in the management of CS and forms the centerpiece of management. The randomized SHOCK Trial demonstrated 132 lives saved per 1000 patients treated with early revascularization with PCI or CABG compared to initial medical therapy including IABP with fibrinolytics followed by delayed revascularization (Fig. 255-3). The greatest benefit was in patients <75 years. Early revascularization with PCI or CABG is a class I recommendation for such patients with ST elevation or left bundle branch block MI who develop CS within 36 h of MI and who can be revascularized within 18 h of development of shock. When mechanical revascularization is not possible, IABP and fibrinolytic therapy are recommended. Older patients should be managed on an individual basis.

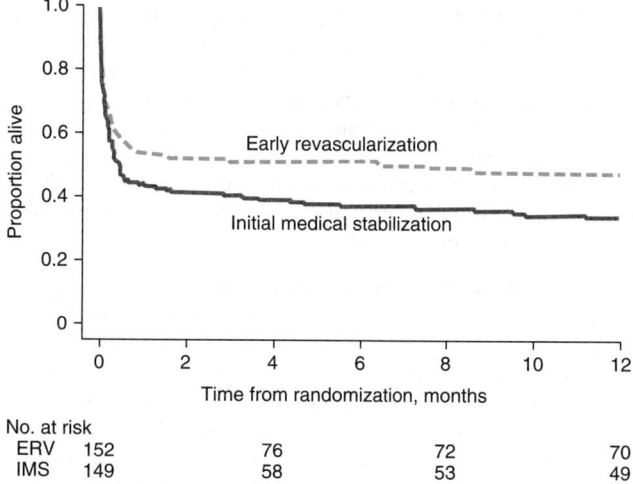

No. at risk				
ERV	152	76	72	70
IMS	149	58	53	49

FIGURE 255-3 Early revascularization (ERV) (percutaneous coronary intervention or coronary artery bypass graft) for cardiogenic shock complicating acute myocardial infarction resulted in substantially improved 1-year survival compared to initial mechanical stabilization (IMS), including intraaortic balloon pumping and fibrinolytic agents, followed by selective delayed revascularization in the SHOCK Trial (SHould we emergently revascularize Occluded coronaries for Cardiogenic shocK?) *(Reprinted with permission from JAMA.)*

PROGNOSIS   Within this high-risk condition, there is a wide range of expected death rates based on age, severity of hemodynamic abnormalities, severity of the clinical manifestations of hypoperfusion, and the performance of early revascularization. Independent risk factors are advanced age; depressed cardiac index, ejection fraction, and arterial pressure; elevated PCWP; more extensive coronary artery disease; and renal insufficiency.

SHOCK SECONDARY TO RIGHT VENTRICULAR INFARCTION   Although transient hypotension is common in patients with RV infarction and inferior MI (Chap. 228), persistent CS due to RV failure accounts for only 3% of CS complicating MI. The salient features of RV shock are absence of pulmonary congestion, high right atrial pressure (which may be seen only after volume loading), RV dilatation and dysfunction, only mildly or moderately depressed LV function, and predominance of single-vessel proximal right coronary artery occlusion. Management includes intravenous fluid administration to optimize right atrial pressure (10 to 15 mmHg); avoidance of excess fluids, which cause a shift of the interventricular septum into the LV; sympathomimetic amines; IABP; and the early reestablishment of infarct-artery flow.

MITRAL REGURGITATION (See also Chap 228)   Acute severe MR may complicate MI and result in CS and/or pulmonary edema. This complication most often occurs on the first day, with a second peak several days later. The diagnosis is confirmed by echo-Doppler. Rapid stabilization with IABP is recommended, with administration of dobutamine as needed to raise cardiac output. Reducing the load against which the left ventricle pumps (afterload) reduces the volume of regurgitant flow of blood into the left atrium. Mitral valve surgery is the definitive therapy and should be performed early in the course in suitable candidates.

VENTRICULAR SEPTAL RUPTURE (See also Chap 228)   Echo-Doppler demonstrates shunting of blood from the left to the right ventricle and may visualize the opening in the interventricular septum. Timing and management are similar to that for MR with IABP support and surgical correction for suitable candidates.

FREE WALL RUPTURE   Myocardial rupture is a dramatic complication of STEMI that is most likely to occur during the first week after the onset of symptoms; its frequency increases with the age of the patient. First infarction, a history of hypertension, no history of angina pectoris, and a relatively large Q-wave infarct are associated with a higher incidence of cardiac rupture. The clinical presentation typically is a sudden loss of pulse, blood pressure, and consciousness while the ECG continues to show sinus rhythm (apparent electromechanical dissociation or pulseless electrical activity). The myocardium continues to contract, but forward flow is not maintained as blood escapes into the pericardium. Cardiac tamponade (Chap. 222) ensues, and closed-chest massage is ineffective. This condition is almost universally fatal, although dramatic cases of urgent pericardiotensis followed by successful surgical repair have been reported.

ACUTE FULMINANT MYOCARDITIS (See also Chap 221)   Myocarditis can mimic acute MI with ST deviation or bundle branch block on the electrocardiogram and marked elevation of cardiac markers. Acute myocarditis causes CS in ~15% of cases. These patients are typically younger than those with CS due to acute MI and often do not have typical ischemic chest pain. Echocardiography typically shows global LV dysfunction. Initial management is the same as for CS complicating acute MI (Fig. 255-2) but of course does not involve coronary revascularization.

PULMONARY EDEMA

→*The etiologies and pathophysiology of pulmonary edema are discussed in Chap. 29.*

DIAGNOSIS

Acute pulmonary edema usually presents with the rapid onset or aggravation of dyspnea at rest, tachypnea, tachycardia, and severe hypoxemia. In addition to rales, wheezing due to airway compression from peribronchial cuffing may be audible. Hypertension is usually present due to endogenous release of catecholamines.

It is often difficult to distinguish cardiogenic and noncardiogenic causes of acute pulmonary edema. *Echocardiography* with color flow Doppler may identify systolic and diastolic ventricular dysfunction and valvular lesions and aid in the differentiation of these two causes. Pulmonary edema associated with electrocardiographic ST elevation and evolving Q waves is usually diagnostic of acute MI and should prompt immediate institution of MI protocols and coronary artery reperfusion therapy (Chap. 228). Brain natriuretic peptide levels, when elevated, support heart failure as the etiology of acute dyspnea with pulmonary edema (Chap. 216).

The use of a *balloon flotation catheter* permits measurement of PCWP and helps to differentiate high pressure (cardiogenic) and normal pressure (noncardiogenic) causes of pulmonary edema. Pulmonary artery catheterization (see p. 1614) is indicated when the etiology of the pulmonary edema is uncertain, when it is refractory to therapy, or when it is accompanied by hypotension.

℞ TREATMENT

The treatment of pulmonary edema depends upon the specific etiology. Given the acute, life-threatening nature of the condition, a number of measures must be applied immediately to support the circulation, gas exchange, and lung mechanics as outlined in Fig. 255-2. In addition, conditions that frequently complicate pulmonary edema, such as infection, acidemia, anemia, and renal failure, must be corrected.

Support of Oxygenation and Ventilation   Patients with acute cardiogenic pulmonary edema often have an identifiable cause of acute LV failure such as arrhythmia, ischemia, or myocardial decompensation (Chap. 216) that can be rapidly treated, with improvement in gas exchange. In contrast, noncardiogenic edema usually resolves much less quickly, and most patients require mechanical ventilation.

OXYGEN THERAPY   Support of oxygenation is essential to ensure adequate O_2 delivery to peripheral tissues, including the heart.

POSITIVE PRESSURE VENTILATION   The work of breathing and the O_2 requirements of this work are increased and may pose a significant physiologic stress on the heart. For patients with inadequate oxygenation or ventilation in spite of supplemental O_2, assisted ventilation should be initiated. This can be accomplished either by noninvasive ventilation using a face or nasal mask or by endotracheal intubation and ventilation. Continuous or bilevel positive airway pressure (Chap. 252) can rest the respiratory muscles, improve oxygenation and cardiac function, and reduce the need for intubation. In refractory cases, mechanical ventilation can relieve the work of breathing more completely than noninvasive ventilation. Mechanical ventilation with positive end-expiratory pressure can have multiple beneficial effects on pulmonary edema: (1) it can decrease both preload and afterload, thereby improving cardiac function; (2) it can redistribute lung water from the intraalveolar to the extraalveolar space where it does not interfere as much with gas exchange; and (3) it can increase lung volume to avoid atelectasis.

Reduction of Preload   In most forms of pulmonary edema, the quantity of extravascular lung water is related to both the PCWP and the intravascular volume status.

DIURETICS   The "loop diuretics" furosemide, bumetanide, and torsemide are effective in most forms of pulmonary edema, even in the presence of hypoalbuminemia, hyponatremia, or hypochloremia. Furosemide is also a venodilator that can reduce preload rapidly, prior to any diuresis, and is the diuretic of choice. The initial dose of furosemide should be ≤0.5 mg/kg, but a higher dose (1 mg/kg) is required in patients with renal insufficiency, chronic diuretic use, or hypervolemia or after failure of a lower dose.

NITRATES   Nitroglycerin and isosorbide dinitrate act predominantly as venodilators, with coronary vasodilating properties as well. They are rapid in onset and effective when administered by a variety of routes. Sublingual nitroglycerin (0.4 mg × 3 every 5 min) is first-line therapy for acute cardiogenic pulmonary edema. If pulmonary edema persists and in the absence of hypotension, sublingual may be followed by intravenous nitroglycerin, commencing at 5 to 10 μg/min. Intravenous nitroprusside (0.1 to 5 μg/kg per min) is a potent and predominantly arterial vasodilator that is useful for patients with pulmonary edema and hypertension and for cautious afterload and preload reduction if systolic pressure >100 mmHg. It requires close monitoring and titration, including the use of an arterial catheter for continuous blood pressure measurement in the intensive care unit.

MORPHINE   Given in 2- to 4-mg intravenous boluses, morphine is a transient venodilator that reduces preload while relieving dyspnea and anxiety. These effects can diminish stress, catecholamine levels, tachycardia, and ventricular afterload in patients with pulmonary edema and systemic hypertension.

ANGIOTENSIN-CONVERTING ENZYME (ACE) INHIBITORS   ACE inhibitors reduce both afterload and preload and are recommended in hypertensive patients. A low dose of a short-acting agent may be initiated and followed by increasing oral doses. In acute MI with heart failure, ACE inhibitors reduce short- and long-term mortality.

OTHER PRELOAD-REDUCING AGENTS   Intravenous recombinant brain natriuretic peptide (nesiritide) is a potent vasodilator with diuretic properties and is effective in the treatment of pulmonary edema. The starting dose is a 2-μg/kg intravenous bolus, followed by a 0.01-μg/kg per min infusion.

PHYSICAL METHODS   Reduction of venous return reduces preload. Patients without hypotension should be maintained in the sitting position with the legs dangling along the side of the bed.

INOTROPIC AND INODILATOR DRUGS   The sympathomimetic amines dopamine and dobutamine (see above) are potent inotropic agents. The bipyridine phosphodiesterase-3 inhibitors (inodilators), such as amrinone (0.75-mg/kg loading dose followed by 5 to 20 μg/kg per min) or milrinone (50 μg/kg followed by 0.25 to 0.75 μg/kg per min) stimulate myocardial contractility while promoting peripheral and pulmonary vasodilation. Such agents are indicated in patients with cardiogenic pulmonary edema and severe LV dysfunction.

DIGITALIS GLYCOSIDES   Once a mainstay of treatment because of their positive inotropic action (Chap. 216), digitalis glycosides are rarely used at present. However, they may be useful for control of ventricular rate in patients with rapid atrial fibrillation or flutter and LV dysfunction, since they do not have the negative inotropic effects of other drugs that inhibit atrioventricular nodal conduction.

INTRAAORTIC COUNTERPULSATION   IABP may help to relieve cardiogenic pulmonary edema. It is indicated as a stabilizing measure when acute severe mitral regurgitation or ventricular septal rupture cause refractory pulmonary edema, especially in preparation for surgical repair. IABP or LV-assist devices (Chap. 217) are useful as bridging therapy to cardiac transplantation in patients with refractory pulmonary edema secondary to myocarditis or cardiomyopathy.

TREATMENT OF TACHYARRHYTHMIAS AND ATRIAL-VENTRICULAR RESYNCHRONIZATION   (See also Chap. 214)   Sinus tachycardia or atrial fibrillation results from elevated left atrial pressure and sympathetic stimulation. Tachycardia itself can also limit LV filling time and raise left atrial pressure further. While relief of pulmonary congestion will slow the sinus rate or ventricular response in atrial fibrillation, a primary tachyarrhythmia may require cardioversion. In patients with reduced LV function and without atrial contraction or with lack of synchronized atrioventricular

contraction, placement of an atrioventricular sequential pacemaker should be considered (Chap. 213).

Special Considerations ■ *THE RISK OF IATROGENIC CARDIOGENIC SHOCK*   In the treatment of pulmonary edema vasodilators lower blood pressure, and, particularly when used in combination, their use may lead to hypotension, coronary artery hypoperfusion, and shock (Fig. 255-1). In general, patients with a *hypertensive* response to pulmonary edema tolerate and are benefited by these medications. In normotensive patients, low doses of single agents should be instituted sequentially, as needed.

ACUTE CORONARY SYNDROMES   Acute ST-segment elevation MI complicated by pulmonary edema is associated with in-hospital mortality rates of 20 to 40%. After immediate stabilization, coronary artery blood flow must be rapidly reestablished. When available, primary PCI is preferable; alternatively, a fibrinolytic agent should be administered. Early coronary angiography and revascularization by PCI or CABG are also indicated for patients with non-ST elevation acute coronary syndrome. IABP use may be required to stabilize patients for coronary angiography if hypotension develops or for refractory pulmonary edema in patients with LV failure who are candidates for revascularization (Chap. 228).

UNUSUAL TYPES OF EDEMA   Specific etiologies of pulmonary edema may require particular therapy. One type is reexpansion pulmonary edema that develops after removal of air or fluid that has been in the pleural space for some time. These patients may develop hypotension or oliguria resulting from rapid fluid shifts into the lung. Diuretics and preload reduction are contraindicated, and intravascular volume repletion is often needed while supporting oxygenation and gas exchange.

The risk of development of high-altitude pulmonary edema can be prevented by use of dexamethasone, calcium channel-blocking drugs, or long-acting inhaled β_2-adrenergic agonists. Treatment includes descent from altitude, bed rest, oxygen, and, if feasible, inhaled nitric oxide; nifedipine may also be effective.

For pulmonary edema resulting from upper airway obstruction, recognition of the obstructing cause is key, since treatment then is to relieve or bypass the obstruction.

FURTHER READING

ANTMAN EM: Treatment of ST elevation myocardial infarction, in *Braunwald's Heart Disease*, 7th ed, D Zipes et al (eds). Philadelphia, Saunders, 2005

ANTMAN EM et al: ACC/AHA guidelines for the management of patients with ST-segment elevation myocardial infarction. J Am Coll Cardiol (In press)

COTTER G et al: Randomised trial of high-dose isosorbide dinitrate plus low-dose furosemide versus high-dose furosemide plus low-dose isosorbide dinitrate in severe pulmonary oedema. Lancet 351:389, 1998

——— et al: The role of cardiac power and systemic vascular resistance in the pathophysiology and diagnosis of patients with acute congestive heart failure. Eur J Heart Fail (In press)

GOLDBERG RJ et al: Temporal trends in cardiogenic shock complicating acute myocardial infarction. N Engl J Med 340:1162, 1999

HOCHMAN JS: Cardiogenic shock complicating acute myocardial infarction: Expanding the paradigm. Circulation 107:2998, 2003

——— et al: Early revascularization in acute myocardial infarction complicated by cardiogenic shock. N Engl J Med 341:625, 1999

——— et al: One-year survival following early revascularization for cardiogenic shock. JAMA 285:190, 2001

JACOBS AK et al: Cardiogenic shock caused by right ventricular infarction: A report from the SHOCK Registry. J Am Coll Cardiol 41:159, 2003

MAISEL AS et al: Rapid measurement of B-type natriuretic peptide in the emergency diagnosis of heart failure. N Engl J Med 347:161, 2002

MASIP J et al: Non-invasive pressure support ventilation versus conventional oxygen therapy in acute cardiogenic pulmonary oedema. Lancet 356:2126, 2000

MENON V et al: Acute myocardial infarction complicated by systemic hypoperfusion without hypotension: Report of the SHOCK Trial Registry. Am J Med 108:374, 2000

OVERVIEW AND DEFINITIONS

The vast majority of naturally occurring sudden deaths are caused by cardiac disorders. The magnitude of sudden *cardiac* death (SCD) as a public health problem is highlighted by estimates that more than 400,000 deaths occur each year in the United States by this mechanism, accounting for 50% of all cardiac deaths. SCD is a direct consequence of cardiac arrest, which is potentially reversible if responded to promptly. Since resuscitation techniques and emergency rescue systems are available to respond to and save victims of out-of-hospital cardiac arrest, which was uniformly fatal in the past, understanding the SCD problem has practical importance.

SCD must be defined carefully. In the context of time, "sudden" is defined, for most clinical and epidemiologic purposes, as 1 h or less between a change in clinical status heralding the onset of the terminal clinical event, and the cardiac arrest itself. An exception is unwitnessed deaths in which pathologists may expand the definition of time to 24 h after the victim was last seen to be alive and stable.

Because of community-based interventions, victims may remain biologically alive for days or even weeks after a cardiac arrest that has resulted in irreversible central nervous system damage. Confusion in terms can be avoided by adhering strictly to definitions of cardiovascular collapse, cardiac arrest, and death (Table 256-1). Death is biologically, legally, and literally an absolute and irreversible event. Death may be delayed in a survivor of cardiac arrest, but "survival after sudden death" is an irrational term. A generally accepted definition of SCD is *natural death due to cardiac causes*, heralded by abrupt loss of consciousness within *1 h* of the onset of acute symptoms, in an individual who may have known *preexisting* heart disease but in whom the *time* and *mode* of death are *unexpected*. When biologic death of the cardiac arrest victim is delayed because of interventions, the relevant pathophysiologic event remains the sudden and unexpected cardiac arrest that leads ultimately to death, even though delayed by artificial methods. The language used should reflect the fact that the index event was a cardiac arrest and that death was due to its delayed consequences.

CLINICAL DEFINITION OF FORMS OF CARDIOVASCULAR COLLAPSE

Cardiovascular collapse is a general term connoting loss of effective blood flow due to acute dysfunction of the heart and/or peripheral vasculature. Cardiovascular collapse may be caused by vasodepressor syncope (vasovagal syncope, postural hypotension with syncope, neurocardiogenic syncope; Chap. 20), a transient severe bradycardia, or cardiac arrest. The latter is distinguished from the transient forms of cardiovascular collapse in that it usually requires an intervention to achieve resuscitation. In contrast, vasodepressor syncope and many primary bradyarrhythmic syncopal events are transient and non-life-threatening, with spontaneous return of consciousness.

The most common electrical mechanism for true cardiac arrest is ventricular fibrillation (VF), which is responsible for 65 to 80% of cardiac arrests. Severe persistent bradyarrhythmias, asystole, and pulseless electrical activity (PEA; an organized electrical activity without mechanical response, formerly called electromechanical dissociation) cause another 20 to 30%. Sustained ventricular tachycardia (VT) with hypotension is a less common cause. Acute low cardiac output states, having precipitous onset, may also present clinically as a cardiac arrest. These hemodynamic causes include massive acute pulmonary emboli, internal blood loss from ruptured aortic aneurysm, intense anaphylaxis, and cardiac rupture after myocardial infarction (MI).

ETIOLOGY, INITIATING EVENTS, AND CLINICAL EPIDEMIOLOGY

Clinical and epidemiologic studies have identified population subgroups at high risk for SCD. In addition, a large body of pathologic data provides information on the underlying *structural abnormalities* in victims of SCD, and studies of clinical physiology have begun to identify a group of *transient functional factors* that may convert a long-standing underlying structural abnormality from a stable to an unstable state (Table 256-2). This information has developed into an understanding of the causes and mechanisms of SCD.

Cardiac disorders constitute the most common causes of sudden *natural* death. After an initial peak incidence of sudden death between birth and 6 months of age (the sudden infant death syndrome), the incidence of sudden death declines sharply and remains low through childhood and adolescence. Among adolescents and young adults, the incidence of SCD is approximately 1 per 100,000 population per year. The incidence begins to increase in adults over the age of 30 years, reaching a second peak in the age range of 45 to 75 years, when the incidence approximates 1 to 2 per 1000 per year among the unselected adult population. Increasing age within this range is associated with increasing risk for sudden *cardiac* death, and the proportion of cardiac causes among all sudden natural deaths increases dramatically with advancing years. From 1 to 13 years of age, only one of five sudden *natural* deaths is due to cardiac causes. Between 14 and 21 years of age, the proportion increases to 30%, and then to 88% in the middle-aged and elderly.

Young and middle-aged men and women have very different susceptibilities to SCD, but the gender differences decrease with advancing age. In the 45- to 64-year-old age group, the male SCD excess is nearly 7:1. It falls to less than 2:1 in the 65- to 74-year-old age group. The difference in risk for SCD parallels the differences in age-related risks for other manifestations of coronary heart disease (CHD) between men and women. As the gender gap for manifestations of CHD closes in the seventh and eighth decades of life, the excess risk of SCD in males also narrows. Despite the lower incidence among younger women, coronary risk factors such as cigarette smoking, diabetes, hyperlipidemia, and hypertension are highly influential, and SCD remains an important clinical and epidemiologic problem. The inci-

TABLE 256-1 *Distinction Between Cardiovascular Collapse, Cardiac Arrest, and Death*

Term	Definition	Qualifiers or Exceptions
Cardiovascular collapse	A sudden loss of effective blood flow due to cardiac and/or peripheral vascular factors which may reverse spontaneously (e.g., neurocardiogenic syncope; vasovagal syncope) or only with interventions (e.g., cardiac arrest)	Nonspecific term that includes cardiac arrest and its consequences and also events that characteristically revert spontaneously
Cardiac arrest	Abrupt cessation of cardiac pump function which may be reversible by a prompt intervention but will lead to death in its absence	Rare spontaneous reversions; likelihood of successful interventions relates to mechanism of arrest, clinical setting, and prompt return of circulation
Death	Irreversible cessation of all biologic functions	None

TABLE 256-2 *Cardiac Arrest and Sudden Cardiac Death*

STRUCTURAL CAUSES

I. Coronary heart disease
   A. Coronary artery abnormalities
      1. Chronic atherosclerotic lesions
      2. Acute (active) lesions (plaque fissuring, platelet aggregation, acute thrombosis)
      3. Anomalous coronary artery anatomy
   B. Myocardial infarction
      1. Healed
      2. Acute
II. Myocardial hypertrophy
   A. Secondary
   B. Hypertrophic cardiomyopathy
      1. Obstructive
      2. Nonobstructive
III. Dilated cardiomyopathy—primary muscle disease
IV. Inflammatory and infiltrative disorders
   A. Myocarditis
   B. Noninfectious inflammatory diseases
   C. Infiltrative diseases
   D. Right ventricular dysplasia
V. Valvular heart disease
VI. Electrophysiologic abnormalities, structural
   A. Anomalous pathways in Wolff-Parkinson-White syndrome
   B. Conducting system disease
VII. Inherited disorders of molecular structure associated with electro-physiologic abnormalities (e.g., congenital long QT syndromes, Brugada syndrome)

FUNCTIONAL CONTRIBUTING FACTORS

I. Alterations of coronary blood flow
   A. Transient ischemia
   B. Reperfusion after ischemia
II. Low cardiac output states
   A. Heart failure
      1. Chronic
      2. Acute decompensation
   B. Shock
III. Systemic metabolic abnormalities
   A. Electrolyte imbalance (e.g., hypokalemia)
   B. Hypoxemia, acidosis
IV. Neurophysiologic disturbances
   A. Autonomic fluctuations: central, neural, humoral
   B. Receptor function
V. Toxic responses
   A. Proarrhythmic drug effects
   B. Cardiac toxins (e.g., cocaine, digitalis intoxication)
   C. Drug interactions

dence of SCD among the African-American population appears to be higher than among the white population, but the reasons remain uncertain.

Hereditary factors contribute to the risk of SCD. In a nonspecific sense, they represent expressions of the hereditary predisposition to CHD. In addition, however, there are recent data suggesting a familial predisposition to SCD as a specific form of expression of CHD. In a few syndromes, such as hypertrophic cardiomyopathy, congenital long QT interval syndromes, right ventricular dysplasia, and the syndrome of right bundle branch block and non-ischemic ST-segment elevations (Brugada syndrome), there is a specific inherited risk of SCD (Chap. 214).

The structural causes of and functional factors contributing to the SCD syndrome are listed in Table 256-2. Worldwide, and especially in western cultures, coronary atherosclerotic heart disease is the most common structural abnormality associated with SCD in middle-aged and older adults. Up to 80% of all SCDs in the United States are due to the consequences of coronary atherosclerosis. The cardiomyopathies (dilated and hypertrophic, collectively; Chap. 221) account for another 10 to 15% of SCDs, and all the remaining diverse etiologies cause only 5 to 10% of all SCDs. The inherited arrhythmia syndromes

(see above and Table 256-2) are more common causes in adolescents and young adults.

Transient ischemia in the previously scarred or hypertrophied heart, hemodynamic and fluid and electrolyte disturbances, fluctuations in autonomic nervous system activity, and transient electrophysiologic changes caused by drugs or other chemicals (e.g., proarrhythmia) have all been implicated as mechanisms responsible for transition from electrophysiologic stability to instability. In addition, reperfusion of ischemic myocardium may cause transient electrophysiologic instability and arrhythmias.

PATHOLOGY

Data from postmortem examinations of SCD victims parallel the clinical observations on the prevalence of CHD as the major structural etiologic factor. More than 80% of SCD victims have pathologic findings of CHD. The pathologic description often includes a combination of long-standing, extensive atherosclerosis of the epicardial coronary arteries and unstable coronary artery lesions, which include a combination of fissured or ruptured plaques, platelet aggregates, hemorrhage, and thombosis. In one study, chronic coronary atherosclerosis involving two or more major vessels with ≥75% stenosis was observed in 75% of the victims. In another study, atherosclerotic plaque fissuring, platelet aggregates, and/or acute thrombosis were observed in 95 of 100 individuals who had pathologic studies after SCD.

As many as 70 to 75% of males who die suddenly have preexisting healed MIs, while only 20 to 30% have recent acute MIs, despite the prevalence of unstable plaques and thrombi. Regional or global left ventricular (LV) hypertrophy coexists with prior MIs.

PREDICTION AND PREVENTION OF CARDIAC ARREST AND SUDDEN CARDIAC DEATH

SCD accounts for approximately one-half the total cardiovascular mortality rate. As shown in Fig. 256-1A, the very high risk subgroups provide more focused populations ("percent per year") for predicting cardiac arrest or SCD; but the impact of such subgroups on the overall problem of SCD, indicated by the absolute number of preventable events ("events per year"), is relatively small. The requirements for achieving a major population impact are effective prevention of underlying diseases and/or new epidemiologic probes that will allow better resolution of subgroups at specific risk within the large general populations.

Strategies for predicting and preventing SCD are categorized as primary and secondary, in addition to responses intended to abort cardiac arrests. *Primary prevention* refers to the attempt to identify individual patients at specific risk for SCD and institute preventive strategies. *Secondary prevention* refers to measures taken to prevent recurrent cardiac arrest or death in individuals who have survived a previous cardiac arrest. The primary prevention strategies currently used depend upon magnitude of risk among the various population subgroups. Because the annual incidence of SCD among the unselected adult population is limited to 1 to 2 per 1000 population per year (Fig. 256-1A), and more than 30% of all SCDs due to coronary artery disease occur as the first clinical manifestation of the disease (Fig. 256-2A), the only practical strategies are profiling for risk of developing CHD and risk factor control (Fig. 256-2B). The most powerful long-term risk factors include age, cigarette smoking, elevated serum cholesterol, diabetes mellitus, elevated blood pressure, LV hypertrophy, and nonspecific electrocardiographic abnormalities. Markers of inflammation (e.g., C-reactive protein levels) that may predict plaque destabilization, have recently been added to risk classifications. The presence of multiple risk factors progressively increases incidence, but not sufficiently or specifically enough to warrant therapies targeted to potentially fatal arrhythmias (Fig. 256-1A). However, recent studies offer the hope that genetic markers for specific risk may

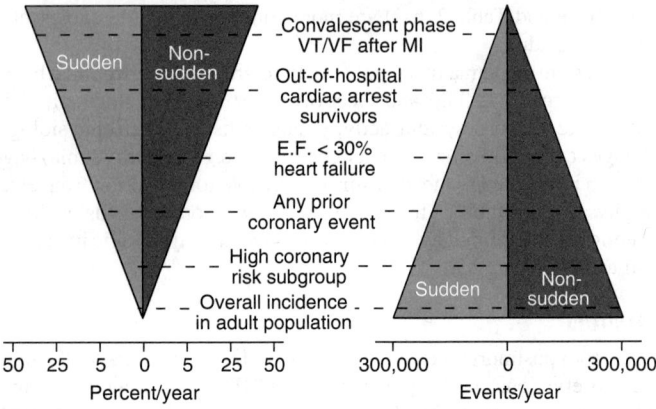

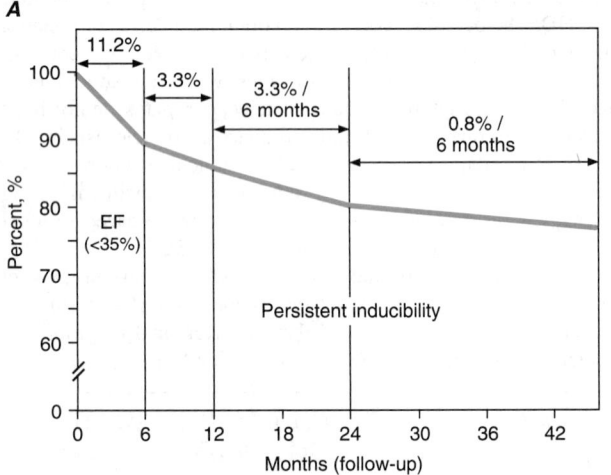

FIGURE 256-1 *A.* Incidence of sudden and nonsudden cardiac deaths in population subgroups, and the relation of total number of events per year to incidence figures. Approximations of subgroup incidence figures, and the related population pool from which they are derived, are presented. Approximately 50% of all cardiac deaths are sudden and unexpected. The incidence triangle on the left ("Percent/Year") indicates the approximate percentage of sudden and nonsudden deaths in each of the population subgroups indicated, ranging from the lowest percentage in unselected adult populations (0.1 to 2% per year) to the highest percentage in patients with VT or VF during convalescence after an MI (approximately 50% per year). The triangle on the right indicates the total number of events per year in each of these groups, to reflect incidence in context with the size of the population subgroups. The highest risk categories identify the smallest number of total annual events, and the lowest incidence category accounts for the largest number of events per year. (EF, ejection fraction; VT, ventricular tachycardia; VF, ventricular fibrillation; MI, myocardial infarction.) *B.* Time dependence of risk among survivors of out-of-hospital cardiac arrest. Recurrence risk is highest in the first 6 months of the index event. Survival is expressed as a percentage. High risk is best predicted initially by an ejection fraction ≤ 35% during the first 6 months, and subsequently persistent inducibility of VT during electrophysiologic testing becomes an added major risk. *n* = 101 at *t* = 0. [*After T Furukawa et al, in RJ Myerburg et al, Circulation 85(Suppl 1):2, 1992. Reproduced with permission of the American Heart Association.*]

be available in the future. These studies suggest that a family history of SCD associated with acute coronary syndromes predicts a higher likelihood of cardiac arrest as the initial manifestation of coronary artery disease in first-degree family members.

After coronary artery disease has been identified in a patient, additional strategies for risk profiling become available (Fig. 256-2*B*), but the majority of SCDs occur among the large unselected groups rather than in the specific high-risk subgroups that become evident among populations with established disease (compare events per year with percent per year in Fig. 256-1*A*). Under most conditions of higher level of risk, particularly those indexed to a major recent cardiovascular event (e.g., MI, recent onset of heart failure, survival after out-of-hospital cardiac arrest), the highest risk of SCD occurs during the

initial 6 to 18 months and then plateaus towards the baseline risk of the underlying disease (Fig. 256-1*B*). Accordingly, preventive interventions are more likely to be effective when initiated early.

Among patients in the acute, convalescent, and chronic phases of myocardial infarction (Chap. 228), subgroups at high absolute risk of SCD can be identified. During the acute phase, the potential risk of cardiac arrest from onset through the first 48 hours may be as high as 15 to 20%, emphasizing the importance for patients to respond promptly to the onset of symptoms. Those who survive acute-phase VF, however, are not at continuing risk for recurrent cardiac arrest indexed to that event. During the convalescent phase after MI (3 days to ~6 weeks), an episode of sustained VT or VF predicts a mortality risk of up to 50% at 12 months. At least 50% of the deaths are sudden. Aggressive intervention techniques may reduce this incidence.

After passage into the chronic phase of MI, the longer-term risk for total and SCD mortality is predicted by a number of factors (Fig. 256-2*B*). The most important for both SCD and non-sudden death is the extent of myocardial damage sustained as a result of the acute MI. This is measured by the magnitude of reduction of the ejection fraction (EF), functional capacity, and/or the occurrence of heart failure. Various studies have demonstrated that an EF < 40% contributes significantly to this risk. In addition, inducibility of VT or VF during electrophysiologic testing of patients who have ambient ventricular arrhythmias [premature ventricular contractions (PVCs) and nonsustained VT] and an EF < 35 or 40% is a strong predictor of SCD risk. Patients in this subgroup are now considered candidates for implantable cardioverter defibrillators (ICDs) (see below). Risk falls off sharply with EFs > 40% after MI and the absence of ambient arrhythmias, and conversely continues to rise with EFs < 30% even without the ambient arrhythmia markers.

The cardiomyopathies (dilated and hypertrophic) are the second most common category of diseases associated with risk of SCD, following CHD (Table 256-2). Some risk factors have been identified, largely related to extent of disease, documented ventricular arrhythmias, and symptoms of arrhythmias (e.g., unexplained syncope). The rare diseases associated with SCD in younger populations (adolescents, young adults, competitive athletes), such as the long QT interval syndromes, right ventricular dysplasia, hypertrophic cardiomyopathy, and Brugada syndrome, may be recognized or suspected based on symptoms, family history of premature sudden death or known presence of the specific entity, or incidental clinical data. Despite the low absolute incidence of SCD among the younger population (<1/ 100,000 per year), routine electrocardiographic (ECG) screening has been suggested for identifying individuals at risk.

Secondary prevention strategies are applied to surviving victims of a cardiac arrest that was not associated with an acute MI or a transient risk of SCD (e.g., drug exposures, correctable electrolyte imbalances). The extent of underlying disease (CHD, dilated cardiomyopathy), or merely its presences in association with life-threatening arrhythmias (e.g., long QT syndromes, right ventricular dysplasia) predicts a 1- to 2-year SCD or cardiac arrest recurrence risk of up to 30% in the absence of specific interventions (see below).

CLINICAL CHARACTERISTICS OF CARDIAC ARREST

PRODROME, ONSET, ARREST, DEATH

SCD may be presaged by days, weeks, or months of increasing angina, dyspnea, palpitations, easy fatigability, and other nonspecific complaints. However, these *prodromal complaints* are generally predictive of any major cardiac event; they are not specific for predicting SCD.

The *onset of the terminal event*, leading to cardiac arrest, is defined as an acute change in cardiovascular status preceding cardiac arrest by up to 1 h. When the onset is instantaneous or abrupt, the probability that the arrest is cardiac in origin is >95%. Continuous ECG recordings, fortuitously obtained at the onset of a cardiac arrest, commonly demonstrate changes in cardiac electrical activity during the minutes or hours before the event. There is a tendency for the heart rate to increase and for advanced grades of PVCs to evolve. Most cardiac arrests that are caused by VF begin with a run of sustained or nonsustained VT, which then degenerates into VF.

Sudden unexpected loss of effective circulation may be separated into "arrhythmic events" and "circulatory failure." Arrhythmic events are characterized by a high likelihood of patients being awake and active immediately prior to the event, are dominated by VF as the electrical mechanism, and have a short duration of terminal illness (<1 h). In contrast, circulatory failure deaths occur in patients who are inactive or comatose, have a higher incidence of asystole than VF, have a tendency to a longer duration of terminal illness, and are dominated by noncardiac events preceding the terminal illness.

The onset of cardiac arrest may be characterized by typical symptoms of an acute cardiac event, such as prolonged angina or the pain of onset of MI; acute dyspnea or orthopnea; or the sudden onset of palpitations, sustained tachycardia, or light-headedness. However, in many patients, the onset is precipitous, with minimal forewarning.

Cardiac arrest is, by definition, abrupt. Mentation may be impaired in patients with sustained VT during the onset of the terminal event. However, complete loss of consciousness is *a sine qua non* in cardiac arrest. Although rare spontaneous reversions occur, it is usual that cardiac arrest progresses to death within minutes (i.e., SCD has occurred) if active interventions are not undertaken promptly.

The probability of achieving successful resuscitation from cardiac arrest is related to the interval from onset to institution of resuscitative efforts, the

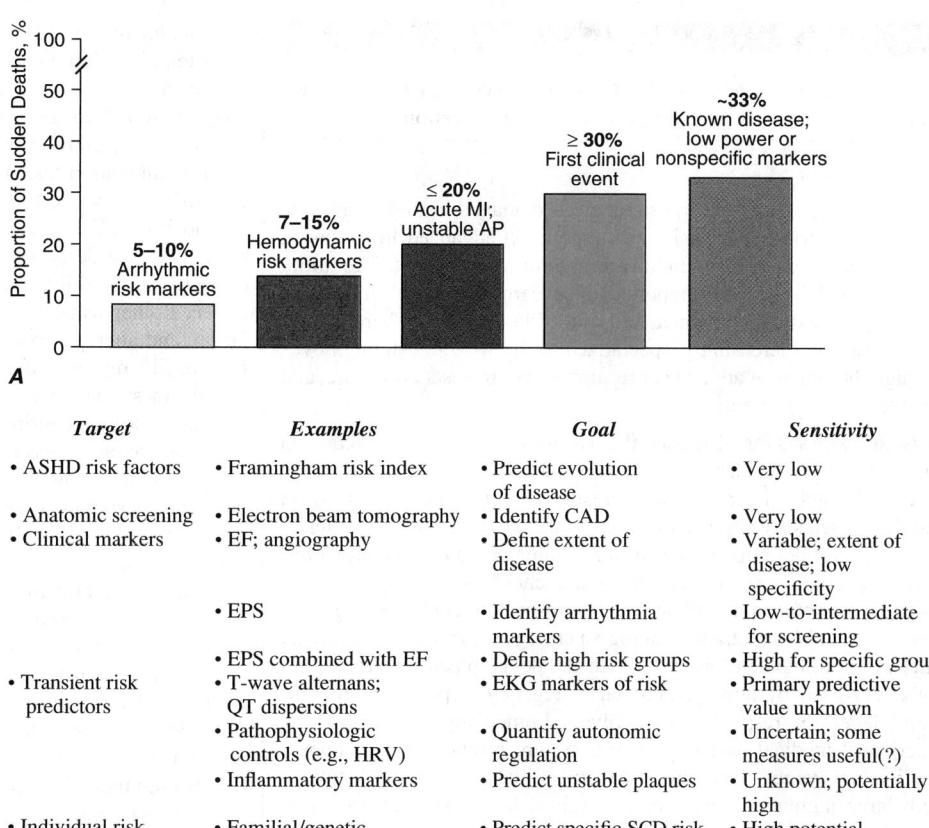

Target	Examples	Goal	Sensitivity
• ASHD risk factors	• Framingham risk index	• Predict evolution of disease	• Very low
• Anatomic screening	• Electron beam tomography	• Identify CAD	• Very low
• Clinical markers	• EF; angiography	• Define extent of disease	• Variable; extent of disease; low specificity
	• EPS	• Identify arrhythmia markers	• Low-to-intermediate for screening
	• EPS combined with EF	• Define high risk groups	• High for specific groups
• Transient risk predictors	• T-wave alternans; QT dispersions	• EKG markers of risk	• Primary predictive value unknown
	• Pathophysiologic controls (e.g., HRV)	• Quantify autonomic regulation	• Uncertain; some measures useful(?)
	• Inflammatory markers	• Predict unstable plaques	• Unknown; potentially high
• Individual risk predictors	• Familial/genetic profiles	• Predict specific SCD risk before disease expression	• High potential for future profiling

B

FIGURE 256-2 Population subsets, risk predictors, and distribution of sudden cardiac deaths (SCDs) according to clinical circumstances. *A.* The population subset with high-risk arrhythmia markers in conjunction with low ejection fraction is a group at high risk of SCD, but accounts for <10% of the total SCD burden attributable to coronary artery disease. In contrast, nearly two-thirds of all SCD victims present with SCD as the first and only manifestation of underlying disease or have known disease but are considered relatively low-risk, because of the absence of high-risk markers. *B.* Risk profile for prediction and prevention of SCD is difficult. The highest absolute numbers of events occur among the general population who may have risk factors for coronary heart disease or expressions of disease that do not predict high risk. This results in a low sensitivity for predicting and preventing SCD. New approaches that include epidemiologic modeling of transient risk factors and methods of predicting individual patient risk offer hope for greater sensitivity in the future. AP, angina pectoris; ASHD, arteriosclerotic heart disease; CAD, coronary artery disease; EPS, electrophysiologic study; HRV, heart rate variability. (*From Myerburg, reproduced with permission of the publisher*).

setting in which the event occurs, the mechanism (VF, VT, pulseless electrical activity, asystole), and the clinical status of the patient prior to the cardiac arrest. Return of circulation and survival rates as a result of defibrillation decrease linearly from the first minute to 10 minutes. By 5 minutes, survival rates are no better than 25 to 30% in out-of-hospital settings. Those settings in which it is possible to institute prompt cardiopulmonary resuscitation (CPR) with rapid defibrillation of VF provide a better chance of a successful outcome. However, the outcome in intensive care units and other in-hospital environments is heavily influenced by the patient's preceding clinical status. The immediate outcome is good for cardiac arrest occurring in the intensive care unit in the presence of an acute cardiac event or transient metabolic disturbance, but survival among patients with far-advanced chronic cardiac disease or advanced noncardiac diseases (e.g., renal failure, pneumonia, sepsis, diabetes, cancer) is low, and not much more successful in the in-hospital than in the out-of-hospital setting.

The success rate for initial resuscitation and survival to hospital discharge after an out-of-hospital cardiac arrest depends heavily on the mechanism of the event. When the mechanism is VT, the outcome is best; VF is the next most successful; and asystole and PEA generate dismal outcome statistics. Advanced age also influences adversely the chances of successful resuscitation.

Progression to biologic death is a function of the mechanism of cardiac arrest and the length of the delay before interventions. VF or

asystole without CPR within the first 4 to 6 min has a poor outcome even if defibrillation is successful, because of superimposed brain damage; and there are few survivors among patients who had no life support activities for the first 8 min after onset. Outcome statistics are improved by lay bystander intervention (basic life support—see below) prior to definitive interventions (advanced life support), and even more by early defibrillation. In regard to the latter, evaluations of deployment of automatic external defibrillators (AEDs) in communities (e.g., police vehicles, large buildings, stadiums) are beginning to generate encouraging data.

Death during the hospitalization after a successfully resuscitated cardiac arrest relates closely to the severity of central nervous system injury. Anoxic encephalopathy and infections subsequent to prolonged respirator dependence account for 60% of the deaths. Another 30% occur as a consequence of low cardiac output states that fail to respond to interventions. Recurrent arrhythmias are the least common cause of death, accounting for only 10% of in-hospital deaths.

In the setting of acute MI, it is important to distinguish between primary and secondary cardiac arrests. *Primary cardiac arrests* refer to those that occur in the absence of hemodynamic instability, and *secondary cardiac arrests* are those that occur in patients in whom abnormal hemodynamics dominate the clinical picture before cardiac arrest. The success rate for immediate resuscitation in primary cardiac arrest during acute MI in a monitored setting should approach 100%.

In contrast, as many as 70% of patients with secondary cardiac arrest succumb immediately or during the same hospitalization.

℞ TREATMENT

The individual who collapses suddenly is managed in four stages: (1) the initial response and basic life support, (2) advanced life support, (3) postresuscitation care, and (4) long-term management. The initial response and basic life support can be carried out by physicians, nurses, paramedical personnel, and trained lay persons. There is a requirement for increasingly specialized skills as the patient moves through the stages of advanced life support, postresuscitation care, and long-term management.

Initial Response and Basic Life Support The initial evaluation will confirm whether a sudden collapse is indeed due to a cardiac arrest. Observations of the state of consciousness, respiratory movements, skin color, and the presence or absence of pulses in the carotid or femoral arteries will promptly determine whether a life-threatening cardiac arrest has occurred. For lay responders, the pulse check is no longer recommended. As soon as a cardiac arrest is suspected, confirmed, or even considered to be impending, calling an emergency rescue system (e.g., 911) is the immediate priority. With the development of AEDs that are easily used by nonconventional emergency responders, an additional layer for response has evolved. Immediate defibrillation by emergency medical rescue personnel on fire rescue vehicles, police, public conveyance personnel, security officers in various locations with large numbers of people, and trained lay persons is becoming available to save more cardiac arrest victims.

Agonal respiratory movements may persist for a short time after the onset of cardiac arrest, but it is important to observe for severe stridor with a persistent pulse as a clue to aspiration of a foreign body or food. If this is suspected, a Heimlich maneuver (see below) may dislodge the obstructing body. A precordial blow, or "thump," delivered firmly by the clenched fist to the junction of the middle and lower third of the sternum may occasionally revert VT or VF, but there is concern about converting VT to VF. Therefore, it has been recommended to use precordial thumps as an advanced life support technique when monitoring and defibrillation are available. This conservative application of the technique remains controversial.

The third action during the initial response is to clear the airway. The head is tilted back and chin lifted so that the oropharynx can be explored to clear the airway. Dentures or foreign bodies are removed, and the Heimlich maneuver is performed if there is reason to suspect that a foreign body is lodged in the oropharynx. If respiratory arrest precipitating cardiac arrest is suspected, a second precordial thump is delivered after the airway is cleared.

Basic life support, more popularly known as CPR, is intended to maintain organ perfusion until definitive interventions can be instituted. The elements of CPR are the maintenance of ventilation of the lungs and compression of the chest. Mouth-to-mouth respiration may be used if no specific rescue equipment is immediately available (e.g., plastic oropharyngeal airways, esophageal obturators, masked Ambu bag). Conventional ventilation techniques during CPR require the lungs to be inflated twice in succession every 15 chest compressions.

Chest compression is based on the assumption that cardiac compression allows the heart to maintain a pump function by sequential filling and emptying of its chambers, with competent valves maintaining forward direction of flow. The palm of one hand is placed over the lower sternum, with the heel of the other resting on the dorsum of the lower hand. The sternum is depressed, with the arms remaining straight, at a rate of approximately 100 per minute. Sufficient force is applied to depress the sternum 4 to 5 cm, and relaxation is abrupt.

Advanced Life Support Advanced life support is intended to achieve adequate ventilation, control cardiac arrhythmias, stabilize blood pressure and cardiac output, and restore organ perfusion. The activities carried out to achieve these goals include (1) defibrillation/cardiover-sion and/or pacing, (2) intubation with an endotracheal tube, and (3) insertion of an intravenous line. The speed with which defibrillation/cardioversion is carried out is an important element for successful resuscitation, both for restoration of spontaneous circulation and protection of the central nervous system. Immediate defibrillation should precede intubation and insertion of an intravenous line; CPR should be carried out while the defibrillator is being charged. As soon as a diagnosis of VF or VT is established, a shock of at least 200 J should be delivered. Additional shocks at higher energies, up to a maximum of 360 J, are tried if the initial shock does not successfully abolish VT or VF. Epinephrine, 1 mg intravenously, is given after failed defibrillation, and attempts to defibrillate are repeated. The dose of epinephrine may be repeated after intervals of 3 to 5 min (Fig. 256-3A). Vasopressin (a single 40 Unit dose given IV) has been suggested as an alternative to epinephrine.

If the patient is less than fully conscious upon reversion, or if two or three attempts fail, prompt intubation, ventilation, and arterial blood gas analysis should be carried out. Ventilation with O_2 (room air if O_2 is not immediately available) may promptly reverse hypoxemia and acidosis. The patient who is persistently acidotic after successful defibrillation and intubation should be given 1 meq/kg $NaHCO_3$ initially and an additional 50% of the dose repeated every 10 to 15 min. However, it should not be used routinely.

After initial unsuccessful defibrillation attempts, or with persistent/recurrent electrical instability, antiarrhythmic therapy should be instituted. Intravenous amiodarone has emerged as the initial treatment of choice (150 mg over 10 min, followed by 1 mg/min for up to 6 h and 0.5 mg/min thereafter) (Fig. 256-3A). A bolus of 1 mg/kg of lidocaine may be given intravenously (Chap. 228), and the dose repeated in 2 min, in those patients in whom amiodarone is unsuccessful, and possibly in those who clearly have an acute MI as the triggering mechanism for the cardiac arrest. Intravenous procainamide (loading infusion of 100 mg/5 min to a total dose of 500 to 800 mg, followed by continuous infusion at 2 to 5 mg/min) is rarely used in this setting any longer but may be tried for persisting, hemodynamically stable arrhythmias. Intravenous calcium gluconate is no longer considered safe or necessary for routine administration. It is used only in patients in whom acute hyperkalemia is known to be the triggering event for resistant VF, in the presence of known hypocalcemia, or in patients who have received toxic doses of calcium channel antagonists.

Cardiac arrest secondary to bradyarrhythmias or asystole is managed differently (Fig. 256-3B). The patient is promptly intubated, CPR is continued, and an attempt is made to control hypoxemia and acidosis. Epinephrine and/or atropine are given intravenously or by an intracardiac route. External pacing devices are now available to attempt to establish a regular rhythm, but the prognosis is generally very poor in this form of cardiac arrest, even with successful electrical pacing. PEA is treated similarly to bradyarrhythmias, but its outcome is also dismal. The one exception is bradyarrhythmic/asystolic cardiac arrest secondary to airway obstruction. This form of cardiac arrest may respond promptly to removal of foreign bodies by the Heimlich maneuver or, in hospitalized patients, by intubation and suctioning of obstructing secretions in the airway.

Postresuscitation Care This phase of management is determined by the clinical setting of the cardiac arrest. Primary VF in acute MI (Chap. 228) is generally very responsive to life-support techniques and easily controlled after the initial event. In the in-hospital setting, respirator support is usually not necessary or is needed for only a short time, and hemodynamics stabilize promptly after defibrillation or cardioversion. In secondary VF in acute MI (those events in which hemodynamic abnormalities predispose to the potentially fatal arrhythmia), resuscitative efforts are less often successful; and in those patients who are successfully resuscitated, the recurrence rate is high. The clinical picture and outcome are dominated by hemodynamic instability and the ability to control hemodynamic dysfunction. Bradyarrhythmias, asystole, and PEA are commonly secondary events in hemodynamically unstable patients. The in-hospital phase of care of the out-of-hospital

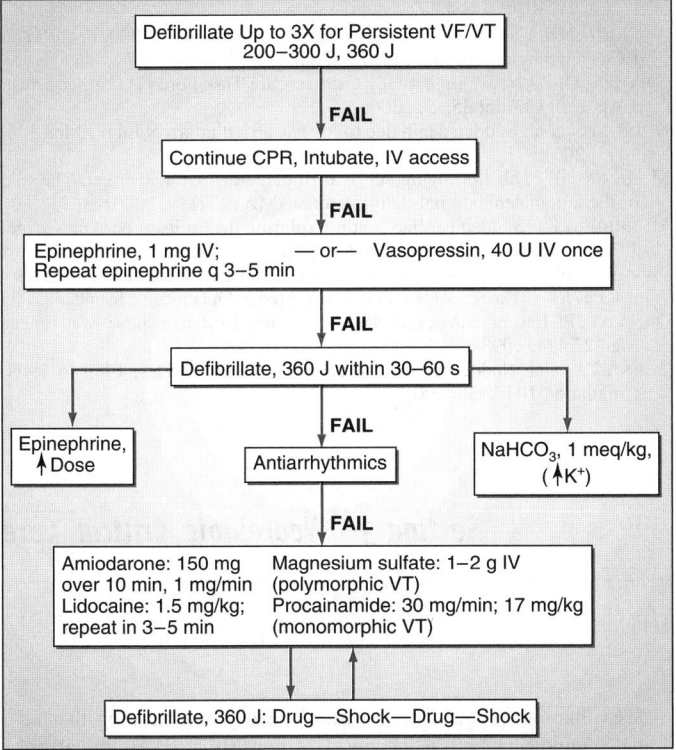

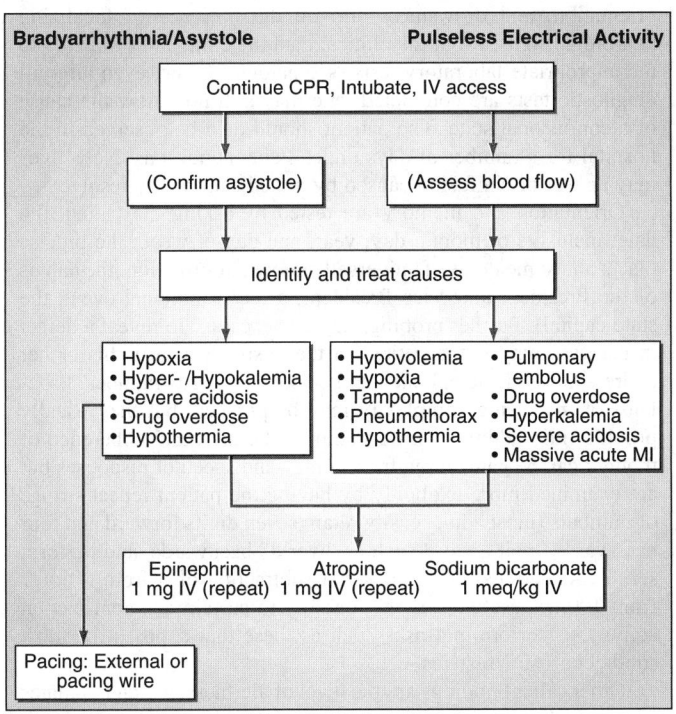

FIGURE 256-3 Management of cardiac arrest. *A.* The algorithm of ventricular fibrillation or hypotensive ventricular tachycardia begins with defibrillation attempts. If that fails, it is followed by epinephrine and then antiarrhythmic drugs. See text for details. *B.* The algorithms for bradyarrhythmia/asystole (left) or pulseless electrical activity (right) is dominated first by continued life support and a search for reversible causes. Subsequent therapy is nonspecific and accompanied by a low success rate. See text for details. CPR, cardiopulmonary resuscitation; MI, myocardial infarction.

cardiac arrest survivor is dictated by specific clinical circumstances. The most difficult is the presence of anoxic encephalopathy which is a strong predictor of in-hospital death. A recent addition to the management of this condition is induced hypothermia to reduce metabolic demands and cerebral edema.

The outcome after in-hospital cardiac arrest associated with non-cardiac diseases is poor, and in the few successfully resuscitated patients, the postresuscitation course is dominated by the nature of the underlying disease. Patients with cancer, renal failure, acute central nervous system disease, and uncontrolled infections, as a group, have a survival rate of less than 10% after in-hospital cardiac arrest. Some major exceptions are patients with transient airway obstruction, electrolyte disturbances, proarrhythmic effects of drugs, and severe metabolic abnormalities, most of whom may have an excellent chance of survival if they can be resuscitated promptly and maintained while the transient abnormalities are being corrected.

Long-Term Management after Survival of Out-of-Hospital Cardiac Arrest Patients who survive cardiac arrest without irreversible damage to the central nervous system, and who achieve hemodynamic stability, should have extensive diagnostic testing and appropriate therapeutic interventions for their long-term management. This aggressive approach is driven by the fact that survival after out-of-hospital cardiac arrest was followed by a 25 to 30% mortality rate during the first 2 years after the event, and there are data suggesting that significant reductions in risk can be achieved by appropriate therapy.

Among patients in whom an acute transmural MI is identified as the specific mechanism triggering an out-of-hospital cardiac arrest, the management is dictated in part by the known transient nature of life-threatening arrhythmia risk in the acute phase of MI, and in part by the extent of permanent myocardial damage that results. Several clinical trials have now documented an improved mortality among cardiac arrest survivors who have EFs < 40% and receive ICDs. It is not clear whether ICDs provide a benefit over aminodarone therapy when the EF is between 35 and 40% or >40%, but the data support the use of ICDs when the EF < 35%. Since is is usually not possible to determine whether the EF reduction was preexisting or a consequence of the MI, the cut-offs described are those generally used as ICD indications. Earlier studies had suggested that inducibility of ventricular arrhythmias during programmed electrical stimulation (E-P) studies in the electrophysiology laboratory could stratify risk prediction, but this is not universally used any longer for patients with low EFs, since even without inducible arrhythmias, the risk remains high enough to warrant ICDs in these cardiac arrest survivors.

For patients with cardiac arrest thought to be due to a transient ischemic mechanism, particularly with higher EFs, anti-ischemic therapy by pharmacologic or interventional methods is generally accepted as appropriate management. However, despite the absence of supportive clinical trial evidence, some adopt a more aggressive attitude about the use of ICDs in this group of cardiac arrest survivors as well, given the unpredictability of recurrent ischemia as a triggering mechanism.

The principles guiding therapy for patients with coronary artery disease who survive a cardiac arrest generally apply to the other cardiac disorders as well, with the exception that there is less focus on the extent of disease in certain disorders. Generally, cardiac arrest survivors from other categories of disease, such as the hypertrophic or dilated cardiomyopathies and various rare inherited disorders (e.g., RV dysplasia, long QT syndrome, Brugada syndrome, arrhythmic VF) are all considered ICD candidates.

PREVENTION OF SCD IN HIGH-RISK INDIVIDUALS WITHOUT PRIOR CARDIAC ARREST

Post-MI patients have been the subject of clinical trials for ICD benefit. It is now established that for post-MI patients with EFs < 40%, ambient ventricular arrhythmias, and inducible ventricular tachyarrhythmias in the electrophysiology laboratory, ICDs provide a significant reduction in relative risk of SCD and total mortality. Total mortality benefits in the range of a 20 to 30% reduction over 2 to 3 years have been observed, and ICD has emerged as preferred therapy for such patients. One study suggests that when the EF < 30%, electrophysiologic testing is not necessary to identify ICD benefit (see Chaps. 214 and 216).

Decision-making for primary prevention in disorders other than coronary artery disease is generally driven by observational data and judgment based on clinical observations. Controlled clinical trials providing evidence-based indicators for ICDs are lacking for these smaller population subgroups. In general, for both the cardiomyopathies and the rare disorders listed above, indicators of arrhythmic risk such as syncope, documented ventricular tachyarrhythmias, aborted cardiac arrest or perhaps a family history of SCD, and a number of other clinical or ECG markers, may be used as indicators for ICDs.

FURTHER READING

AMERICAN HEART ASSOCIATION: International Guidelines 2000 for CPR and ECC. Circulation 102(Suppl I):I-1, 2000

EWY GA, ORNATO JP: Emergency Cardiac Care Task Force 1: Cardiac arrest. J Am Coll Cardiol 35:832, 2000

HUIKURI H et al: Sudden death due to cardiac arrhythmias. N Engl J Med 345: 1473, 2001

MARENCO JP et al: Improving survival from sudden cardiac arrest: The role of the automated external defibrillator. JAMA 285:1193, 2001

MYERBURG RJ: Sudden cardiac death: Exploring the limits of our knowledge. J Cardiovasc Electrophysiol 12:369, 2001

———, CASTELLANOS A: Cardiac arrest and sudden cardiac death, in *Braunwald's Heart Disease*, 7th ed, D Zipes et al (eds). Philadelphia, Saunders, 2005

ORNATO JP: Use of adrenergic agonists during CPR in adults. Ann Emerg Med 22:411, 1993

ZHENG ZJ et al: Sudden cardiac death in the United States, 1989 to 1998. Circulation 104:2158, 2001

Section 3   Neurologic Critical Care

257   ACUTE CONFUSIONAL STATES AND COMA
Allan H. Ropper

Confusional states and coma are among the most common problems in general medicine. They account for a substantial portion of admissions to emergency wards and occur frequently on all hospital services. Because confusion and a diminished level of consciousness frequently coexist and are caused by many of the same diseases, they are presented together here, but from a medical perspective they have different clinical characteristics and physiologic explanations.

Almost all instances of diminished alertness can be traced to widespread abnormalities of the cerebral hemispheres or to reduced activity of a special thalamocortical alerting system termed the *reticular activating system* (RAS). The proper functioning of this system, its ascending projections to the cortex, and the cortex itself are required to maintain alertness and coherence of thought.

THE CONFUSIONAL STATE

Confusion is a mental and behavioral state of reduced comprehension, coherence, and capacity to reason. Inattention, as defined by the inability to sustain uninterrupted thought and actions, and disorientation are its earliest outward signs. As the state of confusion worsens, there are more global mental failings, including impairments of memory, perception, comprehension, problem solving, language, praxis, visuospatial function, and various aspects of emotional behavior that are attributable to particular regions of the brain. In some instances an apparent confusional state may be due to an isolated deficit in mental function such as an impairment of language (*aphasia*), loss of memory (*amnesia*), or lack of appreciation of spatial relations of self or the external environment (*agnosia*) (Chap. 23). Confusion is also a feature of dementia (Chap. 350), in which case the chronicity of the process distinguishes it from an acute encephalopathy.

The confused patient is usually subdued, not inclined to speak, and is physically inactive. A state of confusion that is accompanied by agitation, hallucinations, tremor, and illusions (misperceptions of environmental sight, sound, or touch) is termed *delirium*, as typified by delirium tremens from alcohol or drug withdrawal.

APPROACH TO THE PATIENT

Confusion and delirium always signify a disorder of the nervous system. They may be the major manifestations of a head injury; a seizure; drug toxicity (or drug withdrawal); a metabolic disorder resulting from hepatic, renal, pulmonary or cardiac failure; a systemic infection; meningitis or encephalitis; or a chronic dementing disease.

Evaluation begins with a careful history emphasizing the patient's condition before the onset of confusion. The clinical examination should focus on signs of diminished attentiveness, disorientation, and drowsiness and on the presence of localizing neurologic signs. From the clinical data the clinician is directed to the appropriate laboratory tests (see below.). Often, even after all diagnostic tests are completed, one may still not know the cause of a confusional state. The patient should then be observed in the hospital for a number of days under stable conditions. New clues may appear or confusion caused by a medication may resolve.

Orientation and memory are tested by asking the patient the date, inclusive of month, day, year, and day of week; the precise place; and some items of universally known information (the names of the President and Vice President, a recent national event, the state capital). Further probing may be necessary to reveal a defect in clarity—why is the patient in the hospital; what is his or her address, zip code, telephone number, social security number? Problems of increasing complexity may be pursued, but they usually provide little additional information. Attention and coherence of thought can be gauged by the accuracy and speed of responses but are examined more explicitly by having the patient repeat strings of numbers (most adults easily retain seven digits forward and four backward), spell a word such as "world" backwards, and perform serial calculations—tests of serial subtraction of 3 from 30 or 7 from 100 are useful. It is the inability to sustain coherent mental activity in performing tasks such as these that exposes the most subtle confusional states.

Other salient findings are the level of alertness, which fluctuates if there is drowsiness; indications of focal damage of the cerebrum such as hemiparesis, hemianopia, and aphasia; or adventitious movements of myoclonus or partial convulsions. The language of the confused patient may be disorganized and rambling, even to the extent of incorporating paraphasic words. These features, along with impaired comprehension that is due mainly to inattention, may be mistaken for aphasia.

One of the most specific signs of a metabolic encephalopathy is *asterixis*, which is an arrhythmic flapping tremor that is typically elicited by asking the patient to hold the arms outstretched with the wrists and hands fully extended. After a few seconds, there is a large jerking lapse in the posture of the hand and then a rapid return to the original position. The same movements can be found in any tonically held posture, even of the protruded tongue. Bilateral asterixis always signifies a metabolic encephalopathy, e.g., from hepatic failure, hypercapnia, or drug intoxication, especially with anticonvulsant medications. Myoclonic jerking and tremor are typical of uremic encephalopathy or exposure to antipsychotic drugs such as lithium, phenothiazines, or butyrophenones; myoclonus is also common with severe anoxic cerebral damage.

Confusion in the postoperative period, particularly after cardiac and extensive orthopedic procedures, is common but at times so subtle as to escape attention. Often a careful history will reveal that a mild but compensated dementia existed prior to the operation. Medications, particularly those with anticholinergic activity (including meperidine), inadvertent withdrawal from sleeping pills or alcohol, fever, and any of the endogenous metabolic derangements listed above may be responsible, or a stroke may have occurred. In many cases, particularly in the elderly, transient confusion and drowsiness arise with a febrile infection of the urinary tract, lungs, blood, or peritoneum. The term *septic encephalopathy* is used to describe this association, but the mechanism by which systemic infection leads to cerebral dysfunction is unknown.

Distinguishing dementia from an acute confusional state is a problem in the elderly. The two may coexist if an acute medical problem or a poorly tolerated medication supervenes in a mildly demented patient, producing a so-called beclouded dementia. The memory loss of dementia brings about a confusional state that varies little in severity from day to day. Poor mental performance in dementia is manifested primarily as incomplete recollection; inadequate access to names and words, and ideas; and the inability to retain new information, thus affecting orientation and factual knowledge. In contrast to the acute confusional states, attention, alertness, and coherence are preserved until the most advanced stages. Dementia in its advanced stages produces a chronic confusion with breakdown of all types of mental performance; the distinction from an acute encephalopathy then depends mainly on the longstanding nature of the condition.

Treatment of the confused patient requires that all unnecessary medication be stopped, metabolic alterations be rectified, and infection be treated. Skilled nursing and a quiet room with a window are important. Careful explanations should be given at regular intervals to the family. In the elderly, regular reorientation and active measures to lessen risk factors (sleep deprivation, immobility, and vision and hearing impairments) have been shown to reduce the number and severity of episodes of delirium in hospitalized patients.

COMA AND RELATED DISORDERS OF CONSCIOUSNESS

States of reduced alertness and responsiveness represent a continuum that in its severest form is called *coma*, a deep sleeplike state from which the patient cannot be aroused. *Stupor* refers to lesser degrees of unarousability in which the patient can be awakened only by vigorous stimuli, accompanied by motor behavior that leads to avoidance of uncomfortable or aggravating stimuli. *Drowsiness*, which is familiar to all persons, simulates light sleep and is characterized by easy arousal and the persistence of alertness for brief periods. Drowsiness and stupor are usually attended by some degree of confusion. A narrative description of the level of arousal and of the type of responses evoked by various stimuli precisely as observed at the bedside is preferable to ambiguous terms such as semicoma or obtundation.

Several other neurologic conditions render patients apparently unresponsive and simulate coma, and certain subsyndromes of coma must be considered separately because of their special significance. Among the latter, the *vegetative state* signifies an awake but unresponsive state. These patients have emerged from coma after a period of days or weeks to an unresponsive state in which the eyelids are open, giving the appearance of wakefulness. Yawning, coughing, swallowing, as well as limb and head movements persist, but there are few, if any, meaningful responses to the external and internal environment—in essence, an "awake coma." Respiratory and autonomic func-

tions are retained. The term "vegetative" is unfortunate as it is subject to misinterpretation by lay persons. There are always accompanying signs that indicate extensive damage in both cerebral hemispheres, e.g., decerebrate or decorticate limb posturing and absent responses to visual stimuli (see below). In the closely related *minimally conscious state* the patient may make intermittent rudimentary vocal or motor responses. Cardiac arrest and head injuries are the most common causes of the vegetative state (Chaps. 258 and 357). The prognosis for regaining mental faculties once the vegetative state has supervened for several months is almost nil, hence the term *persistent vegetative state*. Most reports of dramatic recovery, when investigated carefully, are found to yield to the usual rules for prognosis, but there have been rare instances of awakening to a demented condition.

Certain clinical states are prone to be misinterpreted as stupor or coma. *Akinetic mutism* refers to a partially or fully awake patient who is able to form impressions and think but remains immobile and mute, particularly when unstimulated. The condition results from damage in the regions of the medial thalamic nuclei, the frontal lobes (particularly situated deeply or on the orbitofrontal surfaces), or from hydrocephalus. The term *abulia* is used to describe a mental and physical slowness and diminished ability to initiate activity that is in essence a mild form of akinetic mutism, with the same anatomic origins. *Catatonia* is a curious hypomobile and mute syndrome associated with a major psychosis. In the typical form patients appear awake with eyes open but make no voluntary or responsive movements, although they blink spontaneously, swallow, and may not appear distressed. Often, the eyes are half-open as if the patient is in a fog or light sleep. There are signs that indicate the patient is responsive, though it may take some ingenuity on the part of the examiner to demonstrate these. For example, eyelid elevation is actively resisted, blinking occurs in response to a visual threat, and the eyes move concomitantly with head rotation, all of which are inconsistent with a brain lesion. It is characteristic but not invariable in catatonia for the limbs to retain the posture, no matter how bizarre, in which they have been placed by the examiner ("waxy flexibility," or catalepsy.) Upon recovery, such patients have some memory of events that occurred during their catatonic stupor. The appearance is superficially similar to akinetic mutism, but clinical evidence of cerebral damage is lacking.

The *locked-in state* describes a pseudocoma in which an awake patient has no means of producing speech or volitional movement in order to indicate that he is awake, but vertical eye movements and lid elevation remain unimpaired, thus allowing the patient to signal. Such individuals have written entire treatises using Morse code. Infarction or hemorrhage of the ventral pons, which transects all descending corticospinal and corticobulbar pathways, is the usual cause. A similar awake but de-efferented state occurs as a result of total paralysis of the musculature in severe cases of Guillain-Barré syndrome (Chap. 365), critical illness neuropathy (Chap. 258), and pharmacologic neuromuscular blockade.

THE ANATOMY AND PHYSIOLOGY OF UNCONSCIOUSNESS To the extent that all complex waking behaviors require the widespread participation of the cerebral cortex, consciousness cannot exist without the activity of this structure. The RAS, a loosely grouped aggregation of neurons located in the upper brainstem and medial thalamus, maintains the cerebral cortex in a state of wakeful consciousness. It follows that the principal causes of coma are (1) lesions that damage the RAS or its projections; (2) destruction of large portions of both cerebral hemispheres; and (3) suppression of reticulo-cerebral function by drugs, toxins, or metabolic derangements such as hypoglycemia, anoxia, azotemia, or hepatic failure.

The regions of the reticular formation that are critical to the maintenance of wakefulness extend from the caudal midbrain to the lower thalamus. The neurons of the RAS project rostrally to the cortex primarily via thalamic relay nuclei that in turn exert a tonic influence on the activity of the entire cerebral cortex. The behavioral arousal ef-

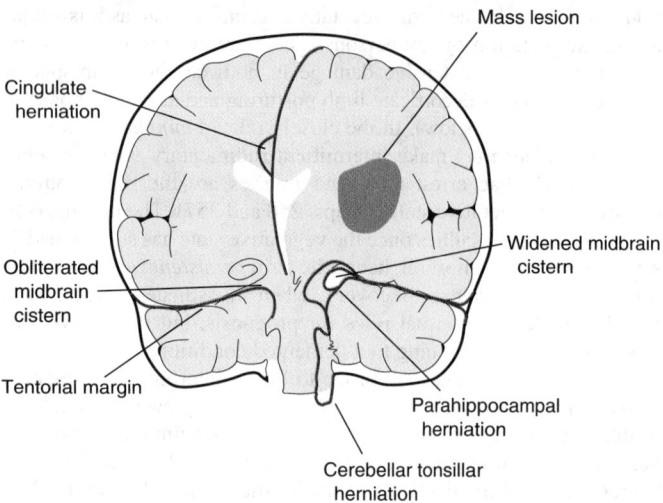

FIGURE 257-1   Types of cerebral herniation.

fected by somesthetic, auditory, and visual stimuli depends upon the rich reciprocal innervation that the RAS receives from these sensory systems. A most important practical consideration derives from the anatomic proximity of the RAS to structures that control pupillary function and eye movements. Pupillary enlargement and loss of vertical and adduction movements of the globes suggest that upper brainstem damage may be the source of coma.

Coma due to Cerebral Mass Lesions and Herniations   The cranial cavity is separated into compartments by infoldings of the dura—the two cerebral hemispheres are separated by the falx, and the anterior and posterior fossae by the tentorium. *Herniation* refers to displacement of brain tissue into a compartment that it normally does not occupy. Many of the signs associated with coma, and indeed coma itself, can be attributed to these tissue shifts (Fig. 257-1).

Uncal transtentorial herniation refers to impaction of the anterior medial temporal gyrus (the uncus) into the anterior portion of the tentorial opening. The displaced tissue compresses the third nerve as it traverses the subarachnoid space and results in enlargement of the ipsilateral pupil (putatively because the fibers subserving parasympathetic pupillary function are located peripherally in the nerve). The coma that follows may be due to lateral compression of the midbrain

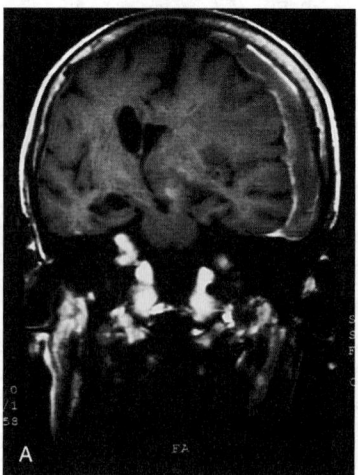
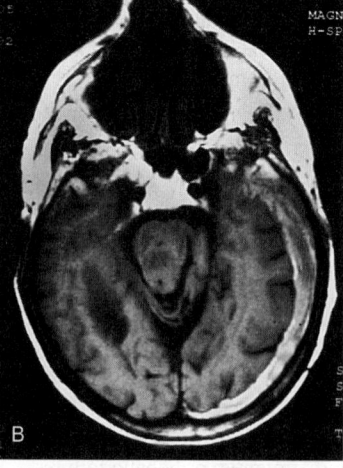

FIGURE 257-2   Coronal *(A)* and axial *(B)* magnetic resonance images from a stuporous patient with a left third nerve palsy as a result of a large left-sided subdural hematoma (seen as a gray-white rim). The upper midbrain and lower thalamic regions are compressed and displaced horizontally away from the mass, and there is transtentorial herniation of the medial temporal lobe structures, including the uncus anteriorly. The lateral ventricle opposite to the hematoma has become enlarged as a result of compression of the third ventricle.

against the opposite tentorial edge by the displaced parahippocampal gyrus (Fig. 257-2). In some cases the lateral displacement causes compression of the opposite cerebral peduncle, producing a Babinski response and hemiparesis contralateral to the original hemiparesis (the Kernohan-Woltman sign). In addition to compressing the upper brainstem, tissue shifts, including herniations, may compress major blood vessels, particularly the anterior and posterior cerebral arteries as they pass over the tentorial reflections, thus producing brain infarctions. The distortions may also entrap portions of the ventricular system, resulting in regional hydrocephalus.

Central transtentorial herniation denotes a symmetric downward movement of the upper thalamic region through the tentorial opening. Miotic pupils and drowsiness are the heralding signs. Both temporal and central herniations are thought to cause progressive compression of the brainstem from above: first the midbrain, then the pons, and finally the medulla. The result is a sequential appearance of neurologic signs that correspond to the affected level. Other forms of herniation are *transfalcial herniation* (displacement of the cingulate gyrus under the falx and across the midline), and *foraminal herniation* (downward forcing of the cerebellar tonsils into the foramen magnum).

A direct relationship between the various configurations of transtentorial herniations and coma is not always found. Displacement of deep brain structures by a mass in any direction, with or without herniation, is adequate to compress the region of the RAS and result in coma. Furthermore, drowsiness and stupor typically occur with moderate horizontal shifts at the level of the diencephalon (thalami) well before transtentorial or other herniations are evident. Lateral shift is easily quantified on axial images of computed tomography (CT) and magnetic resonance imaging (MRI) scans (Fig. 257-2). In cases of *acutely appearing masses*, a fairly consistent relationship exists between the degree of horizontal displacement of midline structures and the level of consciousness. Specifically, horizontal displacement of the pineal calcification of 3 to 5 mm is generally associated with drowsiness, 6 to 8 mm with stupor, and >9 mm with coma. At the same time, intrusion of the medial temporal lobe into the tentorial opening may be apparent on MRI and CT scan by an obliteration of the cisterns that surround the upper brainstem.

Coma and Confusional States due to Metabolic Disorders   Many systemic metabolic abnormalities cause coma by interrupting the delivery of energy substrates (hypoxia, ischemia, hypoglycemia) or by altering neuronal excitability (drug and alcohol intoxication, anesthesia, and epilepsy). The same metabolic abnormalities that produce coma may in milder form induce widespread cortical dysfunction and an acute confusional state. Thus, in metabolic encephalopathies, clouded consciousness and coma are in a continuum. Neuropathologic changes are variable—prominent in hypoxia-ischemia, evident as astrocytic changes in hepatic coma, and negligible in renal and other metabolic encephalopathies.

Cerebral neurons are fully dependent on cerebral blood flow (CBF) and the related delivery of oxygen and glucose. CBF approximates 75 mL per 100 g/min in gray matter and 30 mL per 100 g/min in white matter (mean = 55 mL per 100 g/min); oxygen consumption is 3.5 mL per 100 g/min, and glucose utilization is 5 mg per 100 g/min. Brain stores of glucose provide energy for approximately 2 min after blood flow is interrupted, and oxygen stores last 8 to 10 s after the cessation of blood flow. Simultaneous hypoxia and ischemia exhaust glucose more rapidly. The electroencephalogram (EEG) rhythm in these circumstances becomes diffusely slowed, typical of metabolic encephalopathies, and as conditions of substrate delivery worsen, eventually all recordable brain electrical activity ceases. In almost all instances of metabolic encephalopathy, the global metabolic activity of the brain is reduced in proportion to the degree of unconsciousness.

Conditions such as hypoglycemia, hyponatremia, hyperosmolarity, hypercapnia, hypercalcemia, and hepatic and renal failure are associated with a variety of alterations in neurons and astrocytes. The reversible effects of these conditions on the brain are not understood, but may result from impaired energy supplies, changes in ion fluxes across neuronal membranes, and neurotransmitter abnormalities. For example, the high brain ammonia concentration of hepatic coma interferes with cerebral energy metabolism and with the Na^+, K^+-ATPase pump, increases the number and size of astrocytes, alters nerve cell function, and causes increased concentrations of potentially toxic products of ammonia metabolism; it may also result in abnormalities of neurotransmitters, including putative "false" neurotransmitters that are active at receptor sites. Apart from hyperammonemia, which of these mechanisms is of critical importance is not clear. The mechanism of the encephalopathy of renal failure is also not known. Unlike ammonia, urea itself does not produce central nervous system (CNS) toxicity. A multifactorial causation has been proposed, including increased permeability of the blood-brain barrier to toxic substances such as organic acids and an increase in brain calcium or cerebrospinal fluid (CSF) phosphate content.

Coma and seizures are a common accompaniment of any large shifts in sodium and water balance. These changes in osmolarity arise from systemic medical disorders including diabetic ketoacidosis, the nonketotic hyperosmolar state, and hyponatremia from any cause (e.g., water intoxication, excessive secretion of antidiuretic hormone or atrial natriuretic peptides). The volume of brain water correlates with the level of consciousness in these states, but other factors also play a role. Sodium levels below 125 mmol/L induce confusion, and below 115 mmol/L are associated with coma and convulsions. In hyperosmolar coma the serum osmolarity generally exceeds 350 mosmol/L. *As in most other metabolic encephalopathies, the severity of neurologic change depends to a large degree on the rapidity with which the serum changes occur.* Hypercapnia depresses the level of consciousness in proportion to the rise in CO_2 tension in the blood; the level of consciousness also depends on the rapidity of change. The pathophysiology of other metabolic encephalopathies such as hypercalcemia, hypothyroidism, vitamin B_{12} deficiency, and hypothermia are incompletely understood but must also reflect derangements of CNS biochemistry and membrane function.

Epileptic Coma   Continuous, generalized electrical discharges of the cortex (*seizures*) are associated with coma even in the absence of epileptic motor activity (*convulsions*). The self-limited coma that follows seizures, termed the *postictal state*, may be due to exhaustion of energy reserves or effects of locally toxic molecules that are the byproduct of seizures. The postictal state produces a pattern of continuous, generalized slowing of the background EEG activity similar to that of other metabolic encephalopathies.

Pharmacologic Coma   This class of encephalopathy is in large measure reversible and leaves no residual damage providing hypoxia does not supervene. Many drugs and toxins are capable of depressing nervous system function. Some produce coma by affecting both the brainstem nuclei, including the RAS, and the cerebral cortex. The combination of cortical and brainstem signs, which occurs in certain drug overdoses, may lead to an incorrect diagnosis of structural brainstem disease.

APPROACH TO THE PATIENT

Acute respiratory and cardiovascular problems should be attended to prior to neurologic assessment. In most instances, a complete medical evaluation, except for vital signs, funduscopy, and examination for nuchal rigidity, may be deferred until the neurologic evaluation has established the severity and nature of coma. →*The approach to the patient with trauma is discussed in Chap. 357.*

History   In many cases, the cause of coma is immediately evident (e.g., trauma, cardiac arrest, or known drug ingestion). In the remainder, certain points are especially useful: (1) the circumstances and rapidity with which neurologic symptoms developed; (2) the antecedent symptoms (confusion, weakness, headache, fever, seizures, dizziness, double vision, or vomiting); (3) the use of medications, illicit drugs, or alcohol; and (4) chronic liver, kidney, lung, heart, or other medical disease. Direct interrogation or telephone calls to family and observers on the scene are an important part of the initial evaluation. Ambulance technicians often provide the most useful information.

General Physical Examination   The temperature, pulse, respiratory rate and pattern, and blood pressure should be measured quickly. Fever suggests a systemic infection, bacterial meningitis, or encephalitis; only rarely is it attributable to a brain lesion that has disturbed temperature-regulating centers. A slight elevation in temperature may follow vigorous convulsions. High body temperature, 42 to 44°C, associated with dry skin should arouse the suspicion of heat stroke or anticholinergic drug intoxication. Hypothermia is observed with alcoholic, barbiturate, sedative, or phenothiazine intoxication; hypoglycemia; peripheral circulatory failure; or hypothyroidism. Hypothermia itself causes coma only when the temperature is <31°C. Tachypnea may indicate acidosis or pneumonia. Aberrant respiratory patterns that reflect brainstem disorders are discussed below. Marked hypertension indicates hypertensive encephalopathy or a rapid rise in intracranial pressure (ICP) and may occur acutely after head injury. Hypotension is characteristic of coma from alcohol or barbiturate intoxication, internal hemorrhage, myocardial infarction, sepsis, profound hypothyroidism, or Addisonian crisis. The funduscopic examination can detect subarachnoid hemorrhage (subhyaloid hemorrhages), hypertensive encephalopathy (exudates, hemorrhages, vessel-crossing changes, papilledema), and increased ICP (papilledema). Petechiae suggest thrombotic thrombocytopenic purpura, meningococcemia, or a bleeding diathesis from which an intracerebral hemorrhage arises.

Neurologic Assessment   First, the patient should be observed without intervention by the examiner. Patients who toss about, reach up toward the face, cross their legs, yawn, swallow, cough, or moan are close to being awake. Lack of restless movements on one side or an outturned leg suggests a hemiplegia. Intermittent twitching movements of a foot, finger, or facial muscle may be the only sign of seizures. Multifocal myoclonus almost always indicates a metabolic disorder, particularly uremia, anoxia, or drug intoxication (lithium and haloperidol are particularly likely to cause this sign), or the rarer conditions of spongiform encephalopathy and Hashimoto disease. In a drowsy and confused patient bilateral asterixis is a certain sign of metabolic encephalopathy or drug intoxication.

The terms *decorticate rigidity* and *decerebrate rigidity*, or "posturing," describe stereotyped arm and leg movements occurring spontaneously or elicited by sensory stimulation. Flexion of the elbows and wrists and supination of the arm (decortication) suggests bilateral damage rostral to the midbrain, whereas extension of the elbows and wrists with pronation (decerebration) indicates damage to motor tracts in the midbrain or caudal diencephalon. The less frequent combination of arm extension with leg flexion or flaccid legs is associated with lesions in the pons. These concepts have been adapted from animal work and cannot be applied with the same precision to coma in humans. In fact, acute and widespread cerebral disorders of any type, regardless of location, frequently cause limb extension, and almost all such extensor posturing becomes predominantly flexor as time passes. Posturing may also be unilateral and may coexist with purposeful limb movements, usually reflecting incomplete damage to the motor system.

Level of Arousal and Elicited Movements   If the patient is not aroused by a conversational volume of voice, a sequence of increasingly intense stimuli is used to determine the threshold for arousal and the optimal motor response of each side of the body. The results of testing may vary from minute to minute and serial examinations are most useful. Tickling the nostrils with a cotton wisp is a moderate stimulus to arousal—all but deeply stuporous and comatose patients will move the head away and rouse to some degree. Using the hand to remove the offending stimulus represents an even greater degree of responsiveness.

Responses to noxious stimuli should be appraised critically. Stereotyped posturing indicates severe dysfunction of the corticospinal system. Abduction-avoidance movement of a limb is usually purposeful and denotes an intact corticospinal system. Pressure on the knuckles or bony prominences and pinprick are humane forms of noxious stimuli; pinching the skin causes unsightly ecchymoses and is generally not necessary but may be useful in eliciting abduction withdrawal movements of the limbs.

Brainstem Reflexes   Assessment of brainstem function is essential to localization of the lesion in coma (Fig. 257-3). The brainstem reflexes that are conveniently examined are pupillary responses to light, spontaneous and elicited eye movements, corneal responses, and the respiratory pattern. As a rule, when these brainstem activities are preserved, particularly the pupil reactions and eye movements, coma must be ascribed to bilateral hemispheral disease. The converse, however, is not always true as a mass in the hemispheres may be the underlying cause of coma but nonetheless produce brainstem signs.

PUPILS   Pupillary reactions are examined with a bright, diffuse light (not an ophthalmoscope); if the response is absent, this should be confirmed by observation through a magnifying lens. Normally reactive and round pupils of midsize (2.5 to 5 mm) essentially exclude midbrain damage, either primary or secondary to compression. Reaction to light is often difficult to appreciate in pupils <2 mm in diameter, and bright room lighting mutes pupillary reactivity. One unreactive and enlarged pupil (>6 mm) or one that is poorly reactive signifies a compression or stretching of the third nerve from the effects of a mass above. Enlargement of the pupil contralateral to a mass may occur first but is infrequent. An oval and slightly eccentric pupil is a transitional sign that accompanies early midbrain–third nerve compression. The most extreme pupillary sign, bilaterally dilated and unreactive pupils, indicates severe midbrain damage, usually from compression by a mass. Ingestion of drugs with anticholinergic activity, the use of mydriatic eye drops, and direct ocular trauma are among the causes of misleading pupillary enlargement.

Unilateral miosis in coma has been attributed to dysfunction of sympathetic efferents originating in the posterior hypothalamus and descending in the tegmentum of the brainstem to the cervical cord. It is an occasional finding with a large cerebral hemorrhage that affects the thalamus. Reactive and bilaterally small (1 to 2.5 mm) but not pinpoint pupils are seen in metabolic encephalopathies or in deep bilateral hemispheral lesions such as hydrocephalus or thalamic hemorrhage. Very small but reactive pupils (<1 mm) characterize narcotic or barbiturate overdoses but also occur with extensive pontine hemorrhage. The response to naloxone and the presence of reflex eye movements (see below) distinguish these.

OCULAR MOVEMENTS   The eyes are first observed by elevating the lids and noting the resting position and spontaneous movements of the globes. Lid tone, tested by lifting the eyelids and noting their resistance to opening and the speed of closure, is reduced progressively as coma deepens. Horizontal divergence of the eyes at rest is normal in drowsiness. As coma deepens, the ocular axes may become parallel again.

Spontaneous eye movements in coma often take the form of conjugate horizontal roving. This finding alone exonerates the midbrain and pons and has the same significance as normal reflex eye movements (see below). Conjugate horizontal ocular deviation to one side indicates damage to the pons on the opposite side or a lesion in the frontal lobe on the same side. This phenomenon may

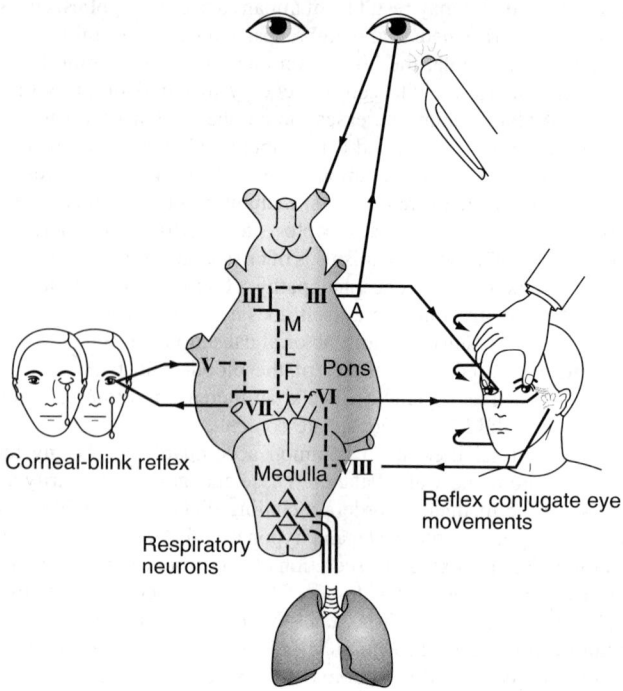

FIGURE 257-3   Examination of brainstem reflexes in coma. Midbrain and third nerve function are tested by pupillary reaction to light, pontine function by spontaneous and reflex eye movements and corneal responses, and medullary function by respiratory and pharyngeal responses. Reflex conjugate, horizontal eye movements are dependent on the medial longitudinal fasciculus (MLF) interconnecting the sixth and contralateral third nerve nuclei. Head rotation (oculocephalic reflex) or caloric stimulation of the labyrinths (oculovestibular reflex) elicits contraversive eye movements (for details see text).

be summarized by the following maxim: *The eyes look toward a hemispheral lesion and away from a brainstem lesion.* Seizures also drive the eyes to one side. On rare occasions, the eyes may turn paradoxically away from the side of a deep hemispheral lesion ("wrong-way eyes"). The eyes turn down and inward as a result of thalamic and upper midbrain lesions, typically with thalamic hemorrhage. "Ocular bobbing" describes a brisk downward and slow upward movement of the eyes associated with loss of horizontal eye movements and is diagnostic of bilateral pontine damage, usually from thrombosis of the basilar artery. "Ocular dipping" is a slower, arrhythmic downward movement followed by a faster upward movement in patients with normal reflex horizontal gaze; it indicates diffuse cortical anoxic damage. Many other complex eye movements are known but do not have the same significance as the ones already mentioned.

The oculocephalic reflexes depend on the integrity of the ocular motor nuclei and their interconnecting tracts that extend from the midbrain to the pons and medulla. These reflexes are elicited by moving the head from side to side or vertically and observing evoked eye movements in the direction opposite to the head movement (Fig. 257-3). These movements, called somewhat inappropriately "doll's eyes" (which refers more accurately to the reflex elevation of the eyelids with flexion of the neck), are normally suppressed in the awake patient by visual fixation. Their presence therefore indicates a reduced cortical influence on the brainstem. Furthermore, preservation of evoked reflex eye movements signifies the integrity of the brainstem and, by implication, that the origin of unconsciousness lies in the cerebral hemispheres. The opposite—the absence of reflex eye movements—signifies damage within the brainstem but can be produced infrequently by profound overdoses of certain drugs. Normal pupillary size and light reaction distinguishes most drug-induced comas from structural brainstem damage.

Thermal, or "caloric," stimulation of the vestibular apparatus (oculovestibular response) provides a more intense stimulus for the oculocephalic reflex but gives fundamentally the same information. The test is performed by irrigating the external auditory canal with cool water in order to induce convection currents in the labyrinths. After a brief latency, the result is tonic deviation of both eyes to the side of cool-water irrigation and nystagmus in the opposite direction. (The acronym "COWS" has been used to remind generations of medical students of the direction of nystagmus—"cold water opposite, warm water same"). The absence of nystagmus despite conjugate deviation of the globes signifies that the cerebral hemispheres are damaged or suppressed. The loss of conjugate ocular movements indicates brainstem damage.

By touching the cornea with a wisp of cotton, a response consisting of brief bilateral lid closure is normally observed. The corneal reflexes depend on the integrity of pontine pathways between the fifth (afferent) and both seventh (efferent) cranial nerves; although rarely useful alone, in conjunction with reflex eye movements they are important clinical tests of pontine function. CNS depressant drugs diminish or eliminate the corneal responses soon after reflex eye movements are paralyzed but before the pupils become unreactive to light. The corneal (and pharyngeal) response may be lost for a time on the side of an acute hemiplegia.

RESPIRATION Respiratory patterns are of less localizing value in comparison to other brainstem signs. Shallow, slow, but regular breathing suggests metabolic or drug depression. Cheyne-Stokes respiration in its classic cyclic form, ending with a brief apneic period, signifies bihemispheral damage or metabolic suppression and commonly accompanies light coma. Rapid, deep (Kussmaul) breathing usually implies metabolic acidosis but may also occur with pontomesencephalic lesions. Agonal gasps reflect bilateral lower brainstem damage and are well known as the terminal respiratory pattern of severe brain damage. A number of other cyclic breathing variations are of lesser significance.

LABORATORY STUDIES AND IMAGING The studies that are most useful in the diagnosis of confusional states and coma are: chemical-toxicologic analysis of blood and urine, cranial CT or MRI, EEG, and CSF examination. Arterial blood-gas analysis is helpful in patients with lung disease and acid-base disorders. The metabolic aberrations commonly encountered in clinical practice require measurements of electrolytes, glucose, calcium, osmolarity, and renal (blood urea nitrogen) and hepatic (NH_3) function. Toxicologic analysis is necessary in any case of coma where the diagnosis is not immediately clear. However, the presence of exogenous drugs or toxins, especially alcohol, does not exclude the possibility that other factors, particularly head trauma, are also contributing to the clinical state. An ethanol level of 43 mmol/L (200 mg/dL) in nonhabituated patients generally causes impaired mental activity and of >65 mmol/L (300 mg/dL) is associated with stupor. The development of tolerance may allow the chronic alcoholic to remain awake at levels >87 mmol/L (400 mg/dL).

The availability of CT and MRI has focused attention on causes of coma that are radiologically detectable (e.g., hemorrhages, tumors, or hydrocephalus). Resorting primarily to this approach, although at times expedient, is imprudent because most cases of coma (and confusion) are metabolic or toxic in origin. The notion that a normal CT scan excludes anatomic lesions as the cause of coma is also erroneous. Bilateral hemisphere infarction, small brainstem lesions, encephalitis, meningitis, mechanical shearing of axons as a result of closed head trauma, sagittal sinus thrombosis, and subdural hematomas that are isodense to adjacent brain are some of the disorders that may not be detected. Nevertheless, if the source of coma remains unknown, a scan should be obtained.

The EEG is useful in metabolic or drug-induced confusional states but is rarely diagnostic, except when coma is due to clinically unrecognized seizures, to herpesvirus encephalitis, or to Creutzfeldt-Jakob disease. The amount of background slowing of the EEG is a reflection of the severity of any diffuse encephalopathy. Predominant high-voltage slowing (δ or triphasic waves) in the frontal regions is typical of metabolic coma, as from hepatic failure, and widespread fast (β) activity implicates sedative drugs (e.g., diazepines, barbiturates). A special pattern of "α coma," defined by widespread, variable 8- to 12-Hz activity, superficially resembles the normal α rhythm of waking but is unresponsive to environmental stimuli. It results from pontine or diffuse cortical damage and is associated with a poor prognosis. Most importantly, EEG recordings may reveal clinically inapparent epileptic discharges in a patient with coma. Normal α activity on the EEG also alerts the clinician to the locked-in syndrome or to hysteria or catatonia.

Lumbar puncture is performed less frequently than in the past because neuroimaging scans effectively exclude intracerebral and subarachnoid hemorrhages that are severe enough to cause coma. However, examination of the CSF is indispensable in the diagnosis of meningitis and encephalitis. Lumbar puncture should therefore not be deferred if meningitis is a possibility.

DIFFERENTIAL DIAGNOSIS OF COMA (Table 257-1) The causes of coma can be conceptualized in three broad categories: those without focal neurologic signs (e.g., metabolic encephalopathies); meningitis syndromes, characterized by fever or stiff neck and an excess of cells in the spinal fluid (e.g., bacterial meningitis, subarachnoid hemorrhage);

TABLE 257-1 *Differential Diagnosis of Coma*

1. Diseases that cause no focal or lateralizing neurologic signs, usually with normal brainstem functions; CT scan and cellular content of the CSF are normal
   a. Intoxications: alcohol, sedative drugs, opiates, etc.
   b. Metabolic disturbances: anoxia, hyponatremia, hypernatremia, hypercalcemia, diabetic acidosis, nonketotic hyperosmolar hyperglycemia, hypoglycemia, uremia, hepatic coma, hypercarbia, addisonian crisis, hypo- and hyperthyroid states, profound nutritional deficiency
   c. Severe systemic infections: pneumonia, septicemia, typhoid fever, malaria, Waterhouse-Friderichsen syndrome
   d. Shock from any cause
   e. Postseizure states, status epilepticus, subclinical epilepsy
   f. Hypertensive encephalopathy, eclampsia
   g. Severe hyperthermia, hypothermia
   h. Concussion
   i. Acute hydrocephalus
2. Diseases that cause meningeal irritation with or without fever, and with an excess of WBCs or RBCs in the CSF, usually without focal or lateralizing cerebral or brainstem signs; CT or MRI shows no mass lesion
   a. Subarachnoid hemorrhage from ruptured aneurysm, arteriovenous malformation, trauma
   b. Acute bacterial meningitis
   c. Viral encephalitis
   d. Miscellaneous: Fat embolism, cholesterol embolism, carcinomatous and lymphomatous meningitis, etc.
3. Diseases that cause focal brainstem or lateralizing cerebral signs, with or without changes in the CSF; CT and MRI are abnormal
   a. Hemispheral hemorrhage (basal ganglionic, thalamic) or infarction (large middle cerebral artery territory) with secondary brainstem compression
   b. Brainstem infarction due to basilar artery thrombosis or embolism
   c. Brain abscess, subdural empyema
   d. Epidural and subdural hemorrhage, brain contusion
   e. Brain tumor with surrounding edema
   f. Cerebellar and pontine hemorrhage and infarction
   g. Widespread traumatic brain injury
   h. Metabolic coma (see above) with preexisting focal damage
   i. Miscellaneous: cortical vein thrombosis, herpes simplex encephalitis, multiple cerebral emboli due to bacterial endocarditis, acute hemorrhagic leukoencephalitis, acute disseminated (postinfectious) encephalomyelitis, thrombotic thrombocytopenic purpura, cerebral vasculitis, gliomatosis cerebri, pituitary apoplexy, intravascular lymphoma, etc.

Note: CT, computed tomography; CSF, cerebrospinal fluid; WBCs, white blood cells; RBCs, red blood cells; MRI, magnetic resonance imaging.

and those with prominent focal signs (e.g., stroke, cerebral hemorrhage). In most instances confusion and coma are part of an obvious medical problem such as drug ingestion, hypoxia, stroke, trauma, or liver or kidney failure. Conditions that cause sudden coma include drug ingestion, cerebral hemorrhage, trauma, cardiac arrest, epilepsy, or basilar artery embolism. Coma that appears subacutely is usually related to a preceding medical or neurologic problem, including the secondary brain swelling of a mass lesion such as tumor or cerebral infarction.

Cerebrovascular diseases cause the greatest difficulty in coma diagnosis (Chap. 349). These may be summarized as follows: (1) basal ganglia and thalamic hemorrhage (acute but not instantaneous onset, vomiting, headache, hemiplegia, and characteristic eye signs); (2) pontine hemorrhage (sudden onset, pinpoint pupils, loss of reflex eye movements and corneal responses, ocular bobbing, posturing, hyperventilation, and excessive sweating); (3) cerebellar hemorrhage (occipital headache, vomiting, gaze paresis, and inability to stand); (4) basilar artery thrombosis (neurologic prodrome or warning spells, diplopia, dysarthria, vomiting, eye movement and corneal response abnormalities, and asymmetric limb paresis); and (5) subarachnoid hemorrhage (precipitous coma after headache and vomiting). The most common stroke, infarction in the territory of the middle cerebral artery, does not cause coma, but edema surrounding large infarcts may expand during the first few days and act as a mass. The syndrome of acute hydrocephalus accompanies many intracranial diseases, particularly subarachnoid hemorrhage. It is characterized by headache and sometimes vomiting that may progress quickly to coma, with extensor posturing of the limbs, bilateral Babinski signs, small nonreactive pupils, and impaired oculocephalic movements in the vertical direction.

If the history and examination do not indicate the cause of coma, then information obtained from CT or MRI may be needed. As mentioned earlier, the majority of medical causes of coma can be established without a neuroimaging study.

BRAIN DEATH   This is a state in which there has been cessation of cerebral blood flow; as a result there is global loss of brain function while respiration is maintained by artificial means and the heart continues to pump. It is the only type of brain damage that is recognized as equivalent to death. Many roughly equivalent criteria have been advanced for the diagnosis of brain death, and it is essential to adhere to those standards endorsed by the local medical community. Ideal criteria are simple, can be conducted at the bedside, and allow no chance of diagnostic error. They contain three essential elements: (1) widespread cortical destruction shown by deep coma—unresponsiveness to all forms of stimulation; (2) global brainstem damage demonstrated by absent pupillary light reaction and the loss of oculovestibular and corneal reflexes; and (3) destruction of the medulla manifested by complete apnea. The pulse rate is invariant and unresponsive to atropine. Diabetes insipidus is often present, but may develop hours or days after the other clinical signs of brain death. The pupils are often enlarged but may be mid-sized; they should not be constricted. The absence of deep tendon reflexes is not required because the spinal cord remains functional.

Demonstration that apnea is due to irreversible medullary damage requires that the P_{CO_2} be high enough to stimulate respiration during a test of spontaneous breathing (apnea test). This can be done safely by the use, prior to removing the ventilator, of diffusion oxygenation. This is accomplished by preoxygenation with 100% oxygen, which is then sustained during the test by oxygen administered through a tracheal cannula. CO_2 tension increases approximately 0.3 to 0.4 kPa/min (2 to 3 mmHg/min) during apnea. At the end of the period of observation, typically several minutes in duration, arterial P_{CO_2} should be at least >6.6 to 8.0 kPa (50 to 60 mmHg) for the test to be valid. Complete apnea is considered to be present if no respiratory effort is observed in the presence of a sufficiently elevated P_{CO_2}.

The possibility of profound drug-induced or hypothermic depression of the nervous system should be excluded, and some period of observation, usually 6 to 24 h, is desirable during which this state is shown to be sustained. It is particularly advisable to delay clinical testing for at least 24 h if a cardiac arrest has caused brain death or if the inciting disease is not known. An isoelectric EEG may be used as a confirmatory test for total cerebral damage but is not absolutely necessary. Radionuclide brain scanning, cerebral angiography, or transcranial Doppler measurements may also be used to demonstrate the absence of cerebral blood flow but they have not been extensively correlated with pathologic changes.

There is no compelling reason to embark on the demonstration of brain death except when organ transplantation is involved. Although it is largely accepted in western society that the respirator can be disconnected from a brain-dead patient, problems frequently arise because of poor communication and inadequate preparation of the family by the physician. Reasonable medical practice allows the removal of support or transfer out of an intensive care unit of patients who are not brain dead but whose condition is nonetheless hopeless and are likely to live for only a brief time.

℞ TREATMENT

The immediate goal is prevention of further nervous system damage. Hypotension, hypoglycemia, hypercalcemia, hypoxia, hypercapnia, and hyperthermia should be corrected rapidly. An oropharyngeal airway is adequate to keep the pharynx open in drowsy patients who are breathing normally. Tracheal intubation is indicated if there is apnea, upper airway obstruction, hypoventilation, or emesis, or if the patient is liable to aspirate because of coma. Mechanical ventilation is required if there is hypoventilation or a need to induce hypocapnia in order to lower ICP as described below. Intravenous access is established, and naloxone and dextrose are administered if narcotic overdose or hypoglycemia are even remote possibilities; thiamine is given along with glucose to avoid provoking Wernicke disease in malnourished patients. In cases of suspected basilar thrombosis with brainstem ischemia, intravenous heparin or a thrombolytic agent is often utilized, after cerebral hemorrhage is excluded by a neuroimaging study. Physostigmine may awaken patients with anticholinergic-type drug overdose, but must be used only by experienced physicians and with careful monitoring; many physicians believe that it should only be used to treat anticholinergic overdose–associated cardiac arrhythmias. The use of benzodiazepine antagonists offers some prospect of improvement after overdoses of soporific drugs and has transient benefit in hepatic encephalopathy. Intravenous administration of hypotonic solutions should be monitored carefully in any serious acute brain illness because of the potential for exacerbating brain swelling. Cervical spine injuries must not be overlooked, particularly prior to attempting intubation or evaluating of oculocephalic responses. Headache accompanied by fever and meningismus indicates an urgent need for examination of the CSF to diagnose meningitis. If the lumbar puncture in a case of suspected meningitis is delayed for any reason, an antibiotic such as a third-generation cephalosporin should be administered as soon as possible, preferably after obtaining blood cultures. The management of raised ICP is discussed in Chap. 258.

PROGNOSIS   The prediction of the outcome of coma must be considered in reference to long-term care and medical resources. One hopes to avoid the emotionally painful, hopeless outcome of a patient who is left severely disabled or vegetative. The uniformly pessimistic outcome of the persistent vegetative state has already been mentioned. Children and young adults may have ominous early clinical findings such as abnormal brainstem reflexes and yet recover, so that temporization in offering a prognosis in this group of patients is wise. Metabolic comas have a far better prognosis than traumatic comas. All schemes for prognosis in adults should be taken as approximations, and medical judgments must be tempered by factors such as age, underlying systemic disease, and general medical condition. In an attempt to collect prognostic information from large numbers of patients with head injury, the Glasgow Coma Scale was devised; empirically it has predictive value in cases of brain trauma (Chap. 357). For anoxic and metabolic coma, clinical signs such as the pupillary and motor responses after 1 day, 3 days, and 1 week have been shown to have predictive value (Chap. 258). The absence of the cortical waves of the somatosensory evoked potentials has also proved a strong indicator of poor outcome in coma from any cause.

FURTHER READING

PARVIZI J, DAMASIO AR: Neuroanatomical correlates of brainstem coma. Brain 126:1524, 2003

ROPPER AH: *Neurological and Neurosurgical Intensive Care*, 4th ed. New York, Lippincott, Williams & Wilkins, 2004

258 | CRITICAL CARE NEUROLOGY
J. Claude Hemphill

Life-threatening neurologic illness may be caused by a primary disorder affecting any region of the neuroaxis or may occur as a consequence of a systemic disorder such as hepatic failure, multisystem organ failure, or cardiac arrest (Table 258-1). Neurologic critical care focuses on preservation of neurologic tissue and prevention of secondary brain injury caused by ischemia, edema, and elevated intracranial pressure (ICP).

PATHOPHYSIOLOGY ■ Brain Edema

Swelling, or edema, of brain tissue occurs with many types of brain injury. The two principal types of edema are vasogenic and cytotoxic. *Vasogenic edema* refers to the influx of fluid and solutes into the brain through an incompetent blood-brain barrier (BBB). In the normal cerebral vasculature, endothelial tight junctions associated with astrocytes create an impermeable barrier (the BBB), through which access into the brain interstitium is dependent upon specific transport mechanisms (Chap. 345). The BBB may be compromised in ischemia, trauma, infection, and metabolic derangements. Typically, vasogenic edema develops rapidly following injury. *Cytotoxic edema* refers to cellular swelling and occurs in a variety of settings including brain ischemia and trauma. Early astrocytic swelling is a hallmark of ischemia. Brain edema that is clinically significant usually represents a combination of vasogenic and cellular components. Edema can lead to increased ICP as well as tissue shifts and brain displacement from focal processes. These tissue shifts can cause injury by mechanical distraction and compression in addition to the ischemia of impaired perfusion consequent to the elevated ICP.

Ischemic Cascade and Cellular Injury

When delivery of substrates, principally oxygen and glucose, is inadequate to sustain cellular function, a series of interrelated biochemical reactions known as the *ischemic cascade* is initiated. The release of excitatory amino acids, especially glutamate, leads to influx of calcium and sodium ions, which disrupt cellular homeostasis. An increased intracellular calcium concentration may activate proteases and lipases, which then lead to lipid peroxidation and free radical–mediated cell membrane injury. Cytoxic edema ensues, and ultimately necrotic cell death and tissue infarction occur. This pathway to irreversible cell death is common to ischemic stroke, global cerebral ischemia, and traumatic brain injury. *Penumbra* refers to ischemic brain tissue that has not yet undergone irreversible infarction, implying that the region is potentially salvagable if ischemia can be reversed. Factors that may exacerbate ischemic

TABLE 258-1 *Neurologic Disorders in Critical Illness*

Localization Along Neuroaxis	Syndrome
CENTRAL NERVOUS SYSTEM	
Brain: Cerebral hemispheres	Global encephalopathy
	Sepsis
	Organ failure—hepatic, renal
	Medication related
	Sedatives/hypnotics/analgesics
	H_2 blockers, antihypertensives
	Drug overdose
	Electrolyte disturbance—hyponatremia; hypoglycemia
	Hypotension/hypoperfusion
	Hypoxia
	Meningitis
	Subarachnoid hemorrhage
	Wernicke's disease
	Seizure—postictal or nonconvulsive status
	Hypertensive encephalopathy
	Hypothyroidism—myxedema
	Focal deficits
	Ischemic stroke
	Tumor
	Abscess, subdural empyema
	Subdural/epidural hematoma
Brainstem	Mass effect and compression
	Ischemic stroke, intraparenchymal hemorrhage
	Hypoxia
Spinal cord	Mass effect and compression
	Disc herniation
	Epidural hematoma
	Ischemia—hypotension/embolic
	Subdural empyema
	Trauma, central cord syndrome
PERIPHERAL NERVOUS SYSTEM	
Peripheral nerve	
Axonal	Critical illness polyneuropathy
	Possible neuromuscular blocking agent complication
	Metabolic disturbances, uremia—hyperglycemia
	Medication effects—chemotherapeutic, antiretroviral
Demyelinating	Guillian-Barré syndrome
	Chronic inflammatory demyelinating polyneuropathy
Neuromuscular junction	Prolonged effect of neuromuscular blockade
	Medication effects—aminoglycosides
	Myasthenia-gravis, Lambert-Eaton syndrome
Muscle	Septic myopathy
	Cachectic myopathy—with or without disuse atrophy
	Electrolyte disturbances—hypokalemia/hyperkalemia; hypophosphatemia
	Acute quadriplegic myopathy

brain injury include systemic hypotension and hypoxia, which further reduce substrate delivery to vulnerable brain tissue, and fever, seizures, and hyperglycemia, which can increase cellular metabolism outstripping compensatory processes. Clinically, these events are known as *secondary brain insults* because they lead to exacerbation of the primary brain injury. Prevention, identification, and treatment of secondary brain insults are fundamental goals of management.

An alternative pathway of cellular injury is *apoptosis*. This process implies programmed cell death, which may occur in the setting of ischemic stroke, global cerebral ischemia, traumatic brain injury, and possibly intracerebral hemorrhage. Apoptotic cell death can be distinguished histologically from the necrotic cell death of ischemia and is mediated through a different set of biochemical pathways. At present, interventions for prevention and treatment of apoptotic cell death remain less well defined than those for ischemia. →*Excitotoxicity and mechanisms of cell death are discussed in more detail in Chap. 345.*

Cerebral Perfusion and Autoregulation   Brain tissue requires constant perfusion in order to ensure adequate delivery of substrate. The hemodynamic response of the brain has the capacity to preserve perfusion across a wide range of systemic blood pressures. Cerebral perfusion pressure (CPP), defined as the mean systemic arterial pressure (MAP) minus the ICP, provides the driving force for circulation across the capillary beds of the brain. *Autoregulation* refers to the physiologic response whereby cerebral blood flow (CBF) remains relatively constant over a wide range of blood pressures as a consequence of alterations of cerebrovascular resistance (Fig. 258-1). If systemic blood pressure drops, cerebral perfusion is preserved through vasodilatation of arterioles in the brain; likewise, arteriolar vasoconstriction occurs at high systemic pressures to prevent hyperperfusion. At the extreme limits of MAP or CPP (high or low), flow becomes directly related to perfusion pressure. These autoregulatory changes occur in the microcirculation and are mediated by vessels below the resolution of those seen on angiography. CBF is also strongly influenced by pH and P_{CO_2}. CBF increases with hypercapnia and acidosis and decreases with hypocapnia and alkalosis. This forms the basis for the use of hyperventilation to lower ICP, and this effect on ICP is mediated through a decrease in intracranial blood volume. Cerebral autoregulation is critical to the normal homeostatic functioning of the brain, and this process may be disordered focally and unpredictably in disease states such as traumatic brain injury and severe focal cerebral ischemia.

Cerebrospinal Fluid and Intracranial Pressure   The cranial contents consist essentially of brain, cerebrospinal fluid (CSF), and blood. CSF is produced principally in the choroid plexus of each lateral ventricle, exits the brain via the foramina of Luschka and Magendi, and flows over the cortex to be absorbed into the venous system along the superior sagittal sinus. Approximately 150 mL of CSF are contained within the ventricles and surrounding the brain and spinal cord; the cerebral blood volume is also ~150 mL. The bony skull offers excellent protection for the brain but allows little tolerance for additional volume. Significant increases in volume eventually result in increased ICP. Obstruction of CSF outflow, edema of cerebral tissue, or increases in volume from tumor or hematoma may increase ICP. Elevated ICP diminishes cerebral perfusion and can lead to tissue ischemia. Ischemia in turn may lead to vasodilatation via autoregulatory mechanisms designed to restore cerebral perfusion. However, vasodilatation also increases cerebral blood volume, which in turn then increases ICP, lowers CPP, and provokes further ischemia (Fig. 258-2). This vicious cycle is commonly seen in traumatic brain injury, massive intracerebral hemorrhage, and large hemispheric infarcts with significant tissue shift.

APPROACH TO THE PATIENT

Critically ill patients with severe central nervous system dysfunction require rapid evaluation and intervention in order to limit primary and secondary brain injury. Initial neurologic evaluation should be performed concurrent with stabilization of basic respiratory, cardiac, and hemodynamic parameters. Significant barriers may exist to neurologic assessment in the critical care unit. Endotracheal intubation and the use of sedative or paralytic agents to facilitate critical care procedures can make clinical assessment challenging.

An impaired level of consciousness is frequent in critically ill patients. The essential first task in assessment is to determine whether the cause of dysfunction is related to a diffuse, usually metabolic, process or whether a focal, usually structural, process is implicated. Examples of diffuse processes include metabolic encephalopathies related to organ failure, drug overdose, or hypoxia-ischemia. Focal processes include ischemic and hemorrhagic stroke and traumatic brain injury, especially with intracranial hematomas. Since these two categories of disorders have fundamentally different causes, treatments, and prognoses, the initial focus is on making this distinction rapidly and accurately. →*The approach to the confused or comatose patient is discussed in Chap. 257; etiologies are listed in Table 257-1.*

Minor focal deficits may be present on the neurologic examination in patients with metabolic encephalopathies. However, the finding of prominent focal signs such as pupillary asymmetry, hemiparesis, gaze palsy, or paraplegia should alert the examiner to the possibility of a structural lesion. All patients with a decreased level of consciousness associated with focal findings should undergo an urgent neuroimaging procedure, as should all patients

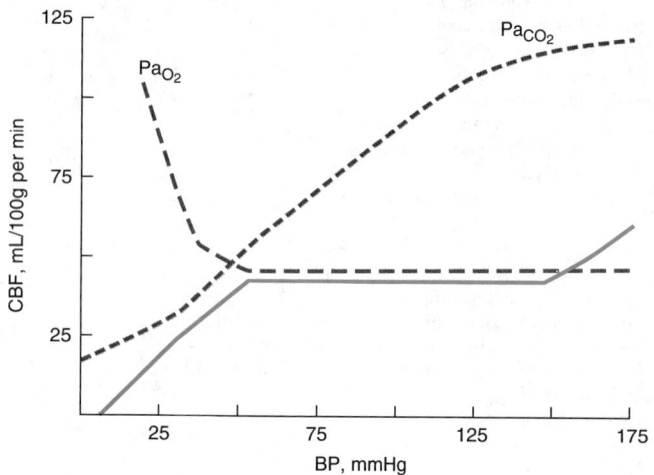

FIGURE 258-1   Autoregulation of cerebral blood flow (solid line). Cerebral perfusion is constant over a wide range of systemic blood pressure. Perfusion is increased in the setting of hypoxia or hypercarbia. BP, blood pressure; CBF, cerebral blood flow. (*Reprinted with permission from Anesthesiology 43:447, 1975. Copyright 1975, Lippincott Company.*)

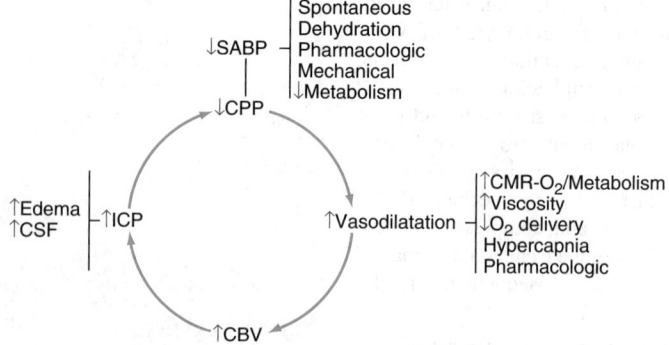

FIGURE 258-2   Ischemia and vasodilatation. Reduced cerebral perfusion pressure (CPP) leads to increased ischemia, vasodilatation, increased intracranial pressure (ICP), and further reductions in CPP, a cycle leading to further neurologic injury. CBV, cerebral blood volume; CMR, cerebral metabolic rate; CSF, cerebrospinal fluid; SABP, systolic arterial blood pressure. (*From MJ Rosner et al: J Neurosurg 83:949, 1995; with permission.*)

with coma of unknown etiology. Computed tomographic (CT) scanning is usually the most appropriate initial study because it can be performed quickly in critically ill patients and demonstrates hemorrhage, hydrocephalus, and intracranial tissue shifts well. Magnetic resonance imaging (MRI) may provide more specific information in some situations, such as acute ischemic stroke (diffusion-weighted imaging, DWI) and cerebral venous sinus thrombosis (magnetic resonance venography, MRV). Any suggestion of trauma from the history or examination should alert the examiner to the possibility of cervical spine injury and prompt an imaging evaluation using plain x-rays, MRI, or CT.

Other diagnostic studies are best utilized in specific circumstances, usually when neuroimaging studies fail to reveal a structural lesion and the etiology of the altered mental state remains uncertain. Electroencephalography (EEG) can be important in the evaluation of critically ill patients with severe brain dysfunction. The EEG of metabolic encephalopathy typically reveals generalized slowing. One of the most important uses of EEG is to help exclude inapparent seizures, especially nonconvulsive status epilepticus. Untreated continuous or frequently recurrent seizures may cause neuronal injury, making the diagnosis and treatment of seizure crucial in this patient group. Lumbar puncture (LP) may be necessary to exclude infectious processes, and an elevated opening pressure may be an important clue to cerebral venous sinus thrombosis. In patients with coma or profound encephalopathy, it is preferable to perform a neuroimaging study prior to LP. If bacterial meningitis is suspected, an LP may be performed first or antibiotics may be empirically administered before the diagnostic studies are completed. Standard laboratory evaluation of critically ill patients should include assessment of serum electrolytes (especially sodium and calcium), glucose, renal and hepatic function, complete blood counts, and coagulation. Serum or urine toxicology screens should be performed in patients with encephalopathy of unknown cause. EEG, LP, and other specific laboratory tests are most useful when the mechanism of the altered level of consciousness is uncertain; they are not routinely performed in clear-cut cases of stroke or traumatic brain injury.

Monitoring of ICP can be an important tool in selected patients. Indications for ICP monitoring, as well as specific types of monitors, vary. In general, patients who should be considered for ICP monitoring are those with primary neurologic disorders, such as stroke or traumatic brain injury, who are at significant risk for secondary brain injury due to elevated ICP and decreased CPP. Such patients include those with severe traumatic brain injury resulting in coma [Glasgow Coma Scale (GCS) score of ≤8 (Table 357-1)]; those with large tissue shifts from supratentorial ischemic or hemorrhagic stroke resulting in decreased consciousness; and those with (or at risk for) hydrocephalus from subarachnoid hemorrhage, intraventricular hemorrhage, or posterior fossa stroke. An additional disorder in which ICP monitoring can add important information is fulminant hepatic failure, in which elevated ICP may be treated with barbiturates or, eventually, liver transplantation. In general, ventriculostomy is preferable to ICP monitoring devices that are placed in brain parenchyma, because ventriculostomy allows CSF drainage as a method of treating elevated ICP. However, parenchymal ICP monitoring is most appropriate for patients with diffuse edema and small ventricles (which may make ventriculostomy placement more difficult) or any degree of coagulopathy (in which ventriculostomy carries a higher risk of hemorrhagic complications).

Treatment of Elevated ICP Elevated ICP may occur in a wide range of disorders including head trauma, intracerebral hemorrhage, subarachnoid hemorrhage with hydrocephalus, and fulminant hepatic failure. Because CSF and blood volume can be redistributed initially, by the time elevated ICP occurs intracranial compliance is severely impaired. At this point, small changes in the volume of CSF, intravascular blood, edema, or a mass lesion may result in significant changes in ICP. Elevated ICP then diminishes cerebral

perfusion. This is a fundamental mechanism of secondary ischemic brain injury and constitutes an emergency that requires immediate attention. Specific thresholds of ICP vary, but in general, ICP should be maintained at <20 mmHg and CPP should be maintained at ≥70 mmHg.

A number of different interventions may lower ICP, and ideally the selection of treatment will be based on the underlying mechanism responsible for the elevated ICP (Table 258-2). For example, in hydrocephalus from subarachnoid hemorrhage, the principal cause of elevated ICP is impairment of CSF drainage. In this setting, ventricular drainage of CSF is likely to be sufficient and most appropriate. In head trauma and stroke, cytotoxic edema may be most responsible, and the use of osmotic diuretics such as mannitol becomes an appropriate early step. As described above, elevated ICP may cause tissue ischemia, and, if cerebral autoregulation is intact, the resulting vasodilatation can lead to a cycle of worsening ischemia. Paradoxically, administration of vasopressor agents to increase mean arterial pressure may actually lower ICP by improving perfusion, thereby allowing autoregulatory vasoconstriction as ischemia is relieved and ultimately decreasing intracranial blood volume.

Early signs of elevated ICP include drowsiness and a diminished level of consciousness. Neuroimaging studies may reveal evidence of edema and mass effect. Hypotonic intravenous fluids should be avoided, and elevation of the head of the bed is recommended. Patients must be carefully observed for risk of aspiration and compromise of the airway as the level of alertness declines. Coma and unilateral pupillary changes are late signs and require immediate intervention. Emergent treatment of elevated ICP is most quickly achieved by intubation and hyperventilation, which causes vasoconstriction and reduces cerebral blood volume. Because of the concern of provoking or worsening cerebral ischemia, hyperventilation is best used for short periods of time until a more definitive treatment can be instituted. Furthermore, the effects of continued hyperventilation on ICP are short-lived, often only for several hours because of the buffering capacity of the cerebral interstitium, and rebound elevated ICP may accompany abrupt discontinuation of hyperventilation. As the level of consciousness declines to coma, the ability to follow the neurologic status of the patient by examination deteriorates and measurement of ICP must be considered. If a ventriculostomy device is in place, direct drain-

---

TABLE 258-2 Stepwise Approach to Treatment of Elevated Intracranial Pressure[a]

Insert ICP monitor—ventriculostomy versus parenchymal device
General goals: maintain ICP < 20 mmHg and CPP > 70 mmHg

For ICP > 20–25 mmHg for >5 min:
1. Drain CSF via ventriculostomy (if in place)
2. Elevate head of the bed
3. Osmotherapy—mannitol 25–100 g q4h as needed (maintain serum osmolality <320 mosmol)
4. Glucocorticoids—dexamethasone 4 mg q6h for vasogenic edema from tumor, abscess (avoid glucocorticoids in head trauma, ischemic and hemorrhagic stroke)
5. Sedation (e.g., morphine, propofol, or midazolam); add neuromuscular paralysis if necessary (patient will require endotracheal intubation and mechanical ventilation at this point, if not before)
6. Hyperventilation—to Pa_{CO_2} 30–35 mmHg
7. Pressor therapy—phenylephrine, dopamine, or norepinephrine to maintain adequate MAP to ensure CPP > 70 mmHg (maintain euvolemia to minimize deleterious systemic effects of pressors)
8. Consider second-tier therapies for refractory elevated ICP
   a. High-dose barbiturate therapy ("pentobarb coma")
   b. Aggressive hyperventilation to Pa_{CO_2} < 30 mmHg
   c. Hemicraniectomy

[a] Throughout ICP treatment algorithm, consider repeat head CT to identify mass lesions amenable to surgical evacuation.

Note: CPP, cerebral perfusion pressure; MAP, mean arterial pressure; Pa_{CO_2}, arterial partial pressure of carbon dioxide.

age of CSF to reduce ICP is possible. Finally, high-dose barbiturates or hypothermia are sometimes used for refractory elevated ICP, although these have significant side effects and have not been shown to improve outcome.

Secondary Brain Insults Patients with primary brain injuries, whether trauma or stroke, are at significant risk for ongoing secondary ischemic brain injury. Because secondary brain injury can be a major determinant of a poor outcome, strategies for minimizing secondary brain insults are an integral part of the critical care of all patients. While elevated ICP may lead to secondary ischemia, most secondary brain injury is mediated through other clinical events that exacerbate the ischemic cascade already initiated by the primary brain injury. Episodes of secondary brain insults are usually not associated with apparent neurologic worsening. Rather, they lead to cumulative injury, which manifests as higher mortality or worsened long-term functional outcome. Thus, clinical strategies involve close monitoring of vital signs and early intervention to prevent secondary ischemia. Avoiding hypotension and hypoxia is critical, as significant hypotensive events (systolic blood pressure < 90 mmHg) as short as 10 min in duration have been shown to adversely influence outcome after traumatic brain injury. Even in patients with stroke or head trauma who do not require ICP monitoring, close attention to adequate cerebral perfusion is warranted. Hypoxia (percutaneous oxygen saturation < 90%), alone or in combination with hypotension, also leads to secondary brain injury. Likewise, fever and hyperglycemia both worsen experimental ischemia and have been associated with worsened clinical outcome after stroke and head trauma. Aggressive control of fever with a goal of normothermia is warranted and can usually be achieved with antipyretic medications and cooling blankets. The use of intravenous insulin infusion is encouraged for control of hyperglycemia as this allows better regulation of serum glucose levels than subcutaneous insulin. A reasonable goal is to maintain the serum glucose level at <160 mg/dL, although some experts believe that even tighter control is appropriate. New cerebral monitoring tools that allow continuous evaluation of brain tissue oxygen tension, CBF, and metabolism (via microdialysis) may further improve the management of secondary brain injury.

CRITICAL CARE DISORDERS OF THE CENTRAL NERVOUS SYSTEM ASSOCIATED WITH SYSTEMIC DISEASE

HYPOXIC-ISCHEMIC ENCEPHALOPATHY This occurs from lack of delivery of oxygen to the brain because of hypotension or respiratory failure. The most common causes are myocardial infarction, cardiac arrest, shock, asphyxiation, paralysis of respiration, and carbon monoxide or cyanide poisoning. In some circumstances, hypoxia may predominate. Carbon monoxide and cyanide poisoning are termed *histotoxic hypoxia* since they cause a direct impairment of the respiratory chain.

Clinical Manifestations Mild degrees of pure hypoxia, such as occur at high altitudes, cause impaired judgment, inattentiveness, motor incoordination, and, at times, euphoria. However, with hypoxia-ischemia, such as occurs with circulatory arrest, consciousness is lost within seconds. If circulation is restored within 3 to 5 min, full recovery may occur, but if hypoxia-ischemia lasts beyond 3 to 5 min, some degree of permanent cerebral damage is the rule. Except in extreme cases, it may be difficult to judge the precise degree of hypoxia-ischemia, and some patients make a relatively full recovery after even 8 to 10 min of global cerebral ischemia. The distinction between pure hypoxia and hypoxia-ischemia is important, since a Pa_{O_2} as low as 20 mmHg (2.7 kPa) can be well tolerated if it develops gradually and normal blood pressure is maintained, but short durations of very low or absent cerebral circulation may result in permanent impairment.

Clinical examination at different time points after a hypoxic-ischemic insult (especially cardiac arrest) is useful in assessing prognosis

for long-term neurologic outcome. The prognosis is better for patients with intact brainstem function, as indicated by normal pupillary light responses and intact oculocephalic (doll's-eyes), oculovestibular (caloric), and corneal reflexes (Fig. 258-3). Absence of these reflexes and the presence of persistently dilated pupils that do not react to light are grave prognostic signs. A uniformly dismal prognosis from hypoxic-ischemic coma is conveyed by the clinical findings of absence of pupillary light reflex or absence of a motor response to pain on day 3 following the injury. Electrophysiologically, the finding of bilateral absence of the early cortical somatosensory evoked response (SSEPs) in the first week also conveys a poor prognosis. Whether administration of mild hypothermia after cardiac arrest (see "Treatment") will alter the usefulness of these clinical and electrophysiologic predictors is unknown. Long-term consequences of hypoxic-ischemic encepha-

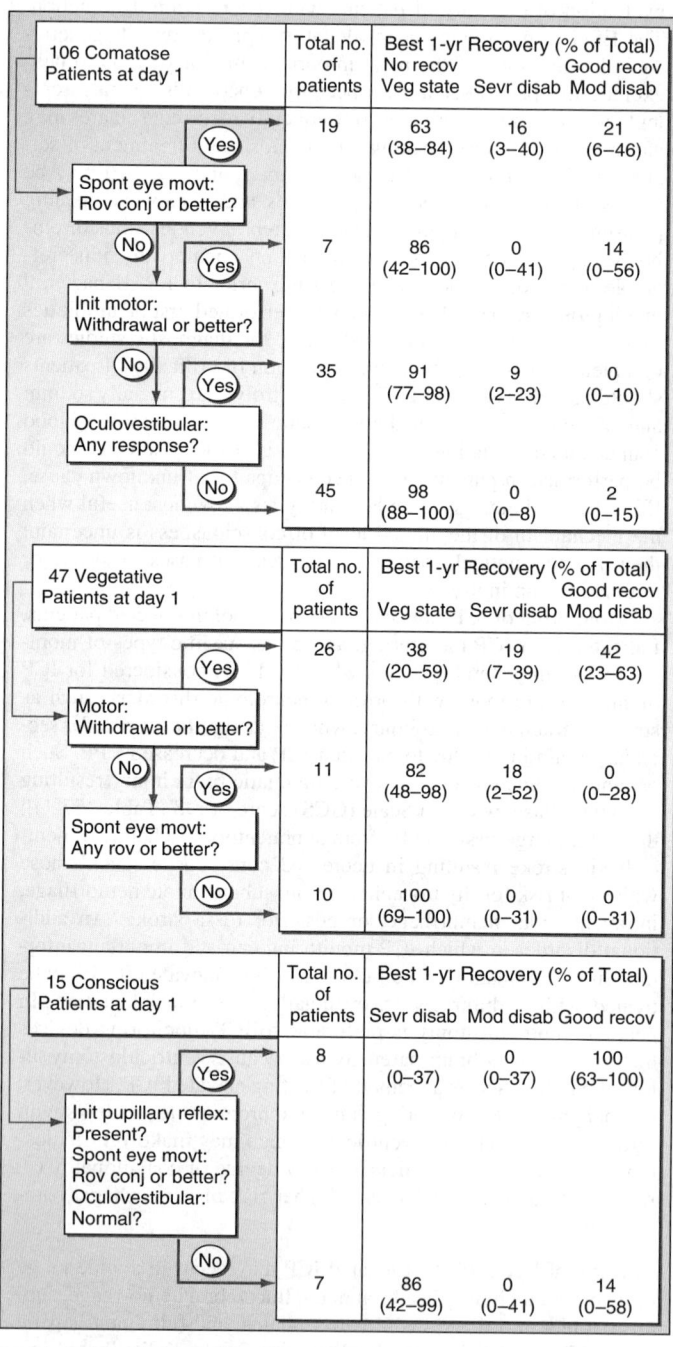

FIGURE 258-3 Clinical examination at day 1 provides useful prognostic information in hypoxic-ischemic encephalopathy. Numbers in parentheses represent 95% confidence intervals. Recov, recovery; veg, vegetative; sev, severe; mod, moderate; spont eye movt, spontaneous eye movement; rov conj, roving conjugate. *(From DE Levy et al: JAMA 253:1420, 1985; with permission.)*

lopathy include persistent coma or vegetative state (Chap. 257), dementia, visual agnosia (Chap. 23), parkinsonism, choreoathetosis, cerebellar ataxia, myoclonus, seizures, and an amnestic state, which may be a consequence of selective damage to the hippocampus.

Pathologic Findings Principal histologic findings are extensive multifocal or diffuse laminar cortical necrosis (Fig. 258-4), with almost invariable involvement of the hippocampus. The hippocampal CA1 neurons (Fig. 350-1) are vulnerable to even brief episodes of hypoxia-ischemia, perhaps explaining why selective persistent memory deficits may occur after brief cardiac arrest. Scattered small areas of infarction or neuronal loss may be present in the basal ganglia, hypothalamus, or brainstem. In some cases, extensive bilateral thalamic scarring may affect pathways that mediate arousal, and this pathology may be responsible for the persistent vegetative state. A specific form of hypoxic-ischemic encephalopathy, so-called watershed infarcts, occurs at the distal territories between the major cerebral arteries and can cause cognitive deficits, including visual agnosia, and weakness that is greater in proximal than in distal muscle groups.

Diagnosis Diagnosis is based upon the history of a hypoxic-ischemic event such as cardiac arrest. Blood pressure <70 mmHg systolic or $Pa_{O_2} < 40$ mmHg is usually necessary, although both absolute levels as well as duration of exposure are important determinants of cellular injury. Occasionally the clinical and radiographic features of a hypoxic-ischemic syndrome are seen without documented profound hypotension or hypoxia. Carbon monoxide intoxication can be confirmed by measurement of carboxyhemoglobin and is suggested by a cherry red color of the skin, although the latter is an inconsistent clinical finding.

℞ TREATMENT

Treatment should be directed at restoration of normal cardiorespiratory function. This includes securing a clear airway, ensuring adequate oxygenation and ventilation, and restoring cerebral perfusion, whether by cardiopulmonary resuscitation, fluid, pressors, or cardiac pacing. Hypothermia may target the neuronal cell injury cascade and has substantial neuroprotective properties in experimental models of brain injury. In two recently reported clinical trials, mild hypothermia (33°C) improved functional outcome in patients who remained comatose after resuscitation from a cardiac arrest. Treatment was initiated within minutes of cardiac resuscitation and continued for 12 h in one study and 24 h in the other. Potential complications of hypothermia treatment include coagulopathy and an increased risk of infection.

Severe carbon monoxide intoxication may be treated with hyper-

baric oxygen. Anticonvulsants may be needed to control seizures, although these are not usually given prophylactically. Posthypoxic myoclonus may respond to oral administration of clonazepam at doses of 1.5 to 10 mg daily or valproate at doses of 300 mg to 1200 mg daily in divided doses. Myoclonic status epilepticus after a severe hypoxic-ischemic insult portends a universally poor prognosis, even if seizures are controlled.

DELAYED POSTANOXIC ENCEPHALOPATHY Delayed postanoxic encephalopathy is an uncommon phenomenon in which patients appear to make an initial recovery from hypoxic-ischemic insult but then develop a relapse characterized by apathy, confusion, and agitation. Progressive neurologic deficits may include shuffling gait, diffuse rigidity and spasticity, persistent parkinsonism or myoclonus, and, on occasion, coma and death after 1 to 2 weeks. Widespread cerebral demyelination may be present.

Carbon monoxide and cyanide intoxication can also cause a delayed encephalopathy. Little clinical impairment is evident when the patient first regains consciousness, but a parkinsonian syndrome characterized by akinesia and rigidity without tremor may develop. Symptoms can worsen over months, accompanied by increasing evidence of damage in the basal ganglia as seen on both CT and MRI.

METABOLIC ENCEPHALOPATHIES Altered mental states, variously described as confusion, delirium, disorientation, and encephalopathy, are present in many patients with severe illness in an intensive care unit (ICU). Older patients are particularly vulnerable to delirium, a confusional state characterized by disordered perception, frequent hallucinations, delusions, and sleep disturbance. This is often attributed to medication effects, sleep deprivation, pain, and anxiety. The term *ICU psychosis* has been used to describe a mental state with profound agitation occurring in this setting. The presence of family members in the ICU may help to calm and orient agitated patients, and in severe cases, low doses of neuroleptics (e.g., haloperidol 0.5 to 1 mg) can be useful. Ultimately, the psychosis resolves with improvement in the underlying illness and a return to familiar surroundings.

In the ICU setting, several metabolic causes of an altered level of consciousness predominate. Hypercarbic encephalopathy can present with headache, confusion, stupor, or coma. Hypoventilation syndrome occurs most frequently in patients with a history of chronic CO_2 retention who are receiving oxygen therapy for emphysema or chronic pulmonary disease (Chap. 246). The elevated Pa_{CO_2} leading to CO_2 narcosis may have a direct anesthetic effect, and cerebral vasodilatation from increased Pa_{CO_2} can lead to increased ICP. Hepatic encephalopathy is suggested by asterixis and can occur in chronic liver failure or acute fulminant hepatic failure. Both hyperglycemia and hypoglycemia can cause encephalopathy, as can hypernatremia and hyponatremia. Confusion, impairment of eye movements, and gait ataxia are the hallmarks of acute Wernicke's disease (see below).

SEPTIC ENCEPHALOPATHY ■ Pathogenesis In patients with sepsis, the systemic response to infectious agents leads to the release of circulating inflammatory mediators that appear to contribute to encephalopathy. Critical illness, in association with the systemic inflammatory response syndrome (SIRS), can lead to multisystem organ failure. This syndrome can occur in the setting of apparent sepsis, severe burns, or trauma, even without clear identification of an infectious agent. Many patients with critical illness, sepsis, or SIRS develop encephalopathy without obvious explanation. This condition is broadly termed *septic encephalopathy*. While the specific mediators leading to neurologic dysfunction remain uncertain, it is clear that the encephalopathy is not simply the result of metabolic derangements of multiorgan failure. The cytokines tumor necrosis factor α, interleukin (IL) 1, IL-2, and IL-6 are thought to play a role in this syndrome.

Diagnosis Septic encephalopathy presents clinically as a diffuse dysfunction of the brain without prominent focal findings. Confusion, disorientation, agitation, and fluctuations in level of alertness are typ-

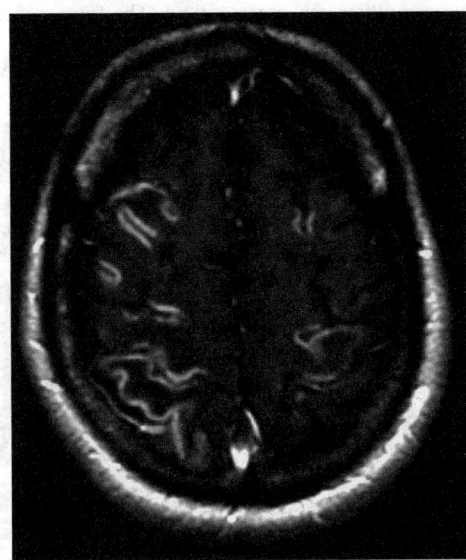

FIGURE 258-4   Cortical laminar necrosis in hypoxic-ischemic encephalopathy. T1-weighted postcontrast magnetic resonance image shows cortical enhancement in a watershed distribution consistent with laminar necrosis.

ical. In more profound cases, especially with hemodynamic compromise, the decrease in level of alertness can be more prominent, at times resulting in coma. Hyperreflexia and frontal release signs such as a grasp or snout reflex (Chap. 23) can be seen. Abnormal movements such as myoclonus, tremor, or asterixis can occur. Septic encephalopathy is quite common, occurring in the majority of patients with sepsis and multisystem organ failure. Diagnosis is often difficult because of the multiple potential causes of neurologic dysfunction in critically ill patients, and requires exclusion of structural, metabolic, toxic, and infectious (e.g., meningitis or encephalitis) causes. Although the mortality of patients with septic encephalopathy severe enough to produce coma approaches 50%, this reflects the severity of the underlying critical illness and is not a direct result of the septic encephalopathy. Neurologically, successful treatment of the underlying critical illness almost always results in complete resolution of the encephalopathy, without significant residua.

CENTRAL PONTINE MYELINOLYSIS This disorder typically presents in a devastating fashion as quadriplegia and pseudobulbar palsy. Predisposing factors include severe underlying medical illness or nutritional deficiency; most cases are associated with rapid correction of hyponatremia or with hyperosmolar states. The pathology consists of demyelination without inflammation in the base of the pons, with relative sparing of axons and nerve cells. MRI is useful in establishing the diagnosis (Fig. 258-5) and may also identify partial forms that present as confusion, dysarthria, and/or disturbances of conjugate gaze without quadriplegia. Therapeutic guidelines for the restoration of severe hyponatremia should aim for gradual correction, i.e., by ≤10 mmol/L (10 meq/L) within 24 h and 20 mmol/L (20 meq/L) within 48 h.

WERNICKE'S DISEASE Wernicke's disease is a common and preventable disorder due to a deficiency of thiamine (Chap. 61). In the United States, alcoholics account for most cases, but patients with malnutrition due to hyperemesis, starvation, renal dialysis, cancer, or AIDS are also at risk. The characteristic clinical triad is that of ophthalmoplegia, ataxia, and global confusion. However, only one-third of patients with acute Wernicke's disease present with the classic clinical triad. Most patients are profoundly disoriented, indifferent, and inattentive, although rarely they have an agitated delirium related to ethanol withdrawal. If the disease is not treated, stupor, coma, and death may ensue. Ocular motor abnormalities include horizontal nystagmus on lateral gaze, lateral rectus palsy (usually bilateral), conjugate gaze palsies, and rarely ptosis. Gait ataxia probably results from a combination of polyneuropathy, cerebellar involvement, and vestibular paresis. The pupils are usually spared, but they may become miotic with advanced disease.

Wernicke's disease is usually associated with other manifestations of nutritional disease, such as polyneuropathy. Rarely, amblyopia or myelopathy occurs. Tachycardia and postural hypotension may be related to impaired function of the autonomic nervous system or to the coexistence of cardiovascular beriberi. Patients who recover show improvement in ocular palsies within hours after the administration of thiamine, but horizontal nystagmus may persist. Ataxia improves more slowly than the ocular motor abnormalities. Approximately half recover incompletely and are left with a slow, shuffling, wide-based gait and an inability to tandem walk. Apathy, drowsiness, and confusion improve more gradually. As these symptoms recede, an amnestic state with impairment in recent memory and learning may become more apparent (*Korsakoff's psychosis*). Korsakoff's psychosis is frequently persistent; the residual mental state is characterized by gaps in memory, confabulation, and disordered temporal sequencing.

Pathology Lesions in the periventricular regions of the diencephalon, midbrain, and brainstem as well as the superior vermis of the cerebellum consist of symmetric discoloration of structures surrounding the third ventricle, aqueduct, and fourth ventricle, with petechial hemorrhages in occasional acute cases and atrophy of the mamillary bodies in most chronic cases. There is frequently endothelial proliferation,

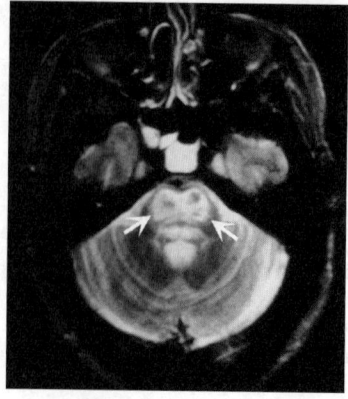

FIGURE 258-5 Central pontine myelinolysis. Axial T2-weighted magnetic resonance scan through the pons reveals a symmetric area of abnormal high signal intensity within the basis pontis (*arrows*).

demyelination, and some neuronal loss. These changes may be detected by MRI scanning (Fig. 258-6). The amnestic defect is related to lesions in the dorsal medial nuclei of the thalamus.

Pathogenesis Thiamine is a cofactor of several enzymes, including transketolase, pyruvate dehydrogenase, and α-ketoglutarate dehydrogenase. Thiamine deficiency produces a diffuse decrease in cerebral glucose utilization and results in mitochondrial damage. Glutamate accumulates owing to impairment of α-ketoglutarate dehydrogenase activity and, in combination with the energy deficiency, may result in excitotoxic cell damage.

℞ TREATMENT

Wernicke's disease is a medical emergency and requires immediate administration of thiamine, in a dose of 100 mg either intravenously or intramuscularly. The dose should be given daily until the patient resumes a normal diet and should be begun prior to treatment with intravenous glucose solutions. Glucose infusions may precipitate Wernicke's disease in a previously unaffected patient or cause a rapid worsening of an early form of the disease. For this reason, thiamine should be administered to all alcoholic patients requiring parenteral glucose.

CRITICAL CARE DISORDERS OF THE PERIPHERAL NERVOUS SYSTEM ASSOCIATED WITH SYSTEMIC DISEASE

Critical illness with disorders of the peripheral nervous system (PNS) arises in two contexts: (1) primary neurologic diseases that require critical care interventions such as intubation and mechanical ventilation, and (2) secondary PNS manifestations of systemic critical illness, often involving multisystem organ failure. The former include acute polyneuropathies such as Guillain-Barré syndrome (Chap. 365), neuromuscular junction disorders including myasthenia gravis (Chap.

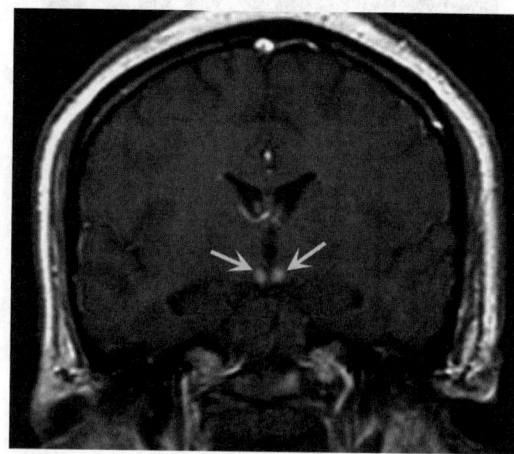

FIGURE 258-6 Wernicke's disease. Coronal T1-weighted postcontrast magnetic resonance image reveals abnormal enhancement of the mammillary bodies (*arrows*), typical of acute Wernicke's encephalopathy.

366) and botulism (Chap. 125), and primary muscle disorders such as polymyositis (Chap. 369). The latter result either from the systemic disease itself or as a consequence of interventions.

General principles of respiratory evaluation in patients with PNS involvement, regardless of cause, include assessment of pulmonary mechanics, such as maximal inspiratory force (MIF) and vital capacity (VC), and evaluation of strength of bulbar muscles. Regardless of the cause of weakness, endotracheal intubation should be considered when the MIF falls to < -25 cmH$_2$O or the VC is <1 L. Also, patients with severe palatal weakness may require endotracheal intubation in order to prevent acute upper airway obstruction or recurrent aspiration. Arterial blood gases and percutaneous oxygen saturation are used to follow patients with potential respiratory compromise from PNS dysfunction. However, intubation and mechanical ventilation should be undertaken based on clinical assessment rather than waiting until oxygen saturation drops or CO$_2$ retention develops from hypoventilation. →*Principles of mechanical ventilation are discussed in Chap. 252.*

NEUROPATHY While encephalopathy may be the most obvious neurologic dysfunction in critically ill patients, dysfunction of the PNS is also quite common. It is typically present in patients with prolonged critical illnesses lasting several weeks and involving sepsis; clinical suspicion is aroused when there is failure to wean from mechanical ventilation despite improvement of the underlying sepsis and critical illness. *Critical illness polyneuropathy* refers to the most common PNS complication related to critical illness; it is seen in the setting of prolonged critical illness, sepsis, and multisystem organ failure. Neurologic findings include diffuse weakness, decreased reflexes, and distal sensory loss. Electrophysiologic studies demonstrate a diffuse, symmetric, distal axonal sensorimotor neuropathy, and pathologic studies have confirmed axonal degeneration. The precise mechanism of critical illness polyneuropathy remains unclear, but circulating factors such as cytokines, which are associated with sepsis and SIRS, are thought to play a role. It has been reported that up to 70% of patients with the sepsis syndrome have some degree of neuropathy, although far fewer have a clinical syndrome profound enough to cause severe respiratory muscle weakness requiring prolonged mechanical ventilation or resulting in failure to wean. Treatment is supportive, with specific intervention directed at treating the underlying illness. While spontaneous recovery is usually seen, the time course may extend over weeks to months and necessitate long-term ventilatory support and care even after the underlying critical illness has resolved.

DISORDERS OF NEUROMUSCULAR TRANSMISSION A defect in neuromuscular transmission may be a source of weakness in critically ill patients. Myasthenia gravis may be a consideration; however, persistent weakness secondary to impaired neuromuscular junction transmission is almost always due to administration of drugs. A number of medications impair neuromuscular transmission; these include antibiotics, especially aminoglycosides, and beta-blocking agents. In the ICU, the nondepolarizing neuromuscular blocking agents (nd-NMBAs), also known as muscle relaxants, are most commonly responsible. Included in this group of drugs are such agents as pancuronium, vecuronium, rocuronium, and atracurium. They are often used to facilitate mechanical ventilation or other critical care procedures, but with prolonged use persistent neuromuscular blockade may result in weakness even after discontinuation of these agents hours or days earlier. Risk factors for this prolonged action of neuromuscular blocking agents include female sex, metabolic acidosis, and renal failure.

Prolonged neuromuscular blockade does not appear to produce permanent damage to the PNS. Once the offending medications are discontinued, full strength is restored, although this may take days. In general, the lowest dose of neuromuscular blocking agent should be used to achieve the desired result, and, when these agents are used in the ICU, a peripheral nerve stimulator should be used to monitor neuromuscular junction function.

MYOPATHY Critically ill patients, especially those with sepsis, frequently develop muscle wasting, often in the face of seemingly adequate nutritional support. The assumption has been that this represents a catabolic myopathy brought about as a result of multiple factors, including elevated cortisol and catecholamine release and other circulating factors induced by the SIRS. In this syndrome, known as *cachectic myopathy*, serum creatine kinase levels and electromyography (EMG) are normal. Muscle biopsy shows type II fiber atrophy. Panfascicular muscle fiber necrosis may also occur in the setting of profound sepsis. This so-called *septic myopathy* is characterized clinically by weakness progressing to a profound level over just a few days. There may be associated elevations in serum creatine kinase and urine myoglobin. Both EMG and muscle biopsy may be normal initially but eventually show abnormal spontaneous activity and panfascicular necrosis with an accompanying inflammatory reaction.

Acute quadriplegic myopathy describes a clinical syndrome of severe weakness seen in the setting of glucocorticoid and nd-NMBA use. The most frequent scenario in which this is encountered is the asthmatic patient who requires high-dose glucocorticoids and nd-NMBA to facilitate mechanical ventilation. This muscle disorder is not due to prolonged action of nd-NMBAs at the neuromuscular junction but, rather, is an actual myopathy with muscle damage; it has occasionally been described with high-dose glucocorticoid use alone. Clinically this syndrome is most often recognized when a patient fails to wean from mechanical ventilation despite resolution of the primary pulmonary process. Pathologically, there may be vacuolar changes in both type I and type II muscle fibers with evidence of regeneration. Acute quadriplegic myopathy has a good prognosis. If patients survive their underlying critical illness, the myopathy invariably improves and patients usually return to normal. However, because this syndrome is a result of true muscle damage, not just prolonged blockade at the neuromuscular junction, this process may take weeks or months, and tracheostomy with prolonged ventilatory support may be necessary. At present, it is unclear how to prevent this myopathic complication, except by avoiding use of nd-NMBAs, a strategy not always possible. Monitoring with a peripheral nerve stimulator can help to avoid the overuse of these agents. However, this is more likely to prevent the complication of prolonged neuromuscular junction blockade than it is to prevent this myopathy.

FURTHER READING

THE HYPOTHERMIA AFTER CARDIAC ARREST STUDY GROUP: Mild therapeutic hypothermia to improve the neurologic outcome after cardiac arrest. N Engl J Med 346:549, 2002

LIOU AK et al: To die or not to die for neurons in ischemia, traumatic brain injury and epilepsy: A review on the stress-activated signaling pathways and apoptotic pathways. Prog Neurobiol 69:103, 2003

VAN MOOK WN and HULSEWE-EVERS RP: Critical illness polyneuropathy. Curr Opin Crit Care 8:302, 2002

259 | ADAPTATION TO RENAL INJURY
Robert M. Brenner, Barry M. Brenner

Near constancy of the internal environment, including the volume, composition, and compartmental distribution of the body fluids, is essential to survival. With normal day-to-day variations in the intake of food and water, preservation of the internal environment requires the excretion in amounts that balance the quantities ingested. While losses from intestines, lungs, and skin contribute, the greatest responsibility for solute and water excretion is borne by the kidneys. This chapter reviews the excretory functions of the kidney and examines how these functions are affected by chronic renal disease.

EFFECTS OF NEPHRON LOSS ON RENAL EXCRETORY MECHANISMS

GLOMERULAR ULTRAFILTRATION Urine production begins at the glomerulus where an ultrafiltrate of plasma is formed. The rate of glomerular ultrafiltration (glomerular filtration rate, GFR) is governed chiefly by forces favoring filtration on the one hand (hydraulic pressure in the glomerular capillaries) and forces opposing filtration on the other (the sum of hydraulic pressure in Bowman's space and colloid osmotic pressure of blood in the glomerular capillaries). The rate of glomerular plasma flow and the total surface area of the glomerular capillaries are also determinants of GFR. Decreased GFR can therefore be expected when (1) glomerular hydraulic pressure is reduced (as in circulatory shock); (2) tubule (hence Bowman's space) hydraulic pressure is elevated, as in urinary tract obstruction; (3) plasma colloid osmotic pressure rises to high levels (hemoconcentration due to severe volume depletion, or myeloma, other dysproteinemias); (4) renal, and hence glomerular, blood flow is reduced (severe hypovolemia, cardiac failure); (5) permeability is reduced (diffuse glomerular disease); or (6) filtration surface area is diminished, through nephron loss in progressive renal failure.

The glomerular capillary wall is specially adapted to allow passage of extremely large volumes of water while retaining all but the smallest solute molecules. Molecules the size of inulin (approximately 5200 mol wt) pass freely across the glomerular filtration barrier, appearing at approximately the same concentration in Bowman's space as in plasma. The passage of solutes across the glomerular barrier decreases progressively with increasing molecular size such that, as the molecular weight of albumin is approached, most of the solute is retained in the plasma. Albumin, a polyanionic molecule in plasma, is further retarded at the glomerular filtration barrier by *electrostatic forces* imparted by negatively charged cell-surface molecules on the epithelial foot processes that form the *filtration slits* and the *slit diaphragms*. With disruption of these structural and electrostatic barriers, as in many forms of glomerular injury (Chap. 264), large quantities of plasma proteins gain access to the glomerular filtrate.

GLOMERULAR ADAPTATIONS TO NEPHRON LOSS With loss of nephron mass, the remaining functional (or least injured) nephrons tend to hypertrophy and take on an increased workload so that the overall loss of function is minimized. For example, a patient with a unilateral nephrectomy loses one-half of the nephron mass, resulting in a 50% reduction in GFR at the time of surgery. However, within several months total GFR may rise to 80% of the preoperative value. This indicates that the GFR of the individual remaining nephrons has increased above normal, a state known as *hyperfiltration*. Increases in single-nephron GFR may be achieved by renal hemodynamic adjustments (increased glomerular plasma flow and increased glomerular capillary hydraulic pressure), which augment the forces driving ultra-filtration, and by glomerular hypertrophy, which increases the maximum surface area available for filtration. These structural adaptations are evident from the enlargement of glomeruli (and tubules) seen on histologic sections from persons with single kidneys. Similar structural changes are observed in kidneys damaged by chronic disease processes; foci of hypertrophied glomeruli and tubules are interspersed with areas of atrophic or scarred parenchyma. Although direct measurements of single-nephron GFR cannot be made in humans, it is reasonable to conclude that focal nephron enlargement as occurs in chronically diseased kidneys generally signifies focally increased single-nephron GFR, and that these dynamic adaptations represent compensatory adjustments for the effects of nephron loss through disease.

GLOMERULOTUBULAR BALANCE The close integration of glomerular and tubular functions (*glomerulotubular balance*) seen in chronic renal failure (CRF) supports the notion that progressive nephron obliteration is the usual mode of GFR reduction in CRF. Preservation of glomerulotubular balance until the terminal stages of CRF is fundamental to the *intact-nephron hypothesis*, which states that as CRF advances, kidney function is supported by a diminishing pool of functioning (or hyperfunctioning) nephrons, rather than relatively constant numbers of nephrons, each with diminishing function. This hypothesis has important implications for the mechanisms of disease progression in CRF. A considerable amount of evidence suggests that nephrons subjected to increased excretory burdens for prolonged periods actually sustain injury as a result of these adaptations: thus the cost of these compensatory adaptations to nephron loss may ultimately be relentless destruction of the remaining nephron pool.

The magnitude of the single-nephron hyperfiltration induced by loss of 50% of the total nephron mass usually has no serious adverse clinical consequences, even when sustained over two to three decades. When more than 50% of the total nephron mass is lost, however, as in renal-sparing surgery for bilateral trauma or neoplasm or from a renal disease whose activity has abated, the remaining nephrons are forced to the limits of their compensatory capacity. While these adaptations achieve remarkable short-term success at offsetting the tendency for GFR to fall, over time, proteinuria and focal and segmental glomerulosclerosis develop, the more so where greater amounts of nephrons are lost or removed. As a result, a progressive decline in GFR ensues. Experimental study of the processes that advance glomerular injury show that the adverse long-term consequences of severe nephron deficits are invariably preceded by increases in glomerular capillary hydraulic pressure (glomerular capillary hypertension), glomerular hyperperfusion, and hypertrophy. Interventions directed against these compensatory and maladaptive responses can greatly ameliorate the subsequent development of renal failure. In particular, drugs (e.g., angiotensin-converting enzyme inhibitors and angiotensin II receptor blockers) and other interventions (such as dietary protein restriction) that lower glomerular pressure can slow the rate of progression of experimental and human renal disease. In the absence of such interventions, more and more glomeruli cease to function through advancing glomerulosclerosis and disruption of tubule structure and function, leading eventually to marked or even total loss of GFR (i.e., end-stage renal disease). This *final common pathway* for chronic renal injury helps to explain the observed progressive nature of chronic renal failure resulting from many different kidney diseases.

BIOLOGIC CONSEQUENCES OF SUSTAINED REDUCTIONS IN GFR

Figure 259-1 depicts the major types of response to impaired GFR. The degree of reduction in total GFR is plotted on the abscissa, expressed as a percentage of normal (100%). The renal handling of most solutes normally present in glomerular filtrate conforms to one of three

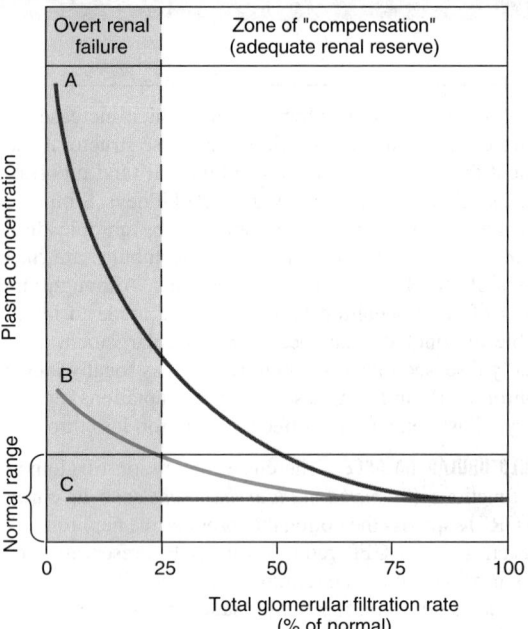

FIGURE 259-1   Representative patterns of adaptation for different types of solutes in body fluids in chronic renal failure. *[After NS Bricker et al, in BM Brenner (ed): Brenner and Rector's The Kidney, 6th ed. Philadelphia, Saunders, 2000.]*

patterns. Curve *A* describes the pattern with substances such as creatinine and urea that normally depend largely on glomerular filtration for urinary excretion, i.e., secretion contributes little to overall excretion. Therefore, as illustrated, gradual reductions in GFR are accompanied by progressive increases in plasma levels of creatinine, urea, and other substances normally excreted primarily by filtration.

The clinical course of CRF usually also approximates the pattern described by curve *A*. Patients with CRF usually pass from a long asymptomatic period of "compensation" to a more accelerated and clinically overt terminal phase. In other words, despite chronic injury leading to destruction of more than 50% of nephrons, plasma elevations of creatinine and urea may still lie within the normal limits for these substances. With further nephron loss and reduction in GFR, however, the limits of renal reserve are exceeded and continued accumulations of curve *A*–type solutes lead to abnormally elevated plasma concentrations (Fig. 259-1). Because some of these retained solutes are thought to exert "toxic" effects on all organ systems, clinical manifestations of CRF may now become apparent.

The accumulation of curve *A*–type solutes with chronic loss of renal function proceeds until external balance is restored, i.e., intake and/or production rates exactly match excretion rates. In the case of creatinine, for example, assuming a constant rate of creatinine production, a 50% reduction in GFR results in an approximate doubling of the plasma creatinine concentration. The latter restores the filtered load of creatinine (i.e., the product of GFR and plasma creatinine concentration) to normal, and the urinary excretion rate once again is equivalent to creatinine production. *In practice, so long as the net rates of acquisition and production (i.e., liver function and muscle mass) remain reasonably constant, the inverse relationship between plasma concentrations of solutes such as creatinine and urea and GFR is sufficiently reliable to serve as clinical indices of GFR.* However, where muscle mass is low, as with severe weight loss, even normal plasma levels of creatinine may belie substantial reductions in GFR.

In contrast to solutes of the curve *A* type, plasma levels of phosphate (PO_4^{3-}), urate, and potassium (K^+) and hydrogen (H^+) ions usually do not rise until the GFR falls to a small percentage of normal. With progressive renal failure this pattern of response (curve *B* in Fig. 259-1) reflects the participation of tubule transport mechanisms in the excretion of these substances. In other words, as *GFR declines, the*

tubules facilitate greater elimination of these substances, by enhancing secretion and/or by diminishing reabsorption, so that a greater fraction of the filtered load is excreted. Plasma levels of curve *B*–type solutes, therefore, rise less than those of curve *A* because, with progressive reductions in GFR, *excretion rate per nephron* and therefore *fractional excretion* both increase. Eventually, however, with further loss of GFR, enhanced fractional excretion can no longer mitigate the reduction in net filtered load of these solutes and plasma levels rise (Fig. 259-1). For urate, PO_4^{3-}, and K^+, at least, increased fractional excretion serves to maintain normal plasma levels until GFR falls to less than one-fourth of normal.

Finally, for certain solutes, such as sodium chloride (NaCl), plasma concentrations remain normal throughout the course of CRF, despite unrestricted intake of these substances (curve *C* in Fig. 259-1). The compensatory mechanism required to achieve this represents a fundamental adaptation to chronic renal injury. To illustrate the magnitude of this adaptation, it is useful to compare the excretion of sodium (Na^+) in a normal individual (GFR of 125 mL/min) with that of a patient with advanced renal failure (GFR of 2 mL/min). Both individuals consume a conventional diet containing 7 g/d of salt (120 mmol Na^+). With a serum Na^+ concentration of 140 mmol/L, external Na^+ balance is achieved in the normal subject by excreting approximately 0.5% of the filtered load. By contrast, for external balance to be maintained in the patient with CRF, fractional excretion of Na^+ must rise to 30%. In other words, *to maintain external Na^+ balance*, the same amount of Na^+ must be excreted into the urine each day in the patient with CRF as in the normal individual. Given the drastic reduction in GFR in CRF, external balance can only be maintained by marked adaptations in the reabsorptive processes in surviving tubules. In this manner, a progressively larger fraction of the filtered load escapes reabsorption and appears in the final urine.

ADAPTATIONS IN TUBULE TRANSPORT MECHANISMS IN RESPONSE TO NEPHRON LOSS

Despite progressive nephron loss, many mechanisms that regulate renal solute and water balance differ only quantitatively, and not qualitatively, from those that operate normally. Thus, glomerulotubular balance is maintained. The most important of these mechanisms are considered below.

TUBULAR TRANSPORT OF SODIUM CHLORIDE AND WATER   Most of the filtered water and sodium salts are reabsorbed by the tubules, leaving small and variable amounts, equivalent on average to the quantities ingested, to reach the final urine. About two-thirds of the glomerular ultrafiltrate is reabsorbed in the *proximal tubule* with little change in the osmolality or Na^+ concentration of the unreabsorbed fraction (Fig. 259-2). In other words, fluid reabsorption in the proximal tubule is nearly *isosmotic* and is coupled to the active transport of Na^+. Since chloride (Cl^-) and bicarbonate (HCO_3^-) are the primary anions in the extracellular fluid, they constitute the main solutes that accompany Na^+ reabsorption in the renal tubules. In the earliest portion of the proximal tubule, bicarbonate is the principal anion that accompanies the reabsorption of Na^+. This process occurs via a Na^+/H^+ exchanger at the luminal brush border and is dependent on the activity of carbonic anhydrase. Glucose, amino acids, and other organic solutes (e.g., lactate) are also extensively reabsorbed in the proximal tubule by cotransport mechanisms that link the cellular entry of these organic molecules with Na^+.

The coupling of water absorption (i.e., volume) with solute absorption appears to be dependent upon three processes. First, given the remarkably high water permeability of this segment, very small transepithelial osmolality differences, i.e., *luminal hypotonicity* of the order of 2 to 3 mosmol/L produced by solute absorption, could drive water absorption. Second, due to preferential absorption of HCO_3^- and organic solutes in the early portions of the proximal tubule, the concentrations of these substances decrease along the proximal tubule while that of chloride increases. Volume reabsorption would then occur if the diffusion of Na^+ and Cl^- down their respective electrochemical gradients across the proximal tubule epithelium occurred more easily than the back-diffusion of sodium bicarbonate into the lumen, creating an *effective osmotic pressure gradient*. Finally, *lateral interstitial space hypertonicity* produced by differences in the rates at which solutes are transported into the spaces or exit them by diffusion may also contribute to the coupling of water and solute reabsorption.

Reabsorption of Fluid from Proximal Convoluted Tubules This is sensitive to *Starling forces*, i.e., the hydraulic and colloid osmotic (or oncotic) pressures acting across the walls of the peritubular capillaries. Because the plasma proteins in glomerular capillaries are concentrated by ultrafiltration, oncotic pressure rises along the glomerular capillary network. This step-up in oncotic pressure is transmitted largely unchanged to the first branches of the peritubular capillaries via the efferent arterioles. These resistance vessels cause a substantial drop in hydraulic pressure, however, so that when the plasma reaches the peritubular capillaries, oncotic pressure greatly exceeds hydraulic pressure. The Starling forces are therefore oriented in an *uptake* mode, in contrast to their configuration at the glomerulus where hydraulic pressure exceeds oncotic pressure, favoring *filtration*. The extent to which oncotic pressure exceeds hydraulic pressure in the peritubular capillary network modulates the overall rate of fluid absorption by the peritubular capillaries. Therefore, when peritubular capillary oncotic pressure falls, or hydraulic pressure rises, uptake of fluid by these capillaries is reduced. As a result, fluid is retained in the interstitial space, tending to increase hydraulic pressure, ultimately retarding the egress of fluid from the lateral intercellular channels.

Without an adequate route of drainage, fluid in the intercellular channels leaks back into the tubule lumen, thereby *diminishing net fluid reabsorption* from this tubule segment. The opposite occurs in states where peritubular oncotic pressure is increased (increased filtration fraction) or hydraulic pressure is decreased (enhanced efferent arteriolar tone). Under these circumstances, peritubular capillary uptake of reabsorbate is augmented, leading ultimately to *enhanced net fluid reabsorption* by the proximal tubule. Although physical factors appear to be the major determinants of fluid reabsorption in the proximal tubule, hormones (e.g., angiotensin II) may also modulate fluid reabsorption directly, by enhancing luminal Na^+ entry into proximal tubule cells via an apical Na^+/H^+ exchanger.

The Limbs of Henle's Loop In contrast to the proximal tubule, active outward transport of Na^+ has not been established for the *thin descending or ascending limbs of Henle's loop*. However, passive outward salt transport does occur, as indicated in Fig. 259-2. In the next nephron segment, the *medullary thick ascending limb of Henle*, the concentration of NaCl is reduced as fluid traverses this segment. Here Cl^- absorption occurs by an active process involving a $Na^+:K^+:2Cl^-$ cotransport mechanism in the luminal membrane, with one-half of Na^+ absorption pro-

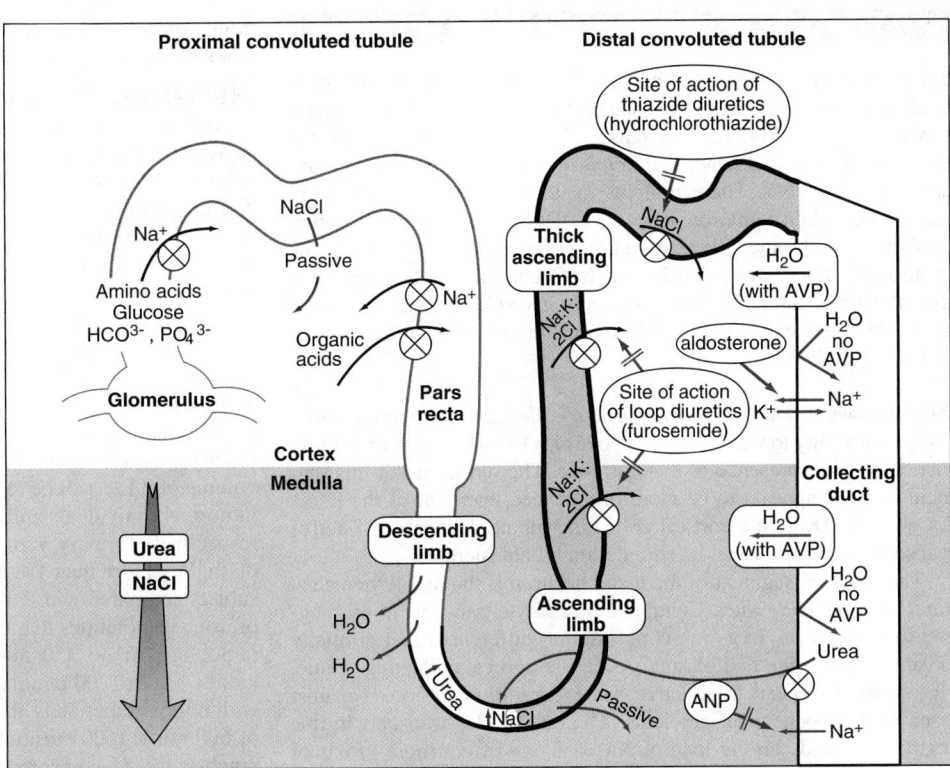

FIGURE 259-2 Transport functions of the various anatomic segments of the mammalian nephron. Fluid reabsorption across the proximal tubule is isosmotic and accounts for reabsorption of approximately two-thirds of the filtered Na^+ and H_2O. The major portions of the filtered HCO_3^-, amino acids, glucose, and phosphate are reabsorbed in the early proximal convoluted tubule. Reabsorption of glucose and amino acids is coupled to Na^+ transport and thereby generates a negative potential difference within the tubule lumen. At the same time, HCO_3^- is reabsorbed by a nonelectrogenic mechanism, via H^+ secretion. The active transport of these solutes results in transepithelial concentration and effective osmotic pressure gradients promoting H_2O flow across the proximal tubule, into the peritubular capillaries. The rise in tubule fluid Cl^- concentration is a necessary reciprocal consequence of the decreased luminal HCO_3^- concentration. The resultant high concentration of Cl^- becomes an important force for the outward passive transport of Cl^- down its concentration gradient, resulting in a lumen-positive potential difference in the late proximal convoluted tubule.

The pars recta of the proximal tubule is capable of active electrogenic transport of Na^+ independent of organic solute transport. Under normal conditions, approximately one-third of the glomerular filtrate enters the descending limb of Henle's loop. This segment is incapable of active outward NaCl transport and is characterized by low permeability to Na^+ but high H_2O permeability. H_2O is abstracted passively as the fluid approaches the bend of Henle's loop. Hypertonic fluid with a greater NaCl concentration but lower urea concentration than the surrounding medullary interstitium thus enters the thin ascending limb of Henle, which is largely impermeable to H_2O and urea but highly permeable to NaCl. This permits passive outward diffusion of NaCl. Active $Na:K:2Cl$ transport across the water-impermeable thick ascending limb of Henle enables tubule fluid to become dilute and the medullary interstitium hypertonic.

Irrespective of the final osmolality of the urine, the fluid that enters the distal convoluted tubule (DCT) is always hypoosmotic. This segment exhibits active Na^+ reabsorption. All but the terminal portion of the DCT is water-impermeable, even in the presence of arginine vasopressin (AVP). Aldosterone exerts its effect in this segment by enhancing Na^+ reabsorption, which is variably coupled to K^+ and H^+ secretion. The cortical and papillary portions of the collecting duct are sites where AVP exerts its principal effect. The permeability of these segments to H_2O in the absence of AVP is very low but can be greatly enhanced in the presence of AVP. These segments are also characterized by active Na^+ reabsorption, which appears to depend on the presence of mineralocorticoid. In the absence of AVP, the collecting tubule is water-impermeable so that hypotonic tubule fluid courses through it. However, in the presence of AVP, water is avidly reabsorbed here, resulting in hypertonic final urine. Sites of action of furosemide and thiazide diuretics and of aldosterone and atrial natriuretic peptide (ANP) are shown.

ceeding passively, driven by the lumen positive transepithelial voltage difference. This cotransporter is the site of action of the powerful loop diuretics, and mutations give rise to Bartter's syndrome. Since the ascending limb of Henle is impermeable to water, net NaCl reabsorption generates a hypotonic tubule fluid and gives rise to the high NaCl concentration of the outer medullary interstitium (Fig. 259-2).

Distal Tubule The fluid leaving the thick ascending limb of Henle is normally of low NaCl concentration, a characteristic independent of the organism's hydration status. In the *distal tubule*, water reabsorption is variable, depending on the state of hydration or, specifically, on the presence or absence of arginine vasopressin (AVP) in plasma. In the absence of AVP, this and more distal nephron segments are impermeable to water, so that hypotonic fluid entering this segment is excreted as *dilute urine*. Indeed, continued salt reabsorption along the distal convoluted tubule (DCT) and connecting tubule segments, a process that can be inhibited by thiazide diuretics, results in further dilution of the urine. In the presence of AVP, the permeability of these nephron segments to water increases. This is made possible by the insertion of proteins known as *aquaporins* into the luminal cell membrane of DCT cells. These proteins facilitate water movement from the low-osmolality environment of the DCT lumen into the higher osmolality of the medullary interstitium, thereby contributing to the creation of a concentrated final urine. NaCl continues to be reabsorbed from the tubule lumen against moderately steep chemical and electrical gradients. The reabsorption of NaCl at the collecting tubule is enhanced by *aldosterone*.

Collecting Tubules and Ducts The *cortical collecting tubule* possesses a low permeability to water in the absence of AVP, whereas permeability increases in the presence of this hormone. The sensitivity of this segment to AVP appears to be more pronounced than that of the DCT. As with the DCT, the cortical collecting tubule is capable of active reabsorption of NaCl and its stimulation by aldosterone.

The terminal segment of the distal nephron is the highly branched *papillary collecting duct*. Continued electrolyte transport in this segment results in the large ion concentration differences that normally exist between urine and plasma. As in the cortical collecting tubule, Na^+ transport appears to be active, since reabsorption proceeds against sizeable electrochemical gradients. The rate of Na^+ transport in this segment depends on the load of Na^+ delivered from more proximal segments and is also affected by aldosterone. The permeability to water is also increased markedly in the presence of AVP.

EFFECTS OF NEPHRON LOSS ON SODIUM CHLORIDE TRANSPORT IN SURVIVING NEPHRONS With progressive nephron loss, *maintenance of external balance for NaCl requires that fractional salt excretion increases in concert with the decline in GFR.* Several mechanisms contribute to this adaptive increase in fractional Na^+ excretion. With loss of functioning nephrons, peritubular capillary Starling forces are altered in directions that serve to reduce proximal tubule reabsorption of NaCl and water. For example, a rise in peritubular capillary hydraulic pressure, which tends to inhibit net proximal fluid reabsorption, might be anticipated with systemic hypertension, a common feature of CRF. Similarly, reductions in peritubular capillary oncotic pressures may be anticipated due to reductions in both filtration fraction and hypoalbuminemia.

Several factors that regulate NaCl transport across tubules under normal conditions are also likely to contribute to the enhanced fractional excretion of NaCl in renal insufficiency. Atrial natriuretic peptides are released from the heart in response to elevated cardiac (atrial) filling pressures as seen with increased plasma volume or atrial tachyarrhythmias. These peptides affect natriuresis by reducing net Na^+ reabsorption through complementary actions on Na^+ transport in the collecting duct and by altering Starling forces in the adjacent vasa recta. Other modulators of tubule transport processes may also contribute to increased single-nephron natriuresis in the setting of nephron loss. Vasodilator prostaglandins are present at increased plasma levels in CRF, as are other inhibitors of transport, including inhibitor(s) of the Na^+,K^+-ATPase. Serum and urine from patients with uremia contain retained toxins capable of inhibiting this enzyme.

The obligatory high rate of solute excretion per surviving nephron (so-called osmotic diuresis due to urea and other retained solutes) also contributes to enhancing fractional NaCl excretion, much as occurs in normal individuals after the administration of mannitol or other nonreabsorbable solutes. Finally, certain forms of CRF are associated with unusually large losses of salt in the urine. These *salt-wasting nephropathies* include chronic pyelonephritis and other tubulointerstitial diseases (Chap. 266) as well as polycystic and medullary cystic diseases. These disorders have in common greater destruction of medullary and tubulointerstitial, rather than cortical and glomerular, portions of the renal parenchyma. →*For discussion of clinical derangements that alter renal handling of NaCl in CRF (including hypo- and hypervolemia, hypertension, etc.), see Chap. 261.*

EFFECTS OF NEPHRON LOSS ON WATER REABSORPTION IN SURVIVING NEPHRONS
As with NaCl, there is a progressive increase in the fractional excretion of water with advancing renal insufficiency, so that external water balance can be maintained even with a total GFR of 5 mL/min or less. The adaptations of water handling by the diseased kidney are of importance in the defects in urinary concentration and dilution and hence the polyuria, nocturia, and tendency to develop water retention encountered in CRF (Chap. 40). To appreciate the mechanisms involved, the responses of a normal individual and a patient with CRF maintaining external water balance need to be considered. Assuming both individuals have the same dietary and fluid intakes, total solute and volume excretion in both should be identical as well. If the *obligatory solute load* to be excreted by each is 600 mmol/d (600 mosmol/d) and the urine osmolality is 300 mmol/kg water (300 mosmol/kg), a urine volume of 2 L/d will be required to excrete the total solute. If the GFR in normal individuals and the patient with CRF totals 180 and 4 L/d, respectively, urinary volume excretion of 2 L/d represents excretion of slightly more than 1% of the total glomerular filtrate in the normal subject compared with 50% in the patient with CRF. Since the range of urine osmolalities that the diseased kidney can achieve [250 to 350 mmol/kg (250 to 350 mosmol/kg)] is narrower than in the normal kidney [40 to 1200 mmol/kg (40 to 1200 mosmol/kg)], the individual with normal function is able to excrete the obligatory daily solute load of 600 mmol (600 mosmol) in as little as 500 mL urine per day or as much as 15 L/d, compared with the narrower range in CRF, from about 1.7 to 2.4 L/d.

In CRF, the limited capacity to concentrate the urine often correlates with other measures of impaired renal function. Isosthenuria (urine of similar osmolality to plasma) is therefore an almost universal finding when the GFR falls below 25 mL/min. At this level of GFR and below, urine osmolality does not rise even when supraphysiologic doses of AVP are administered, suggesting that the concentrating defect relates to impaired concentrating capacity in surviving nephrons. The associated increased fractional excretion per nephron of a variety of solutes produces an obligatory water loss (solute diuresis) at roughly isotonic proportions. Consequently, formation of a concentrated urine is prevented. Disease-induced abnormalities of the architecture of the renal medulla (loops of Henle, vasa recta), aberrations in medullary blood flow, and defective transport of NaCl in the ascending limb of Henle also contribute to this defect in urine concentration.

Since patients with CRF are unable to excrete concentrated or dilute urine, they must have access to adequate, and to some extent, relatively constant amounts of water per day to ensure that they have adequate water to eliminate total daily solute loads. For this reason, restriction of fluid intake may be hazardous in patients with CRF. Likewise, impairment of diluting capacity may prevent many patients from excreting excess ingested fluid. →*For discussion of the consequences of the abnormal patterns of water excretion, and the attendant susceptibilities to develop hypo- and hypernatremia, see Chaps. 41 and 261.*

TUBULE TRANSPORT OF PHOSPHATE WITH NORMAL AND REDUCED NEPHRON MASS
Under normal physiologic conditions, about 80 to 90% of phosphate is reabsorbed, mainly in the proximal tubule. *Parathyroid hormone* (PTH), by augmenting phosphate excretion via inhibition of this proximal reabsorptive process (Chap. 331), plays a central role in phosphate homeostasis. When dietary phosphate intake increases, a *transient* rise in plasma phosphate concentration is usually observed. This results in a similarly transient reduction in the plasma ionized calcium level (due largely to deposition of calcium phosphate in bone), which is sensed by a specific receptor on parathyroid cells, stimulating PTH secretion. By enhancing fractional phosphate excretion, PTH restores external phosphate balance and normophosphatemia. This enables plasma ionized calcium and hence phosphate levels to return to normal, thereby removing the stimulus to PTH release.

With advancing renal failure and constant dietary intake of phosphate, external phosphate balance is achieved by progressive reduction in fractional phosphate reabsorption. Enhanced PTH secretion is an important determinant of this phosphaturic response. With succeeding decrements in total GFR, the amount of phosphate filtered by surviving glomeruli is reduced, leading to transient phosphate retention and, therefore, a rise (albeit small) in plasma phosphate concentration. This leads to a small, reciprocal decline in plasma levels of ionized calcium and a corresponding increase in PTH secretion. Although the phosphaturic response of surviving tubules to this elevation in circulating PTH restores plasma phosphate and calcium to normal levels (at least in the "compensated" stage of CRF described by curve *B* in Fig. 259-1), the new steady-state conditions are only achieved at the cost of *persistently elevated plasma PTH levels*. With progressive reductions in GFR, the process is repeated, resulting in substantially elevated PTH levels.

Alterations in Vitamin D Metabolism The kidney is normally the major site of *conversion of vitamin D to its active metabolites*. As discussed in Chap. 331, vitamin D, synthesized in skin or acquired in the diet, undergoes initial hydroxylation in the liver to form 25-hydroxyvitamin D [25(OH)D]. The kidney is the site of a second important conversion to 1,25-dihydroxyvitamin D [1,25(OH$_2$)D]. This active form of vitamin D acts directly on the parathyroid gland to suppress PTH secretion as well as to enhance intestinal absorption of calcium and promote its resorption from bone. With advancing renal disease, nephron loss reduces the renal capacity for vitamin D hydroxylation; phosphate retention also impairs this reaction. Not only are the circulating levels of 1,25(OH$_2$)D diminished in CRF, but the receptors that mediate its action at the parathyroid gland are also diminished. These two effects remove inhibitory influences on PTH secretion, leading again to increased plasma PTH levels. Reduction in circulating 1,25(OH$_2$)D levels, by suppressing intestinal calcium absorption, contributes to the development of the hypocalcemia and hyperparathyroidism of CRF (Chap. 261). →*For a discussion of hyperparathyroidism in chronic renal failure, see Chap. 261.*

HYDROGEN AND BICARBONATE TRANSPORT WITH NORMAL AND REDUCED RENAL MASS As discussed in Chap. 42, the pH of extracellular fluid is normally maintained within a narrow range (7.36 to 7.44) despite day-to-day fluctuations in the quantity of acids added to the extracellular fluid from dietary and metabolic sources (approximately 1 mmol H$^+$ per kilogram of body weight per day). These acids consume buffers from both extracellular and intracellular fluid, of which HCO$_3^-$ is the most important in the intracellular compartment. Such buffering minimizes changes in pH. Long-term effectiveness of the HCO$_3^-$ buffer system, however, requires mechanisms for replenishment, otherwise unrelenting acquisition of nonvolatile acids from dietary and metabolic sources would ultimately exhaust buffering capacity, culminating in fatal acidosis. The kidneys normally function to prevent this eventuality by *regenerating* bicarbonate, thereby maintaining plasma concentrations of HCO$_3^-$. In addition, the kidneys also *reclaim* HCO$_3^-$ in the glomerular ultrafiltrate.

The *reabsorption* of filtered HCO$_3^-$ occurs by the following mechanism. Filtered bicarbonate combines with H$^+$ secreted from proximal tubule cells via the Na$^+$/H$^+$ exchange, to form carbonic acid (H$_2$CO$_3$). Dehydration of carbonic acid under the influence of *luminal* carbonic anhydrase yields H$_2$O and CO$_2$, which is free to diffuse from lumen to peritubular blood. In the proximal tubule cell, the OH$^-$ left behind by the H$^+$ secretion reacts with CO$_2$, under the influence of *intracellular* carbonic anhydrase, forming HCO$_3^-$. This ion is transported across the contraluminal proximal tubule cell membrane, via an electrogenic Na/HCO$_3^-$ cotransporter, to reenter the extracellular HCO$_3^-$ pool. The net result is *reclamation of a filtered bicarbonate ion*. Hydrogen ions in the urine are bound to filtered buffers (e.g., phosphate) in amounts equivalent to the amounts of alkali required to titrate the pH of the urine up to the pH of the blood (the so-called titratable acid). It is not usually possible to excrete all the daily acid load in the form of titratable acid due to limits of urinary pH. Metabolism of glutamine by proximal tubule cells to yield ammonium (ammoniagenesis) serves as an additional mechanism for H$^+$ elimination and bicarbonate re-

generation. Glutamine metabolism forms not only NH$_4^+$ (i.e., NH$_3$ plus H$^+$) but also HCO$_3^-$, which is transported across the proximal tubule (HCO$_3^-$ regeneration). The NH$_4^+$ must be excreted in the urine for this process to be effective in bicarbonate regeneration. *Ammoniagenesis* is responsive to the acid-base needs of the individual. When faced with an acute acid burden and an increased need for HCO$_3^-$ regeneration, the rate of renal ammonia synthesis increases sharply.

The quantity of hydrogen ions excreted as titratable acid and NH$_4^+$ is equal to the quantity of HCO$_3^-$ regenerated in tubule cells and added to plasma. Under steady-state conditions, the net quantity of acid excreted into the urine (the sum of titratable acid and NH$_4^+$ less HCO$_3^-$) must equal the quantity of acid gained by the extracellular fluid from all sources. Metabolic acidosis and alkalosis result when this delicate balance is perturbed, the former the result of insufficient net acid excretion, and the latter due to excessive acid excretion (Chap. 42).

Progressive loss of renal function usually causes little or no change in arterial pH, plasma bicarbonate concentration, or arterial carbon dioxide tension (P$_{CO_2}$) until GFR falls below 25% of normal. Thereafter, all three tend to decline as *metabolic acidosis* ensues. In general, the metabolic acidosis of CRF is not due to overproduction of acids but is rather a reflection of nephron loss, which limits the amount of NH$_3$ (and therefore also HCO$_3^-$) that can be generated. Although surviving nephrons appear to be capable of generating supranormal amounts of NH$_3$ *per nephron*, the diminished nephron population causes overall production to be reduced to an extent that is insufficient to permit adequate buffering of H$^+$ in urine. As a result, although patients with CRF may be able to acidify their urine normally (i.e., urine pH as low as 4.5), the defect in NH$_3$ production limits daily net acid excretion to 30 to 40 mmol, or one-half to two-thirds the quantity of nonvolatile acid added to the extracellular fluid in the same time period. Metabolic acidosis resulting from this daily positive balance of H$^+$ is seldom florid in CRF of mild to moderate severity. Relative stability of plasma bicarbonate (albeit at reduced levels of 14 to 18 mmol/L) is maintained at the expense of buffering by bone. Because it contains large reserves of alkaline salts (calcium phosphate and calcium bicarbonate), bone constitutes a major reserve of buffering capacity. Dissolution of these buffers contributes to the osteodystrophy of CRF (see Fig. 261-1).

Although the acidosis of CRF is due to loss of tubule mass, it nevertheless depends to a large part on the level of GFR. When GFR is reduced to only a moderate extent (i.e., to about 50% of normal), retention of anions, principally sulfates and phosphates, is not pronounced. Therefore, as the plasma HCO$_3^-$ falls owing to dysfunction or loss of tubules, retention of Cl$^-$ by the kidneys leads to a *hyperchloremic acidosis*. At this stage *the anion gap is normal*. With further reductions in GFR and progressive azotemia, however, the retention of phosphates, sulfates, and other *unmeasured* anions ensues and plasma Cl$^-$ falls to normal levels despite the reduction in plasma HCO$_3^-$ concentration. *An elevated anion gap therefore develops.*

TUBULE POTASSIUM TRANSPORT WITH NORMAL AND REDUCED NEPHRON MASS As with H$^+$, the concentration of K$^+$ in extracellular fluid is normally maintained within a relatively narrow range, 4 to 5 mmol/L. At least 95% of total-body K$^+$ is in the intracellular compartment, where the intracellular concentration is approximately 160 mmol/L. Normal individuals maintain external K$^+$ balance by excreting amounts into the urine that equal the intake, less the relatively small losses in stool and sweat. K$^+$ is freely filtered at the glomerulus, although the amount excreted usually represents no more than about 20% of the quantity filtered. The great bulk of the K$^+$ filtered is reabsorbed in the early portions of the nephron, about two-thirds in the proximal tubule, and an additional 20 to 25% in the loop of Henle. A *K$^+$ secretory process* operates in the distal tubule and terminal nephron segments. This process is largely dependent on Na$^+$ reabsorption and the accompanying lumen-negative voltage creating an electrical gradient across the tubule wall, favoring K$^+$ secretion into the lumen of the distal tubule and collecting duct.

The ability to maintain external K^+ balance and normal plasma K^+ concentration until relatively late in the course of CRF is a consequence primarily of a progressive increase in fractional excretion of K^+. Greatly enhanced rates of K^+ secretion occur in distal portions of surviving tubules. The augmented secretion rate of aldosterone contributes to enhanced tubule secretion of K^+. In addition, both the increased distal tubule flow rates in surviving nephrons, due to the osmotic diuresis, and enhanced luminal electronegativity, created by the increased presence of highly impermeable anions such as phosphate and sulfate, enhance K^+ secretion. Aldosterone also stimulates net entry of K^+ into the lumen of the colon, a mechanism known to be enhanced in CRF. →*For more detailed discussions of abnormal K^+ homeostasis in acute and chronic forms of renal failure, see Chaps. 260 and 261.*

FURTHER READING

BRENNER BM et al: Diverse biological actions of atrial natriuretic peptides. Physiol Rev 70:665, 1990

O'CALLAGHAN CA, BRENNER BM: *The Kidney at a Glance.* Oxford, Blackwell Science Ltd., 2000

TAAL MW et al: Adaptation to nephron loss, in *Brenner and Rector's The Kidney,* 7th ed, BM Brenner, (ed). Philadelphia, Saunders, 2004

TAAL MW, BRENNER BM: Renoprotective benefits of RAS inhibition: From ACEI to angiotensin II antagonists. Kidney Int 57:1803, 2000

260 ACUTE RENAL FAILURE
Hugh R. Brady, Barry M. Brenner

Acute renal failure (ARF) is a syndrome characterized by rapid decline in glomerular filtration rate (hours to days), retention of nitrogenous waste products, and perturbation of extracellular fluid volume and electrolyte and acid-base homeostasis. ARF complicates approximately 5% of hospital admissions and up to 30% of admissions to intensive care units. Oliguria (urine output < 400 mL/d) is a frequent but not invariable clinical feature (~50%). ARF is usually asymptomatic and diagnosed when biochemical monitoring of hospitalized patients reveals a recent increase in blood urea and creatinine concentrations. It may complicate a wide range of diseases, which for purposes of diagnosis and management are conveniently divided into three categories: (1) diseases that cause renal hypoperfusion without compromising the integrity of renal parenchyma (*prerenal ARF*, prerenal azotemia) (~55%); (2) diseases that directly involve renal parenchyma (*intrinsic renal ARF*, renal azotemia) (~40%); and (3) diseases associated with urinary tract obstruction (*postrenal ARF*, postrenal azotemia) (~5%). Most ARF is reversible, the kidney being relatively unique among major organs in its ability to recover from almost complete loss of function. Nevertheless, ARF is associated with major in-hospital morbidity and mortality, in large part due to the serious nature of the illnesses that precipitate the ARF.

ETIOLOGY AND PATHOPHYSIOLOGY

PRERENAL ARF (PRERENAL AZOTEMIA) Prerenal ARF is the most common form of ARF and represents a physiologic response to mild to moderate renal hypoperfusion. Prerenal ARF is by definition rapidly reversible upon restoration of renal blood flow and glomerular ultrafiltration pressure. Renal parenchymal tissue is not damaged; indeed, kidneys from individuals with prerenal ARF function well when transplanted into recipients with normal cardiovascular function. More severe hypoperfusion may lead to ischemic injury of renal parenchyma and intrinsic renal ARF (see below). Thus, prerenal ARF and intrinsic renal ARF due to ischemia are part of a spectrum of manifestations of renal hypoperfusion. As shown in Table 260-1, prerenal ARF can complicate any disease that induces hypovolemia, low cardiac output, systemic vasodilatation, or selective intrarenal vasoconstriction.

Hypovolemia leads to a fall in mean systemic arterial pressure, which is detected as reduced stretch by arterial (e.g., carotid sinus) and cardiac baroreceptors. Activated baroreceptors trigger a coordinated series of neural and humoral responses designed to restore blood volume and arterial pressure. These include activation of the sympathetic nervous system and renin-angiotensin-aldosterone system and release of arginine vasopressin (AVP; formerly called antidiuretic hormone). Norepinephrine, angiotensin II, and AVP act in concert in an attempt to preserve cardiac and cerebral perfusion by stimulating vasoconstriction in relatively "nonessential" vascular beds, such as the musculocutaneous and splanchnic circulations, by inhibiting salt loss through sweat glands, by stimulating thirst and salt appetite, and by promoting renal salt and water retention. Glomerular perfusion, ultrafiltration pressure, and filtration rate are preserved during mild hypoperfusion through several compensatory mechanisms. Stretch receptors in afferent arterioles, in response to a reduction in perfusion pressure, trigger afferent arteriolar vasodilatation through a local myogenic reflex (autoregulation). Biosynthesis of vasodilator prostaglandins (e.g., prostaglandin E_2 and prostacyclin) is also enhanced, and these compounds preferentially dilate afferent arterioles. In addition, angiotensin II induces preferential constriction of efferent arterioles. As a result, intraglomerular pressure is maintained, the fraction of plasma flowing through glomerular capillaries that is filtered is increased (filtration fraction), and glomerular filtration rate (GFR) is preserved. During states of more severe hypoperfusion, these compensatory responses are overwhelmed and GFR falls, leading to prerenal ARF.

Autoregulatory dilatation of afferent arterioles is maximal at mean systemic arterial blood pressures of ~80 mmHg, and hypotension below this level is associated with a precipitous decline in GFR. Lesser degrees of hypotension may provoke prerenal ARF in the elderly and in patients with diseases affecting the integrity of afferent arterioles (e.g., hypertensive nephrosclerosis, diabetic vasculopathy). In addition, drugs that interfere with adaptive responses in the renal microcirculation may convert compensated renal hypoperfusion into overt prerenal ARF or trigger progression of prerenal ARF to ischemic intrinsic renal ARF (see below). Pharmacologic inhibitors of either renal prostaglandin biosynthesis [*cyclooxygenase inhibitors*; nonsteroidal anti-inflammatory drugs (NSAIDs)] or angiotensin-converting enzyme (ACE) activity (ACE inhibitors) and angiotensin II receptor blockers are the major culprits and should be used judiciously in the setting of suspected renal hypoperfusion. NSAIDs do not compromise GFR in healthy individuals but may precipitate prerenal ARF in patients with volume depletion or in those with chronic renal insufficiency in whom GFR is maintained, in part, through prostaglandin-mediated hyperfiltration by the remaining functional nephrons. ACE inhibitors should be used with special care in patients with bilateral renal artery stenosis or unilateral stenosis in a solitary functioning kidney. In these settings glomerular perfusion and filtration may be exquisitely dependent on the actions of angiotensin II. Angiotensin II preserves glomerular filtration pressure distal to stenoses by elevating systemic arterial pressure and by triggering selective constriction of efferent arterioles. ACE inhibitors blunt these responses and precipitate ARF, usually reversible, in ~30% of these patients.

Hepatorenal Syndrome This is a particularly aggressive form of ARF, with many of the features of prerenal ARF, that frequently complicates hepatic failure due to advanced cirrhosis or other liver diseases, including malignancy, hepatic resection, and biliary obstruction. In full-blown hepatorenal syndrome, ARF progresses even after optimization

TABLE 260-1 *Classification and Major Causes of Acute Renal Failure (ARF)*

PRERENAL ARF
I. Hypovolemia
  A. Hemorrhage, burns, dehydration
  B. Gastrointestinal fluid loss: vomiting, surgical drainage, diarrhea
  C. Renal fluid loss: diuretics, osmotic diuresis (e.g., diabetes mellitus), hypoadrenalism
  D. Sequestration in extravascular space: pancreatitis, peritonitis, trauma, burns, severe hypoalbuminemia
II. Low cardiac output
  A. Diseases of myocardium, valves, and pericardium; arrhythmias; tamponade
  B. Other: pulmonary hypertension, massive pulmonary embolus, positive pressure mechanical ventilation
III. Altered renal systemic vascular resistance ratio
  A. Systemic vasodilatation: sepsis, antihypertensives, afterload reducers, anesthesia, anaphylaxis
  B. Renal vasoconstriction: hypercalcemia, norepinephrine, epinephrine, cyclosporine, tacrolimus, amphotericin B
  C. Cirrhosis with ascites (hepatorenal syndrome)
IV. Renal hypoperfusion with impairment of renal autoregulatory responses
  Cyclooxygenase inhibitors, angiotensin-converting enzyme inhibitors
V. Hyperviscosity syndrome (rare)
  Multiple myeloma, macroglobulinemia, polycythemia

INTRINSIC RENAL ARF
I. Renovascular obstruction (bilateral or unilateral in the setting of one functioning kidney)
  A. Renal artery obstruction: atherosclerotic plaque, thrombosis, embolism, dissecting aneurysm, vasculitis
  B. Renal vein obstruction: thrombosis, compression
II. Disease of glomeruli or renal microvasculature
  A. Glomerulonephritis and vasculitis
  B. Hemolytic uremic syndrome, thrombotic thrombocytopenic purpura, disseminated intravascular coagulation, toxemia of pregnancy, accelerated hypertension, radiation nephritis, systemic lupus erythematosus, scleroderma
III. Acute tubular necrosis
  A. Ischemia: as for prerenal ARF (hypovolemia, low cardiac output, renal vasoconstriction, systemic vasodilatation), obstetric complications (abruptio placentae, postpartum hemorrhage)
  B. Toxins
    1. Exogenous: radiocontrast, cyclosporine, antibiotics (e.g., aminoglycosides), chemotherapy (e.g., cisplatin), organic solvents (e.g., ethylene glycol), acetaminophen, illegal abortifacients
    2. Endogenous: rhabdomyolysis, hemolysis, uric acid, oxalate, plasma cell dyscrasia (e.g., myeloma)
IV. Interstitial nephritis
  A. Allergic: antibiotics (e.g., β-lactams, sulfonamides, trimethoprim, rifampicin), nonsteroidal anti-inflammatory agents, diuretics, captopril
  B. Infection: bacterial (e.g., acute pyelonephritis, leptospirosis), viral (e.g., cytomegalovirus), fungal (e.g., candidiasis)
  C. Infiltration: lymphoma, leukemia, sarcoidosis
  D. Idiopathic
V. Intratubular deposition and obstruction
  Myeloma proteins, uric acid, oxalate, acyclovir, methotrexate, sulphonamides
VI. Renal allograft rejection

POSTRENAL ARF (OBSTRUCTION)
I. Ureteric
  Calculi, blood clot, sloughed papillae, cancer, external compression (e.g., retroperitoneal fibrosis)
II. Bladder neck
  Neurogenic bladder, prostatic hypertrophy, calculi, cancer, blood clot
III. Urethra
  Stricture, congenital valve, phimosis

of systemic hemodynamics and carries a mortality rate of >90%. →*The diagnosis and management of this condition are discussed in Chaps. 289 and 291.*

INTRINSIC RENAL ARF (INTRINSIC RENAL AZOTEMIA) Intrinsic renal ARF can complicate many diverse diseases of the renal parenchyma. From a clinicopathologic viewpoint, it is useful to divide the causes of intrinsic renal ARF into (1) diseases of larger renal vessels, (2) diseases of the renal microcirculation and glomeruli, (3) ischemic and nephrotoxic ARF, and (4) tubulointerstitial inflammation (Table 260-1). Most intrinsic renal ARF is triggered by ischemia (ischemic ARF) or nephrotoxins (nephrotoxic ARF), insults that classically induce acute tubular necrosis (ATN). Accordingly, the terms ARF and ATN are usually used interchangeably in these settings. However, as many as 20 to 30% of patients with ischemic or nephrotoxic ARF do not have clinical (granular or tubular cell urinary casts) or morphologic evidence of tubular necrosis, underscoring the role of sublethal injury to tubular epithelium and injury to other renal cells (e.g., endothelial cells) in the pathophysiology of this syndrome.

Etiology and Pathophysiology of Ischemic ARF Prerenal ARF and ischemic ARF are part of a spectrum of manifestations of renal hypoperfusion. Ischemic ARF differs from prerenal ARF in that the hypoperfusion induces ischemic injury to renal parenchymal cells, particularly tubular epithelium, and recovery typically takes 1 to 2 weeks after normalization of renal perfusion as it requires repair and regeneration of renal cells. In its most extreme form, ischemia leads to bilateral renal cortical necrosis and irreversible renal failure. Ischemic ARF occurs most frequently in patients undergoing major cardiovascular surgery or suffering severe trauma, hemorrhage, sepsis, and/or volume depletion (Table 260-1). Ischemic ARF can also complicate milder forms of true hypovolemia or reduced "effective" arterial blood volume if they occur in the presence of other insults (e.g., nephrotoxins or sepsis) or in patients with compromised autoregulatory defense mechanisms or preexisting renal disease.

The course of ischemic ARF is typically characterized by three phases: the initiation, maintenance, and recovery phases. The *initiation phase* (hours to days) is the initial period of renal hypoperfusion during which ischemic injury is evolving. GFR declines because (1) glomerular ultrafiltration pressure is reduced as a consequence of the fall in renal blood flow, (2) the flow of glomerular filtrate within tubules is obstructed by casts comprised of epithelial cells and necrotic debris derived from ischemic tubule epithelium, and (3) there is backleak of glomerular filtrate through injured tubular epithelium (Fig. 260-1). Ischemic injury is most prominent in the terminal medullary portion of the proximal tubule (S_3 segment, pars recta) and the medullary portion of the thick ascending limb of the loop of Henle. Both segments have high rates of active (ATP-dependent) solute transport and oxygen consumption and are located in a zone of the kidney (the outer medulla) that is relatively ischemic, even under basal conditions, by virtue of the unique countercurrent arrangement of the medullary vasculature. Cellular ischemia results in a series of alterations in energetics, ion transport, and membrane integrity that ultimately lead to cell injury and, if severe, cell apoptosis or necrosis. These alterations include depletion of ATP, inhibition of active sodium transport and transport of other solutes, impairment of cell volume regulation and cell swelling, cytoskeletal disruption and loss of cell polarity, cell-cell and cell-matrix attachment, accumulation of intracellular calcium, altered phospholipid metabolism, oxygen free radical formation, and peroxidation of membrane lipids. Importantly, renal injury can be limited by restoration of renal blood flow during this period.

The initiation phase is followed by a *maintenance phase* (typically 1 to 2 weeks) during which renal cell injury is established, GFR stabilizes at its nadir (typically 5 to 10 mL/min), urine output is lowest, and uremic complications arise (see below). The reasons why the GFR remains low during this phase, despite correction of systemic hemodynamics, are still being defined. Putative mechanisms include persistent intrarenal vasoconstriction and medullary ischemia triggered by dysregulated release of vasoactive mediators from injured endothelial cells (e.g., decreased nitric oxide, increased endothelin-1, adenosine, and platelet-activating factor), congestion of medullary blood vessels, and reperfusion injury induced by reactive oxygen species and other mediators derived from leukocytes or renal parenchymal cells

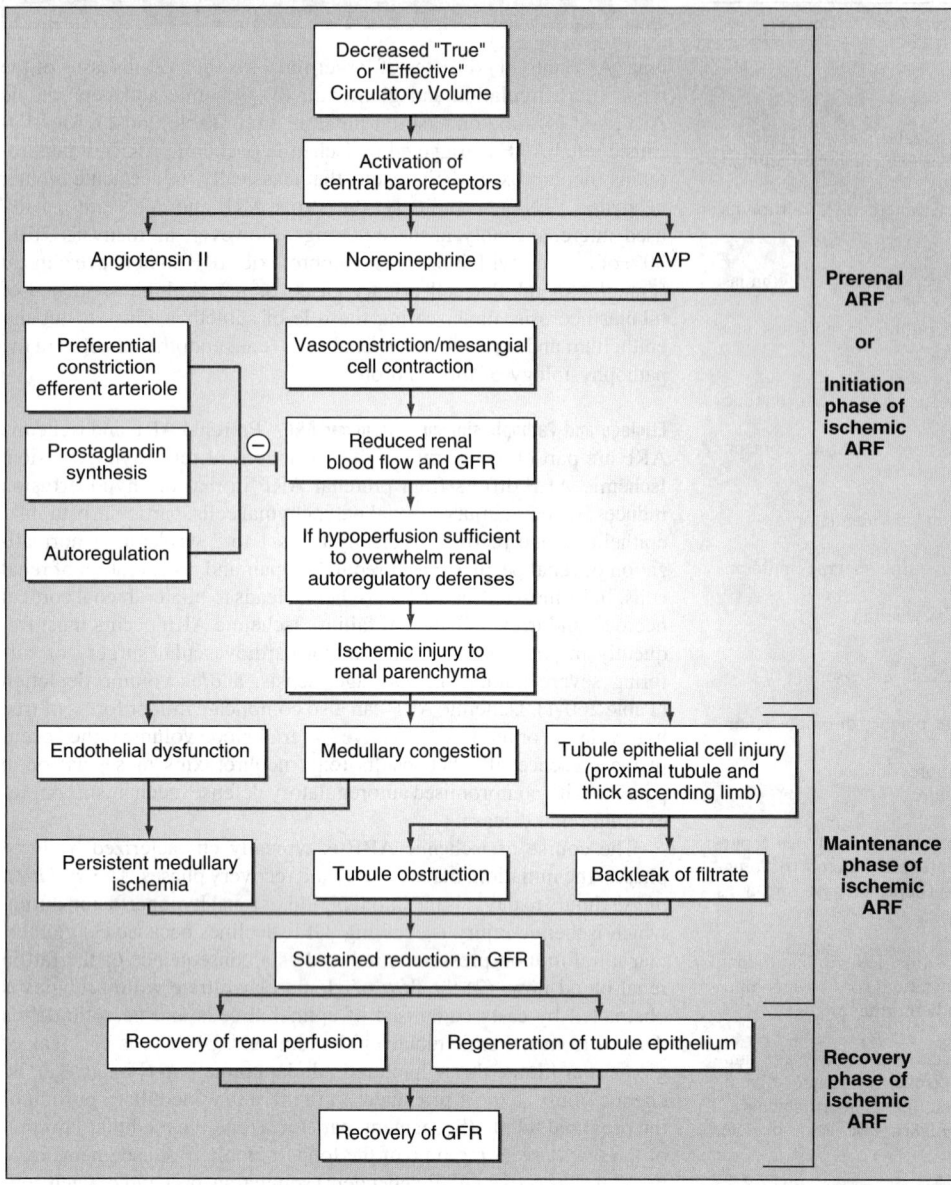

FIGURE 260-1 Overview of the pathophysiology of prerenal ARF and ischemic intrinsic renal ARF: A spectrum of manifestations of renal hypoperfusion. ARF, acute renal failure; AVP, arginine vasopressin; GFR, glomerular filtration rate.

(Fig. 260-1). In addition, epithelial cell injury per se may contribute to persistent intrarenal vasoconstriction by a process termed *tubuloglomerular feedback*. Specialized epithelial cells in the macula densa region of distal tubules detect increases in distal salt (probably chloride) delivery that occur as a consequence of impaired reabsorption by more proximal nephron segments. Macula densa cells in turn stimulate constriction of adjacent afferent arterioles by a poorly defined mechanism and further compromise glomerular perfusion and filtration, thereby contributing to a vicious cycle. A *recovery phase* is characterized by renal parenchymal cell, particularly tubule epithelial cell, repair and regeneration and a gradual return of GFR to or towards premorbid levels. The recovery phase may be complicated by a marked diuretic phase due to excretion of retained salt and water and other solutes, continued use of diuretics, and/or delayed recovery of epithelial cell function (solute and water reabsorption) relative to glomerular filtration (see below).

Etiology and Pathophysiology of Nephrotoxic ARF Acute intrinsic renal ARF can complicate exposure to many structurally diverse pharmacologic agents (Table 260-1). With most nephrotoxins, the incidence of ARF is increased in the elderly and in patients with preexisting chronic renal insufficiency, true or "effective" hypovolemia, or concomitant exposure to other toxins.

Intrarenal vasoconstriction is a pivotal event in ARF that is triggered by *radiocontrast agents* (contrast nephropathy), *cyclosporine*, and *tacrolimus (FK506)*. In keeping with this pathophysiology, both agents induce ARF that shares features with prerenal ARF: namely, an acute fall in renal blood flow and GFR, a relatively benign urine sediment, and a low fractional excretion of sodium (see below). Severe cases may show clinical or pathologic evidence of ATN. Contrast nephropathy classically presents as an acute (onset within 24 to 48 h) but reversible (peak 3 to 5 days, resolution within 1 week) rise in blood urea nitrogen and creatinine and is most common in individuals with preexisting chronic renal insufficiency, diabetes mellitus, congestive heart failure, hypovolemia, or multiple myeloma. The syndrome appears to be dose-related, and its incidence is only slightly reduced in high-risk individuals by use of more expensive low osmolality, nonionic contrast agents.

Direct toxicity to tubule epithelial cells and/or intratubular obstruction are major pathophysiologic events in ARF induced by many antibiotics and anticancer drugs. Frequent offenders are the antimicrobial agents, such as acyclovir, foscarnet, aminoglycosides, amphotericin B, and pentamidine, and chemotherapeutic agents, such as cisplatin, carboplatin, and ifosfamide. ARF complicates 10 to 30% of courses of *aminoglycoside antibiotics*, even in the presence of therapeutic levels. *Amphotericin B* causes dose-related ARF through intrarenal vasoconstriction and direct toxicity to proximal tubule epithelium. Cisplatin and carboplatin, like the aminoglycosides, are accumulated by proximal tubule cells and typically provoke ARF after 7 to 10 days of exposure by inducing mitochondrial injury, inhibition of ATPase activity and solute transport, free radical–mediated injury to cell membranes, apoptosis, and/or necrosis.

The most common endogenous nephrotoxins are calcium, myoglobin, hemoglobin, urate, oxalate, and myeloma light chains. Hypercalcemia can compromise GFR, predominantly by inducing intrarenal vasoconstriction. Calcium phosphate deposition within the kidney may also contribute. Both *rhabdomyolysis* and *hemolysis* can induce ARF, particularly in hypovolemic or acidotic individuals. Myoglobinuric ARF complicates approximately 30% of cases of rhabdomyolysis. Common causes of the latter include traumatic crush injury, acute muscle ischemia, seizures, excessive exercise, heat stroke or malignant hyperthermia, intoxications (e.g., alcohol, cocaine), and infectious or metabolic disorders. ARF due to hemolysis is relatively rare and is observed following massive blood transfusion reactions. It has been postulated that myoglobin and hemoglobin or other compounds released from muscle or red blood cells cause ARF via toxic effects on tubule epithelial cells, by promoting intrarenal oxidative stress and by inducing intratubular cast formation. Hypovolemia or acidosis may contribute to the pathogenesis of ARF in this setting by promoting intratubular cast formation. In addition, both hemoglobin and myoglobin are potent inhibitors of nitric oxide bioactivity and may trigger intrarenal vasoconstriction and ischemia in patients with borderline renal hypoperfusion. The formation of intratubular casts containing filtered immunoglobulin light chains and other proteins, including Tamm-Horsfall protein produced by thick ascending limb cells, is the major trigger for ARF in patients with *multiple myeloma* (myeloma cast nephropathy). In addition, light chains are directly toxic to tubule epithelial cells. Intratubular obstruction is also an important cause of ARF in patients with severe *hyperuricosuria* or *hyperoxaluria*. Acute uric acid nephropathy typically complicates treatment of lymphoproliferative or myeloproliferative disorders but occasionally occurs in other forms of primary or secondary hyperuricemia if the urine is concentrated.

Pathology of Ischemic and Nephrotoxic ARF The classic pathologic features of ischemic ARF are patchy and focal necrosis of tubule epithelium with detachment from its basement membrane and occlusion of tubule lumens with casts composed of intact or degenerating epithelial cells, cellular debris, Tamm-Horsfall mucoprotein, and pigments. Leukocyte accumulation is frequently observed in vasa recta; however, the morphology of the glomeruli and renal vasculature is characteristically normal. Necrosis is most severe in the straight portion (pars recta) of proximal tubules but may also affect the medullary thick ascending limb of the loop of Henle.

In nephrotoxic ARF, morphologic changes tend to be most prominent in both the convoluted and straight portions of proximal tubules. Tubule cell necrosis is less pronounced than in ischemic ARF.

Other Causes of Intrinsic Renal ARF Patients with advanced atherosclerosis can develop ARF after manipulation of the aorta or renal arteries at surgery or angiography, following trauma, or, rarely, spontaneously due to embolization of cholesterol crystals to the renal vasculature (atheroembolic ARF). Cholesterol crystals lodge in small- and medium-sized arteries and incite a giant cell and fibrotic reaction in the vessel wall with narrowing or obstruction of the vessel lumen. Atheroembolic ARF is frequently irreversible. A myriad of structurally diverse pharmacologic agents induce ARF by triggering allergic interstitial nephritis, a disease characterized by infiltration of the tubulointerstitium by granulocytes (typically but not invariably eosinophils), macrophages, and/or lymphocytes and by interstitial edema. The most common offenders are antibiotics (e.g., penicillins, cephalosporins, trimethoprim, sulfonamides, rifampicin) and NSAIDs (Table 260-1).

POSTRENAL ARF (See also Chap. 270) Urinary tract obstruction accounts for fewer than 5% of cases of ARF. Because one kidney has sufficient clearance capacity to excrete the nitrogenous waste products generated daily, ARF from obstruction requires obstruction to urine flow between the external urethral meatus and bladder neck, bilateral ureteric obstruction, or unilateral ureteric obstruction in a patient with one functioning kidney or with preexisting chronic renal insufficiency. Bladder neck obstruction represents the most common cause of postrenal ARF and is usually due to prostatic disease (e.g., hypertrophy, neoplasia, or infection), neurogenic bladder, or therapy with anticholinergic drugs. Less common causes of acute lower urinary tract obstruction include blood clots, calculi, and urethritis with spasm. Ureteric obstruction may result from intraluminal obstruction (e.g., calculi, blood clots, sloughed renal papillae), infiltration of the ureteric wall (e.g., neoplasia), or external compression (e.g., retroperitoneal fibrosis, neoplasia or abscess, inadvertent surgical ligature). During the early stages of obstruction (hours to days), continued glomerular filtration leads to increased intraluminal pressure upstream to the site of obstruction. As a result there is gradual distention of the proximal ureter, renal pelvis, and calyces and a fall in GFR. Acute obstruction is initially associated with modest increase in renal blood flow, but arteriolar vasoconstriction soon supervenes, leading to a further decline in glomerular filtration.

CLINICAL FEATURES AND DIFFERENTIAL DIAGNOSIS

Patients presenting with renal failure should be assessed initially to determine if the decline in GFR is acute or chronic. An acute process

is easily established if a review of laboratory records reveals a recent rise in blood urea and creatinine levels, but previous measurements are not always available. Findings that suggest chronic renal failure (Chap. 261) include anemia, neuropathy, and radiologic evidence of renal osteodystrophy or small scarred kidneys. However, it should be noted that anemia may also complicate ARF (see below), and renal size may be normal or increased in several chronic renal diseases (e.g., diabetic nephropathy, amyloidosis, polycystic kidney disease). Once a diagnosis of ARF has been established, several issues should be addressed promptly: (1) the identification of the cause of ARF, (2) the elimination of the triggering insult (e.g., nephrotoxin) and/or institution of disease-specific therapies, and (3) the prevention and management of uremic complications.

CLINICAL ASSESSMENT Clinical clues to *prerenal* ARF are symptoms of thirst and orthostatic dizziness and physical evidence of orthostatic hypotension and tachycardia, reduced jugular venous pressure, decreased skin turgor, dry mucous membranes, and reduced axillary sweating. Case records should be reviewed for documentation of a progressive fall in urine output and body weight and recent initiation of treatment with NSAIDs, ACE inhibitors, or angiotensin II receptor blockers. Careful clinical examination may reveal stigmata of chronic liver disease and portal hypertension, advanced cardiac failure, sepsis, or other causes of reduced "effective" arterial blood volume (Table 260-1).

Intrinsic renal ARF due to ischemia is likely following severe renal hypoperfusion complicating hypovolemic or septic shock or following major surgery. The likelihood of ischemic ARF is increased further if ARF persists despite normalization of systemic hemodynamics. Diagnosis of nephrotoxic ARF requires careful review of the clinical data and pharmacy, nursing, and radiology records for evidence of recent exposure to nephrotoxic medications or radiocontrast agents or to endogenous toxins (e.g., myoglobin, hemoglobin, uric acid, myeloma protein, or elevated levels of serum calcium).

Although ischemic and nephrotoxic ARF account for more than 90% of cases of intrinsic renal ARF, other renal parenchymal diseases must be considered (Table 260-2). Flank pain may be a prominent symptom following occlusion of a renal artery or vein and with other parenchymal diseases distending the renal capsule (e.g., severe glomerulonephritis or pyelonephritis). Subcutaneous nodules, livedo reticularis, bright orange retinal arteriolar plaques, and digital ischemia, despite palpable pedal pulses, are clues to atheroembolization. ARF in association with oliguria, edema, hypertension, and an "active" urine sediment (nephritic syndrome) suggests acute glomerulonephritis or vasculitis. Malignant hypertension is a likely cause of ARF in patients with severe hypertension and evidence of hypertensive injury to other organs (e.g., left ventricular hypertrophy and failure, hypertensive retinopathy and papilledema, neurologic dysfunction). Fever, arthralgias, and a pruritic erythematous rash following exposure to a new drug suggest allergic interstitial nephritis, although systemic features of hypersensitivity are frequently absent.

Postrenal ARF presents with suprapubic and flank pain due to distention of the bladder and of the renal collecting system and capsule, respectively. Colicky flank pain radiating to the groin suggests acute ureteric obstruction. Prostatic disease is likely if there is a history of nocturia, frequency, and hesitancy and enlargement or induration of the prostate on rectal examination. Neurogenic bladder should be suspected in patients receiving anticholinergic medications or with physical evidence of autonomic dysfunction. Definitive diagnosis of postrenal ARF hinges on judicious use of radiologic investigations and rapid improvement in renal function following relief of obstruction.

URINALYSIS Anuria suggests complete urinary tract obstruction but may complicate severe cases of prerenal or intrinsic renal ARF. Wide fluctuations in urine output raise the possibility of intermittent obstruction, whereas patients with partial urinary tract obstruction can present with polyuria due to impairment of urine concentrating mechanisms.

Cause of Acute Renal Failure	Suggestive Clinical Features	Typical Urinalysis	Some Confirmatory Tests
I. Prerenal ARF	Evidence of true volume depletion (thirst, postural or absolute hypotension and tachycardia, low jugular venous pressure, dry mucous membranes/axillae, weight loss, fluid output > input) or decreased "effective" circulatory volume (e.g., heart failure, liver failure), treatment with NSAIDs or ACE inhibitors	Hyaline casts FE_{Na} <1% U_{Na} <10 mmol/L SG >1.018	Occasionally requires invasive hemodynamic monitoring; rapid resolution of ARF upon restoration of renal perfusion
II. Intrinsic renal ARF			
A. Diseases involving large renal vessels			
1. Renal artery thrombosis	History of atrial fibrillation or recent myocardial infarct; flank or abdominal pain	Mild proteinuria Occasionally red cells	Elevated LDH with normal transaminases, renal arteriogram
2. Atheroembolism	Age usually > 50 years, recent manipulation of aorta, retinal plaques, subcutaneous nodules, palpable purpura, livedo reticularis, vasculopathy, hypertension, anticoagulation	Often normal, eosinophiluria, rarely casts	Eosinophilia, hypocomplementemia, skin biopsy, renal biopsy
3. Renal vein thrombosis	Evidence of nephrotic syndrome or pulmonary embolism, flank pain	Proteinuria, hematuria	Inferior vena cavagram and selective renal venogram
B. Diseases of small vessels and glomeruli			
1. Glomerulonephritis/vasculitis	Compatible clinical history (e.g., recent infection), sinusitis, lung hemorrhage, skin rash or ulcers, arthralgias, new cardiac murmur, history of hepatitis B or C infection	Red cell or granular casts, red cells, white cells, mild proteinuria	Low C3, ANCA, anti-GBM Ab, ANA, ASO, anti-DNase, cryoglobulins, blood cultures, renal biopsy
2. Hemolytic-uremic syndrome/thrombotic thrombocytopenic purpura	Compatible clinical history (e.g., recent gastrointestinal infection, cyclosporine, anovulants), fever, pallor, ecchymoses, neurologic abnormalities	May be normal, red cells, mild proteinuria, rarely red cell/granular casts	Anemia, thrombocytopenia, schistocytes on blood smear, increased LDH, renal biopsy
3. Malignant hypertension	Severe hypertension with headaches, cardiac failure, retinopathy, neurologic dysfunction, papilledema	Red cells, red cell casts, proteinuria	LVH by echocardiography/ECG, resolution of ARF with control of blood pressure
C. ARF mediated by ischemia or toxins (ATN)			
1. Ischemia	Recent hemorrhage, hypotension (e.g., cardiac arrest), surgery	Muddy brown granular or tubular epithelial cell casts FE_{Na} >1% U_{Na} >20 mmol/L SG <1.015	Clinical assessment and urinalysis usually sufficient for diagnosis
2. Exogenous toxins	Recent radiocontrast study, nephrotoxic antibiotics or anticancer agents often coexistent with volume depletion, sepsis, or chronic renal insufficiency	Muddy brown granular or tubular epithelial cell casts FE_{Na} >1% U_{Na} >20 mmol/L SG <1.015	Clinical assessment and urinalysis usually sufficient for diagnosis
3. Endogenous toxins	History suggestive of rhabdomyolysis (seizures, coma, ethanol abuse, trauma)	Urine supernatant positive for heme	Hyperkalemia, hyperphosphatemia, hypocalcemia, increased circulating myoglobin, CPK (MM), and uric acid
	History suggestive of hemolysis (blood transfusion)	Urine supernatant pink and positive for heme	Hyperkalemia, hyperphosphatemia, hypocalcemia, hyperuricemia, pink plasma positive for hemoglobin
	History suggestive of tumor lysis (recent chemotherapy), myeloma (bone pain), or ethylene glycol ingestion	Urate crystals, dipstick-negative proteinuria, oxalate crystals, respectively	Hyperuricemia, hyperkalemia, hyperphosphatemia (for tumor lysis); circulating or urinary monoclonal spike (for myeloma); toxicology screen, acidosis, osmolal gap (for ethylene glycol)
D. Acute diseases of the tubulointerstitium			
1. Allergic interstitial nephritis	Recent ingestion of drug, and fever, rash, or arthralgias	White cell casts, white cells (frequently eosinophiluria), red cells, rarely red cell casts, proteinuria (occasionally nephrotic)	Systemic eosinophilia, skin biopsy of rash (leukocytoclastic vasculitis), renal biopsy
2. Acute bilateral pyelonephritis	Flank pain and tenderness, toxic, febrile	Leukocytes, proteinuria, red cells, bacteria	Urine and blood cultures
III. Postrenal ARF	Abdominal or flank pain, palpable bladder	Frequently normal, hematuria if stones, hemorrhage, malignancy, or prostatic hypertrophy	Plain film, renal ultrasound, IVP, retrograde or anterograde pyelography, CT scan

Note: U_{Na}, urine sodium concentration; SG, specific gravity; LDH, lactate dehydrogenase; C3, complement component; ANCA, antineutrophil cytoplasmic autoantibody; anti-GBM Ab, anti-glomerular basement membrane antibody; ANA, antinuclear antibody; ASO, antistreptolysin O; LVH, left ventricular hypertrophy; ECG, electrocardiogram; CK, creatine kinase; IVP, intravenous pyelogram; CT, computed tomography.
Source: Adapted with permission from Brady et al.

In prenatal ARF, the sediment is characteristically acellular and contains transparent hyaline casts ("bland," "benign," "inactive" urine sediment). Hyaline casts are formed in concentrated urine from normal constitutents of urine—principally Tamm-Horsfall protein, which is secreted by epithelial cells of the loop of Henle. Postrenal ARF may also present with an inactive sediment, although hematuria and pyuria are common in patients with intraluminal obstruction or prostatic disease. Pigmented "muddy brown" granular casts and casts containing tubule epithelial cells are characteristic of ATN and suggest ischemic or nephrotoxic ARF. They are usually found in association with microscopic hematuria and mild "tubular" proteinuria (<1 g/d); the latter reflects impaired reabsorption and processing of filtered proteins by injured proximal tubules. Casts are absent, however, in 20 to 30% of patients with ischemic or nephrotoxic ARF and are not a requisite for diagnosis. In general, red blood cell casts indicate glomerular injury or, less often, acute tubulointerstitial nephritis. White cell casts and nonpigmented granular casts suggest interstitial nephritis, whereas broad granular casts are characteristic of chronic renal disease and probably reflect interstitial fibrosis and dilatation of tubules. Eosinophiluria (>5% of urine leukocytes) is a common finding (~90%) in antibiotic-induced allergic interstitial nephritis when studied using Hansel's stain; however, lymphocytes may predominate in allergic interstitial nephritis induced by NSAIDs. Eosinophiluria is also a feature of atheroembolic ARF. Occasional uric acid crystals (pleomorphic in shape) are common in the concentrated urine of prenatal ARF but suggest acute urate nephropathy if seen in abundance. Oxalate (envelope-shaped) and hippurate (needle-shaped) crystals raise the possibility of ethylene glycol ingestion and toxicity.

Proteinuria of >1 g/d suggests injury to the glomerular ultrafiltration barrier ("glomerular proteinuria") or excretion of myeloma light chains. The latter are not detected by conventional dipsticks (which detect albumin) and must be sought by other means (e.g., sulfosalicylic acid test, immunoelectrophoresis). Heavy proteinuria is also a frequent finding (~80%) in patients who develop combined allergic interstitial nephritis and minimal change glomerulopathy when treated with NSAIDs. A similar syndrome can be triggered by ampicillin, rifampicin, or interferon α. Hemoglobinuria or myoglobinuria should be suspected if urine is strongly positive for heme by dipstick, but contains few red cells, and if the supernatant of centrifuged urine is positive for free heme. Bilirubinuria may provide a clue to the presence of hepatorenal syndrome.

RENAL FAILURE INDICES Analysis of urine and blood biochemistry is particularly useful for distinguishing prenatal ARF from ischemic or nephrotoxic intrinsic renal ARF (Table 260-3). The fractional excretion of sodium (FE$_{Na}$) is most useful in this regard. The FE$_{Na}$ relates sodium clearance to creatinine clearance. Sodium is reabsorbed avidly from glomerular filtrate in patients with prenatal ARF, in an attempt to restore intravascular volume, but not in patients with ischemic or nephrotoxic intrinsic ARF, as a result of tubular epithelial cell injury. In contrast, creatinine is not reabsorbed in either setting. Consequently, patients with prenatal ARF typically have a FE$_{Na}$ of <1.0% (frequently <0.1%), whereas the FE$_{Na}$ in patients with ischemic or nephrotoxic ARF is usually >1.0%. The *renal failure index* (Table 260-3) provides comparable information, since clinical variations in serum sodium concentration are relatively small. *Urine sodium concentration* is a less sensitive index for distinguishing prenatal ARF from ischemic and nephrotoxic ARF as values overlap between groups. Similarly, indices of urinary concentrating ability such as urine specific gravity, urine osmolality, urine-to-plasma urea ratio, and blood urea-to-creatinine ratio are of limited value in differential diagnosis.

Many caveats apply when interpreting biochemical renal failure indices. FE$_{Na}$ may be >1.0% in prenatal ARF if patients are receiving diuretics or have bicarbonaturia (accompanied by sodium to maintain electroneutrality), preexisting chronic renal failure complicated by salt wasting, or adrenal insufficiency. In contrast, the FE$_{Na}$ is <1.0% in approximately 15% of patients with nonoliguric ischemic or nephrotoxic ARF, probably reflecting patchy injury to tubular epithelium with preservation of reabsorptive function in some areas. The FE$_{Na}$ is also often <1.0% in ARF due to urinary tract obstruction, glomerulonephritis, and vascular diseases.

LABORATORY FINDINGS Serial measurements of serum creatinine can provide useful pointers to the cause of ARF. Prenatal ARF is typified by fluctuating levels that parallel changes in hemodynamic function. Creatinine rises rapidly (within 24 to 48 h) in patients with ARF following renal ischemia, atheroembolization, and radiocontrast exposure. Peak creatinine levels are observed after 3 to 5 days with contrast nephropathy and return to baseline after 5 to 7 days. In contrast, creatinine levels typically peak later (7 to 10 days) in ischemic ARF and atheroembolic disease. The initial rise in serum creatinine is characteristically delayed until the second week of therapy with many tubule epithelial cell toxins (e.g., aminoglycosides, cisplatin) and probably reflects the need for accumulation of these agents within cells before GFR falls.

Hyperkalemia, hyperphosphatemia, hypocalcemia, and elevations in serum uric acid and creatine kinase (MM isoenzyme) levels at presentation suggest a diagnosis of rhabdomyolysis. Hyperuricemia [>890 μmol/L (>15 mg/dL)] in association with hyperkalemia, hyperphosphatemia, and increased circulating levels of intracellular enzymes such as lactate dehydrogenase may indicate acute urate nephropathy and tumor lysis syndrome following cancer chemotherapy. A wide serum anion and osmolal gap (measured serum osmolality minus the serum osmolality calculated from serum sodium, glucose, and urea concentrations) indicate the presence of an unusual anion or osmole in the circulation and are clues to diagnosis of ethylene glycol or methanol ingestion. Severe anemia in the absence of hemorrhage raises the possibility of hemolysis, multiple myeloma, or thrombotic microangiopathy. Systemic eosinophilia suggests allergic interstitial nephritis but is also a feature of atheroembolic disease and polyangiitis nodosa.

RADIOLOGIC FINDINGS Imaging of the urinary tract by ultrasonography is useful to exclude postrenal ARF. Computed tomography and magnetic resonance imaging are alternative imaging modalities. Whereas pelvicalyceal dilatation is usual with urinary tract obstruction (98% sensitivity), dilatation may be absent immediately following obstruc-

TABLE 260-3 *Urine Diagnostic Indices in Differentiation of Prenatal versus Intrinsic Renal ARF*

Diagnostic Index	Typical Findings in ARF	
	Prenatal	Intrinsic Renal
Fractional excretion of sodium (%)^a	<1	>1
$\dfrac{U_{Na} \times P_{Cr}}{P_{Na} \times U_{Cr}} \times 100$		
Urine sodium concentration (mmol/L)	<10	>20
Urine creatinine to plasma creatinine ratio	>40	<20
Urine urea nitrogen to plasma urea nitrogen ratio	>8	<3
Urine specific gravity	>1.020	~1.010
Urine osmolality (mosmol/kg H$_2$O)	>500	~300
Plasma BUN/creatinine ratio	>20	<10–15
Renal failure index^a	<1	>1
$\dfrac{U_{Na}}{U_{Cr}/P_{Cr}}$		
Urinary sediment	Hyaline casts	Muddy brown granular casts

^{a} Most sensitive indices.
Note: U$_{Na}$, urine sodium concentration; P$_{Cr}$, plasma creatinine concentration; P$_{Na}$, plasma sodium concentration; U$_{Cr}$, urine creatinine concentration; BUN, blood urea nitrogen.

tion or in patients with ureteric encasement (e.g., retroperitoneal fibrosis, neoplasia). Retrograde or anterograde pyelography are more definitive investigations in complex cases and provide precise localization of the site of obstruction. A plain film of the abdomen, with tomography if necessary, is a valuable initial screening technique in patients with suspected nephrolithiasis. Doppler ultrasonography and magnetic resonance angiography are useful for assessment of patency of renal arteries and veins in patients with suspected vascular obstruction; however, contrast angiography is usually required for definitive diagnosis.

RENAL BIOPSY   Biopsy is reserved for patients in whom prerenal and postrenal ARF have been excluded and the cause of intrinsic renal ARF is unclear. Renal biopsy is particularly useful when clinical assessment and laboratory investigations suggest diagnoses other than ischemic or nephrotoxic injury that may respond to disease-specific therapy. Examples include glomerulonephritis, vasculitis, hemolytic-uremic syndrome, thrombotic thrombocytopenic purpura, and allergic interstitial nephritis.

COMPLICATIONS

ARF impairs renal excretion of sodium, potassium, and water and perturbs divalent cation homeostasis and urinary acidification mechanisms. As a result, ARF is frequently complicated by intravascular volume overload, hyponatremia, hyperkalemia, hyperphosphatemia, hypocalcemia, hypermagnesemia, and metabolic acidosis. In addition, patients are unable to excrete nitrogenous waste products and are prone to develop the uremic syndrome (Chap. 261). The speed of development and the severity of these complications reflect the degree of renal impairment and catabolic state of the patient.

Expansion of extracellular fluid volume is an inevitable consequence of diminished salt and water excretion in oliguric or anuric individuals. Whereas milder forms are characterized by weight gain, bibasilar lung rales, raised jugular venous pressure, and dependent edema, continued volume expansion may precipitate life-threatening pulmonary edema. Hypervolemia may be particularly problematic in patients receiving multiple intravenous medications and enteral or parenteral nutrition. Excessive administration of free water either through ingestion and nasogastric administration or as hypotonic saline or isotonic dextrose solutions (dextrose being metabolized) can induce *hypoosmolality* and *hyponatremia*, which, if severe, lead to cerebral edema and neurologic abnormalities, including seizures.

Hyperkalemia is a frequent complication of ARF. Serum potassium typically rises by 0.5 mmol/L per day in oliguric and anuric patients due to impaired excretion of ingested or infused potassium and potassium released from injured tissue. Coexistent metabolic acidosis may exacerbate hyperkalemia by promoting potassium efflux from cells. Hyperkalemia may be particularly severe, even at the time of diagnosis, in patients with rhabdomyolysis, hemolysis, and tumor lysis syndrome. Mild hyperkalemia (<6.0 mmol/L) is usually asymptomatic. Higher levels may trigger electrocardiographic abnormalities and/or arrythmias (Chap. 210).

Metabolism of dietary protein yields between 50 and 100 mmol/d of fixed nonvolatile acids that are normally excreted by the kidneys. Consequently, ARF is typically complicated by *metabolic acidosis*, often with an increased serum anion gap (Chap. 42). Acidosis can be particularly severe when endogenous production of hydrogen ions is increased by other mechanisms (e.g., diabetic or fasting ketoacidosis; lactic acidosis complicating generalized tissue hypoperfusion, liver disease, or sepsis; metabolism of ethylene glycol or methanol).

Mild *hyperphosphatemia* is an almost invariable complication of ARF. Severe hyperphosphatemia may develop in highly catabolic patients or following rhabdomyolysis, hemolysis, or tumor lysis. Metastatic deposition of calcium phosphate can lead to *hypocalcemia*, particularly when the product of serum calcium (mg/dL) and phosphate (mg/dL) concentrations exceeds 70. Other factors that contribute

to hypocalcemia include tissue resistance to the actions of parathyroid hormone and reduced levels of 1,25-dihydroxyvitamin D. Hypocalcemia is often asymptomatic but can cause perioral paresthesia, muscle cramps, seizures, hallucinations and confusion, and prolongation of the QT interval and nonspecific T-wave changes on electrocardiography (Chap. 332).

Anemia develops rapidly in ARF and is usually mild and multifactorial in origin. Contributing factors include impaired erythropoiesis, hemolysis, bleeding, hemodilution, and reduced red cell survival time. Prolongation of the *bleeding time* and *leukocytosis* are also common. Common contributors to the bleeding diathesis include mild thrombocytopenia, platelet dysfunction, and/or clotting factor abnormalities (e.g., factor VIII dysfunction), whereas leukocytosis usually reflects sepsis, a stress response, or other concurrent illness. *Infection* is a common and serious complication of ARF, occurring in 50 to 90% of cases and accounting for up to 75% of deaths. It is unclear whether patients with ARF have a clinically significant defect in host immune responses or whether the high incidence of infection reflects repeated breaches of mucocutaneous barriers (e.g., intravenous cannulae, mechanical ventilation, bladder catheterization). *Cardiopulmonary complications* of ARF include arrhythmias, myocardial infarction, pericarditis and pericardial effusion, pulmonary edema, and pulmonary embolism. Mild *gastrointestinal bleeding* is common (10 to 30%) and is usually due to stress ulceration of gastric or small intestinal mucosa.

Protracted periods of severe ARF are invariably associated with the development of the *uremic syndrome* (Chap. 261).

A *vigorous diuresis* can occur during the recovery phase of ARF (see above), which may on occasions be inappropriate and lead to intravascular volume depletion and delayed recovery of GFR by causing secondary prerenal ARF. *Hypernatremia* can also complicate recovery if water losses via hypotonic urine are not replaced or if losses are inappropriately replaced by relatively hypertonic saline solutions. *Hypokalemia, hypomagnesemia, hypophosphatemia,* and *hypocalcemia* are less common metabolic complications during this period.

℞ TREATMENT

Prevention   Because there are no specific therapies for ischemic or nephrotoxic ARF, prevention is of paramount importance. Many cases of ischemic ARF can be avoided by close attention to cardiovascular function and intravascular volume in high-risk patients, such as the elderly and those with preexisting renal insufficiency. Indeed, aggressive restoration of intravascular volume has been shown to reduce dramatically the incidence of ischemic ARF after major surgery or trauma, burns, or cholera. The incidence of nephrotoxic ARF can be reduced by tailoring the dosage of nephrotoxic drugs to body size and GFR; for example, reducing the dose or frequency of administration of drugs in patients with preexisting renal impairment. In this regard, it should be noted that serum creatinine is a relatively insensitive index of GFR and may overestimate GFR considerably in small or elderly patients. For purposes of drug dosing, it is advisable to estimate the GFR using the Cockcroft-Gault formula, which factors in the variables of age and weight (Chap. 40). Adjusting drug dosage according to circulating drug levels also appears to limit renal injury in patients receiving aminoglycoside antibiotics, cyclosporine, or tacrolimus. Diuretics, cyclooxygenase inhibitors, ACE inhibitors, angiotensin II receptor blockers, and other vasodilators should be used with caution in patients with suspected true or "effective" hypovolemia or renovascular disease as they may precipitate prerenal ARF or convert the latter to ischemic ARF. Allopurinol and forced alkaline diuresis are useful prophylactic measures in patients at high risk for acute urate nephropathy (e.g., cancer chemotherapy in hematologic malignancies) to limit uric acid generation and prevent precipitation of urate crystals in renal tubules. Forced alkaline diuresis may also prevent or attenuate ARF in patients receiving high-dose methotrexate or suffering from rhabdomyolysis. *N*-acetylcysteine limits acetaminophen-induced renal injury if given within 24 h of ingestion. Dimercaprol, a chelating agent, may prevent heavy metal nephrotoxicity. Ethanol inhibits ethylene glycol metabolism to oxalic acid and other toxic metabolites and is an important adjunct to hemodialysis in the emergency management of ethylene glycol intoxication.

Specific Therapies By definition, prerenal ARF is rapidly reversible upon correction of the primary hemodynamic abnormality, and postrenal ARF resolves upon relief of obstruction. To date, there are no specific therapies for established intrinsic renal ARF due to ischemia or nephrotoxicity. Management of these disorders should focus on elimination of the causative hemodynamic abnormality or toxin, avoidance of additional insults, and prevention and treatment of complications. Specific treatment of other causes of intrinsic renal ARF depends on the underlying pathology.

PRERENAL ARF The composition of replacement fluids for treatment of prerenal ARF due to hypovolemia must be tailored according to the composition of the lost fluid. Severe hypovolemia due to hemorrhage should be corrected with packed red cells, whereas isotonic saline is usually appropriate replacement for mild to moderate hemorrhage or plasma loss (e.g., burns, pancreatitis). Urinary and gastrointestinal fluids can vary greatly in composition but are usually hypotonic. Hypotonic solutions (e.g., 0.45% saline) are usually recommended as initial replacement in patients with prerenal ARF due to increased urinary or gastrointestinal fluid losses, although isotonic saline may be more appropriate in severe cases. Subsequent therapy should be based on measurements of the volume and ionic content of excreted or drained fluids. Serum potassium and acid-base status should be monitored carefully, and potassium and bicarbonate supplemented as appropriate. Cardiac failure may require aggressive management with positive inotropes, preload and afterload reducing agents, antiarrhythmic drugs, and mechanical aids such as intraaortic balloon pumps. Invasive hemodynamic monitoring may be required to guide therapy for complications in patients in whom clinical assessment of cardiovascular function and intravascular volume is difficult.

Fluid management may be particularly challenging in patients with cirrhosis complicated by ascites. In this setting, it is important to distinguish between full-blown hepatorenal syndrome (Chap. 289), which carries a grave prognosis, and reversible ARF due to true or "effective" hypovolemia induced by overzealous use of diuretics or sepsis (e.g., spontaneous bacterial peritonitis). The contribution of hypovolemia to ARF can be definitively assessed only by administration of a fluid challenge. Fluids should be administered slowly and titrated against jugular venous pressure and, if necessary, central venous and pulmonary capillary wedge pressure, abdominal girth, and urine output. Patients with a reversible prerenal component typically have an increase in urine output and fall in serum creatinine, whereas patients with hepatorenal syndrome do not and may suffer increased ascites formation and pulmonary compromise if not monitored closely. Large volumes of ascitic fluid can usually be drained by paracentesis without deterioration in renal function if intravenous albumin is administered simultaneously. Indeed, "large-volume paracentesis" may afford an increase in GFR, possibly by lowering intraabdominal pressure and improving flow in renal veins. Shunting of ascitic fluid from the peritoneum to a central vein (peritoneojugular shunt, LeVeen or Denver shunts) is an alternative approach in refractory cases but has not been shown to improve survival in controlled trials. The efficacy of the newer technique of transjugular intrahepatic portosystemic shunting (TIPS procedure) is currently undergoing rigorous clinical assessment. Shunting can also improve GFR and sodium excretion transiently, probably because the increase in central blood volume stimulates release of atrial natriuretic peptides (ANPs) and inhibits secretion of aldosterone and norepinephrine.

INTRINSIC RENAL ARF Many different approaches have been tested for their ability to attenuate injury or hasten recovery in ischemic and nephrotoxic ARF. These include ANP, low-dose dopamine, endothelin antagonists, loop-blocking diuretics, calcium channel blockers, α-adrenoreceptor blockers, prostaglandin analogues, antioxidants, antibodies against leukocyte adhesion molecules, and insulin-like growth

factor type I. Whereas many of these are beneficial in experimental models of ischemic or nephrotoxic ARF, they have either failed to confer consistent benefit or proved ineffective in humans.

ARF due to other intrinsic renal diseases such as acute glomerulonephritis or vasculitis may respond to glucocorticoids, alkylating agents, and/or plasmapheresis, depending on the primary pathology. Glucocorticoids also hasten remission in some cases of allergic interstitial nephritis. Aggressive control of systemic arterial pressure is of paramount importance in limiting renal injury in malignant hypertensive nephrosclerosis, toxemia of pregnancy, and other vascular diseases. Hypertension and ARF due to scleroderma may be exquisitely sensitive to treatment with ACE inhibitors.

POSTRENAL ARF Management of postrenal ARF requires close collaboration between nephrologist, urologist, and radiologist. Obstruction of the urethra or bladder neck is usually managed initially by transurethral or suprapubic placement of a bladder catheter, which provides temporary relief while the obstructing lesion is identified and treated definitively. Similarly, ureteric obstruction may be treated initially by percutaneous catheterization of the dilated renal pelvis or ureter. Indeed, obstructing lesions can often be removed percutaneously (e.g., calculus, sloughed papilla) or bypassed by insertion of a ureteric stent (e.g., carcinoma). Most patients experience an appropriate diuresis for several days following relief of obstruction. Approximately 5% of patients develop a transient salt-wasting syndrome that may require administration of intravenous saline to maintain blood pressure.

Supportive Measures (Table 260-4) Following correction of hypovolemia, salt and water intake are tailored to match losses. Hypervolemia can usually be managed by restriction of salt and water intake and diuretics. Indeed, there is, as yet, no proven rationale for administration of diuretics in ARF except to treat this complication. High doses of loop-blocking diuretics such as furosemide (up to 200 to 400 mg intravenously) or bumetanide (up to 10 mg intravenously administered as a bolus or by continuous infusion) may promote diuresis in patients who fail to respond to conventional doses. Despite the fact that subpressor doses of dopamine may transiently promote salt and water excretion by increasing renal blood flow and GFR and by inhibiting tubule sodium reabsorption, subpressor ("low-dose," "renal-dose,") dopamine has proved ineffective in clinical trials, may trigger arrythmias and sudden cardiac death in critically ill patients, and should not be used as a renoprotective agent in this setting. Ultrafiltration or dialysis is used to treat severe hypervolemia when conservative measures fail. Hyponatremia and hypoosmolality can usually be controlled by restriction of free water intake. Conversely, hypernatremia is treated by administration of water or intravenous hypotonic saline or isotonic dextrose-containing solutions. →*The management of hyperkalemia is described in Chap. 41.*

Metabolic acidosis is not usually treated unless serum bicarbonate concentration falls below 15 mmol/L or arterial pH falls below 7.2. More severe acidosis is corrected by oral or intravenous sodium bicarbonate. Initial rates of replacement are guided by estimates of bicarbonate deficit and adjusted thereafter according to serum levels (Chap. 42). Patients are monitored for complications of sodium bicarbonate administration such as hypervolemia, metabolic alkalosis, hypocalcemia, and hypokalemia. From a practical point of view, most patients requiring sodium bicarbonate need emergency dialysis within days. Hyperphosphatemia is usually controlled by restriction of dietary phosphate and by oral aluminum hydroxide or calcium carbonate, which reduce gastrointestinal absorption of phosphate. Hypocalcemia does not usually require treatment unless severe, as may occur with rhabdomyolysis or pancreatitis or following admininstration of bicarbonate. Hyperuricemia is typically mild [<890 μmol/L (< 15 mg/dL)] and does not require intervention.

The objective of *nutritional management* during the maintenance phase of ARF is to provide sufficient calories to avoid catabolism and starvation ketoacidosis, while minimizing production of nitrogenous

TABLE 260-4 *Management of Ischemic and Nephrotoxic Acute Renal Failure*[a]

Management Issue	Therapy
REVERSE CAUSATIVE RENAL INSULT	
Ischemic ARF	Restore systemic hemodynamics and renal perfusion
Nephrotoxic ARF	Eliminate nephrotoxins
	Consider specific measures (e.g., forced alkaline diuresis, chelators: see text)
PREVENTION AND TREATMENT OF COMPLICATIONS	
Intravascular volume overload	Salt (1–2 g/d) and water (usually <1 L/d) restriction
	Diuretics (usually loop blockers ± thiazide)
	Ultrafiltration or dialysis
Hyponatremia	Restriction of enteral free water intake (<1 L/d)
	Avoid hypotonic intravenous solutions (including dextrose solutions)
Hyperkalemia	Restriction of dietary K^+ intake (usually <40 mmol/d)
	Eliminate K^+ supplements and K^+-sparing diuretics
	Potassium-binding ion-exchange resins (e.g., sodium polystyrene sulphonate)
	Glucose (50 mL of 50% dextrose) and insulin (10 units regular)
	Sodium bicarbonate (usually 50–100 mmol)
	Calcium gluconate (10 mL of 10% solution over 5 min)
	Dialysis (with low K^+ dialysate)
Metabolic acidosis	Restriction of dietary protein (usually 0.6 g/kg per day of high biologic value)
	Sodium bicarbonate (maintain serum bicarbonate >15 mmol/L or arterial pH >7.2)
	Dialysis
Hyperphosphatemia	Restriction of dietary phosphate intake (usually <800 mg/d)
	Phosphate binding agents (calcium carbonate, aluminum hydroxide)
Hypocalcemia	Calcium carbonate (if symptomatic or if sodium bicarbonate to be administered)
	Calcium gluconate (10–20 mL of 10% solution)
Hypermagnesemia	Discontinue Mg^{2+}-containing antacids
Hyperuricemia	Treatment usually not necessary [if <890 μmol/L (<15 mg/dL)]
Nutrition	Restriction of dietary protein (~0.6 g/kg per day)
	Carbohydrate (~100 g/d)
	Enteral or parenteral nutrition (if recovery prolonged or patient very catabolic)
Indications for dialysis	Clinical evidence (symptoms or signs) of uremia
	Intractable intravascular volume overload
	Hyperkalemia or severe acidosis resistant to conservative measures
	?Prophylactic dialysis when urea >100–150 mg/dL or creatinine >8–10 mg/dL
PRESCRIBING OF MEDICATIONS	
Choice of agents	Avoid other nephrotoxins, ACE inhibitors, cyclooxygenase inhibitors, and radiocontrast unless absolute indication and no alternative agent
Drug dosing	Adjust doses and frequency of administration for degree of renal impairment

[a] These are general recommendations and must be tailored to needs of individual patients.

waste. This is best achieved by restricting dietary protein to approximately 0.6 g/kg per day of protein of high biologic value (i.e., rich in essential amino acids) and to provide most calories as carbohydrate (approximately 100 g daily). Nutritional management is easier in non-oliguric patients and following institution of dialysis. Vigorous parenteral hyperalimentation is claimed to improve prognosis; however, convincing benefit has yet to be demonstrated in controlled trials.

Anemia may necessitate blood transfusion if severe or if recovery is delayed. In contrast to chronic renal failure, recombinant human erythropoietin is rarely used in ARF because bone marrow resistance to erythropoietin is common, more immediate treatment of anemia (if any) is required, and renal failure is usually self-limiting. Uremic bleeding usually responds to correction of anemia, administration of desmopressin or estrogens, or dialysis. Regular doses of antacids appear to reduce the incidence of gastrointestinal hemorrhage significantly and may be more effective in this regard than H_2 antagonists or proton pump inhibitors. Meticulous care of intravenous cannulae, bladder catheters, and other invasive devices is mandatory to avoid infections. Unfortunately, prophylactic antibiotics have not been shown to reduce the incidence of infection in these high-risk patients.

INDICATIONS AND MODALITIES OF DIALYSIS (See also Chap. 262) Dialysis replaces renal function until regeneration and repair restore renal function. Hemodialysis and peritoneal dialysis appear equally effective for management of ARF. Thus, the dialysis modality is chosen according to the needs of individual patients (e.g., peritoneal dialysis may be preferable if the patient is hemodynamically unstable, and hemodialysis after abdominal surgery involving the peritoneum), the expertise of the nephrologist, and the facilities of the institution. Vascular access for conventional intermittent hemodialysis is best achieved by insertion of a temporary double-lumen hemodialysis catheter into the internal jugular vein. The subclavian and femoral veins are alternative access sites. Peritoneal dialysis is achieved by insertion of a cuffed catheter into the peritoneal cavity. Absolute indications for dialysis include symptoms or signs of the uremic syndrome and management of refractory hypervolemia, hyperkalemia, or acidosis. Most nephrologists also initiate dialysis empirically for blood urea levels of >100 mg/dL, even in the absence of clinical uremia; however, this approach has yet to be validated in controlled clinical trials. Recent evidence suggests that more intensive hemodialysis (e.g., daily rather than alternate-day intermittent dialysis) is clinically superior and confers improved survival in ARF once dialysis is required. This conclusion may not be as intuitive as it first appears as dialysis itself has been postulated to prolong the period of oliguria in some cases by inducing hypotension and further renal ischemia and through activation of leukocytes on the dialysis membrane, which may then proceed to aggravate renal injury.

Continuous renal replacement therapies (CRRTs) are alternatives to conventional intermittent hemodialysis techniques for treatment of ARF. They are particularly valuable techniques in patients in whom intermittent hemodialysis fails to control hypervolemia or uremia and for those who do not tolerate intermittent hemodialysis and in whom peritoneal dialysis is not possible. Continuous arteriovenous hemodiafiltration (CAVHD) requires both arterial and venous access. The patient's own blood pressure generates an ultrafiltrate of plasma across a porous biocompatible dialysis membrane. A physiologic crystalloid solution is passed along the other side of the membrane to achieve diffusive clearance. Continuous venovenous hemodiafiltration (CVVHD), in contrast, requires only a double-lumen venous catheter as a blood pump generates ultrafiltration pressure across the dialysis membrane. In the more simple techniques of continuous arteriovenous hemofiltration (CAVH) and continuous venovenous hemofiltration (CVVH) the dialysis step is eliminated and an ultrafiltrate of plasma is removed across the dialysis membrane and replaced by a physiologic crystalloid solution. The bulk of evidence to date suggests that intermittent and continuous dialytic therapies are equally effective in the context of ARF. The choice of technique is currently tailored to the specific needs of the patient, the resources of the institution, and the expertise of the physician. Potential disadvantages of continuous hemodialysis techniques are the need for prolonged immobilization in bed, systemic anticoagulation, arterial cannulation (in CAVH), and prolonged exposure of blood to synthetic, albeit relatively biocompatible, dialysis membranes.

OUTCOME AND LONG-TERM PROGNOSIS

The mortality rate among patients with ARF approximates 50% and has changed little over the past 30 years. It should be stressed, however, that patients usually die from sequelae of the primary illness that induced ARF and not from ARF itself. Indeed, the kidney is one of the few organs whose function can be replaced artificially (i.e., by dialysis) for protracted periods of time. In agreement with this interpretation, mortality rates vary greatly depending on the cause of ARF: ~15% in obstetric patients, ~30% in toxin-related ARF, and ~60% following trauma or major surgery. Oliguria (<400 mL/d) at time of presentation and a rise in serum creatinine of >265 μmol/L (>3 mg/dL) are associated with a poor prognosis and probably reflect the severity of renal injury and of the primary illness. Mortality rates are higher in older debilitated patients and in those with multiple organ failure. Most patients who survive an episode of ARF recover sufficient renal function to live normal lives. However, 50% have subclinical impairment of renal function or residual scarring on renal biopsy. Approximately 5% of patients never recover function and require long-

term renal replacement with dialysis or transplantation. An additional 5% suffer progressive decline in GFR, following an initial recovery phase, probably due to hemodynamic stress and sclerosis of remnant glomeruli (Chap. 264).

FURTHER READING

BRADY HR et al: Acute renal failure, in *Brenner and Rector's The Kidney*, 7th ed., BM Brenner (ed). Philadelphia, Saunders, 2004

DAUGIRDAS JT et al: (eds): *Handbook of Dialysis*. New York, Little, Brown, 2001

DENTON MD et al: "Renal-dose" dopamine for the treatment of acute renal failure: Scientific rationale, experimental studies and clinical trials. Kidney Int 49:4, 1996

RONCO C et al: Effect of different doses of continuous veno-venous haemofiltration on outcomes of acute renal failure: A prospective randomised trial. Lancet 355:26, 2000

SCHIFFL H et al: Daily hemodialysis and the outcome of acute renal failure. N Engl J Med 346:305; 2002

261 CHRONIC RENAL FAILURE
Karl Skorecki, Jacob Green,[†] Barry M. Brenner

MECHANISMS OF CHRONIC RENAL FAILURE

DEFINITIONS *Chronic renal disease* (CRD) is a pathophysiologic process with multiple etiologies, resulting in the inexorable attrition of nephron number and function and frequently leading to *end-stage renal disease* (ESRD). In turn, ESRD represents a clinical state or condition in which there has been an irreversible loss of endogenous renal function, of a degree sufficient to render the patient permanently dependent upon renal replacement therapy (dialysis or transplantation) in order to avoid life-threatening *uremia*. Uremia is the clinical and laboratory syndrome, reflecting dysfunction of all organ systems as a result of untreated or undertreated acute or chronic renal failure. Given the capacity of the kidneys to regain function following acute injury (Chap. 260), the vast majority (>90%) of patients with ESRD have reached this state as a result of CRD.

PATHOPHYSIOLOGY OF CRD (See also Chap. 259) The pathophysiology of CRD involves initiating mechanisms specific to the underlying etiology as well as a set of progressive mechanisms that are a common consequence following long-term reduction of renal mass, irrespective of etiology. Such reduction of renal mass causes structural and functional hypertrophy of surviving nephrons. This compensatory hypertrophy is mediated by vasoactive molecules, cytokines, and growth factors and is due initially to adaptive hyperfiltration, in turn mediated by increases in glomerular capillary pressure and flow. Eventually, these short-term adaptations prove maladaptive, in that they predispose to sclerosis of the remaining viable nephron population. Increased intrarenal activity of the renin-angiotensin axis appears to contribute both to the initial adaptive hyperfiltration and to the subsequent maladaptive hypertrophy and sclerosis.

The definition of CRD requires that the pathophysiologic process described above last more than 3 months. A recently widely accepted international classification divides CRD into a number of stages (Table 261-1) defined by clinical estimation of the glomerular filtration rate (GFR). These stages help guide clinical diagnostic and management approaches. First, it is important to identify factors that increase the risk for CRD, even in individuals with normal GFR. Such factors include family history of heritable renal disease, hypertension, diabetes, autoimmune disease, older age, past episode of acute renal failure, and current evidence of kidney damage with normal or even

increased GFR. Such evidence of kidney damage in the face of normal or increased GFR places affected individuals into stage 1 CRD and includes proteinuria, abnormal urinary sediment, or urinary tract structural abnormalities (e.g., vesicoureteric reflux) evident on imaging studies. Even at this stage, when baseline GFR is normal, there is often a characteristic loss of renal reserve. This early stage is particularly well documented in diabetic nephropathy. Further stages in the pathogenesis of CRD are characterized by a progressive decline in estimated GFR with mild, moderate, and severe stages defined at GFR levels (mL/min per 1.73 m²) of 60 to 89, 30 to 59, and 15 to 29, respectively. At a GFR < 15 mL/min per 1.73 m², renal replacement therapy may be indicated if uremia is present. For purposes of staging CRD, current guidelines recommend estimating GFR using one of the two equations shown in Table 261-2, based on measured plasma creatinine concentration, age, gender, and ethnic origin. The normal annual mean decline in GFR with age beginning at age 20 to 30 years is 1 mL/min per 1.73 m², reaching a mean value in males of 70 at age 70. GFR is slightly lower in women than men. By the time plasma creatinine concentration is even mildly elevated, substantial chronic nephron injury has already occurred.

Albuminuria serves as a key adjunctive tool for monitoring nephron injury and response to therapy in many forms of CRD. Current guidelines recommend use of albumin-specific dipstick measurement or quantitation by measurement of albumin-to-creatinine ratio in a spot first morning urine sample. Persistence of >17 mg albumin per gram of creatinine in adult males and 25 mg albumin per gram of creatinine in adult females usually signifies chronic renal damage, irrespective of GFR, and can be followed in monitoring natural history and response to therapy, especially in CRD consequent to diabetes, hypertension, or glomerulonephritis. →*Further considerations in the overall clinical approach to proteinuria are provided in Chap. 40.*

During stages 1 and 2 CRD, patients often remain free of symp-

TABLE 261-1 *Stages of Chronic Renal Disease CRD*

Stage	Description	GFR, mL/min per 1.73 m²
	At increased risk	90 (with CRD risk factors)
1	Kidney damage with normal or increased GFR	90
2	Kidney damage with mildly decreased GFR	60–89
3	Moderately decreased GFR	30–59
4	Severely decreased GFR	15–29
5	Renal failure	<15 (or dialysis)

Note: GFR, glomerular filtration rate.
Source: Adapted from Levey, with permission.

---

†Deceased

TABLE 261-2 *Recommended Equations for Estimation of Glomerular Filtration Rate (GFR) from Laboratory-Validated Plasma Creatinine Concentration (P_{Cr})*

1. Equation from the Modification of Diet in Renal Disease study[a]
   Estimated GFR (mL/min per 1.73 m²) = $1.86 \times (P_{Cr})^{-1.154} \times (\text{age})^{-0.203}$
   Multiply by 0.742 for women
   Multiply by 1.21 for African Americans
2. Cockcroft-Gault equation
   Estimated creatinine clearance (mL/min) =
   $$\frac{(140 - \text{age}) \times \text{body weight (kg)}}{72 \times P_{Cr} \text{ (mg/dL)}}$$
   Multiply by 0.85 for women

[a] Equation is *available* in hand-held calculators and in tabular form.
Source: Adapted from Levey, with permission.

TABLE 261-3 *Summary of Clinical Presentations That may Suggest Given Major Categories of Causes of Chronic Renal Disease*

Cause	Clinical Presentation
Diabetic kidney disease	History of diabetes, proteinuria, retinopathy
Hypertension	Elevated blood pressure, normal urinalysis, family history.
Nondiabetic glomerular disease	Nephritic or nephrotic presentations (Chap. 264)
Cystic kidney disease	Urinary tract symptoms, abnormal urinary sediment, radiologic imaging abnormalities
Tubulointerstitial disease	History of urinary tract infections and reflux, chronic medication and drug exposure, abnormalities in urinary tract imaging, tubular syndromes including urine-concentrating defect, abnormal urinalysis

Source: Adapted from Levey, with permission.

toms, other than those that might accompany the underlying etiologic process causing renal disease. As the decline in GFR progresses to stages 3 and 4 (GFR < 60 mL/min per 1.73 m²), clinical and laboratory complications of CRD become progressively more prominent. Virtually all organ systems are affected, but the most evident complications include anemia and loss of energy; decreasing appetite and disturbances in nutritional status; abnormalities in calcium and phosphorus metabolism accompanied by metabolic bone disease; and abnormalities in sodium, water, potassium, and acid-base homeostasis. When GFR falls to <15 mL/min per 1.73 m², patients usually experience a severe disturbance in their activities of daily living, sense of well-being, nutritional status, and water and electrolyte homeostasis, eventuating in an overtly uremic state wherein continued survival without renal replacement therapy becomes impossible.

ETIOLOGY AND EPIDEMIOLOGY It has been estimated that at least 6% of the adult U.S. population have chronic renal damage with a GFR > 60 mL/min per 1.73 m² (stages 1 and 2 CRD) and hence are at imminent risk of a progressive further decline in GFR. An additional ~4.5% of the U.S. population are in stages 3 and 4 CRD. Diabetic and hypertensive nephropathy are the leading underlying etiologies of both CRD and ESRD. Hypertension is a particularly common cause and consequence of CRD in the elderly, in whom chronic renal ischemia due to renovascular disease may be an underrecognized additional contribution to the pathophysiologic process. It should be noted that cardiovascular mortality precludes most patients with CRD from reaching the stage of ESRD. Identification of CRD as a major risk factor for cardiovascular morbidity and mortality, and the expectation of effective interventions to diminish premature cardiovascular mortality, and increasing longevity overall, will increase the cohort of patients reaching ESRD.

Although the clinical manifestations of the declining GFR per se dominate the clinical presentation in all forms of CRD, in many cases the underlying etiology can be presumed from associated additional clinical information (Table 261-3).

GENETIC CONSIDERATIONS Disorders with clear-cut monogenic inheritance comprise a small but important component among the etiologies of CRD. Among these, autosomal dominant polycystic kidney disease is the most common on a world-wide basis (Chap. 265). Alport's hereditary nephritis (Chap. 264) is a less common cause of both benign hematuria without progression to CRD and more severe nephron injury with progression to ESRD, and it most often displays an X-linked pattern of inheritance. Several genetic loci have been identified that encode important components of the glomerular podocyte-associated filtration barrier, and mutations in these genes cause inherited forms of focal segmental glomerular sclerosis with glucocorticoid nonresponsive nephrotic syndrome and progression to ESRD. Nephronopthisis, medullary cystic kidney disease, and Fabry's disease are among other rare causes of progressive CRD with monogenic inheritance based on well-characterized genetic loci. In contrast, the two most common etiologies of CRD, diabetes mellitus (both types

1 and 2) and essential hypertension, display complex polygenic patterns of inheritance.

The striking interindividual variability in the rate of progression to ESRD has an important heritable component, and a number of genetic loci that contribute to the progression of CRD have been identified. Most extensively studied has been an insertion/deletion polymorphism of the angiotensin-converting enzyme (ACE) gene. The homozygous deletion (D/D) variant is associated with the highest expression of endogenous ACE activity and a greater risk of CRD progression. This finding leads to the prediction that ACE inhibitor therapy might be most effective in patients who are homozygous for the "at-risk" allele. Similar conclusions have been reached with respect to genes encoding other components of the renin-angiotensin axis. More recent studies of genetic association with renal failure progression have focused on a region of human chromosome 10, homologous to a well-characterized rodent renal failure susceptibility gene (*Rf1*).

PATHOPHYSIOLOGY AND BIOCHEMISTRY OF UREMIA *Azotemia* refers to the retention of nitrogenous waste products as renal insufficiency develops. *Uremia* refers to the more advanced stages of progressive renal insufficiency when the complex, multiorgan system derangements become clinically manifest.

Although not the major cause of overt uremic toxicity, urea may contribute to some of the clinical abnormalities, including anorexia, malaise, vomiting, and headache. Additional categories of nitrogenous excretory products include guanido compounds, urates and hippurates, end products of nucleic acid metabolism, polyamines, myoinositol, phenols, benzoates, and indoles, among others. Nitrogenous compounds with a molecular mass of 500 to 12,000 Da (so-called middle molecules) are also retained in CRD and similarly are believed to contribute to morbidity and mortality in uremic subjects. However, uremia involves more than renal excretory failure alone. A host of metabolic and endocrine functions normally subserved by the kidney are also impaired, resulting in anemia; malnutrition; impaired metabolism of carbohydrates, fats, and proteins; defective utilization of energy; and metabolic bone disease. Furthermore, plasma levels of many polypeptide hormones, including parathyroid hormone (PTH), insulin, glucagon, luteinizing hormone, and prolactin, rise with renal failure, not only because of impaired renal catabolism but also because of enhanced endocrine secretion, occurring as a secondary consequence of primary excretory or synthetic renal dysfynction. On the other hand, the renal production of erythropoietin (EPO) and 1,25-dihydroxycholecalciferol is impaired. Thus, the pathophysiology of the uremic syndrome can be divided into two sets of abnormalities: (1) those consequent to the accumulation of products of protein metabolism; and (2) those consequent to the loss of other renal functions, such as fluid and electrolyte homeostasis and hormonal abnormalities.

Uremia leads to disturbances in the function of every organ system. Chronic dialysis (Chap. 262) reduces the incidence and severity of these disturbances, so that, where modern medicine is practiced, the overt and florid manifestations of uremia have largely disappeared. Unfortunately, as indicated in Table 261-4, even optimal dialysis therapy is not a panacea, because some disturbances resulting from impaired renal function fail to respond fully, while others continue to progress.

FLUID, ELECTROLYTE, AND ACID-BASE DISORDERS (See also Chaps. 41, 42, and 259) ■ **Sodium and Water Homeostasis** In most patients with stable CRD, the total body contents of Na^+ and H_2O are increased modestly, although this may not be clinically apparent. The underlying etiologic disease process may itself disrupt glomerulotubular balance and promote Na^+ retention (e.g., glomerulonephritis), or excessive Na^+ ingestion may lead to cumulative positive Na^+ balance and attendant extracellular fluid volume (ECFV) expansion. Such ECFV expansion contributes to hypertension, which in turn accelerates further the progression of nephron injury. As long as water intake does not exceed the capacity for free water clearance, the ECFV expansion will be isotonic and the patient will remain normonatremic. Hyponatremia is an uncommon complication in predialysis patients, and water restriction is only necessary when hyponatremia is documented. Weight gain usually associated with volume expansion may be offset in patients with CRD by concomitant loss of lean body mass. In the CRD patient who is not yet on dialysis but has clear evidence of ECFV expansion, administration of loop diuretics coupled with restriction of salt intake are the mainstays of therapy. It should be noted that resistance to loop diuretics in renal failure often mandates use of higher doses than those usually used when GFR is well preserved. The combination of loop diuretics with metalozone, which inhibits the Na^+Cl^- cotransporter of the distal convoluted tubule, can sometimes overcome diuretic resistance. When the GFR falls to <5 to 10 mL/min per 1.73 m^2, even high doses of combination diuretics are ineffective. ECFV expansion under these circumstances usually means that dialysis is indicated.

Patients with CRD also have impaired renal mechanisms for conserving Na^+ and H_2O (Chap. 259). When an *extrarenal* cause for fluid loss is present (e.g., vomiting, diarrhea, sweating, fever), these patients are prone to volume depletion. Depletion of ECFV may compromise residual renal function with resulting signs and symptoms of overt uremia. Because of impaired renal Na^+ and H_2O conservation, the usual indices of prerenal azotemia (oliguria, high urine osmolality, low urinary Na^+ concentration, and low fractional excretion of Na^+) are not useful. Cautious volume repletion, usually with normal saline, returns ECFV to normal and usually restores renal function to prior levels.

Potassium Homeostasis (See also Chap. 41) In CRD, the decline in GFR is not necessarily accompanied by a concomitant and proportionate decline in urinary K^+ excretion. In addition, K^+ excretion in the gastrointestinal tract is augmented in patients with CRD. However, hyperkalemia may be precipitated in a number of clinical situations, including constipation, augmented dietary intake, protein catabolism, hemolysis, hemorrhage, transfusion of stored red blood cells, metabolic acidosis, and following the exposure to a variety of medications that inhibit K^+ entry into cells or K^+ secretion in the distal nephron. Most commonly encountered medications in this regard are beta blockers, ACE inhibitors and angiotensin receptor blockers, K^+-sparing diuretics (amiloride, triamterene, spironolactone), and nonsteroidal anti-inflammatory drugs (NSAIDs). In addition, certain etiologies of CRD may be associated with earlier and more severe disruption of K^+ secretory mechanisms in the distal nephron, relative to the reduction in GFR. Most important are conditions associated with hyporeninemic hypoaldosteronism (e.g., diabetic nephropathy and certain forms of distal renal tubular acidosis; Chaps. 264 and 265).

Hypokalemia is uncommon in CRD and usually reflects markedly reduced dietary K^+ intake, in association with excessive diuretic therapy or gastrointestinal losses. Hypokalemia occurs as a result of primary renal K^+ wasting in association with other solute transport abnormalities, as in Fanconi's syndrome, renal tubular acidosis, or other forms of hereditary or acquired tubulointerstitial diseases. However, even under these circumstances, as GFR declines, the tendency

---

TABLE 261-4 Clinical Abnormalities in Uremia[a]

Fluid and electrolyte disturbances	Neuromuscular disturbances	Dermatologic disturbances
Volume expansion and contraction (I)	Fatigue (I)[b]	Pallor (I)[b]
Hypernatremia and hyponatremia (I)	Sleep disorders (P)	Hyperpigmentation (I, P,
Hyperkalemia and hypokalemia (I)	Headache (I or P)	or D)
Metabolic acidosis (I)	Impaired mentation (I)[b]	Pruritus (P)
Hyperphosphatemia (I)	Lethargy (I)[b]	Ecchymoses (I)
Hypocalcemia (I)	Asterixis (I)	Uremic frost (I)
	Muscular irritability (I)	
Endocrine-metabolic disturbances	Peripheral neuropathy (I or P)	**Gastrointestinal disturbances**
Secondary hyperparathyroidism (I or P)	Restless legs syndrome (I or P)	Anorexia (I)
Adynamic osteomalacia (D)	Paralysis (I or P)	Nausea and vomiting (I)
Vitamin D–deficient osteomalacia (I)	Myoclonus (I)	Uremic fetor (I)
Carbohydrate intolerance (I)	Seizures (I or P)	Gastroenteritis (I)
Hyperuricemia (I or P)	Coma (I)	Peptic ulcer (I or P)
Hypertriglyceridemia (I or P)	Muscle cramps (P or D)	Gastrointestinal bleeding
Increased Lp(a) level (P)	Dialysis disequilibrium syndrome (D)	(I, P, or D)
Decreased high-density lipoprotein level (P)	Myopathy (P or D)	Hepatitis (D)
Protein-energy malnutrition (I or P)		Idiopathic ascites (D)
Impaired growth and development (P)	**Cardiovascular and pulmonary disturbances**	Peritonitis (D)
Infertility and sexual dysfunction (P)	Arterial hypertension (I or P)	
Amenorrhea (P)	Congestive heart failure or pulmonary edema (I)	**Hematologic and immunologic**
Hypothermia (I)	Pericarditis (I)	**disturbances**
β_2-Microglobulin deposition (P or D)	Cardiomyopathy (I or P)	Anemia (I)[b]
Associated amyloidosis (P)	Uremic lung (I)	Lymphocytopenia (P)
	Accelerated atherosclerosis	Bleeding diathesis (I or D)[b]
	(P or D)	Increased susceptibility to infection (I or P)
	Hypotension and arrhythmias (D)	Splenomegaly and hypersplenism (P)
	Vascular calcification (P or D)	Leukopenia (D)
		Hypocomplementemia (D)

[a] Virtually all abnormalities in this table are completely reversed in time by successful renal transplantation. The response of these abnormalities to hemodialysis or peritoneal dialysis therapy is more variable. (I) denotes an abnormality that usually improves with an optimal program of dialysis and related therapy; (P) denotes an abnormality that tends to persist or even progress, despite an optimal program; (D) denotes an abnormality that develops only after initiation of dialysis therapy.

[b] Improves with dialysis and erythropoietin therapy.

Note: Lp(a), lipoprotein A.

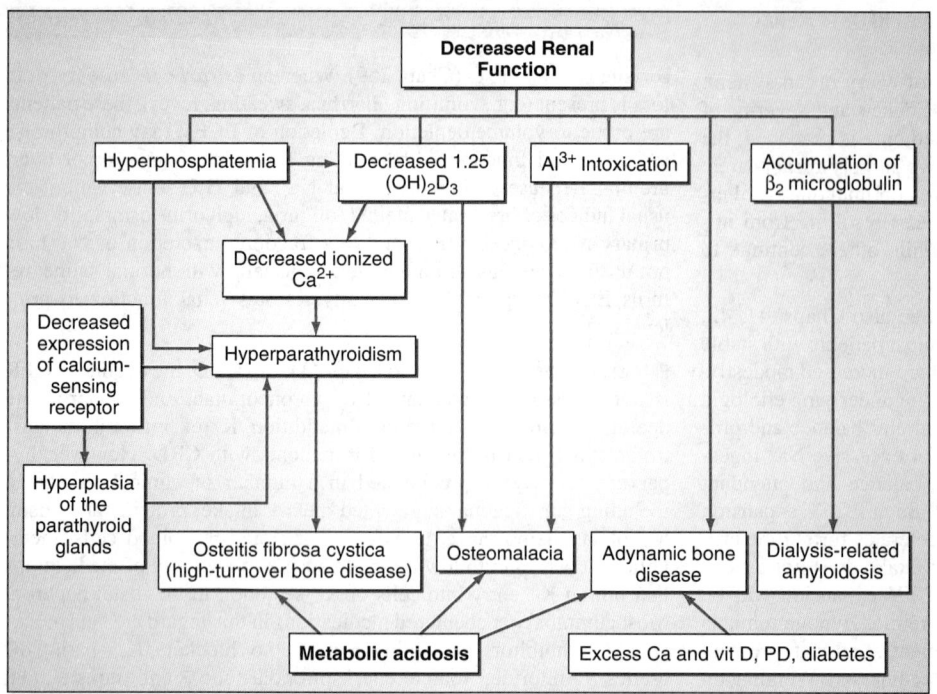

FIGURE 261-1 Flowchart for the development of bone, phosphate, and calcium abnormalities in chronic renal disease. (PD, peritoneal dialysis).

the use of diuretics if they are also indicated for management of sodium balance. Many salt substitutes contain potassium instead of sodium, and patients with CRD seeking to avoid sodium should be cautioned accordingly as part of their dietary counseling. Potassium-binding resins taken with cathartics can promote gastrointestinal potassium losses and thus are useful as temporizing measures in the treatment or avoidance of hyperkalemia in CRD patients. However, the need for such treatment over a prolonged period, in the absence of other reversible causes of hyperkalemia, usually signifies the need to initiate renal replacement therapy.

BONE DISEASE AND DISORDERS OF CALCIUM AND PHOSPHATE METABOLISM (Fig. 261-1; see also Chaps. 331 and 332) The major disorders of bone disease in CRD can be classified into those associated with high bone turnover and high PTH levels (including osteitis fibrosa, the hallmark lesion of secondary hyperparathyroidism) and low bone turnover with low or normal PTH levels (osteomalacia and adynamic bone disease).

The pathophysiology of bone disease due to secondary hyperparathyroidism is related to abnormal mineral metabolism. (1) Decreased GFR leads to reduced inorganic phosphate (PO_4^{3-}) excretion and consequent PO_4^{3-} retention, (2) retained PO_4^{3-} has a direct stimulatory effect on PTH synthesis and on cellular mass of the parathyroid glands, (3) retained PO_4^{3-} also indirectly causes excessive production and secretion of PTH through lowering of ionized Ca^{2+} and by suppression of calcitriol (1,25-dihydroxycholecalciferol) production, and (4) reduced calcitriol production in CRD results both from decreased synthesis due to reduced kidney mass and from hyperphosphatemia. Low calcitriol levels, in turn, lead to hyperparathyroidism via both direct and indirect mechanisms. Calcitriol is known to have a direct suppressive effect on PTH transcription (i.e., a genomic effect), and therefore reduced calcitriol in CRD causes elevated levels of PTH. In addition, reduced calcitriol leads to impaired Ca^{2+} absorption from the gastrointestinal tract, thereby leading to hypocalcemia, which then increases PTH secretion and production. Taken together, hyperphosphatemia, hypocalcemia, and reduced calcitriol synthesis all promote the production of PTH and the proliferation of parathyroid cells, resulting in secondary hyperparathyroidism.

In addition to excessive release of PTH from individual parathyroid cells, the mass of parathyroid cells increases progressively with CRD. Excessive parathyroid gland cellular mass may assume one of the following patterns: (1) diffuse hyperplasia (polyclonal), (2) nodular growth (monoclonal) within diffuse hyperplastic tissue, or (3) diffuse monoclonal hyperplasia ("adenoma" or tertiary autonomous hyperparathyroidism). Patients with monoclonal ("autonomous") hyperplasia are especially prone to develop hypercalcemia following successful kidney transplantation, often necessitating parathyroidectomy. High PTH levels stimulate osteoblasts and result in high bone turnover, which leads to *osteitis fibrosa cystica*. The latter is characterized by irregularly woven abnormal osteoid, fibrosis, and cyst formation, which result in decreased cortical bone and bone strength and an increased risk of fracture.

Low-turnover bone disease can be classified into two categories—osteomalalcia and adynamic bone disease. Both lesions are characterized by a reduced number of osteoclasts and osteoblasts and decreased activity of the latter. In *osteomalacia* there is an accumulation of unmineralized bone matrix, or increased osteoid volume, which may be caused by vitamin D deficiency, excess aluminum deposition, or meta-

to hypokalemia diminishes and hyperkalemia may supervene. Accordingly, K^+ supplementation and K^+-sparing diuretics should generally be avoided as GFR declines.

Metabolic Acidosis (See also Chap. 42) Acidosis is a common disturbance during the advanced stages of CRD. Although in a majority of patients with CRD the urine can be acidified normally, these patients have a reduced ability to produce ammonia. Hyperkalemia further depresses urinary ammonium excretion. The combination of hyperkalemia and hyperchloremic metabolic acidosis (known as type IV renal tubular acidosis, or hyporeninemic hypoaldosteronism) is most characteristically seen in patients with diabetes or in those with predominantly tubulointerstitial disease. Treatment of the hyperkalemia frequently improves the acidosis as well.

With advancing renal failure, total urinary net daily acid excretion is usually limited to 30 to 40 mmol, and an anion gap of ~20 mmol/L with a reciprocal fall in plasma [HCO_3^-] may develop. In most patients, the metabolic acidosis is mild; the pH is rarely <7.35 and can usually be corrected by treating the patient with 20 to 30 mmol of $NaHCO_3$ or sodium citrate daily. However, the concomitant Na^+ load mandates careful attention to volume status and the potential need for diuretic agents. Also, citrate enhances aluminum absorption in the large bowel, and citrate-containing agents should be avoided if aluminum-containing drugs are also administered. Severe symptomatic manifestations of acid-base imbalance may occur when the patient is challenged with an excessive endogenous or exogenous acid load or loses excessive alkali (e.g., with diarrhea).

℞ TREATMENT

Adjustments in dietary intake and use of loop diuretics, occasionally in combination with metalozone, may be needed to maintain salt and hence extracellular fluid volume balance. In contrast, overzealous salt restriction and diuretic use may cause hypovolemia and precipitate a further decline in GFR. Occasional patients with salt-wasting states need to be given sodium-rich diets or sodium supplements. Water restriction is indicated only if there is a demonstrated propensity to hyponatremia. Intractable ECFV expansion, despite dietary restriction and diuretic use, indicates the need to initiate renal replacement therapy. Hyperkalemia often responds to dietary restriction of potassium, avoidance of potassium-containing or -retaining medications, and to

bolic acidosis. Adynamic bone disease is now recognized to be as prevalent as the hyperparathyroid bone lesion in patients with CRD and ESRD, and is especially common among diabetic patients. *Adynamic bone disease* is characterized by reduced bone volume and mineralization and may result in part from excessive suppression of PTH production with calcitriol treatment or, currently less common, from aluminium exposure.

Irrespective of the cause for skeletal abnormalities in CRD, bone disease can lead to pain, increased incidence of fractures, and severe incapacity. Bone fractures complicate both the high- and low-turnover types of bone disease, and it is now appreciated that patients with adynamic bone may be more predisposed to fractures than those with osteitis fibrosa cystica. In the latter disorder, however, a PTH-associated proximal myopathy often coexists, giving rise to gait abnormalities and impaired ambulation.

Other Complications of Abnormal Calcium-Phosphate Product Metabolism

In addition to abnormalities in bone metabolism, abnormal calcium-phosphate product metabolism may lead to *calciphylaxis*, i.e., extraosseous ("metastatic") calcification of soft tissue and blood vessels. Electron beam computed tomography in patients with CRD has revealed highly elevated coronary calcification scores, which likely represent a major factor in the predisposition to occlusive coronary vascular disease in the CRD and ESRD populations. The pathogenesis remains unclear, but hyperphosphatemia, hypercalcemia, elevated calcium-phosphate product, and increased PTH levels are all thought to contribute to this process. Calciphylaxis represents a severe and systemic form of vascular and soft tissue calcium-phosphate product deposition associated with skin and soft tissue necrosis, which can lead to extremity loss.

℞ TREATMENT

Secondary hyperparathyroidism and osteitis fibrosa are best prevented and treated by reducing the plasma PO_4^{3-} concentration through the use of a phosphate-restricted diet as well as oral phosphate-binding agents. Calcium carbonate and calcium acetate are useful phosphate-binding agents. Sevelamer, a nonabsorbable, non-calcium-containing polymer has been recently added to the phosphate-lowering armamentarium. It has an advantage over the calcium-based phosphate chelating agents in that it does not predispose CRD patients to hypercalcemia and attenuates calcium deposition in the coronary arteries and aorta.

Daily oral calcitriol, or intermittent oral or intravenous pulses, appears to exert a direct suppressive effect on PTH secretion, in addition to the indirect effect mediated through raising plasma Ca^{2+} concentration. The use of calcitriol and calcium preparations in the predialysis population must take into account potential effects of increased PO_4^{3-} and Ca^{2+} on the rate of progression of CRD. The recommended target plasma PO_4^{3-} concentration is approximately 1.4 mmol/L (4.5 mg/dL), with a corresponding plasma Ca^{2+} concentration of approximately 2.5 mmol/L (10 mg/dL) in an attempt to suppress parathyroid hyperplasia, thus avoiding or reversing osteitis fibrosa cystica, osteomalacia, and myopathy. It is particularly important to maintain the calcium-phosphate product in the normal range to avoid metastatic calcification. Recognition of the role of the extracellular calcium–sensing receptor has led to the development of calcimimetic agents that enhance the sensitivity to Ca^{2+}-suppressive effects on PTH secretion. The first-generation calcimimetic agent tested produced a dose-dependent reduction in PTH and plasma Ca^{2+} concentration, and subsequent formulations with improved pharmacokinetic profiles show great promise as effective and safe treatments for secondary hyperparathyroidism. However, since adynamic bone disease is often a consequence of overzealous treatment of secondary hyperparathyroidism, suppression of PTH levels to <120 pg/mL in CRD patients may not be desirable.

The incidence of aluminum-induced osteomalacia has been greatly reduced with the recognition of aluminum as the principal culprit. Therapy for this disorder is based on the complete cessation of the use of aluminum combined with the use of a chelating agent such as deferoxamine.

Management of metabolic acidosis should aim to maintain a nearly normal level of plasma bicarbonate with the administration of calcium acetate or calcium carbonate, with the addition of sodium bicarbonate (limited by considerations of sodium load) if necessary. Excessive administration of alkali should be avoided to minimize risk of urinary precipitation of Ca^{2+} phosphate.

CARDIOVASCULAR ABNORMALITIES Cardiovascular disease is the leading cause of morbidity and mortality in patients with CRD at all stages. Estimates of the increase in cardiovascular disease risk attributable to CRD range from 10- to 200-fold, depending on the stage of CRD, other risk factors, and comorbid conditions. Between 30 and 45% of patients reaching ESRD already have advanced cardiovascular complications. Thus the management of patients with CRD should emphasize prevention of cardiovascular complications as well as measures aimed at alleviating the progression and complications of CRD itself.

Ischemic Cardiovascular Disease CRD at all stages constitutes a major risk factor for ischemic cardiovascular disease, including occlusive coronary heart, cerebrovascular, and peripheral vascular diseases. Increased prevalence of coronary heart disease in CRD derives from both traditional ("classic") and CRD-related ("nontraditional") risk factors. The former include hypertension (see below), hypervolemia, dyslipidemia, sympathetic overactivitiy, and hyperhomocysteinemia. The CRD-related risks include anemia, hyperphosphatemia, hyperparathyroidism, and a state of "microinflammation" that can be found at all stages of CRD but is undoubtedly aggravated by dialysis. The inflammatory state elicits a rise in acute-phase reactants such as interleukin 6 and C-reactive protein, which contribute to the coronary occlusive process and are predictors of cardiovascular disease risk. Other abnormalities augment myocardial ischemia. These include reduced myocardial tolerance to ischemia due to left ventricular hypertrophy (see below) and microvascular disease. Also, coronary reserve, defined as the increase in coronary blood flow in response to greater demand, is attenuated. Nitric oxide is an important mediator for vascular dilatation. Its availability in CRD is decreased because of increased concentrations of asymmetric dimethyl-l-arginine, even at early stages of CRD, and also because nitric oxide is scavenged by reactive oxygen species. In addition, coronary arteriolar hypertrophy/hyperplasia limits vasodilatory capacity.

Congestive Heart Failure (See also Chap. 216) Abnormal cardiac function secondary to myocardial ischemic disease and/or left ventricular hypertrophy, together with salt and water retention in uremia, often result in congestive heart failure and/or pulmonary edema. A unique form of pulmonary congestion and edema may occur even in the absence of volume overload and is associated with normal or mildly elevated intracardiac and pulmonary capillary wedge pressures. This entity, characterized radiologically by peripheral vascular congestion giving rise to a "butterfly wing" distribution, is due to increased permeability of alveolar capillary membranes. This "low-pressure" pulmonary edema as well as cardiopulmonary abnormalities associated with circulatory overload usually respond promptly to vigorous dialysis.

Hypertension and Left Ventricular Hypertrophy (See also Chap. 230) Hypertension is the most common complication of CRD and ESRD. It may develop early during the course of CRD and is associated with adverse outcomes—in particular, more rapid loss of renal function and development of cardiovascular disease. Numerous epidemiologic studies and clinical trials have shown a relationship between the level of blood pressure and rate of progression of diabetic and non-diabetic kidney disease (see below).

Administration of EPO (p. 1658) may raise blood pressure and increase the requirement for antihypertensive drugs in CRD patients. Left ventricular hypertrophy and dilated cardiomyopathy are among the most ominous risk factors for excess cardiovascular morbidity and mortality in patients with CRD and ESRD and are thought to be related primarily to prolonged hypertension and ECFV overload. In addition, anemia and the surgical placement of an arteriovenous anastomosis for future or ongoing dialysis access may generate a high cardiac output state and pulmonary hypertension, which also intensify the burden placed on the left ventricle. *Absence* of hypertension may signify the presence of a salt-wasting form of renal disease (e.g., medullary cystic disease, chronic tubulointerstitial disease, or papillary necrosis), ongoing antihypertensive therapy, volume-depletion due to gastrointestinal causes or diuretic therapy, or reduced cardiac index.

Since volume overload is the major cause of hypertension in uremia, the normotensive state can often be restored by appropriate (not overzealous) use of salt restriction and natriuretic drugs or ultrafiltration in the dialysis setting. Nevertheless, because of hyperreninemia and other disturbances in renal vasoconstrictors and vasodilators, some patients remain hypertensive despite rigorous salt and water restriction and ultrafiltration. Rarely, such patients may develop accelerated or malignant hypertension. Intravenous labetolol, or more recently approved agents such as fenoldopam or urapidil, together with control of ECFV generally control such hypertension. Enalaprilat or other ACE inhibitors may also be considered, but in the face of bilateral renovascular disease they have the potential to further reduce GFR abruptly.

℞ TREATMENT

Management of Hypertension (See also Chap. 230)   There are two overall goals: to slow the progression of CRD itself and to prevent the extrarenal complications of hypertension, such as cardiovascular disease and stroke. In all patients with CRD, blood pressure should be controlled to at least the level established in the guidelines of the Sixth Joint National Commission on Hypertension Detection Education and Follow-up Program (130/80 to 85 mmHg). In CRD patients with diabetes or proteinuria >1 g per 24 h, blood pressure should be further reduced to 125/75 mmHg. Volume control with salt restriction and diuretics is the mainstay of therapy. When volume management is not sufficient, the choice of antihypertensive agent is similar to that in the general population, with the added consideration of cardioprotective benefit provided by ACE inhibition, or angiotensin receptor blockade. The choice of antihypertensive agents may come from all the major classes, with careful consideration of comorbid conditions. However, powerful direct-acting vasodilators, such as hydralazine or minoxidil, may perpetuate the tendency to cardiac hypertrophy, despite the lowering of blood pressure. Therefore, prolonged use of such agents should be reserved for those very rare patients in whom severe refractory hypertension persists, despite adequate volume reduction and compliance with all other classes of antihypertensives.

Management of Cardiovascular Disease   Hypertension, hyperhomocysteinemia, and lipid abnormalities promote atherosclerosis but are potentially treatable complications of CRD. Ongoing or prior nephrotic syndrome is also associated with hyperlipidemia and hypercoagulability, which increase the risk of occlusive vascular disease. Since diabetes mellitus and hypertension are themselves the two most frequent etiologies of CRD, it is not surprising that cardiovascular disease is the most frequent cause of death in ESRD patients. Therefore, accepted life-style changes and therapeutic measures for cardiac risk reduction (Chap. 225) are especially important in this group of patients. Hyperhomocysteinemia may respond to vitamin therapy, which includes folate supplementation to between 1 and 5 mg/d. Hyperlipidemia in patients with CRD and ESRD should be managed aggressively according to the guidelines of the National Cholesterol Education Program (Chap. 335). If dietary measures are inadequate, the preferred lipid-lowering medications are gemfibrozil and an HMG-CoA reductase inhibitor. However, caution should be exercised in combining these two classes of agents because of an increased risk of myositis and rhabdomyolysis in CRD and ESRD patients.

Pericarditis (See also Chap. 222)   With the advent of early initiation of renal replacement therapy, pericarditis is now observed more often in underdialyzed patients than in predialysis CRD patients. Pericardial pain with respiratory accentuation, accompanied by a friction rub, are the hallmarks of uremic pericarditis. The finding of a multicomponent friction rub strongly supports the diagnosis. Classic electrocardiographic abnormalities include PR-interval depression and diffuse ST-segment elevation. Pericarditis may be accompanied by the accumulation of pericardial fluid that is readily detected by echocardiography and that sometimes leads to cardiac tamponade. Pericardial fluid in uremic pericarditis is more often hemorrhagic than in viral pericarditis.

℞ TREATMENT

Uremic pericarditis is an absolute indication for initiation of dialysis or for intensification of the dialysis prescription in those already on dialysis. Because of the propensity to hemorrhagic pericardial fluid, heparin-free dialysis is indicated. Pericardiectomy should be considered only if more conservative measures fail. Nonuremic causes of pericarditis and pericardial effusion include viral, malignant, and tuberculous pericarditis and pericarditis associated with myocardial infarction; these are also more frequent in patients with ESRD and should be managed according to the dictates of the underlying disease process.

HEMATOLOGIC ABNORMALITIES ■ Anemia   A normocytic, normochromic anemia attributable to CRD is observed beginning at stage 3 CRD and is almost universal at stage 4. If untreated, the anemia of CRD is associated with a number of physiologic abnormalities, including decreased tissue oxygen delivery and utilization, increased cardiac output, cardiac enlargement, ventricular hypertrophy, angina, congestive heart failure, decreased cognition and mental acuity, altered menstrual cycles, and impaired host defense against infection. In addition, anemia may play a role in growth retardation in children with CRD. The primary cause of anemia in patients with CRD is insufficient production of EPO by the diseased kidneys. Additional factors include iron and folate deficiency, severe hyperparathyroidism, acute and chronic inflammation, aluminum toxicity, shortened red cell survival, and associated comorbid conditions such as hemoglobinopathies. These potential contributing factors should be considered and addressed, especially in EPO-resistant patients.

℞ TREATMENT

The anemia of CRD is due to several factors including chronic blood loss, hemolysis, marrow suppression by retained uremic factors and reduced renal production of EPO. The availability of recombinant human EPO, epoetin alfa, has made possible one of the most significant advances in the care of renal patients since the introduction of dialysis and transplantation. More recently, a novel erythropoiesis-stimulating protein has been introduced for the treatment of anemia in CRD patients. This protein, darbopoetin alfa, is a hyperglycosylated analogue of recombinant human EPO that possesses greater biologic activity and prolonged half-life. Thus, dose intervals can be extended and still effectively correct renal anemia in both predialysis and dialysis patients. Guidelines for using epoetin and darbopoetin alfa for the management of anemia of CRD are provided in Table 261-5.

The iron status of the patient with CRD must be assessed, and adequate iron stores should be available before treatment with EPO is initiated. Iron supplementation is usually essential to ensure an adequate response to EPO in patients with CRD, because the demands for iron by the erythroid marrow frequently exceed the amount of iron that is immediately available for erythropoiesis (as measured by percent transferrin saturation) as well as iron stores (as measured by serum ferritin). In most cases, intravenous iron is required to achieve and/or maintain adequate iron. However, excessive iron therapy may be associated with a number of complications, including hemosiderosis, accelerated atherosclerosis, increased susceptibility to infection, and possibly an increased propensity to the emergence of malignancies. In addition to iron, an adequate supply of the other major substrates and cofactors for erythrocyte production must be assured, especially vitamin B_{12} and folate. Anemia resistant to recommended doses of EPO in the face of adequate availability of iron and vitamin factors often suggests inadequate dialysis; uncontrolled hyperparathyroidism; aluminum toxicity; chronic blood loss or hemolysis; associated hemoglobinopathy, malnutrition, chronic infection, multiple myeloma, or another malignancy. Blood transfusions may contribute to suppression of erythropoiesis in CRD; because they increase the risk of hepatitis, hemosiderosis, and transplant sensitization, they should be avoided unless the anemia fails to respond to erythropoietin and the patient is symptomatic.

TABLE 261-5 *Management Guidelines for Correction of Anemia of Chronic Renal Disease*

Erythropoietin	
Starting dosage:	50–150 units/kg per week IV or SC (once, twice, or three times per week)
Target hemoglobin (Hb):	11–12 g/dL
Optimal rate of correction[a]	Increase Hb by 1–2 g/dL over 4-week period
Darbepoetin alfa	
Starting dosage:	0.45 μg/kg administered as a single IV or SC injection once weekly
	0.75 μg/kg administered as a single IV or SC injection once every 2 weeks
Target Hb:	≤12 g/dL
Optimal rate of correction	Increase Hb by 1–2 g/dL over 4-week period
Iron	

1. Monitor iron stores by percent transferrin saturation (TSat) and serum ferritin.
2. If patient is iron-deficient (TSat <20%; serum ferritin <100 μg/L), administer iron, 50–100 mg IV twice per week for 5 weeks; if iron indices are still low, repeat the same course.
3. If iron indices are normal yet Hb is still inadequate, administer IV iron as outlined above; monitor Hb, TSat, and ferritin.
4. Withhold iron therapy when TSat > 50% and/or ferritin > 800 ng/mL (>800 μg/L).

[a] If correction of anemia is inadequate, consider causes for refractoriness as outlined in text. Recent reports of pure red blood cell aplasia, may lead to preferences for IV route for some EPO formulations.

Abnormal Hemostasis This is common in CRD and is associated with prolongation of bleeding time, decreased activity of platelet factor III, abnormal platelet aggregation and adhesiveness, and impaired prothrombin consumption. Clinical manifestations include an increased tendency to abnormal bleeding and bruising; bleeding from surgical wounds; and spontaneous bleeding into the gastrointestinal tract, pericardial sac, or intracranial vault (in the form of subdural hematoma or intracerebral hemorrhage). Notwithstanding these abnormalities in hemostasis, CRD patients have a greater susceptibility to thromboembolic complications, particularly if their underlying disease was characterized by a nephrotic presentation.

℞ TREATMENT

Abnormal bleeding times and coagulopathy in patients with renal failure may be reversed with desmopressin, cryoprecipitate, conjugated estrogens, and blood transfusions, as well as EPO. On the other hand, patients with CRD should also be viewed as being at greater risk for thromboembolic complications and receive appropriate anticoagulant prophylaxis when indicated. Avoidance or dose adjustment of certain anticoagulants, such as fractionated low-molecular-weight heparin, is necessary in CRD patients.

NEUROMUSCULAR ABNORMALITIES Central, peripheral, and autonomic neuropathy, as well as abnormalities in muscle composition and function, are all common complications in CRD. Retained nitrogenous metabolites and middle molecules as well as PTH all contribute to the pathophysiology of neuromuscular abnormalities. Subtle clinical manifestations of uremic neuromuscular disease usually become evident beginning at stage 3 CRD. Early manifestations of central nervous system complications include mild disturbances in memory and concentration and sleep disturbance. Neuromuscular irritability, including hiccups, cramps, and fasciculations/twitching of muscles, becomes evident at later stages. Asterixis, myoclonus, and chorea are common in terminal uremia, which may also be associated with seizures and coma.

Peripheral neuropathy usually becomes clinically evident when the patient has been at stage 4 CRD for >6 months, although electrophysiologic and histologic evidence of peripheral neuropathy occurs earlier. Initially, sensory nerves are involved more than motor nerves, lower extremities more than upper, and distal portions of the extremities more than proximal. The "restless legs syndrome" is characterized by ill-defined sensations of discomfort in the legs and feet requiring frequent leg movement. If dialysis is not instituted soon after onset of sensory abnormalities, motor involvement follows, including muscle weakness and loss of deep tendon reflexes. Accordingly, evidence of peripheral neuropathy is a firm indication for renal replacement therapy. Some of the central nervous system and neuromuscular complications of advanced uremia resolve with dialysis, although nonspecific electroencephalographic abnormalities may persist. Successful transplantation may reverse residual peripheral neuropathy.

GASTROINTESTINAL AND NUTRITIONAL ABNORMALITIES *Uremic fetor*, a uriniferous odor to the breath, derives from the breakdown of urea to ammonia in saliva and is often associated with an unpleasant metallic taste sensation. Gastritis, peptic disease, and mucosal ulcerations at any level of the gastrointestinal tract occur in uremic patients and can lead to abdominal pain, nausea, vomiting, and blood loss. Other gastrointestinal complications of CRD include an increased incidence of diverticulosis, particularly in patients with polycystic kidney disease, and an increased incidence of pancreatitis. In addition, central nervous system effects of uremia contribute to anorexia, hiccups, nausea, and vomiting. Protein restriction is useful in diminishing nausea and vomiting late in the course of renal failure. However, protein restriction should not be implemented in patients with signs of protein-energy malnutrition, which is a consequence of low protein and caloric intake, resistance to anabolic actions of insulin and other hormones and growth factors, disturbed dietary protein utilization, proinflammatory cytokine activation, and metabolic acidosis. Assessment for protein-energy malnutrition should begin at stage 3 CRD (GFR < 60 mL/min per 1.73 m^2). A number of indices are useful in this assessment and include dietary history, edema-free body weight, measurement of urinary protein nitrogen appearance, and plasma markers, of which albumin is the most useful. Guidelines for calorie and protein intake in patients with CRD are provided below (p. 1661).

ENDOCRINE-METABOLIC DISTURBANCES Disturbances in parathyroid function have already been considered (p. 1656).

Glucose metabolism is impaired in CRD, as evidenced by a slowing of the rate at which blood glucose levels decline after a glucose load. Fasting blood glucose is usually normal or only slightly elevated, and the mild glucose intolerance related to uremia per se, when present, does not require specific therapy. Because the kidney contributes significantly to insulin removal from the circulation, plasma levels of insulin are slightly to moderately elevated in most uremic subjects, both in the fasting and postprandial states. However, the response to insulin and glucose utilization is impaired in CRD. Many hypoglycemic drugs require dose reduction in renal failure, and some, such as metformin, are contraindicated when the GFR has diminished by more than approximately 25 to 50%.

In women, *estrogen levels* are low, and amenorrhea and inability to carry pregnancies to term are common manifestations of uremia. When the GFR has declined by ~30%, pregnancy may hasten the progression of CRD. In men with CRD, including those receiving chronic dialysis, impotence, oligospermia, and germinal cell dysplasia are common, as are reduced plasma testosterone levels. Like growth, sexual maturation is often impaired in adolescent children with CRD, even among those treated with chronic dialysis. Many of these abnormalities improve or reverse with successful renal transplantation.

DERMATOLOGIC ABNORMALITIES   The skin may show evidence of anemia (pallor), defective hemostasis (ecchymoses and hematomas), calcium-phosphate deposition and secondary hyperparathyroidism (pruritus, excoriations), and deposition of pigmented metabolites or *urochromes* (yellow discoloration) or urea itself (uremic frost). Although many of these cutaneous abnormalities improve with dialysis, *uremic pruritus* often remains a problem. The first lines of management are to rule out unrelated skin disorders and to control PO_4^{3-} concentration with avoidance of an elevated calcium-phosphate product. Occasionally, pruritus remains refractory to these measures and to other nonspecific systemic and topical therapies. Skin necrosis can occur as part of the calciphylaxis syndrome, which also includes subcutaneous, vascular, joint, and visceral calcification in patients with poorly controlled calcium-phosphate product.

EVALUATION AND MANAGEMENT OF PATIENTS WITH CRD

INITIAL APPROACH ■ History and Physical Examination   Complaints referred to the kidneys themselves are often conspicuously absent in CRD, and this often surprises patients and is a cause of skepticism and denial. Of special importance in establishing the etiology of CRD are a history of hypertension; diabetes; systemic infectious, inflammatory, or metabolic diseases; exposure to drugs and toxins; and a family history of renal and urologic disease. Drugs of particular importance include analgesics (usage frequently underestimated or denied by the patient), NSAIDs, gold, penicillamine, antimicrobials, lithium, and ACE inhibitors. In evaluating the uremic syndrome, questions about appetite, diet, nausea, vomiting, hiccupping, shortness of breath, edema, weight change, muscle cramps, pruritus, mental acuity, and activities of daily living are especially helpful.

On physical examination, particular attention should be paid to blood pressure, fundoscopy, precordial examination, examination of the abdomen for bruits and palpable renal masses, examination for edema, and neurologic examination for the presence of asterixis, muscle weakness, and neuropathy. In addition the evaluation of prostate size in men, and potential pelvic masses in women should be undertaken.

Laboratory Investigations   These should also focus on a search for clues to an underlying disease process and its continued activity. Therefore, if the history and physical examination warrant, immunologic tests for systemic lupus erythematosus and vasculitis might be considered. Serum and urinary protein electrophoresis should be undertaken in all patients >40 years with unexplained CRD and anemia, to rule out paraproteinemia. Other tests to determine the stage and chronicity of the disease, including complications of the uremic syndrome, include serial measurements of plasma creatinine and estimation of GFR, urea, electrolytes (including HCO_3^-, Ca^{2+}, and PO_4^{3-}), and alkaline phosphatase to assess metabolic bone disease as well as hemoglobin. Urinalysis may be helpful in assessing the presence of ongoing activity of the underlying inflammatory or proteinuric disease process and, when indicated, should be supplemented by a 24-h urine collection for protein excretion. The latter is particularly helpful in guiding management strategies aimed at ameliorating the progression of CRD. The presence of broad casts on examination of the urinary sediment is a nonspecific finding seen with all underlying etiologies and reflects chronic tubulointerstitial scarring and tubular atrophy with widened tubule diameter, usually signifying an advanced stage of CRD.

Imaging Studies   The most useful imaging study is renal ultrasonography. An ultrasound examination of the kidneys can verify the presence of two symmetric kidneys, provide an estimate of kidney size, and rule out renal masses and obstructive uropathy. The documentation of symmetric small kidneys supports the diagnosis of progressive CRD with an irreversible component of scarring. Normal kidney size suggests the possibility of an acute rather than chronic process. However, polycystic kidney disease, amyloidosis, diabetes, and HIV-associated renal disease (Chap. 173) may lead to CRD with normal kidney size. Documentation of asymmetric kidney size suggests either a unilateral developmental abnormality or chronic renovascular disease. In the latter case, a vascular imaging procedure, such as duplex doppler sonography of the renal arteries, radionuclide scintigraphy, or magnetic resonance angiography should be strongly considered if the possibility of revascularization is feasible. A spiral computed tomographic scan without contrast may be useful in assessing kidney stone activity. Voiding cystourethrography to rule out reflux may be indicated in some patients with a history of enuresis or with a family history of reflux. However, in most cases by the time CRD is established, reflux has resolved, and even if present, its repair does not stabilize renal function. In any case, imaging studies should avoid exposure to intravenous radiocontrast dye where possible because of its nephrotoxicity.

Renal Biopsy   This procedure should be reserved for patients with near-normal kidney size, in whom a clear-cut diagnosis cannot be made by less invasive means and when the possibility of a reversible underlying disease process remains tenable, such that clarification of the underlying etiology may alter management. The extent of tubulointerstitial scarring on kidney biopsy generally provides the most reliable pathologic correlate indicating prognosis for continued deterioration toward ESRD. Contraindications to renal biopsy include bilateral small kidneys, polycystic kidney disease, uncontrolled hypertension, urinary tract or perinephric infection, bleeding diathesis, respiratory distress, and morbid obesity. Ultrasound-guided percutaneous biopsy is the favored approach, but surgical approaches, including laparoscopic biopsy, may be considered in special circumstances such as biopsy of a solitary kidney.

ESTABLISHING THE DIAGNOSIS AND ETIOLOGY OF CRD   The most important initial step in the evaluation of a patient presenting de novo with biochemical or clinical evidence of renal failure is to distinguish newly diagnosed CRD from acute renal failure. Availability of past medical records documenting serial measurements of the plasma urea and/or creatinine concentrations can be of great help in this regard. In the absence of such information, some of the laboratory tests and imaging studies outlined above can be useful. In particular, a urinary sediment that is inactive or reveals proteinuria and broad casts; the demonstration of evidence of chronic metabolic bone disease with hyperphosphatemia, hypocalcemia, elevated PTH levels, and radiologic bone disease; normocytic and normochromic anemia; and the finding of bilaterally reduced kidney size (< 8.5 cm) by imaging studies, strongly favor a long-standing process consistent with CRD. However, these findings do not rule out the superimposition of an acute and reversible exacerbating factor that may have accelerated the decline in GFR (see below).

In the early stages of CRD it is often possible to establish the underlying etiology. Integration of a particular constellation of clinical, laboratory, and imaging findings based on the approach noted above strongly supports a particular presumed underlying etiologic disease process. For example, in a patient with insulin-dependent type 1 diabetes mellitus of 15 to 20 years duration, diabetic retinopathy, and nephrotic-range albuminuria without hematuria, the diagnosis of *diabetic nephropathy* is likely. The diagnosis of *chronic hypertensive nephrosclerosis* requires a history of long-standing hypertension, in the absence of evidence for another renal disease process, and hence it is usually a diagnosis of exclusion. Usually proteinura is mild to moderate (< 3 g/d) and the urine sediment inactive. It should be noted that in many cases of presumed hypertensive nephrosclerosis, renovascular disease not only may be the cause of hypertension but also may cause ischemic renal damage. In this regard, bilateral renovascular ischemic disease may be a greatly underdiagnosed cause of CRD. This is of therapeutic significance from two points of view: (1) documentation of ischemic renal disease secondary to occlusive vascular disease may prompt revascularization therapy in some subgroups of patients, with occasional stabilization and improvement in renal function; (2) renovascular ischemic disease is a contraindication to ACE inhibitor therapy in most cases. *Analgesic-associated chronic tubulointerstitial nephropathy* is also an underdiagnosed cause of CRD. Imaging studies, including computed tomography, often reveal pathognomonic features such as papillary calcification and necrosis. Under such circumstances, cessation of analgesic exposure may dramatically stabilize renal function.

In the absence of an etiologically suggestive clinical constellation, renal biopsy may be the only recourse to establish etiology in early CRD. However, in advanced stages of CRD, definitively establishing an underlying etiology becomes less feasible and is also of less therapeutic significance.

Rx TREATMENT

Specific treatments aimed at selected underlying etiologies of CRD are provided in the respective chapters describing these disease states. The optimal time for such therapy is usually well before there has been a measurable decline in baseline GFR and usually well before CRD is established. It is of benefit to follow and plot the rate of decline in GFR in all patients. Any acceleration in the rate of decline should prompt a search for superimposed acute processes that may lead to an acute and reversible decline in GFR in patients with CRD. These include superimposed volume depletion, accelerated and uncontrolled hypertension, urinary tract infection, superimposed obstructive uropathy (e.g., due to stone disease, papillary necrosis), nephrotoxic effect of medications (e.g., NSAIDs) and radiocontrast agents, and reactivation or flare of the original underlying etiologic disease process.

SLOWING THE PROGRESSION OF CRD While there is great interindividual variation in the rate of decline of GFR in patients with CRD, a series of therapeutic interventions should be pursued that aim to stabilize the GFR or reduce the annual rate of decline.

Protein Restriction (Table 261-6) A major goal of protein restriction in CRD, beyond ameliorating the complications of uremia, is to slow the rate of nephron injury. This concept is based on clinical and experimental evidence demonstrating the role of protein-mediated hyperfiltration in progressive nephron injury. The effectiveness of protein restriction in slowing the progression of CRD has been shown in controlled clinical trials in patients with both diabetic and nondiabetic renal disease.

Protein restriction should be carried out in the context of an overall dietary program that optimizes nutritional status and avoids malnutrition, especially as patients near dialysis or transplantation. Metabolic and nutritional studies indicate that protein requirements for patients with CRD are similar to those for normal adults and are in the range

of 0.6 g/kg per day. However, there is a particular requirement in patients with CRD that the composition of dietary protein be higher in essential amino acids, and that this be combined with an overall energy supply sufficient to mitigate a catabolic state. Energy requirements in the range of 35 kcal/kg per day are recommended. Fortunately, even patients with advanced CRD (GFR ~ 10 to 15 mL/min per 1.73 m²) are able to activate the same adaptive responses to dietary protein restriction as healthy individuals, i.e., a postprandial suppression of whole-body protein degradation and a marked inhibition of amino acid oxidation. These compensatory responses to dietary protein restriction and nutritional indices are sustained during long-term therapy.

Reducing Intraglomerular Hypertension and Proteinuria (See also p. 1657) In addition to reduction of cardiovascular disease risk, antihypertensive therapy in patients with CRD also aims to slow the progression of nephron injury, by ameliorating intraglomerular hypertension and hypertrophy. Progressive renal injury in CRD appears to be most closely related to the height of intraglomerular pressure and/or the extent of glomerular hypertrophy. Control of hypertension is as at least as important as dietary protein restriction in slowing the progression of CRD. Furthermore, the target for pharmacologic therapy is highly dependent on the level of proteinuria. Indeed, proteinuria is now considered a risk factor for both progressive nephron injury as well cardiovascular disease. Elevated blood pressure increases proteinuria due to the transmission to the glomeruli of the elevated systemic pressure. Conversely, the renoprotective effect of antihypertensive medications is evident through the curtailment of proteinuria. Thus, the more effective a given treatment is in lowering proteinuria, the greater the subsequent impact on protection from GFR decline. This is the basis for the treatment guideline establishing 125/75 mmHg as the target blood pressure value in proteinuric CRD patients.

Owing to their unique effect on the glomerular microcirculation (i.e., dilatation of the efferent arteriole), which is related to inhibition of the renin-angiotensin system, ACE inhibitors and angiotensin receptor blockers are now clearly established as effective, antiproteinuric agents. Several multicenter studies have shown that these drugs are effective in slowing the progression of renal failure in patients with both diabetic and nondiabetic renal failure. The slowing in the progression of renal failure by these drugs is strongly related to their proteinuria-lowering effect. In the absence of a significant antiproteinuric response, combined treatment with both an ACE inhibitor and angiotensin receptor blocker can be tried. Contraindications to or adverse effects of the use of these classes of agents (e.g., intractable cough, anaphylaxis, hyperkalemia not controlled by dietary restriction) may prompt the choice of calcium channel blockers as a second-line therapeutic approach. Among the calcium channel blockers, diltiazem and verapamil may exhibit superior antiproteinuric and renal protective effects. Available clinical studies have indicated that calcium antagonists as a group do not adversely affect renal function in patients with nondiabetic renal insufficiency, and also indicate that they may be more effective in preventing or ameliorating progressive renal injury than some other classes of antihypertensive drugs in this group of patients. Thus, it appears that at least two different categories of responses may exist: one in which progression is strongly associated with systemic and intraglomerular hypertension and with proteinuria (e.g., diabetic nephropathy, glomerular diseases) and in which ACE inhibitors and angiotensin receptor blockers are likely to be the first choice; and the second in which proteinuria is mild or absent (e.g., adult polycystic kidney disease), probably with a less prominent role for intraglomerular hypertension, and which might respond as well to calcium entry blockers.

SLOWING DIABETIC RENAL DISEASE (See also Chap. 323) Diabetic nephropathy is now the leading cause of CRD eventuating in ESRD in many parts of the world. Furthermore, the prognosis of diabetic patients on chronic renal replacement therapy is very poor, owing to

TABLE 261-6 *Management Guidelines for Dietary Protein Restriction in CRD*

CRD Stage	Protein, g/kg per d	Phosphorus, g/kg per d
Stages 1 and 2	Protein restriction not usually recommended	No restriction
Stage 3	0.6 g/kg per d including ≥0.35 g/kg per d of HBV	≤10
Stages 4 and 5	0.6 g/kg per d including ≥0.35 g/kg per d of HBV *or*	≤10
	0.3 g/kg per d supplemented with EAA or KA	≤9
GFR <60 mL/ min per 1.73 m² (nephrotic syndrome)	0.8 g/kg per d (plus 1 g protein/g proteinuria) *or*	≤12
	0.3 g/kg per d supplemented with EAA or KA (plus 1 g protein/g proteinuria)	≤9

Note: CRD, chronic renal disease; GFR, glomerular filtration rate; HBV, high biologic value protein; EAA, essential amino acid supplement; KA, ketoanalogue supplement.

accelerated cardiovascular disease. Therefore, it is particularly compelling to search for strategies whose aim is to prevent or slow the progression of this complication of diabetes mellitus.

Glucose Control　Although tight glycemic control reduces the risk of kidney disease in patients with type 1 diabetes, there has been prolonged controversy over whether the same is true in patients with type 2 diabetes. The results of recent controlled prospective studies provide incontrovertible evidence that in type 2 diabetes mellitus the risk of the development and progression of albuminuria and CRD can also be substantially reduced by improving glycemic control. The United Kingdom Prospective Diabetes Study showed that the way in which glycemic control was achieved, whether by insulin or oral antihyperglycemic agents such as sulfonylureas or metformin, was far less important than success in achieving control. Achieving a target hemoglobin A_{1C} level of $<7.2\%$, as compared to $>9\%$, is associated with an approximately 50% reduction in the occurrence of indices of progressive nephropathy. As a result of these findings, recommendations for glucose control aim to achieve plasma values for preprandial glucose in the range of 90 to 130 mg/dL, and for average bedtime glucose of 110 to 150 mg/dL and hemoglobin $A_{1C} < 7\%$. Reduction in GFR mandates dose adjustment of many antihyperglycemic agents, and in particular the discontinuation of metformin when the plasma creatinine is >133 μmol/L (1.5 mg/dL).

Control of Blood Pressure and Proteinuria　Hypertension or an abnormal circadian blood pressure profile is found in 80% of type 2 diabetic patients at the time of diagnosis. Both of these findings correlate with the presence of albuminuria and are powerful predictors of cardiovascular and renal events. The onset of microalbuminuria precedes the decline in GFR in diabetic patients and heralds renal as well as cardiovascular complications. Therefore, microalbuminuria testing is recommended in all diabetic patients at least annually, and more frequently to follow therapeutic interventions. Antihypertensive treatment reduces albuminuria and diminishes the risk of progression of albuminuria even in normotensive patients with diabetes. There is now compelling evidence that ACE inhibitors and angiotensin receptor blockers have specific renoprotective properties in diabetic patients with microalbuminuria or overt proteinuria. These salutary effects are almost certainly mediated by reducing intraglomerular pressure and inhibition of transforming growth factor β–mediated sclerosing pathways.

MANAGING OTHER COMPLICATIONS OF CHRONIC RENAL FAILURE ▪ Impending Uremic Symptomatology　Temporary relief of symptoms and signs of impending uremia, such as anorexia, nausea, vomiting, asterixis, lassitude, and other central nervous system manifestations, may be achieved with protein restriction. However, this must be associated with careful monitoring of nutritional status, so as to avoid protein-energy malnutrition, evidence of which serves as a clear-cut indication for initiation of renal replacement therapy.

Medication Dose Adjustment　(See also Chap. 3)　Although the loading dose of most drugs is not affected by CRD, maintenance doses of many drugs need to be adjusted. For those drugs in which $>70\%$ excretion is by a nonrenal (e.g., hepatic or intestinal) route, dosage adjustment may not be needed. Some drugs that should be entirely avoided include meperidine, metformin, and other oral hypoglycemics with a renal route of elimination. Commonly used medications that require either a reduction in dosage or changes in interval include allopurinol, many antibiotics, several antihypertensives, and antiarrhythmics. For a comprehensive detailed and authoritative listing of the recommended dose adjustment for most of the commonly used medications, the reader is referred to the American College of Physicians' handbook "*Drug Prescribing in Renal Failure*" (see *www.acponline.org*). In addition to dose adjustment requirements, many drugs have nephrotoxicity as a prominent side effect, to which patients with CRD are more susceptible. Of particular notoriety in this regard are NSAIDs, because of

their widespread availability and usage. These drugs aggravate the tendency to sodium retention, hypertension, hyperkalemia, and hyponatremia and further reduce GFR in patients with CRD. In this regard, there is no advantage to more selective inhibitors of cyclooxygenase-2.

Preparation for Renal Replacement Therapy　(See also Chaps. 262 and 263)　Over the past 40 years, renal replacement therapy using dialysis and transplantation has prolonged the lives of hundreds of thousands of patients with ESRD. Renal replacement therapy should *not* be initiated when the patient is totally asymptomatic; however, dialysis and/or transplantation should be started sufficiently early to prevent serious complications of the uremic state. Clear indications for initiation of renal replacement therapy include pericarditis, progressive neuropathy attributable to uremia, encephalopathy, muscle irritability, anorexia and nausea that are not ameliorated by reasonable protein restriction, evidence of protein-energy malnutrition, and fluid and electrolyte abnormalities that are refractory to conservative measures. The latter include volume overload unresponsive to diuretic therapy, hyperkalemia unresponsive to dietary potassium restriction, and progressive metabolic acidosis that cannot be managed with alkali therapy. Clinical clues indicating the imminent development of uremic complications are a history of hiccupping, intractable pruritus, morning nausea and vomiting, muscle twitching and cramps, and the presence of asterixis on physical examination. In addition, the patient whose follow-up and compliance with conservative management are questionable should be considered for earlier initiation of renal replacement therapy, lest potentially life-threatening uremic complications or electrolyte disturbances supervene.

Since there is considerable interindividual variability in the severity of uremic symptoms and renal function, it is ill-advised to assign a certain "usual" level of blood urea nitrogen, serum creatinine, or GFR to the need to start dialysis. Nevertheless, in the United States, the Health Care Financing Administration has assigned levels of serum creatinine and creatinine clearance to qualify for reimbursement from Medicare for patients receiving dialysis. Serum creatinine must be ≥ 700 μmol/L (≥ 8.0 mg/dL) and the creatinine clearance must be ≤ 10 mL/min. Recent controlled studies have failed to show a survival advantage for early initiation of renal replacement therapy prior to onset of clinical indications.

Patient Education and Adjustment　Social, psychological, and physical preparation for the transition to renal replacement therapy and choice of the optimal initial modality is best accomplished with a gradual approach involving a multidisciplinary team. While conservative measures are being carried out in patients with CRD, it is important to prepare them with an intensive educational program, explaining the likelihood and timing of initiation of renal replacement therapy and the various forms of therapy available. The more knowledgable patients are concerning hemodialysis, peritoneal dialysis, and transplantation, the easier and more appropriate will be their decisions at a later time. Exploration of social service support resources is of great importance. In those who may perform home dialysis or undergo transplantation, early education of family members for selection and preparation as a home dialysis helper or a related donor for transplantation should occur long before the onset of symptomatic renal failure.

Selection of patients to be treated with various modalities of dialysis or transplantation is a matter of some debate, with considerable variation in different parts of the world. In general, in the United States and some other countries, nearly all patients who have reached ESRD are accepted for dialysis if they or their families desire prolongation of life, irrespective of age.

Only kidney transplantation (Chap. 263) offers the potential for nearly complete rehabilitation. This is because dialysis techniques replace only 10 to 15% of normal kidney function at the level of small-solute removal and are even less efficient at the removal of larger solutes. Generally, kidney transplantation follows a prior period of dialysis treatment. All patients in whom an acute reversible component of renal failure has not been completely excluded should be supported with dialysis first, at least for some period of time, to allow for possible return of renal function before consideration of transplantation. Recovery of endogenous renal function in patients treated with dialysis for >6 months is a rare occurrence. For patients approaching ESRD in whom a reversible component has been excluded, and who have a good antigenic match with a willing donor, consideration should be given to preemptive or primary transplantation without intervening dialysis.

FURTHER READING

ALJAMA P et al: New insights in ESRD. Kidney Int (Suppl) No. 80, 2002

BRENNER BM et al: For the RENAAL Study Investigators: Effects of Losartan on renal and cardiovascular outcomes in patients with type 2 diabetes and nephropathy. N Engl J Med 345:861, 2001

COZZOLINO M et al: Role of calcium-phosphate product and bone-associated proteins on vascular calcification in renal failure. J Am Soc Nephrol 12: 2511, 2001

GOODMAN WG: Recent developments in the management of secondary hyperparathyroidism. Kidney Int 59:1187, 2001

LEVEY AS et al: National Kidney Foundation K/DOQI *Clinical Practice Guidelines for Chronic Kidney Disease: Evaluation, Classification and Stratification.* Am J Kidney Dis 39(Suppl 1):S1, 2002

LIM VS et al: Protein metabolism in patients with chronic renal failure: Role of uremia and dialysis. Kidney Int 58:1, 2000

MAXWELL AP: Novel erythropoiesis-stimulating protein in the management of the anemia of chronic renal failure. Kidney Int 62:720, 2002

262 DIALYSIS IN THE TREATMENT OF RENAL FAILURE
Ajay K. Singh, Barry M. Brenner

With the widespread availability of dialysis, the lives of hundreds of thousands of patients with end-stage renal disease (ESRD) have been prolonged. In the United States alone, there are now approximately 400,000 patients with ESRD. The overall incidence of ESRD is 260 cases per million population per year. The incident population of patients with ESRD is increasing at approximately 6% each year. The incidence of ESRD is disproportionately higher in African Americans (843 per million population per year) as compared with white Americans (189 per million population per year). In the United States, the leading cause of ESRD is diabetes mellitus, currently accounting for nearly 45% of newly diagnosed cases of ESRD. The second most common cause is hypertension, which is estimated to cause 28% of ESRD cases. Other causes of ESRD include glomerulonephritis, polycystic kidney disease, and obstructive uropathy. The mortality of patients with ESRD is lowest in Europe and Japan but is very high in the developing world because of the limited availability of dialysis. In the United States, the mortality rate of patients on dialysis is approximately 18% per year. Deaths are due mainly to cardiovascular diseases and infections (approximately 50% and 15% of deaths, respectively).

TREATMENT OPTIONS FOR ESRD PATIENTS

Commonly accepted criteria for placing patients on dialysis include the presence of the uremic syndrome; the presence of hyperkalemia unresponsive to conservative measures; extracellular volume expansion; acidosis refractory to medical therapy; a bleeding diathesis; and a creatinine clearance of 10 mL/min per 1.73 m². Early referral to a nephrologist for advanced planning and creation of a dialysis access, education about ESRD treatment options, and the aggressive management of the complications of chronic renal failure, including acidosis, anemia, and hyperparathyroidism, are important. In addition to carefully evaluating patients for the onset of uremia (Chap. 261), regular measurement of renal function is important.

Renal function can be assessed indirectly by measurement of serum creatinine and blood urea nitrogen or of creatinine and urea clearance, or directly by measurement of glomerular filtration rate (GFR) using a radioisotope such as iothalamate. Creatinine clearance usually overestimates GFR because a substantial fraction of creatinine excretion in advanced renal failure occurs as a consequence of proximal tubular secretion. On the other hand, urea clearance invariably underestimates GFR because urea is reabsorbed in the distal nephron. Thus, when measurement of GFR by a direct test is not available, the average of the sum of the creatinine and urea clearance, or a cimetidine-blocked creatinine clearance (cimetidine blocks proximal tubular secretion), is recommended. Alternatively, the GFR can be estimated using a prediction equation that computes a calculated value for GFR. Examples of such equations include the Cockcroft-Gault equation and the Modification of Diet in Renal Disease (MDRD) equation.

The treatment options available for patients with renal failure depend on whether it is acute or chronic (Fig. 262-1). In acute renal failure, treatments include hemodialysis, continuous renal replacement therapies (Chap. 260), and peritoneal dialysis. In chronic renal failure (ESRD) the options include hemodialysis (in center or at home); peritoneal dialysis, as either continuous ambulatory peritoneal dialysis (CAPD) or continuous cyclic peritoneal dialysis (CCPD); or transplantation (Chap. 263). Although there are geographic variations, hemodialysis remains the most common therapeutic modality for ESRD (>80% of patients in the United States). The choice between hemodialysis and peritoneal dialysis involves the interplay of various factors that include the patient's age, the presence of comorbid conditions, the ability to perform the procedure, and the patient's own conceptions about the therapy. Peritoneal dialysis is favored in younger patients because of their better manual dexterity and greater visual acuity, and because younger patients prefer the independence and flexibility of home-based peritoneal dialysis treatment. In contrast, larger patients (>80 kg), patients with no residual renal function, and patients who have truncal obesity with or without prior abdominal surgery may be more suited to hemodialysis. Larger patients with no residual renal function are more appropriate for hemodialysis because these patients have a large volume of distribution of urea and require significantly higher amounts of peritoneal dialysis, which may be difficult to achieve because of the limited willingness of patients to perform more than four exchanges each day. In some patients, the inability to obtain vascular access necessitates a switch from hemodialysis to peritoneal dialysis.

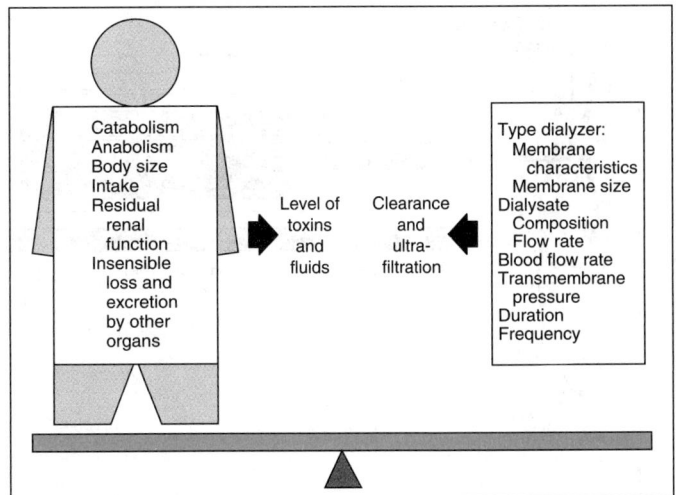

FIGURE 262-1 Factors in the development of the uremic syndrome and considerations in its treatment.

HEMODIALYSIS

Hemodialysis relies on the principles of solute diffusion across a semipermeable membrane. Movement of metabolic waste products takes place down a concentration gradient from the circulation into the dialysate. The rate of diffusive transport increases in response to several factors, including the magnitude of the concentration gradient, the membrane surface area, and the mass transfer coefficient of the membrane. The latter is a function of the porosity and thickness of the membrane, the size of the solute molecule, and the conditions of flow on the two sides of the membrane. According to the laws of diffusion, the larger the molecule, the slower its rate of transfer across the membrane. A small molecule such as urea (60 Da) undergoes substantial clearance, whereas a larger molecule such as creatinine (113 Da) is cleared less efficiently. In addition to diffusive clearance, movement of toxic materials such as urea from the circulation into the dialysate may occur as a result of ultrafiltration. Convective clearance occurs because of solvent drag with solutes getting swept along with water across the semipermeable dialysis membrane.

THE DIALYZER   There are three essential components to dialysis: the dialyzer, the composition and delivery of the dialysate, and the blood delivery system (Fig. 262-2). The dialyzer consists of a plastic device with the facility to perfuse blood and dialysate compartments at very high flow rates. The surface area of dialysis membranes in adult patients is usually in the range of 0.8 to 1.2 m².

There are currently two geometric configurations for dialyzers: hollow fiber and flat plate. The hollow fiber dialyzer is the most common in use in the United States. These dialyzers are composed of bundles of capillary tubes through which blood circulates while dialysate travels on the outside of the fiber bundle. In contrast, the less frequently utilized flat plate dialyzers are composed of sandwiched sheets of membrane in a parallel plate configuration. The advantage of the hollow fiber construction is the lower priming volume (60 to 90 mL vs 100 to 120 mL for the flat plate) and easier reprocessing of the filter for reuse in future dialysis treatments.

Recent advances have led to the development of many different types of membrane material. Broadly, there are four categories of dialysis membranes: cellulose, substituted cellulose, cellulosynthetic, and synthetic. Over the past two decades, there has been a gradual switch from cellulose-derived to synthetic membranes, because the latter are more biocompatible. Bioincompatibility may be defined as the ability of the membrane to activate the complement cascade. Cellulosic membranes are bioincompatible because of the presence of free hydroxyl groups on the membrane surface. In contrast, with the substituted cellulose membranes (e.g., cellulose acetate) or the cellulosynthetic membranes, the hydroxyl groups are chemically bonded to either acetate or tertiary amino groups, resulting in limited complement activation. Synthetic membranes, such as polysulfone, polymethylmethacrylate, and polyacrylonitrile membranes, are more biocompatible because of the absence of these hydroxyl groups. Polysulfone membranes are now used in over 60% of the dialysis treatments in the United States.

Reprocessing and reuse of hemodialyzers are employed for patients on chronic hemodialysis in nearly 80% of dialysis centers in the United States, in large part because of the expense of individual dialyzers. Evidence also suggests that reuse reduces complement activation, the incidence of anaphylactoid reactions to the membrane (first-use syndrome), and, in some studies, mortality rates among dialysis patients. In most centers, only the dialyzer unit is reprocessed and reused, whereas in the developing world blood lines are also frequently reused. The reprocessing procedure can be either manual or automated. It consists of the sequential rinsing of the blood and dialysate compartments with water, a chemical cleansing step with reverse ultrafiltration from the dialysate to the blood compartment, the testing of the patency of the dialyzer, and, finally, disinfection of the dialyzer. Formaldehyde, peracetic acid–hydrogen peroxide, and glutaraldehyde are the most frequently used reprocessing agents, with peracetic acid–hydrogen peroxide being the most common.

DIALYSATE   The composition of dialysate is listed in Table 262-1. Bicarbonate has replaced acetate as the preferred buffer in the United States. This change has resulted in fewer episodes of hypotension dur-

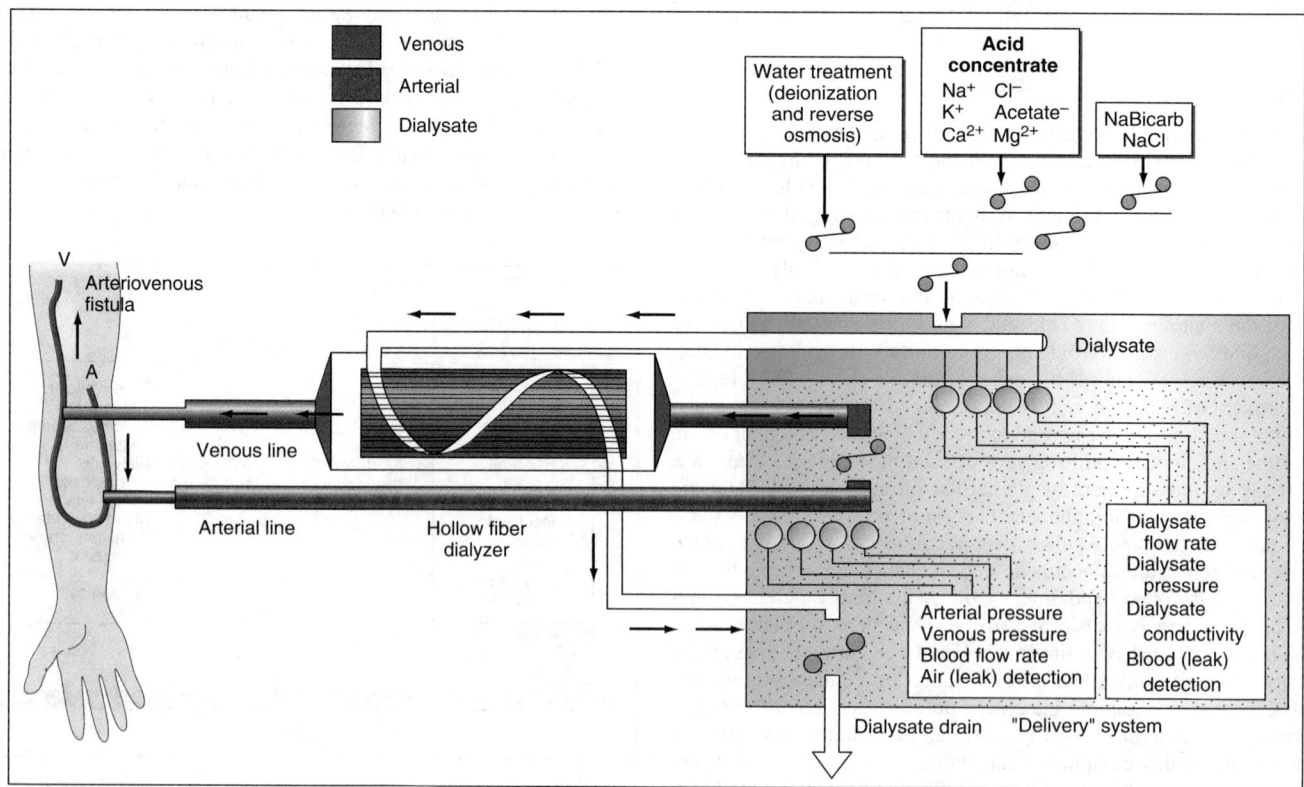

FIGURE 262-2   *Schema for hemodialysis.*

TABLE 262-1 *Composition of Commercial Dialysate for Hemodialysate*

Solute	Bicarbonate Dialysate
Sodium (meq/L)	137–143
Potassium (meq/L)	0–4.0
Chloride (meq/L)	100–111
Calcium (meq/L)	0–3.5
Magnesium (meq/L)	0.75–1.5
Acetate (meq/L)	2.0–4.5
Bicarbonate (meq/L)	30–35
Glucose (mg/dL)	0–0.25

ing dialysis. The potassium concentration of dialysate may be varied from 0 to 4 mmol/L depending on the predialysis plasma potassium concentration. The usual dialysate calcium concentration is 1.25 mmol/L (2.5 meq/L). The usual dialysate sodium concentration is 140 mmol/L. Lower dialysate sodium concentrations are associated with a higher frequency of hypotension, cramping, nausea, vomiting, fatigue, and dizziness. In patients who frequently develop hypotension during their dialysis run, sodium modeling to counterbalance urea-related osmolar gradients is now widely used. In this technique, the dialysate sodium concentration is gradually lowered from the range of 148 to 160 meq/L to isotonic levels (140 meq/L) near the end of the dialysis treatment. A dialysate glucose concentration of 200 mg/dL (11 mmol/L) is used to optimize blood glucose concentrations. Because patients are exposed to approximately 120 L of water during each dialysis treatment, untreated water could expose them to a variety of environmental contaminants. Therefore, in 98% of U.S. dialysis centers, water used for the dialysate is subjected to filtration, softening, deionization, and, ultimately, reverse osmosis. During the reverse osmosis process, water is forced through a semipermeable membrane at very high pressure to remove microbiologic contaminants and more than 90% of dissolved ions.

BLOOD DELIVERY SYSTEM The blood delivery system is composed of the extracorporeal circuit in the dialysis machine and the dialysis access. The dialysis machine consists of a blood pump, dialysis solution delivery system, and various safety monitors. The blood pump, using a roller mechanism, moves blood from the access site, through the dialyzer, and back to the patient. The blood flow rate may range from 250 to 500 mL/min. Negative hydrostatic pressure on the dialysate side can be manipulated to achieve desirable fluid removal: so-called *ultrafiltration*. Dialysis membranes have different ultrafiltration coefficients (i.e., mL removed/min per mmHg) so that along with hydrostatic changes, fluid removal can be varied. The dialysis solution delivery system dilutes the dialysate concentrate with water and monitors the temperature, conductivity, and flow of dialysate. The dialysate may be delivered to the dialyzer from a storage tank or a proportioning system that manufactures dialysate online.

Dialysis Access The fistula, graft, or catheter through which blood is obtained for hemodialysis is often referred to as a *dialysis access*. A native fistula created by the anastomosis of an artery to a vein (e.g., the Cimino-Breschia fistula, in which the cephalic vein is anastomosed to the radial artery) results in arterialization of the vein. This facilitates its subsequent use in the placement of large needles (typically 15 gauge) to access the circulation. Although fistulas have a high patency rate (approximately 60% are patent at 3 years following creation), fistulas are created in only approximately 30% of patients in the United States. In the majority of U.S. dialysis patients, the dialysis access consists of an arteriovenous graft that interposes prosthetic material, such as polytetrafluoroethylene, between an artery and a vein. Reasons for the higher rates of graft placement include the late referral of patients to vascular access surgeons so that by the time surgery is planned, the patient's arm veins have already been obliterated through multiple blood draws; the high prevalence of patients with diabetes mellitus and its associated microvascular disease; and the greater surgical skill required in creating a fistula. However, by 3 years most grafts fail because of thrombosis or infection. Fortunately, grafts may

be inserted in one of several locations: the arm (brachial artery to basilic vein), the chest wall (axillary artery to axillary vein), or the leg (femoral artery to femoral vein). The most common access-related complication is thrombosis due to intimal hyperplasia, which results in stenosis 2 to 3 cm proximal to the venous anastomosis.

A double-lumen cuffed catheter is used in approximately 20% of patients on chronic hemodialysis in the United States. These catheters are used as an alternative to either a native arteriovenous fistula or a graft in selected patients in whom dialysis is required relatively urgently, such as patients who manifest delayed recovery from acute renal failure, or where a further permanent access procedure (e.g., arteriovenous fistula or arteriovenous graft) is not feasible for anatomical reasons. Although double-lumen catheters may permit blood flows comparable to a permanent arteriovenous access, these catheters are prone to infection and to occlusion because of thrombosis. Temporary double-lumen catheters in either the femoral vein or the internal jugular or subclavian vein are usually employed in patients with acute renal failure. The jugular is preferred to the subclavian vein because, for unclear reasons, a catheter placed in a subclavian vein appears to be associated with a higher rate of venous stenosis. Temporary access can be used for 2 to 3 weeks. Thrombosis, low blood flow, and infection limit the life of the catheter.

GOALS OF DIALYSIS The hemodialysis procedure is targeted at removing both low- and high-molecular-weight solutes. The procedure consists of pumping heparinized blood through the dialyzer at a flow rate of 300 to 500 mL/min, while dialysate flows in an opposite *countercurrent* direction at 500 to 800 mL/min. The clearance of urea ranges from 200 to 350 mL/min, while the clearance of α_2 microglobulin is more modest and ranges from 20 to 25 mL/min. The efficiency of dialysis is determined by blood and dialysate flow through the dialyzer, as well as dialyzer characteristics (i.e., its efficiency in removing solute). The *dose* of dialysis, which is defined as the magnitude of urea clearance during a single dialysis treatment, is further governed by patient size, residual renal function, dietary protein intake, the degree of anabolism or catabolism, and the presence of comorbid conditions.

Since the landmark studies of Sargent and Gatch relating the measurement of the dose of dialysis using urea concentration with patient outcome, the *delivered* dose of dialysis has been correlated with morbidity and mortality. This has led to the development of two major models for assessing the adequacy of the dialysis dose. Fundamentally, these two widely used measures of the adequacy of dialysis are calculated from the decrease in the blood urea nitrogen concentration during the dialysis treatment—that is, the urea reduction ratio (URR), and KT/V, an index based on the urea clearance rate, K, and the size of the urea pool, represented as the urea distribution volume, V. K, which is the sum of clearance by the dialyzer plus renal clearance, is multiplied by the time spent on dialysis, T. Increasingly, KT/V has become the preferred marker for dialysis adequacy. Currently, a URR of 65% and a KT/V of 1.2 per treatment are minimal standards for adequacy among ESRD patients; lower levels of dialysis treatment are associated with increased morbidity and mortality. The HEMO study examined the effect of dialysis dose and the level of flux of the dialyzer membrane on mortality and morbidity and found that a higher dialysis dose (single pool KT/V of 1.71 ± 0.11) did not confer a benefit over a standard dialysis dose (single pool KT/V of 1.32 ± 0.09). Thus, the study supported the continued use of current US Practice Guidelines, which recommend a KT/V of at least 1.2. Furthermore, since no benefit of a high flux dialyzer was demonstrated in the study, the use of a high flux dialyzer was also not supported.

For the majority of patients with chronic renal failure, between 9 and 12 h of dialysis is required each week, usually divided into three equal sessions. However, the dialysis dose must be individualized. Recently there has been much interest in the possibility that more frequent dialysis may be associated with improved outcomes in patients with acute or chronic renal failure. Indeed, it has been suggested that among patients with acute renal failure, daily dialysis may better control uremia, reduce hypotensive episodes, more rapidly resolve acute renal failure, and significantly lower mortality. Therefore, the measurement of dialysis adequacy using KT/V or the URR should serve only as a guide; body size, residual renal function, dietary intake, complicating illness, degree of anabolism or catabolism, and the presence of large interdialytic fluid gains should be important factors that are taken into consideration in the dialysis prescription.

COMPLICATIONS DURING HEMODIALYSIS   Hypotension is the most common acute complication of hemodialysis, particularly among diabetics. Numerous factors appear to increase the risk of hypotension, including excessive ultrafiltration with inadequate compensatory vascular filling, impaired vasoactive or autonomic responses, osmolar shifts, food ingestion, impaired cardiac reserve, diastolic dysfunction, the use of antihypertensive drugs, anemia, and vasodilation due to the use of warm dialysate. Because of the vasodilatory and cardiodepressive effects of acetate, the use of acetate as the buffer in dialysate was once a common cause of hypotension. Since the introduction of bicarbonate-containing dialysate, dialysis-associated hypotension has become less common. The management of hypotension during dialysis consists of discontinuing ultrafiltration, the administration of 100 to 250 mL of isotonic saline or 10 mL of 23% saturated hypertonic saline, and administration of salt-poor albumin. Hypotension during dialysis can frequently be prevented by careful evaluation of the dry weight, withholding of antihypertensive medications on the day prior to and on the day of dialysis, and avoiding heavy meals during dialysis. Additional maneuvers include ultrafiltration modeling, such that more fluid is ultrafiltered at the beginning rather than the end of the dialysis procedure; the performance of sequential ultrafiltration followed by dialysis; the use of midodrine, a selective α_1-adrenergic pressor agent; and cooling of the dialysate during dialysis treatment.

Muscle cramps during dialysis are also a common complication of the procedure. However, since the introduction of volumetric controls on dialysis machines and sodium modeling, the incidence of cramps has fallen. The etiology of dialysis-associated cramps remains obscure. Changes in muscle perfusion because of excessively aggressive volume removal, particularly below the estimated dry weight, and the use of low-sodium-containing dialysate, have been proposed as precipitants of dialysis-associated cramps. Strategies that may be used to prevent cramps include reducing volume removal during dialysis, the use of higher concentrations of sodium in the dialysate, and the use of quinine sulfate (260 mg 2 h before treatment).

Anaphylactoid reactions to the dialyzer, particularly on its first use, have been reported most frequently with the bioincompatible cellulosic-containing membranes. With the gradual phasing out of cuprophane membranes in the United States, the first-use syndrome has become relatively uncommon. The first-use syndrome consists of either an intermediate hypersensitivity reaction due to an IgE-mediated reaction to ethylene oxide used in the sterilization of new dialyzers, or a symptom complex of nonspecific chest and back pain, which appears to result from complement activation and cytokine release.

The major cause of death in patients with ESRD receiving chronic dialysis is cardiovascular disease. The rate of death from cardiac disease is higher in patients on hemodialysis as compared to patients on peritoneal dialysis and renal transplantation. The underlying cause of cardiovascular disease is unclear but may be related to the inadequate treatment of hypertension; the presence of hyperlipidemia, homocystinemia and anemia; the calcification of coronary arteries in patients with an elevated calcium-phosphorus product; and perhaps alterations in cardiovascular dynamics during the dialysis treatment. Intensive investigation of the mechanisms and potential interventions that could impact on reducing the mortality from cardiovascular causes is currently underway.

CONTINUOUS RENAL REPLACEMENT THERAPY   Continuous renal replacement therapies (CRRT) have become increasingly prevalent in the intensive care unit (ICU) setting for management of acute renal failure. The advantages of CRRT over intermittent hemodialysis are that it is usually better tolerated hemodynamically; it facilitates gradual correction of biochemical abnormalities; it is highly effective in removing fluid; and it is technically simple to perform. Clearance of toxic materials (using urea as the marker) can occur with CRRT from convective clearance alone if the ultrafiltration rate is high and with diffusive clearance if dialysis accompanies ultrafiltration. CRRT techniques include continuous arteriovenous hemodiafiltration (CAVH/D) with or without dialysis, and continuous veno-venous hemodiafiltration (CVVH/D) with or without dialysis.

Veno-venous therapies differ fundamentally from arteriovenous therapies in that veno-venous therapies do not require arterial access. This allows obtaining less risky and easier vascular access. However, because there is no systemic arterial pressure to drive hemofiltration, veno-venous therapies require a blood pump in the extracorporeal circuit. Veno-venous therapies such as CVVH provide substantial flexibility because changing the blood flow rate in the pump can change the ultrafiltration and clearance rates. In contrast, arteriovenous therapies such as CAVH are associated with variable efficiency because the systemic blood pressure is frequently low or unstable in patients with acute renal failure. Furthermore, low blood flow with CAVH may also result in clotting of the extracorporeal circuit. CAVH often results in clearance rates as low as 10 to 15 mL/min, whereas CVVH may generate clearances in the range of 30 to 40 mL/min. Thus, in light of these advantages of CVVH, many centers have completely switched from arteriovenous to veno-venous therapies in patients with acute renal failure in the ICU setting.

Vascular access in patients on CVVH is usually achieved by the insertion of a double-lumen catheter into the femoral vein. The blood pump is typically set to deliver approximately 150 to 180 mL/min. In automated systems, (e.g., the Cobe Prisma system), the treatment is volumetrically governed by continuously weighing the effluent and replacement solutions and using a servomechanism to drive the replacement fluid pump at a rate computed either to balance the inflow and loss of fluid or to maintain a predetermined rate of fluid loss. Anticoagulation of the extracorporeal circuit is via a heparin infusion (200 to 1600 U/h) through the inflow side of the circuit. Alternatively, citrate can be used to chelate calcium in the extracorporeal circuit to provide regional anticoagulation in selected patients who cannot undergo systemic heparinization. The replacement solution in continuous therapies is designed specifically to replace calcium, magnesium, and bicarbonate. In place of bicarbonate, lactate or citrate is the buffer in the replacement solution. However, bicarbonate-based replacement fluid is the preferred option in patients with liver failure because of the impaired ability of the liver to metabolize either lactate or acetate into bicarbonate.

PERITONEAL DIALYSIS

Peritoneal dialysis consists of infusing 1 to 3 L of a dextrose-containing solution into the peritoneal cavity and allowing the fluid to dwell for 2 to 4 h. As with hemodialysis, toxic materials are removed through a combination of convective clearance generated through ultrafiltration, and diffusive clearance down a concentration gradient. The clearance of solute and water during a peritoneal dialysis exchange depends on the balance between the movement of solute and water into the peritoneal cavity versus absorption from the peritoneal cavity. The rate of diffusion diminishes with time and eventually stops when equilibration between plasma and dialysate is reached. Absorption of solutes and water from the peritoneal cavity occurs across the peritoneal membrane into the peritoneal capillary circulation and via peritoneal lymphatics into the lymphatic circulation. The rate of peritoneal solute transport varies from patient to patient and may be altered by the presence of infection (peritonitis), drugs such as beta blockers and calcium channel blockers, and physical factors such as position and exercise.

FORMS OF PERITONEAL DIALYSIS   Peritoneal dialysis may be carried out as continuous ambulatory peritoneal dialysis (CAPD), continuous cyclic peritoneal dialysis (CCPD), or nocturnal intermittent peritoneal dialysis (NIPD). In CAPD, dialysis solution is manually infused into the peritoneal cavity during the day and exchanged three to four times daily. A nighttime dwell is frequently instilled at bedtime and remains in the peritoneal cavity through the night. The drainage of spent dialysate (effluence) is performed manually with the assistance of gravity to move fluid out of the abdomen. In CCPD, exchanges are performed in an automated fashion, usually at night; the patient is connected to the automated cycler, which then performs four to five exchange cycles while the patient sleeps. Peritoneal dialysis cyclers automatically cycle dialysate in and out of the abdominal cavity. In the morning the patient, with the last exchange remaining in the abdomen, is disconnected from the cycler and goes about his regular daily activities. In NIPD, the patient is given approximately 10 h of cycling each night, with the abdomen left dry during the day.

Peritoneal dialysis solutions are available in various volumes ranging from 0.5 to 3.0 L. The electrolyte composition is shown in Table 262-2. Lactate is the preferred buffer in peritoneal dialysis solutions. Acetate in peritoneal dialysis solutions appears to accelerate peritoneal sclerosis, whereas use of bicarbonate results in precipitation of calcium and caramelization of glucose. The most common additives to peritoneal dialysis solutions are heparin and antibiotics during an episode of acute peritonitis. Insulin may also be added in patients with diabetes mellitus.

ACCESS TO THE PERITONEAL CAVITY   This is obtained through a peritoneal catheter. These are either *acute* catheters, used to perform acute continuous peritoneal dialysis, usually in an emergency setting, or *chronic* catheters, which have either one or two Dacron cuffs and are tunneled under the skin into the peritoneal cavity. An acute catheter consists of a straight or slightly curved rigid tube with several holes at its distal end. Catheters can be inserted at the bedside by making a small incision in the anterior abdominal wall; the catheter is inserted with the assistance of a guidewire or stylet. Acute catheters are anchored externally with adhesives or sutures and are usually reserved for temporary use because of the risk of infection, which increases after 72 h of use. In contrast, chronic catheters are flexible and made of silicon rubber with numerous side holes at the distal end. These chronic catheters usually have two Dacron cuffs to promote fibroblast proliferation, granulation, and invasion of the cuff. The scarring that occurs around the cuffs anchors the catheter and seals it from bacteria tracking from the skin surface into the peritoneal cavity; it also prevents the external leakage of fluid from the peritoneal cavity. The cuffs are placed in the preperitoneal plane and approximately 2 cm from the skin surface. The most common chronic peritoneal dialysis catheter in use is the Tenckhoff catheter, which contains two cuffs.

The initial CAPD prescription consists of the infusion of a 2-L volume of a 1.5% dextrose concentration peritoneal dialysis solution into the peritoneal cavity over 10 min and allowing it to dwell for 2.5 h. The effluent solution is then drained over 20 min before the next exchange. Three daytime exchanges are accompanied by a 2-L nighttime dwell as the standard prescription. Because peritoneal membrane characteristics vary from one individual to another, the peritoneal equilibrium test should be employed within 2 months of a patient initiating peritoneal dialysis. This test measures the peritoneal membrane transfer rate for solutes (usually urea and creatinine) based on the ratio of their concentration in dialysate and plasma at specific times during the dialysate dwell. It allows patients to be classified as low, low–average, high–average, and high transporters. Approximately 10 to 17% of patients are high transporters, 50% high–average transporters, 25 to 30% low–average transporters, and 1 to 5% low transporters. Identifying the high transporters early is important, since these patients not only demonstrate excellent solute removal, they also absorb glucose rapidly; maximum ultrafiltration occurs early in the dwell, followed by reabsorption of water back into the circulation over the course of the dwell. Such patients benefit from either NIPD or CAPD without a nighttime dwell.

The dose of peritoneal dialysis required to provide adequate or optimal dialysis as measured by patient outcomes is not known. However, there is emerging consensus that the weekly KT/V should be >2.0 and the creatinine clearance >65 L/week per 1.73 m^2. The most frequently utilized approach to calculating a weekly KT/V and creatinine clearance is to collect the spent dialysate and urine over a 24-h period. The peritoneal dialysis prescription can be tailored to improve suboptimal clearance values by increasing the volume of individual exchanges, increasing the number of exchanges, or combining the CAPD and CCPD techniques. In combining these techniques, the CAPD patient hooks up to a cycler at night and the machine automatically performs one or two nocturnal exchanges, whereas the CCPD patient makes an additional manual daytime exchange.

FURTHER READING

BURKART JM et al: Peritoneal dialysis, in *Brenner and Rector's The Kidney*, 7th ed, BM Brenner (ed). Philadelphia, Saunders, 2004

DIAZ-BUXO JA: Early referral and selection of peritoneal dialysis as a treatment modality. Nephrol Dial Transplant 15:147, 2000

EKNOYAN G et al: Effect of dialysis dose and membrane flux in maintenance hemodialysis. N Engl J Med 346:2010, 2002

EKNOYAN G, LEVIN N: NKF-DOQ1 clinical practice guidelines: Update 2000. Am J Kidney Dis 37(Suppl 1):55, 2001

FORNI LG, HILTON PJ: Current concepts: Continuous hemofiltration in the treatment of acute renal failure. N Engl J Med 336:1303, 1997

IFUDU O: Care of patients undergoing hemodialysis. N Engl J Med 339:1054, 1998

MEYER MM: Renal replacement therapies. Crit Care Clin 16:29, 2000

SCHIFFL H et al: Daily hemodialysis and the outcome of acute renal failure. N Engl J Med 346:305, 2002

U.S. RENAL DATA SYSTEM: USRDS 2001 Annual Data Report: Atlas of End-Stage Renal Disease in the United States. Bethesda, National Institutes of Health, National Institute of Diabetes and Digestive and Kidney Disease, 2001

TABLE 262-2 *Composition of Peritoneal Dialysate*

Solute	Dianeal (PD-2)
Sodium (meq/L)	132
Potassium (meq/L)	0
Chloride (meq/L)	96
Calcium (meq/L)	3.5
Magnesium (meq/L)	0.5
D,L-Lactate (meq/L)	40
Glucose (g%)	
1.5	
2.5	
4.25	
pH	5.2

Transplantation of the human kidney is frequently the most effective treatment of advanced chronic renal failure. Worldwide, tens of thousands of such procedures have been performed. When azathioprine and prednisone were initially used as immunosuppressive drugs in the 1960s, the results with properly matched familial donors were superior to those with organs from cadaveric donors, namely, 75 to 90% compared with 50 to 60% graft survival rates at 1 year. During the 1970s and 1980s, the success rate at the 1-year mark for cadaveric transplants rose progressively. By the time cyclosporine was introduced in the early 1980s, cadaveric donor grafts had a 70% 1-year survival and reached the 82% level in the mid-1990s and 88% by 1998 (Fig. 263-1). After the first year, graft survival curves show an exponential decline in numbers of functioning grafts from which a half-life ($t_{1/2}$) in years is calculated; this has increased by 2 years since the 1980s (Fig. 263-1).

Mortality rates after transplantation are highest in the first year and are age-related: 2% for ages 18 to 34 years, 3% for ages 35 to 49 years, and 6.8% for ages over 50 to 60 years. These rates compare favorably to those in the chronic dialysis population, even after risk adjustments for age, diabetes, and cardiovascular status. Occasionally, acute irreversible rejection may occur after many months of good function, especially if the patient neglects to take the immunosuppressive drugs. Most grafts, however, succumb at varying rates to a chronic vascular and interstitial obliterative process termed *chronic rejection*, although its pathogenesis is incompletely understood. Overall, transplantation returns the majority of patients to an improved lifestyle and an improved life expectancy, as compared to patients on dialysis; however, careful prospective cohort studies have yet to be reported.

RECIPIENT SELECTION There are few absolute contraindications to renal transplantation. The transplant procedure is relatively noninvasive, as the organ is placed in the inguinal fossa without entering the peritoneal cavity. Recipients without perioperative complications can often be discharged from the hospital in excellent condition within 5 days of the operation.

Virtually all end-stage renal disease (ESRD) patients who receive a transplant have a higher life expectancy than risk-matched patients who remain on dialysis. Even though diabetics or older candidates have a higher mortality rate than other transplant recipients, their survival is improved with transplantation compared to remaining on dialysis. This global benefit of transplantation as a treatment modality poses substantial ethical issues for policy makers, as the number of cadaveric kidneys available is far from sufficient to meet the current needs of the candidates. Waiting lists continue to grow, and the average wait time for a cadaver kidney is now >4 years in many locales. The current standard of care is that the candidate should have a life expectancy of >5 years to be put on a cadaver organ wait list. Even for living donation, the candidate should have >5 years of life expectancy. This is because the benefits of kidney transplantation over dialysis are only realized after a perioperative period in which the mortality is higher in transplanted patients than in dialysis patients with comparable risk profile.

All candidates must have a thorough risk/benefit evaluation prior to being approved for transplantation. In particular, an aggressive approach to diagnosis of correctable coronary artery disease, presence of latent or indolent infection (HIV, hepatitis B or C, tuberculosis), and neoplasm should be a routine part of the candidate workup. Most transplant centers consider overt AIDS and active hepatitis to be an absolute contraindication to transplantation because of the high risk of opportunistic infection. Some centers are now transplanting individuals with hepatitis and even HIV infection under strict protocols to determine whether the risks and benefits favor transplantation over dialysis.

Among the few absolute contraindications to transplantation is the presence of potentially harmful antibody against the donor kidney at the time of the anticipated transplant. Harmful antibodies that can cause very early graft loss include natural antibodies against the ABO blood group antigens and antibodies against HLA-class I (A, B, C) or class II (DR) antigens. These antibodies are routinely excluded by proper pretransplant screening of the candidates, ABO and HLA typing of donor and recipient, and cross-matching of candidate serum with that of the donor.

DONOR SELECTION Donors can be cadavers or volunteer living donors. The latter are usually family members selected to have at least partial compatibility for HLA antigens. Living volunteer donors should be normal on physical examination and of the same major ABO blood group, because crossing major blood group barriers prejudices survival of the allograft. It is possible, however, to transplant a kidney of a type O donor into an A, B, or AB recipient. Selective renal arteriography should be performed on donors to rule out the presence of multiple or abnormal renal arteries, because the surgical procedure is difficult and the ischemic time of the transplanted kidney long when vascular abnormalities exist. Transplant surgeons are now using a laparoscopic method to isolate and remove the living donor kidney. This operation has the advantage of less evident surgical scars, and, because there is less tissue trauma, the laparoscopic donors have a substantially shorter hospital stay and less discomfort than those who have the traditional surgery. Cadaveric donors should be free of malignant neoplastic disease, hepatitis, and HIV because of possible transmission to the recipient. Increased risk of graft failure exists when the donor is elderly or has renal failure and when the kidney has a prolonged period of ischemia and storage.

In the United States, there is a coordinated national system of regulations, allocation support, and outcomes analysis for kidney transplantation called the Organ Procurement Transplant Network. It is now possible to remove cadaver kidneys and to maintain them for up to 48 h on cold pulsatile perfusion or simple flushing and cooling. This permits adequate time for typing, cross-matching, transportation, and selection problems to be solved.

TISSUE TYPING AND CLINICAL IMMUNOGENETICS Matching for antigens of the HLA major histocompatibility gene complex (Chap. 296) is an

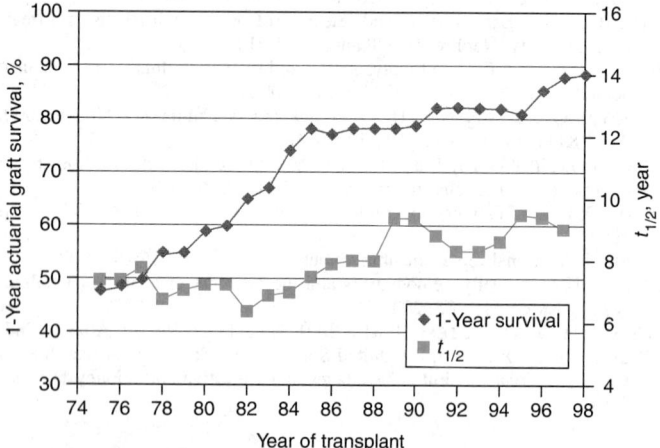

FIGURE 263-1 One-year actuarial graft survival of cohorts of first cadaver kidney transplants performed from 1975 through 1998 is displayed (in purple) along with $t_{1/2}$ or post-year-one half-life of the same cohorts (green). These registry data are derived from the U.S. Renal Data System 2002 Annual Report. The upper curve represents the 1-year actual graft survival, which approaches 90% by 1998. From 1982 to 1985 there was an impressive rise in the 1-year survival, partially attributable to the introduction of cyclosporine. Since 1985, there has been a consistent, slow increase in 1-year survival. The lower curve represents long-term graft survival, expressed as the half-life ($t_{1/2}$), which has been relatively stable over the past decade.

important criterion for selection of donors for renal allografts. Each mammalian species has a single chromosomal region that encodes the strong, or major, transplantation antigens, and this region on the human sixth chromosome is called *HLA*. HLA antigens have been classically defined by serologic techniques, but methods to define specific nucleotide sequences in genomic DNA are increasingly being used. Other antigens, called "minor," may nevertheless play crucial roles, in addition to the ABH(O) blood groups and endothelial antigens that are not shared with lymphocytes. The Rh system is not expressed on graft tissue. Evidence for designation of HLA as the genetic region encoding major transplantation antigens comes from the success rate in living related donor renal and bone marrow transplantation, with superior results in HLA-identical sibling pairs. Nevertheless, 5% of HLA-identical renal allografts are rejected, often within the first weeks after transplantation. These failures represent states of prior sensitization to non-HLA antigens. Non-HLA minor antigens are relatively weak when initially encountered and are therefore suppressible by conventional immunosuppressive therapy. Once priming has occurred, however, secondary responses are much more refractory to treatment. ABO incompatibilities are hazardous because of the presence of natural anti-A and anti-B antibodies in recipients and the normal expression of A and B blood group substances on endothelium, resulting in immediate vascular injury.

Living Donors When first-degree relatives are donors, graft survival rates at 1 year are 5 to 7% greater than those for cadaver grafts. The 5-year survival rates still favor the partially matched (3/6 HLA mismatched) family donor over a randomly selected cadaver donor (Table 263-1). In addition, living donors provide the advantage of immediate availability. For both living and cadaveric donors, the 5-year outcomes are poor if there is a complete (6/6) HLA mismatch. Waiting lists for cadaveric kidneys have grown faster than the available organ supply, to the point where most new patients with ESRD wait for >4 years. In response to this increasing disparity between cadaver donor supply and patient demand, living unrelated volunteers, usually spouses or close friends, are being accepted as donors in increasing numbers. The survival rate of living unrelated renal allografts is as good or better than that of perfectly HLA matched cadaver renal transplants and comparable to that of kidneys from living relatives. This is likely to be a consequence both of short cold ischemia time and the extra care taken to document that the condition and renal function of the donor are optimal before proceeding with a living unrelated donation (Table 263-1). It is illegal in the United States to purchase organs for transplantation.

Concern has been expressed regarding the potential risk to a volunteer kidney donor of premature renal failure after several years of increased blood flow and hyperfiltration per nephron in the remaining kidney. There are a few reports of the development of hypertension, proteinuria, and even lesions of focal segmental sclerosis in donors under long-term follow-up. Difficulties in donors followed for ≥20 years are unusual, however, and it may be that having a single kidney becomes significant only when another condition, such as hyperten-

sion, is superimposed. It is also desirable to consider the risk of development of type 1 diabetes mellitus in a family member who is a potential donor to a diabetic renal failure patient. Anti-insulin and anti-islet antibodies should be measured, and glucose tolerance tests should be performed in such donors to rule out a prediabetic state.

HLA Matching and Cadaveric Donors The question of whether matching of HLA antigens in unrelated donor-recipient pairs would approximate the high initial success rates and slow rates of subsequent graft loss with HLA-identical sib pairs could not be answered until the late 1980s when reliable class II histocompatibility (DR) typing became widely available. Now that pooled data on tens of thousands of cadaveric renal transplants from all over the world are available, the HLA-matching effect can be clearly seen, especially in the long-term survival figures. It is shown in Table 263-1 that there is an overall beneficial effect of HLA matching in cadaveric grafts. With increasing numbers of mismatches for cadaveric donors, the 5-year survival drops from 68.2% to 55.3%. The survival rates at the 10-year mark are projected to range from 65 (zero mismatches) to 34% (six mismatches). There is controversy regarding the value of cadaveric organ-sharing rules that are based entirely upon the numbers of HLA mismatches. Giving preference to HLA zero-mismatched candidates (Table 263-1) is a top priority in the United States, however, and 20% of kidneys are transplanted on this basis. Table 263-1 also shows the interaction of HLA matching and graft ischemia on results; namely, kidneys from HLA-incompatible unrelated or spousal donors do better than those from similarly mismatched cadaver donors, suggesting that the additional ischemic injury of organ storage is important. Nevertheless, when such a cadaveric donor is HLA-compatible, the benefit of matching can still be seen.

Presensitization A positive cross match of recipient serum with donor T lymphocytes representing anti-HLA class I is usually predictive of an acute vasculitic event termed *hyperacute rejection*. Patients with anti-HLA antibodies can be safely transplanted if careful cross-matching of donor blood lymphocytes with recipient serum is performed. Patients sustained by dialysis often show fluctuating antibody titers and specificity patterns. At the time of assignment of a cadaveric kidney, cross matches are performed with at least a current serum. Previously analyzed antibody specificities and additional cross matches are performed accordingly. Techniques for cross-matching are not universally standardized; however, at least two techniques are employed in most laboratories. The minimal purpose for the cross match is avoidance of hyperacute rejection mediated by recipient antibodies to donor HLA class I antigens. Sensitive tests, such as the use of flow cytometry, can be useful for avoidance of accelerated, and often untreatable, early graft rejection in patients receiving second or third transplants. Donor T lymphocytes, which express only class I antigens, are used as targets for detection of anti-class I (HLA-A and -B) antibodies. Preformed anti-class II (HLA-DR) antibodies against the donor carry a higher risk of graft loss as well, particularly in recipients who have suffered early loss of a prior kidney transplant. B lymphocytes expressing both class I and class II antigens are used in these assays. Non-HLA antigens restricted in expression to endothelium and sometimes monocytes have been described, but clinical relevance is not well established. A series of minor histocompatibility antigens do not elicit antibodies, and sensitization to these is detectable only by cytotoxic T cells, an assay too cumbersome for routine use.

Blood Transfusions Exposure to leukocyte HLA antigens during transfusions is a major cause of sensitization that limits transplantation access and increases the risk of early graft rejection. In the 1970s, attempts to avoid all blood exposure in dialysed patients paradoxically increased the risk of graft rejection. The beneficial "transfusion effect" was never fully explained, and it almost disappeared in the 1980s as overall management of patients improved with the use of cyclosporine and more effective means of rejection treatment. Currently, with the use of erythropoietin the need for transfusion is much reduced. It has

TABLE 263-1 *Effect of HLA-A, -B, -DR Mismatching on Kidney Graft Survival*[b]

Degree of Donor Mismatch	1-Year Survival, %	5-Year Survival, %
Cadaver donor (all)	89.2	61.3
0/6-HLA mismatch	91.3	68.2
3/6-HLA mismatch	90.1	60.8
6/6-HLA mismatch	85.2	55.3
Living related donor (all)	94.7	76.0
0/6-HLA mismatch	96.7	87.0
3/6-HLA mismatch	94.3	73.2
6/6-HLA mismatch	92.7	57.7
Living unrelated donor	95.3	77.4

Note: 0-mismatched related donor transplants are virtually all from HLA-identical siblings, while 3/6-mismatched transplants can be one haplotype mismatched (1-A, 1-B, and 1-DR antigen) from parent, child or sibling; 6/6-HLA-mismatched living related kidneys are derived from siblings or relatives outside of the nuclear family.

been noted, however, that nontransfused patients do have more rejection activity.

IMMUNOLOGY OF REJECTION   Both cellular and humoral (antibody-mediated) effector mechanisms can play roles in kidney transplant rejection. Antibodies directed against ABO blood group antigens and HLA class I or class II antigens can cause hyperacute rejection within minutes to hours of engraftment if they are present in the recipient at the time of engraftment. Such antibodies bind to vascular endothelium, cause activation of the complement cascade, and direct endothelial damage, platelet aggregation, microvascular thrombi, and in the most severe cases ischemic necrosis of the organ. Antibodies against ABO are naturally found in humans. Anti-HLA antibodies are produced as a consequence of prior blood transfusions, multiple pregnancies, or rejection of a prior HLA-incompatible transplant. Antibodies that bind to cells within the transplant can also initiate a form of antibody-dependent cell death mediated by recipient cells that bear receptors for the Fc portion of immunoglobulin.

Cellular rejection is mediated by lymphocytes that respond to HLA antigens expressed within the organ. The CD4+ lymphocyte responds to class II (HLA-DR) incompatibility by proliferating and releasing proinflammatory cytokines that augment the proliferative response of both CD4+ and CD8+ cells. CD8+ cytotoxic lymphocyte precursors respond primarily to class I (HLA-A, -B) antigens and mature into cytotoxic effector cells. The cytotoxic effector, or "killer" T, cells cause organ damage through direct contact and lysis of donor target cells. The natural role of HLA antigens is to present processed peptide fragments of antigen to T lymphocytes, the fragments residing in a "groove" of the HLA molecule distal to the cell surface. T cells can be directly stimulated by non-self HLA antigen expressed on donor parenchymal cells and residual donor leukocytes residing in the kidney interstitium. In addition, donor HLA molecules can be processed by a variety of donor or recipient cells capable of antigen presentation and then presented to T cells in the same manner as most other antigens. The former mode of stimulation is sometimes called *direct presentation* and the latter mode called *indirect presentation* (Fig. 263-2). There is evidence that non-HLA antigens can also play a role in renal transplant rejection episodes. Recipients who receive a kidney from an HLA-identical sibling can have rejection episodes and require maintenance immunosuppression, while identical twin transplants require no immunosuppression. There are documented non-HLA antigens, such as an endothelial-specific antigen system with limited polymorphism and a tubular antigen, which can be targets of humoral or cellular rejection responses, respectively.

IMMUNOSUPPRESSIVE TREATMENT   Immunosuppressive therapy, as presently available, generally suppresses all immune responses, including those to bacteria, fungi, and even malignant tumors. In the 1950s when clinical renal transplantation began, sublethal total-body irradiation was employed. We have now reached the point where sophisticated pharmacologic immunosuppression is available, but it still has the hazard of promoting infection and malignancy. In general, all clinically useful drugs are more selective to primary than to memory immune responses. Agents to suppress the immune response are discussed in the following paragraphs, and those currently in clinical use are listed in Table 263-2.

Drugs   *Azathioprine,* an analogue of mercaptopurine, was for two decades the keystone to immunosuppressive therapy in humans. This agent can inhibit synthesis of DNA, RNA, or both. Because cell division and proliferation are a necessary part of the immune response to antigenic stimulation, suppression by this agent may be mediated by the inhibition of mitosis of immunologically competent lymphoid cells, interfering with synthesis of DNA. Alternatively, immunosuppression may be brought about by blocking the synthesis of RNA (possibly messenger RNA), inhibiting processing of antigens prior to lymphocyte stimulation. Therapy with azathioprine in doses of 1.5 to

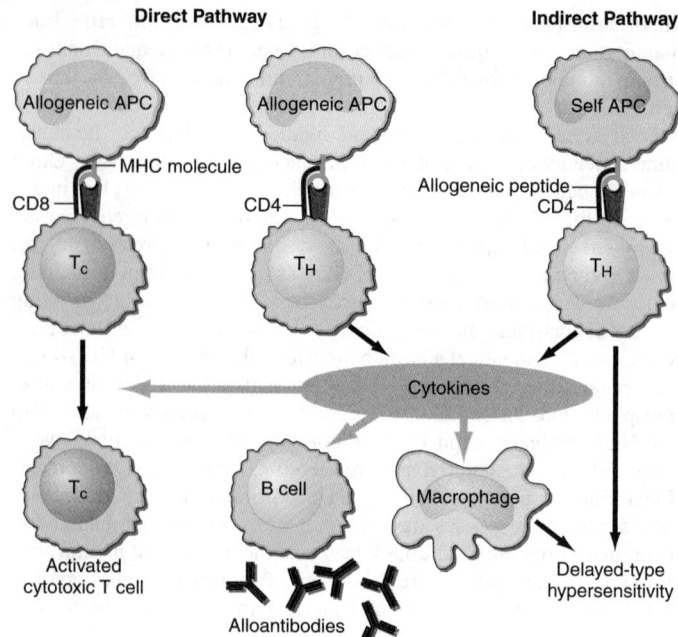

FIGURE 263-2   Recognition pathways for major histocompatibility complex (MHC) antigens. Graft rejection is initiated by CD4 helper T lymphocytes (T_H) having antigen receptors that bind to specific complexes of peptides and MHC class II molecules on antigen-presenting cells (APC). In transplantation, in contrast to other immunologic responses, there are two sets of T cell clones involved in rejection. In the direct pathway the class II MHC of donor allogeneic APCs is recognized by CD4 T_H cells that bind to the intact MHC molecule, and class I MHC allogeneic cells are recognized by CD8 T cells. The latter generally proliferate into cytotoxic cells (T_C). In the indirect pathway, the incompatible MHC molecules are processed into peptides that are presented by the self-APCs of the recipient. The indirect, but not the direct, pathway is the normal physiologic process in T cell recognition of foreign antigens. Once T_H cells are activated, they proliferate, and by secretion of cytokines and direct contact exert strong helper effects on macrophages, T_C, and B cells. *(From Sayegh and Turka, Copyright 1998, Massachusetts Medical Society. All rights reserved.)*

2.0 mg/kg per day is generally added to cyclosporine as a means of decreasing the requirements for the latter. Because azathioprine is rapidly metabolized by the liver, its dosage need not be varied directly in relation to renal function, even though renal failure results in retention of the metabolites of azathioprine. Reduction in dosage is required because of leukopenia and occasionally thrombocytopenia. Excessive amounts of azathioprine may also cause jaundice, anemia, and alopecia. If it is essential to administer allopurinol concurrently, the azathioprine dose must be reduced, since inhibition of xanthine oxidase delays degradation. This combination is best avoided.

Mycophenolate mofetil is now used in place of azathioprine in many centers. It has a similar mode of action and a mild degree of gastrointestinal toxicity but produces minimal bone marrow suppression. Its advantage is its increased potency in preventing or reversing rejection. Patients with hyperuricemia can be given allopurinol without adjustment of the mycophenylate dose.

Glucocorticoids are important adjuncts to immunosuppressive therapy. Of all the agents employed, prednisone has effects that are easiest to assess, and in large doses it is usually effective for the reversal of rejection. In general, 200 to 300 mg prednisone is given immediately prior to or at the time of transplantation, and the dosage is reduced to 30 mg within a week. The side effects of the glucocorticoids, particularly impairment of wound healing and predisposition to infection, make it desirable to taper the dose as rapidly as possible in the immediate postoperative period. Customarily, methylprednisolone, 0.5 to 1.0 g intravenously, is administered immediately upon diagnosis of beginning rejection and continued once daily for 3 days. When the drug is effective, the results are usually apparent within 96 h. Such "pulse" doses are not effective in chronic rejection. Most patients whose renal function is stable after 6 months or a year do not require large doses of prednisone; maintenance doses of 10 to 15 mg/d are the rule. Many patients tolerate an alternate-day course of steroids without an increased risk of rejection.

A major effect of steroids is on the monocyte-macrophage system, preventing the release of interleukin (IL) 6 and IL-1. Lymphopenia after large doses of glucocorticoids is primarily due to sequestration of recirculating blood lymphocytes to lymphoid tissue.

Cyclosporine is a fungal peptide with potent immunosuppressive activity. It acts on the calcineurin pathway to block transcription of mRNA for IL-2 and other proinflammatory cytokines, thereby inhibiting T cell proliferation. Although it works alone, cyclosporine is more effective in conjunction with glucocorticoids. Since cyclosporine blocks production of IL-2 by T cells, its combination with steroids is expected to produce a double block in the macrophage → IL-6/IL-1 → T cell → IL-2 sequence. Clinical results with tens of thousands of renal transplants have been impressive. Of its toxic effects (nephrotoxicity, hepatotoxicity, hirsutism, tremor, gingival hyperplasia, diabetes), only nephrotoxicity presents a serious management problem and is further discussed below.

TABLE 263-2 *Maintenance Immunosuppressive Drugs*

Agent	Pharmacology	Mechanisms	Side Effects
Glucocorticoids	Increased bioavailability with hypoalbuminemia and liver disease; prednisone/prednisolone generally used	Binds cytosolic receptors and heat shock proteins. Blocks transcription of IL-1,-2,-3,-6, TNF-α, and IFN-γ	Hypertension, glucose intolerance, dyslipidemia, osteoporosis
Cyclosporine (CsA)	Lipid-soluble polypeptide, variable absorption, microemulsion more predictable	Trimolecular complex with cyclophilin and calcineurin → block in cytokine (e.g., IL-2) production; however, stimulates TGF-β production	Nephrotoxicity, hypertension, dyslipidemia, glucose intolerance, hirsutism/hyperplasia of gums
Tacrolimus (FK506)	Macrolide, well absorbed	Trimolecular complex with FKBP-12 and calcineurin → block in cytokine (e.g., IL-2) production; may stimulate TGF-β production	Similar to CsA, but hirsutism/hyperplasia of gums unusual, and diabetes more likely
Azathioprine	Mercaptopurine analogue	Hepatic metabolites inhibit purine synthesis	Marrow suppression (WBC > RBC > platelets)
Mycophenolate mofetil (MMF)	Metabolized to mycophenolic acid	Inhibits purine synthesis via inosine monophosphate dehydrogenase	Diarrhea/cramps; dose-related liver and marrow suppression is uncommon
Sirolimus	Macrolide, poor oral bioavailability	Complexes with FKBP-12 and then blocks p70 S6 kinase in the IL-2 receptor pathway for proliferation	Hyperlipidemia, thrombocytopenia

Note: IL, interleukin; TNF, tumor necrosis factor; IFN, interferon; TGF, transforming growth factor; FKBP-12, FK506 binding protein 12; WBC, white blood cells; RBC, red blood cells.

Tacrolimus (FK-506) is a fungal macrolide that has the same mode of action, and a similar side effect profile, as cyclosporine. It does not produce hirsutism or gingival hyperplasia, however. De novo induction of diabetes mellitus is more common with tacrolimus. The drug was first used in liver transplantation and may substitute for cyclosporine entirely or be tried as an alternative in renal patients whose rejections are poorly controlled by cyclosporine.

Sirolimus (previously called rapamycin) is another fungal macrolide but has a different mode of action, i.e., it inhibits T cell growth factor pathways, preventing the response to IL-2 and other cytokines. Sirolimus can be used in conjunction with cyclosporine or tacrolimus as an alternative immunosuppressive regimen. Its use with tacrolimus alone shows promise as a steroid-sparing regimen, especially in patients who would benefit from pancreatic islet transplantation, where steroids have an adverse effect on islet survival.

Antibodies to Lymphocytes When serum from animals made immune to host lymphocytes is injected into the recipient, a marked suppression of cellular immunity to the tissue graft results. The action on cell-mediated immunity is greater than on humoral immunity. A globulin fraction of serum [antilymphocyte globulin (ALG)] is the agent generally employed. For use in humans, peripheral human lymphocytes, thymocytes, or lymphocytes from spleens or thoracic duct fistulas have been injected into horses, rabbits, or goats to produce antilymphocyte serum, from which the globulin fraction is then separated. Monoclonal antibodies against defined lymphocyte subsets offer a more precise and standardized form of therapy. OKT3 is directed to the CD3 molecules that form a portion of the T cell antigen-receptor complex; hence CD3 is expressed on all mature T cells. CD4 or CD8 molecules also form part of the fully activated cluster of molecules, and monoclonal antibodies to these offer the potential for more selective targeting of T cell subsets.

Another approach to more selective therapy is to target the 55-kDa alpha chain of the IL-2 receptor, expressed only on T cells that have been recently activated. The problem with such mouse antibodies is the potential for developing human antimouse antibodies (HAMA), an event that limits the effective period of use. Genetically engineered monoclonal antibodies can solve this problem. Two such antibodies to the IL-2 receptor, in which either a chimeric protein has been made between mouse Fab with human Fc (basiliximab) or "humanized" by splicing the combining sites of the mouse into a molecule that is 90% human IgG (daclizumab), have been approved for prophylaxis of acute rejection in the immediate posttransplant period. They are effective at decreasing the acute rejection rate and have few adverse side effects.

CLINICAL COURSE AND MANAGEMENT OF THE RECIPIENT Adequate hemodialysis should be performed within 48 h of surgery, and care should be taken that the serum potassium level is not markedly elevated so that intraoperative cardiac arrhythmias can be averted. The diuresis that commonly occurs postoperatively must be carefully monitored; in some instances it may be massive, reflecting the inability of ischemic tubules to regulate sodium and water excretion; with large diureses, massive potassium losses may occur. Most chronically uremic patients have some excess of extracellular fluid, and it is useful to maintain an expanded fluid volume in the immediate postoperative period. Acute tubular necrosis (ATN) may cause immediate oliguria or may follow an initial short period of graft function. ATN is most likely when cadaveric donors have been hypotensive or if the interval between cessation of blood flow and organ harvest (warm ischemic time) is more than a few minutes. Recovery usually occurs within 3 weeks, although periods as long as 6 weeks have been reported. Superimposition of rejection on ATN is common, and the differential diagnosis may be difficult without a graft biopsy. Cyclosporine therapy prolongs ATN, and some patients do not diurese until the dose is drastically reduced. Many centers avoid starting cyclosporine for the first several days, using ALG or a monoclonal antibody along with mycophenolate mofetil and prednisone until renal function is established. Fig. 263-3 illustrates an algorithm followed by many transplant centers for early

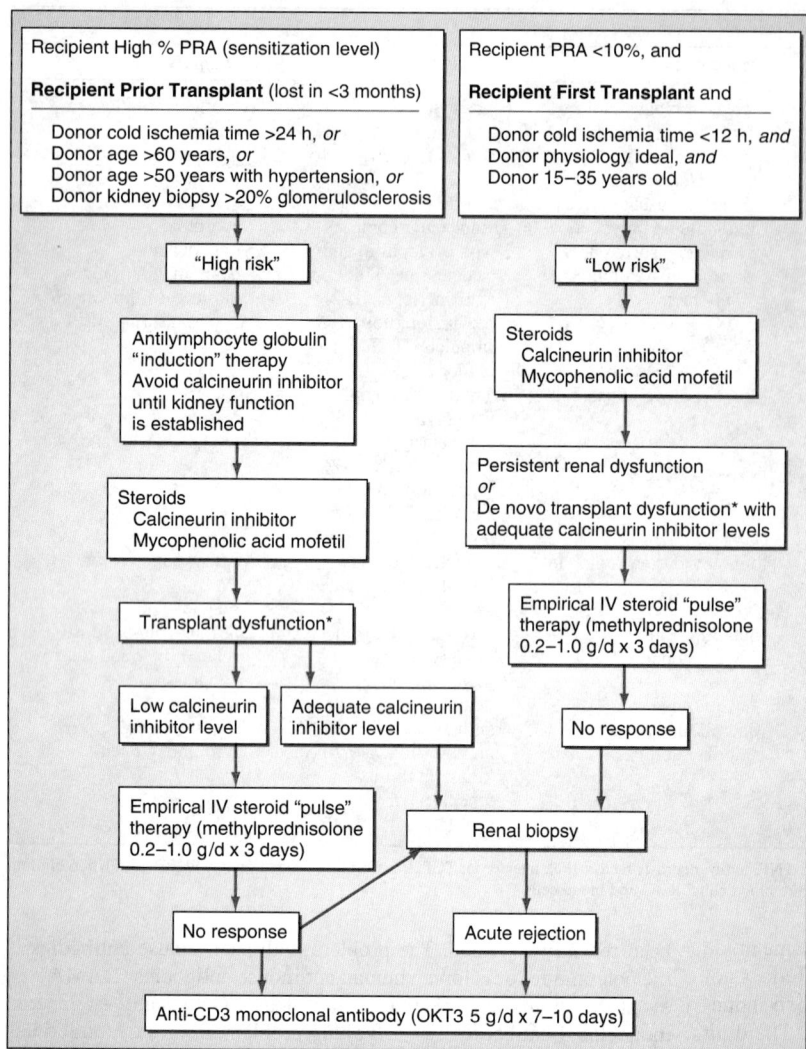

FIGURE 263-3 A typical algorithm for early posttransplant care of the kidney recipient. If any of the recipient or donor "high-risk" factors exist, more aggressive management is called for. Low-risk patients can be treated with a standard immunosuppressive regimen. Patients at higher risk of rejection or early ischemic and nephrotoxic transplant dysfunction are often induced with an antilymphocyte globulin to provide more potent early immunosuppression or to spare calcineurin nephrotoxicity. *When there is early transplant dysfunction, prerenal, obstructive, and vascular causes must be ruled out by ultrasonographic examination. The panel reactive antibody (PRA) is a quantitation of how much antibody is present in a candidate against a panel of cells representing the distribution of antigens in the donor pool.

The figure boxes contain:

Recipient High % PRA (sensitization level)
Recipient Prior Transplant (lost in <3 months)
Donor cold ischemia time >24 h, or
Donor age >60 years, or
Donor age >50 years with hypertension, or
Donor kidney biopsy >20% glomerulosclerosis

Recipient PRA <10%, and
Recipient First Transplant and
Donor cold ischemia time <12 h, and
Donor physiology ideal, and
Donor 15–35 years old

"High risk"

"Low risk"

Antilymphocyte globulin "induction" therapy
Avoid calcineurin inhibitor until kidney function is established

Steroids
Calcineurin inhibitor
Mycophenolic acid mofetil

Steroids
Calcineurin inhibitor
Mycophenolic acid mofetil

Persistent renal dysfunction
or
De novo transplant dysfunction* with adequate calcineurin inhibitor levels

Transplant dysfunction*

Empirical IV steroid "pulse" therapy (methylprednisolone 0.2–1.0 g/d × 3 days)

Low calcineurin inhibitor level

Adequate calcineurin inhibitor level

No response

Empirical IV steroid "pulse" therapy (methylprednisolone 0.2–1.0 g/d × 3 days)

Renal biopsy

No response

Acute rejection

Anti-CD3 monoclonal antibody (OKT3 5 g/d × 7–10 days)

---

posttransplant management of recipients at high or low risk of early renal dysfunction.

The Rejection Episode Early diagnosis of rejection allows prompt institution of therapy to preserve renal function and prevent irreversible damage. Clinical evidence of rejection is rarely characterized by fever, swelling, and tenderness over the allograft. Rejection may present only with a rise in serum creatinine, with or without a reduction in urine volume. The focus should be on ruling out other causes of functional deterioration.

Arteriography and radioactive iodohippurate sodium renograms of the transplanted kidney may be useful in ascertaining changes in the renal vasculature and in renal blood flow, even in the absence of urinary flow. Thrombosis of the renal vein occurs rarely; it may be reversible if caused by technical factors and intervention is prompt. Diagnostic ultrasound is the procedure of choice to rule out urinary obstruction or to confirm the presence of perirenal collections of urine, blood, or lymph. When renal function has been good initially, a rise in the serum creatinine level is the most sensitive and reliable indicator of possible rejection and may be the only sign.

Calcineurin inhibitors (cyclosporine or tacrolimus) may cause de-

terioration in renal function in a manner similar to a rejection episode. In fact, rejection processes tend to be more indolent with these inhibitors, and the only way to make a diagnosis may be by renal biopsy. Calcineurin inhibitors have an afferent arteriolar constrictor effect on the kidney and may produce permanent vascular and interstitial injury after sustained high-dose therapy. Addition of angiotensin-converting enzyme (ACE) inhibitors or nonsteroidal anti-inflammatory drugs are likely to raise serum creatinine levels. The former are generally safe to use after the early months, while the latter are best avoided in all renal transplant patients. There is no universally accepted lesion(s) that makes a diagnosis of calcineurin inhibitor toxicity, although interstitial fibrosis, isometric tubular vacuolization, and thickening of arteriolar walls have been noted by some. Basically, if the biopsy does not reveal moderate and active cellular rejection activity, the serum creatinine will most likely respond to a reduction in dose. Blood levels of drug can be useful if very high or very low but do not correlate precisely with renal function, although serial changes in a patient can be useful. If rejection activity is present in the biopsy, appropriate therapy is indicated. The first rejection episode is usually treated with intravenous administration of methylprednisolone, 500 to 1000 mg daily for 3 days. Failure to respond is indication for antibody therapy, usually with OKT3.

OKT3 monoclonal antibody, given intravenously for 10 to 14 days, is effective in >90% of first rejections but less so if methylprednisolone pulses have failed and in cases of severe recurrent rejection activity. A major problem with OKT3 is that severe systemic reactions may be produced during the first day or two of therapy. Chills, fever, hypotension, and headache are the direct result of the antibody effects on the targeted T cells, most likely related to the known potential of OKT3 to activate T cells nonspecifically with release of cytokines, especially tumor necrosis factor α. If the antibody is administered to overhydrated oliguric patients, pulmonary edema may be induced. These reactions are not characteristic of other monoclonal antibodies, such as those to the IL-2 receptor. Recurrent or rebound rejection activity may require additional therapy. In such circumstances, methylprednisolone may be effective even though it failed initially. Second courses of OKT3 may be given in spite of HAMA generated in response to the first course if the titers are low and the human antibodies are not directed to the combining-site region (idiotype) of the OKT3.

Management Problems The usual clinical manifestations of infection in the posttransplant period are blunted by immunosuppressive therapy. The major toxic effect of azathioprine is bone marrow suppression, which is less likely with mycophenolate mofetil, while calcineurin inhibitors have no marrow effects. All drugs predispose to unusual opportunistic infections, however. The typical times posttransplant when the most common opportunistic infections occur are tabulated in Table 263-3. The signs and symptoms of infection may be masked or distorted. Fever without obvious cause is common and only after days or weeks may it become apparent that it has a viral or fungal origin. Bacterial infections are most common during the first month after transplantation. The importance of blood cultures in such patients cannot be overemphasized, because systemic infection without obvious foci is frequent, although wound infections with or without urinary fistulas are most common. Particularly ominous are rapidly occurring pulmonary lesions, which may result in death within 5 days of onset. When these become apparent, immunosuppressive agents should be discontinued, except for maintenance doses of prednisone.

TABLE 263-3 *The Most Common Opportunistic Infections in the Renal Transplant Recipient*

Peritransplant (<1 month)	Late (>6 months)
Wound infections	*Aspergillus*
Herpesvirus	*Nocardia*
Oral candidiasis	BK virus (polyoma)
Urinary tract infection	Herpes zoster
Early (1–6 months)	Hepatitis B
Pneumocystis carinii	Hepatitis C
Cytomegalovirus	
Legionella	
Listeria	
Hepatitis B	
Hepatitis C	

Aggressive diagnostic procedures, including transbronchial and open lung biopsy, are frequently indicated. In the case of *Pneumocystis carinii* (Chap. 191) infection, trimethoprim-sulfamethoxazole is the treatment of choice; amphotericin B has been used effectively in systemic fungal infections. Prophylaxis against *P. carinii* with daily or alternate day low-dose trimethoprim-sulfamethoxazole is very effective. Involvement of the oropharynx with *Candida* (Chap. 187) may be treated with local nystatin. Tissue-invasive fungal infections require treatment with systemic agents such as fluconazole. Small doses (a total of 300 mg) of amphotericin given over a period of 2 weeks may be effective in fungal infections refractory to fluconazole. Macrolide antibiotics, especially ketoconazole and erythromycin, and some calcium channel blockers (diltiazem, verapamil) compete with calcineurin inhibitors for P450 catabolism and cause elevated levels of these immunosuppressive drugs. Analeptics, such as phenytoin and carbamazepine, will increase catabolism to result in low levels. *Aspergillus* (Chap. 188), *Nocardia* (Chap. 146), and cytomegalovirus (CMV) (Chap. 166) infections also occur.

CMV is a common and dangerous infection in transplant recipients. It does not generally appear until the end of the first posttransplant month. Active CMV infection is sometimes associated, or occasionally confused, with rejection episodes. Patients at highest risk for severe CMV disease are those without anti-CMV antibodies who receive a graft from a CMV antibody–positive donor (15% mortality). Serial intravenous administration of high-titer CMV immune globulin is effective in reducing this risk. Prophylactic use of ganciclovir is an effective alternative. Valganciclovir is a cost-effective and bioavailable oral form of ganciclovir that has proven effective in both prophylaxis and treatment of CMV disease. Early diagnosis in a febrile patient can be made by detecting CMV antigens in the blood. A rise in IgM antibodies to CMV is also diagnostic. Culture of CMV from blood may be less sensitive. Tissue invasion of CMV is common in the gastrointestinal tract and lungs. CMV retinopathy occurs late in the course, if untreated. Treatment of active CMV disease with valganciclovir is always indicated. Many patients immune to CMV can activate the virus after heavy immunosuppression, such as with OKT3. Concurrent treatment with ganciclovir during OKT3 administration appears to be effective for prophylaxis of CMV activation. The complications of glucocorticoid therapy are well known and include gastrointestinal bleeding, impairment of wound healing, osteoporosis, diabetes mellitus, cataract formation, and hemorrhagic pancreatitis. The treatment of unexplained jaundice in transplant patients should include cessation or reduction of immunosuppressive drugs if hepatitis or drug toxicity is suspected. It is surprising that cessation of azathioprine or calcineurin inhibitor therapy in such circumstances often does not result in rejection of a graft, at least for several weeks. Acyclovir is effective in therapy of herpes simplex virus infections.

Chronic Lesions of the Transplanted Kidney While 1-year transplant survival is excellent, most recipients experience progressive decline in kidney function over time thereafter. The chronic renal transplant dysfunction can be caused by recurrent disease, hypertension, cyclosporine or tacrolimus nephrotoxicity, chronic immunologic rejection, secondary focal glomerulosclerosis, or a combination of these pathophysiologies. Chronic vascular changes with intimal proliferation and medical hypertrophy are commonly found. Control of systemic and intrarenal hypertension with ACE inhibitors is thought to have a beneficial influence on the rate of progression of chronic renal transplant dysfunction. Renal biopsy can distinguish subacute cellular rejection from recurrent disease or secondary focal sclerosis.

Malignancy The incidence of tumors in patients on immunosuppressive therapy is 5 to 6%, or approximately 100 times greater than that in the general population of the same age range. The most common lesions are cancer of the skin and lips and carcinoma in situ of the cervix, as well as lymphomas, such as non-Hodgkin's lymphomas. The risks are increased in proportion to the total immunosuppressive load administered and time elapsed since transplantation. Surveillance for skin and cervical cancers is necessary.

Other Complications *Hypercalcemia* after transplantation may indicate failure of hyperplastic parathyroid glands to regress. Aseptic necrosis of the head of the femur is probably due to preexisting hyperparathyroidism, with aggravation by glucocorticoid treatment. With improved management of calcium and phosphorus metabolism during chronic dialysis, the incidence of parathyroid-related complications has fallen dramatically. Persistent hyperparathyroid activity may require subtotal parathyroidectomy.

Hypertension may be caused by (1) native kidneys; (2) rejection activity in the transplant; (3) renal artery stenosis, if an end-to-end anastomosis was constructed with an iliac artery branch; and (4) renal calcineurin inhibitor toxicity. The latter may improve with reduction in dose. Whereas ACE inhibitors may be useful, calcium channel blockers are more frequently used initially. Amelioration of hypertension to the 120 to 130/70 to 80 mmHg range should be the goal in all patients.

While most transplant patients have a robust production of erythropoietin and normalization of the hemoglobin without exogenous erythropoietin administration, *anemia* is commonly seen in the posttransplant period. Often the anemia is attributable to bone marrow–suppressant immunosuppressive medications such as azathioprine, mycophenolate mofetil, or sirolimus. Gastrointestinal bleeding is a common side effect of high-dose and long-term steroid administration. Many transplant patients have creatinine clearances of 30 to 50 mL/min and can be considered in the same way as other patients with chronic renal insufficiency for anemia management, including supplemental erythropoietin.

Chronic hepatitis, particularly when due to hepatitis B virus, can be a progressive, fatal disease over a decade or so. Patients who are persistently hepatitis B surface antigen–positive are at higher risk, according to some studies, but the presence of hepatitis C virus is also a concern when one embarks on a course of immunosuppression in a transplant recipient.

Both chronic dialysis and renal transplant patients have a higher incidence of death from myocardial infarction and stroke than in the population at large, and this is particularly true in diabetic patients. Contributing factors are the use of glucocorticoids, hypertension, and hypertriglyceridemia. Increased low-density lipoprotein cholesterol and depressed high-density lipoprotein cholesterol concentrations may be exaggerated after transplantation and require treatment, particularly in patients receiving sirolimus. Recipients of renal transplants have a high prevalence of coronary artery and peripheral vascular diseases. The percentage of deaths from these causes has been slowly rising as the numbers of transplanted diabetic patients and the average age of all recipients increase. More than 50% of renal recipient mortality is attributable to cardiovascular disease. In addition to strict control of blood pressure and blood lipid levels, close monitoring of patients for indications of further medical or surgical intervention is an important part of management.

FURTHER READING

CHANDRAKER A et al: Transplantation immunobiology, in *Brenner and Rector's The Kidney*, 7th ed, B Brenner (ed). Philadelphia, Saunders, 2004, pp 2759–84

LIMAYE AP et al: Quantitation of BK virus load in serum for the diagnosis of BK virus–associated nephropathy in renal transplant recipients. J Infect Dis 183:1669, 2001

MACDONALD AS: A worldwide, phase III, randomized, controlled, safety and efficacy study of a sirolimus/cyclosporine regimen for prevention of acute rejection in recipients of primary mismatched renal allografts. Transplantation 71:271, 2001

MAHONEY RJ et al: B-Cell crossmatching and kidney allograft outcome in 9031 United States transplant recipients. Hum Immunol 63:324, 2002

PESCOVITZ MD, GOVANI M: Sirolimus and mycophenolate mofetil for calcineurin-free immunosuppression in renal transplant recipients. Am J Kidney Dis 38:S16, 2001

SAYEGH MH, TURKA LA: The role of T-cell costimulatory activation pathways in transplant rejection. N Engl J Med 338:1813, 1998

VELIDEDEOGLU E et al: Comparison of open, laparoscopic, and hand-assisted approaches to live-donor nephrectomy. Transplantation 74:169, 2002

264 GLOMERULAR DISEASES
Hugh R. Brady, Yvonne M. O'Meara,
Barry M. Brenner

PATHOGENESIS

The glomerulus is a modified capillary network that delivers an ultrafiltrate of plasma to Bowman's space, the most proximal portion of the renal tubule. Approximately 1.6 million glomeruli are present in two mature kidneys (range 0.5 to 2.4 million) and collectively they produce 120 to 180 L of ultrafiltrate daily. Glomerular filtration rate (GFR) is dependent on glomerular blood flow, ultrafiltration pressure, and the area and composition of the filtration barrier. These parameters are tightly regulated through changes in afferent and efferent arteriolar tone (for blood flow and ultrafiltration pressure) and mesangial cell contractility (for filtration surface area). Arteriolar tone and mesangial cell contractility are, in turn, modulated by neurohumoral factors, local myenteric reflexes, and endothelium-derived vasoactive substances, such as nitric oxide, prostanoids, and endothelins. In health, glomerular endothelium is also antithrombotic and antiadhesive for leukocytes and platelets, thereby preventing inappropriate vascular thrombosis and inflammation during the filtration process. Filtration of most plasma proteins and all blood cells is normally prevented as a consequence of the physiochemical and electrostatic charge characteristics of the glomerular filtration barrier, the latter being composed of fenestrated glomerular endothelium, basement membrane, and the foot processes and slit diaphragms of visceral epithelial cells (podocytes). Parietal epithelium facilitates glomerular filtration by maintaining the integrity of Bowman's space. In keeping with the physiologic functions of the glomerulus outlined above, virtually all glomerular injury results in impairment of glomerular filtration and/or the inappropriate appearance of plasma proteins and blood cells in the urine.

CLINICOPATHOLOGIC CORRELATES IN GLOMERULAR DISEASE The major morphologic patterns of glomerular disease and their clinical features are summarized in Table 264-1. These clinicopathologic entities can be induced by a variety of mechanisms. Prompt diagnosis, optimal management, and accurate prognostication is a multistep process that requires (1) recognition of the presenting clinical syndrome, (2) delineation of the underlying morphologic pattern of glomerular injury, and (3) elucidation of the specific renal-limited or systemic disease that triggered glomerular dysfunction.

Nomenclature The terms *glomerulonephritis* and *glomerulopathy* are usually used interchangeably to denote glomerular injury, although some authorities reserve the former term for injury with evidence of inflammation such as leukocyte infiltration, antibody deposition, and complement activation. Glomerular diseases are classified as *primary* when the pathology is confined to the kidney and any systemic features are a direct consequence of glomerular dysfunction (e.g., pulmonary edema, hypertension, the uremic syndrome). Usually, but not always, the term primary is synonymous with *idiopathic*. Glomerular diseases are classified as *secondary* when part of a multisystem disorder. In general, *acute* refers to glomerular injury occurring over days or weeks, *subacute* or *rapidly progressive* over weeks or a few months, and *chronic* over many months or years. Lesions are classified as *focal* or *diffuse* when they involve the minority (<50%) or majority (≥50%) of glomeruli, respectively. Lesions are termed *segmental* or *global* when they involve part of or almost all of the glomerular tuft, respectively. *Proliferative* is used to describe an increase in glomerular cell number, which can be either true proliferation of resident glomerular cells or glomerular hypercellularity caused by infiltration by leukocytes.

Proliferation of resident glomerular cells is classified as *intracapillary* or *endocapillary* when referring to endothelial or mesangial cells and *extracapillary* when referring to cells in Bowman's space. A *crescent* is a half-moon-shaped collection of cells in Bowman's space, usually composed of proliferating parietal epithelial cells and infiltrating macrophages. Because crescentic glomerulonephritis is often associated with renal failure that progresses rapidly over weeks to months, the clinical term *rapidly progressive glomerulonephritis* and pathologic term *crescentic glomerulonephritis* are often used interchangeably. The description *membranous* is applied to glomerulonephritis dominated by expansion of the glomerular basement membrane (GBM) by immune deposits. *Sclerosis* refers to an increase in the amount of homogeneous nonfibrillar extracellular material of similar composition to GBM and mesangial matrix. This process is distinct from *fibrosis*, which involves deposition of collagens type I and III and is more commonly a consequence of healing of crescents or tubulointerstitial inflammation.

Major Clinicopathologic Entities In the absence of comprehensive knowledge of disease etiology, most glomerulopathies are still classified and named according to their morphologic features (Table 264-1). The major inflammatory glomerulopathies are *focal proliferative glomerulonephritis* (termed *mesangial proliferative glomerulonephritis* if the proliferating cells are predominantly mesangial cells), *diffuse proliferative glomerulonephritis*, and *crescentic glomerulonephritis*. These diseases typically present with a *nephritic-type* "active" urine sediment characterized by the presence of red blood cells, red blood cell casts, leukocytes, and *subnephrotic* proteinuria of <3 g/24 h. The severity of renal insufficiency varies in proportion to the degree of glomerular inflammation.

The major morphologic patterns affecting the glomerular filtration barrier for proteins, namely the GBM and visceral epithelial cells, are *membranous glomerulopathy*, *minimal change disease* (MCD), and *focal and segmental glomerulosclerosis* (FSGS). These entities typically present with *nephrotic-range* proteinuria of ≥3 g/24 h and the presence of relatively few red blood cells, leukocytes, or cellular casts. As a consequence of the heavy proteinuria, nephrotic syndrome is associated with hypoalbuminemia, edema, hyperlipidemia, and lipiduria, and a prothrombotic state. *Membranoproliferative glomerulonephritis*, as the name suggests, is a hybrid lesion that presents with a combination of nephritic and nephrotic features.

The *glomerular deposition diseases* are a group of disorders characterized by prominent extravascular deposition of a paraprotein or fibrillar material. These diseases can trigger either nephritic-type or nephrotic-type responses (or a combination of both) and thus show marked clinical and morphologic overlap with the entities described above.

TABLE 264-1 *Major Clinicopathologic Presentation of Glomerular Disease*

Structural Pattern	Typical Clinical Presentation	Typical Pathology Findings	Most Common Etiologies
Diffuse proliferative GN	Acute nephritic syndrome: Acute renal failure over days to weeks, hypertension, edema, oliguria, active urine sediment, subnephrotic proteinuria	Diffuse increase in cellularity of tufts of most glomeruli due to infiltration by neutrophils and monocytes, and proliferation of glomerular endothelial and mesangial cells	Immune complex GN: idiopathic, postinfectious, SLE, SBE, cryoglobulinemia, HSP Pauci-immune GN and anti-GBM disease (crescentic GN common—see below)
Crescentic GN	Rapidly progressive glomerulonephritis (RPGN): Subacute renal failure over weeks to months, active urine sediment, variable amount of hypertension, edema, oliguria, and proteinuria	Majority of glomeruli contain areas of fibrinoid necrosis and crescents in Bowman's space, composed of proliferating parietal epithelial cells, infiltrating macrophages, and fibrin	Immune complex GN (as above) Pauci-immune GN: Wegener's granulomatosis, microscopic polyarteritis nodosa, renal-limited crescentic GN Anti-GBM disease (Goodpasture's syndrome if lung hemorrhage)
Focal proliferative GN	Mild to moderate glomerular inflammation: Active urine sediment and mild to moderate decline in GFR	Segmental areas of proliferation and necrosis in less than 50% of glomeruli, occasionally with crescent formation	Early and milder forms, or recovery phase of most diseases causing diffuse proliferative and crescentic GN IgA nephropathy/HSP
Mesangial proliferative GN	Chronic glomerular inflammation: Proteinuria, hematuria, hypertension, variable effect on GFR	Proliferation of mesangial cells and matrix	IgA nephropathy/HSP Early and milder forms, or recovery phases of most diseases that cause diffuse proliferative and crescentic GN (see above) In association with minimal change glomerulopathy and FSGS
Membranoproliferative GN	Variable combination of nephritic and nephrotic features: Acute or subacute decline in GFR, active urine sediment, proteinuria often in nephrotic range	Diffuse proliferation of mesangial cells and infiltration of glomeruli by macrophages; increased mesangial matrix and thickening and reduplication of glomerular basement membrane	Immune complex GN (as for diffuse proliferative GN) In association with thrombotic microangiopathies (see below) In association with deposition diseases (see below) Postrenal or -marrow transplantation
Minimal change GN	Nephrotic syndrome: Proteinuria of >3–3.5 g/d, hypoalbuminemia, edema, hyperlipidemia, lipiduria, thrombotic diathesis, slow decline in GFR in 10–30%.	Light microscopy normal, but electron microscopy (EM) shows foot process effacement	Idiopathic In association with drug-induced interstitial nephritis, HIV infection, heroin, Hodgkin's and other lymphomas
Focal segmental glomerulosclerosis	Nephrotic syndrome: Proteinuria of >3–3.5 g/d, hypoalbuminemia, edema, hyperlipidemia, lipiduria, thrombotic diathesis, slow decline in GFR in 10–30%.	Segmental capillary collapse affecting <50% of glomeruli with entrapment of amorphous hyaline material. EM shows foot process effacement	Primary FSGS: idiopathic, HIV, heroin, lysosomal diseases, Charcot-Marie-Tooth Secondary response to reduction in nephron number from any cause (hyperfiltration injury)
Nodular or global sclerosis	Proteinuria and chronic renal failure	Sclerosis of most glomeruli with interstitial fibrosis	Diabetic nephropathy Potential long-term consequence of most glomerulopathies listed above
Membranous GN	Nephrotic syndrome: Proteinuria of >3–3.5 g/d, hypoalbuminemia, edema, hyperlipidemia, lipiduria, thrombotic diathesis, slow decline in GFR in 10–30%	Diffuse thickening of the glomerular basement membrane with subepithelial projections ("spikes") around immune deposits	Idiopathic Infections (e.g., hepatitis B & C, syphilis, schistasomiasis, malaria, leprosy) Drugs (e.g., gold, penicillamine, captopril) Autoimmune diseases (SLE, rheumatoid arthritis) Paraneoplastic
Deposition diseases	Combination of nephritic and nephrotic features: Renal failure over months to years, proteinuria, hematuria, and hypertension.	Mesangial expansion and thickening of glomerular capillary wall; variable cellular proliferation and crescent formation	Amyloid Cryoglobulinemia Light chain deposition disease Fibrillary/immunotactoid GN
Thrombotic microangiopathy	Acute or subacute renal failure: Variable degree of hypertension, edema and proteinuria, urine sediment usually contains red blood cells, but less activity than patients with nephritic syndrome or RPGN	Microthrombi in glomerular capillaries ± endothelial injury	Idiopathic In association with gastrointestinal infections, or drugs such as anovulants, mitomycin C, cyclosporine Other diseases: SLE, scleroderma, toxemia, malignant hypertension
Nonimmune basement membrane abnormalities	Asymptomatic hematuria and variable renal failure	Alport's syndrome—mesangial hypercellularity with focal sclerosis and interstitial fibrosis; splintering of GBM on EM.	Alport's syndrome, Thin basement membrane disease. Nail-patella syndrome, Lecithin–cholesterol acyltransferase deficiency

Note: Diffuse, affecting ≥50% of glomeruli; focal, affecting <50% of glomeruli; global, affecting ≥50% of glomerular tuft; segmental, affecting <50% of glomerular tuft; GN, glomerulonephritis; FSGS, focal segmental glomerulosclerosis; HSP, Henoch-Schönlein purpura; SLE, systemic lupus erythematosus; SBE, subacute bacterial endocarditis; GBM, glomerular basement membrane; GFR, glomerular filtration rate.

TABLE 264-2 *Primary Mechanisms of Glomerular Injury*

Mechanism of Injury	Some Renal Insults/Defects	Glomerular Disease
Immunologic[a]	Immunoglobulin[b]	Immune complex–mediated glomerulonephritis
	Cell-mediated injury[b]	Pauci-immune glomerulonephritis
	Cytokine (or other soluble factor)	Primary focal segmental glomerulosclerosis
	Persistent complement activation	Membranoproliferative glomerulonephritis (type II)
Metabolic[a]	Hyperglycemia[b]	Diabetic nephropathy
	Fabry's disease and sialidosis	Focal segmental glomerulosclerosis
Hemodynamic[a]	Systemic hypertension[b]	Hypertensive nephrosclerosis
	Intraglomerular hypertension[b]	Secondary focal segmental glomerulosclerosis
Toxic	E. coli–derived verotoxin	Thrombotic microangiopathy
	Therapeutic drugs (e.g., NSAIDs)	Minimal change disease
	Recreational drugs (heroin)	Focal segmental glomerulosclerosis
Deposition	Amyloid fibrils	Amyloid nephropathy
Infectious	HIV	HIV nephropathy
	Subacute bacterial endocarditis	Immune complex glomerulonephritis
Inherited	Defect in gene for α5 chain of type IV collagen	Alport's syndrome
	Abnormally thin basement membrane	Thin basement membrane disease

[a] Most common categories.
[b] Most common insults within these categories.

Note: NSAIDs, nonsteroidal anti-inflammatory drugs.

The *thrombotic microangiopathies* are a family of diseases in which the pathologic presentation is dominated by coagulation disturbances or endothelial cell injury that result in the formation of thrombi within the renal microvasculature, often leading to renal insufficiency. →*For further discussion of this category of glomerular diseases see Chap. 267.*

MAJOR DETERMINANTS OF GLOMERULAR INJURY The important determinants of the extent and severity of glomerular injury, and accordingly of the clinical presentation, include (1) the nature of the primary insult and the secondary mediator systems that it invokes; (2) the site of injury within the glomerulus; and (3) the speed of onset, the extent, and intensity of disease.

Primary Insult Glomeruli are susceptible to a variety of inflammatory, metabolic, hemodynamic, toxic, and infectious insults (Table 264-2). Most human glomerular disease is triggered by either immune attack (e.g., most forms of inflammatory glomerulonephritis), metabolic stress (e.g., diabetic nephropathy), or mechanical stress (e.g., hypertension). Diverse insults can induce similar clinicopathologic presentations, suggesting marked overlap among downstream molecular and cellular responses. For example, immune complex deposition triggered by streptococcal pharyngitis and antibody-independent glomerular injury in microscopic polyarteritis can each induce proliferative glomerulonephritis. Similarly, metabolic (e.g., diabetes mellitus) and deposition diseases (e.g., amyloid) can each induce glomerulosclerosis with nephrotic syndrome.

Site of Injury The consequences of injury at different sites within the glomerulus can be predicted from the physiologic functions of the cells within the local milieu. In health the renal endothelium is antiadhesive for leukocytes and antithrombotic and maintains the diameter of the vascular lumen through release of nitric oxide and prostacyclin. The major sequelae of injury to the endothelium and subendothelial aspect of the GBM are (1) recruitment of leukocytes leading to inflammatory glomerulonephritis, or (2) perturbed hemostasis leading to thrombotic microangiopathy. It is usual for one of these phenotypes to dominate; however, hybrid lesions may occur (e.g., in lupus nephritis; see below). Intrarenal vasoconstriction and mesangial cell contraction can complicate each phenotype and thereby contribute to renal failure. Injury localized to the mesangial area typically presents as asymptomatic abnormalities of the urinary sediment and mild renal insufficiency. Proteinuria dominates the clinical presentation of injury to the subepithelial aspect of the GBM and visceral epithelial cells. As with mesangial injury, GFR is often only mildly compromised in this setting unless there is concomitant tubulointerstitial injury. The classic pathologic manifestation of parietal epithelial cell injury is crescent formation, which typically presents with acute or subacute renal failure. Crescents can be the dominant morphologic presentation of glomerular disease or complicate proliferative or membranous lesions.

Speed of Onset, Intensity, and Extent of Injury To illustrate the importance of the speed of onset, extent, and intensity of glomerular injury, it is instructive to compare two forms of immune complex glomerulonephritis, i.e., acute postinfectious glomerulonephritis and IgA nephropathy. Poststreptococcal glomerulonephritis is characterized by rapid deposition of immune complexes throughout the glomerular capillary wall, which often provokes acute diffuse proliferative glomerulonephritis with the classic hallmarks of acute inflammation (i.e., complement activation, leukocyte recruitment, lysosomal enzyme release, free radical generation, and perturbation of vascular tone and permeability) with resultant acute renal failure. In contrast, IgA nephropathy is characterized by slow, but sustained, formation of IgA-containing immune complexes, largely confined to the mesangium; less dramatic activation of complement and other mediator systems; and either stability of GFR or progressive renal insufficiency over decades.

MAJOR MECHANISMS OF GLOMERULAR INJURY

Hereditary defects accounts for a minority of glomerular disease. Most acquired glomerular disease is triggered by immune-mediated injury, metabolic stress, or mechanical stress.

INHERITED GLOMERULAR DISEASES *Alport's syndrome* (hereditary nephritis; p. 1691 and Chap. 342), the prototypical inherited glomerular disease, is usually transmitted as an X-linked dominant trait, although autosomal dominant and recessive forms have been reported. Patients afflicted with the classic X-linked form have a mutation in the COL4A5 gene that encodes the α5 chain of type IV collagen located on the X chromosome. As a result, the GBM is irregular with longitudinal layering, splitting, or thickening, and patients develop hematuria, progressive glomerulosclerosis, and renal failure. Other inherited glomerular diseases include *thin basement membrane disease* (p. 1690), *nail-patella syndrome* (osteoonychodysplasia), *partial lipodystrophy*, and *familial lecithin–cholesterol acyltransferase deficiency*. These will be discussed later in this chapter.

IMMUNOLOGIC GLOMERULAR INJURY Immune-mediated glomerulonephritis accounts for a large fraction of acquired renal disease (Fig. 264-1). The majority of cases are associated with the deposition of antibodies, often autoantibodies, within the glomerular tuft, indicating dysregulation of humoral immunity. Cellular immune mechanisms contribute to the pathogenesis of antibody-mediated glomerulonephritis by modulating antibody production and through antibody-dependent cell cytotoxicity (see below). Cellular immune mechanisms also play a dominant role in the pathophysiology of "pauci-immune" glomerulonephritis, notable for robust glomerular inflammation without immunoglobulin deposition.

Humoral Antibody-Mediated Injury Most antibody-mediated glomerulonephritis in humans is initiated by reactivity of circulating antibodies with glomerular antigens. The major mechanisms of antibody deposition within the glomerulus are (1) reactivity of circulating autoantibodies with intrinsic autoantigens that are components of normal glomerular parenchyma, as occurs in anti-GBM disease (Goodpasture's syndrome); (2) in situ formation of immune complexes within glomeruli through interaction of circulating antibodies with extrinsic antigens that have been trapped, or "planted," within the glomerulus, as occurs in postinfectious glomerulonephritis; and (3) intraglomerular trapping of immune complexes that have formed in the systemic circulation, as occurs in cryoglobulinemia-associated glomerulonephritis. Circulating autoantibodies against neutrophil cytoplasmic antigens (antineutrophil cytoplasmic antibodies, ANCA) and endothelial antigens (antiendothelial cell antibodies, AECA) may represent additional mechanisms of antibody-mediated glomerular injury in patients without discernible immune complexes in the glomerular parenchyma.

GENERATION OF NEPHRITOGENIC ANTIBODIES Exposure of the host to a foreign antigen (e.g., a prodromal infection) has been implicated as the trigger for the generation of nephritogenic autoantibodies in several forms of glomerulonephritis. Foreign antigens can provoke autoantibody formation through several mechanisms. First, a foreign antigen, whose structure resembles that of a host glomerular antigen, may stimulate the production of autoantibodies that cross-react with the intrinsic glomerular antigen (*molecular mimickry*). Second, the foreign antigen may trigger aberrant expression of major histocompatibility complex (MHC) class II molecules on glomerular cells, which present previously "invisible" autoantigens to T lymphocytes and thereby generate an autoimmune response. Third, the foreign antigen can trigger polyclonal activation of B lymphocytes, some of which generate nephritogenic antibodies. Alternatively, individuals may suffer a breakdown of immune tolerance through other mechanisms (e.g., genetically programmed).

Autoreactive B cells are usually deleted in the thymus during development (*clonal deletion*) or rendered anergic in peripheral lymphoid tissue (*clonal anergy*). Similar tolerogenic mechanisms exist for deleting or anergizing autoreactive T helper cells that modulate immunoglobulin production by autoreactive B cells. Perturbation of these tolerogenic mechanisms could drive immunoglobulin production in some forms of autoimmune glomerulonephritis. Indeed, defective clonal deletion of autoreactive T cells has been demonstrated in experimental lupus nephritis due to defective synthesis of Fas, a cell-surface receptor that modulates T cell deletion through *apoptosis* (programmed cell death) within the thymus.

DEPOSITION OF NEPHRITOGENIC ANTIBODIES WITHIN THE GLOMERULUS (Fig. 264-1) The site of antibody deposition within the glomerulus is a critical determinant of the clinicopathologic presentation and is determined by the avidity, affinity, and quantity of the antibody; the size, charge, and site of the antigen; the size of the immune complexes; the efficiency of the clearance mechanisms for immune complexes; and local hemodynamic factors. Relatively anionic antigens are repelled by the GBM, which is negatively charged, and tend to be trapped in the subendothelial cell space and mesangium. In contrast, relatively cationic antigens tend to permeate the GBM and deposit within the GBM or in the subepithelial space.

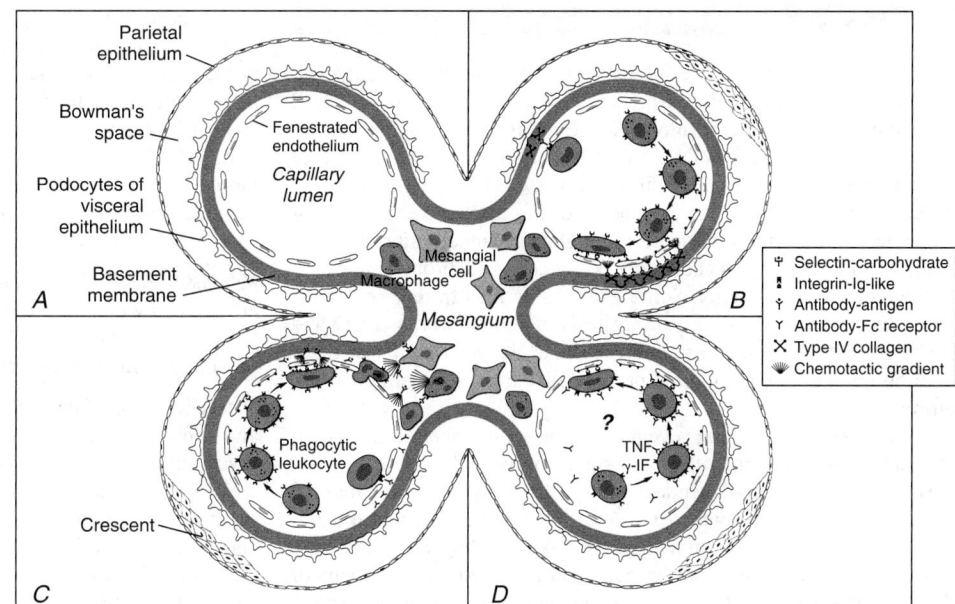

FIGURE 264-1 Major mechanisms of antibody-mediated injury in glomerulonephritis. *A.* Normal glomerulus. Key components of "healthy" glomerular capillary loop. *B.* Antiglomerular basement membrane antibody-mediated glomerulonephritis. Linear deposition of IgG against the Goodpasture antigen. The latter autoantigen is a normal constituent of the non-collagenous domain of $\alpha 3$ chain of type IV collagen, whose "chicken wire"–like structure is essential for maintenance of normal glomerular basement membrane architecture and function. *C.* Immune complex–mediated glomerulonephritis. Immune complexes scattered throughout the glomerular capillary wall, e.g., as can occur in lupus nephritis or postinfectious glomerulonephritis. In mechanisms *B* and *C*, leukocyte chemotaxis is triggered by complement components, chemokines, and other inflammatory mediators. Leukocyte–endothelial cell adhesion is supported by four major classes of adhesion molecules: the selectins and their diverse carbohydrate-bearing ligands, the leukocyte integrins, and immunoglobulin-like molecules such as intercellular adhesion molecule-1. Leukocytes also adhere through binding of their Fc receptors to the Fc domains of immunoglobulin. *D.* Antineutrophil cytoplasmic antibody (ANCA)-associated glomerulonephritis. In diseases such as Wegener's granulomatosis, ANCA are postulated to induce glomerular injury by interacting with neutrophil granule components that have migrated to the cell surface following priming of neutrophils by cytokines, as may occur during a prodromal viral illness. Reactivity of ANCA with neutrophil granule components in vitro triggers neutrophil activation and endothelial cell injury. This mechanism of glomerular injury remains to be established definitively in vivo, however, hence the symbol "?" in the cartoon. Crescents are formed by proliferation of parietal epithelial cells and migration of monocyte-macrophages into the glomerulus from the glomerular capillary lumen and tubulointerstitial space. As they expand, crescents compress the glomerular capillary tuft and are a rich source of mediators that further amplify the inflammatory response. TNF, tumor necrosis factor; γ-IF, interferon γ.

Acute deposition of antibody in the subendothelial cell space (e.g., poststreptococcal glomerulonephritis) or mesangium (e.g., Henoch-Schönlein purpura) typically triggers a nephritic-type response characterized by rapid recruitment of leukocytes and platelets, probably because inflammatory mediators generated at these sites are strategically positioned to activate endothelial and hematogenous cells. Leukocyte-derived products, such as reactive oxygen species, lysosomal enzymes and cytokines, complement components, and other toxic moieties generated in the local inflammatory milieu are both injurious to the glomerular vascular wall and filtration barrier and attract subsequent waves of leukocytes from the circulation. Antibody deposition in the subepithelial cell space (e.g., membranous nephropathy) typically induces a nephrotic-type response characterized by proteinuria without a pronounced inflammatory cell infiltrate, probably because the immune complexes are shielded from circulating inflammatory cells by the GBM and because the large fluid flux from blood to Bowman's space minimizes back-diffusion of inflammatory mediators towards the endothelium and vascular lumen. In this setting, complement components such as the membrane attack complex (C5b-9) appear to be the major effectors of glomerular injury.

Cellular Antibody-Independent Glomerular Injury Although cell-mediated injury is, as yet, less well defined than antibody-mediated glomerular injury, T cells have also been implicated as independent mediators of glomerular injury and as modulators of the production of nephritogenic antibodies. T cells may be particularly important as initiators of injury in pauci-immune glomerulonephritis. T cells interact, through their cell-surface T cell receptor/CD3 complex, with antigens presented in the groove of MHC molecules of resident glomerular endothelial, mesangial, and epithelial cells, a process that is facilitated by cell-cell adhesion and costimulatory molecules. Cytokines and other mediators released by activated T cells are potent stimuli for further leukocyte recruitment, cytotoxicity, and fibrogenesis. CD4 T lymphocytes are important recruiters of macrophages and trigger clonal expansion of autoreactive B cells; they also promote glomerular cell injury by CD8 cytotoxic T lymphocytes and natural killer cells and through antibody-dependent cell cytotoxicity. Soluble factors derived from T cells have also been implicated in the pathogenesis of proteinuria in MCD and primary FSGS. The identity and molecular characterization of these nonimmunoglobulin circulating permeability factors remain to be determined.

Whereas the initiating events in antibody-independent pauci-immune forms of glomerular injury are poorly understood by comparison with antibody-dependent injury, there appears to be marked overlap between the downstream mediator systems that perturb glomerular morphology and function. Thus key pathogenic roles have already been defined in pauci-immune glomerular disease for many of the mediator systems discussed above including leukocyte-derived toxic moieties, such as reactive oxygen species, proteases, cytokines, chemokines, and other inflammatory mediators derived from recruited and resident renal cells.

Cell Proliferation and Accumulation of Extracellular Matrix A hallmark of the nephritic-type proliferative glomerulopathies is an increase in glomerular cell number. Initially, this hypercellularity is due predominantly to infiltration of the glomerular tuft by leukocytes. Subsequently, resident glomerular cells proliferate in response to growth factors [e.g., epidermal growth factor (EGF), platelet-derived growth factor (PDGF)] released into the local inflammatory milieu. The proliferating cells are typically mesangial in mesangioproliferative glomerulonephritis and both endothelial and mesangial cells in diffuse proliferative glomerulonephritis. The visceral epithelial cell is, for the most part, a terminally differentiated cell that does not proliferate rapidly, even when injured.

Whereas acute antibody-mediated glomerulonephritis typically induces acute diffuse proliferative glomerulonephritis and acute renal failure over days to weeks (nephritic syndrome), subacute immune injury often induces the formation of glomerular crescents and renal failure over weeks to months (termed *rapidly progressive glomerulonephritis* (RPGN). As discussed above, crescents are extracapillary proliferations of cells in Bowman's space, composed of infiltrating monocytes, proliferating parietal epithelial cells, and fibrin.

Sustained low-level immune complex deposition over months to years can provoke a marked increase in basement membrane or mesangial matrix production. Mild to moderate accumulation of matrix usually manifests as proteinuria due to disruption of the glomerular filtration barrier; however, in its most severe form, matrix accumulation causes glomerulosclerosis and chronic renal insufficiency.

Determinants of Resolution, Repair, and Scarring Glomerular inflammation can resolve with complete recovery of renal function or with a variable amount of scarring and chronic renal insufficiency. Acute poststreptococcal glomerulonephritis, for example, usually resolves spontaneously and fully in children, whereas adults may be left with residual renal impairment. The resolution process requires cessation of further antibody production and immune complex formation, removal of deposited and circulating immune complexes, inhibition of further recruitment of inflammatory cells, dissipation of the gradients of inflammatory mediators, restoration of normal endothelial adhesiveness and permeability, normalization of vascular tone, and clearance of infiltrating inflammatory cells and proliferating resident glomerular cells. Putative pro-resolution signals in spontaneously resolving glomerular inflammation include the lipoxygenase-derived eicosanoids, the lipoxins, and cytokines such as interleukin (IL)-4, -10, and -13.

Unfortunately, the resolution phase of most inflammatory glomerulopathies in adults terminates in some glomerular scarring. This is particularly true in patients with crescentic glomerulopathies who may be left with end-stage renal failure requiring dialysis or transplantation. Transforming growth factor (TGF) β and connective tissue growth factor (CTGF) stimulate production of extracellular matrix by most glomerular cells, inhibits synthesis of tissue proteases that normally degrade matrix proteins, and appear to be important stimuli for scar formation immediately following glomerular injury.

NONIMMUNOLOGIC GLOMERULAR INJURY While many glomerular diseases are driven by immunologic events, a variety of nonimmunologic metabolic, hemodynamic, and toxic stresses can each induce glomerular pathology, either alone or in concert with immunologic processes.

Metabolic Injury Glomerulopathy complicates a variety of inherited and acquired diseases of carbohydrate and lipid metabolism. Hyperglycemia is a central event in the injury process. The mechanisms by which hyperglycemia perturbs renal function in diabetes are still being appreciated and include (1) the interactions of advanced glycosylation end-products (AGEs) with renal cells; (2) direct effects of high glucose on renal cells mediated through the generation of reactive oxygen species, cell sorbitol accumulation, activation of protein kinase C, and mitogen-activated protein kinases; and (3) high glucose–triggered glomerular hypertension. Important functional consequences of these high glucose–triggered events include mesangial cell hypertrophy, increased mesangial cell matrix production, reduced matrix catabolism, and glomerulosclerosis.

Several rare inherited lysosomal enzyme defects induce focal segmental glomerulosclerosis, probably by allowing accumulation of toxic metabolites in renal cells. *Fabry's disease* (α-galactosidase deficiency) and *sialidosis* (*N*-acetylneuraminic acid hydrolase deficiency) are the major culprits in this regard.

Hemodynamic Glomerular Injury High intraglomerular pressure is a major cause of glomerular injury and can result from systemic hypertension or from local change in glomerular hemodynamics leading to glomerular hypertension.

Systemic Hypertension (See also Chap. 230) Although the kidneys have evolved sophisticated mechanisms for autoregulating glomerular blood flow and pressure, marked or sustained increments in systemic blood pressure can overwhelm these compensatory systems and perturb glomerular morphology and function. In its most dramatic form, namely malignant hypertension, hemodynamic stress causes massive fibrinoid necrosis of afferent arterioles and glomeruli, thrombotic microangiopathy, a nephritic urinary sediment, and acute renal failure. Chronic sustained hypertension typically leads to arteriolar vasoconstriction and sclerosis, which, in turn, cause secondary atrophy and sclerosis of glomeruli and the tubulointerstitium. A variety of molecular signals appear to couple elevations in intravascular pressure to myointimal proliferation and eventually sclerosis of the vessel wall. These include growth factors such as angiotensin II, EGF, PDGF, and CTGF; cytokines such as TGF-β; and activation of stretch-activated ion channels and early response genes.

Glomerular Hypertension As discussed below, glomerular hypertension is also a key factor in the pathogenesis of the progressive glomerulosclerosis and renal failure. Glomerular hypertension is an adaptive response to increased workload in the remaining functioning nephrons following loss of other nephrons from any cause, including chronic allograft failure. While appropriate in the short term, sustained glomerular hypertension is a stimulus for increased mesangial matrix production and glomerulosclerosis. Importantly, glomerular hypertension appears to precede the development of systemic hypertension in many forms of glomerular disease where it is an independent risk factor for glomerular injury.

Miscellaneous Mechanisms of Nonimmunologic Glomerular Injury In addition to the major immune, metabolic, and mechanical mechanisms of glomeruli injury described above, glomerulopathy can be precipitated by a variety of infectious and toxic agents; the latter include both exogenous (e.g., drugs) and endogenous (e.g., fibril deposition) toxins.

FINAL COMMON PATHWAYS OF INJURY IN GLOMERULAR DISEASE Two pathologic features dominate most cases of chronic progressive glomerular disease, i.e., focal segmental glomerulosclerosis and tubulointerstitial fibrosis. By elucidating the molecular events that contribute to these final common pathways of injury, it should be possible to design new renoprotective therapies. Indeed, the identification of glomerular hypertension as a major stimulus for secondary focal segmental glomerulosclerosis has already led to the use of angiotensin-converting enzyme (ACE) inhibitors and angiotensin II receptor blockers (ARBs) as specific renoprotective agents in clinical practice.

Secondary Focal Segmental Glomerulosclerosis Nephron loss, from any cause, is followed by compensatory vasodilation of afferent arterioles, increased glomerular pressure (*glomerular hypertension*), and increased filtration (*glomerular hyperfiltration*) in the remaining functional glomeruli. This adaptive response is appropriate in the short term and maintains GFR. Over years, however, sustained glomerular hypertension and hyperfiltration induce focal and segmental glomerulosclerosis and eventually global sclerosis, which manifests clinically as proteinuria, hypertension, and progressive renal insufficiency. Glomerular hypertension, in particular, has been implicated as a major stimulus for glomerulosclerosis in this setting. Increased glomerular blood flow and ultrafiltration pressure are early findings in remnant nephrons in most experimental models in which the function of >50% of nephron mass has been lost through surgical ablation, immunologic or toxic injury, or other mechanisms.

Sustained glomerular hypertension is thought to stimulate the accumulation of extracellular matrix by perturbing the function of visceral epithelial and mesangial cells, either directly or by increasing the flux of circulating macromolecules through the glomerular capillary wall. As with most forms of glomerulosclerosis, TGF-β may be an important regulator of matrix accumulation in remnant nephrons. Angiotensin II, PDGF, CTGF, and endothelins are other potential modulators of this process. Maneuvers that lower intraglomerular pressure, such as a low-protein diet or treatment with ACE inhibitors or ARBs, slow the development of glomerulosclerosis and renal failure. Glomerular hypertrophy, intracapillary microthrombi, recruited macrophages, and hyperlipidemia are other potential stimuli for glomerulosclerosis. Indeed, glomerular capillary hypertension and hypertrophy appear to be independent risk factors that could act synergistically to cause progressive renal insufficiency. Intriguingly, angiotensin II may trigger TGF-β production, and engagement of angiotensin II receptors may trigger activation of growth factor receptor signaling pathways (so-called *receptor transactivation*) in remnant nephrons, suggesting that ACE inhibitors and ARBs may be renoprotective through complementary effects on glomerular hemodynamics and matrix production.

Tubulointerstitial Inflammation and Fibrosis Downstream from Glomerular Injury Moderate-to-severe glomerulonephritis is usually associated with a variable degree of tubulointerstitial inflammation and scarring in addition to glomerular injury. Indeed, the severity of tubulointerstitial injury usually correlates closely with long-term impairment of renal function. The pathogenesis of tubulointerstitial inflammation in this setting is unclear. Potential mechanisms include: (1) primary involvement of both the glomeruli and the tubulointerstitium in autoimmune disease; (2) induction of tubulointerstitial inflammation by mediators generated by diseased glomeruli, which then diffuse into the tubulointerstitium via blood, tubular fluid, or the interstitial space; (3) injury to tubule epithelial cells by excessive filtered proteins ("protein overload" hypothesis); and (4) ischemia to areas of the tubulointerstitium downstream to areas of vigorous glomerular inflammation or severe glomerulosclerosis.

CLINICAL PRESENTATIONS

ACUTE NEPHRITIC SYNDROME AND RAPIDLY PROGRESSIVE GLOMERULONEPHRITIS

CLINICAL FEATURES AND CLINICOPATHOLOGIC CORRELATES The *acute nephritic syndrome* is the clinical correlate of acute glomerular inflammation. In its most dramatic form, the acute nephritic syndrome is characterized by sudden onset (i.e., over days to weeks) of acute renal failure and oliguria (400 mL/day of urine). Renal blood flow and GFR fall as a result of obstruction of the glomerular capillary lumen by infiltrating inflammatory cells and proliferating resident glomerular cells. Renal blood flow and GFR are further compromised by intrarenal vasoconstriction and mesangial cell contraction that result from local imbalances of vasoconstrictor (e.g., leukotrienes, platelet-activating factor, thromboxanes, endothelins) and vasodilator substances (e.g., nitric oxide, prostacyclin) within the renal microcirculation. Extracellular fluid volume expansion, edema, and hypertension develop because of impaired GFR and enhanced tubular reabsorption of salt and water. As a result of injury to the glomerular capillary wall, urinalysis typically reveals red blood cell casts, dysmorphic red blood cells, leukocytes, and subnephrotic proteinuria of <3.0 g per 24 h ("nephritic urinary sediment"). Hematuria is often macroscopic.

The classic pathologic correlate of the nephritic syndrome is *proliferative glomerulonephritis*. The proliferation of glomerular cells is due initially to infiltration of the glomerular tuft by neutrophils and monocytes and subsequently to true proliferation of resident glomerular endothelial and mesangial cells (endocapillary proliferation). In its most severe form, the nephritic syndrome is associated with acute inflammation of most glomeruli, i.e., *acute diffuse proliferative glomerulonephritis*. When less vigorous, <50% of glomeruli may be involved, i.e., *focal proliferative glomerulonephritis*. In milder forms of nephritic injury, cellular proliferation may be confined to the mesangium, i.e., *mesangioproliferative glomerulonephritis*.

RPGN is the clinical correlate of more subacute glomerular inflammation. Patients develop renal failure over weeks to months in association with a nephritic urinary sediment, subnephrotic proteinuria and variable oliguria, hypervolemia, edema, and hypertension. The classic pathologic correlate of RPGN is crescent formation involving most glomeruli (*crescentic glomerulonephritis*). In practice, the clinical term *rapidly progressive glomerulonephritis* and the pathologic term *crescentic glomerulonephritis* are often used interchangeably. In addition to classic crescentic glomerulonephritis, in which crescents dominate the glomerular pathology, crescents can also develop concomitantly with proliferative glomerulonephritis or as a complication of membranous glomerulopathy and other more indolent forms of glomerular inflammation.

The acute nephritic syndrome and RPGN are part of a spectrum of presentations of immunologically mediated proliferative glomerulonephritis. Studies of experimental models suggest that nephritic syndrome and diffuse proliferative glomerulonephritis represent an acute immune response to a sudden large antigen load, whereas RPGN and crescentic glomerulonephritis represent a more subacute immune response to a smaller antigen load in presensitized individuals. At the other end of the spectrum, chronic low-grade immune injury presents with slowly progressive renal insufficiency or asymptomatic hematuria in association with focal proliferative or mesangioproliferative glomerulonephritis. These more indolent forms of immune-mediated glomerulonephritis are discussed later in this chapter.

ETIOLOGY AND DIFFERENTIAL DIAGNOSIS Acute nephritic syndrome and RPGN can result from renal-limited *primary* glomerulopathy or from *secondary* glomerulopathy complicating systemic disease. Figure 264-2 highlights the histopathologic and serologic features that help distinguish among the major causes of nephritic syndrome and RPGN. In general, rapid diagnosis and prompt treatment are critical to avoid

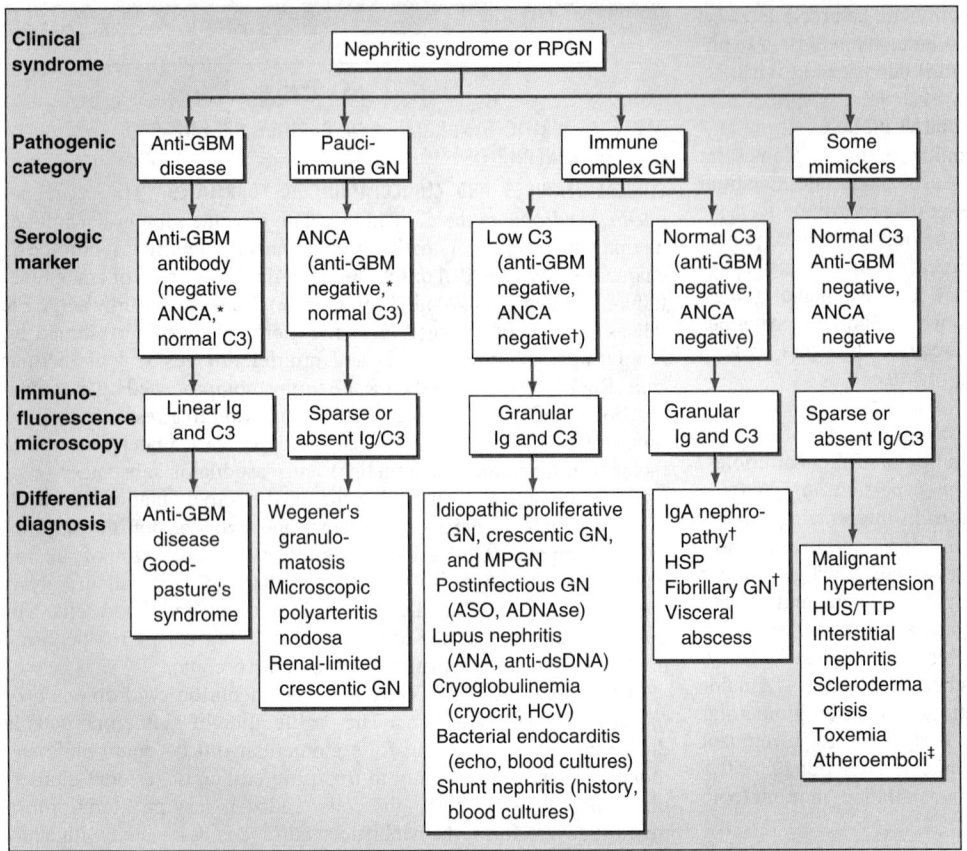

FIGURE 264-2 Differential diagnosis of nephritic syndrome and rapidly progressive glomerulonephritis. Abbreviations: GN, glomerulonephritis; RPGN, rapidly progressive glomerulonephritis; MPGN, membranoproliferative glomerulonephritis; GBM, glomerular basement membrane; ANCA, antineutrophil cytoplasmic antibodies; Ig, immunoglobulin; C3, third component of complement; ASO, antistreptolysin O antibody titer; ADNAse, anti-deoxyribonuclease antibody titer; ANA, antinuclear antibody; anti-dsDNA, anti-double-stranded DNA antibody; HCV, hepatitis C virus; echo, echocardiogram; HSP, Henoch-Schönlein purpura; HUS, hemolytic-uremic syndrome; TTP, thrombotic thrombocytopenic purpura. *Approximately 20% of patients with anti-GBM disease have ANCA, which may portend a better prognosis. †Nephritic syndrome and RPGN are unusual presentations of IgA nephropathy and fibrillary GN. ‡Atheroembolic renal disease may cause transient hypocomplementemia.

the development of irreversible renal failure. Renal biopsy remains the "gold standard" for diagnosis. *Immunofluorescence microscopy* is particularly helpful and identifies three major patterns of deposition of immunoglobulin that define three broad diagnostic categories: (1) scattered *granular* deposits of immunoglobulin, a hallmark of *immune-complex glomerulonephritis*; (2) more discrete *linear* deposition of immunoglobulin along the GBM, characteristic of *anti-GBM disease*; and (3) paucity or absence of immunoglobulin—*pauci-immune glomerulonephritis* (Figs. 264-1 and 264-3). Most patients (≥70%) with full-blown acute nephritic syndrome have immune-complex glomerulonephritis. Pauci-immune glomerulonephritis is less common in this setting (<30%), and anti-GBM disease is rare (<1%). Among patients with RPGN, immune-complex glomerulonephritis and pauci-immune glomerulonephritis are equally prevalent (~45% each), whereas anti-GBM disease again accounts for a minority of cases (<10%).

Three *serologic markers* often predict the immunofluorescence microscopy findings in nephritic syndrome and RPGN and may obviate the need for renal biopsy in classic cases. They are the serum C3 level and titers of anti-GBM antibody and ANCA. As discussed in previous sections, the kidney is host to immune attack in immune-complex glomerulonephritis, most cases being initiated either by in situ formation of immune complexes or less commonly by glomerular trapping of circulating immune complexes. These patients typically have hypocomplementemia (low C3 in 90%) and negative anti-GBM and ANCA serology, the major exception being IgA nephropathy/Henoch Schönlein purpura where complement levels are typically normal. The glomerulus is the direct target of immune attack in anti-GBM disease, glomerular inflammation being initiated by an autoantibody directed at a 28-kDa autoantigen on the α3 chain of type IV collagen. Approx-

imately 90 to 95% of patients with anti-GBM disease have circulating anti-GBM autoantibodies detectable by immunoassay; serum complement levels are typically normal, and ANCA are usually not detected. The pathogenesis of pauci-immune glomerulonephritis is still being defined; however, most patients have circulating ANCA. Serum complement levels are typically normal, and anti-GBM titers are usually negative in ANCA-associated renal disease. It should be noted, however, that there may be some serologic overlap, with as many as 20% of patients with immune complex or anti-GBM glomerulonephritis also having at least low levels of circulating ANCA.

NEPHRITIC SYNDROME AND RPGN DUE TO IMMUNE-COMPLEX GLOMERULONEPHRITIS

Nephritic syndrome induced by immune-complex glomerulonephritis may be (1) be idiopathic, (2) represent a response to a known antigenic stimulus (e.g., glomerulonephritis triggered by bacterial endocarditis or streptococcal infection, or hepatitis B or C infection in cryoglobulinemic glomerulonephritis), or (3) form part of a multisystem immune-complex disorder (e.g., lupus nephritis, Henoch-Schönlein purpura; Table 264-1, Figs. 264-1 to 264-3).

INFECTION-ASSOCIATED GLOMERULONEPHRITIS INCLUDING GLOMERULONEPHRITIS ASSOCIATED WITH STREPTOCOCCAL INFECTION AND INFECTIVE ENDOCARDITIS A variety of infections can precipitate immune-complex glomerulonephritis. The most common clinicopathologic lesion in this setting is acute diffuse proliferative glomerulonephritis presenting as the acute nephritic syndrome; however, depending on the speed of onset and site and extent of immune complex formation, infection-associated immune complex formation can trigger mesangioproliferative, focal proliferative, membranoproliferative, or membranous glomerulopathy.

Poststreptococcal glomerulonephritis is the prototypical *postinfectious glomerulonephritis* and a leading cause of acute nephritic syndrome. Most cases are sporadic, though the disease can occur as an epidemic. Glomerulonephritis develops, on average, 10 days after pharyngitis or 2 weeks after a skin infection (impetigo) with a nephritogenic strain of group A β-hemolytic streptococcus. The known nephritic strains include M types 1, 2, 4, 12, 18, 25, 49, 55, 57, and 60. Immunity to these strains is type-specific and long-lasting, and repeated infection and nephritis are rare. Epidemic poststreptococcal glomerulonephritis is most commonly encountered in children of 2 to 6 years of age with pharyngitis during the winter months. This entity appears to be decreasing in frequency, possibly due to more widespread and prompt use of antibiotics. Poststreptococcal glomerulonephritis in association with cutaneous infections usually occurs in a setting of poor personal hygiene or streptococcal superinfection of another skin disease.

The classic clinical presentation of poststreptococcal glomerulonephritis is full-blown nephritic syndrome with oliguric acute renal failure; however, most patients have milder disease. Indeed, subclinical cases outnumber overt cases by four- to tenfold during epidemics. Patients with overt disease present with gross hematuria (red or

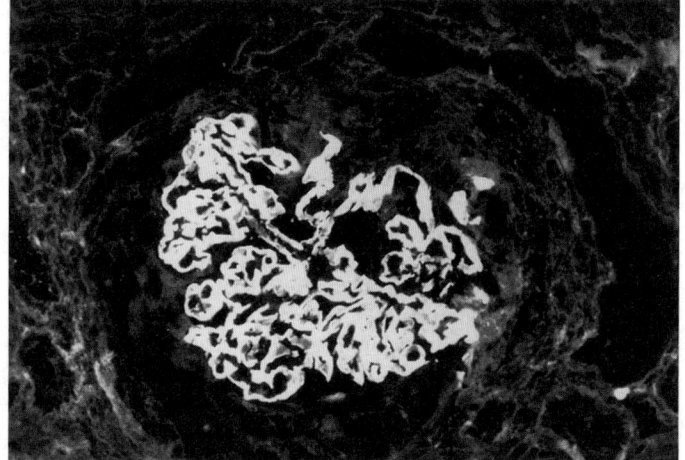

A

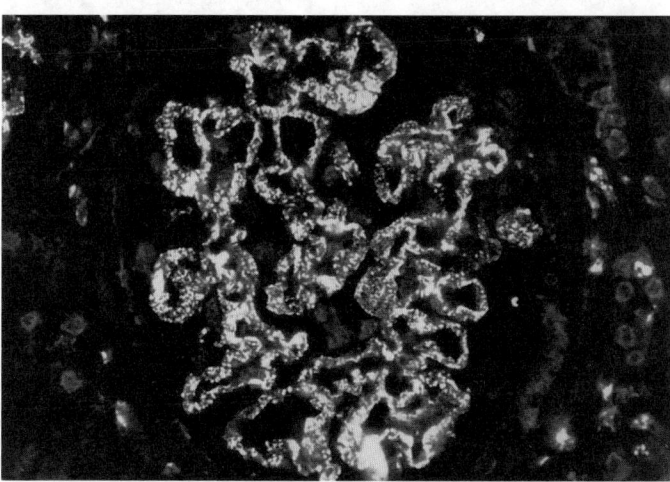

B

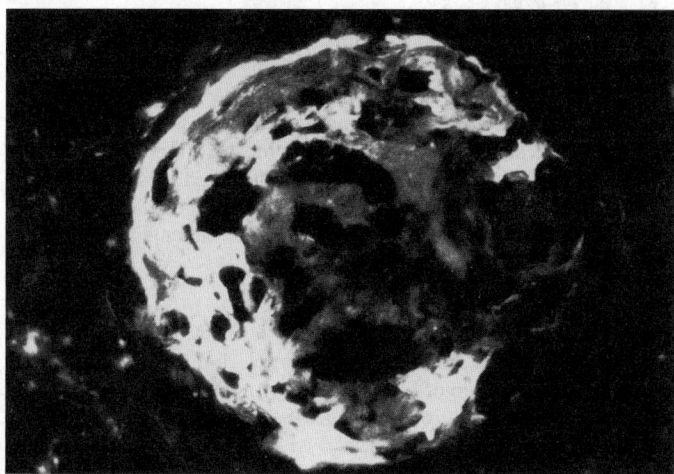

C

FIGURE 264-3 Typical findings on immunofluorescence microscopy of renal biopsy specimens from patients with anti-glomerular basement membrane antibody disease, immune complex–mediated glomerulonephritis, and pauci-immune glomerulonephritis. Specimens in the upper and middle panels were stained for immunoglobulin and show the classic linear "ribbon-like" pattern of anti-GBM disease (*A*) and granular pattern of immune complex–mediated glomerulonephritis (*B*). Immunoglobulin is sparse or absent in patients with pauci-immune glomerulonephritis (not shown); however, abundant fibrin is detected in crescents (*C*). (*Micrographs courtesy of Dr. Helmut Rennke.*)

morphic red blood cells, red cell casts, leukocytes, occasionally leukocyte casts, and subnephrotic proteinuria. Fewer than 5% of patients develop nephrotic-range proteinuria. The latter may only manifest as acute nephritis resolves and renal blood flow and GFR recover. Coexistent rheumatic fever is extremely rare.

The serum creatinine is often mildly elevated at presentation. Serum C3 levels and CH_{50} are depressed within 2 weeks in ~90% of cases. C4 levels are characteristically normal, indicating activation of the alternate pathway of complement. Complement levels usually return to normal within 6 to 8 weeks. Persistently depressed levels after this period should suggest another cause, such as the presence of a C3 nephritic factor (see "Membranoproliferative Glomerulonephritis," p. 1687). The majority of patients (>75%) have transient hypergammaglobulinemia and mixed cryoglobulinemia. The antecedent streptococcal infection may still be evident or may have resolved either spontaneously or in response to antibiotic therapy. Most patients (>90%) have circulating antibodies against streptococcal exoenzymes such as antistreptolysin O (ASO), anti-deoxyribonuclease B (anti-DNAse B), antistreptokinase (ASKase), anti-nicotinyl adenine dinucleotidase (anti-NADase), and antihyaluronidase (AHase).

Acute poststreptococcal glomerulonephritis is usually diagnosed on clinical and serologic grounds, without resort to renal biopsy, especially in children with a typical antecedent history. The characteristic lesion on light microscopy is diffuse proliferative glomerulonephritis. Crescents are uncommon, and extraglomerular involvement is usually mild. Immunofluorescence microscopy reveals diffuse granular deposition of IgG and C3, giving rise to a "starry sky" appearance (Figs. 264-1 and 264-3). The characteristic finding on electron microscopy is the presence of large electron-dense immune deposits in the subendothelial, subepithelial, and mesangial areas.

In addition to poststreptococcal glomerulonephritis, the nephritic syndrome and RPGN can complicate acute immune-complex glomerulonephritis due to other viral, bacterial, fungal, and parasitic infections. Diffuse proliferative immune-complex glomerulonephritis is a well-described complication of acute and *subacute infective endocarditis* and is usually associated with hypocomplementemia. The glomerular lesion typically resolves following eradication of the cardiac infection.

℞ TREATMENT

Treatment of poststreptococcal glomerulonephritis focuses on eliminating the streptococcal infection with antibiotics and providing supportive therapy until spontaneous resolution of glomerular inflammation occurs. Patients are usually confined to bed during the acute inflammatory phase. Diuretics and antihypertensive agents are employed to control extracellular fluid volume and blood pressure. Dialysis is rarely needed to control hypervolemia or the uremic syndrome. Poststreptococcal glomerulonephritis carries an excellent prognosis and rarely causes end-stage renal disease (ESRD). Whereas spontaneous resolution of the glomerular lesion and nephritic syndrome is the norm in children within 6 to 8 weeks, >20% of adults may have some degree of persistent proteinuria and/or compromise of GFR 1 year after presentation. As with poststreptoccal glomerulonephritis, treatment of immune complex glomerulonephritis in association with bacterial endocarditis and other forms of infection is supportive until the causative infection is eliminated.

SYSTEMIC LUPUS ERYTHEMATOSUS (SLE) (LUPUS NEPHRITIS) (See also Chap. 300)   Renal involvement is clinically evident in 40 to 85% of patients with SLE; it varies from isolated abnormalities of the urinary sediment to full-blown nephritic or nephrotic syndrome or chronic renal failure. Most glomerular injury is triggered by the formation of immune complexes within the glomerular capillary wall; however, thrombotic microangiopathy may be the dominant reason for renal dysfunction in a small subset of patients with the antiphospholipid antibody syndrome. Renal biopsy has proven very useful for identifying the different pat-

"smoky" urine), headache, and generalized symptoms such as anorexia, nausea, vomiting, and malaise. Swelling of the renal capsule can cause flank or back pain. Physical examination reveals hypervolemia, edema, and hypertension. The urinary sediment is nephritic, with dys-

terns of immune-complex glomerulonephritis in SLE, which are diverse, portend different prognoses, and do not necessarily correlate with the clinical findings. Indeed, clinically silent lupus nephritis is well described as having a urinalysis virtually normal but renal biopsy demonstrating varying degrees of injury.

Patients with active lupus nephritis have a range of serologic abnormalities. Hypocomplementemia is present in 75 to 90% of patients and is most striking with diffuse proliferative glomerulonephritis. Antinuclear antibodies (ANA) are usually detected (95 to 99%), although not specific for SLE. ANA titers tend to fall with treatment, and ANA may not be detected during remissions. Anti-double-stranded DNA (dsDNA) antibodies are highly specific for SLE, and changes in their titers correlate with the activity of lupus nephritis.

Patients with the lupus-related antiphospholipid antibody syndrome can develop a variable degree of renal impairment due to thrombotic microangiopathy. The latter typically affects the interlobular arteries, arterioles, and glomerular capillaries and is characterized by intravascular microthrombi and swelling of endothelial cells. Decreased levels of tissue plasminogen activator and increased levels of α_2-antiplasmin, both of which would tend to promote thrombosis, have been described in this syndrome.

℞ TREATMENT

The treatment of lupus nephritis is controversial and based largely on the class of injury and disease activity. Because there is relatively poor correlation between clinical features (urinalysis findings, serum creatinine) and histologic class, the renal biopsy findings are an important guide to therapy. Treatment is not indicated for those with a normal biopsy or only mesangial deposits of immunoglobulins, as these histologic patterns portend an excellent prognosis (100% and 90% 5-year survival rates, respectively). Extrarenal manifestations may warrant treatment with glucocorticoids, salicylates, or antimalarials. Glucocorticoids and cyclophosphamide are the mainstays of therapy for patients with proliferative nephritis. High-dose steroids given as intravenous boluses (pulse therapy) are usually effective at rapidly controlling acute glomerular inflammation. Cyclophosphamide and azathioprine are important adjuncts to steroid therapy and appear to afford better long-term preservation of renal function than steroids alone. Intravenous pulse cyclophosphamide is as efficacious as oral therapy and appears to be less toxic. An initial regimen of monthly intravenous boluses of cyclophosphamide for 6 months should be administered. Subsequent therapy is tailored to disease activity and typically involves dosing every 3 to 6 months for a total treatment period of 12 to 24 months.

The initial dose of cyclophosphamide is 0.5 g/m², and the dose is increased gradually to a maximum of 1 g/m² unless patients develop leukopenia or other side effects. Steroids are usually started simultaneously at 1 mg/kg per day and are tapered over the first 6 months to a maintenance dose of 5 to 10 mg/d for the duration of cyclophosphamide therapy. Cyclophosphamide may be stopped after 6 months and replaced with either azathioprine or mycophenolate provided that partial or complete remission has been achieved. Five-year renal survival rates of 60 to 90% have been obtained with these regimens. Mycophenolate mofetil has also been used as a therapeutic option in patients resistant to cyclophosphamide. A large randomized, prospective trial indicated that plasmapheresis does not offer additional benefit in patients with severe proliferative lupus nephritis.

The management of membranous lupus nephritis (see "Nephrotic Syndrome," below) is less well defined. As with idiopathic membranous glomerulopathy, the incidence of spontaneous remission approaches 50% in membranous lupus nephritis, and the course of the disease is generally indolent, with a 70 to 90% renal survival rate at 5 years. Some authorities advocate steroids at the time of diagnosis, whereas others reserve them for patients with progressive renal insufficiency or severe nephrotic syndrome. Useful parameters for monitoring the response to therapy and predicting relapse include the activity of the urine sediment, proteinuria, GFR, serum complement levels, and anti-dsDNA titers. As in other proteinuric renal diseases, ACE inhibitors or ARBs are usually prescribed as adjunctive treatment. Despite maximal immunosuppressive therapy, about 20% of patients with aggressive lupus nephritis develop ESRD requiring dialysis. SLE tends to become quiescent with advanced uremia, and patients rarely develop systemic flares once they commence dialysis. Recurrence of nephritis and systemic flares are also very uncommon after renal transplantation, and allograft survival rates are comparable to those in patients with other causes of ESRD.

In patients with thrombotic microangiopathy due to lupus-related antiphospholipid antibody syndrome, anticoagulation to maintain the Internalized Normal Ratio (INR) at 3.0 may be beneficial in reducing the incidence of recurrent thromboses. There are uncontrolled reports of a benefit of plasmapheresis in the setting of acute renal failure secondary to thrombotic microangiopathy.

CRYOGLOBULINEMIA GLOMERULOPATHY (See also Chap. 306) Renal involvement is most common with the mixed cryoglobulinemias (types II and III), which are more common in females and usually begin in the sixth decade. Most patients present with a variable combination of leukocytoclastic vasculitis, skin ulcerations, arthralgias, fatigue, and Raynaud's phenomenon. Renal disease is a complication in 50% of patients and usually develops after 12 to 24 months. The typical clinical renal manifestations are nephrotic-range proteinuria, microscopic hematuria, and hypertension. Acute nephritic syndrome occurs in 20 to 30%, and oliguric acute renal failure in about 5% of patients with renal disease.

Circulating levels of C3, C4, and CH50 are depressed in about 80% of patients with renal involvement, and a transient ANA (speckled pattern) is sometimes detected. Hepatitis C virus (HCV) RNA has been isolated from the serum of patients with essential mixed cryoglobulinemia (EMC).

℞ TREATMENT

Traditionally, glucocorticoids, with or without cyclophosphamide, and plasmapheresis were the standard treatment for EMC, with poor results. With the recognition that many cases are triggered by HCV infection, interferon α has been employed to successfully control viral replication and stabilize renal function in most HCV-positive patients. Unfortunately, relapse is common when interferon α is discontinued, a major problem given the cost of this agent. In general, patient and renal survival are good in EMC, with 75% of patients being alive at 10 years.

IGA NEPHROPATHY AND HENOCH-SCHÖNLEIN PURPURA IgA nephropathy (Berger's disease) is a renal-limited form of glomerulonephritis characterized by deposition of IgA-containing immune deposits in the glomerular mesangium (p. 1690). Henoch-Schönlein purpura (Chap. 306) is a systemic disease characterized by a petechial rash on the extremities, arthropathy, abdominal pain, and glomerulonephritis. Because the glomerular lesion is identical to that found in IgA nephropathy, Henoch-Schönlein nephritis and IgA nephropathy may be part of a spectrum of manifestations of a single disease. Nephritis is present in 80% of patients and manifests as a nephritic urine sediment and moderate proteinuria. Macroscopic hematuria and nephrotic-range proteinuria are uncommon. Light-microscopic appears can vary from mild mesangial proliferation and expansion to diffuse proliferation with glomerular crescents. The sine qua non for diagnosis is the presence of mesangial IgA deposition on immunofluorescence microscopy. IgG and C3 are also detected. Electron microscopy reveals mesangial immune deposits. Immune complexes may also be present in the peripheral glomerular capillary wall and paramesangial areas. Biopsy of involved skin reveals dermal IgA deposition and leukocytoclastic vasculitis. IgA deposition is also seen in areas of uninvolved skin.

℞ TREATMENT

Since there is no proven therapy for Henoch-Schönlein nephritis, treatment is supportive. Steroids and/or cytotoxic agents are often tried in patients with severe disease, but without compelling scientific evidence to support their use. The disease typically undergoes clinical exacerbations and remissions in the first year and then enters long-term remission. The prognosis is generally excellent; chronic renal failure and persistent hypertension occur in <10% of patients. The treatment of IgA nephropathy will be discussed later.

NEPHRITIC SYNDROME AND RPGN DUE TO ANTI-GLOMERULAR BASEMENT MEMBRANE DISEASE (GOODPASTURE'S SYNDROME)   Anti-GBM disease is an autoimmune disease in which autoantibodies directed against type IV collagen induce RPGN and crescentic glomerulonephritis (Figs. 264-1 to 264-3). Acute nephritic syndrome is rare. Between 50 and 70% of patients have lung hemorrhage; the clinical complex of anti-GBM nephritis and lung hemorrhage is referred to as *Goodpasture's syndrome*. Patients with this syndrome are typically young males (5 to 40 years; male-female ratio of 6:1). In contrast, patients presenting during the second peak in the sixth decade rarely suffer lung hemorrhage and have an almost equal sex distribution. The target antigen is a component of the noncollagenous (NCI) domain of the $\alpha 3$ chain of type IV collagen, the $\alpha 3$ chain being preferentially expressed in glomerular and pulmonary alveolar basement membrane.

Anti-GBM disease commonly presents with hematuria, nephritic urinary sediment, subnephrotic proteinuria, and rapidly progressive renal failure over weeks, with or without pulmonary hemorrhage. When pulmonary hemorrhage occurs, it usually predates nephritis by weeks or months. Hemoptysis can vary from fluffy pulmonary infiltrates on chest x-ray and mild dyspnea on exertion to life-threatening pulmonary hemorrhage; hypertension is unusual.

The diagnostic serologic marker is circulating anti-GBM antibodies with a specificity for the NCI domain of the $\alpha 3$ chain of type IV collagen. Anti-GBM antibodies are detected in the serum of >90% of patients with anti-GBM nephritis by specific immunoassay. Renal biopsy is the gold standard for diagnosis of anti-GBM nephritis. The typical morphologic pattern on light microscopy is diffuse proliferative glomerulonephritis, with focal necrotizing lesions and crescents in >50% of glomeruli (crescentic glomerulonephritis). Immunofluorescence microscopy reveals linear ribbon-like deposition of IgG along the GBM (Fig. 264-3).

℞ TREATMENT

Prior to the introduction of immunosuppressive therapy, >80% of patients with anti-GBM nephritis developed ESRD within 1 year, and many patients died from pulmonary hemorrhage or complications of uremia. With early and aggressive use of plasmapheresis, glucocorticoids, cyclophosphamide, and azathioprine, renal and patient survival have improved dramatically. In general, emergency plasmapheresis is performed daily or on alternate days until anti-GBM antibodies are not detected in the circulation (usually 1 to 2 weeks). Prednisone (1 mg/kg per day) is started simultaneously, in combination with either cyclophosphamide (2 to 3 mg/kg per day) or azathioprine (1 to 2 mg/kg per day) to suppress new synthesis of anti-GBM antibodies. The speed of initiation of therapy is a critical determinant of outcome. One-year renal survival approaches 90% if treatment is started before serum creatinine exceeds 442 μmol/L (5 mg/dL) and falls to about 10% if renal failure is more advanced. Patients who require dialysis at presentation rarely recover renal function. Serial anti-GBM titers are monitored to gauge response to therapy. Relapses are not unusual and are often heralded by rising antibody titers. In patients with ESRD, renal transplantation is a viable treatment option. Recurrence of anti-GBM nephritis in the allograft is extremely unusual provided that anti-GBM antibody titers have been consistently negative for 6 to 12 months prior to transplantation. However, in occasional patients with Alport's syndrome, when the allograft presents normal GBM components to the immune system of the recipient for the first time, anti-GBM nephritis can occur de novo in renal allografts.

NEPHRITIC SYNDROME AND RPGN DUE TO PAUCI-IMMUNE GLOMERULONEPHRITIS   The major pauci-immune glomerulonephritides are *idiopathic renal-limited crescentic glomerulonephritis*, *microscopic polyangiitis nodosa* (PAN), and *Wegener's granulomatosis* (Figs. 264-1 to 264-3). Significant glomerular disease may also complicate the Churg-Strauss syndrome and classic forms of PAN, albeit less frequently than the aforementioned three conditions. RPGN is a more common clinical presentation than acute nephritic syndrome, and the usual pathology is necrotizing glomerulonephritis with crescents affecting 50% of glomeruli (crescentic glomerulonephritis). The marked overlap of clinical features and glomerular histopathology, and the presence of circulating ANCA in most patients, suggest that these entities are a spectrum of a single disease. Indeed this group of diseases is frequently categorized under the all-encompassing term *ANCA-associated small vessel vasculitis*. They are more common in whites and older patients (mean age 57 years) and typically present with nonspecific constitutional symptoms and signs such as lethargy, malaise, anorexia, weight loss, fever, arthralgias, and myalgias. Nonspecific laboratory abnormalities include a rapid sedimentation rate, elevated C-reactive protein, leukocytosis, thrombocytosis, and normochromic, normocytic anemia. Serum complement levels are typically normal.

ANCA-Associated Renal Disease   Patients with ANCA-associated renal disease usually present with a nephritic urine sediment and subnephrotic proteinuria. Renal dysfunction can vary from a mild decrement in GFR to RPGN. Renal biopsy typically reveals focal, segmental, necrotizing glomerulonephritis with crescent formation. Immunofluorescence and electron microscopy are remarkable for the paucity or absence of immunoglobulin, complement, and immune deposits; hence the term *pauci-immune glomerulonephritis*.

Idiopathic Renal-Limited Crescentic Glomerulonephritis   This is more common in middle-aged and older patients and shows a slight male preponderance. Patients typically present with RPGN, nephritic syndrome being rare. ANCA, usually a perinuclear ANCA IgG with specificity for myeloperoxidase, are detected in 70 to 90% of patients. The erythrocyte sedimentation rate and C-reactive protein levels may be elevated; however, C3 levels are typically normal, and circulating immune complexes, cryoglobulins, and anti-GBM antibodies are not detected. Most patients have crescents on light microscopy, often associated with necrotizing glomerulonephritis. Immune deposits are scanty or absent. Immunofluorescence microscopy reveals abundant fibrin deposits within crescents (Fig. 264-3).

Wegener's Granulomatosis (See also Chap. 306)   Renal injury occurs in 80% of patients with Wegener's granulomatosis and varies from indolent smoldering inflammation to rapidly progressive renal failure. Cytoplasmic ANCA are detected at presentation in 80% of patients with renal disease and in 10% more on follow-up. Renal biopsy typically reveals focal, segmental, necrotizing pauci-immune glomerulonephritis with crescent formation. In contrast to the lung, granulomas are rarely seen in the kidney.

Microscopic Polyangiitis Nodosa (See also Chap. 306)   Microscopic PAN is a systemic disease characterized by leukocytoclastic vasculitis involving multiple organ systems including the lungs, skin, joints, and kidneys. Clinical renal disease ranges from a nephritic urinary sediment with mild impairment of GFR to RPGN. The usual histopathologic lesion is pauci-immune focal segmental necrotizing and crescentic glomerulonephritis. Circulating ANCA are detected in 70 to 80% of patients at presentation, with cANCA or pANCA being equally prevalent.

Churg-Strauss Syndrome (See also Chap. 306)   Clinical renal involvement in Churg-Strauss syndrome is relatively infrequent and usually limited to mild proteinuria and hematuria. Evolution to chronic renal failure is rare. Renal biopsy most frequently reveals extraglomerular pathology, with involvement of the renal vasculature and tubulointerstitium by granulomatous vasculitis. Focal segmental glomerulonephritis with crescents is also seen. A minority of patients have focal segmental necrotizing glomerulonephritis.

CLASSIC POLYANGIITIS NODOSA AND LARGE VESSEL VASCULITIDES

(See also Chap. 306) In contrast to the small vessel vasculitides discussed above, it is unusual to detect ANCA in classic PAN and the major large-vessel vasculitides. The typical glomerular lesion in classic PAN is ischemic collapse and obsolescence. Characteristic clinical and serologic features are hypertension, a bland urine sediment with subnephrotic proteinuria, slowly progressive renal insufficiency, normal serum complement levels, and absence of ANCA. Glomerular involvement is exceedingly rare in the major large vessel vasculitides such as Takayasu's disease and giant cell arteritis.

℞ TREATMENT

Glucocorticoids and cyclophosphamide are the mainstays of treatment and dramatically ameliorate glomerular injury in pauci-immune glomerulonephritis. Steroids are usually administered initially by pulse intravenous therapy on three consecutive days, followed by a daily oral dose of about 1 mg/kg body weight tapered to a maintenance doses of 5 to 10 mg every day or alternate day over 3 to 6 months. Cyclophosphamide is typically administered orally at a daily dose of 1 to 2 mg/kg or as six monthly intravenous pulses of 1 g/m² of body surface area followed by pulses every 3 months for a maximum of 1 to 2 years. Alternatively, patients are switched from cyclophosphamide to either azathioprine or mycophenolate after 6 months in an effort to avoid cyclophosphamide toxicity and treatment is continued for a total duration of at least 1 year. Plasmapheresis may be a useful adjunct in patients with severe nephritis requiring dialysis. As many as 30% of patients relapse after treatment-induced remission. As with all patients receiving potent immunosuppressive therapy, the benefits of immunosuppression must be balanced against the risk of toxicity, and factors such as patient age co-morbidity, and the intensity of the vasculitic process must be taken into account. A persistently elevated or rising ANCA titer may predict relapse in individual patients; however, this relationship is not strong enough to justify treatment based on titers alone. Recent studies demonstrate that administration of trimethoprim-sulfamethoxazole reduces the relapse rate, possibly by eradicating nasal carriage of *Staphylococcus aureus*. Dialysis and renal transplantation afford excellent survival in patients with ESRD. Recurrence of Wegener's granulomatosis in the allograft is rare. ACE inhibitors may help to slow the progression to end-stage renal failure.

NEPHROTIC SYNDROME

Proteinuria >150 mg per 24 h is abnormal and can result from a number of mechanisms. *Glomerular proteinuria* results from leakage of plasma proteins through a perturbed glomerular filtration barrier; *tubular proteinuria* results from failure of tubular reabsorption of low-molecular-weight plasma proteins that are normally filtered and then reabsorbed and metabolized by tubular epithelium; *overflow proteinuria* results from filtration of proteins, usually immunoglobulin light chains, that are present in excess in the circulation. Tubular proteinuria virtually never exceeds 2 g per 24 h and thus, by definition, never causes nephrotic syndrome. Overflow proteinuria should be suspected in patients with clinical or laboratory evidence of multiple myeloma or other lymphoproliferative malignancy. Suspicion is heightened when there is a discrepancy between proteinuria detected by dipstick, the latter being sensitive to albumin but not light chains, and the sulfosalicylic acid precipitation method, which detects both.

DEFINITION The *nephrotic syndrome* is a clinical complex characterized by a number of renal and extrarenal features, the most prominent of which are proteinuria of >3.5 g per 1.73 m² per 24 h (in practice, >3.0 to 3.5 g per 24 h), hypoalbuminemia, edema, hyperlipidemia, lipiduria, and hypercoagulability. Nephrotic syndrome can complicate any disease that perturbs the negative electrostatic charge or architecture of the GBM and the podocytes and their slit diaphragms. Recent attention has focused on several key molecules that mediate GBM-podocyte-slit diaphragm interactions such as nephrin, podocin, and alpha-actinin-4. Six entities account for >90% of cases of nephrotic syndrome in adults: minimal change disease (MCD), focal and segmental glomerulosclerosis (FSGS), membranous glomerulopathy, membranoproliferative glomerulonephritis (MPGN), diabetic nephropathy, and amyloidosis. *Renal biopsy* is a valuable tool in adults with nephrotic syndrome for establishing a definitive diagnosis, guiding therapy, and assessing prognosis. Renal biopsy is not required in the majority of children with nephrotic syndrome as most cases are due to MCD and respond to empirical treatment with glucocorticoids.

It should be stressed that the key component of nephrotic syndrome is *proteinuria*, which results from altered permeability of the glomerular filtration barrier for protein, namely the GBM and the podocytes and their slit diaphragms. The other components of the nephrotic syndrome and the ensuing metabolic complications are all secondary to urine protein loss and can occur with lesser degrees of proteinuria or may be absent even in patients with massive proteinuria.

PATHOPHYSIOLOGY In general, the greater the proteinuria, the lower the serum albumin level. *Hypoalbuminemia* is compounded further by increased renal catabolism and inadequate, albeit usually increased, hepatic synthesis of albumin. The pathophysiology of *edema* formation in nephrotic syndrome is poorly understood. The *underfilling hypothesis* postulates that hypoalbuminemia results in decreased intravascular oncotic pressure, leading to leakage of extracellular fluid from blood to the interstitium. Intravascular volume falls, thereby stimulating activation of the renin-angiotensin-aldosterone axis and the sympathetic nervous system and release of vasopressin (antidiuretic hormone), and suppressing atrial natriuretic peptide release. These neural and hormonal responses promote renal salt and water retention, thereby restoring intravascular volume and triggering further leakage of fluid to the interstitium. This hypothesis does not, however, explain the occurrence of edema in many patients in whom plasma volume is expanded and the renin-angiotensin-aldosterone axis is suppressed. The latter finding suggests that *primary renal salt and water retention may also contribute to edema formation in some cases.

Hyperlipidemia is believed to be a consequence of increased hepatic lipoprotein synthesis that is triggered by reduced oncotic pressure and may be compounded by increased urinary loss of proteins that regulate lipid homeostasis. Defective lipid catabolism is also thought to play an important role. Low-density lipoproteins and cholesterol are increased in the majority of patients, whereas very low density lipoproteins and triglycerides tend to rise in patients with severe disease. Although not proven conclusively, hyperlipidemia may accelerate atherosclerosis and progression of renal disease.

Hypercoagulability is probably multifactorial in origin and is caused, at least in part, by increased urinary loss of antithrombin III, altered levels and/or activity of proteins C and S, hyperfibrinogenemia due to increased hepatic synthesis, impaired fibrinolysis, and increased platelet aggregability. As a consequence of these perturbations, patients can develop spontaneous *peripheral arterial or venous thrombosis*, *renal vein thrombosis*, and *pulmonary embolism*. Clinical features that suggest acute renal vein thrombosis include sudden onset of flank or abdominal pain, gross hematuria, a left-sided varicocele (the left testicular vein drains into the renal vein), increased proteinuria, and an acute decline in GFR. Chronic renal vein thrombosis is usually asymptomatic. Renal vein thrombosis is particularly common (up to 40%) in patients with nephrotic syndrome due to membranous glomerulopathy, membranoproliferative glomerulonephritis, and amyloidosis.

Other metabolic complications of nephrotic syndrome include *protein malnutrition* and iron-resistant *microcytic hypochromic anemia* due to transferrin loss. *Hypocalcemia* and secondary hyperparathyroidism can occur as a consequence of vitamin D deficiency due to enhanced urinary excretion of cholecalciferol-binding protein, whereas loss of thyroxine-binding globulin can result in *depressed thyroxine levels*. An increased *susceptibility to infection* may reflect low levels of IgG that result from urinary loss and increased catabolism. In addition, patients are prone to unpredictable changes in the *pharmacokinetics* of therapeutic agents that are normally bound to plasma proteins.

℞ TREATMENT

GENERAL MANAGEMENT OF NEPHROTIC SYNDROME AND COMPLICATIONS The treatment of nephrotic syndrome involves (1) specific treatment of the underlying morphologic entity and, when possible, causative disease (see above); (2) general measures to control proteinuria if remission is not achieved through immunosuppressive therapy and other specific measures; and (3) general measures to control nephrotic complications.

General measures may be warranted to control proteinuria in nephrotic syndrome if patients do not respond to immunosuppressive therapy and other specific measures and suffer progressive renal failure or severe nephrotic complications. Nonspecific measures that may reduce proteinuria include ACE inhibitors, ARBs, and nonsteroidal anti-inflammatory drugs (NSAIDs). ACE inhibitors and ARBs reduce proteinuria and slow the rate of progression of renal failure by lowering intraglomerular pressure and preventing the development of hemodynamically mediated focal segmental glomerulosclerosis. There is conclusive evidence that these drugs are renoprotective in human diabetic nephropathy and many other proteinuric glomerulopathies, including secondary FSGS. NSAIDs also reduce proteinuria in some patients with nephrotic syndrome, probably by altering glomerular hemodynamics and GBM permeability characteristics. This potential benefit must be balanced against the risk of inducing acute renal failure, hyperkalemia, salt and water retention, and other side effects.

Complications of nephrotic syndrome that may require treatment include edema, hyperlipidemia, thromboembolism, malnutrition, and vitamin D deficiency. Edema should be managed cautiously by moderate *salt restriction*, usually 1 to 2 g per day, and the judicious use of *loop diuretics*. It is unwise to remove >1.0 kg of edema per day without close monitoring as more aggressive diuresis may precipitate intravascular volume depletion and prerenal azotemia. Administration of salt-poor albumin is not recommended as most is excreted within 24 to 48 h. Whereas many nephrologists advocate lowering low-density lipoproteins and cholesterol levels with *lipid-lowering drugs*, specifically HMG CoA reductase inhibitors to prevent accelerated atherosclerosis and possibly slow the rate of decline of GFR, the value of such interventions in this setting has not been conclusively shown.

Anticoagulation is indicated for patients with deep venous thrombosis, arterial thrombosis, and pulmonary embolism. Patients may be relatively resistant to heparin as a consequence of antithrombin III deficiency. Renal vein and vena caval angiography are probably indicated only when embolization occurs on anticoagulation and insertion of a caval filter is contemplated. There is no consensus regarding the optimal *diet* for patients with nephrotic syndrome. High-protein diets to prevent protein malnutrition are now in disfavor, since protein supplements have little, if any, effect on serum albumin levels and may hasten the progression of renal disease by increasing urinary protein excretion. The potential value of dietary protein restriction for reducing proteinuria must be balanced against the risk of contributing to malnutrition. *Vitamin D* supplementation is advisable in patients with clinical or biochemical evidence of vitamin D deficiency.

MINIMAL CHANGE DISEASE (MINIMAL CHANGE GLOMERULOPATHY)
MCD accounts for about 80% of nephrotic syndrome in children younger than 16 years and 20% in adults (Table 264-3). The peak incidence is between 6 and 8 years. Patients typically present with nephrotic syndrome and benign urinary sediment. Microscopic hematuria is present in 20 to 30%. Hypertension and renal insufficiency are very rare.

MCD (also called nil disease, lipoid nephrosis, or foot process disease) is so named because glomerular size and architecture are normal by light microscopy. Immunofluorescence studies are typically nega-

TABLE 264-3	*Major Causes of Minimal Change Disease (Nil Disease, Lipoid Nephrosis)*

Idiopathic (majority)
In association with systemic diseases or drugs
  Drug-induced interstitial nephritis induced by NSAIDs, rifampin,
    interferon α
  Hodgkin's disease and other lymphoproliferative malignancy
  HIV infection

Note: NSAIDs, nonsteroidal anti-inflammatory drugs.

tive for immunoglobulin and C3. The findings of mesangial hypercellularity and sparse deposits of C3 and IgM portend a worse prognosis. Electron microscopy reveals characteristic *diffuse effacement of the foot processes of visceral epithelial cells* (Fig. 264-4). This morphologic finding is referred to as foot process fusion in the older literature.

The etiology of MCD is unknown, and the vast majority of cases are idiopathic (Table 264-3). MCD occasionally develops after upper respiratory tract infection, immunizations, and atopic attacks. Patients with atopy and MCD have an increased incidence of HLA-B12, suggesting a genetic predisposition. MCD, often in association with interstitial nephritis, is a rare side effect of NSAIDs, rifampin, and interferon α. The occasional association with lymphoproliferative malignancies (such as Hodgkin's lymphoma), the tendency for idiopathic MCD to remit during intercurrent viral infection such as measles, and the good response of idiopathic forms to immunosuppressive agents (see below) suggest an immune etiology. In children, the urine contains albumin principally and minimal amounts of higher molecular weight proteins such as IgG and α$_2$-macroglobulin. This *selective proteinuria* in conjunction with foot process effacement suggests injury to podocytes and loss of the fixed *negative charge* in the glomerular filtration barrier for protein. Proteinuria is typically nonselective in adults, suggesting more extensive perturbation of membrane permeability. Mutations in nephrin, α-actinin-4, and podocin, molecules that pay central roles in the anchoring of podocytes together through their slit diaphragms and to the GBM, cause proteinuria and glomerular morphologic changes that are virtually identical to those observed with acquired MCD and FSGS. There is increasing evidence that the expression and/or function of these and related molecules is also perturbed in acquired MCD and FSGS.

℞ TREATMENT

MCD is highly steroid-responsive and carries an excellent prognosis. Spontaneous remission occurs in 30 to 40% of childhood cases but is less common in adults. Approximately 90% of children and 50% of adults enter remission following 8 weeks of high-dose oral glucocorticoids. In a typical regimen using prednisone, children receive 60 mg/m^2 of body surface area daily for 4 weeks, followed by 40 mg/m^2 on alternate days for an additional 4 weeks; adults receive 1 to 1.5 mg/kg body weight per day for 4 weeks, followed by 1 mg/kg per day on alternate days for 4 weeks. Up to 90% of adults enter remission if therapy is extended for 20 to 24 weeks. Nephrotic syndrome relapses in over >50% of cases following withdrawal of glucocorticoids. Alkylating agents are reserved for the small number of patients who fail to achieve lasting remission. These include patients who relapse during or shortly after withdrawal of steroids (steroid-dependent) and those who relapse more than three times per year (frequently relapsing). In these settings, cyclophosphamide (2 to 3 mg/kg per day) or chlorambucil (0.1 to 0.2 mg/kg per day) is started after steroid-induced remission and continued for 8 to 12 weeks. Cytotoxic agents may also induce remission in occasional steroid-resistant cases. These benefits must be balanced against the risk of infertility, cystitis, alopecia, infection, and secondary malignancies, particularly in children and young adults. Azathioprine has not been proven to be a useful adjunct to steroid therapy. Cyclosporine induces remission in 60 to 80% of patients; it is an alternative to cytotoxic agents and an option in patients who are resistant to cytotoxic agents. Unfortunately, relapse is usual

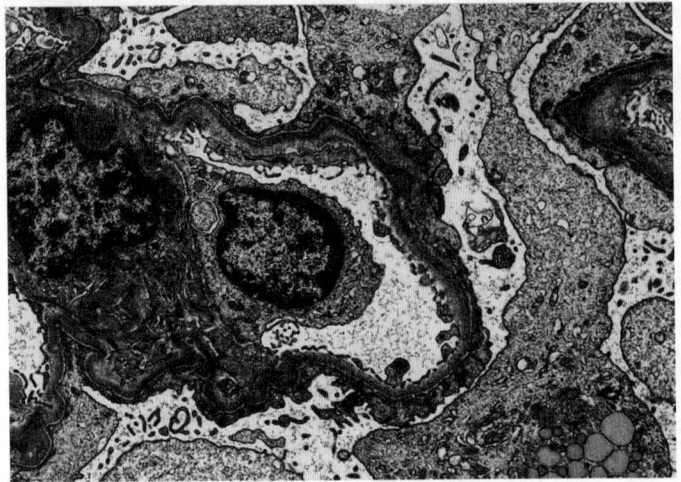

A

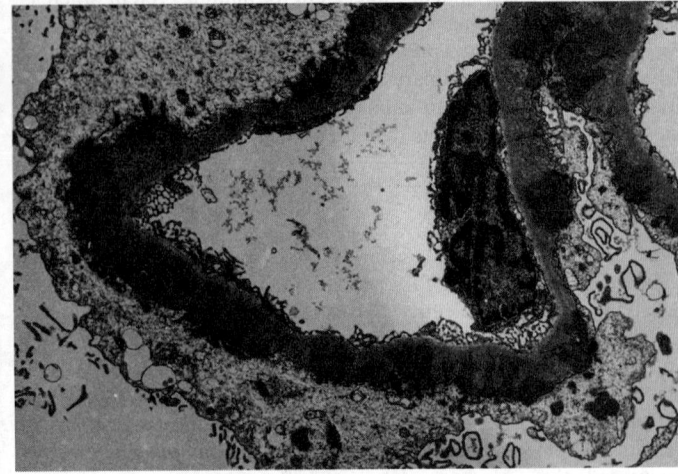

B

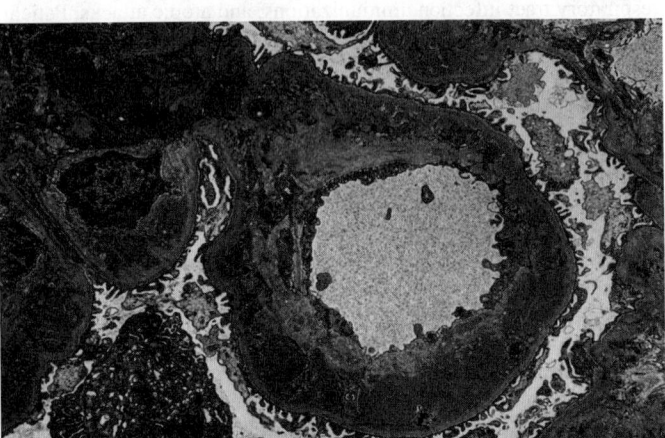

C

FIGURE 264-4 Typical findings on electron microscopy of renal biopsy specimens from patients with minimal change glomerulopathy, membranous glomerulopathy, and membranoproliferative glomerulonephritis. The pathognomonic feature of minimal change glomerulopathy (*A*) is effacement of foot processes of visceral epithelial cells (podocytes), giving the impression of foot process fusion. Foot process effacement is also evident in focal and segmental glomerulosclerosis (not shown here); in addition, there is typically detachment of podocytes from basement membrane, areas of glomerular capillary collapse, deposits of hyaline material, and sclerosis. Membranous nephropathy (*B*) is characterized by immune complexes in the subepithelial space. These electron-dense immune deposits stimulate production of new GBM, which eventually surrounds and incorporates the immune deposits into the GBM. The hallmarks of type I membranoproliferative glomerulonephritis (*C*) are increased mesangial cellularity and matrix and thickening and reduplication of the GBM. The latter is initiated by formation of electron-dense immune complexes on the subendothelial aspect of the GBM, which are subsequently covered by a new layer of GBM, probably produced by regenerating endothelial cells. (*Micrographs courtesy of Dr. Helmut Rennke.*)

when cyclosporine is withdrawn, and long-term therapy carries the risk of nephrotoxicity and other side effects. Long-term renal and patient survival is excellent in MCD.

FOCAL AND SEGMENTAL GLOMERULOSCLEROSIS The pathognomonic morphologic lesion in FSGS is sclerosis with hyalinosis involving portions (segmental) of fewer than 50% (focal) of glomeruli on a tissue section. The incidence of idiopathic (primary) FSGS has increased over the past two decades so that it now accounts for about one-third of cases of nephrotic syndrome in adults and as many as one-half of cases of nephrotic syndrome in blacks. Secondary FSGS can complicate a number of systemic diseases and sustained glomerular capillary hypertension following nephron loss from any cause (Table 264-4).

Idiopathic FSGS typically presents as nephrotic syndrome (~66%) or subnephrotic proteinuria (~33%) in association with hypertension, mild renal insufficiency, and an abnormal urine sediment that contains red blood cells and leukocytes. Proteinuria is nonselective in most cases.

Light microscopy of renal biopsy tissue reveals FSGS with entrapment of amorphous hyaline material, a process that shows a predilection for juxtamedullary glomeruli. Electron microscopy reveals evidence of damage to visceral epithelial cell.

The etiology of primary FSGS is unclear, but appears to be, at least in part, immunologic. There is evidence that a circulating nonimmunoglobulin permeability factor, possibly a lymphokine, triggers FSGS in at least a subgroup of patients. Plasmapharesis has been employed with variable success to control the nephrotic syndrome in this group. Secondary FSGS is a potential long-term consequence of nephron loss from any cause. It can complicate congenital renal diseases such as congenital oligomeganephronia, in which both kidneys have a reduced complement of nephrons, and congenital unilateral agenesis. In addition, FSGS may develop following acquired loss of nephrons from extensive surgical ablation of renal mass; reflux nephropathy; glomerulonephritis; interstitial nephritis; sickle cell disease; and the combined effects of ischemia, cyclosporine nephrotoxicity, and rejection on renal allograft function (Table 264-4). It appears that >50% of nephrons must be lost for development of secondary FSGS.

TABLE 264-4 *Etiology of Focal and Segmental Glomerulosclerosis*

Idiopathic (majority)
In association with systemic diseases or drugs
  HIV infection
  Diabetes mellitus
  Fabry's disease
  Sialidosis
  Charcot-Marie-Tooth disease
As consequence of sustained glomerular capillary hypertension
  Congenital oligonephropathies
    Unilateral renal agenesis
    Oligomeganephronia
  Acquired nephron loss
    Surgical resection
    Reflux nephropathy
    Glomerulonephritis or tubulointerstitial nephritis
  Other adaptive responses
    Sickle cell nephropathy
    Obesity with sleep apnea syndrome
    Familial dysautonomia
Miscellaneous
  Heroin use

℞ TREATMENT

Spontaneous remission of primary FSGS is rare and renal prognosis is relatively poor. Proteinuria remits in only 20 to 40% of patients treated with glucocorticoids for 8 weeks. Uncontrolled studies suggest that up to 70% respond when steroid therapy is prolonged for 16 to 24 weeks. Cyclophosphamide and cyclosporine, when used at doses described above for MCD, induce partial or complete remission in 50 to 60% of steroid-responsive patients but are generally ineffective in steroid-resistant cases. Mycophenolate mofetil is another option in resistant cases. Poor prognostic factors at presentation include hypertension, abnormal renal function, black race, and persistent heavy proteinuria. Renal transplantation is complicated by recurrence of FSGS in the allograft in about 50% of cases and graft loss in about 10%. Factors associated with an increased risk of recurrence include a short time interval between the onset of the FSGS and ESRD, young age at onset, and possibly the presence of mesangial hypercellularity on renal biopsy.

MEMBRANOUS GLOMERULOPATHY (MEMBRANOUS NEPHROPATHY) This morphologic lesion is a leading cause of idiopathic nephrotic syndrome in adults (30 to 40%) and a rare cause in children (<5%). It has a peak incidence between the ages of 30 to 50 years and a male-female ratio of 2:1 (Fig. 264-4 and Table 264-5). Membranous glomerulopathy derives its name from the characteristic light-microscopic appearance on renal biopsy, namely diffuse thickening of the GBM, which is most apparent upon staining with periodic acid–Schiff (PAS). Most patients (>80%) present with nephrotic syndrome, proteinuria usually being nonselective. Microscopic hematuria is present in up to 50% of cases. Hypertension is documented in only 10 to 30% of patients at the outset but is common later in patients with progressive renal failure. Serologic tests such as antinuclear antibody, ANCA, anti-GBM antibody, cryoglobulin titers, and complement levels are normal in the idiopathic form.

Light microscopy of renal biopsy sections reveals diffuse thickening of the GBM without evidence of inflammation or cellular proliferation. Immunofluorescence reveals granular deposition of IgG, C3, and the terminal components of complement (C5b–9) along the glomerular capillary wall.

The pathogenesis of idiopathic human membranous glomerulopathy is incompletely understood. The presence of electron-dense immune deposits that contain IgG and C3 suggest an immune process. About one-third of adult membranous nephropathy occurs in association with systemic diseases such as SLE, infections such as hepatitis B, malignancy, and drug therapy with gold and penicillamine (Table 264-5).

Nephrotic syndrome remits spontaneously and completely in up to 40% of patients. The natural history of another 30 to 40% is characterized by repeated relapses and remissions. The final 10 to 20% suffer a slow progressive decline in GFR that typically culminates in ESRD after 10 to 15 years. Presenting features that predict a poor prognosis include male gender, older age, hypertension, severe proteinuria and hyperlipidemia, and impaired renal function. Controlled trials of glucocorticoids have failed to show consistent improvement in proteinuria or renal protection. Cyclophosphamide, chlorambucil, and cyclosporine have each been shown to reduce proteinuria and/or slow the decline in GFR in patients with progressive disease in small or uncontrolled studies. These observations need to be confirmed in controlled prospective studies. Transplantation is a successful treatment option for patients who reach ESRD.

MEMBRANOPROLIFERATIVE GLOMERULONEPHRITIS This morphologic entity, also known as mesangiocapillary glomerulonephritis, is characterized by thickening of the GBM and proliferative changes on light microscopy (Fig. 264-4 and Table 264-6). Two major types are identified; both are characterized by a diffuse increase in mesangial cellularity and matrix, and by thickening and reduplication of the GBM such that the lobular pattern of the glomerular tuft is exaggerated. The hallmark of type I MPGN is the presence of subendothelial and mesangial deposits on electron microscopy that contain C3 and IgG or IgM; rarely, IgA deposits are demonstrated by immunofluorescence microscopy. The hallmark of type II MPGN (dense deposit disease) is the presence of electron-dense deposits within the GBM and other renal basement membranes (shown by electron microscopy) that stain for C3, but little or no immunoglobulin.

Most patients with type I MPGN present with heavy proteinuria or nephrotic syndrome, active urinary sediment, and normal or mildly impaired GFR. C3 levels are usually depressed, and C1q and C4 levels are borderline or low. Type I MPGN is an immune-complex glomerulonephritis and can be associated with a variety of chronic infections (e.g., bacterial endocarditis, HIV, hepatitis B and C), systemic immune-complex diseases (e.g., SLE, cryoglobulinemia), and malignancies (e.g., leukemias, lymphomas). Type I MPGN usually has a protracted course, and as many as 50% of patients reach ESRD by 10 years. There is no proven therapy for patients with progressive disease beyond eradicating the underlying infection, malignancy, or systemic disease, when possible. The incidence of type I MPGN appears to be falling, possibly because the overall incidence of HCV infection has fallen dramatically in western society over the past decade.

TABLE 264-5 *Conditions Associated with Membranous Glomerulopathy*

Idiopathic (majority)
In association with systemic diseases or drugs
  Infection
    Hepatitis B and C, secondary and congenital syphilis, malaria, schistosomiasis, leprosy, hydatid disease, filariasis, enterococcal endocarditis
  Systemic autoimmune diseases
    SLE, rheumatoid disease, Sjögren's syndrome, Hashimoto's disease, Graves' disease, mixed connective tissue disease, primary biliary cirrhosis, ankylosing spondylitis, dermatitis herpetiformis, bullous pemphigoid, myasthenia gravis
  Neoplasia
    Carcinoma of the breast, lung, colon, stomach, and esophagus; melanoma; renal cell carcinoma; neuroblastoma; carotid body tumor
  Drugs
    Gold, penicillamine, captopril, NSAIDs, probenecid, trimethadione, chlormethiazole, mercury
  Miscellaneous
    Sarcoidosis, diabetes mellitus, sickle cell disease, Crohn's disease, Guillain-Barré syndrome, Weber-Christian disease, Fanconi's syndrome, α_1 antitrypsin deficiency, angiofollicular lymph node hyperplasia

Note: SLE, systemic lupus erythematosus; NSAIDs, nonsteroidal anti-inflammatory drugs.

TABLE 264-6 *Causes of Membranoproliferative (Mesangiocapillary) Glomerulonephritis (MPGN)*

Idiopathic	
Type I	With subendothelial and mesangial immune deposits
Type II	With intramembranous dense deposits containing sparse or no Ig; associated with C3 nephritic factor
Type III	Features of type I MPGN and membranous nephropathy
In association with systemic diseases or drugs[a]	
Systemic immune-complex disease	SLE, mixed cryoglobulinemia, Sjögren's syndrome
Chronic infections	Hepatitis B and C, HIV, bacterial endocarditis, ventriculoatrial shunts, visceral abscess
Malignancy	Leukemias, lymphomas
Liver disease	Chronic active hepatitis and cirrhosis (usually associated with hepatitis B or C)
Miscellaneous	Partial lipodystrophy, heroin use, sarcoidosis, inherited C2 deficiency, thrombotic microangiopathies

[a] Usual with morphologic features of idiopathic type I MPGN (see above).
Note: SLE, systemic lupus erythematosus.

Type II MPGN can also present with proteinuria and nephrotic syndrome; however, some patients present with nephritic syndrome, RPGN, or recurrent macroscopic hematuria. Type II MPGN is an autoimmune disease in which patients have an IgG autoantibody, termed *C3 nephritic factor*, that binds to C3 convertase, the enzyme that metabolizes C3, and renders it resistant to inactivation. Type II MPGN runs a variable course; the GFR remains stable in some patients and declines gradually to ESRD over 5 to 10 years in others. There is no effective therapy for this disease, which may be associated with partial lipodystrophy, although corticosteroids are sometimes used.

A third, rarer form of MPGN is associated with subepithelial immune deposits. It should be noted that a membranoproliferative pattern of glomerular injury may also complicate thrombotic microangiopathies (e.g., antiphospholipid antibody syndrome, chronic allograft rejection, healing phase of hemolytic-uremic syndrome, or thrombotic thrombocytopenic purpura) and glomerular deposition disease (e.g., fibrillary glomerulopathy—see below).

MESANGIOPROLIFERATIVE GLOMERULONEPHRITIS   In 5 to 10% of patients with idiopathic nephrotic syndrome, renal biopsy reveals a diffuse increase in glomerular cellularity, predominantly due to proliferation of mesangial and endothelial cells, and infiltration by monocytes. Findings on immunofluorescence microscopy vary and include deposits of IgA, IgG, IgM, and/or complement, or absence of immune reactants. It is likely that this morphologic entity is, in fact, a heterogeneous group of diseases that includes atypical forms of MCD and FSGS and milder or resolving forms of the immune-complex and pauci-immune glomerulopathies described above under nephritic syndrome and RPGN. In keeping with the heterogeneity of this diagnosis, the prognosis is variable. In general, persistent nephrotic-range proteinuria signals a poor prognosis, with many patients progressing to ESRD over 10 to 20 years despite immunosuppressive therapy.

DIABETIC NEPHROPATHY   (See also Chap. 323)   Diabetic nephropathy is the leading cause of ESRD in western societies and accounts for 30 to 35% of patients on renal replacement therapy in North America. Type 1 diabetes mellitus (DM; formerly, insulin-dependent diabetes mellitus) and type 2 DM (formerly, non-insulin-dependent diabetes mellitus) affect approximately 0.5 and 4% of the population, respectively. Nephropathy complicates 30% of cases of type 1 DM and approximately 20% of cases of type 2 DM. However, most diabetic patients with ESRD have type 2 DM because of the greater prevalence of type 2 DM worldwide (90% of all individuals with diabetes). Risk factors for the development of diabetic nephropathy include hyperglycemia, systemic hypertension, glomerular hypertension and hyperfiltration, proteinuria, and possibly cigarette smoking, hyperlipidemia, and gene polymorphisms affecting the activity of the renin-angiotensin-aldosterone axis. For reasons that are unclear, ESRD from diabetic nephropathy is more common in blacks with type 2 DM than in whites (4:1 ratio), whereas the reverse is true for type 1 DM.

Pathophysiology   The pathophysiology, clinical features, and morphology of diabetic nephropathy appears similar in type 1 and type 2 DM, although the true incidence and precise time course of nephropathy in type 2 DM is still debated. Glomerular hypertension and hyperfiltration are the earliest renal abnormalities in experimental and human diabetes and are observed within days to weeks of diagnosis. Microalbuminuria, so named because the abnormal albumin excretion of 30 to 300 mg/24 h is below the limits of detection of standard dipsticks, develops after approximately 5 years of sustained glomerular hypertension and hyperfiltration in type 1 DM.

Microalbuminuria is the first manifestation of injury to the glomerular filtration barrier and predicts the development of overt nephropathy. Dipstick-positive proteinuria, ultimately reaching nephrotic levels, typically develops 5 to 10 years after the onset of microalbuminuria (i.e., 10 to 15 years after the onset of diabetes) and is associated with hypertension and progressive loss of renal function.

In addition, patients can display features of tubulointerstitial disease such as hyperkalemia and type IV renal tubular acidosis. ESRD typically develops 5 to 10 years after the development of overt nephropathy. As noted above, the course of diabetic nephropathy may be shorter in type 2 DM, and many patients present with established nephropathy and hypertension. Diabetic nephropathy is usually diagnosed on clinical grounds without a renal biopsy. Supportive clues are the presence of normal sized or enlarged kidneys, evidence of proliferative diabetic retinopathy, and a bland urinary sediment. Retinopathy is found in 90% and 60% of patients with type 1 and type 2 DM, respectively, who develop nephropathy.

Pathologic Changes   The earliest morphologic abnormalities in diabetic nephropathy are thickening of the GBM and expansion of the mesangium due to accumulation of extracellular matrix. With time, matrix accumulation becomes diffuse and is evident as eosinophilic, PAS-positive glomerulosclerosis on renal biopsy. Prominent areas of nodular matrix expansion (nodular glomerulosclerosis, the classic Kimmelstiel-Wilson lesion) are often superimposed on this background. The glomeruli and kidneys are typically normal or increased in size, distinguishing diabetic nephropathy from most other forms of chronic renal insufficiency (renal amyloidosis and polycystic kidney disease being other important exceptions). Immunofluorescence microscopy may reveal deposition of IgG along the GBM in a linear pattern, but this does not appear to be immunopathogenetic as in anti-GBM disease. Immune deposits are not seen. The renal vasculature typically displays evidence of atherosclerosis, as a consequence of hyperlipidemia, and hypertensive arteriosclerosis.

Factors implicated as triggers for increased matrix production in DM include glomerular hypertension; the direct effects of hyperglycemia on mesangial cells; advanced glycosylation end-products; growth factors such as growth hormone, insulin-like growth factor 1, angiotensin II, CTGF; cytokines such as TGF-β; hyperlipidemia; and cell sorbitol accumulation. Complementary clinical and laboratory approaches suggest an important role for hemodynamic factors. Glomerular hydrostatic pressure and GFR increase within months of the development of hyperglycemia. The mechanism by which DM induces glomerular hypertension is still being defined and appears to involve circulating factors such as atrial natriuretic peptide acting in concert with the direct effects of high glucose on the actin cytoskeleton of renal mesangial and vascular smooth-muscle cells.

In this framework, glycosuria triggers increased reabsorption of glucose coupled to sodium in the proximal tubule, thereby increasing total-body sodium and extracellular fluid volume. As a compensatory response, atrial natriuretic peptide is released from cardiac myocytes and induces natriuresis in part by triggering afferent arteriolar dilatation and thereby increasing intraglomerular pressure and GFR. Whereas this compensatory response is appropriate in the short term, sustained glomerular hypertension provokes thickening of the GBM, increased mesangial matrix production, and glomerulosclerosis and disruption of barrier function. Exposure of mesangial cells and vascular smooth-muscle cells to high glucose in vitro and in vivo results in disruption of the actin cytoskeleton, possibly through the action of reactive oxygen species, rendering the cells relatively unresponsive to vasoconstrictors and further contributing to afferent arteriolar vasodilatation and glomerular hypertension. In keeping with a central role for intraglomerular pressure in the pathogenesis of diabetic nephropathy, ACE inhibitors and ARBs, which lower intraglomerular pressure, slow the progression of diabetic nephropathy, even in normotensive patients.

It remains to be determined why DM and glomerular hypertension induce glomerulosclerosis in some but not all individuals. Epidemiologic studies and studies of disease concordance in identical twins suggest that important, but as yet unidentified, genetic factors may play a role. It is likely that hemodynamic and metabolic factors act in concert to generate the final glomerulosclerotic phenotype in genetically predisposed patients.

℞ TREATMENT

Therapy is aimed at retarding the progression of nephropathy through control of blood sugar, systemic blood pressure, and glomerular capillary pressure. Glycemic control is achieved through regulation of diet and administration of oral hypoglycemic agents and insulin. ACE inhibitors and ARBs are the drugs of choice as they control both systemic hypertension and intraglomerular hypertension by inhibiting the actions of angiotensin II on the systemic vasculature and renal efferent arterioles. In addition, these agents also attenuate the stimulatory effect of angiotensin II on glomerular cell growth and matrix production. Because ACE inhibitors conclusively delayed the time to ESRD by 50% in patients with type 1 DM in several randomized controlled trials and probably delay progression in type 2 DM, it is recommended that all patients with diabetes over the age of 12 should be screened annually for microalbuminuria and should receive an ACE inhibitor on the development of microalbuminuria, even in the absence of systemic hypertension. ARBs slowed the rate of progression of diabetic nephropathy in patients with type 2 DM in two recent randomized controlled trials and are an alternative to ACE inhibitors for renoprotection. Approximately 80% of patients with DM require more than one drug to control systemic hypertension, and aggressive lowering of blood pressure in these patients retards the rate of progression of nephropathy and other diabetic complications.

Diabetic nephropathy is the most common cause of ESRD requiring renal replacement therapy, and patients with DM have the highest annual mortality rate (20 to 30%) of any group on dialysis, in large part as a result of accelerated atherosclerosis. The survival rates of younger patients undergoing either peritoneal dialysis or hemodialysis are comparable; however, older patients with DM appear to have a higher mortality rate on peritoneal dialysis. Renal transplantation, with or without pancreas transplantation, is the preferred mode of renal replacement therapy in patients who are otherwise medically suitable.

GLOMERULAR DEPOSITION DISEASES The glomerular deposition diseases are characterized by deposition of abnormal proteins, usually immunoglobulins or fragments thereof, within the glomerulus. They include amyloidosis, light and heavy chain deposition disease, cryoglobulinemia, and fibrillary/immunotactoid glomerulonephritis below.

Renal Amyloidosis Amyloidosis is classified according to the major component of its fibrils (Chap. 310). There is substantial overlap in the renal clinicopathologic presentations of amyloid (AL) and amyloid A (AA) disease. Glomeruli are involved in 75 to 90% of patients, usually in association with involvement of other organs. The clinical correlate of glomerular amyloid deposition is nephrotic-range proteinuria. In addition, >50% of patients have impaired glomerular filtration at diagnosis. Hypertension is present in about 20 to 25%. Renal size is usually normal or slightly enlarged. A minority of patients present with renal failure due to amyloid deposition in the renal vasculature or with Fanconi's syndrome, nephrogenic diabetes insipidus, or renal tubular acidosis due to involvement of the tubulointerstitium. Rectal biopsy and abdominal fat pad biopsy reveal amyloid deposits in about 70% of patients and may obviate the need for renal biopsy.

Renal biopsy gives a very high yield if there is clinical evidence of renal involvement. The earliest pathologic changes are mesangial expansion by amorphous hyaline material and thickening of the GBM. Further amyloid deposition results in the development of large nodular eosinophilic masses. When stained with Congo red, these deposits show apple-green birefringence under polarized light. Electron microscopy reveals the characteristic nonbranching extracellular amyloid fibrils of 7.5 to 10 nm in diameter. Tubulointerstitial and vascular deposits of amyloid are also seen and may occasionally be more prominent than glomerular deposits.

℞ TREATMENT

Most patients with renal involvement by AL amyloidosis develop ESRD within 2 to 5 years. No treatment has been shown consistently to improve this prognosis; however, some success has been reported with a combination of melphalan and prednisone. Preliminary studies have reported a benefit of high-dose melphalan with autologous stem cell transplantation. Colchicine delays the onset of nephropathy in patients with familial Mediterranean fever but has not proved useful in patients with established disease or with other forms of amyloid. Remissions may be achieved in AA amyloidosis by eradication of the underlying cause. Renal replacement therapy is offered to patients who reach ESRD; however, the 1-year survival rate on dialysis is low (~66%) by comparison with other causes of ESRD. Most patients die from extrarenal complications, particularly cardiovascular disease. Renal transplantation is a viable option in patients with AA amyloidosis whose primary disease has been eradicated. Transplantation is also an option for patients with AL amyloidosis, although a poor prognosis because of extrarenal organ involvement may preclude them as candidates. Here again, the survival rate is lower by comparison with other causes of ESRD; most of the excess mortality is due to infectious and cardiovascular complications. Recurrence of amyloidosis in the allograft is common but rarely leads to graft loss.

LIGHT CHAIN DEPOSITION DISEASE (LCDD) (See also Chap. 98) Renal involvement is a complication in 90% of patients with LCDD and is often the dominant feature. Nephrotic syndrome and renal impairment are the usual presenting features. Microscopic hematuria occurs in about 20% of patients. Defective hydrogen ion and potassium excretion and urinary concentration may be evident if light chains are deposited predominantly in the tubules. The most common pathologic lesion on renal biopsy is ribbon-like thickening of the tubular basement membrane due to light chain deposition. Mesangial expansion and nodular glomerulosclerosis are found in about 33% of patients. This light-microscopic appearance resembles that of idiopathic membranoproliferative glomerulonephritis and diabetic nephropathy. Superimposed crescentic change is occasionally seen. Immunofluorescence studies are strongly positive for monoclonal light chains, in contrast to AL amyloid, because the constant region of the immunoglobulin is typically deposited. The tissue deposits in LCDD are granular rather than fibrillar on electron microscopy, appear more amorphous in character, do not stain with Congo red, and seem to have a greater affinity for basement membranes.

The prognosis of LCDD is poor when it is associated with multiple myeloma, and most patients progress rapidly to ESRD. Treatment with melphalan and prednisone has been reported to reduce proteinuria and stabilize renal function in uncontrolled studies. In the absence of myeloma, the prognosis is somewhat more variable, and several patients have undergone successful renal transplantation.

WALDENSTRÖM'S MACROGLOBULINEMIA (See also Chap. 98) This disorder is characterized by monoclonal proliferation of an IgM-secreting clone of plasma cells. The circulating IgM paraprotein frequently gives rise to the hyperviscosity syndrome, which may compromise renal blood flow and GFR. Direct renal involvement is rare and, when present, involves deposition of large amorphous deposits of eosinophilic material in the glomerular capillaries. Renal amyloidosis can also occur.

FIBRILLARY-IMMUNOTACTOID GLOMERULOPATHY This emerging clinicopathologic entity accounts for 1% of diagnoses in most large renal biopsy series. Virtually all patients present with proteinuria, and ~50% have nephrotic syndrome. The majority of patients also have hematuria, hypertension, and renal insufficiency. The light-microscopic appearances vary from mesangial expansion and basement membrane thickening with PAS-positive material to proliferative and crescentic glomerulonephritis. On electron microscopy, this PAS-positive material is observed to be composed of randomly arranged (fibrillary glomerulopathy) or organized bundles (immunotactoid glomerulopathy) of microfibrils and microtubules, the composition of which has yet to be defined. The etiology of fibrillary-immunotactoid glomerulopathy remains to be determined. Patients with the immunotactoid variant have an increased incidence of lymphoproliferative malignancy. There is no proven therapy for fibrillary-immunotactoid glomerulopathy, and many patients progress to ESRD over 1 to 10 years. Transplantation appears to be a viable option in the latter setting.

ASYMPTOMATIC ABNORMALITIES OF THE URINARY SEDIMENT

Many cases of glomerular disease are diagnosed when asymptomatic hematuria or proteinuria are detected on routine examination of the urinary sediment as part of preemployment or insurance-related medical assessments.

HEMATURIA   Most asymptomatic glomerular hematuria is due to IgA nephropathy (Berger's disease) or thin basement membrane (TBM) disease (benign hematuria). A rarer but more ominous cause of isolated hematuria is Alport's syndrome (p. 1691). The latter is the most common form of hereditary nephritis, is usually transmitted as an X-linked dominant trait, and is associated with sensorineural deafness, ophthalmologic abnormalities, and progressive renal insufficiency. TBM disease is sometimes familial but, in contrast to Alport's syndrome, is usually a benign disorder. Asymptomatic hematuria may also be the presenting feature of indolent forms of most other primary and secondary proliferative glomerulopathies. Glomerular hematuria must be distinguished from a variety of renal parenchymal and extrarenal causes of hematuria. It is particularly important to exclude malignancy of the kidney or urinary tract, particularly in older male patients. Other potential diagnoses include vascular, cystic, and tubulointerstitial diseases; papillary necrosis; hypercalciuria and hyperuricosuria; benign prostatic hypertrophy; and renal calculi. Important clues to the presence of glomerular hematuria are the presence of urinary red blood cell casts; dysmorphic urinary red blood cells; proteinuria >2.0 g per 24 h; and clinical or serologic evidence of nephritic syndrome, RPGN, or a compatible systemic disease.

IGA NEPHROPATHY (BERGER'S DISEASE)   IgA nephropathy is the most common glomerulopathy worldwide and accounts for 10 to 40% of glomerulonephritis in most series (Table 264-7). The disease is particularly common in southern Europe and Asia and appears to be more common in blacks than whites. Familial clustering has been reported but is rare. Most cases are idiopathic. The renal and serologic abnormalities in IgA nephropathy and Henoch-Schönlein purpura are indistinguishable, and most authorities consider these to be a spectrum of a single disease. Less commonly, IgA nephropathy is found in association with systemic diseases, including chronic liver disease, Crohn's

TABLE 264-7   *Diseases Associated with IgA Nephropathy*

Idiopathic (majority)	
Renal-limited or as component of Henoch-Schönlein purpura	
In association with systemic diseases or drugs[a]	
Liver	Chronic liver disease with involvement of biliary tree
Gastrointestinal	Celiac disease, Crohn's disease, adenocarcinoma
Respiratory	Idiopathic interstitial pneumonitis, obstructive bronchiolitis, adenocarcinoma
Skin	Dermatitis herpetiformis, mycosis fungoides, leprosy
Eyes	Episcleritis, anterior uveitis
Miscellaneous	Ankylosing spondylitis, relapsing polychondritis, Sjögren's syndrome, monoclonal IgA gammopathy, schistosomiasis

[a] Although prominent deposition of IgA has been reported with each of these conditions, significant glomerular inflammation and dysfunction are rare.

disease, gastrointestinal adenocarcinoma, chronic obstructive bronchiolitis, idiopathic interstitial pneumonia, dermatitis herpetiformis, mycosis fungoides, leprosy, ankylosing spondylitis, relapsing polychondritis, and Sjögren's syndrome. In many of these conditions, IgA is deposited in the glomerulus without inducing inflammation, and this may be a clinically insignificant consequence of perturbed IgA homeostasis.

Patients with IgA nephropathy typically present with gross hematuria, often 24 to 48 h after a pharyngeal or gastrointestinal infection, vaccination, or strenuous exercise. Other cases are diagnosed upon detection of microscopic hematuria during routine physical examinations. Hypertension (20 to 30%) and nephrotic syndrome (~10%) are unusual at presentation. Light microscopy of renal biopsy specimens typically shows mesangial expansion by increased matrix and cells. Diffuse proliferation, cellular crescents, interstitial inflammation, and areas of glomerulosclerosis may be evident in severe cases. The diagnostic finding, for which the disease is named, is mesangial deposition of IgA, detected by immunofluorescence microscopy. C3 is usually detected in the area of immune deposits, and IgG is observed in 50% of cases. Electron microscopy reveals electron-dense deposits in the mesangium and, in severe cases, these extend into the paramesangial subendothelial space. The pathogenesis of IgA nephropathy is incompletely understood. Among the major abnormalities in IgA metabolism described in this setting are increased IgA production, abnormal IgA glycosylation, and impaired IgA clearance. Although IgA nephropathy is associated with altered mucosal immunity, most IgA deposited in the kidney appears to be derived from bone marrow cells.

℞ TREATMENT

The optimal treatment of IgA nephropathy is a subject of ongoing debate and controversy. Most authorities advise observation only in patients whose GFR is not compromised and whose proteinuria is <1 g/day. ACE inhibitors are usually prescribed for their renoprotective effect in patients with more severe disease. One trial has suggested a role for prolonged (6 months) high-dose glucocorticoids in patients presenting with impaired GFR and >1 g of proteinuria. Randomized controlled trials evaluating the efficacy of daily fish oils have yielded conflicting results. The case for other immunosuppressive agents such as cyclophosphamide and mycophenolate mofetil is unproven, and such agents are usually reserved for the minority of patients presenting with nephritic syndrome or RPGN, and with aggressive crescent formation and marked glomerular inflammation on renal biopsy.

IgA nephropathy typically smolders for decades, with patients often suffering exacerbations of hematuria and renal impairment during intercurrent infections. As many as 20 to 50% of patients develop ESRD within 20 years. Clinical predictors of a poor prognosis include older age, male sex, hypertension, nephrotic-range proteinuria, and renal insufficiency at presentation. Histologic features that predict an aggressive course include diffuse severe disease, extracapillary proliferation (crescents), extension of immune attack into the paramesangial subendothelial space, glomerulosclerosis, interstitial fibrosis, and arteriolar hyalinosis.

THIN BASEMENT MEMBRANE DISEASE (BENIGN HEMATURIA)   This disorder can be heredofamilial or sporadic and is as common as IgA nephropathy in some series of asymptomatic hematuria. When familial, it is usually inherited as an autosomal dominant trait and is due to a defect in the gene encoding the $\alpha 4$ chain of type IV collagen. The molecular basis for the sporadic form of TBM disease has not been determined. TBM disease typically manifests in childhood as persistent hematuria. Intermittent hematuria and exacerbation of hematuria during upper respiratory tract infections have also been reported. The kidney is normal on light and immunofluorescence microscopy. The GBM is thin by comparison with normal subjects. TBM disease is usually a benign condition, and progressive renal impairment or proteinuria should prompt a search for an alternative diagnosis. A small proportion of patients do, however, appear to develop hypertension and focal glomerulosclerosis upon long-term follow-up, and ACE inhibitors are usually prescribed in this group in an effort to attenuate renal injury.

ALPORT'S SYNDROME (HEREDITARY NEPHRITIS) Alport's syndrome is the most common hereditary nephritis and is usually transmitted as an X-linked dominant trait. The genetic defect resides in the gene for the $\alpha 5$ chain of type IV collagen located on the long arm of the X chromosome; type IV collagen is a major structural component of the GBM. Numerous genetic mutations have been detected (Chap. 342).

Typical light-microscopic features on renal biopsy include mesangial hypercellularity, focal and segmental glomerulosclerosis, chronic tubulointerstitial fibrosis, atrophy, and accumulation of foam cells. Electron microscopy reveals thickening, fragmentation, and lamellation of the lamina densa of the GBM.

Males with the disease tend to progress to ESRD and are suitable candidates for dialysis and transplantation. ACE inhibitors are typically prescribed in the predialysis phase in an effort to slow the decline in GFR. About 5% of transplant recipients develop anti-GBM disease in the renal allograft; their immune system recognizes normal GBM of the transplanted kidney as a foreign antigen. These patients can have antibodies against the $\alpha 3$ (Goodpasture antigen) or $\alpha 5$ chains of type IV collagen, probably because defective synthesis of the $\alpha 5$ chain results in defective incorporation or orientation of the $\alpha 3$ chain in the GBM. In the majority of patients this posttransplant anti-GBM disease does not significantly compromise GFR.

PROTEINURIA Between 0.5 and 10% of the population have isolated proteinuria, defined as proteinuria in the presence of an otherwise normal urinary sediment, a radiologically normal urinary tract, and the absence of known renal disease. The majority of these patients excrete <2 g of protein per day, and more than 80% have an excellent prognosis (*benign isolated proteinuria*). A minority (10 to 25%) are found to have persistent proteinuria (*persistent isolated proteinuria*), some of whom develop progressive renal insufficiency over 10 to 20 years.

Benign Isolated Proteinuria The major categories of benign isolated proteinuria are idiopathic transient proteinuria, functional proteinuria, intermittent proteinuria, and postural proteinuria. *Idiopathic transient proteinuria* is usually observed in young adults and refers to dipstick-positive proteinuria in an otherwise healthy individual that disappears spontaneously by the next clinic visit. *Functional proteinuria* refers to transient proteinuria during fever, exposure to cold, emotional stress, congestive cardiac failure, or obstructive sleep apnea. This phenomenon is presumed to be mediated through changes in glomerular ultrafiltration pressure and/or membrane permeability. Patients with *intermittent proteinuria* have proteinuria in approximately half of their urine samples in the absence of other renal or systemic abnormalities. *Postural proteinuria* is proteinuria (usually <2.0 g per 24 h) that is evident only in the upright position. This disorder affects 2 to 5% of adolescents and may be transient (~80%) or fixed (~20%). Fixed postural proteinuria resolves within 10 to 20 years in most cases. In each of these conditions, renal biopsy reveals either normal renal parenchyma or mild and nonspecific changes involving podocytes or the mesangium. All carry an excellent prognosis.

Persistent Isolated Proteinuria Isolated proteinuria detected on multiple ambulatory clinic visits in both the recumbent and upright position usually signals a structural renal lesion. Virtually all glomerulopathies that induce nephrotic syndrome (see above) can cause persistent isolated proteinuria. The most common lesion on renal biopsy is mild mesangial proliferative glomerulonephritis with or without focal and segmental glomerulosclerosis (30 to 70%), followed by focal or diffuse proliferative glomerulonephritis (~15%) and interstitial nephritis (~5%). Although this clinical entity carries a worse prognosis than benign isolated proteinuria, the prognosis is still relatively good, with only 20 to 40% of patients developing renal insufficiency after 20 years. Furthermore, progression to ESRD is extremely rare. It is wise to exclude monoclonal gammopathy by urinary electrophoresis in older patients.

CHRONIC GLOMERULONEPHRITIS AND OTHER GLOMERULAR ABNORMALITIES

This syndrome is characterized by persistent proteinuria and/or hematuria and renal insufficiency that progresses slowly over years. Chronic glomerulonephritis usually comes to light either (1) upon routine urinalysis, (2) when routine blood tests reveal unexplained anemia or elevated blood urea nitrogen and creatinine, (3) following discovery of bilateral small kidneys on abdominal imaging, (4) during evaluation for secondary causes of hypertension, or (5) during a clinical exacerbation of glomerulonephritis triggered by pharyngitis (synpharyngitic) or other infections. Chronic glomerulonephritis can be a manifestation of virtually all of the major glomerulopathies. While renal biopsy may reveal the causative glomerular lesion, glomerular scarring and sclerosis are frequently so advanced by the time patients present that it may be impossible to define the primary diagnosis. Tubulointerstitial inflammation and scarring are frequent additional findings and portend a poor prognosis. Glomerular hypertension and hyperfiltration through remnant functioning nephrons can hasten progression to ESRD. Treatment is directed at lowering systemic and glomerular hypertension, usually with an ACE inhibitor or ARB, and controlling extracellular fluid volume, anemia, metabolic abnormalities, and the uremic syndrome through judicious use of diuretics, erythropoietin, and dietary modification. Some patients develop ESRD and require renal replacement therapy with dialysis or transplantation.

GLOMERULAR DISEASES IN SPECIFIC CLINICAL SITUATIONS

When considering the clinical approach to patients presenting with abnormalities of the urinary sediment, it is worth considering several specific clinical scenarios: (1) patients whose presentation or family history suggests a hereditary disease, (2) patients on therapeutic or recreational drugs, (3) glomerular disease in the setting of a systemic infection, (4) glomerular disease in a patient with neoplasia, and (5) glomerular disease in patients with arthritis and connective tissue diseases.

HEREDITARY DISEASE WITH GLOMERULAR INVOLVEMENT Although relatively rare, hereditary glomerular diseases are an important category of glomerular disease because of their propensity to cause progressive loss of renal function and for transmission down the generations. Furthermore, studies into the pathogenesis of these disorders have shed important new insights on renal physiology and pathophysiology that are relevant to a wider group of glomerulopathies.

Alport's Syndrome Alport's syndrome is the most common form of hereditary glomerular disease (Chap. 342).

Sickle Cell Disease (See also Chap. 91) Glomerular disease is common (15 to 30%) in homozygotes for sickle cell disease. Glomerular hyperfiltration and hypertrophy occur within the first 5 years of life. Approximately 15 to 30% of patients develop proteinuria in the first three decades, and 5% develop ESRD. The glomerular pathology is usually focal segmental glomerulosclerosis, probably due to sustained glomerular capillary hypertension. MPGN is also seen on occasion. Predictors of chronic renal failure are worsening anemia, proteinuria, nephrotic syndrome, and hypertension. ACE inhibitors and ARBs may slow the progression of renal disease by lowering systemic and glomerular capillary hypertension.

Fabry's Disease (See also Chap. 340) In patients with Fabry's disease, renal biopsy reveals accumulation of neutral glycosphingolipids with terminal α-galactosyl moieties in lysosomes of glomerular, tubular, vascular, and interstitial cells. Focal and global glomerulosclerosis are later features. Electron microscopy reveals stacked, concentric lamellar profiles known as "myeloid" bodies, which are characteristic. Renal disease manifests in the late teens to early twenties with lipiduria, proteinuria with minimal hematuria, nephrotic syndrome, hypertension, and progressive renal insufficiency. The renal lesion is progressive, and these patients often tolerate hemodynamic changes during dialysis poorly because of progressive vascular disease. Significant slowing of disease progression has been demonstrated in early trials of enzyme replacement with recombinant human α-galactosidase A. Successful renal transplantation has been reported despite recurrence in the allograft.

Nail-Patella Syndrome The nail-patella syndrome is a rare hereditary disorder transmitted as an autosomal dominant trait. The abnormal gene is located on the long arm of chromosome 9 and encodes transcription factor of the LIM-homeodomain type, namely LMX1B. The phenotype is characterized by multiple osseous abnormalities, primarily affecting the elbows and knees, and nail dysplasia. About 50% of patients have clinically evident nephropathy. The light-microscopic features on renal biopsy include local GBM thickening, tubular atrophy, interstitial fibrosis, and varying degrees of glomerular sclerosis. The disease usually manifests clinically as asymptomatic hematuria and proteinuria, occasionally in the nephrotic range, but it may be silent. The renal lesion is relatively benign, and progression to ESRD occurs in 10 to 30% of patients.

Lipodystrophy MPGN type II (dense deposit disease) is the most frequent glomerular lesion in patients with lipodystrophy (80%), whereas MPGN type I affects the remainder (20%). The disease occurs mostly in females between the ages of 5 and 15 years, and the clinical presentation and course are similar to those of idiopathic MPGN, namely nephrotic-range proteinuria and progressive renal insufficiency. Low C3 levels are common in association with C3 nephritic factor (p. 1680).

Lecithin-Cholesterol Acyltransferase Deficiency (See also Chap. 335) Renal manifestations of this disease include proteinuria, microscopic hematuria, and progressive renal insufficiency. Renal biopsy typically reveals focal and segmental glomerulosclerosis. Endothelial cell detachment is also evident, and capillary lumens may be occluded by vacuolated foam cells. Recurrence of the disease has been documented in the renal allograft but without marked impairment of graft function.

DRUG-INDUCED GLOMERULAR DISEASE A variety of drugs damage the glomerular filtration barrier and induce proteinuria and nephrotic syndrome (Table 264-8). In contrast, drug-induced proliferative glomerulonephritis is rare. The more common drug-induced glomerulopathies are discussed here.

NSAIDs have a variety of renal side effects, including hemodynamically mediated acute renal failure, salt and water retention, hyponatremia, hyperkalemia, papillary necrosis, acute interstitial nephritis, nephrotic syndrome, and ESRD. Nephrotic syndrome and acute renal failure frequently coexist due to a combination of acute interstitial nephritis and a glomerular lesion that is identical to that of MCD. This entity occurs most commonly in patients on propionic acid derivatives such as fenoprofen, ibuprofen, and naproxen but can occur with other NSAIDs, ampicillin, rifampin, and interferon α. Withdrawal of the drug usually results in resolution of renal disease. Membranous nephropathy is also described as an idiosyncratic reaction to NSAIDs. While the more selective inhibitors of cyclooxygenase (COX)-2 appear to have less renal toxicity, many of the renal syndromes described for NSAIDs have also been reported with COX-2 inhibitors.

Gold therapy, administered by injection or orally, induces proteinuria in 5 to 25% of patients with rheumatoid arthritis. Proteinuria develops after 4 to 6 months of therapy, and up to 33% of patients develop full-blown nephrotic syndrome. Renal biopsy typically reveals membranous glomerulopathy, though MCD or mesangial proliferative lesions have also been described. Progressive renal impairment is rare. Nephrotic syndrome is more common in patients who are HLA-B8/DR3 positive, suggesting a genetic susceptibility. Withdrawal of the drug leads to gradual resolution of the proteinuria.

Penicillamine also induces proteinuria in 5 to 30% of patients. As with gold, the underlying glomerular lesion is usually membranous glomerulopathy, and proteinuria gradually resolves after withdrawal

TABLE 264-8 *Drug-Induced Glomerular Disease*

Morphologic Lesion	Causative Agent
Minimal change diseases (usually with interstitial nephritis)	Nonsteroidal anti-inflammatory agents Recombinant interferon α Rifampin Ampicillin
Membranous nephropathy	Penicillamine Gold Mercury Trimethadione Captopril Chlormethiazole
Focal segmental glomerulosclerosis	Heroin
Pauci-immune necrotizing GN	Ciprofloxacin Hydralazine
Proliferative GN with vasculitis	Allopurinol Penicillin Sulfonamides Thiazides Intravenous amphetamines
RPGN	Rifampin Warfarin Carbimazole Amoxicillin Penicillamine

Note: GN, glomerulonephritis; RPGN, rapidly progressive glomerulonephritis.

of the drug. Acute renal failure secondary to crescentic glomerulonephritis with immune deposits has also been described.

Intravenous heroin use is associated with an increased incidence of focal and segmental glomerulosclerosis (heroin-associated nephropathy). It is not clear whether the nephrotoxin in this setting is heroin itself or a contaminant. Heroin-associated nephropathy occurs predominantly in blacks and is characterized by nephrotic syndrome, hypertension, and a gradual progression to ESRD over a period of 3 to 5 years. The pathologic features are similar to those of idiopathic FSGS, although mesangial deposition of IgM and C3 may be more prominent. The incidence of this disease appears to be declining steadily. Potential reasons for the decline include increased purity of street heroin and a bias to attribute FSGS to HIV infection when both risk factors coexist. Intravenous *amphetamine* abuse is a rare cause of systemic necrotizing vasculitis.

GLOMERULAR LESIONS ASSOCIATED WITH INFECTIOUS DISEASES Infectious organisms can induce glomerular disease through several different mechanisms: (1) by direct infection of renal cells, (2) by elaborating nephrotoxins such as *Escherichia coli*–derived verotoxin, (3) by inciting intraglomerular deposition of immune complexes (e.g., postinfectious glomerulonephritis) or cryoglobulins (e.g., hepatitis B or C), and (4) by providing a chronic stimulus for amyloid fibril formation, as in AA amyloidosis. Direct infection of glomerular cells is a relatively rare mechanism of injury but has been implicated in the pathogenesis of nephropathy associated with HIV (Chap. 173 and below).

Viral Infections ■ *HEPATITIS B VIRUS (HBV) INFECTION* (See also Chap. 285) Infectious HBV, HCV, and HIV are strongly associated with glomerular disease. Glomerular lesions associated with HBV infection include membranous glomerulopathy, MPGN, IgA nephropathy, essential mixed cryoglobulinemia, and polyarteritis nodosa. Membranous glomerulopathy is most common. In endemic areas, such as Asia and Africa, 80 to 100% of children and 30 to 45% of adults with membranous glomerulopathy have HBV surface antigenemia. HBV antigens have been identified in renal immune deposits, suggesting in situ immune-complex formation after planting of HBV antigens or trapping of circulating immune complexes containing HBV antigens. Patients typically present with nephrotic syndrome and microscopic hematuria. Hypertension and renal impairment are rare. The most common associated hepatic lesion is chronic persistent or chronic active hepatitis. In nonendemic areas there is a male preponderance, and many patients are intravenous drug users or have other risk factor for acquisition of HBV. The asymptomatic carrier state of HBV is frequently associated with MPGN in endemic areas. Hypertension and azotemia are more common with this morphologic pattern than with membranous glomerulopathy. Children with HBV-associated membranous glomerulonephritis have a good prognosis, and almost two-thirds enter spontaneous remission within 3 years. ESRD is rare. In contrast, 30% of adults develop progressive renal failure within 5 years, with 10% reaching ESRD. Steroids and cytotoxic agents are contraindicated as they may lead to increased viral replication and worsening of liver disease. Interferon α may reduce proteinuria and stabilize renal function in patients with progressive disease.

HEPATITIS C VIRUS INFECTION (See also Chap. 285) This should be considered in all patients with cryoglobulinemic proliferative glomerulonephritis, MPGN, and membranous glomerulopathy. These three clinicopathologic entities may represent a spectrum of morphologic manifestations of the same pathogenetic process, namely HCV-induced immune-complex disease. Up to 30% of patients with chronic HCV infection have an abnormal urinary sediment. HCV infection accounts for 10 to 20% of type I MPGN and is a major cause of essential mixed cryoglobulinemia. Renal biopsy reveals typical features of type I MPGN and IgG, IgM, C3, and/or cryoglobulin deposits. Most patients present with nephrotic syndrome and microscopic hematuria and may have red blood cell casts. Liver function tests are usually abnormal, and C3 levels are typically depressed. Anti-HCV antibodies are detected in most patients, and viral RNA has been documented in blood and cryoglobulins. Various treatments have been reported to be useful in HCV-induced renal disease including steroids, cytotoxic agents, and plasmapheresis; however, controlled trials to support their use are lacking. Interferon α has been demonstrated to clear antigenemia, lower cryoglobulin levels, and stabilize renal disease. Unfortunately, relapse is usual once the drug is discontinued.

HIV INFECTION (See also Chap. 173) This condition has been associated with focal segmental glomerulosclerosis, acute diffuse proliferative glomerulonephritis, and mesangioproliferative glomerulonephritis, including IgA nephropathy, MPGN, and membranous glomerulopathy. The classic and most common HIV-associated glomerulopathy is an aggressive form of focal segmental glomerulosclerosis, an entity that is termed *HIV-associated nephropathy* (HIVAN). This disease may be the first manifestation of infection in otherwise asymptomatic patients. HIVAN is more common in blacks than in other ethnic groups and is more frequent in intravenous drug abusers with HIV infection than in homosexuals. The disease has been described in all high-risk groups, however, including infants of HIV-positive mothers. Renal biopsy typically reveals visceral epithelial cell swelling, collapse of the glomerular capillary tuft, severe tubulointerstitial inflammation, and microcystic dilatation of renal tubules. The presence of tubuloreticular inclusions and the aggressive clinical course distinguish HIVAN from idiopathic focal segmental glomerulosclerosis. The mechanisms of renal cell injury are still being defined. Viral DNA has been demonstrated in the renal epithelia of HIV-infected patients with and without nephropathy, suggesting that pathogenetic factors, other than infection of cells, are required for induction of disease. The typical clinical correlates of HIVAN are severe nephrotic syndrome and rapid progression to ESRD, occurring in weeks to months. Despite early reports of poor survival of patients on dialysis, more recent studies indicate improved survival for both asymptomatic patients with HIV and patients with full-blown AIDS.

There is no proven therapy for HIVAN. The initial experience with combined highly active antiretroviral therapy (triple therapy) suggests that these regimens have reduced the incidence of nephropathy in HIV-infected patients and improved prognosis in patients with established nephropathy. A number of retrospective studies of glucocorticoids alone or in combination with triple therapy have demonstrated a reduction in proteinuria and slowing of renal progression in some patients with established nephropathy. The precise role of steroids requires further study. ACE inhibitors may confer renoprotection as in other proteinuric renal diseases.

Bacterial Infections Immune-complex glomerulonephritis is a relatively frequent complication of *infective endocarditis* (Chap. 109). Other mechanisms of renal injury in bacterial endocarditis include embolic renal infarction, septic abscesses, acute tubular necrosis secondary to septicemia and drug therapy, disseminated intravascular coagulation, and antibiotic-induced acute interstitial nephritis. Patients typically present with microscopic hematuria, urinary red blood cell casts, pyuria and modest proteinuria (nephrotic range in 25% of patients), and variable degrees of renal failure. Rheumatoid factor is present in 10 to 70%, and circulating immune complexes in 90%. Serum complement levels are usually depressed. Renal biopsy reveals mild focal proliferative glomerulonephritis with mesangial and capillary wall deposition of IgG and C3 by immunofluorescence microscopy and subendothelial, mesangial, and subepithelial electron-dense deposits by electron microscopy. Occasional patients develop diffuse necrotizing glomerulonephritis with crescent formation and present with nephritic syndrome or RPGN. Endocarditis-associated glomerulonephritis typically has a good prognosis and resolves with eradication of the underlying infection.

Suppurative infections such as intrathoracic and intraabdominal abscesses, osteomyelitis, and dental abscesses have been associated with glomerulonephritis. The usual presentation is hematuria, urinary red blood cell casts, proteinuria, and acute renal failure. Oliguria and hypertension are common. Pathologic renal lesions include mesangial proliferative, membranoproliferative, and diffuse proliferative glomerulonephritis with crescents. Immunofluorescence reveals mesangial and capillary wall deposition predominantly of C3, although IgG and IgM may also be seen.

Nephrotic syndrome is a complication in 0.3% of patients with secondary *syphilis* and 8% of patients with congenital syphilis. The usual pathology is membranous glomerulopathy.

Leprosy most commonly causes AA amyloidosis; however, a syndrome resembling acute poststreptococcal glomerulonephritis has also been described.

Protozoan and Parasitic Infections Transient proteinuria (50% of patients) and nephrotic syndrome (<1% of patients) are complications of infection with *Plasmodium falciparum*. Membranoproliferative glomerulonephritis is the usual pathologic lesion and may respond to eradication of infection. *P. malariae* has been associated with diffuse or focal proliferative glomerulonephritis, membranous glomerulopathy, and minimal change disease. Eradication of the malarial infection does not consistently induce remission of the nephrotic syndrome. *Schistosoma mansoni* causes nephrotic syndrome in 5 to 10% of patients, and progression to ESRD is common. The usual pathology is MPGN or mesangial proliferative glomerulonephritis, although membranous glomerulonephritis and amyloidosis are occasionally seen. *Filariasis* can trigger membranous glomerulonephritis (*Loa loa*) and occasionally induces proliferative glomerulonephritis (*Onchocerca volvulus*). *Congenital toxoplasmosis* infection occasionally induces immune-complex glomerulonephritis characterized by mesangial and subendothelial immune deposits that contain *Toxoplasma* antigens. Membranous glomerulopathy and proliferative glomerulonephritis are occasional complications of *hydatid disease* and *trichinosis*, respectively.

GLOMERULAR LESIONS ASSOCIATED WITH NEOPLASIA Infectious glomerulopathies associated with neoplasia include membranous glomerulopathy, MCD, FSGS, immune-complex glomerulonephritis, fibrillary/immunotactoid glomerulonephritis, LCDD, and amyloidosis. Mild proteinuria is common in patients with *solid tumors*, but overt glomerulonephritis is rare. Occasional patients with solid tumors of the lung, gastrointestinal tract, breast, kidney, and ovary develop full-blown nephrotic syndrome, usually due to a membranous glomerulopathy. Estimates of the incidence of occult malignancy in patients presenting with membranous glomerulopathy range from 0.1 to 10%. Most authorities agree that an extensive search for malignancy is not indicated, unless there are other suggestive clinical features. As many as 35% of patients with renal cell carcinoma have mesangial deposition of IgG and C3 visible on immunofluorescence; however, morphologic abnormalities are detected in only 50% of these patients, and clinically significant glomerulopathy is rare. Glomerular amyloidosis has also been described in association with this tumor.

An array of glomerular disease has been reported in patients with lymphoproliferative malignancy. Nephrotic syndrome is a recognized complication of *Hodgkin's lymphoma*, with 70% of cases due to MCD. The latter may occur concurrently with (40 to 45%), precede (10 to 15%), or follow (40 to 50%) diagnosis of the malignancy. It is postulated that a lymphokine or other mediator released by malignant T lymphocytes perturbs podocyte function and alters glomerular permeability in this setting. Nephrotic syndrome typically resolves with successful treatment and relapses with recurrence of disease. Less frequent associations with Hodgkin's lymphoma include FSGS, membranous glomerulopathy, MPGN, proliferative glomerulonephritis, and crescentic glomerulonephritis. MCD, membranous glomerulopathy, MPGN, and crescentic glomerulonephritis have also been reported in patients with *non-Hodgkin's lymphoma*. Glomerulopathy in the context of leukemia is rare. MPGN can complicate *chronic lymphatic leukemia* and related *B cell lymphomas*, particularly when associated with cryoglobulinemia. Other glomerular lesions associated with *paraproteinemia* include primary amyloid, LCDD, proliferative glomerulonephritis induced by cryoglobulinemia, and fibrillary/immunotactoid glomerulopathy. Here again, the renal lesion frequently improves or resolves with successful treatment of the underlying malignancy.

GLOMERULAR LESIONS ASSOCIATED WITH ARTHRITIS AND OTHER FORMS OF CONNECTIVE TISSUE DISEASE Although extraarticular manifestations are present in 35% of patients with rheumatoid arthritis, direct involvement of the kidney by rheumatoid disease is rare, and glomerular injury is usually secondary to AA amyloidosis or a side effect of drug therapy. AA amyloidosis is a complication experienced by 10 to 20% of patients with rheumatoid arthritis, and renal involvement is evident clinically in 3 to 10% of these patients (nephrotic syndrome, renal insufficiency). Amyloidosis is more frequent in patients with rheumatoid arthritis of long duration (>10 years), with circulating rheumatoid factor, and with destructive arthropathy. Less frequent glomerular lesions include mesangial proliferative glomerulonephritis and basement membrane thickening by subepithelial immune deposits. Gold and penicillamine may cause nephrotic syndrome by inducing membranous glomerulopathy, whereas NSAIDs can trigger the nephrotic syndrome by inducing minimal change nephropathy, usually in association with acute interstitial nephritis (see above). Tubulointerstitial injury is the most common form of renal involvement in Sjögren's syndrome and usually presents as either Fanconi's syndrome, distal renal tubular acidosis, or impairment of renal concentrating ability. Glomerulonephritis is relatively rare and should prompt a search for other causes. Membranous glomerulopathy and MPGN are the most common lesions. Anecdotal reports describe successful therapy with glucocorticoids and cytotoxic agents. Occasional cases of focal mesangial proliferative glomerulonephritis with mesangial deposition of IgG and complement have been described in polymyositis/dermatomyositis. Membranous glomerulopathy has also been reported, particularly when polymyositis/dermatomyositis is associated with malignancy. Mixed connective tissue disease is a syndrome that includes features of SLE, scleroderma, and polymyositis and is associated with high titers of anti-ribonucleoprotein antibodies and negative anti-smooth-muscle antibodies. Renal involvement occurs in fewer than 15% of patients and manifests as hematuria and subnephrotic proteinuria. The usual pathologic lesion is membranous glomerulopathy or MPGN. The prognosis is usually excellent, and steroid therapy may be useful in rare patients with progressive renal disease.

FURTHER READING

APPEL G et al: Secondary glomerular diseases, in *Brenner & Rector's The Kidney*, 7th ed, BM Brenner (ed). Philadelphia, Saunders, 2004, p 1381

BRENNER BM et al: Effects of losartan on renal and cardiovascular outcomes in patients with type 2 diabetes and nephropathy. N Engl J Med 345:861, 2001

DAGHESTANI L et al: Renal manifestations of hepatitis C infection. Am J Med 106:347, 1999

FALK R et al: Primary glomerular diseases, in *Brenner & Rector's The Kidney*, 7th ed, BM Brenner (ed). Philadelphia, Saunders, 2004, pp 1293–1380

LEWIS EJ et al: Renoprotective effect of the angiotensin receptor antagonist irbesartan in patients with nephropathy due to type 2 diabetes. N Engl J Med 345:851, 2001

ORTH SR, RITZ E: The nephrotic syndrome. N Engl J Med 338:1202, 1998

PARVING HH et al: Diabetic nephropathy, in *Brenner & Rector's The Kidney*, 7th ed, BM Brenner (ed). Philadelphia, Saunders, 2004, pp 1777–1818

STEHMAN-BREEN C, JOHNSON RJ: Hepatitis C virus–associated glomerulonephritis. Adv Intern Med 43:79, 1998

TAAL MW, BRENNER BM: Renoprotective effects of RAS inhibition: From ACEI to angiotensin II antagonists. Kidney Int 57:1803, 2000

265   TUBULAR DISORDERS
John R. Asplin, Fredric L. Coe

The renal tubular disorders and their morphologic and functional abnormalities, mode of inheritance, and associated abnormalities are summarized in Table 265-1. The individual disorders are discussed in detail below.

AUTOSOMAL DOMINANT POLYCYSTIC KIDNEY DISEASE

Etiology and Pathology Autosomal dominant polycystic kidney disease (ADPKD) has a prevalence of 1:300 to 1:1000 and accounts for ~4% of end-stage renal disease (ESRD) in the United States. Some 90% of cases are inherited as an autosomal dominant trait, and ~10% are spontaneous mutations.

GENETIC CONSIDERATIONS Three forms of ADPKD have been identified. ADPKD-1 accounts for 85% of cases, and the gene has been mapped to chromosome 16p13.3. The gene for ADPKD-2 has been mapped to chromosome 4q21-23. The protein products of the two genes form the polycystin complex, which may regulate cell-cell or cell-matrix interactions. A defect in either of these proteins interrupts the normal function of the polycystin complex, resulting in the same phenotype for two distinct genetic abnormalities. ADPKD-2 appears to have a later age of onset of symptoms and renal failure than ADPKD-1. A rare third form has been described but has not been mapped to a gene at this point.

The kidneys are grossly enlarged, with multiple cysts studding the surface of the kidney. The cysts contain straw-colored fluid that may become hemorrhagic. The cysts are spherical, vary in size from a few millimeters to centimeters, and are distributed evenly throughout the cortex and medulla. Only 1 to 5% of nephrons will develop cysts. Cysts form when a "second hit" causes a somatic mutation in the normal allele of a tubule cell, leading to monoclonal proliferation of the tubular epithelium. The remaining renal parenchyma reveals varying degrees of tubular atrophy, interstitial fibrosis, and nephrosclerosis.

TABLE 265-1 Renal Tubule Defects

Disease	Renal Morphologic Abnormalities	Renal Functional Abnormalities	Mode of Inheritance	Associated Abnormalities
Autosomal dominant polycystic disease	Cortical and medullary cysts	Chronic renal failure, >20 yr	AD	Hepatic cysts, intracranial aneurysms, colonic diverticula
Autosomal recessive polycystic disease	Distal tubule and collecting duct cysts	Chronic renal failure, <20 yr	AR	Congenital hepatic fibrosis
Tuberous sclerosis	Renal cysts and angiomyolipomas	None	AD, S	Skin lesions, hamartomas of the central nervous system
Von Hippel–Lindau disease	Renal cysts, increased risk of renal cell cancer	None	AD	Hemangioblastoma of the retina and central nervous system
Medullary sponge kidney	Dilated collecting ducts	Nephrocalcinosis, hematuria	AD, S	None
Nephronophthisis	Medullary cysts, small kidneys	Chronic renal failure, <20 yr polyuria, salt wasting	AR	Hepatic fibrosis, retinal abnormalities
Medullary cystic disease	Medullary cysts, small kidneys	Chronic renal failure, >20 yr polyuria, salt wasting	AD	None
Liddle's syndrome	None	Hypokalemia, alkalosis, low aldosterone levels	AD	Hypertension
Bartter's syndrome	Juxtaglomerular apparatus hyperplasia	Hypokalemia, alkalosis, high aldosterone levels	AR	None
Gitelman's syndrome	Juxtaglomerular apparatus hypertrophy	Hypokalemia, alkalosis, hypocalciuria	AR	None
Congenital nephrogenic diabetes insipidus	None	Vasopressin renal concentrating defect	XL, AR	None
Renal tubular acidosis, type 1	Nephrocalcinosis	Impaired proton secretion in distal tubule, non-anion-gap metabolic acidosis	AD, AR, S, ACQ	Rickets, osteomalacia, nephrolithiasis
Renal tubular acidosis, type 2	None	Reduced bicarbonate reabsorption, non-anion-gap metabolic acidosis	AR, AD, ACQ	Fanconi syndrome, rickets
Renal tubular acidosis, type 4	Chronic renal insufficiency	Reduced proton and potassium secretion	ACQ	Renal insufficiency
X-linked hypophosphatemia	None	Reduced phosphate reabsorption	XL	Rickets, osteomalacia, normal serum $1,25(OH)_2D_3$
Autosomal dominant hypophosphatemic rickets	None	Reduced phosphate reabsorption	AD	Rickets, osteomalacia
Vitamin D–dependent rickets, type 1	None	Defective renal $1,25(OH)_2D_3$ production	AR	Rickets, osteomalacia, low serum $1,25(OH)_2D_3$
Vitamin D–dependent rickets, type 2	None	Renal resistance to $1,25(OH)_2D_3$	AR, S	Rickets, osteomalacia, high serum $1,25(OH)_2D_3$
Oncogenic osteomalacia	None	Reduced phosphate reabsorption	ACQ	Osteomalacia, mesenchymal tumors
Dent's disease	Interstitial fibrosis, medullary calcifications	Hypercalciuria, low-molecular-weight proteinuria	XL	Renal failure
Isolated hyperuricemia	None	Reduced urate reabsorption	AR	Variable hypercalciuria
Hartnup disorder	None	Reduced reabsorption of neutral amino acids	AR	Dermatitis, diarrhea, dementia
Cystinuria	Cystine stones	Reduced reabsorption of dibasic amino acids	AR	Short stature
Iminoglycinuria	None	Reduced reabsorption of proline, hydroxyproline, and glycine	AR	None
Fanconi syndrome	Swan neck deformity of proximal tubule	Reduced reabsorption of bicarbonate, glucose, phosphate, uric acid, and amino acids	AR	Rickets, osteomalacia, hypokalemia, metabolic acidosis

Note: AD, autosomal dominant; AR, autosomal recessive; S, sporadic; XL, X-linked; ACQ, acquired

Clinical Features The disease may present at any age but most frequently causes symptoms in the third or fourth decade. Patients may develop chronic flank pain from the mass effect of the enlarged kidneys. Acute pain indicates infection, urinary tract obstruction by clot or stone, or sudden hemorrhage into a cyst. Gross and microscopic hematuria are common, and impaired renal concentrating ability frequently leads to nocturia. Nephrolithiasis occurs in 15 to 20% of patients, calcium oxalate and uric acid stones being most common. Low urine pH, low urine citrate, and urinary stasis from distortion of the collecting system by cysts all play a role in stone formation. Hypertension is found in 20 to 30% of children and up to 75% of adults. It is secondary to intrarenal ischemia from distortion of the renal architecture, leading to activation of the renin-angiotensin system. Patients with hypertension have a much more rapid progression to ESRD. Urinary tract infection is common and may involve the bladder or renal interstitium (pyelonephritis) or infect a cyst (pyocyst). Pyocysts can be difficult to diagnose but are more likely to be present if the patient has positive blood cultures, new renal pain, or failed to improve clinically after a standard course of antibiotic therapy.

Progressive decline in renal function is common, with ~50% of patients developing ESRD by age 60. However, there is considerable variation in age of onset of renal failure, even within the same family. Hypertension, recurrent infections, male sex, and early age of diagnosis are related to early onset renal failure. Renal failure usually progresses slowly; if a sudden decrement in kidney function occurs, ureteral obstruction from stone, clot, or compression by a cyst are likely causes. Patients usually have high hematocrits for their level of renal function, as erythropoietin production is high. Fluid overload is uncommon because of a tendency for renal salt wasting.

Extrarenal manifestations of this disease are frequent and underscore the systemic nature of the defect. Hepatic cysts occur in 50 to 70% of patients. Cysts are generally asymptomatic, and liver function is normal, though women may develop massive hepatic cystic disease on occasion. Cyst formation has also been observed in the spleen, pancreas, and ovaries. Intracranial aneurysms are present in 5 to 10% of asymptomatic patients, with potential for permanent neurologic injury or death from subarachnoid hemorrhage. Screening of all ADPKD patients for aneurysms is not recommended, but patients with a family history of subarachnoid hemorrhage should be studied noninvasively with magnetic resonance imaging angiography. Colonic diverticular disease is common, and patients are more likely to develop perforation than the general population with colonic diverticula. Mitral valve prolapse is found in 25% of patients, and the prevalence of aortic and tricuspid valve insufficiency is increased.

Diagnosis Ultrasound is the preferred technique for diagnosis of symptomatic patients and for screening asymptomatic family members. The ability to detect cysts increases with the subject's age: 80 to 90% of ADPKD patients over the age of 20 will have detectable cysts, and almost 100% over the age of 30 will have cysts. At least three to five cysts in each kidney is the standard diagnostic criteria for ADPKD. Computed tomography (CT) scan may be more sensitive than ultrasound in detection of small cysts. Genetic linkage analysis is now available for diagnosis of ADPKD but is reserved for cases where radiographic imaging is negative and the need for definitive diagnosis critical, such as screening family members for potential kidney donation.

℞ TREATMENT

The goals of treatment are to slow the rate of progression of renal disease and minimize symptoms. Hypertension and renal infection should be treated aggressively to maintain renal function. Converting enzyme inhibitors are effective antihypertensive agents, though patients should be closely monitored as some develop renal insufficiency and hyperkalemia. Urinary infection is treated in a standard manner unless a pyocyst is suspected, in which case antibiotics that penetrate cysts should be used, such as trimethoprim-sulfamethoxazole, ciprofloxacin, and chloramphenicol. Chronic pain from cysts can be managed by cyst puncture and sclerosis with ethanol.

AUTOSOMAL RECESSIVE POLYCYSTIC KIDNEY DISEASE

GENETIC CONSIDERATIONS Autosomal recessive polycystic kidney disease (ARPKD) is a rare genetic disease with an incidence of 1:20,000 births. The gene for ARPKD has been localized to chromosome 6p21 and encodes a large novel protein whose function has not yet been determined. In the past, ARPKD was categorized as being of neonatal, infantile, or juvenile form depending on the age of onset and the relative degree of involvement of the kidneys and liver. However, variable clinical presentations within siblings in the same family, as well as the localization of the disease to chromosome 6 in multiple families, support the premise that this is a single genetic disease with variable phenotypic presentation.

At birth the kidneys are enlarged with a smooth external surface. The distal tubules and collecting ducts are dilated into elongated cysts that are arranged in a radial fashion. As the patient ages, the cysts may become more spherical and the disease can be confused with ADPKD. Interstitial fibrosis is also seen as renal function deteriorates. Liver involvement includes proliferation and dilation of intrahepatic bile ducts as well as periportal fibrosis.

Clinical Features The majority of cases are diagnosed in the first year of life, presenting as bilateral abdominal masses. Death in the neonatal period is most commonly due to pulmonary hypoplasia. Hypertension and impaired urinary concentrating ability are common. The time course to ESRD is variable, though many children maintain adequate kidney function for years. Older children present with complications secondary to congenital hepatic fibrosis and generally have less severe kidney disease. Hepatosplenomegaly, portal hypertension, and esophageal varices are frequent complications of ARPKD.

Diagnosis Ultrasound is the most common technique used to diagnose ARPKD, prenatally and in childhood. Ultrasound examination reveals enlarged kidneys with increased echogenicity. At times spherical cysts may be seen, potentially leading to an incorrect diagnosis of ADPKD. A thorough family history and imaging the kidneys of the parents aids in differentiation from other cystic diseases. Hepatic fibrosis seen on imaging studies in association with cystic kidneys supports the diagnosis of ARPKD.

℞ TREATMENT

Aggressive treatment of hypertension and urinary tract infection are the major goals of therapy in order to maintain native renal function as long as possible. Dialysis and transplant are appropriate when kidney failure occurs. Hepatic fibrosis may lead to life-threatening variceal hemorrhage, requiring sclerotherapy or portosystemic shunts.

TUBEROUS SCLEROSIS

Patients with this multisystem disease most commonly present with skin lesions and benign tumors of the central nervous system (Chap. 358). Renal involvement is common; angiomyolipomas are the most frequent abnormality and are usually bilateral. Renal cysts may be present as well and can give an appearance similar to that of ADPKD. Histologically, the cysts are unique—the cyst lining cells are large with an eosinophilic staining cytoplasm and may form hyperplastic nodules that can fill the cyst space.

 GENETIC CONSIDERATIONS One-third of cases are inherited as an autosomal dominant trait, the rest are due to sporadic mutations. Mutations of tumor-suppression genes have been identified on chromosomes 9q34 (*TSC1*) and 16p13 (*TSC2*). Mutations of *TSC2* account for the majority of cases and are more likely to be associated with mental retardation and polycystic kidneys. Tuberous sclerosis may be confused with ADPKD if extrarenal manifestations are minimal.

VON HIPPEL–LINDAU DISEASE

This autosomal dominant disease is characterized by hemangioblastomas of the retina and the central nervous system (Chap. 358). Renal cysts occur in the majority of cases and are usually bilateral. The *VHL* gene, located on chromosome 3p25, is a tumor-suppressor gene that regulates hypoxia-induced transcription factors. It is the same gene that is mutated in sporadic renal cell carcinoma. Renal cell carcinoma may be found in 40 to 70% of patients with von Hippel–Lindau disease and is frequently multifocal. Yearly screening of adults using CT scans has been recommended in an attempt to diagnose renal cell cancers at an early stage.

MEDULLARY SPONGE KIDNEY

Etiology and Pathology Medullary sponge kidney (MSK) is a congenital disorder. Although some cases have apparent autosomal dominant inheritance, most are sporadic. It is found in 0.5 to 1% of all intravenous pyelograms. Males and females are affected equally. The pathologic lesion is cystic dilation of the inner medullary and papillary collecting ducts. Bilateral renal involvement is present in 70% of cases, but not all papillae are equally affected. The dilated ducts are lined by cuboidal epithelium with areas of pseudostratified and stratified squamous epithelium. Calculi are frequently found in the dilated collecting ducts.

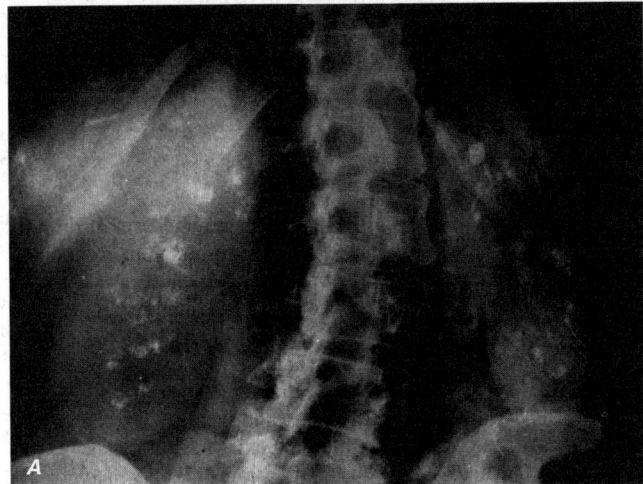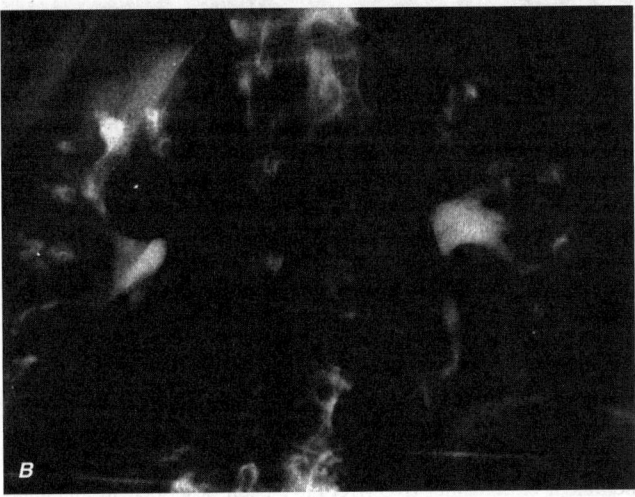

FIGURE 265-1   *A.* Radiographic appearance of medullary sponge kidney. Abdominal flat plate reveals multiple bilateral calcifications. *B.* Radiographic contrast material accumulates in the dilated and cystic terminal collecting ducts and obscures the calcifications.

Clinical Features   Patients generally present in the third or fourth decade with kidney stones, infection, or recurrent hematuria. The disease is most commonly diagnosed by intravenous pyelogram, which shows linear striations radiating into the renal papillae or small cystic collections of contrast in the dilated ducts (Fig. 265-1). Approximately 60% of patients with MSK have stones, and 12% of all stone formers will have MSK. Hypercalciuria occurs with the same frequency in MSK as it does in random stone formers. Papillary nephrocalcinosis occurs more frequently in patients with MSK than in the random stone former. Proteinuria is minimal, if present at all, and renal function is normally preserved unless there is renal damage from recurrent infection or severe stone disease.

℞ TREATMENT

Asymptomatic patients require no specific therapy except to maintain high fluid intake to reduce the risk of nephrolithiasis. If stones are present, standard laboratory evaluation should be done and metabolic abnormalities treated as in any stone former (Chap. 268). Infection should be treated aggressively, and instrumentation of the urinary tract should be minimized to avoid introducing infection.

NEPHRONOPHTHISIS/MEDULLARY CYSTIC DISEASE

GENETIC CONSIDERATIONS   Nephronophthisis (NPH) and medullary cystic disease (MCD) have similar pathologic findings but differ in inheritance pattern and age of onset. NPH is inherited as an autosomal recessive disease. Three forms have been identified, the most common is juvenile (NPH1), which maps to a gene on chromosome 2q13. The infantile form (NPH2) maps to chromosome 9, and the adolescent form (NPH3) maps to chromosome 3. MCD is an autosomal dominant disease. Two loci have been associated with MCD, one on chromosome 1q21 and the other on 16p12. In both NPH and MCD the kidneys tend to be small, with cysts throughout the medulla; the cortex and papilla rarely have cysts. The cysts originate in the collecting ducts, distal convoluted tubules, and loops of Henle and range in size from 1 to 10 mm. Sclerotic glomeruli, tubule atrophy, and interstitial fibrosis are frequent findings on biopsy.

Clinical Features   Patients with NPH present during childhood with symptoms of polyuria, growth retardation, anemia, and progressive renal insufficiency. ESRD develops at an average age of 2 years in NPH2, 13 years in NPH1, and 19 years in NPH3. NPH accounts for 2 to 10% of renal failure in children. Hepatic fibrosis and cerebellar ataxia have been reported in association with NPH. MCD presents in the third or fourth decade, though some cases may be diagnosed in the elderly population. Presenting symptoms in MCD are the same as in NPH except for growth retardation. In addition, MCD does not have extrarenal abnormalities. Severe salt wasting can be seen, though this is usually a transient phase that resolves as the disease progresses to ESRD. Other features of tubule damage are often found, including hyperkalemia and hyperchloremic metabolic acidosis. Proteinuria is mild, and hematuria is rare.

Diagnosis   The diagnosis is suggested by a family history of renal disease. The pattern of inheritance and age of onset aid in distinguishing NPH/MCD from other inherited diseases. Radiographic studies show small kidneys, loss of the corticomedullary junction, and multiple cysts in the medulla. CT scan is more sensitive than ultrasound in making the diagnosis. The majority of cases of NPH can be diagnosed using molecular genetics techniques. Open renal biopsy, including medullary tissue, may be required for diagnosis in some cases.

℞ TREATMENT

Treatment is mainly supportive, as there is no specific therapy to prevent loss of renal function. Patients with salt wasting require a large oral intake of salt and water to maintain adequate extracellular volume. Alkali replacement and erythropoietin are required for acidosis and anemia, respectively. Renal transplantation has been performed in numerous patients, and the disease does not recur.

LIDDLE'S SYNDROME

Liddle's syndrome is a rare autosomal dominant disorder with a clinical presentation of hyperaldosteronism, consisting of hypertension, hypokalemia, and metabolic alkalosis. However, aldosterone levels are undetectable and renin levels are suppressed. The syndrome is caused by activating mutations in the amiloride-sensitive sodium channel, which leads to increased distal tubule sodium reabsorption and potassium wasting. Potassium-sparing diuretics that block the sodium channel, such as amiloride and triamterene, used in conjunction with a low-sodium diet, are effective in treating the hypertension and electrolyte abnormalities. Spironolactone is ineffective, since the disease is not mediated via the aldosterone receptor.

BARTTER'S SYNDROME

Clinical Features   Hypokalemia secondary to renal potassium wasting, metabolic alkalosis, and normal to low blood pressure are the clinical features of Bartter's syndrome. Two variants of Bartter's syndrome have been described. *Antenatal Bartter's syndrome* (also known as *hyperprostaglandin E syndrome*) is characterized by polyhydramnios and premature delivery. During infancy, episodes of fever and dehydration are common and can lead to growth retardation. Nephrocalcinosis secondary to hypercalciuria is frequent. Prostaglandin E production is very high. Most cases of *classic Bartter's syndrome* present during childhood. Symptoms such as weakness and cramps are secondary to the hypokalemia. Polyuria and nocturia are common due to the hypokalemia-induced nephrogenic diabetes insipidus. Nephrocalcinosis is less common than in the antenatal form. Both forms are inherited as autosomal recessive traits. Although rarely required for diagnosis, renal biopsy reveals hyperplasia of the juxtaglomerular apparatus and prominence of medullary interstitial cells, with variable degrees of interstitial fibrosis, though these are not pathognomonic for the syndrome.

GENETIC CONSIDERATIONS Abnormalities in three renal tubule transport proteins have been shown to cause Bartter's syndrome. Mutations in either the bumetanide-sensitive Na-K-2Cl cotransporter or the apical K^+ channel (ROMK) have been described in antenatal Bartter's. Mutations of a basolateral chloride channel (CLC-Kb) are found in patients with classic Bartter's syndrome. All of these mutations lead to a loss of Na^+ and Cl^- reabsorption in the loop of Henle. The resultant volume depletion activates the renin-angiotensin system. Distal delivery of NaCl and water are high in the presence of high aldosterone, promoting secretion of K^+ and H^+ ions. Prostaglandin overproduction is mediated by volume depletion, hypokalemia, and high angiotensin II and kallikrein levels. Increased prostaglandin production contributes to the severity of disease by inducing resistance to the pressor effects of angiotensin II and reducing reabsorption in the thick ascending limb of the loop of Henle.

Diagnosis Hypokalemia, metabolic alkalosis, and normal to low blood pressure are the clinical findings characteristic of Bartter's syndrome. The differential diagnosis includes vomiting, surreptitious diuretic abuse, and magnesium deficiency. Chronic vomiting can be diagnosed by a low urine Cl^- concentration. Magnesium deficiency causes kaluresis and alkalosis, simulating Bartter's syndrome. Serum and urine magnesium will be low in such cases. Diuretic abuse produces metabolic abnormalities indistinguishable from Bartter's syndrome. Urine should be screened for diuretics multiple times before the diagnosis of Bartter's is made in a patient without a family history of the disorder.

℞ **TREATMENT**

Dietary intake of sodium and potassium should be liberal. Potassium supplements are usually required. Spironolactone will reduce potassium wasting. Nonsteroidal antiinflammatory drugs (NSAIDs) are useful, particularly in patients with antenatal Bartter's syndrome, since they reduce prostaglandin production. Angiotensin-converting enzyme (ACE) inhibitors may be beneficial in some patients.

GITELMAN'S SYNDROME

Gitelman's syndrome shares many features with Bartter's syndrome including hypokalemia, metabolic alkalosis, salt wasting, elevated renin and aldosterone levels, and normal blood pressure. Clinically it is distinguished from Bartter's by hypomagnesemia and hypocalciuria. Gitelman's syndrome is usually diagnosed during adolescence or adulthood, with weakness, fatigue, muscle cramps, and nocturia being the most common symptoms. The syndrome is inherited as an autosomal recessive trait and is due to mutations in the thiazide-sensitive Na-Cl transporter. The reduced Na^+ reabsorption in the distal convoluted tubule leads to volume depletion and hypokalemia. Loss of activity of the thiazide-sensitive transporter increases tubule calcium reabsorption, leading to the classic finding of hypocalciuria in Gitelman's syndrome. Treatment consists of liberal dietary sodium intake, potassium and magnesium supplements, and potassium sparing diuretics. Unlike in Bartter's syndrome, NSAIDs and ACE inhibitors are not effective.

CONGENITAL NEPHROGENIC DIABETES INSIPIDUS

GENETIC CONSIDERATIONS This rare genetic disorder is most commonly inherited as an X-linked disease, with full expression in males and variable penetrance in females. Vasopressin acts through two receptors; type 1 receptors are located in the vasculature, while type 2 receptors are found in the collecting ducts of the kidney. In X-linked nephrogenic diabetes insipidus (NDI), only the actions requiring type 2 receptors are abnormal. Mutations of the type 2 vasopressin receptor lead to misfolding and trapping of the receptor in the endoplasmic reticulum, with no receptor present on the cell surface. Less frequently, NDI may be inherited as an autosomal trait, either recessive or dominant, in which mutations in the gene for the water channels in collecting duct cells (aquaporin 2) lead to abnormal cell routing of aquaporin 2.

Clinical Features The clinical presentation is that of persistent polyuria, dehydration, and hypotonic urine in the presence of hypernatremia. Vasopressin levels are appropriately elevated in the hypertonic state, but renal response is lacking. About 90% of cases are diagnosed in the first 2.5 years of life. Recurrent hypernatremia may lead to seizures or mental retardation. Once old enough to satisfy their thirst, children will be clinically stable though in a chronic state of polyuria and polydypsia. Renal function is normal, and radiographic studies of the urinary system reveal dilated ureters and bladder secondary to the chronically high urine flow. Since the most common form of the disease is X-linked, most patients are male. Heterozygous females generally have mild concentrating defects, though a few have phenotypic expression similar to males due to skewed X-chromosome inactivation.

℞ **TREATMENT**

Treatment is aimed at maintaining adequate hydration. In the infant, low-solute feedings and high water intake are generally adequate. Addition of a thiazide diuretic reduces urine flow by inhibiting sodium reabsorption in the distal convoluted tubule. This lowers free water production and, by causing extracellular volume contraction, increases proximal salt and water reabsorption, reducing delivery to the distal nephron. Amiloride or indomethacin are frequently used to potentiate the effects of thiazide diuretics. Administration of vasopressin and its analogues has no role in the management of this disorder.

RENAL TUBULAR ACIDOSIS

Renal tubular acidosis (RTA) is a disorder of renal acidification out of proportion to the reduction in glomerular filtration rate. RTA is characterized by hyperchloremic metabolic acidosis with a normal serum anion gap $[Na^+ - (Cl^- + HCO_3^-)]$. There are multiple forms of RTA, depending on which aspects of renal acid handling have been affected. Defective bicarbonate reabsorption in the proximal tubule, suppressed renal ammoniagenesis, and inadequate distal tubule proton secretion are the abnormalities that produce RTA. Three major forms of RTA exist (Table 265-2). Types 1 and 2 may be inherited or acquired. Type 4 is usually acquired and is associated with either hypoaldosteronism or tubular hyporesponsiveness to mineralocorticoids. *Type 3 is a very rare form of RTA with features of both type 1 and type 2 RTA.* It is due to deficiency carbonic anhydrase II, an enzyme present in both the proximal and distal tubules. It is an autosomal recessive disease associated with osteopetrosis and mental retardation.

TYPE 1 (DISTAL) RTA In this disorder the distal nephron does not lower urine pH normally, either because the collecting ducts permit excessive back-diffusion of hydrogen ions from lumen to blood or because there is inadequate transport of hydrogen ions. Excretion of titratable acid is low, as inadequate proton secretion prevents titration of urinary buffers such as phosphate. Urine ammonium excretion is inappropriately low for the level of acidosis, as the defect in acidification reduces the ion trapping required for ammonium excretion. Urinary concentration and potassium conservation also tend to be impaired.

Chronic acidosis lowers tubule reabsorption of calcium, causing renal hypercalciuria and mild secondary hyperparathyroidism. Buffering of bone by the daily metabolic acid load contributes to hypercalciuria. Urine citrate excretion is low, as acidosis and hypokalemia stimulate proximal tubule reabsorption of citrate. The hypercalciuria, alkaline urine, and low levels of urine citrate cause calcium phosphate stones and nephrocalcinosis. Growth retardation is common and improves with correction of the acidosis by alkali. In both children and adults, bone diseases may result, in part, from acidosis-induced loss of bone material and inadequate production of 1,25-dihydroxyvitamin D_3 [1,25$(OH)_2D_3$]. Since the kidney does not conserve potassium or concentrate the urine normally, polyuria and hypokalemia occur. With the stress of an intercurrent illness, acidosis and hypokalemia can be life-threatening.

TABLE 265-2 Comparison of Normal Anion-Gap Acidoses

Finding	Type 1 RTA	Type 2 RTA	Type 4 RTA	GI Bicarbonate Loss
Normal anion-gap acidosis	Yes	Yes	Yes	Yes
Minimum urine pH	>5.5	<5.5	<5.5	5 to 6
% Filtered bicarbonate excreted	<10	>15	<10	<10
Serum potassium	Low	Low	High	Low
Fanconi syndrome	No	Yes	No	No
Stones/nephrocalcinosis	Yes	No	No	No
Daily acid excretion	Low	Normal	Low	High
Urine anion gap	Positive	Positive	Positive	Negative
Daily bicarbonate replacement needs	<4 mmol/kg	>4 mmol/kg	<4 mmol/kg	Variable

Note: RTA, renal tubular acidosis.

GENETIC CONSIDERATIONS Type 1 RTA can be familial, with autosomal dominant as the most common mode of inheritance. Autosomal recessive and sporadic cases have been reported. Mutations in the basolateral chloride-bicarbonate exchanger (*AE1*) of intercalated cells have been identified in the autosomal dominant form. The autosomal recessive form has been associated with mutations in the H^+-ATPase in some families. Sensorineural deafness frequently accompanies the H^+-ATPase mutation. Other hereditary diseases that cause type 1 RTA include galactosemia, Ehler-Danlos syndrome, Fabry's disease, MSK, Wilson's disease, and hereditary elliptocytosis. The majority of cases of type 1 RTA are secondary to a systemic disorder such as Sjögren's syndrome, hypergammaglobulinemia, chronic active hepatitis, or lupus.

Diagnosis The diagnosis of type 1 RTA is suggested by a normal anion gap metabolic acidosis with a simultaneous urine pH > 5.5. Calcium phosphate stones or nephrocalcinosis support the diagnosis, though they are not present in all cases. Bicarbonaturia is not present, which distinguishes this disorder from type 2 RTA. If acidosis is not severe and urine pH is equivocal, an oral ammonium chloride loading test may confirm the diagnosis. As systemic acidosis worsens with ammonium chloride, urine pH does not fall below 5.5 in patients with type I RTA.

Chronic diarrheal states cause normal anion gap acidosis and hypokalemia; urine pH may be >5.5 if ammonium production is very high. The urine anion gap ($Na^+ + K^+ - Cl^-$) can be used to estimate renal ammonium production and distinguish RTA from gastrointestinal bicarbonate loss. Normally the urine anion gap is positive, as unmeasured anions exceed unmeasured cations. If urine ammonium levels are high, urine chloride concentration increases to balance the charge. Unmeasured cation (predominantly ammonium) now exceeds unmeasured anion, and the urine anion gap is negative. During metabolic acidosis, a negative urine anion gap suggests an extrarenal cause of acidosis, whereas a positive urine anion gap suggests RTA. The urine anion gap cannot be used if there are large amounts of unmeasured anions, such as bicarbonate or ketones, in the urine.

Rx **TREATMENT**

Alkali supplements are the standard therapy. Enough alkali is prescribed to titrate the daily metabolic acid production, usually in the range of 0.5 to 2.0 mmol/kg body weight in four to six divided doses per day. Sodium bicarbonate and Shohl's solution are common treatments. Potassium alkali salts can be used if hypokalemia is a persistent problem. Citrate requires less frequent dosing than bicarbonate salts as it is metabolized to bicarbonate after absorption. The dose of alkali should be raised until acidosis and hypercalciuria are both eliminated.

Requirements for alkali may rise during intercurrent illnesses but are <4 mmol/kg body weight per day. The relatives of patients with idiopathic type 1 RTA should be screened for this disorder, as timely treatment can prevent growth retardation in children. Incomplete RTA secondary to idiopathic hypercalciuria is best treated using thiazide diuretics in conjunction with potassium citrate (Chap. 268).

TYPE 2 (PROXIMAL) RTA Type 2 RTA usually occurs as part of a generalized disorder of proximal tubule function, presenting as hyperchloremic acidosis with other features of Fanconi syndrome. Bicarbonate reabsorption in the proximal tubule is defective. At normal concentrations of plasma bicarbonate, large amounts of bicarbonate are delivered to the distal tubule, overwhelming the absorptive capacity of the distal tubule and resulting in bicarbonaturia. As plasma bicarbonate levels fall, the lower filtered load of bicarbonate can be reabsorbed by the proximal tubule, resulting in normal distal delivery of bicarbonate. At this point the distal nephron can acidify the urine normally, resulting in normal excretion of daily metabolic acid production, albeit at a low serum bicarbonate level. Hypophosphatemia and low calcitriol levels are common and may lead to rickets or osteomalacia. Hypercalciuria occurs, but stone formation is unusual since urine citrate levels are normal or high because of reduced proximal tubule citrate reabsorption. Type 2 RTA without Fanconi syndrome may be inherited as an autosomal dominant or recessive disorder. Mutations in the Na^+-HCO_3^- cotransporter (NBC-1) have been reported in some families with the autosomal recessive form. Type 2 RTA may be acquired in association with other diseases (see "Fanconi Syndrome," below) or be secondary to drugs that inhibit carbonic anhydrase activity, such as acetazolamide.

Type 2 RTA may be distinguished from type 1 RTA by the ability to normally acidify urine during spontaneous or ammonium chloride–induced acidosis. Correction of acidosis with bicarbonate will result in bicarbonaturia in type 2 RTA but not in type 1 RTA. Fractional excretion of bicarbonate is >15% at normal or near-normal serum bicarbonate levels. In distal RTA it is <10%. It is unusual for serum bicarbonate levels to fall below 15 mmol/L in proximal RTA. The urine anion gap will be positive, as ammonium excretion is normal to handle daily acid production but is not elevated as in nonrenal causes of acidosis.

Rx **TREATMENT**

Children should be treated to prevent growth retardation. Alkali must be given in large amounts daily, 5 to 15 mmol/kg body weight per day, because bicarbonate is rapidly excreted in the urine. A thiazide diuretic can be used in conjunction with a low-salt diet to reduce the amount of bicarbonate required. Potassium requirements increase during alkali therapy due to increased renal loss of potassium from bicarbonaturia.

TYPE 4 RTA In type 4 RTA, also called *hyperkalemic distal RTA*, distal tubule secretion of both potassium and hydrogen ions is abnormal, resulting in hyperchloremic acidosis with hyperkalemia. Type 4 RTA is an acquired disorder; a moderate degree of renal insufficiency is present in the majority of patients. Patients with type 4 RTA can be differentiated from patients with type 1 since they have an acid urine (pH < 5.5) during periods of acidosis (Table 265-2) and hyperkalemia. They differ from type 2 patients by having a fractional excretion of bicarbonate <10% and a daily bicarbonate requirement of 1 to 3 mmol/kg body weight per day. Because potassium and hydrogen ion excretion are abnormal, such patients are considered to have generalized distal nephron dysfunction due to either insufficient aldosterone production or intrinsic renal disease causing aldosterone resistance. The resulting hyperkalemia reduces proximal tubule ammonia production, in addition to the inadequate proton secretion, leading to inadequate excretion of the daily metabolic proton load. These patients have an acid urine despite reduced proton secretion because there is inadequate ammonia to buffer protons in the distal tubule. If buffer delivery to the distal nephron is increased, urine pH will rise despite persistent acidosis.

Type 4 RTA due to inadequate aldosterone production has multiple etiologies. Hyporeninemic hypoaldosteronism is the most common cause of type 4 RTA and is usually associated with diabetic nephropathy. Plasma levels of renin and aldosterone are subnormal, even during extracellular volume depletion. NSAIDs, ACE inhibitors, trimethoprim, and heparin can reduce aldosterone production and produce a type 4 RTA. Drug-induced type 4 RTA is usually seen in patients with preexisting renal insufficiency. Reduced aldosterone production may be due to adrenal disease, occurring as either an isolated defect or as part of a more generalized adrenal disorder (Chap. 321). Renin levels are normal to high in adrenal disorders.

Patients with tubular resistance to aldosterone present with the same clinical features as those with hyporeninemic hypoaldosteronism. A tubulointerstitial process damages the distal tubule, restricting potassium and hydrogen ion excretion, despite adequate aldosterone levels. Obstructive uropathy and sickle cell disease are the most common causes of acquired tubular resistance to aldosterone. Hyporeninemic hypoaldosteronism can be found in addition to tubular aldosterone resistance in many patients. Potassium-sparing diuretics can cause a type 4 RTA by producing an aldosterone resistant state.

Rx TREATMENT

The main goal of therapy is to reduce serum potassium, as acidosis will usually improve once the hyperkalemic block of ammonium production is removed. All patients should be placed on a low-potassium diet. Any drug that suppresses aldosterone production or blocks aldosterone effect should be discontinued. Mineralocorticoid supplementation with fludrocortisone, 0.1 to 0.2 mg/d, will improve hyperkalemia and acidosis; however, the patients who also have a partial tubule resistance to mineralocorticoid will require a higher dose. Mineralocorticoid replacement may not be appropriate for patients with hypertension or a history of heart failure. In such situations, a loop diuretic with a liberal sodium intake can usually promote adequate potassium excretion. Exchange resins will reduce potassium levels but are usually not tolerated well enough to be used for long-term treatment.

PSEUDOHYPOALDOSTERONISM

GENETIC CONSIDERATIONS Type I pseudohyperaldosteronism is transmitted as either an autosomal dominant or recessive trait. The autosomal dominant form is caused by mutations in the mineralocorticoid receptor gene; the autosomal recessive disease is caused by inactivating mutations in the amiloride-sensitive epithelial sodium channel. The aldosterone resistance leads to hyperkalemia, metabolic acidosis, salt wasting, and volume depletion, which present during childhood. Plasma renin and aldosterone levels are elevated. Treatment includes salt supplements, alkali, and potassium restriction.

Type II pseudohypoaldosteronism (also known as *Gordon syn-*

drome) presents as hypertension, hyperkalemia, and metabolic acidosis with normal renal function. The disease is inherited as an autosomal dominant trait and appears to be secondary to overactivity of the thiazide sensitive Na-Cl cotransporter. Two genes have been linked to the disease and both encode WNK kinases that are expressed in the distal tubule. Thiazide diuretics control the hypertension and correct the electrolyte disorders.

VITAMIN D DISORDERS

X-LINKED HYPOPHOSPHATEMIC RICKETS (See also Chap. 331) This disorder is an X-linked dominant disorder characterized by hypophosphatemia with renal phosphate wasting, rickets, and short stature. Hypophosphatemia is present soon after birth; rachitic bowing of the legs develops when the child begins to walk. Children have growth retardation, which is limited almost entirely to the lower extremities. Dentition is delayed, and skull abnormalities are common. Presentation in adults ranges from disabling bone pain to no active symptoms, but generally some physical sign of childhood disease, such as short stature or bowed legs, is present. Overgrowth of bone at joints or sites of muscle attachment may reduce the mobility of the joint or cause nerve entrapment.

Hypophosphatemia secondary to reduced renal phosphate reabsorption is the hallmark of the disease. Serum calcium levels are usually normal, with low intestinal absorption and renal excretion of calcium. Serum alkaline phosphatase and osteocalcin levels are elevated. Parathyroid hormone levels are normal, as would be expected with normal serum calcium. $1,25(OH)_2D_3$ levels are usually normal, though in the setting of hypophosphatemia $1,25(OH)_2D_3$ levels should be elevated. The disease is caused by inactivating mutations in the PHEX gene, located on chromosome Xp22.1, which codes for a membrane-bound endopeptidase. Circulating humoral factors, phosphatonins, that are normally inactivated by the PHEX endopeptidase accumulate in the serum and reduce proximal tubule phosphate reabsorption and $1,25(OH)_2D_3$ production.

Rx TREATMENT

The goal of therapy is to raise serum phosphorous to normal or near-normal levels to improve bone mineralization. Oral neutral phosphate, 1 to 4 g/d in four to six doses, combined with calcitriol is an effective therapy that improves growth rate, reduces bone pain, and leads to radiographically evident improvement of the bone disease. Patients should be closely monitored during therapy as they may develop nephrocalcinosis and renal insufficiency.

AUTOSOMAL DOMINANT HYPOPHOSPHATEMIC RICKETS This disorder usually presents during childhood with low serum phosphate from renal phosphate wasting, rickets, and dental abnormalities. There is significant phenotypic variability with some subjects not presenting until adulthood and other cases spontaneously correcting metabolic abnormalities after puberty. The disorder has been linked to a locus on chromosome 12p13, and mutations have been identified in the gene product, fibroblast growth factor (FGF-23). FGF-23 may act as a phosphatonin and promote renal phosphate wasting.

VITAMIN D–DEPENDENT RICKETS TYPE I

GENETIC CONSIDERATIONS This is an autosomal recessive disorder in which $1,25(OH)_2D_3$ levels are very low but 25-hydroxy-vitamin D levels are normal. The disease is caused by inactivating mutations in the gene encoding the 1α-hydroxylase enzyme, leading to a clinical syndrome of vitamin D deficiency.

Symptoms usually appear before the age of 2, including rickets and growth retardation. Levels of serum calcium and phosphorous are low, but that of alkaline phosphatase is elevated. Intestinal calcium absorption and urinary calcium excretion are low. Parathyroid hormone is elevated in response to the hypocalcemia, resulting in increased urinary phosphate losses.

℞ TREATMENT

Calcitriol (0.5 to 1 μg/d) leads to rapid correction of the biochemical abnormalities and resolution of the bone disease. Calcium and phosphorous supplementation are usually not required.

VITAMIN D–DEPENDENT RICKETS TYPE II (See also Chap. 331)　End-organ resistance to 1,25(OH)$_2$D$_3$ is the pathogenesis of this disorder. Serum calcium and phosphate levels are low, secondary hyperparathyroidism is present, and 1,25(OH)$_2$D$_3$ levels are elevated. Inheritance is usually autosomal recessive, though sporadic cases have been reported. Most patients present during childhood with rickets, though some have a milder form of disease not recognized until adulthood. Alopecia is common and tends to be associated with the more severe childhood form of the disease. Mutations in the vitamin D receptor reduce tissue response to 1,25(OH)$_2$D$_3$. Pharmacologic doses of calcitriol (5 to 30 μg/d) along with mineral supplementation will improve the biochemical disorders and bone disease, though some patients have no response to massive doses of calcitriol.

ONCOGENIC OSTEOMALACIA　This syndrome generally occurs in adults with highly vascular mesenchymal tumors. Patients present with bone pain and muscle weakness. Symptoms may be present for years before the correct diagnosis is made. Over 90% of the tumors are benign, and most are found in the extremities or maxillofacial region. Hypophosphatemia secondary to renal phosphate wasting and low levels of 1,25(OH)$_2$D$_3$ are the major biochemical abnormalities. Serum calcium and parathyroid hormone levels are normal. The tumors produce humoral agents, phosphatonins, that reduce proximal tubule phosphate reabsorption and 1α-hydroxylase activity. FGF-23 is a fibroblast growth factor that has been identified as a potential phosphatonin. Removal of the tumor leads to rapid resolution of the disease. Octreotide therapy reduces secretion of phosphatonins and improves serum phosphorus in some patients with oncogenic osteomalacia.

DENT'S DISEASE

This disorder presents as hypercalciuria, low-molecular-weight proteinuria, calcium nephrolithiasis, and nephrocalcinosis in male children. Progression to renal failure is common. Phosphaturia, glycosuria, aminoaciduria, and other features of Fanconi's syndrome may be present. Females carrying the gene are asymptomatic except for low-molecular-weight proteinuria. Kidney biopsy reveals tubular atrophy, interstitial fibrosis, and medullary calcifications. The gene has been mapped to the short arm of the X chromosome and encodes a voltage-gated chloride channel (CLC-5). Treatment with thiazide diuretics improves the hypercalciuria, but whether thiazides help preserve renal function is not known.

ISOLATED HYPOURICEMIA (See also Chap. 338)

This disorder is generally inherited as an autosomal recessive trait. Most commonly there is deficient urate reabsorption in the proximal tubule, though some patients have been demonstrated to oversecrete urate. Serum uric acid is usually <120 μmol/L (2 mg/dL) and hyperuricosuria is common, possibly due to decreased intestinal urate excretion. Hypouricemia is usually an incidental finding, as patients with this disorder are asymptomatic except for an increased risk of nephrolithiasis. Other disorders associated with hypouricemia include Fanconi syndrome, Wilson's disease, Hodgkin's disease, and Hartnup disease. No treatment is required except for high fluid intake to prevent kidney stones. Alkali and allopurinol may be used to prevent stones if fluids alone are not sufficient.

SELECTED DISORDERS OF AMINO ACID TRANSPORT

HARTNUP DISEASE　This disorder is characterized by reduced intestinal absorption and renal reabsorption of neutral amino acids. The defect involves an amino acid transporter on the brush border of the jejunum and the proximal tubule. Intestinal absorption of free amino acids is reduced, though the neutral amino acids can be absorbed when present in di- and tripeptides. Degradation of unabsorbed tryptophan by intestinal bacteria produces indolic acids that are absorbed and subsequently excreted at high levels in the urine of these patients. The disorder is inherited as an autosomal recessive trait with an estimated incidence of 1 in 24,000 live births. Linkage analysis suggests a locus on chromosome 5.

The majority of individuals with this disorder are asymptomatic. Approximately 10 to 20% present with clinical symptoms similar to those seen in pellagra, including a photosensitive erythematous scaly rash, intermittent cerebral ataxia, delirium, and diarrhea. Short stature is noted in some patients. The symptoms are thought to be due to deficiency in the essential amino acid tryptophan and resultant inadequate synthesis of nicotinamide. Though the inheritance of the disorder is autosomal recessive, the development of symptomatic disease appears to be multifactorial. Diet, environment, and polygenic traits controlling plasma amino acid levels all contribute to development of symptoms.

Clinically affected patients can be differentiated from patients with pellagra by dietary history and the presence of aminoaciduria. Diagnosis is made by the characteristic finding of large amounts of neutral amino acids in the urine. It can easily be distinguished from generalized aminoaciduria by the normal excretion of proline. There are no other renal tubule defects as in Fanconi syndrome. Heterozygotes have normal urinary amino acid excretion.

℞ TREATMENT

Symptomatic individuals should receive oral nicotinamide, 40 to 200 mg/d, and a high-protein diet to compensate for the poor amino acid absorption. Some patients who do not respond to nicotinamide may improve with tryptophan ethyl ester, which is lipid soluble and can be absorbed without an active transport system.

FANCONI SYNDROME

 GENETIC CONSIDERATIONS　Fanconi syndrome is a generalized defect in proximal tubule transport involving amino acids, glucose, phosphate, uric acid, sodium, potassium, bicarbonate, and proteins. Idiopathic Fanconi syndrome may be inherited as an autosomal dominant, autosomal recessive, or X-linked trait. The autosomal dominant form has been mapped to chromosome 15. Sporadic cases are also seen. A variety of inherited systemic disorders are also associated with Fanconi syndrome including Wilson's disease, galactosemia, tyrosinemia, cystinosis, fructose intolerance, and Lowe's oculocerebral syndrome. The syndrome may be acquired in multiple myeloma, amyloid, heavy metal toxicity, and from chemotherapeutic drugs.

The patients may present with a wide array of laboratory abnormalities including proximal renal tubular acidosis, glucosuria with a normal serum glucose, hypophosphatemia, hypouricemia, hypokalemia, generalized aminoaciduria, and low-molecular-weight proteinuria. Some patients do not have abnormalities in all proximal tubule transporters and may present with only a few of the laboratory findings. Rickets and osteomalacia are common findings secondary to the hypophosphatemia; production of calcitriol may also be abnormal. Metabolic acidosis also contributes to the bone disease. Polyuria, salt wasting, and hypokalemia may be quite severe.

℞ TREATMENT

Treatment includes phosphate supplements and calcitriol to heal the bone lesions, alkali for the acidosis, and liberal intake of salt and water. Alkali in the form of potassium salts may be particularly useful in the patient with RTA and hypokalemia. Aminoaciduria, glucosuria, hypouricemia, and low-molecular-weight proteinuria do not require treatment.

FURTHER READING

CRUZ DN et al: Gitelman's syndrome revisited: An evaluation of symptoms and health-related quality of life. Kidney Int 59:710, 2001

HILDEBRANDT F, OTTO E: Molecular genetics of nephronophthisis and medullary cystic kidney disease. J Am Soc Nephrol 11:1753, 2000

IGARISH P, SOMLO S: Genetics and pathogenesis of polycystic kidney disease. J Am Soc Nephrol 13:2384, 2002

JAN SM, LEVINE MA: Molecular pathogenesis of hypophosphatemic rickets. J Clin Endocrinol Metab 87:2467, 2002

PIRSON Y et al: Management of cerebral aneurysms in autosomal dominant polycystic kidney disease. J Am Soc Nephrol 13:269, 2002

SEUFERT J et al: Octreotide therapy for tumor-induced osteomalacia. N Engl J Med 345:1883, 2001

SORIANO JR: Renal tubular acidosis: The clinical entity. J Am Soc Nephrol 13:2160, 2002

WARD CJ et al: The gene mutated in autosomal recessive polycystic kidney disease encodes a large, receptor-like protein. Nat Genet 30:259, 2002

WILSON FH et al: Human hypertension caused by mutations in WNK kinases. Science 293:1107, 2001

266 TUBULOINTERSTITIAL DISEASES OF THE KIDNEY
Alan S. L. Yu, Barry M. Brenner

Primary tubulointerstitial diseases of the kidney, as distinct from the disorders considered in Chaps. 264 and 267, are characterized by histologic and functional abnormalities that involve the tubules and interstitium to a greater degree than the glomeruli and renal vasculature (Table 266-1). Secondary tubulointerstitial disease occurs as a consequence of progressive glomerular or vascular injury. Morphologically, acute forms of these disorders are characterized by interstitial edema, often associated with cortical and medullary infiltration by both mononuclear cells and polymorphonuclear leukocytes, and patchy areas of tubule cell necrosis. In more chronic forms, interstitial fibrosis predominates, inflammatory cells are typically mononuclear, and abnormalities of the tubules tend to be more widespread, as evidenced by atrophy, luminal dilatation, and thickening of tubule basement membranes. Because of the nonspecific nature of the histology, particularly in chronic tubulointerstitial diseases, biopsy specimens rarely provide a specific diagnosis. The urine sediment is also unlikely to be diagnostic, except in allergic forms of acute tubulointerstitial disease, in which eosinophils may predominate in the urinary sediment.

Defects in renal function often accompany these alterations of tubule and interstitial structure (Table 266-2). Proximal tubule dysfunction may be manifested as selective reabsorptive defects leading to hypokalemia, aminoaciduria, glycosuria, phosphaturia, uricosuria, or bicarbonaturia [proximal or type II renal tubular acidosis (RTA); Chap. 265]. In combination, these defects constitute the *Fanconi syndrome*. Proteinuria, predominantly of low-molecular-weight proteins, is usually modest, rarely exceeding 2 g/d.

Defects in urinary acidification and concentrating ability often represent the most troublesome of the tubule dysfunctions encountered in patients with tubulointerstitial disease. Hyperchloremic metabolic acidosis often develops at a relatively early stage in the course. Patients with this finding generally elaborate urine of maximal acidity (pH $\leq$ 5.3). In such patients the defect in acid excretion is usually caused by a reduced capacity to generate and excrete ammonia due to the reduction in renal mass. Preferential damage to the collecting ducts, as in amyloidosis or chronic obstructive uropathy, may also predispose to distal or type I RTA, characterized by high urine pH ($\geq$5.5) during spontaneous or NH_4Cl-induced metabolic acidosis. Patients with tubulointerstitial diseases affecting predominantly medullary and papillary structures may also exhibit concentrating defects, with resultant nocturia and polyuria. Analgesic nephropathy and sickle cell disease are prototypes of this form of injury.

TOXINS

Although the kidney is vulnerable to toxic injury, renal damage by a variety of nephrotoxins often goes unrecognized because the manifestations of such injury are usually nonspecific in nature and insidious in onset. Diagnosis largely depends on a history of exposure to a certain toxin. Particular attention should be paid to the occupational history, as well as to an assessment of exposure—current and remote—to drugs, especially antibiotics and analgesics, and to dietary supplements or herbal remedies. The recognition of a potential asso-

TABLE 266-1 *Principal Causes of Tubulointerstitial Disease of the Kidney*

ACUTE INTERSTITIAL NEPHRITIS

Drugs[a]
  Antibiotics (β-lactams, sulfonamides, quinolones, vancomycin, erythromycin, minocycline, rifampin, ethambutol, acyclovir)
  Nonsteroidal anti-inflammatory drugs
  Diuretics (thiazides, furosemide, triamterene)
  Anticonvulsants (phenytoin, phenobarbital, carbamazepine, valproic acid)
  Miscellaneous (captopril, H_2 receptor blockers, omeprazole, mesalazine, indinavir, allopurinol)
Infection
  Bacteria (*Streptococcus, Staphylococcus, Legionella, Salmonella, Brucella, Yersinia, Corynebacterium diphtheriae*)
  Viruses (Epstein-Barr virus, cytomegalovirus, Hantavirus, HIV)
  Miscellaneous (*Leptospira, Rickettsia, Mycoplasma*)
Idiopathic
  Tubulointerstitial nephritis–uveitis syndrome
  Anti-tubule basement membrane disease
  Sarcoidosis

CHRONIC TUBULOINTERSTITIAL DISEASES

Hereditary renal diseases
  Polycystic kidney disease[a] (Chap. 276)
  Medullary cystic disease (Chap. 276)
  Medullary sponge kidney (Chap. 276)
Exogenous toxins
  Analgesic nephropathy[a]
  Lead nephropathy
  Miscellaneous nephrotoxins (e.g. lithium[a], cyclosporine[a], heavy metals, slimming regimens with Chinese herbs)
Metabolic toxins
  Hyperuricemia[a]
  Hypercalcemia
  Miscellaneous metabolic toxins (e.g., hypokalemia, hyperoxaluria, cystinosis, Fabry's disease)
Autoimmune disorders
  Sjögren's syndrome
Neoplastic disorders
  Leukemia
  Lymphoma
  Multiple myeloma[a]
Miscellaneous disorders
  Sickle cell nephropathy
  Chronic pyelonephritis
  Chronic urinary tract obstruction
  Vesicoureteral reflux[a]
  Radiation nephritis
  Balkan nephropathy
  Tubulointerstitial disease secondary to glomerular and vascular disease

[a] Common

ciation between a patient's renal disease and exposure to a nephrotoxin is crucial, because, unlike many other forms of renal disease, progression of the functional and morphologic abnormalities associated with toxin-induced nephropathies may be prevented, and even reversed, by eliminating additional exposure.

TABLE 266-2 *Functional Consequences of Tubulointerstitial Disease*

Defect	Cause(s)
Reduced glomerular filtration rate[a]	Obliteration of microvasculature and obstruction of tubules
Fanconi syndrome	Damage to proximal tubular reabsorption of glucose, amino acids, phosphate, and bicarbonate
Hyperchloremic acidosis[a]	1. Reduced ammonia production 2. Inability to acidify the collecting duct fluid (distal renal tubular acidosis) 3. Proximal bicarbonate wasting
Tubular or small-molecular-weight proteinuria[a]	Failure of proximal tubule protein reabsorption
Polyuria, isothenuria[a]	Damage to medullary tubules and vasculature
Hyperkalemia[a]	Potassium secretory defects including aldosterone resistance
Salt wasting	Distal tubular damage with impaired sodium reabsorption

[a] Common

EXOGENOUS TOXINS ■ **Analgesic Nephropathy** A distinct clinicopathologic syndrome has been described in heavy users of analgesic mixtures containing phenacetin in combination with aspirin, acetaminophen, or caffeine. Morphologically, analgesic nephropathy is characterized by papillary necrosis and tubulointerstitial inflammation. At an early stage, damage to the vascular supply of the inner medulla (vasa recta) leads to a local interstitial inflammatory reaction and, eventually, to papillary ischemia, necrosis, fibrosis, and calcification. The susceptibility of the renal papillae to damage by phenacetin is believed to be related to the establishment of a renal gradient for its acetaminophen metabolite, resulting in papillary tip concentrations tenfold higher than those in renal cortex. Aspirin in these analgesic compounds contributes to renal injury by uncoupling oxidative phosphorylation in renal mitochondria and by inhibiting the synthesis of renal prostaglandins, which are potent endogenous renal vasodilator hormones.

In analgesic nephropathy, renal function usually declines gradually. Occasionally, papillary necrosis may be associated with hematuria and even renal colic owing to obstruction of a ureter by necrotic tissue. More than half of patients with analgesic nephropathy have pyuria, which, if persistently associated with sterile urine, provides an important clue to the diagnosis. Nonetheless, active pyelonephritis may coexist in patients with analgesic nephropathy. Proteinuria, if present, is typically mild (< 1 g/d). Patients with analgesic nephropathy are usually unable to generate maximally concentrated urine, reflecting the underlying medullary and papillary damage. An acquired form of distal RTA (Chap. 265) may contribute to the development of *nephrocalcinosis*. The occurrence of anemia out of proportion to the degree of azotemia may also provide a clue to the diagnosis of analgesic nephropathy. When analgesic nephropathy has progressed to renal insufficiency, the kidneys usually appear bilaterally shrunken on intravenous pyelography, and the calyces are deformed. A "ring sign" on the pyelogram is pathognomonic of papillary necrosis and represents the radiolucent sloughed papilla surrounded by the radiodense contrast material in the calyx. Computed tomography may reveal papillary calcifications surrounding the central sinus complex in a "garland" pattern. Transitional cell carcinoma may develop in the urinary pelvis or ureters as a late complication of analgesic abuse.

Whether non-phenacetin analgesics, alone or in combination, cause renal disease is controversial. A recent cohort study of men with normal baseline renal function found no association between moderate analgesic use and subsequent renal dysfunction, suggesting that the risk, if any, is low. Until conclusive evidence is available, however, physicians should consider screening heavy users of acetaminophen and nonsteroidal anti-inflammatory drugs (NSAIDs) for evidence of renal disease, and discouraging their use of these drugs.

Lead Nephropathy (See also Chap. 376) Lead intoxication may produce a chronic tubulointerstitial renal disease. Children who repeatedly ingest lead-based paints (pica) may develop kidney disease as adults. Significant occupational exposure may occur in workplaces where lead-containing metals or paints are heated to high temperatures, such as battery factories, smelters, salvage yards, and weapon firing ranges. Alcohol, illegally distilled in an apparatus constructed from automobile radiators (so-called moonshine), is another cause of lead poisoning. Environmental lead exposure, particularly in industrial regions, may be great enough to produce changes in renal function.

Tubule transport processes enhance the accumulation of lead within renal cells, particularly in the proximal convoluted tubule, leading to cell degeneration, mitochondrial swelling, and eosinophilic intranuclear inclusion bodies rich in lead. In addition, lead nephropathy is associated with ischemic changes in the glomeruli, fibrosis of the adventitia of small renal arterioles, and focal areas of cortical scarring. Eventually, the kidneys become atrophic. Urinary excretion of lead, porphyrin precursors such as δ-aminolevulinic acid and coproporphyrin, and urobilinogen may be increased. Patients with chronic lead nephropathy are characteristically *hyperuricemic*, a consequence of enhanced reabsorption of filtered urate. Acute gouty arthritis (so-called saturnine gout) develops in about 50% of patients with lead nephropathy, in striking contrast to other forms of chronic renal failure in which de novo gout is rare (Chap. 338). Hypertension is also a complication. Therefore, in any patient with slowly progressive renal failure, atrophic kidneys, gout, and hypertension, the diagnosis of lead intoxication should be considered. Features of acute lead intoxication (abdominal colic, anemia, peripheral neuropathy, and encephalopathy) are usually absent.

The diagnosis may be suspected by finding elevated serum levels of lead. However, because blood levels may not be elevated even in the presence of a toxic total-body burden of lead, the quantitation of lead excretion following infusion of the chelating agent calcium disodium edetate is a more reliable indicator of serious lead exposure. While urinary excretion of more than 0.6 mg/d of lead is generally considered to be indicative of overt or potential toxicity, recent evidence suggests that even lead burdens of 0.15 to 0.6 mg/d may cause progressive loss of renal function.

℞ TREATMENT

Treatment includes removing the patient from the source of exposure and augmenting lead excretion with a chelating agent such as calcium disodium edetate.

Lithium Use of lithium salts for bipolar disorder (Chap. 371) is associated with chronic tubulointerstitial nephropathy, generally manifest as the insidious development of chronic renal insufficiency. Nephrogenic diabetes insipidus, which may occur alone or in association with the renal insufficiency, is common. It manifests as polyuria and polydipsia, and is due to lithium-induced downregulation of the vasopressin-regulated water channels in the collecting duct. Mild proteinuria can occur. The predominant finding on renal biopsy is tubular atrophy and interstitial fibrosis out of proportion to the extent of glomerular or vascular disease. Tubular cysts are common, and concomitant focal segmental glomerulosclerosis can be observed.

Renal function should be followed in patients taking this drug, and caution should be exercised if lithium is employed in patients with underlying renal disease. Once renal impairment occurs, lithium therapy should be stopped and an alternative agent substituted. Despite discontinuation of lithium, chronic renal disease in such patients is often irreversible and can progress to end-stage renal failure.

Miscellaneous Nephrotoxins The immunosuppressant *cyclosporine* causes both acute and chronic renal injury. The acute injury and the use of cyclosporine in transplantation are discussed in Chap. 263. The chronic injury results in an irreversible reduction in glomerular filtration rate (GFR), with mild proteinuria and arterial hypertension. Hyperkalemia is a relatively common complication and results in part from tubule resistance to aldosterone. The histologic changes in renal tissue include patchy interstitial fibrosis and tubular atrophy. In addition, the intrarenal vasculature often demonstrates hyalinosis, and focal segmental glomerular sclerosis can be present as well. Fibrosis may be the result of a cyclosporine-induced increase in renal collagen production. Vasoconstrictive mediators, such as angiotensin II, may also play a role in chronic cyclosporine toxicity. In patients receiving this drug for renal transplantation (Chap. 263), chronic graft dysfunction and recurrence of the primary disease may coincide with chronic cyclosporine injury, and on clinical grounds, distinction among these may be difficult. Cyclosporine nephrotoxicity is also seen in patients undergoing heart or lung transplantation, as well as in patients receiving cyclosporine as an immunosuppressant in a variety of inflammatory and autoimmune disorders. Dose reduction appears to mitigate cyclosporine-associated renal fibrosis but may increase the risk of rejection and graft loss. Treatment of any associated arterial hypertension may lessen renal injury.

Chinese herbs nephropathy is characterized by rapidly progressive interstitial renal fibrosis in young women due to ingestion of slimming pills containing Chinese herbs. At least one of the culprit ingredients is aristolochic acid. Clinically, patients present with progressive chronic renal insufficiency with sterile pyuria and anemia that is disproportionately severe relative to the level of renal function. The pathologic findings are interstitial fibrosis and tubular atrophy that affects the cortex in preference to the medulla, fibrous intimal thickening of the interlobular arteries, and a relative paucity of cellular infiltrates.

Many agents that commonly lead to acute renal failure are also capable of producing tubulointerstitial injury (Chap. 260). These include antibiotics (e.g., aminoglycosides, amphotericin B), radiographic contrast agents, various hydrocarbons (e.g., carbon tetrachloride), and heavy metals (e.g., mercury, cadmium, and bismuth).

METABOLIC TOXINS ▪ Acute Uric Acid Nephropathy (See also Chap. 313) Acute overproduction of uric acid and extreme hyperuricemia often lead to a rapidly progressive renal insufficiency, so-called acute uric acid nephropathy. This tubulointerstitial disease is usually seen as part of the tumor lysis syndrome in patients given cytotoxic drugs for the treatment of lymphoproliferative or myeloproliferative disorders but may also occur in these patients before such treatment is begun. The pathologic changes are largely the result of deposition of uric acid crystals in the kidneys and their collecting systems, leading to partial or complete obstruction of collecting ducts, renal pelvis, or ureter. Since obstruction is often bilateral, patients typically follow the clinical course of acute renal failure, characterized by oliguria and rapidly rising serum creatinine concentration. In the early phase uric acid crystals can be found in urine, usually in association with microscopic or gross hematuria. Hyperuricemia can also be a consequence of renal failure of any etiology. The finding of a urine/uric acid creatinine ratio greater than 1 mg/mg (0.7 mol/mol) distinguishes acute uric acid nephropathy from other causes of renal failure.

Prevention of hyperuricemia in patients at risk by treatment with allopurinol in doses of 200 to 800 mg/d prior to cytotoxic therapy reduces the danger of acute uric acid nephropathy. Once hyperuricemia develops, however, efforts should be directed to preventing deposition of uric acid within the urinary tract. Increasing urine volume with potent diuretics (furosemide or mannitol) effectively lowers intratubular uric acid concentrations, and alkalinization of the urine to pH 7 or greater with sodium bicarbonate and/or a carbonic anhydrase inhibitor (acetazolamide) enhances uric acid solubility. If these efforts, together with allopurinol therapy, are ineffective in preventing acute renal failure, dialysis should be instituted to lower the serum uric acid concentration as well as to treat the acute manifestations of uremia.

Gouty Nephropathy (See also Chap. 313) Patients with less severe but prolonged forms of hyperuricemia are predisposed to a more chronic tubulointerstitial disorder, often referred to as *gouty nephropathy*. The severity of renal involvement correlates with the duration and magnitude of the elevation of the serum uric acid concentration. Histologically, the distinctive feature of gouty nephropathy is the presence of crystalline deposits of uric acid and monosodium urate salts in kidney parenchyma. These deposits not only cause intrarenal obstruction but also incite an inflammatory response, leading to lymphocytic infiltration, foreign-body giant cell reaction, and eventual fibrosis, especially of medullary and papillary regions of the kidney. Bacteriuria and pyelonephritis occur in about one-fourth of cases, presumably as complications of intrarenal urinary stasis. Since patients with gout frequently suffer from hypertension and hyperlipidemia, degenerative changes of the renal arterioles may constitute a striking feature of the histologic abnormality, often out of proportion to other morphologic defects. Clinically, gouty nephropathy is an insidious cause of renal insufficiency. Early in its course, GFR may be near normal, often despite focal morphologic changes in medullary and cortical interstitium, proteinuria, and diminished urinary concentrating ability. Whether reducing serum uric acid levels with allopurinol exerts a beneficial effect on the kidney remains to be demonstrated. Although such undesirable consequences of hyperuricemia as gout and uric acid stones respond well to allopurinol, use of this drug in asymptomatic hyperuricemia has not been shown to improve renal function consistently. On the other hand, uricosuric agents such as probenecid, which may increase uric acid stone production, clearly have no role in the treatment of renal disease associated with hyperuricemia.

Hypercalcemic Nephropathy (See also Chap. 332) Chronic hypercalcemia, as occurs in primary hyperparathyroidism, sarcoidosis, multiple myeloma, vitamin D intoxication, or metastatic bone disease, can cause tubulointerstitial damage and progressive renal insufficiency. The earliest lesion is a focal degenerative change in renal epithelia, primarily in collecting ducts, distal convoluted tubules, and loops of Henle. Tubule cell necrosis leads to nephron obstruction and stasis of intrarenal urine, favoring local precipitation of calcium salts and infection. Dilatation and atrophy of tubules eventually occur, as do interstitial fibrosis, mononuclear leukocyte infiltration, and interstitial calcium deposition (nephrocalcinosis). Calcium deposition may also occur in glomeruli and the walls of renal arterioles.

Clinically, the most striking defect is an inability to concentrate the urine maximally, resulting in polyuria and nocturia. Reduced collecting duct responsiveness to vasopressin and defective transport of NaCl in the ascending limb of Henle's loop are responsible for this concentrating defect. Reductions in GFR and renal blood flow also occur, both in acute severe hypercalcemia and with prolonged hypercalcemia of lesser severity. Distal RTA and sodium and potassium wasting have also been described in these chronic states. Eventually, uncontrolled hypercalcemia leads to severe tubulointerstitial damage and overt renal failure. Abdominal x-rays may demonstrate nephrocalcinosis as well as nephrolithiasis, the latter due to the hypercalciuria that often accompanies hypercalcemia.

℞ TREATMENT

This consists of reducing the serum calcium concentration toward normal and correcting the primary abnormality of calcium metabolism. The management of hypercalcemia is discussed in Chap. 332. Prognosis for recovery of renal function depends on the severity of the renal lesion at the time hypercalcemia is corrected. Renal dysfunction of acute hypercalcemia may be completely reversible. Gradual, progressive renal insufficiency related to chronic hypercalcemia, however, may not improve with correction of the calcium disorder. Nonetheless, every effort should be made to return serum calcium concentration to normal to minimize further loss of renal function.

RENAL PARENCHYMAL DISEASE ASSOCIATED WITH EXTRARENAL NEOPLASM

Except for the glomerulopathies associated with lymphomas and several solid tumors (Chap. 264), the renal manifestations of primary extrarenal neoplastic processes are confined mainly to the interstitium and tubules. Although metastatic renal involvement by solid tumors is unusual, the kidneys are often invaded by neoplastic cells in hematologic malignancies. In postmortem studies of patients with *lymphoma* and *leukemia*, renal involvement is found in approximately half. Diffuse infiltration of the renal parenchyma with malignant cells is seen most commonly. There may be flank pain, and x-rays may show enlargement of one or both kidneys. Renal insufficiency occurs in a minority of cases, and overt uremia is rare. Treatment of the primary disease may improve renal function in these cases.

PLASMA CELL DYSCRASIAS Several glomerular and tubulointerstitial disorders may occur in association with plasma cell dyscrasias (Chap. 98). Infiltration of the kidneys with myeloma cells is infrequent. When it occurs, the process is usually focal, so renal insufficiency from this cause is also uncommon. The more usual lesion is *myeloma kidney*, characterized histologically by atrophic tubules, many with eosinophilic intraluminal casts, and numerous multinucleated giant cells within tubule walls and in the interstitium. The frequent occurrence of myeloma kidney in patients with Bence Jones proteinuria has suggested a causal relation. Bence Jones proteins are thought to cause myeloma kidney through direct toxicity to renal tubule cells. In addition, Bence Jones proteins may precipitate within the distal nephron where the high concentrations of these proteins and the acid composition of the tubule fluid favor intraluminal cast formation and intrarenal obstruction. Occasionally, acute renal failure occurs after intravenous pyelography in patients with multiple myeloma and is believed to result from the further precipitation of Bence Jones proteins induced by dehydration prior to radiographic study. Dehydration of the patient with myeloma in preparation for intravenous pyelography should therefore be avoided. Multiple myeloma may also affect the kidneys indirectly. Hypercalcemia or hyperuricemia may lead to the nephropathies described above. Proximal tubule disorders are also seen occasionally, including type II proximal RTA and the Fanconi syndrome.

AMYLOIDOSIS (See also Chaps. 264 and 310) Glomerular pathology usually predominates and leads to heavy proteinuria and azotemia. However, tubule function may also be deranged, giving rise to a nephrogenic diabetes insipidus and to distal (type I) RTA. In several cases these functional abnormalities correlated with peritubular deposition of amyloid, particularly in areas surrounding vasa rectae, loops of Henle, and collecting ducts. Bilateral enlargement of the kidneys, especially in a patient with massive proteinuria and tubule dysfunction, should raise the possibility of amyloid renal disease.

IMMUNE DISORDERS

ALLERGIC INTERSTITIAL NEPHRITIS An acute diffuse tubulointerstitial reaction may result from hypersensitivity to a number of drugs, including sulfonamides, many penicillins and cephalosporins, the fluoroquinolone antibiotics ciprofloxacin and norfloxacin, and the antituberculous drugs isoniazid and rifampin. Acute tubulointerstitial damage has also occurred after use of thiazide and loop diuretics, antiulcer medications (cimetidine, ranitidine, and omeprazole), allopurinol, and NSAIDs. Of note, the tubulointerstitial nephropathy that develops in some patients taking NSAIDs may be associated with nephrotic-range proteinuria and histologic evidence of either minimal change or membranous glomerulopathy. The use of mesalazine for the treatment of inflammatory bowel disease is associated with a more subacute disorder in which a severe indolent interstitial nephritis occurs several months after the initiation of the drug. Grossly, the kidneys are usually enlarged. Histologically, the glomeruli appear normal. The principal pathologic abnormalities are in the interstitium of the kidney, which reveals pronounced edema and infiltration with polymorphonuclear leukocytes, lymphocytes, plasma cells, and, in some cases, large numbers of eosinophils. If the process is severe, tubule cell necrosis and regeneration may also be apparent. Immunofluorescence studies have either been unrevealing or demonstrated a linear pattern of immunoglobulin and complement deposition along tubule basement membranes.

Most patients require several weeks of drug exposure before developing evidence of renal injury. Rare cases have occurred after only a few doses or after a year or more of use. Azotemia is usually present; a diagnostic triad of fever, skin rash, and peripheral blood eosinophilia is highly suggestive of acute tubulointerstitial nephritis but is often absent. Examination of the urine sediment reveals hematuria and often pyuria; occasionally, eosinophils may be present. Proteinuria is usually mild to moderate, except in cases of NSAID-induced tubulointerstitial nephritis with minimal change glomerulopathy. The clinical picture may be confused with acute glomerulonephritis, but when acute azotemia and hematuria are accompanied by eosinophilia, skin rash, and a history of drug exposure, a hypersensitivity reaction leading to acute tubulointerstitial nephritis should be regarded as the leading diagnostic possibility. Discontinuation of the drug usually results in complete reversal of the renal injury; rarely, renal damage may be irreversible. Glucocorticoids may accelerate renal recovery, but their value has not been definitively established.

SJÖGREN'S SYNDROME (See also Chap. 304) When the kidneys are involved in this disorder, the predominant histologic findings are those of chronic tubulointerstitial disease. Interstitial infiltrates are composed primarily of lymphocytes, causing the histology of the renal parenchyma in these patients to resemble that of the salivary and lacrimal glands. Renal functional defects include diminished urinary concentrating ability and distal (type I) RTA. Urinalysis may show pyuria (predominantly lymphocyturia) and mild proteinuria.

TUBULOINTERSTITIAL ABNORMALITIES ASSOCIATED WITH GLOMERULONEPHRITIS Primary glomerulopathies are often associated with damage to tubules and the interstitium. Occasionally, the primary disorder may affect glomeruli and tubules directly. For example, in more than half of patients with the nephropathy of systemic lupus erythematosus, deposits of immune complexes can be identified in tubule basement membranes, usually accompanied by an interstitial mononuclear inflammatory reaction. Similarly, in many patients with glomerulonephritis associated with anti-glomerular basement membrane antibody, the same antibody is reactive against tubule basement membranes as well. More frequently, tubulointerstitial damage is a secondary consequence of glomerular dysfunction. The extent of tubulointerstitial fibrosis correlates closely with the degree of renal impairment. Potential mechanisms by which glomerular disease might cause tubulointerstitial injury include glomerular leak of plasma proteins toxic to epithelial cells, activation of tubule epithelial cells by glomerulus-derived cytokines, reduced peritubular blood flow leading to downstream tubulointerstitial ischemia, and hyperfunction of remnant tubules.

MISCELLANEOUS DISORDERS

VESICOURETERAL REFLUX (See also Chap. 270) When the function of the ureterovesical junction is impaired, urine may reflux into the ureters due to the high intravesical pressure that develops during voiding. Clinically, reflux is often detected on the voiding and postvoiding films obtained during intravenous pyelography, although voiding cystourethrography may be required for definitive diagnosis. Bladder infection may ascend the urinary tract to the kidneys through incompetent ureterovesical sphincters. Not surprisingly, therefore, reflux is often discovered in patients with acute and/or chronic urinary tract infections. With more severe degrees of reflux, characterized by dilatation of ureters and renal pelves, progressive renal damage often appears, and although active infection may also be present, uncertainty exists as to the necessity of infection in producing the scarred kidney of reflux nephropathy. Substantial proteinuria is often present, and glomerular lesions similar to those of idiopathic focal glomerulosclerosis (Chap. 264) are often found in addition to the changes of chronic tubulointerstitial disease. Surgical correction of reflux is usually necessary only with the more severe degrees of reflux since renal damage correlates with the extent of reflux. Obviously, if extensive glomerulosclerosis already exists, urologic repair may no longer be warranted.

RADIATION NEPHRITIS   Renal dysfunction can be expected to occur if 23 Gy (2300 rad) or more of x-ray irradiation is administered to both kidneys during a period of 5 weeks or less. Histologic examination of the kidneys reveals hyalinized glomeruli, atrophic tubules, extensive interstitial fibrosis, and hyalinization of the media of renal arterioles. Radiation-induced renal ischemia is believed to be the main pathogenic factor responsible for the tubulointerstitial damage, which may not become evident clinically for months after completion of radiation. The presentation of acute radiation nephritis includes rapidly progressive azotemia, moderate to malignant hypertension, anemia, and proteinuria that may reach the nephrotic range. More than 50% progress to chronic renal failure. A more insidious form is characterized by slower development of azotemia, anemia, and nephrotic syndrome. Malignant hypertension may follow unilateral renal irradiation and resolve with ipsilateral nephrectomy. Radiation nephritis has all but vanished because of heightened awareness of its pathogenesis by radiotherapists.

FURTHER READING

GOBEL U et al: The protean face of renal sarcoidosis. J Am Soc Nephrol 12: 616, 2001

HARRIS DC: Tubulointerstitial renal disease. Curr Opin Nephrol Hypertens 10: 303, 2001

KELLY CJ, NEILSON EG: Tubulointerstitial diseases, in BM Brenner (ed): *Brenner and Rector's The Kidney*, 7th ed. Philadelphia, Saunders, 2004, pp 1483–1512

MARKOWITZ GS et al: Lithium nephrotoxicity: A progressive combined glomerular and tubulointerstitial nephropathy. J Am Soc Nephrol 11:1439, 2000

REXRODE KM et al: Analgesic use and renal function in men. JAMA 286:315, 2001

SKOPOULI FN: Kidney injury in Sjogren's syndrome. Nephrol Dial Transplant 16:63, 2001

267   VASCULAR INJURY TO THE KIDNEY
Kamal F. Badr, Barry M. Brenner

Adequate delivery of blood to the glomerular capillary network is crucial for glomerular filtration and overall salt and water balance. Thus, in addition to the threat to the viability of renal tissue, vascular injury to the kidney may compromise the maintenance of body fluid volume and composition. Involvement of the renal vessels by atherosclerotic, hypertensive, embolic, inflammatory, and hematologic disorders is usually a manifestation of generalized vascular pathology. The morphologic and clinical responses to these insults are considered in this chapter.

THROMBOEMBOLIC DISEASES OF THE RENAL ARTERIES

Thrombosis of the major renal arteries or their branches is an important cause of deterioration of renal function, especially in the elderly. It is often difficult to diagnose and therefore requires a high index of suspicion. Thrombosis may occur as a result of intrinsic pathology in the renal vessels (posttraumatic, atherosclerotic, or inflammatory) or as a result of emboli originating in distant vessels, most commonly fat emboli, emboli originating in the left heart (mural thrombi following myocardial infarction, bacterial endocarditis, or aseptic vegetations), or "paradoxical" emboli passing from the right side of the circulation via a patent foramen ovale or atrial septal defect. Renal emboli are bilateral in 15 to 30% of cases.

The clinical presentation is variable, depending on the time course and the extent of the occlusive event. Acute thrombosis and infarction, such as follows embolization, may result in sudden onset of flank pain and tenderness, fever, hematuria, leukocytosis, nausea, and vomiting. If infarction occurs, renal enzymes may be elevated, namely aspartate aminotransferase (AST), lactate dehydrogenase (LDH), and alkaline phosphatase, which rise and fall in the order listed. Urinary LDH and alkaline phosphatase may also increase after infarction. Renal function deteriorates acutely, leading in bilateral thrombosis to acute oliguric renal failure. More gradual (i.e., atherosclerotic) occlusion of a single renal artery may go undetected. A spectrum of clinical presentations lies between these two extremes. Hypertension usually follows renal infarction and results from renin release in the peri-infarction zone. Hypertension is usually transient but may be persistent. Diagnosis is established by renal arteriography.

℞ TREATMENT

Management of *acute* renal arterial thrombosis includes surgical intervention, anticoagulant therapy, conservative and supportive therapy, and control of hypertension. The choice of treatment depends mainly on (1) the condition of the patient, in particular the patient's ability to withstand major surgery, and (2) the extent of renovascular occlusion and amount of renal mass at risk of infarction. In general, supportive care and anticoagulant therapy are indicated in unilateral disease. In *acute* bilateral thrombosis, medical and surgical therapies yield comparable results. Twenty-five percent of patients die during the acute episode, usually from extrarenal complications. In *chronic* ischemic renal disease, surgical revascularization is more likely to preserve and improve renal function (see below).

ATHEROEMBOLIC DISEASE OF THE RENAL ARTERIES

Atheroembolic renal disease is part of a systemic syndrome characterized by cholesterol crystal embolization. Renal damage results from embolization of cholesterol crystals from atherosclerotic plaques present in large arteries, such as the aorta, to small arteries in the renal vasculature. Atheroembolic renal disease is an increasingly common and often underdiagnosed cause of renal insufficiency in the elderly. A review of 372 autopsies identified cholesterol emboli in 2.4% of renal tissue samples. Male gender, older age, hypertension, and diabetes mellitus are important predisposing factors, present in 85% of cases. Patients with cholesterol embolization syndrome also often have a history of ischemic cardiovascular disease, aortic aneurysm, cerebrovascular disease, congestive heart failure, or renal insufficiency. A significant association is present between renal artery stenosis and atheroembolic renal disease. Inciting events, which include vascular surgery, arteriography, angioplasty, anticoagulation with heparin, and thrombolytic therapy, can be identified in about 50% of cases. Arteriographic procedures constitute the most common cause of cholesterol embolization.

Clinical manifestations usually appear 1 to 14 days after an inciting event, but their onset can be more insidious. Systemic manifestations occur in fewer than half of the patients and include fever, myalgias, headaches, and weight loss. Cutaneous manifestations such as livedo reticularis, "purple" toes, and toe gangrene occur in 50 to 90% of patients and constitute the most common extrarenal findings. Other targets of cholesterol embolization include the retina, musculoskeletal system, nervous system, and gut. Accelerated or labile hypertension is present in one-half of patients. Malignant hypertension has been described. Renal insufficiency is usually subacute and advances in a stepwise fashion over a period of several weeks. Renal failure, however, can be acute and oliguric. Uremic signs and symptoms requiring dialytic therapy develop in 40% of patients, only half of whom recover sufficient renal function to stop dialysis after 1 year. More recent data suggest less inexorable deterioration with a possibility of recovery of renal function in about one-third of patients after variable periods of dialytic support. Renal infarction secondary to cholesterol embolization is rare. Cholesterol embolic disease in renal allografts has been reported and can be of donor or of recipient origin.

Antemortem diagnosis of atherosclerotic renal emboli is difficult. The demonstration of cholesterol emboli in the retina is helpful, but a firm diagnosis is established only by demonstration of cholesterol crystals in the smaller arteries and arterioles on renal biopsy. These may also be seen in asymptomatic skeletal muscle or skin. Atheroembolic renal disease is associated with a 64 to 81% mortality rate.

TREATMENT

No effective therapy for atheroembolic renal disease is available. Withdrawal of anticoagulation may be beneficial. In some patients, kidney function improved even after a prolonged period of renal insufficiency. Cholesterol-lowering agents may also improve outcome. An aggressive therapeutic approach with patient-tailored supportive measures may be associated with more favorable clinical outcome.

RENAL VEIN THROMBOSIS (RVT)

Thrombosis of one or both main renal veins occurs in a variety of settings (Table 267-1). Nephrotic syndrome accompanying membranous glomerulopathy and certain carcinomas seems to predispose to the development of RVT, which occurs in 10 to 50% of patients with these disorders. RVT may exacerbate preexisting proteinuria but is infrequently the cause of the nephrotic syndrome.

The clinical manifestations depend on the severity and abruptness of its occurrence. Acute cases occur typically in children and are characterized by sudden loss of renal function, often accompanied by fever, chills, lumbar tenderness (with kidney enlargement), leukocytosis, and hematuria. Hemorrhagic infarction and renal rupture may lead to hypovolemic shock. In young adults RVT is usually suspected from an unexpected and relatively acute or subacute deterioration of renal function and/or exacerbation of proteinuria and hematuria in the appropriate clinical setting. In cases of gradual thrombosis, usually occurring in the elderly, the only manifestation may be recurrent pulmonary emboli or development of hypertension. A Fanconi-like syndrome and proximal renal tubular acidosis have been described.

The definitive diagnosis can only be established through selective renal venography with visualization of the occluding thrombus. Short of angiography, Doppler ultrasound, contrast-enhanced computed tomography (CT), and magnetic resonance imaging (MRI) often provides definitive evidence of thrombus.

TREATMENT

Treatment consists of anticoagulation, the main purpose of which is prevention of pulmonary embolization, although some authors have also claimed improvement in renal function and proteinuria. Encouraging reports have appeared concerning the use of streptokinase. Spontaneous recanalization with clinical improvement has also been observed. Anticoagulant therapy is more rewarding in the acute thrombosis seen in younger individuals. Nephrectomy is advocated in infants with life-threatening renal infarction. Thrombectomy is effective in some cases.

RENAL ARTERY STENOSIS (RAS)/ISCHEMIC RENAL DISEASE

Ischemic renal disease underlies end-stage renal disease in 15 to 20% of uremic patients over 50 years of age. Stenosis of the main renal artery and/or its major branches is causative in 2 to 5% of patients with hypertension (Chap. 230). The common cause in the middle-aged and elderly is an atheromatous plaque at the origin of the renal artery. In a large unselected autopsy series, stenosis producing >50% renal artery diameter reduction was found in 18% of those between 65 and 74 years of age and in 42% of those older than 75 years. Bilateral

involvement is present in half of the affected cases in both age groups. It should be considered seriously in elderly individuals, particularly in those with evidence of hypertension, diabetes, and atherosclerotic arterial disease elsewhere. In this population, the incidence of renal arterial stenosis can be as high as 40%. Established plaques progress in >50% of cases over 5 years (15% to total occlusion). Renal hypertrophy is detectable in 20% of affected kidneys. In younger women, stenosis is due to intrinsic structural abnormalities of the arterial wall caused by a heterogeneous group of lesions termed *fibromuscular dysplasia*. Clinical settings in which RAS should be considered are listed in Table 267-2.

DIAGNOSIS Diagnostic evaluation for significant RAS should begin with noninvasive approaches. An initial screening test is Doppler ultrasonography, which provides information on blood-flow velocity and pressure waveforms in the renal arteries and, when positive, is helpful. Its limitations, however, include significant operator dependence, technical difficulty in obese patients, and poor sensitivity in the presence of multiple renal arteries, distal stenoses, and total occlusion. Measurement of the intrarenal resistance index (RI) by Doppler ultrasonography provides valuable information on the extent of parenchymal tissue loss in stenosed and nonstenosed kidneys and hence on the prognosis for functional recovery following revascularization procedures.

Absence of compensatory hypertrophy in the contralateral kidney should raise the suspicion of bilateral stenosis or superimposed parenchymal renal disease, most commonly hypertensive or diabetic nephropathy. Because angiotensin-converting enzyme (ACE) inhibitors magnify the impairment in renal blood flow and glomerular filtration rate (GFR) caused by functionally significant renal artery stenosis, use of these drugs in association with ^{99m}Tc-labeled pentetic acid (DTPA) or ^{99m}Tc-labeled mertiatide (MAG$_3$) renography enhances diagnostic precision and is of additional predictive value. Gadolinium-enhanced three-dimensional magnetic resonance angiography (MRA) has replaced previous modalities as the most sensitive (>90%) and specific (95%) test for the diagnosis of RAS. The most definitive diagnostic procedure is contrast-enhanced arteriography. Intraarterial digital subtraction techniques minimize the requirements for contrast, reducing the risk of renal toxicity.

TREATMENT

Interventional therapy RAS (i.e., surgery or angioplasty) is superior to medical therapy. Success rates with conventional percutaneous transluminal angioplasty in young patients with fibromuscular dysplasia are 50% cure and improvement in blood pressure control in another

---

TABLE 267-1   Conditions Associated with Renal Vein Thrombosis

Trauma
Extrinsic compression (lymph nodes, aortic aneurysm, tumor)
Invasion by renal cell carcinoma
Dehydration (infants)
Nephrotic syndrome
Pregnancy or oral contraceptives

TABLE 267-2   Clinical Findings Associated with Renal Artery Stenosis

Hypertension
  Abrupt onset of hypertension before the age of 50 years (suggestive of fibromuscular dysplasia)
  Abrupt onset of hypertension at or after the age of 50 years (suggestive of atherosclerotic renal artery stenosis)
  Accelerated or malignant hypertension
  Refractory hypertension (not responsive to therapy with ≥3 drugs)
Renal abnormalities
  Unexplained azotemia (suggestive of atherosclerotic renal artery stenosis)
  Azotemia induced by treatment with an angiotensin-converting enzyme inhibitor
  Unilateral small kidney
  Unexplained hypokalemia
Other findings
  Abdominal bruit, flank bruit, or both
  Severe retinopathy
  Carotid, coronary, or peripheral vascular disease
  Unexplained congestive heart failure or acute pulmonary edema

Source: From Safian and Textor, reprinted with permission.

30%. For atherosclerotic lesions, conventional balloon angioplasty is associated with high restenosis rates (up to 47%) and either stent placement or surgery is recommended. About half of those with reduced renal function as a result of RAS improve following angioplasty or surgery, even when preintervention arteriography shows little evidence of cortical perfusion. In the presence of unilateral RAS and normal overall GFR, the decision for angiographic or surgical revascularization may depend on the results of fractional flow and filtration rate studies to each kidney with ^{99m}TC-DTPA or ^{99m}Tc-MAG$_3$. These techniques can also be used to assess the response to revascularization. Three-year survival is influenced by baseline renal function, being 94% in the presence of normal baseline renal function and falling to 52% in patients with serum creatinine >177 μmol/L (>2.0 mg/dL). Renal parenchymal damage, as reflected in noninvasive imaging and degree of proteinuria, is the major predictor of functional outcome and should be used for risk stratification. Rapid decline in renal function is associated with a favorable response to intervention.

Despite the risks associated with surgery, long-term follow-up studies demonstrate an advantage of surgery over angioplasty both with regard to the incidence of restenosis and to the preservation or improvement in GFR. Surgery, however, is restricted to those patients in whom angioplasty and stenting are not feasible. As with coronary angioplasty, stenting of renal arteries following balloon angioplasty is being used increasingly. Results are highly encouraging, with reste-

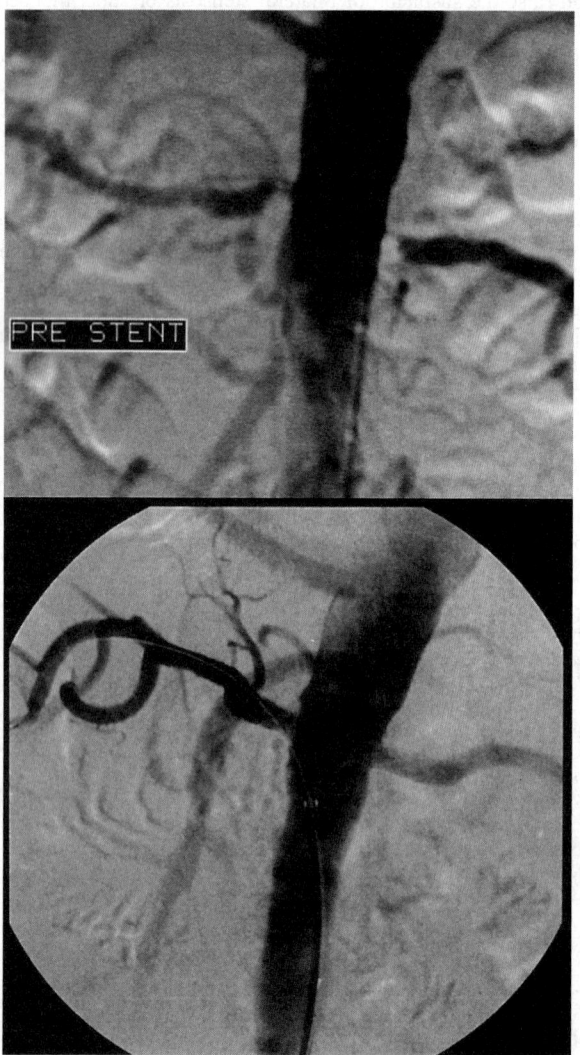

FIGURE 267-1 Bilateral severe ostial renal artery stenosis prior to and following balloon dilatation and stent placement in a patient with severe hypertension and renal insufficiency.

nosis rates <15% at 1 year. Renal functional recovery or stabilization of renal function is seen in approximately 70% of patients. An illustrative example of renal artery stenting is shown in Fig. 267-1.

HEMOLYTIC UREMIC SYNDROME (HUS) AND THROMBOTIC THROMBOCYTOPENIC PURPURA (TTP) (See also Chap. 101)

HUS and TTP, consumptive coagulopathies characterized by microangiopathic hemolytic anemia and thrombocytopenia, have a particular predilection for the kidney and the central nervous system, the latter especially in TTP. The kidneys of patients with HUS or TTP often exhibit a "flea-bitten" appearance, the result of multiple cortical hemorrhagic infarcts. The major sites of pathology are the small renal arteries and afferent arterioles, which are nearly occluded as a result of marked intimal hyperplasia (particularly in TTP) and fibrin deposits in the subintimal regions. When the vasoocclusive process is extensive, bilateral cortical necrosis may occur. In addition, arteriolar microaneurysms, glomerular infarction, or nonspecific focal changes may be seen. In keeping with the focal nature of the vascular lesions, patchy areas of interstitial edema, tubular necrosis, and, eventually, fibrosis occur. By immunofluorescence staining, complement components and immunoglobulins may be demonstrated in the arterioles, and fibrinogen deposits are present in arteries, arterioles, and glomerular capillary loops.

Endothelial cell injury appears to be the initiating pathophysiologic event in HUS/TTP. Injurious agents include bacterial toxins (Shiga toxin–like) mostly from specific *Escherichia coli* genotypes, endotoxin (lipopolysaccharides, LPS), bacterial neuraminidases, immune complexes, and drugs. Among the latter, most commonly associated with HUS/TTP are chemotherapeutic agents, cyclosporine, clopidogrel, and quinine. Also implicated in endothelial cell injury are intrinsic abnormalities of the complement sytem and the von Willebrand factor pathways, which may account for the genetic predisposition observed in familial forms of the disease.

Renal failure is common in both HUS and TTP, usually manifested by azotemia, mild proteinuria, and microscopic and/or gross hematuria. Patients with HUS have more severe renal failure, often marked by oligoanuria and hypertension and commonly progressing to chronic renal failure. The prognosis in HUS is better in children than in adults. In TTP, the course of which may span days to months, renal failure is usually less severe.

℞ TREATMENT

In TTP, high-dose glucocorticoids and plasma exchange often provide complete remission or cure. Plasma exchange should be initiated as early as possible, and the treatment cycles can be repeated if thrombocytopenia recurs. Splenectomy and antiplatelet therapy have also been used with varying degrees of success. The success of plasma exchange in adult HUS is less well established than in TTP.

ARTERIOLAR NEPHROSCLEROSIS (See also Chaps. 224 and 230)

Whether hypertension is "essential" or of known etiology, persistent exposure of the renal circulation to elevated intraluminal pressures results in development of intrinsic lesions of the renal arterioles (hyaline arteriolosclerosis) that eventually lead to loss of function (nephrosclerosis). Nephrosclerosis is divided into two distinct entities: "benign" and "malignant" (or accelerated).

BENIGN ARTERIOLAR NEPHROSCLEROSIS Benign arteriolar nephrosclerosis is seen in patients who are hypertensive for an extended period of time (blood pressure >150/90 mmHg) but whose hypertension has not progressed to a malignant form (described below). Such patients, usually in the older age group, are often discovered to be hypertensive on routine physical examination or as a result of nonspecific symptomatology (e.g., headaches, weakness, palpitations).

Kidney size is normal to reduced, with loss of cortical mass leading to a fine granularity. Although the larger arteries may show atherosclerotic changes, the characteristic pathology is in the afferent arterioles, which have thickened walls due to deposition of homogeneous eosinophilic material (hyaline arteriolosclerosis). Narrowing of vascular lumina results, with consequent ischemic injury to glomeruli and tubules.

Nephrosclerosis accompanying long-standing systemic arterial hypertension is only one manifestation of a generalized process affecting the cardiovascular system. Physical examination, therefore, may reveal changes in retinal vessels (arteriolar narrowing and/or flame-shaped hemorrhages), cardiac hypertrophy, and possibly signs of congestive heart failure. Renal disease may manifest as a mild to moderate elevation of serum creatinine concentration and/or mild proteinuria. In general, clinical evaluation does not reveal significant renal abnormalities. More specialized examination may disclose elevated urinary albumin excretion, tapering and loss of caliber of intrarenal vessels on arteriography, and an exaggerated natriuresis in response to a fluid challenge. Patients with benign nephrosclerosis generally maintain a near-normal GFR despite a reduction in renal blood flow.

MALIGNANT ARTERIOLAR NEPHROSCLEROSIS Patients with long-standing benign hypertension or patients not previously known to be hypertensive may develop malignant hypertension characterized by a sudden (accelerated) elevation of blood pressure (diastolic often >130 mmHg) accompanied by papilledema, central nervous system manifestations, cardiac decompensation, and acute progressive deterioration of renal function. The absence of papilledema does not rule out the diagnosis in a patient with markedly elevated blood pressure and rapidly declining renal function. The kidneys are characterized by a flea-bitten appearance resulting from hemorrhages in surface capillaries. Histologically, two distinct vascular lesions can be seen. The first, affecting arterioles, is fibrinoid necrosis, i.e., infiltration of arteriolar walls with eosinophilic material including fibrin, thickening of vessel walls and, occasionally, an inflammatory infiltrate (necrotizing arteriolitis). The second lesion, involving the interlobular arteries, is a concentric hyperplastic proliferation of the cellular elements of the vascular wall with deposition of collagen to form a hyperplastic arteriolitis (onionskin lesion). Fibrinoid necrosis occasionally extends into the glomeruli, which may also undergo proliferative changes or total necrosis. Most glomerular and tubular changes are secondary to ischemia and infarction. The sequence of events leading to the development of malignant hypertension is poorly defined. Two pathophysiologic alterations appear central in its initiation and/or perpetuation: (1) increased permeability of vessel walls to invasion by plasma components, particularly fibrin, which activates clotting mechanisms leading to a microangiopathic hemolytic anemia, thus perpetuating the vascular pathology; and (2) activation of the renin-angiotensin-aldosterone system at some point in the disease process, which contributes to the acceleration and maintenance of blood pressure elevation and, in turn, to vascular injury.

Malignant hypertension is most likely to develop in a previously hypertensive individual, usually in the third or fourth decade of life. There is a higher incidence among men, particularly black men. The presenting symptoms are usually neurologic (dizziness, headache, blurring of vision, altered states of consciousness, and focal or generalized seizures). Cardiac decompensation and renal failure appear thereafter. Renal abnormalities include a rapid rise in serum creatinine, hematuria (at times macroscopic), proteinuria, and red and white blood cell casts in the sediment. Nephrotic syndrome may be present. Elevated plasma aldosterone levels cause hypokalemic metabolic alkalosis in the early phase. Uremic acidosis and hyperkalemia eventually obscure these early findings. Hematologic indices of microangiopathic hemolytic anemia (i.e., schistocytes) are often seen.

℞ TREATMENT

Control of hypertension is the principal goal of therapy for both benign and malignant forms. The time of initiation of therapy, its effectiveness, and patient compliance are crucial factors in arresting the progression of benign nephrosclerosis. Untreated, most of these patients succumb to the extrarenal complications of hypertension. In contrast, malignant hypertension is a medical emergency; its natural course includes a death rate of 80 to 90% within 1 year of onset, almost always due to uremia. Supportive measures should be instituted to control the neurologic, cardiac, and other complications of acute renal failure, but the mainstay of therapy is prompt and aggressive reduction of blood pressure, which, if successful, can reverse all complications in the majority of patients. Presently, 5-year survival is 50%, and some patients have evidence of partial reversal of the vascular lesions and a return of renal function to near-normal levels.

SCLERODERMA (PROGRESSIVE SYSTEMIC SCLEROSIS)
(See also Chap. 303)

Renal involvement can present in one of two ways, depending on whether malignant hypertension is superimposed on the renal pathology: (1) *Persistent urinary abnormalities* with or without hypertension tend to follow an indolent course with mild proteinuria, occasional casts, cellular elements in the urinary sediment, and a propensity for development of hypertension. Azotemia is absent initially, but when it develops, dialysis is required within 1 year. (2) *Scleroderma renal crisis* (SRC) is a rapid deterioration in renal function, usually accompanied by malignant hypertension, oliguria, fluid retention, microangiopathic hemolytic anemia, and central nervous system involvement. It occurs in 5 to 15% of patients, most commonly in the first 5 years following diagnosis, particularly in patients with diffuse cutaneous involvement. SRC may occur in patients with previously undemonstrable or slowly progressive renal disease. Untreated, it leads to chronic renal failure within days to months.

℞ TREATMENT

The prognosis of scleroderma renal disease is generally poor, particularly following the onset of azotemia. Aggressive antihypertensive therapy may be effective in delaying the progression of renal failure. In SRC, prompt treatment with ACE inhibitors may reverse acute renal failure. Recently, a prospective study on short- and long-term outcomes of SRC in patients who received ACE inhibitors showed that 61% of patients had favorable outcomes (no dialysis or temporary dialysis) with a survival rate at 8 years of 80 to 85%, similar to that of patients with diffuse scleroderma who did not have renal crisis. Moreover, more than half of patients with SRC who initially required dialysis and were treated aggressively with ACE inhibitors were able to discontinue dialysis 3 to 18 months later, suggesting that patients should continue to take ACE inhibitors even after beginning dialysis, in hope of discontinuing it. A significant association exists between antecedent high-dose glucocorticoid therapy and the development of SRC.

SICKLE CELL NEPHROPATHY (See also Chap. 91)

Sickle cell disease causes renal complications that arise mainly as a result of sickling of red blood cells in the microvasculature. The hypertonic and relatively hypoxic environment of the renal medulla, coupled with the slow blood flow in the vasa recta, favors the sickling of red blood cells, with resultant local infarction (papillary necrosis). Functional tubule defects in patients with sickle cell disease are likely the result of partial ischemic injury to the renal tubules.

In addition to the intrarenal microvascular pathology described above, young patients with sickle cell disease are characterized by renal hyperperfusion, glomerular hypertrophy, and hyperfiltration. Many of these individuals eventually develop a glomerulopathy leading to glomerular proteinuria (present in as many as 30%) and, in some, the nephrotic syndrome. Co-inheritance of microdeletions in the α-globin gene (α thalassemia) appear to protect against the development of nephropathy, associated with lower mean arterial pressure and less proteinuria.

Mild azotemia and hyperuricemia can also develop. Advanced renal failure and uremia occur in 4 to 18% of cases. Pathologic examination reveals the typical lesion of "hyperfiltration nephropathy," namely, focal segmental glomerular sclerosis. This finding has led to the suggestion that anemia-induced hyperfiltration in childhood is the principal cause of the adult glomerulopathy. Nephron loss secondary to ischemic injury also contributes to the development of azotemia in these patients.

In addition to the glomerulopathy described above, renal complications of sickle cell disease include the following: *Cortical infarcts* can cause loss of function, persistent hematuria, and perinephric hematomas. *Papillary infarcts*, demonstrated radiographically in 50% of patients with sickle trait, lead to an increased risk of bacterial infection in the scarred renal tissues and functional tubule abnormalities. Painless gross hematuria occurs with a higher frequency in sickle trait than in sickle cell disease and likely results from infarctive episodes in the renal medulla. *Functional tubule abnormalities* such as nephrogenic diabetes insipidus result from marked reduction in vasa recta blood flow, combined with ischemic tubule injury. This concentrating defect places these patients at increased risk of dehydration and, hence, sickling crises. The concentrating defect also occurs in individuals with sickle trait. Other tubule defects involve potassium and hydrogen ion excretion, occasionally leading to hyperkalemic metabolic acidosis and a defect in uric acid excretion which, combined with increased purine synthesis in the bone marrow, results in hyperuricemia.

Management of sickle nephropathy is not separate from that of overall patient management (Chap. 91). In addition, however, the use of ACE inhibitors has been associated with improvement of the hyperfiltration glomerulopathy. Three-year graft and patient survival in renal transplant recipients with sickle nephropathy is diminished as compared to those with other causes of end-stage renal disease.

TOXEMIAS OF PREGNANCY See also Chap. 6

BILATERAL CORTICAL NECROSIS

Acute bilateral cortical necrosis is associated with septic abortions, abruptio placentae, and preeclampsia. Coagulation in cortical vessels and arterioles leads to renal tissue necrosis. Anuria and renal failure ensue and may be irreversible. In other cases, renal function returns partially, but on long-term follow-up most patients slowly progress to uremia.

FURTHER READING

BOUDEWIJN G et al: Diagnostic tests for renal artery stenosis in patients suspected of having renovascular hypertension: A meta-analysis. Ann Intern Med 135:401, 2001

CAREY RM et al: Role of the angiotensin type 2 receptor in the regulation of blood pressure and renal function. Hypertension 35:155, 2000

CHATZIANTONIOU C, DUSSAULE JC: Endothelin and renal vascular fibrosis: Of mice and men. Curr Opin Nephrol Hypertens 9:31, 2000

GHANIOUS VE et al: Evaluating patients with renal failure for renal artery stenosis with gadolinium-enhanced magnetic resonance angiography. Am J Kidney Dis 33:36, 1999

GREENBERG A et al: Focal segmental glomerulosclerosis associated with nephrotic syndrome in cholesterol atheroembolism. Clinicopathologic correlations. Am J Kidney Dis 29:344, 1997

MODI KS et al: Atheroembolic renal disease. J Am Soc Nephrol 12:1781, 2001

MURAY S et al: Rapid decline in renal function reflects reversibility and predicts the outcome after angioplasty in renal artery stenosis. Am J Kidney Dis 39:60, 2002

PHUONG-THU T. PHAM et al: Renal abnormalities in sickle cell disease. Kidney Intl 157:1, 2000

RADERMACHER J et al: Techniques for predicting a favourable response to renal angioplasty in patients with renovascular disease. Curr Opin Nephrol Hypertens 10:799, 2001

RUGGENENTI P et al: Thrombotic microangiopathy, hemolytic uremic syndrome, and thrombotic thrombocytopenic purpura. Kidney Intl 60:831, 2001

SABORIO P et al: Sickle cell nephropathy. J Am Soc Nephrol 10:187, 1999

SAFIAN RD, TEXTOR SC: Renal-artery stenosis. N Engl J Med 344:431, 2001

SCOLARI F et al: Cholesterol crystal embolism: A recognizable cause of renal disease. Am J Kidney Dis 36:1089, 2000

TUTTLE KR, RAABE RD: Endovascular stents for renal artery revascularization. Curr Opin Nephrol Hypertens 7:695, 1998

WRIGHT JR et al: A prospective study of the determinants of renal functional outcome and mortality in atherosclerotic renovascular disease. Am J Kidney Dis 39:1153, 2002

YUDD M, LLACH F: Disorders of the renal arteries and veins in BM Brenner (ed): *The Kidney*, 7th ed. Philadelphia, Saunders, 2004, pp 1571–1600

268 NEPHROLITHIASIS
John R. Asplin, Fredric L. Coe, Murray J. Favus

TYPES OF STONES

Calcium salts, uric acid, cystine, and struvite ($MgNH_4PO_4$) are the basic constituents of most kidney stones in the western hemisphere. Calcium oxalate and calcium phosphate stones make up 75 to 85% of the total (Table 268-1) and may be admixed in the same stone. Calcium phosphate in stones is usually hydroxyapatite [$Ca_5(PO_4)_3OH$] or, less commonly, brushite ($CaHPO_4H_2O$).

Calcium stones are more common in men; the average age of onset is the third to fourth decade. Approximately 50% of people who form a single calcium stone eventually form another within the next 10 years. The average rate of new stone formation in recurrent stone formers is about one stone every 2 or 3 years. Calcium stone disease is frequently familial. *Uric acid stones* are radiolucent and are also more common in men. Half of patients with uric acid stones have gout; uric acid lithiasis is usually familial whether or not gout is present. *Cystine stones* are uncommon; their radiopacity is due to the sulfur content. Cystine crystals appear in the urine as flat, hexagonal plates. *Struvite stones* are common and potentially dangerous. These stones occur mainly in women or patients who require chronic bladder catheterization and result from urinary tract infection with urease-producing bacteria, usually *Proteus* species. The stones can grow to a large size and fill the renal pelvis and calyces to produce a "staghorn" appearance. They are radiopaque and have a variable internal density. In urine, struvite crystals are rectangular prisms said to resemble coffin lids.

MANIFESTATIONS OF STONES

As stones grow on the surfaces of the renal papillae or within the collecting system, they need not produce symptoms. Asymptomatic stones may be discovered during the course of radiographic studies undertaken for unrelated reasons. Stones rank, along with benign and malignant neoplasms, and renal cysts, among the common causes of isolated hematuria. Much of the time, however, stones break loose and enter the ureter or occlude the ureteropelvic junction, causing pain and obstruction.

STONE PASSAGE A stone can traverse the ureter without symptoms, but passage usually produces pain and bleeding. The pain begins gradually, usually in the flank, but increases over the next 20 to 60 min to become so severe that narcotic drugs may be needed for its control. The pain may remain in the flank or spread downward and anteriorly toward the ipsilateral loin, testis, or vulva. Pain that migrates downward indicates that the stone has passed to the lower third of the ureter, but if the pain does not migrate, the position of the stone cannot be predicted. A stone in the portion of the ureter within the bladder wall causes frequency, urgency, and dysuria that may be confused with urinary tract infection. The vast majority of ureteral stones less than 0.5 cm in diameter will pass spontaneously.

It has been standard practice to diagnose acute renal colic by intravenous pyelography; however, helical computed tomography (CT) scan without radiocontrast enhancement is now the preferred proce-

TABLE 268-1 *Major Causes of Renal Stones*

Stone Type and Causes	Percent of all Stones[a]	Percent Occurrence of Specific Causes[a]	Ratio of Males to Females	Etiology	Diagnosis	Treatment
Calcium stones	75–85		2:1 to 3:1			
Idiopathic hypercalciuria		50–55	2:1	Hereditary (?)	Normocalcemia, unexplained hypercalciuria[b]	Thiazide diuretic agents
Hyperuricosuria		20	4:1	Diet	Urine uric acid >750 mg per 24 h (women), >800 mg per 24 h (men)	Allopurinol or diet
Primary hyperparathyroidism		5	3:10	Neoplasia	Unexplained hypercalcemia	Surgery
Distal renal tubular acidosis		Rare	1:1	Hereditary	Hyperchloremic acidosis, minimum urine pH >5.5	Alkali replacement
Dietary hyperoxaluria		10–30	1:1	High oxalate diet or low calcium diet	Urine oxalate >50 mg per 24 h	Low oxalate diet
Enteric hyperoxaluria		~1–2	1:1	Bowel surgery	Urine oxalate >75 mg per 24 h	Cholestyramine or oral calcium loading
Hereditary hyperoxaluria		Rare	1:1	Hereditary	Urine oxalate and glycolic or l-glyceric acid increased	Fluids and pyridoxine
Hypocitraturia		15–60	2:1 to 5:1	Hereditary (?), diet	Urine citrate <320 mg per 24 h	Alkali supplements
Idiopathic stone disease		20	2:1	Unknown	None of the above present	Oral phosphate, fluids
Uric acid stones	5–8					
Gout		~50	3:1 to 4:1	Hereditary	Clinical diagnosis	Alkali and allopurinol
Idiopathic		~50	1:1	Hereditary (?)	Uric acid stones, no gout	Alkali and allopurinol if daily urine uric acid above 1000 mg
Dehydration		?	1:1	Intestinal, habit	History, intestinal fluid loss	Alkali, fluids, reversal of cause
Lesch-Nyhan syndrome		Rare	Males only	Hereditary	Reduced hypoxanthine-guanine phosphoribosyltransferase level	Allopurinol
Malignant tumors		Rare	1:1	Neoplasia	Clinical diagnosis	Allopurinol
Cystine stones	1		1:1	Hereditary	Stone type; elevated cystine excretion	Massive fluids, alkali, D-penicillamine if needed
Struvite stones	10–15		2:10	Infection	Stone type	Antimicrobial agents and judicious surgery

[a] Values are percent of patients who form a particular type of stone and who display each specific cause of stones.

[b] Urine calcium above 300 mg/24 h (men), 250 mg/24 h (women), or 4 mg/kg per 24 h either sex. Hyperthyroidism, Cushing syndrome, sarcoidosis, malignant tumors, immobilization, vitamin D intoxication, rapidly progressive bone disease, and Paget's disease all cause hypercalciuria and must be excluded in diagnosis of idiopathic hypercalciuria.

dure. The advantages of CT include detection of uric acid stones in addition to the traditional radiopaque stones, no exposure to the risk of radiocontrast agents, and possible diagnosis of other causes of abdominal pain in a patient suspected of having renal colic from stones. Ultrasound is not as sensitive as CT in detecting renal or ureteral stones.

OTHER SYNDROMES ▪ Staghorn Calculi Struvite, cystine, and uric acid stones often grow too large to enter the ureter. They gradually fill the renal pelvis and may extend outward through the infundibula to the calyces themselves.

Nephrocalcinosis Calcium stones grow on the papillae. Most break loose and cause colic, but they may remain in place so that multiple papillary calcifications are found by x-ray, a condition termed *nephrocalcinosis*. Papillary nephrocalcinosis is common in hereditary distal renal tubular acidosis (RTA) and in other types of severe hypercalciuria. In medullary sponge kidney disease (Chap. 265), calcification may occur in dilated distal collecting ducts.

Sludge Sufficient uric acid or cystine in the urine may plug both ureters with precipitate. Calcium oxalate crystals do not do this because less than 100 mg oxalate usually is excreted daily in the urine even in severe hyperoxaluric states, compared with 1000 mg uric acid in patients with hyperuricosuria and 400 to 800 mg cystine in patients with cystinuria. Calcium phosphate crystals can render the urine milky but do not plug the urinary tract.

INFECTION Although urinary tract infection is not a direct consequence of stone disease, it can occur after instrumentation and surgery of the urinary tract, which are frequent in the treatment of stone disease. Stone disease and urinary tract infection can enhance their respective seriousness and interfere with treatment. Obstruction of an infected kidney by a stone may lead to sepsis and extensive damage of renal tissue, since it converts the urinary tract proximal to the obstruction into a closed, or partially closed, space that can become an abscess. Stones may harbor bacteria in the stone matrix, leading to recurrent urinary tract infection. On the other hand, infection due to bacteria that possess the enzyme urease can cause stones composed of struvite.

ACTIVITY OF STONE DISEASE Active disease means that new stones are forming or that preformed stones are growing. Sequential radiographs of the renal areas are needed to document the growth or appearance of new stones and to ensure that passed stones are actually newly formed, not preexistent ones.

PATHOGENESIS OF STONES

Urinary stones usually arise because of the breakdown of a delicate balance. The kidneys must conserve water, but they must excrete materials that have a low solubility. These two opposing requirements must be balanced during adaptation to diet, climate, and activity. The problem is mitigated to some extent by the fact that urine contains substances that inhibit crystallization of calcium salts and others that bind calcium in soluble complexes. These protective mechanisms are less than perfect. When the urine becomes supersaturated with insoluble materials, because excretion rates are excessive and/or because water conservation is extreme, crystals form and may grow and aggregate to form a stone.

SUPERSATURATION   In a solution in equilibrium with crystals of calcium oxalate, the product of the chemical activities of the calcium and oxalate ions in the solution is termed the *equilibrium solubility product*. If crystals are removed, and if either calcium or oxalate ions are added to the solution, the activity product increases, but no new crystals form. Such a solution is *metastably supersaturated*. If new calcium oxalate seed crystals are now added, they will grow in size. Ultimately, as calcium or oxalate are added to the solution, the activity product reaches a critical value at which a solid phase begins to develop spontaneously. This value is called the *upper limit of metastability*. Stone growth in the urinary tract requires a urine that, on average, is above the equilibrium solubility product. Excessive supersaturation is common in stone formation.

Calcium, oxalate, and phosphate form many stable soluble complexes among themselves and with other substances in urine, such as citrate. As a result, their free ion activities are below their chemical concentrations and can be measured only by indirect techniques. Reduction in ligands such as citrate can increase ion activity, and therefore supersaturation, without changing total urinary calcium. Urine supersaturation can be increased by dehydration or by overexcretion of calcium, oxalate, phosphate, cystine, or uric acid. Urine pH is also important; phosphate and uric acid are weak acids that dissociate readily over the physiologic range of urine pH. Alkaline urine contains more dibasic phosphate, favoring deposits of brushite and apatite. Below a urine pH of 5.5, uric acid crystals (pK 5.47) predominate, whereas phosphate crystals are rare. The solubility of calcium oxalate, on the other hand, is not influenced by changes in urine pH. Measurements of supersaturation in a pooled 24-h urine sample probably underestimate the risk of precipitation. Transient dehydration, variation of urine pH, and postprandial bursts of overexcretion may cause values considerably above average.

NUCLEATION   In urine that is supersaturated with respect to calcium oxalate, these two ions form clusters. Most small clusters eventually disperse because the internal forces that hold them together are too weak to overcome the random tendency of ions to move away. Large ion clusters can remain stable because attractive forces balance surface losses. Once they are stable, nuclei can grow at levels of supersaturation below that needed for their creation. Cell debris, calcifications on the renal papillae, and other urinary crystals can serve as templates for crystal formation, a process known as *heterogeneous nucleation*. Heterogeneous nucleation lowers the level of supersaturation required for crystal formation and is likely the mechanism by which stones form in human urine.

INHIBITORS OF CRYSTAL FORMATION   Stable nuclei must grow and aggregate to produce a stone of clinical significance. Urine contains potent inhibitors of nucleation, growth, and aggregation for calcium oxalate and calcium phosphate but not for uric acid, cystine, or struvite. Inorganic pyrophosphate is a potent inhibitor that appears to affect calcium phosphate more than calcium oxalate crystals. Citrate inhibits crystal growth and nucleation, though most of the stone inhibitory activity of citrate is due to lowering urine supersaturation via complexation of calcium. Other urine components such as glycoproteins inhibit all three processes of calcium oxalate stone formation. As a consequence of the presence of these inhibitors, crystal growth in urine is slow compared with growth in simple salt solutions, and the upper limit of metastability is higher.

EVALUATION AND TREATMENT OF PATIENTS WITH NEPHROLITHIASIS

Most patients with nephrolithiasis have remediable metabolic disorders that cause stones and can be detected by chemical analyses of serum and urine. Adults with recurrent kidney stones and children with

even a single kidney stone should be evaluated. A practical outpatient evaluation consists of two or three 24-h urine collections, with a corresponding blood sample; measurements of serum and urine calcium, uric acid, electrolytes, and creatinine, and urine pH, volume, oxalate, and citrate should be made. Since stone risks vary with diet, activity, and environment, at least one urine collection should be made on a weekend when the patient is at home and another on a work day. When possible, the composition of kidney stones should be determined because treatment depends on stone type (Table 268-1). No matter what disorders are found, every patient should be counseled to avoid dehydration and to drink copious amounts of water. The efficacy of high fluid intake was confirmed in a prospective study of first-time stone formers. Increasing urine volume to 2.5 L per day resulted in a 50% reduction of stone recurrence compared to the control group. Because treatment is prolonged, the use of medications must be justified by the activity and severity of stone disease and the importance of protection against new stones.

 TREATMENT

The management of stones already present in the kidneys or urinary tract requires a combined medical and surgical approach. The specific treatment depends on the location of the stone, the extent of obstruction, the function of the affected and unaffected kidney, the presence or absence of urinary tract infection, the progress of stone passage, and the risks of operation or anesthesia given the clinical state of the patient. In general, severe obstruction, infection, intractable pain, and serious bleeding are indications for removal of a stone.

In the past, stones were removed by operation or by passing a flexible basket retrograde up the ureter from the bladder during cystoscopy. There are now three alternatives. *Extracorporeal lithotripsy* causes the in situ fragmentation of stones in the kidney, renal pelvis, or ureter by exposing them to shock waves. The kidney stone is centered at a focal point of parabolic reflectors, and high-intensity shock waves are created by high-voltage discharge. The waves are transmitted to the patient using water as a conduction medium, either by placing the patient in a water tank or by placing water-filled cushions between the patient and the shock wave generators. After multiple discharges, most stones are reduced to powder that moves through the ureter into the bladder. *Percutaneous nephrolithotomy* requires the passage of a cystoscope-like instrument into the renal pelvis through a small incision in the flank. Stones are then disrupted by a small ultrasound transducer or holmium laser. The last method is *lithotripsy via a ureteroscope* for removal of ureteral stones. These various forms of lithotripsy have largely replaced pyelolithotomy and ureterolithotomy.

CALCIUM STONES ■ Idiopathic Hypercalciuria (See also Chap. 332)   This condition appears to be hereditary, and its diagnosis is straightforward (Table 268-1). In some patients, primary intestinal hyperabsorption of calcium causes transient postprandial hypercalcemia that suppresses secretion of parathyroid hormone. The renal tubules are deprived of the normal stimulus to reabsorb calcium at the same time that the filtered load of calcium is increased. In other patients, reabsorption of calcium by the renal tubules appears to be defective, and secondary hyperparathyroidism is evoked by urinary losses of calcium. Renal synthesis of 1,25-dihydroxyvitamin D is increased, enhancing intestinal absorption of calcium. In the past, the separation of "absorptive" and "renal" forms of hypercalciuria was used to guide treatment. However, these may not be distinct entities but the extremes of a continuum of behavior. Vitamin D overactivity, either through high calcitriol levels or excess vitamin D receptor, is a likely explanation for the hypercalciuria in many of these patients. Hypercalciuria contributes to stone formation by raising urine saturation with respect to calcium oxalate and calcium phosphate.

TREATMENT

For many years the standard therapy for hypercalciuria was dietary calcium restriction. However, recent studies have shown that low-calcium diets increase the risk of incident stone formation. In addition, hypercalciuric stone formers have reduced bone mineral density and an increased risk of fracture compared to the non-stone-forming population. Low calcium intake likely contributes to the low bone mineral density. A recent prospective trial compared the efficacy of a low-calcium diet to a low-protein, low-sodium, normal-calcium diet in preventing stone recurrence in male calcium stone formers. The group on the low-calcium diet had a significantly greater rate of stone relapse. As a whole, low-calcium diets do not appear to be efficacious and carry a long-term risk of bone disease in the stone-forming population. Low-sodium and low-protein diets are a superior option in stone formers. If diet therapy is not sufficient to prevent stones, then thiazide diuretics may be used. Thiazide diuretics lower urine calcium and are effective in preventing the formation of stones. Three 3-year randomized trials have shown a 50% decrease in stone formation in the thiazide-treated groups as compared to the placebo-treated controls. The drug effect requires slight contraction of the extracellular fluid volume, and massive use of NaCl reduces its therapeutic effect. Thiazide-induced hypokalemia should be aggressively treated since hypokalemia will reduce urine citrate, increasing urine calcium ion levels.

Hyperuricosuria About 20% of calcium oxalate stone formers are hyperuricosuric, primarily because of an excessive intake of purine from meat, fish, and poultry. The mechanism of stone formation is probably due to salting out calcium oxalate by urate. A low-purine diet is desirable but difficult for many patients to achieve. The alternative is allopurinol, which has been shown to be effective in a randomized, controlled trial. A dose of 100 mg bid is usually sufficient.

Primary Hyperparathyroidism (See also Chap. 332) The diagnosis of this condition is established by documenting that hypercalcemia that cannot be otherwise explained is accompanied by inappropriately elevated serum concentrations of parathyroid hormone. Hypercalciuria, usually present, raises the urine supersaturation of calcium phosphate and/or calcium oxalate (Table 268-1). Prompt diagnosis is important because parathyroidectomy should be carried out before renal damage or bone disease occurs.

Distal Renal Tubular Acidosis (See also Chap. 265) The defect in this condition seems to reside in the distal nephron, which cannot establish a normal pH gradient between urine and blood, leading to hyperchloremic acidosis. The diagnosis is suggested by a minimum urine pH above 5.5 in the presence of systemic acidosis. If the diagnosis is in doubt because metabolic abnormalities are mild, oral challenge with NH_4Cl, 1.9 mmol/kg of body weight, will not lower urine pH below 5.5 in patients with distal RTA. Hypercalciuria, an alkaline urine, and a low urine citrate level cause supersaturation with respect to calcium phosphate. Calcium phosphate stones form, nephrocalcinosis is common, and osteomalacia or rickets may occur. Renal damage is frequent, and glomerular filtration rate falls gradually.

Treatment with supplemental alkali reverses hypercalciuria and limits the production of new stones. The usual dose of sodium bicarbonate is 0.5 to 2.0 mmol/kg of body weight per day in four to six divided doses. An alternative is potassium citrate supplementation, given at the same dose per day but needing to be given only three to four times per day. In incomplete distal RTA, systemic acidosis is absent, but urine pH cannot be lowered below 5.5 after an exogenous acid load such as ammonium chloride. Incomplete RTA may develop in some patients who form calcium oxalate stones because of idiopathic hypercalciuria; the importance of RTA in producing stones in this situation is uncertain, and thiazide treatment is a reasonable alternative. Some patients with incomplete RTA form calcium phosphate stones because of low urine citrate and an alkaline urine and are best treated with alkali as if RTA were complete. When treating patients with alkali it is prudent to monitor changes in urine citrate and pH. If urine pH increases without an increase in citrate then calcium phosphate supersaturation will increase and stone disease may worsen.

Hyperoxaluria Oxalate is a metabolic end product in humans. Urine oxalate comes from diet and endogenous metabolic production, with approximately 40 to 50% originating from dietary sources. The upper limit of normal for oxalate excretion is generally considered to be 40 to 50 mg per day. Mild hyperoxaluria (50 to 80 mg/d) is usually caused by excessive intake of high-oxalate foods such as spinach, nuts, and chocolate. In addition, low-calcium diets may promote hyperoxaluria as there is less calcium binding oxalate in the intestine, increasing the amount of oxalate available for absorption. Enteric hyperoxaluria is a consequence of small bowel disease resulting in fat malabsorption. Oxalate excretion is often over 100 mg per day. Enteric hyperoxaluria may be caused by jejunoileal bypass for obesity, bacterial overgrowth syndromes, pancreatic insufficiency, or extensive small intestine involvement from Crohn's disease. With fat malabsorption, calcium in the bowel lumen is bound by fatty acids instead of oxalate, which is left free for absorption in the colon. Delivery of unabsorbed fatty acids and bile salts to the colon may injure the colonic mucosa and enhance oxalate absorption. Hereditary hyperoxaluria states are rare causes of severe hyperoxaluria, often greater than 150 mg per day. Patients usually present with recurrent calcium oxalate stones during childhood. Type I hereditary hyperoxaluria is inherited as an autosomal recessive trait and is due to a deficiency in the peroxisomal enzyme alanine: glyoxylate aminotransferase. Type II is due to a deficiency of D-glyceric dehydrogenase. Severe hyperoxaluria from any cause can produce tubulointerstitial nephropathy (Chap. 266) and lead to stone formation.

℞ TREATMENT

Patients with mild to moderate hyperoxaluria should be treated with a diet low in oxalate and with a normal intake of calcium and magnesium to reduce oxalate absorption. Enteric hyperoxaluria can be treated with the oxalate-binding resin cholestyramine at a dose of 8 to 16 g/d, correction of fat malabsorption, and a low-fat, low-oxalate diet. Calcium supplements, given with meals, precipitate oxalate in the gut lumen, providing an additional form of therapy. Treatment for hereditary hyperoxaluria includes a high fluid intake, neutral phosphate, and pyridoxine (25 to 200 mg/d). Citrate supplementation may also have some benefit. Even with aggressive therapy, irreversible renal failure secondary to recurrent stone formation often occurs. Segmental liver transplant, to correct the enzyme defect, combined with a kidney transplant has been successfully utilized in patients with hereditary hyperoxaluria.

Hypocitraturia Urine citrate prevents calcium stone formation by creating a soluble complex with calcium, effectively reducing free urine calcium. Hypocitraturia is found in 15 to 60% of stone formers, either as a single disorder or in combination with other metabolic abnormalities. It can be secondary to systemic disorders, such as RTA, chronic diarrheal illness, or hypokalemia, or it may be a primary disorder, in which case it is called *idiopathic hypocitraturia*.

℞ TREATMENT

Treatment is with alkali, which increases urine citrate excretion; generally bicarbonate or citrate salts are used. Potassium salts are preferred as sodium loading increases urinary excretion of calcium, reducing the effectiveness of treatment. Two randomized, placebo-controlled trials have demonstrated the effectiveness of citrate supplements in calcium oxalate stone formers.

Idiopathic Calcium Lithiasis Some patients have no metabolic cause for stones despite a thorough metabolic evaluation (Table 268-1). The best treatment appears to be high fluid intake so that the urine specific gravity remains at 1.005 or below throughout the day and night. Thiazide diuretics, allopurinol, and citrate therapy may help reduce crystallization of calcium salts, but there are no prospective trials in this patient population. Oral phosphate at a dose of 2 g phosphorus daily may lower urine calcium and increase urine pyrophosphate and thereby reduce the rate of recurrence. Orthophosphate causes mild nausea and diarrhea, but tolerance may improve with continued intake.

URIC ACID STONES   These stones form because the urine becomes supersaturated with undissociated uric acid that is protonated at its N-9 position. In gout, idiopathic uric acid lithiasis, and dehydration, the average pH is usually below 5.4 and often below 5.0. Undissociated uric acid therefore predominates and is soluble in urine only in concentrations of 100 mg/L. Concentrations above this level represent supersaturation that causes crystals and stones to form. Hyperuricosuria, when present, increases supersaturation, but urine of low pH can be supersaturated with undissociated uric acid even though the daily excretion rate is normal. Myeloproliferative syndromes, chemotherapy of malignant tumors, and Lesch-Nyhan syndrome cause such massive production of uric acid and consequent hyperuricosuria that stones and uric acid sludge form even at a normal urine pH. Plugging of the renal collecting tubules by uric acid crystals can cause acute renal failure.

TREATMENT

The two goals of treatment are to raise urine pH and to lower excessive urine uric acid excretion to less than 1 g/d. Supplemental alkali, 1 to 3 mmol/kg of body weight per day, should be given in three or four evenly spaced, divided doses, one of which should be given at bedtime. The form of the alkali may be important. Potassium citrate may reduce the risk of calcium salts crystallizing when urine pH is increased, whereas sodium citrate or sodium bicarbonate may increase the risk. If the overnight urine pH is below 5.5, the evening dose of alkali may be raised or 250 mg acetazolamide added at bedtime. A low-purine diet should be instituted in those uric acid stone formers with hyperuricosuria. Patients who continue to form uric acid stones despite treatment with fluids, alkali, and a low-purine diet should have allopurinol added to their regimen. If hypercalciuria is also present, it should be specifically treated, as alkali alone could lead to calcium phosphate stone formation.

CYSTINURIA AND CYSTINE STONES (See also Chap. 343)   In this autosomal recessive disorder, proximal tubular and jejunal transport of the dibasic amino acids cystine, lysine, arginine, and ornithine are defective, and excessive amounts are lost in the urine. Clinical disease is due solely to the insolubility of cystine, which forms stones.

Pathogenesis   Cystinuria occurs because of defective transport of dibasic amino acids by the brush borders of renal tubule and intestinal epithelial cells. The disease classically has been broken into three types based on differences in intestinal and renal amino acid handling in families. However, genomic studies suggest type II and type III cystinuria are due to defects in the same protein. Disease-causing mutations have been identified in both the heavy and light chain of a heteromeric amino acid transporter found in the proximal tubule of the kidney. A gene located on chromosome 2 and designated *SLC3A1* encodes the heavy chain of the transporter and has been found to be abnormal in type I cystinuria. Non-type-I cystinuria is due to mutations in the *SLC7A9* gene on chromosome 19, which encodes the light chain of the heteromeric transporter.

Diagnosis   Cystine stones are formed only by patients with cystinuria, but 10% of stones in cystinuric patients do not contain cystine; therefore, every stone former should be screened for the disease. The sediment from a first morning urine specimen in many patients with homozygous cystinuria reveals typical flat, hexagonal, platelike cystine crystals. Cystinuria also can be detected using the urine sodium nitroprusside test. Because the test is sensitive, it is positive in many asymptomatic heterozygotes for cystinuria. A positive nitroprusside

test or the finding of cystine crystals in the urine sediment should be evaluated by measurement of daily cystine excretion. Normal adults excrete 40 to 60 mg cystine per gram of creatinine, heterozygotes usually excrete less than 300 mg/g, and homozygotes almost always excrete greater than 250 mg/g.

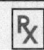 TREATMENT

High fluid intake, even at night, is the cornerstone of therapy. Daily urine volume should exceed 3 L. Raising urine pH with alkali is helpful, provided the urine pH exceeds 7.5. A low-salt diet (100 mmol/d) can reduce cystine excretion up to 40%. Because side effects are frequent, drugs such as penicillamine and tiopronin, which form the soluble disulfide cysteine-drug complexes, should be used only when fluid loading, salt reduction, and alkali therapy are ineffective. Captopril, which has a free sulfhydryl group to bind cysteine, has been used in a limited number of patients with some success. Low-methionine diets have not proved to be practical for clinical use, but patients should avoid protein gluttony.

STRUVITE STONES   These stones are a result of urinary infection with bacteria, usually *Proteus* species, which possess urease, an enzyme that degrades urea to NH_3 and CO_2. The NH_3 hydrolyzes to NH_4^+ and raises urine pH to 8 or 9. The CO_2 hydrates to H_2CO_3 and then dissociates to CO_3^{2-} that precipitates with calcium as $CaCO_3$. The NH_4^+ precipitates PO_4^{3-} and Mg^{2+} to form $MgNH_4PO_4$ (struvite). The result is a stone of calcium carbonate admixed with struvite. Struvite does not form in urine in the absence of infection, because NH_4^+ concentration is low in urine that is alkaline in response to physiologic stimuli. Chronic *Proteus* infection can occur because of impaired urinary drainage, urologic instrumentation or surgery, and especially with chronic antibiotic treatment, which can favor the dominance of *Proteus* in the urinary tract.

TREATMENT

Complete removal of the stone with subsequent sterilization of the urinary tract is the treatment of choice for patients who can tolerate the procedures. Open surgery is successful in debulking the stone and improving renal function if obstruction is present; however, there is recurrence of stone in 25% of the patients. Irrigation of the renal pelvis and calyces with hemiacidrin, a solution that dissolves struvite, can reduce recurrence after surgery. Newer procedures such as lithotripsy and percutaneous nephrolithotomy, alone or in combination, have largely replaced open surgery. Stone-free rates of 50 to 90% have been reported after these procedures. Antimicrobial treatment is best reserved for dealing with acute infection and for maintenance of a sterile urine after surgery. Urine cultures and culture of stone fragments removed at surgery should guide the choice of antibiotic. For patients who are not candidates for surgical removal of stone, acetohydroxamic acid, an inhibitor of urease, can be used. Though effective in treating the stones, acetohydroxamic acid has many side effects, such as headache, tremor, and thrombophlebitis, that limit its use.

FURTHER READING

BUSHINSKY DA: Kidney stones. Adv Intern Med 47:219, 2001

CHILLARON J et al: Heteromeric amino acid transporters: Biochemistry, genetics, and physiology. Am J Physiol Renal Physiol 281:F995, 2001

FOWLER KA et al: Ultrasound for detecting renal calculi with nonenhanced CT as a reference standard. Radiology 222:09, 2002

HOLMES RP et al: Contribution of dietary oxalate to urinary oxalate excretion. Kidney Int 59:270, 2001

LAUDERDALE DS et al: Bone mineral density and fracture among prevalent kidney stone cases in the Third National Health and Nutrition Examination Survey. J Bone Miner Res 16:1893, 2001

PARKS JH et al: A single 24-hour urine collection is inadequate for the medical evaluation of nephrolithiasis. J Urol 167:1607, 2002

DEFINITIONS Acute infections of the urinary tract can be subdivided into two general anatomic categories: lower tract infection (urethritis and cystitis) and upper tract infection (acute pyelonephritis, prostatitis, and intrarenal and perinephric abscesses). Infections at these various sites may occur together or independently and may either be asymptomatic or present as one of the clinical syndromes described below. Infections of the urethra and bladder are often considered superficial (or mucosal) infections, while prostatitis, pyelonephritis, and renal suppuration signify tissue invasion.

From a microbiologic perspective, urinary tract infection (UTI) exists when pathogenic microorganisms are detected in the urine, urethra, bladder, kidney, or prostate. In most instances, growth of $>10^5$ organisms per milliliter from a properly collected midstream "clean-catch" urine sample indicates infection. However, significant bacteriuria is lacking in some cases of true UTI. Especially in symptomatic patients, a smaller number of bacteria (10^2 to 10^4/mL) may signify infection. In urine specimens obtained by suprapubic aspiration or "in-and-out" catheterization and in samples from a patient with an indwelling catheter, colony counts of 10^2 to 10^4/mL generally indicate infection. Conversely, colony counts of $>10^5$/mL of midstream urine are occasionally due to specimen contamination, which is especially likely when multiple bacterial species are found.

Infections that recur after antibiotic therapy can be due to the persistence of the originally infecting strain (as judged by species, antibiogram, serotype, and molecular type) or to reinfection with a new strain. "Same-strain" recurrent infections that become evident within 2 weeks of cessation of therapy can be the result of unresolved renal or prostatic infection (termed *relapse*) or of persistent vaginal or intestinal colonization leading to rapid reinfection of the bladder.

Symptoms of dysuria, urgency, and frequency that are unaccompanied by significant bacteriuria have been termed the *acute urethral syndrome*. Although widely used, this term lacks anatomic precision because many cases so designated are actually bladder infections. Moreover, since the causative agent can usually be identified in these patients, the term *syndrome*—implying unknown causation—is inappropriate.

Chronic pyelonephritis refers to chronic interstitial nephritis believed to result from bacterial infection of the kidney (Chap. 266). Many noninfectious diseases also cause an interstitial nephritis that is indistinguishable pathologically from chronic pyelonephritis.

ACUTE UTIs: URETHRITIS, CYSTITIS, AND PYELONEPHRITIS

EPIDEMIOLOGY Epidemiologically, UTIs are subdivided into catheter-associated (or nosocomial) infections and non-catheter-associated (or community-acquired) infections. Infections in either category may be symptomatic or asymptomatic. Acute community-acquired infections are very common and account for more than 7 million office visits annually in the United States. These infections occur in 1 to 3% of schoolgirls and then increase markedly in incidence with the onset of sexual activity in adolescence. The vast majority of acute symptomatic infections involve young women; a prospective study demonstrated an annual incidence of 0.5 to 0.7 infections per patient-year in this group. Acute symptomatic UTIs are unusual in men under the age of 50. The development of asymptomatic bacteriuria parallels that of symptomatic infection and is rare among men under 50 but common among women between 20 and 50. Asymptomatic bacteriuria is more common among elderly men and women, with rates as high as 40 to 50% in some studies.

ETIOLOGY Many different microorganisms can infect the urinary tract, but by far the most common agents are the gram-negative bacilli. *Escherichia coli* causes ~80% of acute infections in patients without catheters, urologic abnormalities, or calculi. Other gram-negative rods, especially *Proteus* and *Klebsiella* and occasionally *Enterobacter*,

account for a smaller proportion of uncomplicated infections. These organisms, plus *Serratia* and *Pseudomonas*, assume increasing importance in recurrent infections and in infections associated with urologic manipulation, calculi, or obstruction. They play a major role in nosocomial, catheter-associated infections (see below). *Proteus* spp., by virtue of urease production, and *Klebsiella* spp., through the production of extracellular slime and polysaccharides, predispose to stone formation and are isolated more frequently from patients with calculi.

Gram-positive cocci play a lesser role in UTIs. However, *Staphylococcus saprophyticus*—a novobiocin-resistant, coagulase-negative species—accounts for 10 to 15% of acute symptomatic UTIs in young females. Enterococci occasionally cause acute uncomplicated cystitis in women. More commonly, enterococci and *Staphylococcus aureus* cause infections in patients with renal stones or previous instrumentation or surgery. Isolation of *S. aureus* from the urine should arouse suspicion of bacteremic infection of the kidney.

About one-third of women with dysuria and frequency have either an insignificant number of bacteria in midstream urine cultures or completely sterile cultures and have been previously defined as having the urethral syndrome. About three-quarters of these women have pyuria, while one-quarter have no pyuria and little objective evidence of infection. In the women with pyuria, two groups of pathogens account for most infections. Low counts (10^2 to 10^4/mL) of typical bacterial uropathogens such as *E. coli, S. saprophyticus, Klebsiella*, or *Proteus* are found in midstream urine specimens from most of these women. These bacteria are probably the causative agents in these infections because they can usually be isolated from a suprapubic aspirate, are associated with pyuria, and respond to appropriate antimicrobial therapy. In other women with acute urinary symptoms, pyuria, and urine that is sterile (even when obtained by suprapubic aspiration), sexually transmitted urethritis-producing agents such as *Chlamydia trachomatis, Neisseria gonorrhoeae*, and herpes simplex virus are etiologically important. These agents are found most frequently in young, sexually active women with new sexual partners.

The causative role of several more unusual bacterial and nonbacterial pathogens in UTIs remains poorly defined. *Ureaplasma urealyticum* has frequently been isolated from the urethra and urine of patients with acute dysuria and frequency but is also found in specimens from many patients without urinary symptoms. Ureaplasmas probably account for some cases of urethritis and cystitis. *U. urealyticum* and *Mycoplasma hominis* have been isolated from prostatic and renal tissues of patients with acute prostatitis and pyelonephritis, respectively, and are probably responsible for some of these infections as well. Adenoviruses cause acute hemorrhagic cystitis in children and in some young adults, often in epidemics. Although other viruses can be isolated from urine (e.g., cytomegalovirus), they are thought not to cause acute UTI. Colonization of the urine of catheterized or diabetic patients by *Candida* and other fungal species is common and sometimes progresses to symptomatic invasive infection (Chap. 187). →*Mycobacterial infection of the genitourinary tract is discussed in Chap. 150.*

PATHOGENESIS AND SOURCES OF INFECTION The urinary tract should be viewed as a single anatomic unit that is united by a continuous column of urine extending from the urethra to the kidney. In the vast majority of UTIs, bacteria gain access to the bladder via the urethra. Ascent of bacteria from the bladder may follow and is probably the pathway for most renal parenchymal infections.

The vaginal introitus and distal urethra are normally colonized by diphtheroids, streptococcal species, lactobacilli, and staphylococcal species but not by the enteric gram-negative bacilli that commonly cause UTIs. In females prone to the development of cystitis, however, enteric gram-negative organisms residing in the bowel colonize the introitus, the periurethral skin, and the distal urethra before and during episodes of bacteriuria. The factors that predispose to periurethral colonization with gram-negative bacilli remain poorly understood, but alteration of the normal vaginal flora by antibiotics, other genital infections, or contraceptives (especially spermicide) appears to play an important role. Loss of the normally dominant H_2O_2-producing lactobacilli in the vaginal flora appears to facilitate colonization by *E. coli*. Small numbers of periurethral bacteria probably gain entry to the bladder frequently, a process that is facilitated in some cases by urethral massage during intercourse. Whether bladder infection ensues depends on interacting effects of the pathogenicity of the strain, the inoculum size, and the local and systemic host defense mechanisms.

Under normal circumstances, bacteria placed in the bladder are rapidly cleared, partly through the flushing and dilutional effects of voiding but also as a result of the antibacterial properties of urine and the bladder mucosa. Owing mostly to a high urea concentration and high osmolarity, the bladder urine of many normal persons inhibits or kills bacteria. Prostatic secretions possess antibacterial properties as well. Polymorphonuclear leukocytes enter the bladder epithelium and the urine soon after infection arises and play a role in clearing bacteriuria. The role of locally produced antibody remains unclear.

Hematogenous pyelonephritis occurs most often in debilitated patients who are either chronically ill or receiving immunosuppressive therapy. Metastatic staphylococcal or candidal infections of the kidney may follow bacteremia or fungemia, spreading from distant foci of infection in the bone, skin, vasculature, or elsewhere.

CONDITIONS AFFECTING PATHOGENESIS ■ **Gender and Sexual Activity** The female urethra appears to be particularly prone to colonization with colonic gram-negative bacilli because of its proximity to the anus, its short length (~4 cm), and its termination beneath the labia. Sexual intercourse causes the introduction of bacteria into the bladder and is temporally associated with the onset of cystitis; it thus appears to be important in the pathogenesis of UTIs in younger women. Voiding after intercourse reduces the risk of cystitis, probably because it promotes the clearance of bacteria introduced during intercourse. Use of spermicidal compounds with a diaphragm or cervical cap or use of spermicide-coated condoms dramatically alters the normal introital bacterial flora and has been associated with marked increases in vaginal colonization with *E. coli* and in the risk of UTI.

In males who are <50 years old and who have no history of heterosexual or homosexual rectal intercourse, UTI is exceedingly uncommon, and this diagnosis should be questioned in the absence of clear documentation. An important factor predisposing to bacteriuria in men is urethral obstruction due to prostatic hypertrophy. Insertive rectal intercourse is also associated with an increased risk of cystitis in men. Men (and women) who are infected with HIV and who have CD4+ T cell counts of <200/μL are at increased risk of both bacteriuria and symptomatic UTI. Finally, lack of circumcision has been identified as a risk factor for UTI in both neonates and young men.

Pregnancy UTIs are detected in 2 to 8% of pregnant women. Symptomatic upper tract infections, in particular, are unusually common during pregnancy; fully 20 to 30% of pregnant women with asymptomatic bacteriuria subsequently develop pyelonephritis. This predisposition to upper tract infection during pregnancy results from decreased ureteral tone, decreased ureteral peristalsis, and temporary incompetence of the vesicoureteral valves. Bladder catheterization during or after delivery causes additional infections. Increased incidences of low-birth-weight infants, premature delivery, and newborn mortality result from UTIs during pregnancy, particularly those infections involving the upper tract.

Obstruction Any impediment to the free flow of urine—tumor, stricture, stone, or prostatic hypertrophy—results in hydronephrosis and a greatly increased frequency of UTI. Infection superimposed on urinary tract obstruction may lead to rapid destruction of renal tissue. It is of utmost importance, therefore, when infection is present, to identify and repair obstructive lesions. On the other hand, when an obstruction is minor and is not progressive or associated with infection, great caution should be exercised in attempting surgical correction. The introduction of infection in such cases may be more damaging than an uncorrected minor obstruction that does not significantly impair renal function.

Neurogenic Bladder Dysfunction Interference with bladder enervation, as in spinal cord injury, tabes dorsalis, multiple sclerosis, diabetes, and other diseases, may be associated with UTI. The infection may be initiated by the use of catheters for bladder drainage and is favored by the prolonged stasis of urine in the bladder. An additional factor often operative in these cases is bone demineralization due to immobilization, which causes hypercalciuria, calculus formation, and obstructive uropathy.

Vesicoureteral Reflux Defined as reflux of urine from the bladder cavity up into the ureters and sometimes into the renal pelvis, vesicoureteral reflux occurs during voiding or with elevation of pressure in the bladder. In practice, this condition is demonstrated by the finding of retrograde movement of radiopaque or radioactive material during a voiding cystourethrogram. An anatomically impaired vesicoureteral junction facilitates reflux of bacteria and thus upper tract infection. However, since a fluid connection between the bladder and the kidney always exists, even in the normal urinary system, some retrograde movement of bacteria probably takes place during infection but is not detected by radiologic techniques.

Vesicoureteral reflux is common among children with anatomic abnormalities of the urinary tract as well as among children with anatomically normal but infected urinary tracts. In the latter group, reflux disappears with advancing age and is probably attributable to factors other than UTI. Long-term follow-up of children with UTI who have reflux has established that renal damage correlates with marked reflux, not with infection.

The routine search for reflux would be aided by the development of noninvasive tests applicable to young children, in whom the need for an effective technique is greatest. In the meantime, it appears reasonable to search for reflux in anyone with unexplained failure of renal growth or with renal scarring, because UTI per se is an insufficient explanation for these abnormalities. On the other hand, it is doubtful that all children who have recurrent UTIs but whose urinary tract appears normal on pyelography should be subjected to voiding cystoureterography merely for the detection of the rare patient with marked reflux not revealed by the intravenous pyelogram.

Bacterial Virulence Factors Not all strains of *E. coli* are equally capable of infecting the intact urinary tract. Bacterial virulence factors markedly influence the likelihood that a given strain, once introduced into the bladder, will cause UTI. Most *E. coli* strains that cause symptomatic UTIs in noncatheterized patients belong to a small number of specific O, K, and H serogroups. These uropathogenic clones have accumulated a number of virulence genes that are often closely linked on the bacterial chromosome in "virulence islands." Adherence of bacteria to uroepithelial cells is a critical first step in the initiation of infection. For both *E. coli* and *Proteus*, fimbriae (hairlike proteinaceous surface appendages) mediate the attachment of bacteria to specific receptors on epithelial cells. The attachment of bacteria to uroepithelial cells initiates a number of important events in the mucosal epithelial cell, including secretion of interleukin (IL) 6 and IL-8 (with subsequent chemotaxis of leukocytes to the bladder mucosa) and induction of apoptosis and epithelial cell desquamation. Besides fimbriae, uropathogenic *E. coli* strains usually produce hemolysin and aerobactin (a siderophore for scavenging iron) and are resistant to the bactericidal action of human serum. Nearly all *E. coli* strains causing acute pyelonephritis and most of those causing acute cystitis are uropathogenic. In contrast, infections in patients with structural or functional abnormalities of the urinary tract are generally caused by bacterial strains that lack these uropathogenic properties; the implication is that these properties are not needed for infection of the compromised urinary tract.

Genetic Factors   Increasing evidence suggests that host genetic factors influence susceptibility to UTI. A maternal history of UTI is more often found among women who have experienced recurrent UTIs than among controls. The number and type of receptors on uroepithelial cells to which bacteria may attach are at least in part genetically determined. Many of these structures are components of blood group antigens and are present on both erythrocytes and uroepithelial cells. For example, P fimbriae mediate attachment of *E. coli* to P-positive erythrocytes and are found on nearly all strains causing acute uncomplicated pyelonephritis. Conversely, P blood group–negative individuals, who lack these receptors, have a decreased likelihood of pyelonephritis. It has also been demonstrated that nonsecretors of blood group antigens are at increased risk of recurrent UTI; this predisposition may relate to a different profile of genetically determined glycolipids on uroepithelial cells. Mutations in host genes integral to the immune response (interferon γ receptors and others) may also affect susceptibility to UTI.

LOCALIZATION OF INFECTION   Unfortunately, currently available methods of distinguishing renal parenchymal infection from cystitis are neither reliable nor convenient enough for routine clinical use. Fever or an elevated level of C-reactive protein often accompanies acute pyelonephritis and is found in rare cases of cystitis but also occurs in infections other than pyelonephritis.

CLINICAL PRESENTATION ■ Cystitis   Patients with cystitis usually report dysuria, frequency, urgency, and suprapubic pain. The urine often becomes grossly cloudy and malodorous, and it is bloody in ~30% of cases. White cells and bacteria can be detected by examination of unspun urine in most cases. However, some women with cystitis have only 10^2 to 10^4 bacteria per milliliter of urine, and in these instances bacteria cannot be seen in a Gram-stained preparation of unspun urine. Physical examination generally reveals only tenderness of the urethra or the suprapubic area. If a genital lesion or a vaginal discharge is evident, especially in conjunction with $<10^5$ bacteria per milliliter on urine culture, then pathogens that may cause urethritis, vaginitis, or cervicitis, such as *C. trachomatis, N. gonorrhoeae, Trichomonas, Candida*, and herpes simplex virus, should be considered. Prominent systemic manifestations, such as a temperature of $>38.3°C$ ($>101°F$), nausea, and vomiting, usually indicate concomitant renal infection, as does costovertebral angle tenderness. However, the absence of these findings does not ensure that infection is limited to the bladder and urethra.

Acute Pyelonephritis   Symptoms of acute pyelonephritis generally develop rapidly over a few hours or a day and include a fever, shaking chills, nausea, vomiting, and diarrhea. Symptoms of cystitis may or may not be present. Besides fever, tachycardia, and generalized muscle tenderness, physical examination reveals marked tenderness on deep pressure in one or both costovertebral angles or on deep abdominal palpation. In some patients, signs and symptoms of gram-negative sepsis predominate. Most patients have significant leukocytosis and bacteria detectable in Gram-stained unspun urine. Leukocyte casts are present in the urine of some patients, and the detection of these casts is pathognomonic. Hematuria may be demonstrated during the acute phase of the disease; if it persists after acute manifestations of infection have subsided, a stone, a tumor, or tuberculosis should be considered.

Except in individuals with papillary necrosis, abscess formation, or urinary obstruction, the manifestations of acute pyelonephritis usually respond to therapy within 48 to 72 h. However, despite the absence of symptoms, bacteriuria or pyuria may persist. In severe pyelonephritis, fever subsides more slowly and may not disappear for several days, even after appropriate antibiotic treatment has been instituted.

Urethritis   Approximately 30% of women with acute dysuria, frequency, and pyuria have midstream urine cultures that show either no growth or insignificant bacterial growth. Clinically, these women cannot always be readily distinguished from those with cystitis. In this situation, a distinction should be made between women infected with sexually transmitted pathogens, such as *C. trachomatis, N. gonorrhoeae*, or herpes simplex virus, and those with low-count *E. coli* or staphylococcal infection of the urethra and bladder. Chlamydial or gonococcal infection should be suspected in women with a gradual onset of illness, no hematuria, no suprapubic pain, and >7 days of symptoms. The additional history of a recent sex-partner change, especially if the patient's partner has recently had chlamydial or gonococcal urethritis, should heighten the suspicion of a sexually transmitted infection, as should the finding of mucopurulent cervicitis (Chap. 115). Gross hematuria, suprapubic pain, an abrupt onset of illness, a duration of illness of <3 days, and a history of UTIs favor the diagnosis of *E. coli* UTI.

Catheter-Associated UTIs   (See also Chap. 116)   Bacteriuria develops in at least 10 to 15% of hospitalized patients with indwelling urethral catheters. The risk of infection is ~3 to 5% per day of catheterization. *E. coli, Proteus, Pseudomonas, Klebsiella, Serratia*, staphylococci, enterococci, and *Candida* usually cause these infections. Many infecting strains display markedly greater antimicrobial resistance than organisms that cause community-acquired UTIs. Factors associated with an increased risk of catheter-associated UTI include female sex, prolonged catheterization, severe underlying illness, disconnection of the catheter and drainage tube, other types of faulty catheter care, and lack of systemic antimicrobial therapy.

Infection occurs when bacteria reach the bladder by one of two routes: by migrating through the column of urine in the catheter lumen (intraluminal route) or by moving up the mucous sheath outside the catheter (periurethral route). Hospital-acquired pathogens reach the patient's catheter or urine-collecting system on the hands of hospital personnel, in contaminated solutions or irrigants, and via contaminated instruments or disinfectants. Bacteria usually enter the catheter system at the catheter–collecting tube junction or at the drainage bag portal. The organisms then ascend intraluminally into the bladder within 24 to 72 h. Alternatively, the patient's own bowel flora may colonize the perineal skin and periurethral area and reach the bladder via the external surface of the catheter. This route is particularly common in women. Studies have demonstrated the importance of the attachment and growth of bacteria on the surfaces of the catheter in the pathogenesis of catheter-associated UTI. Such bacteria growing in biofilms on the catheter eventually produce encrustations consisting of bacteria, bacterial glycocalyces, host urinary proteins, and urinary salts. These encrustations provide a refuge for bacteria and may protect them from antimicrobial agents and phagocytes.

Clinically, most catheter-associated infections cause minimal symptoms and no fever and often resolve after withdrawal of the catheter. The frequency of upper tract infection associated with catheter-induced bacteriuria is unknown. Gram-negative bacteremia, which follows catheter-associated bacteriuria in 1 to 2% of cases, is the most significant recognized complication of catheter-induced UTIs. The catheterized urinary tract has repeatedly been demonstrated to be the most common source of gram-negative bacteremia in hospitalized patients, generally accounting for ~30% of cases.

Catheter-associated UTIs can sometimes be prevented in patients catheterized for <2 weeks by use of a sterile closed collecting system, by attention to aseptic technique during insertion and care of the catheter, and by measures to minimize cross-infection. Other preventive approaches, including short courses of systemic antimicrobial therapy, topical application of periurethral antimicrobial ointments, use of preconnected catheter–drainage tube units, use of catheters impregnated with antimicrobial agents, and addition of antimicrobial drugs to the drainage bag, have all been protective in at least one controlled trial but are not recommended for general use. Despite precautions, the majority of patients catheterized for >2 weeks eventually develop bacteriuria. For example, because of spinal cord injury, incontinence, or other factors, some patients in hospitals or nursing homes require long-term or semipermanent bladder catheterization. Measures intended to prevent infection have been largely unsuccessful, and essentially all such chronically catheterized patients develop bacteriuria. If feasible, intermittent catheterization by a nurse or by the patient appears to reduce the incidence of bacteriuria and associated complications in such patients. Treatment should be provided when symptomatic infections arise, but treatment of asymptomatic bacteriuria in such patients has no apparent benefit.

DIAGNOSTIC TESTING   Determination of the number and type of bacteria in the urine is an extremely important diagnostic procedure. In symptomatic patients, bacteria are usually present in the urine in large numbers ($\geq 10^5$/mL). In asymptomatic patients, two consecutive urine specimens should be examined bacteriologically before therapy is instituted, and $\geq 10^5$ bacteria of a single species per milliliter should be demonstrable in both specimens. Since the large number of bacteria in the bladder urine is due in part to bacterial multiplication during residence in the bladder cavity, samples of urine from the ureters or renal pelvis may contain $< 10^5$ bacteria per milliliter and yet indicate infection. Similarly, the presence of bacteriuria of any degree in suprapubic aspirates or of $\geq 10^2$ bacteria per milliliter of urine obtained by catheterization usually indicates infection. In some circumstances (antibiotic treatment, high urea concentration, high osmolarity, low pH), urine inhibits bacterial multiplication, resulting in relatively low bacterial colony counts despite infection. For this reason, antiseptic solutions should not be used in washing the periurethral area before collection of the urine specimen. Water diuresis or recent voiding also reduces bacterial counts in urine.

Microscopy of urine from symptomatic patients can be of great diagnostic value. Microscopic bacteriuria, which is best assessed with Gram-stained uncentrifuged urine, is found in >90% of specimens from patients whose infections are associated with colony counts of at least 10^5/mL, and this finding is very specific. However, bacteria cannot usually be detected microscopically in infections with lower colony counts (10^2 to 10^4/mL). The detection of bacteria by urinary microscopy thus constitutes firm evidence of infection, but the absence of microscopically detectable bacteria does not exclude the diagnosis. When carefully sought by means of chamber-count microscopy, pyuria is a highly sensitive indicator of UTI in symptomatic patients. Pyuria is demonstrated in nearly all acute bacterial UTIs, and its absence calls the diagnosis into question. The leukocyte esterase "dipstick" method is less sensitive than microscopy in identifying pyuria but is a useful alternative where microscopy is not feasible. Pyuria in the absence of bacteriuria (sterile pyuria) may indicate infection with unusual bacterial agents such as *C. trachomatis*, *U. urealyticum*, and *Mycobacterium tuberculosis* or with fungi. Alternatively, sterile pyuria may be demonstrated in noninfectious urologic conditions such as calculi, anatomic abnormality, nephrocalcinosis, vesicoureteral reflux, interstitial nephritis, or polycystic disease.

Although many authorities have recommended that urine culture and antimicrobial susceptibility testing be performed for any patient with a suspected UTI, it may be more practical and cost-effective to manage women who have symptoms characteristic of acute uncomplicated cystitis without an initial urine culture. Two approaches to presumptive therapy have generally been used. In the first, treatment is initiated solely on the basis of a typical history and/or typical findings on physical examination. In the second, women with symptoms and signs of acute cystitis and without complicating factors are managed with urinary microscopy (or, alternatively, with a leukocyte esterase test). A positive result for pyuria and/or bacteriuria provides enough evidence of infection to indicate that urine culture and susceptibility testing can be omitted and the patient treated empirically. Urine should be cultured, however, when a woman's symptoms and urine-examination findings leave the diagnosis of cystitis in question. Pretherapy cultures and susceptibility testing are also essential in the management of all patients with suspected upper tract infections and of those with complicating factors, as in these situations any of a variety

of pathogens may be involved and antibiotic therapy is best tailored to the individual organism.

℞ TREATMENT

The following principles underlie the treatment of UTIs:

1. Except in acute uncomplicated cystitis in women, a quantitative urine culture or a comparable alternative diagnostic test should be performed to confirm infection before empirical treatment is begun. When culture results become available, antimicrobial sensitivity testing should be used to further direct therapy.
2. Factors predisposing to infection, such as obstruction and calculi, should be identified and corrected if possible.
3. Relief of clinical symptoms does not always indicate bacteriologic cure.
4. Each course of treatment should be classified after its completion as a failure (symptoms and/or bacteriuria not eradicated during therapy or in the immediate posttreatment culture) or a cure (resolution of symptoms and elimination of bacteriuria). Recurrent infections should be classified as same-strain or different-strain and as early (occurring within 2 weeks of the end of therapy) or late.
5. In general, uncomplicated infections confined to the lower urinary tract respond to short courses of therapy, while upper tract infections require longer treatment. After therapy, early recurrences due to the same strain may result from an unresolved upper tract focus of infection but often (especially after short-course therapy for cystitis) result from persistent vaginal colonization. Recurrences >2 weeks after the cessation of therapy nearly always represent reinfection with a new strain or with the previously infecting strain that has persisted in the vaginal and rectal flora.
6. Despite increasing resistance, community-acquired infections, especially initial infections, are usually due to more antibiotic-sensitive strains.
7. In patients with repeated infections, instrumentation, or recent hospitalization, the presence of antibiotic-resistant strains should be suspected. Although many antimicrobial agents reach high concentrations in urine, in vitro resistance usually predicts a substantially higher failure rate.

The anatomic location of a UTI greatly influences the success or failure of a therapeutic regimen. Bladder bacteriuria (cystitis) can usually be eliminated with nearly any antimicrobial agent to which the infecting strain is sensitive; in the past, it was demonstrated that as little as a single dose of 500 mg of intramuscular kanamycin eliminated bladder bacteriuria in most cases. With upper tract infections, however, single-dose therapy fails in the majority of cases, and even a 7-day course is unsuccessful in many instances. Longer periods of treatment (2 to 6 weeks) aimed at eradicating a persistent focus of infection may be necessary in some cases.

In *acute uncomplicated cystitis*, more than 90 to 95% of infections are due to one of two organisms: *E. coli* or *S. saprophyticus*. Although resistance patterns vary geographically and resistance has increased in many areas, most strains are sensitive to many antibiotics. In most parts of the United States, more than one-quarter of *E. coli* strains causing acute cystitis are resistant to amoxicillin, sulfa drugs, and cephalexin; resistance to trimethoprim (TMP) and trimethoprim-sulfamethoxazole (TMP-SMX) is now approaching these levels as well in many areas. Substantially higher rates of resistance to TMP-SMX have been documented in some other countries, as has resistance to fluoroquinolones.

Many have advocated single-dose treatment for acute cystitis. The advantages of single-dose therapy include less expense, ensured compliance, fewer side effects, and perhaps less intense pressure favoring the selection of resistant organisms in the intestinal, vaginal, or perineal flora. However, more frequent recurrences develop shortly after single-dose therapy than after 3-day treatment, and single-dose therapy does not eradicate vaginal colonization with *E. coli* as effectively as do longer regimens. A 3-day course of therapy with TMP-SMX, TMP, norfloxacin, ciprofloxacin, or ofloxacin appears to preserve the low rate of side effects of single-dose therapy while improving efficacy (Table 269-1); thus 3-day regimens are currently preferred for acute cystitis. In areas where TMP-SMX resistance exceeds 20%, either a fluoroquinolone or nitrofurantoin can be used (Table 269-1). Neither single-dose nor 3-day therapy should be used for women with symptoms or signs of pyelonephritis, urologic abnormalities or stones, or previous infections due to antibiotic-resistant organisms. Males with UTI often have urologic abnormalities or prostatic involvement and hence are not candidates for single-dose or 3-day therapy. For empirical therapy, they should generally receive a 7- to 14-day course of a fluoroquinolone (Table 269-1).

The choice of treatment for women with acute urethritis depends on the etiologic agent involved. In chlamydial infection, azithromycin (1 g in a single oral dose) or doxycycline (100 mg twice daily by mouth for 7 days) should be used. Women with acute dysuria and frequency, negative urine cultures, and no pyuria usually do not respond to antimicrobial agents.

In women, *acute uncomplicated pyelonephritis* without accompanying clinical evidence of calculi or urologic disease is due to *E. coli* in most cases. Although the optimal route and duration of therapy have not been established, a 7- to 14-day course of a fluoroquinolone, an aminoglycoside, or a third-generation cephalosporin is usually adequate. Neither ampicillin nor TMP-SMX should be used as initial therapy because >25% of strains of *E. coli* causing pyelonephritis are now resistant to these drugs in vitro. For at least the first few days of treatment, antibiotics should probably be given intravenously to most patients, but patients with mild symptoms can be treated for 7 to 14 days with an oral antibiotic (usually ciprofloxacin or ofloxacin), with or without an initial single parenteral dose (Table 269-1). Patients who fail to respond to treatment within 72 h or who relapse after therapy should be evaluated for unrecognized suppurative foci, calculi, or urologic disease.

Complicated UTIs (those arising in a setting of catheterization, instrumentation, urologic anatomic or functional abnormalities, stones, obstruction, immunosuppression, renal disease, or diabetes) are typically due to hospital-acquired bacteria, including *E. coli, Klebsiella, Proteus, Serratia, Pseudomonas*, enterococci, and staphylococci. Many of the infecting strains are antibiotic-resistant. Empirical antibiotic therapy ideally provides broad-spectrum coverage against these pathogens. In patients with minimal or mild symptoms, oral therapy with a fluoroquinolone, such as ciprofloxacin or ofloxacin, can be administered until culture results and antibiotic sensitivities are known. In patients with more severe illness, including acute pyelonephritis or suspected urosepsis, hospitalization and parenteral therapy should be undertaken. Commonly used empirical regimens include imipenem alone, a penicillin or cephalosporin plus an aminoglycoside, and (when the involvement of enterococci is unlikely) ceftriaxone or ceftazidime. When information on the antimicrobial sensitivity pattern of the infecting strain becomes available, a more specific antimicrobial regimen can be selected. Therapy should generally be administered for 10 to 21 days, with the exact duration depending on the severity of the infection and the susceptibility of the infecting strain. Follow-up cultures 2 to 4 weeks after cessation of therapy should be performed to demonstrate cure.

The need for treatment as well as the optimal type and duration of treatment for *catheterized patients with asymptomatic bacteriuria* have not been established. Removal of the catheter in conjunction with a

TABLE 269-1 *Treatment Regimens for Bacterial Urinary Tract Infections*

Condition	Characteristic Pathogens	Mitigating Circumstances	Recommended Empirical Treatment[a]
Acute uncomplicated cystitis in women	*Escherichia coli, Staphylococcus saprophyticus, Proteus mirabilis, Klebsiella pneumoniae*	None	3-Day regimens: oral TMP-SMX, TMP, quinolone; 7-day regimen: macrocrystalline nitrofurantoin[b]
		Diabetes, symptoms for >7 d, recent UTI, use of diaphragm, age >65 years	Consider 7-day regimen: oral TMP-SMX, TMP, quinolone[b]
		Pregnancy	Consider 7-day regimen: oral amoxicillin, macrocrystalline nitrofurantoin, cefpodoxime proxetil, or TMP-SMX[b]
Acute uncomplicated pyelonephritis in women	*E. coli, P. mirabilis, S. saprophyticus*	Mild to moderate illness, no nausea or vomiting; outpatient therapy	Oral[c] quinolone for 7–14 d (initial dose given IV if desired); or single-dose ceftriaxone (1 g) or gentamicin (3–5 mg/kg) IV followed by oral TMP-SMX[b] for 14 d
		Severe illness or possible urosepsis: hospitalization required	Parenteral[d] quinolone, gentamicin (± ampicillin), ceftriaxone, or aztreonam until defervescence; then oral[c] quinolone, cephalosporin, or TMP-SMX for 14 d
Complicated UTI in men and women	*E. coli, Proteus, Klebsiella, Pseudomonas, Serratia*, enterococci, staphylococci	Mild to moderate illness, no nausea or vomiting: outpatient therapy	Oral[c] quinolone for 10–14 d
		Severe illness or possible urosepsis: hospitalization required	Parenteral[d] ampicillin and gentamicin, quinolone, ceftriaxone, aztreonam, ticarcillin/clavulanate, or imipenem-cilastatin until defervescence; then oral[c] quinolone or TMP-SMX for 10–21 d

[a] Treatments listed are those to be prescribed before the etiologic agent is known; Gram's staining can be helpful in the selection of empirical therapy. Such therapy can be modified once the infecting agent has been identified. Fluoroquinolones should not be used in pregnancy. TMP-SMX, although not approved for use in pregnancy, has been widely used. Gentamicin should be used with caution in pregnancy because of its possible toxicity to eighth-nerve development in the fetus.

[b] Multiday oral regimens for cystitis are as follows: TMP-SMX, 160/800 mg q12h; TMP, 100 mg q12h; norfloxacin, 400 mg q12h; ciprofloxacin, 250 mg q12h; ofloxacin, 200 mg q12h; levofloxacin, 250 mg/d; gatifloxacin, 200 or 400 mg/d; moxifloxacin, 400 mg/d; lomefloxacin, 400 mg/d; enoxacin, 400 mg q12h; macrocrystalline nitrofurantoin, 100 mg qid; amoxicillin, 250 mg q8h; cefpodoxime proxetil, 100 mg q12h.

[c] Oral regimens for pyelonephritis and complicated UTI are as follows: TMP-SMX, 160/800 mg q12h; ciprofloxacin, 500 mg q12h; ofloxacin, 200–300 mg q12h; lomefloxacin, 400 mg/d; enoxacin, 400 mg q12h; gatifloxacin, 400 mg/d; levofloxacin, 200 mg q12h; moxifloxacin, 400 mg/d; amoxicillin, 500 mg q8h; cefpodoxime proxetil, 200 mg q12h.

[d] Parenteral regimens are as follows: ciprofloxacin, 400 mg q12h; ofloxacin, 400 mg q12h; gatifloxacin, 400 mg/d; levofloxacin, 500 mg/d; gentamicin, 1 mg/kg q8h; ceftriaxone, 1–2 g/d; ampicillin, 1 g q6h; imipenem-cilastatin, 250–500 mg q6–8h; ticarcillin/clavulanate, 3.2 g q8h; aztreonam, 1 g q8–12h.

Note: UTI, urinary tract infection; TMP, trimethoprim; TMP-SMX, trimethoprim-sulfamethoxazole.

short course of antibiotics to which the organism is susceptible probably constitutes the best course of action and nearly always eradicates bacteriuria. Treatment of asymptomatic catheter-associated bacteriuria may be of greatest benefit to elderly women, who most often develop symptoms if left untreated. If the catheter cannot be removed, antibiotic therapy usually proves to be unsuccessful and may in fact result in infection with a more resistant strain. In this situation, the bacteriuria should be ignored unless the patient develops symptoms or is at high risk of developing bacteremia. In these cases, use of systemic antibiotics or urinary bladder antiseptics may reduce the degree of bacteriuria and the likelihood of bacteremia.

In *pregnancy*, acute cystitis can be managed with 7 days of treatment with amoxicillin, nitrofurantoin, or a cephalosporin. All pregnant women should be screened for asymptomatic bacteriuria during the first trimester and, if bacteriuric, should be treated with one of the regimens listed in Table 269-1. After treatment, a culture should be performed to ensure cure, and cultures should be repeated monthly thereafter until delivery. Acute pyelonephritis in pregnancy should be managed with hospitalization and parenteral antibiotic therapy, generally with a cephalosporin or an extended-spectrum penicillin. Continuous low-dose prophylaxis with nitrofurantoin should be given to women who have recurrent infections during pregnancy.

Asymptomatic bacteriuria in noncatheterized patients is common, especially among elderly patients, but has not been linked to adverse outcomes in most circumstances other than pregnancy. Thus antimicrobial therapy is unnecessary and may in fact promote the emergence of resistant strains in most patients with asymptomatic bacteriuria. High-risk patients with neutropenia, renal transplants, obstruction, or other complicating conditions may require treatment when asymptomatic bacteriuria occurs. Seven days of therapy with an oral agent to which the organism is sensitive should be given initially. If bacteriuria persists, it can be monitored without further treatment in most patients. Longer-term therapy (4 to 6 weeks) may be necessary in high-risk patients with persistent asymptomatic bacteriuria.

UROLOGIC EVALUATION   Very few women with recurrent UTIs have correctable lesions discovered at cystoscopy or upon intravenous pyelography, and these procedures should not be undertaken routinely in such cases. Urologic evaluation should be performed in selected instances—namely, in women with relapsing infection, a history of childhood infections, stones or painless hematuria, or recurrent pyelonephritis. Most males with UTI should be considered to have complicated infection and thus should be evaluated urologically. Possible exceptions include young men who have cystitis associated with sexual activity, who are uncircumcised, or who have AIDS. Men or women presenting with acute infection and signs or symptoms suggestive of an obstruction or stones should undergo prompt urologic evaluation, generally by means of ultrasound.

PROGNOSIS   In patients with uncomplicated cystitis or pyelonephritis, treatment ordinarily results in complete resolution of symptoms. Lower tract infections in women are of concern mainly because they cause discomfort, morbidity, loss of time from work, and substantial health care costs. Cystitis may also result in upper tract infection or in bacteremia (especially during instrumentation), but little evidence suggests that renal impairment follows. When repeated episodes of cystitis occur, they are more commonly reinfections rather than relapses.

Acute uncomplicated pyelonephritis in adults rarely progresses to renal functional impairment and chronic renal disease. Repeated upper tract infections often represent relapse rather than reinfection, and a vigorous search for renal calculi or an underlying urologic abnormality should be undertaken. If neither is found, 6 weeks of chemotherapy may be useful in eradicating an unresolved focus of infection.

Repeated symptomatic UTIs in children and in adults with obstructive uropathy, neurogenic bladder, structural renal disease, or diabetes progress to chronic renal disease with unusual frequency. Asymptomatic bacteriuria in these groups as well as in adults without urologic disease or obstruction predisposes to increased numbers of episodes of symptomatic infection but does not result in renal impairment in most instances.

PREVENTION   Women who experience frequent symptomatic UTIs (≥ 3 per year on average) are candidates for long-term administration of low-dose antibiotics directed at preventing recurrences. Such women should be advised to avoid spermicide use and to void soon after intercourse. Daily or thrice-weekly administration of a single dose of TMP-SMX (80/400 mg), TMP alone (100 mg), or nitrofurantoin (50 mg) has been particularly effective. Norfloxacin and other fluoroquinolones have also been used for prophylaxis. Prophylaxis should be initiated only after bacteriuria has been eradicated with a full-dose treatment regimen. The same prophylactic regimens can be used after sexual intercourse to prevent episodes of symptomatic infection in women in whom UTIs are temporally related to intercourse. Other patients for whom prophylaxis appears to have some merit include men with chronic prostatitis; patients undergoing prostatectomy, both during the operation and in the postoperative period; and pregnant women with asymptomatic bacteriuria. All pregnant women should be screened for bacteriuria in the first trimester and should be treated if bacteriuria is demonstrated.

PAPILLARY NECROSIS

When infection of the renal pyramids develops in association with vascular diseases of the kidney or with urinary tract obstruction, renal papillary necrosis is likely to result. Patients with diabetes, sickle cell disease, chronic alcoholism, and vascular disease seem peculiarly susceptible to this complication. Hematuria, pain in the flank or abdomen, and chills and fever are the most common presenting symptoms. Acute renal failure with oliguria or anuria sometimes develops. Rarely, sloughing of a pyramid may take place without symptoms in a patient with chronic UTI, and the diagnosis is made when the necrotic tissue is passed in the urine or identified as a "ring shadow" on pyelography. If renal function deteriorates suddenly in a diabetic individual or a patient with chronic obstruction, the diagnosis of renal papillary necrosis should be entertained, even in the absence of fever or pain. Renal papillary necrosis is often bilateral; when it is unilateral, however, nephrectomy may be a life-saving approach to the management of overwhelming infection.

EMPHYSEMATOUS PYELONEPHRITIS AND CYSTITIS

These unusual clinical entities almost always occur in diabetic patients, often in concert with urinary obstruction and chronic infection. Emphysematous pyelonephritis is usually characterized by a rapidly progressive clinical course, with high fever, leukocytosis, renal parenchymal necrosis, and accumulation of fermentative gases in the kidney and perinephric tissues. Most patients also have pyuria and glucosuria. *E. coli* causes most cases, but occasionally other Enterobacteriaceae are isolated. Gas in tissues can often be seen on plain films and can best be confirmed and localized by computed tomography. Surgical resection of the involved tissue in addition to systemic antimicrobial therapy is usually needed to prevent a fatal outcome in emphysematous pyelonephritis.

Emphysematous cystitis also occurs primarily in diabetic patients, usually in association with *E. coli* or other facultative gram-negative rods and often in relation to bladder outlet obstruction. Patients with this condition are generally less severely ill and have less rapidly progressive disease than those with emphysematous pyelonephritis. The patient typically reports abdominal pain, dysuria, frequency, and (in some cases) pneumaturia. Computed tomography shows gas within both the bladder lumen and the bladder wall. Generally, conservative therapy with systemic antimicrobial agents and relief of outlet obstruction are effective, but some patients do not respond to these measures and require cystectomy.

RENAL AND PERINEPHRIC ABSCESS

See Chap. 112.

PROSTATITIS

The term *prostatitis* has been used for various inflammatory conditions affecting the prostate, including acute and chronic infections with specific bacteria and, more commonly, instances in which signs and symptoms of prostatic inflammation are present but no specific organisms can be detected. Patients with acute bacterial prostatitis can usually be readily identified on the basis of typical symptoms and signs, pyuria, and bacteriuria. To classify a patient with suspected chronic prostatitis correctly, first-void and midstream urine specimens, a prostatic expressate, and a postmassage urine specimen should be quantitatively cultured and evaluated for numbers of leukocytes. On the basis of the results of these studies and other considerations, a panel of the National Institutes of Health has recommended that patients with suspected chronic prostatitis be categorized as having chronic bacterial prostatitis, chronic pelvic pain syndrome, or asymptomatic inflammatory prostatitis. Each of these groups is discussed below.

ACUTE BACTERIAL PROSTATITIS When it occurs spontaneously, this disease generally affects young men; however, it may also be associated with an indwelling urethral catheter in older men. It is characterized by fever, chills, dysuria, and a tense or boggy, extremely tender prostate. Although prostatic massage usually produces purulent secretions with a large number of bacteria on culture, bacteremia may result from manipulation of the inflamed gland. For this reason and because the etiologic agent can usually be identified by Gram's staining and culture of urine, vigorous prostatic massage should be avoided. In non-catheter-associated cases, the infection is generally due to common gram-negative urinary tract pathogens (*E. coli* or *Klebsiella*). Initially, an intravenous fluoroquinolone, third-generation cephalosporin, or aminoglycoside can be administered. The response to antibiotics in acute bacterial prostatitis is usually prompt, perhaps because drugs penetrate more readily into the acutely inflamed prostate. In catheter-associated cases, the spectrum of etiologic agents is broader, including hospital-acquired gram-negative rods and enterococci. The urinary Gram stain may be particularly helpful in such cases. Imipenem, an aminoglycoside, a fluoroquinolone, or a third-generation cephalosporin should be used for initial therapy until the organism has been isolated and its susceptibilities have been determined. The long-term prognosis is good, although in some instances acute infection may result in abscess formation, epididymoorchitis, seminal vesiculitis, septicemia, and residual chronic bacterial prostatitis. Since the advent of antibiotics, the frequency of acute bacterial prostatitis has diminished markedly.

CHRONIC BACTERIAL PROSTATITIS This entity is now infrequent but should be considered in men with a history of recurrent bacteriuria. Symptoms are often lacking between episodes, and the prostate usually feels normal on palpation. Obstructive symptoms or perineal pain develops in some patients. Intermittently, infection spreads to the bladder, producing frequency, urgency, and dysuria. A pattern of relapsing infection in a middle-aged man strongly suggests chronic bacterial prostatitis. Classically, the diagnosis is established by culture of *E. coli*, *Klebsiella*, *Proteus*, or other uropathogenic bacteria from the expressed prostatic secretion or postmassage urine in higher quantities than are found in first-void or midstream urine. Antibiotics promptly relieve the symptoms associated with acute exacerbations but have been less effective in eradicating the focus of chronic infection in the prostate. The relative ineffectiveness of antimicrobial agents in achieving long-term cure has in part been due to the poor penetration into the prostate by most of these drugs. Fluoroquinolones have been considerably more successful than other antimicrobials, but even they must generally be given for at least 12 weeks to be effective. Patients with frequent episodes of acute cystitis in whom attempts at curative therapy fail can be managed with prolonged courses of low-dose antimicrobial agents (usually a sulfonamide, TMP, or nitrofurantoin), with a view toward suppressing symptoms and keeping the bladder urine sterile. Total prostatectomy obviously results in the cure of chronic prostatitis but is associated with considerable morbidity. Transurethral prostatectomy is safer but cures only one-third of patients.

CHRONIC PELVIC PAIN SYNDROME (FORMERLY NONBACTERIAL PROSTATITIS)
Patients who present with symptoms of prostatitis (intermittent perineal and low-back pain, obstructive voiding symptoms), few signs on examination, no bacterial growth in cultures, and no history of recurrent episodes of bacterial prostatitis are classified as having chronic pelvic pain syndrome (CPPS). Patients with CPPS are divided into inflammatory and noninflammatory subgroups based on the presence or absence of prostatic inflammation. Prostatic inflammation can be considered present when the expressed prostatic secretion and postmassage urine contain at least tenfold more leukocytes than the first-void and midstream urine specimens or when the expressed prostatic secretion contains ≥1000 leukocytes per microliter.

The likely etiology of CPPS associated with inflammation would be an infectious agent, but the agent has not yet been identified. Evidence for a causative role of both *U. urealyticum* and *C. trachomatis* has been presented but is not conclusive. Since most cases of inflammatory CPPS occur in young, sexually active men and since many cases follow an episode of nonspecific urethritis, the causative agent may well be sexually transmitted. The effectiveness of antimicrobial agents in this condition remains uncertain. Some patients benefit from a 4- to 6-week course of treatment with erythromycin, doxycycline, TMP-SMX, or a fluoroquinolone, but controlled trials are lacking. Patients who have symptoms and signs of prostatitis but who have no evidence of prostatic inflammation (normal leukocyte counts) and negative urine cultures are classified as having noninflammatory CPPS. Despite their symptoms, these patients most likely do not have prostatic infection and should not be given antimicrobial agents.

FURTHER READING

FIHN SD et al: Clinical practice: Acute uncomplicated urinary tract infection in women. N Engl J Med 349:259, 2003

GUPTA K et al: Increasing antimicrobial resistance and the management of uncomplicated community-acquired urinary tract infections. Ann Intern Med 135:41, 2001

HOOTON TM, STAMM WE: Diagnosis and treatment of uncomplicated urinary tract infection. Infect Dis Clin North Am 11:551, 1997

——— et al: Randomized comparative trial and cost analysis of 3-day antimicrobial regimens for treatment of acute cystitis in women. JAMA 273: 41, 1995

——— et al: A prospective study of risk factors for symptomatic urinary tract infection in young women. N Engl J Med 335:468, 1996

SAINT S et al: Enhancing the safety of critically ill patients by reducing urinary and central venous catheter–related infections. Am J Respir Crit Care Med 165:1475, 2002

STAMM WE, SCHAEFFER AJ (eds): *The State of the Art in the Management of Urinary Tract Infections.* Am J Med 113(Suppl 1A):1S–84S, 2002

TALAN DA et al: Comparison of ciprofloxacin (7 days) and trimethoprim-sulfamethoxazole (14 days) for acute uncomplicated pyelonephritis in women. JAMA 283:1583, 2000

WARREN JW et al: Guidelines for antimicrobial therapy of uncomplicated acute bacterial cystitis and acute pyelonephritis in women. Clin Infect Dis 29:745, 1999

Obstruction to the flow of urine, with attendant stasis and elevation in urinary tract pressure, impairs renal and urinary conduit functions and is a common cause of acute and chronic renal failure. With early relief of obstruction, the defects in function usually disappear completely. However, chronic obstruction may produce permanent loss of renal mass (renal atrophy) and excretory capability, as well as enhanced susceptibility to local infection and stone formation. Early diagnosis and prompt therapy are therefore essential to minimize the otherwise devastating effects of obstruction on kidney structure and function.

ETIOLOGY Obstruction to urine flow can result from *intrinsic* or *extrinsic mechanical blockade* as well as from *functional defects* not associated with fixed occlusion of the urinary drainage system. Mechanical obstruction can occur at any level of the urinary tract, from the renal calyces to the external urethral meatus. Normal points of narrowing, such as the ureteropelvic and ureterovesical junctions, bladder neck, and urethral meatus, are common sites of obstruction. When blockage is above the level of the bladder, unilateral dilatation of the ureter (*hydroureter*) and renal pyelocalyceal system (*hydronephrosis*) occur; lesions at or below the level of the bladder cause bilateral involvement.

Common forms of obstruction are listed in Table 270-1. Childhood causes include *congenital malformations* such as narrowing of the ureteropelvic junction and anomalous (retrocaval) location of the ureter. Posterior urethral valves are the most common cause of bilateral hydronephrosis in boys. Bladder dysfunction may be secondary to congenital urethral stricture, urethral meatal stenosis, or bladder neck obstruction. In adults, urinary tract obstruction is due mainly to *acquired defects*. Pelvic tumors, calculi, and urethral stricture predominate. Ligation of, or injury to, the ureter during pelvic or colonic surgery can lead to hydronephrosis which, if unilateral, may remain relatively silent and undetected. *Schistosoma haematobium* and genitourinary tuberculosis are infectious causes of ureteral obstruction. Obstructive uropathy may also result from extrinsic neoplastic (carcinoma of cervix or colon) or inflammatory disorders. Retroperitoneal fibrosis, an inflammatory condition in middle-aged men, must be distinguished from other retroperitoneal causes of ureteral obstruction, particularly lymphomas and pelvic neoplasms.

Functional impairment of urine flow usually results from disorders that involve both the ureter and bladder. Causes include neurogenic bladder, often with adynamic ureter, and vesicoureteral reflux. Reflux of urine from bladder to ureter(s) is more common in children, may result in severe unilateral or bilateral hydroureter and hydronephrosis. Abnormal insertion of the ureter into the bladder is the most common cause. Vesicoureteral reflux in the absence of urinary tract infection or bladder neck obstruction usually does not lead to renal parenchymal damage and often resolves with age. Reinsertion of the ureter into the bladder is indicated if reflux is severe and unlikely to improve spontaneously, if renal function deteriorates, or if urinary tract infections recur despite chronic antimicrobial therapy. Hydronephrosis is common in pregnancy, due both to ureteral compression by the enlarged uterus and to functional effects of progesterone.

CLINICAL FEATURES The pathophysiology and clinical features of urinary tract obstruction are summarized in Table 270-2. *Pain*, the symptom that most commonly leads to medical attention, is due to distention of the collecting system or renal capsule. Pain severity is influenced more by the rate at which distention develops than by the degree of distention. Acute supravesical obstruction, as from a stone lodged in a ureter (Chap. 268), is associated with excruciatingly severe pain, usually called *renal colic*. This pain is relatively steady and continuous, with little fluctuation in intensity, and often radiates to the lower abdomen, testes, or labia. By contrast, more insidious causes of obstruction, such as chronic narrowing of the ureteropelvic junction, may produce little or no pain yet result in total destruction of the affected kidney. Flank pain that occurs only with micturition is pathognomonic of vesicoureteral reflux.

Azotemia develops when overall excretory function is impaired, often in the setting of bladder outlet obstruction, bilateral renal pelvic or ureteric obstruction, or unilateral disease in a patient with a solitary functioning kidney. Complete bilateral obstruction should be suspected when acute renal failure is accompanied by anuria. Any patient with renal failure otherwise unexplained, or with a history of nephrolithiasis, hematuria, diabetes mellitus, prostatic enlargement, pelvic surgery, trauma, or tumor should be evaluated for urinary tract obstruction.

In the acute setting, bilateral obstruction may mimic prerenal azotemia. However, with more prolonged obstruction, symptoms of *polyuria* and *nocturia* commonly accompany partial urinary tract obstruction and result from impaired renal concentrating ability. This defect usually does not improve with administration of vasopressin and is therefore a form of acquired nephrogenic diabetes insipidus. Disturbances in sodium chloride transport in the ascending limb of Henle and, in azotemic patients, the osmotic (urea) diuresis per nephron lead to decreased medullary hypertonicity and hence a concentrating defect. Partial obstruction, therefore, may be associated with increased rather than decreased urine output. Indeed, wide fluctuations in urine output in a patient with azotemia should always raise the possibility of intermittent or partial urinary tract obstruction. If fluid intake is inadequate, severe dehydration and hypernatremia may develop. Hesitancy and straining to initiate the urinary

TABLE 270-1 Common Mechanical Causes of Urinary Tract Obstruction		
Ureter	**Bladder Outlet**	**Urethra**
CONGENITAL		
Ureteropelvic junction narrowing or obstruction	Bladder neck obstruction	Posterior urethral valves
Ureterovesical junction narrowing or obstruction	Ureterocele	Anterior urethral valves
Ureterocele		Stricture
Retrocaval ureter		Meatal stenosis
		Phimosis
ACQUIRED INTRINSIC DEFECTS		
Calculi	Benign prostatic hyperplasia	Stricture
Inflammation	Cancer of prostate	Tumor
Trauma	Cancer of bladder	Calculi
Sloughed papillae	Calculi	Trauma
Tumor	Diabetic neuropathy	Phimosis
Blood clots	Spinal cord disease	
Uric acid crystals	Anticholinergic drugs and α-adrenergic antagonists	
ACQUIRED EXTRINSIC DEFECTS		
Pregnant uterus	Carcinoma of cervix, colon	Trauma
Retroperitoneal fibrosis	Trauma	
Aortic aneurysm		
Uterine leiomyomata		
Carcinoma of uterus, prostate, bladder, colon, rectum		
Lymphoma, pelvic inflammatory disease		
Accidental surgical ligation		

stream, postvoid dribbling, urinary frequency, and incontinence are common with obstruction at or below the level of the bladder.

Partial bilateral urinary tract obstruction often results in *acquired distal renal tubular acidosis, hyperkalemia,* and *renal salt wasting.* These defects in tubule function are often accompanied by renal tubulointerstitial damage. Initially the interstitium becomes edematous and infiltrated with mononuclear inflammatory cells. Later, interstitial fibrosis and atrophy of the papillae and medulla occur and precede these processes in the cortex.

Urinary tract obstruction must always be considered in patients with urinary tract infections or urolithiasis. Urinary stasis encourages the growth of organisms. Urea-splitting bacteria are associated with magnesium ammonium phosphate (struvite) calculi. *Hypertension* is frequent in acute and subacute unilateral obstruction and is usually a consequence of increased release of renin by the involved kidney. Chronic hydronephrosis, in the presence of extracellular volume expansion, may result in significant hypertension. *Erythrocytosis,* an infrequent complication of obstructive uropathy, is probably secondary to increased erythropoietin production.

DIAGNOSIS A history of difficulty in voiding, pain, infection, or changes in urinary volume is common. Evidence for distention of the kidney or urinary bladder can often be obtained by palpation and percussion of the abdomen. A careful rectal examination may reveal enlargement or nodularity of the prostate, abnormal rectal sphincter tone, or a rectal or pelvic mass. The penis should be inspected for evidence of meatal stenosis or phimosis. In the female, vaginal, uterine, and rectal lesions responsible for urinary tract obstruction are usually revealed by inspection and palpation.

Urinalysis may reveal hematuria, pyuria, and bacteriuria. The urine sediment is often normal, even when obstruction leads to marked azotemia and extensive structural damage. An abdominal scout film may detect nephrocalcinosis or a radiopaque stone. As indicated in Fig. 270-1, if urinary tract obstruction is suspected, a bladder catheter should be inserted. If diuresis does not follow, then abdominal ultrasonography should be performed to evaluate renal and bladder size, as well as pyelocalyceal contour. Ultrasonography is approximately 90% specific and sensitive for detection of hydronephrosis. False-positive results are associated with diuresis, renal cysts, or presence of an extrarenal pelvis, a normal congenital variant. Hydronephrosis may be absent on ultrasound when obstruction is associated with volume contraction, staghorn calculi, retroperitoneal fibrosis, or infiltrative renal disease.

In some cases, the intravenous urogram may define the site of obstruction. In the presence of obstruction, the appearance time of the nephrogram is delayed. Eventually the renal image becomes more dense than normal because of slow tubular fluid flow rate, which results in greater concentration of contrast medium. The kidney involved by an acute obstructive process is usually slightly enlarged, and there is dilatation of the calyces, renal pelvis, and ureter above the obstruction. The ureter is not tortuous as in chronic obstruction. In comparison with the nephrogram, the urogram may be faint, especially if the dilated renal pelvis is voluminous, causing dilution of the contrast medium. The radiographic study should be continued until the site of obstruction is determined or the contrast medium is excreted. Radionuclide scans, though sensitive for the detection of obstruction, define less anatomic detail than intravenous urography and, like the urogram, are of limited value when renal function is poor. They have a role in patients at high risk for reaction to intravenous contrast. Patients suspected of having intermittent ureteropelvic obstruction should have radiologic evaluation while in pain, since a normal urogram is commonly seen during asymptomatic periods. Hydration often helps to provoke a symptomatic attack.

To facilitate visualization of a suspected lesion in a ureter or renal pelvis, *retrograde* or *antegrade urography* should be attempted. These diagnostic studies may be preferable to the intravenous urogram in the azotemic patient, in whom poor excretory function precludes adequate visualization of the collecting system. Furthermore, intravenous urography carries the risk of contrast-induced acute renal failure in patients with proteinuria, renal insufficiency, diabetes mellitus, or mul-

TABLE 270-2 *Pathophysiology of Bilateral Ureteral Obstruction*

Hemodynamic Effects	Tubule Effects	Clinical Features
ACUTE		
↑Renal blood flow	↑Ureteral and tubule pressures	Pain (capsule distention)
↓GFR	↑Reabsorption of Na⁺, urea, water	Azotemia
↓Medullary blood flow	water	Oliguria or anuria
↑Vasodilator prostaglandins		
CHRONIC		
↓Renal blood flow	↓Medullary osmolarity	Azotemia
↓↓GFR	↓Concentrating ability	Hypertension
↑Vasoconstrictor prostaglandins	Structural damage; parenchymal atrophy	ADH-insensitive polyuria
↑Renin-angiotensin production	↓Transport functions for Na⁺, K⁺, H⁺	Natriuresis
		Hyperkalemic, hyperchloremic acidosis
RELEASE OF OBSTRUCTION		
Slow ↑ in GFR (variable)	↓Tubule pressure	Postobstructive diuresis
	↑Solute load per nephron (urea, NaCl)	Potential for volume depletion and electrolyte imbalance due to losses of Na⁺, K⁺, PO₄³⁻, Mg²⁺, and water
	Natriuretic factors present	

Note: GFR, glomerular filtration rate.

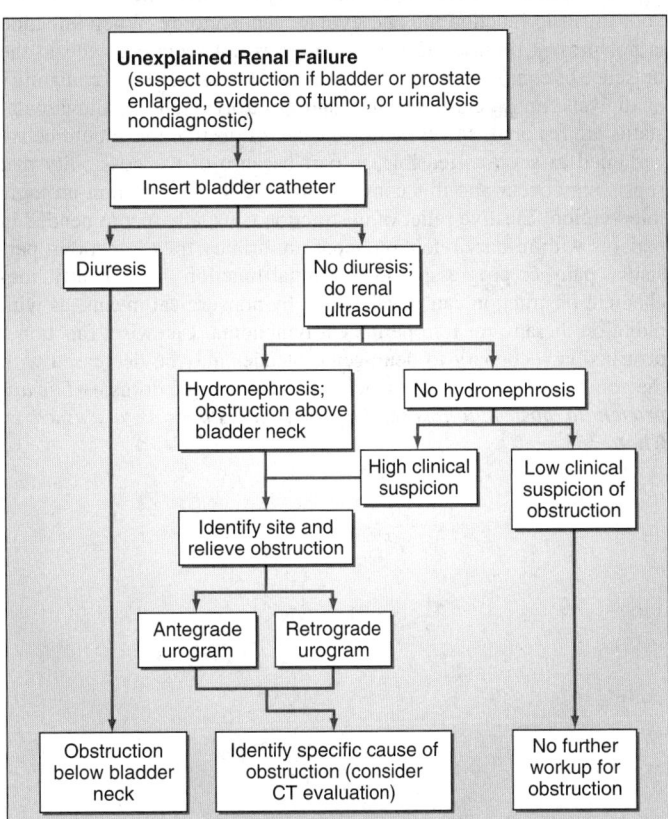

FIGURE 270-1 Diagnostic approach for urinary tract obstruction in unexplained renal failure. CT, computed tomography.

tiple myeloma, particularly if they are dehydrated. The retrograde approach involves catheterization of the involved ureter under cystoscopic control, while the antegrade technique necessitates placement of a catheter into the renal pelvis via a needle inserted percutaneously under ultrasonic or fluoroscopic guidance. While the antegrade approach may provide immediate decompression of a unilateral obstructing lesion, many urologists initially attempt the retrograde approach unless the catheterization is unsuccessful or general anesthesia is contraindicated.

Voiding cystourethrography is of value in the diagnosis of vesicoureteral reflux and bladder neck and urethral obstructions. Patients with obstruction at or below the level of the bladder exhibit thickening, trabeculation, and diverticula of the bladder wall. Postvoiding films reveal residual urine. If these radiographic studies fail to provide adequate information for diagnosis, endoscopic visualization by the urologist often permits precise identification of lesions involving the urethra, prostate, bladder, and ureteral orifices.

Computed tomography (CT) is useful in the diagnosis of specific intraabdominal and retroperitoneal causes of obstruction. The spiral CT is the preferred study to image urinary calculi. Magnetic resonance imaging may also be useful in the identification of specific obstructive causes.

℞ TREATMENT

Urinary tract obstruction complicated by infection requires relief of obstruction as soon as possible to prevent development of generalized sepsis and progressive renal damage. On a temporary basis, drainage is often satisfactorily achieved by nephrostomy, ureterostomy, or ureteral, urethral, or suprapubic catheterization. The patient with acute urinary tract infection and obstruction should be given appropriate antibiotics based on in vitro bacterial sensitivity and the ability of the drug to concentrate in the urine. Treatment may be required for 3 to 4 weeks. Chronic or recurrent infections in an obstructed kidney with poor intrinsic function may necessitate nephrectomy. When infection is not present, immediate surgery often is not required, even in the presence of complete obstruction and anuria because of the availability of dialysis, until acid-base, fluid and electrolyte, and cardiovascular status are restored. Nevertheless, the site of obstruction should be ascertained as soon as feasible, in part because of the possibility that sepsis may occur and this complication necessitates prompt urologic intervention. Elective relief of obstruction is usually recommended in patients with urinary retention, recurrent urinary tract infections, persistent pain, or progressive loss of renal function. Infrequently, mechanical obstruction can be alleviated by nonsurgical means, as with radiation therapy for retroperitoneal lymphoma. Likewise, functional obstruction secondary to neurogenic bladder may be decreased with the combination of frequent voiding and cholinergic drugs. →*The approach to obstruction secondary to renal stones is discussed in Chap. 268.*

PROGNOSIS   With relief of obstruction, the prognosis regarding return of renal function depends largely on whether irreversible renal damage has occurred. When obstruction is not relieved, the course will depend mainly on whether the obstruction is complete or incomplete, bilateral or unilateral, and whether urinary tract infection is also present. Complete obstruction with infection can lead to total destruction of the kidney within days. Partial return of glomerular filtration rate may follow relief of complete obstruction of 1 and 2 weeks' duration but after 8 weeks of obstruction, recovery is unlikely. In the absence of definitive evidence of irreversibility, every effort should be made to decompress the obstruction in the hope of restoring renal function at least partially. A renal radionuclide scan, performed after a prolonged period of decompression, may be used to predict reversible renal function.

POSTOBSTRUCTIVE DIURESIS   Relief of bilateral, but not unilateral, complete obstruction commonly results in polyuria, which may be massive. The urine is usually hypotonic and may contain large amounts of sodium chloride, potassium, and magnesium. The natriuresis is due in part to the excretion of retained urea (osmotic diuresis). The increase in intratubular pressure very likely also contributes to the impairment in net sodium chloride reabsorption, especially in the terminal nephron segments. Natriuretic factors may also accumulate during uremia and depress salt and water reabsorption when urine flow is reestablished. In the majority of patients this diuresis results in the *appropriate* excretion of the excesses of retained salt and water. When extracellular volume and composition return to normal, the diuresis usually abates spontaneously. Therefore, replacement of urinary losses should only be done in the setting of hypovolemia, hypotension, or disturbances in serum electrolyte concentrations. Occasionally, iatrogenic expansion of extracellular volume is responsible for, or sustains, the diuresis observed in the postobstructive period. Replacement of no more than two-thirds of urinary volume losses per day is usually effective in avoiding this complication. The loss of electrolyte-free water with urea may result in hypernatremia. Serum and urine sodium and osmolal concentrations should guide the use of appropriate intravenous replacement. Often replacement with 0.45% saline is required. In a rare patient, relief of obstruction may be followed by urinary salt and water losses severe enough to provoke profound dehydration and vascular collapse. In these patients, an intrinsic defect in tubule reabsorptive function is probably responsible for the marked diuresis. Appropriate therapy in such patients includes intravenous administration of salt-containing solutions to replace sodium and volume deficits.

FURTHER READING

GULMI FA et al: Pathophysiology of urinary tract obstruction, in PC Walsh et al (eds): *Campbell's Urology*, 8th ed. Philadelphia, Saunders, 2002, pp 411–463

KLAHR S: Urinary tract obstruction, in RW Schrier, CW Gottschalk (eds): *Diseases of the Kidney*, 7th ed. Boston, Little, Brown, 2001, pp 751–787

WILSON DR: Renal function during and following obstruction. Ann Rev Med 28:329, 1977

ZEIDEL ML, PIRTSKHALAISHVILI G: Urinary tract obstruction, in BM Brenner (ed): *Brenner and Rector's The Kidney*, 7th ed. Philadelphia, Saunders, 2004, pp 1867–1894

271 | APPROACH TO THE PATIENT WITH GASTROINTESTINAL DISEASE
William L. Hasler, Chung Owyang

ANATOMIC CONSIDERATIONS

The gastrointestinal (GI) tract extends from the mouth to the anus and comprises several organs with distinct functions. The organs are separated by specialized independently controlled thickened sphincters that assist in gut compartmentalization. The gut wall is organized into well-defined layers that contribute to the functional activities in each region. The mucosa serves as a barrier to luminal contents or as a site for transfer of fluids or nutrients. Gut smooth muscle mediates propulsion from one region to the next. Many GI organs possess a serosal layer that not only provides a supportive foundation but also permits external input.

Interactions with other organ systems serve the needs both of the gut and the body. Pancreaticobiliary conduits deliver bile and enzymes into the duodenum. A rich vascular supply is modulated by GI tract activity. Lymphatic channels assist in gut immune activities. Intrinsic gut wall nerves provide the basic controls for propulsion and fluid regulation. Extrinsic neural input provides volitional or involuntary control to degrees that are specific for each gut region.

FUNCTIONS OF THE GASTROINTESTINAL TRACT

The GI tract serves two main functions—assimilation of nutrients and elimination of waste. The gut anatomy is organized to serve these functions. In the mouth, food is processed, mixed with salivary amylase, and delivered to the luminal GI tract. The esophagus propels the bolus into the stomach, and the lower esophageal sphincter prevents oral reflux of gastric contents. The esophageal mucosa has a protective squamous histology that does not permit significant diffusion or absorption. The propulsive activities of the esophagus are exclusively aboral and are coordinated with relaxation of the upper and lower esophageal sphincters upon swallowing.

The stomach furthers food preparation by triturating and mixing the bolus with pepsin and acid. Gastric acid also sterilizes the upper gut. Gastric motor activities exhibit regional variability: (1) the proximal stomach serves a storage function by relaxing to accommodate the meal; (2) the distal stomach exhibits phasic contractions that propel solid food residue against the pylorus, where it is repeatedly propelled proximally for further mixing before it is emptied into the duodenum; and (3) finally, the stomach secretes intrinsic factor for vitamin B_{12} absorption.

The small intestine serves most of the nutrient absorptive function of the gut. The intestinal mucosa exhibits villous architecture to provide maximal surface area for absorption and is endowed with specialized enzymes and transporters. Triturated food from the stomach is mixed with pancreatic juice and bile in the proximal duodenum to facilitate digestion. Pancreatic juice contains the main enzymes for carbohydrate, protein, and fat digestion as well as bicarbonate to optimize the pH for activation of these enzymes. Bile secreted by the liver and stored in the gallbladder is essential for intestinal lipid digestion. The proximal intestine is optimized for rapid absorption of nutrient breakdown products and most minerals, while the ileum is better suited for absorption of vitamin B_{12} and bile acids. The small intestine also aids in waste elimination. Bile contains byproducts of erythrocyte degradation, toxins, metabolized and unmetabolized medications, and cholesterol. Motor function of the small intestine delivers indigestible food residue and sloughed enterocytes into the colon for further processing. The small intestine terminates in the ileocecal junc-

tion, a sphincteric structure that prevents coloileal reflux and maintains small-intestinal sterility.

The colon prepares the waste material for controlled evacuation. The colonic mucosa dehydrates the stool, decreasing daily fecal volumes from the 1000 to 1500 mL delivered from the ileum to the 100 to 200 mL expelled from the rectum. The colonic lumen possesses a dense bacterial colonization that ferments undigested carbohydrates and short-chain fatty acids. Whereas transit times in the esophagus are on the order of seconds and times in the stomach and small intestine range from minutes to a few hours, propagation through the colon takes >1 day in most individuals. Colonic motor patterns exhibit a to-and-fro character that facilitates slow fecal desiccation. The proximal colon serves to mix and absorb fluid, while the distal colon exhibits peristaltic contractions and mass actions that function to expel the stool. The colon terminates in the anus, a structure with volitional and involuntary controls to permit retention of the fecal bolus until it can be released in a socially convenient setting.

EXTRINSIC MODULATION OF GUT FUNCTION

GI function is modified by influences outside of the gut. Unlike other organ systems, the gut is in physical continuity with the outside environment. Thus, protective mechanisms are vigilant against the deleterious effects of consumed foods, medications, toxins, and infectious organisms. Mucosal immune mechanisms include a lymphocyte and plasma cell population that resides in the epithelial layer and lamina propria backed up by lymph node chains to prevent noxious agents from entering the circulation. All substances absorbed into the bloodstream are filtered through the liver via the portal venous circulation. In the liver, many drugs and toxins are detoxified by a variety of mechanisms. Although intrinsic nerves control most basic gut activities, extrinsic neural input modulates a number of functions. The two activities under voluntary control are swallowing and defecation. Many normal GI reflexes involve extrinsic vagus or splanchnic nerve pathways. An active brain-gut axis further alters function in regions not under volitional regulation. As an example, stress alters GI transit as well as gut immune function.

OVERVIEW OF GASTROINTESTINAL DISEASES

GI diseases develop as a consequence of abnormalities within or outside of the gut and range in severity from those that produce mild symptoms and no long-term morbidity to those with intractable symptoms or an adverse outcome. Diseases may be localized to a single organ or exhibit diffuse involvement at a number of sites.

CLASSIFICATION OF GI DISEASES   GI diseases are manifestations of alterations in nutrient assimilation or waste evacuation or in the activities supporting these main functions.

Impaired Digestion and Absorption   Diseases of the stomach, intestine, biliary tree, and pancreas can disrupt nutrient digestion and absorption. Gastric hypersecretory conditions such as Zollinger-Ellison syndrome damage the intestinal mucosa and accelerate transit due to excess gastric acid. The most common intestinal maldigestion syndrome, lactase deficiency, produces flatus and diarrhea after dairy product ingestion and has no other adverse outcomes. Other intestinal enzyme deficiencies produce similar symptoms with ingestion of other simple sugars. Conversely, celiac disease, bacterial overgrowth, infectious enteritis, Crohn's ileitis, and radiation damage produce anemia, dehydration, electrolyte disorders, or malnutrition. Biliary obstruction from stricture or neoplasm may impair fat digestion. Impaired release of pancreatic enzymes in chronic pancreatitis or pancreatic cancer decreases intraluminal digestion and can lead to profound malnutrition.

Altered Secretion   Selected GI diseases result from dysregulation of gut secretion. Gastric acid hypersecretion occurs in Zollinger-Ellison syndrome, G-cell hyperplasia, retained antrum syndrome, and in some individuals with duodenal ulcer disease. Conversely, patients with atrophic gastritis or pernicious anemia release little or no gastric acid. Inflammatory and infectious small-intestinal and colonic diseases produce fluid loss through impaired absorption or enhanced secretion but do not usually cause malnutrition. Common intestinal and colonic hypersecretory conditions include acute viral infection, chronic *Giardia* or cryptosporidia infections, small-intestinal bacterial overgrowth, microscopic colitis, diabetic diarrhea, and abuse of certain laxatives. Less common causes include large colonic villous adenomas and endocrine neoplasias with tumor overproduction of secretagogue transmitters such as vasoactive intestinal polypeptide.

Altered Gut Transit   Alterations in gut transit are commonly secondary to mechanical obstruction. Esophageal occlusion often results from acid-induced stricture or neoplasm. Gastric outlet obstruction develops from peptic ulcer disease or gastric cancer. Small-intestinal obstruction most commonly results from adhesions but may also occur with Crohn's disease, radiation- or drug-induced strictures, and, less likely, malignancy. The most common cause of colonic obstruction is colon cancer, although inflammatory strictures develop in patients with inflammatory bowel disease, after certain infections, or with some drugs.

Retardation of propulsion also develops from disordered gut motor function. *Achalasia* is characterized by impaired esophageal body peristalsis and incomplete lower esophageal sphincter relaxation. *Gastroparesis* is the symptomatic delay in gastric emptying of solid or liquid meals. Intestinal pseudoobstruction causes marked delays in smallbowel transit due to injury to enteric nerves or intestinal smooth muscle. Slow transit constipation is produced by diffusely impaired colonic propulsion. Constipation is also produced by outlet abnormalities such as rectal prolapse, intussusception, or failure of anal relaxation upon attempted defecation.

Disorders of rapid propulsion are less common than those with delayed transit. Rapid gastric emptying occurs in postvagotomy dumping syndrome and with gastric hypersecretion. Exaggerated intestinal or colonic motor patterns are minor factors in symptoms with selected diarrheal conditions. Accelerated transit with hyperdefecation is noted in hyperthyroidism.

Immune Dysregulation   Many inflammatory GI conditions are consequences of altered gut immune function. The mucosal inflammation of *celiac disease* results from dietary ingestion of gluten-containing grains. Some patients with food allergy also exhibit altered immune populations. *Eosinophilic gastroenteritis* is an inflammatory condition with prominent mucosal eosinophils. *Ulcerative colitis* and *Crohn's disease* are disorders of uncertain etiology that produce mucosal injury primarily in the lower gut. The microscopic colitides, lymphocytic and collagenous colitis, exhibit colonic subepithelial infiltrates without visible mucosal damage. Bacterial, viral, and protozoal organisms may produce ileitis or colitis in selected patient populations.

Impaired Gut Blood Flow   Different GI regions are at variable risk for ischemic damage from impaired blood flow. Rare cases of gastroparesis result from blockage of the celiac and superior mesenteric arteries. More commonly encountered are intestinal and colonic ischemia, which are consequences of arterial embolus; arterial thrombosis; venous thrombosis; or hypoperfusion from dehydration, sepsis, hemorrhage, or reduced cardiac output. These may produce mucosal injury, hemorrhage, or even perforation. Some cases of radiation enterocolitis exhibit reduced mucosal blood flow.

Neoplastic Degeneration   All GI regions are susceptible to malignant degeneration to varying degrees. In the United States, colorectal cancer is most common and typically presents after age 50. Worldwide, gastric cancer is especially prevalent in certain Asian regions. Esophageal cancer develops with chronic acid reflux or in those with an extensive alcohol or tobacco use history. Small-intestinal neoplasms are rare and occur with underlying inflammatory disease. Anal cancers may arise with prior anal infection or inflammation. Pancreatic and biliary cancers elicit severe pain, weight loss, and jaundice and have poor prognoses. Hepatocellular carcinoma usually arises in the setting of chronic viral hepatitis or cirrhosis secondary to other causes. Most GI cancers are epithelial-derived; however, lymphomas and other cell types are also observed.

Disorders without Obvious Organic Abnormalities   The most common GI disorders show no abnormalities on biochemical or structural testing and include irritable bowel syndrome (IBS), functional dyspepsia, noncardiac chest pain, and functional heartburn. These functional bowel disorders exhibit altered gut motor function; however, the pathogenic relevance of these abnormalities is uncertain. Exaggerated visceral sensory responses to noxious stimulation may cause discomfort in these disorders. Symptoms in some patients result from altered processing of visceral pain sensations in the central nervous system. Patients with functional bowel abnormalities with severe symptoms may exhibit significant emotional disturbances on psychometric testing.

Genetic Influences   Although many GI diseases result from environmental factors, others exhibit hereditary components. Family members of inflammatory bowel disease (IBD) patients show a genetic predisposition to disease development themselves. Colonic and esophageal malignancies arise in certain inherited disorders. Hereditary pancreatitis is caused by mutation in the cationic trypsinogen gene. Rare genetic dysmotility syndromes are described. Familial clustering is even observed in the functional bowel disorders, although this may be secondary to learned familial illness behavior rather than a true hereditary factor.

SYMPTOMS OF GASTROINTESTINAL DISEASE   The most common GI symptoms are abdominal pain, heartburn, nausea and vomiting, altered bowel habits, GI bleeding, and jaundice (Table 271-1). Others are dysphagia, anorexia, weight loss, fatigue, and extraintestinal symptoms.

Abdominal Pain   Abdominal pain results from GI disease and extraintestinal conditions involving the genitourinary tract, abdominal wall, thorax, or spine. Visceral pain is generally midline in location and vague in character, while parietal pain is localized and precisely described. Common inflammatory diseases with pain include peptic ulcer, appendicitis, diverticulitis, IBD, and infectious enterocolitis. Other intraabdominal causes of pain include gallstone disease and pancreatitis. Noninflammatory visceral sources include mesenteric ischemia and neoplasia. The most common causes of abdominal pain are IBS and functional dyspepsia.

Heartburn   Heartburn, a burning substernal sensation, is reported intermittently by at least 40% of the population. Classically, heartburn is felt to result from excess gastroesophageal reflux of acid. However, some cases exhibit normal esophageal acid exposure and may result from heightened sensitivity of esophageal mucosal nerves.

Nausea and Vomiting   Nausea and vomiting are caused by GI diseases, medications, toxins, acute and chronic infection, endocrine disorders, labyrinthine conditions, and central nervous system disease. The best-characterized GI etiologies relate to mechanical obstruction of the upper gut; however, disorders of propulsion including gastroparesis and intestinal pseudoobstruction also elicit prominent symptoms. As with abdominal pain, IBS and functional dyspepsia commonly present with nausea and vomiting.

Altered Bowel Habits   Altered bowel habits are common complaints of patients with GI disease. Constipation is reported as infrequent defecation, straining with defecation, passage of hard stools, or a sense of

TABLE 271-1 *Common Causes of Common GI Symptoms*

Abdominal Pain	Nausea and Vomiting	Diarrhea	GI Bleeding	Obstructive Jaundice
Appendicitis	Medications	Infection	Ulcer disease	Bile duct stones
Gallstone disease	GI obstruction	Poorly absorbed sugars	Esophagitis	Cholangiocarcinoma
Pancreatitis	Motor disorders	Inflammatory bowel disease	Varices	Cholangitis
Diverticulitis	Functional bowel disorder	Microscopic colitis	Vascular lesions	Sclerosing cholangitis
Ulcer disease	Enteric infection	Functional bowel disorder	Neoplasm	Ampullary stenosis
Esophagitis	Pregnancy	Celiac disease	Diverticula	Ampullary carcinoma
GI obstruction	Endocrine disease	Pancreatic insufficiency	Hemorrhoids	Pancreatitis
Inflammatory bowel disease	Motion sickness	Hyperthyroidism	Fissures	Pancreatic tumor
Functional bowel disorder	Central nervous system disease	Ischemia	Inflammatory bowel disease	
Vascular disease		Endocrine tumor	Infectious colitis	
Gynecologic causes				
Renal stone				

incomplete fecal evacuation. Causes of constipation include obstruction, motor disorders of the colon, medications, and endocrine diseases such as hypothyroidism and hyperparathyroidism. Diarrhea is reported as frequent defecation, passage of loose or watery stools, fecal urgency, or a similar sense of incomplete evacuation. The differential diagnosis of diarrhea is broad and includes infections, inflammatory causes, malabsorption, and medications. IBS produces constipation, diarrhea, or an alternating bowel pattern. Fecal mucus is common in IBS, while pus characterizes inflammatory disease. Steatorrhea develops with malabsorption.

GI Bleeding Hemorrhage may develop from any gut organ. Most commonly, upper GI bleeding presents with melena or hematemesis, whereas lower GI bleeding produces passage of bright red or maroon stools. However, briskly bleeding upper sites can elicit voluminous red rectal bleeding, while slowly bleeding ascending colon sites may produce melena. Chronic slow GI bleeding may present with iron-deficiency anemia. The most common upper GI causes of bleeding are ulcer disease, gastroduodenitis, and esophagitis. Other etiologies include portal hypertensive causes, malignancy, tears across the gastroesophageal junction, and vascular lesions. The most prevalent lower GI sources of hemorrhage include hemorrhoids, anal fissures, diverticula, and arteriovenous malformations. Other causes include neoplasm, IBD, ischemia, infectious colitis, and other vascular lesions.

Jaundice Jaundice results from prehepatic, intrahepatic, or posthepatic disease. Posthepatic causes of jaundice include biliary diseases such as choledocholithiasis, cholangitis, stricture, and neoplasm and pancreatic disorders such as acute and chronic pancreatitis, stricture, and malignancy.

Other Symptoms Other symptoms are manifestations of GI disease. Dysphagia, odynophagia, and unexplained chest pain suggest esophageal disease. A globus sensation is reported with esophagopharyngeal conditions but also occurs with functional GI disorders. Weight loss, anorexia, and fatigue are nonspecific symptoms of neoplastic, inflammatory, gut motor, pancreatic, small bowel mucosal, and psychiatric conditions. Fever is reported with inflammatory illness, but malignancies also evoke febrile responses. GI disorders also produce extraintestinal symptoms. IBD is associated with hepatobiliary dysfunction, skin and eye lesions, and arthritis. Celiac disease may present with dermatitis herpetiformis. Jaundice can produce pruritus. Conversely, systemic diseases can have GI consequences. Systemic lupus may cause gut ischemia, presenting with pain or bleeding. Overwhelming stress or severe burns may lead to gastric ulcer formation.

EVALUATION OF THE PATIENT WITH GASTROINTESTINAL DISEASE

Evaluation of the patient with GI disease begins with a careful history and physical examination. Subsequent investigation with a variety of tools designed to test the structure or function of the gut are indicated in selected cases. Some patients exhibit normal findings on diagnostic testing. In these individuals, validated symptom profiles are employed for confident diagnosis of a functional bowel disorder.

HISTORY The history of the patient with suspected GI disease has several components. Symptom timing can suggest specific etiologies. Symptoms of short duration commonly result from acute infection, toxin exposure, or abrupt inflammation or ischemia. Long-standing symptoms point to an underlying chronic inflammatory or neoplastic condition or a functional bowel disorder. Symptoms from mechanical obstruction, ischemia, IBD, and functional bowel disorders are worsened by meal ingestion. Conversely, ulcer symptoms may be relieved by eating or antacids. The symptom pattern and duration may suggest underlying etiologies. Ulcer pain occurs at intermittent intervals lasting weeks to months, whereas biliary colic has a sudden onset and lasts up to several hours. Pain from acute inflammation, as with acute pancreatitis, is severe and persists for days to weeks. Meals elicit diarrhea in some cases of IBD and IBS, while defecation relieves discomfort in these conditions. Functional bowel disorders are exacerbated by stress. Sudden awakening from sleep suggests organic disease rather than a functional bowel disorder. Diarrhea from malabsorption usually improves with fasting, while secretory diarrhea persists without oral intake.

Symptom relation to other factors narrows the list of diagnostic possibilities. Obstructive symptoms with prior abdominal surgery raise concern for adhesions, whereas loose stools after gastrectomy or gallbladder excision suggest dumping syndrome or post-cholecystectomy diarrhea. Symptom onset after travel prompts a search for enteric infection. Medications produce pain, altered bowel habits, or GI bleeding. Lower GI bleeding likely results from neoplasm, diverticula, or vascular lesions in an older person and anorectal abnormalities or IBD in a younger individual. Celiac disease is prevalent in people of Irish descent, whereas IBD is more common in certain Jewish populations. A sexual history may raise concern for sexually transmitted diseases or immunodeficiency.

Over the past two decades, working groups have been convened to devise symptom criteria to improve the confident diagnosis of the functional bowel disorders and to minimize the number of unnecessary diagnostic tests performed. The most widely accepted symptom-based criteria are the *Rome criteria*. When tested against findings of structural investigations, the Rome criteria exhibit diagnostic specificities >90% for many of the functional bowel disorders.

PHYSICAL EXAMINATION The physical examination complements information from the history. Abnormal vital signs provide diagnostic clues and determine the need for acute intervention. Fever suggests inflammation or neoplasm. Orthostasis is found with significant blood loss, dehydration, sepsis, or autonomic neuropathy. Skin, eye, or joint findings may point to specific diagnoses. Neck examination with swallowing assessment evaluates dysphagia. Cardiopulmonary disease may present with abdominal pain or nausea; thus lung and cardiac examinations are important. Pelvic examination tests for a gynecologic source of abdominal pain. Rectal examination may detect blood, indicating gut mucosal injury or neoplasm, or a palpable inflammatory mass in appendicitis. Metabolic conditions and gut motor disorders have associated peripheral neuropathy.

Inspection of the abdomen may reveal distention from obstruction, tumor, or ascites or vascular abnormalities with liver disease. Ecchymoses develop with severe pancreatitis. Auscultation can detect bruits or friction rubs from vascular disease or hepatic tumors. Loss of bowel sounds signifies ileus, while high-pitched, hyperactive sounds characterize intestinal obstruction. Percussion assesses liver size and can detect shifting dullness from ascites. Palpation assesses for hepatosplenomegaly as well as neoplastic or inflammatory masses. Abdominal examination is helpful in evaluating unexplained pain. Intestinal ischemia elicits severe pain but little tenderness. Patients with visceral pain may exhibit generalized discomfort, while those with parietal pain or peritonitis have directed pain often with involuntary guarding, rigidity, or rebound. Patients with musculoskeletal abdominal wall pain may note tenderness exacerbated by Valsalva or straight leg lift maneuvers.

TOOLS FOR PATIENT EVALUATION   Laboratory, radiographic, and scintigraphic tests can assist in diagnosis of suspected GI disease. The GI tract is also amenable to internal evaluation with upper and lower endoscopy and to examination of luminal contents. Histopathologic examinations of gastrointestinal tissues complement these tests.

Laboratory   Selected laboratory tests facilitate the diagnosis of GI disease. Iron-deficiency anemia suggests mucosal blood loss, whereas vitamin B_{12} deficiency results from small-intestinal, gastric, or pancreatic disease. Either can also result from inadequate oral intake. Leukocytosis and increased erythrocyte sedimentation rates are found in inflammatory conditions, while leukopenia is seen in viremic illness. Severe vomiting or diarrhea elicits electrolyte disturbances, acid-base abnormalities, and elevated blood urea nitrogen. Pancreaticobiliary or liver disease is suggested by elevated pancreatic or liver chemistries. Thyroid chemistries, cortisol, and calcium levels are obtained to exclude endocrinologic causes of GI symptoms. Pregnancy testing is considered for young women with unexplained nausea. Serologic tests are available for rheumatologic diseases such as systemic lupus erythematosus or scleroderma. Hormone levels are obtained for suspected endocrine neoplasia. Intraabdominal malignancies produce tumor markers including carcinoembryonic antigen, while paraneoplastic dysmotility is associated with antineuronal antibodies. Other body fluids are sampled under certain circumstances. Ascitic fluid is analyzed for infection, malignancy, or findings of portal hypertension. Cerebrospinal fluid is obtained for suspected central nervous system causes of vomiting. Urine samples screen for carcinoid, porphyria, and heavy metal intoxication.

Luminal Contents   Luminal contents can be examined for diagnostic clues. Stool samples are cultured for bacterial pathogens or examined for leukocytes or parasites. Duodenal aspirates can be examined for parasites or cultured for bacterial overgrowth. Fecal fat is quantified in possible malabsorption. Stool electrolytes and osmolarity can be measured in diarrheal conditions. A stool osmotic gap >100 mosmol/L indicates osmotic diarrhea. Laxative screens are done when laxative abuse is suspected. Gastric acid is quantified to rule out Zollinger-Ellison syndrome. Esophageal pH testing is done for refractory symptoms of acid reflux. Pancreatic juice is analyzed for enzyme or bicarbonate content to exclude pancreatic exocrine insufficiency.

Endoscopy   The gut is accessible by means of endoscopy, which can provide the diagnosis of the causes of bleeding, pain, nausea and vomiting, weight loss, altered bowel function, and fever. Table 271-2 lists the most common indications for the major endoscopic procedures. Upper endoscopy evaluates the esophagus, stomach, and duodenum, while colonoscopy assesses the colon and distal ileum. Upper endoscopy is advocated as the initial structural test performed in patients with upper GI bleeding, suspected ulcer disease, esophagitis, neoplasm, malabsorption, and Barrett's metaplasia because of its ability both to visualize the abnormality directly and to biopsy it. Colonoscopy is the procedure of choice for colon cancer screening and surveillance; diagnosis of colitis secondary to infection, ischemia, radiation, and IBD; and characterization of causes of lower GI bleeding. Sigmoidoscopy examines the colon up to the splenic flexure and is currently used to exclude distal colonic inflammation or obstruction in young patients not at significant risk for colon cancer. For elusive GI bleeding secondary to arteriovenous malformations or superficial ulcers, small-intestinal examination is performed with push enteroscopy or capsule endoscopy. Endoscopic retrograde cholangiopancreaticography (ERCP) provides diagnoses of pancreatic and biliary disease. Endoscopic ultrasound is useful for evaluating the extent of disease in GI malignancy as well as exclusion of choledocholithiasis, evaluation of pancreatitis, drainage of pancreatic pseudocysts, and assessment of anal continuity.

Radiography/Nuclear Medicine   Radiographic tests evaluate diseases of the gut and extraluminal structures. Oral or rectal contrast agents such as barium provide mucosal definition from the esophagus to the rectum. Contrast radiography also assesses gut transit and pelvic floor dysfunction. Barium swallow is the initial procedure for evaluation of dysphagia to exclude subtle rings or strictures and assess for achalasia, whereas small-bowel contrast radiology reliably diagnoses intestinal tumors and Crohn's ileitis. Contrast enemas are performed when colonoscopy is unsuccessful or contraindicated. Ultrasound and computed tomography (CT) evaluate regions not accessible by endoscopy or contrast studies, including the liver, pancreas, gallbladder, kidneys, and retroperitoneum. These tests are useful for diagnosis of mass lesions, fluid collections, and organ enlargement. Ultrasound is the initial test to evaluate for gallstone disease. Virtual CT colonoscopy is being evaluated as a method of colon cancer screening. Magnetic res-

TABLE 271-2   *Common Indications for Endoscopy*

Upper Endoscopy	Colonoscopy	Endoscopic Retrograde Cholangiopancreatography	Endoscopic Ultrasound
Dyspepsia despite treatment	Cancer screening	Jaundice	Staging of malignancy
Dyspepsia with signs of organic disease	Lower bleeding	Postbiliary surgery complaints	Characterize and biopsy submucosal mass
Refractory vomiting	Anemia	Cholangitis	Bile duct stones
Dysphagia	Diarrhea	Gallstone pancreatitis	Chronic pancreatitis
Upper bleeding	Polypectomy	Pancreatic/biliary/ampullary tumor	Drain pseudocyst
Anemia	Obstruction	Unexplained pancreatitis	Large gastric folds
Weight loss	Biopsy radiologic abnormality	Pancreatitis with unrelenting pain	Anal continuity
Malabsorption	Cancer surveillance:	Fistulas	
Biopsy radiologic abnormality	Family history, prior polyp/cancer, colitis	Biopsy radiologic abnormality	
Polypectomy	Palliate neoplasm	Pancreaticobiliary drainage	
Place gastrostomy	Remove foreign body	Sample bile	
Barrett's metaplasia surveillance		Sphincter of Oddi manometry	
Palliate neoplasm			
Sample duodenal tissue/fluid			
Remove foreign body			

onance imaging assesses the mesenteric circulation to screen for arterial exclusion; the pancreaticobiliary ducts to exclude neoplasm, stones, and sclerosing cholangitis; and the liver to characterize benign and malignant tumors. Angiography excludes mesenteric ischemia and determines spread of malignancy. Angiographic techniques also access the biliary tree in obstructive jaundice. Positron emission tomography may become useful in distinguishing malignant from benign pancreatic disease.

Scintigraphy both evaluates structural abnormalities and quantifies luminal transit. Radionuclide bleeding scans localize bleeding sites in patients with brisk hemorrhage so that therapy with endoscopy, angiography, or surgery may be directed. Radiolabeled leukocyte scans can search for intraabdominal abscesses not visualized on CT. Biliary scintigraphy is complementary to ultrasound in the assessment of cholecystitis. Scintigraphy to quantify esophageal and gastric emptying are well established, while techniques to measure small-intestinal or colonic transit are less widely used.

Histopathology Gut mucosal biopsies obtained at endoscopy evaluate for inflammatory, infectious, and neoplastic disease. Deep rectal biopsies assist with diagnosis of Hirschsprung's disease or amyloid. Liver biopsy is indicated in cases with abnormal liver chemistries, unexplained jaundice, following liver transplant to exclude rejection, and to characterize the degree of inflammation in patients with chronic viral hepatitis prior to initiating antiviral therapy. Biopsies obtained during CT or ultrasound can evaluate for other intraabdominal conditions not accessible by endoscopy.

Functional Testing Tests of gut function provide important data when structural testing is nondiagnostic. In addition to gastric acid and pancreatic function testing, functional testing of motor activity is provided by regional manometric techniques. Esophageal manometry is useful for suspected achalasia, whereas small-intestinal manometry tests for pseudoobstruction. Anorectal manometry is employed for unexplained incontinence or constipation from outlet dysfunction. Biliary manometry tests for sphincter of Oddi dysfunction with unexplained biliary pain. Electrogastrography measures gastric electrical activity in individuals with nausea and vomiting, whereas electromyography assesses anal function in fecal incontinence.

Rx TREATMENT

Management options for the patient with GI disease depend on the cause of symptoms. Available treatments include modifications in dietary intake, medications, interventional endoscopy or radiology techniques, surgery, and therapies directed to external influences.

Nutritional Manipulation Dietary modifications for GI disease include treatments that only reduce symptoms, therapies that correct pathologic defects, and measures that replace normal food intake with enteral or parenteral formulations. Changes that improve symptoms but do not reverse an organic abnormality include lactose restriction for lactase deficiency, liquid meals in gastroparesis, carbohydrate restrictions in dumping syndrome, and high-fiber diets in IBS. The gluten-free diet for celiac disease exemplifies a modification that serves as primary therapy to reduce mucosal inflammation. Enteral medium-chain triglycerides replace normal fats in patients with short-gut syndrome or severe ileal disease. Perfusion of liquid meals through a gastrostomy is performed in those who cannot swallow safely. Enteral feeding through a jejunostomy is considered for gastric dysmotility syndromes that preclude feeding into the stomach. Intravenous hyperalimentation is employed for individuals with generalized gut malfunction who cannot tolerate or who cannot be sustained with enteral nutrition.

Pharmacotherapy Several medications are available to treat GI diseases. Considerable health care resources are expended on over-the-counter (OTC) remedies. Many prescription drug classes are offered as short-term or continuous therapy of GI illness. A plethora of alternative treatments have gained popularity in GI conditions for which traditional therapies provide incomplete relief.

OVER-THE-COUNTER AGENTS OTC agents are reserved for mild GI symptoms. Antacids and histamine H_2 antagonists decrease symptoms in gastroesophageal reflux and dyspepsia, whereas antiflatulents and adsorbents reduce gaseous symptoms. Fiber supplements, stool softeners, enemas, and laxatives are used for constipation. Laxatives are categorized as stimulants, saline cathartics, and poorly absorbed sugars. Nonprescription antidiarrheal agents include kaolin-pectin combinations and loperamide. Supplemental enzymes include lactase pills for lactose intolerance and bacterial α-galactosidase to treat excess gas. In general, use of a nonprescription drug for more than a short time should be supervised by a health care provider.

PRESCRIPTION DRUGS Prescription drugs for GI diseases are a major focus of attention from pharmaceutical companies. Potent acid suppressants, including drugs that inhibit the proton pump, are advocated for acid reflux when OTC preparations are inadequate. Cytoprotective agents are sometimes used for upper gut ulcers. Prokinetic drugs stimulate GI propulsion in gastroparesis, pseudoobstruction, and constipation as well as the functional bowel disorders. Isotonic solutions containing polyethylene glycol are prescribed for constipation refractory to other agents. Prescription antidiarrheals include opiate drugs, anticholinergic antispasmodics, tricyclics, bile acid binders, and serotonin antagonists. Antispasmodics, tricyclic antidepressants, and selective serotonin reuptake inhibitors are also useful for functional abdominal pain and IBS, whereas narcotics are used for organic conditions such as disseminated malignancy and chronic pancreatitis. Antiemetics in several classes reduce nausea and vomiting. Potent pancreatic enzymes decrease malabsorption and pain from pancreatic disease. Antisecretory drugs such as somatostatin analogue, octreotide, treat hypersecretory states. Antibiotics treat ulcer disease secondary to *Helicobacter pylori*, infectious diarrhea, diverticulitis, intestinal bacterial overgrowth, and Crohn's disease. Anti-inflammatory and immunosuppressive drugs are used in ulcerative colitis, Crohn's disease, microscopic colitis, and refractory celiac disease. Chemotherapy with or without radiotherapy is offered for GI malignancies. Most GI carcinomas respond poorly to therapy, whereas lymphomas may be cured with appropriate intervention.

ALTERNATIVE THERAPIES Alternative treatments are marketed to treat selected GI symptoms. Ginger, acupressure, and acustimulation have been advocated for nausea, while pyridoxine has been investigated for nausea of first trimester pregnancy. Probiotics containing active bacterial cultures are used as adjuncts in some cases of refractory infectious diarrhea and have been used as primary therapy of IBS. Low-potency pancreatic enzyme preparations are sold as general digestive aids but have little evidence to support their efficacy.

Enteric Therapies/Interventional Endoscopy and Radiology Simple luminal interventions are commonly performed for GI diseases. Nasogastric tube suction decompresses the upper gut in ileus or mechanical obstruction. Nasogastric lavage using saline or water in the patient with upper GI hemorrhage determines the rate of bleeding and helps evacuate blood prior to endoscopy. Enteral feedings can be initiated through a nasogastric or nasoenteric tube. Enemas relieve fecal impaction or assist in gas evacuation in acute colonic pseudoobstruction. A rectal tube can be left in place to vent the distal colon.

In addition to its diagnostic role, endoscopy has therapeutic capabilities in certain settings. Cautery techniques can stop hemorrhage from ulcers, vascular malformations, and tumors. Injection with vasoconstrictor substances or sclerosants is used for bleeding ulcers, vascular malformations, varices, and hemorrhoids. Endoscopic encirclement of varices and hemorrhoids with constricting bands stops hemorrhage from these sites. Endoscopy can remove polyps or debulk lumen-narrowing malignancies. Endoscopic sphincterotomy of the ampulla of Vater relieves symptoms of choledocholithiasis. Obstructions of the gut lumen and pancreaticobiliary tree are relieved by endoscopic dilation or placement of plastic or expandable metal stents. In cases of acute colonic pseudoobstruction, colonoscopy is employed to withdraw luminal gas. Finally, endoscopy is commonly used to insert feeding tubes.

Radiologic measures are also useful in GI disease. Angiographic embolization or vasoconstriction decreases bleeding from sites not amenable to endoscopic intervention. Dilation or stenting with fluoroscopic guidance relieves luminal strictures. Contrast enemas can reduce volvulus and evacuate air in acute colonic pseudoobstruction. CT and ultrasound help drain abdominal fluid collections, in many cases obviating the need for surgery. Percutaneous transhepatic cholangiography relieves biliary obstruction when ERCP is contraindicated. Lithotripsy can fragment gallstones in patients who are not candidates for surgery. In some instances, radiologic approaches offer advantages over endoscopy for gastrostomy placement. Finally, central venous catheters for parenteral nutrition may be placed using radiographic techniques.

Surgery   Surgery is performed to cure GI disease, control symptoms without cure, maintain nutrition, or palliate unresectable neoplasm. Medication-unresponsive ulcerative colitis, diverticulitis, cholecystitis, appendicitis, and intraabdominal abscess are curable with surgery, whereas only symptom control without cure is possible with Crohn's disease. Surgery is mandated for ulcer complications such as bleeding, obstruction, or perforation and intestinal obstructions that do not resolve with conservative care. Fundoplication of the gastroesophageal junction is performed for presentations ranging from ulcerative esophagitis to drug-refractory symptoms of acid reflux. Achalasia responds to operations to relieve lower esophageal sphincter pressure. Surgery may be needed to place a jejunostomy for long-term enteral feedings. The threshold for performing surgery depends on the clinical setting. In all cases, the benefits of operation must be weighed against the potential for post-operative complications.

Therapy Directed to External Influences   In some conditions, GI symptoms respond to treatments directed outside the gut. Systemic anti-inflammatory or immunosuppressive drugs decrease GI manifestations of gut vasculitis. Plasma expanders may improve gut perfusion in bowel ischemia secondary to hypoperfusion. Finally, psychological therapies including psychotherapy, behavior modification, hypnosis, and biofeedback have shown efficacy in functional bowel disorders. Patients with significant psychological dysfunction and those with little response to treatments targeting the gut are likely to benefit from this form of therapy.

FURTHER READING

AMERICAN SOCIETY FOR GASTROINTESTINAL ENDOSCOPY: *Appropriate Use of Gastrointestinal Endoscopy Consensus Statement.* Manchester, MA, ASGE, 1992

FELMAN M et al: *Sleisenger and Fordtran's Gastrointestinal and Liver Disease,* 7th ed. Philadelphia, Saunders, 2002

YAMADA T (ed): *Textbook of Gastroenterology and Hepatology,* 4th ed. Philadelphia, Lippincott Williams & Wilkins, 2003

272 GASTROINTESTINAL ENDOSCOPY
Mark Topazian

Gastrointestinal endoscopy has been attempted for over 200 years, but the introduction of semi-rigid gastroscopes in the middle of the twentieth century marked the dawn of the modern endoscopic era. Since then, rapid advances in endoscopic technology have led to dramatic changes in the diagnosis and treatment of many digestive diseases. Innovative endoscopic devices and new endoscopic treatment modalities continue to expand the use of endoscopy in patient care.

Flexible endoscopes provide either an optical image (transmitted over fiberoptic bundles) or an electronic video image (generated by a charge-coupled device in the tip of the endoscope). Operator controls permit deflection of the endoscope tip; fiberoptic bundles bring light to the tip of the endoscope; and working channels allow washing, suctioning, and the passage of instruments. Progressive changes in the diameter and stiffness of endoscopes have improved the ease and patient tolerance of endoscopy.

ENDOSCOPIC PROCEDURES

Upper Endoscopy   Upper endoscopy, also referred to as esophagogastroduodenoscopy (EGD), is performed by passing a flexible endoscope through the mouth into the esophagus (Figs. 272-1 to 272-5), stomach (Figs. 272-6 to 272-10), bulb (Figs. 272-11, -12), and second duodenum. The procedure is the best method of examining the upper gastrointestinal mucosa. While the upper gastrointestinal radiographic series has similar accuracy for diagnosis of duodenal ulcer, EGD is superior for detection of gastric ulcers, detects flat mucosal lesions such as those of Barrett's esophagus, and permits directed biopsy and endoscopic therapy, if needed. Topical pharyngeal anesthesia is used, and intravenous conscious sedation is given to most patients in the United States to ease the anxiety and discomfort of the procedure, although in many countries EGD is routinely performed without sedation. Patient tolerance of unsedated EGD is improved by the use of an ultrathin, 5-mm diameter endoscope.

Colonoscopy   Colonoscopy is performed by passing a flexible colonoscope through the anal canal into the rectum and colon. The cecum is reached in >95% of cases, and the terminal ileum can often be examined. Colonoscopy is the "gold standard" for diagnosis of colonic mucosal disease (Figs. 272-13 to 272-21). Barium enema is more accurate for evaluation of diverticula and for accurate measurement of colonic strictures, but colonoscopy has greater sensitivity for colitis, polyps, and cancers. Conscious sedation is usually given before colonoscopy in the United States, although a willing patient and a skilled examiner can complete the procedure without sedation in many cases.

Flexible Sigmoidoscopy   Flexible sigmoidoscopy is similar to colonoscopy but visualizes only the rectum and a variable portion of the left colon, typically to 60 cm from the anal verge. This procedure causes abdominal cramping, but it is brief and is almost always performed without sedation. Flexible sigmoidoscopy is used for colorectal cancer screening and for evaluation of diarrhea and hematochezia.

Small-Bowel Enteroscopy   Two techniques are currently used to evaluate the small intestine, most often in patients with unexplained small-bowel bleeding. *Push enteroscopy* is performed with a long endoscope similar in design to an upper endoscope. The enteroscope is pushed down the small bowel with the help of a stiffening overtube that extends from the mouth to the duodenum. The mid-jejunum is usually reached, and the endoscope's instrument channel allows for biopsies or endoscopic therapy.

Capsule endoscopy involves the patient swallowing a disposable capsule containing a charge-coupled device chip. Color still images (Fig. 272-22) are transmitted wirelessly to an external receiver at fixed intervals until the capsule's battery is exhausted or it is passed into the toilet. Much of the jejunal and ileal mucosa is usually visualized.

Endoscopic Retrograde Cholangiopancreatography (ERCP)   During ERCP, a side-viewing endoscope is passed through the mouth to the duodenum, the ampulla of Vater is identified and cannulated with a thin plastic catheter, and radiographic contrast material is injected into the bile duct and pancreatic duct under fluoroscopic guidance (Fig. 272-23 to 272-25). When indicated, the sphincter of Oddi can be opened using the technique of endoscopic sphincterotomy (Fig. 272-26). Stones can be retrieved from the ducts, and strictures of the ducts can be biopsied, dilated, and stented. ERCP is often performed for therapy but remains important in diagnosis, especially for bile duct stones.

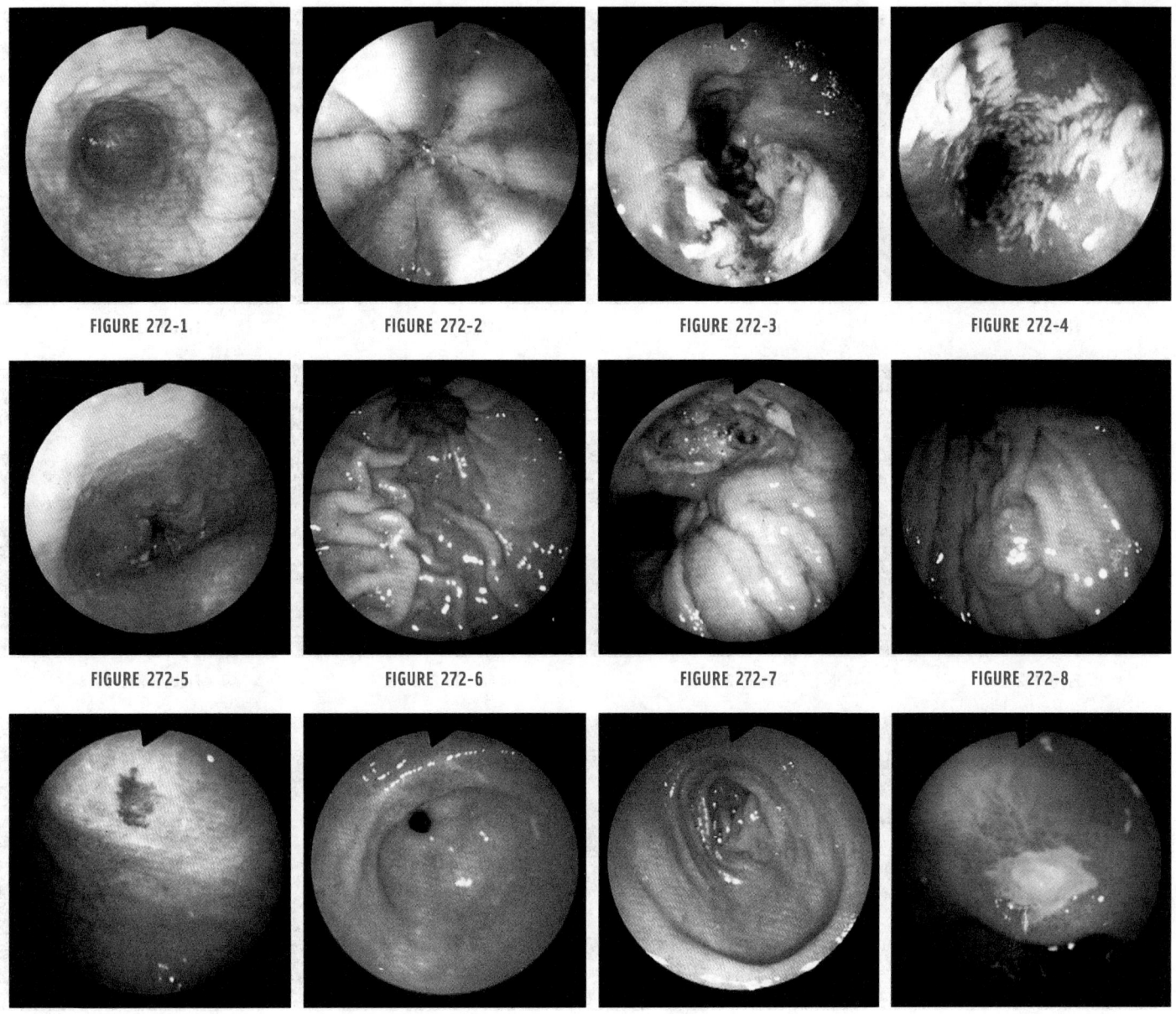

FIGURE 272-1   FIGURE 272-2   FIGURE 272-3   FIGURE 272-4

FIGURE 272-5   FIGURE 272-6   FIGURE 272-7   FIGURE 272-8

FIGURE 272-9   FIGURE 272-10   FIGURE 272-11   FIGURE 272-12

FIGURES 272-1   Normal esophagus where fine vasculature can be seen.   **272-2**   Linear red streaks with a central white streak extend up the esophagus in a peptic regurgitant esophagitis.   **272-3**   Ulcerated squamous cell carcinoma, with a depressed center, involving one wall of the esophagus.   **272-4**   Moniliasis of the esophagus—a white exudate is seen with underlying erythematous mucosa.   **272-5**   Barrett's metaplasia of the esophagus with an adenocarcinoma. The squamocolumnar junction is noted in the proximal esophagus. A mucosal irregularity in the center of the photograph was an adenocarcinoma.   **272-6**   Normal body of the stomach with rugal folds.   **272-7**   Large, benign, lesser curve gastric ulcer—the folds end at the ulcer margin.   **272-8**   The histologic type of this gastric polyp must be determined by excision and pathologic examination.   **272-9**   An arteriovenus malformation of the gastric mucosa.   **272-10**   A normal pylorus. Note the absence of gastric rugal folds in the antrum proximal to the pylorus.   **272-11**   A normal duodenal bulb.   **272-12**   A typical duodenal ulcer with a clean base is seen on the anterior surface of the duodenal bulb.

Endoscopic Ultrasound (EUS)   EUS utilizes high-frequency ultrasound transducers incorporated into the tip of a flexible endoscope. Ultrasound images are obtained of the gut wall and adjacent organs, vessels, and lymph nodes. By sacrificing depth of ultrasound penetration and bringing the ultrasound transducer close to the area of interest via endoscopy, very high resolution images are obtained. EUS provides the most accurate preoperative local staging of esophageal, pancreatic, and rectal malignancies, although it does not detect most distant metastases. Examples of EUS tumor staging are shown in Fig. 272-27. EUS is also highly sensitive for diagnosis of bile duct stones, gallbladder disease, submucosal gastrointestinal lesions, and chronic pancreatitis. Fine-needle aspiration of masses and lymph nodes in the posterior mediastinum, abdomen, and pelvis can be performed under EUS guidance (Fig. 272-28).

RISKS OF ENDOSCOPY

All endoscopic procedures carry some risk of bleeding and gastrointestinal perforation. These risks are quite low with diagnostic upper endoscopy and colonoscopy (<1:1000 procedures), although the risk is as high as 2:100 when therapeutic procedures such as polypectomy, control of hemorrhage, or stricture dilation are performed. Bleeding and perforation are rare with flexible sigmoidoscopy. The risks for diagnostic EUS (without needle aspiration) are similar to the risks for diagnostic upper endoscopy.

Infectious complications are unusual with most endoscopic procedures. Some procedures carry a higher incidence of postprocedure bacteremia, and prophylactic antibiotics may be indicated for these procedures in some patients (Table 272-1).

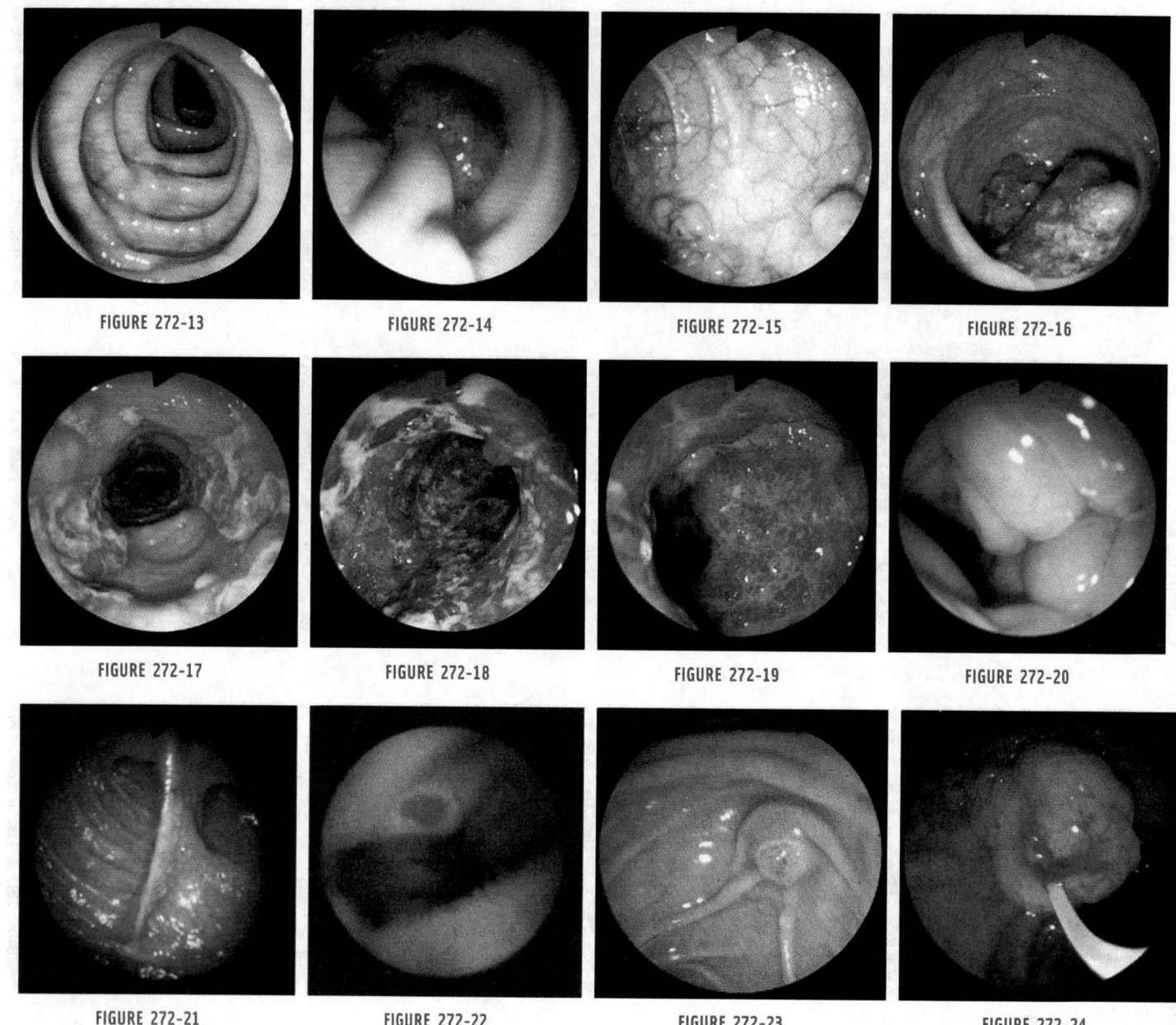

FIGURE 272-13

FIGURE 272-14

FIGURE 272-15

FIGURE 272-16

FIGURE 272-17

FIGURE 272-18

FIGURE 272-19

FIGURE 272-20

FIGURE 272-21

FIGURE 272-22

FIGURE 272-23

FIGURE 272-24

FIGURES 272-13 Typical folds and vascular pattern can be seen in a normal colon. **272-14** This colonic adenomatous polyp is erythematous; a stalk is seen covered with normal mucosa. **272-15** Multiple, small, colonic adenomatous polyps in a case of familial polyposis coli. This colon was removed to prevent the development of cancer. **272-16** Colon adenocarcinoma—the cancer is multilobed and growing into the lumen. **272-17** Crohn's colitis with linear, serpiginous, white-based ulcers surrounded by colonic mucosa which is relatively normal. **272-18** Severe ulcerative colitis with diffuse ulceration, bleeding, and exudation. **272-19** Kaposi's sarcoma involving the colon in a patient with AIDS. The erythematous lesions involve most of the colonic mucosa in the photograph. **272-20** In this case of colonic varices, multiple, serpiginous, subepithelial structures impinge on the colonic lumen. **272-21** The mucosa appears normal in this pouch reconstructed from ileum to provide a reservoir after total proctocolectomy and ileoanal anastomosis. **272-22** Capsule endoscopy image of a jejunal vascular ectasia. (*Courtesy of Dr. Blair Lewis.*) **272-23** Normal papilla of Vater—bile is seen adjacent to the papilla. **272-24** Periampullary carcinoma—the mass at the papilla of Vater has been catheterized during ERCP.

ERCP carries additional risks. Pancreatitis occurs in about 5% of patients undergoing ERCP and is seen in up to 25% of patients with sphincter of Oddi dysfunction. Young anicteric patients with normal ducts are at increased risk. Post-ERCP pancreatitis is usually mild and self-limited but may infrequently result in prolonged hospitalization, surgery, diabetes, or death. Bleeding occurs after 1% of endoscopic sphincterotomies. Ascending cholangitis, pseudocyst infection, and retroperitoneal perforation and abscess may all occur as a result of ERCP.

The conscious sedation administered during endoscopy may cause respiratory depression or allergic reactions. Percutaneous gastrostomy tube placement during EGD is associated with a 10 to 15% incidence of complications, most often wound infections. Fasciitis, pneumonia, bleeding, and colonic injury may result from gastrostomy placement.

URGENT ENDOSCOPY

ACUTE GASTROINTESTINAL HEMORRHAGE Endoscopy is an important diagnostic and therapeutic technique for patients with acute gastrointestinal hemorrhage. Although most gastrointestinal bleeding stops spontaneously, a minority of patients will have persistent or recurrent hemorrhage that may be life-threatening. Clinical predictors of rebleeding help identify patients most likely to benefit from urgent endoscopy and endoscopic, angiographic, or surgical hemostasis.

Initial Evaluation The initial evaluation of the bleeding patient focuses on the magnitude of hemorrhage as reflected by the postural vital signs, the frequency of hematemesis or melena, and (in some cases) findings on nasogastric lavage. Decreases in hematocrit and hemoglobin lag the clinical course and are not reliable gauges of the magnitude of acute bleeding. This initial evaluation, completed well before the bleeding source is confidently identified, guides immediate supportive care of the patient and helps determine the timing of endoscopy. The magnitude of the initial hemorrhage is probably the most important indication for urgent endoscopy, since a large initial bleed increases the likelihood of ongoing or recurrent bleeding. Patients with resting hypotension, repeated hematemesis, nasogastric aspirate that does not clear with large volume lavage, orthostatic change in vital signs, or those requiring blood transfusions should be considered for urgent endoscopy. In addition, patients with cirrhosis, coagulopathy, or respiratory or renal failure and those over 70 years are more likely to have significant rebleeding.

Bedside evaluation also suggests an upper or lower gastrointestinal source of bleeding in most patients. Over 95% of patients with melena are bleeding proximal to the ligament of Treitz, and about 90% of patients with hematochezia are bleeding from the colon. Melena can result from bleeding in the small bowel or right colon, especially in older patients with slow colonic transit. Conversely, some patients with massive hematochezia are bleeding from a duodenal ulcer, with rapid intestinal transit. Early upper endoscopy should be considered in such patients.

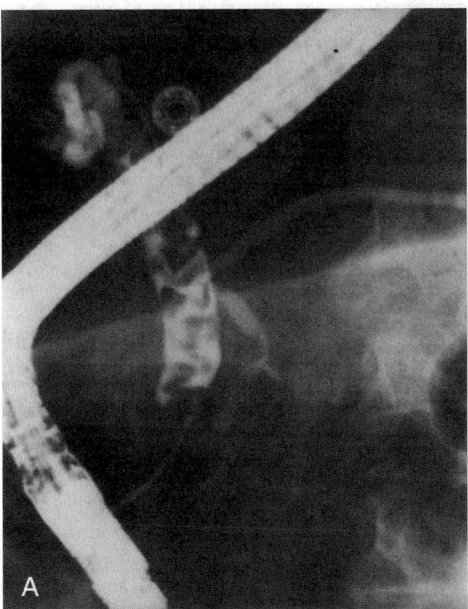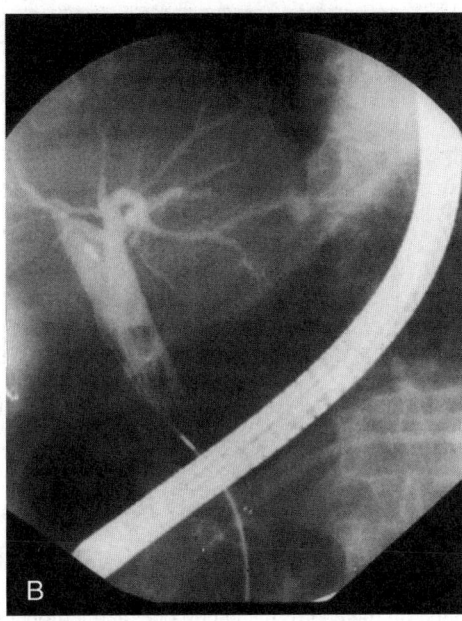

FIGURE 272-25 Endoscopic retrograde cholangiopancreatography (ERCP) for bile duct stones with cholangitis. *A.* Faceted bile duct stones are demonstrated in the common bile duct. *B.* After endoscopic sphincterotomy, the stones are extracted with a Dormia basket. A small abscess communicates with the left intrahepatic duct.

Endoscopy should be performed after the patient has been resuscitated with intravenous fluids and transfusions as necessary. Marked coagulopathy or thrombocytopenia is usually treated before endoscopy, since correction of these abnormalities may lead to resolution of bleeding, and techniques for endoscopic hemostasis are limited in such patients. Metabolic derangements should also be addressed. Tracheal intubation for airway protection should be considered before upper endoscopy in patients with repeated hematemesis and suspected variceal hemorrhage.

Most patients with impressive hematochezia can undergo colonoscopy after a rapid colonic purge with a polyethylene glycol solution; the preparation fluid is often administered via a nasogastric tube. Colonoscopy has a higher diagnostic yield than angiography in lower gastrointestinal bleeding, and endoscopic therapy is appropriate in some cases. In a small minority of cases, persistent bleeding and recurrent hemodynamic instability prevent endoscopic visualization of the colonic mucosa, and other techniques (such as bleeding scans, angiography, or emergency subtotal colectomy) must be employed. Even in these cases, the anal and rectal mucosa should be visualized endoscopically early in the course, since bleeding lesions in or close to the anal canal are often amenable to surgical transanal hemostatic techniques.

Peptic Ulcer The endoscopic appearance of peptic ulcers provides useful prognostic information in patients with acute hemorrhage. When a platelet plug is seen protruding from a vessel wall in the base of an ulcer (a so-called sentinel clot or visible vessel), risk of major rebleeding from the ulcer is 40%. This finding often leads to local endoscopic therapy to decrease the rebleeding rate. A clean-based ulcer is associated with low (3 to 5%) risk of rebleeding; patients with melena and a clean-based duodenal ulcer are often discharged home from the emergency room or endoscopy suite if they are young, reliable, and otherwise healthy. Other findings have an intermediate risk of rebleeding: flat red or purple spots in the ulcer base have a 10% risk, and large adherent clots covering the ulcer base have a 20% risk. Occasionally, active spurting from an ulcer is seen (with >90% risk of ongoing bleeding). Examples of endoscopic stigmata of recent hemorrhage are shown in Fig. 272-29.

Patients with a visible vessel or active bleeding are usually treated endoscopically, decreasing rebleeding rates by about half. Hemostatic techniques include "coaptive coagulation" of the vessel in the base of the ulcer, using a thermal probe that is pressed against the site of bleeding, or injection of epinephrine or sclerosant into and around the vessel.

Varices Two complementary strategies guide therapy of bleeding varices: local treatment of the bleeding vessel and treatment of underlying portal hypertension. Local therapies (including endoscopic sclerotherapy, endoscopic band ligation, and balloon tamponade with a Sengstaken-Blakemore tube) effectively control acute hemorrhage in most patients and are the mainstay of acute treatment, although therapies that decrease portal pressures (pharmacologic treatment, surgical

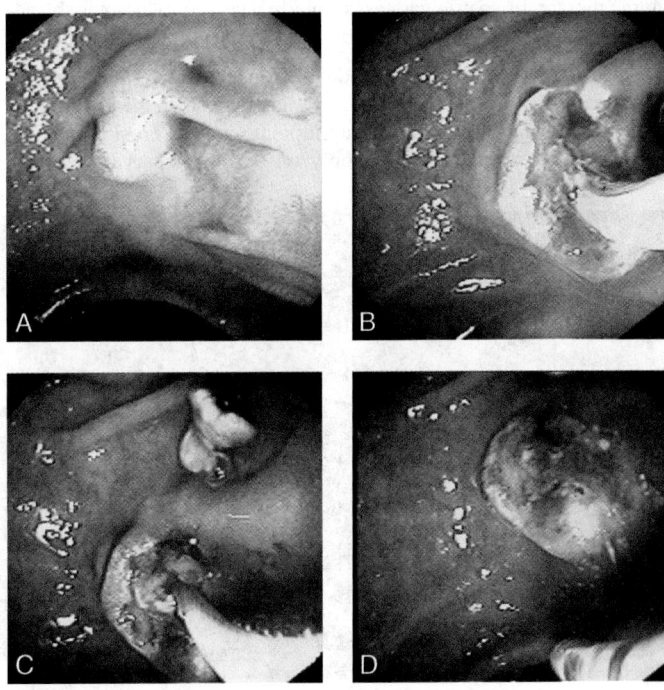

FIGURE 272-26 Endoscopic sphincterotomy. *A.* A normal-appearing ampulla of Vater. *B.* Sphincterotomy is performed with electrocautery. *C.* Bile duct stones are extracted with a balloon catheter. *D.* Final appearance of the sphincterotomy.

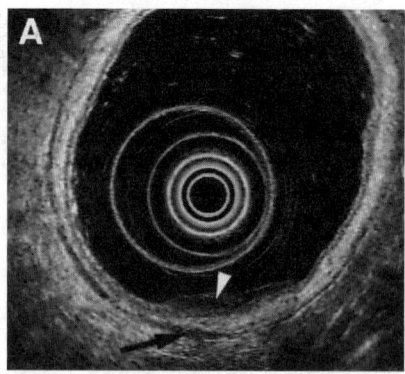 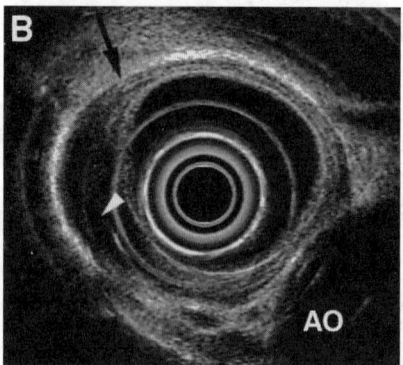 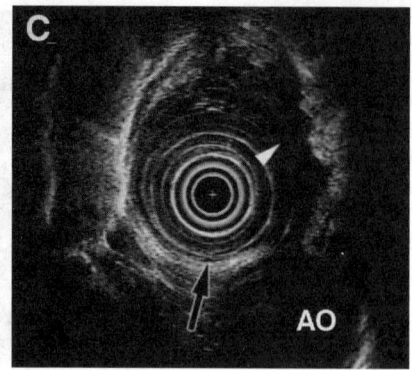

FIGURE 272-27 Local staging of gastrointestinal cancers with endoscopic ultrasound. In each example the white arrowhead marks the primary tumor and the black arrow indicates the muscularis propria (mp) of the intestinal wall. "AO" indicates aorta. *A.* T1 gastric cancer. The tumor does not invade the mp. *B.* T2 esophageal cancer. The tumor invades the mp. *C.* T3 esophageal cancer. The tumor extends through the mp into the surrounding tissue, and focally abuts the aorta.

shunts, or radiologically placed intrahepatic shunts) also play an important role.

Endoscopic band ligation is the preferred local therapy for bleeding esophageal varices. In this technique a varix is suctioned into a cap fitted on the end of the endoscope, and a rubber band is then released from the cap, ligating the varix. Acute hemorrhage can be controlled in up to 90% of patients, and complications (such as sepsis, symptomatic esophageal ulceration, or esophageal stenosis) are uncommon. Endoscopic sclerotherapy is another technique in which a sclerosing, thrombogenic solution is injected into or next to esophageal varices. Sclerotherapy also controls acute hemorrhage in most patients but has higher complication rates. These techniques are used when varices are actively bleeding during endoscopy or (more commonly) when varices are the only identifiable cause of acute hemorrhage.

After treatment of the acute hemorrhage, an elective course of endoscopic therapy can be undertaken with the goal of eradicating esophageal varices and preventing rebleeding months to years later. This chronic therapy is less successful, preventing long-term rebleeding in ~50% of patients. Pharmacologic therapies that decrease portal pressure have similar efficacy, and the two modalities may be combined.

Gastric varices are less amenable to endoscopic therapy and are best treated with a portal decompressive procedure (surgical portosystemic shunt or radiologic transjugular portosystemic shunt). Endoscopic therapy of gastric varices is usually reserved for actively bleeding varices or for patients with thrombosis of the portal venous system.

Dieulafoy's Lesion This lesion, also called *persistent caliber artery*, is a large-caliber arteriole that runs immediately beneath the gastrointestinal mucosa and bleeds through a pinpoint mucosal erosion. Dieulafoy's lesion is seen most commonly on the lesser curvature of the

proximal stomach, causes impressive arterial hemorrhage, and is difficult to diagnose; it is often recognized only after repeated endoscopy for recurrent bleeding. Endoscopic therapy with a thermal probe usually controls acute bleeding and successfully ablates the underlying vessel once the bleeding site has been identified. Embolization or surgical oversewing are sometimes required.

Mallory-Weiss Tear A Mallory-Weiss tear is a linear mucosal rent near or across the gastroesophageal junction that is often associated with retching or vomiting. When the tear disrupts a submucosal arteriole, brisk hemorrhage may result. Endoscopy is the best method of diagnosis, and an actively bleeding tear can be treated endoscopically with coaptive coagulation using a thermal probe or by injection of dilute epinephrine. Since Mallory-Weiss tears only rarely rebleed, a sentinel clot in the base of the tear is usually not treated endoscopically.

Vascular Ectasias Vascular ectasias are flat mucosal vascular anomalies best diagnosed by endoscopy. They usually cause slow intestinal blood loss and have several characteristic distributions in the gastrointestinal tract. When limited to the cecum, where they occur as senile lesions, or the gastric antrum (gastric antral vascular ectasias, or "watermelon stomach"), ectasias are often responsive to local endoscopic ablative therapy. Patients with diffuse small-bowel vascular ectasias (associated with chronic renal failure and with hereditary hemorrhagic telangiectasia) often continue to bleed despite endoscopic treatment of accessible lesions and may benefit from octreotide or estrogen/progesterone therapy.

Colonic Diverticula Diverticula form where nutrient arteries penetrate the muscular wall of the colon en route to the colonic mucosa. The artery found in the base of a diverticulum may bleed, causing painless and impressive hematochezia. Colonoscopy is indicated in patients with hematochezia and suspected diverticular hemorrhage, since other causes of bleeding (such as vascular ectasias, colitis, and colonic cancer) must be excluded. In addition, an actively bleeding diverticulum is occasionally seen and treated during colonoscopy.

GASTROINTESTINAL OBSTRUCTION AND PSEUDO-OBSTRUCTION Endoscopy is useful for evaluation and treatment of some forms of gastrointestinal obstruction. An important exception is small-bowel obstruction, which is generally not diagnosed by endoscopy or amenable to endoscopic therapy. Esophageal, gastroduodenal, and colonic obstruction or pseudoobstruction can all be diagnosed and often managed endoscopically.

Acute Esophageal Obstruction Esophageal obstruction by impacted food or an ingested foreign body is a potentially life-threatening

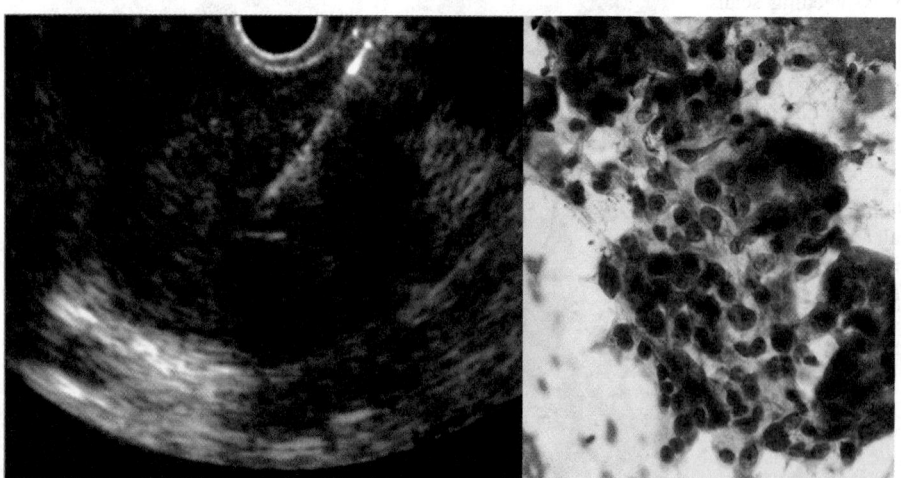

FIGURE 272-28 Endoscopic ultrasound (EUS)–guided needle aspiration. *A.* Ultrasound image of a 22-gauge needle passed through the duodenal wall and positioned in a hypoechoic pancreatic head mass. *B.* Micrograph of aspirated malignant cells. (*Image B courtesy of Dr. Mary Chacho.*)

TABLE 272-1 *Antibiotic Prophylaxis for Selected Endoscopic Procedures*

Patient Condition	Procedure Contemplated	Antibiotic Prophylaxis[a]
Prosthetic valve, history of endocarditis, systemic-pulmonary shunt, synthetic vascular graft (<1 year old)	High risk[b]	Recommended
	Low risk[c]	Optional[d] (insufficient data)
Rheumatic valvular disease, mitral valve prolapse with insufficiency, congenital cardiac malformations, hypertrophic cardiomyopathy	High risk	Optional[d] (insufficient data)
	Low risk	Not recommended[d]
Pacemakers, implantable defibrillators, prior coronary artery bypass grafts; prosthetic joints	High or low risk	Not recommended

[a] Acceptable antibiotic regimens for esophageal procedures include amoxicillin, 2 g PO, 1 h before, or ampicillin, 2 g IV, 30 min before upper endoscopy; clindamycin, 600 mg PO, may be substituted in penicillin-allergic patients. Acceptable regimens for colonic procedures in high-risk patients include gentamicin, 1.5 mg/kg (not to exceed 120 mg), and ampicillin, 2 g IV, within 30 min of colonoscopy, with or without amoxicillin, 1 g orally, 6 h later; vancomycin, 1 g IV, may be substituted for penicillins in penicillin-allergic patients. For colonic procedures in moderate-risk patients, amoxicillin, 2 g PO, 1 h before the procedure or vancomycin, 1 g IV, are sufficient.

[b] High-risk endoscopic procedures: stricture dilation, variceal sclerosis, endoscopic ultrasound with fine-needle aspiration, endoscopic retrograde cholangiopancreatography with an obstructed biliary tree.

[c] Low-risk endoscopic procedures: esophagogastroduodenoscopy and colonoscopy with or without biopsy and polyp removal, variceal ligation.

[d] Controversy exists and recommendations vary. For more detailed discussion, see Dajani AS et al: Clin Infect Dis 25:1448, 1997.

Source: Adapted from *Antibiotic Prophylaxis for Endoscopic Procedures*, American Society for Gastrointestinal Endoscopy, 1998.

event. Left untreated, the patient may develop esophageal ulceration, ischemia, and perforation. Patients with persistent esophageal obstruction often have hypersalivation and are usually unable to swallow water; endoscopy is generally the best initial test in such patients, since endoscopic removal of the obstructing material is usually possible, and the presence of an underlying esophageal stricture can often be determined. Radiographs of the chest and neck should be considered before endoscopy in patients with fever, obstruction for ≥24 h, or ingestion of a sharp object such as a fishbone. Radiographic contrast studies interfere with subsequent endoscopy and are not advisable in most patients with a clinical picture of esophageal obstruction. Occasionally, sublingual nifedipine or nitrates, or intravenous glucagon, may resolve an esophageal food impaction, but in most patients an underlying web, ring, or stricture is present and endoscopic removal of the obstructing food bolus is necessary.

Gastric Outlet Obstruction Obstruction of the gastric outlet is commonly caused by malignancy of the prepyloric gastric antrum or chronic peptic ulceration with stenosis of the pylorus. Patients vomit partially digested food many hours after eating. Gastric decompression with a nasogastric tube and subsequent lavage for removal of retained ma-

terial is the first step in treatment. The diagnosis can then be confirmed with a saline load test, if desired. Endoscopy is useful for diagnosis and treatment. Patients with pyloric stenosis may be treated with endoscopic balloon dilation of the pylorus, and a course of endoscopic dilation results in long-term relief of symptoms in about 50% of patients. Malignant pyloric obstruction can be treated with endoscopically placed expandable stents if the patient is deemed a poor surgical candidate.

Colonic Obstruction and Pseudoobstruction These both present with abdominal distention and discomfort; tympany; and a dilated, air-filled colon on plain abdominal radiography. Both conditions may lead to colonic perforation if untreated. Acute colonic pseudoobstruction is a form of colonic ileus that is usually attributable to electrolyte disorders, narcotic and anticholinergic medications, immobility (as after surgery), and retroperitoneal hemorrhage or mass. Multiple causative factors are often present. Either colonoscopy or a water-soluble contrast enema may be used to look for an obstructing lesion and differentiate obstruction from pseudoobstruction. One of these diagnostic studies should be strongly considered if the patient does not have clear risk factors for pseudoobstruction, if radiographs do not show air in the rectum, or if the patient fails to improve when the underlying causes of pseudoobstruction have been addressed. The risk of cecal perforation in pseudoobstruction rises when the cecal diameter exceeds 12 cm, and in such patients decompression of the colon may be achieved using intravenous neostigmine, colonoscopic decompression, or placement of a cecostomy tube. Most patients should receive a trial of conservative therapy (with correction of electrolyte disorders, removal of offending medications, and increased mobilization) before undergoing an invasive decompressive procedure.

Colonic obstruction is an indication for urgent intervention. Emergency diverting colostomy is often performed with a subsequent operation after bowel preparation to address the underlying cause. Colonscopic placement of an expandable stent is an alternative that can relieve malignant obstruction without emergency surgery and permit bowel preparation for elective surgery.

ACUTE BILIARY OBSTRUCTION The steady, severe pain that occurs when a gallstone acutely obstructs the common bile duct often brings patients to a hospital. The diagnosis of a ductal stone is suspected when the patient is jaundiced or when serum liver tests or pancreatic enzyme levels are elevated, and confirmed by direct cholangiography (performed endoscopically, percutaneously, or during surgery). ERCP is currently the primary means of diagnosing and treating common bile duct stones in most hospitals in the United States.

Bile Duct Imaging While transabdominal ultrasound and biliary scintigraphy are not sufficiently accurate for reliable diagnosis of bile duct stones, newer imaging modalities such as spiral computed tomography (CT), magnetic resonance cholangiopancreatography (MRCP), and EUS are more accurate and have an emerging role in diagnosis. Ex-

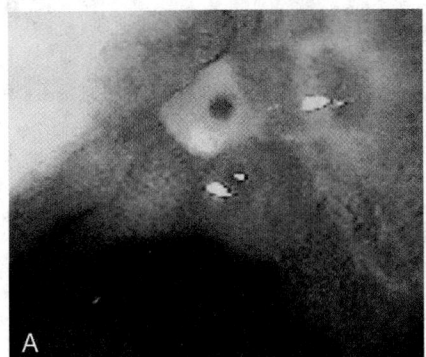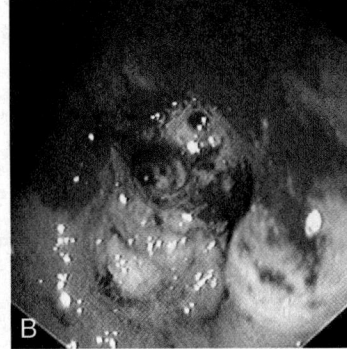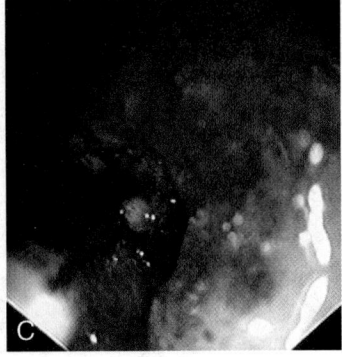

FIGURE 272-29 Endoscopic stigmata of recent bleeding in peptic ulcers. *A.* A flat red spot in an ulcer base. *B.* A sentinel clot protruding from an ulcer base. *C.* Coagulation of the sentinel clot shown in (*B*) with a thermal probe. (*Courtesy of American Society for Gastrointestinal Endoscopy.*)

amples of these modalities are shown in Fig. 272-30. During MRCP, images are obtained that demonstrate stagnant or slowly flowing fluid and subtract all other tissue. The resulting images of the right upper quadrant are strikingly similar to a direct cholangiogram, although with less resolution. MRCP can be performed rapidly without sedation and does not require any radiographic contrast. When an echo-endoscope is passed into the duodenum, detailed EUS views of the adjacent bile duct are readily obtained. While this procedure requires intravenous sedation, it has a very low incidence of complications, in contradistinction to ERCP. Spiral CT has a sensitivity of 85% for diagnosis of bile duct stones, MRCP has a sensitivity of 85 to 95%, and EUS has a sensitivity of 88 to 98%. EUS is more accurate than ERCP in some hands.

When a bile duct stone is highly likely and urgent treatment is required (as in a patient with jaundice and biliary sepsis), ERCP is the procedure of choice, since it remains the gold standard for diagnosis and provides immediate treatment. When a persistent bile duct stone is relatively unlikely (as in a patient with gallstone pancreatitis), less-invasive imaging techniques may supplant ERCP or intraoperative cholangiography.

Ascending Cholangitis   Charcot's triad of jaundice, abdominal pain, and fever is present in about 70% of patients with ascending cholangitis and biliary sepsis. Initially, such patients are managed with fluid resuscitation and intravenous antibiotics. Abdominal ultrasound is often done to look for gallbladder stones and bile duct dilation. The bile duct may not be dilated early in the course of acute biliary obstruction, however. Medical management usually improves the patient's clinical status, providing a window of approximately 24 h during which biliary drainage should be established, typically by ERCP. Undue delay can result in recrudesence of overt sepsis and increased morbidity. If, in addition to Charcot's triad, shock and confusion are present (Reynolds's pentad), urgent attempts to restore biliary drainage are usually indicated.

Gallstone Pancreatitis   Gallstones may cause acute pancreatitis as they pass through the ampulla of Vater. The occurrence of gallstone pancreatitis usually implies passage of a stone into the duodenum, and only about 20% of patients harbor a persistent stone in the ampulla or the common bile duct. Retained stones are more common in patients with jaundice, severe pancreatitis, or superimposed ascending cholangitis.

Urgent ERCP decreases the morbidity of gallstone pancreatitis in some subsets of patients. It remains unclear whether the benefit of ERCP is mainly attributable to treatment and prevention of ascending cholangitis or to relief of pancreatic duct obstruction. ERCP is warranted early in the course of gallstone pancreatitis if ascending cho-

langitis is also suspected, especially in a jaundiced patient. Urgent ERCP appears to benefit patients predicted to have severe pancreatitis using a clinical index of severity (such as the Glasgow or Ranson score).

ELECTIVE ENDOSCOPY

Dyspepsia and Reflux   Dyspepsia is a chronic or recurrent burning discomfort or pain in the upper abdomen that may be caused by diverse processes such as gastroesophageal reflux, peptic ulcer disease, and "nonulcer dyspepsia," a heterogeneous category that includes disorders of motility, sensation, and somatization. Gastric and esophageal malignancies are less common causes of dyspepsia. Careful history-taking allows accurate differential diagnosis of dyspepsia in only about half of patients. In the remainder, endoscopy can be a useful diagnostic tool, especially in those patients whose symptoms are not resolved by an empirical trial of symptomatic treatment.

Gastroesophageal Reflux Disease (GERD)   When classic symptoms of gastroesophageal reflux are present, such as water brash and substernal heartburn, presumptive diagnosis and empirical treatment are often sufficient. Although endoscopy is sensitive for diagnosis of esophagitis, it can miss cases of reflux, since some patients have symptomatic reflux without esophagitis. The most sensitive test for diagnosis of GERD is 24-h ambulatory pH monitoring. Endoscopy is indicated in patients with resistant reflux symptoms and in those with recurrent dyspepsia after treatment that is not clearly due to reflux on clinical grounds alone, to assess the esophagus and exclude other diseases. Endoscopy is also advised in a patient with reflux and dysphagia, to look for a stricture or malignancy. Endoscopy may be indicated in patients with long-standing ($\geq$10 years) frequent heartburn, who are at sixfold increased risk of Barrett's esophagus compared to a patient with <1 year of reflux symptoms. Patients with Barrett's esophagus usually enter a program of periodic endoscopy with biopsies, to detect dysplasia or early carcinoma.

Peptic Ulcer   Peptic ulcer classically causes epigastric gnawing or burning, often occurring nocturnally and promptly relieved by food or antacids. Although endoscopy is the most sensitive diagnostic test for peptic ulcer, immediate endoscopy is not a cost-effective strategy in young patients with ulcer-like dyspeptic symptoms unless endoscopy is available at low cost. Patients with suspected peptic ulcer should be evaluated for *Helicobacter pylori* infection. Serology (past or present infection), urea breath testing (current infection), and stool tests are less invasive and costly than endoscopy with biopsy. Patients with ulcer-like symptoms despite treatment should undergo endoscopy to exclude gastric malignancy, and patients with "alarm symptoms" (weight loss, anemia, bleeding) should also undergo endoscopy.

Nonulcer Dyspepsia   This may be associated with bloating and, unlike peptic ulcer, tends not to remit and recur. Most patients do not respond

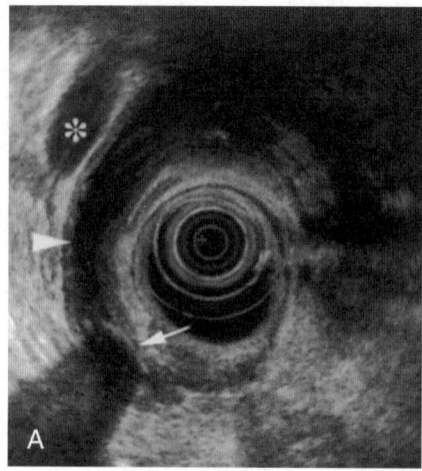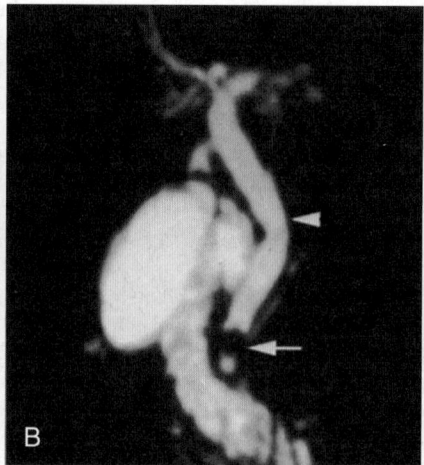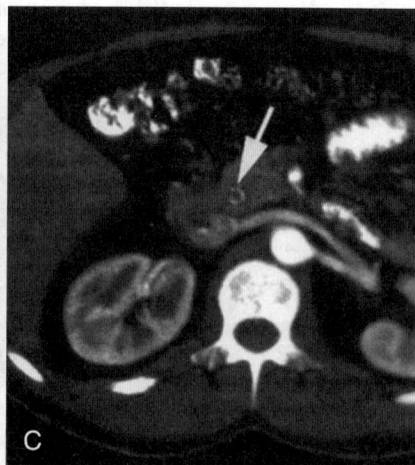

FIGURE 272-30   Methods of bile duct imaging. Arrows mark bile duct stones. Arrowheads indicate the common bile duct, and the asterisk marks the portal vein.   *A.* Endoscopic ultrasonography (EUS). *B.* Magnetic resonance cholangiography (MRCP). *C.* Helical computed tomography.

to acid-reducing, prokinetic, or anti-*Helicobacter* therapy and are referred for endoscopy to exclude a refractory ulcer. While endoscopy usefully excludes other diagnoses, it generally does little to improve the treatment of patients with nonulcer dyspepsia.

Dysphagia About 50% of patients with difficulty swallowing have a mechanical obstruction; the remainder have a motor disorder. Careful history-taking often suggests a diagnosis and leads to the appropriate use of diagnostic tests. Esophageal strictures typically cause progressive dysphagia, first for solids, then liquids; motor disorders often cause intermittent dysphagia for both solids and liquids. Some underlying disorders have characteristic historic features: Schatzki's ring causes episodic dysphagia for solids, typically at the beginning of a meal; pharyngeal motor disorders are associated with difficulty initiating deglutition ("transfer dysphagia") and nasal reflux with swallowing; and achalasia may cause nocturnal regurgitation of undigested food.

When mechanical obstruction is suspected, endoscopy is a useful initial diagnostic test, since it permits immediate biopsy and dilation of strictures, masses, or rings. Blind or forceful passage of an endoscope may lead to perforation in a patient with stenosis of the cervical esophagus or a Zenker's diverticulum, but gentle passage of an endoscope under direct visual guidance is reasonably safe. Endoscopy can miss a subtle stricture or ring in some patients.

When a motor disorder is suspected, esophageal radiography is the best initial diagnostic test. The pharyngeal swallowing mechanism, esophageal peristalsis, and the lower esophageal sphincter can all be assessed. In some disorders, subsequent esophageal manometry may also be important for diagnosis.

Anemia and Occult Blood in the Stool Iron-deficiency anemia may be attributed to poor iron absorption (as in celiac sprue) or, more commonly, chronic blood loss. Intestinal bleeding should be strongly suspected in men and postmenopausal women with iron-deficiency anemia, and colonoscopy is indicated in such patients, even in the absence of detectable occult blood in the stool. Some 30% will have large colonic polyps, 10% will have colorectal cancer, and additional patients will have colonic vascular lesions. When a convincing source of blood loss is not found in the colon, upper gastrointestinal endoscopy should also be performed; if no lesion is found, duodenal biopsies should be obtained to exclude sprue. Small-bowel evaluation may be appropriate if both EGD and colonoscopy are unrevealing.

Tests for occult blood in the stool detect hemoglobin or the heme moiety and are most sensitive for colonic blood loss, although they will also detect larger amounts of upper gastrointestinal bleeding. Patients over 50 with occult blood in normal-appearing stool should undergo colonoscopy to diagnose or exclude colorectal neoplasia. The diagnostic yield is lower than in iron-deficiency anemia. Whether upper endoscopy is also indicated largely depends on the patient's symptoms.

The small intestine may be the source of chronic intestinal bleeding, especially if colonoscopy and upper endoscopy are not diagnostic. The utility of small-bowel evaluation varies with the clinical setting and is most important in patients whose bleeding causes chronic or recurrent anemia. While small-bowel radiography is usually normal, capsule endoscopy yields a specific diagnosis in about 50% of such patients. The most common finding is mucosal vascular ectasias.

Colorectal Cancer Screening Most colon cancers develop from preexisting colonic adenomas, and colorectal cancer can be largely prevented by the detection and removal of adenomatous polyps. Screening for polyps and early, asymptomatic cancers can be accomplished both by testing stool specimens for occult blood and by directly examining the colonic mucosa. Since tests for occult blood are insensitive, detecting only about one-fourth of colon cancers and large polyps, visualization of at least a part of the colon is an important component of colorectal cancer screening.

The choice of screening strategy for an asymptomatic patient depends in part on their personal and family history. Patients at increased risk for colon cancer include those with a past history of inflammatory bowel disease, colorectal polyps, a family history of first-degree family members with adenomatous polyps or cancer, or certain familial cancer syndromes. These considerations alter screening recommendations. An individual without these factors is generally considered at average risk.

Screening strategies are summarized in Table 272-2. Either sigmoidoscopy or colonoscopy may be used for cancer screening in asymptomatic average-risk patients. Use of sigmoidoscopy was based on the historic finding that the majority of colorectal cancers occurred in the rectum and left colon, and that patients with right-sided colon cancers had left-sided polyps. Over the past several decades, however, the distribution of colon cancers has changed, with proportionally fewer rectal and left-sided cancers than in the past. Large studies of colonoscopy for screening of average-risk individuals show that cancers are roughly equally distributed between left and right colon and half of patients with right-sided lesions have no polyps in the left colon. In addition, the new imaging technique of "virtual colonoscopy" holds considerable promise. This modality uses data from helical CT to generate a graphic display of a "flight" down the colonic lumen.

TABLE 272-2 *Colorectal Cancer Screening Strategies*

	Recommendation
AVERAGE-RISK PATIENTS	
Asymptomatic individuals ≥ 50 years of age	Colonscopy every 10 years, *or* Annual fecal occult blood test and flexible sigmoidoscopy every 5 years, or Double-contrast barium enema every 5 to 10 years
HIGH-RISK PATIENTS[a]	
Personal history History of colon cancer	Evaluate entire colon around the time of resection, then colonoscopy every 3 to 5 years
History of colonic adenomas	Colonoscopy every 3 to 5 years
Ulcerative pancolitis of 8 years' duration, left-sided colitis >15 years' duration	Colonoscopy with biopsies every 1 to 3 years
Family history Familial adenomatous polyposis	Consider genetic testing Annual sigmoidoscopy beginning at age 10 to 12; consider colectomy when polyps develop; if no polyps, annual sigmoidoscopy until age 40, then every 3 to 5 years
Hereditary nonpolyposis colorectal cancer (HNPCC)	Consider genetic testing Colonoscopy every 2 years beginning at 25 or when 5 years younger than the youngest affected relative; annual colonoscopy after age 40
Two first-degree relatives with colorectal cancer or adenomas	Colonoscopy every 3 to 5 years, beginning when 10 years younger than the youngest affected relative
One first-degree relative with sporadic colorectal cancer or adenoma before age 60	Same as above

a High-risk patients: Past history of inflammatory bowel disease, colorectal adenomatous polyps, or colorectal cancer; family history of colorectal adenomatous polyps, colorectal cancer, or certain familial cancer syndromes.

Source: Adapted from *Recommendations for Colorectal Cancer Screening and Surveillance in People at Average and at Increased Risk*, American Medical Association Council on Scientific Affairs, 2001; and *Screening and Surveillance Colonoscopy in Individuals at Increased Risk for Colorectal Cancer*, American Society for Gastrointestinal Endoscopy, 1998.

This technique is not yet sufficiently sensitive for routine clinical use, but further refinement may result in a useful noninvasive screening method.

Diarrhea   Most cases of diarrhea are acute, self-limited, and due to infections or medication. Chronic diarrhea (lasting >6 weeks) is more often due to a primary inflammatory or malabsorptive disorder, is less likely to resolve spontaneously, and generally requires diagnostic evaluation. Patients with chronic diarrhea or severe, unexplained acute diarrhea often undergo endoscopy if stool tests for pathogens are unrevealing. The choice of endoscopic test depends on the clinical setting.

Patients with colonic symptoms and findings such as bloody diarrhea, tenesmus, fever, or leukocytes in stool generally undergo sigmoidoscopy or colonoscopy to look for colitis. Sigmoidoscopy is often adequate and is the best initial test in most such patients. On the other hand, patients with symptoms and findings suggesting small-bowel disease such as large-volume watery stools, substantial weight loss, and malabsorption of iron, calcium, or fat may undergo upper endoscopy with duodenal biopsies.

Many patients with chronic diarrhea do not fit either of these patterns. When there is a long-standing history of alternating constipation and diarrhea dating to early adulthood, without findings such as blood in the stool or anemia, a diagnosis of irritable bowel syndrome may be made without direct visualization of the bowel. Steatorrhea and upper abdominal pain may prompt evaluation of the pancreas rather than the gut. Patients whose chronic diarrhea is not easily categorized often undergo initial colonoscopy to examine the entire colon (and terminal ileum) for inflammatory or neoplastic disease.

Minor Hematochezia   Bright red blood passed with or on formed brown stool usually has a rectal, anal, or distal sigmoid source. Patients with even trivial amounts of hematochezia should be investigated with flexible sigmoidoscopy to exclude large polyps or cancers in the distal bowel. Patients who report red blood on the toilet tissue only, without blood in the toilet or on the stool, are bleeding from a lesion in the anal canal, and careful external and digital examinations and anoscopy are sufficient for diagnosis in most cases.

Unexplained Pancreatitis   About 20% of patients with pancreatitis have no identified cause after routine clinical investigation (including a review of medication and alcohol use, measurement of serum triglyceride and calcium levels, abdominal ultrasonography, and CT). Endoscopic techniques lead to a specific diagnosis in the majority of such patients, often altering clinical management. Endoscopic investigation is particularly appropriate if the patient has had more than one episode of pancreatitis.

Microlithiasis, or the presence of microscopic crystals in bile, is a leading cause of previously unexplained acute pancreatitis and is sometimes seen during abdominal ultrasonography as layering sludge or flecks of floating, echogenic material in the gallbladder. Gallbladder bile can be obtained for microscopic analysis by administering a cholecystokinin analogue during endoscopy, causing contraction of the gallbladder. Bile is suctioned from the duodenum as it drains from the papilla, and the darkest fraction is examined for cholesterol crystals or bilirubinate granules. Combined EUS of the gallbladder and bile microscopy is probably the most sensitive means of diagnosing microlithiasis.

Previously undetected chronic pancreatitis, pancreatic malignancy, or pancreas divisum may be diagnosed by either ERCP or EUS. Sphincter of Oddi dysfunction probably causes some cases of pancreatitis and can be diagnosed by manometric studies performed during ERCP.

Cancer Staging   Local staging of esophageal, gastric, pancreatic, bile duct, and rectal cancers can be obtained with EUS. EUS with fine-needle aspiration (Fig. 272-28) currently provides the most accurate preoperative assessment of local tumor and nodal staging, but it does not detect distant metastases. Details of the local tumor stage can guide treatment decisions including resectability and need for neoadjuvant therapy. EUS with transesophageal needle biopsy may also be used to assess the presence of non-small cell lung cancer in mediastinal nodes.

OPEN-ACCESS ENDOSCOPY

While gastroenterologists have traditionally seen patients in consultation before arranging an endoscopic procedure, direct scheduling of endoscopic procedures by primary care physicians, or *open-access endoscopy*, is an increasingly common practice. When the indications for endoscopy are clear cut and appropriate, the procedural risks are low, and the patient understands what to expect, open-access endoscopy streamlines patient care and decreases costs.

Patients referred for open-access endoscopy should have a recent history, physical examination, and medication review. A copy of such an evaluation should be available when the patient comes to the endoscopy suite. Patients with unstable cardiovascular or respiratory conditions should not be referred directly for open-access endoscopy. Patients with selected cardiac conditions undergoing certain procedures should be prescribed prophylactic antibiotics prior to endoscopy, as described in Table 272-1. In addition, patients taking anticoagulants may need changes in treatment before endoscopy, as detailed in Table 272-3. While many endoscopists recommend discontinuing aspirin for 5 days before elective endoscopic procedures, most evidence suggests that in the absence of a preexisting bleeding disorder it is safe to perform endoscopic procedures in patients taking aspirin and nonsteroidal anti-inflammatory drugs.

Common indications for open-access EGD include dyspepsia resistant to a trial of appropriate therapy; gastrointestinal bleeding; and persistent anorexia, or early satiety. Open-access colonoscopy is often requested in men or postmenopausal women with iron-deficiency anemia, patients over age 50 with occult blood in the stool, patients with a previous history of colorectal adenomatous polyps or cancer, and for colorectal cancer screening. Flexible sigmoidoscopy is commonly performed as an open-access procedure.

When patients are referred for open-access colonoscopy, the primary care provider may need to choose a colonic preparation. Commonly used oral preparations include polyethelene glycol lavage solution and sodium phosphate. Sodium phosphate may cause fluid and electrolyte abnormalities, especially in patients with renal failure, congestive heart failure, and patients over 70 years of age.

TABLE 272-3   *Management of Anticoagulation before Endoscopic Procedures*

	High Patient Risk of Thromboembolism[a]	Low Patient Risk of Thromboembolism[b]
High-risk procedure[c]	Stop warfarin 3–5 days before the procedure; consider heparin when INR is below the therapeutic range	Stop warfarin 3–5 days before the procedure; restart warfarin after the procedure
Low-risk procedure[d]	No change in anticoagulation; elective procedures should be delayed while INR is above the therapeutic range	No change in anticoagulation; elective procedures should be delayed while INR is above the therapeutic range

[a] High-risk conditions: atrial fibrillation associated with valvular heart disease, mechanical valve in the mitral position, mechanical valve and prior thromboembolic event.
[b] Low-risk conditions: Uncomplicated or paroxysmal nonvalvular atrial fibrillation, mechanical valve in the aortic position, bioprosthetic valve, deep vein thrombosis.
[c] High-risk procedures: Polypectomy, stricture dilation, treatment of varices, gastrostomy placement, biliary sphincterotomy, endoscopic ultrasound with needle aspiration.
[d] Low-risk procedures: Diagnostic upper endoscopy, colonoscopy, sigmoidoscopy with or without biopsy, diagnostic endoscopic retrograde cholangiopancreatography, endoscopic ultrasound without needle aspiration.

Note: INR, international normalized ratio.
Source: Adapted from *The Management of Anticoagulants and Anti-Inflammatory Medications in Patients Undergoing Endoscopic Procedures*, American Society for Gastrointestinal Endoscopy, 1998.

FURTHER READING

BARON TH: Expandable metal stents for the treatment of cancerous obstruction of the gastrointestinal tract. N Engl J Med 344:1681, 2001

DAJANI AS et al: Prevention of bacterial endocarditis: Recommendations by the American Heart Association. Clin Infect Dis 25:1448, 1997

IMPERIALE TF et al: Risk of advanced proximal neoplasms in asymptomatic adults according to the distal colorectal findings. N Engl J Med 343:169, 2000

JENSEN DM et al: Urgent colonoscopy for the diagnosis and treatment of severe diverticular hemorrhage. N Engl J Med 342:78, 2000

LIEBERMAN DA et al: Use of colonoscopy to screen asymptomatic adults for colorectal cancer. N Engl J Med 343:162, 2000

OFMAN JJ, RABENECK L: The effectiveness of endoscopy in the management of dyspepsia: A qualitative systematic review. Am J Med 106:335, 1999

273 DISEASES OF THE ESOPHAGUS
Raj K. Goyal

The two major functions of the esophagus are the transport of the food bolus from the mouth to the stomach and the prevention of retrograde flow of gastrointestinal contents. The transport function is achieved by peristaltic contractions in the pharynx and esophagus associated with relaxation of upper and lower esophageal sphincters (Chap. 33). Retrograde flow is prevented by the two esophageal sphincters, which remain closed between swallows. The upper esophageal sphincter (UES) consists of the cricopharyngeus and inferior pharyngeal constrictor muscles, both of which are striated muscles innervated by excitatory somatic lower motor neurons. These muscles exhibit no myogenic tone and receive no inhibitory innervation. The UES remains closed owing to the elastic properties of its wall and to neurogenic tonic contraction of the sphincter muscles. Inhibition in the central nervous system opens the sphincter muscles in concert with forward displacement of the larynx by the suprahyoid muscles. In contrast, the lower esophageal sphincter (LES) is composed of smooth muscle and is innervated by parallel sets of parasympathetic excitatory and inhibitory pathways. It remains closed because of its intrinsic myogenic tone, which is modulated by the excitatory and inhibitory nerves. It opens in response to the activity of the inhibitory nerves. The neurotransmitters of the excitatory nerves are acetylcholine and substance P, and those of the inhibitory nerves are vasoactive intestinal peptide (VIP) and nitric oxide. The function of the LES is supplemented by the striated muscle of the diaphragmatic crura, which surrounds the LES and acts as an external LES. Relaxation of the LES without esophageal contraction occurs during belching and gastric distention. Gastric distention–evoked transient lower esophageal sphincter relaxation (tLESR) is a vasovagal reflex. Fatty meals, smoking, and beverages with a high xanthine content (tea, coffee, cola) also cause a reduction in sphincter pressure. Many hormones and neurotransmitters can modify LES pressure. Muscarinic M_2 and M_3 receptor agonists, α-adrenergic agonists, gastrin, substance P, and prostaglandin $F_{2\alpha}$ cause contraction. Nicotine, β-adrenergic agonists, dopamine, cholecystokinin, secretin, VIP, calcitonin gene–related peptide (CGRP), adenosine, prostaglandin E, and nitric oxide donors such as nitrates reduce sphincter pressure.

SYMPTOMS

DYSPHAGIA See Chap. 33

ESOPHAGEAL PAIN *Heartburn*, or pyrosis, is characterized by burning retrosternal discomfort that may move up and down the chest like a wave. When severe, it may radiate to the sides of the chest, the neck, and the angles of the jaw. Heartburn is a characteristic symptom of reflux esophagitis and may be associated with regurgitation or a feeling of warm fluid climbing up the throat. It is aggravated by bending forward, straining, or lying recumbent and is worse after meals. It is relieved by an upright posture, by the swallowing of saliva or water, and, more reliably, by antacids. Heartburn is produced by heightened mucosal sensitivity and can be reproduced by infusion of dilute (0.1 *N*) hydrochloric acid (Bernstein test) or neutral hyperosmolar solutions into the esophagus.

Odynophagia, or painful swallowing, is characteristic of nonreflux esophagitis, particularly monilial and herpes esophagitis. Odynophagia

may occur with peptic ulcer of the esophagus (Barrett's ulcer), carcinoma with periesophageal involvement, caustic damage of the esophagus, and esophageal perforation. Odynophagia is unusual in uncomplicated reflux esophagitis. Crampy chest pain associated with impaction of a food bolus should be distinguished from odynophagia.

Atypical chest pain other than heartburn and odynophagia occurs in reflux esophagitis or esophageal motility disorders such as diffuse esophageal spasm. Spasm may occur spontaneously or during a meal. Chest pain due to periesophageal involvement with carcinoma or peptic ulcer may be constant and agonizing. Sometimes different types of esophageal pains exist together in the same patient, and frequently patients are not able to describe the pain accurately enough to allow its classification. Coronary artery disease should always be excluded before the esophagus is considered as the cause of atypical chest pain. The most frequent esophageal cause of chest pain is reflux esophagitis. Some patients with atypical chest pain have nonspecific esophageal motor abnormalities of uncertain significance. Many of these patients have behavioral abnormalities, psychosomatic disorders, depression, anxiety, panic reactions, and other psychological disorders.

REGURGITATION *Regurgitation* is the effortless appearance of gastric or esophageal contents in the mouth. In distal esophageal obstruction and stasis, as in achalasia or the presence of a large diverticulum, the regurgitated material consists of tasteless mucoid fluid or undigested food. Regurgitation of sour or bitter-tasting material occurs in severe gastroesophageal reflux and is associated with incompetence of both the UES and the LES. Regurgitation may result in laryngeal aspiration, with spells of coughing and choking that awaken the patient from sleep, and in aspiration pneumonia. Water brash is reflex salivary hypersecretion that occurs in response to peptic esophagitis and should not be confused with regurgitation.

DIAGNOSTIC TESTS

RADIOLOGIC STUDIES Barium swallow with fluoroscopy and an esophagogram is a widely used test for the diagnosis of esophageal disease and can be used to evaluate both structural and motor disorders. Spontaneous reflux of barium from the stomach into the esophagus suggests gastroesophageal reflux. Esophageal peristalsis is best studied in the recumbent position, because in the upright position barium passage occurs largely by gravity alone. A double-contrast esophagogram, obtained by coating the esophageal mucosa with barium and distending the esophageal lumen with air using effervescent granules, is particularly useful in demonstrating mucosal ulcers and early cancers. A barium-soaked piece of bread or a 13-mm barium tablet is sometimes used to demonstrate an obstructive lesion. Figures 273-1 and 273-2 illustrate the radiographic appearance of some esophageal disorders. Since the oropharyngeal phase of swallowing lasts no more than a second, videofluoroscopy is necessary to permit detection and analysis of abnormalities of oral and pharyngeal function. The pharynx is examined to detect stasis of barium in the valleculae and piriform sinuses and regurgitation of barium into the nose and tracheobronchial tree.

ESOPHAGOSCOPY Esophagoscopy is the direct method of establishing the cause of mechanical dysphagia and of identifying mucosal lesions that may not be identified by the usual barium swallow. If the lumen is markedly narrowed, use of a smaller-caliber endoscope may be needed; on occasion a stricture must be dilated before the examination can be completed. Endoscopic biopsies are useful in diagnosing car-

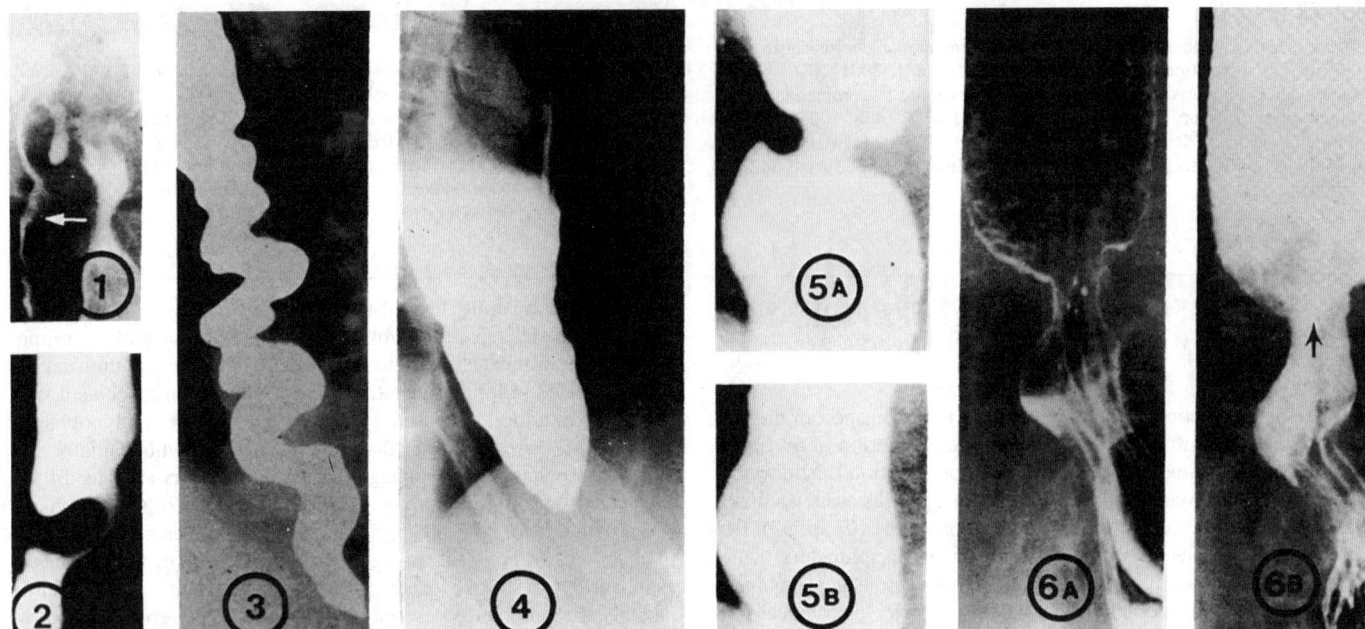

FIGURE 273-1 Radiographic appearance of some motor disorders of the pharynx and esophagus. (1) Pharyngeal paralysis with tracheal aspiration (*arrow*). (2) Cricopharyngeal achalasia. Note the prominent cricopharyngeus, which is recognized by its smoothness and location in the posterior wall. (3) Diffuse esophageal spasm. Note the typical corkscrew appearance of the lower part of the esophagus. (4) Achalasia, showing a dilated esophageal body with an air-fluid level and a closed lower esophageal sphincter. (5) Muscular (contractile) lower esophageal ring. The asymmetric contraction visible in (5A) has disappeared in (5B), obtained during the same examination. (6) Scleroderma esophagus showing dilated esophagus with a stricture (6A) and reflux of barium from the stomach into the esophagus (6B). (Courtesy of Dr. Harvey Goldstein.)

cinoma, reflux esophagitis, and other mucosal diseases. Cells obtained by a cytology balloon or brushing the mucosa can be evaluated for carcinoma. Endoscopic ultrasonography permits evaluation of intramural masses and staging of esophageal cancer.

ESOPHAGEAL MOTILITY The study of esophageal motility entails simultaneous recording of pressures from different sites in the esophageal lumen with an assembly of pressure sensors positioned 5 cm apart. The UES and LES appear as zones of high pressure that relax on swallowing. The pharynx and esophagus normally show peristaltic waves with each swallow.

Esophageal motility studies are helpful in the diagnosis of esophageal motor disorders (achalasia, spasm, scleroderma) (Fig. 273-3) but are of little value in the diagnosis of mechanical dysphagia. In patients with reflux esophagitis, esophageal manometry is useful in quantitating lower esophageal competence and providing information on the status of the esophageal body motor activity. Manometry provides quantitative data that cannot be obtained by barium swallow or endoscopy. Tests for reflux esophagitis are described later.

MOTOR DISORDERS

STRIATED MUSCLE ■ Oropharyngeal Paralysis Paralysis of oral muscles leads to difficulty initiating swallowing and drooling of food out of the mouth. Pharyngeal paralysis, characterized by dysphagia, nasal regurgitation, and aspiration during swallowing, occurs in a variety of

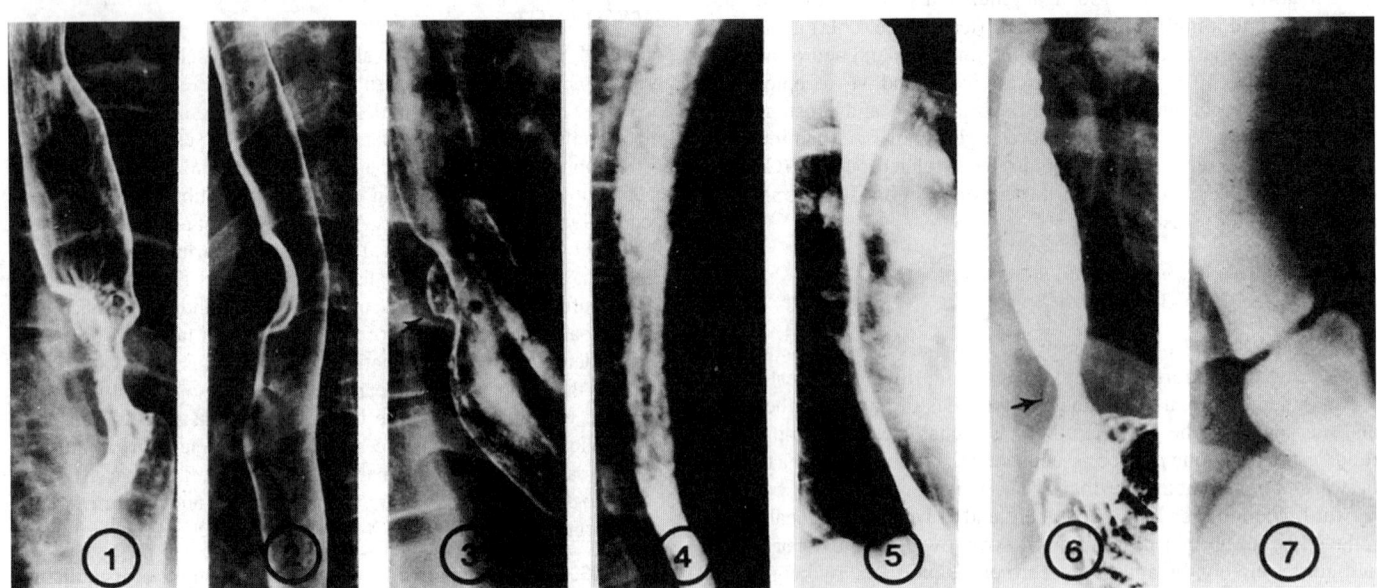

FIGURE 273-2 Selected structural lesions of the esophagus. (1) Carcinoma of the esophagus, with typical annular narrowing with overhanging margins and destruction of the mucosa. (2) Leiomyoma of the esophagus, with a smooth filling defect and right angles of origin from the esophageal wall. (3) Esophageal ulcer in columnar cell–lined esophagus (Barrett's esophagus). (4) Monilial esophagitis, with irregular plaquelike filling defects. (5) Long stricture secondary to lye ingestion. (6) Peptic stricture, short and tubular, with associated hiatal hernia. (7) Lower esophageal mucosal (Schatzki) ring. A thin, weblike annular constriction at the esophagogastric junction is associated with a small hiatal hernia. (Courtesy of Dr. Harvey Goldstein.)

neuromuscular disorders (see Table 33-1). Some of these disorders also involve laryngeal muscles, causing hoarseness. When the suprahyoid muscles are paralyzed, the UES does not open with swallowing, leading to paralytic achalasia of the UES and severe dysphagia.

Videofluoroscopy with barium of various consistencies may reveal difficulties in the oral phase of swallowing. The test may show stasis of barium in the valleculae and piriform sinuses, nasal and tracheal aspiration, failure of the upper sphincter to open, and/or abnormal movement of the hyoid bone and the larynx with a swallow (Fig. 273-1 panel 1). Motility studies demonstrate a reduced amplitude of pharyngeal and upper esophageal contractions and reduced basal upper esophageal sphincter pressure without further relaxation on swallowing (Fig. 273-3). Patients with myasthenia gravis (Chap. 366) and polymyositis (Chap. 369) respond to treatment. Dysphagia resulting from a cerebrovascular accident improves with time, although often not completely. Treatment consists of maneuvers to reduce pharyngeal stasis and enhance airway protection under the direction of a trained swallow therapist. Feeding by a nasogastric tube or an endoscopically placed gastrostomy tube may be necessary for nutritional support; however, these maneuvers do not provide protection against aspiration of salivary secretions. Cricopharyngeal myotomy is sometimes performed, but its usefulness is unproven. Extensive operative procedures to prevent aspiration are rarely needed. Death is often due to pulmonary complications.

Cricopharyngeal Bar Failure of the cricopharyngeus to relax on swallowing appears as a prominent bar on the posterior wall of the pharynx on barium swallow (Fig. 273-1 panel 2). A transient cricopharyngeal bar is seen in up to 5% of individuals without dysphagia undergoing upper gastrointestinal studies; it can be produced in normal individuals during a Valsalva maneuver. A persistent cricopharyngeal bar may be caused by fibrosis in the cricopharyngeus. Some of these patients complain of food sticking in their throats. Cricopharyngeal myotomy may be helpful but is contraindicated in the presence of gastroesophageal reflux because it may lead to pharyngeal and pulmonary aspiration.

Globus Pharyngeus A sensation of a constant lump in the throat, but no difficulty in swallowing, occurs especially in individuals with emotional disorders, particularly women. Results of barium studies and manometry are normal. Treatment consists primarily of reassurance. Some patients with globus pharyngeus have associated reflux esophagitis, and they may respond to treatment of the esophagitis.

SMOOTH MUSCLE ■ Achalasia Achalasia is a motor disorder of the esophageal smooth muscle in which the LES does not relax normally with swallowing, and the esophageal body undergoes nonperistaltic contractions.

PATHOPHYSIOLOGY The underlying abnormality is the loss of intramural neurons. Inhibitory neurons containing VIP and nitric oxide synthase are predominantly involved, but cholinergic neurons are also affected in advanced disease. Primary idiopathic achalasia accounts for most of the patients seen in the United States. Secondary achalasia may be caused by gastric carcinoma that infiltrates the esophagus, lymphoma, Chagas' disease, certain viral infections, eosinophilic gastroenteritis, and neurodegenerative disorders.

CLINICAL FEATURES Achalasia affects patients of all ages and both sexes. Dysphagia, chest pain, and regurgitation are the main symptoms. Dysphagia appears early, occurs with both liquids and solids, and is worsened by emotional stress and hurried eating. Various maneuvers designed to increase intraesophageal pressure, including the Valsalva

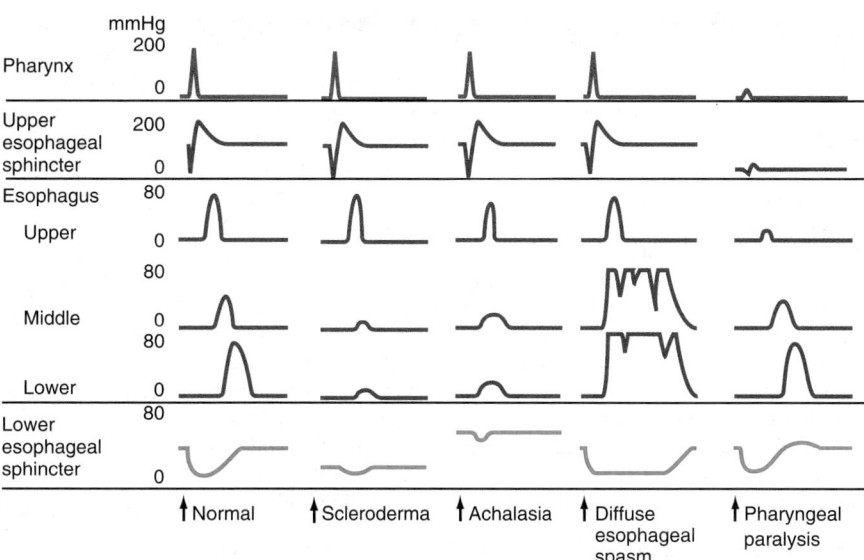

FIGURE 273-3 Motility patterns in selected esophageal and pharyngeal disorders. In normal individuals, the upper and lower esophageal sphincters (UES and LES) appear as zones of high pressure. With a swallow (indicated by ↑), pressure in the sphincters falls and a contraction wave starts in the pharynx and progresses down the esophagus. In scleroderma, the lower part of the esophagus (smooth muscle) shows a reduced amplitude of contractions, which may be peristaltic or simultaneous in onset, and hypotension of the LES. In achalasia, the lower part of the esophagus shows contractions that are reduced in amplitude and simultaneous in onset. In contrast to scleroderma, the LES in achalasia is hypertensive and fails to relax in response to a swallow. In diffuse esophageal spasm, the lower part of the esophagus shows simultaneous-onset, large-amplitude, prolonged, repetitive contractions. In pharyngeal paralysis, the smooth-muscle part of the esophagus is normal. The skeletal muscle part shows a reduced amplitude of contractions. The UES is hypotensive and may not relax normally on swallowing due to associated weakness of the suprahyoid muscles.

maneuver, may aid the passage of the bolus into the stomach. Regurgitation and pulmonary aspiration occur because of retention of large volumes of saliva and ingested food in the esophagus. Patients may complain of difficulty belching. The presence of gastroesophageal reflux argues against achalasia; in patients with long-standing heartburn, cessation of heartburn and appearance of dysphagia suggest development of achalasia on top of reflux esophagitis. The course is usually chronic, with progressive dysphagia and weight loss over months to years. Achalasia associated with carcinoma is characterized by severe weight loss and a rapid downhill course if untreated.

DIAGNOSIS A chest x-ray shows absence of the gastric air bubble and sometimes a tubular mediastinal mass beside the aorta. An air-fluid level in the mediastinum in the upright position represents retained food in the esophagus. Barium swallow shows esophageal dilation, and in advanced cases the esophagus may become sigmoid. On fluoroscopy, normal peristalsis is lost in the lower two-thirds of the esophagus. The terminal part of the esophagus shows a persistent beaklike narrowing representing the nonrelaxing LES (Fig. 273-1 panel 4).

Manometry shows the basal LES pressure to be normal or elevated, and swallow-induced relaxation either does not occur or is reduced in degree, duration, and consistency. The esophageal body shows an elevated resting pressure. In response to swallows, primary peristaltic waves are replaced by simultaneous-onset contractions (Fig. 273-3). These contractions may be of poor amplitude (classic achalasia) or of large amplitude and long duration (vigorous achalasia). Cholecystokinin (CCK), which normally causes a fall in the sphincter pressure, paradoxically causes contraction of the LES (the CCK test). This paradoxical response occurs because, in achalasia, the neurally transmitted inhibitory effect of CCK is absent owing to the loss of inhibitory neurons. Endoscopy is helpful in excluding the secondary causes of achalasia, particularly gastric carcinoma.

℞ **TREATMENT**

Treatment with soft foods, sedatives, and anticholinergic drugs is usually unsatisfactory. Nitrates and calcium channel blockers provide short-term benefit, but their use may be limited by side effects. Nitroglycerin, 0.3 to 0.6 mg, is used sublingually before meals and as needed for chest pain. Isosorbide dinitrate, 2.5 to 5 mg sublingually or 10 to 20 mg orally, is used before meals. Nitrates are associated with headache and postural hypotension. The calcium channel blocker nifedipine, 10 to 20 mg orally or sublingually before meals, is also effective. Endoscopic intrasphincteric injection of botulinum toxin is effective over a short period in some patients. Repeated injections may lead to fibrosis, complicating further operative therapy. Botulinum toxin acts by blocking cholinergic excitatory nerves in the sphincter. Balloon dilatation reduces the basal LES pressure by tearing muscle fibers. In experienced hands, this technique is effective in ~85% of patients. Perforation and bleeding are potential complications. Heller's extramucosal myotomy of the LES, in which the circular muscle layer is incised, is equally effective. Laparoscopic myotomy is the procedure of choice. Reflux esophagitis and peptic stricture may follow successful treatment (more often with myotomy than with balloon dilatation).

Diffuse Esophageal Spasm and Related Motor Disorders These disorders present with clinical symptoms of chest pain and dysphagia and are recognized by their manometric features. In pure form, they all show normal relaxation to swallows. Diffuse esophageal spasm is characterized by nonperistaltic contractions, usually of large amplitude and long duration. An esophageal motility pattern showing hypertensive but peristaltic contractions has been called "nutcracker esophagus."

PATHOPHYSIOLOGY Nonperistaltic contractions are due to dysfunction of inhibitory nerves. Histopathologic studies show patchy neural degeneration localized to nerve processes, rather than the prominent degeneration of nerve cell bodies seen in achalasia. Diffuse esophageal spasm may progress to achalasia. Hypertensive peristaltic contractions and hypertensive or hypercontracting LES may represent cholinergic or myogenic hyperactivity.

CLINICAL FEATURES Diffuse spasm and related motor disorders (hypertensive peristaltic contraction, hypertensive LES, and hypercontracting LES) cannot be distinguished clinically. They all present with chest pain, dysphagia, or both. Chest pain is particularly marked in patients with esophageal contractions of large amplitude and long duration. Chest pain usually occurs at rest but may be brought on by swallowing or by emotional stress. The pain is retrosternal; it may radiate to the back, the sides of the chest, both arms, or the sides of the jaw and may last from a few seconds to several minutes. Pain may be acute and severe, mimicking the pain of myocardial ischemia. Dysphagia for solids and liquids may occur with or without chest pain and is correlated with simultaneous-onset contractions.

Diffuse esophageal spasm and related esophageal motor disorders must be differentiated from other causes of chest pain, particularly ischemic heart disease with atypical angina. A complete cardiac workup should be done before a noncardiac etiology is considered seriously. The presence of dysphagia in association with pain should point to the esophagus as the site of disease. Esophageal motility disorders are an uncommon cause of noncardiac chest pain, which is more commonly due to reflux esophagitis or visceral hypersensitivity.

DIAGNOSIS In diffuse esophageal spasm, barium swallow shows that normal sequential peristalsis below the aortic arch is replaced by uncoordinated simultaneous contractions that produce the appearance of curling or multiple ripples in the wall, sacculations, and pseudodiverticula—the "corkscrew" esophagus (Fig. 273-1 panel 3). Sometimes an esophageal contraction obliterates the lumen, and barium is pushed away in both directions. The barium swallow is frequently normal in diffuse esophageal spasm and mostly normal in the related disorders.

Diffuse esophageal spasm (Fig. 273-3) and related motor disorders are manometric diagnoses. Because these abnormalities may be episodic, the results of manometry may be normal at the time of the study. Several techniques are used to provoke esophageal spasm. Cold swallows produce chest pain but do not produce spasm on manometric studies. Solid boluses and pharmacologic agents, particularly edro-

phonium, induce both chest pain and motor abnormalities. However, correlation between induction of pain and motility changes is poor. The usefulness of pharmacologic provocative tests is limited.

℞ TREATMENT

Anticholinergics are usually of limited value. Agents that relax smooth muscle, such as sublingual nitroglycerin (0.3 to 0.6 mg) or longer-acting agents such as isosorbide dinitrate (10 to 30 mg orally before meals) and nifedipine (10 to 20 mg orally before meals), are helpful. Sublingual forms of these agents can also be used. Reassurance and tranquilizers are helpful in allaying apprehension.

SCLERODERMA ESOPHAGUS The esophageal lesions in systemic sclerosis consist of atrophy of smooth muscle, manifested by weakness in the lower two-thirds of the esophageal body and incompetence of the LES. The esophageal wall is thin and atrophic and may exhibit areas of patchy fibrosis. Patients usually present with dysphagia to solids. Liquids may cause dysphagia when the patient is recumbent. These patients usually also complain of heartburn, regurgitation, and other symptoms of gastroesophageal reflux disease (GERD). Barium swallow shows dilation and loss of peristaltic contractions in the middle and distal portions of the esophagus. The LES is patulous, and gastroesophageal reflux may occur freely (Fig. 273-1 panel 6). Mucosal changes due to esophageal ulceration and esophageal stricture may be present. Motility studies show a marked reduction in the amplitude of smooth-muscle contractions, which may be peristaltic or nonperistaltic. The resting pressure of the LES is subnormal, but sphincter relaxation is normal (Fig. 273-3). Similar esophageal motor abnormalities are found in other collagen vascular diseases and in Raynaud's syndrome alone. Dietary adjustments with the use of soft foods are helpful in management. GERD and its complications should be treated aggressively.

GASTROESOPHAGEAL REFLUX DISEASE

GERD is one of the most prevalent gastrointestinal disorders. Population-based studies show that up to 15% of individuals have heartburn and/or regurgitation at least once a week and 7% have symptoms daily. Symptoms are caused by backflow of gastric acid and other gastric contents into the esophagus due to incompetent barriers at the gastroesophageal junction.

Pathophysiology The normal antireflux mechanisms consist of the LES, the crural diaphragm, and the anatomical location of the gastroesophageal junction below the diaphragmatic hiatus. Reflux occurs only when the gradient of pressure between the LES and the stomach is lost. It can be caused by a sustained or transient decrease in LES tone. A sustained hypotension of the LES may be due to muscle weakness that is often without apparent cause. Secondary causes of sustained LES incompetence include scleroderma-like diseases, myopathy associated with chronic intestinal pseudo-obstruction, pregnancy, smoking, anticholinergic drugs, smooth-muscle relaxants [β-adrenergic agents, aminophylline, nitrates, calcium channel blockers, phosphodiesterase inhibitors that increase cyclic AMP or cyclic GMP (including sildenafil)], surgical damage to the LES, and esophagitis. tLESR without associated esophageal contraction is due to a vagal reflex in which LES relaxation is elicited by gastric distention. Increased episodes of tLESR are associated with GERD. A similar reflex operates during belching. Apart from incompetent barriers, gastric contents are most likely to reflux (1) when gastric volume is increased (after meals, in pyloric obstruction, in gastric stasis, during acid hypersecretion states), (2) when gastric contents are near the gastroesophageal junction (in recumbency, bending down, hiatal hernia), and (3) when gastric pressure is increased (obesity, pregnancy, ascites, tight clothes). Incompetence of the diaphragmatic crural muscle, which surrounds the esophageal hiatus in the diaphragm and functions as an external LES, also predisposes to GERD.

Exposure of the esophagus to refluxed acid correlates with potential for mucosal damage. Exposure depends on the amount of refluxed material per episode, frequency of episodes, and rate of clearing the esophagus by gravity and peristaltic contractions. When peristaltic contractions are impaired, esophageal clearance is impaired. Acid refluxed into the esophagus is neutralized by saliva. Thus, impaired salivary secretion also increases esophageal exposure time. If the refluxed material extends to the cervical esophagus and breaches the upper sphincter, it can enter the pharynx, larynx, and trachea.

Reflux esophagitis is a complication of reflux and develops when mucosal defenses are unable to counteract the damage done by acid, pepsin, and bile. *Mild esophagitis* involves microscopic changes of mucosal infiltration with granulocytes or eosinophils, hyperplasia of basal cells, and elongation of dermal pegs. In nonerosive reflux disease, endoscopic appearance may be normal or show mild erythema. *Erosive esophagitis* shows endoscopically apparent mucosal damage, redness, friability, bleeding, superficial linear ulcers, and exudates. Histology shows polymorphic infiltrates and granulation tissue. *Peptic stricture* results from fibrosis that causes luminal constriction. These strictures occur in ~10% of patients with untreated GERD. Short strictures caused by spontaneous reflux are usually 1 to 3 cm long and are present in the distal esophagus near the squamocolumnar junction (Fig. 273-2 panel 6). Long, tubular peptic strictures can result from persistent vomiting or prolonged nasogastric intubation. Erosive esophagitis may heal by intestinal metaplasia (*Barrett's esophagus*), which is a risk factor for adenocarcinoma.

Clinical Features Regurgitation of sour material in the mouth and heartburn are the characteristic symptoms of GERD. Reflux into the pharynx, larynx, and tracheobronchial tree can cause chronic cough, bronchoconstriction, pharyngitis, laryngitis, bronchitis, or pneumonia. Morning hoarseness may be noted. Recurrent pulmonary aspiration can cause aspiration pneumonia, pulmonary fibrosis, or chronic asthma. Heartburn is produced by the contact of refluxed material with the sensitized or ulcerated esophageal mucosa. Angina-like or atypical chest pain occurs in some patients, while others experience no heartburn or chest pain. Persistent dysphagia suggests development of a peptic stricture. Most patients with peptic stricture have a history of several years of heartburn preceding dysphagia. However, in one-third of patients, dysphagia is the presenting symptom. Rapidly progressive dysphagia and weight loss may indicate the development of adenocarcinoma in Barrett's esophagus. Bleeding occurs due to mucosal erosions or Barrett's ulcer. Many patients with GERD remain asymptomatic or self-treated and do not seek attention until severe complications occur.

Diagnosis The diagnosis is easily made by history alone. Diagnostic studies are indicated in patients with persistent symptoms or complications or those who do not respond to therapy. The diagnostic approach to GERD can be divided into three categories:

1. documentation of mucosal injury,
2. documentation and quantitation of reflux, and
3. definition of the pathophysiology.

Mucosal damage is documented by the use of barium swallow, esophagoscopy, and mucosal biopsy. The results of barium swallow are usually normal in uncomplicated esophagitis but may reveal a stricture or ulcer. A high esophageal peptic stricture, a deep ulcer, or adenocarcinoma suggest Barrett's esophagus. Esophagoscopy may reveal the presence of erosive esophagitis, distal peptic stricture, or columnar cell–lined lower esophagus with or without a proximally located peptic stricture, ulcer, or adenocarcinoma. Results of esophagoscopy are normal in patients with nonerosive esophagitis; in such patients, mucosal biopsies and the Bernstein test are helpful. The mucosal biopsies should be performed at least 5 cm above the LES, as the esophageal mucosal changes of chronic esophagitis are quite frequent in the most distal esophagus in otherwise normal individuals. The Bernstein test involves the infusion of solutions of 0.1 N HCl or normal saline into the esophagus. In patients with symptomatic esophagitis, infusion of acid, but not of saline, reproduces the symptoms of heartburn. Infusion of acid in normal individuals usually produces no

symptoms. Supraesophageal manifestations are diagnosed by careful otolaryngologic exam.

A therapeutic trial with a proton pump inhibitor (PPI) (such as omeprazole, 40 mg bid) for 1 week provides strong support for the diagnosis of GERD.

Documentation and quantitation of reflux, when necessary, can be done by ambulatory long-term (24-h) esophageal pH recording. For evaluation of pharyngeal reflux, a system of recording simultaneously from pharyngeal and esophageal sites may be useful. The pH recordings are helpful only in the evaluation of acid reflux. Documentation of reflux is necessary only when the role of reflux in the symptom complex is unclear, particularly in evaluation of supraesophageal symptoms and chest pain without endoscopic evidence of esophagitis.

Definition of pathophysiologic factors in GERD is sometimes indicated for management decisions such as antireflux surgery. Esophageal motility studies may provide useful quantitative information on the competence of the LES and on esophageal motor function.

 TREATMENT

The goals of treatment are to provide symptom relief, heal erosive esophagitis, and prevent complications. The management of mild cases includes weight reduction, sleeping with the head of the bed elevated by about 4 to 6 in. with blocks, and elimination of factors that increase abdominal pressure. Patients should not smoke and should avoid consuming fatty foods, coffee, chocolate, alcohol, mint, orange juice, and certain medications (such as anticholinergic drugs, calcium channel blockers, and other smooth-muscle relaxants). They should also avoid ingesting large quantities of fluids with meals. In mild cases, lifestyle changes and over-the-counter antisecretory agents may be adequate. H_2 receptor blocking agents (cimetidine, 300 mg; ranitidine, 150 mg bid; famotidine, 20 mg bid; nizatidine, 150 mg bid) are effective in symptom relief. PPIs are more effective in symptom relief and more commonly used.

The PPIs are comparably effective: omeprazole (20 mg/d), lansoprazole (30 mg/d), pantoprazole (40 mg/d), esomeprazole (40 mg/d), or rabeprazole (20 mg/d) for 8 weeks can heal erosive esophagitis in up to 90% of patients. The drug is taken 15 to 30 min before breakfast and can be maintained indefinitely. Refractory patients can double the dose and administer it twice a day before meals. Side effects are minimal. Aggressive acid suppression causes hypergastrinemia but does not increase the risk for carcinoid tumors or gastrinomas. Vitamin B_{12} absorption is compromised by the treatment. Patients who have Barrett's esophagus with concomitant esophagitis should be similarly treated; however, acid suppression does not lead to resolution of the Barrett's metaplasia or cancer prevention. Patients who have an associated peptic stricture are treated with dilators to relieve dysphagia, and such patients are provided with vigorous treatment for reflux. Esophagoscopy should be performed in patients suspected of complications such as bleeding, stricture, or development of cancer.

Antireflux surgery, in which the gastric fundus is wrapped around the esophagus (fundoplication), increases the LES pressure and should be considered as an alternative for patients who require long-term, high-dose PPIs. Laparoscopic fundoplication is the surgery of choice. Ideal candidates for fundoplication are those in whom motility studies show persistently inadequate LES pressure but normal peristaltic contractions in the esophageal body.

Patients with alkaline esophagitis are treated with general antireflux measures and neutralization of bile salts with cholestyramine, aluminum hydroxide, or sucralfate. Sucralfate is particularly useful in these cases, as it also serves as a mucosal protector.

BARRETT'S ESOPHAGUS The metaplasia of esophageal squamous epithelium to columnar epithelium (Barrett's esophagus) is a complication of severe reflux esophagitis, and it is a risk factor for esophageal adenocarcinoma (Chap. 77). Metaplastic columnar epithelium develops during healing of erosive esophagitis with continued acid reflux because columnar epithelium is more resistant to acid-pepsin damage than is squamous epithelium. The metaplastic epithelium is a mosaic of different epithelial types including goblet cells and columnar cells that have features of both secretory and absorptive cells (incomplete or type III metaplasia). Barrett's esophagus is arbitrarily divided into long-segment (>2–3 cm) or short-segment (<2–3 cm) groups; long-segment disease is present in 0.5% of the population and short-segment disease may occur in up to 15%.

Barrett's epithelium progresses through a dysplastic stage before developing into adenocarcinoma. The rate of cancer development is 0.5% per year; those with long-segment disease have a risk of developing esophageal cancer that is 30 to 125 times the risk of the general population. Barrett's esophagus can also lead to chronic peptic ulcer of the esophagus with high (midesophageal) and long strictures.

Given the natural history, erosive esophagitis should be aggressively treated. The prevalence of intestinal metaplasia is estimated at 4 to 10% of patients with significant heartburn. Barrett's esophagus is more common in men, particularly white men, and prevalence increases with age. A one-time esophagoscopy is recommended in patients with persistent GERD symptoms at age 50 to identify patients with Barrett's esophagus. Established metaplasia does not regress with treatment; thus, acid suppression and fundoplication are indicated only when active esophagitis is also present.

The need and frequency of surveillance endoscopies in patients with established Barrett's esophagus are debated. The risk of developing esophageal adenocarcinoma is related to the length of involved esophageal mucosa. People with short segments of Barrett's esophagus (distal 2 to 3 cm) account for up to 25% of unselected patients undergoing endoscopy with or without GERD symptoms and appear to be at low risk. They are not routinely surveyed. However, those with long-segment Barrett's esophagus are advised to have endoscopic surveillance at 1-year intervals for 2 years and then every 2 to 3 years. The frequency is increased if dysplasia is detected independent of the length of the metaplasia. Optical methods of recognizing dysplasia during the endoscopy (laser-induced fluorescence spectroscopy, optical coherence tomography) are being developed. Once high-grade dysplasia is detected, treatment of choice is esophagectomy of the Barrett's segment. Photodynamic laser or thermocoagulative mucosal ablation and endoscopic mucosal resection are being evaluated as alternatives.

INFLAMMATORY DISORDERS

INFECTIOUS ESOPHAGITIS   Infectious esophagitis can be due to viral, bacterial, fungal, or parasitic organisms. In severely immunocompromised patients, multiple organisms may coexist.

Viral Esophagitis   *Herpes simplex virus* (HSV) type 1 occasionally causes esophagitis in immunocompetent individuals, but either HSV type 1 or HSV type 2 may afflict patients who are immunosuppressed (Chap. 163). Patients complain of an acute onset of chest pain, odynophagia, and dysphagia. Bleeding may occur in severe cases; tracheoesophageal fistula and food impaction have been noted. Systemic manifestations such as nausea, vomiting, fever, chills, and mild leukocytosis may be present. Herpetic vesicles on the nose and lips may provide a clue to the diagnosis. Barium swallow is inadequate to detect early lesions and cannot reliably distinguish HSV infection from other types of infections. Endoscopy shows vesicles and small, discrete, punched-out ("volcano-like") superficial ulcerations with or without a fibrinous exudate. In later stages, a diffuse erosive esophagitis develops from enlargement and coalescence of the ulcers. Mucosal cells from a biopsy sample taken at the edge of an ulcer or from a cytologic smear show ballooning degeneration, ground-glass changes in the nuclei with eosinophilic intranuclear inclusions (Cowdry type A), and giant cell formation on routine stains. Culture for HSV becomes positive within days and is helpful in diagnosis and to identify acyclovir-resistant virus. Acyclovir (400 mg 5 times a day for 14 to 21 days) is

effective. In patients with severe odynophagia, intravenous acyclovir, 5 mg/kg every 8 h for 7 to 14 days is used. Symptoms usually resolve in 1 week, but large ulcerations may take longer to heal. Foscarnet (90 mg/kg intravenously bid for 2 to 4 weeks) is used if resistance to acyclovir occurs.

Varicella-zoster virus (VZV) (Chap. 164) sometimes produces esophagitis in children with chickenpox and adults with herpes zoster. Esophageal VZV also can be the source of disseminated VZV infection without skin involvement. In an immunocompromised host, VZV esophagitis causes vesicles and confluent ulcers and usually resolves spontaneously, but it may cause necrotizing esophagitis in a severely compromised host. On routine histologic examination of mucosal biopsy samples or cytology specimens, VZV is difficult to distinguish from HSV, but the distinction can be made immunohistologically or by culture. Acyclovir reduces the duration of symptoms in VZV esophagitis.

Cytomegalovirus (CMV) infections (Chap. 166) occur only in immunocompromised patients. CMV is usually activated from a latent stage or may be acquired from blood product transfusions. CMV lesions initially appear as serpiginous ulcers in an otherwise normal mucosa. These may coalesce to form giant ulcers, particularly in the distal esophagus.

Patients present with odynophagia, persistent and focal chest pain, hematemesis, nausea, and vomiting. Diagnosis requires endoscopy and biopsies of the ulcer. Mucosal brushings are not useful. Routine histologic examination shows intranuclear and small intracytoplasmic inclusions in large fibroblasts and endothelial cells. Immunohistology with monoclonal antibodies to CMV and in situ hybridization of CMV DNA on centrifugation culture and are useful for early diagnosis. Ganciclovir, 5 mg/kg every 12 h intravenously, is the treatment of choice. Valganciclovir (900 mg bid) is an oral formulation of ganciclovir. Foscarnet (90 mg/kg every 12 h intravenously) is used in resistant cases. Therapy is continued until healing occurs, which may take 2 to 4 weeks.

HIV (Chap. 173) may be associated with a self-limited syndrome of acute esophageal ulceration associated with oral ulcers and a maculopapular skin rash, which occurs at the time of HIV seroconversion. Some patients with advanced disease have deep, persistent esophageal ulcers requiring treatment with oral glucocorticoids or thalidomide. Some ulcers respond to local steroid injection.

Bacterial and Fungal Esophagitis   *Bacterial esophagitis* is unusual, but esophagitis caused by *Lactobacillus* and β-hemolytic streptococci can occur in the immunocompromised host. In patients with profound granulocytopenia and patients with cancer, bacterial esophagitis is often overlooked because it is commonly present with other organisms, including viruses and fungi. In patients with AIDS, infection with *Cryptosporidium* or *Pneumocystis carinii* may cause nonspecific inflammation, and *Mycobacterium tuberculosis* infection may cause deep ulcerations of the distal esophagus. Very rarely, other types of fungi may cause esophagitis.

CANDIDA ESOPHAGITIS

Candida species are normal commensals in the throat but become pathogenic and produce esophagitis in immunodeficiency states. Candida esophagitis can occur without any predisposing factors. Patients may be asymptomatic or complain of odynophagia and dysphagia. Oral thrush or other evidence of mucocutaneous candidiasis may be absent. Rarely, Candida esophagitis is complicated by esophageal bleeding, perforation, and stricture or by systemic invasion. Barium swallow may be normal or show multiple nodular filling defects of various sizes (Fig. 273-2 panel 4). Large nodular defects may resemble grape clusters. Endoscopy shows small, yellow-white raised plaques with surrounding erythema in mild disease. Confluent linear and nodular plaques reflect extensive disease. Diagnosis is made by demonstration of yeast or hyphal forms in plaque smears and exudate stained with periodic acid–Schiff or Gomori silver stains. Histologic examination is often negative. Culture is not useful in diagnosis but may define the species and the drug sensitivities of the yeast; *Candida albicans* is most common (Chap. 187). Empirical therapy with fluconazole for 7 days is appropriate for suspected cases. Oral fluconazole (200 mg on the first day, followed by 100 mg daily) is the preferred treatment. Patients refractory to fluconazole often respond to itraconazole. Patients who respond poorly or cannot swallow oral medications are treated with amphotericin B (10 to 15 mg as an intravenous infusion for 6 h daily to a total dose of 300 to 500 mg) or intravenous fluconazole. Nystatin oral suspension (100,000 units per mL) in doses of 10 to 20 mL every 6 h is effective for oral thrush. In resistant cases, amphotericin lozenges are used for 7 to 10 days followed by nystatin or fluconazole for as long as the host resistance remains low.

OTHER TYPES OF ESOPHAGITIS *Radiation esophagitis* is a common occurrence during radiation treatment for thoracic cancers. The frequency and severity of esophagitis increase with the amount of radiation delivered and may be enhanced by radiosensitizing drugs like doxorubicin, bleomycin, cyclophosphamide, and cisplatin. Dysphagia and odynophagia may last several weeks to several months after therapy. The esophageal mucosa becomes erythematous, edematous, and friable. Superficial erosions coalesce to form larger superficial ulcers. Submucosal fibrosis and degenerative changes in the blood vessels, muscles, and myenteric neurons may occur. The treatment is relief of pain with viscous lidocaine during the acute phase; indomethacin treatment may reduce radiation damage. Esophageal stricture may develop.

Corrosive esophagitis is caused by the ingestion of caustic agents, such as strong alkali or acid. Severe corrosive injury may lead to esophageal perforation, bleeding, and death. Glucocorticoids are not useful in acute corrosive esophagitis. Healing is usually associated with stricture formation. Caustic strictures are usually long and rigid (Fig. 273-2 panel 5) and generally require dilatation with dilators passed over a guidewire through the stricture. *Pill-induced esophagitis* is associated with the ingestion of certain types of pills and occurs most often in bedridden patients. Antibiotics such as doxycycline, tetracycline, oxytetracycline, minocycline, penicillin, and clindamycin account for more than half the cases. Nonsteroidal anti-inflammatory agents such as aspirin, indomethacin, and ibuprofen may cause injury. Other commonly prescribed pills that cause esophageal injury include potassium chloride, ferrous sulfate or succinate, quinidine, alprenolol, theophylline, ascorbic acid, and pinaverium bromide. Bisphosphonates, particularly alendronate and pamidronate, are more common offenders. Pill esophagitis can be prevented by avoiding the offending agents or by having patients take pills in the upright position and wash them down with copious amounts of fluids.

Sclerotherapy for bleeding esophageal varices usually produces transient retrosternal chest pain and dysphagia; esophageal ulcer, stricture, hematoma, or perforation may occur. Variceal banding causes similar complications but less frequently. *Esophagitis* associated with mucocutaneous and systemic diseases is usually associated with blister and bulla formation, epithelial desquamation, and thin, weblike, or dense esophageal strictures. Pemphigus vulgaris and bullous pemphigoid form intraepithelial and subepithelial bullae, respectively, and can be distinguished by specific immunohistology; both are characterized by sloughing of epithelium or the presence of esophageal casts. Glucocorticoid treatment is usually effective. Cicatricial pemphigoid, Stevens-Johnson syndrome, and toxic epidermolysis bullosa can produce esophageal bullous lesions and strictures requiring gentle dilatation. Graft-versus-host disease occurs in patients who have received allogeneic bone marrow transplants and is associated with generalized desquamation and esophageal strictures. Behçet's disease and eosinophilic gastroenteritis may involve the esophagus and may respond to glucocorticoid therapy. An erosive lichen planus also can involve the esophagus. Crohn's disease may cause inflammatory strictures, sinus tracts, filiform polyps, and fistulas in the esophagus.

OTHER ESOPHAGEAL DISORDERS

DIVERTICULA Diverticula are outpouchings of the wall of the esophagus. A *Zenker's diverticulum* appears in the natural zone of weakness in the posterior hypopharyngeal wall (Killian's triangle) and causes halitosis and regurgitation of saliva and food particles consumed several days previously. When it becomes large and filled with food, such a diverticulum can compress the esophagus and cause dysphagia or complete obstruction. Nasogastric intubation and endoscopy should be performed with utmost care in these patients, since they may cause perforation of the diverticulum. A *midesophageal diverticulum* may be caused by traction from old adhesions or by propulsion associated with esophageal motor abnormalities. An *epiphrenic diverticulum* may be associated with achalasia. Small or medium-sized diverticula and midesophageal and epiphrenic diverticula are usually asymptomatic. *Diffuse intramural diverticulosis* of the esophagus is due to dilation of the deep esophageal glands and may lead to chronic candidiasis or to the development of a stricture high up in the esophagus. These patients may present with dysphagia. Symptomatic Zenker's diverticula are treated by cricopharyngeal myotomy with or without diverticulectomy. Large symptomatic esophageal diverticula are removed surgically. When they are associated with motor abnormalities, distal myotomy is performed. Strictures associated with diffuse intramural diverticulosis are treated with rubber dilators.

WEBS AND RINGS Weblike constrictions of the esophagus are usually congenital or inflammatory in origin. Asymptomatic hypopharyngeal webs are demonstrated in <10% of normal individuals. When concentric, they cause intermittent dysphagia to solids. The combination of symptomatic hypopharyngeal webs and iron-deficiency anemia in middle-aged women constitutes *Plummer-Vinson syndrome*. The clinical importance of this syndrome is uncertain. Midesophageal webs are rare. A *lower esophageal mucosal ring* (Schatzki ring) is a thin, weblike constriction located at the squamocolumnar mucosal junction at or near the border of the LES (Fig. 273-2 panel 7). It invariably produces dysphagia when the lumen diameter is <1.3 cm. Dysphagia to solids is the only symptom, and it is usually episodic. Asymptomatic rings may be present in ~10% of normal individuals. A lower esophageal ring is one of the common causes of dysphagia. Symptomatic webs and mucosal lower esophageal rings are easily treated by dilatation. A *lower esophageal muscular ring* (contractile ring) is located proximal to the site of mucosal rings and may represent an abnormal uppermost segment of the LES. These rings can be recognized by the fact that they are not constant in size and shape. They also may cause dysphagia and should be differentiated from peptic strictures, achalasia, and lower esophageal mucosal rings. Muscular rings do not respond well to dilatation.

HIATAL HERNIA A *hiatal hernia* is a herniation of part of the stomach into the thoracic cavity through the esophageal hiatus in the diaphragm. A *sliding hiatal hernia* is one in which the gastroesophageal junction and fundus of the stomach slide upward. A sliding hernia may result from weakening of the anchors of the gastroesophageal junction to the diaphragm, from longitudinal contraction of the esophagus, or from increased intra-abdominal pressure. Small sliding hernias can be demonstrated commonly during barium studies if intra-abdominal pressure is increased. Incidence increases with age; in individuals in the sixth decade of life, the prevalence of such hernias is ~60%. Small sliding hiatal hernias alone probably produce no symptoms but can contribute to reflux esophagitis. A *paraesophageal hernia* is one in which the esophagogastric junction remains fixed in its normal location and a pouch of stomach is herniated beside the gastroesophageal junction through the esophageal hiatus. A paraesophageal or mixed paraesophageal and sliding hernia may become incarcerated and strangulate, leading to acute chest pain, dysphagia, and a mediastinal mass and requiring surgery. A herniated gastric pouch may cause dysphagia, develop gastritis, or ulcerate, causing chronic blood loss. Large paraesophageal hernias should be surgically repaired.

MECHANICAL TRAUMA *Esophageal rupture* may be caused by (1) iatrogenic damage from instrumentation of the esophagus or external trauma, (2) increased intraesophageal pressure associated with forceful vomiting or retching (*spontaneous rupture* or *Boerhaave's syndrome*), or (3) diseases of the esophagus such as corrosive esophagitis, esophageal ulcer, and neoplasm. The site of perforation depends on the cause. Instrumental perforation usually occurs in the pharynx or lower esophagus, just above the diaphragm in the posterolateral wall. Esophageal perforation causes severe retrosternal chest pain, which may be worsened by swallowing and breathing. Free air enters the mediastinum and spreads to neighboring structures, causing palpable subcutaneous emphysema in the neck, mediastinal crackling sounds on auscultation, and pneumothorax. With time, secondary infection supervenes, and mediastinal abscess may develop. Esophageal perforation associated with vomiting usually deposits gastric contents in the mediastinum and causes severe mediastinal complications. By contrast, instrumental perforation may be clinically mild and free of severe complications. Spontaneous rupture of the esophagus may mimic myocardial infarction, pancreatitis, or rupture of an abdominal viscus. Symptoms of chest pain may be mild, particularly in the elderly. Mediastinal emphysema may develop late. An x-ray of the chest shows abnormalities in most patients, but computed tomography (CT) of the chest is more sensitive in detecting mediastinal air. Fluid from pleural effusions may have a high content of (salivary) amylase. The diagnosis is confirmed by swallow of radiopaque contrast material. Gastrografin is used initially, and if no leak is found, a small amount of thin barium is used to confirm the diagnosis. Treatment includes esophageal and gastric suction and parenteral broad-spectrum antibiotics. Surgical drainage and repair of the laceration should be performed as soon as possible. In patients with terminal carcinoma, surgical repair may not be feasible, and patients with minor instrumental perforation can be treated conservatively. Extensive corrosive damage may require esophageal diversion and excision of the damaged portion.

Mucosal Tear (Mallory-Weiss Syndrome)   This tear is usually caused by vomiting, retching, or vigorous coughing. The tear usually involves the gastric mucosa near the squamocolumnar mucosal junction. Patients present with upper gastrointestinal bleeding, which may be severe. In most patients bleeding ceases spontaneously; continued bleeding may respond to vasopressin therapy or angiographic embolization. Surgery is rarely needed.

Intramural Hematoma   Emetogenic injury, particularly in patients with bleeding abnormalities, can cause bleeding between the mucosal and muscle layers of the esophagus. The patients develop sudden dysphagia. The diagnosis is made by barium swallow and CT. Resolution is usually spontaneous.

FOREIGN BODIES   Foreign bodies may lodge in the cervical esophagus just beyond the UES, near the aortic arch, or above the LES. Impaction of a bolus of food, particularly a piece of meat or bread, may occur when the esophageal lumen is narrowed due to stricture, carcinoma, or a lower esophageal ring. Acute impaction causes a complete inability to swallow and severe chest pain. Both foreign bodies and food boluses may be removed endoscopically. Use of a meat tenderizer to facilitate passage of a meat bolus is discouraged because of potential esophageal perforation and aspiration pneumonia.

FURTHER READING

DEMEESTER SR et al: Barrett's esophagus. Curr Probl Surg 38:558, 2001

HIRANO I: Pathophysiology of achalasia. Curr Gastroenterol Rep 1:198, 1999

ORLANDO RC: Pathogenesis of gastroesophageal reflux disease. Gastroenterol Clin North Am 31:S35, 2002

PATERSON WG: Extraesophageal manifestations of reflux disease: Myths and reality. Chest Surg Clin N Am 11:523, 2001

RAMAKRISHNAN A, KATZ PO: Pharmacologic management of gastroesophageal reflux disease. Curr Gastroenterol Rep 4:218, 2002

SPECHLER SJ: Barrett's esophagus and esophageal adenocarcinoma: Pathogenesis, diagnosis and therapy. Med Clin North Am 86:1423, 2002

————: AGA technical review on treatment of patients with dysphagia caused by benign disorders of the distal esophagus. Gastroenterology 117:233, 1999

WARING JP: Surgical and endoscopic treatment of gastroesophageal reflux disease. Gastroenterol Clin North Am 31:S89, 2002

274 PEPTIC ULCER DISEASE AND RELATED DISORDERS
John Del Valle

PEPTIC ULCER DISEASE

Burning epigastric pain exacerbated by fasting and improved with meals is a symptom complex associated with peptic ulcer disease (PUD). An *ulcer* is defined as disruption of the mucosal integrity of the stomach and/or duodenum leading to a local defect or excavation due to active inflammation. Ulcers occur within the stomach and/or duodenum and are often chronic in nature. Acid peptic disorders are very common in the United States, with 4 million individuals (new cases and recurrences) affected per year. Lifetime prevalence of PUD in the United States is ~12% in men and 10% in women. Moreover, an estimated 15,000 deaths per year occur as a consequence of complicated PUD. The financial impact of these common disorders has been substantial, with an estimated burden on direct and indirect health care costs of ~$10 billion per year in the United States.

GASTRIC PHYSIOLOGY   Despite the constant attack on the gastroduodenal mucosa by a host of noxious agents (acid, pepsin, bile acids, pancreatic enzymes, drugs, and bacteria), integrity is maintained by an intricate system that provides mucosal defense and repair.

Gastric Anatomy   The gastric epithelial lining consists of rugae that contain microscopic gastric pits, each branching into four or five gastric glands made up of highly specialized epithelial cells. The makeup of gastric glands varies with their anatomic location. Glands within the gastric cardia comprise <5% of the gastric gland area and contain mucous and endocrine cells. The majority of gastric glands (75%) are found within the oxyntic mucosa and contain mucous neck, parietal, chief, endocrine, and enterochromaffin cells (Fig. 274-1). Pyloric glands contain mucous and endocrine cells (including gastrin cells) and are found in the antrum.

The parietal cell, also known as the oxyntic cell, is usually found in the neck, or isthmus, or the oxyntic gland. The resting, or unstimulated, parietal cell has prominent cytoplasmic tubulovesicles and intracellular canaliculi containing short microvilli along its apical surface (Fig. 274-2). H^+, K^+-ATPase is expressed in the tubulovesicle membrane; upon cell stimulation, this membrane, along with apical membranes, transforms into a dense network of apical intracellular canaliculi containing long microvilli. Acid secretion, a process requiring high energy, occurs at the apical canalicular surface. Numerous mitochondria (30 to 40% of total cell volume) generate the energy required for secretion.

Gastroduodenal Mucosal Defense   The gastric epithelium is under a constant assault by a series of endogenous noxious factors including HCl, pepsinogen/pepsin, and bile salts. In addition, a steady flow of exogenous substances such as medications, alcohol, and bacteria encounter the gastric mucosa. A highly intricate biologic system is in place to provide defense from mucosal injury and to repair any injury that may occur.

The mucosal defense system can be envisioned as a three-level barrier, composed of preepithelial, epithelial, and subepithelial elements (Fig. 274-3). The first line of defense is a mucus-bicarbonate

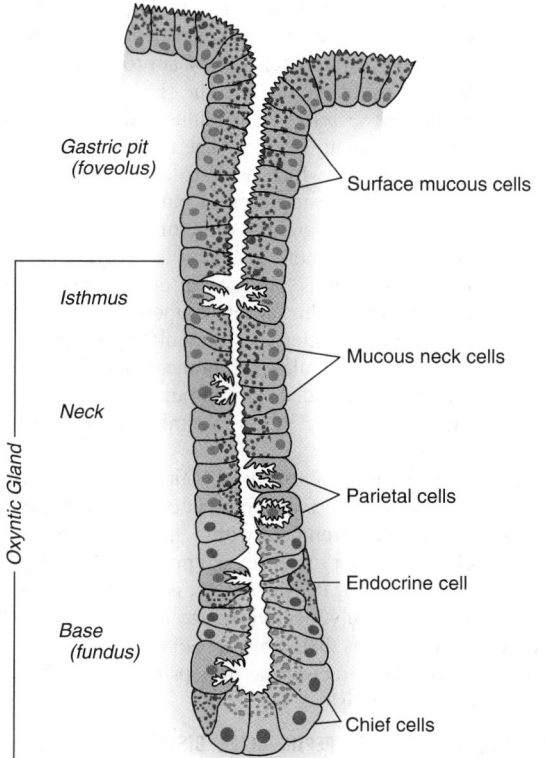

FIGURE 274-1 Diagramatic representation of the oxyntic gastric gland. *(Adapted from S Ito, RJ Winchester: Cell Biol 16:541, 1963.)*

layer, which serves as a physicochemical barrier to multiple molecules including hydrogen ions. Mucus is secreted in a regulated fashion by gastroduodenal surface epithelial cells. It consists primarily of water (95%) and a mixture of lipids and glycoproteins. Mucin is the constituent glycoprotein that, in combination with phospholipids (also secreted by gastric mucous cells), forms a hydrophobic surface with fatty acids that extend into the lumen from the cell membrane. The mucous gel functions as a nonstirred water layer impeding diffusion of ions and molecules such as pepsin. Bicarbonate, secreted by surface epithelial cells of the gastroduodenal mucosa into the mucous gel, forms a pH gradient ranging from 1 to 2 at the gastric luminal surface and reaching 6 to 7 along the epithelial cell surface. Bicarbonate secretion is stimulated by calcium, prostaglandins, cholinergic input, and luminal acidification.

Surface epithelial cells provide the next line of defense through several factors, including mucus production, epithelial cell ionic transporters that maintain intracellular pH and bicarbonate production, and intracellular tight junctions. If the preepithelial barrier were breached,

gastric epithelial cells bordering a site of injury can migrate to restore a damaged region (*restitution*). This process occurs independent of cell division and requires uninterrupted blood flow and an alkaline pH in the surrounding environment. Several growth factors including epidermal growth factor (EGF), transforming growth factor (TGF) α, and basic fibroblast growth factor (FGF) modulate the process of restitution. Larger defects that are not effectively repaired by restitution require cell proliferation. Epithelial cell regeneration is regulated by prostaglandins and growth factors such as EGF and TGF-α. In tandem with epithelial cell renewal, formation of new vessels (*angiogenesis*) within the injured microvascular bed occurs. Both FGF and vascular endothelial growth factor (VEGF) are important in regulating angiogenesis in the gastric mucosa.

An elaborate microvascular system within the gastric submucosal layer is the key component of the subepithelial defense/repair system. A rich submucosal circulatory bed provides HCO_3^-, which neutralizes the acid generated by parietal cell secretion of HCl. Moreover, this microcirculatory bed provides an adequate supply of micronutrients and oxygen while removing toxic metabolic by-products.

Prostaglandins play a central role in gastric epithelial defense/repair (Fig. 274-4). The gastric mucosa contains abundant levels of prostaglandins. These metabolites of arachidonic acid regulate the release of mucosal bicarbonate and mucus, inhibit parietal cell secretion, and are important in maintaining mucosal blood flow and epithelial cell restitution. Prostaglandins are derived from esterified arachidonic acid, which is formed from phospholipids (cell membrane) by the action of phospholipase A_2. A key enzyme that controls the rate-limiting step in prostaglandin synthesis is cyclooxygenase (COX), which is present in two isoforms (COX-1, COX-2), each having distinct characteristics regarding structure, tissue distribution, and expression. COX-1 is expressed in a host of tissues including the stomach, platelets, kidneys, and endothelial cells. This isoform is expressed in a constitutive manner and plays an important role in maintaining the integrity of renal function, platelet aggregation, and gastrointestinal mucosal integrity. In contrast, the expression of COX-2 is inducible by inflammatory stimuli, and it is expressed in macrophages, leukocytes, fibroblasts, and synovial cells. The beneficial effects of nonsteroidal anti-inflammatory drugs (NSAIDs) on tissue inflammation are due to inhibition of COX-2; the toxicity of these drugs (e.g., gastrointestinal mucosal ulceration and renal dysfunction) is related to inhibition of the COX-1 isoform. The highly COX-2-selective NSAIDs have the potential to provide the beneficial effect of decreasing tissue inflammation while minimizing toxicity in the gastrointestinal tract.

Physiology of Gastric Secretion Hydrochloric acid and pepsinogen are the two principal gastric secretory products capable of inducing mucosal injury. Acid secretion should be viewed as occurring under basal and stimulated conditions. Basal acid production occurs in a circadian pattern, with highest levels occurring during the night and lowest levels during the morning hours. Cholinergic input via the vagus nerve and histaminergic input from local gastric sources are the principal contributors to basal acid secretion. Stimulated gastric acid secretion occurs primarily in three phases based on the site where the signal originates (cephalic, gastric, and intestinal). Sight, smell, and taste of food are the components of the cephalic phase, which stimulates gastric secretion via the vagus nerve. The gastric phase is activated once food enters the stomach. This component of secretion is driven by nutrients (amino acids and amines) that directly stimulate the G cell to release gastrin, which in turn activates the parietal cell via direct and indirect mechanisms. Distention of the stomach wall also leads to gastrin release and acid production. The last phase of gastric acid secretion is initiated as food enters the intestine and is mediated by luminal distention and nutrient assimilation. A series of pathways that inhibit gastric acid production are also set into motion during these phases. The gastrointestinal hormone somatostatin is released from endocrine cells found in the gastric mucosa (D cells) in response to HCl. Somatostatin can inhibit acid production by both direct (parietal

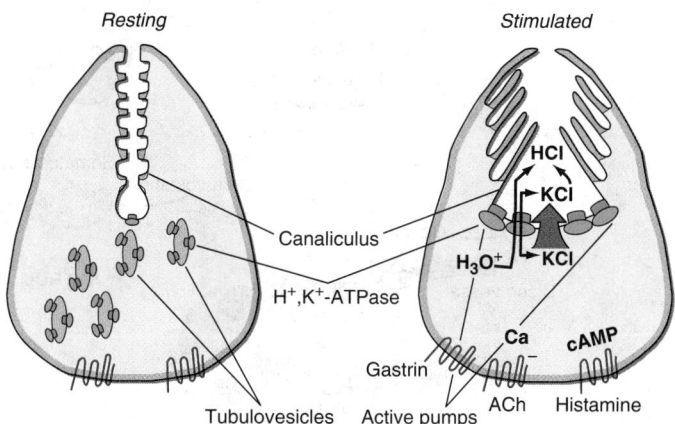

FIGURE 274-2 Gastric parietal cell undergoing transformation after secretagogue-mediated stimulation. *(Adapted from SJ Hersey, G Sachs: Physiol Rev 75:155, 1995.)*

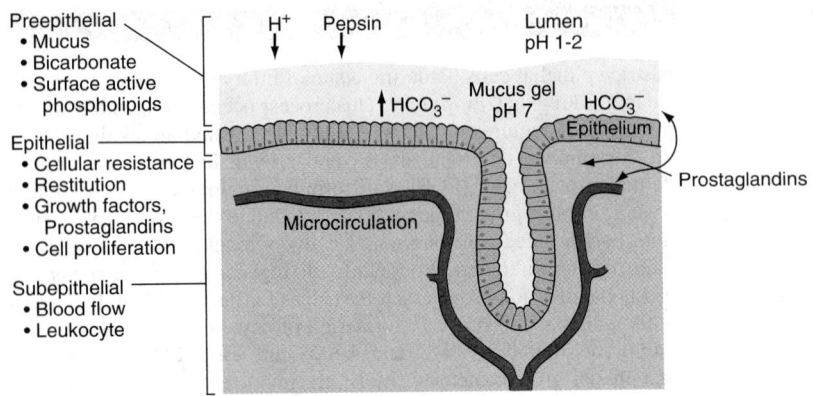

FIGURE 274-3 Components involved in providing gastroduodenal mucosal defense and repair.

cell) and indirect mechanisms [decreased histamine release from enterochromaffin-like (ECL) cells and gastrin release from G cells. Additional neural (central and peripheral) and hormonal (secretin, cholecystokinin) factors play a role in counterbalancing acid secretion. Under physiologic circumstances, these phases are occurring simultaneously.

The acid-secreting parietal cell is located in the oxyntic gland, adjacent to other cellular elements (ECL cell, D cell) important in the gastric secretory process (Fig. 274-5). This unique cell also secretes intrinsic factor (IF). The parietal cell expresses receptors for several stimulants of acid secretion including histamine (H_2), gastrin (cholecystokinin B/gastrin receptor), and acetylcholine (muscarinic, M_3). Each of these are G protein–linked, seven transmembrane–spanning receptors. Binding of histamine to the H_2 receptor leads to activation of adenylate cyclase and an increase in cyclic AMP. Activation of the gastrin and muscarinic receptors results in activation of the protein kinase C/phosphoinositide signaling pathway. Each of these signaling pathways in turn regulates a series of downstream kinase cascades, which control the acid-secreting pump, H^+, K^+-ATPase. The discovery that different ligands and their corresponding receptors lead to activation of different signaling pathways explains the potentiation of acid secretion that occurs when histamine and gastrin or acetylcholine are combined. More importantly, this observation explains why blocking one receptor type (H_2) decreases acid secretion stimulated by agents that activate a different pathway (gastrin, acetylcholine). Parietal cells also express receptors for ligands that inhibit acid production (prostaglandins, somatostatin, and EGF).

The enzyme H^+, K^+-ATPase is responsible for generating the large concentration of H^+. It is a membrane-bound protein that consists of two subunits, α and β. The active catalytic site is found within the α

subunit; the function of the β subunit is unclear. This enzyme uses the chemical energy of ATP to transfer H^+ ions from parietal cell cytoplasm to the secretory canaliculi in exchange for K^+. The H^+, K^+-ATPase is located within the secretory canaliculus and in nonsecretory cytoplasmic tubulovesicles. The tubulovesicles are impermeable to K^+, which leads to an inactive pump in this location. The distribution of pumps between the nonsecretory vesicles and the secretory canaliculus varies according to parietal cell activity (Fig. 274-2). Under resting conditions, only 5% of pumps are within the secretory canaliculus, whereas upon parietal cell stimulation, tubulovesicles are immediately transferred to the secretory canalicular membrane, where 60 to 70% of the pumps are activated. Proton pumps are recycled back to the inactive state in cytoplasmic vesicles once parietal cell activation ceases.

The chief cell, found primarily in the gastric fundus, synthesizes and secretes pepsinogen, the inactive precursor of the proteolytic enzyme pepsin. The acid environment within the stomach leads to cleavage of the inactive precursor to pepsin and provides the low pH (<2.0) required for pepsin activity. Pepsin activity is significantly diminished at a pH of 4 and irreversibly inactivated and denatured at a pH of ≥ 7. Many of the secretagogues that stimulate acid secretion also stimulate pepsinogen release. The precise role of pepsin in the pathogenesis of PUD remains to be established.

PATHOPHYSIOLOGIC BASIS OF PEPTIC ULCER DISEASE PUD encompasses both gastric and duodenal ulcers. Ulcers are defined as a break in the mucosal surface >5 mm in size, with depth to the submucosa. Duodenal ulcers (DUs) and gastric ulcers (GUs); share many common features in terms of pathogenesis, diagnosis, and treatment, but several factors distinguish them from one another.

Epidemiology ■ *DUODENAL ULCERS* DUs are estimated to occur in 6 to 15% of the western population. The incidence of DUs declined steadily from 1960 to 1980 and has remained stable since then. The death rates, need for surgery, and physician visits have decreased by $>50\%$ over the past 30 years. The reason for the reduction in the frequency of DUs is likely related to the decreasing frequency of *Helicobacter pylori*. Before the discovery of *H. pylori*, the natural history of DUs was typified by frequent recurrences after initial therapy. Eradication of *H. pylori* has greatly reduced these recurrence rates.

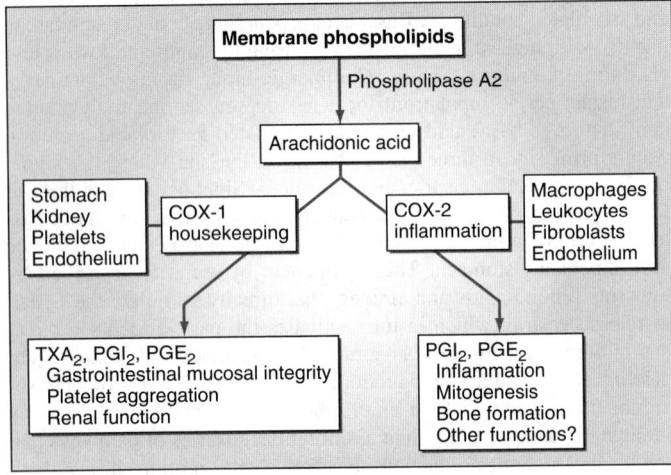

FIGURE 274-4 Schematic representation of the steps involved in synthesis of prostaglandin E_2 (PGE_2) and prostacyclin (PGI_2). Characteristics and distribution of the cyclooxgenase (COX) enzymes 1 and 2 are also shown. TXA_2, thromboxane A_2.

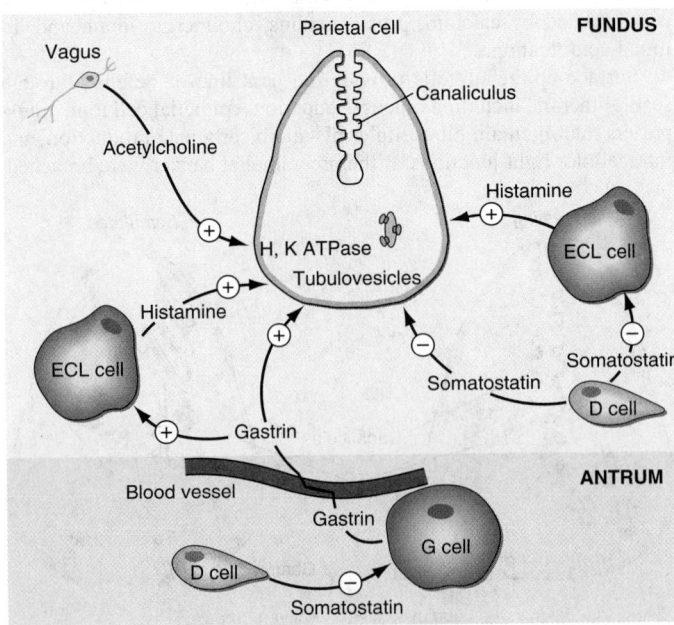

FIGURE 274-5 Regulation of gastric acid secretion at the cellular level. ECL cell, enterochromaffin-like cell.

GASTRIC ULCERS GUs tend to occur later in life than duodenal lesions, with a peak incidence reported in the sixth decade. More than half of GUs occur in males and are less common than DUs, perhaps due to the higher likelihood of GUs being silent and presenting only after a complication develops. Autopsy studies suggest a similar incidence of DUs and GUs.

Pathology ■ *DUODENAL ULCERS* DUs occur most often in the first portion of duodenum (>95%), with ~90% located within 3 cm of the pylorus. They are usually ≤1 cm in diameter but can occasionally reach 3 to 6 cm (giant ulcer). Ulcers are sharply demarcated, with depth at times reaching the muscularis propria. The base of the ulcer often consists of a zone of eosinophilic necrosis with surrounding fibrosis. Malignant duodenal ulcers are extremely rare.

GASTRIC ULCERS In contrast to DUs, GUs can represent a malignancy. Benign GUs are most often found distal to the junction between the antrum and the acid secretory mucosa. This junction is variable, but in general the antral mucosa extends about two-thirds of the distance of the lesser curvature and one-third the way up the greater curvature. Benign GUs are quite rare in the gastric fundus and are histologically similar to DUs. Benign GUs associated with *H. pylori* are associated with antral gastritis. In contrast, NSAID-related GUs are not accompanied by chronic active gastritis but may instead have evidence of a chemical gastropathy.

Pathophysiology It is now clear that *H. pylori* and NSAID-induced injury account for the majority of DUs. Gastric acid contributes to mucosal injury but does not play a primary role.

DUODENAL ULCERS Many acid secretory abnormalities have been described in DU patients. Of these, average basal and nocturnal gastric acid secretion appear to be increased in DU patients as compared to control; however, the level of overlap between DU patients and control subjects is substantial. The reason for this altered secretory process is unclear, but *H. pylori* infection may contribute to this finding. Accelerated gastric emptying of liquids has been noted in some DU patients but is not consistently observed; its role in DU formation, if any, is unclear. Bicarbonate secretion is significantly decreased in the duodenal bulb of patients with an active DU as compared to control subjects. *H. pylori* infection may also play a role in this process.

GASTRIC ULCERS As in DUs, the majority of GUs can be attributed to either *H. pylori* or NSAID-induced mucosal damage. GUs that occur in the prepyloric area or those in the body associated with a DU or a duodenal scar are similar in pathogenesis to DUs. Gastric acid output (basal and stimulated) tends to be normal or decreased in GU patients. When GUs develop in the presence of minimal acid levels, impairment of mucosal defense factors may be present.

Abnormalities in resting and stimulated pyloric sphincter pressure with a concomitant increase in duodenal gastric reflux have been implicated in some GU patients. Although bile acids, lysolecithin, and pancreatic enzymes may injure gastric mucosa, a definite role for these in GU pathogenesis has not been established. Delayed gastric emptying of solids has been described in GU patients but has not been reported consistently. The observation that patients who have undergone disruption of the normal pyloric barrier (pyloroplasty, gastroenterostomy) often have superficial gastritis without frank ulceration decreases enthusiasm for duodenal gastric reflux as an explanation for GU pathogenesis.

H. PYLORI AND ACID PEPTIC DISORDERS Gastric infection with the bacterium *H. pylori* accounts for the majority of PUD. This organism also plays a role in the development of gastric mucosal-associated lymphoid tissue (MALT) lymphoma and gastric adenocarcinoma. Although the entire genome of *H. pylori* has been sequenced, it is still not clear how this organism, which is in the stomach, causes ulceration in the duodenum, or whether its eradication will lead to a decrease in gastric cancer.

The Bacterium The bacterium, initially named *Campylobacter pyloridis*, is a gram-negative microaerophilic rod found most commonly in the deeper portions of the mucous gel coating the gastric mucosa or between the mucous layer and the gastric epithelium. It may attach to gastric epithelium but under normal circumstances does not appear to invade cells. It is strategically designed to live within the aggressive environment of the stomach. It is S-shaped (~0.5 × 3 μm in size) and contains multiple sheathed flagella. Initially, *H. pylori* resides in the antrum but, over time, migrates toward the more proximal segments of the stomach. The organism is capable of transforming into a coccoid form, which represents a dormant state that may facilitate survival in adverse conditions. The genome of *H. pylori* has been sequenced (1.65 million base pairs) and encodes ~1500 proteins. Amongst this multitude of proteins there are factors that are essential determinants of *H. pylori*–mediated pathogenesis and colonization such as the outer membrane protein (Hop proteins), urease, and the vacuolating cytotoxin (Vac A). Moreover, the majority of *H. pylori* strains contain a genomic fragment, which encodes the cag pathogenicity island (cag-PAI). Several of the genes that make up cag-PAI encode components of a type IV secretion island that translocates Cag A into host cells. Once in the cell, Cag A activates a series of cellular events important in cell growth and cytokine production. The first step in infection by *H. pylori* is dependent on the bacteria's motility and its ability to produce urease. Urease produces ammonia from urea, an essential step in alkalinizing the surrounding pH. Additional bacterial factors include catalase, lipase, adhesins, platelet-activating factor, and pic B (induces cytokines). Multiple strains of *H. pylori* exist and are characterized by their ability to express several of these factors (Cag A, Vac A, etc.). It is possible that the different diseases related to *H. pylori* infection can be attributed to different strains of the organism with distinct pathogenic features.

Epidemiology The prevalence of *H. pylori* varies throughout the world and depends to a great extent on the overall standard of living in the region. In developing parts of the world, 80% of the population may be infected by the age of 20, whereas the prevalence is 20 to 50% in industrialized countries. In contrast, in the United States, this organism is rare in childhood. The overall prevalence of *H. pylori* in the United States is ~30%, with individuals born before 1950 having a higher rate of infection than those born later. About 10% of Americans <30 are colonized with the bacteria. The rate of infection with *H. pylori* in industrialized countries has decreased substantially in recent decades. The steady increase in the prevalence of *H. pylori* noted with increasing age is due primarily to a cohort effect, reflecting higher transmission during a period in which the earlier cohorts were children. It has been calculated, through mathematical models, that improved sanitation during the latter half of the nineteenth century dramatically decreased transmission of *H. pylori*. Moreover, with the present rate of intervention, it is predicted that the organism will be ultimately eliminated from the United States. Two factors that predispose to higher colonization rates include poor socioeconomic status and less education. These factors, not race, are responsible for the rate of *H. pylori* infection in blacks and Hispanic Americans being double the rate seen in whites of comparable age. Other risk factors for *H. pylori* infection are (1) birth or residence in a developing country, (2) domestic crowding, (3) unsanitary living conditions, (4) unclean food or water, and (5) exposure to gastric contents of an infected individual.

Transmission of *H. pylori* occurs from person to person, following an oral-oral or fecal-oral route. The risk of *H. pylori* infection is declining in developing countries. The rate of infection in the United States has fallen by >50% when compared to 30 years ago.

Pathophysiology *H. pylori* infection is virtually always associated with a chronic active gastritis, but only 10 to 15% of infected individuals develop frank peptic ulceration. The basis for this difference is unknown. Initial studies suggested that >90% of all DUs were associated with *H. pylori*, but *H. pylori* is present in only 30 to 60% of individuals with GUs and 70% of patients with DUs. The pathophysiology of ulcers not associated with *H. pylori* or NSAID ingestion [or the rare Zollinger-Ellison syndrome (ZES)] is unclear.

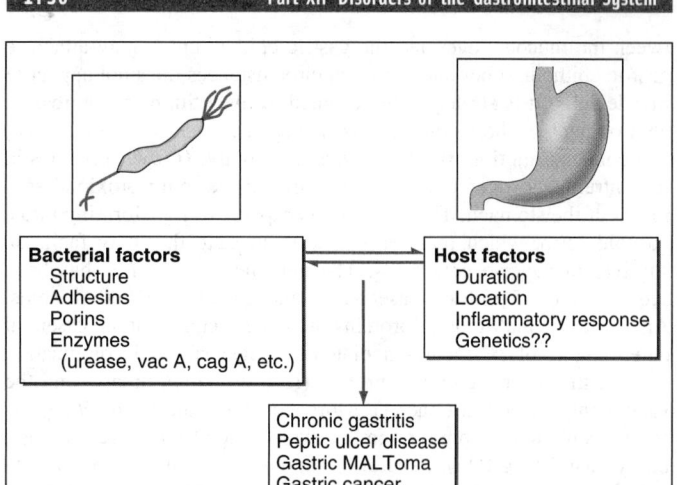

FIGURE 274-6 Outline of the bacterial and host factors important in determining *H. pylori*–induced gastrointestinal disease. MALT, mucosal-associated lymphoid tissue.

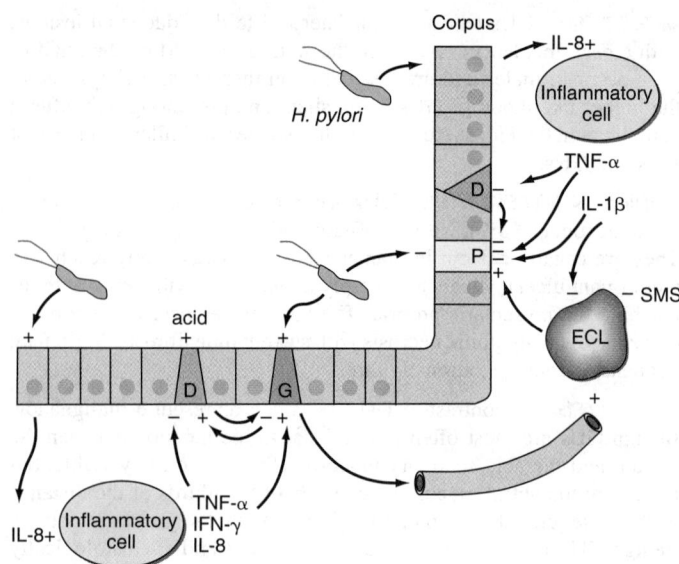

FIGURE 274-7 Summary of potential mechanisms by which *H. pylori* may lead to gastric secretory abnormalities. D, somatostatin cell; ECL, enterochromaffin-like; G, G cell; IFN, interferon; IL, interleukin; P, parietal cell; SMS, somatostatin; TNF, tumor necrosis factor. *(Adapted from J Calam et al: Gastroenterology 113:543, 1997.)*

The particular end result of *H. pylori* infection (gastritis, PUD, gastric MALT lymphoma, gastric cancer) is determined by a complex interplay between bacterial and host factors (Fig. 274-6).

1. *Bacterial factors*: *H. pylori* is able to facilitate gastric residence, induce mucosal injury, and avoid host defense. Different strains of *H. pylori* produce different virulence factors. A specific region of the bacterial genome, the pathogenicity island, encodes the virulence factors Cag A and pic B. Vac A also contributes to pathogenicity, though it is not encoded within the pathogenicity island. These virulence factors, in conjunction with additional bacterial constituents, can cause mucosal damage. Urease, which allows the bacteria to reside in the acidic stomach, generates NH_3, which can damage epithelial cells. The bacteria produce surface factors that are chemotactic for neutrophils and monocytes, which in turn contribute to epithelial cell injury (see below). *H. pylori* makes proteases and phospholipases that break down the glycoprotein lipid complex of the mucous gel, thus reducing the efficacy of this first line of mucosal defense. *H. pylori* expresses adhesins, which facilitate attachment of the bacteria to gastric epithelial cells. Although lipopolysaccharide (LPS) of gram-negative bacteria often plays an important role in the infection, *H. pylori* LPS has low immunologic activity compared to that of other organisms. It may promote a smoldering chronic inflammation.

2. *Host factors*: The inflammatory response to *H. pylori* includes recruitment of neutrophils, lymphocytes (T and B), macrophages, and plasma cells. The pathogen leads to local injury by binding to class II MHC molecules expressed on gastric epithelial cells leading to cell death (*apoptosis*). Moreover, bacterial strains that encode cag-PAI can introduce Cag A into the host cells, leading to further cell injury and activation of cellular pathways involved in cytokine production. Elevated concentrations of multiple cytokines are found in the gastric epithelium of *H. pylori*–infected individuals, including interleukin (IL) $1\alpha/\beta$, IL-2, IL-6, IL-8, tumor necrosis factor (TNF) α and interferon (IFN) γ. *H. pylori* infection also leads to both a mucosal and systemic humoral response, which does not lead to eradication of the bacteria but further compounds epithelial cell injury. Additional mechanisms by which *H. pylori* may cause epithelial cell injury include: activated neutrophil-mediated production of reactive oxygen or nitrogen species and enhanced epithelial cell turnover and apoptosis related to interaction with T cells (T helper 1, or T_H1, cells) and interferon-γ.

The reason for *H. pylori*–mediated duodenal ulceration remains unclear. One potential explanation is that gastric metaplasia in the duodenum of DU patients permits *H. pylori* to bind to it and produce local injury secondary to the host response. Another hypothesis is that *H. pylori* antral infection could lead to increased acid production, in-creased duodenal acid, and mucosal injury. Basal and stimulated [meal, gastrin-releasing peptide (GRP)] gastrin release are increased in *H. pylori*–infected individuals, and somatostatin-secreting D cells may be decreased. *H. pylori* infection might induce increased acid secretion through both direct and indirect actions of *H. pylori* and proinflammatory cytokines (IL-8, TNF, and IL-1) on G, D, and parietal cells (Fig. 274-7). *H. pylori* infection has also been associated with decreased duodenal mucosal bicarbonate production. Data supporting and contradicting each of these interesting theories have been demonstrated. Thus, the mechanism by which *H. pylori* infection of the stomach leads to duodenal ulceration remains to be established.

In summary, the final effect of *H. pylori* on the gastrointestinal tract is variable and determined by microbial and host factors. The type and distribution of gastritis correlate with the ultimate gastric and duodenal pathology observed. Specifically, the presence of antral-predominant gastritis is associated with DU formation; gastritis involving primarily the corpus predisposes to the development of GUs, gastric atrophy, and ultimately gastric carcinoma (Figure 274-8).

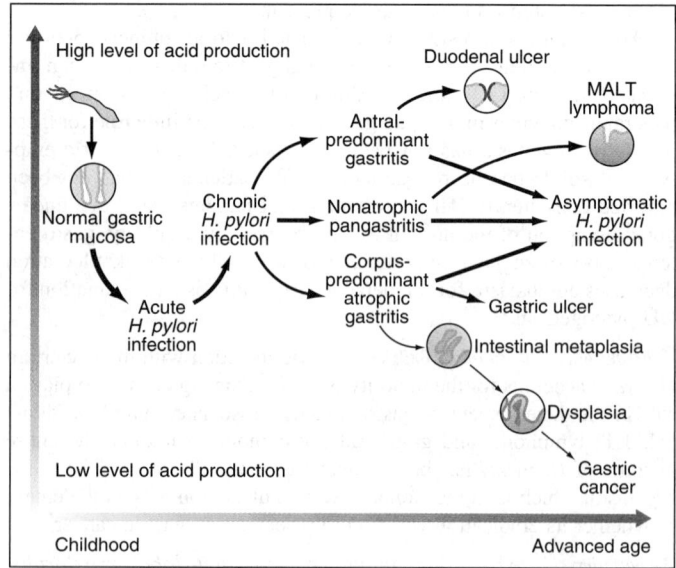

FIGURE 274-8 Natural history of *H. pylori* infection. *(Used with permission from Suerbaum and Michetti.)*

NSAIDS-INDUCED DISEASE ■ *Epidemiology* NSAIDs represent one of the most commonly used medications in the United States. More than 30 billion over-the-counter tablets and 70 million prescriptions are sold yearly in the United States alone. In fact, after the introduction of COX-2 inhibitors in the year 2000, the number of prescriptions written for NSAIDs was >111 million at a cost of $4.8 billion. The spectrum of NSAID-induced morbidity ranges from nausea and dyspepsia (prevalence reported as high as 50 to 60%) to a serious gastrointestinal complication such as frank peptic ulceration (3 to 4%) complicated by bleeding or perforation in as many as 1.5% of users per year. About 20,000 patients die each year from serious gastrointestinal complications from NSAIDs. Unfortunately, dyspeptic symptoms do not correlate with NSAID-induced pathology. Over 80% of patients with serious NSAID-related complications did not have preceding dyspepsia. In view of the lack of warning signs, it is important to identify patients who are at increased risk for morbidity and mortality related to NSAID usage. Even 75 mg/d of aspirin may lead to serious gastrointestinal ulceration, thus no dose of NSAID is completely safe. Established risk factors include advanced age, history of ulcer, concomitant use of glucocorticoids, high dose NSAIDs, multiple NSAIDs, concomitant use of anticoagulants, and serious or multisystem disease. Possible risk factors include concomitant infection with *H. pylori*, cigarette smoking, and alcohol consumption.

Pathophysiology Prostaglandins play a critical role in maintaining gastroduodenal mucosal integrity and repair. It therefore follows that interruption of prostaglandin synthesis can impair mucosal defense and repair, thus facilitating mucosal injury via a systemic mechanism. A summary of the pathogenetic pathways by which systemically administered NSAIDs may lead to mucosal injury is shown in Fig. 274-9.

Injury to the mucosa also occurs as a result of the topical encounter with NSAIDs. Aspirin and many NSAIDs are weak acids that remain in a nonionized lipophilic form when found within the acid environment of the stomach. Under these conditions, NSAIDs migrate across lipid membranes of epithelial cells, leading to cell injury once trapped intracellularly in an ionized form. Topical NSAIDs can also alter the surface mucous layer, permitting back diffusion of H⁺ and pepsin, leading to further epithelial cell damage. Moreover, enteric-coated or buffered preparations are also associated with risk of peptic ulceration.

MISCELLANEOUS PATHOGENETIC FACTORS IN ACID PEPTIC DISEASE Cigarette smoking has been implicated in the pathogenesis of PUD. Not only have smokers been found to have ulcers more frequently than do nonsmokers, but smoking appears to decrease healing rates, impair response to therapy, and increase ulcer-related complications such as perforation. The mechanism responsible for increased ulcer diathesis in smokers is unknown. Theories have included altered gastric emptying, decreased proximal duodenal bicarbonate production, increased risk for

H. pylori infection, and cigarette-induced generation of noxious mucosal free radicals. Acid secretion is not abnormal in smokers. Despite these interesting theories, a unifying mechanism for cigarette-induced peptic ulcer diathesis has not been established.

Genetic predisposition has also been considered to play a role in ulcer development. First-degree relatives of DU patients are three times as likely to develop an ulcer; however, the potential role of *H. pylori* infection in contacts is a major consideration. Increased frequency of blood group O and of the nonsecretor status have also been implicated as genetic risk factors for peptic diathesis. However, *H. pylori* preferentially binds to group O antigens. Therefore, the role of genetic predisposition in common PUD has not been established.

Psychological stress has been thought to contribute to PUD, but studies examining the role of psychological factors in its pathogenesis have generated conflicting results. Although PUD is associated with certain personality traits (neuroticism), these same traits are also present in individuals with nonulcer dyspepsia (NUD) and other functional and organic disorders. Although more work in this area is needed, no typical PUD personality has been found.

Diet has also been thought to play a role in peptic diseases. Certain foods can cause dyspepsia, but no convincing studies indicate an association between ulcer formation and a specific diet. This is also true for beverages containing alcohol and caffeine. Specific chronic disorders have been associated with PUD. Those with a strong association are (1) systemic mastocytosis, (2) chronic pulmonary disease, (3) chronic renal failure, (4) cirrhosis, (5) nephrolithiasis, and (6) α_1-antitrypsin deficiency. Those with a possible association are (1) hyperparathyroidism, (2) coronary artery disease, (3) polycythemia vera, and (4) chronic pancreatitis.

Multiple factors play a role in the pathogenesis of PUD. The two predominant causes are *H. pylori* infection and NSAID ingestion. PUD not related to *H. pylori* or NSAIDs may be increasing. Independent of the inciting or injurious agent, peptic ulcers develop as a result of an imbalance between mucosal protection/repair and aggressive factors. Gastric acid plays an essential role in mucosal injury.

CLINICAL FEATURES ■ **History** Abdominal pain is common to many gastrointestinal disorders, including DU and GU, but has a poor predictive value for the presence of either DU or GU. Up to 10% of patients with NSAID-induced mucosal disease can present with a complication (bleeding, perforation, and obstruction) without antecedent symptoms. Despite this poor correlation, a careful history and physical examination are essential components of the approach to a patient suspected of having peptic ulcers.

Epigastric pain described as a burning or gnawing discomfort can be present in both DU and GU. The discomfort is also described as an ill-defined, aching sensation or as hunger pain. The typical pain pattern in DU occurs 90 min to 3 h after a meal and is frequently relieved by antacids or food. Pain that awakes the patient from sleep (between midnight and 3 A.M.) is the most discriminating symptom, with two-thirds of DU patients describing this complaint. Unfortunately, this symptom is also present in one-third of patients with NUD. The pain pattern in GU patients may be different from that in DU patients, where discomfort may actually be precipitated by food. Nausea and weight loss occur more commonly in GU patients. In the United States, endoscopy detects ulcers in <30% of patients who have dyspepsia. Despite this, 40% of these individuals with typical ulcer symptoms had an ulcer crater, and 40% had gastroduodenitis on endoscopic examination.

The mechanism for development of abdominal pain in ulcer patients is unknown. Several possible explanations include acid-induced activation of chemical receptors in the duodenum, enhanced duodenal sensitivity to bile acids and pepsin, or altered gastroduodenal motility.

Variation in the intensity or distribution of the abdominal pain, as well as the onset of associated symptoms such as nausea and/or vomiting, may be indicative of an ulcer complication. Dyspepsia that be-

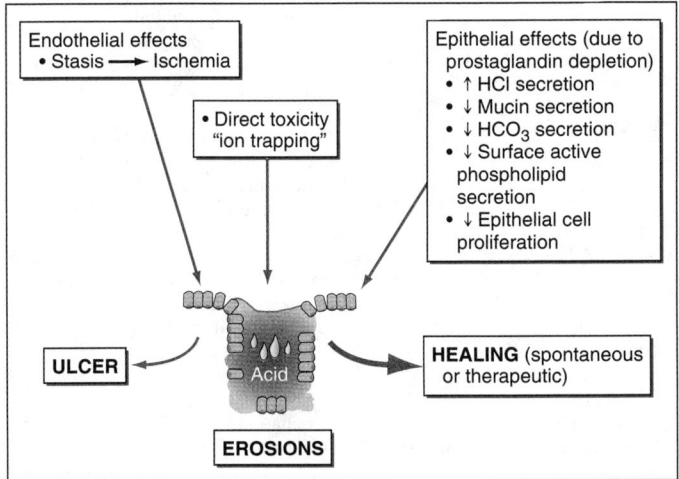

FIGURE 274-9 Mechanisms by which NSAIDs may induce mucosal injury. *(Adapted from J Scheiman et al: J Clin Outcomes Management 3:23, 1996.)*

comes constant, is no longer relieved by food or antacids, or radiates to the back may indicate a penetrating ulcer (pancreas). Sudden onset of severe, generalized abdominal pain may indicate perforation. Pain worsening with meals, nausea, and vomiting of undigested food suggest gastric outlet obstruction. Tarry stools or coffee ground emesis indicate bleeding.

Physical Examination Epigastric tenderness is the most frequent finding in patients with GU or DU. Pain may be found to the right of the midline in 20% of patients. Unfortunately, the predictive value of this finding is rather low. Physical examination is critically important for discovering evidence of ulcer complication. Tachycardia and orthostasis suggest dehydration secondary to vomiting or active gastrointestinal blood loss. A severely tender, boardlike abdomen suggests a perforation. Presence of a succussion splash indicates retained fluid in the stomach, suggesting gastric outlet obstruction.

PUD-Related Complications ■ *GASTROINTESTINAL BLEEDING* Gastrointestinal bleeding is the most common complication observed in PUD. It occurs in ~15% of patients and more often in individuals >60 years old. The higher incidence in the elderly is likely due to the increased use of NSAIDs in this group. As many as 20% of patients with ulcer-related hemorrhage bleed without any preceding warning signs or symptoms.

PERFORATION The second most common ulcer-related complication is perforation, being reported in as many as 6 to 7% of PUD patients. As in the case of bleeding, the incidence of perforation in the elderly appears to be increasing secondary to increased use of NSAIDs. Penetration is a form of perforation in which the ulcer bed tunnels into an adjacent organ. DUs tend to penetrate posteriorly into the pancreas, leading to pancreatitis, whereas GUs tend to penetrate into the left hepatic lobe. Gastrocolic fistulas associated with GUs have also been described.

GASTRIC OUTLET OBSTRUCTION Gastric outlet obstruction is the least common ulcer-related complication, occurring in 1 to 2% of patients. A patient may have relative obstruction secondary to ulcer-related inflammation and edema in the peripyloric region. This process often resolves with ulcer healing. A fixed, mechanical obstruction secondary to scar formation in the peripyloric areas is also possible. The latter requires endoscopic (balloon dilation) or surgical intervention. Signs and symptoms relative to mechanical obstruction may develop insidiously. New onset of early satiety, nausea, vomiting, increase of postprandial abdominal pain, and weight loss should make gastric outlet obstruction a possible diagnosis.

Differential Diagnosis The list of gastrointestinal and nongastrointestinal disorders that can mimic ulceration of the stomach or duodenum is quite extensive. The most commonly encountered diagnosis among patients seen for upper abdominal discomfort is NUD. NUD, also known as *functional dyspepsia* or *essential dyspepsia*, refers to a group of heterogeneous disorders typified by upper abdominal pain without the presence of an ulcer. Dyspepsia has been reported to occur in up to 30% of the U.S. population. Up to 60% of patients seeking medical care for dyspepsia have a negative diagnostic evaluation. The etiology of NUD is not established, and the potential role of *H. pylori* in NUD remains controversial.

Several additional disease processes that may present with "ulcer-like" symptoms include proximal gastrointestinal tumors, gastroesophageal reflux, vascular disease, pancreaticobiliary disease (biliary colic, chronic pancreatitis), and gastroduodenal Crohn's disease.

Diagnostic Evaluation In view of the poor predictive value of abdominal pain for the presence of a gastroduodenal ulcer and the multiple disease processes that can mimic this disease, the clinician is often confronted with having to establish the presence of an ulcer. Documentation of an ulcer requires either a radiographic (barium study) or an endoscopic procedure. However, a large percentage of patients with symptoms suggestive of an ulcer have NUD; empirical therapy is appropriate for individuals who are otherwise healthy and <45, before embarking on a diagnostic evaluation (Chap. 34).

Barium studies of the proximal gastrointestinal tract are still commonly used as a first test for documenting an ulcer. The sensitivity of older single-contrast barium meals for detecting a DU is as high as 80%, with a double-contrast study providing detection rates as high as 90%. Sensitivity for detection is decreased in small ulcers (<0.5 cm), presence of previous scarring, or in postoperative patients. A DU appears as a well-demarcated crater, most often seen in the bulb. A GU may represent benign or malignant disease. Typically, a benign GU also appears as a discrete crater with radiating mucosal folds originating from the ulcer margin. Ulcers >3 cm in size or those associated with a mass are more often malignant. Unfortunately, up to 8% of GUs that appear to be benign by radiographic appearance are malignant by endoscopy or surgery. Radiographic studies that show a GU must be followed by endoscopy and biopsy.

Endoscopy provides the most sensitive and specific approach for examining the upper gastrointestinal tract. In addition to permitting direct visualization of the mucosa, endoscopy facilitates photographic documentation of a mucosal defect and tissue biopsy to rule out malignancy (GU) or *H. pylori*. Endoscopic examination is particularly helpful in identifying lesions too small to detect by radiographic examination, for evaluation of atypical radiographic abnormalities, or to determine if an ulcer is a source of blood loss.

Although the methods for diagnosing *H. pylori* are outlined in Chap. 135, a brief summary will be included here (Table 274-1). Several biopsy urease tests have been developed (PyloriTek, Clotest, Hpfast, Pronto Dry) and have a sensitivity and specificity of >90 to 95%. Several noninvasive methods for detecting this organism have been developed. Three types of studies routinely used include serologic testing, the ^{13}C- or ^{14}C-urea breath test (UBT), and the fecal *H. pylori* antigen test.

Occasionally, specialized testing such as serum gastrin and gastric acid analysis or sham feeding may be needed in individuals with complicated or refractory PUD (see "Zollinger-Ellison Syndrome," below). Screening for aspirin or NSAIDS (blood or urine) may also be necessary in refractory *H. pylori*–negative PUD patients.

℞ TREATMENT

Before the discovery of *H. pylori*, the therapy of PUD disease was centered on the old dictum by Schwartz of "no acid, no ulcer." Al-

TABLE 274-1 *Tests for Detection of H. pylori*

Test	Sensitivity/ Specificity, %	Comments
INVASIVE (ENDOSCOPY/BIOPSY REQUIRED)		
Rapid urease	80–95/95–100	Simple, false negative with recent use of PPIs, antibiotics, or bismuth compounds
Histology	80–90/>95	Requires pathology processing and staining; provides histologic information
Culture	—/—	Time-consuming, expensive, dependent on experience; allows determination of antibiotic susceptibility
NON-INVASIVE		
Serology	>80/>90	Inexpensive, convenient; not useful for early follow-up
Urea breath test	>90/>90	Simple, rapid; useful for early follow-up; false negatives with recent therapy (see rapid urease test); exposure to low-dose radiation with ^{14}C test
Stool antigen	>90/>90	Inexpensive, convenient; not established for eradication but promising

Note: PPIs, proton pump inhibitors.

though acid secretion is still important in the pathogenesis of PUD, eradication of *H. pylori* and therapy/prevention of NSAID-induced disease is the mainstay. A summary of commonly used drugs for treatment of acid peptic disorders is shown in Table 274-2.

Acid Neutralizing/Inhibitory Drugs ■ *ANTACIDS* Before we understood the important role of histamine in stimulating parietal cell activity, neutralization of secreted acid with antacids constituted the main form of therapy for peptic ulcers. They are now rarely, if ever, used as the primary therapeutic agent but instead are often used by patients for symptomatic relief of dyspepsia. The most commonly used agents are mixtures of aluminum hydroxide and magnesium hydroxide. Aluminum hydroxide can produce constipation and phosphate depletion; magnesium hydroxide may cause loose stools. Many of the commonly used antacids (e.g., Maalox, Mylanta) have a combination of both aluminum and magnesium hydroxide in order to avoid these side effects. The magnesium-containing preparation should not be used in chronic renal failure patients because of possible hypermagnesemia, and aluminum may cause chronic neurotoxicity in these patients.

Calcium carbonate and sodium bicarbonate are potent antacids with varying levels of potential problems. The long-term use of calcium carbonate (converts to calcium chloride in the stomach) can lead to milk-alkali syndrome (hypercalcemia, hyperphosphatemia with possible renal calcinosis and progression to renal insufficiency). Sodium bicarbonate may induce systemic alkalosis.

H₂ RECEPTOR ANTAGONISTS Four of these agents are presently available (cimetidine, ranitidine, famotidine, and nizatidine), and their structures share homology with histamine. Although each has different potency, all will significantly inhibit basal and stimulated acid secretion to comparable levels when used at therapeutic doses. Moreover, similar ulcer-healing rates are achieved with each drug when used at the correct dosage. Presently, this class of drug is often used for treatment of active ulcers (4 to 6 weeks) in combination with antibiotics directed at eradicating *H. pylori* (see below).

Cimetidine was the first H_2 receptor antagonist used for the treatment of acid peptic disorders. The initial recommended dosing profile for cimetidine was 300 mg four times per day. Subsequent studies have documented the efficacy of using 800 mg at bedtime for treatment of active ulcer, with healing rates approaching 80% at 4 weeks. Cimetidine may have weak antiandrogenic side effects resulting in reversible gynecomastia and impotence, primarily in patients receiving high doses for prolonged periods of time (months to years, as in ZES). In view of cimetidine's ability to inhibit cytochrome P450, careful monitoring of drugs such as warfarin, phenytoin, and theophylline is indicated with long-term usage. Other rare reversible adverse effects reported with cimetidine include confusion and elevated levels of serum aminotransferases, creatinine, and serum prolactin. Ranitidine, famotidine, and nizatidine are more potent H_2 receptor antagonists than cimetidine. Each can be used once a day at bedtime. Comparable nighttime dosing regimens are ranitidine, 300 mg, famotidine, 40 mg, and nizatidine, 300 mg.

Additional rare, reversible systemic toxicities reported with H_2 receptor antagonists include pancytopenia, neutropenia, anemia, and thrombocytopenia, with a prevalence rate varying from 0.01 to 0.2%. Cimetidine and rantidine (to a lesser extent) can bind to hepatic cytochrome P450; famotidine and nizatidine do not.

PROTON PUMP (H⁺,K⁺-ATPASE) INHIBITORS Omeprazole, esomeprazole, lansoprazole, rabeprazole, and pantoprazole are substituted benzimidazole derivatives that covalently bind and irreversibly inhibit H⁺,K⁺-ATPase. Esomeprazole, the newest member of this drug class, is the S-enantiomer of omeprazole, which is a racemic mixture of both S- and R-optical isomers. These are the most potent acid inhibitory agents available. Omeprazole and lansoprazole are the proton pump inhibitors (PPIs) that have been used for the longest time. Both are acid labile and are administered as enteric-coated granules in a sustained-release capsule that dissolves within the small intestine at a pH of 6. Pantoprazole and rabeprazole are available as enteric-coated tablets. Pantoprazole is also available as a parenteral formulation for intravenous use. These agents are lipophilic compounds; upon entering the parietal cell, they are protonated and trapped within the acid environment of the tubulovesicular and canalicular system. These agents potently inhibit all phases of gastric acid secretion. Onset of action is rapid, with a maximum acid inhibitory effect between 2 and 6 h after administration and duration of inhibition lasting up to 72 to 96 h. With repeated daily dosing, progressive acid inhibitory effects are observed, with basal and secretagogue-stimulated acid production being inhibited by >95% after 1 week of therapy. The half-life of PPIs is ~18 h; thus it can take between 2 and 5 days for gastric acid secretion to return to normal levels once these drugs have been discontinued. Because the pumps need to be activated for these agents to be effective, their efficacy is maximized if they are administered before a meal (e.g., in the morning before breakfast). Standard dosing for omeprazole and lansoprazole is 20 mg and 30 mg once per day, respectively. Mild to moderate hypergastrinemia has been observed in patients taking these drugs. Carcinoid tumors developed in some animals given the drugs preclinically; however, extensive experience has failed to demonstrate gastric carcinoid tumor development in humans. Serum gastrin levels return to normal levels within 1 to 2 weeks after drug cessation. As with any agent that leads to significant hypochlorhydria, PPIs may interfere with absorption of drugs such as ketoconazole, ampicillin, iron, and digoxin. Hepatic cytochrome P450 can be inhibited by the earlier PPIs (omeprazole, lansoprazole). Rabeprazole, pantoprazole, and esomeprazole do not appear to interact significantly with drugs metabolized by the cytochrome P450 system. The overall clinical significance of this observation is not definitely established. Caution should be taken when using warfarin, diazepam, and phenytoin concomitantly with PPIs.

Cytoprotective Agents ■ *SUCRALFATE* Sucralfate is a complex sucrose salt in which the hydroxyl groups have been substituted by aluminum hydroxide and sulfate. This compound is insoluble in water and becomes a viscous paste within the stomach and duodenum, binding primarily to sites of active ulceration. Sucralfate may act by several mechanisms. In the gastric environment, aluminum hydroxide dissociates, leaving the polar sulfate anion, which can bind to positively charged tissue proteins found within the ulcer bed, and providing a physicochemical barrier impeding further tissue injury by acid and pepsin. Sucralfate may also induce a trophic effect by binding growth factors such as EGF, enhance prostaglandin synthesis, stimulate mucous and bicarbonate secretion, and enhance mucosal defense and repair. Toxicity from this drug is rare, with constipation being the most common one reported (2 to 3%). It should be avoided in patients with chronic renal

TABLE 274-2 Drugs Used in the Treatment of Peptic Ulcer Disease

Drug Type/Mechanism	Examples	Dose
Acid-suppressing drugs		
Antacids	Mylanta, Maalox, Tums, Gaviscon	100–140 meq/L 1 and 3 h after meals and hs
H_2 receptor antagonists	Cimetidine	400 mg bid
	Ranitidine	300 mg hs
	Famotidine	40 mg hs
	Nizatidine	300 mg hs
Proton pump inhibitors	Omeprazole	20 mg/d
	Lansoprazole	30 mg/d
	Rabeprazole	20 mg/d
	Pantoprazole	40 mg/d
	Esomeprazole	20 mg/d
Mucosal protective agents		
Sucralfate	Sucralfate	1 g qid
Prostaglandin analogue	Misoprostol	200 μg qid
Bismuth-containing compounds	Bismuth subsalicylate (BSS)	See anti-*H. pylori* regimens (Table 274-3)

insufficiency to prevent aluminum-induced neurotoxicity. Hypophosphatemia and gastric bezoar formation have also been rarely reported. Standard dosing of sucralfate is 1 g four times per day.

BISMUTH-CONTAINING PREPARATIONS Sir William Osler considered bismuth-containing compounds the drug of choice for treating PUD. The resurgence in the use of these agents is due to their effect against *H. pylori*. Colloidal bismuth subcitrate (CBS) and bismuth subsalicylate (BSS, Pepto-Bismol) are the most widely used preparations. The mechanism by which these agents induce ulcer healing is unclear. Potential mechanisms include ulcer coating; prevention of further pepsin/HCl-induced damage; binding of pepsin; and stimulation of prostaglandins, bicarbonate, and mucous secretion. Adverse effects with short-term usage are rare with bismuth compounds. Long-term usage with high doses, especially with the avidly absorbed CBS, may lead to neurotoxicity. These compounds are commonly used as one of the agents in an anti-*H. pylori* regimen (see below).

PROSTAGLANDIN ANALOGUES In view of their central role in maintaining mucosal integrity and repair, stable prostaglandin analogues were developed for the treatment of PUD. The prostaglandin E_1 derivative misoprostal is the only agent of this class approved by the U.S. Food and Drug Administration for clinical use in the prevention of NSAID-induced gastroduodenal mucosal injury (see below). The mechanism by which this rapidly absorbed drug provides its therapeutic effect is through enhancement of mucosal defense and repair. Prostaglandin analogues enhance mucous bicarbonate secretion, stimulate mucosal blood flow, and decrease mucosal cell turnover. The most common toxicity noted with this drug is diarrhea (10 to 30% incidence). Other major toxicities include uterine bleeding and contractions; misoprostal is contraindicated in women who may be pregnant, and women of childbearing age must be made clearly aware of this potential drug toxicity. The standard therapeutic dose is 200 μg four times per day.

MISCELLANEOUS DRUGS A number of drugs aimed at treating acid peptic disorders have been developed over the years. In view of their limited utilization in the United States, if any, they will only be listed briefly. Anticholinergics, designed to inhibit activation of the muscarinic receptor in parietal cells, met with limited success due to their relatively weak acid-inhibiting effect and significant side effects (dry eyes, dry mouth, urinary retention). Tricyclic antidepressants have been suggested by some, but again the toxicity of these agents in comparison to the safe, effective drugs already described precludes their utility. Finally, the licorice extract carbenoxolone has aldosterone-like side effects with fluid retention and hypokalemia, making it an undesirable therapeutic option.

Therapy of *H. pylori* Extensive effort has been placed into determining who of the many individuals with *H. pylori* infection should be treated. The common conclusion arrived at by multiple consensus conferences (National Institutes of Health Consensus Development, American Digestive Health Foundation International Update Conference, European Maastricht Consensus, and Asia Pacific Consensus Conference) is that *H. pylori* should be eradicated in patients with documented PUD. This holds true independent of time of presentation (first episode or not), severity of symptoms, presence of confounding factors such as ingestion of NSAIDs, or whether the ulcer is in remission. Some have advocated treating patients with a history of documented PUD who are found to be *H. pylori*–positive by serology or breath testing. Over half of patients with gastric MALT lymphoma experience complete remission of the tumor in response to *H. pylori* eradication. Treating patients with NUD to prevent gastric cancer or patients with gastroesophageal reflux disease requiring long-term acid suppression remains controversial.

Multiple drugs have been evaluated in the therapy of *H. pylori*. No single agent is effective in eradicating the organism. Combination therapy for 14 days provides the greatest efficacy. A short-time course administration (7 to 10 days), although attractive, has not proved as

successful as the 14-day regimens. The agents used with the greatest frequency include amoxicillin, metronidazole, tetracycline, clarithromycin, and bismuth compounds.

The physician's goal in treating PUD is to provide relief of symptoms (pain or dyspepsia), promote ulcer healing, and ultimately prevent ulcer recurrence and complications. The greatest impact of understanding the role of *H. pylori* in peptic disease has been the ability to prevent recurrence of what was often a recurring disease. Documented eradication of *H. pylori* in patients with PUD is associated with a dramatic decrease in ulcer recurrence to 4% (as compared to 59%) in GU patients and 6% (compared to 67%) in DU patients. Eradication of the organism may lead to diminished recurrent ulcer bleeding. The impact of its eradication on ulcer perforation is unclear.

Suggested treatment regimens for *H. pylori* are outlined in Table 274-3. Choice of a particular regimen will be influenced by several factors including efficacy, patient tolerance, existing antibiotic resistance, and cost of the drugs. The aim for initial eradication rates should be 85 to 90%. Dual therapy [PPI plus amoxicillin, PPI plus clarithromycin, ranitidine bismuth citrate (Tritec) plus clarithromycin] are not recommended in view of studies demonstrating eradication rates of <80 to 85%. The combination of bismuth, metronidazole, and tetracycline was the first triple regimen found effective against *H. pylori*. The combination of two antibiotics plus either a PPI, H_2 blocker, or bismuth compound has comparable success rates. Addition of acid suppression assists in providing early symptom relief and may enhance bacterial eradication.

Triple therapy, although effective, has several drawbacks, including the potential for poor patient compliance and drug-induced side effects. Compliance is being addressed somewhat by simplifying the regimens so that patients can take the medications twice a day. Simpler (dual therapy) and shorter regimens (7 and 10 days) are not as effective as triple therapy for 14 days. Two anti-*H. pylori* regimens are available in prepackaged formulation: Prevpac (lansoprazole, clarithromycin, and amoxicillin) and Helidac (bismuth subsalicylate, tetracycline, and metronidazole). The contents of the Prevpac are to be taken twice per day for 14 days, whereas Helidac constituents are taken four times per day with an antisecretory agent (PPI or H_2 blocker), also taken for at least 14 days.

Side effects have been reported in up to 20 to 30% of patients on triple therapy. Bismuth may cause black stools, constipation, or darkening of the tongue. The most feared complication with amoxicillin is pseudomembranous colitis, but this occurs in <1 to 2% of patients. Amoxicillin can also lead to antibiotic-associated diarrhea, nausea, vomiting, skin rash, and allergic reaction. Tetracycline has been reported to cause rashes and very rarely hepatotoxicity and anaphylaxis.

TABLE 274-3   *Regimens Recommended for Eradication of H. pylori Infection*

Drug	Dose
TRIPLE THERAPY	
1. Bismuth subsalicylate *plus*	2 tablets qid
Metronidazole *plus*	250 mg qid
Tetracycline[a]	500 mg qid
2. Ranitidine bismuth citrate *plus*	400 mg bid
Tetracycline *plus*	500 mg bid
Clarithromycin or metronidazole	500 mg bid
3. Omeprazole (lansoprazole) *plus*	20 mg bid (30 mg bid)
Clarithromycin *plus*	250 or 500 mg bid
Metronidazole[b] *or*	500 mg bid
Amoxicillin[c]	1 gr bid
QUADRUPLE THERAPY	
Omeprazole (lansoprazole)	20 mg (30 mg) daily
Bismuth subsalicylate	2 tablets qid
Metronidazole	250 mg qid
Tetracycline	500 mg qid

[a] Alternative: use prepacked Helidac (see text).
[b] Alternative: use prepacked Prevpac (see text).
[c] Use either metronidazole or amoxicillin, not both.

One important concern with treating patients who may not need treatment is the potential for development of antibiotic-resistant strains. The incidence and type of antibiotic-resistant *H. pylori* strains vary worldwide. Strains resistant to metronidazole, clarithromycin, amoxicillin, and tetracycline have been described, with the latter two being uncommon. Antibiotic-resistant strains are the most common cause for treatment failure in compliant patients. Unfortunately, in vitro resistance does not predict outcome in patients. Culture and sensitivity testing of *H. pylori* is not performed routinely. Although resistance to metronidazole has been found in as many as 30% and 95% of isolates in North America and Asia, respectively, triple therapy is effective in eradicating the organism in >50% of patients infected with a resistant strain. Clarithromycin resistance is seen in about 10% of persons in the United States.

Failure of *H. pylori* eradication with triple therapy is usually due to infection with a resistant organism. Quadruple therapy (Table 274-3), where clarithromycin is substituted for metronidazole (or vice versa), should be the next step. The combination of pantoprazole, amoxicillin, and rifabutin for 10 days has also been used successfully (86% cure rate) in patients infected with resistant strains. If eradication is still not achieved in a compliant patient, then culture and sensitivity of the organism should be considered.

Reinfection after successful eradication of *H. pylori* is rare in the United States (<1%/year). If recurrent infection occurs within the first 6 months after completing therapy, the most likely explanation is recrudescence as opposed to reinfection, which occurs later in time.

Therapy of NSAID-Related Gastric or Duodenal Injury Medical intervention for NSAID-related mucosal injury includes treatment of an active ulcer and prevention of future injury. Recommendations for the treatment and prevention of NSAID-related mucosal injury are in Table 274-4. Ideally the injurious agent should be stopped as the first step in the therapy of an active NSAID-induced ulcer. If that is possible, then treatment with one of the acid inhibitory agents (H_2 blockers, PPIs) is indicated. Cessation of NSAIDs is not always possible because of the patient's severe underlying disease. Only PPIs can heal GUs or DUs, independent of whether NSAIDs are discontinued.

Prevention of NSAID-induced ulceration can be accomplished by misoprostol (200 μg qid) or a PPI. High-dose H_2 blockers (famotidine, 40 mg bid) have also shown some promise, although PPIs are superior. The use of COX-2-selective NSAIDs may also reduce injury to gastric mucosa. Two highly selective COX-2 inhibitors, celecoxib and rofecoxib, are 100 times more selective inhibitors of COX-2 than standard NSAIDs, leading to gastric or duodenal mucosal injury that is comparable to placebo. However, several issues regarding the safety of these selective COX-2 inhibitors require clarification. Specifically, the CLASS study demonstrates that the advantage of celecoxib in preventing gastrointestinal complications was offset when low-dose aspirin was used simultaneously. Therefore, gastric protection therapy is required in individuals taking COX-2 inhibitors and aspirin prophylaxis. In addition, COX-2 inhibitors delay experimental ulcer healing in animal models and may promote cardiovascular thrombosis. Finally, much of the work performed demonstrating the benefit of COX-2 inhibitors and PPIs on gastrointestinal injury has been performed in individuals of average risk; it is unclear if the same level of benefit will be achieved in high-risk patients.

Approach and Therapy: Summary Controversy continues regarding the best approach to the patient who presents with dyspepsia (Chap. 34). The discovery of *H. pylori* and its role in pathogenesis of ulcers has added a new variable to the equation. Previously, if a patient <50 presented with dyspepsia and without alarming signs or symptoms suggestive of an ulcer complication or malignancy, an empirical therapeutic trial with acid suppression was commonly recommended. Although this approach is practiced by some today, an approach presently gaining approval for the treatment of patients with dyspepsia is outlined in Fig. 274-10. The referral to a gastroenterologist is for the potential need of endoscopy and subsequent evaluation and treatment if the endoscopy is negative.

TABLE 274-4 *Recommendations for Treatment of NSAID-Related Mucosal Injury*

Clinical Setting	Recommendation
Active ulcer	
NSAID discontinued	H_2 receptor antagonist or PPI
NSAID continued	PPI
Prophylactic therapy	Misoprostol
	PPI
	Selective COX-2 inhibitor
H. pylori infection	Eradication if active ulcer present or there is a past history of peptic ulcer disease

Note: PPI, proton pump inhibitor; COX-2, isoenzyme of cyclooxygenase.

Once an ulcer (GU or DU) is documented, then the main issue at stake is whether *H. pylori* or an NSAID is involved. With *H. pylori* present, independent of the NSAID status, triple therapy is recommended for 14 days, followed by continued acid-suppressing drugs (H_2 receptor antagonist or PPIs) for a total of 4 to 6 weeks. Selection of patients for documentation of *H. pylori* eradication (organisms gone at least 4 weeks after completing antibiotics) is an area of some debate. The test of choice for documenting eradication is the UBT. The stool antigen study may also hold promise for this purpose, but the data have not been as clear cut as in the case of using the stool antigen test for primary diagnosis. Further studies are warranted, but if the UBT is not available, a stool antigen should be considered to document eradication. Serologic testing is not useful for the purpose of documenting eradication since antibody titers fall slowly and often do not become undetectable. Two approaches toward documentation of eradication exist: (1) test for eradication only in individuals with a complicated course or in individuals who are frail or with multisystem disease who would do poorly with an ulcer recurrence, and (2) test all patients for successful eradication. Some recommend that patients with complicated ulcer disease or who are frail should be treated with long-term acid suppression, thus making documentation of *H. pylori* eradication a moot point. In view of this discrepancy in practice, it would be best to discuss with the patient the different options available.

Several issues differentiate the approach to a GU versus a DU. GUs,

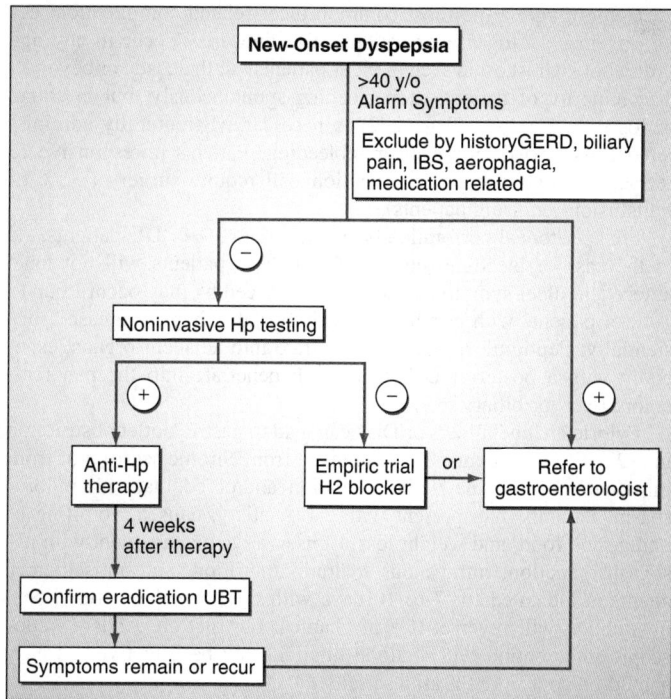

FIGURE 274-10 Overview of new-onset dyspepsia. Hp, *H. pylori*; UBT, urea breath test; IBS, irritable bowel syndrome. (*Adapted from BS Anand and DY Graham: Endoscopy 31:215, 1999.*)

especially of the body and fundus, have the potential of being malignant. Multiple biopsies of a GU should be taken initially; even if these are negative for neoplasm, repeat endoscopy to document healing at 8 to 12 weeks should be performed, with biopsy if the ulcer is still present. About 70% of GUs eventually found to be malignant undergo significant (usually incomplete) healing.

The majority (>90%) of GUs and DUs heal with the conventional therapy outlined above. A GU that fails to heal after 12 weeks and a DU that does not heal after 8 weeks of therapy should be considered refractory. Once poor compliance and persistent *H. pylori* infection have been excluded, NSAID use, either inadvertent or surreptitious, must be excluded. In addition, cigarette smoking must be eliminated. For a GU, malignancy must be meticulously excluded. Next, consideration should be given to a gastric hypersecretory state, which can be excluded with gastric acid analysis. Although a subset of patients have gastric acid hypersecretion of unclear etiology as a contributing factor to refractory ulcers, ZES should be excluded with a fasting gastrin or secretin stimulation test (see below). More than 90% of refractory ulcers (either DUs or GUs) heal after 8 weeks of treatment with higher doses of PPI (omeprazole, 40 mg/d; lansoprazole 30 to 60 mg/d). This higher dose is also effective in maintaining remission. Surgical intervention may be a consideration at this point; however, other rare causes of refractory ulcers must be excluded before recommending surgery. Rare etiologies of refractory ulcers that may be diagnosed by gastric or duodenal biopsies include: ischemia, Crohn's disease, amyloidosis, sarcoidosis, lymphoma, eosinophilic gastroenteritis, or infection [cytomegalovirus (CMV), tuberculosis, or syphilis].

Surgical Therapy   Surgical intervention in PUD can be viewed as being either elective, for treatment of medically refractory disease, or as urgent/emergent, for the treatment of an ulcer-related complication. The development of pharmacologic and endoscopic approaches for the treatment of peptic disease has led to a substantial decrease in the number operations needed for this disorder. Refractory ulcers are an exceedingly rare occurrence. Surgery is more often required for treatment of an ulcer-related complication. Gastrointestinal bleeding (Chap. 37), perforation, and gastric outlet obstruction are the three complications that may require surgical intervention.

Hemorrhage is the most common ulcer-related complication, occurring in ~15 to 25% of patients. Bleeding may occur in any age group but is most often seen in older patients (sixth decade or beyond). The majority of patients stop bleeding spontaneously, but in some, endoscopic therapy (Chap. 272) is necessary. Parenterally administered PPIs also decrease ulcer rebleeding. Patients unresponsive or refractory to endoscopic intervention will require surgery (~5% of transfusion-requiring patients).

Free peritoneal perforation occurs in ~2 to 3% of DU patients. As in the case of bleeding, up to 10% of these patients will not have antecedent ulcer symptoms. Concomitant bleeding may occur in up to 10% of patients with perforation, with mortality being increased substantially. Peptic ulcer can also penetrate into adjacent organs, especially with a posterior DU, which can penetrate into the pancreas, colon, liver, or biliary tree.

Pyloric channel ulcers or DUs can lead to gastric outlet obstruction in ~2 to 3% of patients. This can result from chronic scarring or from impaired motility due to inflammation and/or edema with pylorospasm. Patients may present with early satiety, nausea, vomiting of undigested food, and weight loss. Conservative management with nasogastric suction, intravenous hydration/nutrition, and antisecretory agents is indicated for 7 to 10 days with the hope that a functional obstruction will reverse. If a mechanical obstruction persists, endoscopic intervention with balloon dilation may be effective. Surgery should be considered if all else fails.

Specific Operations for Duodenal Ulcers   Surgical treatment is designed to decrease gastric acid secretion. Operations most commonly performed include (1) vagotomy and drainage (by pyloroplasty, gastroduodenos-

tomy, or gastrojejunostomy), (2) highly selective vagotomy (which does not require a drainage procedure), and (3) vagotomy with antrectomy. The specific procedure performed is dictated by the underlying circumstances: elective vs. emergency, the degree and extent of duodenal ulceration, and the expertise of the surgeon.

Vagotomy is a component of each of these procedures and is aimed at decreasing acid secretion through ablating cholinergic input to the stomach. Unfortunately, both truncal and selective vagotomy (preserves the celiac and hepatic branches) result in gastric atony despite successful reduction of both basal acid output (BAO, decreased by 85%) and maximal acid output (MAO, decreased by 50%). Drainage through pyloroplasty or gastroduodenostomy is required in an effort to compensate for the vagotomy-induced gastric motility disorder. This procedure has an intermediate complication rate and a 10% ulcer recurrence rate. To minimize gastric dysmotility, highly selective vagotomy (also known as parietal cell, super selective, and proximal vagotomy) was developed. Only the vagal fibers innervating the portion of the stomach that contains parietal cells is transected, thus leaving fibers important for regulating gastric motility intact. Although this procedure leads to an immediate decrease in both BAO and stimulated acid output, acid secretion recovers over time. By the end of the first postoperative year, basal and stimulated acid output are ~30 and 50%, respectively, of preoperative levels. Ulcer recurrence rates are higher with highly selective vagotomy (≥10%), although the overall complication rates are the lowest of the three procedures.

The procedure that provides the lowest rates of ulcer recurrence (1%) but has the highest complication rate is vagotomy (truncal or selective) in combination with antrectomy. Antrectomy is aimed at eliminating an additional stimulant of gastric acid secretion, gastrin. Gastrin originates from G cells found in the antrum. Two principal types of reanastomoses are used after antrectomy, gastroduodenostomy (Billroth I) or gastrojejunostomy (Billroth II) (Fig. 274-11). Although Billroth I is often preferred over II, severe duodenal inflammation or scarring may preclude its performance.

Of these procedures, highly selective vagotomy may be the one of choice in the elective setting, except in situations where ulcer recurrence rates are high (prepyloric ulcers and those refractory to H$_2$ therapy). Selection of vagotomy and antrectomy may be more appropriate in these circumstances.

These procedures have been traditionally performed by standard laparotomy. The advent of laparoscopic surgery has led several surgical teams to successfully perform highly selective vagotomy, truncal vagotomy/pyloroplasty, and truncal vagotomy/antrectomy through

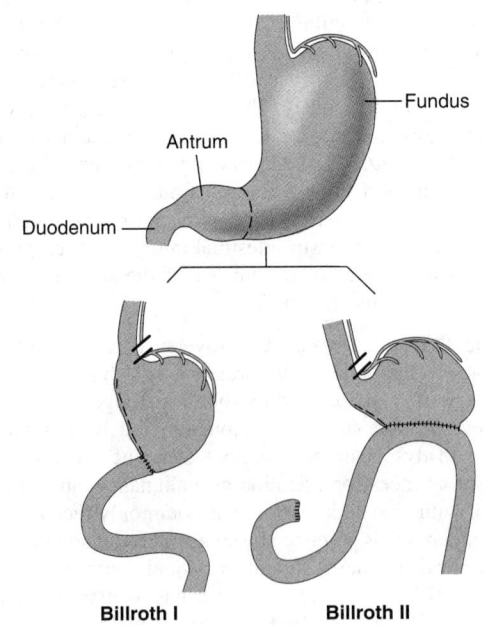

FIGURE 274-11   Schematic representation of Billroth I and II procedures.

this approach. An increase in the number of laparoscopic procedures for treatment of PUD is expected.

Specific Operations for Gastric Ulcers The location and the presence of a concomitant DU dictate the operative procedure performed for a GU. Antrectomy (including the ulcer) with a Billroth I anastomosis is the treatment of choice for an antral ulcer. Vagotomy is performed only if a DU is present. Although ulcer excision with vagotomy and drainage procedure has been proposed, the higher incidence of ulcer recurrence makes this a less desirable approach. Ulcers located near the esophagogastric junction may require a more radical approach, a subtotal gastrectomy with a Roux-en-Y esophagogastrojejunostomy (Csende's procedure). A less aggressive approach including antrectomy, intraoperative ulcer biopsy, and vagotomy (Kelling-Madlener procedure) may be indicated in fragile patients with a high GU. Ulcer recurrence approaches 30% with this procedure.

Surgery-Related Complications Complications seen after surgery for PUD are related primarily to the extent of the anatomical modification performed. Minimal alteration (highly selective vagotomy) is associated with higher rates of ulcer recurrence and less gastrointestinal disturbance. More aggressive surgical procedures have a lower rate of ulcer recurrence but a greater incidence of gastrointestinal dysfunction. Overall, morbidity and mortality related to these procedures are quite low. Morbidity associated with vagotomy and antrectomy or pyloroplasty is ≤5%, with mortality ~1%. Highly selective vagotomy has lower morbidity and mortality rates of 1 and 0.3%, respectively.

In addition to the potential early consequences of any intraabdominal procedure (bleeding, infection, thromboembolism), gastroparesis, duodenal stump leak, and efferent loop obstruction can be observed.

RECURRENT ULCERATION The risk of ulcer recurrence is directly related to the procedure performed. Ulcers that recur after partial gastric resection tend to develop at the anastomosis (stomal or marginal ulcer). Epigastric abdominal pain is the most frequent presenting complaint. Severity and duration of pain tend to be more progressive than observed with DUs before surgery.

Ulcers may recur for several reasons including incomplete vagotomy, retained antrum, and, less likely, persistent or recurrent *H. pylori* infection. ZES should have been excluded preoperatively. More recently, surreptitious use of NSAIDs has been found to be a reason for recurrent ulcers after surgery, especially if the initial procedure was done for an NSAID-induced ulcer. Once *H. pylori* and NSAIDs have been excluded as etiologic factors, the question of incomplete vagotomy or retained gastric antrum should be explored. For the latter, fasting plasma gastrin levels should be determined. If elevated, retained antrum or ZES (see below) should be considered. A combination of acid secretory analysis and secretin stimulation (see below) can assist in this differential diagnosis. Incomplete vagotomy can be ruled out by gastric acid analysis coupled with sham feeding. In this test, gastric acid output is measured while the patient sees, smells, and chews a meal (without swallowing). The cephalic phase of gastric secretion, which is mediated by the vagus, is being assessed with this study. An increase in gastric acid output in response to sham feeding is evidence that the vagus nerve is intact.

Medical therapy with H$_2$ blockers will heal postoperative ulceration in 70 to 90% of patients. The efficacy of PPIs has not been fully assessed in this group, but one may anticipate greater rates of ulcer healing compared to those obtained with H$_2$ blockers. Repeat operation (complete vagotomy, partial gastrectomy) may be required in a small subgroup of patients who have not responded to aggressive medical management.

AFFERENT LOOP SYNDROMES Two types of afferent loop syndrome can occur in patients who have undergone partial gastric resection with Billroth II anastomosis. The most common of the two is bacterial overgrowth in the afferent limb secondary to stasis. Patients may experience postprandial abdominal pain, bloating, and diarrhea with concomitant malabsorption of fats and vitamin B$_{12}$. Cases refractory to antibiotics may require surgical revision of the loop. The less common

afferent loop syndrome can present with severe abdominal pain and bloating that occur 20 to 60 min after meals. Pain is often followed by nausea and vomiting of bile-containing material. The pain and bloating may improve after emesis. The cause of this clinical picture is theorized to be incomplete drainage of bile and pancreatic secretions from an afferent loop that is partially obstructed. Cases refractory to dietary measures may need surgical revision.

DUMPING SYNDROME Dumping syndrome consists of a series of vasomotor and gastrointestinal signs and symptoms and occurs in patients who have undergone vagotomy and drainage (especially Billroth procedures). Two phases of dumping, early and late, can occur. Early dumping takes place 15 to 30 min after meals and consists of crampy abdominal discomfort, nausea, diarrhea, belching, tachycardia, palpitations, diaphoresis, light-headedness, and, rarely, syncope. These signs and symptoms arise from the rapid emptying of hyperosmolar gastric contents into the small intestine, resulting in a fluid shift into the gut lumen with plasma volume contraction and acute intestinal distention. Release of vasoactive gastrointestinal hormones (vasoactive intestinal polypeptide, neurotensin, motilin) is also theorized to play a role in early dumping.

The late phase of dumping typically occurs 90 min to 3 h after meals. Vasomotor symptoms (light-headedness, diaphoresis, palpitations, tachycardia, and syncope) predominate during this phase. This component of dumping is thought to be secondary to hypoglycemia from excessive insulin release.

Dumping syndrome is most noticeable after meals rich in simple carbohydrates (especially sucrose) and high osmolarity. Ingestion of large amounts of fluids may also contribute. Up to 50% of postvagotomy and drainage patients will experience dumping syndrome to some degree. Signs and symptoms often improve with time, but a severe protracted picture can occur in up to 1% of patients.

Dietary modification is the cornerstone of therapy for patients with dumping syndrome. Small, multiple (six) meals devoid of simple carbohydrates coupled with elimination of liquids during meals is important. Antidiarrheals and anticholinergic agents are complementary to diet. Guar and pectin, which increase the viscosity of intraluminal contents, may be beneficial in more symptomatic individuals. Acarbose, an α-glucosidase inhibitor that delays digestion of ingested carbohydrates, has also been shown to be beneficial in the treatment of the late phases of dumping. The somatostatin analogue octreotide has been successful in diet-refractory cases. This drug is administered subcutaneously (50 μg tid), titrated according to clinical response. Recently a long-acting formulation has become available, but its use in dumping syndrome has not been examined.

POSTVAGOTOMY DIARRHEA Up to 10% of patients may seek medical attention for the treatment of postvagotomy diarrhea. This complication is most commonly observed after truncal vagotomy. Patients may complain of intermittent diarrhea that occurs typically 1 to 2 h after meals. Occasionally the symptoms may be severe and relentless. This is due to a motility disorder from interruption of the vagal fibers supplying the luminal gut. Other contributing factors may include decreased absorption of nutrients (see below), increased excretion of bile acids, and release of luminal factors that promote secretion. Diphenoxylate or loperamide is often useful in symptom control. The bile salt–binding agent cholestyramine may be helpful in severe cases. Surgical reversal of a 10-cm segment of jejunum may yield a substantial improvement in bowel frequency in a subset of patients.

BILE REFLUX GASTROPATHY A subset of post-partial gastrectomy patients will present with abdominal pain, early satiety, nausea, and vomiting, who have as the only finding mucosal erythema of the gastric remnant. Histologic examination of the gastric mucosa reveals minimal inflammation but the presence of epithelial cell injury. This clinical picture is categorized as bile or alkaline reflux gastropathy/gastritis. Although reflux of bile is implicated as the reason for this disorder, the mechanism is unknown. Prokinetic agents (cisapride, 10 to 20 mg before meals and at bedtime) and cholestyramine have been effective treatments. Cisapride is no longer available because it induces cardiac arrhythmias. Severe refractory symptoms may require using either nuclear scanning with ^{99m}Tc-HIDA, to document reflux, or an alkaline challenge test, where 0.1 N NaOH is infused into the stomach in an effort to reproduce the patient's symptoms. Surgical diversion of pancreaticobiliary secretions away from the gastric remnant with a Roux-en-Y gastrojejunostomy consisting of a long (50 to 60 cm) Roux limb has been used in severe cases. Bilious vomiting improves, but early satiety and bloating may persist in up to 50% of patients.

MALDIGESTION AND MALABSORPTION   Weight loss can be observed in up to 60% of patients after partial gastric resection. A significant component of this weight reduction is due to decreased oral intake. However, mild steatorrhea can also develop. Reasons for maldigestion/malabsorption include decreased gastric acid production, rapid gastric emptying, decreased food dispersion in the stomach, reduced luminal bile concentration, reduced pancreatic secretory response to feeding, and rapid intestinal transit.

Decreased serum vitamin B_{12} levels can be observed after partial gastrectomy. This is usually not due to deficiency of IF, since a minimal amount of parietal cells (source of IF) are removed during antrectomy. Reduced vitamin B_{12} may be due to competition for the vitamin by bacterial overgrowth or inability to split the vitamin from its protein-bound source due to hypochlorhydria.

Iron-deficiency anemia may be a consequence of impaired absorption of dietary iron in patients with a Billroth II gastrojejunostomy. Absorption of iron salts is normal in these individuals; thus a favorable response to oral iron supplementation can be anticipated. Folate deficiency with concomitant anemia can also develop in these patients. This deficiency may be secondary to decreased absorption or diminished oral intake.

Malabsorption of vitamin D and calcium resulting in osteoporosis and osteomalacia is common after partial gastrectomy and gastrojejunostomy (Billroth II). Osteomalacia can occur as a late complication in up to 25% of post-partial gastrectomy patients. Bone fractures occur twice as commonly in men after gastric surgery as in a control population. It may take years before x-ray findings demonstrate diminished bone density. Elevated alkaline phosphatase, reduced serum calcium, bone pain, and pathologic fractures may be seen in patients with osteomalacia. The high incidence of these abnormalities in this subgroup of patients justifies treating them with vitamin D and calcium supplementation indefinitely. Therapy is especially important in females.

GASTRIC ADENOCARCINOMA   The incidence of adenocarcinoma in the gastric stump is increased 15 years after resection. Some have reported a four- to fivefold increase in gastric cancer 20 to 25 years after resection. The pathogenesis is unclear but may involve alkaline reflux, bacterial proliferation, or hypochlorhydria. Endoscopic screening every other year may detect surgically treatable disease.

RELATED CONDITIONS

ZOLLINGER–ELLISON SYNDROME   Severe peptic ulcer diathesis secondary to gastric acid hypersecretion due to unregulated gastrin release from a non-β cell endocrine tumor (gastrinoma) defines the components of the ZES. Initially, ZES was typified by aggressive and refractory ulceration in which total gastrectomy provided the only chance for enhancing survival. Today ZES can be cured by surgical resection in up to 30% of patients.

Epidemiology   The incidence of ZES varies from 0.1 to 1% of individuals presenting with PUD. Males are more commonly affected than females, and the majority of patients are diagnosed between ages 30 and 50. Gastrinomas are classified into sporadic tumors (more common) and those associated with multiple endocrine neoplasia (MEN) type I (see below).

Pathophysiology   Hypergastremia originating from an autonomous neoplasm is the driving force responsible for the clinical manifestations in ZES. Gastrin stimulates acid secretion through gastrin receptors on parietal cells and by inducing histamine release from ECL cells. Gastrin also has a trophic action on gastric epithelial cells. Long-standing hypergastrinemia leads to markedly increased gastric acid secretion through both parietal cell stimulation and increased parietal cell mass. The increased gastric acid output leads to the peptic ulcer diathesis, erosive esophagitis, and diarrhea.

Tumor Distribution   Although early studies suggested that the vast majority of gastrinomas occurred within the pancreas, a significant number of these lesions are extrapancreatic. Over 80% of these tumors are found within the hypothetical gastrinoma triangle (confluence of the cystic and common bile ducts superiorly, junction of the second and third portions of the duodenum inferiorly, and junction of the neck and body of the pancreas medially). Duodenal tumors constitute the most common nonpancreatic lesion; up to 50% of gastrinomas are found here. Less common extrapancreatic sites include stomach, bones, ovaries, heart, liver, and lymph nodes. More than 60% of tumors are considered malignant, with up to 30 to 50% of patients having multiple lesions or metastatic disease at presentation. Histologically, gastrin-producing cells appear well differentiated, expressing markers typically found in endocrine neoplasms (chromogranin, neuron-specific enolase).

Clinical Manifestations   Gastric acid hypersecretion is responsible for the signs and symptoms observed in patients with ZES. Peptic ulcer is the most common clinical manifestation, occurring in >90% of gastrinoma patients. Initial presentation and ulcer location (duodenal bulb) may be indistinguishable from common PUD. Clinical situations that should create suspicion of gastrinoma are ulcers in unusual locations (second part of the duodenum and beyond), ulcers refractory to standard medical therapy, ulcer recurrence after acid-reducing surgery, ulcers presenting with frank complications (bleeding, obstruction, and perforation), or ulcers in the absence of *H. pylori* or NSAID ingestion. Symptoms of esophageal origin are present in up to two-thirds of patients with ZES, with a spectrum ranging from mild esophagitis to frank ulceration with stricture and Barrett's mucosa.

Diarrhea is the next most common clinical manifestation, in up to 50% of patients. Although diarrhea often occurs concomitantly with acid peptic disease, it may also occur independent of an ulcer. Etiology of the diarrhea is multifactorial, resulting from marked volume overload to the small bowel, pancreatic enzyme inactivation by acid, and damage of the intestinal epithelial surface by acid. The epithelial damage can lead to a mild degree of maldigestion and malabsorption of nutrients. The diarrhea may also have a secretory component due to the direct stimulatory effect of gastrin on enterocytes or the cosecretion of additional hormones from the tumor, such as vasoactive intestinal peptide.

Gastrinomas can develop in the presence of MEN I syndrome (Chap. 329) in ~25% of patients. This autosomal dominant disorder involves primarily three organ sites: the parathyroid glands (80 to 90%), pancreas (40 to 80%), and pituitary gland (30 to 60%). The genetic defect in MEN I is in the long arm of chromosome 11 (11q11-q13). In view of the stimulatory effect of calcium on gastric secretion, the hyperparathyroidism and hypercalcemia seen in MEN I patients may have a direct effect on ulcer disease. Resolution of hypercalcemia by parathyroidectomy reduces gastrin and gastric acid output in gastrinoma patients. An additional distinguishing feature in ZES patients with MEN I is the higher incidence of gastric carcinoid tumor development (as compared to patients with sporadic gastrinomas). Gastrinomas tend to be smaller, multiple, and located in the duodenal wall more often than is seen in patients with sporadic ZES. Establishing the diagnosis of MEN I is critical not only from the standpoint of providing genetic counseling to the patient and his or her family but also from the surgical approach recommended.

TABLE 274-5	When to Obtain a Fasting Serum Gastrin Level

Multiple ulcers
Ulcers in unusual locations; associated with severe esophagitis; resistant
   to therapy with frequent recurrences; in the absence of NSAID
   ingestion or *H. pylori* infection
Ulcer patients awaiting surgery
Extensive family history for peptic ulcer disease
Postoperative ulcer recurrence
Basal hyperchlorhydria
Unexplained diarrhea or steatorrhea
Hypercalcemia
Family history of pancreatic islet, pituitary, or parathyroid tumor
Prominent gastric or duodenal folds

Diagnosis The first step in the evaluation of a patient suspected of having ZES is to obtain a fasting gastrin level. A list of clinical scenarios that should arouse suspicion regarding this diagnosis is shown in Table 274-5. Fasting gastrin levels are usually <150 pg/mL. Virtually all gastrinoma patients will have a gastrin level >150 to 200 pg/mL. Measurement of fasting gastrin should be repeated to confirm the clinical suspicion.

Multiple processes can lead to an elevated fasting gastrin level: gastric hypochlorhydria or achlorhydria (the most frequent), with or without pernicious anemia; retained gastric antrum; G cell hyperplasia; gastric outlet obstruction; renal insufficiency; massive small-bowel obstruction; and conditions such as rheumatoid arthritis, vitiligo, diabetes mellitus, and pheochromocytoma. Gastric acid induces feedback inhibition of gastrin release. A decrease in acid production will subsequently lead to failure of the feedback inhibitory pathway, resulting in net hypergastrinemia. Gastrin levels will thus be high in patients using antisecretory agents for the treatment of acid peptic disorders and dyspepsia. *H. pylori* infection can also cause hypergastrinemia.

The next step in establishing a biochemical diagnosis of gastrinoma is to assess acid secretion. Nothing further needs to be done if decreased acid output is observed. In contrast, normal or elevated gastric acid output suggests a need for additional tests. Gastric acid analysis is performed by placing a nasogastric tube in the stomach and drawing samples at 15-min intervals for 1 h during unstimulated or basal state (BAO), followed by continued sampling after administration of intravenous pentagastrin (MAO). Up to 90% of gastrinoma patients may have a BAO of ≥15 meq/h (normal, <4 meq/h). Up to 12% of patients with common PUD may have comparable levels of acid secretion. A BAO/MAO ratio >0.6 is highly suggestive of ZES, but a ratio <0.6 does not exclude the diagnosis. Pentagastrin is no longer available in the United States, making measurement of MAO virtually impossible. If the technology for measuring gastric acid secretion is not available, a basal gastric pH ≥3 virtually excludes a gastrinoma.

Gastrin provocative tests have been developed in an effort to differentiate between the causes of hypergastrinemia and are especially helpful in patients with indeterminant acid secretory studies. The tests are the secretin stimulation test, the calcium infusion study, and a standard meal test. In each of these, a fasted patient has an indwelling intravenous catheter in place for serial blood sampling and an intravenous line in place for secretin or calcium infusion. The patient receives either secretin (intravenous bolus of 2 μg/kg) or calcium (calcium gluconate, 5 mg/kg body weight over 3 h) or is fed a meal. Blood is then drawn at predetermined intervals (10 min and 1 min before and at 2, 5, 10, 15, 20, and 30 min after injection for secretin stimulation and at 30-min intervals during the calcium infusion). The most sensitive and specific gastrin provocative test for the diagnosis of gastrinoma is the secretin study. An increase in gastrin of ≥200 pg within 15 min of secretin injection has a sensitivity and specificity of >90% for ZES. The calcium infusion study is less sensitive and specific than the secretin test, with a rise of >400 pg/mL observed in ~80% of gastrinoma patients. The lower accuracy, coupled with it being a more cumbersome study with greater potential for adverse effects, makes calcium infusion less useful and therefore rarely, if ever,

utilized. Rarely, one may observe increased BAO and hypergastrinemia in a patient who in the past has been categorized as having G cell hyperplasia or hyperfunction. This set of findings may have been due to *H. pylori*. The standard meal test was devised to assist in making the diagnosis of G cell–related hyperactivity, by observing a dramatic increase in gastrin after a meal (>200%). This test is not useful in differentiating between G cell hyperfunction and ZES.

Tumor Localization Once the biochemical diagnosis of gastrinoma has been confirmed, the tumor must be located. Multiple imaging studies have been utilized in an effort to enhance tumor localization (Table 274-6). The broad range of sensitivity is due to the variable success rates achieved by the different investigative groups. Endoscopic ultrasound (EUS) permits imaging of the pancreas with a high degree of resolution (<5 mm). This modality is particularly helpful in excluding small neoplasms within the pancreas and in assessing the presence of surrounding lymph nodes and vascular involvement. Several types of endocrine tumors express cell-surface receptors for somatostatin. This permits the localization of gastrinomas by measuring the uptake of the stable somatostatin analogue ¹¹¹In-pentreotide (octreoscan) with sensitivity and specificity rates of >75%.

Up to 50% of patients have metastatic disease at diagnosis. Success in controlling gastric acid hypersecretion has shifted the emphasis of therapy towards providing a surgical cure. Detecting the primary tumor and excluding metastatic disease are critical in view of this paradigm shift. Once a biochemical diagnosis has been confirmed, the patient should first undergo an abdominal computed tomographic scan, magnetic resonance imaging, or octreoscan (depending on availability) to exclude metastatic disease. Once metastatic disease has been excluded, an experienced endocrine surgeon may opt for exploratory laparotomy with intraoperative ultrasound or transillumination. In other centers, careful examination of the peripancreatic area with EUS, accompanied by endoscopic exploration of the duodenum for primary tumors, will be performed before surgery. Selective arterial secretin injection may be a useful adjuvant for localizing tumors in a subset of patients.

℞ TREATMENT

Treatment of functional endocrine tumors is directed at ameliorating the signs and symptoms related to hormone overproduction, curative resection of the neoplasm, and attempts to control tumor growth in metastatic disease.

PPIs are the treatment of choice and have decreased the need for total gastrectomy. Initial doses of omeprazole or lansoprazole should be in the range of 60 mg/d. Dosing can be adjusted to achieve a BAO <10 meq/h (at the drug trough) in surgery-naive patients and to <5 meq/h in individuals who have previously undergone an acid-reducing operation. Although the somatostatin analogue has inhibitory effects on gastrin release from receptor-bearing tumors and inhibits gastric

TABLE 274-6	Sensitivity of Imaging Studies in Zollinger Ellison Syndrome	
	Sensitivity, %	
Study	Primary Gastrinoma	Metastatic Gastrinoma
Ultrasound	21–28	14
CT scan	35–59	35–72
Selective angiography	35–68	33–86
Portal venous sampling	70–90	N/A
SASI	55–78	41
MRI	30–60	71
Octreoscan	67–86	80–100
EUS	80–100	N/A

Note: CT, computed tomography; SASI, selective arterial secretin injection; MRI, magnetic resonance imaging; octreoscan, imaging with ¹¹¹In-pentreotide; EUS, endoscopic ultrasonography.

acid secretion to some extent, PPIs have the advantage of reducing parietal cell activity to a greater degree.

The ultimate goal of surgery would be to provide a definitive cure. Improved understanding of tumor distribution has led to 10-year disease-free intervals as high as 34% in sporadic gastrinoma patients undergoing surgery. A positive outcome is highly dependent on the experience of the surgical team treating these rare tumors. Surgical therapy of gastrinoma patients with MEN I remains controversial because of the difficulty in rendering these patients disease free with surgery. In contrast to the encouraging postoperative results observed in patients with sporadic disease, only 6% of MEN I patients are disease free 5 years after an operation. Some groups suggest surgery only if a clearly identifiable, nonmetastatic lesion is documented by structural studies. Others advocate a more aggressive approach, where all patients free of hepatic metastasis are explored and all detected tumors in the duodenum are resected; this is followed by enucleation of lesions in the pancreatic head, with a distal pancreatectomy to follow. The outcome of the two approaches has not been clearly defined.

Therapy of metastatic endocrine tumors in general remains suboptimal; gastrinomas are no exception. A host of medical therapeutic approaches including chemotherapy (streptozotocin, 5-fluorouracil, and doxorubicin), IFN-α, and hepatic artery embolization lead to significant toxicity without a substantial improvement in overall survival. ^{111}In-pentetreotide has been utilized in the therapy of metastatic neuroendocrine tumors; further studies are needed. Surgical approaches including debulking surgery and liver transplantation for hepatic metastasis have also produced limited benefit. Therefore, early recognition and surgery are the only chances for curing this disease.

The 5- and 10-year survival rates for gastrinoma patients are 62 to 75% and 47 to 53%, respectively. Individuals with the entire tumor resected or those with a negative laparotomy have 5- and 10-year survival rates >90%. Patients with incompletely resected tumors have 5- and 10-year survival of 43% and 25%, respectively. Patients with hepatic metastasis have <20% survival at 5 years. Favorable prognostic indicators include primary duodenal wall tumors, isolated lymph node tumor, and undetectable tumor upon surgical exploration. Poor outcome is seen in patients with shorter disease duration, higher gastrin levels (>10,000 pg/mL); large pancreatic primary tumors (>3 cm), metastatic disease to lymph nodes, liver, and bone; and Cushing's syndrome. Rapid growth of hepatic metastases is also predictive of poor outcome.

STRESS-RELATED MUCOSAL INJURY Patients suffering from shock, sepsis, massive burns, severe trauma, or head injury can develop acute erosive gastric mucosal changes or frank ulceration with bleeding. Classified as stress-induced gastritis or ulcers, injury is most commonly observed in the acid-producing (fundus and body) portions of the stomach. The most common presentation is gastrointestinal bleeding, which is usually minimal but can occasionally be life-threatening. Respiratory failure requiring mechanical ventilation and underlying coagulopathy are risk factors for bleeding, which tends to occur 48 to 72 h after the acute injury or insult.

Histologically, stress injury does not contain inflammation or *H. pylori*; thus "gastritis" is a misnomer. Although elevated gastric acid secretion may be noted in patients with stress ulceration after head trauma (Cushing's ulcer) and severe burns (Curling's ulcer), mucosal ischemia and breakdown of the normal protective barriers of the stomach also play an important role in the pathogenesis. Acid must contribute to injury in view of the significant drop in bleeding noted when acid inhibitors are used as a prophylactic measure for stress gastritis.

Improvement in the general management of intensive care unit patients has led to a significant decrease in the incidence of gastrointestinal bleeding due to stress ulceration. The estimated decrease in bleeding is from 20 to 30% to <5%. This improvement has led to some debate regarding the need for prophylactic therapy. The limited benefit of medical (endoscopic, angiographic) and surgical therapy in

a patient with hemodynamically compromising bleeding associated with stress ulcer/gastritis supports the use of preventive measures in high-risk patients (mechanically ventilated, coagulopathy, multiorgan failure, or severe burns). Maintenance of gastric pH > 3.5 with continuous infusion of H_2 blockers or liquid antacids administered every 2 to 3 h are viable options. Sucralfate slurry (1 g every 4 to 6 h) has also been successful. If bleeding occurs despite these measures, endoscopy, intraarterial vasopressin, or embolization are options. If all else fails, then surgery should be considered. Although vagotomy and antrectomy may be used, the better approach would be a total gastrectomy, which has an exceedingly high mortality rate in this setting.

GASTRITIS The term *gastritis* should be reserved for histologically documented inflammation of the gastric mucosa. Gastritis is not the mucosal erythema seen during endoscopy and is not interchangeable with "dyspepsia." The etiologic factors leading to gastritis are broad and heterogeneous. Gastritis has been classified based on time course (acute vs. chronic), histologic features, and anatomical distribution or proposed pathogenic mechanism (Table 274-7).

The correlation between the histologic findings of gastritis, the clinical picture of abdominal pain or dyspepsia, and endoscopic findings noted on gross inspection of the gastric mucosa is poor. Therefore, there is no typical clinical manifestation of gastritis.

Acute Gastritis The most common causes of acute gastritis are infectious. Acute infection with *H. pylori* induces gastritis. However, *H. pylori* acute gastritis has not been extensively studied. Reported as presenting with sudden onset of epigastric pain, nausea, and vomiting, limited mucosal histologic studies demonstrate a marked infiltrate of neutrophils with edema and hyperemia. If not treated, this picture will evolve into one of chronic gastritis. Hypochlorhydria lasting for up to 1 year may follow acute *H. pylori* infection.

The highly acidic gastric environment may be one reason why infectious processes of the stomach are rare. Bacterial infection of the stomach or phlegmonous gastritis is a rare potentially life-threatening disorder, characterized by marked and diffuse acute inflammatory infiltrates of the entire gastric wall, at times accompanied by necrosis. Elderly individuals, alcoholics, and AIDS patients may be affected. Potential iatrogenic causes include polypectomy and mucosal injection with India ink. Organisms associated with this entity include streptococci, staphylococci, *Escherichia coli*, *Proteus*, and *Haemophilus* sp. Failure of supportive measures and antibiotics may result in gastrectomy.

Other types of infectious gastritis may occur in immunocompromised individuals such as AIDS patients. Examples include herpetic (herpes simplex) or CMV gastritis. The histologic finding of intranuclear inclusions would be observed in the latter.

Chronic Gastritis Chronic gastritis is identified histologically by an inflammatory cell infiltrate consisting primarily of lymphocytes and plasma cells, with very scant neutrophil involvement. Distribution of the inflammation may be patchy, initially involving superficial and glandular portions of the gastric mucosa. This picture may progress to more severe glandular destruction, with atrophy and metaplasia.

TABLE 274-7   Classification of Gastritis

I. Acute gastritis	II. Chronic atrophic gastritis
A. Acute *H. pylori* infection	A. Type A: Autoimmune, body-predominant
B. Other acute infectious gastritides	B. Type B: *H. pylori*–related, antral-predominant
1. Bacterial (other than *H. pylori*)	C. Indeterminant
2. *Helicobacter helmanni*	III. Uncommon Forms of Gastritis
3. Phlegmonous	A. Lymphocytic
4. Mycobacterial	B. Eosinophilic
5. Syphilitic	C. Crohn's disease
6. Viral	D. Sarcoidosis
7. Parasitic	E. Isolated granulomatous gastritis
8. Fungal	

Chronic gastritis has been classified according to histologic characteristics. These include superficial atrophic changes and gastric atrophy.

The early phase of chronic gastritis is *superficial gastritis*. The inflammatory changes are limited to the lamina propria of the surface mucosa, with edema and cellular infiltrates separating intact gastric glands. Additional findings may include decreased mucus in the mucous cells and decreased mitotic figures in the glandular cells. The next stage is *atrophic gastritis*. The inflammatory infiltrate extends deeper into the mucosa, with progressive distortion and destruction of the glands. The final stage of chronic gastritis is *gastric atrophy*. Glandular structures are lost; there is a paucity of inflammatory infiltrates. Endoscopically the mucosa may be substantially thin, permitting clear visualization of the underlying blood vessels.

Gastric glands may undergo morphologic transformation in chronic gastritis. Intestinal metaplasia denotes the conversion of gastric glands to a small intestinal phenotype with small-bowel mucosal glands containing goblet cells. The metaplastic changes may vary in distribution from patchy to fairly extensive gastric involvement. Intestinal metaplasia is an important predisposing factor for gastric cancer (Chap. 77).

Chronic gastritis is also classified according to the predominant site of involvement. Type A refers to the body-predominant form (autoimmune) and type B is the central-predominant form (*H. pylori*-related). This classification is artificial in view of the difficulty in distinguishing these two entities. The term *AB gastritis* has been used to refer to a mixed antral/body picture.

TYPE A GASTRITIS The less common of the two forms involves primarily the fundus and body, with antral sparing. Traditionally, this form of gastritis has been associated with pernicious anemia (Chap. 92) in the presence of circulating antibodies against parietal cells and IF; thus it is also called *autoimmune gastritis*. *H. pylori* infection can lead to a similar distribution of gastritis. The characteristics of an autoimmune picture are not always present.

Antibodies to parietal cells have been detected in >90% of patients with pernicious anemia and in up to 50% of patients with type A gastritis. The parietal cell antibody is directed against H^+,K^+-ATPase. T cells are also implicated in the injury pattern of this form of gastritis.

Parietal cell antibodies and atrophic gastritis are observed in family members of patients with pernicious anemia. These antibodies are observed in up to 20% of individuals over age 60 and in ~20% of patients with vitiligo and Addison's disease. About half of patients with pernicious anemia have antibodies to thyroid antigens, and about 30% of patients with thyroid disease have circulating anti-parietal cell antibodies. Anti-IF antibodies are more specific than parietal cell antibodies for type A gastritis, being present in ~40% of patients with pernicious anemia. Another parameter consistent with this form of gastritis being autoimmune in origin is the higher incidence of specific familial histocompatibility haplotypes such as HLA-B8 and -DR3.

The parietal cell–containing gastric gland is preferentially targeted in this form of gastritis, and achlorhydria results. Parietal cells are the source of IF, lack of which will lead to vitamin B_{12} deficiency and its sequelae (megaloblastic anemia, neurologic dysfunction).

Gastric acid plays an important role in feedback inhibition of gastrin release from G cells. Achlorhydria, coupled with relative sparing of the antral mucosa (site of G cells), leads to hypergastrinemia. Gastrin levels can be markedly elevated (>500 pg/mL) in patients with pernicious anemia. ECL cell hyperplasia with frank development of gastric carcinoid tumors may result from gastrin trophic effects. The role of gastrin in carcinoid development is confirmed by the observation that antrectomy leads to regression of these lesions. Hypergastrinemia and achlorhydria may also be seen in non-pernicious anemia–associated type A gastritis.

TYPE B GASTRITIS Type B, or antral-predominant, gastritis is the more common form of chronic gastritis. *H. pylori* infection is the cause of this entity. Although described as "antral-predominant," this is likely a misnomer in view of studies documenting the progression of the inflammatory process towards the body and fundus of infected indi-

viduals. The conversion to a pan-gastritis is time-dependent—estimated to require 15 to 20 years. This form of gastritis increases with age, being present in up to 100% of persons over age 70. Histology improves after *H. pylori* eradication. The number of *H. pylori* organisms decreases dramatically with progression to gastric atrophy, and the degree of inflammation correlates with the level of these organisms. Early on, with antral-predominant findings, the quantity of *H. pylori* is highest and a dense chronic inflammatory infiltrate of the lamina propria is noted accompanied by epithelial cell infiltration with polymorphonuclear leukocytes (Fig. 274-12).

Multifocal atrophic gastritis, gastric atrophy with subsequent metaplasia, has been observed in chronic *H. pylori*–induced gastritis. This may ultimately lead to development of gastric adenocarcinoma (Fig. 274-8; Chap. 77). *H. pylori* infection is now considered an independent risk factor for gastric cancer. Worldwide epidemiologic studies have documented a higher incidence of *H. pylori* infection in patients with adenocarcinoma of the stomach as compared to control subjects. Seropositivity for *H. pylori* is associated with a three- to sixfold increased risk of gastric cancer. This risk may be as high as ninefold after adjusting for the inaccuracy of serologic testing in the elderly. The mechanism by which *H. pylori* infection leads to cancer is unknown. However, eradication of *H. pylori* as a general preventative measure for gastric cancer is not recommended.

Infection with *H. pylori* is also associated with development of a low-grade B cell lymphoma, gastric MALT lymphoma (Chap. 97).

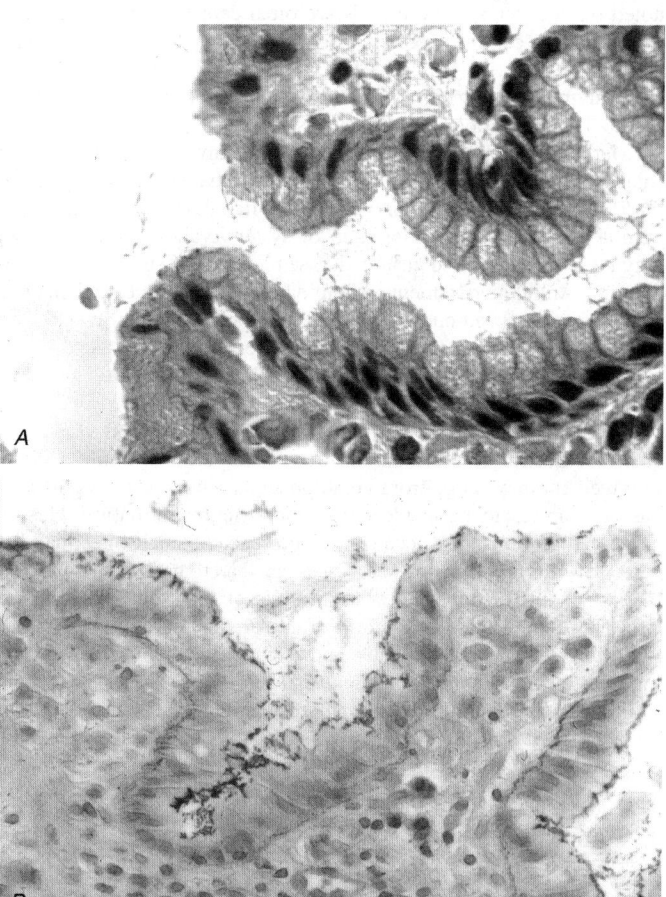

FIGURE 274-12 Chronic gastritis and *Helicobacter pylori* organisms. *A*. H&E stain of gastric mucosa showing surface foveolar cells, adherent mucus, and scattered bacillary forms within the mucus. *B*. Steiner silver stain of superficial gastric mucosa, showing abundant darkly staining microorganisms layered over the apical portion of the surface epithelium. Note that there is no tissue invasion. [*Courtesy of James M. Crawford, M.D., Ph.D. Reprinted with permission from JM Crawford, in V Kumar et al (eds): Basic Pathology. Philadelphia, Saunders, 1997.*]

The chronic T cell stimulation caused by the infection leads to production of cytokines that promote the B cell tumor. Tumor growth remains dependent upon the presence of *H. pylori* in that its eradication is often associated with complete regression of the tumor. The tumor may take more than a year to regress after treating the infection. Such patients should be followed by EUS every 2 to 3 months. If the tumor is stable or decreasing in size, no other therapy is necessary. If the tumor grows, it may have become a high-grade B cell lymphoma. When the tumor becomes a high-grade aggressive lymphoma histologically, it loses responsiveness to *H. pylori* eradication.

Rx TREATMENT

Treatment in chronic gastritis is aimed at the sequelae and not the underlying inflammation. Patients with pernicious anemia will require parenteral vitamin B_{12} supplementation on a long-term basis. Eradication of *H. pylori* is not routinely recommended unless PUD or a low-grade MALT lymphoma is present.

Miscellaneous Forms of Gastritis Lymphocytic gastritis is characterized histologically by intense infiltration of the surface epithelium with lymphocytes. The infiltrative process is primarily in the body of the stomach and consists of mature T cells and plasmacytes. The etiology of this form of chronic gastritis is unknown. It has been described in patients with celiac sprue, but whether there is a common factor associating these two entities is unknown. No specific symptoms suggest lymphocytic gastritis. A subgroup of patients have thickened folds noted on endoscopy. These folds are often capped by small nodules that contain a central depression or erosion; this form of the disease is called *varioliform gastritis*. *H. pylori* probably plays no significant role in lymphocytic gastritis. Therapy with glucocorticoids or sodium cromoglycate has obtained unclear results.

Marked eosinophilic infiltration involving any layer of the stomach (mucosa, muscularis propria, and serosa) is characteristic of *eosinophilic gastritis*. Affected individuals will often have circulating eosinophilia with clinical manifestation of systemic allergy. Involvement may range from isolated gastric disease to diffuse eosinophilic gastroenteritis. Antral involvement predominates, with prominent edematous folds being observed on endoscopy. These prominent antral folds can lead to outlet obstruction. Patients can present with epigastric discomfort, nausea, and vomiting. Treatment with glucocorticoids has been successful.

Several systemic disorders may be associated with *granulomatous gastritis*. Gastric involvement has been observed in Crohn's disease. Involvement may range from granulomatous infiltrates noted only on gastric biopsies to frank ulceration and stricture formation. Gastric Crohn's disease usually occurs in the presence of small-intestinal disease. Several rare infectious processes can lead to granulomatous gastritis, including histoplasmosis, candidiasis, syphilis, and tuberculosis. Other unusual causes of this form of gastritis include sarcoidosis, idiopathic granulomatous gastritis, and eosinophilic granulomas involving the stomach. Establishing the specific etiologic agent in this form of gastritis can be difficult, at times requiring repeat endoscopy with biopsy and cytology. Occasionally, a surgically obtained full-thickness biopsy of the stomach may be required to exclude malignancy.

MÉNÉTRIER'S DISEASE Ménétrier's disease is a rare entity characterized by large, tortuous gastric mucosal folds. The differential diagnosis of large gastric folds includes ZES, malignancy, infectious etiologies (CMV, histoplasmosis, syphilis), and infiltrative disorders such as sarcoidosis. The mucosal folds in Ménétrier's disease are often most prominent in the body and fundus. Histologically, massive foveolar hyperplasia (hyperplasia of surface and glandular mucous cells) is noted, which replaces most of the chief and parietal cells. This hyperplasia produces the prominent folds observed. The pits of the gastric glands elongate and may become extremely tortuous. Although the lamina propria may contain a mild chronic inflammatory infiltrate, Ménétrier's disease is not considered a form of gastritis. The etiology of this unusual clinical picture is unknown. Overexpression of growth factors such as TGF-α may be involved in the process.

Epigastric pain at times accompanied by nausea, vomiting, anorexia, and weight loss are signs and symptoms in patients with Ménétrier's disease. Occult gastrointestinal bleeding may occur, but overt bleeding is unusual and, when present, is due to superficial mucosal erosions. Twenty to 100% of patients (depending on time of presentation) develop a protein-losing gastropathy accompanied by hypoalbuminemia and edema. Gastric acid secretion is usually reduced or absent because of the replacement of parietal cells. Large gastric folds are readily detectable by either radiographic (barium meal) or endoscopic methods. Endoscopy with deep mucosal biopsy (and cytology) is required to establish the diagnosis and exclude other entities that may present similarly. A nondiagnostic biopsy may lead to a surgically obtained full-thickness biopsy to exclude malignancy.

Rx TREATMENT

Medical therapy with anticholinergic agents, prostaglandins, PPIs, prednisone, and H_2 receptor antagonists has obtained varying results. Anticholinergics decrease protein loss. A high-protein diet should be recommended to replace protein loss in patients with hypoalbuminemia. Ulcers should be treated with a standard approach. Severe disease with persistent and substantial protein loss may require total gastrectomy. Subtotal gastrectomy is performed by some; it may be associated with higher morbidity and mortality secondary to the difficulty in obtaining a patent and long-lasting anastomosis between normal and hyperplastic tissues.

ACKNOWLEDGMENT
The author acknowledges the contribution of material to this chapter by Dr. Lawrence Friedman and Dr. Walter Peterson from their chapter on this subject in the 14th edition of Harrison's.

FURTHER READING

CHAN FK et al: Preventing recurrent upper gastrointestinal bleeding in patients with *Helicobacter pylori* infection who are taking low-dose aspirin or naproxen. N Engl J Med 344:967, 2001

CHAN FKL, LEUNG WK: Peptic-ulcer disease. Lancet 360:933, 2002

——— et al: Celecoxib versus diclofenac and omeprazole in reducing the risk of recurrent ulcer bleeding in patients with arthritis. N Engl J Med 347:2104, 2002

LAI KC et al: Lansoprazole for the prevention of recurrences of ulcer complications from long-term low-dose aspirin use. N Engl J Med 346:2033, 2002

LAINE L: Approaches to nonsteroidal anti-inflammatory drug use in the high-risk patient. Gastroenterology 120:594, 2001

———: Gastrointestinal effects of NSAIDs and coxibs. J Pain Symptom Manage 25 (suppl 2):532, 2003

MOAYYEDI P et al: An update of the Cothrane systematic review of *Helicobacter pylori* eradication therapy in nonulcer dyspepsia: Resolving the discrepancy between systematic reviews. Am J Gastroenterol 98:2621, 2003

ROY PK et al: Gastric secretion in Zollinger-Ellison syndrome. Correlation with clinical expression, tumor extent and role in diagnosis—a prospective NIH study of 235 patients and a review of 984 cases in the literature. Medicine (Baltimore) 80:189, 2001

SUERBAUM S, MICHETTI P: *Helicobacter pylori* infection. N Engl J Med 347:1175, 2002

UEMURA N et al: *Helicobacter pylori* infection and the development of gastric cancer. N Engl J Med 345:784, 2001

275 DISORDERS OF ABSORPTION
Henry J. Binder

Disorders of absorption constitute a broad spectrum of conditions with multiple etiologies and varied clinical manifestations. Almost all of these clinical problems are associated with *diminished* intestinal absorption of one or more dietary nutrients and are often referred to as the *malabsorption syndrome*. This latter term is not ideal as it represents a pathophysiologic state, does *not* provide an etiologic explanation for the underlying problem, and should not be considered an adequate final diagnosis. The only clinical situations in which absorption is *increased* are hemochromatosis and Wilson's disease, in which there is increased absorption of iron and copper, respectively.

Most, but not all, of these clinical conditions are associated with *steatorrhea*, an increase in stool fat excretion of >6% of dietary fat intake. Some disorders of absorption are not associated with steatorrhea: Primary lactase deficiency, which represents a congenital absence of the small intestinal brush border disaccharidase enzyme lactase, is associated with lactose "malabsorption," and pernicious anemia is associated with a marked decrease in intestinal absorption of cobalamin (vitamin B_{12}) due to an absence of gastric parietal cell intrinsic factor required for cobalamin absorption.

Disorders of absorption must be included in the differential diagnosis of diarrhea (Chap. 35). First, diarrhea is frequently associated with and/or is a consequence of the diminished absorption of one or more dietary nutrients. The diarrhea may be secondary either to the intestinal process that is responsible for the steatorrhea or to steatorrhea per se. Thus, celiac sprue (see below) is associated with both extensive morphologic changes in the small intestinal mucosa and reduced absorption of several dietary nutrients; in contrast, the diarrhea of steatorrhea is the result of the effect of nonabsorbed dietary fatty acids on intestinal, usually colonic, ion transport. For example, oleic acid and ricinoleic acid (a bacterially hydroxylated fatty acid that is also the active ingredient in castor oil, a widely used laxative) induce active colonic Cl ion secretion, most likely secondary to increasing intracellular Ca. In addition, diarrhea per se may result in mild steatorrhea (<11 g fat excretion while on a 100-g fat diet). Second, as diarrhea is both a symptom and a sign, most patients will indicate that they have diarrhea, not that they have fat malabsorption. Third, many intestinal disorders that have diarrhea as a prominent symptom (e.g., ulcerative colitis, traveler's diarrhea secondary to an enterotoxin produced by *Escherichia coli*) do not necessarily have diminished absorption of any dietary nutrient.

Diarrhea as a *symptom* (i.e., when used by patients to describe their bowel movement pattern) may be either a decrease in stool consistency, an increase in stool volume, an increase in number of bowel movements, or any combination of these three changes. In contrast, diarrhea as a *sign* is a quantitative increase in stool water or weight of >200 to 225 mL, or gram per 24 h, when a western-type diet is consumed. Individuals consuming a diet with a higher fiber content may normally have a stool weight of up to 400 g per 24 h. Thus, the clinician must clarify what an individual patient means by diarrhea. Some 10% of patients referred to gastroenterologists for further evaluation of unexplained diarrhea do not have an increase in stool water when it is determined quantitatively. Such patients may have small, frequent, somewhat loose bowel movements with stool urgency that is indicative of proctitis but do not have an increase in stool weight or volume.

It is also critical to establish whether a patient's diarrhea is secondary to diminished absorption of one or more dietary nutrients, in contrast to diarrhea that is due to small- and/or large-intestinal fluid and electrolyte secretion. The former has often been termed *osmotic diarrhea*, while the latter has been referred to as *secretory diarrhea*. Unfortunately, both secretory and osmotic elements can be present simultaneously in the same disorder; thus, this separation is not always precise. Nonetheless, two studies—determination of stool electrolytes and observation of the effect of a fast on stool output—can help make this distinction.

The demonstration of the effect of prolonged (>24 h) fasting on stool output can be very effective in suggesting that a *dietary nutrient* is responsible for the individual's diarrhea. A secretory diarrhea associated with enterotoxin-induced traveler's diarrhea would not be affected by prolonged fasting, as enterotoxin-induced stimulation of intestinal fluid and electrolyte secretion is not altered by eating. In contrast, diarrhea secondary to lactose malabsorption in primary lactase deficiency would undoubtedly cease during a prolonged fast. Thus, a substantial decrease in stool output while fasting during a quantitative stool collection of at least 24 h is presumptive evidence that the diarrhea is related to malabsorption of a dietary nutrient. The persistence of stool output while fasting indicates that the diarrhea is likely secretory and that the cause of diarrhea is *not* due to a dietary nutrient. Either a luminal (e.g., *E. coli* enterotoxin) or circulating (e.g., vasoactive intestinal peptide) secretagogue could be responsible for the patient's diarrhea persisting unaltered during a prolonged fast. The observed effects of fasting can be compared and correlated with stool electrolyte and osmolality determinations.

Measurement of stool electrolytes and osmolality requires the comparison of stool Na^+ and K^+ concentrations determined in liquid stool to the stool osmolality to determine the presence or absence of a so-called stool osmotic gap. The following formula is used:

$$2 \times (\text{stool } [Na^+] + \text{stool } [K^+]) \leq \text{stool osmolality}$$

The cation concentrations are doubled to estimate stool anion concentrations. The presence of a significant osmotic gap suggests the presence in stool water of a substance (or substances) other than Na/K/ anions that presumably is responsible for the patient's diarrhea. Originally, stool osmolality was measured, but it is almost invariably greater than the required 290 to 300 mosmol/kg H_2O, reflecting bacterial degradation of nonabsorbed carbohydrate either immediately before defecation or in the stool jar while awaiting chemical analysis, even when the stool is refrigerated. As a result, the stool osmolality should be assumed to be 300 mosmol/kg H_2O. When the calculated difference is >50, an osmotic gap is present, suggesting that the diarrhea is due to a nonabsorbed dietary nutrient, e.g., a fatty acid and/ or carbohydrate. When this difference is <25, it is presumed that a dietary nutrient is not responsible for the diarrhea. Since elements of both osmotic (i.e., malabsorption of a dietary nutrient) and secretory diarrhea may be present, this separation at times is less clear-cut at the bedside than when used as a teaching example. Ideally, the presence of an osmotic gap will be associated with a marked decrease in stool output during a prolonged fast, while the absence of an osmotic gap will likely be present in an individual whose stool output had not been reduced substantially during a period of fasting.

NUTRIENT DIGESTION AND ABSORPTION

The lengths of the small intestine and colon are ~300 cm and ~80 cm, respectively. However, the effective functional surface area is approximately 600-fold greater than that of a hollow tube as a result of the presence of folds, villi (in the small intestine), and microvilli. The functional surface area of the small intestine is somewhat greater than that of a doubles tennis court. In addition to nutrient digestion and absorption, the intestinal epithelia have several other functions:

1. *Barrier and immune defense.* The intestine is exposed to a large number of potential antigens and enteric and invasive microorganisms, and it is extremely effective preventing the entry of almost all these agents. The intestinal mucosa also synthesizes and secretes secretory IgA.
2. *Fluid and electrolyte absorption and secretion.* The intestine absorbs ~7 to 8 L of fluid daily, comprising dietary fluid intake (1 to 2 L/d) and salivary, gastric, pancreatic, biliary, and intestinal fluid (6 to 7 L/d). The intestine also responds to several stimuli, especially bacteria and bacterial enterotoxins, that induce fluid and electrolyte secretion, often leading to diarrhea (Chap. 113).
3. *Synthesis and secretion of several proteins.* The intestinal mucosa

is a major site for the production of proteins, including apolipo-proteins.

4. *Production of several bioactive amines and peptides*. The intestine is one of the largest endocrine organs in the body and produces several amines and peptides that serve as paracrine and hormonal mediators of intestinal function.

The small and large intestine are anatomically distinct in that villi are present in the small intestine but are absent in the colon and functionally distinct in that nutrient digestion and absorption take place in the small intestine but not in the colon. No precise anatomical characteristics separate duodenum, jejunum, and ileum, although certain nutrients are absorbed exclusively in specific areas of the small intestine. However, villus cells in the small intestine (and surface epithelial cells in the colon) and crypt cells have distinct anatomical and functional characteristics. Intestinal epithelial cells are continuously renewed, with new proliferating epithelial cells at the base of the crypt migrating over 48 to 72 h to the tip of the villus (or surface of the colon), where they are well-developed epithelial cells with digestive and absorptive function. This high rate of cell turnover explains the relatively rapid resolution of diarrhea and other digestive tract side effects during chemotherapy as new cells not exposed to these toxic agents are produced. Equally important is the paradigm of separation of villus/surface cell and crypt cell function: digestive hydrolytic enzymes are present primarily in the brush border of villus epithelial cells. Absorptive and secretory functions are also separated, with villus/surface cells primarily, but not exclusively, being the site for absorptive function, while secretory function is present in crypts of both the small and large intestine.

Nutrients, minerals, and vitamins are absorbed by one or more active transport mechanisms. (The mechanisms of intestinal fluid and electrolyte absorption and secretion are discussed in Chap. 35.) Active transport mechanisms are energy-dependent and mediated by membrane transport proteins. These transport processes will result in the *net* movement of a substance against or in the absence of an electrochemical concentration gradient. Intestinal absorption of amino acids and monosaccharides, e.g., glucose, is also a specialized form of active transport—*secondary active transport*. The movement of these actively transported nutrients against a concentration gradient is Na^+-dependent and is due to a Na^+ gradient across the apical membrane. The Na^+ gradient is maintained by Na^+,K^+-ATPase, the so-called Na^+ pump located on the basolateral membrane, which extrudes Na^+ and maintains a low intracellular [Na] as well as the Na^+ gradient across the apical membrane. As a result, active glucose absorption and glucose-stimulated Na^+ absorption require both the apical membrane transport protein, SGLT, and the basolateral Na^+,K^+-ATPase. In addition to glucose absorption being Na^+-dependent, glucose also stimulates Na^+ and fluid absorption, which is the physiologic basis of oral rehydration therapy for the treatment of diarrhea (Chap. 35).

Although the intestinal epithelial cells are crucial mediators of absorption and ion and water flow, the several cell types in the lamina propria (e.g., mast cells, macrophages, myofibroblasts) and the enteric nervous system interact with the epithelium to regulate mucosal cell function. The function of the intestine is the result of the integrated responses of and interactions between both intestinal epithelial cells and intestinal muscle.

ENTEROHEPATIC CIRCULATION OF BILE ACIDS Bile acids are not present in the diet but are synthesized in the liver by a series of enzymatic steps that also include cholesterol catabolism. Indeed, interruption of the enterohepatic circulation of bile acids can reduce serum cholesterol levels by 10% before a new steady state is established. Bile acids are either primary or secondary: primary bile acids are synthesized in the liver from cholesterol, and secondary bile acids are synthesized from primary bile acids in the intestine by colonic bacterial enzymes. The two primary bile acids in humans are cholic acid and chenodeoxycholic acid; the two most abundant secondary bile acids are deoxycholic

acid and lithocholic acid. Approximately 500 mg bile acids are synthesized in the liver daily, conjugated to either taurine or glycine to form tauro-conjugated or glyco-conjugated bile acids, respectively, and are secreted into the duodenum in bile. The primary functions of bile acids are (1) to promote bile flow, (2) to solubilize cholesterol and phospholipid in the gallbladder by mixed micelle formation, and (3) to enhance dietary lipid digestion and absorption by forming mixed micelles in the proximal small intestine.

Bile acids are primarily absorbed by an active, Na^+-dependent process that is located exclusively in the ileum, though bile acids can also be absorbed to a lesser extent by non-carrier-mediated transport processes in the jejunum, ileum, and colon. Conjugated bile acids that enter the colon are deconjugated by colonic bacterial enzymes to unconjugated bile acids and are rapidly absorbed. Colonic bacterial enzymes also dehydroxylate bile acids to secondary bile acids.

Bile acids absorbed from the intestine return to the liver via the portal vein where they are resecreted (Fig. 275-1). Bile acid synthesis is largely autoregulated by 7α-hydroxylase, the initial enzyme in cholesterol degradation. A decrease in the amount of bile acids returning to the liver from the intestine is associated with an increase in bile acid synthesis/cholesterol catabolism, which helps keep the bile acid pool size relatively constant. However, there is a relatively limited capacity for an increase in bile acid synthesis—about two to two and one-half times (see below). The bile acid pool size is approximately 4 g and is circulated via the enterohepatic circulation about twice during each meal, or six to eight times during a 24-h period. A relatively small quantity of bile acids is not absorbed and is excreted in stool daily; this fecal loss is matched by hepatic bile acid synthesis.

Defects in any of the steps of the enterohepatic circulation of bile acids can result in a decrease in duodenal concentration of conjugated bile acids and, as a result, steatorrhea. Thus, steatorrhea can be caused by abnormalities in bile acid synthesis and excretion, their physical state in the intestinal lumen, and reabsorption (Table 275-1).

Synthesis Decreased bile acid synthesis and steatorrhea have been demonstrated in chronic liver disease, but steatorrhea is often not a major component of the illness of these patients.

Secretion Although bile acid secretion may be reduced or absent in biliary obstruction, steatorrhea is rarely a significant medical problem in these patients. In contrast, primary biliary cirrhosis represents a

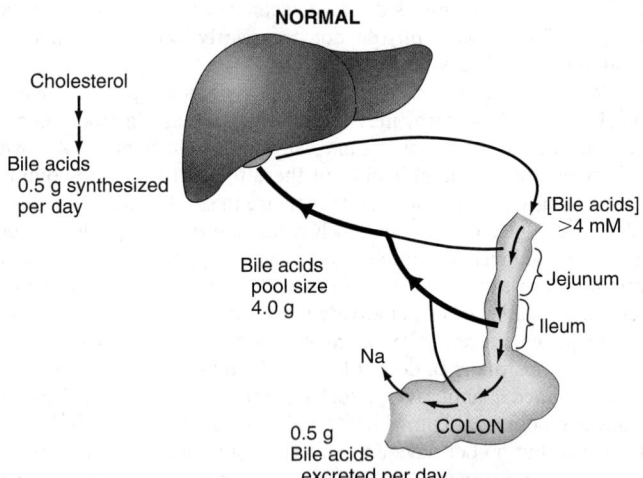

FIGURE 275-1 Schematic representation of the enterohepatic circulation of bile acids. Bile acid synthesis is cholesterol catabolism and occurs in the liver. Bile acids are secreted in bile and are stored in the gallbladder between meals and at night. Food in the duodenum induces the release of cholecystokinin, which is a potent stimulus for gallbladder contraction resulting in bile acid entry into the duodenum. Bile acids are primarily absorbed via a Na-dependent transport process that is located only in the ileum. A relatively small quantity of bile acids (~500 mg) is not absorbed in a 24-h period and is lost in stool. Fecal bile acid losses are matched by bile acid synthesis. The bile acid pool, i.e., the total amount of bile acids in the body at any time, is ~4 g and is circulated twice during each meal or six to eight times in a 24-h period.

TABLE 275-1 Defects in Enterohepatic Circulation of Bile Acids

Process	Pathophysiologic Defect	Disease Example
Synthesis	Decreased hepatic function	Cirrhosis
Biliary secretion	Altered canalicular function	Primary biliary cirrhosis
Maintenance of conjugated bile acids	Bacterial overgrowth	Jejunal diverticulosis
Reabsorption	Abnormal ileal function	Crohn's disease

defect in canalicular excretion of organic anions, including bile acids, and not infrequently is associated with steatorrhea and its consequences, e.g., chronic bone disease. Thus, the osteomalacia and other chronic bone abnormalities often present in patients with primary biliary cirrhosis and other cholestatic syndromes are secondary to steatorrhea that then leads to calcium and vitamin D malabsorption.

Maintenance of Conjugated Bile Acids In bacterial overgrowth syndromes associated with diarrhea, steatorrhea, and macrocytic anemia, there is an increase in a colonic type of bacterial flora in the small intestine. The steatorrhea is primarily a result of the decrease in conjugated bile acids secondary to their deconjugation by colonic-type bacteria. Two complementary explanations account for the resulting impairment of micelle formation: (1) unconjugated bile acids are rapidly absorbed in the jejunum by nonionic diffusion, resulting in a reduced concentration of duodenal bile acids; and (2) the critical micellar concentration (CMC) of unconjugated bile acids is higher than that of conjugated bile acids, and therefore unconjugated bile acids are less effective than conjugated bile acids in micelle formation.

Reabsorption Ileal dysfunction caused by either Crohn's disease or surgical resection results in a decrease in bile acid reabsorption in the ileum and an *increase* in the delivery of bile acids to the large intestine. The resulting clinical consequences—diarrhea with or without steatorrhea—are determined by the *degree* of ileal dysfunction and the *response* of the enterohepatic circulation to bile acid losses (Table 275-2). Patients with limited ileal disease or resection will often have diarrhea, but not steatorrhea. The diarrhea, a result of bile acids in the colon stimulating active Cl secretion, has been called *bile acid diarrhea*, or cholorrheic enteropathy, and responds promptly to cholestyramine, an anion-binding resin. Such patients do not develop steatorrhea because hepatic synthesis of bile acids increases to compensate for the rate of fecal bile acid losses, resulting in maintenance of both the bile acid pool size and the intraduodenal concentrations of bile acids. In contrast, patients with greater degrees of ileal disease and/or resection will often have diarrhea and steatorrhea that do not respond to cholestyramine. In this situation, ileal disease is also associated with increased amounts of bile acids entering the colon; however, hepatic synthesis can no longer increase sufficiently to maintain the bile acid pool size. As a consequence, the intraduodenal concentration of bile acids is also reduced to less than the CMC, resulting in impaired micelle formation and steatorrhea. This second situation is often called *fatty acid diarrhea*. Although cholestyramine may not be effective (and may even increase the diarrhea by further depleting the intraduodenal bile acid concentration), a low-fat diet to reduce fatty acids entering the colon can be effective. Two clinical features, the length

TABLE 275-2 Comparison of Bile Acid and Fatty Acid Diarrhea

	Bile Acid Diarrhea	Fatty Acid Diarrhea
Extent of ileal disease	Limited	Extensive
Ileal bile acid absorption	Reduced	Reduced
Fecal bile acid excretion	Increased	Increased
Fecal bile acid loss compensated by hepatic synthesis	Yes	No
Bile acid pool size	Normal	Reduced
Intraduodenal [bile acid]	Normal	Reduced
Steatorrhea	None or mild	>20 g
Response to cholestyramine	Yes	No
Response to low-fat diet	No	Yes

TABLE 275-3 Comparison of Different Types of Fatty Acids

	Long-Chain	Medium-Chain	Short-Chain
Carbon chain length	>12	8–12	<8
Present in diet	In large amounts	In small amounts	No
Origin	In diet as triglycerides	Only in small amounts in diet as triglycerides	Bacterial degradation in colon of nonabsorbed carbohydrate to fatty acids
Primary site of absorption	Small intestine	Small intestine	Colon
Requires pancreatic lipolysis	Yes	No	No
Requires micelle formation	Yes	No	No
Presence in stool	Minimal	No	Substantial

of ileum removed and the degree of steatorrhea, can predict whether an individual patient will respond to cholestyramine. Unfortunately, these predictors are imperfect, and a therapeutic trial of cholestyramine is often necessary to establish whether an individual patient will benefit from cholestyramine. Table 275-2 contrasts the characteristics of bile acid diarrhea (small ileal dysfunction) and fatty acid diarrhea (large ileal dysfunction).

LIPIDS Steatorrhea is caused by one or more defects in the digestion and absorption of dietary fat. Average intake of dietary fat in the United States is approximately 120 to 150 g/d, and fat absorption is linear to dietary fat intake. The total load of fat presented to the small intestine is considerably greater, as substantial amounts of lipid are secreted in bile each day. (See above for discussion of enterohepatic circulation of bile acids.) Three types of fatty acids compose fats: long-chain fatty acids (LCFAs), medium-chain fatty acids (MCFAs), and short-chain fatty acids (SCFAs) (Table 275-3). Dietary fat is exclusively composed of long-chain triglycerides (LCTs), i.e., glycerol that is bound via ester-linkages to three LCFAs. While the majority of dietary LCFAs have carbon chain lengths of 16 or 18, fatty acids of carbon chain length >12 are metabolized in the same manner; saturated and unsaturated fatty acids are handled identically.

Assimilation of dietary lipid requires several integrated processes that can be divided into (1) an intraluminal, or digestive, phase; (2) a mucosal, or absorptive, phase; and (3) a delivery, or postabsorptive, phase. An abnormality at any site of this process can cause steatorrhea (Table 275-4). Therefore, it is essential that any patient with steatorrhea be evaluated to identify the specific physiologic defect in overall

TABLE 275-4 Defects in Lipid Digestion and Absorption in Steatorrhea

Phase: Process	Pathophysiologic Defect	Disease Example
Digestive		
Lipolysis formation	Decrease lipase secretion	Chronic pancreatitis
Micelle formation	Decreased intraduodenal [bile acids]	See Table 275-1
Absorptive		
Mucosal uptake and resterification	Mucosal dysfunction	Celiac sprue
Post-absorptive		
Chylomicron formation	Absent betalipoproteins	Abetalipoproteinemia
Delivery from intestine	Abnormal lymphatics	Intestinal lymphangiectasia

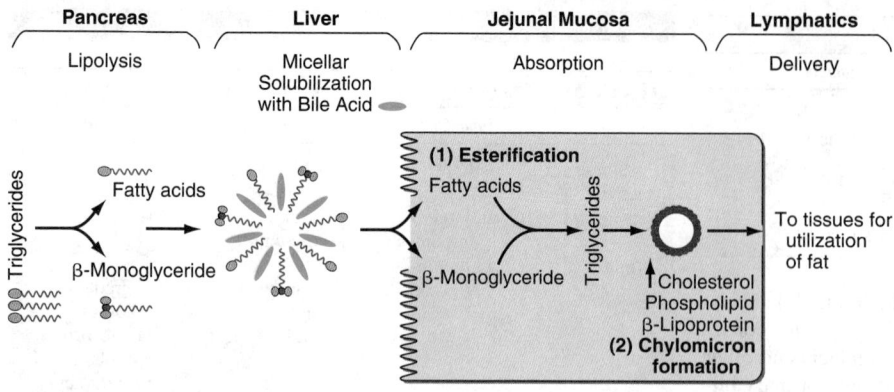

Pancreas	Liver	Jejunal Mucosa	Lymphatics
Lipolysis	Micellar Solubilization with Bile Acid	Absorption	Delivery

FIGURE 275-2 Schematic representation of lipid digestion and absorption. Dietary lipid is in the form of long-chain triglycerides (LCTs). The overall process can be divided into (1) a digestive phase that includes both lipolysis and micelle formation requiring pancreatic lipase and conjugated bile acids, respectively, in the duodenum; (2) an absorptive phase for mucosal uptake and reesterification; and (3) a postabsorptive phase that includes chylomicron formation and exit from the intestinal epithelial cell via lymphatics. *(Courtesy of John M. Dietschy, MD.)*

lipid digestion-absorption as therapy will be determined by the specific cause responsible for the steatorrhea.

The digestive phase has two components, *lipolysis* and *micellar formation*. Although dietary lipid is in the form of LCTs, the intestinal mucosa does not absorb triglycerides; they must first be hydrolyzed (Fig. 275-2). The initial step in lipid digestion is the formation of emulsions of finely dispersed lipid, which is accomplished by mastication and gastric contractions. Lipolysis, the hydrolysis of triglycerides to free fatty acids, monoglycerides, and glycerol by lipase, is initiated in the stomach by a gastric lipase that has a pH optimum of 4.5 to 6.0. About 20 to 30% of total lipolysis occurs in the stomach. Lipolysis is completed in the duodenum and jejunum by pancreatic lipase, which is inactivated by pH <7.0. Pancreatic lipolysis is greatly enhanced by the presence of a second pancreatic enzyme, colipase, which facilitates the movement of lipase to the triglyceride.

Impaired lipolysis can lead to steatorrhea and can occur in the presence of pancreatic insufficiency due to chronic pancreatitis in adults or cystic fibrosis in children and adolescents. Normal lipolysis can be maintained by approximately 5% of maximal pancreatic lipase secretion; thus, steatorrhea is a late manifestation of these disorders. A reduction in intraduodenal pH can also result in altered lipolysis as pancreatic lipase is inactivated at pH <7. Thus, ~15% of patients with gastrinoma (Chap. 274) with substantial increases in gastric acid secretion from ectopic production of gastrin (usually from an islet cell adenoma) have diarrhea, and some will have steatorrhea believed secondary to acid-inactivation of pancreatic lipase. Similarly, patients with chronic pancreatitis (who have reduced lipase secretion) often have a decrease in pancreatic bicarbonate secretion, which will also result in a decrease in intraduodenal pH and inactivation of endogenous pancreatic lipase or of therapeutically administered lipase.

Overlying the microvillus membrane of the small intestine is the so-called unstirred water layer, a relatively stagnant aqueous phase that must be traversed by the products of lipolysis that are primarily water-insoluble. Water-soluble mixed micelles provide a mechanism for the water-insoluble products of lipolysis to reach the luminal plasma membrane of villus epithelial cells, the site for lipid absorption. Mixed micelles are molecular aggregates composed of fatty acids, monoglycerides, phospholipids, cholesterol, and conjugated bile acids. Mixed micelles are formed when the concentration of conjugated bile acids is greater than its CMC, which differs among the several bile acids present in the small intestinal lumen. Conjugated bile acids, synthesized in the liver and excreted into the duodenum in bile, are regulated by the enterohepatic circulation (see above). Steatorrhea can result from impaired movement of fatty acids across the unstirred aqueous fluid layer in two situations: (1) an increase in the relative thickness of the unstirred water layer that occurs in bacterial overgrowth syndromes (see below) secondary to functional jejunal stasis (e.g., scleroderma), and (2) a decrease in the *duodenal* concentration of con-

jugated bile acids below its CMC, resulting in impaired micelle formation. Thus, steatorrhea can be caused by one or more defects in the enterohepatic circulation of bile acids.

Uptake and reesterification constitute the *absorptive phase* of lipid digestion-absorption. Although passive diffusion has been thought responsible, a carrier-mediated process may mediate fatty acid and monoglyceride uptake. Regardless of the uptake process, fatty acids and monoglycerides are reesterified by a series of enzymatic steps in the endoplasmic reticulum and Golgi to form triglycerides, the form in which lipid exits from the intestinal epithelial cell. Impaired lipid absorption as a result of either mucosal inflammation (e.g., celiac sprue) and/or intestinal resection can also lead to steatorrhea.

The reesterified triglycerides require the formation of *chylomicrons* to permit their exit from the small-intestinal epithelial cell and their delivery to the liver via the *lymphatics*. Chylomicrons are composed of β-lipoprotein and contain triglycerides, cholesterol, cholesterol esters, and phospholipids and enter the lymphatics, not the portal vein. Defects in the *postabsorptive phase* of lipid digestion-absorption can also result in steatorrhea, but these disorders are uncommon. Abetalipoproteinemia, or acanthocytosis, is a rare disorder of impaired synthesis of β-lipoprotein associated with abnormal erythrocytes (acanthocytes), neurologic problems, and steatorrhea. Lipolysis, micelle formation, and lipid uptake are all normal in patients with abetalipoproteinemia, but the reesterified triglyceride cannot exit from the epithelial cell because of the failure to produce chylomicrons. Small-intestinal biopsies of these rare patients in the postprandial state reveal lipid-laden small-intestinal epithelial cells that become perfectly normal in appearance following a 72- to 96-h fast. Similarly, abnormalities of intestinal lymphatics (e.g., intestinal lymphangiectasia) may also be associated with steatorrhea as well as protein loss (see below). Steatorrhea can result from defects at any of the several steps in lipid digestion-absorption. The mechanism of lipid digestion-absorption outlined above is limited to *dietary* lipid that is almost exclusively in the form of LCTs (Table 275-3). Medium-chain triglycerides (MCTs), composed of fatty acids with carbon chain lengths of 8 to 10, are present in large amounts in coconut oil and are used as a nutritional supplement. MCTs can be digested and absorbed by a different pathway from LCTs and at one time held promise as an important treatment of steatorrhea of almost all etiologies. Unfortunately, their therapeutic effects have been less than expected because their use is often not associated with an increase in body weight for reasons that are not completely understood.

MCTs, in contrast to LCTs, do not require pancreatic lipolysis as the triglyceride can be absorbed intact by the intestinal epithelial cell. Further, micelle formation is not necessary for the absorption of MCTs or medium-chain fatty acids, if hydrolyzed by pancreatic lipase. MCTs are absorbed more efficiently than LCTs for the following reasons: (1) the rate of MCT absorption is greater than that of long-chain fatty acids; (2) medium-chain fatty acids following absorption are not reesterified; (3) following absorption, MCTs are hydrolyzed to medium-chain fatty acids; (4) MCTs do not require chylomicron formation for their exit from the intestinal epithelial cells; and (5) their route of exit is via the portal vein and not via lymphatics. Thus, the absorption of MCTs is greater than that of LCTs in pancreatic insufficiency, conditions with reduced intraduodenal bile acid concentrations, small-intestinal mucosal disease, abetalipoproteinemia, and intestinal lymphangiectasia.

SCFAs are not dietary lipids but are synthesized by colonic bacterial enzymes from nonabsorbed carbohydrate and are the anions in highest concentration in stool (between 80 and 130 mM). The SCFAs present in stool are primarily acetate, propionate, and butyrate, whose carbon chain lengths are 2, 3, and 4, respectively. Butyrate is the primary nutrient for colonic epithelial cells, and its deficiency may be associated with one or more colitides. SCFAs conserve calories and carbohydrate, because carbohydrates not completely absorbed in the small intestine will not be absorbed in the large intestine due to the absence of both disaccharidases and SGLT, the transport protein that mediates monosaccharide absorption. In contrast, SCFAs are rapidly absorbed and stimulate colonic Na-Cl and fluid absorption. Most non–*Clostridium difficile* antibiotic-associated diarrhea is due to antibiotic suppression of colonic microflora, with a resulting decrease in SCFA production. As *C. difficile* accounts for about 10 to 15% of all antibiotic-associated diarrhea, a relative decrease in colonic production of SCFAs is likely the cause of most antibiotic-associated diarrhea.

The clinical manifestations of steatorrhea are a consequence of both the underlying disorder responsible for the development of steatorrhea and steatorrhea per se. Depending on the degree of steatorrhea and the level of dietary intake, significant fat malabsorption may lead to weight loss. Steatorrhea per se can be responsible for diarrhea; if the primary cause of the steatorrhea has not been identified, a low-fat diet can often ameliorate the diarrhea by decreasing fecal fat excretion. Steatorrhea is often associated with fat-soluble vitamin deficiency, which will require replacement with water-soluble preparations of these vitamins.

Disorders of absorption may also be associated with malabsorption of other dietary nutrients, most often carbohydrates, with or without a decrease in dietary lipid digestion and absorption. Therefore, knowledge of the mechanism of the digestion and absorption of carbohydrates, proteins, and other minerals and vitamins is useful in the evaluation of patients with altered intestinal nutrient absorption.

CARBOHYDRATES Carbohydrates in the diet are present in the form of starch, disaccharides (sucrose and lactose), and glucose. Carbohydrates are absorbed only in the small intestine and only in the form of monosaccharides. Therefore, before their absorption, starch and disaccharides must first be digested by pancreatic amylase and intestinal brush border disaccharidases to monosaccharides. Monosaccharide absorption occurs by a Na-dependent process mediated by the brush border transport protein SGLT.

Lactose malabsorption is the only clinically important disorder of carbohydrate absorption. Lactose, the disaccharide present in milk, requires digestion by brush border lactase to its two constituent monosaccharides, glucose and galactose. Lactase is present in almost all species in the postnatal period but then disappears throughout the animal kingdom, except in humans. Lactase activity persists in many individuals throughout life. Two different types of lactase deficiency exist—primary and secondary. In *primary lactase deficiency*, a genetically determined decrease or absence of lactase is noted, while all other aspects of both intestinal absorption and brush border enzymes are normal. In a number of non-Caucasian groups, primary lactase deficiency is common in adulthood. Table 275-5 presents the incidence of primary lactase deficiency in several different ethnic groups. Northern European and North American Caucasians are the only population group to maintain small-intestinal lactase activity throughout adult life. The persistence of lactase is the abnormality due to a defect in the regulation of its maturation. In contrast, *secondary lactase deficiency* occurs in association with small-intestinal mucosal disease with abnormalities in both structure and function of other brush border enzymes and transport processes. Secondary lactase deficiency is often seen in celiac sprue.

As lactose digestion is rate-limiting compared to glucose/galactose absorption, lactase deficiency is associated with significant lactose malabsorption. Some individuals with lactose malabsorption develop symptoms such as diarrhea, abdominal pain, cramps, and/or flatus. Most individuals with primary lactase deficiency do not have symptoms. Since lactose intolerance may be associated with symptoms suggestive of an irritable bowel syndrome, persistence of such symptoms in an individual with lactose intolerance while on a strict lactose-free diet would suggest that the individual's symptoms were related to irritable bowel syndrome.

Development of symptoms of lactose intolerance is related to several factors:

1. *Amount of lactose in the diet.*
2. *Rate of gastric emptying.* Symptoms are more likely when gastric emptying is rapid than when gastric emptying is slower. Therefore, it is more likely that skim milk will be associated with symptoms of lactose intolerance than will whole milk, as the rate of gastric emptying following skim milk intake is more rapid. Similarly, the diarrhea observed following subtotal gastrectomy is often a result of lactose intolerance, as gastric emptying is accelerated in patients with a gastrojejunostomy.
3. *Small-intestinal transit time.* Although the small and large intestine contribute to the development of symptoms, many of the symptoms of lactase deficiency are related to the interaction of colonic bacteria and nonabsorbed lactose. More rapid small-intestinal transit makes symptoms more likely.
4. *Colonic compensation by production of SCFAs* from nonabsorbed lactose. Reduced levels of colonic microflora, which can occur following antibiotic use, will also be associated with increased symptoms following lactose ingestion, especially in a lactase-deficient individual.

Glucose-galactose or monosaccharide malabsorption may also be associated with diarrhea and is due to a congenital absence of SGLT. Diarrhea is present when individuals with this disorder ingest carbohydrates that contain actively transported monosaccharides (e.g., glucose, galactose) but not monosaccharides that are not actively transported (e.g., fructose). Fructose is absorbed by the brush border transport protein GLUT 5, a facilitated diffusion process that is not Na-dependent and is distinct from SGLT. In contrast, some individuals develop diarrhea as a result of consuming large quantities of sorbitol, a sugar used in diabetic candy; sorbitol is only minimally absorbed due to the absence of an intestinal absorptive transport mechanism for sorbitol.

PROTEINS Protein is present in food almost exclusively as polypeptides and requires extensive hydrolysis to di- and tripeptides and amino acids before absorption. Proteolysis occurs in both the stomach and small intestine; it is mediated by pepsin secreted as pepsinogen by gastric chief cells and trypsinogen and other peptidases from pancreatic acinar cells. These proenzymes, pepsinogen and trypsinogen, must be activated to pepsin (by pepsin in the presence of a pH <5) and trypsin (by the intestinal brush border enzyme enterokinase, and subsequently by trypsin). Proteins are absorbed by separate transport systems for di- and tripeptides and for different types of amino acids, e.g., neutral and dibasic. Alterations in either protein or amino acid digestion and absorption are rarely observed clinically, even in the presence of extensive small-intestinal mucosal inflammation. However, three rare genetic disorders involve protein digestion-absorption: (1) *enterokinase deficiency* is due to an absence of the brush border enzyme that converts the proenzyme trypsinogen to trypsin and is associated with diarrhea, growth retardation, and hypoproteinemia; (2) *Hartnup syndrome*, a defect in neutral amino acid transport, is characterized by a pellagra-like rash and neuropsychiatric symptoms; and (3) *cystinu-*

TABLE 275-5 *Primary Lactase Deficiency in Different Adult Ethnic Groups*

Ethnic Group	Prevalence of Lactase Deficiency, %
Northern European	5–15
Mediterranean	60–85
African black	85–100
American black	45–80
American Caucasian	10–25
Native American	50–95
Mexican American	40–75
Asian	90–100

Source: From FJ Simons: Am J Dig Dis 23:963, 1978.

ria, a defect in dibasic amino acid transport, is associated with renal calculi and chronic pancreatitis.

EVALUATION OF MALABSORPTION

The clues provided by the history, symptoms, and initial preliminary observations will serve to limit extensive, ill-focused, and expensive laboratory and imaging studies. For example, a clinician evaluating a patient with symptoms suggestive of malabsorption who recently had extensive small-intestinal resection for mesenteric ischemia should direct the initial assessment almost exclusively to define whether a short bowel syndrome might explain the entire clinical picture. Similarly, the development of a pattern of bowel movements suggestive of steatorrhea in a patient with long-standing alcohol abuse and chronic pancreatitis should lead toward assessing pancreatic exocrine function.

The classic picture of malabsorption described in textbooks >30 years ago is rarely seen today in most parts of the United States. As a consequence, diseases with malabsorption must be suspected in individuals with less severe symptoms and signs and with subtle evidence of the altered absorption of only a *single* nutrient rather than obvious evidence of the malabsorption of multiple nutrients.

Although diarrhea can be caused by changes in fluid and electrolyte movement in either the small or the large intestine, dietary nutrients are absorbed almost exclusively in the small intestine. Therefore, the demonstration of diminished absorption of a dietary nutrient provides unequivocal evidence of small-intestinal disease, although colonic dysfunction may also be present (e.g., Crohn's disease may involve both small and large intestine). Dietary nutrient absorption may be segmental or diffuse along the small intestine and is site-specific. Thus, for example, calcium, iron, and folic acid are exclusively absorbed by active transport processes in the proximal small intestine, especially the duodenum; in contrast, the active transport mechanisms for both cobalamin and bile acids are present only in the ileum. Therefore, in an individual who years previously had had an intestinal resection, the details of which are not presently available, a presentation with evidence of calcium, folic acid, and iron malabsorption but without cobalamin deficiency would make it likely that the duodenum and jejunum, but not ileum, had been resected.

Some nutrients, e.g., glucose, amino acids, and lipids, are absorbed throughout the small intestine, though there is evidence that their rate of absorption is greater in the proximal than in the distal segments. However, following segmental resection of the small intestine, the remaining segments will undergo both morphologic and functional "adaptation" to enhance absorption. Such adaptation is secondary to the presence of luminal nutrients and hormonal stimuli and may not be complete in humans for several months following the resection. Adaptation is critical for individuals who have undergone massive resection of the small intestine and/or colon to help ensure survival.

Establishing the presence of steatorrhea and identifying its specific cause are often quite difficult for several reasons. Despite attempts to develop tests that do *not* require the collection of stool to document the presence of steatorrhea, the "gold standard" still remains a timed, quantitative stool fat determination. On a practical basis, stool collections are invariably difficult and often incomplete as nobody wants to handle stool. A qualitative test—Sudan III stain—has long been available to establish the presence of an increase in stool fat. This test is rapid and inexpensive but, as a qualitative test, does not establish the degree of fat malabsorption and is best used as a preliminary screening study. Many of the blood, breath, and isotopic tests that have been developed either (1) do not directly measure fat absorption, (2) have excellent sensitivity when steatorrhea is obvious and severe but have poor sensitivity when steatorrhea is mild, or (3) have not survived the transition from their development in a laboratory to commercial utilization and dissemination.

Despite this situation, the use of routine laboratory studies (i.e., complete blood count, prothrombin time, serum protein determination, alkaline phosphatase) may suggest the presence of dietary nutrient depletion, especially iron, folate, cobalamin, and vitamins D and K. Additional studies include measurement of serum carotene, cholesterol, albumin, iron, folate, and cobalamin levels. The serum carotene level can also be reduced if the patient has poor dietary intake of leafy vegetables.

If steatorrhea and/or altered absorption of other nutrients are suspected, the history, clinical observations, and laboratory testing can help detect deficiency of a dietary nutrient, especially the fat-soluble vitamins A, D, E, or K. Thus, evidence of metabolic bone disease with elevated alkaline phosphatase and/or reduced serum calcium levels would suggest vitamin D malabsorption. A deficiency of vitamin K would be suggested by an elevated prothrombin time in an individual without liver disease who was not taking anticoagulants. Macrocytic anemia would lead to evaluation of whether cobalamin or folic acid malabsorption was present. The presence of iron-deficiency anemia in the absence of occult bleeding from the gastrointestinal tract in either a male or a nonmenstruating female would require evaluation of iron malabsorption and the exclusion of celiac sprue, as iron is absorbed exclusively in the proximal small intestine.

At times, however, a timed (72-h) quantitative stool collection, preferably on a defined diet, must be obtained to determine stool fat content and establish the presence of steatorrhea. The presence of steatorrhea then requires further assessment to establish the pathophysiologic process(es) responsible for the defect in dietary lipid digestion-absorption (Table 275-4). Some of the other studies include the Schilling test, D-xylose test, duodenal mucosal biopsy, small-intestinal radiologic examination, and tests of pancreatic exocrine function.

THE SCHILLING TEST   This test is performed to determine the cause for cobalamin malabsorption. Since cobalamin absorption requires multiple steps, including gastric, pancreatic, and ileal processes, the Schilling test can also be used to assess the integrity of these other organs (Chap. 92). Cobalamin is present primarily in meat. Except in strict vegans, *dietary* cobalamin deficiency is exceedingly uncommon. Dietary cobalamin is bound in the stomach to a glycoprotein called *R-binder protein*, which is synthesized in both the stomach and salivary glands. This cobalamin–R binder complex is formed in the acid milieu of the stomach. Cobalamin absorption has an absolute requirement for intrinsic factor, another glycoprotein synthesized and released by gastric parietal cells, to promote its uptake by specific cobalamin receptors on the brush border of ileal enterocytes. Pancreatic protease enzymes split the cobalamin–R binder complex to release cobalamin in the proximal small intestine, where cobalamin is then bound by intrinsic factor.

As a consequence, cobalamin absorption may be abnormal in the following:

1. Pernicious anemia, a disease in which immunologically mediated atrophy of gastric parietal cells leads to an absence of both gastric acid and intrinsic factor secretion.
2. Chronic pancreatitis as a result of deficiency of pancreatic proteases to split the cobalamin–R binder complex. Although 50% of patients with chronic pancreatitis have been reported to have an abnormal Schilling test that was corrected by pancreatic enzyme replacement, the presence of a cobalamin-responsive macrocytic anemia in chronic pancreatitis is extremely rare. Although this probably reflects a difference in the digestion/absorption of cobalamin in food versus that in a crystalline form, the Schilling test can still be used to assess pancreatic exocrine function.
3. Achlorhydria or absence of another factor secreted with acid that is responsible for splitting cobalamin away from the proteins in food to which it is bound. Up to one-third of individuals >60 years of age have marginal vitamin B_{12} absorption because of the inability to release cobalamin from food; these people have no defects in absorbing crystalline vitamin B_{12}.
4. Bacterial overgrowth syndromes, which are most often secondary to stasis in the small intestine, leading to bacterial utilization of cobalamin (often referred to as *stagnant bowel syndrome*) (see below).

5. Ileal dysfunction (as a result of either inflammation or prior intestinal resection) due to impaired function of the mechanism of cobalamin–intrinsic factor uptake by ileal intestinal epithelial cells.

The Schilling test is performed by administering ^{58}Co-labeled cobalamin and collecting urine for 24 h and is dependent on normal renal and bladder function. Urinary excretion of cobalamin will reflect cobalamin absorption provided that intrahepatic binding sites for cobalamin are fully occupied. To ensure saturation of hepatic cobalamin binding sites so that all absorbed radiolabeled cobalamin will be excreted in urine, 1 mg cobalamin is administered intramuscularly 1 h following ingestion of the radiolabeled cobalamin. The Schilling test may be abnormal (usually defined as <10% excretion in 24 h) in pernicious anemia, chronic pancreatitis, blind loop syndrome, and ileal disease (Table 275-6). Therefore, whenever an abnormal Schilling test is found, ^{58}Co-labeled cobalamin should be administered on another occasion either bound to intrinsic factor, with pancreatic enzymes, or following a 5-day course of antibiotics (often tetracycline). A variation of the Schilling test can detect failure to split cobalamin from food proteins. The labeled cobalamin is cooked together with a scrambled egg and administered orally. People with achlorydria will excrete <10% of the labeled cobalamin in the urine. In addition to establishing the etiology for cobalamin deficiency, the Schilling test can be used to help delineate the pathologic process responsible for steatorrhea by assessing ileal, pancreatic, and small-intestinal luminal function. Unfortunately, in recent years the Schilling test has been infrequently performed because radiolabeled cobalamin is often not available.

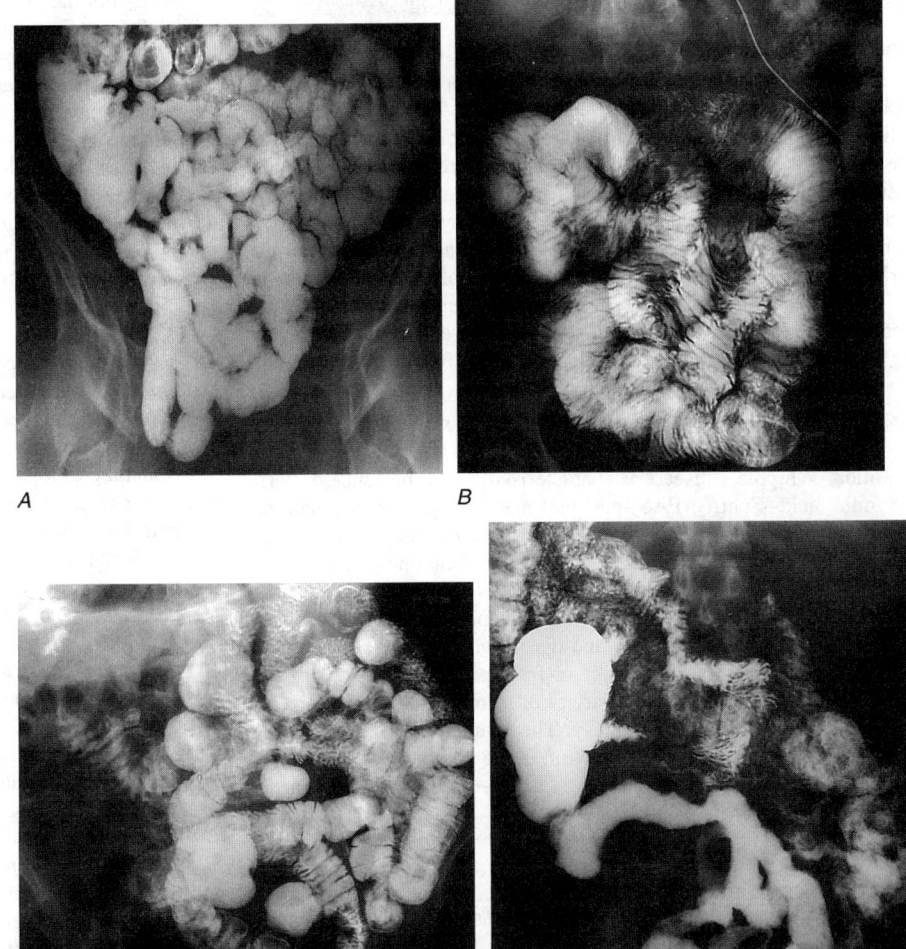

FIGURE 275-3 Barium contrast small-intestinal radiologic examinations. *A.* Normal individual. *B.* Celiac sprue. *C.* Jejunal diverticulosis. *D.* Crohn's disease. *(Courtesy of Morton Burrell, MD, Yale University.)*

URINARY D-XYLOSE TEST The urinary D-xylose test for carbohydrate absorption provides an assessment of proximal small-intestinal mucosal function. D-Xylose, a pentose, is absorbed almost exclusively in the proximal small intestine. The D-xylose test is usually performed by giving 25 g D-xylose and collecting urine for 5 h. An abnormal test (<4.5 g excretion) primarily reflects the presence of duodenal/jejunal mucosal disease. The D-xylose test can also be abnormal in patients with blind loop syndrome (as a consequence primarily of abnormal intestinal mucosa) and, as a false-positive study, in patients with large collections of fluid in a third space (i.e., ascites, pleural fluid). The ease of obtaining a mucosal biopsy of the small intestine by endoscopy and the false-negative rate of the D-xylose test have led to its diminished use. When small-intestinal mucosal disease is suspected, a small-intestinal mucosal biopsy should be performed.

RADIOLOGIC EXAMINATION Radiologic examination of the small intestine using barium contrast (small-bowel series or study) can provide important information in the evaluation of the patient with presumed or suspected malabsorption. These studies are most often performed in conjunction with the examination of the esophagus, stomach, and duodenal bulb, and insufficient barium is given to the patient to permit an adequate examination of the small-intestinal mucosa, especially the ileum. As a result, many gastrointestinal radiologists alter the procedure of a barium contrast examination of the small intestine by performing either a small-bowel series in which a large amount of barium is given by mouth without concurrent examination of the esophagus and stomach or an enteroclysis study in which a large amount of barium is introduced into the duodenum via a fluoroscopically placed tube. In addition, many of the diagnostic features initially described by radiologists to denote the presence of small-intestinal disease (e.g., flocculation, segmentation) are rarely seen with current barium suspensions. Nonetheless, in skilled hands barium contrast examination of the small intestine can yield important information. For example, with extensive mucosal disease, dilation of intestine can be seen, as candilution of barium from increased intestinal fluid secretion (Fig. 275-3). A normal barium contrast study does *not* exclude the possibility of small-intestinal disease. However, a small-bowel series remains a very useful examination to assess for the presence of anatomical abnormalities, such as strictures and fistulas (as in Crohn's disease) or blind loop syndrome (e.g., multiple jejunal diverticula), and to define the extent of a previous surgical resection.

TABLE 275-6 *Differential Results of Schilling Test in Several Diseases Associated with Cobalamin (Cbl) Malabsorption*

	^{58}Co-Cbl	With Intrinsic Factor	With Pancreatic Enzymes	After 5 Days of Antibiotics
Pernicious anemia	Reduced	Normal	Reduced	Reduced
Chronic pancreatitis	Reduced	Reduced	Normal	Reduced
Bacterial overgrowth	Reduced	Reduced	Reduced	Normal
Ileal disease	Reduced	Reduced	Reduced	Reduced

BIOPSY OF SMALL-INTESTINAL MUCOSA   A small-intestinal mucosal biopsy is essential in the evaluation of a patient with documented steatorrhea or chronic diarrhea (lasting >3 weeks) (Chap. 35). The ready availability of endoscopic equipment to examine the stomach and duodenum has led to its almost uniform use as the preferred method to obtain histologic material of proximal small-intestinal mucosa. The primary indications for a small-intestinal biopsy are (1) evaluation of a patient either with documented or suspected steatorrhea or with chronic diarrhea, and (2) diffuse or focal abnormalities of the small intestine defined on a small-intestinal series. Lesions seen on small-bowel biopsy can be classified into three different categories (Table 275-7): (1) diffuse, specific; (2) patchy, specific; and (3) diffuse, nonspecific.

1. *Diffuse, specific lesions.* Relatively few diseases associated with altered nutrient absorption have specific histopathologic abnormalities on small-intestinal mucosal biopsy, and they are uncommon. Whipple's disease is characterized by the presence of periodic acid–Schiff (PAS)-positive macrophages in the lamina propria, while the bacilli that are also present may require electron-microscopic examination for identification (Fig. 275-4). *Abetalipoproteinemia* is characterized by a normal mucosal appearance except for the presence of mucosal absorptive cells that contain lipid postprandially and disappear following a prolonged period of either fat-free intake or fasting. *Immune globulin deficiency* is associated with a variety of histopathologic findings on small-intestinal mucosal biopsy. The characteristic feature is the absence of or substantial reduction in the number of plasma cells in the lamina propria; the mucosal architecture may be either per-

fectly normal or flat, i.e., villus atrophy. As patients with immune globulin deficiency are often infected with *Giardia lamblia*, *Giardia* trophozoites may also be seen in the biopsy.

2. *Patchy, specific lesions.* Several diseases are associated with abnormal small-intestinal mucosal biopsies, but the characteristic features that are present have a patchy distribution. As a result, biopsies obtained randomly or in the absence of abnormalities visualized endoscopically may not reveal these diagnostic features. Intestinal *lymphoma* can at times be diagnosed on mucosal biopsy by the identification of malignant lymphoma cells in the lamina propria and submucosa (Chap. 97). The presence of dilated lymphatics in the submucosa and sometimes in the lamina propria indicates the presence of *lymphangiectasia* associated with hypoproteinemia secondary to protein loss into the intestine. *Eosinophilic gastroenteritis* comprises a heterogeneous group of disorders with a spectrum of presentations and symptoms with an eosinophilic infiltrate of the lamina propria, with or without peripheral eosinophilia. The patchy nature of the infiltrate as well as its presence in the submucosa often leads to an absence of histopathologic findings on mucosal biopsy. As the involvement of the duodenum in *Crohn's disease* is also submucosal and not necessarily continuous, mucosal biopsies are not the most direct approach to the diagnosis of duodenal Crohn's disease (Chap. 276). Amyloid deposition can be identified by Congo Red stain in some patients with *amyloidosis* involving the duodenum (Chap. 310).

    Several microorganisms can be identified on small-intestinal biopsies, establishing a correct diagnosis. Many of these microorganisms are associated with diarrhea that occurs in immunodeficient individuals, especially those with HIV infection, and include *Cryptosporidium*, *Isospora belli*, cytomegalovirus, *Mycobacterium avium-intracellulare*, and *G. lamblia*.

3. *Diffuse, nonspecific lesions. Celiac sprue* presents with a characteristic mucosal appearance on duodenal/proximal jejunal mucosal biopsy that is not diagnostic of the disease. The diagnosis of celiac sprue is established by clinical, histologic, and immunologic response to a gluten-free diet. *Tropical sprue* is associated with histopathologic findings similar to those of celiac sprue after a tropical or subtropical exposure but does not respond to gluten restriction; most often symptoms improve with antibiotics and folate administration.

Patients with steatorrhea require assessment of *pancreatic exocrine function*, which is often abnormal in chronic pancreatitis. No test assesses pancreatic exocrine function well. Endoscopic approaches provide excellent assessment of pancreatic duct anatomy but do **not** assess exocrine function (Chap. 293). One noninvasive study (bentiromide test) of pancreatic exocrine function is based on the feeding of a tripeptide containing *p*-aminobenzoic acid (PABA). Following splitting of PABA by pancreatic proteases, PABA is liberated, absorbed, and excreted in urine. Reduced proteolysis results in reduced urinary excretion of PABA. This test is neither sensitive nor specific.

Table 275-8 summarizes the results of the D-xylose test, Schilling test, and small-intestinal mucosal biopsy in patients with five different causes of steatorrhea.

SPECIFIC DISEASE ENTITIES

CELIAC SPRUE   Celiac sprue is a common cause of malabsorption of one or more nutrients in Caucasians, especially those of European descent. Estimated incidence in the United States may be as high as 1:13 people. Celiac sprue has had several other names including nontropical sprue, celiac disease (in children), adult celiac disease, and gluten-sensitive enteropathy. The etiology of celiac sprue is not known, but environmental, immunologic, and genetic factors are important. Celiac sprue has protean manifestations, almost all of which are secondary to nutrient malabsorption, and a varied natural history, with the onset of symptoms occurring at ages ranging from the first year of life through the eighth decade.

The hallmark of celiac sprue is the presence of an abnormal small-intestinal biopsy (Fig. 275-4) and the response of both symptoms—

TABLE 275-7 *Disease that Can be Diagnosed by Small-Intestinal Mucosal Biopsies*

Lesions	Pathologic Findings
Diffuse, specific	
Whipple's disease	Lamina propria contains macrophages containing PAS+ material
Agammaglobulinemia	No plasma cells; either normal or absent villi ("flat mucosa");
Abetalipoproteinemia	Normal villi; epithelial cells vacuolated with fat postprandially
Patchy, specific	
Intestinal lymphoma	Malignant cells in lamina propria and submucosa
Intestinal lymphangiectasia	Dilated lymphatics; clubbed villi
Eosinophilic gastroenteritis	Eosinophil infiltration of lamina propria and mucosa
Amyloidosis	Amyloid deposits
Crohn's disease	Noncaseating granulomas
Infection by one or more microorganisms (see text)	Specific organisms
Mastocytosis	Mast cell infiltration of lamina propria
Diffuse, nonspecific	
Celiac sprue	Short or absent villi; mononuclear infiltrate; epithelial cell damage; hypertrophy of crypts
Tropical sprue	Similar to celiac sprue
Bacterial overgrowth	Patchy damage to villi; lymphocyte infiltration
Folate deficiency	Short villi; decreased mitosis in crypts; megalocytosis
Vitamin B_{12} deficiency	Similar to folate deficiency
Radiation enteritis	Similar to folate deficiency
Zollinger-Ellison syndrome	Mucosal ulceration and erosion from acid
Protein-calorie malnutrition	Villous atrophy; secondary bacterial overgrowth
Drug-induced enteritis	Variable histology

Note: PAS+, periodic acid–Schiff positive.

evidence of malabsorption and the histopathologic changes on the small-intestinal biopsy—to the elimination of gluten from the diet. The histopathologic changes have a proximal to distal intestinal distribution of severity, which probably reflects the exposure of the intestinal mucosa to varied amounts of dietary gluten; the degree of symptoms is often related to the extent of these histopathologic changes.

The symptoms of celiac sprue may appear with the introduction of cereals in an infant's diet, although there is frequently a spontaneous remission during the second decade of life that may be either permanent or followed by the reappearance of symptoms over several years. Alternatively, the symptoms of celiac sprue may first become evident at almost any age throughout adulthood. In many patients, frequent spontaneous remissions and exacerbations occur. The symptoms range from significant malabsorption of multiple nutrients with diarrhea, steatorrhea, weight loss, and the consequences of nutrient depletion (i.e., anemia and metabolic bone disease) to the absence of any gastrointestinal symptoms but with evidence of the depletion of a single nutrient (e.g., iron or folate deficiency, osteomalacia, edema from protein loss). Asymptomatic relatives of patients with celiac sprue have been identified as having this disease either by small-intestinal biopsy or by serologic studies (e.g., antiendomysial antibodies).

Etiology The etiology of celiac sprue is not known, but environmental, immunologic, and genetic factors all appear to contribute to the disease.

One *environmental* factor is the clear association of the disease with gliadin, a component of gluten that is present in wheat, barley, rye, and, in smaller amounts, oats. In addition to the role of gluten restriction in treatment, the instillation of gluten into both normal-appearing rectum and distal ileum of patients with celiac sprue results within hours in morphologic changes.

An *immunologic* component to etiology is suspected for three reasons. First, serum antibodies—IgA antigliadin, IgA antiendomysial, and IgA anti-tissue transglutaminase (tTG) antibodies—are present, but it is also not known whether such antibodies are primary or secondary to the tissue damage. The antiendomysial antibody has 90 to 95% sensitivity and 90 to 95% specificity, and the antigen recognized by the antiendomysial antibody test is tissue transglutaminase. Antibody studies are frequently used to identify patients with celiac sprue; patients with these antibodies should undergo duodenal biopsy. The relationship of this autoantibody to a pathogenetic mechanism (or mechanisms) responsible for celiac sprue remains to be established. Nonetheless, this antibody will undoubtedly prove extremely useful in establishing the true prevalence of celiac sprue in the general population and may provide important clues to its etiology. Second, treatment with prednisolone for 4 weeks of a patient with celiac sprue who continues to eat gluten will induce a remission and convert the "flat" abnormal duodenal biopsy to a more normal-appearing one. Third, gliadin peptides may interact with gliadin-specific T cells that may either mediate tissue injury or induce the release of one or more cytokines that are responsible for the tissue injury.

Genetic factor(s) also appear to be involved in celiac sprue. The incidence of celiac sprue varies widely in different population groups (high in Caucasians, low in blacks and Asians) and is 10% in first-

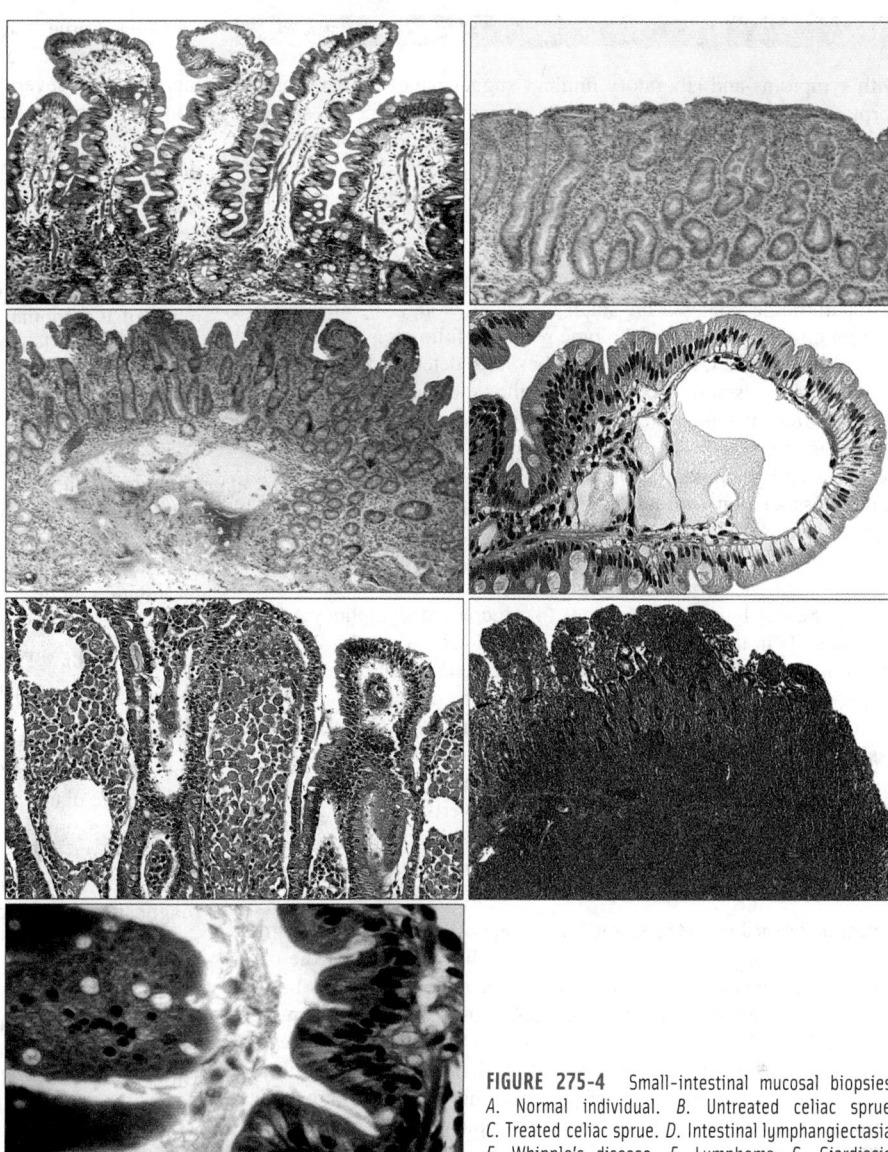

FIGURE 275-4 Small-intestinal mucosal biopsies. *A.* Normal individual. *B.* Untreated celiac sprue. *C.* Treated celiac sprue. *D.* Intestinal lymphangiectasia. *E.* Whipple's disease. *F.* Lymphoma. *G.* Giardiasis. *(Courtesy of Marie Robert, MD, Yale University.)*

degree relatives of celiac sprue patients. Furthermore, about 95% of patients with celiac sprue express the HLA-DQ2 allele, though only a minority of all persons expressing DQ2 have celiac sprue.

Diagnosis A small-intestinal biopsy is required to establish a diagnosis of celiac sprue (Fig. 275-4). A biopsy should be performed in patients

TABLE 275-8 *Results of Diagnostic Studies in Different Causes of Steatorrhea*

	D-*Xylose Test*	*Schilling Test*	*Duodenal Mucosal Biopsy*
Chronic pancreatitis	Normal	50% abnormal; if abnormal, normal with pancreatic enzymes	Normal
Bacterial overgrowth syndrome	Normal or only modestly abnormal	Often abnormal; if abnormal, normal after antibiotics	Usually normal
Ileal disease	Normal	Abnormal	Normal
Celiac sprue	Decreased	Normal	Abnormal: probably "flat"
Intestinal lymphangiectasia	Normal	Normal	Abnormal: "dilated lymphatics"

with symptoms and laboratory findings suggestive of nutrient malabsorption and/or deficiency. Since the presentation of celiac sprue is often subtle, without overt evidence of malabsorption or nutrient deficiency, it is important to have a relatively low threshold to perform a biopsy. It is more prudent to perform a biopsy than to obtain another test of intestinal absorption, which can never completely exclude or establish this diagnosis.

The diagnosis of celiac sprue requires the presence of characteristic histopathologic changes on small-intestinal biopsy together with a prompt clinical and histopathologic response following the institution of a gluten-free diet. If serologic studies have detected the presence of IgA antiendomysial or tTG antibodies, they too should disappear after a gluten-free diet is started. The changes seen on duodenal/jejunal biopsy are restricted to the mucosa and include (1) absence or reduced height of villi, resulting in a flat appearance; (2) increased loss of villus cells in association with increased crypt cell proliferation resulting in crypt hyperplasia and loss of villus structure, with consequent villus, but not mucosal, atrophy; (3) cuboidal appearance and nuclei that are no longer oriented basally in surface epithelial cells and increased intraepithelial lymphocytes; and (4) increased lymphocytes and plasma cells in the lamina propria (Fig. 275-4*B*). Although these histopathologic features are characteristic of celiac sprue, they are *not* diagnostic because a similar appearance can be seen in tropical sprue, eosinophilic enteritis, and milk-protein intolerance in children and occasionally in lymphoma, bacterial overgrowth, Crohn's disease, and gastrinoma with acid hypersecretion. However, the presence of a characteristic histopathologic appearance that reverts toward normal following the initiation of a gluten-free diet establishes the diagnosis of celiac sprue (Fig. 275-4*C*). Readministration of gluten with or without an additional small-intestinal biopsy is not necessary.

Failure to Respond to Gluten Restriction   The most common cause of persistent symptoms in a patient who fulfills all the criteria of the diagnosis of celiac sprue is continued intake of gluten. Gluten is ubiquitous, and significant effort must be made to exclude all gluten from the diet. Use of rice in place of wheat flour is very helpful, and several support groups provide important aid to patients with celiac sprue and to their families. About 90% of patients who have the characteristic findings of celiac sprue will respond to complete dietary gluten restriction. The remainder constitute a heterogeneous group (whose condition is often called *refractory sprue*) that includes some patients who (1) respond to restriction of other dietary protein, e.g., soy; (2) respond to glucocorticoids; (3) are "temporary," i.e., the clinical and morphologic findings disappear after several months or years; or (4) fail to respond to all measures and have a fatal outcome, with or without documented complications of celiac sprue, such as development of intestinal T cell lymphoma.

Mechanism of Diarrhea   The diarrhea in celiac sprue has several pathogenetic mechanisms. Diarrhea may be secondary to (1) steatorrhea, which is primarily a result of the changes in jejunal mucosal function; (2) secondary lactase deficiency, a consequence of changes in jejunal brush border enzymatic function; (3) bile acid malabsorption resulting in bile acid–induced fluid secretion in the colon, in cases with more extensive disease involving the ileum; and (4) endogenous fluid secretion resulting from the crypt hyperplasia. Patients with more severe involvement with celiac sprue may obtain temporary improvement with *dietary lactose and fat restriction* while awaiting the full effects of total gluten restriction, which is primary therapy.

Associated Diseases   Celiac sprue is associated with dermatitis herpetiformis (DH), though the association has not been explained. Patients with DH have characteristic papulovesicular lesions that respond to dapsone. Almost all patients with DH have histopathologic changes in the small intestine consistent with celiac sprue, although usually much milder and less diffuse in distribution. Most patients with DH have mild, or no, gastrointestinal symptoms. In contrast, relatively few patients with celiac sprue have DH.

Celiac sprue is also associated with diabetes mellitus type 1 and IgA deficiency. The clinical importance of the former association is that although severe watery diarrhea without evidence of malabsorption is most often seen in patients with "diabetic diarrhea" (Chap. 323), assay of antiendomysial antibodies and/or a small-intestinal biopsy must at times be considered to exclude this association.

Complications   The most important complication of celiac sprue is the development of cancer. An increased incidence of both gastrointestinal and nongastrointestinal neoplasms as well as intestinal lymphoma exists in patients with celiac sprue. For unexplained reasons the occurrence of lymphoma in patients with celiac sprue is higher in Ireland and the United Kingdom than in the United States. The possibility of lymphoma must be considered whenever a patient with celiac sprue previously doing well on a gluten-free diet is no longer responsive to gluten restriction or a patient who presents with clinical and histopathologic features consistent with celiac sprue does not respond to a gluten-free diet. Other complications of celiac sprue include the development of intestinal ulceration independent of lymphoma and so-called refractory sprue (see above) and collagenous sprue. In *collagenous sprue*, a layer of collagen-like material is present beneath the basement membrane; patients with collagenous sprue generally do not respond to a gluten-free diet and often have a poor prognosis.

TROPICAL SPRUE   Tropical sprue is a poorly understood syndrome that affects both expatriates and natives in certain but not all tropical areas and is manifested by chronic diarrhea, steatorrhea, weight loss, and nutritional deficiencies, including those of both folate and cobalamin. This disease affects 5 to 10% of the population in some tropical areas.

Chronic diarrhea in a tropical environment is most often caused by infectious agents including *G. lamblia*, *Yersinia enterocolitica*, *C. difficile*, *Cryptosporidium parvum*, and *Cyclospora cayetanensis*, among other organisms. Tropical sprue should not be entertained as a possible diagnosis until the presence of cysts and trophozoites has been excluded in three stool samples. →*Chronic infections of the gastrointestinal tract and diarrhea in patients with or without AIDS are discussed in Chaps. 113 and 173.*

The small-intestinal mucosa in individuals living in tropical areas is not identical to that of individuals who reside in temperate climates. Biopsies reveal a mild alteration of villus architecture with a modest increase in mononuclear cells in the lamina propria, which on occasion can be as severe as that seen in celiac sprue. These changes are observed both in native residents and in expatriates living in tropical regions and are usually associated with mild decreases in absorptive function, but revert to "normal" when an individual moves or returns to a temperate area. Some have suggested that the changes seen in tropical enteropathy and in tropical sprue represent different ends of the spectrum of a single entity, but convincing evidence to support this concept is lacking.

Etiology   The etiology of tropical sprue is not known, though because tropical sprue responds to antibiotics, the consensus is that tropical sprue may be caused by one or more infectious agents. Nonetheless, there are multiple uncertainties regarding the etiology and pathogenesis of tropical sprue. First, its occurrence is not evenly distributed in all tropical areas; rather, it is found in specific locations including South India, the Philippines, and several Caribbean islands (e.g., Puerto Rico, Haiti) but is rarely observed in Africa, Jamaica, or Southeast Asia. Second, an occasional individual will not develop symptoms of tropical sprue until long after having left an endemic area. This is the reason why the original term for celiac sprue was *nontropical sprue* to distinguish it from tropical sprue. Third, multiple microorganisms have been identified on jejunal aspirate with relatively little consistency among studies. *Klebsiella pneumoniae*, *Enterobacter cloacae*, or *E. coli* have been implicated in some studies of tropical sprue, while other investigations have favored a role for a toxin produced by one or more of these bacteria. Fourth, the incidence of tropical sprue appears to have decreased substantially during the past decade. One speculation for this reduced occurrence of tropical sprue is the wider use of antibiotics in acute diarrhea, especially in travelers to tropical areas from temperate countries. Fifth, the role of folic acid deficiency in the pathogenesis of tropical sprue requires clarification. Folic acid is absorbed exclusively in the duodenum and proximal jejunum, and most patients with tropical sprue have evidence of folate malabsorption and depletion. Although folate deficiency can cause changes in small-intestinal mucosa that are corrected by folate replacement, the several earlier studies reporting that tropical sprue could be cured by folic acid did not provide an explanation for the "insult" that was initially responsible for folate malabsorption.

The clinical pattern of tropical sprue varies in different areas of the world (e.g., India vs Puerto Rico). Not infrequently, individuals in South India initially will report the occurrence of an acute enteritis before the development of steatorrhea and malabsorption. In contrast, in Puerto Rico, a most insidious onset of symptoms and a more dramatic response to antibiotics is seen when compared to some other locations. Tropical sprue in different areas of the world may not be the same disease; similar clinical entities may have different etiologies.

Diagnosis   The diagnosis of tropical sprue is best made by the presence of an abnormal small-intestinal mucosal biopsy in an individual with chronic diarrhea and evidence of malabsorption who is either residing or has recently lived in a tropic country. The small-intestinal biopsy in tropical sprue does not have pathognomonic features but resembles, and can often be indistinguishable from, that seen in celiac sprue (Fig. 275-4). The biopsy in tropical sprue will have less villus architectural alteration and more mononuclear cell infiltrate in the lamina propria. In contrast to celiac sprue, the histopathologic features of tropical sprue are present with a similar degree of severity throughout the small intestine, and a gluten-free diet does not result in either clinical or histopathologic improvement in tropical sprue.

℞ TREATMENT

Broad-spectrum antibiotics and folic acid are most often curative, especially if the patient leaves the tropical area and does not return. Tetracycline should be used for up to 6 months and may be associated with improvement within 1 to 2 weeks. Folic acid alone will induce a hematologic remission as well as improvement in appetite, weight gain, and some morphologic changes in small intestinal biopsy. Because of the presence of marked folate deficiency, folic acid is most often given together with antibiotics.

SHORT BOWEL SYNDROME   This is a descriptive term for the myriad clinical problems that often occur following resection of varying lengths of small intestine. The factors that determine both the type and degree of symptoms include (1) the specific segment (jejunum vs ileum) resected, (2) the length of the resected segment, (3) the integrity of the ileocecal valve, (4) whether any large intestine has also been removed, (5) residual disease in the remaining small and/or large intestine (e.g., Crohn's disease, mesenteric artery disease), and (6) the degree of adaptation in the remaining intestine. Short bowel syndrome can occur at any age from neonates through the elderly.

Three different situations in adults demand intestinal resections: (1) mesenteric vascular disease including atherosclerosis, thrombotic phenomena, and vasculitides; (2) primary mucosal and submucosal disease, e.g., Crohn's disease; and (3) operations without preexisting small intestinal disease, such as trauma and jejunoileal bypass for obesity.

Following resection of the small intestine, the residual intestine undergoes adaptation of both structure and function that may last for up to 6 to 12 months. Continued intake of dietary nutrients and calories is required to stimulate adaptation via direct contact with intestinal mucosa, the release of one or more intestinal hormones, and pancreatic and biliary secretions. Thus, enteral nutrition and calorie administration must be maintained, especially in the early postoperative period, even if an extensive intestinal resection requiring total parenteral nutrition (TPN) was performed. The subsequent ability of such patients to absorb nutrients will not be known for several months, until adaptation is completed.

Multiple factors besides the absence of intestinal mucosa (required

for lipid, fluid, and electrolyte absorption) contribute to the diarrhea and steatorrhea in these patients. Removal of the ileum and especially the ileocecal valve is often associated with more severe diarrhea than jejunal resection. Without part or all of the ileum, diarrhea can be caused by an increase in bile acids entering the colon, leading to their stimulation of colonic fluid and electrolyte secretion. Absence of the ileocecal valve is also associated with a decrease in intestinal transit time and bacterial overgrowth from the colon. Lactose intolerance as a result of the removal of lactase-containing mucosa as well as gastric hypersecretion will also contribute to the diarrhea.

In addition to diarrhea and/or steatorrhea, a range of nonintestinal symptoms is also observed in some patients. A significant increase in renal calcium oxalate calculi is observed in patients with a small-intestinal resection with an intact colon and is due to an increase in oxalate absorption by the large intestine, with subsequent hyperoxaluria (called *enteric hyperoxaluria*). Since oxalate is high in relatively few foods (e.g., spinach, rhubarb, tea), dietary restrictions alone are not adequate treatment. Cholestyramine, an anion-binding resin, and calcium have proved useful in reducing the hyperoxaluria. Similarly, an increase in cholesterol gallstones is related to a decrease in the bile acid pool size, which results in the generation of cholesterol supersaturation in gallbladder bile. Gastric hypersecretion of acid occurs in many patients following large resections of the small intestine. The etiology is unclear but may be related to either reduced hormonal inhibition of acid secretion or increased gastrin levels due to reduced small-intestinal catabolism of circulating gastrin. The resulting gastric acid secretion may be an important factor contributing to the diarrhea and steatorrhea. A reduced pH in the duodenum can inactivate pancreatic lipase and/or precipitate duodenal bile acids, thereby increasing steatorrhea, and an increase in gastric secretion can create a volume overload relative to the reduced small-intestinal absorptive capacity. Inhibition of gastric acid secretion with either proton pump inhibitors or H_2 receptor antagonists can help in reducing the diarrhea and steatorrhea.

℞ TREATMENT

Treatment of short bowel syndrome depends on the severity of symptoms and whether the individual is able to maintain caloric and electrolyte balance with oral intake alone. Initial treatment includes judicious use of opiates (including codeine) to reduce stool output and to establish an effective diet. An initial diet should be low-fat and high-carbohydrate to minimize the diarrhea from fatty acid stimulation of colonic fluid secretion. MCTs (see above), a low-lactose diet, and various fiber-containing diets should also be tried. In the absence of an ileocecal valve, the possibility of bacterial overgrowth must be considered and treated. If gastric acid hypersecretion is contributing to the diarrhea and steatorrhea, a proton pump inhibitor may be helpful. Usually none of these therapeutic approaches will provide an instant solution but they can reduce disabling diarrhea.

The patient's vitamin and mineral status must also be monitored; replacement therapy should be initiated if indicated. Fat-soluble vitamins, folate, cobalamin, calcium, iron, magnesium, and zinc are the most critical factors to monitor on a regular basis. If these approaches are not successful, home TPN is an established therapy that can be maintained for many years. Intestinal transplantation is becoming established as a possible approach for individuals with extensive intestinal resection who cannot be maintained without TPN.

BACTERIAL OVERGROWTH SYNDROME   Bacterial overgrowth syndrome comprises a group of disorders with diarrhea, steatorrhea, and macrocytic anemia whose common feature is the proliferation of colon-type bacteria within the small intestine. This bacterial proliferation is due to stasis caused by impaired peristalsis (i.e., *functional stasis*), changes in intestinal anatomy (i.e., *anatomic stasis*), or direct communication between the small and large intestine. These conditions have also been referred to as *stagnant bowel syndrome* or *blind loop syndrome*.

Pathogenesis   The manifestations of bacterial overgrowth syndromes are a direct consequence of the presence of increased amounts of a colonic-type bacterial flora, such as *E. coli* or *Bacteroides*, in the small intestine. *Macrocytic anemia* is due to cobalamin, not folate, deficiency. Most bacteria require cobalamin for growth, and increasing concentrations of bacteria use up the relatively small amounts of dietary cobalamin. *Steatorrhea* is due to impaired micelle formation as a consequence of a reduced intraduodenal concentration of conjugated bile acids and the presence of unconjugated bile acids. Certain bacteria, e.g., *Bacteroides*, deconjugate conjugated bile acids to unconjugated bile acids. In the presence of bacterial overgrowth, unconjugated bile acids will be absorbed more rapidly than conjugated bile acids, and, as a result, the intraduodenal concentration of bile acids will be reduced. In addition, the CMC of unconjugated bile acids is higher than that of conjugated bile acids, resulting in a decrease in micelle formation. *Diarrhea* is due, at least in part, to the steatorrhea, when it is present. However, some patients manifest diarrhea *without* steatorrhea, and it is assumed that the colonic-type bacteria in these patients are producing one or more bacterial enterotoxins that are responsible for fluid secretion and diarrhea.

Etiology   The etiology of these different disorders is bacterial proliferation in the small intestinal lumen secondary to either anatomical or functional stasis or to a communication between the relatively sterile small intestine and the colon with its high levels of aerobic and anaerobic bacteria. Several examples of anatomical stasis have been identified: (1) one or more diverticula (both duodenal and jejunal) (Fig. 275-3*C*); (2) fistulas and strictures related to Crohn's disease (Fig. 275-3*D*); (3) a proximal duodenal afferent loop following a subtotal gastrectomy and gastrojejunostomy; (4) a bypass of the intestine, e.g., jejunoileal bypass for obesity; and (5) dilation at the site of a previous intestinal anastomosis. These anatomical derangements are often associated with the presence of a segment (or segments) of intestine out of continuity of propagated peristalsis, resulting in stasis and bacterial proliferation. Bacterial overgrowth syndromes can also occur in the absence of an anatomical blind loop when functional stasis is present. Impaired peristalsis and bacterial overgrowth in the absence of a blind loop occur in scleroderma, where motility abnormalities exist in both the esophagus and small intestine (Chap. 303), and in small-intestinal stricture associated with either Crohn's disease or an intestinal anastomosis. Functional stasis and bacterial overgrowth can also occur in association with diabetes mellitus and in the small intestine when a direct connection exists between the small and large intestine, including an ileocolonic resection, or occasionally following an enterocolic anastomosis that permits entry of bacteria into the small intestine as a result of bypassing the ileocecal valve.

Diagnosis   The diagnosis may be suspected from the combination of a low serum cobalamin level and an elevated serum folate level as enteric bacteria frequently produce folate compounds that will be absorbed in the duodenum. Ideally, the diagnosis of the bacterial overgrowth syndrome is the demonstration of increased levels of aerobic and/or anaerobic colonic-type bacteria in a jejunal aspirate obtained by intubation. This specialized test is rarely available, and bacterial overgrowth is best established by a Schilling test (Table 275-6), which should be abnormal following the administration of ^{58}Co-labeled cobalamin, with or without the administration of intrinsic factor. Following the administration of tetracycline for 5 days, the Schilling test will become normal, confirming the diagnosis of bacterial overgrowth. Breath hydrogen testing following lactose administration has also been used to detect bacterial overgrowth.

℞ TREATMENT

Primary treatment should be directed, if at all possible, to the surgical correction of an anatomical blind loop. In the absence of functional stasis, it is important to define the anatomical relationships responsible for stasis and bacterial overgrowth. For example, bacterial overgrowth

secondary to strictures, one or more diverticula, or a proximal afferent loop can potentially be cured by surgical correction of the anatomical state. In contrast, the functional stasis of scleroderma or certain anatomical stasis states (e.g., multiple jejunal diverticula), cannot be corrected surgically, and these conditions should be treated with broad-spectrum antibiotics. Tetracycline used to be the initial treatment of choice but, due to increasing resistance, other antibiotics such as metronidazole, amoxicillin/clavulanic acid, and cephalosporins have been employed. The antibiotic should be given for approximately 3 weeks or until symptoms remit. Since the natural history of these conditions is chronic, antibiotics should not be given continuously, and symptoms usually remit within 2 to 3 weeks of initial antibiotic therapy. Therapy need not be repeated until symptoms recur. In the presence of frequent recurrences several treatment strategies exist, but the use of antibiotics for 1 week per month whether or not symptoms are present is often most effective.

Unfortunately, therapy for bacterial overgrowth syndrome is largely empirical, with an absence of clinical trials on which to base decisions regarding the antibiotic to be used, the duration of treatment, and/or the best approach for treating recurrences. Bacterial overgrowth may also occur as a component of another chronic disease, e.g., Crohn's disease, radiation enteritis, or short bowel syndrome. Treatment of the bacterial overgrowth in these settings will not cure the underlying problem but may be very important in ameliorating a subset of clinical problems that are related to bacterial overgrowth.

WHIPPLE'S DISEASE   Whipple's disease is a chronic multisystem disease associated with diarrhea, steatorrhea, weight loss, arthralgia, and central nervous system and cardiac problems; it is caused by the bacteria *Tropheryma whipplei*. Until the identification of *T. whipplei* by polymerase chain reaction, the hallmark of Whipple's disease had been the presence of PAS-positive macrophages in the small intestine (Fig. 275-4*E*) and other organs with evidence of disease.

Long before the establishment of *T. whipplei* as the causative agent of Whipple's disease, gram-positive bacilli had been identified both within and outside of macrophages.

Etiology   Whipple's disease is caused by a small gram-positive bacillus, *T. whipplei*. The bacillus, an actinobacterium, has low virulence but high infectivity, and relatively minimal symptoms are observed compared to the extent of the bacilli in multiple tissues.

Clinical Presentation   The onset of Whipple's disease is insidious and is characterized by diarrhea, steatorrhea, abdominal pain, weight loss, migratory large-joint arthropathy, and fever as well as ophthalmologic and central nervous system symptoms. The development of dementia is a relatively late symptom and is an extremely poor prognostic sign, especially in patients who relapse following the induction of a remission with antibiotics. For unexplained reasons, the disease occurs primarily in middle-aged Caucasian men. The steatorrhea in these patients is generally believed secondary to both small-intestinal mucosal injury and lymphatic obstruction secondary to the increased number of PAS-positive macrophages in the lamina propria of the small intestine.

Diagnosis   The diagnosis of Whipple's disease is suggested by a multisystem disease in a man with diarrhea and steatorrhea. Obtaining tissue biopsies from the small intestine and/or other organs that may be involved (e.g., liver, lymph nodes, heart, eyes, central nervous system, or synovial membranes), based on the patient's symptoms, is the primary approach to establish the diagnosis of Whipple's disease. The presence of PAS-positive macrophages containing the characteristic small (0.25 × 1 to 2 mm) bacilli is suggestive of this diagnosis. However, Whipple's disease can be confused with the PAS-positive macrophages containing *M. avium* complex, which may be a cause of diarrhea in AIDS. The presence of the *T. whipplei* bacillus outside of macrophages is a more important indicator of active disease than is their presence within the macrophages. *T. whipplei* has now been successfully grown in culture.

TABLE 275-9 *Classification of Malabsorption Syndromes*

Inadequate digestion
  Postgastrectomy[a]
  Deficiency or inactivation of pancreatic lipase
    Exocrine pancreatic insufficiency
      Chronic pancreatitis
      Pancreatic carcinoma
      Cystic fibrosis
      Pancreatic insufficiency—congenital or acquired
    Gastrinoma—acid inactivation of lipase[a]
    Drugs—orlistat
Reduced intraduodenal bile acid concentration/impaired micelle
  formation
  Liver disease
    Parenchymal liver disease
    Cholestatic liver disease
  Bacterial overgrowth in small intestine:

Anatomic stasis	Functional stasis
Afferent loop stasis/blind	Diabetes[a]
loop/strictures/fistulae	Scleroderma[a]
	Intestinal pseudoobstruction

  Interrupted enterohepatic circulation of bile salts
    Ileal resection
    Crohn's disease[a]
  Drugs (bind or precipitate bile salts)—neomycin, cholestyramine,
    calcium carbonate
Impaired mucosal absorption/mucosal loss or defect
  Intestinal resection or bypass[a]
  Inflammation, infiltration, or infection:

Crohn's disease[a]	Celiac sprue
Amyloidosis	Collagenous sprue
Scleroderma[a]	Whipple's disease[a]
Lymphoma[a]	Radiation enteritis[a]
Eosinophilic enteritis	Folate and vitamin B_{12} deficiency
Mastocytosis	Infections—giardiasis
Tropical sprue	Graft-vs.-host disease

  Genetic disorders
    Disaccharidase deficiency
    Agammaglobulinemia
    Abetalipoproteinemia
    Hartnup disease
    Cystinuria
Impaired nutrient delivery to and/or from intestine:

Lymphatic obstruction	Circulatory disorders
Lymphoma[a]	Congestive heart failure
Lymphangiectasia	Constrictive pericarditis
	Mesenteric artery atherosclerosis
	Vasculitis

Endocrine and metabolic disorders
  Diabetes[a]
  Hypoparathyroidism
  Adrenal insufficiency
  Hyperthyroidism
  Carcinoid syndrome

[a] Malabsorption caused by more than one mechanism.

℞ TREATMENT

The treatment for Whipple's disease is prolonged use of antibiotics. The current drug of choice is double-strength trimethoprim/sulfamethoxazole for approximately 1 year. PAS-positive macrophages can persist following successful treatment, and the presence of bacilli outside of macrophages is indicative of persistent infection or an early sign of recurrence. Recurrence of disease activity, especially with dementia, is an extremely poor prognostic sign and requires an antibiotic that crosses the blood-brain barrier. If trimethoprim/sulfamethoxazole is not tolerated, chloramphenicol is an appropriate second choice.

PROTEIN-LOSING ENTEROPATHY Protein-losing enteropathy is not a specific disease but rather describes a group of gastrointestinal and nongastrointestinal disorders with hypoproteinemia and edema in the absence of either proteinuria or defects in protein synthesis, e.g., chronic liver disease. These diseases are characterized by excess protein loss into the gastrointestinal tract. Normally, about 10% of the total protein

catabolism occurs via the gastrointestinal tract. Evidence of increased protein loss into the gastrointestinal tract has been established in more than 65 different diseases, which can be classified into three primary groups: (1) mucosal ulceration such that the protein loss primarily represents exudation across damaged mucosa, e.g., ulcerative colitis, gastrointestinal carcinomas, and peptic ulcer; (2) nonulcerated mucosa but with evidence of mucosal damage so that the protein loss represents loss across epithelia with altered permeability, e.g., celiac sprue and Ménétrier's disease in the small intestine and stomach, respectively; and (3) lymphatic dysfunction, either representing primary lymphatic disease or secondary to partial lymphatic obstruction that may occur as a result of enlarged lymph nodes or cardiac disease.

Diagnosis The diagnosis of protein-losing enteropathy is suggested by the presence of peripheral edema and low serum albumin and globulin levels in the absence of renal and hepatic disease. It is extremely rare for an individual with protein-losing enteropathy to have selective loss of *only* albumin or *only* globulins. Therefore, marked reduction of serum albumin with normal serum globulins should not initiate an evaluation for protein-losing enteropathy but should suggest the presence of renal and/or hepatic disease. Likewise, reduced serum globulins with normal serum albumin levels are more likely a result of reduced globulin synthesis rather than enhanced globulin loss into the intestine. Documentation of an increase in protein loss into the gastrointestinal tract has been established by the administration of one of several radiolabeled proteins and its quantitation in stool during a 24- or 48-h period. Unfortunately, none of these radiolabeled proteins is available for routine clinical use. α_1 Antitrypsin, a protein that amounts to approximately 4% of total serum proteins and is resistant to proteolysis, can be used to document enhanced rates of serum protein loss into the intestinal tract but cannot be used to assess gastric protein loss due to its degradation in an acid milieu. α_1 Antitrypsin clearance is measured by determining stool volume and both stool and plasma α_1 antitrypsin concentrations. In addition to the loss of protein via abnormal and distended lymphatics, peripheral lymphocytes may also be lost via lymphatics, resulting in a relative lymphopenia. Thus, the pres-

TABLE 275-10 *Pathophysiology of Clinical Manifestations of Malabsorption Disorders*

Symptom or Sign	Mechanism
Weight loss/malnutrition	Anorexia, malabsorption of nutrients
Diarrhea	Impaired absorption or secretion of water and electrolytes; colonic fluid secretion secondary to unabsorbed dihydroxy bile acids and fatty acids
Flatus	Bacterial fermentation of unabsorbed carbohydrate
Glossitis, cheilosis, stomatitis	Deficiency of iron, vitamin B_{12}, folate, and vitamin A
Abdominal pain	Bowel distention or inflammation, pancreatitis
Bone pain	Calcium, vitamin D malabsorption, protein deficiency, osteoporosis
Tetany, paresthesia	Calcium and magnesium malabsorption
Weakness	Anemia, electrolyte depletion (particularly K^+)
Azotemia, hypotension	Fluid and electrolyte depletion
Amenorrhea, decreased libido	Protein depletion, decreased calories, secondary hypopituitarism
Anemia	Impaired absorption of iron, folate, vitamin B_{12}
Bleeding	Vitamin K malabsorption, hypoprothrombinemia
Night blindness/ xerophthalmia	Vitamin A malabsorption
Peripheral neuropathy	Vitamin B_{12} and thiamine deficiency
Dermatitis	Deficiency of vitamin A, zinc, and essential fatty acid

ence of lymphopenia in a patient with hypoproteinemia supports the presence of increased loss of protein into the gastrointestinal tract.

Patients with increased protein loss into the gastrointestinal tract from lymphatic obstruction often have steatorrhea and diarrhea. The steatorrhea is a result of altered lymphatic flow as lipid-containing chylomicrons exit from intestinal epithelial cells via intestinal lymphatics (Table 275-4; Fig. 275-4). In the absence of mechanical or anatomical lymphatic obstruction, intrinsic intestinal lymphatic dysfunction, with or without lymphatic dysfunction in the peripheral extremities, has been named *intestinal lymphangiectasia*. Similarly, about 50% of individuals with intrinsic peripheral lymphatic disease (Milroy disease) will also have intestinal lymphangiectasia and hypoproteinemia. Other than steatorrhea and enhanced protein loss into the gastrointestinal tract, all other aspects of intestinal absorptive function are normal in intestinal lymphangiectasia.

Other Causes   Patients who appear to have idiopathic protein-losing enteropathy without any evidence of gastrointestinal disease should be examined for cardiac disease—especially right-sided valvular disease and chronic pericarditis (Chaps. 219 and 222). On occasion, hypoproteinemia can be the only presentation for these two types of heart disease. Ménétrier's disease (also called *hypertrophic gastropathy*) is an uncommon entity that involves the body and fundus of the stomach and is characterized by large gastric folds, reduced gastric acid secretion, and, at times, enhanced protein loss into the stomach.

℞ TREATMENT

As excess protein loss into the gastrointestinal tract is most often secondary to a specific disease, treatment should be directed primarily to the underlying disease process and not to the hypoproteinemia. For example, if significant hypoproteinemia with resulting peripheral edema is present secondary to either celiac sprue or ulcerative colitis, a gluten-free diet or mesalamine, respectively, would be the initial

therapy. When enhanced protein loss is secondary to lymphatic obstruction, it is critical to establish the nature of this obstruction. Identification of mesenteric nodes or lymphoma may be possible by imaging studies. Similarly, it is important to exclude cardiac disease as a cause of protein-losing enteropathy either by echosonography or, on occasion, by a right-heart catheterization.

The increased protein loss that occurs in intestinal lymphangiectasia is a result of distended lymphatics associated with lipid malabsorption. Treatment of the hypoproteinemia is accomplished by a low-fat diet and the administration of MCTs (Table 275-3), which do not exit from the intestinal epithelial cells via lymphatics but are delivered to the body via the portal vein.

SUMMARY

A pathophysiologic classification of the many conditions that can produce malabsorption is given in Table 275-9. A summary of the pathophysiology of the various clinical manifestations of malabsorption is given in Table 275-10.

FURTHER READING

AMERICAN GASTROENTEROLOGICAL ASSOCIATION: AGA technical review on the evaluation and management of chronic diarrhea. Gastroenterology 116:1464, 1999

COOK SI, SELLIN JH: Short chain fatty acids in health and disease. Aliment Pharmacol Ther 12:499, 1998

CRAIG RM, EHRENPREIS ED: D-Xylose testing. J Clin Gastroenterol 29:143, 1999

FENOLLAR F, RAOULT D: Whipple's disease. Curr Gastroenterol Rep 5:379, 2003

GREEN PH, JABRI B: Coeliac disease. Lancet 362:383, 2003

GREENBERGER NJ: Enzymatic therapy in patients with chronic pancreatitis. Gastroenterol Clin North Am 28:687, 1999

HAREWOOD GC, MURRAY JA: Approaching the patient with chronic malabsorption syndrome. Semin Gastrointest Dis 10:138, 1999

SHAW AD, DAVIES GJ: Lactose intolerance: Problems in diagnosis and treatment. J Clin Gastroenterol 28:208, 1999

276 | INFLAMMATORY BOWEL DISEASE
Sonia Friedman, Richard S. Blumberg

Inflammatory bowel disease (IBD) is an idiopathic and chronic intestinal inflammation. Ulcerative colitis (UC) and Crohn's disease (CD) are the two major types of IBD.

EPIDEMIOLOGY

The incidence of IBD varies within different geographic areas. Northern countries, such as the United States, United Kingdom, Norway, and Sweden, have the highest rates. The incidence rates of UC and CD in the United States are about 11 per 100,000 and 7 per 100,000, respectively (Table 276-1). Countries in southern Europe, South Africa, and Australia have lower incidence rates: 2 to 6.3 per 100,000 for UC, and 0.9 to 3.1 per 100,000 for CD. In Asia and South America, IBD is rare; incidence rates of UC and CD are 0.5 and 0.08 per 100,000, respectively. The highest mortality in IBD patients is during the first years of disease and in long-duration disease due to the risk of colon cancer. In a Swedish population study, the standardized mortality ratios for CD and UC were 1.51 and 1.37, respectively.

The peak age of onset of UC and CD is between 15 and 30 years. A second peak occurs between the ages of 60 and 80. The male to female ratio for UC is 1:1 and for CD is 1.1 to 1.8:1. A two- to fourfold increased frequency of UC and CD in Jewish populations has been described in the United States, Europe, and South Africa. Furthermore, disease frequency differs within the Jewish populations. The prevalence of IBD in Ashkenazi Jews is about twice that of Israeli-born, Sephardic, or Oriental Jews. The prevalence decreases progressively

TABLE 276-1	Epidemiology of IBD	
	Ulcerative Colitis	**Crohn's Disease**
Incidence (U.S.)	11/100,000	7/100,000
Age of onset	15–30 & 60–80	15–30 & 60–80
Ethnicity	Jewish > Non-Jewish Caucasian > African American > Hispanic > Asian	
Male:female ratio	1:1	1.1–1.8:1
Smoking	May prevent disease	May cause disease
Oral contraceptives	No increased risk	Relative risk 1.9
Appendectomy	Protective	Not protective
Monozygotic twins	20% concordance	67% concordance
Dizygotic twins	0% concordance	8% concordance

in non-Jewish Caucasian, African-American, Hispanic, and Asian populations. Urban areas have a higher prevalence of IBD than rural areas, and high socioeconomic classes have a higher prevalence than lower socioeconomic classes.

The effects of cigarette smoking are different in UC and CD. The risk of UC in smokers is 40% that of nonsmokers. Additionally, former smokers have a 1.7-fold increased risk for UC than people who have never smoked. In contrast, smoking is associated with a twofold increased risk of CD. Oral contraceptives are also linked to CD; the relative risk of CD for oral contraceptive users is about 1.9. Appendectomy appears to be protective against UC, but no studies have applied this as a preventive intervention.

IBD runs in families. If a patient has IBD, the lifetime risk that a first-degree relative will be affected is ~10%. If two parents have IBD, each child has a 36% chance of being affected. In twin studies, 67% of monozygotic twins are concordant for CD and 20% are concordant for UC, whereas 8% of dizygotic twins are concordant for CD and none are concordant for UC. Anatomic site and clinical type of CD is also concordant within families.

Additional evidence for genetic predisposition to IBD comes from its association with certain genetic syndromes. UC and CD are both associated with Turner's syndrome, and Hermansky-Pudlak syndrome is associated with a granulomatous colitis. Glycogen storage disease type 1b can present with Crohn's-like lesions of the large and small bowel. Other immunodeficiency disorders, such as hypogammaglobulinemia, selective IgA deficiency, and hereditary angioedema, also exhibit an increased association with IBD.

ETIOLOGY AND PATHOGENESIS

Although IBD has been described as a clinical entity for over 100 years, its etiology and pathogenesis have not been defined. A consensus hypothesis is that in genetically predisposed individuals, both exogenous factors (e.g., infectious agents, normal lumenal flora) and host factors (e.g., intestinal epithelial cell barrier function, vascular supply, neuronal activity) cause a chronic state of dysregulated mucosal immune function that is further modified by specific environmental factors (e.g., smoking). Although it is possible that the chronic activation of the mucosal immune system may represent an appropriate response to an unidentified infectious agent, a search for such an agent has thus far been unrewarding. As such, IBD is currently considered an inappropriate response to either the endogenous microbial flora within the intestine, with or without some component of autoimmunity. Importantly, the normal intestine contains a large number of immune cells in a chronic state of so-called physiologic inflammation, in which the gut is poised for, but actively restrained from, full immunologic responses. During the course of infections in the normal host, full activation of the gut-associated lymphoid tissue occurs but is rapidly superceded by dampening the immune response and tissue repair. In IBD this process is not regulated normally.

GENETIC CONSIDERATIONS IBD is a polygenic disorder that gives rise to multiple clinical subgroups within UC and CD. Genome-wide searches have shown potential disease-associated loci on chromosomes 16, 12, 7, 5, 3, and 1, although the specific gene associations are mostly undefined. The disease-related gene on chromosome 16 is *NOD-2*, an intracellular molecule that senses bacterial peptidoglycan and regulates NF-κB signaling. Homozygosity for mutant alleles confers up to a 40-fold increased risk for fibrostenosing CD, especially in the ileum. HLA alleles may also play a role. UC patients disproportionately express DR2-related alleles, whereas in CD an increased use of the DR5 DQ1 haplotype or the DRB*0301 allele has been described. In UC patients with pancolitis undergoing total proctocolectomy, 14.3% versus 3.2% of non-IBD controls express the HLA DRB1*0103 allele. This allele is associated with extensive disease and extraintestinal manifestations such as mouth ulcers, arthritis, and uveitis. Other associations with immunoregulatory genes include the intercellular adhesion molecule R241 allele in UC and CD and the interleukin (IL) 1 receptor antagonist allele 2 in UC patients that is associated with total colonic inflammation. Patients with IBD and their first-degree relatives may also exhibit diminished intestinal epithelial cell barrier function.

DEFECTIVE IMMUNE REGULATION IN IBD The normal state of the mucosal immune system is one of inhibited immune responses to lumenal contents due to oral tolerance that occurs in the normal individual. When soluble antigens are administered orally rather than subcutaneously or intramuscularly, antigen-specific non-responsiveness is induced. Multiple mechanisms are involved in the induction of oral tolerance and include deletion or anergy of antigen-reactive T cells or activation of CD4+ T cells that suppress gut inflammation through secretion of inhibitory cytokines, such as IL-10 and transforming growth factor β (TGF-β). Oral tolerance may be responsible for the lack of immune responsiveness to dietary antigens and the commensal flora in the in-

testinal lumen. In IBD this suppression of inflammation is altered, leading to uncontrolled inflammation. The mechanisms that maintain this regulated immune suppression are unknown.

Gene knockout (-/-) or transgenic (Tg) mouse models of colitis have revealed that deleting specific cytokines (e.g., IL-2, IL-10, TGF-β) or their receptors, deleting molecules associated with T cell antigen recognition (e.g., T cell antigen receptors, MHC class II), or interfering with intestinal epithelial cell barrier function (e.g., blocking N-cadherin, deleting multidrug resistance gene 1a or trefoil factor) leads to colitis. Thus, a variety of specific alterations can lead to autoimmunity directed at the colon in mice.

In both UC and CD, activated CD4+ T cells in the lamina propria and peripheral blood secrete inflammatory cytokines. Some activate other inflammatory cells (macrophages and B cells) and others act indirectly to recruit other lymphocytes, inflammatory leukocytes, and mononuclear cells from the peripheral vasculature into the gut through interactions between homing receptors on leukocytes (e.g., $\alpha4\beta7$ integrin) and addressins on vascular endothelium (e.g., MadCAM1). CD4+ T cells are of two major types, both of which may be associated with colitis in animal models and humans: T_H1 cells [interferon (IFN) γ, tumor necrosis factor (TNF)] and T_H2 cells (IL-4, IL-5, IL-13). T_H1 cells appear to induce transmural granulomatous inflammation that resembles CD, and T_H2 cells appear to induce superficial mucosal inflammation resembling UC. The T_H1 cytokine pathway is initiated by IL-12, a key cytokine in the pathogenesis of experimental models of mucosal inflammation. Thus, use of antibodies to block proinflammatory cytokines (e.g., anti-TNF-α, anti-IL-12) or molecules associated with leukocyte recruitment (e.g., anti-$\alpha4\beta7$) or use of cytokines that inhibit inflammation (e.g., IL-10) or promote intestinal barrier function (e.g., IL-11) may be beneficial to humans with colitis.

THE INFLAMMATORY CASCADE IN IBD Once initiated in IBD, the immune inflammatory response is perpetuated as a consequence of T cell activation. A sequential cascade of inflammatory mediators acts to extend the response; each step is a potential target for therapy. Inflammatory cytokines, such as IL-1, IL-6, and TNF, have diverse effects on tissue. They promote fibrogenesis, collagen production, activation of tissue metalloproteinases, and the production of other inflammatory mediators; they also activate the coagulation cascade in local blood vessels (e.g., increased production of von Willebrand's factor). These cytokines are normally produced in response to infection, but are usually turned off or inhibited at the appropriate time to limit tissue damage. In IBD their activity is not regulated, resulting in an imbalance between the proinflammatory and anti-inflammatory mediators. Therapies such as the 5-ASA (5-aminosalicylic acid) compounds are potent inhibitors of these inflammatory mediators through inhibition of transcription factors such as NF-κB that regulate their expression.

EXOGENOUS FACTORS IBD may have an as yet undefined infectious etiology. Three specific agents have received the greatest attention, *Mycobacterium paratuberculosis*, Paramyxovirus, and *Helicobacter* species. The immune response to a specific organism could be expressed differently, depending upon the individual's genetic background. *M. paratuberculosis* does not have a confirmed disease association, and antimycobacterial agents are not effective in treating CD. A role for the measles virus or paramyxoviruses in the development of CD has been suggested based on an increase in the incidence of CD in England that paralleled use of the measles vaccine. However, studies in the United States have not substantiated this finding. In an animal model of IBD, *H. hepaticus* has been implicated as a trigger for the inflammatory response; evidence in humans is lacking.

Multiple pathogens (e.g., *Salmonella*, *Shigella* sp., *Campylobacter* sp.) may initiate IBD by triggering an inflammatory response that the mucosal immune system may fail to control. However, in an IBD patient the normal flora is likely perceived as if it were a pathogen. Anaerobic organisms, particularly *Bacteroides* species, may be responsible for the induction of inflammation. Such a notion is supported by the response in patients with CD to agents that alter the intestinal flora, such as metronidazole, ciprofloxacin, and elemental diets. CD also responds to fecal diversion, demonstrating the ability of lumenal contents to exacerbate disease. On the other hand, other bacteria, so-called probiotics (*Lactobacillus* sp.), inhibit inflammation in animal models and humans.

Psychosocial factors can contribute to worsening of symptoms. Major life events such as illness or death in the family, divorce or separation, interpersonal conflict, or other major loss are associated with an increase in IBD symptoms such as pain, bowel dysfunction, and bleeding. Acute daily stress can worsen bowel symptoms even after controlling for major life events. When the sickness-impact profile, a measurement of overall psychological and physical functioning, is used, IBD patients have functional impairment greater than that of a normal population but less than that of patients with chronic back pain or amyotrophic lateral sclerosis. IBD patients have been hypothesized to have a characteristic personality that renders them susceptible to emotional stresses. However, emotional dysfunction could also be the result of chronic illness rather than a cause.

PATHOLOGY

ULCERATIVE COLITIS: MACROSCOPIC FEATURES   UC is a mucosal disease that usually involves the rectum and extends proximally to involve all or part of the colon. About 40 to 50% of patients have disease limited to the rectum and rectosigmoid, 30 to 40% have disease extending beyond the sigmoid but not involving the whole colon, and 20% have a total colitis. Proximal spread occurs in continuity without areas of uninvolved mucosa. When the whole colon is involved, the inflammation extends 1 to 2 cm into the terminal ileum in 10 to 20% of patients. This is called *backwash ileitis* and is of little clinical significance. Although variations in macroscopic activity may suggest skip areas, biopsies from normal-appearing mucosa are usually abnormal. Thus, it is important to obtain multiple biopsies from apparently uninvolved mucosa, whether proximal or distal, during endoscopy.

With mild inflammation, the mucosa is erythematous and has a fine granular surface that looks like sandpaper. In more severe disease, the mucosa is hemorrhagic, edematous, and ulcerated (Fig. 276-1). In long-standing disease, inflammatory polyps (pseudopolyps) may be present as a result of epithelial regeneration. The mucosa may appear normal in remission, but in patients with many years of disease it appears atrophic and featureless and the entire colon becomes narrowed and shortened. Patients with fulminant disease can develop a toxic colitis or megacolon where the bowel wall thins and the mucosa is severely ulcerated; this may lead to perforation.

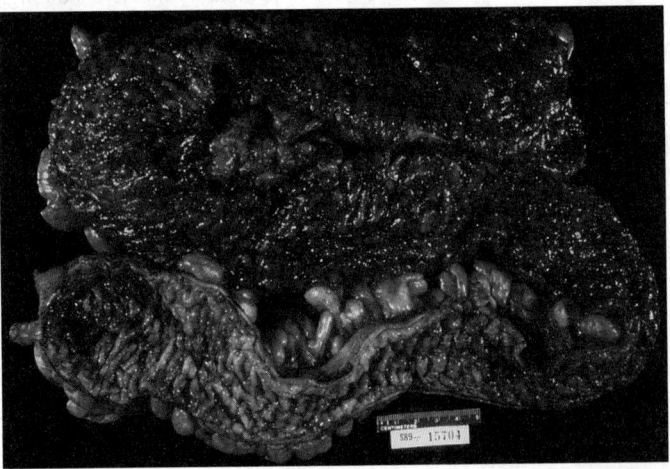

FIGURE 276-1   Pan-ulcerative colitis. Mucosa has a lumpy, bumpy appearance because of areas of inflamed but intact mucosa separated by ulcerated areas. (*Courtesy of Dr. EK Rosado and Dr. CA Perkos, Division of Gastrointestinal Pathology, Department of Pathology, Emory University, Atlanta, Georgia.*)

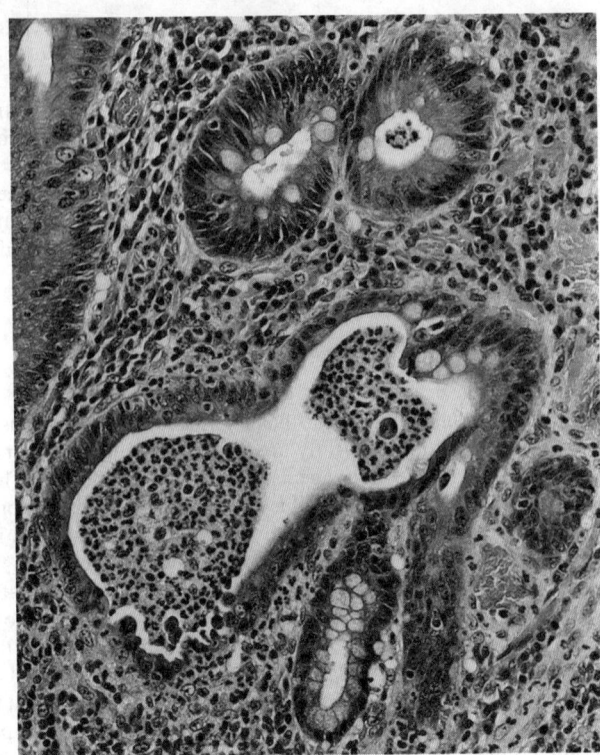

FIGURE 276-2   Characteristic findings of IBD in a case of ulcerative colitis: crypt distortion, cryptitis, and crypt abscess. (*Courtesy of Dr. EK Rosado and Dr. CA Perkos, Division of Gastrointestinal Pathology, Department of Pathology, Emory University, Atlanta, Georgia.*)

ULCERATIVE COLITIS: MICROSCOPIC FEATURES   Histologic findings correlate well with the endoscopic appearance and clinical course of UC. The process is limited to the mucosa and superficial submucosa, with deeper layers unaffected except in fulminant disease. In UC, two major histologic features are indicative of chronicity and help distinguish it from infectious or acute self-limited colitis. First, the crypt architecture of the colon is distorted; crypts may be bifid and reduced in number, often with a gap between the crypt bases and the muscularis mucosae. Second, some patients have basal plasma cells and multiple basal lymphoid aggregates. Mucosal vascular congestion with edema and focal hemorrhage, and an inflammatory cell infiltrate of neutrophils, lymphocytes, plasma cells, and macrophages may be present. The neutrophils invade the epithelium, usually in the crypts, and give rise to cryptitis and, ultimately, to crypt abscesses (Fig. 276-2).

CROHN'S DISEASE: MACROSCOPIC FEATURES   CD can affect any part of the gastrointestinal tract from the mouth to the anus. Some 30 to 40% of patients have small-bowel disease alone, 40 to 55% have disease involving both the small and large intestines, and 15 to 25% have colitis alone. In the 75% of patients with small-intestinal disease, the terminal ileum is involved in 90%. Unlike UC, which almost always involves the rectum, the rectum is often spared in CD. CD is segmental, with skip areas in the midst of diseased intestine (Fig. 276-3). Perirectal fistulas, fissures, abscesses, and anal stenosis are present in one-third

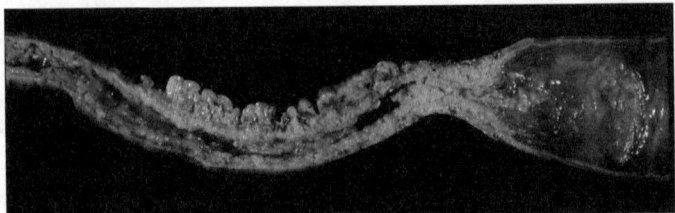

FIGURE 276-3   Portion of colon with stricture in patient with CD. (*Courtesy of Dr. EK Rosado and Dr. CA Perkos, Division of Gastrointestinal Pathology, Department of Pathology, Emory University, Atlanta, Georgia.*)

of patients with CD, particularly those with colonic involvement. CD may also involve the liver and the pancreas.

Unlike UC, CD is a transmural process. Endoscopically, aphthous or small superficial ulcerations characterize mild disease; in more active disease, stellate ulcerations fuse longitudinally and transversely to demarcate islands of mucosa that frequently are histologically normal. This "cobblestone" appearance is characteristic of CD, both endoscopically and by barium radiography. As in UC, pseudopolyps can form in CD.

Active CD is characterized by focal inflammation and formation of fistula tracts, which resolve by fibrosis and stricturing of the bowel. The bowel wall thickens and becomes narrowed and fibrotic, leading to chronic, recurrent bowel obstructions. Projections of thickened mesentery encase the bowel ("creeping fat"), and serosal and mesenteric inflammation promote adhesions and fistula formation.

CROHN'S DISEASE: MICROSCOPIC FEATURES The earliest lesions are aphthoid ulcerations and focal crypt abscesses with loose aggregations of macrophages, which form noncaseating granulomas in all layers of the bowel wall from mucosa to serosa (Fig. 276-4). Granulomas can be seen in lymph nodes, mesentery, peritoneum, liver, and pancreas. Although granulomas are a pathognomonic feature of CD, they are rarely found on mucosal biopsies. Surgical resection reveals granulomas in about half of cases. Other histologic features of CD include submucosal or subserosal lymphoid aggregates, particularly away from areas of ulceration, gross and microscopic skip areas, and transmural inflammation that is accompanied by fissures that penetrate deeply into the bowel wall and sometimes form fistulous tracts or local abscesses.

CLINICAL PRESENTATION

ULCERATIVE COLITIS ■ Signs and Symptoms The major symptoms of UC are diarrhea, rectal bleeding, tenesmus, passage of mucus, and crampy abdominal pain. The severity of symptoms correlates with the extent of disease. Although UC can present acutely, symptoms usually have been present for weeks to months. Occasionally, diarrhea and bleeding are so intermittent and mild that the patient does not seek medical attention.

Patients with proctitis usually pass fresh blood or blood-stained mucus, either mixed with stool or streaked onto the surface of a normal or hard stool. They also have tenesmus, or urgency with a feeling of incomplete evacuation. They rarely have abdominal pain. With proctitis or proctosigmoiditis, proximal transit slows, which may account

TABLE 276-2 Ulcerative Colitis: Disease Presentation

	Mild	Moderate	Severe
Bowel movements	<4 per day	4–6 per day	>6 per day
Blood in stool	Small	Moderate	Severe
Fever	None	<37.5°C mean	>37.5°C mean
Tachycardia	None	<90 mean pulse	>90 mean pulse
Anemia	Mild	>75%	≤75%
Sedimentation rate	<30 mm		>30 mm
Endoscopic appearance	Erythema, decreased vascular pattern, fine granularity	Marked erythema, coarse granularity, absent vascular markings, contact bleeding, no ulcerations	Spontaneous bleeding, ulcerations

for the constipation that is commonly seen in patients with distal disease.

When the disease extends beyond the rectum, blood is usually mixed with stool or grossly bloody diarrhea may be noted. Colonic motility is altered by inflammation with rapid transit through the inflamed intestine. When the disease is severe, patients pass a liquid stool containing blood, pus, and fecal matter. Diarrhea is often nocturnal and/or postprandial. Although severe pain is not a prominent symptom, some patients with active disease may experience vague lower abdominal discomfort or mild central abdominal cramping. Severe cramping and abdominal pain can occur in association with severe attacks of the disease. Other symptoms in moderate to severe disease include anorexia, nausea, vomiting, fever, and weight loss.

Physical signs of proctitis include a tender anal canal and blood on rectal examination. With more extensive disease, patients have tenderness to palpation directly over the colon. Patients with a toxic colitis have severe pain and bleeding, and those with megacolon have hepatic tympany. Both may have signs of peritonitis if a perforation has occurred. The classification of disease activity is shown in Table 276-2.

Laboratory, Endoscopic, and Radiographic Features Active disease can be associated with a rise in acute-phase reactants (C-reactive protein, orosomucoid levels), platelet count, erythrocyte sedimentation rate (ESR), and a decrease in hemoglobin. In severely ill patients, the serum albumin level will fall rather quickly. Leukocytosis may be present but is not a specific indicator of disease activity. Proctitis or proctosigmoiditis rarely causes a rise in C-reactive protein. Diagnosis relies upon the patient's history; clinical symptoms, negative stool examination for bacteria, *Clostridium difficile* toxin, and ova and parasites; sigmoidoscopic appearance (see Fig. 272-18); and histology of rectal or colonic biopsy specimens.

Sigmoidoscopy is used to assess disease activity and is often performed before treatment. If the patient is not having an acute flare, colonoscopy is used to assess disease extent and activity. Histologic features change more slowly than clinical features but can also be used to grade disease activity.

Patients with a severe attack of UC should have a plain, supine film of the abdomen. In the presence of severe disease, the margin of the colon becomes edematous and irregular. Colon thickening and toxic dilation can both be seen on a plain radiograph.

The earliest radiologic change of UC seen on single-contrast barium enema is a fine mucosal granularity (Fig. 276-5). With increasing severity, the mucosa becomes thickened and superficial ulcers are seen. Deep ulcerations can appear as "collar-button" ulcers, which indicate that the ulceration has penetrated the mucosa. Haustral folds may be normal in mild disease, but as activity progresses they become edematous and thickened. Loss of haustration can occur, especially in patients with long-standing disease. In addition, the colon becomes shortened and narrowed. Polyps in the colon may be postinflammatory polyps or pseudopolyps, adenomatous polyps, or carcinoma.

Computed tomography (CT) scanning is not as helpful as endoscopy and barium enema in making the diagnosis of UC, but typical findings include mild mural thickening (<1.5 cm), inhomogeneous

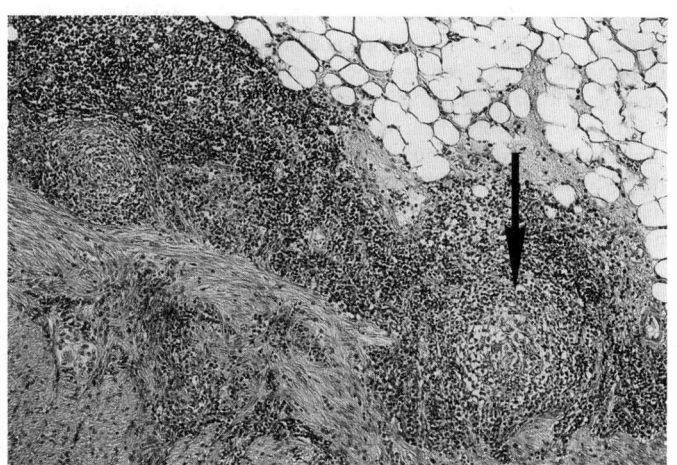

FIGURE 276-4 Granulomas (*arrow*) in bowel wall and serosa of colon, CD. (*Courtesy of Dr. EK Rosado and Dr. CA Perkos, Division of Gastrointestinal Pathology, Department of Pathology, Emory University, Atlanta, Georgia.*)

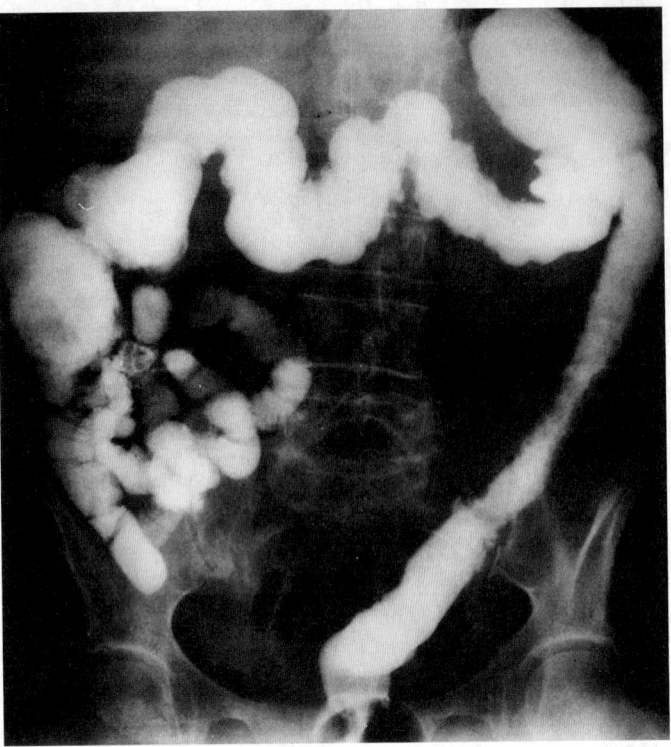

FIGURE 276-5   Barium enema in a patient with acute ulcerative colitis: inflammation of the entire colon. *(Courtesy of Dr. JM Braver, Gastrointestinal Radiology, Department of Radiology, Brigham and Women's Hospital, Boston, Massachusetts.)*

wall density, absence of small-bowel thickening, increased perirectal and presacral fat, target appearance of the rectum, and adenopathy.

Complications   Only 15% of patients with UC present initially with catastrophic illness. Massive hemorrhage occurs with severe attacks of disease in 1% of patients, and treatment for the disease usually stops the bleeding. However, if a patient requires 6 to 8 units of blood within 24 to 48 h, colectomy is indicated. Toxic megacolon is defined as a transverse colon with a diameter of >5 to 6 cm, with loss of haustration in patients with severe attacks of UC. It occurs in about 5% of attacks and can be triggered by electrolyte abnormalities and narcotics. About 50% of acute dilations will resolve with medical therapy alone, but urgent colectomy is required for those that do not improve. Perforation is the most dangerous of the local complications, and the physical signs of peritonitis may not be obvious, especially if the patient is receiving glucocorticoids. Although perforation is rare, the mortality rate for perforation complicating a toxic megacolon is about 15%. In addition, patients can develop a toxic colitis and such severe ulcerations that the bowel may perforate without first dilating.

Obstructions caused by benign stricture formation occur in 10% of patients, with one-third of the strictures occurring in the rectum. These should be surveyed endoscopically for carcinoma. UC patients occasionally develop anal fissures, perianal abscesses, or hemorrhoids, but the occurrence of extensive perianal lesions should suggest CD.

CROHN'S DISEASE ■ Signs and Symptoms   Although CD usually presents as acute or chronic bowel inflammation, the inflammatory process evolves toward one of two patterns of disease: a fibrostenotic-obstructing pattern or a penetrating-fistulous pattern, each with different treatments and prognoses. The site of disease influences the clinical manifestations.

ILEOCOLITIS   Because the most common site of inflammation is the terminal ileum, the usual presentation of ileocolitis is a chronic history of recurrent episodes of right lower quadrant pain and diarrhea. Sometimes the initial presentation mimics acute appendicitis with pronounced right lower quadrant pain, a palpable mass, fever, and leukocytosis. Pain is usually colicky; it precedes and is relieved by defecation. A low-grade fever is usually noted. High-spiking fever suggests intraabdominal abscess formation. Weight loss is common—typically 10 to 20% of body weight—and develops as a consequence of diarrhea, anorexia, and fear of eating.

An inflammatory mass may be palpated in the right lower quadrant of the abdomen. The mass is composed of inflamed bowel, adherent and indurated mesentery, and enlarged abdominal lymph nodes. Extension of the mass can cause obstruction of the right ureter or bladder inflammation, manifested by dysuria and fever. Edema, bowel wall thickening, and fibrosis of the bowel wall within the mass account for the radiographic "string sign" of a narrowed intestinal lumen.

Bowel obstruction may take several forms. In the early stages of disease, bowel wall edema and spasm produce intermittent obstructive manifestations and increasing symptoms of postprandial pain. Over several years, persistent inflammation gradually progresses to fibrostenotic narrowing and stricture. Diarrhea will decrease and be replaced by chronic bowel obstruction. Acute episodes of obstruction occur as well, precipitated by bowel inflammation and spasm or sometimes by impaction of undigested food or medication. These episodes usually resolve with intravenous fluids and gastric decompression.

Severe inflammation of the ileocecal region may lead to localized wall thinning, with microperforation and fistula formation to the adjacent bowel, the skin, the urinary bladder, or to an abscess cavity in the mesentery. Enterovesical fistulas typically present as dysuria or recurrent bladder infections or less commonly as pneumaturia or fecaluria. Enterocutaneous fistulas follow tissue planes of least resistance, usually draining through abdominal surgical scars. Enterovaginal fistulas are rare and present as dyspareunia or as a feculent or foul-smelling, often painful vaginal discharge. They are unlikely to develop without a prior hysterectomy.

JEJUNOILEITIS   Extensive inflammatory disease is associated with a loss of digestive and absorptive surface, resulting in malabsorption and steatorrhea. Nutritional deficiencies can also result from poor intake and enteric losses of protein and other nutrients. Intestinal malabsorption can cause hypoalbuminemia, hypocalcemia, hypomagnesemia, coagulopathy, and hyperoxaluria with nephrolithiasis. Vertebral fractures are caused by a combination of vitamin D deficiency, hypocalcemia, and prolonged glucocorticoid use. Pellagra from niacin deficiency can occur in extensive small-bowel disease, and malabsorption of vitamin B_{12} can lead to a megaloblastic anemia and neurologic symptoms.

Diarrhea is characteristic of active disease; its causes include: (1) bacterial overgrowth in obstructive stasis or fistulization, (2) bile-acid malabsorption due to a diseased or resected terminal ileum, and (3) intestinal inflammation with decreased water absorption and increased secretion of electrolytes.

COLITIS AND PERIANAL DISEASE   Patients with colitis present with low-grade fevers, malaise, diarrhea, crampy abdominal pain, and sometimes hematochezia. Gross bleeding is not as common as in UC and appears in about half of patients with exclusively colonic disease. Only 1 to 2% bleed massively. Pain is caused by passage of fecal material through narrowed and inflamed segments of large bowel. Decreased rectal compliance is another cause for diarrhea in Crohn's colitis patients. Toxic megacolon is rare but may be seen with severe inflammation and short-duration disease.

Stricturing can occur in the colon and produce symptoms of bowel obstruction. Also, colonic disease may fistulize into the stomach or duodenum, causing feculent vomiting, or to the proximal or mid small bowel, causing malabsorption by "short circuiting" and bacterial overgrowth. Ten percent of women with Crohn's colitis will develop a rectovaginal fistula.

Perianal disease affects about one-third of patients with Crohn's colitis and is manifested by incontinence, large hemorrhoidal tags, anal strictures, anorectal fistulae, and perirectal abscesses. Not all patients with perianal fistula will have endoscopic evidence of colonic inflammation.

GASTRODUODENAL DISEASE Symptoms and signs of upper gastrointestinal tract disease include nausea, vomiting, and epigastric pain. Patients usually have a *H. pylori*–negative gastritis. The second portion of the duodenum is more commonly involved than the bulb. Fistulas involving the stomach or duodenum arise from the small or large bowel and do not necessarily signify the presence of upper gastrointestinal tract involvement. Patients with advanced gastroduodenal CD may develop a chronic gastric outlet obstruction.

Laboratory, Endoscopic, and Radiographic Features Laboratory abnormalities include elevated ESR and C-reactive protein. In more severe disease, findings include hypoalbuminemia, anemia, and leukocytosis.

Endoscopic features of CD include rectal sparing, aphthous ulcerations, fistulas, and skip lesions. Endoscopy is useful for biopsy of mass lesions or strictures, or for visualization of filling defects seen on barium enema. Colonoscopy allows examination and biopsy of the terminal ileum, and upper endoscopy is useful in diagnosing gastroduodenal involvement in patients with upper tract symptoms. Ileal or colonic strictures may be dilated with balloons introduced through the colonoscope. Endoscopic appearance correlates poorly with clinical remission; thus, repeated endoscopy is not used to monitor the inflammation.

In CD early radiographic findings in the small bowel include thickened folds and aphthous ulcerations. "Cobblestoning" from longitudinal and transverse ulcerations most frequently involves the small bowel (Fig. 276-6). In more advanced disease, strictures, fistulas (Fig. 276-7), inflammatory masses, and abscesses may be detected. The earliest macroscopic findings of colonic CD are aphthous ulcers. These small ulcers are often multiple and separated by normal intervening mucosa. As disease progresses, aphthous ulcers become enlarged, deeper, and occasionally connected to one another, forming longitudinal stellate, serpiginous, and linear ulcers (see Fig. 272-17).

The transmural inflammation of CD leads to decreased luminal diameter and limited distensibility. As ulcers progress deeper, they can lead to fistula formation. The radiographic "string sign" represents long areas of circumferential inflammation and fibrosis, resulting in long segments of luminal narrowing. The segmental nature of CD

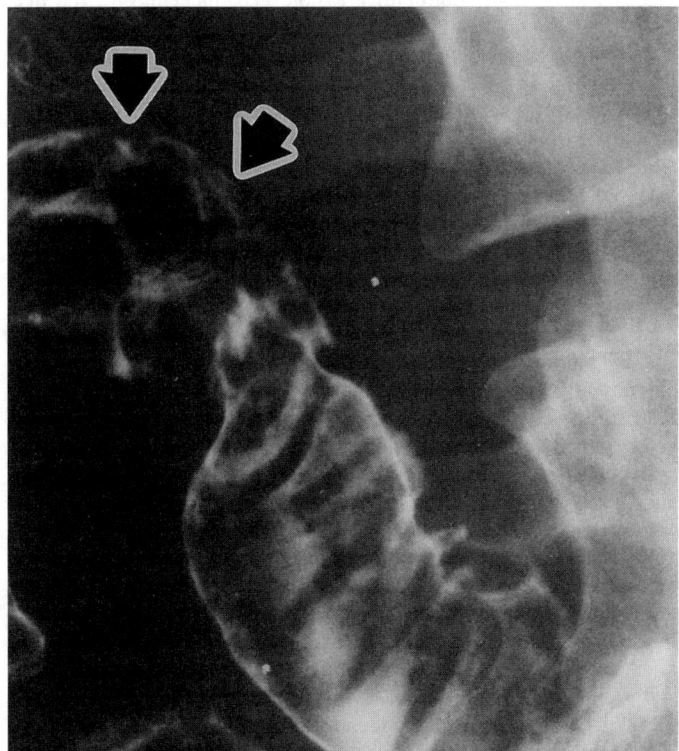

FIGURE 276-6 Crohn's disease: small bowel series demonstrating "cobblestoning" of the terminal ileum (*arrows*). (*Courtesy of Dr. JM Braver, Gastrointestinal Radiology, Department of Radiology, Brigham and Women's Hospital, Boston, Massachusetts.*)

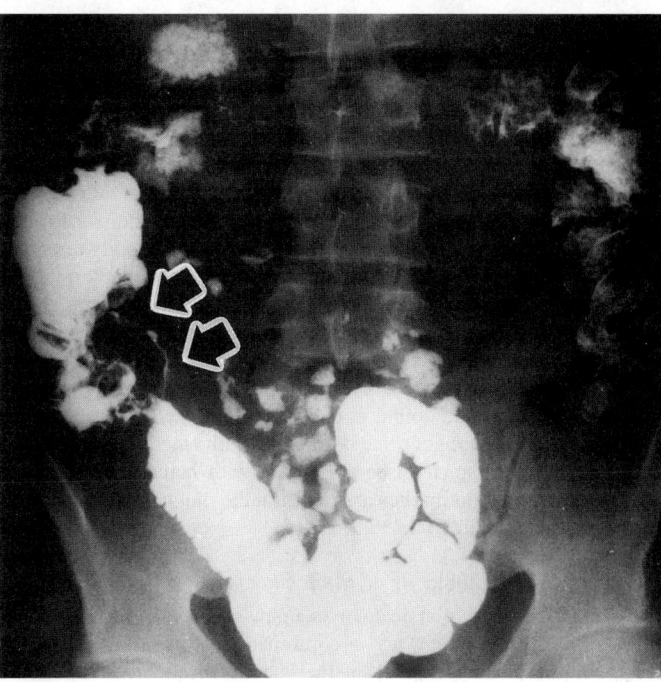

FIGURE 276-7 Small bowel series demonstrating distal ileal inflammation and fistulization (*arrows*) in a patient with CD. (*Courtesy of Dr. JM Braver, Gastrointestinal Radiology, Department of Radiology, Brigham and Women's Hospital, Boston, Massachusetts.*)

results in wide gaps of normal or dilated bowel between involved segments.

CT findings include mural thickening >2 cm, homogeneous wall density, mural thickening of small bowel, mesenteric fat stranding, perianal disease, and adenopathy. CT scanning can help identify abscesses, fistulas, and sinus tracts. Magnetic resonance imaging (MRI) may prove superior for demonstrating pelvic lesions such as ischiorectal abscesses.

Complications Because CD is a transmural process, serosal adhesions develop that provide direct pathways for fistula formation and reduce the incidence of free perforation. Free perforation occurs in 1 to 2% of patients, usually in the ileum but occasionally in the jejunum or as a complication of toxic megacolon. The peritonitis of free perforation, especially colonic, may be fatal. Generalized peritonitis may also result from the rupture of an intraabdominal abscess. Other complications include intestinal obstruction in 40%, massive hemorrhage, malabsorption, and severe perianal disease.

Serologic Markers Several serologic markers may be used to differentiate between CD and UC and help to predict the course of disease. Two antibodies that can be detected in the serum of IBD patients are perinuclear antineutrophil cytoplasmic antibodies (pANCAs) and anti-*Saccharomyces cerevisiae* antibodies (ASCAs). A distinct set of antineutrophil cytoplasmic antibodies with perinuclear staining by indirect immunofluorescence is associated with UC. The antigens to which these antibodies are directed have not been identified, but they are distinct from those associated with vasculitis and may be a marker for reactivity to enteric bacteria. pANCA positivity is found in about 60 to 70% of UC patients and 5 to 10% of CD patients; 5 to 15% of first-degree relatives of UC patients are pANCA positive, whereas only 2 to 3% of the general population is pANCA positive. pANCA may also identify specific disease phenotypes. pANCA positivity is more often associated with pancolitis, early surgery, pouchitis, or inflammation of the pouch after ileal pouch–anal anastamosis (IPAA) and primary sclerosing cholangitis. pANCA in CD is associated with colonic disease that resembles UC.

ASCA antibodies recognize mannose sequences in the cell wall mannan of *S. cerevisiae*; 60 to 70% of CD patients, 10 to 15% of UC patients, and up to 5% of non-IBD controls are ASCA positive. About 55% of CD patients are seroreactive to outer-membrane porin C (OMPC), a bacterial antigen. The combined measurement of pANCA and ASCA has been advocated as a valuable diagnostic approach to IBD. In one report, pANCA+ with ASCA− results showed a 57% sensitivity and 97% specificity for UC, whereas pANCA− with ASCA+ results showed a 49% sensitivity and 97% specificity for CD. ASCA was associated with small-bowel CD. These antibody tests may help decide whether a patient with indeterminate colitis should undergo an IPAA, because patients with predominant features of CD often have a more difficult postoperative course.

Other serologic markers in IBD patients include anti-goblet cell autoantibodies, pancreatic autoantibodies, and an autoantibody against tropomyosin isoform 5 found in colon epithelial cells. Antibodies to red cell membrane antigens that cross-react with enteropathogens such as *Campylobacter* sp. may be associated with hemolytic anemia in CD. None of these antibodies are useful in the diagnosis and management of patients with IBD.

DIFFERENTIAL DIAGNOSIS OF UC AND CD

UC and CD have similar features to many other diseases. In the absence of a key diagnostic test, a combination of clinical, laboratory, histopathologic, radiographic, and therapeutic observations is required (Table 276-3). Once a diagnosis of IBD is made, distinguishing between UC and CD is impossible in 10 to 15% of cases. These are termed *indeterminate colitis*.

INFECTIOUS DISEASE Infections of the small intestines and colon can mimic CD or UC. They may be bacterial, fungal, viral, or protozoal in origin (Table 276-4). *Campylobacter* colitis can mimic the endoscopic appearance of severe UC and can cause a relapse of established UC. *Salmonella* can cause watery or bloody diarrhea, nausea, and vomiting. Shigellosis causes watery diarrhea, abdominal pain, and fe-

TABLE 276-3 *Different Clinical, Endoscopic, and Radiographic Features*

	Ulcerative Colitis	Crohn's Disease
CLINICAL		
Gross blood in stool	Yes	Occasionally
Mucus	Yes	Occasionally
Systemic symptoms	Occasionally	Frequently
Pain	Occasionally	Frequently
Abdominal mass	Rarely	Yes
Significant perineal disease	No	Frequently
Fistulas	No	Yes
Small-intestinal obstruction	No	Frequently
Colonic obstruction	Rarely	Frequently
Response to antibiotics	No	Yes
Recurrence after surgery	No	Yes
ANCA-positive	Frequently	Rarely
ASCA-positive	Rarely	Frequently
ENDOSCOPIC		
Rectal sparing	Rarely	Frequently
Continuous disease	Yes	Occasionally
"Cobblestoning"	No	Yes
Granuloma on biopsy	No	Occasionally
RADIOGRAPHIC		
Small bowel significantly abnormal	No	Yes
Abnormal terminal ileum	Occasionally	Yes
Segmental colitis	No	Yes
Asymmetric colitis	No	Yes
Stricture	Occasionally	Frequently

Note: ANCA, antineutrophil cytoplasm antibody; ASCA, anti-Saccharomyces cerevisiae antibody.

TABLE 276-4 *Diseases that Mimic IBD*

INFECTIOUS ETIOLOGIES

Bacterial	**Mycobacterial**	**Viral**
Salmonella	Tuberculosis	Cytomegalovirus
Shigella	*Mycobacterium*	Herpes simplex
Toxigenic	*avium*	HIV
Escherichia coli	**Parasitic**	**Fungal**
Campylobacter	Amebiasis	Histoplasmosis
Yersinia	*Isospora*	*Candida*
Clostridium	*Trichuris trichura*	*Aspergillus*
difficile	Hookworm	
Gonorrhea	*Strongyloides*	
Chlamydia		
trachomatis		

NONINFECTIOUS ETIOLOGIES

Inflammatory	**Neoplastic**	**Drugs and Chemicals**
Appendicitis	Lymphoma	NSAIDs
Diverticulitis	Metastatic	Phosphasoda
Diversion colitis	carcinoma	Cathartic colon
Collagenous/	Carcinoma of the	Gold
lymphocytic	ileum	Oral contraceptives
colitis	Carcinoid	Cocaine
Ischemic colitis	Familial polyposis	Chemotherapy
Radiation colitis/		
enteritis		
Solitary rectal ulcer		
Eosinophilc		
gastroenteritis		
Neutropenic colitis		
Beçhet's syndrome		
Graft-versus-host		
disease		

Note: NSAIDs, nonsteroidal anti-inflammatory drugs.

ver followed by rectal tenesmus and by the passage of blood and mucus per rectum. All three are usually self-limited, but 1% of patients infected with *Salmonella* become asymptomatic carriers. *Yersinia enterocolitica* infection occurs mainly in the terminal ileum and causes mucosal ulceration, neutrophil invasion, and thickening of the ileal wall. Other bacterial infections that may mimic IBD include *C. difficile*, which presents with watery diarrhea, tenesmus, nausea, and vomiting; and *Escherichia coli*, three categories of which can cause colitis. These are enterohemorrhagic, enteroinvasive, and enteroadherent *E. coli*, all of which can cause bloody diarrhea and abdominal tenderness. Diagnosis of bacterial colitis is made by sending stool specimens for bacterial culture and *C. difficile* toxin analysis. Gonorrhea, *Chlamydia*, and syphilis can also cause proctitis.

Gastrointestinal involvement with mycobacterial infection occurs primarily in the immunosuppressed patient but may occur in patients with normal immunity. Distal ileal and cecal involvement predominates, and patients present with symptoms of small-bowel obstruction and a tender abdominal mass. The diagnosis is made most directly by colonoscopy with biopsy and culture. *Mycobacterium avium-intracellulare* complex infection occurs in advanced stages of HIV infection and in other immunocompromised states and usually manifests as a systemic infection with diarrhea, abdominal pain, weight loss, fever, and malabsorption. Diagnosis is established by acid-fast smear and culture of mucosal biopsies.

Although most of the patients with viral colitis are immunosuppressed, cytomegalovirus (CMV) and herpes simplex proctitis may occur in immunocompetent individuals. CMV occurs most commonly in the esophagus, colon, and rectum but may also involve the small intestine. Symptoms include abdominal pain, bloody diarrhea, fever, and weight loss. With severe disease, necrosis and perforation can occur. Diagnosis is made by identification of intranuclear inclusions in mucosal cells on biopsy. Herpes simplex infection of the gastrointestinal tract is limited to the oropharynx, anorectum, and perianal areas. Symptoms include anorectal pain, tenesmus, constipation, inguinal adenopathy, difficulty with urinary voiding, and sacral paresthesias. Diagnosis is made by rectal biopsy. HIV itself can cause diarrhea, nausea, vomiting, and anorexia. Small-intestinal biopsies show partial villus atrophy; small-bowel bacterial overgrowth and fat malabsorption may also be noted.

Protozoan parasites include *Isospora belli*, which can cause a self-limited infection in healthy hosts but causes a chronic profuse, watery diarrhea and weight loss in AIDS patients. *Entamoeba histolytica* or related species infect about 10% of the world's population; symptoms include abdominal pain, tenesmus, frequent loose stools containing blood and mucus, and abdominal tenderness. Colonoscopy reveals focal punctate ulcers with normal intervening mucosa; diagnosis is made by biopsy or serum amebic antibodies. Fulminant amebic colitis is rare but has a mortality rate of >50%.

Other parasitic infections that may mimic IBD include hookworm (*Necator americanus*), whipworm (*Trichuris trichiura*), and *Strongyloides stercoralis*. In severely immunocompromised patients *Candida* or *Aspergillus* can be identified in the submucosa. Disseminated histoplasmosis can involve the ileocecal area.

NONINFECTIOUS DISEASE Many diseases may mimic IBD (Table 276-4). Diverticulitis can be confused with CD clinically and radiographically. Both diseases cause fever, abdominal pain, tender abdominal mass, leukocytosis, elevated ESR, partial obstruction, and fistulas. Perianal disease or ileitis on small-bowel series favors the diagnosis of CD. Significant endoscopic mucosal abnormalities are more likely in CD than in diverticulitis. Endoscopic or clinical recurrence following segmental resection favors CD. Diverticular-associated colitis is similar to CD, but mucosal abnormalities are limited to the sigmoid and descending colon.

Ischemic colitis is commonly confused with IBD. The ischemic process can be chronic and diffuse as in UC, or segmental as in CD. Colonic inflammation due to ischemia may resolve quickly or may persist and result in transmural scarring and stricture formation. Ischemic bowel disease should be considered in the elderly following abdominal aortic aneurysm repair or when a patient has a hypercoagulable state or a severe cardiac or peripheral vascular disorder. Patients usually present with sudden onset of left lower quadrant pain, urgency to defecate, and the passage of bright red blood per rectum. Endoscopic examination often demonstrates a normal-appearing rectum and a sharp transition to an area of inflammation in the descending colon and splenic flexure.

The effects of radiation therapy on the gastrointestinal tract can be difficult to distinguish from IBD. Acute symptoms can occur within 1 to 2 weeks of starting radiotherapy. When the rectum and sigmoid are irradiated, patients develop bloody, mucoid diarrhea and tenesmus, as in distal UC. With small-bowel involvement, diarrhea is common. Late symptoms include malabsorption and weight loss. Stricturing with obstruction and bacterial overgrowth may occur. Fistulas can penetrate the bladder, vagina, or abdominal wall. Flexible sigmoidoscopy reveals mucosal granularity, friability, numerous telangiectasias, and occasionally discrete ulcerations. Biopsy can be diagnostic.

Solitary rectal ulcer syndrome is uncommon and can be confused with IBD. It occurs in persons of all ages and may be caused by impaired evacuation and failure of relaxation of the puborectalis muscle. Ulceration may arise from anal sphincter overactivity, higher intrarectal pressures during defecation, and digital removal of stool. Patients complain of constipation with straining and pass blood and mucus per rectum. Other symptoms include abdominal pain, diarrhea, tenesmus, and perineal pain. The ulceration, which can be as large as 5 cm in diameter, is usually seen anteriorly or anteriorlaterally 3 to 15 cm from the anal verge. Biopsies can be diagnostic.

Several types of colitis have been associated with nonsteroidal anti-inflammatory drugs (NSAIDs), including de novo colitis, reactivation of IBD, and proctitis caused by use of suppositories. Most patients with NSAID-related colitis present with diarrhea and abdominal pain and complications include stricture, bleeding, obstruction, perforation,

and fistulization. Withdrawal of these agents is crucial, and in cases of reactivated IBD, standard therapies are indicated.

INDETERMINATE COLITIS Cases of IBD that cannot be categorized as UC or CD are called *indeterminate colitis*. Long-term follow-up reduces the number of cases labeled indeterminate to about 10%. The disease course of indeterminate colitis is unclear and surgical recommendations are difficult, especially since up to 20% of pouches fail, requiring ileosotomy. A multistage IPAA (the initial stage consisting of a subtotal colectomy with Hartmann pouch) with careful histologic evaluation of the resected specimen to exclude CD is advised. Medical therapy is similar to that for UC and CD; most clinicians use 5-ASA drugs, glucocorticoids, and immunomodulators as necessary.

THE ATYPICAL COLITIDIES Two atypical colitides—collagenous colitis and lymphocytic colitis—have completely normal endoscopic appearances. Collagenous colitis has two main histologic components: increased subepithelial collagen deposition and colitis with increased intraepithelial lymphocytes. Female to male ratio is 9:1, and most patients present in the sixth or seventh decades of life. The main symptom is chronic watery diarrhea. Treatments range from sulfasalazine or mesalamine and Lomotil to bismuth to glucocorticoids for refractory disease.

Lymphocytic colitis has features similar to collagenous colitis including age at onset and clinical presentation, but it has almost equal incidence in men and women and no subepithelial collagen deposition on pathologic section. However, intraepithelial lymphocytes are increased. Diarrhea stops in most patients treated with 5-ASA or prednisone.

Diversion colitis is an inflammatory process that arises in segments of the large intestine that are excluded from the fecal stream. It usually occurs in patients with ileostomy or colostomy when a mucus fistula or a Hartmann's pouch has been created. Diversion colitis is reversible by surgical reanastamosis. Clinically, patients have mucus or bloody discharge from the rectum. Erythema, granularity, friability, and, in more severe cases, ulceration can be seen on endoscopy. Histopathology shows areas of active inflammation with foci of cryptitis and crypt abscesses. Crypt architecture is normal and this differentiates it from UC. It may be impossible to distinguish it from CD. Short-chain fatty acid enemas will help in diversion colitis, but the definitive therapy is surgical reanastamosis.

EXTRAINTESTINAL MANIFESTATIONS

IBD is associated with a variety of extraintestinal manifestations; up to one-third of patients have at least one. Patients with perianal CD are at higher risk for developing extraintestinal manifestations than other IBD patients.

DERMATOLOGIC Erythema nodosum (EN) occurs in up to 15% of CD patients and 10% of UC patients. Attacks usually correlate with bowel activity; skin lesions develop after the onset of bowel symptoms, and patients frequently have concomitant active peripheral arthritis. The lesions of EN are hot, red, tender nodules measuring 1 to 5 cm in diameter and are found on the anterior surface of the lower legs, ankles, calves, thighs, and arms. Therapy is directed toward the underlying bowel disease.

Pyoderma gangrenosum (PG) is seen in 1 to 12% of UC patients and less commonly in Crohn's colitis. Although it usually presents after the diagnosis of IBD, PG may occur years before the onset of bowel symptoms, run a course independent of the bowel disease, respond poorly to colectomy, and even develop years after proctocolectomy. It is usually associated with severe disease. Lesions are commonly found on the dorsal surface of the feet and legs but may occur on the arms, chest, stoma, and even the face. PG usually begins as a pustule and then spreads concentrically to rapidly undermine healthy skin. Lesions then ulcerate, with violaceous edges surrounded by a margin of erythema. Centrally, they contain necrotic tissue with blood and exudates. Lesions may be single or multiple and grow as large as 30 cm. They are sometimes very difficult to treat and often require intravenous antibiotics, intravenous glucocorticoids, dapsone, azathioprine, thalidomide, intravenous cyclosporine, or infliximab.

Other dermatologic manifestations include pyoderma vegetans that occurs in intertriginous areas, pyostomatitis vegetans that involves the mucous membranes, Sweet's syndrome, a neutrophilic dermatosis, and metastatic CD, a rare disorder defined by cutaneous granuloma formation. Psoriasis affects 5 to 10% of patients with IBD and is unrelated to bowel activity. Perianal skin tags are found in 75 to 80% of patients with CD, especially those with colon involvement. Oral mucosal lesions are seen often in CD and rarely in UC and include aphthous stomatitis and "cobblestone" lesions of the buccal mucosa.

RHEUMATOLOGIC   Peripheral arthritis develops in 15 to 20% of IBD patients, is more common in CD, and worsens with exacerbations of bowel activity. It is asymmetric, polyarticular, and migratory and most often affects large joints of the upper and lower extremities. Treatment is directed at reducing bowel inflammation. In severe UC, colectomy frequently cures the arthritis.

Ankylosing spondylitis (AS) occurs in about 10% of IBD patients and is more common in CD than UC. About two-thirds of IBD patients with AS test positive for the HLA-B27 antigen. The activity of AS is not related to bowel activity and does not remit with glucocorticoids or colectomy. It most often affects the spine and pelvis, producing symptoms of diffuse low-back pain, buttock pain, and morning stiffness. The course is continuous and progressive, leading to permanent skeletal damage and deformity.

Sacroiliitis is symmetric, occurs equally in UC and CD, is often asymptomatic, does not correlate with bowel activity, and does not always progress to AS. Other rheumatic manifestations include hypertrophic osteoarthropathy, pelvic/femoral osteomyelitis, and relapsing polychondritis.

OCULAR   The incidence of ocular complications in IBD patients is 1 to 10%. The most common are conjunctivitis, anterior uveitis/iritis, and episcleritis. Uveitis is associated with both UC and Crohn's colitis, may be found during periods of remission, and may develop in patients following bowel resection. Symptoms include ocular pain, photophobia, blurred vision, and headache. Prompt intervention, sometimes with systemic glucocorticoids, is required to prevent scarring and visual impairment. Episcleritis is a benign disorder that presents with symptoms of mild ocular burning. It occurs in 3 to 4% of IBD patients, more commonly in Crohn's colitis, and is treated with topical glucocorticoids.

HEPATOBILIARY   Hepatic steatosis is detectable in about half of the abnormal liver biopsies from patients with CD and UC; patients usually present with hepatomegaly. Fatty liver usually results from a combination of chronic debilitating illness, malnutrition, and glucocorticoid therapy. Cholelithiasis is more common in CD than UC and occurs in 10 to 35% of patients with ileitis or ileal resection. Gallstone formation is caused by malabsorption of bile acids resulting in depletion of the bile salt pool and the secretion of lithogenic bile.

Primary sclerosing cholangitis (PSC) is characterized by both intrahepatic and extrahepatic bile duct inflammation and fibrosis, frequently leading to biliary cirrhosis and hepatic failure; 1 to 5% of patients with IBD have PSC, but 50 to 75% of patients with PSC have IBD. Although it can be recognized after the diagnosis of IBD, PSC can be detected earlier or even years after proctocolectomy. Most patients have no symptoms at the time of diagnosis; when symptoms are present they consist of fatigue, jaundice, abdominal pain, fever, anorexia, and malaise. Diagnosis is made by endoscopic retrograde cholangiopancreatography (ERCP), which demonstrates multiple bile duct strictures alternating with relatively normal segments. The bile acid ursodeoxycholic acid (ursodiol) may reduce alkaline phosphatase and serum aminotransferase levels, but histologic improvement has been marginal. High doses (25 to 30 mg/kg per day) may have long-term benefit. Endoscopic stenting may be palliative for cholestasis secondary to bile duct obstruction. Patients with symptomatic disease develop cirrhosis and liver failure over 5 to 10 years and eventually require liver transplantation. Ten percent of PSC patients develop cholangiocarcinoma and cannot be transplanted. Pericholangitis is a subset of PSC found in about 30% of IBD patients; it is confined to small bile ducts and is usually benign.

UROLOGIC   The most frequent genitourinary complications are calculi, ureteral obstruction, and fistulas. The highest frequency of nephrolithiasis (10 to 20%) occurs in patients with CD following small-bowel resection. Calcium oxalate stones develop secondary to hyperoxaluria, which results from increased absorption of dietary oxalate. Normally, dietary calcium combines with luminal oxalate to form insoluble calcium oxalate, which is eliminated in the stool. In patients with ileal dysfunction, however, nonabsorbed fatty acids bind calcium and leave oxalate unbound. The unbound oxalate is then delivered to the colon, where it is readily absorbed, especially in the presence of colonic inflammation.

OTHER   The risk of thromboembolic disease increases when IBD becomes active, and patients may present with deep vein thrombosis, pulmonary embolism, cerebrovascular accidents, and arterial emboli. Factors responsible for the hypercoagulable state include reactive thrombocytosis; increased levels of fibrinopeptide A, factor V, factor VIII, and fibrinogen; accelerated thromboplastin generation; antithrombin III deficiency secondary to increased gut losses or increased catabolism; and free protein S deficiency. A spectrum of vasculitidies involving small, medium, and large vessels has also been observed in IBD patients.

Patients with IBD have an increased prevalence of osteoporosis and osteomalacia from vitamin D deficiency, calcium malabsorption, malnutrition, glucocorticoid use, and the intestinal inflammation itself. Deficiencies of vitamin B_{12} and fat-soluble vitamins may occur after ileal resection or with ileal disease.

More common cardiopulmonary manifestations include endocarditis, myocarditis, pleuropericarditis, and interstitial lung disease. A secondary or reactive amyloidosis can occur in patients with longstanding IBD, especially in patients with CD. Amyloid material is deposited systemically and can cause diarrhea, constipation, and renal failure. The renal disease can be successfully treated with colchicine. Pancreatitis is a rare extraintestinal manifestation of IBD and results from duodenal fistulas, ampullary CD, gallstones, PSC, drugs such as 6-mercaptopurine, azathioprine, or very rarely, 5-ASA agents, autoimmune pancreatitis, and primary CD of the pancreas.

℞ TREATMENT

5-ASA AGENTS   The mainstay of therapy for mild to moderate UC and Crohn's colitis is sulfasalazine and the other 5-ASA agents. These agents are effective at inducing remission in both UC and CD and in maintaining remission in UC; it remains unclear whether they have a role in remission maintenance in CD.

Sulfasalazine was originally developed to deliver both antibacterial (sulfapyridine) and anti-inflammatory (5-ASA) therapy into the connective tissues of joints and the colonic mucosa. The molecular structure provides a convenient delivery system to the colon by allowing the intact molecule to pass through the small intestine after only partial absorption, and to be broken down in the colon by bacterial azo reductases that cleave the azo bond linking the sulfa and 5-ASA moieties. Sulfasalazine is effective treatment for mild to moderate UC and Crohn's ileocolitis and colitis, but its high rate of side effects limits its use. Although sulfasalazine is more effective at higher doses, at 6 or 8 g/d up to 30% of patients experience allergic reactions or intolerable side effects such as headache, anorexia, nausea, and vomiting that are attributable to the sulfapyridine moiety. Hypersensitivity reactions, independent of sulfapyridine levels, include rash, fever, hepatitis, agranulocytosis, hypersensitivity pneumonitis, pancreatitis, worsening of colitis, and reversible sperm abnormalities. Sulfasalazine can also impair folate absorption, and patients should be given folic acid supplements.

Newer sulfa-free aminosalicylate preparations deliver increased amounts of the pharmacologically active ingredient of sulfasalazine (5-ASA, mesalamine) to the site of active bowel disease while limiting systemic toxicity. 5-ASA may function through inhibition of NF-κB activity. Sulfa-free aminosalicylate formulations include alternative azo-bonded carriers, 5-ASA dimers, pH-dependent tablets, and continuous-release preparations. Each has the same efficacy as sulfasalazine when equimolar concentrations are used. Olsalazine is composed of two 5-ASA radicals linked by an azo bond, which is split in the colon by bacterial reduction and two 5-ASA molecules are released. Olsalazine is similar in effectiveness to sulfasalazine in treating CD and UC, but up to 17% of patients experience non-bloody diarrhea caused by increased secretion of fluid in the small bowel. Balsalazide contains an azo bond binding mesalamine to the carrier molecule 4-aminobenzoyl-β-alanine; it is effective in the colon. Claversal is an enteric-coated form of 5-ASA that consists of mesalamine surrounded by an acrylic-based polymer resin and a cellulose coating that releases mesalamine at pH > 6.0, a level that is present from the mid-jejunum continuously to the distal colon.

The most commonly used drugs besides sulfasalazine in the United States are Asacol and Pentasa. Asacol is also an enteric-coated form of mesalamine, but it has a slightly different release pattern, with 5-ASA liberated at pH > 7.0. The disintegration of Asacol is variable, with complete breakup of the tablet occurring in many different parts of the gut ranging from the small intestine to the splenic flexure; it has increased gastric residence when taken with a meal. Asacol is used to induce and maintain remission in UC and to induce remission in CD ileitis, ileocolitis, and colitis. Appropriate doses of Asacol and the other 5-ASA compounds are shown in Table 276-5. Some 50 to 75% of patients with mild to moderate UC and CD improve when treated with 2 g/d of 5-ASA; the dose response continues up to at least 4.8 g/d. Doses of 1.5 to 4 g/d maintain remission in 50 to 75% of patients with UC.

Pentasa is another mesalamine formulation that uses an ethylcellulose coating to allow water absorption into small beads containing the mesalamine. Water dissolves the 5-ASA, which then diffuses out of the bead into the lumen. Disintegration of the capsule occurs in the stomach. The microspheres then disperse throughout the entire gastrointestinal tract from the small intestine through the distal colon in both fasted or fed conditions. Controlled trials of Pentasa and Asacol in active CD demonstrate a 40 to 60% clinical improvement or remission, but the data are not conclusive that these agents maintain remission in CD. 5-ASA agents may be effective in postoperative prophylaxis of CD.

Topical mesalamine enemas are effective in mild-to-moderate distal UC and CD. Clinical response occurs in up to 80% of UC patients with colitis distal to the splenic flexure. Mesalamine suppositories are effective in treating proctitis.

Glucocorticoids The majority of patients with moderate to severe UC benefit from oral or parenteral glucocorticoids. Prednisone is usually started at doses of 40 to 60 mg/d for active UC that is unresponsive to 5-ASA therapy. Parenteral glucocorticoids may be administered as intravenous hydrocortisone, 300 mg/d, or methylprednisolone, 40 to 60 mg/d. Adrenocorticotropic hormone (ACTH) is occasionally preferred for glucocorticoid-naïve patients despite a risk of adrenal hemorrhage. ACTH has equivalent efficacy to intravenous hydrocortisone in both glucocorticoid-naïve and -experienced CD patients.

Topically applied glucocorticoids are also beneficial for distal colitis and may serve as an adjunct in those who have rectal involvement plus more proximal disease. Hydrocortisone enemas or foam may control active disease, although they have no proven role as maintenance therapy. These glucocorticoids are significantly absorbed from the rectum and can lead to adrenal suppression with prolonged administration.

Glucocorticoids are also effective for treatment of moderate-to-severe CD and induce a 60 to 70% remission rate compared to a 30% placebo response. The systemic effects of standard glucocorticoid formulations have led to the development of more potent formulations that are less well absorbed and have increased first-pass metabolism. Controlled ileal-release budesonide has been nearly equal to prednisone for ileocolonic CD with fewer glucocorticoid side effects. Budesonide is used for 2 to 3 months at a dose of 9 mg/d, then tapered.

Glucocorticoids play no role in maintenance therapy in either UC or CD. Once clinical remission has been induced, they should be tapered according to the clinical activity, normally at a rate of no more than 5 mg per week. They can usually be tapered to 20 mg/d within 4 to 5 weeks but often take several months to be discontinued altogether. The side effects are numerous, including fluid retention, abdominal striae, fat redistribution, hyperglycemia, subcapsular cataracts, osteonecrosis, myopathy, emotional disturbances, and withdrawal symptoms. Most of these side effects, aside from osteonecrosis, are related to the dose and duration of therapy.

ANTIBIOTICS Antibiotics have no role in the treatment of active or quiescent UC. However, pouchitis, which occurs in about a third of UC patients after colectomy and IPAA, usually responds to treatment with metronidazole or ciprofloxacin.

Metronidazole is effective in active inflammatory, fistulous, and perianal CD and may prevent recurrence after ileal resection. The most effective dose is 15 to 20 mg/kg per day in three divided doses; it is usually continued for several months. Common side effects include nausea, metallic taste, and disulfiram-like reaction. Peripheral neuropathy can occur with prolonged administration (several months) and on rare occasions is permanent despite discontinuation. Ciprofloxacin (500 mg bid) is also beneficial for inflammatory, perianal, and fistulous CD. These two antibiotics should be used as second-line drugs in active CD after 5-ASA agents and as first-line drugs in perianal and fistulous CD.

AZATHIOPRINE AND 6-MERCAPTOPURINE Azathioprine and 6-mercaptopurine (6-MP) are purine analogues commonly employed in the management of glucocorticoid-dependent IBD. Azathioprine is rapidly absorbed and converted to 6-MP, which is then metabolized to the active end product, thioinosinic acid, an inhibitor of purine ribonucleotide synthesis and cell proliferation. These agents also inhibit the immune response. Efficacy is seen at 3 to 4 weeks. Compliance can

TABLE 276-5 *Oral 5-ASA Preparations*

Preparation	Formulation	Delivery	Dosing, g/d
AZO-BOND			
Sulfasalazine (500 mg)	Sulfapyridine-5-ASA	Colon	4–8 (acute) 2–6 (maintenance)
Olsalazine (250 mg)	5-ASA-5-ASA	Colon	1–3
Balsalazide (500–750 mg)	Aminobenzoyl-alanine-5-ASA	Colon	2.25–6.75
DELAYED-RELEASE			
Asacol (400 mg)	Eudragit S (pH 7)	Distal ileum-colon	2.4–4.8 (acute) 1.6–4.8 (maintenance)
Claversal (250–500 mg)	Eudragit L (pH 6)	Ileum-colon	1.5–3 (acute) 0.75–3 (maintenance)
SUSTAINED-RELEASE			
Pentasa (250 mg)	Ethylcellulose microgranules	Stomach-colon	2–4 (acute) 1.5–4 (maintenance)

TABLE 276-6 *Medical Management of IBD*

Ulcerative Colitis: Active Disease

	Mild	Moderate	Severe	Fulminant
Distal	5-ASA oral and/or enema	5-ASA oral and/or enema Glucocorticoid enema Oral glucocorticoid	5-ASA oral and/or enema Glucocorticoid enema Oral or IV glucocorticoid	Intravenous glucocorticoid Intravenous CSA
Extensive	5-ASA oral and/or enema	5-ASA oral and/or enema Glucocorticoid enema Oral glucocorticoid	5-ASA oral and/or enema Glucocorticoid enema Oral or IV glucocorticoid	Intravenous glucocorticoid Intravenous CSA

Ulcerative Colitis: Maintenance Therapy

Distal	5-ASA oral and/or enema 6-MP or azathioprine
Extensive	5-ASA oral and/or enema 6-MP or azathioprine

Crohn's Disease: Active Disease

Mild–Moderate	Severe	Perianal or Fistulizing Disease
5-ASA oral and/or enema Metronidazole and/or ciprofloxacin Oral glucocorticoids Infliximab Budesonide	5-ASA oral and/or enema Metronidazole and/or ciprofloxacin Oral or IV glucocorticoids Infliximab TPN or elemental diet	Metronidazole and/or ciprofloxacin Azathioprine or 6-MP Infliximab Intravenous CSA

Crohn's Disease: Maintenance Therapy

Inflammatory	Perianal or Fistulizing Disease
5-ASA oral and/or enema Azathioprine or 6-MP Infliximab	Metronidazole and/or ciprofloxacin Azathioprine or 6-MP Infliximab

Note: CSA, cyclosporine; 6-MP, 6-mercaptopurine; TPN, total parenteral nutrition.

be monitored by measuring the levels of 6-thioguanine and 6-methylmercaptopurine, end products of 6-MP metabolism. Azathioprine (2.0 to 2.5 mg/kg per day) or 6-MP (1.0 to 1.5 mg/kg per day) have been employed successfully as glucocorticoid-sparing agents in up to two-thirds of UC and CD patients previously unable to be weaned from glucocorticoids. The role of these immunomodulators as maintenance therapy in UC and CD and for treating active perianal disease and fistulas in CD appears promising. In addition, 6-MP or azathioprine may be effective for postoperative prophylaxis of CD.

Although azathioprine and 6-MP are usually well tolerated, pancreatitis occurs in 3 to 4% of patients, typically presents within the first few weeks of therapy, and is completely reversible when the drug is stopped. Other side effects include nausea, fever, rash, and hepatitis. Bone marrow suppression (particularly leukopenia) is dose-related and often delayed, necessitating regular monitoring of the complete blood count. Additionally, 1 in 300 individuals lacks thiopurine methyltransferase, the enzyme responsible for drug metabolism; an additional 11% of the population are heterozygotes with intermediate enzyme activity. Both are at increased risk of toxicity because of increased accumulation of thioguanine metabolites. No increased risk of cancer has been documented in IBD patients chronically taking these medications.

METHOTREXATE Methotrexate (MTX) inhibits dihydrofolate reductase, resulting in impaired DNA synthesis. Additional anti-inflammatory properties may be related to decreased IL-1 production. Intramuscular or subcutaneous MTX (25 mg per week) is effective in inducing remission and reducing glucocorticoid dosage, and 15 mg per week is effective in maintaining remission in active CD. Potential toxicities include leukopenia and hepatic fibrosis, necessitating periodic evaluation of complete blood counts and liver enzymes. The role of liver biopsy in patients on long-term MTX is uncertain. Hypersensitivity pneumonitis is a rare but serious complication of therapy.

CYCLOSPORINE Cyclosporine (CSA) alters the immune response by acting as a potent inhibitor of T cell–mediated responses. Although CSA acts primarily via inhibition of IL-2 production from T helper cells, it also decreases recruitment of cytotoxic T cells and blocks other cytokines, including IL-3, IL-4, IFN-γ, and TNF. It has a more rapid onset of action than 6-MP and azathioprine.

CSA is most effective given at 2 to 4 mg/kg per day intravenously in severe UC that is refractory to intravenous glucocorticoids, with 82% of patients responding. CSA can be an alternative to colectomy. The long-term success of oral CSA is not as dramatic, but if patients are started on 6-MP or azathioprine at the time of hospital discharge, remission can be maintained. Intravenous CSA is effective in 80% of patients with refractory fistulas, but 6-MP or azathioprine must be used to maintain remission. Oral CSA alone is effective only at a higher dose (7.5 mg/kg per day) in active disease but is not effective in maintaining remission without 6-MP/azathioprine. Serum levels should be monitored and kept in the range of 200 to 400 ng/mL.

CSA may cause significant toxicity; renal function should be monitored frequently. Hypertension, gingival hyperplasia, hypertrichosis, paresthesias, tremors, headaches, and electrolyte abnormalities are common side effects. Creatinine elevation calls for dose reduction or discontinuation. Seizures may also complicate therapy, especially if the patient is hypomagnesemic or if serum cholesterol levels are <3.1 mmol/L (<120 mg/dL). Opportunistic infections, most notably *Pneumocystis carinii* pneumonia, may occur with combination immunosuppressive treatment; prophylaxis should be given.

NUTRITIONAL THERAPIES Dietary antigens may stimulate the mucosal immune response. Patients with active CD respond to bowel rest, along with total enteral or total parenteral nutrition (TPN). Bowel rest and TPN are as effective as glucocorticoids at inducing remission of active CD but are not effective as maintenance therapy. Enteral nutrition in the form of elemental or peptide-based preparations are also as effective as glucocorticiods or TPN, but these diets are not palatable. Enteral diets may provide the small intestine with nutrients vital to cell growth and do not have the complications of TPN. In contrast to CD, active UC is not effectively treated with either elemental diets or TPN. Standard medical management of UC and CD is reviewed in Table 276-6.

NEWER MEDICAL THERAPIES ■ Anti-Tumor Necrosis Factor Antibody TNF is a key inflammatory cytokine and mediator of intestinal inflammation. The expression of TNF is increased in IBD. Infliximab is a chimeric mouse-human monoclonal antibody against TNF that is extremely effective in CD. It blocks TNF in the serum and at the cell surface and likely lyses TNF-producing macrophages and T cells through complement fixation and antibody-dependent cytotoxicity. Of active CD patients refractory to glucocorticoids, 6-MP, or 5-ASA, 65% will respond to intravenous infliximab (5 mg/kg); one-third will enter complete remission. Of the patients who experience an initial response, 40% will maintain remission for at least 1 year with repeated infusions of infliximab every 8 weeks.

Infliximab is also effective in CD patients with refractory perianal and enterocutaneous fistulas, with a 68% response rate (50% reduction in fistula drainage) and a 50% complete remission rate. Reinfusion, typically every 8 weeks, is necessary to continue therapeutic benefits in many patients.

The development of antibodies to infliximab (ATI) is associated with an increased risk of infusion reactions and a decreased response to treatment. Patients who receive on-demand or episodic infusions rather than periodic (every 8 weeks) infusions are more likely to develop ATI. A humanized antibody to TNF also shows some promise in early clinical testing.

Among 120,000 patients treated with infliximab, 8 developed lymphoma: 5 patients with CD and 3 with rheumatoid arthritis. As the risk of lymphoma is already increased in these conditions, it is unclear whether infliximab is the cause. Thus, infliximab is extremely effective in refractory inflammatory and fistulous CD but should be used only when necessary. Results on the efficacy of infliximab in UC are mixed.

Newer Immunosuppressive Agents   Tacrolimus has a mechanism of action similar to cyclosporine. It has shown efficacy in children with refractory IBD and in adults with extensive involvement of the small bowel.

Mycophenolate mofetil is another immunomodulator that may be effective in CD patients resistant to or intolerant of 6-MP azathioprine. Patients with CD who received 15 mg/kg per day have tolerated the drug well and have experienced benefit with reduction of glucocorticoid requirements.

6-Thioguanine is the active metabolite of 6-MP and has shown activity in patients resistant to or intolerant of 6-MP/azathioprine.

Thalidomide has been shown to inhibit TNF production by monocytes and other cells. Thalidomide is effective in glucocorticoid-refractory and fistulous CD, but randomized controlled trials still need to be performed.

The $\alpha 4$ integrin-specific humanized monoclonal antibody, natalizumab, prevents the migration of leukocytes into the parenchyma and blocks their activation in inflammatory sites. It seems to be effective in CD, but more trials are needed.

SURGICAL THERAPY ▪ Ulcerative Colitis   Nearly half of patients with extensive chronic UC undergo surgery within the first 10 years of their illness. The indications for surgery are listed in Table 276-7. Morbidity is about 20% in elective, 30% for urgent, and 40% for emergency proctocolectomy. The risks are primarily hemorrhage, contamination and sepsis, and neural injury. Although single-stage total proctocolec-

tomy with ileostomy has been the operation of choice, newer operations maintain continence while surgically removing the involved rectal mucosa.

The IPAA is the most frequent continence-preserving operation performed. Because UC is a mucosal disease, the rectal mucosa can be dissected out and removed down to the dentate line of the anus or about 2 cm proximal to it. The ileum is fashioned into a pouch that serves as a neorectum. This ileal pouch is then sutured circumferentially to the anus in an end-to-end fashion. If performed carefully, this operation preserves the anal sphincter and maintains continence. The overall operative morbidity is 10%, with the major complication being bowel obstruction. Pouch failure necessitating conversion to permanent ileostomy occurs in 5 to 10% of patients. Some inflamed rectal mucosa is usually left behind, and thus endoscopic surveillance is necessary. Primary dysplasia of the ileal mucosa of the pouch has occurred rarely.

Patients with IPAAs usually have about six to eight bowel movements a day. On validated quality-of-life indices, they report better performance in sports and sexual activities than ileostomy patients. The most frequent late complication of IPAA is pouchitis in about one-third of patients with UC. This syndrome consists of increased stool frequency, watery stools, cramping, urgency, nocturnal leakage of stool, arthralgias, malaise, and fever. Pouch biopsies and pANCA/ ASCA/OMPC serologies can distinguish true pouchitis from underlying CD. Although it usually responds to antibiotics, in 3 to 5% of patients it is refractory and requires pouch take-down.

Crohn's Disease   Most patients with CD require at least one operation in their lifetime. The need for surgery is related to duration of disease and the site of involvement. Patients with small-bowel disease have an 80% chance of requiring surgery. Those with colitis alone have a 50% chance. The indications for surgery are shown in Table 276-7.

SMALL INTESTINAL DISEASE   Because CD is chronic and recurrent with no clear surgical cure, as little intestine as possible is resected. Current surgical alternatives for treatment of obstructing CD include resection of the diseased segment and strictureplasty. Surgical resection of the diseased segment is the most frequently performed operation, and in most cases primary anastomosis can be done to restore continuity. If much of the small bowel has already been resected and the strictures are short with intervening areas of normal mucosa, strictureplasties should be done to avoid a functionally insufficient length of bowel. The strictured area of intestine is incised longitudinally and the incision sutured transversely, thus widening the narrowed area. Complications of strictureplasty include prolonged ileus, hemorrhage, fistula, abscess, leak, and restricture.

COLORECTAL DISEASE   A greater percentage of patients with Crohn's colitis require surgery for intractability, fulminant disease, and anorectal disease. Several alternatives are available, ranging from the use of a temporary loop ileostomy to resection of segments of diseased colon or even the entire colon and rectum. For patients with segmental involvement, segmental colon resection with primary anastomosis can be performed. In 20 to 25% of patients with extensive colitis, the rectum is spared sufficiently to consider rectal preservation. Most surgeons believe that an IPAA is contraindicated in CD due to the high incidence of pouch failure. A diverting colostomy may help heal severe perianal disease or rectovaginal fistulas, but disease almost always recurs with reanastomosis. Often, these patients require a total proctocolectomy and ileostomy.

INFLAMMATORY BOWEL DISEASE AND PREGNANCY

Patients with quiescent UC and CD have normal fertility rates; the fallopian tubes can be scarred by the inflammatory process of CD, especially on the right side because of the proximity of the terminal ileum. In addition, perirectal, perineal, and rectovaginal abscesses and fistulae can result in dyspareunia. Infertility in men can be caused by sulfasalazine but reverses when treatment is stopped.

TABLE 276-7 *Indications for Surgery*	
Ulcerative Colitis	**Crohn's Disease**
Intractable disease	CD of Small Intestine
Fulminant disease	Stricture and obstruction
Toxic megacolon	unresponsive to medical
Colonic perforation	therapy
Massive colonic hemorrhage	Massive hemorrhage
Extracolonic disease	Refractory fistula
Colonic obstruction	Abscess
Colon cancer prophylaxis	CD of Colon and Rectum
Colon dysplasia or cancer	Intractable disease
	Fulminant disease
	Perianal disease unresponsive to
	medical therapy
	Refractory fistula
	Colonic obstruction
	Cancer prophylaxis
	Colon dysplasia or cancer

In mild or quiescent UC and CD, fetal outcome is nearly normal. Spontaneous abortions, stillbirths, and developmental defects are increased with increased disease activity, not medications. The courses of CD and UC during pregnancy mostly correlate with disease activity at the time of conception. Patients should be in remission for 6 months before conceiving. Most CD patients can deliver vaginally, but cesarean section may be the preferred route of delivery for patients with anorectal and perirectal abscesses and fistulas to reduce the likelihood of fistulas developing or extending into the episiotomy scar.

Sulfasalazine, mesalamine, and balsalazide are safe for use in pregnancy and nursing, but folate supplementation must be given with sulfasalazine. Topical 5-ASA agents are also safe during pregnancy and nursing. Glucocorticoids are generally safe for use during pregnancy and are indicated for patients with moderate to severe disease activity. The amount of glucocorticoids received by the nursing infant is minimal. The safest antibiotics to use for CD in pregnancy for short periods of time (weeks, not months) are ampicillin, cephalosporin, or flagyl. Ciprofloxacin causes cartilage lesions in immature animals and should be avoided because of the absence of data on its effects on growth and development in humans.

6-MP and azathioprine pose minimal or no risk during pregnancy, but experience is limited. If the patient cannot be weaned from the drug or has an exacerbation that requires 6-MP/azathioprine during pregnancy, she should continue the drug with informed consent. Their effects during nursing are unknown.

Little data exist on cyclosporine in pregnancy. In a small number of patients with severe IBD treated with intravenous cyclosporine during pregnancy, 80% of pregnancies were successfully completed without development of renal toxicity, congenital malformations, or developmental defects. However, because of the lack of data, cyclosporine should probably be avoided unless the patient would otherwise require surgery. Methotrexate is contraindicated in pregnancy and nursing. Based on 35 reported pregnancies, infliximab does not appear to present a risk to the mother or baby.

Surgery in UC should be performed only for emergency indications, including severe hemorrhage, perforation, and megacolon refractory to medical therapy. Total colectomy and ileostomy carry a 60% risk of postoperative spontaneous abortion. Fetal mortality is also high in CD requiring surgery. Patients with IPAAs have increased nighttime stool frequency during pregnancy that resolves post-partum. Transient small-bowel obstruction or ileus has been noted in up to 8% of patients with ileostomies.

INFLAMMATORY BOWEL DISEASE IN THE ELDERLY

The most common presenting symptoms in the elderly are diarrhea, weight loss, and abdominal pain. CD in the elderly mostly affects the colon with a distal distribution and occurs predominantly in women. Proctitis has been documented in 50% of elderly patients, and the diagnosis is often delayed. Diseases that can mimic CD in the elderly are ischemic colitis, diverticular disease, irritable bowel, infectious colitides, and malignancies, including carcinoma, lymphoma, and carcinoid. The incidence of surgery is high in elderly patients, with up to 50% of patients with ileitis, ileocolitis, or extensive colitis requiring urgent or early surgery for first-time disease. In addition, surgery has a much higher morbidity than in younger patients, although the rate of postoperative recurrence is less. Most elderly patients respond as well as younger individuals to medical management.

UC in the elderly is more common in men, presents usually with diarrhea and weight loss, and may have a more distal distribution than in younger patients. Most elderly patients have a favorable response to medical therapy, especially 5-ASA agents, and immunosuppressives used in conjunction with low doses of glucocorticoids. Cyclosporine has been used more frequently in the elderly, but the age-related decreases in renal clearance may affect dosing. Glucocorticoid complications such as osteoporosis and hyperglycemia are also increased in the elderly. 6-MP and azathioprine are well tolerated in the elderly.

Surgery also has a higher morbidity and mortality in UC, and elderly patients have a longer hospital stay than younger patients. The risk of colon cancer in UC and Crohn's colitis is no greater than that in the general population since the duration of disease is short and the extent of disease is often distal.

CANCER IN INFLAMMATORY BOWEL DISEASE

ULCERATIVE COLITIS   Patients with long-standing UC are at increased risk for developing colonic epithelial dysplasia and carcinoma (Fig. 276-8). Several features distinguish sporadic colon cancer (SCC) and colitis-associated colon cancer (CAC). First, SCCs usually arise from an adenomatous polyp; CACs typically arise from either flat dysplasia or a dysplasia-associated lesion or mass (DALM). Second, multiple synchronous colon cancers occur in 3 to 5% of SCC but in 12% of CAC. Third, the mean age of individuals with SCC is in the sixties; the mean age of those with CAC is in the thirties. Fourth, SCC exhibits a left-sided predominance, whereas CAC is distributed more uniformly throughout the colon. Fifth, mucinous and anaplastic cancers are more common in CAC than SCC. At the molecular level, p53 mutations occur much earlier and *APC* gene mutations much later in CAC than in SCC.

The risk of neoplasia in chronic UC increases with duration and extent of disease. For patients with pancolitis, the risk of cancer rises 0.5 to 1% per year after 8 to 10 years of disease. This observed increase in cancer rates has led to the endorsement of surveillance colonoscopy with biopsies for patients with chronic UC as the standard of care. Annual or biennial colonoscopy with multiple biopsies has been advocated for patients with >8 to 10 years of pancolitis or 12 to 15 years of left-sided colitis and has been widely employed to screen and survey for subsequent dysplasia and carcinoma.

CROHN'S DISEASE   Risk factors for developing colorectal cancer in CD are a history of colonic (or ileocolonic) involvement and long disease duration. The cancer risks in CD and UC are probably equivalent for similar extent and duration of disease. In patients with extensive

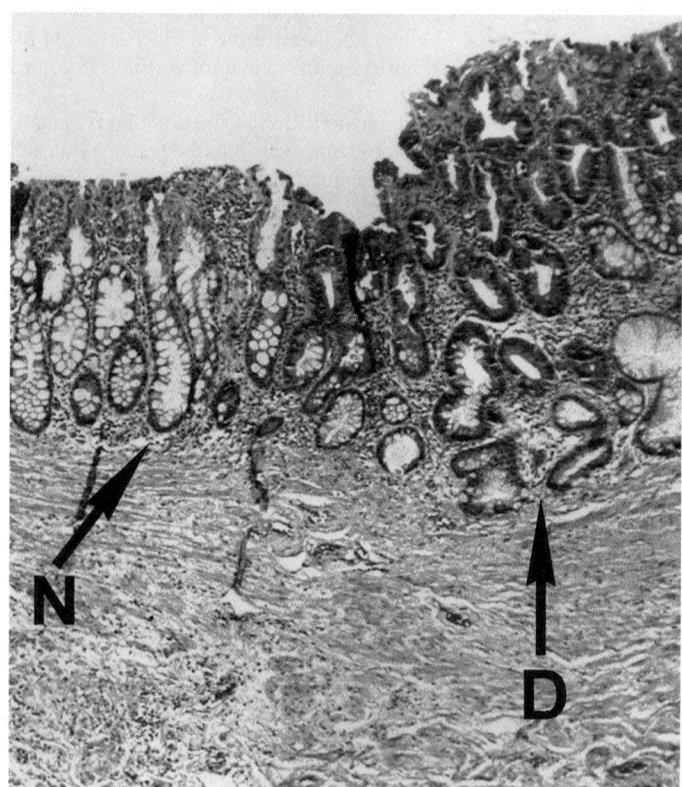

FIGURE 276-8   Low-power transition between dysplasia (D) and nondysplastic (N) mucosa in a case of ulcerative colitis. *(Courtesy of Dr. EK Rosado and Dr. CA Perkos, Division of Gastrointestinal Pathology, Department of Pathology, Emory University, Atlanta, Georgia.)*

Crohn's colitis, 22% developed dysplasia or cancer by the fourth surveillance exam after a negative screening colonoscopy. Thus, the same endoscopic surveillance strategy used for UC is recommended for patients with chronic Crohn's colitis. A pediatric colonoscope can be used to pass narrow strictures in CD patients, but surgery should be considered in symptomatic patients with impassable strictures.

MANAGEMENT OF DYSPLASIA AND CANCER Dysplasia can be flat or polypoid. If flat high-grade dysplasia (HGD) is encountered on colonoscopic surveillance, the usual treatment for UC is colectomy and for CD is either colectomy or segmental resection. If flat low-grade dysplasia (LGD) is found, most investigators recommend immediate colectomy. Adenomas may occur coincidently in UC and CD patients with chronic colitis and can be removed endoscopically provided that biopsies of the surrounding mucosa are free of dysplasia.

IBD patients are also at greater risk for other malignancies. Patients with CD may have an increased risk of developing non-Hodgkin's lymphoma and squamous cell carcinoma of the skin. Although CD patients have a twelvefold increased risk of developing small-bowel cancer, this type of carcinoma is extremely rare.

QUALITY OF LIFE IN INFLAMMATORY BOWEL DISEASE

The assessment of health-related quality of life plays an important role in the evaluation and treatment of IBD patients. Although clinical trials have generally relied upon traditional disease activity indices such as the Crohn's Disease Activity Index (CDAI) to measure therapeutic efficacy, these measures do not reflect quality of life. The Inflammatory Bowel Disease Questionnaire (IBDQ) is a validated, disease-specific instrument that has been used to measure quality of life. It is a 32-item questionnaire that measures global function, systemic and bowel symptoms, functional and social impairment, and emotional function. When compared to the general population, IBD patients have an impaired quality of life in all six categories. The most frequent concerns of UC patients are having an ostomy bag, developing cancer, effects of medication, the uncertain nature of the disease, and having surgery. The most frequent concerns of CD patients are the uncertain nature of the disease, energy level, effects of medication, having surgery, and having an ostomy bag.

FURTHER READING

CHEUNG O, REGUEIRO D: Inflammatory bowel disease emergencies. Gastroenterol Clin North Am 32:1269, 2003

FRASER AG et al: The efficacy of azathioprine for the treatment of inflammatory bowel disease: A 30-year review. Gut 50:485, 2002

FRIEDMAN S et al: Screening and surveillance colonoscopy in chronic Crohn's colitis. Gastroenterology 120:820, 2001

HANAUER SB, SANBORN W: Management of Crohn's disease in adults. Am J Gastroenterol 96:635, 2001

HUGOT JP et al: Association of NOD2 leucine-rich repeat variants with susceptibility to Crohn's disease. Nature 411:599, 2001

ITZKOWITZ SH: Cancer prevention in patients with inflammatory bowel disease. Gastroenterol Clin North Am 31:1133, 2002

KORNBLUTH A, SACHAR DB: Ulcerative colitis practice guidelines in adults. Am J Gastroenterol 92:204, 1997

NAVARRO F, HANAUER SB: Treatment of inflammatory bowel disease: Safety and tolerability issues. Am J Gastroenterol 98(Suppl 12):518, 2003

277 IRRITABLE BOWEL SYNDROME
Chung Owyang

Irritable bowel syndrome (IBS) is a gastrointestinal (GI) disorder characterized by altered bowel habits and abdominal pain in the absence of detectable structural abnormalities. No clear diagnostic markers exist for IBS, thus all definitions of the disease are based on the clinical presentation. The Rome II criteria for the diagnosis of IBS are summarized in Table 277-1. It is one of the most common conditions encountered in clinical practice but one of the least well understood. Until recently, many physicians did not consider IBS to be a disease at all; they viewed it as nothing more than a somatic manifestation of psychological stress. With the availability of better techniques to study colonic and GI motility and visceral sensory function, along with the development of newer concepts on the importance of the brain in regulating gut function, significant progress has been made toward a better understanding of the pathogenesis of IBS. This may result in improved methods of treatment.

CLINICAL FEATURES IBS is a disorder of the young, with most new patients presenting before age 45. However, some reports suggest that the elderly are troubled by IBS symptoms up to 92% as often as middle-aged persons. Indeed, many of the diagnoses of "painful diverticular disease" given to elderly patients may represent IBS. Women are diagnosed with IBS two to three times as often as men. Moreover, women make up 80% of the population with severe IBS. Patients with IBS fall into two broad clinical groups. Most commonly, patients have abdominal pain associated with altered bowel habits that consist of constipation, diarrhea, or both. In the second group, patients have painless diarrhea. This symptom in this group, who account for <20% of patients with IBS, may be caused by a separate entity. In fact, painless diarrhea does not strictly fulfill the Rome II criteria to be classified as IBS.

Abdominal Pain According to the Rome II criteria, abdominal pain or discomfort is a prerequisite clinical feature of IBS. Abdominal pain in IBS is highly variable in intensity and location; it is localized to the hypogastrium in 25%, the right side in 20%, to the left side in 20%, and the epigastrium in 10% of patients. It is frequently episodic and crampy, but it may be superimposed on a background of constant ache. Pain may be mild enough to be ignored or it may interfere with daily activities. Despite this, malnutrition due to inadequate caloric intake is exceedingly rare with IBS. Sleep deprivation is also unusual because abdominal pain is almost uniformly present only during waking hours. However, patients with severe IBS often wake repeatedly during the night, and, hence, nocturnal pain is a poor discriminating factor between organic and functional bowel disease. Pain is often exacerbated by eating or emotional stress and relieved by passage of flatus or stools. Female patients with IBS commonly report worsening symptoms during the premenstrual and menstrual phases.

Altered Bowel Habits Alteration in bowel habits is the most consistent clinical feature in IBS. It usually begins in adult life. The most common pattern is constipation alternating with diarrhea, usually with one of these symptoms predominating. At first, constipation may be episodic, but eventually it becomes continuous and increasingly intractable to treatment with laxatives. Stools are usually hard with narrowed caliber, possibly reflecting excessive dehydration caused by prolonged colonic retention and spasm. Most patients also experience a sense of incomplete evacuation, leading to repeated attempts at defecation in a short time span. Patients whose predominant symptom is constipation may have weeks or months of constipation interrupted with brief periods of diarrhea. In other patients, diarrhea may be the predominant symptom. Diarrhea resulting from IBS usually consists of small volumes of loose stools. Most patients have stool volumes of <200 mL.

TABLE 277-1 *Rome II Criteria for the Diagnosis of IBS*

At least 12 weeks, which need not be consecutive, in the preceding 12 months of abdominal discomfort or pain that has two of following three features:
1. Relieved by defecation
2. Onset associated with changes in stool frequency
3. Onset associated with changes in stool form

Nocturnal diarrhea does not occur in IBS. Diarrhea may be aggravated by emotional stress or eating. Stool may be accompanied by passage of large amounts of mucus; hence, the term *mucous colitis* has been used to describe IBS. This is a misnomer, since inflammation is not present. Bleeding is not a feature of IBS unless hemorrhoids are present, and malabsorption or weight loss does not occur.

Gas and Flatulence   Patients with IBS frequently complain of abdominal distention and increased belching or flatulence, all of which they attribute to increased gas. Although some patients with these symptoms actually may have a larger amount of gas, quantitative measurements reveal that most patients who complain of increased gas generate no more than a normal amount of intestinal gas. Studies have shown that most IBS patients have impaired transit and tolerance of intestinal gas loads. In addition, patients with IBS tend to reflux gas from the distal to the more proximal intestine, which may explain the belching.

Upper Gastrointestinal Symptoms   Between 25 and 50% of patients with IBS complain of dyspepsia, heartburn, nausea, and vomiting. This suggests that other areas of the gut apart from the colon may be involved. Prolonged ambulant recordings of small-bowel motility in patients with IBS show a high incidence of abnormalities in the small bowel during the diurnal (waking) period; nocturnal motor patterns are no different from those of healthy controls. A great deal of overlap is seen between dyspepsia and IBS. The prevalence of IBS is higher among individuals with dyspepsia (31.7%) than among those who report no symptoms of dyspepsia (7.9%). Conversely among those with IBS, 55.6% report symptoms of dyspepsia. In addition, the functional abdominal symptoms can change over time. Those with predominant dyspepsia or IBS can fluctuate between the two. Thus, functional dyspepsia and IBS may be two manifestations of a single, more extensive digestive system disorder. Furthermore, IBS symptoms are prevalent in noncardiac chest pain patients, suggesting overlap with other functional gut disorders.

PATHOPHYSIOLOGY   The pathogenesis of IBS is poorly understood, although roles for abnormal gut motor and sensory activity, central neural dysfunction, psychological disturbances, stress, and luminal factors have been proposed.

Studies of colonic myoelectrical and motor activity under unstimulated conditions have not shown consistent abnormalities in IBS. In contrast, colonic motor abnormalities are more prominent under stimulated conditions in IBS. IBS patients may exhibit increased rectosigmoid motor activity for up to 3 h after eating. Provocative stimuli also induce exaggerated colonic motor responses in IBS patients compared with healthy volunteers. For example, inflation of rectal balloons both in diarrhea- and constipation-predominant IBS patients leads to marked distention-evoked contractile activity, which may be prolonged. Recording from the transverse, descending, and sigmoid colon shows that the motility index and peak amplitude of high-amplitude propagating contractions in diarrhea-prone IBS patients are greatly increased compared to healthy subjects. These contractions are associated with rapid colonic transit and accompanied by abdominal pain.

As with studies of motor activity, IBS patients frequently exhibit exaggerated sensory responses to visceral stimulation. Postprandial pain has been temporally related to the entry of the food bolus into the cecum in 74% of patients. Exaggerated symptoms can be induced by visceral distention in IBS patients. Rectal balloon inflation produces nonpainful and painful sensations at lower volumes in IBS patients than in healthy controls without altering rectal tension, suggestive of visceral afferent dysfunction in IBS. The visceral hyperalgesia of IBS appears to be selective for mechanoreceptor-activated stimuli, as perception of intestinal mucosal electrical stimulation is normal in IBS. Similar studies show gastric and esophageal hypersensitivity in patients with nonulcer dyspepsia and noncardiac chest pain, raising the possibility that these conditions have a similar pathophysiologic basis. Lipids lower the thresholds for the first sensation of gas, discomfort, and pain in IBS patients. Furthermore, IBS patients have an increased

area of referred pain after lipid ingestion that is not observed in healthy subjects. Hence, postprandial symptoms in IBS patients may be explained in part by a nutrient-dependent exaggerated sensory component of the gastrocolonic response. In contrast to enhanced gut sensitivity, IBS patients do not exhibit heightened sensitivity elsewhere in the body. Thus the afferent pathway disturbances in IBS appear to be selective for visceral innervation, with sparing of somatic pathways. The mechanisms responsible for visceral hypersensitivity are still under investigation. These exaggerated responses may be due to (1) increased end-organ sensitivity with recruitment of "silent" nociceptors, (2) spinal hyperexcitability with activation of nitric oxide and possibly other neurotransmitters, (3) endogenous (cortical and brainstem) modulation of caudad nociceptive transmission, and (4) over time, the possible development of long-term hyperalgesia due to development of neuroplasticity, resulting in permanent or semipermanent changes in neural responses to chronic or recurrent visceral stimulation (Table 277-2).

The role of central nervous system (CNS) factors in the pathogenesis of IBS is strongly suggested by the clinical association of emotional disorders and stress with symptom exacerbation and the therapeutic response to therapies that act on cerebral cortical sites. Positron emission tomography has been employed to quantify regional cerebral blood flow in IBS. In healthy individuals, rectal distention increases blood flow in the anterior cingulate cortex, a region with an abundance of opiate receptors, which, when activated, may help to reduce sensory input. In contrast, IBS patients exhibit no increased blood flow in the anterior cingulate gyrus but show activation of the prefrontal cortex, either in response to rectal activation or in anticipation of rectal distention. Activation of the frontal lobes may activate a vigilance network within the brain that increases alertness. The anterior cingulate cortex and the prefrontal cortex appear to have reciprocal inhibitory associations. Thus, in patients with IBS, the preferential activation of the prefrontal lobe, without activation of the anterior cingulate cortex, may represent a form of cerebral dysfunction leading to the increased perception of visceral pain.

Abnormal psychiatric features are recorded in up to 80% of IBS patients, especially in referral centers; however, no single psychiatric diagnosis predominates. Most of these patients demonstrate exaggerated symptoms in response to visceral distention, and this abnormality persists even after exclusion of psychological factors. Psychological factors also influence pain thresholds in IBS patients; stress alters sensory thresholds. An association between prior sexual or physical abuse and development of IBS has been reported. Forms of sexual abuse associated with IBS include verbal aggression, exhibitionism, sexual harassment, sexual touching, and rape. The pathophysiologic relationship between IBS and sexual or physical abuse is unknown. Sexual abuse is not associated with a lower pain threshold in IBS patients.

Thus, patients with IBS frequently demonstrate increased motor reactivity of the colon and small bowel to a variety of stimuli and altered visceral sensation associated with lowered sensation thresholds. These may result from CNS or enteric nervous system dysregulation.

IBS may be induced by gastrointestinal infection. In an investigation of 544 patients with confirmed bacterial gastroenteritis, one-quarter subsequently developed IBS. Conversely, about a third of IBS patients experienced an acute "gastroenteritis-like" illness at the onset of their chronic IBS symptomatology. This "postinfective" IBS occurs more commonly in women and affects younger, rather than older, patients and those who have a protracted acute diarrheal illness. The

TABLE 277-2 *Proposed Mechanisms for Visceral Hypersensitivity*	
End-organ sensitivity	Long-term hyperalgesia
"Silent" nociceptors	Tonic cortical regulation
CNS modulation	Neuroplasticity
Cortex	
Brainstem	

Note: CNS, central nervous system.

microbes involved in the initial infection are *Campylobacter*, *Salmonella*, and *Shigella*. Those patients infected with *Campylobacter* who are toxin-positive are more likely to develop postinfective IBS. Increased rectal mucosal enteroendocrine cells, T lymphocytes, and gut permeability are acute changes following *Campylobacter* enteritis that could persist for more than a year and may contribute to postinfective IBS.

The serotonin (5HT)-containing enterochromaffin cells in the colon are increased in diarrhea-predominant IBS patients compared to healthy subjects or to patients with ulcerative colitis. Furthermore, postprandial plasma 5HT plasma levels are significantly higher in diarrhea-predominant IBS patients compared to healthy controls. As 5HT plays an important role in the regulation of GI motility and visceral perception, the increased release of 5HT may contribute to the postprandial symptoms of these patients and provides a rationale for the use of 5HT antagonists in the treatment of this disorder.

APPROACH TO THE PATIENT

Because IBS is a disorder for which no pathognomonic abnormalities have been identified, its diagnosis relies on recognition of positive clinical features and elimination of other organic diseases. A careful history and physical examination are frequently helpful in establishing the diagnosis. Clinical features suggestive of IBS include the following: recurrence of lower abdominal pain with altered bowel habits over a period of time without progressive deterioration, onset of symptoms during periods of stress or emotional upset, absence of other systemic symptoms such as fever and weight loss, and small-volume stool without any evidence of blood.

On the other hand, the appearance of the disorder for the first time in old age, a progressive course from time of onset, persistent diarrhea after a 48-h fast, and presence of nocturnal diarrhea or steatorrheal stools argue against the diagnosis of IBS.

Because the major symptoms of IBS—abdominal pain, abdominal bloating, and alteration in bowel habits—are common complaints of many GI organic disorders, the list of differential diagnoses is long. The quality, location, and timing of pain may be helpful in suggesting specific disorders. Pain due to IBS that occurs in the epigastric or periumbilical area must be differentiated from biliary tract disease, peptic ulcer disorders, intestinal ischemia, and carcinoma of the stomach and pancreas. If pain occurs mainly in the lower abdomen, the possibility of diverticular disease of the colon, inflammatory bowel disease (including ulcerative colitis and Crohn's disease), and carcinoma of the colon must be considered. Postprandial pain accompanied by bloating, nausea, and vomiting suggests gastroparesis or partial intestinal obstruction. Intestinal infestation with *Giardia lamblia* or other parasites may cause similar symptoms. When diarrhea is the major complaint, the possibility of lactase deficiency, laxative abuse, malabsorption, hyperthyroidism, inflammatory bowel disease, or infectious diarrhea must be ruled out. On the other hand, constipation may be a side effect of many different drugs, such as anticholinergic, antihypertensive, and antidepressant medications. Endocrinopathies such as hypothyroidism and hypoparathyroidism must also be considered in the differential diagnosis of constipation, particularly if other systemic signs or symptoms of these endocrinopathies are present. In addition, acute intermittent porphyria and lead poisoning may present in a fashion similar to that of IBS, with painful constipation as the major complaint. These possibilities are suspected on the basis of their clinical presentations and are confirmed by appropriate serum and urine tests.

Because IBS is in part a diagnosis of exclusion, certain diagnostic tests should be performed routinely; others may be required depending on the specific presenting symptoms. The American Gastroenterological Association has delineated factors to be considered when determining the aggressiveness of the diagnostic evaluation. These include the duration of symptoms, the change in symptoms over time, the age and sex of the patient, the referral status of the patient, prior diagnostic studies, a family history of colorectal malignancy, and the degree of psychosocial dysfunction. Thus, a younger individual with mild symptoms requires a minimal diagnostic evaluation, while an older person or an individual with rapidly progressive symptoms should undergo a more thorough exclusion of organic disease. Most patients should have a complete blood count and sigmoidoscopic examination; in addition, stool specimens should be examined for ova and parasites. In those older than 40 years, an air-contrast barium enema or colonoscopy should also be performed. If the main symptoms are diarrhea and increased gas, the possibility of lactase deficiency should be ruled out with a hydrogen breath test or with evaluation after a 3-week lactose-free diet. In patients with concurrent symptoms of dyspepsia, upper GI radiographs or esophagogastroduodenoscopy may be advisable. In patients with postprandial right upper quadrant pain, an ultrasonogram of the gallbladder should be obtained. Laboratory features that argue against IBS include evidence of anemia, elevated sedimentation rate, presence of leukocytes or blood in stool, and stool volume >200 to 300 mL/d. These findings would necessitate other diagnostic considerations.

R_X TREATMENT

Patient Counseling and Dietary Alterations Reassurance and careful explanation of the functional nature of the disorder and of how to avoid obvious food precipitants are important first steps in patient counseling and dietary change. Occasionally, a meticulous dietary history may reveal substances (such as coffee, disaccharides, legumes, and cabbage) that aggravate symptoms. As a therapeutic trial, patients should be encouraged to eliminate any foodstuffs that appear to produce symptoms.

Stool-Bulking Agents High-fiber diets and bulking agents, such as bran or hydrophilic colloid, are frequently used in treating IBS. Dietary fiber has multiple effects on colonic physiology. The water-holding action of fiber may contribute to increased stool bulk because of the ability of fiber to increase fecal output of bacteria. Fiber also speeds up colonic transit in most persons. In diarrhea-prone patients, whole colonic transit is faster than average; however, dietary fiber can delay transit. Furthermore, because of their hydrophilic properties, stool-bulking agents bind water and thus prevent both excessive hydration or dehydration of stool. The latter observation may explain the clinical experience that a high-fiber diet relieves diarrhea in some IBS patients. More recently, fiber supplementation with psyllium has been shown to reduce perception of rectal distention, indicating that fiber may have a positive affect on visceral afferent function.

The beneficial effects of dietary fiber on colonic physiology suggest that dietary fiber should be an effective treatment for IBS patients, but controlled trials of dietary fiber have produced variable results. This is not surprising since IBS is a heterogeneous disorder, with some patients being constipated and others having predominant diarrhea. Most investigations report increases in stool weight, decreases in colonic transit times, and improvement in constipation. Others have noted benefits in patients with alternating diarrhea and constipation, pain, and bloating; however, most studies observe no responses in patients with diarrhea- or pain-predominant IBS. Different fiber preparations may have dissimilar effects on selected symptoms in IBS. A crossover comparison of different fiber preparations found that psyllium produced greater improvements in stool pattern and abdominal pain than bran. Furthermore, psyllium preparations tend to produce less bloating and distention. Despite the equivocal data regarding efficacy, most gastroenterologists consider stool-bulking agents worth trying in patients with IBS.

Antispasmodics Clinicians have observed that anticholinergic drugs may provide temporary relief for symptoms such as painful cramps related to intestinal spasm. Although controlled clinical trials have produced mixed results, evidence generally supports beneficial effects of anticholinergic drugs for pain. A meta-analysis of 26 double-blind clinical trials of antispasmodic agents in IBS reported better global improvement (62%) and abdominal pain reduction (64%) compared to placebo (35% and 45%, respectively), indicative of their symptomatic efficacy. The drugs are most effective when prescribed in anticipation of predictable pain. Physiologic studies demonstrate that anticholinergic drugs inhibit the gastrocolic reflex; hence, postprandial pain is best managed by giving antispasmodics 30 min before meals so that effective blood levels are achieved shortly before the anticipated onset of pain. Most anticholinergics contain natural belladonna alkaloids, which may cause xerostomia, urinary hesitancy and retention, blurred vision, and drowsiness. Some physicians prefer to use synthetic anticholinergics such as dicyclomine that have less effect on mucous membrane secretions and therefore produce fewer undesirable side effects.

Antidiarrheal Agents Peripherally acting opiate-based agents are the initial therapy of choice for diarrhea-predominant IBS. Physiologic studies demonstrate increases in segmenting colonic contractions, delays in fecal transit, increases in anal pressures, and reductions in rectal perception with these drugs. When diarrhea is severe, especially in the painless diarrhea variant of IBS, small doses of diphenoxylate (Lomotil), 2.5 to 5 mg every 4 to 6 h, can be prescribed. These agents are less addictive than paregoric, codeine, or tincture of opium. In general, the intestines do not become tolerant of the antidiarrheal effect of opiates, and increasing doses are not required to maintain antidiarrheal potency. These agents are most useful if taken before anticipated stressful events that are known to cause diarrhea. Treatment with antidiarrheals, however, should be considered only as temporary management; the final goal of treatment is gradual withdrawal of medication with substitution of a high-fiber diet.

Antidepressant Drugs In addition to their mood-elevating effects, antidepressent medications have several physiologic effects that may be beneficial in IBS. In diarrhea-predominant IBS patients, the tricyclic antidepressant imipramine slows jejunal migrating motor complex transit propagation and delays orocecal and whole-gut transit, indicative of a motor inhibitory effect. Tricyclic agents may also alter visceral afferent neural function.

Tricyclic antidepressants may be effective in some IBS patients. In a 2-month study of desipramine, abdominal pain improved in 86% of patients compared to 59% given a placebo. Another study of desipramine in 28 IBS patients showed improvement in stool frequency, diarrhea, pain, and depression. Improvements were observed mainly in diarrhea-predominant patients, with no improvement being noted in constipated patients. The beneficial effects of the tricyclic compounds in the treatment of IBS appear to be independent of their antidepression actions. The therapeutic benefits for the bowel symptoms occur faster and at a lower dosage. The efficacy of other classes of antidepressant agents in the management of IBS is less well evaluated. The selective serotonin reuptake inhibitor (SSRI) paroxetine accelerates orocecal transit, raising the possibility that this drug class may be useful in constipation-predominant patients. The SSRI citalopram blunts perception of rectal distention and reduces the magnitude of the gastrocolonic response in healthy volunteers. A small placebo-controlled study of citalopram in IBS patients reported reductions in pain. An

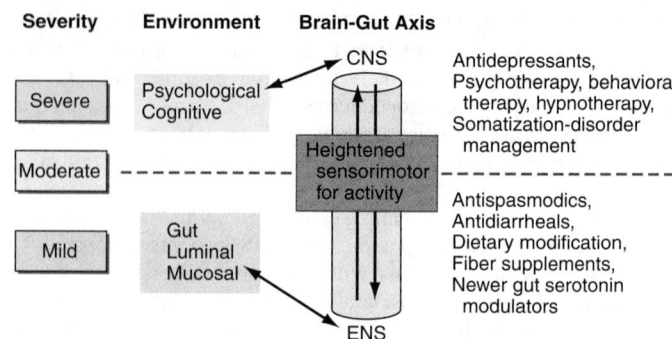

FIGURE 277-1 Therapeutic targets for irritable bowel syndrome. Patients with mild to moderate symptoms usually have intermittent symptoms that correlate with altered gut physiology. Treatments include gut-acting pharmacologic agents such as antispasmodics, antidiarrheals, fiber supplements, and gut serotonin modulators. Patients who have severe symptoms usually have constant pain and psychosocial difficulties. This group of patients are best managed with antidepressants and other psychological treatments. CNS, central nervous system; ENS, enteric nervous system.

investigation of mianserin, with serotonin $5HT_2$ and $5HT_3$ receptor antagonist and α_2-adrenoceptor antagonist effects, reported reductions in pain, distress, and functional disability compared to placebo. Despite these preliminary results, the efficacy of SSRIs in the treatment of IBS still needs further confirmation.

Antiflatulence Therapy The management of excessive gas is seldom satisfactory, except in obvious aerophagia or disaccharidase deficiency. Patients should be advised to eat slowly; avoid chewing gum or drinking carbonated beverages; and avoid consuming artificial sweeteners, legumes, and foods of the cabbage family. Simethicone, antacids, and activated charcoal have all been tried, usually with disappointing results.

Serotonin Receptor Agonists and Antagonists Serotonin receptor antagonists have been evaluated as therapies for diarrhea-predominant IBS. Serotonin acting on $5HT_3$ receptors enhances the sensitivity of afferent neurons projecting from the gut. In humans, a $5HT_3$ receptor antagonist such as alosetron reduces perception of painful visceral stimulation in IBS. It also induces rectal relaxation, increases rectal compliance, and delays colonic transit. Large, 12-week, placebo-controlled trials of alosetron reported reductions in discomfort and improvements in stool frequency, consistency, and urgency in nonconstipated IBS patients. A follow-up 48-week study confirmed the long-term efficacy of alosetron. For unclear reasons, women with IBS derived greater benefit than men. However, in postrelease surveillance, 70 cases of ischemic colitis were observed, including 10 cases requiring surgery and 3 deaths. As a consequence, the medication was voluntarily withdrawn by the manufacturer. Preliminary studies in nonconstipated IBS patients of a newer $5HT_3$ receptor antagonist, cilansetron, have shown similar improvements in abdominal pain and diarrhea as alosetron. Follow-up investigation will determine if side effects also undermine the utility of this agent.

Novel $5HT_4$ receptor agonists exhibit prokinetic activity by stimulating peristalsis. In IBS patients with constipation, tegaserod accelerated intestinal and ascending colon transit. Clinical trials involving >4000 constipation-predominant IBS patients have reported reductions in discomfort and improvements in constipation and bloating compared to placebo. Other than diarrhea, no other significant side effects were noted. Tegaserod has been approved for the treatment of constipation-predominant IBS.

Summary The treatment strategy of IBS depends on the severity of the disorder (Table 277-3). Most IBS patients have mild symptoms. They are usually cared for in primary care practices and have little or no psychosocial difficulties and do not seek health care often. Treatment usually involves education, reassurance, and dietary/lifestyle changes. A smaller proportion have moderate symptoms that are usually intermittent and correlate with altered gut physiology, such as worsening with eating or stress and relieved by defecation. Treatments include

TABLE 277-3 *Spectrum of Severity in IBS*

	Mild	Moderate	Severe
Clinical features			
Prevalence	70%	25%	5%
Correlation with gut physiology	+++	++	+
Symptoms constant	0	+	+++
Psychosocial difficulties	0	+	+++
Health care issues	+	++	+++
Practice type	Primary	Specialty	Referral

gut-acting pharmacologic agents such as antispasmodics, antidiarrheals, fiber supplements, and the newer gut serotonin modulators (Fig. 277-1). A small proportion of IBS patients have severe and refractory symptoms. They are usually seen in referral centers and frequently have constant pain and psychosocial difficulties (Fig. 277-1). This group of patients are best managed with antidepressants and other psychological treatments.

FURTHER READING

AMERICAN GASTROENTEROLOGICAL ASSOCIATION MEDICAL POSITION STATEMENT: Irritable bowel syndrome. Gastroenterology 112:2118, 1997

BUENO L et al: Mediators and pharmacology of visceral sensitivity: from basic to clinical investigations. Gastroenterology 112:1714, 1997

HASLER WL, OWYANG C: Irritable bowel syndrome, in *Textbook of Gastroenterology*, 4th ed, T Yamada (ed). Philadelphia, Lippincott Williams & Wilkins, 2003, pp 1817–1842

JACKSON JL et al: Treatment of functional gastrointestinal disorders with antidepressant medications: A meta-analysis. Am J Med 108:65, 2000

MERTZ H: Irritable bowel syndrome. N Engl J Med 349:2136, 2003

SPILLER RC et al: Increased rectal mucosal enteroendocrine cells, T lymphocytes, and increased gut permeability following acute *Campylobacter* enteritis and in post-dysenteric irritable bowel syndrome. Gut 47:804, 2000

TALLEY NJ: Evaluation of drug treatment for irritable bowel syndrome. Br J Clin Pharmacol 56:362, 2003

278 | FAMILIAL MEDITERRANEAN FEVER AND OTHER HEREDITARY RECURRENT FEVERS
Daniel L. Kastner

FAMILIAL MEDITERRANEAN FEVER

Familial Mediterranean fever (FMF) is the prototype of a group of inherited diseases (Table 278-1) that are characterized by recurrent episodes of fever with serosal, synovial, or cutaneous inflammation and, in some individuals, the eventual development of systemic AA amyloidosis (Chap. 310). Because of the relative infrequency of high-titer autoantibodies or antigen-specific T cells, the term *autoinflammatory* has been proposed to describe these disorders.

BACKGROUND AND PATHOPHYSIOLOGY FMF was first recognized among Armenians, Arabs, Turks, and non-Ashkenazi (primarily North African and Iraqi) Jews. With the advent of genetic testing, FMF has been documented with increasing frequency among Ashkenazi Jews and

TABLE 278-1 *The Hereditary Periodic Fever Syndromes*

	FMF	TRAPS	HIDS	MWS	FCAS	NOMID
Ethnicity	Jewish, Arab, Turkish, Armenian, Italian	Any ethnic group	Predominantly Dutch, northern European	Any ethnic group	Any ethnic group	Any ethnic group
Inheritance	Recessive	Dominant	Recessive	Dominant	Dominant	Usually de novo mutations
Gene/chromosome	*MEFV*/16p13.3	*TNFRSF1A*/12p13	*MVK*/12q24	*CIAS1*/1q44	*CIAS1*/1q44	*CIAS1*/1q44
Protein	Pyrin	p55 TNF receptor	Mevalonate kinase	Cryopyrin	Cryopyrin	Cryopyrin
Attack length	1–3 days	Often >7 days	3–7 days	1–2 days	Minutes–3 days	Continuous, with flares
Serosa	Pleurisy, peritonitis; asymptomatic pericardial effusions	Pleurisy, peritonitis, pericarditis	Abd pain, but seldom peritonitis; pleurisy, pericarditis uncommon	Abd pain common; pleurisy, pericarditis rare	Rare	Rare
Skin	Erysipeloid erythema	Centrifugally migrating erythema	Diffuse maculopapular rash; oral, vaginal ulcers	Diffuse urticaria-like rash	Cold-induced urticaria-like rash	Diffuse urticaria-like rash
Joints	Acute monoarthritis; chronic hip arthritis (rare)	Acute monoarthritis, arthralgia	Arthralgia, oligoarthritis	Arthralgia, large-joint oligoarthritis	Polyarthralgia	Epiphyseal, patellar overgrowth, clubbing
Muscle	Exercise-induced myalgia common; protracted febrile myalgia rare	Migratory myalgia	Uncommon	Myalgia common	Sometimes myalgia	Sometimes myalgia
Eyes, ears	Uncommon	Periorbital edema, conjunctivitis, rarely uveitis	Uncommon	Conjunctivitis, episcleritis, optic disc edema; sensorineural hearing loss	Conjunctivitis	Conjunctivitis, uveitis, optic disc edema, blindness, sensorineural hearing loss
CNS	Aseptic meningitis rare	Headache	Headache	Headache	Headache	Aseptic meningitis, seizures
Amyloidosis	Most common in M694V homozygotes	~15% of cases	Not described	~25% of cases	Uncommon	Late complication
Treatment	Oral colchicine prophylaxis	Glucocorticoids, etanercept	NSAIDs for fever; etanercept investigational	NSAIDs, prednisone; anakinra investigational	NSAIDs	Anakinra investigational

Abbreviations: FMF, familial Mediterranean fever; TNF, tumor necrosis factor; TRAPS, TNF receptor-associated periodic syndrome; HIDS, hyperimmunoglobulin D with periodic fever syndrome; MWS, Muckle-Wells syndrome; FCAS, familial cold autoinflammatory syndrome; NOMID; neonatal onset multisystem inflammatory disease; Abd, abdominal; CNS, central nervous system; NSAID, nonsteroidal anti-inflammatory drug.

Italians, and occasional cases have been confirmed even in the absence of known Mediterranean ancestry. FMF is recessively inherited, but, particularly in countries where families are small, a positive family history can be elicited only in ~50% of cases. DNA testing demonstrates carrier frequencies as high as 1:3 among affected populations, suggesting a heterozygote advantage.

The FMF gene was identified by positional cloning in 1997. It encodes a 781-amino acid, ~95-kDa protein denoted *pyrin* (or *marenostrin*) that is expressed in association with the cytoskeleton in granulocytes, eosinophils, and cytokine-activated monocytes. The N-terminal 92 amino acids of pyrin define a motif, the PYRIN domain, similar in structure to death domains, death effector domains, and caspase recruitment domains. PYRIN domains mediate homotypic protein-protein interactions and have been found in several other proteins, including cryopyrin, which is mutated in three other recurrent fever syndromes. Through the interaction of this domain with an intermediary adaptor protein, pyrin regulates caspase-1 [interleukin (IL) 1β-converting enzyme], and thereby IL-1β secretion. Pyrin-deficient mice exhibit heightened sensitivity to endotoxin, excessive IL-1β production, and impaired monocyte apoptosis.

ACUTE ATTACKS   Febrile episodes in FMF may begin even in early infancy; 90% of patients have had their first attack by age 20. Typical FMF episodes generally last 24 to 72 h, with arthritic attacks tending to last somewhat longer. In some patients the episodes occur with great regularity, but more often the frequency of attacks varies over time, ranging from as often as once every few days to remissions lasting several years. Attacks are often unpredictable, although some patients relate them to physical exertion, emotional stress, or menses; pregnancy may be associated with remission.

If measured, temperature elevation is nearly always present throughout FMF attacks. Severe hyperpyrexia and even febrile seizures may be seen in infants, and fever is sometimes the only manifestation of FMF in young children.

Over 90% of FMF patients experience abdominal attacks at some time. Episodes range in severity from dull, aching pain and distention with mild tenderness on direct palpation to severe generalized pain with absent bowel sounds, rigidity, rebound tenderness, and air-fluid levels on upright radiographs. Computed tomography (CT) scanning may demonstrate a small amount of fluid in the abdominal cavity. If such patients undergo exploratory laparotomy, a sterile, neutrophil-rich peritoneal exudate is present, sometimes with adhesions from previous episodes. Ascites is rare.

Pleural attacks are usually manifested by unilateral, sharp, stabbing chest pain. Radiographs may show atelectasis and sometimes an effusion; thoracentesis demonstrates an exudative fluid rich in neutrophils. After repeated attacks, pleural thickening may develop.

FMF arthritis is most frequent among individuals homozygous for the M694V mutation, which is especially common in the non-Ashkenazi Jewish population. Acute arthritis in FMF is usually monoarticular, affecting the knee, ankle, or hip, although other patterns can be seen, particularly in children. Large sterile effusions rich in neutrophils are frequent, without commensurate erythema or warmth. Even after repeated arthritic attacks, radiographic changes are rare. Before the advent of colchicine prophylaxis, chronic arthritis of the knee or hip was seen in ~5% of FMF patients with arthritis. Chronic sacroiliitis can occur in FMF irrespective of the HLA-B27 antigen, even in the face of colchicine therapy. In the United States, FMF patients are much more likely to have arthralgia than arthritis.

The most characteristic cutaneous manifestation of FMF is erysipelas-like erythema, a flat, raised erythematous rash that most commonly occurs on the dorsum of the foot, ankle, or lower leg, alone or in combination with abdominal pain, pleurisy, or arthritis. Biopsy demonstrates perivascular infiltrates of granulocytes and monocytes. This rash is seen most often in M694V homozygotes and is relatively rare in the United States.

Exercise-induced (nonfebrile) myalgia is common in FMF, and a small percentage of patients develop a protracted febrile myalgia that can last several weeks. Symptomatic pericardial disease is rare, although some patients have small pericardial effusions as an incidental echocardiographic finding. Unilateral acute scrotal inflammation may occur in prepubertal boys. Aseptic meningitis has been reported, but the causal connection is controversial. Vasculitis, including Henoch-Schönlein purpura and periarteritis nodosum (Chap. 306), may be seen at increased frequency in FMF.

Laboratory features of FMF attacks are consistent with acute inflammation and include an elevated erythrocyte sedimentation rate; leukocytosis; thrombocytosis (in children); and elevations in the C-reactive protein, fibrinogen, haptoglobin, and serum immunoglobulins. Transient albuminuria and hematuria may also be seen.

AMYLOIDOSIS   Before the advent of colchicine prophylaxis, systemic amyloidosis was a common complication of FMF. It is caused by deposition of a fragment of serum amyloid A, an acute-phase reactant, in the kidneys, adrenals, intestine, spleen, lung, and testes. Amyloidosis should be suspected in patients who have proteinuria between attacks; renal or rectal biopsy is most often used to establish the diagnosis. Risk factors include the M694V homozygous genotype, positive family history (independent of FMF mutational status), the SAA 1 genotype, male gender, noncompliance with colchicine therapy, and having grown up in the Middle East.

DIAGNOSIS   For typical cases, experienced physicians can often make the diagnosis on clinical grounds alone. Clinical criteria for FMF have been shown to have high sensitivity and specificity in parts of the world where the pretest probability of FMF is high. Genetic testing can provide a useful adjunct in ambiguous cases or for physicians not experienced in FMF. Most of the disease-associated FMF mutations are in exon 10 of the gene, with a smaller group of mutations in exon 2. An updated list of mutations for FMF and other hereditary periodic fevers can be found online at *http://fmf.igh.cnrs.fr/infevers/*.

Genetic testing has permitted a broadening of the clinical spectrum and geographic distribution of FMF and may be of prognostic value. Most studies indicate that M694V homozygotes have an earlier age of onset and a higher frequency of arthritis, rash, and amyloidosis. In contrast, the E148Q mutation is usually associated with milder disease. E148Q is sometimes found in *cis* with exon 10 mutations, which complicates the interpretation of genetic test results. Only ~70% of patients with clinically typical FMF have two identifiable mutations in *trans*, suggesting either that current screening methods do not detect all of the relevant mutations or that one mutation may be sufficient for disease under some circumstances. In these cases clinical judgment is very important, and sometimes a therapeutic trial of colchicine may help to confirm the diagnosis. Genetic testing of unaffected individuals is usually inadvisable because of the possibility of nonpenetrance and the potential impact of a positive test on future insurability.

If a patient is seen during their first attack, the differential diagnosis may be broad, although delimited by the specific organ involvement. After several attacks the differential diagnosis may include the other hereditary periodic fever syndromes (Table 278-1); the syndrome of periodic fever with aphthous ulcers, pharyngitis, and cervical adenopathy (PFAPA); systemic-onset juvenile rheumatoid arthritis or adult Still's disease; porphyria; hereditary angioedema; inflammatory bowel disease; and, in women, gynecologic disorders.

Rx TREATMENT

The treatment of choice for FMF is daily oral colchicine, which decreases the frequency and intensity of attacks and prevents the development of amyloidosis in compliant patients. Intermittent dosing at the onset of attacks is not as effective as daily prophylaxis and is of unproven value in preventing amyloidosis. The usual adult dose of colchicine is 1.2 to 1.8 mg/d, which causes substantial reduction in symptoms in two-thirds of patients and some improvement in >90%. Children may require lower doses, although not proportionately to body weight.

Common side effects of colchicine include bloating, abdominal cramps, lactose intolerance, and diarrhea. They can be minimized by starting at a low dose and gradually advancing as tolerated, splitting the dose, use of simethicone for flatulence, and avoidance of dairy products. If taken by either parent at the time of conception, colchicine may cause a small increase in the risk of trisomy 21 (Down syndrome). In elderly patients with renal insufficiency, colchicine can cause a myoneuropathy characterized by proximal muscle weakness and elevation of the creatine kinase. Cyclosporine inhibits hepatic excretion of colchicine by its effects on the MDR-1 transport system, sometimes leading to colchicine toxicity in patients who have undergone renal transplantation for amyloidosis. Intravenous colchicine should generally not be administered to patients already taking oral colchicine, because severe, sometimes fatal, toxicity can occur in this setting.

No alternatives have been established for the small number of patients who do not respond to colchicine or cannot tolerate therapeutic dosages, although interferon-α and tumor necrosis factor (TNF) inhibitors are investigational. Bone marrow transplantation has been suggested for refractory FMF, but the risk-benefit ratio is currently regarded as unacceptable.

OTHER HEREDITARY RECURRENT FEVERS

Within 5 years of the discovery of the FMF gene, three additional genes causing five other hereditary periodic fever syndromes were identified, catalyzing a paradigm shift in diagnosis and treatment of these disorders.

TNF RECEPTOR–ASSOCIATED PERIODIC SYNDROME (TRAPS) TRAPS is caused by dominantly inherited mutations in the extracellular domains of the 55-kDa TNF receptor (TNFRSF1A, p55). Although originally described in a large Irish family (and hence the name *familial Hibernian fever*), TRAPS has a broad ethnic distribution. TRAPS episodes often begin in childhood. The duration of attacks ranges from 1 to 2 days to as long as several weeks, and in severe cases symptoms may be nearly continuous. In addition to peritoneal, pleural, and synovial attacks similar to those in FMF, TRAPS patients frequently have ocular inflammation (most often conjunctivitis and/or periorbital edema) and a distinctive migratory myalgia with overlying painful erythema. TRAPS patients generally respond better to glucocorticoids than to prophylactic colchicine. About 15% develop amyloidosis. The diagnosis of TRAPS is based on the demonstration of *TNFRSF1A* mutations in the presence of characteristic symptoms. Leukocytes from patients with certain TRAPS mutations exhibit a defect in TNF receptor shedding, possibly impairing normal homeostasis and explaining autoinflammatory manifestations. Etanercept, a TNF inhibitor, has been shown to ameliorate TRAPS attacks, although its effect on amyloidosis is unproven.

HYPERIMMUNOGLOBULINEMIA D WITH PERIODIC FEVER SYNDROME (HIDS) HIDS is a recessively inherited recurrent fever syndrome found primarily in individuals of northern European ancestry. It is caused by mutations in mevalonate kinase (*MVK*), encoding an enzyme involved in the synthesis of cholesterol and nonsterol isoprenoids. Attacks usually begin in infancy, and last 3 to 7 days. Clinically distinctive features include painful cervical lymphadenopathy, a diffuse maculopapular rash sometimes affecting the palms and soles, and aphthous ulcers; pleurisy is rare, and amyloidosis has not yet been reported. Although originally defined by the persistent elevation of serum IgD, disease activity is not related to IgD level, and some patients with FMF or TRAPS may have modestly increased serum IgD. Moreover, occasional patients with *MVK* mutations and periodic fever have normal IgD levels. No treatment for HIDS has been established.

THE CRYOPYRINOPATHIES Three hereditary febrile syndromes, familial cold autoinflammatory syndrome (FCAS), Muckle-Wells syndrome (MWS), and neonatal onset multisystem inflammatory disease (NOMID), are all caused by mutations in *CIAS1*, the gene encoding cryopyrin, and represent a clinical spectrum of disease. FCAS patients develop chills, fever, headache, arthralgia, conjunctivitis, and an urticaria-like rash in response to generalized cold exposure. In MWS there is a similar rash, but it is not usually induced by cold. MWS patients also develop fevers, abdominal pain, limb pain, arthritis, conjunctivitis, and, over time, sensorineural hearing loss. NOMID is the most severe of the three disorders, with chronic aseptic meningitis, a characteristic arthropathy, and urticarial rash. Like the FMF protein, pyrin, cryopyrin has an N-terminal PYRIN domain and regulates IL-1β production. Initial therapeutic experience with anakinra, the IL-1 receptor antagonist, in MWS has been encouraging.

FURTHER READING

AKSENTIJEVICH I et al: De novo *CIAS1* mutations, cytokine activation, and evidence for genetic heterogeneity in patients with neonatal-onset multisystem inflammatory disease (NOMID). A new member of the expanding family of pyrin-associated autoinflammatory diseases. Arthritis Rheum 46: 3340, 2002

DRENTH JPH, VAN DER MEER JWM: Hereditary periodic fever. N Engl J Med 345:1748, 2001

HAWKINS PN et al: Interleukin-1-receptor antagonist in the Muckle-Wells syndrome. N Engl J Med 348:2583, 2003

HOFFMAN HM et al: Mutation of a new gene encoding a putative pyrin-like protein causes familial cold autoinflammatory syndrome and Muckle-Wells syndrome. Nat Genet 29:301, 2001

HULL KM et al: The TNF receptor-associated periodic syndrome (TRAPS). Emerging concepts of an autoinflammatory disorder. Medicine (Baltimore) 81:349, 2002

———: The expanding spectrum of systemic autoinflammatory disorders and their rheumatic manifestations. Curr Opin Rheumatol 15:61, 2003

LA REGINA M et al: Familial Mediterranean fever is no longer a rare disease in Italy. Eur J Hum Genet 11:50, 2003

279 COMMON DISEASES OF THE COLON AND ANORECTUM AND MESENTERIC VASCULAR INSUFFICIENCY
Susan L. Gearhart, Gregory Bulkley

COLON

DIVERTICULAR DISEASE ■ Incidence and Epidemiology Among western populations, diverticulosis affects nearly one-half of individuals over age 60. The prevalence among females and males is similar. However, males tend to present at a younger age. Fortunately, only 20% of patients with diverticulosis develop symptomatic disease. Diverticulosis is rare in underdeveloped countries, where diets include more fiber and roughage.

Anatomy and Pathophysiology Two types of diverticula occur in the intestine: true and false, or pseudodiverticula. The most common type of diverticulum affecting the colon is the pseudodiverticulum. This is a herniation or saclike projection of the mucosa through the muscularis propria. The protrusion occurs commonly at the point where the nutrient artery penetrates through the muscularis propria, resulting in a break in the integrity of the colonic wall. Diverticulosis commonly affects the sigmoid colon; only 5% of persons exhibit pancolonic diverticula. This may be a result of the relative high-pressure zone within the sigmoid colon. Thus, higher amplitude contractions combined with constipated, high-fat content stool within the sigmoid lumen results in the creation of these diverticula. *Diverticulitis*, or inflammation of a diverticulum, is related to the retention of particulate material within the diverticular sac and the formation of a fecalith. Consequently, the blood vessel is either compressed or eroded, leading to either perforation or bleeding.

Presentation, Evaluation, and Management of Diverticular Bleeding   Hemorrhage from a colonic diverticulum is the most common cause of hematochezia in patients over the age of 60, yet only 20% of patients with diverticulosis will have gastrointestinal bleeding. Patients at increased risk for bleeding tend to be hypertensive, have atherosclerosis, and regularly use nonsteroidal anti-inflammatory agents. Most bleeds are self-limited and stop spontaneously with bowel rest. The lifetime risk of rebleeding is 25%.

Localization of diverticular bleeding should include colonoscopy, which may be both diagnostic and therapeutic in the management of mild to moderate diverticular bleeding. If the patient is stable, massive bleeding is best managed by angiography. Mesenteric angiography can localize the bleeding site and occlude it successfully with a coil in 80% of cases. The patient can then be followed closely with or without repetitive endoscopy looking for evidence of colonic ischemia. With newer techniques of highly selective coil embolization, the rate of colonic ischemia is <10% and the risk of acute rebleeding is <25%. Alternatively, a selective infusion of vasopressin can be given to stop the hemorrhage. However, this has been associated with significant complications, including myocardial infarction and intestinal ischemia in >40% of patients. Furthermore, bleeding recurs in 50% of patients once the infusion is stopped. Localization studies indicate that bleeding as a result of colonic diverticulosis is more often seen from the right colon. For this reason, patients with presumed bleeding from diverticular disease requiring emergent surgery without localization should undergo a total abdominal colectomy. Current recommendations state that if the patient is unstable or has had a 6-unit bleed within 24 h, surgery should be performed. In patients without severe comorbidities, surgical resection can be performed with a primary anastomosis. A higher anastomotic leak rate has been reported in patients undergoing primary anastomosis who received >10 units of blood.

Presentation and Evaluation of Diverticulitis   Acute diverticulitis characteristically presents with fever, anorexia, left lower quadrant abdominal pain, and diarrhea. In severe cases, patients may have generalized peritonitis and obstipation. Diverticular perforation with a fistula to the bladder presents with pneumaturia or recurrent urinary tract infections. On examination, the patient may have abdominal distention and signs of localized or generalized peritonitis. Laboratory investigations will demonstrate a leukocytosis. Rarely, a patient may present with an air-fluid level in the left lower quadrant on plain abdominal film. This is a giant diverticulum of the sigmoid colon and is managed with resection to avoid impending perforation.

The diagnosis of diverticulitis is best made on computed tomography (CT) with the following findings: sigmoid diverticula; thickened colonic wall >4 mm; inflammation within the pericolic fat ± the collection of contrast material or fluid. Symptoms of irritable bowel syndrome (IBS) may mimic those of diverticulitis. Therefore, suspected diverticulitis that does not meet CT criteria or is not associated with a leukocytosis or fever is not diverticular disease. A gastrograffin enema may also be useful in the evaluation of patients with presumed diverticular disease. If the patient has diverticular disease with a contained perforation (abscess), this study will differentiate whether the abscess is communicating with the bowel lumen or not. The latter can be managed acutely with antimicrobial therapy, whereas the former has a higher rate of failure of medical management. Repeated use of CT imaging in mild disease is not recommended as the rate of perforation with abscess formation from left-sided diverticular disease is only 16%.

Barium enema or colonoscopy should not be performed in the acute setting because of the higher risk of colonic perforation associated with insufflation or insertion of barium-based contrast material under pressure. A sigmoid malignancy can masquerade as diverticular disease.

Therefore, a barium enema or colonoscopy should be performed before surgical resection.

Staging of Complicated Diverticulitis   In contrast to uncomplicated diverticulitis, *complicated diverticular disease* is defined as diverticular disease associated with a stricture, abscess, or fistula requiring surgical intervention to cure. Complicated diverticular disease is staged using the Hinchey classification system (Fig. 279-1). This staging system was developed to predict outcomes following the surgical management of complicated diverticular disease. Other preoperative risk factors influencing postoperative mortality rates include higher American Society of Anesthesia (ASA) class and preexisting organ failure.

℞ TREATMENT

Medical Management   Asymptomatic diverticular disease discovered on imaging studies or at the time of endoscopy is best managed by diet alterations. Patients should be instructed to eat a fiber-enriched diet. This diet requires that 15 to 30 g of fiber be consumed each day, best accomplished with supplementary fiber products such as Metamucil, Fibercon, or Citrucel. The patient should also be instructed to avoid nuts and popcorn.

Symptomatic diverticular disease, defined as radiographic and hematologic confirmation of inflammation and infection within the colon, should be treated initially with antibiotics and bowel rest. Nearly 75% of patients hospitalized for acute diverticulitis will respond to nonoperative treatment with a suitable antimicrobial regiment. The current recommended antimicrobial coverage is trimethoprim/sulfamethoxazole or ciprofloxacin and metronidazole targeting aerobic gram-negative rods and anaerobic bacteria. Unfortunately, this does not cover enterococci, and the addition of ampicillin to this regimen for nonresponders is recommended. Single-agent therapy with a third-generation penicillin such as piperacillin may be effective. The usual course of antibiotics is 7 to 10 days. Current recommendations concerning bowel rest suggest that patients should remain on nothing by mouth or on clear liquids until their pain resolves. A role for parenteral nutrition has not been established.

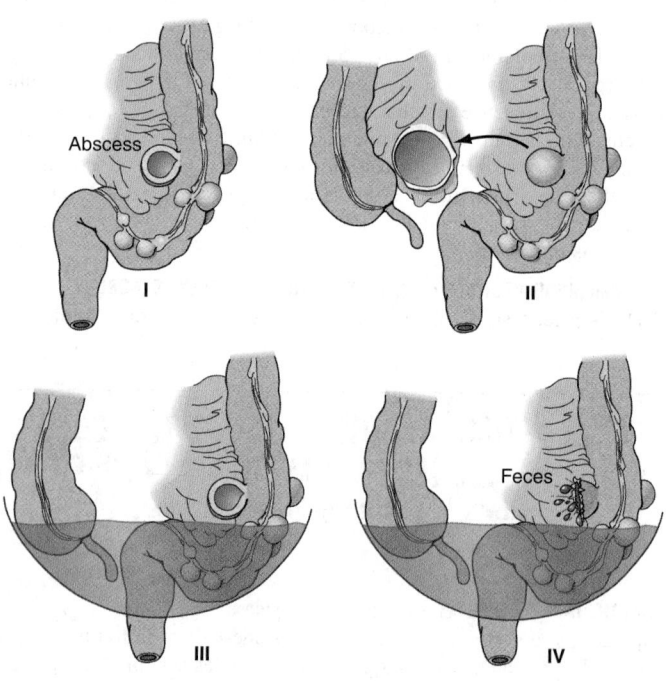

FIGURE 279-1   Hinchey classification of diverticulitis. Stage I: perforated diverticulitis with a confined paracolic abscess. Stage II: perforated diverticulitis that has closed spontaneously with distant abscess formation. Stage III: noncommunicating perforated diverticulitis with fecal peritonitis (the diverticular neck is closed off and therefore contrast will not freely expel on radiographic images). Stage IV: perforation and free communication with the peritoneum, resulting in fecal peritonitis.

Surgical Management Surgical therapy should be offered to patients who have had at least two documented attacks of diverticulitis or those who do not rapidly improve on medical therapy. Surgical therapy is indicated in all patients with complicated diverticular disease. In contrast to older patients, younger patients may experience a more aggressive form of the disease. Nearly 30% of people with diverticular disease are <40 years old. Surgical intervention is required in >70% of these patients. Patients under age 40 should undergo surgical excision following the first episode of documented diverticulitis.

The goals of surgical management of diverticular disease include controlling sepsis, eliminating complications such as fistula or obstruction, removing the diseased colonic segment, and restoring intestinal continuity. These goals must be obtained while minimizing morbidity, length of hospitalization, and cost and maximizing survival and quality of life. The options for the surgical management of diverticular disease include: (1) proximal diversion of the fecal stream with an ileostomy or colostomy and sutured omental patch with drainage, (2) resection with colostomy and mucus fistula or closure of distal bowel with formation of a Hartmann's pouch, (3) resection with anastomosis (coloproctostomy), or (4) resection with anastomosis and diversion (coloproctostomy with loop ileostomy or colostomy).

Patients with Hinchey stages I and II disease are managed with percutaneous drainage followed by resection with anastomosis about 6 weeks later. Percutaneous drainage is recommended for abscesses that are ≥5 cm with a well-defined wall that is accessible. Paracolic abscesses that are <5 cm in size will usually resolve with bowel rest and antibiotics alone. Contraindications to percutaneous drainage are pneumoperitoneum and fecal peritonitis. Urgent operative intervention is undertaken if patients develop generalized peritonitis, and most will need to be managed with a Hartmann's procedure. In selected cases, nonoperative therapy may be considered. Nonoperative management of isolated paracolic abscesses (Hinchey stage I) is associated with only a 20% recurrence rate at 2 years. Over 80% of patients with distant abscesses (Hinchey stage II) require surgical resection for recurrent symptoms.

Hinchey stage III disease is managed with a Hartman's procedure or with primary anastomosis and proximal diversion. If the patient has significant comorbidities, making operative intervention risky, a limited procedure including intraoperative peritoneal lavage (irrigation), omental patch to the oversewn perforation, and proximal diversion of the fecal stream with either an ileostomy or transverse colostomy can be performed. No anastomosis of any type should be attempted in Hinchey stage IV disease. A limited approach to these patients is associated with a decreased mortality (Table 279-1). Other important modalities in the surgical management of diverticular disease include newer minimally invasive surgical techniques. Patients undergoing successful laparoscopic resection for diverticular disease have shorter hospital stays and return to work earlier. However, conversion rates from laparoscopic to open resection are higher in patients with complicated diverticular disease.

Recurrent Symptoms Recurrent abdominal symptoms following surgical resection for diverticular disease occurs in 10% of patients. Recurrent diverticular disease develops in patients following inadequate surgical resection. A retained segment of diseased rectosigmoid colon is associated with twice the incidence of recurrence. IBS may also cause symptom recurrence. Patients undergoing surgical resection for presumed diverticulitis and symptoms of abdominal cramping and irregular loose bowel movements consistent with IBS have functionally poorer outcomes.

MESENTERIC VASCULAR INSUFFICIENCY

INTESTINAL ISCHEMIA ■ Incidence and Epidemiology Intestinal ischemia may result from either arterial occlusive and vasospastic disease or from venoocclusive disease. The most common form of intestinal ischemia is acute arterial ischemia. Risk factors for acute arterial ischemia include atrial fibrillation, recent myocardial infarction, valvular heart disease, and recent cardiac or vascular catheterization. The increased incidence of intestinal ischemia seen among western countries

TABLE 279-1 *Outcome Following Surgical Therapy for Complicated Diverticular Disease*

Hinchey Stage	Operative Procedure	Anastomotic Leak Rate, %	Overall Morbidity, %
I	Resection with primary anastomosis without diverting stoma	3.8	22
II	Resection with primary anastomosis +/− diversion	3.8	30
III	Hartmann's procedure vs. diverting colostomy and omental pedal graft	—	0 vs. 6 mortality
IV	Hartmann's procedure vs. diverting colostomy and omental pedicle graft	—	6 vs. 2 mortality

parallels atherosclerosis and the aging population. With the exception of strangulated small-bowel obstruction, ischemic colitis is the most common form of acute ischemia and the most prevalent gastrointestinal disease complicating cardiovascular surgery. The incidence of ischemic colitis following elective aortic repair is 5 to 9%, and the incidence triples in patients following emergent repair. Other less common forms of intestinal ischemia include chronic mesenteric angina associated with atherosclerotic disease and mesenteric venous thrombosis. Mesenteric venous thrombosis is associated with the presence of a hypercoaguable state including proteins C and S deficiency, antithrombin III deficiency, polycythema vera, and carcinoma.

Anatomy and Pathophysiology Intestinal ischemia occurs when insufficient perfusion to intestinal tissue produces ischemic tissue injury. The blood supply to the intestines is depicted in Fig. 279-2. To prevent ischemic injury, extensive collateralization occurs between major mesenteric trunks and branches of the mesenteric arcades (Table 279-2). Collateral vessels within the small bowel are numerous and meet

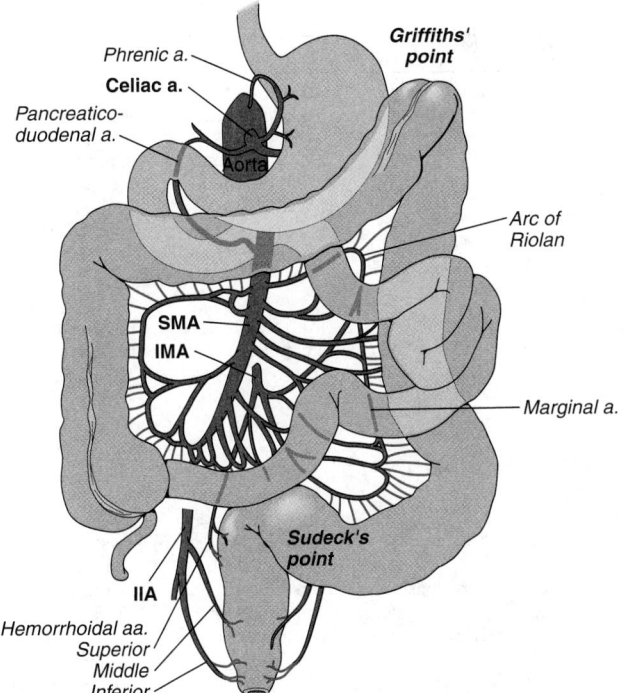

FIGURE 279-2 Blood supply to the intestines includes the celiac artery, superior mesenteric artery (SMA), inferior mesenteric artery (IMA), and branches of the internal iliac artery (IIA). Sudeck's and Griffiths' points, indicated by shaded area, are watershed areas within the colonic blood supply and common locations for ischemia.

TABLE 279-2 *Collateral Arterial Intestinal Blood Flow*

Involved Circulation	Mesenteric Artery	Adjoining Artery	Collateral Artery
Systemic	Celiac	Descending aorta	Phrenic
Systemic	IMA	Hypogastric	Middle hemorrhoidal
Mesenteric	Celiac	SMA	Superior/inferior pancreaticoduodenal
Mesenteric	SMA	IMA	Arch of Riolan
Mesenteric	SMA	Celiac/IMA	Intramesenteric
Mesenteric	SMA	IMA	Marginal

Note: IMA, inferior mesenteric artery; SMA, superior mesenteric artery.

within the duodenum and the bed of the pancreas. Collateral vessels within the colon meet at the splenic flexure and descending/sigmoid colon. These areas, which are inherently at risk for decreased blood flow, are known as *Sudek's point* and *Griffiths' point*, respectively, and are the most common locations for colonic ischemia (Fig. 279-2, shaded area). The splanchnic circulation can receive up to 30% of the cardiac output. Protective responses to prevent intestinal ischemia include abundant collateralization, autoregulation of blood flow, and the ability to increase oxygen extraction.

Intestinal ischemia may result from arterial occlusive disease, arterial nonocclusive or vasospastic disease, and venous thrombosis. Occlusive ischemia is a result of disruption of blood flow by an embolus or progressive thrombosis in a major artery supplying the intestine. Emboli originate from the heart in >75% of cases and lodge preferentially just distal to the origin of the middle colic artery from the superior mesenteric artery. Progressive thrombosis of at least two of the major vessels supplying the intestine is required for the development of chronic intestinal angina. Nonocclusive ischemia is disproportionate mesenteric vasoconstriction (arteriolar vasospasm) in response to a severe physiologic stress such as dehydration or shock. If left untreated, early mucosal stress ulceration will progress to full-thickness injury.

Presentation, Evaluation, and Management Intestinal ischemia remains one of the most challenging diagnoses. The mortality rate with intes-

tinal ischemia is >50%. The most significant indicator of survival is the timeliness of diagnosis and treatment. An overview of diagnosis and management of each form of intestinal ischemia is given in Table 279-3.

Acute mesenteric ischemia resulting from arterial embolus or thrombosis presents with severe acute, nonremitting abdominal pain strikingly out of proportion to the physical findings. Associated symptoms may include nausea and vomiting, transient diarrhea, and bloody stools. With the exception of minimal abdominal distention and hypoactive bowel sounds, early abdominal examination is unimpressive. Later findings will demonstrate peritonitis and cardiovascular collapse. In the evaluation of acute intestinal ischemia, routine laboratory tests should be obtained, including complete blood count, serum chemistry, coagulation profile, arterial blood gas, amylase, lipase, lactic acid, blood type and cross match, and cardiac enzymes. Regardless of the need for urgent surgery, emergent admission to a monitored bed or intensive care unit is recommended for resuscitation and further evaluation. If the diagnosis of intestinal ischemia is being considered, consultation with a surgical service is necessary.

Other diagnostic modalities that may be useful in diagnosis but should not delay surgical therapy include electrocardiogram (ECG), abdominal radiographs, CT, and mesenteric angiography. The ECG may demonstrate an arrhythmia, indicating the possible source of the emboli. A plain abdominal film may show evidence of free intraperitoneal air, indicating a perforated viscus and the need for emergent exploration. Earlier features of intestinal ischemia seen on abdominal radiographs include bowel-wall edema, known as "thumbprinting." If the ischemia progresses, air can be seen within the bowel wall (*pneumatosis intestinalis*) and within the portal venous system. Other features include calcifications of the aorta and its tributaries, indicating atherosclerotic disease. With the administration of oral and intravenous contrast, dynamic CT with three-dimensional reconstruction is a highly sensitive test for intestinal ischemia. Other common causes of abdominal pain that may be identified on CT and alter the management of the patient are pancreatitis, diverticulitis, appendicitis, and small-bowel obstruction. In acute embolic disease, mesenteric angiography is best performed intraoperatively.

The "gold standard" for the diagnosis and management of acute arterial occlusive disease is laparotomy. Surgical exploration should not be delayed if suspicion of acute occlusive mesenteric ischemia is high or evidence of clinical deterioration or frank peritonitis is present. The goal of operative exploration is to resect compromised bowel and restore blood supply. Intraoperative or preoperative arteriography and systemic heparinization may assist the vascular surgeon in restoring blood supply to compromised bowel. The entire length of the small and large bowel beginning at the ligament of Treitz should be evaluated. The pattern of intestinal ischemia may indicate the level of arterial occlusion. In the case of superior mesenteric artery occlusion where the embolus usually lies just proximal to the origin of the middle colic artery, the proximal jejunum is often spared while the remainder of the small bowel to the transverse colon will be ischemic. The surgical management of acute mesenteric ischemia of the small bowel is attempted embolectomy via intra-

TABLE 279-3 *Overview of the Management of Acute Intestinal Ischemia*

Condition	Key to Early Diagnosis	Treatment of Underlying Cause	Treatment of Specific Lesion	Treatment of Systemic Consequences
Arterial embolus	Early laparotomy	Anticoagulation Cardioversion Proximal thrombectomy Aneurysmectomy	Laparotomy Embolectomy Vascular bypass Assess viability and resect dead bowel	Ensure hydration Give antibiotics Reverse acidosis Optimize oxygen delivery Support cardiac output Treat other embolic sites Avoid vasoconstrictors
Arterial thrombosis	Duplex ultrasound Angiography	Anticoagulation Hydration	Endovascular stent Endarterectomy/ thrombectomy or vascular bypass Assess viability and resect dead bowel	Give antibiotics Reverse acidosis Optimize oxygen delivery Support cardiac output Avoid vasoconstrictors
Venous thrombosis	Spiral CT	Anticoagulation Massive hydration	Anticoagulation +/− laparotomy/thrombectomy/ portasystemic shunt Assess viability and resect dead bowel	Give antibiotics Reverse acidosis Optimize oxygen delivery Support cardiac output Avoid vasoconstrictors
Nonocclusive mesenteric ischemia	Vasospasm: Angiography Hypoperfusion: Spiral CT or colonoscopy	Ensure hydration Support cardiac output Avoid vasoconstrictors Ablate renin-angiotensin axis	Vasospasm: Intraarterial vasodilators Hypoperfusion: Delayed laparotomy Assess viability and resect dead bowel	Ensure hydration Give antibiotics Reverse acidosis Optimize oxygen delivery Support cardiac output Avoid vasoconstrictors

Note: CT, computed tomography.
Source: Modified from GB Bulkley, in JL Cameron (ed): *Current Surgical Therapy*, 2d ed. Toronto, BC Decker, 1986.

operative angiography or arteriotomy. Although more commonly applied to chronic disease, acute thrombosis may be managed with angioplasty, with or without endovascular stent placement. If this is unsuccessful, a bypass from the aorta to the superior mesenteric artery is performed.

Nonocclusive or vasospastic mesenteric ischemia presents with generalized abdominal pain, anorexia, bloody stools, and abdominal distention. Often these patients are obtunded, and physical findings may not assist in the diagnosis. The presence of a leukocytosis, metabolic acidosis, elevated amylase or creatinine phosphokinase levels, and/or lactic acidosis are useful in support of the diagnosis of advanced intestinal ischemia; however, these markers may not be indicative of either reversible ischemia or frank necrosis. Newer investigational markers for intestinal ischemia that have been used include D-dimer, glutathione S-transferase, platelet-activating factor (PAF), and mucosal pH monitoring. Regardless of the need for urgent surgery, emergent admission to a monitored bed or intensive care unit is recommended for resuscitation and further evaluation. Early manifestations of intestinal ischemia include fluid sequestration within the bowel wall. This may lead to a loss of interstitial volume, and aggressive fluid resuscitation may be necessary. To optimize oxygen delivery, blood transfusions may be given. Broad-spectrum antibiotics to provide sufficient coverage for enteric pathogens, including gram-negative and anaerobic organisms, should be administered. Frequent monitoring of the patient's vital signs, urine output, blood gases, and lactate levels is paramount, as is frequent abdominal examination. All vasoconstriction agents should be avoided, allowing fluid resuscitation to maintain hemodynamics.

If ischemic colitis is a concern, colonscopy should be performed to assess the integrity of the colon mucosa (Fig. 279-3). Visualization of the rectosigmoid region may demonstrate decreased mucosal integrity, associated more commonly with nonocclusive mesenteric ischemia, or, on occasion, occlusive disease as a result of acute loss of inferior mesenteric arterial flow following aortic surgery. Ischemia of the colonic mucosa is graded as *mild* with minimal mucosal erythema or as *moderate* with pale mucosal ulcerations and evidence of exten-

sion to the muscular layer of the bowel wall. *Severe* ischemic colitis presents with severe ulcerations resulting in black or green discoloration of the mucosa, consistent with full-thickness bowel-wall necrosis. The degree of reversibility can be predicted from the mucosal findings: mild erythema is nearly 100% reversible, moderate ~50%, and frank necrosis is simply dead bowel. Follow-up colonoscopy can be performed to rule out progression of ischemic colitis.

Laparotomy for nonocclusive mesenteric ischemia is warranted for signs of peritonitis or worsening endoscopic findings and if the patient's condition does not improve with aggressive resuscitation. Ischemic colitis is optimally treated with resection of the ischemic bowel and formation of a proximal stoma. Primary anastomosis should not be performed in patients with acute intestinal ischemia.

Patients with mesenteric venous thrombosis may present with a gradual or sudden onset. Symptoms include vague abdominal pain, nausea, and vomiting. Examination findings include abdominal distention with mild to moderate tenderness and signs of dehydration. The gold standard for the diagnosis of mesenteric thrombosis is the abdominal spiral CT with oral and intravenous contrast. Findings on CT include bowel-wall thickening and ascites. Intravenous contrast will demonstrate a delayed arterial phase and clot within the superior mesenteric vein. The goal of management is to optimize hemodynamics and correct electrolyte abnormalities with massive fluid resuscitation. Intravenous antibiotics as well as anticoagulation should be initiated. If laparotomy is performed and mesenteric venous thrombosis is suspected, heparin anticoagulation is immediately initiated and clearly compromised bowel is resected.

Chronic intestinal ischemia presents with intestinal angina or abdominal pain associated with need for increased blood flow to the intestine. Patients report abdominal cramping and pain following ingestion of a meal. Weight loss and chronic diarrhea may also be noted. Abdominal pain without weight loss is not chronic mesenteric angina. Physical examination will often reveal the presence of an abdominal bruit as well as other manifestations of atherosclerosis. Duplex ultrasound evaluation of the mesenteric vessels has gained in popularity. In the absence of obesity and an increased bowel gas pattern, the radiologist may be able to identify flow disturbances within the vessels or the lack of a vasodilation response to feeding. This tool is frequently used as a screening test for patients with symptoms suggestive of chronic mesenteric ischemia. The gold standard for confirmation of mesenteric arterial occlusion is mesenteric angiography. Evaluation with mesenteric angiography allows for identification and possible intervention for the treatment of thrombus within the vessel lumen and will also evaluate the patency of remaining mesenteric vessels. The use of mesenteric angiography may be limited in the presence of renal failure or contrast allergy. Magnetic resonance angiography is an alternative if the administration of contrast dye is contraindicated.

The management of chronic intestinal ischemia includes medical management of atherosclerotic disease by lipid-lowering medications, exercise, and cessation of smoking. A full cardiac evaluation should be performed before intervention. Newer endovascular procedures may avoid an operative intervention in selective patient populations. Angioplasty with endovascular stenting in the treatment of chronic mesenteric ischemia is associated with an 80% long-term success rate. In patients requiring surgical exploration, the approach used is determined by the mesenteric angiogram. The entire length of the small and large bowel should be evaluated, beginning at the ligament of Treitz. Restoration of blood flow at the time of laparotomy is accomplished with mesenteric bypass.

Determination of intestinal viability intraoperatively in patients with suspected intestinal ischemia can be challenging. After revascularization, the bowel wall should be observed for return of a pink color and peristalsis. Palpation of major arterial vessels can be performed as well as applying a doppler flowmeter to the antimesenteric border of the bowel wall, but neither is a definitive indicator of viability. In equivocal cases, 1 g of intravenous sodium fluorescein is administered

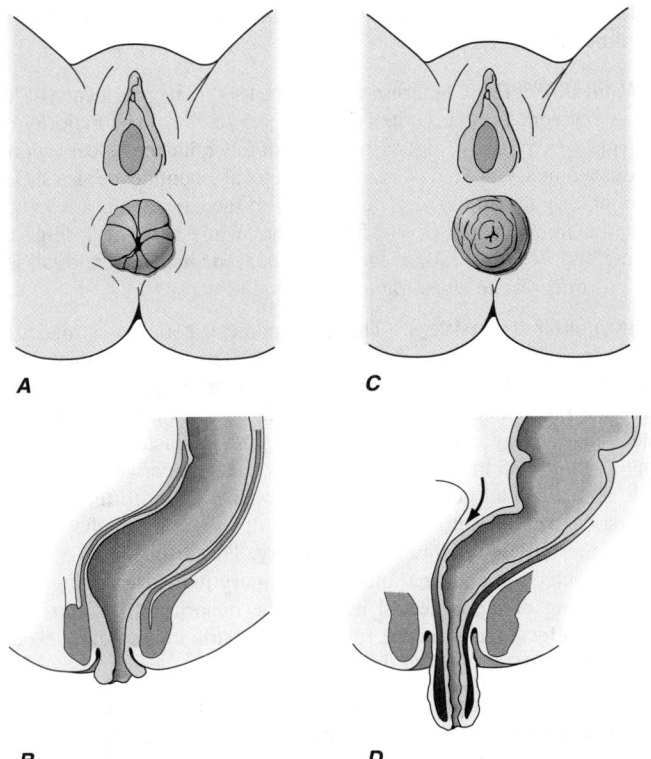

FIGURE 279-3 Degree of rectal prolapse. Mucosal prolapse only (A, B, sagittal view). Full-thickness prolapse associated with redundant rectosigmoid and deep pouch of Douglas (C, D, sagittal view).

and the pattern of bowel reperfusion is observed under ultraviolet illumination with a standard (3600 A) Wood's lamp. An area of nonfluorescence >5 mm in diameter is indicative of nonviability. If doubt still persists, reexploration should be performed 24 to 48 h following surgery. This will allow demarcation of nonviable bowel. Primary intestinal anastomosis in patients with ischemic bowel is always worrisome, and reanastomosis should be deferred to the time of second-look laparotomy.

ANORECTUM

RECTAL PROLAPSE (PROCIDENTIA) ■ Incidence and Epidemiology
The incidence of rectal prolapse peaks in women >60 years. Rectal prolapse is six times more common in women than in men. The incidence of rectal prolapse peaks in women >60 years. Women with rectal prolapse have a higher incidence of associated pelvic floor disorders including urinary incontinence, rectocele, cystocele, and enterocele. Nearly one-third of male patients with rectal prolapse suffer from a neurologic or psychiatric disorders. About 20% of children with rectal prolapse will have cystic fibrosis. All children presenting with prolapse should undergo a sweat chloride test. Less common associations include Ehlers-Danlos syndrome, solitary rectal ulcer syndrome, congenital hypothyroidism, and Hirschsprung's disease.

Anatomy and Pathophysiology   Rectal prolapse (procidentia) is a circumferential, full-thickness protrusion of the rectal wall through the anal orifice. It is often associated with a redundant sigmoid colon, pelvic laxity, and a deep pouch of Douglas. Initially, rectal prolapse was considered to be the result of early internal rectal intussusception, the first step in an inevitable progression to full-thickness external prolapse. However, only 1 of 38 patients with internal prolapse followed for >5 years developed full-thickness prolapse. Others have suggested that full-thickness prolapse is the result of damage to the pudendal nerves from repeated stretching with straining to defecate. Damage to the pudendal nerves would weaken the pelvic floor muscles, including the anal sphincters.

Presentation and Evaluation   Patients are often concerned that the symptoms they are experiencing may be a cancer. The majority of complaints include anal mass, bleeding per rectum, and a change in bowel habits. Prolapse of the rectum usually occurs following defecation. It is often associated with mild bleeding and inability to maintain good perianal hygiene. Constipation and differing degrees of fecal incontinence are common complaints associated with rectal prolapse.

To evaluate a patient's prolapse in the office, it is best to give the patient an enema in the bathroom and to have them signal when the prolapse protrudes. An important distinction should be made between full-thickness rectal prolapse and isolated mucosal prolapse associated with hemorrhoidal disease (Fig. 279-4). Mucosal prolapse is known for radial grooves rather than circumferential folds around the anus and is due to increased laxity of the connective tissue between the submucosa and underlying muscle of the anal canal. The evaluation of prolapse should also include cystoproctography and colonoscopy. These examinations evaluate for associated pelvic floor disorders and rule out a malignancy or a polyp as the lead point for prolapse. If rectal prolapse is associated with constipation, the patient should undergo a sitzmark study. For patients with fecal incontinence, endoanal ultrasound and manometric evaluation, including pudendal nerve testing of their anal sphincter muscles, should be performed before surgery for prolapse (see "Fecal Incontinence," below).

℞ TREATMENT

The medical approach to the management of rectal prolapse is limited and includes stool-bulking agents or fiber supplementation to ease the process of evacuation. Surgical correction of rectal prolapse is the mainstay of therapy. Two approaches are commonly considered, transabdominal and transperineal. Transabdominal approaches have been

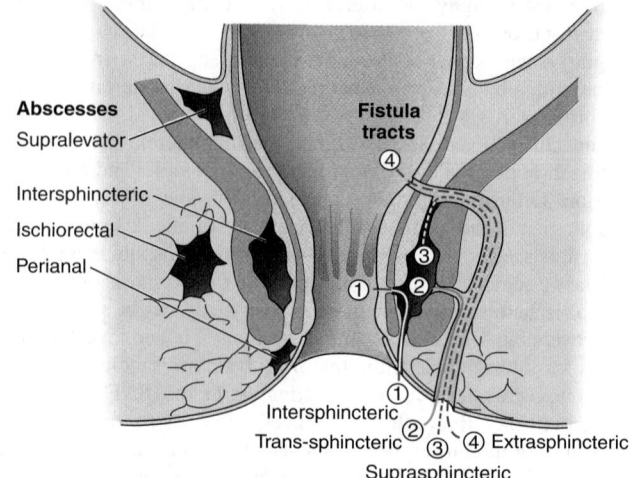

FIGURE 279-4   Common locations of anorectal abscess (*left*) and fistula in ano (*right*).

associated with lower recurrence rates, but some patients with significant comorbidities are better served by a transperineal approach.

Common transperineal approaches include a transanal proctectomy (Altmeier procedure), mucosal proctectomy (Delorme procedure), or placement of a Tirsch wire encircling the anus. The goal of the transperineal approach is to remove the redundant rectosigmoid colon. Common transabdominal approaches include presacral suture or mesh rectopexy (Ripstein) with (Frykman-Goldberg) or without resection of the redundant sigmoid. The goal of the transabdominal approach is to attempt to restore normal anatomy by removing redundant bowel and reattaching the supportive tissue of the rectum to the presacral fascia. The final alternative is abdominal proctectomy with end-sigmoid colostomy. Colon resection, in general, is reserved for patients with constipation and outlet obstruction. If total colonic inertia is present, as defined by a history of constipation and a positive sitzmark study (retention of >20% of markers 5 days after swallowing), a subtotal colectomy with an ileosigmoid or rectal anastomosis may be required at the time of rectopexy.

FECAL INCONTINENCE ■ Incidence and Epidemiology
The prevalence of fecal incontinence in the United States is 0.5 to 11%. The majority of patients are women. A higher incidence of incontinence is seen among parous women. One-half of patients with fecal incontinence also suffer from urinary incontinence. The majority of incontinence is a result of obstetric injury to the pelvic floor, either while carrying a fetus or during the delivery. Other causes include congenital abnormalities such as imperforate anus, trauma, or rectal prolapse.

Anatomy and Pathophysiology   The anal sphincter complex is made up of the internal and external anal sphincter. The internal sphincter is smooth muscle and a continuation of the circular fibers of the rectal wall. It is innervated by the intestinal myenteric plexus and is therefore under involuntary control. The external anal sphincter is formed in continuation with the levator ani muscles and is under voluntary control. The pudendal nerve supplies motor innervation to the external anal sphincter. Obstetric injury may result in tearing of the muscle fibers anteriorly at the time of the delivery. This results in an obvious anterior defect on endoanal ultrasound. Injury may also be the result of stretching of the pudendal nerves. The majority of patients who suffer with fecal incontinence following obstetric injury do so several years following the birth of their last child.

Presentation and Evaluation   Patients may suffer with varying degrees of fecal incontinence. Minor incontinence includes incontinence to flatus and occasional seepage of liquid stool. Major incontinence is frequent inability to control solid waste. As a result of fecal incontinence, patients suffer from poor perianal hygiene. Beyond the immediate problems associated with fecal incontinence, these patients are often withdrawn and suffer from depression. For this reason, quality-of-life measures have become an important component in the evaluation of patients with fecal incontinence.

The evaluation of fecal incontinence should include a thorough history and physical examination, anal manometry, pudendal nerve terminal motor latency (PNTML), and endoanal ultrasound. Anal manometry determines the resting and squeeze pressures within the anal canal. Pudendal nerves studies evaluate the function of the nerves innervating the anal canal. Stretch injuries to these nerves will result in a delayed response of the sphincter muscle to a stimulus, indicating a prolonged latency. Finally, ultrasound will evaluate the extent of the injury to the sphincter muscles. Only PNTML has been able to predict outcome following surgical intervention.

Rarely does a pelvic floor disorder exist alone. The majority of patients with fecal incontinence will have a degree of urinary incontinence. Similarly, fecal incontinence is a part of the spectrum of pelvic organ prolapse. For this reason, patients may present with symptoms of obstructed defecation as well as fecal incontinence. Careful evaluation including cinedefography should be performed to search for other associated defects. Surgical repair of incontinence without attention to other associated defects may decrease the success of the repair.

TABLE 279-4   *The Staging and Treatment of Hemorrhoids*

Stage	Description of Classification	Treatment
I	Enlargement with bleeding	Fiber supplementation Cortisone suppository Sclerotherapy
II	Protrusion with spontaneous reduction	Fiber supplementation Cortisone suppository
III	Protrusion requiring manual reduction	Fiber supplementation Cortisone suppository Banding Operative hemorrhoidectomy (stapled or traditional)
IV	Irreducible protrusion	Fiber supplementation Cortisone suppository Operative hemorrhoidectomy

℞ TREATMENT

The gold standard for the treatment of fecal incontinence with an isolated sphincter defect is overlapping sphincteroplasty. The external anal sphincter muscle and scar tissue as well as any identifiable internal sphincter muscle are dissected free from the surrounding adipose and connective tissue anteriorly and then an overlapping repair is performed in an attempt to rebuild the muscular ring and restore its function. Other newer approaches include radiofrequency therapy to the anal canal to aid in the development of collagen fibers and provide tensile strength to the sphincter muscles. Sacral nerve stimulation and the artificial bowel sphincter are both adaptations of procedures developed for the management of urinary incontinence. Sacral nerve stimulation is ideally suitable for patients with intact but weak anal sphincters. The artificial bowel sphincter allows the patient to manually close off the anal canal unless defecation is necessary.

Long-term results following overlapping sphincteroplasty show about a 50% failure rate over 5 years. Poorer outcome has been seen in patients with prolonged PNTML. Long-term results for sacral stimulation and the artificial bowel sphincter have not been reported. However, the artificial bowel sphincter has been associated with a 30% infection rate.

HEMORRHOIDAL DISEASE ■ **Incidence and Epidemiology** Symptomatic hemorrhoids affect >1 million individuals in western civilization per year. The prevalence of hemorrhoidal disease is not selective for age or sex. However, age is known to have a deleterious effect on the anal canal. The prevalence of hemorrhoidal disease is less in underdeveloped countries. The typical low-fiber, high-fat western diet is associated with constipation and straining, and the development of symptomatic hemorrhoids.

Anatomy and Pathophysiology Hemorrhoidal cushions are a normal part of the anal canal. The vascular structures contained within this tissue aid in continence by preventing damage to the sphincter muscle. Three main hemorrhoidal complexes traverse the anal canal—the left lateral, the right anterior, and the right posterior. Engorgement and straining results in prolapse of this tissue into the anal canal. Over time, the anatomic support system of the hemorrhoidal complex weakens, exposing this tissue to the outside of the anal canal where it is susceptible to injury. Hemorrhoids are commonly classified as internal or external. Although small external cushions do exist, the standard classification of hemorrhoidal disease is based on the progression of the disease from their normal internal location to the prolapsing external position (Table 279-4).

Presentation and Evaluation Patients commonly present to a physician for two reasons: bleeding and protrusion. Pain is less common than with fissures and, if present, is described as a dull ache from engorgement of the hemorrhoidal tissue. Severe pain may indicate a thrombosed hemorrhoid. Hemorrhoidal bleeding is described as bright red blood seen either in the toilet or upon wiping. Occasional patients can present with significant bleeding, which may be a cause of anemia; however, the presence of a colonic neoplasm must be ruled out. Patients who present with a protruding mass complain about inability to maintain perianal hygiene and are often concerned about the presence of a malignancy.

The diagnosis of hemorrhoidal disease is made on physical examination. Inspection of the perianal region for evidence of thrombosis or excoriation is performed, followed by a careful digital examination. Anoscopy is performed paying particular attention to the known position of hemorrhoidal disease. The patient is asked to strain. If this is difficult for the patient, the maneuver can be performed while sitting on a toilet. The physician is notified when the tissue prolapses. It is important to differentiate the circumferential appearance of a full-thickness rectal prolapse from the radial nature of prolapsing hemorrhoids (see "Rectal Prolapse," above). The stage and location of the hemorrhoidal complexes are defined.

℞ TREATMENT

The treatment for bleeding hemorrhoids is based upon the stage of the disease (Table 279-4). In all patients with bleeding, the possibility of other causes must be considered. In young patients without a family history of colorectal cancer, the hemorrhoidal disease may be treated first and a colonoscopic examination performed if the bleeding continues. Older patients who have not had colorectal cancer screening should undergo colonoscopy or flexible sigmoidoscopy.

With rare exceptions, the acutely thrombosed hemorrhoid should be excised with an elliptical excision. Sitz baths, fiber, and stool softeners are prescribed. Additional therapy for bleeding hemorrhoids includes banding, sclerotherapy, excisional hemorrhoidectomy, and stapled hemorrhoidectomy. Sensation begins at the dentate line; therefore, banding or sclerotherapy can be performed without discomfort in the office. Two bands (doubled) are placed around the engorged tissue, causing ischemia and fibrosis. The aids in fixing the tissue proximally in the anal canal. During sclerotherapy, 1 to 2 mL of a sclerosant (usually sodium tetradechol sulfate) is injected using a 25-gauge needle into the submucosa of the hemorrhoidal complex. Care must be taken not to inject the anal canal circumferentially or stenosis may occur. The stapled hemorrhoidectomy is associated with less discomfort. It is currently recommended that no procedures on hemorrhoids should be done in patients who are immunocompromised or who have active proctitis. Furthermore, emergent hemorrhoidectomy for bleeding hemorrhoids is associated with a higher complication rate.

Acute complications associated with the treatment of hemorrhoids include pain, infection, recurrent bleeding, and urinary retention. Care should be taken to place bands properly and to avoid overhydration in patients undergoing operative hemorrhoidectomy. Late complications include fecal incontinence as a result of injury to the sphincter during the dissection. Anal stenosis may develop from overzealous excision, with loss of mucosal skin bridges for reepithelialization. Finally, an *ectropion* (prolapse of rectal mucosa from the anal canal) may develop. Patients with an ectropion complain of a "wet" anus as a result of inability to prevent soiling once the rectal mucosa is exposed below the dentate line.

ANORECTAL ABSCESS ■ Incidence and Epidemiology The development of a perianal abscess is more common in men than women by a ratio of 3:1. The peak incidence is in the third to fifth decade of life. Perianal pain associated with the presence of an abscess accounts for 15% of office visits to a colorectal surgeon. The disease is more prevalent in immunocompromised patients such as diabetics, those with hematologic disorders or inflammatory bowel disease (IBD), and persons who are HIV positive. These disorders should be considered in patients with recurrent perianal infections.

Anatomy and Pathophysiology An anorectal abscess is an abnormal fluid-containing cavity in the anorectal region. Anorectal abscess results from an infection involving the glands surrounding the anal canal. Normally, these glands release mucus into the anal canal, which aids in defecation. When stool accidentally enters the anal glands, the glands become infected and an abscess develops. Anorectal abscesses are perianal in 40 to 50% of patients, ischiorectal in 20 to 25%, intersphincteric in 2 to 5%, and supralevator in 2.5% (Fig. 279-4).

Presentation and Evaluation Perianal pain and fever are the hallmarks of an abscess. Patients may have difficulty voiding and have blood in the stool. A prostatic abscess may present with similar complaints including dysuria. Patients with a prostatic abscess will often have a history of recurrent sexually transmitted diseases. On physical examination, a large fluctuant area is usually readily visible. Routine laboratory evaluation shows an elevated white blood cell count. Diagnostic procedures are rarely necessary unless evaluating a recurrent abscess. A CT scan or magnetic resonance imaging (MRI) has an accuracy of 80% in determining incomplete drainage. If there is a concern about the presence of IBD, a rigid or flexible sigmoidoscopic examination may be done at the time of drainage to evaluate for inflammation within the rectosigmoid region. A more complete evaluation for Crohn's disease would include a full colonoscopy and small-bowel series.

℞ TREATMENT

Office drainage of an uncomplicated anorectal abscess may suffice. A small incision close to the anal verge is made and a Mallenkot drain is advanced into the abscess cavity. For patients who have a complicated abscess or who are diabetic or immunocompromised, drainage should be performed in a operating room under anesthesia. These patients are at greater risk for developing necrotizing fasciitis. The course of antibiotics is controversial but should be at least 2 weeks in patients who are immunocompromised or have prosthetic heart valves, artificial joints, diabetes, or IBD.

FISTULA IN ANO ■ Incidence and Epidemiology The incidence and prevalence of fistulating perianal disease parallels the incidence of anorectal abscess. Some 30 to 40% of abscesses will give rise to fistula in ano. While the majority of the fistulas are cryptoglandular in origin, 10% are associated with IBD, tuberculosis, malignancy, and radiation.

Anatomy and Pathophysiology A fistula in ano is defined as a communication of an abscess cavity with an identifiable internal opening within the anal canal. This identifiable opening is most commonly located at the dentate line where the anal glands enter the anal canal. Patients experiencing continuous drainage following the treatment of a perianal abscess likely have a fistula in ano. These fistulas are classified by their relationship to the anal sphincter muscles, with 70%

being intersphincteric, 23% transsphincteric, 5% suprasphincteric, and 2% extrasphincteric (Fig. 279-4).

Presentation and Evaluation A patient with a fistula in ano will complain of constant drainage from the perianal region. The drainage may increase with defecation. Perianal hygiene is difficult to maintain. Examination under anesthesia is the best way to evaluate a fistula. At the time of the examination, anoscopy is performed to look for an internal opening. Diluted hydrogen peroxide will aid in identifying such an opening. In lieu of anesthesia, MRI with an endoanal coil will also identify tracts in 80% of the cases. After drainage of an abscess with insertion of a Mallenkot catheter, a fistulagram through the catheter can be obtained in search of an occult fistula tract. Goodsale's rule states that a posterior external fistula will enter the anal canal in the posterior midline, whereas an anterior fistula will enter at the nearest crypt. A fistula exiting >3 cm from the anal verge may have a complicated upward extension and may not obey Goodsale's rule.

℞ TREATMENT

A newly diagnosed draining fistula is best managed with placement of a seton, a vessel loop or silk tie placed through the fistula tract, which maintains the tract open and quietens the surrounding inflammation that occurs from repeated blockage of the tract (Fig. 279-4). Once the inflammation is quieted, the exact relationship of the fistula tract to the anal sphincters can be ascertained. A simple fistulotomy can be performed for intersphincteric and low (less than one-third of the muscle) transphincteric fistulas without compromising continence. For a higher transphincteric fistula, an anorectal advancement flap in combination with a drainage catheter or fibrin glue may be used. Very long (>2 cm) and narrow tracts respond better to fibrin glue than shorter tracts. Patients should be maintained on stool-bulking agents, nonnarcotic pain medication, and sitz baths. Early complications from these procedures include urinary retention and bleeding. Later complications include temporary and permanent incontinence. Recurrence following fistulotomy is 0 to 18% and following anorectal advancement flap is 20 to 30% and is related to failure to excise and close the internal opening.

ANAL FISSURE ■ Incidence and Epidemiology Anal fissures occur at all ages but are more common in the third through the fifth decades. A fissure is the most common cause of rectal bleeding in infancy. The prevalence is equal in males and females. It is associated with constipation, diarrhea, infectious etiologies, perianal trauma, and Crohn's disease.

Anatomy and Pathophysiology Trauma to the anal canal occurs following defecation. This injury occurs in the anterior or, more commonly, the posterior anal canal. Irritation caused by the trauma to the anal canal results in an increased resting pressure of the internal sphincter. The blood supply to the sphincter and anal mucosa enters laterally. Therefore, increased anal sphincter tone results in a relative ischemia in the region of the fissure and leads to poor healing of the anal injury. A fissure that is not in the posterior or anterior position should raise suspicion for other causes including tuberculosis, syphilis, Crohn's disease, and malignancy.

Presentation and Evaluation A fissure can be easily diagnosed on history alone. The classic complaint is pain, which is strongly associated with defecation and is relentless. The bright red bleeding that can be associated with a fissure is less extensive than that associated with hemorrhoids. On examination, most fissures are located in either the posterior or anterior position. A lateral fissure is worrisome as it may have a less benign nature, and systemic disorders should be ruled out. A chronic fissure is indicated by the presence of a hypertrophied anal papilla at the proximal end of the fissure and a sentinel pile or skin tag at the distal end. Often the circular fibers of the hypertrophied internal sphincter are visible within the base of the fissure. If anal manometry is performed, elevation in anal resting pressure and a sawtooth deformity with paradoxical contractions of the sphincter muscles are pathognomonic.

℞ TREATMENT

The management of the acute fissure is conservative. Stool softeners for those with constipation, increased dietary fiber, topical anesthetics, glucocorticoids, and sitz baths are prescribed and will heal 60 to 90% of fissures. Chronic fissures are those present for >6 weeks. These can be treated with modalities aimed at decreasing the anal canal resting pressure including nitroglycerin ointment (0.2%), applied three times a day, and botulinum toxin type A, up to 20 units, injected into the internal sphincter on each side of the fissure. Surgical management includes anal dilation and lateral internal sphincterotomy. Usually, one-third of the internal sphincter muscle is divided; it is easily identified because it is hypertrophied. Recurrence rates from medical therapy are higher, but this is offset by a risk of incontinence following sphincterotomy. Lateral internal sphincterotomy more commonly leads to incontinence in women.

ACKNOWLEDGMENT
We would like to thank Cory Sandore for providing the illustrations for this chapter.

FURTHER READING

AMBROSETTI P et al: Incidence, outcome, and proposed management of isolated abscesses complicating acute left-sided colonic diverticulitis. A prospective study of 140 patients. Dis Colon Rectum 35:1072, 1992

COLECCHIA A et al: Diverticular disease of the colon: New perspectives in symptom development and treatment. World J Gastroenterol 9:1385, 2003

JENSEN DM et al: Urgent colonoscopy for the diagnosis and treatment of severe diverticular hemorrhage. N Engl J Med 342:78, 2000

KARULF R et al: Rectal prolapse. Curr Probl Surg 38:757, 2001

LINDSEY I et al: A randomized, controlled trial of fibrin glue vs. conventional treatment for anal fistula. Dis Colon Rectum 45:1608, 2002

MATSUMOTO AH et al: Percutaneous transluminal angioplasty and stenting in the treatment of chronic mesenteric ischemia: Results and long-term follow-up. J Am Coll Surg 194 (Suppl):S22, 2002

STEIN E: Botulinum toxin and anal fissure. Curr Probl Dermatol 30:218, 2002

SUTHERLAND LM et al: A systematic review of stapled hemorrhoidectomy. Arch Surg 137:1395, 2002

WONG WD et al: Practice parameters for the treatment of sigmoid diverticulitis—supporting documentation. Dis Colon Rectum 43:290, 2000

280 ACUTE INTESTINAL OBSTRUCTION
William Silen

ETIOLOGY AND CLASSIFICATION   Intestinal obstruction may be *mechanical* or *nonmechanical* (resulting from neuromuscular disturbances that produce either adynamic or dynamic ileus). The causes of mechanical obstruction of the lumen are conveniently divided into (1) lesions *extrinsic* to the intestine, e.g., adhesive bands, internal and external hernias; (2) lesions *intrinsic* to the wall of the intestine, e.g., diverticulitis, carcinoma, regional enteritis; and (3) obturation of the lumen, e.g., gallstone obstruction, intussusception. Clinically, however, it is most useful to consider whether the obstructive mechanism involves the small or large intestine, because the causes, symptoms, and treatments are different (see below). Adhesions and external hernias are the most common causes of obstruction of the small intestine, constituting 70 to 75% of cases of this type. Adhesions, however, almost never produce obstruction of the colon, whereas carcinoma, sigmoid diverticulitis, and volvulus, in that order, are the most common causes and together account for about 90% of the cases. Primary intestinal pseudoobstruction (Chap. 279) is a chronic motility disorder that frequently mimics mechanical obstruction. Unnecessary operations in such patients should be avoided.

Adynamic ileus is probably the most common overall cause of obstruction. The development of this condition is mediated via the hormonal component of the sympathoadrenal system. Adynamic ileus may occur after any peritoneal insult, and its severity and duration will be dependent to some degree on the type of peritoneal injury. Hydrochloric acid, colonic contents, and pancreatic enzymes are among the most irritating substances, whereas blood and urine are less so. Adynamic ileus occurs to some degree after any abdominal operation. Retroperitoneal hematomas, particularly associated with vertebral fracture, commonly cause severe adynamic ileus, and the latter may occur with other retroperitoneal conditions, such as ureteral calculus or severe pyelonephritis. Thoracic diseases, including lower-lobe pneumonia, fractured ribs, and myocardial infarction, frequently produce adynamic ileus, as do electrolyte disturbances, particularly potassium depletion. Finally, intestinal ischemia, whether the result of vascular occlusion or intestinal distention itself, may perpetuate an adynamic ileus.

Spastic ileus, or *dynamic ileus*, is very uncommon and results from extreme and prolonged contraction of the intestine. It has been observed in heavy metal poisoning, uremia, porphyria, and extensive intestinal ulcerations.

PATHOPHYSIOLOGY   Distention of the intestine is caused by the accumulation of gas and fluid proximal to and within the obstructed segment. Between 70 and 80% of intestinal gas consists of swallowed air, and because this is composed mainly of nitrogen, which is poorly absorbed from the intestinal lumen, removal of air by continuous gastric suction is a useful adjunct in the treatment of intestinal distention. The accumulation of fluid proximal to the obstructing mechanism results not only from ingested fluid, swallowed saliva, gastric juice, and biliary and pancreatic secretions but also from interference with normal sodium and water transport. During the first 12 to 24 h of obstruction, there is a marked depression of flux from lumen to blood of sodium and consequently water in the distended proximal intestine. After 24 h, there is movement of sodium and water into the lumen, contributing further to the distention and fluid losses. Intraluminal pressure rises from a normal of 2 to 4 cmH$_2$O to 8 to 10 cmH$_2$O. During peristalsis, when simple obstruction or a "closed loop" is present, pressures reach 30 to 60 cmH$_2$O. Closed-loop obstruction of the small intestine results when the lumen is occluded at two points by a single mechanism such as a hernial ring or adhesive band, thus producing a closed loop whose blood supply is often obstructed at the same time. Strangulation of the loop itself is thus common in association with marked distention proximal to the involved loop. A form of closed-loop obstruction is encountered when complete obstruction of the colon exists in the presence of a competent ileocecal valve (85% of individuals). Although the blood supply of the colon is not entrapped within the obstructing mechanism, distention of the cecum is extreme because of its greater diameter (Laplace's law), and impairment of the intramural blood supply is considerable with consequent gangrene of the cecal wall, usually anteriorly. Necrosis of the small intestine may occur by the same mechanism of interference with intramural blood flow when distention is extreme, but this sequence is uncommon in the small intestine. Once impairment of blood supply occurs, bacterial invasion supervenes, and peritonitis develops. The systemic effects of extreme distention include elevation of the diaphragm with restricted ventilation and subsequent atelectasis. Venous return via the inferior vena cava may also be impaired.

The loss of fluids and electrolytes may be extreme and, unless replacement is prompt, leads to hemoconcentration, hypovolemia, renal insufficiency, shock, and death. Vomiting, accumulation of fluids within the lumen by the mechanisms described above, and the sequestration of fluid into the edematous intestinal wall and peritoneal cavity as a result of impairment of venous return from the intestine all contribute to massive loss of fluid and electrolytes, especially potassium. As soon as significant impedance to venous return is present, the intestine becomes severely congested, and blood begins to seep into the intestinal lumen. Blood loss may reach significant levels when long segments of intestine are involved.

SYMPTOMS *Mechanical small-intestinal obstruction* is characterized by cramping midabdominal pain, which tends to be more severe the higher the obstruction. The pain occurs in paroxysms, and the patient is relatively comfortable in the intervals between the pains. Audible borborygmi are often noted by the patient simultaneously with the paroxysms of pain. The pain may become less severe as distention progresses, probably because motility is impaired in the edematous intestine. When strangulation is present, the pain is usually more localized and may be steady and severe without a colicky component, a fact that often causes delay in diagnosis of obstruction. Vomiting is almost invariable, and it is earlier and more profuse the higher the obstruction. The vomitus initially contains bile and mucus and remains as such if the obstruction is high in the intestine. With low ileal obstruction, the vomitus becomes feculent, i.e., orange-brown in color with a foul odor, which results from the overgrowth of bacteria proximal to the obstruction. Hiccups (singultus) are common. Obstipation and failure to pass gas by rectum are invariably present when the obstruction is complete, although some stool and gas may be passed spontaneously or after an enema shortly after onset of the complete obstruction. Diarrhea is occasionally observed in partial obstruction. Blood in the stool is rare but does occur in cases of intussusception. Other than some minor but inconsistent differences in pain patterns noted above, the symptoms of strangulating obstructions cannot be distinguished from those of nonstrangulating obstructions.

Mechanical colonic obstruction produces colicky abdominal pain similar in quality to that of small-intestinal obstruction but of much lower intensity. Complaints of pain are occasionally absent in stoic elderly patients. Vomiting occurs late, if at all, particularly if the ileocecal valve is competent. Paradoxically, feculent vomitus is very rare. A history of recent alterations in bowel habits and blood in the stool is common because carcinoma and diverticulitis are the most frequent causes. Constipation becomes progressive, and obstipation with failure to pass gas ensues. Acute symptoms may develop over a period of a week. Cecal volvulus more closely resembles obstruction of the small intestine clinically, whereas patients with sigmoid volvulus more typically have the picture of colonic obstruction in which marked distention predominates, with relatively less pain.

In *adynamic ileus*, colicky pain is absent, and only discomfort from distention is evident. Vomiting may be frequent but is rarely profuse. It usually consists of gastric contents and bile and is almost never feculent. Complete obstipation may or may not occur. Singultus (hiccups) is common.

PHYSICAL FINDINGS *Abdominal distention* is the hallmark of all forms of intestinal obstruction. It is least marked in cases of obstruction high in the small intestine and most marked in colonic obstruction. Early, especially in closed-loop strangulating small-bowel obstruction, distention may be barely perceptible or absent. Tenderness and rigidity are usually minimal; the temperature is rarely >37.8°C (100°F) in nonstrangulating obstruction of the small and large intestine. Contrary to popular belief, the same is true of strangulating obstruction until very late, a fact that has often resulted in unfortunate delay in treatment. Signs and symptoms of shock also occur *very late* in strangulating obstruction. The appearance of shock, tenderness, rigidity, and fever often means that contamination of the peritoneum with infected intestinal content has occurred. Hernial orifices should always be carefully examined for the presence of a mass. The presence of a palpable abdominal mass usually signifies a closed-loop strangulating small-bowel obstruction because the tense fluid-filled loop is the palpable lesion. Auscultation may reveal loud, high-pitched borborygmi coincident with the colicky pain, but this finding is often absent late in strangulating or nonstrangulating obstruction. A quiet abdomen does

not eliminate the possibility of obstruction, nor does it necessarily establish the diagnosis of adynamic ileus.

LABORATORY AND X-RAY FINDINGS Leukocytosis, with shift to the left, usually occurs when strangulation is present, but a normal white blood cell count does not exclude strangulation. Elevation of the serum amylase level is encountered occasionally in all forms of intestinal obstruction, especially the strangulating variety.

The x-ray is extremely valuable but under certain circumstances may also be misleading. In nonstrangulating complete small-bowel obstruction, x-rays are almost completely reliable. Distention of fluid- and gas-filled loops of small intestine usually arranged in a "stepladder" pattern with air-fluid levels and an absence or paucity of colonic gas are pathognomonic (Fig. 280-1). These findings, however, are absent in slightly over half the cases of strangulating small-bowel obstruction, especially early in the disease. A general haze due to peritoneal fluid and sometimes a "coffee bean"–shaped mass are seen in strangulating obstruction. Occasionally, the films are normal, but when symptoms are consistent with obstruction of the small intestine, a normal film should suggest strangulation. In these circumstances, computed tomography may be very useful. Roentgenographic differentiation of partial mechanical small-bowel obstruction from adynamic ileus may be impossible because gas is present in both the small and large intestines; however, colonic distention is usually more prominent in adynamic ileus. A radiopaque dye given by mouth is useful in making this distinction.

Colonic obstruction with a competent ileocecal valve is easily recognized because distention with gas is mainly confined to the colon. Barium enema, sigmoidoscopy, or colonoscopy, depending on the suspected site of obstruction, is usually advisable to determine the nature of the lesion, except when concomitant perforation is suspected, a rare occurrence. Sigmoidoscopy may be therapeutic in cases of sigmoid volvulus. When the ileocecal valve is incompetent, the films resemble those of partial small-bowel obstruction or adynamic ileus, and barium enema or colonoscopy is necessary to establish the correct diagnosis. Barium given by mouth is perfectly safe when obstruction is in the small intestine, since the barium sulfate does not become inspissated

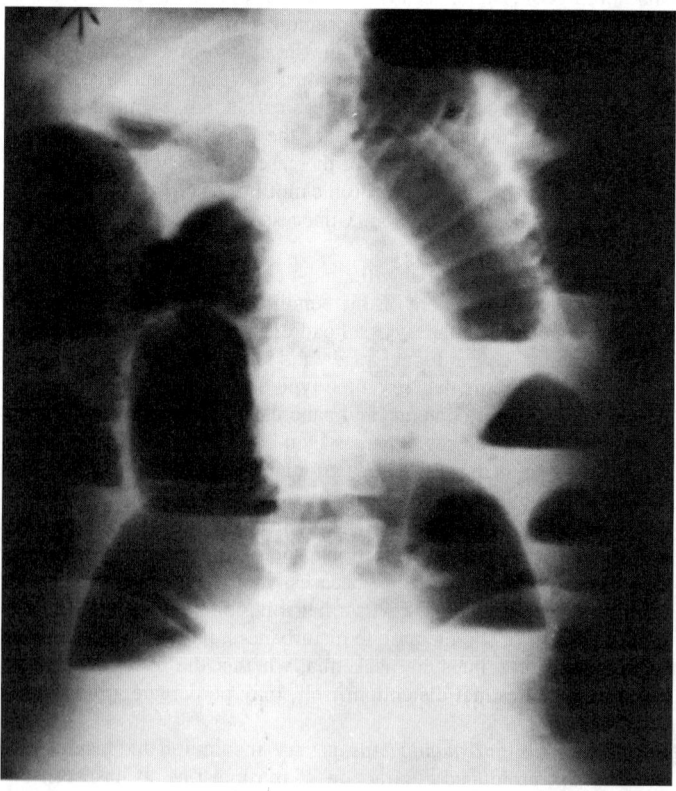

FIGURE 280-1 Acute mechanical obstruction of small intestine (upright film). Note air-fluid levels, marked distention of bowel loops, and absence of colonic gas.

in this location. *Barium should never be given by mouth to a patient with possible colonic obstruction* until that possibility has been excluded.

℞ TREATMENT

Small-Intestinal Obstruction   The overall mortality rate for obstruction of the small intestine is about 10%, even under the most optimal conditions. While the mortality rate for nonstrangulating obstruction is as low as 5 to 8%, that for strangulating obstruction has been reported to be between 20 and 75%. Well over half the deaths from small-bowel obstruction occur in those with strangulation; however, the latter constitute only one-fourth to one-third of the cases. Careful studies indicate that the clinical, laboratory, and x-ray findings are not reliable in distinguishing strangulating from nonstrangulating obstruction when obstruction is complete. Complete obstruction is suggested when passage of gas or stool per rectum has ceased and when gas is absent in the distal intestine by x-ray. Since strangulating small-bowel obstruction is always complete, operation should always be undertaken in such patients after suitable preparation. Before operation, fluid and electrolyte balance should be restored and decompression instituted by means of a nasogastric tube. Replacement of potassium is especially important because intake is nil and losses in vomitus are large. From 6 to 8 h of preparation may be necessary. During this period, broad-spectrum antibiotics are indicated if strangulation is felt to be likely, but operation should not be delayed unless there is unequivocal clinical and roentgenographic evidence of resolution of the obstruction during the period of preparation. Attempts to pass a long tube into the small intestine usually fail while putting the patient through uncomfortable, unproductive manipulations that delay appropriate fluid replacement and decompression. *There are few, if any, indications for the use of a long intestinal tube.* Procrastination of operation because of improvement in well-being of the patient during resuscitation and gastric decompression usually leads to unnecessary and hazardous delay in proper treatment. Purely nonoperative therapy is safe only in the presence of incomplete obstruction and is best utilized in patients with (1) repeated episodes of partial obstruction, (2) recent postoperative partial obstruction, and (3) partial obstruction following a recent episode of diffuse peritonitis.

Colonic Obstruction   The mortality rate for colonic obstruction is about 20%. As in small-bowel obstruction, nonoperative treatment is contraindicated unless the obstruction is incomplete. Occasionally, but not always, when the obstruction is incomplete, nonoperative therapy may result in sufficient decompression that a definitive operative procedure can be undertaken at a later date. This can usually be accomplished by discontinuation of all oral intake and perhaps by nasogastric suction, although attempts to decompress a *completely* obstructed colon by intubation are almost invariably futile. A long intestinal tube will not decompress an obstructed colon with a competent ileocecal valve. When obstruction is complete, early operation is mandatory, especially when the ileocecal valve is competent; cecal gangrene is likely if the cecal diameter is >10 cm on plain abdominal film. For obstruction on the left side of the colon, the most common site, preliminary operative decompression by cecostomy or transverse colostomy followed by definitive resection of the primary lesion has been the treatment of choice. Recently, primary resection of obstructing left-sided lesions with on-table washout of the colon has been accomplished safely. For a lesion of the right or transverse colon, primary resection and anastomosis can be performed safely because distention of the ileum with consequent discrepancy in size and hazard in suture are not present.

Adynamic Ileus   This type of ileus usually responds to nonoperative continuous decompression and adequate treatment of the primary disease. The prognosis is usually good. Successful decompression of severe colonic ileus has been accomplished by colonoscopy, but this should be avoided if tenderness in the right lower quadrant suggests possible cecal gangrene. Neostigmine is effective in cases of colonic ileus that have not responded to other conservative treatment. Rarely, adynamic colonic distention may become so great that cecostomy is required if cecal gangrene is feared. Spastic ileus usually responds to treatment of the primary disease.

FURTHER READING

BULKLEY GB et al: Intraoperative determination of small intestinal viability following ischemic injury: Prospective controlled trial of two adjuvant methods (Doppler and fluorescein) compared with standard clinical judgement. Ann Surg 193:628, 1981

DUBOIS A et al: Postoperative ileus: Physiopathology, etiology and treatment. Ann Surg 178:781, 1973

ESKELINEN M et al: Contributions of history-taking, physical examination, and computer assistance to diagnosis of acute small-bowel obstruction. A prospective study of 1333 patients with acute abdominal pain. Scand J Gastroenterol 29:715, 1994

FEVANG BT et al: Complications and death after surgical treatment of small bowel obstruction: A 35-year institutional experience. Ann Surg 231:529, 2000

JACKSON BR: The diagnosis of colonic obstruction. Dis Colon Rectum 25: 603, 1982

SILEN W: *Cope's Early Diagnosis of the Acute Abdomen*, 20th ed. London, Oxford, 2000

281 | ACUTE APPENDICITIS AND PERITONITIS
William Silen

ACUTE APPENDICITIS

INCIDENCE AND EPIDEMIOLOGY   The peak incidence of acute appendicitis is in the second and third decades of life; it is relatively rare at the extremes of age. Males and females are equally affected, except between puberty and age 25, when males predominate in a 3:2 ratio. Perforation is more common in infancy and in the aged, during which periods mortality rates are highest. The mortality rate has decreased steadily in Europe and the United States from 8.1 per 100,000 of the population in 1941 to <1 per 100,000 in 1970 and subsequently. The absolute incidence of the disease also decreased by about 40% between 1940 and 1960 but since then has remained unchanged. Although various factors such as changing dietary habits, altered intestinal flora, and better nutrition and intake of vitamins have been suggested to explain the reduced incidence, the exact reasons have not been elucidated. The overall incidence of appendicitis is much lower in underdeveloped countries, especially parts of Africa, and in lower socioeconomic groups.

PATHOGENESIS   Luminal obstruction has long been considered the pathogenetic hallmark. However, obstruction can be identified in only 30 to 40% of cases; ulceration of the mucosa is the initial event in the majority. The cause of the ulceration is unknown, although a viral etiology has been postulated. Infection with *Yersinia* organisms may cause the disease, since high complement fixation antibody titers have been found in up to 30% of cases of proven appendicitis. Whether the inflammatory reaction seen with ulceration is sufficient to obstruct the tiny appendiceal lumen even transiently is not clear. Obstruction, when present, is most commonly caused by a fecalith, which results from accumulation and inspissation of fecal matter around vegetable fibers. Enlarged lymphoid follicles associated with viral infections (e.g., measles), inspissated barium, worms (e.g., pinworms, *Ascaris*, and *Tae-*

nia), and tumors (e.g., carcinoid or carcinoma) may also obstruct the lumen. Secretion of mucus distends the organ, which has a capacity of only 0.1 to 0.2 mL, and luminal pressures rise as high as 60 cmH$_2$O. Luminal bacteria multiply and invade the appendiceal wall as venous engorgement and subsequent arterial compromise result from the high intraluminal pressures. Finally, gangrene and perforation occur. If the process evolves slowly, adjacent organs such as the terminal ileum, cecum, and omentum may wall off the appendiceal area so that a localized abscess will develop, whereas rapid progression of vascular impairment may cause perforation with free access to the peritoneal cavity. Subsequent rupture of primary appendiceal abscesses may produce fistulas between the appendix and bladder, small intestine, sigmoid, or cecum. Occasionally, acute appendicitis may be the first manifestation of Crohn's disease.

While chronic infection of the appendix with tuberculosis, amebiasis, and actinomycosis may occur, a useful clinical aphorism states that *chronic appendiceal inflammation is not usually the cause of prolonged abdominal pain of weeks' or months' duration.* In contrast, recurrent acute appendicitis does occur, often with complete resolution of inflammation and symptoms between attacks. Recurrent acute appendicitis may become more frequent as antibiotics are dispensed more freely and if a long appendiceal stump is left after laparoscopic appendectomy.

CLINICAL MANIFESTATIONS   The history and sequence of symptoms are important diagnostic features of appendicitis. The initial symptom is almost invariably *abdominal pain* of the visceral type, resulting from appendiceal contractions or distention of the lumen. It is usually poorly localized in the periumbilical or epigastric region with an accompanying urge to defecate or pass flatus, neither of which relieves the distress. This visceral pain is mild, often cramping, and rarely catastrophic in nature, usually lasting 4 to 6 h, but it may not be noted by stoic individuals or by some patients during sleep. As inflammation spreads to the parietal peritoneal surfaces, the pain becomes somatic, steady, and more severe, aggravated by motion or cough, and usually located in the *right lower quadrant. Anorexia* is very common; a hungry patient does not have acute appendicitis. *Nausea* and *vomiting* occur in 50 to 60% of cases, but vomiting is usually self-limited. The development of nausea and vomiting before the onset of pain is extremely rare. Change in bowel habit is of little diagnostic value, since any or no alteration may be observed, although the presence of diarrhea caused by an inflamed appendix in juxtaposition to the sigmoid may cause serious diagnostic difficulties. Urinary frequency and dysuria occur if the appendix lies adjacent to the bladder. The typical sequence of symptoms (poorly localized periumbilical pain followed by nausea and vomiting with subsequent shift of pain to the right lower quadrant) occurs in only 50 to 60% of patients.

Physical findings vary with time after onset of the illness and according to the location of the appendix, which may be situated deep in the pelvic cul-de-sac; in the right lower quadrant in any relation to the peritoneum, cecum, and small intestine; in the right upper quadrant (especially during pregnancy); or even in the left lower quadrant. *The diagnosis cannot be established unless tenderness can be elicited.* While tenderness is sometimes absent in the early visceral stage of the disease, it ultimately always develops and is found in any location corresponding to the position of the appendix. Abdominal tenderness may be completely absent if a retrocecal or pelvic appendix is present, in which case the sole physical finding may be tenderness in the flank or on rectal or pelvic examination. Percussion, rebound tenderness, and referred rebound tenderness are often, but not invariably, present; they are most likely to be absent early in the illness. Flexion of the right hip and guarded movement by the patient are due to parietal peritoneal involvement. Hyperesthesia of the skin of the right lower quadrant and a positive psoas or obturator sign are often late findings and are rarely of diagnostic value. When the inflamed appendix is in close proximity to the anterior parietal peritoneum, muscular rigidity is present yet is often minimal early.

The temperature is usually normal or slightly elevated [37.2 to 38°C (99 to 100.5°F)], but a temperature >38.3°C (101°F) should suggest perforation. Tachycardia is commensurate with the elevation of the temperature. Rigidity and tenderness become more marked as the disease progresses to perforation and localized or diffuse peritonitis. Distention is rare unless severe diffuse peritonitis has developed. The disappearance of pain and tenderness just before perforation is extremely unusual. A mass may develop if localized perforation has occurred but will not usually be detectable before 3 days after onset. Earlier presence of a mass suggests carcinoma of the cecum or Crohn's disease. Perforation is rare before 24 h after onset of symptoms, but the rate may be as high as 80% after 48 h.

Diagnosis is based primarily on clinical grounds. Although moderate leukocytosis of 10,000 to 18,000 cells/μL is frequent (with a concomitant left shift), the absence of leukocytosis does not rule out acute appendicitis. Leukocytosis of >20,000 cells/μL suggests probable perforation. Anemia and blood in the stool suggest a primary diagnosis of carcinoma of the cecum, especially in elderly individuals. The urine may contain a few white or red blood cells without bacteria if the appendix lies close to the right ureter or bladder. Urinalysis is most useful in excluding genitourinary conditions that may mimic acute appendicitis.

Radiographs are rarely of value except when an opaque fecalith (5% of patients) is observed in the right lower quadrant (especially in children). Consequently, abdominal films are not routinely obtained unless other conditions such as intestinal obstruction or ureteral calculus may be present. In some patients with recurrent or prolonged symptoms, computed tomography (CT) may reveal an extrinsic defect on the medial wall of the cecum or a calcified fecalith. The predictive value of CT scan in acute appendicitis is being evaluated. The diagnosis may also be established by the ultrasonic demonstration of an enlarged and thick-walled appendix. Ultrasound is most useful to exclude ovarian cysts, ectopic pregnancy, or tuboovarian abscess.

While the typical historic sequence and physical findings are present in 50 to 60% of cases, a wide variety of atypical patterns of disease are encountered, especially at the age extremes and during pregnancy. Infants under 2 years of age have a 70 to 80% incidence of perforation and generalized peritonitis. Any infant or child with diarrhea, vomiting, and abdominal pain is highly suspect. Fever is much more common in this age group, and abdominal distention is often the only physical finding. In the elderly, pain and tenderness are often blunted, and thus the diagnosis is frequently delayed and leads to a 30% incidence of perforation in patients over 70. Elderly patients often present initially with a slightly painful mass (a primary appendiceal abscess) or with adhesive intestinal obstruction 5 or 6 days after a previously undetected perforated appendix.

Appendicitis occurs about once in every 1000 pregnancies and is the most common extrauterine condition requiring abdominal operation. The diagnosis may be missed or delayed because of the frequent occurrence of mild abdominal discomfort and nausea and vomiting during pregnancy. During the last trimester, when the mortality rate from appendicitis is highest, uterine displacement of the appendix to the right upper quadrant and laterally leads to confusion in diagnosis because pain and tenderness are similarly displaced.

DIFFERENTIAL DIAGNOSIS   Appendicitis can be confused with any condition that causes abdominal pain. Diagnostic accuracy is about 75 to 80% for experienced clinicians based solely on the clinical criteria outlined. It is probably better to err slightly in the direction of overdiagnosis, since delay is associated with perforation and increased morbidity and mortality. In unperforated appendicitis, the mortality rate is 0.1%, little more than that associated with general anesthesia; for perforated appendicitis, overall mortality is 3% (15% in the elderly). In doubtful cases, 4 to 6 h of observation is always more beneficial than harmful. The most common conditions discovered at operation when acute appendicitis is erroneously diagnosed are, in order of frequency, mesenteric lymphadenitis, no organic disease, acute pelvic inflammatory disease, ruptured graafian follicle or corpus luteum cyst, and acute gastroenteritis. In addition, acute cholecystitis, perforated ulcer, acute pancreatitis, acute diverticulitis, strangulating intestinal obstruction, ureteral calculus, and pyelonephritis may present diagnostic difficulties.

Differentiation of *pelvic inflammatory disease* from acute appendicitis on clinical grounds may be virtually impossible. Gram-negative intracellular diplococci on cervical smear are not pathognomonic unless *Neisseria gonorrhoeae* can be cultured. Pain on movement of the cervix is not specific and may occur in appendicitis if perforation has occurred or if the appendix lies adjacent to the uterus or adnexa. *Rupture of a graafian follicle* (mittelschmerz) occurs at midcycle and will spill off blood and fluid to produce pain and tenderness more diffuse and usually of a less severe degree than in appendicitis. Fever and leukocytosis are usually absent. *Rupture of a corpus luteum cyst* is identical clinically to rupture of a graafian follicle but develops about the time of menstruation. The presence of an adnexal mass, evidence of blood loss, and a positive pregnancy test help differentiate *ruptured tubal pregnancy*, but a negative pregnancy test is present when tubal abortion has occurred. *Twisted ovarian cyst* and *endometriosis* are occasionally difficult to distinguish from appendicitis. In all these female conditions, ultrasonography, laparoscopy, and occasionally CT may be of great value.

Acute mesenteric lymphadenitis is the diagnosis usually given when enlarged, slightly reddened lymph nodes at the root of the mesentery and a normal appendix are encountered at operation in a patient who usually has right lower quadrant tenderness. Whether this is a single, discrete entity is unclear, since the causative factor is not known. Some of these patients have infection with *Y. pseudotuberculosis* or *Y. enterocolitica*, in which case the diagnosis can be established by culture of the mesenteric nodes or by serologic titers (Chap. 143). The diagnosis is essentially impossible clinically, although retrospectively these patients may have a higher temperature and more diffuse pain and tenderness. Children seem to be affected more frequently than adults. *Acute gastroenteritis* usually causes profuse watery diarrhea, often with nausea and vomiting, but without localized findings. Between cramps, the abdomen is completely relaxed. In *Salmonella* gastroenteritis, the abdominal findings are similar, although the pain may be more severe and more localized, and fever and chills are common. The occurrence of similar symptoms among other members of the family may be helpful. When the diagnosis of acute pelvic appendicitis with perforation has been missed, gastroenteritis is the most common previous working diagnosis. Persistent abdominal or rectal tenderness should eliminate the diagnosis of gastroenteritis. *Regional enteritis* (Crohn's disease) is usually associated with a more prolonged history, often with previous exacerbations regarded as episodes of gastroenteritis unless the diagnosis has been established previously. *Meckel's diverticulitis* usually cannot be distinguished from acute appendicitis but is very rare.

℞ TREATMENT

Cathartics and enemas should be avoided if appendicitis is under consideration, and antibiotics should not be administered when the diagnosis is in question, since they will only mask the perforation. The treatment is early operation and appendectomy as soon as the patient can be prepared. Appendectomy is increasingly accomplished laparoscopically and may have some benefits over the open technique. Preparation for operation rarely takes more than 1 to 2 h in early appendicitis but may require 6 to 8 h in cases of severe sepsis and dehydration associated with late perforation. The *only* circumstance in which operation is *not* indicated is the presence of a palpable mass 3 to 5 days after the onset of symptoms. Should operation be undertaken at that time, a phlegmon rather than a definitive abscess will be found, and complications from its dissection are frequent. Such patients treated with broad-spectrum antibiotics, parenteral fluids, and rest usually show resolution of the mass and symptoms within 1 week. *Interval appendectomy* should be done safely 3 months later. Should the mass enlarge or the patient become more toxic, drainage of the abscess is

necessary. The complications of subphrenic, pelvic, or other intraabdominal abscesses usually follow perforation with generalized peritonitis and can be avoided by early diagnosis of the disease.

ACUTE PERITONITIS

Peritonitis is an inflammation of the peritoneum; it may be localized or diffuse in location, acute or chronic in natural history, infectious or aseptic in pathogenesis. Acute peritonitis is most often infectious and is usually related to a perforated viscus (and called secondary peritonitis). When no bacterial source is identified, infectious peritonitis is called primary or spontaneous. Acute peritonitis is associated with decreased intestinal motor activity resulting in distention of the intestinal lumen with gas and fluid. The accumulation of fluid in the bowel together with the lack of oral intake leads to rapid intravascular volume depletion with effects on cardiac, renal, and other systems.

ETIOLOGY Infectious agents gain access to the peritoneal cavity through a perforated viscus, a penetrating wound of the abdominal wall, or external introduction of a foreign object that is or becomes infected (for example, a chronic peritoneal dialysis catheter). In the absence of immune compromise, host defenses are capable of eradicating small contaminations. Large numbers of mixed aerobic and anaerobic bacteria, particularly when persistently infused, can lead to peritonitis. The conditions that most commonly result in the introduction of bacteria into the peritoneum are ruptured appendix, ruptured diverticulum, perforated peptic ulcer, incarcerated hernia, gangrenous gall bladder, volvulus, bowel infarction, cancer, inflammatory bowel disease, or intestinal obstruction. However, a wide range of mechanisms may play a role (Table 281-1). Bacterial peritonitis can also occur in the apparent absence of an intraperitoneal source of bacteria (primary or spontaneous bacterial peritonitis). This condition occurs in the setting of ascites and liver cirrhosis in 90% of the cases, usually in patients with ascites with low protein concentration (<1 g/L) (Chap. 289). →*Bacterial peritonitis is discussed in detail in Chap. 112.*

Aseptic peritonitis may be due to peritoneal irritation by abnormal presence of physiologic fluids (e.g., gastric juice, bile, pancreatic enzymes, blood, or urine) or sterile foreign bodies (e.g., surgical sponges or instruments, starch from surgical gloves) in the peritoneal cavity or as a complication of rare systemic diseases such as lupus erythematosus, porphyria, or familial Mediterranean fever (Chap. 278). Chemical irritation of the peritoneum is greatest for acidic gastric juice and pancreatic enzymes. In chemical peritonitis, a major risk of secondary bacterial infection exists.

TABLE 281-1 *Conditions Leading to Secondary Bacterial Peritonitis*

Perforations of bowel	Perforations or leaking of other organs
Trauma, blunt or penetrating	Pancreas—pancreatitis
Inflammation	Gall bladder—cholecystitis
Appendicitis	Urinary bladder—trauma, rupture
Diverticulitis	Liver—bile leak after biopsy
Peptic ulcer disease	Fallopian tubes—salpingitis
Inflammatory bowel disease	Bleeding into the peritoneal cavity
Iatrogenic	**Disruption of integrity of peritoneal cavity**
Endoscopic perforation	
Anastomotic leaks	Trauma
Catheter perforation	Continuous ambulatory peritoneal dialysis (indwelling catheter)
Vascular	
Embolus	Intraperitoneal chemotherapy
Ischemia	Perinephric abscess
Obstructions	Iatrogenic—postoperative, foreign body
Adhesions	
Strangulated hernias	
Volvulus	
Intussusception	
Neoplasms	
Ingested foreign body, toothpick, fish bone	

CLINICAL FEATURES   The cardinal manifestations of peritonitis are acute abdominal pain and tenderness, usually with fever. The location of the pain depends on the underlying cause and whether the inflammation is localized or generalized. Localized peritonitis is most common in uncomplicated appendicitis and diverticulitis and physical findings are limited to the area of inflammation. Generalized peritonitis is associated with widespread inflammation and diffuse abdominal tenderness and rebound. Rigidity of the abdominal wall is common in both localized and generalized peritonitis. Bowel sounds are usually absent. Tachycardia, hypotension, and signs of dehydration are common. Leukocytosis and acidosis are common laboratory findings. Plain abdominal films may show dilation of large and small bowel with edema of the bowel wall. Free air under the diaphragm is associated with a perforated viscus. CT and/or ultrasonography can identify the presence of free fluid or an abscess. When ascites is present, diagnostic paracentesis with cell count (>250 neutrophils/μL is usual in peritonitis), protein and lactate dehydrogenase levels, and culture is essential. In elderly and immunosuppressed patients, signs of peritoneal irritation may be more difficult to detect.

THERAPY AND PROGNOSIS   Treatment relies on rehydration, correction of electrolyte abnormalities, antibiotics, and surgical correction of the underlying defect. Mortality rates are $<10\%$ for uncomplicated peritonitis associated with a perforated ulcer or ruptured appendix or diverticulum in an otherwise healthy person. Mortality rates of $\geq40\%$ have been reported for elderly people, those with underlying illnesses, and when peritonitis has been present for >48 h.

FURTHER READING

CHEADLE WG, SPAIN DA: The continuing challenge of intraabdominal infection. Am J Surg 186(Suppl 1):15, 2003

FLUM DR et al: Has misdiagnosis of appendicitis decreased over time? A population-based analysis. JAMA 286:1748, 2001

GRONROOS JM, GRONROOS P: Leucocyte count and C-reactive protein in the diagnosis of acute appendicitis. Br J Surg 86:501, 1999

GWYNN LK: The diagnosis of acute appendicitis: Clinical assessment versus computed tomography evaluation. J Emerg Med 21:119, 2001

RAO P et al: Effect of computed tomography of the appendix on treatment of patients and use of hospital resources. N Engl J Med 338:141, 1998

WADE DS et al: Accuracy of ultrasound in the diagnosis of acute appendicitis compared with the surgeon's clinical impression. Arch Surg 128:1039, 1993

Section 2   Liver and Biliary Tract Disease

282 | APPROACH TO THE PATIENT WITH LIVER DISEASE
Marc Ghany, Jay H. Hoofnagle

In most instances, a diagnosis of liver disease can be made accurately by a careful history, physical examination, and application of a few laboratory tests. In some circumstances, radiologic examinations are helpful or, indeed, diagnostic. Liver biopsy is considered the "gold standard" in evaluation of liver disease but is now needed less for diagnosis than for grading and staging disease. This chapter provides an introduction to diagnosis and management of liver disease, briefly reviewing the structure and function of the liver; the major clinical manifestations of liver disease; and the use of clinical history, physical examination, laboratory tests, imaging studies, and liver biopsy.

LIVER STRUCTURE AND FUNCTION   The liver is the largest organ of the body, weighing 1 to 1.5 kg and representing 1.5 to 2.5% of the lean body mass. The size and shape of the liver vary and generally match the general body shape—long and lean or squat and square. The liver is located in the right upper quadrant of the abdomen under the right lower rib cage against the diaphragm and projects for a variable extent into the left upper quadrant. The liver is held in place by ligamentous attachments to the diaphragm, peritoneum, great vessels, and upper gastrointestinal organs. It receives a dual blood supply; approximately 20% of the blood flow is oxygen-rich blood from the hepatic artery, and 80% is nutrient-rich blood from the portal vein arising from the stomach, intestines, pancreas, and spleen.

The majority of cells in the liver are hepatocytes, which constitute two-thirds of the mass of the liver. The remaining cell types are Kupffer cells (members of the reticuloendothelial system), stellate (Ito or fat-storing) cells, endothelial cells and blood vessels, bile ductular cells, and supporting structures. Viewed by light microscopy, the liver appears to be organized in lobules, with portal areas at the periphery and central veins in the center of each lobule. However, from a functional point of view, the liver is organized into acini, with both hepatic arterial and portal venous blood entering the acinus from the portal areas (zone 1) and then flowing through the sinusoids to the terminal hepatic veins (zone 3); the intervening hepatocytes constituting zone 2. The advantage of viewing the acinus as the physiologic unit of the liver is that it helps to explain the morphologic patterns and zonality of many vascular and biliary diseases not explained by the lobular arrangement.

Portal areas of the liver consist of small veins, arteries, bile ducts, and lymphatics organized in a loose stroma of supporting matrix and small amounts of collagen. Blood flowing into the portal areas is distributed through the sinusoids, passing from zone 1 to zone 3 of the acinus and draining into the terminal hepatic veins ("central veins"). Secreted bile flows in the opposite direction, in a counter current pattern from zone 2 to zone 1. The sinusoids are lined by unique endothelial cells that have prominent fenestrae of variable size, allowing the free flow of plasma but not cellular elements. The plasma is thus in direct contact with hepatocytes in the subendothelial space of Disse.

Hepatocytes have distinct polarity. The basolateral side of the hepatocyte lines the space of Disse and is richly lined with microvilli; it demonstrates endocytotic and pinocytotic activity, with passive and active uptake of nutrients, proteins, and other molecules. The apical pole of the hepatocyte forms the cannicular membranes through which bile components are secreted. The cannicular of hepatocytes form a fine network, which fuses into the bile ductular elements near the portal areas. Kupffer cells usually lie within the sinusoidal vascular space and represent the largest group of fixed macrophages in the body. The stellate cells are located in the space of Disse but are not usually prominent unless activated, when they produce collagen and matrix. Red blood cells stay in the sinusoidal space as blood flows through the lobules, but white blood cells can migrate through or around endothelial cells into the space of Disse and from there to portal areas, where they can return to the circulation through lymphatics.

Hepatocytes perform numerous and vital roles in maintaining homeostasis and health. These functions include the synthesis of most essential serum proteins (albumin, carrier proteins, coagulation factors, many hormonal and growth factors), the production of bile and its carriers (bile acids, cholesterol, lecithin, phospholipids), the regulation of nutrients (glucose, glycogen, lipids, cholesterol, amino acids), and metabolism and conjugation of lipophilic compounds (bilirubin, anions, cations, drugs) for excretion in the bile or urine. Measurement of these activities to assess liver function is complicated by the multiplicity and variability of these functions. The most commonly used liver "function" tests are measurements of serum bilirubin, albumin, and prothrombin time. The serum bilirubin level is a measure of hepatic conjugation and excretion, and the serum albumin level and prothrombin time are measures of protein synthesis. Abnormalities of bilirubin, albumin, and prothrombin time are typical of hepatic dysfunction. Frank liver failure is incompatible with life, and the functions of the liver are too complex and diverse to be subserved by a mechanical pump; dialysis membrane; or concoction of infused hormones, proteins, and growth factors.

LIVER DISEASES While there are many causes of liver disease (Table 282-1), they generally present clinically in a few distinct patterns, usually classified as hepatocellular, cholestatic (obstructive), or mixed. In *hepatocellular diseases* (such as viral hepatitis or alcoholic liver disease), features of liver injury, inflammation, and necrosis predominate. In *cholestatic diseases* (such as gall stone or malignant obstruction, primary biliary cirrhosis, some drug-induced liver diseases), features of inhibition of bile flow predominate. In a mixed pattern, features of both hepatocellular and cholestatic injury are present (such as in cholestatic forms of viral hepatitis and many drug-induced liver diseases). The pattern of onset and prominence of symptoms can rapidly suggest a diagnosis, particularly if major risk factors are considered, such as the age and sex of the patient and a history of

TABLE 282-1 *Liver Diseases*

Inherited hyperbilirubinemia	Liver involvement in systemic diseases
Gilbert's syndrome	Sarcoidosis
Crigler-Najjar syndrome, types I and II	Amyloidosis
Dubin-Johnson syndrome	Glycogen storage diseases
Rotor syndrome	Celiac disease
Viral hepatitis	Tuberculosis
Hepatitis A	*Myobacterium avium intracellulare*
Hepatitis B	Cholestatic syndromes
Hepatitis C	Benign postoperative cholestasis
Hepatitis D	Jaundice of sepsis
Hepatitis E	Total parenteral nutrition (TPN)–induced
Others (mononucleosis, herpes, adenovirus	jaundice
hepatitis)	Cholestasis of pregnancy
Cryptogenic hepatitis	Cholangitis and cholecystitis
Immune and autoimmune liver diseases	Extrahepatic biliary obstruction (stone, stricture,
Primary biliary cirrhosis	cancer)
Autoimmune hepatitis	Biliary atresia
Sclerosing cholangitis	Caroli's disease
Overlap syndromes	Cryptosporidiosis
Graft-vs-host disease	Drug-induced liver disease
Allograft rejection	Hepatocellular patterns (isoniazid, acetaminophen)
Genetic liver diseases	Cholestatic patterns (methyltestosterone)
α_1 Antitrypsin deficiency	Mixed patterns (sulfonamides, phenytoin)
Hemochromatosis	Micro- and macrovesicular steatosis
Wilson's disease	(methotrexate, fialuridine)
Benign recurrent intrahepatic cholestasis	Vascular injury
(BRIC)	Venoocclusive disease
Familial intrahepatic cholestasis (FIC),	Budd-Chiari syndrome
types I–III	Ischemic hepatitis
Others (galactosemia, tyrosinemia, cystic	Passive congestion
fibrosis, Newman-Pick disease,	Portal vein thrombosis
Gaucher's disease)	Nodular regenerative hyperplasia
Alcoholic liver disease	Mass lesions
Acute fatty liver	Hepatocellular carcinoma
Acute alcoholic hepatitis	Cholangiocarcinoma
Laennec's cirrhosis	Adenoma
Nonalcoholic fatty liver	Focal nodular hyperplasia
Steatosis	Metastatic tumors
Steatohepatitis	Abscess
Acute fatty liver of pregnancy	Cysts

exposure or risk behaviors.

Typical presenting symptoms of liver disease include jaundice, fatigue, itching, right upper quadrant pain, abdominal distention, and intestinal bleeding. At present, however, many patients are diagnosed with liver disease who have no symptoms and who have been found to have abnormalities in biochemical liver tests as a part of a routine physical examination or screening for blood donation or for insurance or employment. The wide availability of batteries of liver tests makes it relatively simple to demonstrate the presence of liver injury as well as to rule it out in someone suspected of liver disease.

Evaluation of patients with liver disease should be directed at (1) establishing the etiologic diagnosis, (2) estimating the disease severity (grading), and (3) establishing the disease stage (staging). *Diagnosis* should focus on the category of disease, such as hepatocellular, cholestatic, or mixed injury, as well as on the specific etiologic diagnosis. *Grading* refers to assessing the severity or activity of disease—active or inactive, and mild, moderate, or severe. *Staging* refers to estimating the place in the course of the natural history of the disease, whether acute or chronic; early or late; precirrhotic, cirrhotic, or end-stage.

The goal of this chapter is to introduce general, salient concepts in the evaluation of patients with liver disease that help lead to the diagnoses discussed in subsequent chapters.

CLINICAL HISTORY The clinical history should focus on the symptoms of liver disease—their nature, pattern of onset, and progression—and on potential risk factors for liver disease. The symptoms of liver disease include constitutional symptoms such as fatigue, weakness, nausea, poor appetite, and malaise and the more liver-specific symptoms

of jaundice, dark urine, light stools, itching, abdominal pain, and bloating. Symptoms can also suggest the presence of cirrhosis, end-stage liver disease, or complications of cirrhosis such as portal hypertension. Generally, the constellation of symptoms and their pattern of onset rather than a specific symptom points to an etiology.

Fatigue is the most common and most characteristic symptom of liver disease. It is variously described as lethargy, weakness, listlessness, malaise, increased need for sleep, lack of stamina, and poor energy. The fatigue of liver disease typically arises after activity or exercise and is rarely present or severe in the morning after adequate rest (afternoon versus morning fatigue). Fatigue in liver disease is often intermittent and variable in severity from hour to hour and day to day. In some patients, it may not be clear whether fatigue is due to the liver disease or to other problems such as stress, anxiety, sleep disturbance, or a concurrent illness.

Nausea occurs with more severe liver disease and may accompany fatigue or be provoked by odors of food or eating fatty foods. Vomiting can occur but is rarely persistent or prominent. Poor appetite with weight loss occurs commonly in acute liver diseases but is rare in chronic disease, except when cirrhosis is present and advanced. Diarrhea is uncommon in liver disease, except with severe jaundice, where lack of bile acids reaching the intestine can lead to steatorrhea.

Right upper quadrant discomfort or ache ("liver pain") occurs in many liver diseases and is usually marked by tenderness over the liver area. The pain arises from stretching or irritation of Glisson's capsule, which surrounds the liver and is rich in nerve endings. Severe pain is most typical of gall bladder disease, liver abscess, and severe venoocclusive disease but is an occasional accompaniment of acute hepatitis.

Itching occurs with acute liver disease, appearing early in obstructive jaundice (from biliary obstruction or drug-induced cholestasis) and somewhat later in hepatocellular disease (acute hepatitis). Itching also occurs in chronic liver diseases, typically the cholestatic forms such as primary biliary cirrhosis and sclerosing cholangitis where it is often the presenting symptom, occurring before the onset of jaundice. However, itching can occur in any liver disease, particularly once cirrhosis is present.

Jaundice is the hallmark symptom of liver disease and perhaps the most reliable marker of severity. Patients usually report darkening of the urine before they notice scleral icterus. Jaundice is rarely detectable with a bilirubin level <43 μmol/L (2.5 mg/dL). With severe cholestasis there will also be lightening of the color of the stools and steatorrhea. Jaundice without dark urine usually indicates indirect (unconjugated) hyperbilirubinemia and is typical of hemolytic anemia and the genetic disorders of bilirubin conjugation, the common and benign form being Gilbert's syndrome and the rare and severe form being Crigler-Najjar syndrome. Gilbert's syndrome affects up to 5% of the population; the jaundice is more noticeable after fasting and with stress.

Major risk factors for liver disease that should be sought in the clinical history include details of alcohol use, medications (including herbal compounds, birth control pills, and over-the-counter medications), personal habits, sexual activity, travel, exposure to jaundiced or other high-risk persons, injection drug use, recent surgery, remote or recent transfusion with blood and blood products, occupation, accidental exposure to blood or needlestick, and familial history of liver disease.

For assessing the risk of viral hepatitis, a careful history of sexual activity is of particular importance and should include number of lifetime sexual partners and, for men, a history of having sex with men. Sexual exposure is a common mode of spread of hepatitis B but is rare for hepatitis C. A family history of hepatitis, liver disease, and liver cancer is also important. Maternal-infant transmission occurs with both hepatitis B and C. Vertical spread of hepatitis B can now be prevented by passive and active immunization of the infant at birth. Vertical spread of hepatitis C is uncommon, but there are no reliable means of prevention. A history of injection drug use, even in the remote past, is of great importance in assessing the risk for hepatitis B and C. Injection drug use is now the single most common risk factor for hepatitis C. Transfusion with blood or blood products is no longer an important risk factor for acute viral hepatitis. However, blood transfusions received before the introduction of sensitive enzyme immunoassays for antibody to hepatitis C virus (anti-HCV) in 1992 is an important risk factor for chronic hepatitis C. Blood transfusion before 1986, when screening for antibody to hepatitis B core antigen (anti-HBc) was introduced, is also a risk factor for hepatitis B. Travel to an underdeveloped area of the world, exposure to persons with jaundice, and exposure to young children in day-care centers are risk factors for hepatitis A. Tattooing and body piercing (for hepatitis B and C) and eating shellfish (for hepatitis A) are frequently mentioned but actually quite rate types of exposure for acquiring hepatitis.

A history of alcohol intake is important in assessing the cause of liver disease and also in planning management and recommendations. In the United States, for example, at least 70% of adults drink alcohol to some degree, but significant alcohol intake is less common; in population-based surveys, only 5% have more than two drinks per day, the average drink representing 11 to 15 g alcohol. Alcohol consumption associated with an increased rate of alcoholic liver disease is probably more than two drinks (22 to 30 g) per day in women and three drinks (33 to 45 g) in men. Most patients with alcoholic cirrhosis have a much higher daily intake and have drunk excessively for 10 years or more before onset of liver disease. In assessing alcohol intake, the history should also focus upon whether alcohol abuse or dependence is present. Alcoholism is usually defined on the behavioral patterns and consequences of alcohol intake, not on the basis of the amount of alcohol intake. *Abuse* is defined by a repetitive pattern of drinking alcohol that has adverse effects on social, family, occupational, or health status. *Dependence* is defined by alcohol-seeking behavior, despite its adverse effects. Many alcoholics demonstrate both dependence and abuse, and dependence is considered the more serious and advanced form of alcoholism. A clinically helpful approach to diagnosis of alcohol dependence and abuse is the use of the CAGE questionnaire (Table 282-2), which is recommended in all medical history taking.

Family history can be helpful in assessing liver disease. Familial causes of liver disease include Wilson's disease; hemochromatosis and α_1 antitrypsin (α_1AT) deficiency; and the more uncommon inherited pediatric liver diseases of familial intrahepatic cholestasis, benign recurrent intrahepatic cholestasis, and Alagille's syndrome. Onset of severe liver disease in childhood or adolescence with a family history of liver disease or neuropsychiatric disturbance should lead to investigation for Wilson's disease. A family history of cirrhosis, diabetes, or endocrine failure and the appearance of liver disease in adulthood should suggest hemochromatosis and lead to investigation of iron status. Patients with abnormal iron studies warrant genotyping of the *HFE* gene for the C282Y and H63D mutations typical of genetic hemochromatosis. A family history of emphysema should provoke investigation of α_1AT levels and, if low, for Pi genotype.

PHYSICAL EXAMINATION　The physical examination rarely demonstrates evidence of liver dysfunction in a patient without symptoms or laboratory findings, nor are most signs of liver disease specific to one diagnosis. Thus, the physical examination usually complements rather than replaces the need for other diagnostic approaches. In many patients, the physical examination is normal unless the disease is acute or severe and advanced. Nevertheless, the physical examination is important in that it can be the first evidence for the presence of hepatic failure, portal hypertension, and liver decompensation. In addition, the physical examination can reveal signs that point to a specific diagnosis, either in risk factors or in associated diseases or findings.

Typical physical findings in liver disease are icterus, hepatomegaly, hepatic tenderness, splenomegaly, spider angiomata, palmar erythema, and excoriations. Signs of advanced disease include muscle-wasting, ascites, edema, dilated abdominal veins, hepatic fetor, asterixis, mental confusion, stupor, and coma. In males with cirrhosis, particularly when related to alcohol, signs of hyperestrogenemia such as gynecomastia, testicular atrophy, and loss of male-pattern hair distribution may be found.

Icterus is best appreciated by inspecting the sclera under natural light. In fair-skinned individuals, a yellow color of the skin may be obvious. In dark-skinned individuals, the mucous membranes below the tongue can demonstrate jaundice. Jaundice is rarely detectable if the serum bilirubin level is <43 μmol/L (2.5 mg/dL) but may remain detectable below this level during recovery from jaundice (because of protein and tissue binding of conjugated bilirubin).

Spider angiomata and palmar erythema occur in both acute and chronic liver disease and may be especially prominent in persons with cirrhosis, but they can occur in normal individuals and are frequently present during pregnancy. Spider angiomata are superficial, tortuous arterioles and, unlike simple telangiectases, typically fill from the center outwards. Spider angiomata occur only on the arms, face, and upper torso; they can be pulsatile and may be difficult to detect in dark-skinned individuals.

TABLE 282-2　CAGE Questions[a]

Acronym	Question
C	Have you ever felt you ought to *C*ut down on your drinking?
A	Have people *A*nnoyed you by criticizing your drinking?
G	Have you ever felt *G*uilty or bad about your drinking?
E	Have you ever had a drink first thing in the morning to steady your nerves or get rid of a hangover (*E*yeopener)?

[a] One "yes" response should raise suspicion of an alcohol use problem, and more than one is a strong indication that abuse or dependence exists.

Hepatomegaly is not a very reliable sign of liver disease, because of the variability of the size and shape of the liver and the physical impediments to assessing liver size by percussion and palpation. Marked hepatomegaly is typical of cirrhosis, venoocclusive disease, metastatic or primary cancers of the liver, and alcoholic hepatitis. Careful assessment of the liver edge may also demonstrate unusual firmness, irregularity of the surface, or frank nodules. Perhaps the most reliable physical finding in examining the liver is hepatic tenderness. Discomfort on touching or pressing on the liver should be carefully sought with percussive comparison of the right and left upper quadrants.

Splenomegaly occurs in many medical conditions but can be a subtle but significant physical finding in liver disease. The availability of ultrasound (US) assessment of the spleen allows for confirmation of the physical finding.

Signs of advanced liver disease include muscle-wasting and weight loss as well as hepatomegaly, bruising, ascites, and edema. Ascites is best appreciated by attempts to detect shifting dullness by careful percussion. US examination will confirm the finding of ascites in equivocal cases. Peripheral edema can occur with or without ascites. In patients with advanced liver disease, other factors frequently contribute to edema formation, including hypoalbuminemia, venous insufficiency, heart failure, and medications.

Hepatic failure is defined as the occurrence of signs or symptoms of hepatic encephalopathy in a person with severe acute or chronic liver disease. The first signs of hepatic encephalopathy can be subtle and nonspecific—change in sleep patterns, change in personality, irritability, and mental dullness. Thereafter, confusion, disorientation, stupor, and eventually coma supervene. Physical findings include asterixis and flapping tremors of the body and tongue. *Fetor hepaticus* refers to the slightly sweet, ammoniacal odor that is common in patients with liver failure, particularly if there is portal-venous shunting of blood around the liver. Other causes of coma and confusion should be excluded, mainly electrolyte imbalances, sedative use, and renal or respiratory failure. A helpful measure of hepatic encephalopathy is a careful mental status examination and use of the trail-making test, which consists of a series of 25 numbered circles that the patient is asked to connect as rapidly as possible using a pencil. The normal range for the connect-the-dot test is 15 to 30 s; it is considerably delayed in patients with early hepatic encephalopathy. Other tests include drawing abstract objects or comparison of a signature to previous examples.

Other signs of advanced liver disease include umbilical hernia from ascites, prominent veins over the abdomen, and *caput medusa*, which consists of collateral veins seen radiating from the umbilicus and resulting from the recanulation of the umbilical vein. Widened pulse pressure and signs of a hyperdynamic circulation can occur in patients with cirrhosis as a result of fluid and sodium retention, increased cardiac output, and reduced peripheral resistance. Patients with long-standing cirrhosis and portal hypertension are prone to develop the hepatopulmonary syndrome, defined by the triad of liver disease, with hypoxemia, and pulmonary arteriovenous shunting. The hepatopulmonary syndrome is characterized by platypnea and orthodeoxia, representing shortness of breath and oxygen desaturation that occur paradoxically upon assuming an upright position.

Several skin disorders and changes occur commonly in liver disease. Hyperpigmentation is typical of advanced chronic cholestatic diseases such as primary biliary cirrhosis and sclerosing cholangitis. In these same conditions, xanthelasma and tendon xanthomata occur as a result of retention and high serum levels of lipids and cholesterol. A slate-gray pigmentation to the skin also occurs with hemochromatosis if iron levels are high for a prolonged period. Mucocutaneous vasculitis with palpable purpura, especially on the lower extremities, is typical of cryoglobulinemia of chronic hepatitis C but can also occur in chronic hepatitis B.

Some physical signs point to specific liver diseases. Kayser-Fleischer rings occur in Wilson's disease and consist of a golden-brown copper pigment deposited in Disemet's membrane at the periphery of the cornea; they are best seen by slit-lamp examination. In metastatic liver disease or primary hepatocellular carcinoma, signs of cachexia and wasting may be prominent, as well as firm hepatomegaly and a hepatic bruit.

LABORATORY TESTING Diagnosis in liver disease is greatly aided by the availability of reliable and sensitive tests of liver injury and function. Use and interpretation of liver function tests is summarized in Chap. 283. A typical battery of blood tests used for initial assessment of liver disease includes measuring levels of serum alanine and aspartate aminotransferases (ALT and AST), alkaline phosphatase, direct and total serum bilirubin, and albumin and assessing prothrombin time. The pattern of abnormalities generally points to hepatocellular versus cholestatic liver disease and will help to decide whether the disease is acute or chronic and whether cirrhosis and hepatic failure are present. Based on these results, further testing over time may be necessary. Other laboratory tests may be helpful, such as γ-glutamyl transpeptidase (GGT) to define whether alkaline phosphatase elevations are due to liver disease; hepatitis serology to define the type of viral hepatitis; and autoimmune markers to diagnose primary biliary cirrhosis (antimitochondrial antibody; AMA), sclerosing cholangitis (peripheral antineutrophil cytoplasmic antibody; P-ANCA), and autoimmune hepatitis (antinuclear, smooth-muscle, and liver-kidney microsomal antibody). A simple delineation of laboratory abnormalities and common liver diseases is given in Table 282-3.

DIAGNOSTIC IMAGING There have been great advances made in hepatic imaging, although no method is suitably accurate in demonstrating underlying cirrhosis. There are many modalities available for imaging the liver. US, computed tomography (CT), and magnetic resonance imaging (MRI) are the most commonly employed and are complementary to each other. In general, US and CT have a high sensitivity for detecting biliary duct dilatation and are the first-line options for investigating the patient with suspected obstructive jaundice. Both US and CT can detect a fatty liver, which appears bright on both studies. Magnetic resonance cholangiopancreatography (MRCP) and endo-

TABLE 282-3 *Important Diagnostic Tests in Common Liver Diseases*

Disease	Diagnostic Test
Hepatitis A	Anti-HAV IgM
Hepatitis B	
Acute	HBsAg and anti-HBc IgM
Chronic	HBsAg and HBeAg and/or HBV DNA
Hepatitis C	Anti-HCV and HCV RNA
Hepatitis D (delta)	HBsAg and anti-HDV
Hepatitis E	Anti-HEV
Autoimmune hepatitis	ANA or SMA, elevated IgG levels, and compatible histology
Primary biliary cirrhosis	Mitochondrial antibody, elevated IgM levels, and compatible histology
Primary sclerosing cholangitis	P-ANCA, cholangiography
Drug-induced liver disease	History of drug ingestion
Alcoholic liver disease	History of excessive alcohol intake and compatible histology
Nonalcoholic steatohepatitis	Ultrasound or CT evidence of fatty liver and compatible histology
α_1 Antitrypsin disease	Reduced α_1 antitrypsin levels, phenotypes PiZZ or PiSZ
Wilson's disease	Decreased serum ceruloplasmin and increased urinary copper; increased hepatic copper level
Hemochromatosis	Elevated iron saturation and serum ferritin; genetic testing for *HFE* gene mutations
Hepatocellular cancer	Elevated α-fetoprotein level >500; ultrasound or CT image of mass

Note: HAV, HBV, HCV, HDV, HEV: hepatitis A, B, C, D, or E virus; HBsAg, hepatitis B surface antigen; anti-HBc, antibody to hepatitis B core (antigen); HBeAg, hepatitis e antigen; ANA, antinuclear antibodies; SMA, smooth-muscle antibody; P-ANCA, peripheral antineutrophil cytoplasmic antibody; CT, computed tomography.

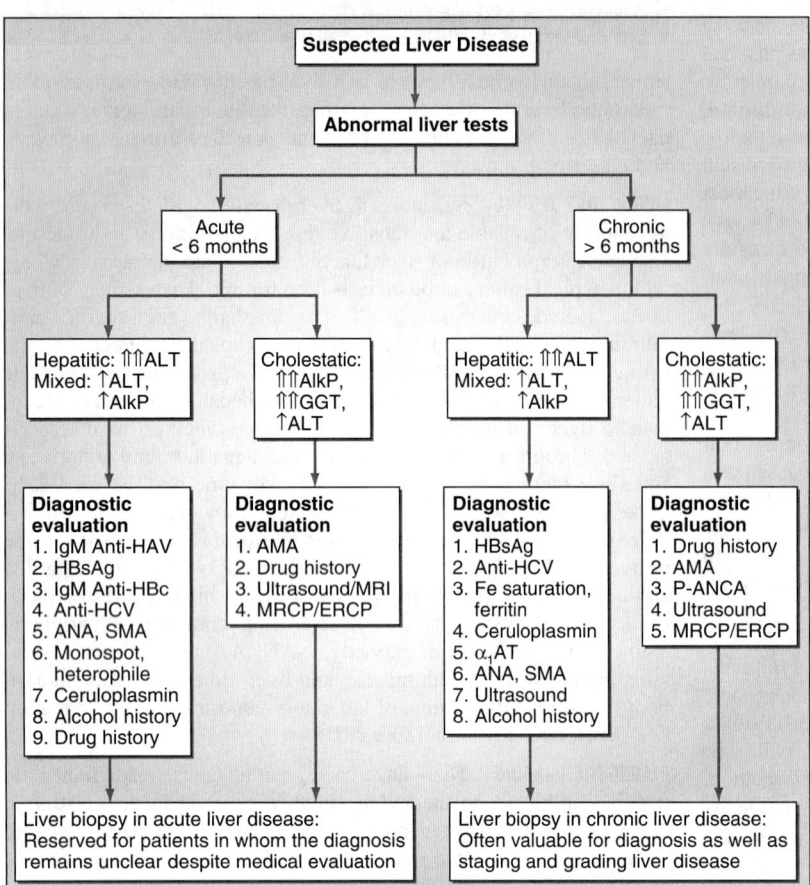

```
                    ┌──────────────────────┐
                    │ Suspected Liver Disease │
                    └──────────────────────┘
                              │
                    ┌──────────────────────┐
                    │   Abnormal liver tests │
                    └──────────────────────┘
                              │
              ┌───────────────┴───────────────┐
        ┌──────────┐                     ┌──────────┐
        │  Acute   │                     │ Chronic  │
        │ < 6 months│                     │ > 6 months│
        └──────────┘                     └──────────┘
```

Hepatitic: ⇈⇈ALT Mixed: ↑ALT, ↑AlkP	Cholestatic: ⇈⇈AlkP, ⇈⇈GGT, ↑ALT	Hepatitic: ⇈⇈ALT Mixed: ↑ALT, ↑AlkP	Cholestatic: ⇈⇈AlkP, ⇈⇈GGT, ↑ALT
Diagnostic evaluation 1. IgM Anti-HAV 2. HBsAg 3. IgM Anti-HBc 4. Anti-HCV 5. ANA, SMA 6. Monospot, heterophile 7. Ceruloplasmin 8. Alcohol history 9. Drug history	**Diagnostic evaluation** 1. AMA 2. Drug history 3. Ultrasound/MRI 4. MRCP/ERCP	**Diagnostic evaluation** 1. HBsAg 2. Anti-HCV 3. Fe saturation, ferritin 4. Ceruloplasmin 5. α₁AT 6. ANA, SMA 7. Ultrasound 8. Alcohol history	**Diagnostic evaluation** 1. Drug history 2. AMA 3. P-ANCA 4. Ultrasound 5. MRCP/ERCP

Liver biopsy in acute liver disease: Reserved for patients in whom the diagnosis remains unclear despite medical evaluation	Liver biopsy in chronic liver disease: Often valuable for diagnosis as well as staging and grading liver disease

FIGURE 282-1 Algorithm for evaluation of abnormal liver tests. For patients with suspected liver disease, an appropriate approach to evaluation is initial testing for routine liver tests such as bilirubin, albumin, alanine aminotransferase (ALT), aspartate aminotransferase (AST), and alkaline phosphatase (AlkP). These results (sometimes complemented by testing of γ-glutamyl transpeptidase; GGT) will establish whether the pattern of abnormalities is hepatic, cholestatic, or mixed. In addition, the duration of symptoms or abnormalities will show whether the disease is acute or chronic. If the disease is acute and if history, laboratory tests, and imaging studies do not reveal a diagnosis, liver biopsy is appropriate to help to establish the diagnosis. If the disease is chronic, liver biopsy can be helpful not only for diagnosis, but also to grade the activity and stage the progression of disease. This approach is largely applicable to patients without immune deficiency. In patients with HIV infection or after bone marrow or solid organ transplantation, diagnostic evaluation should also include evaluation of opportunistic infections (adenovirus, cytomegalovirus, coccidioidomycosis, etc.) as well as vascular and immunologic conditions (venoocclusive disease, graft-vs-host disease). HAV, HCV: hepatitis A or C virus; HBsAg, hepatitis B sulface antigen; anti-HBc, antibody to hepatitis B core (antigen); ANA, antinuclear antibodies; SMA, smooth-muscle antibody; MRI, magnetic resonance imaging; MRCP; magnetic resonance cholangiopancreatography; ERCP, endoscopic retrograde cholangiopancreatography; α₁AT, α₁ antitrypsin; AMA; antimitochondrial antibody; P-ANCA, peripheral antineutrophil cytoplasmic antibody.

scopic retrograde cholangiopancreatography (ERCP) are the procedures of choice for visualization of the biliary tree. MRCP offers several advantages over ERCP; there is no need for contrast media or ionizing radiation, images can be acquired faster, it is less operator dependent, and it carries no risk of pancreatitis. MRCP is superior to US and CT for detecting choledocholithiasis but less specific. It is useful in the diagnosis of bile duct obstruction and congenital biliary abnormalities, but ERCP is more valuable in evaluating ampullary lesions and primary sclerosing cholangitis. ERCP allows for biopsy, direct visualization of the ampulla and common bile duct, and intraductal ultrasonography. It also provides several therapeutic options in patients with obstructive jaundice, such as sphincterotomy, stone extraction, and placement of nasobiliary catheters and biliary stents. Doppler US and MRI are used to assess hepatic vasculature and hemodynamics and to monitor surgically or radiologically placed vascular shunts such as transjugular intrahepatic portosystemic shunts. CT and MRI are indicated for the identification and evaluation of hepatic masses, staging of liver tumors, and preoperative assessment. With regard to mass lesions, sensitivity of hepatic imaging continues to increase; unfortunately, specificity remains a problem, and often two

and sometimes three studies are needed before a diagnosis can be reached. Finally, interventional radiologic techniques allow the biopsy of solitary lesions, insertion of drains into hepatic abscesses, and creation of vascular shunts in patients with portal hypertension. Which modality to use depends on factors such as availability, cost, and experience of the radiologist with each technique.

LIVER BIOPSY Liver biopsy remains the gold standard in the evaluation of patients with liver disease, particularly in patients with chronic liver diseases. In selected instances, liver biopsy is necessary for diagnosis but is more often useful in assessing the severity (grade) and stage of liver damage, in predicting prognosis, and in monitoring response to treatment.

Diagnosis of Liver Disease The major causes of liver disease and key diagnostic features are outlined in Table 282-3, and an algorithm for evaluation of the patient with suspected liver disease is given in Fig. 282-1. Specifics of diagnosis are discussed in later chapters. The most common causes of acute liver disease are viral hepatitis (particularly hepatitis A, B, and C), drug-induced liver injury, cholangitis, and alcoholic liver disease. Liver biopsy is usually not needed in the diagnosis and management of acute liver disease, exceptions being situations where the diagnosis remains unclear despite thorough clinical and laboratory investigation. Liver biopsy can be helpful in the diagnosis of drug-induced liver disease and in establishing the diagnosis of acute alcoholic hepatitis.

The most common causes of chronic liver disease in general order of frequency are chronic hepatitis C, alcoholic liver disease, nonalcoholic steatohepatitis, chronic hepatitis B, autoimmune hepatitis, sclerosing cholangitis, primary biliary cirrhosis, hemochromatosis, and Wilson's disease. Strict diagnostic criteria have not been developed for most liver diseases, but liver biopsy plays an important role in the diagnosis of autoimmune hepatitis, primary biliary cirrhosis, nonalcoholic and alcoholic steatohepatitis, and Wilson's disease (with a quantitative hepatic copper level).

Grading and Staging of Liver Disease Grading refers to an assessment of the severity or activity of liver disease, whether acute or chronic; active or inactive; and mild, moderate, or severe. Liver biopsy is the most accurate means of assessing severity, particularly in chronic liver disease. Serum aminotransferase levels are used as a convenient and noninvasive means to follow disease activity, but aminotransferases are not always reliable in reflecting disease severity. Thus, normal serum aminotransferases in patients with hepatitis B surface antigen (HBsAg) in serum may indicate the inactive HBsAg carrier state or may reflect mild chronic hepatitis B or hepatitis B with fluctuating disease activity. Serum testing for hepatitis B e antigen and hepatitis B virus DNA can help resolve these different patterns, but these markers can also fluctuate and change over time. Similarly, in chronic hepatitis C, serum aminotransferases can be normal despite moderate activity of disease. Finally, in both alcoholic and nonalcoholic steatohepatitis, aminotransferases are quite unreliable in reflecting severity. In these conditions, liver biopsy is helpful in guiding management and recommending therapy, particularly if therapy is difficult, prolonged, and expensive as is often the case in chronic viral hepatitis. There are several well-verified numerical scales for grading activity in chronic liver disease, the most common being the histology activity index and the Ishak histology scale.

Liver biopsy is also the most accurate means of assessing stage of disease as early or advanced, precirrhotic, and cirrhotic. Staging of disease pertains largely to chronic liver diseases in which progression

TABLE 282-4 *Child-Pugh Classification of Cirrhosis*

Factor	Units	1	2	3
Serum bilirubin	μmol/L	<34	34–51	>51
	mg/dL	<2.0	2.0–3.0	>3.0
Serum albumin	g/L	>35	30–35	<30
	g/dL	>3.5	3.0–3.5	<3.0
Prothrombin time	second prolonged	0–4	4–6	>6
	INR	<1.7	1.7–2.3	>2.3
Ascites		None	Easily controlled	Poorly controlled
Hepatic encephalopathy		None	Minimal	Advanced

Note: The Child-Pugh score is calculated by adding the scores of the five factors and can range from 5 to 15. Child-Pugh class is either A (a score of 5 to 6), B (7 to 9), or C (10 or above). Decompensation indicates cirrhosis with a Child-Pugh score of 7 or more (Class B). This level has been the accepted criterion for listing for liver transplantation.

to cirrhosis and end-stage liver disease can occur, but which may require years or decades to develop. Clinical features, biochemical tests, and hepatic imaging studies are helpful in assessing stage but generally become abnormal only in the middle to late stages of cirrhosis. Noninvasive tests that suggest advanced fibrosis include mild elevations of bilirubin, prolongation of prothrombin time, slight decreases in serum albumin, and mild thrombocytopenia (which is often the first indication of worsening fibrosis). Early stages of cirrhosis are generally detectable only by liver biopsy. In assessing stage, the degree of fibrosis is usually used as its quantitative measure. The amount of fibrosis is generally staged on a 0 to 4+ (histology activity index) or 0 to 6+ scale (Ishak scale). The importance of staging relates primarily to prognosis and to guiding management of complications. Patients with cirrhosis are candidates for screening and surveillance for esophageal varices and hepatocellular carcinoma. Patients without advanced fibrosis need not undergo screening.

Cirrhosis can also be staged clinically. A reliable staging system is the modified Child-Pugh classification with a scoring system of 5 to 15: scores of 5 and 6 being Child-Pugh class A (consistent with "compensated cirrhosis"), scores of 7 to 9 indicating class B, and 10 to 15 class C (Table 282-4). This scoring system was initially devised to stratify patients into risk groups prior to undergoing portal decompressive surgery. The Child-Pugh score is a reasonably reliable predictor of survival in many liver diseases and predicts the likelihood of major complications of cirrhosis such as bleeding from varices and spontaneous bacterial peritonitis. It was used to assess prognosis in cirrhosis and to provide the standard criteria for listing for liver transplantation (Child-Pugh class B). Recently the Child-Pugh system has been replaced by the model for end-stage liver disease (MELD) score for assessing the need for liver transplantation. The MELD score is a prospectively derived scoring system designed to predict prognosis of patients with liver disease and portal hypertension. It is calculated using three noninvasive variables—the prothrombin time expressed as international normalized ratio (INR), serum bilirubin, and serum creatinine (www.mayo.edu/int-med/gi/model/). MELD provides a more objective means of assessing disease severity and has less center-to-center variation than the Child-Pugh score and has a wider range of values. MELD is currently used to establish priority listing for liver transplantation in the United States.

Thus, liver biopsy is helpful not only in diagnosis but also in management of chronic liver disease and assessment of prognosis. Because liver biopsy is an invasive procedure and not without complications, it should be used only when it will contribute materially to management and therapeutic decisions.

NONSPECIFIC ISSUES IN MANAGEMENT OF PATIENTS WITH LIVER DISEASE

Specifics on management of different forms of acute or chronic liver disease are given in subsequent chapters, but certain issues are applicable to any patient with liver disease. These include advice regarding alcohol use, medications, vaccination, and surveillance for complications of liver disease. Alcohol should be used sparingly, if at all, by patients with liver disease. Abstinence from alcohol should be encouraged for all patients with alcohol-related liver disease and in patients with cirrhosis and those receiving interferon-based therapy for hepatitis B or C. Regarding vaccinations, all patients with liver disease should receive hepatitis A vaccine and those with risk factors should receive hepatitis B vaccination as well. Influenza and pneumococcal vaccination should also be encouraged. Patients with liver disease should be careful in use of any medications, other than the most necessary. Drug-induced hepatotoxicity can mimic many forms of liver disease and can cause exacerbations of chronic hepatitis and cirrhosis; drugs should be suspected in any situation where the cause of exacerbation is unknown. Finally, consideration should be given to surveillance for complications of chronic liver disease such as variceal hemorrhage and hepatocellular carcinoma. Patients with cirrhosis warrant upper endoscopy to assess the presence of varices and should be given chronic therapy with beta blockers if large varices are found. Patients with cirrhosis also warrant screening and long-term surveillance for development of hepatocellular carcinoma. While the optimal regimen for such surveillance has not been established, an appropriate approach is US of the liver at 6- to 12-month intervals.

FURTHER READING

DESMET VJ et al: Classification of chronic hepatitis: Diagnosis, grading and staging. Hepatology 19:1513, 1994

ISHAK K et al: Histological grading and staging of chronic hepatitis. J Hepatol 22:696, 1995

KAMATH PS et al: A model to predict survival in patients with end-stage liver disease. Hepatology 33:464, 2001

SCHIFF ER et al (eds): *Schiff's Diseases of the Liver*, 9th ed. Philadelphia, Lippincott Williams & Wilkins, 2002

ZAKIM D, BOYER TD (eds): *Hepatology: A Textbook of Liver Disease*, 4th ed. Philadelphia, Saunders, 2003

ZIMMERMAN HJ: *Hepatotoxicity: The Adverse Effects of Drugs and Other Chemicals on the Liver*, 2d ed. Philadelphia, Lippincott Williams & Wilkins, 1999

283 EVALUATION OF LIVER FUNCTION
Daniel S. Pratt, Marshall M. Kaplan

Several biochemical tests are useful in the evaluation and management of patients with hepatic dysfunction. These tests can be used to (1) detect the presence of liver disease, (2) distinguish among different types of liver disorders, (3) gauge the extent of known liver damage, and (4) follow the response to treatment.

Liver tests have shortcomings. They can be normal in patients with serious liver disease and abnormal in patients with diseases that do not affect the liver. Liver tests rarely suggest a specific diagnosis; rather, they suggest a general category of liver disease, such as hepatocellular or cholestatic, which then further directs the evaluation.

The liver carries out thousands of biochemical functions, most of which cannot be easily measured by blood tests. Laboratory tests measure only a limited number of these functions. In fact, many tests, such as the aminotransferases or alkaline phosphatase, do not measure liver function at all. Rather, they detect liver cell damage or interference with bile flow. Thus, no one test enables the clinician to accurately assess the liver's total functional capacity.

To increase both the sensitivity and the specificity of laboratory tests in the detection of liver disease, it is best to use them as a battery. Those tests usually employed in clinical practice include the bilirubin,

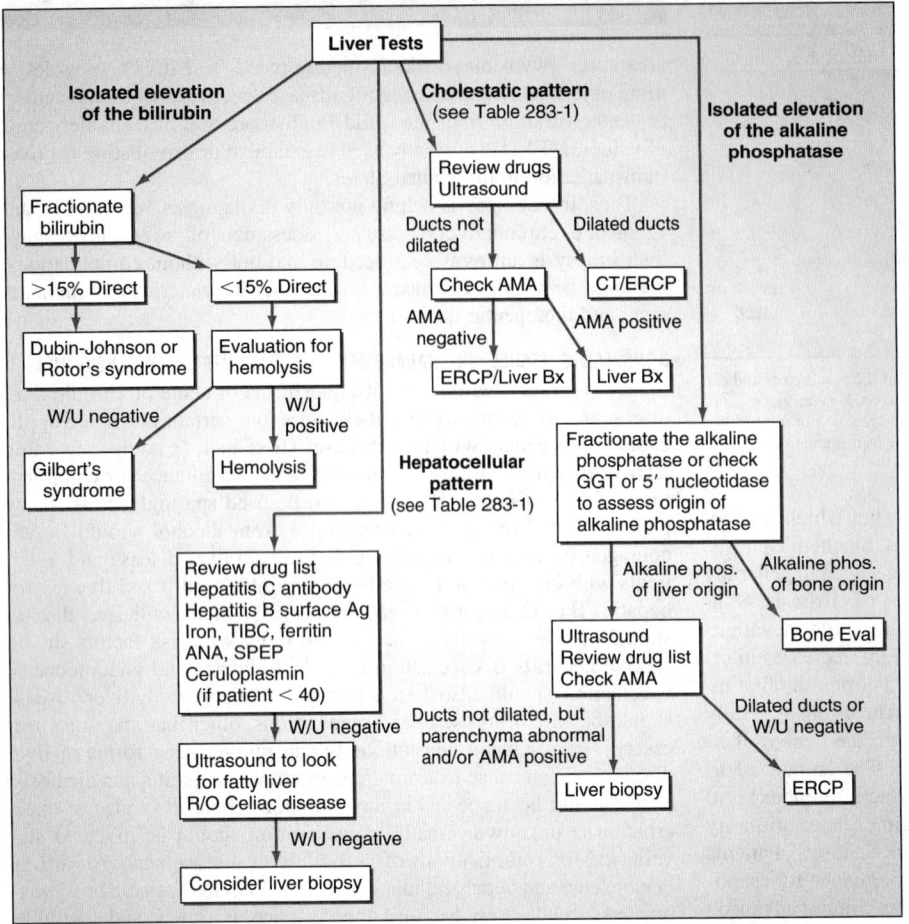

FIGURE 283-1 Algorithm for the evaluation of chronically abnormal liver tests. ERCP, endoscopic retrograde cholangiopancreatography; CT, computed tomography; AMA, antimitochondrial antibody; ANA, antinuclear antibody; SPEP, serum protein electrophoresis; TIBC, total iron-binding capacity; GGT, gamma glutamyl transpeptidase.

aminotransferases, alkaline phosphatase, albumin, and prothrombin time tests. When more than one of these tests provide abnormal findings, or the findings are persistently abnormal on serial determinations, the probability of liver disease is high. When all test results are normal, the probability of missing occult liver disease is low.

When evaluating patients with liver disorders, it is helpful to group these tests into general categories. The classification we have found most useful is given below.

TESTS BASED ON DETOXIFICATION AND EXCRETORY FUNCTIONS ■ **Serum Bilirubin** (See also Chap. 38) Bilirubin, a breakdown product of the porphyrin ring of heme-containing proteins, is found in the blood in two fractions—conjugated and unconjugated. The unconjugated fraction, also termed the *indirect fraction*, is insoluble in water and is bound to albumin in the blood. The conjugated (direct) bilirubin fraction is water soluble and can therefore be excreted by the kidney. When measured by the original van den Bergh method, the normal total serum bilirubin concentration is <17 μmol/L (1 mg/dL). Up to 30%, or 5.1 μmol/L (0.3 mg/dL), of the total is direct-reacting (or conjugated) bilirubin.

Elevation of the unconjugated fraction of bilirubin is rarely due to liver disease. An isolated elevation of unconjugated bilirubin is seen primarily in hemolytic disorders and in a number of genetic conditions such as Crigler-Najjar and Gilbert's syndromes (Chap. 38). Isolated unconjugated hyperbilirubinemia (bilirubin elevated, but less than 15% direct) should prompt a workup for hemolysis (Fig. 283-1). In the absence of hemolysis, an isolated unconjugated hyperbilirubinemia in an otherwise healthy patient can be attributed to Gilbert's syndrome and no further evaluation is required.

In contrast, conjugated hyperbilirubinemia almost always implies liver or biliary tract disease. The rate-limiting step in bilirubin metab-

olism is not conjugation of bilirubin, but rather the transport of conjugated bilirubin into the bile canaliculi. Thus, elevation of the conjugated fraction may be seen in any type of liver disease. In most liver diseases, both conjugated and unconjugated fractions of the bilirubin tend to be elevated. Except in the presence of a purely unconjugated hyperbilirubinemia, fractionation of the bilirubin is rarely helpful in determining the cause of jaundice.

Urine Bilirubin Unconjugated bilirubin always binds to albumin in the serum and is not filtered by the kidney. Therefore, any bilirubin found in the urine is conjugated bilirubin; the presence of bilirubinuria implies the presence of liver disease. A urine dipstick test can theoretically give the same information as fractionation of the serum bilirubin. This test is almost 100% accurate. Phenothiazines may give a false-positive reading with the Ictotest tablet.

Blood Ammonia Ammonia is produced in the body during normal protein metabolism and by intestinal bacteria, primarily those in the colon. The liver plays a role in the detoxification of ammonia by converting it to urea, which is excreted by the kidneys. Striated muscle also plays a role in detoxification of ammonia, which is combined with glutamic acid to form glutamine. Patients with advanced liver disease typically have significant muscle wasting, which likely contributes to hyperammonemia in these patients. Some physicians use the blood ammonia for detecting encephalopathy or for monitoring hepatic synthetic function, although its use for either of these indications has problems. There is very poor correlation between either the presence or the degree of acute encephalopathy and elevation of blood ammonia; it can be occasionally useful for identifying the occult liver disease in patients with mental status changes. There is also a poor correlation of the blood serum ammonia and hepatic function. The ammonia can be elevated in patients with severe portal hypertension and portal blood shunting around the liver even in the presence of normal or near normal hepatic function.

Serum Enzymes The liver contains thousands of enzymes, some of which are also present in the serum in very low concentrations. These enzymes have no known function in the serum and behave like other serum proteins. They are distributed in the plasma and in interstitial fluid and have characteristic half-lives, usually measured in days. Very little is known about the catabolism of serum enzymes, although they are probably cleared by cells in the reticuloendothelial system. The elevation of a given enzyme activity in the serum is thought to primarily reflect its increased rate of entrance into serum from damaged liver cells.

Serum enzyme tests can be grouped into three categories: (1) enzymes whose elevation in serum reflects damage to hepatocytes, (2) enzymes whose elevation in serum reflects cholestasis, and (3) enzyme tests that do not fit precisely into either pattern.

ENZYMES THAT REFLECT DAMAGE TO HEPATOCYTES The aminotransferases (transaminases) are sensitive indicators of liver cell injury and are most helpful in recognizing acute hepatocellular diseases such as hepatitis. They include the aspartate aminotransferase (AST) and the alanine aminotransferase (ALT). AST is found in the liver, cardiac muscle, skeletal muscle, kidneys, brain, pancreas, lungs, leukocytes, and erythrocytes in decreasing order of concentration. ALT is found primarily in the liver. The aminotransferases are normally present in the serum in low concentrations. These enzymes are released into the blood in greater amounts when there is damage to the liver cell membrane resulting in increased permeability. Liver cell necrosis is not required for the release of the aminotransferases, and there is a poor correlation between the degree of liver cell damage and the level of the aminotransferases. Thus, the absolute elevation of the aminotransferases is of no prognostic significance in acute hepatocellular disorders.

Any type of liver cell injury can cause modest elevations in the serum aminotransferases. Levels of up to 300 U/L are nonspecific and may be found in any type of liver disorder. Striking elevations—i.e., aminotransferases >1000 U/L—occur almost exclusively in disorders associated with extensive hepatocellular injury such as (1) viral hepatitis, (2) ischemic liver injury (prolonged hypotension or acute heart failure), or (3) toxin or drug-induced liver injury.

The pattern of the aminotransferase elevation can be helpful diagnostically. In most acute hepatocellular disorders, the ALT is higher than or equal to the AST. An AST:ALT ratio > 2:1 is suggestive while a ratio > 3:1 is highly suggestive of alcoholic liver disease. The AST in alcoholic liver disease is rarely >300 U/L and the ALT is often normal. A low level of ALT in the serum is due to an alcohol-induced deficiency of pyridoxal phosphate.

The aminotransferases are usually not greatly elevated in obstructive jaundice. One notable exception occurs during the acute phase of biliary obstruction caused by the passage of a gallstone into the common bile duct. In this setting, the aminotransferases can briefly be in the 1000 to 2000 U/L range. However, aminotransferase levels decrease quickly, and the liver function tests rapidly evolve into one typical of cholestasis.

ENZYMES THAT REFLECT CHOLESTASIS   The activities of three enzymes—alkaline phosphatase, 5′-nucleotidase, and gamma glutamyl transpeptidase (GGT)—are usually elevated in cholestasis. Alkaline phosphatase and 5′-nucleotidase are found in or near the bile canalicular membrane of hepatocytes, while GGT is located in the endoplasmic reticulum and in bile duct epithelial cells. Reflecting its more diffuse localization in the liver, GGT elevation in serum is less specific for cholestasis than are elevations of alkaline phosphatase or 5′-nucleotidase. Some have advocated the use of GGT to identify patients with occult alcohol use. Its lack of specificity makes its use in this setting questionable.

The normal serum alkaline phosphatase consists of many distinct isoenzymes found in the liver, bone, placenta, and, less commonly, small intestine. Patients over age 60 can have a mildly elevated alkaline phosphatase (1 to 1½ times normal), while individuals with blood types O and B can have an elevation of the serum alkaline phosphatase after eating a fatty meal due to the influx of intestinal alkaline phosphatase into the blood. It is also nonpathologically elevated in children and adolescents undergoing rapid bone growth because of bone alkaline phosphatase, and late in normal pregnancies due to the influx of placental alkaline phosphatase.

Elevation of liver-derived alkaline phosphatase is not totally specific for cholestasis, and a less than threefold elevation can be seen in almost any type of liver disease. Alkaline phosphatase elevations greater than four times normal occur primarily in patients with cholestatic liver disorders, infiltrative liver diseases such as cancer, and bone conditions characterized by rapid bone turnover (e.g., Paget's disease). In bone diseases, the elevation is due to increased amounts of the bone isoenzymes. In liver diseases, the elevation is almost always due to increased amounts of the liver isoenzyme.

If an elevated serum alkaline phosphatase is the only abnormal finding in an apparently healthy person, or if the degree of elevation is higher than expected in the clinical setting, identification of the source of elevated isoenzymes is helpful (Fig. 283-1). This problem can be approached in several ways. First, and most precise, is the fractionation of the alkaline phosphatase by electrophoresis. The second approach is based on the observation that alkaline phosphatases from individual tissues differ in susceptibility to inactivation by heat.

The finding of an elevated serum alkaline phosphatase level in a patient with a heat-stable fraction strongly suggests that the placenta or a tumor is the source of the elevated enzyme in serum. Susceptibility to inactivation by heat increases, respectively, for the intestinal, liver, and bone alkaline phosphatases, bone being by far the most sensitive. The third, best substantiated, and most available approach involves the measurement of serum 5′-nucleotidase or GGT. These enzymes are rarely elevated in conditions other than liver disease.

In the absence of jaundice or elevated aminotransferases, an elevated alkaline phosphatase of liver origin often, but not always, suggests early cholestasis and, less often, hepatic infiltration by tumor or granulomata. Other conditions that cause isolated elevations of the alkaline phosphatase include Hodgkin's disease, diabetes, hyperthyroidism, congestive heart failure, and inflammatory bowel disease.

The level of serum alkaline phosphatase elevation is not helpful in distinguishing between intrahepatic and extrahepatic cholestasis. There is essentially no difference among the values found in obstructive jaundice due to cancer, common duct stone, sclerosing cholangitis, or bile duct stricture. Values are similarly increased in patients with intrahepatic cholestasis due to drug-induced hepatitis, primary biliary cirrhosis, rejection of transplanted livers, and, rarely, alcohol-induced steatonecrosis. Values are also greatly elevated in hepatobiliary disorders seen in patients with AIDS (e.g., AIDS cholangiopathy due to cytomegalovirus or cryptosporidial infection and tuberculosis with hepatic involvement).

TESTS THAT MEASURE BIOSYNTHETIC FUNCTION OF THE LIVER ■ Serum Albumin
Serum albumin is synthesized exclusively by hepatocytes. Serum albumin has a long half-life: 15 to 20 days, with approximately 4% degraded per day. Because of this slow turnover, the serum albumin is not a good indicator of acute or mild hepatic dysfunction; only minimal changes in the serum albumin are seen in acute liver conditions such as viral hepatitis, drug-related hepatoxicity, and obstructive jaundice. In hepatitis, albumin levels <3 g/dL should raise the possibility of chronic liver disease. Hypoalbuminemia is more common in chronic liver disorders such as cirrhosis and usually reflects severe liver damage and decreased albumin synthesis. One exception is the patient with ascites in whom synthesis may be normal or even increased, but levels are low because of the increased volume of distribution. However, hypoalbuminemia is not specific for liver disease and may occur in protein malnutrition of any cause, as well as protein-losing enteropathies, nephrotic syndrome, and chronic infections that are associated with prolonged increases in levels of serum interleukin 1 and/or tumor necrosis factor, cytokines that inhibit albumin synthesis. Serum albumin should not be measured for screening in patients in whom there is no suspicion of liver disease. A general medical clinic study of consecutive patients in whom no indications were present for albumin measurement showed that while 12% of patients had abnormal test results, the finding was of clinical importance in only 0.4%.

Serum Globulins
Serum globulins are a group of proteins made up of gamma globulins (immunoglobulins) produced by B lymphocytes and alpha and beta globulins produced primarily in hepatocytes. Gamma globulins are increased in chronic liver disease, such as chronic hepatitis and cirrhosis. In cirrhosis, the increased serum gamma globulin concentration is due to the increased synthesis of antibodies, some of which are directed against intestinal bacteria. This occurs because the cirrhotic liver fails to clear bacterial antigens that normally reach the liver through the hepatic circulation.

Increases in the concentration of specific isotypes of gamma globulins are often helpful in the recognition of certain chronic liver diseases. Diffuse polyclonal increases in IgG levels are common in autoimmune hepatitis; increases >100% should alert the clinician to this possibility. Increases in the IgM levels are common in primary biliary cirrhosis, while increases in the IgA levels occur in alcoholic liver disease.

TABLE 283-1 Liver Test Patterns in Hepatobiliary Disorders

Type of Disorder	Bilirubin	Aminotransferases	Alkaline Phosphatase	Albumin	Prothrombin Time
Hemolysis/Gilbert's syndrome	Normal to 86 μmol/L (5 mg/dl) 85% due to indirect fractions No bilirubinuria	Normal	Normal	Normal	Normal
Acute hepatocellular necrosis (viral and drug hepatitis, hepatotoxins, acute heart failure)	Both fractions may be elevated Peak usually follows aminotransferases Bilirubinuria	Elevated, often >500 IU ALT >AST	Normal to <3 times normal elevation	Normal	Usually normal. If >5X above control and not corrected by parenteral vitamin K, suggests poor prognosis
Chronic hepatocellular disorders	Both fractions may be elevated Bilirubinuria	Elevated, but usually <300 IU	Normal to <3 times normal elevation	Often decreased	Often prolonged Fails to correct with parenteral vitamin K
Alcoholic hepatitis Cirrhosis	Both fractions may be elevated Bilirubinuria	AST:ALT > 2 suggests alcoholic hepatitis or cirrhosis	Normal to <3 times normal elevation	Often decreased	Often prolonged Fails to correct with parenteral vitamin K
Intra- and extra-hepatic cholestasis (Obstructive jaundice)	Both fractions may be elevated Bilirubinuria	Normal to moderate elevation Rarely >500 IU	Elevated, often >4 times normal elevation	Normal, unless chronic	Normal If prolonged, will correct with parenteral vitamin K
Infiltrative diseases (tumor, granulomata); partial bile duct obstruction	Usually normal	Normal to slight elevation	Elevated, often >4 times normal elevation Fractionate, or confirm liver origin with 5' nucleotidase or gamma glutamyl transpeptidase	Normal	Normal

COAGULATION FACTORS   With the exception of factor VIII, the blood clotting factors are made exclusively in hepatocytes. Their serum half-lives are much shorter than albumin, ranging from 6 h for factor VII to 5 days for fibrinogen. Because of their rapid turnover, measurement of the clotting factors is the single best acute measure of hepatic synthetic function and helpful in both the diagnosis and assessing the prognosis of acute parenchymal liver disease. Useful for this purpose is the *serum prothrombin time*, which collectively measures factors II, V, VII, and X. Biosynthesis of factors II, VII, IX, and X depends on vitamin K. The prothrombin time may be elevated in hepatitis and cirrhosis as well as in disorders that lead to vitamin K deficiency such as obstructive jaundice or fat malabsorption of any kind. Marked prolongation of the prothrombin time, >5 s above control and not corrected by parenteral vitamin K administration, is a poor prognostic sign in acute viral hepatitis and other acute and chronic liver diseases.

OTHER DIAGNOSTIC TESTS   While tests may direct the physician to a category of liver disease, additional radiologic testing and procedures are often necessary to make the proper diagnosis, as shown in Fig. 283-1. The two most commonly used ancillary tests are reviewed here.

Percutaneous Liver Biopsy   Percutaneous biopsy of the liver is a safe procedure that can be easily performed at the bedside with local anesthesia. Liver biopsy is of proven value in the following situations: (1) hepatocellular disease of uncertain cause, (2) prolonged hepatitis with the possibility of chronic active hepatitis, (3) unexplained hepatomegaly, (4) unexplained splenomegaly, (5) hepatic filling defects by radiologic imaging, (6) fever of unknown origin, (7) staging of malignant lymphoma. Liver biopsy is most accurate in disorders causing diffuse changes throughout the liver and is subject to sampling error in focal infiltrative disorders such as hepatic metastases. Liver biopsy should not be the initial procedure in the diagnosis of cholestasis. The biliary tree should first be assessed for signs of obstruction.

Ultrasonography   Ultrasonography is the first diagnostic test to use in patients whose liver tests suggest cholestasis, to look for the presence of a dilated intrahepatic or extrahepatic biliary tree or to identify gallstones. In addition, it shows space-occupying lesions within the liver, enables the clinician to distinguish between cystic and solid masses, and helps direct percutaneous biopsies. Ultrasound with Doppler imaging can detect the patency of the portal vein, hepatic artery, and hepatic veins and determine the direction of blood flow. This is the first test ordered in patients suspected of having Budd-Chiari syndrome.

USE OF LIVER TESTS   As previously noted, the best way to increase the sensitivity and specificity of laboratory tests in the detection of liver disease is to employ a battery of tests that include the aminotransferases, alkaline phosphatase, bilirubin, albumin, and prothrombin time along with the judicious use of the other tests described in this chapter. Table 283-1 shows how patterns of liver tests can lead the clinician to a category of disease that will direct further evaluation. However, it is important to remember that no single set of liver tests will necessarily provide a diagnosis. It is often necessary to repeat these tests on several occasions over days to weeks for a diagnostic pattern to emerge. Figure 283-1 is an algorithm for the evaluation of chronically abnormal liver tests.

FURTHER READING

BOSMA PJ et al: The genetic basis of the reduced expression of bilirubin UDP-glucoronosyltransferase 1 in Gilbert's syndrome. N Engl J Med 333:1171, 1995

BRENSILVER HL, KAPLAN MM: Significance of elevated liver alkaline phosphatase in serum. Gastroenterology 68:1556, 1975

COHEN JA, KAPLAN MM: The SGOT/SGPT ratio: An indicator of alcoholic liver disease. Dig Dis Sci 24:835, 1979

PRATT DS, KAPLAN MM: Laboratory tests, in *Schiff's Diseases of the Liver*, 9th ed, ER Schiff et al (eds). Philadelphia, Lippincott Williams & Wilkins, 2003

WEISS JS et al: The clinical importance of a protein bound fraction of serum bilirubin in patients with hyperbilirubinemia. N Engl J Med 309:147, 1983

BILIRUBIN METABOLISM

The details of bilirubin metabolism are presented in Chap. 38, "Jaundice." However, the hyperbilirubinemias are best understood in terms of perturbations of specific aspects of bilirubin metabolism and transport, and these will be briefly reviewed here as depicted in Fig. 284-1.

Bilirubin is the end product of heme degradation. From 70 to 90% of bilirubin is derived from degradation of the hemoglobin of senescent red blood cells. Bilirubin produced in the periphery is transported to the liver within the plasma, where, due to its insolubility in aqueous solutions, it is tightly bound to albumin. Under normal circumstances, bilirubin is removed from the circulation rapidly and efficiently by hepatocytes. Transfer of bilirubin from blood to bile involves four distinct but interrelated steps (Fig. 284-1):

1. *Hepatocellular uptake*: Uptake of bilirubin by the hepatocyte has carrier-mediated kinetics. Although a number of candidate bilirubin transporters have been proposed, the actual transporter remains elusive.

2. *Intracellular binding*: Within the hepatocyte, bilirubin is kept in solution by binding as a nonsubstrate ligand to several of the glutathione-S-transferases, formerly called ligandins.

3. *Conjugation*: Bilirubin is conjugated with one or two glucuronic acid moieties by a specific UDP-glucuronosyltransferase to form bilirubin mono- and diglucuronide, respectively. Conjugation disrupts the internal hydrogen bonding that limits aqueous solubility of bilirubin, and the resulting glucuronide conjugates are highly soluble in water. Conjugation is obligatory for excretion of bilirubin across the bile canalicular membrane into bile. The UDP-glucuronosyltransferases have been classified into gene families based on the degree of homology among the mRNAs for the various isoforms. Those that conjugate bilirubin and certain other substrates have been designated the *UGT1* family. These are expressed from a single gene complex by alternative promoter usage. This gene complex contains multiple substrate-specific first exons, designated A1, A2, etc. (Fig. 284-2), each with its own promoter and each encoding the amino-terminal half of a specific isoform. In addition, there are four common exons (exons 2 to 5) that encode the shared carboxyl-terminal half of all of the *UGT1* isoforms. The various first exons encode the specific aglycone substrate–binding sites for each isoform, while the shared exons encode the binding site for the sugar donor, UDP-glucuronic acid, and the transmembrane domain. Exon A1 and the four common exons, collectively designated the *UGT1A1* gene (Fig. 284-2), encode the physiologically critical enzyme bilirubin-UDP-glucuronosyltransferase (UGT1A1). A functional corollary of the organization of the *UGT1* gene is that a mutation in one of the first exons will affect only a single enzyme isoform. By contrast, a mutation in exons 2 to 5 will alter all isoforms encoded by the *UGT1* gene complex.

4. *Biliary excretion*: Bilirubin mono- and diglucuronides are excreted across the canalicular plasma membrane into the bile canaliculus by an ATP-dependent transport process mediated by a canalicular membrane protein called *multidrug resistance–associated protein 2* (MRP2). Mutations of MRP2 result in the Dubin-Johnson syndrome (see below).

EXTRAHEPATIC ASPECTS OF BILIRUBIN DISPOSITION ■ Bilirubin in the Gut

Following secretion into bile, conjugated bilirubin reaches the duodenum and passes down the gastrointestinal tract without reabsorption by the intestinal mucosa. An appreciable fraction is converted by bacterial metabolism in the gut to the water-soluble colorless compound, urobilinogen. Urobilinogen undergoes enterohepatic cycling. Urobilinogen not taken up by the liver reaches the systemic circulation, from which some is cleared by the kidneys. Unconjugated bilirubin ordinarily does not reach the gut except in neonates or, by ill-defined alternative pathways, in the presence of severe unconjugated hyperbilirubinemia [e.g., Crigler-Najjar syndrome, type I (CN-I)]. Unconjugated bilirubin that reaches the gut is partly reabsorbed, amplifying any underlying hyperbilirubinemia.

Renal Excretion of Bilirubin Conjugates Unconjugated bilirubin is not excreted in urine as it is too tightly bound to albumin for effective glomerular filtration and there is no tubular mechanism for its renal secretion. In contrast, the bilirubin conjugates are readily filtered at the glomerulus and can appear in urine in disorders characterized by increased bilirubin conjugates in the circulation.

DISORDERS OF BILIRUBIN METABOLISM LEADING TO UNCONJUGATED HYPERBILIRUBINEMIA

INCREASED BILIRUBIN PRODUCTION ■ Hemolysis Increased destruction of erythrocytes leads to increased bilirubin turnover and unconjugated hyperbilirubinemia; the hyperbilirubinemia is usually modest in the presence of normal liver function. In particular, the bone marrow is only capable of a sustained eightfold increase in erythrocyte production in response to a hemolytic stress. Therefore, hemolysis alone cannot result in a sustained hyperbilirubinemia of more than approximately 68 μmol/L (4 mg/dL). Higher values imply concomitant hepatic dysfunction. When hemolysis is the only abnormality in an otherwise healthy individual, the result is a purely unconjugated hyperbilirubinemia, with the direct-reacting fraction as measured in a typical clinical laboratory being ≤15% of the total serum bilirubin. In the presence of systemic disease, which may include a degree of hepatic dysfunction, hemolysis may produce a component of conjugated hyperbilirubinemia in addition to an elevated unconjugated bilirubin concentration. Prolonged hemolysis may lead to the precipitation of bilirubin salts within the gall bladder or biliary tree, resulting in the formation of gallstones in which bilirubin, rather than cholesterol, is the major component. Such pigment stones may lead to acute or chronic cholecystitis, biliary obstruction, or any other biliary tract consequence of calculous disease.

Ineffective Erythropoiesis During erythroid maturation, small amounts of hemoglobin may be lost at the time of nuclear extrusion, and a fraction of developing erythroid cells is destroyed within the marrow. These processes normally account for a small proportion of bilirubin that is produced. In various disorders, including thalassemia major, megaloblastic anemias due to folate or vitamin B$_{12}$ deficiency, congenital erythropoietic porphyria, lead poisoning, and various congenital and acquired dyserythropoietic anemias, the fraction of total bilirubin production derived from ineffective erythropoiesis is increased,

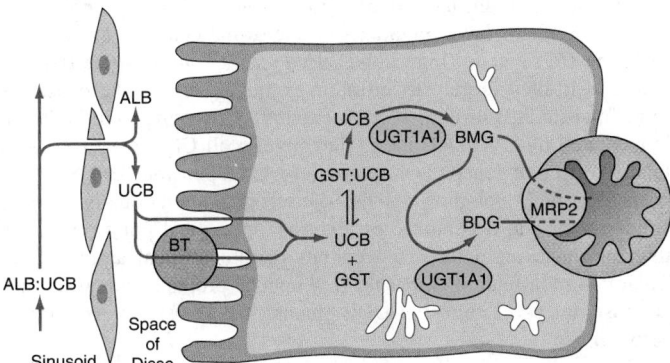

FIGURE 284-1 Hepatocellular bilirubin transport. Albumin-bound bilirubin in sinusoidal blood passes through endothelial cell fenestrae to reach the hepatocyte surface, entering the cell by both facilitated and simple diffusional processes. Within the cell it is bound to glutathione-S-transferases and conjugated by bilirubin-UDP-glucuronosyltransferase (UGT1A1) to mono- and diglucuronides, which are actively transported across the canalicular membrane into the bile. ALB, albumin; UCB, unconjugated bilirubin; UGT1A1, bilirubin-UDP-glucuronosyltransferase; BMG, bilirubin monoglucuronide; GST, glutathione-S-transferase; MRP2, multidrug resistance–associated protein 2; BDG, bilirubin diglucuronide; BT, proposed bilirubin transporter.

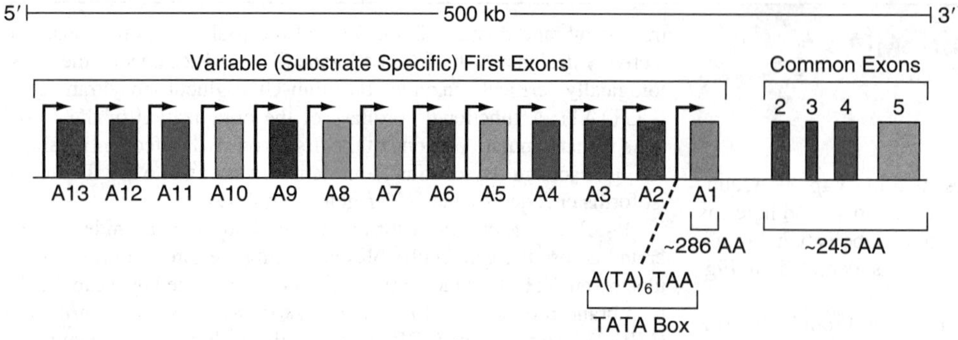

FIGURE 284-2 Structural organization of the human *UGT1* gene complex. This large complex on chromosome 2 contains at least 13 substrate-specific first exons (A1, A2, etc.). Since four of these are pseudogenes, nine UGT1 isoforms with differing substrate specificities are expressed. Each exon 1 has its own promoter and encodes the amino-terminal substrate-specific ~286 amino acids of the various *UGT1*-encoded isoforms, and common exons 2 to 5 that encode the 245 carboxyl-terminal amino acids common to all of the isoforms. mRNAs for specific isoforms are assembled by splicing a particular first exon such as the bilirubin-specific exon A1 to exons 2 to 5. The resulting message encodes a complete enzyme, in this particular case bilirubin-UDP-glucuronosyltransferase (UGT1A1). Mutations in a first exon affect only a single isoform. Those in exons 2 to 5 affect all enzymes encoded by the UGT1 complex.

reaching as much as 70% of the total. This may be sufficient to produce modest degrees of unconjugated hyperbilirubinemia.

Miscellaneous Degradation of the hemoglobin of extravascular collections of erythrocytes, such as those seen in massive tissue infarctions or large hematomas, may lead transiently to unconjugated hyperbilirubinemia.

DECREASED HEPATIC BILIRUBIN CLEARANCE ■ Decreased Hepatic Uptake Decreased hepatic bilirubin uptake is believed to contribute to the unconjugated hyperbilirubinemia of Gilbert's syndrome (GS), although the molecular basis for this finding remains unclear (see below). Several drugs, including flavaspidic acid, novobiocin, and various cholecystographic contrast agents, have been reported to inhibit bilirubin uptake. The resulting unconjugated hyperbilirubinemia resolves with cessation of the medication.

Impaired Conjugation ■ *PHYSIOLOGIC NEONATAL JAUNDICE* Bilirubin produced by the fetus is cleared by the placenta and eliminated by the maternal liver. Immediately after birth, the neonatal liver must assume responsibility for bilirubin clearance and excretion. However, many hepatic physiologic processes are incompletely developed at birth. Levels of UGT1A1 are low, and alternative excretory pathways allow passage of unconjugated bilirubin into the gut. Since the intestinal flora that convert bilirubin to urobilinogen are also undeveloped, an enterohepatic circulation of unconjugated bilirubin ensues. As a consequence, most neonates develop mild unconjugated hyperbilirubinemia between days 2 and 5 after birth. Peak levels are typically <85 to 170 μmol/L (5 to 10 mg/dL) and decline to normal adult concentrations within 2 weeks, as mechanisms required for bilirubin disposition mature. Prematurity, with more profound immaturity of hepatic function, or hemolysis, result in higher levels of unconjugated hyperbilirubinemia. A rapidly rising unconjugated bilirubin concentration, or absolute levels >340 μmol/L (20 mg/dL), puts the infant at risk for bilirubin encephalopathy, or kernicterus. Under these circumstances, bilirubin crosses an immature blood-brain barrier and precipitates in the basal ganglia and other areas of the brain. The consequences range from appreciable neurologic deficits to death. Treatment options include phototherapy, which converts bilirubin into water-soluble photoisomers that are excreted directly into bile, and exchange transfusion. The canalicular mechanisms responsible for bilirubin excretion are also immature at birth, and their maturation may lag behind that of UGT1A1; this can lead to transient conjugated neonatal hyperbilirubinemia, especially in infants with hemolysis.

ACQUIRED CONJUGATION DEFECTS A modest reduction in bilirubin-conjugating capacity may be observed in advanced hepatitis or cirrhosis. However, in this setting, conjugation is better preserved than other aspects of bilirubin disposition, such as canalicular excretion. Various drugs, including pregnanediol, novobiocin, chloramphenicol, and gentami-

cin, may produce unconjugated hyperbilirubinemia by inhibiting UGT1A1 activity. Finally, bilirubin conjugation may be inhibited by certain fatty acids that are present in breast milk but not serum of mothers whose infants have excessive neonatal hyperbilirubinemia (*breast milk jaundice*). The pathogenesis of breast milk jaundice appears to differ from that of transient familial neonatal hyperbilirubinemia (Lucey-Driscoll syndrome), in which there is a UGT1A1 inhibitor in maternal serum.

HEREDITARY DEFECTS IN BILIRUBIN CONJUGATION Three familial disorders characterized by differing degrees of unconjugated hyperbilirubinemia have long been recognized. The defining clinical features of each are described below (Table 284-1). While these disorders have been recognized for decades to reflect differing degrees of deficiency in the ability to conjugate bilirubin, recent advances in the molecular biology of the *UGT1* gene complex have elucidated their interrelationships and clarified previously puzzling features.

Crigler-Najjar Syndrome, Type I CN-I is characterized by striking unconjugated hyperbilirubinemia of about 340 to 765 μmol/L (20 to 45 mg/dL) that appears in the neonatal period and persists for life. Other conventional hepatic biochemical tests such as serum aminotransferases and alkaline phosphatase are normal, and there is no evidence of hemolysis. Hepatic histology is also essentially normal except for the occasional presence of bile plugs within canaliculi. Bilirubin glucuronides are virtually absent from the bile, and there is no detectable constitutive expression of UGT1A1 activity in hepatic tissue. Neither UGT1A1 activity nor the serum bilirubin concentration responds to administration of phenobarbital or other enzyme inducers. In the absence of conjugation, unconjugated bilirubin accumulates in plasma, from which it is eliminated very slowly by alternative pathways that include direct passage into the bile and small intestine. These account for the small amounts of urobilinogen found in feces. No bilirubin is found in the urine. First described in 1952, the disorder is rare (estimated prevalence of 0.6 to 1.0 per million). Many patients are from geographically or socially isolated communities in which consanguinity is common, and pedigree analyses show an autosomal recessive pattern of inheritance. The majority of patients (type IA) exhibit defects in the glucuronide conjugation of a spectrum of substrates in addition to bilirubin, including various drugs and other xenobiotics. These individuals have mutations in one of the common exons (2 to 5) of the *UGT1* gene (Fig. 284-2). In a smaller subset (type IB), the defect is limited largely to bilirubin conjugation, and the causative mutation is in the bilirubin-specific exon A1. Estrogen glucuronidation is mediated by UGT1A1 and is defective in all CN-I patients. More than 30 different genetic lesions of *UGT1A1* responsible for CN-I have been identified, including deletions, insertions, alterations in intronic splice donor and acceptor sites, exon skipping, and point mutations that introduce premature stop codons or alter critical amino acids. Their common feature is that they all encode proteins with absent or, at most, traces of bilirubin-UDP-glucuronosyltransferase enzymatic activity.

Prior to the availability of phototherapy, most patients with CN-I died of bilirubin encephalopathy (*kernicterus*) in infancy or early childhood. A few lived as long as early adult life without overt neurologic damage, although more subtle testing usually indicated mild but progressive brain damage. In the absence of liver transplantation, death eventually supervened from late-onset bilirubin encephalopathy, which often followed a nonspecific febrile illness. Recent data suggest that the best hope for survival of a neurologically intact patient involves the following treatment options: (1) about 12 h/d of phother-

Feature	Crigler-Najjar Syndrome Type I	Crigler-Najjar Syndrome Type II	Gilbert's Syndrome
Total serum bilirubin, μmol/L [mg/dL]	310–755 (usually >345) [18–45 (usually >20)]	100–430 (usually ≤345) [6–25 (usually ≤20)]	Typically ≤70 μmol/L [≤4 mg/dL] in absence of fasting or hemolysis
Routine liver tests	Normal	Normal	Normal
Response to phenobarbital	None	Decreases bilirubin by >25%	Decreases bilirubin to normal
Kernicterus	Usual	Rare	No
Hepatic histology	Normal	Normal	Usually normal; increased lipofuscin pigment in some
Bile characteristics			
Color:	Pale or colorless	Pigmented	Normal dark color
Bilirubin fractions:	>90% unconjugated	Largest fraction (mean:57%) monoconjugates	Mainly diconjugates but monoconjugates increased (mean 23%)
Bilirubin UDP-glucuronosyl-transferase activity	Typically absent; traces in some patients	Markedly reduced: 0 to 10% of normal	Reduced: typically 10–33% of normal
Inheritance (all autosomal)	Recessive	Predominantly recessive	Promoter mutation: recessive. Missense mutations: 7 of 8 dominant; 1 reportedly recessive

apy from birth throughout childhood, perhaps supplemented by exchange transfusion in the immediate neonatal period; (2) use of tin-protoporphyrin, an inhibitor of heme oxygenase, to blunt transient exacerbations of hyperbilirubinemia; (3) oral administration of a combination of calcium phosphate and calcium carbonate to sequester unconjugated bilirubin in the gut; and (4) liver transplantation prior to the onset of brain damage. In a single patient, transplantation with isolated allogeneic hepatocytes produced a clinically significant reduction in serum bilirubin concentration.

Crigler-Najjar Syndrome, Type II (CN-II) This condition was recognized as a distinct entity in 1962 and is characterized by marked unconjugated hyperbilirubinemia in the absence of abnormalities of other conventional hepatic biochemical tests, hepatic histology, or hemolysis. It differs from CN-I in several specific ways (Table 284-1): (1) Although there is considerable overlap, average bilirubin concentrations are lower in CN-II; (2) accordingly, CN-II is only infrequently associated with kernicterus; (3) bile is deeply colored, and bilirubin glucuronides are present, with a striking, characteristic increase in the proportion of monoglucuronides; (4) UGT1A1 in liver is usually present at reduced levels (typically ≤10% of normal) but may be undetectable by older, less sensitive assays; (5) while typically detected in infancy, hyperbilirubinemia was not recognized in some cases until later in life and, in one instance, at age 34. As with CN-I, most CN-II cases exhibit abnormalities in the conjugation of other compounds, such as salicylamide and menthol, but in some instances the defect appears limited to bilirubin. Reduction of serum bilirubin concentrations by >25% in response to enzyme inducers such as phenobarbital distinguishes CN-II from CN-I, although this response may not be elicited in early infancy and often is not accompanied by measurable UGT1A1 induction. Bilirubin concentrations during phenobarbital administration do not return to normal but are typically in the range of 51 to 86 μmol/L (3 to 5 mg/dL). Although the incidence of kernicterus in CN-II is low, instances have occurred, not only in infants but also in adolescents and adults, often in the setting of an intercurrent illness, fasting, or another factor that temporarily raises the serum bilirubin concentration above baseline and reduces serum albumin levels. For this reason, phenobarbital therapy is widely recommended, a single bedtime dose often sufficing to maintain clinically safe plasma bilirubin concentrations.

At least 10 different mutations of *UGT1* have been identified that are associated with CN-II. Their common feature is that they encode for a bilirubin-UDP-glucuronosyltransferase with markedly reduced but detectable enzymatic activity. The spectrum of residual enzyme activity explains the spectrum of phenotypic severity of the resulting hyperbilirubinemia. Molecular analysis has established that a large majority of CN-II patients are either homozygotes or compound het-

erozygotes for CN-II mutations and that individuals carrying one mutated and one entirely normal allele have normal bilirubin concentrations. Possible inheritance of a dominant negative mutation in one case remains to be confirmed.

Gilbert's Syndrome This syndrome is characterized by mild unconjugated hyperbilirubinemia, normal values for standard hepatic biochemical tests, and normal hepatic histology other than a modest increase of lipofuscin pigment in some patients. Serum bilirubin concentrations are most often <51 μmol/L (<3 mg/dL), although both higher and lower values are frequent. The clinical spectrum of hyperbilirubinemia fades into that of CN-II at serum bilirubin concentrations of 86 to 136 μmol/L (5 to 8 mg/dL). At the other end of the scale, the distinction between mild cases of GS and a normal state is often blurred. Bilirubin concentrations may fluctuate substantially in any given individual, and at least 25% of patients will exhibit temporarily normal values during prolonged follow-up. More elevated values are associated with stress, fatigue, alcohol use, reduced caloric intake, and intercurrent illness, while increased caloric intake or administration of enzyme-inducing agents produce lower bilirubin levels. GS is most often diagnosed at or shortly after puberty or in adult life during routine examinations that include multichannel biochemical analyses. UGT1A1 activity is typically reduced to 10 to 35% of normal, and bile pigments exhibit a characteristic increase in bilirubin monoglucuronides. Studies of radiobilirubin kinetics indicate that hepatic bilirubin clearance is reduced to an average of one-third of normal. Administration of phenobarbital normalizes both the serum bilirubin concentration and hepatic bilirubin clearance; however, failure of UGT1A1 activity to improve in many such instances suggests the possible coexistence of an additional defect. Compartmental analysis of bilirubin kinetic data suggests that GS patients have a defect in bilirubin uptake as well as in conjugation. Defect(s) in the hepatic uptake of other organic anions that at least partially share an uptake mechanism with bilirubin, such as sulfobromophthalein and indocyanine green (ICG), are observed in a minority of patients. The metabolism and transport of bile acids, which do not utilize the bilirubin uptake mechanism, are normal. The magnitude of changes in the plasma bilirubin concentration induced by provocation tests such as 48 h of fasting or the intravenous administration of nicotinic acid have been reported to be of help in separating GS patients from normal individuals. Other studies dispute this assertion. Moreover, on theoretical grounds, the results of such studies should provide no more information than simple measurements of the baseline plasma bilirubin concentration. Family studies indicate that GS and hereditary hemolytic anemias such as hereditary spherocytosis, glucose-6-phosphate dehydrogenase deficiency, and β-thalassemia trait sort independently. Reports of hemolysis in up to 50% of GS patients are believed to reflect better case finding, since patients with both GS and hemolysis have higher bilirubin concentrations, and are more likely to be jaundiced, than patients with either defect alone.

GS is common, with many series placing its prevalence at ≥8%. Males predominate over females by reported ratios ranging from 1.5:1 to >7:1. However, these ratios may have a large artifactual component since normal males have higher mean bilirubin levels than normal females, but the diagnosis of GS is often based on comparison to normal ranges established in men. The high prevalence of GS in the general population may explain the reported frequency of mild unconjugated hyperbilirubinemia in liver transplant recipients. The disposition of most xenobiotics metabolized by glucuronidation appears to be normal in GS, as is oxidative drug metabolism in the majority of reported studies. The principal exception is the metabolism of the antitumor agent irinotecan (CPT-11), whose active metabolite (SN-38) is glucuronidated specifically by bilirubin-UDP-glucuronosyltransferase. Administration of CPT-11 to patients with GS has resulted in several toxicities, including intractable diarrhea and myelosuppression. Some reports also suggest abnormal disposition of menthol, estradiol benzoate, acetaminophen, tolbutamide, and rifamycin SV. Although some of these studies have been disputed, and there have been no reports of clinical complications from use of these agents in GS, prudence should be exercised in prescribing them, or any agents metabolized primarily by glucuronidation, in this condition.

Most older pedigree studies of GS were consistent with autosomal dominant inheritance with variable expressivity. However, studies of the *UGT1* gene in GS have indicated a variety of molecular genetic bases for the phenotypic picture and several different patterns of inheritance. Studies in Europe and the United States found that nearly all patients had normal coding regions for UGT1A1 but were homozygous for the insertion of an extra TA (i.e., A[TA]$_7$TAA rather than A[TA]$_6$TAA) in the promoter region of the first exon. This appeared to be necessary, but not sufficient, for clinically expressed GS, since 15% of normal controls were also homozygous for this variant. While normal by standard criteria, these individuals had somewhat higher bilirubin concentrations than the rest of the controls studied. Heterozygotes for this abnormality had bilirubin concentrations identical to those homozygous for the A[TA]$_6$TAA allele. The prevalence of the A[TA]$_7$TAA allele in a general western population is 30%, in which case 9% would be homozygotes. This is slightly higher than the prevalence of GS based on purely phenotypic parameters. It was suggested that additional variables, such as mild hemolysis or a defect in bilirubin uptake, might be among the factors enhancing phenotypic expression of the defect.

Phenotypic expression of GS due solely to the A[TA]$_7$TAA promoter abnormality is inherited as an autosomal recessive trait. A number of CN-II kindreds have been identified in which there is also an allele containing a normal coding region but the A[TA]$_7$TAA promoter abnormality. CN-II heterozygotes who have the A[TA]$_6$TAA promoter are phenotypically normal, whereas those with the A[TA]$_7$TAA promoter express the phenotypic picture of GS. GS in such kindreds may also result from homozygosity for the A[TA]$_7$TAA promoter abnormality. Seven different missense mutations in the *UGT1* gene that reportedly cause GS with dominant inheritance have been found in Japanese individuals. Another Japanese patient with mild unconjugated hyperbilirubinemia was homozygous for a missense mutation in exon 5. GS in her family appeared to be recessive. Missense mutations causing GS have not been reported outside of certain Asian populations.

DISORDERS OF BILIRUBIN METABOLISM LEADING TO MIXED OR PREDOMINANTLY CONJUGATED HYPERBILIRUBINEMIA

In hyperbilirubinemia due to acquired liver disease (e.g., acute hepatitis, common bile duct stone), there are usually elevations in the serum concentrations of both conjugated and unconjugated bilirubin. Although biliary tract obstruction or hepatocellular cholestatic injury may present on occasion with a predominantly conjugated hyperbilirubinemia, it is generally not possible to differentiate intrahepatic from extrahepatic causes of jaundice based upon the serum levels or relative proportions of unconjugated and conjugated bilirubin. The major reason for determining the amounts of conjugated and unconjugated bilirubin in the serum is for the initial differentiation of hepatic parenchymal and obstructive disorders (mixed conjugated and unconjugated hyperbilirubinemia) from the inheritable and hemolytic disorders discussed above that are associated with unconjugated hyperbilirubinemia.

FAMILIAL DEFECTS IN HEPATIC EXCRETORY FUNCTION ■ Dubin-Johnson Syndrome (DJS)

This benign, relatively rare disorder is characterized by low-grade, predominantly conjugated hyperbilirubinemia (Table 284-2). Total bilirubin concentrations are typically between 34 and 85 μmol/L (2 and 5 mg/dL) but on occasion can be in the normal range or as high as 340 to 430 μmol/L (20 to 25 mg/dL) and can fluctuate widely in any given patient. The degree of hyperbilirubinemia may be increased by intercurrent illness, oral contraceptive use, and pregnancy. As the hyperbilirubinemia is due to a predominant rise in conjugated bilirubin, bilirubinuria is characteristically present. Aside from elevated serum bilirubin levels, other routine laboratory tests are normal. Physical examination is usually normal except for jaundice, although an occasional patient may have hepatosplenomegaly.

Patients with DJS are usually asymptomatic, although some may have vague constitutional symptoms. These latter patients have usually undergone extensive and often unnecessary diagnostic examinations for unexplained jaundice and have high levels of anxiety. In women, the condition may be subclinical until the patient becomes pregnant

TABLE 284-2 *Principal Differential Characteristics of Inheritable Disorders of Bile Canalicular Function*

	DJS	Rotor	PFIC1	BRIC	PFIC2	PFIC3
Gene	*ABCCA*	?	*ATP8B1*	*ATP8B1*	*ABCB11*	*ABCB4*
Protein	MRP2	?	FIC1	FIC1	BSEP	MDR3
Cholestasis	No	No	Yes	Episodic	Yes	Yes
Serum γ-GT	Normal	Normal	Normal	Normal	Normal	↑↑
Serum bile acids	Normal	Normal	↑↑	↑↑ during episodes	↑↑	↑↑
Clinical features	Mild conjugated hyperbilirubinemia; otherwise normal liver function; dark pigment in liver; characteristic pattern of urinary coproporphyrins	Mild conjugated hyperbilirubinemia; otherwise normal liver function; liver without abnormal pigmentation	Severe cholestasis beginning in childhood	Recurrent episodes of cholestasis beginning at any age	Severe cholestasis beginning in childhood	Severe cholestasis beginning in childhood; decreased phospholipids in bile

Note: DJS, Dubin-Johnson syndrome; PFIC, progressive familial intrahepatic cholestasis; MRP2, multidrug resistance–associated protein 2; BSEP, bile salt excretory protein; γ-GT, γ-glutamyltransferase; ↑↑, increased.

or receives oral contraceptives, at which time chemical hyperbilirubinemia becomes frank jaundice. Even in these situations, other routine liver function tests, including serum alkaline phosphatase and transaminase activities, are normal.

A cardinal feature of DJS is the accumulation in the lysosomes of centrilobular hepatocytes of dark, coarsely granular pigment. As a result, the liver may be grossly black in appearance. This pigment is thought to be derived from epinephrine metabolites that are not excreted normally. The pigment may disappear during bouts of viral hepatitis, only to reaccumulate slowly after recovery.

Biliary excretion of a number of anionic compounds is compromised in DJS. These include various cholecystographic agents, as well as sulfobromophthalein (Bromsulphalein, BSP), a synthetic dye formerly used in a test of liver function. In this test, the rate of disappearance of BSP from plasma was determined following bolus intravenous administration. BSP is conjugated with glutathione in the hepatocyte; the resulting conjugate is normally excreted rapidly into the bile canaliculus. Patients with DJS exhibit a characteristic rise in its plasma concentration at 90 min after injection, due to reflux of conjugated BSP into the circulation from the hepatocyte. Dyes such as ICG that are taken up by hepatocytes but are not further metabolized prior to biliary excretion do not show this reflux phenomenon. Continuous BSP infusion studies suggest a reduction in the t_{max} for biliary excretion. Bile acid disposition, including hepatocellular uptake and biliary excretion, is normal in DJS. These patients have normal serum and biliary bile acid concentrations and do not have pruritus.

By analogy with findings in several mutant rat strains, the selective defect in biliary excretion of bilirubin conjugates and certain other classes of organic compounds, but not of bile acids, that characterizes DJS in humans was found to reflect defective expression of MRP2, an ATP-dependent canalicular membrane transporter. Several different mutations in the *MRP2* gene produce the Dubin-Johnson phenotype, which has an autosomal recessive pattern of inheritance. Although MRP2 is undoubtedly important in the biliary excretion of conjugated bilirubin, the fact that this pigment is still excreted in the absence of MRP2 suggests that other, as yet uncharacterized, transport proteins may serve in a secondary role in this process.

Patients with DJS also have a diagnostic abnormality in urinary coproporphyrin excretion. There are two naturally occurring coproporphyrin isomers, I and III. Normally, approximately 75% of the coproporphyrin in urine is isomer III. In urine from DJS patients, total coproporphyrin content is normal, but >80% is isomer I. Heterozygotes for the syndrome show an intermediate pattern. The molecular basis for this phenomenon remains unclear.

Rotor Syndrome   This benign, autosomal recessive disorder is clinically similar to DJS (Table 284-2), although it is seen even less frequently. A major phenotypic difference is that the liver in patients with Rotor syndrome has no increased pigmentation and appears totally normal. The only abnormality in routine laboratory tests is an elevation of total serum bilirubin, due to a predominant rise in conjugated bilirubin. This is accompanied by bilirubinuria. Several additional features differentiate Rotor syndrome and DJS. In Rotor syndrome, the gallbladder is usually visualized on oral cholecystography, in contrast to the nonvisualization that is typical of DJS. The pattern of urinary coproporphyrin excretion also differs. The pattern in Rotor syndrome resembles that of many acquired disorders of hepatobiliary function, in which coproporphyrin I, the major coproporphyrin isomer in bile, refluxes from the hepatocyte back into the circulation and is excreted in urine. Thus, total urinary coproporphyrin excretion is substantially increased in Rotor syndrome, in contrast to the normal levels seen in DJS. Although the fraction of coproporphyrin I in urine is elevated, it is usually <70% of the total, as compared to 80% or more in DJS. The disorders also can be distinguished by their patterns of BSP excretion. Although clearance of BSP from plasma is delayed in Rotor syndrome, there is no reflux of conjugated BSP back into the circulation as seen in DJS. Kinetic analysis of plasma BSP infusion studies suggests the presence

of a defect in intrahepatocellular storage of this compound. This has never been demonstrated directly, and the molecular basis of Rotor syndrome remains unknown.

Benign Recurrent Intrahepatic Cholestasis (BRIC)   This rare disorder is characterized by recurrent attacks of pruritus and jaundice. The typical episode begins with mild malaise and elevations in serum aminotransferase levels, followed rapidly by rises in alkaline phosphatase and conjugated bilirubin and onset of jaundice and itching. The first one or two episodes may be misdiagnosed as acute viral hepatitis. The cholestatic episodes, which may begin in childhood or adulthood, can vary in duration from several weeks to months, following which there is complete clinical and biochemical resolution. Intervals between attacks may vary from several months to years. Between episodes, physical examination is normal, as are serum levels of bile acids, bilirubin, transaminases, and alkaline phosphatase. The disorder is familial and has an autosomal recessive pattern of inheritance. BRIC is considered a benign disorder in that it does not lead to cirrhosis or end-stage liver disease. However, the episodes of jaundice and pruritus can be prolonged and debilitating, and some patients have undergone liver transplantation to relieve the intractable and disabling symptoms. Treatment during the cholestatic episodes is symptomatic; there is no specific treatment to prevent or shorten the occurrence of episodes.

A gene termed *FIC1* was recently identified and found to be mutated in patients with BRIC. Curiously, this gene is expressed strongly in the small intestine but only weakly in the liver. The protein encoded by *FIC1* shows little similarity to genes that have been shown to play a role in bile canalicular excretion of various compounds. Rather, it appears to be a member of a P-type ATPase family that transports aminophospholipids from the outer to the inner leaflet of a variety of cell membranes. Its relationship to the pathobiology of this disorder remains unclear.

Progressive Familial Intrahepatic Cholestasis (FIC)   This name is applied to three phenotypically related syndromes (Table 284-2). Progressive FIC type 1 (Byler disease) presents in early infancy as cholestasis that may be initially episodic. However, in contrast to BRIC, Byler disease progresses to malnutrition, growth retardation, and end-stage liver disease during childhood. This disorder is also a consequence of a *FIC1* mutation. The functional relationship of the FIC1 protein to the pathogenesis of cholestasis in these disorders is unknown. Two other types of progressive FIC (types 2 and 3) have been described. Type 2 is associated with a mutation in the protein named *sister of p-glycoprotein*, which is the major bile canalicular exporter of bile acids and is also known as *bile salt excretory protein* (BSEP). Type 3 has been associated with a mutation of MDR3, a protein that is essential for normal hepatocellular excretion of phospholipids across the bile canaliculus. Although all three types of progressive FIC have similar clinical phenotypes, only type 3 is associated with high serum levels of γ-glutamyltransferase activity. In contrast, activity of this enzyme is normal or only mildly elevated in symptomatic BRIC and progressive FIC types 1 and 2.

FURTHER READING

BOSMA P et al: The genetic basis of the reduced expression of bilirubin-UDP-glucuronosyltransferase 1 in Gilbert's syndrome. N Engl J Med 333:1171, 1995

IYANAGI T et al: Biochemical and molecular aspects of genetic disorders of bilirubin metabolism. Biochim Biophys Acta 1407:173, 1998

JANSEN PL: Diagnosis and management of Crigler-Najjar syndrome. Eur J Pediatr 158:S89, 1999

ROY CHOWDHURY J et al: Hereditary jaundice and disorders of bilirubin metabolism, in *The Metabolic and Molecular Bases of Inherited Disease*, 8th ed. CR Scriver et al (eds.) New York, McGraw-Hill, 2001, pp 3063–3101

THOMPSON R et al: Genetic defects in hepatocanalicular transport. Semin Liver Dis 20:365, 2000

Acute viral hepatitis is a systemic infection affecting the liver predominantly. Almost all cases of acute viral hepatitis are caused by one of five viral agents: hepatitis A virus (HAV), hepatitis B virus (HBV), hepatitis C virus (HCV), the HBV-associated delta agent or hepatitis D virus (HDV), and hepatitis E virus (HEV). Other transfusion-transmitted agents, e.g., "hepatitis G" virus and "TT" virus, have been identified but do not cause hepatitis. All these human hepatitis viruses are RNA viruses, except for hepatitis B, which is a DNA virus. Although these agents can be distinguished by their molecular and antigenic properties, all types of viral hepatitis produce clinically similar illnesses. These range from asymptomatic and inapparent to fulminant and fatal acute infections common to all types, on the one hand, and from subclinical persistent infections to rapidly progressive chronic liver disease with cirrhosis and even hepatocellular carcinoma, common to the bloodborne types (HBV, HCV, and HDV), on the other.

VIROLOGY AND ETIOLOGY ■ Hepatitis A Hepatitis A virus is a nonenveloped 27-nm, heat-, acid-, and ether-resistant RNA virus in the hepatovirus genus of the picornavirus family (Fig. 285-1). Its virion contains four capsid polypeptides, designated VP1 to VP4, which are cleaved posttranslationally from the polyprotein product of a 7500-nucleotide genome. Inactivation of viral activity can be achieved by boiling for 1 min, by contact with formaldehyde and chlorine, or by ultraviolet irradiation. Despite nucleotide sequence variation of up to 20% among isolates of HAV, all strains of this virus are immunologically indistinguishable and belong to one serotype. Hepatitis A has an incubation period of approximately 4 weeks. Its replication is limited to the liver, but the virus is present in the liver, bile, stools, and blood during the late incubation period and acute preicteric phase of illness. Despite persistence of virus in the liver, viral shedding in feces, viremia, and infectivity diminish rapidly once jaundice becomes apparent. HAV can be cultivated reproducibly in vitro.

Antibodies to HAV (anti-HAV) can be detected during acute illness when serum aminotransferase activity is elevated and fecal HAV shedding is still occurring. This early antibody response is predominantly of the IgM class and persists for several months, rarely for 6 to 12 months. During convalescence, however, anti-HAV of the IgG class becomes the predominant antibody (Fig. 285-2). Therefore, the diagnosis of hepatitis A is made during acute illness by demonstrating anti-HAV of the IgM class. After acute illness, anti-HAV of the IgG class remains detectable indefinitely, and patients with serum anti-HAV are immune to reinfection. Neutralizing antibody activity parallels the appearance of anti-HAV, and the IgG anti-HAV present in immune globulin accounts for the protection it affords against HAV infection.

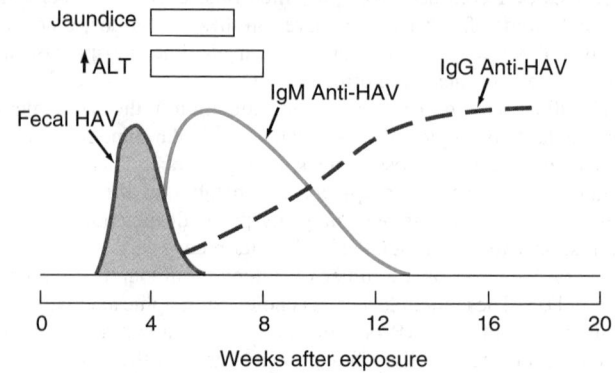

FIGURE 285-2 Scheme of typical clinical and laboratory features of viral hepatitis A.

Hepatitis B Hepatitis B virus is a DNA virus with a remarkably compact genomic structure; despite its small, circular, 3200-basepair size, HBV DNA codes for four sets of viral products with a complex, multiparticle structure. HBV achieves its genomic economy by relying on an efficient strategy of encoding proteins from four overlapping genes: S, C, P, and X (Fig. 285-3), as detailed below. Once thought to be unique among viruses, HBV is now recognized as one of a family of animal viruses, hepadnaviruses (hepatotropic DNA viruses), and is classified as hepadnavirus type 1. Similar viruses infect certain species of woodchucks, ground and tree squirrels, and Pekin ducks, to mention the most carefully characterized. Like HBV, all have the same distinctive three morphologic forms, have counterparts to the envelope and nucleocapsid virus antigens of HBV, replicate in the liver but exist in extrahepatic sites, contain their own endogenous DNA polymerase, have partially double-stranded and partially single-stranded genomes, are associated with acute and chronic hepatitis and hepatocellular carcinoma, and rely on a replicative strategy unique among DNA viruses but typical of retroviruses. Instead of DNA replication directly from a DNA template, hepadnaviruses rely on reverse transcription (effected by the DNA polymerase) of minus-strand DNA from a "pregenomic" RNA intermediate. Then plus-strand DNA is transcribed from the minus-strand DNA template by the DNA-dependent DNA polymerase and converted in the hepatocyte nucleus to a covalently closed circular DNA, which serves as a template for messenger RNA and pregenomic RNA. Viral proteins are translated by the messenger RNA, and the proteins and genome are packaged into virions and secreted from the hepatocyte. Although HBV is difficult to cultivate in vitro in the conventional sense from clinical material, several cell lines have been transfected with HBV DNA. Such transfected cells support in vitro replication of the intact virus and its component proteins.

VIRAL PROTEINS AND PARTICLES Of the three particulate forms of HBV (Table 285-1), the most numerous are the 22-nm particles, which appear as spherical or long filamentous forms; these are antigenically indistinguishable from the outer surface or envelope protein of HBV and are thought to represent excess viral envelope protein. Outnumbered in serum by a factor of 100 or 1000 to 1 compared with the spheres and tubules are large, 42-nm, double-shelled spherical particles, which represent the intact hepatitis B virion (Fig. 285-1) . The envelope protein expressed on the outer surface of the virion and on the smaller spherical and tubular structures is referred to as *hepatitis B surface antigen* (HBsAg). The concentration of HBsAg and virus particles in the blood may reach 500 μg/mL and 10 trillion particles per milliliter, respectively. The envelope protein, HBsAg, is the product of the S gene of HBV.

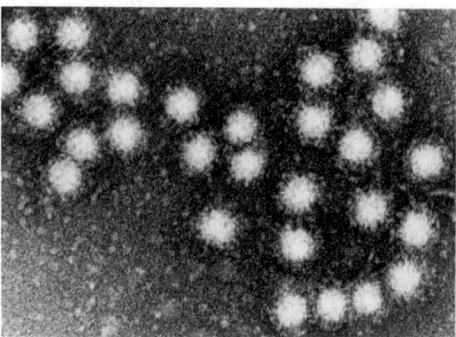 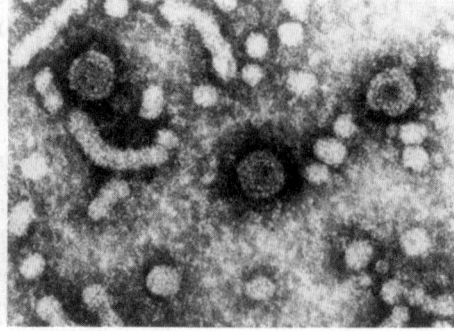

FIGURE 285-1 *Left.* Electron micrograph of 27-nm hepatitis A virus particles purified from stool of a patient with acute hepatitis A virus infection and aggregated by hepatitis A antibody. *Right.* Electron micrograph of concentrated serum from a patient with hepatitis B infection, demonstrating the 42-nm virions, tubular forms, and spherical 22-nm particles of hepatitis B surface antigen. 132,000×. (Hepatitis D resembles 42-nm virions of hepatitis B but is smaller, 35 to 37 nm; hepatitis E resembles hepatitis A virus but is slightly larger, 32 to 34 nm; hepatitis C has not been visualized definitively.)

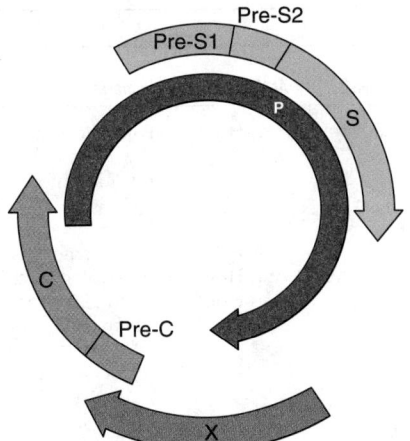

FIGURE 285-3 Its compact genomic structure, with overlapping genes, permits HBV to code for multiple proteins. The S gene codes for the "major" envelope protein, HBsAg. Pre-S1 and pre-S2, upstream of S, combine with S to code for two larger proteins, "middle" protein, the product of pre-S2 + S, and "large" protein, the product of pre-S1 + pre-S2 + S. The largest gene, P, codes for DNA polymerase. The C gene codes for two nucleocapsid proteins, HBeAg, a soluble, secreted protein (initiation from the pre-C region of the gene) and HBcAg, the intracellular core protein (initiation after pre-C). The X gene codes for HBxAg, which can transactivate the transcription of cellular and viral genes; its clinical relevance is not known, but it may contribute to carcinogenesis by binding to p53.

A number of different HBsAg subdeterminants have been identified. There is a common group-reactive antigen, *a*, shared by all HBsAg isolates. In addition, HBsAg may contain one of several subtype-specific antigens, namely, *d* or *y*, *w* or *r*, as well as other more recently characterized specificities. Hepatitis B isolates fall into one of at least eight subtypes and seven genotypes (A–G). Geographic distribution of genotypes and subtypes varies; genotypes A (corresponding to subtype *adw* and D (*ayw*) predominate in the United States and Europe, while genotypes B (*adw*) and C (*adr*) predominate in Asia. Clinical course and outcome are independent of subtype, but preliminary reports suggest that genotype B is associated with less rapidly progressive liver disease and a lower likelihood, or delayed appearance, of hepatocellular carcinoma than genotype C. In addition, "precore" mutations are favored by certain genotypes (see below).

Upstream of the S gene are the pre-S genes (Fig. 285-3), which code for pre-S gene products, including receptors on the HBV surface for polymerized human serum albumin and for hepatocyte membrane proteins. The pre-S region actually consists of both pre-S1 and pre-S2. Depending on where translation is initiated, three potential HBsAg gene products are synthesized. The protein product of the S gene is HBsAg (*major protein*), the product of the S region plus the adjacent pre-S2 region is the *middle protein*, and the product of the pre-S1 plus pre-S2 plus S regions is the *large protein*. Compared with the smaller spherical and tubular particles of HBV, complete 42-nm virions are enriched in the large protein. Both pre-S proteins and their respective antibodies can be detected during HBV infection, and the period of pre-S antigenemia appears to coincide with other markers of virus replication, as detailed below.

The intact 42-nm virion contains a 27-nm nucleocapsid core particle. Nucleocapsid proteins are coded for by the C gene. The antigen expressed on the surface of the nucleocapsid core is referred to as *hepatitis B core antigen* (HBcAg), and its corresponding antibody is anti-HBc. A third HBV antigen is *hepatitis B e antigen* (HBeAg), a soluble, nonparticulate, nucleocapsid protein that is immunologically distinct from intact HBcAg but is a product of the same C gene. The C gene has two initiation codons, a precore and a core region (Fig. 285-3). If translation is initiated at the precore region, the protein product is HBeAg, which has a signal peptide that binds it to the smooth endoplasmic reticulum and leads to its secretion into the circulation. If translation begins with the core region, HBcAg is the protein product; it has no signal peptide, it is not secreted, but it assembles into

nucleocapsid particles, which bind to and incorporate RNA and which, ultimately, contain HBV DNA. Also packaged within the nucleocapsid core is a DNA polymerase, which directs replication and repair of HBV DNA. When packaging within viral proteins is complete, synthesis of the incomplete plus strand stops; this accounts for the single-stranded gap and for differences in the size of the gap. HBcAg particles remain in the hepatocyte, where they are readily detectable by immunohistochemical staining, and are exported after encapsidation by an envelope of HBsAg. Therefore, naked core particles do not circulate in the serum. The secreted nucleocapsid protein, HBeAg, provides a convenient, readily detectable, qualitative marker of HBV replication and relative infectivity.

HBsAg-positive serum containing HBeAg is more likely to be highly infectious and to be associated with the presence of hepatitis B virions (and detectable HBV DNA, see below) than HBeAg-negative or anti-HBe-positive serum. For example, HBsAg carrier mothers who are HBeAg-positive almost invariably (>90%) transmit hepatitis B infection to their offspring, whereas HBsAg carrier mothers with anti-HBe rarely (10 to 15%) infect their offspring.

Early during the course of acute hepatitis B, HBeAg appears transiently; its disappearance may be a harbinger of clinical improvement and resolution of infection. Persistence of HBeAg in serum beyond the first 3 months of acute infection may be predictive of the development of chronic infection, and the presence of HBeAg during chronic hepatitis B is associated with ongoing viral replication, infectivity, and inflammatory liver injury.

The third of the HBV genes is the largest, the P gene (Fig. 285-3), which codes for the DNA polymerase; as noted above, this enzyme has both DNA-dependent DNA polymerase and RNA-dependent reverse transcriptase activities. The fourth gene, X, codes for a small, nonparticulate protein, hepatitis B x antigen (HBxAg), that is capable of transactivating the transcription of both viral and cellular genes (Fig. 285-3). In the cytoplasm, HBxAg effects calcium release (possibly from mitochrondria), which activates signal-transduction pathways that lead to stimulation of HBV reverse transcription and HBV DNA replication. Such transactivation may enhance the replication of HBV, leading to the clinical association observed between the expression of HBxAg and antibodies to it in patients with severe chronic hepatitis and hepatocellular carcinoma. The transactivating activity can enhance the transcription and replication of other viruses besides HBV, such as HIV. Cellular processes transactivated by X include the human interferon γ gene and class I major histocompatibility genes; potentially, these effects could contribute to enhanced susceptibility of HBV-infected hepatocytes to cytolytic T cells. The expression of X can also induce programmed cell death (apoptosis).

SEROLOGIC AND VIROLOGIC MARKERS After a person is infected with HBV, the first virologic marker detectable in serum is HBsAg (Fig. 285-4). Circulating HBsAg precedes elevations of serum aminotransferase activity and clinical symptoms and remains detectable during the entire icteric or symptomatic phase of acute hepatitis B and beyond. In typical cases, HBsAg becomes undetectable 1 to 2 months after the onset of jaundice and rarely persists beyond 6 months. After HBsAg disappears, antibody to HBsAg (anti-HBs) becomes detectable in serum and remains detectable indefinitely thereafter. Because HBcAg is sequestered within an HBsAg coat, HBcAg is not detectable routinely in the serum of patients with HBV infection. By contrast, anti-HBc is readily demonstrable in serum, beginning within the first 1 to 2 weeks after the appearance of HBsAg and preceding detectable levels of anti-HBs by weeks to months. Because variability exists in the time of appearance of anti-HBs after HBV infection, occasionally a gap of several weeks or longer may separate the disappearance of HBsAg and the appearance of anti-HBs. During this "gap" or "window" period, anti-HBc may represent serologic evidence of current or recent HBV infection, and blood containing anti-HBc in the absence of HBsAg and anti-HBs has been implicated in the development of transfusion-as-

TABLE 285-1 *Nomenclature and Features of Hepatitis Viruses*

Hepatitis Type	Virus Particle	Morphology	Genome[a]	Classification	Antigen(s)	Antibodies	Remarks
HAV	27 nm	Icosahedral nonenveloped	7.5-kb RNA, linear, ss, +	Hepatovirus	HAV	Anti-HAV	Early fecal shedding; Diagnosis: IgM anti-HAV; Previous infection: IgG anti-HAV
HBV	42 nm	Double-shelled virion (surface and core) spherical	3.2-kb DNA, circular, ss/ds	Hepadnavirus	HBsAg HBcAg HBeAg	Anti-HBs Anti-HBc Anti-HBe	Bloodborne virus; carrier state; Acute diagnosis: HBsAg, IgM anti-HBc; Chronic diagnosis: IgG anti-HBc, HBsAg; Markers of replication: HBeAg, HBV DNA; Liver, lymphocytes, other organs
	27 nm	Nucleocapsid core			HBcAg HBeAg	Anti-HBc Anti-HBe	Nucleocapsid contains DNA and DNA polymerase; present in hepatocyte nucleus; HBcAg does not circulate; HBeAg (soluble, nonparticulate) and HBV DNA circulate—correlate with infectivity and complete virions
	22 nm	Spherical and filamentous; represents excess virus coat material			HBsAg	Anti-HBs	HBsAg detectable in >95% of patients with acute hepatitis B; found in serum, body fluids, hepatocyte cytoplasm; anti-HBs appears following infection—protective antibody
HCV	Approx. 40–60 nm	Enveloped	9.4-kb RNA, linear, ss, +	Hepacivirus	HCV C100-3 C33c C22-3 NS5	Anti-HCV	Bloodborne agent, formerly labeled non-A, non-B hepatitis; Acute diagnosis: anti-HCV (C33c, C22-3, NS5), HCV RNA; Chronic diagnosis: anti-HCV (C100-3, C33c, C22-3, NS5) and HCV RNA; cytoplasmic location in hepatocytes
HDV	35–37 nm	Enveloped hybrid particle with HBsAg coat and HDV core	1.7-kb RNA, circular, ss, −	Resembles viroids and plant satellite viruses	HBsAg HDV antigen	Anti-HBs Anti-HDV	Defective RNA virus, requires helper function of HBV (hepadnaviruses); HDV antigen present in hepatocyte nucleus; Diagnosis: anti-HDV, HDV RNA; HBV/HDV coinfection—IgM anti-HBc and anti-HDV; HDV superinfection—IgG anti-HBc and anti-HDV
HEV	32–34 nm	Nonenveloped icosahedral	7.6-kb RNA, linear, ss, +	Alphavirus-like	HEV antigen	Anti-HEV	Agent of enterically transmitted hepatitis; rare in USA; occurs in Asia, Mediterranean countries, Central America; Diagnosis: IgM/IgG anti-HEV (assays being developed); virus in stool, bile, hepatocyte cytoplasm

[a] ss, single-strand; ss/ds, partially single-strand, partially double-strand; −, minus-strand; +, plus-strand.

sociated hepatitis B. In part because the sensitivity of immunoassays for HBsAg and anti-HBs has increased, however, this window period is rarely encountered. In some persons, years after HBV infection, anti-HBc may persist in the circulation longer than anti-HBs. Therefore, isolated anti-HBc does not necessarily indicate active virus replication; most instances of isolated anti-HBc represent hepatitis B infection in the remote past. Rarely, however, isolated anti-HBc represents low-level hepatitis B viremia, with HBsAg below the detection threshold; occasionally, isolated anti-HBc represents a cross-reacting or false-positive immunologic specificity. Recent and remote HBV infections can be distinguished by determination of the immunoglobulin class of anti-HBc. Anti-HBc of the IgM class (IgM anti-HBc) predominates during the first 6 months after acute infection, whereas IgG anti-HBc is the predominant class of anti-HBc beyond 6 months. Therefore,

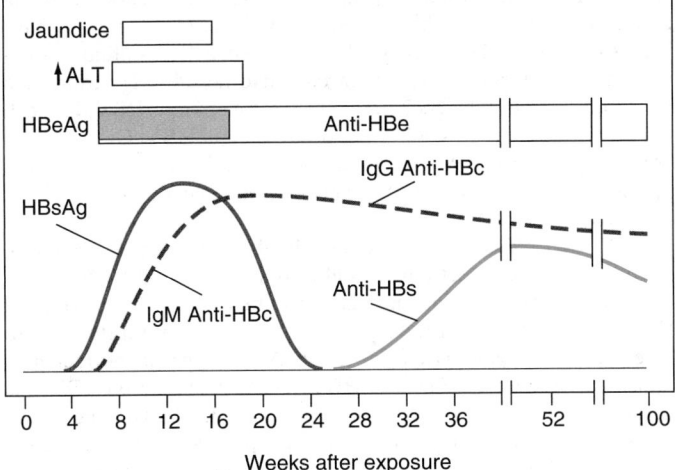

FIGURE 285-4 *Scheme of typical clinical and laboratory features of acute viral hepatitis B.*

patients with current or recent acute hepatitis B, including those in the anti-HBc window, have IgM anti-HBc in their serum. In patients who have recovered from hepatitis B in the remote past as well as those with chronic HBV infection, anti-HBc is predominantly of the IgG class. Infrequently, in no more than 1 to 5% of patients with acute HBV infection, levels of HBsAg are too low to be detected; in such cases, the presence of IgM anti-HBc establishes the diagnosis of acute hepatitis B. When isolated anti-HBc occurs in the rare patient with chronic hepatitis B whose HBsAg level is below the sensitivity threshold of contemporary immunoassays (a low-level carrier), the anti-HBc is of the IgG class. Generally, in persons who have recovered from hepatitis B, anti-HBs and anti-HBc persist indefinitely.

The temporal association between the appearance of anti-HBs and resolution of HBV infection as well as the observation that persons with anti-HBs in serum are protected against reinfection with HBV suggest that *anti-HBs is the protective antibody*. Therefore, strategies for prevention of HBV infection are based on providing susceptible persons with circulating anti-HBs (see below). Occasionally, in 10 to 20% of patients with chronic hepatitis B, low-level, low-affinity anti-HBs can be detected. This antibody is directed against a subtype determinant different from that represented by the patient's HBsAg; its presence is thought to reflect the stimulation of a related clone of antibody-forming cells, but it has no clinical relevance and does not signal imminent clearance of hepatitis B.

The other readily detectable serologic marker of HBV infection, HBeAg, appears concurrently with or shortly after HBsAg. Its appearance coincides temporally with high levels of virus replication and reflects the presence of circulating intact virions and detectable HBV DNA. Pre-S1 and pre-S2 proteins are also expressed during periods of peak replication, but assays for these gene products are not routinely available. In self-limited HBV infections, HBeAg becomes undetectable shortly after peak elevations in aminotransferase activity, before the disappearance of HBsAg, and anti-HBe then becomes detectable, coinciding with a period of relatively lower infectivity (Fig. 285-4). Because markers of HBV replication appear transiently during acute infection, testing for such markers is of little clinical utility in typical cases of acute HBV infection. In contrast, markers of HBV replication provide valuable information in patients with protracted infections.

Departing from the pattern typical of acute HBV infections, in chronic HBV infection, HBsAg remains detectable beyond 6 months, anti-HBc is primarily of the IgG class, and anti-HBs is either undetectable or detectable at low levels (see "Laboratory Features," below) (Fig. 285-5). During early chronic HBV infection, HBV DNA can be detected both in serum and in hepatocyte nuclei, where it is present in free or episomal form. This *replicative stage* of HBV infection is the time of maximal infectivity and liver injury; HBeAg is a qualitative marker and HBV DNA a quantitative marker of this replicative phase,

during which all three forms of HBV circulate, including intact virions. Over time, the replicative phase of chronic HBV infection gives way to a relatively *nonreplicative phase*. This occurs at a rate of approximately 10% per year and is accompanied by seroconversion from HBeAg-positive to anti-HBe-positive. In most cases, this seroconversion coincides with a transient, acute hepatitis-like elevation in aminotransferase activity, believed to reflect cell-mediated immune clearance of virus-infected hepatocytes. In the nonreplicative phase of chronic infection, when HBV DNA is demonstrable in hepatocyte nuclei, it tends to be integrated into the host genome. In this phase, only spherical and tubular forms of HBV, *not intact virions*, circulate, and liver injury tends to subside. Most such patients would be characterized as *inactive HBV carriers*. In reality, the designations *replicative* and *nonreplicative* are only relative; even in the so-called nonreplicative phase, HBV replication can be detected with highly sensitive amplification probes such as the polymerase chain reaction (PCR). Still, the distinctions are pathophysiologically and clinically meaningful. Occasionally, nonreplicative HBV infection converts back to replicative infection. Such spontaneous reactivations are accompanied by reexpression of HBeAg and HBV DNA, and sometimes of IgM anti-HBc, as well as by exacerbations of liver injury.

MOLECULAR VARIANTS Variation occurs throughout the HBV genome, and clinical isolates of HBV that do not express typical viral proteins have been attributed to mutations in individual or even multiple gene locations. For example, variants have been described that lack nucleocapsid proteins, envelope proteins, or both. Two categories of HBV have attracted the most attention. One of these was identified initially in Mediterranean countries among patients with an unusual serologic-clinical profile. They have severe chronic HBV infection and detectable HBV DNA but with anti-HBe instead of HBeAg. These patients were found to be infected with an HBV mutant that contained an alteration in the precore region rendering the virus incapable of encoding HBeAg. Although several potential mutation sites exist in the pre-C region, the region of the C gene necessary for the expression of HBeAg (see "Virology and Etiology," above), the most commonly encountered in such patients is a single base substitution, from G to A, which occurs in the second to last codon of the pre-C gene at nucleotide 1896. This substitution results in the replacement of the TGG tryptophan codon by a stop codon (TAG), which prevents the translation of HBeAg. Another mutation, in the core promoter region, prevents transcription of the coding region for HBeAg and yields an

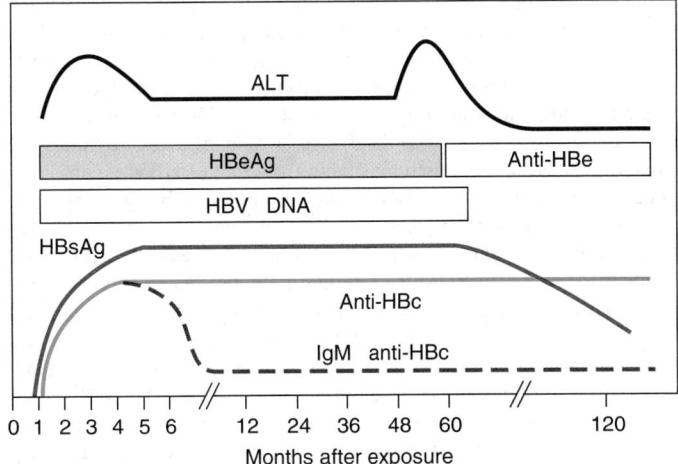

FIGURE 285-5 *Scheme of typical laboratory features of chronic viral hepatitis B. HBeAg and HBV DNA can be detected in serum during the replicative phase of chronic infection, which is associated with infectivity and liver injury. Seroconversion from the replicative phase to the nonreplicative phase occurs at a rate of approximately 10 to 15% per year and is heralded by an acute hepatitis–like elevation of ALT activity; during the nonreplicative phase, infectivity and liver injury are limited.*

HBeAg-negative phenotype. Patients with such precore mutants that are unable to secrete HBeAg tend to have severe liver disease that progresses more rapidly to cirrhosis. Both "wild-type" HBV and precore-mutant HBV can coexist in the same patient, or mutant HBV may arise late during wild-type HBV infection. In addition, clusters of fulminant hepatitis B in Israel and Japan have been attributed to common-source infection with a precore mutant. Fulminant hepatitis B in North America and western Europe, however, occurs in patients infected with wild-type HBV, in the absence of precore mutants, and both precore mutants and other mutations throughout the HBV genome occur commonly even in patients with typical, self-limited, milder forms of HBV infection. Precore-mutant hepatitis B is now the most frequently encountered form of hepatitis B in Mediterranean countries and in Europe. In the United States, where HBV genotype A (less prone to G1896A mutation) is prevalent, precore-mutant HBV is much less common. Characteristic of such HBeAg-negative chronic hepatitis B are lower levels of HBV DNA and periodic fluctuations in hepatic necroinflammatory activity.

The second important category of HBV mutants consists of *escape mutants*, in which a single amino acid substitution, from glycine to arginine, occurs at position 145 of the immunodominant *a* determinant common to all subtypes of HBsAg. This change in HBsAg leads to a critical conformational change that results in a loss of neutralizing activity by anti-HBs. This specific HBV/*a* mutant has been observed in two situations, active and passive immunization, in which humoral immunologic pressure may favor evolutionary change ("escape") in the virus—in a small number of hepatitis B vaccine recipients who acquired HBV infection despite the prior appearance of neutralizing anti-HBs and in liver transplant recipients who underwent the procedure for hepatitis B and who were treated with a high-potency human monoclonal anti-HBs preparation. Although such mutants have not been recognized frequently, their existence raises a concern that may complicate vaccination strategies and serologic diagnosis.

EXTRAHEPATIC SITES   Hepatitis B antigens and HBV DNA have been identified in extrahepatic sites, including lymph nodes, bone marrow, circulating lymphocytes, spleen, and pancreas. Although the virus does not appear to be associated with tissue injury in any of these extrahepatic sites, its presence in these "remote" reservoirs has been invoked to explain the recurrence of HBV infection after orthotopic liver transplantation. A more complete understanding of the clinical relevance of extrahepatic HBV remains to be defined.

Hepatitis D   The delta hepatitis agent, or HDV, is a defective RNA virus that coinfects with and requires the helper function of HBV (or other hepadnaviruses) for its replication and expression. Slightly smaller than HBV, delta is a formalin-sensitive, 35- to 37-nm virus with a hybrid structure. Its nucleocapsid expresses delta antigen, which bears no antigenic homology with any of the HBV antigens, and contains the virus genome. The delta core is "encapsidated" by an outer envelope of HBsAg, indistinguishable from that of HBV except in its relative compositions of major, middle, and large HBsAg component proteins. The genome is a small, 1700-nucleotide, circular, single-stranded RNA (minus strand) that is nonhomologous with HBV DNA (except for a small area of the polymerase gene) but that has features and the rolling circle model of replication common to genomes of plant satellite viruses or viroids. HDV RNA contains many areas of internal complementarity; therefore, it can fold on itself by internal base pairing to form an unusual, very stable, rodlike structure. HDV RNA requires host RNA polymerase II for its replication via RNA-directed RNA synthesis by transcription of genomic RNA to a complementary antigenomic (plus strand) RNA; the antigenomic RNA, in turn, serves as a template for subsequent genomic RNA synthesis. Between the genomic and antigenomic RNAs of HDV, there are coding regions for nine proteins. Delta antigen, which is a product of the antigenomic strand, exists in two forms, a small, 195-amino-acid species, which plays a role in facilitating HDV RNA replication, and a large, 214-

amino-acid species, which appears to suppress replication but is required for assembly of the antigen into virions. Delta antigens have been shown to bind directly to RNA polymerase II, resulting in stimulation of transcription. Although complete hepatitis D virions and liver injury require the cooperative helper function of HBV, intracellular replication of HDV RNA can occur without HBV. Genomic heterogeneity among HDV isolates has been described; however, pathophysiologic and clinical consequences of this genetic diversity have not been recognized.

HDV can either infect a person simultaneously with HBV (*coinfection*) or superinfect a person already infected with HBV (*superinfection*); when HDV infection is transmitted from a donor with one HBsAg subtype to an HBsAg-positive recipient with a different subtype, the HDV agent assumes the HBsAg subtype of the recipient, rather than the donor. Because HDV relies absolutely on HBV, the duration of HDV infection is determined by the duration of (and cannot outlast) HBV infection. HDV antigen is expressed primarily in hepatocyte nuclei and is occasionally detectable in serum. During acute HDV infection, anti-HDV of the IgM class predominates, and 30 to 40 days may elapse after symptoms appear before anti-HDV can be detected. In self-limited infection, anti-HDV is low titer and transient, rarely remaining detectable beyond the clearance of HBsAg and HDV antigen. In chronic HDV infection, anti-HDV circulates in high titer, and both IgM and IgG anti-HDV can be detected. HDV antigen in the liver and HDV RNA in serum and liver can be detected during HDV replication.

Hepatitis C   Hepatitis C virus, which, before its identification was labeled "non-A, non-B hepatitis," is a linear, single-strand, positive-sense, 9600-nucleotide RNA virus, the genome of which is similar in organization to that of flaviviruses and pestiviruses; HCV is the only member of the genus *Hepacivirus* in the family Flaviviridae. The HCV genome contains a single large open reading frame (gene) that codes for a virus polyprotein of approximately 3000 amino acids. The 5' end of the genome consists of an untranslated region (containing an internal ribosomal entry site) adjacent to the genes for structural proteins, the nucleocapsid core protein and two envelope glycoproteins, E1 and E2/NS1. The 5' untranslated region and core gene are highly conserved among genotypes, but the envelope proteins are coded for by the hypervariable region, which varies from isolate to isolate and may allow the virus to evade host immunologic containment directed at accessible virus-envelope proteins. The 3' end of the genome contains the genes for nonstructural (NS) proteins. The first reported HCV clone, 5-1-1, and the nucleotide sequence coding for C100-3, the recombinant virus protein used in the first immunoassay for antibodies to HCV, reside within the NS4 gene, and the RNA-dependent RNA polymerase, through which HCV replicates, is encoded by the NS5 region (Fig. 285-6). Because HCV does not replicate via a DNA intermediate, it does not integrate into the host genome. Because HCV tends to circulate in relatively low titer, visualization of virus particles, estimated to be 40 to 60 nm in diameter, has been difficult. Still, the replication rate of HCV is very high, 10^{12} virions per day; its half-life is 2.7 h. The chimpanzee is a helpful but cumbersome animal model. Although in vitro replication has been difficult, hepatocellular carcinoma–derived cell lines have been described (replicon systems) that support replication of genetically manipulated, truncated or full-length HCV RNA (but not intact virions). Although a robust, reproducible, small-animal model is lacking, HCV replication has been documented in an immunodeficient-mouse model containing explants of human liver.

At least six distinct genotypes, as well as subtypes within genotypes, of HCV have been identified by nucleotide sequencing. Genotypes differ one from another in sequence homology by ≥30%. Because divergence of HCV isolates within a genotype or subtype, and within the same host, may vary insufficiently to define a distinct genotype, these intragenotypic differences are referred to as *quasispecies* and differ in sequence homology by only a few percent. The genotypic and quasispecies diversity of HCV, resulting from its high mutation

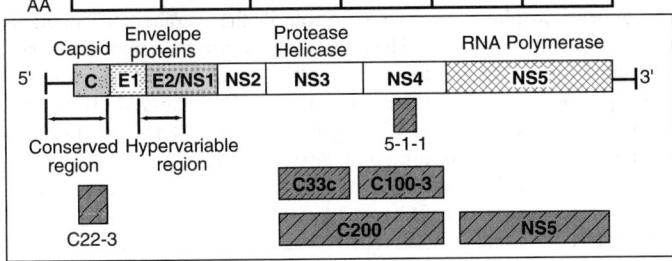

= viral proteins

FIGURE 285-6 *Organization of the hepatitis C virus genome and its associated proteins. Structural genes at the 5' end include the nucleocapsid region, C, and the envelope regions, E1 and E2. The 5' untranslated region and the C region are highly conserved among isolates, while the envelope domain E2/NS1 contains the hypervariable region. At the 3' end are five nonstructural (NS) regions. Viral proteins included in the first-generation (C100-3), second-generation (C200, a fusion protein of C100-3 and C33c, and C22-3), and third-generation (C22-3, C200, or C33c and C100-3, and NS5) immunoassays and in the recombinant immunoblot assay (5-1-1, C100-3, C33c, C22-3, NS5) are presented below their corresponding genes (AA, amino acid).*

rate, interferes with effective humoral immunity. Neutralizing antibodies to HCV have been demonstrated, but they tend to be short-lived; and HCV infection does not induce lasting immunity against reinfection with different virus isolates or even the same virus isolate. Thus, neither *heterologous* nor *homologous* immunity appears to develop commonly after acute HCV infection. Some HCV genotypes are distributed worldwide, while others are more geographically confined. In addition, differences exist among genotypes in responsiveness to antiviral therapy; however, early reports of differences in pathogenicity among genotypes have not been corroborated.

As noted above, the first assay detected antibodies to C100-3, a recombinant polypeptide derived from the NS4 region of the genome. In most patients with acute hepatitis C, antibody detected with this assay appears between 1 to 3 months after the onset of acute hepatitis but sometimes not for a year or longer. Second-generation assays incorporate recombinant proteins from the nucleocapsid core region, C22-3, and the NS3 region, C33c (expressed in combination with C100-3 as C200); these assays are more sensitive (by approximately 20%) and detect anti-HCV 30 to 90 days earlier, during the period of acute hepatitis. A third-generation immunoassay, which incorporates proteins from the NS5 region and replaces some recombinant proteins with synthetic peptides, may detect anti-HCV even earlier. Because nonspecificity has been encountered in clinical samples tested for anti-HCV, a supplementary recombinant immunoblot assay was introduced. Reactivity in an immunoassay is "confirmed" by incubation with a nitrocellulose strip that contains individual bands of recombinant or synthetic HCV proteins. This approach allows the demonstration of individual antibodies to nonstructural and structural viral proteins and identifies false-positive reactivity associated with nonviral specificities. Although useful to support the validity of anti-HCV-reactive samples, especially in patients with a low prior probability of true infection (e.g., blood donors) or in patients with confounding activity in serum (such as a rheumatoid factor) that may yield false-positive antibody reactivity, immunoblotting assays have been supplanted by tests for HCV RNA. The most sensitive indicator is the presence of HCV RNA, which requires molecular amplification by (PCR) or transcription-mediated amplification (TMA) (Fig. 285-7). An alternative method for detection of HCV RNA, more easily automated but one or two orders of magnitude less sensitive, is branched-chain complementary DNA hybridization. HCV RNA can be detected within a few days of exposure to HCV, well before the appearance of anti-HCV, and tends to persist for the duration of HCV infection; however, occasionally in patients with chronic HCV infection, HCV RNA may be detectable only intermittently. Application of sensitive molecular probes for HCV RNA has revealed the presence of replicative HCV in peripheral blood lymphocytes of infected persons; however, as is

the case for HBV in lymphocytes, the clinical relevance of HCV lymphocyte infection is not known.

Hepatitis E Previously labeled *epidemic* or *enterically transmitted non-A, non-B hepatitis*, HEV is an enterically transmitted virus that occurs primarily in India, Asia, Africa, and Central America. This agent, with epidemiologic features resembling those of hepatitis A, is a 32- to 34-nm, nonenveloped, HAV-like virus with a 7600-nucleotide, single-stranded, positive-sense RNA genome. HEV has three open reading frames (genes), the largest of which encodes nonstructural proteins involved in virus replication. A middle-sized gene encodes the nucleocapsid protein, and the smallest, whose function is not known, encodes protein specificities to which antibodies appear in human serum. All HEV isolates appear to belong to a single serotype, despite genomic heterogeneity of up to 25%. There is no genomic or antigenic homology, however, between HEV and HAV or other picornaviruses; and HEV, although resembling caliciviruses, appears to be sufficiently distinct from any known agent to merit a new classification of its own within the alphavirus group. The virus has been detected in stool, bile, and liver and is excreted in the stool during the late incubation period; immune responses to viral antigens occur very early during the course of acute infection. Both IgM anti-HEV and IgG anti-HEV can be detected, but both fall rapidly after acute infection, reaching low levels within 9 to 12 months. Currently, serologic testing for HEV infection is not available routinely.

PATHOGENESIS   Under ordinary circumstances, none of the hepatitis viruses is known to be directly cytopathic to hepatocytes. Evidence suggests that the clinical manifestations and outcomes after acute liver injury associated with viral hepatitis are determined by the immunologic responses of the host.

HEPATITIS B   Among the viral hepatitides, the immunopathogenesis of hepatitis B has been studied most extensively. Certainly for this agent, the existence of inactive hepatitis B carriers with normal liver histology and function suggests that the virus is not directly cytopathic. The fact that patients with defects in cellular immune competence are more likely to remain chronically infected rather than to clear the virus is cited to support the role of cellular immune responses in the pathogenesis of hepatitis B–related liver injury. The model that has the most experimental support involves cytolytic T cells sensitized specifically to recognize host and hepatitis B viral antigens on the liver cell surface. Laboratory observations suggest that nucleocapsid proteins (HBcAg and possibly HBeAg), present on the cell membrane in minute quantities, are the viral target antigens that, with host antigens, invite cytolytic T cells to destroy HBV-infected hepatocytes. Differences in the

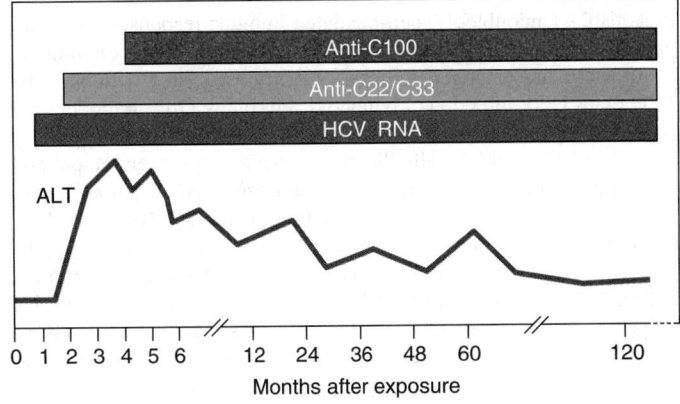

FIGURE 285-7 *Scheme of typical laboratory features during acute hepatitis C progressing to chronicity. HCV RNA is the first detectable event, preceding ALT elevation and the appearance of anti-HCV. The appearance of antibody to C100, detectable with first-generation assays, is delayed from 1 to 3 months after the appearance of antibody to C22 and C33, antibodies that are included in second-generation immunoassays. Anti-HCV detectable with second-generation assays appears during acute hepatitis C.*

robustness of cytolytic T cell responsiveness and in the elaboration of antiviral cytokines by T cells have been invoked to explain differences in outcomes between those who recover after acute hepatitis and those who progress to chronic hepatitis or between those with mild and those with severe (fulminant) acute HBV infection.

Although a robust cytolytic T cell response occurs and eliminates virus-infected liver cells during acute hepatitis B, >90% of HBV DNA has been found in experimentally infected chimpanzees to disappear from the liver and blood before maximal T cell infiltration of the liver and before most of the biochemical and histologic evidence of liver injury. This observation suggests that inflammatory cytokines, independent of cytopathic antiviral mechanisms, participate in early viral clearance; this effect has been shown to represent elimination of HBV replicative intermediates from the cytoplasm and covalently closed circular viral DNA from the nucleus of infected hepatocytes.

Debate continues over the relative importance of viral and host factors in the pathogenesis of HBV-associated liver injury and its outcome. As noted above, precore genetic mutants of HBV have been associated with the more severe outcomes of HBV infection (severe chronic and fulminant hepatitis), suggesting that, under certain circumstances, relative pathogenicity is a property of the virus, not the host. The fact that concomitant HDV and HBV infections are associated with more severe liver injury than HBV infection alone and the fact that cells transfected in vitro with the gene for HDV (delta) antigen express HDV antigen and then become necrotic in the absence of any immunologic influences are also consistent with a viral effect on pathogenicity. Similarly, in patients who undergo liver transplantation for end-stage chronic hepatitis B, occasionally, rapidly progressive liver injury appears in the new liver. This clinical pattern is associated with an unusual histologic pattern in the new liver, *fibrosing cholestatic hepatitis*, which, ultrastructurally, appears to represent a choking of the cell with overwhelming quantities of HBsAg. This observation suggests that under the influence of the potent immunosuppressive agents required to prevent allograft rejection, HBV may have a direct cytopathic effect on liver cells, independent of the immune system.

Although the precise mechanism of liver injury in HBV infection remains elusive, studies of nucleocapsid proteins have shed light on the profound immunologic tolerance to HBV of babies born to mothers with highly replicative (HBeAg-positive), chronic HBV infection. In HBeAg-expressing transgenic mice, in utero exposure to HBeAg, which is sufficiently small to traverse the placenta, induces T cell tolerance to both nucleocapsid proteins. This, in turn, may explain why, when infection occurs so early in life, immunologic clearance does not occur, and protracted, lifelong infection ensues.

Hepatitis C Undoubtedly, cell-mediated immune responses and elaboration by T cells of antiviral cytokines contribute to the containment of infection and pathogenesis of liver injury associated with hepatitis C. Perhaps HCV infection of lymphoid cells plays a role in moderating immune responsiveness to the virus, as well. Intrahepatic HLA class-I-restricted cytolytic T cells directed at nucleocapsid, envelope, and NS viral protein antigens have been demonstrated in patients with chronic hepatitis C: however, such virus-specific cytolytic T cell responses do not correlate adequately with the degree of liver injury or with recovery. Yet, a consensus has emerged supporting a role in the pathogenesis of HCV-associated liver injury of virus-activated CD4 helper T cells that stimulate, via the cytokines they elaborate, HCV-specific CD8 cytotoxic T cells. These responses appear to be more robust in those who recover from HCV than in those who have chronic infection. Several HLA alleles have been linked with self-limited hepatitis C, but such associations do not apply universally. Finally, cross-reactivity between viral and host autoantigens has been invoked to explain the association between hepatitis C and a subset of patients with autoimmune hepatitis and antibodies to liver-kidney microsomal (LKM) antigen (anti-LKM) (Chap. 287).

EXTRAHEPATIC MANIFESTATIONS Immune complex–mediated tissue damage appears to play a pathogenetic role in the extrahepatic manifestations of acute hepatitis B. The occasional prodromal serum sickness–like syndrome observed in acute hepatitis B appears to be related to the deposition in tissue blood vessel walls of HBsAg-anti-HBs circulating immune complexes, leading to activation of the complement system and depressed serum complement levels.

In patients with chronic hepatitis B, other types of immune-complex disease may be seen. Glomerulonephritis with the nephritic syndrome is occasionally observed; HBsAg, immunoglobulin, and C3 deposition has been found in the glomerular basement membrane. While polyarteritis nodosa develops in considerably fewer than 1% of patients with chronic HBV infection, 20 to 30% of patients with polyarteritis nodosa have HBsAg in serum (Chap. 306). In these patients, the affected small and medium-sized arterioles have been shown to contain HBsAg, immunoglobulins, and complement components. Another extrahepatic manifestation of viral hepatitis, essential mixed cryoglobulinemia (EMC), was reported initially to be associated with hepatitis B. The disorder is characterized clinically by arthritis, cutaneous vasculitis (palpable purpura), and occasionally with glomerulonephritis and serologically by the presence of circulating cryoprecipitable immune complexes of more than one immunoglobulin class (Chaps. 264 and 306). Many patients with this syndrome have chronic liver disease, but the association with HBV infection is limited; instead, a substantial proportion have chronic HCV infection, with circulating immune complexes containing HCV RNA. Immune-complex glomerulonephritis is another recognized extrahepatic manifestation of chronic hepatitis C.

PATHOLOGY The typical morphologic lesions of all types of viral hepatitis are similar and consist of panlobular infiltration with mononuclear cells, hepatic cell necrosis, hyperplasia of Kupffer cells, and variable degrees of cholestasis. Hepatic cell regeneration is present, as evidenced by numerous mitotic figures, multinucleated cells, and "rosette" or "pseudoacinar" formation. The mononuclear infiltration consists primarily of small lymphocytes, although plasma cells and eosinophils occasionally are present. Liver cell damage consists of hepatic cell degeneration and necrosis, cell dropout, ballooning of cells, and acidophilic degeneration of hepatocytes (forming so-called Councilman or apoptotic bodies). Large hepatocytes with a ground-glass appearance of the cytoplasm may be seen in chronic but not in acute HBV infection; these cells contain HBsAg and can be identified histochemically with orcein or aldehyde fuchsin. In uncomplicated viral hepatitis, the reticulin framework is preserved.

In hepatitis C, the histologic lesion is often remarkable for a relative paucity of inflammation, a marked increase in activation of sinusoidal lining cells, lymphoid aggregates, the presence of fat (more frequent in genotype 3 and linked to increased fibrosis), and, occasionally, bile duct lesions in which biliary epithelial cells appear to be piled up without interruption of the basement membrane. Occasionally, microvesicular steatosis occurs in hepatitis D. In hepatitis E, a common histologic feature is marked cholestasis. A cholestatic variant of slowly resolving acute hepatitis A also has been described.

A more severe histologic lesion, *bridging hepatic necrosis*, also termed *subacute* or *confluent necrosis*, is occasionally observed in some patients with acute hepatitis. "Bridging" between lobules results from large areas of hepatic cell dropout, with collapse of the reticulin framework. Characteristically, the bridge consists of condensed reticulum, inflammatory debris, and degenerating liver cells that span adjacent portal areas, portal to central veins, or central vein to central vein. This lesion had been thought to have prognostic significance; in many of the originally described patients with this lesion, a subacute course terminated in death within several weeks to months or severe chronic hepatitis and postnecrotic cirrhosis developed. Subsequent investigations have failed to uphold the association between bridging necrosis and such a poor prognosis in patients with acute hepatitis. Therefore, although demonstration of this lesion in patients with chronic hepatitis has prognostic significance (Chap. 287), its demonstration during acute hepatitis is less meaningful, and liver biopsies to identify this lesion are no longer undertaken routinely in patients with acute hepatitis. In *massive hepatic necrosis* (fulminant hepatitis, acute yellow atrophy), the striking feature at postmortem examination is the finding of a small, shrunken, soft liver. Histologic examination reveals massive necrosis and dropout of liver cells of most lobules with extensive collapse and condensation of the reticulin framework. When histologic documentation is required in the management of fulminant or very severe hepatitis, a biopsy can be done by the angiographically guided transjugular route, which permits the performance of this invasive procedure in the presence of severe coagulopathy.

Immunohistochemical and electron-microscopic studies have localized HBsAg to the cytoplasm and plasma membrane of infected liver cells. In contrast, HBcAg predominates in the nucleus, but occasionally, scant amounts are also seen in the cytoplasm and on the cell membrane. HDV antigen is localized to the hepatocyte nucleus, while HAV, HCV, and HEV antigens are localized to the cytoplasm.

EPIDEMIOLOGY Before the availability of serologic tests for hepatitis viruses, all viral hepatitis cases were labeled either as "infectious" or "serum" hepatitis. Modes of transmission overlap, however, and *a clear distinction among the different types of viral hepatitis cannot be made solely on the basis of clinical or epidemiologic features* (Table 285-2). The most accurate means to distinguish the various types of viral hepatitis involves specific serologic testing.

Hepatitis A *This agent is transmitted almost exclusively by the fecal-oral route.* Person-to-person spread of HAV is enhanced by poor personal hygiene and overcrowding; large outbreaks as well as sporadic cases have been traced to contaminated food, water, milk, frozen raspberries and strawberries, and shellfish. Intrafamily and intrainstitutional spread are also common. Early epidemiologic observations suggested that there is a predilection for hepatitis A to occur in late fall and early winter. In temperate zones, epidemic waves have been recorded every 5 to 20 years as new segments of nonimmune population appeared; however, in developed countries, the incidence of hepatitis A has been declining, presumably as a function of improved sanitation,

and these cyclic patterns are no longer being observed. No HAV carrier state has been identified after acute hepatitis A; perpetuation of the virus in nature depends presumably on nonepidemic, inapparent subclinical infection.

In the general population, anti-HAV, a marker for previous HAV infection, increases in prevalence as a function of increasing age and of decreasing socioeconomic status. In the 1970s, serologic evidence of prior hepatitis A infection occurred in about 40% of urban populations in the United States, most of whose members never recalled having had a symptomatic case of hepatitis. In subsequent decades, however, the prevalence of anti-HAV has been declining in the United States. In developing countries, exposure, infection, and subsequent immunity are almost universal in childhood. As the frequency of subclinical childhood infections declines in developed countries, a susceptible cohort of adults emerges. Hepatitis A tends to be more symptomatic in adults; therefore, paradoxically, as the frequency of HAV infection declines, the likelihood of clinically apparent, even severe, HAV illnesses increases in the susceptible adult population. Travel to endemic areas is a common source of infection for adults from nonendemic areas. More recently recognized epidemiologic foci of HAV infection include child-care centers, neonatal intensive care units, promiscuous homosexual men, and injection drug users. Although hepatitis A is rarely bloodborne, several outbreaks have been recognized in recipients of clotting factor concentrates.

Hepatitis B Percutaneous inoculation has long been recognized as a major route of hepatitis B transmission, but the outmoded designation "serum hepatitis" is an inaccurate label for the epidemiologic spectrum of HBV infection recognized today. As detailed below, most of the hepatitis transmitted by blood transfusion is not caused by HBV; moreover, in approximately two-thirds of patients with acute type B hepatitis, there is no history of an identifiable percutaneous exposure. We now recognize that many cases of hepatitis B result from less obvious modes of nonpercutaneous or covert percutaneous transmission.

TABLE 285-2 *Clinical and Epidemiologic Features of Viral Hepatitis*

Feature	HAV	HBV	HCV	HDV	HEV
Incubation (days)	15–45, mean 30	30–180, mean 60–90	15–160, mean 50	30–180, mean 60–90	14–60, mean 40
Onset	Acute	Insidious or acute	Insidious	Insidious or acute	Acute
Age preference	Children, young adults	Young adults (sexual and percutaneous), babies, toddlers	Any age, but more common in adults	Any age (similar to HBV)	Young adults (20–40 years)
Transmission					
Fecal-oral	+++	–	–	–	+++
Percutaneous	Unusual	+++	+++	+++	–
Perinatal	–	+++	±[a]	+	–
Sexual	±	++	±[a]	++	–
Clinical					
Severity	Mild	Occasionally severe	Moderate	Occasionally severe	Mild
Fulminant	0.1%	0.1–1%	0.1%	5–20%[b]	1–2%[e]
Progression to chronicity	None	Occasional (1–10%) (90% of neonates)	Common (50–70% chronic hepatitis; 80–90% chronic infection)	Common[d]	None
Carrier	None	0.1–30%[c]	1.5–3.2%	Variable[f]	None
Cancer	None	+ (neonatal infection)	+	±	None
Prognosis	Excellent	Worse with age, debility	Moderate	Acute, good Chronic, poor	Good
Prophylaxis	IG Inactivated vaccine	HBIG Recombinant vaccine	None	HBV vaccine (none for HBV carriers)	Unknown
Therapy	None	Interferon Lamivudine Adefovir	Pegylated interferon plus ribavirin	Interferon ±	None

[a] Primarily with HIV co-infection and high-level viremia in index case; risk ~5%.
[b] Up to 5% in acute HBV/HDV co-infection; up to 20% in HDV superinfection of chronic HBV infection.
[c] Varies considerably throughout the world and in subpopulations within countries; see text.
[d] In acute HBV/HDV co-infection, the frequency of chronicity is the same as that for HBV; in HDV superinfection, chronicity is invariable.
[e] 10–20% in pregnant women.
[f] Common in Mediterranean countries, rare in North America and western Europe.

HBsAg has been identified in almost every body fluid from infected persons, and at least some of these body fluids—most notably semen and saliva—are infectious, albeit less so than serum, when administered percutaneously or nonpercutaneously to experimental animals. Among the nonpercutaneous modes of HBV transmission, oral ingestion has been documented as a potential but inefficient route of exposure. By contrast, the two nonpercutaneous routes considered to have the greatest impact are intimate (especially sexual) contact and perinatal transmission.

In sub-Saharan Africa, intimate contact among toddlers is considered instrumental in contributing to the maintenance of the high frequency of hepatitis B in the population. Perinatal transmission occurs primarily in infants born to HBsAg carrier mothers or mothers with acute hepatitis B during the third trimester of pregnancy or during the early postpartum period. Perinatal transmission is uncommon in North America and western Europe but occurs with great frequency and is the most important mode of HBV perpetuation in the Far East and developing countries. Although the precise mode of perinatal transmission is unknown, and although approximately 10% of infections may be acquired in utero, epidemiologic evidence suggests that most infections occur approximately at the time of delivery and are not related to breast feeding. The likelihood of perinatal transmission of HBV correlates with the presence of HBeAg; 90% of HBeAg-positive mothers but only 10 to 15% of anti-HBe-positive mothers transmit HBV infection to their offspring. In most cases, acute infection in the neonate is clinically asymptomatic, but the child is very likely to become an HBsAg carrier.

The more than 350 million HBsAg carriers in the world constitute the main reservoir of hepatitis B in human beings. Serum HBsAg is infrequent (0.1 to 0.5%) in normal populations in the United States and western Europe. However, a prevalence of up to 5 to 20% has been found in the Far East and in some tropical countries; in persons with Down's syndrome, lepromatous leprosy, leukemia, Hodgkin's disease, polyarteritis nodosa; in patients with chronic renal disease on hemodialysis; and in injection drug users.

Other groups with high rates of HBV infection include spouses of acutely infected persons, sexually promiscuous persons (especially promiscuous men who have sex with men), health care workers exposed to blood, persons who require repeated transfusions especially with pooled blood product concentrates (e.g., hemophiliacs), residents and staff of custodial institutions for the developmentally handicapped, prisoners, and, to a lesser extent, family members of chronically infected patients. In volunteer blood donors, the prevalence of anti-HBs, a reflection of previous HBV infection, ranges from 5 to 10%, but the prevalence is higher in lower socioeconomic strata, older age groups, and persons—including those mentioned above—exposed to blood products.

Prevalence of infection, modes of transmission, and human behavior conspire to mold geographically different epidemiologic patterns of HBV infection. In the Far East and Africa, hepatitis B, a disease of the newborn and young children, is perpetuated by a cycle of maternal-neonatal spread. In North America and western Europe, hepatitis B is primarily a disease of adolescence and early adulthood, the time of life when intimate sexual contact as well as recreational and occupational percutaneous exposures tend to occur.

Hepatitis D   Infection with HDV has a worldwide distribution, but two epidemiologic patterns exist. In Mediterranean countries (northern Africa, southern Europe, the Middle East), HDV infection is endemic among those with hepatitis B, and the disease is transmitted predominantly by nonpercutaneous means, especially close personal contact. In nonendemic areas, such as the United States and northern Europe, HDV infection is confined to persons exposed frequently to blood and blood products, primarily injection drug users and hemophiliacs. HDV infection can be introduced into a population through drug users or by migration of persons from endemic to nonendemic areas. Thus, pat-

terns of population migration and human behavior facilitating percutaneous contact play important roles in the introduction and amplification of HDV infection. Occasionally, the migrating epidemiology of hepatitis D is expressed in explosive outbreaks of severe hepatitis, such as those that have occurred in remote South American villages as well as in urban centers in the United States. Ultimately, such outbreaks of hepatitis D—either of coinfections with acute hepatitis B or of superinfections in those already infected with HBV—may blur the distinctions between endemic and nonendemic areas. On a global scale, HDV infection is declining. Even in Italy, an HDV-endemic area, public health measures introduced to control HBV infection resulted during the 1990s in a 1.5%/year reduction in the prevalence of HDV infection.

Hepatitis C   Routine screening of blood donors for HBsAg and the elimination of commercial blood sources in the early 1970s reduced the frequency of, but did not eliminate, transfusion-associated hepatitis. During the 1970s, the likelihood of acquiring hepatitis after transfusion of voluntarily donated, HBsAg-screened blood was approximately 10% per patient (up to 0.9% per unit transfused); 90 to 95% of these cases were classified, based on serologic exclusion of hepatitis A and B, as "non-A, non-B" hepatitis. For patients requiring transfusion of pooled products, such as clotting factor concentrates, the risk was even higher, up to 20 to 30%.

During the 1980s, voluntary self-exclusion of blood donors with risk factors for AIDS and then the introduction of donor screening for anti-HIV reduced further the likelihood of transfusion-associated hepatitis to under 5%. During the late 1980s and early 1990s, the introduction first of "surrogate" screening tests for non-A, non-B hepatitis [alanine aminotransferase (ALT) and anti-HBc, both shown to identify blood donors with a higher likelihood of transmitting non-A, non-B hepatitis to recipients] and, subsequently, after the discovery of HCV, first-generation immunoassays for anti-HCV reduced the frequency of transfusion-associated hepatitis even further. A prospective analysis of transfusion-associated hepatitis conducted between 1986 and 1990 showed that the incidence of transfusion-associated hepatitis at one urban university hospital fell from a baseline of 3.8% per patient (0.45% per unit transfused) to 1.5% per patient (0.19% per unit) after the introduction of surrogate testing and to 0.6% per patient (0.03% per unit) after the introduction of first-generation anti-HCV assays. The introduction of second-generation anti-HCV assays reduced the frequency of transfusion-associated hepatitis C to almost imperceptible levels, 1 in 100,000, and these gains are being reinforced by the application of automated PCR testing of donated blood for HCV RNA.

In addition to being transmitted by transfusion, hepatitis C can be transmitted by other percutaneous routes, such as injection drug use. In addition, this virus can be transmitted by occupational exposure to blood, and the likelihood of infection is increased in hemodialysis units. Although the frequency of transfusion-associated hepatitis C fell as a result of blood donor screening, the overall frequency of hepatitis C remained the same until the early 1990s, when the overall frequency fell by 80%, in parallel with a reduction in the number of new cases in injection drug users. After the exclusion of anti-HCV-positive plasma units from the donor pool, rare, sporadic instances have occurred of hepatitis C among recipients of immune globulin (IG) preparations for intravenous (but not intramuscular) use.

Serologic evidence for HCV infection occurs in 90% of patients with a history of transfusion-associated hepatitis (almost all occurring before 1992, when second-generation HCV-screening tests were introduced), hemophiliacs and others treated with clotting factors, and injection drug users; 60 to 70% of patients with sporadic "non-A, non-B" hepatitis who lack identifiable risk factors; 0.5% of volunteer blood donors; and 1.8% of the general population in the United States, which translates into 4 million persons. Comparable frequencies of HCV infection occur in most countries around the world, with 170 million persons infected worldwide, but extraordinarily high prevalences of HCV infection occur in certain countries, such as Egypt, where more than 20% of the population in some cities is infected. The high frequency in Egypt is attributable to contaminated equipment used for medical procedures and unsafe injection practices. In the United States, African Americans and Mexican Americans have higher frequencies of HCV infection than whites, and 30- to 49-year-old adult males have the highest frequencies of infection. Hepatitis C accounts for 40% of chronic liver disease, is the most frequent indication for liver transplantation, and is estimated to account for 8000 to 10,000 deaths per year in the United States.

Most asymptomatic blood donors found to have anti-HCV and approximately 20 to 30% of persons with reported cases of acute hepatitis C do not fall into a recognized risk group; however, many such blood donors do recall risk-associated behaviors when questioned carefully.

As a bloodborne infection, HCV potentially can be transmitted sexually and perinatally; however, both of these modes of transmission are inefficient for hepatitis C. Although 10 to 15% of patients with acute hepatitis C report having potential sexual sources of infection, most studies have failed to identify sexual transmission of this agent. The chances of sexual and perinatal transmission have been estimated to be approximately 5%, well below comparable rates for HIV and HBV infections. Moreover, sexual transmission appears to be confined to such subgroups as persons with multiple sexual partners and sexually transmitted diseases; transmission of HCV infection is rare between stable, monogamous sexual partners. Breast feeding does not increase the risk of HCV infection between an infected mother and her infant. Infection of health workers is not dramatically higher than among the general population; however, health workers are more likely to acquire HCV infection through accidental needle punctures, the efficiency of which is ~3%. Infection of household contacts is rare as well.

Other groups with an increased frequency of HCV infection include patients who require hemodialysis and organ transplantation and those who require transfusions in the setting of cancer chemotherapy. In immunosuppressed individuals, levels of anti-HCV may be undetectable, and a diagnosis may require testing for HCV RNA. Although new acute cases of hepatitis C are rare, newly diagnosed cases are common among otherwise healthy persons who experimented briefly with injection drugs two or three decades earlier. Such instances usually remain unrecognized for years, until unearthed by laboratory screening for routine medical examinations, insurance applications, and attempted blood donation.

Hepatitis E This type of hepatitis, identified in India, Asia, Africa, and Central America, resembles hepatitis A in its primarily enteric mode of spread. The commonly recognized cases occur after contamination of water supplies such as after monsoon flooding, but sporadic, isolated cases occur. An epidemiologic feature that distinguishes HEV from other enteric agents is the rarity of secondary person-to-person spread from infected persons to their close contacts. Infections arise in populations that are immune to HAV and favor young adults. It is not known if hepatitis E occurs outside of recognized endemic areas, for example, in the United States, but preliminary studies suggest that HEV does not account for any of the sporadic "non-A, non-B" cases in nonendemic areas. Cases imported from endemic areas have been found in the United States. Several reports suggest a zoonotic reservoir for HEV in swine.

CLINICAL AND LABORATORY FEATURES ■ Symptoms and Signs Acute viral hepatitis occurs after an incubation period that varies according to the responsible agent. Generally, incubation periods for hepatitis A range from 15 to 45 days (mean 4 weeks), for hepatitis B and D from 30 to 180 days (mean 4 to 12 weeks), for hepatitis C from 15 to 160 days (mean 7 weeks), and for hepatitis E from 14 to 60 days (mean 5 to 6 weeks). The *prodromal symptoms* of acute viral hepatitis are systemic and quite variable. Constitutional symptoms of anorexia, nausea and vomiting, fatigue, malaise, arthralgias, myalgias, headache, photophobia, pharyngitis, cough, and coryza may precede the onset of jaundice by 1 to 2 weeks. The nausea, vomiting, and anorexia are frequently associated with alterations in olfaction and taste. A low-grade fever between 38 and 39°C (100 to 102°F) is more often present in hepatitis

A and E than in hepatitis B or C, except when hepatitis B is heralded by a serum sickness–like syndrome; rarely, a fever of 39.5 to 40°C (103 to 104°F) may accompany the constitutional symptoms. Dark urine and clay-colored stools may be noticed by the patient from 1 to 5 days before the onset of clinical jaundice.

With the onset of *clinical jaundice*, the constitutional prodromal symptoms usually diminish, but in some patients mild weight loss (2.5 to 5 kg) is common and may continue during the entire icteric phase. The liver becomes enlarged and tender and may be associated with right upper quadrant pain and discomfort. Infrequently, patients present with a cholestatic picture, suggesting extrahepatic biliary obstruction. Splenomegaly and cervical adenopathy are present in 10 to 20% of patients with acute hepatitis. Rarely, a few spider angiomas appear during the icteric phase and disappear during convalescence. During the *recovery phase*, constitutional symptoms disappear, but usually some liver enlargement and abnormalities in liver biochemical tests are still evident. The duration of the posticteric phase is variable, ranging from 2 to 12 weeks, and is usually more prolonged in acute hepatitis B and C. Complete clinical and biochemical recovery is to be expected 1 to 2 months after all cases of hepatitis A and E and 3 to 4 months after the onset of jaundice in three-quarters of uncomplicated cases of hepatitis B and C. In the remainder, biochemical recovery may be delayed. A substantial proportion of patients with viral hepatitis never become icteric.

Infection with HDV can occur in the presence of acute or chronic HBV infection; the duration of HBV infection determines the duration of HDV infection. When acute HDV and HBV infection occur simultaneously, clinical and biochemical features may be indistinguishable from those of HBV infection alone, although occasionally they are more severe. As opposed to patients with *acute* HBV infection, patients with *chronic* HBV infection can support HDV replication indefinitely. This can happen when acute HDV infection occurs in the presence of a nonresolving acute HBV infection. More commonly, acute HDV infection becomes chronic when it is superimposed on an underlying chronic HBV infection. In such cases, the HDV superinfection appears as a clinical exacerbation or an episode resembling acute viral hepatitis in someone already chronically infected with HBV. Superinfection with HDV in a patient with chronic hepatitis B often leads to clinical deterioration (see below).

In addition to superinfections with other hepatitis agents, acute hepatitis-like clinical events in persons with chronic hepatitis B may accompany spontaneous HBeAg-to–anti-HBe seroconversion or spontaneous reactivation, i.e., reversion from nonreplicative to replicative infection. Such reactivations can occur as well in therapeutically immunosuppressed patients with chronic HBV infection when cytotoxic-immunosuppressive drugs are withdrawn; in these cases, restoration of immune competence is thought to allow resumption of previously checked cell-mediated immune cytolysis of HBV-infected hepatocytes. Occasionally, acute clinical exacerbations of chronic hepatitis B may represent the emergence of a precore mutant (see "Virology and Etiology," above), and the subsequent course in such patients may be characterized by periodic exacerbations.

Laboratory Features The serum aminotransferases aspartate aminotransferase (AST) and ALT (previously designated SGOT and SGPT) show a variable increase during the prodromal phase of acute viral hepatitis and precede the rise in bilirubin level (Figs. 285-2 and 285-4). The acute level of these enzymes, however, does not correlate well with the degree of liver cell damage. Peak levels vary from 400 to 4000 IU or more; these levels are usually reached at the time the patient is clinically icteric and diminish progressively during the recovery phase of acute hepatitis. The diagnosis of anicteric hepatitis is based on clinical features and on aminotransferase elevations.

Jaundice is usually visible in the sclera or skin when the serum bilirubin value exceeds 43 μmol/L (2.5 mg/dL). When jaundice appears, the serum bilirubin typically rises to levels ranging from 85 to

HBsAg	Anti-HBs	Anti-HBc	HBeAg	Anti-HBe	Interpretation
+	−	IgM	+	−	Acute hepatitis B, high infectivity
+	−	IgG	+	−	Chronic hepatitis B, high infectivity
+	−	IgG	−	+	1. Late acute or chronic hepatitis B, low infectivity 2. HBeAg-negative ("precore-mutant") hepatitis B (chronic or, rarely, acute)
+	+	+	+/−	+/−	1. HBsAg of one subtype and heterotypic anti-HBs (common) 2. Process of seroconversion from HBsAg to anti-HBs (rare)
−	−	IgM	+/−	+/−	1. Acute hepatitis B 2. Anti-HBc "window"
−	−	IgG	−	+/−	1. Low-level hepatitis B carrier 2. Hepatitis B in remote past
−	+	IgG	−	+/−	Recovery from hepatitis B
−	+	−	−	−	1. Immunization with HBsAg (after vaccination) 2. Hepatitis B in the remote past (?) 3. False-positive

TABLE 285-3 *Commonly Encountered Serologic Patterns of Hepatitis B Infection*

340 μmol/L (5 to 20 mg/dL). The serum bilirubin may continue to rise despite falling serum aminotransferase levels. In most instances, the total bilirubin is equally divided between the conjugated and unconjugated fractions. Bilirubin levels >340 μmol/L (20 mg/dL) extending and persisting late into the course of viral hepatitis are more likely to be associated with severe disease. In certain patients with underlying hemolytic anemia, however, such as glucose-6-phosphate dehydrogenase deficiency and sickle cell anemia, a high serum bilirubin level is common, resulting from superimposed hemolysis. In such patients, bilirubin levels >513 μmol/L (30 mg/dL) have been observed and are not necessarily associated with a poor prognosis.

Neutropenia and lymphopenia are transient and are followed by a relative lymphocytosis. Atypical lymphocytes (varying between 2 and 20%) are common during the acute phase. Measurement of the prothrombin time (PT) is important in patients with acute viral hepatitis, for a prolonged value may reflect a severe hepatic synthetic defect, signify extensive hepatocellular necrosis, and indicate a worse prognosis. Occasionally, a prolonged PT may occur with only mild increases in the serum bilirubin and aminotransferase levels. Prolonged nausea and vomiting, inadequate carbohydrate intake, and poor hepatic glycogen reserves may contribute to hypoglycemia noted occasionally in patients with severe viral hepatitis. Serum alkaline phosphatase may be normal or only mildly elevated, while a fall in serum albumin is uncommon in uncomplicated acute viral hepatitis. In some patients, mild and transient steatorrhea has been noted as well as slight microscopic hematuria and minimal proteinuria.

A diffuse but mild elevation of the gamma globulin fraction is common during acute viral hepatitis. Serum IgG and IgM levels are elevated in about one-third of patients during the acute phase of viral hepatitis, but the serum IgM level is elevated more characteristically during acute hepatitis A. During the acute phase of viral hepatitis, antibodies to smooth muscle and other cell constituents may be present, and low titers of rheumatoid factor, nuclear antibody, and heterophil antibody can also be found occasionally. In hepatitis C and D, antibodies to LKM may occur; however, the species of LKM antibodies in the two types of hepatitis are different from each other as well as from the LKM antibody species characteristic of autoimmune chronic hepatitis type 2 (Chap. 287). The autoantibodies in viral hepatitis are nonspecific and can also be associated with other viral and systemic diseases. In contrast, virus-specific antibodies, which appear during and after hepatitis virus infection, are serologic markers of diagnostic importance.

As described above, serologic tests are available with which to establish a diagnosis of hepatitis A, B, D, and C. Tests for fecal or serum HAV are not routinely available. Therefore, a diagnosis of hepatitis A is based on detection of IgM anti-HAV during acute illness

(Fig. 285-2). Rheumatoid factor can give rise to false-positive results in this test.

A diagnosis of HBV infection can usually be made by detection of HBsAg in serum. Infrequently, levels of HBsAg are too low to be detected during acute HBV infection, even with the current generation of highly sensitive immunoassays. In such cases, the diagnosis can be established by the presence of IgM anti-HBc.

The titer of HBsAg bears little relation to the severity of clinical disease. Indeed, there may be an inverse correlation between the serum concentration of HBsAg and the degree of liver cell damage. For example, titers are highest in immunosuppressed patients, lower in patients with chronic liver disease (but higher in mild chronic than in severe chronic hepatitis), and very low in patients with acute fulminant hepatitis. These observations suggest that in hepatitis B the degree of liver cell damage and the clinical course are probably related to variations in the patient's immune response to HBV rather than to the amount of circulating HBsAg. In immunocompetent persons, however, there is a correlation between markers of HBV *replication* and liver injury (see below).

Another serologic marker that may be of value in patients with hepatitis B is HBeAg. Its principal clinical usefulness is as an indicator of relative infectivity. Because HBeAg is invariably present during early acute hepatitis B, HBeAg testing is indicated primarily during follow-up of chronic infection.

In patients with hepatitis B surface antigenemia of unknown duration, e.g., blood donors found to be HBsAg-positive and referred to a physician for evaluation, testing for IgM anti-HBc may be useful to distinguish between acute or recent infection (IgM anti-HBc-positive) and chronic HBV infection (IgM anti-HBc-negative, IgG anti-HBc-positive). A false-positive test for IgM anti-HBc may be encountered in patients with high-titer rheumatoid factor.

Anti-HBs is rarely detectable in the presence of HBsAg in patients with *acute* hepatitis B, but 10 to 20% of persons with *chronic* HBV infection may harbor low-level anti-HBs. This antibody is directed not against the common group determinant, *a*, but against the heterotypic subtype determinant (e.g., HBsAg of subtype *ad* with anti-HBs of subtype *y*). In most cases, this serologic pattern cannot be attributed to infection with two different HBV subtypes, and the presence of this antibody is not a harbinger of imminent HBsAg clearance. When such antibody is detected, its presence is of no recognized clinical significance (see "Virology and Etiology," above).

After immunization with hepatitis B vaccine, which consists of HBsAg alone, anti-HBs is the only serologic marker to appear. The commonly encountered serologic patterns of hepatitis B and their interpretations are summarized in Table 285-3. Tests for the detection of HBV DNA in liver and serum are now available. Like HBeAg, serum HBV DNA is an indicator of HBV replication, but tests for HBV DNA are more sensitive and quantitative. Hybridization assays for HBV DNA have a sensitivity of approximately 10^5 to 10^6 virions/mL, a relative threshold below which infectivity and liver injury are limited and HBeAg is usually undetectable. Currently, testing for HBV DNA has shifted from insensitive hybridization assays to amplification assays, e.g., the PCR-based assay, which can detect as few as 100 or 1000 virions/mL. With increased sensitivity, amplification assays remain reactive well below the threshold for infectivity and liver injury. These markers are useful in following the course of HBV replication in patients with chronic hepatitis B receiving antiviral chemotherapy, e.g., with interferon or lamivudine (Chap. 287). In immunocompetent persons, a general correlation does appear to exist between the level of HBV replication, as reflected by the level of HBV DNA in serum, and the degree of liver injury. High serum HBV DNA levels, increased expression of viral antigens, and necroinflammatory activity in the liver go hand in hand unless immunosuppression interferes with cytolytic T cell responses to virus-infected cells; reduction of HBV replication with antiviral drugs tends to be accompanied by an improvement in liver histology.

In patients with hepatitis C, an episodic pattern of aminotransferase elevation is common. A specific serologic diagnosis of hepatitis C can be made by demonstrating the presence in serum of anti-HCV. When a second- or third-generation immunoassay (that detects antibodies to nonstructural and nucleocapsid proteins) is used, anti-HCV can be detected in acute hepatitis C during the initial phase of elevated aminotransferase activity. This antibody may never become detectable in 5 to 10% of patients with acute hepatitis C, and levels of anti-HCV may become undetectable after recovery from acute hepatitis C. In patients with chronic hepatitis C, anti-HCV is detectable in >95% of cases. Nonspecificity can confound immunoassays for anti-HCV, especially in persons with a low prior probability of infection, such as volunteer blood donors, or in persons with circulating rheumatoid factor, which can bind nonspecifically to assay reagents. A supplementary recombinant immunoblot assay (RIBA), in which serum is incubated with a nitrocellulose strip containing viral protein bands, can be used to establish the specific viral proteins to which anti-HCV is directed (see "Virology and Etiology," above). Such RIBA determinations were used to confirm anti-HCV reactivity in blood donors, but determinations of HCV RNA have supplanted RIBA in most clinical settings. Assays for HCV RNA are the most sensitive tests for HCV infection and represent the "gold standard" in establishing a diagnosis of hepatitis C. HCV RNA can be detected even before acute elevation of aminotransferase activity and before the appearance of anti-HCV in patients with acute hepatitis C. In addition, HCV RNA remains detectable indefinitely, continuously in most but intermittently in some, in patients with chronic hepatitis C (even detectable in some persons with normal liver tests, i.e., asymptomatic carriers). In the small minority of patients with hepatitis C who lack anti-HCV, a diagnosis can be supported by detection of HCV RNA. If all these tests are negative and the patient has a well-characterized case of hepatitis after percutaneous exposure to blood or blood products, a diagnosis of hepatitis caused by another agent, as yet unidentified, can be entertained.

Amplification techniques are required to detect HCV RNA, and two are available. One is a branched-chain complementary DNA (bDNA) assay, in which the detection signal (a colorimetrically detectable enzyme bound to a complementary DNA probe) is amplified. The other involves target amplification, i.e., synthesis of multiple copies of the viral genome. This can be done by PCR or TMA, in which the viral RNA is reverse transcribed to complementary DNA and then amplified by repeated cycles of DNA synthesis. Both can be used as quantitative assays and a measurement of relative "viral load"; PCR and TMA, with a sensitivity of 10^2 IU/mL, are more sensitive than bDNA, with a sensitivity of 10^5. Determination of viral load is not a reliable marker of disease severity or prognosis but is helpful in predicting relative responsiveness to antiviral therapy. The same is true for determinations of HCV genotype (Chap. 287).

A proportion of patients with hepatitis C have isolated anti-HBc in their blood, a reflection of a common risk in certain populations to multiple bloodborne hepatitis agents. The anti-HBc in such cases is almost invariably of the IgG class and usually represents HBV infection in the remote past, rarely current HBV infection with low-level virus carriage.

The presence of HDV infection can be identified by demonstrating intrahepatic HDV antigen or, more practically, an anti-HDV seroconversion (a rise in titer of anti-HDV or de novo appearance of anti-HDV). Circulating HDV antigen, also diagnostic of acute infection, is detectable only briefly, if at all. Because anti-HDV is often undetectable once HBsAg disappears, retrospective serodiagnosis of acute self-limited, simultaneous HBV and HDV infection is difficult. Early diagnosis of acute infection may be hampered by a delay of up to 30 to 40 days in the appearance of anti-HDV.

When a patient presents with acute hepatitis and has HBsAg and

anti-HDV in serum, determination of the class of anti-HBc is helpful in establishing the relationship between infection with HBV and HDV. Although IgM anti-HBc does not distinguish *absolutely* between acute and chronic HBV infection, its presence is a reliable indicator of recent infection and its absence a reliable indicator of infection in the remote past. In simultaneous acute HBV and HDV infections, IgM anti-HBc will be detectable, while in acute HDV infection superimposed on chronic HBV infection, anti-HBc will be of the IgG class.

Tests for the presence of HDV RNA are useful for determining the presence of ongoing HDV replication and relative infectivity. Currently, probes for this marker are restricted to a limited number of research laboratories. Diagnostic tests for hepatitis E are commercially available in several countries outside the United States; in the United States, diagnostic assays can be performed at the Centers for Disease Control and Prevention.

Liver biopsy is rarely necessary or indicated in acute viral hepatitis, except when there is a question about the diagnosis or when there is clinical evidence suggesting a diagnosis of chronic hepatitis.

A diagnostic algorithm can be applied in the evaluation of cases of acute viral hepatitis. A patient with acute hepatitis should undergo four serologic tests, HBsAg, IgM anti-HAV, IgM anti-HBc, and anti-HCV (Table 285-4). The presence of HBsAg, with or without IgM anti-HBc, represents HBV infection. If IgM anti-HBc is present, the HBV infection is considered acute; if IgM anti-HBc is absent, the HBV infection is considered chronic. A diagnosis of acute hepatitis B can be made in the absence of HBsAg when IgM anti-HBc is detectable. A diagnosis of acute hepatitis A is based on the presence of IgM anti-HAV. If IgM anti-HAV coexists with HBsAg, a diagnosis of simultaneous HAV and HBV infections can be made; if IgM anti-HBc (with or without HBsAg) is detectable, the patient has simultaneous acute hepatitis A and B, and if IgM anti-HBc is undetectable, the patient has acute hepatitis A superimposed on chronic HBV infection. The presence of anti-HCV supports a diagnosis of acute hepatitis C. Occasionally, testing for HCV RNA or repeat anti-HCV testing later during the illness is necessary to establish the diagnosis. Absence of all serologic markers is consistent with a diagnosis of "non-A, non-B, non-C" hepatitis, if the epidemiologic setting is appropriate.

In patients with chronic hepatitis, initial testing should consist of HBsAg and anti-HCV. Anti-HCV supports and HCV RNA testing establishes the diagnosis of chronic hepatitis C. If a serologic diagnosis of chronic hepatitis B is made, testing for HBeAg and anti-HBe is indicated to evaluate relative infectivity. Testing for HBV DNA in such patients provides a more quantitative and sensitive measure of the level of virus replication and, therefore, is very helpful during antiviral therapy (Chap. 287). In patients with hepatitis B, testing for anti-HDV is useful under the following circumstances: patients with

TABLE 285-4 *Simplified Diagnostic Approach in Patients Presenting with Acute Hepatitis*

	Serologic Tests of Patient's Serum			
HBsAg	IgM Anti-HAV	IgM Anti-HBc	Anti-HCV	Diagnostic Interpretation
+	−	+	−	Acute hepatitis B
+	−	−	−	Chronic hepatitis B
+	+	−	−	Acute hepatitis A superimposed on chronic hepatitis B
+	+	+	−	Acute hepatitis A and B
−	+	−	−	Acute hepatitis A
−	+	+	−	Acute hepatitis A and B (HBsAg below detection threshold)
−	−	+	−	Acute hepatitis B (HBsAg below detection threshold)
−	−	−	+	Acute hepatitis C

severe and fulminant diseases, patients with severe chronic disease, patients with chronic hepatitis B who have acute hepatitis-like exacerbations, persons with frequent percutaneous exposures, and persons from areas where HDV infection is endemic.

PROGNOSIS Virtually all previously healthy patients with hepatitis A recover completely from their illness with no clinical sequelae. Similarly, in acute hepatitis B, 95 to 99% of previously healthy adults have a favorable course and recover completely. Certain clinical and laboratory features, however, suggest a more complicated and protracted course. Patients of advanced age and with serious underlying medical disorders may have a prolonged course and are more likely to experience severe hepatitis. Initial presenting features such as ascites, peripheral edema, and symptoms of hepatic encephalopathy suggest a poorer prognosis. In addition, a prolonged PT, low serum albumin level, hypoglycemia, and very high serum bilirubin values suggest severe hepatocellular disease. Patients with these clinical and laboratory features deserve prompt hospital admission. The case-fatality rate in hepatitis A and B is very low (approximately 0.1%) but is increased by advanced age and underlying debilitating disorders. Among patients ill enough to be hospitalized for acute hepatitis B, the fatality rate is 1%. Hepatitis C is less severe during the acute phase than hepatitis B and is more likely to be anicteric; fatalities are rare, but the precise case-fatality rate is not known. In outbreaks of waterborne hepatitis E in India and Asia, the case-fatality rate is 1 to 2% and up to 10 to 20% in pregnant women. Patients with simultaneous acute hepatitis B and hepatitis D do not necessarily experience a higher mortality rate than do patients with acute hepatitis B alone; however, in several recent outbreaks of acute simultaneous HBV and HDV infection among injection drug users, the case-fatality rate has been approximately 5%. In the case of HDV superinfection of a person with chronic hepatitis B, the likelihood of fulminant hepatitis and death is increased substantially. Although the case-fatality rate for hepatitis D has not been defined adequately, in outbreaks of severe HDV superinfection in isolated populations with a high hepatitis B carrier rate, the mortality rate has been recorded in excess of 20%.

COMPLICATIONS AND SEQUELAE A small proportion of patients with hepatitis A experience *relapsing hepatitis* weeks to months after apparent recovery from acute hepatitis. Relapses are characterized by recurrence of symptoms, aminotransferase elevations, occasionally jaundice, and fecal excretion of HAV. Another unusual variant of acute hepatitis A is *cholestatic hepatitis*, characterized by protracted cholestatic jaundice and pruritus. Rarely, liver test abnormalities persist for many months, even up to a year. Even when these complications occur, hepatitis A remains self-limited and does not progress to chronic liver disease. During the prodromal phase of acute hepatitis B, a serum sickness–like syndrome characterized by arthralgia or arthritis, rash, angioedema, and rarely hematuria and proteinuria may develop in 5 to 10% of patients. This syndrome occurs before the onset of clinical jaundice, and these patients are often erroneously diagnosed as having rheumatologic diseases. The diagnosis can be established by measuring serum aminotransferase levels, which are almost invariably elevated, and serum HBsAg. As noted above, EMC is an immune-complex disease that can complicate chronic hepatitis C and is part of a spectrum of B cell lymphoproliferative disorders, which, in rare instances, can evolve to B cell lymphoma (Chap. 97). Attention has been drawn as well to associations between hepatitis C and such cutaneous disorders as porphyria cutanea tarda and lichen planus. A mechanism for these associations is unknown.

The most feared complication of viral hepatitis is *fulminant hepatitis* (massive hepatic necrosis); fortunately, this is a rare event. Fulminant hepatitis is primarily seen in hepatitis B and D, as well as hepatitis E, but rare fulminant cases of hepatitis A occur primarily in older adults and in persons with underlying chronic liver disease, including, according to some reports, chronic hepatitis B and C. Hepatitis B accounts for >50% of fulminant hepatitis cases, a sizable proportion of which are associated with HDV infection and another proportion with underlying chronic hepatitis C. Fulminant hepatitis is seen rarely in hepatitis C, but hepatitis E, as noted above, can be complicated by fatal fulminant hepatitis in 1 to 2% of all cases and in up to 20% of cases occurring in pregnant women. Patients usually present with signs and symptoms of encephalopathy that may evolve to deep coma. The liver is usually small and the PT excessively prolonged. The combination of rapidly shrinking liver size, rapidly rising bilirubin level, and marked prolongation of the PT, even as aminotransferase levels fall, together with clinical signs of confusion, disorientation, somnolence, ascites, and edema, indicates that the patient has hepatic failure with encephalopathy. Cerebral edema is common; brainstem compression, gastrointestinal bleeding, sepsis, respiratory failure, cardiovascular collapse, and renal failure are terminal events. The mortality rate is exceedingly high (>80% in patients with deep coma), but patients who survive may have a complete biochemical and histologic recovery. If a donor liver can be located in time, liver transplantation may be life-saving in patients with fulminant hepatitis (Chap. 291).

It is particularly important to document the disappearance of HBsAg after apparent clinical recovery from acute hepatitis B. Before laboratory methods were available to distinguish between acute hepatitis and acute hepatitis–like exacerbations (*spontaneous reactivations*) of chronic hepatitis B, observations suggested that approximately 10% of patients remained HBsAg-positive for >6 months after the onset of clinically apparent acute hepatitis B. Half these persons cleared the antigen from their circulations during the next several years, but the other 5% remained chronically HBsAg-positive. More recent observations suggest that the true rate of chronic infection after clinically apparent acute hepatitis B is as low as 1% in normal, immunocompetent, young adults. Earlier, higher estimates may have been biased by inadvertent inclusion of acute exacerbations in chronically infected patients; these patients, chronically HBsAg-positive before exacerbation, were unlikely to seroconvert to HBsAg-negative thereafter. Whether the rate of chronicity is 10 or 1%, such patients have anti-HBc in serum; anti-HBs is either undetected or detected at low titer against the opposite subtype specificity of the antigen (see "Laboratory Features," above). These patients may (1) be inactive carriers; (2) have low-grade, mild chronic hepatitis; or (3) have moderate to severe chronic hepatitis with or without cirrhosis. The likelihood of becoming an HBsAg carrier after acute HBV infection is especially high among neonates, persons with Down's syndrome, chronically hemodialyzed patients, and immunosuppressed patients, including persons with HIV infection.

Chronic hepatitis is an important late complication of acute hepatitis B occurring in a small proportion of patients with acute disease but more common in those who present with chronic infection without having experienced an acute illness (Chap. 287). Certain clinical and laboratory features suggest progression of acute hepatitis to chronic hepatitis: (1) lack of complete resolution of clinical symptoms of anorexia, weight loss, and fatigue and the persistence of hepatomegaly; (2) the presence of bridging or multilobular hepatic necrosis on liver biopsy during protracted, severe acute viral hepatitis; (3) failure of the serum aminotransferase, bilirubin, and globulin levels to return to normal within 6 to 12 months after the acute illness; and (4) the persistence of HBeAg beyond 3 months or HBsAg beyond 6 months after acute hepatitis.

Although acute hepatitis D infection does not increase the likelihood of chronicity of simultaneous acute hepatitis B, hepatitis D has the potential for contributing to the severity of chronic hepatitis B. Hepatitis D superinfection can transform asymptomatic or mild chronic hepatitis B into severe, progressive chronic hepatitis and cirrhosis; it also can accelerate the course of chronic hepatitis B. Some HDV superinfections in patients with chronic hepatitis B lead to fulminant hepatitis. Although HDV and HBV infections are associated with severe liver disease, mild hepatitis and even asymptomatic carriage have been identified in some patients, and the disease may become indolent beyond the early years of infection. After acute HCV infection, the likelihood of remaining chronically *infected* approaches 85 to 90%. Although many patients with chronic hepatitis C have no symptoms, cirrhosis may develop in as many as 20% within 10 to 20 years of acute illness; in some series of cases, cirrhosis has been reported in as many as 50% of patients with chronic hepatitis C. Although chronic hepatitis C accounts for at least 40% of cases of chronic liver disease and of patients undergoing liver transplantation for end-stage liver disease in the United States and Europe, in the majority of patients with chronic hepatitis C, morbidity and mortality are limited during the initial 20 years after the onset of infection. Progression of chronic hepatitis C may be influenced by hepatitis C genotype, age of acquisition, duration of infection, immunosuppression, coexisting excessive alcohol use, other hepatitis virus infection, or HIV co-infection. In fact, instances of severe and rapidly progressive chronic hepatitis B and C are being recognized with increasing frequency in patients with HIV infection (Chap. 173). In contrast, neither HAV nor HEV causes chronic liver disease.

Rare complications of viral hepatitis include pancreatitis, myocarditis, atypical pneumonia, aplastic anemia, transverse myelitis, and peripheral neuropathy. Persons with chronic hepatitis B, particularly those infected in infancy or early childhood and especially those with HBeAg, have an enhanced risk of hepatocellular carcinoma. The risk of hepatocellular carcinoma is increased as well in patients with chronic hepatitis C, almost exclusively in patients with cirrhosis, and almost always after at least several decades, usually after three decades of disease (Chap. 78). In children, hepatitis B may present rarely with anicteric hepatitis, a nonpruritic papular rash of the face, buttocks, and limbs, and lymphadenopathy (papular acrodermatitis of childhood or Gianotti-Crosti syndrome).

DIFFERENTIAL DIAGNOSIS Viral diseases such as infectious mononucleosis; those due to cytomegalovirus, herpes simplex, and coxsackieviruses; and toxoplasmosis may share certain clinical features with viral hepatitis and cause elevations in serum aminotransferase and less commonly in serum bilirubin levels. Tests such as the differential heterophile and serologic tests for these agents may be helpful in the differential diagnosis if HBsAg, anti-HBc, IgM anti-HAV, and anti-HCV determinations are negative. Aminotransferase elevations can accompany almost any systemic viral infection; other rare causes of liver injury confused with viral hepatitis are infections with *Leptospira*, *Candida*, *Brucella*, *Mycobacteria*, and *Pneumocystis*. A complete drug history is particularly important, for many drugs and certain anesthetic agents can produce a picture of either acute hepatitis or cholestasis (Chap. 286). Equally important is a past history of unexplained "repeated episodes" of acute hepatitis. This history should alert the physician to the possibility that the underlying disorder is chronic hepatitis. Alcoholic hepatitis must also be considered, but usually the serum aminotransferase levels are not as markedly elevated and other stigmata of alcoholism may be present. The finding on liver biopsy of fatty infiltration, a neutrophilic inflammatory reaction, and "alcoholic hyaline" would be consistent with alcohol-induced rather than viral liver injury. Because acute hepatitis may present with right upper quadrant abdominal pain, nausea and vomiting, fever, and icterus, it is often confused with acute cholecystitis, common duct stone, or ascending cholangitis. Patients with acute viral hepatitis may tolerate surgery poorly; therefore, it is important to exclude this diagnosis, and in confusing cases, a percutaneous liver biopsy may be necessary before laparotomy. Viral hepatitis in the elderly is often misdiagnosed as obstructive jaundice resulting from a common duct stone or carcinoma of the pancreas. Because acute hepatitis in the elderly may be quite severe and the operative mortality high, a thorough evaluation including biochemical tests, radiographic studies of the biliary tree, and even liver biopsy may be necessary to exclude primary parenchymal liver disease. Another clinical constellation that may mimic acute hepatitis is right ventricular failure with passive hepatic congestion or hypoperfusion syndromes, such as those associated with shock, severe hypotension, and severe left ventricular failure. Also included in this general category is any disorder that interferes with venous return to the heart, such as right atrial myxoma, constrictive pericarditis, hepatic vein occlusion (Budd-Chiari syndrome), or venoocclusive disease. Clinical features are usually sufficient to distinguish between these vascular disorders and viral hepatitis. Acute fatty liver of pregnancy, cholestasis of pregnancy, eclampsia, and the HELLP syndrome (hemolysis, elevated liver tests, and low platelets) can be confused with viral hepatitis during pregnancy. Very rarely, malignancies metastatic to the liver can mimic acute or even fulminant viral hepatitis. Occasionally, genetic or metabolic liver disorders (e.g., Wilson's disease, α_1-antitrypsin deficiency) as well as nonalcoholic fatty liver disease are confused with viral hepatitis.

℞ TREATMENT

Treatment of Acute Attack In hepatitis B, among previously healthy adults who present with clinically apparent acute hepatitis, recovery occurs in approximately 99%; therefore, antiviral therapy is not likely to improve the rate of recovery and is not required. In rare instances of severe acute hepatitis B, treatment with a nucleoside analogue, such as lamivudine, at the 100-mg/d oral dose used to treat chronic hepatitis B (Chap. 287), has been attempted successfully. However, clinical trials have not been done to establish the efficacy of this approach, severe acute hepatitis B is not an approved indication for therapy, and the duration of therapy has not been determined. In typical cases of acute hepatitis C, recovery is rare, progression to chronic hepatitis is the rule, and meta-analyses of small clinical trials suggest that antiviral therapy with interferon α monotherapy (3 million units subcutaneously three times a week) is beneficial, reducing the rate of chronicity considerably by inducing sustained responses in 30 to 70% of patients. In a German multicenter study of 44 patients with acute symptomatic hepatitis C, initiation of intensive interferon α therapy (5 million units subcutaneously daily for 4 weeks, then three times a week for another 20 weeks) within an average of 3 months after infection resulted in a sustained virologic response rate of 98%. Although treatment of acute hepatitis C is recommended, the optimum regimen, duration of therapy, and time to initiate therapy remain to be determined. Many authorities now opt for the best regimen identified for the treatment of chronic hepatitis C, long-acting pegylated interferon plus the nucleoside analogue ribavirin, the efficacy of which is superior to that of standard interferon monotherapy regimens (Chap. 287). Because of the marked reduction over the last two decades in the frequency of acute hepatitis C, opportunities to identify and treat patients with acute hepatitis C are rare indeed. Hospital epidemiologists, however, will encounter health workers who sustain hepatitis C–contaminated needle sticks; when monitoring for ALT elevations and HCV RNA after these accidents identifies acute hepatitis C, therapy should be initiated.

Notwithstanding these specific therapeutic considerations, in most cases of typical acute viral hepatitis, specific treatment generally is not necessary. Although hospitalization may be required for clinically severe illness, most patients do not require hospital care. Forced and prolonged bed rest is not essential for full recovery, but many patients will feel better with restricted physical activity. A high-calorie diet is desirable, and because many patients may experience nausea late in the day, the major caloric intake is best tolerated in the morning. Intravenous feeding is necessary in the acute stage if the patient has persistent vomiting and cannot maintain oral intake. Drugs capable of producing adverse reactions such as cholestasis and drugs metabolized by the liver should be avoided. If severe pruritus is present, the use of the bile salt–sequestering resin cholestyramine is helpful. Glucocorticoid therapy has no value in acute viral hepatitis, even in severe cases associated with *bridging necrosis*, and may be hazardous.

Physical isolation of patients with hepatitis to a single room and bathroom is rarely necessary except in the case of fecal incontinence for hepatitis A and E or uncontrolled, voluminous bleeding for hepatitis B (with or without concomitant hepatitis D) and hepatitis C. Because most patients hospitalized with hepatitis A excrete little if any

HAV, the likelihood of HAV transmission from these patients during their hospitalization is low. Therefore, burdensome *enteric precautions are no longer recommended*. Although gloves should be worn when the bedpans or fecal material of patients with hepatitis A are handled, these precautions do not represent a departure from sensible procedure for all hospitalized patients. For patients with hepatitis B and hepatitis C, emphasis should be placed on blood precautions, i.e., avoiding direct, ungloved hand contact with blood and other body fluids. Enteric precautions are unnecessary. The importance of simple hygienic precautions, such as hand washing, cannot be overemphasized. Universal precautions that have been adopted for all patients apply to patients with viral hepatitis.

Hospitalized patients may be discharged when there is substantial symptomatic improvement, a significant downward trend in the serum aminotransferase and bilirubin values, and a return to normal of the PT. Mild aminotransferase elevations should not be considered contraindications to the gradual resumption of normal activity.

In *fulminant hepatitis*, the goal of therapy is to support the patient by maintenance of fluid balance, support of circulation and respiration, control of bleeding, correction of hypoglycemia, and treatment of other complications of the comatose state in anticipation of liver regeneration and repair. Protein intake should be restricted, and oral lactulose or neomycin administered. Glucocorticoid therapy has been shown in controlled trials to be ineffective. Likewise, exchange transfusion, plasmapheresis, human cross-circulation, porcine liver cross-perfusion, and hemoperfusion have not been proven to enhance survival; however, the efficacy of extracorporeal liver-assist devices, involving hollow-fiber chambers containing hepatocytes, is being evaluated in clinical trials. Meticulous intensive care is the one factor that does appear to improve survival. Orthotopic liver transplantation is resorted to with increasing frequency, with excellent results, in patients with fulminant hepatitis (Chap. 291).

PROPHYLAXIS   Because application of therapy for acute viral hepatitis is limited, and because antiviral therapy for chronic viral hepatitis is effective in only a proportion of patients (Chap. 287), emphasis is placed on prevention through immunization. The prophylactic approach differs for each of the types of viral hepatitis. In the past, immunoprophylaxis relied exclusively on passive immunization with antibody-containing globulin preparations purified by cold ethanol fractionation from the plasma of hundreds of normal donors. Currently, for hepatitis A and B, active immunization with vaccines is available as well.

Hepatitis A   Both passive immunization with IG and active immunization with killed vaccines are available. All preparations of IG contain anti-HAV concentrations sufficient to be protective. When administered before exposure or during the early incubation period, IG is effective in preventing clinically apparent hepatitis A. For postexposure prophylaxis of intimate contacts (household, sexual, institutional) of persons with hepatitis A, the administration of 0.02 mL/kg is recommended as early after exposure as possible; it may be effective even when administered as late as 2 weeks after exposure. Prophylaxis is not necessary for casual contacts (office, factory, school, or hospital), for most elderly persons, who are very likely to be immune, or for those known to have anti-HAV in their serum. In day-care centers, recognition of hepatitis A in children or staff should provide a stimulus for immunoprophylaxis in the center and in the children's family members. By the time most common-source outbreaks of hepatitis A are recognized, it is usually too late in the incubation period for IG to be effective; however, prophylaxis may limit the frequency of secondary cases. For travelers to tropical countries, developing countries, and other areas outside standard tourist routes, IG prophylaxis had been recommended, before a vaccine became available. When such travel lasted less than 3 months, 0.02 mL/kg was given; for longer travel or residence in these areas, a dose of 0.06 mL/kg every 4 to 6 months was recommended. Administration of plasma-derived globulin is safe;

all contemporary lots of IG are subjected to viral inactivation steps and must be free of HCV RNA as determined by PCR testing. Administration of intramuscular lots of IG has not been associated with transmission of HBV, HCV, or HIV.

Formalin-inactivated vaccines made from strains of HAV attenuated in tissue culture have been shown to be safe, immunogenic, and effective in preventing hepatitis A. Hepatitis A vaccines are approved for use in persons who are at least 2 years old and appear to provide adequate protection 4 weeks after a primary inoculation. If it can be given within 4 weeks of an expected exposure, such as by travel to an endemic area, hepatitis A vaccine is the preferred approach to *preexposure* immunoprophylaxis. If travel is more imminent, IG (0.02 mL/kg) should be administered at a different injection site, along with the first dose of vaccine. Because vaccination provides long-lasting protection (protective levels of anti-HAV should last 20 years after vaccination), persons whose risk will be sustained (e.g., frequent travelers or those remaining in endemic areas for prolonged periods) should be vaccinated, and vaccine should supplant the need for repeated IG injections. Other groups who are candidates for hepatitis A vaccination include military personnel, populations with cyclic outbreaks of hepatitis A (e.g., Alaskan natives), employees of day-care centers, primate handlers, laboratory workers exposed to hepatitis A or fecal specimens, children in communities with a high frequency of hepatitis A, and patients with chronic liver disease. Because of an increased risk of fulminant hepatitis A—observed in some experiences but not confirmed in others—among patients with chronic hepatitis C, patients with chronic hepatitis C have been singled out as candidates for hepatitis A vaccination. Other populations whose recognized risk of hepatitis A is increased should be vaccinated, including men who have sex with men, injection drug users, and persons with clotting disorders who require frequent administration of clotting-factor concentrates. Recommendations for dose and frequency differ for the two approved vaccine preparations (Table 285-5); all injections are intramuscular. Hepatitis A vaccine has been reported to be effective in preventing secondary household cases of acute hepatitis A, but its role in other instances of postexposure prophylaxis remains to be demonstrated.

Hepatitis B   Until 1982, prevention of hepatitis B was based on *passive* immunoprophylaxis either with standard IG, containing modest levels of anti-HBs, or hepatitis B immune globulin (HBIG), containing high-titer anti-HBs. The efficacy of standard IG has never been established and remains questionable; even the efficacy of HBIG, demonstrated in several clinical trials, has been challenged, and its contribution appears to be in reducing the frequency of clinical *illness*, not in preventing *infection*. The first vaccine for *active* immunization, introduced in 1982, was prepared from purified, noninfectious 22-nm spherical forms of HBsAg derived from the plasma of healthy HBsAg carriers. In 1987, the plasma-derived vaccine was supplanted by a genetically engineered vaccine derived from recombinant yeast. The latter vaccine consists of HBsAg particles that are nonglycosylated but are otherwise indistinguishable from natural HBsAg; two recombinant vaccines are licensed for use in the United States. Current recommendations can be divided into those for preexposure and postexposure prophylaxis.

For *preexposure* prophylaxis against hepatitis B in settings of frequent exposure (health workers exposed to blood; hemodialysis pa-

TABLE 285-5 *Hepatitis A Vaccination Schedules*			
Age, years	No. of Doses	Dose	Schedule, months
HAVRIX (GLAXOSMITHKLINE)			
2–18	2	720 ELU[a] (0.5 mL)	0, 6–12
>18	2	1440 ELU (1.0 mL)	0, 6–12
VAQTA (MERCK)			
2–17	2	25 units (0.5 mL)	0, 6
>17	2	50 units (1.0 mL)	0, 6–18

[a] Enzyme-linked immunoassay units.

tients and staff; residents and staff of custodial institutions for the developmentally handicapped; injection drug users; inmates of long-term correctional facilities; persons with multiple sexual partners; persons such as hemophiliacs who require long-term, high-volume therapy with blood derivatives; household and sexual contacts of HBsAg carriers; persons living in or traveling extensively in endemic areas; unvaccinated children under the age of 18; and unvaccinated children who are Alaskan natives, Pacific Islanders, or residents in households of first-generation immigrants from endemic countries), three intramuscular (deltoid, not gluteal) injections of hepatitis B vaccine are recommended at 0, 1, and 6 months. Pregnancy is *not* a contraindication to vaccination. In areas of low HBV endemicity such as the United States, despite the availability of safe and effective hepatitis B vaccines, a strategy of vaccinating persons in high-risk groups has not been effective. The incidence of new hepatitis B cases continued to increase in the United States after introduction of vaccines; fewer than 10% of all targeted persons in high-risk groups have actually been vaccinated, and approximately 30% of persons with sporadic acute hepatitis B do not fall into any high-risk-group category. Therefore, to have an impact on the frequency of HBV infection in an area of low endemicity such as the United States, universal hepatitis B vaccination in childhood has been recommended. For unvaccinated children born after the implementation of universal infant vaccination, vaccination during early adolescence, at age 11 to 12 years, was recommended, and this recommendation has been extended to include all unvaccinated children age 0 to 18 years. In HBV-hyperendemic areas, e.g., Asia, universal vaccination of children has resulted in a marked 10- to 15-year decline in hepatitis B and its complications.

The two available recombinant hepatitis B vaccines are comparable, one containing 10 μg of HBsAg (Recombivax-HB) and the other containing 20 μg of HBsAg (Engerix-B), and recommended doses for each injection vary for the two preparations (Table 285-6).

For unvaccinated persons sustaining an exposure to HBV, *postexposure* prophylaxis with a combination of HBIG (for rapid achievement of high-titer circulating anti-HBs) and hepatitis B vaccine (for achievement of long-lasting immunity as well as its apparent efficacy in attenuating clinical illness after exposure) is recommended. For *perinatal* exposure of infants born to HBsAg-positive mothers, a single dose of HBIG, 0.5 mL, should be administered intramuscularly in the thigh *immediately after birth*, followed by a complete course of three injections of recombinant hepatitis B vaccine (see doses above) to be started within the first 12 h of life. For those experiencing a direct percutaneous inoculation or transmucosal exposure to HBsAg-positive blood or body fluids (e.g., accidental *needle stick*, other mucosal penetration, or ingestion), a single intramuscular dose of HBIG, 0.06 mL/kg, administered as soon after exposure as possible, is followed by a complete course of hepatitis B vaccine to begin within the first week. For those exposed by *sexual* contact to a patient with acute hepatitis B, a single intramuscular dose of HBIG, 0.06 mL/kg, should be given within 14 days of exposure, to be followed by a complete course of hepatitis B vaccine. When both HBIG and hepatitis B vaccine are

recommended, they may be given at the same time but at separate sites.

The precise duration of protection afforded by hepatitis B vaccine is unknown; however, approximately 80 to 90% of immunocompetent vaccinees retain protective levels of anti-HBs for at least 5 years, and 60 to 80% for 10 years. Thereafter and even after anti-HBs becomes undetectable, protection persists against clinical hepatitis B, hepatitis B surface antigenemia, and chronic HBV infection. Currently, *booster* immunizations are not recommended routinely, except in immunosuppressed persons who have lost detectable anti-HBs or immunocompetent persons who sustain percutaneous HBsAg-positive inoculations after losing detectable antibody. Specifically, for hemodialysis patients, annual anti-HBs testing is recommended after vaccination; booster doses are recommended when anti-HBs levels fall below 10 mIU/mL. For people at risk of both hepatitis A and B, a combined vaccine is available containing 720 enzyme-linked immunoassay units of inactivated HAV and 20 μg of recombinant HBsAg (at 0, 1, and 6 months).

Hepatitis D Infection with hepatitis D can be prevented by vaccinating susceptible persons with hepatitis B vaccine. No product is available for immunoprophylaxis to prevent HDV superinfection in HBsAg carriers; for them, avoidance of percutaneous exposures and limitation of intimate contact with persons who have HDV infection are recommended.

Hepatitis C IG is ineffective in preventing hepatitis C and is no longer recommended for postexposure prophylaxis in cases of perinatal, needle stick, or sexual exposure. Although a prototype vaccine that induces antibodies to HCV envelope protein has been developed, currently, hepatitis C vaccination is not feasible practically. Genotype and quasispecies viral heterogeneity, as well as rapid evasion of neutralizing antibodies by this rapidly mutating virus, conspire to render HCV a difficult target for immunoprophylaxis with a vaccine. Prevention of transfusion-associated hepatitis C has been accomplished by the following successively introduced measures: Exclusion of commercial blood donors and reliance on a volunteer blood supply; screening donor blood with surrogate markers such as ALT (no longer recommended) and anti-HBc, markers that identify segments of the blood donor population with an increased risk of bloodborne infections; exclusion of blood donors in high-risk groups for AIDS and the introduction of anti-HIV screening tests; and progressively sensitive serologic screening tests for HCV infection. Chemical and heat treatment of blood products used for large-pool and concentrated blood derivates are being pursued.

In the absence of active or passive immunization, prevention of hepatitis C includes behavior changes and precautions to limit exposures to infected persons. Recommendations designed to identify patients with clinically inapparent hepatitis as candidates for medical management have as a secondary benefit the identification of persons whose contacts could be at risk of becoming infected. A so-called "look-back" program has been recommended to identify persons who were transfused before 1992 with blood from a donor found subsequently to have hepatitis C. In addition, anti-HCV testing is recommended for anyone who received a blood transfusion or a transplanted organ before the introduction of second-generation screening tests in 1992, people who ever used injection drugs, chronically hemodialyzed patients, persons with clotting disorders who received clotting factors made before 1987 from pooled blood products, persons with elevated aminotransferase levels, health workers exposed to HCV-positive blood or contaminated needles, and children born to HCV-positive mothers.

For stable, monogamous sexual partners, sexual transmission of hepatitis C is unlikely, and sexual barrier precautions are not recommended. For persons with multiple sexual partners or with sexually transmitted diseases, the risk of sexual transmission of hepatitis C is increased, and barrier precautions (latex condoms) are recommended.

TABLE 285-6 *Preexposure Hepatitis B Vaccination Schedules*

Target Group	No. of Doses	Dose	Schedule, months
RECOMBIVAX-HB (MERCK)			
Infants, children (<11 years)	3	5 μg (0.5 mL)	0–2, 1–4, 6–18
Adolescents (11–19 years)	3	5 μg (0.5 mL)	0–2, 1–4, 4–6
Adults (≥20 years)	3	10 μg (1.0 mL)	0–2, 1–4, 4–6
Hemodialysis patients[a]	3	40 μg (1.0 mL)	0, 1, 6
ENGERIX-B (GLAXOSMITHKLINE)			
Infants, children (<10 years)	3	10 μg (0.5 mL)	0–2, 1–4, 6–18
Adolescents (10–19 years)	3	10 μg (0.5 mL)	0–2, 1–4, 4–6
Adults (≥ 20 years)	3	20 μg (1.0 mL)	0–2, 1–4, 4–6
Hemodialysis patients[a]	3	40 μg (1.0 mL)	0, 1, 6

[a] Includes other immunocompromised persons.

A person with hepatitis C should avoid sharing such items as razors, toothbrushes, and nail clippers with sexual partners and family members. No special precautions are recommended for babies born to mothers with hepatitis C, and breast feeding does not have to be restricted.

Hepatitis E   Whether IG prevents hepatitis E remains undetermined. A recombinant vaccine has been developed and is undergoing clinical testing.

FURTHER READING

BRANCH AD, SEEFF LB (eds): Hepatitis C: State of the art at the millennium. Semin Liver Dis 20:1, 127, 2000

CENTERS FOR DISEASE CONTROL AND PREVENTION: Updated U.S. Public Health Service guidelines for the management of occupational exposures to HBV, HCV, and HIV and recommendations for postexposure prophylaxis. Morb Mort Week Rep 50(RR-11):1, 2001

———: General recommendations on immunization: Recommendations of the Advisory Committee on Immunization Practices and the American Academy of Family Physicians. Morb Mort Week Rep 51(RR-2):1, 2002

CHU C-J et al: Hepatitis B virus genotype B is associated with earlier HBeAg seroconversion compared with hepatitis B virus genotype C. Gastroenterology 122:1756, 2002

CONSENSUS STATEMENT: EASL International Consensus Conference on Hepatitis C. J Hepatol 30:956, 1999

EL-SERAG HB et al: Extrahepatic manifestation of hepatitis C among United States male veterans. Hepatology 36:1439, 2002

JAECKEL E et al: Treatment of acute hepatitis C with interferon alfa-2b. N Engl J Med 345:1452, 2001

KOFF RS et al: Hepatitis A. Lancet 341:1643, 1998

LAUER GM, WALKER BD: Medical progress: Hepatitis C virus infection. N Engl J Med 345:41, 2001

LOK ASF, MCMAHON BJ: Chronic hepatitis B. Hepatology 34:1225, 2001

MARGOLIS HS et al (eds): *Viral Hepatitis and Liver Disease*. Atlanta/London: International Medical Press, 2002

ORLAND JR et al: Acute hepatitis C. Hepatology 33:321, 2001

PAWLOTSKY J-M: Molecular diagnosis of viral hepatitis. Gastroenterology 122:1554, 2002

SCHREIBER GB et al: The risk of transfusion-transmitted viral infection. N Engl J Med 334:1685, 1996

SEEFF LB (ed) et al: Long-term mortality and morbidity of transfusion-associated non-A, non-B, and type C hepatitis: A National Heart, Lung, and Blood Institute collaborative study. Hepatology 33:455, 2001

THIMME R et al: Viral and immunological determinants of hepatitis C virus clearance, persistence, and disease. Proc Natl Acad Sci USA 99:15661, 2002

TONG MJ et al: Clinical outcomes after transfusion-associated hepatitis C. N Engl J Med 332:1463, 1995

YANG H-I et al: Hepatitis B e antigen and the risk of hepatocellular carcinoma. N Engl J Med 347:168, 2002

286   TOXIC AND DRUG-INDUCED HEPATITIS
Jules L. Dienstag, Kurt J. Isselbacher

Liver injury may follow the inhalation, ingestion, or parenteral administration of a number of pharmacologic and chemical agents. These include industrial toxins (e.g., carbon tetrachloride, trichloroethylene, and yellow phosphorus), the heat-stable toxic bicyclic octapeptides of certain species of *Amanita* and *Galerina* (hepatotoxic mushroom poisoning), and, more commonly, pharmacologic agents used in medical therapy. It is essential that any patient presenting with jaundice or altered biochemical liver tests be questioned carefully about exposure to chemicals used in work or at home, drugs taken by prescription or bought "over the counter," and herbal or alternative medicines. Hepatotoxic drugs can injure the hepatocyte directly, e.g., via a free-radical or metabolic intermediate that causes peroxidation of membrane lipids and that results in liver cell injury. Alternatively, the drug or its metabolite can distort cell membranes or other cellular molecules, activate apoptotic pathways, or block biochemical pathways or cellular integrity. Such injuries, in turn, may lead to necrosis of hepatocytes; injure bile ducts, producing cholestasis; or block pathways of lipid movement, inhibit protein synthesis, or impair mitochondrial oxidation of fatty acids, resulting in lactic acidosis and fat accumulation (steatosis). In some cases, drug metabolites sensitize hepatocytes to toxic cytokines, and differences between susceptible and nonsusceptible drug recipients may be attributable to polymorphisms in elaboration of competing, protective cytokines, as has been suggested for acetaminophen hepatotoxicity (see below). In addition, a role has been shown for activation of nuclear transporters, such as the constitutive androstane receptor (CAR), in the induction of drug hepatotoxicity. In general, two major types of chemical hepatotoxicity have been recognized: (1) direct toxic type and (2) idiosyncratic type.

Most drugs, which are water-insoluble, undergo a series of metabolic transformation steps, culminating in a water-soluble form appropriate for renal or biliary excretion. This process begins with oxidation or methylation initially mediated by the mixed-function oxygenases cytochrome P450 (phase I reaction), followed by glucuronidation or sulfation (phase II reaction) or inactivation by glutathione. Most drug hepatotoxicity is mediated by a phase I toxic metabolite, but glutathione depletion, precluding inactivation of harmful compounds by glutathione S-transferase, can contribute as well.

As shown in Table 286-1, direct toxic hepatitis occurs with predictable regularity in individuals exposed to the offending agent and is dose-dependent. The latent period between exposure and liver injury is usually short (often several hours), although clinical manifestations may be delayed for 24 to 48 h. Agents producing toxic hepatitis are generally systemic poisons or are converted in the liver to toxic metabolites. The direct hepatotoxins result in morphologic abnormalities

TABLE 286-1   *Some Features of Toxic and Drug-Induced Hepatic Injury*

| Features | Direct Toxic Effect[a] | | Idiosyncratic[a] | | | Other[a] |
	(Carbon Tetrachloride)	(Acetaminophen)	(Halothane)	(Isoniazid)	(Chlorpromazine)	(Oral Contraceptive Agents)
Predictable and dose-related toxicity	+	+	0	0	0	+
Latent period	Short	Short	Variable	Variable	Variable	Variable
Arthralgia, fever, rash, eosinophilia	0	0	+	0	+	0
Liver morphology	Necrosis, fatty infiltration	Centrilobular necrosis	Similar to viral hepatitis	Similar to viral hepatitis	Cholestasis *with* portal inflammation	Cholestasis *without* portal inflammation, vascular lesions

[a] The drugs listed are typical samples.

that are reasonably characteristic and reproducible for each toxin. For example, carbon tetrachloride and trichloroethylene characteristically produce a centrilobular zonal necrosis, whereas yellow phosphorus poisoning typically results in periportal injury. The hepatotoxic octapeptides of *Amanita phalloides* usually produce massive hepatic necrosis. The lethal dose of the toxin is about 10 mg, the amount found in a single deathcap mushroom. Tetracycline, when administered in intravenous doses >1.5 g daily, leads to microvesicular fat deposits in the liver. Liver injury, which is often only one facet of the toxicity produced by the direct hepatotoxins, may go unrecognized until jaundice appears.

In idiosyncratic drug reactions the occurrence of hepatitis is usually infrequent and unpredictable, the response is not dose-dependent, and it may occur at any time during or shortly after exposure to the drug. Adding to the difficulty of predicting or identifying idiosyncratic drug hepatotoxicity is the occurrence of mild, transient, nonprogressive serum aminotransferase elevations that resolve with continued drug use. Such "adaptation," the mechanism of which is unknown, occurs in such drugs as isoniazid, valproate, phenytoin, and HMG-CoA reductase inhibitors (statins). Extrahepatic manifestations of hypersensitivity, such as rash, arthralgias, fever, leukocytosis, and eosinophilia, occur in about one-quarter of patients with idiosyncratic hepatotoxic drug reactions; this observation and the unpredictability of idiosyncratic drug hepatototoxicity contributed to the hypothesis that this category of drug reactions is immunologically mediated. More recent evidence, however, suggests that, in most cases, even idiosyncratic reactions represent direct hepatotoxity but are caused by drug metabolites rather than by the intact compound. Even the prototypes of idiosyncratic hepatoxicity reactions, halothane hepatitis and isoniazid hepatotoxicity, associated frequently with hypersensitivity manifestations, are now recognized to be mediated by toxic metabolites that damage liver cells directly. Currently, most idiosyncratic reactions are thought to result from differences in metabolic reactivity to specific agents; host susceptibility is mediated by the kinetics of toxic metabolite generation, which differs among individuals. Occasionally, however, the clinical features of an allergic reaction (prominent tissue eosinophilia, autoantibodies, etc.) are difficult to ignore. In vitro models have been described in which lymphocyte cytotoxicity can be demonstrated against rabbit hepatocytes altered by incubation with the potential offending drug. Furthermore, several instances of drug hepatotoxicity are associated with the appearance of autoantibodies, including a class of antibodies to liver-kidney microsomes, anti-LKM2, directed against a cytochrome P450 enzyme. Similarly, in selected cases, a drug or its metabolite has been shown to bind to a host cellular component forming a hapten; the immune response to this "neoantigen" is postulated to play a role in the pathogenesis of liver injury. Therefore, some authorities subdivide idiosyncratic drug hepatotoxicity into hypersensitivity (allergic) and "metabolic" categories. Several unusual exceptions notwithstanding, true drug allergy is difficult to support in most cases of idiosyncratic drug-induced liver injury.

Idiosyncratic reactions lead to a morphologic pattern that is more variable than those produced by direct toxins; a single agent is often capable of causing a variety of lesions, although certain patterns tend to predominate. Depending on the agent involved, idiosyncratic hepatitis may result in a clinical and morphologic picture indistinguishable from that of viral hepatitis (e.g., halothane) or may simulate extrahepatic bile duct obstruction clinically with morphologic evidence of cholestasis. Drug-induced cholestasis ranges from mild to increasingly severe: (1) bland cholestasis with limited hepatocellular injury (e.g., estrogens, 17,α-substituted androgens); (2) inflammatory cholestasis (e.g., phenothiazines, amoxicillin–clavulanic acid, oxacillin, erythromcyin estolate); (3) sclerosing cholangitis (e.g., after intrahepatic infusion of the chemotherapeutic agent floxuridine for hepatic metastases from a primary colonic carcinoma); (4) disappearance of bile ducts, "ductopenic" cholestasis, similar to that observed in chronic rejection following liver transplantation (e.g., carbamazepine, chlorpromazine, tricyclic antidepressant agents). Cholestasis may result

from binding of drugs to canalicular membrane transporters, accumulation of toxic bile acids resulting from canalicular pump failure, or genetic defects in canalicular transporter proteins. Morphologic alterations may also include bridging hepatic necrosis (e.g., methyldopa), or, infrequently, hepatic granulomas (e.g., sulfonamides). Some drugs result in macrovesicular or microvesicular steatosis or steatohepatitis, which in some cases has been linked to mitochondrial dysfunction and lipid peroxidation. Severe hepatotoxicity associated with steatohepatitis, most likely a result of mitochondrial toxicity, is being recognized with increasing frequency among patients receiving antiretroviral therapy with reverse transcriptase inhibitors (e.g., zidovudine, didanosine) or protease inhibitors (e.g., indinavir, ritonavir) for HIV infection (Chap. 173). Generally, such mitochondrial hepatotoxicity of these antiretroviral agents is reversible, but dramatic, nonreversible hepatotoxicity associated with mitochondrial injury (inhibition of DNA polymerase γ) was the cause of acute liver failure encountered during early clinical trials of fialuridine, a fluorinated pyrimidine analogue with potent antiviral activity against hepatitis B virus. Another potential target for idiosyncratic drug hepatotoxicity is sinusoidal lining cells; when these are injured, such as by high-dose chemotherapeutic agents (e.g., cyclophosphamide, melphalan, busulfan) administered prior to bone marrow transplantation, venoocclusive disease can result.

Not all adverse hepatic drug reactions can be classified as either toxic or idiosyncratic in type. For example, oral contraceptives, which combine estrogenic and progestational compounds, may result in impairment of hepatic tests and occasionally in jaundice. However, they do not produce necrosis or fatty change, manifestations of hypersensitivity are generally absent, and susceptibility to the development of oral contraceptive–induced cholestasis appears to be genetically determined. Such estrogen-induced cholestasis is more common in women with cholestasis of pregnancy, a disorder linked to genetic defects in multidrug resistance–associated canalicular transporter proteins. Other instances of genetically determined drug hepatotoxicity have been identified. For example, approximately 10% of the population have an autosomally recessive trait associated with the absence of cytochrome P450 enzyme 2D6 and have impaired debrisoquine-4-hydroxylase enzyme activity. As a result, they cannot metabolize, and are at increased risk of hepatotoxicity resulting from, certain compounds such as desipramine, propranolol, and quinidine.

Some forms of drug hepatotoxicity are so rare, e.g., occurring in <1:10,000 recipients, that they do not become apparent during clinical trials, involving only several thousand recipients, conducted to obtain drug registration. An example of such rare, but serious, idiosyncratic drug hepatotoxicity followed the approval and generalized use of troglitazone, a peroxisomal, proliferator activator–receptor γ agonist, the first-introduced example of a thiazolidinedione insulin-sensitizing agent. This instance of drug hepatotoxicity was not recognized until well after the drug was introduced, underlining the importance of postmarketing surveillance in identifying toxic drugs and in leading to their withdrawal from use.

Because drug-induced hepatitis is often a presumptive diagnosis and many other disorders produce a similar clinicopathologic picture, evidence of a causal relationship between the use of a drug and subsequent liver injury may be difficult to establish. The relationship is most convincing for the direct hepatotoxins, which lead to a high frequency of hepatic impairment after a short latent period. Idiosyncratic reactions may be reproduced, in some instances, when rechallenge, after an asymptomatic period, results in a recurrence of signs, symptoms, and morphologic and biochemical abnormalities. Rechallenge, however, is often ethically unfeasible, because severe reactions may occur.

Generally, drug hepatotoxicity is not more frequent in persons with underlying chronic liver disease. Reported exceptions include hepatotoxicity of aspirin, methotrexate, isoniazid (only in certain experiences), and antiretroviral therapy for HIV infection.

Principal Morphologic Change	Class of Agent	Example
Cholestasis	Anabolic steroid	Methyl testosterone
	Anti-inflammatory	Sulindac
	Antithyroid	Methimazole
	Antibiotic	Erythromycin estolate, nitrofurantoin, rifampin, amoxicillin–clavulanic acid, oxacillin
	Oral contraceptive	Norethynodrel with mestranol
	Oral hypoglycemic	Chlorpropamide
	Tranquilizer	Chlorpromazine[b]
	Oncotherapeutic	Anabolic steroids, busulfan, tamoxifen
	Immunosuppressive	Cyclosporine
	Anticonvulsant	Carbamazepine
	Calcium channel blocker	Nifedipine, verapamil
Fatty liver	Antibiotic	Tetracycline
	Anticonvulsant	Sodium valproate
	Antiarrhythmic	Amiodarone
	Antiviral	Dideoxynucleosides (e.g., zidovudine) protease inhibitors (e.g., indinavir, ritonavir)
	Oncotherapeutic	Asparaginase, methotrexate
Hepatitis	Anesthetic	Halothane[c]
	Anticonvulsant	Phenytoin, carbamazepine
	Antihypertensive	Methyldopa,[c] captopril, enalapril
	Antibiotic	Isoniazid,[c] rifampin, nitrofurantoin
	Diuretic	Chlorothiazide
	Laxative	Oxyphenisatin[c]
	Antidepressant	Iproniazid, amitriptyline, imipramine, trazodone, venlafaxine
	Anti-inflammatory	Ibuprofen, indomethacin, diclofenac, sulindac, bomfenac
	Antifungal	Ketoconazole, fluconazole, itraconazole
	Antiviral	Zidovudine, didanosine, nevirapine
	Calcium channel blocker	Nifedipine, verapamil, diltiazem
	Cholinesterase inhibitor	Tacrine
	Oral hypoglycemic	Troglitazone
	Antiandrogen	Flutamide
Mixed hepatitis/ cholestatic	Immunosuppressive	Azathioprine
	Lipid-lowering	Nicotinic acid, lovastatin and other statins
	Antibiotic	Amoxicillin–clavulanic acid, trimethoprim-sulfamethoxazole
	Antifungal	Terbinafine
Toxic (necrosis)	Hydrocarbon	Carbon tetrachloride
	Metal	Yellow phosphorus
	Mushroom	*Amanita phalloides*
	Analgesic	Acetaminophen
	Solvent	Dimethylformamide
Granulomas	Anti-inflammatory	Phenylbutazone
	Antibiotic	Sulfonamides
	Xanthine oxidase inhibitor	Allopurinol
	Antiarrhythmic	Quinidine, diltiazem
	Anticonvulsant	Carbamazepine

[a] Several agents cause more than one type of liver lesion and appear under more than one category.
[b] Rarely associated with primary biliary cirrhosis–like lesion.
[c] Occasionally associated with chronic hepatitis or bridging hepatic necrosis or cirrhosis.

Rx TREATMENT

Treatment of toxic and drug-induced hepatic disease is largely supportive, except in acetaminophen hepatotoxicity (see below). In patients with fulminant hepatitis resulting from drug hepatotoxicity, liver transplantation may be life-saving (Chap. 291). Withdrawal of the suspected agent is indicated at the first sign of an adverse reaction. In the case of the direct toxins, liver involvement should not divert attention from renal or other organ involvement, which may also threaten survival. Glucocorticoids for drug hepatotoxicity with allergic features, silibinin for hepatotoxic mushroom poisoning, and ursodeoxycholic acid for cholestatic drug hepatotoxicity have never been shown to be effective and are not recommended.

In Table 286-2, several classes of chemical agents are listed, together with examples of the pattern of liver injury produced by them.

Certain drugs appear to be responsible for the development of chronic as well as acute hepatic injury. For example, oxyphenisatin, methyldopa, and isoniazid have been associated with moderate to severe chronic hepatitis, and halothane and methotrexate have been implicated in the development of cirrhosis. A syndrome resembling primary biliary cirrhosis has been described following treatment with chlorpromazine, methyl testosterone, tolbutamide, and other drugs. Portal hypertension in the absence of cirrhosis may result from alterations in hepatic architecture produced by vitamin A or arsenic intoxication, industrial exposure to vinyl chloride, or administration of thorium dioxide. The latter three agents have also been associated with angiosarcoma of the liver. Oral contraceptives have been implicated in the development of hepatic adenoma and, rarely, hepatocellular carcinoma and hepatic vein occlusion (Budd-Chiari syndrome). Another unusual lesion, peliosis hepatis (blood cysts of the liver), has been observed in some patients treated with anabolic steroids. The existence of these hepatic disorders expands the spectrum of liver injury induced by chemical agents and emphasizes the need for a thorough drug history in all patients with liver dysfunction.

The following are the patterns of adverse hepatic reactions for some prototypic agents.

ACETAMINOPHEN HEPATOTOXICITY (DIRECT TOXIN)

Acetaminophen can cause severe centrilobular hepatic necrosis when ingested in large amounts in suicide attempts or accidentally by children. A single dose of 10 to 15 g, occasionally less, may produce clinical evidence of liver injury. Fatal fulminant disease is usually (although not invariably) associated with ingestion of ≥ 25 g. Blood levels of acetaminophen correlate with the severity of hepatic injury (levels >300 μg/mL 4 h after ingestion are predictive of the development of severe damage; levels <150 μg/mL suggest that hepatic injury is highly unlikely). Nausea, vomiting, diarrhea, abdominal pain, and shock are early manifestations occurring 4 to 12 h after ingestion. Then 24 to 48 h later, when these features are abating, hepatic injury becomes apparent. Maximal abnormalities and hepatic failure may not be evident until 4 to 6 days after ingestion, and aminotransferase levels approaching 10,000 units are not uncommon. Renal failure and myocardial injury may be present.

Acetaminophen is metabolized predominantly by a phase II reaction to innocuous sulfate and glucuronide metabolites; however, a small proportion of acetaminophen is metabolized by a phase I reaction to a hepatotoxic metabolite formed from the parent compound by the cytochrome P450 2E1. This metabolite, *N*-acetyl-benzoquinone-imide (NAPQI), is detoxified by binding to "hepatoprotective" glutathione to become harmless, water-soluble mercapturic acid, which undergoes renal excretion. When excessive amounts of NAPQI are formed, or when glutathione levels are low, glutathione levels are depleted and overwhelmed, permitting covalent binding to nucleophilic hepatocyte macromolecules. This process is believed to lead to hepatocyte necrosis; the precise sequence and mechanism are unknown. Hepatic injury may be potentiated by prior administration of alcohol, phenobarbital, or other drugs, by conditions that stimulate the mixed-function oxidase system, or by conditions such as starvation that reduce hepatic glutathione levels. The xenobiotic (environmental, exogenous substance) receptor CAR has been shown in a mouse model of acetaminophen hepatotoxicity to induce acetaminophen-metabolizing enzymes and, thereby, regulate and increase hepatotoxicity. Cimetidine, which inhibits P450 enzymes, has the potential to reduce generation of the toxic metabolite. Alcohol induces cytochrome P450 2E1; consequently, increased levels of the toxic metabolite NAPQI are produced in chronic alcoholics after acetaminophen ingestion. In addition, alcohol suppresses hepatic glutathione production. Therefore, in chronic alcoholics, the toxic dose of acetaminophen may be as low as 2 g, and alcoholic patients should be warned specifically about the dangers of even standard doses of this commonly used drug. Such "therapeutic misadventures" also occur occasionally in patients with severe, febrile illnesses or pain syndromes; in such a setting, several days of anorexia and near-fasting coupled with regular administration of extra-strength acetaminophen formulations result in a combination of glutathione depletion and relatively high NAPQI levels in the absence of a history of recognized acetaminophen overdose.

℞ TREATMENT

Treatment of acetaminophen overdosage includes gastric lavage, supportive measures, and oral administration of activated charcoal or cholestyramine to prevent absorption of residual drug. Neither of these agents appears to be effective if given >30 min after acetaminophen ingestion; if they are used, the stomach lavage should be done before other agents are administered orally. The chances of possible-, probable-, and high-risk hepatotoxicity can be derived from a nomogram plot (Fig. 286-1), readily available in emergency departments, of acetaminophen plasma levels as a function of hours after ingestion. In patients with high acetaminophen blood levels (>200 μg/mL measured at 4 h or >100 μg/mL at 8 h after ingestion), the administration of sulfhydryl compounds (e.g., cysteamine, cysteine, or N-acetylcysteine) appears to reduce the severity of hepatic necrosis. These agents appear to act by providing a reservoir of sulfhydryl groups to bind the toxic metabolites or by stimulating synthesis and repletion of hepatic glutathione. Therapy should be begun within 8 h of ingestion but may be effective even if given as late as 24 to 36 h after overdose. Later administration of sulfhydryl compounds is of uncertain value. Routine use of N-acetylcysteine has substantially reduced the occurrence of fatal acetaminophen hepatotoxicity. When given orally, N-acetylcysteine is diluted to yield a 5% solution. A loading dose of 140 mg/kg is given, followed by 70 mg/kg every 4 h for 15 to 20 doses. Whenever a patient with potential acetaminophen hepatotoxicity is encountered, a local poison control center should be contacted. Treatment can be stopped when plasma acetaminophen levels indicate that the risk of liver damage is low. If signs of hepatic failure (e.g., progressive jaundice, coagulopathy, confusion) occur despite N-acetylcysteine therapy for acetaminophen hepatotoxicity, liver transplantation may be the only option. Preliminary data suggest that early arterial blood lactate levels among such patients with acute liver failure may distinguish patients highly likely to require liver transplantation (lactate levels > 3.5 mmol/L) from those likely to survive without liver replacement.

Survivors of acute acetaminophen overdose usually have no evidence of hepatic sequelae. In a few patients, prolonged or repeated administration of acetaminophen in therapeutic doses appears to have led to the development of chronic hepatitis and cirrhosis.

HALOTHANE HEPATOTOXICITY (IDIOSYNCRATIC REACTION) Although currently quite rare, halothane hepatotoxicity was one of the prototypical, and most intensively studied, examples of idiosyncratic drug hepatotoxicity. Administration of halothane, a nonexplosive fluorinated hydrocarbon anesthetic agent that is structurally similar to chloroform, results in severe hepatic necrosis in a small number of individuals, many of whom have previously been exposed to this agent. The failure to produce similar hepatic lesions reliably in animals, the rarity of hepatic impairment in human beings, and the delayed appearance of hepatic injury suggest that halothane is not a direct hepatotoxin but rather a sensitizing agent. However, manifestations of hypersensitivity are seen in <25% of cases. A genetic predisposition leading to an idiosyncratic metabolic reactivity has been postulated and appears to be the most likely mechanism of halothane hepatotoxicity. Adults (rather than children), obese people, and women appear to be particularly susceptible. Fever, moderate leukocytosis, and eosinophilia may occur in the first week following halothane administration. Jaundice is usually noted 7 to 10 days after exposure but may occur earlier in previously exposed patients. Nausea and vomiting may precede the onset of jaundice. Hepatomegaly is often mild, but liver tenderness is common. The serum aminotransferase levels are elevated. The pathologic changes at autopsy are indistinguishable from massive hepatic necrosis resulting from viral hepatitis. The case-fatality rate of halothane hepatitis is not known but may vary from 20 to 40% in cases with severe liver involvement. Patients in whom unexplained spiking fever, especially delayed fever, or jaundice develops after halothane anesthesia should not receive this agent again. Because cross-reactions between halothane and methoxyflurane have been reported, the latter agent should not be used after halothane reactions. Later-generation halogenated hydrocarbon anesthetics, which have supplanted halothane except in rare instances (e.g., certain types of thoracic surgery), are felt to be associated with a lower risk of hepatotoxicity.

METHYLDOPA HEPATOTOXICITY (TOXIC AND IDIOSYNCRATIC REACTION) Minor alterations in liver tests are reported in about 5% of patients treated with this antihypertensive agent. These trivial abnormalities typically resolve despite continued drug administration. In <1% of patients, acute liver injury resembling viral or chronic hepatitis or, rarely, a cholestatic reaction is seen 1 to 20 weeks after methyldopa is started.

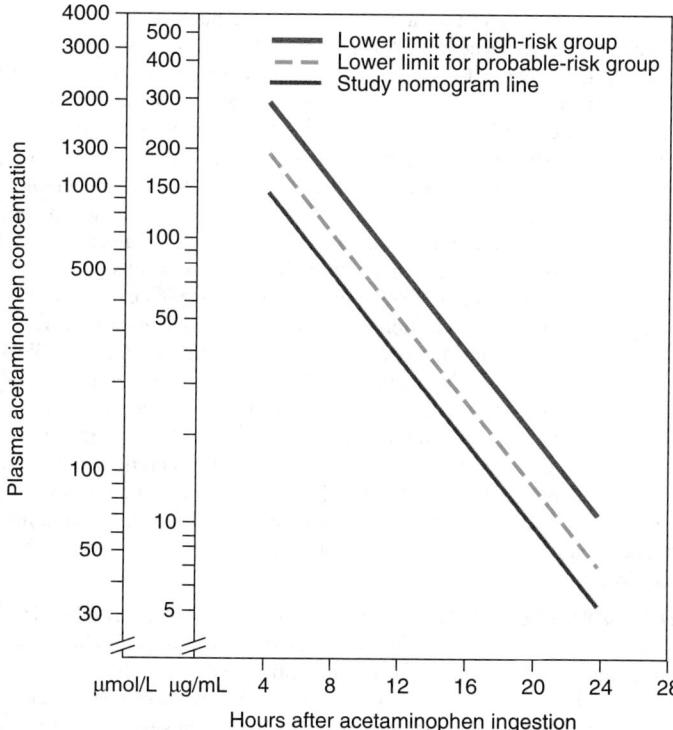

FIGURE 286-1 Nomogram to define risk of acetaminophen hepatotoxicity according to initial plasma acetaminophen concentration. *(After BH Rumack, H Matthew, Pediatrics 55:871, 1975.)*

In 50% of cases the interval is <4 weeks. A prodrome of fever, anorexia, and malaise may be noted for a few days before the onset of jaundice. Rash, lymphadenopathy, arthralgia, and eosinophilia are rare. Serologic markers of autoimmunity are detected infrequently, and <5% of patients have a Coombs-positive hemolytic anemia. In about 15% of patients with methyldopa hepatotoxicity, the clinical, biochemical, and histologic features are those of moderate to severe chronic hepatitis, with or without bridging necrosis and macronodular cirrhosis. With discontinuation of the drug, the disorder usually resolves. Although methyldopa is currently used infrequently, its hepatotoxicity is very well characterized. Among the currently popular antihypertensive agents, angiotensin-converting enzyme (ACE) inhibitors, such as captopril and enalapril, have been blamed, albeit rarely, for hepatotoxicity (primarily cholestasis and cholestatic hepatitis, but also hepatocellular injury). Angiotensin-II receptor antagonists, such as losartan, are unlikely hepatotoxins, although rare reports of liver injury in their recipients have appeared.

ISONIAZID HEPATOTOXICITY (TOXIC AND IDIOSYNCRATIC REACTION)

In approximately 10% of adults treated with the antituberculosis agent isoniazid, elevated serum aminotransferase levels develop during the first few weeks of therapy; this appears to represent an adaptive response to a toxic metabolite of the drug. Whether or not isoniazid is continued, these values (usually <200 units) return to normal in a few weeks. In about 1% of treated patients, an illness develops that is indistinguishable from viral hepatitis; approximately half of these cases occur within the first 2 months of treatment, while in the remainder, clinical disease may be delayed for many months. Liver biopsy reveals morphologic changes similar to those of viral hepatitis or bridging hepatic necrosis. The disease may be severe, with a case-fatality rate of 10%. Important liver injury appears to be age-related, increasing substantially after age 35; the highest frequency is in patients over age 50, the lowest under the age of 20. Even for patients >50 years monitored carefully during therapy, hepatotoxicity occurs in only approximately 2%, well below the risk estimate derived from earlier experiences. Isoniazid hepatotoxicity is enhanced by alcohol, rifampin and pyrazinamide. Fever, rash, eosinophilia, and other manifestations of drug allergy are distinctly unusual. A reactive metabolite of acetylhydrazine, a metabolite of isoniazid, may be responsible for liver injury, and patients who are rapid acetylators would be more prone to such injury. Counterintuitively, in some reports, the opposite is true; slow acetylators are more likely to experience hepatotoxicity and more severe hepatotoxicity than rapid acetylators. Contrary to past reports, several recent studies suggest that hepatotoxicity due to isoniazid as well as to combination antituberculous therapy that includes isoniazid is more likely in patients with underlying chronic hepatitis B. A picture resembling chronic hepatitis has been observed in a few patients. Careful liver-test monitoring is advisable in patients being treated with isoniazid.

SODIUM VALPROATE HEPATOTOXICITY (TOXIC AND IDIOSYNCRATIC REACTION)

Sodium valproate, an anticonvulsant useful in the treatment of petit mal and other seizure disorders, has been associated with the development of severe hepatic toxicity and, rarely, fatalities, predominantly in children but also in adults. Asymptomatic elevations of serum aminotransferase levels have been recognized in as many as 45% of treated patients. These "adaptive" changes, however, appear to have no clinical importance, for major hepatotoxicity is not seen in the majority of patients despite continuation of drug therapy. In those rare patients in whom jaundice, encephalopathy, and evidence of hepatic failure are found, examination of liver tissue reveals microvesicular fat and bridging hepatic necrosis, predominantly in the centrilobular zone. Bile duct injury may also be apparent. It seems likely that sodium valproate is not directly hepatotoxic but that its metabolite, 4-pentenoic acid, may be responsible for hepatic injury. Valproate hepatotoxicity is more common in persons with mitochondrial enzyme deficiencies and may be ameliorated by administration of carnitine, which valproate therapy can deplete.

PHENYTOIN HEPATOTOXICITY (IDIOSYNCRATIC REACTION)

Phenytoin, formerly diphenylhydantoin, a mainstay in the treatment of seizure disorders, has been associated in rare instances with the development of severe hepatitis-like liver injury leading to fulminant hepatic failure. In many patients the hepatitis is associated with striking fever, lymphadenopathy, rash (Stevens-Johnson syndrome or exfoliative dermatitis), leukocytosis, and eosinophilia, suggesting an immunologically mediated hypersensitivity mechanism. Despite these observations, there is also evidence that metabolic idiosyncrasy may be responsible for hepatic injury. In the liver, phenytoin is converted by the cytochrome P450 system to metabolites, which include the highly reactive electrophilic arene oxides. These metabolites are normally metabolized further by epoxide hydrolases. A defect (genetic or acquired) in epoxide hydrolase activity could permit covalent binding of arene oxides to hepatic macromolecules, thereby leading to hepatic injury. Regardless of the mechanism, hepatic injury is usually manifest within the first 2 months after beginning phenytoin therapy. With the exception of an abundance of eosinophils in the liver, the clinical, biochemical, and histologic picture resembles that of viral hepatitis. In rare instances, bile duct injury may be the salient feature of phenytoin hepatotoxicity, with striking features of intrahepatic cholestasis. Asymptomatic elevations of aminotransferase and alkaline phosphatase levels have been observed in a sizable proportion of patients receiving long-term phenytoin therapy. These liver changes are believed by some authorities to represent the potent hepatic enzyme–inducing properties of phenytoin and are accompanied histologically by swelling of hepatocytes in the absence of necroinflammatory activity or evidence of chronic liver disease.

AMIODARONE HEPATOTOXICITY (TOXIC AND IDIOSYNCRATIC REACTION)

Therapy with this potent antiarrhythmic drug is accompanied in 15 to 50% of patients by modest elevations of serum aminotransferase levels that may remain stable or diminish despite continuation of the drug. Such abnormalities may appear days to many months after beginning therapy. A proportion of those with elevated aminotransferase levels have detectable hepatomegaly, and clinically important liver disease develops in <5% of patients. Features that represent a direct effect of the drug on the liver and that are common to the majority of long-term recipients are ultrastructural phospholipidosis, unaccompanied by clinical liver disease, and interference with hepatic mixed-function oxidase metabolism of other drugs. The cationic amphiphilic drug and its major metabolite desethylamiodarone accumulate in hepatocyte lysosomes and mitochondria and in bile duct epithelium. The relatively common elevations in aminotransferase levels are also considered a predictable, dose-dependent, direct hepatotoxic effect. On the other hand, in the rare patient with clinically apparent, symptomatic liver disease, liver injury resembling that seen in alcoholic liver disease is observed. The so-called pseudoalcoholic liver injury can range from steatosis, to alcoholic hepatitis-like neutrophilic infiltration and Mallory's hyaline, to cirrhosis. Electron-microscopic demonstration of phospholipid-laden lysosomal lamellar bodies can help to distinguish amiodarone hepatotoxicity from typical alcoholic hepatitis. This category of liver injury appears to be a metabolic idiosyncrasy that allows hepatotoxic metabolites to be generated. Rarely, an acute idiosyncratic hepatocellular injury resembling viral hepatitis or cholestatic hepatitis occurs. Hepatic granulomas have occasionally been observed. Because amiodarone has a long half-life, liver injury may persist for months after the drug is stopped.

ERYTHROMYCIN HEPATOTOXICITY (CHOLESTATIC IDIOSYNCRATIC REACTION)

The most important adverse effect associated with erythromycin, more common in children than adults, is the infrequent occurrence of a cholestatic reaction. Although most of these reactions have been associated with erythromycin estolate, other erythromycins may also be responsible. The reaction usually begins during the first 2 or 3 weeks of therapy and includes nausea, vomiting, fever, right upper quadrant abdominal pain, jaundice, leukocytosis, and moderately elevated aminotransferase levels. The clinical picture can resemble acute cholecystitis or bacterial cholangitis. Liver biopsy reveals variable cholestasis; portal inflammation comprising lymphocytes, polymorphonuclear leukocytes, and eosinophils; and scattered foci of hepatocyte necrosis. Symptoms and laboratory findings usually subside within a few days of drug withdrawal, and evidence of chronic liver disease has not been found on follow-up. The precise mechanism remains ill-defined.

ORAL CONTRACEPTIVE HEPATOTOXICITY (CHOLESTATIC REACTION) The administration of oral contraceptive combinations of estrogenic and progestational steroids leads to intrahepatic cholestasis with pruritus and jaundice in a small number of patients weeks to months after taking these agents. Especially susceptible seem to be patients with recurrent idiopathic jaundice of pregnancy, severe pruritus of pregnancy, or a family history of these disorders. With the exception of liver biochemical tests, laboratory studies are normal, and extrahepatic manifestations of hypersensitivity are absent. Liver biopsy reveals cholestasis with bile plugs in dilated canaliculi and striking bilirubin staining of liver cells. In contrast to chlorpromazine-induced cholestasis, portal inflammation is absent. The lesion is reversible on withdrawal of the agent. The two steroid components appear to act synergistically on hepatic function, although the estrogen may be primarily responsible. Oral contraceptives are contraindicated in patients with a history of recurrent jaundice of pregnancy. Primarily benign, but rarely malignant, neoplasms of the liver, hepatic vein occlusion, and peripheral sinusoidal dilatation have also been associated with oral contraceptive therapy. Focal nodular hyperplasia of the liver is not more frequent among users of oral contraceptives.

17,α-ALKYL-SUBSTITUTED ANABOLIC STEROIDS (CHOLESTATIC REACTION) In the majority of patients receiving these agents, used therapeutically mainly in the treatment of bone marrow failure but used surreptitiously and without medical indication by athletes to improve their performance, mild hepatic dysfunction develops. Impaired excretory function is the predominant defect, but the precise mechanism is uncertain. Jaundice, which appears to be dose-related, develops in only a minority of patients and may be the sole clinical manifestation of hepatotoxicity, although anorexia, nausea, and malaise may occur. Pruritus is not a prominent feature. Serum aminotransferase levels are usually <100 units, and serum alkaline phosphatase levels are normal, mildly elevated, or, in <5% of patients, three or more times the upper limit of normal. Examination of liver tissue reveals cholestasis without inflammation or necrosis. Hepatic sinusoidal dilatation and peliosis hepatis have been found in a few patients. The cholestatic disorder is usually reversible on cessation of treatment, although fatalities have been linked to peliosis. An association with hepatic adenoma and hepatocellular carcinoma has been reported.

TRIMETHOPRIM-SULFAMETHOXAZOLE HEPATOTOXICITY (IDIOSYNCRATIC REACTION) This antibiotic combination is used routinely for urinary tract infections in immunocompetent persons and for prophylaxis against and therapy of *Pneumocystis carinii* pneumonia in immunosuppressed persons (transplant recipients, patients with AIDS). With its increasing use, its occasional hepatotoxicity is being recognized with growing frequency. Its likelihood is unpredictable, but when it occurs, trimethoprim-sulfamethoxazole hepatotoxicity follows a relatively uniform latency period of several weeks and is often accompanied by eosinophilia, rash, and other features of a hypersensitivity reaction. Biochemically and histologically, acute hepatocellular necrosis predominates, but cholestatic features are quite frequent. Occasionally, cholestasis without necrosis occurs, and very rarely, a severe cholangiolytic pattern of liver injury is observed. In most cases, liver injury is self-limited, but rare fatalities have been recorded. The hepatotoxicity is attributable to the sulfamethoxazole component of the drug and is similar in features to that seen with other sulfonamides; tissue eosinophilia and granulomas may be seen. The risk of trimethoprim-sulfamethoxazole hepatotoxicity is increased in persons with HIV infection.

HMG-COA REDUCTASE INHIBITORS (STATINS) (IDIOSYNCRATIC MIXED HEPATOCELLULAR AND CHOLESTATIC REACTION) Between 1 and 2% of patients taking lovastatin, simvastatin, pravastatin, fluvastatin, or one of the newer statin drugs for the treatment of hypercholesterolemia experience asymptomatic, reversible elevations (> threefold) of aminotransferase activity. Acute hepatitis-like histologic changes, centrilobular necrosis, and centrilobular cholestasis have been described in several cases. In a larger proportion, minor aminotransferase elevations appear during the first several weeks of therapy. Careful laboratory monitoring can distinguish between patients with minor, transitory changes, who may continue therapy, and those with more profound and sustained abnormalities, who should discontinue therapy.

TOTAL PARENTERAL NUTRITION (STEATOSIS, CHOLESTASIS) Total parenteral nutrition (TPN) is often complicated by cholestatic hepatitis attributable to either steatosis, cholestasis, or gallstones (or gallbladder sludge). Steatosis or steatohepatitis may result from the excess carbohydrate calories in these nutritional supplements and is the predominant form of TPN-associated liver disorder in adults. The frequency of this complication has been reduced substantially by the introduction of balanced TPN formulas that rely on lipid as an alternative caloric source. Cholestasis and cholelithiasis, caused by the absence of stimulation of bile flow and secretion resulting from the lack of oral intake, is the predominant form of TPN-associated liver disease in infants, especially in premature neonates. Often, cholestasis in such neonates is multifactorial, contributed to by other factors such as sepsis, hypoxemia, and hypotension; occasionally, TPN-induced cholestasis in neonates culminates in chronic liver disease and liver failure. When TPN-associated liver test abnormalities occur in adults, balancing the TPN formula with more lipid is the intervention of first recourse. In infants with TPN-associated cholestasis, the addition of oral feeding may ameliorate the problem. Therapeutic interventions suggested, but not yet shown to be of proven benefit, include cholecystokinin, ursodeoxycholic acid, S-adenosyl methionine, and taurine.

"ALTERNATIVE MEDICINES" (IDIOSYNCRATIC HEPATITIS, STEATOSIS) The misguided popularity of herbal medications that are of scientifically unproven efficacy and that lack prospective safety oversight by regulatory agencies has resulted in occasional instances of hepatotoxicity. Included among the herbal remedies associated with toxic hepatitis are Jin Bu Huan (Chap. 10), xiao-chai-hu-tang, germander, chaparral, senna, mistletoe, skullcap, gentian, comfrey (containing pyrrolizidine alkaloids), Ma huang, bee pollen, valerian root, pennyroyal oil, kava, celandine, Impila (*Callilepsis laureaola*), LipoKinetix, and herbal teas. Recently well characterized are the acute hepatitis-like histologic lesions following Jin Bu Huan use: focal hepatocellular necrosis, mixed mononuclear portal tract infiltration, coagulative necrosis, apoptotic hepatocyte degeneration, tissue eosinophilia, and microvesicular steatosis. Megadoses of vitamin A can injure the liver, as can pyrrolizidine alkaloids, which often contaminate Chinese herbal preparations and can cause a venoocclusive injury leading to sinusoidal hepatic vein obstruction. Because some alternative medicines induce toxicity via active metabolites, alcohol and drugs that stimulate cytochrome P450 enzymes may enhance the toxicity of some of these products. Conversely, some alternative medicines also stimulate cytochrome P450 and may result in or amplify the toxicity of recognized drug hepatotoxins. Given the widespread use of such poorly defined herbal preparations, hepatotoxicity is likely to be encountered with increasing frequency; therefore, a drug history in patients with acute and chronic liver disease should include use of "alternative medicines" and other nonprescription preparations sold in so-called health food stores.

HIGHLY ACTIVE ANTIRETROVIRAL THERAPY (HAART) FOR HIV INFECTION (MITOCHONDRIAL TOXIC, IDIOSYNCRATIC, STEATOSIS; HEPATOCELLULAR, CHOLESTATIC, AND MIXED) The recognition of drug hepatotoxicity in persons with HIV infection is complicated in this population by the many alternative causes of liver injury (chronic viral hepatitis, fatty infiltration, infiltrative disorders, mycobacterial infection, etc.), but drug hepatotoxicity associated with HAART is an emerging and common type of liver injury in HIV-infected persons (Chap. 173). Although no one antiviral agent is recognized as a potent hepatotoxin, combination regimens including reverse transcriptase and protease inhibitors cause hepatotoxicity in ~10% of treated patients. Implicated most frequently are combinations including nucleoside analogue reverse transcriptase inhibitors zidovudine, didanosine, and, to a lesser extent, stavudine; protease inhibitors ritonavir and indinavir; and nonnucleoside reverse transcriptase inhibitors nevirapine and, to a lesser extent, efavirenz. These drugs cause predominantly hepatocellular injury but cholestatic injury as well, and prolonged (>6 months) use of reverse transcriptase inhibitors has been associated with mitochondrial injury, steatosis, and lactic acidosis. Distinguishing the impact of HAART hepatotoxicity in patients with HIV and hepatitis virus co-infection is made challenging by the following: (1) both chronic hepatitis B and hepatitis C can affect the natural history of HIV infection and the response to HAART, and (2) HAART can have an impact on chronic viral hepatitis. For example, immunologic reconstitution with HAART can result in immunologically mediated liver-cell injury in patients with chronic hepatitis B co-infection if lamivudine is withdrawn or if lamivudine resistance emerges. Infection with HIV, especially with low CD4+ T

cell counts, has been reported to increase the rate of hepatic fibrosis associated with chronic hepatitis C, and HAART therapy can increase levels of serum aminotransferases and hepatitis C virus RNA in patients with hepatitis C co-infection.

FURTHER READING

BISSELL DM et al: Drug-induced liver injury: Mechanisms and test systems. Hepatology 33:1009, 2001

FARRELL GC, LIDDLE C (guest eds.): Hepatotoxicity in the twenty-first century. Semin Liver Dis 22:109, 2002

MORGAN DJ, SMALLWOOD RA: Drug-induced liver disease. Curr Opin Gastroenterol 12:246, 1996

NOLAN CM et al: Hepatotoxicity associated with isoniazid preventive therapy. JAMA 281:1014, 1999

SCHMIDT LE et al: Acute versus chronic alcohol consumption in acetaminophen-induced hepatotoxicity. Hepatology 35:876, 2002

SULKOWSKI MS et al: Hepatotoxicity associated with antiretroviral therapy in adults infected with human immunodeficiency virus and the role of hepatitis C or B virus infection. JAMA 283:74, 2000

ZHANG J et al: Modulation of acetaminophen-induced hepatotoxicity by the xenobiotic receptor CAR. Science 298:422, 2002

ZIMMERMAN HJ et al: Drug-induced liver disease, in *Schiff's Diseases of the Liver*, 8th ed. E Schiff et al (eds). Philadelphia, Lippincott-Raven, 1999, p 973

287   CHRONIC HEPATITIS
Jules L. Dienstag, Kurt J. Isselbacher

Chronic hepatitis represents a series of liver disorders of varying causes and severity in which hepatic inflammation and necrosis continue for at least 6 months. Milder forms are nonprogressive or only slowly progressive, while more severe forms may be associated with scarring and architectural reorganization, which, when advanced, lead ultimately to cirrhosis. Several categories of chronic hepatitis have been recognized. These include chronic viral hepatitis (Chap. 285), drug-induced chronic hepatitis (Chap. 286), and autoimmune chronic hepatitis. In many cases, clinical and laboratory features are insufficient to allow assignment into one of these three categories; these "idiopathic" cases are also believed to represent autoimmune chronic hepatitis. Finally, clinical and laboratory features of chronic hepatitis are observed occasionally in patients with such hereditary/metabolic disorders as Wilson's disease (copper overload) and even occasionally in patients with alcoholic liver injury (Chap. 288). Although all types of chronic hepatitis share certain clinical, laboratory, and histopathologic features, chronic viral and chronic autoimmune hepatitis are sufficiently distinct to merit separate discussions.

CLASSIFICATION OF CHRONIC HEPATITIS   Common to all forms of chronic hepatitis are histopathologic distinctions based on localization and ex-

tent of liver injury. These vary from the milder forms, previously labeled chronic persistent hepatitis and chronic lobular hepatitis, to the more severe form, formerly called chronic active hepatitis. When first defined, these designations were felt to have prognostic implications, which have been challenged by more recent observations. Compared to the time three decades ago when the histologic designations chronic persistent, chronic lobular, and chronic active hepatitis were adopted, much more information is currently available about the causes, natural history, pathogenesis, serologic features, and therapy of chronic hepatitis. Therefore, categorization of chronic hepatitis based primarily upon histopathologic features has been replaced by a more informative classification based upon a combination of clinical, serologic, and histologic variables. Classification of chronic hepatitis is based upon (1) its *cause*, (2) its histologic activity, or *grade*, and (3) its degree of progression, or *stage*. Thus, neither clinical features alone nor histologic features—requiring liver biopsy—alone are sufficient to characterize and distinguish among the several categories of chronic hepatitis.

Classification by Cause   Clinical and serologic features allow the establishment of a diagnosis of *chronic viral hepatitis*, caused by hepatitis B, hepatitis B plus D, hepatitis C, or potentially other unknown viruses; *autoimmune hepatitis*, including several subcategories, types 1, 2, and 3, based on serologic distinctions; *drug-associated chronic hepatitis*; and a category of unknown cause, or *cryptogenic chronic hepatitis* (Table 287-1). These are addressed in more detail below.

Classification by Grade   Grade, a histologic assessment of necroinflammatory activity, is based upon examination of the liver biopsy. An assessment of important histologic features includes the degree of *periportal necrosis* and the disruption of the limiting plate of periportal hepatocytes by inflammatory cells (so-called *piecemeal necrosis* or *interface hepatitis*); the degree of confluent necrosis that links or forms bridges between vascular structures—between portal tract and portal tract or even more important bridges between portal tract and central vein—referred to as *bridging necrosis*; the degree of

TABLE 287-1   *Clinical and Laboratory Features of Chronic Hepatitis*

Type of Hepatitis	Diagnostic Test(s)	Autoantibodies	Therapy
Chronic hepatitis B	HBsAg, IgG anti-HBc, HBeAg, HBV DNA	Uncommon	IFN-α, lamivudine
Chronic hepatitis C	Anti-HCV, HCV RNA	Anti-LKM1[a]	PEG-IFN-α plus ribavirin
Chronic hepatitis D	Anti-HDV, HDV RNA, HBsAg, IgG anti-HBc	Anti-LKM3	IFN-α (?)
Autoimmune hepatitis	ANA[b] (homogeneous), anti-LKM1(±), hyperglobulinemia	ANA, anti-LKM1, anti-SLA[c]	Prednisone, azathioprine
Drug-associated	—	Uncommon	Withdraw drug
Cryptogenic	All negative	None	Prednisone (?), azathioprine (?)

[a] Antibodies to liver-kidney microsomes type 1 (autoimmune hepatitis type II and some cases of hepatitis C).
[b] Antinuclear antibody (autoimmune hepatitis type I).
[c] Antibodies to soluble liver antigen (autoimmune hepatitis type III).
Note: HBsAg, hepatitis B surface antigen; IFN-α, interferon α; PEG-IFN-α, pegylated interferon α.

hepatocyte degeneration and focal necrosis within the lobule; and the degree of *portal inflammation*. Several scoring systems that take these histologic features into account have been devised, and the most popular is the numerical histologic activity index (HAI), based on the work of Knodell and Ishak (Table 287-2). Technically, the HAI, which is primarily a measure of *grade*, also includes an assessment of fibrosis, which is currently used to categorize *stage* of the disease, as described below. Based on the presence and degree of these features of histologic activity, chronic hepatitis can be graded as mild, moderate, or severe.

Classification by Stage The stage of chronic hepatitis, which reflects the level of progression of the disease, is based on the degree of fibrosis. When fibrosis is so extensive that fibrous septa surround parenchymal nodules and alter the normal architecture of the liver lobule, the histologic lesion is defined as cirrhosis. Staging is based on the degree of fibrosis as categorized by one of several numerical scales (Table 287-2).

Reconciliation between Histologic Classification and New Classification For historic purposes, and to provide the basis for navigating several decades worth of literature on chronic hepatitis, the histologic categories of chronic persistent hepatitis, chronic lobular hepatitis, and chronic active hepatitis are correlated with their contemporary counterparts in Table 287-3. When the early classification was devised, chronic persistent and lobular hepatitis were felt to have a good prognosis, while chronic active hepatitis was considered a progressive disorder with a poor prognosis. The prognostic value of these histologic distinctions, however, was found to be limited, and this classification scheme has been supplanted by distinctions in grade and stage.

CHRONIC VIRAL HEPATITIS Both the enterically transmitted forms of viral hepatitis, hepatitis A and E, are self-limited and do not cause chronic hepatitis (rare reports notwithstanding in which acute hepatitis A serves as a trigger for the onset of autoimmune hepatitis in genetically susceptible patients). In contrast, the entire clinicopathologic spectrum of chronic hepatitis occurs in patients with chronic viral hepatitis B and C as well as in patients with chronic hepatitis D superimposed on chronic hepatitis B.

Chronic Hepatitis B The likelihood of chronicity after acute hepatitis B varies as a function of age. Infection at birth is associated with a clinically silent acute infection but a 90% chance of chronic infection, while infection in young adulthood in immunocompetent persons is typically associated with clinically apparent acute hepatitis but a risk of chronicity of only approximately 1%. Most cases of chronic hepatitis B among adults, however, occur in patients who never had a recognized episode of clinically apparent acute viral hepatitis. The degree of liver injury (grade) in patients with chronic hepatitis B is variable, ranging from none in inactive carriers, to mild, to severe. Among adults with chronic hepatitis B, histologic features are of prognostic importance. In one long-term study of patients with chronic hepatitis B, investigators found a 5-year survival of 97% for patients with mild chronic hepatitis, of 86% for patients with moderate to severe chronic hepatitis, and of only 55% for patients with chronic hepatitis and postnecrotic cirrhosis. The 15-year survival in these cohorts

TABLE 287-2 Histologic Activity Index (HAI) (Knodell-Ishak Score) in Chronic Hepatitis

Histologic Feature	HAI[a] Severity	Score	Modified HAI[b] Severity		Score
1. Perioportal necrosis, including piecemeal necrosis (PN) and/or bridging necrosis (BN)	None	0	None		0
	Mild PN	1	Mild		1
	Moderate PN	3	Mild/moderate		2
	Marked PN	4	Moderate		3
	Moderate PN + BN	5	Severe		4
	Marked PN + BN	6			
	Multilobular necrosis	10			
2. Intralobular necrosis	None	0	Confluent	None	0
	Mild	1		Focal	1
	Moderate	3		Zone 3 some	2
	Marked	4		Zone 3 most	3
				Zone 3 + BN few	4
				Zone 3 + BN multiple	5
				Panacinar/multiacinar	6
			Focal	None	0
				≤ 1 focus/10× field	1
				2–4 foci/10× field	2
				5–10 foci/10× field	3
				>10 foci/10× field	4
3. Portal inflammation	None	0			0
	Mild	1			1
	Moderate	3			2
	Moderate/marked	3			3
	Marked	4			4
4. Fibrosis	None	0			0
	Portal fibrosis—some	1			1
	Portal fibrosis—most	1			2
	Bridging fibrosis—few	3			3
	Bridging fibrosis—many	3			4
	Incomplete cirrhosis	4			5
	Cirrhosis				6
Maximum score		22			Grade 18/Stage 6

[a] "Knodell Score," *Hepatology* 1:431, 1981   [b] "Ishak Score," *Hepatology* 24:289, 1996

were 77, 66, and 40%, respectively. On the other hand, more recent observations do not allow us to be so sanguine about the prognosis in patients with mild chronic hepatitis; among such patients followed for 1 to 13 years, progression to more severe chronic hepatitis and cirrhosis has been observed in more than a quarter of cases.

Probably more important to consider than histology alone in patients with chronic hepatitis B is the degree of hepatitis B virus (HBV) replication. As reviewed in Chap. 285, chronic hepatitis B can be divided into two phases based on the relative level of HBV replication. The relatively *replicative phase* is characterized by the presence in the serum of markers of HBV replication [hepatitis B e antigen (HBeAg) HBV DNA], by the presence in the liver of detectable intrahepatocyte nucleocapsid antigens [primarily hepatitis B core antigen (HBcAg)], by high infectivity, and by accompanying liver injury; HBV DNA can

TABLE 287-3 Correlation Between Earlier and Contemporary Nomenclature of Chronic Hepatitis

Old Classification	Contemporary Classification Grade (Activity)	Stage (Fibrosis)
Chronic persistent hepatitis[a]	Minimal or mild	None or mild
Chronic lobular hepatitis[b]	Mild or moderate	Mild
Chronic active hepatitis[c]	Mild, moderate, or severe	Mild, moderate, or severe

[a] Inflammatory infiltrate localized to, and confined within, portal tracts.
[b] Portal inflammation confined within portal tracts plus foci of necrosis and inflammation in the liver lobule, resembling slowly resolving acute hepatitis.
[c] Erosion of the limiting plate of periportal hepatocytes by inflammatory cells ("piecemeal necrosis" or "interface hepatitis"), usually with periportal connective tissue septa extending into the liver lobule. More severe instances involve hepatocellular dropout and collapse spanning liver lobules ("bridging necrosis"), and, in the most severe form, multilobular collapse, bridging necrosis, and collapse of lobules are extensive and associated with rapid clinical deterioration.

be detected in the liver but is extrachromosomal. In contrast, the relatively *nonreplicative phase* is characterized by the absence of conventional markers of HBV replication (HBeAg and HBV DNA detectable by hybridization) but an association with anti-HBe, the absence of intrahepatocytic HBcAg, limited infectivity, and minimal liver injury; HBV DNA can be detected in the liver but is integrated into the host genome. Those in the replicative phase tend to have more severe chronic hepatitis, while those in the nonreplicative phase tend to have minimal or mild chronic hepatitis or to be inactive hepatitis B carriers; however, distinctions in HBV replication and in histologic category do not always coincide. The likelihood of converting spontaneously from relatively replicative to nonreplicative chronic HBV infection is approximately 10 to 15% per year. As noted in Chap. 285, the conversion from replicative to nonreplicative chronic hepatitis B is associated with a transient elevation in aminotransferase activity resembling acute hepatitis; occasionally, spontaneous resumptions of replicative activity occur in nonreplicative infection; and occasionally, HBV variants occur in which serologic markers of replication (HBeAg) are absent, despite the presence of replicative infection (see below). Chronic HBV infection, especially when acquired at birth or in early childhood, is associated with an increased risk of hepatocellular carcinoma (Chap. 78). →*A discussion of the pathogenesis of liver injury in patients with chronic hepatitis B appears in Chap. 285.*

As noted in Chap. 285, *HBeAg-negative chronic hepatitis B*, i.e., chronic HBV infection with active virus replication, readily detectable HBV DNA (by insensitive hybridization assays with sensitivity thresholds of 10^5 to 10^6 virions/mL) but without HBeAg (anti-HBe-reactive), is more common than HBeAg-reactive chronic hepatitis B in Mediterranean and European countries and in Asia (and, correspondingly, in HBV genotypes other than A). Most such cases represent precore or core-promoter mutations acquired late in the natural history of the disease (mostly early-life onset; age range 40 to 55 years, older than that for HBeAg-reactive chronic hepatitis B); these mutations prevent translation of HBeAg from the precore component of the HBV genome (precore mutants) or are characterized by down-regulated transcription of precore mRNA (core-promoter mutants; Chap. 285). Although their levels of HBV DNA tend to be lower than among patients with HBeAg-reactive chronic hepatitis B, patients with HBeAg-negative chronic hepatitis B tend to have progressive liver injury (complicated more frequently by cirrhosis and hepatocellular carcinoma), to experience episodic reactivation of liver disease reflected in fluctuating levels of aminotransferase activity ("flares"), and, generally, to be more refractory to antiviral therapy (see below).

The spectrum of *clinical features* of chronic hepatitis B is broad, ranging from asymptomatic infection to debilitating disease or even end-stage, fatal hepatic failure. As noted above, the onset of the disease tends to be insidious in most patients, with the exception of the very few in whom chronic disease follows failure of resolution of clinically apparent acute hepatitis B. The clinical and laboratory features associated with progression from acute to chronic hepatitis B are discussed in Chap. 285. *Fatigue* is a common symptom, and persistent or intermittent *jaundice* is a common feature in severe or advanced cases. Intermittent deepening of jaundice and recurrence of malaise and anorexia, as well as worsening fatigue, are reminiscent of acute hepatitis; such exacerbations may occur spontaneously, often coinciding with evidence of virologic reactivation, may lead to progressive liver injury, and, when superimposed on well-established cirrhosis, may cause hepatic decompensation. Complications of cirrhosis occur in end-stage chronic hepatitis and include ascites, edema, bleeding gastroesophageal varices, hepatic encephalopathy, coagulopathy, or hypersplenism. Occasionally, these complications bring the patient to initial clinical attention. Extrahepatic complications of chronic hepatitis B, similar to those seen during the prodromal phase of acute hepatitis B, are associated with deposition of circulating hepatitis B antigen–antibody immune complexes. These include arthralgias and arthritis, which are

common, and the more rare purpuric cutaneous lesions (leukocytoclastic vasculitis), immune-complex glomerulonephritis, and generalized vasculitis (polyarteritis nodosa) (Chaps. 285 and 306).

Laboratory features of chronic hepatitis B do not distinguish adequately between histologically mild and severe hepatitis. Aminotransferase elevations tend to be modest for chronic hepatitis B but may fluctuate in the range of 100 to 1000 units. As is true for acute viral hepatitis B, alanine aminotransferase (ALT) tends to be more elevated than aspartate aminotransferase (AST); however, once cirrhosis is established, AST tends to exceed ALT. Levels of alkaline phosphatase activity tend to be normal or only marginally elevated. In severe cases, moderate elevations in serum bilirubin [51.3 to 171 μmol/L (3 to 10 mg/dL)] occur. Hypoalbuminemia and prolongation of the prothrombin time occur in severe or end-stage cases. Hyperglobulinemia and detectable circulating autoantibodies are distinctly absent in chronic hepatitis B (in contrast to autoimmune hepatitis). →*Viral markers of chronic HBV infection are discussed in Chap. 285.*

℞ TREATMENT

Although progression to cirrhosis is more likely in severe than in mild or moderate chronic hepatitis B, all forms of chronic hepatitis B can be progressive, and progression occurs primarily in patients with active HBV replication. Moreover, in populations of patients with chronic hepatitis B who are at risk for hepatocellular carcinoma (Chap. 78), the risk is highest for those with continued, high-level HBV replication. Therefore, management of chronic hepatitis B is directed at suppressing the level of virus replication. Early in its development, antiviral therapy for hepatitis B was confined to patients with HBeAg-reactive chronic hepatitis B; however, HBeAg-negative chronic hepatitis B has emerged as an important target for antiviral therapy as well. To date, three drugs have been approved for treatment of chronic hepatitis B: injectable interferon (IFN) α and two oral agents, lamivudine and adefovir dipivoxil; several other drugs are in the process of efficacy testing in clinical trials.

Interferon   Interferon-α was the first approved therapy for chronic hepatitis B. For immunocompetent adults with HBeAg-reactive chronic hepatitis B (who tend to have HBV DNA detectable by hybridization assay and histologic evidence of chronic hepatitis on liver biopsy), a 16-week course of IFN given subcutaneously at a daily dose of 5 million units, or three times a week at a dose of 10 million unit, results in a loss of HBeAg and hybridization-detectable HBV DNA (i.e., a reduction to levels below 10^5 to 10^6 virions/mL) in ~30% of patients, with a concomitant improvement in liver histology. Seroconversion from HBeAg to anti-HBe occurs in approximately 20%, and, in early trials, approximately 8% lost hepatitis B surface antigen (HBsAg). Successful interferon therapy and seroconversion are often accompanied by an acute hepatitis-like elevation in aminotransferase activity, which has been postulated to result from enhanced cytolytic T cell clearance of HBV-infected hepatocytes. Relapse after successful therapy is rare (1 or 2%). The likelihood of responding to IFN is higher in patients with lower levels of HBV DNA and substantial elevations of ALT. Although children can respond as well as adults, IFN therapy has not been effective in very young children infected at birth. Similarly, IFN therapy has not been effective in immunosuppressed persons, Asian patients with minimal-to-mild ALT elevations, or in patients with decompensated chronic hepatitis B (in whom such therapy can actually be detrimental, sometimes precipitating decompensation, often associated with severe adverse effects). Among patients with HBeAg loss during therapy, long-term follow-up has demonstrated that 80% experience eventual loss of HBsAg, i.e., all serologic markers of infection, and normalization of ALT over a 9-year posttreatment period. In addition, improved long-term and complication-free survival as well as a reduction in the frequency of hepatocellular carcinoma have been documented among interferon responders, supporting the conclusion that successful interferon therapy improves the natural history of chronic hepatitis B.

Retreatment of IFN nonresponders with another course of IFN may enhance response rates somewhat; however, currently, most would opt to address IFN nonresponders by offering them one of the newer, oral therapies.

Initial trials of brief-duration IFN therapy in patients with *HBeAg-negative chronic hepatitis B* were disappointing, suppressing HBV replication transiently during therapy but almost never resulting in sustained antiviral responses. In subsequent IFN trials among patients with HBeAg-negative chronic hepatitis B, however, more protracted courses, lasting up to a year and a half, have been reported to result in sustained remissions, with suppressed HBV DNA and aminotransferase activity, in ~20%.

Complications of IFN therapy include systemic "flulike" symptoms, marrow suppression, emotional lability (irritability commonly, depression rarely), autoimmune reactions (especially autoimmune thyroiditis), and miscellaneous side effects such as alopecia, rashes, diarrhea, and numbness and tingling of the extremities. With the possible exception of autoimmune thyroiditis, all these side effects are reversible upon dose lowering or cessation of therapy.

Whether or not IFN remains competitive with the newer generation of antivirals, it did represent the first successful antiviral approach, and it set the standard against which subsequent drugs are measured—the achievement of durable virologic, serologic, biochemical, and histologic responses; consolidation of virologic and biochemical benefit in the ensuing years after therapy; and improvement in the natural history of chronic hepatitis B. Indications for IFN therapy in patients with chronic hepatitis B are summarized in Table 287-4.

In patients with chronic hepatitis B, long-term therapy with glucocorticoids is not only ineffective but also detrimental. Short-term glucocorticoid therapy, however, which increases HBV replication and expression in hepatocytes but depresses cytolytic T cells, has been advocated as a potential antiviral approach. A brief course of glucocorticoids, followed by their abrupt withdrawal, permits steroid therapy–suppressed T cells to resume their function against hepatocytes enriched in HBV expression by the recent burst of steroid exposure. An acute hepatitis-like flare of aminotransferase activity follows and may be accompanied by a dramatic drop, or even loss of, HBV replication. Such glucocorticoid "priming" prior to interferon therapy has not been shown to be more effective than interferon alone and has been abandoned.

Lamivudine Several nucleoside analogues active against HBV are being evaluated and developed. The first of these to be approved, the dideoxynucleoside lamivudine, inhibits reverse transcriptase activity of both HIV and HBV and is a potent and effective agent for patients with chronic hepatitis B. Lamivudine suppresses HBV DNA by a median of four orders of magnitude at oral daily doses of 100 mg. In clinical trials, lamivudine therapy for 12 months was associated with almost universal suppression of HBV DNA detectable by hybridization assays; loss of HBeAg in 32 to 33%; HBeAg seroconversion (i.e., conversion from HBeAg-reactive to anti-HBe-reactive) in 16 to 20%;

normalization of ALT in approximately 40%; improvement in histology in over 50%; retardation in fibrosis in 20 to 30%; and prevention of progresstion to cirrhosis. HBeAg responses can occur even in subgroups who are resistant (e.g., those with high-level HBV DNA), or who failed in the past to respond, to IFN. As is true for IFN therapy of chronic hepatitis B, patients with near-normal ALT activity do not experience HBeAg responses (despite suppression of HBV DNA), and those with ALT levels exceeding five times the upper limit of normal can expect 1-year HBeAg seroconversion rates of 50 to 60%. Generally, HBeAg seroconversions are confined to patients who achieve suppression of HBV DNA to $<10^4$ genomes/mL. Among patients who undergo HBeAg responses during therapy, the response is sustained in the vast majority (~70 to 80%) for 4 to 6 months after cessation of therapy; therefore, the achievement of an HBeAg response represents a viable stopping point in therapy. Moreover, for patients with such several-month-sustained HBeAg responses, the durability of these responses over the next 2 years (the limit of follow-up monitoring in current trials) is ~80%, accompanied, at least in western patients, by a >20% HBsAg seroconversion rate, comparable to that seen at 2 years after IFN-induced HBeAg responses. If HBeAg is unaffected by lamivudine therapy, the current approach is to continue therapy until an HBeAg response occurs, but long-term therapy may be required to suppress HBV replication and, in turn, limit liver injury. Preliminary observations indicate that HBeAg seroconversions can increase to a level of 50% after 5 years of therapy. Histologic improvement continues to accrue with therapy beyond the first year; after a cumulative course of 3 years of lamivudine therapy, necroinflammatory activity is reduced in the majority of patients, and cirrhosis has been shown to regress to precirrhotic stages.

Losses of HBsAg have been few during the first year of lamivudine therapy, and this observation had been cited as an advantage of IFN over lamivudine; however, in head-to-head comparisons between IFN and lamivudine monotherapy, HBsAg losses were rare in both groups. Trials in which lamivudine and interferon were administered in combination failed to show a benefit of combination therapy over lamivudine monotherapy for either treatment-naive patients or prior interferon nonresponders; however, trials are currently underway to assess the potential value of combination lamivudine plus long-active pegylated IFN (developed for treatment of chronic hepatitis C, see below).

In patients with *HBeAg-negative chronic hepatitis B*, i.e., in those with precore and core-promoter HBV mutations, 1 year of lamivudine therapy results in HBV DNA suppression and normalization of ALT in three-quarters of patients and in histologic improvement in approximately two-thirds. Therapy has been shown to suppress HBV DNA to undetectable levels in 39%, as measured by sensitive polymerase chain reaction (PCR) amplification assays. Lacking HBeAg at the outset, patients with HBeAg-negative chronic hepatitis B cannot achieve an HBeAg response—a stopping point in HBeAg-reactive patients; invariably, when therapy is discontinued, reactivation is the rule. Therefore, these patients require long-term therapy; with successive years, the proportion with suppressed HBV DNA and normal ALT increases.

Clinical and laboratory side effects of lamivudine are negligible, indistinguishable from those observed in placebo recipients. During lamivudine therapy, transient ALT elevations, resembling those seen during IFN therapy and during spontaneous HBeAg-to-anti-HBe seroconversions, occur in a quarter of patients. These ALT elevations may result from restored cytolytic T cell activation permitted by suppression of HBV replication. Similar ALT elevations, however, occur at an identical frequency in placebo recipients, but ALT elevations associated with HBeAg seroconversion are confined to lamivudine-treated patients. When therapy is stopped after a year of therapy, two- to threefold ALT elevations occur in 20 to 30% of lamivudine-treated patients, representing renewed liver-cell injury as HBV replication returns. Although these posttreatment flares are almost always transient and mild, rare severe exacerbations, especially in cirrhotic patients,

TABLE 287-4 *Patients with Chronic Hepatitis B Who Are Candidates for Antiviral Therapy*

Clinical Feature	Interferon	Lamivudine	Adefovir
Detectable markers of HBV replication	Yes	Yes	Yes
Normal ALT activity	No	No	No
ALT <2 × upper limit of normal	No	No	No
ALT >2 × upper limit of normal	Yes	Yes	Yes
Immunocompetent	Yes	Yes	Yes
Immunocompromised	No	Yes	Yes
Adult acquisition (western)	Yes	Yes	Yes
Childhood acquisition (Asian)	No	Yes	Yes
Compensated liver disease	Yes	Yes	Yes
Decompensated liver disease	No	Yes	Yes
"Wild-type" HBeAg-reactive	Yes	Yes	Yes
HBeAg-negative chronic hepatitis	Yes	Yes	Yes
Interferon-refractory	No	Yes	Yes

Note: HBV, hepatitis B virus; ALT, alanine aminotransferase; HBeAg, hepatitis B e antigen.

have been observed, mandating close and careful clinical and virologic monitoring after discontinuation of treatment.

Long-term monotherapy with lamivudine is associated with methionine-to-valine or methionine-to-isoleucine mutations in the YMDD (tyrosine-methionine-aspartate-aspartate) motif of HBV DNA polymerase, analogous to mutations that occur in patients with HIV infection treated with this drug. During a year of therapy, YMDD mutations occur in 15 to 30% of patients; the frequency increases with each year of therapy, reaching 70% at year 5. Although transient elevations in ALT and HBV DNA levels occur when such variants emerge, YMDD-variant HBV appears to be less replicatively competent and a less robust pathogen. Even after YMDD mutations occur, HBV DNA and ALT levels as well as histologic scores tend to remain lower than baseline levels in immunocompetent patients. In immunosuppressed patients, a proportion of patients with YMDD mutations experience hepatic decompensation. Even in immunocompetent persons, ultimately, after 2 to 3 years, YMDD-variant HBV leads to a deterioration in histology. Therefore, if therapy is begun with lamivudine monotherapy, the emergence of a YMDD variant, reflected clinically by a breakthrough from suppressed levels of HBV DNA and ALT, is managed by adding another antiviral to which YMDD variants are sensitive (e.g., adefovir, see below).

Because lamivudine monotherapy can result universally in the rapid emergence of YMDD variants in persons with HIV infection, patients with chronic hepatitis B should be tested for anti-HIV prior to therapy; if HIV infection is identified, lamivudine monotherapy at the HBV daily dose of 100 mg is contraindicated. These patients should be treated with triple-drug antiretroviral therapy, including a lamivudine daily dose of 300 mg (Chap. 173). The safety of lamivudine during pregnancy has not been established.

Adefovir Dipivoxil The acyclic nucleotide analogue adefovir dipivoxil, the prodrug of adevovir, is a potent antiviral that, at an oral daily dose of 10 mg, reduces HBV DNA by approximately 3.5 to 4 logs and is equally effective in treatment-naïve patients and IFN nonresponders. In HBeAg-reactive chronic hepatitis B, a 48-week course of adefovir dipivoxil was shown to achieve histologic improvement (and reduce the progression of fibrosis) and normalization of ALT in half the patients, HBeAg seroconversion in 12%, HBeAg loss in 23%, and suppression to an undetectable level of HBV DNA in 21%, as measured by PCR. Similar to IFN and lamivudine, adefovir dipivoxil is more likely to achieve an HBeAg response in patients with high baseline ALT; for example, among adefovir-treated patients with ALT level >5 times the upper limit of normal, HBeAg seroconversions occurred in 25%. Although the durability of adefovir-induced HBeAg responses remains to be documented, expectations are that they will be as durable as those seen during lamivudine therapy and that HBeAg responses can be relied upon as a stopping point for adefovir therapy.

In patients with *HBeAg-negative chronic hepatitis B,* a 48-week course of 10 mg/d of adefovir dipivoxil resulted in histologic improvement in two-thirds, normalization of ALT in three-quarters, and suppression of HBV DNA to PCR-undetectable levels in half. As was true for lamivudine, because HBeAg responses—a potential stopping point—cannot be achieved in this group, reactivation is the rule when adefovir therapy is discontinued, and indefinite, long-term therapy is anticipated.

Adevofir contains a flexible acyclic linker instead of the L-nucleoside ring of lamivudine, avoiding steric hindrance by mutated amino acids. In addition, the molecular structure of phosphorylated adefovir is very similar to that of its natural substrate; therefore mutations to adefovir would also affect binding of the natural substrate, dATP. Hypothetically, these are among the reasons that resistance to adefovir dipivoxil has not been encountered in 1 year of clinical-trial therapy and in only 2.5% after 2 years of therapy, in both immunocompetent and immunocompromised patients. Among patients co-infected with HBV and HIV and who have normal CD4+ T cell counts, adefovir

dipivoxil is effective in suppressing HBV dramatically (in one study, by 5 logs). Moreover, adefovir dipivoxil is effective in lamivudine-associated YMDD-variant HBV and can be used when such lamivudine-induced variants emerge. When, in the past, this drug had been evaluated as therapy for HIV infection, doses of 60 to 120 mg were required to suppress HIV, and at these doses, the drug was nephrotoxic. Even at 30 mg/d, creatinine elevations of 44 μmol/L (0.5 mg/dL) occur in 10% of patients; however, at the HBV-effective dose of 10 mg, such elevations of creatinine are rarely encountered. If any nephrotoxicity does occur, it rarely appears before 6 to 8 months of therapy. Although renal tubular injury is a rare potential side effect, and although creatinine monitoring is recommended during treatment, the therapeutic index of adefovir dipivoxil is high, and the nephrotoxicity observed in clinical trials at higher doses was reversible. For patients with underlying renal disease, adefovir dipivoxil dose reductions are recommended: administration reduced to every 48 h for creatinine clearances of 20 to 49 mL/min, to every 72 h for creatinine clearances of 10 to 19 mL/min, and once a week, following dialysis, for patients undergoing hemodialysis. Adevofir dipivoxil is very well tolerated, and ALT elevations during and after withdrawal of therapy are similar to those observed and described above in clinical trials of lamivudine.

No treatment is recommended or available for inactive "nonreplicative" hepatitis B carriers. For patients with ALT levels less than twice the upper limit of normal, in whom sustained responses are not likely and who would require multiyear therapy, antiviral therapy is not currently recommended. For patients with ALT more than twice the upper limit, any one of the three available drugs is recommended, but in patients with HBeAg-negative chronic hepatitis B, the requirement for indefinite-duration therapy favors a drug such as adefovir dipivoxil, which is complicated only rarely by the emergence of resistance. Either lamivudine or adefovir is recommended for interferon-refractory patients. Whereas patients with decompensated chronic hepatitis B are not candidates for IFN therapy, they may respond to lamivudine or adefovir dipivoxil, with reversal of the signs of decompensation. Table 287-4 summarizes indications for antiviral therapy in patients with chronic hepatitis B. Interferon, lamivudine, and adefovir can each be used as first-line therapy (Table 287-5). Interferon requires only brief-duration therapy, too limited in duration to support viral variants, but requires subcutaneous injections and is associated with a high level of intolerability. Lamivudine requires long-term therapy in most patients and, when used alone, fosters the emergence of viral variants. On the other hand, lamivudine is taken orally, is very well tolerated, leads to improved histology even in the absence of HBeAg responses, and is effective even in patients who fail to respond to interferon. Adefovir, like lamivudine, is taken orally, is well tolerated, and is effective in IFN nonresponders. Its major advantage is the near absence of resistance. Although the drug is safe, creatinine monitoring is recommended. Although some prefer to begin with IFN, most physicians and patients prefer lamivudine or adefovir as first-line therapy.

For patients with end-stage chronic hepatitis B, liver transplantation is the only potential lifesaving intervention. In the absence of antiviral therapy, reinfection of the new liver is almost universal; however, the likelihood of liver injury associated with hepatitis B in the new liver is variable. The majority of patients become high-level viremic carriers with minimal liver injury. Unfortunately, an unpredictable proportion experience severe hepatitis B–related liver injury, sometimes a fulminant-like hepatitis, sometimes a rapid recapitulation of the original severe chronic hepatitis B (Chap. 291). Prevention of recurrent hepatitis B after liver transplantation has been achieved by *prophylaxis* with hepatitis B immune globulin and with the nucleoside analogues lamivudine and adefovir; in addition, nucleoside analogues have been used successfully to *reverse* posttransplantation liver injury associated with recurrent hepatitis B (Chap. 291).

Novel Antivirals and Strategies In addition to the three approved antiviral drugs for hepatitis B, several others are being evaluated in clinical trials, as listed in Table 287-6. Preliminary indications are that entecavir and is telbivudine can reduce HBV DNA levels by five and six logs, respectively, and that entecavir and is active against lamivudine-associated YMDD variants. Tenofovir, similar to adefovir, was developed for HIV infection but appears to have activity against wild-type and YMDD-variant HBV similar to that of adefovir; however, to date, it has not been studied extensively in patients with HBV infection.

Initial emphasis in the development of antiviral therapy for hepatitis B was placed on monotherapy; however, in the future, combination therapies will be studied. If combination therapies reduce HBV replication more substantially than monotherapies and avoid resistance, combination therapy regimens will become the norm.

Chronic Hepatitis D (Delta Hepatitis) The clinical and laboratory features of chronic hepatitis D virus (HDV) infection are summarized in Chap. 285. Chronic hepatitis D may follow acute co-infection with HBV but at a rate no higher than the rate of chronicity of hepatitis B. That is, although HDV co-infection can increase the severity of acute hepatitis B, HDV does not increase the likelihood of progression to chronic hepatitis B. However, when HDV superinfection occurs in a person who is already chronically infected with HBV, long-term HDV infection is the rule and a worsening of the liver disease the expected consequence. Except for severity, chronic hepatitis B plus D has similar clinical and laboratory features to those seen in chronic hepatitis B alone. Relatively severe chronic hepatitis, with or without cirrhosis, is the rule, and mild chronic hepatitis the exception. Occasionally, mild hepatitis, or even, rarely, inactive carriage, occurs in patients with chronic hepatitis B plus D, and recent observations suggest that the disease may become indolent after several years of infection. A distinguishing serologic feature of chronic hepatitis D is the presence in the circulation of antibodies to liver-kidney microsomes (anti-LKM); however, the anti-LKM seen in hepatitis D are designated anti-LKM3, are directed against uridine diphosphate glucuronosyltransferase, and are distinct from anti-LKM1 seen in patients with autoimmune hepatitis and in a subset of patients with chronic hepatitis C (see below).

℞ TREATMENT

Management is not well defined. Glucocorticoids are ineffective and are not used. Preliminary experimental trials of IFN-α suggested that conventional doses and durations of therapy lower levels of HDV RNA and aminotransferase activity only transiently during treatment but have no impact on the natural history of the disease. Although high-dose IFN-α (9 million units) three times a week for 12 months may be associated with a sustained loss of HDV replication and clinical improvement in up to 50% of patients, ultimately recurrent HDV replication becomes universal after cessation of therapy. Antiviral therapy for chronic hepatitis D remains the subject of experimental trials; lamivudine is not effective, but preliminary indications are that clevudine (L-FMAU) may be. In patients with end-stage liver disease secondary to chronic hepatitis D, liver transplantation has been effective. If hepatitis D recurs in the new liver without the expression of hepatitis B (an unusual serologic profile in immunocompetent persons,

but common in transplant patients), liver injury is limited. In fact, the outcome of transplantation for chronic hepatitis D is superior to that for chronic hepatitis B (Chap. 291).

Chronic Hepatitis C Regardless of the epidemiologic mode of acquisition of hepatitis C virus (HCV) infection, chronic hepatitis follows acute hepatitis C in 50 to 70% of cases; even in those with a return to normal in aminotransferase levels after acute hepatitis C, chronic infection is common, adding up to an 85 to 90% likelihood of chronic HCV infection after acute hepatitis C. Furthermore, in patients with chronic transfusion-associated hepatitis followed for 10 to 20 years, progression to cirrhosis occurs in about 20%. Such is the case even for patients with relatively clinically mild chronic hepatitis, including those without symptoms, with only modest elevations of aminotransferase activity, and with mild chronic hepatitis on liver biopsy. Even in cohorts of well-compensated patients with chronic hepatitis C referred for clinical research trials (no complications of chronic liver

TABLE 287-5 *Comparison of Interferon, Lamivudine, and Adefovir Dipivoxil Therapy for Chronic Hepatitis B[a]*

Feature	Interferon	Lamivudine	Adefovir
Route of administration	Injection	Oral	Oral
Duration of therapy[b]	4 months	≥52 weeks	≥48 weeks
Tolerability	Poorly tolerated	Well tolerated	Well tolerated
Nephrotoxicity	None	None	Creatinine monitoring recommended
HBeAg loss	33%	32–33%	23%
HBeAg seroconversion	18–20%	16–20%	12%
HBeAg seroconversion if ALT >5 × normal	Not reported	>50%	21%
Log$_{10}$ HBV DNA reduction	?	4	3.5–4
HBV DNA PCR-negative	Unlikely	~30% HBeAg+ 39% HBeAg−	21% HBeAg+ 51% HBeAg−
ALT normalization	Confined to HBeAg responders	>40% HBeAg+ >70% HBeAg−	50% HBeAg+ 72% HBeAg−
HBsAg loss during Rx	3–8%	2–4%	Unlikely
HBsAg loss after Rx	80% over 9 years	23% over 2 years	To be determined
Histologic improvement	Confined to HBeAg responders	>50% HBeAg+ >66% HBeAg−	>50% HBeAg+ >66% HBeAg−
Retardation of fibrosis	Not demonstrated	20–30%	20–30%
Viral resistance	None	15–30% @ 1 year 70% @ 5 years	None @ 1 year 2.5% @ 2 years
Natural history	Reduced mortality, decompensation, HCC	To be determined	To be determined
HBeAg-negative chronic hepatitis B	~20% sustained response after ≥1 year of Rx	>60–70% virologic and histologic response; relapse likely after Rx	Same as lamivudine
Candidate range[c]	Narrow	Broad	Broad
Cost (U.S. $)	~$5000/4 months	~$1700/year	~$5600/year

[a] Generally, these comparisons are based upon data on each drug tested individually versus placebo in registration clinical trials; because, with rare exception, these comparisons are not based on head-to-head testing of these drugs, relative advantages and disadvantages should be interpreted cautiously.
[b] Duration of therapy in clinical efficacy trials; use in clinical practice may vary.
[c] See Table 287-4.
Note: HBeAg, hepatitis B e antigen; ALT, alanine aminotransferase; HBV, hepatitis B virus; PCR, polymerase chain reaction; HBsAg, hepatitis B surface antigen; HCC, hepatocellular carcinoma.

TABLE 287-6 *New Antiviral Drugs Being Developed for the Treatment of Chronic Hepatitis B*

Entecavir[a]
Telbivudine (L-dT)
Clevudine (L-FMAU)
Emtricitabine (FTC)
Pegylated alpha interferons

[a] Reported to have activity against lamivudine-associated YMDD-variant HBV.
Note: YMDD, tyrosine-methionine-aspartate-aspartate.

disease and with normal hepatic synthetic function), the prevalence of cirrhosis may be as high as 50%. Many cases of hepatitis C are identified in asymptomatic patients who have no history of acute hepatitis C, e.g., those discovered while attempting to donate blood or as a result of routine laboratory screening tests. The source of HCV infection in most of these cases is not defined, although a long-forgotten percutaneous exposure in the remote past can be elicited in a substantial proportion. Approximately a third of patients with chronic hepatitis C have normal or near-normal aminotransferase activity; although a third to a half of these patients have chronic hepatitis on liver biopsy, the grade of liver injury and stage of fibrosis tend to be mild in the vast majority. In some cases, more severe liver injury has been reported, even, rarely, cirrhosis, most likely the result of previous histologic activity. Among patients with persistent normal aminotransferase activity sustained over ≥5 years, histologic progression has been shown not to occur; however, approximately a quarter of patients with normal aminotransferase activity experience subsequent aminotransferase elevations, and histologic injury can be progressive once abnormal biochemical activity resumes. Therefore, continued clinical monitoring is indicated, even for patients with normal aminotransferase activity.

Despite this substantial rate of progression of chronic hepatitis C, and despite the fact that liver failure can result from end-stage chronic hepatitis C, the long-term prognosis for chronic hepatitis C in a majority of patients is relatively benign. Mortality over 10 to 20 years among patients with transfusion-associated chronic hepatitis C has been shown not to differ from mortality in a matched population of transfused patients in whom hepatitis C did not develop. Although death in the hepatitis group is more likely to result from liver failure, and although hepatic decompensation may occur in ~15% of such patients over the course of a decade, the majority (almost 60%) of patients remain asymptomatic and well compensated, with no clinical sequelae of chronic liver disease. Overall, then, chronic hepatitis C tends to be very slowly and insidiously progressive, if at all, in the vast majority of patients, while in approximately a quarter of cases, chronic hepatitis C will progress eventually to end-stage cirrhosis. Referral bias may account for the more severe outcomes described in cohorts of patients reported from tertiary-care centers versus the more benign outcomes in cohorts of patients monitored from initial blood-product-associated acute hepatitis. Still unexplained, however, are the wide ranges in reported progression to cirrhosis, from 2% over 17 years in a population of women with hepatitis C infection acquired from contaminated anti-D immune globulin to 30% over ≤11 years in recipients of contaminated intravenous immune globulin.

Progression of liver disease in patients with chronic hepatitis C has been reported to be more likely in patients with older age, longer duration of infection, advanced histologic stage and grade, genotype 1, more complex quasispecies diversity, and increased hepatic iron. Among these variables, however, duration of infection appears to be the most important, and many of the others probably reflect disease duration to some extent (e.g., quasispecies diversity, hepatic iron accumulation).

Perhaps the best prognostic indicator in chronic hepatitis C is liver histology. Patients with mild necrosis and inflammation as well as those with limited fibrosis have an excellent prognosis and limited progression to cirrhosis. In contrast, among patients with moderate to severe necroinflammatory activity or fibrosis, including septal or bridging fibrosis, progression to cirrhosis is highly likely over the course of 10 to 20 years. Among patients with compensated cirrhosis associated with hepatitis C, the 10-year survival is close to 80%; mortality occurs at a rate of 2 to 6% per year, decompensation at a rate of 4 to 5% per year, and hepatocellular carcinoma at a rate of 1 to 4% per year.

In addition, severity of chronic hepatitis is greater and progression of chronic liver disease is more accelerated in patients who have chronic hepatitis C as well as other liver processes, including alcoholic liver disease, chronic hepatitis B, HIV infection, hemochromatosis, and α_1-antitrypsin deficiency. No other epidemiologic or clinical features of chronic hepatitis C (e.g., severity of acute hepatitis, level of aminotransferase activity, level of HCV RNA, presence or absence of jaundice during acute hepatitis) are predictive of eventual outcome. Despite the relative benignity of chronic hepatitis C over time, cirrhosis following chronic hepatitis C has been associated with the late development, after several decades, of hepatocellular carcinoma (HCC) (Chap. 78). As noted above, the annual rate of HCC in cirrhotic patients with hepatitis C is 1 to 4%.

Clinical features of chronic hepatitis C are similar to those described above for chronic hepatitis B. Generally, *fatigue* is the most common symptom; jaundice is rare. Immune complex–mediated extrahepatic complications of chronic hepatitis C are less common than in chronic hepatitis B, with the exception of essential mixed cryoglobulinemia (Chap. 285). This is the case despite the fact that assays for immune complex–like activity are often positive in patients with chronic hepatitis C. In addition, chronic hepatitis C has been associated with extrahepatic complications unrelated to immune-complex injury. These include Sjögren's syndrome, lichen planus, and porphyria cutanea tarda. *Laboratory features* of chronic hepatitis C are similar to those in patients with chronic hepatitis B, but aminotransferase levels tend to fluctuate more (the characteristic episodic pattern of aminotransferase activity) and to be lower, especially in patients with long-standing disease. An interesting and occasionally confusing finding in patients with chronic hepatitis C is the presence of autoantibodies. Rarely, patients with autoimmune hepatitis (see below) and hyperglobulinemia have false-positive enzyme immunoassays for anti-HCV. On the other hand, some patients with serologically confirmable chronic hepatitis C have circulating anti-LKM. These antibodies are anti-LKM1, as seen in patients with autoimmune hepatitis *type 2* (see below), and are directed against a 33-amino-acid sequence of P450 IID6. The occurrence of anti-LKM1 in some patients with chronic hepatitis C may result from the partial sequence homology between the epitope recognized by anti-LKM1 and two segments of the HCV polyprotein. In addition, the presence of this autoantibody in some patients with chronic hepatitis C suggests that autoimmunity may be playing a role in the pathogenesis of chronic hepatitis C. →*Histopathologic features of chronic hepatitis C, especially those that distinguish hepatitis C from hepatitis B, are described in Chap. 285.*

℞ **TREATMENT**

Therapy for chronic hepatitis C has evolved substantially in the decade and a half since IFN-α was introduced for this indication. When first approved, IFN-α was administered via subcutaneous injection three times a week for 6 months but achieved a sustained virologic response (a reduction of HCV RNA to undetectable levels by PCR when measured ≥6 months after completion of therapy) below 10%. Doubling the duration of therapy—but not increasing the dose or changing IFN preparations—increased the sustained virologic response rate to ~20%, and addition to the regimen of daily ribavirin, an oral guanosine nucleoside, increased sustained virologic responses to 40%. When used alone, ribavirin is ineffective and does not reduce HCV RNA levels, but ribavirin enhances the efficacy of IFN by reducing the likelihood of virologic relapse after the achievement of an end-treatment response (response measured during, and maintained to the end of, treatment). Proposed mechanisms to explain the role of ribavirin include subtle direct reduction of HCV replication, immune modulation, and induction of virologic mutational catastrophe.

Many important lessons about antiviral therapy for chronic hepatitis C were learned from the experience with IFN monotherapy and combination IFN-ribavirin therapy. Even in the absence of biochemical and virologic responses, histologic improvement occurs in approximately three-quarters of all treated patients. Unlike the case in hepatitis B, in chronic hepatitis C, responses to therapy are not accompanied by transient, acute hepatitis–like aminotransferase elevations; instead, ALT levels fall precipitously during therapy. Up to 90% of virologic responses are achieved within the first 12 weeks of therapy; responses thereafter are rare. Sustained virologic responses are very durable; normal ALT, improved histology, and absence of HCV RNA in serum and liver have been documented 5 to 6 years after successful therapy, and "relapses" 2 years after sustained responses are almost unheard of. Thus, sustained virologic responses to antiviral therapy of chronic hepatitis C are tantamount to cures.

Patient variables that tend to correlate with sustained virologic responsiveness to IFN include low baseline HCV RNA level (<2 million copies/mL), histologically mild hepatitis and minimal fibrosis, favorable genotype (genotypes 2 and 3 as opposed to genotyptes 1 and 4), age <40, absence of obesity, and female gender. Patients with cirrhosis can respond, but they are less likely to do so. Studies of combination IFN-ribavirin therapy showed conclusively that, in patients with genotype 1, therapy should last a full year, while in those with genotypes 2 and 3, a 6-month course of therapy suffices. The response rate in African Americans is disappointingly low for reasons that remain obscure. Finally, the likelihood of a sustained response is best if adherence to the treatment regimen is high, i.e., if patients receive ≥80% of the IFN and ribavirin doses, and if they continue treatment for ≥80% of the anticipated duration of therapy. Other variables reported to correlate with increased responsiveness include brief duration of infection, low HCV quasispecies diversity, immunocompetence, and low liver iron levels. High levels of HCV RNA, more histologically advanced liver disease, and high quasispecies diversity all go hand in hand with advanced duration of infection, which may be the single most important variable determining IFN responsiveness. The ironic fact, then, is that patients whose disease is *least* likely to progress are the ones *most* likely to respond to interferon and vice versa. Finally, among patients with genotype 1b, responsiveness to IFN is enhanced in those with amino-acid-substitution mutations in the nonstructural protein 5A gene.

Side effects of IFN therapy are described above in the section on treatment of chronic hepatitis B. The most pronounced side effect of ribavirin therapy is hemolysis; a reduction in hemoglobin of up to 2 to 3 g or in hematocrit of 5 to 10% can be anticipated. A small, unpredictable proportion of patients experience profound, brisk hemolysis, resulting in symptomatic anemia; therefore, close monitoring of blood counts is crucial, and ribavirin should be avoided in patients with anemia or hemoglobinopathies and in patients with coronary artery disease or cerebrovascular disease, in whom anemia can precipitate an ischemic event. When symptomatic anemia occurs, ribavirin dose reductions or addition of erythropoietin to boost red blood cell levels may be required. In addition, ribavirin, which is renally excreted, should not be used in patients with renal insufficiency; the drug is teratogenic, precluding its use during pregnancy and mandating the use of efficient contraception during therapy.

Ribavirin can also cause nasal and chest congestion, pruritus, and precipitation of gout. Combination IFN-ribavirin therapy is more difficult to tolerate than IFN monotherapy. In one large clinical trial of combination therapy versus monotherapy, among those in the 1-year treatment group, 21% of the combination group (but only 14% of the monotherapy group) had to discontinue treatment, while 26% of the combination group (but only 9% of the monotherapy group) required dose reductions.

Studies of viral kinetics have shown that despite a virion half-life in serum of only 2 to 3 h, the level of HCV is maintained by a high replication rate of 10^{12} hepatitis C virions per day. IFN-α blocks virion production or release with an efficacy that increases with increasing drug doses; moreover, the calculated death rate for infected cells during IFN therapy is inversely related to viral load; patients with the most rapid death rate of infected hepatocytes are more likely to achieve undetectable HCV RNA at 3 months; achieving this landmark is predictive of a subsequent sustained response. Therefore, to achieve rapid viral clearance from serum and the liver, *high-dose induction therapy* has been advocated. In practice, however, high-dose induction therapy has not yielded higher sustained response rates.

Treatment of Choice For the treatment of chronic hepatitis C, standard IFNs have now been supplanted by "pegylated" IFNs, long-acting IFNs bound to polyethylene glycol (PEG). Such pegylated IFNs have elimination times up to sevenfold longer than standard IFNs, i.e., a substantially longer half-life, and achieve prolonged concentrations, permitting administration once, rather than three times, a week. Instead of the frequent drug peaks (linked to side effects) and troughs (when drug is absent) associated with frequent administration of short-acting IFNs, administration of pegylated IFNs results in drug concentrations that are more stable and sustained over time. Early studies showed that once-a-week pegylated IFN monotherapy is twice as effective as monotherapy with its standard IFN counterpart, approaches the efficacy of combination standard IFN plus ribavirin, and is as well tolerated as standard IFNs, without more difficult-to-manage thrombocytopenia and leukopenia than standard IFNs. The current standard of care, however, is a combination of pegylated IFN plus ribavirin.

Two pegylated IFNs are available, pegylated IFN-α2b and -α2a. In the registration trial for pegylated IFN-α2b plus ribavirin, the best regimen was 48 weeks of 1.5 μg per kilogram of pegylated IFN once a week plus 800 mg of ribavirin daily. A posthoc analysis suggested that weight-based dosing of ribavirin would have been more effective than the fixed 800-mg dose used in the study. In the first registration trial for pegylated IFN-α2a plus ribavirin, the best regimen was 48 weeks of 180 μg of pegylated IFN plus 1000 mg (for patients < 75 kg) to 1200 mg (for patients ≥ 75 kg) of ribavirin. Sustained virologic responses of 54% and 56% were reported in these two studies, respectively. A subsequent study of pegylated IFN-α2a plus ribavirin showed that, for patients with genotypes 2 and 3, a duration of 6 months and a ribavirin dose of 800 mg was sufficient. Among the three studies, for patients in the optimal treatment arm, sustained response rates for patients with genotype 1 were 42 to 51%, and for patients with genotypes 2 and 3 rates were 76 to 82%.

In the initial registration trials for combination pegylated IFN plus ribavirin, both combination pegylated IFN regimens were compared to standard IFN-α2b plus ribavirin. Side effects of the combination pegylated IFN-α2b regimen were comparable to those for the combination standard-IFN regimen; however, when the combination pegylated IFN-α2a regimen was compared to the combination standard IFN-α2b regimen, flulike symptoms and depression were less common in the combination pegylated IFN group. Although the two combination pegylated IFN regimens were not tested head-to-head, when each was tested against standard IFN-α2b plus ribavirin, combination pegylated IFN-α2a plus ribavirin appeared to be better tolerated. Recommended doses for the two pegylated IFNs plus ribavirin and other comparisons between the two therapies are shown in Table 287-7.

Unless ribavirin is contraindicated (see above), combination pegylated IFN plus ribavirin is the recommended course of therapy—24 weeks for genotypes 2 and 3 and 48 weeks for genotype 1. Measurement of quantitative HCV RNA levels at 12 weeks is helpful in guiding therapy; if a 2-log drop in HCV RNA has not been achieved by this time, chances for a sustained virologic response are negligible. If the goal of therapy is sustained virologic response, failure to achieve a 12-week 2-log drop in HCV RNA may be used as a signal to discontinue therapy, especially in those who do not tolerate the drugs well. Still, conceivably, some may achieve histologic benefit in the absence of a virologic response, and some clinicians choose to continue therapy even in the absence of a 2-log HCV RNA reduction at 12 weeks. Studies are underway to determine whether, even in the absence of a virologic response, maintenance therapy with pegylated IFN can slow histologic and clinical progression of hepatitis C.

Indications for Antiviral Therapy Patients with chronic hepatitis C who have elevated ALT levels, detectable HCV RNA, and chronic hepatitis of at least moderate grade and stage (portal or bridging fibrosis) are

TABLE 287-7 *Comparison of Pegylated Interferon α2a and α2b for Chronic Hepatitis C[a]*

	PEG IFN-α2b	PEG IFN-α2a
PEG size	12 kDa linear	40 kDa branched
Mean terminal half-life	40 h	80 h
Mean clearance	94 mL/h per kg	22 mL/h per kg
Best-dose monotherapy	1.0 μg/kg (weight-based)	180 μg
Best-dose combination therapy	1.5 μg/kg (weight-based)	180 μg
Storage	Room temperature	Refrigerated
Ribavirin		
Genotype 1	800 mg[b]	1000–1200 mg[c]
Genotype 2/3	800 mg	800 mg
Duration of therapy		
Genotype 1	48 weeks	48 weeks
Genotype 2/3	48 weeks[d]	24 weeks
Efficacy of combination Rx	54%	56%
Genotype 1	42%	46–51%
Genotype 2/3	82%	76–78%
Side effects of pegylated interferon/ribavirin vs standard interferon/ribavirin[e]		
Fever	46% vs 33%	43% vs 56%
Myalgias	56% vs 50%	42% vs 50%
Rigors	48% vs 41%	24% vs 35%
Depression	31% vs 34%	22% vs 30%
Irritability	35% vs 34%	24% vs 28%

[a] These comparisons are based upon data on each drug tested individually versus other regimens in registration trials; because these comparisons are not based on head-to-head comparisons between the two drugs, and because the populations tested are not entirely analogous, relative advantages and disadvantages should be interpreted with caution.

[b] In the registration trial for pegylated IFN-α2b plus ribavirin, the optimal regimen was 1.5 μg of pegylated IFN plus 800 mg of ribavirin; however, a posthoc analysis of this study as well as data from other studies suggest that 1000 (for patients < 75 kg)–1200 (for patients ≥ 75 kg) mg of ribavirin might be better, certainly for genotype 1, and many clinicians prescribe the higher ribavirin doses.

[c] 1000 mg for patients < 75 kg; 1200 mg for patients ≥ 75 kg.

[d] In the registration trial for pegylated IFN-α2b plus ribavirin, all patients were treated for 48 weeks; however, data from other trials of standard IFNs and the other pegylated IFN suggest that 24 weeks should suffice for patients with genotypes 2 and 3.

[e] These comparisons show the frequency in registration trials of the listed side effects for the respective pegylated IFN plus ribavirin as compared to the listed side effects in comparitor groups who received standard IFN-α2b plus ribavirin. As noted above, these comparisons do not represent head-to-head tests of the two pegylated IFNs.

Note: PEG, polyethylene glycol; IFN, interferon.

candidates for antiviral therapy with pegylated IFN plus ribavirin, unless ribavirin is contraindicated (Table 287-8). Therapy with IFN has been shown to improve survival and complication-free survival and to slow progression of fibrosis. Prior to therapy, HCV genotype should be determined, and the genotype dictates the duration of therapy, 1 year (48 weeks) for patients with genotype 1 and 6 months (24 weeks) for those with genotypes 2 and 3. As noted above, the absence of a 2-log drop in HCV RNA at week 12 (an "early virologic response") weighs heavily against the likelihood of a sustained virologic response even if therapy is continued for the remainder of the planned full year; therefore, measuring HCV RNA at baseline and at 12 weeks is recommended routinely, especially for patients with genotype 1. The consensus view is that therapy can be discontinued if an early virologic response is not achieved; however, histologic benefit may occur even in the absence of a virologic response. In addition, if current trials show that maintenance therapy can slow the progression of chronic hepatitis C, early virologic nonresponders may be identified as candidates for maintenance therapy; the results of these trials are awaited. Although response rates are lower in patients with certain pretreatment variables, selection for treatment should not be based on symptoms, genotype, HCV RNA level, mode of acquisition of hepatitis C, or advanced hepatic fibrosis. Patients with cirrhosis can respond and should not be excluded as candidates for therapy.

Patients who have relapsed after a course of IFN monotherapy are candidates for retreatment with pegylated IFN plus ribavirin. For non-responders to a prior course of IFN monotherapy, retreatment with IFN monotherapy or combination IFN plus ribavirin therapy is unlikely to achieve a sustained virologic response; however, a trial of combination pegylated IFN plus ribavirin may be worthwhile. End-treatment virologic responses as high as 40% can occur in this setting, but a sustained virologic response is the outcome in <20% of patients. Sustained virologic responses to retreatment of nonresponders are

TABLE 287-8 *Indications and Recommendations for Antiviral Therapy of Chronic Hepatitis C*

STANDARD INDICATIONS FOR THERAPY

Elevated ALT activity
Portal/bridging fibrosis or moderate to severe hepatitis on liver biopsy
Detectable HCV RNA

RETREATMENT RECOMMENDED

Relapsers after a previous course of standard IFN monotherapy or combination standard IFN/ribavirin therapy
  A course of pegylated IFN plus ribavirin
Nonresponders to a previous course of standard IFN monotherapy or combination standard IFN/ribavirin therapy
  A course of pegylated IFN plus ribavirin—more likely to achieve a sustained virologic response in Caucasian patients without previous ribavirin therapy, with low baseline HCV RNA levels, with a substantial reduction in HCV RNA during previous therapy, with genotypes 2 and 3, and without reduction in ribavirin dose.

ANTIVIRAL THERAPY NOT RECOMMENDED ROUTINELY BUT MANAGEMENT DECISIONS MADE ON AN INDIVIDUAL BASIS

Children (age <18 years)
Age >60
Normal ALT
Mild hepatitis on liver biopsy
Compensated cirrhosis
Patients with HIV infection and normal CD4+ counts

LONG-TERM MAINTENANCE THERAPY RECOMMENDED

Cutaneous vasculitis and glomerulonephritis associated with chronic hepatitis C

LONG-TERM MAINTENANCE THERAPY BEING ASSESSED IN CLINICAL TRIALS

Relapsers
Nonresponders

ANTIVIRAL THERAPY NOT RECOMMENDED

Decompensated cirrhosis

THERAPEUTIC REGIMENS

First-line treatment: Pegylated IFN subcutaneously once a week plus daily ribavirin orally
1. HCV genotype 1—48 weeks of therapy
  Pegylated IFN-α2a, 180 μg, plus ribavirin, 1000 mg/d (weight <75 kg) to 1200 mg/d (weight ≥75 kg) *or*
  Pegylated IFN-α2b, 1.5 μg/kg, plus ribavirin, 800 mg/d (although higher, weight-based ribavirin doses above are preferred by many)
2. HCV genotypes 2 and 3—24 weeks of therapy
  Pegylated IFN-α2a, 180 μg, plus ribavirin, 800 mg/d *or*
  Pegylated IFN-α2b, 1.5 μg/kg, plus ribavirin, 800 mg/d
Alternative regimen: Pegylated IFN (α2a, 180 μg, or α2b, 1.0 μg/kg) subcutaneously once a week (primarily for patients in whom ribavirin is contraindicated or not tolerated) for 24 (genotypes 2 and 3) or 48 (genotype 1) weeks

FEATURES ASSOCIATED WITH REDUCED RESPONSIVENESS

Advanced fibrosis (e.g., cirrhosis)
Long-duration disease
Genotype 1
High-level HCV RNA (>2 million copies/mL)
High HCV quasispecies diversity
Immunosuppression
African American
Obesity
Reduced adherence (lower drug doses and reduced duration of therapy)

Note: ALT, alanine aminotransferase; HCV, hepatitis C virus; IFN, interferon.

more frequent in those who had never received ribavirin in the past, in those with genotypes 2 and 3, in those with low pretreatment HCV RNA levels, but less frequent in African Americans, in those who failed to achieve a substantial reduction in HCV RNA during their previous course of therapy, and in those who required ribavirin-dose reductions.

Early treatment is indicated for persons with acute hepatitis C (Chap. 285). In patients with persistently normal or near-normal ALT levels, long-term monitoring studies have shown the absence of histologic progression, and the same applies to patients with histologically mild hepatitis C; however, patients with normal ALT and histologically mild hepatitis C respond just as well as those with elevated ALT and more histologically severe hepatitis to combination IFN plus ribavirin therapy (and, although not reported yet, probably to combination pegylated IFN plus ribavirin). Therefore, therapy for these patients should be considered and the decision made based upon such factors as patient motivation, genotype, stage of fibrosis, age, and comorbid conditions. A pretreatment liver biopsy is recommended in most cases to assess pretreatment histologic grade and stage.

Patients with compensated cirrhosis can respond to therapy, although their likelihood of a sustained response is lower than in noncirrhotics. Whether survival is improved after successful antiviral therapy in cirrhotics is controversial. Similarly, although several retrospective studies have suggested that antiviral therapy in cirrhotics with chronic hepatitis C reduces the frequency of HCC, less advanced disease in the treated cirrhotics, not treatment itself, may have accounted for the reduced frequency of HCC observed in the treated cohort; prospective studies to address this question are in progress. Patients with decompensated cirrhosis are not candidates for IFN-based antiviral therapy but should be referred for liver transplantation. After liver transplantation, recurrent hepatitis C is the rule, and the pace of disease progression is more accelerated than in immunocompetent patients (Chap. 291); current therapy with pegylated IFN and ribavirin is unsatisfactory in most patients, but attempts to minimize immunosuppression are beneficial. The cutaneous and renal vasculitis of HCV-associated essential mixed cryoglobulinemia (Chap. 285) may respond to antiviral therapy, but sustained responses are rare after discontinuation of therapy; therefore, prolonged, perhaps indefinite, therapy is recommended in this group.

Anecdotal reports suggest that antiviral therapy may be effective in porphyria cutanea tarda or lichen planus associated with hepatitis C. In patients with HCV/HIV co-infection, responses similar to those seen in other groups have been reported in patients with normal CD4+ T cell counts; careful monitoring for side effects of IFN/ribavirin and antiretroviral drugs is advisable. Persons with a history of injection-drug use and alcoholism can be treated successfully for chronic hepatitis C, preferably in conjunction with drug and alcohol treatment programs.

AUTOIMMUNE HEPATITIS ■ **Definition** Autoimmune hepatitis is a chronic disorder characterized by continuing hepatocellular necrosis and inflammation, usually with fibrosis, which tends to progress to cirrhosis and liver failure. When fulfilling criteria of severity, this type of chronic hepatitis may have a 6-month mortality of as high as 40%. The prominence of extrahepatic features of autoimmunity as well as seroimmunologic abnormalities in this disorder supports an autoimmune process in its pathogenesis; this concept is reflected in the labels "lupoid," plasma cell, or autoimmune hepatitis. Because autoantibodies and other typical features of autoimmunity do not occur in all cases, however, a broader, more appropriate designation for this type of chronic hepatitis is "idiopathic" or cryptogenic. Cases in which hepatotropic viruses, metabolic/genetic derangements, and hepatotoxic drugs have been excluded merit this designation and probably include a spectrum of heterogeneous liver disorders of unknown cause, a proportion of which have characteristic autoimmune features.

Immunopathogenesis The weight of evidence suggests that the progressive liver injury in patients with idiopathic/autoimmune hepatitis is the result of a cell-mediated immunologic attack directed against liver cells; in all likelihood, predisposition to autoimmunity is inherited, while the liver specificity of this injury is triggered by environmental (e.g., chemical or viral) factors. For example, patients have been described in whom apparently self-limited cases of acute hepatitis A or B led to autoimmune hepatitis, presumably because of genetic susceptibility or predisposition. Evidence to support an autoimmune pathogenesis in this type of hepatitis includes the following: (1) In the liver, the histopathologic lesions are composed predominantly of cytotoxic T cells and plasma cells; (2) circulating autoantibodies (nuclear, smooth muscle, thyroid, etc.; see below), rheumatoid factor, and hyperglobulinemia are common; (3) other autoimmune disorders—such as thyroiditis, rheumatoid arthritis, autoimmune hemolytic anemia, ulcerative colitis, proliferative glomerulonephritis, juvenile diabetes mellitus, and Sjögren's syndrome—occur with increased frequency in patients who have autoimmune hepatitis and in their relatives; (4) histocompatibility haplotypes associated with autoimmune diseases, such as HLA-B1, -B8, -DR3, and -DR4, are common in patients with autoimmune hepatitis; and (5) this type of chronic hepatitis is responsive to glucocorticoid/immunosuppressive therapy, effective in a variety of autoimmune disorders.

Cellular immune mechanisms appear to be important in the pathogenesis of autoimmune hepatitis. In vitro studies have suggested that in patients with this disorder, lymphocytes are capable of becoming sensitized to hepatocyte membrane proteins and of destroying liver cells. Abnormalities of immunoregulatory control over cytotoxic lymphocytes (impaired suppressor cell influences) may play a role as well. Studies of genetic predisposition to autoimmune hepatitis demonstrate that certain haplotypes are associated with the disorder, as enumerated above. The precise triggering factors, genetic influences, and cytotoxic and immunoregulatory mechanisms involved in this type of liver injury remain poorly defined.

Intriguing clues into the pathogenesis of autoimmune hepatitis come from the observation that circulating autoantibodies are prevalent in patients with this disorder. Among the autoantibodies described in these patients are antibodies to nuclei [so-called antinuclear antibodies (ANA), primarily in a homogeneous pattern] and smooth muscle (so-called anti-smooth-muscle antibodies, directed at actin), anti-LKM (see below), antibodies to "soluble liver antigen" (directed at a member of the glutathione S-transferase gene family), as well as antibodies to the liver-specific asialoglycoprotein receptor (or "hepatic lectin") and other hepatocyte membrane proteins. Although some of these provide helpful diagnostic markers, their involvement in the pathogenesis of autoimmune hepatitis has not been established.

Humoral immune mechanisms have been shown to play a role in the extrahepatic manifestations of autoimmune/idiopathic hepatitis. Arthralgias, arthritis, cutaneous vasculitis, and glomerulonephritis occurring in patients with autoimmune hepatitis appear to be mediated by the deposition in affected tissue vessels of circulating immune complexes, followed by complement activation, inflammation, and tissue injury. While specific viral antigen-antibody complexes can be identified in acute and chronic viral hepatitis, the nature of the immune complexes in autoimmune hepatitis has not been defined.

Many of the *clinical features* of autoimmune hepatitis are similar to those described for chronic viral hepatitis. The onset of disease may be insidious or abrupt; the disease may present initially like, and be confused with, acute viral hepatitis; a history of recurrent bouts of what had been labeled acute hepatitis is not uncommon. A subset of patients with autoimmune hepatitis has distinct features. Such patients are predominantly young to middle-aged women with marked hyperglobulinemia and high-titer circulating ANA. This is the group with positive LE preparations (initially labeled "lupoid" hepatitis) in whom other autoimmune features are common. Fatigue, malaise, anorexia, amenorrhea, acne, arthralgias, and jaundice are common. Occasionally, arthritis, maculopapular eruptions (including cutaneous vasculitis), erythema nodosum, colitis, pleurisy, pericarditis, anemia, azotemia, and sicca syndrome (keratoconjunctivitis, xerostomia) occur. In some patients, complications of cirrhosis, such as ascites and edema (associated with hypoalbuminemia), encephalopathy, hypersplenism, coagulopathy, or variceal bleeding may bring the patient to initial medical attention.

The course of autoimmune hepatitis may be variable. In those with mild disease or limited histologic lesions (e.g., piecemeal necrosis without bridging), progression to cirrhosis is limited. In those with severe symptomatic autoimmune hepatitis (aminotransferase levels >10 times normal, marked hyperglobulinemia, "aggressive" histologic lesions—bridging necrosis or multilobular collapse, cirrhosis), the 6-month mortality without therapy may be as high as 40%. Such severe disease accounts for only 20% of cases; the natural history of milder disease is variable, often accentuated by spontaneous remissions and exacerbations. Especially poor prognostic signs include multilobular collapse at the time of initial presentation and failure of the bilirubin to improve after 2 weeks of therapy. Death may result from hepatic failure, hepatic coma, other complications of cirrhosis (e.g., variceal hemorrhage), and intercurrent infection. In patients with established cirrhosis, hepatocellular carcinoma may be a late complication (Chap. 78).

Laboratory features of autoimmune hepatitis are similar to those seen in chronic viral hepatitis. Liver biochemical tests are invariably abnormal but may not correlate with the clinical severity or histopathologic features in individual cases. Many patients with autoimmune hepatitis have normal serum bilirubin, alkaline phosphatase, and globulin levels with only minimal aminotransferase elevations. Serum AST and ALT levels are increased and fluctuate in the range of 100 to 1000 units. In severe cases, the serum bilirubin level is moderately elevated [51 to 171 μmol/L (3 to 10 mg/dL)]. Hypoalbuminemia occurs in patients with very active or advanced disease. Serum alkaline phosphatase levels may be moderately elevated or near normal. In a small proportion of patients, marked elevations of alkaline phosphatase activity occur; in such patients, clinical and laboratory features overlap with those of primary biliary cirrhosis (Chap. 289). The prothrombin time is often prolonged, particularly late in the disease or during active phases.

Hypergammaglobulinemia (>2.5 g/dL) is common in autoimmune hepatitis. Rheumatoid factor is common as well. As noted above, circulating autoantibodies are also common. The most characteristic are ANA in a homogeneous staining pattern. Smooth-muscle antibodies are less specific, seen just as frequently in chronic viral hepatitis. Because of the high levels of globulins achieved in the circulation of some patients with autoimmune hepatitis, occasionally the globulins may bind nonspecifically in solid-phase binding immunoassays for viral antibodies. This has been recognized most commonly in tests for antibodies to hepatitis C virus, as noted above. In fact, studies of autoantibodies in autoimmune hepatitis have led to the recognition of new categories of autoimmune hepatitis. *Type I autoimmune hepatitis* is the classic syndrome occurring in young women, associated with marked hyperglobulinemia, lupoid features, and circulating ANA. *Type II autoimmune hepatitis*, often seen in children and more common in Mediterranean populations, is associated not with ANA but with anti-LKM. Actually, anti-LKM represent a heterogeneous group of antibodies. In type II autoimmune hepatitis, the antibody is anti-LKM1, directed against P450 IID6. This is the same anti-LKM seen in some patients with chronic hepatitis C. Anti-LKM2 is seen in drug-induced hepatitis, and anti-LKM3 is seen in patients with chronic hepatitis D. Type II autoimmune hepatitis has been subdivided by some authorities into two categories, one more typically autoimmune and the other associated with viral hepatitis type C. Autoimmune hepatitis type IIa is felt to be autoimmune, is more likely to occur in young women, is associated with hyperglobulinemia, is associated with high-titer anti-LKM1, responds to glucocorticoid therapy, and is seen commonly in western Europe and the United Kingdom. Type IIb autoimmune hepatitis is associated with HCV infection, tends to occur in older men, is associated with normal globulin levels and low-titer anti-

LKM1, responds to IFN, and occurs most commonly in Mediterranean countries. In addition, another type of autoimmune hepatitis has been recognized, *autoimmune hepatitis type III*. These patients lack ANA and anti-LKM1 and have circulating antibodies to soluble liver antigen, which are directed at hepatocyte cytoplasmic cytokeratins 8 and 18. Most of these patients are women and have clinical features similar to those of patients with type I autoimmune hepatitis.

Liver biopsy abnormalities are similar to those described for chronic viral hepatitis. Expanding portal tracts and extending beyond the plate of periportal hepatocytes into the parenchyma (designated "interface hepatitis" or "piecemeal necrosis") is a mononuclear cell infiltrate that, in autoimmune hepatitis, may include the presence of plasma cells. Necroinflammatory activity characterizes the lobular parenchyma, and evidence of hepatocellular regeneration is reflected by "rosette" formation, the occurrence of thickened liver cell plates, and regenerative "pseudolobules." Septal fibrosis, bridging fibrosis, and cirrhosis are frequent. Bile duct injury and granulomas are uncommon; however, a subgroup of patients with autoimmune hepatitis have histologic, biochemical, and serologic features overlapping those of primary biliary cirrhosis (Chap. 289).

Diagnostic Criteria   An international group has suggested a set of criteria for establishing a diagnosis of autoimmune hepatitis. Exclusion of liver disease caused by genetic disorders, viral hepatitis, drug hepatotoxicity, and alcohol are linked with such inclusive diagnostic criteria as hyperglobulinemia, autoantibodies, and characteristic histologic features. This international group has also suggested a comprehensive diagnostic scoring system that, rarely required for typical cases, may be helpful when typical features are not present. Factors that weigh in favor of the diagnosis include female gender; predominant aminotransferase elevation; presence and level of globulin elevation; presence of nuclear, smooth muscle, and LKM1 autoantibodies; concurrent other autoimmune diseases; characteristic histologic features (interface hepatitis, plasma cells, rosettes); HLA DR3 or DR4 markers; and response to treatment (see below). Weighing against the diagnosis are predominant alkaline phosphatase elevation; mitochondrial antibodies, markers of viral hepatitis, history of hepatotoxic drugs or excessive alcohol, histologic biliary changes, or such atypical histologic features as fatty infiltration, iron overload, and viral inclusions.

℞ TREATMENT

The mainstay of management in autoimmune or idiopathic (nonviral) hepatitis is glucocorticoid therapy. Several controlled clinical trials have documented that such therapy leads to symptomatic, clinical, biochemical, and histologic improvement as well as increased survival. A therapeutic response can be expected in up to 80% of patients. Unfortunately, therapy has not been shown to prevent ultimate progression to cirrhosis; however, instances of reversal of fibrosis and cirrhosis have been reported in patients responding to treatment. Although some advocate the use of prednisolone (the hepatic metabolite of prednisone), prednisone is just as effective and is favored by most authorities. Therapy may be initiated at 20 mg/d, but a popular regimen in the United States relies on an initiation dose of 60 mg/d. This high dose is tapered successively over the course of a month down to a maintenance level of 20 mg/d. An alternative but equally effective approach is to begin with half the prednisone dose (30 mg/d) along with azathioprine (50 mg/d). With azathioprine maintained at 50 mg/d, the prednisone dose is tapered over the course of a month down to a maintenance level of 10 mg/d. The advantage of the combination approach is a reduction, over the span of an 18-month course of therapy, in serious, life-threatening complications of steroid therapy from 66% down to under 20%. Azathioprine alone, however, is not effective in achieving remission, nor is alternate-day glucocorticoid therapy. Although therapy has been shown to be effective for severe autoimmune hepatitis (AST $\geq$ 10 times the upper limit of normal or $\geq$5 times the upper limit of normal in conjunction with serum globulin $\geq$ twice normal; bridging necrosis or multilobular necrosis on liver biopsy;

presence of symptoms), therapy is not indicated for mild forms of chronic hepatitis (which used to be labeled chronic persistent hepatitis or chronic lobular hepatitis), and the efficacy of therapy in mild or asymptomatic autoimmune hepatitis has not been established.

Improvement of fatigue, anorexia, malaise, and jaundice tends to occur within days to several weeks; biochemical improvement occurs over the course of several weeks to months, with a fall in serum bilirubin and globulin levels and an increase in serum albumin. Serum aminotransferase levels usually drop promptly, but improvements in AST and ALT alone do not appear to be a reliable marker of recovery in individual patients; histologic improvement, characterized by a decrease in mononuclear infiltration and in hepatocellular necrosis, may be delayed for 6 to 24 months. Still, if interpreted cautiously, aminotransferase levels are valuable indicators of relative disease activity, and many authorities do *not* advocate serial liver biopsies to assess therapeutic success or to guide decisions to alter or stop therapy. Therapy should continue for at least 12 to 18 months. After tapering and cessation of therapy, the likelihood of relapse is at least 50%, even if posttreatment histology has improved to show mild chronic hepatitis, and the majority of patients require therapy at maintenance doses indefinitely. Continuing azathioprine alone (2 mg per kg body weight daily) after cessation of prednisone therapy may reduce the frequency of relapse.

In medically refractory cases, an attempt should be made to intensify treatment with high-dose glucocorticoid monotherapy (60 mg daily) or combination glucocorticoid (30 mg daily) plus high-dose azathioprine (150 mg daily) therapy. After a month, doses of prednisone can be reduced by 10 mg a month, and doses of azathioprine can be reduced by 50 mg a month towards ultimate, conventional maintenance doses. Patients refractory to this regimen may be treated with cyclosporine, tacrolimus, or mycophenolate mofetil; however, to date, only limited anectodal reports support these approaches. If medical therapy fails, or when chronic hepatitis progresses to cirrhosis and is associated with life-threatening complications of liver decompensation, liver transplantation is the only recourse (Chap. 291). Recurrence of autoimmune hepatitis in the new liver occurs rarely in most experiences but in as many as a third of cases in others.

DIFFERENTIAL DIAGNOSIS   Early during the course of chronic hepatitis, the disease may resemble typical *acute viral hepatitis*. Without histologic assessment, severe chronic hepatitis cannot be readily distinguished based on clinical or biochemical criteria from mild chronic hepatitis. In adolescence, *Wilson's disease* may present with features of chronic hepatitis long before neurologic manifestations become apparent and before the formation of Kayser-Fleischer rings; in this age group, serum ceruloplasmin and serum and urinary copper determinations plus measurement of liver copper levels will establish the correct diagnosis. *Postnecrotic* or *cryptogenic cirrhosis* and *primary biliary cirrhosis* share clinical features with autoimmune hepatitis; biochemical, serologic, and histologic assessments are usually suffi-

cient to allow these entities to be distinguished from autoimmune hepatitis. Of course, the distinction between autoimmune ("idiopathic") and chronic viral hepatitis is not always straightforward, especially when viral antibodies occur in patients with autoimmune disease or when autoantibodies occur in patients with viral disease. Finally, the presence of extrahepatic features such as arthritis, cutaneous vasculitis, or pleuritis—not to mention the presence of circulating autoantibodies—may cause confusion with *rheumatologic disorders* such as rheumatoid arthritis and systemic lupus erythematosus. The existence of clinical and biochemical features of progressive necroinflammatory liver disease distinguishes chronic hepatitis from these other disorders, which are not associated with severe liver disease.

Finally, occasionally, features of autoimmune hepatitis overlap with features of autoimmune biliary disorders such as primary biliary cirrhosis, primary sclerosing cholangitis, or, even more rarely, mitochondrial-antibody-negative autoimmune cholangitis. Such overlap syndromes are difficult to categorize, and often response to therapy may be the distinguishing factor that establishes the diagnosis.

FURTHER READING

ALTER HJ, SEEFF LB: Recovery, persistence, and sequelae in hepatitis C virus infection: A perspective on long-term outcome. Semin Liver Dis 20:17, 2000

CZAJA AJ, FREESE DK: Diagnosis and treatment of autoimmune hepatitis. Hepatology 36:479, 2002

DIENSTAG JL et al: Histologic outcome during long-term lamivudine therapy. Gastroenterology 124:105, 2003

ESTEBAN R (guest ed): Advancing HBV therapy to overcome treatment challenges. Semin Liver Dis 22(Suppl 1):1, 2002

FRIED MV et al: Peginterferon alfa-2a plus ribavirin for chronic hepatitis C virus infection. N Engl J Med 347:975, 2002

GHANY MG et al: Progression of fibrosis in chronic hepatitis C. Gastroenterology 124:97, 2003

HADZIYANNIS SJ et al: Adefovir dipivoxil for the treatment of hepatitis B e antigen-negative chronic hepatitis B. N Engl J Med 348:800, 2003

MANNS MP (guest ed): Autoimmune hepatitis. Semin Liver Dis 22:1, 2002

MARCELLIN P et al: Adefovir dipivoxil for the treatment of hepatitis B e antigen-positive chronic hepatitis B. N Engl J Med 348:808, 2003

NATIONAL DIGESTIVE DISEASES INFORMATION CLEARINGHOUSE: *Chronic Hepatitis C: Current Disease Management.* NIH Publication No. 02-4230, 2002 (www.niddk.nih.gov/health/digest/pubs/chrnhepc.htm)

NATIONAL INSTITUTES OF HEALTH CONSENSUS DEVELOPMENT CONFERENCE: Management of hepatitis C. Hepatology 36(Suppl 1):1S, 2002

PAPATHEODORIDIS GV, HADZIYANNIS SJ: Diagnosis and management of pre-core mutant chronic hepatitis B. J Viral Hepatitis 8:311, 2001

POYNARD T et al: Impact of pegylated interferon alfa-2b and ribavirin on liver fibrosis in patients with chronic hepatitis C. Gastroenterology 122:1303, 2002

SULKOWSKI MS, THOMAS DL: Hepatitis C in the HIV-infected person. Ann Intern Med 138:197, 2003

YOSHIDA H et al: Interferon therapy prolonged life expectancy among chronic hepatitis C patients. Gastroenterology 123:483, 2002

288 ALCOHOLIC LIVER DISEASE
Mark E. Mailliard, Michael F. Sorrell

Chronic and excessive alcohol ingestion is one of the major causes of liver disease in the western world. The pathology of alcoholic liver injury comprises three major lesions, rarely existing in a pure form: (1) fatty liver, (2) alcoholic hepatitis, and (3) cirrhosis. Fatty liver is present in over 90% of binge and chronic drinkers. A much smaller percentage of heavy drinkers will progress to alcoholic hepatitis, thought to be a precursor to cirrhosis. The prognosis of severe alcoholic liver disease is dismal; the mortality of patients with alcoholic hepatitis concurrent with cirrhosis is nearly 60% at 4 years. Although alcohol is considered a direct hepatotoxin, only between 10 and 20% of alcoholics will develop alcoholic hepatitis. The explanation for this

apparent paradox is unclear but involves the interaction of facilitating and comorbid factors such as gender, heredity, and immunity.

ETIOLOGY AND PATHOGENESIS   Quantity and duration of alcohol intake are the most important risk factors involved in the development of alcoholic liver disease (Table 288-1). The roles of beverage type and pattern of drinking are less clear. Progress of the hepatic injury beyond the fatty liver stage seems to require additional risk factors that remain incompletely defined. Women are more susceptible to alcoholic liver injury when compared to men. They develop advanced liver disease with substantially less alcohol intake. In general, the time it takes to develop liver disease is directly related to the amount of alcohol consumed. It is useful in estimating alcohol consumption to understand that one beer, four ounces of wine, or one ounce of 80% spirits all contain approximately 12 g of alcohol. The threshold for developing

TABLE 288-1   *Risk Factors for Alcoholic Liver Disease*

Risk Factor	Comment
Quantity	In men, 40–80 g/d of ethanol produces fatty liver; 160 g/d for 10–20 years causes hepatitis or cirrhosis. Only 15% of alcoholics develop alcoholic liver disease.
Gender	Women exhibit increased susceptibility to alcoholic liver disease at quantities >20 g/d; two drinks per day probably safe.
Hepatitis C	HCV infection concurrent with alcoholic liver disease is associated with younger age for severity, more advanced histology, decreased survival.
Genetics	Gene polymorphisms may include alcohol dehydrogenase, cytochrome P4502E1, and those associated with alcoholism (twin studies).
Malnutrition	Alcohol injury does not require malnutrition, but obesity and fatty liver from the effect of carbohydrate on the transcriptional control of lipid synthesis and transport may be factors. Patients should receive vigorous attention to nutritional support.

severe alcoholic liver disease in men is an intake of >60 to 80 g/d of alcohol for 10 years, while women are at increased risk for developing similar degrees of liver injury by consuming 20 to 40 g/d. Gender-dependent differences in the gastric and hepatic metabolism of alcohol, in addition to poorly understood hormonal factors, likely contribute to the increased susceptibility of women to alcohol-induced liver injury. Social, nutritional, immunologic, and host factors have all been postulated to play a part in the development of the pathogenic process.

Chronic infection with hepatitis C (HCV) (Chap. 287) is an important comorbidity in the progression of alcoholic liver disease to cirrhosis in chronic and excessive drinkers. Alcohol intake >50 g/d more than doubles the risk of cirrhosis in HCV-infected individuals. Patients with both alcoholic liver injury and HCV infection develop decompensated liver disease at a younger age and have poorer overall survival. As a consequence of the overlapping injurious processes secondary to alcohol abuse and HCV infection, patients can develop an increased liver iron burden and, rarely, porphyria cutanea tarda. In addition, alcohol intake in HCV-infected patients with cirrhosis increases the risk for the development of hepatocellular carcinoma.

Our understanding of the pathogenesis of alcoholic liver injury is incomplete. Alcohol is a direct hepatotoxin, but ingestion of alcohol initiates a variety of metabolic responses that influence the final hepatotoxic response. The initial concept of malnutrition as the major pathogenic mechanism has given way to the present understanding that the metabolism of alcohol by the hepatocyte initiates a pathogenic process involving production of protein-aldehyde adducts, lipid peroxidation, immunologic activity, and cytokine release (Fig. 288-1). The complex interaction of distinct hepatic cell types is crucial to alcohol-mediated liver injury. Stellate cell activation and collagen production are key events in hepatic fibrogenesis. The resulting fibrosis determines the extent of architectural derangement of the liver following chronic alcohol ingestion.

PATHOLOGY   The liver has a limited repertoire in response to injury. Fatty liver is the initial and most common histologic response to hepatotoxic stimuli, including excessive alcohol ingestion. The accumulation of fat within the perivenular hepatocytes coincides with the location of alcohol dehydrogenase, the major enzyme responsible for alcohol metabolism. Continuing alcohol ingestion results in fat accumulation throughout the entire hepatic lobule. Despite extensive fatty change and distortion of the hepatocytes with macrovesicular fat, the cessation of drinking results in normalization of hepatic architecture and fat content within the liver. Alcoholic fatty liver has traditionally been regarded as entirely benign, but similar to the spectrum of nonalcoholic steatohepatitis, certain pathologic features such as giant mitochondria, perivenular fibrosis, and macrovesicular fat may be associated with progressive liver injury.

The transition between fatty liver and the development of alcoholic hepatitis is blurred. The hallmark of alcoholic hepatitis is hepatocyte injury characterized by ballooning degeneration, spotty necrosis, polymorphonuclear infiltrate, and fibrosis in the perivenular and perisinusoidal space of Disse. Mallory bodies are often present in florid cases but are neither specific nor necessary to establishing the diagnosis. Alcoholic hepatitis is thought to be a precursor to the development of cirrhosis. However, like fatty liver, it is potentially reversible with cessation of drinking. Cirrhosis is present in up to 50% of patients with biopsy-proven alcoholic hepatitis and its repair is difficult, even with abstention.

CLINICAL FEATURES   The clinical manifestations of alcoholic fatty liver are subtle and characteristically detected as a consequence of the patient's visit for a seemingly unrelated matter. Previously unsuspected hepatomegaly is often the only clinical finding. Occasionally, patients with fatty liver will present with right upper quadrant discomfort, tender hepatomegaly, nausea, and jaundice. Differentiation of alcoholic fatty liver from nonalcoholic fatty liver is difficult unless an accurate drinking history is ascertained. Alcoholism does not respect social and economic class. In every instance where liver disease is present, a thoughtful and sensitive drinking history should be obtained. Alcoholic hepatitis is associated with a wide gamut of clinical features. Cytokine production is thought to be responsible for the systemic manifestations of alcoholic hepatitis. Fever, spider nevi, jaundice, and abdominal pain simulating an acute abdomen represent the extreme end of the spectrum, while many patients will be entirely asymptomatic. Recognition of the clinical features of alcoholic hepatitis is central to the initiation of an effective and appropriate diagnostic and therapeutic strategy.

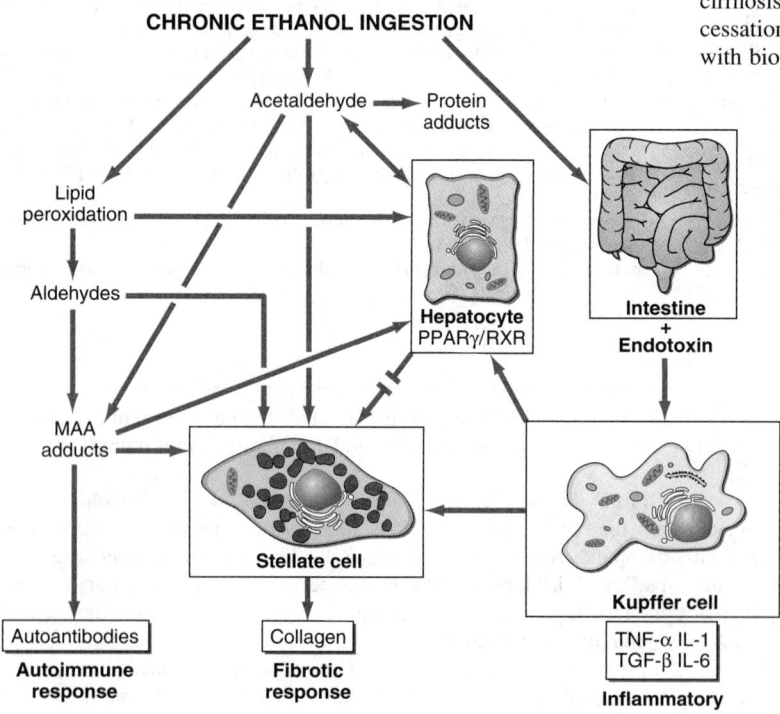

CHRONIC ETHANOL INGESTION

FIGURE 288-1   Biomedical and cellular pathogenesis of liver injury secondary to chronic ethanol ingestion. MAA, malondialdehyde-acetaldehyde; TNF, tumor necrosis factor; TGF, transforming growth factor; IL, interleukin; PPAR, peroxisome proliferator-activated receptor; RXR, retinoid X receptor.

LABORATORY FEATURES   Patients with alcoholic fatty liver are often identified through routine screening tests. The typical laboratory abnormalities are nonspecific and in-

TABLE 288-2 *Laboratory Diagnosis of Alcoholic Fatty Liver and Alcoholic Hepatitis*

Test	Comment
AST	Increased two- to sevenfold, less than 400 U/L, greater than ALT
ALT	Increased two- to sevenfold, less than 400 U/L
AST/ALT	Usually >1
GGTP	Not specific to alcohol, easily inducible, elevated in all forms of fatty liver
Bilirubin	May be markedly increased in alcoholic hepatitis despite modest elevation in alkaline phosphatase
PMN	If > 5500/μL, predicts severe alcoholic hepatitis when discriminant function > 32

Note: AST, aspartate aminotransferase; ALT, alanine aminotransferase; GGTP, gamma-glutamyl transpeptidase; PMN, polymorphonuclear cells.

clude modest elevations of the aspartate aminotransferase (AST), alanine aminotransferase (ALT), and gamma-glutamyl transpeptidase (GGTP), accompanied by hypertriglyceridemia, hypercholesterolemia, and occasionally hyperbilirubinemia. In alcoholic hepatitis and in contrast to other causes of fatty liver, the AST and ALT are usually elevated two- to sevenfold. They are rarely >400 IU, and the AST/ALT ratio >1 (Table 288-2). Hyperbilirubinemia is common and is accompanied by modest increases in the alkaline phosphatase level. Derangement in hepatocyte synthetic function indicates more serious disease. Hypoalbuminemia and coagulopathy are common in advanced liver injury. An increase in the circulating polymorphonuclear cell number >5500/μL parallels the occurrence of the lobular infiltration of neutrophils observed in the florid lesion of alcoholic hepatitis. Ultrasonography is useful in detecting fatty infiltration of the liver and determining liver size. The demonstration by ultrasound of portal vein flow reversal, ascites, and intraabdominal collaterals indicates serious liver injury with less potential for complete reversal of liver disease.

PROGNOSIS Critically ill patients with alcoholic hepatitis have short-term mortality rates approaching 70%. Severe alcoholic hepatitis is heralded by coagulopathy (prothrombin time > 5 s), anemia, serum albumin concentrations below <25 g/L (2.5 mg/dL), serum bilirubin levels > 137 μmol/L (8 mg/dL), renal failure, and ascites. A discriminant function calculated as 4.6 × [prothrombin time − control (seconds)] + serum bilirubin (mg/dL) can identify patients with a poor prognosis (discriminant function > 32). The presence of ascites, variceal hemorrhage, deep encephalopathy, or hepatorenal syndrome predicts a dismal prognosis. The pathologic stage of the injury can be helpful in predicting prognosis. Liver biopsy should be performed whenever possible to confirm the diagnosis, to establish potential

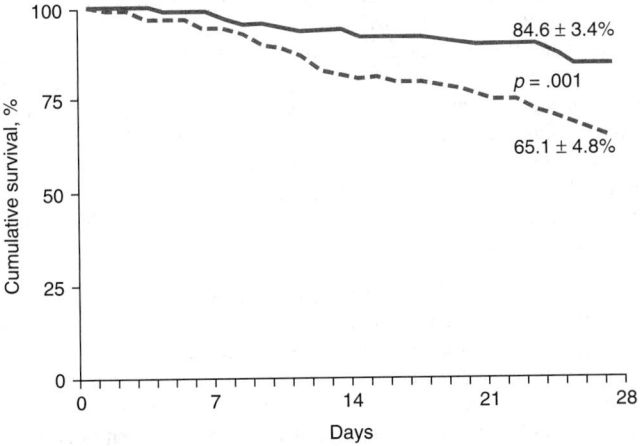

FIGURE 288-2   Effect of glucocorticoid therapy of severe alcoholic hepatitis on short-term survival: the result of a meta-analysis of individual data from three studies. Prednisolone, solid line; placebo, dotted line. *(Adapted from Mathurin et al., with permission from Elsevier Science)*

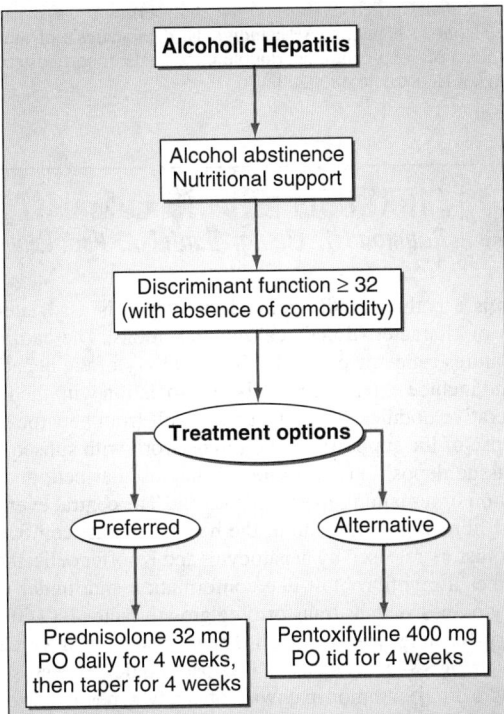

FIGURE 288-3   Treatment algorithm for alcoholic hepatitis. As identified by a calculated discriminant function > 32 (see text), patients with severe alcoholic hepatitis, without the presence of gastrointestinal bleeding or infection, would be candidates for either glucocorticoids or pentoxifylline administration.

reversibility of the liver disease, and to guide the therapeutic decisions.

℞ TREATMENT

Complete abstinence from alcohol is the cornerstone in the treatment of alcoholic liver disease. Improved survival and the potential for reversal of histologic injury regardless of the initial clinical presentation are associated with total avoidance of alcohol ingestion. Referral of patients to experienced alcohol counselors and/or alcohol treatment programs should be routine in the management of patients with alcoholic liver disease. Attention should be directed to the nutritional and psychosocial states during the evaluation and treatment periods. Because of data suggesting that the pathogenic mechanisms in alcoholic hepatitis involve cytokine release and the perpetuation of injury by immunologic processes, glucocorticoids have been extensively evaluated in the treatment of alcoholic hepatitis. Patients with severe alcoholic hepatitis, defined as a discriminant function > 32, were given prednisone, 40 mg/d, or prednisolone, 32 mg/d, for 4 weeks followed by a steroid taper (Fig. 288-2). Exclusion criteria included active gastrointestinal bleeding, sepsis, renal failure, or pancreatitis. Newer understanding of the role of cytokines in alcoholic liver injury and emerging experience with pharmacologic inhibition of tumor necrosis factor by pentoxifylline has led to the recent inclusion of this agent as an alternative to glucocorticoids in the therapy of severe alcoholic hepatitis (Fig. 288-3). Because of inordinate surgical mortality and the high rates of recidivism following transplantation, patients with alcoholic hepatitis are not candidates for immediate liver transplantation. The transplant candidacy of these patients should be reevaluated after a defined period of sobriety.

FURTHER READING

AKRIVIADIS E et al: Pentoxifylline improves short-term survival in severe acute alcoholic hepatitis: A double blind placebo controlled trial. Gastroenterology 119:1637, 2000

MATHURIN P et al: Corticosteroids improve short-term survival in patients with severe alcoholic hepatitis (AH): Individual data analysis of the last three randomized placebo controlled double blind trials of corticosteroids in severe AH. J Hepatol 36:480, 2002

PETERS MG, TERRAULT NA: Alcohol use and hepatitis C. Hepatology 36: S220, 2002

TELI MR et al: Determinants of progression to cirrhosis or fibrosis in pure alcoholic fatty liver. Lancet 346:987, 1995

TUYNS A, PEQUIGNOT G: Greater risk of ascitic cirrhosis in females in relation to alcohol consumption. Int J Epidemiol 13:53, 1984

289 CIRRHOSIS AND ITS COMPLICATIONS
Raymond T. Chung, Daniel K. Podolsky

Cirrhosis is a pathologically defined entity that is associated with a spectrum of characteristic clinical manifestations. The cardinal pathologic features reflect irreversible chronic injury of the hepatic parenchyma and include extensive fibrosis in association with the formation of regenerative nodules. These features result from hepatocyte necrosis, collapse of the supporting reticulin network with subsequent connective tissue deposition, distortion of the vascular bed, and nodular regeneration of remaining liver parenchyma. The central event leading to hepatic fibrosis is activation of the hepatic stellate cell. Upon activation by factors released by hepatocytes and Kupffer cells, the stellate cell assumes a myofibroblast-like conformation and, under the influence of cytokines such as transforming growth factor β (TGF-β), produces fibril-forming type I collagen. The precise point at which fibrosis becomes irreversible is unclear. The pathologic process should be viewed as a final common pathway of many types of chronic liver injury. Clinical features of cirrhosis derive from the morphologic alterations and often reflect the severity of hepatic damage rather than the etiology of the underlying liver disease. Loss of functioning hepatocellular mass may lead to jaundice, edema, coagulopathy, and a variety of metabolic abnormalities; fibrosis and distorted vasculature lead to portal hypertension and its sequelae, including gastroesophageal varices and splenomegaly. Ascites and hepatic encephalopathy result from both hepatocellular insufficiency and portal hypertension.

Classification of the various types of cirrhosis based on either etiology or morphology alone is unsatisfactory. A single pathologic pattern may result from a variety of insults, while the same insult may produce several morphologic patterns. Nevertheless, most types of cirrhosis may be usefully classified by a mixture of etiologically and morphologically defined entities as follows: (1) alcoholic; (2) cryptogenic and posthepatitic; (3) biliary; (4) cardiac; and (5) metabolic, inherited, and drug-related. This chapter considers the various types of cirrhosis and their complications.

ALCOHOLIC CIRRHOSIS

Definition *Alcoholic cirrhosis* is only one of many consequences resulting from chronic alcohol ingestion, and it often accompanies other forms of alcohol-induced liver injury, including alcoholic fatty liver and alcoholic hepatitis (Chap. 288). Alcoholic cirrhosis, historically referred to as *Laennec's cirrhosis*, is the most common type of cirrhosis encountered in North America and many parts of western Europe and South America. It is characterized by diffuse fine scarring, fairly uniform loss of liver cells, and small regenerative nodules, and therefore it is sometimes referred to as *micronodular cirrhosis*. However, micronodular cirrhosis may also result from other types of liver injury (e.g., following jejunoileal bypass), and thus alcoholic cirrhosis and micronodular cirrhosis are not necessarily synonymous. Conversely, alcoholic cirrhosis may progress to macronodular cirrhosis with time.

Etiology See Chap. 288, "Alcoholic Liver Disease."

Pathology and Pathogenesis With continued alcohol intake and destruction of hepatocytes, fibroblasts (including activated hepatic stellate cells that have transformed into myofibroblasts with contractile properties) appear at the site of injury and deposit collagen. Weblike septa of connective tissue appear in periportal and pericentral zones and eventually connect portal triads and central veins. This fine connective tissue network surrounds small masses of remaining liver cells, which regenerate and form nodules. Although regeneration occurs within the small remnants of parenchyma, cell loss generally exceeds replacement. With continuing hepatocyte destruction and collagen deposition, the liver shrinks in size, acquires a nodular appearance, and becomes hard as "end-stage" cirrhosis develops. Although alcoholic cirrhosis is usually a progressive disease, appropriate therapy and strict avoidance of alcohol may arrest the disease at most stages and permit functional improvement. In addition, there is strong evidence that concomitant chronic hepatitis C virus (HCV) infection significantly accelerates development of alcoholic cirrhosis.

Clinical Features ■ *SIGNS AND SYMPTOMS* Alcoholic cirrhosis may be clinically silent, and many cases (10 to 40%) are discovered incidentally at laparotomy or autopsy. In many cases symptoms are insidious in onset, occurring usually after $\geq$10 years of excessive alcohol use and progressing slowly over subsequent weeks and months. Anorexia and malnutrition lead to weight loss and a reduction in skeletal muscle mass. The patient may experience easy bruising, increasing weakness, and fatigue. Eventually the clinical manifestations of hepatocellular dysfunction and portal hypertension ensue, including progressive jaundice, bleeding from gastroesophageal varices, ascites, and encephalopathy. The abrupt onset of one of these complications may be the first event prompting the patient to seek medical attention. In other cases, cirrhosis first becomes evident when the patient requires treatment of symptoms related to alcoholic hepatitis.

A firm, nodular liver may be an early sign of disease; the liver may be either enlarged, normal, or decreased in size. Other frequent findings include jaundice, palmar erythema, spider angiomas, parotid and lacrimal gland enlargement, clubbing of fingers, splenomegaly, muscle wasting, and ascites with or without peripheral edema. Men may have decreased body hair and/or gynecomastia and testicular atrophy, which, like the cutaneous findings, result from disturbances in hormonal metabolism, including increased peripheral formation of estrogen due to diminished hepatic clearance of the precursor androstenedione. Testicular atrophy may reflect hormonal abnormalities or the toxic effect of alcohol on the testes. In women, signs of virilization or menstrual irregularities may occasionally be encountered. Dupuytren's contractures resulting from fibrosis of the palmar fascia with resulting flexion contracture of the digits are associated with alcoholism but are not specifically related to cirrhosis.

Although the cirrhotic patient may stabilize if drinking is discontinued, over a period of years, the patient may become emaciated, weak, and chronically jaundiced. Ascites and other signs of portal hypertension may become increasingly prominent. Ultimately, most patients with advanced cirrhosis die in hepatic coma, commonly precipitated by hemorrhage from esophageal varices or intercurrent infection. Progressive renal dysfunction often complicates the terminal phase of the illness.

LABORATORY FINDINGS In advanced alcoholic liver disease, abnormalities of laboratory tests are more common. Anemia may result from acute and chronic gastrointestinal blood loss, coexistent nutritional deficiency (notably of folic acid and vitamin B_{12}), hypersplenism, and a direct suppressive effect of alcohol on the bone marrow. Hemolytic anemia, presumably due to effects of hypercholesterolemia or erythrocyte membranes resulting in unusual spurlike projections (acanthocytosis), has been described in some alcoholics with cirrhosis. Mild or pronounced hyperbilirubinemia may be found, usually in association with varying elevations of serum alkaline phosphatase levels. Levels of serum AST (asparate aminotransferase) are frequently elevated, but levels >5 μkat (300 units) are unusual and should prompt one to look for other coincident or complicating factors. In contrast to viral hepatitis, the serum AST is usually disproportionately elevated relative to ALT (alanine aminotransferase), i.e., AST/ALT ratio >2. This discrepancy in alcoholic liver disease may result from the proportionally greater inhibition of ALT synthesis by ethanol, which may be partially reversed by pyridoxal phosphate.

The serum prothrombin time is frequently prolonged, reflecting reduced synthesis of clotting proteins, most notably the vitamin K–dependent factors (see "Coagulopathy," below). The serum albumin level is usually depressed, while serum globulins are increased. Hypoalbuminemia reflects in part overall impairment in hepatic protein synthesis, while hyperglobulinemia is thought to result from nonspecific stimulation of the reticuloendothelial system. Elevated blood ammonia levels in patients with hepatic encephalopathy reflect diminished hepatic clearance because of impaired liver function and shunting of portal venous blood around the cirrhotic liver into the systemic circulation (see "Hepatic Encephalopathy," below).

A variety of metabolic disturbances may be detected. Glucose intolerance due to endogenous insulin resistance may be present; however, clinical diabetes is uncommon. Central hyperventilation may lead to respiratory alkalosis in patients with cirrhosis. Dietary deficiency and increased urinary losses lead to hypomagnesemia and hypophosphatemia. In patients with ascites and dilutional hyponatremia, hypokalemia may occur from increased urinary potassium losses due in part to hyperaldosteronism. Prerenal azotemia is also observed in such patients.

Diagnosis Alcoholic cirrhosis should be strongly suspected in patients with a history of prolonged or excessive alcohol intake and physical signs of chronic liver disease. However, since only 10 to 15% of individuals with excessive alcohol intake develop cirrhosis, other causes and types of liver disease may have to be excluded. The clinical features and laboratory findings are usually sufficient to provide reasonable indication of the presence and extent of hepatic injury. Although a percutaneous needle biopsy of the liver is not usually necessary to confirm the typical findings of alcoholic hepatitis or cirrhosis, it may be helpful in distinguishing patients with less advanced liver disease from those with cirrhosis and in excluding other forms of liver injury such as viral hepatitis. Biopsy may also be helpful as a diagnostic tool in evaluating patients with clinical findings suggestive of alcoholic liver disease who deny alcohol intake. In patients with features of cholestasis, ultrasonography may be appropriate to exclude the presence of extrahepatic biliary obstruction. When the clinical status of an otherwise stable cirrhotic patient deteriorates without an obvious explanation, complicating conditions, such as infection, portal vein thrombosis, and hepatocellular carcinoma, should be sought.

Prognosis Abstinence from alcohol as well as early and appropriate medical care can decrease long-term morbidity and mortality and delay or prevent the appearance of further complications. Patients who have had a major complication of cirrhosis and who continue to drink have a 5-year survival of <50%. However, those patients who remain abstinent have a substantially better prognosis. In general, the overall outlook in patients with advanced liver disease remains poor; most of these patients eventually die as a result of massive variceal hemorrhage and/or profound hepatic encephalopathy.

℞ TREATMENT

Alcoholic cirrhosis is a serious illness that requires long-term medical supervision and careful management. Therapy of the underlying liver disease is largely supportive. Specific treatment is directed at particular complications such as variceal bleeding and ascites (see below). While some studies suggest that administration of glucocorticoids in moderately large doses for 4 weeks is helpful in patients with severe alcoholic hepatitis and encephalopathy, these drugs have no role in the treatment of established alcoholic cirrhosis. One study has suggested

survival benefit in alcoholic cirrhosis patients receiving S-adenosyl methionine, which may act to decrease proinflammatory cytokines.

The patient should be made to realize that there is no medication that will protect the liver against the effects of further alcohol ingestion. Therefore, alcohol should be absolutely forbidden. An important component of the complete care of such patients is encouragement to become involved in an appropriate alcohol counseling program.

All medicines must be administered with caution in the patient with cirrhosis, especially those eliminated or modified through hepatic metabolism or biliary pathways. In particular, care must be taken to avoid overzealous use of drugs that may directly or indirectly precipitate complications of cirrhosis. For example, vigorous treatment of ascites with diuretics may result in electrolyte abnormalities or hypovolemia, which can lead to coma. Similarly, even modest doses of sedatives can lead to deepening encephalopathy. Aspirin should be avoided in patients with cirrhosis because of its effects on coagulation and gastric mucosa. Acetaminophen should be used with caution and in doses of less than 2 g/d. Patients who drink alcohol are more sensitive to the hepatotoxic effects of acetaminophen, probably due to increased metabolism of the drug to toxic intermediates and decreased glutathione levels.

POSTHEPATITIC AND CRYPTOGENIC CIRRHOSIS

Definition Posthepatitic or postnecrotic cirrhosis represents the final common pathway of many types of chronic liver disease. *Coarsely nodular cirrhosis* and *multilobular cirrhosis* are terms synonymous with posthepatitic cirrhosis. The term *cryptogenic cirrhosis* has been used interchangeably with posthepatitic cirrhosis, but this designation should be reserved for those cases in which the etiology of cirrhosis is unknown (approximately 10% of all patients with cirrhosis).

Etiology Posthepatitic cirrhosis is a morphologic term referring to a defined stage of advanced chronic liver injury of either specific or unknown (cryptogenic) causes. Epidemiologic and serologic evidence suggest that in one-fourth to three-fourths of cases of posthepatitic cirrhosis, viral hepatitis (hepatitis B or hepatitis C) may be an antecedent factor. In areas where hepatitis B virus (HBV) infection is endemic (e.g., Southeast Asia, sub-Saharan Africa), up to 15% of the population may acquire the infection in early childhood, and cirrhosis may ultimately develop in one-fourth of these chronic carriers. Although HBV infection is much less prevalent in the United States, it is relatively common among certain high-risk groups (e.g., persons with multiple sexual partners, especially men who have sex with men, injection drug users) and contributes to an increased incidence of cirrhosis. In the United States, HCV infection accounts for many cases of cirrhosis following blood transfusions. Before routine screening of blood donors was introduced, hepatitis C occurred in 5 to 10% of blood recipients. Following infection, cirrhosis may ultimately develop in >20% of individuals after 20 years. Increasing recognition of the progressive nature of nonalcoholic fatty liver disease (NAFLD) has revealed that many cases previously designated cryptogenic cirrhosis may be attributable to this disorder (Chap. 290). Posthepatitic cirrhosis may also develop in patients with autoimmune hepatitis (Chap. 287).

The most common causes of cirrhosis in the United States that ultimately lead to liver transplantation include chronic HCV infection, alcohol, primary biliary cirrhosis, primary sclerosing cholangitis, and NAFLD. Less common causes of posthepatitic cirrhosis, including drugs and toxins, are listed in Table 289-1.

Pathology The posthepatitic liver is typically shrunken in size, distorted in shape, and composed of nodules of liver cells separated by dense and broad bands of fibrosis. The microscopic picture is consistent with the gross impression. Posthepatitic cirrhosis is characterized morphologically by (1) extensive confluent loss of liver cells, (2) stromal collapse and fibrosis resulting in broad bands of connective tissue containing the remains of many portal triads, and (3) irregular

TABLE 289-1 *Causes of Cirrhosis and/or Chronic Liver Disease*

Infectious Diseases	Drugs and Toxins (Chap. 286)
Brucellosis (Chap. 141)	Alcohol (Chap. 288)
Capillariasis (Chap. 201)	Amioradone
Echinococcosis (Chap. 240)	Arsenicals
Schistosomiasis (Chap. 203)	Oral contraceptives (Budd-Chiari)
Toxoplasmosis (Chap. 198)	Pyrrolidizine alkaloids and
Viral hepatitis [hepatitis B, C, D;	antineoplastic agents
cytomegalovirus; Epstein-Barr	(venoocclusive disease)
virus (Chaps. 285, 165, 166)]	**Other Causes**
Inherited and Metabolic	Biliary obstruction (chronic)
Disorders (Chap. 290)	(Chap. 292)
α_1-Antitrypsin deficiency	Cystic fibrosis (Chap. 241)
(Chap. 290)	Graft-versus-host disease
Alagille's syndrome (Chap. 282)	(Chap. 100)
Biliary atresia (Chap. 292)	Jejunoileal bypass (Chap. 36)
Familial intrahepatic cholestasis	Nonalcoholic fatty liver disease
(FIC) types 1–3 (Chap. 292)	(Chap. 290)
Fanconi's syndrome (Chap. 340)	Primary biliary cirrhosis (Chap.
Galactosemia (Chap. 341)	289)
Gaucher's disease (Chap. 340)	Primary sclerosing cholangitis
Glycogen storage disease	(Chap. 292)
(Chap. 341)	Sarcoidosis (Chap. 309)
Hemochromatosis (Chap. 336)	
Hereditary fructose intolerance	
(Chap. 341)	
Hereditary tyrosinemia (Chap.	
343)	
Wilson's disease (Chap. 339)	

nodules of regenerating hepatocytes, varying in size from microscopic to several centimeters in diameter.

Clinical Features In patients with cirrhosis of known etiology in whom there is progression to a posthepatitic stage, the clinical manifestations are an extension of those resulting from the initial disease process. Usually clinical symptoms are related to portal hypertension and its sequelae, such as ascites, splenomegaly, hypersplenism, encephalopathy, and bleeding gastroesophageal varices. The hematologic and liver function abnormalities resemble those seen with other types of cirrhosis. In a few patients with posthepatitic cirrhosis, the diagnosis may be made incidentally at operation, at postmortem, or by a needle biopsy of the liver performed to investigate abnormal liver function tests or hepatomegaly.

Diagnosis and Prognosis Posthepatitic cirrhosis should be suspected in patients with signs and symptoms of cirrhosis or portal hypertension. Needle or operative liver biopsies confirm the diagnosis, although nonuniformity of the pathologic process may result in sampling errors. The diagnosis of cryptogenic cirrhosis is reserved for those patients in whom no known etiology can be demonstrated. About 75% of patients have progressive disease despite supportive therapy and die within 1 to 5 years from complications, including variceal hemorrhage, hepatic encephalopathy, or superimposed hepatocellular carcinoma.

℞ TREATMENT

Management is usually limited to treatment of the complications of portal hypertension, including control of ascites, avoidance of drugs or excessive protein intake that may induce hepatic coma, and prompt treatment of infections (see below). In patients with asymptomatic cirrhosis, expectant management alone is appropriate. In those patients in whom posthepatitic cirrhosis has developed as a result of a treatable condition, therapy directed at the primary disorder may limit further progression (e.g., Wilson's disease, hemochromatosis).

BILIARY CIRRHOSIS

Biliary cirrhosis results from injury to or prolonged obstruction of either the intrahepatic or extrahepatic biliary system. It is associated with impaired biliary excretion, destruction of hepatic parenchyma, and progressive fibrosis. Primary biliary cirrhosis (PBC) is characterized by chronic inflammation and fibrous obliteration of intrahepatic bile ductules. Secondary biliary cirrhosis (SBC) is the result of long-standing obstruction of the larger extrahepatic ducts. Although primary and secondary biliary cirrhosis are separate pathophysiologic entities with respect to the initial insult, many clinical features are similar.

PRIMARY BILIARY CIRRHOSIS ■ Etiology and Pathogenesis The cause of PBC remains unknown. Several observations suggest that a disordered immune response may be involved. PBC is frequently associated with a variety of disorders presumed to be autoimmune in nature, such as the syndrome of *c*alcinosis, *R*aynaud's phenomenon, *e*sophageal dysmotility, *s*clerodactyly, *t*elangiectasia (CREST); the sicca syndrome (dry eyes and dry mouth); autoimmune thyroiditis; type 1 diabetes mellitus; and IgA deficiency.

Most important, a circulating IgG antimitochondrial antibody (AMA) is detected in >90% of patients with PBC and only rarely in other forms of liver disease. It has been demonstrated that these autoantibodies recognize inner mitochondrial membrane proteins identified as enzymes of the pyruvate dehydrogenase complex (PDC), the branched chain–2-oxoacid dehydrogenase complex (BCOADC), and the 2-oxoglutarate dehydrogenase complex (OGDC). The major autoantigen in PBC (found in 90% of patients) has been identified as the 74-kDa E2 component of the PDC, dihydrolipoamide acetyltransferase. The antibodies are directed to a region essential for binding of a lipoic acid cofactor and inhibit the overall enzymatic activity of the PDC. Other AMA autoantibodies in PBC patients are directed to similar constituents of BCOADC and OGDC and also inhibit their enzymatic function. It remains unclear whether these properties have a direct pathogenetic role in the development of PBC. In addition to AMA, elevated serum levels of IgM and cryoproteins consisting of immune complexes capable of activating the alternative complement pathway are found in 80 to 90% of patients. Aberrant expression of major histocompatibility complex class II molecules has been found on biliary epithelium in association with PBC, suggesting that these cells may serve as antigen-presenting cells in this setting. Lymphocytes are prominent in the portal regions and surround damaged bile ducts. These histologic findings resemble those noted in graft-versus-host disease following bone marrow transplantation and suggest that damage to bile ducts may be immunologically mediated, perhaps reflecting a defect in a suppressor cell population. While it has been suggested that PBC may be initiated by molecular mimicry following infection or xenobiotic exposure, definitive evidence is lacking.

Pathology PBC is divided into four stages based on morphologic findings. The earliest recognizable lesion (stage I), termed *chronic nonsuppurative destructive cholangitis*, is a necrotizing inflammatory process of the portal triads. It is characterized by destruction of medium and small bile ducts, a dense infiltrate of acute and chronic inflammatory cells, mild fibrosis, and occasionally, bile stasis. At times, periductal granulomas and lymph follicles are found adjacent to affected bile ducts. Subsequently, the inflammatory infiltrate becomes less prominent, the number of bile ducts is reduced, and smaller bile ductules proliferate (stage II). Progression over a period of months to years leads to a decrease in interlobular ducts, loss of liver cells, and expansion of periportal fibrosis into a network of connective tissue scars (stage III). Ultimately, cirrhosis, which may be micronodular or macronodular, develops (stage IV).

Clinical Features ■ *SIGNS AND SYMPTOMS* Most patients with PBC are asymptomatic, and the disease is initially detected on the basis of elevated serum alkaline phosphatase levels during routine screening. The majority of such patients remain asymptomatic for prolonged periods, although many ultimately develop progressive liver injury.

Among patients with symptomatic disease, 90% are women age 35 to 60. Often the earliest symptom is pruritus, which may be either generalized or limited initially to the palms and soles. In addition, fatigue is commonly a prominent early symptom. After several months or years, jaundice and gradual darkening of the exposed areas of the skin (melanosis) may ensue. Other early clinical manifestations of PBC reflect impaired bile excretion. These include steatorrhea and the malabsorption of lipid-soluble vitamins. Protracted elevation of serum lipids, especially cholesterol, leads to subcutaneous lipid deposition around the eyes (xanthelasmas) and over joints and tendons (xanthomas). Over a period of months to years, the itching, jaundice, and hyperpigmentation slowly worsen. Eventually, signs of hepatocellular failure and portal hypertension develop and ascites appears. Progression may be quite variable. Whereas a proportion of asymptomatic patients may show no signs of progression for a decade or longer, in others, death due to hepatic insufficiency may occur within 5 to 10 years after the first signs of the illness. Such decompensation is often precipitated by uncontrolled variceal hemorrhage or infection.

Physical examination may be entirely normal in the early phase of the disease, when patients are asymptomatic or pruritus is the sole complaint. Later, there may be jaundice of varying intensity, hyperpigmentation of the exposed skin areas, xanthelasmas and tendinous and planar xanthomas, moderate to striking hepatomegaly, splenomegaly, and clubbing of the fingers. Bone tenderness, signs of vertebral compression, ecchymoses, glossitis, and dermatitis may all be noted. Clinical evidence of the sicca syndrome can be found in as many as 75% of patients, and serologic evidence of autoimmune thyroid disease in 25%. Other conditions encountered with increased frequency include rheumatoid arthritis, CREST syndrome, keratoconjunctivitis sicca, IgA deficiency, type 1 diabetes mellitus, scleroderma, pernicious anemia, and renal tubular acidosis. Bone disease is often a significant problem encountered over the course of the disease. While osteomalacia occurs due to diminished vitamin D absorption, accelerated osteoporosis in this patient population (the majority of whom are postmenopausal women) is even more common.

LABORATORY FINDINGS PBC is increasingly diagnosed at a presymptomatic stage, prompted by the finding of a twofold or greater elevation of the serum alkaline phosphatase during routine screening. Serum 5'-nucleotidase activity and γ-glutamyl transpeptidase levels are also elevated. In this setting, serum bilirubin is usually normal and aminotransferase levels minimally increased. The diagnosis is supported by a positive AMA test (titer > 1:40). The latter is both relatively specific and sensitive; a positive test is found in >90% of symptomatic patients and is present in <5% of patients with other liver diseases. As the disease evolves, the serum bilirubin level rises progressively and may reach 510 μmol/L (30 mg/dL) or more in the final stages. Serum aminotransferase values rarely exceed 2.5 to 3.3 μkat (150 to 200 units). Hyperlipidemia is common, and a striking increase of the serum unesterified cholesterol is often noted. An abnormal serum lipoprotein (lipoprotein X) may be present in PBC but is not specific and appears in other cholestatic conditions. A deficiency of bile salts in the intestine leads to moderate steatorrhea and impaired absorption of the fat-soluble vitamins and hypoprothrombinemia. Patients with PBC have elevated liver copper levels, but this finding is not specific and is found in all disorders in which there is prolonged cholestasis.

Diagnosis PBC should be considered in middle-aged women with unexplained pruritus or an elevated serum alkaline phosphatase and in whom there may be other clinical or laboratory features of protracted impairment of biliary excretion. Although a positive serum AMA determination provides important diagnostic evidence, false-positive results do occur; therefore, liver biopsy should be performed to confirm the diagnosis. Rarely, the AMA test may be negative in patients with histologic features of PBC. Frequently, patients have antibodies to the E2 protein in tests using these specific antigens. In some cases with histologic features of PBC and a negative AMA, antinuclear or smooth-muscle antibodies are present (as in autoimmune hepatitis), and the designation *autoimmune cholangitis* is applied. The natural history of this entity, however, appears to resemble that of PBC. If the AMA test is negative, the biliary tract should be evaluated to exclude primary sclerosing cholangitis and remediable extrahepatic biliary tract obstruction, especially in view of the frequent presence of coexisting cholelithiasis.

℞ TREATMENT

While there is no specific therapy for PBC, ursodiol has been shown to improve biochemical and histologic features and might improve survival, particularly liver transplantation–free survival (although this remains unproven). Ursodiol should be given in doses of 13 to 15 mg/kg per day, but lower doses are sometimes just as effective in reducing serum alkaline phosphatase and aminotransferase levels. Ursodiol should be given with food and can be taken in a single dose daily. Side effects are rare: gastrointestinal intolerance (diarrhea) and skin rashes occur but are uncommon. Isolated instances of severe exacerbation of pruritus have been reported in patients with advanced disease. Ursodiol probably works by replacing the endogenously produced hydrophobic bile acids with urosdeoxycholate, a hydrophilic and relatively nontoxic bile acid.

Unfortunately, ursodiol may not prevent ultimate progression of PBC, which is effectively predicted by the Mayo risk score, and the only established "cure" is liver transplantation. Results of liver transplantation for PBC are excellent, survival exceeding that for patients receiving transplantation for most other forms of end-stage liver disease. Recurrence of PBC after liver transplantation has been reported but is uncommon, and the recurrent disease is only slowly progressive. Most patients remain AMA positive after transplantation, and as many as 25% will have histologic features of PBC on liver biopsy after 5 years. Other therapies such as glucocorticoids, colchicine, methotrexate, azathioprine, cyclosporine, and tacrolimus have been reported as effective in small case series, but none have shown to be effective in adequately controlled trials.

Relief of symptoms is also an important part of management of PBC. As noted, ursodiol may be helpful in controlling symptoms and improving the patient's sense of well-being. Although the mechanism of the protracted pruritus is not entirely clear, cholestyramine, an oral bile salt–sequestering resin, may be helpful in doses of 12 to 16 g/d to decrease both pruritus and hypercholesterolemia. Rifampin, opiate antagonists (naloxone or naltrexone), ondansetron, plasmapheresis, and ultraviolet light have all been tried for control of pruritus, with varying results. Steatorrhea can be reduced by a low-fat diet and substituting medium-chain triglycerides for dietary long-chain triglycerides. Fat-soluble vitamins A, D, E, and K should be given at regular intervals. Zinc supplementation may be necessary if night blindness is refractory to vitamin A therapy. An important part of management of PBC and any cholestatic liver disease is assessment and treatment of osteoporosis and osteomalacia. Patients should be screened periodically by bone densitometry and treated as needed with calcium supplements (1500 mg/d), vitamin D (1000 IU/d), and/or bisphosphonate agents (e.g., alendronate) when osteoporosis is present. Progression of PBC leads to the typical complications of advanced liver disease (see below).

SECONDARY BILIARY CIRRHOSIS ■ **Etiology** SBC results from prolonged partial or total obstruction of the common bile duct or its major branches. In adults, obstruction is most frequently caused by postoperative strictures or gallstones, usually with superimposed infectious cholangitis. Chronic pancreatitis may lead to biliary stricture and secondary cirrhosis. SBC is also an important complication of primary sclerosing cholangitis, a progressive immunologic disorder of the intrahepatic and extrahepatic biliary tree (Chap. 292). Patients with malignant tumors of the common bile duct or pancreas rarely survive long enough to develop SBC. In children, congenital biliary atresia and cystic fibrosis are common causes of SBC. Choledochal cysts, if unrecognized, may also be a rare cause of SBC.

Pathology and Pathogenesis Unrelieved obstruction of the extrahepatic bile ducts leads to (1) bile stasis and focal areas of centrilobular necrosis followed by periportal necrosis, (2) proliferation and dilatation of the portal bile ducts and ductules, (3) sterile or infected cholangitis with accumulation of polymorphonuclear infiltrates around bile ducts, and (4) progressive expansion of portal tracts by edema and fibrosis. Extravasation of bile from ruptured interlobular bile ducts into areas of periportal necrosis leads to the formation of "bile lakes" surrounded by cholesterol-rich pseudoxanthomatous cells. As in other forms of cirrhosis, injury is accompanied by regeneration in residual parenchyma. These changes gradually lead to a finely nodular cirrhosis. In general, at least 3 to 12 months is required for biliary obstruction to result in cirrhosis. Relief of the obstruction is frequently accompanied by biochemical and morphologic improvement and may even ameliorate cirrhosis.

Clinical Features   The symptoms, signs, and biochemical findings of SBC are similar to those of PBC. Jaundice and pruritus are usually the most prominent features. In addition, fever and/or right upper quadrant pain, reflecting bouts of cholangitis or biliary colic, are typical. The manifestations of portal hypertension are found only in advanced cases. SBC should be considered in any patient with clinical and laboratory evidence of prolonged obstruction to bile flow, especially when there is a history of previous biliary tract surgery or gallstones, bouts of ascending cholangitis, or right upper quadrant pain. Cholangiography (either percutaneous or endoscopic) usually demonstrates the underlying pathologic process. Liver biopsy, although not always necessary from a clinical standpoint, can document the development of cirrhosis.

℞ TREATMENT

Relief of obstruction to bile flow, by either endoscopic or surgical means, is the most important step in the prevention and therapy of SBC. Effective decompression of the biliary tract results in a significant improvement in both symptoms and survival, even in patients with established cirrhosis. When obstruction cannot be relieved, as in sclerosing cholangitis, antibiotics may be helpful acutely in controlling superimposed infection or, when administered on a chronic basis, as prophylactic therapy in suppressing recurring episodes of ascending cholangitis. Without relief of obstruction, there is a steady progression to end-stage cirrhosis and its terminal manifestations.

CARDIAC CIRRHOSIS

Definition   Prolonged, severe right-sided congestive heart failure may lead to chronic liver injury and cardiac cirrhosis. The characteristic pathologic features of fibrosis and regenerative nodules distinguish cardiac cirrhosis from both reversible passive congestion of the liver due to acute heart failure and acute hepatocellular necrosis ("ischemic hepatitis" or "shock liver") resulting from systemic hypotension and hypoperfusion of the liver.

Etiology and Pathology   In right-sided heart failure, retrograde transmission of elevated venous pressure via the inferior vena cava and hepatic veins leads to congestion of the liver. Hepatic sinusoids become dilated and engorged with blood, and the liver becomes tensely swollen. With prolonged passive congestion and ischemia from poor perfusion secondary to reduced cardiac output, necrosis of centrilobular hepatocytes ensues and leads to fibrosis in these central areas. Ultimately, centrilobular fibrosis develops, with collagen extending outward in a characteristic stellate pattern from the central vein. Gross examination of the liver shows alternating red (congested) and pale (fibrotic) areas, a pattern often referred to as "nutmeg liver." Improvement in management of cardiac disorders, particularly advances in surgical treatment, has reduced the frequency of cardiac cirrhosis.

Clinical Features   A range of abnormalities of liver function tests may be found, though none is uniformly present. The serum bilirubin is usually only mildly increased and may be predominantly either conjugated or unconjugated. Mild to moderate elevation in alkaline phosphatase level and prothrombin time prolongation are sometimes present. The AST level is typically mildly elevated but may be transiently very high following a period of marked systemic hypotension

(shock liver), when the clinical picture can mimic acute viral or drug-induced hepatitis. In cases of tricuspid insufficiency the liver may be pulsatile, but this finding disappears as cirrhosis develops. With prolonged right-sided heart failure the liver becomes enlarged, firm, and usually nontender. The signs and symptoms of heart failure usually overshadow the liver disease. Bleeding from esophageal varices is rare, but chronic encephalopathy may be prominent, with a waxing and waning course reflecting variations in the severity of right-sided heart failure. Ascites and peripheral edema, often primarily related to the underlying cardiac dysfunction, may be worsened by the superimposed liver disease.

Diagnosis   The presence of a firm, enlarged liver with signs of chronic liver disease in a patient with valvular heart disease, constrictive pericarditis, or cor pulmonale of long duration (>10 years) should suggest cardiac cirrhosis. Liver biopsy can confirm the diagnosis but is often contraindicated because of coagulopathy or ascites. Coexistent chronic heart and liver disease should also raise the possibility of hemochromatosis (Chap. 336), amyloidosis (Chap. 310), or other infiltrative diseases.

Budd-Chiari syndrome resulting from the occlusion of the hepatic veins or inferior vena cava may be confused with acute congestive hepatomegaly. In this condition the liver is grossly enlarged and tender, and severe intractable ascites is present. However, signs and symptoms of heart failure are notably absent. The most common cause is thrombosis of the hepatic veins, often in the setting of polycythemia rubra vera, myeloproliferative syndromes, paroxysmal nocturnal hemoglobinuria, oral contraceptive use, or other hypercoagulable states; it may also result from invasion of the inferior vena cava by tumor, such as renal cell or hepatocellular carcinoma. Idiopathic membranous obstruction of the inferior vena cava is the most common cause of this syndrome in Japan. Hepatic venography or liver biopsy showing centrilobular congestion and sinusoidal dilatation in the absence of right-sided heart failure establishes the diagnosis of Budd-Chiari syndrome. Venoocclusive disease affecting the sublobular branches of the hepatic veins and the hepatic venues may result from hepatic irradiation, treatment with certain antineoplastic agents as preparation for stem cell transplantation, or ingestion of pyrrolidizine alkaloids present in some herbal teas ("bush tea disease") and can mimic congestive hepatomegaly.

℞ TREATMENT

Prevention or treatment of cardiac cirrhosis depends on the diagnosis and therapy of the underlying cardiovascular disorder. Improvement in cardiac function frequently results in improvement of liver function and stabilization of the liver disease.

METABOLIC, HEREDITARY, DRUG-RELATED, AND OTHER TYPES OF CIRRHOSIS (See Table 289-1)

Cirrhosis or hepatitis may result from a wide variety of other processes encompassing the spectrum of etiologic factors listed in Table 289-2. Although some of these disorders have distinctive clinical or morphologic features, the manifestations of cirrhosis are largely independent of the underlying pathogenic mechanism.

NONCIRRHOTIC FIBROSIS OF THE LIVER

Several diseases, either congenital or acquired, may be associated with localized or generalized hepatic fibrosis. They are distinguished from

TABLE 289-2   *Some Causes of Noncirrhotic Hepatic Fibrosis*

Idiopathic portal hypertension (noncirrhotic portal fibrosis, Banti's syndrome); three variants:
   Intrahepatic phlebosclerosis and fibrosis
   Portal and splenic vein sclerosis
   Portal and splenic vein thrombosis
Schistosomiasis ("pipe-stem" fibrosis with presinusoidal portal hypertension)
Congenital hepatic fibrosis (may be associated with polycystic disease of liver and kidneys)

cirrhosis by the absence of hepatocellular damage and the lack of nodular regenerative activity. The clinical manifestations in such cases are largely secondary to portal hypertension. The different types of these disorders are indicated in Table 289-2; with the exception of schistosomiasis in some regions of the world, all these conditions are relatively rare.

MAJOR COMPLICATIONS OF CIRRHOSIS

The clinical course of patients with advanced cirrhosis is often complicated by a number of important sequelae that are independent of the etiology of the underlying liver disease. These include portal hypertension and its consequences (e.g., gastroesophageal varices and splenomegaly), ascites, hepatic encephalopathy, spontaneous bacterial peritonitis, hepatorenal syndrome, and hepatocellular carcinoma.

PORTAL HYPERTENSION ■ **Definition and Pathogenesis**   Normal pressure in the portal vein is low (5 to 10 mmHg) because vascular resistance in the hepatic sinusoids is minimal. Portal hypertension (>10 mmHg) most commonly results from increased resistance to portal blood flow. Because the portal venous system lacks valves, resistance at any level between the right side of the heart and splanchnic vessels results in retrograde transmission of an elevated pressure. Increased resistance can occur at three levels relative to the hepatic sinusoids: (1) presinusoidal, (2) sinusoidal, and (3) postsinudoidal. Obstruction in the *presinusoidal* venous compartment may be anatomically outside the liver (e.g., portal vein thrombosis) or within the liver itself but at a functional level proximal to the hepatic sinusoids so that the liver parenchyma is not exposed to the elevated venous pressure (e.g., schistosomiasis).

Postsinusoidal obstruction may also occur outside the liver at the level of the hepatic veins (e.g., Budd-Chiari syndrome), the inferior vena cava, or, less commonly, within the liver (e.g., venoocclusive disease). When cirrhosis is complicated by portal hypertension, the increased resistance is usually *sinusoidal*. While distinctions between pre-, post-, and sinusoidal processes are conceptually appealing, functional resistance to portal flow in a given patient may occur at more than one level. Portal hypertension may also arise from increased blood flow (e.g., massive splenomegaly or arteriovenous fistulas), but the low outflow resistance of the normal liver makes this a rare clinical problem.

Cirrhosis is the most common cause of portal hypertension in the United States. Clinically significant portal hypertension is present in >60% of patients with cirrhosis. *Portal vein obstruction* is the second most common cause; it may be idiopathic or occur in association with cirrhosis, infection, pancreatitis, or abdominal trauma. Idiopathic portal vein thrombosis may develop in a variety of hypercoagulable states including polycythemia vera; essential thrombocythemia; deficiencies of protein C, protein S, or antithrombin III; resistance to activated protein C (factor V Leiden); and a mutation of the prothrombin gene (G20210A). Most of the remaining patients with idiopathic cases have a subclinical myeloproliferative disorder. Hepatic vein thrombosis (Budd-Chiari syndrome) and hepatic venoocclusive disease are relatively infrequent causes of portal hypertension (see above). Portal vein occlusion may result in massive hematemesis from gastroesophageal varices, but ascites is usually found only when cirrhosis is present. Noncirrhotic portal fibrosis (Table 289-2) accounts for only a few cases of portal hypertension.

Clinical Features   The major clinical manifestations of portal hypertension include hemorrhage from gastroesophageal varices, splenomegaly with hypersplenism, ascites, and acute and chronic hepatic encephalopathy. These are related, at least in part, to the development of portal-systemic collateral channels. The absence of valves in the portal venous system facilitates retrograde (hepatofugal) blood flow from the high-pressure portal venous system to the lower-pressure systemic venous circulation. Major sites of collateral flow involve the veins around the cardioesophageal junction (esophagogastric varices), the rectum (hemorrhoids), retroperitoneal space, and the falciform ligament of the liver (periumbilical or abdominal wall collaterals). Abdominal wall collaterals appear as tortuous epigastric vessels that radiate from the umbilicus toward the xiphoid and rib margins (caput medusae).

A frequent marker of the presence of cirrhosis in a patient being followed for chronic liver disease is a progressive decrease in platelet count. A low-normal platelet count can be the first clue to progression to cirrhosis. Ultimately, a marked decrease in platelets (to 30,000 to 60,000/μL) and white blood cells can occur.

Diagnosis   In patients with known liver disease, the development of portal hypertension is usually revealed by the appearance of splenomegaly, ascites, encephalopathy, and/or esophageal varices. Conversely, the finding of any of these features should prompt evaluation of the patient for the presence of underlying portal hypertension and liver disease. Varices are most reliably documented by fiberoptic esophagoscopy; their presence lends indirect support to the diagnosis of portal hypertension. Magnetic resonance imaging and intravenous contrast computed tomography are also sensitive tools for detection of the collateral circulation of portal hypertension. Although rarely necessary, portal venous pressure may be measured directly by percutaneous transhepatic "skinny needle" catheterization or indirectly through transjugular cannulation of the hepatic veins. Both free and wedged hepatic vein pressure should be measured. While the latter is elevated in sinusoidal and postsinusoidal portal hypertension, including cirrhosis, this measurement is usually normal in presinusoidal portal hypertension. In patients in whom additional information is necessary (e.g., preoperative evaluation before portal-systemic shunt surgery) or when percutaneous catheterization is not feasible, mesenteric and hepatic angiography may be helpful. Particular attention should be directed to the venous phase to assess the patency of the portal vein and the direction of portal blood flow.

℞ TREATMENT

Although treatment is usually directed toward a specific complication of portal hypertension, attempts are sometimes made to reduce the pressure in the portal venous system. Surgical decompression procedures have been used for many years to lower portal pressure in patients with bleeding esophageal varices (see below). However, portal-systemic shunt surgery does not result in improved survival rates in patients with cirrhosis. Decompression can now be accomplished without surgery through the percutaneous placement of a portal-systemic shunt, termed a *transjugular intrahepatic portosystemic shunt* (TIPS). *β-Adrenergic blockade* with nonselective agents such as propranolol or nadolol reduces portal pressure through vasoconstrictive effects on both the splanchnic arterial bed and the portal venous system in combination with reduced cardiac output. Such therapy has been shown to be effective in preventing both a first variceal bleed and subsequent episodes after an initial bleed. Treatment of patients with clinically significant sequelae of portal hypertension, especially variceal bleeding, is titrated to reduce the hepatic venous pressure gradient (HVPG = wedged hepatic venous pressure − free hepatic venous pressure) to <12 mmHg or by 20% from baseline. When the HVPG is not available or feasible, reduction of resting pulse by 25% is reasonable if no contraindications to therapy exist.

Vigorous treatment of patients with alcoholic hepatitis and cirrhosis, chronic active hepatitis, or other liver diseases may lead to a fall in portal pressure and to a reduction in variceal size. In general, however, portal hypertension due to cirrhosis is not reversible. In appropriately selected patients, hepatic transplantation will be beneficial.

VARICEAL BLEEDING ■ **Pathogenesis**   While vigorous hemorrhage may arise from any portal-systemic venous collaterals, bleeding is most common from varices in the region of the gastroesophageal junction. The factors contributing to bleeding from gastroesophageal varices are not entirely understood but include the degree of portal hypertension (>12 mmHg) and the size of the varices.

Clinical Features and Diagnosis   Variceal bleeding often occurs without obvious precipitating factors and usually presents with painless but massive hematemesis with or without melena. Associated signs range from mild postural tachycardia to profound shock, depending on the extent of blood loss and degree of hypovolemia. Because patients with varices may bleed just as frequently from other gastrointestinal lesions (e.g., peptic ulcer, gastritis), exclusion of other bleeding sources is important even in patients with prior variceal hemorrhage. Endoscopy is the best approach to evaluate upper gastrointestinal hemorrhage in patients with known or suspected portal hypertension.

℞ TREATMENT

Management of Acute Bleeding   (See Fig. 289-1) Variceal bleeding is a life-threatening emergency. Prompt estimation and vigorous replacement of blood loss to maintain intravascular volume are essential and take precedence over diagnostic studies and more specific intervention to stop the bleeding. However, excessive fluid administration can increase portal pressure with resultant further bleeding and should therefore be avoided. Replacement of clotting factors with fresh-frozen plasma is important in patients with coagulopathy. Patients are best managed in an intensive care unit and require close monitoring of central venous or pulmonary capillary wedge pressures, urine output, and mental status. When the patient is hemodynamically stable, attention should be directed toward specific diagnostic studies (especially endoscopy) and other therapeutic modalities to prevent further or recurrent bleeding.

About half of all episodes of variceal hemorrhage cease without intervention, although the risk of rebleeding is very high. The medical management of acute variceal hemorrhage includes the use of vasoconstrictors (somatostatin/octreotide or vasopressin), balloon tamponade, and endoscopic variceal ligation (EVL) or sclerosis of varices (sclerotherapy). Intravenous infusion of *vasopressin* at a rate of 0.1 to 0.4 U/min results in generalized vasoconstriction leading to diminished blood flow in the portal venous system. Intravenous infusion of vasopressin is as effective as selective intraarterial administration.

Control of bleeding can be achieved in up to 80% of cases, but bleeding recurs in more than half after the vasopressin is tapered and discontinued. Furthermore, a number of serious side effects, including cardiac and gastrointestinal tract ischemia, acute renal failure, and hyponatremia, may be associated with vasopressin therapy. Concurrent use of venodilators such as nitroglycerin as an intravenous infusion or isosorbide dinitrate sublingually may enhance the effectiveness of vasopressin and reduce complications. *Somatostatin* and its analogue, *octreotide*, are direct splanchnic vasoconstrictors. In some studies somatostatin, given as an initial 250-μg bolus followed by constant infusion (250 μg/h), has been found to be as effective as vasopressin. Octreotide at doses of 50 to 100 μg/h is also effective. These agents are preferable to vasopressin, offering equivalent efficacy with fewer complications. If bleeding is too vigorous or endoscopy is not available, *balloon tamponade* of the bleeding varices may be accomplished with a triple-lumen (Sengstaken-Blakemore) or four-lumen (Minnesota) tube with esophageal and gastric balloons. Because of the high risk of aspiration, endotracheal intubation should be performed prior to placing one of these tubes. After the tube is introduced into the stomach, the gastric balloon is inflated and pulled back into the cardia of the stomach. If bleeding does not stop, the esophageal balloon is inflated for additional tamponade. Complications occur in 15% or more of patients and include aspiration pneumonitis as well as esophageal rupture.

Where available, *endoscopic intervention* should be employed as the first-line treatment to control bleeding acutely (Chaps. 37 and 272). EVL, in which esophageal varices are ligated and strangulated by endoscopically placed small elastic O-rings, has generally supplanted endoscopic injection of sclerosants in the control of acute variceal bleeding. EVL controls acute bleeding in up to 90% of cases and should be repeated until obliteration of all varices is accomplished.

Surgical treatment of portal hypertension and variceal bleeding involves the creation of a portal-systemic shunt to permit decompression of the portal system. Two types of portal systemic shunts have been used: nonselective shunts, to decompress the entire portal system, and selective shunts, intended to decompress only the varices while maintaining blood flow to the liver itself. Nonselective shunts include end-to-side or side-to-side portacaval and proximal splenorenal anastomoses; selective shunts include the distal splenorenal shunt. Nonselective shunts are more likely to be complicated by encephalopathy than selective shunts. Emergency portal-systemic nonselective shunts may control acute hemorrhage, but such surgery is usually used only as a last resort because early operative mortality can be high.

In TIPS, a technique developed to create a portal-systemic shunt by a percutaneous approach, an expandable metal stent is advanced under angiographic guidance to the hepatic veins and then through the substance of the liver to create a direct portacaval channel. This technique offers an alternative to surgery for refractory bleeding due to portal hypertension. However, stents frequently undergo stenosis or become occluded over a period of months, necessitating revision, a second TIPS, or an alternative approach. Encephalopathy may occur after TIPS, just as in the surgical shunts, and is especially problematic in the elderly and those patients with preexisting encephalopathy. TIPS should be reserved for those individuals who fail endoscopic or medical management and are poor surgical risks. TIPS sometimes serves a useful role as a "bridge" for those patients with end-stage cirrhosis awaiting liver transplantation. Procedures such as esophageal transection have also been advocated for the management of acute variceal bleeding, but their efficacy remains unproven, and these procedures are usually considered a last resort.

The management of bleeding gastric fundal varices, found either alone or in conjunction with esophageal varices, is more problematic, since banding and sclerotherapy are generally not effective. Vasoactive pharmacologic therapy should be instituted, but TIPS or shunt surgery should be considered because of high failure and rebleeding rates. For isolated gastric varices, splenic vein thrombosis should be specifically sought, since splenectomy is curative.

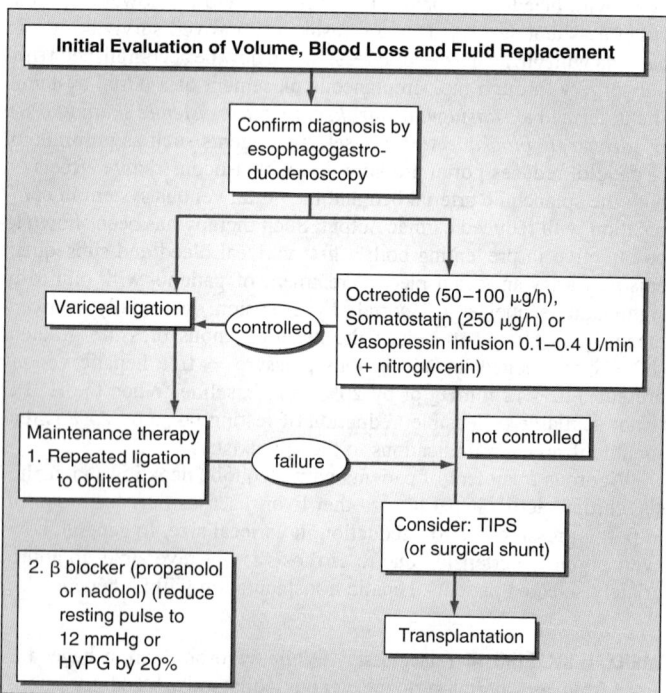

FIGURE 289-1   Approach to the patient with bleeding esophageal varices. Use of a beta blocker is the only intervention demonstrated to offer prophylactic benefit in a patient who has never bled. TIPS, transjugular intrahepatic portosystemic shunt; HVPG, hepatic venous pressure gradient.

Prevention of First Hemorrhage Prophylactic treatment with nonselective β-adrenergic antagonists (propranolol or nadolol) in patients with large ("high-risk") varices that have never bled appears to decrease the incidence of bleeding by 40 to 50% and prolong survival. Thus, endoscopic screening for varices in patients with cirrhosis is desirable; some have suggested this should be repeated every other year.

Although prophylactic banding of esophageal varices in the absence of proven bleeding cannot yet be recommended, one report suggests that banding may be more effective than beta-blockade in primary prevention of variceal bleeding in high-risk patients.

Prevention of Recurrent Hemorrhage Obliteration of varices by endoscopic band ligation reduces risk of recurrent hemorrhage by >50%. Pharmacologic agents also have demonstrated benefit. While the utility of beta blockers can be limited by concomitant hypotension, a number of studies demonstrate their value in secondary prevention of recurrent variceal hemorrhage. Pharmacologic and endoscopic therapy are comparable in overall reduction of rebleeding risk, but the subgroup of patients who achieve hemodynamic response to pharmacologic therapy appears to experience survival benefit.

Patients with portal hypertension in the absence of specific contraindications should be given propranolol or nadolol in doses that produce a 25% reduction in the resting heart rate or a reduction in the HVPG to 12 mmHg or 20% below baseline, where available. Propranolol may also prevent recurrent bleeding from severe portal hypertensive gastropathy in patients with cirrhosis. The optimal combination of endoscopic and pharmacologic therapy for prevention of recurrent hemorrhage remains to be established.

The role of portal-systemic shunt surgery after initial control of bleeding by nonoperative means is also uncertain. Surgically created shunts effectively reduce the risk of recurrent hemorrhage, but the overall mortality of patients undergoing such surgery is comparable to that of unoperated patients. Although patients who have undergone portal-systemic surgery succumb to recurrent bleeding less commonly than unoperated patients, this improvement is counterbalanced by increased morbidity from encephalopathy and death from progressive liver failure. Increasingly, therapeutic portal-systemic shunts have been reserved for patients who experience further bleeding despite serial endoscopic therapy.

Portal Hypertensive Gastropathy Although variceal hemorrhage is the most commonly encountered bleeding complication of portal hypertension, many patients will develop a congestive gastropathy due to the venous hypertension. In this condition, identified by endoscopic examination, the mucosa appears engorged and friable. Indolent mucosal bleeding occurs rather than the brisk hemorrhage typical of a variceal source. β-Adrenergic blockade with propranolol (reducing splanchnic arterial pressure as well as portal pressure) is sometimes effective in ameliorating this condition. Proton pump inhibitors or other agents useful in the treatment of peptic disease are usually not helpful.

SPLENOMEGALY ■ Definition and Pathogenesis Congestive splenomegaly is common in patients with severe portal hypertension. Rarely, massive splenomegaly from nonhepatic disease leads to portal hypertension due to increased blood flow in the splenic vein.

Clinical Features Although usually asymptomatic, splenomegaly may be massive and contribute to the thrombocytopenia or pancytopenia of cirrhosis. In the absence of cirrhosis, splenomegaly in association with variceal hemorrhage should suggest the possibility of splenic vein thrombosis.

Rx TREATMENT

Splenomegaly usually requires no specific treatment, although massive enlargement of the spleen may occasionally necessitate splenectomy at the time of shunt surgery. However, it should be noted that splenectomy without an accompanying shunt may actually increase portal pressure, and portal vein thrombosis may result from splenectomy.

Splenectomy may also be indicated if splenomegaly is the cause rather than the result of portal hypertension (as in splenic vein thrombosis). Thrombocytopenia alone is rarely severe enough to necessitate removal of the spleen. Splenectomy should be avoided in a patient eligible for liver transplantation.

ASCITES ■ Definition Ascites is the accumulation of excess fluid within the peritoneal cavity. It is most frequently encountered in patients with cirrhosis and other forms of severe liver disease, but a number of other disorders may lead to either transudative or exudative ascites (Chap. 39).

Pathogenesis The accumulation of ascitic fluid represents a state of total-body sodium and water excess, but the event that initiates this imbalance is unclear. Three theories have been proposed (Fig. 289-2). The "underfilling" theory suggests that the primary abnormality is inappropriate sequestration of fluid within the splanchnic vascular bed due to portal hypertension and a consequent decrease in effective circulating blood volume. According to this theory, an apparent decrease in intravascular volume (underfilling) is sensed by the kidney, which responds by retaining salt and water. The "overflow" theory suggests that the primary abnormality is inappropriate renal retention of salt and water in the absence of volume depletion. A third, more attractive theory, the peripheral arterial vasodilation hypothesis, may unify the earlier theories and accounts for the constellation of arterial hypotension and increased cardiac output in association with high levels of vasoconstrictor substances that are routinely found in patients with cirrhosis and ascites. Again, sodium retention is considered secondary to arterial vascular underfilling and the result of a disproportionate increase of the vascular compartment due to arteriolar vasodilation rather than from decreased intravascular volume. According to this theory, portal hypertension results in splanchnic arteriolar vasodilation, mediated by nitric oxide, and leading to underfilling of the arterial vascular space and baroreceptor-mediated stimulation of renin-angiotensin, sympathetic output, and antidiuretic hormone release.

Regardless of the initiating event, a number of factors contribute to accumulation of fluid in the abdominal cavity (Fig. 289-2). Elevated levels of serum epinephrine and norepinephrine have been well documented. *Increased central sympathetic outflow* is found in patients with cirrhosis and ascites but not in those with cirrhosis alone. Increased sympathetic output results in diminished natriuresis by acti-

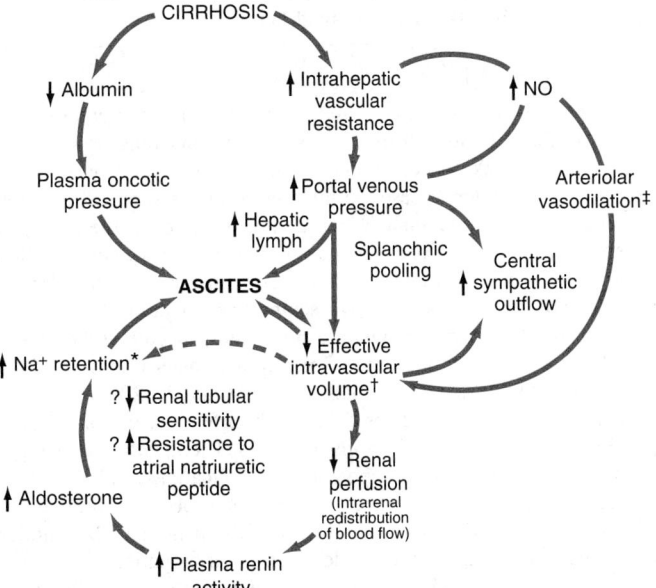

FIGURE 289-2 Multiple factors involved in development of ascites. Current concepts suggest that initiating factor may be primary sodium retention (*"overflow"), diminished effective intravascular volume (†"underfilling"), or arteriolar vasodilation (‡"vasodilation"). NO, nitric oxide.

vation of the renin-angiotensin system and diminished sensitivity to atrial natriuretic peptide. *Portal hypertension* plays an important role in the formation of ascites by raising hydrostatic pressure within the splanchnic capillary bed. *Hypoalbuminemia* and *reduced plasma oncotic pressure* also favor the extravasation of fluid from plasma to the peritoneal cavity, and thus ascites is infrequent in patients with cirrhosis unless both portal hypertension and hypoalbuminemia are present. Hepatic lymph may weep freely from the surface of the cirrhotic liver due to distortion and obstruction of hepatic sinusoids and lymphatics and contributes to ascites formation. In contrast to the contribution of transudative fluid from the portal vascular bed, hepatic lymph may weep into the peritoneal cavity even in the absence of marked hypoproteinemia because the endothelial lining of the hepatic sinusoids is discontinuous. This mechanism may account for the high protein concentration present in the ascitic fluid of some patients with venoocclusive disease or the Budd-Chiari syndrome.

Renal factors also play an important role in perpetuating ascites. Patients with ascites fail to excrete a water load in a normal fashion. They have increased renal sodium reabsorption by both proximal and distal tubules, the latter due largely to increased plasma renin activity and secondary hyperaldosteronism. Insensitivity to circulating atrial natriuretic peptide, often present in elevated concentrations in patients with cirrhosis and ascites, may be an important contributory factor in many patients. This insensitivity has been documented in those patients with the most severely impaired sodium excretion, who typically also exhibit low arterial pressure and marked overactivity of the renin-aldosterone axis. Renal vasoconstriction, perhaps resulting from increased serum prostaglandin or catecholamine levels, may also contribute to sodium retention. Recently a role for endothelin, a potent vasoconstrictor peptide, has been proposed. While elevated levels have been reported by some, this has not been observed by others.

Clinical Features and Diagnosis Usually ascites is first noticed by the patient because of increasing abdominal girth. More pronounced accumulation of fluid may cause shortness of breath because of elevation of the diaphragm. When peritoneal fluid accumulation exceeds 500 mL, ascites may be demonstrated on physical examination by the presence of shifting dullness, a fluid wave, or bulging flanks. Ultrasound examination, preferably with a Doppler study, can detect smaller quantities of ascites and should be performed when physical examination is equivocal or when the cause of the recent onset of ascites is not clear (e.g., exclude Budd-Chiari syndrome).

℞ TREATMENT

(See Fig. 289-3) A thorough search should be made for precipitating factors in the patient with recent onset of or worsening ascites, e.g., excessive salt intake, medication noncompliance, superimposed infection, worsening liver disease, portal vein thrombosis, or development of hepatocellular carcinoma. When ascites develops in the setting of severe, acute liver disease, resolution of ascites is likely to follow improvement in liver function. More commonly, ascites develops in patients with stable or steadily worsening liver function. Paracentesis should usually be performed with a small-gauge needle at the time of initial evaluation or at the time of any clinical deterioration of a cirrhotic patient with ascites. A small amount of fluid (<200 mL) should be obtained and examined for evidence of infection, tumor, or other possible causes and complications of ascites. Therapeutic intervention is indicated both to prevent potential complications and to control progressive increase in ascites, which may become pronounced enough to cause physical discomfort. For the patient with a modest accumulation, therapy can be undertaken as an outpatient and should be gentle and incremental (see below). The goal is the loss of no more than 1.0 kg/d if both ascites and peripheral edema are present and no more than 0.5 kg/d in patients with ascites alone. In some patients, particularly those with a large accumulation of fluid, it may be desirable to hospitalize the patient so that daily weights and frequent serum

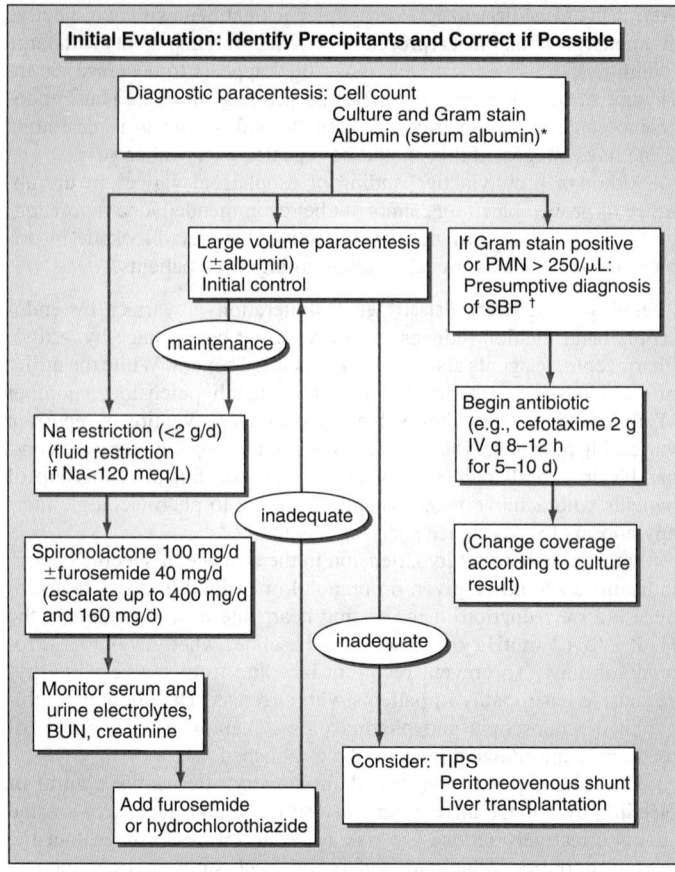

FIGURE 289-3 Approach to the patient with ascites [and spontaneous bacterial peritonitis (SBP)]. PMN, polymorphonuclear leukocytes; TIPS, transjugular intrahepatic portosystemic shunt. *Calculate SAAG [serum ascites albumin gradient = serum albumin − ascites albumin (g/dL)] to confirm high gradient (>1.1 g/dL) in portal hypertension. †If PMN >250/μL but culture is negative = culture negative neutrocytic ascites; begin empirical antibiotic and retap at 48 h; if culture is positive but PMN < 250/μL normal = monomicrobial nonneutrocytic bacterascites; retap; treat if PMN > 250/μL: if polymicrobial infection, exclude secondary peritonitis. U_{Na}, urinary sodium; U_{Ka}, urinary potassium; BUN, blood urea nitrogen.

electrolyte levels can be monitored and compliance ensured. Although abdominal girth measurements are frequently used as an index of fluid loss, they tend to be unreliable.

Salt restriction is the cornerstone of therapy. A diet containing 800 mg sodium (2 g NaCl) is often adequate to induce a negative sodium balance and permit diuresis. Response to salt restriction alone is more likely to occur if the ascites is of recent onset, the underlying liver disease is reversible, a precipitating factor can be corrected, or the patient has a high urinary sodium excretion (>25 mmol/d) and normal renal function. Fluid restriction of approximately 1000 mL/d does little to enhance diuresis but may be necessary to correct hyponatremia. If sodium restriction alone fails to result in diuresis and weight loss, diuretics should be prescribed. Because of the role of hyperaldosteronism in sustaining salt retention, spironolactone or other distal tubule–acting diuretics (triamterene, amiloride) are the drugs of choice. The development of azotemia or hyperkalemia may be limiting or even warrant a reduction in the dose of these medications. In some patients, diuresis does not occur despite maximal doses of distal tubule–acting agents because of avid proximal tubular sodium absorption. More potent, proximally acting diuretics (furosemide, bumetanide, torasemide) may be added to the regimen. Thus, spironolactone is initially given at a dose of 100 mg/d with or without furosemide, 40 mg/d, and both agents may be increased by 100- and 40-mg increments respectively: total dose should not exceed 400 mg/d and 160 mg/d, respectively. An indication of the minimum effective dose of spironolactone may be obtained by monitoring urinary electrolyte concentrations for a rise in sodium and fall in potassium concentrations, reflecting effective competitive inhibition of aldosterone. Great caution should be exercised to avoid plasma volume depletion, azotemia, and hypokalemia, which may lead to encephalopathy.

In patients with pronounced ascites, particularly those requiring hospitalization, large-volume paracentesis has proven to be an effective and less costly approach to initial management than prolonged bed rest and conventional diuretic treatment. In this approach, ascitic fluid is removed by peritoneal cannula using strict aseptic techniques and monitoring hemodynamic and renal function. This can be safely accomplished in a single session. Concomitant albumin replacement by intravenous infusion is prudent in the patient without peripheral edema, to avoid depleting the intravascular space and precipitating hypotension. Maintenance diuretic therapy in conjunction with sodium restriction may then be instituted to avoid recurrent ascites.

A minority of patients with advanced cirrhosis have "refractory ascites" or rapidly reaccumulate fluid after control by paracentesis. In some patients, a side-to-side *portacaval shunt* may result in improvement in ascites, although generally these patients are extremely poor surgical risks. In the past, intractable ascites has also been treated with the surgical implantation of a plastic *peritoneovenous shunt*, which has a pressure-sensitive, one-way valve allowing ascitic fluid to flow from the abdominal cavity to the superior vena cava. However, the usefulness of this technique is limited by a high rate of complications such as infection, disseminated intravascular coagulation, and thrombosis of the shunt. More recently, in selected patients, TIPS has been used effectively to control refractory ascites, although portal decompression, while mobilizing ascitic fluid, has precipitated severe hepatic encephalopathy in some patients. None of these shunts has been shown to extend life expectancy.

SPONTANEOUS BACTERIAL PERITONITIS (SBP) Patients with ascites and cirrhosis may develop acute bacterial peritonitis without an obvious primary source of infection. Patients with advanced liver disease are particularly susceptible to SBP, which portends a poor prognosis (Chap. 112).

HEPATORENAL SYNDROME ■ Definition and Pathogenesis Hepatorenal syndrome is a serious complication in the patient with cirrhosis and ascites and is characterized by worsening azotemia with avid sodium retention and oliguria in the absence of identifiable specific causes of renal dysfunction. The exact basis for this syndrome is not clear, but altered renal hemodynamics appear to be involved. There is evidence for inappropriate intense renal vasoconstriction, perhaps in response to the splanchnic vasodilation accompanying cirrhosis. The kidneys are structurally intact; urinalysis and pyelography are usually normal. Renal biopsy, although rarely needed, is also normal, and in fact, kidneys from such patients have been used successfully for renal transplantation.

Clinical Features and Diagnosis Worsening azotemia, hyponatremia, progressive oliguria, and hypotension are the hallmarks of the hepatorenal syndrome. This syndrome, which is distinct from prerenal azotemia, may be precipitated by severe gastrointestinal bleeding, sepsis, or overly vigorous attempts at diuresis or paracentesis; it may also occur without an obvious cause. It is essential to exclude other causes of renal impairment often seen in these patients. These include prerenal azotemia or acute tubular necrosis due to hypovolemia (e.g., secondary to gastrointestinal bleeding or diuretic therapy) or an increased nitrogen load such as that seen as a result of bleeding. Drug nephrotoxicity is also often a consideration, particularly in the patient who has received agents such as aminoglycosides or contrast dye. The diagnosis rests on the finding of an elevated serum creatinine level [>133 μmol/L (>1.5 g/dL)] that fails to improve with volume expansion or withdrawal of diuretics, together with an unremarkable urine sediment. The diagnosis is supported by the demonstration of avid urinary sodium retention. Typically, the urine sodium concentration is <5 mmol/L, a concentration lower than that generally found in uncomplicated prerenal azotemia.

Rx TREATMENT

Treatment is usually unsuccessful. Although some patients with hypotension and decreased plasma volume may respond to infusions of salt-poor albumin, volume expansion must be undertaken with caution to avoid precipitating variceal bleeding. Vasodilator therapy, including intravenous infusions of low dose dopamine, is not effective. Evidence for the benefit of systemic vasoconstrictors alone or in combination with other agents such as terlipressin, norepinephrine with albumin, and octreotide with midodrine has emerged recently, but additional study is needed. While TIPS has been reported to improve renal function in some patients, its use cannot be recommended. In appropriate candidates, the treatment of choice for hepatorenal syndrome is liver transplantation. In patients with spontaneous bacterial peritonitis, early intravenous albumin infusion can prevent development of hepatorenal syndrome in some patients.

HEPATIC ENCEPHALOPATHY ■ Definition Hepatic (portal-systemic) encephalopathy is a complex neuropsychiatric syndrome characterized by disturbances in consciousness and behavior, personality changes, fluctuating neurologic signs, asterixis or "flapping tremor," and distinctive electroencephalographic changes. Encephalopathy may be *acute* and reversible or *chronic* and progressive. In severe cases, irreversible coma and death may occur. Acute episodes may recur with variable frequency.

Pathogenesis The specific cause of hepatic encephalopathy is unknown. The most important factors in the pathogenesis are severe hepatocellular dysfunction and/or intrahepatic and extrahepatic shunting of portal venous blood into the systemic circulation so that the liver is largely bypassed. As a result of these processes, various toxic substances absorbed from the intestine are not detoxified by the liver and lead to metabolic abnormalities in the central nervous system (CNS). *Ammonia* is the substance most often incriminated in the pathogenesis of encephalopathy. Many, but not all, patients with hepatic encephalopathy have elevated blood ammonia levels, and recovery from encephalopathy is often accompanied by declining blood ammonia levels. Other compounds and metabolites that may contribute to the development of encephalopathy include mercaptans (derived from intestinal metabolism of methionine), short-chain fatty acids, and phenol. *False neurochemical transmitters* (e.g., octopamine), resulting in part from alterations in plasma levels of aromatic and branched-chain amino acids, may also play a role. An increase in the permeability of the blood-brain barrier to some of these substances may be an additional factor involved in the pathogenesis of hepatic encephalopathy. Several observations suggest that excessive concentrations of γ-aminobutyric acid (GABA), an inhibitory neurotransmitter, in the CNS are important in the reduced levels of consciousness seen in hepatic encephalopathy. Increased CNS GABA may reflect failure of the liver to extract precursor amino acids efficiently or to remove GABA produced in the intestine. In support of this, there is also evidence to suggest that endogenous benzodiazepines, which act through the GABA receptor, may contribute to the development of hepatic encephalopathy. This evidence includes isolation of 1,4-benzodiazepines from brain tissue of patients with fulminant hepatic failure as well as the partial response observed in some patients and experimental animals after administration of flumazenil, a benzodiazepine antagonist. However, the inconsistent effect of flumazenil in patients with encephalopathy, as well as potential methodologic pitfalls in the measurement of endogenous benzodiazepines, preclude definitive attribution of a role to these substances in the pathogenesis of hepatic encephalopathy. The finding of direct enhancement of GABA receptor activation by ammonia suggests that several of the factors described above may be operating via a final common pathway to produce the neuronal depression of hepatic encephalopathy. Finally, the observation of hyperintensity in the basal ganglia by magnetic resonance imaging in cirrhotic patients suggests that excessive *manganese* dep-

TABLE 289-3 *Common Precipitants of Hepatic Encephalopathy*

Increased nitrogen load	Drugs
Gastrointestinal bleeding	Narcotics, tranquilizers, sedatives
Excess dietary protein	Diuretics (see "Electrolyte
Azotemia	imbalance")
Constipation	Miscellaneous
Electrolyte and metabolic	Infection
imbalance	Surgery
Hypokalemia	Superimposed acute liver disease
Alkalosis	Progressive liver disease
Hypoxia	Portal-systemic shunts
Hyponatremia	
Hypovolemia	

osition may also contribute to the pathogenesis of hepatic encephalopathy. Further studies are needed to determine whether chelation therapy exerts long-term benefit.

In the patient with otherwise stable cirrhosis, hepatic encephalopathy often follows a clearly identifiable precipitating event (Table 289-3). Perhaps the most common predisposing factor is *gastrointestinal bleeding*, which leads to an increase in the production of ammonia and other nitrogenous substances, which are then absorbed. Similarly, *increased dietary protein* may precipitate encephalopathy as a result of increased production of nitrogenous substances by colonic bacteria. *Electrolyte disturbances*, particularly hypokalemic alkalosis secondary to overzealous use of diuretics, vigorous paracentesis, or vomiting, may precipitate hepatic encephalopathy. Systemic alkalosis causes an increase in the amount of nonionic ammonia (NH_3) relative to ammonium ions (NH_4). Only nonionic (uncharged) ammonia readily crosses the blood-brain barrier and accumulates in the CNS. Hypokalemia also directly stimulates renal ammonia production. Injudicious use of CNS-depressing drugs (e.g., barbiturates, benzodiazepines) and acute infection may trigger or aggravate hepatic encephalopathy, although the mechanisms involved are not clear. Other potential precipitating factors include superimposed acute viral hepatitis, alcoholic hepatitis, extrahepatic bile duct obstruction, constipation, surgery, and other coincidental medical complications.

Hepatic encephalopathy has protean manifestations, and any neurologic abnormality, including focal deficits, may be encountered. In patients with acute encephalopathy, neurologic deficits are completely reversible upon correction of underlying precipitating factors and/or improvement in liver function, but in patients with chronic encephalopathy, the deficits may be irreversible and progressive. Cerebral edema is frequently present and contributes to the clinical picture and overall mortality in patients with both acute and chronic encephalopathy.

The diagnosis of hepatic encephalopathy should be considered when four major factors are present: (1) acute or chronic hepatocellular disease and/or extensive portal-systemic collateral shunts (the latter may be either spontaneous, e.g., secondary to portal hypertension, or mechanically created, e.g., TIPS); (2) disturbances of awareness and mentation, which may progress from forgetfulness and confusion to stupor and finally coma; (3) shifting combinations of neurologic signs,

including asterixis, rigidity, hyperreflexia, extensor plantar signs, and rarely, seizures; and (4) a characteristic (but nonspecific) symmetric, high-voltage, triphasic slow-wave (2 to 5 per second) pattern on the electroencephalogram. Asterixis ("liver flap," "flapping tremor") is a nonrhythmic asymmetric lapse in voluntary sustained position of the extremities, head, and trunk. It is best demonstrated by having the patient extend the arms and dorsiflex the hands. Because elicitation of asterixis depends on sustained voluntary muscle contraction, it is not present in the comatose patient. Asterixis is nonspecific and also occurs in patients with other forms of metabolic brain disease. Disturbances of sleep with reversal of sleep/wake cycles are among the earliest signs of encephalopathy. Alterations in personality, mood disturbances, confusion, deterioration in self-care and handwriting, and daytime somnolence are additional clinical features of encephalopathy. *Fetor hepaticus*, a unique musty odor of the breath and urine believed to be due to mercaptans, may be noted in patients with varying stages of hepatic encephalopathy.

Grading or classifying the stages of hepatic encephalopathy is often helpful in following the course of the illness and assessing response to therapy. One useful classification is shown in Table 289-4.

The diagnosis of hepatic encephalopathy is usually one of exclusion. There are no diagnostic liver function test abnormalities, although an elevated serum ammonia level in the appropriate clinical setting is highly suggestive of the diagnosis. Examination of the cerebrospinal fluid is unremarkable, and computed tomography of the brain shows no characteristic abnormalities until late in stage IV when cerebral edema may supervene. A number of conditions, particularly disorders related to acute and chronic alcoholism, can mimic the clinical features of hepatic encephalopathy. These include acute alcohol intoxication, sedative overdose, delirium tremens, Wernicke's encephalopathy, and Korsakoff's psychosis (Chap. 361). Subdural hematoma, meningitis, and hypoglycemia or other metabolic encephalopathies must also be considered, especially in patients with alcoholic cirrhosis. In young patients with liver disease and neurologic abnormalities, Wilson's disease should be excluded.

℞ TREATMENT

(See Fig. 289-4) Early recognition and prompt treatment of hepatic encephalopathy are essential. Patients with acute, severe hepatic en-

TABLE 289-4 *Clinical Stages of Hepatic Encephalopathy*

Stage	Mental Status	Asterixis	EEG
I	Euphoria or depression, mild confusion, slurred speech, disordered sleep	+/−	Triphasic waves
II	Lethargy, moderate confusion	+	Triphasic waves
III	Marked confusion, incoherent speech, sleeping but arousable	+	Triphasic waves
IV	Coma; initially responsive to noxious stimuli, later unresponsive	−	Delta activity

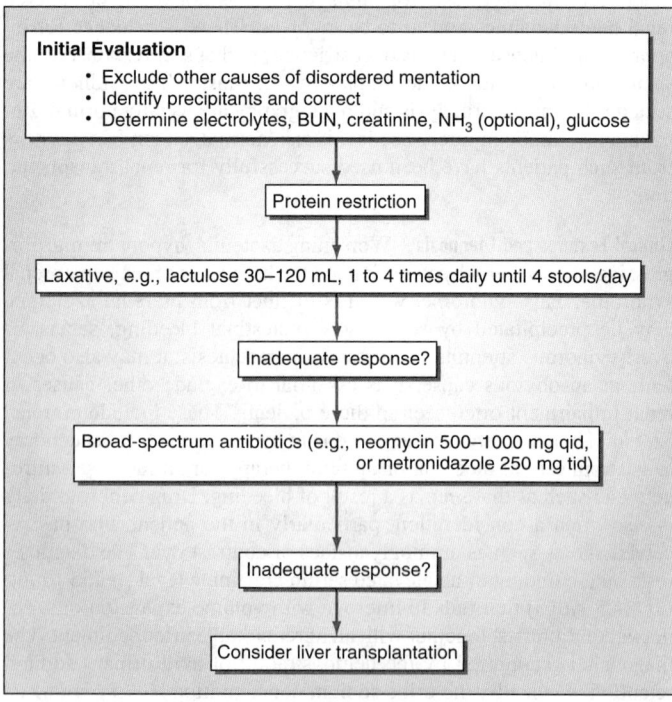

FIGURE 289-4 Approach to the patient with hepatic encephalopathy. BUN, blood urea nitrogen.

cephalopathy (stage IV) require the usual supportive measures for the comatose patient. Specific treatment of hepatic encephalopathy is aimed at (1) elimination or treatment of precipitating factors and (2) lowering of blood ammonia (and other toxin) levels by decreasing the absorption of protein and nitrogenous products from the intestine. In the setting of acute gastrointestinal bleeding, blood in the bowel should be promptly evacuated with laxatives (and enemas if necessary) in order to reduce the nitrogen load. Protein should be excluded from the diet, and constipation should be avoided. Ammonia absorption can be decreased by the administration of lactulose, a nonabsorbable disaccharide that acts as an osmotic laxative. Metabolism of lactulose by colonic bacteria may also result in an acid pH that favors conversion of ammonia to the poorly absorbed ammonium ion. In addition, lactulose may actually diminish ammonia production through its direct effects on bacterial metabolism. Acutely, lactulose syrup can be administered in a dose of 30 to 60 mL every hour until diarrhea occurs; thereafter the dose is adjusted (usually 15 to 30 mL three times daily) so that the patient has two to four soft stools daily. Intestinal ammonia production by bacteria can also be decreased by oral administration of a "nonabsorbable" antibiotic such as neomycin (0.5 to 1.0 g every 6 h). However, despite poor absorption, neomycin may reach sufficient concentrations in the bloodstream to cause renal toxicity. Equal benefits may be achieved with broad-spectrum antibiotics such as metronidazole. Flumazenil, a short-acting benzodiazepine antagonist, may have a role in management of hepatic encephalopathy precipitated by use of benzodiazepines, if there is a need for urgent therapy. Hemoperfusion to remove toxic substances and therapy directed primarily toward coincident cerebral edema in acute encephalopathy are also of unproven value. The efficacy of extracorporeal liver assist devices employing hepatocytes of porcine or human origin to bridge patients to recovery or transplantation is as yet unproven but is currently being studied.

Chronic encephalopathy may be effectively controlled by administration of lactulose. Management of patients with chronic encephalopathy should include dietary protein restriction (usually to 60 g/d) in combination with low doses of lactulose or neomycin. Nephrotoxicity or ototoxicity may be limiting in prolonged usage of neomycin. There are suggestions that vegetable protein may be preferable to animal protein.

OTHER SEQUELAE OF CIRRHOSIS ■ **Coagulopathy** Patients with cirrhosis often demonstrate a variety of abnormalities in both cellular and humoral clotting function. Thrombocytopenia may result from hypersplenism. In the alcoholic patient, there may be direct bone marrow suppression by ethanol. Diminished protein synthesis may lead to reduced production of fibrinogen (factor I), prothrombin (factor II), and factors V, VII, IX, and X. Reduction in levels of all factors except factor V may be worsened by the coincident malabsorption of the fat-soluble cofactor vitamin K due to cholestasis (Chap. 275). Of these, factor VII appears to be pivotal. In cirrhosis, it is the first of the factors to become depleted and, because of its short half-life, replacement with plasma often fails to correct an elevated prothrombin time. Preliminary studies suggest that selective replacement of factor VII can correct the prothrombin time in patients with cirrhosis.

Hepatocellular Carcinoma   See Chap. 78.

HYPOXEMIA AND HEPATOPULMONARY SYNDROME ■ **Definition and Pathogenesis** Mild hypoxemia occurs in approximately one-third of patients with chronic liver disease. The hepatopulmonary syndrome is typically manifest by hypoxemia, platypnea, and orthodeoxia. Hypoxemia usually results from right-to-left intrapulmonary shunts through dilatations in intrapulmonary vessels that can be detected by contrast-enhanced echocardiography or a macroaggregated albumin lung perfusion scan. The mechanisms of shunt formation are unclear, but one animal model suggests that endothelin-1 levels and pulmonary nitric oxide, raised in cirrhosis, correlate with degree of shunting.

℞ TREATMENT

No specific treatment is consistently effective, though large arteriovenous shunts may be embolized. It is now increasingly recognized that liver transplantation may eventually lead to amelioration of the hepatopulmonary syndrome in cases that have not yet been complicated by advanced pulmonary hypertension.

FURTHER READING

DIXON JB et al: Nonalcoholic fatty liver disease: Predictors of nonalcoholic steatohepatitis and liver disease in the severely obese. Gastroenterology 121:91, 2001

DUVOUX C et al: Effects of noradrenaline and albumin in patients with type I hepatorenal syndrome: A pilot study. Hepatology 36:374, 2002

KAPLAN MM et al: Medical progress: Primary biliary cirrhosis. N Engl J Med 335:1570, 1996

MCCULLOUGH AJ, O'CONNOR JFB: Alcoholic liver disease: Recommendations for the American College of Gastroenterology. Am J Gastroenterol 93:2022, 1998

RIORDAN SM, WILLIAMS R: Treatment of hepatic encephalopathy. N Engl J Med 337:473, 1997

RUNYON BA et al: Management of adult patients with ascites caused by cirrhosis. Hepatology 27:264, 1998

SHARARA AI et al: Gastroesophageal variceal hemorrhage. N Engl J Med 345:669, 2001

VILLANUEVA C et al: Endoscopic ligation compared with combined treatment with nadolol and isosorbide mononitrate to prevent recurrent variceal bleeding. N Engl J Med 345:647, 2001

290 | INFILTRATIVE, GENETIC, AND METABOLIC DISEASES AFFECTING THE LIVER
Daniel K. Podolsky

Many disseminated, systemic, or metabolic diseases involve the liver in a diffuse manner by the infiltration of abnormal cells or the accumulation of chemical substances or metabolites. Chemical accumulation may be extracellular or intracellular and may involve hepatocytes, Kupffer cells, or other elements of the reticuloendothelial system. Although infiltrative diseases may vary widely in cause and extrahepatic manifestations, the findings in the liver may be quite similar. Generalized enlargement and firmness of the liver, gradual and nonspecific deterioration of liver function, and, less often, signs of portal hypertension or ascites are typical features of this group of diseases. Differential diagnosis by clinical means may be difficult on occasion, but in patients in whom ancillary clinical findings do not establish the diagnosis, the diffusely infiltrated liver provides an excellent source of tissue for diagnostic purposes.

NONALCOHOLIC FATTY LIVER DISEASE (NAFLD), HEPATIC STEATOSIS (FATTY LIVER), AND NONALCOHOLIC STEATOHEPATITIS (NASH)

Slight to moderate enlargement of the liver due to a diffuse accumulation of neutral fat (triglycerides) in hepatocytes is an important clinical and pathologic finding. Imaging techniques such as computed tomography (CT), ultrasound, and magnetic resonance imaging (MRI) may each yield alterations suggesting increased fat in the liver. Several mechanisms can contribute to lipid accumulation in the liver. Fatty liver can be separated into two categories based on whether the fat droplets in the hepatocytes are macrovesicular or microvesicular (Table 290-1). In addition, fatty infiltration may be accompanied by necroinflammatory activity, a condition designated *nonalcoholic steatohepatitis*, a form of NAFLD. Although prospective data on natural history are limited, there is increasing evidence that patients may pro-

TABLE 290-1 *Causes of Hepatic Steatosis*

Macrovesicular (large fat droplets in hepatocytes)
  Alcohol, alcoholic liver disease[a]
  Insulin resistance
  Syndrome X (obesity, diabetes, hypertriglyceridemia, hypertension)
  Lipodystrophy
  Dysbetalipoproteinemias
  Protein-calorie malnutrition, starvation
  Total parenteral nutrition,[a] jejunoileal bypass
  Rapid weight loss
  Drugs,[a] e.g., methotrexate, aspirin, vitamin A, glucocorticoids,
    amiodarone, calcium channel blocker and synthetic estrogen,
    nucleoside analogues (ddI, AZT)
  Inflammatory bowel disease
Microvascular (small fat droplets in hepatocytes)
  Reye's syndrome
  Acute fatty liver of pregnancy
  Jamaican vomiting sickness
  Drugs, e.g., valproic acid, tetracycline, nucleoside analogues
  Environmental hepatotoxins (e.g., phosphorus, petrochemicals)

[a] May also be associated with necroinflammatory activity.

gress through several histologically distinct stages beginning with fatty liver and culminating in cirrhosis with intervening states of steatohepatitis and steatohepatitis with fibrosis (Fig. 290-1).

MACROVESICULAR FATTY LIVER   This is the most common type of fatty liver and is seen most frequently in alcoholism or alcoholic liver disease, diabetes mellitus, obesity, and prolonged parenteral nutrition. Hematoxylin and eosin-stained liver sections show hepatocytes with large, empty vacuoles with the nucleus "pushed" to the periphery of the cell. In general, fat in the liver is not damaging per se, and the fat will disappear with improvement or elimination of the predisposing condition.

Etiology   The major causes of fatty liver with macrovesicular fat depend on the age, geographic location, and metabolic-nutritional status of the patient population. *Chronic alcoholism* is the most common cause of hepatic steatosis in this country and in other countries with a high alcohol intake. The severity of fatty involvement is roughly proportional to the duration and degree of alcoholic excess. In addition, in western countries NAFLD/NASH is associated with obesity. Many of these patients (up to one-third) have type 2 diabetes and/or hyperlipidemia. The constellation of obesity, diabetes, hypertriglyceridemia, and hypertension has been designated *syndrome X* and has an especially strong association with progressive NAFLD. Age >45, obesity (body mass index ≥30), ratio of aspartate aminotransferase (AST)/ to alanine aminotransferase (ALT) >1, and diabetes are all associated with increased risk for development of significant fibrosis. Inflammatory activity when present may reflect the combined effects of oxidative stress, subsequent lipid peroxidation, and abnormal cytokine expression, especially increased tumor necrosis factor.

Protein malnutrition, especially in infancy and early childhood, accounts for most cases of severe fatty liver in the tropical zones of Africa, South America, and Asia. The hepatic changes may be associated with other clinical and pathologic features of kwashiorkor. *Jejunoileal bypass* for surgical treatment of morbid obesity was sometimes associated with severe fatty liver and hepatic failure that could be fatal. Ironically, patients with rapid weight loss or undergoing gastric bypass surgery for morbid obesity may also develop NAFLD. In patients with Cushing's syndrome and in those receiving large doses of glucocorticoids, fatty infiltration of the liver may occur. In many *chronic illnesses*, especially those complicated by impaired nutrition or malabsorption, increased fat is found in liver cells. For example, patients with severe ulcerative colitis, chronic pancreatitis, or protracted heart failure frequently have moderate hepatic steatosis at the time of death. Patients maintained on prolonged *total parenteral nutrition* may also develop a fatty liver. In some cases, fatty infiltration and steatohepatitis may occur in the absence of an identifiable cause.

Acute fatty liver is caused by a number of hepatotoxins and is frequently accompanied by signs and symptoms of liver failure. Carbon tetrachloride intoxication, DDT poisoning, and ingestion of substances containing yellow phosphorus result in severe hepatic steatosis. Acute and prolonged alcohol ingestion may also be considered in this category and may be associated with a rapidly enlarging and fat-laden liver.

Clinical Features   The signs and symptoms of hepatic steatosis are related to the degree of fat infiltration, the time course of its accumulation, and the underlying cause. The obese or diabetic patient with a chronic fatty liver is usually asymptomatic and has only mild tenderness over the enlarged liver. The liver function tests are normal or show mild elevations of alkaline phosphatase or aminotransferases. In contrast, the rapid accumulation of fat seen in the setting of hyperalimentation may lead to marked tenderness, presumably resulting from stretching of Glisson's capsule. Similarly, alcoholic patients with acute fatty liver following a bout of heavy drinking may have right upper quadrant pain and tenderness, often with laboratory evidence of cholestasis. The clinical presentation of fatty liver from hepatotoxins is similar to that of fulminant hepatic failure arising from any cause, with evidence of hepatic encephalopathy, marked elevations of prothrombin time and aminotransferases, and variable degrees of jaundice. Although steatohepatitis is generally thought to have a benign clinical course with improvement following elimination of the associated precipitant, in some individuals it may result in significant fibrosis and even cirrhosis. Recent studies indicate that substantial fibrosis or cirrhosis may be present in 15 to 50% of patients with NASH. In the only long-term follow-up study, 30% of patients with fibrosis had cirrhosis after 10 years. It is possible that some cases of "cryptogenic" cirrhosis are due to longstanding NASH and that the fat leaves the liver as end-stage liver disease develops.

Diagnosis   The findings of a firm, nontender, and generally enlarged liver with minimal hepatic dysfunction in a patient with chronic alcoholism, malnutrition, poorly controlled diabetes mellitus, or obesity should suggest hepatic steatosis. This can usually be detected by CT, MRI, or ultrasound. Modest elevations of aminotransferases are often found in association with hepatic steatohepatitis. A disproportional elevation in AST leading to an AST/ALT ratio >2 is generally associated with alcoholic hepatitis. When diagnostic uncertainty exists, needle biopsy of the liver will demonstrate the increased fat content, the presence of any fibrosis, and possibly the underlying primary disorder.

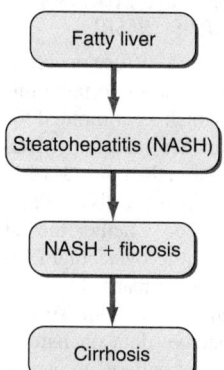

FIGURE 290-1 Hypothetical sequence of nonalcoholic fatty liver disease states. NASH, nonalcoholic steatohepatitis.

℞ TREATMENT

Adequate nutritional intake, removal of alcohol or offending toxins, and correction of any associated metabolic disorders usually result in recovery. There is no clinical rationale for the use of lipotropic agents such as choline. When indicated, attention should be directed to abstinence from alcohol, careful control of diabetes (by insulin therapy or use of oral hypoglycemic agents), weight loss, or correction of intestinal absorptive defects. In the alcoholic fatty liver, there is gradual disappearance of fat from the liver after 4 to 8 weeks of adequate diet and abstinence from alcohol. Similarly, fatty infiltration usually resolves within 2 weeks after discontinuation of parenteral hyperalimentation. Pilot studies in patients with NASH have suggested benefits from ursodiol, betaine (a precursor of S-adenosyl-methonine), and vitamin E and from phlebotomy. Troglitazone has shown some benefit in those patients with concomitant insulin resistance.

MICROVESICULAR FATTY LIVER This is the less common form of fatty liver. On microscopic examination, the fat is present in many small vacuoles. Although the droplets consist of triglycerides in both the macrovesicular and microvesicular forms, the reason for this difference in morphologic appearance is not clear.

Acute fatty liver of pregnancy (AFLP) is a syndrome that occurs late in pregnancy and is often associated with jaundice and hepatic failure. The liver is typically small. AFLP is more common when the mother is carrying a male fetus and may be associated with a deficiency of long-chain-3-hydroxy acyl COH dehydrogenase. AFLP usually necessitates termination of pregnancy due to the risk of rapid and fatal deterioration. Preeclampsia or the syndrome of *h*emolysis, *e*levated *l*iver enzymes, and *l*ow *p*latelet count (HELLP), which may complicate eclampsia, presents in a similar fashion and progresses to severe liver dysfunction, though typically with a normal size liver. Aminotransferase elevations are typically modest in all of these conditions (generally <500). If diagnosed in time, the disease usually resolves with termination of the pregnancy. Recurrence in subsequent pregnancies is rare.

Microvesicular fat accumulation also may be seen as a toxic reaction to valproic acid and with excessive doses of tetracycline. It is a typical finding in *Jamaican vomiting sickness*, which is caused by hypoglycin A present in unripened ackee fruit. The combination of lactic acidosis and severe liver injury with microvesicular fat has been described as a complication of nucleoside analogue therapy.

REYE'S SYNDROME (FATTY LIVER WITH ENCEPHALOPATHY) This acute illness is encountered exclusively in children <15 years. It is characterized clinically by vomiting and signs of progressive central nervous system damage, signs of hepatic injury, and hypoglycemia. Morphologically, there is extensive fatty vacuolization of the liver and renal tubules. There is mitochondrial dysfunction with decreased activity of hepatic mitochondrial enzymes. The cause is unknown, although viral agents and drugs, especially salicylates, have been implicated. Increased aspirin use and much higher serum salicylate levels in children with this illness than in the general population have been described during outbreaks of Reye's syndrome. Recognition of this relationship and reduced aspirin use in this setting may account for the decreasing incidence of Reye's syndrome. However, this illness may occur in the absence of exposure to salicylates. In fatal cases, the liver is enlarged and yellow with striking diffuse fatty microvacuolization of cells. Peripheral zonal hepatic necrosis has also been present in some cases. Fatty changes of the renal tubular cells, cerebral edema, and neuronal degeneration of the brain are the major extrahepatic changes. Electron-microscopic studies show structural alterations of mitochondria in liver, brain, and muscle.

The onset usually follows an upper respiratory tract infection, especially influenza or chickenpox. Within 1 to 3 days, persistent vomiting occurs, together with stupor, which usually progresses rapidly to generalized convulsions and coma. The liver is enlarged, but *jaundice is characteristically absent or minimal*. Elevations in serum aminotransferases and prothrombin time, hypoglycemia, metabolic acidosis, and elevated serum ammonia levels are the major laboratory findings. The mortality rate in Reye's syndrome is approximately 50%. Therapy consists of infusions of 20% glucose and fresh-frozen plasma, as well as intravenous mannitol to reduce the cerebral edema. Chronic liver disease has not been reported in survivors.

STORAGE DISEASES

Lipid storage diseases include the hereditary disorders of Gaucher's and Niemann-Pick diseases. Other rare diseases associated with increased fat in the liver include abetalipoproteinemia, Tangier disease, Fabry's disease, and types I and V hyperlipoproteinemia (Chap. 335).

Hepatic enlargement caused by distention of liver cells with glycogen is present in some poorly controlled diabetics and frequently in juvenile diabetes. More often, however, hepatomegaly is due to fatty infiltration (see above). Ketoacidosis and vigorous insulin therapy may further enhance hepatic enlargement.

HEPATIC MINERAL ACCUMULATION

WILSON'S DISEASE This is an uncommon inherited disorder of copper metabolism. Wilson's disease usually presents clinically in adolescence or young adulthood by which time there is excess copper accumulation in the liver and other tissues. Deficiency of the plasma copper protein ceruloplasmin is a characteristic feature. The accumulation appears to result from impaired copper excretion due to a mutation in a gene that encodes a P-type ATPase copper transporter. Clinically, patients may present in teenage or early adult years with chronic hepatitis, cirrhosis, or their complications. A small number of patients will present with fulminant hepatitis. Liver disease is often accompanied by softening and degeneration of the basal ganglia (hepatolenticular degeneration) due to copper deposition, which results in extrapyramidal neurologic and psychiatric symptoms. Brownish pigmentation of Descemet's membrane in the cornea (Kayser-Fleischer rings) is frequently present. Hemolytic anemia is also common, especially with fulminant disease. Liver biopsy may reveal findings ranging from fulminant hepatitis to chronic hepatitis and macronodular cirrhosis, in addition to excess copper levels. Typically, liver cells are ballooned and show increased glycogen with glycogen vacuolization in the nuclei. All patients under age 40 with unexplained chronic hepatitis or cirrhosis should be evaluated for possible Wilson's disease. Prompt diagnosis is important; treatment, which must be continued throughout life, can prevent progression of end-organ damage. →*For further discussion, see Chap. 339.*

HEMOCHROMATOSIS Hemochromatosis may be the most common genetic disorder of humans; it involves accumulation of abnormal amounts of iron due to inappropriate absorption from the intestine. Between 85 and 95% of patients with genetic hemochromatosis are homozygous for a point mutation (cystine to tyrosine at codon 282: C282). The liver, as a primary site of iron storage, is affected most directly. There is diffuse deposition of excess iron in hepatocytes, in contrast to the characteristic accumulation of iron in the reticuloendothelial compartment typical of secondary iron overload and hemosiderosis. Excess hepatic iron commonly results in hepatomegaly. Although liver function is initially well preserved, if the disease is untreated, progressive impairment is followed by the development of cirrhosis. Prompt diagnosis can permit the institution of effective lifelong therapy to reduce the iron load and halt progression of the disease. → *For further discussion, see Chap. 336.*

OTHER INFILTRATIVE AND METABOLIC DISEASES

α_1-ANTITRYPSIN DEFICIENCY Patients with homozygous deficiency of serum α_1-antitrypsin (α_1AT) are prone to develop emphysema in adult life. The disease is suggested by the absence of α_1-globulin on serum electrophoresis (α_1AT makes up 90% of this fraction normally) and confirmed by direct measurement of α_1AT. The exact phenotype can then be determined by electrophoresis. Although there are approximately 75 recognized alleles, only PiZ and PiS are associated with clinical disease. The molecular bases of these altered products have been related to single nucleic acid substitutions—e.g., PiZ is caused by a G (guanine) to A (adenine) transposition, which results in a substitution of a glutamic acid for lysine at residue 292 in the α_1AT protein. Hepatocytes of some patients with this deficiency contain globules positive with the periodic acid–Schiff reaction. Approximately 10% of children with homozygous deficiency (PiZZ phenotype) of α_1AT will develop significant liver disease, including neonatal hepatitis and progressive cirrhosis. It has been suggested that 15 to 20% of all chronic liver disease in infancy may be attributed to α_1AT deficiency. In adults, the most common manifestation of α_1AT deficiency is asymptomatic cirrhosis, which may progress from a micronodular to a macronodular state and may be complicated by the development of hepatocellular carcinoma. The occurrence of liver disease in these patients is not dependent on the development of lung disease. →*For further discussion, see Chap. 242.*

HURLER'S SYNDROME   This is an uncommon hereditary disease that is characterized by the widespread tissue deposition of mucopolysaccharide (chondroitin sulfate B and heparan sulfate) in many tissues. The liver is frequently enlarged and firm. Microscopically, Kupffer cells and other macrophages are enlarged and filled with metachromatic granular material. Cirrhosis may be a late complication. →*For further discussion, see Chap. 340.*

PORPHYRIAS   See Chap. 337.

RETICULOENDOTHELIAL DISORDERS   (See also Chaps. 52 and 98)

Moderate to massive hepatomegaly and splenomegaly occur frequently in the various types of *leukemia* and *lymphoma*. Jaundice, when present, is usually slight and results from hemolysis, although cholestasis may occasionally be associated with lymphoma as a paraneoplastic syndrome. Deep and protracted jaundice is distinctly rare and is caused by obstruction of the intrahepatic or extrahepatic bile ducts by tumor. Liver biopsy specimens reveal portal and sinusoidal infiltrates in most cases of leukemia, but the cellular pattern may be mixed and nonspecific. Liver biopsy is diagnostic in only 5% of patients with *Hodgkin's disease*. This percentage is increased in those with advanced disease or splenomegaly. Directed biopsy at laparoscopy or laparotomy is more likely to be positive than "blind" needle biopsy. Nonspecific histologic changes in the liver have been described in patients with lymphoma and may contribute to the abnormal liver function tests.

Myeloid metaplasia and other myeloproliferative disorders associated with extramedullary hematopoiesis produce hepatomegaly which may reach huge proportions, especially following splenectomy. Serum alkaline phosphatase elevations are often found. Ascites and portal hypertension, resulting from diffuse involvement of portal venules and lymphatics, are rare complications.

GRANULOMATOUS INFILTRATIONS

Perhaps as a result of the large population of mononuclear phagocytes, a number of systemic granulomatous diseases involve the liver, including sarcoidosis, miliary tuberculosis, histoplasmosis, brucellosis, schistosomiasis, berylliosis, and drug reactions (Table 290-2). In addition, isolated granulomas of no diagnostic importance may be found occasionally in patients with various forms of cirrhosis and hepatitis. The liver infiltrated by granulomas may be slightly enlarged and firm,

TABLE 290-2   *Some Causes of Hepatic Granulomas*

SYSTEMIC DISEASE	
Sarcoidosis	Berylliosis
Hodgkin's and non-Hodgkin's lymphoma	Crohn's disease
	Wegener's granulomatosis
Primary biliary cirrhosis	Granulomatous hepatitis, idiopathic
INFECTIONS	
Bacterial	Parasitic
Tuberculosis	Schistosomiasis
Mycobacterium avium-intracellulare	Rickettsial
Brucellosis	Q fever
Leprosy	Spirochetes
Viral	Syphilis
Epstein-Barr virus	Drugs
Cytomegalovirus	Sulfonamides
Chicken pox	Isoniazid
	Allopurinol

but hepatic dysfunction is usually limited. Increases in serum alkaline phosphatase are common and may range from mild to marked. Occasionally, mild serum elevations in aminotransferases are also present. In a few patients with sarcoidosis or brucellosis, portal hypertension may develop, and extensive postnecrotic scarring or postnecrotic cirrhosis may follow healing of the granulomatous lesions, as in schistosomiasis.

Needle biopsy of the liver often provides the first definite evidence of a systemic or disseminated granulomatous disease. In patients with sarcoidosis who have neither clinical nor laboratory evidence of hepatic involvement, needle biopsy shows sarcoid granulomas in about 80% of cases. In cases of suspected miliary tuberculosis, a portion of the biopsy should be cultured and stained for mycobacteria. The organism can be detected in the majority of cases, particularly when caseating granulomas are present. Serial sections of the biopsy specimen should be examined if granulomas are not apparent. Individual granulomas are rarely specific in their microscopic appearance, and final diagnosis usually requires other clinical, laboratory, or histologic data.

In approximately 20% of patients, it is not possible to identify a cause for the granulomatous infiltration. When these infiltrates are accompanied by fever of unknown origin, the diagnosis of *granulomatous hepatitis* should be considered. This is an uncommon disorder of unknown cause and is diagnosed by exclusion. While granulomatous hepatitis invariably responds to moderate doses of glucocorticoids, relapses are frequent, and such therapy should never be undertaken unless tuberculous disease or other causes of granulomatous infiltration have been excluded. This may include an initial empirical trial of antituberculous therapy.

AMYLOIDOSIS   (See also Chap. 310)   Systemic amyloidosis, whether primary and idiopathic, familial, or secondary to chronic inflammatory or neoplastic diseases, often involves the liver. Grossly, the liver infiltrated with amyloid is enlarged and pale and rubbery in consistency. Microscopically, the birefringent amyloid deposits appear as homogeneous waxy material within the space of Disse, often being concentrated in the periportal areas and associated with atrophy of adjacent liver cell plates. Selective involvement of the walls of blood vessels, especially of the hepatic arterioles, may be a striking feature of primary amyloidosis. With this possible exception, however, the hepatic lesions are the same in all forms of amyloidosis and are present in 60 to 90% of cases.

An enlarged and firm liver is found in about 60% of patients, and ascites occurs in advanced stages of the disease in about 20%. Jaundice, portal hypertension, and other signs of chronic liver disease are usually absent. Liver function changes, although frequent, correlate poorly with the extent of liver infiltration. Hypoalbuminemia and elevated serum alkaline phosphatase are common. Hypoalbuminemia, however, may be related to the presence of nephrosis; the prothrombin time is usually normal. The diagnosis is established by biopsy of rectum, skin, liver, or other involved organs and demonstration of the characteristic Congo red–staining deposits by polarizing microscopy.

AIDS-RELATED LIVER DISEASE

Liver disease has become an important cause of morbidity and mortality in patients with HIV/AIDS, due largely to complications derived from chronic active hepatitis involving co-infection with hepatitis B and/or C viruses (Chaps. 173 and 285). This has become particularly evident in the era of highly active antiretroviral therapy (HAART), which has been successful in decreasing the levels of HIV viremia (Chap. 173). Patients are living longer due to the beneficial effects of HAART, and their liver disease and its complications have assumed a more important role in determining the ultimate clinical course of these patients. The approach to such patients is discussed in detail in Chaps. 173 and 285. Other important sources of liver damage in HIV-infected individuals are the direct hepatotoxic effects of antiretroviral drugs used in the HAART regimens. This is particularly true of the non-nucleoside analogue nevirapine (Chap. 173) as well as certain of the nucleoside analogues and protease inhibitors. Finally, patients with advanced HIV diseases commonly have evidence of secondary liver disease, generally mild, that is due to hepatic involvement with other systemic diseases. In these patients, hepatic granulomatous disease is often present and may be caused by opportunistic infections, with *Mycobacterium avium-intracellulare* being a common pathogen. Cytomegalovirus hepatitis and hepatic mycoses are less common. AIDS cholangiopathy is a well-recognized entity. It exhibits features similar to those found in primary sclerosing cholangitis and is typically associated with cryptosporidia, microsporidia, and/or cytomegalovirus infection in the biliary tree. Papillary stenosis is frequently present.

FURTHER READING

AMERICAN GASTROENTEROLOGICAL ASSOCIATION: Medical Position Statement: Nonalcoholic fatty liver disease. Gastroenterology 123:1702, 2002

ANGULO P: Nonalcoholic fatty liver disease. N Engl J Med 346:1221, 2002

KNOX TA, OLANS LB: Liver disease in pregnancy. N Engl J Med 335:569, 1996

SCRIVER CR et al (eds): *The Metabolic and Molecular Bases of Inherited Disease*, 8th ed. New York, McGraw-Hill, 2001

ZAKIM D, BOYER TD: *Hepatology: A Textbook of Liver Disease*, 3d ed. Philadelphia, Saunders, 1996

291 LIVER TRANSPLANTATION
Jules L. Dienstag

Liver transplantation—the replacement of the native, diseased liver by a normal organ (allograft)—has matured from an experimental procedure reserved for desperately ill patients to an accepted, lifesaving operation applied much earlier in the natural history of end-stage liver disease. The preferred and technically most advanced approach is *orthotopic transplantation*, in which the native organ is removed and the donor organ is inserted in the same anatomic location. Pioneered in the 1960s by Starzl at the University of Colorado and, later, at the University of Pittsburgh and by Calne in Cambridge, England, liver transplantation is now performed routinely by dozens of centers throughout North America and western Europe. Success measured as 1-year survival has improved from ~30% in the 1970s to >85% today. These improved prospects for prolonged survival, dating back to the early 1980s, resulted from refinements in operative technique, improvements in organ procurement and preservation, advances in immunosuppressive therapy, and, perhaps most influentially, more enlightened patient selection and timing. Despite the perioperative morbidity and mortality, the technical and management challenges of the procedure, and its costs, liver transplantation has become the approach of choice for selected patients whose chronic or acute liver disease is progressive, life-threatening, and unresponsive to medical therapy. Based on the current level of success, the number of liver transplants has continued to grow each year; in 2000 to 2002, approximately 4500 patients received liver allografts in the United States. Still, the demand for new livers continues to outpace availability; in the same period, >16,000 patients in the United States were on a waiting list for a donor liver. In response to this drastic shortage of donor organs, many transplantation centers have begun to supplement cadaver-organ liver transplantation with living-donor transplantation.

INDICATIONS Potential candidates for liver transplantation are children and adults who, in the absence of contraindications (see below), suffer from severe, irreversible liver disease for which alternative medical or surgical treatments have been exhausted or are unavailable. *Timing of the operation is of critical importance.* Indeed, improved timing and better patient selection are felt to have contributed more to the increased success of liver transplantation in the 1980s and beyond than all the impressive technical and immunologic advances combined. Although the disease should be advanced, and although opportunities for spontaneous or medically induced stabilization or recovery should be allowed, the procedure should be done sufficiently early to give the surgical procedure a fair chance for success. Ideally, transplantation should be considered in patients with end-stage liver disease who are experiencing or have experienced a life-threatening complication of hepatic decompensation, whose quality of life has deteriorated to unacceptable levels, or whose liver disease will result predictably in irreversible damage to the central nervous system (CNS). If this is done sufficiently early, the patient will not have developed any contraindications or extrahepatic systemic deterioration. Although patients with well-compensated cirrhosis can survive for many years, many patients

with quasi-stable chronic liver disease have much more advanced disease than may be apparent. As discussed below, the better the status of the patient prior to transplantation, the higher will be the anticipated success rate of transplantation. The decision about *when* to transplant is complex and requires the combined judgment of an experienced team of hepatologists, transplant surgeons, anesthesiologists, and specialists in support services, not to mention the well-informed consent of the patient and the patient's family.

Transplantation in Children Indications for transplantation in children are listed in Table 291-1. The most common is *biliary atresia. Inherited or genetic disorders of metabolism* associated with liver failure constitute another major indication for transplantation in children and adolescents. In Crigler-Najjar disease type I and in certain hereditary disorders of the urea cycle and of amino acid or lactate-pyruvate metabolism, transplantation may be the only way to prevent impending deterioration of CNS function, despite the fact that the native liver is structurally normal. Combined heart and liver transplantation has yielded dramatic improvement in cardiac function and in cholesterol levels in children with homozygous familial hypercholesterolemia; combined liver and kidney transplantation has been successful in patients with hereditary oxalosis. In hemophiliacs with transfusion-associated hepatitis and liver failure, liver transplantation has been associated with recovery of normal factor VIII synthesis.

Transplantation in Adults Liver transplantation is indicated for end-stage *cirrhosis* of all causes (Table 291-1). In sclerosing cholangitis and *Caroli's disease* (multiple cystic dilatations of the intrahepatic biliary tree), recurrent infections and sepsis associated with inflammatory and fibrotic obstruction of the biliary tree may be an indication for transplantation. Because prior biliary surgery complicates, and is a relative contraindication for, liver transplantation, surgical diversion of the biliary tree has been all but abandoned for patients with sclerosing cho-

TABLE 291-1 *Indications for Liver Transplantation*

Children	Adults
Biliary atresia	Primary biliary cirrhosis
Neonatal hepatitis	Secondary biliary cirrhosis
Congenital hepatic fibrosis	Primary sclerosing cholangitis
Alagille's disease[a]	Caroli's disease[c]
Byler's disease[b]	Cryptogenic cirrhosis
α_1-Antitrypsin deficiency	Chronic hepatitis with cirrhosis
Inherited disorders of metabolism	Hepatic vein thrombosis
Wilson's disease	Fulminant hepatitis
Tyrosinemia	Alcoholic cirrhosis
Glycogen storage diseases	Chronic viral hepatitis
Lysosomal storage diseases	Primary hepatocellular malignancies
Protoporphyria	Hepatic adenomas
Crigler-Najjar disease type I	
Familial hypercholesterolemia	
Hereditary oxalosis	
Hemophilia	

[a] Arteriohepatic dysplasia, with paucity of bile ducts, and congenital malformations, including pulmonary stenosis.
[b] Intrahepatic cholestasis, progressive liver failure, mental and growth retardation.
[c] Multiple cystic dilatations of the intrahepatic biliary tree.

langitis. In patients who undergo transplantation for *hepatic vein thrombosis (Budd-Chiari syndrome)*, postoperative anticoagulation is essential; underlying myeloproliferative disorders may have to be treated but are not a contraindication to liver transplantation. If a donor organ can be located quickly, before life-threatening complications—including cerebral edema—set in, patients with *fulminant hepatitis* are candidates for liver transplantation. Initially controversial but now routine candidates for liver transplantation are patients with *alcoholic cirrhosis*, *chronic viral hepatitis*, and *primary hepatocellular malignancies*. Although all three of these categories are considered to be high risk, liver transplantation can be offered to carefully selected patients, and, currently chronic hepatitis C and alcoholic liver disease are the most common indications for liver transplantation, accounting for 40% of all adult candidates for the procedure. Patients with alcoholic cirrhosis can be considered as candidates for transplantation if they meet strict criteria for abstinence and reform. Patients with chronic hepatitis C have early allograft and patient survival comparable to those of other subsets of patients after transplantation; however, reinfection in the donor organ is universal, recurrent hepatitis C is insidiously progressive, the impact of antiviral therapy is limited, and cirrhosis and late organ failure (beyond 5 years) are being recognized with increasing frequency. In patients with chronic hepatitis B, in the absence of measures to prevent recurrent hepatitis B, survival after transplantation is reduced by approximately 10 to 20%; however, prophylactic use of hepatitis B immune globulin (HBIg) during and after transplantation increases the success of transplantation to a level comparable to that seen in patients with nonviral causes of liver decompensation. The specific oral antiviral drugs lamivudine and adefovir dipivoxil (Chap. 287) can be used for both prophylaxis against, and treatment of, recurrent hepatitis B, facilitating further the management of patients undergoing liver transplantation for end-stage hepatitis B. Issues of disease recurrence are discussed in more detail below. Patients with nonmetastatic primary hepatobiliary tumors—primary hepatocellular carcinoma, cholangiocarcinoma, hepatoblastoma, angiosarcoma, epithelioid hemangioendothelioma, and multiple or massive hepatic adenomata—have undergone liver transplantation; however, for hepatobiliary malignancies, overall survival is significantly lower than that for other categories of liver disease. To minimize the very high likelihood of recurrent tumor after transplantation, some centers are evaluating experimental adjuvant chemotherapy protocols. Some transplantation centers have reported excellent long-term, recurrence-free survival in patients with unresectable hepatocellular carcinoma for single tumors <5 cm in diameter or for three or fewer lesions all <3 cm. Consequently, most centers restrict liver transplanation to patients whose hepatic malignancies are confined to these limits. Because the likelihood of recurrent cholangiocarcinoma is almost universal, this tumor is no longer considered an indication for transplantation.

CONTRAINDICATIONS *Absolute contraindications* for transplantation include life-threatening systemic diseases, uncontrolled extrahepatic bacterial or fungal infections, preexisting advanced cardiovascular or pulmonary disease, multiple uncorrectable life-threatening congenital anomalies, metastatic malignancy, active drug or alcohol abuse, and HIV infection (Table 291-2). Because carefully selected patients in their sixties and even seventies have undergone transplantation successfully, advanced age per se is no longer considered an absolute contraindication; however, in older patients, a more thorough preoperative evaluation should be undertaken to exclude ischemic cardiac disease. Advanced age (>70 years), however, may be considered a *relative contraindication*—that is, a factor to be taken into account with other relative contraindications. Other relative contraindications include portal vein thrombosis, preexisting renal disease not associated with liver disease, intrahepatic or biliary sepsis, severe hypoxemia resulting from right-to-left intrapulmonary shunts, previous extensive hepatobiliary surgery, and any uncontrolled serious psychiatric disorder. Any one of these relative contraindications is insufficient in and

TABLE 291-2 *Contraindications to Liver Transplantation*

Absolute	Relative
Uncontrolled extrahepatobiliary infection	Age >70
Active, untreated sepsis	Prior extensive hepatobiliary surgery
Uncorrectable, life-limiting congenital anomalies	Portal vein thrombosis
Active substance or alcohol abuse	Renal failure
Advanced cardiopulmonary disease	Previous extrahepatic malignancy
Extrahepatobiliary malignancy	Severe obesity
Metastatic malignancy to the liver	Severe malnutrition/wasting
Cholangiocarcinoma	Medical noncompliance
AIDS	HIV seropositivity
Life-threatening systemic diseases	Intrahepatic sepsis
	Severe hypoxemia secondary to right-to-left intrapulmonary shunts
	Uncontrolled psychiatric disorder

of itself to preclude transplantation. For example, the problem of portal vein thrombosis can be overcome by constructing a graft from the donor liver portal vein to the recipient's superior mesenteric vein. Now that highly active antiretroviral therapy has dramatically improved the survival of persons with HIV infection (Chap. 173), and because chronic hepatitis C has emerged as a serious source of morbidity and mortality in the HIV-infected population, the applicability of liver transplantation to this previously excluded patient group is being reexamined. Clinical trials of liver transplantation for patients with HIV infection are in progress.

TECHNICAL CONSIDERATIONS ■ **Cadaver Donor Selection** Cadaver donor livers for transplantation are procured primarily from victims of head trauma. Organs from brain-dead donors up to age 60 are acceptable if the following criteria are met: hemodynamic stability, adequate oxygenation, absence of bacterial or fungal infection, absence of abdominal trauma, absence of hepatic dysfunction, and serologic exclusion of hepatitis B and C viruses and HIV. Occasionally, organs from donors with hepatitis B and C are used, e.g., for recipients with prior hepatitis B and C, respectively. Donor organs with antibody to hepatitis B core antigen (anti-HBc) are used rarely, when the need is especially urgent, and recipients of these organs are treated prophylactically with HBIg and other antiviral drugs. Cardiovascular and respiratory functions are maintained artificially until the liver can be removed. Compatibility in ABO blood group and organ size between donor and recipient are important considerations in donor selection; however, ABO-incompatible or reduced-donor-organ transplants can be performed in emergency or marked donor-scarcity situations. Tissue typing for HLA matching is not required, and preformed cytotoxic HLA antibodies do not preclude liver transplantation. Following perfusion with cold electrolyte solution, the donor liver is removed and packed in ice. The use of University of Wisconsin (UW) solution, rich in lactobionate and raffinose, has permitted the extension of cold ischemic time up to 20 h; however, 12 h may be a more reasonable limit. Improved techniques for harvesting multiple organs from the same donor have increased the availability of donor livers, but the availability of donor livers is far outstripped by the demand. Currently, in the United States, all donor livers are distributed through a nationwide organ-sharing network [United Network of Organ Sharing (UNOS)] designed to allocate available organs based on regional considerations and recipient acuity. Recipients who require the highest level of care (intensive care) have the highest priority, but allocation strategies that balance highest urgency against best outcomes continue to evolve to distribute cadaver organs most effectively. Allocation based on the Child-Turcotte-Pugh (CTP) score, which uses five clinical variables (encephalopathy stage, ascites, bilirubin, albumin, and prothrombin time) and waiting time, has been supplanted by allocation based upon urgency alone, calculated by the Model for End-Stage Liver Disease (MELD) score. The MELD score is based upon a mathematical model that includes bilirubin, creatinine, and prothrombin time expressed as international normalized ratio (INR) (Table 291-3). Neither waiting time (except as a tie breaker between two potential recipients with the same MELD scores) nor posttransplantation outcome is taken into account, but the MELD score has been shown to be the best predictor of pretransplantation mortality, satisfies the prevailing view that medical need should be the decisive determinant, and eliminates both the subjectivity inherent in the CTP scoring system (presence and degree of ascites and hepatic encephalopathy) and the differences in waiting times among different regions of the country. Because candidates for liver transplantation who have hepatocellular carcinoma may not be sufficiently decompensated to compete for donor organs based upon urgency criteria alone, and because protracted waiting for cadaver donor organs results often in tumor growth beyond acceptable limits for transplantation, such patients are assigned extra MELD points (Table 291-3).

TABLE 291-3 *United Network for Organ Sharing (UNOS) Liver Transplantation Waiting List Criteria*

PREVIOUS ALLOCATION SCHEME (IN ORDER OF DESCENDING URGENCY)

Status 1	Fulminant hepatic failure (including primary graft nonfunction and hepatic artery thrombosis within 7 days after transplantation as well as acute decompensated Wilson's disease)[a]
Status 2A	Chronic liver disease with CTP[b] score ≥ 10, in intensive care unit, predicted <7 days to live, plus one of following: hepatic encephalopathy ≥ stage III, unresponsive variceal bleeding, heptorenal syndrome, refractory ascites or hepatic hydrothorax, coagulopathy with ongoing bleeding (cannot have extrahepatic sepsis, high-dose or double pressor dependency, or multiorgan failure)
Status 2B	Chronic liver disease with CTP score ≥ 10 or CTP score ≥ 7 plus one of following: variceal bleeding, heptorenal syndrome, history of spontaneous bacterial periotonitis, refractory ascites or hepatic hydrothorax, refractory bleeding
Status 3	CTP score ≥ 7
Status 7	Inactive

CURRENT ALLOCATION SCHEME

The Model for End-Stage Liver Disease (MELD) score, on a continuous scale,[c] determines allocation of donor organs. This model is based upon the following calculation:

$3.78 \times \log_e$ bilirubin (mg/100 mL) $+ 11.2 \times \log_e$ international normalized ratio (INR) $+ 9.57 \times \log_e$ creatinine (mg/100 mL) $+ 6.43$ ($\times$ 0 for alcoholic and cholestatic liver disease, $\times$ 1 for all other types of liver disease).[d,e,f]

Online calculators to determine MELD scores are available, such as *www.mayoclinic.org/gi-rst/mayomodel6.htm*

[a] For children < 18 years, status 1 includes acute or chronic liver failure plus hospitalization in an intensive care unit or inborn errors of metabolism.
[b] Child-Turcotte-Pugh (CTP) score components

Points	1	2	3
Encephalopathy	None	Stages I–II	Stages III–IV
Ascites	Absent	Slight, responsive	Moderate-severe
Bilirubin (mg/100 mL)	<2	2–3	>3
Albumin (g/100 mL)	>3.5	2.8–3.5	<2.8
Prothrombin time	<15 s	15–17 s	>17 s

The CTP score is calculated by assigning 1 point for any feature in column 1, 2 points for any feature in column 2, and 3 points for any feature in column 3. Class A = ≤6; class B = 7–9; class C = ≥10. For cholestatic disorders, such as primary biliary cirrhosis, primary sclerosing cholangitic, etc., the bilirubin categories are <4, 4–10, and >10.
[c] Instead of the 4 categories of severity in the previous system and 8 potential CTP scores between 7 and 15, the MELD scale is continuous, with 34 levels ranging between 6 and 40. The MELD scale replaces status 2A, 2B, and 3 (and 7), but status 1 is retained for those with the highest priority. Donor organs rarely become available unless the MELD score exceeds 20 to 30.
[d] Patients with hepatocellular carcinoma receive an extra 20 (for stage T1) or 24 (for stage T2) points. An α-fetoprotein level ≥ 500 ng/mL is considered as stage I hepatocellular carcinoma even without evidence for a tumor on imaging.
[e] Creatinine is included, because renal function is a validated predictor of survival in patients with liver disease. For adults undergoing dialysis twice a week, the creatinine in the equation is set to 4 mg/100 mL.
[f] For children <18 years, the Pediatric End-Stage Liver Disease (PELD) scale is used. This scale is based upon albumin, bilirubin, INR, growth failure, and age. Status 1 is retained, but the PELD replaces status 2 and 3.

Living-Donor Transplantation Occasionally, especially for liver transplantation in children, one cadaver organ can be split between two (one adult and one child) recipients. A more viable alternative, transplantation of the right lobe of the liver from a healthy adult into an adult recipient, is gaining increasing popularity. Living-donor transplantation of the left lobe (left lateral segment), introduced in the early 1990s to alleviate the extreme shortage of donor organs for small children, accounts currently for approximately a third of all liver transplantation procedures in children. Driven by the shortage of cadaver organs, living-donor transplantation involving the more sizable right lobe is being considered with increasing frequency in adults. More than 500 such procedures were done in 2001, representing >5% of all liver transplant operations done in the United States.

Living-donor transplantation can reduce waiting time and cold-ischemia time; is done under elective, rather than emergency, circumstances; and may be lifesaving in recipients who cannot afford to wait for a cadaver donor. The downside, of course, is the risk to the healthy donor (a mean of 10 weeks of medical disability; biliary complications in ~5%; postoperative complications such as wound infection, small-bowel obstruction, and incisional hernias in 9 to 19%; and, even, in 0.2 to 0.4%, death) as well as the increased frequency of biliary (15 to 32%) and vascular (10%) complications in the recipient. Potential donors must participate voluntarily without coercion, and transplantation teams should go to great lengths to exclude subtle coercive or inappropriate psychological factors as well as to outline carefully to both donor and recipient the potential benefits and risks of the procedure. Donors for the procedure should be 18 to 60 years old; have a compatible blood type with the recipient; have no chronic medical problems or history of major abdominal surgery; be related genetically or emotionally to the recipient; and pass an exhaustive series of clinical, biochemical, and serologic evaluations to unearth disqualifying medical disorders. The recipient should meet the same UNOS criteria for liver transplantation as recipients of a cadaver donor allograft.

Surgical Technique Removal of the recipient's native liver is technically difficult, particularly in the presence of portal hypertension with its associated collateral circulation and extensive varices, and even more so in the presence of scarring from previous abdominal operations. The combination of portal hypertension and coagulopathy (elevated prothrombin time and thrombocytopenia) may translate into large blood product transfusion requirements. After the portal vein and infrahepatic and suprahepatic inferior vena cavae are dissected, the hepatic artery and common bile duct are dissected. Then, the native liver is removed and the donor organ inserted. During the anhepatic phase, coagulopathy, hypoglycemia, hypocalcemia, and hypothermia are encountered and must be managed by the anesthesiology team. Caval, portal vein, hepatic artery, and bile duct anastomoses are performed in succession, the last by end-to-end suturing of the donor and recipient common bile ducts or by choledochojejunostomy to a Roux en Y loop if the recipient common bile duct cannot be used for reconstruction (e.g., in sclerosing cholangitis). A typical transplant operation lasts 8 h, with a range of 6 to 18 h. Because of excessive bleeding, large volumes of blood, blood products, and volume expanders may be required during surgery; however, blood requirements have fallen sharply with improvements in surgical technique and experience.

As noted above, emerging alternatives to orthotopic liver transplantation include split-liver grafts, in which one donor organ is divided and inserted into two recipients; and living-donor procedures, in which the left (for children) or the right (for adults) lobe of the liver is harvested from a living donor for transplantation into the recipient. In the adult procedure, once the right lobe is removed from the donor, the donor right hepatic vein is anastomosed to the recipient right hepatic vein remnant, followed by donor-to-recipient anastomoses of the portal vein and then the hepatic artery. Finally, the biliary anastomosis is performed, duct-to-duct if practical or via Roux-en-Y anastomosis. Heterotopic liver transplantation, in which the donor liver is inserted without removal of the native liver, has met with very limited success and acceptance, except in a very small number of centers. To support desperately ill patients until a suitable donor organ can be identified, several transplantation centers are studying extracorporeal perfusion with bioartificial liver cartridges constructed from hepatocytes bound to hollow fiber systems and used as temporary hepatic-assist devices, but their efficacy remains to be established. Areas of research with the potential to overcome the shortage of donor organs include hepatocyte transplantation and xenotransplantation with genetically modified organs of nonhuman origin (e.g., swine).

POSTOPERATIVE COURSE AND MANAGEMENT ■ **Immunosuppressive Therapy**
The introduction in 1980 of cyclosporine as an immunosuppressive agent contributed substantially to the improvement in survival after liver transplantation. Cyclosporine, a calcineurin inhibitor, blocks early activation of T cells and is specific for T cell functions that result from the interaction of the T cell with its receptor and that involve the calcium-dependent signal transduction pathway. As a result, the activity of cyclosporine leads to inhibition of lymphokine gene activation, blocking interleukins 2, 3, and 4, tumor necrosis factor α, as well as other lymphokines. Cyclosporine also inhibits B cell functions. This process occurs without affecting rapidly dividing cells in the bone marrow, which may account for the reduced frequency of posttransplantation systemic infections. The most common and important side effect of cyclosporine therapy is nephrotoxicity. Cyclosporine causes dose-dependent renal tubular injury and direct renal artery vasospasm. Following renal function, therefore, is important in monitoring cyclosporine therapy, perhaps even a more reliable indicator than blood levels of the drug. Nephrotoxicity is reversible and can be managed by dose reduction. Other adverse effects of cyclosporine therapy include hypertension, hyperkalemia, tremor, hirsutism, glucose intolerance, and gum hyperplasia.

Tacrolimus (originally labeled FK 506) is a macrolide lactone antibiotic isolated from a Japanese soil fungus, *Streptomyces tsukubaensis*. It has the same mechanism of action as cyclosporine but is 10 to 100 times more potent. Initially applied as "rescue" therapy for patients in whom rejection occurred despite the use of cyclosporine, tacrolimus was shown in two large, multicenter, randomized trials to be associated with a reduced frequency of acute rejection, refractory rejection, and chronic rejection. Although patient and graft survival are the same with these two drugs, the advantage of tacrolimus in minimizing episodes of rejection, reducing the need for additional glucocorticoid doses, and reducing the likelihood of bacterial and cytomegalovirus infection has simplified the management of patients undergoing liver transplantation. In addition, the oral absorption of tacrolimus is more predictable than that of cyclosporine, especially during the early postoperative period when T-tube drainage interferes with the enterohepatic circulation of cyclosporine. As a result, in most transplantation centers, tacrolimus has now supplanted cyclosporine for primary immunosuppression, and many centers rely on oral, rather than intravenous, administration from the outset. For transplantation centers that prefer cyclosporine, a new, better-absorbed, microemulsion preparation is now available.

Although tacrolimus is more potent than cyclosporine, it is also more toxic and more likely to be discontinued for adverse events. The toxicity of tacrolimus is similar to that of cyclosporine; nephrotoxicity and neurotoxicity are the most commonly encountered adverse effects, and neurotoxicity (tremor, seizures, hallucinations, psychoses, coma) is more likely and more severe in tacrolimus-treated patients. Both drugs can cause diabetes mellitus, but tacrolimus does not cause hirsutism or gingival hyperplasia. Because of overlapping toxicity between cyclosporine and tacrolimus, especially nephrotoxicity, and because tacrolimus reduces cyclosporine clearance, these two drugs should not be used together. Because 99% of tacrolimus is metabolized by the liver, hepatic dysfunction reduces its clearance; in primary graft nonfunction (when, for technical reasons or because of ischemic dam-

age prior to its insertion, the allograft is defective and does not function normally from the outset) tacrolimus doses have to be reduced substantially, especially in children. Both cyclosporine and tacrolimus are metabolized by the cytochrome P450 IIIA system, and, therefore, drugs that induce cytochrome P450 (e.g., phenytoin, phenobarbital, carbamazepine, rifampin) reduce available levels of cyclosporine and tacrolimus; drugs that inhibit cytochrome P450 (e.g., erythromycin, fluconazole, ketoconazole, clotrimazole, itraconazole, verapamil, diltiazem, nicardipine, cimetidine, danazol, metoclopramide, bromocriptine) increase cyclosporine and tacrolimus blood levels. Like azathioprine, cyclosporine and tacrolimus appear to be associated with a risk of lymphoproliferative malignancies (see below), which may occur earlier after cyclosporine or tacrolimus than after azathioprine therapy. Because of these side effects, combinations of cyclosporine or tacrolimus with prednisone and azathioprine—all at reduced doses—are preferable regimens for immunosuppressive therapy.

In patients with pretransplant renal dysfunction or renal deterioration that occurs intraoperatively or immediately postoperatively, tacrolimus or cyclosporine therapy may not be practical; under these circumstances, induction or maintenance of immunosuppression with monoclonal antibodies to T cells, OKT3, may be appropriate. Therapy with OKT3 has been especially effective in reversing acute rejection in the posttransplant period and is the standard treatment for acute rejection that fails to respond to methylprednisolone boluses. Intravenous infusions of OKT3 may be complicated by transient fever, chills, and diarrhea. When this drug is used to induce immunosuppression initially or to provide "rescue" in those who reject despite "conventional" therapy, the incidence of bacterial, fungal, and especially cytomegalovirus infections is increased during and after such therapy. In some centers, ganciclovir antiviral therapy is initiated prophylactically as a routine along with OKT3. Because OKT3 is such a potent immunosuppressive agent, its use is more likely to be complicated by opportunistic infection or lymphoproliferative disorders; therefore, and because of the availability of alternative immunosuppressive drugs, OKT3 is used less often nowadays. Another immunosuppressive drug being used for patients undergoing liver transplantation is mycophenolic acid, a nonnucleoside purine metabolism inhibitor derived as a fermentation product from several *Penicillium* species. Mycophenolate has been shown to be better than azathioprine, when used with other standard immunosuppressive drugs, in preventing rejection after renal transplantation and has been adopted as well for use in liver transplantation. The most common adverse effects of mycophenolate are leukopenia and gastrointestinal complaints. Rapamycin, an inhibitor of later events in T cell activation, is yet another drug undergoing evaluation as an immunosuppressive agent.

The most important principle of immunosuppression is that the ideal approach strikes a balance between immunosuppression and immunologic competence. Given sufficient immunosuppression, acute liver allograft rejection is always reversible; however, if the cumulative dose of immunosuppressive therapy is too large, the patient will succumb to opportunistic infection. Therefore, immunosuppressive drugs must be used judiciously, with strict attention to the infectious consequences of such therapy. In this vein, efforts have been made to minimize the use of glucocorticoids, a mainstay of immunosuppressive regimens, and, in some instances, steroid-free immunosuppression can be achieved.

Postoperative Complications Complications of liver transplantation can be divided into hepatic and nonhepatic categories (Tables 291-4 and 291-5). In addition, both immediately postoperative and late complications are encountered. Patients who undergo liver transplantation as a rule have been chronically ill for protracted periods and may be malnourished and wasted. The impact of such chronic illness and the multisystem failure that accompanies liver failure continues to require attention in the postoperative period. Because of the massive fluid losses and fluid shifts that occur during the operation, patients may remain fluid overloaded during the immediate postoperative period, straining cardiovascular reserve; this effect can be amplified in the face

TABLE 291-4 *Nonhepatic Complications of Liver Transplantation*

Fluid overload	
Cardiovascular instability	Arrhythmias
	Congestive heart failure
	Cardiomyopathy
Pulmonary compromise	Pneumonia
	Pulmonary capillary vascular permeability
	Fluid overload
Renal dysfunction	Prerenal azotemia
	Hypoperfusion injury (acute tubular necrosis)
	Drug nephrotoxicity
	↓ Renal blood flow secondary to ↑ intraabdominal pressure
Hematologic	Anemia 2° to gastrointestinal and/or intraabdominal bleeding
	Hemolytic anemia, aplastic anemia
	Thrombocytopenia
Infection	Bacterial: early, common postoperative infections
	Fungal/parasitic: late, opportunistic infections
	Viral: late, opportunistic infections, recurrent hepatitis
Neuropsychiatric	Seizures
	Encephalopathy
	Depression
	Difficult psychosocial adjustment
Diseases of donor	Infectious
	Malignant
Malignancy	B-cell lymphoma (posttransplantation lymphoproliferative disorders)

of transient renal dysfunction and pulmonary capillary vascular permeability. Continuous monitoring of cardiovascular and pulmonary function, measures to maintain the integrity of the intravascular compartment and to treat extravascular volume overload, and scrupulous attention to potential sources and sites of infection are of paramount importance. Cardiovascular instability may also result from the electrolyte imbalance that may accompany reperfusion of the donor liver. Pulmonary function may be compromised further by paralysis of the right hemidiaphragm associated with phrenic nerve injury. The hyperdynamic state with increased cardiac output that is characteristic of patients with liver failure reverses rapidly after successful liver transplantation.

Other immediate management issues include renal dysfunction; prerenal azotemia, acute kidney injury associated with hypoperfusion (acute tubular necrosis), and renal toxicity caused by antibiotics, tacrolimus, or cyclosporine are frequently encountered in the postoperative period, sometimes necessitating dialysis. Occasionally, postoperative intraperitoneal bleeding may be sufficient to increase intraabdominal pressure, which, in turn, may reduce renal blood flow; this effect is rapidly reversible when abdominal distention is relieved by exploratory laparotomy to identify and ligate the bleeding site and to remove intraperitoneal clot. Anemia may also result from acute upper gastrointestinal bleeding or from transient hemolytic anemia, which may be autoimmune, especially when blood group O livers are transplanted into blood group A or B recipients. This autoimmune hemolytic anemia is mediated by donor intrahepatic lymphocytes that recognize red blood cell A or B antigens on recipient erythrocytes. Transient in nature, this process resolves once the donor liver is repopulated by recipient bone marrow–derived lymphocytes; the hemolysis can be treated by transfusing blood group O red blood cells and/or by administering higher doses of glucocorticoids. Transient thrombocytopenia is also commonly encountered. Aplastic anemia, a late occurrence, is rare but has been reported in almost 30% of patients who underwent liver transplantation for acute, severe hepatitis of unknown cause.

Bacterial, fungal, or viral infections are common and may be life-threatening postoperatively. Early after transplant surgery, common postoperative infections predominate—pneumonia, wound infections, infected intraabdominal collections, urinary tract infections, and intra-

venous line infections—rather than opportunistic infections; these infections may involve the biliary tree and liver as well. Beyond the first postoperative month, the toll of immunosuppression becomes evident, and opportunistic infections—cytomegalovirus, herpes viruses, fungal infections (*Aspergillus*, *Candida*, cryptococcal disease), mycobacterial infections, parasitic infections (*Pneumocystis*, *Toxoplasma*), bacterial infections (*Nocardia*, *Legionella*, and *Listeria*)—predominate. Rarely, early infections represent those transmitted with the donor liver, either infections present in the donor or infections acquired during procurement processing. De novo viral hepatitis infections acquired from the donor organ or, almost unheard of nowadays, from transfused blood products occur after typical incubation periods for these agents (well beyond the first month). Obviously, infections in an immunosuppressed host demand early recognition and prompt management; prophylactic antibiotic therapy is administered routinely in the immediate postoperative period. Use of sulfamethoxazole with trimethoprim reduces the incidence of postoperative *Pneumocystis carinii* pneumonia.

Neuropsychiatric complications include seizures (commonly associated with cyclosporine and tacrolimus toxicity), encephalopathy, depression, and difficult psychosocial adjustment. Rarely, diseases are transmitted by the allograft from the donor to the recipient. In addition to viral and bacterial infections, malignancies of donor origin have occurred. Posttransplantation lymphoproliferative disorders, especially B cell lymphoma, are a recognized complication associated with immunosuppressive drugs such as azathioprine, tacrolimus, and cyclosporine (see above). Epstein-Barr virus has been shown to play a contributory role in some of these tumors, which may regress when immunosuppressive therapy is reduced.

Long-term complications after liver transplantation attributable primarily to immunosuppressive medications include diabetes mellitus (associated with glucocorticoids) as well as hypertension, hyperlipidemia, and chronic renal insufficiency (associated with cyclosporine and tacrolimus). Monitoring and treating these disorders is a routine component of posttransplantation care; in some cases, they respond to changes in immunosuppressive regimen, while in others, specific treatment of the disorder is introduced.

Hepatic Complications Hepatic dysfunction after liver transplantation is similar to the hepatic complications encountered after major abdominal and cardiothoracic surgery; however, in addition, there may be complications such as primary graft failure, vascular compromise, failure or obstruction of the biliary anastomoses, and rejection. As in

TABLE 291-5 *Hepatic Complications of Liver Transplantation*

HEPATIC DYSFUNCTION COMMON AFTER MAJOR SURGERY

Prehepatic	Pigment load
	Hemolysis
	Blood collections (hematomas, abdominal collections)
Intrahepatic	
Early	Hepatotoxic drugs and anesthesia
	Hypoperfusion (hypotension, shock, sepsis)
	Benign postoperative cholestasis
Late	Transfusion-associated hepatitis
	Exacerbation of primary hepatic disease
Posthepatic	Biliary obstruction
	↓ Renal clearance of conjugated bilirubin (renal dysfunction)

HEPATIC DYSFUNCTION UNIQUE TO LIVER TRANSPLANTATION

Primary graft nonfunction	
Vascular compromise	Portal vein obstruction
	Hepatic artery thrombosis
	Anastomotic leak with intraabdominal bleeding
Bile duct disorder	Stenosis, obstruction, leak
Rejection	
Recurrent primary hepatic disease	

nontransplant surgery, postoperative jaundice may result from prehepatic, intrahepatic, and posthepatic sources. *Prehepatic* sources represent the massive hemoglobin pigment load from transfusions, hemolysis, hematomas, ecchymoses, and other collections of blood. *Early intrahepatic* liver injury includes effects of hepatotoxic drugs and anesthesia; hypoperfusion injury associated with hypotension, sepsis, and shock; and benign postoperative cholestasis. *Late intrahepatic* sources of liver injury include posttransfusion hepatitis and exacerbation of primary disease. *Posthepatic* sources of hepatic dysfunction include biliary obstruction and reduced renal clearance of conjugated bilirubin. Hepatic complications unique to liver transplantation include primary graft failure associated with ischemic injury to the organ during harvesting; vascular compromise associated with thrombosis or stenosis of the portal vein or hepatic artery anastomoses; vascular anastomotic leak; stenosis, obstruction, or leakage of the anastomosed common bile duct; recurrence of primary hepatic disorder (see below); and rejection.

Transplant Rejection   Despite the use of immunosuppressive drugs, rejection of the transplanted liver still occurs in a proportion of patients, beginning 1 to 2 weeks after surgery. Clinical signs suggesting rejection are fever, right upper quadrant pain, and reduced bile pigment and volume. Leukocytosis may occur, but the most reliable indicators are increases in serum bilirubin and aminotransferase levels. Because these tests lack specificity, distinguishing among rejection and biliary obstruction, primary graft nonfunction, vascular compromise, viral hepatitis, cytomegalovirus infection, drug hepatotoxicity, and recurrent primary disease may be difficult. Radiographic visualization of the biliary tree and/or percutaneous liver biopsy often helps to establish the correct diagnosis. Morphologic features of acute rejection include portal infiltration, bile duct injury, and/or endothelial inflammation ("endothelialitis"); some of these findings are reminiscent of graft-versus-host disease and primary biliary cirrhosis. As soon as transplant rejection is suspected, treatment consists of intravenous methylprednisolone in repeated boluses; if this fails to abort rejection, many centers use antibodies to lymphocytes, such as OKT3, or polyclonal antilymphocyte globulin.

Chronic rejection is a relatively rare outcome that can follow repeated bouts of acute rejection or that occurs unrelated to preceding rejection episodes. Morphologically, chronic rejection is characterized by progressive cholestasis, focal parenchymal necrosis, mononuclear infiltration, vascular lesions (intimal fibrosis, subintimal foam cells, fibrinoid necrosis), and fibrosis. This process may be reflected as ductopenia—the vanishing bile duct syndrome. Some of the histologic hallmarks of chronic rejection may be so similar to those of chronic viral hepatitis that differentiation between the two may be difficult. Reversibility of chronic rejection is limited; in patients with therapy-resistant chronic rejection, retransplantation has yielded encouraging results.

OUTCOME ■ Survival   The survival rate for patients undergoing liver transplantation has improved steadily since 1983. One-year survival rates have increased from ~70% in the early 1980s to 85 to 90% in the late 1990s. Currently, the 5-year survival rate exceeds 60%. An important observation is the relation between clinical status before transplantation and outcome. For patients who undergo liver transplantation when their level of compensation is high (e.g., still working or only partially disabled), a 1-year survival rate of 85% is common. For those whose level of decompensation mandates continuous in-hospital care prior to transplantation, the 1-year survival rate is about 70%, while for those who are so decompensated that they require life support in an intensive care unit, the 1-year survival rate is ~50%. Indeed, the trend toward transplantation earlier in the natural history of end-stage liver disease is a major factor in the increased success of liver transplantation during the 1980s and 1990s. Another important distinction in survival has been drawn between high-risk and low-risk

patient categories. For patients who do not fit any "high-risk" designations, 1-year and 5-year survival rates of 85 and 80%, respectively, have been recorded. In contrast, among patients in high-risk categories—cancer, fulminant hepatitis, age >65, concurrent renal failure, respirator dependence, portal vein thrombosis, and history of a portacaval shunt or multiple right upper quadrant operations—survival statistics fall into the range of 60% at 1 year and 35% at 5 years. Survival after retransplantation for primary graft nonfunction is ~50%. Causes of failure of liver transplantation vary with time. Failures within the first 3 months result primarily from technical complications, postoperative infections, and hemorrhage. Transplant failures after the first 3 months are more likely to result from infection, rejection, or recurrent disease (such as malignancy or viral hepatitis).

Recurrence of Primary Disease   Features of autoimmune hepatitis, primary sclerosing cholangitis, and primary biliary cirrhosis overlap with those of rejection or posttransplantation bile-duct injury. Whether autoimmune hepatitis and sclerosing cholangitis recur after liver transplantation is controversial; data supporting recurrent autoimmune hepatitis (in up to a third of patients in some series) are more convincing than those supporting recurrent sclerosing cholangitis. Similarly, reports of recurrent primary biliary cirrhosis after liver transplantation have appeared; however, the histologic features of primary biliary cirrhosis and acute rejection are virtually indistinguishable and occur as frequently in patients with primary biliary cirrhosis as in patients undergoing transplantation for other reasons. Hereditary disorders such as Wilson's disease and α_1-antitrypsin deficiency have not recurred after liver transplantation; however, recurrence of disordered iron metabolism has been observed in some patients with hemochromatosis. Hepatic vein thrombosis (Budd-Chiari syndrome) may recur; this can be minimized by treating underlying lymphoproliferative disorders and by anticoagulation. Cholangiocarcinoma recurs almost invariably; therefore, few centers now offer transplantation to such patients. In patients with hepatocellular carcinoma, tumor recurrence in the liver is common after ~1 year, although better success has been reported (1- and 5-year survivals similar to those achieved in patients undergoing liver transplantation for nonmalignant diseases) in patients with an unresectable isolated lesion <5 cm or with three or fewer lesions all <3 cm. Trials are underway to assess the benefit of adjuvant chemotherapy.

Hepatitis A can recur after transplantation for fulminant hepatitis A, but such acute reinfection has no serious clinical sequelae. In fulminant hepatitis B, recurrence is not the rule; however, in the absence of any prophylactic measures, hepatitis B usually recurs after transplantation for end-stage chronic hepatitis B. Before the introduction of prophylactic antiviral therapy, immunosuppressive therapy sufficient to prevent allograft rejection led inevitably to marked increases in hepatitis B viremia, regardless of pretransplantation values. Overall graft and patient survival were poor, and some patients experienced a rapid recapitulation of severe injury—severe chronic hepatitis or even fulminant hepatitis—after transplantation. Also recognized in the era before availability of antiviral regimens was *fibrosing cholestatic hepatitis*, rapidly progressive liver injury associated with marked hyperbilirubinemia, substantial prolongation of the prothrombin time (both out of proportion to relatively modest elevations of aminotransferase activity), and rapidly progressive liver failure. This lesion has been suggested to represent a "choking off" of the hepatocyte by an overwhelming density of hepatitis B virus (HBV) proteins. Complications such as sepsis and pancreatitis were also observed more frequently in patients undergoing liver transplantation for hepatitis B prior to the introduction of antiviral therapy. The introduction of long-term prophylaxis with HBIg revolutionized liver transplantation for chronic hepatitis B. Neither preoperative hepatitis B vaccination, preoperative or postoperative interferon therapy, nor short-term (≤2 months) HBIg prophylaxis has been shown to be effective, but a retrospective analysis of data from several hundred European patients followed for 3 years after transplantation has shown that long-term (≥6 months) prophylaxis with HBIg is associated with a lowering of the risk of HBV reinfection from ~75% to 35% and a reduction in mortality from ~50% to 20%.

As a result of long-term HBIg use following liver transplantation for chronic hepatitis B, similar improvements in outcome have been observed in the United States, with 1-year survival rates between 75 and 90%. Currently, with HBIg prophylaxis, the outcome of liver transplantation for chronic hepatitis B is indistinguishable from that for chronic liver disease unassociated with chronic hepatitis B; essentially, medical concerns regarding liver transplantation for chronic hepatitis B have been eliminated. Passive immunoprophylaxis with HBIg is begun during the anhepatic stage of surgery, repeated daily for the first 6 postoperative days, then continued with infusions that are given either at regular intervals of 4 to 6 weeks or, alternatively, when anti-HBs levels fall below a threshold of 100 mIU/mL. The current approach in most centers is to continue HBIg indefinitely, which can add approximately $20,000 per year to the cost of care; some centers are evaluating regimens that shift to less frequent administration or to intramuscular administration in the late posttransplantation period. Still, occasionally, "breakthrough" HBV infection occurs.

Futher improving the outcome of liver transplantation for chronic hepatitis B is the current availability of such antiviral drugs as lamivudine and adefovir dipivoxil (Chap. 287). When lamivudine is administered to patients with decompensated liver disease, a proportion improve sufficiently to postpone imminent liver transplantation. In addition, lamivudine can be used to prevent recurrence of HBV infection when administered *prior* to transplantation, to treat hepatitis B that recurs *after* transplantation, including in patients who break through HBIg prophylaxis, and to reverse the course of otherwise fatal fibrosing cholestatic hepatitis. Clinical trials have shown that lamivudine monotherapy reduces the level of HBV replication substantially, sometimes even resulting in clearance of hepatitis B surface antigen (HBsAg); reduces alanine aminotransferase (ALT) levels; and improves histologic features of necrosis and inflammation. Long-term use of lamivudine is safe and effective, but, after several months, a proportion of patients become resistant to lamivudine, resulting from YMDD (tyrosine-methionine-aspartate-aspartate) mutations in the HBV polymerase motif (Chap. 287). In approximately half of such resistant patients, hepatic deterioration may ensue. Fortunately, adefovir dipivoxil is available as well and can be used to treat lamivudine-associated YMDD variants, effectively "rescuing" patients experiencing hepatic decompensation after lamivudine breakthrough. Currently, most liver transplantation centers combine HBIg plus lamivudine or adefovir, and additional antivirals are being introduced as well. Clinical trials are underway to define the optimal application of these antiviral agents in the management of patients undergoing liver transplantation for chronic hepatitis B; conceivably, in the future, combinations of oral antiviral drugs may supplant HBIg.

Prophylactic approaches applied to patients undergoing liver transplantation for chronic hepatitis B are being used as well for patients without hepatitis B who receive organs from donors with anti-HBc. Patients who undergo liver transplantation for chronic hepatitis B plus D are less likely to experience recurrent liver injury than patients undergoing liver transplantation for hepatitis B alone; still, such co-infected patients would also be offered standard posttransplantation prophylactic therapy for hepatitis B.

Accounting for up to 40% of all liver transplantation procedures, the most common indication for liver transplantation is end-stage liver disease resulting from chronic hepatitis C. Recurrence of hepatitis C virus (HCV) after liver transplantation can be documented in almost every patient, if sufficiently sensitive virus markers are used. Although acute and chronic liver injury occur after transplantation in patients with chronic hepatitis C, clinical consequences of recurrent hepatitis C are limited during the first 5 years after transplantation. Nonetheless, despite the relative clinical benignity of recurrent hepatitis C in the early years after liver transplantation, and despite the negligible impact

on patient survival during these early years, histologic studies have documented the presence of moderate to severe chronic hepatitis in more than half of all patients and bridging fibrosis or cirrhosis in ~10%. Moreover, progression to cirrhosis within 5 years is even more common, occurring in up to two-thirds of patients, after moderate hepatitis is detected in a 1-year biopsy. Ultimately, such histologic evidence of chronic hepatitis and cirrhosis will be expressed clinically as well, and the expectation is that the outcome beyond 10 years will not be as favorable as the 5-year statistics suggest. In a proportion of patients, even during the early posttransplantation period, recurrent hepatitis C may be sufficiently severe biochemically and histologically to merit antiviral therapy. Treatment with interferon monotherapy can *suppress* HCV-associated liver injury in approximately half of patients but rarely leads to *sustained* benefit. The addition of the nucleoside analogue ribavirin to interferon as well as the substitution of more effective and long-acting pegylated interferons for standard interferons (Chap. 287) have resulted in improved responses to antiviral therapy, and many centers have adopted some form of combination therapy for their patients with recurrent hepatitis C after liver transplantation. Overall, however, current approaches to antiviral therapy for hepatitis C after liver transplantation have been disappointing; sustained virologic responses are the exception, and reduced tolerability is often dose-limiting. Studies are underway to determine whether preemptive therapy immediately after transplantation provides any benefit over therapy introduced after clinical hepatitis occurs. Similarly, although interferon-based antiviral therapy is not recommended for patients with decompensated liver disease, some centers have experimented with pretransplantation antiviral therapy in an attempt to eradicate HCV replication prior to transplantation; preliminary results are promising. Initial trials of hepatitis C immune globulin preparations to prevent recurrent hepatitis C after liver transplantation have not been successful.

A small number succumb to early HCV-associated liver injury, and a syndrome reminiscent of fibrosing cholestatic hepatitis (see above) has been observed rarely. Because patients with more episodes of rejection receive more immunosuppressive therapy, and because immunosuppressive therapy enhances HCV replication, patients with severe or multiple episodes of rejection are more likely to experience early recurrence of hepatitis C after transplantation. Both HCV genotype 1b and high viral load have been linked to recurrent HCV-induced liver disease and to earlier disease recurrence after transplantation; however, the association between genotype and recurrence of HCV-associated liver injury has not been supported by more recent reports.

Patients who undergo liver transplantation for end-stage alcoholic cirrhosis are at risk of resorting to drinking again after transplantation, a potential source of recurrent alcoholic liver injury. Currently, alcoholic liver disease is one of the more common indications for liver transplantation, accounting for 20 to 25% of all liver transplantation procedures, and most transplantation centers screen candidates carefully for predictors of continued abstinence. Recidivism is more likely in patients whose sobriety prior to transplantation was <6 months. For abstinent patients with alcoholic cirrhosis, liver transplantation can be undertaken successfully, with outcomes comparable to those for other categories of patients with chronic liver disease, when coordinated by a team approach that includes substance abuse counseling.

Posttransplantation Quality of Life Full rehabilitation is achieved in the majority of patients who survive the early postoperative months and escape chronic rejection or unmanageable infection. Psychosocial maladjustment interferes with medical compliance in a small number of patients, but most manage to adhere to immunosuppressive regimens, which must be continued indefinitely. In one study, 85% of patients who survived their transplants returned to gainful activities. In fact, some women have conceived and carried pregnancies to term after transplantation without demonstrable injury to their infants.

FURTHER READING

BROWN RS JR et al: A survey of liver transplantation from living adult donors in the United States. N Engl J Med 348:818, 2003

CARITHERS RL JR: Liver transplantation. Liver Transpl 6:122, 2000

FISHMAN JA, RUBIN RH: Infection in organ-transplant recipients. N Engl J Med 338:1741, 1998

HOOFNAGLE JH et al: Liver transplantation for alcoholic liver disease: Executive statement and recommendations. Liver Transpl Surg 3:347, 1997

KEEFFE EB et al: Liver transplantation: Current status and novel approaches to liver replacement. Gastroenterology 120:749, 2001

SORRELL MF (Guest ed): Liver transplantation in the new millennium. Semin Liver Dis 20:409, 2000

VARGAS HE et al: A concise update on the status of liver transplantation for hepatitis B virus: The challenges in 2002. Liver Transpl 8:2, 2002

292 DISEASES OF THE GALLBLADDER AND BILE DUCTS
Norton J. Greenberger, Gustav Paumgartner

PHYSIOLOGY OF BILE PRODUCTION AND FLOW ■ Bile Secretion and Composition Bile formed in the hepatic lobules is secreted into a complex network of canaliculi, small bile ductules, and larger bile ducts that run with lymphatics and branches of the portal vein and hepatic artery in portal tracts situated between hepatic lobules. These interlobular bile ducts coalesce to form larger septal bile ducts that join to form the right and left hepatic ducts, which in turn unite to form the common hepatic duct. The common hepatic duct is joined by the cystic duct of the gallbladder to form the common bile duct (CBD), which enters the duodenum (often after joining the main pancreatic duct) through the ampulla of Vater.

Hepatic bile is an isotonic fluid with an electrolyte composition resembling blood plasma. The electrolyte composition of gallbladder bile differs from that of hepatic bile because most of the inorganic anions, chloride and bicarbonate, have been removed by reabsorption across the gallbladder epithelium. As a result of water reabsorption, total solute concentration of bile increases from 3 to 4 g/dL in hepatic bile and 10 to 15 g/dL in gallbladder bile.

Major solute components of bile by moles percent include bile acids (80%), lecithin and traces of other phospholipids (16%), and unesterified cholesterol (4.0%). In the lithogenic state the cholesterol value can be as high as 8 to 10%. Other constituents include conjugated bilirubin, proteins (IgA, metabolites of hormones, and other proteins metabolized in the liver), electrolytes, mucus, and, often, drugs and their metabolites.

The total daily basal secretion of hepatic bile is approximately 500 to 600 mL. Many substances taken up or synthesized by the hepatocyte are secreted into the bile canaliculi. The canalicular membrane forms microvilli and is associated with microfilaments of actin, microtubules, and other contractile elements. Prior to their secretion into the bile, many substances that are taken up into the hepatocyte are conjugated, while others such as phospholipids, a portion of primary bile acids, and some cholesterol are synthesized de novo in the hepatocyte. Three mechanisms are important in regulating bile flow: (1) active transport of bile acids from hepatocytes into the bile canaliculi, (2) active transport of other organic anions, and (3) cholangiocellular secretion. The last is a secretin-mediated and cyclic AMP–dependent mechanism that results in the secretion of a sodium- and bicarbonate-rich fluid into the bile ducts.

Active vectorial secretion of biliary constituents from the portal blood into the bile canaliculi is driven by a distinct set of polarized transport systems at the basolateral (sinusoidal) and the canalicular plasma membrane domains of the hepatocyte. Two sinusoidal bile salt uptake systems have been cloned in humans, the Na^+/taurocholate cotransporter (NTCP) and the organic anion transporting proteins (OATPs), which also transport a large variety of non-bile salt organic anions. Several ATP-dependent canalicular transport systems ("export pumps") have been identified, the most important of which are: the bile salt export pump (BSEP); the conjugate export pump (MRP2), which mediates the canalicular excretion of various amphiphilic conjugates formed by phase II conjugation (e.g., bilirubin mono- and diglucuronides); the multidrug export pump (MDR1) for hydrophobic cationic compounds; and the phospholipid export pump (MDR3). Indirect evidence suggests that the two hemitransporters ABCG5/G8,

functioning as a couple, constitute the principal canalicular cholesterol transporter. The canalicular membrane also contains ATP-independent transport systems such as the Cl^-/HCO_3^- anion exchanger isoform 2 for canalicular bicarbonate secretion. For some of these transporters, genetic defects have been identified that are associated with various forms of cholestasis or defects of biliary excretion. BSEP is defective in progressive familial intrahepatic cholestasis (PFIC) type 2. Mutations of MRP2 cause the Dubin-Johnson syndrome, an inherited form of conjugated hyperbilirubinemia (Chap. 284). A defective MDR3 results in PFIC-3. ABCG5/G8, the canalicular half transporters for cholesterol and neutral sterols, are defective in sitosterolemia. The cystic fibrosis transmembrane regulator located on bile duct epithelial cells is defective in cystic fibrosis, which is associated with impaired cholangiocellular bile formation and chronic cholestatic liver disease.

The Bile Acids The primary bile acids, cholic acid and chenodeoxycholic acid (CDCA), are synthesized from cholesterol in the liver, conjugated with glycine or taurine, and excreted into the bile. Secondary bile acids, including deoxycholate and lithocholate, are formed in the colon as bacterial metabolites of the primary bile acids. However, lithocholic acid is much less efficiently absorbed from the colon than deoxycholic acid. Another secondary bile acid, found in low concentration, is ursodeoxycholic acid (UDCA), a stereoisomer of CDCA. In normal bile, the ratio of glycine to taurine conjugates is about 3:1.

Bile acids are detergent-like molecules that in aqueous solutions and above a critical concentration of about 2 mM form molecular aggregates called *micelles*. Cholesterol alone is sparingly soluble in aqueous environments, and its solubility in bile depends on both the total lipid concentration and the relative molar percentages of bile acids and lecithin. Normal ratios of these constituents favor the formation of solubilizing *mixed micelles*, while abnormal ratios promote the precipitation of cholesterol crystals in bile.

In addition to facilitating the biliary excretion of cholesterol, bile acids are necessary for the normal intestinal absorption of dietary fats, mainly cholesterol and fat-soluble vitamins, via a micellar transport mechanism (Chap. 275). Bile acids also serve as a major physiologic driving force for hepatic bile flow and aid in water and electrolyte transport in the small bowel and colon.

Enterohepatic Circulation Bile acids are efficiently conserved under normal conditions. Unconjugated, and to a lesser degree also conjugated, bile acids are absorbed by *passive diffusion* along the entire gut. Quantitatively much more important for bile salt recirculation, however, is the *active transport* mechanism for conjugated bile acids in the distal ileum (Chap. 275). The reabsorbed bile acids enter the portal bloodstream and are taken up rapidly by hepatocytes, reconjugated, and resecreted into bile (enterohepatic circulation).

The normal bile acid pool size is approximately 2 to 4 g. During digestion of a meal, the bile acid pool undergoes at least one or more enterohepatic cycles, depending on the size and composition of the meal. Normally, the bile acid pool circulates approximately 5 to 10 times daily. Intestinal absorption of the pool is about 95% efficient, so fecal loss of bile acids is in the range of 0.3 to 0.6 g/d. This fecal loss is compensated by an equal daily synthesis of bile acids by the liver, and thus the size of the bile acid pool is maintained. Bile acids returning to the liver suppress de novo hepatic synthesis of primary bile acids from cholesterol by inhibiting the rate-limiting enzyme cholesterol 7α-hydroxylase. While the loss of bile salts in stool is usually matched by increased hepatic synthesis, the maximum rate of synthesis is approximately 5 g/d, which may be insufficient to replete the bile acid pool size when there is pronounced impairment of intestinal bile salt reabsorption.

Gallbladder and Sphincteric Functions In the fasting state, the sphincter of Oddi offers a high-pressure zone of resistance to bile flow from the CBD into the duodenum. This tonic contraction serves to (1) prevent reflux of duodenal contents into the pancreatic and bile ducts and (2) promote bile filling of the gallbladder. The major factor controlling the evacuation of the gallbladder is the peptide hormone cholecystokinin (CCK), which is released from the duodenal mucosa in response to the ingestion of fats and amino acids. CCK produces (1) powerful contraction of the gallbladder, (2) decreased resistance of the sphincter of Oddi, and (3) enhanced flow of biliary contents into the duodenum.

Hepatic bile is "concentrated" within the gallbladder by energy-dependent transmucosal absorption of water and electrolytes. Almost the entire bile acid pool may be sequestered in the gallbladder following an overnight fast for delivery into the duodenum with the first meal of the day. The normal capacity of the gallbladder is about 30 mL of bile.

DISEASES OF THE GALLBLADDER

CONGENITAL ANOMALIES Anomalies of the biliary tract are not uncommon and include abnormalities in number, size, and shape (e.g., agenesis of the gallbladder, duplications, rudimentary or oversized "giant" gallbladders, and diverticula). *Phrygian cap* is a clinically innocuous entity in which a partial or complete septum (or fold) separates the fundus from the body. Anomalies of position or suspension are not uncommon and include left-sided gallbladder, intrahepatic gallbladder, retrodisplacement of the gallbladder, and "floating" gallbladder. The latter condition predisposes to acute torsion, volvulus, or herniation of the gallbladder.

GALLSTONES ■ Pathogenesis Gallstones are quite prevalent in most western countries. In the United States, autopsy series have shown gallstones in at least 20% of women and in 8% of men over the age of 40. It is estimated that at least 20 million persons in the United States have gallstones and that approximately 1 million new cases of cholelithiasis develop each year.

Gallstones are formed by concretion or accretion of normal or abnormal bile constituents. They are divided into two major types: cholesterol stones account for 80% of the total, with pigment stones comprising the remaining 20%. Cholesterol gallstones usually contain >50% cholesterol monohydrate plus an admixture of calcium salts, bile pigments, proteins, and fatty acids. Pigment stones are composed primarily of calcium bilirubinate; they contain <20% cholesterol.

CHOLESTEROL STONES AND BILIARY SLUDGE Cholesterol is essentially water insoluble and requires aqueous dispersion into either micelles or vesicles, both of which require the presence of a second lipid to solubilize the cholesterol. Cholesterol and phospholipids are secreted into bile as unilamellar bilayered vesicles, which are converted into mixed micelles consisting of bile acids, phospholipids, and cholesterol by the action of bile acids. If there is an excess of cholesterol in relation to phospholipids and bile acids, unstable cholesterol-rich vesicles remain, which aggregate into large multilamellar vesicles from which cholesterol crystals precipitate (Fig. 292-1).

There are several important mechanisms in the formation of lithogenic (stone-forming) bile. The most important is increased biliary secretion of cholesterol. This may occur in association with obesity, high-caloric and cholesterol-rich diets, or drugs (e.g., clofibrate) and may result from increased activity of HMG-CoA reductase, the rate-limiting enzyme of hepatic cholesterol synthesis, and increased hepatic uptake of cholesterol from blood. In patients with gallstones, dietary cholesterol *increases* biliary cholesterol secretion. This does not occur

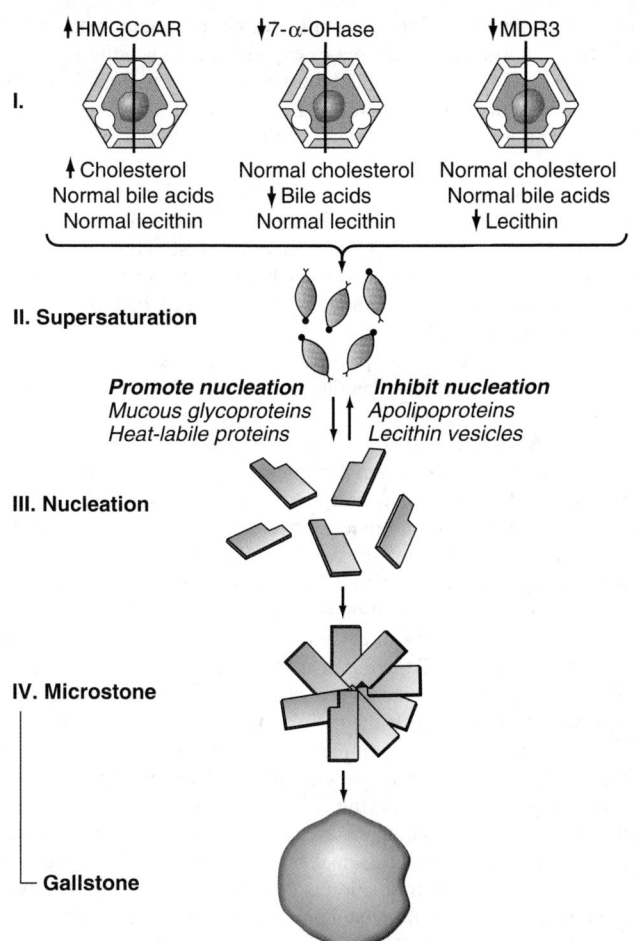

FIGURE 292-1 Scheme showing pathogenesis of cholesterol gallstone formation. Conditions or factors that increase the ratio of cholesterol to bile acids and phospholipids (lecithin) favor gallstone formation. HMG-CoAR, hydroxymethylglutaryl–coenzyme A reductase; 7-α-OHase, cholesterol, 7α-hydroxylase; MDR3, multidrug resistance–associated protein 3, also called phospholipid export pump.

in non-gallstone patients on high-cholesterol diets. In addition to environmental factors such as high-caloric and cholesterol-rich diets, genetic factors play an important role in cholesterol hypersecretion and gallstone formation. A high prevalence of gallstones is found among first-degree relatives of gallstone carriers and in certain ethnic populations such as American Indians as well as Chilean Indians and Chilean Hispanics. A common genetic trait has been identified for some of these populations by mitochondrial DNA analysis. In some patients, impaired hepatic conversion of cholesterol to bile acids may also occur, resulting in an increase of the lithogenic cholesterol/bile acid ratio. Recently, a mutation in the *CYP7A1* gene has been described that results in a deficiency of the enzyme cholesterol 7α-hydroxylase, which catalyzes the initial step in cholesterol catabolism and bile acid synthesis. The homozygous state is associated with hypercholesterolemia and gallstones. Because the phenotype is expressed in the heterozygote state, mutations in the *CYP7A1* gene may contribute to the susceptibility to cholesterol gallstone disease in the population. Mutations in the *MDR3* gene, which encodes the phospholipid export pump in the canalicular membrane of the hepatocyte, may cause defective phospholipid secretion into bile, resulting in cholesterol supersaturation of bile and formation of cholesterol gallstones in the gallbladder and in the bile ducts. Thus an excess of biliary cholesterol in relation to bile acids and phospholipids is primarily due to hypersecretion of cholesterol, but hyposecretion of bile acids or phospholipids may contribute. An additional disturbance of bile acid metabolism that is likely to contribute to supersaturation of bile with cholesterol is enhanced conversion of cholic acid to deoxycholic acid, with replacement of the cholic acid pool by an expanded deoxycholic acid pool. It may result from enhanced dehydroxylation of cholic acid and increased absorption of newly formed deoxycholic acid. An increased deoxycholate secretion is associated with hypersecretion of cholesterol into bile.

While supersaturation of bile with cholesterol is an important prerequisite for gallstone formation, it is generally not sufficient by itself to produce cholesterol precipitation in vivo. Most people with supersaturated bile do not develop stones because the time required for cholesterol crystals to nucleate and grow is longer than the time bile spends in the gallbladder.

An important mechanism is *nucleation* of cholesterol monohydrate crystals, which is greatly accelerated in human lithogenic bile. Accelerated nucleation of cholesterol monohydrate in bile may be due to either an *excess of pronucleating factors* or a *deficiency of antinucleating factors*. Mucin and certain non-mucin glycoproteins appear to be pronucleating factors, while apolipoproteins AI and AII and other glycoproteins appear to be antinucleating factors. Cholesterol monohydrate crystal nucleation and crystal growth probably occur within the mucin gel layer. Vesicle fusion leads to liquid crystals, which, in turn, nucleate into solid cholesterol monohydrate crystals. Continued growth of the crystals occurs by direct nucleation of cholesterol molecules from supersaturated unilamellar or multilamellar biliary vesicles.

A third important mechanism in cholesterol gallstone formation is *gallbladder hypomotility*. If the gallbladder emptied all supersaturated or crystal-containing bile completely, stones would not be able to grow. A high percentage of patients with gallstones exhibits abnormalities of gallbladder emptying. Ultrasonographic studies show that gallstone patients have an increased gallbladder volume during fasting and also after a test meal (residual volume) and that fractional emptying after gallbladder stimulation is decreased. Gallbladder emptying is a major determinant of gallstone recurrence in patients who underwent biliary lithotripsy. Within 3 years, only 13% of patients with good but 53% of patients with poor gallbladder emptying form recurrent stones.

Biliary sludge is a thick mucous material that upon microscopic examination reveals lecithin-cholesterol crystals, cholesterol monohydrate crystals, calcium bilirubinate, and mucin thread or mucous gels. Biliary sludge typically forms a crescent-like layer in the most dependent portion of the gallbladder and is recognized by characteristic echoes on ultrasonography (see below). The presence of biliary sludge implies two abnormalities: (1) the normal balance between gallbladder mucin secretion and elimination has become deranged and (2) nucleation of biliary solutes has occurred. That biliary sludge may be a precursor form of gallstone disease is evident from several observations. In one study, 96 patients with gallbladder sludge were followed prospectively by serial ultrasound studies. In 18%, biliary sludge disappeared and did not recur for at least 2 years. In 60%, biliary sludge disappeared and reappeared; in 14%, gallstones (8% asymptomatic, 6% symptomatic) developed, and in 6%, severe biliary pain with or without acute pancreatitis occurred. In 12 patients, cholecystectomies were performed, 6 for gallstone-associated biliary pain and 3 in symptomatic patients with sludge but without gallstones who had prior attacks of pancreatitis; the latter did not recur after cholecystectomy. It should be emphasized that biliary sludge can develop with disorders that cause gallbladder hypomotility, i.e., surgery, burns, total parenteral nutrition, pregnancy, and oral contraceptives—all of which are associated with gallstone formation.

Two other conditions are associated with cholesterol stone or biliary sludge formation: pregnancy and very low calorie diet. There appear to be two key changes during pregnancy that contribute to a "cholelithogenic state": (1) a marked increase in cholesterol saturation during the third trimester and (2) sluggish gallbladder contraction in response to a standard meal, resulting in impaired gallbladder emptying. That these changes are related to pregnancy per se is supported

by several studies that show reversal of these abnormalities after delivery. During pregnancy, gallbladder sludge develops in 20 to 30% of women and gallstones in 5 to 12%. While biliary sludge is a common finding during pregnancy, it is usually asymptomatic and often resolves spontaneously after delivery. Gallstones, which are less common than sludge and frequently associated with biliary colic, may also disappear after delivery because of spontaneous dissolution related to bile becoming unsaturated with cholesterol post partum.

Approximately 10 to 20% of people with rapid weight reduction achieved through very low calorie dieting develop gallstones. In a study involving 600 patients who completed a 16-week, 520-kcal/d diet, UDCA in a dosage of 600 mg/d proved highly effective in preventing gallstone formation; gallstones developed in only 3% of UDCA recipients compared to 28% of placebo-treated patients.

To summarize, cholesterol gallstone disease occurs because of several defects, which include (1) bile supersaturation with cholesterol, (2) nucleation of cholesterol monohydrate with subsequent crystal retention and stone growth, and (3) abnormal gallbladder motor function with delayed emptying and stasis. Other important factors known to predispose to cholesterol stone formation are summarized in Table 292-1.

PIGMENT STONES Black pigment stones are composed of either pure calcium bilirubinate or polymer-like complexes with calcium and mucin glycoproteins. They are more common in patients who have chronic hemolytic states (with increased conjugated bilirubin in bile), liver

---

TABLE 292-1 *Predisposing Factors for Cholesterol and Pigment Gallstone Formation*

Cholesterol Stones
1. Demographic/genetic factors
   a. Prevalence highest in North American Indians, Chilean Indians, and Chilean Hispanics, greater in Northern Europe and North America than in Asia, lowest in Japan; familial disposition; hereditary aspects
2. Obesity
   a. Normal bile acid pool and secretion but increased biliary secretion of cholesterol
3. Weight loss
   a. Mobilization of tissue cholesterol leads to increased biliary cholesterol secretion while enterohepatic circulation of bile acids is decreased
4. Female sex hormones
   a. Estrogens stimulate hepatic lipoprotein receptors, increase uptake of dietary cholesterol, and increase biliary cholesterol secretion
   b. Natural estrogens, other estrogens, and oral contraceptives lead to decreased bile salt secretion and decreased conversion of cholesterol to cholesteryl esters
5. Increasing age
   a. Increased biliary secretion of cholesterol, decreased size of bile acid pool, decreased secretion of bile salts
6. Gallbladder hypomotility leading to stasis and formation of sludge
   a. Prolonged parenteral nutrition
   b. Fasting
   c. Pregnancy
   d. Drugs such as octreotide
7. Clofibrate therapy
   a. Increased biliary secretion of cholesterol
8. Decreased bile acid secretion
   a. Primary biliary cirrhosis
   b. Genetic defect of the *CYP7A1* gene
9. Decreased phospholipid secretion
   a. Genetic defect of the *MDR3* gene
10. Miscellaneous
    a. High-calorie, high-fat diet
    b. Spinal cord injury

Pigment Stones
1. Demographic/genetic factors: Asia, rural setting
2. Chronic hemolysis
3. Alcoholic cirrhosis
4. Pernicious anemia
5. Cystic fibrosis
6. Chronic biliary tract infection, parasite infections
7. Increasing age
8. Ileal disease, ileal resection or bypass

cirrhosis, Gilbert's syndrome, or cystic fibrosis. Gallbladder stones in patients with ileal diseases, ileal resection, or ileal bypass generally are also black pigment stones. Enthrohepatic recycling of bilirubin contributes to their pathogenesis. Brown pigment stones are composed of calcium salts of unconjugated bilirubin with varying amounts of cholesterol and protein. They are caused by the presence of increased amounts of unconjugated, insoluble bilirubin in bile that precipitates to form stones. Deconjugation of an excess of soluble bilirubin mono- and diglucuronides may be mediated by endogenous β-glucuronidase but may also occur by spontaneous alkaline hydrolysis. Sometimes, the enzyme is also produced when bile is chronically infected by bacteria. Pigment stone formation is especially prominent in Asians and is often associated with infections in the biliary tree (Table 292-1).

Diagnosis Procedures of potential use in the diagnosis of cholelithiasis and other diseases of the gallbladder are detailed in Table 292-2. The plain abdominal film may detect gallstones containing sufficient calcium to be radiopaque (10 to 15% of cholesterol and approximately 50% of pigment stones). Plain radiography may also be of use in the diagnosis of emphysematous cholecystitis, porcelain gallbladder, limey bile, and gallstone ileus.

Ultrasonography of the gallbladder is very accurate in the identification of cholelithiasis and has several advantages over oral cholecystography (Fig. 292-2A). Stones as small as 2 mm in diameter may be confidently identified provided that firm criteria are used [e.g., acoustic "shadowing" of opacities that are within the gallbladder lumen and that change with the patient's position (by gravity)]. In major medical centers, the false-negative and false-positive rates for ultrasound in gallstone patients are about 2 to 4%. Biliary sludge is material of low echogenic activity that typically forms a layer in the most dependent position of the gallbladder. This layer shifts with postural changes but fails to produce acoustic shadowing; these two characteristics distinguish sludges from gallstones. Ultrasound can also be used to assess the emptying function of the gallbladder.

Oral cholecystography (OCG) is a useful procedure for the diagnosis of gallstones but has been largely replaced by ultrasound. It may be used to assess the patency of the cystic duct and gallbladder emptying function. Further, OCG can also delineate the size and number of gallstones and determine whether they are calcified.

Radiopharmaceuticals such as ^{99m}Tc-labeled N-substituted imino-

diacetic acids (HIDA, DIDA, DISIDA, etc.) are rapidly extracted from the blood and are excreted into the biliary tree in high concentration even in the presence of mild to moderate serum bilirubin elevations. Failure to image the gallbladder in the presence of biliary ductal visualization may indicate cystic duct obstruction, acute or chronic cholecystitis, or surgical absence of the organ. Such scans have their greatest application in the diagnosis of acute cholecystitis.

Symptoms of Gallstone Disease Gallstones usually produce symptoms by causing inflammation or obstruction following their migration into the cystic duct or CBD. The most specific and characteristic symptom of gallstone disease is biliary colic. Obstruction of the cystic duct or CBD by a stone produces increased intraluminal pressure and distention of the viscus that cannot be relieved by repetitive biliary contractions. The resultant visceral pain is characteristically a severe, steady ache or fullness in the epigastrium or right upper quadrant (RUQ) of the abdomen with frequent radiation to the interscapular area, right scapula, or shoulder.

Biliary colic begins quite suddenly and may persist with severe intensity for 30 min to 5 h, subsiding gradually or rapidly. It is steady rather than intermittent as would be suggested by the word *colic*, which must be regarded as a misnomer, although in widespread use. An episode of biliary pain persisting beyond 5 h should raise the suspicion of acute cholecystitis (see below). Nausea and vomiting frequently accompany episodes of biliary pain. An elevated level of serum bilirubin and/or alkaline phosphatase suggests a common duct stone. Fever or chills (rigors) with biliary pain usually imply a complication, i.e., cholecystitis, pancreatitis, or cholangitis. Complaints of vague epigastric fullness, dyspepsia, eructation, or flatulence, especially following a fatty meal, should not be confused with biliary pain. Such symptoms are frequently elicited from patients with or without gallstone disease but are not specific for biliary calculi. Biliary colic may be precipitated by eating a fatty meal, by consumption of a large meal following a period of prolonged fasting, or by eating a normal meal; it is frequently nocturnal.

Natural History Gallstone disease discovered in an asymptomatic patient or in a patient whose symptoms are not referable to cholelithiasis

TABLE 292-2 *Diagnostic Evaluation of the Gallbladder*

Diagnostic Advantages	Diagnostic Limitations	Comment
GALLBLADDER ULTRASOUND		
Rapid Accurate identification of gallstones (>95%) Simultaneous scanning of GB, liver, bile ducts, pancreas "Real-time" scanning allows assessment of GB volume, contractility Not limited by jaundice, pregnancy May detect very small stones	Bowel gas Massive obesity Ascites	Procedure of choice for detection of stones
RADIOISOTOPE SCANS (HIDA, DIDA, ETC.)		
Accurate identification of cystic duct obstruction Simultaneous assessment of bile ducts	?Contraindicated in pregnancy Serum bilirubin >103–205 μmol/L (6–12 mg/dL) Cholecystogram of low resolution	Indicated for confirmation of suspected acute cholecystitis; less sensitive and less specific in chronic cholecystitis; useful in diagnosis of acalculous cholecystopathy, especially if given with CCK to assess gallbladder emptying
PLAIN ABDOMINAL X-RAY		

Low cost
Readily available
	Relatively low yield
	?Contraindicated in pregnancy
		Pathognomonic findings in:
		  Calcified gallstones
		  Limey bile, porcelain GB
		  Emphysematous cholecystitis
		  Gallstone ileus

ORAL CHOLECYSTOGRAM		
		Largely replaced by GBUS

Note: GB, gallbladder; CCK, cholecystokinin; GBUS, gallbladder ultrasound.

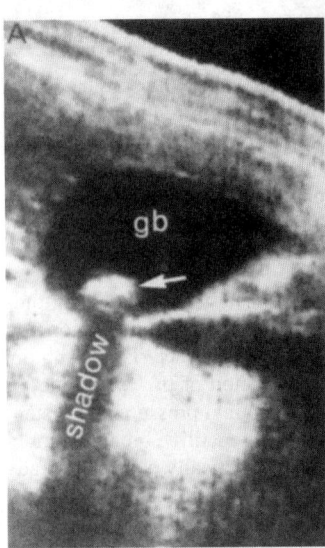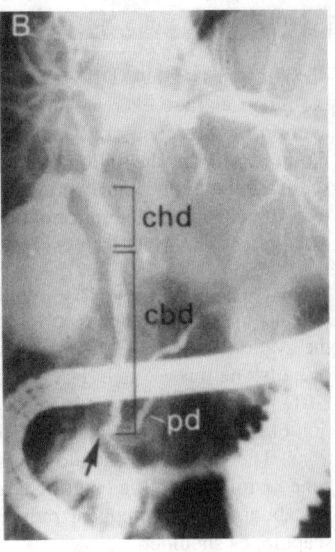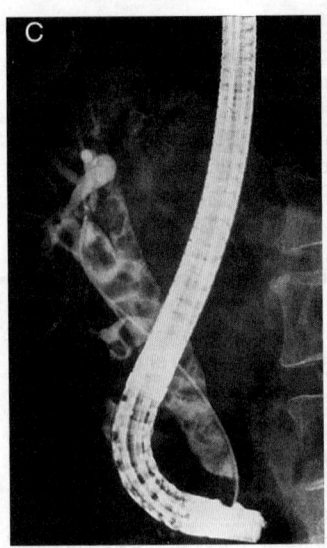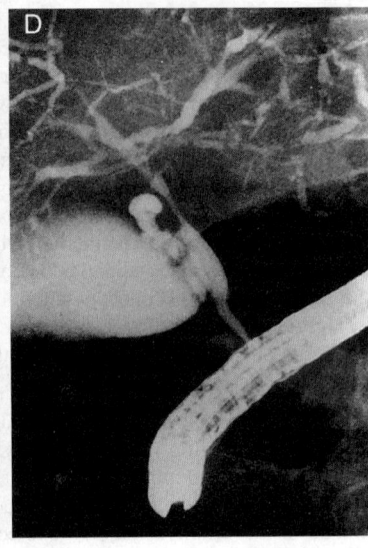

FIGURE 292-2 Examples of ultrasound and radiologic studies of the biliary tract. *A.* An ultrasound study showing a distended gallbladder containing a single large stone (*arrow*) which casts an acoustic shadow. *B.* Endoscopic retrograde cholangiopancreatogram (ERCP) showing normal biliary tract anatomy. In addition to the endoscope and large vertical gallbladder filled with contrast dye, the common hepatic duct (chd), common bile duct (cbd), and pancreatic duct (pd) are shown. The arrow points to the ampulla of Vater. *C.* Endoscopic retrograde cholangiogram (ERC) showing choledocholithiasis. The biliary tract is dilatated and contains multiple radiolucent calculi. *D.* ERCP showing sclerosing cholangitis. The common bile duct shows areas that are strictured and narrowed.

is a common clinical problem. The natural history of "silent" or asymptomatic gallstones has occasioned much debate. A study of predominantly male silent gallstone patients suggests that the cumulative risk for the development of symptoms or complications is relatively low—10% at 5 years, 15% at 10 years, and 18% at 15 years. Patients remaining asymptomatic for 15 years were found to be unlikely to develop symptoms during further follow-up, and most patients who did develop complications from their gallstones experienced *prior* warning symptoms. Similar conclusions apply to diabetic patients with silent gallstones. Decision analysis has suggested that (1) the cumulative risk of death due to gallstone disease while on expectant management is small, and (2) prophylactic cholecystectomy is not warranted.

Complications requiring cholecystectomy are much more common in gallstone patients who have developed symptoms of biliary pain. Patients found to have gallstones at a young age are more likely to develop symptoms from cholelithiasis than are patients older than 60 years at the time of initial diagnosis. Patients with diabetes mellitus and gallstones may be somewhat more susceptible to septic complications, but the magnitude of risk of septic biliary complications in diabetic patients is incompletely defined.

℞ TREATMENT

Surgical Therapy In asymptomatic gallstone patients, the risk of developing symptoms or complications requiring surgery is quite small (in the range of 1 to 2% per year). Thus a recommendation for cholecystectomy in a patient with gallstones should probably be based on assessment of three factors: (1) the presence of symptoms that are frequent enough or severe enough to interfere with the patient's general routine; (2) the presence of a prior complication of gallstone disease, i.e., history of acute cholecystitis, pancreatitis, gallstone fistula, etc.; or (3) the presence of an underlying condition predisposing the patient to increased risk of gallstone complications (e.g., calcified or porcelain gallbladder and/or a previous attack of acute cholecystitis regardless of current symptomatic status). Patients with very large gallstones (>3 cm in diameter) and patients having gallstones in a congenitally anomalous gallbladder might also be considered for prophylactic cholecystectomy. Although young age is a worrisome factor in asymptomatic gallstone patients, few authorities would now recommend routine cholecystectomy in all young patients with silent stones. Laparoscopic cholecystectomy is a minimal-access approach for the removal of the gallbladder together with its stones. Its advantages include a markedly

shortened hospital stay as well as decreased cost, and it is the procedure of choice for most patients referred for elective cholecystectomy.

From several studies involving over 4000 patients undergoing laparoscopic cholecystectomy, the following key points emerge: (1) complications develop in about 4% of patients, (2) conversion to laparotomy occurs in 5%, (3) the death rate is remarkably low (i.e., <0.1%), and (4) bile duct injuries are unusual (i.e., 0.2 to 0.5%). These data indicate why laparoscopic cholecystectomy has become the "gold standard" for treating symptomatic cholelithiasis.

Medical Therapy—Gallstone Dissolution UDCA decreases cholesterol saturation of bile and also appears to produce a lamellar liquid crystalline phase in bile that allows a dispersion of cholesterol from stones by physical-chemical means. UDCA may also retard cholesterol crystal nucleation. In carefully selected patients with a functioning gallbladder and with radiolucent stones <10 mm in diameter, complete dissolution can be achieved in about 50% of patients within 6 months to 2 years with UDCA at a dose of 8 to 10 mg/kg per day. The highest success rate (i.e., >70%) occurs in patients with small (<5 mm) floating radiolucent gallstones. Probably no more than 10% of patients with *symptomatic* cholelithiasis are candidates for such treatment. However, in addition to the vexing problem of recurrent stones (30 to 50% over 3 to 5 years of follow-up), there is also the factor of taking an expensive drug for up to 2 years. The advantages and success of laparoscopic cholecystectomy have largely reduced the role of gallstone dissolution to patients who wish to avoid or are not candidates for elective cholecystectomy.

Gallbladder stones may be fragmented by extracorporeal shock waves. While such shock wave lithotripsy combined with medical litholytic therapy is safe and effective in carefully selected patients with gallbladder calculi (radiolucent, solitary stone <2 cm in well-contracting gallbladder), the procedure is employed infrequently because of the emergence of laparoscopic cholystectomy as the procedure of choice for symptomatic cholelithiasis, the recurrence of gallstones in 30% of patients within 5 years after lithotripsy combined with medical litholytic therapy, and the cost of taking UDCA for a variable period after the procedure.

ACUTE AND CHRONIC CHOLECYSTITIS ■ **Acute Cholecystitis** Acute inflammation of the gallbladder wall usually follows obstruction of the cystic duct by a stone. Inflammatory response can be evoked by three factors: (1) *mechanical inflammation* produced by increased intraluminal pressure and distention with resulting ischemia of the gallbladder mucosa and wall, (2) *chemical inflammation* caused by the release of lysolecithin (due to the action of phospholipase on lecithin in bile) and other local tissue factors, and (3) *bacterial inflammation*, which may play a role in 50 to 85% of patients with acute cholecystitis. The organisms most frequently isolated by culture of gallbladder bile in these patients include *Escherichia coli*, *Klebsiella* spp., *Streptococcus* spp., and *Clostridium* spp.

Acute cholecystitis often begins as an attack of biliary pain that progressively worsens. Approximately 60 to 70% of patients report having experienced prior attacks that resolved spontaneously. As the episode progresses, however, the pain of acute cholecystitis becomes more generalized in the right upper abdomen. As with biliary colic, the pain of cholecystitis may radiate to the interscapular area, right scapula, or shoulder. Peritoneal signs of inflammation such as increased pain with jarring or on deep respiration may be apparent. The patient is anorectic and often nauseated. Vomiting is relatively common and may produce symptoms and signs of vascular and extracellular volume depletion. Jaundice is unusual early in the course of acute cholecystitis but may occur when edematous inflammatory changes involve the bile ducts and surrounding lymph nodes.

A low-grade fever is characteristically present, but shaking chills or rigors are not uncommon. The RUQ of the abdomen is almost invariably tender to palpation. An enlarged, tense gallbladder is palpable in one-quarter to one-half of patients. Deep inspiration or cough during subcostal palpation of the RUQ usually produces increased pain and inspiratory arrest (Murphy's sign). A light thump delivered to the right subcostal area may elicit a marked increase in pain. Localized rebound tenderness in the RUQ is common, as are abdominal distention and hypoactive bowel sounds from paralytic ileus, but generalized peritoneal signs and abdominal rigidity are usually lacking, in the absence of perforation.

The diagnosis of acute cholecystitis is usually made on the basis of a characteristic history and physical examination. The triad of sudden onset of RUQ tenderness, fever, and leukocytosis is highly suggestive. Typically, leukocytosis in the range of 10,000 to 15,000 cells per microliter with a left shift on differential count is found. The serum bilirubin is mildly elevated [<85.5 μmol/L (5 mg/dL)] in fewer than half of patients, while about one-fourth have modest elevations in serum aminotransferases (usually less than a fivefold elevation). The radionuclide (e.g., HIDA) biliary scan may be confirmatory if bile duct imaging is seen without visualization of the gallbladder. Ultrasound will demonstrate calculi in 90 to 95% of cases.

Approximately 75% of patients treated medically have remission of acute symptoms within 2 to 7 days following hospitalization. In 25%, however, a complication of acute cholecystitis will occur despite conservative treatment (see below). In this setting, prompt surgical intervention is required. Of the 75% of patients with acute cholecystitis who undergo remission of symptoms, approximately one-quarter will experience a recurrence of cholecystitis within 1 year, and 60% will have at least one recurrent bout within 6 years. In view of the natural history of the disease, acute cholecystitis is best treated by early surgery whenever possible.

Mirrizzi's syndrome is a rare complication in which a gallstone becomes impacted in the cystic duct or neck of the gallbladder causing compression of the CBD, resulting in CBD obstruction and jaundice. Ultrasound shows gallstone(s) lying outside the hepatic duct. Endoscopic retrograde cholangiopancreatography (ERCP) or percutaneous transhepatic cholangiography (PTC) will usually demonstrate the characteristic extrinsic compression of the CBD. Surgery consists of removing the cystic duct, diseased gallbladder, and the impacted stone. The preoperative diagnosis of Mirrizzi's syndrome is important to avoid CBD injury.

ACALCULOUS CHOLECYSTITIS In 5 to 10% of patients with acute cholecystitis, calculi obstructing the cystic duct are not found at surgery. In over 50% of such cases, an underlying explanation for acalculous inflammation is not found. An increased risk for the development of acalculous cholecystitis is especially associated with serious trauma or

burns, with the postpartum period following prolonged labor, and with orthopedic and other nonbiliary major surgical operations in the postoperative period. It may possibly complicate periods of prolonged parenteral hyperalimentation. For some of these cases, biliary sludge in the cystic duct may be responsible. Other precipitating factors include vasculitis, obstructing adenocarcinoma of the gallbladder, diabetes mellitus, torsion of the gallbladder, "unusual" bacterial infections of the gallbladder (e.g., *Leptospira*, *Streptococcus*, *Salmonella*, or *Vibrio cholerae*), and parasitic infestation of the gallbladder. Acalculous cholecystitis may also be seen with a variety of other systemic disease processes (sarcoidosis, cardiovascular disease, tuberculosis, syphilis, actinomycosis, etc.) and may possibly complicate periods of prolonged parenteral hyperalimentation.

Although the clinical manifestations of acalculous cholecystitis are indistinguishable from those of calculous cholecystitis, the setting of acute gallbladder inflammation complicating severe underlying illness is characteristic of acalculous disease. Ultrasound, computed tomography (CT) scanning, or radionuclide examinations demonstrating a large, tense, static gallbladder without stones and with evidence of poor emptying over a prolonged period may be diagnostically useful in some cases. The complication rate for acalculous cholecystitis exceeds that for calculous cholecystitis. Successful management of acute acalculous cholecystitis appears to depend primarily on early diagnosis and surgical intervention, with meticulous attention to postoperative care.

ACALCULOUS CHOLECYSTOPATHY Disordered motility of the gallbladder can produce recurrent biliary pain in patients without gallstones. Infusion of an octapeptide of CCK can be used to measure the gallbladder ejection fraction during cholescintigraphy. CCK cholescintigraphy using ^{99}Tc-diisopropyl iminodiacetic acid (DIDA) or HIDA may document an abnormal gallbladder ejection fraction (<40% at 45 min). The surgical findings have included abnormalities such as chronic cholecystitis, gallbladder muscle hypertrophy, and/or a markedly narrowed cystic duct. Some of these patients may well have had antecedent gallbladder disease. The following criteria can be used to identify patients with acalculous cholecystopathy: (1) recurrent episodes of typical RUQ pain characteristic of biliary tract pain, (2) abnormal CCK cholescintigraphy demonstrating a gallbladder ejection fraction of <40%, and (3) infusion of CCK reproduces the patient's pain. An additional clue would be the identification of a large gallbladder on ultrasound examination. Finally, it should be noted that sphincter of Oddi dysfunction can also give rise to recurrent RUQ pain and CCK-scintigraphic abnormalities.

EMPHYSEMATOUS CHOLECYSTITIS So-called emphysematous cholecystitis is thought to begin with acute cholecystitis (calculous or acalculous) followed by ischemia or gangrene of the gallbladder wall and infection by gas-producing organisms. Bacteria most frequently cultured in this setting include anaerobes, such as *C. welchii* or *C. perfringens*, and aerobes, such as *E. coli*. This condition occurs most frequently in elderly men and in patients with diabetes mellitus. The clinical manifestations are essentially indistinguishable from those of nongaseous cholecystitis. The diagnosis is usually made on plain abdominal film by finding gas within the gallbladder lumen, dissecting within the gallbladder wall to form a gaseous ring, or in the pericholecystic tissues. The morbidity and mortality rates with emphysematous cholecystitis are considerable. Prompt surgical intervention coupled with appropriate antibiotics is mandatory.

Chronic Cholecystitis Chronic inflammation of the gallbladder wall is almost always associated with the presence of gallstones and is thought to result from repeated bouts of subacute or acute cholecystitis or from persistent mechanical irritation of the gallbladder wall by gallstones. The presence of bacteria in the bile occurs in more than one-quarter of patients with chronic cholecystitis. The presence of infected bile in a patient with *chronic* cholecystitis undergoing elective cholecystectomy probably adds little to the operative risk. Chronic cholecystitis may be asymptomatic for years, may progress to symptomatic gallbladder disease or to acute cholecystitis, or may present with complications (see below).

Complications of Cholecystitis ■ *EMPYEMA AND HYDROPS* Empyema of the gallbladder usually results from progression of acute cholecystitis with persistent cystic duct obstruction to superinfection of the stagnant bile with a pus-forming bacterial organism. The clinical picture resembles that of cholangitis with high fever, severe RUQ pain, marked leukocytosis, and often, prostration. Empyema of the gallbladder carries a high risk of gram-negative sepsis and/or perforation. Emergency surgical intervention with proper antibiotic coverage is required as soon as the diagnosis is suspected.

Hydrops or mucocele of the gallbladder may also result from prolonged obstruction of the cystic duct, usually by a large solitary calculus. In this instance, the obstructed gallbladder lumen is progressively distended, over a period of time, by mucus (mucocele) or by a clear transudate (hydrops) produced by mucosal epithelial cells. A visible, easily palpable, nontender mass sometimes extending from the RUQ into the right iliac fossa may be found on physical examination. The patient with hydrops of the gallbladder frequently remains asymptomatic, although chronic RUQ pain may also occur. Cholecystectomy is indicated, since empyema, perforation, or gangrene may complicate the condition.

GANGRENE AND PERFORATION Gangrene of the gallbladder results from ischemia of the wall and patchy or complete tissue necrosis. Underlying conditions often include marked distention of the gallbladder, vasculitis, diabetes mellitus, empyema, or torsion resulting in arterial occlusion. Gangrene usually predisposes to perforation of the gallbladder, but perforation may also occur in chronic cholecystitis without premonitory warning symptoms. *Localized perforations* are usually contained by the omentum or by adhesions produced by recurrent inflammation of the gallbladder. Bacterial superinfection of the walled-off gallbladder contents results in abscess formation. Most patients are best treated with cholecystectomy, but some seriously ill patients may be managed with cholecystostomy and drainage of the abscess. *Free perforation* is less common but is associated with a mortality rate of approximately 30%. Such patients may experience a sudden transient relief of RUQ pain as the distended gallbladder decompresses; this is followed by signs of generalized peritonitis.

FISTULA FORMATION AND GALLSTONE ILEUS *Fistulization* into an adjacent organ adherent to the gallbladder wall may result from inflammation and adhesion formation. Fistulas into the duodenum are most common, followed in frequency by those involving the hepatic flexure of the colon, stomach or jejunum, abdominal wall, and renal pelvis. Clinically "silent" biliary-enteric fistulas occurring as a complication of acute cholecystitis have been found in up to 5% of patients undergoing cholecystectomy. Asymptomatic cholecystoenteric fistulas may sometimes be diagnosed by finding gas in the biliary tree on plain abdominal films. Barium contrast studies or endoscopy of the upper gastrointestinal tract or colon may demonstrate the fistula. Treatment in the symptomatic patient usually consists of cholecystectomy, CBD exploration, and closure of the fistulous tract.

Gallstone ileus refers to mechanical intestinal obstruction resulting from the passage of a large gallstone into the bowel lumen. The stone customarily enters the duodenum through a cholecystoenteric fistula at that level. The site of obstruction by the impacted gallstone is usually at the ileocecal valve, provided that the more proximal small bowel is of normal caliber. The majority of patients do not give a history of either prior biliary tract symptoms or complaints suggestive of acute cholecystitis or fistulization. Large stones over 2.5 cm in diameter are thought to predispose to fistula formation by gradual erosion through the gallbladder fundus. Diagnostic confirmation may occasionally be found on the plain abdominal film (e.g., small-intestinal obstruction with gas in the biliary tree and a calcified, ectopic gallstone) or following an upper gastrointestinal series (cholecystoduo-

denal fistula with small-bowel obstruction at the ileocecal valve). Laparotomy with stone extraction (or propulsion into the colon) remains the procedure of choice to relieve obstruction. Evacuation of large stones within the gallbladder should also be performed. In general, the gallbladder and its attachment to the intestines should be left alone.

LIMEY (MILK OF CALCIUM) BILE AND PORCELAIN GALLBLADDER Calcium salts may be secreted into the lumen of the gallbladder in sufficient concentration to produce calcium precipitation and diffuse, hazy opacification of bile or a layering effect on plain abdominal roentgenography. This so-called limey bile, or milk of calcium bile, is usually clinically innocuous, but cholecystectomy is recommended, especially when it occurs in a hydropic gallbladder. In the entity called *porcelain gallbladder*, calcium salt deposition within the wall of a chronically inflamed gallbladder may be detected on the plain abdominal film. Cholecystectomy is advised in all patients with porcelain gallbladder because in a high percentage of cases this finding appears to be associated with the development of carcinoma of the gallbladder.

℞ TREATMENT

Medical Therapy Although surgical intervention remains the mainstay of therapy for acute cholecystitis and its complications, a period of in-hospital stabilization may be required before cholecystectomy. Oral intake is eliminated, nasogastric suction may be indicated, and extracellular volume depletion and electrolyte abnormalities are repaired. Meperidine or nonsteroidal anti-inflammatory drugs (NSAIDs) are usually employed for analgesia because they may produce less spasm of the sphincter of Oddi than drugs such as morphine. Intravenous antibiotic therapy is usually indicated in patients with severe acute cholecystitis even though bacterial superinfection of bile may not have occurred in the early stages of the inflammatory process. Antibiotic therapy is guided by the most common organisms likely to be present, which are *E. coli*, *Klebsiella* spp., and *Streptococcus* spp. Effective antibiotics include ureidopenicillins such as piperacillin or mezlocillin, ampicillin sulbactam, and third-generation cephalosporins. Anaerobic coverage by a drug such as metronidazole should be added if gangrenous or emphysematous cholecystitis is suspected. Similarly, combination therapy with an aminoglycoside and other antibiotics may be considered in diabetic or debilitated patients and in those with signs of gram-negative sepsis (Chap. 134). Postoperative complications of wound infection, abscess formation, or sepsis are reduced in antibiotic-treated patients.

Surgical Therapy The optimal timing of surgical intervention in patients with acute cholecystitis depends on stabilization of the patient. The clear trend is toward earlier surgery, and this is due in part to requirements for shorter hospital stays. Urgent (emergency) cholecystectomy or cholecystostomy is probably appropriate in most patients in whom a complication of acute cholecystitis such as empyema, emphysematous cholecystitis, or perforation is suspected or confirmed. In uncomplicated cases of acute cholecystitis, up to 30% of patients fail to resolve their symptoms on appropriate medical therapy, and progression of the attack or a supervening complication leads to the performance of early operation (within 24 to 72 h). The technical complications of surgery are not increased in patients undergoing early as opposed to delayed cholecystectomy. Delayed surgical intervention is probably best reserved for (1) patients in whom the overall medical condition imposes an unacceptable risk for early surgery and (2) patients in whom the diagnosis of acute cholecystitis is in doubt. Early cholecystectomy is the treatment of choice for most patients with acute cholecystitis. Mortality figures for emergency cholecystectomy in most centers approach 3%, while the mortality risk for elective or early cholecystectomy approximates 0.5% in patients under age 60. Of course, the operative risks increase with age-related diseases of other organ systems and with the presence of long- or short-term complications of gallbladder disease. Seriously ill or debilitated patients with cholecystitis may be managed with cholecystostomy and tube drainage of the gallbladder. Elective cholecystectomy may then be done at a later date.

Postcholecystectomy Complications Early complications following cholecystectomy include atelectasis and other pulmonary disorders, abscess formation (often subphrenic), external or internal hemorrhage, biliary-enteric fistula, and bile leaks. Jaundice may indicate absorption of bile from an intraabdominal collection following a biliary leak or mechanical obstruction of the CBD by retained calculi, intraductal blood clots, or extrinsic compression. Routine performance of intraoperative cholangiography during cholecystectomy has helped to reduce the incidence of these early complications.

Overall, cholecystectomy is a very successful operation that provides total or near-total relief of preoperative symptoms in 75 to 90% of patients. The most common cause of persistent postcholecystectomy symptoms is an overlooked symptomatic nonbiliary disorder (e.g., reflux esophagitis, peptic ulceration, pancreatitis, or—most often—irritable bowel syndrome). In a small percentage of patients, however, a disorder of the extrahepatic bile ducts may result in persistent symptomatology. These so-called postcholecystectomy syndromes may be due to (1) biliary strictures, (2) retained biliary calculi, (3) cystic duct stump syndrome, (4) stenosis or dyskinesia of the sphincter of Oddi, or (5) bile salt–induced diarrhea or gastritis.

CYSTIC DUCT STUMP SYNDROME In the absence of cholangiographically demonstrable retained stones, symptoms resembling biliary pain or cholecystitis in the postcholecystectomy patient have frequently been attributed to disease in a long (>1 cm) cystic duct remnant (cystic duct stump syndrome). Careful analysis, however, reveals that postcholecystectomy complaints are attributable to other causes in almost all patients in whom the symptom complex was originally thought to result from the existence of a long cystic duct stump. Accordingly, considerable care should be taken to investigate the possible role of other factors in the production of postcholecystectomy symptoms before attributing them to cystic duct stump syndrome.

PAPILLARY DYSFUNCTION, PAPILLARY STENOSIS, SPASM OF THE SPHINCTER OF ODDI, AND BILIARY DYSKINESIA Symptoms of biliary colic accompanied by signs of recurrent, intermittent biliary obstruction may be produced by papillary stenosis, papillary dysfunction, spasm of the sphincter of Oddi, and biliary dyskinesia. Papillary stenosis is thought to result from acute or chronic inflammation of the papilla of Vater or from glandular hyperplasia of the papillary segment. Five criteria have been used to define papillary stenosis: (1) upper abdominal pain, usually RUQ or epigastric; (2) abnormal liver tests; (3) dilatation of the common bile duct upon ERCP examination; (4) delayed (>45 min) drainage of contrast material from the duct; and (5) increased basal pressure of the sphincter of Oddi, a finding that may be of only minor significance. An alternative to ERCP is magnetic resonance cholangiography (MRC) if ERCP and/or biliary manometry are either unavailable or not feasible. In patients with papillary stenosis, quantitative hepatobiliary scintigraphy has revealed delayed transit from the common bile duct to the bowel, ductal dilatation, and abnormal time-activity dynamics. This technique can also be used before and after sphincterotomy to document improvement in biliary emptying. Treatment consists of endoscopic or surgical sphincteroplasty to ensure wide patency of the distal portions of both the bile and pancreatic ducts. The greater the number of the preceding criteria present, the greater the likelihood that a patient does have a degree of papillary stenosis sufficient to justify correction. The factors usually considered as indications for sphincterotomy include (1) prolonged duration of symptoms, (2) lack of response to symptomatic treatment, (3) presence of severe disability, and (4) the patient's choice of sphincterotomy over surgery (given a clear understanding on his or her part of the risks involved in both procedures).

Criteria for diagnosing dyskinesia of the sphincter of Oddi are even more controversial than those for papillary stenosis. Proposed mechanisms include spasm of the sphincter, denervation sensitivity resulting in hypertonicity, and abnormalities of the sequencing or frequency rates of sphincteric contraction waves. When thorough evaluation has failed to demonstrate another cause for the pain, and when cholangiographic and manometric criteria suggest a diagnosis of biliary dys-

kinesia, medical treatment with nitrites or anticholinergics to attempt pharmacologic relaxation of the sphincter has been proposed. Endoscopic biliary sphincterotomy (EBS) or surgical sphincteroplasty may be indicated in patients who fail to respond to a 2- to 3-month trial of medical therapy, especially if basal sphincter of Oddi pressures are elevated. EBS has become the procedure of choice for removing bile duct stones and for other biliary and pancreatic problems. A study of EBS found four key findings: (1) Dysfunction of the sphincter of Oddi was associated with an increased rise of complications, especially pancreatitis; (2) pancreatitis was more frequent in young patients; (3) difficulty in cannulating the bile duct and the use of "precut" sphincterotomy were important technique-related risk factors for complications; and (4) experience in the volume of procedures proved to be important; endoscopists who perform more than one EBS per week had lower complication rates than endoscopists who performed a smaller number of procedures.

Bile Salt–Induced Diarrhea and Gastritis Postcholecystectomy patients may develop symptoms of dyspepsia, which have been attributed to duodenogastric reflux of bile. However, firm data linking these symptoms to bile gastritis after surgical removal of the gallbladder are lacking. Cholecystectomy induces persistent changes in gut transit, and these changes effect a noticeable modification of bowel habits. Cholecystectomy shortens gut transit time by accelerating passage of the fecal bolus through the colon with marked acceleration in the right colon, thus causing an increase in colonic bile acid output and a shift in bile acid composition toward the more diarrheagenic secondary bile acids. Diarrhea that is severe enough, i.e., three or more watery movements per day, can be classified as postcholecystectomy diarrhea, and this occurs in 5 to 10% of patients undergoing elective cholecystectomy. Treatment with bile acid sequestering agents such as cholestyramine or colestipol is often effective in ameliorating troublesome diarrhea.

THE HYPERPLASTIC CHOLECYSTOSES The term *hyperplastic cholecystoses* is used to denote a group of disorders of the gallbladder characterized by excessive proliferation of normal tissue components.

Adenomyomatosis is characterized by a benign proliferation of gallbladder surface epithelium with glandlike formations, extramural sinuses, transverse strictures, and/or fundal nodule ("adenoma" or "adenomyoma") formation. Outpouchings of mucosa termed *Rokitansky-Aschoff sinuses* may be seen on oral cholecystography in conjunction with hyperconcentration of contrast medium. Characteristic dimpled filling defects also may be seen.

Cholesterolosis is characterized by abnormal deposition of lipid, especially cholesteryl esters within macrophages in the lamina propria of the gallbladder wall. In its diffuse form ("strawberry gallbladder"), the gallbladder mucosa is brick red and speckled with bright yellow flecks of lipid. The localized form shows solitary or multiple "cholesterol polyps" studding the gallbladder wall. Cholesterol stones of the gallbladder are found in nearly half the cases. Cholecystectomy is indicated in both adenomyomatosis and cholesterolosis when symptomatic or when cholelithiasis is present.

The prevalence of gallbladder polyps in the adult population is about 5%, with a marked male predominance. Few significant changes have been found over a 5-year period in asymptomatic patients with gallbladder polyps <10 mm in diameter. Cholecystectomy is recommended in symptomatic patients, as well as in asymptomatic patients over 50 years of age, or in those whose polyps are >10 mm in diameter or associated with gallstones or polyp growth on serial ultrasonography.

DISEASES OF THE BILE DUCTS

CONGENITAL ANOMALIES ■ Biliary Atresia and Hypoplasia Atretic and hypoplastic lesions of the extrahepatic and major intrahepatic bile ducts are the most common biliary anomalies of clinical relevance encountered in infancy. The clinical picture is one of severe obstructive jaundice during the first month of life, with pale stools. When biliary atresia is suspected on the basis of clinical, laboratory, and imaging findings the diagnosis is confirmed by surgical exploration and operative cholangiography. The diagnosis is confirmed by surgical exploration with operative cholangiography. Approximately 10% of cases of biliary atresia are treatable with roux-en-Y choledochojejunostomy, with the Kasai procedure (hepatic portoenterostomy) being attempted in the remainder in an effort to restore some bile flow. Most patients, even those having successful biliary-enteric anastomoses, eventually develop chronic cholangitis, extensive hepatic fibrosis, and portal hypertension.

Choledochal Cysts   Cystic dilatation may involve the free portion of the CBD, i.e., choledochal cyst, or may present as diverticulum formation in the intraduodenal segment. In the latter situation, chronic reflux of pancreatic juice into the biliary tree can produce inflammation and stenosis of the extrahepatic bile ducts leading to cholangitis or biliary obstruction. Because the process may be gradual, approximately 50% of patients present with onset of symptoms after age 10. The diagnosis may be made by ultrasound, abdominal CT, MRC, or cholangiography. Only one-third of patients show the classic triad of abdominal pain, jaundice, and an abdominal mass. Ultrasonographic detection of a cyst separate from the gallbladder should suggest the diagnosis of choledochal cyst, which can be confirmed by demonstrating the entrance of extrahepatic bile ducts into the cyst. Surgical treatment involves excision of the "cyst" and biliary-enteric anastomosis. Patients with choledochal cysts are at increased risk for the subsequent development of cholangiocarcinoma.

Congenital Biliary Ectasia   Dilatation of intrahepatic bile ducts may involve either the major intrahepatic radicles (Caroli's disease), the inter- and intralobular ducts (congenital hepatic fibrosis), or both. In Caroli's disease, clinical manifestations include recurrent cholangitis, abscess formation in and around the affected ducts, and, often, gallstone formation within portions of ectatic intrahepatic biliary radicles. Ultrasound, MRC, and CT are of great diagnostic value in demonstrating cystic dilatation of the intrahepatic bile ducts. Treatment with ongoing antibiotic therapy is usually undertaken in an effort to limit the frequency and severity of recurrent bouts of cholangitis. Progression to secondary biliary cirrhosis with portal hypertension, extrahepatic biliary obstruction, cholangiocarcinoma, or recurrent episodes of sepsis with hepatic abscess formation is common.

CHOLEDOCHOLITHIASIS ■ **Pathophysiology and Clinical Manifestations**   Passage of gallstones into the CBD occurs in approximately 10 to 15% of patients with cholelithiasis. The incidence of common duct stones increases with increasing age of the patient, so that up to 25% of elderly patients may have calculi in the common duct at the time of cholecystectomy. Undetected duct stones are left behind in approximately 1 to 5% of cholecystectomy patients. The overwhelming majority of bile duct stones are cholesterol stones formed in the gallbladder, which then migrate into the extrahepatic biliary tree through the cystic duct. Primary calculi arising de novo in the ducts are usually pigment stones developing in patients with (1) hepatobiliary parasitism or chronic, recurrent cholangitis; (2) congenital anomalies of the bile ducts (especially Caroli's disease); (3) dilated, sclerosed, or strictured ducts; or (4) an *MDR3* gene defect leading to impaired biliary phospholipids secretion. Common duct stones may remain asymptomatic for years, may pass spontaneously into the duodenum, or (most often) may present with biliary colic or a complication.

Complications ■ *CHOLANGITIS*   Cholangitis may be acute or chronic, and symptoms result from inflammation, which usually requires at least partial obstruction to the flow of bile. Bacteria are present on bile culture in approximately 75% of patients with acute cholangitis early in the symptomatic course. The characteristic presentation of acute cholangitis involves biliary pain, jaundice, and spiking fevers with chills (Charcot's triad). Blood cultures are frequently positive, and

leukocytosis is typical. *Nonsuppurative acute cholangitis* is most common and may respond relatively rapidly to supportive measures and to treatment with antibiotics. In *suppurative acute cholangitis*, however, the presence of pus under pressure in a completely obstructed ductal system leads to symptoms of severe toxicity—mental confusion, bacteremia, and septic shock. Response to antibiotics alone in this setting is relatively poor, multiple hepatic abscesses are often present, and the mortality rate approaches 100% unless prompt endoscopic or surgical relief of the obstruction and drainage of infected bile are carried out. Endoscopic management of bacterial cholangitis is as effective as surgical intervention. ERCP with endoscopic sphincterotomy is safe and the preferred initial procedure for both establishing a definitive diagnosis and providing effective therapy.

OBSTRUCTIVE JAUNDICE   Gradual obstruction of the CBD over a period of weeks or months usually leads to initial manifestations of jaundice or pruritus without associated symptoms of biliary colic or cholangitis. Painless jaundice may occur in patients with choledocholithiasis, but this manifestation is much more characteristic of biliary obstruction secondary to malignancy of the head of the pancreas, bile ducts, or ampulla of Vater.

In patients whose obstruction is secondary to choledocholithiasis, associated chronic calculous cholecystitis is very common, and the gallbladder in this setting may be relatively indistensible. The absence of a palpable gallbladder in most patients with biliary obstruction from duct stones is the basis for *Courvoisier's law*, i.e., that the presence of a palpably enlarged gallbladder suggests that the biliary obstruction is secondary to an underlying malignancy rather than to calculous disease. Biliary obstruction causes progressive dilatation of the intrahepatic bile ducts as intrabiliary pressures rise. Hepatic bile flow is suppressed, and reabsorption and regurgitation of conjugated bilirubin into the bloodstream lead to jaundice accompanied by dark urine (bilirubinuria) and light-colored (acholic) stools.

CBD stones should be suspected in any patient with cholecystitis whose serum bilirubin level exceeds 85.5 μmol/L (5 mg/dL). The maximum bilirubin level is seldom over 256.5 μmol/L (15.0 mg/dL) in patients with choledocholithiasis unless concomitant hepatic disease or another factor leading to marked hyperbilirubinemia exists. Serum bilirubin levels of 342.0 μmol/L (20 mg/dL) or more should suggest the possibility of neoplastic obstruction. The serum alkaline phosphatase level is almost always elevated in biliary obstruction. A rise in alkaline phosphatase often precedes clinical jaundice and may be the only abnormality in routine liver function tests. There may be a two- to tenfold elevation of serum aminotransferases, especially in association with acute obstruction. Following relief of the obstructing process, serum aminotransferase elevations usually return rapidly to normal, while the serum bilirubin level may take 1 to 2 weeks to return to normal. The alkaline phosphatase level usually falls slowly, lagging behind the decrease in serum bilirubin.

PANCREATITIS   The most common associated entity discovered in patients with nonalcoholic acute pancreatitis is biliary tract disease. Biochemical evidence of pancreatic inflammation complicates acute cholecystitis in 15% of cases and choledocholithiasis in over 30%, and the common factor appears to be the passage of gallstones through the common duct. Coexisting pancreatitis should be suspected in patients with symptoms of cholecystitis who develop (1) back pain or pain to the left of the abdominal midline, (2) prolonged vomiting with paralytic ileus, or (3) a pleural effusion, especially on the left side. Surgical treatment of gallstone disease is usually associated with resolution of the pancreatitis.

SECONDARY BILIARY CIRRHOSIS   Secondary biliary cirrhosis may complicate prolonged or intermittent duct obstruction with or without recurrent cholangitis. Although this complication may be seen in patients with choledocholithiasis, it is more common in cases of prolonged obstruction from stricture or neoplasm. Once established, secondary biliary cirrhosis may be progressive even after correction of the obstructing process, and increasingly severe hepatic cirrhosis may lead to portal hypertension or to hepatic failure and death. Prolonged biliary obstruction may also be associated with clinically relevant deficiencies of the fat-soluble vitamins A, D, E, and K.

Diagnosis and Treatment The diagnosis of choledocholithiasis is usually made by cholangiography (Table 292-3), either preoperatively by ERCP or intraoperatively at the time of cholecystectomy. As many as 15% of patients undergoing cholecystectomy will prove to have CBD stones. With the advent of laparoscopic cholecystectomy, the management of CBD stones in the presence of gallstones is gradually being

clarified. Preoperative ERCP with endoscopic papillotomy and stone extraction is the preferred approach. It not only provides stone clearance but also defines the anatomy of the biliary tree in relationship to the cystic duct. ERCP is indicated in gallstone patients who have any of the following risk factors: (1) a history of jaundice or pancreatitis, (2) abnormal tests of liver function, and (3) ultrasonographic evidence

TABLE 292-3 *Diagnostic Evaluation of the Bile Ducts*

Diagnostic Advantages	Diagnostic Limitations	Contraindications	Complications	Comment
HEPATOBILIARY ULTRASOUND				
Rapid Simultaneous scanning of GB, liver, bile ducts, pancreas Accurate identification of dilated bile ducts Not limited by jaundice, pregnancy Guidance for fine-needle biopsy	Bowel gas Massive obesity Ascites Barium Partial bile duct obstruction Poor visualization of distal CBD	None	None	Initial procedure of choice in investigating possible biliary tract obstruction
COMPUTED TOMOGRAPHY				
Simultaneous scanning of GB, liver, bile ducts, pancreas Accurate identification of dilated bile ducts, masses Not limited by jaundice, gas, obesity, ascites High-resolution image Guidance for fine-needle biopsy	Extreme cachexia Movement artifact Ileus Partial bile duct obstruction	Pregnancy	Reaction to iodinated contrast, if used	Indicated for evaluation of hepatic or pancreatic masses Procedure of choice in investigating possible biliary obstruction if diagnostic limitations prevent HBUS
MAGNETIC RESONANCE CHOLANGIOPANCREATOGRAPHY				
Useful modality for visualizing pancreatic and biliary ducts Has excellent sensitivity for bile duct dilatation, biliary stricture, and intraductal abnormalities Can identify pancreatic duct dilatation or stricture, pancreatic duct stenosis, and pancreas divisum	Cannot offer therapeutic intervention High cost	Claustrophobia Certain metals (iron)	None	
PERCUTANEOUS TRANSHEPATIC CHOLANGIOGRAM				
Extremely successful when bile ducts dilated Best visualization of proximal biliary tract Bile cytology/culture Percutaneous transhepatic drainage	Nondilated or sclerosed ducts	Pregnancy Uncorrectable coagulopathy Massive ascites ? Hepatic abscess	Bleeding Hemobilia Bile peritonitis Bacteremia, sepsis	Indicated when ERCP is contraindicated or failed
ENDOSCOPIC RETROGRADE CHOLANGIOPANCREATOGRAM				
Simultaneous pancreatography Best visualization of distal biliary tract Bile or pancreatic cytology Endoscopic sphincterotomy and stone removal Biliary manometry	Gastroduodenal obstruction ? Roux en Y biliary-enteric anastomosis	Pregnancy ? Acute pancreatitis ? Severe cardiopulmonary disease	Pancreatitis Cholangitis, sepsis Infected pancreatic pseudocyst Perforation (rare) Hypoxemia, aspiration	Cholangiogram of choice in: Absence of dilated ducts ? Pancreatic, ampullary or gastroduodenal disease Prior biliary surgery Endoscopic sphincterotomy a treatment possibility
ENDOSCOPIC ULTRASOUND				
Most sensitive method to detect ampullary stones				Can be used in pregnancy

Note: GB, gallbladder; CBD, common bile duct; HBUS, hepatobiliary ultrasound; ERCP, endoscopic retrograde cholangiopancreatography. Intravenous cholangiography is an obsolete technique because 40% of common duct stones are missed and there is poor resolution even with tomography. There are few indications for its use, especially since other cholangiographic techniques are usually available.

of a dilated CBD or stones in the duct. Alternatively, if intraoperative cholangiography reveals retained stones, postoperative ERCP can be carried out. The need for preoperative ERCP is expected to decrease further as laparoscopic techniques improve.

The widespread use of laparoscopic cholecystectomy and ERCP has decreased the incidence of complicated biliary tract disease and the need for choledocholithotomy and T-tube drainage of the bile ducts. EBS followed by spontaneous passage or stone extraction is the treatment of choice in the management of patients with common duct stones, especially in elderly or poor-risk patients.

TRAUMA, STRICTURES, AND HEMOBILIA Approximately 95% of benign strictures of the extrahepatic bile ducts result from surgical trauma and occur in about 1 in 500 cholecystectomies. Strictures may present with bile leak or abscess formation in the immediate postoperative period or with biliary obstruction or cholangitis as long as 2 years or more following the inciting trauma. The diagnosis is established by percutaneous or endoscopic cholangiography. Endoscopic brushing of biliary strictures may be helpful in establishing the nature of the lesion and is more accurate than bile cytology alone. When positive exfoliative cytology is obtained, the diagnosis of a neoplastic stricture is established. This procedure is especially important in patients with primary sclerosing cholangitis (PSC) who are predisposed to the development of cholangiocarcinomas. Successful operative correction of non-PSC bile duct strictures by a skillful surgeon with duct-to-bowel anastomosis is usually possible, although mortality rates from surgical complications, recurrent cholangitis, or secondary biliary cirrhosis are high.

Hemobilia may follow traumatic or operative injury to the liver or bile ducts, intraductal rupture of a hepatic abscess or aneurysm of the hepatic artery, biliary or hepatic tumor hemorrhage, or mechanical complications of choledocholithiasis or hepatobiliary parasitism. Diagnostic procedures such as liver biopsy, PTC, and transhepatic biliary drainage catheter placement may also be complicated by hemobilia. Patients often present with a classic triad of biliary pain, obstructive jaundice, and melena or occult blood in the stools. The diagnosis is sometimes made by cholangiographic evidence of blood clot in the biliary tree, but selective angiographic verification may be required. Although minor episodes of hemobilia may resolve without operative intervention, surgical ligation of the bleeding vessel is frequently required.

EXTRINSIC COMPRESSION OF THE BILE DUCTS Partial or complete biliary obstruction may sometimes be produced by extrinsic compression of the ducts. The most common cause of this form of obstructive jaundice is carcinoma of the head of the pancreas. Biliary obstruction may also occur as a complication of either acute or chronic pancreatitis or involvement of lymph nodes in the porta hepatis by lymphoma or metastatic carcinoma. The latter should be distinguished from cholestasis resulting from massive replacement of the liver by tumor.

HEPATOBILIARY PARASITISM Infestation of the biliary tract by adult helminths or their ova may produce a chronic, recurrent pyogenic cholangitis with or without multiple hepatic abscesses, ductal stones, or biliary obstruction. This condition is relatively rare but does occur in inhabitants of southern China and elsewhere in Southeast Asia. The organisms most commonly involved are trematodes or flukes, including *Clonorchis sinensis*, *Opisthorchis viverrini* or *O. felineus*, and *Fasciola hepatica*. The biliary tract also may be involved by intraductal migration of adult *Ascaris lumbricoides* from the duodenum or by intrabiliary rupture of hydatid cysts of the liver produced by *Echinococcus* spp. The diagnosis is made by cholangiography and the presence of characteristic ova on stool examination. When obstruction is present, the treatment of choice is laparotomy under antibiotic coverage, with common duct exploration and a biliary drainage procedure. It should be emphasized that in the Far East, one also sees cholangiohepatitis associated with pigment lithiasis, which may, in fact, be more common than cholangitis due to parasites.

SCLEROSING CHOLANGITIS Primary or idiopathic sclerosing cholangitis is characterized by a progressive, inflammatory, sclerosing, and obliterative process affecting the extrahepatic and/or the intrahepatic bile ducts. The disorder occurs in about 70% in association with inflammatory bowel disease, especially ulcerative colitis. It may also be associated (albeit rarely) with multifocal fibrosclerosis syndromes such as retroperitoneal, mediastinal, and/or periureteral fibrosis; Riedel's struma; or pseudotumor of the orbit.

Patients with primary sclerosing cholangitis often present with signs and symptoms of chronic or intermittent biliary obstruction: RUQ abdominal pain, pruritus, jaundice, or acute cholangitis. Late in the course, complete biliary obstruction, secondary biliary cirrhosis, hepatic failure, or portal hypertension with bleeding varices may occur. The diagnosis is usually established by finding multifocal, diffusely distributed strictures with intervening segments of normal or dilated ducts, producing a beaded appearance on cholangiography (Fig. 292-2D). The cholangiographic technique of choice in suspected cases is ERCP, since intrahepatic ductal involvement may make PTC difficult. When a diagnosis of sclerosing cholangitis has been established, a search for associated diseases, especially for chronic inflammatory bowel disease, should be carried out.

A recent study describes the natural history and outcome for 305 patients of Swedish descent with primary sclerosing cholangitis; 134 (44%) of the patients were asymptomatic at the time of diagnosis and, not surprisingly, had a significantly higher survival rate with a median follow-up time of 63 months. The independent predictors of a bad prognosis were age, serum bilirubin concentration, and liver histologic changes. Cholangiocarcinoma was found in 24 patients (8%). Inflammatory bowel disease was closely associated with primary sclerosing cholangitis and had a prevalence of 81% in this study population.

Small duct PSC is defined by the presence of chronic cholestasis and hepatic histology consistent with PSC but with normal findings on cholangiography. Small duct PSC is found in about 5% of patients with PSC and may represent an earlier stage of PSC associated with a significantly better long-term prognosis. However, such patients may progress to classic PSC and/or end-stage liver disease with consequent necessity of liver transplantation.

In patients with AIDS, cholangiopancreatography may demonstrate a broad range of biliary tract changes as well as pancreatic duct obstruction and occasionally pancreatitis (Chap. 173). Further, biliary tract lesions in AIDS include infection and cholangiopancreatographic changes similar to those of PSC. Changes noted include: (1) diffuse involvement of intrahepatic bile ducts alone, (2) involvement of both intra- and extrahepatic bile ducts, (3) ampullary stenosis, (4) stricture of the intrapancreatic portion of the common bile duct, and (5) pancreatic duct involvement. Associated infectious organisms include *Cryptosporidium*, *Mycobacterium avium-intracellulare*, cytomegalovirus, *Microsporidia*, and *Isospora*. In addition, acalculous cholecystitis occurs in up to 10% of patients. ERCP sphincterotomy, while not without risk, provides significant pain reduction in patients with AIDS-associated papillary stenosis. Secondary sclerosing cholangitis may occur as a long-term complication of choledocholithiasis, cholangiocarcinoma, operative or traumatic biliary injury, or contiguous inflammatory processes.

℞ TREATMENT

Therapy with cholestyramine may help control symptoms of pruritus, and antibiotics are useful when cholangitis complicates the clinical picture. Vitamin D and calcium supplementation may help prevent the loss of bone mass frequently seen in patients with chronic cholestasis. Glucocorticoids, methotrexate, and cyclosporine have not been shown to be efficacious in PSC. UDCA in high dosage (20 mg/kg) improves serum liver tests, but an effect on survival has not been documented. In cases where high-grade biliary obstruction (dominant strictures) has occurred, balloon dilatation or stenting may be appropriate. Only rarely is surgical intervention indicated. Efforts at biliary-enteric anastomosis or stent placement may, however, be complicated by recurrent cholangitis and further progression of the stenosing process. The prognosis is unfavorable, with a median survival of 9 to 12 years following the diagnosis, regardless of therapy. Four variables (age, serum bilirubin level, histologic stage, and splenomegaly) predict survival in patients with PSC and serve as the basis for a risk score. PSC is one of the most common indications for liver transplantation.

FURTHER READING

APSTEIN MD, CAREY MC: Pathogenesis of cholesterol gallstones: A parsimonious hypothesis. Eur J Clin Invest 26:343, 1996

BERR F et al: Disorders of bile acid metabolism in cholesterol gallstone disease. J Clin Invest 90:589, 1992

BROOME U et al: Natural history and outcome in 32 Swedish patients with small duct primary sclerosing cholangitis (PSC). J Hepatol 36:586, 2002

PAULETZKI J et al: Gallbladder emptying and gallstone formation: A prospective study on gallstone recurrence. Gastroenterology 111:765, 1996

PAUMPARTNER G: Nonsurgical management of gallstone disease, in *Sleisenger and Fordtran's Gastrointestinal and Liver Disease*, 7th ed, M Feldman et al (eds). Philadelphia, Saunders, 2002, 1107–1115

RANSOHOFF DF, GRACIE WA: Treatment of gallstones. Ann Intern Med 119: 606, 1993

ZACKS SL et al: A population-based cohort study comparing laparoscopic cholecystectomy and open cholecystectomy. Ann J Gastroenterol 97:334, 2002

Section 3 Disorders of the Pancreas

293 APPROACH TO THE PATIENT WITH PANCREATIC DISEASE
Phillip P. Toskes, Norton J. Greenberger

GENERAL CONSIDERATIONS

Inflammatory disease of the pancreas may be acute or chronic. Although good data exist concerning the frequency of acute pancreatitis (about 5000 new cases per year in the United States, with a mortality rate of about 10%), the number of patients who suffer with recurrent acute pancreatitis or chronic pancreatitis is largely undefined. Only one prospective study on the incidence of chronic pancreatitis is available; it showed an incidence of 8.2 new cases per 100,000 per year and a prevalence of 26.4 cases per 100,000. These numbers probably underestimate considerably the true incidence and prevalence, because non-alcohol-induced pancreatitis was largely ignored. At autopsy, the prevalence of chronic pancreatitis ranges from 0.04 to 5%. The relative inaccessibility of the pancreas to direct examination and the nonspecificity of the abdominal pain associated with pancreatitis make the diagnosis of pancreatitis difficult and usually dependent on elevation of blood amylase levels. Many patients with chronic pancreatitis do not have elevated blood amylase levels. Some patients with chronic pancreatitis develop signs and symptoms of pancreatic exocrine insufficiency, and thus objective evidence for pancreatic disease can be demonstrated. However, there is a very large reservoir of pancreatic exocrine function. More than 90% of the pancreas must be damaged before maldigestion of fat and protein is manifested. Even the secretin stimulation test, which is the most sensitive method of assessing pancreatic exocrine function, is probably abnormal only when >60% of exocrine function has been lost. Noninvasive, indirect tests of pancreatic exocrine function (fecal elastase, serum trypsinogen) are much more likely to give abnormal results in patients with obvious pancreatic disease, i.e., pancreatic calcification, steatorrhea, or diabetes mellitus, than in patients with occult disease. Thus, the number of patients who have subclinical exocrine dysfunction (<90% loss of function) is unknown.

The clinical manifestations of acute and chronic pancreatitis and pancreatic insufficiency are protean. Thus, patients may present with hypertriglyceridemia, vitamin B_{12} malabsorption, hypercalcemia, hypocalcemia, hyperglycemia, ascites, pleural effusions, and chronic abdominal pain with normal blood amylase levels. Indeed, if the clinician considers pancreatitis as a possible diagnosis only when presented with a patient having classic symptoms (i.e., severe, constant epigastric pain that radiates through to the back, along with an elevated blood amylase level), only a minority of patients with pancreatitis will be diagnosed correctly.

As emphasized in Chap. 294, the etiologies as well as the clinical manifestations of pancreatitis are quite varied. Although it is well appreciated that pancreatitis is frequently secondary to alcohol abuse and biliary tract disease, it can also be caused by drugs, trauma, and viral infections and is associated with metabolic and connective tissue disorders. In approximately 30% of patients with acute pancreatitis and 25 to 40% of patients with chronic pancreatitis, the etiology is obscure.

TESTS USEFUL IN THE DIAGNOSIS OF PANCREATIC DISEASE

Several tests have proved of value in the evaluation of pancreatic exocrine function. Examples of specific tests and their usefulness in the diagnosis of acute and chronic pancreatitis are summarized in Table 293-1 and Fig. 293-1. At most institutions, pancreatic function tests are performed if the diagnosis of pancreatic disease remains a possibility after noninvasive tests [ultrasound, computed tomography (CT)] and invasive tests [endoscopic retrograde cholangiopancreatography (ERCP)] have given normal or inconclusive results. In this regard, tests employing *direct* stimulation of the pancreas are the most sensitive.

PANCREATIC ENZYMES IN BODY FLUIDS The serum amylase level is widely used as a screening test for acute pancreatitis in the patient with acute abdominal pain or back pain. A value >65 U/L should raise the question of acute pancreatitis. Levels >130 U/L make the diagnosis more likely, and values greater than three times normal virtually clinch the diagnosis if gut perforation or infarction is excluded. In acute pancreatitis, the serum amylase is usually elevated within 24 h of onset and remains so for 1 to 3 days. Levels return to normal within 3 to 5 days unless there is extensive pancreatic necrosis, incomplete ductal obstruction, or pseudocyst formation. Approximately 85% of patients with acute pancreatitis have an elevated serum amylase level. This index may be normal, however, if (1) there is a delay (of 2 to 5 days) before blood samples are obtained, (2) the underlying disorder is chronic pancreatitis rather than acute pancreatitis, or (3) hypertriglyceridemia is present. Patients with hypertriglyceridemia and proven pancreatitis have been found to have spuriously low levels of amylase and perhaps lipase activity.

The serum amylase is often elevated in other conditions (Table 293-2), in part because the enzyme is found in many organs in addition to the pancreas (salivary glands, liver, small intestine, kidney, fallopian tube) and can be produced by various tumors (carcinomas of the lung, esophagus, breast, and ovary). An assay of serum trypsinogen (performed by several commercial laboratories) is quite helpful in this regard. Since this enzyme is secreted specifically by the pancreas, a normal serum trypsinogen level in a patient with minimal elevation of serum amylase essentially rules out acute pancreatitis. Urinary amylase measurements, including the amylase/creatinine clearance ratio, are no more sensitive or specific than blood amylase levels.

Elevation of ascitic fluid amylase occurs in acute pancreatitis as well as in (1) pancreatogenous ascites due to disruption of the main pancreatic duct or a leaking pseudocyst and (2) other abdominal disorders that simulate pancreatitis (e.g., intestinal obstruction, intestinal infarction, and perforated peptic ulcer). Elevation of pleural fluid am-

Test	Principle	Comment
PANCREATIC ENZYMES IN BODY FLUIDS		
Amylase		
1. Serum	Pancreatic inflammation leads to increased enzyme levels	Simple; 20–40% false negatives and positives; reliable if test results are three times the upper limit of normal
2. Urine	Renal clearance of amylase is increased in acute pancreatitis	May be abnormal when serum levels normal; false negatives and positives
3. Ascitic fluid	Disruption of gland or main pancreatic duct leads to increased amylase concentration	Can establish diagnosis of pancreatitis; false positives occur with intestinal obstruction and perforated ulcer
4. Pleural fluid	Exudative pleural effusion with pancreatitis	False positives occur with carcinoma of the lung and esophageal perforation
5. Isoenzymes	P isoamylases arise from the pancreas; S isoamylases are from other sources	More specific than total serum amylase in diagnosis of acute pancreatitis; useful in identifying nonpancreatic causes of hyperamylasemia
Serum lipase	Pancreatic inflammation leads to increased enzyme levels	New methods have greatly simplified determination; positive in 70–85% of cases
Serum trypsinogen	Pancreatic inflammation leads to increased levels	*Elevated* in acute pancreatitis; *decreased* in chronic pancreatitis *with* steatorrhea; normal in chronic pancreatitis *without* steatorrhea and in steatorrhea with normal pancreatic function
STUDIES PERTAINING TO PANCREATIC STRUCTURE		
Radiologic and radionuclide tests		
1. Plain film of the abdomen	Abnormal in acute and chronic pancreatitis	Simple; normal in >50% of cases of both acute and chronic pancreatitis
2. Upper gastrointestinal x-rays	Abnormally thickened duodenal folds; displacement of stomach or widening of duodenal loop suggests a pancreatic mass (inflammatory, neoplastic, cystic)	Simple; frequently normal; largely superseded by US and CT scanning
3. Ultrasonography (US)	Can provide information on edema, inflammation, calcification, pseudocysts, and mass lesions	Simple, noninvasive; sequential studies quite feasible; useful in diagnosis of pseudocyst
4. CT scan	Permits detailed visualization of pancreas and surrounding structures	Useful in the diagnosis of pancreatic calcification, dilated pancreatic ducts, and pancreatic tumors; may not be able to distinguish between inflammatory and neoplastic mass lesions
5. Selective angiography	Can identify pancreatic neoplasms (1) by sheathing of celiac or superior mesenteric branches by tumor or (2) by tumor staining; displacement of vessels by tumor	Indicated (1) in suspected islet cell tumors and (2) before pancreatic or duodenal resection; most reliable features reflect nonresectable pancreatic cancer
6. Endoscopic retrograde cholangiopancreatography (ERCP)	Cannulation of pancreatic and common bile duct permits visualization of pancreatic-biliary ductal system	Provides diagnostic data in 60–85% of cases; differentiation of chronic pancreatitis from pancreatic carcinoma may be difficult
7. Endoscopic ultrasonography (EUS)	High-frequency transducer employed with EUS can produce very high resolution images and depict changes in the pancreatic duct and parenchyma with better detail	Exact role of EUS versus ERCP and CT not yet fully defined; sensitivity and specificity under study
8. Magnetic resonance cholangiopancreatography	Three-dimensional rendering has been used to produce very good images of the pancreatic duct by a noninvasive technique	May be used to evaluate patients judged to be at high risk for ERCP, such as the elderly; may replace ERCP as a diagnostic test, although large controlled studies need to be done
Pancreatic biopsy with US or CT guidance	Percutaneous biopsy with skinny needle and localization of lesion by US	High diagnostic yield; laparotomy avoided; requires special technical skills
TESTS OF EXOCRINE PANCREATIC FUNCTION		
Direct stimulation of the pancreas with analysis of duodenal contents		
1. Secretin-pancreozymin (CCK) test	Secretin leads to increased output of pancreatic juice and HCO_3^-; CCK leads to increased output of pancreatic enzymes; pancreatic secretory response is related to the functional mass of pancreatic tissue	Sensitive enough to detect occult disease; involves duodenal intubation and fluoroscopy; poorly defined normal enzyme response; overlap in chronic pancreatitis; large secretory reserve capacity of the pancreas
Measurement of intraluminal digestion products		
1. Microscopic examination of stool for undigested meat fibers and fat	Lack of proteolytic and lipolytic enzymes causes decreased digestion of meat fibers and triglycerides	Simple, reliable; not sensitive enough to detect milder cases of pancreatic insufficiency
2. Quantitative stool fat determination	Lack of lipolytic enzymes brings about impaired fat digestion	Reliable, reference standard for defining severity of malabsorption; does not distinguish between maldigestion and malabsorption
3. Fecal nitrogen	Lack of proteolytic enzymes leads to impaired protein digestion, resulting in an increase in stool nitrogen	Does not distinguish between maldigestion and malabsorption; low sensitivity

(continued)

TABLE 293-2— *(Continued)*

Test	Principle	Comment
Measurement of pancreatic enzymes in feces 1. Elastase	Pancreatic secretion of proteolytic enzymes	Excellent specificity; sensitivity similar to that of serum trypsinogen
Miscellaneous tests 1. Dual-labeled Schilling test	Intrinsic factor [^{57}Co]cobalamin and Hog R protein [^{58}Co]cobalamin are given together. Since proteases are necessary to cleave R protein, the ratio of labeled cobalamin excreted in urine is an index of exocrine dysfunction.	Time-consuming and expensive

ylase occurs in acute pancreatitis, chronic pancreatitis, carcinoma of the lung, and esophageal perforation.

Lipase may now be the single best enzyme to measure for the diagnosis of acute pancreatitis. Improvements in substrates and technology offer clinicians improved options, especially when a turbidimetric assay is used. The newer lipase assays have colipase as a cofactor and are fully automated.

An assay for trypsinogen (or for trypsin-like immunoreactivity) has a theoretical advantage over amylase and lipase determinations in that the pancreas is the only organ that contains this enzyme. The test appears to be useful in the diagnosis of both acute and chronic pancreatitis. Sensitivity and specificity are comparable to those of amylase and lipase determinations. Since trypsinogen is also excreted by the kidney, elevated serum values are found in renal failure, as is the case with serum amylase and lipase levels. *No single blood test is reliable for the diagnosis of acute pancreatitis in patients with renal failure.* Determining whether a patient with renal failure and abdominal pain has pancreatitis remains a difficult clinical problem. A recent study found that serum amylase levels were elevated in patients with renal dysfunction only when creatinine clearance was <50 mL/min. In such patients, the serum amylase level was invariably <500 IU/L in the absence of objective evidence of acute pancreatitis. In that study, serum lipase and trypsin levels paralleled serum amylase values.

A recent study evaluated the sensitivity and specificity of five assays used to diagnose acute pancreatitis: two for amylase, one for lipase, one for trypsin-like immunoreactivity (TLI), and one for pancreatic isoamylase. The data obtained (1) show that, if the best cutoff level is used, all these assays have similar specificities and (2) suggest that total serum amylase is as good an indicator of acute pancreatitis as any of the alternatives. However, inherent in many such studies is

the problem that the recognition and diagnosis of acute pancreatitis hinge on the finding of an elevated serum amylase level. The question arises as to whether any diagnostic test result can be proved superior to the total serum amylase level if hyperamylasemia is required for the diagnosis. In other studies, when "objective" confirmation of the clinical diagnosis of pancreatitis was required (ultrasonography, CT, laparotomy), the sensitivity of the serum amylase has been found to be as low as 68%. With these limitations in mind, the recommended screening tests for acute pancreatitis are *total serum amylase* and *serum lipase activities.* Serum amylase values greater than three times normal are highly specific.

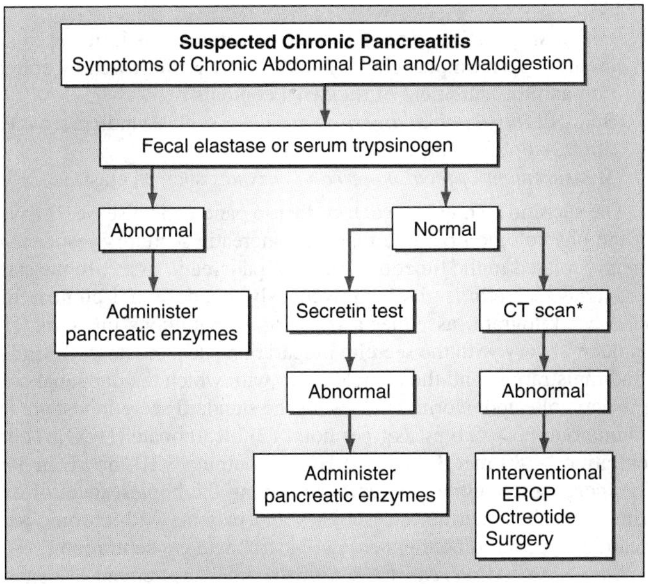

STUDIES PERTAINING TO PANCREATIC STRUCTURE ■ Radiologic Tests Plain films of the abdomen provide useful information in 30 to 50% of patients with acute pancreatitis. The most frequent abnormalities include (1) a localized ileus, usually involving the jejunum ("sentinel loop"); (2) a generalized ileus with air-fluid levels; (3) the "colon cutoff sign," which results from isolated distention of the transverse colon; (4) duodenal distention with air-fluid levels; and (5) a mass, which is frequently a pseudocyst. In chronic pancreatitis, an important radiographic finding is pancreatic calcification, which characteristically is localized adjacent to and superimposed on the second lumbar vertebra (Fig. 294-3*A*).

Suspected Chronic Pancreatitis
Symptoms of Chronic Abdominal Pain and/or Maldigestion

→ Fecal elastase or serum trypsinogen

Abnormal → Administer pancreatic enzymes

Normal → Secretin test / CT scan*

Secretin test → Abnormal → Administer pancreatic enzymes

CT scan* → Abnormal → Interventional ERCP / Octreotide / Surgery

FIGURE 293-1 An approach to the patient with suspected chronic pancreatitis. EUS and MRCP are appropriate diagnostic alternatives.

TABLE 293-2 *Causes of Hyperamylasemia and Hyperamylasuria*

PANCREATIC DISEASE

I. Pancreatitis
  A. Acute
  B. Chronic: ductal obstruction
  C. Complications of pancreatitis
    1. Pancreatic pseudocyst
    2. Pancreatogenous ascites
    3. Pancreatic abscess
    4. Pancreatic necrosis

II. Pancreatic trauma
III. Pancreatic carcinoma

NONPANCREATIC DISORDERS

I. Renal insufficiency
II. Salivary gland lesions
  A. Mumps
  B. Calculus
  C. Irradiation sialadenitis
  D. Maxillofacial surgery
III. "Tumor" hyperamylasemia
  A. Carcinoma of the lung
  B. Carcinoma of the esophagus
  C. Breast carcinoma, ovarian carcinoma

IV. Macroamylasemia
V. Burns
VI. Diabetic ketoacidosis
VII. Pregnancy
VIII. Renal transplantation
IX. Cerebral trauma
X. Drugs: morphine

OTHER ABDOMINAL DISORDERS

I. Biliary tract disease: cholecystitis, choledocholithiasis
II. Intraabdominal disease
  A. Perforated or penetrating peptic ulcer
  B. Intestinal obstruction or infarction
  C. Ruptured ectopic pregnancy
  D. Peritonitis
  E. Aortic aneurysm
  F. Chronic liver disease
  G. Postoperative hyperamylasemia

Upper gastrointestinal x-rays may reveal displacement of the stomach by the retroperitoneal mass (Fig. 294-2A) or widening and effacement of the duodenal C loop, which also suggest the presence of a pancreatic mass, which could be inflammatory, cystic, or neoplastic. However, the use of x-ray films has been largely superseded by ultrasound.

Ultrasonography can provide important information in patients with acute pancreatitis, chronic pancreatitis, pancreatic calcification, pseudocyst, and pancreatic carcinoma. Echographic appearances can indicate the presence of edema, inflammation, and calcification (not obvious on plain films of the abdomen), as well as pseudocysts, mass lesions, and gallstones (Figs. 294-2B and 294-3B). In acute pancreatitis, the pancreas is characteristically enlarged. In pancreatic pseudocyst, the usual appearance is that of an echo-free, smooth, round fluid collection. Pancreatic carcinoma distorts the usual landmarks, and mass lesions >3.0 cm are usually detected as localized, echo-free solid lesions. Ultrasound is often the initial investigation for most patients with suspected pancreatic disease. However, obesity, excess small- and large-bowel gas, and recently performed barium contrast examinations can interfere with ultrasound studies.

CT is the best imaging study for initial evaluation of a suspected chronic pancreatic disorder and for the complications of acute and chronic pancreatitis. It is especially useful in the detection of pancreatic tumors, fluid-containing lesions such as pseudocysts and abscesses, and calcium deposits (Figs. 294-3C and 294-4A). Most lesions are characterized by (1) enlargement of the pancreatic outline, (2) distortion of the pancreatic contour, and/or (3) a fluid filling that has a different attenuation coefficient than normal pancreas. However, it is occasionally difficult to distinguish between inflammatory and neoplastic lesions. Oral water-soluble contrast agents may be used to opacify the stomach and duodenum during CT scans; this strategy permits more precise delineation of various organs as well as mass lesions. Dynamic CT (using rapid intravenous administration of contrast) is useful in estimating the degree of pancreatic necrosis and in predicting morbidity and mortality. Spiral (helical) CT provides clear images much more rapidly and essentially negates artifact caused by patient movement (Fig. 294-2D).

Endoscopic ultrasonography (EUS) produces high-resolution images of the pancreatic parenchyma and pancreatic duct with a transducer fixed to an endoscope that can be directed onto the surface of the pancreas through the stomach or duodenum. EUS is replacing ERCP for diagnostic purposes in many centers. EUS allows one to obtain information about the pancreatic duct as well as the parenchyma and has no complications associated with it, in contrast to the 5 to 20% of post-ERCP pancreatitis observed. EUS is also very good in detecting common bile duct stones. Pancreatic masses can be biopsied via EUS and one can deliver nerve blocks through EUS. Figures 294-2A–C show the value of EUS in demonstrating pancreatic calcification, pancreatic pseudocysts, and dilation of the main pancreatic duct. Although criteria for abnormalities on EUS in severe pancreatic disease have been developed, the true sensitivity and specificity of this procedure has yet to be determined. In particular, it is not clear whether EUS can detect early pancreatic disease before abnormalities appear on more conventional radiograph tests such as ultrasonography or CT. The exact role of EUS versus ERCP and CT has yet to be defined.

Magnetic resonance cholangiopancreatography (MRCP) is now being used to view both the bile duct and the pancreatic duct. Non-breath-holding and three-dimensional turbo spin-echo techniques are being utilized to produce superb MRCP images. The main pancreatic duct and common bile duct can be seen well, but there is still a question as to whether changes can be detected consistently in the secondary ducts. MRCP may be particularly useful to evaluate the pancreatic duct in high-risk patients such as the elderly because this is a noninvasive procedure.

Both EUS and MRCP may replace ERCP in some patients. As these techniques become more refined, they may well be the diagnostic tests of choice to evaluate the pancreatic duct. ERCP is still needed to perform therapy of bile duct and pancreatic duct lesions.

Selective catheterization of the celiac and superior mesenteric arteries combined with superselective catheterization of others arteries, such as the hepatic, splenic, and gastroduodenal arteries, permits visualization of the pancreas and detection of pancreatic neoplasms and pseudocysts. Pancreatic neoplasms can be identified by the sheathing of blood vessels by a mass lesion (Fig. 294-1D). Hormone-producing pancreatic tumors are especially likely to exhibit increased vascularity and tumor staining. Angiographic abnormalities are noted in many patients with pancreatic carcinoma but are uncommon in patients without pancreatic disease. Angiography complements ultrasonography and ERCP in the study of patients with a suspected pancreatic lesion and may be carried out if ERCP is either unsuccessful or nondiagnostic.

ERCP may provide useful information on the status of the pancreatic ductal system and thus aid in the differential diagnosis of pancreatic disease (Figs. 294-1C, 294-3D, and 294-4B). Pancreatic carcinoma is characterized by stenosis or obstruction of either the pancreatic duct or the common bile duct; both ductal systems are often abnormal. In chronic pancreatitis, ERCP abnormalities include (1) luminal narrowing; (2) irregularities in the ductal system with stenosis, dilation, sacculation, and ectasia; and (3) blockage of the pancreatic duct by calcium deposits. The presence of ductal stenosis and irregularity can make it difficult to distinguish chronic pancreatitis from carcinoma. It is important to be aware that ERCP changes interpreted as indicating chronic pancreatitis actually may be due to the effects of aging on the pancreatic duct or to the fact that the procedure was performed within several weeks of an attack of acute pancreatitis. Although aging may cause impressive ductal alterations, it does not affect the results of pancreatic function tests (i.e., the secretin test). Elevated serum and/or urine amylase levels after ERCP have been reported in 25 to 75% of patients, but clinical pancreatitis is uncommon. If no lesion is found in the biliary and/or pancreatic ducts in a patient with repeated attacks of acute pancreatitis, manometric studies of the sphincter of Oddi may be indicated. Such studies, however, do increase the risk of post-ERCP/manometry acute pancreatitis. Such pancreatitis appears to be more common in patients with a nondilated pancreatic duct.

Pancreatic Biopsy with Radiologic Guidance Percutaneous aspiration biopsy of a pancreatic mass often distinguishes a pancreatic inflammatory mass from a pancreatic neoplasm.

TESTS OF EXOCRINE PANCREATIC FUNCTION

Pancreatic function tests (Table 293-1) can be divided into the following:

1. *Direct stimulation of the pancreas* by intravenous infusion of secretin or secretin plus cholecystokinin (CCK) followed by collection and measurement of duodenal contents
2. Study of *intraluminal digestion products*, such as undigested meat fibers, stool fat, and fecal nitrogen
3. *Measurement of fecal pancreatic enzymes* such as elastase

The secretin test, used to detect diffuse pancreatic disease, is based on the physiologic principle that the pancreatic secretory response is directly related to the functional mass of pancreatic tissue. In the standard assay, secretin is given intravenously in a dose of 1 clinical unit (CU) per kilogram, as either a bolus or a continuous infusion. The results will vary with the secretin preparation used, the dose, the mode of administration, and the completeness with which the duodenal contents are collected. Normal values for the standard secretin test are (1) volume output > 2.0 mL/kg per hour, (2) bicarbonate (HCO_3^-) concentration > 80 meq/L, and (3) HCO_3^- output > 10 meq/L in 1 h. The most reproducible measurement, giving the highest level of discrimination between normal subjects and patients with chronic pancreatitis, appears to be the maximal bicarbonate concentration.

The *combined secretin-CCK test* permits measurement of pancreatic amylase, lipase, trypsin, and chymotrypsin. Although there is overlap in the distributions of enzyme output in normal subjects and patients with pancreatitis in response to this test, markedly low enzyme outputs suggest advanced damage and destruction of acinar cells. With frank exocrine pancreatic insufficiency, there is usually an overall reduction in both HCO_3^- concentration and output of several enzymes. However, with lesser degrees of pancreatic damage there may be a dissociation between HCO_3^- concentration and enzyme output. There may also be a dissociation between the results of the secretin test and those of tests of absorptive function. For example, patients with chronic pancreatitis often have abnormally low outputs of HCO_3^- after secretin but have normal fecal fat excretion. Thus the secretin test measures the secretory capacity of ductular epithelium, while fecal fat excretion indirectly reflects intraluminal lipolytic activity. Steatorrhea does not occur until intraluminal levels of lipase are markedly reduced, underscoring the fact that only small amounts of enzymes are necessary for intraluminal digestive activities. An abnormal secretin test result suggests only that chronic pancreatic damage is present; it will not consistently distinguish between chronic pancreatitis and pancreatic carcinoma.

Another test of exocrine pancreatic function is the *bentiromide test.*

This test is an indirect measure of pancreatic function and reflects intraluminal chymotrypsin activity. The test has excellent specificity but is not very sensitive. It no longer is available for clinical use in the United States.

The *serum trypsinogen level,* which is determined by radioimmunoassay, also has excellent specificity but is not very sensitive. It is a simple blood test that can detect severe damage to the exocrine pancreas. The normal values are 28 to 58 ng/mL, and any value <20 ng/mL reflects pancreatic steatorrhea.

Measurement of *intraluminal digestion products,* i.e., undigested muscle fibers, stool fat, and fecal nitrogen, is discussed in Chap. 275. The amount of elastase in stool reflects the pancreatic output of this proteolytic enzyme. Decreased elastase activity in stool has been reported in patients with chronic pancreatitis and cystic fibrosis. →*Tests useful in the diagnosis of exocrine pancreatic insufficiency and the differential diagnosis of malabsorption are also discussed in Chaps. 275 and 294.*

294 | ACUTE AND CHRONIC PANCREATITIS
Norton J. Greenberger, Phillip P. Toskes

BIOCHEMISTRY AND PHYSIOLOGY OF PANCREATIC EXOCRINE SECRETION

GENERAL CONSIDERATIONS   The pancreas secretes 1500 to 3000 mL of isosmotic alkaline (pH > 8.0) fluid per day containing about 20 enzymes and zymogens. The pancreatic secretions provide the enzymes needed to effect the major digestive activity of the gastrointestinal tract and provide an optimal pH for the function of these enzymes.

REGULATION OF PANCREATIC SECRETION   The exocrine pancreas is influenced by intimately interacting hormonal and neural systems. *Gastric acid* is the stimulus for the release of secretin, which stimulates the secretion of pancreatic juice rich in water and electrolytes. Release of cholecystokinin (CCK) from the duodenum and jejunum is largely triggered by long-chain fatty acids, certain essential amino acids (tryptophan, phenylalanine, valine, methionine), and gastric acid itself. CCK evokes an enzyme-rich secretion from the pancreas. The *parasympathetic nervous system* (via the vagus nerve) exerts significant control over pancreatic secretion. Secretion evoked by secretin and CCK depends on permissive roles of vagal afferent and efferent pathways. This is particularly true for enzyme secretion, whereas water and bicarbonate secretion is heavily dependent on the hormonal effects of secretin and CCK. Also, vagal stimulation effects the release of vasoactive intestinal peptide (VIP), a secretin agonist. Bile salts also stimulate pancreatic secretion, thereby integrating the functions of the biliary tract, pancreas, and small intestine.

Pancreatic exocrine secretion is influenced by inhibitory neuropeptides such as somatostatin, pancreatic polypeptide, peptide YY, neuropeptide Y, enkephalin, pancreastatin, calcitonin gene–related peptides, glucagon, and galanin. Although pancreatic polypeptide and peptide YY may act primarily on nerves outside the pancreas, somatostatin acts at multiple sites. Nitric oxide is also an important neurotransmitter. The mechanism of action of these various factors has not been fully defined.

WATER AND ELECTROLYTE SECRETION   Bicarbonate is the ion of primary physiologic importance within pancreatic secretion. The ductal cells secrete bicarbonate predominantly derived from plasma (93%) rather than intracellular metabolism (7%). Bicarbonate enters through the sodium bicarbonate co-transporter with depolarization caused by chloride efflux through the cystic fibrosis transductance regulator (CFTR). Secretin and VIP, both of which increase intracellular cyclic AMP, act on the ductal cells opening the CFTR in promoting secretion. CCK, acting as a neuromodulator, markedly potentiates the stimulatory ef-

fects of secretin. Acetylcholine also plays an important role in ductal cell secretion. Bicarbonate helps neutralize gastric acid and creates the appropriate pH for the activity of pancreatic enzymes.

ENZYME SECRETION   The acinar cell is highly compartmentalized and is concerned with the secretion of pancreatic enzymes. Proteins synthesized by the rough endoplasmic reticulum are processed in the Golgi and then targeted to the appropriate site, whether that be zymogen granules, lysosomes, or other cell compartments. The pancreas secretes amylolytic, lipolytic, and proteolytic enzymes. *Amylolytic enzymes,* such as amylase, hydrolyze starch to oligosaccharides and to the disaccharide maltose. The *lipolytic enzymes* include lipase, phospholipase A, and cholesterol esterase. Bile salts inhibit lipase in isolation; but colipase, another constituent of pancreatic secretion, binds to lipase and prevents this inhibition. Bile salts activate phospholipase A and cholesterol esterase. *Proteolytic enzymes* include endopeptidases (trypsin, chymotrypsin), which act on internal peptide bonds of proteins and polypeptides; exopeptidases (carboxypeptidases, aminopeptidases), which act on the free carboxyl- and amino-terminal ends of peptides, respectively; and elastase. The proteolytic enzymes are secreted as inactive precursors (zymogens). Ribonucleases (deoxyribonucleases, ribonuclease) are also secreted. *Enterokinase,* an enzyme found in the duodenal mucosa, cleaves the lysine-isoleucine bond of trypsinogen to form trypsin. Trypsin then activates the other proteolytic zymogens in a cascade phenomenon. All pancreatic enzymes have pH optima in the alkaline range. The nervous system initiates pancreatic enzyme secretion. The neurologic stimulation is cholinergic, involving extrinsic innervation by the vagus nerve and subsequent innervation by intrapancreatic cholinergic nerves. The stimulatory neurotransmitters are acetylcholine and gastrin-releasing peptides. These neurotransmitters activate calcium-dependent second messenger systems resulting in the release of zymogen granules. VIP is present in intrapancreatic nerves and potentiates the effect of acetylcholine. In contrast to other species, there are no CCK receptors on acinar cells in humans. CCK in physiologic concentrations stimulates pancreatic secretion by stimulating central vagal and intrapancreatic nerves.

AUTOPROTECTION OF THE PANCREAS   Autodigestion of the pancreas is prevented by the packaging of proteases in precursor form and by the synthesis of protease inhibitors. These protease inhibitors are found in the acinar cell, the pancreatic secretions, and the α_1- and α_2-globulin fractions of plasma.

EXOCRINE-ENDOCRINE RELATIONSHIPS   Insulin appears to be needed locally for secretin and CCK to promote exocrine secretion; thus, it acts in a permissive role for these two hormones.

ENTEROPANCREATIC AXIS AND FEEDBACK INHIBITION Pancreatic enzyme secretion is controlled, at least in part, by a negative feedback mechanism induced by the presence of active serine proteases in the duodenum. To illustrate, perfusion of the duodenal lumen with phenylalanine causes a prompt increase in plasma CCK levels as well as increased secretion of chymotrypsin. However, simultaneous perfusion with trypsin blunts both responses. Conversely, perfusion of the duodenal lumen with protease inhibitors actually leads to enzyme hypersecretion. The available evidence supports the concept that the duodenum contains a peptide called *CCK-releasing factor* (CCK-RF) that is involved in stimulating CCK release. It appears that serine proteases inhibit pancreatic secretion by acting on a CCK-releasing peptide in the lumen of the small intestine. Thus the integrative result of both bicarbonate and enzyme secretion depends on a feedback process for both bicarbonate and pancreatic enzymes. Acidification of the duodenum releases secretin, which stimulates vagal-vagal and other neural pathways to activate pancreatic duct cells, which secrete bicarbonate. This bicarbonate then neutralizes the duodenal acid, and the feedback loop is completed. Duodenal proteins lead to a reduction in free proteases, thereby leading to an increase in free CCK-RF. CCK-RF is then released into the blood in physiologic concentrations, acting primarily through the neural pathways (vagal-vagal). This leads to acetylcholine-mediated pancreatic enzyme secretion. Proteases continue to be secreted from the pancreas until the protein within the duodenum and CCK-RF are digested. At this point, the free duodenal proteases rise again, thus completing this step in the feedback process.

ACUTE PANCREATITIS

GENERAL CONSIDERATIONS Pancreatic inflammatory disease may be classified as (1) acute pancreatitis and (2) chronic pancreatitis. The pathologic spectrum of acute pancreatitis varies from *edematous pancreatitis*, which is usually a mild and self-limited disorder, to *necrotizing pancreatitis*, in which the degree of pancreatic necrosis correlates with the severity of the attack and its systemic manifestations. The term *hemorrhagic pancreatitis* is less meaningful in a clinical sense because variable amounts of interstitial hemorrhage can be found in pancreatitis as well as in other disorders such as pancreatic trauma, pancreatic carcinoma, and severe congestive heart failure.

The incidence of pancreatitis varies in different countries and depends on cause, e.g., alcohol, gallstones, metabolic factors, and drugs (Table 294-1). The estimated incidence in England is 5.4/100,000 per year; in the United States it is 79.8/100,000 per year, thus resulting in 185,000 new cases of acute pancreatitis annually.

ETIOLOGY AND PATHOGENESIS There are many causes of acute pancreatitis (Table 294-1), but the mechanisms by which these conditions trigger pancreatic inflammation have not been identified. Gallstones continue to be the leading cause of acute pancreatitis in most series (30 to 60%). Alcohol is the second most common cause, responsible for 15 to 30% of cases in the United States. The incidence of pancreatitis in alcoholics is surprisingly low (5/100,000), indicating that in addition to the amount of alcohol ingested unknown factors affect a person's susceptibility to pancreatic injury. The mechanism of injury is not well understood. Hypertriglyceridemia is the cause of acute pancreatitis in 1.3 to 3.8% of cases; serum triglyceride levels are usually >11.3 mmol/L (>1000 mg/dL). Most patients with hypertriglyceridemia, when subsequently examined, show evidence of an underlying derangement in lipid metabolism, probably unrelated to pancreatitis. Patients with diabetes mellitus or who are on certain medications may also develop high triglyceride levels. Acute pancreatitis occurs in 5 to 20% of patients following endoscopic retrograde cholangiopancreatography (ERCP). Approximately 2 to 5% of cases of acute pancreatitis are drug-related. Drugs cause pancreatitis either by a hypersensitivity reaction or by the generation of a toxic metabolite, although in some cases it is not clear which of these mechanisms is operative. (Table 294-1).

TABLE 294-1 *Causes of Acute Pancreatitis*

Common Causes
   Gallstones (including microlithiasis)
   Alcohol (acute and chronic alcoholism)
   Hypertriglyceridemia
   Endoscopic retrograde cholangiopancreatography (ERCP), especially
      after biliary manometry
   Trauma (especially blunt abdominal trauma)
   Postoperative (abdominal and nonabdominal operations)
   Drugs (azathioprine, 6-mercaptopurine, sulfonamides, estrogens,
      tetracycline, valproic acid, anti-HIV medications)
   Sphincter of Oddi dysfunction
Uncommon causes
   Vascular causes and vasculitis (ischemic-hypoperfusion states after
      cardiac surgery)
   Connective tissue disorders and thrombotic thrombocytopenic purpura
      (TTP)
   Cancer of the pancreas
   Hypercalcemia
   Periampullary diverticulum
   Pancreas divisum
   Hereditary pancreatitis
   Cystic fibrosis
   Renal failure
Rare causes
   Infections (mumps, coxsackievirus, cytomegalovirus, echovirus,
      parasites)
   Autoimmune (e.g., Sjögren's syndrome)
**Causes to consider in patients with recurrent bouts of acute
   pancreatitis without an obvious etiology**
   Occult disease of the biliary tree or pancreatic ducts, especially
      microlithiasis, sludge
   Drugs
   Hypertriglyceridemia
   Pancreas divisum
   Pancreatic cancer
   Sphincter of Oddi dysfunction
   Cystic fibrosis
   Idiopathic

Autodigestion is one pathogenic theory, according to which pancreatitis results when proteolytic enzymes (e.g., trypsinogen, chymotrypsinogen, proelastase, and phospholipase A) are activated in the pancreas rather than in the intestinal lumen. A number of factors (e.g., endotoxins, exotoxins, viral infections, ischemia, anoxia, and direct trauma) are believed to activate these proenzymes. Activated proteolytic enzymes, especially trypsin, not only digest pancreatic and peripancreatic tissues but also can activate other enzymes, such as elastase and phospholipase.

Activation of Pancreatic Enzymes in the Pathogenesis of Acute Pancreatitis Several recent studies have suggested that pancreatitis is a disease that evolves in three phases. The initial phase is characterized by intrapancreatic digestive enzyme activation and acinar cell injury. Zymogen activation appears to be mediated by lysosomal hydrolases such as cathepsin B which become co-localized with digestive enzymes in intracellular organelles; it is currently believed that acinar cell injury is the consequence of zymogen activation. The second phase of pancreatitis involves the activation, chemoattraction, and sequestration of neutrophils in the pancreas resulting in an intrapancreatic inflammatory reaction of variable severity. Neutrophil depletion induced by prior administration of an antineutrophil serum has been shown to reduce the severity of experimentally induced pancreatitis. There is also evidence to support the concept that neutrophil sequestration can activate trypsinogen. Thus, intrapancreatic acinar cell activation of trypsinogen could be a two-step process, i.e., with a neutrophil-independent and a neutrophil-dependent phase. The third phase of pancreatitis is due to the effects of activated proteolytic enzymes and mediators, released by the inflamed pancreas, on distant organs. Activated proteolytic enzymes, especially trypsin, not only digest pancreatic and peripancreatic tissues but also activate other enzymes such as elastase and phospholipase. The active enzymes then digest cellular membranes and cause proteolysis, edema, interstitial hemorrhage, vascular damage, coagulation necrosis, fat necrosis, and parenchymal cell necrosis. Cellular injury and death result in the liberation of bradykinin peptides, vasoactive substances, and histamine that can produce vasodilation, increased vascular permeability, and edema with profound effects on many organs, most notably the lung. The systemic inflammatory response syndrome (SIRS) and acute respiratory distress syndrome (ARDS) as well as multiorgan failure may occur as result of this cascade of local as well as distant effects.

CLINICAL FEATURES *Abdominal pain* is the major symptom of acute pancreatitis. Pain may vary from a mild and tolerable discomfort to severe, constant, and incapacitating distress. Characteristically, the pain, which is steady and boring in character, is located in the epigastrium and periumbilical region and often radiates to the back as well as to the chest, flanks, and lower abdomen. The pain is frequently more intense when the patient is supine, and patients often obtain relief by sitting with the trunk flexed and knees drawn up. Nausea, vomiting, and abdominal distention due to gastric and intestinal hypomotility and chemical peritonitis are also frequent complaints.

Physical examination frequently reveals a distressed and anxious patient. Low-grade fever, tachycardia, and hypotension are fairly common. Shock is not unusual and may result from (1) hypovolemia secondary to exudation of blood and plasma proteins into the retroperitoneal space (a "retroperitoneal burn"); (2) increased formation and release of kinin peptides, which cause vasodilation and increased vascular permeability; and (3) systemic effects of proteolytic and lipolytic enzymes released into the circulation. Jaundice occurs infrequently; when present, it usually is due to edema of the head of the pancreas with compression of the intrapancreatic portion of the common bile duct. Erythematous skin nodules due to subcutaneous fat necrosis may occur. In 10 to 20% of patients, there are pulmonary findings, including basilar rales, atelectasis, and pleural effusion, the latter most frequently left-sided. Abdominal tenderness and muscle rigidity are present to a variable degree, but, compared with the intense pain, these signs may be unimpressive. Bowel sounds are usually diminished or absent. A pancreatic pseudocyst may be palpable in the upper abdomen. A faint blue discoloration around the umbilicus (Cullen's sign) may occur as the result of hemoperitoneum, and a blue-red-purple or green-brown discoloration of the flanks (Turner's sign) reflects tissue catabolism of hemoglobin. The latter two findings, which are uncommon, indicate the presence of a severe necrotizing pancreatitis.

LABORATORY DATA The diagnosis of acute pancreatitis is usually established by the detection of an increased level of serum amylase. Values threefold or more above normal virtually clinch the diagnosis if overt salivary gland disease and gut perforation or infarction are excluded. However, there appears to be no definite correlation between the severity of pancreatitis and the degree of serum amylase elevation. After 48 to 72 h, even with continuing evidence of pancreatitis, total serum amylase values tend to return to normal. However, pancreatic isoamylase and lipase levels may remain elevated for 7 to 14 days. It will be recalled that amylase elevations in serum and urine occur in many conditions other than pancreatitis (Table 293-2). Importantly, patients with *acidemia* (arterial pH ≤ 7.32) may have spurious elevations in serum amylase. In one study, 12 of 33 patients with acidemia had elevated serum amylase, but only 1 had an elevated lipase value; in 9, salivary-type amylase was the predominant serum isoamylase. This finding explains why patients with diabetic ketoacidosis may have marked elevations in serum amylase without any other evidence of acute pancreatitis. Serum lipase activity increases in parallel with amylase activity, and measurement of both enzymes increases the diagnostic yield. An elevated serum lipase or trypsin value is usually diagnostic of acute pancreatitis; these tests are especially helpful in patients with nonpancreatic causes of hyperamylasemia (Table 293-2). Markedly increased levels of peritoneal or pleural fluid amylase [>1500 nmol/L (>5000 U/dL)] are also helpful, if present, in establishing the diagnosis.

Leukocytosis (15,000 to 20,000 leukocytes μL) occurs frequently.

Patients with more severe disease may show hemoconcentration with hematocrit values exceeding 50% because of loss of plasma into the retroperitoneal space and peritoneal cavity. *Hyperglycemia* is common and is due to multiple factors, including decreased insulin release, increased glucagon release, and an increased output of adrenal glucocorticoids and catecholamines. *Hypocalcemia* occurs in approximately 25% of patients, and its pathogenesis is incompletely understood. Although earlier studies suggested that the response of the parathyroid gland to a decrease in serum calcium is impaired, subsequent observations have failed to confirm this idea. Intraperitoneal saponification of calcium by fatty acids in areas of fat necrosis occurs occasionally, with large amounts (up to 6.0 g) dissolved or suspended in ascitic fluid. Such "soap formation" may also be significant in patients with pancreatitis, mild hypocalcemia, and little or no obvious ascites. *Hyperbilirubinemia* [serum bilirubin > 68 μmol/L (>4.0 mg/dL)] occurs in approximately 10% of patients. However, jaundice is transient, and serum bilirubin levels return to normal in 4 to 7 days. Serum alkaline phosphatase and aspartate aminotransferase (AST) levels are also transiently elevated and parallel serum bilirubin values. Markedly elevated serum lactic dehydrogenase (LDH) levels [>8.5 μmol/L (>500 U/dL)] suggest a poor prognosis. Serum albumin is decreased to ≤30 g/L (≤3.0 g/dL) in about 10% of patients; this sign is associated with more severe pancreatitis and a higher mortality rate (Table 294-2). *Hypertriglyceridemia* occurs in 15 to 20% of patients, and serum amylase levels in these individuals are often spuriously normal (Chap. 293). Approximately 25% of patients have *hypoxemia* (arterial P_{O_2} ≤ 60 mmHg), which may herald the onset of ARDS. Finally, the electrocardiogram is occasionally abnormal in acute pancreatitis with ST-segment and T-wave abnormalities simulating myocardial ischemia.

Although one or more radiologic abnormalities are found in >50% of patients, the findings are inconstant and nonspecific. The chief value of conventional x-rays [chest films; kidney, ureter, and bladder (KUB) studies] in acute pancreatitis is to help exclude other diagnoses, especially a perforated viscus. Upper gastrointestinal tract x-rays have been superseded by ultrasonography and computed tomography (CT). A CT scan may confirm the clinical impression of acute pancreatitis even in the face of normal serum amylase levels. Importantly, CT is quite helpful in indicating the severity of acute pancreatitis and the risk of morbidity and mortality (see below). Sonography and radionuclide scanning [N-p-isopropylacetanilide-iminodiacetic acid (PIPIDA) scan; hepatic 2,6-dimethyliminodiacetic acid (HIDA) scan] are useful in acute pancreatitis to evaluate the gallbladder and biliary tree. →*Radiologic studies useful in the diagnosis of acute pancreatitis are discussed in Chap. 293 and listed in Table 293-1.*

DIAGNOSIS Any severe acute pain in the abdomen or back should suggest acute pancreatitis. The diagnosis is usually entertained when a patient with a possible predisposition to pancreatitis presents with se-

TABLE 294-2 *Risk Factors That Adversely Affect Survival in Acute Pancreatitis*

1. Organ failure[a]
   a. Cardiovascular: hypotension (systolic blood pressure < 90 mmHg) or tachycardia > 130 beats/min
   b. Pulmonary: P_{O_2} < 60 mmHg
   c. Renal: oliguria (<50 mL/h) or increasing BUN or creatinine
   d. Gastrointestinal bleeding
2. Pancreatic necrosis[a] (see Table 294-4)
3. Obesity[a] (BMI > 29); age > 70
4. Hemoconcentration[a] (hematocrit > 44%)
5. C-Reactive protein > 150 mg/L
6. Trypsinogen activation peptide
   a. >3 Ranson criteria (not fully utilizable until 48 h)[b]
   b. Apache II score > 8 (cumbersome)[b]

[a] Most useful.
[b] Often cited, but less useful.
Note: BUN, blood urea nitrogen; BMI, body mass index.

vere and constant abdominal pain, nausea, emesis, fever, tachycardia, and abnormal findings on abdominal examination. Laboratory studies frequently reveal leukocytosis, an abnormal appearance on x-rays of the abdomen and chest, hypocalcemia, and hyperglycemia. The diagnosis is usually confirmed by the finding of an elevated level of serum amylase and/or lipase. Not all the above features have to be present for the diagnosis to be established.

The *differential diagnosis* should include the following disorders: (1) perforated viscus, especially peptic ulcer; (2) acute cholecystitis and biliary colic; (3) acute intestinal obstruction; (4) mesenteric vascular occlusion; (5) renal colic; (6) myocardial infarction; (7) dissecting aortic aneurysm; (8) connective tissue disorders with vasculitis; (9) pneumonia; and (10) diabetic ketoacidosis. A penetrating duodenal ulcer can usually be identified by upper gastrointestinal x-rays and/or endoscopy. A perforated duodenal ulcer is readily diagnosed by the presence of free intraperitoneal air. It may be difficult to differentiate acute cholecystitis from acute pancreatitis, since an elevated serum amylase may be found in both disorders. Pain of biliary tract origin is more right-sided and gradual in onset, and ileus is usually absent; sonography and radionuclide scanning are helpful in establishing the diagnosis of cholelithiasis and cholecystitis. Intestinal obstruction due to mechanical factors can be differentiated from pancreatitis by the history of colicky pain, findings on abdominal examination, and x-rays of the abdomen showing changes characteristic of mechanical obstruction. Acute mesenteric vascular occlusion is usually evident in elderly debilitated patients with brisk leukocytosis, abdominal distention, and bloody diarrhea, in whom paracentesis shows sanguineous fluid and arteriography shows vascular occlusion. Serum as well as peritoneal fluid amylase levels are increased, however, in patients with intestinal infarction. Systemic lupus erythematosus and polyarteritis nodosa may be confused with pancreatitis, especially since pancreatitis may develop as a complication of these diseases. Diabetic ketoacidosis is often accompanied by abdominal pain and elevated total serum amylase levels, thus closely mimicking acute pancreatitis. However, the serum lipase and pancreatic isoamylase levels are not elevated in diabetic ketoacidosis.

COURSE OF THE DISEASE AND COMPLICATIONS It is important to identify patients with acute pancreatitis who have an increased risk of dying. Multiple factor scoring systems (Ranson, Imrie, Apache II) are difficult to use, show poor predictive powers, and have not been uniformly embraced by clinicians. The key indicators of a severe attack of pancreatitis are listed in Table 294-2 and include age > 70 years, body mass index (BMI) > 30, hematocrit > 44%, admission C-reactive protein > 150 mg/L, and elevated levels of urine trypsinogen activation peptide (TAP). However, it is organ failure, in which respiratory failure (P_{O_2} < 60 mmHg) dominates, that determines outcome in the majority of difficult to manage cases. The presence of shock (systolic blood pressure < 90 mmHg or tachycardia > 130), renal failure [serum creatinine > 177 μmol/L (>2.0 mg/dL)], and gastrointestinal bleeding (>500 mL/24 h) are also key factors. The high mortality rate of such severely ill patients is due in large part to infection and warrants intensive radiologic intervention and monitoring and/or a combination of radiologic and surgical means, as discussed in detail below.

The local and systemic complications of acute pancreatitis are listed in Table 294-3. In the first 2 to 3 weeks after pancreatitis patients frequently develop an inflammatory mass, which may be due to pancreatic necrosis (with or without infection) or may represent an abscess or pseudocyst (see below). Systemic complications include pulmonary, cardiovascular, hematologic, renal, metabolic, and central nervous system abnormalities. Pancreatitis and hypertriglyceridemia constitute an association in which cause and effect remain incompletely understood. However, several reasonable conclusions can be drawn. First, hypertriglyceridemia can precede and apparently cause pancreatitis. Second, the vast majority (>80%) of patients with acute pancreatitis do not have hypertriglyceridemia. Third, almost all patients

TABLE 294-3   Complications of Acute Pancreatitis

LOCAL

Necrosis	Pancreatic ascites
Sterile	Disruption of main pancreatic
Infected	duct
Pancreatic fluid collections	Leaking pseudocyst
Pancreatic abscess	Involvement of contiguous
Pancreatic pseudocyst	organs by necrotizing
Pain	pancreatitis
Rupture	Massive intraperitoneal
Hemorrhage	hemorrhage
Infection	Thrombosis of blood vessels
Obstruction of gastrointestinal	(splenic vein, portal vein)
tract (stomach, duodenum,	Bowel infarction
colon)	Obstructive jaundice

SYSTEMIC

Pulmonary	Renal
Pleural effusion	Oliguria
Atelectasis	Azotemia
Mediastinal abscess	Renal artery and/or renal vein
Pneumonitis	thrombosis
Adult respiratory distress	Acute tubular necrosis
syndrome	Metabolic
Cardiovascular	Hyperglycemia
Hypotension	Hypertriglyceridemia
Hypovolemia	Hypocalcemia
Sudden death	Encephalopathy
Nonspecific ST-T changes in	Sudden blindness (Purtscher's
electrocardiogram simulating	retinopathy)
myocardial infarction	Central nervous system
Pericardial effusion	Psychosis
Hematologic	Fat emboli
Disseminated intravascular	Fat necrosis
coagulation	Subcutaneous tissues
Gastrointestinal hemorrhage[a]	(erythematous nodules)
Peptic ulcer disease	Bone
Erosive gastritis	Miscellaneous (mediastinum,
Hemorrhagic pancreatic necrosis	pleura, nervous system)
with erosion into major blood	
vessels	
Portal vein thrombosis, variceal	
hemorrhage	

[a] Aggravated by coagulation abnormalities (disseminated intravascular coagulation).

with pancreatitis and hypertriglyceridemia have preexisting abnormalities in lipoprotein metabolism. Fourth, many of the patients with this association have persistent hypertriglyceridemia after recovery from pancreatitis and are prone to recurrent episodes of pancreatitis. Fifth, any factor (e.g., drugs or alcohol) that causes an abrupt increase in serum triglycerides to levels >11 mmol/L (1000 mg/dL) can precipitate a bout of pancreatitis that can be associated with significant complications and even become fulminant. To avert the risk of triggering pancreatitis, a fasting serum triglyceride measurement should be obtained before estrogen replacement therapy is begun in postmenopausal women. Fasting levels < 3.4 mmol/L (300 mg/dL) pose no risk, whereas levels >8.5 mmol/L (750 mg/dL) are associated with a high probability of developing pancreatitis. Finally, patients with a deficiency of apolipoprotein CII have an increased incidence of pancreatitis; apolipoprotein CII activates lipoprotein lipase, which is important in clearing chylomicrons from the bloodstream.

Purtscher's retinopathy, a relatively unusual complication, is manifested by a sudden and severe loss of vision in a patient with acute pancreatitis. It is characterized by a peculiar funduscopic appearance with cotton-wool spots and hemorrhages confined to an area limited by the optic disk and macula; it is believed to be due to occlusion of the posterior retinal artery with aggregated granulocytes.

The two most common causes of acute pancreatitis are biliary tract disease and alcoholism; other causes are listed in Table 294-1. The risk of acute pancreatitis in patients with at least one gallstone <5 mm in diameter is fourfold greater than that in patients with larger stones. However, after a conventional workup, a specific cause is not identified in about 30% of patients. It is important to note that ultrasound examinations fail to detect gallstones, especially microlithiasis and/or sludge, in 4 to 7% of patients. In one series of 31 patients diagnosed initially as having idiopathic acute pancreatitis, 23 were found to have occult gallstone disease. Thus, approximately two-thirds of patients with recurrent acute pancreatitis without an obvious cause actually have occult gallstone disease due to microlithiasis. Examination of duodenal aspirates in such cases often reveals cholesterol crystals, which confirm the diagnosis. Other diseases of the biliary tree and pancreatic ducts that can cause acute pancreatitis include choledochocele; ampullary tumors; pancreas divisum; and pancreatic duct stones, stricture, and tumor. Approximately 2 to 4% of patients with pancreatic carcinoma present with acute pancreatitis.

Recurrent Pancreatitis Approximately 25% of patients who have had an attack of acute pancreatitis have a recurrence. The two most common etiologic factors are alcohol and cholelithiasis. In patients with recurrent pancreatitis without an obvious cause the differential diagnosis should encompass occult biliary tract disease including microlithiasis, hypertriglyceridemia, drugs, pancreatic cancer, sphincter of Oddi dysfunction, pancreas divisum, cystic fibrosis, and pancreatic cancer (Table 294-1).

Pancreatitis in Patients with AIDS The incidence of acute pancreatitis is increased in patients with AIDS for two reasons: (1) the high incidence of infections involving the pancreas, such as infections with cytomegalovirus, *Cryptosporidium*, and the *Mycobacterium avium* complex; and (2) the frequent use by patients with AIDS of medications such as didanosine, pentamidine, and trimethoprim-sulfamethoxazole (Chap. 173).

℞ TREATMENT

In most patients (approximately 85 to 90%) with acute pancreatitis, the disease is self-limited and subsides spontaneously, usually within 3 to 7 days after treatment is instituted. Conventional measures include (1) analgesics for pain, (2) intravenous fluids and colloids to maintain normal intravascular volume, (3) no oral alimentation, and (4) nasogastric suction to decrease gastrin release from the stomach and prevent gastric contents from entering the duodenum. Recent controlled trials, however, have shown that nasogastric suction offers no clearcut advantages in the treatment of mild to moderately severe acute pancreatitis. Its use, therefore, must be considered elective rather than mandatory.

It has been demonstrated that CCK-stimulated pancreatic secretion is almost abolished in four different experimental models of acute pancreatitis. This finding probably explains why drugs to block pancreatic secretion in acute pancreatitis have failed to have any therapeutic benefit. For this and other reasons, anticholinergic drugs are not indicated in acute pancreatitis. In addition to nasogastric suction and anticholinergic drugs, other therapies designed to "rest the pancreas" by inhibiting pancreatic secretion have not changed the course of the disease. Although antibiotics have been used in the treatment of acute pancreatitis, randomized, prospective trials have shown no benefit from their use in acute pancreatitis of mild to moderate severity.

However, current evidence favors the use of prophylactic antibiotics in necrotizing acute pancreatitis. A recent meta-analysis of controlled trials comparing antibiotic prophylaxis with no prophylaxis in patients with acute necrotizing pancreatitis showed significant reduction in sepsis by 21% [number needed to treat (NNT) = 5] and mortality by 12% (NNT = 8). Early antibiotic prophylaxis in patients with documented pancreatic necrosis is recommended; however, the optimal drug(s) and duration of therapy remain incompletely defined. The current recommendation is the use of a systemic antibiotic such as imipenem-cilastatin, 500 mg thrice daily for 2 weeks. In addition, because secondary infection of necrotic pancreatic tissue (abscess, pseudocyst or obstructed biliary passages, ascending cholangitis complicating choledocholithiasis) contributes to many of the late deaths from pancreatitis, appropriate antibiotic therapy of established infections is quite important.

Several other drugs have been evaluated by prospective controlled trials and found ineffective in the treatment of acute pancreatitis. The list, by no means complete, includes glucagon, H_2 blockers, protease inhibitors such as aprotinin, glucocorticoids, calcitonin, nonsteroidal anti-inflammatory drugs (NSAIDs), and lexiplafant, a platelet-activating factor inhibitor. A recent meta-analysis of somatostatin, ocreotide, and the antiprotease gabexate mesilate in therapy of acute pancreatitis suggested (1) a reduced mortality rate but no change in complications with octreotide, and (2) no effect on the mortality rate but reduced pancreatic damage with gabexate.

Intraabdominal *Candida* infection during acute necrotizing pancreatitis is increasing in frequency and is associated with an increased mortality rate. In one representatitve trial, intraabdominal *Candida* infection was found in 13 of 37 cases and was associated with a mortality rate fourfold greater than that associated with intraabdominal bacterial infection alone. Given the impact of *Candida* infection on the mortality rate in acute necrotizing pancreatitis and the apparent benefit of prophylactic chemotherapy, these data suggest earlier use of fungicides.

A CT scan, especially a contrast-enhanced dynamic CT (CECT) scan, provides valuable information on the severity and prognosis of acute pancreatitis (Fig. 294-1 and Table 294-4). In particular, a CECT scan allows estimation of the presence and extent of pancreatic necrosis. Recent studies suggest that the likelihood of prolonged pancreatitis or a serious complication is negligible when the CT severity index is 1 or 2 and low with scores of 3 to 6. However, patients with scores of 7 to 10 had a 92% morbidity rate and a 17% mortality rate. Necrosis is present in 20 to 30% of patients. Those with necrosis have a morbidity rate >20%, whereas those without necrosis have a morbidity rate <10% and a negligible mortality rate. A few retrospective studies have raised concern that the use of intravenous contrast early in the course of acute pancreatitis might intensify pancreatic necrosis. However, since prospective human studies are not available, it is reasonable to reserve CECT scans for patients with severe pancreatitis or suspected local septic complications. The patient with mild to moderate pancreatitis usually requires treatment with intravenous fluids, fasting, and possibly nasogastric suction for 2 to 4 days. A clear liquid diet is frequently started on the third to sixth day, and a regular diet by the fifth to seventh day. The decision to reintroduce oral intake is usually based on the following criteria: (1) a decrease in or resolution of abdominal pain; (2) the patient is hungry; and (3) organ dysfunction, if present, has improved. Elevation of serum amylase/lipase or persistent inflammatory changes seen on CT scans should not discourage feeding a hungry asymptomatic patient. In this regard, persistence of inflammatory changes on CT scans or persistent elevations in serum amylase/lipase may not normalize for weeks to months. The patient with unremitting *fulminant pancreatitis* usually requires inordinate amounts of fluid and close attention to complications such as cardiovascular collapse, respiratory insufficiency, and pancreatic infection. The latter should be managed by a combination of radiologic and surgical means (see below). While earlier uncontrolled studies suggested that *peritoneal lavage* through a percutaneous dialysis catheter was helpful in severe pancreatitis, subsequent studies indicate that this treatment does not influence the outcome of such attacks. Aggressive surgical pancreatic debridement (necrosectomy) should be undertaken soon after confirmation of the presence of infected necrosis, and multiple operations may be required. Since the mortality rate from sterile acute necrotizing pancreatitis is approximately 10%, laparotomy with adequate drainage and removal of necrotic tissue should be considered if conventional therapy does not halt the patient's deterioration. The use of parenteral nutrition makes it possible to give nutritional support to patients with severe, acute, or protracted pancreatitis who are unable to eat normally. Several studies have demonstrated that enteral feeding via a nasojejunal tube infused distal to the ligament of Treitz is associated with a decreased rate of complications, including infection, when compared to total parenteral nutrition. Patients with severe gallstone-induced pancreatitis may improve dramatically if papillotomy is

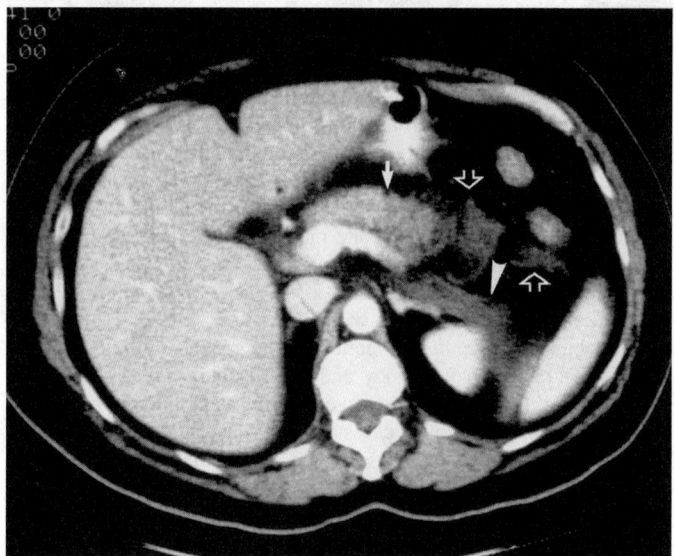

A

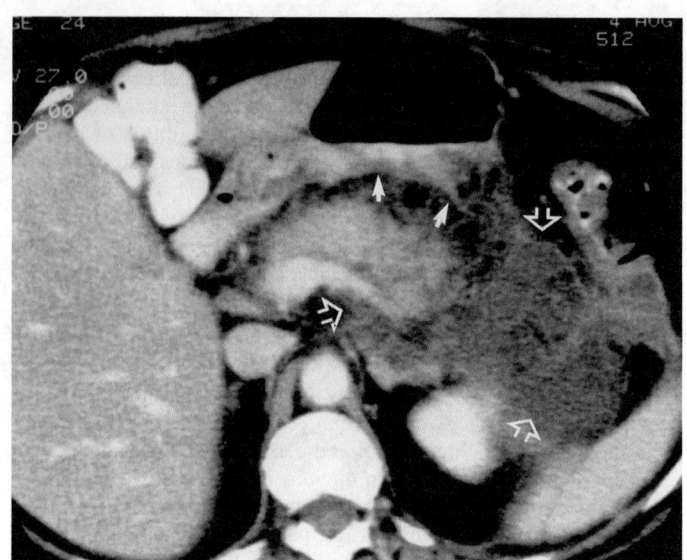

B

FIGURE 294-1 Acute pancreatitis: CT evolution. *A.* Contrast-enhanced CT scan of the abdomen performed on admission of a patient with clinical evidence of acute pancreatitis. Note the mildly decreased density of the body of the pancreas to the left of the midline (*arrow*). There are a few linear strands in the peripancreatic fat, suggesting inflammation (*open arrows*). A small amount of fluid is seen in the anterior pararenal space (*arrowhead*). *B.* Nine days after admission, there is a marked worsening with severe inflammation of the pancreas evidenced by anterior displacement of the posterior gastric wall (*arrows*), increased inflammation of the peripancreatic fat, and increased pancreatic effusion in the anterior perirenal space and around the splenic vein (*open arrows*). (*Courtesy of Dr. PR Ros, University of Florida College of Medicine.*)

carried out within the first 36 to 72 h of the attack. Studies indicate that only those patients with gallstone pancreatitis who are in the very severe group should be considered for urgent ERCP. Finally, the treatment for patients with hypertriglyceridemia-associated pancreatitis includes (1) weight loss to ideal weight, (2) a lipid-restricted diet, (3) exercise, (4) avoidance of alcohol and of drugs that can elevate serum triglycerides (i.e., estrogens, vitamin A, thiazides, and beta-blockers), and (5) control of diabetes.

INFECTED PANCREATIC NECROSIS, ABSCESS, AND PSEUDOCYST Infected pancreatic necrosis should be differentiated from pancreatic abscess. The former is a diffuse infection of an acutely inflamed, necrotic pancreas occurring in the first 1 to 2 weeks after the onset of pancreatitis. In contrast, a pancreatic abscess is an ill-defined, liquid collection of pus that evolves over a longer period, often 4 to 6 weeks. It tends to be less life-threatening and is associated with a lower rate of surgical mortality. Infected pancreatic necrosis should be treated by surgical debridement because the solid component of the infected pancreas is not amenable to effective radiologically guided percutaneous evacuation. Pancreatic abscess can be treated surgically or, in selected cases, by percutaneous drainage. The necrotic pancreas becomes secondarily infected in 40 to 60% of patients, most frequently with gram-negative bacteria of alimentary origin. Whether infection occurs depends on several factors, including the extent of pancreatic and peripancreatic necrosis, the degree of pancreatic ischemia and hypoperfusion, and the presence of organ or multiorgan failure.

The early diagnosis of pancreatic infection can be accomplished by CT-guided needle aspiration. In one study, 60 patients, representing 5% of all admissions for acute pancreatitis, were suspected of harboring a pancreatic infection on the basis of fever, leukocytosis, and an abnormal CT scan (pseudocyst or extrapancreatic fluid collection). Importantly, 60% of these patients had a pancreatic infection, and 55% of these infections developed in the first 2 weeks. These findings suggest that only guided aspiration can reliably distinguish sterile from infected pancreatic necrosis. The following are guidelines for patients meeting the above selection criteria: (1) Pseudocysts should be aspirated promptly, because more than half may be infected; (2) extrapancreatic fluid collections need not be aspirated promptly, because most are sterile; (3) if a necrotic pancreas is found initially to be sterile but fever and leukocytosis persist, several days of observation should be allowed to pass before reaspiration is considered, as clinical improve-

ment frequently occurs; and (4) if fever and leukocytosis recur after an interval of well-being, reaspiration should be considered.

Severe pancreatitis with the presence of key risk factors, postoperative pancreatitis, early oral feeding, early laparotomy, and perhaps injudicious use of antibiotics predispose to the development of pancreatic abscess, which occurs in 3 to 4% of patients with acute pancreatitis. Pancreatic abscess may also develop because of a communication between a pseudocyst and the colon, inadequate surgical drainage of a pseudocyst, or needling of a pseudocyst. The characteristic signs of abscess are fever, leukocytosis, ileus, and rapid deterioration in a patient previously recovering from pancreatitis. Sometimes, however, the only manifestations are persistent fever and signs of continuing pancreatic inflammation. Drainage of pancreatic abscesses by percutaneous catheter techniques, using CT guidance, has been only moderately successful (resolution in 50 to 60% of patients). Accordingly, laparotomy with radical sump drainage and possibly resection of necrotic tissue is usually required, because the mortality rate for undrained pancreatic abscess approaches 100%. Multiple abscesses are common, and reoperation is frequently necessary.

Pseudocysts of the pancreas are collections of tissue, fluid, debris, pancreatic enzymes, and blood which develop over a period of 1 to 4 weeks after the onset of acute pancreatitis; they form in approximately 15% of patients with acute pancreatitis. In contrast to true cysts, pseudocysts do not have an epithelial lining; their walls consist of necrotic tissue, granulation tissue, and fibrous tissue. Disruption of the pancre-

TABLE 294-4 *Severity Index in Acute Pancreatitis*

	Points
Grade of acute pancreatitis	
Normal pancreas	0
Pancreatic enlargement alone	1
Inflammation compared with pancreas and peripancreatic fat	2
One peripancreatic fluid collection	3
Two or more fluid collections	4
Degree of pancreatic necrosis	
No necrosis	0
Necrosis of one-third of pancreas	2
Necrosis of one-half of pancreas	4
Necrosis of more than one-half of pancreas	6
CT severity index (CTSI) = CT grade + necrosis score (0–10)	

atic ductal system is common. However, the subsequent course of this disruption varies widely, ranging from spontaneous healing to continuous leakage of pancreatic juice, which results in tense ascites. Pseudocysts are preceded by pancreatitis in 90% of cases and by trauma in 10%. Approximately 85% are located in the body or tail of the pancreas and 15% in the head. Some patients have two or more pseudocysts. Abdominal pain, with or without radiation to the back, is the usual presenting complaint. A palpable, tender mass may be found in the middle or left upper abdomen. The serum amylase level is elevated in 75% of patients at some point during their illness and may fluctuate markedly.

On x-ray examination, 75% of pseudocysts can be seen to displace some portion of the gastrointestinal tract (Fig. 294-2). Sonography, however, is reliable in detecting pseudocysts. Sonography also permits differentiation between an edematous, inflamed pancreas, which can give rise to a palpable mass, and an actual pseudocyst. Furthermore,

serial ultrasound studies will indicate whether a pseudocyst has resolved. CT complements ultrasonography in the diagnosis of pancreatic pseudocyst (Fig. 294-2), especially when the pseudocyst is infected.

In studies with sonography, pseudocysts were seen to resolve in 25 to 40% of patients. Pseudocysts that are >5 cm in diameter and that persist for >6 weeks should be considered for drainage. Recent natural history studies have suggested that noninterventional, expectant management is the best course in selected patients with minimal symptoms and no evidence of active alcohol use in whom the pseudocyst appears mature by radiography and does not resemble a cystic neoplasm. A significant number of these pseudocysts resolve spontaneously more than 6 weeks after their formation. Also, these studies demonstrate that large pseudocyst size is not an absolute indication for interven-

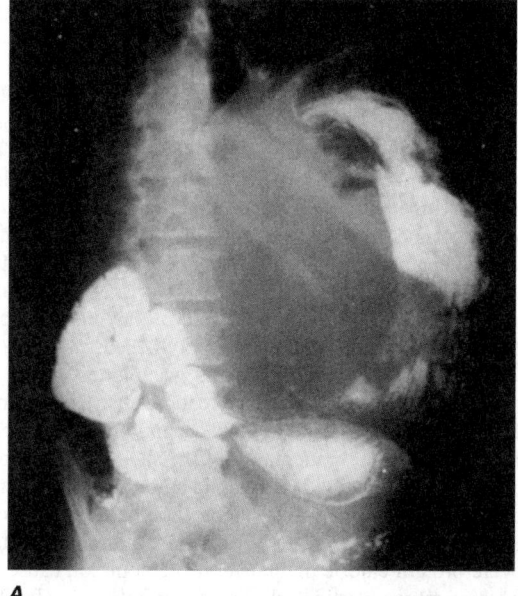

A

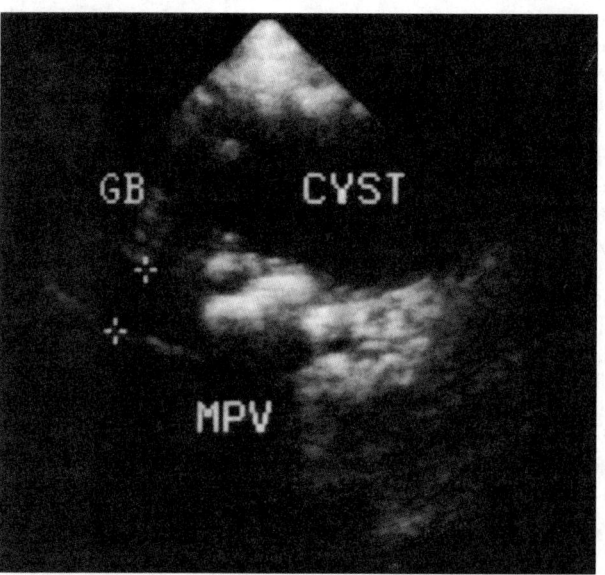

B

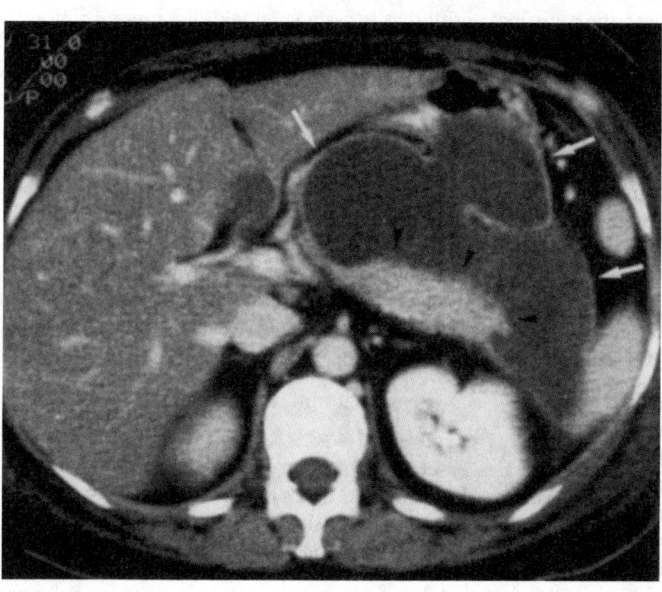

C

D

FIGURE 294-2 Pseudocyst of pancreas. *A.* Upper gastrointestinal x-ray showing displacement of stomach by pseudocyst. *B.* Sonogram showing pseudocyst (*cyst*). GB, gallbladder; MVP, portal vein. Behind the large pseudocyst is seen the calcified head of the pancreas. A dilated common bile duct (*asterisk*) is noted. *C.* CT scan showing pseudocyst. Note the large, lobulated fluid collection (*arrows*) surrounding the tail of the pancreas (*arrowheads*). Note also the dense, thin rim in the periphery representing the fibrous capsule of the pseudocyst. *D.* Spiral CT showing a pseudocyst (*small arrow*) with a pseudoaneurysm (light area in pseudocyst). Note the demonstration of the main pancreatic duct (*big arrow*), even though this duct is minimally dilated by ERCP. (*A, B courtesy of Dr. CE Forsmark, University of Florida College of Medicine; C, D courtesy of Dr. PR Ros, University of Florida College of Medicine.*)

tional therapy and that many peripancreatic fluid collections detected on CT in cases of acute pancreatitis resolve spontaneously. A pseudocyst that does not resolve spontaneously may lead to serious complications, such as (1) pain caused by expansion of the lesion and pressure on other viscera, (2) rupture, (3) hemorrhage, and (4) abscess. Rupture of a pancreatic pseudocyst is a particularly serious complication. Shock almost always supervenes, and mortality rates range from 14% if the rupture is not associated with hemorrhage to over 60% if hemorrhage has occurred. Rupture and hemorrhage are the prime causes of death from pancreatic pseudocyst. A triad of findings—an increase in the size of the mass, a localized bruit over the mass, and a sudden decrease in hemoglobin level and hematocrit without obvious external blood loss—should alert one to the possibility of hemorrhage from a pseudocyst. Thus, in patients who are stable and free of complications and in whom serial ultrasound studies show that the pseudocyst is shrinking, conservative therapy is indicated. Conversely, if the pseudocyst is expanding and is complicated by rupture, hemorrhage, or abscess, the patient should be operated on. With ultrasound or CT guidance, sterile chronic pseudocysts can be treated safely with single or repeated needle aspiration or more prolonged catheter drainage with a success rate of 45 to 75%. The success rate of these techniques for infected pseudocysts is considerably less (40 to 50%). Patients who do not respond to drainage require surgical therapy for internal or external drainage of the cyst.

Pseudoaneurysms develop in up to 10% of patients with acute pancreatitis at sites reflecting the distribution of pseudocysts and fluid collections (Fig. 294-2*D*). The splenic artery is most frequently involved, followed by the inferior and superior pancreatic duodenal arteries. This diagnosis should be suspected in patients with pancreatitis who develop upper gastrointestinal bleeding without an obvious cause or in whom thin-cut CT scanning reveals a contrast-enhanced lesion within or adjacent to a suspected pseudocyst. Arteriography is necessary to confirm the diagnosis.

PANCREATIC ASCITES AND PANCREATIC PLEURAL EFFUSIONS Pancreatic ascites is usually due to disruption of the main pancreatic duct, often by an internal fistula between the duct and the peritoneal cavity or a leaking pseudocyst (Chap. 39). This diagnosis is suggested in a patient with an elevated serum amylase level in whom the ascites fluid has both increased levels of albumin [>30 g/L (>3.0 g/dL)] and a markedly elevated level of amylase. The fluid in true pancreatic ascites usually has an amylase concentration of >20,000 U/L as a result of the ruptured duct or leaking pseudocyst. Lower amylase elevations may be found in the peritoneal fluid of patients with acute pancreatitis. In addition, ERCP often demonstrates passage of contrast material from a major pancreatic duct or a pseudocyst into the peritoneal cavity. As many as 15% of patients with pseudocysts have concurrent pancreatic ascites. The differential diagnosis should include intraperitoneal carcinomatosis, tuberculous peritonitis, constrictive pericarditis, and Budd-Chiari syndrome.

If the pancreatic duct disruption is posterior, an internal fistula may develop between the pancreatic duct and the pleural space, producing a pleural effusion, which is usually left-sided and often massive. This complication often requires thoracentesis or chest tube drainage.

℞ TREATMENT

Treatment usually requires the use of nasogastric suction and parenteral alimentation to decrease pancreatic secretion. In addition, paracentesis is performed to keep the peritoneal cavity free of fluid and, it is hoped, to effect sealing of the leak. The long-acting somatostatin analogue octreotide, which inhibits pancreatic secretion, is useful in cases of pancreatic ascites and pleural effusion. If ascites continues to recur after 2 to 3 weeks of medical management, the patient should be operated on after pancreatography to define the anatomy of the abnormal duct. A disrupted main pancreatic duct can also be treated effectively by stenting. Patients in whom ERCP identifies two or more

sites of extravasation are unlikely to respond to conservative management and/or stenting.

CHRONIC PANCREATITIS AND PANCREATIC EXOCRINE INSUFFICIENCY

GENERAL AND ETIOLOGIC CONSIDERATIONS Chronic inflammatory disease of the pancreas may present as episodes of acute inflammation in a previously injured pancreas or as chronic damage with persistent pain or malabsorption. The causes of relapsing chronic pancreatitis are similar to those of acute pancreatitis (Table 294-1), except that there is an appreciable incidence of cases of undetermined origin. In addition, the pancreatitis associated with gallstones is predominantly acute or relapsing-acute in nature. A cholecystectomy is almost always performed in patients after the first or second attack of gallstone-associated pancreatitis. Patients with chronic pancreatitis may present with persistent abdominal pain, with or without steatorrhea; some (~15%) present with steatorrhea and no pain.

Patients with chronic pancreatitis in whom there is extensive destruction of the pancreas (<10% of exocrine function remaining) have steatorrhea and azotorrhea. Among American adults, alcoholism is the most common cause of clinically apparent pancreatic exocrine insufficiency, while cystic fibrosis is the most frequent cause in children. In up to 25% of American adults with chronic pancreatitis, the cause is not known; that is, they have idiopathic chronic pancreatitis. Indeed, idiopathic chronic pancreatitis is the leading cause of nonalcoholic chronic pancreatitis in adults in the United States. In a recent series, genetic testing was done on 39 patients with idiopathic chronic pancreatitis. Seventeen patients had CFTR mutations and 9 had mutations in a trypsin inhibitor gene (PSTI). Pancreatitis risk was increased 14-fold by having the PSTI mutation, 40-fold by having two abnormal copies of CFTR, and 600-fold by having both. Thus, the risk of pancreatitis showed complex inheritance and was highest in individuals who had abnormalities in both the pancreatic ducts (CFTR) and acini (PSTI). These findings suggest that PSTI is a modifier gene for CFTR-related idiopathic chronic pancreatitis. Current knowledge indicates that about 15% of patients with idiopathic chronic pancreatitis have a genetic basis for this disorder. The therapeutic and prognostic implication of these findings remain to be determined. In other parts of the world, severe protein-calorie malnutrition is a common cause.

In certain countries, particularly Japan and Italy, there has been an increased interest in autoimmune chronic pancreatitis. The Japanese describe a distinct entity that is associated with the presence of autoantibodies in the blood, elevated levels of serum IgG, association with other autoimmune disorders such as primary biliary cirrhosis and inflammatory bowel disease, diffuse enlargement of the pancreas, and irregular narrowing of the main pancreatic duct. Symptoms are usually mild without acute relapsing attacks of pancreatitis, and patients usually experience a good therapeutic response to glucocorticoids. It is noteworthy that pancreatic pseudocysts and calcification within the pancreas are unusual. Although this kind of pancreatitis is not very common in the United States, all major medical centers are seeing examples of autoimmune chronic pancreatitis. Table 294-5 lists other causes of pancreatic exocrine insufficiency, but they are relatively uncommon.

PATHOPHYSIOLOGY The events that initiate an inflammatory process in the pancreas are still not well understood, and the many hypotheses will not be reviewed here. In the case of alcohol-induced pancreatitis, it has been suggested that the primary defect may be the precipitation of protein (inspissated enzymes) in the ducts. The resulting ductal obstruction could lead to duct dilation, diffuse atrophy of the acinar cells, fibrosis, and eventual calcification of some of the protein plugs. However, the fact that some alcoholic patients with recurrent acute pancreatitis show no evidence of chronic pancreatitis does not support this hypothesis. In fact, experimental and clinical observations have shown that alcohol has direct toxic effects on the pancreas. While patients with alcohol-induced pancreatitis generally consume large amounts of alcohol, some consume very little (≤50 g/d). Thus prolonged consumption of "socially acceptable" amounts of alcohol is

TABLE 294-5 Causes of Pancreatic Exocrine Insufficiency

Alcohol, chronic alcoholism
Idiopathic pancreatitis
Cystic fibrosis
Hypertriglyceridemia
Severe protein-calorie malnutrition with hypoalbuminemia
  Tropical pancreatitis (Africa, Asia)
Pancreatic and duodenal neoplasms
Pancreatic resection
Gastric surgery
  Subtotal gastrectomy with Billroth I anastomosis
  Subtotal gastrectomy with Billroth II anastomosis
  Truncal vagotomy and pyloroplasty
Gastrinoma (Zollinger-Ellison syndrome)
Hereditary pancreatitis
Traumatic pancreatitis
Autoimmune pancreatitis
Abdominal radiotherapy
Hemochromatosis
Primary sclerosing cholangitis
Primary biliary cirrhosis
Shwachman's syndrome (pancreatic insufficiency and bone marrow
  dysfunction)
Trypsinogen deficiency
Enterokinase deficiency
Isolated deficiencies of amylase, lipase, or proteases
α_1-Antitrypsin deficiency

compatible with the development of pancreatitis. In addition, the finding of extensive pancreatic fibrosis in patients who died during their first attack of clinical acute alcohol-induced pancreatitis supports the concept that such patients already have chronic pancreatitis.

CLINICAL FEATURES Patients with relapsing chronic pancreatitis may present with symptoms identical to those of acute pancreatitis, but pain may be continuous, intermittent, or absent. The pathogenesis of this pain is poorly understood. Although the classic description is of epigastric pain radiating through the back, the pain pattern is often atypical; the pain may be worst in the right or left upper quadrant of the back or may be diffuse throughout the upper abdomen; it may even be referred to the anterior chest or flank. Characteristically it is persistent, deep-seated, and unresponsive to antacids. It often is worsened by ingestion of alcohol or a heavy meal (especially one rich in fat). Often the pain is severe enough to necessitate the frequent use of narcotics.

Weight loss, abnormal stools, and other signs or symptoms suggestive of malabsorption (Chap. 275) are common in chronic pancreatitis. However, clinically apparent deficiencies of fat-soluble vitamins are surprisingly rare. The physical findings in these patients are usually not impressive, so that there is a disparity between the severity of the abdominal pain and the physical signs (other than some abdominal tenderness and mild temperature elevation).

DIAGNOSTIC EVALUATION (See also Chap. 293) In contrast to relapsing acute pancreatitis, the serum amylase and lipase levels are usually not elevated in chronic pancreatitis. Elevations of serum bilirubin and alkaline phosphatase levels may indicate cholestasis secondary to chronic inflammation around the common bile duct (Fig. 294-3). Many patients demonstrate impaired glucose tolerance, and some have an elevated fasting blood glucose level.

The classic triad of pancreatic calcification, steatorrhea, and diabetes mellitus usually establishes the diagnosis of chronic pancreatitis and exocrine pancreatic insufficiency but is found in fewer than one-third of chronic pancreatitis patients. Accordingly, it is often necessary to perform an intubation test such as the *secretin stimulation test*, which usually gives abnormal results when 60% or more of pancreatic exocrine function has been lost. Approximately 40% of patients with chronic pancreatitis have *cobalamin (vitamin B₁₂)* malabsorption, which can be corrected by the administration of oral pancreatic enzymes. There is usually a marked excretion of fecal fat (Chap. 275), which can be reduced by the administration of oral pancreatic en-

zymes. The serum trypsinogen (Chap. 293) and the D-xylose urinary excretion test are useful in patients with "pancreatic steatorrhea," since the trypsinogen level will be abnormal, and D-xylose excretion is usually normal. A decreased serum trypsinogen (<20 ng/mL) or a fecal elastase level of <100 μg/mg of stool strongly suggests severe pancreatic exocrine insufficiency.

The radiographic hallmark of chronic pancreatitis is the presence of scattered calcification throughout the pancreas (Fig. 294-3). Diffuse pancreatic calcification indicates that significant damage has occurred and obviates the need for a secretin test. While alcohol is by far the most common cause, pancreatic calcification may also be seen in cases of severe protein-calorie malnutrition, hereditary pancreatitis, post-traumatic pancreatitis, hyperparathyroidism, islet cell tumors, and idiopathic chronic pancreatitis. A large prospective study has shown convincingly that pancreatic calcification decreases or even disappears spontaneously in one-third of patients with severe chronic pancreatitis; this outcome may also follow ductal decompression. Pancreatic calcification is a dynamic process that is incompletely understood.

Sonography, CT, and ERCP greatly aid the diagnosis of pancreatic disease. In addition to excluding pseudocysts and pancreatic cancer, sonography and CT may show calcification or dilated ducts associated with chronic pancreatitis (Fig. 294-4). ERCP and endoscopic ultrasound (EUS) are procedures that provide information about the main pancreatic duct and the smaller ducts. EUS is also useful in evaluating the pancreatic parenchyma. In patients with alcohol-induced pancreatitis, ERCP may reveal a pseudocyst missed by sonography or CT.

COMPLICATIONS OF CHRONIC PANCREATITIS The complications of chronic pancreatitis are protean. Cobalamin (vitamin B₁₂) malabsorption occurs in 40% of patients with alcohol-induced chronic pancreatitis and in virtually all with cystic fibrosis. It is consistently corrected by the administration of pancreatic enzymes (containing proteases). It may be due to excessive binding of cobalamin by cobalamin-binding proteins other than intrinsic factor, which ordinarily are destroyed by pancreatic proteases and therefore do not compete with intrinsic factor for cobalamin binding. Although most patients show impaired glucose tolerance, diabetic ketoacidosis and coma are uncommon. Similarly, end-organ damage (retinopathy, neuropathy, nephropathy) is also uncommon, and the appearance of these complications should raise the question of concomitant genetic diabetes mellitus. A nondiabetic retinopathy, peripheral in location and secondary to vitamin A and/or zinc deficiency, is common in these patients. Effusions containing high concentrations of amylase may occur into the pleural, pericardial, or peritoneal space. Gastrointestinal bleeding may occur from peptic ulceration, gastritis, a pseudocyst eroding into the duodenum, or ruptured varices secondary to splenic vein thrombosis due to inflammation of the tail of the pancreas. Icterus may occur, caused either by edema of the head of the pancreas, which compresses the common bile duct, or by chronic cholestasis secondary to a chronic inflammatory reaction around the intrapancreatic portion of the common bile duct (Fig. 294-3). The chronic obstruction may lead to cholangitis and ultimately to biliary cirrhosis. Subcutaneous fat necrosis may appear as tender red nodules on the lower extremities. Bone pain may be secondary to intramedullary fat necrosis. Inflammation of the large and small joints of the upper and lower extremities may occur. The incidence of pancreatic carcinoma is increased in patients with chronic pancreatitis who have been followed for 2 or more years. Twenty years after the diagnosis of chronic pancreatitis, the cumulative risk of pancreatic carcinoma is 4%. Perhaps the most common and troublesome complication is addiction to narcotics.

℞ TREATMENT

Therapy for patients with chronic pancreatitis is directed toward two major problems—pain and maldigestion. Patients with intermittent attacks of pain are treated essentially like those with acute pancreatitis

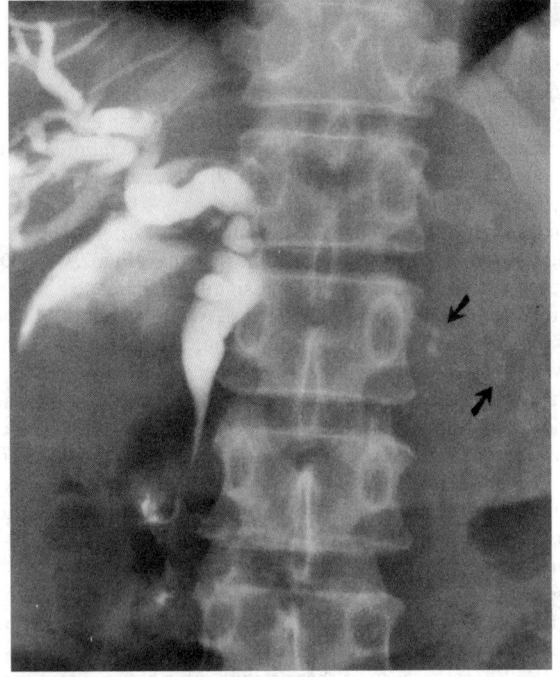

A

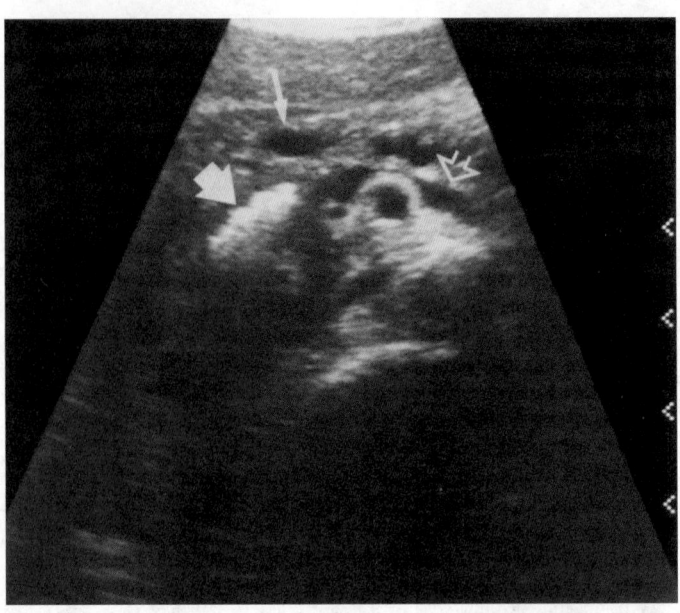

B

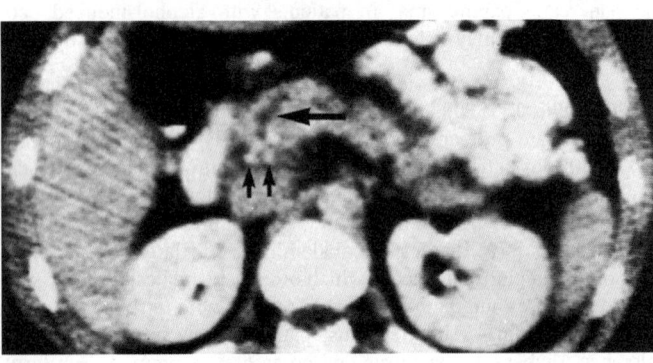

C

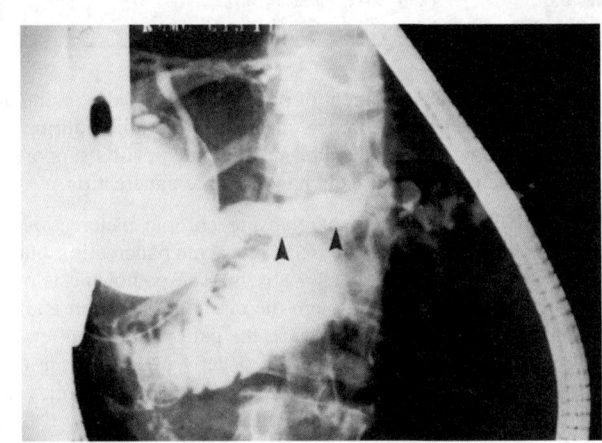

D

FIGURE 294-3 Radiologic abnormalities in chronic pancreatitis. *A*. Pancreatic calcification (*arrows*) and stenosis (tapering) of the intrahepatic portion of the common bile duct demonstrated by percutaneous transhepatic cholangiography. *B*. Pancreatic calcification (*large white arrow*) demonstrated by sonography. Note dilated pancreatic duct (*thin white arrow*) and splenic vein (*open arrow*). *C*. Pancreatic calcification (*vertical arrows*) and dilated pancreatic duct (*horizontal arrow*) demonstrated by CT scan. *D*. Endoscopic retrograde cholangiogram shows grossly dilated pancreatic ducts (*arrows*) in a patient with long-standing pancreatitis.

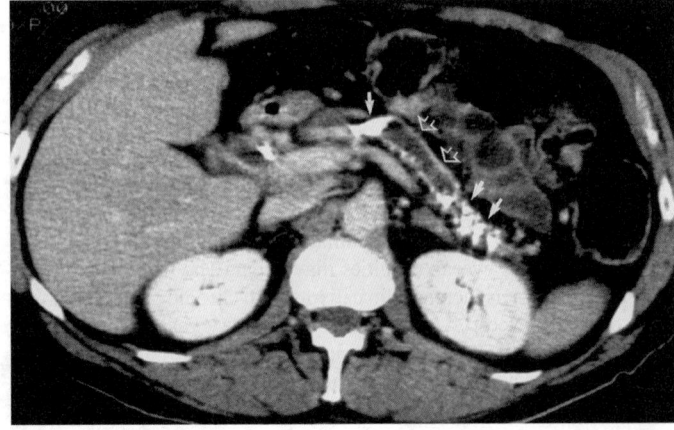

A

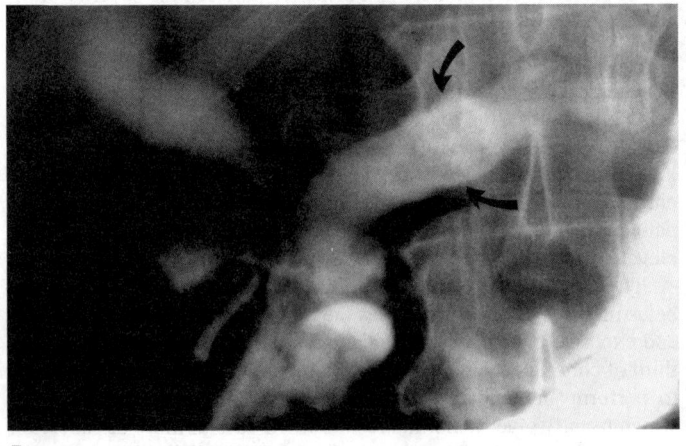

B

FIGURE 294-4 Chronic pancreatitis and pancreatic calculi: CT scan and ERCP appearance. *A*. In this contrast-enhanced CT scan of the abdomen, there is evidence of an atrophic pancreas with multiple calcifications (*arrows*). Note the markedly dilated pancreatic duct seen in this section through the body and tail (*open arrows*). *B*. ERCP in the same patient demonstrates the dilated pancreatic duct as well as an intrapancreatic duct calculus (*arrows*). These findings correlate nicely with the CT scan appearance.

(see above). Patients with severe and persistent pain should avoid alcohol completely and avoid large meals rich in fat. Since the pain is often severe enough to require frequent use of narcotics (and hence addiction), a number of surgical procedures have been developed for pain relief. ERCP allows the surgeon to plan the operative approach. If there is a stricture of the pancreatic duct, a local resection may ameliorate the pain. Unfortunately, isolated localized strictures are not common. In most patients with alcohol-induced disease, the pancreas is diffusely involved, and surgically correctible localized ductal disease is rare. When there is primary ductal obstruction and dilation, ductal decompression may provide effective pain palliation. Short-term pain relief may be achieved in up to 80% of patients, while long-term pain relief occurs in approximately 50%. In some of these patients, however, pain relief can be achieved only by resecting 50 to 95% of the gland. Although pain relief is achieved in three-quarters of these patients, they tend to develop pancreatic endocrine and exocrine insufficiency and must be treated with pancreatic enzyme replacement therapy. It is important to screen patients carefully, for such radical surgery is contraindicated in those who are severely depressed or suicidal or who continue to drink. Procedures such as splanchnicectomy, celiac ganglionectomy, and nerve blocks usually bring only temporary relief and are not recommended. Endoscopic treatment of chronic pancreatitis may involve sphincterotomy of the minor or major pancreatic sphincter, dilatation of strictures, removal of calculi, or stenting of the ventral or dorsal pancreatic duct. Although many of these techniques are technically impressive, none has been subjected to a randomized trial in patients with chronic pancreatitis. In addition, significant complications—acute pancreatitis, pancreatic abscess, damage to the pancreatic duct, and death—have occurred in up to 36% of patients after stent placement.

Three double-blind trials have demonstrated that administration of pancreatic enzymes decreases abdominal pain in selected patients with chronic pancreatitis. In these trials, approximately 75% of the patients evaluated experienced pain relief. The patients most likely to respond are those with mild to moderate exocrine pancreatic dysfunction, as evidenced by an abnormal secretin test, normal fat absorption, and minimal abnormalities on ERCP examination. These clinical observations seem to fit with data from humans and experimental animals demonstrating a negative feedback regulation for pancreatic exocrine secretion controlled by the amount of proteases within the lumen of the proximal small intestine. It seems reasonable to use the following approach for patients with severe, persistent, or continuous abdominal pain thought to be caused by chronic pancreatitis. After other causes of abdominal pain (peptic ulcer, gallstones, etc.) have been excluded, a pancreatic sonogram should be done. If no mass is found, a secretin test may be performed, because its results are usually abnormal in cases of chronic pancreatitis with pain. If the results are abnormal (i.e., decreased bicarbonate concentration or volume output), a 3- to 4-week trial of pancreatic enzyme administration is appropriate. Four to eight conventional tablets or capsules are taken at meals and at bedtime. There are a number of studies suggesting that patients may have small-duct chronic pancreatitis and chronic abdominal pain with a normal appearance on radiographic evaluations (ultrasound, CT, ERCP) but abnormal results on hormone stimulation tests (secretin test) and/or abnormal pancreatic histology. Such minimal-change chronic pancreatitis may respond well to pancreatic enzyme therapy (non-enteric-coated) for relief of abdominal pain. If no relief is obtained, and especially if the volume secreted during the secretin test is very low, ERCP or EUS should be performed. If a pseudocyst or a localized ductal obstruction is found, surgery should be considered. A patient who has dilated ducts may be a candidate for a surgical ductal decompression procedure. This procedure provides short-term relief in up to 80% of patients, although long-term results are closer to 50%. Some studies have shown octreotide to be effective in decreasing abdominal pain in patients with severe large-duct disease. If no surgically remediable lesion is found and severe pain continues despite abstinence from alcohol, subtotal pancreatic resection may be necessary.

The treatment of maldigestion rests on the use of pancreatic enzyme replacement therapy. Diarrhea and steatorrhea are usually improved by this treatment, although the steatorrhea may not be completely corrected. The major problem is delivering enough active enzyme into the duodenum. Steatorrhea could be abolished if 10% of the normal amount of lipase could be delivered to the duodenum at the proper time. This concentration of lipase cannot be achieved with the current preparations of pancreatic enzymes, even if the latter are given in large doses. The reason for these poor results may be that lipase is inactivated by gastric acid, that food empties from the stomach faster than do the pancreatic enzymes, and that batches of commercially available pancreatic extracts vary in enzyme activity.

For the usual patient, two or three enteric-coated capsules or eight conventional (non-enteric-coated) tablets of a potent enzyme preparation should be administered with meals. Some patients using conventional tablets require adjuvant therapy to improve enzyme replacement treatment. H_2 receptor antagonists, sodium bicarbonate, and proton pump inhibitors are effective adjuvants. Antacids containing calcium carbonate or magnesium hydroxide are not effective and may actually result in increased steatorrhea. Several publications have reported colonic strictures in patients with cystic fibrosis receiving extraordinarily high doses of high-potency pancreatic enzyme preparations. Such lesions have not been reported in adults with chronic pancreatitis.

Supportive measures include diet restriction and pain medications. The diet should be moderate in fat (30%), high in protein (24%), and low in carbohydrate (40%). Restriction of long-chain triglyceride intake can help patients who do not respond satisfactorily to pancreatic enzyme therapy. Use of foods containing mainly medium-chain fatty acids, which do not require lipase for digestion, may be beneficial. Nonnarcotic analgesics should be emphasized. Patients taking narcotic drugs for pain relief often become addicted and continue to have pain.

Patients with severe exocrine pancreatic insufficiency secondary to alcohol who continue to drink have a high mortality rate (in one series, 50% of patients who were followed for 5 to 12 years died during this period) and significant morbidity (weight loss, lassitude, vitamin deficiency, and narcotic addiction). Chronic pancreatitis carries significant medical and social costs. A recent study found that pancreatitis led to retirement in 11% of patients with the disease, accounting for 45% of all retirements. In 87% of patients with chronic pancreatitis unable to maintain gainful employment, alcoholism was a contributing factor. Patients with chronic pancreatitis also use substantial medical resources. In 1987 in the United States, this diagnosis accounted for 122,000 recorded outpatient visits and 56,000 hospital admissions. Pain may abate if progressive severe exocrine insufficiency continues. Patients who abstain from alcohol and use vigorous replacement therapy for maldigestion do reasonably well.

HEREDITARY PANCREATITIS Hereditary pancreatitis is a rare disease that is similar to chronic pancreatitis except for an early age of onset and evidence of hereditary factors (involving an autosomal dominant gene with incomplete penetrance). A genome-wide search using genetic linkage analysis identified the hereditary pancreatitis gene on chromosome 7. Mutations in ion codons 29 (exon 2) and 122 (exon 3) of the cationic trypsinogen gene cause autosomal dominant forms of hereditary pancreatitis. The codon 122 mutations lead to a substitution of the corresponding arginine with another amino acid, usually histidine. This substitution, when it occurs, eliminates a fail-safe trypsin self-destruction site necessary to eliminate trypsin that is prematurely activated within the acinar cell. These patients have recurring attacks of severe abdominal pain which may last from a few days to a few weeks. The serum amylase and lipase levels may be elevated during acute attacks but are usually normal. Patients frequently develop pancreatic calcification, diabetes mellitus, and steatorrhea, and, in addition, they have an increased incidence of pancreatic carcinoma, with the cumulative incidence being as high as 40% by age 70. Such patients often require ductal decompression for pain relief. Abdominal complaints in relatives of patients with hereditary pancreatitis should raise the question of pancreatic disease.

Pancreatic Secretory Trypsin Inhibitor (PSTI) Gene Mutations   PSTI, or SPINK1, is a 56-amino-acid peptide that specifically inhibits trypsin by physically blocking its active site. SPINK1 acts as the first line of defense against prematurely activated trypsinogen in the acinar cell. Recently, it has been shown that the frequency of SPINK1 mutations in patients with idiopathic chronic pancreatitis is markedly increased, suggesting that these mutations may be associated with pancreatitis.

PANCREATIC ENDOCRINE TUMORS

→*Pancreatic endocrine tumors are discussed in Chap. 329.*

OTHER CONDITIONS

ANNULAR PANCREAS   When the ventral pancreatic anlage fails to migrate correctly to make contact with the dorsal anlage, the result may be a ring of pancreatic tissue encircling the duodenum. Such an annular pancreas may cause intestinal obstruction in the neonate or the adult. Symptoms of postprandial fullness, epigastric pain, nausea, and vomiting may be present for years before the diagnosis is entertained. The radiographic findings are symmetric dilation of the proximal duodenum with bulging of the recesses on either side of the annular band, effacement but not destruction of the duodenal mucosa, accentuation of the findings in the right anterior oblique position, and lack of change on repeated examinations. The differential diagnosis should include duodenal webs, tumors of the pancreas or duodenum, postbulbar peptic ulcer, regional enteritis, and adhesions. Patients with annular pancreas have an increased incidence of pancreatitis and peptic ulcer. Because of these and other potential complications, the treatment is surgical even if the condition has been present for years. Retrocolic duodeno-jejunostomy is the procedure of choice, although some surgeons advocate Billroth II gastrectomy, gastroenterostomy, and vagotomy.

PANCREAS DIVISUM   Pancreas divisum occurs when the embryologic ventral and dorsal pancreatic anlagen fail to fuse, so that pancreatic drainage is accomplished mainly through the accessory papilla. Pancreas divisum is the most common congenital anatomic variant of the human pancreas. Current evidence indicates that this anomaly does not predispose to the development of pancreatitis in the great majority of patients who harbor it. However, the combination of pancreas divisum and a small accessory orifice could result in dorsal duct obstruction. The challenge is to identify this subset of patients with dorsal duct pathology. Cannulation of the dorsal duct by ERCP is not as easily done as is cannulation of the ventral duct. Patients with pancreatitis and pancreas divisum demonstrated by ERCP should be treated with conservative measures. In many of these patients, pancreatitis is idiopathic and unrelated to the pancreas divisum. Endoscopic or surgical intervention is indicated only when the above methods fail. If marked dilation of the dorsal duct can be demonstrated, surgical ductal decompression should be performed. The appropriate therapy for patients without dilation of the dorsal duct is not yet defined. It should be stressed that the ERCP appearance of pancreas divisum—i.e., a small-caliber ventral duct with an arborizing pattern—may be mistaken as representing an obstructed main pancreatic duct secondary to a mass lesion.

MACROAMYLASEMIA   In macroamylasemia, amylase circulates in the blood in a polymer form too large to be easily excreted by the kidney. Patients with this condition demonstrate an elevated serum amylase value, a low urinary amylase value, and a C_{am}/C_{cr} ratio of $<1\%$. The presence of macroamylase can be documented by chromatography of the serum. The prevalence of macroamylasemia is 1.5% of the nonalcoholic general adult hospital population. Usually macroamylasemia is an incidental finding and is not related to disease of the pancreas or other organs.

Macrolipasemia has now been documented in a few patients with cirrhosis or non-Hodgkin's lymphoma. In these patients, the pancreas appeared normal on ultrasound and CT examination. Lipase was shown to be complexed with immunoglobulin A. Thus, the possibility of *both* macroamylasemia and macrolipasemia should be considered in patients with elevated blood levels of these enzymes.

ACKNOWLEDGMENT
This chapter represents a revised version of the chapter by Dr. Norton J. Greenberger, Dr. Phillip P. Toskes, and Dr. Kurt J. Isselbacher that was in the previous editions of Harrison's.

FURTHER READING

DRAGANOV P, TOSKES PP: Chronic pancreatitis. Curr Opin Gastroenterol 18: 558, 2002

FORSMARK CE: The diagnosis of chronic pancreatitis. Gastrointest Endosc 52: 293, 2000

LOWENFELS AB et al: Prognosis of chronic pancreatitis: An international multicenter study. Am J Gastroenterol 89:1467, 1994

SOMOGYI L et al: Recurrent acute pancreatitis: An algorithmic approach to identification and elimination of inciting factors. Gastroenterology 120:708, 2001

YADAY Y et al: A critical evaluation of laboratory tests in acute pancreatitis. Am J Gastroenterol 97:1309, 2002

Section 1   The Immune System in Health and Disease

295 | INTRODUCTION TO THE IMMUNE SYSTEM
Barton F. Haynes, Anthony S. Fauci

DEFINITIONS

- *Adaptive immune system*—recently evolved system of immune responses mediated by T and B lymphocytes. Immune responses by these cells are based on specific antigen recognition by clonotypic receptors that are products of genes that rearrange during development and throughout the life of the organism. Additional cells of the adaptive immune system include various types of antigen-presenting cells (Table 295-9).

- *Antibody*—B cell–produced molecules encoded by genes that rearrange during B cell development consisting of immunoglobulin heavy and light chains that together form the central component of the B cell receptor for antigen. Antibody can exist as B cell surface antigen-recognition molecules or as secreted molecules in plasma and other body fluids (Table 295-10).

- *Antigens*—foreign or self molecules that are recognized by the adaptive and innate immune systems resulting in immune cell triggering, T cell activation, and/or B cell antibody production.

- *Antimicrobial peptides*—small peptides <100 amino acids in length that are produced by cells of the innate immune system and have anti-infectious agent activity (Table 295-2).

- *Apoptosis*—the process of *programmed cell death* whereby signaling through various "death receptors" on the surface of cells [e.g., tumor necrosis factor (TNF) receptors, CD95] leads to a signaling cascade that involves activation of the caspase family of molecules and leads to DNA cleavage and cell death. Apoptosis, which does not lead to induction of inordinate inflammation, is to be contrasted with *cell necrosis*, which does lead to induction of inflammatory responses.

- *B lymphocytes*—bone marrow–derived or bursal-equivalent lymphocytes that express surface immunoglobulin (the B cell receptor for antigen) and secrete specific antibody after interaction with antigen (Figs. 295-8, 295-10).

- *B cell receptor for antigen*—complex of surface molecules that rearrange during postnatal B cell development, made up of surface immunoglobulin (Ig) and associated Ig $\alpha\beta$ chain molecules that recognize nominal antigen via Ig heavy and light chain variable regions, and signal the B cell to terminally differentiate to make antigen-specific antibody (Figs. 295-7, 295-9).

- *CD classification of human lymphocyte differentiation antigens*—the development of monoclonal antibody technology led to the discovery of a large number of new leukocyte surface molecules. In 1982, the First International Workshop on Leukocyte Differentiation Antigens was held to establish a nomenclature for cell-surface molecules of human leukocytes. From this and subsequent leukocyte differentiation workshops has come the *cluster of differentiation (CD) classification* of leukocyte antigens (Table 295-1).

- *Complement*—cascading series of plasma enzymes and effector proteins whose function is to lyse pathogens and/or target them to be phagocytized by neutrophils and monocyte/macrophage lineage cells of the reticuloendothelial system (Fig. 295-4, Table 295-7).

- *Co-stimulatory molecules*—molecules of antigen-presenting cells (such as B7-1 and B7-2 or CD40) that lead to T cell activation when bound by ligands on activated T cells (such as CD28 or CD40 ligand) (Fig. 295-6).

- *Cytokines*—soluble proteins that interact with specific cellular receptors that are involved in the regulation of the growth and activation of immune cells and mediate normal and pathologic inflammatory and immune responses (Tables 295-5, 295-8).

- *Dendritic cells*—myeloid and/or lymphoid lineage antigen-presenting cells of the adaptive immune system. Immature dendritic cells, or dendritic cell precursors, are key components of the innate immune system by responding to infections with production of high levels of cytokines. Dendritic cells are key initiators both of innate immune responses via cytokine production and of adaptive immune responses via presentation of antigen to T lymphocytes (Figs. 295-10, 295-11, Table 295-4).

- *Innate immune system*—ancient immune recognition system of host cells bearing germ line–encoded pattern recognition receptors (PRRs) that recognize pathogens and trigger a variety of mechanisms of pathogen elimination. Cells of the innate immune system include natural killer (NK) cell lymphocytes, monocytes/macrophages, dendritic cells, neutrophils, basophils, eosinophils, tissue mast cells, and epithelial cells (Tables 295-2, 295-3, 295-4, 295-6, 295-7).

- *Large granular lymphocytes*—lymphocytes of the innate immune system with azurophilic cytotoxic granules that have NK cell activity capable of killing foreign and host cells with little or no self major histocompatibility complex (MHC) class I molecules (Fig. 295-3).

- *Natural killer cells*—large granular lymphocytes that kill target cells that express little or no HLA class I molecules, such as malignantly transformed cells and virally infected cells. NK cells express receptors that inhibit killer cell function when self MHC class I is present (Fig. 295-3).

- *Pathogen-associated molecular patterns* (PAMPs)—Invariant molecular structures expressed by large groups of microorganisms that are recognized by host cellular pattern recognition receptors in the mediation of innate immunity (Fig. 295-2).

- *Pattern recognition receptors* (PRRs)—germ line–encoded receptors expressed by cells of the innate immune system that recognize pathogen-associated molecular patterns (Table 295-3).

- *T cells*—thymus-derived lymphocytes that mediate adaptive cellular immune responses including T helper, T regulatory, and cytotoxic T lymphocyte effector cell functions (Figs. 295-5, 295-6, 295-10, 295-11).

- *T cell receptor for antigen*—complex of surface molecules that rearrange during postnatal T cell development made up of clonotypic T cell receptor (TCR) α and β chains that are associated with the CD3 complex composed of invariant γ, δ, ε, ζ, and η chains. The clonotypic TCR-α and -β chains recognize peptide fragments of protein antigen physically bound in antigen-presenting cell MHC class I or II molecules, leading to signaling via the CD3 complex to mediate effector functions (Fig. 295-6).

- *Tolerance*—B and T cell nonresponsiveness to antigens that results from encounter with foreign or self antigens by B and T lymphocytes in the absence of expression of antigen-presenting cell co-stimulatory molecules. Tolerance to antigens may be induced and maintained by multiple mechanisms either centrally (in the thymus) or peripherally at sites throughout the peripheral immune system.

Surface Antigen (Other Names)	Family	Molecular Mass, kDa	Distribution	Ligand(s)	Function
CD1a (T6, HTA-1)	Ig	49	CD, cortical thymocytes, Langerhans type of dendritic cells	TCRγδ T cells	CD1 molecules present lipid antigens of intracellular bacteria such as *M. leprae* and *M. tuberculosis* to TCRγδ T cells.
CD1b	Ig	45	CD, cortical thymocytes, Langerhans type of dendritic cells	TCRγδ T cells	
CD1c	Ig	43	DC, cortical thymocytes, subset of B cells, Langerhans type of dendritic cells	TCRγδ T cells	
CD1d	Ig	?	Cortical thymocytes, intestinal epithelium, Langerhans type of dendritic cells	TCRγδ T cells	
CD2 (T12, LFA-2)	Ig	50	T, NK	CD58, CD48, CD59, CD15	Alternative T cell activation, T cell anergy, T cell cytokine production, T- or NK-mediated cytolysis, T cell apoptosis, cell adhesion
CD3 (T3, Leu-4)	Ig	γ:25–28, δ:21–28, ε:20–25, η:21–22, ζ:16	T	Associates with the TCR	T cell activation and function; ζ is the signal transduction components of the CD3 complex
CD4 (T4, Leu-3)	Ig	55	T, myeloid	MHC-II, HIV, gp120, IL-16, SABP	T cell selection, T cell activation, signal transduction with p56*lck*, primary receptor for HIV
CD7 (3A1, Leu-9)	Ig	40	T, NK	K-12 (CD7L)	T and NK cell signal transduction and regulation of IFN-γ, TNF-α production
CD8 (T8, Leu-2)	Ig	34	T	MHC-I	T cell selection, T cell activation, signal transduction with p56*lck*
CD14 (LPS-receptor)	LRG	53–55	M, G (weak), not by myeloid progenitors	Endotoxin (lipopolysaccharide), lipoteichoic acid, PI	TLR4 mediates with LPS and other PAMP activation of innate immunity
CD19 B4	Ig	95	B (except plasma cells), FDC	Not known	Associates with CD21 and CD81 to form a complex involved in signal transduction in B cell development, activation, and differentiation
CD20 (B1)	Unassigned	33–37	B (except plasma cells)	Not known	Cell signaling, may be important for B cell activation and proliferation
CD21 (B2, CR2, EBV-R, C3dR)	RCA	145	Mature B, FDC, subset of thymocytes	C3d, C3dg, iC3b, CD23, EBV	Associates with CD19 and CD81 to form a complex involved in signal transduction in B cell development, activation, and differentiation; Epstein-Barr virus receptor
CD22 (BL-CAM)	Ig	130–140	Mature B	CDw75	Cell adhesion, signaling through association with p72*sky*, p53/56*lyn*, PI3 kinase, SHP1, fLCγ
CD23 (FcεRII, B6, Leu-20, BLAST-2)	C-type lectin	45	B, M, FDC	IgE, CD21, CD11b, CD11c	Regulates IgE synthesis, cytokine release by monocytes
CD28	Ig	44	T, plasma cells	CD80, CD86	Co-stimulatory for T cell activation; involved in the decision between T cell activation and anergy
CD40	TNFR	48–50	B, DC, EC, thymic epithelium, MP, cancers	CD154	B cell activation, proliferation, and differentiation, formation of GCs, isotype switching, rescue from apoptosis
CD45 (LCA, T200, B220)	PTP	180, 200, 210, 220	All leukocytes	Galectin-1, CD2, CD3, CD4	T and B activation, thymocyte development, signal transduction, apoptosis
CD45RA	PTP	210, 220	Subset T, medullary thymocytes, "naive" T	Galectin-1, CD2, CD3, CD4	Isoforms of CD45 containing exon 4 (A), restricted to a subset of T cells

(continued)

TABLE 295-1—(Continued)

Surface Antigen (Other Names)	Family	Molecular Mass, kDa	Distribution	Ligand(s)	Function
CD45RB	PTP	200, 210, 220	All leukocytes	Galectin-1, CD2, CD3, CD4	Isoforms of CD45 containing exon 5 (B)
CD45RC	PTP	210, 220	Subset T, medullary thymocytes, "naive" T	Galectin-1, CD2, CD3, CD4	Isoforms of CD45 containing exon 6 (C), restricted to a subset of T cells
CD45RO	PTP	180	Subset T, cortical thymocytes, "memory" T	Galectin-1, CD2, CD3, CD4	Isoforms of CD45 containing no differentially spliced exons, restricted to a subset of T cells
CD80 (B7-1, BB1)	Ig	60	Activated B and T, MP, DC	CD28, CD152	Co-regulator of T cell activation; signaling through CD28 stimulates and through CD152 inhibits T cell activation
CD86 (B7-2, B70)	Ig	80	Subset B, DC, EC, activated T, thymic epithelium	CD28, CD152	Co-regulator of T cell activation; signaling through CD28 stimulates and through CD152 inhibits T cell activation
CD95 (APO-1, Fas)	TNFR	135	Activated T and B	Fas ligand	Mediates apoptosis
CD152 (CTLA-4)	Ig	30–33	Activated T	CD80, CD86	Inhibits T cell proliferation
CD154 (CD40L)	TNF	33	Activated CD4+ T, subset CD8+ T, NK, M, basophil	CD40	Co-stimulatory for T cell activation, B cell proliferation and differentiation

Note: CTLA, cytotoxic T lymphocyte–associated protein; DC, dendritic cells; EBV, Epstein-Barr virus; EC, endothelial cells; ECM, extracellular matrix; Fcγ RIIIA, low-affinity IgG receptor isoform A; FDC, follicular dendritic cells; G, granulocytes; GC, germinal center; GPI, glycosyl phosphotidylinositol; HTA, human thymocyte antigen; IgG, immunoglobulin G; LCA, leukocyte common antigen; LPS, lipopolysaccharide; MHC-I, major histocompatibility complex class I; MP, macrophages; Mr, relative molecular mass; NK, natural killer cells; P, platelets; PBT, peripheral blood T cells; PI, phosphotidylinositol; PI3K, phosphotidylinositol 3-kinase; PLC, phospholipase C; PTP, protein tyrosine phos-

phatase; TCR, T cell receptor; TNF, tumor necrosis factor; TNFR, tumor necrosis factor receptor. For an expanded list of cluster of differentiation (CD) human antigens, see Harrison's Online at *http://harrisons.accessmedicine.com*; and for a full list of CD human antigens from the most recent Human Workshop on Leukocyte Differentiation Antigens (VII), see *http//www.ncbi.nlm.nih.gov/prow/guide*.

Source: Compiled with permission from T Kishimoto et al (eds): *Leukocyte Typing VI*, New York, Garland Publishing 1997; R Brines et al: Immunology Today 18S:1, 1997; and S Shaw ed: *Protein Reviews on the Web* www.ncbi.nlm.nih.gov/prow/guide.

INTRODUCTION The human immune system has evolved over millions of years from both invertebrate and vertebrate organisms to develop sophisticated defense mechanisms to protect the host from microbes and their virulence factors. From invertebrates, humans have inherited the innate immune system, an ancient defense system that uses germ line–encoded proteins to recognize pathogens. Cells of the innate immune system, such as macrophages, dendritic cells, and NK lymphocytes, recognize pathogen molecular motifs that are highly conserved among many microbes (PAMPs) and use a diverse set of receptor molecules (PRRs). Important components of the recognition of microbes by the innate immune system are: (1) recognition by germ line–encoded host molecules, (2) recognition of key microbe virulence factors but not recognition of self molecules, and (3) nonrecognition of benign foreign molecules or microbes. Upon contact with pathogens, macrophages and NK cells may kill pathogens directly or may activate a series of events that both slows the infection and recruits the more recently evolved arm of the human immune system, the adaptive immune system.

Adaptive immunity is found only in vertebrates and is based on the generation of antigen receptors on T and B lymphocytes by germline gene rearrangements, such that individual T or B cells express unique antigen receptors on their surface capable of specifically recognizing diverse antigens of the myriad of infectious agents in the environment. Coupled with finely tuned specific recognition mechanisms that maintain tolerance (nonreactivity) to self antigens, T and B lymphocytes bring both *specificity* and *immune memory* to vertebrate host defenses.

This chapter describes the cellular components, molecules (Table 295-1), and mechanisms that make up the innate and adaptive immune systems, and describes how adaptive immunity is recruited to the defense of the host by innate immune responses. An appreciation of the cellular and molecular bases of innate and adaptive immune responses is critical to understanding the pathogenesis of inflammatory, autoimmune, infectious, and immunodeficiency diseases.

THE INNATE IMMUNE SYSTEM All multicellular organisms, including humans, have developed the use of a limited number of germ line–encoded molecules that recognize large groups of pathogens. Because of the myriad human pathogens, host molecules of the human innate im-

mune system sense "danger signals" and either recognize PAMPs, the common molecular structures shared by many pathogens, or recognize host cell molecules produced in response to infection such as heat shock proteins and fragments of the extracellular matrix. PAMPs must be conserved structures vital to pathogen virulence and survival, such as bacterial endotoxin, so that pathogens cannot mutate molecules of PAMPs to evade human innate immune responses. PPRs are host proteins of the innate immune system that recognize PAMPs or host danger signal molecules (Tables 295-2, 295-3). Thus, recognition of pathogen molecules by hematopoietic and nonhematopoietic cell types leads to activation/production of the complement cascade, cytokines, and antimicrobial peptides as effector molecules. In addition, pathogen PAMPs and host danger signal molecules activate dendritic cells to mature and to express molecules on the dendritic cell surface that optimize antigen presentation to respond to foreign antigens.

PATTERN RECOGNITION Major PRR families of proteins include C-type lectins, leucine-rich proteins, macrophage scavenger receptor proteins, plasma pentraxins, lipid transferase, and integrins (Table 295-3). A major group of PRR collagenous glycoproteins with C-type lectin do-

TABLE 295-2 Major Components of the Innate Immune System

Pattern recognition receptors (PRR)	C type lectins, leucine-rich proteins, scavenger receptors, pentraxins, lipid transferases, integrins
Antimicrobial peptides	α-Defensins, β-defensins, cathelin, protegrin, granulsyin, histatin, secretory leukoprotease inhibitor, and probiotics
Cells	Macrophages, dendritic cells, NK cells, NK-T cells, neutrophils, eosinophils, mast cells, basophils, and epithelial cells
Complement components	Classic and alternative complement pathway, and proteins that bind complement components
Cytokines	Autocrine, paracrine, endocrine cytokines that mediate host defense and inflammation, as well as recruit, direct, and regulate adaptive immune responses

Note: NK cells, natural killer cells.

PRR Protein Family	Sites of Expression	Examples	Ligands (PAMPs)	Functions of PRR
C-type lectins				
Humoral	Plasma proteins	Collectins, mannose-binding lectin	Bacterial and viral carbohydrates	Opsonization of bacteria and virus, activation of complement
Cellular	Macrophages, dendritic cell	Macrophage mannose receptor	Terminal mannose	Phagocytosis of pathogens
	Natural killer (NK) cells	NKG2-A	Carbohydrate on HLA molecules	Inhibits killing of host cells expressing HLA+ self peptides
Leucine-rich proteins	Macrophages, dendritic cells, epithelial cells	CD14	Lipopolysaccharide (LPS)	Binds LPS and Toll proteins
	Macrophages, dendritic cells, epithelial cells, many others	Toll-like receptors 1–9	Lipopolysaccharide	Binds multiple TLR ligands and activates the cell to produce cytokines to activate adaptive immunity. TLR ligands bind macrophages, dendritic cells, or B cell induces B7-1 (CD80) and B7-2 (CD86) co-stimulatory molecules that are required for T and B cell antigen presentation in adaptive immune responses
Scavenger receptors	Macrophage	Macrophage scavenger receptors	Bacterial cell walls	Phagocytosis of bacteria
Pentraxins	Plasma protein	C-creative proteins	Phosphatidyl choline	Opsonization of bacteria, activation of complement
	Plasma protein	Serum amyloid P	Bacterial cell walls	Opsonization of bacteria, activation of complement
Lipid transferases	Plasma protein	LPS binding protein	LPS	Binds LPS, transfers LPS to CD14
Integrins	Macrophages, dendritic cells, NK cells	CD11b,c; CD18	LPS	Signals cells, activates phagocytosis

Note: PAMPs, pathogen-associated molecular patterns.

Source: Adapted with permission from R Medzhitov, CA Janeway, Jr: Curr Opin Immunol 9:4, 1997a.

mains are termed *collectins* and include the serum protein, mannose-binding lectin (MBL). MBL and other collectins, as well as two other protein families—the pentraxins (such as C-reactive protein and serum amyloid P) and macrophage scavenger receptors—all have the property of opsonizing (coating) bacteria for phagocytosis by macrophages and can also activate the complement cascade to lyse bacteria. Integrins are cell-surface adhesion molecules that signal cells after cells bind bacterial lipopolysacchride (LPS) and activate phagocytic cells to ingest pathogens.

A series of recent discoveries has revealed the mechanisms of connection between the innate and adaptive immune systems; these include (1) the plasma protein, LPS-binding protein, which binds and transfers LPS to the macrophage LPS receptor, CD14; and (2) a human family of proteins called *Toll-like receptor proteins* (TLR), which are associated with CD14, bind LPS, and signal epithelial cells, dendritic cells, and macrophages to produce cytokines and upregulate cell-surface molecules that signal the initiation of adaptive immune responses (Fig. 295-1, Table 295-3, and Table 295-4). Proteins in the Toll family (TLR 1–9) can be expressed on macrophages, dendritic cells, and B cells as well as on a variety of non-hematopoietic cell types including respiratory epithelial cells. Upon ligation, these receptors activate a series of intracellular events that lead to the killing of bacteria- and virus-infected cells as well as to the recruitment and ultimate activation of antigen-specific T and B lymphocytes (Fig. 295-1). Importantly, signaling by massive amounts of LPS through TLR4 leads to the release of large amounts of cytokines that mediate LPS-induced shock. Mutations in TLR4 proteins in mice protect from LPS shock, and TLR mutations in humans protect from LPS-induced inflammatory diseases such as LPS-induced asthma (Fig. 295-2).

Cells of invertebrates and vertebrates produce antimicrobial small peptides containing fewer than 100 amino acids that can act as endogenous antibodies (Table 295-2). Some of these peptides are produced by epithelia that line various organs, while others are found in macrophages or neutrophils that ingest pathogens. Antimicrobial peptides have been identified that kill bacteria such as *Pseudomonas* spp., *Escherichia coli*, and *Mycobacterium tuberculosis*.

EFFECTOR CELLS OF INNATE IMMUNITY Cells of the innate immune system and their roles in the first line of host defense are described in Table 295-4. Equally important as their roles in the mediation of innate immune responses are the roles that each cell type plays in recruiting T and B lymphocytes of the adaptive immune system to engage in specific antipathogen responses.

Monocytes-Macrophages Monocytes arise from precursor cells within bone marrow (Fig. 295-2) and circulate with a half-life ranging from 1 to 3 days. Monocytes leave the peripheral circulation by marginating in capillaries and migrating into a vast extravascular pool. Tissue macrophages arise from monocytes that have migrated out of the circulation and by in situ proliferation of macrophage precursors in tissue. Common locations where tissue macrophages (and certain of their specialized forms) are found are lymph node, spleen, bone marrow, perivascular connective tissue, serous cavities such as the peritoneum, pleura, skin connective tissue, lung (alveolar macrophage), liver (Kupffer cell), bone (osteoclast), central nervous system (microglia), and synovium (type A lining cell).

In general, monocytes-macrophages are on the first line of defense associated with innate immunity; however, they also play a major role in recruitment of adaptive immune responses by mediation of functions such as binding LPS, the presentation of antigen to T lymphocytes, and the secretion of factors such as interleukin (IL) 1, TNF, IL-12, and IL-6, which are central to antigen-specific activation of T and B lymphocytes (Fig. 295-1). Although monocytes-macrophages were originally thought to be the major antigen-presenting cells (APCs) of the immune system, it is now clear that dendritic cells are the most potent and effective APCs in the body (see below). Monocytes-macrophages mediate innate immune effector functions such as destruction of antibody-coated bacteria, tumor cells, or even normal hematopoietic cells in certain types of autoimmune cytopenias. Monocytes-macrophages ingest bacteria or are infected by viruses, and in doing so, frequently undergo apoptosis. Macrophages that are "stressed" by intracellular infectious agents are recognized by dendritic cells as infected and apoptotic cells and are phagocytosed by dendritic cells. In this manner, dendritic cells "cross-present" infectious agent antigens of macrophages to T cells. Activated macrophages can also mediate antigen-nonspecific lytic activity and eliminate cell types such as tumor cells in the absence of antibody. This activity is largely mediated by cytokines (i.e., TNF-α and IL-1). Monocytes-macrophages express lineage-specific molecules (e.g., the cell-surface LPS receptor, CD14) as well as surface receptors for a number of molecules, including the Fc region of IgG, activated complement components, and various cytokines (Table 295-5). Finally, macrophage secretory products are more diverse than those of any other cell of the immune system. Among monocyte-macrophage-secreted products are hydrolytic enzymes, products of oxidative metabolism, TNF-α, IL-1, -6, -10, -12, -15, -18, and a number of chemoattractant cytokines (chemokines) involved in the orchestration of an immune response in tissues (Table 295-5).

Dendritic Cells Dendritic cells are bone marrow–derived APCs that are distinct from monocytes-macrophages and are derived from both lymphoid and myeloid lineages. They generally lack the standard T, B, NK, and monocyte cell markers but do express CD83 and other molecules that aid in their identification. They can be expanded in culture, and their function is enhanced by the cytokines granulocyte-macrophage colony-stimulating factor (GM-CSF), IL-1, IL-4, and TNF-α. They are distinguished by an exceptional ability to present antigen, by expression of high levels of MHC class II and co-stimulatory molecules, and by dendritic morphology with multiple thin membrane projections (veils).

Lymphoid dendritic cells are also called *plasmacytoid dendritic cells*. They express some lymphoid markers, are present in T cell zones of lymphoid organs, and circulate in blood. Plasmacytoid dendritic cells are the most potent producers of interferon (IFN)-α and are also important presenters of antigen to T cells. INF-α is a potent antiviral cytokine; it activates NK cells to kill virally infected cells and drives T_H1 helper T cell responses to respond to viral and bacterial infections (see below for T helper types of responses).

There are two types of myeloid dendritic cells: *interstitial dendritic cells* (also called *follicular dendritic cells*) and *Langerhans dendritic cells*. Myeloid interstitial dendritic cells express myeloid markers, secrete IL-12 and IL-10, and are important APCs for both T and B cells. They circulate in blood and are located in T cell zones of lymphoid organs; in germinal centers of B cell follicles; and in tissue interstices of lung, heart, and kidney. Interstitial, or follicular, dendritic cells have extensive, thin, finger-like projections that surround the B cells in the germinal centers, allowing for maximal exposure of trapped antigen. The retention of antigen on the surface of interstitial dendritic cell membranes is critical for the selection and growth of high-affinity

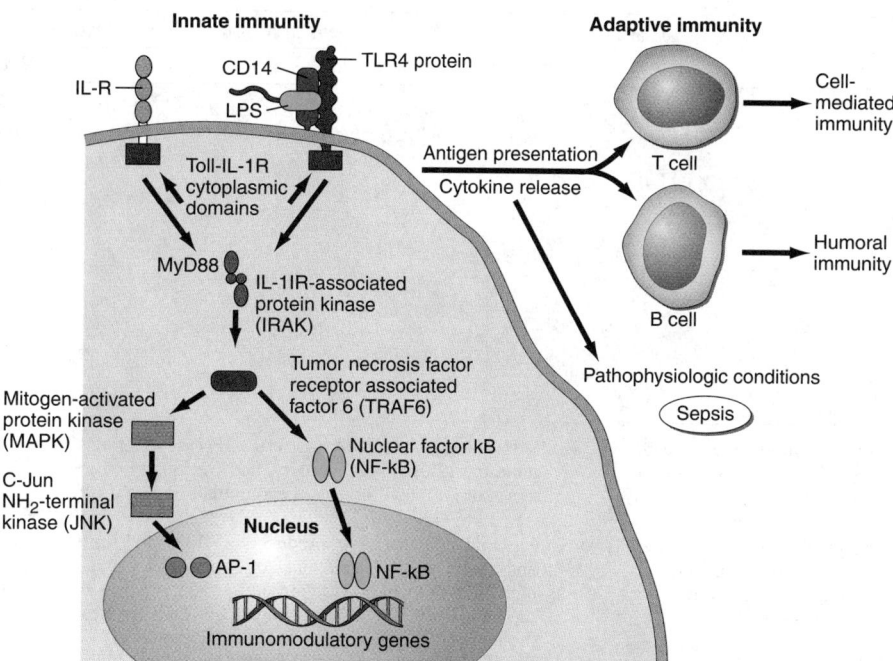

Innate immunity | **Adaptive immunity**

FIGURE 295-1 Role of Toll-like receptors (TLR) in the regulation of the response of macrophages to bacterial lipopolysaccharide (LPS). Lipopolysaccharide, a component of the cell wall of gram-negative bacteria, binds with high affinity to CD14, a glycosyl phosphatidylinositol–linked protein expressed on the surface of macrophages, and to TLR4 protein. This leads to activation of the transmembrane TLR4 protein, initiating an intracellular signaling cascade. Signaling through TLRs goes through the same signaling pathway as does interleukin (IL)1α and β signaling through the IL-1 receptor (R). The cytoplasmic domains of TRLs and IL-1R are highly homologous and are each called Toll-IL-1R cytoplasmic domains (TIR). Signaling by the TLR4 protein to the transcriptional regulatory complex of NF-κB and IκB occurs through the recruitment of MyD88 (a transcription factor) and the IL-1R-associated kinase (IRAK) and involves the adapter tumor necrosis factor receptor–associated factor 6 (TRAF-6) and the transcription factor NF-κB. Mitogen-activated protein kinase (MAPK) activates c-jun NH2-terminal kinase (Jnk), which in turn activates the nuclear transcription factor AP-1. AP-1 and NF-κB pass into the nucleus and bind to specific sequences in the promoter regions of immunomodulatory genes such as cytokine genes. This leads to the expression of immunomodulatory genes, including cytokines and co-stimulatory molecules. These gene products act on T and B cells to initiate the adaptive immune response. Under pathophysiologic conditions, high levels of immune system activation by bacterial LPS may lead to septic shock. *(Adapted from Modlin et al: N Engl J Med 340:1834, 1999; with permission.)*

clones of B cells and for the maintenance of B cell memory. Of note, HIV is trapped in large quantities on the processes of interstitial dendritic cells in lymphoid organs, allowing the lymphoid tissue to serve as a reservoir of virus and a source of infection for CD4+ T cells migrating into the area to provide help to B cells in the initiation and propagation of an HIV-specific humoral response (Chap. 173). Langerhans dendritic cells express the CD1a antigen in addition to myeloid markers; circulate in blood; and populate T cell zones of lymph node, the thymus medulla, and skin and gut epithelial layers. They produce IL-12 and are key APCs for T cell activation at epithelial and other sites.

When dendritic cells come in contact with bacterial products, viral proteins, or host proteins released as danger signals from distressed host cells (Fig. 295-2), they bind to various TLRs and activate dendritic cells to release cytokines that drive cells of the innate immune system to become activated to respond to the invading organism, and recruit T and B cells of the adaptive immune system to respond. TLR engagement on dendritic cells upregulates dendritic cell MHC class II, B7-1 (CD80), and B7-2 (CD86) that enhance specific antigen presentation and induce dendritic cell cytokine production (Table 295-1). Thus, plasmacytoid and myeloid dendritic cells are important bridges between early (innate) and later (adaptive) immunity.

Large Granular Lymphocytes/Natural Killer Cells Large granular lymphocytes (LGLs) account for ~5 to 10% of peripheral blood lymphocytes. LGLs are nonadherent, nonphagocytic cells with large azurophilic cytoplasmic granules. LGLs express surface receptors for the Fc portion of IgG (CD16) and for NCAM-I (CD56), and many LGLs express some T lineage markers, particularly CD8, and proliferate in response

TABLE 295-4 *Cells of the Innate Immune System and Their Major Roles in Triggering Adaptive Immunity*

Cell Type	Major Role in Innate Immunity	Major Role in Adaptive Immunity
Macrophages	Phagocytose and kill bacteria; produce antimicrobial peptides; bind lipopolysaccharide (LPS); produce inflammatory cytokines	Produce interleukin (IL) 1 and tumor necrosis factor (TNF) α to upregulate lymphocyte adhesion molecules and chemokines to attract antigen-specific lymphocytes; produce IL-12 to recruit T_H1 helper T cell responses; upregulate co-stimulatory and MHC molecules to facilitate T and B lymphocyte recognition and activation; macrophages and dendritic cells, after LPS signaling, upregulate co-stimulatory molecules B7-1 (CD80) and B7-2 (CD86) required for activation of antigen-specific antipathogen T cells; there are also Toll-like proteins on B cells and dendritic cells that after LPS ligation induce CD80 and CD86 on these cells for T cell antigen presentation.
Plasmacytoid dendritic cells (DCs) of lymphoid lineage	Produce large amounts of interferon (IFN)α, which has antitumor and antiviral activity, and are found in T cell zones of lymphoid organs; they circulate in blood	IFN-α is a potent activator of macrophage and mature DCs to phagocytose invading pathogens and present pathogen antigens to T and B cells
Myeloid dendritic cells are of two types: interstitial and Langerhans-derived	Interstitial DCs are strong producers of IL-12 and IL-10 and are located in T cell zones of lymphoid organs, circulate in blood, and are present in the interstices of the lung, heart, and kidney; Langerhans DCs are strong producers of IL-12; are located in T cell zones of lymph nodes, skin epithelia, and the thymic medulla; and circulate in blood	Interstitial DCs are potent antigen-presenting cells for T cells and are potent primers of B cell activation for antibody production; Langerhans DCs are potent antigen-presenting cells for T cell priming
Natural killer (NK) cells	Kill foreign and host cells that have low levels of MHC+ self peptides. Express NK receptors that inhibit NK function in the presence of high expression of self-MHC.	Produce TNF-α and IFN-γ that recruit T_H1 helper T cell responses
NK-T cells	Lymphocytes with both T cell and NK surface markers that recognize lipid antigens of intracellular bacteria such as *M. tuberculosis* by CD1 molecules and kill host cells infected with intracellular bacteria.	Produce IL-4 to recruit T_H2 helper T cell responses, IgG1 and IgE production
Neutrophils	Phagocytose and kill bacteria, produce antimicrobial peptides	Produce nitric oxide synthase and nitric oxide that inhibit apoptosis in lymphocytes and can prolong adaptive immune responses
Eosinophils	Kill invading parasites	Produce IL-5 that recruits Ig-specific antibody responses
Mast cells and basophils	Release TNF-α, IL-6, IFN-γ in response to a variety of bacterial PAMPs	Produce IL-4 that recruits T_H2 helper T cell responses and recruit IgG1- and IgE-specific antibody responses
Epithelial cells	Produce anti-microbial peptides; tissue specific epithelia produce mediator of local innate immunity, e.g. lung epithelial cells produce surfactant proteins (proteins within the collectin family) that bind and promote clearance of lung invading microbes	Produce TGF-β that triggers IgA-specific antibody responses

Note: MHC, major histocompatibility complex; PAMP, pathogen-associated molecular patterns.

Source: Adapted with permission from R Medzhitov, CA Janeway, Jr: Curr Opin Immunol 9:4, 1997a.

to IL-2. LGLs arise in both bone marrow and thymic microenvironments.

Functionally, LGLs share features with both monocytes-macrophages and neutrophils in that LGLs mediate both antibody-dependent cellular cytotoxicity (ADCC) and NK activity. ADCC is the binding of an opsonized (antibody-coated) target cell to an Fc receptor–bearing effector cell via the Fc region of antibody, resulting in lysis of the target by the effector cell. NK cell activity is the nonimmune (i.e., effector cell never having had previous contact with the target), MHC-unrestricted, non-antibody-mediated killing of target cells, which are usually malignant cell types, transplanted foreign cells, or virus-infected cells. Thus, LGLs that mediate NK cell activity may play an important role in immune surveillance and destruction of cells that spontaneously undergo malignant transformation in vivo. Subsets of NK cells may play a role in hematopoietic cell engraftment; some subsets stimulate bone marrow stem cells, and others stimulate engraftment. Lymphokine-activated killer (LAK) cells are NK lymphocytes that proliferate in vitro to high concentrations of IL-2 and

develop the ability to kill tumor cells more efficiently than unstimulated NK cells. Rare patients with complete absence of NK cells have been described who lack both NK cell activity and CD56+, CD16+ lymphocytes but have normal T and B cell function. NK cell hyporesponsiveness is also observed in patients with the *Chédiak-Higashi syndrome*, an autosomal recessive disease associated with fusion of cytoplasmic granules and defective degranulation of neutrophil lysosomes.

The ability of NK cells to kill target cells is inversely related to target cell expression of MHC class I molecules. Thus, NK cells kill target cells with low or no levels of MHC class I expression and are prevented from killing target cells with high levels of class I expression. Recent studies have demonstrated the presence of NK receptors (NK-Rs) or killer immunoglobulin-like receptors (KIRs) that bind to either classic MHC class I molecules in a polymorphic way or the MHC-class Ib molecule HLA-E (Fig. 295-3). In every person, NK cells express at least one NK-R that recognizes a self–MHC class I allele. NK-Rs of the Ig superfamily bind specific MHC class I molecules;

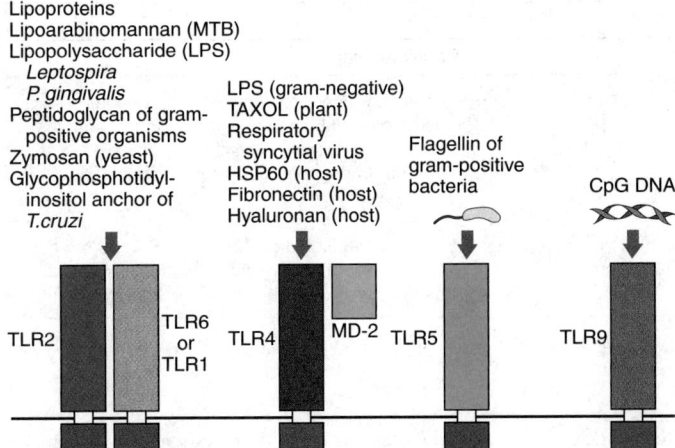

Lipoproteins
Lipoarabinomannan (MTB)
Lipopolysaccharide (LPS)
  Leptospira
  P. gingivalis
Peptidoglycan of gram-
  positive organisms
Zymosan (yeast)
Glycophosphotidyl-
  inositol anchor of
  T.cruzi

LPS (gram-negative)
TAXOL (plant)
Respiratory
  syncytial virus
HSP60 (host)
Fibronectin (host)
Hyaluronan (host)

Flagellin of
gram-positive
bacteria

CpG DNA

TLR2   TLR6 or TLR1   TLR4   MD-2   TLR5   TLR9

FIGURE 295-2 Toll-like receptors and their ligands. Certain pathogen-associated molecular patterns and host-derived products utilize Toll-like receptor (TLR) family members as critical signal transducers. TLR2 recognizes a variety of microbial products. TLR4 is essential for signaling via lipopolysaccharide (LPS) from Gram-negative bacteria; the exceptions are *Leptospira* and *Pseudomonas gingivalis*, the LPS of which is recognized by TLR2. TLR4 recognizes not only viral and plant products, but also endogenous host-derived products, such as heat shock protein 60 (HSP60) and fragments from fibronectin and hyaluronan. Compared with TLR2 and TLR4, recognition by TLR5 and TLR9 is more restricted and is required for flagellin and CpG DNA-mediated signaling, respectively. *(From S Akira et al: Nat Immunol 2:675, 2001; with permission.)*

e.g., the NK-R p140 binds HLA-A3, and NK-R p70 binds HLA-B27 (Fig. 295-3). A second NK-R of the C-type lectin family of proteins is termed *CD94/NKG2A* and binds the MHC-related protein HLA-E (Fig. 295-3). HLA-E has an MHC class I structure but exclusively binds the leader sequence peptides of classic MHC class I molecules in the HLA-E MHC-like "notch" (see "Molecular Basis of T Cell Recognition of Antigen," below). In this manner, CD94/NKG2A NK cell molecules survey and monitor the total level of classic MHC class I molecules on the surface of host cells. When cell-surface levels of host MHC class I molecules decrease, such as occurs during malignant transformation or viral infection of host cells, the altered host cell with diminished MHC class I expression is recognized by NK-Rs, and the NK cell is activated to kill the host tumor or virally infected cells. The ability of NK-Rs to bind to self-MHC and inhibit NK killing of normal host cells is a key protective mechanism for prevention of NK cell–mediated autoimmune disease. In addition, when HLA-E-positive cells become "stressed," such as occurs during viral infections, the leader sequence of heat shock protein-60 (HSP-60) is processed and inserted in the notch of HLA-E, yet this particular peptide/HLA-E complex is not recognized by NK cells. In this manner, NK cells can detect and recognize stressed virally infected cells for elimination.

Some NK cells express CD3 and are termed *NK/T cells*. NK/T cells can also express oligoclonal forms of the TCR for antigen that can recognize lipid molecules of intracellular bacteria when presented in the context of CD1 molecules on APCs. This mode of recognition of intracellular bacteria such as *Listeria monocytogenese* and *M. tuberculosis* by NK/T cells is thought to be an important defense mechanism against these organisms that, via usage of a clonal form of TCRs for antigen, incorporates components of both the innate and adaptive immune systems.

Neutrophils, Eosinophils, and Basophils Granulocytes are present in nearly all forms of inflammation and are amplifiers and effectors of innate immune responses. Unchecked accumulation and activation of granulocytes can lead to host tissue damage, as seen in neutrophil- and eosinophil-mediated *systemic necrotizing vasculitis*. Granulocytes are derived from stem cells in bone marrow. Each type of granulocyte (neutrophil, eosinophil, or basophil) is derived from a different subclass of progenitor cell, which is stimulated to proliferate by colony-stimulating factors (Table 295-5). During terminal maturation of granulocytes, class-specific nuclear morphology and cytoplasmic granules appear that allow for histologic identification of granulocyte type.

Neutrophils express Fc receptors for IgG (CD16) and receptors for activated complement components (C3b or CD35). Upon interaction of neutrophils with opsonized bacteria or immune complexes, azurophilic granules (containing myeloperoxidase, lysozyme, elastase, and other enzymes) and specific granules (containing lactoferrin, lysozyme, collagenase, and other enzymes) are released, and microbicidal superoxide radicals (O_2^-) are generated at the neutrophil surface. The generation of superoxide leads to inflammation by direct injury to tissue and by alteration of macromolecules such as collagen and DNA.

Eosinophils express Fc receptors for IgG (CD32) and are potent cytotoxic effector cells for various parasitic organisms. In *Nippostrongylus brasiliensis* helminth infection, eosinophils are key cytotoxic effector cells in removal of these parasites. Key to regulation of eosinophil cytotoxicity to *N. brasiliensis* worms are antigen-specific T helper cells that produce IL-4, thus providing an example of regulation of innate immune responses by adaptive immunity antigen-specific T cells. Intracytoplasmic contents of eosinophils, such as major basic protein, eosinophil cationic protein, and eosinophil-derived neurotoxin, are capable of directly damaging tissues and may be responsible in part for the organ system dysfunction in the *hypereosinophilic syndromes* (Chap. 55). Since the eosinophil granule contains anti-inflammatory types of enzymes (histaminase, arylsulfatase, phospholipase D), eosinophils may homeostatically downregulate or terminate ongoing inflammatory responses.

The normal functions of basophils and tissue mast cells are not completely understood; they are potent reservoirs of cytokines such as IL-4. The capacity of basophil cytokines and mediators to increase local delivery of antibodies and complement by increasing vascular permeability is hypothetical. Thus, the basophil is identified principally with allergic reactions and some delayed cutaneous hypersensitivity states. Certainly, the promotion of increased vascular permeability by basophils is important in the genesis of inflammatory lesions in some vasculitis syndromes (Chap. 306). Basophils express high-affinity surface receptors for IgE (FcRI) and, upon cross-linking of basophil-bound IgE by antigen, release histamine, eosinophil chemotactic factor of anaphylaxis, and neutral protease—all mediators of immediate (anaphylaxis) hypersensitivity responses (Table 295-6). In addition, basophils express surface receptors for activated complement components (C3a, C5a), through which mediator release can be directly effected. →*For further discussion of tissue mast cells, see Chap. 298.*

THE COMPLEMENT SYSTEM The complement system, an important soluble component of the innate immune system, is a series of plasma enzymes, regulatory proteins, and proteins that are activated in a cascading fashion, resulting in cell lysis. There are four pathways of the complement system: the classic activation pathway activated by antigen/antibody immune complexes, the mannose-binding lectin (a serum collectin; Table 295-3) activation pathway activated by microbes with terminal mannose groups, the alternative activation pathway activated by microbes or tumor cells, and the terminal pathway that is common to the first three pathways and leads to the membrane attack complex that lyses cells (Fig. 295-4). The series of enzymes of the complement system are serine proteases.

Activation of the classic complement pathway via immune complex binding to C1q links the innate and adaptive immune systems via specific antibody in the immune complex. The alternative complement activation pathway is antibody-independent and is activated by binding of C3 directly to pathogens and "altered self" such as tumor cells. In the renal glomerular inflammatory disease, *IgA nephropathy*, IgA activates the alternative complement pathway and causes glomerular damage and decreased renal function. Activation of the classic complement pathway via C1, C4, and C2 and activation of the alternative pathway via factor D, C3, and factor B both lead to cleavage and

TABLE 295-5 Cytokines and Cytokine Receptors

Cytokine	Receptor	Cell Source	Cell Target	Biologic Activity
IL-1α,β	Type 1 IL-1R, type 2 IL-1R	Monocytes/macrophages, B cells, fibroblasts, most epithelial cells including thymic epithelium, endothelial cells	All cells	Upregulates adhesion molecule expression, neutrophil and macrophage emigration; mimics shock, fever; upregulates hepatic acute-phase protein production; facilitates hematopoiesis
IL-2	IL-2R α,β, common γ	T cells	T cells, B cells, NK cells, monocytes/macrophages	T cell activation and proliferation, B cell growth, NK cell proliferation and activation, enhanced monocyte/macrophage cytolytic activity
IL-3	IL-3R, common β	T cells, NK cells, mast cells	Monocytes/macrophages, mast cells, eosinophils, bone marrow progenitors	Stimulation of hematopoietic progenitors
IL-4	IL-4R α, common γ	T cells, mast cells, basophils	T cells, B cells, NK cells, monocytes/macrophages, neutrophils, eosinophils, endothelial cells, fibroblasts	Stimulates T_H2 helper T cell differentiation and proliferation; stimulates B cell Ig class switch to IgG1 and IgE; anti-inflammatory action on T cells, monocytes
IL-5	IL-5R α, common β	T cells, mast cells, and eosinophils	Eosinophils, basophils, murine B cells	Regulates eosinophil migration and activation
IL-6	IL-6R, gp130	Monocytes/macrophages, B cells, fibroblasts, most epithelium including thymic epithelium, endothelial cells	T cells, B cells, epithelial cells, hepatocytes, monocytes/macrophages	Induction of acute-phase protein production, T and B cell differentiation and growth, myeloma cell growth, osteoclast growth and activation
IL-7	IL-7R α, common γ	Bone marrow, thymic epithelial cells	T cells, B cells, bone marrow cells	Differentiation of B, T, and NK cell precursors, activation of T and NK cells
IL-8	CXCR1, CXCR2	Monocytes/macrophages, T cells, neutrophils, fibroblasts, endothelial cells, epithelial cells	Neutrophils, T cells, monocytes/macrophages, endothelial cells, basophils	Induces neutrophil, monocyte, and T cell migration; induces neutrophil adherance to endothelial cells and histamine release from basophils; stimulates angiogenesis; suppresses proliferation of hepatic precursors
IL-10	IL-10R	Monocytes/macrophages, T cells, B cells, keratinocytes, mast cells	Monocytes/macrophages, T cells, B cells, NK cells, mast cells	Inhibits macrophage proinflammatory cytokine production; downregulates cytokine class II antigen and B7-1 and B7-2 expression; inhibits differentiation of T_H1 helper T cells; inhibits NK cell function; stimulates mast cell proliferation and function and B cell activation and differentiation
IL-11	IL-11R, gp130	Bone marrow stromal cells	Megakaryocytes, B cells, hepatocytes	Induces megakaryocyte colony formation and maturation; enhances antibody responses; stimulates acute-phase protein production
IL-12 (35-kDa and 40-kDa subunits)	IL-12R	Activated macrophages, dendritic cells, neutrophils	T cells, NK cells	Induces T_H1 T helper cell formation and lymphokine-activated killer cell formation; increases CD8+ CTL activity
IL-13	IL-13/IL-4R	T cells (T_H2)	Monocytes/macrophages, B cells, endothelial cells, keratinocytes	Upregulation of VCAM-1 and C-C chemokine expression on endothelial cells; B cell activation and differentiation; inhibits macrophage proinflammatory cytokine production
IL-17	IL17R	CD4+ T cells	Fibroblasts, endothelium, epithelium	Enhanced cytokine secretion that promotes a predominant T_H1 response
IL-18	IL-18R (IL-1R-related protein)	Keratinocytes, macrophages	T cells, B cells, NK cells	Upregulated IFN-γ production, enhanced NK cell cytotoxicity
IFN-α	Type I interferon receptor	All cells	All cells	Antiviral activity; stimulates T cell, macrophage, and NK cell activity; direct antitumor effects; upregulates MHC class I antigen expression; used therapeutically in viral and autoimmune conditions

(continued)

TABLE 295-5—(Continued)

Cytokine	Receptor	Cell Source	Cell Target	Biologic Activity
IFN-β	Type I interferon receptor	All cells	All cells	Antiviral activity; stimulates T cell, macrophage, and NK cell activity; direct antitumor effects; upregulates MHC class I antigen expression; used therapeutically in viral and autoimmune conditions
IFN-γ	Type II interferon receptor	T cells, NK cells	All cells	Regulates macrophage and NK cell activation; stimulates immunoglobulin secretion by B cells; induction of class II histocompatibility antigens; T_H1 T cell differentiation
TNF-α	TNF-RI, TNF-RII	Monocytes/macrophages, mast cells, basophils, eosinophils, NK cells, B cells, T cells, keratinocytes, fibroblasts, thymic epithelial cells	All cells except erythrocytes	Fever, anorexia, shock, capillary leak syndrome, enhanced leukocyte cytotoxicity, enhanced NK cell function, acute-phase protein synthesis, proinflammatory cytokine induction
G-CSF	G-CSFR; gp130	Monocytes/macrophages, fibroblasts, endothelial cells, thymic epithelial cells, stromal cells	Myeloid cells, endothelial cells	Regulates myelopoiesis; enhances survival and function of neutrophils; clinical use in reversing neutropenia after cytotoxic chemotherapy
GM-CSF	GM-CSFR; common β	T cells, monocytes/macrophages, fibroblasts, endothelial cells, thymic epithelial cells	Monocytes/macrophages, neutrophils, eosinophils, fibroblasts, endothelial cells	Regulates myelopoiesis; enhances macrophage bactericidal and tumoricidal activity; mediator of dendritic cell maturation and function; upregulates NK cell function; clinical use in reversing neutropenia after cytotoxic chemotherapy
M-CSF	M-CSFR (c-fms proto-oncogene)	Fibroblasts, endothelial cells, monocytes/macrophages, T cells, B cells, epithelial cells including thymic epithelium	Monocytes/macrophages	Regulates monocyte/macrophage production and function
Fractalkine	CX3CR1	Activated endothelial cells	NK cells, T cells, monocytes/macrophages	Cell surface chemokine/mucin hybrid molecule that functions as a chemoattractant, leukocyte activator, and cell adhesion molecule

Note: 1 CSF, colony-stimulating factor; CXCR, CXC-type chemokine receptor; G-CSF, granulocyte CSF; GM-CSF, granulocyte-macrophage CSF; IFN, interferon; IL, interleukin; IP, IFN-γ-inducible protein; M-CSF, macrophage CSF; MDC, macrophage-derived chemokine; MHC, major histocompatibility complex; NK, natural killer; PMBC, peripheral blood mononuclear cells; PF, platelet factor; SCF, stem cell factor; TNF, tumor necrosis factor; VCAM, vascular cell adhesion molecule. For an expanded list of cytokines, see Harrison's Online at *http://harrisons.accessmedicine.com.*
Source: From JS Sundy et al, in J Gallin and R Snyderman (eds): *Inflammation, Basic Principles and Clinical Correlates,* 3d ed. Philadelphia, Lippincott Williams & Wilkins, 1999, with permission.

activation of C3. C3 activation fragments, when bound to target surfaces such as bacteria and other foreign antigens, are critical for opsonization (coating by antibody and complement) in preparation for phagocytosis. The MBL pathway substitutes MBL-associated serine proteases (MASP) 1 and 2 for C1q, C1r, and C1s to activate C4. The MBL activation pathway is activated by mannose on the surface of bacteria and viruses.

The three pathways of complement activation all converge on the final common terminal pathway. C3 cleavage by each pathway results in activation of C5, C6, C7, C8, and C9 resulting in the membrane attack complex that physically inserts into the membranes of target cells or bacteria and lyses them.

Thus, complement activation is a critical component of innate immunity for responding to microbial infection. The functional consequences of complement activation by the three initiating pathways and the terminal pathway are shown in Fig. 295-4 and Table 295-7. In general the cleavage products of complement components facilitate microbe or damaged cell clearance (C1q, C4, C3), promote activation and enhancement of inflammation (anaphylatoxins, C3a, C5a), and promote microbe or opsonized cell lysis (membrane attack complex).

CYTOKINES Cytokines are soluble proteins produced by a wide variety of hematopoietic and nonhematopoietic cell types (Table 295-5). They are critical for both normal innate and adaptive immune responses, and

their expression may be perturbed in most immune, inflammatory, and infectious disease states.

Cytokines are involved in the regulation of the growth, development, and activation of immune system cells and in the mediation of the inflammatory response. In general, cytokines are characterized by considerable redundancy in that different cytokines have similar functions. In addition, many cytokines are pleiotropic in that they are capable of acting on many different cell types. This pleiotropism results from the expression on multiple cell types of receptors for the same cytokine (see below), leading to the formation of "cytokine networks." The action of cytokines may be: (1) autocrine when the target cell is the same cell that secretes the cytokine, (2) paracrine when the target cell is nearby, and (3) endocrine when the cytokine is secreted into the circulation and acts distal to the source.

Cytokines have been named based on presumed targets or based on presumed functions. Those cytokines that are thought to primarily target leukocytes have been named interleukins (IL-1, -2, -3, etc.). Many cytokines that were originally described as having a certain function have retained those names (granulocyte colony-stimulating factor or G-CSF, etc.). Cytokines belong in general to four major structural families, the four α-helix bundle family, the IL-1 family, the IL-17 family, and the chemokine family (Table 295-8). The four α-helix group is the largest family whose members have a three-dimensional core with four bundles of α-helices. Within this family are three sub-

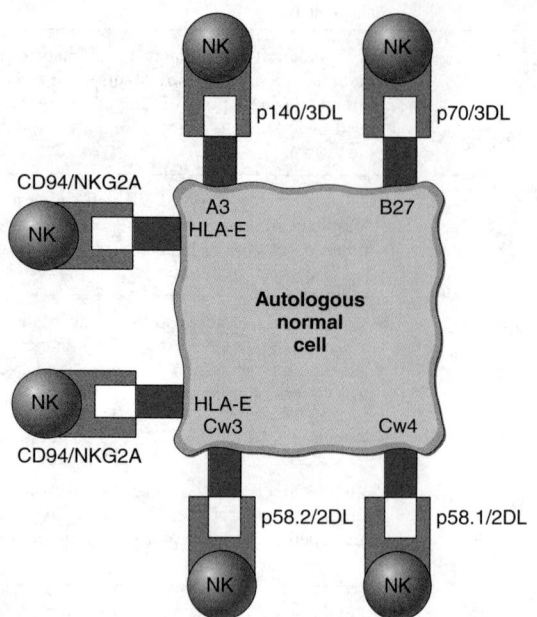

FIGURE 295-3 A schematic representation of the human natural killer (NK) receptor repertoire. The NK cells of a given individual express clonally distributed NK-Rs for self-HLA class I molecules. In this representative donor (HLA haplotype: HLA-A1, A3; HLA-B7, B27; HLA-Cw3, Cw4), NK cells express at least one inhibitory receptor that interacts with self-HLA alleles. The NK-Rs depicted in white are those belonging to the Ig superfamily that recognize allelic forms of HLA class I molecules. CD94/NKG2A receptors (stippled blue) bind to the MHC class I–like molecules, HLA-E, that present leader sequence peptides of classic MHC class I molecules to CD94/NKG2A molecules. The receptors belonging to the Ig superfamily do not cover the whole set of HLA class I alleles and are not expressed by 100% of NK cells. CD94/NKG2A receptors play important roles in monitoring the total level of MHC class I molecules on viral and malignantly transformed cells. (*Adapted from A Moretta et al: Immunol Rev 155:105, 1997; with permission. For nomenclature, see EO Long et al: Protein Rev at www.ncbi.nlm.nih.gov/prow/guide 679664748_g.htm, 1999.*)

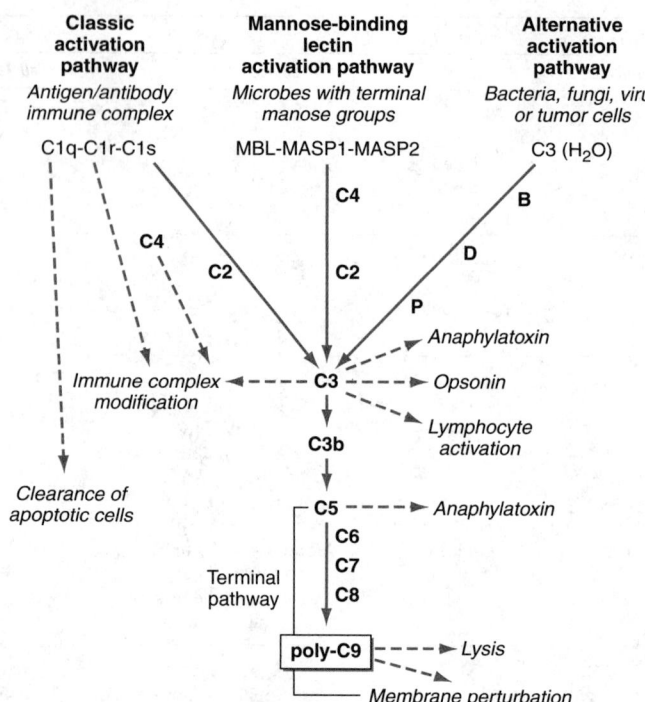

FIGURE 295-4 The four pathways and the effector mechanisms of the complement system. Dashed arrows indicate the functions of pathway components. (*After BJ Morley, MJ Walport: The Complement Facts Books. London, Academic Press, Chap 2, 2000; with permission.*)

families, the IL-2, IFN, and IL-10 subfamilies. The second group of cytokines is the IL-1 family, made up of IL-1α, IL-1β, and IL-18, all of which share about 25% sequence homology to each other. Most of the IL-17 family of cytokines promote $T_H 1$ types of T cell responses that lead to cytotoxic T cell effector function. Finally, chemokines are cytokines that regulate cell movement and trafficking. Chemokines act through G protein–coupled receptors and have a distinctive three-dimensional structure. IL-8 is the only chemokine that early on was named an interleukin.

In general, cytokines exert their effects by influencing gene activation that results in cellular activation, growth, differentiation, functional cell-surface molecule expression, and cellular effector function. In this regard, cytokines can have dramatic effects on the regulation of immune responses and the pathogenesis of a variety of diseases. Indeed, T cells have been categorized on the basis of the pattern of cytokines that they secrete that results in either humoral immune response ($T_H 2$) or a cell-mediated immune response ($T_H 1$).

Cytokine receptors can be grouped into five general families based on similarities in their extracellular amino acid sequences and conserved structural domains. The *immunoglobulin (Ig) superfamily* represents a large number of cell-surface and secreted proteins. The IL-1 receptors (type 1, type 2) are examples of cytokine receptors with extracellular Ig domains.

TABLE 295-6 *Mediators Released from Human Mast Cells and Basophils*

Mediator	Actions
Histamine	Smooth-muscle contraction, increased vascular permeability
Slow-reacting substance of anaphylaxis (SRSA) (leukotriene C4, D4, E4)	Smooth-muscle contraction
Eosinophil chemotactic factor of anaphylaxis (ECF-A)	Chemotactic attraction of eosinophils
Platelet-activating factor	Activates platelets to secrete serotonin and other mediators: smooth-muscle contraction; induces vascular permeability
Neutrophil chemotactic factor (NCF)	Chemotactic attraction of neutrophils
Leukotactic activity (leukotriene B4)	Chemotactic attraction of neutrophils
Heparin	Anticoagulant
Basophil kallikrein of anaphylaxis (BK-A)	Cleaves kininogen to form bradykinin

TABLE 295-7 *Biologic Activities of Some Complement Components*

Component	Activity
C4a weak anaphylatoxin	Evokes histamine release from basophils and mast cells
C3a	Anaphylatoxin; evokes histamine release from basophils and mast cells
C5a	Anaphylatoxin; evokes histamine release from basophils and mast cells; potent chemoattractant for monocytes and neutrophils
C3b, C3bi	Enhancement of phagocytosis by neutrophils and monocytes; promotes immune-complex binding to cells within monocyte-macrophage system, as well as neutrophils; C3b with Bb forms alternative pathway C3 convertase and amplifies alternative pathway; promotes solubilization of immune complexes
C5–9	Membrane attack complex; forms transmembrane channels leading to cell destruction

Source: After S Ruddy, in WN Kelley et al (eds): *Textbook of Rheumatology*, 4th ed. Philadelphia, Saunders, 1993, with permission.

The hallmark of the *hematopoietic growth factor (type 1) receptor* family is that the extracellular regions of each receptor contain two conserved motifs. One motif located at the N terminus is rich in cysteine residues. The other motif is located at the C terminus proximal to the transmembrane region and comprises five amino acid residues, tryptophan-serine-X-tryptophan-serine (WSXWS). This family can be grouped on the basis of the number of receptor subunits they have and on the utilization of shared subunits. A number of cytokine receptors, i.e., IL-6, IL-11, IL-12, and leukemia inhibitory factor, are paired with gp130. There is also a common 150-kDa subunit shared by IL-3, IL-5, and GM-CSF receptors. The gamma chain (γ_c) of the IL-2 receptor is common to the IL-2, IL-4, IL-7, IL-9, and IL-15 receptors. Thus,

TABLE 295-8 *Four Major Structural Families of Cytokines*

Four α-helix bundle family	Interleukin 2 (IL-2) Subfamily Interleukin: IL-2, IL-3, IL-4, IL-5, IL-6, IL-7, IL-9, IL-11, IL-12, IL-13, IL-15, IL-21, IL-23 Not called interleukins: Colony-stimulating factor-1 (CSF1), granulocyte-macrophage colony-stimulating factor (CSF2), Flt-3 ligand, erythropoietin (EPO), thrombopoietin (THPO), leukocyte inhibitory factor (LIF) Not Interleukins: Growth hormone (GH1), prolactin (PRL), leptin (LEP), cardiotrophin (CTF1), ciliary neurotrophic factor (CNTF), cytokine receptor-like factor 1 (CLC or CLF) Interferon (IFN) subfamily IFN-β, IFN-α IL-10 subfamily IL-10, IL-19, IL-20, IL-22, IL-24 and IL-26
IL-1 Family	IL-1α (IL1A), IL-1β, (IL1B), IL-18 (IL-18), and paralogues
IL-17 Family	IL-17A, IL-17B, IL-17C, IL-17D, IL-17E, IL-17F
Chemokines	IL-8, MCP-1, MCP-2, MCP-3, MCP-4, eotaxin, TARC, LARC/MIP-3α, MDC, MIP-1α, MIP-1β, RANTES, MIP-3β, I-309, SLC, PARC, TECK, GROα, GROβ, NAP-2, IP-10, MIG, SDF-1, PF4

Note: GRO, growth-related peptide; IL, interleukin; IP, IFNδ-inducible protein; LARC, liver and activation-regulated chemokine; MCP, monocyte chemotactic protein; MDC, macrophage-derived chemokine; MIG, monoteine-induced by IFNδ; MIP, macrophage inflammatory protein; NAP, neutrophil-activating protein; PARC, pulmonary and activation-regulated chemokine; PF4, platelet factor; RANTES, regulated on activation normally T cell expressed and secreted; SDF, stromal-cell derived factor; SLC, secondary lymphoid tissue chemokine; TARC, thymus and activation-regulated chemokine; TECK, thymus-express chemokine.
Source: Adapted with permission from JW Schrader: Trends Immunol 23:573, 2002.

the specific cytokine receptor is responsible for ligand-specific binding, while the subunits such as gp130, the 150-kDa subunit, and γ_c are important in signal transduction. The γ_c gene is on the X chromosome, and mutations in the γ_c protein result in the *X-linked form of severe combined immune deficiency syndrome (X-SCID)* (Chap. 297).

The members of the *interferon (type II) receptor* family include the receptors for IFN-γ, and -β, which share a similar 210-amino-acid binding domain with conserved cysteine pairs at both the amino and carboxy termini. The members of the *TNF (type III) receptor family* share a common binding domain composed of repeated cysteine-rich regions. Members of this family include the p55 and p75 receptors for TNF (TNFR1 and TNFR2, respectively); CD40 antigen, which is an important B cell–surface marker involved in immunoglobulin isotype switching; fas/Apo-1, whose triggering induces apoptosis; CD27 and CD30, which are found on activated T cells and B cells; and nerve growth factor receptor.

The common motif for the *seven transmembrane helix family* was originally found in receptors linked to GTP-binding proteins. This family includes receptors for chemokines, β-adrenergic receptors, and retinal rhodopsin. It is important to note that two members of the chemokine receptor family, CXC chemokine receptor type 4 (CXCR4) and β chemokine receptor type 5 (CCR5), have recently been found to serve as the two major coreceptors for binding and entry of HIV into CD4-expressing host cells (Chap. 173).

Significant advances have been made in defining the signaling pathways through which cytokines exert their effects intracellularly. The Janus family of protein tyrosine kinases (JAK) is a critical element involved in signaling via the hematopoietin receptors. Four JAK kinases, JAK1, JAK2, JAK3, and Tyk2, preferentially bind different cytokine receptor subunits. Cytokine binding to its receptor brings the cytokine receptor subunits into apposition and allows a pair of JAKs to transphosphorylate and activate one another. The JAKs then phosphorylate the receptor on the tyrosine residues and allow signaling molecules to bind to the receptor, where these molecules become phosphorylated. Signaling molecules bind the receptor because they have domains (SH2, or src homology 2 domains) that can bind phosphorylated tyrosine residues. There are a number of these important signaling molecules that bind the receptor, such as the adapter molecule SHC, which can couple the receptor to the activation of the mitogen-activated protein kinase pathway. In addition, an important class of substrate of the JAKs is the signal transducers and activators of transcription (STAT) family of transcription factors. STATs have SH2

domains that enable them to bind to phosphorylated receptors, where they are then phosphorylated by the JAKs. It appears that different STATs have specificity for different receptor subunits. The STATs then dissociate from the receptor and translocate to the nucleus, bind to DNA motifs that they recognize, and regulate gene expression. The STATs preferentially bind DNA motifs that are slightly different from one another and thereby control transcription of specific genes. The importance of this pathway is particularly relevant to lymphoid development. Mutations of JAK3 itself also result in a disorder identical to X-SCID; however, since JAK3 is found on chromosome 19 and not on the X chromosome, JAK3 deficiency occurs in boys and girls (Chap. 297).

THE ADAPTIVE IMMUNE SYSTEM Adaptive immunity is characterized by antigen-specific responses to a foreign antigen or pathogen. A key feature of adaptive immunity is that following the initial contact with antigen (*immunologic priming*), subsequent antigen exposure leads to more rapid and vigorous immune responses (*immunologic memory*). The adaptive immune system consists of dual limbs of cellular and humoral immunity. The principal effectors of cellular immunity are T lymphocytes, while the principal effectors of humoral immunity are B lymphocytes (Table 295-9). Both B and T lymphocytes derive from a common stem cell.

The proportion and distribution of immunocompetent cells in various tissues reflect cell traffic, homing patterns, and functional capabilities. Bone marrow is the major site of maturation of B cells, monocytes-macrophages, and granulocytes and contains pluripotent stem cells which, under the influence of various colony stimulating factors, are capable of giving rise to all hematopoietic cell types. T cell precursors also arise from hematopoietic stem cells and home to

TABLE 295-9 *Components of the Adaptive Immune System*

Cellular: Thymus-derived (T) lymphocytes—T cell precursors in the thymus; naive mature T lymphocytes before antigen exposure; memory T lymphocytes after antigen contact; helper T lymphocytes for B and T cell responses; cytotoxic T lymphocytes that kill pathogen-infected target cells

Humoral: Bone-marrow-derived (B) lymphocytes—B cell precursors in bone marrow; naive B cells prior to antigen recognition, memory B cells after antigen contact; plasma cells that secrete specific antibody

Cytokines: Soluble proteins that direct, focus, and regulate specific T versus B lymphocyte immune responses

the thymus for maturation. Mature T lymphocytes, B lymphocytes, monocytes, and dendritic/Langerhans cells enter the circulation and home to peripheral lymphoid organs (lymph nodes, spleen) and the gut-associated lymphoid tissue (tonsil, Peyer's patches, and appendix) as well as the skin and mucous membranes and await activation by foreign antigen.

T Cells The pool of effector T cells is established in the thymus early in life and is maintained throughout life both by new T cell production in the thymus and by antigen-driven expansion of virgin peripheral T cells into "memory" T cells that reside in peripheral lymphoid organs. The thymus exports ~2% of the total number of thymocytes per day throughout life, with the total number of daily thymic emigrants decreasing by ~3% per year during the first four decades of life. Thymic emigrants can be identified by the expression of certain combinations of T cell surface markers and by the presence in nuclei of excised (deleted) pieces of rearranged TCR DNA, called *T cell receptor excision circles.*

Mature T lymphocytes constitute 70 to 80% of normal peripheral blood lymphocytes (only 2% of the total-body lymphocytes are contained in peripheral blood), 90% of thoracic duct lymphocytes, 30 to 40% of lymph node cells, and 20 to 30% of spleen lymphoid cells. In lymph nodes, T cells occupy deep paracortical areas around B cell germinal centers, and in the spleen, they are located in periarteriolar areas of white pulp (Chap. 54). T cells are the primary effectors of cell-mediated immunity, with subsets of T cells maturing into CD8+ cytotoxic T cells capable of lysis of virus-infected or foreign cells. In general, CD4+ T cells are also the primary regulatory cells of T and B lymphocyte and monocyte function by the production of cytokines and by direct cell contact. In addition, T cells regulate erythroid cell maturation in bone marrow, and through cell contact (CD40 ligand) have an important role in activation of B cells and induction of Ig isotype switching.

Human T cells express cell-surface proteins that mark stages of intrathymic T cell maturation or identify specific functional subpopulations of mature T cells. Many of these molecules mediate or participate in important T cell functions (Table 295-1; Fig. 295-5).

The earliest identifiable T cell precursors in bone marrow are CD34+ pro-T cells (i.e., cells in which TCR genes are neither rearranged nor expressed). In the thymus, CD34+ T cell precursors begin cytoplasmic (c) synthesis of components of the CD3 complex of TCR-associated molecules (Fig. 295-5.) Within T cell precursors, TCR for antigen gene rearrangement begins under the influence of IL-7 and yields two T cell lineages, expressing either TCRαβ chains or TCRγδ chains. T cells expressing the TCRαβ chains comprise the majority of peripheral T cells in blood, lymph node, and spleen and terminally differentiate into either CD4+ or CD8+ cells. Cells expressing TCRγδ chains circulate as a minor population in blood; their functions, although not fully understood, have been postulated to be those of immune surveillance at epithelial surfaces and cellular defenses against mycobacterial organisms and other intracellular bacteria (see below). Immature cortical thymocytes express both CD4 and CD8 (i.e., they are double positive); however, upon reaching functional maturity, T cell CD4 and CD8 are reciprocally expressed (i.e., T cells become single positive for either CD4 or CD8).

In the thymus, the recognition of self-peptides on thymic epithelial cells, thymic macrophages, and dendritic cells plays an important role in shaping the T cell repertoire to recognize foreign antigen (*positive selection*) and in eliminating highly autoreactive T cells (*negative selection*). As immature cortical thymocytes begin to express surface TCR for antigen, autoreactive thymocytes are destroyed (negative selection), thymocytes with TCRs capable of interacting with foreign antigen peptides in the context of self–MHC antigens are activated and develop to maturity (positive selection), and thymocytes with TCR that are incapable of binding to self–MHC antigens die of attrition (*no selection*). Mature thymocytes that are positively selected are either

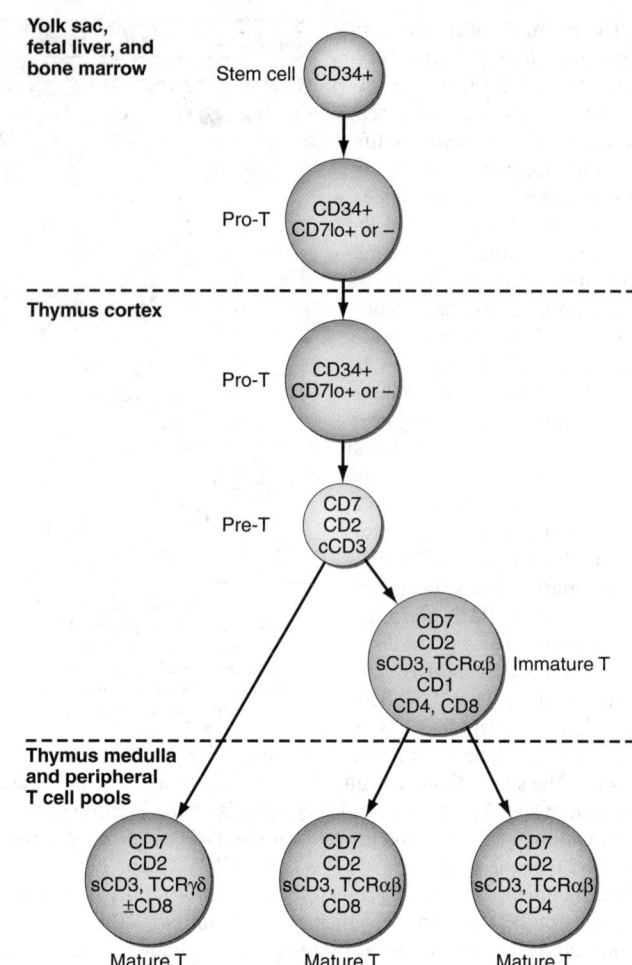

FIGURE 295-5 Human T cell maturation. sCD3, surface CD3 expression; cCD3, cytoplasmic CD3 expression; TCR, T cell receptor.

CD4+ helper T cells or MHC class II–restricted cytotoxic (killer) T cells, or they are CD8+ T cells destined to become MHC class I–restricted cytotoxic T cells. *MHC class I– or class II–restricted* means that T cells recognize antigen peptide fragments only when they are presented in the antigen-recognition site of a class I or class II MHC molecule, respectively (see below).

After thymocyte maturation and selection, CD4 and CD8 thymocytes leave the thymus and migrate to the peripheral immune system. It is important to note that the adult thymus continues to function, albeit with decreasing output, well into adult life. Thus, the thymus continues to be a contributor to the peripheral immune system, both normally and when the peripheral T cell pool is damaged, such as occurs in AIDS and cancer chemotherapy.

MOLECULAR BASIS OF T CELL RECOGNITION OF ANTIGEN The TCR for antigen is a complex of molecules consisting of an antigen-binding heterodimer of either αβ or γδ chains noncovalently linked with five CD3 subunits (γ, δ, ε, ζ, and η) (Fig. 295-6). The CD3 ζ chains are either disulfide-linked homodimers (CD3-ζ₂) or disulfide-linked heterodimers composed of one ζ chain and one η chain. TCRαβ or TCRγδ molecules must be associated with CD3 molecules to be inserted into the T cell surface membrane, TCRα being paired with TCRβ and TCRγ being paired with TCRδ. Molecules of the CD3 complex mediate transduction of T cell activation signals via TCRs, while TCRα and -β or -γ and -δ molecules combine to form the TCR antigen-binding site.

The α, β, γ, and δ TCR for antigen molecules have amino acid sequence homology and structural similarities to immunoglobulin heavy and light chains and are members of the *immunoglobulin gene superfamily* of molecules. The genes encoding TCR molecules are encoded as clusters of gene segments that rearrange during the course of T cell maturation. This creates an efficient and compact mechanism for housing the diversity requirements of antigen receptor molecules. The TCRα chain is on chromosome 14 and consists of a series of V (variable), J (joining), and C (constant) regions. The TCRβ chain is on chromosome 7 and consists of multiple V, D (diversity), J, and C TCRβ loci. The TCRγ chain is on chromosome 7, and the TCRδ chain is in the middle of the TCRα locus on chromosome 14. Thus, molecules of the TCR for antigen have constant (framework) and variable regions, and the gene segments encoding the α, β, γ, and δ chains of these molecules are recombined and selected in the thymus, culminating in synthesis of the completed molecule. In both T and B cell precursors (see below), DNA rearrangements of antigen receptor genes involve the same enzymes, recombinase activating gene (RAG)1 and RAG2, both DNA-dependent protein kinases.

TCR diversity is created by the different V, (D), and J segments that are possible for each receptor chain by the many permutations of V, D, and J segment combinations, by "N-region diversification" due to the addition of nucleotides at the junction of rearranged gene segments, and the pairing of individual chains to form a TCR dimer. As T cells mature in the thymus, the repertoire of antigen-reactive T cells is modified by selection processes that eliminate many autoreactive T cells, enhance the proliferation of cells that function appropriately with self-MHC molecules and antigen, and allow T cells with nonproductive TCR rearrangements to die.

TCRαβ cells do not recognize native protein or carbohydrate antigens. Instead, T cells recognize only short (~9 to 13 amino acids) peptide fragments derived from protein antigens taken up or produced in APCs. Foreign antigens may be taken up by endocytosis into acidified intracellar vesicles or by phagocytosis and degraded into small peptides that associate with MHC class II molecules (exogenous antigen-presentation pathway). Other foreign antigens arise endogenously in the cytosol (such as from replicating viruses) and are broken down into small peptides that associate with MHC class I molecules (endogenous antigen-presenting pathway). Thus, APCs proteolytically degrade foreign proteins and display peptide fragments embedded in the MHC class I or II antigen-recognition site on the MHC molecule surface, where foreign peptide fragments are available to bind to TCRαβ or TCRγδ chains of reactive T cells. CD4 molecules act as an adhesive and, by direct binding to MHC class II (DR, DQ, or DP) molecules, stabilize the interaction of TCR with peptide antigen (Fig. 295-6). Similarly, CD8 molecules also act as adhesives to stabilize the TCR-antigen interaction by direct CD8 molecule binding to MHC class I (A, B, or C) molecules.

Antigens that arise in the cytosol and are processed via the endogenous antigen-presentation pathway are cleaved into small peptides by a 28-subunit complex of proteases called the *proteasome*. From the proteasome, antigen peptide fragments are transported from the cytosol into the lumen of the endoplasmic reticulum by a heterodimeric complex termed *transporters associated with antigen processing*, or TAP proteins. There, MHC class I molecules in the endoplasmic reticulum membrane physically associate with processed cytosolic peptides. Following peptide association with class I molecules, peptide–class I complexes are exported to the Golgi apparatus, and then to the cell surface, for recognition by CD8+ T cells.

Antigens taken up from the extracellular space via endocytosis into

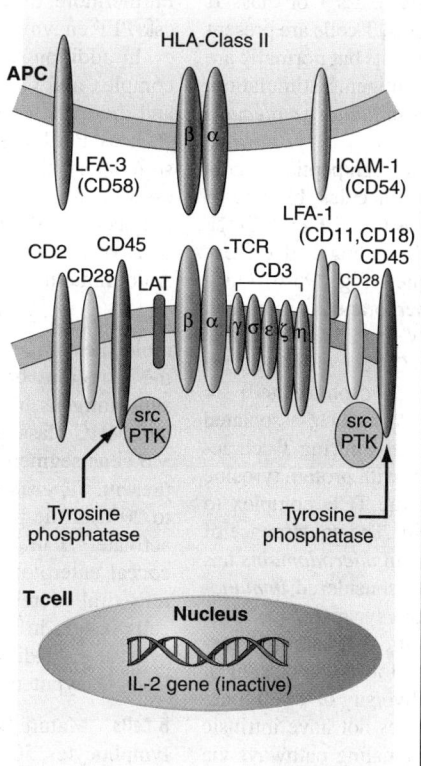
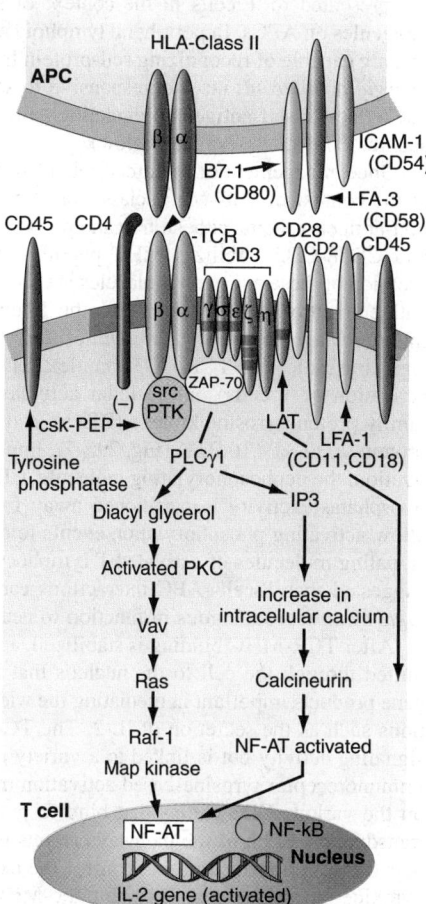

Before MHC-peptide binding to T cell receptor

After MHC-peptide binding to T cell receptor

FIGURE 295-6 Molecules involved in human T cell recognition of antigen and in human T cell activation. *A.* Schematic arrangement of antigen-presenting cell (APC) molecules (top cell) and T cell molecules (bottom cell) before MHC-peptide binding to T cell receptor (TCR). *B.* The changes that occur in T cell and APC molecules after MHC-peptide binding to TCR. The black triangle at the tip of the αβ chains of MHC class II molecules represents a peptide fragment of "processed" protein antigen. After TCR ligation, src protein tyrosine kinase (PTK) is activated via dephosphorylation and the TCR complex is joined by CD4, CD2, and CD28 as well as the linker for activated T lymphocytes (LAT) in a lipid microdomain area (gray area). Activation signals are mediated via immunoreceptor tyrosine-based activation (ITAM) sequences in LAT and CD3 chains (blue bars) that bind to enzymes and transduce activation signals to the nucleus via the indicated intracellular activation pathways. See text for details of the activation and signal transduction process. (*Adapted from A Weiss and DR Littman: Cell 76:263, 1995; with permission.*)

intracellular acidified vesicles are degraded by vesicle proteases into peptide fragments. Intracellular vesicles containing MHC class II molecules fuse with peptide-containing vesicles, thus allowing peptide fragments to physically bind to MHC class II molecules. Peptide–MHC class II complexes are then transported to the cell surface for recognition by CD4+ T cells.

Whereas it is generally agreed that the TCRαβ receptor recognizes peptide antigens in the context of MHC class I or class II molecules, lipids in the cell wall of intracellular bacteria such as *M. tuberculosis* can also be presented to a wide variety of T cells, including subsets of CD4−, CD8− TCRαβ T cells, TCRγδ T cells, and a subset of CD8+ TCRαβ T cells. Importantly, bacterial lipid antigens are not presented in the context of MHC class I or II molecules, but rather are presented in the context of MHC-related CD1 molecules. Some γδ T cells that recognize lipid antigens via CD1 molecules have very restricted TCR usage, do not need antigen priming to respond to bacterial lipids, and may actually be a form of innate rather than acquired immunity to intracellular bacteria.

Just as foreign antigens are degraded and their peptide fragments presented in the context of MHC class I or class II molecules on APCs, endogenous self-proteins are also degraded and self-peptide fragments are presented to T cells in the context of MHC class I or class II molecules on APCs. In peripheral lymphoid organs, T cells are present that are capable of recognizing self-protein fragments but normally are *anergic* or *tolerant*, i.e., nonresponsive to self-antigenic stimulation, due to lack of self-antigen upregulating APC *co-stimulatory molecules* such as B7-1 and B7-2 (see below).

Once engagement of mature T cell TCR by foreign peptide occurs in the context of self–MHC class I or class II molecules, binding of non-antigen-specific adhesion ligand pairs such as CD54-CD11/CD18 and CD58-CD2 stabilizes MHC peptide–TCR binding and the expression of these adhesion molecules is upregulated (Fig. 295-6). Once antigen ligation of the TCR occurs, the T cell membrane is partitioned into *lipid membrane microdomains*, or *lipid rafts*, that coalesce the key signaling molecules TCR/CD3 complex, CD28, CD2, LAT (linker for activation of T cells), intracellular activated (dephosphorylated) src family protein tyrosine kinases (PTKs), and the key CD3ζ-associated protein-70 (ZAP-70) PTK (Fig. 295-7). Importantly, during T cell activation, the dephosphorylating molecule, CD45, with protein tyrosine phosphatase activity is partitioned away from the TCR complex to allow activating phosphorylation events to occur. The coalescence of signaling molecules of activated T lymphocytes in *microdomains* has suggested that T cell–APC interactions can be considered *immunologic synapses*, analogous in function to neuronal synapses.

After TCR-MHC binding is stabilized, activation signals are transmitted through the cell to the nucleus that lead to the expression of gene products important in mediating the wide diversity of T cell functions such as the secretion of IL-2. The TCR does not have intrinsic signaling activity but is linked to a variety of signaling pathways via immunoreceptor tyrosine-based activation motifs (ITAMs) expressed on the various CD3 chains that bind to proteins that mediate signal transduction. Each of the pathways results in the activation of particular transcription factors that control the expression of cytokine and cytokine receptor genes. Thus, antigen-MHC binding to the TCR induces the activation of the src family of PTKs, fyn and lck (lck is associated with CD4 or CD8 co-stimulatory molecules); phosphorylation of CD3ζ chain; activation of the related tyrosine kinases ZAP-70 and syk; and downstream activation of the calcium-dependent calcineurin pathway, the ras pathway, and the protein kinase C pathway. Each of these pathways leads to activation of specific families of transcription factors (including NF-AT, fos and jun, and rel/NF-κB) that form heteromultimers capable of inducing expression of IL-2, IL-2 receptor, IL-4, TNF-α, and other T cell mediators. The src family

kinases require dephosphorylation of an inactivation site by CD45 phosphatase before they can be phosphorylated on an activation site. Furthermore, the activity through the receptor is downregulated by the csk-PEP enzyme, a phosphatase that inactivates the src family kinases.

In addition to the signals delivered to the T cell from the TCR complex and CD4 and CD8, molecules on the T cell such as CD28 and inducible co-stimulator (ICOS) and molecules on dendritic cells such as B7-1 (CD80) and B7-2 (CD86) also deliver important co-stimulatory signals that upregulate T cell cytokine production and are essential for T cell activation. If signaling through CD28 or ICOS does not occur, or if CD28 is blocked, the T cell becomes *anergic* (nonresponsive, or *tolerant*) rather than activated (see "Immune Tolerance and Autoimmunity," below).

T CELL SUPERANTIGENS Conventional antigens bind to MHC class I or II molecules in the groove of the αβ heterodimer and bind to T cells via the V regions of the TCRα and -β chains (Fig. 295-6). In contrast, superantigens bind directly to the lateral portion of the TCRβ chain and MHC class II β chain and stimulate T cells based solely on the Vβ gene segment utilized independent of the D, J, and Vα sequences present. *Superantigens* are protein molecules capable of activating up to 20% of the peripheral T cell pool, whereas conventional antigens activate <1 in 10,000 T cells. T cell superantigens include staphylococcal enterotoxins, other bacterial products, and certain nonhuman retroviral proteins. Superantigen stimulation of human peripheral T cells occurs in the clinical setting of the *staphylococcal toxic shock syndrome*, leading to massive overproduction of T cell cytokines that leads to hypotension and shock (Chap. 120).

B Cells Mature B cells comprise 10 to 15% of human peripheral blood lymphocytes, 50% of splenic lymphocytes, and ~10% of bone marrow lymphocytes. B cells express on their surface intramembrane immunoglobulin (Ig) molecules that function as B cell receptors (BCRs) for antigen in a complex of Ig-associated α and β signaling molecules with properties similar to those described in T cells (Fig. 295-7). Unlike T cells, which recognize only processed peptide fragments of conventional antigens embedded in the notches of MHC class I and class II antigens of APCs, B cells are capable of recognizing and proliferating to whole unprocessed native antigens via antigen binding to B cell surface Ig (sIg) receptors. B cells also express surface receptors for the Fc region of IgG molecules (CD32) as well as receptors for activated complement components (C3d or CD21, C3b or CD35). The primary function of B cells is to produce antibodies. B cells also serve as APCs and are highly efficient at antigen processing. Their antigen-presenting function is enhanced by a variety of cytokines. Mature B cells are derived from bone marrow precursor cells that arise continuously throughout life (Figs. 295-2, 295-10).

B lymphocyte development can be separated into antigen-independent and antigen-dependent phases. Antigen-independent B cell development occurs in primary lymphoid organs and includes all stages of B cell maturation up to the sIg+ mature B cell. Antigen-dependent B cell maturation is driven by the interaction of antigen with the mature B cell sIg, leading to memory B cell induction, Ig class switching, and plasma cell formation. Antigen-dependent stages of B cell maturation occur in secondary lymphoid organs, including lymph node, spleen, and gut Peyer's patches. In contrast to the T cell repertoire that is generated intrathymically before contact with foreign antigen, the repertoire of B cells expressing diverse antigen-reactive sites is modified by further alteration of Ig genes after stimulation by antigen—a process called *somatic mutation*—which occurs in lymph node germinal centers.

During B cell development, diversity of the antigen-binding variable region of Ig is generated by an ordered set of Ig gene rearrangements that are similar to the rearrangements undergone by TCR α, β, γ, and δ genes. For the heavy chain, there is first a rearrangement of D segments to J segments, followed by a second rearrangement between a V gene segment and the newly formed D-J sequence; the C segment is aligned to the V-D-J complex to yield a functional Ig heavy chain gene (V-D-J-C). During later stages, a functional κ or λ light

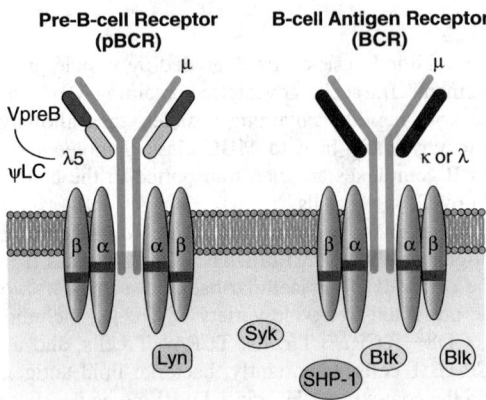

FIGURE 295-7 The pre-B cell receptor and B-cell antigen receptor associate with the signal-transducing heterodimer Igα/Igβ. Solid horizontal bars in α and β chains denote the immunoreceptor tyrosine-based activation motif (ITAM). Signals from the antigen receptors are further propagated downstream by other signaling molecules such as the syk and the src family of tyrosine kinases (fyn, lyn, blk, and btk), as well as by the phosphatase, SHP-1. *(Adapted from K-P Lam, K Rajewsky: Inflammation: Basic Principles and Clinical Correlates, 3d ed., Philadelphia, Lippincott Williams & Wilkins, pp 151–166, 1999; with permission.)*

chain gene is generated by rearrangement of a V segment to a J segment, ultimately yielding an intact Ig molecule composed of heavy and light chains.

The process of Ig gene rearrangement is regulated and results in a single antibody specificity produced by each B cell, with each Ig molecule comprising one type of heavy chain and one type of light chain. Although each B cell contains two copies of Ig light and heavy chain genes, only one gene of each type is productively rearranged and expressed in each B cell, a process termed *allelic exclusion.*

There are ~300 V_κ genes and 5 J_κ genes, resulting in the pairing of V_κ and J_κ genes to create >1500 different light chain combinations. The number of distinct κ light chains that can be generated is increased by somatic mutations within the V_κ and J_κ genes, thus creating large numbers of possible specificities from a limited amount of germ-line genetic information. As noted above, in heavy chain Ig gene rearrangement, the VH domain is created by the joining of three types of germ-line genes called V_H, D_H, and J_H, thus allowing for even greater diversity in the variable region of heavy chains than of light chains.

The most immature B cell precursors (early pro-B cells) lack cytoplasmic Ig (cIg) and sIg (Fig. 295-8). The large pre-B cell is marked by the acquisition of the surface pre-BCR composed of μ heavy (H) chains and a pre-B light chain, termed ψLC (Fig. 295-7). ψLC is a surrogate light chain receptor encoded by the nonrearranged V pre-B and the λ5 light chain locus (the pre-BCR). Pro- and pre-B cells are driven to proliferate and mature by signals from bone marrow stroma, in particular, IL-7. Light chain rearrangement occurs in the small pre-B cell stage such that the full BCR is expressed at the immature B cell stage. Immature B cells have rearranged Ig light chain genes and express sIgM. As immature B cells develop into mature B cells, sIgD is expressed as well as sIgM. At this point, B lineage development in bone marrow is complete, and B cells exit into the peripheral circulation and migrate to secondary lymphoid organs to encounter specific antigens.

Random rearrangements of Ig genes occasionally generate self-reactive antibodies, and mechanisms must be in place to correct these mistakes. One such mechanism is BCR editing, whereby autoreactive BCRs are mutated to not react with self-antigens. If receptor editing is unsuccessful in eliminating autoreactive B cells, then autoreactive B cells undergo negative selection in the bone marrow through induction of apoptosis after BCR engagement of self-antigen.

After leaving the bone marrow, B cells populate peripheral B cell sites, such as lymph node and spleen, and await contact with foreign antigens that react with each B cell's clonotypic receptor. As antigen-driven B cell activation occurs through the BCR, a process known as *somatic hypermutation* takes place whereby point mutations in rearranged H- and L-genes give rise to mutant sIg molecules, some of which bind antigen better than the original sIg molecules. Somatic hypermutation, therefore, is a process whereby memory B cells in peripheral lymph organs have the best binding, or the highest affinity antibodies. This overall process of generating the best antibodies is called *affinity maturation of antibody.*

Lymphocytes that synthesize IgG, IgA, and IgE are derived from sIgM+, sIgD+ mature B cells. Ig class switching occurs in lymph node and other peripheral lymphoid tissue germinal centers. CD40 on B cells and CD40 ligand on T cells comprise a critical co-stimulatory receptor-ligand pair of immune-stimulatory molecules. Pairs of CD40+ B cells and CD40 ligand+ T cells bind and drive B cell Ig switching via T cell–produced cytokines such as IL-4 and transforming growth factor (TGF) β. IL-1, -2, -4, -5, and -6 synergize to drive mature B cells to proliferate and differentiate into Ig-secreting cells.

Humoral Mediators of Adaptive Immunity: Immunoglobulins   Immunoglobulins are the products of differentiated B cells and mediate the humoral arm of the immune response. The primary functions of antibodies are to bind specifically to antigen and bring about the inactivation or removal of the offending toxin, microbe, parasite, or other foreign substance from the body. The structural basis of Ig molecule function and Ig gene organization has provided insight into the role of antibodies in normal protective immunity, pathologic immune-mediated damage by immune complexes, and autoantibody formation against host determinants.

All immunoglobulins have the basic structure of two heavy and two light chains (Figs. 295-7 and 295-9). Immunoglobulin isotype (i.e., G, M, A, D, E) is determined by the type of Ig heavy chain present. IgG and IgA isotypes can be divided further into subclasses (G1, G2, G3, G4, and A1, A2) based on specific antigenic determinants on Ig heavy chains. The characteristics of human immunoglobulins are outlined in Table 295-10. The four chains are covalently linked by disulfide bonds. Each chain is made up of a V region and C regions (also called *domains*), themselves made up of units of ~110 amino

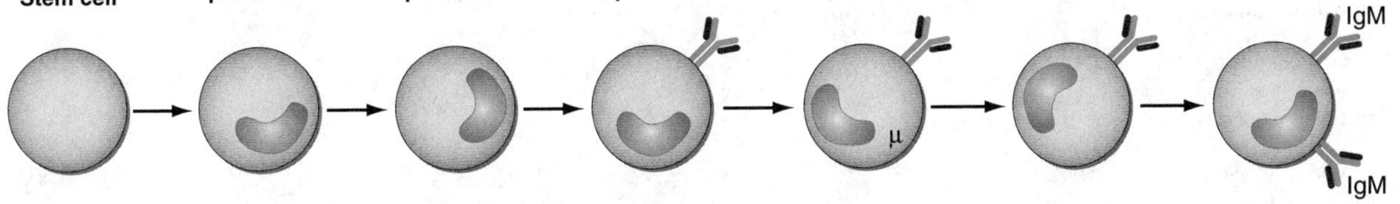

	Stem cell	Early pro-B cell	Late pro-B cell	Large pre-B cell	Small pre-B cell	Immature B cell	Mature B cell
H-chain genes	Germ line	DJ rearranged	VDJ rearranged	VDJ rearranged	VDJ rearranged	VDJ rearranged	VDJ rearranged
L-chain genes	Germ line	Germ line	Germ line	Germ line	VJ rearranged	VJ rearranged	VJ rearranged
Surface Ig	Absent	Absent	Absent	μ H-chain at surface as part of pre-β receptor	μ H-chain in cytoplasm and at surface	IgM expressed on cell surface	IgD and IgM made from alternatively spliced H-chain transcripts
Surface marker proteins	CD34	CD34 CD10 CD19 CD38	CD10 CD19 CD20 CD38 CD40	CD19 CD20 CD38 CD40	CD19 CD20 CD38 CD40	CD19 CD20 CD40	CD19 CD20 CD21 CD40

FIGURE 295-8   Developmental stages of B cells. Elements of the developing B cell receptor for antigen (BCR) are shown schematically. The classification into the various stages of B cell development is primarily defined by rearrangement of the immunoglobulin (Ig), heavy (H), and light (L) chain genes and by the absence or presence of specific surface markers. [Adapted from CA Janeway et al (eds): Immunobiology. The Immune System in Health and Disease, 4th ed, New York, Garland, 1999; with permission.]

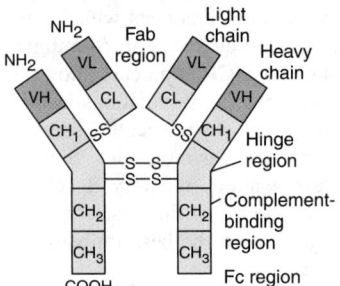

FIGURE 295-9 Schematic structure of the immunoglobulin G (IgG) molecule.

acids. Light chains have one variable (V_L) and one constant (C_L) unit; heavy chains have one variable unit (V_H) and three or four constant (C_H) units, depending on isotype. As the name suggests, the constant, or C, regions of Ig molecules are made up of homologous sequences and share the same primary structure as all other Ig chains of the same isotype and subclass. Constant regions are involved in biologic functions of Ig molecules. The C_{H2} domain of IgG and the C_{H4} units of IgM are involved with the binding of the C1q portion of C1 during complement activation. The C_H region at the carboxy-terminal end of the IgG molecule, the Fc region (Fig. 295-9), binds to surface Fc receptors (CD16, CD32, CD64) of macrophages, LGLs, B cells, neutrophils, and eosinophils.

Variable regions (V_L and V_H) constitute the antibody-binding (Fab) region of the molecule. Within the V_L and V_H regions are hypervariable regions (extreme sequence variability) that constitute the antigen-binding site unique to each Ig molecule. The idiotype is defined as the specific region of the Fab portion of the Ig molecule to which antigen binds. Antibodies against the idiotype portion of an antibody molecule are called *anti-idiotype antibodies*. The formation of such antibodies in vivo during a normal B cell antibody response may generate a negative (or "off") signal to B cells to terminate antibody production.

IgG comprises ~75 to 85% of total serum immunoglobulin. The four IgG subclasses are numbered in order of their level in serum,

IgG1 being found in greatest amounts and IgG4 the least. IgG subclasses have clinical relevance in their varying ability to bind macrophage and neutrophil Fc receptors and to activate complement (Table 295-10). Moreover, selective deficiencies of certain IgG subclasses give rise to clinical syndromes in which the patient is inordinately susceptible to bacterial infections. IgG antibodies are frequently the predominant antibody made after rechallenge of the host with antigen (secondary antibody response).

IgM antibodies normally circulate as a 950-kDa pentamer with 160-kDa bivalent monomers joined by a molecule called the *J chain*, a 15-kDa nonimmunoglobulin molecule that also effects polymerization of IgA molecules. IgM is the first immunoglobulin to appear in the immune response (primary antibody response) and is the initial type of antibody made by neonates. Membrane IgM in the monomeric form also functions as a major antigen receptor on the surface of mature B cells (Fig. 295-9). IgM is an important component of immune complexes in autoimmune diseases. For example, IgM antibodies against IgG molecules (rheumatoid factors) are present in high titers in *rheumatoid arthritis*, other collagen diseases, and some infectious diseases (*subacute bacterial endocarditis*).

IgA comprises only 7 to 15% of total serum immunoglobulin but is the predominant class of immunoglobulin in secretions. IgA in secretions (tears, saliva, nasal secretions, gastrointestinal tract fluid, and human milk) is in the form of secretory IgA (sIgA), a polymer consisting of two IgA monomers, a joining molecule, again called the J chain, and a glycoprotein called the *secretory protein*. Of the two IgA subclasses, IgA1 is primarily found in serum, whereas IgA2 is more prevalent in secretions. IgA fixes complement via the alternative complement pathway and has potent antiviral activity in humans by prevention of virus binding to respiratory and gastrointestinal epithelial cells.

IgD is found in minute quantities in serum and, together with IgM, is a major receptor for antigen on the B cell surface. IgE, which is present in serum in very low concentrations, is the major class of immunoglobulin involved in arming mast cells and basophils by binding to these cells via the Fc region. Antigen cross-linking of IgE molecules on basophil and mast cell surfaces results in release of mediators of the immediate hypersensitivity response (Table 295-6).

TABLE 295-10 *Physical, Chemical, and Biologic Properties of Human Immunoglobulins*

Property	IgG	IgA	IgM	IgD	IgE
Usual molecular form	Monomer	Monomer, dimer	Pentamer, hexamer	Monomer	Monomer
Other chains	None	J chain, SC	J chain	None	None
Subclasses	G1, G2, G3, G4	A1, A2	None	None	None
Heavy chain allotypes	Gm (=30)	No A1, A2m (2)	None	None	None
Molecular mass, kDa	150	160, 400	950, 1150	175	190
Sedimentation constant, Sw20	6.6S	7S, 11S	19S	7S	8S
Carbohydrate content, %	3	7	10	9	13
Serum level in average adult, mg/mL	9.5–12.5	1.5–2.6	0.7–1.7	0.04	0.0003
Percentage of total serum Ig	75–85	7–15	5–10	0.3	0.019
Serum half-life, days	23	6	5	3	2.5
Synthesis rate, mg/kg per day	33	65	7	0.4	0.016
Antibody valence	2	2,4	10,12	2	2
Classical complement activation	+(G1, 2?, 3)	–	++	–	–
Alternate complement activation	+(G4)	+	–	+	–
Binding cells via Fc	Macrophages, neutrophils, large granular lymphocytes	Lymphocytes	Lymphocytes	None	Mast cells, basophils, B cells
Biologic properties	Placental transfer, secondary Ab for most antipathogen responses	Secretory immunoglobulin	Primary Ab responses	Marker for mature B cells	Allergy, antiparasite responses

Source: After L Carayannopoulos and JD Capra, in WE Paul (ed): *Fundamental Immunology*, 2d ed. New York, Raven, 1989; with permission.

CELLULAR INTERACTIONS IN REGULATION OF NORMAL IMMUNE RESPONSES

The net result of activation of the humoral (B cell) and cellular (T cell) arms of the adaptive immune system by foreign antigen is the elimination of antigen directly by specific effector T cells or in concert with specific antibody. Figure 295-10 is a simplified schematic diagram of the T and B cell responses indicating some of these cellular interactions.

The expression of adaptive immune cell function is the result of a complex series of immunoregulatory events that occur in phases. Both T and B lymphocytes mediate immune functions, and each of these cell types, when given appropriate signals, passes through stages, from activation and induction through proliferation, differentiation, and ultimately effector functions. The effector function expressed may be at the end point of a response, such as secretion of antibody by a differentiated plasma cell, or it might serve a regulatory function that modulates other functions, such as is seen with CD4+ and CD8+ T lymphocytes that modulate both differentiation of B cells and activation of CD8+ cytotoxic T cells.

CD4 helper T cells can be subdivided on the basis of cytokines produced (Figs. 295-10 and 295-11). Activated T_H1-type helper T cells secrete IL-2, IFN-γ, IL-3, TNF-α, GM-CSF, and TNF-β, while activated T_H2-type helper T cells secrete IL-3, -4, -5, -6, -10, and -13. T_H1 CD4+ T cells, through elaboration of IFN-γ, have a central role in mediating intracellular killing by a variety of pathogens. T_H1 CD4+ T cells also provide T cell help for generation of cytotoxic T cells and some types of opsonizing antibody, and generally respond to antigens that lead to delayed hypersensitivity types of immune responses for many intracellular viruses and bacteria (such as HIV or *M. tuberculosis*). In contrast, T_H2 cells have a primary role in regulatory humoral immunity and isotype switching. In addition, T_H2 cells, through production of IL-4 and IL-10, have a regulatory role in limiting proinflammatory responses mediated by T_H1 cells (Table 295-5). In addition, T_H2 CD4+ T cells provide help to B cells for specific Ig production and respond to antigens that require high antibody levels for foreign antigen elimination (extracellular encapsulated bacteria such as *Streptococcus pneumoniae* and certain parasite infections). The type of T cell response generated in an immune response is determined by the microbe PAMPs presented to the dentritic cells, the TLRs on the dendritic cells that become activated, the types of dendritic cells that are activated, and the cytokines that are produced. Commonly, myeloid dendritic cells produce IL-12 and activate T_H1 T cell responses that result in IFN-γ and cytotoxic T cell induction, and plasmacytoid dendritic cells product IFN-α and lead to T_H2 responses that result in IL-4 production and enhanced antibody responses.

As shown in Figs. 295-10 and 295-11, upon activation by dendritic cells, T cell subsets that produce IL-2, IL-3, IFN-γ, and/or IL-4, -5, -6, -10, and -13 are generated that exert positive and negative influences on effector T and B cells. For B cells, trophic effects are mediated by a variety of cytokines, particularly T cell–derived IL-3, -4, -5, and -6, that act at sequential stages of B cell maturation, resulting in B cell proliferation, differentiation, and ultimately antibody secretion. For cytotoxic T cells, trophic factors include inducer T cell secretion of IL-2, IFN-γ, and IL-12. In addition, B cells themselves are capable of serving as APCs, processing and presenting antigens to T cells, and secreting TNF-α and IL-6.

An important type of immunomodulatory T cell that controls immune responses are *CD4+ and CD8+ T regulatory cells*. These cells constitutively express the α chain of the IL-2 receptor (CD25), produce large amounts of IL-10, and can suppress both T and B cell responses. T regulatory cells are induced by immature dendritic cells and play key roles in maintaining tolerance to self-antigens in the periphery. Loss of T regulatory cells is the cause of organ-specific autoimmune disease in mice such as autoimmune thyroiditis, adrenalitis, and oophoritis (see "Immune Tolerance and Autoimmunity," below). T regulatory cells also play key roles in controlling the magnitude and duration of immune responses to microbes. Normally, after the initial immune response to a microbe has eliminated the invader, T regulatory cells are activated to suppress the anti-microbe response and prevent host injury. Some microbes have adapted to induce T regulatory cell activation at the site of infection to promote parasite infection and survival. In *Leishmania* infection, the parasite locally induces T regulatory cell accumulation at skin infection sites that dampens anti-*Leishmania* T cell responses and prevents elimination of the parasite.

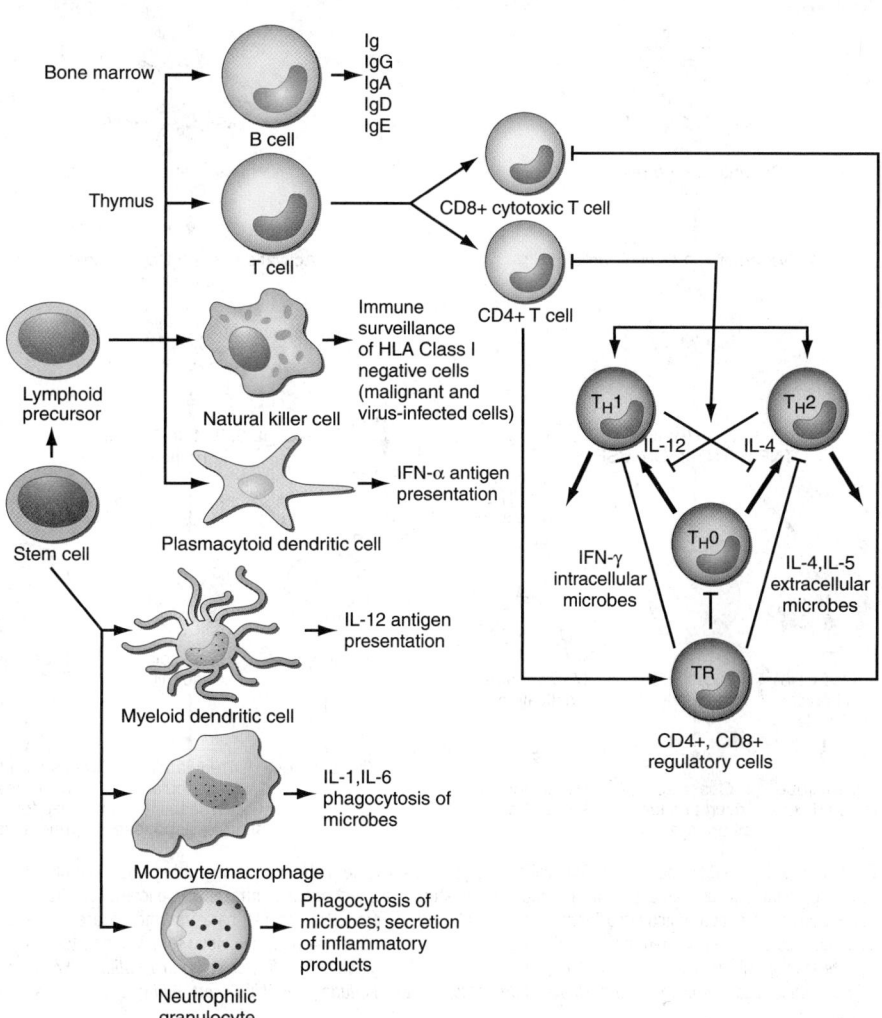

FIGURE 295-10 Schematic model of intercellular interactions of adaptive immune system cells. In this figure the arrows denote that cells develop from precursor cells or produce cytokines or antibodies; lines ending with bars indicate suppressive intercellular interactions. Stem cells differentiate into either T cells, antigen-presenting dendritic cells, natural killer cells, macrophages, granulocytes, or B cells. Foreign antigen is processed by dendritic cells, and peptide fragments of foreign antigen are presented to CD4+ and/or CD8+ T cells. CD8+ T cell activation leads to induction of cytotoxic T lymphocyte (CTL) or killer T cell generation, as well as induction of cytokine-producing CD8+ cytotoxic T cells. For antibody production against the same antigen, active antigen is bound to sIg within the B cell receptor complex and drives B cell maturation into plasma cells that secrete Ig. T_H1 or T_H2 CD4+ T cells producing interleukin (IL) 4, IL-5, or interferon (IFN) γ regulate the Ig class switching and determine the type of antibody produced. CD4+, CD25+ T regulatory cells produce IL-10 and downregulate T and B cell responses once the microbe has been eliminated. GM-CSF, granulocyte-macrophage colony stimulating factor; TNF, tumor necrosis factor.

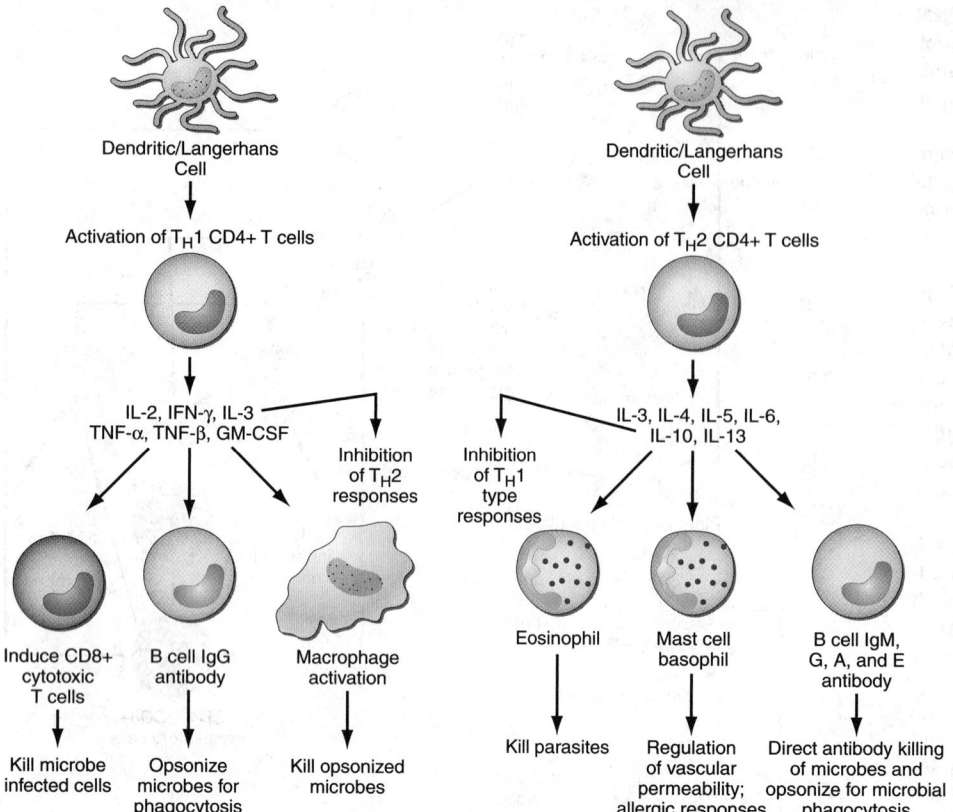

FIGURE 295-11 CD4+ helper T 1 (T_H1) cells and T_H2 T cells secrete distinct but overlapping sets of cytokines. T_H1 CD4+ cells are frequently activated in immune and inflammatory reactions against intracellular bacteria or viruses, while T_H2 CD4+ cells are frequently activated for certain types of antibody production against parasites and extracellular encapsulated bacteria; they are also activated in allergic diseases. GM-CSF, granulocyte-macrophage colony stimulating factor; IFN, interferon; IL, interleukin; TNF, tumor necrosis factor. [*Adapted from S Romagnani: CD4 effector cells, in J Gallin, R Snyderman (eds): Inflammation: Basic Principles and Clinical Correlates, 3d ed. Philadelphia, Lippincott Williams & Wilkins, 1999; with permission.*]

It is thought that many chronic infections such as by *M. tuberculosis* are associated with abnormal T regulatory cell activation that prevents elimination of the microbe.

Although B cells recognize native antigen via B cell surface Ig receptors, B cells require T cell help to produce high-affinity antibody of multiple isotypes that are the most effective in eliminating foreign antigen. This T cell dependence likely functions in the regulation of B cell responses and in protection against excessive autoantibody production. T cell–B cell interactions that lead to high-affinity antibody production require: (1) processing of native antigen by B cells and expression of peptide fragments on the B cell surface for presentation to T_H cells, (2) the ligation of B cells both by the TCR complex and the CD40 ligand, (3) induction of the process termed *antibody isotype switching* in antigen-specific B cell clones, and (4) induction of the process of *affinity maturation* of antibody in the germinal centers of B cell follicles of lymph node and spleen.

Naive B cells express cell-surface IgD and IgM, and initial contact of naive B cells with antigen is via binding of native antigen to B cell–surface IgM. T cell cytokines, released following T_H2 cell contact with B cells or by a "bystander" effect, induce changes in Ig gene conformation that promote recombination of Ig genes. These events then result in the "switching" of expression of heavy chain exons in a triggered B cell, leading to the secretion of IgG, IgA, or, in some cases, IgE antibody with the same V region antigen specificity as the original IgM antibody, for response to a wide variety of extracellular bacteria, protozoa, and helminths. CD40 ligand expression by activated T cells is critical for induction of B cell antibody isotype switching and for B cell responsiveness to cytokines. Patients with mutations in T cell CD40 ligand have B cells that are unable to undergo isotype switching, resulting in lack of memory B cell generation and the immunodeficiency syndrome of *X-linked hyper-IgM syndrome* (Chap. 297).

IMMUNE TOLERANCE AND AUTOIMMUNITY
Immune tolerance is defined as the absence of activation of pathogenic autoreactivity. *Autoimmune diseases* are syndromes caused by the activation of T or B cells or both, with no evidence of other causes such as infections or malignancies (Chap. 299). Once thought to be mutually exclusive, immune tolerance and autoimmunity are now both recognized to be present normally in health, and when abnormal, represent extremes from the normal state. For example, it is now known that low levels of autoreactivity of T and B cells with self-antigens in the periphery are critical to their survival. Similarly, low levels of autoreactivity and thymocyte recognition of self-antigens in the thymus are the mechanisms whereby (1) normal T cells are positively selected to survive and leave the thymus to respond to foreign microbes in the periphery, and (2) T cells highly reactive to self-antigens are negatively selected and die to prevent overly self-reactive T cells from getting into the periphery (central tolerance). However, not all self-antigens are expressed in the thymus to delete highly self-reactive T cells, and there are mechanisms for peripheral tolerance induction of T cells as well. Unlike the presentation of microbial antigens by mature dendritic cells, the presentation of self-antigens by immature dendritic cells neither activates nor matures the dendritic cells to express high levels of co-stimulatory molecules such as B7-1 (CD80) or B7-2 (CD86). When peripheral T cells are stimulated by dendritic cells expressing self-antigens in the context of HLA molecules, sufficient stimulation of T cells occurs to keep them alive, but otherwise they remain anergic, or nonresponsive, until they contact a dendritic cell with high levels of co-stimulatory molecules expressing microbial antigens. In the latter setting, normal T cells then become activated to respond to the microbe. If B cells have high self-reactivity BCRs, they normally undergo receptor editing to express a less autoreactive receptor or are induced to die. Although many autoimmune diseases are characterized by the abnormal or pathogenic autoantibody production (Table 295-11), most autoimmune diseases are caused by a combination of excess T and B cell reactivity.

Multiple factors contribute to the genesis of clinical autoimmune disease syndromes including genetic susceptibility (Table 295-12), environmental immune stimulants such as drugs (e.g., procainamide and dilantin with drug-induced systemic lupus erythematosus), infectious agent triggers (such as Epstein-Barr virus and autoantibody production against red blood cells and platelets), and loss of T regulatory cells (leading to thyroiditis, adrenalitis, and oophoritis).

THE CELLULAR AND MOLECULAR CONTROL OF PROGRAMMED CELL DEATH The process of apoptosis (programmed cell death) plays a crucial role in regulating normal immune responses to antigen. In general, a wide variety of stimuli trigger one of several apoptotic pathways to eliminate microbe-infected cells, eliminate cells with damaged DNA, or eliminate activated immune cells that are no longer needed (Fig. 295-12). The largest known family of "death receptors" are the tumor necrosis factor receptor (TNF-R) family [TNF-R1, TNF-R2, Fas (CD95), death receptor 3 (DR3), death receptor 4 (TRAIL-R1), and death receptor 5 (DR5, TRAIL-R2)]; their ligands are all in the TNF-α family. Binding of ligands to these death receptors leads to a signaling cascade

TABLE 295-11 *Recombinant or Purified Autoantigens Recognized by Autoantibodies Associated with Human Autoimmune Disorders*

Autoantigen	Autoimmune Diseases	Autoantigen	Autoimmune Diseases
CELL- OR ORGAN-SPECIFIC AUTOIMMUNITY			
Acetylcholine receptor	Myasthenia gravis	Insulin receptor	Type B insulin resistance, acanthosis, systemic lupus erythematosus (SLE)
Actin	Chronic active hepatitis, primary bilary cirrhosis	Intrinsic factor type 1	Pernicious anemia
Adenine nucleotide translator (ANT)	Dilated cardiomyopathy, myocarditis	Leukocyte function-associated antigen (LFA-1)	Treatment-resistant Lyme arthritis
β-Adrenoreceptor	Dilated cardiomyopathy	Myelin-associated glycoprotein (MAG)	Polyneuropathy
Aromatic L-amino acid decarboxylase	Autoimmune polyendocrine syndrome type 1 (APS-1)	Myelin-basic protein	Multiple sclerosis, demyelinating diseases
Asialoglycoprotein receptor	Autoimmune hepatitis	Myelin oligodendrocyte glycoprotein (MOG)	Multiple sclerosis
Bactericidal/permeability-increasing protein (Bpi)	Cystic fibrosis vasculitides	Myosin	Rheumatic fever
Calcium-sensing receptor	Acquired hypoparathyroidism	p-80-Collin	Atopic dermatitis
Cholesterol side-chain cleavage enzyme (CYPlla)	Autoimmune polyglandular syndrome-1	Pyruvate dehydrogenase complex-E2 (PDC-E2)	Primary biliary cirrhosis
Collagen type IV-α3-chain	Goodpasture syndrome	Sodium iodide symporter (NIS)	Graves' disease, autoimmune hypothyroidism
Cytochrome P450 2D6 (CYP2D6)	Autoimmune hepatitis	SOX-10	Vitiligo
Desmin	Crohn disease, coronary artery disease	Thyroid and eye muscle shared protein	Thyroid-associated ophthalmopathy
Desmoglein 1	Pemphigus foliaceus	Thyroglobulin	Autoimmune thyroiditis
Desmoglein 3	Pemphigus vulgaris	Thyroid peroxidase	Autoimmune Hashimoto thyroiditis
F-actin	Autoimmune hepatitis	Throtropin receptor	Graves' disease
GM gangliosides	Guillain-Barré syndrome	Tissue transglutaminase	Celiac disease
Glutamate decarboxylase (GAD65)	Type 1 diabetes, stiff man syndrome	Transcription coactivator p75	Atopic dermatitis
Glutamate receptor (GLUR)	Rasmussen encephalitis	Tryptophan hydroxylase	Autoimmune polyglandular syndrome-1
H/K ATPase	Autoimmune gastritis	Tyrosinase	Vitiligo, metastatic melanoma
17-α-Hydroxylase (CYP17)	Autoimmune polyglandular syndrome-1	Tyrosine hydroxylase	Autoimmune polyglandular syndrome-1
21-Hydroxylase (CYP21)	Addison disease		
IA-2 (ICA512)	Type 1 diabetes		
Insulin	Type 1 diabetes, insulin hypoglycemic syndrome (Hirata disease)		
SYSTEMIC AUTOIMMUNITY			
ACTH	ACTH deficiency	Histone H2A-H2B-DNA	SLE
Aminoacyl-tRAN histidyl synthetase	Myositis, dermatomyositis	IgE receptor	Chronic idiopathic urticaria
Aminoacyl-tRNA synthetase (several)	Polymyositis, dermatomyositis	Keratin	RA
Cardiolipin	SLE	Ku-DNA-protein kinase	SLE
Carbonic anhydrase II	SLE, Sjögren syndrome, systemic sclerosis	Ku-nucleoprotein	Connective tissue syndrome
		La phosphoprotein (La 55-B)	Sjögren syndrome
Collagen (multiple types)	Rheumatoid arthritis (RA), SLE, progressive systemic sclerosis	Myeloperoxidase	Necrotizing and crescentic glomerulonephritis (NCGN), systemic vasculitis
Centromere-associated proteins	Systemic sclerosis		
DNA-dependent nucleosine-stimulated ATPase	Dermatomyositis	Proteinase 3 (PR3)	Wegener granulomatosis, Churg-Strauss syndrome
Fibrillarin	Scleroderma	RNA polymerase I–III (RNP)	Systemic sclerosis, SLE
Fibronectin	SLE, RA, morphea	Signal recognition protein (SRP54)	Polymyositis
Glucose-6-phosphate isomerase	RA	Topoisomerase-1 (Scl-70)	Scleroderma, Raynaud syndrome
β2-Glycoprotein I (B2-GPI)	Primary antiphospholipid syndrome	Tublin	Chronic liver disease, visceral leishmaniasis
Golgin (95, 97, 160, 180)	Sjögren syndrome, SLE, RA		
Heat shock protein	Various immune-related disorders	Vimentin	Systemic autoimmune disease
Hemidesmosomal protein 180	Bullous pemphigoid, herpes gastationis, cicatricial pemphigoid		
PLASMA PROTEIN AND CYTOKINE AUTOIMMUNITY			
C1 inhibitor	Autoimmune C1 deficiency	Glycoprotein IIb/IIIg and Ib/IX	Autoimmune thrombocytopenia purpura
C1q	SLE, membrane proliferative glomerulonephritis (MPGN)	IgA	Immunodeficiency associated with SLE, pernicious anemia, thyroiditis, Sjögren's syndrome and chronic active hepatitis
Cytokines (IL-1α, IL-1β, IL-6, IL-10, LIF)	RA, systemic sclerosis, normal subjects		
Factor II, factor V, factor VII, factor VIII, factor IX, factor X, factor XI, thrombin vWF	Prolonged coagulation time	Oxidized LDL (OxLDL)	Atherosclerosis
CANCER AND PARANEOPLASTIC AUTOIMMUNITY			
Amphiphysin	Neuropathy, small-cell lung cancer	p62 (IGF-II mRNA-binding protein)	Hepatocellular carcinoma (China)
Cyclin B1	Hepatocellular carcinoma	Recoverin	Cancer-associated retinopathy
DNA topoisomerase II	Liver cancer	Ri protein	Paraneoplastic opsoclonus myoclonus ataxia
Desmoplakin	Paraneoplastic pemphigus		
Gephyrin	Paraneoplastic stiff man syndrome	βIV spectrin	Lower motor neuron syndrome
Hu proteins	Paraneoplastic encephalomyelitis	Synaptotagmin	Lambert-Eaton myasthenic syndrome
Neuronal nicotinic acetylcholine receptor	Subacute autonomic neuropathy, cancer	Voltage-gated calcium channels	Lambert-Eaton myasthenic syndrome
		Yo protein	Paraneoplastic cerebellar degeneration
p53	Cancer, SLE		

Source: From A Lernmark et al: J Clin Invest 108:1091, 2001; with permission.

Protein	Defect	Disease or Syndrome	Observation in Animal Models or Humans
CYTOKINES AND SIGNALING PROTEINS			
Tumor necrosis factor (TNF) α	Overexpression	Inflammatory bowel disease (IBD), arthritis, vasculitis	Mice
TNF-α	Underexpression	Systemic lupus erythematosus (SLE)	Mice
Interleukin-1-receptor antagonist	Underexpression	Arthritis	Mice
IL-2	Overexpression	IBD	Mice
IL-7	Overexpression	IBD	Mice
IL-10	Overexpression	IBD	Mice
IL-2 receptor	Overexpression	IBD	Mice
IL-10 receptor	Overexpression	IBD	Mice
IL-3	Overexpression	Demyelinating syndrome	Mice
Interferon-δ	Overexpression in skin	SLE	Mice
STAT-3	Underexpression	IBD	Mice
STAT-4	Overexpression	IBD	Mice
Transforming growth factor (TGF) β	Underexpression	Systemic wasting syndrome and IBD	Mice
TGF-β receptor in T cells	Underexpression	SLE	Mice
Programmed death (PD-1)	Underexpression	SLE-like syndrome	Mice
Cytotoxic T lymphocyte, antigen-4 (CTLA-4)	Underexpression	Systemic lymphoproliferative disease	Mice
IL-10	Underexpression	IBD (mouse) Type 1 diabetes, thyroid disease, primary (human)	Mice and humans
MAJOR HISTOCOMPATIBILITY LOCUS MOLECULES[a]			
HLA B27	Allele expression or over-expression	Inflammatory bowel disease	Rats and humans
Complement deficiency of C1,2,3 or 4	Underexpression	See Table 305-13	Humans
LIGHT (TNF superfamily 14)	Overexpression	Systemic lymphoproliferative (mouse) and autoimmunity	Mice
HLA class II DQB10301, DQB10302	Allele expression	Juvenile-onset diabetes	Human
HLA class II DQB10401, DQB10402	Allele expression	Rheumatoid arthritis	Humans
HLA class I B27	Allele expression	Ankylosing spondylitis, IBD	Rats and humans
APOPTOSIS PROTEINS			
TNFactor receptor 1 (TNF-R1)	Underexpression	Familial periodic fever syndrome	Humans
Fas (CD95; Apo-1)	Underexpression	Autoimmune lymphoproliferative syndrome type 1 (ALPS 1); malignant lymphoma; bladder cancer	Humans
Fas ligand	Underexpression	SLE (only one case identified)	Humans
Perforin	Underexpression	Familial hemophagocytic lymphohistiocytosis (FHL)	Humans
Caspase 10	Underexpression	Autoimmune lymphoproliferative syndrome type II (ALPS II)	Humans
bcl-10	Underexpression	Non-Hodgkin's lymphoma	Humans
P53	Underexpression	Various malignant neoplasms	Humans
Bax	Underexpression	Colon cancer; hematopoietic malignancies	Humans
bcl-2	Underexpression	Non-Hodgkin's lymphoma	Humans
c-IAP2	Underexpression	Low-grade MALT lymphoma	Humans
NAIP1	Underexpression	Spinal muscular atrophy	Humans

[a] Many autoimmune diseases are associated with a myriad of major compatibility complex gene allele (HLA) types. There are presented here as examples.

Note: MALT, mucosa-associated lymphoid tissue.

Source: Adopted from L Mullauer et al: Mutat Res 488:211, 2001; A Davidson, B Diamond: N Engl J Med 345:340, 2001; with permission.

that involves activation of the *caspase* family of molecules that leads to DNA cleavage and cell death. Two other pathways of programmed cell death involve nuclear *p53* in the elimination of cells with abnormal DNA and *mitochondrial cytochrome c* to induce cell death in damaged cells (Fig. 295-12). A number of human diseases have now been described that result from, or are associated with, mutated apoptosis genes (Table 295-12). These include mutations in the TNF-R1 in *hereditary periodic fever* (*familial Mediterranean fever*) (Chap. 279), Fas and Fas ligand in autoimmune and lymphoproliferation syndromes, and multiple associations of mutations in genes in the apoptotic pathway with malignant syndromes.

MECHANISMS OF IMMUNE-MEDIATED DAMAGE TO MICROBES OR HOST TISSUES

Several responses by the host innate and adaptive immune systems to foreign microbes culminate in rapid and efficient elimination of microbes. In these scenarios, the classic weapons of the adaptive immune system (T cells, B cells) interface with cells (macrophages, dendritic cells, NK cells, neutrophils, eosinophils, basophils) and soluble products (microbial peptides, pentraxins, complement and coagulation systems) of the innate immune system (Chaps. 55 and 298).

There are five general phases of host defenses: (1) migration of leukocytes to sites of antigen localization; (2) antigen-nonspecific recognition of pathogens by macrophages and other cells and systems of the innate immune system; (3) specific recognition of foreign antigens mediated by T and B lymphocytes; (4) amplification of the inflammatory response with recruitment of specific and nonspecific effector cells by complement components, cytokines, kinins, arachidonic acid metabolites, and mast cell–basophil products; and (5) macrophage, neutrophil, and lymphocyte participation in destruction of antigen with ultimate removal of antigen particles by phagocytosis (by macrophages or neutrophils) or by direct cytotoxic mechanisms (involving macrophages, neutrophils, and lymphocytes). Under normal circumstances, orderly progression of host defenses through these phases results in a well-controlled immune and inflammatory response that protects the host from the offending antigen. However, dysfunction of any of the host defense systems can damage host tissue and produce clinical disease. Furthermore, for certain pathogens or antigens, the normal immune response itself might contribute substantially to the tissue damage. For example, the immune and inflammatory response in the brain to certain pathogens such as *M. tuberculosis* may be responsible for much of the morbidity of this disease in that organ system (Chap. 150). In addition, the morbidity associated with certain pneumonias such as that caused by *Pneumocystis carinii* may be associated more with inflammatory infiltrates than with the tissue destructive effects of the microorganism itself (Chap. 191).

The Molecular Basis of Lymphocyte–Endothelial Cell Interactions The control of lymphocyte circulatory patterns between the bloodstream and peripheral lymphoid organs operates at the level of lymphocyte–endothelial cell interactions to control the specificity of lymphocyte subset entry into organs. Similarly, lymphocyte–endothelial cell interactions regulate the entry of lymphocytes into inflamed tissue. Adhesion molecule expression on lymphocytes and endothelial cells regulates the retention and subsequent egress of lymphocytes within tissue sites of antigenic stimulation, delaying cell exit from tissue and preventing reentry into the circulating lymphocyte pool. All types of lymphocyte migration begin with lymphocyte attachment to specialized regions of vessels, termed *high endothelial venules* (HEVs). An important concept is that adhesion molecules do not generally bind their ligand until a conformational change (ligand activation) occurs in the adhesion molecule that allows ligand binding. Induction of a conformation-dependent determinant on an adhesion molecule can be accomplished by cytokines or via ligation of other adhesion molecules on the cell.

The first stage of lymphocyte–endothelial cell interactions, *attachment and rolling*, occurs when lymphocytes leave the stream of flowing blood cells in a postcapillary venule and roll along venule endothelial cells (Fig. 295-13). Lymphocyte rolling is mediated by the L-selectin molecule (LECAM-1, LAM-1, CD62L) and slows cell transit time through venules, allowing time for activation of adherent cells.

The second stage of lymphocyte–endothelial cell interactions, *firm adhesion with activation-dependent stable arrest*, requires stimulation of lymphocytes by chemoattractants or by endothelial cell–derived cytokines. Cytokines thought to participate in adherent cell activation include members of the IL-8 family, platelet-activation factor, leukotriene B$_4$, and C5a. Following activation by chemoattractants, lymphocytes shed L-selectin from the cell surface and upregulate cell CD11b/18 (MAC-1) or CD11a/18 (LFA-1) molecules, resulting in firm attachment of lymphocytes to HEVs.

Lymphocyte homing to peripheral lymph nodes involves adhesion of L-selectin to carbohydrate of peripheral node HEVs, whereas homing of lymphocytes to intestine Peyer's patches primarily involves adhesion of the $\alpha4,\beta7$ integrin to MAdCAM-1 oligosaccharides on the Peyer's patch HEVs. However, for migration to mucosal Peyer's patch lymphoid aggregates, naive lymphocytes primarily use L-selectin, whereas memory lymphocytes use $\alpha4,\beta7$ integrin. $\alpha4,\beta1$ integrin (CD49d/CD29, VLA-4)–VCAM-1 interactions are important in the initial

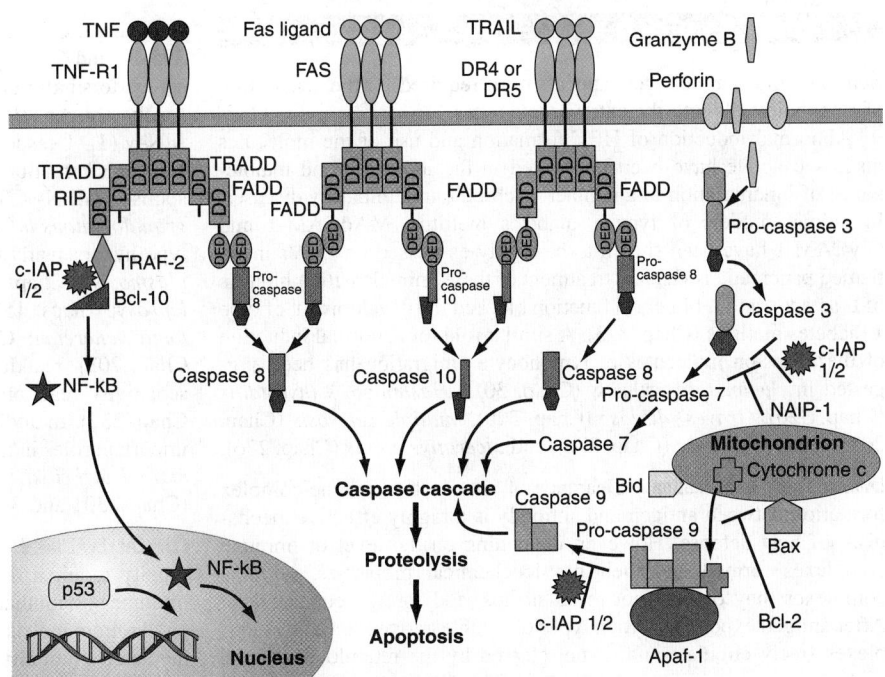

FIGURE 295-12 Scheme of major apoptosis pathways. DD, death domain; DED, death effector domain. (*From L Mullauer et al: Mutat Res 488:211, 2001; with permission.*)

interaction of memory lymphocytes with HEVs of multiple organs in sites of inflammation.

The third stage of leukocyte emigration in HEVs is *sticking and arrest*. Sticking of the lymphocyte to endothelial cells and arrest at the site of sticking are mediated predominantly by ligation of $\alpha L,\beta2$ integrin LFA-1 to the integrin ligand ICAM-1 on HEVs. While the first three stages of lymphocyte attachment to HEVs takes only a few seconds, the fourth stage of lymphocyte emigration, *transendothelial migration*, takes ~10 min. Although the molecular mechanisms that control lymphocyte transendothelial migration are not fully characterized, the HEV CD44 molecule and molecules of the HEV glycocalyx (extracellular matrix) are thought to play important regulatory roles in this process (Fig. 295-13). Finally, expression of matrix metalloproteases capable of digesting the subendothelial basement membrane,

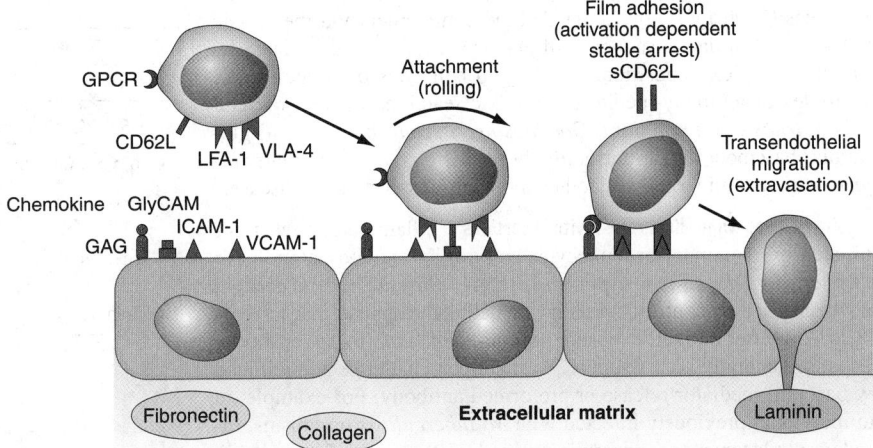

FIGURE 295-13 Schematic of the multistep model of leukocyte migration in high endothelial venules (HEV). The initial interaction of lymphocytes with HEV in peripheral lymph nodes is mediated by L-selectin (CD62L) that recognizes HEV mucin-like counterreceptors such as glycosylation-dependent cell adhesion molecule 1 (GlyCAM-1). Activation of lymphocyte adhesiveness occurs via G protein–coupled receptors (GPCR) that bind to chemokines anchored to endothelial cells by glycoaminoglycans (GAG). The integrin leukocyte function–associated molecule 1 (LFA-1) and very late antigen-4 (VLA-4) and their HEV counterreceptors, intercellular adhesion molecule 1 (ICAM-1; CD54) play a major role in lymphocyte arrest in HEV. The molecular mechanisms of lymphocyte extravasations are not completely worked out. (*From DD Patel, BF Haynes: Curr Dir Autoimmun 3:133, 2001; with permission.*)

rich in nonfibrillar collagen, appears to be required for the penetration of lymphoid cells into the extravascular sites.

Abnormal induction of HEV formation and use of the molecules discussed above have been implicated in the induction and maintenance of inflammation in a number of chronic inflammatory diseases. In animal models of type 1 diabetes mellitus, MAdCAM-1 and GlyCAM-1 have been shown to be highly expressed on HEVs in inflamed pancreatic islets, and treatment of these animals with inhibitors of L-selectin and $\alpha 4$ integrin function blocked the development of type 1 diabetes mellitus (Chap. 323). A similar role for abnormal induction of the adhesion molecules of lymphocyte emigration has been suggested in *rheumatoid arthritis* (Chap. 301), *Hashimoto's thyroiditis* (Chap. 320), *Graves' disease* (Chap. 320), *multiple sclerosis* (Chap. 262), *Crohn's disease* (Chap. 276), and *ulcerative colitis* (Chap. 276).

Immune-Complex Formation Clearance of antigen by immune-complex formation between antigen and antibody is a highly effective mechanism of host defense. However, depending on the level of immune complexes formed and their physicochemical properties, immune complexes may or may not result in host and foreign cell damage. After antigen exposure, certain types of soluble antigen-antibody complexes freely circulate and, if not cleared by the reticuloendothelial system, can be deposited in blood vessel walls and in other tissues such as renal glomeruli and cause *vasculitis* or *glomerulonephritis* syndromes (Chaps. 264 and 306).

Immediate-Type Hypersensitivity Helper T cells that drive anti-allergen IgE responses are usually T_H2-type inducer T cells that secrete IL-4, IL-5, IL-6, and IL-10. Mast cells and basophils have high-affinity receptors for the Fc portion of IgE (FcRI), and cell-bound antiallergen IgE effectively "arms" basophils and mast cells. Mediator release is triggered by antigen (allergen) interaction with Fc receptor–bound IgE; the mediators released are responsible for the pathophysiologic changes of *allergic diseases* (Table 295-6). Mediators released from mast cells and basophils can be divided into three broad functional types: (1) those that increase vascular permeability and contract smooth muscle (histamine, platelet-activating factor, SRS-A, BK-A), (2) those that are chemotactic for or activate other inflammatory cells (ECF-A, NCF, leukotriene B$_4$), and (3) those that modulate the release of other mediators (BK-A, platelet-activating factor) (Chap. 298).

Cytotoxic Reactions of Antibody In this type of immunologic injury, complement-fixing (C1-binding) antibodies against normal or foreign cells or tissues (IgM, IgG1, IgG2, IgG3) bind complement via the classic pathway and initiate a sequence of events similar to that initiated by immune-complex deposition, resulting in cell lysis or tissue injury. Examples of antibody-mediated cytotoxic reactions include red cell lysis in *transfusion reactions*, *Goodpasture's syndrome* with anti-glomerular basement membrane antibody formation, and *pemphigus vulgaris* with antiepidermal antibodies inducing blistering skin disease.

Classic Delayed-Type Hypersensitivity Reactions Inflammatory reactions initiated by mononuclear leukocytes and not by antibody alone have been termed *delayed-type hypersensitivity reactions*. The term *delayed* has been used to contrast a secondary cellular response that appears 48 to 72 h after antigen exposure with an *immediate* hypersensitivity response generally seen within 12 h of antigen challenge and initiated by basophil mediator release or preformed antibody. For example, in an individual previously infected with *M. tuberculosis* organisms, intradermal placement of tuberculin purified-protein derivative as a skin test challenge results in an indurated area of skin at 48 to 72 h, indicating previous exposure to tuberculosis.

The cellular events that result in classic delayed-type hypersensitivity responses are centered around T cells (predominantly, though not exclusively, IFN-γ, IL-2, and TNF-α-secreting T_H1-type helper T cells) and macrophages. First, local immune and inflammatory responses at the site of foreign antigen upregulate endothelial cell adhesion molecule expression, promoting the accumulation of

lymphocytes at the tissue site. In the general scheme outlined in Figs. 295-10 and 295-11, antigen is processed by dendritic cells and presented to small numbers of CD4+ T cells expressing a TCR specific for the antigen. IL-12 produced by APCs induces T cells to produce IFN-γ (T_H-1 response). Macrophages frequently undergo epithelioid cell transformation and fuse to form multinucleated giant cells in response to IFN-γ. This type of mononuclear cell infiltrate is termed *granulomatous inflammation*. Examples of diseases in which delayed-type hypersensitivity plays a major role are fungal infections (*histoplasmosis*; Chap. 183), mycobacterial infections (*tuberculosis, leprosy*; Chaps. 150 and 151), chlamydial infections (*lymphogranuloma venereum*; Chap. 160), helminth infections (*schistosomiasis*; Chap. 203), reactions to toxins (*berylliosis*; Chap. 238), and hypersensitivity reactions to organic dusts (*hypersensitivity pneumonitis*; Chap. 237). In addition, delayed-type hypersensitivity responses play important roles in tissue damage in autoimmune diseases such as *rheumatoid arthritis, temporal arteritis*, and *Wegener's granulomatosis* (Chaps. 301 and 306).

CLINICAL EVALUATION OF IMMUNE FUNCTION Clinical assessment of immunity requires investigation of the four major components of the immune system that participate in host defense and in the pathogenesis of autoimmune diseases: (1) humoral immunity (B cells); (2) cell-mediated immunity (T cells, monocytes); (3) phagocytic cells of the reticuloendothelial system (macrophages), as well as polymorphonuclear leukocytes; and (4) complement. Clinical problems that require an evaluation of immunity include chronic infections, recurrent infection, unusual infecting agents, and certain autoimmune syndromes. The type of clinical syndrome under evaluation can provide information regarding possible immune defects (Chap. 297). Defects in cellular immunity generally result in viral, mycobacterial, and fungal infections. An extreme example of deficiency in cellular immunity is *AIDS* (Chap. 173). Antibody deficiencies result in recurrent bacterial infections, frequently with organisms such as *S. pneumoniae* and *Haemophilus influenzae* (Chap. 297). Disorders of phagocyte function are frequently manifested by recurrent skin infections, often due to *Staphylococcus aureus* (Chap. 55). Finally, deficiencies of early and late complement components are associated with autoimmune phenomena and recurrent *Neisseria* infections (Table 295-13). →*For further discussion of useful initial screening tests of immune function, see Chap. 297.*

IMMUNOTHERAPY Most current therapies for autoimmune and inflammatory diseases involve the use of nonspecific immune-modulating or

TABLE 295-13 *Complement Deficiencies and Associated Diseases*

Component	Associated Diseases
CLASSIC PATHWAY	
C1q, C1r, C1s, C4	Immune-complex syndromes,[a] pyogenic infections
C2	Immune-complex syndromes,[a] few with pyogenic infections
C1 inhibitor	Rare immune-complex disease, few with pyogenic infections
C3 AND ALTERNATIVE PATHWAY C3	
C3	Immune-complex syndromes,[a] pyogenic infections
D	Pyogenic infections
Properdin	*Neisseria* infections
I	Pyogenic infections
H	Hemolytic uremic syndrome
MEMBRANE ATTACK COMPLEX	
C5, C6, C7, C8	Recurrent *Neisseria* infections, immune-complex disease
C9	Rare *Neisseria* infections

[a] Immune-complex syndromes include systemic lupus erythematosus (SLE) and SLE-like syndromes, glomerulonephritis, and vasculitis syndromes.
Source: After JA Schifferli and DK Peters, Lancet 88:957, 1983; with permission.

immunosuppressive agents such as glucocorticoids or cytotoxic drugs. The goal of development of new treatments for immune-mediated diseases is to design ways to specifically interrupt pathologic immune responses, leaving nonpathologic immune responses intact. Novel ways to interrupt pathologic immune responses that are under investigation include: the use of anti-inflammatory cytokines or specific cytokine inhibitors as anti-inflammatory agents; the use of monoclonal antibodies against T or B lymphocytes as therapeutic agents; the induction of anergy by administration of soluble CTLA-4 protein; the use of intravenous Ig for certain infections and immune complex–mediated diseases; the use of specific cytokines to reconstitute components of the immune system; and bone marrow transplantation to replace the pathogenic immune system with a more normal immune system (Table 295-14) (Chaps. 55, 297, and 173).

Cytokines and Cytokine Inhibitors Recently a humanized mouse anti-TNF-α monoclonal antibody (MAb) has been tested in both rheumatoid arthritis and ulcerative colitis. Use of anti-TNF-α antibody therapy has resulted in clinical improvement in patients with these diseases and has opened the way for targeting TNF-α to treat other severe forms of autoimmune and/or inflammatory disease. Blockage of TNF-α has been effective in *rheumatoid arthritis*, *psoriasis*, *Crohn's disease*, and *ankylosing spondylitis*. Anti-TNF-α MAb (infliximab) has been approved for treatment of patients with rheumatoid arthritis.

Other cytokine inhibitors under investigation are recombinant soluble TNF-α receptor (R) fused to human Ig and soluble IL-1 receptor (termed *IL-1 receptor antagonist*, or IL-1 ra). Soluble TNF-αR (etanercept) and IL-1 ra act to inhibit the activity of pathogenic cytokines in rheumatoid arthritis, i.e., TNF-α and IL-1, respectively. Similarly, anti-IL-6, IFN-β, and IL-11 act to inhibit pathogenic proinflammatory cytokines. Anti-IL-6 inhibits IL-6 activity, while IFN-β and IL-11 decrease IL-1 and TNF-α production.

Recent studies have identified mutations in the IL-12 gene in patients susceptible to severe myobacterial infections. IL-12 is a critical cytokine for induction of IFN-γ and cytotoxic T lymphocytes (CTLs) against intracellular organisms; it is under study for treatment of severe infections such as that caused by *M. tuberculosis* and for treatment of various cancers. In this latter setting, IL-12 is being studied for its ability to enhance antitumor cellular immunity by enhancing the induction of antitumor CTL.

Of particular note has been the successful use of IFN-γ in the treat-

TABLE 295-14 *Current Status of Development of Immunomodulatory Agents*

Agents	Rationale	Status
CYTOKINES AND CYTOKINE INHIBITORS TO INHIBIT IMMUNE RESPONSES AND INFLAMMATION		
Anti-TNF-α monoclonal antibody: Humanized mouse chimeric MAb, infliximab Fully humanized MAb, adalimumab	Inhibit TNF-α	FDA approved for rheumatoid arthritis, Crohn's colitis (infliximab); FDA approved for rheumatoid arthritis (adalimumab)
Recombinant TNF-receptor-Ig fusion protein (etanercept)	Inhibit TNF-α	FDA approved for rheumatoid arthritis, juvenile rheumatoid arthritis, psoriasis
Recombinant IL-1 receptor antagonist (IL-1Ra) (anakinra)	Inhibit IL-1α and -β	FDA approved for rheumatoid arthritis
Anti-IL-6 monoclonal antibody	Inhibit IL-6	Tested in phase I trial in rheumatoid arthritis
Inferferon-β	Inhibit IL-1, decrease synovial T cells	In trials for use in rheumatoid arthritis
Interferon-γ	Induce monocyte/macrophage activation	Effective in treating monocyte/macrophage phagocytic defects in chronic granulomatous disease
IL-11	Inhibit TNF-α and IL-1 production	In trials for Crohn's colitis
IL-12	Stimulate anti-tumor and anti-viral or bacterial cytotoxic T lymphocyte responses	Trials underway for use in cancer patients; trials planned in humans to prevent/treat severe infections
MONOCLONAL ANTIBODIES AGAINST T OR B CELLS		
Anti-CD3 anti-T cell monoclonal antibody	Inhibit T cell function; induce T cell lymphopenia	FDA approved for treatment of cardiac and renal allograft rejection
Anti-CD4 monoclonal antibody	Inhibit CD4+ T cell function	In trials for rheumatoid arthritis
Anti-CD40 ligand (CD154) monoclonal antibody	Inhibit CD40-CD40 ligand interaction; induces T cell tolerance	In primate trials for prevention of renal allograft rejection
SOLUBLE T CELL MOLECULE		
Soluble CTLA-4 protein	Inhibit CD28-B7-1 and B7-2 interactions; induce tolerance to organ grafts; inhibit autoimmune T cell reactivity in autoimmune diseases	In trials for preventing GVHD in bone marrow transplantation and for treatment of psoriasis
INTRAVENOUS IMMUNOGLOBULIN		
IVIg	Reticuloendothelial cell blockage; complement inhibition; regulation of idiotype/anti-idiotype antibodies; modulation of cytokine production; modulation of lymphocyte production	FDA approved for Kawasaki's disease and immune thrombocytopenia purpura; treatment of GVHD, multiple sclerosis, myasthenia gravis, Guillain-Barré syndrome, and chronic inflammatory demylenating polyneuropathy supported by clinical trials
CYTOKINES FOR IMMUNE RECONSTITUTION		
IL-2	Induce proliferation of peripheral memory CD4+ and CD8+ T cells	In trial for treatment of HIV infection
IL-7	Induce renewed thymopoiesis	Under consideration for treatment of diseases associated with T cell deficiency
HEMATOPOIETIC STEM CELL TRANSPLANTATION		
Hematopoietic stem transplantation for immune reconstitution	Remove pathologic autoreactive immune system and replace with less autoreactive immunity	In clinical trials for systemic lupus erythematosus, multiple sclerosis, and scleroderma

Note: FDA, US Food and Drug Administration; GVHD, graft-versus-host disease.

ment of the phagocytic cell defect in *chronic granulomatous disease* (Chap. 55). Intermittent infusions of IL-2 in HIV-infected individuals in the early or intermediate stages of disease have resulted in substantial and sustained increases in CD4+ T cells.

Monoclonal Antibodies to T and B Cells   The OKT3 MAb against human T cells has been used for several years as a T cell–specific immunosuppressive agent that can substitute for horse anti-thymocyte globulin (ATG) in the treatment of solid organ transplant rejection. OKT3 produces fewer allergic reactions than ATG but does induce human anti-mouse Ig antibody—thus limiting its use. Anti-CD4 MAb therapy has been used in trials to treat patients with rheumatoid arthritis. While inducing profound immunosuppression, anti-CD4 MAb treatment also induces susceptibility to severe infections. Treatment of patients with a MAb against the T cell molecule CD40 ligand (CD154) is under investigation to induce tolerance to organ transplants, with promising results reported in animal studies.

Tolerance Induction   Specific immunotherapy has moved into a new era with the introduction of soluble CTLA-4 protein into clinical trials. Use of this molecule to block T cell activation via TCR/CD28 ligation during organ or bone marrow transplantation has showed promising results in animals and in early human clinical trials. Specifically, treatment of bone marrow with CTLA-4 protein reduces rejection of the graft in HLA-mismatched bone marrow transplantation. In addition, promising results with soluble CTLA-4 have been reported in the downmodulation of autoimmune T cell responses in the treatment of psoriasis.

Intravenous Immunoglobulin (IVIg)   IVIg has been used successfully to block reticuloendothelial cell function and immune complex clearance in various immune cytopenias such as immune thrombocytopenia (Chap. 101). In addition, IVIg is useful for prevention of tissue damage in certain inflammatory syndromes such as Kawasaki's disease (Chap. 306) and as Ig replacement therapy for certain types of immunoglobulin deficiencies (Chap. 297). In addition, controlled clinical trials support the use of IVIg in selected patients with graft-versus-host disease, multiple sclerosis, myasthenia gravis, Guillain-Barré syndrome, and chronic demyelinating polyneuropathy (Table 295-14).

Stem Cell Transplantation   Hematopoietic stem cell transplantation (SCT) is now being comprehensively studied to treat several autoimmune diseases, including systemic lupus erythematosus, multiple sclerosis, and scleroderma. The goal of immune reconstitution in autoimmune disease syndromes is to replace a dysfunctional immune system with a normally reactive immune cell repertoire. Preliminary results in patients with scleroderma and lupus have showed encouraging results. Controlled clinical trials in these three diseases are now being launched in the United States and Europe to compare the toxicity and efficacy of conventional immunosuppression therapy with that of myeloablative autologous SCT.

Thus, a number of recent insights into immune system function have spawned a new field of interventional immunotherapy and have enhanced the prospect for development of specific and nontoxic therapies for immune and inflammatory diseases.

FURTHER READING

AKIRA S et al: Toll-like receptors: Critical proteins linking innate and acquired immunity. Nat Immunol 2:675, 2001

ARMITAGE RJ et al: CD40L: A multifunctional ligand. Semin Immunol 5:401, 1993

BENSCHOP RJ, CAMBIER JC: B cell development: Signal transduction by antigen receptors and their surrogates. Curr Opin Immunol 11:143, 1999

DAVIDSON A, DIAMOND B: Autoimmune diseases. N Engl J Med 345: 340, 2001

DIAMOND B et al: The immune tolerance network and rheumatic disease: Immune tolerance comes to the clinic. Arthritis Rheum 44:1730, 2001

GLEICH GJ: Eosinophils, basophils and mast cells. J Allergy Clin Immunol 84: 1024, 1989

HAYNES BF et al: The role of the thymus in immune reconstitution in aging bone marrow transplantation and AIDS. Ann Rev Immunol, 18:529, 2000

JANEWAY CA et al (eds): *Immunobiology. The Immune System in Health and Disease*, 4th ed. New York, Garland, 1999

KOPP EB, MEDZHITOV R: The Toll-receptor family and control of innate immunity. Curr Opin Immunol 11:13, 1999

LAM K-P, RAJEWSKY K: B cell development, in *Inflammation: Basic Principles and Clinical Correlates*, 3d ed. J Gallin, R Snyderman (eds). Philadelphia, Lippincott Williams & Wilkins, 1999, pp 151–166

LIU Y-J et al: Dendritic cell lineage, plasticity and cross-regulation. Nat Immunol 2:585:2001

LONG EO et al: KIR, in Protein Reviews on the Web, at *http://www.ncbi.nlm.nih.gov/prow/guide679664748_g.htm*, 1999

MEDZHITOV R, JANEWAY CA Jr.: Innate immunity: Impact on the adaptive immune response. Curr Opin Immunol 9:4, 1997a

———, ———: Innate immunity: The virtues of a nonclonal system of recognition. Cell 91:295, 1997b

MICHAELSSON J et al: A signal peptide derived from hsp60 binds HLA-E and interferes with CD94/NKG2A Recognition. J Exp Med 196:1403, 2002

MODLIN RL et al: The Toll of innate immunity on microbial pathogens. N Engl J Med 340:1834, 1999

MORETTA A et al: Major histocompatibility complex class I–specific receptors on human natural killer and T lymphocytes. Immunol Rev 155:105, 1997

MORLEY BJ, WALPORT MJ: *The Complement Facts Books*. London, Academic Press, Chap 2, 2000

PATEL DD, HAYNES BF: Leukocyte homing to synovium. Curr Dir Autoimmun 3:133, 2001

PULENDRAN B et al: Modulating the immune response with dendritic cells and their growth factors. Trends Immunol 22:41, 2001

SAKAGUCHI S: Regulatory T cells: Mediating compromises between host and parasite. Nature Immunol 4:10, 2003

SCHRADER JW: Interleukin is as interleukin does. Trends Immunol 23:573, 2002

SHEVACH EM: Regulatory T cells in autoimmunity. Annu Rev Immunol 18: 423, 2000

SHINKAI K et al: Helper T cells regulate type-2 innate immunity in vivo. Nature 420:825, 2002

---

296 | THE MAJOR HISTOCOMPATIBILITY GENE COMPLEX
Gerald T. Nepom, Joel D. Taurog

THE HLA COMPLEX AND ITS PRODUCTS

The human major histocompatibility complex (MHC), commonly called the human leukocyte antigen (HLA) complex, is a 4-megabase (Mb) region on chromosome 6 (6p21.3) that is densely packed with expressed genes. The best known of these genes are the HLA class I and class II genes, whose products are critical for immunologic specificity and transplantation histocompatibility, and they play a major role in susceptibility to a number of autoimmune diseases. Many other genes in the HLA region are also essential to the innate and antigen-specific functioning of the immune system. The HLA region shows extensive conservation with the MHC of other mammals in terms of genomic organization, gene sequence, and protein structure and function. Much of our understanding of the MHC has come from investigation of the MHC in mice, which is termed the *H-2 complex*, and to a lesser degree from other species as well. Nonetheless, in this chapter discussion will be confined to information applicable to the MHC in humans.

The *HLA class I genes* are located in a 2-Mb stretch of DNA at the telomeric end of the HLA region (Fig. 296-1). The classic (MHC class Ia) HLA-A, -B, and -C loci, the products of which are integral participants in the immune response to intracellular infections, tumors, and allografts, are expressed in all nucleated cells and are highly polymorphic in the population. *Polymorphism* refers to a high degree of allelic variation within a genetic locus that leads to extensive variation between different individuals expressing different alleles. Over 260 alleles at HLA-A, 500 at HLA-B, and 125 at HLA-C have been identified in different human populations, making this the most highly polymorphic segment known within the human genome. Each of the alleles at these loci encodes a *heavy chain* (also called an *α chain*) that associates noncovalently with the nonpolymorphic light chain *β₂-microglobulin*, encoded on chromosome 15.

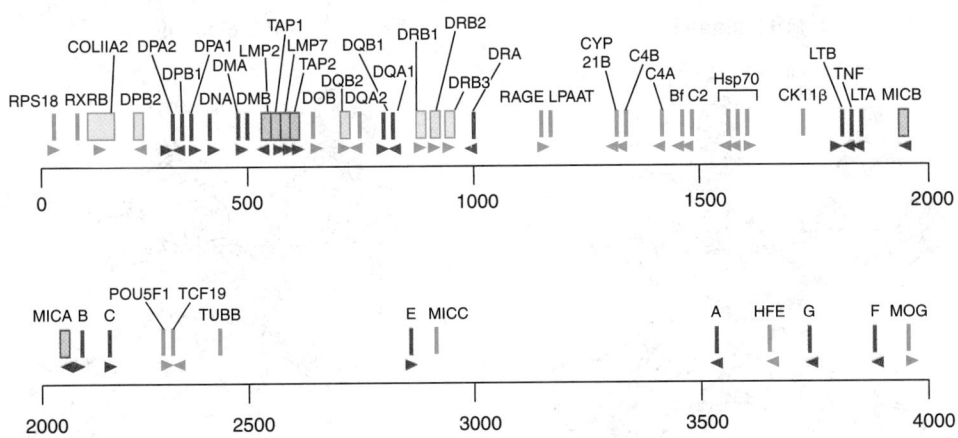

FIGURE 296-1 Physical map of the HLA region, showing the class I and class II loci, other immunologically important loci, and a sampling of other genes mapped to this region. Gene orientation is indicated by arrowheads. Scale is in kilobase (kb). The approximate genetic distance from DP to A is 3.2 cM. This includes 0.8 cM between A and B (including 0.2 cM between C and B), 0.4 to 0.8 cM between B and DR-DQ, and 1.6 to 2.0 cM between DR-DQ and DP.

The nomenclature of HLA genes and their products reflects the grafting of newer DNA sequence information on an older system based on serology. Among class I genes, alleles of the HLA-A, -B, and -C loci were originally identified in the 1950s, 1960s, and 1970s by alloantisera, derived primarily from multiparous women, who in the course of normal pregnancy produce antibodies against paternal antigens expressed on fetal cells. The serologic allotypes were designated by consecutive numbers, e.g., HLA-A1, HLA-B8. Currently, under World Health Organization (WHO) nomenclature, class I alleles are given a single designation that indicates locus, serologic specificity, and sequence-based subtype. For example, HLA-A*0201 indicates subtype 1 of the serologically defined allele HLA-A2. Subtypes that differ from each other at the nucleotide but not the amino acid sequence level are designated by an extra numeral, e.g., HLA-B*07021 and HLA-B*07022 are two variants of the HLA-B7 subtype of HLA-B*0702. The nomenclature of class II genes, discussed below, is made more complicated by the fact that both chains of a class II molecule are encoded by closely linked HLA-encoded loci, both of which may be polymorphic, and by the presence of differing numbers of isotypic DRB loci in different individuals. It has become clear that accurate HLA genotyping requires DNA sequence analysis, and the identification of alleles at the DNA sequence level has contributed greatly to the understanding of the role of HLA molecules as peptide-binding ligands, to the analysis of associations of HLA alleles with certain diseases, to the study of the populations genetics of HLA, and to a clearer understanding of the contribution of HLA differences to allograft rejection and graft-vs-host disease. Current databases of HLA class I and class II sequences can be accessed by internet (e.g., from the IMGT/HLA Database, *http://www.ebi.ac.uk/imgt/hla*), and frequent updates of HLA gene lists are published in several journals.

As shown in Fig. 296-2 and discussed below in detail, two characteristic structural features in particular define the functional properties of class I and class II HLA molecules. First is the *peptide-binding groove* that enables these molecules to form highly stable complexes with a wide array of peptide sequences that can be recognized as antigens by T cells. Second is a site for binding either the CD8 (in the case of class I HLA molecules) or the CD4 (in the case of HLA class II) molecules, which are expressed on mature T lymphocytes. In the case of class I molecules, peptide binding provides a display on the cell surface of peptides derived from intracellular proteins and thus serve as a readout to CD8+ T cells of the proteins being produced within somatic cells. The polymorphism at the loci encoding these molecules predominantly affects the amino acid residues that make up the peptide-binding groove, further amplifying the array of peptides that can be bound by different HLA molecules and generating important functional immune differences and transplantation incompatibility among different individuals.

The nonclassic, or class Ib, MHC molecules, HLA-E, -F, and -G, are much less polymorphic than MHC Ia and appear to have distinct functions. The HLA-E molecule, which has a peptide repertoire restricted to signal peptides cleaved from classic MHC class I molecules, is the major self-recognition target for the natural killer (NK) cell inhibitory receptors NKG2A or NKG2C paired with CD94 (see below and Chap. 295); four HLA-E alleles are known. HLA-G is expressed selectively in extravillous trophoblasts, the fetal cell population directly in contact with maternal tissues. It binds a wide array of peptides, is expressed in six different alternatively spliced forms, and provides inhibitory signals to both NK cells and T cells, presumably in the service of maintaining maternofetal tolerance. The function of HLA-F remains largely unknown. Although HLA-C is considered a classic class I molecule, its degree of polymorphism and level of surface expression are significantly lower than those of HLA-A and HLA-B. Moreover, unlike HLA-A and -B molecules, which function primarily by presenting antigen to CD8+ T cells expressing αβ T cell receptors, the primary function of HLA-C molecules appears to be to serve as targets of NK cell recognition (see below).

Additional class I–like genes have been identified, some HLA-linked and some encoded on other chromosomes, that show only distant homology to the class Ia and Ib molecules, but which share the three-dimensional class I structure. Those on chromosome 6p21 include MIC-A and MIC-B, which are encoded centromeric to HLA-B, and HLA-HFE, located 3 to 4 cM (centi-Morgan) telomeric of HLA-F. MIC-A and MIC-B do not bind peptide but are expressed on gut and other epithelium in a stress-inducible manner and serve as activation signals for certain γδ T cells, NK cells, CD8 T cells, and activated macrophages, acting through the activating NKG2D receptors. Fifty-four MIC-A and seventeen MIC-B alleles are known, and additional diversification comes from variable alanine repeat sequences in the transmembrane domain. HLA-HFE encodes the gene defective in hereditary hemochromatosis (Chap. 336). Among the non-HLA, class I–like genes, CD1 refers to a family of molecules that present glycolipids or other nonpeptide ligands to certain T cells, including T cells with NK activity; FcRn binds IgG within lysosomes and protects it from catabolism (Chap. 295); and Zn-α₂-glycoprotein 1 binds a nonpeptide ligand and promotes catabolism of triglycerides in adipose tissue. Like the HLA-A, -B, -C, -E, -F, and -G heavy chains, each of which forms a heterodimer with β₂-microglobulin (Fig. 296-2), the class I–like molecules, HLA-HFE, FcRn, and CD1 also bind to β₂-microglobulin, but MIC-A, MIC-B, and Zn-α₂-glycoprotein 1 do not.

The *HLA class II region* is also illustrated in Fig. 296-1. Multiple class II genes are arrayed within the centromeric 1 Mb of the HLA region, forming distinct haplotypes. A *haplotype* refers to an array of alleles at polymorphic loci along a chromosomal segment. Multiple class II genes are present on a single haplotype, clustered into three major subregions: HLA-DR, -DQ, and -DP. Each of these subregions contains at least one functional alpha (A) locus and one functional beta (B) locus. Together these encode proteins which form the α and β polypeptide chains of a mature class II HLA molecule. Thus, the DRA and DRB genes encode an HLA-DR molecule; products of the DQA1

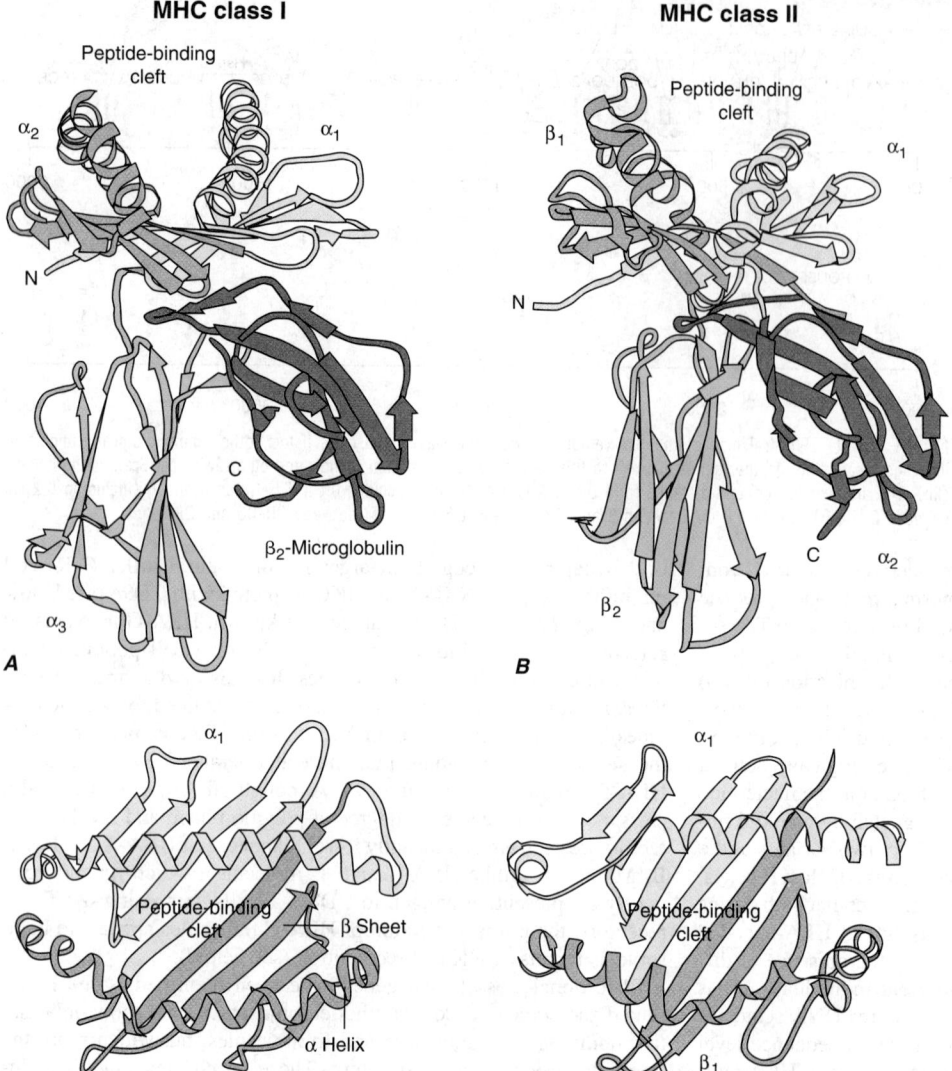

MHC class I

Peptide-binding cleft

α_2 α_1

N

C

β_2-Microglobulin

α_3

A

MHC class II

Peptide-binding cleft

β_1 α_1

N

C α_2

β_2

B

α_1

Peptide-binding cleft

β Sheet

α Helix

C α_2

α_1

Peptide-binding cleft

β_1

D

FIGURE 296-2   Side (*A, B*) and top (*C, D*) views of the MHC class I and class II molecules. The α_1 and α_2 domains of class I and the α_1 and β_1 domains of class II form a β-sheet platform that forms the floor of the peptide-binding groove, and α helices that form the sides of the groove. The α_3 (*A*) and β_2 domains (*B*) project from the cell surface and form the contact sites for CD8 and CD4, respectively. (*Adapted from C. Janeway et al, Immunobiology Bookshelf, 2d ed., Garland Publishing, New York, 1997, with permission.*)

and DQB1 genes form an HLA-DQ molecule; and the DPA1 and DPB1 genes encode an HLA-DP molecule. There are several DRB genes (DRB1, DRB2, DRB3, etc.), so that two expressed DR molecules are encoded on most haplotypes by combining the α-chain product of the DRA gene with separate β chains. More than 325 alleles have been identified at the HLA-DRB1 locus, with most of the variation occurring within limited segments encoding residues that interact with antigens. Detailed analysis of sequences and population distribution of these alleles strongly suggests that this diversity is actively selected by environmental pressures associated with pathogen diversity.

The class II region was originally termed the *D-region*. The allelic gene products were first detected by their ability to stimulate lymphocyte proliferation by *mixed lymphocyte reaction*, and were named Dw1, Dw2, etc. Subsequently, serology was used to identify gene products on peripheral blood B cells, and the antigens were termed *DR* (D-related). After additional class II loci were identified, these came to be known as DQ and DP. In the DQ region, both DQA1 and DQB1 are polymorphic, with 22 DQA1 alleles and >50 DQB1 alleles. The current nomenclature is largely analogous to that discussed above for class I, using the convention "locus * allele." Thus, for example, subtypes of the serologically defined specificity DR4, encoded by the DRB1 locus, are termed DRB1*0401, -0402, etc. In addition to allelic

polymorphism, products of different DQA1 alleles can, with some limitations, pair with products of different DQB1 alleles through both *cis* and *trans* pairing to create combinatorial complexity and expand the number of expressed class II molecules. Because of the enormous allelic diversity in the general population, most individuals are heterozygous at all of the class I and class II loci. Thus, most individuals express six classic class I molecules (two each of HLA-A, -B, and -C) and around eight class II molecules—two DP, two DR (more in the case of haplotypes with additional functional DRB genes), and up to four DQ (two *cis* and two *trans*).

The localization of polymorphic residues in class II molecules is similar to that for class I, i.e, it is predominantly in sites that affect peptide binding (see below). In the case of class II molecules, the peptides displayed on the cell surface are primarily derived from proteins acquired from the extracellular environment, processed through the endosomal-lysosomal pathway, and presented to CD4+ T cells.

OTHER GENES IN THE MHC   In addition to the class I and class II genes themselves, there are numerous genes interspersed among the HLA loci that have interesting and important immunologic functions. Our current concept of the function of MHC genes now encompasses many of these additional genes. As discussed in more detail below, TAP and LMP genes are also polymorphic and encode molecules that participate in intermediate steps in the HLA class I biosynthetic pathway. Another set of HLA genes, DMA and DMB, perform an analogous function for the class II pathway. These genes encode an intracellular molecule that facilitates the proper complexing of HLA class II molecules with antigen (see below). The *HLA class III region* is a name given to a cluster of genes between the class I and class II complexes, which includes genes for the two closely related cytokines tumor necrosis factor (TNF)-α and lymphotoxin (TNF-β); the complement components C2, C4, and Bf; heat shock protein (HSP)70; and the enzyme 21-hydroxylase.

The class I genes HLA-A, -B, and -C are expressed in all nucleated cells, although generally to a higher degree on leukocytes than on nonleukocytes. In contrast, the class II genes show a more restricted distribution: HLA-DR and HLA-DP genes are constitutively expressed on most cells of the myeloid cell lineage, whereas all three class II gene families (HLA-DR, -DQ, and -DP) are inducible by certain stimuli provided by inflammatory cytokines such as interferon γ. Within the lymphoid lineage, expression of these class II genes is constitutive on B cells and inducible on human T cells. Most endothelial and epithelial cells in the body, including the vascular endothelium and the intestinal epithelium, are also inducible for class II gene expression. Thus, while these somatic tissues normally express only class I and not class II genes, during times of local inflammation they are recruited by cytokine stimuli to express class II genes as well, thereby becoming active participants in ongoing immune responses. Class II expression is controlled largely at the transcriptional level through a conserved set of promoter elements that interact with a protein known as *CIITA*. Cytokine-mediated induction of CIITA is a principal method by which tissue-specific expression of HLA gene expression is controlled. Other HLA genes involved in the immune response, such as TAP and LMP, are also susceptible to upregulation by signals such as interferon γ. Sequence data for the entire HLA region can be accessed on the internet (e.g., *http://www.sanger.ac.uk/HGP/Chr6*). Many new genes have been discovered, the functions of which remain to be determined, as well as numerous microsatellite regions and other genetic elements. The gene density of the class II region is high, with approximately one protein encoded every 30 kb, and that of the class I and class III regions is even higher, with approximately one protein encoded every 15 kb.

LINKAGE DISEQUILIBRIUM In addition to extensive polymorphism at the class I and class II loci, another characteristic feature of the HLA complex is *linkage disequilibrium*. This is formally defined as a deviation from Hardy-Weinberg equilibrium for alleles at linked loci. This is reflected in the very low recombination rates between certain loci within the HLA complex. For example, recombination between DR and DQ loci is almost never observed in family studies, and characteristic haplotypes with particular arrays of DR and DQ alleles are found in every population. Similarly, the complement components C2, C4, and Bf are almost invariably inherited together, and the alleles at these loci are found in characteristic haplotypes. In contrast, there is a recombinational hotspot between DQ and DP, which are separated by 1 to 2 cM of genetic distance, despite their close physical proximity. Certain extended haplotypes encompassing the interval from DQ into the class I region are commonly found, the most notable being the haplotype DR3-B8-A1, which is found, in whole or in part, in 10 to 30% of northern European Caucasians. The genetic mechanisms that account for linkage disequilibrium in HLA have not been determined. It has been hypothesized that selective pressures may maintain certain haplotypes, but this remains to be determined. As discussed below under HLA and immunologic disease, one consequence of the phenomenon of linkage disequilibrium has been the resulting difficulty in assigning HLA-disease associations to a single allele at a single locus.

MHC STRUCTURE AND FUNCTION

Class I and class II molecules display a distinctive structural architecture, which contains specialized functional domains responsible for the unique genetic and immunologic properties of the HLA complex. The principal known function of both class I and class II HLA molecules is to bind antigenic peptides in order to present antigen to an appropriate T cell. The ability of a particular peptide to satisfactorily bind to an individual HLA molecule is a direct function of the molecular fit between the amino acid residues on the peptide with respect to the amino acid residues of the HLA molecule. The bound peptide forms a tertiary structure called the *MHC-peptide complex*, which communicates with T lymphocytes through binding to the T cell receptor (TCR) molecule. The first site of TCR-MHC-peptide interaction in the life of a T cell occurs in the thymus, where self-peptides are presented to developing thymocytes by MHC molecules expressed on thymic epithelium and hematopoietically derived antigen-presenting cells, which are primarily responsible for positive and negative selection, respectively (Chap. 295). Mature T cells encounter MHC molecules in the periphery both in the maintenance of tolerance (Chap. 299) and in the initiation of immune responses. Because most antibody responses and all T cell responses are T cell dependent (Chap. 295), the MHC-peptide-TCR interaction is the central event in the initiation of most antigen-specific immune responses, since it is the event that actually confers the specificity. Thus, the population of MHC–T cell complexes expressed in the thymus shapes the TCR repertoire. For potentially immunogenetic peptides, the ability of a given peptide to be generated and bound by an HLA molecule is a primary determinant of whether or not an immune response to that peptide can be generated, and the repertoire of peptides that a particular individual's HLA molecules can bind exerts a major influence over the specificity of that individual's immune response.

When a TCR molecule binds to an HLA-peptide complex, it forms intermolecular contacts with both the antigenic peptide and with the HLA molecule itself. The outcome of this recognition event depends on the density and duration of the binding interaction, accounting for a dual specificity requirement for activation of the T cell. That is, the TCR must be specific both for the antigenic peptide and for the HLA molecule. The polymorphic nature of the presenting molecules, and the influence that this exerts on the peptide repertoire of each molecule, results in the phenomenon of *MHC restriction* of the T cell specificity for a given peptide. The binding of CD8 or CD4 molecules to the class I or class II molecule, respectively, also contributes to the interaction between T cell and the HLA-peptide complex, by providing for the selective activation of the appropriate T cell.

CLASS I STRUCTURE (Fig. 296-2*A*) As noted above, MHC class I molecules provide a cell-surface display of peptides derived from intracellular proteins, and they also provide the signal for self-recognition by NK cells. Surface-expressed class I molecules consist of an MHC-encoded 44-kD glycoprotein heavy chain, a non-MHC-encoded 12-kD light chain β_2-microglobulin, and an antigenic peptide, typically 8 to 11 amino acids in length and derived from intracellularly produced protein. The heavy chain displays a prominent peptide-binding groove. In HLA-A and -B molecules, the groove is approximately 3 nm in length by 1.2 nm in maximum width (30 Å $\times$ 12 Å), whereas it is apparently somewhat wider in HLA-C. Antigenic peptides are noncovalently bound in an extended conformation within the peptide-binding groove, with both N- and C-terminal ends anchored in pockets within the groove (A and F pockets, respectively) and, in many cases, with a prominent kink, or arch, approximately one-third of the way from the N-terminus that elevates the peptide main chain off the floor of the groove.

A remarkable property of peptide binding by MHC molecules is the ability to form highly stable complexes with a wide array of peptide sequences. This is accomplished by a combination of peptide sequence–independent and peptide sequence–dependent bonding. The former consists of hydrogen bond and van der Waals interactions between conserved residues in the peptide-binding groove and charged or polar atoms along the peptide backbone. The latter is dependent upon the six side pockets that are formed by the irregular surface produced by protrusion of amino acid side chains from within the binding groove. The side chains lining the pockets interact with some of the peptide side chains. The sequence polymorphism among different class I alleles and isotypes predominantly affects the residues that line these pockets, and the interactions of these residues with peptide residues constitute the sequence-dependent bonding that confers a particular sequence "motif" on the range of peptides that can bind any given MHC molecule.

CLASS I BIOSYNTHESIS (Fig. 296-3*A*). The biosynthesis of the classic MHC class I molecules reflects their role in presenting endogenous peptides. The heavy chain is cotranslationally inserted into the membrane of the endoplasmic reticulum (ER), where it becomes glycosylated and associates sequentially with the chaperone proteins calnexin and ERp57. It then forms a complex with β_2-microglobulin, and this complex associates with the chaperone calreticulin and the MHC-encoded molecule tapasin, which physically links the class I complex to TAP, the MHC-encoded transporter associated with antigen processing. Meanwhile, peptides generated within the cytosol from intracellular proteins by the multisubunit, multicatalytic proteasome complex are actively transported into the ER by TAP, where they are trimmed by a peptidase known as *ERAAP* (ER aminopeptidase associated with antigen processing). At this point, peptides with appropriate sequence complementarity bind specific class I molecules to form complete, folded heavy chain–β_2-microglobulin–peptide trimer complexes. These are transported rapidly from the ER, through the *cis*- and *trans*-Golgi where the N-linked oligosaccharide is further processed, and thence to the cell surface.

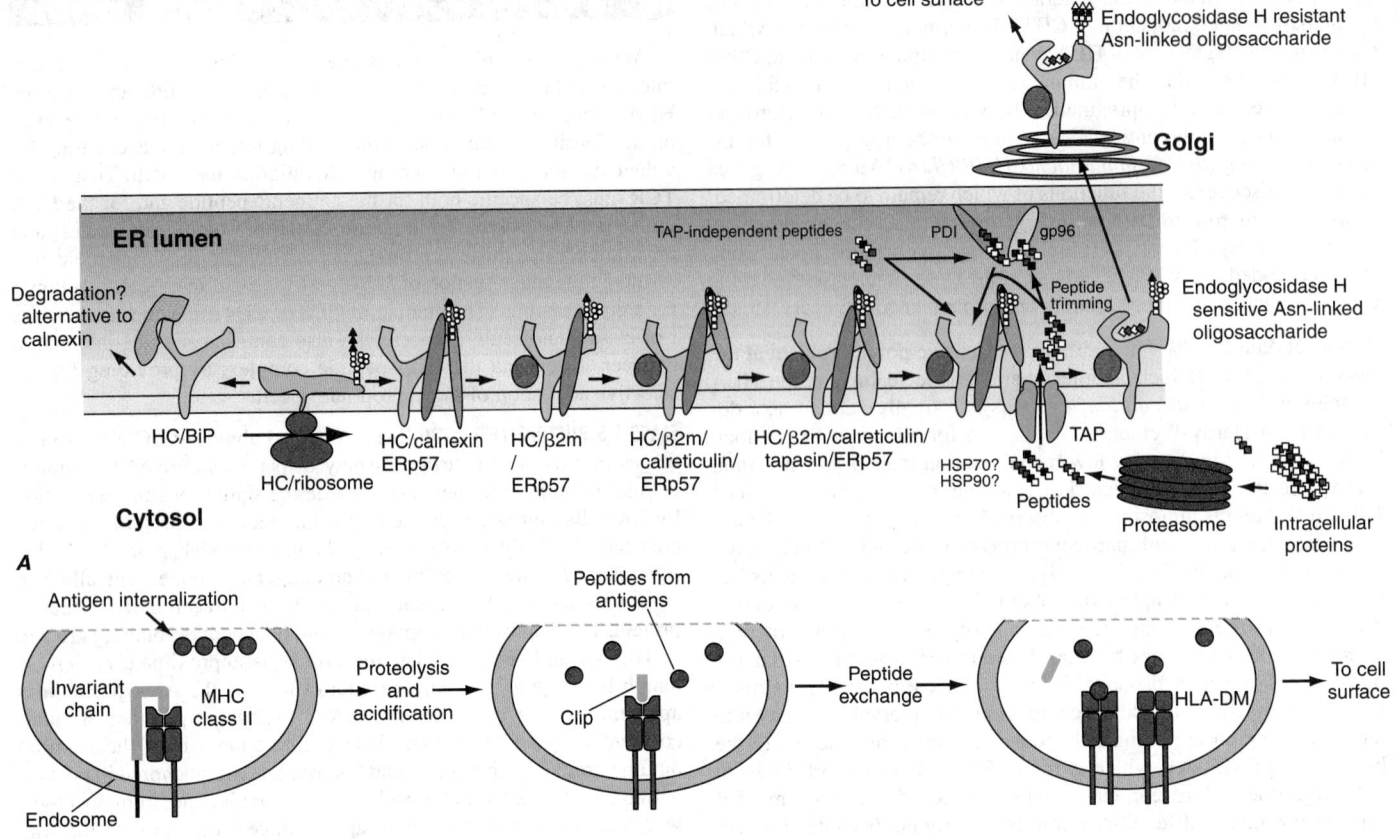

FIGURE 296-3 Biosynthesis of class I (*A*) and class II (*B*) molecules. *A*. Nascent heavy chain (HC) becomes associated with β_2-microglobulin (β2m) and peptide through interactions with a series of chaperones. Peptides generated by the proteasome are transported into the endoplasmic reticulum (ER) by TAP. Peptides undergo N-terminal trimming in the ER and become associated with chaperones, including gp96 and PDI. Once peptide binds to HC–β2m, the HC–β2m-peptide trimeric complex exits the ER and is transported by the secretory pathway to the cell surface. In the Golgi, the N– linked oligosaccharide undergoes maturation, with addition of sialic acid residues. Molecules are not necessarily drawn to scale. *B*. Pathway of HLA class II molecule assembly and antigen processing. After transport through the Golgi and post-Golgi compartment, the class II–invariant chain complex moves to an acidic endosome, where the invariant chain is proteolytically cleaved into fragments and displaced by antigenic peptides, facilitated by interactions with the DMA-DMB chaperone protein. This class II molecule– peptide complex is then transported to the cell surface.

Most of the peptides transported by TAP are produced in the cytosol by proteolytic cleavage of intracellular proteins by the multisubunit, multicatalytic protesasome, and inhibitors of the proteasome dramatically reduce expression of class I–presented antigenic peptides. A thiol-dependent oxidoreductase Erp57, which mediates disulfide bond rearrangements, also appears to play an important role in folding the class I–peptide complex into a stable multicomponent molecule. The MHC-encoded proteasome subunits LMP2 and LMP7 may influence the spectrum of peptides produced but are not essential for proteasome function.

CLASS I FUNCTION ■ **Peptide Antigen Presentation**   On any given cell, a class I molecule occurs in 100,000 to 200,000 copies and binds several hundred to several thousand distinct peptide species. The vast majority of these peptides are self-peptides to which the host immune system is tolerant by one or more of the mechanisms that maintain tolerance, e.g., clonal deletion in the thymus or clonal anergy or clonal ignorance in the periphery (Chaps. 295 and 299). However, class I molecules bearing foreign peptides expressed in a permissive immunologic context activate CD8 T cells, which, if naïve, will then differentiate into cytolytic T lymphocytes (CTLs). These T cells and their progeny, through their $\alpha\beta$ TCRs, are then capable of Fas/CD95- and/or perforin-mediated cytotoxicity and/or cytokine secretion (Chap. 295) upon further encounter with the class I–peptide combination that originally activated it, and also with other combinations of class I molecule plus peptide that present a similar immunochemical stimulus to the TCR. As alluded to above, this phenomenon by which T cells recognize foreign antigens in the context of specific MHC alleles is termed *MHC restriction*, and the specific MHC molecule is termed the *restriction element*. The most common source of foreign peptides presented by

class I molecules is viral infection, in the course of which peptides from viral proteins enter the class I pathway. The generation of a strong CTL response that destroys virally infected cells represents an important antigen-specific defense against many viral infections (Chap. 295). In the case of some viral infections—hepatitis B, for example—CTL-induced target cell apoptosis is thought to be a more important mechanism of tissue damage than any direct cytopathic effect of the virus itself. The importance of the class I pathway in the defense against viral infection is underscored by the identification of a number of viral products that interfere with the normal class I biosynthetic pathway and thus block the immunogenetic expression of viral antigens.

Other examples of intracellularly generated peptides that can be presented by class I molecules in an immunogenic manner include peptides derived from nonviral intracellular infectious agents (e.g., *Listeria*, *Plasmodium*), tumor antigens, minor histocompatibility antigens, and certain autoantigens. There are also situations in which cell surface–expressed class I molecules are thought to acquire and present exogenously derived peptides.

HLA Class I Receptors and NK Cell Recognition (Chap. 295)   NK cells, which play an important role in innate immune responses, are activated to cytotoxicity and cytokine secretion by contact with cells that lack MHC class I expression, and NK cell activation is inhibited by cells that express MHC class I. In humans, the recognition of class I molecules by NK cells is carried out by three classes of receptor families, the killer cell–inhibitory cell receptor (KIR) family, the leukocyte Ig-like receptor (LIR) family, and the CD94/NKG2 family. The KIR family, also called CD158, is encoded on chromosome 19q13.4 and consists of glycoproteins of the immunoglobulin (Ig) superfamily, currently divided into two types, the inhibitor (L) and stimulatory (S)

KIRs. KIR molecules of the L class bind HLA class I molecules and inhibit NK cell–mediated cytotoxicity and are also expressed on subsets of T lymphocytes. An estimated 40 genes are divided into two subfamilies, 2DL and 3DL, which contain, respectively, either two or three Ig domains. The KIR2DL1 molecules primarily recognize alleles of HLA-C, which possess a lysine at position 80 (HLA-Cw2, -4, -7 and -8), while the KIR2DL2 and KIR2DL3 families primarily recognize alleles of HLA-C with asparagine at this position (HLA-Cw1, -3, -5 and -6). The KIR3D molecules predominantly recognize HLA-B alleles that fall into the HLA-Bw4 class determined by residues 77 to 83 in the α_1 domain of the heavy chain. Less is known about the stimulatory KIR receptors, and their primary specificity may be for nonclassic class I molecules or for related structures present on some pathogens. The most common KIR haplotype in Caucasians contains one activating KIR and six inhibitory KIR genes, although there is a great deal of diversity in the population, with at least 15 different haplotypes. It appears that most individuals have at least one inhibitory KIR for a self-HLA class I molecule, providing a structural basis for NK cell target specificity.

The LIR gene family (CD85, also called ILT) is encoded centromeric of the KIR locus on 19q13.4, and it encodes a variety of inhibitory immunoglobulin-like receptors expressed on many lymphocyte and other hematopoietic lineages. Interaction of LIR-1 (ILT2) with NK or T cells inhibits activation and cytotoxicity, mediated by many different HLA class I molecules, including HLA-G. HLA-F also appears to interact with LIR molecules, although the functional context for this is not understood.

The third family of NK receptors for HLA is encoded in the NK complex on chromosome 12p12.3-13.1 and consists of CD94 and five NKG2 genes, A/B, C, E/H, D, and F. These molecules are C-type (calcium-binding) lectins and most function as disulfide-bonded heterodimers between CD94 and one of the NKG2 glycoproteins. The principle ligand of CD94/NKG2A receptors is the HLA-E molecule, complexed to a peptide derived from the signal sequence of classic HLA class I molecules and HLA-G. Thus, analogous to the way in which KIR receptors recognize HLA-C, the NKG2 receptor monitors self–class I expression, albeit indirectly through peptide recognition in the context of HLA-E. NKG2C, -E, and -H appear to have similar specificities but act as activating receptors. NKG2D is expressed as a homodimer and functions as an activating receptor expressed on NK cells, $\gamma\delta$ TCR T cells, and activated CD8 T cells. When complexed with an adaptor called DAP10, NKG2D recognizes MIC-A and MIC-B molecules and activates the cytolytic response. NKG2D also binds a class of molecules known as *ULBP*, structurally related to class I molecules but not encoded in the MHC. **→*The function of NK cells in immune responses is discussed in Chap. 295.***

CLASS II STRUCTURE (Fig. 296-2*B*)   A specialized functional architecture similar to that of the class I molecules can be seen in the example of a class II molecule depicted in Fig. 296-2*B*, with an antigen-binding cleft arrayed above a supporting scaffold that extends the cleft toward the external cellular environment. However, in contrast to the HLA class I molecular structure, β_2-microglobulin is not associated with class II molecules. Rather, the class II molecule is a heterodimer, composed of a 29-kD α chain and a 34-kD β chain. The amino-terminal domains of each chain form the antigen-binding elements which, like the class I molecule, cradle a bound peptide in a groove bounded by extended α-helical loops, one encoded by the A (α chain) gene and one by the B (β chain) gene. Like the class I groove, the class II antigen-binding groove is punctuated by pockets that contact the side chains of amino acid residues of the bound peptide, but unlike the class I groove, it is open at both ends. Therefore, peptides bound by class II molecules vary greatly in length, since both the N- and C-terminal ends of the peptides can extend through the open ends of this groove. Approximately 11 amino acids within the bound peptide form intimate contacts with the class II molecule itself, with backbone hydrogen bonds and specific side chain interactions combining to provide, respectively, stability and specificity to the binding (Fig. 296-4).

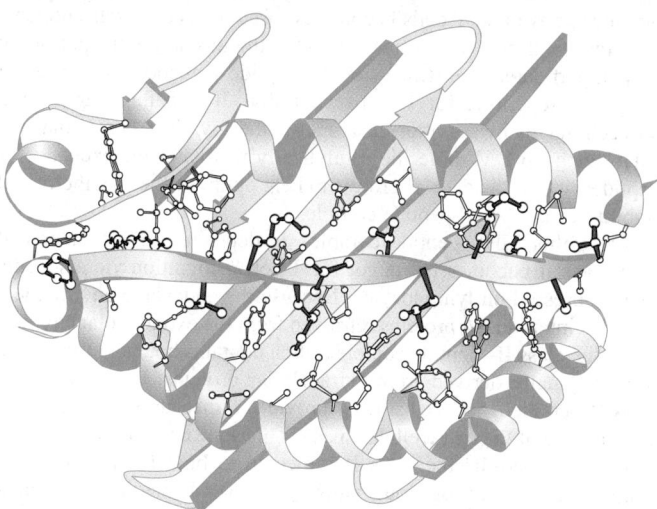

FIGURE 296-4   Top view of the HLA-DR1 molecule containing the peptide 296-318 from influenza hemagglutinin. The N terminus of the peptide is at left, and the peptide lies relatively flat within the peptide-binding groove in an extended conformation with a pronounced twist. Some 35% of the peptide surface is potentially available for interaction with the antigen receptor on T cells. Pockets in the peptide-binding site accommodate 5 of the 13 side chains of the bound peptide, manifesting the peptide specificity of HLA-DR1. Twelve hydrogen bonds between conserved HLA-DR1 residues and the main chain of the peptide provide a universal mode of peptide binding. The ends of the binding groove are open, and longer variants of the peptide can extend out from each end. In contrast, peptides bound to class I molecules are anchored into pockets at their N and C termini by conserved residues, and the middle portion of the peptide is typically kinked upwards out of the groove. (*Adapted from LJ Stern et al: Nature 368:215, 1994. Copyright 1994 Macmillan Magazines Ltd, with permission.*)

The genetic polymorphisms that distinguish different class II genes correspond to changes in the amino acid composition of the class II molecule, and these variable sites are clustered predominantly around the pocket structures within the antigen-binding groove. As with class I, this is a critically important feature of the class II molecule, which explains how genetically different individuals have functionally different HLA molecules.

As noted above, the class I–peptide complex is preferentially recognized by CD8 T cells, and the class II–peptide complex is preferentially recognized by CD4 T cells. These interactions provide an important signal for activation of specific T cell lineages during antigen-recognition events. The CD8 recognition site is located on the α_3 domain of the MHC class I molecule, and the CD4 recognition site is located on the β_2 domain of the class II molecule, in both cases remote from the peptide-binding site.

BIOSYNTHESIS AND FUNCTION OF CLASS II MOLECULES (Fig. 296-3*B*)   The intracellular assembly of class II molecules occurs within a specialized compartmentalized pathway that differs dramatically from the class I pathway described above. As illustrated in Fig. 296-3*B*, the class II molecule assembles in the ER in association with a chaperone molecule, known as the *invariant chain*. The invariant chain performs at least two roles. First, it binds to the class II molecule and blocks the peptide-binding groove, thus preventing antigenic peptides from binding. This role of the invariant chain appears to account for one of the important differences between class I and class II MHC pathways, since it can explain why class I molecules present endogenous peptides from proteins newly synthesized in the ER but class II molecules generally do not. Second, the invariant chain contains molecular localization signals that direct the class II molecule to traffic into post-Golgi compartments known as *endosomes*, which develop into specialized acidic compartments where proteases cleave the invariant chain, and antigenic peptides can now occupy the class II groove. The specificity and tissue distribution of these proteases appear to be an important way in which the immune system regulates access to the peptide-binding groove and T cells become exposed to specific self-antigens. Differences in protease expression in the thymus and in the periphery may in part determine which specific peptide sequences comprise the peripheral repertoire for T cell recognition. It is at this stage in the intracellular pathway, after cleavage of the invariant chain, that the MHC-encoded DM molecule catalytically facilitates the exchange of peptides within the class II groove to help optimize the specificity and stability of the MHC-peptide complex.

Once this MHC-peptide complex is deposited in the outer cell membrane it becomes the target for T cell recognition via a specific TCR expressed on lymphocytes. Because the endosome environment contains internalized proteins retrieved from the extracellular environment, the class II–peptide complex often contains bound antigens that were originally derived from extracellular proteins. In this way, the class II peptide–loading pathway provides a mechanism for immune surveillance of the extracellular space. This appears to be an important feature that permits the class II molecule to bind foreign peptides, distinct from the endogenous pathway of class I–mediated presentation.

ROLE OF HLA IN TRANSPLANTATION

The development of modern clinical transplantation in the decades since the 1950s provided a major impetus for elucidation of the HLA system, as allograft survival is highest when donor and recipient are HLA-identical. Although many molecular events participate in transplantation rejection, allogeneic differences at class I and class II loci play a major role. Class I molecules can promote T cell responses in several different ways. In the cases of allografts in which the host and donor are mismatched at one or more class I loci, host T cells can be activated by classic *direct alloreactivity*, in which the antigen receptors on the host T cells react with the foreign class I molecule expressed on the allograft. In this situation, the response of any given TCR may be dominated by the allogeneic MHC molecule, the peptide bound to it, or some combination of the two. Another type of host antigraft T cell response involves the uptake and processing of donor MHC antigens by host antigen-presenting cells and the subsequent presentation of the resulting peptides by host MHC molecules. This mechanism is termed *indirect alloreactivity*.

In the case of class I molecules on allografts that are shared by the host and the donor, a host T cell response may still be triggered because of peptides that are presented by the class I molecules of the graft but not of the host. The most common basis for the existence of these endogenous antigen peptides, called *minor histocompatibility antigens*, is a genetic difference between donor and host at a non-MHC locus encoding the structural gene for the protein from which the peptide is derived. These loci are termed *minor histocompatibility loci*, and nonidentical individuals typically differ at many such loci. CD4 T cells react to analogous class II variation, both direct and indirect, and class II differences alone are sufficient to drive allograft rejection.

ASSOCIATION OF HLA ALLELES WITH SUSCEPTIBILITY TO DISEASE

It has long been postulated that infectious agents provide the driving force for the allelic diversification seen in the HLA system. An important corollary of this hypothesis is that resistance to specific pathogens may differ between individuals, based on HLA genotype. Observations of specific HLA genes associated with resistance to malaria or dengue fever, persistence of hepatitis B, and to disease progression in HIV infection are consistent with this model. Pathogen diversity is probably also the major selective pressure favoring HLA heterozygosity. The extraordinary scope of HLA allelic diversity increases the likelihood that most new pathogens will be recognized by some HLA molecules, helping to assure immune fitness to the host. However, another consequence of diversification is that some alleles may become preferentially selective for recognition of self-antigens as well. Indeed, particular HLA alleles are strongly associated with certain disease states, particularly for some common autoimmune diseases (Chap. 299). By comparing allele frequencies in patients with any particular disease and in control

populations, a large number of such associations have been identified, some of which are listed in Table 296-1. The strength of genetic association is reflected in the term *relative risk*, which is a statistical odds ratio representing the risk of disease for an individual carrying a particular genetic marker compared with the risk for individuals in that population without that marker. The nomenclature shown in Table 296-1 reflects both the HLA serotype (e.g., DR3, DR4) and the HLA genotype (e.g., DRB1*0301, DRB1*0401). It very likely the class I and class II alleles themselves are the true susceptibility alleles for most of these associations. However, as discussed below, because of the extremely strong linkage disequilibrium between the DR and DQ loci, in some cases it has been difficult to determine the specific locus or combination of class II loci involved. In some cases, the susceptibility gene may be one of the HLA-linked genes located near the class I or class II region, but not the HLA gene itself, and in other cases the susceptibility gene may be a non-HLA gene, such as TNF-α, which is nearby.

As might be predicted from the known function of the class I and class II gene products, almost all of the diseases associated with specific HLA alleles have an immunologic component to their pathogenesis. It should be stressed that even the strong HLA associations with disease (those associations with relative risk of $\geq$10) implicate normal, rather than defective, alleles. Most individuals who carry these susceptibility genes do not express the associated disease; in this way the particular HLA gene is permissive for disease but requires other environmental (e.g., the presence of specific antigens) or genetic factors for full penetrance. In each case studied, even in diseases with very strong HLA associations, the concordance of disease in monozygotic twins is higher than in HLA-identical dizygotic twins or other sibling pairs, indicating that non-HLA genes contribute to susceptibility and can significantly modify the risk attributable to HLA.

Another group of diseases is genetically linked to HLA, not because of the immunologic function of HLA alleles, but rather because they are caused by autosomal dominant or recessive abnormal alleles at loci that happen to reside in or near the HLA region. Examples of these are 21-hydroxylase deficiency (Chap. 321), hemochromatosis (Chap. 336), and spinocerebellar ataxia (Chap. 353).

CLASS I ASSOCIATIONS WITH DISEASE

Although the associations of human disease with particular HLA alleles or haplotypes predominantly involve the class II region, there are also several prominent disease associations with class I alleles. These include the association of Behçet's disease (Chap. 307) with HLA-B51, psoriasis vulgaris (Chap. 47) with HLA-Cw6, and, most notably, the spondyloarthropathies (Chap. 305) with HLA-B27. Twenty-five HLA-B locus alleles, designated HLA-B*2701 to B*2725, encode the family of B27 class I molecules. All of the subtypes share a common B pocket in the peptide-binding groove, a deep, negatively charged pocket that shows a strong preference for binding the arginine side chain. In addition, B27 is among the most negatively charged of HLA class I heavy chains, and the overall preference is for positively charged peptides. HLA-B*2705 is the predominant subtype in Caucasians and most other non-Oriental populations, and this subtype is very highly associated with ankylosing spondylitis (AS) (Chap. 305), both in its idiopathic form and in association with chronic inflammatory bowel disease or psoriasis vulgaris. It is also associated with reactive arthritis (ReA) (Chap. 305), with other idiopathic forms of peripheral arthritis (undifferentiated spondyloarthropathy), and with recurrent acute anterior uveitis. B27 is found in 50 to 90% of individuals with these conditions, compared with a prevalence of ~7% in North American Caucasians. The prevalence of B27 in patients with idiopathic AS is 90%, and in AS complicated by iritis or aortic insufficiency it is close to 100%. The absolute risk of spondyloarthropathy in unselected B27+ individuals has been variously estimated at 2 to 13% and >20% if a B27+ first-degree relative is affected. The concordance rate of AS in identical twins is very high, at least 65%. It can be concluded that the B27 molecule itself is involved in disease pathogenesis, based on strong evidence from clinical epidemiology and on the occurrence of a spondyloarthropathy-like disease in HLA-B27 transgenic rats. Both AS and ReA are associated with the B27 subtypes B*2702, -04, and -05, and anecdotal association has been reported for subtypes B*2701, -03, -07, -08, -10, and -11.

The association of B27 with these diseases may derive from the specificity of a particular peptide or family of peptides bound to B27 or through another mechanism that is independent of the peptide specificity of B27. The first alternative can be further subdivided into mechanisms that involve T cell recognition of B27-peptide complexes and those that do not. A variety of other roles for B27 in disease pathogenesis have been postulated, including molecular or antigenic mimicry between B27 and certain bacteria and reduced killing of intracellular bacteria in cells expressing B27. HLA-B27 has been shown to form heavy chain homodimers, utilizing the cysteine residue at position 67 of the B57 α chain. These homodimers are expressed on the surface of lymphocytes and monocytes from patients with AS, and receptors including KIR3DL1, KIR3DL2, and ILT4 are capable of binding to them. Whether these interactions contribute to disease susceptibility or pathogenesis is currently unknown.

CLASS II DISEASE ASSOCIATIONS As can be seen in Table 296-1, the majority of associations of HLA and disease are with class II alleles. Several diseases have complex HLA genetic associations.

Celiac Disease In the case of celiac disease (Chap. 275), it is probable that the HLA-DQ genes are the primary basis for the disease association. HLA-DQ genes present on both the celiac-associated DR3 and DR7 haplotypes include the DQB1*0201 gene, and further detailed studies have documented a specific class II $\alpha\beta$ dimer encoded by the DQA1*0501 and DQB1*0201 genes, which appears to account for the HLA genetic contribution to celiac disease susceptibility. This specific HLA association with celiac disease may have a straightforward explanation: peptides derived from the wheat gluten component gliaden are bound to the molecule encoded by DQA1*0501 and DQB1*0201 and presented to T cells. A gliaden-derived peptide that has been implicated in this immune activation binds the DQ class II dimer best when the peptide contains a glutamine to glutamic acid substitution. It has been proposed that tissue transglutaminase, an enzyme present at increased levels in the intestinal cells of celiac patients, converts glutamine to glutamic acid in gliadin, creating peptides that are capable of being bound by the DQ2 molecule and presented to T cells.

Pemphigus Vulgaris In the case of pemphigus vulgaris (Chap. 49), there are two HLA haplotypes associated with disease, DRB1*0402-DQB1*0302 and DRB1*1401-DQB1*0503. Peptides derived from epidermal autoantigens have been implicated that preferentially bind to the DRB1*0402-encoded molecule, suggesting that specific peptide binding by this disease-associated class II molecule is important in disease. However, there are no class II genes in common between the disease-associated DR4 and DR14 haplotypes, and there is no evidence for any interaction of the latter haplotype interacting with the epidermal peptides that bind the DRB1*0402-encoded molecule. Thus, the

most likely interpretation is that each of these class II associations with pemphigus represents a different pathway to a comparable clinical outcome.

Juvenile Arthritis Pauciarticular juvenile arthritis (Chap. 301) is an autoimmune disease associated with genes at the DRB1 locus and also with genes at the DPB1 locus. Patients with both DPB1*0201 and a DRB1 susceptibility allele (usually DRB1*08 or -*05) have a higher relative risk than expected from the additive effect of those genes alone. In juvenile patients with rheumatoid factor–positive polyarticular disease, heterozygotes carrying both DRB1*0401 and -*0404 have a relative risk >100, reflecting an apparent synergy in individuals inheriting both of these susceptibility genes.

Type I Diabetes Mellitus There are several aspects of the genetics of type I diabetes (Chap. 323) that illustrate the complex nature of HLA associations with autoimmune diseases. First, type 1 (autoimmune) diabetes mellitus is associated with both DR3 and DR4 serotypes and

TABLE 296-1 *Significant HLA Class I and Class II Associations with Disease*[a]

	Marker	Gene	Strength of Association
SPONDYLOARTHROPATHIES			
Ankylosing spondylitis	B27	B*2702, -04, -05	++++
Reiter's syndrome	B27		++++
Acute anterior uveitis	B27		+++
Reactive arthritis (*Yersinia, Salmonella, Shigella, Chlamydia*)	B27		+++
Psoriatic spondylitis	B27		+++
COLLAGEN-VASCULAR DISEASES			
Juvenile arthritis, pauciarticular	DR8		++
	DR5		++
Rheumatoid arthritis	DR4	DRB1*0401, -04, -05	+++
Sjögren's syndrome	DR3		++
Systemic lupus erythematosus			
Caucasian	DR3		+
Japanese	DR2		++
AUTOIMMUNE GUT AND SKIN			
Gluten-sensitive enteropathy (celiac disease)	DR3	DQA1*0501 DQB1*0201	+++
Chronic active hepatitis	DR3		++
Dermatitis herpetiformis	DR3		+++
Psoriasis vulgaris	Cw6		++
Pemphigus vulgaris	DR4	DRB1*0402	+++
	DR6	DQB1*0503	
AUTOIMMUNE ENDOCRINE			
Type 1 diabetes mellitus	DR4	DQB1*0302	+++
	DR3		++
	DR2	DQB1*0602	—[b]
Hyperthyroidism (Graves')	B8		+
	DR3		+
Hyperthyroidism (Japanese)	B35		+
Adrenal insufficiency	DR3		++
AUTOIMMUNE NEUROLOGIC			
Myasthenia gravis	B8		+
	DR3		+
Multiple sclerosis	DR2	DRB1*1501 DRB5*0101	++
OTHER			
Behçet's disease	B51		++
Congenital adrenal hyperplasia	B47	21·OH (Cyp21B)	+++
Narcolepsy	DR2		++++
Goodpasture's syndrome (anti-GBM)	DR2		++

[a] Various diseases associated with HLA genes are listed, with the HLA serotype or linked marker most frequently found related to disease. Genes are listed for cases where specific alleles have been identified as responsible for this association. The strength of association reflects the likelihood of disease in individuals with the marker compared to individuals who do not carry the marker; ++++, relative risk > 10; +++, relative risk > 5; ++, relative risk > 3; +, relative risk > 1.5.

[b] Strong negative association, i.e., genetic association with protection from diabetes.

their corresponding genes. The presence of both the DR3 and DR4 haplotypes in one individual confers the highest known genetic risk for type 1 diabetes, and individuals carrying either of these haplotypes also carry some increased risk. Specific class II genes on each haplotype have been thoroughly studied, and the strongest association is with DQB1*0302, a specific gene on the diabetes-associated DR4 haplotypes. Thus, all DR4 haplotypes that carry a DQB1*0302 gene are associated with type 1 diabetes, whereas related DR4 haplotypes that carry a different DQB1 gene are not. The primary class II determinant of susceptibility, therefore, is HLA-DQB1*0302. However, the relative risk associated with inheritance of this gene can be modified, depending on other HLA genes present either on the same or a second haplotype. For example, just as the presence of a second haplotype containing DR3 is associated with increased diabetes risk, the presence of a DR2-positive haplotype containing a DQB1*0602 gene is associated with decreased risk. This gene, DQB1*0602, is considered "protective" for type 1 diabetes. Even some DRB1 genes that can occur on the same haplotype as DQB1*0302 may modulate risk, so that individuals with the DR4 haplotype that contains DRB1*0403 are less susceptible to type 1 diabetes than individuals with other DR4-DQB1*0302 haplotypes.

Although the presence of a DR3 haplotype in combination with the DR4-DQB1*0302 haplotype is a very high risk combination for diabetes susceptibility, the specific gene on the DR3 haplotype that is responsible for this synergy is not yet identified. This is because the predominant HLA-DR3 haplotype in Caucasians has very tight linkage with other genes within the MHC, including HLA-A1, -B8, -Cw7, and -C4A, as discussed above. Thus, any of a large variety of genes within the HLA region on this DR3 haplotype may be the primary gene(s) responsible for contributing to diabetes susceptibility. An example that more directly implicates other genes linked to DR3 is the association between HLA genes and systemic lupus erythematosus (SLE) (Chap. 300). The C4A null alleles that are present on the HLA-DR3 haplotypes in SLE are also often present in patients without DR3, notably those with HLA-DR2. This implicates the presence of a C4A silent allele, which is a defective structural gene for the C4 complement component, rather than the expression of any particular class II gene, as a potential susceptibility gene within HLA associated with SLE.

HLA and Rheumatoid Arthritis The HLA genes associated with rheumatoid arthritis (RA) (Chap. 301) are DRB1*0401 and DRB1*0404. These genes encode a distinctive sequence of amino acids from codons 67 to 74 of the DRβ molecule: RA-associated class II molecules carry the sequence LeuLeuGluGlnArgArgAlaAla or LeuLeuGlu-GlnLysArgAlaAla in this region, while non-RA-associated genes carry one or more differences in this region. These residues form a portion of the molecule that lies in the middle of the α-helical portion of the DRB1-encoded class II molecule, termed the *shared epitope*.

These DR4-positive RA-associated alleles are most frequent among patients with more severe, erosive disease. The frequency of these DR4-positive alleles is lower among rheumatoid factor–negative patients with RA, as well as among patients with nonerosive forms of the disease. It is important to note that, although the frequency of these DRB1 susceptibility alleles in RA patients is high, the same genes are also prevalent in the unaffected population, and thus the absolute risk associated with these susceptibility alleles is low. The highest risk for susceptibility to RA comes in individuals who carry both a DRB1*0401 and DRB1*0404 gene. Some forms of RA are associated with other HLA genes, such as DRB1*01, -*1001, and -*1402, which also carry the shared epitope sequence, strongly suggesting that this part of the class II molecule contributes directly to disease pathogenesis.

MOLECULAR MECHANISMS FOR HLA-DISEASE ASSOCIATIONS As noted above, HLA molecules play a key role in the selection and establishment of the antigen-specific T cell repertoire and a major role in the subsequent activation of those T cells during the initiation of an immune response. Precise genetic polymorphisms characteristic of individual alleles dictate the specificity of these interactions and thereby instruct and guide antigen-specific immune events. These same genetically determined pathways are therefore implicated in disease pathogenesis when specific HLA genes are responsible for autoimmune disease susceptibility.

The fate of developing T cells within the thymus is determined by the affinity of interaction between T cell receptor and HLA molecules bearing self-peptides, and thus the particular HLA types of each individual control the precise specificity of the T cell repertoire (Chap. 295). The primary basis for HLA-associated disease susceptibility may well lie within this thymic maturation pathway. The positive selection of potentially autoreactive T cells, based on the presence of specific HLA susceptibility genes, may establish the threshold for disease risk in a particular individual.

At the time of onset of a subsequent immune response, the primary role of the HLA molecule is to bind peptide and present it to antigen-specific T cells. The HLA complex can therefore be viewed as encoding genetic determinants of precise immunologic activation events. Antigenic peptides that bind particular HLA molecules are capable of stimulating T cell immune responses; peptides that do not bind are not presented to T cells and are not immunogenic. This genetic control of the immune response is mediated by the polymorphic sites within the HLA antigen–binding groove that interact with the bound peptides. In autoimmune and immune-mediated diseases, it is likely that specific tissue antigens that are targets for pathogenic lymphocytes are complexed with the HLA molecules encoded by specific susceptibility alleles. In autoimmune diseases with an infectious etiology, it is likely that immune responses to peptides derived from the initiating pathogen are bound and presented by particular HLA molecules to activate T lymphocytes that play a triggering or contributory role in disease pathogenesis. The concept that early events in disease initiation are triggered by specific HLA-peptide complexes offers some prospects for therapeutic intervention, since it may be possible to design compounds that interfere with the formation or function of specific HLA-peptide–T cell receptor interactions.

When considering mechanisms of HLA associations with immune response and disease, it is well to remember that just as HLA genetics are complex, so are the mechanisms likely to be heterogeneous. Immune-mediated disease is a multistep process in which one of the HLA-associated functions is to establish a repertoire of potentially reactive T cells, while another HLA-associated function is to provide the essential peptide-binding specificity for T cell recognition. For diseases with multiple HLA genetic associations, it is possible that both of these interactions occur and synergize to advance an accelerated pathway of disease.

FURTHER READING

BRAUD VM et al: Functions of nonclassical MHC and non-MHC-encoded class I molecules. Curr Opin Immunol 11:100, 1999

HAMMER J et al: HLA class II peptide binding specificity and autoimmunity. Adv Immunol 66:67, 1997

HILL AV: The immunogenetics of human infectious diseases. Annu Rev Immunol 16:593, 1998

NEPOM GT: Major histocompatibility complex–directed susceptibility to rheumatoid arthritis. Adv Immunol 68:315, 1998

———, KWOK WW: Molecular basis for HLA-DQ associations with IDDM. Diabetes 47:117, 1998

PAMER E, CRESSWELL P: Mechanisms of MHC class I–restricted antigen processing. Annu Rev Immunol 16:323, 1998

STERN LJ, WILEY DC: Antigenic peptide binding by class I and class II histocompatibility proteins. Structure 2:245, 1994

TAUROG JD et al: Inflammatory disease in HLA-B27 transgenic rats. Immunol Rev 169:209, 1999

Specific adaptive immune responses are mediated by developmentally independent, but functionally interacting, families of lymphocytes. T lymphocytes mediate cellular immunity, while B lymphocytes and their plasma cell progeny produce antibodies to provide humoral immunity. The activities of B and T cells and their products in host defense are closely integrated with innate immune functions of other cells of the reticuloendothelial system. Dendritic cells, Langerhans' cells in the skin, and macrophages play an important role in the trapping and presentation of antigens to T and B cells to initiate the immune response. Macrophages also become effector cells, especially when activated by cytokine products of lymphocytes. The scavenger activity of macrophages and polymorphonuclear leukocytes is directed and made specific by antibodies in concert with cytokines and the complement system. Natural killer (NK) cells, a population of granular lymphocytes with receptors specific for major histocompatibility complex (MHC) class I molecules, may spontaneously kill tumor and virus-infected cells, activities that are enhanced by the cytokine products of immune and inflammatory cells. Killing by NK cells can also be targeted by IgG antibodies for which NK cells have cell-surface receptors. The interaction of basophils and tissue mast cells with IgE antibodies in causation of immediate-type hypersensitivity is discussed in Chap. 298. Consideration of these interrelationships is an important part of the analysis of patients with suspected immune deficiency.

DIFFERENTIATION OF T AND B CELLS The functional deficits that occur in both congenital and acquired immunodeficiencies are usefully viewed as being caused by defects at various points along the differentiation pathways of immunocompetent cells. Lymphoid progenitors derived from hematopoietic stem cells may migrate to the thymus to begin T cell development or remain in the fetal liver or bone marrow where they enter the B and NK cell pathways of development (Fig. 297-1). Immature T and B cells then migrate through the circulation to the spleen, lymph nodes, intestine, and other peripheral lymphoid organs. In these sites, they may encounter antigens presented by dendritic cells or macrophages and respond with proliferation, differentiation, and mediation of immune responses. →*Chap. 295 provides a general account of their roles in cellular and humoral immunity.*

Differentiation of T or B cells may be arrested at either the primary or secondary stages. Reflecting the complex cellular interactions involved in immune responses and the pivotal role played by T lymphocytes, immune deficiencies primarily involving T cells are usually also associated with abnormal B cell function.

CLINICAL DISEASE FEATURES COMMON TO IMMUNE DEFICIENCY Immunodeficiency syndromes, whether congenital, spontaneously acquired, or iatrogenic, are characterized by unusual susceptibility to infection and not infrequently to autoimmune disease and lymphoreticular

malignancies. The types of infection often provide the first clue to the nature of the immunologic defect.

Patients with *defects in humoral immunity* have recurrent or chronic sinopulmonary infection, meningitis, and bacteremia, most commonly caused by pyogenic bacteria such as *Haemophilus influenzae*, *Streptococcus pneumoniae*, and *Staphylococcus aureus*. These and other pyogenic organisms also cause frequent infections in individuals who have either neutropenia or a deficiency of the pivotal third component of complement (C3). The tripartite collaboration of antibody, complement, and phagocytes in host defense against pyogenic organisms makes it important to assess all three systems in individuals with unusual susceptibility to bacterial infections.

Antibody-deficient patients in whom cell-mediated immunity is intact have an interesting response to viral infections. The clinical course of primary infection with viruses such as varicella zoster or rubeola, unless complicated by bacterial infection, does not differ significantly from that of the normal host. However, multiple bouts of chickenpox and measles may occur. Such observations suggest that intact T cells may be sufficient for control of established viral infections, while antibodies play an important role in limiting the initial dissemination of virus and in providing long-lasting protection. Exceptions to this generalization are becoming more widely recognized. Agammaglobulinemic patients fail to clear hepatitis B virus from their circulation and

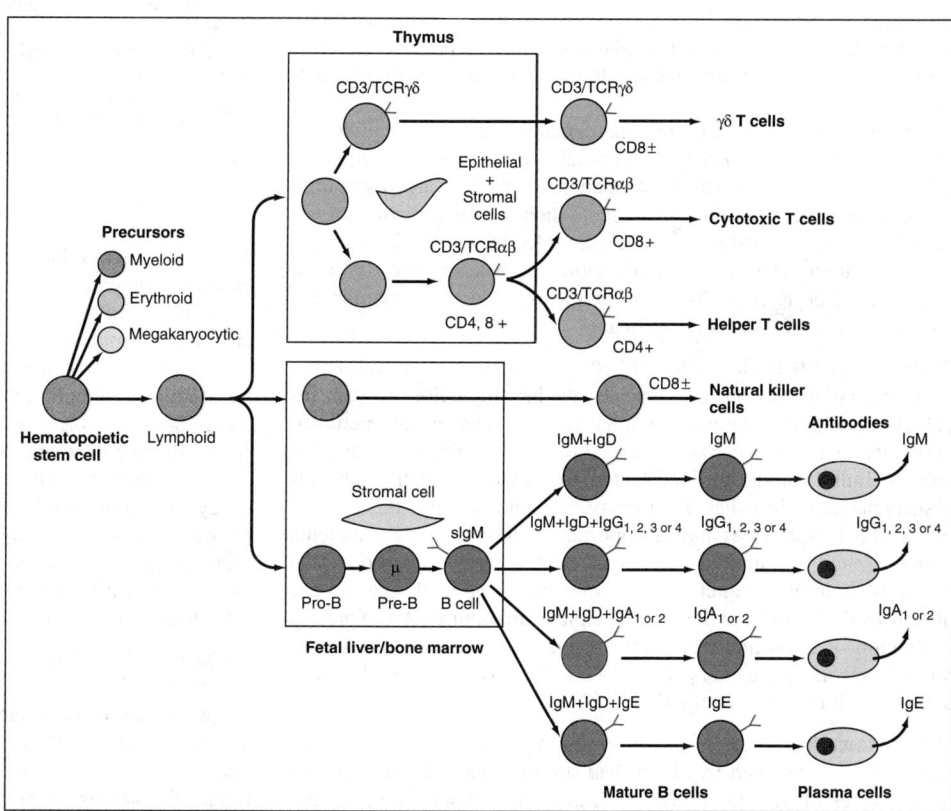

FIGURE 297-1 Hypothetical model outlining the differentiation of hematopoietic stem cells along T, B, and NK cell lineages. The antigen presenting dendritic cells, not shown here, are derived from both lymphoid and myeloid progenitors. Failure to develop T and B cells may result from defective stem cells or from inborn metabolic errors affecting both cell types. Rarely, other hematopoietic cell lines are also absent. Absence of either T or B cells suggests malfunction of central lymphoid tissues, including the thymus and the fetal liver–bone marrow complex. B cell deficiency may result from failure to generate pre-B cells from their stem cell precursors or from failure of pre-B cells to give rise to their B lymphocyte progeny. Similarly, differentiation may be arrested at several levels within the T cell lineage; arrests at the thymocyte level and failure to develop the helper subset have been observed in immunodeficient patients. Agammaglobulinemia and deficiencies of some T cell functions may occur despite the presence of normal numbers of B or T cells in the circulation. Failure of B lymphocytes to differentiate to plasma cells can be due to intrinsic cellular abnormalities or to faulty T cell regulation.

have a progressive, and often fatal, course. Poliomyelitis has occurred following live-virus vaccination in some patients. Chronic encephalitis, which may progress over a period of months to years, is a particular threat in congenitally agammaglobulinemic boys. Echoviruses and adenoviruses have been isolated from brain, spinal fluid, or other sites in such patients.

The occurrence of an unusually serious infection, for example, *H. influenzae* meningitis in an older child or adult, warrants consideration of humoral immune deficiency. Recurrent bacterial pneumonias also suggest this possibility. Chronic otitis media occurs frequently in patients with hypogammaglobulinemia and is significant because of its relative rarity in normal adults. Pansinusitis, although almost invariably present in immunoglobulin deficiency, is a less helpful finding because it is not rare in apparently normal people. Bacterial infections of the skin or urinary tract are less frequent problems in hypogammaglobulinemic patients. Infestation with the intestinal parasite *Giardia lamblia* is a frequent cause of diarrhea in antibody-deficient patients.

Abnormalities of cell-mediated immunity predispose to disseminated virus infections, particularly with latent viruses such as herpes simplex (Chap. 163), varicella zoster (Chap. 164), and cytomegalovirus (Chap. 166). In addition, patients so affected almost invariably develop mucocutaneous candidiasis and frequently acquire systemic fungal infections. Pneumonia caused by *Pneumocystis carinii* is also common (Chap. 191). Severe enteritis caused by *Cryptosporidium* infection may extend to the biliary tract to result in sclerosing cholangitis.

T cell deficiency is always accompanied by some abnormality of antibody responses (Fig. 297-1), although this may not be reflected by hypogammaglobulinemia. This explains in part why patients with primary T cell defects are also subject to overwhelming bacterial infection.

The most severe form of immune deficiency occurs in individuals who lack both cell-mediated and humoral immune functions. Individuals with severe combined immunodeficiency (SCID) are susceptible to the whole range of infectious agents including organisms not ordinarily considered pathogenic. Multiple infections with viruses, bacteria, and fungi occur, often simultaneously. Because donor lymphocytes cannot be rejected by these recipients, blood transfusions can produce fatal graft-versus-host disease.

EVALUATION OF IMMUNODEFICIENT PATIENTS A careful history and physical examination will usually indicate whether the major problem involves the antibody-complement-phagocyte system or cell-mediated immunity. A history of contact dermatitis due to poison ivy suggests intact cellular immunity. Persistent mucocutaneous candidiasis suggests deficient cell-mediated immunity. Lymphopenia and the absence of palpable lymph nodes may be important findings. However, patients with profound immunodeficiency may have diffuse lymphoid hyperplasia. Most immunodeficiencies may be diagnosed by thoughtful use of tests available in local or regional clinical laboratories. More precise evaluation of immunologic functions and treatment may require referral to specialized centers. Table 297-1 presents a résumé of widely available laboratory investigations.

Humoral Immunity With rare exceptions, deficiency of humoral immunity is accompanied by diminished serum concentration of one or more classes of immunoglobulin. Normal values vary with age, and adult concentrations of IgM (1.0 ± 0.4 g/L) are reached at about 1 year, of IgG (10.0 ± 3.0 g/L) at 5 to 6 years, and of IgA (2.5 ± 1.0 g/L) by puberty (Chap. 295). The wide range of values among normal adults creates difficulty in defining the lower limits of normal. Reasonable estimates for low values are below 0.4 g/L for IgM, 5 g/L for IgG, and 0.5 g/L for IgA. In the presence of borderline hypogammaglobulinemia, assessing the patient's capacity to produce specific antibodies becomes particularly important. Isohemagglutinins and "febrile agglutinins" are valuable standard assays, and measurements of pre- and postimmunization titers to tetanus toxoid, diphtheria toxoid,

TABLE 297-1 *Laboratory Evaluation of Host Defense Status*

Initial Screening Assays[a]
Complete blood count with differential smear
Serum immunoglobulin levels: IgM, IgG, IgA, IgD, IgE
Other Readily Available Assays
Quantification of blood mononuclear cell populations by
 immunofluorescence assays employing monoclonal antibody markers[b]
 T cells: CD3, CD4, CD8, TCR$\alpha\beta$, TCR$\gamma\delta$
 B cells: CD19, CD20, CD21, Ig($\mu, \delta, \gamma, \alpha, \kappa, \lambda$), Ig-associated
   molecules (α, β)
 Activation markers: HLA-DR, CD25, CD80 (B cells), CD154 (T cells)
 NK cells: CD16/CD56
 Monocytes: CD15
T cell functional evaluation
 1. Delayed hypersensitivity skin tests (PPD, *Candida*, histoplasmin,
   tetanus toxoid)
 2. Proliferative response to mitogens (anti-CD3 antibody,
   phytohemagglutinin, concanavalin A) and allogeneic cells (mixed
   lymphocyte response)
 3. Cytokine production
B cell functional evaluation
 1. Natural or commonly acquired antibodies: isohemagglutinins;
   antibodies to common viruses (influenza, rubella, rubeola) and
   bacterial toxins (diphtheria, tetanus)
 2. Response to immunization with protein (tetanus toxoid) and
   carbohydrate (pneumococcal vaccine, *H. influenzae* B vaccine)
   antigens
 3. Quantitative IgG subclass determinations
Complement
 1. CH$_{50}$ assays (classic and alternative pathways)
 2. C3, C4, and other components
Phagocyte function
 1. Reduction of nitroblue tetrazolium
 2. Chemotaxis assays
 3. Bactericidal activity

[a] Together with a history and physical examination, these tests will identify more than
95% of patients with primary immunodeficiencies.
[b] The menu of monoclonal antibody markers may be expanded or contracted to focus on
particular clinical questions.

H. influenzae capsular polysaccharide, and *S. pneumoniae* serotypes provide a comprehensive assessment of humoral responsiveness.

Estimation of numbers of circulating B and T lymphocytes is of value in determining the pathogenesis of certain types of immune deficiency. B lymphocytes are identified by the presence of membrane-bound immunoglobulins, their associated α- and β-chain units, and other lineage-specific molecules on the B cell surface (Table 297-1), which can be identified and enumerated by specific monoclonal antibodies.

Since antibody deficiency may be mimicked clinically by deficiency of complement components, measurement of total hemolytic complement (CH$_{50}$) should be a part of the evaluation of host defense. Measurement of C3 alone is inadequate for screening, since deficiencies of both early and late complement components may predispose to bacterial infection (Chap. 295).

Cellular Immunity T lymphocytes may be enumerated by their expression of the TCR/CD3 complex of surface molecules (TCR; T cell receptor). The CD4 molecule serves as a marker for helper T cells, although macrophages also express this molecule in relatively low levels. Conversely, CD8$\alpha\beta$ heterodimers are expressed by cytotoxic T cells. CD8 is also expressed by some $\gamma\delta$ T cells and by NK cells as CD8$\alpha\alpha$ homodimeric molecules.

Normal levels of serum immunoglobulins and antibody responsiveness are reliable indices of intact helper T cell function. T lymphocyte function can be measured directly by delayed hypersensitivity skin testing using a variety of antigens to which the majority of older children and adults have been sensitized. A generally useful skin test antigen is a 1:5 dilution of tetanus toxoid injected intradermally, since almost all individuals will have been sensitized. Purified protein derivative (PPD), histoplasmin, mumps antigen, and extracts of *Candida* or *Trichophyton* also may be used.

T lymphocyte function may be estimated in vitro by the capacity of cells to proliferate in response to antigens to which the patient has been sensitized, to lymphocytes from an unrelated donor, to antibodies that cross-link the CD3/TCR complex, or to the T cell mitogens, such as phytohemagglutinin and concanavalin A. The response is usually quantified 3 days later by measurement of incorporation of radioactive thymidine into newly synthesized DNA. The production of cytokines (or interleukins) by activated T cells can be measured, as can the ability of T cells activated in mixed lymphocyte culture to lyse target cells. Finally, assays exist for detection of defects in T cell surface receptors and specific elements of their signal transduction pathways.

CLASSIFICATION *Primary immunodeficiencies* may be either congenital or manifested later in life and are currently classified according to mode of inheritance and whether the genetic defect affects T cells, B cells, or both (Table 297-2). The following discussion emphasizes three related concepts: (1) that immunodeficiencies are logically viewed as defects of cellular differentiation; (2) that these defects may involve either primary development of T or B cells or the antigen-dependent phase of their differentiation; and (3) that defects of B cell differentiation may in some instances reflect faulty T-B collaboration.

Secondary immunodeficiencies are those not caused by intrinsic

TABLE 297-2 *Primary Immunodeficiencies—Laboratory and Clinical Features*

| | Lymphocytes | | | Cellular Immunity | Humoral Immunity | | | | | |
| | | | | | Serum Immunoglobulins | | | | Antibody Responses | Common Infections |
	B	T	NK		M	G	A	E		
Severe combined immunodeficiency (SCID)										
Adenosine deaminse (ADA) deficiency	−	−	+	−	↓	↓	↓	↓	−	Bacteria, viruses, fungi
Artemis deficiency (SCIDA)	−	−	+	−	↓	↓	↓	↓	−	Bacteria, viruses, fungi
CD45 deficiency	+	−	−	−	↓	↓	↓	↓	−	Bacteria, viruses, fungi
Interleukin receptor γ chain deficiency (X-linked SCID)	+	−	−	−	N	↓	↓	↓	−	Bacteria, viruses, fungi
Janus-associated kinase 3 (JAK3) deficiency	+	−	−	−	N	↓	↓	↓	−	Bacteria, viruses, fungi
Recombinase activating gene (RAG 1/2) deficiency	−	−	+	−	↓	↓	↓	↓	−	Bacteria, viruses, fungi
Reticular dysgenesis	−	−	−	−	↓	↓	↓	↓	−	Bacteria, viruses, fungi
TAP-1 or TAP-2 deficiency (MHC class I deficiency)	+	±	+	−	N	N	N	N	+	Bacteria, viruses, fungi
Primary T Cell Deficiency										
CD8 deficiency	+	±	+	±	N	N	N	N	+	Bacteria
DiGeorge syndrome	+	−	+	−	N	N	N	N	±	Bacteria, viruses, fungi
MHC class II deficiency	+	±	+	+	N	↓	↓	↓	±	Bacteria, viruses, fungi
Nude syndrome (wing helix nude deficiency)	+	−	+	−	N	N/↓	N/↓	N/↓	±	Bacteria, viruses, fungi
Purine nucleotide phosphorylase (PNP) deficiency	+	−	+	−	N	↓	↓	↓	±	Bacteria, viruses, fungi
T cell receptor deficiency (CD3ε or CD3ε deficiency)	+	+	+	−	N	N	N	N	±	Bacteria, viruses, fungi
Zap70 tyrosine kinase deficiency	+	±	+	−	N	N/↓	N/↓	N/↓	±	Bacteria, viruses, fungi
Predominantly antibody deficiency										
IgG subclass deficiency	+	+	+	+	N	N/↓	N/↓	N/↓	±	Bacteria
Autosomal recessive agammaglobulinemia (λ5, Igβ, or BLNK deficiency)	−	+	+	+	↓	↓	↓	↓	−	Bacteria, *Giardia lamblia*
Common variable immune deficiency	+	+	+	+	N/↓	↓	↓	↓	−	Bacteria, *Giardia lamblia*
Selective IgA deficiency	+	+	+	+	N	N	↓	N	±	Bacteria, *Giardia lamblia*
X-linked agammaglobulinemia	−	+	+	+	↓	↓	↓	↓	−	Bacteria, *Giardia lamblia*
Hyper IgM syndrome										
Activation-induced cytidine deaminase deficiency	+	+	+	+	N/↑	↓	↓	↓	±	Bacteria
X-linked CD40 ligand deficiency	+	+	+	+	N/↑	↓	N/↓	↓	±	Bacteria, viruses, fungi
X-linked IKK-gamma (NEMO) deficiency	+	+	+	+	N/↑	↓	↓	↓	±	Bacteria, viruses, fungi
CD40 deficiency	+	+	+	+	N/↑	↓	N/↓	↓	±	Bacteria, viruses, fungi
Other well-defined immunodeficiency syndromes										
Ataxia telangiectasia	+	+	+	+	N/↑	N/↓	N/↓	↓	±	Bacteria
Hyper IgE syndrome	+	+	+	+	N	N	N	↑↑↑	+	Bacteria
Immunodeficiency with thymoma	−	+	+	±	↓	↓	↓	↓	±	Bacteria
Wiskott-Aldrich syndrome	+	±	+	±	↓	N	↑	↑	±	Bacteria
Interferon γ receptor deficiency	+	+	+	+	N	N	N	N	+	Mycobacteria, viruses
Interleukin 12 and interleukin 12 receptor deficiency	+	+	+	+	N	N	N	N	+	Mycobacteria, *Salmonella*
X-linked lymphoproliferative syndrome	+	+	+	+	N	N/↓	N/↓	N/↓	±	Epstein-Barr virus

Note: B, B cells; T, T cells; NK, natural killer lymphocytes; +, normal levels; −, reduced or absent levels; N, ↑, ↓, normal, elevated, or reduced serum immunoglobulins.

abnormalities in development or function of T and B cells. The best known of these is AIDS, which may follow infection with the human immunodeficiency virus (Chap. 173). Other examples are immune deficiency associated with malnutrition, protein-losing enteropathy, and intestinal lymphangiectasia. Also considered secondary are immunodeficiencies resulting from hypercatabolic states such as occur in myotonic dystrophy; immunodeficiency associated with lymphoreticular malignancy; and immunodeficiency resulting from treatment with x-rays, antilymphocyte antibodies, or immunosuppressive drugs.

Incidence   As a group, the primary immunodeficiencies are relatively common. The most frequent, isolated IgA deficiency, occurs in approximately 1 in 600 individuals in Europe and North America. Common variable immunodeficiency, a related disorder characterized by pan-hypogammaglobulinemia, is the next most common disorder. Both of these immunodeficiency states often become clinically evident in young adults.

The more severe forms of primary immunodeficiency are relatively rare, have their onset early in life, and all too frequently result in death during childhood. However, patients with congenital hypogammaglobulinemia may lead relatively healthy lives with adequate antibody-replacement therapy. In a referral center for patients with immunodeficiency diseases, approximately two-thirds of the immunodeficient patients will be adults.

Severe Combined Immunodeficiency   The SCID syndrome is characterized by gross functional impairment of both humoral and cell-mediated immunity and by susceptibility to devastating fungal, bacterial, and viral infections. Inherited either as an X-linked or autosomal recessive defect, affected infants rarely survive beyond 1 year without treatment.

The overall incidence of SCID is 1 in 100,000 to 1 in 1,000,000. The syndrome has been associated with a diversity of defects in development of immunocompetent cells, which are caused by mutations in genes whose products are necessary for the normal differentiation of T, B, and, sometimes, NK cells.

In one autosomal recessive form of SCID characterized by severe lymphopenia, the failure in T and B cell development is due to mutations in the *RAG-1* or *RAG-2* genes, the combined activities of which are needed for V(D)J recombination. A function-loss mutation in either the DNA-dependent tyrosine kinase or the *Artemis* genes may cause SCID, since they also encode essential enzymes for the V(D)J gene rearrangement process. About half of patients with autosomal recessive SCID are deficient in an enzyme involved in purine metabolism, adenosine deaminase (ADA), due to mutations in the *ADA* gene. The abortive lymphoid differentiation associated with ADA deficiency is due to intracellular accumulation of adenosine and deoxyadenosine nucleotides that trigger apoptosis of immature T and B lineage cells.

SCID may also occur with an X-linked inheritance pattern. Aborted thymocyte differentiation and an absence of peripheral T cells and NK cells is seen in X-linked SCID. B lymphocytes are present in normal numbers but are functionally defective. The defective gene encodes a common γ chain of the receptors for interleukin (IL) 2, -4, -7, -9, and -15, thus disrupting the action of this important set of lymphokines. The same $T^- NK^- B^+$ SCID phenotype seen in X-linked SCID can be inherited as an autosomal recessive disease due to mutations in the gene for JAK3 protein kinase deficiency. This enzyme associates with the common γ chain of the receptors for IL-2, -4, -7, -9, and -15 to serve as a key element in their signal transduction pathways.

℞ TREATMENT

The cellular defects in SCID patients logically rest with the pluripotent hematopoietic stem cells or their lymphoid progenitor progeny. Accordingly, the immunologic deficits in all of the different types of SCID patients have been repaired by transplantation of histocompatible bone marrow as a source of stem cells, thereby implying that the stromal microenvironments of these individuals are intact and capable of supporting T and B cell development. However, antibody deficiency

requiring immunoglobulin replacement therapy may persist for years in the γc-deficient and JAK3-deficient patients, unless the defective B cells are eliminated prior to bone marrow transplantation to allow their replacement with normal B cells of donor origin. *Ex vivo* insertion of a γc transgene into bone marrow progenitors has successfully corrected the immune deficiency of X-linked SCID patients. Notably, however, chance insertion of the γc transgene near a tumor-suppressor gene was associated with development of a $\gamma \delta$ T cell lymphoproliferative disorder in two patients so treated. In ADA-deficient patients without histocompatible bone marrow donors, the administration of exogenous ADA (conjugated to polyethylene glycol to prolong its half-life) may improve immunologic function and clinical status. Hematopoietic stem cell gene therapy has also been used successfully in treating ADA-deficient SCID patients; myeloablative conditioning was required to clear a space in the bone marrow for the ADA transduced cells. Treatment of SCID patients should be performed in centers with a strong research interest in this problem. It is crucial that these patients be recognized and treated early. Live viral vaccines or blood transfusions must be avoided since they can cause fatal infections and graft-versus-host disease in SCID patients.

Primary T Cell Immunodeficiency   Reflecting the diversity of T cell functions, abnormalities of T cell development may be responsible for a wide spectrum of immune deficiencies, including combined immunodeficiency, selective defects in cell-mediated immunity, and syndromes presenting as antibody deficiency. These defects may be acquired (Chap. 173) as well as congenital.

THE DIGEORGE SYNDROME   This classic example of isolated T cell deficiency results from maldevelopment of thymic epithelial elements derived from the third and fourth pharyngeal pouches. The gene defect has been mapped to chromosome 22q11 in most patients with the DiGeorge syndrome, and to chromosome 10p in others. Defective development of organs dependent on cells of embryonic neural crest origin includes: congenital cardiac defects, particularly those involving the great vessels; hypocalcemic tetany, due to failure of parathyroid development; and absence of a normal thymus. Facial abnormalities may include abnormal ears, shortened philtrum, micrognathia, and hypertelorism. Serum immunoglobulin concentrations are frequently normal, but antibody responses, particularly of IgG and IgA isotypes, are usually impaired. T cell levels are reduced, whereas B cell levels are normal. Affected individuals usually have a small, histologically normal thymus located near the base of the tongue or in the neck, allowing most patients to develop functional T cells in numbers that may or may not be adequate for host defense.

THE NUDE SYNDROME   The human disease counterpart to the *nude* mouse is caused by mutations of the *whn* (winged-helix-nude) gene that result in impairment of hair follicle and epithelial thymic development. The human *nude* phenotype is characterized by congenital baldness, nail dystrophy, and severe T cell immunodeficiency.

T CELL RECEPTOR DEFICIENCY   Since the expression and function of antigen-specific TCRs is dependent on their signal transducing CD3γ, δ, ϵ, and ζ-η chains, defective genes for any of these receptor components can impair T cell development and function. Immunodeficiencies due to inherited CD3γ and CD3ϵ mutations have been identified. CD3γ mutations result in a selective deficit in CD8 T cells, whereas CD3ϵ mutations lead to a preferential reduction in CD4 T cells, thus implying differences in the signal transduction roles for each CD3 component.

MHC CLASS II DEFICIENCY   Because T cells are required for B cell responses to most antigens, any gene defect (or acquired disorder) that interferes with T cell development and cell-mediated immunity will also compromise antibody production and humoral immunity. MHC class II deficiency results in one such immunodeficiency in that the TCR$\alpha\beta$ must see protein antigens as peptide fragments held within the α helical grooves of class II and class I molecules encoded by the MHC. Antigen-presenting cells in individuals with this relatively rare disorder fail to express the class II molecules DP, DQ, and DR on their surface. Limited numbers of helper CD4 T cells are therefore generated in the thymus, and they fail to see antigen in the periphery. Affected individuals experience recurrent bronchopulmonary infections, chronic diarrhea, and severe viral infections that usually prove fatal before 4 years of age. The defect is caused by mutations in genes that encode essential transcriptional factors that bind to promoter elements for the MHC class II genes. The class II transactivator (*CIITA*) gene is mutated in one subgroup of MHC class II–deficient patients, whereas mutations in *RFX* genes encoding additional transcriptional factors for MHC class II genes are responsible for the defective development and function of CD4 T cells in other families: *RFXANK* in subgroup B, *RFX5* in subgroup C, and *RFXAP* in subgroup D.

ZAP70 TYROSINE KINASE DEFICIENCY Recurrent and opportunistic infections begin within the first year of life in individuals with a deficiency in ZAP70 tyrosine kinase, a pivotal component in the TCR/CD3 signal transduction cascade. The rare inheritance of mutations in both alleles of the *ZAP70* gene results in a selective deficiency of CD8 T cells and dysfunction of CD4 T cells, which are present in normal numbers. Severe immunodeficiency is the inevitable consequence.

PURINE NUCLEOSIDE PHOSPHORYLATION DEFICIENCY Function-loss mutations of the *purine nucleoside phosphorylase (PNP)* gene are associated with an often severe and selective deficiency of T lymphocyte function. This enzyme functions in the same purine salvage pathway as ADA; toxic effects of the PNP deficiency may result from the intracellular accumulation of deoxyguanosine triphosphate.

ATAXIA-TELANGIECTASIA Ataxia-telangiectasia (AT) is an autosomal recessive genetic disorder characterized by cerebellar ataxia, oculocutaneous telangiectasia, and immunodeficiency. The mutant *ATM* gene has sequence similarity to the phosphatidyl-inositol-3 kinases that are involved in signal transduction. The *ATM* gene belongs to a conserved family of genes that monitor DNA repair and coordinate DNA synthesis with cell division. The deleterious effects of the *ATM* gene are widespread. Truncal ataxia may become evident when walking begins and is progressive. Telangiectasia, primarily represented by dilated blood vessels in the ocular sclera, in a butterfly area of the face, and on the ears, is an early diagnostic feature. Immunodeficiency may be clinically manifest by recurrent and chronic sinopulmonary infection leading to bronchiectasis, although not all patients have overt immunodeficiency. Ovarian agenesis is a frequent occurrence. Persistence of very high serum levels of oncofetal proteins, including α fetoprotein and carcinoembryonic antigen, may be of diagnostic value. Frequent causes of death are chronic pulmonary disease and malignancy. Lymphomas are most common, although carcinomas also occur.

The immunologic abnormalities seem to be related to maldevelopment of the thymus. The markedly hypoplastic thymus is similar in appearance to an embryonic thymus. The peripheral T cell pool is reduced in size, especially in lymphoid tissue compartments. Cutaneous anergy and delayed rejection of skin grafts are common. Although B lymphocyte development is normal, most patients are deficient in serum IgE and IgA, and a smaller number have reduced serum levels of IgG, particularly of the IgG2, IgG4 subclasses.

The defect in DNA repair mechanisms in AT patients renders their cells highly susceptible to radiation-induced chromosomal damage and resultant tumor development. AT is a rare disorder, one in 10,000 to 100,000 incidence, but 1% of the population is heterozygous for an AT mutation. This is important because the heterozygous state also predisposes to enhanced cellular radiosensitivity and cancer, especially breast cancer in females (Chap. 353).

℞ TREATMENT

Therapeutic options other than symptomatic treatment are limited for this group of patients. Live vaccines and blood transfusions containing viable T cells should be assiduously avoided. Exposure to x-irradiation should also be avoided in patients with AT. Therapeutic intervention in the form of an epithelial thymic transplant should repair the T cell deficiency in patients with the *nude* syndrome and in the most severe

cases of the DiGeorge syndrome where T cells are absent. Treatment by bone marrow transplantation is sometimes successful after myeloablative conditioning in patients with PNP and MHC class II deficiencies. Preventive therapy for *P. carinii* in the form of trimethoprimsulfamethoxazole should be considered. Immunoglobulin infusions are also recommended for those T cell–deficient individuals with severe antibody deficiency reflected by low serum levels of IgG.

Immunoglobulin Deficiency Syndromes ■ *X-LINKED AGAMMAGLOBULINEMIA* Males with this syndrome often begin to have recurrent bacterial infections in the first year of life when maternally derived immunoglobulins have disappeared. Although B cell progenitors are found in the bone marrow, affected individuals have very few immunoglobulin-bearing B lymphocytes in their circulation and lack primary and secondary lymphoid follicles. The developmental block is evident at the pre-B cell level (Fig. 297-1). Mutations of *Bruton's tyrosine kinase (Btk)* gene are responsible for X-linked agammaglobulinemia. B cells in heterozygous female carriers exclusively utilize the X chromosome with the normal *Btk* gene, while T cells and myeloid cells express either X chromosome. A variant disorder, *X-linked agammaglobulinemia with growth hormone deficiency*, has been associated with *Btk* mutations that result in truncated messages.

Agammaglobulinemia is a misnomer, since most of these patients synthesize some immunoglobulins. Within the same family, some affected males may have substantial levels of IgM, IgG, and IgA, while others are nearly agammaglobulinemic. Btk-deficient patients typically are very deficient in circulating B lymphocytes. The few B lymphocytes that escape the block in pre-B cell differentiation are impaired in their responsiveness to antigenic stimulation, making antibody replacement therapy essential in these patients.

Sinopulmonary bacterial infections constitute the most frequent clinical problem. *Mycoplasma* infections also cause arthritis in some of these patients. Chronic encephalitis of viral etiology, sometimes associated wtih dermatomyositis, can be a fatal complication. These complications are reduced by treatment with intravenous immunoglobulin.

AUTOSOMAL RECESSIVE AGAMMAGLOBULINEMIA This syndrome can result from mutations in a variety of genes whose products are required for B lineage differentiation. For example, signals induced via pre-B receptors are essential for pre-B cell development. Consequently, mutations in any of the genes coding pre-B receptor components—*μ heavy chain, surrogate light chain (VpreB and λ5/14.1), Igα, and Igβ*—can block B lineage differentiation. Congenital absence of B cells, agammaglobulinemia, and recurrent bacterial infections have been seen in children with function-loss mutations in both alleles of the *μ heavy chain* gene or the *λ5/14.1* and *Igβ* genes. Disruption of B cell development may also occur as a consequence of mutations in genes coding transcription factors for pre-B receptor genes or for key elements in the pre-B receptor signaling pathway. For example, mutations in the *BLNK* gene can cause agammaglobulinemia because this gene encodes a cytoplasmic adaptor protein that is essential for B cell development.

TRANSIENT HYPOGAMMAGLOBULINEMIA OF INFANCY This diagnosis is reserved for those rare instances in which normal physiologic hypogammaglobulinemia of infancy is unusually prolonged and severe. IgG levels normally drop to 3.0 to 4.0 g/L between 3 and 6 months of age as maternally derived IgG is catabolized. The IgG levels subsequently rise, reflecting the infants' increased synthetic capacity. Periodic immunologic assessment is needed to differentiate transient hypogammaglobulinemia from other forms of antibody deficiency. Antibody replacement therapy is recommended only in the face of severe or recurrent infections.

IgA DEFICIENCY An inability to produce antibodies of the IgA1 and IgA2 subclasses occurs in approximately 1 in 600 individuals of European origin, a much higher incidence than is seen for other primary immunodeficiencies. IgA deficiency is much less common in people of

Asian and African origin. In Japan, for example, the incidence is approximately 1 in 18,500. While the precise genetic basis for this difference in incidence is unknown, IgA deficiency is frequently associated with certain MHC haplotypes that are more common in Caucasians.

Individuals with isolated IgA deficiency may appear healthy or present with an increased number of respiratory infections of varying severity, and a few have progressive pulmonary disease leading to bronchiectasis. Chronic diarrheal diseases also occur. Reductions in the IgG2 and IgG4 subclasses are associated with the increased infections in some IgA-deficient individuals. The incidence of asthma and other atopic diseases among IgA-deficient patients is high. Conversely, the incidence of IgA deficiency among atopic children has been found to be more than 20 times that in the normal population. IgA deficiency is also significantly associated with arthritis (Chap. 301) and systemic lupus erythematosus (Chap. 300). IgA-deficient patients frequently produce autoantibodies. Some of them produce antibodies to IgA, which make them vulnerable to severe anaphylactic reactions when transfused with normal blood or blood products containing IgA.

An accurate picture of the clinical consequences of IgA deficiency requires lifelong study of affected individuals. Among 204 healthy young adults whose IgA deficiency was identified when they served as blood donors, 80% were found to experience episodes of infections, drug allergy, autoimmune disorders, or atopic disease during the next 20 years of their life. They had an increased susceptibility to pneumonia, recurrent episodes of respiratory infections, and a higher incidence of autoimmune diseases, including vitiligo, autoimmune thyroiditis, and possibly rheumatoid arthritis.

IgA deficiency is often familial. It can also occur in association with congenital intrauterine infections, such as toxoplasmosis, rubella, and cytomegalovirus infection, or following treatment with phenytoin, penicillamine, or other medications in genetically susceptible individuals. The pathogenesis of IgA deficiency, whether genetic or triggered by environmental insult, involves a block in B cell differentiation that may reflect defective interaction between T and B cells.

Treatment of IgA deficiency is essentially symptomatic. IgA cannot be effectively replaced by exogenous immunoglobulin or plasma, and use of either can increase the risk of development of antibodies to IgA. IgA-deficient patients in need of transfusion should be screened for the presence of antibodies to IgA and ideally should be given blood only from IgA-deficient donors. Immunoglobulin infusions may benefit the exceptional IgA-deficient person in whom IgG2 and IgG4 subclass deficiencies are associated with severe infections, but the risk of anaphylactic reactions to contaminating IgA must always be considered in treating these patients.

IgG SUBCLASS DEFICIENCIES Selective deficiencies in one or more of the four IgG subclasses are seen in some patients with repeated infections. The IgG subclass deficiency may easily go undetected when the total serum IgG level is measured, because IgG2, IgG3, and IgG4 together account for only 30 to 40% of the IgG antibodies. Even a deficiency in IgG1 may be masked by increases in the remaining IgG isotypes. However, the availability of subclass-specific monoclonal antibodies allows precise measurement of IgG subclass levels.

Homozygous deletions of genes encoding the constant region of the different γ chains are the basis for the IgG subclass deficiency in some individuals. For example, deletion of the $C_{\alpha1}$, $C_{\gamma2}$, $C_{\gamma4}$, and C_{ϵ} genes in the heavy chain locus on both chromosomes 14 was responsible for one individual's inability to make IgA1, IgG2, IgG4, and IgE. Because other components of their immune system are intact, individuals with this and other patterns of C_H-gene deletions may not have unusual infections.

Most of the IgG subclass–deficient individuals with repeated infections appear to have regulatory defects that prevent normal B cell differentiation. The defect may extend to other isotypes. IgA deficiency may accompany IgG2 and IgG4 subclass deficiencies (see "IgA

Deficiency," above); an inability to produce IgM antibodies to polysaccharide antigens often reflects a broader defect in antibody responsiveness. While patients with IgG subclass deficiency may benefit from administration of immunoglobulin, a thorough assessment of humoral immunity is needed to identify the relatively few who need this therapy.

COMMON VARIABLE IMMUNODEFICIENCY This diagnostic category includes a heterogeneous group, mostly adults, who have in common the clinical manifestations of deficient production of all the different classes of antibodies. The majority of these hypogammaglobulinemic patients have normal numbers of B lymphocytes that are clonally diverse but phenotypically immature. B lymphocytes in these patients are able to recognize antigens and can proliferate in response, but they largely fail to become memory B cells and mature plasma cells. This abortive differentiation pattern leads to the frequent occurrence of nodular B lymphocyte hyperplasia, resulting in splenomegaly and intestinal lymphoid hyperplasia, sometimes of massive proportion.

It is important to note that common variable immunodeficiency and IgA deficiency represent polar ends of a clinical spectrum due to the same underlying gene defect(s) in a large subset of these patients. The two disorders feature similar B cell differentiation arrests, differing only in the numbers of immunoglobulin classes involved. Over a period of years, IgA-deficient patients may progress to the pan-hypogammaglobulinemia phenotype characteristic of common variable immunodeficiency, and vice versa. Both disorders occur frequently within the same family, and the same MHC haplotypes are associated with both immunodeficiency patterns. Family studies suggest an underlying susceptibility gene in the MHC class III region for both disorders.

It is important to consider the diagnosis of common variable immunodeficiency in adults with chronic pulmonary infections, some of whom will present with bronchiectasis. Intestinal diseases—including chronic giardiasis, intestinal malabsorption, and atrophic gastritis with pernicious anemia—are common in this group of patients. Patients with common variable immunodeficiency may also present with signs and symptoms highly suggestive of lymphoid malignancy, including fever, weight loss, anemia, thrombocytopenia, splenomegaly, generalized lymphadenopathy, and lymphocytosis. Histologic examination of lymphoid tissues usually reveals germinal center hyperplasia that may be difficult to distinguish from nodular lymphoma (Chap. 97). Demonstration of a normal distribution of immunoglobulin isotypes and light chain classes for circulating and tissue B lymphocytes can serve to distinguish these patients from those having a monoclonal B cell malignancy with secondary hypogammaglobulinemia. The administration of intravenous immunoglobulin in adequate doses (see below) is an essential part of the prevention and treatment of all these complications.

X-LINKED IMMUNODEFICIENCY WITH HYPER IgM In this syndrome, typically the IgG and IgA levels are very low, while IgM levels may be very high, normal, or even low. The development of B lymphocytes bearing IgM and IgD and the absence of IgG and IgA B lymphocytes indicate a defect in isotype switching. The defective *CD40L* gene in these patients encodes a transiently expressed molecule on activated T cells that is the ligand for the CD40 molecule on dendritic (D) cells and B cells. Gene mutations that preclude normal CD40 ligand expression prevent normal T and B cell cooperation, germinal center formation, V-region diversification by somatic hypermutation, and isotype switching. T cell responses are also compromised in these CD40 ligand–deficient patients because their T cells are deprived of an important activation stimulus as a consequence of the defective T, D, and B cell interactions (Chap. 295). Consequently, these patients experience more severe infections than those occurring with other hypogammaglobulinemic states. In addition to recurrent bacterial infections, pneumonia may be caused by *P. carinii*, cytomegalovirus, *Aspergillus*, *Cryptosporidium*, and other unusual organisms. Enteritis due to cryptosporidial infection may extend into the biliary tract to result in a sclerosing cholangitis and hepatic cirrhosis. Neutropenia is frequent in affected males and increases their vulnerability to infections.

Immunodeficiency with hyper IgM is also seen in patients of both sexes who lack mutations in their *CD40L* gene. One such hyper IgM syndrome is caused by deficiency of activation-induced cytidine deaminase (AID). Patients with AID mutations make IgM antibodies of relatively low affinity because this nuclear enzyme is essential for immunoglobulin isotype switching and somatic hypermutation. The non-X-linked form of immunodeficiency with hyper IgM can also be caused by *CD40* mutation or by mutations of genes coding components of the CD40/CD40L signaling pathways. Impaired signaling through the nuclear factor–kappa B (NF-kB) pathway due to *I Kappa–B kinase gamma IKBKG* mutations can cause an X-linked hyper-IgM and anhidrotic ectodermal dysplasia (XHM-ED) syndrome with or without osteopetrosis and lymphedema.

R̞x TREATMENT

Replacement therapy with human immunoglobulin is the therapeutic cornerstone for antibody-deficient patients who have recurrent infections and who are deficient in IgG. Maintenance of serum IgG levels above 5.0 g/L will prevent most systemic infections in the patients. These serum levels can usually be achieved by intravenous administration of immunoglobulin, 400 to 500 mg/kg, at 3- to 4-week intervals. In patients with mild to moderate IgG deficiency (3.0 to 5.0 g/L) or isolated IgG subclass deficiencies, the decision to treat should be based on evaluation of clinical symptoms and antibody responses to antigenic challenge. Since immunoglobulin preparations are composed almost entirely of IgG antibodies, they are of no value for repairing deficiencies of immunoglobulins other than IgG. Infusions of immunoglobulin are also not benign. While HIV transmission has not been reported, previous epidemics of hepatitis C virus infections in hypogammaglobulinemic patients receiving contaminated immunoglobulin preparations have led to improved safety measures for current commercial preparations. Some antibody-deficient patients develop symptoms of diaphoresis, tachycardia, flank pain, and hypotension during immunoglobulin infusion. This reaction may be resolved by slowing the rate of immunoglobulin infusion. Thrombotic complications, including stroke, myocardial infarction, and pulmonary emboli, have also been reported to be associated with rapid immunoglobulin infusion. Serious anaphylactic reactions may occur as a consequence of antibodies produced by the patient against donor immunoglobulins, particularly IgA (Chap. 99). The potential for severe adverse reactions merits administration of the initial immunoglobulin infusion under medical supervision in a hospital or clinic setting.

A heightened index of suspicion of infection is essential for antibody-deficient patients. Identification of infectious agents in order to select appropriate antibiotic, antiparasitic, or antiviral therapy is also very important. Immunoglobulin infusions usually do not suffice to eliminate chronic sinopulmonary infections with *H. influenzae* and other microorganisms, and a prolonged course of antibiotic therapy may be required to treat these infections effectively and prevent progression to pulmonary fibrosis and bronchiectasis. Maintenance of good pulmonary toilet with regular postural drainage and chest percussion can be especially important in management of these patients. Infestation with *G. lamblia*, a common cause of chronic diarrhea in antibody-deficient patients, usually responds to therapy with metronidazole.

Cryptosporidial infections in CD40 ligand–deficient patients may respond to long-term treatment with amphotericin B and flucytosine. The neutropenia frequently associated with infections in these patients may or may not resolve with improvement of infections and antibody replacement therapy. Bone marrow transplantation following myeloablative pretransplantation therapy can be curative for boys with this devastating immunodeficiency. This treatment has a much greater chance of success when performed during childhood.

Miscellaneous Immunodeficiency Syndromes Infection with *Candida albicans* is the almost universal accompaniment of severe deficiencies in cell-mediated immunity. *Chronic mucocutaneous candidiasis* is different because superficial candidiasis is usually the only major manifestation of immunodeficiency in this syndrome. These patients rarely develop systemic infection with *Candida* or other fungal agents and are not unusually susceptible to virus or bacterial disease. No uniformity of immunologic defects has been identified in these patients, although defects of antibody formation have been detected occasionally. Humoral immunity, including ability to make specific anti-*Candida* antibodies, is usually normal. Many patients are anergic, some to a variety of antigens and some only to *Candida*. The syndrome is often congenital and may be associated with single or multiple endocrinopathies as well as iron deficiency. One well-defined genetic disorder, *autoimmune polyendocrinopathy-candidiasis-ectodermal dystrophy* (APECED) is caused by autoimmune regulator (*AIRE*) mutations. The AIRE transcription factor upregulates ectopic expression of many tissue-specific proteins in the thymus to promote the development of immunologic tolerance to self-antigens. Treatment of associated con-

TABLE 297-3 *Primary Immunodeficiencies Associated with or Secondadry to Other Diseases*[a]

Chromosomal instability or defective repair
  Bloom syndrome (*BLM* helicase)
  DNA ligase IV deficiency
  Fanconi anemia (multiple complementation groups)
  ICF syndrome (*DNMT3B* DNA methyltransferase)
  Nijmegen breakage syndrome (*Nibrin*)
  Seckel syndrome
  Xeroderma pigmentosum (multiple complementation groups)
Chromosomal defects
  Down syndrome (trisomy 21)
  Turner syndrome (X chromosome monosomy)
  Deletions or rings of chromosome 18 (18p- and 18q-)
Immunodeficiency with generalized growth retardation
  Schimke immuno-osseous dysplasia (*SMARCAL1*)
  Dubowitz syndrome
  Kyphomelic dysplasia with SCID
  Mulibrey nannism (*TRIM37*)
  Growth retardation, facial anomalies, and immunodeficiency
  Progeria (Hutchinson-Gilford syndrome)
  Thumb agenesis, short stature, and immunodeficiency
  X-linked agammaglobulinemia with growth hormone deficiency (*BTK*)
Immunodeficiency with dermatologic defects
  Dyskeratosis congenita
    Autosomal dominant (*TERC*)
    Autosomal recessive
    X-linked, Zinsser-Cole-Engman syndrome (*dyskerin*)
  Ectrodactyly-ectodermal dysplasia-clefting syndrome
  Erythroderma desquamative of Leiner
  Griscelli syndrome, partial albinism (*RAB27A*)
  Netherton syndrome (*SPINK5*)
  Omenn syndrome (*RAG 1/2*)
  Trichothiodystrophy, congenital ichthyosis (*ERCC2/XPD* or *ERCC3/XPB*)
Hereditary metabolic defects
  α-Mannosidosis (*MAN2B1*)
  Acrodermatitis enteropathica, zinc deficiency type (*SLC39A4*)
  Propionyl-CoA carboxylase, beta subunit, deficiency (*PCCB*)
  Glycogen storage disease, type 1b (*G6PT1*)
  Hyperzincemia with functional zinc depletion
  Oroticaciduria I (*UMPS*)
  Transcobalamin 2 deficiency (*TCN2*)
Hypercatabolism of immunoglobulin
  Familial hypercatabolism
  Intestinal lymphangiectasia
Other
  Chédiak-Higashi syndrome (*CHS1*)
  Cartilage-hair hypoplasia (endoribonuclease *RMRP*)
  Chronic mucocutaneous candidiasis
  Autoimmune polyendocrinopathy-candidiasis-ectodermal dystrophy (APECED)
  Hereditary or congenital hyposplenia or asplenia
  Ivermark syndrome

[a] Mutant genes indicated in parentheses.

TABLE 297-4 *Genes or Genetic Loci Associated with Primary Immunodeficiencies*

Disorder	Gene or Locus	Chromosome
Severe combined immunodeficiency (SCID)		
Adenosine deaminase deficiency	*ADA*	20q13.11
Artemis deficiency	*ARTEMIS*	10p
CD45 deficiency	*CD45*	1q31-32
DNA-dependent protein kinase deficiency	*PRKDC*	8q11
Interleukin receptor γ chain deficiency	IL2RG	Xq13
Janus-associated kinase 3 deficiency	JAK3	19p13.1
Recombinase activating gene deficiency	*RAG1, RAG2*	11p13
Primary T cell immunodeficiency		
Antigen peptide transporter deficiency	*TAP1, TAP2*	6p21.3
CD8 deficiency	*CD8*	2p12
DiGeorge syndrome	*DGCR1*	22q11
	DGCR2	10p13
Nude syndrome	*WHN*	17q11-q12
T cell receptor deficiency:		
CD3γ	*CD3G*	7q35
CD3ε	CD3E	11q23
MHC class II deficiency:		
MHC class II transactivator (group A)	*CIITA*	16p13
Regulatory factor X, ankyrin-repeat containing (group B)	*RFXANK*	19p12
Regulatory factor X, 5 (group C)	*RFX5*	1q21.1-q21.3
Regulatory factor X-associated protein (group D)	*RFXAP*	13q14
Zeta-chain-associated protein kinase deficiency	*ZAP70*	2q12
Purine nucleotide phosphorylase deficiency	*NP*	14q13.1
Predominantly antibody deficiencies		
Activation-induced cytidine deaminase deficiency	*HIGM2*	12p13
CD40 deficiency	*HIGM3*	20 q12-q13.2
IgA deficiency/common variable immunodeficiency	*MHC*	6p21.3
Immunoglobulin-associated beta (Igβ) deficiency	*CD79B*	17q23
Immunoglobulin heavy chain deficiencies	*IGHG11*	14q32.33
BLNK deficiency	*BLNK*	10q23.2
Surrogate light chain deficiency	*IGLL55*	22q11.21
X-linked agammaglobulinemia	*BTK*	Xq21.3-q22
X-linked hyper-IgM syndrome	*HIGM1*	Xq26
XHM with ectodermal dysplasia (XHM-ED)	*IKBKG*	Xq28
Other well-defined immunodeficiency syndromes		
Ataxia telangiectasia	*ATM*	11q22.3
Interferon γ receptor deficiency	*IFNGR1*	6q23-q24
	IFNGR2	21q22.1-22.2
Interleukin 12 deficiency	*IL12B*	5q31-q33
Interleukin 12 receptor deficiency	*IL12RB1*	19p13.1
Mannose binding lectin deficiency	*MBL2*	10q11.2-q21
Wiskott-Aldrich syndrome	*WAS*	Xp11.23-p11.22
X-linked lymphoproliferative syndrome	*SH2D1A/SAP*	Xq25

ditions may lead to improvement or even cure of *Candida* infection. In other patients, intensive treatment with amphotericin B coupled with surgical removal of infected nails has led to sustained improvement. Oral antifungal agents, such as fluconazole and itraconazole, may also be effective.

INTERFERON γ RECEPTOR DEFICIENCY This immunodeficiency is characterized by serious infections caused by bacille Calmette-Guérin vaccine and environmental non-tuberculous mycobacteria. Associated salmonella infections occur in a minority of the cases. This syndrome can be caused by mutations in the interferon γ receptor signal-transducing chain (*IFNGR2*). Two additional forms of this syndrome are caused by different types of mutations in the interferon γ receptor 1 (*IFNGR1*) gene that encodes the ligand binding chain of the interferon γ receptor. Null mutations in both *IFNGR1* alleles are responsible for a more severe autosomal recessive form. A less severe form, inherited in an autosomal dominant pattern, is caused by *IFNGR1* mutations in a small deletional hotspot that result in a truncated receptor chain lacking the cytoplasmic tail. Accumulation of the truncated receptor on the surface of macrophages compromises their response to interferon γ and the killing of ingested mycobacterium.

INTERLEUKIN 12 RECEPTOR DEFICIENCY Mutations in the gene coding the β_1 subunit of the IL-12 receptor can also result in disseminated mycobacterial infections attributable to bacille Calmette-Guérin and non-tuberculous mycobacteria, and in some cases non-typhi salmonella

infections. Although the clinical manifestations are usually less severe than in patients with complete IFNGR1 deficiency, IL-12 receptor deficiency may predispose individuals to clinical tuberculosis as well. Deficient interferon γ production by the otherwise normal NK and T cells is seen in IL-12 receptor deficient patients, and therapeutic use of interferon γ may cure their mycobacterial infection.

IMMUNODEFICIENCY WITH THYMOMA The association of hypogammaglobulinemia with spindle cell thymoma usually occurs relatively late in adult life. Bacterial infections and severe diarrhea often reflect the antibody deficiency, whereas fungal and viral infections are infrequent complications. T cell numbers and cell-mediated immunity are usually intact, but these patients are very deficient in circulating B lymphocytes and pre-B cells in the bone marrow. They also frequently have eosinopenia and may develop erythroid aplasia. Complete bone marrow failure sometimes occurs. The relationship between the usually benign thymoma and apparent abnormalities of hematopoietic stem cells remains conjectural, and treatment is limited to immunoglobulin administration and symptomatic therapy.

WISKOTT-ALDRICH SYNDROME This X-linked disease characterized by eczema, thrombocytopenia, and repeated infections is caused by mutations in the *WASP* gene. The WASP protein is expressed in cells of all hematopoietic lineages. It may serve a cytoskeletal organizing role for signaling elements that are particularly important in platelets and T cells. The platelets are small and have a shortened half-life. Affected male infants often present with bleeding, and most do not survive childhood, dying of complications of bleeding, infection, or lymphoreticular malignancy. The immunologic defects include low serum concentrations of IgM, while IgA and IgG are normal and IgE is frequently increased. The number and class distribution of B lymphocytes are usually normal. Functionally, these patients are unable to make antibodies to polysaccharide antigens normally; responses to protein antigens may also be impaired late in the course of the disease. Most patients eventually acquire T cell deficiencies. Affected boys frequently become anergic, and their T cells do not respond normally to antigenic challenge. This results in vulnerability to overwhelming infections with herpes simplex virus and other infectious agents.

Transplantation of histocompatible bone marrow from a sibling donor following myeloablative therapy can correct both the hematologic and immunologic abnormalities. In patients lacking a suitable donor, intravenous immunoglobulin infusions or splenectomy may improve platelet counts and reduce the risk of serious hemorrhage. Because of the increased risk of pneumococcal bacteremia, splenectomized patients should receive prophylactic penicillin.

X-LINKED LYMPHOPROLIFERATIVE SYNDROME This disease involves a selective impairment in immune elimination of Epstein-Barr virus (EBV). A fulminant and fatal outcome is the consequence of EBV infection in approximately half of the affected males. Hypogammaglobulinemia is the outcome in 30%, and B cell malignancies are acquired in approximately 25% of EBV-infected patients. The disease may be manifested from early childhood onward, depending on the time of EBV infection. Carrier females handle EBV infections normally. Cytotoxic T cells and NK appear to be primarily responsible for control of EBV infection in normal persons. In males with the X-linked lymphoproliferative syndrome, this process is impaired as a consequence of mutations in a gene coding a T cell and NK cell signaling element called SH2D1A or SAP. Intravenous immunoglobulins should be administered to affected males who develop hypogammaglobulinemia. Bone marrow transplantation from an HLA-matched donor may be curative, especially in younger children with this syndrome. However, myeloablative chemotherapy is a necessary prerequisite to successful bone marrow transplantation, thereby increasing the risk of this procedure.

HYPER-IgE SYNDROME The hyper IgE syndrome (Chap. 55) is characterized by recurrent abscesses involving skin, lungs, and other organs and very high IgE levels. IgE levels may decline with time to reach normal levels in approximately 20% of affected adults. Staphylococcal infection is common to all patients, but most have infections with other pyogenic organisms as well. Abnormal neutrophil chemotaxis is an inconsistent finding, and diminished antibody responses to secondary immunization have been noted. Non-immunologic features include impaired shedding of the primary teeth, recurrent bone fractures, hyperextensible joints, and scoliosis. Males and females are affected in an inheritance pattern suggesting an autosomal dominant defect with variable penetrance, but the gene defect has not been identified. Prophylaxis with penicillinase-resistant penicillins or cephalosporins is highly recommended to prevent staphylococcal infections. Pneumatoceles, a frequent complication of pneumonias, may require surgical excision.

Metabolic Abnormalities Associated with Immunodeficiency The relation of deficiencies of the purine salvage enzymes adenosine deaminase and purine nucleoside phosphorylase to immunodeficiency was discussed earlier. The syndrome of *acrodermatitis enteropathica* includes severe desquamating skin lesions, intractable diarrhea, bizarre neurologic symptoms, variable combined immunodeficiency, and an often fatal outcome. This disease is apparently caused by an inborn error of metabolism resulting in malabsorption of dietary zinc and can be treated effectively by parenteral or large oral doses of zinc. Zinc deficiency

might in part account for the immunodeficiency that accompanies severe malnutrition. Inherited *deficiency of transcobalamin II*, the serum carrier molecule responsible for transport of vitamin B$_{12}$ to tissues, is associated with failure of immunoglobulin production as well as megaloblastic anemia, leukopenia, thrombocytopenia, and severe malabsorption. All abnormalities of this rare disorder are reversed by administration of vitamin B$_{12}$. Finally, primary immunodeficiencies are associated with or are secondary to a number of diverse diseases (Table 297-3).

CONCLUSION Defective genes have been identified for most of the primary immunodeficiency diseases that are currently recognized (Table 297-4). It can be anticipated that many different gene mutations will be identified in other individuals with increased susceptibility to infection. Identification of the mutant genes is the first step toward a better understanding of the pathogenesis of immunodeficiency disease and improved therapeutic strategies. Successful gene repair is the ultimate goal for these individuals.

FURTHER READING

AIUTI A et al: Correction of ADA-SCID by stem cell gene therapy combined with non-ablative conditioning. Science 296:2410, 2002

BUCKLEY RH: Primary cellular immunodeficiencies. J Allergy Clin Immunol 109:747, 2002

BURROWS PD, COOPER MD: IgA deficiency. Adv Immunol 65:245, 1997

FISCHER A: Primary immunodeficiency diseases: Natural mutant models for the study of the immune system. Scand J Immunol 55:238, 2002

GELFAND EW: Antibody-directed therapy: Past, present, and future. J Allergy Clin Immunol 108:S111, 2001

HACIEN-BEY AS et al: Sustained correction of X-linked severe combined immunodeficiency by *ex vivo* gene therapy. N Engl J Med 346:1185, 2002

OCHS HD et al: *Primary Immunodeficiency Diseases.* New York, Oxford University Press, 1999

ROSEN FS et al: Primary immunodeficiency diseases. Report of an IUIS Scientific Committee. Clin Exp Immunol 119(Suppl 1):1, 1999

Section 2   Disorders of Immune-Mediated Injury

298 ALLERGIES, ANAPHYLAXIS, AND SYSTEMIC MASTOCYTOSIS
K. Frank Austen

The term *atopic allergy* implies a familial tendency to manifest such conditions as asthma, rhinitis, urticaria, and eczematous dermatitis (atopic dermatitis) alone or in combination. However, individuals without an atopic background may also develop hypersensitivity reactions, particularly urticaria and anaphylaxis, associated with the same class of antibody, IgE, found in atopic individuals. Inasmuch as the mast cell is the key effector cell of the biologic response in allergic rhinitis, urticaria, anaphylaxis, and systemic mastocytosis, the introduction to these clinical problems will consider the developmental biology, activation pathway, product profile, and target tissues for this cell type.

The fixation of IgE to human mast cells and basophils, a process termed *sensitization*, prepares these cells for subsequent antigen-specific activation. The sensitization of the high-affinity Fc receptor for IgE, designated FcεRI, also stabilizes the cellular expression of the receptor. FcεRI is composed of one α, one β, and two disulfide-linked γ chains, which together cross the plasma membrane seven times. The α chain is responsible for IgE binding, and the β and γ chains provide for signal transduction that follows the aggregation of the sensitized tetrameric receptors by polymeric antigen. Signal transduction is initiated through the action of a *src* family–related tyrosine kinase, termed *Lyn*, that is constitutively associated with the β chain. Lyn transphosphorylates the canonical immunoreceptor tyrosine-based ac-

tivation motifs (ITAMs) of the β and γ chains of the receptor, resulting in recruitment of more active Lyn to the β chain and of the Syk/zap-70 family tyrosine kinases. The phosphorylated tyrosines in the ITAMs function as binding sites for the tandem *src* homology two (SH2) domains within these kinases. Syk activates not only phospholipase Cγ but also phosphatidylinositol-3-kinase to provide phosphatidyl-3,4,5-triphosphate, which allows membrane targeting of the Tec family kinases (Btk and Itk) and their activation by Lyn. The phospholipase Cγ cleavage of the phospholipid membrane substrate provides inositol-1,4,5-triphosphate (IP$_3$) and 1,2-diacylglycerols (1,2-DAGs) so as to mobilize intracellular calcium and activate protein kinase C. The subsequent opening of calcium-regulated activated channels provides the sustained elevations of intracellular calcium required to recruit the mitogen-activated protein kinases, JNK and p38 (serine/threonine kinases), which provide cascades to augment arachidonic acid release and to mediate nuclear translocation of transcription factors for various cytokines. The calcium ion–dependent activation of phospholipases cleaves membrane phospholipids to generate lysophospholipids, which, like 1,2-DAG, are fusogenic and may facilitate the fusion of the secretory granule perigranular membrane with the cell membrane, a step that releases the membrane-free granules containing the preformed mediators of mast cell effects.

The secretory granule of the human mast cell has a crystalline structure, unlike mast cells of lower species. IgE-dependent cell activation results in solubilization and swelling of the granule contents within the first minute of receptor perturbation; this reaction is followed by the ordering of intermediate filaments about the swollen granule, movement of the granule toward the cell surface, and fusion of the perigranular membrane with that of other granules and with the plasmalemma to form extracellular channels for mediator release while maintaining cell viability.

In addition to exocytosis, aggregation of FcεRI initiates two other pathways for generation of bioactive products, namely, lipid mediators and cytokines. The biochemical steps involved in expression of such cytokines as tumor necrosis factor α (TNF-α), interleukin (IL) 6, IL-4, IL-5, IL-13, granulocyte-macrophage colony-stimulating factor (GM-CSF), and others have not been specifically defined for mast cells. Nonetheless, inhibition studies of cytokine production (IL-1β, TNF-α, and IL-6) in mouse mast cells with cyclosporine or FK506 reveal binding to the ligand-specific immunophilin and attenuation of the calcium ion– and calmodulin-dependent serine/threonine phosphatase, calcineurin.

Lipid mediator generation (Fig. 298-1) involves translocation of calcium ion–dependent cytosolic phospholipase A_2 to the outer nuclear membrane, with subsequent release of arachidonic acid for metabolic processing by the distinct prostanoid and leukotriene pathways. The constitutive prostaglandin endoperoxide synthase (PGHS-1/cyclooxygenase-1) and the de novo inducible PGHS-2 (cyclooxygenase-2) convert released arachidonic acid to the sequential intermediates, prostaglandins G_2 and H_2. The glutathione-dependent hematopoietic prostaglandin D_2 (PGD$_2$) synthase then converts PGH$_2$ to PGD$_2$, the predominant mast cell prostanoid.

For the leukotriene biosynthetic pathway, the released arachidonic acid is metabolized by 5-lipoxygenase (5-LO) in the presence of an integral nuclear membrane protein, the 5-LO activating protein (FLAP). The calcium ion–dependent translocation of 5-LO to the nuclear membrane converts the arachidonic acid to the sequential intermediates, 5-hydroperoxyeicosatetraenoic acid and leukotriene (LT)

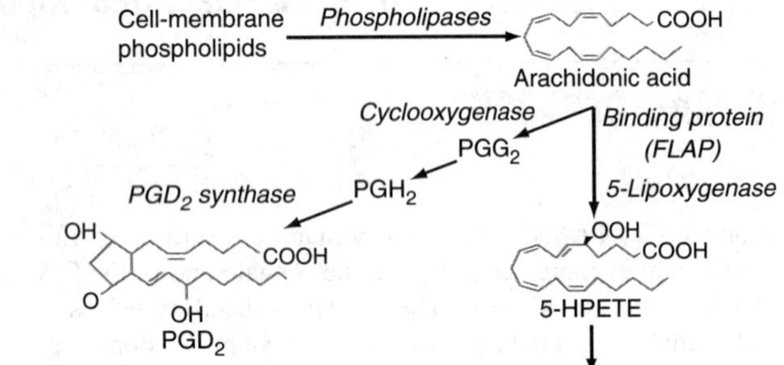

FIGURE 298-1 Pathways for biosynthesis and release of membrane-derived lipid mediators from mast cells. In the 5-lipoxygenase pathway leukotriene A$_4$ (LTA$_4$) is the intermediate from which the terminal-pathway enzymes generate the distinct final products, leukotriene C$_4$ (LTC$_4$) and leukotriene B$_4$ (LTB$_4$), which leave the cell by separate saturable transport systems. Gamma glutamyl transpeptidase and a dipeptidase then cleave glutamic acid and glycine from LTC$_4$ to form LTD$_4$ and LTE$_4$, respectively. The only mast cell product of the cyclooxygenase system is PGD$_2$.

A_4. LTA$_4$ is conjugated with reduced glutathione by LTC$_4$ synthase, an integral nuclear membrane protein homologous to FLAP. Intracellular LTC$_4$ is released by a carrier-specific export step for extracellular conversion to LTD$_4$ and LTE$_4$ by sequential removal of glutamic acid and glycine. Alternatively, cytosolic LTA$_4$ hydrolase converts some LTA$_4$ to the dihydroxy leukotriene LTB$_4$, which also undergoes specific export. Two receptors for LTB$_4$, LTB$_1$R and LTB$_2$R, mediate chemotaxis of human neutrophils. Two receptors for the cysteinyl leukotrienes, CysLT$_1$R and CysLT$_2$R, are present on smooth muscle of the airways and the microvasculature and on hematopoietic cells such as eosinophils and mast cells. Whereas CysLT$_1$R has a preference for LTD$_4$ and is blocked by the receptor antagonists in clinical use, CysLT$_2$R is equally responsive to LTC$_4$ and is unaffected by these antagonists. The lysophospholipid formed during release of arachidonic acid from 1-O-alkyl-2-acyl-sn-glyceryl-3-phosphorylcholine can be acetylated in the second position to form platelet-activating factor (PAF).

Unlike most other cells of bone marrow origin, mast cells leave the marrow and circulate as committed progenitors lacking their definitive secretory granules and characteristic FcεRI. These committed progenitors express the receptor, c-*kit*, for stem cell factor (SCF), and unlike other lineages, they retain and increase its expression with maturation. The SCF interaction with c-*kit* is an absolute requirement for the development of constitutive tissue mast cells residing in skin and connective tissue sites and for the T cell–dependent comitogenesis providing mast cells to mucosal surfaces. Indeed, in clinical T cell deficiencies, mast cells are absent from the intestinal mucosa but are present in the submucosa. Based on the immunodetection of secretory granule neutral proteases, mast cells in the lung parenchyma and intestinal mucosa selectively express tryptase, and those in the intestinal and airway submucosa, skin, lymph nodes, and breast parenchyma express tryptase, chymase, and carboxypeptidase A (CPA). The secretory granules of mast cells selectively positive for tryptase exhibit closed scrolls with a periodicity suggestive of a crystalline structure by electron microscopy; whereas the secretory granules of mast cells with multiple proteases are scroll-poor, with an amorphous or lattice-like appearance.

Mast cells are distributed at cutaneous and mucosal surfaces and in submucosal tissues about venules and could influence the entry of foreign substances by their rapid response capability (Fig. 298-2). Upon stimulus-specific activation and secretory granule exocytosis, histamine and acid hydrolases are solubilized, whereas the neutral proteases, which are cationic, remain largely complexed to the anionic proteoglycans, heparin and chrondroitin sulfate E, so as to function in concert. Histamine and the various lipid mediators (PGD$_2$, LTC$_4$/D$_4$/E$_4$, PAF) alter venular permeability, thereby allowing influx of plasma proteins such as complement and immunoglobulins, whereas LTB$_4$ mediates leukocyte–endothelial cell adhesion and subsequent directed migration (chemotaxis). The accumulation of leukocytes and plasma opsonins would facilitate defense of the microenvironment. The inflammatory response can also be detrimental, as in bronchial asthma, where the smooth-muscle constrictor activity of the cysteinyl leukotrienes is evident and much more potent than that of histamine.

The cellular component of the mast cell–mediated inflammatory response would be augmented and sustained by cytokines and chemokines of mast cell origin. IgE-dependent activation of human skin mast cells in situ elicits TNF-α production and release, which in turn induces endothelial cell responses favoring leukocyte adhesion. Similarly, activation of purified human lung mast cells or cord blood–derived cultured mast cells in vitro results in substantial production of proinflammatory (TNF-α) and immunomodulatory cytokines (IL-4, IL-5, IL-13) and chemokines. Bronchial biopsies of patients with bronchial asthma reveal that mast cells are immunohistochemically positive for IL-4 and IL-5, but that the predominant localization of IL-4, IL-5, and GM-CSF is to T cells, defined as T$_H$2 by this profile. IL-4 modulates the T cell phenotype to the T$_H$2 subtype, determines the isotype switch to IgE (as does IL-13), and upregulates FcεRI-mediated expression of cytokines by mast cells.

An immediate and late cellular phase of allergic inflammation can be induced in the skin, nose, or lung of some allergic humans with local allergen challenge. In the immediate phase of a local challenge, there is pruritus and watery discharge from the nose, bronchospasm and mucus secretion in the lungs, and a wheal-and-flare response with pruritus in the skin. The reduced nasal patency, reduced pulmonary function, or evident erythema with swelling at the skin site in a late-phase response at 6 to 8 h is associated with biopsy findings of infiltrating and activated T_H2 type T cells, eosinophils, basophils, and even some neutrophils. This allergic inflammation proceeding from early mast cell activation to late cellular infiltration has been used as an experimental surrogate of perennial rhinitis or bronchial asthma. However, in bronchial asthma there is a separate variable, intrinsic hyperreactivity of the airways.

Consideration of the mechanism of immediate-type hypersensitivity diseases in the human has focused largely on the IgE-dependent recognition of otherwise nontoxic substances. A region of chromosome 5 (5q23-31) contains genes implicated in the control of IgE levels including IL-4 and IL-13, as well as IL-3 and IL-9 involved in reactive mast cell hyperplasia and IL-5 and GM-CSF central to eosinophil development and their enhanced tissue viability. Genes with linkage to the specific IgE response to particular allergens include those encoding the major histocompatibility complex (MHC) and certain chains of the T cell receptor (TCR-$\alpha\delta$). The complexity of atopy and the associated diseases includes susceptibility, severity, and therapeutic responses, each of which is among the separate variables modulated by both innate and adaptive immune stimuli.

The induction of allergic disease requires sensitization of a predisposed individual to specific allergen. This sensitization can occur anytime in life, although the greatest propensity for the development of allergic disease appears to occur in childhood and early adolescence. Exposure of a susceptible individual to an allergen results in processing of the allergen by antigen-presenting cells of the monocytic lineage located throughout the body at surfaces that contact the outside environment, such as the nose, lungs, eyes, skin, and intestine. These antigen-presenting cells process the allergen protein and present the epitope-bearing peptides via their MHC to particular T cell helper subsets. The T cell response depends both on cognate recognition through various ligand/receptor interactions and on the cytokine microenvironment, with IL-4 directing a T_H2 response and interferon (IFN)γ a T_H1 profile. T cells can potentially induce several responses to an allergen, including those typical of contact dermatitis, known as the T_H1 type response, and those mediated by IgE, known as the T_H2 allergic response. The T_H2 response is associated with activation of specific B cells that can also present allergens or that transform into plasma cells for antibody production. Synthesis and release into the serum of allergen-specific IgE by plasma cells result in sensitization of IgE Fc receptor–bearing cells including mast cells and basophils, which subsequently are capable of becoming activated upon exposure to the specific allergen. In certain diseases, including those associated with atopy, the monocyte and eosinophil populations can express a trimeric high-affinity receptor, FcϵRI, which lacks the β chain, and yet respond to its aggregation.

ANAPHYLAXIS

DEFINITION The life-threatening anaphylactic response of a sensitized human appears within minutes after administration of specific antigen and is manifested by respiratory distress, laryngeal edema, and/or intense bronchospasm, often followed by vascular collapse or by shock without antecedent respiratory difficulty. Cutaneous manifestations exemplified by pruritus and urticaria with or without angioedema are characteristic of such systemic anaphylactic reactions. Gastrointestinal

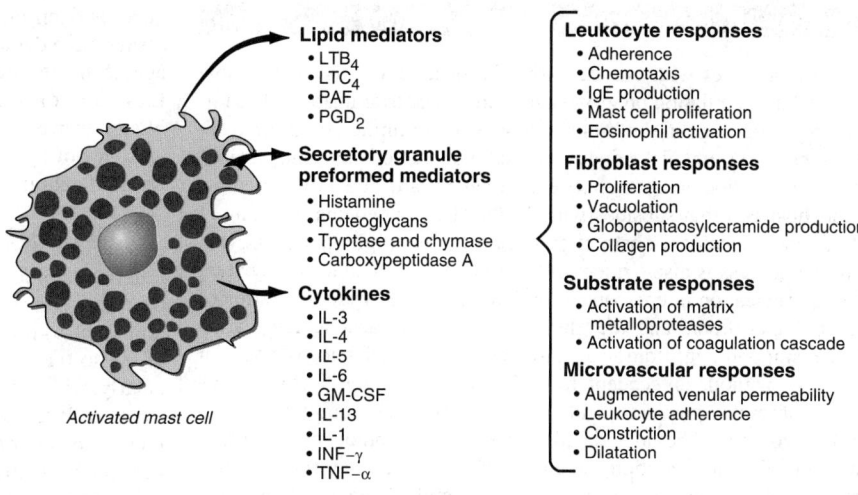

Lipid mediators
• LTB$_4$
• LTC$_4$
• PAF
• PGD$_2$

Secretory granule preformed mediators
• Histamine
• Proteoglycans
• Tryptase and chymase
• Carboxypeptidase A

Cytokines
• IL-3
• IL-4
• IL-5
• IL-6
• GM-CSF
• IL-13
• IL-1
• INF-γ
• TNF-α

Leukocyte responses
• Adherence
• Chemotaxis
• IgE production
• Mast cell proliferation
• Eosinophil activation

Fibroblast responses
• Proliferation
• Vacuolation
• Globopentaosylceramide production
• Collagen production

Substrate responses
• Activation of matrix metalloproteases
• Activation of coagulation cascade

Microvascular responses
• Augmented venular permeability
• Leukocyte adherence
• Constriction
• Dilatation

Activated mast cell

FIGURE 298-2 Bioactive mediators of three categories generated by IgE-dependent activation of murine mast cells can elicit common but sequential target cell effects leading to acute and sustained inflammatory responses. LT, leukotriene; PAF, platelet-activating factor; PGD$_2$, prostaglandin D$_2$; IL, interleukin; GM-CSF, granulocyte-macrophage colony-stimulating factor; INF, interferon; TNF, tumor necrosis factor.

manifestations include nausea, vomiting, crampy abdominal pain, and diarrhea.

PREDISPOSING FACTORS AND ETIOLOGY There is no convincing evidence that age, sex, race, occupation, or geographic location predisposes a human to anaphylaxis except through exposure to some immunogen. According to most studies, atopy does not predispose individuals to anaphylaxis from penicillin therapy or venom of a stinging insect but is a risk factor for allergens in food or latex.

The materials capable of eliciting the systemic anaphylactic reaction in humans include the following: heterologous proteins in the form of hormones (insulin, vasopressin, parathormone), enzymes (trypsin, chymotrypsin, penicillinase, streptokinase), pollen extracts (ragweed, grass, trees), nonpollen extracts (dust mites, dander of cats, dogs, horses, and laboratory animals), food (milk, eggs, seafood, nuts, grains, beans, gelatin in capsules), antiserum (antilymphocyte gamma globulin), occupation-related proteins (latex rubber products), and Hymenoptera venom (yellow jacket, yellow and baldfaced hornets, paper wasp, honey bee, imported fire ants); polysaccharides such as dextran and thiomerosal as a vaccine preservative; and most commonly drugs such as protamine and antibiotics (penicillins, cephalosporins, amphotericin B, nitrofurantoin, quinolones), local anesthetics (procaine, lidocaine), muscle relaxants (suxamethonium, gallamine, pancuronium), vitamins (thiamine, folic acid), diagnostic agents (sodium dehydrocholate, sulfobromophthalein), and occupation-related chemicals (ethylene oxide), which are considered to function as haptens that form immunogenic conjugates with host proteins. The conjugating hapten may be the parent compound, a nonenzymatically derived storage product, or a metabolite formed in the host.

PATHOPHYSIOLOGY AND MANIFESTATIONS Individuals differ in the time of appearance of symptoms and signs, but the hallmark of the anaphylactic reaction is the onset of some manifestation within seconds to minutes after introduction of the antigen, generally by injection or less commonly by ingestion. There may be upper or lower airway obstruction or both. Laryngeal edema may be experienced as a "lump" in the throat, hoarseness, or stridor, while bronchial obstruction is associated with a feeling of tightness in the chest and/or audible wheezing. Patients with bronchial asthma are predisposed to severe involvement of the lower airways. A characteristic feature is the eruption of well-circumscribed, discrete cutaneous wheals with erythematous, raised, serpiginous borders and blanched centers. These urticarial eruptions are intensely pruritic and may be localized or disseminated. They may coalesce to form giant hives, and they seldom persist beyond 48 h. A localized, nonpitting, deeper edematous cutaneous process, angioedema, may also be present. It may be asymptomatic or cause a burning or stinging sensation.

In fatal cases with clinical bronchial obstruction, the lungs show marked hyperinflation on gross and microscopic examination. The microscopic findings in the bronchi, however, are limited to luminal secretions, peribronchial congestion, submucosal edema, and eosinophilic infiltration, and the acute emphysema is attributed to intractable bronchospasm that subsides with death. The angioedema resulting in death by mechanical obstruction occurs in the epiglottis and larynx, but the process is also evident in the hypopharynx and to some extent in the trachea; on microscopic examination there is wide separation of the collagen fibers and the glandular elements; vascular congestion and eosinophilic infiltration are also present. Patients dying of vascular collapse without antecedent hypoxia from respiratory insufficiency have visceral congestion with a presumptive loss of intravascular blood volume. The associated electrocardiographic abnormalities, with or without infarction, noted in some patients may reflect a primary cardiac event or be secondary to a critical reduction in blood volume.

The angioedematous and urticarial manifestations of the anaphylactic syndrome have been attributed to release of endogenous histamine. A role for the cysteinyl leukotrienes in altering pulmonary mechanics by causing marked bronchiolar constriction seems likely. Vascular collapse without respiratory distress in response to experimental challenge with the sting of a hymenopteran was associated not only with marked and prolonged elevations in blood histamine but also with evidence of intravascular coagulation and kinin generation. The finding that patients with systemic mastocytosis and episodic hypotension proceeding to vascular collapse excrete large amounts of PGD_2 metabolites in addition to histamine suggests that PGD_2 is also of importance in the hypotensive anaphylactic reactions. The cysteinyl leukotrienes may be involved in the pathobiologic process in patients with myocardial ischemia without or with infarction.

DIAGNOSIS The diagnosis of an anaphylactic reaction depends largely on an accurate history revealing the onset of the appropriate symptoms and signs within minutes after the responsible material is encountered. When only a portion of the full syndrome is present, such as isolated urticaria, sudden bronchospasm in a patient with asthma, or vascular collapse after intravenous administration of an agent, it may be appropriate to consider a complement-mediated immune complex reaction, an idiosyncratic response to any of the nonsteroidal anti-inflammatory agents, or the direct effect of certain drugs or diagnostic agents on mast cells. Intravenous administration of a chemical mast cell–degranulating agent, including opiate derivatives and radiographic contrast media, may elicit generalized urticaria, angioedema, and a sensation of retrosternal oppression with or without clinically detectable bronchoconstriction or hypotension. Aspirin and other nonsteroidal anti-inflammatory agents such as indomethacin, aminopyrine, and mefenamic acid may precipitate a life-threatening episode of obstruction of upper or lower airways, especially in patients with asthma, that is clinically reminiscent of anaphylaxis but is not associated with a detectable IgE response. This syndrome, which is commonly associated with nasal polyposis, is due to inhibition of PGHS-1 with corresponding unregulated, amplified generation of the cysteinyl leukotrienes via the 5-LO/LTC$_4$ synthase pathway. In the transfusion anaphylactic reaction that occurs in patients with IgA deficiency, the responsible specificity resides in IgG or IgE anti-IgA; the mechanism of the reaction mediated by IgG anti-IgA is presumed to be complement activation with secondary mast cell participation.

The presence of specific IgE in the heart blood of patients dying of systemic anaphylaxis has been demonstrated at postmortem by passive transfer of the serum intradermally into a normal recipient, followed in 24 h by antigen challenge into the same site, with subsequent development of a wheal and flare, the *Prausnitz-Küstner reaction*. To avoid the hazards of transferring hepatitis or other infections to a recipient, it is preferable to use the serum to seek passive sensitization of a human leukocyte suspension enriched with basophils for subsequent antigen-induced histamine release. Furthermore, radioimmunoassays have demonstrated specific IgE antibodies in patients with anaphylactic reactions, but such approaches require purified antigens. Elevations of β-tryptase levels in serum implicate mast cell activation in an adverse systemic reaction and are particularly informative with episodes of hypotension during general anesthesia or when there has been a fatal outcome.

℞ TREATMENT

Early recognition of an anaphylactic reaction is mandatory, since death occurs within minutes to hours after the first symptoms. Mild symptoms such as pruritus and urticaria can be controlled by administration of 0.3 to 0.5 mL of 1:1000 epinephrine subcutaneously or intramuscularly, with repeated doses as required at 20-min intervals for a severe reaction. If the antigenic material was injected into an extremity, the rate of absorption may be reduced by prompt application of a tourniquet proximal to the reaction site, administration of 0.2 mL of 1:1000 epinephrine into the site, and removal without compression of an insect stinger, if present. An intravenous infusion should be initiated to provide a route for administration of 2.5 mL epinephrine, diluted 1:10,000, at 5- to 10-min intervals, volume expanders such as normal saline, and vasopressor agents such as dopamine if intractable hypotension occurs. Replacement of intravascular volume due to postcapillary venular leakage may require several liters of saline. Epinephrine provides both α- and β-adrenergic effects, resulting in vasoconstriction, bronchial smooth-muscle relaxation, and attenuation of enhanced venular permeability. Beta blockers are relatively contraindicated in persons at risk for anaphylactic reactions, especially those sensitive to Hymenoptera venom or those undergoing immunotherapy for respiratory system allergy. When epinephrine fails to control the anaphylactic reaction, hypoxia due to airway obstruction or related to a cardiac arrhythmia, or both, must be considered. Oxygen via a nasal catheter or intermittent positive-pressure breathing of oxygen with inhaled or nebulized albuterol may be helpful, but either endotracheal intubation or a tracheostomy is mandatory for oxygen delivery if progressive hypoxia develops. Ancillary agents such as the antihistamine diphenhydramine, 50 to 100 mg intramuscularly or intravenously, and aminophylline, 0.25 to 0.5 g intravenously, are appropriate for urticaria-angioedema and bronchospasm, respectively. Intravenous glucocorticoids are not effective for the acute event but may alleviate later recurrence of bronchospasm, hypotension, or urticaria. Furthermore, in a syndrome termed *idiopathic anaphylaxis* with recurrent angioedema of the upper airways, glucocorticoid administration may be beneficial by reducing the frequency of attacks and/or the severity of episodes.

PREVENTION Prevention of anaphylaxis must take into account the sensitivity of the recipient, the dose and character of the diagnostic or therapeutic agent, and the effect of the route of administration on the rate of absorption. If there is a definite history of a past anaphylactic reaction, even though mild, it is advisable to select another agent or procedure. A knowledge of cross-reactivity among agents is critical since, for example, cephalosporins share a common β-lactam ring with the penicillins. A prick or scratch skin test should precede an intradermal skin test, since the latter has a higher risk of causing anaphylaxis. These tests should be performed before the administration of certain materials that are likely to elicit anaphylactic reactions, such as allergenic extracts, or when the nature of the past adverse reaction is unknown. With regard to penicillin, two-thirds of patients with a positive reaction history and positive skin tests to benzylpenicilloyl-polylysine (BPL) and/or the minor determinant mixture (MDM) of benzylpenicillin products experience allergic reactions with treatment, and these are almost uniformly of the anaphylactic type in those patients with minor determinant reactivity. Even patients without a history of previous clinical reactions have a 2 to 6% incidence of positive skin tests to the two test materials, and about 3 per 1000 with a negative history experience anaphylaxis with therapy, with a mortality of about 1 per 100,000. Skin testing for antibiotics should be performed only on patients with a positive clinical history consistent with an IgE-mediated reaction and in imminent need of the antibiotic in question; skin testing is of no value for non-IgE-mediated eruptions. Desensitization with most antibiotics can proceed by the intravenous, subcutaneous, or oral route. Typically, graded quantities of the antibiotic are given by the selected route using double doses until a therapeutic dosage is achieved. Due to the risk of systemic anaphylaxis during the course of desensitization, such a procedure should be performed only in a setting in which resuscitation equipment is at hand and an intravenous line is in place. It is critical to give the therapeutic agent at regular intervals to prevent the reestablishment of a sensitized cell pool of large size.

A different form of protection involves the development of blocking antibody of the IgG class, which is protective against Hymenoptera venom—induced anaphylaxis by interacting with antigen so that less reaches the sensitized tissue mast cells; to be effective, this immunotherapy requires the use of specific or cross-reacting Hymenoptera venom. Because sensitization can be transient, the maximal risk for systemic anaphylactic reactions in persons with Hymenoptera sensitivity occurs in association with a currently positive skin test. Although there is only low-grade cross-reactivity between honey bee and yellow jacket venoms, there is a high degree of cross-reactivity between yellow jacket venom and the rest of the vespid venoms (yellow or bald-faced hornets and wasps). Prevention involves modification of outdoor activities to exclude bare feet, wearing perfumed toiletries, eating in areas attractive to insects, clipping hedges or grass, and hauling away trash or fallen fruit. As with each anaphylactic sensitivity, the individual should wear an informational bracelet and have immediate access to an unexpired epinephrine kit. The limitations of lifestyle and the psychological duress can be addressed by venom immunotherapy to achieve a venom-specific IgG titer. Although it has been recommended that venom therapy be continued indefinitely or until the skin and specific serum IgE tests are unremarkable, there is evidence that 5 years of treatment induces a state of resistance to sting reactions that is independent of serum levels of specific IgG or IgE. This contrasts with the definite relation of sting immunity to specific IgG earlier in the treatment regime. For children with a systemic reaction limited to skin, the likelihood of progression to more serious respiratory or vascular manifestations is low, and thus immunotherapy is not recommended.

URTICARIA AND ANGIOEDEMA

DEFINITION Urticaria and angioedema may appear separately or together as cutaneous manifestations of localized nonpitting edema; a similar process may occur at mucosal surfaces of the upper respiratory or gastrointestinal tract. *Urticaria* involves only the superficial portion of the dermis, presenting as well-circumscribed wheals with erythematous raised serpiginous borders with blanched centers that may coalesce to become giant wheals. *Angioedema* is a well-demarcated localized edema involving the deeper layers of the skin, including the subcutaneous tissue. Recurrent episodes of urticaria and/or angioedema of less than 6 weeks' duration are considered acute, whereas attacks persisting beyond this period are designated chronic.

PREDISPOSING FACTORS AND ETIOLOGY The occurrence of urticaria and angioedema is probably more frequent than usually described because of the evanescent, self-limited nature of such eruptions, which seldom require medical attention when limited to the skin. Although persons in any age group may experience acute or chronic urticaria and/or angioedema, these lesions increase in frequency after adolescence, with the highest incidence occurring in persons in the third decade of life; indeed, one survey of college students indicated that 15 to 20% had experienced a pruritic wheal reaction.

The classification of urticaria-angioedema presented in Table 298-1 focuses on the different mechanisms for eliciting clinical disease and can be useful for differential diagnosis; nonetheless, most cases of chronic urticaria are idiopathic. Urticaria and/or angioedema occurring

TABLE 298-1 *Classification of Urticaria and/or Angioedema*

1. IgE-dependent
   a. Specific antigen sensitivity (pollens, foods, drugs, fungi, molds, Hymenoptera venom, helminths)
   b. Physical: dermographism, cold, solar, cholinergic, vibratory, exercise-related
   c. Autoimmune
2. Bradykinin-mediated
   a. Hereditary angioedema: C1 inhibitor deficiency: null (type 1) and dysfunctional (type 2)
   b. Acquired angioedema: C1 inhibitor deficiency: anti-idiotype and anti-C1 inhibitor
   c. Angiotensin-converting enzyme inhibitors
3. Complement-mediated
   a. Necrotizing vasculitis
   b. Serum sickness
   c. Reactions to blood products
4. Nonimmunologic
   a. Direct mast cell—releasing agents (opiates, antibiotics, curare, D-tubocurarine, radiocontrast media)
   b. Agents that alter arachidonic acid metabolism (aspirin and nonsteroidal anti-inflammatory agents, azo dyes, and benzoates)
5. Idiopathic

during the appropriate season in patients with seasonal respiratory allergy or as a result of exposure to animals or molds is attributed to inhalation or physical contact with pollens, animal dander, and mold spores, respectively. However, urticaria and angioedema secondary to inhalation are relatively uncommon compared to urticaria and angioedema elicited by ingestion of fresh fruits, shellfish, fish, milk products, chocolate, legumes including peanuts, and various drugs that may elicit not only the anaphylactic syndrome with prominent gastrointestinal complaints but also chronic urticaria.

Additional etiologies include physical stimuli such as cold, heat, solar rays, exercise, and mechanical irritation. The physical urticarias can be distinguished by the precipitating event and other aspects of the clinical presentation. *Dermographism*, which occurs in 1 to 4% of the population, is defined by the appearance of a linear wheal at the site of a brisk stroke with a firm object or by any configuration appropriate to the eliciting event. Dermographism has a prevalence that peaks in the second to third decades. It is not influenced by an atopic diathesis and has a duration generally of less than 5 years. *Pressure urticaria*, which often accompanies dermographism or chronic idiopathic urticaria, presents in response to a sustained stimulus such as a shoulder strap or belt, running (feet), or manual labor (hands). *Cholinergic urticaria* is distinctive in that the pruritic wheals are of small size (1 to 2 mm) and are surrounded by a large area of erythema; attacks are precipitated by fever, a hot bath or shower, or exercise and are presumptively attributed to a rise in core body temperature. *Exercise-related anaphylaxis* can be precipitated by exertion alone or can be dependent on prior food ingestion. The clinical presentation can be limited to erythema and pruritic urticaria but may progress to angioedema of the face, oropharynx, larynx, or intestine or to vascular collapse; it is distinguished from cholinergic urticaria by presenting with wheals of conventional size and by not occurring with fever or a hot bath. *Cold urticaria*, either acquired or hereditary, is local at body areas exposed to low ambient temperature or cold objects (ice cube) but can progress to vascular collapse with immersion in cold water (swimming). *Solar urticaria* is subdivided into three groups by the response to specific portions of the light spectrum. *Vibratory angioedema* may occur after years of occupational exposure or can be idiopathic; it may be accompanied by cholinergic urticaria. Other rare forms of physical allergy, always defined by stimulus-specific elicitation, include *local heat urticaria*, *aquagenic urticaria* from contact with water of any temperature (sometimes associated with polycythemia vera), and *contact urticaria* from direct interaction with some chemical substance.

Angioedema without urticaria due to generation of bradykinin occurs with C1 inhibitor (C1INH) deficiency that may be inborn as an autosomal dominant characteristic or may be acquired. The angiotensin-converting enzyme (ACE) inhibitors can provoke a similar clinical presentation in 0.1 to 0.5% of hypertensive patients due to attenuated degradation of bradykinin. The urticaria and angioedema associated with classic serum sickness or with hypocomplementemic cutaneous necrotizing angiitis are believed to be immune-complex diseases. The drug reactions to mast cell granule–releasing agents and to nonsteroidal anti-inflammatory drugs may be systemic, resembling anaphylaxis, or limited to cutaneous sites.

PATHOPHYSIOLOGY AND MANIFESTATIONS Urticarial eruptions are distinctly pruritic, involve any area of the body from the scalp to the soles of the feet, and appear in crops of 24- to 72-h duration, with old lesions fading as new ones appear. The most common sites for urticaria are the extremities and face, with angioedema often being periorbital and in the lips. Although self-limited in duration, angioedema of the upper respiratory tract may be life-threatening due to laryngeal obstruction, while gastrointestinal involvement may present with abdominal colic, with or without nausea and vomiting, and may precipitate unnecessary surgical intervention. No residual discoloration occurs with either urticaria or angioedema unless there is an underlying process leading to superimposed extravasation of erythrocytes.

The pathology of urticaria and angioedema is usually characterized by edema of the dermis in urticaria and of the subcutaneous tissue as well as the dermis in angioedema. Collagen bundles in affected areas are widely separated, and the venules are sometimes dilated. The perivenular infiltrate may consist of lymphocytes, eosinophils, and neutrophils that are present in varying combination and number throughout the dermis.

Perhaps the best-studied example of IgE- and mast cell–mediated urticaria and angioedema is *cold urticaria*. Cryoglobulins may be recognized, but not in the majority of patients. Immersion of an extremity in an ice bath precipitates angioedema of the distal portion with urticaria at the air interface within minutes of the challenge. Histologic studies reveal marked mast cell degranulation with associated edema of the dermis and subcutaneous tissues. The venous effluent of the cold-challenged and angioedematous extremity reveals a marked rise in plasma content of histamine, whereas the venous effluent of the contralateral normal extremity contains no increment of this mediator. Elevated levels of histamine have been found in the plasma of venous effluent and in the fluid of suction blisters at experimentally induced lesional sites in patients with dermographism, pressure urticaria, vibratory angioedema, light urticaria, and heat urticaria. By ultrastructural analysis, the pattern of mast cell degranulation in cold urticaria resembles an IgE-mediated response with solubilization of granule contents, fusion of the perigranular and cell membranes, and discharge of granule contents, whereas in a dermographic lesion there is an additional superimposed zonal (piecemeal) degranulation. Elevations of plasma histamine levels with biopsy-proven mast cell degranulation have also been demonstrated with systemic attacks of *cholinergic urticaria* and *exercise-related anaphylaxis* precipitated experimentally in subjects exercising on a treadmill while wearing a wet suit; however, only in cholinergic urticaria is there a concomitant decrease in pulmonary function.

Up to one-third of patients with chronic urticaria have autoantibodies to IgE or to the α chain of the FcϵRI. In these patients, autologous serum injected into their own skin can induce a wheal and flare involving mast cell activation, but the relationship of such antibodies to the clinical course remains to be defined. In vitro studies reveal that these autoantibodies can mediate basophil degranulation with enhancement by serum as a source of the anaphylatoxic fragment, C5a.

Hereditary angioedema is an autosomal dominant disease due to a deficiency of C1INH (type 1) in about 85% of patients and to a dysfunctional protein (type 2) in the remainder. In the acquired form there is excessive consumption of C1INH due either to immune complexes formed between anti-idiotypic antibody and monoclonal IgG presented by B cell lymphomas or to an autoantibody directed to C1INH. C1INH blocks the catalytic function of activated factor XII (Hageman factor) and of kallikrein, as well as the C1r/C1s components of C1. During clinical attacks of angioedema, C1INH-deficient patients have elevated plasma levels of bradykinin, particularly in the venous effluent of an involved extremity, and reduced levels of prekallikrein and high-molecular-weight kinnogen, from which bradykinin is cleaved. The parallel decline in the complement substrates, C4 and C2, reflect the action of activated C1 during such attacks. Mice with targeted disruption of the gene for C1INH exhibit a chronic increase in vascular permeability. The pathobiology is aggravated by administration of an ACE inhibitor (captopril) and is attenuated by breeding the C1INH null strain to a bradykinin 2 receptor (Bk2R) null strain. As ACE is also described as kininase II, the use of blockers results in impaired bradykinin degradation and explains the angioedema occurring idiosyncratically in hypertensive patients with a normal C1INH.

DIAGNOSIS The rapid onset and self-limited nature of urticarial and angioedematous eruptions are distinguishing features. Additional characteristics are the occurrence of the urticarial crops in various stages of evolution and the asymmetric distribution of the angioedema. Urticaria and/or angioedema involving IgE-dependent mechanisms are often appreciated by historic considerations implicating specific allergens or physical stimuli, by seasonal incidence, and by exposure to certain environments. Direct reproduction of the lesion with physical stimuli is particularly valuable because it so often establishes the cause of the lesion. The diagnosis of an environmental allergen based on the clinical history can be confirmed by skin testing or assay for allergen-specific IgE in serum. IgE-mediated urticaria and/or angioedema may or may not be associated with an elevation of total IgE or with peripheral eosinophilia. Fever, leukocytosis, and an elevated sedimentation rate are absent.

The classification of urticarial and angioedematous states noted in Table 298-1 in terms of possible mechanisms necessarily includes some differential diagnostic points. Hypocomplementemia is not observed in IgE-mediated mast cell disease and may reflect either an acquired abnormality generally attributed to the formation of immune complexes or a genetic deficiency of C1INH. Chronic recurrent urticaria, generally in females, associated with arthralgias, an elevated sedimentation rate, and normo- or hypocomplementemia suggests an underlying cutaneous necrotizing angiitis. Vasculitic urticaria typically persists longer than 72 h, whereas conventional urticaria often has a duration of less than 24 to 48 h. Confirmation depends on a biopsy that reveals cellular infiltration, nuclear debris, and fibrinoid necrosis of the venules. The same pathobiologic process accounts for the urticaria in association with such diseases as systemic lupus erythematosus or viral hepatitis with or without an associated arteritis. Serum sickness per se or a similar clinical entity due to drugs includes not only urticaria but also pyrexia, lymphadenopathy, myalgia, and arthralgia or arthritis. Urticarial reactions to blood products or intravenous administration of immunoglobulin are defined by the event and generally are not progressive unless the recipient is IgA-deficient in the former case or the reagent is aggregated in the latter.

The diagnosis of hereditary angioedema is suggested not only by family history but also by the lack of pruritus and of urticarial lesions, the prominence of recurrent gastrointestinal attacks of colic, and episodes of laryngeal edema. Laboratory diagnosis depends on demonstrating a deficiency of C1INH antigen (type 1) or a nonfunctional protein (type 2) by a catalytic inhibition assay. While levels of C1 are normal, its substrates, C4 and C2, are chronically depleted and fall further during attacks due to the activation of additional C1. The acquired forms of C1INH deficiency have the same clinical manifestations but differ in the lack of a familial element and exhibit a reduction of C1 function and C1q protein as well as C1INH, C4, and C2. Inborn and acquired C1INH deficiency and ACE inhibitor–elicited angioedema are associated with elevated levels of bradykinin.

Urticaria and angioedema must be differentiated from contact sensitivity, a vesicular eruption that progresses to chronic thickening of the skin with continued allergenic exposure. They must also be differentiated from atopic dermatitis, a condition that may present as erythema, edema, papules, vesiculation, and oozing proceeding to a subacute and chronic stage in which vesiculation is less marked or absent and scaling, fissuring, and lichenification predominate in a distribution that characteristically involves the flexor surfaces. In cutaneous mastocytosis, the reddish brown macules and papules, characteristic of urticaria pigmentosa, urticate with pruritus upon trauma; and in systemic mastocytosis, without or with urticaria pigmentosa, there is an episodic systemic flushing with or without urticaria but no angioedema.

℞ TREATMENT

Identification of the etiologic factor(s) and their elimination provide the most satisfactory therapeutic program; this approach is feasible to varying degrees with IgE-mediated reactions to allergens or physical stimuli. For most forms of urticaria, H_1 antihistamines such as chlorpheniramine or diphenhydramine, and including the nonsedating class such as loratadine or cetirizine, are effective in attenuating both urtication and pruritus. Cyproheptadine and especially hydroxyzine have proven effective when H_1 antihistamines have been inadequate. Doxepin, a dibenzoxepin tricyclic compound with both H_1 and H_2 receptor antagonist activity, is yet another alternative. Terbutaline, an α-adrenergic agonist, or a $CysLT_1R$ antagonist may be added to the treatment regimen. Topical glucocorticoids are of no value, and systemic glucocorticoids are generally avoided in idiopathic, allergen-induced, or physical urticarias due to their long-term toxicity. Systemic glucocorticoids are useful in the management of patients with pressure urticaria, with vasculitic urticaria (especially with eosinophil prominence), with idiopathic angioedema with or without urticaria, or with chronic urticaria that responds poorly to conventional treatment. With persistent vasculitic urticaria, hydroxychloroquine or colchicine may be added to the regimen after hydroxyzine and before or along with systemic glucocorticoids.

The therapy of inborn C1INH deficiency has been simplified by the finding that attenuated androgens correct the biochemical defect and afford prophylactic protection; their efficacy is attributed to production by the normal gene of an amount of functional C1INH sufficient to control the spontaneous activation of C1. The antifibrinolytic agent ϵ-aminocaproic acid may be used for preoperative prophylaxis but is contraindicated in patients with thrombotic tendencies or ischemia due to arterial atherosclerosis. Infusion of isolated C1INH protein appears useful in prophylaxis and to ameliorate an attack.

SYSTEMIC MASTOCYTOSIS

DEFINITION *Systemic mastocytosis* is defined by mast cell hyperplasia that in most instances is indolent and nonneoplastic. The hyperplasia is generally recognized only in bone marrow and in the normal peripheral distribution sites of the cells, such as skin, gastrointestinal mucosa, liver, and spleen. Mastocytosis occurs at any age and has a slight preponderance in males. The prevalence of systemic mastocytosis is not known, a familial occurrence has not been established, and atopy is not increased.

CLASSIFICATION AND PATHOPHYSIOLOGY A recent consensus classification for mastocytosis recognizes cutaneous mastocytosis with variants and four systemic forms (Table 298-2). The form designated as *indolent systemic mastocytosis* (ISM) accounts for the majority of patients; it implies that there is no evidence of an associated hematologic disorder, liver disease, or lymphadenopathy and is not known to alter life expectancy. In *systemic mastocytosis associated with clonal hematologic non-mast cell lineage disease* (SM-AHNMD), the prognosis is determined by the nature of the associated disorder, which can range from dysmyelopoiesis to leukemia. In *aggressive systemic mastocytosis* (ASM), mast cell proliferation in parenchymal organs causing impaired liver function, hypersplenism, and/or malabsorption has a poor

TABLE 298-2 *Classification of Mastocytosis*

Cutaneous mastocytosis (CM)
   Urticaria pigmentosa (UP)/maculopapular cutaneous mastocytosis (MPCM)
     Variants: plaque form, nodular form; telangiectasia macularis eruptive perstans (TMEP); diffuse cutaneous mastocytosis (DCM)
     Solitary mastocytoma of skin
Indolent systemic mastocytosis (ISM)
Systemic mastocytosis with an associated clonal hematologic non-mast cell lineage disease (SM-AHNMD)
Aggressive systemic mastocytosis (ASM)
     Variant: lymphadenopathic mastocytosis with eosinophilia
Mast cell leukemia (MCL)
Mast cell sarcoma (MCS)

Source: Modified from P Valent et al, in ES Jaffee et al (eds): *World Health Organization Classification of Tumors: Pathology and Genetics in Tumors of Hematopoietic and Lymphoid Tissues*, Lyon, IARC Press, 2001.

prognosis in the absence of a hematologic disorder; a subset of these patients have prominent eosinophilia with hepatosplenomegaly and lymphadenopathy. *Mast cell leukemia* is the rarest form of the disease and is invariably fatal at present; the peripheral blood contains circulating, metachromatically staining, atypical mast cells.

A point mutation of A to T at codon 816 that causes an aspartic acid to valine substitution is found in multiple cell lineages in patients with mastocytosis, indicating a somatic gain-in-function mutation. This substitution, as well as others at 816, is characteristic of adults with SM-AHNMD but is also detected in patients with ISM and cutaneous mastocytosis, as might be anticipated because mast cells at any site are of bone marrow lineage. In infants and children with cutaneous manifestations, namely, urticaria pigmentosa or bullous lesions, visceral involvement is usually lacking, and resolution is common because gain-in-function mutations are infrequent.

CLINICAL MANIFESTATIONS The clinical manifestations of systemic mastocytosis, distinct from a leukemic complication, are due to tissue occupancy by the mast cell mass, the tissue response to that mass, and the release of bioactive substances acting at both local and distal sites. The pharmacologically induced manifestations are pruritus, flushing, palpitations and vascular collapse, gastric distress, lower abdominal crampy pain, and recurrent headache. The increase in cell burden is evidenced by the lesions of urticaria pigmentosa at skin sites, but it also contributes to bone pain and malabsorption. The mast cell—mediated fibrotic changes are limited to liver, spleen, and bone marrow and presumably relate to the functional characteristics of mast cells developing at those sites, as opposed to those at sites without fibrosis, such as the gastrointestinal tissue or skin. Immunofluorescent analysis of bone marrow and skin lesions in ISM and of spleen, lymph node, and skin in ASM has revealed only one mast cell phenotype, namely, scroll-poor cells expressing tryptase, chymase, and CPA.

The cutaneous lesions of urticaria pigmentosa are reddish-brown macules or papules that respond to trauma with urtication and erythema (Darier's sign). The apparent incidence of these lesions is ≥90% in patients with ISM and <50% in those with SM-AHNMD or ASM. Approximately 1% of patients with ISM have skin lesions that appear as tan-brown macules with striking patchy erythema and associated telangiectasia (telangiectasia macularis eruptiva perstans). In the upper gastrointestinal tract, histamine-mediated hypersecretion is the most common problem, with resultant gastritis and peptic ulcer. In the lower intestinal tract, the occurrence of diarrhea and abdominal pain is attributed to increased motility due to mast cell mediators, and this can be aggravated by malabsorption with secondary nutritional insufficiency and osteomalacia. The periportal fibrosis associated with mast cell infiltration and a prominence of eosinophils may lead to portal hypertension and ascites. In some patients, flushing and recurrent vascular collapse are markedly aggravated by an idiosyncratic response to a minimal dosage of nonsteroidal anti-inflammatory agents. The neuropsychiatric disturbances are clinically most evident as impaired recent memory, decreased attention span, and "migraine-like" headaches. Patients in every category of systemic mastocytosis may experience exacerbation of a specific clinical sign or symptom with alcohol ingestion, use of mast cell–interactive narcotics, or ingestion of nonsteroidal anti-inflammatory agents.

DIAGNOSIS Although the diagnosis of mastocytosis is generally suspected on the basis of the clinical history and physical findings, and can be supported by laboratory procedures, it can be established only by a tissue diagnosis. By recent convention, the diagnosis of systemic mastocytosis is facilitated by bone marrow biopsy to meet the criteria of one major plus one minor or three minor findings (Table 298-3). The bone marrow provides the major criterion by revealing aggregates of mast cells, often in paratrabecular and perivascular locations with lymphocytes and eosinophils, as well as the minor criteria of an abnormal mast cell morphology, an aberrant mast cell membrane immunophenotype, or a codon 816 mutation in any cell type. A serum total tryptase level and/or a 24-h urine collection for measurement of histamine, histamine metabolites, or metabolites of PGD_2 are useful common noninvasive approaches to consider before bone marrow biopsy. The α form of tryptase is elevated in more than one-half of patients with systemic mastocytosis and provides a minor criterion; the β form is increased in patients undergoing an anaphylactic reaction. Additional studies directed by the presentation include a bone scan or skeletal survey; contrast studies of the upper gastrointestinal tract with small-bowel follow-through, computed tomography scan, or endoscopy; and a neuropsychiatric evaluation, including an electroencephalogram.

The differential diagnosis requires the exclusion of other flushing disorders. The 24-h urine assessment of 5-hydroxy-indoleacetic acid and metanephrines should exclude a carcinoid tumor or a pheochromocytoma. Most patients with recurrent anaphylaxis, including the idiopathic group, present with angioedema and/or wheezing, which are not manifestations of systemic mastocytosis.

℞ TREATMENT

The management of systemic mastocytosis uses a stepwise and symptom/sign–directed approach that includes an H_1 antihistamine for flushing and pruritus, an H_2 antihistamine or proton pump inhibitor for gastric acid hypersecretion, oral cromolyn sodium for diarrhea and abdominal pain, and aspirin for severe flushing with or without associated vascular collapse, despite use of H_1 and H_2 antihistamines, to block biosynthesis of PGD_2. Systemic glucocorticoids appear to alleviate the malabsorption. Headaches are generally managed with tricyclic antidepressants and other neurotransmitter-modifying agents. Ketotifen has been used to alleviate flushing in patients with gastric intolerance to nonsteroidal anti-inflammatory agents and in patients with bone pain or intractable headaches. The efficacy of IFN-α in ASM is controversial, and this may relate to dosage limitations due to side effects. Treatment with hydroxyurea to reduce the mast cell lineage progenitors may have merit in ASM. Chemotherapy is appropriate for the frank leukemias.

TABLE 298-3 *Diagnostic Criteria for Systemic Mastocytosis*[a]

Major: Multifocal dense infiltrates of mast cells in bone marrow or other extracutaneous tissues with confirmation by immunodetection of tryptase or metachromasia

Minor: Abnormal mast cell morphology with a spindle shape and/or multilobed or eccentric nucleus

Aberrant mast cell surface phenotype with expression of CD25 and CD2 (IL-2 receptor) in addition to C117 (c-*kit*)

Detection of codon 816 mutation in peripheral blood cells, bone marrow cells, or lesional tissue

Total serum tryptase (mostly alpha) greater than 20 ng/mL

[a] Diagnosis requires either major and one minor or three minor criteria.

ALLERGIC RHINITIS

DEFINITION Allergic rhinitis is characterized by sneezing; rhinorrhea; obstruction of the nasal passages; conjunctival, nasal, and pharyngeal itching; and lacrimation, all occurring in a temporal relationship to allergen exposure. Although commonly seasonal due to elicitation by airborne pollens, it can be perennial in an environment of chronic exposure. The incidence of allergic rhinitis in North America is about 7%, with the peak occurring in childhood and adolescence.

PREDISPOSING FACTORS AND ETIOLOGY Allergic rhinitis generally presents in atopic individuals, i.e., in persons with a family history of a similar or related symptom complex and a personal history of collateral allergy expressed as eczematous dermatitis, urticaria, and/or asthma (Chap. 236). Up to 40% of patients with rhinitis manifest asthma, whereas ~70% of individuals with asthma experience rhinitis. Symptoms generally appear before the fourth decade of life and tend to diminish gradually with aging, although complete spontaneous remissions are uncommon. A relatively small number of weeds that depend on wind rather than insects for cross-pollination, as well as grasses and some trees, produce sufficient quantities of pollen suitable for wide distribution by air currents to elicit seasonal allergic rhinitis. The dates of pollination of these species generally vary little from year to year in a particular locale but may be quite different in another climate. In the temperate areas of North America, trees typically pollinate from March through May, grasses in June and early July, and ragweed from mid-August to early October. Molds, which are widespread in nature because they occur in soil or decaying organic matter, may propagate spores in a pattern dependent on climatic conditions. Perennial allergic rhinitis occurs in response to allergens that are present throughout the year, including desquamating epithelium in animal dander, cockroach-derived proteins, mold spores, or dust, which has mites such as *Dermatophagoides farinae* and *D. pteronyssinus*. Dust mites are scavengers of flecks of human skin and coat the digestate with mite-specific protein for excretion. In up to one-half of patients with perennial rhinitis, no clear-cut allergen can be demonstrated as causative. The ability of allergens to cause rhinitis rather than lower respiratory symptoms may be attributed to their large size, 10 to 100 μm, and retention within the nose.

PATHOPHYSIOLOGY AND MANIFESTATIONS Episodic rhinorrhea, sneezing, obstruction of the nasal passages with lacrimation, and pruritus of the conjunctiva, nasal mucosa, and oropharynx are the hallmarks of allergic rhinitis. The nasal mucosa is pale and boggy, the conjunctiva congested and edematous, and the pharynx is generally unremarkable. Swelling of the turbinates and mucous membranes with obstruction of the sinus ostia and eustachian tubes precipitates secondary infections of the sinuses and middle ear, respectively. Nasal polyps, representing mucosal protrusions containing edema fluid with variable numbers of eosinophils, can arise concurrently with infection within the nasopharynx or sinuses and increase obstructive symptoms.

The nose presents a large mucosal surface area through the folds of the turbinates and serves to adjust the temperature and moisture content of inhaled air and to filter out particulate materials above 10 μm in size by impingement in a mucous blanket; ciliary action moves the entrapped particles toward the pharynx. Entrapment of pollen and digestion of the outer coat by mucosal enzymes such as lysozymes release protein allergens generally of 10,000 to 40,000 molecular weight. The initial interaction occurs between the allergen and intraepithelial mast cells and then proceeds to involve deeper perivenular mast cells, both of which are sensitized with specific IgE. During the symptomatic season when the mucosae are already swollen and hyperemic, there is enhanced adverse reactivity to the seasonal pollen as well as to antigenically unrelated pollens for which there is underlying hypersensitivity due to improved penetration of the allergens. Biopsy specimens of nasal mucosa during seasonal rhinitis show submucosal edema with infiltration by eosinophils, along with some basophils and neutrophils.

The mucosal surface fluid contains IgA that is present because of its secretory piece and also IgE, which apparently arrives by diffusion from plasma cells in proximity to mucosal surfaces. IgE fixes to mucosal and submucosal mast cells, and the intensity of the clinical response to inhaled allergens is quantitatively related to the naturally occurring pollen dose. In sensitive individuals, the introduction of allergen into the nose is associated with sneezing, "stuffiness," and discharge, and the fluid contains histamine, PGD_2, and leukotrienes. Thus the mast cells of the nasal mucosa and submucosa generate and release mediators through IgE-dependent reactions that are capable of producing tissue edema and eosinophilic infiltration.

DIAGNOSIS The diagnosis of seasonal allergic rhinitis depends largely on an accurate history of occurrence coincident with the pollination of the offending weeds, grasses, or trees. The continuous character of perennial allergic rhinitis due to contamination of the home or place of work makes historic analysis difficult, but there may be a variability in symptoms that can be related to exposure to animal dander, dust mite and/or cockroach allergens, or work-related allergens such as latex. Patients with perennial rhinitis commonly develop the problem in adult life, and manifest nasal congestion and a postnasal discharge, often associated with thickening of the sinus membranes demonstrated by radiography. The term *vasomotor rhinitis* designates a condition of enhanced reactivity of the nasopharynx in which a symptom complex resembling perennial allergic rhinitis occurs with nonspecific stimuli. Other entities to be excluded are structural abnormalities of the nasopharynx; exposure to irritants; upper respiratory infection; pregnancy with prominent nasal mucosal edema; prolonged topical use of α-adrenergic agents in the form of nose drops (rhinitis medicamentosa); and the use of certain therapeutic agents such as rauwolfia, β-adrenergic antagonists, or estrogens.

The nasal secretions of allergic patients are rich in eosinophils, and a modest peripheral eosinophilia is a common feature. Local or systemic neutrophilia implies infection. Total serum IgE is frequently elevated, but the demonstration of immunologic specificity for IgE is critical to an etiologic diagnosis. A skin test by the intracutaneous route (puncture or prick) with the allergens of interest provides a rapid and reliable approach to identifying allergen-specific IgE that has sensitized cutaneous mast cells. A positive intracutaneous skin test with 1:10 to 1:20 weight/volume of extract has a high predictive value for the presence of allergy. An intradermal test with a 1:500 to 1:1000 dilution of 0.05 mL may follow if indicated by history when the intracutaneous test is negative; but while more sensitive, it is less reliable due to the reactivity of some asymptomatic individuals at the test dose. Skin testing by the intracutaneous route for food allergens can be supportive of the clinical history. A double-blind, placebo-controlled challenge may document a food allergy, but such a procedure does bear the risk of an anaphylactic reaction. An elimination diet is safer but is tedious and less definitive. Food allergy is uncommon as a cause of allergic rhinitis.

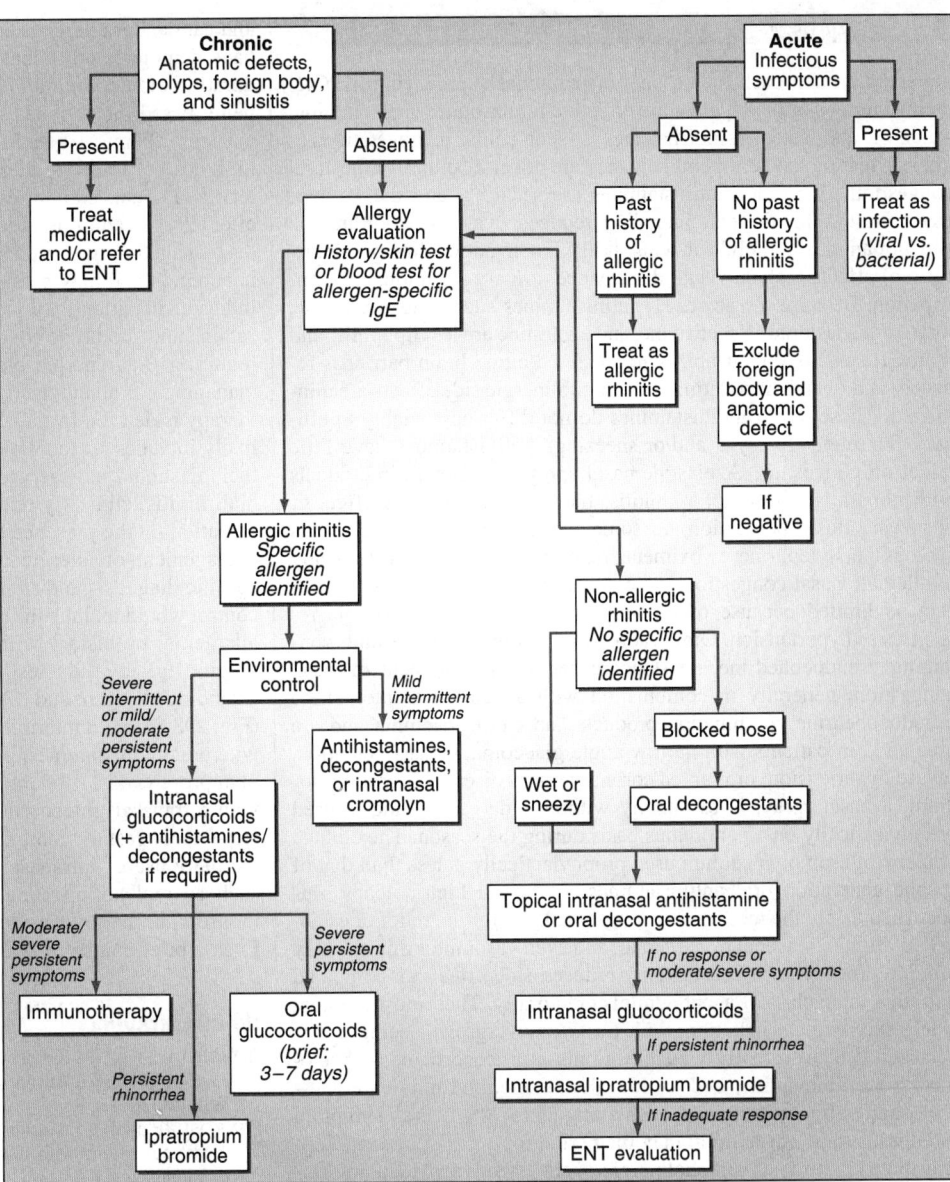

FIGURE 298-3 Algorithm for the diagnosis and management of rhinitis. ENT, ear, nose, and throat surgeon.

Newer methodology for detecting total IgE, including the development of enzyme-linked immunosorbent assays (ELISA) employing anti-IgE bound to either a solid-phase or a liquid-phase particle, provides rapid and cost-effective determinations. Measurements of specific anti-IgE in serum are obtained by its binding to an allergen and quantitation by subsequent uptake of labeled anti-IgE. As compared to the skin test, the assay of specific IgE in serum is less sensitive but has high specificity.

PREVENTION Avoidance of exposure to the offending allergen is the most effective means of controlling allergic diseases; removal of pets from the home to avoid animal danders, utilization of air filtration devices to minimize the concentrations of airborne pollens, elimination of cockroach-derived proteins by chemical destruction of the pest and careful food storage, travel to nonpollinating areas during the critical periods, and even a change of domicile to eliminate a mold spore problem may be necessary. Control of dust mites by allergen avoidance includes use of plastic-lined covers for mattresses, pillows, and comforters, and elimination of carpets and drapes.

℞ TREATMENT

Although allergen avoidance is the most cost-effective means of managing allergic rhinitis, treatment with pharmacologic agents represents the standard approach to seasonal or perennial allergic rhinitis. Oral antihistamines of the H_1 class are effective for nasopharyngeal itching, sneezing, and watery rhinorrhea and for such ocular manifestations as itching, tearing, and erythema, but they are not efficacious for the nasal congestion. The older antihistamines are sedating, and they induce psychomotor impairment, including reduced eye-hand coordination and impaired automobile driving skills. Their anticholinergic (muscarinic) effects include visual disturbance, urinary retention, and constipation. Because the newer H_1 antihistamines such as fexofenadine, loratadine, desloradine, cetirizine, and azelastine are less lipophilic and more H_1 selective, their ability to cross the blood-brain barrier is reduced, and thus their sedating and anticholinergic side effects are minimized. These newer antihistamines do not differ appreciably in efficacy for relief of coryza and/or sneezing. Antihistamines have little effect on congestion. Azelastine nasal spray may benefit individuals with nonallergic vasomotor rhinitis, but it has an adverse effect of dysgeusia (taste perversion) in some patients. α-Adrenergic agents such as phenylephrine or oximetazoline are generally used topically to alleviate nasal congestion and obstruction, but the duration of efficacy is limited because of rebound rhinitis and such systemic responses as hypertension. Oral α-adrenergic agonist decongestants containing pseudoephedrine are standard for the management of nasal congestion, generally in combination with an antihistamine. These pseudoephedrine combination products can cause insomnia and are precluded in patients with narrow angle glaucoma, urinary retention, severe hypertension, or marked coronary artery disease. Cromolyn sodium, a nasal spray, is essentially without side effects and is used prophylactically on a continuous basis during the season. The clinical efficacy of cromolyn sodium used prophylactically is less than that of second-generation oral antihistamines. Intranasal high-potency glucocorticoids are the most potent drugs available for the relief of established rhinitis, seasonal or perennial, and even vasomotor rhinitis; they provide efficacy with substantially reduced side effects as compared with this same class of agent administered orally. Their most frequent side effect is local irritation, with *Candida* overgrowth being a rare occurrence. The currently available intranasal glucocorticoids—beclomethasone, flunisolide, budesonide, fluticasone, and mometasone—are equally effective clinically, achieving up to 70% overall symptom relief with some variation in the time period for onset of benefit. Topical ipratropium is an anticholinergic agent effective in reducing rhinorrhea, including that in patients with perennial symptoms, and it can be additionally efficacious when combined with intranasal steroids. For systemic symptoms not related to the nasopharynx, such as allergic conjunctivitis, treatment may be local.

Immunotherapy, often termed *hyposensitization*, consists of repeated subcutaneous injections of gradually increasing concentrations of the allergen(s) considered to be specifically responsible for the symptom complex. Controlled studies of ragweed, grass, dust mite,

and cat dander allergens administered for treatment of allergic rhinitis have demonstrated at least partial relief of symptoms and signs. The duration of such immunotherapy is 3 to 5 years, with discontinuation being based on minimal symptoms over two consecutive seasons of exposure. Clinical benefit appears related to the administration of a high dose of relevant allergen advancing from weekly to monthly intervals. Patients should remain at the treatment site for at least 20 min after allergen administration so that any anaphylactic consequence can be managed. Local reactions with erythema and induration are not uncommon and may persist for 1 to 3 days. Immunotherapy is contraindicated in patients with significant cardiovascular disease or unstable asthma and should be conducted with particular caution in any patient requiring β-adrenergic blocking therapy because of the difficulty in managing an anaphylactic complication. The response to immunotherapy is derived from a complex of cellular and humoral effects that likely includes a modulation in T cell cytokine production. Immunotherapy should be reserved for clearly documented seasonal or perennial rhinitis, clinically related to defined allergen exposure with confirmation by the presence of allergen-specific IgE. A sequence for the management of allergic or perennial rhinitis based on an allergen-specific diagnosis and stepwise management as required for symptom control would include the following: (1) identification of the offending allergen(s) by history with confirmation of the presence of allergen-specific IgE by skin test and/or serum assay; (2) avoidance of the offending allergen; and (3) medical management in a stepwise fashion (Fig. 298-3). Mild intermittent symptoms of allergic rhinitis are treated with oral antihistamines, intranasal antihistamines, or intranasal cromolyn prophylaxis. Moderate to more severe allergic rhinitis is managed with intranasal glucocorticoids plus oral antihistamines or antihistamine-decongestant combinations. Persistent allergic rhinitis requiring the daily use of intranasal glucocorticoids with add-on interventions such as oral antihistamines, decongestant combinations, or topical ipratropium merits consideration of allergen-specific immunotherapy. Even a brief course of oral prednisone can be indicated.

FURTHER READING

BOYCE JA, AUSTEN KF: The biology of the mast cell, in *Immunologic Diseases*, 6th ed, KF Austen et al (eds). Philadelphia, Lippincott Williams & Wilkins, 2001

PENROSE JF et al: Leukotrienes: Biosynthetic pathways, release, and receptor-mediated actions with relevance to disease states, in *Inflammation: Basic Principles and Clinical Correlates*, 3d ed, JI Gallin and R Snyderman (eds). Philadelphia, Lippincott Williams & Wilkins, 1999

SOTER NA, KAPLAN AP: Urticaria and angioedema, in *Fitzpatrick's Dermatology in General Medicine*, 6th ed, IM Freedberg et al (eds). New York, McGraw-Hill, 2003, pp 1129–1139

VALENTINE MD: Insect venom allergy, in *Immunologic Diseases*, 6th ed, KF Austen et al (eds). Philadelphia, Lippicott Williams & Wilkins, 2001

WOROBEC A, METCALFE DD: Anaphylactic syndrome, in *Immunologic Diseases*, 6th ed, KF Austen et al (eds). Philadelphia, Lippincott Williams & Wilkins, 2001

299 AUTOIMMUNITY AND AUTOIMMUNE DISEASES

Peter E. Lipsky, Betty Diamond

One of the classically accepted features of the immune system is the capacity to distinguish self from non-self. Although they are able to recognize and generate reactions to a vast array of foreign materials, most animals do not mount immune responses to self-antigens under ordinary circumstances and thus are tolerant to self. Whereas recognition of self plays an important role in shaping both the T cell and B cell repertoires of immune receptors and plays an essential role in the recognition of nominal antigen by T cells, the development of potentially harmful immune responses to self-antigens is, in general, precluded. Autoimmunity, therefore, represents the end result of the breakdown of one or more of the basic mechanisms regulating immune tolerance.

The essential feature of an autoimmune disease is that tissue injury is caused by the immunologic reaction of the organism with its own tissues. Autoimmunity, on the other hand, refers merely to the presence of antibodies or T lymphocytes that react with self-antigens and does not necessarily imply that the development of self-reactivity has pathogenic consequences.

Autoimmunity may be seen in normal individuals and in higher frequency in normal older people. In addition, autoreactivity may develop during various infectious conditions. The expression of autoimmunity may be self-limited, as occurs with many infectious processes, or persistent. When autoimmunity is induced by an inciting event, such as infection or tissue damage from trauma or infarction, there may or may not be ensuing pathology. Even in the presence of organ pathology, it may be difficult to determine whether the damage is mediated by autoreactivity. Thus, the presence of self-reactivity may be either the cause or a consequence of an ongoing pathologic process.

MECHANISMS OF AUTOIMMUNITY Since Ehrlich first postulated the existence of mechanisms to prevent the generation of self-reactivity in 1900, ideas concerning the nature of this inhibition have developed in parallel with the progressive increase in understanding of the immune system. Burnet's clonal selection theory included the idea that interaction of lymphoid cells with their specific antigens during fetal or early postnatal life would lead to elimination of such "forbidden clones." This idea became untenable, however, when it was shown by a number of investigators that autoimmune diseases could be induced by simple immunization procedures, that autoantigen-binding cells could be demonstrated easily in the circulation of normal individuals, and that self-limited autoimmune phenomena frequently developed during infections. These observations indicated that clones of cells capable of responding to autoantigens were present in the repertoire of antigen-reactive cells in normal adults and suggested that mechanisms in addition to clonal deletion were responsible for preventing their activation.

Currently, three general processes are thought to be involved in the maintenance of selective unresponsiveness to autoantigens (Table 299-1): (1) sequestration of self-antigens, rendering them inaccessible to the immune system; (2) specific unresponsiveness (tolerance or anergy) of relevant T or B cells; and (3) limitation of potential reactivity by regulatory mechanisms.

Derangements of these normal processes may predispose to the development of autoimmunity (Table 299-2). In general, these abnormal responses relate to stimulation by exogenous agents, usually bacterial or viral, or endogenous abnormalities in the cells of the immune system. Microbial superantigens, such as staphylococcal protein A and staphylococcal enterotoxins, are substances that can stimulate a broad range of T and B cells based upon specific interactions with selected families of immune receptors irrespective of their antigen specificity. If autoantigen reactive T and/or B cells express these receptors, autoimmunity might develop. Alternatively, molecular mimicry or crossreactivity between a microbial product and a self-antigen might lead to activation of autoreactive lymphocytes. One of the best examples of autoreactivity and autoimmune disease resulting from molecular mimicry is rheumatic fever, in which antibodies to the M protein of streptococci cross-react with myosin, laminin, and other matrix proteins. Deposition of these autoantibodies in the heart initiates an inflammatory response. Molecular mimicry between microbial proteins and host tissues has been reported in type 1 diabetes mellitus, rheumatoid arthritis, and multiple sclerosis. The capacity of nonspecific stimulation of the immune system to predispose to the development of autoimmunity has been explored in a number of models; one is provided by the effect of adjuvants on the production of autoimmunity. Autoantigens become much more immunogenic when administered with adjuvant. It is presumed that infectious agents may be able to overcome self-tolerance because they possess molecules, such as bacterial endotoxin, that have adjuvant-like effects on the immune system by stimulating cells through Toll-like receptors.

Endogenous derangements of the immune system may also contribute to the loss of immunologic tolerance to self-antigens and the development of autoimmunity (Table 299-2). Many autoantigens re-

side in immunologically privileged sites, such as the brain or the anterior chamber of the eye. These sites are characterized by the inability of engrafted tissue to elicit immune responses. Immunologic privilege results from a number of events, including the limited entry of proteins from those sites into lymphatics, the local production of immunosuppressive cytokines such as transforming growth factor (TGF) β, and the local expression of molecules such as Fas ligand that can induce apoptosis of activated T cells. Lymphoid cells remain in a state of immunologic ignorance (neither activated nor anergized) to proteins expressed uniquely in immunologically privileged sites. If the privileged site is damaged by trauma or inflammation, or if T cells are activated elsewhere, proteins expressed at this site can become the targets of immunologic assault. Such an event may occur in multiple sclerosis and sympathetic ophthalmia, in which antigens uniquely expressed in the brain and eye, respectively, become the target of activated T cells.

Alterations in antigen presentation may also contribute to autoimmunity. This may occur by epitope spreading, in which protein determinants (*epitopes*) not routinely seen by lymphocytes (*cryptic epitopes*) are recognized as a result of immunologic reactivity to associated molecules. For example, animals immunized with one protein component of a multimolecular complex may be induced to produce antibodies to the other components of the complex. Finally, inflammation, drug exposure, or normal senescence may cause a primary chemical alteration in proteins, resulting in the generation of immune responses that cross-react with normal self-proteins. Alterations in the availability and presentation of autoantigens may be important components of immunoreactivity in certain models of organ-specific autoimmune diseases. In addition, these factors may be relevant in understanding the pathogenesis of various drug-induced autoimmune conditions. However, the diversity of autoreactivity manifest in nonorgan-specific systemic autoimmune diseases suggests that these conditions might result from a more general activation of the immune system rather than from an alteration in individual self-antigens.

A number of experimental models have suggested that intense stimulation of T lymphocytes can produce nonspecific signals that bypass the need for antigen-specific helper T cells and lead to polyclonal B cell activation with the formation of multiple autoantibodies. For example, antinuclear, antierythrocyte, and antilymphocyte antibodies are produced during the chronic graft-versus-host reaction. In addition, true autoimmune diseases, including autoimmune hemolytic anemia and immune complex–mediated glomerulonephritis, can also be induced in this manner. While it is clear that such diffuse activation of helper T cell activity can cause autoimmunity, nonspecific stimulation of B lymphocytes can also lead to the production of autoantibodies. Thus, the administration of polyclonal B cell activators, such as bac-

TABLE 299-2 *Mechanisms of Autoimmunity*

I. Exogenous
  A. Molecular mimicry
  B. Superantigenic stimulation
  C. Microbial adjuvanticity
II. Endogenous
  A. Altered antigen presentation
    1. Loss of immunologic privilege
    2. Presentation of novel or crytic epitopes (epitope spreading)
    3. Alteration of self-antigen
    4. Enhanced function of antigen-presenting cells
      a. Costimulatory molecule expression
      b. Cytokine production
  B. Increased T cell help
    1. Cytokine production
    2. Costimulatory molecules
  C. Increased B cell function
  D. Apoptotic defects
  E. Cytokine imbalance
  F. Altered immunoregulation

TABLE 299-1 *Mechanisms Preventing Autoimmunity*

1. Sequestration of self-antigen
2. Generation and maintenance of tolerance
   a. Central deletion of autoreactive lymphocytes
   b. Peripheral anergy of autoreactive lymphocytes
   c. Receptor replacement by autoreactive lymphocytes
3. Regulatory mechanisms

TABLE 299-3 *Mechanisms of Tissue Damage in Autoimmune Disease*

Effector	Mechanism	Target	Disease
Autoantibody	Blocking or inactivation	α Chain of the nicotinic acetylcholine receptor	Myasthenia gravis
		Phospholipid–β_2-glycoprotein 1 complex	Antiphospholipid syndrome
		Insulin receptor	Insulin-resistant diabetes mellitus
		Intrinsic factor	Pernicious anemia
	Stimulation	TSH receptor (LATS)	Graves' disease
		Proteinase-3 (ANCA)	Wegener's granulomatosis
		Epidermal cadherin, Desmoglein 3	Pemphigus vulgaris
	Complement activation	α_3 Chain of collagen IV	Goodpasture's syndrome
	Immune-complex formation	Double-strand DNA	Systemic lupus erythematosus
		Ig	Rheumatoid arthritis
	Opsonization	Platelet GpIIb:IIIa	Autoimmune thrombocytopenic purpura
		Rh antigens, I antigen	Autoimmune hemolytic anemia
	Antibody-dependent cellular cytotoxicity	Thyroid peroxidase, thyroglobulin	Hashimoto's thyroiditis
T cells	Cytokine production	?	Rheumatoid arthritis, multiple sclerosis, type 1 diabetes mellitus
	Cellular cytotoxicity	?	Type 1 diabetes mellitus

Note: ANCA, antineutrophil cytoplasmic antibody; LATS, long-acting thyroid stimulator; TSH, thyroid-stimulating hormone.

terial endotoxin, to normal mice leads to the production of a number of autoantibodies, including those directed to DNA and IgG (rheumatoid factor).

Primary alterations in the activity of T and/or B cells, cytokine imbalances, or defective immunoregulatory circuits may also contribute to the emergence of autoimmunity. For example, decreased apoptosis, as can be seen in animals with defects in Fas (CD95) or Fas ligand or in patients with related abnormalities, can be associated with the development of autoimmunity. Similarly, diminished production of tumor necrosis factor (TNF) and interleukin (IL) 10 has been reported to be associated with the development of autoimmunity.

Autoimmunity may also result from an abnormality of immunoregulatory mechanisms. Observations made in both human autoimmune disease and animal models suggest that defects in the generation and expression of regulatory T cell activity may allow for the production of autoimmunity. Administration of normal regulatory T cells or factors derived from them can prevent the development of autoimmune disease in rodent models of autoimmunity.

It should be apparent that no single mechanism can explain all the varied manifestations of autoimmunity. Furthermore, genetic evaluation has shown that a number of abnormalities often need to converge to induce an autoimmune disease. Additional factors that appear to be important determinants in the induction of autoimmunity include age, sex (many autoimmune diseases are far more common in women), genetic background, exposure to infectious agents, and environmental contacts. How all of these disparate factors affect the capacity to develop self-reactivity is currently being intensively investigated.

GENETIC CONSIDERATIONS Evidence in humans that there are susceptibility genes for autoimmunity comes from family studies and especially from studies of twins. Studies in type 1 diabetes mellitus, rheumatoid arthritis, multiple sclerosis, and systemic lupus erythematosus (SLE) have shown that approximately 15 to 30% of pairs of monozygotic twins show disease concordance, compared with <5% of dizygotic twins. The occurrence of different autoimmune diseases within the same family has suggested that certain susceptibility genes may predispose to a variety of autoimmune diseases. Genetic mapping

has begun to identify chromosomal regions that predispose to specific autoimmune diseases. In addition to this evidence from humans, certain inbred mouse strains reproducibly develop specific spontaneous or experimentally induced autoimmune diseases, whereas others do not. These findings have led to an extensive search for genes that determine susceptibility to autoimmune disease.

The most consistent association for susceptibility to autoimmune disease has been with particular alleles of the major histocompatibility complex (MHC). It has been suggested that the association of MHC genotype with autoimmune disease relates to differences in the ability of different allelic variations of MHC molecules to present autoantigenic peptides to autoreactive T cells. An alternative hypothesis involves the role of MHC alleles in shaping the T cell receptor repertoire during T cell ontogeny in the thymus. Additionally, specific MHC gene products themselves may be the source of peptides that can be recognized by T cells. Cross-reactivity between such MHC peptides and peptides derived from proteins produced by common microbes may trigger autoimmunity by molecular mimicry. However, MHC genotype alone does not determine the development of autoimmunity. Identical twins are far more likely to develop the same autoimmune disease than MHC-identical nontwin siblings, suggesting that genetic factors other than the MHC also affect disease susceptibility. Recent studies of the genetics of type 1 diabetes, SLE, rheumatoid arthritis, and multiple sclerosis in humans and mice have shown that there are several independently segregating disease susceptibility loci in addition to the MHC.

There is evidence that several other genes are important in increasing susceptibility to autoimmune disease. In humans, inherited homozygous deficiency of the early proteins of the classic pathway of complement (C1, C4, or C2) is very strongly associated with the development of SLE. In mice and humans, abnormalities in the genes encoding proteins involved in the regulation of apoptosis, including Fas (CD95) and Fas ligand (CD95 ligand), are strongly associated with the development of autoimmunity. There is also evidence that inherited variation in the level of expression of certain cytokines, such as $TNF\alpha$ or IL-10, may also increase susceptibility to autoimmune disease.

A further important factor in disease susceptibility is the hormonal status of the patient. Many autoimmune diseases show a strong sex bias, which appears in most cases to relate to the hormonal status of women.

IMMUNOPATHOGENIC MECHANISMS IN AUTOIMMUNE DISEASES The mechanisms of tissue injury in autoimmune diseases can be divided into antibody-mediated and cell-mediated processes. Representative examples are listed in Table 299-3.

The pathogenicity of autoantibodies can be mediated through several mechanisms, including opsonization of soluble factors or cells, activation of an inflammatory cascade via the complement system, and interference with the physiologic function of soluble molecules or cells.

In autoimmune thrombocytopenic purpura, opsonization of platelets targets them for elimination by phagocytes. Likewise, in autoimmune hemolytic anemia, binding of immunoglobulin to red cell membranes leads to phagocytosis and lysis of the opsonized cell. Goodpasture's syndrome, a disease characterized by lung hemorrhage and severe glomerulonephritis, represents an example of antibody binding leading to local activation of complement and neutrophil accumulation and activation. The autoantibody in this disease binds to the α_3 chain of type IV collagen in the basement membrane. In SLE, activation of the complement cascade at sites of immunoglobulin deposition in renal glomeruli is considered to be a major mechanism of renal damage.

Autoantibodies can also interfere with normal physiologic functions of cells or soluble factors. Autoantibodies against hormone receptors can lead to stimulation of cells or to inhibition of cell function through interference with receptor signaling. For example, long-acting thyroid stimulators, which are autoantibodies that bind to the receptor for thyroid-stimulating hormone, are present in Graves' disease and function as agonists, causing the thyroid to respond as if there were an excess of thyroid-stimulating hormone. Alternatively, antibodies to the insulin receptor can cause insulin-resistant diabetes mellitus through receptor blockade. In myasthenia gravis, autoantibodies to the acetylcholine receptor can be detected in 85 to 90% of patients and are responsible for muscle weakness. The exact location of the antigenic epitope, the valence and affinity of the antibody, and perhaps other characteristics determine whether activation or blockade results from antibody binding.

Antiphospholipid antibodies are associated with thromboembolic events in primary and secondary antiphospholipid syndrome and have also been associated with fetal wastage. The major antibody is directed to the phospholipid–β_2-glycoprotein I complex and appears to exert a procoagulant effect. In pemphigus vulgaris, autoantibodies bind to a component of the epidermal cell desmosome, desmoglein 3, and play a role in the induction of the disease. They exert their pathologic effect by disrupting cell-cell junctions through stimulation of the production of epithelial proteases, leading to blister formation. Cytoplasmic antineutrophil cytoplasmic antibody (c-ANCA), found in Wegener's granulomatosis, is an antibody to an intracellular antigen, the 29-kDa serine protease (proteinase-3). In vitro experiments have shown that IgG anti-c-ANCA causes cellular activation and degranulation of primed neutrophils.

It is important to note that autoantibodies of a given specificity may cause disease only in genetically susceptible hosts, as has been shown in experimental models of myasthenia gravis. Finally, some autoantibodies seem to be markers for disease but have as yet no known pathogenic potential.

AUTOIMMUNE DISEASE   Manifestations of autoimmunity are found in a large number of pathologic conditions. However, their presence does not necessarily imply that the pathologic process is an autoimmune disease. A number of attempts to establish formal criteria for the diagnosis of autoimmune diseases have been made, but none is universally accepted. One set of criteria is shown in Table 299-4; however, this should be viewed merely as a guide in consideration of the problem.

To classify a disease as autoimmune, it is necessary to demonstrate that the immune response to a self-antigen causes the observed pathology. Initially, the demonstration that antibodies against the affected tissue could be detected in the serum of patients suffering from various diseases was taken as evidence that these diseases had an autoimmune basis. However, such autoantibodies are also found when tissue damage is caused by trauma or infection, and the autoantibody is secondary to tissue damage. Thus, it is necessary to show that autoimmunity is pathogenic before classifying a disease as autoimmune.

If the autoantibodies are pathogenic, it may be possible to transfer disease to experimental animals by the administration of autoantibodies, with the subsequent development of pathology in the recipient similar to that seen in the patient from whom the antibodies were obtained. This has been shown, for example, in Graves' disease. Some autoimmune diseases can be transferred from mother to fetus and are observed in the newborn babies of diseased mothers. The symptoms of the disease in the newborn usually disappear as the levels of the

TABLE 299-4 *Human Autoimmune Disease: Presumptive Evidence for an Immunologic Pathogenesis*

Major Criteria
1. Presence of autoantibodies or evidence of cellular reactivity to self
2. Documentation of relevant autoantibody or lymphocytic infiltrate in the pathologic lesion.
3. Demonstration that relevant autoantibody or T cells can cause tissue pathology
   a. Transplacental transmission
   b. Adaptive transfer into animals
   c. In vitro impact on cellular function

Supportive Evidence
1. Reasonable animal model
2. Beneficial effect from immunosuppressive agents
3. Association with other evidence of autoimmunity
4. No evidence of infection or other obvious cause

maternal antibody decrease. An exception is congenital heart block, in which damage to the developing conducting system of the heart as a result of transfer of anti-Ro antibody from the mother results in permanent heart block.

In most situations, the critical factors that determine when the development of autoimmunity results in autoimmune disease have not been delineated. The relationship of autoimmunity to the development of autoimmune disease may relate to the fine specificity of the antibodies or T cells or their specific effector capabilities. In many circumstances a mechanistic understanding of the pathogenic potential of autoantibodies has not been established. In some autoimmune diseases, biased production of cytokines by helper T (T_H) cells may play a role in pathogenesis. In this regard, T cells can differentiate into specialized effector cells that predominantly produce interferon γ (T_H1) or IL-4 (T_H2) (Chap. 295). The former facilitate macrophage activation and classic cell-mediated immunity, whereas the latter are thought to have regulatory functions and are involved in the resolution of normal immune responses and also the development of responses to a variety of parasites. In a number of autoimmune diseases, such as rheumatoid arthritis, multiple sclerosis, type 1 diabetes mellitus, and Crohn's disease, there appears to be biased differentiation of T_H1 cells, with resultant organ damage.

ORGAN-SPECIFIC VERSUS SYSTEMIC AUTOIMMUNE DISEASES   Autoimmune diseases form a spectrum, from those specifically affecting a single organ to systemic disorders with involvement of many organs (Table 299-5). Hashimoto's autoimmune thyroiditis is an example of an organ-specific autoimmune disease (Chap. 320). In this disorder, there is a specific lesion in the thyroid associated with infiltration of mono-

TABLE 299-5   *Some Autoimmune Diseases*

ORGAN SPECIFIC

Graves' disease	Autoimmune hemolytic anemia
Hashimoto's thyroiditis	
Autoimmune polyglandular syndrome	Autoimmune thrombocytopenic purpura
Type 1 diabetes mellitus	Pernicious anemia
Insulin-resistant diabetes mellitus	Myasthenia gravis
Immune-mediated infertility	Multiple sclerosis
Autoimmune Addison's disease	Guillain-Barré syndrome
Pemphigus vulgaris	Stiff-man syndrome
Pemphigus foliaceus	Acute rheumatic fever
Dermatitis herpetiformis	Sympathetic ophthalmia
Autoimmune alopecia	Goodpasture's syndrome
Vitiligo	

ORGAN NONSPECIFIC (SYSTEMIC)

Systemic lupus erythematosus	Wegener's granulomatosis
Rheumatoid arthritis	Antiphospholipid syndrome
Systemic necrotizing vasculitis	Sjögren's syndrome

nuclear cells and damage to follicular cells. Antibody to thyroid constituents can be demonstrated in nearly all cases. Other organ- or tissue-specific autoimmune disorders include pemphigus vulgaris, autoimmune hemolytic anemia, idiopathic thrombocytopenic purpura, Goodpasture's syndrome, myasthenia gravis, and sympathetic ophthalmia. One important feature of some organ-specific auto-immune diseases is the tendency for overlap, such that an individual with one specific syndrome is more likely to develop a second syndrome. For example, there is a high incidence of pernicious anemia in individuals with autoimmune thyroiditis. More striking is the tendency for individuals with an organ-specific autoimmune disease to develop multiple other manifestations of autoimmunity without the development of associated organ pathology. Thus, as many as 50% of individuals with pernicious anemia have non-cross-reacting antibodies to thyroid constituents, whereas patients with myasthenia gravis may develop antinuclear antibodies, antithyroid antibodies, rheumatoid factor, antilymphocyte antibodies, and polyclonal hypergammaglobulinemia. Part of the explanation for this may relate to the genetic elements shared by individuals with these different diseases.

Systemic autoimmune diseases differ from organ-specific diseases in that pathologic lesions are found in multiple, diverse organs and tissues. The hallmark of these conditions is the demonstration of associated relevant autoimmune manifestations that are likely to be etiologic in the organ pathology. SLE represents the prototype of these disorders because of its abundance of autoimmune manifestations.

SLE is a disease of protean manifestations that characteristically involves the kidneys, joints, skin, serosal surfaces, blood vessels, and central nervous system (Chap. 300). The disease is associated with a vast array of autoantibodies whose production appears to be a part of a generalized hyperreactivity of the humoral immune system. Other features of SLE include generalized B cell hyperresponsiveness, polyclonal hypergammaglobulinemia, and increased titers of antibodies to commonly encountered viral antigens.

℞ TREATMENT

Treatment of autoimmune diseases can focus on either suppressing the induction of autoimmunity, restoring normal regulatory mechanisms, or inhibiting the effector mechanisms. To eliminate autoreactive cells, immunosuppressive or ablative therapies are most commonly used. In recent years, cytokine blockade has been demonstrated to be effective in preventing immune activation in some diseases. New therapies are currently in clinical trials to target lymphoid cells more specifically, either by blocking a costimulatory signal needed for T or B cell activation, by eliminating the effector T cells or B cells, or by using autoantigen itself to induce tolerance. The major advance in inhibiting effector mechanisms has been the introduction of cytokine blockade, targeting at TNF or IL-1, that appears to limit organ damage in some diseases. Therapies that prevent target organ damage or support target organ function remain an important therapeutic approach to autoimmune disease.

FURTHER READING

DAVIDSON A, DIAMOND B: Autoimmune diseases. N Engl J Med 345:340, 2001

GREEN EA, FLAVELL RA: The initiation of autoimmune diabetes. Curr Opin Immunol 11:663, 1999

LIPSKY PE: Systemic lupus erythematosus: An autoimmune disease of B cell hyperactivity. Nat Immunol 2:764, 2001

MARRACK P et al: Autoimmune disease: Why and where it occurs. Nat Med 7:889, 2001

McDEVITT HO: The role of MHC class II molecules in susceptibility and resistance to autoimmunity. Curr Opin Immunol 10:677, 1998

ROSE NR: The role of infection in the pathogenesis of autoimmune disease. Semin Immunol 10:5, 1998

SHEVACH EM: Suppressor T cells: Rebirth, function and homeostasis. Curr Biol 10:R572, 2000

300 | SYSTEMIC LUPUS ERYTHEMATOSUS
Bevra Hannahs Hahn

DEFINITION AND PREVALENCE Systemic lupus erythematosus (SLE) is an autoimmune disease in which organs, tissues, and cells undergo damage mediated by tissue-binding autoantibodies and immune complexes. Ninety percent of patients are women of child-bearing years; people of both genders, all ages, and all ethnic groups are susceptible. Prevalence of SLE in the United States is 15 to 50 per 100,000; the highest prevalence among ethnic groups is in African Americans.

PATHOGENESIS AND ETIOLOGY SLE is caused by interactions between susceptibility genes and environmental factors, resulting in abnormal immune responses. The immune responses include hyperreactivity and hypersensitivity of T and B lymphocytes and ineffective regulation of antigen availability and of ongoing antibody responses. Hyperreactivity of T and B cells is indicated by increased surface expression of molecules such as HLA-D and CD40L, showing that cells are easily activated by antigens that induce first-activating signals and by molecules that drive cells to full activation via second signals. The end result of these abnormalities is sustained production of pathogenic autoantibodies and formation of immune complexes that bind target tissues, resulting in (1) sequestration and destruction of Ig-coated circulating cells; (2) fixation and cleaving of complement proteins; and (3) release of chemotaxins, vasoactive peptides, and destructive enzymes into tissues. Many autoantibodies in persons with SLE are directed against DNA/protein or RNA/protein complexes such as nucleosomes, some nucleolar RNA, and spliceosomal RNA (Table 300-1). During apoptosis these antigens migrate to cell surfaces, where they are enclosed in blebs, and membrane phospholipids change orientation so that antigenic portions are near the surface. Intracellular molecules altered during cell activation or damage migrate to the cell surface. All these antigens near or in cell surfaces probably activate the immune system to produce autoantibodies. In individuals with SLE, phagocytosis and removal of apoptotic cells and of immune complexes are impaired. Thus, in SLE, antigens are available; they are presented in locations recognized by the immune system; and the antigens, autoantibodies, and immune complexes persist for prolonged periods of time, allowing tissue damage to accumulate to the point of clinical illness.

SLE is a multigenic disease. It is likely that alleles of multiple normal genes each contribute a small amount to the abnormal immune responses; if enough variations accumulate, disease results. Some predisposing genes are located in the HLA region (particularly HLA class II DR and DQ genes, and HLA class III genes encoding C'2 and C'4). The relevant HLA DR/DQ genes increase risk for SLE by approximately twofold if one susceptibility haplotype is present and by four- to sixfold if two or more are present. Some proteins important in clearing apoptotic cells play a role in genetic susceptibility; for example, homozygous deficiencies of early components of complement Clq, C'2, and C'4 and certain alleles of mannose-binding ligand increase the risk for SLE. Clq deficiency confers the highest genetic risk known but is rare. There are at least five chromosomal regions independent of HLA that contain susceptibility genes. Within one of these regions on chromosome 1 are alleles encoding Fcγ receptors that bind subsets of IgG (IgG1, -2, or -3): African Americans inheriting one allele of FcγRIIA have a receptor that binds the Ig in immune complexes weakly; those persons have increased risk for lupus nephritis. Caucasians and Asians in some populations with alleles of FcγRIIIA that bind Ig weakly are predisposed to SLE. A region on chromosome 16 contains genes that predispose to SLE, rheumatoid arthritis, psoriasis, and Crohn's disease, suggesting the presence of "autoimmunity genes" that, when interacting with other genes, predispose to different autoimmune diseases. Thus, SLE is modified by multiple susceptibility genes, some of which interact. There are likely to be protective gene alleles as well. These gene combinations influence immune responses to the external and internal environment; when such responses are too high and/or too prolonged, autoimmunity results.

Female gender is permissive for SLE; females of many mammalian species make higher antibody responses than males. Women exposed to estrogen-containing oral contraceptives or hormone replacement have an increased risk of developing SLE (approximately twofold). Estradiol binds to receptors on T and B lymphocytes, increasing activation and survival of those cells, thus favoring prolonged immune responses.

Several environmental stimuli may influence SLE. Exposure to ultraviolet light causes SLE flares in approximately 70% of patients, possibly by increasing apoptosis in keratinocytes and other cells or by altering DNA and intracellular proteins to make them antigenic. It is likely that various infections that stimulate immune responses (antibodies and activated T lymphocytes)

TABLE 300-1 *Autoantibodies of SLE*

Antibody	Prevalence, %	Antigen Recognized	Clinical Utility
Antinuclear antibodies	98	Multiple nuclear	Best screening test; repeated negative tests make SLE unlikely
Anti-dsDNA	70	DNA (double-stranded)	High titers are SLE-specific and in some patients correlate with disease activity, nephritis, vasculitis
Anti-Sm	25	Protein complexed to 6 species of nuclear U1 RNA	Specific for SLE; no definite clinical correlations; most patients also have anti-RNP; more common in African Americans and Asians than Caucasians
Anti-RNP	40	Protein complexed to U1 RNAγ	Not specific for SLE; high titers associated with syndromes that have overlap features of several rheumatic syndromes including SLE; more common in African Americans than Caucasians
Anti-Ro (SS-A)	30	Protein complexed to hY RNA, primarily 60 kDa and 52 kDa	Not specific for SLE; associated with sicca syndrome, subacute cutaneous lupus, and neonatal lupus with congenital heart block; associated with decreased risk for nephritis
Anti-La (SS-B)	10	47-kDa protein complexed to hY RNA	Usually associated with anti-Ro; associated with decreased risk for nephritis
Antihistone	70	Histones associated with DNA (in nucleosome, chromatin)	More frequent in drug-induced lupus than in SLE
Antiphospholipid	50	Phospholipids, β_2 glycoprotein 1 cofactor, prothrombin	Three tests available—ELISAs for cardiolipin and B2G1, sensitive prothrombin time (DRVVT); predisposes to clotting, fetal loss, thrombocytopenia
Antierythrocyte	60	Erythrocyte membrane	Measured as direct Coombs' test; a small proportion develop overt hemolysis
Antiplatelet	30	Surface and altered cytoplasmic antigens in platelets	Associated with thrombocytopenia but sensitivity and specificity are not good; this is not a useful clinical test
Antineuronal	60	Neuronal and lymphocyte surface antigens	In some series a positive test in CSF correlate with active CNS lupus
Antiribosomal P	20	Protein in ribosomes	In some series a positive test in serum correlates with depression or psychosis due to CNS lupus

Note: ELISA, enzyme-linked immunosorbent assay; DRVVT, dilute Russell viper venom time; CSF, cerebrospinal fluid; CNS, central nervous system.

that cross-react with self or responses that, as they mature, develop the ability to recognize self can promote autoimmune responses that lead to SLE. The observation that children and adults with SLE are more likely to be infected by Epstein-Barr Virus (EBV) than age-, gender-, and ethnically matched controls without SLE is intriguing, because EBV activates B lymphocytes and also contains amino acid sequences that mimic sequences on human spliceosomes—a common autoantibody specificity in people with SLE. Thus, interplay between genetic susceptibility, gender, and environmental stimuli may result in autoimmunity.

For maximal production of harmful autoantibodies, B cells require help from T cells, and those functions of T and B cells are normally downregulated by several mechanisms. In murine SLE models, many downregulating networks are abnormal, including generation of multiple types of regulatory and natural killer T cells and of humoral idiotypic downregulating networks.

PATHOLOGY In SLE, biopsies of affected skin show deposition of Ig at the dermal-epidermal junction (DEJ), injury to basal keratinocytes, and inflammation dominated by T lymphocytes in the DEJ and around blood vessels and dermal appendages. Clinically unaffected skin may also show Ig deposition at the DEJ. In renal biopsies, the pattern of injury is important in diagnosis and in selecting the best therapy. The World Health Organization (WHO) has classified lupus nephritis as grade I (no histologic changes), II (proliferative changes confined to the mesangium), III (proliferative changes in tufts of 10 to 50% of glomeruli; higher proportions of glomeruli affected suggest worse

prognosis), IV [diffuse proliferative glomerulonephritis (DPGN) affecting >50% of glomeruli], V (predominantly membranous changes with various degrees of proliferation), and VI (end stage, scarred glomeruli). In addition, pathologists report the extent of inflammatory (potentially reversible) and chronic (irreversible scarring in glomeruli, renal tubules, and blood vessels) changes. In general, treatment for lupus nephritis is not recommended in patients with class I or II disease or with extensive irreversible changes. In contrast, aggressive immunosuppression is recommended for patients with class III, IV, or V inflammatory proliferative lesions because the majority of those individuals, if untreated, develop end-stage renal disease (ESRD) within 2 years. In children, a diagnosis of SLE can be established on the basis of renal histology without meeting additional diagnostic criteria (Table 300-2). Histologic abnormalities in blood vessels are not specific for SLE: leukocytoclastic vasculitis is most common (Chap. 306). Lymph node biopsies show nonspecific diffuse chronic inflammation.

DIAGNOSIS The diagnosis of SLE is based on characteristic clinical features and autoantibodies. Criteria for classification are listed in Table 300-2, and an algorithm for diagnosis and initial therapy is shown in Fig. 300-1. The criteria are intended for confirming the diagnosis of SLE in patients included in studies; the author uses them in individual patients for estimating the probability that a disease is SLE. Any combination of 4 or more of 11 criteria, well-documented at any time during a patient's history, makes it likely that the patient has SLE (specificity and sensitivity are ~95% and 75%, respectively). In many

TABLE 300-2 *Classification Criteria for the Diagnosis of SLE*[a]

Malar rash	Fixed erythema, flat or raised, over the malar eminences
Discoid rash	Erythematous circular raised patches with adherent keratotic scaling and follicular plugging; atrophic scarring may occur
Photosensitivity	Exposure to ultraviolet light causes rash
Oral ulcers	Includes oral and nasopharyngeal ulcers, observed by physician
Arthritis	Nonerosive arthritis of two or more peripheral joints, with tenderness, swelling, or effusion
Serositis	Pleuritis or pericarditis documented by ECG or rub or evidence of effusion
Renal disorder	Proteinuria >0.5 g/d or ≥3+, or cellular casts
Neurologic disorder	Seizures or psychosis without other causes
Hematologic disorder	Hemolytic anemia or leukopenia ($<4000/\mu L$) or lymphopenia ($<1500/\mu L$) or thrombocytopenia ($<100,000/\mu L$) in the absence of offending drugs
Immunologic disorder	Anti-dsDNA, anti-Sm, and/or anti-phospholipid
Antinuclear antibodies	An abnormal titer of ANA by immunofluorescence or an equivalent assay at any point in time in the absence of drugs known to induce ANAs

[a] If ≥4 of these criteria, well documented, are present at any time in a patient's history, the diagnosis is likely to be SLE. Specificity is ~95%: sensitivity is ~75%.
Note: ECG, electrocardiography; dsDNA, double-stranded DNA; ANA, antinuclear antibodies.
Source: Criteria published by EM Tan et al: Arthritis Rheum 25:1271, 1982; updated by MC Hochberg, Arthritis Rheum 40:1725, 1997.

patients, additional criteria accrue over time. Antinuclear antibodies (ANA) are positive in >95% of patients during the course of disease; repeated negative tests suggest that the diagnosis is not SLE. High-titer IgG antibodies to double-stranded DNA and antibodies to the Sm antigen are both specific for SLE and, therefore, favor the diagnosis in the presence of compatible clinical manifestations. The presence in an individual of multiple autoantibodies without clinical symptoms should not be considered diagnostic for SLE, although such persons are at increased risk.

INTERPRETATION OF CLINICAL MANIFESTATIONS When a diagnosis of SLE is made, it is important to establish the severity and potential reversibility of the illness and estimate the possible consequences of various therapeutic interventions. In the following paragraphs, descriptions of some disease manifestations begin with relatively mild problems and progress to those more life-threatening.

Overview and Systemic Manifestations At its onset, SLE may involve one or several organ systems; over time, additional manifestations of disease may occur (Table 300-3). Most of the autoantibodies characteristic of each person are present at the time clinical manifestations appear (Tables 300-1 and 300-2). Severity of SLE varies from mild and intermittent to severe and fulminant. Most patients experience exacerbations interspersed with periods of relative quiescence; however, permanent complete remissions (absence of symptoms with no treatment) are rare. Systemic symptoms, particularly fatigue and myalgias/arthralgias, are present most of the time. Severe systemic illness requiring glucocorticoid therapy can occur with fever, prostration, weight loss, and anemia in addition to any other organ-targeted manifestations.

Musculoskeletal Manifestations Most people with SLE have intermittent polyarthritis, varying from mild to disabling, characterized by soft tissue swelling and tenderness in joints, most commonly in hands, wrists, and knees. Presence of visible synovitis suggests active systemic disease. Joint deformities (hands and feet) develop in only 10%. Erosions on joint x-rays are rare; their presence suggests a non-lupus inflammatory arthropathy such as rheumatoid arthritis (Chap. 301). If pain persists in a single joint, such as knee, shoulder, or hip, a diagnosis of ischemic necrosis of bone should be considered, particularly if there are no other manifestations of active SLE. The prevalence of ischemic necrosis of bone is increased in SLE, especially in patients treated with systemic glucocorticoids. Myositis with clinical muscle weakness, elevated creatine kinase levels, and biopsy evidence of muscle necrosis and inflammation can occur, although most patients have myalgias without frank myositis. Glucocorticoid and, rarely, antimalarial therapies can also cause muscle weakness; these adverse effects must be distinguished from active disease.

Cutaneous Manifestations Lupus dermatitis can be classified as discoid lupus erythematosus (DLE), systemic rash, subacute cutaneous lupus erythematosus (SCLE), or "other." Discoid lesions are roughly circular with slightly raised, scaly hyperpigmented erythematous rims and depigmented, atrophic centers in which all dermal appendages are permanently destroyed. Lesions can be disfiguring, partic-

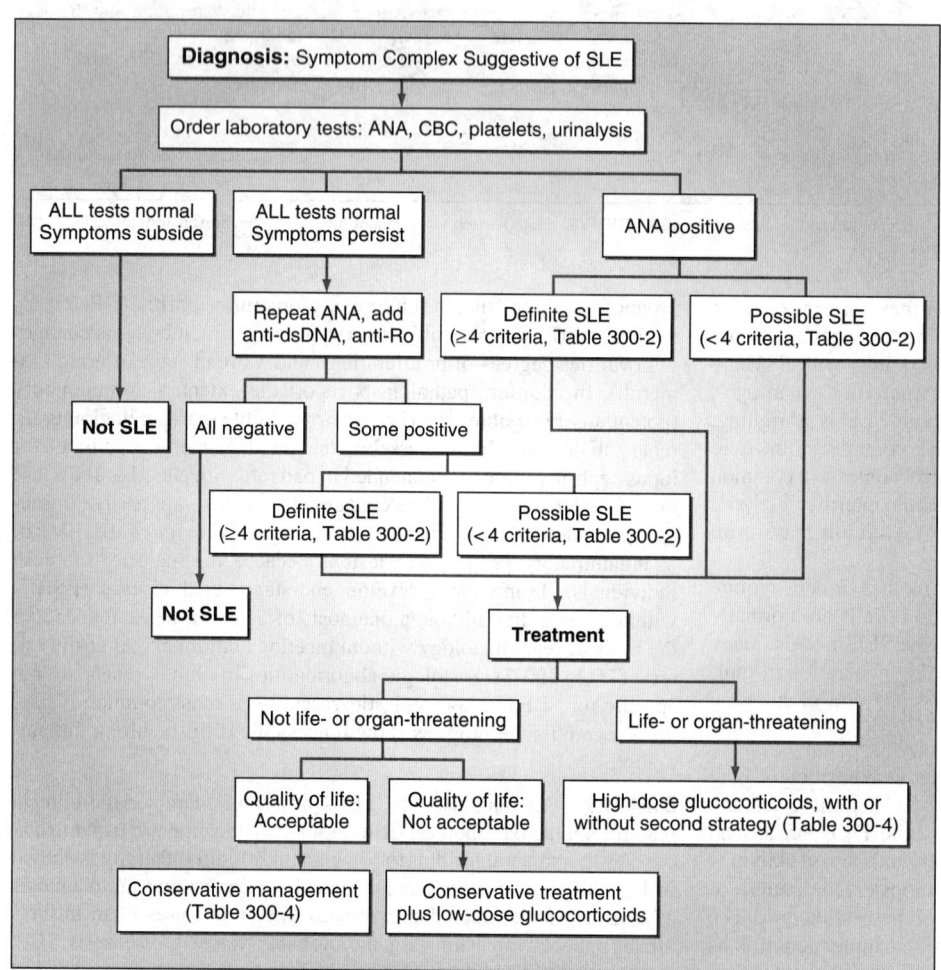

FIGURE 300-1 Algorithm for diagnosis and initial therapy of SLE. ANA, antinuclear antibodies; CBC, complete blood count.

TABLE 300-3 *Clinical Manifestations of SLE and Prevalence over the Entire Course of Disease*[a]

Systemic: Fatigue, malaise, fever, anorexia, weight loss	95
Musculoskeletal	95
Arthralgias/myalgias	95
Nonerosive polyarthritis	60
Hand deformities	10
Myopathy/myositis	25/5
Ischemic necrosis of bone	15
Cutaneous	80
Photosensitivity	70
Malar rash	50
Oral ulcers	40
Alopecia	40
Discoid rash	20
Vasculitis rash	20
Other (e.g., urticaria, subacute cutaneous lupus)	15
Hematologic	85
Anemia (chronic disease)	70
Leukopenia ($<4000/\mu L$)	65
Lymphopenia ($<1500/\mu L$)	50
Thrombocytopenia ($<100,000/\mu L$)	15
Lymphadenopathy	15
Splenomegaly	15
Hemolytic anemia	10
Neurologic	60
Cognitive disorder	50
Mood disorder	40
Headache	25
Seizures	20
Mono-, polyneuropathy	15
Stroke, TIA	10
Acute confusional state or movement disorder	2–5
Aseptic meningitis, myelopathy	<1
Cardiopulmonary	60
Pleurisy, pericarditis, effusions	30–50
Myocarditis, endocarditis	10
Lupus pneumonitis	10
Coronary artery disease	10
Interstitial fibrosis	5
Pulmonary hypertension, ARDS, hemorrhage	<5
Renal	30–50
Proteinuria >500 mg/24 h, cellular casts	30–50
Nephrotic syndrome	25
End-stage renal disease	5–10
Gastrointestinal	40
Nonspecific (nausea, mild pain, diarrhea)	30
Abnormal liver enzymes	40
Vasculitis	5
Thrombosis	15
Venous	10
Arterial	5
Ocular	15
Sicca syndrome	15
Conjunctivitis, episcleritis	10
Vasculitis	5

[a] Numbers indicate percent of patients who have the manifestation sometime during the course of illness.

Note: TIA, transient ischemic attack; ARDS, acute respiratory distress syndrome.

ularly on the face and scalp. Treatment consists primarily of local glucocorticoids and systemic antimalarials. Only 5% of people with DLE have SLE (although half have positive ANA); however, among people with SLE, as many as 20% have DLE. The most common SLE rash is a photosensitive, slightly raised erythema, occasionally scaly, on the face (particularly the cheeks and nose—the "butterfly" rash), ears, chin, V region of the neck, upper back, and extensor surfaces of the arms. Worsening of this rash often accompanies flare of systemic disease. SCLE consists of scaly red patches similar to psoriasis or attacks of circular red-rimmed lesions. Patients with these manifestations are exquisitely photosensitive; most have antibodies to Ro (SS-A). Many other rashes are seen less frequently in SLE, including recurring urticaria, lichen planus–like dermatitis, bullae, and panniculitis ("lupus profundus"). Rashes of SLE can be minor or very severe;

they may be the major disease manifestation. Small, painful ulcerations on the oral or nasal mucosa are common in SLE: the lesions resemble aphthous ulcers and usually indicate systemic disease activity.

Renal Manifestations Nephritis is usually the most serious manifestation of SLE, particularly since nephritis and infection are the leading causes of mortality in the first decade of disease. Since nephritis is asymptomatic in most lupus patients, urinalysis should be ordered in any person suspected of having SLE. The classification of lupus nephritis is primarily histologic (see "Pathology," above). Renal biopsy is useful in planning current and near-future therapies. Patients with dangerous proliferative forms of glomerular damage usually have microscopic hematuria and proteinuria (>500 mg per 24 h); approximately one-half develop nephrotic syndrome, and most develop hypertension. If DPGN is untreated, virtually all patients develop ESRD within 2 years of diagnosis. Therefore, aggressive immunosuppression is indicated (usually systemic glucocorticoids plus a cytotoxic drug), unless damage is irreversible. African-American individuals are more likely to develop ESRD than are Caucasians, even with the most current therapies. Overall in the United States, ~20% of individuals with DPGN die or develop ESRD within 10 years of diagnosis. Such individuals require aggressive control of SLE and of the complications of renal disease and of therapy. A small proportion of SLE patients with proteinuria (usually nephrotic) have membranous glomerular changes without proliferation on renal biopsy. Their outcome is better than for those with DPGN, but proteinuria is less likely to improve on lupus nephritis immunosuppressive therapies. Lupus nephritis tends to be an ongoing disease, with flares requiring re-treatment over many years. For most people with lupus nephritis, accelerated atherosclerosis becomes important after several years of disease; attention must be given to control of blood pressure, hyperlipidemia, and hyperglycemia.

Nervous System Manifestations There are many central nervous system (CNS) and peripheral nervous system manifestations of SLE; in some patients these are the major cause of morbidity and mortality. It is useful to approach this diagnostically by asking first whether the symptoms result from SLE or another condition (such as infection in immunosuppressed individuals). If symptoms are related to SLE, it should be determined whether they are caused by a diffuse process or vascular occlusive disease. The most common manifestation of diffuse CNS lupus is cognitive dysfunction, particularly difficulties with memory and reasoning. Headaches are also common; when excruciating, they often indicate SLE flare; when milder, they are difficult to distinguish from migraine or tension headaches. Seizures of any type may be caused by lupus; treatment often requires both anti-seizure and immunosuppressive therapies. Psychosis can be the dominant manifestation of SLE; it must be distinguished from glucocorticoid-induced psychosis. The latter usually occurs in the first weeks of glucocorticoid therapy, at doses of ≥40 mg of prednisone or equivalent; psychosis resolves over several days after glucocorticoids are decreased or stopped. Myelopathy is not rare and is often disabling; high-dose glucocorticoid therapy is recommended and should be started within hours or a few days of the onset of symptoms.

Vascular Occlusions The prevalence of transient ischemic attacks, strokes, and myocardial infarctions is increased in patients with SLE. These vascular events are increased in, but not exclusive to, SLE patients with antibodies to phospholipids (aPL). Ischemia in the brain can be caused by focal occlusion (either noninflammatory or associated with vasculitis) or by embolization from carotid artery plaque or from fibrinous vegetations of Libman-Sachs endocarditis. Appropriate tests for aPL (see below) and for sources of emboli should be ordered in such patients to estimate the need for, intensity of, and duration of anti-inflammatory and/or anticoagulant therapies. In SLE, myocardial infarctions are primarily manifestations of accelerated atherosclerosis. The increased risk for vascular events is as much as 50-fold in women with SLE <45 years old compared to healthy women. Characteristics associated with increased risk for atherosclerosis include older age, hypertension, dyslipidemia, aPL, repeated high scores for disease activity, and high cumulative doses of glucocorticoids. When it is most likely that an event results from clotting, long-term anticoagulation is the therapy of choice. Two processes can occur at once—vasculitis plus bland vascular occlusions—in which case it is appropriate to treat with anticoagulation plus immunosuppression.

Pulmonary Manifestations The most common pulmonary manifestation of SLE is pleuritis with or without pleural effusion. This manifestation, when mild, may respond to treatment with nonsteroidal anti-inflammatory drugs (NSAIDs); when more severe, patients require a brief course of glucocorticoid therapy. Pulmonary infiltrates also occur as a manifestation of active SLE and are difficult to distinguish from infection on imaging studies. Life-threatening pulmonary manifestations include interstitial inflammation, leading to fibrosis, and intraalveolar hemorrhage; both of these probably require aggressive immunosuppressive and supportive treatments early after their onset.

Cardiac Manifestations Pericarditis is the most frequent cardiac manifestation; it usually responds to anti-inflammatory therapy and infrequently leads to tamponade. More serious cardiac manifestations are myocarditis and fibrinous endocarditis of Libman-Sachs. The endocardial involvement can lead to valvular insufficiencies, most commonly of the mitral or aortic valves, or to embolic events. It has not been proved that glucocorticoid or other immunosuppressive therapies lead to improvement of lupus myocarditis or endocarditis, but it is usual practice to administer a trial of high-dose steroids along with appropriate supportive therapy for heart failure, arrhythmia, or embolic events. As discussed above, patients with SLE are at increased risk for myocardial infarction, usually due to accelerated atherosclerosis.

Hematologic Manifestations The most frequent hematologic manifestation of SLE is anemia, usually normochromic normocytic, reflecting chronic illness. Hemolysis can be rapid in onset and severe, requiring high-dose glucocorticoid therapy, which is effective in most patients. Leukopenia is also common and almost always consists of lymphopenia, not granulocytopenia; this rarely predisposes to infections and by itself usually does not require therapy. Thrombocytopenia may be a recurring problem. If platelet counts are >40,000/μL and abnormal bleeding is absent, therapy may not be required. High-dose glucocorticoid therapy (e.g., 1 mg/kg per day of prednisone or equivalent) is usually effective for the first few episodes of severe thrombocytopenia. Recurring or prolonged hemolytic anemia or thrombocytopenia, or disease requiring an unacceptably high dose of daily glucocorticoids, should be treated with an additional strategy (see "Treatment," below).

Gastrointestinal Manifestations Nausea, sometimes with vomiting, and diarrhea can be manifestations of an SLE flare, as can diffuse abdominal pain caused by autoimmune peritonitis. Increases in serum AST and ALT are common when SLE is active. These manifestations usually improve promptly during systemic glucocorticoid therapy. Vasculitis involving the intestine may be life-threatening; perforations, ischemia, bleeding, and sepsis are frequent complications. Aggressive immunosuppressive therapy with high-dose glucocorticoids is recommended for short-term control; evidence of recurrence is an indication for additional therapies.

Ocular Manifestations Sicca syndrome (Sjögren's syndrome; Chap. 304) and nonspecific conjunctivitis are common in SLE and rarely threaten vision. In contrast, retinal vasculitis and optic neuritis are serious manifestations: blindness can develop over days to weeks. Aggressive immunosuppression is recommended, although there are no controlled trials to prove effectiveness. Complications of glucocorticoid therapy include cataracts (common) and glaucoma.

LABORATORY TESTS Laboratory tests serve (1) to establish or rule out the diagnosis; (2) to follow the course of disease, particularly to suggest that a flare is occurring or organ damage is developing; and (3) to identify adverse effects of therapies.

Tests for Autoantibodies (See Tables 300-1 and 300-2) Diagnostically, the most important autoantibodies to detect are ANA since the test is positive in >95% of patients, usually at the onset of symptoms. A few patients develop ANA within 1 year of symptom onset; repeated testing may then be useful. ANA-negative lupus exists but is very rare in adults and is usually associated with other autoantibodies (anti-Ro or anti-DNA). High-titer IgG antibodies to double-stranded DNA (dsDNA) (but not to single-stranded DNA) are specific for SLE. There is no international standardized test for ANA; variability between different service laboratories is high. Enzyme-linked immunosorbent assays (ELISA) and immunofluorescent reactions of sera with the dsDNA in the flagellate *Crithidia lucilliae* have ~60% sensitivity for SLE; identification of high-avidity anti-dsDNA in the Farr assay is not as sensitive but may correlate better with risk for nephritis. Titers of anti-dsDNA vary over time. In some patients, increase in quantities of anti-dsDNA herald a flare, particularly of nephritis or vasculitis. Antibodies to Sm are also specific for SLE and assist in diagnosis; anti-Sm antibodies do not usually correlate with disease activity or clinical manifestations. aPL are not specific for SLE, but their presence fulfills one classification criterion and they identify patients at increased risk for venous or arterial clotting, thrombocytopenia, and fetal loss. There are two widely accepted tests that measure different antibodies (anticardiolipin and the lupus anticoagulant): (1) ELISA for anticardiolipin (internationally standardized with good reproducibility) and (2) a sensitive phospholipid-based activated prothrombin time such as the dilute Russell venom viper test. Some centers also recommend measurement of antibodies to β_2 glycoprotein 1, a serum protein cofactor that is the target of most antibodies to cardiolipin and some lupus anticoagulants. High titers of IgG anticardiolipin (>50 IU) indicate high risk for a clinical episode of clotting. Quantities of aPL may vary markedly over time; repeated testing is justified if clinical manifestations of the antiphospholipid antibody syndrome (APS) appear. To make a diagnosis of APS, with or without SLE, requires the presence of clotting and/or repeated fetal losses plus at least two positive tests for aPL, at least 6 weeks apart.

An additional autoantibody test with predictive value (not used for diagnosis) detects anti-Ro, which indicates increased risk for neonatal lupus, sicca syndrome, and SCLE. Women with child-bearing potential and SLE should be screened for aPL and anti-Ro.

Standard Tests for Diagnosis Screening tests for complete blood count, platelet count, and urinalysis may detect abnormalities that contribute to the diagnosis and influence management decisions.

Tests for Following Disease Course It is useful to follow tests that indicate the status of organ involvement known to be present during SLE flares. These might include hemoglobin levels, platelet counts, urinalysis, and serum levels of creatinine or albumin. There is great interest in identification of additional markers of disease activity. Candidates include levels of anti-DNA antibodies, several components of complement (C'3 is most widely available), activated complement products, soluble interleukin (IL) 2, and urinary monocyte chemotactic protein 1. None are uniformly agreed upon as reliable indicators of response or flare. The physician should determine for each patient whether certain laboratory test changes predict flare. If so, altering therapy in response to these changes is acceptable to prevent flares. In addition, given the increased prevalence of atherosclerosis in SLE, it is advisable to follow the recommendations of the National Cholesterol Education Program for testing.

℞ TREATMENT

There is no cure for SLE, and complete sustained remissions are rare. Therefore, the physician should plan to control acute, severe flares then develop maintenance strategies that suppress symptoms to an acceptable level and prevent organ damage. Usually patients will endure some adverse effects of medications. Therapeutic choices depend on: (1) whether disease manifestations are life-threatening or likely to cause organ damage, justifying aggressive therapies; (2) whether manifestations are potentially reversible; and (3) the best approaches to preventing complications of disease and its treatments. Therapies, doses, and adverse effects are listed in (Table 300-4).

Conservative Therapies for Management of Non-Life-Threatening Disease
Among patients with fatigue, pain, and autoantibodies of SLE, but

without major organ involvement, management can be directed to suppression of symptoms. Analgesics and antimalarials are mainstays. NSAIDs are useful analgesics/anti-inflammatories, particularly for arthritis/arthralgias; however, SLE patients compared to the general population are at increased risk for NSAID-induced aseptic meningitis, elevated serum transaminases, hypertension, and renal dysfunction. Cyclooxygenase-2 specific inhibitors, compared to nonspecific

TABLE 300-4 *Medications for the Management of SLE*

Medication	Dose Range	Drug Interactions	Serious or Common Adverse Effects
NSAIDs, salicylates (Ecotrin[a] and St. Joseph's aspirin[a] approved by FDA for use in SLE)	Doses toward upper limit of recommended range usually required	A2R/ACE inhibitors, glucocorticoids, fluconazole, methotrexate, thiazides	NSAIDs: Higher incidence of aseptic meningitis, transaminitis, decreased renal function, vasculitis of skin
Salicylates: ototoxicity, tinnitus
Both: GI events and symptoms, allergic reactions, dermatitis, dizziness, acute renal failure, edema, hypertension
Topical glucocorticoids	Mid-potency for face; mid to high potency other areas	None known	Atrophy of skin, contact dermatitis, folliculitis, hypopigmentation, infection
Topical sunscreens	SPF 15 at least; 30+ preferred	None known	Contact dermatitis
Hydroxychloroquine[a] (quinacrine can be added or substituted)	200–400 mg qd (100 mg qd)	None known	Retinal damage, agranulocytosis, aplastic anemia, ataxia, cardiomyopathy, dizziness, myopathy, ototoxicity, peripheral neuropathy, pigmentation of skin, seizures, thrombocytopenia
Quinacrine usually causes diffuse yellow skin coloration
DHEA (dehydroepiandrosterone)	200 mg qd	Unclear	Acne, menstrual irregularities, high serum levels of testosterone
Methotrexate (for dermatitis, arthritis)	10–25 mg once a week, with folic acid; decrease dose if CrCl < 60 mL/min	Acitretin, leflunomide, NSAIDs and salicylates, penicillins, probenecid, sulfonamides, trimethoprim	Anemia, bone marrow suppression, leukopenia, thrombocytopenia, hepatotoxicity, nephrotoxicity, infections, neurotoxicity, pulmonary fibrosis, pneumonitis, severe dermatitis, seizures
Glucocorticoids, oral[a] (several specific brands are approved by FDA for use in SLE)	Prednisone, prednisolone: 0.5–1 mg/kg per day for severe SLE 0.07–0.3 mg/kg per day or qod for milder disease	A2R/ACE antagonists, antiarrhythmics class III, β_2 cyclosporine, NSAIDs and salicylates, phenothiazines, phenytoins, quinolones, rifampin, risperidone, thiazides, sulfonylureas, warfarin	Infection, VZV infection, hypertension, hyperglycemia, hypokalemia, acne, allergic reactions, anxiety, aseptic necrosis of bone, Cushingoid changes, CHF, fragile skin, insomnia, menstrual irregularities, mood swings, osteoporosis, psychosis
Methylprednisolone sodium succinate, intravenous[a] (approved for lupus nephritis)	For severe disease, 1 g IV qd × 3 days	As for oral glucocorticoids	As for oral glucocorticoids (if used repeatedly); anaphylaxis
Cyclophosphamide[b]		Allopurinol, bone marrow suppressants, colony-stimulating factors, doxorubicin, rituximab, succinylcholine, zidovudine	Infection, VZV infection, bone marrow suppression, leukopenia, anemia, thrombocytopenia, hemorrhagic cystitis (less with IV), carcinoma of the bladder, alopecia, nausea, diarrhea, malaise, malignancy, sterility
Intravenous	7–25 mg/kg q month × 6; consider mesna administration with dose		
Oral	1.5–3 mg/kg per day Decrease dose for CrCl < 25 mL/min		
Mycophenolate mofetil[b] (approved for lupus nephritis)	2–3 g/d PO	Acyclovir, antacids, azathioprine, bile acid–binding resins, ganciclovir, iron salts, probenecid, oral contraceptives	Infection, leukopenia, anemia, thrombocytopenia, lymphoma, lymphoproliferative disorders, malignancy
Alopecia, cough, diarrhea, fever, GI symptoms, headache, hypertension, hypercholesterolemia, hypokalemia, insomnia peripheral edema, transaminitis, tremor, rash
Azathioprine[b]	2–3 mg/kg per day PO; decrease frequency of dose if CrCl < 50 mL/min	ACE inhibitors, allopurinol, bone marrow suppressants, interferons, mycophenolate mofetil, rituximab, warfarin, zidovudine	Infection, VZV infection, bone marrow suppression, leukopenia, anemia, thrombocytopenia, pancreatitis, hepatotoxicity, malignancy, alopecia, fever, flulike illness, GI symptoms

[a] Indicates medication is approved for use in SLE by the U.S. Food and Drug Administration.
[b] Indicates the medication has been used with glucocorticoids in the trials showing efficacy.

Note: NSAIDs, nonsteroidal anti-inflammatory drugs; FDA, U.S. Food and Drug Administration; A2R, angiotensin 2 receptor; ACE, angiotensin-converting enzyme; GI, gastrointestinal; SPF, sun protection factor; CrCl, creatinine clearance; VZV, varicella-zoster virus; CHF, congestive heart failure.

NSAIDs, are no safer in this regard, although they may cause fewer adverse gastrointestinal events (studies are not available in SLE). Antimalarials (hydroxychloroquine, chloroquine, and quinacrine) often reduce dermatitis, arthritis, and fatigue; a randomized placebo-controlled prospective trial has shown that hydroxychloroquine reduces the number of disease flares. Because of potential retinal toxicity, patients receiving antimalarials should undergo opthalmologic examinations at least annually. A recent placebo-controlled prospective trial suggests that administration of dehydroepiandrosterone may reduce disease activity. If quality of life is inadequate in spite of these conservative measures, treatment with low doses of systemic glucocorticoids may be necessary.

Life-Threatening SLE: Proliferative Forms of Lupus Nephritis The mainstay of treatment for any inflammatory life-threatening or organ-threatening manifestations of SLE is systemic glucocorticoids (0.5 to 2 mg/kg per day orally or 1000 mg of methylprednisolone sodium succinate intravenously daily for 3 days followed by 0.5–1 mg/kg of daily prednisone or equivalent). Evidence that glucocorticoid therapy is life-saving comes from retrospective studies from the predialysis era; survival is significantly better in people with DPGN treated with high-dose daily glucocorticoids (40 to 60 mg of prednisone daily for 4 to 6 months) versus lower doses. Currently, high doses are recommended for much shorter periods; recent trials of interventions for severe SLE employ 4 to 6 weeks of these doses. Thereafter, doses are tapered as rapidly as the clinical situation permits, usually to a maintenance dose varying from 5 to 10 mg of prednisone, prednisolone, or equivalent per day or 10 to 20 mg every other day. Most patients with an episode of severe lupus require many years of maintenance therapy with low-dose glucocorticoids, which can be increased to prevent or treat disease flares. However, frequent attempts to gradually reduce the glucocorticoid requirement are recommended because virtually everyone develops important adverse effects (Table 300-4). Prospective controlled trials in active lupus nephritis show that administration of high doses of glucocorticoids (1000 mg of methylprednisolone daily for 3 days) by intravenous routes compared to daily oral routes shortens the time to maximal improvement by a few weeks but does not result ultimately in better renal function. It has become standard practice to initiate therapy for active, potentially life-threatening SLE with high-dose intravenous glucocorticoid pulses, based on studies in lupus nephritis. This approach must be tempered by safety considerations, such as the presence of conditions adversely affected by glucocorticoids (infection, hyperglycemia, hypertension, osteoporosis, etc).

Cytotoxic drugs are another important class of drugs used to treat serious SLE. Almost all prospective controlled trials in SLE involving cytotoxic agents have been conducted in patients with lupus nephritis. The alkylating agent cyclophosphamide has become the standard drug used for controlling life-threatening active lupus nephritis, particularly in patients whose renal biopsies show WHO grades III, IV, and V proliferative or membranoproliferative forms of nephritis. All successful studies with cyclophosphamide have also used concomitant glucocorticoid therapy; cyclophosphamide responses begin 3 to 16 weeks after treatment is initiated, whereas glucocorticoid responses may begin within 24 h. Cyclophosphamide should be administered to patients whose severe lupus is likely to be reversible (Table 300-4); those with high serum creatinine levels [e.g., $\geq$265 μmol/L $\geq$3.0 mg/dL)] of many months duration and high chronicity scores on renal biopsy are not likely to respond. Prospective studies suggest that ESRD is significantly less frequent in patients treated with cyclophosphamide (intermittent intravenous or daily oral) compared to patients treated with glucocorticoids alone or azathioprine plus glucocorticoids. This benefit becomes measurable 5 years or more following initiation of therapy. Short-term results of any intervention (e.g., 1 to 2 years) are useful but may not adequately describe the overall utility of that approach. The recommended duration of cyclophosphamide therapy

is controversial; one prospective controlled trial (from the U.S. National Institutes of Health) comparing 6 months of intermittent intravenous treatment (monthly doses) to 30 months of treatment (6 monthly doses followed by quarterly doses) showed fewer disease flares in the 30-month group. However, a recent prospective controlled trial suggests that similar good improvement occurs if 6 monthly doses of intravenous cyclophosphamide (500 mg/m^2) plus 2 quarterly doses are followed by daily azathioprine for 2 years; equally effective was intravenous cyclophosphamide, 500 mg total, every 2 weeks for six doses, followed by daily azathioprine. Approximately 90% of this group were Caucasian. Response of lupus nephritis to cyclophosphamide and glucocorticoids is better in Caucasian groups than in African Americans. Therefore, interpretation of studies using different therapeutic approaches must include considerations of ethnicity as well as duration of follow-up and differences in inclusion and exclusion criteria for entry. The adverse effects most likely to influence patient choice against the use of cyclophosphamide are a high rate of irreversible ovarian or testicular failure with increasing cumulative doses, nausea and malaise that often accompany each intravenous dose, alopecia, and frequent infections.

Since glucocorticoid-plus-cyclophosphamide therapy has many adverse effects and is often disliked by patients, there has been a search for other cytotoxic agents and for different approaches that are less toxic. Azathioprine (a purine antagonist) added to glucocorticoids probably reduces the number of SLE flares and the maintenance glucocorticoid requirement; however, this approach requires several months to be effective, and cyclophosphamide is effective in a higher proportion of patients. Daily oral azathioprine may have fewer adverse effects than daily oral cyclophosphamide; intermittent intravenous cyclophosphamide probably has fewer adverse effects than daily oral cyclophosphamide. Mycophenolate mofetil (a relatively lymphocyte-specific inhibitor of inosine monophosphate dehydrogenase) is an effective cytotoxic agent in some patients with severe SLE. A recent prospective study in Chinese patients with lupus nephritis comparing daily oral mycophenolate plus prednisolone for 12 months to daily oral cyclophosphamide plus prednisolone for 6 months followed by oral daily azathioprine plus prednisolone showed good improvement in ~80% of patients in both groups at 1 year of follow-up and fewer adverse effects with mycophenolate. Chlorambucil is an alkylating agent that can be substituted for cyclophosphamide; the risk of irreversible bone marrow suppression may be greater with this agent. Methotrexate (a folinic acid antagonist) may have a role in the treatment of arthritis and dermatitis but probably not in life-threatening disease. The role of leflunomide, a relatively lymphocyte-specific pyrimidine antagonist, is being studied in patients with SLE. Cyclosporine, which inhibits production of IL-2 and inhibits T lymphocyte functions, has not been studied in prospective controlled trials in SLE but is nonetheless used by some clinicians. Since it has potential nephrotoxicity, but no bone marrow toxicity, the author uses it (in doses of 3 to 5 mg/kg per day orally) in patients with steroid-resistant cytopenias of SLE or in steroid-resistant patients who have developed bone marrow suppression from standard cytotoxic agents.

Special Conditions in SLE that May Require Additional or Different Therapies

■ *PREGNANCY AND LUPUS* Fertility rates for men and women with SLE are probably normal. However, rate of fetal loss is increased (approximately two- to threefold) in women with SLE. Fetal demise is higher in mothers with high disease activity, antiphospholipid antibodies, and/or nephritis. Suppression of disease activity can be achieved by administration of systemic glucocorticoids. A placental enzyme 11-β-dehydrogenase 2 deactivates glucocorticoids; it is more effective in deactivating prednisone and prednisolone than the fluorinated glucocorticoids dexamethasone and betamethasone. Therefore, maternal SLE should be controlled with prednisone/prednisolone at the lowest effective doses for the shortest time required. Adverse effects of prenatal glucocorticoid exposure (primarily betamethasone) on offspring may include low birth weight, developmental abnormalities in the

CNS, and predeliction toward adult metabolic syndrome. In SLE patients with aPL (on at least two occasions) and prior fetal losses, treatment with heparin (standard or low-molecular-weight) plus low-dose aspirin has been shown in prospective controlled trials to increase significantly the proportion of live births. An additional potential problem for the fetus is the presence of antibodies to Ro, sometimes associated with neonatal lupus (rash and congenital heart block). The latter can be life-threatening; therefore the presence of anti-Ro requires vigilant monitoring of fetal heart rates with prompt intervention if distress occurs. Women with SLE usually tolerate pregnancy without disease flares. However, a small proportion develop severe flares requiring aggressive glucocorticoid therapy or early delivery. Poor maternal outcomes are highest in women with active nephritis or irreversible organ damage in kidneys, brain, or heart.

LUPUS AND APS Patients with SLE who have venous or arterial clotting, and/or repeated fetal losses, and at least two positive tests for aPL have APS and should be managed with long-term anticoagulation. A target INR of 3.0 is recommended, based on reduction of new clotting events in patients treated to this target INR compared to patients treated to lower INR levels, in retrospective analyses of cohorts with primary or secondary APS.

MICROVASCULAR THROMBOTIC CRISIS (THROMBOTIC THROMBOCYTOPENIC PURPURA, HEMOLYTIC UREMIC SYNDROME) This syndrome of hemolysis, thrombocytopenia, and microvascular thrombosis in kidneys, brain, and other tissues carries a high mortality rate and occurs most commonly in young individuals with lupus nephritis. The most useful laboratory tests are identification of schistocytes on peripheral blood smears and elevated serum levels of lactate dehydrogenase. Plasma exchange or extensive plasmapheresis is usually life-saving; there is no evidence that glucocorticoids or cytotoxic drugs are effective.

LUPUS DERMATITIS Patients with any form of lupus dermatitis should minimize exposure to ultraviolet light, employing appropriate clothing and sunscreens with a sun protection factor of at least 15. Topical glucocorticoids and antimalarials (such as hydroxychloroquine) are effective in reducing lesion severity in most patients and are relatively safe. Systemic treatment with retinoic acid is a useful strategy in patients with inadequate improvement on topical glucocorticoids and antimalarials; adverse effects are potentially severe (particularly fetal abnormalities). Extensive, pruritic, bullous, or ulcerating dermatitides usually improve promptly after institution of systemic glucocorticoids; tapering may be accompanied by flare of lesions, thus necessitating use of a second medication such as hydroxychloroquine, retinoids, or cytotoxic medications such as methotrexate or azathioprine. In therapy-resistant lupus dermatitis there are reports of success with topical tacrolimus or with systemic dapsone or thalidomide (the extreme danger of fetal deformities from thalidomide requires permission from and supervision by the supplier).

Preventive Therapies Prevention of complications of SLE and its therapy include providing appropriate vaccinations (the administration of influenza and pneumococcal vaccines has been studied in patients with SLE; flare rates are similar to those receiving placebo) and suppressing recurrent urinary tract infections. In addition, strategies to prevent osteoporosis should be initiated in most patients likely to require long-term glucocorticoid therapy and/or with other predisposing factors. Control of hypertension and appropriate prevention strategies for atherosclerosis, including monitoring and treatment of dyslipidemias, management of hyperglycemia, and obesity, are recommended.

Experimental Therapies Several new biologics and selective cytotoxic medications are in various phases of clinical trials in the United States. Most strategies target T or B lymphocytes, particularly those under-

going activation, rather than entire cell populations. These include LJP394 (may tolerize B cells making anti-DNA), antibodies to CD40L and CTLA4-Ig fusion protein (interrupt T/B second signals), antibody to complement C′5, and antibody to CD20 (depletes some B cells). Several studies have employed transplantation of hematopoietic stem cells for the treatment of severe and refractory SLE.

PATIENT OUTCOMES, PROGNOSIS, AND SURVIVAL Survival in patients with SLE is 90 to 95% at 2 years, 82 to 90% at 5 years, 71 to 80% at 10 years, and 63 to 75% at 20 years. Poor prognosis (approximately 50% mortality in 10 years) is associated with (at the time of diagnosis) high serum creatinine levels [>124 μmol/L (>1.4 mg/dL)], hypertension, nephrotic syndrome (24-h urine protein excretion >2.6 g), anemia [hemoglobin <124 g/L (<12.4 g/dL)], hypoalbuminemia, hypocomplementemia, and aPL. Prognosis is worse in African Americans than in Caucasians. Patients who require renal transplantation have a relatively high incidence of graft rejection (approximately twice that of patients with other causes of ESRD), but overall patient survival is comparable (85% at 2 years). Lupus nephritis occurs in 10% of transplanted kidneys. Disability in patients with SLE is common due primarily to chronic renal disease, fatigue, arthritis, and pain. As many as 25% of patients may experience remissions, sometimes for a few years, but these are rarely permanent. The leading causes of death in the first decade of disease are systemic disease activity, renal failure, and infections; subsequently, thromboembolic events become increasingly frequent causes of mortality.

DRUG-INDUCED LUPUS This is a syndrome of positive ANA associated with symptoms such as fever, malaise, arthritis or intense arthralgias/myalgias, serositis, and/or rash. The syndrome appears during therapy with certain medications and biologic agents, is predominant in Caucasians, has less female predilection than SLE, rarely involves kidneys or brain, is rarely associated with anti-dsDNA, is commonly associated with antibodies to histones, and usually resolves over several weeks after discontinuation of the offending medication. The list of substances that can induce lupus-like disease is long. Among the most frequent are the anti-arrhythmics procaineamide, disopyramide, propafenone; the antihypertensives hydralazine, several angiotensin-converting enzyme inhibitors and beta-blockers; the antithyroid propylthiouracil; the antipsychotics chlorpromazine and lithium; the anticonvulsants carbamazepine and phenytoin; the antibiotics isoniazid, minocycline, and macrodantin; the antirheumatic sulfasalazine; the diuretic hydrochlorothiazide; the antihyperlipidemics lovastatin and simvastatin; and the biologics interferons and tumor necrosis factor inhibitors. ANA usually appears before symptoms; however, many of the medications mentioned above induce ANA in patients who never develop symptoms of drug-induced lupus. It is appropriate to test for ANA at the first hint of relevant symptoms and to use test results to help decide whether to withdraw the suspect agent.

FURTHER READING

DAVIDSON A, DIAMOND B: Autoimmune diseases. N Engl J Med 354:340, 2001

GAFFNEY PM et al: Recent advances in the genetics of systemic lupus erythematosus. Rheum Dis Clin North Am 28:111, 2002

HAHN BH: Mechanisms of disease: Antibodies to DNA. N Engl J Med 338: 1359, 1998

HOUSSIAU FA et al: Immunosuppressive therapy in lupus nephritis: the Euro-Lupus Nephritis Trial, a randomized trial of low-dose versus high-dose cyclophosphamide therapy. Arthritis Rheum 46:2121, 2002

LEVINE JS et al: The antiphospholipid syndrome. N Engl J Med 346:752, 2002

WALLACE DJ, HAHN BH (eds): *Dubois' Lupus Erythematosus*, 6th ed. Philadelphia, Lippincott Williams & Wilkins, 2002

Rheumatoid arthritis (RA) is a chronic multisystem disease of unknown cause. Although there are a variety of systemic manifestations, the characteristic feature of RA is persistent inflammatory synovitis, usually involving peripheral joints in a symmetric distribution. The potential of the synovial inflammation to cause cartilage damage and bone erosions and subsequent changes in joint integrity is the hallmark of the disease. Despite its destructive potential, the course of RA can be quite variable. Some patients may experience only a mild oligoarticular illness of brief duration with minimal joint damage, whereas others will have a relentless progressive polyarthritis with marked functional impairment.

EPIDEMIOLOGY AND GENETICS The prevalence of RA is approximately 0.8% of the population (range 0.3 to 2.1%); women are affected approximately three times more often than men. The prevalence increases with age, and sex differences diminish in the older age group. RA is seen throughout the world and affects all races. However, the incidence and severity seem to be less in rural sub-Saharan Africa and in Caribbean blacks. The onset is most frequent during the fourth and fifth decades of life, with 80% of all patients developing the disease between the ages of 35 and 50. The incidence of RA is more than six times greater in 60- to 64-year-old women compared to 18- to 29-year-old women. Recent data indicate that the incidence of RA may be diminishing.

Family studies indicate a genetic predisposition. For example, severe RA is found at approximately four times the expected rate in first-degree relatives of individuals with disease associated with the presence of the autoantibody, rheumatoid factor; approximately 10% of patients with RA will have an affected first-degree relative. Moreover, monozygotic twins are at least four times more likely to be concordant for RA than dizygotic twins, who have a similar risk of developing RA as nontwin siblings. Only 15 to 20% of monozygotic twins are concordant for RA, however, implying that factors other than genetics play an important etiopathogenic role. Of note, the highest risk for concordance of RA is noted in twins who have two HLA-DRB1 alleles known to be associated with RA. The class II major histocompatibility complex allele HLA-DR4 (DRβ1*0401) and related alleles are known to be major genetic risk factors for RA. Early studies showed that as many as 70% of patients with classic or definite RA express HLA-DR4 compared with 28% of control individuals. An association with HLA-DR4 has been noted in many populations, including North American and European whites, Chippewa Indians, Japanese, and native populations in India, Mexico, South America, and southern China. In a number of groups, including Israeli Jews, Asian Indians, and Yakima Indians of North America, however, there is no association between the development of RA and HLA-DR4. In these individuals, there is an association between RA and the closely related HLA-DR1 (DRβ1*0101) in the former two groups and HLA-Dw16 (DRβ1*1402) in the latter. It has been estimated that the risk of developing RA in a person with DRβ1*0401 or the closely related DRβ1*0404 is 1 in 35 and 1 in 20, respectively, whereas the presence of both alleles puts persons at an even greater risk. In certain groups of patients, there does not appear to be a clear association between HLA-DR4–related epitopes and RA. Thus, nearly 75% of African-American RA patients do not have this genetic element. Moreover, there is an association with HLA-DR10 (DRβ1*1001) in Spanish and Italian patients, with HLA-DR9 (DRβ1*0901) in Chileans, and with HLA-DR3 (DRβ1*0301) in Arab populations.

Additional genes in the HLA-D complex may also convey altered susceptibility to RA. Certain HLA-DR alleles, including HLA-DR5 (DRβ1*1101), HLA-DR2 (DRβ1*1501), HLA-DR3 (DRβ1*0301), and HLA-DR7 (DRβ1*0701), may protect against the development of RA in that they tend to be found at lower frequency in RA patients

than in controls. Moreover, the HLA-DQ alleles, DQβ1*0301 and DQβ1*0302, that are in linkage disequilibrium with HLA-DR4 and DQβ1*0501, have also been associated with RA. This has raised the possibility that HLA-DQ alleles may represent the actual RA susceptibility genes, whereas specific HLA-DR alleles may convey protection. In this model, the complement of HLA-DR and DQ alleles determines RA susceptibility. Disease manifestations have also been associated with HLA phenotype. Thus, early aggressive disease and extraarticular manifestations are more frequent in patients with DRβ1*0401 or DRβ1*0404, and more slowly progressive disease in those with DRβ1*0101. The presence of both DRβ1*0401 and DRβ1*0404 appears to increase the risk for both aggressive articular and extraarticular disease. It has been estimated that HLA genes contribute only a portion of the genetic susceptibility to RA. Thus genes outside the HLA complex also contribute. These include genes controlling the expression of the antigen receptor on T cells and both immunoglobulin heavy and light chains. Moreover, polymorphisms in the tumor necrosis factor (TNF) and the interleukin (IL) 10 genes are also associated with RA, as is a region on chromosome 3 (3q13). In addition, a number of other genetic regions appear to confer risk for RA.

Genetic risk factors do not fully account for the incidence of RA, suggesting that environmental factors also play a role in the etiology of the disease. This is emphasized by epidemiologic studies in Africa that have indicated that climate and urbanization have a major impact on the incidence and severity of RA in groups of similar genetic background.

ETIOLOGY The cause of RA remains unknown. It has been suggested that RA might be a manifestation of the response to an infectious agent in a genetically susceptible host. Because of the worldwide distribution of RA, it has been hypothesized that if an infectious agent is involved, the organism must be ubiquitous. A number of possible causative agents have been suggested, including *Mycoplasma*, Epstein-Barr virus (EBV), cytomegalovirus, parvovirus, and rubella virus, but convincing evidence that these or other infectious agents cause RA has not emerged. The process by which an infectious agent might cause chronic inflammatory arthritis with a characteristic distribution also remains a matter of controversy. One possibility is that there is persistent infection of articular structures or retention of microbial products in the synovial tissues that generates a chronic inflammatory response. Alternatively, the microorganism or response to the microorganism might induce an immune response to components of the joint by altering its integrity and revealing antigenic peptides. In this regard, reactivity to type II collagen and heat shock proteins has been demonstrated. Another possibility is that the infecting microorganism might prime the host to cross-reactive determinants expressed within the joint as a result of "molecular mimicry." Recent evidence of similarity between products of certain gram-negative bacteria and EBV and the HLA-DR4 molecule itself has supported this possibility. Finally, products of infecting microorganisms, such as superantigens, might induce the disease. Superantigens are proteins with the capacity to bind to HLA-DR molecules and particular V$_\beta$ segments of the heterodimeric T cell receptor and stimulate specific T cells expressing the V$_\beta$ gene products (Chap. 295). The role of superantigens in the etiology of RA remains speculative. Of all the potential environmental triggers, the only one clearly associated with the development of RA is cigarette smoking.

PATHOLOGY AND PATHOGENESIS Microvascular injury and an increase in the number of synovial lining cells appear to be the earliest lesions in rheumatoid synovitis. The nature of the insult causing this response is not known. Subsequently, an increased number of synovial lining cells is seen along with perivascular infiltration with mononuclear cells. Before the onset of clinical symptoms, the perivascular infiltrate is predominantly composed of myeloid cells, whereas in symptomatic arthritis, T cells can also be found, although their number does not appear to correlate with symptoms. As the process continues, the synovium becomes edematous and protrudes into the joint cavity as villous projections.

Light-microscopic examination discloses a characteristic constellation of features, which include hyperplasia and hypertrophy of the synovial lining cells; focal or segmental vascular changes, including microvascular injury, thrombosis, and neovascularization; edema; and infiltration with mononuclear cells, often collected into aggregates around small blood vessels (Fig. 301-1). The endothelial cells of the rheumatoid synovium have the appearance of high endothelial venules of lymphoid organs and have been altered by cytokine exposure to facilitate entry of cells into tissue. Rheumatoid synovial endothelial cells express increased amounts of various adhesion molecules involved in this process. Although this pathologic picture is typical of RA, it can also be seen in a variety of other chronic inflammatory arthritides. The mononuclear cell collections are variable in composition and size. The predominant infiltrating cell is the T lymphocyte. CD4+ T cells predominate over CD8+ T cells and are frequently found in close proximity to HLA-DR+ macrophages and dendritic cells. Increased numbers of a separate population of T cells expressing the $\gamma\delta$ form of the T cell receptor have also been found in the synovium, although they remain a minor population there and their role in RA has not been delineated. The major population of T cells in the rheumatoid synovium is composed of CD4+ memory T cells that form the majority of cells aggregated around postcapillary venules. Scattered throughout the tissue are CD8+ T cells. Both populations express the early activation antigen, CD69. Besides the accumulation of T cells, rheumatoid synovitis is also characterized by the infiltration of variable numbers of B cells and antibody-producing plasma cells. In advanced disease, structures similar to germinal centers of secondary lymphoid organs may be observed in the synovium. Both polyclonal immunoglobulin and the autoantibody rheumatoid factor are produced within the synovial tissue, which leads to the local formation of immune complexes. Antibodies to synovial tissue components may also contribute to inflammation. Increased numbers of activated mast cells are also found in the rheumatoid synovium. Local release of the contents of their granules may contribute to inflammation. Finally, the synovial fibroblasts in RA manifest evidence of activation in that they produce a number of enzymes such as collagenase and cathepsins that can degrade components of the articular matrix. These activated fibroblasts are particularly prominent in the lining layer and at the interface with bone and cartilage. Osteoclasts are also prominent at sites of bone erosion. Activated mesenchymal stromal cells, similar to those found in normal bone marrow, can also be found in the rheumatoid synovium.

The rheumatoid synovium is characterized by the presence of a number of secreted products of activated lymphocytes, macrophages, and fibroblasts. The local production of these cytokines and chemokines appears to account for many of the pathologic and clinical manifestations of RA. These effector molecules include those that are derived from T lymphocytes, those originating from activated myeloid cells, and those secreted by other cell types in the synovium, such as fibroblasts and endothelial cells. The activity of these chemokines and cytokines appears to account for many of the features of rheumatoid synovitis, including the synovial tissue inflammation, synovial fluid inflammation, synovial proliferation, and cartilage and bone damage, as well as the systemic manifestations of RA. In addition to the production of effector molecules that propagate the inflammatory process, local factors are produced that tend to slow the inflammation, including specific inhibitors of cytokine action and additional cytokines, such as transforming growth factor (TGF-β), which inhibits many of the features of rheumatoid synovitis including T cell activation and proliferation, B cell differentiation, and migration of cells into the inflammatory site.

These findings have suggested that the propagation of RA is an immunologically mediated event, although the original initiating stimulus has not been characterized. One view is that the inflammatory process in the tissue is driven by the CD4+ T cells infiltrating the synovium. Evidence for this includes (1) the predominance of CD4+ T cells in the synovium; (2) the increase in soluble IL-2 receptors, a product of activated T cells, in blood and synovial fluid of patients with active RA; and (3) amelioration of the disease by removal of T cells by thoracic duct drainage or peripheral lymphapheresis or suppression of their proliferation or function by drugs, such as cyclosporine, leflunomide, or nondepleting monoclonal antibodies to CD4, or inhibitors of T cell activation, such as the T cell co-stimulation competitor, CTLA-4·Ig. In addition, the association of RA with certain HLA-DR or -DQ alleles, whose only known functions are to shape the repertoire of CD4+ T cells during ontogeny in the thymus and bind and present antigenic peptides to CD4+ T cells in the periphery, strongly implies a role for CD4+ T cells in the pathogenesis of the disease. Finally, patients with established RA who become infected with HIV have also been noted to improve, although this has not been a uniform finding. Within the rheumatoid synovium, the CD4+ T cells differentiate predominantly into T_H1-like effector cells producing the proinflammatory cytokine interferon (IFN) γ and appear to be deficient in differentiation into T_H2-like effector cells capable of producing the anti-inflammatory cytokine IL-4. As a result of the ongoing secretion of IFN-γ without the regulatory influences of IL-4, macrophages are activated to produce the proinflammatory cytokines IL-1 and TNF and also increase expression of HLA molecules. Direct contact between activated T cells and myeloid cells may also lead to the production of proinflammatory cytokines by the latter. Moreover, T lymphocytes express surface molecules such as CD154 (CD40 ligand) and also produce a variety of cytokines that promote B cell proliferation and differentiation into antibody-forming cells and therefore may also promote local B cell stimulation. The resultant production of immunoglobulin and rheumatoid factor can lead to immune-complex formation with consequent complement activation and exacerbation of the inflammatory process by the production of the anaphylatoxins, C3a and C5a, and the chemotactic factor C5a. In addition, antibodies may be produced to other self-antigens than can contribute to disease pathogenesis. The tissue inflammation is reminiscent of chronic inflammatory responses to persistent microorganisms, although it has become clear that the number of T cells producing cytokines such as IFN-γ is less than is found in typical delayed-type hypersensitivity reactions, perhaps owing to the large amount of reactive oxygen species produced locally in the synovium that can dampen T cell function. It remains unclear whether the persistent T cell activity represents a response to a persistent exogenous antigen or to altered autoantigens such as collagen, immunoglobulin, or one of the heat shock proteins, or perhaps both. Alternatively, it could represent persistent responsiveness to activated autologous cells such as might occur as a result

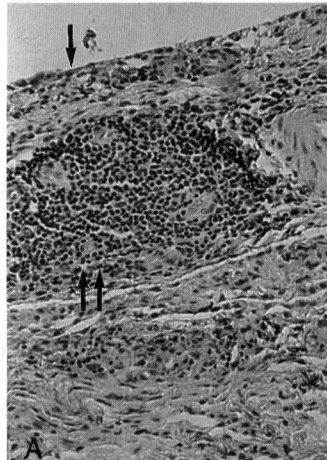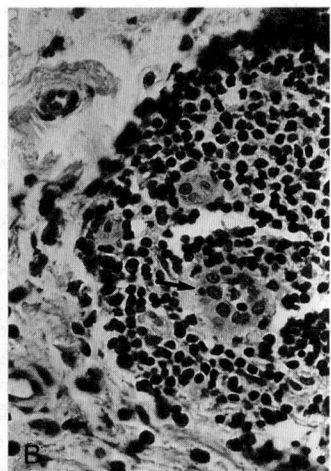

FIGURE 301-1 Histology of rheumatoid synovitis. *A.* The characteristic features of rheumatoid inflammation with hyperplasia of the lining layer (*arrow*) and mononuclear infiltrates in the sublining layer (*double arrow*). *B.* A higher magnification of the largely CD4+ T cell infiltrate around postcapillary venules (*arrow*).

of EBV infection or persistent response to a foreign antigen or super-antigen in the synovial tissue. Finally, rheumatoid inflammation could reflect persistent stimulation of T cells by synovial-derived antigens that cross-react with determinants introduced during antecedent exposure to foreign antigens or infectious microorganisms. The important contribution of B lymphocytes to the chronic inflammatory process has been emphasized by the observation that treatment with a monoclonal antibody to the B cell marker, CD20, caused prompt depletion of B lymphocytes and an amelioration of signs and symptoms of inflammation.

Overriding the chronic inflammation in the synovial tissue is an acute inflammatory process in the synovial fluid. The exudative synovial fluid contains more polymorphonuclear leukocytes than mononuclear cells. A number of mechanisms play a role in stimulating the exudation of synovial fluid. Locally produced antibodies to tissue components and immune complexes can activate complement and generate anaphylatoxins and chemotactic factors. Local production of chemokines and cytokines with chemotactic activity as well as inflammatory mediators such as leukotriene B_4 and products of complement activation can attract neutrophils. Moreover, many of these same agents can also stimulate the endothelial cells of postcapillary venules to become more efficient at binding circulating cells. The net result is the enhanced migration of polymorphonuclear leukocytes into the synovial site. In addition, vasoactive mediators such as histamine produced by the mast cells that infiltrate the rheumatoid synovium may also facilitate the exudation of inflammatory cells into the synovial fluid. Finally, the vasodilatory effects of locally produced prostaglandin E_2 may also facilitate entry of inflammatory cells into the inflammatory site. Once in the synovial fluid, the polymorphonuclear leukocytes can ingest immune complexes, with the resultant production of reactive oxygen metabolites and other inflammatory mediators, further adding to the inflammatory milieu. Locally produced cytokines and chemokines can additionally stimulate polymorphonuclear leukocytes. The production of large amounts of cyclooxygenase and lipoxygenase pathway products of arachidonic acid metabolism by cells in the synovial fluid and tissue further accentuates the signs and symptoms of inflammation.

The precise mechanism by which bone and cartilage destruction occurs has not been completely resolved. Although the synovial fluid contains a number of enzymes potentially able to degrade cartilage, the majority of destruction occurs in juxtaposition to the inflamed synovium, or pannus, that spreads to cover the articular cartilage. This vascular granulation tissue is composed of proliferating fibroblasts, small blood vessels, and a variable number of mononuclear cells and produces a large amount of degradative enzymes, including collagenase and stromelysin, that may facilitate tissue damage. The cytokines IL-1 and TNF play an important role by stimulating the cells of the pannus to produce collagenase and other neutral proteases. These same two cytokines also activate chondrocytes in situ, stimulating them to produce proteolytic enzymes that can degrade cartilage locally and also inhibiting synthesis of new matrix molecules. Finally, these two cytokines may contribute to the local demineralization of bone by activating osteoclasts that accumulate at the site of local bone resorption. Prostaglandin E_2 produced by fibroblasts and macrophages may also contribute to bone demineralization. The common final pathway of bone erosion is likely to involve the activation of osteoclasts that are present in large numbers at these sites. Systemic manifestations of RA can be accounted for by release of inflammatory effector molecules from the synovium. These include IL-1, TNF, and IL-6, which account for many of the manifestations of active RA, including malaise, fatigue, and elevated levels of serum acute-phase reactants. The importance of TNF in producing these manifestations is emphasized by the prompt amelioration of symptoms following administration of a monoclonal antibody to TNF or a soluble TNF receptor Ig construct to patients with RA. In addition, immune complexes produced within the synovium and entering the circulation may account for other features of the disease, such as systemic vasculitis.

As shown in Fig. 301-2, the pathology of RA evolves over the duration of this chronic disease. The earliest event appears to be a nonspecific inflammatory response initiated by an unknown stimulus and characterized by accumulation of macrophages and other mononuclear cells within the sublining layer of the synovium. The activity of these cells is demonstrated by the increased appearance of macrophage-derived cytokines, including TNF, IL-1β, and IL-6. Subsequently, activation and differentiation of memory CD4+ T cells is induced, presumably in response to antigenic peptides displayed by a variety of antigen-presenting cells in the synovial tissue. The activated memory T cells are capable of producing cytokines, especially IFN-γ, which amplify and perpetuate the inflammation. The presence of activated T cells expressing CD154 (CD40 ligand) can induce polyclonal B cell stimulation and differentiation of memory B cells and plasma cells that produce autoantibodies locally. The cascade of cytokines produced in the synovium activates a variety of cells in the synovium, bone, and cartilage to produce effector molecules that can cause tissue damage characteristic of chronic inflammation. It is important to emphasize that there is no current way to predict the progress from one stage of inflammation to the next, and once established, each can influence the other. Important features of this model include the following: (1) the major pathologic events vary with time in this chronic disease; (2) the time required to progress from one step to the next may vary in different patients, and the events, once established, may persist simultaneously; (3) once established, the major pathogenic events operative in an individual patient, may vary at different times; (4) the process is chronic and reiterative, with successive events stimulating progressive amplification of inflammation; and (5) once memory T cells and B cells have been generated, anti-inflammatory and anti-cytokine therapy may be capable of suppressing disease manifestations but not preventing recrudescence of disease activity once therapy is discontinued. These considerations have important implications with regard to appropriate treatment.

CLINICAL MANIFESTATIONS ■ Onset Characteristically, RA is a chronic polyarthritis. In approximately two-thirds of patients, it begins insidiously with fatigue, anorexia, generalized weakness, and vague musculoskeletal symptoms until the appearance of synovitis becomes apparent. This prodrome may persist for weeks or months and defy diagnosis. Specific symptoms usually appear gradually as several joints, especially those of the hands, wrists, knees, and feet, become affected in a symmetric fashion. In approximately 10% of individuals, the onset is more acute, with a rapid development of polyarthritis, often accompanied by constitutional symptoms, including fever, lymphadenopathy, and splenomegaly. In approximately one-third of patients, symptoms may initially be confined to one or a few joints. Although the pattern of joint involvement may remain asymmetric in a few patients, a symmetric pattern is more typical.

Signs and Symptoms of Articular Disease Pain, swelling, and tenderness may initially be poorly localized to the joints. Pain in affected joints, aggravated by movement, is the most common manifestation of established RA. It corresponds in pattern to the joint involvement but does not always correlate with the degree of apparent inflammation. Generalized stiffness is frequent and is usually greatest after periods of inactivity. Morning stiffness of greater than 1-h duration is an almost invariable feature of inflammatory arthritis and may serve to distinguish it from various noninflammatory joint disorders. Notably, however, the presence of morning stiffness may not reliably distinguish between chronic inflammatory and noninflammatory arthritides, as it is also found frequently in the latter. The majority of patients will experience constitutional symptoms such as weakness, easy fatigability, anorexia, and weight loss. Although fever to 40°C occurs on occasion, temperature elevation in excess of 38°C is unusual and suggests the presence of an intercurrent problem such as infection.

Clinically, synovial inflammation causes swelling, tenderness, and limitation of motion. Initially, impairment in physical function is caused by pain and inflammation, and disability owing to this is a frequent early feature of aggressive RA. Warmth is usually evident on examination, especially of large joints such as the knee, but erythema is infrequent. Pain originates predominantly from the joint capsule, which is abundantly supplied with pain fibers and is markedly sensitive to stretching or distention. Joint swelling results from accumulation of synovial fluid, hypertrophy of the synovium, and thickening of the joint capsule. Initially, motion is limited by pain. The inflamed joint is usually held in flexion to maximize joint volume and minimize distention of the capsule. Later, fibrous or bony ankylosis or soft tissue contractures lead to fixed deformities.

Although inflammation can affect any diarthrodial joint, RA most often causes symmetric arthritis with characteristic involvement of certain specific joints such as the proximal interphalangeal and metacarpophalangeal joints. The distal interphalangeal joints are rarely involved. Synovitis of the wrist joints is a nearly uniform feature of RA and may lead to limitation of motion, deformity, and median nerve entrapment (carpal tunnel syndrome). Synovitis of the elbow joint often leads to flexion contractures that may develop early in the disease. The knee joint is commonly involved with synovial hypertrophy, chronic effusion, and frequently ligamentous laxity. Pain and swelling behind the knee may be caused by extension of inflamed synovium into the popliteal space (Baker's cyst). Arthritis in the forefoot, ankles, and subtalar joints can produce severe pain with ambulation as well as a number of deformities. Axial involvement is usually limited to the upper cervical spine. Involvement of the lumbar spine is not seen, and lower back pain cannot be ascribed to rheumatoid inflammation. On occasion, inflammation from the synovial joints and bursae of the upper cervical spine leads to atlantoaxial subluxation. This usually presents as pain in the occiput but on rare occasions may lead to compression of the spinal cord.

With persistent inflammation, a variety of characteristic joint changes develop. These can be attributed to a number of pathologic events, including laxity of supporting soft tissue structures; damage or weakening of ligaments, tendons, and the joint capsule; cartilage degradation; muscle imbalance; and unopposed physical forces associated with the use of affected joints. Characteristic changes of the hand include (1) radial deviation at the wrist with ulnar deviation of the digits, often with palmar subluxation of the proximal phalanges ("Z" deformity); (2) hyperextension of the proximal interphalangeal joints, with compensatory flexion of the distal interphalangeal joints (swanneck deformity); (3) flexion contracture of the proximal interphalangeal joints and extension of the distal interphalangeal joints (boutonnière deformity); and (4) hyperextension of the first interphalangeal joint and flexion of the first metacarpophalangeal joint with a consequent loss of thumb mobility and pinch. Typical joint changes may also develop in the feet, including eversion at the hindfoot (subtalar joint), plantar subluxation of the metatarsal heads, widening of the forefoot, hallux valgus, and lateral deviation and dorsal subluxation of the toes. Later in the disease, disability is more related to structural damage to articular structures.

Extraarticular Manifestations RA is a systemic disease with a variety of extraarticular manifestations. Although these occur frequently, not all of them have clinical significance. However, on occasion, they may be the major evidence of disease activity and source of morbidity and require management per se. As a rule, these manifestations occur in individuals with high titers of autoantibodies to the Fc component of immunoglobulin G (rheumatoid factors).

Rheumatoid nodules develop in 20 to 30% of persons with RA.

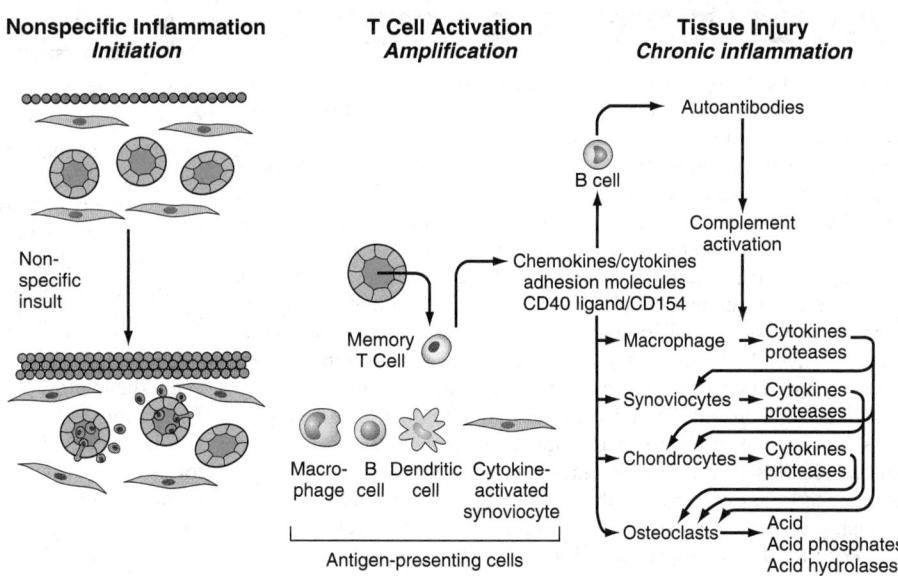

FIGURE 301-2 *The progression of rheumatoid synovitis. This figure depicts the evolution of the pathogenic mechanisms and ultimate pathologic changes involved in the development of rheumatoid synovitis. The stages of rheumatoid arthritis are proposed to be an initiation phase of nonspecific inflammation, followed by an amplification phase resulting from T cell activation, and finally a stage of chronic inflammation with tissue injury. A variety of stimuli may initiate the initial phase of nonspecific inflammation, which may last for a protracted period of time with no or moderate symptoms. When activation of memory T cells in response to a variety of peptides presented by antigen-presenting cells occurs in genetically susceptible individuals, amplification of inflammation occurs with the promotion of local rheumatoid factor production and enhanced capacity to mediate tissue damage.*

They are usually found on periarticular structures, extensor surfaces, or other areas subjected to mechanical pressure, but they can develop elsewhere, including the pleura and meninges. Common locations include the olecranon bursa, the proximal ulna, the Achilles tendon, and the occiput. Nodules vary in size and consistency and are rarely symptomatic, but on occasion they break down as a result of trauma or become infected. They are found almost invariably in individuals with circulating rheumatoid factor. Histologically, rheumatoid nodules consist of a central zone of necrotic material including collagen fibrils, noncollagenous filaments, and cellular debris; a midzone of palisading macrophages that express HLA-DR antigens; and an outer zone of granulation tissue. Examination of early nodules has suggested that the initial event may be a focal vasculitis. In some patients, treatment with methotrexate can increase the number of nodules dramatically.

Clinical weakness and atrophy of skeletal muscle are common. Muscle atrophy may be evident within weeks of the onset of RA and is usually most apparent in musculature approximating affected joints. Muscle biopsy may show type II fiber atrophy and muscle fiber necrosis with or without a mononuclear cell infiltrate.

Rheumatoid vasculitis (Chap. 306), which can affect nearly any organ system, is seen in patients with severe RA and high titers of circulating rheumatoid factor. Rheumatoid vasculitis is very uncommon in African Americans. In its most aggressive form, rheumatoid vasculitis can cause polyneuropathy and mononeuritis multiplex, cutaneous ulceration and dermal necrosis, digital gangrene, and visceral infarction. While such widespread vasculitis is very rare, more limited forms are not uncommon, especially in white patients with high titers of rheumatoid factor. Neurovascular disease presenting either as a mild distal sensory neuropathy or as mononeuritis multiplex may be the only sign of vasculitis. Cutaneous vasculitis usually presents as crops of small brown spots in the nail beds, nail folds, and digital pulp. Larger ischemic ulcers, especially in the lower extremity, may also develop. Myocardial infarction secondary to rheumatoid vasculitis has been reported, as has vasculitic involvement of lungs, bowel, liver, spleen, pancreas, lymph nodes, and testes. Renal vasculitis is rare.

Pleuropulmonary manifestations, which are more commonly observed in men, include pleural disease, interstitial fibrosis, pleuropulmonary nodules, pneumonitis, and arteritis. Evidence of pleuritis is found commonly at autopsy, but symptomatic disease during life is infrequent. Typically, the pleural fluid contains very low levels of glucose in the absence of infection. Pleural fluid complement is also low compared with the serum level when these are related to the total protein concentration. Pulmonary fibrosis can produce impairment of the diffusing capacity of the lung. Pulmonary nodules may appear singly or in clusters. When they appear in individuals with pneumoconiosis, a diffuse nodular fibrotic process (Caplan's syndrome) may develop. On occasion, pulmonary nodules may cavitate and produce a pneumothorax or bronchopleural fistula. Rarely, pulmonary hypertension secondary to obliteration of the pulmonary vasculature occurs. In addition to pleuropulmonary disease, upper airway obstruction from cricoarytenoid arthritis or laryngeal nodules may develop.

Clinically apparent heart disease attributed to the rheumatoid process is rare, but evidence of asymptomatic pericarditis is found at autopsy in 50% of cases. Pericardial fluid has a low glucose level and is frequently associated with the occurrence of pleural effusion. Although pericarditis is usually asymptomatic, on rare occasions death has occurred from tamponade. Chronic constrictive pericarditis may also occur.

RA tends to spare the central nervous system directly, although vasculitis can cause peripheral neuropathy. *Neurologic manifestations* may also result from atlantoaxial or midcervical spine subluxations. Nerve entrapment secondary to proliferative synovitis or joint deformities may produce neuropathies of median, ulnar, radial (interosseous branch), or anterior tibial nerves.

The rheumatoid process involves the *eye* in fewer than 1% of patients. Affected individuals usually have long-standing disease and nodules. The two principal manifestations are episcleritis, which is usually mild and transient, and scleritis, which involves the deeper layers of the eye and is a more serious inflammatory condition. Histologically, the lesion is similar to a rheumatoid nodule and may result in thinning and perforation of the globe (scleromalacia perforans). From 15 to 20% of persons with RA may develop Sjögren's syndrome with attendant keratoconjunctivitis sicca.

Felty's syndrome consists of chronic RA, splenomegaly, neutropenia, and, on occasion, anemia and thrombocytopenia. It is most common in individuals with long-standing disease. These patients frequently have high titers of rheumatoid factor, subcutaneous nodules, and other manifestations of systemic rheumatoid disease. Felty's syndrome is very uncommon in African Americans. It may develop after joint inflammation has regressed. Circulating immune complexes are often present, and evidence of complement consumption may be seen. The leukopenia is a selective neutropenia with polymorphonuclear leukocyte counts of <1500 cells/μL and sometimes <1000 cell/μL. Bone marrow examination usually reveals moderate hypercellularity with a paucity of mature neutrophils. However, the bone marrow may be normal, hyperactive, or hypoactive; maturation arrest may be seen. Hypersplenism has been proposed as one of the causes of leukopenia, but splenomegaly is not invariably found and splenectomy does not always correct the abnormality. Excessive margination of granulocytes caused by antibodies to these cells, complement activation, or binding of immune complexes may contribute to granulocytopenia. Patients with Felty's syndrome have increased frequency of infections usually associated with neutropenia. The cause of the increased susceptibility to infection is related to the defective function of polymorphonuclear leukocytes as well as the decreased number of cells.

Osteoporosis secondary to rheumatoid involvement is common and may be aggravated by glucocorticoid therapy. Glucocorticoid treatment may cause significant loss of bone mass, especially early in the course of therapy, even when low doses are employed. Osteopenia in RA involves both juxtaarticular bone and long bones distant from involved joints. RA is associated with a modest decrease in mean bone mass and a moderate increase in the risk of fracture. Bone mass appears to be adversely affected by functional impairment and active inflammation, especially early in the course of the disease.

RA is associated with an increased incidence of lymphoma, especially large B cell lymphoma. Notably, this is particularly observed in those with persistent inflammatory disease.

RA in the Elderly   The incidence of RA continues to increase past age 60. It has been suggested that elderly-onset RA might have a poorer prognosis, as manifested by more persistent disease activity, more frequent radiographically evident deterioration, more frequent systemic involvement, and more rapid functional decline. Aggressive disease is largely restricted to those patients with high titers of rheumatoid factor. By contrast, elderly patients who develop RA without elevated titers of rheumatoid factor (seronegative disease) generally have less severe, often self-limited disease.

LABORATORY FINDINGS   No tests are specific for diagnosing RA. However, rheumatoid factors, which are autoantibodies reactive with the Fc portion of IgG, are found in more than two-thirds of adults with the disease. Widely utilized tests largely detect IgM rheumatoid factors. The presence of rheumatoid factor is not specific for RA. Rheumatoid factor is found in 5% of healthy persons. The frequency of rheumatoid factor in the general population increases with age, and 10 to 20% of individuals over 65 years old have a positive test. In addition, a number of conditions besides RA are associated with the presence of rheumatoid factor. These include systemic lupus erythematosus, Sjögren's syndrome, chronic liver disease, sarcoidosis, interstitial pulmonary fibrosis, infectious mononucleosis, hepatitis B, tuberculosis, leprosy, syphilis, subacute bacterial endocarditis, visceral leishmaniasis, schistosomiasis, and malaria. In addition, rheumatoid factor may appear transiently in normal individuals after vaccination or transfusion and may also be found in relatives of individuals with RA.

The presence of rheumatoid factor does not establish the diagnosis of RA as the predictive value of the presence of rheumatoid factor in determining a diagnosis of RA is poor. Thus fewer than one-third of unselected patients with a positive test for rheumatoid factor will be found to have RA. Therefore, the rheumatoid factor test is not useful as a screening procedure. However, the presence of rheumatoid factor can be of prognostic significance because patients with high titers tend to have more severe and progressive disease with extraarticular manifestations. Rheumatoid factor is uniformly found in patients with nodules or vasculitis. In summary, a test for the presence of rheumatoid factor can be employed to confirm a diagnosis in individuals with a suggestive clinical presentation and, if present in high titer, to designate patients at risk for severe systemic disease. A number of additional autoantibodies may be found in patients with RA, including antibodies to filaggrin, citrullinated proteins, calpastatin, components of the spliceosome (RA-33), and an unknown antigen, Sa. Some of these may be useful in diagnosis in that they may occur early in the disease before rheumatoid factor is present or may be associated with aggressive disease.

Normochromic, normocytic anemia is frequently present in active RA. It is thought to reflect ineffective erythropoiesis; large stores of iron are found in the bone marrow. In general, anemia and thrombocytosis correlate with disease activity. The white blood cell count is usually normal, but a mild leukocytosis may be present. Leukopenia may also exist without the full-blown picture of Felty's syndrome. Eosinophilia, when present, usually reflects severe systemic disease.

The erythrocyte sedimentation rate is increased in nearly all patients with active RA. The levels of a variety of other acute-phase reactants including ceruloplasmin and C-reactive protein are also elevated, and generally such elevations correlate with disease activity and the likelihood of progressive joint damage.

Synovial fluid analysis confirms the presence of inflammatory arthritis, although none of the findings is specific. The fluid is usually turbid, with reduced viscosity, increased protein content, and a slightly decreased or normal glucose concentration. The white cell count varies between 5 and 50,000/μL; polymorphonuclear leukocytes predominate. A synovial fluid white blood cell count >2000/μL with more than 75% polymorphonuclear leukocytes is highly characteristic of inflammatory arthritis, although not diagnostic of RA. Total hemolytic complement, C3, and C4 are markedly diminished in synovial fluid relative to total protein concentration as a result of activation of the classic complement pathway by locally produced immune complexes.

RADIOGRAPHIC EVALUATION Early in the disease, radiographic evaluations of the affected joints are usually not helpful in establishing a diagnosis. They reveal only that which is apparent from physical examination, namely, evidence of soft tissue swelling and joint effusion. As the disease progresses, abnormalities become more pronounced, but none of the radiographic findings is diagnostic of RA. The diagnosis, however, is supported by a characteristic pattern of abnormalities, including the tendency toward symmetric involvement. Juxtaarticular osteopenia may become apparent within weeks of onset. Loss of articular cartilage and bone erosions develop after months of sustained activity. The primary value of radiography is to determine the extent of cartilage destruction and bone erosion produced by the disease, particularly when one is attempting to estimate the aggressive nature of the disease, monitoring the impact of therapy with disease-modifying drugs, or determining the need for surgical intervention. Other means of imaging bones and joints, including ^{99m}Tc bisphosphonate bone scanning and magnetic resonance imaging, may be capable of detecting early inflammatory changes that are not apparent from standard radiography but are rarely necessary in the routine evaluation of patients with RA.

CLINICAL COURSE AND PROGNOSIS The course of RA is quite variable and difficult to predict in an individual patient. Most patients experience persistent but fluctuating disease activity, accompanied by a variable degree of joint abnormalities and functional impairment. After 10 to 12 years, <20% of patients will have no evidence of disability or joint abnormalities. Within 10 years, ~50% of patients will have work disability. A number of features are correlated with a greater likelihood of developing joint abnormalities or disabilities. These include the presence of >20 inflamed joints, a markedly elevated erythrocyte sedimentation rate, radiographic evidence of bone erosions, the presence of rheumatoid nodules, high titers of serum rheumatoid factor, the presence of functional disability, persistent inflammation, advanced age at onset, the presence of comorbid conditions, low socioeconomic status or educational level, or the presence of HLA-DRβ1*0401 or -DRβ*0404. The presence of one or more of these implies the presence of more aggressive disease with a greater likelihood of developing progressive joint abnormalities and disability. Persistent elevation of the erythrocyte sedimentation rate, disability, and pain on longitudinal follow-up are good predictors of work disability. Patients who lack these features have more indolent disease with a slower progression to joint abnormalities and disability. The pattern of disease onset does not appear to predict the development of disabilities. Approximately 15% of patients with RA will have a short-lived inflammatory process that remits without major disability. These individuals tend to lack the aforementioned features associated with more aggressive disease.

Several features of patients with RA appear to have prognostic significance. Remissions of disease activity are most likely to occur during the first year. White females tend to have more persistent synovitis and more progressively erosive disease than males. Persons who present with high titers of rheumatoid factor, C-reactive protein, and haptoglobin also have a worse prognosis, as do individuals with subcutaneous nodules or radiographic evidence of erosions at the time of initial evaluation. Sustained disease activity of more than 1 year's duration portends a poor outcome, and persistent elevation of acute-phase reactants appears to correlate strongly with radiographic progression. A large proportion of inflamed joints manifest erosions within 2 years, whereas the subsequent course of erosions is highly variable; however, in general, radiographic damage appears to progress at a constant rate in patients with RA. Foot joints are affected more frequently than hand joints. Despite the decrease in the rate of progressive joint damage with time, functional disability, which develops early in the course of the disease, continues to worsen at the same rate, although the most rapid rate of functional loss occurs within the first 2 years of disease.

The median life expectancy of persons with RA is shortened by 3 to 7 years. Of the 2.5-fold increase in mortality rate, RA itself is a contributing feature in 15 to 30%. The increased mortality rate seems to be limited to patients with more severe articular disease and can be attributed largely to infection and gastrointestinal bleeding. Recent evidence has also shown an important role of cardiovascular disease in the increased mortality of RA patients, and this appears to diminish with effective anti-inflammatory therapy. Drug therapy may also play a role in the increased mortality rate seen in individuals with RA. Factors correlated with early death include disability, disease duration or severity, glucocorticoid use, age at onset, and low socioeconomic or educational status.

DIAGNOSIS The mean delay from disease onset to diagnosis is 9 months. This is often related to the nonspecific nature of initial symptoms. The diagnosis of RA is easily made in persons with typical established disease. In a majority of patients, the disease assumes its characteristic clinical features within 1 to 2 years of onset. The typical picture of bilateral symmetric inflammatory polyarthritis involving small and large joints in both the upper and lower extremities with sparing of the axial skeleton except the cervical spine suggests the diagnosis. Constitutional features indicative of the inflammatory nature of the disease, such as morning stiffness, support the diagnosis. Demonstration of subcutaneous nodules is a helpful diagnostic feature. Additionally, the presence of rheumatoid factor, inflammatory synovial fluid with increased numbers of polymorphonuclear leukocytes, and radiographic findings of juxtaarticular bone demineralization and erosions of the affected joints substantiate the diagnosis.

The diagnosis is somewhat more difficult early in the course when only constitutional symptoms or intermittent arthralgias or arthritis in an asymmetric distribution may be present. A period of observation may be necessary before the diagnosis can be established. A definitive diagnosis of RA depends predominantly on characteristic clinical features and the exclusion of other inflammatory processes. The isolated finding of a positive test for rheumatoid factor or an elevated erythrocyte sedimentation rate, especially in an older person with joint pains, should not itself be used as evidence of RA.

In 1987, the American College of Rheumatology developed revised criteria for the classification of RA (Table 301-1). These criteria demonstrate a sensitivity of 91 to 94% and a specificity of 89% when used

---

TABLE 301-1 *The 1987 Revised Criteria for the Classification of RA*

1. Guidelines for classification
   a. Four of seven criteria are required to classify a patient as having rheumatoid arthritis (RA).
   b. Patients with two or more clinical diagnoses are not excluded.
2. Criteria[a]
   a. Morning stiffness: Stiffness in and around the joints lasting 1 h before maximal improvement.
   b. Arthritis of three or more joint areas: At least three joint areas, observed by a physician simultaneously, have soft tissue swelling or joint effusions, not just bony overgrowth. The 14 possible joint areas involved are right or left proximal interphalangeal, metacarpophalangeal, wrist, elbow, knee, ankle, and metatarsophalangeal joints.
   c. Arthritis of hand joints: Arthritis of wrist, metacarpophalangeal joint, or proximal interphalangeal joint.
   d. Symmetric arthritis: Simultaneous involvement of the same joint areas on both sides of the body.
   e. Rheumatoid nodules: Subcutaneous nodules over bony prominences, extensor surfaces, or juxtaarticular regions observed by a physician.
   f. Serum rheumatoid factor: Demonstration of abnormal amounts of serum rheumatoid factor by any method for which the result has been positive in less than 5% of normal control subjects.
   g. Radiographic changes: Typical changes of RA on posteroanterior hand and wrist radiographs that must include erosions or unequivocal bony decalcification localized in or most marked adjacent to the involved joints.

[a] Criteria a–d must be present for at least 6 weeks. Criteria b–e must be observed by a physician.
Source: From FC Arnett et al: Arthritis Rheum 31:315, 1988.

to classify patients with RA compared with control subjects with rheumatic diseases other than RA. Although these criteria were developed as a means of disease classification for investigational purposes, they can be useful as guidelines for establishing the diagnosis. Failure to meet these criteria, however, especially during the early stages of the disease, does not exclude the diagnosis. Indeed, these criteria do not effectively differentiate patients with new-onset RA from those with a variety of other forms of early inflammatory arthritis. Moreover, in patients with early arthritis, the criteria do not discriminate effectively between patients who subsequently develop persistent, disabling, or erosive disease and those who do not.

℞ TREATMENT

General Principles The goals of therapy of RA are (1) relief of pain, (2) reduction of inflammation, (3) protection of articular structures, (4) maintenance of function, and (5) control of systemic involvement. Since the etiology of RA is unknown, the pathogenesis is not completely delineated, and the mechanisms of action of some of the therapeutic agents employed are uncertain, therapy remains somewhat empirical. None of the therapeutic interventions is curative, and therefore all must be viewed as palliative, aimed at relieving the signs and symptoms of the disease. The various therapies employed are directed at nonspecific suppression of the inflammatory or immunologic process in the hope of ameliorating symptoms and preventing progressive damage to articular structures.

Management of patients with RA involves an interdisciplinary approach, which attempts to deal with the various problems that these individuals encounter with functional as well as psychosocial interactions. A variety of physical therapy modalities may be useful in decreasing the symptoms of RA. Rest ameliorates symptoms and can be an important component of the total therapeutic program. In addition, splinting to reduce unwanted motion of inflamed joints may be useful. Exercise directed at maintaining muscle strength and joint mobility without exacerbating joint inflammation is also an important aspect of the therapeutic regimen. A variety of orthotic and assistive devices can be helpful in supporting and aligning deformed joints to reduce pain and improve function. Education of the patient and family is an important component of the therapeutic plan to help those involved become aware of the potential impact of the disease and make appropriate accommodations in life-style to maximize satisfaction and minimize stress on joints.

Medical management of RA involves five general approaches. The first is the use of aspirin, other nonsteroidal anti-inflammatory drugs (NSAIDs), and simple analgesics to control the symptoms and signs of the local inflammatory process. These agents are rapidly effective at mitigating signs and symptoms, but they appear to exert minimal effect on the progression of the disease. Recently, specific inhibitors of the isoform of cyclooxygenase (COX) that is upregulated at inflammatory sites (COX-2) have been developed. COX inhibitors (known as Coxibs), which selectively inhibit COX-2 and not COX-1, have been shown to be as effective as classic NSAIDs, which inhibit both isoforms of COX, but to cause significantly less gastroduodenal ulceration. The second line of therapy involves use of low-dose oral glucocorticoids. Although low-dose glucocorticoids have been widely used to suppress signs and symptoms of inflammation, recent evidence suggests that they may also retard the development and progression of bone erosions. Intraarticular glucocorticoids can often provide transient symptomatic relief when systemic medical therapy has failed to resolve inflammation. The third line of agents includes a variety of agents that have been classified as the disease-modifying or slow-acting antirheumatic drugs. These agents appear to have the capacity to decrease elevated levels of acute-phase reactants in treated patients and, therefore, are thought to modify the inflammatory component of RA and thus its destructive capacity. Recently, combinations of dis-

ease-modifying antirheumatic drugs (DMARDs) have shown promise in controlling the signs and symptoms of RA. A fourth group of agents are the cytokine-neutralizing agents, which have been shown to have a major impact on the signs and symptoms of RA and also to slow progressive damage to articular structures. A fifth group of agents are the immunosuppressive and cytotoxic drugs that have been shown to ameliorate the disease process in some patients. Additional approaches have been employed in an attempt to control the signs and symptoms of RA. Substituting omega-3 fatty acids such as eicosapentaenoic acid found in certain fish oils for dietary omega-6 essential fatty acids found in meat has also been shown to provide symptomatic improvement in patients with RA. A variety of nontraditional approaches have also been claimed to be effective in treating RA, including diets, plant and animal extracts, vaccines, hormones, and topical preparations of various sorts. Many of these are costly, and none has been shown to be effective. However, belief in their efficacy ensures their continued use by some patients.

Drugs ■ *NONSTEROIDAL ANTI-INFLAMMATORY DRUGS* Besides aspirin, many NSAIDs are available to treat RA. As a result of the capacity of these agents to block the activity of the COX enzymes and therefore the production of prostaglandins, prostacyclin, and thromboxanes, they have analgesic, anti-inflammatory, and antipyretic properties. In addition, the agents may exert other anti-inflammatory effects. These agents are all associated with a wide spectrum of toxic side effects. Some, such as gastric irritation, azotemia, platelet dysfunction, and exacerbation of allergic rhinitis and asthma, are related to the inhibition of cyclooxygenase activity, whereas a variety of others, such as rash, liver function abnormalities, and bone marrow depression, may not be. None of the NSAIDs has been shown to be more effective than aspirin in the treatment of RA. However, these nonaspirin drugs are associated with a lower incidence of gastrointestinal intolerance. None of the newer NSAIDs appears to show significant therapeutic advantages over the other available agents. In addition, there is no consistent advantage of any of these newer agents over the others with respect to the incidence or severity of toxic manifestations. Recent evidence indicates that two separate enzymes, COX-1 and -2, are responsible for the initial metabolism of arachidonic acid into various inflammatory mediators. The former is constitutively present in many cells and tissues, including the stomach and the platelet, whereas the latter is specifically induced in response to inflammatory stimuli and is absent from the normal stomach and platelet. Inhibition of COX-2 accounts for the anti-inflammatory effects of NSAIDs, whereas inhibition of COX-1 induces much of the mechanism-based toxicity. As the currently available NSAIDs inhibit both enzymes, therapeutic benefit and toxicity are intertwined. Coxibs have been approved for the treatment of RA. Clinical trials have shown that Coxibs suppress the signs and symptoms of RA as effectively as classic COX-nonspecific NSAIDs but are associated with a significantly reduced incidence of gastroduodenal ulceration and appear to reduce the incidence of gastrointestinal bleeding, perforations, and obstruction to a variable degree compared with classic NSAIDs. However, the use of Coxibs is associated with sodium retention, hypertension, and peripheral edema in a fraction of patients, and the use of some Coxibs may be associated with an increased frequency of myocardial infarction. This suggests that Coxibs might be considered instead of classic COX-nonspecific NSAIDs, especially in persons with increased risk of NSAID-induced major upper gastrointestinal side effects, including persons over 65, those with a history of peptic ulcer disease, persons receiving glucocorticoids or anticoagulants, or those requiring high doses of NSAIDs.

DISEASE-MODIFYING ANTIRHEUMATIC DRUGS Clinical experience has delineated a number of agents that appear to have the capacity to alter the course of RA. This group of agents includes methotrexate, gold compounds, D-penicillamine, the antimalarials, and sulfasalazine. Despite having no chemical or pharmacologic similarities, in practice these agents share a number of characteristics. They exert minimal direct nonspecific anti-inflammatory or analgesic effects, and therefore NSAIDs must be continued during their administration, except in a few cases when true remissions are induced with them. The appearance of benefit from DMARD therapy is usually delayed for weeks or months. As many as two-thirds of patients develop some clinical improvement as a result of therapy with any of these agents, although the induction of true remissions is unusual. In addition to clinical improvement, there is frequently an improvement in serologic evidence of disease activity, and titers of rheumatoid factor and C-reactive protein and the erythrocyte sedimentation rate frequently decline. Moreover, emerging evidence suggests that DMARDs actually retard the development of bone erosions or facilitate their healing. Furthermore, developing evidence suggests that early aggressive treatment with DMARDs may be effective at slowing the appearance of bone erosions.

Which DMARD should be the drug of first choice remains controversial, and trials have failed to demonstrate a consistent advantage of one over the other. Despite this, methotrexate has emerged as the DMARD of choice because of its relatively rapid onset of action, its capacity to effect sustained improvement with ongoing therapy, and the higher level of patient retention on therapy. Each of the DMARDs is associated with considerable toxicity, and therefore careful patient monitoring is necessary. Toxicity of the various agents also becomes important in determining the drug of first choice. Of note, failure to respond or development of toxicity to one DMARD does not preclude responsiveness to another. Thus, a similar percentage of RA patients who have failed to respond to one DMARD will respond to another when it is given as the second disease-modifying drug.

No characteristic features of patients have emerged that predict responsiveness to a DMARD. Moreover, the indications for the initiation of therapy with one of these agents are not well defined. Recently, evidence has emerged that the initiation of DMARD therapy early in the course of RA clearly has a major impact on the development of bone erosions and the progression to disability. It is now felt that DMARD therapy should be begun as soon as the diagnosis of RA is established, especially in those with any evidence of aggressive disease with a poor prognosis.

The folic acid antagonist methotrexate, given in an intermittent low dose (7.5 to 30 mg once weekly), is currently a frequently utilized DMARD. Most rheumatologists recommend use of methotrexate as the initial DMARD, especially in individuals with evidence of aggressive RA. Recent trials have documented the efficacy of methotrexate and have indicated that its onset of action is more rapid than other DMARDs, and patients tend to remain on therapy with methotrexate longer than they remain on other DMARDs because of better clinical responses and less toxicity. Long-term trials have indicated that methotrexate does not induce remission but rather suppresses symptoms while it is being administered. Maximal improvement is observed after 6 months of therapy, with little additional improvement thereafter. Major toxicity includes gastrointestinal upset, oral ulceration, and liver function abnormalities that appear to be dose-related and reversible and hepatic fibrosis that can be quite insidious, requiring liver biopsy for detection in its early stages. Drug-induced pneumonitis has also been reported. Liver biopsy is recommended for individuals with persistent or repetitive liver function abnormalities. Concurrent administration of folic acid or folinic acid may diminish the frequency of some side effects without diminishing effectiveness.

Glucocorticoid Therapy Systemic glucocorticoid therapy can provide effective symptomatic therapy in patients with RA. Low-dose (<7.5 mg/d) prednisone has been advocated as useful additive therapy to control symptoms. Moreover, recent evidence suggests that low-dose glucocorticoid therapy may retard the progression of bone erosions. Monthly pulses with high-dose glucocorticoids may be useful in some patients and may hasten the response when therapy with a DMARD is initiated.

Anti-Cytokine Agents Recently, biologic agents that bind and neutralize TNF have become available. One of these is a TNF type II receptor fused to IgG1 (etanercept), the second is a chimeric mouse/human monoclonal antibody to TNF (infliximab), and the third is a fully human antibody to TNF (adalimumab). Clinical trials have shown that parenteral administration of any of these TNF neutralizing agents is remarkably effective at controlling signs and symptoms of RA in patients who have failed DMARD therapy, as well as in DMARD naïve patients. Repetitive therapy with these agents is effective with or without concomitant methotrexate. These agents not only are effective in persistently controlling signs and symptoms of RA in a majority of patients, but they have also been shown to slow the rate of progression of joint damage assessed radiographically and to improve disability. Side effects include the potential for an increased risk of serious infections. Particularly notable is the capacity of TNF blockade to increase the risk of developing reactivation of dormant tuberculosis. It is prudent to carry out tuberculin skin testing and, if necessary, further evaluation with chest radiographs before beginning therapy with an anti-TNF agent to limit the chance of inciting reactivation of tuberculosis. TNF-neutralizing therapy can also induce the development of anti-DNA antibodies, but rarely is there associated evidence of signs and symptoms of systemic lupus erythematosus. Other side effects include infusion or injection site reactions and rarely the development of demyelinating central nervous system disease. Although these side effects are uncommon, their occurrence mandates that TNF-neutralizing therapy be supervised by physicians with experience in their use.

Anakinra is a recombinant IL-1 receptor antagonist that competitively blocks the binding of IL-1β and IL-1α to the IL-1 receptor and thereby inhibits the activity of these two related proinflammatory cytokines. Anakinra has been shown to improve the signs and symptoms of RA, to decrease disability, and to slow progression of articular damage associated radiographically. It can be given as monotherapy or in combination with methotrexate. The major side effects are injection site reactions.

Immunosuppressive Therapy The immunosuppressive drugs azathioprine, leflunomide, cyclosporine, and cyclophosphamide have been shown to be effective in the treatment of RA and to exert therapeutic effects similar to those of the DMARDs. However, these agents appear to be no more effective than the DMARDs. Moreover, they cause a variety of toxic side effects, and cyclophosphamide appears to predispose the patient to the development of malignant neoplasms. Therefore, these drugs have been reserved for patients who have clearly failed therapy with DMARDs and anti-cytokine therapy. On occasion, extraarticular disease such as rheumatoid vasculitis may require cytotoxic immunosuppressive therapy.

Leflunomide is metabolized to an active metabolite that acts to inhibit dihydroorotate dehydrogenase, an essential enzyme in the pyrimidine biosynthetic pathway. Its predominant action is to inhibit the proliferation of T lymphocytes. Leflunomide has been shown to control the signs and symptoms of RA and to slow the progression of joint damage as effectively as methotrexate. Leflunomide can be given alone or with methotrexate and is the most frequently employed immunosuppressive agent used to treat patients with RA. It is used as monotherapy in patients who have had adverse reactions to methotrexate or inadequate responses to it. The major side effect is the associated increase in liver function enzymes that occurs in 5% of patients receiving leflunomide alone and in >50% of individuals taking leflunomide with methotrexate.

Surgery Surgery plays a role in the management of patients with severely damaged joints. Although arthroplasties and total joint replacements can be done on a number of joints, the most successful procedures are carried out on hips, knees, and shoulders. Realistic goals of these procedures are relief of pain and reduction of disability. Reconstructive hand surgery may lead to cosmetic improvement and some functional benefit. Open or arthroscopic synovectomy may be useful in some patients with persistent monarthritis, especially of the knee.

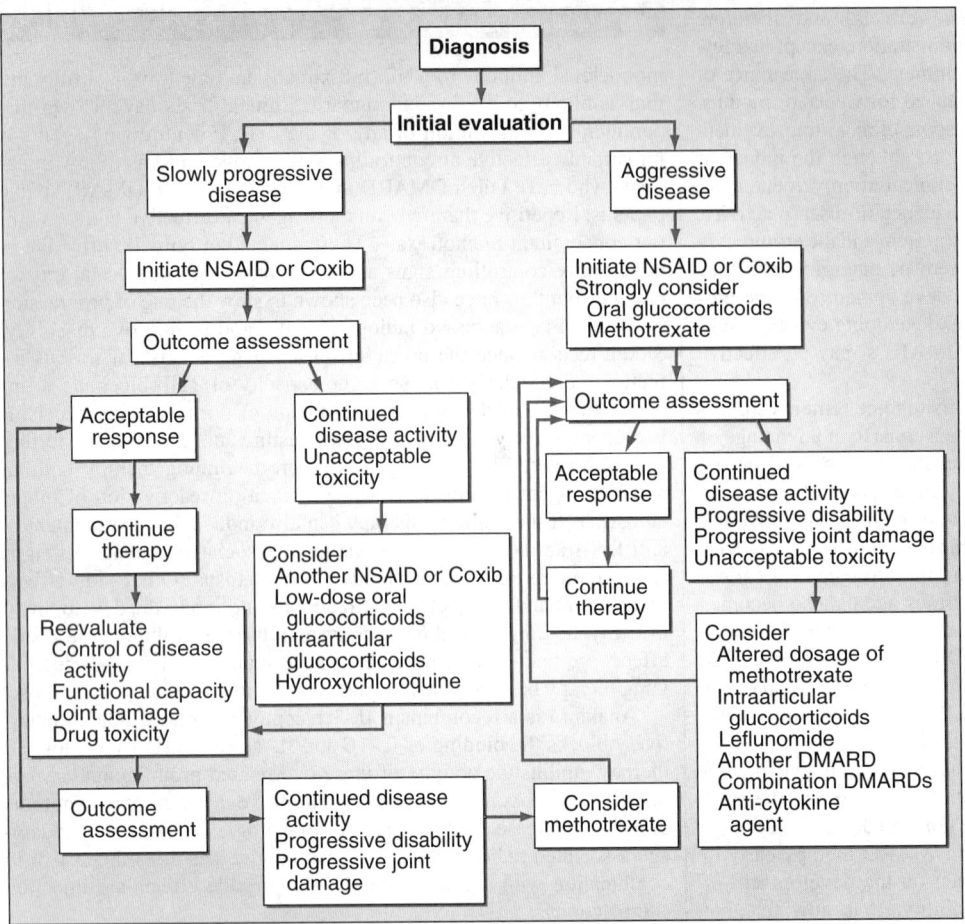

FIGURE 301-3 Algorithm for the medical management of rheumatoid arthritis. NSAID, nonsteroidal anti-inflammatory drug; Coxib, COX-2 inhibitors; DMARD, disease-modifying antirheumatic drug.

graphic evidence of cartilage loss is clear-cut evidence of the destructive potential of the inflammatory process and indicates the need for DMARD therapy. The other indications as outlined above, including persistent pain, joint swelling, or functional impairment, are much more subjective, however. As persistent inflammation, involvement of multiple joints, elevated levels of acute-phase reactants, and rheumatoid factor titers correlate with the development of disability and/or bony erosions, some have advocated the use of these prognostic indicators of aggressive disease in the decision to employ DMARDs early in the course of RA. The decision to begin use of a DMARD and/or low-dose oral glucocorticoids requires experience and clinical judgment as well as the ability to assess joint swelling and functional activity and the patient's pain tolerance and expectation of therapy accurately. In this setting, the fully informed patient must play an active role in the decision to begin DMARD and/or low-dose oral glucocorticoid therapy, after careful review of the therapeutic and toxic potential of the various drugs. If DMARD therapy, usually methotrexate, fails to control signs and symptoms of RA, a decision to add or switch to an anti-cytokine agent is considered. These are quite potent at controlling signs and symptoms of RA, slowing damage to articular structures, and limiting disability but are very expensive and associated with serious adverse events. The decision to employ these agents requires considerable experience, judgment, and the agreement of a fully informed patient.

If a patient responds to a DMARD, therapy is continued with careful monitoring to avoid toxicity. All DMARDs provide a suppressive effect and therefore require prolonged administration. Even with successful therapy, local injection of glucocorticoids may be necessary to diminish inflammation that may persist in a limited number of joints. In addition, NSAIDs or Coxibs may be necessary to mitigate symptoms. Even after inflammation has totally resolved, symptoms from loss of cartilage and supervening degenerative joint disease or altered joint function may require additional treatment. Surgery may also be necessary to relieve pain or diminish the functional impairment secondary to alterations in joint function. Recently an alternative approach to treat patients with RA has been suggested. This involves the initiation of therapy with multiple agents early in the course of disease in an attempt to control inflammation, followed by maintenance on one or more agents as necessary to control disease activity.

Although synovectomy may offer short-term relief of symptoms, it does not appear to retard bone destruction or alter the natural history of the disease. In addition, early tenosynovectomy of the wrist may prevent tendon rupture.

APPROACH TO THE PATIENT

An approach to the medical management of patients with RA is depicted in Fig. 301-3. The principles underlying care of these patients reflect the variability of the disease, the frequent persistent nature of the inflammation and its potential to cause disability, the relationship between sustained inflammation and bone erosions, and the need to reevaluate the patient frequently for symptomatic response to therapy, progression of disability and joint damage, and side effects of treatment. At the onset of disease it is difficult to predict the natural history of an individual patient's illness. Therefore, the usual approach is to attempt to alleviate the patient's symptoms with NSAIDs or Coxibs. Some patients may have mild disease that requires no additional therapy. However, if the patient has any evidence of aggressive disease, as described above, initiation of DMARD therapy should be considered as early as feasible. In RA patients there appears to be a window of opportunity early in the course of the disease, during which initiation of aggressive therapy can have a major impact on subsequent damage to articular structures and disability.

At some time during most patients' course, the possibility of initiating DMARD therapy and/or low-dose oral glucocorticoids is entertained. With aggressive disease this might occur sooner, often within 1 to 3 months of diagnosis, whereas in patients with more indolent disease, smoldering activity may not require such therapy for many years. The development of bone erosions or radio-

FURTHER READING

ARNETT FC et al: The American Rheumatism Association 1987 Revised Criteria for the Classification of Rheumatoid Arthritis. Arthritis Rheum 31: 315, 1988

CHOI HK et al: Methotrexate and mortality in patients with rheumatoid arthritis: A prospective study. Lancet 359:1173, 2002

DROSSAERS-BAKKER KW et al: Long-term outcome in rheumatoid arthritis: A simple algorithm of baseline parameters can predict radiographic damage, disability, and disease course at 12-year followup. Arthritis Rheum 47: 383, 2002

GOLDBACH-MANSKY R, LIPSKY PE: New concepts in the treatment of rheumatoid arthritis. Annu Rev Med 54:197, 2003

KWOH CK et al: Guidelines for the management of rheumatoid arthritis. 2002 Update. Arthritis Rheum 46:328, 2002

LIPSKY PE, DAVIS LS: The central involvement of T cells in rheumatoid arthritis. Immunologist 6:121, 1998

———— et al: Infliximab and methotrexate in the treatment of rheumatoid ar-

thritis. Anti-Tumor Necrosis Factor Trial in Rheumatoid Arthritis with Concomitant Therapy Study Group. N Engl J Med 343:1594, 2000

VAN EVERDINGEN AA et al: Low-dose prednisone therapy for patients with early active rheumatoid arthritis: Clinical efficacy, disease-modifying properties, and side effects: A randomized, double-blind, placebo-controlled clinical trial. Ann Intern Med 136:1, 2002

302 | RHEUMATIC FEVER
Edward L. Kaplan

In many parts of the world, especially in industrialized countries, acute rheumatic fever (ARF) is less common than it was during the early and mid-years of the twentieth century. In the late 1940s, patients with rheumatic fever (RF) and rheumatic heart disease accounted for more than half of schoolchildren recognized to have cardiovascular problems in the United States. During World War II, there were >20,000 cases of ARF in U.S. Navy personnel alone. The incidence of RF has declined remarkably in the industrialized countries of the world, where the disease has become rare. However, in many developing countries, which account for almost two-thirds of the world's population, streptococcal infections, RF, and rheumatic heart disease remain a very significant public health problem. The magnitude of the problem in these countries today is similar to that in North America 60 years ago.

The decreased incidence of ARF and the low prevalence of rheumatic heart disease in industrialized countries have led many physicians and public health authorities to the incorrect conclusion that these conditions are no longer a problem. However, starting in the 1980s, unexpected scattered outbreaks of ARF among both adults and children in North America have confirmed the capacity for this potentially serious illness to reappear and pose significant public health problems. As an example, >600 cases of ARF were seen in middle-class populations in Salt Lake City, Utah, between 1985 and the end of 2002. The disease continues to be a major public health problem in many developing countries of the world. Neither antimicrobial agents nor other public health measures have been totally effective in the control of RF in the industrialized or industrializing world.

EPIDEMIOLOGY   The epidemiology of ARF is identical to that of group A streptococcal upper respiratory tract infections (Chap. 121). As is the case for streptococcal sore throat, ARF most often occurs in children; the peak age-related incidence is between 5 and 15 years. Most initial attacks in adults take place at the end of the second and beginning of the third decades of life. Rarely, initial attacks occur as late as the fourth decade, and recurrent attacks have been documented as late as the fifth decade.

Epidemiologic risk factors classically associated with individual attacks and especially with outbreaks of ARF include lower standards of living, especially crowding; the disease has been more common among socially and economically disadvantaged populations. However, the outbreaks in the United States in the late 1980s and early 1990s cannot be explained entirely by these factors. The large Utah outbreak of >600 cases during 17 years has affected primarily middle-class patients with ready access to medical care. Therefore, one can conclude that the organism itself as well as the degree of host/herd immunity to the prevalent M-types in an affected community are equally important risk factors.

Studies have shown that ~3% of individuals with untreated group A streptococcal pharyngitis will develop RF. The epidemiology of RF is also influenced by the serotypes of group A streptococci present in a population. The concept of "rheumatogenecity" of specific strains is largely based upon epidemiologic evidence associating certain sero-

types with RF (serotypes 1, 3, 5, 6, 18, etc.). Mucoid isolates are frequently associated with virulence and with RF.

PATHOGENESIS   More than half a century ago the pioneering studies of Lancefield differentiated β-hemolytic streptococci into serologic groups (Chap. 121). This ultimately led to the association of infection by the group A organism of the pharynx and tonsils (not of the skin) and the subsequent development of ARF. However, the mechanism(s) responsible for the development of RF after an infection remains incompletely defined. Historically, approaches to understanding the pathogenesis of RF have been grouped into three major categories: (1) direct infection by the group A streptococcus, (2) a toxic effect of streptococcal extracellular products on the host tissues, and (3) an abnormal or dysfunctional immune response to one or more as yet unidentified somatic or extracellular antigens produced by all (or perhaps only by some) group A streptococci ("antigenic mimicry.")

There is insufficient evidence to support direct infection of the heart as the inciting event. Additionally, while toxins such as streptolysin O and others have been postulated to have a pathogenetic role, there is relatively little convincing evidence of this at the present time. Major efforts have focused on an abnormal immune response by the human host to one or more group A streptococcal antigens.

The hypothesis of "antigenic mimicry" between human and group A streptococcal antigens has been studied extensively and has concentrated on two interactions. The first is the similarity between the group-specific carbohydrate of the group A streptococcus and the glycoprotein of heart valves; the second involves the molecular similarity among the streptococcal cell membrane, streptococcal M protein sarcolemma, and other moieties of the human myocardial cell. Investigators have studied tissue-specific antigens as well as major histocompatibility antigens in an attempt to define the pathogenesis.

The possibility of a predisposing genetic influence in some individuals is one of the most tantalizing of the incompletely understood factors that might contribute to susceptibility to RF. The precise genetic factors influencing the attack rate have never been adequately defined. Observations have been described that support the concept that this nonsuppurative sequel to a group A streptococcal upper respiratory tract infection results from an abnormal immune response by the human host. Thus, differences in immune responses to streptococcal antigens have been reported. Further, new data suggest that a unique surface marker on non-T lymphocytes in patients with RF and rheumatic heart disease may be associated with individuals who are susceptible to developing RF after a streptococcal infection because of abnormal immune responses; conclusive proof gained by prospective studies is not yet available.

DIAGNOSIS   There is no specific laboratory test that can establish a diagnosis of RF. The diagnosis, therefore, is a clinical one but requires supporting evidence from the clinical microbiology and clinical immunology laboratories. Because of the variety of signs and symptoms associated with the RF syndrome, in 1944 Jones first proposed criteria to assist the clinician in standardizing the diagnosis of RF. The most recent modification of the *Jones criteria* (Updated Jones Criteria) was published in 1992 by a Special Writing Group of the American Heart Association (Table 302-1). A recent consideration of the Jones criteria by the American Heart Association has basically not resulted in change.

TABLE 302-1 *The Jones Criteria for Rheumatic Fever, Updated 1992*

Major Criteria	Minor Criteria
Carditis	Clinical
Migratory polyarthritis	Fever
Sydenham's chorea	Arthralgia
Subcutaneous nodules	Laboratory
Erythema marginatum	Elevated acute phase reactants
	Prolonged PR interval
plus	

Supporting evidence of a recent group A streptococcal infection (e.g., positive throat culture or rapid antigen detection test; and/or elevated or increasing streptococcal antibody test)

Source: Modified from the Special Writing Group of the American Heart Association: JAMA 268:2069, 1992.

There are five criteria termed *major* because they are most commonly found in patients with RF: carditis, migratory polyarthritis, Sydenham's chorea, subcutaneous nodules, and erythema marginatum.

The *carditis* of ARF is a pancarditis involving the pericardium, myocardium, and endocardium. In most published series, between 40 and 60% of patients with ARF have evidence of carditis, which is characterized by one or more of the following: sinus tachycardia, the murmur of mitral regurgitation, an S_3 gallop, a pericardial friction rub, and cardiomegaly. The introduction of echocardiography has assisted in the identification of subtle abnormalities of the mitral valve, and these may be present in an additional 20% of patients who do not have an audible heart murmur. A prolonged PR interval and evidence of heart failure may be present as well, but these are nonspecific and may be found in a number of other diseases. Among the more controversial aspects of diagnosing RF has been the several reports of significant valvular (particularly of the mitral valve) involvement in the absence of audible murmurs. Although there are suggestions in the literature that echocardiographic criteria be included with the Jones criteria, the long-term follow-ups remain inadequate at the present time.

Healing of the rheumatic valvulitis may cause fibrous thickening and adhesion, resulting in the most serious complication of RF, i.e., valvular stenosis and/or regurgitation (Chap. 219). The mitral valve is involved most frequently, followed by the aortic valve. However, isolated aortic valve disease as a consequence of ARF is quite rare. In patients with aortic valve disease due to RF, the mitral valve is almost always simultaneously affected. Even minor degrees of rheumatic valvular involvement can lead to susceptibilities to infective endocarditis (Chap. 109). Although rheumatic pericarditis can cause a serous effusion, fibrin deposits, and even pericardial calcification, it does not lead to constrictive pericarditis.

A *migratory polyarthritis* is present in as many as 75% of cases, most often affecting the ankles, wrists, knees, and elbows over a period of days. It usually does not affect the small joints of the hands or feet and seldom involves the hip joints. Since salicylates and other anti-inflammatory drugs usually cause prompt resolution of joint symptoms, it is important that the clinician *not* prescribe these medications until it is determined whether the arthritis is migratory. The arthritis of ARF is extremely painful. Pain can be controlled with codeine or similar analgesics until the diagnosis is established. The difference between arthralgia (subjective joint pain) and arthritis (joint pain and swelling) must be understood. Too often, arthralgia is used (incorrectly) as a major criterion. An inflammatory reactive arthritis associated with streptococcal pharyngitis is often confused with the arthritis or arthralgias of ARF. Currently, several antibiotics have been promoted to be used in a <10-day course of therapy. The data at the present time are inconclusive as regards short-course therapy, and most recommendations at the present time recommend a full 10-day course of antibiotics orally for treatment of streptococcal pharyngitis.

Sydenham's chorea occurs in <10% of patients with RF. The latent period between the onset of the initiating streptococcal infection and the onset of Sydenham's chorea may be as long as several months. While differing from the other manifestations, this central nervous system disorder is a part of the RF complex and should be managed as such. Many patients who appear to have only chorea may present several decades later with evidence of typical rheumatic valvular disease. There is no definitive laboratory test for establishing a diagnosis of Sydenham's chorea, and the diagnosis is one of exclusion. Patients with Sydenham's chorea should be given secondary prophylaxis for prevention of recurrent attacks, even if they do not appear to have rheumatic heart disease.

Subcutaneous nodules and *erythema marginatum* are rare major manifestations, usually present in <10% of cases. Subcutaneous nodules are found over extensor surfaces of joints, are seen most often in patients with long-standing rheumatic heart disease, and are extremely rare in patients experiencing an initial attack. Erythema marginatum is an uncommon manifestation. It is an evanescent macular eruption with rounded borders—usually concentrated on the trunk.

The *minor criteria* (Table 302-1) are nonspecific and may be present in many clinical conditions.

To fulfill the Jones criteria, either two major criteria, or one major criterion and two minor criteria, *plus* evidence of an antecedent streptococcal infection are required. The latter may be provided by recovery of the organism on culture or by evidence of an immune response to one of the commonly measured group A streptococcal antibodies (e.g., anti-streptolysin O, anti-deoxyribonuclease B). Since the accurate diagnosis of RF has future medical and financial implications, the clinician is obligated to evaluate any patient completely until the suspected diagnosis is either established or excluded.

Both the clinical microbiology and the clinical immunology laboratories have important roles in confirming the diagnosis of RF. An attempt should be made to recover the organism from a throat culture, although group A streptococci can be recovered from the upper respiratory tract of only 25 to 40% of patients at the time the diagnosis is made. If a rapid antigen detection test is used but is negative, a confirmatory throat culture must be performed. It is helpful to obtain two or three cultures from the throat at the time the diagnosis is suspected, but before initiating antibiotic therapy, in order to confirm the presence of the organism.

At least 80% of patients with ARF have an elevated anti-streptolysin O titer at presentation. If one employs two additional streptococcal antibody tests such as the anti-DNAse B or anti-hyaluronidase test, the percentage of patients who show evidence of a preceding group A streptococcal infection will rise to >95%. While an initially elevated titer is convincing, being able to demonstrate a rise in titer from the acute to the convalescent phase is a more reliable means of documenting the recent infection. If three antibody tests are done and there is no evidence of a preceding infection, the diagnosis must be seriously reconsidered.

℞ TREATMENT

There are two necessary therapeutic approaches to patients with ARF: anti-streptococcal antibiotic therapy and therapy for the clinical manifestations of the disease. At the time of diagnosis, *all* patients with ARF should be treated as if they have a group A streptococcal infection, whether or not the organism is recovered by culture. In addition to the relatively large percentage of such patients who may have a negative throat culture at the time of diagnosis, others may have only a few organisms present in the throat. Conventional antibiotic treatment should be started immediately: a complete 10-day course in adults of either oral penicillin V (500 mg twice daily) or erythromycin (250 mg four times daily) for those with penicillin allergy. Many choose intramuscular benzathine penicillin G (a single intramuscular injection of 1.2 million units) for the treatment of the presumed streptococcal infection; this will also serve as the first dose of secondary prophylaxis for the prevention of recolonization of the upper respiratory tract in the future. Intramuscular benzathine penicillin G has been reported to result in a transient elevation of the erythrocyte sedimentation rate, which can prove confusing in the acute phase of the disease.

Following the initial anti-streptococcal therapy, secondary prophylaxis should be initiated to prevent subsequent infection of the upper respiratory tract with group A streptococci. Recommendations of the American Heart Association and of the World Health Organization are for intramuscular injection of 1.2 million units of benzathine penicillin G every 4 weeks or for oral penicillin V (250 mg twice daily) or oral sulfadiazine (1.0 g daily). Recent studies have shown that in those individuals who are at high risk for recurrence of RF, intramuscular benzathine penicillin G given every 3 weeks is more effective in reducing the risk of recurrence. Since it is known that the risk of recurrence of RF is highest during the first 5 years after the attack, secondary prophylaxis is always given for at least this period. After that the decision to continue or discontinue secondary prophylaxis is dependent upon whether the patient has documented rheumatic heart disease and whether the patient is at high risk of exposure to streptococci (e.g., students, school teachers, medical and military personnel). Many believe that those with documented recurrences and/or documented rheumatic valvular heart disease should receive secondary prophylaxis for life. The duration of prophylaxis is often individualized for specific patients.

Medical therapy for the manifestations of RF depends on the clinical status of the patient. For adult patients with the arthritis of RF, salicylates in doses escalating to 2 g four times daily are very effective and will result in marked clinical improvement, often within 12 h. When this prompt relief does not occur, one should reexamine the original diagnosis. Salicylates may be given for 4 to 6 weeks and gradually tapered so as to prevent a rebound. The erythrocyte sedimentation rate is one method for determining the rate of taper for salicylates. Usually this requires at least 2 weeks. There are no conclusive data to support using nonsteroidal anti-inflammatory drugs for ARF. There is no indication for the use of steroids (usually prednisone) solely for the treatment of the arthritis of RF.

Most experienced physicians believe that there is a role for steroids in patients with severe carditis accompanied by congestive heart failure. However, neither salicylates nor glucocorticoids influence the future development of valvular heart disease. In adults, prednisone can be started in doses as high as 30 mg four times daily in especially severe cases, and, as the patient improves, salicylates can be added during the tapering of the steroid dose; this may require 4 to 6 weeks.

In the presence of congestive heart failure, conventional medical measures (Chap. 216) are indicated. In the past, patients with ARF were kept at complete bed rest for months. This is inappropriate unless there is a specific reason such as persistent active carditis or severe heart failure. Patients with arthritis will begin to feel better very soon after anti-inflammatory therapy with salicylates is begun. They may be released from bed rest but should not resume full activity until signs of inflammatory process have abated and the acute-phase reactants have returned to normal.

FURTHER READING

BISNO AL et al: Practice guidelines for the diagnosis and management of group A streptococcal pharyngitis. (Infectious Disease Society of America.) Clin Infect Dis 35:113, 2002

COMMITTEE ON RHEUMATIC FEVER, ENDOCARDITIS AND KAWASAKI DISEASE OF THE COUNCIL ON CARDIOVASCULAR DISEASE IN THE YOUNG OF THE AMERICAN HEART ASSOCIATION: Treatment of acute streptococcal pharyngitis and prevention of rheumatic fever: A statement for health professionals. Pediatrics 96:758, 1995

DAJANI A: Rheumatic fever, in *Braunwald's Heart Disease*, 7th ed, DP Zipes et al (eds). Philadelphia, Saunders, 2005

FERRIERI P et al: Proceedings of the Jones Criteria Workshop. Special writing group of the American Heart Association. Circulation 106:2521, 2002

SHET A, KAPLAN EL: The clinical use and interpretation of group A streptococcal antibody tests: A practical approach for the pediatrician or primary care physician. Pediatr Infect Dis J 21:420, 2002

STEVENS DL, KAPLAN EL (eds): *Streptococcal Infections: Clinical Aspects, Microbiology, and Molecular Pathogenesis*. New York, Oxford Univ Press, 2000

303 SYSTEMIC SCLEROSIS (SCLERODERMA) AND RELATED DISORDERS
Bruce C. Gilliland

DEFINITION Systemic sclerosis (SSc) is a chronic multisystem disorder of unknown etiology characterized clinically by thickening of the skin caused by accumulation of connective tissue and by structural and functional abnormalities of visceral organs, including the gastrointestinal tract, lungs, heart, and kidneys. Classification of SSc and scleroderma-like disorders is shown in Table 303-1. Vascular damage, immune activation, and excessive synthesis and deposition of extracellular matrix are prominent features of SSc. The degree and rate of skin and internal organ involvement vary among patients. Two subsets, however, can be identified, even though there is some overlap (Table 303-2). One subset is referred to as *diffuse cutaneous scleroderma* and is characterized by the rapid development of symmetric skin thickening of proximal and distal extremities, face, and trunk. These patients are at greater risk for developing kidney and other visceral disease early in their course. The other subset is *limited cutaneous scleroderma*, which is defined by symmetric skin thickening limited to distal extremities and face. This subset frequently has features of the *CREST syndrome*, standing for *c*alcinosis, *R*aynaud's phenomenon, *e*sophageal dysmotility, *s*clerodactyly, and *t*elangiectasia. The prognosis in limited cutaneous scleroderma is better except for those patients who, after many years, develop pulmonary arterial hypertension or biliary cirrhosis. Involvement of visceral organs may also occur in the absence of any skin involvement, which is referred to as *systemic sclerosis sine scleroderma*. Survival is determined by the severity of visceral disease, especially involving the lungs, heart, and/or kidneys.

TABLE 303-1 *Classification of Scleroderma/Systemic Sclerosis and Scleroderma-Like Disorders*

Systemic sclerosis
    Limited cutaneous disease
    Diffuse cutaneous disease
    Sine scleroderma
    Undifferentiated connective tissue disease
    Overlap syndromes
Localized scleroderma
    Morphea
    Linear scleroderma
    En coup de sabre
Chemically induced scleroderma-like disorders
    Toxic-oil syndrome
    Vinyl chloride–induced disease
    Bleomycin-induced fibrosis
    Pentazocine-induced fibrosis
    Epoxy- and aromatic hydrocarbons–induced fibrosis
    Eosinophilia-myalgia syndrome
Other scleroderma-like disorders
    Scleredema adultorum of Buschke
    Scleromyxedema
    Chronic graft-vs.-host disease
    Eosinophilic fasciitis
    Digital sclerosis in diabetes
    Primary amyloidosis and amyloidosis associated with multiple myeloma

TABLE 303-2 Subsets of Systemic Sclerosis

	Diffuse	Limited[a]
Skin involvement	Distal and proximal extremities, face, trunk	Distal to elbows, face
Raynaud's phenomenon	Onset within 1 year or at time of skin changes	May precede skin disease by years
Organ involvement	Pulmonary (interstitial fibrosis); renal (renovascular hypertensive crisis); gastrointestinal; cardiac	Gastrointestinal; pulmonary arterial hypertension after 10–15 years of disease in <10% of patients; biliary cirrhosis
Nail fold capillaries	Dilatation and dropout	Dilatation without significant dropout
Antinuclear antibodies	Anti-topoisomerase 1	Anticentromere

[a] Also referred to as CREST (calcinosis, Raynaud's, esophageal dysmotility, sclerodactyly, telangiectasia).

Preliminary criteria for the classification of systemic sclerosis were developed by the American Rheumatism Association (now called the American College of Rheumatology) for the purpose of uniformity in clinical studies. A major criterion was the presence of sclerodermatous involvement proximal to the digits, affecting proximal portions of the extremities, face, neck, or trunk usually in a bilateral and symmetrical pattern. Sclerodactyly was almost always present. This single major criterion was present in 91% if SSc patients and in less than 1% of comparison disorders. Minor criteria were sclerodactyly, digital pitting scars or tissue loss of the volar pads of the fingertips, and bibasilar pulmonary fibrosis. The diagnosis of SSc was based on the presence of the major criterion or two or more minor criteria. The sensitivity of these criteria was 97%, and the specificity 98%. These criteria are not, however, applicable to clinical practice as some patients with limited cutaneous SSc do not meet these criteria. These patients may have esophageal and/or bowel dysmotility or pulmonary arterial hypertension without pulmonary fibrosis. Scleroderma can also occur in a localized form limited to the skin, subcutaneous tissue, and muscle and without systemic involvement. Localized scleroderma occurs most often in children and young women but can affect any age group. The two localized forms are *morphea*, which occurs as single or multiple plaques of skin induration, and *linear scleroderma*, which involves an extremity or the face. Linear scleroderma of one side of the forehead and scalp produces a disfiguration referred to as *en coup de sabre* because it resembles a wound from a sword. It may be associated with hemiatrophy of the same side of the face.

SSc also occurs in association with features of other connective tissue diseases. The term *overlap syndrome* has been used to describe such patients. Undifferentiated connective tissue disease has been suggested as a designation for patients who do not have diagnostic criteria for any one connective tissue disease. *Mixed connective tissue disease* (MCTD), a syndrome involving features of systemic lupus erythematosus (SLE), SSc, polymyositis, and rheumatoid arthritis and very high titers of circulating antibody to nuclear ribonucleoprotein (RNP) antigen, will be discussed later in the chapter. *Eosinophilic fasciitis* and the *eosinophilia-myalgia syndrome* (EMS) associated with contaminated L-tryptophan ingestion (Chap. 369) are scleroderma-like illnesses and will also be discussed in this chapter.

EPIDEMIOLOGY   SSc has a worldwide distribution and affects all races. The onset of disease is unusual in childhood and young men. The incidence increases with age, peaking in the third to fifth decade. Women overall are affected approximately three times as often as men and even more often during the mid to late childbearing years (≥8:1). African Americans are affected approximately twice as frequently, have a lower age of onset, and more often have diffuse cutaneous involvement and pulmonary fibrosis than Caucasians. Hispanics and Native Americans may also have more severe disease than Caucasians. The annual incidence has been estimated to be 19 cases per million population. The reported prevalence of SSc is between 19 and 75 per 100,000 persons. An exceptionally high prevalence of SSc (469 per

100,000 persons) has been noted in the Choctaw Native Americans in Oklahoma—the highest found to date in any ethnic group. Both incidence and prevalence may be underestimated because patients with early and atypical disease may be overlooked in surveys. Genetic factors play a role in the susceptibility and expression of SSc. Familial aggregation for SSc has been reported in ~1.5% of SSc families. SSc in a first-degree relative is a very strong relative risk factor for SSc. There is also an increased incidence of other autoimmune diseases, including SLE and rheumatoid arthritis, as well as antinuclear antibodies in first-degree relatives of SSc patients. In a recent study, the rate of concordance of SSc in monozygotic twins was only 4.7%, the same as in dizygotic twins. The concordance for the presence of antinuclear antibodies was significantly greater in monozygotic twins (90%) than in dizygotic twins (40%). SSc-associated serum autoantibodies (see Laboratory Findings below) were found only in twins with SSc. The finding of antinuclear antibodies in spouses of SSc patients suggests that environmental factors are also involved in the development of antinuclear antibodies. Studies have not shown a strong association between human leukocyte antigens (HLA) and susceptibility to SSc. C4A null alleles (C4AQ0) and HLA-DQA2 have been reported by some investigators to be markers for disease susceptibility. In a recent study, the frequency of HLA-DQA1*0501 was increased in Caucasian men with SSc over healthy controls from the same geographic area. No one HLA type has been shown to be associated with disease susceptibility in all ethnic groups. A more consistent relationship has been found between certain HLA types and the occurrence of specific autoantibodies in SSc patients. Anticentromere antibodies have been shown to be associated with HLA-DRβ1*0101 and -DQβ1*0501 in Caucasians, African Americans, and Hispanics. Antitopoisomerase 1 antibodies, on the other hand, are associated most frequently with HLA-DRβ1*1101, *1104 and -DQβ1*0301 in Caucasians and African Americans, -DRβ1*1502 in Japanese, and -DRβ1*1602 in Choctaw Native Americans.

Stronger evidence for a genetic role in SSc comes from studies of the Chocktaw Native Americans in Oklahoma who have a very high incidence of SSc. Affected individuals have in common diffuse cutaneous disease, pulmonary fibrosis, and antitopoisomerase antibodies. These autoantibodies are associated with the haplotype DQ 7, DR2 (DRβ1*1602) in this population of Native Americans. The association is stronger for the presence of antitopoisomerase antibodies than for the presence of SSc, as many individuals with autoantibodies do not have SSc. The extracellular fibrillin-1 matrix gene, FBN1, has also been found to be strongly associated with SSc in Chocktaw Native Americans. Not all SSc-affected individuals express the gene, and vice versa. The majority of Chocktaws were shown to produce autoantibodies to recombinant fibrillin-1 proteins. Of interest is that a tandem duplication of the murine gene, *fbn1*, in the tight-skin mouse (murine model of SSc) is thought to be responsible for the tight-skin mouse phenotype.

Infectious agents may play a role in the pathogenesis of SSc in the genetically susceptible individual. Latent cytomegalovirus (CMV) infection has been implicated in the vascular injury of SSc either by direct vascular injury or by immune-mediated mechanisms involving molecular mimicry in which viral and host proteins share similar amino acid sequences. Sera from SSc patients were shown to have antibodies that recognized an epitope contained within human CMV late protein UL94. This epitope is similar to a protein expressed in human endothelial cells. Incubation of SSc serum containing this antibody with endothelial cells was shown to induce apoptosis of endothelial cells, which is a feature of the vascular pathology observed in SSc. Parvovirus B19 has also been implicated in the development of SSc. In one study parvovirus B19 was detected in the bone marrow of >50% of SSc patients, compared to none in normal controls. Also, the frequency of anti-parvovirus B19 antibody was shown to be increased in SSc patients. The actual role of this virus or other micro-organisms in the pathogenesis of SSc awaits further studies.

Several environmental factors have been associated with the development of SSc and scleroderma-like illnesses. SSc appears to be more common in coal and gold miners, especially in those with more extensive exposure, suggesting that silica dust may be a predisposing factor. Workers exposed to polyvinyl chloride may develop Raynaud's phenomenon, acroosteolysis, scleroderma-like skin lesions, pulmonary fibrosis, and nail fold capillary abnormalities similar to those observed in SSc. These workers may also develop hepatic fibrosis and angiosarcoma. The observation that individuals exposed to similar amounts of vinyl chloride do not develop the same degree of disease suggests that a genetic factor may determine susceptibility and disease severity. The development of scleroderma has also been associated with exposure to epoxy resins and aromatic hydrocarbons such as benzine, toluene, and trichloroethylene. In 1981, in Spain, a multisystem disease resembling scleroderma occurred following the ingestion of aniline-adulterated cooking oil (rapeseed oil). Approximately 20,000 people were affected. The patients initially developed interstitial pneumonitis, eosinophilia, arthralgias, arthritis, and myositis, followed subsequently by joint contractures, skin thickening, Raynaud's phenomenon, pulmonary hypertension, sicca syndrome, and resorption of the distal fingertips. Extensive sclerosis of the dermis and subcutaneous tissue has been noted in patients receiving pentazocine, a nonnarcotic analgesic agent. Bleomycin, an anticancer agent, produces fibrotic skin nodules, linear hyperpigmentation, alopecia, Raynaud's phenomenon, gangrene of fingers, and pulmonary fibrosis affecting mainly the lower lobes. Scleroderma and other connective tissue diseases have been reported in women who have had silicone breast implants. Recent studies have not shown that women with these implants carry an increased risk for developing scleroderma or other connective tissue diseases. Localized fibrosis, however, can occur around the implant. While environmental factors or undefined infectious agents may be of etiologic significance, the cause of SSc remains unknown.

PATHOGENESIS The outstanding feature of SSc is overproduction and accumulation of collagen and other extracellular matrix proteins, including fibronectin, tenascin, fibrillin-1, and glycosaminoglycans, in skin and other organs. The disease process involves immunologic mechanisms, vascular endothelial cell activation and/or injury, and activation of fibroblasts resulting in production of excessive collagen (Fig. 303-1).

An early event in SSc that precedes fibrosis is vascular injury involving small arteries, arterioles, and capillaries in the skin, gastrointestinal tract, kidneys, heart, and lungs. Raynaud's phenomenon, the initial symptom of SSc in the majority of patients, is a clinical ex-

pression of the abnormal regulation of blood flow resulting from vascular injury. Injury to endothelial cells and basal lamina occurs early and is followed by proliferation of the intima and smooth-muscle cells, with deposition of matrix and perivascular fibrosis leading to narrowing of the lumen and eventual obliteration of the vessel. As vascular damage progresses, the microvascular bed in the skin and other sites is diminished, producing a state of chronic ischemia. Vascular abnormalities can be observed in the nail folds by wide-field microscopy, which shows drop-out of capillaries with dilatation and tortuosity of remaining ones. In the skin, remaining capillaries may proliferate and dilate to become visible telangiectasia. Endothelial cell damage is reflected in elevated levels of factor VIII/von Willebrand factor in the sera of some patients with SSc.

Several mechanisms for endothelial injury or activation have been proposed in SSc. Any or all of these mechanisms may be involved in a given patient; some evidence for each exists. A cytotoxic factor for endothelium has been identified in some patients that degrades the basal lamina, releasing fragments of type IV collagen and laminin. This factor, a type IV collagenase, is secreted by activated T cells and is referred to as *granzyme 1* because of its location in cytolytic T cells. Type IV collagen and laminin fragments may stimulate an immune response to the basal lamina. Both antibodies and cell-mediated immunity to type IV collagen and laminin have been observed in some SSc patients and may be involved in endothelial injury or may be an epiphenomenon. Anti-endothelial cell antibodies (AECA) may be another mechanism for microvascular damage. In 25% of SSc patients, AECA have been shown to mediate antibody-dependent cell cytotoxicity against human endothelial cells. Circulating AECA in general have been reported in the sera of SSc patients in amounts ranging from 21 to 85%. This wide variation reflects patient selection, type of assay, and the source of endothelium. These antibodies are not specific for SSc and are found in other connective tissue diseases. The frequency of AECA is higher in patients with diffuse cutaneous SSc. They have also been shown to be associated with digital infarcts, pulmonary hypertension, and impaired alveolocapillary diffusion. Studies have shown that AECA initiate programmed cell death (apoptosis) of endothelial cells, which may be an important event in the pathogenesis of SSc. These antibodies also induce expression of vascular cell adhesion molecule-1 (VCAM-1), intercellular adhesion molecule-1 (ICAM-1), E-selectin, and P-selectin on endothelial cells in SSc and stimulate the production of chemoattractants [interleukin (IL) 1, IL-8, monocyte chemotactic protein (MCP)], leading to the binding of T and B cells, natural killer cells, and monocytes to the endothelium and their migration into the perivascular tissue. Elevated serum levels of VCAM-1, ICAM-1, and P-selectin are observed in early stages of SSc.

The injury to the endothelium leads to a state favoring vasoconstriction and tissue ischemia. The damaged endothelium produces decreased amounts of prostacylin, which is an important vasodilator and inhibitor of platelet aggregation. Platelets are activated on binding to the damaged endothelium and release thromboxane, a potent vasoconstrictor. Activated platelets also release platelet-derived growth factor (PDGF), which is chemotactic and mitogenic for both smooth-muscle cells and fibroblasts, and transforming growth factor (TGF) β, which stimulates fibroblast collagen synthesis. These and other cytokines stimulate intimal fibrosis and, with their passage through the injured endothelium, may produce adventitial and perivascular fibrosis. Endothelin-1, a vasoconstricting factor released from endothelial cells on cold exposure, is also increased in SSc patients. In addition, it stimulates fibroblasts and smooth-muscle cells. The vasoconstriction action of endothelin-1 is normally opposed by endothelium-derived relaxation factor (EDRF, nitric oxide), also secreted by endothelial cells. The normal compensatory increase in EDRF is not seen in some patients with SSc, suggesting impairment of its synthesis. An increased α_2 adrenergic–mediated vasoconstriction has been demonstrated in SSc dermal arterioles. A deficiency of vasodilatory neuropeptides resulting from sensory system nerve damage may also produce a

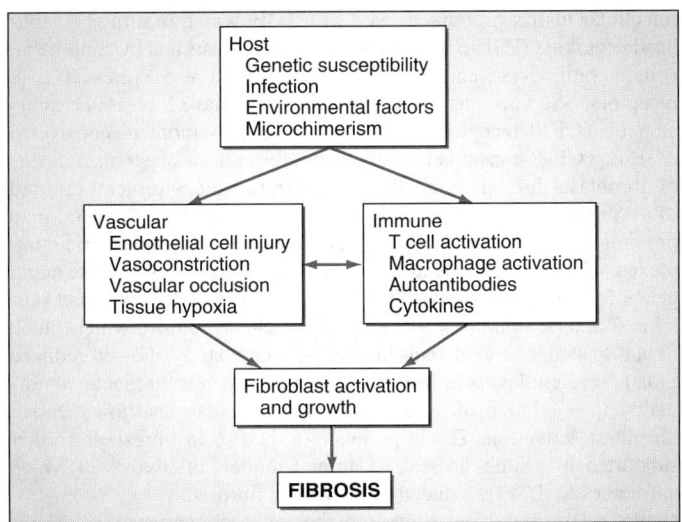

FIGURE 303-1 Algorithm for the multifactorial pathogenic mechanisms of systemic sclerosis.

condition favoring vasoconstriction. Vasoconstriction itself also contributes to endothelial damage through a mechanism of reperfusion injury. Following hypoxic endothelial injury from vasoconstriction, reperfusion can lead to release of oxygen free radicals, causing further tissue damage.

Existing evidence indicates that cell-mediated immunity plays a central role in the development of fibrosis in SSc. T cells, macrophages, endothelial cells, and other cells along with cytokines and growth factors interact in a complex manner to stimulate fibrosis. The vascular endothelium has been proposed as a target for cell-mediated immunity. Laminin and type IV collagen, components of the subendothelial basement membrane, induce in vitro transformation of lymphocytes from SSc patients. In the early stages of SSc, a mononuclear cell infiltrate consisting predominantly of activated helper-inducer T cells (T$_H$2 type) surrounds small blood vessels in the dermis. Subsequently, mononuclear cell infiltrates are found in macroscopically normal-appearing skin adjacent to areas of fibrosis. T cell hyperactivity is reflected by increased serum levels of CD4+ T cells. The ratio of CD4+ to CD8+ T cells is also increased. Elevated circulating levels of IL-2, a product of activated T cells, and IL-2 receptors have been shown to be associated with active fibrosis. In addition, serum levels of IL-4 are increased in SSc patients. IL-4, a product of activated T cells, stimulates fibroblast chemotaxis and proliferation and collagen production. In a recent study, CD8+ T cells isolated from bronchoalveolar lavage fluid from SSc patients made IL-4 and/or IL-5 mRNA. SSc patients with these type 2 cytokines were more likely to have alveolitis and a lower forced vital capacity. Although larger studies are needed, the findings suggest that these cytokines are involved in the pathogenesis of interstitial pulmonary fibrosis. Another cytokine, interferon γ, is produced by activated T cells (T$_H$1 type) and stimulates macrophages but inhibits collagen synthesis by fibroblasts. Reduced serum levels of interferon γ are found in some SSc patients. In vitro stimulation of T cells from SSc patients did not show an increased production of interferon γ compared to normal individuals, suggesting an inability in SSc patients to suppress fibrosis normally.

Macrophages are present in increased numbers in the infiltrates of SSc lesions, including the pulmonary alveoli. Activated macrophages secrete several important products involved in the pathogenesis of SSc including IL-1, IL-6, tumor necrosis factor (TNF) α, TGF-β, and PDGF. IL-1 has been shown to stimulate fibroblast proliferation and collagen synthesis. The important role for IL-6 may be in stimulating the local release of tissue inhibitor of metalloproteinase (TIMP) by fibroblasts and thereby limiting the breakdown of collagen. The role of TGF-β and PDGF secreted by macrophages and other cells is discussed below. In addition to the above cytokines, macrophages secrete *fibronectin*, a large matrix protein that is increased in SSc lesions. Fibronectin is also secreted by fibroblasts. Fibronectin interacts with collagen in the SSc lesions where it binds fibroblasts and mononuclear cells through receptors called *integrins*. Fibronectin functions as a chemoattractant and mitogen for fibroblasts.

Additional support for involvement of cell-mediated immunity in the pathogenesis of SSc is the appearance of scleroderma-like lesions in patients with graft-versus-host disease (GVHD) after bone marrow transplantation and in a murine model of chronic GVHD, conditions known to be associated with activated T cells. GVHD and SSc are both associated with progressive skin induration, joint contractures, and gastrointestinal and pulmonary involvement and are frequently accompanied by Sjögren's syndrome. Antinuclear antibodies are present in both diseases. Raynaud's phenomenon and kidney involvement are infrequent in GVHD.

Mast cells may also be involved in the development of fibrosis. Increased numbers of mast cells are found in the dermis in both involved and uninvolved skin. Mast cell degranulation has been noted in skin that subsequently became fibrosed. Interaction with T cells may be one mechanism for mast cell degranulation resulting in release of tryptase that stimulates fibroblast collagen synthesis. Release of his-

tamine from mast cells may also contribute to edema observed in early disease.

Fibroblast growth and synthesis of collagen, fibronectin, and glycosaminoglycans are increased in SSc. The number of α-smooth muscle actin-positive fibroblasts is greatly increased in SSc lesions. Fibroblasts from SSc appear to have aberrant regulation of growth compared with fibroblasts from normal persons. When fibroblasts from affected SSc skin are removed and cultured in vitro, they continue to produce excessive quantities of collagen. The collagen is biochemically normal, and the proportion of type I to type III is the same as in normal skin. Fibroblasts from SSc patients appear to be in a state of permanent activation, due in part to autocrine and paracrine stimulation by TGF-β and connective tissue growth factor (CTGF). These activated cells are thought to represent an expanded subpopulation of fibroblasts that inherently express increased matrix genes. Studies have revealed a subpopulation of SSc fibroblasts that produces two to three times more collagen than other cells from the same tissue. Fibroblasts with a high-collagen-producing phenotype may be clonally selected by cytokines or other immune stimuli. Another explanation for the subpopulation of high-collagen-producing fibroblasts is that fibroblasts with low-collagen-producing phenotype may be selectively removed by apoptosis. Fibroblasts expressing elevated levels of mRNA for types I and III collagen have been demonstrated by in situ hybridization, particularly around dermal blood vessels in affected SSc skin. Collagen deposition is also initially perivascular in other organs including myocardium, muscle, and kidney. A small number of fibroblasts express increased levels of mRNA for types VI and VII collagen. Type VII collagen is normally found at the dermal-epidermal basement membrane zone and is the major component of anchoring fibrils that act to stabilize the attachment of the basement membrane to the underlying dermis. In SSc patients, type VII collagen is found throughout the dermis and may account for the indurated, tightly bound skin in this disease. PDGF receptors are expressed on SSc fibroblasts not only from affected areas but also from macroscopically normal-appearing skin. Fibroblasts from normal persons lack expression of these receptors. TGF-β has been shown to upregulate the expression of these receptors in SSc fibroblasts but not in normal cells and, in conjunction with PDGF, stimulates SSc fibroblast proliferation. Macrophages and fibroblasts are capable of secreting PDGF and TGF-β, and activated T cells release TGF-β. TGF-β also induces the synthesis of CTGF by fibroblasts, which further stimulates fibroblast proliferation and extracellular matrix proteins including collagen synthesis. CTGF mRNA and protein expression in SSc tissue are increased, and serum levels of CTGF have been found to be elevated in SSc and correlate with the degree of dermal and pulmonary fibrosis.

TGF-β is considered to play an essential role in mediating fibrosis in SSc. TGF-β stimulates fibroblast proliferation and synthesis of extracellular matrix proteins as well as CTGF, which in turn is a profibrotic cytokine. TGF-β is synthesized by fibroblasts and by endothelial cells, keratinocytes, and inflammatory cells that also express TGF-β receptors. SSc fibroblasts have been shown to have increased expression of TGF-β receptors, rendering these cells more responsive to TGF-β. TGF-β transmits its signal from the cell surface to the nucleus of fibroblasts through intracellular transcription factor proteins referred to as *Smads*. When the TGF-β receptor is engaged by TGF-β, Smad proteins 2, 3, and 4 are activated and assemble into multimeric complexes, which are translocated to the nucleus where they activate target genes for matrix synthesis. This pathway is controlled by Smad proteins 6 and 7, inhibitory proteins of the Smad family, which block Smad-dependent signal transduction. A recent study showed reduced Smad 7 protein levels in involved SSc skin, suggesting that an abnormality in regulation of intracellular signaling may lead to excessive fibroblast activation. The importance of TGF-β in fibrosis is further supported by studies in several animal models of fibrosis in which antibodies to TGF-β reduced or prevented fibrosis.

Recent studies have suggested that microchimerism may be involved in the pathogenesis of SSc. Microchimerism in SSc is of interest because of the clinical similarities between SSc and GVHD after allogeneic bone marrow transplantation. Also relevant are the predilection for women in SSc and the increased incidence of SSc in women after the childbearing years. Fetal progenitor cells can persist in the serum of normal women for many years after childbirth. Microchimerism can also occur in nulligravid women and in men with SSc as non-host cells may come from blood transfusion, engraftment of cells from a twin, or from maternal cells in utero. Two-directional traffic of cells occurs during pregnancy. Compared to normal controls, both the quantity and frequency of immune fetal cells have been found to be increased in the serum of SSc patients. The mechanism by which microchimerism is involved in the pathogenesis is not known, but it is conceivable that these small numbers of non-host cells alter immune regulation, leading to autoimmunity.

Chromosomal abnormalities have been noted in >90% of SSc patients. These acquired abnormalities include chromatid breaks, acentric fragments, and ring chromosomes and are found in ~30% of mitotic cells. A chromosomal breakage factor has been found in the serum of SSc patients and their first-degree relatives. The significance of these chromosomal abnormalities is unknown.

PATHOLOGY ■ Skin   In the skin, a thin epidermis overlies compact bundles of collagen that lie parallel to the epidermis. Fingerlike projections of collagen extend from the dermis into the subcutaneous tissue and bind the skin to the underlying tissue. Dermal appendages are atrophied, and rete pegs are lost. In early stages of disease, a mononuclear cell infiltrate of predominantly T cells surrounds small dermal blood vessels. Increased numbers of T cells, monocytes, plasma cells, and mast cells are found, particularly in the lower dermis of involved skin.

Gastrointestinal Tract   In the lower two-thirds of the esophagus, the histologic findings consist of a thin mucosa and increased collagen in the lamina propria, submucosa, and serosa. The degree of fibrosis is less than in the skin. Atrophy of the muscularis in the esophagus and throughout the involved portions of the gastrointestinal tract is more prominent than the amount of fibrotic replacement of muscle. Ulceration of the mucosa is often present and may be due to either SSc or superimposed peptic esophagitis. Chronic esophageal reflux can lead to metaplasia of the lower esophagus (Barrett's esophagus), which is a premalignant lesion. Striated muscles in the upper third of the esophagus are relatively spared. Similar changes may be found throughout the gastrointestinal tract, especially in the second and third portions of the duodenum, in the jejunum, and in the large intestine. Atrophy of the muscularis of the large intestine may lead to the development of large-mouth diverticula. In the later stages of the disease, the involved portions of the gastrointestinal tract become dilated. Infiltration of lymphocytes and plasma cells in the lamina propria is also present.

Lung   With pulmonary involvement, diffuse interstitial fibrosis, thickening of the alveolar membrane, and peribronchial and pleural fibrosis are observed. Bronchiolar epithelial proliferation accompanies the pulmonary fibrosis. Rupture of septa produces small cysts and areas of bullous emphysema. Small pulmonary arteries and arterioles show intimal thickening, fragmentation of the elastica, and muscular hypertrophy; this may occur without interstitial pulmonary fibrosis and produce pulmonary hypertension, particularly in a subset of patients with limited cutaneous SSc.

Musculoskeletal System   The synovium in patients with arthritis is similar to that seen in early rheumatoid arthritis and shows edema with infiltration of lymphocytes and plasma cells. A characteristic finding is a thick layer of fibrin overlying and within the synovium. Later in the disease the synovium may become fibrotic. Fibrinous deposits appear on the surfaces of tendon sheaths and in the overlying fascia and may lead to audible creaking over moving tendons.

Histologic features of primary myopathy consist of interstitial and perivascular lymphocytic infiltrations, degeneration of muscle fibers, and interstitial fibrosis. Arterioles may be thickened, and capillaries may be decreased in number. Pathologic and electrophysiologic findings of polymyositis in proximal muscles are present in the few pa-

tients who are considered to have the overlap syndrome of SSc and polymyositis.

Heart   Cardiac involvement consists of degeneration of myocardial fibers and irregular areas of interstitial fibrosis that are most prominent around blood vessels. Intermittent spasm of blood vessels may result in contraction band necrosis, similar to changes observed in myocardial infarction in patients with atherosclerotic coronary artery disease. Fibrosis also involves the conduction system, leading to atrioventricular conduction defects and arrhythmias. The wall of smaller coronary arteries may be thickened. Fibrinous pericarditis and pericardial effusions are found in some patients.

Kidney   Renal involvement is found in over half the patients and consists of intimal hyperplasia of the interlobular arteries; fibrinoid necrosis of the afferent arterioles, including the glomerular tuft; and thickening of the glomerular basement membrane. Small cortical infarctions and glomerulosclerosis may be present. The renal pathologic change is often indistinguishable from that observed in malignant hypertension. Renal vascular lesions, however, may be present in the absence of hypertension. Immunofluorescence studies of kidney have shown IgM, complement components, and fibrinogen in the walls of affected vessels. Angiographic renal studies in patients with SSc may show constriction of the interlobular arteries, a finding that simulates the vasospasm of the digital arteries observed in Raynaud's phenomenon. Cold-induced Raynaud's phenomenon has been shown to decrease renal blood flow.

Other Organs   Primary liver involvement is not common. Primary biliary cirrhosis occurs in some patients, particularly in those with the limited cutaneous form of SSc. Fibrosis of the thyroid gland may develop in the presence or absence of autoimmune thyroiditis.

Thickening of the periodontal membrane with replacement of the lamina dura is demonstrated radiographically as widening of the periodontal space and may cause gingivitis and loosening of the teeth. The decreased oral aperture and mucosal dryness make eating and oral hygiene difficult.

CLINICAL MANIFESTATIONS (See Table 303-3) **■ Raynaud's Phenomenon** SSc usually begins insidiously; the first symptoms are frequently Raynaud's phenomenon and puffy fingers. Some 95% of patients will experience Raynaud's phenomenon, which is defined as episodic vasoconstriction of small arteries and arterioles of fingers, toes, and sometimes the tip of the nose and earlobes. Episodes are brought on by cold exposure, vibration, or emotional stress. Patients experience pallor and/or cyanosis followed by rubor on rewarming. Pallor and/or cyanosis are usually associated with coldness and numbness of fingers and/or toes, and rubor with pain and tingling. Not all patients appreciate the three color phases. A history of digit pallor appears to be the most reliable symptom for the presence of Raynaud's phenomenon.

TABLE 303-3   *Clinical Features of Systemic Sclerosis*

Clinical Feature	% Patients during Course of Disease	
	Limited[a]	Diffuse[a]
Raynaud's phenomenon	95–100	90–95
Skin thickening	98[b]	100
Subcutaneous calcinosis	50	10
Telangiectasia	85	40
Arthralgias/arthritis	40	70
Myopathy	5	50
Esophageal dysmotility	80	80
Pulmonary fibrosis	35	40
Isolated pulmonary arterial hypertension	<10	<1
Congestive heart failure	<1	30
Renal crisis	<1	15

[a] Limited cutaneous and diffuse cutaneous subsets of SSc.
[b] 2% or fewer of patients have SSc sine scleroderma.

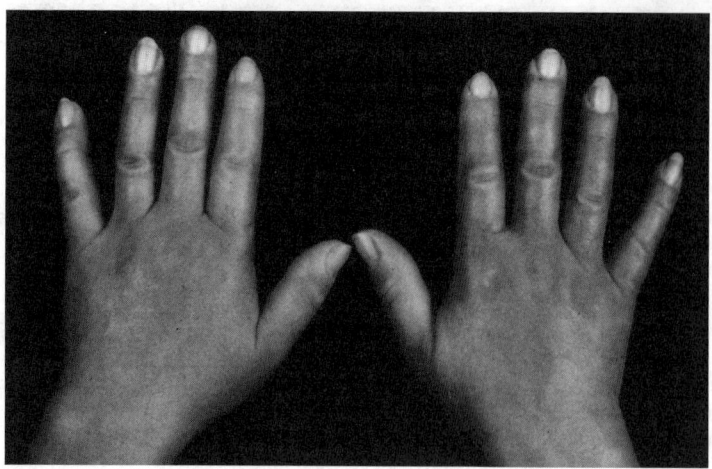

FIGURE 303-2 Swollen hands and fingers in early systemic sclerosis. Swelling may also involve forearms, distal lower extremities, and face. Edematous phase may last weeks to months or even longer.

Raynaud's phenomenon may precede skin changes by several months or even years in those patients who subsequently develop the limited cutaneous form of SSc. In diffuse cutaneous SSc, skin changes are seen typically within a year of the onset of Raynaud's phenomenon. After 2 or more years of Raynaud's phenomenon, few patients who have this as their only symptom will subsequently develop SSc.

Skin Features   In early disease, fingers and hands are swollen (Fig. 303-2). Swelling may also involve forearms, feet, lower legs, and face. However, lower extremities are relatively spared. This edematous phase may last for a few weeks, months, or even longer. The edema may be pitting or nonpitting and accompanied by erythema. The skin changes begin distally in the extremities and advance proximally. The skin gradually becomes firm, thickened, and eventually tightly bound to underlying subcutaneous tissue (indurative phase). In patients with diffuse cutaneous scleroderma, skin changes will become generalized, involving initially the extremities, followed by the face and trunk over a period of time, varying from months to a few years. In some patients, the skin changes may develop gradually over several years. Rapid progression of these changes over a 1- to 3-year period is associated with a greater risk of visceral disease, particularly of the lungs, heart, or kidneys. Also in diffuse cutaneous SSc, the skin changes usually peak in 3 to 5 years and then slowly improve. On the other hand, patients with limited cutaneous scleroderma will usually have a more gradual progression of skin changes, which are restricted to fingers or distal extremity and face and may continue to worsen. In both subsets of SSc, skin thickening is usually greater in the distal extremity. After many years of disease, the skin may soften and return to normal thickness or become thin and atrophic.

In the extremities, the taut skin over fingers gradually limits full extension, and flexion contractures develop (Fig. 303-3). Ulcers may appear on the volar pads of the fingertips and over bony prominences such as elbows, malleoli, and the extensor surface of the proximal interphalangeal joints of the hands. These ulcers may become secondarily infected. The volar pads of the fingertips develop pitting scars and lose soft tissue. In some instances, resorption of the terminal phalanges occurs. Skin over the extremities, face, and trunk may become darkly pigmented, even without exposure to the sun. Hyperpigmentation of the skin may occur over superficial blood vessels and tendons. Areas of hypopigmentation may also develop, similar to vitiligo, involving the eyebrows, scalp, and trunk. The sparing of pigment around hair follicles gives the skin a "salt-and-pepper" appearance. Other patients may develop a diffuse tanning of the skin. The skin loses hair, oil, and sweat glands and so becomes dry and coarse. Vaginal dryness occurs and may cause dyspareunia.

In some patients, particularly those with the limited cutaneous form of disease, calcific deposits develop in intracutaneous and subcutaneous tissue. The sites commonly involved are periarticular tissue, digital

pads, olecranon and prepatellar bursae, and skin along the extensor surface of the forearms. The overlying skin may break down, with drainage of calcific material. Involvement of the face results in thinning of the lips, loss of skin wrinkles and facial expression, as well as microstomia, which may make eating and dental hygiene difficult (Fig. 303-4). The nose takes on a pinched or beaklike appearance. Wrinkles appear around the mouth perpendicular to the lips. Small telangiectatic mats may appear on the fingers, face, lips, tongue, and buccal mucosa after several years. They are seen more frequently in patients with limited cutaneous SSc but are also observed in patients with long-standing diffuse cutaneous SSc. The capillary beds of nail folds of the fingers may show enlargement of capillaries with little or no capillary loss, usually indicative of limited cutaneous scleroderma. In diffuse cutaneous scleroderma, there is disorganization of the capillary beds with dilated capillaries interspersed with areas where capillaries have disappeared (Fig. 303-5). These capillary changes, which are observed by wide-angle microscopy or with an ophthalmoscope used as a magnifier, are not found in patients who have only Raynaud's phenomenon.

Musculoskeletal Features   More than half the patients with SSc complain of pain, swelling, and stiffness of the fingers and knees. A symmetric polyarthritis resembling rheumatoid arthritis may be seen. In more advanced stages of the disease, leathery crepitation can be palpated over moving joints, especially the knee. Extensive fibrotic thickening of the tendon sheaths in the wrist can produce a carpal tunnel syndrome. Muscle weakness is usually present in patients with severe skin involvement and, in most cases, is due to disuse atrophy. There is a distinctive histologic myopathy that accompanies SSc that is not associated with muscle enzyme abnormalities. A few patients develop a myositis characterized by proximal muscle weakness and muscle enzyme elevations that are identical to polymyositis (overlap syndrome). In addition to terminal phalanges, resorption of bone may involve ribs, clavicle, and angle of mandible.

Gastrointestinal Features   The majority of patients from both subsets of SSc have gastrointestinal involvement. Symptoms attributable to esophageal involvement are present in >50% of patients and include epigastric fullness, burning pain in the epigastric or retrosternal regions, and regurgitation of gastric contents. These symptoms, most noticeable when the patient is lying flat or bending over, are due to the reduced tone of the gastroesophageal sphincter and to dilatation of the distal esophagus. Peptic esophagitis frequently occurs and may lead to strictures and narrowing of the lower esophagus. However, it seldom results in bleeding. Barrett's metaplasia may develop, but transition to adenocarcinoma is uncommon. Dysphagia, particularly of solid foods, may occur independent of other esophageal symptoms and is caused by loss of esophageal motility due to neuromuscular dys-

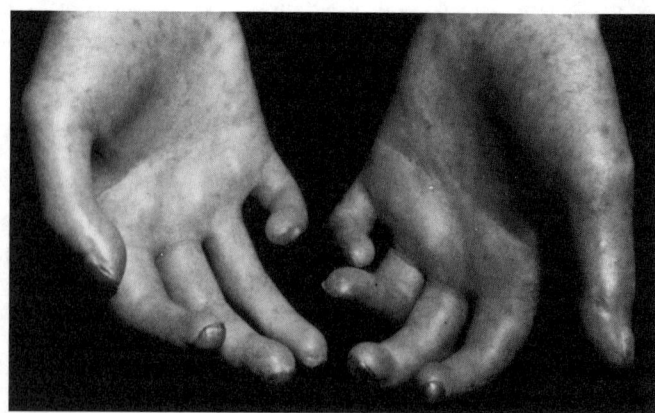

FIGURE 303-3   Flexion deformities of the fingers and sclerodactlyly. The skin over the fingers and hands is taunt and indurated. There is shortening and bony resorption of distal phalanges of the second and third fingers. Ulcers may develop over the distal phalanges and dorsal surfaces of the metacarpal phalangeal and proximal interphalangeal joints.

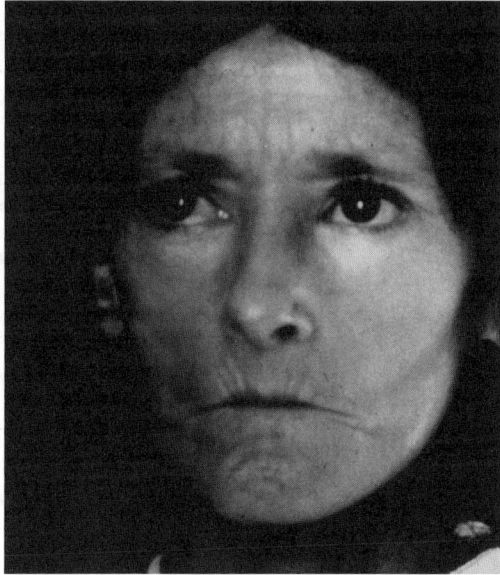

FIGURE 303-4   Skin over cheeks and forehead is tight and shiny with loss of wrinkles and facial expression. There are furrows around the mouth perpendicular to the lips and the lips are thin. The nose has a pinched appearance.

function. Manometry or cineradiography reveals decreased amplitude or disappearance of peristaltic waves in the lower two-thirds of the esophagus. Raynaud's phenomenon in the absence of a connective tissue disease is also associated with esophageal dysmotility. Later in the course of the illness, dilatation and atony of the lower portion of the esophagus as well as reflux are seen. With gastric involvement, barium studies show dilatation, atony, and delayed gastric emptying. Patients may complain of early satiety. Gastric outlet obstruction can also occur.

Hypomotility of the small intestine produces symptoms of bloating and abdominal pain and may suggest an intestinal obstruction or paralytic ileus (pseudoobstruction). Malabsorption syndrome with weight loss, diarrhea, and anemia is due to bacterial overgrowth in the atonic intestine or possibly to obliteration of lymphatics by fibrosis. Roentgenographic features of the second and third portions of the duodenum and of the jejunum include dilatation, loss of the usual feathery pattern, and delayed disappearance of barium. Pneumatosis intestinalis occasionally occurs and appears as radiolucent cysts or linear streaks within the wall of the small intestine. Benign pneumoperitoneum may result from the rupture of these cysts. Involvement of the large intestine may cause chronic constipation and fecal impaction with episodes of bowel obstruction. A segment of atonic bowel may act as a fulcrum for intussusception to occur. Barium studies of the large intestine may show dilatation, atony, and large-mouth diverticula. Laxity of the anal sphincter may cause incontinence or rarely anal prolapse. Some patients may have gastrointestinal features of SSc with little or no cutaneous or other organ involvement, referred to as *SSc sine*

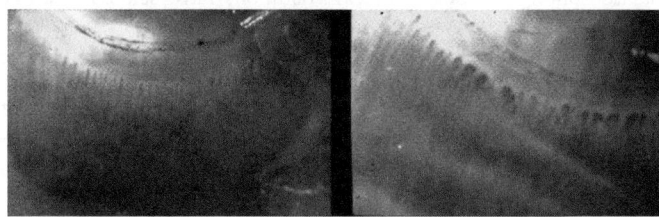

FIGURE 303-5   Nail fold capillaries in normal person (*left panel*) and in scleroderma patient (*right panel*). Capillary loops are found just proximal to the cuticle using a wide angle microscope, a dermatoscope, or an ophthalmoscope serving as a magnifier. Immersion oil is placed over the nail fold to reduce reflection of light. *Left panel*: Capillary loops are small and well organized being parallel to each other and perpendicular to the nail. *Right panel*: Enlarged dilated capillary loops are interspersed with areas where capillaries have disappeared.

scleroderma. Vascular ectasia may develop in the stomach and intestine and can be the source of gastrointestinal bleeding. These dilated submucosal capillaries in the stomach appear on endoscopy as broad stripes—hence the term *watermelon stomach*.

Pulmonary Features   Pulmonary involvement occurs in at least two-thirds of SSc patients and is now the leading cause of death in SSc, replacing renal disease, which can usually be treated effectively. The most common symptom is exertional dyspnea, often accompanied by a dry, nonproductive cough. Bilateral basilar rales may be present. In the majority of patients, symptoms usually correlate with radiologic evidence of pulmonary fibrosis and with restrictive lung disease on pulmonary function tests.

Pulmonary function tests are frequently abnormal and show a reduction in vital capacity and decreased lung compliance. Impairment of gas exchange is reflected by a low diffusing capacity and low P_{O_2} with exercise. These abnormalities may be present even when the chest radiograph is normal. Chest film may show a pattern of linear densities, mottling, and honeycombing involving most prominently the lower two-thirds of the lung. Early interstitial pulmonary disease can be detected by high-resolution computed tomography (HRCT) and bronchoalveolar lavage (BAL). Active inflammatory alveolitis gives a "ground glass" appearance on HRCT. The recovery by BAL of increased numbers of cells, mostly alveolar macrophages accompanied by neutrophils or eosinophils, is evidence for alveolitis.

Both interstitial fibrosis and vascular lesions are found in the lungs of patients with SSc. Interstitial pulmonary fibrosis may be the predominant lesion in patients with diffuse or limited cutaneous SSc. Patients with diffuse cutaneous involvement who have antitopoisomerase 1 antibodies are particularly at risk of developing severe pulmonary fibrosis. In the absence of significant interstitial fibrosis, a severe form of pulmonary arterial hypertension may develop after many years of disease in a subset of patients with limited cutaneous SSc. Fewer than 10% of patients will develop this complication, which is caused by narrowing and obliteration of pulmonary arteries and arterioles by intimal fibrosis and medial hypertrophy. Pulmonary hypertension is manifested initially by exertional dyspnea and eventually by the appearance of right-sided heart failure. Pulmonary artery pressure can be measured noninvasively by two-dimensional echocardiography. The prognosis is extremely poor with the development of pulmonary hypertension; the mean duration of survival is ~2 years.

A less common pulmonary problem is aspiration pneumonia resulting from gastric reflux due to lower esophageal atony. Restriction of chest movement caused by extensive fibrotic skin involvement of the thorax rarely occurs. Superimposed bacterial or viral infection can be a serious complication in patients with pulmonary fibrosis. An increased frequency of alveolar cell and bronchogenic carcinoma is seen in patients with pulmonary fibrosis.

Cardiac Features   Primary cardiac involvement in SSc includes pericarditis with or without effusions, heart failure, and varying degrees of heart block or arrhythmias. The majority of patients with diffuse cutaneous SSc have cardiac abnormalities. Cardiomyopathy attributable to myocardial fibrosis appears in <10% of patients and involves primarily those patients with diffuse cutaneous scleroderma. Radionuclide studies have shown abnormalities of left ventricular function due to myocardial fibrosis. Cold-induced vasospasm of the hands produces defects in myocardial thallium perfusion. The characteristic pathologic feature of contraction band necrosis results from cardiac muscle damage caused by intermittent vasospasm of coronary vessels. Patients may experience angina pectoris even though coronary angiograms are normal. Patients can also develop left ventricular failure secondary to systemic hypertension or cor pulmonale secondary to pulmonary arterial hypertension.

Renal Features   Renal failure was the leading cause of death in SSc until the advent of effective treatment. Significant renal disease occurs mostly in those patients with diffuse cutaneous scleroderma. A high risk of renal crisis is present in those patients who have rapidly progressive widespread skin thickening in their first 2 to 3 years of disease. Renal crisis is characterized by malignant hypertension, which can progress rapidly to renal failure. These patients manifest hypertensive encephalopathy, severe headache, retinopathy, seizures, and left ventricular failure. Hematuria and proteinuria are followed by oliguria and renal failure. The mechanism for the hypertensive crisis is activation of the renin-angiotensin system. Before the advent of effective antihypertensive drugs, the majority of these patients died within 6 months. A small number of patients may develop renal crises in the absence of hypertension. Renal failure can also develop insidiously later in the course of disease in the setting of mild to moderate hypertension and proteinuria. In these patients or those with clinically unrecognized renal disease, reduction of renal plasma flow secondary to heart failure or volume depletion resulting from overdiuresis may precipitate renal crisis. An indicator of impending renal failure is microangiopathic anemia, which may occur in a normotensive patient. The presence of a large chronic pericardial effusion may also herald subsequent renal failure.

Other Features Symptoms of dry eyes and/or dry mouth are frequently present in patients with SSc. Lip biopsy may show lymphocytic infiltration of minor salivary glands characteristic of Sjögren's syndrome or intraglandular or periglandular fibrosis secondary to SSc. Antibodies to SS-A (Ro) and/or SS-B (La) are found in those patients with lip biopsies consistent with Sjögren's syndrome (overlap syndrome-SSc and Sjögren's syndrome) and not in those with salivary gland fibrosis.

Hypothyroidism occurs in a significant number of patients and may be associated with high levels of antithyroid antibodies. Fibrosis of the thyroid gland may be present but also occurs in the absence of autoimmune thyroiditis. Other manifestations of SSc include trigeminal neuralgia and male impotence secondary to decreased penile tumescence. These men have normal serum levels of testosterone and gonadotropins. Pathogenesis of this abnormality has been considered to be caused by vascular and/or autonomic nervous system abnormalities. Biliary cirrhosis is occasionally observed in patients with limited cutaneous SSc.

LABORATORY FINDINGS The erythrocyte sedimentation rate may be elevated. Hypoproliferative anemia related to chronic inflammation is the most common cause of anemia in SSc. Anemia may also be caused by iron deficiency secondary to gastrointestinal bleeding. Bacterial overgrowth due to atony of the small bowel may lead to vitamin B_{12} and/or folic acid–deficiency anemia. Microangiopathic hemolytic anemia is most often associated with renal involvement and is caused by the presence of intravascular fibrin in renal arterioles. Polyclonal hypergammaglobulinemia, consisting mostly of IgG, is found in approximately half the patients. Rheumatoid factor, in low titer, is present in 25% of patients. Cryoglobulins may be present in the serum. Antinuclear antibodies detected by using a cultured human laryngeal carcinoma cell line (HEp-2) substrate are present in 95% of patients (Table 303-4). Antinuclear antibodies that have a high specificity for SSc are antitopoisomerase 1 (Scl-70), antinucleolar, and anticentromere. Antitopoisomerase 1, originally called anti-Scl-70, recognizes the nuclear enzyme DNA topoisomerase 1, a nuclear enzyme involved in the unwinding of DNA for replication and RNA transcription. These antibodies are found in ~20% of all SSc patients and in ~40% of those with diffuse cutaneous SSc. They are associated with diffuse cutaneous involvement, interstitial pulmonary disease, and renal and other visceral organ involvement. A very high frequency of these antibodies has been reported in Choctaw Native Americans in association with diffuse cutaneous SSc. They are seldom present in other disorders or in conjunction with anticentromere antibodies. Anticentromere antibodies react with protein antigens located in the kinetochore region of chromosomes and are present in 40 to 80% of patients with limited cutaneous scleroderma or CREST syndrome. Anticentromere antibod-

TABLE 303-4 *Autoantibodies in Systemic Sclerosis*

Autoantibody	Clinical Association	Percent[a]
Anti-topoisomerase 1	Diffuse cutaneous SSc	40
Anticentromere	Limited cutaneous SSc	60–80
Anti-RNA polymerase I, II, III	Diffuse cutaneous SSc	5–40
Anti-Th RNP	Limited cutaneous SSc	14
Anti-U₁ RNP	Limited cutaneous SSc	5–10
	Mixed connective tissue disease	95–100
Anti-U₃ RNP[b]	Diffuse and limited cutaneous SSc, skeletal myopathy, pulmonary arterial hypertension	5
Anti-PM/Scl	Overlap (SSc, polymyositis)	25

[a] Approximate percentages for the predominant clinical association.
[b] Anti-fibrillarin.

ies are found in only about 2 to 5% of patients with diffuse cutaneous scleroderma and rarely in other connective tissue diseases. They are found occasionally in patients with only Raynaud's phenomenon and may indicate subsequent development of limited cutaneous disease. Antinucleolar antibodies are relatively specific for SSc and are present in ~20 to 30% of patients. Several antinucleolar antibodies have been associated with SSc: Anti-RNA polymerases I, II, and III are found in patients with diffuse cutaneous SSc who have a higher prevalence of renal and cardiac involvement. Anti-Th RNP has been found in patients with limited cutaneous SSc, and anti-PM-Scl, formerly referred to as anti-PM1, along with anti-Ku, may be found in a subset of patients with overlapping features of limited cutaneous SSc and polymyositis. Anti-U₃ RNP (anti-fibrillarin) is also highly specific for SSc and may be associated with skeletal muscle disease, bowel involvement, and pulmonary arterial hypertension. Anti-U₁ RNP is found in ~5 to 10% of SSc patients and in 95 to 100% of those patients with the overlap syndrome of MCTD. The titers in MCTD are usually high (see below). Anti-SS-A (Ro) and/or anti-SS-B (La) are present in those patients with overlap syndrome of SSc and Sjögren's syndrome.

DIAGNOSIS The diagnosis of SSc presents no difficulty in the presence of Raynaud's phenomenon, with typical skin lesions and visceral involvement. Although Raynaud's phenomenon may be the first symptom of SSc, most patients with Raynaud's phenomenon alone do not develop a connective tissue disease. Other causes of Raynaud's phenomenon include thoracic outlet (scalenus anticus and cervical rib) syndromes, shoulder-hand syndrome, trauma (jackhammer or vibratory machine operators), previous cold injury, vinyl chloride exposure, and circulating cryoglobulins or cold agglutinins. Linear scleroderma and morphea are localized forms of scleroderma that can usually be distinguished clinically. In early disease, SSc may initially be confused with rheumatoid arthritis, SLE, or polymyositis when articular or muscle involvement is prominent. SSc without cutaneous involvement should be considered in patients with unexplained pulmonary fibrosis, pulmonary hypertension, cardiomyopathies, heart block, dysphagia, or malabsorption syndrome. Several conditions have scleroderma-like features but lack the visceral involvement. Scleredema (scleredema adultorum of Buschke) occurs predominantly in children and is characterized by painless edematous induration involving the face, scalp, neck, trunk, and proximal portions of the extremities. Involvement of the hands and feet usually does not occur. Scleredema may be associated with previous streptococcal infection and is usually self-limited, resolving in 6 to 12 months. Histology reveals accumulation of mucopolysaccharides in the dermis and skeletal muscle. A rare entity, scleromyxedema is manifested by yellowish or pale red papules in association with diffuse skin thickening that may involve the face and hands. Acid mucopolysaccharide deposits are found in the dermis. Monoclonal IgG may be detected in some of these patients. Patients with insulin-dependent diabetes mellitus may develop digital sclerosis and contractures (prayer hand deformity). Primary amyloidosis and amyloidosis associated with multiple myeloma may involve the skin of the extremities and face diffusely to give the appearance of scleroderma. Biopsy will clearly differentiate these entities.

COURSE AND PROGNOSIS The course of SSc is quite variable. Until the disease differentiates into recognizable subsets, prognosis in early disease is difficult to predict. Patients with limited cutaneous scleroderma, especially those with anticentromere antibodies, have a good prognosis, with the notable exception of those few patients, <10%, who after ≥10 to 20 years develop pulmonary arterial hypertension. Malabsorption syndrome and primary biliary cirrhosis are the causes of morbidity and mortality in some patients with limited cutaneous disease. On the other hand, the prognosis is generally worse in patients with diffuse cutaneous disease, particularly when the onset occurs at an older age. In addition, males have a worse prognosis. Renal and other visceral organ disease may develop early in the course of those patients with rapidly progressive generalized skin thickening. Death occurs most often from pulmonary, cardiac, and renal involvement. With the advent of effective therapy for renal crisis along with renal dialysis for those patients with renal failure, survival has greatly improved. In patients with diffuse cutaneous disease, the 5-year cumulative survival rate is ~70% and the 10-year is ~55%. In limited cutaneous disease the 5-year is ~90% and the 10-year is ~75%.

Skin may spontaneously soften after years of disease. Softening occurs in the reverse order of original skin involvement, beginning with the trunk and followed by the proximal and then the distal extremities. Sclerodactyly and flexion contractures may persist. Skin thickness may eventually approach normal; however, the skin may be atrophic.

℞ TREATMENT

Even though SSc cannot be cured, treatment of involved organ systems can relieve symptoms and improve function. The doctor-patient relationship is extremely important in caring for patients with this chronic debilitating illness. Once the diagnosis of SSc has been made, the patient and family should be instructed about this disorder. The patient will need repeated explanations and reassurances throughout his or her illness. Depending on the severity of illness, the patient will require monitoring of blood pressure, blood counts, urinalysis, and monitoring of renal and pulmonary function on a regular basis.

Effectiveness of drug therapy in SSc is difficult to evaluate because of the variable course and severity of disease especially within its subsets. Controlled drug studies have been difficult to achieve because of this variability and the relative few number of SSc patients. Several drugs with antifibrotic, immunosuppressive, or both properties have been tried in the treatment of SSc without any consistent or prolonged benefit. These drugs have included D-penicillamine, colchicine, IFN-γ, IFN-α, and recombinant human relaxin. In the past, high-dose D-penicillamine (750–1000 mg/d) has been used in patients with early diffuse cutaneous SSc, but a recent study showed no benefit of high versus low doses of this drug (see below). The rationale for using D-penicillamine was that it interfered with inter- and intramolecular cross-linking of collagen and was also thought to be immunosuppressive. Several earlier uncontrolled studies with D-penicillamine showed a reduction in skin thickening and prevention of significant internal organ involvement when compared to historic controls. Five-year cumulative survival rates of 80% had been reported in D-penicillamine–treated patients. A recent study did not show an advantage of high-dose D-penicillamine treatment in SSc. The results of a 2-year double-blind randomized study comparing high-dose D-penicillamine (750–1000 mg/d) with low-dose D-penicillamine (125 mg every other day) in patients with early diffuse cutaneous SSc did not show a significant difference between the groups as to the degree of skin thickening, occurrence of renal crises, other organ involvement and mortality. The majority of adverse or toxic effects occurred in the high dosage group. This study, however, did not compare patients on low-dose D-penicillamine versus placebo. It is possible that this drug in low dose might have some beneficial effect in SSc. Its therapeutic value, however, in

SSc remains in question. Open uncontrolled trials with colchicine showed skin improvement, but other studies were negative. Randomized controlled multicenter trials with recombinant human IFN-γ demonstrated modest improvement in skin sclerosis. Worsening of Raynaud's phenomenon and development of renal crisis as well as influenza-like symptoms were noted in patients treated with recombinant human IFN-γ, and follow-up studies have not been done. IFN-α in a controlled trial showed no benefit. In a randomized, double-blind, placebo-controlled trial, recombinant human relaxin given by continuous subcutaneous infusion for 24 weeks was associated with reduced skin thickening and improved mobility in patients with moderate to severe diffuse cutaneous scleroderma. A subsequent follow-up, however, did not demonstrate any significant benefit. It is unlikely that further studies with this agent will be done.

Several immunosuppressive agents have been tried in SSc. The rationale for using these agents is based on the cellular and humoral immunologic abnormalities that have been demonstrated in SSc. The results of immunosuppressive therapy have been disappointing and, as of now, no agent has been clearly shown in a controlled prospective study to fully suppress or reverse the disease process of SSc. A controlled randomized, double-blind trial with chlorambucil versus control was negative. Earlier reports of benefit with azathioprine have not been confirmed in controlled studies. Cyclosporine was shown to decrease skin induration without improvement in pulmonary or cardiac manifestations. Concern regarding nephrotoxicity has limited its use in SSc. Randomized controlled trials of methotrexate in early diffuse cutaneous SSc have shown mixed results, with one study showing improvement and others showing marginal, if any, clinical benefit. Extracorporeal photopheresis employing ultraviolet A irradiation after the patient has received oral 6-methoxypsoralen has been tried in SSc with the initial report showing skin improvement. The methodology of this study has been challenged and other studies did not show efficacy. Treatment with 5-fluorouracil led to some skin improvement but caused significant gastrointestinal toxicity. Several uncontrolled studies using cyclophosphamide in treating early sclerodermal interstitial lung disease have shown improvement or stabilization of pulmonary function. Improvement of skin induration was also noted in some patients. A controlled study in patients with early and active alveolitis is currently in progress. Because of the poor prognosis in SSc patients who have a rapid onset of diffuse cutaneous disease and early visceral organ involvement (pulmonary, cardiac, or renal), clinical trials are in progress using high-dose immunosuppressive therapy followed by autologous stem cell transplantation. The rationale is that high doses of an immunosuppressive drug such as cyclophosphamide may reverse or modify the disease course. The autologous stem cell transplantation permits the rapid reconstitution of hematopoiesis. Initial results of a multicenter study involving 19 patients with poor prognoses showed improvement of skin and disability scores exceeding those reported with other therapies. Internal organ function was the same or slightly worse following treatment. Four patients had progressive or nonresponsive disease. Two patients died of treatment complications and one of progressive SSc. The role of high-dose immunosuppressive therapy in SSc needs further evaluation in prospective controlled studies before its clinical efficacy can be determined. This treatment is at present experimental.

Several other agents including minocyline, thalidomide and etanercept have been reported to improve skin involvement in small uncontrolled studies. Randomized controlled studies will need to be performed to know whether these agents are effective.

Antiplatelet therapy may play a role in the treatment of SSc, since the biologic products of platelets affect blood vessels. Low doses of aspirin block the formation of thromboxane A_2, a powerful vasoconstrictor and platelet aggregator. In addition, dipyridamole, 200 to 400 mg in divided daily doses, also decreases platelet adhesion to damaged vessel walls. While these drugs have a reasonable therapeutic rationale, a 2-year double-blind study did not show any benefit from their use.

Glucocorticoids are not effective in improving or preventing skin induration and the progression of SSc. They can be beneficial in certain situations. Short courses of low-dose prednisone (10 mg/d or less) may decrease edema associated with the edematous phase of early skin involvement and may also be useful in relieving joint and tendon pain. Higher doses of a glucocorticoid such as prednisone 20–30 mg/d are indicated in only those patients with inflammatory myositis, pericarditis, and possibly in patients with early active alveolitis. The dose should be reduced as soon as possible to the lowest effective dose, which in some patients may require the addition of a steroid-sparing agent such as methotrexate or azathioprine. Glucocorticoids should not be used for the indolent primary form of muscle disease of SSc (see Musculoskeletal System, above). Glucocorticoids have been associated with the development of renal crisis. A retrospective case-control study in patients with early diffuse cutaneous SSc showed a significant association between prior high-dose glucocorticoids (prednisone ≥ 15 mg/d) and the development of scleroderma renal crisis. For this reason, glucocorticoids should be used cautiously in SSc.

The management of Raynaud's phenomenon is directed at control of vasospasm. Patients should be advised to dress warmly and wear mittens and socks, not to smoke, to remove causes of external stress, and to avoid drugs such as amphetamine and ergotamine. Cold drafts should be avoided. Air-conditioned rooms in warm climates can also be a problem for patients with Raynaud's phenomenon. Beta-blocking drugs may make Raynaud's phenomenon worse. Warmth of the central body induces peripheral vasodilatation. Drugs that block sympathetic vasoconstriction, such as reserpine, α-methyldopa, phenoxybenzamine, and prazosin, may be useful in the treatment of Raynaud's phenomenon, but their side effects often curtail extended use. The calcium channel blockers nifedipine, diltiazem, and the longer acting amlodipine can be effective in alleviating Raynaud's phenomenon, but side effects of light-headedness and palpitations may limit their use. The sustained-release form of nifedipine is better tolerated; the dose is 30 mg/d up to 60 or 90 mg/d as required to control symptoms. Nitroglycerin paste, applied to an affected digit, may improve local blood flow. Sildenafil, a phosphodiesterase inhibitor used primarily for erectile dysfunction, is a vasodilator and may be helpful in treating Raynaud's phenomenon. In a 12-week pilot study, losartan (50 mg/d), a specific nonpeptide angiotensen II type 1 receptor antagonist, reduced the severity and frequency of Raynaud's phenomenon episodes. Ketanserin (40 mg TID), an oral serotonin antagonist, has also been shown to be effective. Selective serotonin reuptake inhibitors (e.g., fluoxetine, 20 mg/d) may be beneficial in some patients. These drugs decrease platelet 5-hydroxytryptamine, which is thought to play a role in the pathogenesis of Raynaud's phenomenon. Studies with intravenous iloprost, a prostacyclin analogue, have shown a decrease in frequency and severity of Raynaud's phenomenon and healing of digital ulcers in some patients. Iloprost is still not available in the United States for general use. Intravenous alprostadil, a prostaglandin, can be effective in treating severe Raynaud's phenomenon with digital ulcers. Intravenous epoprostenol and oral Bosentan, an endothelin-1 receptor antagonist, used in the treatment of pulmonary hypertension, also improves Raynaud's phenomenon. Pentoxifylline (400 mg TID) may also improve perfusion by increasing the deformability of the red cell plasma membranes. Techniques of biofeedback have also been used with variable success for teaching patients to control the temperature of their hands. Stellate ganglion blockage may be useful in temporarily alleviating severe ischemic pain in the fingers. Surgical cervical sympathectomy usually provides only temporary improvement, and it, along with other forms of therapy, does not prevent progression of the vascular lesion. Digital sympathectomy can be effective in some patients. The response to any therapy for Raynaud's phenomenon is limited by the degree of existing structural narrowing of digital arteries. In patients with severe Raynaud's phenomenon and refractory digital ulcers, distal ulnar artery occlusion should be considered. A positive Allen test is suggestive, and the diagnosis is confirmed by angiography. When ulnar artery occlusion is present, revascularization and a digital sympathectomy may be beneficial. Gangrene of distal digits may occur and require surgical amputation.

Skin care is very important in SSc. Dryness of the skin may be reduced by avoiding frequent use of detergent soaps and by regularly applying hydrophilic ointments and bath oils. Regular exercise helps to maintain flexibility of extremities and pliability of skin. Massaging the skin several times a day may also be beneficial. Fingertip ulcerations can be protected by applying a guard or cage over the end of the finger. The use of an occlusive dressing, such as the hydrocolloid duoDERM or other membranes, over a noninfected ulcer may promote healing and protect the finger. Skin ulcers should be kept clean by soaking or by surgical or chemical debridement. Sympatholytic drugs or local nitroglycerin paste applied to or adjacent to the ulcer may be beneficial in promoting healing. Infected ulcers can usually be treated with topical antibiotics but may require systemic antibiotics, especially when there is a question of underlying osteomyelitis. The development of calcinosis cannot be prevented, nor can deposits be dissolved. Warfarin has been reported to reduce calcinosis in a few patients.

In patients experiencing dry mouth, frequent sips of water help to relieve symptoms. Pilocarpine hydrochloride tablets may increase salivary secretions in some patients. Patients with dry eyes should use artificial tears regularly.

Patients with reflux esophagitis are treated with small, frequent meals, antacids between meals, and elevation of the head of the bed. Patients should be advised not to lie down for a few hours after a meal and to avoid coffee, tea, alcohol, peppermint, and chocolate, which reduce the pressure of the lower esophageal sphincter. Fatty foods and late-evening snacks should be avoided. Cimetidine, ranitidine, or other newer H_2 blockers may be beneficial. Gastric acid (proton) pump inhibitors are more effective in treating erosive esophagitis than are H_2 blockers. Metoclopramide does not significantly improve esophageal motility; it increases lower esophageal sphincter tone and promotes gastric emptying and can be of help in some patients. The dose is 10 mg given 15–20 min before each meal up to 4 times a day. Nifedipine and, to a lesser extent, diltiazem reduce lower esophageal sphincter tone resulting in esophageal reflux. Patients with dysphagia should be instructed to chew their food thoroughly and wash it down with fluids. Malabsorption syndrome due to duodenal hypomotility and bacterial overgrowth causes bloating and diarrhea, which may improve with intermittent use of appropriate antibiotics. Antibiotics are rotated every 2 weeks. Commonly used antibiotics are metronidazole, vancomycin, erythromycin, ciprofloxacin, neomycin, and tetracycline. Patients with severe debilitating malabsorption may benefit from parenteral hyperalimentation. Patients with chronic intestinal pseudoobstruction might respond to octreotide. Stool softeners and mild laxatives are usually adequate for treating constipation caused by hypomotility of the colon.

Articular symptoms are treated with nonsteroidal anti-inflammatory agents. Low-dose prednisone (≤10 mg/d) may improve symptoms in those not responding to these agents. Physical therapy may help to reduce the loss of joint mobility that occurs in SSc.

In patients with diffuse cutaneous SSc, the early recognition of alveolitis as previously described (see "Pulmonary Features") may allow treatment that might slow or prevent the development of pulmonary fibrosis. Cyclophosphamide has been reported in uncontrolled studies to be beneficial, and a controlled study is presently being done. The role of glucocorticoids in preventing progression of interstitial lung disease is not clear but may be of benefit in early disease. N acetylcysteine has been used as an antioxidant to reduce lung damage in patients with respiratory distress syndromes and may help in SSc lung disease. Pulmonary fibrosis is not reversible, and therefore treatment is directed at symptoms or complications. Pulmonary infection requires prompt treatment with antibiotics. Hypoxia necessitates giving low concentrations of oxygen. Patients should receive polyvalent pneumoccal vaccine (Pneumovax) and yearly influenza immunizations.

For patients with limited cutaneous SSc who develop isolated pulmonary arterial hypertension, treatment is limited. The usual treatment is supplemental oxygen, anticoagulation, and the administration of a vasodilator. A calcium channel blocker such as nifedipine lowers pulmonary arterial resistance and improves cardiac function, but in most patients this is only for a short period of time. Few patients survive more than 5 years. Heart-lung or single-lung transplantation may be a therapeutic option only in those patients without other significant systemic involvement. Intravenous epoprostenol (prostacyclin) is now given to treat SSc-associated pulmonary hypertension. Epoprostenol is infused continuously via a central line with a portable pump. Improvement in symptoms of right heart failure and exercise tolerance occurred. Also hemodynamic tests showed a decrease in the pulmonary vascular resistance and pulmonary artery pressure both in the short term and in a few patients after 1 or 2 years. Bosentan, an orally administered endothelin-1 receptor antagonist, has been shown to improve exercise capacity and cardiopulmonary hemodynamics in patients with pulmonary arterial hypertension, both primary and secondary to SSc. In some treated SSc patients, Raynaud's phenomenon also improved.

Recognition of early signs of renal hypertensive crisis is important in order to preserve renal function and prevent hypertensive encephalopathy. Renal involvement is often accompanied by hypertension and mild to moderate proteinuria. An occasional patient may be normotensive. Antihypertensive agents are often effective in lowering blood pressure and stabilizing or reversing renal failure. These drugs include propranolol, clonidine, and minoxidil. Particularly effective are the angiotensin-converting enzyme inhibitors, which include captopril, enalapril, and lisinopril. Dialysis may be required in patients with progressive renal failure. Some patients, however, have a slow return of renal function after several months and may no longer require dialysis. Patients are usually not candidates for kidney transplantation because of the other systemic manifestations of SSc.

Patients with cardiac failure require careful monitoring of digitalis and diuretic administration. Noninflammatory pericardial effusions may also improve with diuretics. Care should be taken to avoid overdiuresis, which may lead to decreased renal blood flow, decreased cardiac output, and renal failure.

MIXED CONNECTIVE TISSUE DISEASE

MCTD is an overlap syndrome characterized by combinations of clinical features of SLE (Chap. 300), SSc, polymyositis (Chap. 370), and rheumatoid arthritis (Chap. 301) and the presence of very high titers of circulating autoantibodies to nuclear RNP antigen. This antibody in high titer, now referred to as *anti-U₁ RNP*, has been a justification for considering MCTD as a distinct clinical entity. MCTD has been challenged as a distinct disorder by those who consider it as a subset of SLE or scleroderma. Others prefer to classify MCTD as an undifferentiated connective tissue disease. MCTD occurs worldwide and in all races. The peak onset of disease is in the second and third decades, but MCTD is seen in children and the elderly. Women are predominantly affected. The pathogenic mechanisms in MCTD reflect the disorders making up this syndrome.

Clinical Features   The presenting symptoms of MCTD are most often Raynaud's phenomenon, puffy hands, arthralgias, myalgias, and fatigue. Occasionally, patients may present with the acute onset of high fever, polymyositis, arthritis, and neurologic features such as trigeminal neuralgia and aseptic meningitis. The various features of the connective tissue disorders making up MCTD develop over months and years.

The fingers as well as the entire hand may be puffy, followed later by sclerodactyly. Sclerodermal changes are usually limited to the distal extremities and sometimes the face but spare the trunk. Telangiectasia and calcinosis may develop. Some patients have mucocutaneous features of SLE including a classic malar rash, photosensitivity, discoid lesions, alopecia, and painful oral ulcerations. An erythematous rash over the knuckles, elbows, and knees and heliotropic eyelids, typical of dermatomyositis, are uncommon.

Joint pain, stiffness, and swelling involving the peripheral joints occur frequently. Deformities of the hands similar to those of rheumatoid arthritis may develop but usually without bony erosions. A destructive polyarthritis is occasionally observed. Myalgias are a frequent symptom. Some patients develop typical symptoms of polymyositis with proximal muscle weakness, abnormal electromyographic findings, elevated levels of muscle enzymes, and inflammatory changes on muscle biopsy.

Approximately 85% of patients have pulmonary involvement, which is often asymptomatic. Diffusing capacity for carbon monoxide may be the only abnormality. Pleurisy commonly occurs but is seldom associated with large pleural effusions. Some patients develop interstitial lung disease. Pulmonary arterial hypertension is the most common cause of death in MCTD.

Approximately 25% of patients develop renal disease. Membranous glomerulonephritis is most common and usually mild but can cause nephrotic syndrome. Diffuse proliferative glomerulonephritis is unusual in MCTD, perhaps because of the protective role believed to be played by the high titers of anti-U₁ RNP. Renal crisis secondary to malignant renovasculature hypertension, as occurs in scleroderma, is seen in a few patients.

Gastrointestinal involvement is seen in ∼70% of patients. The most common manifestations are esophageal dysmotility, lower esophageal sphincter laxity, and gastroesophageal reflux. Bowel manifestations mimic those of scleroderma bowel disease.

Pericarditis occurs in 30% of patients. Other cardiac features include myocarditis, arrhythmia, conduction disturbances, and mitral valve prolapse. Other clinical features of MCTD include trigeminal neuropathy, peripheral neuropathy, aseptic meningitis, lymphadenopathy, and Sjögren's syndrome. The majority of patients have developed, or will develop within 5 years of presentation, diagnostic clinical criteria for one of the overlapping connective tissue diseases, most often SLE or SSc.

Laboratory Findings   Anemia of chronic inflammation is seen in the majority of patients. A positive direct Coombs' test is found in many patients, but hemolytic anemia is unusual. Leukopenia, thrombocytopenia, or both are present in some patients. Hypergammaglobulinemia is common, and rheumatoid factor is present in 50% of patients.

All patients, by definition of MCTD, have antibodies to U₁ RNP. The specificity of this antibody is to the 70-kDa protein complexed to small nuclear RNA. The anti-U₁ RNP antibodies are associated with HLA-DR4 but not with -DR2 and -DR3 as found in SLE. Molecular mimicry has been demonstrated between U₁ RNP and retroviral antigens by some laboratories.

℞ TREATMENT

The treatment of MCTD is essentially the same as would be indicated for the respective connective tissue diseases defining this syndrome. More than half the patients have a favorable course. The 10-year survival rate overall is ∼80% but varies depending on the connective tissue disease that may eventually develop.

EOSINOPHILIC FASCIITIS

Eosinophilic fasciitis is a scleroderma-like syndrome of unknown cause characterized by inflammation followed later by sclerosis of the dermis, subcutis, and deep fascia. The disease affects adults and often occurs after strenuous physical activity. Patients do not have Raynaud's phenomenon or internal organ involvement. Several immunologic abnormalities have been associated with eosinophilic fasciitis and include aplastic anemia, myelodysplastic syndrome, and thrombocytopenia. Patients usually have the abrupt onset of symmetric tenderness and swelling of the extremities, rapidly followed by induration of the skin and subcutaneous tissue. The skin takes on a cobblestone or puckered appearance. Carpal tunnel syndrome appears early in the course, and flexion contractures develop later. A low-grade myositis is often present, but creatinine kinase levels are usually normal. A marked eosinophilia is found in the early stage of disease and subsequently decreases. Increased levels of polyclonal IgG and immune complexes are often present in the serum. A full-thickness biopsy consisting of skin, fascia, and superficial muscle shows perivascular infiltration of histiocytes, eosinophils, lymphocytes, and plasma cells. Biopsies later in the course show sclerosis. Spontaneous improvement and occasionally complete remission may occur after 2 to 5 years of disease. Some patients have persistent disease, while others are left with flexion contractures. Administration of glucocorticoids may provide symptomatic improvement and will decrease the eosinophilia. Improvement has been reported with the use of the H$_2$ blocker cimetidine.

EOSINOPHILIA-MYALGIA SYNDROME

In 1989, reports of patients with scleroderma-like skin changes, myalgias, and eosinophilia dramatically increased. Most, but not all, of these cases were associated with ingestion of L-tryptophan manufactured by a single Japanese company. Batches of L-tryptophan implicated in EMS were found to contain trace amounts of a contaminant identified as a dimer of L-tryptophan that appeared in 1988 after changes were made in the method of manufacturing this drug. It is not clear whether this chemical contaminant is the etiologic agent or whether another unidentified substance is responsible. *L-Tryptophan products were taken off the market in 1990.* The onset of EMS can be either abrupt or insidious. In the early phases of the disease, clinical manifestations include low-grade fever, fatigue, dyspnea, cough, arthralgias/arthritis, evanescent erythematous rashes, muscle cramping, and severe myalgias. Pulmonary infiltrates may be present. Over the next 2 to 3 months, scleroderma-like skin changes appear. Some patients develop a peripheral neuropathy, which may persist. An ascending polyneuropathy may lead to paralysis and respiratory failure requiring ventilatory assistance. Cognitive dysfunction with impairment of memory and concentration has been recognized in this syndrome. Myocarditis and cardiac arrhythmias occur in some patients, and a few patients develop pulmonary hypertension. Approximately a third of patients have features of eosinophilic fasciitis. EMS most closely resembles toxic oil syndrome; however, Raynaud's phenomenon does not occur, and there is a lower prevalence of pulmonary hypertension and thromboembolic disease. The peripheral eosinophil count is >1000/μL in most patients. The histologic findings on biopsy of skin, fascia, and superficial muscle are similar to those found in eosinophilic fasciitis. The clinical features of EMS may persist after L-tryptophan has been discontinued. EMS may run a chronic course, and response to therapy has been variable. Treatment has included glucocorticoids, antimalarial drugs, immunosuppressive drugs, and plasmapheresis. Prednisone was beneficial during the acute inflammatory phase of the disease in the majority of patients and resulted in resolution of pulmonary infiltrates, peripheral edema, and eosinophilia. In the later phase of the illness, no treatment was found to be of particular value. The pathogenesis of this disease is not known. A followup of patients 2 years after their onset of illness showed that most symptoms and physical findings had resolved or improved except for cognitive dysfunction, which became worse in approximately one-third of the patients, and peripheral neuropathy, which remained unchanged (Chap. 370).

FURTHER READING

CLEMENTS PJ et al: High-dose versus low-dose D-penicillamine in early diffuse systemic sclerosis: Analysis of a two-year, double-blind, randomized, controlled clinical trial. Arthritis Rheum 42:1194, 1999

DEMARCO PJ et al: Predictors and outcomes of scleroderma renal crisis: The high-dose versus low-dose D-penicillamine in early diffuse system sclerosis trial. Arthritis Rheum 46:2836, 2002

FEGHALI-BOSTWICK C et al: Analysis of systemic sclerosis in twins reveals low concordance for disease and high concordance for the presence of antinuclear antibodies. Arthritis Rheum 48:1956, 2003

HAMAMDZIC D et al: Role of infectious agents in the pathogenesis of systemic sclerosis. Curr Opin Rheumatol 14:694, 2002

HERTZMAN PA et al: The eosinophilia-myalgia syndrome: Status of 205 patients and results of treatment 2 years after onset. Ann Intern Med 122:851, 1995

MCSWEENEY PA et al: High-dose immunosuppressive therapy for severe systemic sclerosis: Initial outcomes. Blood 100:1602, 2002

NELSON JL et al: Microchimerism and human autoimmune disease. Lupus 11:651, 2002

ROSE S et al: Gastrointestinal manifestations of scleroderma. Gastroenterol Clin North Am 27:563, 1998

RUBIN LJ et al: Bosentan therapy for pulmonary arterial hypertension. N Engl J Med 346:896, 2002

STEEN VD, MEDSGER TA: Case-control study of corticosteroids and other drugs that either precipitate or protect from the development of scleroderma renal crisis. Arthritis Rheum 41:1613, 1998

304 SJÖGREN'S SYNDROME
Haralampos M. Moutsopoulos

DEFINITION

Sjögren's syndrome is a chronic, slowly progressive autoimmune disease characterized by lymphocytic infiltration of the exocrine glands resulting in xerostomia and dry eyes. Approximately one-third of patients present with systemic manifestations. A small but significant number of patients may develop malignant lymphoma. The disease can be seen alone (primary Sjögren's syndrome) or in association with other autoimmune rheumatic diseases (secondary Sjögren's syndrome) (Table 304-1).

INCIDENCE AND PREVALENCE

The disease affects predominantly middle-age women (female-to-male ratio 9:1), although it occurs in all ages, including childhood. The prevalence of primary Sjögren's syndrome is approximately 0.5 to 1.0%. In addition, 30% of patients with autoimmune rheumatic diseases suffer from secondary Sjögren's syndrome.

PATHOGENESIS

Sjögren's syndrome is characterized by lymphocytic infiltration of the exocrine glands and B lymphocyte hyperreactivity, as illustrated by circulating autoantibodies. In one-fourth of the patients, it is accompanied by an oligomonoclonal B cell process, which is characterized by cryoprecipitable monoclonal immunoglobulins with rheumatoid factor activity.

Sera of patients with Sjögren's syndrome often contain a number of autoantibodies directed against non-organ-specific antigens such as immunoglobulins (rheumatoid factors) and extractable nuclear and cytoplasmic antigens (Ro/SS-A, La/SS-B). Ro/SS-A autoantigen consists of two polypeptides (52 and 60 kDa) in conjunction with cytoplasmic RNAs, whereas the 48-kDa La/SS-B protein is bound to RNA III polymerase transcripts. Autoantibodies to Ro/SS-A and La/SS-B antigens are usually detected at the time of diagnosis and are associated with earlier disease onset, longer disease duration, salivary gland enlargement, severity of lymphocytic infiltration of minor salivary glands, and certain extraglandular manifestations. Antibodies to α-fodrin (120 kDa), a salivary gland–specific protein, have been found

TABLE 304-1 *Association of Sjögren's Syndrome with Other Autoimmune Diseases*

Rheumatoid arthritis	Primary biliary cirrhosis
Systemic lupus erythematosus	Vasculitis
Scleroderma	Chronic active hepatitis
Mixed connective tissue disease	

TABLE 304-2 *Incidence of Extraglandular Manifestations in Primary Sjögren's Syndrome*

Clinical Manifestation	Percent
Arthralgias/arthritis	60
Raynaud's phenomenon	37
Lymphadenopathy	14
Lung involvement	14
Vasculitis	11
Kidney involvement	9
Liver involvement	6
Lymphoma	6
Splenomegaly	3
Peripheral neuropathy	2
Myositis	1

in sera of patients with Sjögren's syndrome. The major infiltrating cells in the affected exocrine glands are activated B and T lymphocytes. Macrophages and natural killer cells are rarely detected. In chronic lesions, a small but persistent number of dendritic cells are apparent in lymphoid follicle–like formations. In contrast to the infiltrating lymphocytes, the glandular epithelial cells undergo apoptotic death. Ductal and acinar epithelial cells appear to play a significant role in the initiation and perpetuation of the autoimmune injury since they inappropriately produce proinflammatory cytokines and lympho-attractant chemokines and express on their surface nuclear autoantigens. Further, they express class II major histocompatibility complex (MHC) and co-stimulatory molecules and are able to provide the second signal for lymphocyte activation. Redistribution of the water-channel protein aquaporin-5 from the apical membranes to the cytoplasm of acinar epithelial cells has also been observed.

Immunogenetic studies have demonstrated that HLA-B8, -DR3, and -DRw52 are prevalent in patients with primary Sjögren's syndrome as compared with the normal control population. Molecular analysis of HLA class II genes has revealed that patients with Sjögren's syndrome, regardless of their ethnic origin, are highly associated with the HLA DQA1*0501 allele.

CLINICAL MANIFESTATIONS

The majority of Sjögren's syndrome patients have symptoms related to diminished lacrimal and salivary gland function. In most patients, the primary syndrome runs a slow and benign course. The initial manifestations can be mucosal dryness or nonspecific, and 8 to 10 years

TABLE 304-3 *Differential Diagnosis of Sicca Symptoms*

Xerostomia	Dry Eye	Bilateral Parotid Gland Enlargement
Viral infections	Inflammation	Viral infections
Drugs	Stevens-Johnson	Mumps
Psychotherapeutic	syndrome	Influenza
Parasympatholytic	Pemphigoid	Epstein-Barr
Antihypertensives	Chronic conjunctivitis	Coxsackievirus A
Psychogenic	Chronic blepharitis	Cytomegalovirus
Irradiation	Sjögren's syndrome	HIV
Diabetes mellitus	Toxicity	Sarcoidosis
Trauma	Burns	Amyloidosis
Sjögren's	Drugs	Sjögren's syndrome
syndrome	Neurologic conditions	Metabolic
	Impaired lacrimal	Diabetes mellitus
	gland function	Hyperlipoprotein-
	Impaired eyelid	emias
	function	Chronic
	Miscellaneous	pancreatitis
	Trauma	Hepatic cirrhosis
	Hypovitaminosis A	Endocrine
	Blink abnormality	Acromegaly
	Lid scarring	Gonadal
	Anesthetic cornea	hypofunction
	Epithelial irregularity	

TABLE 304-4 *Differential Diagnosis of Sjögren's Syndrome*

HIV Infection and Sicca Syndrome	Sjögren's Syndrome	Sarcoidosis
Predominant in young males	Predominant in middle-aged women	Invariable
Lack of autoantibodies to Ro/SS-A and/or La/SS-B	Presence of autoantibodies	Lack of autoantibodies to Ro/SS-A and/or La/SS-B
Lymphoid infiltrates of salivary glands by CD8+ lymphocytes	Lymphoid infiltrates of salivary glands by CD4+ lymphocytes	Granulomas in salivary glands
Association with HLA-DR5	Association with HLA-DR3 and -DRw52	Unknown
Positive serologic tests for HIV	Negative serologic tests for HIV	Negative serologic tests for HIV

elapse from the initial symptoms to full-blown development of the disease.

The principal oral symptom of Sjögren's syndrome is dryness (xerostomia). Patients complain of difficulty in swallowing dry food, inability to speak continuously, a burning sensation, increase in dental caries, and problems in wearing complete dentures. Physical examination shows a dry, erythematous, sticky oral mucosa. There is atrophy of the filiform papillae on the dorsum of the tongue, and saliva from the major glands is either not expressible or cloudy. Enlargement of the parotid or other major salivary glands occurs in two-thirds of patients with primary Sjögren's syndrome but is uncommon in those with the secondary syndrome. Diagnostic tests include sialometry, sialog-

TABLE 304-5 *Revised International Classification Criteria for Sjögren's Syndrome[a,b,c]*

I. Ocular symptoms: a positive response to at least one of three validated questions.
  1. Have you had daily, persistent, troublesome dry eyes for more than 3 months?
  2. Do you have a recurrent sensation of sand or gravel in the eyes?
  3. Do you use tear substitutes more than three times a day?
II. Oral symptoms: a positive response to at least one of three validated questions.
  1. Have you had a daily feeling of dry mouth for more than 3 months?
  2. Have you had recurrent or persistently swollen salivary glands as an adult?
  3. Do you frequently drink liquids to aid in swallowing dry foods?
III. Ocular signs: objective evidence of ocular involvement defined as a positive result to at least one of the following two tests:
  1. Shirmer's I test, performed without anesthesia (≤5 mm in 5 min)
  2. Rose Bengal score or other ocular dye score (≥4 according to van Bijsterveld's scoring system)
IV. Histopathology: In minor salivary glands focal lymphocytic sialoadenitis, with a focus score ≥ 1.
V. Salivary gland involvement: objective evidence of salivary gland involvement defined by a positive result to at least one of the following diagnostic tests:
  1. Unstimulated whole salivary flow (≤1.5 mL in 15 min)
  2. Parotid sialography
  3. Salivary scintigraphy
VI. Antibodies in the serum to Ro/SS-A or La/SS-B antigens, or both

[a] Exclusion criteria: Past head and neck radiation treatment, hepatitis C infection, AIDS, preexisting lymphoma, sarcoidosis, graft versus host disease, use of anticholinergic drugs.
[b] Primary Sjögren's syndrome: any four of the six items, as long as item IV (histopathology) or VI (serology) is positive, or any three of the four objective criteria items (items III, IV, V, VI).
[c] In patients with a potentially associated disease (e.g., another well-defined connective tissue disease), the presence of item I or item II plus any two from among items III, IV, and V may be considered as indicative of secondary Sjögren's syndrome.
Source: From Vitali C et al.

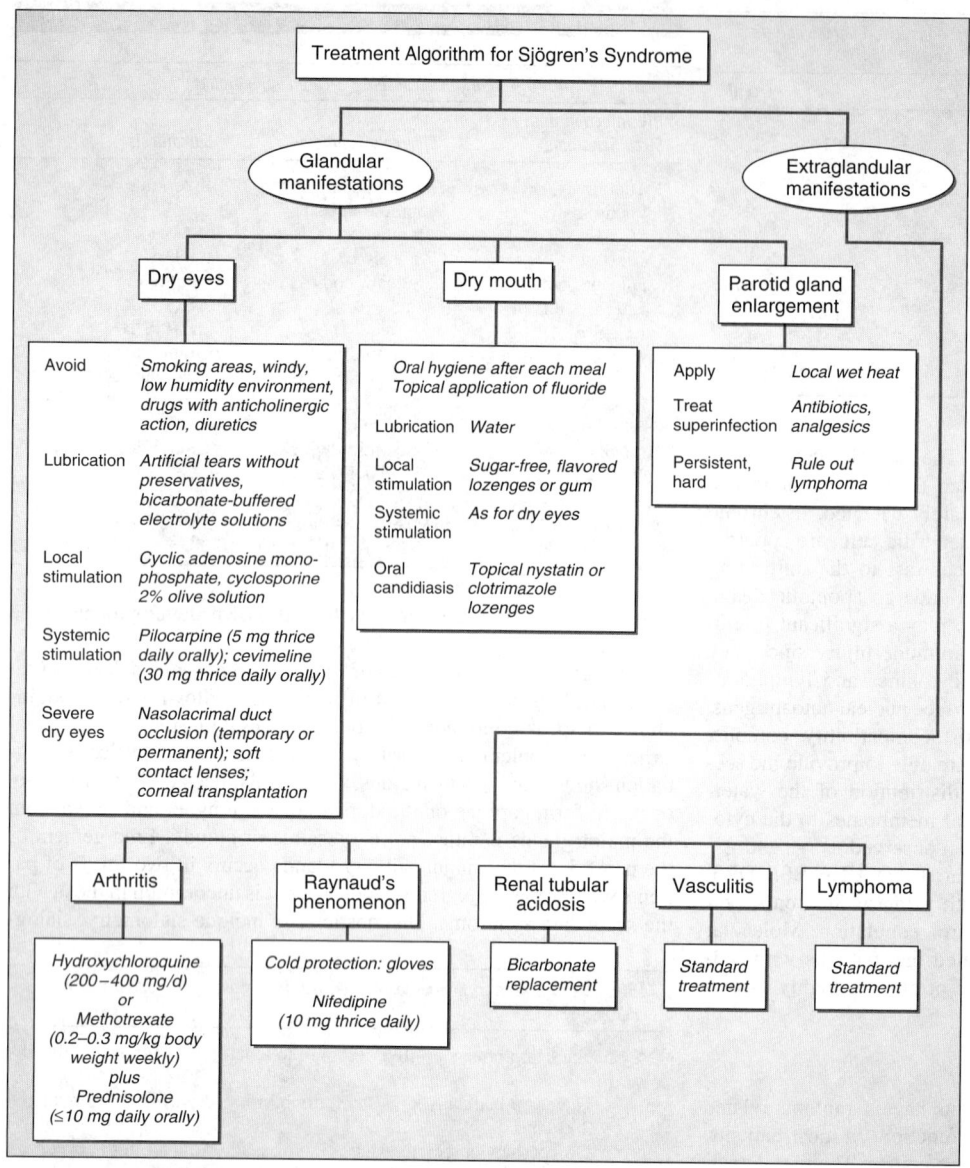

FIGURE 304-1 Treatment algorithm for Sjögren's syndrome.

raphy, and scintigraphy. The labial minor salivary gland biopsy permits histopathologic confirmation of the focal lymphocytic infiltrates.

Ocular involvement is the other major manifestation of Sjögren's syndrome. Patients usually complain of a sandy or gritty feeling under the eyelids. Other symptoms include burning, accumulation of thick strands at the inner canthi, decreased tearing, redness, itching, eye fatigue, and increased photosensitivity. These symptoms are attributed to the destruction of corneal and bulbar conjunctival epithelium, defined as *keratoconjunctivitis sicca*. Diagnostic evaluation of keratoconjunctivitis sicca includes measurement of tear flow by Schirmer's I test and tear composition as assessed by the tear breakup time or tear lysozyme content. Slit-lamp examination of the cornea and conjunctiva after rose Bengal staining reveals punctate corneal ulcerations and attached filaments of corneal epithelium.

Involvement of other exocrine glands occurs less frequently and includes a decrease in mucous gland secretions of the upper and lower respiratory tree, resulting in dry nose, throat, and trachea (xerotrachea), and diminished secretion of the exocrine glands of the gastrointestinal tract, leading to esophageal mucosal atrophy, atrophic gastritis, and subclinical pancreatitis. Dyspareunia due to dryness of the external genitalia and dry skin may also occur.

Extraglandular (systemic) manifestations are seen in one-third of patients with Sjögren's syndrome (Table 304-2), while they are very rare in patients with Sjögren's syndrome associated with rheumatoid arthritis. These patients complain more often of easy fatigability, low-grade fever, Raynaud's phenomenon, myalgias, and arthralgias. Most patients with primary Sjögren's syndrome experience at least one episode of nonerosive arthritis during the course of their disease. Manifestations of pulmonary involvement are frequent but rarely important clinically. Dry cough is the major manifestation that is attributed to small airway disease. Renal involvement includes interstitial nephritis, clinically manifested by hyposthenuria and renal tubular dysfunction with or without acidosis. Untreated acidosis may lead to nephrocalcinosis. Glomerulonephritis is a rare finding that occurs in patients with mixed cryoglobulinemia, or systemic lupus erythematosus overlapping with Sjögren's syndrome. Vasculitis affects small and medium-sized vessels. The most common clinical features are purpura, recurrent urticaria, skin ulcerations, glomerulonephritis, and mononeuritis multiplex. Sensorineural hearing loss was found in one-half of patients with Sjögren's syndrome and correlated with the presence of anticardiolipin antibodies.

It has been suggested that primary Sjögren's syndrome with vasculitis may also present with multifocal, recurrent, and progressive nervous system disease, such as hemiparesis, transverse myelopathy, hemisensory deficits, seizures, and movement disorders. Aseptic meningitis and multiple sclerosis have also been reported in these patients.

Lymphoma is a well-known manifestation of Sjögren's syndrome that usually presents later in the illness. Persistent parotid gland enlargement, purpura, leukopenia, cryoglobulinemia, and low C4 complement levels are manifestations suggesting the development of lymphoma. Most lymphomas are extranodal, marginal zone B cell, and low grade. Usually the low-grade lymphomas are detected incidentally upon evaluating the labial biopsy.

The affected lymph nodes are usually peripheral. Survival is decreased in patients with B symptoms, lymph node mass >7 cm in diameter, and high or intermediate histologic grade.

Routine laboratory tests reveal mild normochromic, normocytic anemia. An elevated erythrocyte sedimentation rate is found in approximately 70% of patients.

DIAGNOSIS AND DIFFERENTIAL DIAGNOSIS

The diagnosis of primary Sjögren's syndrome is obtained if the patient presents with eye and/or mouth dryness, the eye tests disclose keratoconjunctivitis sicca, the mouth evaluation reveals the classic manifestations of the syndrome, and the patient's serum reacts with Ro/SS-A and/or La/SS-B autoantigens. Labial biopsy is needed when the diagnosis is uncertain or to rule out conditions that may cause dry mouth or eyes or parotid gland enlargement (Tables 304-3, 304-4). Validated diagnostic criteria have been established by a European study and have now been further improved by a European-American study group (Table 304-5).

℞ TREATMENT

Treatment of Sjögren's syndrome is aimed at symptomatic relief and limiting the damaging local effects of chronic xerostomia and keratoconjunctivitis sicca by substituting or simulating the missing secretions (Fig. 304-1).

To replace deficient tears, there are several readily available ophthalmic preparations (Tearisol; Liquifilm; 0.5% methylcellulose; Hypo Tears). If corneal ulcerations are present, eye patching and boric acid ointments are recommended. Certain drugs that may increase lacrimal and salivary hypofunction such as diuretics, antihypertensive drugs, and antidepressants should be avoided.

For xerostomia the best replacement is water. Propionic acid gels may be used to treat vaginal dryness. To stimulate secretions, pilocarpine (5 mg thrice daily) or cevimeline (30 mg thrice daily) administered orally appears to improve sicca manifestations and both are well tolerated. Hydroxychloroquine (200 mg) is helpful for arthralgias.

Patients with renal tubular acidosis should receive sodium bicarbonate orally (0.5 to 2.0 mmol/kg in four divided doses). Glucocorticoids (1 mg/kg per day) and/or immunosuppressive agents (e.g., cyclophosphamide) are indicated only for the treatment of systemic vasculitis.

FURTHER READING

IOANNIDIS JP et al: Long-term risk of mortality and lymphoproliferative disease and predictive classification of primary Sjögren's syndrome. Arthritis Rheum 46:741, 2002

MANOUSSAKIS MN, MOUTSOPOULOS HM: Sjögren's syndrome: Current concepts. Adv Intern Med 47:191, 2001

MOUTSOPOULOS NM, MOUTSOPOULOS HM: Therapy of Sjögren's syndrome. Springer Semin Immunopathol 23:131, 2001

SKOPOULI FN et al: Clinical evolution, and morbidity and mortality of primary Sjögren's syndrome. Semin Arthritis Rheum 29:296, 2000

VITALI C et al: Classification criteria for Sjögren's syndrome: A revised version of the European criteria proposed by the American-European Consensus Group. Ann Rheum Dis 61:554, 2002

---

305 | THE SPONDYLOARTHRITIDES
Joel D. Taurog

The spondyloarthritides are a group of disorders that share certain clinical features and an association with the HLA-B27 allele. These disorders include ankylosing spondylitis, reactive arthritis, psoriatic arthritis and spondylitis, enteropathic arthritis and spondylitis, juvenile-onset spondyloarthritis, and undifferentiated spondyloarthritis. The similarities in clinical manifestations and genetic predisposition suggest that these disorders share pathogenic mechanisms.

ANKYLOSING SPONDYLITIS

Ankylosing spondylitis (AS) is an inflammatory disorder of unknown cause that primarily affects the axial skeleton; peripheral joints and extraarticular structures may also be involved. The disease usually begins in the second or third decade; the male to female prevalence is approximately 3:1. Older names include *Marie-Strümpell disease* or *Bechterew's disease*.

EPIDEMIOLOGY   AS shows a striking correlation with the histocompatibility antigen HLA-B27 and occurs worldwide roughly in proportion to the prevalence of this antigen (Chap. 296). In North American Caucasians, the general prevalence of B27 is 7%, whereas >90% of patients with AS have inherited this antigen. The association with B27 is independent of disease severity.

In population surveys, 1 to 6% of adults inheriting B27 have been found to have AS. In contrast, in families of patients with AS, the prevalence is 10 to 30% among adult first-degree relatives inheriting B27. The concordance rate in identical twins is approximately 65%. It is currently believed that susceptibility to AS is determined almost entirely by genetic factors, with B27 comprising about one-third of the genetic component.

PATHOLOGY   The enthesis, the site of ligamentous attachment to bone, is thought to be the primary site of pathology in AS, particularly in the lesions around the pelvis and spine. Enthesitis is associated with prominent edema of the adjacent bone marrow and is often characterized by erosive lesions that eventually undergo ossification.

Sacroiliitis is usually one of the earliest manifestations of AS, with features of both enthesitis and synovitis. The early lesions consist of subchondral granulation tissue, infiltrates of lymphocytes and macrophages in ligamentous and periosteal zones, and subchondral bone marrow edema. Synovitis follows and may progress to pannus formation with islands of new bone formation. The eroded joint margins are gradually replaced by fibrocartilage regeneration and then by ossification. Ultimately, the joint may be totally obliterated.

In the spine, early in the process there is inflammatory granulation tissue at the junction of the annulus fibrosus of the disk cartilage and the margin of vertebral bone. The outer annular fibers are eroded and eventually replaced by bone, forming the beginning of a bony syndesmophyte, which then grows by continued enchondral ossification, ultimately bridging the adjacent vertebral bodies. Ascending progression of this process leads to the "bamboo spine" observed radiographically. Other lesions in the spine include diffuse osteoporosis, erosion of vertebral bodies at the disk margin, "squaring" of vertebrae, and inflammation and destruction of the disk-bone border. Inflammatory arthritis of the apophyseal joints is common, with erosion of cartilage by pannus, often followed by bony ankylosis.

Bone mineral density is significantly diminished in the spine and proximal femur early in the course of the disease, before the advent of significant immobilization.

Peripheral arthritis in AS can show synovial hyperplasia, lymphoid infiltration, and pannus formation, but the process lacks the exuberant synovial villi, fibrin deposits, ulcers, and accumulations of plasma cells seen in rheumatoid arthritis (RA) (Chap. 301). Central cartilaginous erosions caused by proliferation of subchondral granulation tissue are common in AS but rare in RA.

PATHOGENESIS   The pathogenesis of AS is incompletely understood but is almost certainly immune mediated. The dramatic response of all aspects of the disease to therapeutic blockade of tumor necrosis factor α (TNF-α) indicates that this cytokine plays a central role in the immunopathogenesis of AS. The inflamed sacroiliac joint is infiltrated with CD4+ and CD8+ T cells and macrophages and shows high levels of TNF-α. No specific event or exogenous agent that triggers the onset of disease has been identified, although overlapping features with reactive arthritis and inflammatory bowel disease (IBD) suggest that enteric bacteria may play a role. Elevated serum titers of antibodies to certain enteric bacteria are common in AS patients, but no role for these antibodies in the pathogenesis of AS has been identified. Evidence that B27 plays a direct role is provided by the finding that rats transgenic for B27 spontaneously develop spondylitis, along with colitis, peripheral arthritis, and other lesions characteristic of the spondyloarthritides.

Some evidence has accumulated for autoimmunity to the cartilage proteoglycan aggrecan. Sharing of proteoglycan antigenic epitopes may be a possible explanation for the distribution of pathologic sites in AS.

CLINICAL MANIFESTATIONS   The symptoms of the disease are usually first noticed in late adolescence or early adulthood; the median age in western countries is 23. In 5% of patients, symptoms begin after age 40.

The initial symptom is usually dull pain, insidious in onset, felt deep in the lower lumbar or gluteal region, accompanied by low-back morning stiffness of up to a few hours' duration that improves with activity and returns following periods of inactivity. Within a few months of onset, the pain has usually become persistent and bilateral. Nocturnal exacerbation of pain that forces the patient to rise and move around may be frequent.

In some patients, bony tenderness (presumably reflecting enthesitis) may accompany back pain or stiffness, while in others it may be the predominant complaint. Common sites include the costosternal junctions, spinous processes, iliac crests, greater trochanters, ischial tuberosities, tibial tubercles, and heels. Occasionally, bony chest pain is the presenting complaint. Arthritis in the hips and shoulders ("root" joints) occurs in 25 to 35% of patients, in many cases early in the disease course. Arthritis of peripheral joints other than the hips and shoulders, usually asymmetric, occurs in up to 30% of patients and can occur at any stage of the disease. Neck pain and stiffness from involvement of the cervical spine are usually relatively late manifestations. Occasional patients, particularly in the older age group, present with predominantly constitutional symptoms such as fatigue, anorexia, fever, weight loss, or night sweats.

AS often has a juvenile onset in developing countries. In these individuals, peripheral arthritis and enthesitis usually predominate, with axial symptoms supervening in late adolescence.

Initially, physical findings mirror the inflammatory process. The most specific findings involve loss of spinal mobility, with limitation of anterior and lateral flexion and extension of the lumbar spine and of chest expansion. Limitation of motion is usually out of proportion to the degree of bony ankylosis, reflecting muscle spasm secondary to pain and inflammation. Pain in the sacroiliac joints may be elicited either with direct pressure or with maneuvers that stress the joints. In addition, there is commonly tenderness upon palpation at the sites of symptomatic bony tenderness and paraspinous muscle spasm.

The Schober test is a useful measure of lumbar spine flexion. The patient stands erect, with heels together, and marks are made directly over the spine 5 cm below and 10 cm above the lumbosacral junction (identified by a horizontal line between the posterosuperior iliac spines.) The patient then bends forward maximally, and the distance between the two marks is measured. The distance between the two marks increases by ≥5 cm in the case of normal mobility and by <4 cm in the case of decreased mobility. Chest expansion is measured as the difference between maximal inspiration and maximal forced expiration in the fourth intercostal space in males or just below the breasts in females. Normal chest expansion is ≥5 cm.

Limitation or pain with motion of the hips or shoulders is usually present if either of these joints is involved. It should be emphasized that early in the course of mild cases, symptoms may be subtle and nonspecific, and the physical examination may be completely normal.

The course of the disease is extremely variable, ranging from the individual with mild stiffness and radiographically equivocal sacroiliitis to the patient with a totally fused spine and severe bilateral hip arthritis, possibly accompanied by severe peripheral arthritis and extraarticular manifestations. Pain tends to be persistent early in the disease and then becomes intermittent, with alternating exacerbations and quiescent periods. In a typical severe untreated case with progression of the spondylitis to syndesmophyte formation, the patient's posture undergoes characteristic changes, with obliterated lumbar lordosis, buttock atrophy, and accentuated thoracic kyphosis. There may be a forward stoop of the neck or flexion contractures at the hips, compensated by flexion at the knees. The progression of the disease may be followed by measuring the patient's height, chest expansion, Schober test, and occiput-to-wall distance. Occasional individuals are encountered with advanced physical findings who report having never had significant symptoms.

In some but not all studies, onset of the disease in adolescence correlates with a worse prognosis. Early severe hip involvement is an indication of progressive disease. The disease in women tends to progress less frequently to total spinal ankylosis, although there is some evidence for an increased prevalence of isolated cervical ankylosis and peripheral arthritis in women. In industrialized countries, peripheral arthritis (distal to hips and shoulders) occurs overall in about 25% of patients, usually as a late manifestation, whereas in developing countries, the prevalence is much higher, with onset typically early in the disease course. Pregnancy has no consistent effect on AS, with symptoms improving, remaining the same, or deteriorating in about one-third of pregnant patients, respectively.

The most serious complication of the spinal disease is spinal fracture, which can occur with even minor trauma to the rigid, osteoporotic spine. The cervical spine is most commonly involved. These fractures are often displaced and cause spinal cord injury.

The most common extraarticular manifestation is acute anterior uveitis, which occurs in 30% of patients and can antedate the spondylitis. Attacks are typically unilateral, causing pain, photophobia, and increased lacrimation. These tend to recur, often in the opposite eye. Cataracts and secondary glaucoma are not uncommon sequelae. Up to 60% of patients have inflammation in the colon or ileum. This is usually asymptomatic, but in 5 to 10% of patients with AS, frank IBD will develop. Aortic insufficiency, sometimes producing symptoms of congestive heart failure, occurs in a few percent of patients, occasionally early in the course of the spinal disease but usually after prolonged disease. Third-degree heart block may occur alone or together with aortic insufficiency. Subclinical pulmonary lesions and cardiac dysfunction may be relatively common. Cauda equina syndrome and slowly progressive upper pulmonary lobe fibrosis are rare complications of long-standing AS. Retroperitoneal fibrosis is a rare associated condition. Prostatitis has been reported to have an increased prevalence in men with AS. Amyloidosis is rare (Chap. 310).

Several validated measures of disease activity and functional outcome have recently been developed for AS. Despite the persistence of the disease, most patients remain gainfully employed. The effect of AS on survival is controversial. Some, but not all, studies have suggested that AS shortens life span, compared with the general population. Mortality attributable to AS is largely the result of spinal trauma, aortic insufficiency, respiratory failure, amyloid nephropathy, or complications of therapy such as upper gastrointestinal hemorrhage.

LABORATORY FINDINGS No laboratory test is diagnostic of AS. In most ethnic groups, B27 is present in approximately 90% of patients with AS. Erythrocyte sedimentation rate (ESR) and C-reactive protein (CRP) are often, but not always, elevated. Mild anemia may be present. Patients with severe disease may show an elevated alkaline phosphatase level. Elevated serum IgA levels are common. Rheumatoid factor and antinuclear antibodies are largely absent unless caused by a coexistent disease. Synovial fluid from peripheral joints in AS is nonspecifically inflammatory. In cases with restriction of chest wall motion, decreased vital capacity and increased functional residual capacity are common, but airflow measurements are normal and ventilatory function is usually well maintained.

RADIOGRAPHIC FINDINGS Radiographically demonstrable sacroiliitis is usually present in AS. The earliest changes by standard radiography are blurring of the cortical margins of the subchondral bone, followed by erosions and sclerosis. Progression of the erosions leads to "pseudowidening" of the joint space; as fibrous and then bony ankylosis supervene, the joints may become obliterated. The changes and progression of the lesions are usually symmetric.

In the lumbar spine, progression of the disease leads to straightening, caused by loss of lordosis, and reactive sclerosis, caused by osteitis of the anterior corners of the vertebral bodies with subsequent erosion, leading to "squaring" of the vertebral bodies. Progressive ossification leads to eventual formation of marginal syndesmophytes, visible on plain films as bony bridges connecting successive vertebral bodies anteriorly and laterally.

In mild cases, years may elapse before unequivocal sacroiliac abnormalities are evident on plain radiographs. Computed tomography

(CT) and magnetic resonance imaging (MRI) can detect abnormalities reliably at an earlier stage than plain radiography. MRI is highly sensitive and specific for identifying early intraarticular inflammation, cartilage changes, and underlying bone marrow edema in sacroiliitis (Fig. 305-1). In suspected cases in which conventional radiography does not reveal definite sacroiliac abnormalities or is undesirable (e.g., in young women or children), dynamic MRI is the procedure of choice for establishing a diagnosis of sacroiliitis.

Reduced bone mineral density can be detected by dual-energy x-ray absorptiometry of the femoral neck and the lumbar spine. Falsely elevated readings related to spinal ossification can be avoided by using a lateral projection of the L3 vertebral body.

DIAGNOSIS It is important to establish the diagnosis of early AS before the development of irreversible deformity. Modified New York criteria (1984) are widely used for diagnosis. These consist of the following: (1) a history of inflammatory back pain (see below); (2) limitation of motion of the lumbar spine in both the sagittal and frontal planes; (3) limited chest expansion, relative to standard values for age and sex; and (4) definite radiographic sacroiliitis. The presence of radiographic sacroiliitis plus any one of the other three criteria is sufficient for a diagnosis of definite AS. The use of MRI to demonstrate sacroiliitis significantly increases the sensitivity of these criteria (Fig. 305-1).

The presence of B27 is neither necessary nor sufficient for the diagnosis, but the B27 test can be helpful in patients with suggestive clinical findings who have not yet developed radiographic sacroiliitis. Moreover, the absence of B27 in a typical case of AS significantly increases the probability of coexistent IBD.

AS must be differentiated from numerous other causes of low-back pain, some of which are far more common than AS. The inflammatory back pain of AS is usually distinguished by the following five features: (1) age of onset below 40, (2) insidious onset, (3) duration >3 months before medical attention is sought, (4) morning stiffness, and (5) improvement with exercise or activity. The most common causes of back pain other than AS are primarily mechanical or degenerative rather than inflammatory and do not show these features. Less common metabolic, infectious, and malignant causes of back pain must also be differentiated from AS. Ochronosis can produce a phenotype that is clinically and radiographically similar to AS.

Marked calcification and ossification of paraspinous ligaments occur in *diffuse idiopathic skeletal hyperostosis* (DISH). Ligamentous calcification and ossification are usually most prominent in the anterior spinal ligament and give the appearance of "flowing wax" on the anterior bodies of the vertebrae. Intervertebral disk spaces are preserved, and sacroiliac and apophyseal joints appear normal, helping to differentiate DISH from spondylosis and from AS, respectively.

DISH occurs in the middle-aged and elderly. Patients are frequently asymptomatic but may have stiffness. Radiographic changes are generally much more dramatic than symptoms.

℞ TREATMENT

The publication in 2000 of dramatic responses to anti-TNF-α therapy heralded a revolution in the management of AS and other spondyloarthritides. Patients with AS treated with either infliximab (chimeric human/mouse anti-TNF-α monoclonal antibody) or etanercept (soluble p75 TNF-α receptor–IgG fusion protein) have shown rapid, profound, and sustained reductions in all clinical and laboratory measures of disease activity. Patients with long-standing disease and even complete spinal ankylosis have shown striking improvement in both objective and subjective indicators of disease activity and function, including morning stiffness, pain, spinal mobility, peripheral joint swelling, CRP, and ESR. MRI studies indicate substantial resolution of bone marrow edema, enthesitis, and joint effusions in the sacroiliac joints, spine, and peripheral joints. Overall, 10 studies published from 2000 to 2002 (9 with infliximab, 1 with etanercept; 7 open label, 3 randomized controlled trials; duration 8 to 54 weeks) have reported a median 60% reduction in the Bath Ankylosing Spondylitis Disease Activity Index (BASDAI), the most commonly used measure of disease activity (range 45 to 93%, vs. 3 to 10% in the three placebo groups). At present, it is not definitely known whether this therapy will halt the progression of the disease, but it seems likely to do so. Whether this therapy can reverse ankylosis or other damage is less clear but also not improbable.

The administration of these agents to AS patients has been similar to that in RA. Infliximab is given as an intravenous infusion, typically at a dose of 5 mg per kg body weight, and then repeated 2 weeks later, again 6 weeks later, and then at 8-week intervals. Etanercept is given in a dose of 25 mg by subcutaneous injection twice weekly.

Although these potent immunosuppressive agents have so far been remarkably safe, six types of side effects have been seen: (1) serious infections, including disseminated tuberculosis; (2) hematologic disorders such as pancytopenia; (3) demyelinating disorders; (4) exacerbation of congestive heart failure; (5) systemic lupus erythematosus–related autoantibodies and clinical features; and (6) hypersensitivity infusion or injection site reactions. Increased incidence of malignancy is of theoretical concern.

Although serious complications have been uncommon, neither the incidence of side effects nor the long-term effects of these agents are yet known. Moreover, the currently available anti-TNF-α agents are quite expensive. Thus, uncertainty remains as to which patients with AS and other spondyloarthritides should be given this form of therapy. Previously, the mainstay of treatment for AS was nonsteroidal antiinflammatory drug (NSAID) therapy with drugs such as indomethacin or more recently COX-2 inhibitors, combined with exercise programs designed to maintain posture and range of motion. Sulfasalazine, in doses of 2 to 3 g/d, and methotrexate, in doses of 10 to 25 mg/wk, have been shown to be of modest benefit, primarily for peripheral arthritis. No therapeutic role for gold or oral glucocorticoids has been documented in AS. Recent studies suggest potential benefit in AS from three diverse agents: the bisphosphonate pamidronate, at

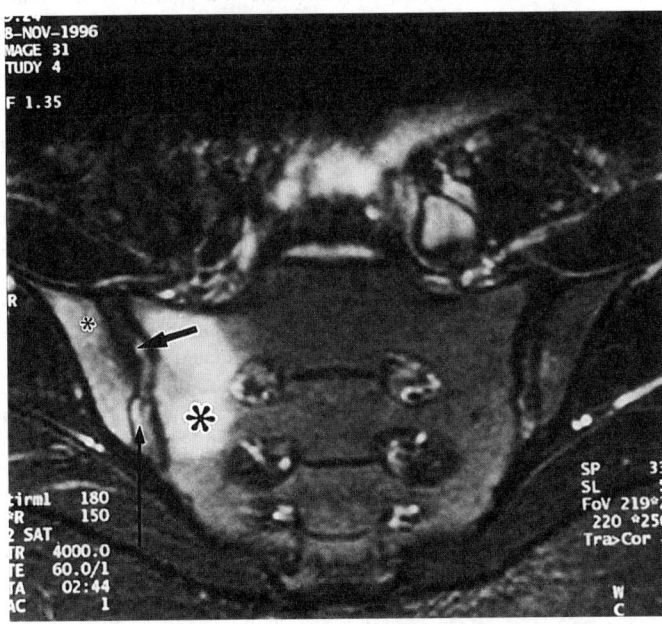

FIGURE 305-1 Early sacroiliitis of ankylosing spondylitis. Magnetic resonance imaging of the sacroiliac joints of a 23-year-old woman with progressive right-sided inflammatory back pain of 6 months' duration. Conventional radiographs were normal. A fat-suppressed image employing a short tau inversion recovery (STIR) sequence shows acute sacroiliitis on the right side, with edema in the juxtaarticular bone marrow (*asterisks*), in the region of the synovium and joint capsule (*thin arrow*), and in the region of the interosseous ligaments (*thick arrow*). Early chronic changes, including cortical erosions and joint space widening, were evident in the right sacroiliac joint in T1-, contrast-enhanced T1-, and T2*-weighted images (not shown). The patient subsequently developed radiographically evident bilateral sacroiliitis, fulfilling the criteria for ankylosing spondylitis. (*Photo provided by Dr. Jürgen Braun; previously published in Zeitschrift für Rheumatologie 58:61, 1999. Reproduced with permission.*)

a dose of 60 mg given monthly by intravenous infusion; thalidomide, 200 mg/d, perhaps also acting through inhibition of TNF-α; and the α-emitting isotope ^{224}Ra, at a dose of 1 MBq given weekly by intravenous infusion.[1]

AS is a chronic progressive disease with a significant impact on productivity and quality of life. Although there are patients with mild AS whose pain is well controlled with NSAID therapy and whose disease shows little radiographic progression, many, if not most, patients have axial pain, stiffness, and disease progression despite conventional therapy. Thus, should anti-TNF-α agents, or similarly potent biologicals, prove reasonably safe and continuously effective, it can be predicted that eventually these agents will become standard therapy for most patients with AS.

The most common indication for surgery in patients with AS is severe hip joint arthritis, the pain and stiffness of which are usually dramatically relieved by total hip arthroplasty. A small number of patients may benefit from surgical correction of extreme flexion deformities of the spine or of atlantoaxial subluxation.

Attacks of uveitis are usually managed effectively with local glucocorticoid administration in conjunction with mydriatic agents, although systemic glucocorticoids or even immunosuppressive drugs may be required in some cases. The response of uveitis to anti-TNF-α therapy has not been as predictable as that of other features of AS. Coexistent cardiac disease may require pacemaker implantation and/or aortic valve replacement. Management of osteoporosis of the axial skeleton is at present similar to that used for primary osteoporosis, since data specific for AS are not available.

REACTIVE ARTHRITIS

Reactive arthritis (ReA) refers to acute nonpurulent arthritis complicating an infection elsewhere in the body. In recent years, the term has been used primarily to refer to spondyloarthritides following enteric or urogenital infections and occurring predominantly in individuals with the histocompatibility antigen HLA-B27. In the setting of HIV infection, the association with B27 is not necessarily found. →*Other forms of reactive and infection-related arthritis not associated with B27 and showing a different spectrum of clinical features, such as rheumatic fever or Lyme disease, are discussed in Chaps. 302 and 157.*

HISTORIC BACKGROUND The association of acute arthritis with episodes of diarrhea or urethritis has been recognized for centuries. A large number of cases during World Wars I and II focused attention on the triad of arthritis, urethritis, and conjunctivitis, which became known as *Reiter's syndrome*, often occurring with additional mucocutaneous lesions. This eponym is now of historic interest only.

The identification of bacterial species capable of triggering the clinical syndrome and the finding that up to 85% of the patients possess the B27 antigen have led to the unifying concept of ReA as a clinical syndrome triggered by specific etiologic agents in a genetically susceptible host. A similar spectrum of clinical manifestations can be triggered by enteric infection with any of several *Shigella*, *Salmonella*, *Yersinia*, and *Campylobacter* species; by genital infection with *Chlamydia trachomatis*; and possibly by other agents as well. The triad of arthritis, urethritis, and conjunctivitis represents one part of the spectrum of the clinical manifestations of ReA, particularly that induced by *Shigella* or *Chlamydia*. For the purposes of this chapter, the use of the term *ReA* will be restricted to those cases of spondyloarthritis in which there is at least presumptive evidence for a related antecedent infection. Patients with clinical features of ReA who lack evidence of an antecedent infection will be considered to have *undifferentiated spondyloarthritis*, discussed below.

---

[1]Azathioprine, methotrexate, sulfasalazine, infliximab, etanercept, pamidronate, thalidomide, and ^{224}Ra have not been approved for this purpose by the U.S. Food and Drug Administration at the time of publication.

EPIDEMIOLOGY Outside the setting of HIV infection, ReA occurs predominantly in individuals who have inherited the B27 gene; in most series in which *Shigella*, *Yersinia*, or *Chlamydia* are the triggering infectious agents, 60 to 85% of patients are B27 positive. The prevalence of B27 tends to be much lower ($\leq$50%) in ReA triggered by *Salmonella* and even lower for *Campylobacter*. The disease is most common in individuals 18 to 40 years of age, but it can occur both in children over 5 years of age and in older adults.

The sex ratio in ReA following enteric infection is nearly 1:1, whereas venereally acquired ReA occurs predominantly in men. The overall prevalence and incidence of ReA are difficult to assess because of the variable prevalence of the triggering infections and genetic susceptibility factors in different populations. The spondyloarthritides were previously almost unknown in sub-Saharan Africa, where <1% of the population carries B27. However, ReA and other peripheral spondyloarthritides have now become the most common rheumatic diseases in Africans in the wake of the AIDS epidemic, with no association to B27. Spondyloarthritis in Africans with HIV infection usually occurs in individuals with stage I disease (as classified by the World Health Organization). It is often the first manifestation of infection and often remits with disease progression. In contrast, western Caucasian patients with HIV and spondyloarthritis are predominantly B27 positive, and the arthritis flares as AIDS advances.

PATHOLOGY Synovial histology is similar to that of other inflammatory arthropathies. Enthesitis shows increased vascularity and macrophage infiltration of fibrocartilage. Microscopic histopathologic evidence of inflammation has occasionally been noted in the colon and ileum of patients with postvenereal ReA, but much less commonly than in postenteric ReA. The skin lesions of keratoderma blenorrhagica, which is associated mainly with venereally acquired ReA, are histologically indistinguishable from psoriatic lesions.

ETIOLOGY AND PATHOGENESIS Of the four *Shigella* species *S. sonnei*, *S. boydii*, *S. flexneri*, and *S. dysenteriae*, *S. flexneri* has most often been implicated in cases of ReA, both sporadic and epidemic. *S. sonnei*, although responsible for the majority of cases of shigellosis in the United States, has only rarely been implicated in cases of ReA.

Other bacteria identified definitively as triggers of ReA include several *Salmonella* spp., *Y. enterocolitica*, *C. jejuni*, and *C. trachomatis*. There is evidence implicating several other microorganisms, including *Y. pseudotuberculosis*, *Clostridium difficile*, and *Ureaplasma urealyticum*. There are also numerous isolated reports of acute arthritis preceded by other bacterial, viral, or parasitic infections, but whether the microorganisms involved are actual triggers of ReA remains to be determined.

It has not been determined whether ReA occurs by the same pathogenic mechanism following infection with each of these microorganisms, nor has the mechanism been fully elucidated in the case of any one of the known bacterial triggers. Most, if not all, of the triggering organisms produce lipopolysaccharide (LPS) and share a capacity to attack mucosal surfaces, to invade host cells, and to survive intracellularly. Antigens from *Chlamydia*, *Yersinia*, *Salmonella*, and *Shigella* have been shown to be present in the synovium and/or synovial fluid leukocytes of patients with ReA for long periods following the acute attack. In ReA triggered by *Y. enterocolitica*, bacterial LPS and heat shock protein antigens have been found in peripheral blood cells years after the triggering infection. In the case of *C. trachomatis*, synovial persistence of microbial DNA and RNA suggests the presence of viable organisms, despite uniform failure to culture the organism from these specimens. ReA, at least in some cases, thus may be a form of chronic infection, rather than solely "reactive." T cells that specifically respond to antigens of the inciting organism have been found in inflamed synovium but not in peripheral blood of patients with ReA. These T cells are predominantly CD4+, but CD8+ B27-restricted bacteria-specific cytolytic T cells have also been isolated in *Yersinia*- and *C. trachomatis*-induced ReA. A unique conserved T cell antigen receptor sequence has been identified in B27-restricted synovial T cells in ReA. Unlike the synovial CD4 T cells in RA, which are predominantly of the T_H1 phenotype, those in ReA also show a T_H2 phenotype. It is likely that antigen-specific T cells play an important role in the pathogenesis of ReA, but the mechanisms remain to be determined.

The role of HLA-B27 in ReA also remains to be determined. The presence of HLA-B27 significantly prolongs the intracellular survival of *Y. enterocolitica* and *S. enteritidis* in human and mouse cell lines. Prolonged intracellular bacterial survival, promoted by B27, other factors, or both, may permit trafficking of infected leukocytes from the site of primary infection to joints, where a T cell response to persistent bacterial antigens may then promote arthritis.

CLINICAL FEATURES The clinical manifestations of ReA constitute a spectrum that ranges from an isolated, transient monarthritis to severe multisystem disease. Usually, a careful history will elicit evidence of an antecedent infection 1 to 4 weeks before onset of symptoms of the reactive disease. However, in a sizable minority, no clinical or laboratory evidence of an antecedent infection can be found. In many cases of presumed venereally acquired reactive disease, there is a history of a recent new sexual partner, even in the absence of laboratory evidence of infection.

Constitutional symptoms are common, including fatigue, malaise, fever, and weight loss. The musculoskeletal symptoms are usually acute in onset. Arthritis is usually asymmetric and additive, with involvement of new joints occurring over a period of a few days to 1 to 2 weeks. The joints of the lower extremities, especially the knee, ankle, and subtalar, metatarsophalangeal, and toe interphalangeal joints, are the most common sites of involvement, but the wrist and fingers can be involved as well. The arthritis is usually quite painful, and tense joint effusions are not uncommon, especially in the knee. Patients often cannot walk without support. Dactylitis, or "sausage digit," a diffuse swelling of a solitary finger or toe, is a distinctive feature of ReA and other peripheral spondyloarthritides but can be seen in polyarticular gout and sarcoidosis. Tendinitis and fasciitis are particularly characteristic lesions, producing pain at multiple insertion sites (entheses), especially the Achilles insertion, the plantar fascia, and sites along the axial skeleton. Spinal and low-back pain are quite common and may be caused by insertional inflammation, muscle spasm, acute sacroiliitis, or, presumably, arthritis in intervertebral articulations.

Urogenital lesions may occur throughout the course of the disease. In males, urethritis may be marked or relatively asymptomatic and may be either an accompaniment of the triggering infection or a result of the reactive phase of the disease. Prostatitis is also common. Similarly, in females, cervicitis or salpingitis may be caused either by the infectious trigger or by the sterile reactive process.

Ocular disease is common, ranging from transient, asymptomatic conjunctivitis to an aggressive anterior uveitis that occasionally proves refractory to treatment and may result in blindness.

Mucocutaneous lesions are frequent. Oral ulcers tend to be superficial, transient, and often asymptomatic. The characteristic skin lesions, *keratoderma blenorrhagica*, consist of vesicles that become hyperkeratotic, ultimately forming a crust before disappearing. They are most common on the palms and soles but may occur elsewhere as well. In patients with HIV infection, these lesions are often extremely severe and extensive, to the point of dominating the clinical picture (Chap. 173). Lesions on the glans penis, termed *circinate balanitis*, are common; these consist of vesicles that quickly rupture to form painless superficial erosions, which in circumcised individuals can form crusts similar to those of keratoderma blenorrhagica. Nail changes are common and consist of onycholysis, distal yellowish discoloration, and/or heaped-up hyperkeratosis.

Less frequent or rare manifestations of ReA include cardiac conduction defects, aortic insufficiency, central or peripheral nervous system lesions, and pleuropulmonary infiltrates.

Long-term follow-up studies suggest that some joint symptoms persist in 30 to 60% of patients with ReA. Recurrences of the acute syndrome are common, and as many as 25% of patients either become unable to work or are forced to change occupations because of per-

sistent joint symptoms. Chronic heel pain is often particularly distressing. Some aspects of AS are also common sequelae. In most studies, HLA-B27-positive patients have shown a worse outcome than B27-negative patients. The extent to which the long-term prognosis varies with different inciting agents is not known. However, patients with *Yersinia*-induced arthritis appear to have less chronic disease than those whose initial episode follows epidemic shigellosis.

LABORATORY AND RADIOGRAPHIC FINDINGS The ESR is usually elevated during the acute phase of the disease. Mild anemia may be present, and acute-phase reactants tend to be increased. Synovial fluid is nonspecifically inflammatory. In most ethnic groups, 50 to 85% of the patients are B27 positive, although the prevalence of B27 can be much lower in cases triggered by *Campylobacter* or *Salmonella* infections. It is unusual for the triggering infection to persist at the site of primary mucosal infection through the time of onset of the reactive disease, but it may occasionally be possible to culture the organism, e.g., in the case of *Yersinia*- or *Chlamydia*-induced disease. Serologic evidence of a recent infection may be present, such as a marked elevation of antibodies to *Yersinia*, *Salmonella*, or *Chlamydia*.

In early or mild disease, radiographic changes may be absent or confined to juxtaarticular osteoporosis. With long-standing persistent disease, marginal erosions and loss of joint space can be seen in affected joints. Periostitis with reactive new bone formation is characteristic of the disease, as it is with all the spondyloarthritides. Spurs at the insertion of the plantar fascia are common.

Sacroiliitis and spondylitis may be seen as late sequelae. The sacroiliitis is more commonly asymmetric than in AS, and the spondylitis, rather than ascending symmetrically from the lower lumbar segments, can begin anywhere along the lumbar spine. The syndesmophytes may be coarse and nonmarginal, arising from the middle of a vertebral body, a pattern rarely seen in primary AS. Progression to spinal fusion is uncommon.

DIAGNOSIS ReA is a clinical diagnosis, there being no definitively diagnostic laboratory test or radiographic finding. The diagnosis should be entertained in any patient with an acute inflammatory, asymmetric, additive arthritis or tendinitis. The evaluation should include questioning regarding possible triggering events such as an episode of diarrhea or dysuria. On physical examination, attention must be paid to the distribution of the joint and tendon involvement and to possible sites of extraarticular involvement, such as the eyes, mucous membranes, skin, nails, and genitalia. Synovial fluid analysis may be helpful in excluding septic or crystal-induced arthritis. Culture, serology, or molecular methods may help to identify a triggering infection.

Although typing for B27 is not needed to secure the diagnosis in clear-cut cases, it may have prognostic significance in terms of severity, chronicity, and the propensity for spondylitis and uveitis. Furthermore, it can be helpful diagnostically in atypical cases, a positive test increasing and a negative test decreasing the probability of ReA. HIV testing is often indicated and may be necessary in order to select appropriate therapy.

It is important to differentiate ReA from disseminated gonococcal disease (Chap. 128), both of which can be venereally acquired and associated with urethritis. Unlike ReA, gonococcal arthritis and tenosynovitis tend to involve both upper and lower extremities equally, to lack back symptoms, and to be associated with characteristic vesicular skin lesions. A positive gonococcal culture from the urethra or cervix does not exclude a diagnosis of ReA; however, culturing gonococci from blood, skin lesion, or synovium establishes the diagnosis of disseminated gonococcal disease. Polymerase chain reaction (PCR) assay for *Neisseria gonorrheae* and *C. trachomatis* may be helpful. Occasionally, only a therapeutic trial of antibiotics can distinguish the two.

ReA shares many features in common with psoriatic arthropathy. However, psoriatic arthritis is usually gradual in onset; the arthritis tends to affect primarily the upper extremities; there is less associated periarthritis; and there are usually no associated mouth ulcers, urethritis, or bowel symptoms.

℞ TREATMENT

Most patients with ReA are benefitted to some degree by NSAIDs, although rarely are symptoms of the acute arthritis completely ameliorated, and some patients fail to respond at all. Indomethacin, 75 to 150 mg/d in divided doses, is the initial treatment of choice. Other NSAIDs may be tried, with phenylbutazone, 100 mg tid or qid, being the NSAID of last resort, to be used only in severe, refractory cases because of its potentially serious side effects. There are no published data on the use of selective COX-2 inhibitors, but these may be tried in patients who do not tolerate conventional NSAIDs.

Several controlled trials have failed to demonstrate any benefit for antibiotic therapy in ReA. However, prompt, appropriate antibiotic treatment of acute chlamydial urethritis may prevent subsequent ReA.

Multicenter trials have suggested that sulfasalazine, up to 3 g/d in divided doses, may be beneficial to patients with persistent ReA.[1] Patients with persistent disease may respond to azathioprine, 1 to 2 mg/kg per day, or to methotrexate, 7.5 to 15 mg per week. Although no trials of anti-TNF-α in ReA have been reported, anecdotal evidence supports the use of these agents in severe chronic cases, although lack of response has also been observed.

Tendinitis and other enthesitic lesions may benefit from intralesional glucocorticoids. Uveitis may require aggressive treatment with glucocorticoids to prevent serious sequelae. Skin lesions ordinarily require only symptomatic treatment. In patients with HIV infection and ReA, many of whom have severe skin lesions, the skin lesions in particular respond to anti-retroviral therapy. Cardiac complications are managed conventionally; management of neurologic complications is symptomatic.

Comprehensive management includes counseling of patients in the avoidance of sexually transmitted disease and exposure to enteropathogens, as well as appropriate use of physical therapy, vocational counseling, and continued surveillance for long-term complications such as ankylosing spondylitis.

PSORIATIC ARTHRITIS

Psoriatic arthritis (PsA) refers to an inflammatory arthritis that characteristically occurs in individuals with psoriasis.

HISTORIC BACKGROUND The association between arthritis and psoriasis was noted in the nineteenth century. In the 1960s, on the basis of epidemiologic and clinical studies, it became clear that unlike RA the arthritis associated with psoriasis was usually seronegative, often involved the distal interphalangeal (DIP) joints of the fingers and the spine and sacroiliac joints, had distinctive radiographic features, and showed considerable familial aggregation. In the 1970s, PsA was included in the broader category of the spondyloarthritides because of features similar to those of AS and ReA.

EPIDEMIOLOGY A recent consensus has emerged that, among individuals with psoriasis, the prevalence of PsA is about 5 to 10%, but figures as high as 30% continue to be reported. In Caucasian populations, psoriasis is estimated to have a prevalence of 1 to 3%. Psoriasis and PsA are less common in other races in the absence of HIV infection. First-degree relatives of PsA patients have an elevated risk for psoriasis, for PsA itself, and for other forms of spondyloarthritis. Of patients with psoriasis, 30% have an affected first-degree relative. In monozygotic twins, the concordance for psoriasis is $\geq$65%, and for PsA $\geq$30%. A variety of HLA associations have been found. HLA-Cw6 is highly associated with psoriasis, particularly familial juvenile onset (type I) psoriasis. HLA-B27 is highly associated with psoriatic spondylitis (see below). HLA-DR7, -DQ3, and -B57 are associated with PsA because of linkage disequilibrium with Cw6. Other associations include HLA-B13, -B37, -B38, -B39, and DR4. The MIC-A-A9 allele at the HLA-B-linked MIC-A locus has also recently been reported associated with PsA, as have certain killer immunoglobulin-like receptor (KIR) alleles. The complex inheritance patterns of psoriasis and PsA suggest that several unlinked allelic loci are required for susceptibility. However, only the MHC has shown consistent linkage from study to study.

PATHOLOGY The inflamed synovium in PsA resembles that of RA, although with somewhat less hyperplasia and cellularity than in RA, and somewhat greater vascularity. Some studies have indicated a higher tendency to synovial fibrosis in PsA. Unlike RA, PsA shows prominent enthesitis, with histology similar to that of the other spondyloarthritides.

PATHOGENESIS PsA is almost certainly immune mediated, although the mechanism is as yet not well understood. PsA synovium shows infiltration with T cells, B cells, and macrophages, and upregulation of leukocyte homing receptors. CD8+ T cells are more frequent in PsA. Cytokine production in the synovium in PsA resembles that in psoriatic skin lesions and in RA synovium, having predominantly a T_H1 pattern. Interleukin (IL) 2, interferon γ, TNF-α, and IL-1β, -6, -8, -10, -12, -13, and -15 are found in PsA synovium or synovial fluid. Differences between PsA and RA in this regard are primarily quantitative, not qualitative.

CLINICAL FEATURES In 60 to 70% of cases, psoriasis precedes joint disease. In 15 to 20%, the two manifestations appear within 1 year of each other. In about 15 to 20% of cases, the arthritis precedes the onset of psoriasis and can present a diagnostic challenge. The frequency in men and women is almost equal, although the frequency of disease patterns differs somewhat in the two sexes. The disease can begin in childhood or late in life, but typically begins in the fourth or fifth decade, at an average age of 37 years.

The spectrum of arthropathy associated with psoriasis is quite broad. Several classification schemes have been proposed, but the most widely accepted is that of Wright and Moll, who described five patterns: (1) arthritis of the DIP joints; (2) asymmetric oligoarthritis; (3) symmetric polyarthritis similar to RA; (4) axial involvement (spine and sacroiliac joints); and (5) arthritis mutilans, a highly destructive form of disease. These patterns are not fixed, and in many patients the pattern that persists chronically differs from that of the initial presentation.

Nail changes in the fingers or toes occur in 90% of patients with PsA, compared with 40% of psoriatic patients without arthritis, and pustular psoriasis is said to be associated with more severe arthritis. Several articular features distinguish PsA from other joint disorders. Dactylitis occurs in >30%; enthesitis and tenosynovitis are also common, and are probably present in most patients, although often not appreciated on physical examination. Shortening of digits because of underlying osteolysis is particularly characteristic of PsA, and there is a much greater tendency than in RA for both fibrous and bony ankylosis of small joints. Rapid ankylosis of one or more PIP joints early in the course of disease is not uncommon. Back and neck pain and stiffness are also common in PsA.

Arthropathy confined to the DIP joints predominates in about 15% of cases. Accompanying nail changes in the affected digits are almost always present. These joints are also often affected in the other patterns of PsA. Approximately 30% of patients have asymmetric oligoarthritis. This pattern commonly involves a knee or another large joint with a few small joints in the fingers or toes, often with dactylitis. Symmetric polyarthritis occurs in about 40% of PsA patients. It may be indistinguishable from RA in terms of the joints involved, but other features characteristic of PsA are usually also present. In general, peripheral joints in PsA tend to be somewhat less tender than in RA, although signs of inflammation are usually present. Almost any peripheral joint can be involved. Axial arthropathy without peripheral involvement is found in about 5% of PsA patients. It may be indistinguishable from idiopathic AS, although more neck involvement and less thoracolumbar spinal involvement is characteristic, and nail changes are not found in idiopathic AS. About 5% of PsA patients have arthritis mutilans, in which there can be widespread shortening of digits ("telescoping"), sometimes coexisting with ankylosis and contractures in other digits.

Six patterns of nail involvement are identified: pitting, horizontal ridging, onycholysis, yellowish discoloration of the nail margins, dystrophic hyperkeratosis, and combinations of these findings. Other extraarticular manifestations of the spondyloarthritides are common. Eye involvement, either conjunctivitis or uveitis, is reported in 7 to 33% of PsA patients. Unlike the uveitis associated with AS, the uveitis in PsA shows more tendency to be bilateral, chronic, and/or posterior. Aortic valve insufficiency has been found in <4% of patients, usually after long-standing disease.

Widely varying estimates of clinical outcome have been reported in PsA. At its worst, severe PsA with arthritis mutilans is at least as crippling and ultimately fatal as severe RA. Unlike RA, however, many patients with PsA experience temporary remissions. Overall, erosive disease develops in the majority of patients, progressive disease with deformity and disability is common, and in some large published series mortality was found to be significantly increased compared with the general population.

The psoriasis and associated arthropathy seen in individuals infected with HIV both tend to be severe and can occur in populations with very little psoriasis in noninfected individuals. Severe enthesopathy, dactylitis, and rapidly progressive joint destruction are seen, but axial involvement is very rare. This condition is prevented by or responds well to anti-retroviral therapy.

LABORATORY AND RADIOGRAPHIC FINDINGS   There are no diagnostic laboratory tests for PsA. ESR and CRP are often, but not always, elevated. A small percentage of patients may have low titers of rheumatoid factor or antinuclear antibodies. Uric acid may be elevated in the presence of extensive psoriasis. HLA-B27 is found in 50 to 70% of patients with axial disease, but in ≤15 to 20% in patients with only peripheral joint involvement.

The peripheral and axial arthropathies in PsA show a number of radiographic features that distinguish them from RA and AS, respectively. Characteristics of peripheral PsA include DIP involvement, including the classic "pencil-in-cup" deformity; marginal erosions with adjacent bony proliferation ("whiskering"); small joint ankylosis; osteolysis of phalangeal and metacarpal bone, with telescoping of digits; and periostitis and proliferative new bone at sites of enthesitis. Characteristics of axial PsA include asymmetric sacroiliitis; compared with idiopathic AS, less zygoapophyseal joint arthritis, fewer and less symmetric and delicate syndesmophytes; fluffy hyperperiostosis on anterior vertebral bodies; severe cervical spine involvement, with a tendency to atlantoaxial subluxation but relative sparing of the thoracolumbar spine; and paravertebral ossification. Ultrasound and MRI both readily demonstrate enthesitis and tendon sheath effusions that can be difficult to assess on physical examination.

DIAGNOSIS   The diagnosis of PsA is primarily clinical and can be challenging when the arthritis precedes psoriasis, the psoriasis is undiagnosed or obscure, or the joint involvement closely resembles another form of arthritis. A high index of suspicion is needed in any patient with an undiagnosed inflammatory arthropathy. The history should include inquiry about psoriasis in the patient and family members. Patients should be asked to disrobe for the physical examination, and psoriasiform lesions should be sought in the scalp, ears, umbilicus, and gluteal folds in addition to more accessible sites, and the finger and toe nails should be carefully examined. Axial symptoms or signs, dactylitis, enthesitis, ankylosis, the pattern of joint involvement, and characteristic radiographic changes can be helpful clues. The differential diagnosis of isolated DIP involvement is short. Osteoarthritis (Heberden's nodes) is usually not inflammatory; gout involving more than one DIP joint often involves other sites and is accompanied by

tophi; the very rare entity multicentric reticulohistiocytosis involves other joints and has characteristic small pearly periungual skin nodules; and the uncommon entity inflammatory osteoarthritis, like the others, lacks the nail changes of PsA. Radiography can be helpful in all of these cases and in distinguishing between psoriatic spondylitis and idiopathic AS. A history of trauma to an affected joint preceding the onset of arthritis is said to occur more frequently in PsA than in other types of arthritis, perhaps reflecting the Koebner phenomenon in which psoriatic skin lesions can arise at sites of the skin trauma.

℞ TREATMENT

Ideally, coordinated therapy is directed at both the skin and joints in PsA. As described above for AS, use of the anti-TNF-α agents promises to revolutionize the treatment of PsA. Prompt and dramatic resolution of both arthritis and skin lesions has been observed in at least five trials of etanercept and infliximab. Many of the responding patients had long-standing disease that was resistant to all previous therapy, as well as extensive skin disease. Although the effect on disease progression has not yet been reported, the clinical response is even more dramatic than in RA, in which both etanercept and infliximab have been shown to halt the progression of joint erosions.

Other treatment for PsA has been based on drugs that have efficacy in RA and/or in psoriasis. Although methotrexate in doses of 15 to 25 mg/wk and sulfasalazine (usually given in doses of 2 to 3 g/d) have each been found to have clinical efficacy in controlled trials, neither effectively halts progression of erosive joint disease. Other agents with efficacy in psoriasis reported to benefit PsA are cyclosporine, retinoic acid derivatives, and psoralen plus ultraviolet light (PUVA). There is controversy regarding the efficacy in PsA of gold and antimalarials, which have been widely used in RA. The new antirheumatic agent leflunomide is currently being evaluated.

All of these treatments require careful monitoring. Use of immunosuppressive therapy, including anti-TNF-α agents, methotrexate, and cyclosporine, is largely contraindicated in HIV-associated PsA.

In one large prospective series, 7% of patients with PsA required musculoskeletal surgery beginning at a mean of 13 years' disease duration. Indications for surgery are similar to those in RA, although there is an impression that outcomes in PsA may be less satisfactory.

SAPHO SYNDROME

The syndrome of synovitis, acne, pustulosis, hyperostosis, and osteitis (SAPHO) is characterized by a variety of skin and musculoskeletal manifestations. Dermatologic manifestations include palmoplantar pustulosis, acne conglobata, acne fulminans, and hidradenitis suppurativa. The main musculoskeletal findings are sternoclavicular and spinal hyperostosis, chronic recurrent foci of sterile osteomyelitis, and occasionally peripheral arthritis. Cases with one or a few manifestations are probably the rule. Granulomas may be present on bone biopsy. The ESR is usually elevated, sometimes dramatically. In some series, B27 is present in about 30% of the cases. Either bone scan or CT scan is helpful diagnostically. Therapy has been inadequate, with high dose NSAIDs, including phenylbutazone, providing the most relief from bone pain. Response to pamidronate and to anti-TNF-α therapy has been observed anecdotally.

UNDIFFERENTIATED AND JUVENILE-ONSET SPONDYLOARTHRITIS

Many patients, usually young adults, present with some features of one or more of the spondyloarthritides discussed above but lack criteria for these diagnoses. For example, a patient may present with inflammatory synovitis of one knee, Achilles tendinitis, and dactylitis of one digit, or sacroiliitis in the absence of other criteria for AS. Such patients are said to have undifferentiated spondyloarthritis, or simply spondyloarthritis, as defined by the European Spondyloarthropathy Study Group (ESSG criteria, Fig. 305-2). Some of these patients may

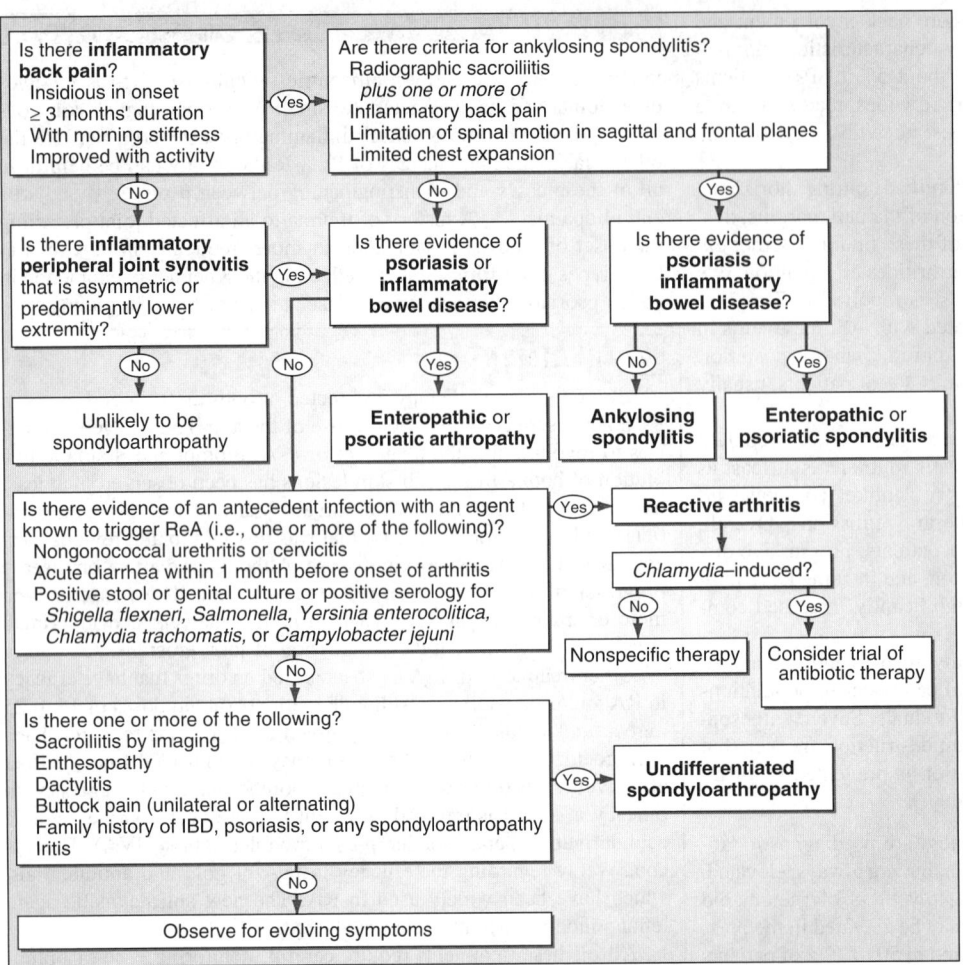

FIGURE 305-2 Algorithm for diagnosis of the spondyloarthritides, adapted from the European Spondyloarthropathy Study Group criteria. If a diagnosis of psoriatic arthropathy, reactive arthritis, or undifferentiated spondyloarthritis is made on the basis of peripheral arthropathy, then HIV infection needs to be considered.

EPIDEMIOLOGY Both of the common forms of IBD, ulcerative colitis (UC) and Crohn's disease (CD) (Chap. 276), are associated with spondyloarthritis. UC and CD both have an estimated prevalence of 0.05 to 0.1%, and the incidence of each is thought to have increased in recent decades. AS and peripheral arthritis are both associated with UC and with CD. Wide variations have been reported in the estimated frequencies of these associations. In three recent European series encompassing almost 2000 patients with IBD for a median 5 to 10 years, overall, AS was diagnosed in 2%, inflammatory back pain in 9%, enthesopathy in 7%, and peripheral arthritis in 10%, with somewhat higher frequencies found in CD than in UC. The combined total frequency of spondyloarthritis was 19%. These figures are somewhat lower than earlier estimates. Asymptomatic radiographic sacroiliitis was found in an additional 5%.

The prevalence of UC or CD in patients with AS is thought to be 5 to 10%. However, investigation of unselected spondyloarthritis patients by ileocolonoscopy has revealed that from one-third to two-thirds of patients with AS have subclinical intestinal inflammation that is evident either macroscopically or histologically. These lesions have also been found in patients with undifferentiated spondyloarthritis or ReA (both enterically and urogenitally acquired).

Both UC and CD have a tendency to familial aggregation, more so for CD. HLA associations have been weak and inconsistent. HLA-B27 is found in about 70% of patients with IBD and AS, but in ≤15% of patients with IBD and peripheral arthritis or IBD alone. Certain alleles of the *NOD2/CARD15* gene on chromosome 16 have recently been found in up to half of patients with CD. It appears that these alleles are not associated with the spondyloarthritides, either occurring alone or in association with CD, but the data are not yet conclusive.

PATHOLOGY Available data for IBD-associated peripheral arthritis suggest a nonspecific inflammatory synovitis, although one study found granulomas associated with CD. Association with arthropathy does not affect the gut histology of UC or CD (Chap. 276). The subclinical inflammatory lesions in the colon and distal ileum associated with spondyloarthritis have been classified as either acute or chronic. The former resemble acute bacterial enteritis, with largely intact architecture and neutrophilic infiltration in the lamina propria. The latter resemble the lesions of CD, with distortion of villi and crypts, aphthoid ulceration, and mononuclear cell infiltration in the lamina propria.

PATHOGENESIS Both IBD and the spondyloarthropathies are immune mediated, but the specific pathogenic mechanisms are poorly understood, and the connection between the two is obscure. IBD is a common phenotype in a number of rodent lines with transgenic overexpression or targeted deletion of genes involved in immune processes. Arthritis is an accompanying prominent feature in two of these IBD models, HLA-B27 transgenic rats and mice with constitutive overexpression of TNF-α, and immune dysregulation is prominent in both. Several lines of evidence indicate trafficking of leukocytes between the gut and the joint. Mucosal leukocytes from IBD patients have been

have ReA in which the triggering infection remains clinically silent. In some other cases, the patient subsequently develops IBD or psoriasis or the process eventually meets criteria for AS. Approximately half the patients with undifferentiated spondyloarthritis are HLA-B27 positive, and thus the absence of B27 is not useful in establishing or excluding the diagnosis. In familial cases, which are almost always B27 positive, there is often eventual progression to AS.

In juvenile-onset spondyloarthritis, which begins between ages 7 and 16, most commonly in boys (60 to 80%), an asymmetric, predominantly lower extremity oligoarthritis and enthesitis without extraarticular features is the typical mode of presentation. The prevalence of B27 in this condition, which has been termed the seronegative, enthesopathy, arthropathy (SEA) syndrome, is approximately 80%. Many, but not all, of these patients go on to develop AS in late adolescence or adulthood.

Management of undifferentiated spondyloarthritis is similar to that of the other spondyloarthritides. Response to anti-TNF-α therapy has been documented, and this therapy is indicated in severe, persistent cases not responsive to other treatment. Current pediatric textbooks and journals should be consulted for information on management of juvenile-onset spondyloarthritis. An algorithm for the diagnosis of the spondyloarthritides in adults is presented in Fig. 305-2.

ENTEROPATHIC ARTHRITIS

HISTORIC BACKGROUND A relationship between arthritis and IBD was observed in the 1930s. The relationship was further defined by the epidemiologic studies in the 1950s and '60s and included in the concept of the spondyloarthritides in the 1970s.

shown to bind avidly to synovial vasculature through several different adhesion molecules, and T cells with identical antigen receptor sequences have been isolated from both the gut and the synovium in the same patient. Macrophages expressing CD163 are prominent in the inflammatory lesions of both gut and synovium in the spondyloarthritides.

CLINICAL FEATURES   AS associated with IBD is clinically indistinguishable from idiopathic AS. It runs a course independent of the bowel disease, and in many patients it precedes the onset of IBD, sometimes by many years. In contrast, peripheral arthritis has generally been reported to parallel the activity of the bowel disease, although it not infrequently begins before onset of overt bowel disease. A recent large study classified the peripheral arthritis of IBD patients into two types. Type 1 involved fewer than five joints, was associated with acute self-limited attacks, and often coincided with relapses of IBD. Type 2 involved five or more joints, tended to be symmetric, and ran a chronic course independent of IBD. The patterns of joint involvement were similar in UC and CD. Type 1 arthritis involved primarily the knee and ankle, whereas type 2 involved these joints but also tended to involve joints in the hand and upper extremity. This dichotomy has yet to be confirmed, but both types are characteristic of the spectrum of peripheral arthritis previously described in IBD. In general, erosions and deformities are infrequent in IBD-associated peripheral arthritis, and joint surgery is rarely required. Dactylitis and enthesopathy are occasionally found. In addition to the ~20% of IBD patients with spondyloarthritis, a comparable percentage have arthralgias or fibromyalgia symptoms.

Other extraintestinal manifestations of IBD are seen in addition to arthropathy, including uveitis, pyoderma gangrenosum, erythema nodosum, and finger clubbing, all somewhat more common in CD than UC. The uveitis shares the features described above for PsA-associated uveitis.

LABORATORY AND RADIOGRAPHIC FINDINGS   Laboratory findings reflect the inflammatory and metabolic manifestations of IBD. Joint fluid is usually at least mildly inflammatory. Of patients with AS and IBD, about 70% carry the HLA-B27 gene, compared with >90% of patients with AS alone and 50 to 70% of those with AS and psoriasis. Hence, definite or probable AS in a B27-negative individual in the absence of psoriasis should prompt a search for occult IBD. Radiographic changes in the axial skeleton are the same as in uncomplicated AS. Erosions are uncommon in peripheral arthritis but may occur, particularly in the metatarsophalangeal joints. Isolated destructive hip disease has been described.

DIAGNOSIS   Diarrhea and arthritis are both common conditions that can coexist for a variety of reasons. When etiopathogenically related, reactive arthritis and IBD-associated arthritis are the most common causes. Rare causes include celiac disease, blind loop syndromes, and Whipple's disease. In most cases, diagnosis depends upon investigation of the bowel disease.

[Rx] **TREATMENT**

As with the spondyloarthritides, treatment of CD is being revolutionized by therapy with infliximab, particularly in patients with fistulas or refractory disease. Recent anecdotal evidence suggests that associated arthritis responds promptly to infliximab. It is of interest that the spondyloarthritides respond to both infliximab and etaner

cept, whereas only infliximab has efficacy in CD and neither agent is effective in UC. Other treatment for IBD, including sulfasalazine and related drugs, systemic glucocorticoids, and immunosuppressive drugs, are also usually of benefit for associated peripheral arthritis. NSAIDs are generally helpful and well tolerated, but they can precipitate flares of IBD.

WHIPPLE'S DISEASE

Whipple's disease (Chap. 275) is a rare chronic bacterial infection, mostly of middle-aged Caucasian men, caused by *Tropheryma whippelii*. At least 75% of affected individuals develop an oligo- or polyarthritis. The joint manifestations usually precede other symptoms of the disease by 5 years or more; they are particularly important because antibiotic therapy is curative, whereas the untreated disease is fatal. Large and small peripheral joints and sacroiliac joints may be involved. The arthritis is abrupt in onset, migratory, usually lasts hours to a few days and then resolves completely. Chronic polyarthritis and joint space loss, visible on x-ray, can occur but are not typical. Eventually, prolonged diarrhea, malabsorption, and weight loss occur. Other manifestations of systemic disease include fever, edema, serositis, endocarditis, pneumonia, hypotension, lymphadenopathy, hyperpigmentation, subcutaneous nodules, clubbing, and uveitis. Central nervous system involvement eventually develops in 80% of untreated patients, with cognitive changes, headache, diplopia, and papilledema, and may be appreciated by abnormalities on MRI. Oculomasticatory and oculo-facial-skeletal myorhythmia, accompanied by supranuclear vertical gaze palsy, are said to be pathognomonic. Laboratory abnormalities include anemia and changes from malabsorption. There may be a weak association with HLA-B27. Synovial fluid is usually inflammatory. Radiography rarely shows joint erosions but may show sacroiliitis. Abdominal CT may reveal lymphadenopathy. Foamy macrophages containing PAS-staining bacterial remnants can be seen in biopsies of small intestine, synovium, lymph node, and other tissues. Diagnosis is established by PCR amplification of the 16S ribosomal gene sequences of *T. whippelii* in biopsied tissue. The organism has recently been isolated, and serologic tests may become available. The syndrome responds best to therapy with penicillin (or ceftriaxone) and streptomycin for 2 weeks followed by trimethoprim-sulfamethoxazole for 1 to 2 years. Monitoring for central nervous system relapse is critical.

FURTHER READING

BOWNESS P: HLA B27 in health and disease: A double-edged sword? Rheumatology (Oxford) 41:857, 2002

BRANDT J et al: Successful short term treatment of severe undifferentiated spondyloarthropathy with the anti-tumor necrosis factor-alpha monoclonal antibody infliximab. J Rheumatol 29:118, 2002

BRAUN J et al: Treatment of active ankylosing spondylitis with infliximab: A randomised controlled multicentre trial. Lancet 359:1187, 2002

BROWN MA et al: Genetic aspects of susceptibility, severity, and clinical expression in ankylosing spondylitis. Curr Opin Rheumatol 14:354, 2002

DOUGADOS M et al: The European Spondyloarthropathy Study Group preliminary criteria for the classification of spondyloarthropathy. Arthritis Rheum 34:1218, 1991

GLADMAN DD: Current concepts in psoriatic arthritis. Curr Opin Rheumatol 14:361, 2002

GORMAN JD et al: Treatment of ankylosing spondylitis by inhibition of tumor necrosis factor alpha. N Engl J Med 346:1349, 2002

DEFINITION *Vasculitis* is a clinicopathologic process characterized by inflammation of and damage to blood vessels. The vessel lumen is usually compromised, and this is associated with ischemia of the tissues supplied by the involved vessel. A broad and heterogeneous group of syndromes may result from this process, since any type, size, and location of blood vessel may be involved. Vasculitis and its consequences may be the primary or sole manifestation of a disease; alternatively, vasculitis may be a secondary component of another primary disease. Vasculitis may be confined to a single organ, such as the skin, or it may simultaneously involve several organ systems.

CLASSIFICATION A major feature of the vasculitic syndromes as a group is the fact that there is a great deal of heterogeneity at the same time as there is considerable overlap among them. This heterogeneity and overlap in addition to a lack of understanding of the pathogenesis of these syndromes have been major impediments to the development of a coherent classification system for these diseases. Table 306-1 lists the major vasculitis syndromes. The distinguishing and overlapping features of these syndromes are discussed below.

PATHOPHYSIOLOGY AND PATHOGENESIS Generally, most of the vasculitic syndromes are assumed to be mediated at least in part by immunopathogenic mechanisms that occur in response to certain antigenic stimuli (Table 306-2). However, evidence supporting this hypothesis is for the most part indirect and may reflect epiphenomena as opposed to true causality. Furthermore, it is unknown why some individuals might develop vasculitis in response to certain antigenic stimuli, whereas others do not. It is likely that a number of factors are involved in the ultimate expression of a vasculitic syndrome. These include the genetic predisposition, environmental exposures, and the regulatory mechanisms associated with immune response to certain antigens.

Pathogenic Immune-Complex Formation Vasculitis is generally considered within the broader category of *immune-complex diseases* that include serum sickness and certain of the connective tissue diseases, of which systemic lupus erythematosus (Chap. 300) is the prototype. Although deposition of immune complexes in vessel walls is the most widely accepted pathogenic mechanism of vasculitis, the causal role of immune complexes has not been clearly established in most of the vasculitic syndromes. Circulating immune complexes need not result in deposition of the complexes in blood vessels with ensuing vasculitis, and many patients with active vasculitis do not have demonstrable circulating or deposited immune complexes. The actual antigen contained in the immune complex has only rarely been identified in vasculitic syndromes. In this regard, hepatitis B antigen has been identified in both the circulating and deposited immune complexes in

TABLE 306-1 *Vasculitis Syndromes*

Primary Vasculitis Syndromes	Secondary Vasculitis Syndromes
Wegener's granulomatosis	Drug-induced vasculitis
Churg-Strauss syndrome	Serum sickness
Polyarteritis nodosa	Vasculitis associated with other
Microscopic polyangiitis	primary diseases
Giant cell arteritis	Infection
Takayasu's arteritis	Malignancy
Henoch-Schönlein purpura	Rheumatic disease
Idiopathic cutaneous vasculitis	
Essential mixed cryoglobulinemia	
Behçet's syndrome	
Isolated vasculitis of the central nervous system	
Cogan's syndrome	
Kawasaki disease	

TABLE 306-2 *Potential Mechanisms of Vessel Damage in Vasculitis Syndromes*

Pathogenic immune complex formation and/or deposition
    Henoch-Schönlein purpura
    Vasculitis associated with collagen vascular diseases
    Serum sickness and cutaneous vasculitis syndromes
    Hepatitis C–associated essential mixed cryoglobulinemia
    Hepatitis B–associated polyarteritis nodosa
Production of antineutrophilic cytoplasmic antibodies
    Wegener's granulomatosis
    Churg-Strauss syndrome
    Microscopic polyangiitis
Pathogenic T lymphocyte responses and granuloma formation
    Giant cell arteritis
    Takayasu's arteritis
    Wegener's granulomatosis
    Churg-Strauss syndrome

Source: Adapted from Sneller and Fauci.

a subset of patients with systemic vasculitis, most notably in polyarteritis nodosa (see below). The syndrome of essential mixed cryoglobulinemia is strongly associated with hepatitis C virus infection; hepatitis C virions and hepatitis C virus antigen-antibody complexes have been identified in the cryoprecipitates of these patients (see below).

The mechanisms of tissue damage in immune complex–mediated vasculitis resemble those described for serum sickness. In this model, antigen-antibody complexes are formed in antigen excess and are deposited in vessel walls whose permeability has been increased by vasoactive amines such as histamine, bradykinin, and leukotrienes released from platelets or from mast cells as a result of IgE-triggered mechanisms. The deposition of complexes results in activation of complement components, particularly C5a, which is strongly chemotactic for neutrophils. These cells then infiltrate the vessel wall, phagocytose the immune complexes, and release their intracytoplasmic enzymes, which damage the vessel wall. As the process becomes subacute or chronic, mononuclear cells infiltrate the vessel wall. The common denominator of the resulting syndrome is compromise of the vessel lumen with ischemic changes in the tissues supplied by the involved vessel. Several variables may explain why only certain types of immune complexes cause vasculitis and why only certain vessels are affected in individual patients. These include the ability of the reticuloendothelial system to clear circulating complexes from the blood, the size and physicochemical properties of immune complexes, the relative degree of turbulence of blood flow, the intravascular hydrostatic pressure in different vessels, and the preexisting integrity of the vessel endothelium.

Antineutrophil Cytoplasmic Antibodies (ANCA) ANCA are antibodies directed against certain proteins in the cytoplasmic granules of neutrophils and monocytes. These autoantibodies are present in a high percentage of patients with certain systemic vasculitis syndromes, particularly Wegener's granulomatosis and microscopic polyangiitis, and in patients with necrotizing and crescentic glomerulonephritis. There are two major categories of ANCA based on different targets for the antibodies. The terminology of *cytoplasmic ANCA* (c-ANCA) refers to the diffuse, granular cytoplasmic staining pattern observed by immunofluorescence microscopy when serum antibodies bind to indicator neutrophils. Proteinase-3, the 29-kDa neutral serine proteinase present in neutrophil azurophilic granules, is the major c-ANCA antigen. More than 90% of patients with typical active Wegener's granulomatosis have detectable antibodies to proteinase-3 (see below). The terminology of *perinuclear ANCA* (p-ANCA) refers to the more localized perinuclear or nuclear staining pattern of the indicator neutrophils. The major target for p-ANCA is the enzyme myeloperoxidase; other targets that can produce a p-ANCA pattern of staining include elastase, cathepsin G, lactoferrin, lysozyme, and bactericidal/permeability-increasing protein. However, only antibodies to myeloperoxidase have been convincingly associated with vasculitis. Antimyeloperoxidase antibodies have been reported to occur in variable percentages of patients with microscopic polyangiitis, Churg-Strauss syndrome, crescentic glomerulonephritis, Goodpasture's syndrome, and Wegener's granulomatosis (see below). A p-ANCA pattern of staining that is not due to antimyeloperoxidase antibodies has been associated with nonvasculitic entities such as rheumatic and nonrheumatic autoimmune diseases, inflammatory bowel disease, certain drugs, and infections such as endocarditis and bacterial airway infections in patients with cystic fibrosis.

It is unclear why patients with these vasculitis syndromes develop antibodies to myeloperoxidase or proteinase-3, whereas such antibodies are rare in other inflammatory diseases and autoimmune diseases. There are a number of in vitro observations that suggest possible mechanisms whereby these antibodies can contribute to the pathogenesis of the vasculitis syndromes. Proteinase-3 and myeloperoxidase reside in the azurophilic granules and lysosomes of resting neutrophils and monocytes, where they are apparently inaccessible to serum antibodies. However, when neutrophils or monocytes are primed by tumor necrosis factor (TNF) α or interleukin (IL) 1, proteinase-3 and myeloperoxidase translocate to the cell membrane where they can interact with extracellular ANCA. The neutrophils then degranulate and produce reactive oxygen species that can cause tissue damage. Furthermore, ANCA-activated neutrophils can adhere to and kill endothelial cells in vitro. Activation of neutrophils and monocytes by ANCA also induces the release of proinflammatory cytokines such as IL-1 and IL-8. Recent adoptive transfer experiments in genetically engineered mice provide further evidence for a direct pathogenic role of ANCA in vivo. In contradiction, however, a number of clinical and laboratory observations argue against a primary pathogenic role for ANCA. Patients may have active Wegener's granulomatosis in the absence of ANCA; the absolute height of the antibody titers does not correlate well with disease activity; and patients with Wegener's granulomatosis in remission may continue to have high antiproteinase-3 (c-ANCA) titers for years (see below). Thus, the role of these autoantibodies in the pathogenesis of systemic vasculitis remains unclear.

Pathogenic T Lymphocyte Responses and Granuloma Formation In addition to the classic immune complex–mediated mechanisms of vasculitis as well as ANCA, other immunopathogenic mechanisms may be involved in damage to vessels. The most prominent of these are delayed hypersensitivity and cell-mediated immune injury as reflected in the histopathologic feature of granulomatous vasculitis. However, immune complexes themselves may induce granulomatous responses. Vascular endothelial cells can express HLA class II molecules following activation by cytokines such as interferon (IFN) γ. This allows these cells to participate in immunologic reactions such as interaction with CD4+ T lymphocytes in a manner similar to antigen-presenting macrophages. Endothelial cells can secrete IL-1, which may activate T lymphocytes and initiate or propagate in situ immunologic processes within the blood vessel. In addition, IL-1 and TNF-α are potent inducers of endothelial-leukocyte adhesion molecule 1 (ELAM-1) and vascular cell adhesion molecule 1 (VCAM-1), which may enhance the adhesion of leukocytes to endothelial cells in the blood vessel wall. Other mechanisms such as direct cellular cytotoxicity, antibody directed against vessel components, or antibody-dependent cellular cytotoxicity have been suggested in certain types of vessel damage. However, there is no convincing evidence to support their causal contribution to the pathogenesis of any of the recognized vasculitis syndromes.

APPROACH TO THE PATIENT

The diagnosis of vasculitis is often considered in any patient with an unexplained systemic illness. However, there are certain clinical abnormalities that when present alone or in combination should suggest a diagnosis of vasculitis. These include palpable purpura, pulmonary infiltrates and microscopic hematuria, chronic inflammatory sinusitis, mononeuritis multiplex, unexplained ischemic

events, and glomerulonephritis with evidence of multisystem disease. A number of nonvasculitic diseases may also produce some or all of these abnormalities. Thus, the first step in the workup of a patient with suspected vasculitis is to exclude other diseases that produce clinical manifestations that can mimic vasculitis (Table 306-3). It is particularly important to exclude infectious diseases with features that overlap those of vasculitis, especially if the patient's clinical condition is deteriorating rapidly and empirical immunosuppressive treatment is being contemplated.

Once diseases that mimic vasculitis have been excluded, the workup should follow a series of progressive steps that establish the diagnosis of vasculitis and determine, where possible, the category of the vasculitis syndrome (Fig. 306-1). This approach is of considerable importance since several of the vasculitis syndromes require aggressive therapy with glucocorticoids and cytotoxic agents, while other syndromes usually resolve spontaneously and require symptomatic treatment only. The definitive diagnosis of vasculitis is made upon biopsy of involved tissue. The yield of "blind" biopsies of organs with no subjective or objective evidence of involvement is very low and should be avoided. When syndromes such as polyarteritis nodosa, Takayasu's arteritis, or isolated central nervous system vasculitis are suspected, angiogram of organs with suspected involvement should be performed. However, angiograms should not be performed routinely when patients present with localized cutaneous vasculitis with no clinical indication of visceral involvement.

The constellation of clinical, laboratory, biopsy, and radiographic findings usually allows proper categorization to a specific syndrome, and therapy where appropriate should be initiated according to this information (see individual syndromes below). If an offending antigen that precipitates the vasculitis is recognized, the antigen should be removed where possible. If the vasculitis is associated with an underlying disease such as an infection, neoplasm, or connective tissue disease, the underlying disease should be treated. If the syndrome does not resolve following removal of an offending antigen or treatment of an underlying disease, or if there is no recognizable underlying disease, treatment should be initiated according to the category of the vasculitis syndrome.

TABLE 306-3 Conditions That Can Mimic Vasculitis

Infectious diseases
  Bacterial endocarditis
  Disseminated gonococcal infection
  Pulmonary histoplasmosis
  Coccidioidomycosis
  Syphilis
  Lyme disease
  Rocky Mountain spotted fever
  Whipple's disease
Coagulopathies/thrombotic microangiopathies
  Antiphospholipid antibody syndrome
  Thrombotic thrombocytopenic purpura
Neoplasms
  Atrial myxoma
  Lymphoma
  Carcinomatosis
Drug toxicity
  Cocaine
  Amphetamines
  Ergot alkaloids
  Methysergide
  Arsenic
Sarcoidosis
Atheroembolic disease
Goodpasture's syndrome
Amyloidosis
Migraine
Cryofibrinogenemia

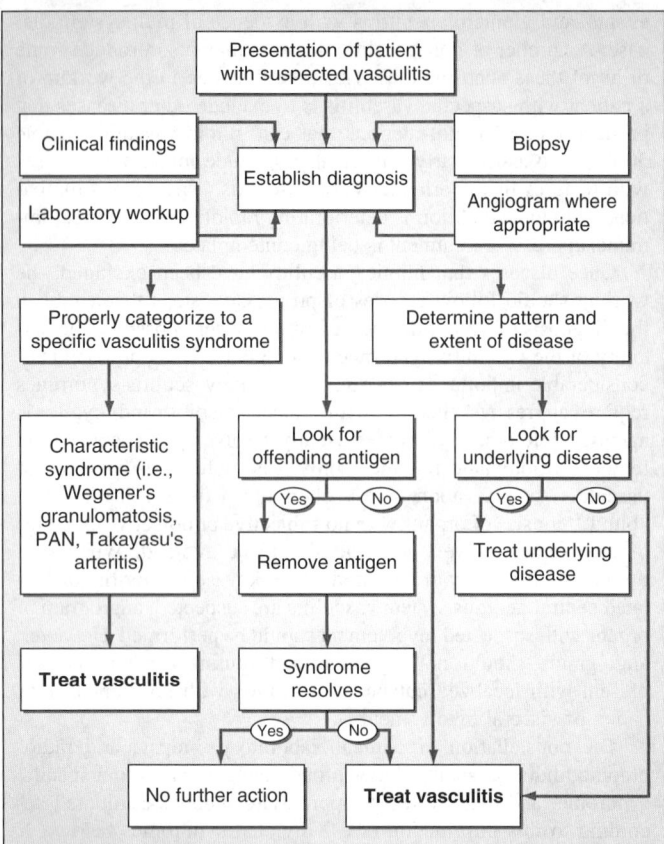

FIGURE 306-1 Algorithm for the approach to a patient with suspected diagnosis of vasculitis.

Treatment options will be considered under the individual syndromes (see below), and general principles of therapy will be considered at the end of the chapter.

WEGENER'S GRANULOMATOSIS

DEFINITION *Wegener's granulomatosis* is a distinct clinicopathologic entity characterized by granulomatous vasculitis of the upper and lower respiratory tracts together with glomerulonephritis. In addition, variable degrees of disseminated vasculitis involving both small arteries and veins may occur.

INCIDENCE AND PREVALENCE Wegener's granulomatosis is an uncommon disease with an estimated prevalence of 3 per 100,000. It is extremely rare in blacks compared with whites; the male-to-female ratio is 1:1. The disease can be seen at any age; approximately 15% of patients are <19 years of age, but only rarely does the disease occur before adolescence; the mean age of onset is approximately 40 years.

PATHOLOGY AND PATHOGENESIS The histopathologic hallmarks of Wegener's granulomatosis are necrotizing vasculitis of small arteries and veins together with granuloma formation, which may be either intravascular or extravascular (Fig. 306-2). Lung involvement typically appears as multiple, bilateral, nodular cavitary infiltrates (Fig. 306-3), which on biopsy almost invariably reveal the typical necrotizing granulomatous vasculitis. Upper airway lesions, particularly those in the sinuses and nasopharynx, typically reveal inflammation, necrosis, and granuloma formation, with or without vasculitis.

In its earliest form, renal involvement is characterized by a focal and segmental glomerulitis that may evolve into a rapidly progressive crescentic glomerulonephritis. Granuloma formation is only rarely seen on renal biopsy. In contrast to other forms of glomerulonephritis, evidence of immune complex deposition is not found in the renal lesion of Wegener's granulomatosis. In addition to the classic triad of

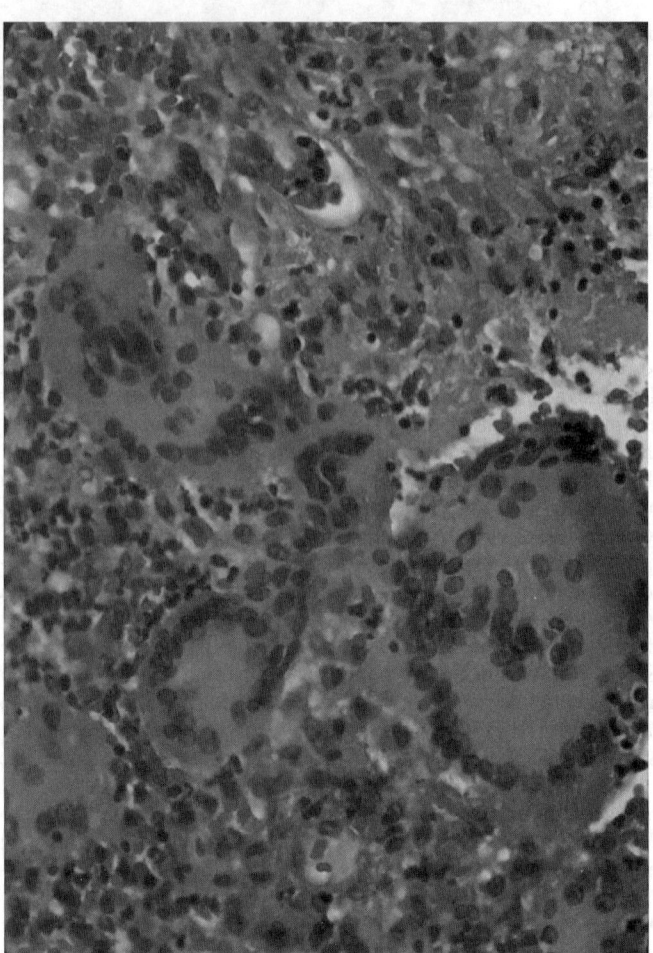

FIGURE 306-2 Lung biopsy in a patient with Wegener's granulomatosis. Biopsy revealed necrotizing vasculitis with granuloma formation. This section demonstrates several well-formed multinucleated giant cells in an area of granulomatous inflammation.

disease of the upper and lower respiratory tracts and kidney, virtually any organ can be involved with vasculitis, granuloma, or both.

The immunopathogenesis of this disease is unclear, although the involvement of upper airways and lungs with granulomatous vasculitis suggests an aberrant cell-mediated immune response to an exogenous or even endogenous antigen that enters through or resides in the upper airway. Chronic nasal carriage of *Staphylococcus aureus* has been reported to be associated with a higher relapse rate of Wegener's gran-

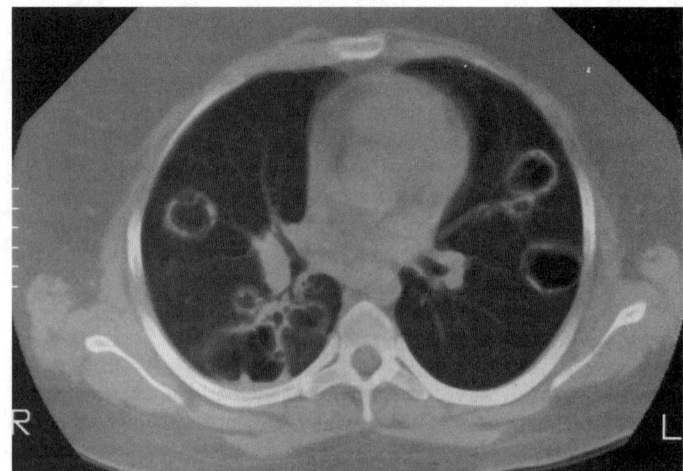

FIGURE 306-3 Computed tomography scan of a patient with Wegener's granulomatosis. The patient developed multiple, bilateral, and cavitary infiltrates.

ulomatosis; however, there is no evidence for a role of this organism in the pathogenesis of the disease.

Peripheral blood mononuclear cells obtained from patients with Wegener's granulomatosis manifest increased secretion of IFN-γ but not of IL-4, IL-5, or IL-10 compared to normal controls. In addition, TNF-α production from peripheral blood mononuclear cells and CD4+ T cells is elevated. Furthermore, monocytes from patients with Wegener's granulomatosis produce increased amounts of IL-12. These findings indicate an unbalanced T_H1-type T-cell cytokine pattern in this disease that may have pathogenic and perhaps ultimately therapeutic implications.

A high percentage of patients with Wegener's granulomatosis develop ANCA and these autoantibodies may play a role in the pathogenesis of this disease (see above).

CLINICAL AND LABORATORY MANIFESTATIONS Involvement of the upper airways occurs in 95% of patients with Wegener's granulomatosis. Patients often present with severe upper respiratory tract findings such as paranasal sinus pain and drainage and purulent or bloody nasal discharge, with or without nasal mucosal ulceration (Table 306-4). Nasal septal perforation may follow, leading to saddle nose deformity. Serous otitis media may occur as a result of eustachian tube blockage. Subglottic tracheal stenosis resulting from active disease or scarring occurs in approximately 16% of patients and may result in severe airway obstruction.

Pulmonary involvement may be manifested as asymptomatic infiltrates or may be clinically expressed as cough, hemoptysis, dyspnea, and chest discomfort. It is present in 85 to 90% of patients. Endo-

bronchial disease, either in its active form or as a result of fibrous scarring, may lead to obstruction with atelectasis.

Eye involvement (52% of patients) may range from a mild conjunctivitis to dacryocystitis, episcleritis, scleritis, granulomatous sclerouveitis, ciliary vessel vasculitis, and retroorbital mass lesions leading to proptosis.

Skin lesions (46% of patients) appear as papules, vesicles, palpable purpura, ulcers, or subcutaneous nodules; biopsy reveals vasculitis, granuloma, or both. Cardiac involvement (8% of patients) manifests as pericarditis, coronary vasculitis, or, rarely, cardiomyopathy. Nervous system manifestations (23% of patients) include cranial neuritis, mononeuritis multiplex, or, rarely, cerebral vasculitis and/or granuloma.

Renal disease (77% of patients) generally dominates the clinical picture and, if left untreated, accounts directly or indirectly for most of the mortality in this disease. Although it may smolder in some cases as a mild glomerulitis with proteinuria, hematuria, and red blood cell casts, it is clear that once clinically detectable renal functional impairment occurs, rapidly progressive renal failure usually ensues unless appropriate treatment is instituted.

While the disease is active, most patients have nonspecific symptoms and signs such as malaise, weakness, arthralgias, anorexia, and weight loss. Fever may indicate activity of the underlying disease but more often reflects secondary infection, usually of the upper airway.

Characteristic laboratory findings include a markedly elevated erythrocyte sedimentation rate (ESR), mild anemia and leukocytosis, mild hypergammaglobulinemia (particularly of the IgA class), and mildly elevated rheumatoid factor. Thrombocytosis may be seen as an acute-phase reactant. Approximately 90% of patients with active Wegener's granulomatosis have a positive antiproteinase-3 ANCA. However, in the absence of active disease, the sensitivity drops to approximately 60 to 70%. A small percentage of patients with Wegener's granulomatosis may have antimyeloperoxidase rather than antiproteinase-3 antibodies.

DIAGNOSIS The diagnosis of Wegener's granulomatosis is made by the demonstration of necrotizing granulomatous vasculitis on tissue biopsy in a patient with compatible clinical features. Pulmonary tissue offers the highest diagnostic yield, almost invariably revealing granulomatous vasculitis. Biopsy of upper airway tissue usually reveals granulomatous inflammation with necrosis but may not show vasculitis. Renal biopsy can confirm the presence of pauci-immune glomerulonephritis.

The specificity of a positive antiproteinase-3 ANCA for Wegener's granulomatosis is very high, especially if active glomerulonephritis is present. However, the presence of ANCA should be adjunctive and, with very rare exceptions, should not substitute for a tissue diagnosis. False-positive ANCA titers have been reported in certain infectious and neoplastic diseases.

In its typical presentation, the clinicopathologic complex of Wegener's granulomatosis usually provides ready differentiation from other disorders. However, if all the typical features are not present at once, it needs to be differentiated from the other vasculitides, Goodpasture's syndrome (Chap. 264), tumors of the upper airway or lung, and infectious diseases such as histoplasmosis (Chap. 183), mucocutaneous leishmaniasis (Chap. 196), and rhinoscleroma (Chap. 27) as well as noninfectious granulomatous diseases.

Of particular note is the differentiation from *midline granuloma* and *upper airway neoplasms*, which are part of the spectrum of *midline destructive diseases*. These diseases lead to extreme tissue destruction and mutilation localized to the midline upper airway structures including the sinuses; erosion through the skin of the face commonly occurs, a feature that is extremely rare in Wegener's granulomatosis. Although blood vessels may be involved in the intense inflammatory reaction and necrosis, primary vasculitis is seen rarely. When systemic involvement occurs, it usually declares itself as a neoplastic process.

TABLE 306-4 *Wegener's Granulomatosis: Frequency of Clinical Manifestations in 158 Patients Studied at the National Institutes of Health*

Manifestation	Percent at Disease Onset	Percent Throughout Course of Disease
Kidney		
Glomerulonephritis	18	77
Ear/nose/throat	73	92
Sinusitis	51	85
Nasal disease	36	68
Otitis media	25	44
Hearing loss	14	42
Subglottic stenosis	1	16
Ear pain	9	14
Oral lesions	3	10
Lung	45	85
Pulmonary infiltrates	25	66
Pulmonary nodules	24	58
Hemoptysis	12	30
Pleuritis	10	28
Eyes		
Conjunctivitis	5	18
Dacryocystitis	1	18
Scleritis	6	16
Proptosis	2	15
Eye pain	3	11
Visual loss	0	8
Retinal lesions	0	4
Corneal lesions	0	1
Iritis	0	2
Other[a]		
Arthralgias/arthritis	32	67
Fever	23	50
Cough	19	46
Skin abnormalities	13	46
Weight loss (>10% body weight)	15	35
Peripheral neuropathy	1	15
Central nervous system disease	1	8
Pericarditis	2	6
Hyperthyroidism	1	3

[a] Fewer than 1% had parotid, pulmonary artery, breast, or lower genitourinary (urethra, cervix, vagina, testicular) involvement.
Source: Hoffman et al.

In this regard, it is likely that midline granuloma is part of the spectrum of *angiocentric immunoproliferative lesions*. The latter are considered to represent a spectrum of postthymic T cell proliferative lesions and should be treated as such (Chap. 97). The term *idiopathic* has been applied to midline granuloma when extensive diagnostic workup including multiple biopsies has failed to reveal anything other than inflammation and necrosis. Under these circumstances, it is possible that the tumor cells were masked by the intensive inflammatory response. Such cases have responded to local irradiation with 50 Gy (5000 rad). Upper airway lesions should never be irradiated in Wegener's granulomatosis.

Wegener's granulomatosis must also be differentiated from *lymphomatoid granulomatosis*, which is an Epstein-Barr virus–positive B cell proliferation that is associated with an exuberant T cell reaction. Lymphomatoid granulomatosis is characterized by lung, skin, central nervous system, and kidney involvement in which atypical lymphocytoid and plasmacytoid cells infiltrate nonlymphoid tissue in an angioinvasive manner. In this regard, it clearly differs from Wegener's granulomatosis in that it is not an inflammatory vasculitis in the classic sense but an infiltration of vessels with atypical mononuclear cells; granuloma may be present in involved tissues. Up to 50% of patients may develop a true malignant lymphoma.

℞ TREATMENT

Wegener's granulomatosis was formerly universally fatal, usually within a few months after the onset of clinically apparent renal disease. Glucocorticoids alone led to some symptomatic improvement, with little effect on the ultimate course of the disease. It has been well established that the most effective therapy in this disease is cyclophosphamide given in doses of 2 mg/kg per day orally together with glucocorticoids. The leukocyte count should be monitored closely during therapy, and the dosage of cyclophosphamide should be adjusted in order to maintain the count above $3000/\mu L$, which generally maintains the neutrophil count at approximately $1500/\mu L$. With this approach, clinical remission can usually be induced and maintained without causing severe leukopenia with its associated risk of infection. As it was originally studied, cyclophosphamide was continued for 1 year following the induction of complete remission and gradually tapered and discontinued thereafter.

At the initiation of therapy, glucocorticoids should be administered together with cyclophosphamide. This can be given as prednisone, 1 mg/kg per day initially (for the first month of therapy) as a daily regimen, with gradual conversion to an alternate-day schedule followed by tapering and discontinuation after approximately 6 months.

Using the above regimen, the prognosis of this disease is excellent; marked improvement is seen in >90% of patients, and complete remissions are achieved in 75% of patients. A number of patients who developed irreversible renal failure but who achieved subsequent remission on appropriate therapy have undergone successful renal transplantation.

Despite the dramatic remissions induced by the therapeutic regimen described above, long-term follow-up of patients has revealed that approximately 50% of remissions are later associated with one or more relapses. Reinduction of remission is almost always achieved; however, a high percentage of patients ultimately have some degree of morbidity from irreversible features of their disease, such as varying degrees of renal insufficiency, hearing loss, tracheal stenosis, saddle nose deformity, and chronically impaired sinus function. The determination of relapse should be based on objective evidence of disease activity taking care to rule out other features that may have a similar appearance such as infection, medication toxicity, or chronic disease sequelae. The ANCA titer can be misleading. Many patients who achieve remission continue to have elevated titers for years. In addition, one study found that >40% of patients who were in remission and had a fourfold increase in ANCA titer did not have a relapse in

disease. Patients who relapse may not do so until many months or years after the rise in ANCA titer. Thus, a rise in ANCA titer by itself is not a harbinger of immediate disease relapse and should not lead to reinstitution or increase in immunosuppressive therapy. However, such a finding should prompt the clinician to examine the patient carefully for any objective evidence of active disease and to monitor that patient closely.

Certain types of morbidity are related to toxic side effects of treatment. Glucocorticoid-related side effects can include diabetes mellitus, cataracts, life-threatening infectious disease complications, serious osteoporosis, and severe cushingoid features. The risk of such toxicities can be reduced with the use of an alternate-day glucocorticoid regimen as outlined in the preceding regimen. Cyclophosphamide-related toxicities are more frequent and severe. Cystitis to varying degrees occurs in at least 30% of patients, bladder cancer in 6%, myelodysplasia in 2%, and there is a high risk of permanent infertility in both men and women.

Some reports have indicated therapeutic success with less frequent and severe toxic side effects using intermittent boluses of intravenous cyclophosphamide (1 g/m^2 per month) in place of daily administration. However, we and others have found an increased rate of relapse with bolus intravenous cyclophosphamide. We therefore strongly recommend that the drug be given as daily oral therapy.

In patients with immediately life-threatening disease, such as rapidly progressive glomerulonephritis, a regimen of daily cyclophosphamide and glucocorticoids is clearly the treatment of choice to induce remission. However, after patients have achieved remission, consideration can be given to stopping cyclophosphamide and beginning methotrexate or azathioprine for remission maintenance. This approach is aimed at lessening the toxicity associated with chronic cyclophosphamide therapy. Methotrexate is administered orally starting at a dosage of 0.3 mg/kg as a single weekly dose, not to exceed 15 mg/week. If the treatment is well tolerated after 1 to 2 weeks, the dosage should be increased by 2.5 mg weekly up to a dosage of 20 to 25 mg/week and maintained at that level. This regimen is given for 2 years past remission, after which time it is tapered by 2.5 mg each month until discontinuation. To lessen toxicity, methotrexate is often given together with folic acid, 1 mg daily, or folinic acid, 5 to 10 mg once a week 24 h following methotrexate. Azathioprine, 2 mg/kg per day, has also proven effective in some patients in maintaining remission following induction with daily cyclophosphamide. There have been no studies to date comparing methotrexate to azathioprine for remission maintenance. In the absence of such data, the choice of agent is often based on toxicity profile, as methotrexate cannot be given to patients with renal insufficiency or chronic liver disease.

For selected patients whose disease is not immediately life threatening or in those patients who have experienced significant cyclophosphamide toxicity, methotrexate together with glucocorticoids given at the dosages described above may be considered as an alternative for initial therapy.

Although certain reports have indicated that trimethoprim-sulfamethoxazole (TMP-SMX) may be of benefit in the treatment of Wegener's granulomatosis, there are no firm data to substantiate this, particularly in patients with serious renal and pulmonary disease. In a study examining the effect of trimethoprim-sulfamethoxazole on relapse, decreased relapses were shown only with regard to upper airway disease, and no differences in major organ relapses were observed. Trimethoprim-sulfamethoxazole alone should never be used to treat active Wegener's granulomatosis outside of the upper airway.

Not all manifestations of Wegener's granulomatosis require or respond to cytotoxic therapy. In managing non-major organ disease, such as that isolated to the sinus, joints, or skin, the risks of treatment should be carefully weighed against the benefits. Given the potential toxicities of this agent, treatment with cyclophosphamide is rarely if ever justified for the treatment of isolated sinus disease in Wegener's granulomatosis. Although patients with non-major organ disease may be effectively treated without cytotoxic therapy, these individuals must be monitored closely for the development of disease activity affecting the lungs, kidneys, or other major organs. Subglottic tracheal stenosis and endobronchial stenosis are examples of disease manifestations that do not typically respond to systemic immunosuppressive treatment.

CHURG-STRAUSS SYNDROME

DEFINITION Churg-Strauss syndrome, also referred to as *allergic angiitis and granulomatosis*, was described in 1951 by Churg and Strauss and is characterized by asthma, peripheral and tissue eosinophilia, extravascular granuloma formation, and vasculitis of multiple organ systems.

INCIDENCE AND PREVALENCE Churg-Strauss syndrome is an uncommon disease with an estimated annual incidence of 1 to 3 per million. The disease can occur at any age with the possible exception of infants. The mean age of onset is 48 years, with a female-to-male ratio of 1.2:1.

PATHOLOGY AND PATHOGENESIS The necrotizing vasculitis of Churg-Strauss syndrome involves small and medium-sized muscular arteries, capillaries, veins, and venules. A characteristic histopathologic feature of Churg-Strauss syndrome are granulomatous reactions that may be present in the tissues or even within the walls of the vessels themselves. These are usually associated with infiltration of the tissues with eosinophils. This process can occur in any organ in the body; lung involvement is predominant, with skin, cardiovascular system, kidney, peripheral nervous system, and gastrointestinal tract also commonly involved. Although the precise pathogenesis of this disease is uncertain, its strong association with asthma and its clinicopathologic manifestations, including eosinophilia, granuloma, and vasculitis, point to aberrant immunologic phenomena.

CLINICAL AND LABORATORY MANIFESTATIONS Patients with Churg-Strauss syndrome often exhibit nonspecific manifestations such as fever, malaise, anorexia, and weight loss, which are characteristic of a multisystem disease. The pulmonary findings in Churg-Strauss syndrome clearly dominate the clinical picture with severe asthmatic attacks and the presence of pulmonary infiltrates. Mononeuritis multiplex is the second most common manifestation and occurs in up to 72% of patients. Allergic rhinitis and sinusitis develop in up to 61% of patients and are often observed early in the course of disease. Clinically recognizable heart disease occurs in approximately 14% of patients and is an important cause of mortality. Skin lesions occur in approximately 51% of patients and include purpura in addition to cutaneous and subcutaneous nodules. The renal disease in Churg-Strauss syndrome is less common and generally less severe than that of Wegener's granulomatosis and microscopic polyangiitis.

The characteristic laboratory finding in virtually all patients with Churg-Strauss syndrome is a striking eosinophilia, which reaches levels >1000 cells/μL in >80% of patients. Evidence of inflammation as evidenced by elevated ESR, fibrinogen, or α_2-globulins can be found in 81% of patients. The other laboratory findings reflect the organ systems involved. Approximately 48% of patients with Churg-Strauss syndrome have circulating ANCA that is usually antimyeloperoxidase.

DIAGNOSIS Although the diagnosis of Churg-Strauss syndrome is optimally made by biopsy in a patient with the characteristic clinical manifestations (see above), histologic confirmation can be challenging as the pathognomonic features often do not occur simultaneously. In order to be diagnosed with Churg-Strauss syndrome, a patient should have evidence of asthma, peripheral blood eosinophilia, and clinical features consistent with vasculitis.

Rx TREATMENT

The prognosis of untreated Churg-Strauss syndrome is poor, with a reported 5-year survival of 25%. With treatment, prognosis is favorable, with one study finding a 78-month actuarial survival rate of 72%. Myocardial involvement is the most frequent cause of death and is responsible for 39% of patient mortality. Glucocorticoids alone appear to be effective in many patients. Dosage tapering is often limited by

asthma, and many patients require low-dose prednisone for persistent asthma many years after clinical recovery from vasculitis. In glucocorticoid failure or in patients who present with fulminant multisystem disease, the treatment of choice is a combined regimen of daily cyclophosphamide and prednisone (see "Wegener's Granulomatosis" for a detailed description of this therapeutic regimen).

POLYARTERITIS NODOSA

DEFINITION *Polyarteritis nodosa* (PAN), also referred to as *classic PAN*, was described in 1866 by Kussmaul and Maier. It is a multisystem, necrotizing vasculitis of small and medium-sized muscular arteries in which involvement of the renal and visceral arteries is characteristic. PAN does not involve pulmonary arteries, although bronchial vessels may be involved; granulomas, significant eosinophilia, and an allergic diathesis are not observed.

INCIDENCE AND PREVALENCE It is difficult to establish an accurate incidence of PAN because previous reports have included PAN and microscopic polyangiitis as well as other related vasculitides. PAN as currently defined, is felt to be a very uncommon disease.

PATHOLOGY AND PATHOGENESIS The vascular lesion in PAN is a necrotizing inflammation of small and medium-sized muscular arteries. The lesions are segmental and tend to involve bifurcations and branchings of arteries. They may spread circumferentially to involve adjacent veins. However, involvement of venules is not seen in PAN and, if present, suggests microscopic polyangiitis (see below). In the acute stages of disease, polymorphonuclear neutrophils infiltrate all layers of the vessel wall and perivascular areas, which results in intimal proliferation and degeneration of the vessel wall. Mononuclear cells infiltrate the area as the lesions progress to the subacute and chronic stages. Fibrinoid necrosis of the vessels ensues with compromise of the lumen, thrombosis, infarction of the tissues supplied by the involved vessel, and, in some cases, hemorrhage. As the lesions heal, there is collagen deposition, which may lead to further occlusion of the vessel lumen. Aneurysmal dilatations up to 1 cm in size along the involved arteries are characteristic of PAN. Granulomas and substantial eosinophilia with eosinophilic tissue infiltrations are not characteristically found and suggest Churg-Strauss syndrome (see above).

Multiple organ systems are involved, and the clinicopathologic findings reflect the degree and location of vessel involvement and the resulting ischemic changes. As mentioned above, pulmonary arteries are not involved in PAN, and bronchial artery involvement is uncommon. The pathology in the kidney in classic PAN is that of arteritis without glomerulonephritis. In patients with significant hypertension, typical pathologic features of glomerulosclerosis may be seen alone or superimposed on lesions of glomerulonephritis. In addition, pathologic sequelae of hypertension may be found elsewhere in the body.

The presence of hepatitis B antigenemia in approximately 10 to 30% of patients with systemic vasculitis, particularly of the PAN type, together with the isolation of circulating immune complexes composed of hepatitis B antigen and immunoglobulin, and the demonstration by immunofluorescence of hepatitis B antigen, IgM, and complement in the blood vessel walls, strongly suggest the role of immunologic phenomena in the pathogenesis of this disease. Hairy cell leukemia can be associated with PAN; the pathogenic mechanisms of this association are unclear.

CLINICAL AND LABORATORY MANIFESTATIONS Nonspecific signs and symptoms are the hallmarks of PAN. Fever, weight loss, and malaise are present in over one-half of cases. Patients usually present with vague symptoms such as weakness, malaise, headache, abdominal pain, and myalgias that can rapidly progress to a fulminant illness. Specific complaints related to the vascular involvement within a particular organ system may also dominate the presenting clinical picture as well as the entire course of the illness (Table 306-5). In PAN, renal involvement most commonly manifests as hypertension, renal insufficiency, or hemorrhage due to microaneurysms.

TABLE 306-5 *Clinical Manifestations Related to Organ System Involvement in Classic Polyarteritis Nodosa*

Organ System	Percent Incidence	Clinical Manifestations
Renal	60	Renal failure, hypertension
Musculoskeletal	64	Arthritis, arthralgia, myalgia
Peripheral nervous system	51	Peripheral neuropathy, mononeuritis multiplex
Gastrointestinal tract	44	Abdominal pain, nausea and vomiting, bleeding, bowel infarction and perforation, cholecystitis, hepatic infarction, pancreatic infarction
Skin	43	Rash, purpura, nodules, cutaneous infarcts, livedo reticularis, Raynaud's phenomenon
Cardiac	36	Congestive heart failure, myocardial infarction, pericarditis
Genitourinary	25	Testicular, ovarian, or epididymal pain
Central nervous system	23	Cerebral vascular accident, altered mental status, seizure

Source: From TR Cupps, AS Fauci: *The Vasculitides*. Philadelphia, Saunders, 1981.

There are no diagnostic serologic tests for PAN. In >75% of patients, the leukocyte count is elevated with a predominance of neutrophils. Eosinophilia is seen only rarely and, when present at high levels, suggests the diagnosis of Churg-Strauss syndrome. The anemia of chronic disease may be seen, and an elevated ESR is almost always present. Other common laboratory findings reflect the particular organ involved. Hypergammaglobulinemia may be present, and up to 30% of patients have a positive test for hepatitis B surface antigen. Antibodies against myeloperoxidase or proteinase-3 (ANCA) are rarely found in patients with PAN.

DIAGNOSIS   The diagnosis of PAN is based on the demonstration of characteristic findings of vasculitis on biopsy material of involved organs. In the absence of easily accessible tissue for biopsy, the angiographic demonstration of involved vessels, particularly in the form of aneurysms of small and medium-sized arteries in the renal, hepatic, and visceral vasculature, is sufficient to make the diagnosis. Aneurysms of vessels are not pathognomonic of PAN; furthermore, aneurysms need not always be present, and angiographic findings may be limited to stenotic segments and obliteration of vessels. Biopsy of symptomatic organs such as nodular skin lesions, painful testes, and nerve/muscle provides the highest diagnostic yields.

℞ TREATMENT

The prognosis of untreated PAN is extremely poor, with a reported 5-year survival rate between 10 and 20%. Death usually results from gastrointestinal complications, particularly bowel infarcts and perforation, and cardiovascular causes. Intractable hypertension often compounds dysfunction in other organ systems, such as the kidneys, heart, and central nervous system, leading to additional late morbidity and mortality in PAN. With the introduction of treatment, survival rate has increased substantially. Favorable therapeutic results have been reported in PAN with the combination of prednisone and cyclophosphamide (see "Wegener's Granulomatosis" for a detailed description of this therapeutic regimen). In less severe cases of PAN, glucocorticoids alone have resulted in disease remission. Favorable results have also been reported in the treatment of PAN related to hepatitis B virus with IFN-α in combination with glucocorticoids and plasma exchange. Careful attention to the treatment of hypertension can lessen the acute and late morbidity and mortality associated with renal, cardiac, and central nervous system complications of PAN. Following successful treatment, relapse of PAN has been estimated to occur in only 10% of patients.

MICROSCOPIC POLYANGIITIS

DEFINITION   The term *microscopic polyarteritis* was introduced into the literature by Davson in 1948 in recognition of the presence of glomerulonephritis in patients with PAN. In 1992, the Chapel Hill Consensus Conference on the Nomenclature of Systemic Vasculitis adopted the term *microscopic polyangiitis* to connote a necrotizing vasculitis with few or no immune complexes affecting small vessels (capillaries, venules, or arterioles). Glomerulonephritis is very common in microscopic polyangiitis, and pulmonary capillaritis often occurs. The absence of granulomatous inflammation in microscopic polyangiitis is said to differentiate it from Wegener's granulomatosis.

INCIDENCE AND PREVALENCE   The incidence of microscopic polyangiitis has not yet been reliably established due to its previous inclusion as part of PAN. The mean age of onset is approximately 57 years of age, and males are slightly more frequently affected than females.

PATHOLOGY AND PATHOGENESIS   The vascular lesion in microscopic polyangiitis is histologically similar to that in PAN. Unlike PAN, the vasculitis seen in microscopic polyangiitis has a predilection to involve capillaries and venules in addition to small and medium-sized arteries. Immunohistochemical staining reveals a paucity of immunoglobulin deposition in the vascular lesion of microscopic polyangiitis, suggesting that immune complex formation does not play a role in the pathogenesis of this syndrome. The renal lesion seen in microscopic polyangiitis is identical to that of Wegener's granulomatosis. Like Wegener's granulomatosis, microscopic polyangiitis is highly associated with the presence of ANCA, which may play a role in pathogenesis of this syndrome (see above).

CLINICAL AND LABORATORY MANIFESTATIONS   Because of its predilection to involve the small vessels, microscopic polyangiitis and Wegener's granulomatosis share similar clinical features. Disease onset may be gradual with initial symptoms of fever, weight loss, and musculoskeletal pain; however, it is often acute. Glomerulonephritis occurs in at least 79% of patients and can be rapidly progressive, leading to renal failure. Hemoptysis may be the first symptom of alveolar hemorrhage, which occurs in 12% of patients. Other manifestations include mononeuritis multiplex and gastrointestinal tract and cutaneous vasculitis. Upper airways disease and pulmonary nodules are not typically found in microscopic polyangiitis and, if present, suggest Wegener's granulomatosis.

Features of inflammation may be seen, including an elevated ESR, anemia, leukocytosis, and thrombocytosis. ANCA are present in 75% of patients with microscopic polyangiitis, with antimyeloperoxidase antibodies being the predominant ANCA associated with this disease.

DIAGNOSIS   The diagnosis is based on histologic evidence of vasculitis or pauci-immune glomerulonephritis in a patient with compatible clinical features of multisystem disease. Although microscopic polyangiitis is strongly ANCA-associated, no studies have as yet established the sensitivity and specificity of ANCA in this disease.

℞ TREATMENT

The 5-year survival rate for patients with treated microscopic polyangiitis is 74% with disease-related mortality occurring from alveolar hemorrhage or gastrointestinal, cardiac, or renal disease. To date there has been limited disease-specific information on the treatment of microscopic polyangiitis. Available data together with a predilection for this disease to affect the small vessels support a therapeutic approach similar to that used in Wegener's granulomatosis. Patients with immediately life-threatening disease should be treated with the combination of prednisone and daily cyclophosphamide (see "Wegener's Granulomatosis" for a detailed description of this therapeutic regimen). Disease relapse has been observed in at least 34% of patients. Treatment for such relapses would be similar to that used at the time of initial presentation and based upon site and severity of disease.

GIANT CELL ARTERITIS

DEFINITION   *Giant cell arteritis*, also referred to as *cranial arteritis* or *temporal arteritis*, is an inflammation of medium- and large-sized arteries. It characteristically involves one or more branches of the carotid artery, particularly the temporal artery. However, it is a systemic disease that can involve arteries in multiple locations.

INCIDENCE AND PREVALENCE Giant cell arteritis occurs almost exclusively in individuals >50 years. It is more common in women than in men and is rare in blacks. The incidence of giant cell arteritis varies widely in different studies and in different geographic regions. A high incidence has been found in Scandinavia and in regions of the United States with large Scandinavian populations, compared to a lower incidence in southern Europe. The annual incidence rates in individuals ≥50 years range from 6.9 to 32.8 per 100,000 population. Familial aggregation has been reported, as has an association with HLA-DR4. In addition, genetic linkage studies have demonstrated an association of temporal arteritis with alleles at the HLA-DRB1 locus, particularly HLA-DRB1*04 variants. The disease is closely associated with *polymyalgia rheumatica*, which is more common than giant cell arteritis. In Olmsted County, Minnesota, the annual incidence of polymyalgia rheumatica in individuals ≥50 years is 58.7 per 100,000 population.

PATHOLOGY AND PATHOGENESIS Although the temporal artery is most frequently involved in this disease, patients often have a systemic vasculitis of multiple medium- and large-sized arteries, which may go undetected. Histopathologically, the disease is a panarteritis with inflammatory mononuclear cell infiltrates within the vessel wall with frequent giant cell formation. There is proliferation of the intima and fragmentation of the internal elastic lamina. Pathophysiologic findings in organs result from the ischemia related to the involved vessels. Distinct cytokine patterns as well as T lymphocytes expressing specific antigen receptors have been described, suggesting the involvement of immunopathogenic mechanisms in temporal arteritis. IL-6 and IL-1β expression have been detected in a majority of circulating monocytes of patients with temporal arteritis and polymyalgia rheumatica. T cells recruited to vasculitic lesions in patients with temporal arteritis produce predominantly IL-2 and IFN-γ, and the latter has been suggested to be involved in the progression to overt arteritis. Sequence analysis of the T cell receptor of tissue-infiltrating T cells in lesions of temporal arteritis indicates restricted clonal expansion, suggesting that an antigen residing in the arterial wall is recognized by a small fraction of T cells.

CLINICAL AND LABORATORY MANIFESTATIONS The disease is characterized clinically by the complex of fever, anemia, high ESR, and headaches in a patient over the age of 50 years. Other manifestations include malaise, fatigue, anorexia, weight loss, sweats, and arthralgias. The polymyalgia rheumatica syndrome is characterized by stiffness, aching, and pain in the muscles of the neck, shoulders, lower back, hips, and thighs.

In patients with involvement of the temporal artery, headache is the predominant symptom and may be associated with a tender, thickened, or nodular artery, which may pulsate early in the disease but may become occluded later. Scalp pain and claudication of the jaw and tongue may occur. A well-recognized and dreaded complication of giant cell arteritis, particularly in untreated patients, is ischemic optic neuropathy, which may lead to serious visual symptoms, even sudden blindness in some patients. However, most patients have complaints relating to the head or eyes before visual loss. Attention to such symptoms with institution of appropriate therapy (see below) will usually avoid this complication. Claudication of the extremities, strokes, myocardial infarctions, and infarctions of visceral organs have been reported. Of note, giant cell arteritis is associated with an increased risk of aortic aneurysm, which is usually a late complication and may lead to dissection and death.

Characteristic laboratory findings in addition to the elevated ESR include a normochromic or slightly hypochromic anemia. Liver function abnormalities are common, particularly increased alkaline phosphatase levels. Increased levels of IgG and complement have been reported. Levels of enzymes indicative of muscle damage such as serum creatine kinase are not elevated.

DIAGNOSIS The diagnosis of giant cell arteritis and its associated clinicopathologic syndrome can often be suggested clinically by the demonstration of the complex of fever, anemia, and high ESR with or without symptoms of polymyalgia rheumatica in a patient >50 years. The diagnosis is confirmed by biopsy of the temporal artery. Since involvement of the vessel may be segmental, positive yield is increased by obtaining a biopsy segment of 3 to 5 cm together with serial sectioning of biopsy specimens. Ultrasonography of the temporal artery has been reported to be helpful in diagnosis. A temporal artery biopsy should be obtained as quickly as possible in the setting of ocular signs and symptoms, and under these circumstances therapy should not be delayed pending a biopsy. In this regard, it has been reported that temporal artery biopsies may show vasculitis even after more than 14 days of glucocorticoid therapy. A dramatic clinical response to a trial of glucocorticoid therapy can further support the diagnosis.

℞ TREATMENT

Disease-related mortality from giant cell arteritis is very uncommon with fatalities occurring from cerebrovascular events, myocardial infarction, or aortic aneurysms. The goals of treatment are to reduce symptoms and, most importantly, to prevent visual loss. Giant cell arteritis and its associated symptoms are exquisitely sensitive to glucocorticoid therapy. Treatment should begin with prednisone, 40 to 60 mg/d for approximately 1 month, followed by a gradual tapering. When ocular signs and symptoms occur, it is important that therapy be initiated or adjusted to control them. Although the optimal duration of glucocorticoid therapy has not been established, most series have found that patients require treatment for ≥2 years. The ESR can serve as a useful indicator of inflammatory disease activity in monitoring and tapering therapy and can be used to judge the pace of the tapering schedule. However, minor increases in the ESR can occur as glucocorticoids are being tapered and do not necessarily reflect an exacerbation of arteritis, particularly if the patient remains symptom-free. Under these circumstances, the tapering should continue with caution. Glucocorticoid toxicity occurs in 35 to 65% of patients and represents an important cause of patient morbidity. The use of weekly methotrexate as a glucocorticoid-sparing agent has been examined in two randomized placebo-controlled trials that reached conflicting conclusions.

TAKAYASU'S ARTERITIS

DEFINITION *Takayasu's arteritis* is an inflammatory and stenotic disease of medium- and large-sized arteries characterized by a strong predilection for the aortic arch and its branches. For this reason, it is often referred to as the *aortic arch syndrome*.

INCIDENCE AND PREVALENCE Takayasu's arteritis is an uncommon disease with an estimated annual incidence rate of 1.2 to 2.6 cases per million. It is most prevalent in adolescent girls and young women. Although it is more common in Asia, it is neither racially nor geographically restricted.

PATHOLOGY AND PATHOGENESIS The disease involves medium- and large-sized arteries, with a strong predilection for the aortic arch and its branches; the pulmonary artery may also be involved. The most commonly affected arteries seen by angiography are listed in Table 306-6. The involvement of the major branches of the aorta is much more marked at their origin than distally. The disease is a panarteritis with inflammatory mononuclear cell infiltrates and occasionally giant cells. There are marked intimal proliferation and fibrosis, scarring and vascularization of the media, and disruption and degeneration of the elastic lamina. Narrowing of the lumen occurs with or without thrombosis. The vasa vasorum are frequently involved. Pathologic changes in various organs reflect the compromise of blood flow through the involved vessels.

Immunopathogenic mechanisms, the precise nature of which is uncertain, are suspected in this disease. As with several of the vasculitis

TABLE 306-6 *Frequency of Arteriographic Abnormalities and Potential Clinical Manifestations of Arterial Involvement in Takayasu's Arteritis*

Artery	Percent of Arteriographic Abnormalities	Potential Clinical Manifestations
Subclavian	93	Arm claudication, Raynaud's phenomenon
Common carotid	58	Visual changes, syncope, transient ischemic attacks, stroke
Abdominal aorta[a]	47	Abdominal pain, nausea, vomiting
Renal	38	Hypertension, renal failure
Aortic arch or root	35	Aortic insufficiency, congestive heart failure
Vertebral	35	Visual changes, dizziness
Coeliac axis[a]	18	Abdominal pain, nausea, vomiting
Superior mesenteric[a]	18	Abdominal pain, nausea, vomiting
Iliac	17	Leg claudication
Pulmonary	10–40	Atypical chest pain, dyspnea
Coronary	<10	Chest pain, myocardial infarction

[a] Arteriographic lesions at these locations are usually asymptomatic but may potentially cause these symptoms.
Source: Kerr et al.

syndromes, circulating immune complexes have been demonstrated, but their pathogenic significance is unclear.

CLINICAL AND LABORATORY MANIFESTATIONS Takayasu's arteritis is a systemic disease with generalized as well as vascular symptoms. The generalized symptoms include malaise, fever, night sweats, arthralgias, anorexia, and weight loss, which may occur months before vessel involvement is apparent. These symptoms may merge into those related to vascular compromise and organ ischemia. Pulses are commonly absent in the involved vessels, particularly the subclavian artery. The frequency of arteriographic abnormalities and the potentially associated clinical manifestations are listed in Table 306-6. Hypertension occurs in 32 to 93% of patients and contributes to renal, cardiac, and cerebral injury.

Characteristic laboratory findings include an elevated ESR, mild anemia, and elevated immunoglobulin levels.

DIAGNOSIS The diagnosis of Takayasu's arteritis should be suspected strongly in a young woman who develops a decrease or absence of peripheral pulses, discrepancies in blood pressure, and arterial bruits. The diagnosis is confirmed by the characteristic pattern on arteriography, which includes irregular vessel walls, stenosis, poststenotic dilatation, aneurysm formation, occlusion, and evidence of increased collateral circulation. Complete aortic arteriography should be obtained, unless this is renally contraindicated, in order to fully delineate the distribution and degree of arterial disease. Histopathologic demonstration of inflamed vessels adds confirmatory data; however, tissue is rarely readily available for examination.

Rx TREATMENT

The long-term outcome of patients with Takayasu's arteritis has varied widely between studies. Although two North American reports found overall survival to be ≥94%, or the 5-year mortality rate from other studies has ranged from 0 to 35%. Disease-related mortality most often occurs from congestive heart failure, cerebrovascular events, myocardial infarction, aneurysm rupture, or renal failure. Even in the absence of life-threatening disease Takayasu's arteritis can be associated with significant morbidity. The course of the disease is variable, and although spontaneous remissions may occur, Takayasu's arteritis is most often chronic and relapsing. Although glucocorticoid therapy in doses of 40 to 60 mg prednisone per day alleviates symptoms, there are no convincing studies that indicate that they increase survival. The combination of glucocorticoid therapy for acute signs and symptoms and an aggressive surgical and/or angioplastic approach to stenosed vessels has markedly improved outcome and decreased morbidity by lessening

the risk of stroke, correcting hypertension due to renal artery stenosis, and improving blood flow to ischemic viscera and limbs. Unless it is urgently required, surgical correction of stenosed arteries should be undertaken only when the vascular inflammatory process is well controlled with medical therapy. In individuals who are refractory to or unable to taper glucocorticoids, methotrexate in doses up to 25 mg per week has yielded encouraging results.

HENOCH-SCHÖNLEIN PURPURA

DEFINITION *Henoch-Schönlein purpura*, also referred to as *anaphylactoid purpura*, is a distinct systemic vasculitis syndrome that is characterized by palpable purpura (most commonly distributed over the buttocks and lower extremities), arthralgias, gastrointestinal signs and symptoms, and glomerulonephritis. It is a small-vessel vasculitis.

INCIDENCE AND PREVALENCE Henoch-Schönlein purpura is usually seen in children; most patients range in age from 4 to 7 years; however, the disease may also be seen in infants and adults. It is not a rare disease; in one series it accounted for between 5 and 24 admissions per year at a pediatric hospital. The male-to-female ratio is 1.5:1. A seasonal variation with a peak incidence in spring has been noted.

PATHOLOGY AND PATHOGENESIS The presumptive pathogenic mechanism for Henoch-Schönlein purpura is immune-complex deposition. A number of inciting antigens have been suggested including upper respiratory tract infections, various drugs, foods, insect bites, and immunizations. IgA is the antibody class most often seen in the immune complexes and has been demonstrated in the renal biopsies of these patients.

CLINICAL AND LABORATORY MANIFESTATIONS In pediatric patients, palpable purpura is seen in virtually all patients; most patients develop polyarthralgias in the absence of frank arthritis. Gastrointestinal involvement, which is seen in almost 70% of pediatric patients, is characterized by colicky abdominal pain usually associated with nausea, vomiting, diarrhea, or constipation and is frequently accompanied by the passage of blood and mucus per rectum; bowel intussusception may occur. Renal involvement occurs in 10 to 50% of patients and is usually characterized by mild glomerulonephritis leading to proteinuria and microscopic hematuria, with red blood cell casts in the majority of patients (Chap. 264); it usually resolves spontaneously without therapy. Rarely, a progressive glomerulonephritis will develop. In adults, presenting symptoms are most frequently related to the skin and joints, while initial complaints related to the gut are less common. Although certain studies have found that renal disease is more frequent and more severe in adults, this has not been a consistent finding. However, the course of renal disease in adults may be more insidious and thus requires close follow-up. Myocardial involvement can occur in adults but is rare in children.

Laboratory studies generally show a mild leukocytosis, a normal platelet count, and occasionally eosinophilia. Serum complement components are normal, and IgA levels are elevated in about one-half of patients.

DIAGNOSIS The diagnosis of Henoch-Schönlein purpura is based on clinical signs and symptoms. Skin biopsy specimen can be useful in confirming leukocytoclastic vasculitis with IgA and C3 deposition by immunofluorescence. Renal biopsy is rarely needed for diagnosis but may provide prognostic information in some patients.

Rx TREATMENT

The prognosis of Henoch-Schönlein purpura is excellent. Mortality is exceedingly rare, and 1 to 5% of children progress to end-stage renal disease. Most patients recover completely, and some do not require therapy. Treatment is similar for adults and children. When glucocorticoid therapy is required, prednisone, in doses of 1 mg/kg per day and tapered according to clinical response, has been shown to be useful in decreasing tissue edema, arthralgias, and abdominal discomfort; however, it has not proven beneficial in the treatment of skin or renal disease and does not appear to shorten the duration of active disease or lessen the chance of recurrence. Patients with rapidly progressive glomerulonephritis have been anecdotally reported to benefit from intensive plasma exchange combined with cytotoxic drugs. Disease recurrences have been reported in 10 to 40% of patients.

IDIOPATHIC CUTANEOUS VASCULITIS

DEFINITION The term *cutaneous vasculitis* is defined broadly as inflammation of the blood vessels of the dermis. Due to its heterogeneity, cutaneous vasculitis has been described by a variety of terms including *hypersensitivity vasculitis* and *cutaneous leukocytoclastic angiitis*. However, cutaneous vasculitis is not one specific disease but a manifestation that can be seen in a variety of settings. In >70% of cases, cutaneous vasculitis occurs either as part of a primary systemic vasculitis or as a secondary vasculitis related to an inciting agent or an underlying disease (see "Secondary Vasculitis"). In the remaining 30% of cases, cutaneous vasculitis occurs idiopathically.

INCIDENCE AND PREVALENCE Cutaneous vasculitis represents the most commonly encountered vasculitis in clinical practice. The exact incidence of idiopathic cutaneous vasculitis has not been determined due to the predilection for cutaneous vasculitis to be associated with an underlying process and the variability of its clinical course.

PATHOLOGY AND PATHOGENESIS The typical histopathologic feature of cutaneous vasculitis is the presence of vasculitis of small vessels. Postcapillary venules are the most commonly involved vessels; capillaries and arterioles may be involved less frequently. This vasculitis is characterized by a *leukocytoclasis*, a term that refers to the nuclear debris remaining from the neutrophils that have infiltrated in and around the vessels during the acute stages. In the subacute or chronic stages, mononuclear cells predominate; in certain subgroups, eosinophilic infiltration is seen. Erythrocytes often extravasate from the involved vessels, leading to palpable purpura.

CLINICAL AND LABORATORY MANIFESTATIONS The hallmark of idiopathic cutaneous vasculitis is the predominance of skin involvement. Skin lesions may appear typically as palpable purpura; however, other cutaneous manifestations of the vasculitis may occur, including macules, papules, vesicles, bullae, subcutaneous nodules, ulcers, and recurrent or chronic urticaria. The skin lesions may be pruritic or even quite painful, with a burning or stinging sensation. Lesions most commonly occur in the lower extremities in ambulatory patients or in the sacral area in bedridden patients due to the effects of hydrostatic forces on the postcapillary venules. Edema may accompany certain lesions, and hyperpigmentation often occurs in areas of recurrent or chronic lesions.

There are no specific laboratory tests diagnostic of idiopathic cutaneous vasculitis. A mild leukocytosis with or without eosinophilia is characteristic, as is an elevated ESR. Laboratory studies should be aimed towards ruling out features to suggest an underlying disease or a systemic vasculitis.

DIAGNOSIS The diagnosis of cutaneous vasculitis is made by the demonstration of vasculitis on biopsy. An important diagnostic principle in patients with cutaneous vasculitis is to search for an etiology of the vasculitis—be it an exogenous agent, such as a drug or an infection, or an endogenous condition, such as an underlying disease (Fig. 306-1). In addition, a careful physical and laboratory examination should be performed to rule out the possibility of systemic vasculitis. This should start with the least invasive diagnostic approach and proceed to the more invasive only if clinically indicated.

℞ TREATMENT

When an antigenic stimulus is recognized as the precipitating factor in the cutaneous vasculitis, it should be removed; if this is a microbe, appropriate antimicrobial therapy should be instituted. If the vasculitis is associated with another underlying disease, treatment of the latter often results in resolution of the former. In situations where disease is apparently self-limited, no therapy, except possibly symptomatic therapy, is indicated. When cutaneous vasculitis persists and when there is no evidence of an inciting agent, an associated disease, or an un-

derlying systemic vasculitis, the decision to treat should be based on weighing the balance between the degree of symptoms and the risk of treatment. Some cases of idiopathic cutaneous vasculitis resolve spontaneously, while others remit and relapse. In those patients with persistent vasculitis, a variety of therapeutic regimens have been tried with variable results. In general, the treatment of idiopathic cutaneous vasculitis has not been satisfactory. Fortunately, since the disease is generally limited to the skin, this lack of consistent response to therapy usually does not lead to a life-threatening situation. Glucocorticoids are often used in the treatment of idiopathic cutaneous vasculitis. Therapy is usually instituted as prednisone, 1 mg/kg per day, with rapid tapering where possible, either directly to discontinuation or by conversion to an alternate-day regimen followed by ultimate discontinuation. In cases that prove refractory to glucocorticoids, a trial of a cytotoxic agent may be indicated. Patients with chronic vasculitis isolated to cutaneous venules rarely respond dramatically to any therapeutic regimen, and cytotoxic agents should be used only as a last resort in these patients. Methotrexate and azathioprine have been used in such situations in anecdotal reports. Although cyclophosphamide is the most effective therapy for the systemic vasculitides, it should almost never be used for idiopathic cutaneous vasculitis because of the potential toxicity. Other agents with which there have been anecdotal reports of success include dapsone, colchicine, and nonsteroidal anti-inflammatory agents.

ESSENTIAL MIXED CRYOGLOBULINEMIA

DEFINITION Cryoglobulins are cold-precipitable monoclonal or polyclonal immunoglobulins. Cryoglobulinemia may be associated with a systemic vasculitis characterized by palpable purpura, arthralgias, weakness, neuropathy, and glomerulonephitis. Although this can be observed in association with a variety of underlying disorders including multiple myeloma, lymphoproliferative disorders, connective tissue diseases, infection, and liver disease, in many instances it appeared to be idiopathic. Because of the apparent absence of an underlying disease and the presence of cryoprecipitate containing oligoclonal/polyclonal immunoglobulins, this entity was referred to as *essential mixed cryoglobulinemia*. Since the discovery of hepatitis C, it has been established that in the vast majority of patients, essential mixed cryoglobulinemia is related to an aberrant immune response to chronic hepatitis C infection.

INCIDENCE AND PREVALENCE The incidence of essential mixed cryoglobulinemia has not been established. It has been estimated, however, that 5% of patients with chronic hepatitis C will develop the syndrome of essential mixed cryoglobulinemia.

PATHOLOGY AND PATHOGENESIS Skin biopsies in essential mixed cryoglobulinemia reveal an inflammatory infiltrate surrounding and involving blood vessel walls, with fibrinoid necrosis, endothelial cell hyperplasia, and hemorrhage. Deposition of immunoglobulin and complement is common. Abnormalities of uninvolved skin including basement membrane alterations and deposits in vessel walls may be found. Membranoproliferative glomerulonephritis is responsible for 80% of all renal lesions in essential mixed cryoglobulinemia.

The association between hepatitis C and essential mixed cryoglobulinemia has been supported by the high frequency of documented hepatitis C infection, the presence of hepatitis C RNA and anti–hepatitis C antibodies in serum cryoprecipitates, evidence of hepatitis C antigens in vasculitic skin lesions, and the effectiveness of antiviral therapy (see below). Current evidence suggest that in the majority of cases, essential mixed cryoglobulinemia occurs when an aberrant immune response to hepatitis C infection leads to the formation of immune complexes consisting of hepatitis C antigens, polyclonal hepatitis C–specific IgG, and monoclonal IgM rheumatoid factor. The deposition of these immune complexes in blood vessel walls triggers an inflammatory cascade that results in the clinical syndrome of essential mixed cryoglobulinemia.

CLINICAL AND LABORATORY MANIFESTATIONS The most common clinical manifestations of essential mixed cryoglobulinemia are cutaneous vasculitis, arthritis, peripheral neuropathy, and glomerulonephritis. Renal disease develops in 10 to 30% of patients. Life-threatening rapidly progressive glomerulonephritis or vasculitis of the central nervous system, gastrointestinal tract, or heart occurs infrequently.

The presence of circulating cryoprecipitates is the fundamental finding in essential mixed cryoglobulinemia. Rheumatoid factor is almost always found and may be a useful clue to the disease when cryoglobulins are not detected. Hypocomplementemia occurs in 90% of patients. An elevated ESR and anemia occur frequently. Evidence for hepatitis C infection must be sought in all patients by testing for hepatitis C antibodies and hepatitis C RNA.

℞ TREATMENT

Acute mortality from essential mixed cryoglobulinemia is uncommon, but the presence of glomerulonephritis is a poor prognostic sign for overall outcome. In such patients, 15% progress to end-stage renal disease with 40% later experiencing fatal cardiovascular disease, infection, or liver failure. As indicated above, the majority of cases are associated with hepatitis C infection. In such patients, treatment with IFN-α and ribavirin (Chap. 285) can prove beneficial. Clinical improvement with IFN-α and ribavirin is dependent on the virologic response. Patients who clear hepatitis C from the blood have objective improvement in their vasculitis along with significant reductions in levels of circulating cryoglobulins, IgM, and rheumatoid factor. However, substantial portions of patients with hepatitis C do not have a sustained virologic response to such therapy, and the vasculitis typically relapses with the return of viremia. While transient improvement can be observed with glucocorticoids, a complete response is seen in only 7% of patients. Plasmapheresis and cytotoxic agents have been used in anecdotal reports. These observations have not been confirmed, and such therapies carry significant risks.

BEHÇET'S SYNDROME

Behçet's Syndrome is a clinicopathologic entity characterized by recurrent episodes of oral and genital ulcers, iritis, and cutaneous lesions. The underlying pathologic process is a leukocytoclastic venulitis, although vessels of any size and in any organ can be involved. →*This disorder is described in detail in Chap. 307.*

ISOLATED VASCULITIS OF THE CENTRAL NERVOUS SYSTEM

Isolated vasculitis of the central nervous system is an uncommon clinicopathologic entity characterized by vasculitis restricted to the vessels of the central nervous system without other apparent systemic vasculitis. Although the arteriole is most commonly affected, vessels of any size can be involved. The inflammatory process is usually composed of mononuclear cell infiltrates with or without granuloma formation.

Patients may present with severe headaches, altered mental function, and focal neurologic defects. Systemic symptoms are generally absent. Devastating neurologic abnormalities may occur depending on the extent of vessel involvement. The diagnosis is generally made by demonstration of characteristic vessel abnormalities on angiography (Fig. 306-4) and confirmed by biopsy of the brain parenchyma and leptomeninges. In the absence of a brain biopsy, care should be taken not to misinterpret as true primary vasculitis angiographic abnormalities that might actually be related to another cause. The differential diagnosis includes infection, atherosclerosis, emboli, connective tissue disease, sarcoidosis, malignancy, vasospasm, and drug-associated causes. The prognosis of this disease is poor; however, some reports indicate that glucocorticoid therapy, alone or together with cyclophosphamide administered as described above, has induced sustained clinical remissions in a small number of patients.

COGAN'S SYNDROME

Cogan's syndrome is characterized by interstitial keratitis together with vestibuloauditory symptoms. It may be associated with a systemic

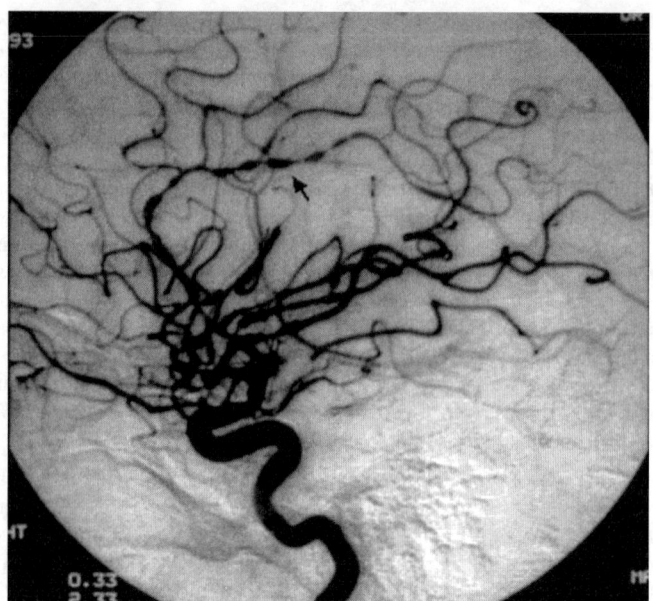

FIGURE 306-4 Cerebral angiogram from a 32-year-old male with central nervous system vasculitis. Dramatic beading (*arrow*) typical of vasculitis is seen.

vasculitis, particularly aortitis with involvement of the aortic valve. Glucocorticoids are the mainstay of treatment. Initiation of treatment as early as possible after the onset of hearing loss improves the likelihood of a favorable outcome.

KAWASAKI DISEASE

Kawasaki disease, also referred to as *mucocutaneous lymph node syndrome,* is an acute, febrile, multisystem disease of children. Some 80% of cases occur prior to the age of 5, with the peak incidence occurring at ≤2 years. It is characterized by nonsuppurative cervical adenitis and changes in the skin and mucous membranes such as edema; congested conjunctivae; erythema of the oral cavity, lips, and palms; and desquamation of the skin of the fingertips. Although the disease is generally benign and self-limited, it is associated with coronary artery aneurysms in approximately 25% of cases, with an overall case-fatality rate of 0.5 to 2.8%. These complications usually occur between the third and fourth weeks of illness during the convalescent stage. Vasculitis of the coronary arteries is seen in almost all the fatal cases that have been autopsied. There is typical intimal proliferation and infiltration of the vessel wall with mononuclear cells. Beadlike aneurysms and thromboses may be seen along the artery. Other manifestations include pericarditis, myocarditis, myocardial ischemia and infarction, and cardiomegaly.

Apart from the up to 2.8% of patients who develop fatal complications, the prognosis of this disease for uneventful recovery is excellent. High-dose intravenous γ globulin (2 g/kg as a single infusion over 10 h) together with aspirin (100 mg/kg per day for 14 days followed by 3 to 5 mg/kg per day for several weeks) have been shown to be effective in reducing the prevalence of coronary artery abnormalities when administered early in the course of the disease.

POLYANGIITIS OVERLAP SYNDROMES

Some patients with systemic vasculitis manifest clinicopathologic characteristics that do not fit precisely into any specific disease but have overlapping features of different vasculitides. Active systemic vasculitis in such settings has the same potential for causing irreversible organ system damage as when it occurs in one of the defined syndromes listed in Table 306-1. The diagnostic and therapeutic considerations as well as the prognosis for these patients depend on the sites and severity of active vasculitis. Patients with vasculitis that could potentially cause irreversible damage to a major organ system should be treated as described under "Wegener's granulomatosis."

Drug-Induced Vasculitis Vasculitis associated with drug reactions usually presents as palpable purpura that may be generalized or limited to the lower extremities or other dependent areas; however, urticarial lesions, ulcers, and hemorrhagic blisters may also occur (Chap. 50). Signs and symptoms may be limited to the skin, although systemic manifestations such as fever, malaise, and polyarthralgias may occur. Although the skin is the predominant organ involved, systemic vasculitis may result from drug reactions. Drugs that have been implicated in vasculitis include allopurinol, thiazides, gold, sulfonamides, phenytoin, and penicillin (Chap. 50).

An increasing number of drugs have been reported to cause vasculitis associated with antimyeloperoxidase ANCA. Of these, the best evidence of causality exists for hydralazine and propylthiouracil. The clinical manifestations in ANCA-positive drug-induced vasculitis can range from cutaneous lesions to glomerulonephritis and pulmonary hemorrhage. Outside of drug discontinuation, treatment should be based on the severity of the vasculitis. Patients with immediately life-threatening small-vessel vasculitis should initially be treated with glucocorticoids and cyclophosphamide as described for Wegener's granulomatosis. Following clinical improvement, consideration may be given for tapering such agents along a more rapid schedule.

Serum Sickness and Serum Sickness–Like Reactions These reactions are characterized by the occurrence of fever, urticaria, polyarthralgias, and lymphadenopathy 7 to 10 days after primary exposure and 2 to 4 days after secondary exposure to a heterologous protein (classic serum sickness) or a nonprotein drug such as penicillin or sulfa (serum sickness–like reaction). Most of the manifestations are not due to a vasculitis; however, occasional patients will have typical cutaneous venulitis that may progress rarely to a systemic vasculitis.

Vasculitis Associated with Other Underlying Primary Diseases Certain *infections* may directly trigger an inflammatory vasculitic process. For example, rickettsias can invade and proliferate in the endothelial cells of small blood vessels causing a vasculitis (Chap. 158). In addition, the inflammatory response around blood vessels associated with certain systemic fungal diseases such as histoplasmosis (Chap. 183) may mimic a primary vasculitic process. A leukocytoclastic vasculitis predominantly involving the skin with occasional involvement of other organ systems may be a minor component of many other infections. These include *subacute bacterial endocarditis, Epstein-Barr virus infection, HIV infection,* as well as a number of other infections.

Vasculitis can be associated with certain *malignancies,* particularly lymphoid or reticuloendothelial neoplasms. Leukocytoclastic venulitis confined to the skin is the most common finding; however, widespread systemic vasculitis may occur. Of particular note is the association of *hairy cell leukemia* (Chap. 97) with PAN.

A number of *connective tissue diseases* have vasculitis as a secondary manifestation of the underlying primary process. Foremost among these are *systemic lupus erythematosus* (Chap. 300), *rheumatoid arthritis* (Chap. 301), *inflammatory myositis* (Chap. 370), *relapsing polychondritis* (Chap. 308), and *Sjögren's syndrome* (Chap. 304). The most common form of vasculitis in these conditions is the small-vessel venulitis isolated to the skin. However, certain patients may develop a fulminant systemic necrotizing vasculitis.

Secondary vasculitis has also been observed in association with *ulcerative colitis, congenital deficiencies of various complement components, retroperitoneal fibrosis, primary biliary cirrhosis,* α_1-antitrypsin deficiency, and *intestinal bypass surgery.*

PRINCIPLES OF TREATMENT

Once a diagnosis of vasculitis has been established, a decision regarding therapeutic strategy must be made (Fig. 306-1). The vasculitis syndromes represent a wide spectrum of diseases with varying degrees of severity. Since the potential toxic side effects of certain therapeutic regimens may be substantial, the risk-versus-benefit ratio of any therapeutic approach should be weighed carefully. Specific therapeutic

regimens are discussed above for the individual vasculitis syndromes; however, certain general principles regarding therapy should be considered. On the one hand, glucocorticoids and/or cytotoxic therapy should be instituted immediately in diseases where irreversible organ system dysfunction and high morbidity and mortality have been clearly established. Wegener's granulomatosis is the prototype of a severe systemic vasculitis requiring such a therapeutic approach (see above). On the other hand, when feasible, aggressive therapy should be avoided for vasculitic manifestations that rarely result in irreversible organ system dysfunction and that usually do not respond to such therapy. For example, idiopathic cutaneous vasculitis usually resolves with symptomatic treatment, and prolonged courses of glucocorticoids uncommonly result in clinical benefit. Cytotoxic agents have not proved to be beneficial in idiopathic cutaneous vasculitis, and their toxic side effects generally outweigh any potential beneficial effects. Glucocorticoids should be initiated in those systemic vasculitides that cannot be specifically categorized or for which there is no established standard therapy; cytotoxic therapy should be added in these diseases only if an adequate response does not result or if remission can only be achieved and maintained with an unacceptably toxic regimen of glucocorticoids. When remission is achieved, one should continually attempt to taper glucocorticoids to an alternate-day regimen and discontinue when possible. When using cytotoxic regimens, one should base the choice of agent upon the available therapeutic data supporting efficacy in that disease, the site and severity of organ involvement, and the toxicity profile of the drug.

Physicians should be thoroughly aware of the toxic side effects of therapeutic agents employed (Table 306-7). Many of the side effects of glucocorticoid therapy are markedly decreased in frequency and duration in patients on alternate-day regimens compared to daily regimens. When cyclophosphamide is administered chronically in doses of 2 mg/kg per day for substantial periods of time (one to several years), the incidence of cystitis is at least 30% and the incidence of bladder cancer is at least 6%. Bladder cancer can occur several years after discontinuation of cyclophosphamide therapy; therefore, monitoring for bladder cancer should continue indefinitely in patients who have received prolonged courses of daily cyclophosphamide. Instructing the patient to take cyclophosphamide all at once in the morning with a large amount of fluid throughout the day in order to maintain

TABLE 306-7 *Major Toxic Side Effects of Drugs Commonly Used in the Treatment of Systemic Vasculitis*

GLUCOCORTICOIDS	
Osteoporosis	Growth suppression in children
Cataracts	Hypertension
Glaucoma	Avascular necrosis of bone
Diabetes mellitus	Myopathy
Electrolyte abnormalities	Alterations in mood
Metabolic abnormalities	Psychosis
Suppression of inflammatory and immune responses leading to opportunistic infections	Pseudotumor cerebri
	Peptic ulcer diathesis
	Pancreatitis
Cushingoid features	

CYCLOPHOSPHAMIDE	
Bone marrow suppression	Hypogammaglobulinemia
Cystitis	Pulmonary fibrosis
Bladder carcinoma	Myelodysplasia
Gonadal suppression	Oncogenesis
Gastrointestinal intolerance	

METHOTREXATE	
Gastrointestinal intolerance	Pneumonitis
Stomatitis	Teratogenicity
Neutropenia	Opportunistic infections
Hepatotoxicity (may lead to fibrosis or cirrhosis)	

a dilute urine can reduce the risk of bladder injury. Significant alopecia is unusual in the chronically administered, low-dose regimen. Permanent infertility can occur in both men and women. Bone marrow suppression is an important toxicity of cyclophosphamide and can be observed during glucocorticoid tapering or over time, even after periods of stable measurements. Monitoring of the complete blood count every 1 to 2 weeks for as long as the patient receives cyclophosphamide can effectively prevent cytopenias. When the white blood count (WBC) is maintained at >3000/μL, and the patient is not receiving daily glucocorticoids, the incidence of life-threatening opportunistic infections is low. However, the WBC is not an accurate predictor of risk of all opportunistic infections; and infections with *Pneumocystis carinii* and certain fungi can be seen in the face of WBCs that are within normal limits, particularly in patients receiving glucocorticoids. All vasculitis patients who are not allergic to sulfa and who are receiving daily glucocorticoids in combination with a cytotoxic drug should receive trimethoprim-sulfamethoxazole as prophylaxis against *P. carinii* infection.

Finally, it should be emphasized that each patient is unique and requires individual decision-making. The above outline should serve as a framework to guide therapeutic approaches; however, flexibility should be practiced in order to provide maximal therapeutic efficacy with minimal toxic side effects in each patient.

FURTHER READING

GUILLEVIN L et al: Microscopic polyangiitis. Clinical and laboratory findings in eighty-five patients. Arthritis Rheum 42:421, 1999

HOFFMAN GS SPECKS U: Antineutrophil cytoplasmic antibodies. Arthritis Rheum 41:1521, 1998

——— et al: Wegener's granulomatosis: An analysis of 158 patients. Ann Intern Med 116:488, 1992

JENNETTE JC et al: Nomenclature of systemic vasculitis. Proposal of an international consensus conference. Arthritis Rheum 37:187, 1994

KERR G et al: Takayasu arteritis. Ann Intern Med 120:919, 1994

LANGFORD CA et al: Use of cytotoxic agents and cyclosporine in the treatment of autoimmune disease. Part 2: Inflammatory bowel disease, systemic vasculitis, and therapeutic toxicity. Ann Intern Med 129:49, 1998

——— et al: A staged approach to the treatment of Wegener's granulomatosis: Induction of remission with glucocorticoids and daily cyclophosphamide switching to methotrexate for remission maintenance. Arthritis Rheum 42:2666, 1999

LUDVIKSSON BR et al: Active Wegener's granulomatosis is associated with HLA-DR+ CD4+ T cells exhibiting an unbalanced Th-1 type T cell cytokine pattern: Reversal with IL-10. J Immunol 160:3602, 1998

SNELLER MC, FAUCI AS: Pathogenesis of vasculitis syndromes. Med Clin North Am 81:221, 1997

307 | BEHÇET'S SYNDROME
Haralampos M. Moutsopoulos

DEFINITION

Behçet's syndrome is a multisystem disorder presenting with recurrent oral and genital ulcerations as well as ocular involvement. Internationally agreed diagnostic criteria have been proposed (Table 307-1).

PREVALENCE, PATHOGENESIS, AND PATHOLOGY

The syndrome affects young males and females from the Mediterranean region, the Middle East, and the Far East, suggesting a link with the ancient Silk Route. Males and females are affected equally, but males often have more severe disease. Blacks are not affected.

The etiology and pathogenesis of this syndrome remain obscure; vasculitis is the main pathologic lesion with a tendency to venous thrombus formation, and circulating autoantibodies to human oral mucous membranes are found in approximately 50% of the patients. In endemic areas the syndrome is associated with HLA-B5 (B51) alloantigen, and approximately 1 in 10 patients has an affected relative.

CLINICAL FEATURES

The recurrent aphthous ulcerations are a sine qua non for the diagnosis. The ulcers are usually painful, shallow or deep with a central yellowish necrotic base, appear singly or in crops, and are located anywhere in the oral cavity. The ulcers persist for 1 to 2 weeks and subside without leaving scars. The genital ulcers are less common, more specific, do not affect the glans penis or urethra, and produce scrotal scars.

Skin involvement includes folliculitis, erythema nodosum, an acne-like exanthem, and infrequently vasculitis. Nonspecific skin inflammatory reactivity to any scratches or intradermal saline injection (pathergy test) is a common and specific manifestation.

TABLE 307-1 *Diagnostic Criteria of Behçet's Disease*

Recurrent oral ulceration plus two of the following:
  Recurrent genital ulceration
  Eye lesions
  Skin lesions
  Pathergy test

Eye involvement with scarring, bilateral panuveitis is the most dreaded complication, since it occasionally progresses rapidly to blindness. The eye disease is usually present at the onset but may also develop within the first few years. In addition to iritis, posterior uveitis, retinal vessel occlusions, and optic neuritis can be seen in some patients with the syndrome. Hypopyon uveitis, a specific but rare manifestation, is a layer of inflammatory cells visible because of the effects of gravity; it usually indicates severe retinal vascular disease.

The arthritis of Behçet's syndrome is not deforming and affects the knees and ankles.

Superficial or deep peripheral vein thrombosis is seen in one-fourth of the patients. Pulmonary emboli are a rare complication. The superior vena cava is obstructed occasionally, producing a dramatic clinical picture. Arterial involvement occurs infrequently and presents with aortitis or peripheral arterial aneurysm and arterial thrombosis. Pulmonary artery vasculitis presenting with dyspnea, cough, chest pain, hemoptysis, and infiltrates on chest roentgenograms has been reported recently in 5% of patients.

Neurologic involvement (5 to 10%) appears mainly in the parenchymal form (80%); it is associated with brain stem involvement and has a serious prognosis. Dural sinus thrombi (20%) are associated with headache and increased intracranial pressure.

Gastrointestinal involvement consists of mucosal ulcerations of the gut.

Laboratory findings are mainly nonspecific indices of inflammation, such as leukocytosis and elevated erythrocyte sedimentation rate, as well as C-reactive protein levels; antibodies to the human oral mucosa are also found.

℞ TREATMENT

The severity of the syndrome usually abates with time. Apart from the patients with parenchymal neurologic involvement, the life expectancy seems to be normal, and the only serious complication is blindness.

Mucous membrane involvement may respond to topical glucocorticoids in the form of mouthwash or paste. In more serious cases thalidomide (100 mg/d) is effective. Thrombophlebitis is treated with aspirin, 325 mg/d. Colchicine or interferon α can be beneficial for the mucocutaneous manifestations of the syndrome. Uveitis and central nervous system involvement require systemic glucocorticoid therapy (prednisone, 1 mg/kg per day) and azathioprine, 2 to 3 mg/kg per day, or cyclosporine, 5 to 10 mg/kg per day. Preliminary data suggest that anti-tumor necrosis factor block may be an alternative therapeutic modality for panuveitis. Early initiation of azathioprine tends to favorably affect the long-term prognosis of Behçet's syndrome.

FURTHER READING

MEADOR R et al: Behçet's disease: Immunopathologic and therapeutic aspects. Curr Rheumatol Rep 4:47, 2002

SFIKAKIS PP. Behçet's disease: a new target for anti-tumour necrosis factor treatment. Ann Rheum Dis 61 (Suppl 2):51, 2002
YAZICI H et al: Behçet's disease. Curr Opin Rheumatol 13:18, 2001
——— et al: Behçet's syndrome: Where do we stand? Am J Med 112:75, 2002

308 RELAPSING POLYCHONDRITIS
Bruce C. Gilliland

Relapsing polychondritis is an uncommon inflammatory disorder of unknown cause characterized by an episodic and generally progressive course affecting predominantly the cartilage of the ears, nose, and laryngotracheobronchial tree. Other manifestations include scleritis, neurosensory hearing loss, polyarthritis, cardiac abnormalities, skin lesions, and glomerulonephritis. The peak age of onset is between the ages of 40 to 50 years, but relapsing polychondritis may affect children and the elderly. It is found in all races, and both sexes are equally affected. No familial tendency is apparent. A significantly higher frequency of HLA-DR4 has been found in patients with relapsing polychondritis than in normal individuals. A predominant subtype allele(s) of HLA-DR4 was not found. Approximately 30% of patients with relapsing polychondritis will have another rheumatologic disorder, the most frequent being systemic vasculitis, followed by rheumatoid arthritis, systemic lupus erythematosus (SLE), Sjögren's syndrome, or ankylosing spondylitis. Nonrheumatic disorders associated with relapsing polychondritis include inflammatory bowel disease, primary biliary cirrhosis, and myelodysplastic syndrome (Table 308-1).

Diagnostic criteria were suggested over 20 years ago by McAdam et al. and modified by Damiani and Levine a few years later. These criteria continue to be generally used in clinical practice. McAdam et al. proposed the following: (1) recurrent chondritis of both auricles; (2) nonerosive inflammatory arthritis; (3) chondritis of nasal cartilage; (4) inflammation of ocular structures including conjunctivitis, keratitis, scleritis/episcleritis, and/or uveitis; (5) chondritis of the laryngeal and/or tracheal cartilages; and (6) cochlear and/or vestibular damage manifested by neurosensory hearing loss, tinnitus, and/or vertigo. The diagnosis is certain when three or more of these features are present along with a positive biopsy from the ear, nasal, or respiratory cartilage. Damiani and Levine later suggested that the diagnosis could be made when one or more of the above features and a positive biopsy were present, when two or more separate sites of cartilage inflammation were present that responded to glucocorticoids or dapsone, or when three or more of the above features were present. A biopsy is not necessary in most patients with clinically evident disease.

PATHOLOGY AND PATHOPHYSIOLOGY The earliest abnormality of hyaline and elastic cartilage noted histologically is a focal or diffuse loss of basophilic staining indicating depletion of proteoglycan from the cartilage matrix. Inflammatory infiltrates are found adjacent to involved cartilage and consist predominantly of mononuclear cells and occasional plasma cells. In acute disease, polymorphonuclear white cells may also be present. Destruction of cartilage begins at the outer edges

and advances centrally. There is lacunar breakdown and loss of chondrocytes. Degenerating cartilage is replaced by granulation tissue and later by fibrosis and focal areas of calcification. Small loci of cartilage regeneration may be present. Immunofluorescence studies have shown immunoglobulins and complement at sites of involvement. Extracellular granular material observed in the degenerating cartilage matrix by electron microscopy has been interpreted to be enzymes, immunoglobulins, or proteoglycans.

Immunologic mechanisms play a role in the pathogenesis of relapsing polychondritis. Immunoglobulin and complement deposits are found at sites of inflammation. In addition, antibodies to type II collagen and to matrilin-1 and immune complexes are detected in the sera of some patients. The possibility that an immune response to type II collagen may be important in the pathogenesis is supported experimentally by the occurrence of auricular chondritis in rats immunized with type II collagen. Antibodies to type II collagen are found in the sera of these animals, and immune deposits are detected at sites of ear inflammation. Humoral immune responses to type IX and type XI collagen, matrilin-1, and cartilage oligomeric matrix protein have been demonstrated in some patients. In a study, rats immunized with matrilin-1 were found to develop severe inspiratory stridor and swelling of the nasal septum. The rats had severe inflammation with erosions of the involved cartilage, which was characterized by increased numbers of CD 4+ and CD 8+ T cells in the lesions. The cartilage of the joints and ear pinna was not involved. All had IgG antibodies to matrilin-1. Matrilin-1 is a noncollagenous protein present in the extracellular matrix in cartilage. It is present in high concentrations in the trachea and is also present in the nasal septum but not in articular cartilage. A subsequent study demonstrated serum anti-matrilin-1 antibodies in approximately 13% of patients with relapsing polychondritis; approximately 70 of these patients had respiratory symptoms. Cell-mediated immunity may also be operative in causing tissue injury, since lymphocyte transformation can be demonstrated when lymphocytes of patients are exposed to cartilage extracts. T cells specific for type II collagen have been found in some patients, and CD 4+ T cells have been observed at sites of cartilage inflammation. The accumulating data strongly suggest that both humoral and cell-mediated immunity play an important role in the pathogenesis of relapsing polychondritis.

Dissolution of cartilage matrix can be induced by the intravenous injection of crude papain, a proteolytic enzyme, into young rabbits, which results in collapse of their normally rigid ears within 4 h. Reconstitution of the matrix occurs in about 7 days. In relapsing polychondritis, loss of cartilage matrix also most likely results from action of proteolytic enzymes released from chondrocytes, polymorphonuclear white cells, and monocytes that have been activated by inflammatory mediators.

CLINICAL MANIFESTATIONS The onset of relapsing polychondritis is frequently abrupt with the appearance of one or two sites of cartilagenous inflammation. Fever, fatigue, and weight loss occur and may precede the clinical signs of relapsing polychondritis by several weeks. Relapsing polychondritis may go unrecognized for several months or even years in patients who only initially manifest intermittent joint pain and/or swelling, or who have unexplained eye inflammation, hearing loss, valvular heart disease, or pulmonary symptoms. The pattern of cartilagenous involvement and the frequency of episodes vary widely among patients.

TABLE 308-1 *Disorders Associated with Relapsing Polychondritis[a]*

Systemic vasculitis	Behçet's syndrome
Rheumatoid arthritis	Inflammatory bowel disease
Systemic lupus erythematosus	Primary biliary cirrhosis
Sjögren's syndrome	Myelodysplastic syndrome
Spondyloarthropathies	

[a] Systemic vasculitis is the most common association followed by rheumatoid arthritis, systemic lupus erythematosus, and Sjögren's syndrome.
Source: Modified from Michet.

TABLE 308-2 *Clinical Manifestations of Relapsing Polychondritis*

Clinical Feature	Frequency, % Presenting	Frequency, % Cumulative
Auricular chondritis	40	85
Hearing loss	10	30
Nasal chondritis	25	55
Saddle nose deformity	20	30
Ocular deformities	20	50
Respiratory disease	25	50
Arthritis	35	50
Aortic regurgitation	—	5
Vasculitis	3	10

Source: Modified from Isaak et al.

Auricular chondritis is the most frequent presenting manifestation of relapsing polychondritis in 40% of patients and eventually affects about 85% of patients (Table 308-2). One or both ears are involved, either sequentially or simultaneously. Patients experience the sudden onset of pain, tenderness, and swelling of the cartilaginous portion of the ear (Fig. 308-1). Earlobes are spared because they do not contain cartilage. The overlying skin has a beefy red or violaceous color. Prolonged or recurrent episodes result in a flabby or droopy ear as a sequela of cartilage destruction. Swelling may close off the eustachian tube (causing otitis media) or the external auditory meatus, either of which can impair hearing. Inflammation of the internal auditory artery or its cochlear branch produces hearing loss, vertigo, ataxia, nausea, and vomiting. Vertigo is almost always accompanied by hearing loss. The cartilage of the nose becomes inflamed during the first or subsequent attacks. Approximately 50% of patients will eventually have nose involvement. Patients may experience nasal stuffiness, rhinorrhea, and epistaxis. The bridge of the nose becomes red, swollen, and tender and may collapse, producing a saddle deformity (Fig. 308-2). In some patients, the saddle deformity develops insidiously without overt inflammation. Saddle nose is observed more frequently in younger patients, especially in women.

Arthritis is the presenting manifestation in relapsing polychondritis in approximately one-third of patients and may be present for several months before other features appear. Eventually, more than half the patients will have arthritis. The arthritis is usually asymmetric and oligo- or polyarticular, and involves both large and small peripheral joints. An episode of arthritis lasts from a few days to several weeks and resolves spontaneously without residual joint deformity. Attacks

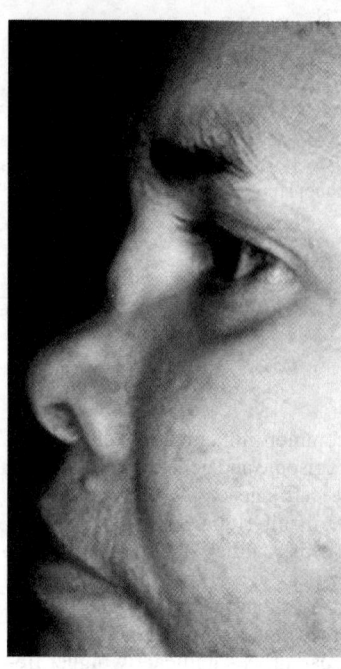

FIGURE 308-2 Saddle nose results from destruction and collapse of the nasal cartilage. (*Reprinted from the Clinical Slide Collection on the Rheumatic Diseases,* © *1991, 1995, 1997, 1998, 1999. Used by permission of the American College of Rheumatology.*)

of arthritis may not be temporally related to other manifestations of relapsing polychondritis. The joints are warm, tender, and swollen. Joint fluid has been reported to be noninflammatory. In addition to peripheral joints, inflammation may involve the costochondral, sternomanubrial, and sternoclavicular cartilages. Destruction of these cartilages may result in a pectus excavatum deformity or even a flail anterior chest wall. Relapsing polychondritis may occur in patients with preexisting rheumatoid arthritis, Reiter's syndrome, psoriatic arthritis, or ankylosing spondylitis.

Eye manifestations occur in more than half of patients and include conjunctivitis, episcleritis, scleritis, iritis, and keratitis. Eye involvement is seldom the presenting feature. Ulceration and perforation of the cornea may occur and cause blindness. Other manifestations include eyelid and periorbital edema, proptosis, cataracts, optic neuritis, extraocular muscle palsies, retinal vasculitis, and renal vein occlusion.

Laryngotracheobronchial involvement occurs in ~50% of patients. Symptoms include hoarseness, a nonproductive cough, and tenderness over the larynx and proximal trachea. Mucosal edema, strictures, and/or collapse of laryngeal or tracheal cartilage may cause stridor and life-threatening airway obstruction necessitating tracheostomy. Collapse of cartilage in bronchi leads to pneumonia and, when extensive, to respiratory insufficiency.

Aortic regurgitation occurs in about 5% of patients and is due to progressive dilation of the aortic ring or to destruction of the valve cusps. Mitral and other heart valves are less often affected. Other cardiac manifestations include pericarditis, myocarditis, and conduction abnormalities. Aneurysms of the proximal, thoracic, or abdominal aorta may occur even in the absence of active chondritis and occasionally rupture.

Systemic vasculitis may occur in association with relapsing polychondritis. Vasculitides include leukocytoclastic vasculitis, polyarteritis, temporal arteritis, and Takayasu's arteritis (Chap. 306). Neurologic abnormalities usually occur as a result of underlying vasculitis, manifesting as seizures, strokes, ataxia, and peripheral and cranial nerve neuropathies. Cranial nerves II, III, VI, and VII are most often involved. Approximately 25% of patients have skin lesions, none of which is characteristic for relapsing polychondritis, that reflect associated vasculitis. These include purpura, erythema nodosum, erythema multiforme, angioedema/urticaria, livedo reticularis, and panniculitis. Segmental necrotizing glomerulonephritis with crescent formation has been noted in some patients, usually in association with microscopic polyangiitis, but may occur in the absence of systemic vasculitis.

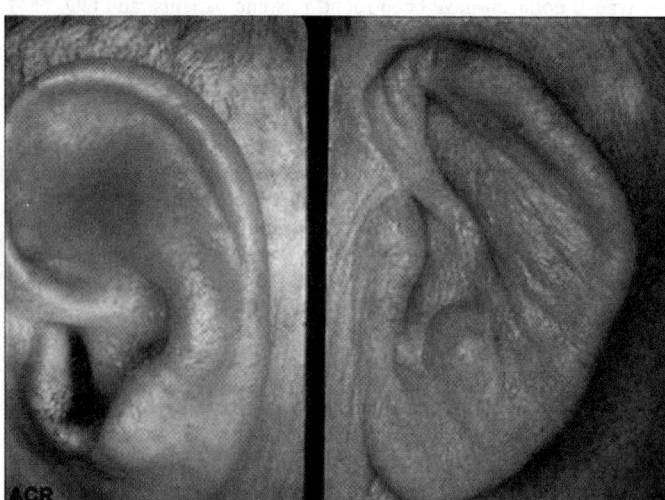

FIGURE 308-1 *Left.* The pinna is erythematous, swollen, and tender. Not shown is the ear lobule that is spared as there is no underlying cartilage. *Right.* The pinna is thickened and deformed. The destruction of the underlying cartilage results in a floppy ear. (*Reprinted from the Clinical Slide Collection on the Rheumatic Diseases,* © *1991, 1995, 1997, 1998, 1999. Used by permission of the American College of Rheumatology.*)

The course of disease is highly variable, with episodes lasting from a few days to several weeks and then subsiding spontaneously. Attacks may recur at intervals varying from weeks to months. In other patients, the disease has a chronic, smoldering course. In a few patients, the disease may be limited to one or two episodes of cartilage inflammation. In one study, the 5-year estimated survival rate was 74% and the 10-year survival rate 55%. In contrast to earlier series, only about half the deaths could be attributed to relapsing polychondritis or complications of treatment. Pulmonary complications accounted for only 10% of all fatalities. In general, patients with more widespread disease have a worse prognosis.

LABORATORY FINDINGS Mild leukocytosis and normocytic, normochromic anemia are often present. Eosinophilia is observed in 10% of patients. The erythrocyte sedimentation rate and C-reactive protein are usually elevated. Rheumatoid factor and antinuclear antibody tests are occasionally positive in low titers. Antibodies to type II collagen are present in fewer than half the patients and are specific. Circulating immune complexes may be detected, especially in patients with early active disease. Elevated levels of γ globulin may be present. Antineutrophil cytoplasmic antibodies (ANCA), either cytoplasmic (C-ANCA) or perinuclear (P-ANCA), are found in some patients with active disease. The upper and lower airways can be evaluated by imaging techniques such as linear tomography, laryngotracheography, and computed tomography, and by bronchoscopy. Magnetic resonance imaging (MRI) is helpful in evaluation of the larynx and trachea. Bronchography is performed to demonstrate bronchial narrowing. Intrathoracic airway obstruction can also be evaluated by inspiratory-expiratory flow studies. The chest film may show narrowing of the trachea and/or the main bronchi, widening of the ascending or descending aorta due to an aneurysm, and cardiomegaly when aortic insufficiency is present. MRI can be used in assessing aortic aneurysmal dilatation. Radiographs may show calcification at previous sites of cartilage damage involving ear, nose, larynx, or trachea.

DIAGNOSIS Diagnosis is based on recognition of the typical clinical features. Biopsies of the involved cartilage from the ear, nose, or respiratory tract will confirm the diagnosis but are only necessary when clinical features are not typical. Patients with Wegener's granulomatosis may have a saddle nose and pulmonary involvement but can be distinguished by the absence of auricular involvement and the presence of granulomatous lesions in the tracheobronchial tree. Patients with Cogan's syndrome have interstitial keratitis and vestibular and auditory abnormalities, but this syndrome does not involve the respiratory tract or ears. Reiter's syndrome may initially resemble relapsing polychondritis because of oligoarticular arthritis and eye involvement, but it is distinguished in time by the appearance of urethritis and typical mucocutaneous lesions and the absence of nose or ear cartilage involvement. Rheumatoid arthritis may initially suggest relapsing polychondritis because of arthritis and eye inflammation. The arthritis in rheumatoid arthritis, however, is erosive and symmetric. In addition, rheumatoid factor titers are usually high compared with those in relapsing polychondritis. Bacterial infection of the pinna may be mistaken for relapsing polychondritis but differs by usually involving only one ear, including the earlobe. Auricular cartilage may also be damaged by trauma or frostbite.

Relapsing polychondritis may develop in patients with a variety of autoimmune disorders, including SLE, rheumatoid arthritis, Sjögren's syndrome, and vasculitis. In most cases, these disorders antedate the appearance of polychondritis, usually by months or years. It is likely that these patients have an immunologic abnormality that predisposes them to development of this group of autoimmune disorders.

℞ TREATMENT

In patients with active chondritis, prednisone, 40 to 60 mg/d, is often effective in suppressing disease activity; it is tapered gradually once disease is controlled. In some patients, prednisone can be stopped, while in others low doses in the range of 10 to 15 mg/d are required for continued suppression of disease. Dapsone instead of prednisone has been effective in suppressing inflammation in some patients. Immunosuppressive drugs such as methotrexate, cyclophosphamide, azathioprine, or cyclosporine should be reserved for patients who fail to respond to prednisone or who require high doses for control of disease activity. Patients with significant ocular inflammation often require intraocular steroids as well as high doses of prednisone. Heart valve replacement or repair of an aortic aneurysm may be necessary. In patients with early subglottic disease, intralesional injection of glutocorticoids may be beneficial. When obstruction is severe, tracheostomy is required. Stents may be necessary in patients with tracheobronchial collapse.

FURTHER READING

HOCHBERG MC: Relapsing polychondritis, in *Kelley's Textbook of Rheumatology*, 6th ed, S Ruddy et al (eds). Philadelphia, Saunders, 2001, pp 1463–1467

ISAAK BL et al: Ocular and systemic findings in relapsing polychondritis. Ophthalmology 93:681, 1986

LETKO E et al: Relapsing polychondritis: A clinical review. Semin Arthritis Rheum 31:384, 2002

MICHET CT: Relapsing polychondritis, in *Arthritis and Allied Conditions*, 14th ed, WJ Koopman (ed). Philadelphia, Lippincott Williams & Wilkins, 2001, pp 1774–1783

ZEUNER M et al: Relapsing polychondritis: Clinical and immunogenic analysis of 62 patients. J Rheumatol 24:96, 1997

309 | SARCOIDOSIS
Ronald G. Crystal

DEFINITION Sarcoidosis is a chronic, multisystem disorder of unknown cause characterized in affected organs by an accumulation of T lymphocytes and mononuclear phagocytes, noncaseating epithelioid granulomas, and derangements of the normal tissue architecture. Although there are usually skin anergy and depressed cellular immune processes in the blood, sarcoidosis is characterized at the sites of disease by exaggerated T helper 1 (T_H1) lymphocyte immune processes. All parts of the body can be involved, but the organ most frequently affected is the lung. Involvement of the skin, eye, liver, and lymph nodes is also common. The disease is often acute or subacute and self-limiting, but in many individuals it is chronic, waxing and waning over many years.

ETIOLOGY The cause of sarcoidosis is unknown. Various infectious and noninfectious agents have been implicated, but there is no proof that any specific agent is responsible. However, all available evidence is consistent with the concept that the disease results from an exaggerated cellular immune response (acquired, inherited, or both) to a limited class of persistent antigens or self-antigens.

INCIDENCE AND PREVALENCE Sarcoidosis is a relatively common disease affecting individuals of both sexes and almost all ages, races, and geographic locations. Females appear to be slightly more susceptible than males. Cases of sarcoidosis have been described in all of the major races, and the disease is found throughout the world. It has been suggested that sarcoidosis is more common in certain geographic areas such as the southeastern part of the United States, but when case-matched controls have been used, these geographic differences are less convincing. There is a remarkable diversity of the prevalence of sarcoidosis among certain ethnic and racial groups, with a range of <1 to 64 per 100,000 worldwide. The prevalence of sarcoidosis is from 10 to 40 per 100,000 in the United States and Europe. In the United States, most patients are black, with a ratio of blacks to whites ranging from 10:1 to 17:1. In Europe, however, the disease affects mostly whites. Furthermore, while the prevalence per 100,000 in Sweden is 64, in France it is 10, in Poland 3, yet for Irish females living in London it is 200. In contrast, the disease is very rare among Inuit, Canadian Indians, New Zealand Maoris, and Southeast Asians.

Most patients present with sarcoidosis between the ages of 20 and 40, but the disease can occur in children and in the elderly. Several hundred kindred groups with familial sarcoidosis have been described, and the disease has been observed in twins, more commonly in monozygotic than in dizygotic pairs. There have also been several instances of husband-wife pairs identified, and geographic foci of sarcoidosis among unrelated individuals living closely within a community, arguing for some environmental factors in the pathogenesis of the disease. Although the disease is believed to result from exaggerated cellular immune responses to a limited class of antigens, no clear patterns in any HLA locus have emerged. Unlike many diseases in which the lung is involved, sarcoidosis favors nonsmokers.

PATHOPHYSIOLOGY AND IMMUNOPATHOGENESIS The first manifestation of the disease is an accumulation of mononuclear inflammatory cells, mostly CD4+ T_H1 lymphocytes and mononuclear phagocytes, in affected organs. This inflammatory process is followed by the formation of granulomas, aggregates of macrophages and their progeny, epithelioid cells, and multinucleated giant cells. The typical sarcoid granuloma is a compact structure composed of an aggregate of mononuclear phagocytes surrounded by a rim of CD4+ T lymphocytes and, to a far lesser extent, B lymphocytes. The overall structure is relatively discrete and is interspersed with fine collagen fibrils, presumably remnants of the underlying connective tissue matrix. The giant cells within the granuloma can be of the Langhans' or foreign-body variety and often contain inclusions such as Schaumann bodies (conchlike struc-

tures), asteroid bodies (stellate-like structures), and residual bodies (refractile calcium-containing inclusions).

Together the accumulated T cells, mononuclear phagocytes, and granulomas represent the active disease. Other than the fact that they take up space and thus their bulk modifies the local architecture, for all except late-stage cases, there is no evidence that the mononuclear inflammatory cells dispersed in the tissue or in the granuloma injure the affected organ by releasing mediators that damage the normal parenchymal cells or the extracellular matrix. Rather, organ dysfunction in sarcoidosis results mostly from the accumulated inflammatory cells distorting the architecture of the affected tissue; if a sufficient number of structures vital to the function of the tissue are involved, the disease becomes clinically apparent in that organ. Thus, while autopsy series show that, to some extent, sarcoidosis involves most organs in the majority of patients, the disease manifests clinically only in organs where it affects function (such as the lung and eye) or in organs where it is readily observed (such as the skin or, by x-ray, the hilar nodes). For example, in the lung, the inflammatory cells and granulomas distort the walls of the alveoli, bronchi, and blood vessels (Fig. 309-1A), thus altering the intimate relationships between air and blood necessary for normal gas exchange. When a sufficient amount of pulmonary tissue is involved, it is sensed by the individual as dyspnea. In contrast, most individuals with sarcoidosis have granulomatous mononuclear cell inflammation in the liver but usually do not have symptoms or significant functional derangements referable to that organ, likely because the disease process does not modify the local structures sufficiently to affect function.

If the disease is suppressed, either spontaneously or with therapy, the mononuclear inflammation is reduced in intensity and the number of granulomas is reduced. The granulomas resolve either by dispersion of the cells or by centripetal proliferation of fibroblasts from the periphery of the granuloma inward, to form a small scar. In chronic cases,

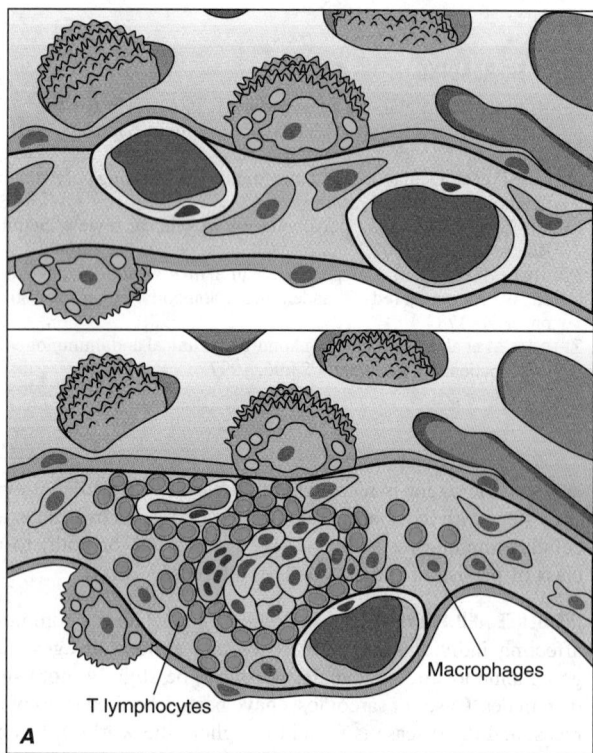

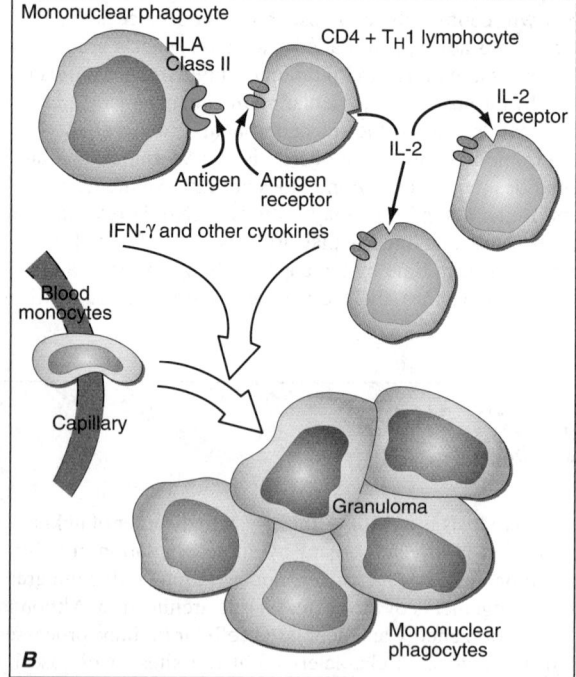

FIGURE 309-1 Pathogenesis of sarcoidosis. *A.* Histologic abnormalities. Normal alveoli (*top*) and alveoli in active sarcoidosis (*bottom*). The latter are distorted by the accumulated CD4+ T_H1 lymphocytes, alveolar macrophages, and macrophages aggregated into granulomas. There is mild damage to alveolar epithelial and endothelial cells. *B.* The exaggerated processes of T_H1 lymphocytes in affected organs result in the accumulation of these cells along with macrophages and macrophages aggregated into granulomas. The trigger for the T_H1 lymphocytes is unknown. It may be a limited class of antigens or self-antigens presented in the context of class II HLA surface molecules by mononuclear phagocytes to the T_H1 lymphocyte. The antigen class II HLA complex is identified by the T cell antigen receptor, and the T cell is activated. Consequent to this process the immune response is exaggerated and skewed to produce activated T_H1 lymphocytes that release IL-2, which drives the accumulation of more T lymphocytes. The activated T_H1 lymphocytes also release interferon γ (INF-γ). Together with cytokines such as IL-12, macrophage inflammatory protein 1α and granulocyte-macrophage colony-stimulating factor released in the local milieu, there is recruitment and activation of blood monocytes and subsequent granuloma formation.

the mononuclear cell inflammation persists for years. If the intensity of the inflammation is sufficiently high for a sufficiently long period, the derangements to the affected tissues result in extensive damage, the development of fibrosis, and permanent loss of organ function.

The available evidence suggests that active sarcoidosis results from an exaggerated cellular immune response to a variety of antigens or self-antigens, in which the process of T lymphocyte triggering, proliferation, and activation is skewed in the direction of CD4+ T_H1 lymphocyte processes (Fig. 309-1B). The result is an exaggerated T_H1 T lymphocyte response and thus the accumulation of large numbers of activated T_H1 cells in the affected organs. Since the activated T_H1 lymphocyte releases mediators that attract and activate mononuclear phagocytes, it is likely that the process of granuloma formation is a secondary phenomenon that is a consequence of the exaggerated T_H1 cell process. In this context, the current hypotheses of the cause of sarcoidosis, not mutually exclusive, include the following: (1) The disease is caused by a class of persistent antigens, nonself or self, that trigger only the T_H1 cell arm of the immune response; (2) the disease results from an inadequate suppressor arm of the immune response, such that T_H1 cell processes cannot be shut down in a normal fashion; or (3) the disease results from inherited (and/or acquired) differences in immune response genes, such that the response to a variety of antigens is an exaggerated, T_H1 cell process.

Independent of the inciting agent(s) or the reason why there is an exaggerated T_H1 cell response, there is a general understanding of the processes responsible for the maintenance of the inflammation and the development of the granuloma. The T_H1 lymphocytes accumulate at the sites of disease, at least in part, because they proliferate in these sites at an exaggerated rate. This T cell proliferation is maintained by the spontaneous release of interleukin (IL) 2, the T cell growth factor, by activated T_H1 cells in the local milieu. In this regard, sarcoidosis is a remarkable example of compartmentalization of the immune system and a dramatic illustration of why disease activity of sarcoidosis cannot be assessed by evaluating the immune system only in the blood. Whereas the T_H1 cells in the involved organs are releasing IL-2 and proliferating at an enhanced rate, the T cells in other sites, such as blood, are quiescent. Furthermore, while there is a marked enhancement of the number of T_H1 cells at the sites of disease, the numbers of T_H1 cells in the blood are normal or slightly reduced. In the involved organs, the ratio of CD4+ to CD8+ T cells may be as high as 10:1 compared to the ratio of 2:1 found in normal tissues or in the blood of affected individuals.

In addition to driving other T_H1 cells in the affected organs to proliferate, the T_H1 cells at the sites of disease are activated and release mediators that both recruit and activate mononuclear phagocytes. The activated T_H1 cells accomplish this by releasing a variety of mediators (lymphokines) including proteins capable of recruiting blood monocytes to the local milieu of the activated T cells and interferon γ, a protein that, among its many actions, activates mononuclear phagocytes. Together with cytokines such as IL-12 and others released locally, these mediators recruit blood monocytes to the affected organs and activate them, providing the building blocks for the formation of the granuloma.

In addition to these exaggerated cellular immune processes, active sarcoidosis is also characterized by hyperglobulinemia. Included among the immunoglobulins are antibodies against a variety of infectious agents as well as IgM anti-T cell antibodies. However, there is no evidence that any of these antibodies plays a role in the pathogenesis of the disease, and they are thought to result from the nonspecific polyclonal stimulation of B cells by the activated T cells at the site of disease.

If the damage in the affected organs is sufficiently extensive that the remaining parenchymal cells cannot reestablish the normal tissue architecture, the usual result is fibrosis, the proliferation of mesenchymal cells, and deposition of their connective tissue products. There is convincing evidence that the fibroblast proliferation is directed by tissue macrophages spontaneously releasing growth signals for fibroblasts, including platelet-derived growth factor, fibronectin, and insulin-like growth factor 1. It is not known, however, why this fibrotic process occurs only in a relatively small proportion of individuals with sarcoidosis.

CLINICAL MANIFESTATIONS Sarcoidosis is a systemic disease, and thus the clinical manifestations may be generalized or focused on one or more organs. However, because the lung is almost always involved, most patients have symptoms referable to the respiratory system. Independent of the site, the clinical manifestations of the disease relate directly to the exaggerated T_H1 lymphocyte–mononuclear phagocyte granulomatous inflammatory process itself or to the sequelae resulting from the permanent damage caused by this process.

Sarcoidosis is occasionally discovered in a completely asymptomatic individual, but more commonly it presents abruptly over 1 to 2 weeks or the affected individual develops symptoms insidiously over several months. Independent of the mode of presentation, ~75% of all cases present in individuals younger than 40 years.

The asymptomatic form is usually detected by a routine examination, such as a chest film. In the United States, this form represents about 10 to 20% of all cases, but in countries where chest films are mandatory in preemployment screening programs, the proportion of asymptomatic patients is higher.

So-called acute or subacute sarcoidosis develops abruptly over a period of a few weeks and represents 20 to 40% of all cases. These individuals usually have constitutional symptoms such as fever, fatigue, malaise, anorexia, or weight loss. These symptoms are usually mild, but in ~25% of the acute cases the constitutional complaints are extensive. Many patients have respiratory symptoms, including cough, dyspnea, a vague retrosternal chest discomfort, and/or polyarthritis. Two syndromes have been identified in the acute group. *Löfgren's syndrome*, frequent in Scandinavian, Irish, and Puerto Rican females, includes the complex of erythema nodosum (Fig. 309-2) and x-ray findings of bilateral hilar adenopathy, often accompanied by joint symptoms, including arthritis at the ankles, knees, wrists, or elbows. The *Heerfordt-Waldenström syndrome* describes individuals with fever, parotid enlargement, anterior uveitis, and facial nerve palsy.

The insidious form of sarcoidosis develops over months and is usually associated with respiratory complaints without constitutional symptoms. In the United States, 40 to 70% of all patients with sarcoidosis patients are in this category. About 10% of these individuals have symptoms referable to organs other than the lung. It is the individuals who present with the insidious form of sarcoidosis who most commonly go on to develop chronic sarcoidosis, with permanent damage to the lung and other organs.

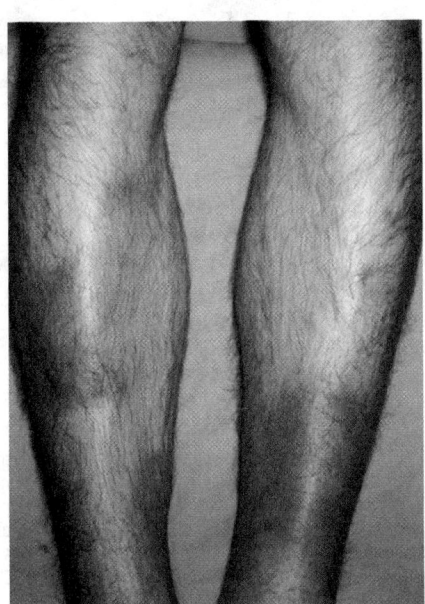

FIGURE 309-2 Erythema nodosum is a panniculitis characterized by tender deep-seated nodules and plaques usually located on the lower extremities.

Despite the fact that sarcoidosis is a systemic disease and some evidence of inflammation can be detected in most organs in the majority of patients, sarcoidosis is important clinically because of the pulmonary abnormalities and, to a lesser extent, lymph node, skin, liver, and eye involvement. Far less commonly, other organs are involved significantly.

Lung Of individuals with sarcoidosis, 90% have abnormal findings on chest x-ray at some time during their course (Fig. 309-3A). Overall, ~50% develop permanent pulmonary abnormalities, and 5 to 15% have progressive fibrosis of the lung parenchyma. Sarcoidosis of the lung is primarily an interstitial lung disease (Chap. 243) in which the inflammatory process involves the alveoli, small bronchi, and small blood vessels. These individuals typically have symptoms of dyspnea, particularly with exercise, and a dry cough. In acute and subacute cases, physical examination usually reveals dry rales. Hemoptysis is rare, as is production of sputum. Occasionally, the large airways are involved to a degree sufficient to cause dysfunction. Distal atelectasis can result from endobronchial sarcoidosis or from external compression from enlarged intrathoracic nodes. Rarely, wheezing is heard, incorrectly suggesting asthma. Large-vessel pulmonary granulomatous arteritis is common, but it rarely causes major problems. If it dominates the pulmonary lesions, it is sometimes called *necrotizing sarcoidal granulomatosis*. The pleura is involved in 1 to 5% of cases, almost always manifesting as a unilateral pleural effusion with characteristics of an exudate containing lymphocytes. The effusions usually clear within a few weeks, but chronic pleural thickening can result. Pneumothorax or hydropneumothorax is observed in sarcoid but is very rare.

Lymph Nodes Lymphadenopathy is very common in sarcoidosis. Intrathoracic nodes are enlarged in 75 to 90% of all patients; usually this involves the hilar nodes, but the paratracheal nodes are commonly involved ((Fig. 309-3A). Less frequently, there is enlargement of subcarinal, anterior mediastinal, or posterior mediastinal nodes. Peripheral lymphadenopathy is very common, particularly involving the cervical, axillary, epitrochlear, and inguinal nodes. The nodes in the retroperitoneal area and in the mesenteric chain also can enlarge. All these nodes are nonadherent, with a firm, rubbery texture. Palpation causes no pain. Unlike nodes in tuberculosis, the nodes do not ulcerate. The lymphadenopathy rarely causes a problem for the affected individual; however, if it is massive, it can be disfiguring and can impinge on other organs and lead to functional impairment.

Skin Sarcoidosis involves the skin in ~25% of patients. The most common lesions are erythema nodosum (Fig. 309-2), plaques, maculopapular eruptions, subcutaneous nodules, and lupus pernio (Fig. 309-4). Erythema nodosum, comprising bilateral, tender red nodules on the anterior surface of the legs, is not specific for sarcoidosis but is common, particularly in acute sarcoidosis, in combination with systemic symptoms and polyarthralgias. Treatment is not required, since the lesions resolve spontaneously in 2 to 4 weeks. Erythema nodosum is much more common among patients with sarcoidosis in Europe than in the United States. Skin plaques associated with sarcoidosis are purple, indolent lesions, often raised, and usually occur on the face, buttocks, and extremities. The maculopapular eruptions occur on the face around the eyes and nose, on the back, and on the extremities. These are elevated lesions <1 cm in diameter with a flat, waxy top. Subcutaneous nodules are most common on the trunk and extremities. Lupus pernio is characterized by indurated blue-purple, swollen, shiny lesions on the nose, cheeks, lips, ears, fingers, and knees. The lesions on the tip of the nose cause a bulbous appearance, sometimes associated with varicosities. The nasal mucosa is usually involved, and underlying bone can be destroyed. Sarcoidosis can also involve old surgical scars and tattoos. Although it may be disfiguring, cutaneous sarcoidosis rarely causes major problems. Clubbing of the fingers is occasionally observed in sarcoidosis, usually in association with extensive pulmonary fibrosis.

Eye Eye involvement occurs in ~25% of patients with sarcoidosis, and it can cause blindness. The usual lesions involve the uveal tract, iris, ciliary body, and choroid. Of those patients with eye involvement, ~75% have anterior uveitis and 25 to 35% have posterior uveitis. There is blurred vision, tearing, and photophobia. The uveitis can develop rapidly and may clear spontaneously over a 6- to 12-month period. It also can develop insidiously and be chronic. The uveitis often occurs in association with retinal vasculitis. Conjunctival involvement is also common, usually with small, yellow nodules. When the lacrimal gland is involved, a keratoconjunctivitis sicca syndrome, with dry, sore eyes, can result.

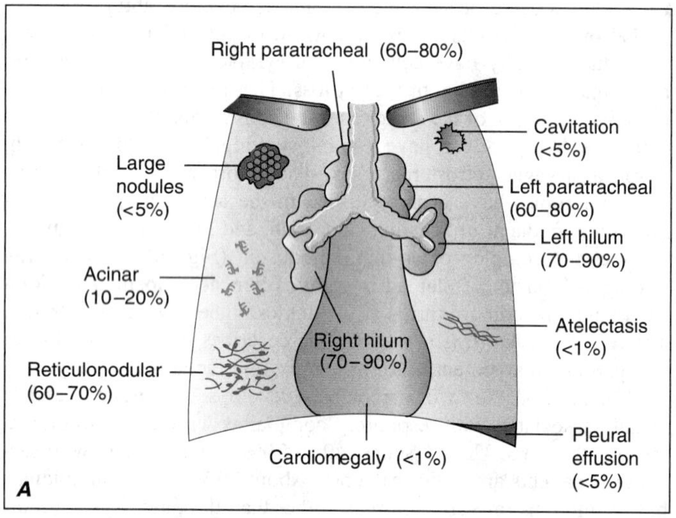

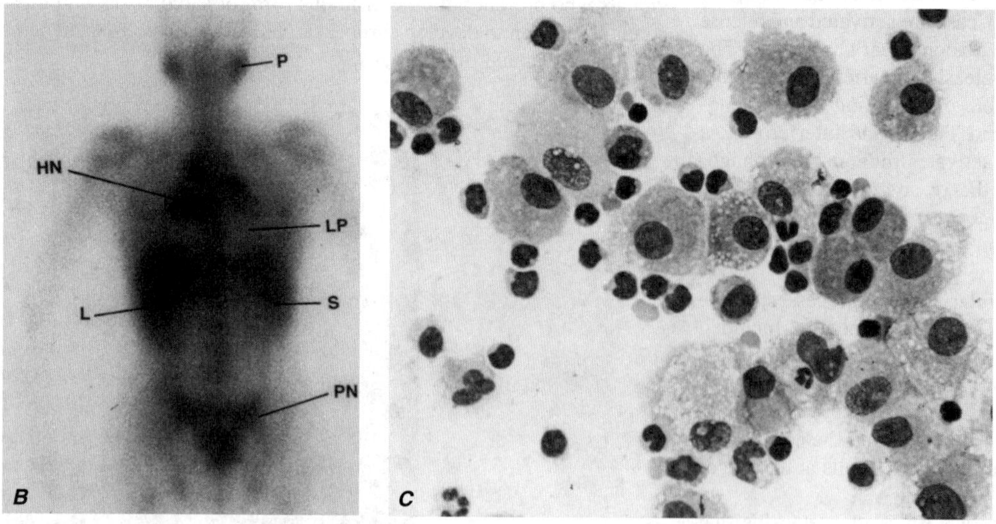

FIGURE 309-3 Common laboratory findings of sarcoidosis. *A.* Schematic view of the abnormal findings on the chest x-ray. Shown are changes observed with the average frequency of occurrence. *B.* Typical gallium-67 scan of an individual with active sarcoidosis. The isotope has accumulated in the lung parenchyma (LP), liver (L), spleen (S), parotid (P), hilar nodes (HN), and pelvic nodes (PN). *C.* Cells recovered by bronchoalveolar lavage of an individual with active pulmonary sarcoidosis. The lavage analysis reflects the inflammation in the tissue. Shown are alveolar macrophages (*large cells*) and lymphocytes (*small cells*). The cell population is dominated by the T_H1 subset of CD4+ lymphocytes, in contrast to normal individuals, in whom lymphocytes represent <20% of the cell population.

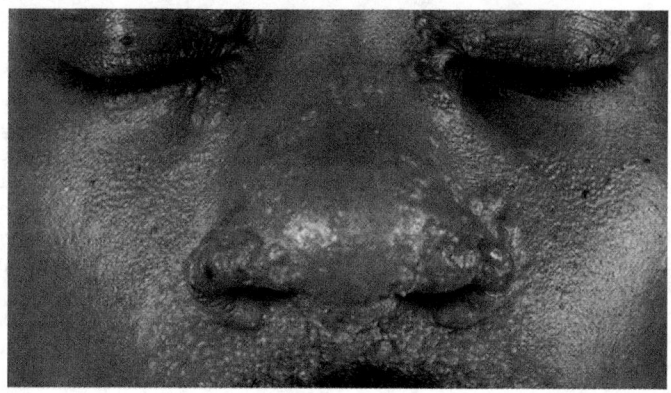

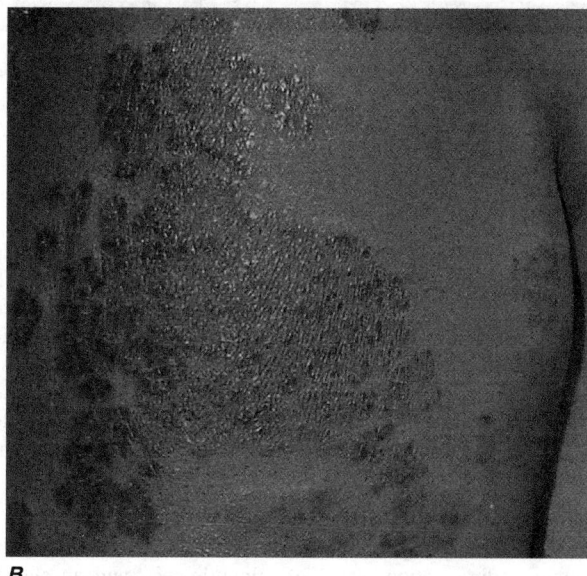

FIGURE 309-4 Sarcoid. *A.* Infiltrated papules and plaques of variable color are seen in a typical paranasal and periorbital location. *B.* Infiltrated, hyperpigmented, and erythematous coalescent papules and plaques on the upper area.

Upper Respiratory Tract The nasal mucosa is involved in up to 20% of patients, usually presenting with nasal stuffiness. Any of the structures of the mouth can be involved, particularly the tonsils but also the tongue. Sarcoidosis involves the larynx in ~5% of patients. The epiglottis and areas around the true vocal cords are usually involved, but the cords themselves are not. These individuals are usually hoarse, and they have dyspnea, wheezing, and stridor; complete obstruction can occur.

Bone Marrow and Spleen Sarcoidosis of the marrow is reported in 15 to 40% of patients, but it rarely causes hematologic abnormalities other than a mild anemia, neutropenia, eosinophilia, and occasionally, thrombocytopenia. Although splenomegaly occurs in only 5 to 10% of patients, celiac angiography or splenic biopsy reveals involvement in 50 to 60% of patients. The presentation and complications of splenomegaly in sarcoidosis are similar to those of splenomegaly in general.

Liver Although liver biopsy reveals liver involvement in 60 to 90% of patients, liver dysfunction is usually not important clinically. Sarcoidosis generally involves the periportal areas. Isolated granulomatous hepatitis can occur. Approximately 20 to 30% have hepatomegaly and/or biochemical evidence of liver involvement. Usually these changes reflect a cholestatic pattern and include an elevated alkaline phosphatase level; the bilirubin and aminotransferase levels are only mildly elevated, and jaundice is rare. Rarely, portal hypertension can develop, as can intrahepatic cholestasis with cirrhosis. There are several reports of the development of sarcoidosis in association of the treatment of chronic hepatitis C with interferon α.

Kidney Clinically apparent primary renal involvement in sarcoidosis is rare, although tubular, glomerular, and renal artery diseases have been reported. More commonly, but still in only 1 to 2% of all patients, there is a disorder of calcium metabolism with hypercalciuria, with or without hypercalcemia. If chronic, nephrocalcinosis and nephrolithiasis can result. It is believed that the calcium abnormalities are associated with enhanced calcium absorption in the gut, which is related to an abnormally high level of circulating 1,25-dihydroxyvitamin D produced by mononuclear phagocytes in the granulomas.

Nervous System All components of the nervous system can be involved in sarcoidosis. Neurologic findings are observed in about 5% of patients. Seventh nerve involvement with unilateral facial paralysis is most common. It occurs suddenly and is usually transient. Other common manifestations of neurosarcoid include optic nerve dysfunction, papilledema, palate dysfunction, hearing abnormalities, hypothalamic and pituitary abnormalities, chronic meningitis, and, occasionally, space-occupying lesions. Psychiatric disturbances have been described, and seizures can occur. Rarely, multiple lesions occur that mimic multiple sclerosis, spinal cord abnormalities, and peripheral neuropathy.

Musculoskeletal System The bones, joints, and/or muscles can be involved in sarcoidosis. Bone lesions are observed in 3 to 13% of patients and include variable-sized cysts in areas of expanded bone, with well-defined, round, punched-out lesions or lattice-like changes, often at the ends of the affected bones. The lesions are cortical, with the periostium preserved. Hand and foot bones are the common sites, but most bones can be involved. Occasionally, the bone lesions are tender and painful. Dactylitis with soft tissue swelling can be present over the affected digit. Joint involvement is more common, with an incidence of 25 to 50% in known cases of sarcoidosis. Arthralgias and frank arthritis occur mostly in large joints; they can be migratory and are usually transient, but they can be chronic and result in deformities. Although muscle biopsy frequently demonstrates granulomatous inflammation, muscle dysfunction is rare. However, nodules, polymyositis, and chronic myopathy have been described.

Heart Approximately 5% of patients have significant heart involvement, with clinical evidence of cardiac dysfunction. Left ventricular wall involvement is common. Arrhythmias are frequent, and serious conduction disturbances, including complete heart block, can occur. Sudden death has been associated with cardiac sarcoid. Papillary muscle dysfunction, pericarditis, and congestive heart failure are also observed. Cor pulmonale secondary to chronic pulmonary fibrosis may occur but is uncommon.

Endocrine and Reproductive System The hypothalamic-pituitary axis is the part of the endocrine system most commonly involved; this condition usually presents as diabetes insipidus. Anterior pituitary dysfunction is also seen, manifesting as a deficiency in one or more pituitary hormones. Complete hypopituitarism is rare. Much less frequently, sarcoidosis can cause primary dysfunction of other endocrine glands. Adrenal cortical involvement resulting in Addison's syndrome has been described. The reproductive organs may be involved, but infertility is rare. Pregnancy is not affected by sarcoidosis, and women with sarcoidosis who become pregnant usually improve during pregnancy. However, the disease may flare post partum; presumably this variation results from fluctuations in endogenous glucocorticoid production.

Exocrine Glands Parotid enlargement is a classic feature of sarcoidosis, but clinically apparent parotid involvement occurs in <10% of patients. Bilateral involvement is the rule. The gland is usually nontender, firm, and smooth. Xerostomia can occur; other exocrine glands are affected only rarely.

Gastrointestinal Tract Although sarcoidosis involvement of the gastrointestinal tract is found occasionally at autopsy, it rarely has clinical importance. Occasionally, patients have esophageal or gastric symptoms. Rarely, the peritoneum is involved with accompanying ascites.

Sarcoid can present as an isolated pancreatic lesion mimicking pancreatic carcinoma.

COMPLICATIONS The respiratory tract abnormalities cause most of the morbidity and mortality associated with sarcoidosis. The major problems are those characteristic of interstitial lung disease (Chap. 243), particularly dyspnea and insufficient oxygen delivery to vital organs. Respiratory failure with carbon dioxide retention is rare. In some patients, lung destruction results in formation of bullae that may harbor mycetomas, which are usually aspergillomas; erosion into the parenchyma can result in massive bleeding. The most common complications apart from the lung are associated with the eye; however, with therapy, blindness is rare. Complications of other organs include a gamut of abnormalities. The most serious are central nervous system (CNS) lesions or cardiac involvement leading to congestive heart failure or sudden death.

LABORATORY ABNORMALITIES Common abnormalities in the blood include lymphocytopenia, an occasional mild eosinophilia, an increased erythrocyte sedimentation rate, hyperglobulinemia, and an elevated level of angiotensin-converting enzyme (ACE). False-positive tests for rheumatoid factor or antinuclear antibodies can be observed. Hypercalcemia is rare. Other serum abnormalities relate to involvement of specific organs such as liver, kidney, or endocrine glands.

Because the lung is involved so commonly, the routine chest film is almost always abnormal (Fig. 309-3*A*). The three classic x-ray patterns of pulmonary sarcoidosis are type I—bilateral hilar adenopathy with no parenchymal abnormalities; type II—bilateral hilar adenopathy with diffuse parenchymal changes; and type III—diffuse parenchymal changes without hilar adenopathy. The type III pattern is sometimes split into two categories, with films that show fibrosis and upper lobe retraction classified separately. Although patients with type I x-ray patterns tend to have the acute or subacute, reversible form of the disease while those with types II and III often have the chronic, progressive disease, these patterns do not represent consecutive "stages" of sarcoidosis. Thus, except for epidemiologic purposes, this x-ray categorization is mostly of historic interest. The hilar adenopathy is almost always bilateral, but unilateral node enlargement can be seen. Nodes are also common in the paratracheal region. The diffuse paren-

chymal changes are typically reticulonodular infiltrates, but an acinar pattern is observed occasionally. Large nodules, similar to those of metastatic disease, are unusual but can occur. When there is massive fibrosis, the hila are pulled upward and there are conglomerate masses in the midlung zones. Some of the unusual chest x-ray findings in sarcoidosis include "egg shell" calcification of hilar nodes, pleural effusions, cavitation, atelectasis, pulmonary hypertension, pneumothorax, and cardiomegaly. Computed tomography of the chest is rarely helpful for either diagnosis or prognosis but can identify early fibrosis. A "ground-glass" appearance is often associated with an active alveolitis but more likely results from the granulomas.

The lung function abnormalities of sarcoidosis are typical for interstitial lung disease (Chap. 243) and include decreased lung volumes and diffusing capacity with a normal or supernormal ratio of the forced expiratory volume in 1 s to the forced vital capacity. Occasionally there is evidence of airflow limitation. There is usually mild hypoxemia and a mild, compensated hypocarbia.

The gallium-67 lung scan is usually abnormal, showing a pattern of diffuse uptake. If present, enlarged nodes are detected in these scans, as is inflammation in a variety of extrathoracic sites that usually have no clinical importance (Fig. 309-3*B*). Bronchoalveolar lavage typically demonstrates an increased proportion of lymphocytes, most of which are members of the activated T_H1 subset of CD4+ T lymphocytes (Fig. 309-3*C*). The remaining cells are mostly alveolar macrophages. In patients with significant fibrosis, a few neutrophils are also found. Eosinophils are rare.

The other laboratory features of sarcoidosis depend on the specific organ involved.

DIAGNOSIS For a typical case, the diagnosis of sarcoidosis is made by a combination of clinical, radiographic, and histologic findings (Fig. 309-5*A*). In a young adult with constitutional complaints, respiratory symptoms, erythema nodosum, blurred vision, and bilateral hilar adenopathy, the diagnosis is almost always sarcoidosis. Commonly, however, the findings are more subtle. Because sarcoidosis can occur in almost any place in the body, like tuberculosis or syphilis, it can be confused with many other disorders. In this context, the differential diagnosis of sarcoidosis must cover a wide range. However, it is confused most commonly with neoplastic diseases such as lymphoma or with disorders also characterized by a mononuclear cell granulomatous inflammatory process, such as the mycobacterial and fungal disorders.

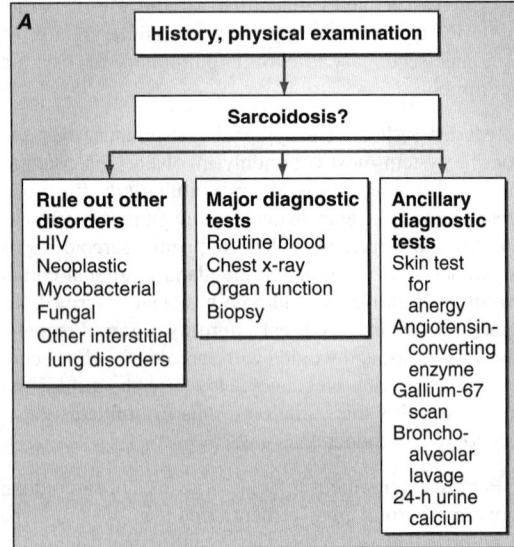

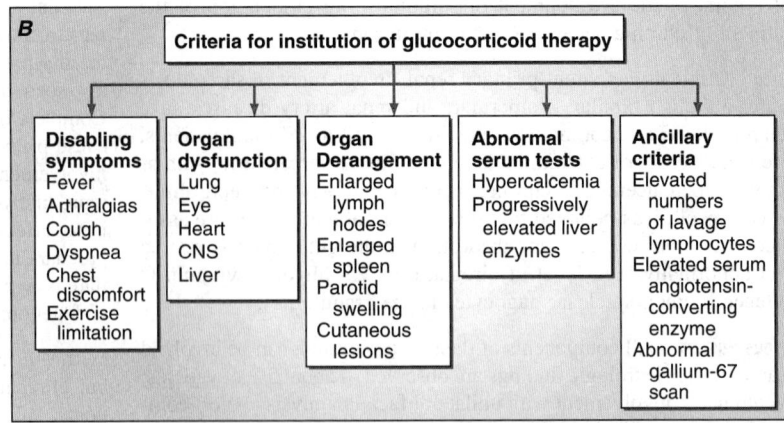

FIGURE 309-5 Diagnostic and therapeutic algorithms relevant to sarcoidosis. *A.* Diagnosis of sarcoidosis. If the history and physical examination suggest sarcoidosis, the diagnosis is made by a combination of history, physical examination, and diagnostic test. No tests are definitive for sarcoidosis; the diagnosis is made by a combination of findings. The major diagnostic tests carry the most weight, with biopsy and histologic assessment of the relevant organ the most important. Assessment of function of the organ systems that appear to be affected help with diagnosis and decisions about therapy. *B.* Therapy of sarcoidosis. Once the definitive diagnosis is made, the decision to not treat or to institute treatment with glucocorticoids is based on the presence or absence of disabling symptoms, organ dysfunction, organ derangement, and results of various tests of disease activity. Any organ can be threatened by sarcoidosis, but lung, eye, heart, liver, and central nervous system are at greatest risk. The disease can wax and wane, and periodic assessments at 3- to 6-month intervals are used to reevaluate decisions regarding therapy.

The presence of skin anergy is typical but not diagnostic of sarcoidosis. Individuals with sarcoidosis who develop active tuberculosis react strongly to skin tests with purified protein derivative. The Kveim-Siltzbach skin test, the intradermal injection of a heat-treated suspension of a sarcoidosis spleen extract which is biopsied 4 to 6 weeks later, yields sarcoidosis-like lesions in 70 to 80% of individuals with sarcoidosis, with <5% false-positive results. The Kveim-Siltzbach material is no longer available, and with the use of the transbronchial biopsy to obtain lung parenchyma for diagnostic purposes, the Kveim-Siltzbach test is only of historic interest.

No blood findings are diagnostic of the disease. Serum levels of ACE are elevated in approximately two-thirds of patients with sarcoidosis. Approximately 5% of all positive tests are not sarcoidosis and are seen in a variety of disorders, including asbestosis, silicosis, berylliosis, fungal infection, granulomatous hepatitis, hypersensitivity pneumonitis, leprosy, lymphoma, and tuberculosis. Hypercalcemia or an elevated 24-h urine calcium level is consistent with the diagnosis but is not specific.

The chest x-ray cannot be used as the sole criterion for the diagnosis of sarcoidosis. While the finding of bilateral hilar adenopathy is the hallmark of this disease, a similar pattern is occasionally observed in lymphoma, tuberculosis, coccidioidomycosis, brucellosis, and bronchogenic carcinoma.

The pattern of the gallium-67 scan is not diagnostic for sarcoidosis, nor is the finding of an increased proportion of lymphocytes among the cells recovered by bronchoalveolar lavage. However, the typical patterns of these tests (Fig. 309-3*B* and *C*) put the diagnosis in the general category of granulomatous lung disorders.

Whether or not the presentation is "classic," biopsy evidence of a mononuclear cell granulomatous inflammatory process is mandatory to make a definitive diagnosis of sarcoidosis. Because the lung is involved so frequently, it is the most common site to be biopsied, usually through a fiberoptic bronchoscope. Less common, but acceptable, sites for biopsy are the hilar nodes (by mediastinoscopy), the skin, conjunctiva, or lip. Rarely, the spleen, intraabdominal nodes, muscle, parotid or other salivary glands, upper respiratory tract, or the heart is biopsied for diagnostic purposes. At any of these sites, the findings must include the typical noncaseating granulomas. However, although histologic evidence is mandatory for a definitive diagnosis of sarcoidosis, the histologic findings are not sufficiently specific to make the diagnosis by themselves, since noncaseating granulomas are found in a number of other diseases, including infections and malignancy. Furthermore, although the liver or scalene nodes often reveal "positive" biopsies in cases of sarcoidosis, noncaseating granulomas from other causes are so frequent in these sites that they are not considered acceptable sites for establishing the diagnosis. Thus the definitive diagnosis of sarcoidosis is based on the biopsy in the context of the history, physical examination, blood tests, x-ray, lung function, and, if available, gallium-67 scan and bronchoalveolar lavage. Patients with HIV infection commonly have lymphocytopenia, chest x-ray abnormalities, positive gallium-67 chest scans, and increased proportions of lavage lymphocytes (early in the course of the disease), and they can have lung granulomas; thus, serologic testing for HIV infection should always be done in individuals suspected of having sarcoidosis.

PROGNOSIS Overall, the prognosis in sarcoidosis is good. Most individuals who present with the acute disease are left with no significant sequelae. Approximately half of all patients have some permanent organ dysfunction, but for most this is mild, stable, and progresses rarely. In ~15 to 20% of patients, the disease remains active or recurs intermittently. Death is attributable directly to the disease in ~10% of all those affected.

℞ TREATMENT

The therapy of choice for sarcoidosis is glucocorticoids (Fig. 309-5*B*). Methotrexate is usually the second-line medication. Various other drugs have been used in refractory cases, including indomethacin, oxyphenbutazone, chloroquine, hydroxychloroquine, thalidomide, infliximab, etanercept, pentoxifylline, tacrolimus, *p*-aminobenzoate, allopurinol, levamisole, azathioprine, and cyclophosphamide; but there is no evidence, apart from anecdotal, uncontrolled reports, to support their efficacy. Cyclosporine is ineffective for the pulmonary manifestations of the disease; anecdotal reports suggest that it may be useful in extrathoracic sarcoid not responding to glucocorticoids.

The major problem in treating sarcoidosis is in deciding when to treat. Because the disease clears spontaneously in ~50% of patients, and because the permanent organ derangements often do not improve with glucocorticoid treatment, there is controversy among clinicians as to the criteria for treatment. However, there is no question that glucocorticoids effectively suppress the activated T_H1 lymphocyte processes occurring at the sites of disease. Thus, the major problem in making decisions concerning therapy in sarcoidosis is to determine the extent and activity of the inflammatory process in the organs at greatest risk, such as the lung, eye, heart, and CNS.

For the lung, this is based on a combination of history, physical findings, chest x-ray, and pulmonary function tests. Centers that see large numbers of these individuals sometimes use criteria based on gallium-67 lung scans and bronchoalveolar lavage findings to help define active disease. Computed tomography is not usually helpful in treatment decisions. The serum level of ACE has been suggested as a criterion for disease activity, but it is not specific for the lung. Unless the respiratory impairment is devastating, active pulmonary sarcoidosis is observed usually without therapy for 2 to 3 months; if the inflammation does not subside spontaneously, therapy is instituted. For the eye, decisions concerning therapy are based on slit-lamp examination and tests for visual acuity. For the heart and CNS, decisions are based on an estimate of the severity of the involvement; patients with minor dysfunction are usually observed, while patients with significant cardiac or neurologic abnormalities are treated. Usually, it is not necessary to treat the systemic symptoms, but occasionally the extent of the fevers, fatigue, and/or weight loss necessitate therapy.

The usual therapy for sarcoidosis is prednisone, 1 mg/kg, for 4 to 6 weeks, followed by a slow taper over 2 to 3 months. This regimen is repeated if the disease again becomes active. Alternate-day therapy is used by some clinicians, but there is no evidence that it is as effective. High-dose bolus intravenous glucocorticoids are used occasionally but are probably not as effective as oral therapy. There is no evidence that inhaled glucocorticoids are efficacious. Mild ocular disease responds usually to local therapy, but suppression of the uveitis often requires systemic glucocorticoids. Methotrexate, 5 to 15 mg/week in a single oral dose, is often used when glucocorticoids are contraindicated or in refractory cases, but there is a cumulative risk for side effects, paricularly hepatotoxicity. There is often a 6-month time lag before improvement is seen with methotrexate. Lung transplant, usually unilateral, is reserved for end-stage disease. The presence of mycetomas is usually a contraindication for transplant. There is a 30 to 80% incidence of recurrence of sarcoid in the transplanted lung, but it is rarely significant.

FURTHER READING

BAUGHMAN RP et al:: Sarcoidosis. Lancet 361, 1111, 2003

CRYSTAL RG: Interstitial lung disease of unknown etiology: Disorders characterized by chronic inflammation of the lower respiratory tract. N Engl J Med 310:154, 235, 1984

JOHNS CJ, MICHELE TM: The clinical management of sarcoidosis. A 50-year experience at the Johns Hopkins Hospital. Medicine 78:65, 1999

ROBINSON DS et al: Granulomatous processes, in *The Lung: Scientific Foundations*, 2d ed, RG Crystal et al (eds). Philadelphia, Lippincott-Raven, 1996, pp 2395–2410

ZIEGENHAGEN MW, MÜLLER-QUERNHEIM J: The cytokine network in sarcoidosis and its clinical relevance. J Intern Med 253:18, 2003

DEFINITION AND CLASSIFICATION *Amyloidosis* results from a sequence of changes in protein folding that leads to the deposition of insoluble amyloid fibrils, mainly in the extracellular spaces of organs and tissues. Depending upon the biochemical nature of the amyloid precursor protein, amyloid fibrils can be deposited locally or may involve virtually every organ system of the body. Amyloid fibril deposition may have no apparent clinical consequences or may be associated with severe pathophysiologic changes. Named by Virchow in 1854 on the basis of color after staining with iodine and sulfuric acid, all amyloid fibrils share an identical secondary structure, the β-pleated sheet conformation, and a unique ultrastructure. All amyloid deposits contain the pentraxin serum amyloid P (SAP) and glycosaminoglycans. Abnormal protein folding and assembly can also result in protein deposition (e.g., in brain or kidney) that lacks the classic fibrillar morphology of amyloid and the presence of SAP.

The amyloidoses are classified according to the identity of the fibril-forming protein (Table 310-1). *Systemic amyloidoses* are neoplastic, inflammatory, genetic, or iatrogenic in origin, while *localized amyloidoses* or *organ-limited amyloidoses* are associated with aging and diabetes and occur in isolated organs without evidence of systemic involvement.

Despite their biochemical and clinical differences, the various amyloidoses share common pathophysiologic features: (1) an amyloidogenic precursor in appropriate concentration; (2) appropriate host genetic background; (3) abnormalities in proteolysis of fibril precursors and nascent amyloid fibrils; and (4) alterations in extracellular matrix constituents such as glycosaminoglycans and Apo E. The guidelines for nomenclature and classification of amyloid and amyloidosis were updated in 2001 by the Nomenclature Committee of the International Society of Amyloidosis (Table 310-1). Amyloid deposits should be classified using the capital letter A as the first letter of designation followed by the protein designation without any open space; for example, AL for amyloidosis involving immunoglobulin light chains.

ETIOLOGY AND PATHOGENESIS OF THE SYSTEMIC AMYLOIDOSES ■ **Light Chain Amyloidosis (AL)** The most common form of systemic amyloidosis seen in current clinical practice is AL (primary idiopathic amyloidosis, or that associated with multiple myeloma) resulting from fibril formation by fragments of monoclonal antibody light chains in primary amyloidosis and in some cases of multiple myeloma (Chap. 98). Fewer than 20% of patients with AL have myeloma. The rest have other monoclonal gammopathies, light chain disease, or even agammaglobulinemia (producing light chains, but not intact immunoglobulin). About 15 to 20% of patients with myeloma have amyloidosis. A monoclonal population of bone marrow plasma cells is present and consistently produces either small lambda or kappa fragments or immunoglobulins that are processed (cleaved) in an abnormal fashion by macrophage enzymes to produce the partially degraded light chains responsible for AL amyloidosis. Lambda chain class predominates over kappa in AL by a 2:1 ratio, whereas in multiple myeloma and normal immunoglobulin synthesis, the reverse is true. Indeed, almost all lambda VI family chains have been associated with amyloid. The primary structure of each amyloid-forming light chain is unique, reflecting the features of the B cell clone that produced it. Also, nonfibrillar deposition diseases have been described. There are three forms of human light chain–associated renal and systemic diseases: AL amyloidosis, cast nephropathy, and light chain deposition disease. Rarely, heavy chain amyloid deposition (AH) has been reported.

Amyloid A Amyloidosis (AA) AA amyloidosis (secondary, reactive, or acquired amyloidosis) occurs most frequently as a complication of chronic inflammatory disease. Effective treatment of the underlying inflammatory condition has reduced incidence in developed countries. In the past in the United States, tuberculosis (Chap. 150), osteomyelitis (Chap. 111), and leprosy (Chap. 151) were the most common precipitating diseases, and they remain so in developing countries. During inflammation, the cytokines interleukin (IL) 1, IL-6, and tumor necrosis factor (TNF) stimulate hepatic synthesis of serum amyloid A, the AA fibril precursor. Thus, effective treatment of the underlying inflammatory disorder blocks the stimulus for precursor synthesis. Familial deposition of the AA protein occurs in patients with the hereditary periodic fever syndromes familial Mediterranean fever (FMF), TNF receptor–associated periodic syndrome (TRAPS), Muckle-Wells syndrome (MWS), and familial cold uticaria (FCU) (Chap. 279). Colchicine treatment effectively blocks attacks of FMF and reduces the incidence of AA amyloidosis in association with FMF. FMF is an autosomal recessive disorder subdivided into phenotype I, with irregularly occurring fever and abdominal, chest, or joint pain, preceding or accompanying renal amyloid; and phenotype

TABLE 310-1 *Amyloid Fibril Proteins and Their Precursors*

Amyloid Protein	Precursor	Systemic (S) or Localized (L)	Syndrome or Involved Tissues
AL	Immunoglobulin light chain	S, L	Primary
			Myeloma-associated
AH	Immunoglobulin heavy chain	S, L	Primary
			Myeloma-associated
ATTR	Transthyretin	S	Familial
			Senile systemic
		L?	Tenosynovium
$A\beta_2M$	β_2-microglobulin	S	Hemodialysis
		L?	Joints
AA	(Apo)serum AA	S	Secondary, reactive
AApoAI	Apolipoprotein AI	S	Familial
		L	Aortic
AApoAII	Apolipoprotein AII	S	Familial
AGel	Gelsolin	S	Familial
ALys	Lysozyme	S	Familial
AFib	Fibrinogen α-chain	S	Familial
ACys	Cystatin C	S	Familial
ABri[a]	ABriPP	L, S?	Familial dementia, British
ADan[a]	*ADanPP*	*L*	*Familial dementia, Danish*
$A\beta$	$A\beta$ protein precursor ($A\beta$PP)	L	Alzheimer's disease, aging
APrP	Prion protein	L	Spongiform encephalopathies
ACal	(Pro)calcitonin	L	C-cell thyroid tumors
AIAPP	Islet amyloid polypeptide	L	Islets of Langerhans
			Insulinomas
AANF	Atrial natriuretic factor	L	Cardiac atria
APro	Prolactin	L	Aging pituitary
			Prolactinomas
AIns	Insulin	L	Iatrogenic
AMed	Lactadherin	L	Senile aortic, media
AKer	Kerato-epithelin	L	Cornea; familial
A(tbn)[b]	*tbn*[b]	*L*	*Pindborg tumors*
ALac	*Lactoferrin*	*L*	*Cornea; familial*

[a] ADan is coming from the same gene as ABri and has identical N-terminal sequence. It will be a matter of further discussion whether ADan should be included in the nomenclature as a separate protein (see text)
[b] To be named.
Note: Proteins in italics are preliminary.
Source: Reprinted from P Westermark et al: Amyloid 9:197, 2002, with permission.

II, in which renal amyloidosis is the first or only manifestation of the disease (Chap. 279). FMF is caused by mutations (17 identified to date) in the gene designated *MEFV* that encodes a 781-amino-acid protein named *pyrin* that appears to be a transcription factor. There is a strong correlation between the M694V mutation in MEFV and development of amyloidosis. TRAPS is an autosomal dominant disorder characterized by mutations in the TNF receptor that lead to defective shedding of the receptor and thus an impediment to the return to homeostasis. Remarkably, AA amyloidosis is not seen as a complication of the hyper IgD periodic fever syndrome (HIDS) that is associated with mutations in the mevalonate kinase gene.

Heredofamilial Amyloidoses   There are a number of types of familial amyloidosis that are dominantly transmitted in association with a mutation that enhances protein misfolding and fibril formation. The protein precursors and the amyloidoses are: transthyretin (ATTR), apolipoprotein AI (AApoAI), apolipoprotein AII (AApoAII), cystatin C (ACys), gelsolin (AGel), fibrinogen alpha chain (AFib), and lysozyme (ALys). The mutant proteins, although present from birth, are associated with a delayed onset of disease symptoms, usually after three to seven decades of life. The familial amyloidoses present as neuropathy, nephropathy, cardiomyopathy, hepatomegaly, visceral pathology, lattice corneal dystrophy, and dementia. The familial amyloidoses are less commonly seen in clinical practice than AL amyloidosis, but the overlap in clinical symptoms and organ involvement makes the chemical identification of the fibril-forming protein imperative.

ATTR   The most frequently occurring form of familial amyloidosis involves transthyretin (TTR), a 14-kDa protein originally described as prealbumin, that transports thyroxine and retinol-binding protein in the blood. The first mutation to be identified in Portuguese families and in families of Swedish origin was a single amino acid substitution, methionine for valine at position 30 (V30M). To date, more than 80 TTR variants have been defined, most of which are amyloidogenic. Variant TTR gene carriers exhibit clinically heterogeneous amyloidoses according to the nature of the amino acid substitution. Patients with the V30M mutation are symptomatic in the third to fifth decades of life with progressive polyneuropathy, postural hypotension, and little myocardial infiltration. Patients with the T60A mutation are symptomatic at an older age than V30M patients and exhibit peripheral and autonomic peripheral neuropathies and progressive myocardial amyloid infiltration. Nearly 4% of the African-American population carries the V122I allele that is associated with infiltrative cardiomyopathy and carpal tunnel syndrome. The disease is late in onset, and recognition requires a high degree of clinical suspicion.

AApoAI   Deposition of apolipoprotein AI variants (G26R, W50R, L60R, L75P, L90P, L174S, and deletion mutations) can be associated with peripheral neuropathy that is clinically similar to the type of familial amyloidosis that is caused by variants of TTR. In some kindreds, the clinical presentation is kidney or liver failure without neurologic symptoms.

AApoAII   A variant of apolipoprotein AII with an extension of the coding region that results in a 25% larger molecule than the wild-type protein is associated with a familial amyloidosis with involvement of kidney glomeruli.

AGel   Two mutations, D187N and D187Y, within the actin-binding region of gelsolin lead to deposition of a 71-residue fragment encompassing the mutation in blood vessels and basement membrane. AGel has been reported primarily in Finland, but also in Denmark, Japan, the Netherlands, and the United States. Clinical manifestations of lattice corneal dystrophy and cranial neuropathy are followed by peripheral neuropathy, dystrophic skin changes, and involvement of other organs.

ALys   Hereditary nonneuropathic systemic amyloidosis has been described in English and French families in which lysozyme is the major fibril protein. Three mutations have been described—I56T, W64R, and D67H. Clinical manifestations include visceral involvement and, in some kindreds, nephropathy.

AFib   Hereditary nonneuropathic renal amyloidosis has been described in families with one of three mutations in the fibrinogen A α chains, R524L, E526V, or R554L.

Aβ_2M   In long-term hemodialysis, amyloidosis is now well recognized as a serious bone and joint complication. β_2-microglobulin is the major constituent of the amyloid fibrils, and formation of advanced glycation end products of β_2-microglobulin has been implicated in the pathogenesis of Aβ_2M.

ETIOLOGY AND PATHOGENESIS OF THE LOCALIZED AMYLOIDOSES ■ Polypeptide Hormone–Derived Amyloidosis   Amyloid deposits are common in polypeptide hormone–producing tissues and tumors. Calcitonin is deposited in the hereditary amyloid syndrome, medullary carcinoma of the thyroid (ACal) (Chap. 320). Prolactin is commonly deposited in the aging pituitary (APro). In AIAPP, islet amyloid polypeptide, also referred to as amylin, is deposited as amyloid fibrils in 90% of individuals with type 2 diabetes (Chap. 323), in endocrine tumors (Chap. 329), and in insulinoma (Chap. 329). AIAPP is thought to play an important role in the beta cell failure associated with type 2 diabetes. Human insulin does not naturally form amyloid fibrils, although fibrils of porcine insulin, AIns, are sometimes found as subcutaneous nodules at sites of insulin injection in diabetic individuals. The form of amyloid that occurs in Pindborg tumors, odontogenic tumors, has been identified as a fragment of a protein of unknown function (FLJ20513) and is thus designated as an amyloid to be named A(*tbn*) (Table 310-1).

Localized Corneal Amyloid   AKer (kerato-epithelin) is deposited as a corneal amyloid fibril protein in association with mutations in the *BIGH3* gene. Lactoferrin, without significant size truncation, is apparently deposited as corneal amyloid with trichiasis.

Localized Cardiovascular Amyloid   Localized deposits of AApoAI in atheromatous plaques, AMed (derived from medin, a fragment of aortic smooth muscle cell–derived lactoadherin) in the aortic media and AANF (atrial natriuretic factor–derived amyloid) in cardiac atria, were initially thought to be clinically insignificant but are now being viewed as potentially pathogenic.

Amyloidosis Associated with Alzheimer's Disease   A novel protein, β-amyloid protein (Aβ), is the major fibril protein in the amyloid deposits of the cerebrovascular walls and the cores of the neuritic plaques of Alzheimer's disease (AD) patients and also in individuals with Down's syndrome (Chap. 57). The intracellular neurofibrillary tangles (ATau) are composed of paired helical filaments arranged in a twisted conformation and have as their major component an abnormally phosphorylated τ-protein, a microtubule-associated protein. Aβ varies in length from 39 to 43 amino acids and is derived from a large transmembrane glycoprotein called amyloid β-precursor protein (AβPP). Mutations in AβPP are associated with familial AD and also with a different type of amyloidosis, hereditary cerebral hemorrhage with amyloidosis (Dutch type). Other forms of familial AD are associated with mutations in genes that encode presenilin proteins. Familial dementias have also been found to be associated with deposition of a newly characterized amyloid fibril protein in families of British and Danish origin (Table 310-1). The 40-amino-acid residue fibril protein is composed of the 22 C-terminal amino acids of the wild-type protein and a 12-amino-acid extension that is due to a mutation in the stop codon.

Prion Diseases   Prions are a unique class of infectious proteins associated with a group of neurodegenerative diseases, the transmissible spongiform encephalopathies. In humans, these diseases include kuru, Creutzfeldt-Jakob disease, Gerstmann-Straussler-Scheinker syndrome, and fatal familial insomnia (Chap. 363); in animals, scrapie and bovine spongiform encephalopathy (mad cow disease). PrP^{Sc} is a pathogenic, transmissible spongiform encephalopathy–specific form of the host-encoded prion protein (PrP); PrP^{Sc} differs from PrP in that it contains a high amount of β-pleated sheet structure and is insoluble and resistant to proteolytic enzymes. PrP^{Sc} deposits either consist of or can be readily converted to amyloid fibrils. APrP is similar to Aβ and ATTR in that both familial and sporadic forms occur. In addition, infectious prion diseases have resulted from the transmission of PrP^{Sc} by ritualistic cannibalism, corneal transplantation, treatment with cadaveric human growth hormone, and a variety of neurosurgical procedures. It has been suggested that the earlier onset familial forms of amyloidosis are due to accelerated fibril formation from mutant precursors, whereas in sporadic cases, amyloid fibrils are formed more slowly from normal precursor molecules. The mutant PrP molecules are nearer the thermodynamic threshold for transition to the amyloidogenic PrP^{Sc} conformation than are the normal. The transition from normal to amyloidogenic PrP^{Sc} is essentially irreversible but very slow. The disease progresses because, once formed, amyloidogenic PrP^{Sc} can seed the conversion of normal molecules into an amyloidogenic form.

Localized Deposition of Systemic Amyloid Proteins The AL and ATTR forms of amyloidosis are usually systemic but are also observed in localized deposits. For example, AL is found in skin, lung, and other sites of the body. Cardiac amyloidosis involving wild-type TTR is considered to be localized but in some cases also to have a systemic component with predominant cardiac involvement, i.e., senile systemic amyloidosis.

CLINICAL MANIFESTATIONS The clinical manifestations of amyloidosis are varied and depend entirely on the biochemical nature of the fibril protein (Table 310-2). Proteinuria is often the first symptom associated with systemic amyloidosis, particularly of the AA and AL type; peripheral neuropathies are associated with familial amyloidoses, and dementia and cognitive dysfunction with amyloid deposits in brain. Organ enlargement, especially of the liver, kidney, spleen, and heart, may be prominent in the case of AL and AA amyloidosis; however, this does not occur in familial amyloidosis, AD, or PrP diseases.

Kidney Renal involvement may consist of mild proteinuria or frank nephrosis (Chaps. 40 and 261). In some cases, the urinary sediment may show a few red blood cells. The renal lesion is usually not reversible and in time leads to progressive azotemia and death. The

prognosis does not appear to be related to the degree of the proteinuria; when azotemia finally develops, the prognosis is grave. Treatment by peritoneal dialysis or hemodialysis or kidney transplantation improves the prognosis considerably (Chaps. 262 and 263). Hypertension is rare, except in long-standing amyloidosis. Renal tubular acidosis or renal vein thrombosis may occur. Localized accumulation of amyloid may be noted in the ureter, bladder, or other parts of the genitourinary tract.

Heart Cardiac amyloidosis can present as intractable heart failure (Chap. 216). Electrocardiographic abnormalities include a low-voltage QRS complex and abnormalities in atrioventricular and intraventricular conduction, often resulting in varying degrees of heart block (Chap. 210). Owing to their propensity to develop conduction defects and arrhythmias, patients with cardiac amyloidosis appear to be especially sensitive to digitalis, and this drug should be used with caution.

With respect to systemic amyloidoses, cardiac amyloidosis is common in primary (AL) and heredofamilial amyloidosis and very rare in the secondary (AA) form. With respect to localized amyloidosis, cardiac amyloidosis of the wild type or nonvariant TTR type is common after 80 years of age; also AANF may be present in the atria and AMed in the aortic media. In systemic amyloidosis, cardiac manifestations consist primarily of congestive failure and cardiomegaly (with or without murmurs) and a variety of arrhythmias and are comparable in AL and the familial amyloidoses, the predominant forms with cardiomyopathy (Chap. 221). Although these manifestations predominantly reflect diffuse myocardial amyloid, the endocardium, valves, and pericardium may also be involved. Pericarditis with effusion is rare, although the differential diagnosis of constrictive pericarditis versus restrictive cardiomyopathy frequently arises. Echocardiography has demonstrated symmetric thickening of the left ventricular wall, hypokinesia and decreased systolic contraction and thickening of the interventricular septum and left ventricular posterior wall, and left ventricular cavities of small to normal size (Chap. 211). Two-dimensional echocardiography produces the characteristic findings of thickened right and left ventricles, a normal left ventricular cavity, and, especially, a diffuse hyperrefractile "granular sparkling" appearance. Hearts that are heavily infiltrated with amyloid may or may not show an enlarged silhouette. Fluoroscopy usually shows decreased mobility of the ventricular wall; angiographic studies usually demonstrate thickened ventricular wall, decreased ventricular mobility, and absence of rapid ventricular filling in early diastole.

Liver While hepatic involvement is common except in heredofamilial amyloidosis of the TTR type, liver function abnormalities are minimal and occur late in the disease (Chap. 290). Portal hypertension occurs but is uncommon. Intrahepatic cholestasis has been noted in about 5% of patients with AL (primary) amyloidosis. Hepatomegaly is common, and AL hepatic amyloid is usually accompanied by the nephrotic syndrome and congestive heart failure with poor prognosis. Amyloidosis of the spleen characteristically is not associated with leukopenia and anemia.

Skin Involvement of the skin is one of the most characteristic manifestations of primary (AL) amyloidosis (Chap. 48). Other forms of amyloidosis such as lichen amyloidosis are thought to involve forms of keratin. In AL amyloidosis, the usually nonpruritic lesions may consist of slightly raised, waxy papules or plaques that are usually clustered in the folds of the axillae, anal, or inguinal regions; the face and neck; or mucosal areas such as ear or tongue. Periorbital ecchymoses ("black eye" or "raccoon syndrome") have been reported.

Gastrointestinal Tract Gastrointestinal symptoms are common in all systemic types of amyloidosis either from direct involvement of the gastrointestinal tract at any level or from infiltration of the autonomic nervous system with amyloid (Chap. 271). Symptoms include obstruction, ulceration, malabsorption, hemorrhage, protein loss, and diarrhea (Chap. 275). Infiltration of the tongue is characteristic of primary amyloidosis (AL) or amyloidosis accompanying multiple myeloma and occasionally leads to macroglossia. When not enlarged, the tongue

---

TABLE 310-2 Clinical Presentation of Systemic Amyloidosis

Disease	Symptoms
AL (primary)	Monoclonal immunoglobulin in urine or serum plus any of the following: Unexplained nephrotic syndrome Hepatomegaly Carpal tunnel syndrome Macroglossia Malabsorption or unexplained diarrhea or constipation Peripheral neuropathy Cardiomyopathy
AA (secondary)	Chronic infection (osteomyelitis, tuberculosis) or chronic inflammation (rheumatoid arthritis, granulomatous ileitis) plus development of any of the following: Proteinuria Hepatomegaly Unexplained gastrointestinal disease
Hereditary amyloidosis	Family history of neuropathy plus any of the following: Early sensorimotor disassociation Vitreous opacities Renal disease Autonomic nervous system symptoms Cardiovascular disease Gastrointestinal disease No family history of neuropathy but Idiopathic cardiomyopathy Idiopathic renal disease

may become stiffened and firm to palpation. Gastrointestinal bleeding may occur from any of a number of sites, notably the esophagus, stomach, or large intestine, and may be severe. Amyloid infiltration of the esophagus may lead to an incompetent or nonrelaxing lower esophageal sphincter, nonspecific motility disorders of the esophageal body, or rarely achalasia. Small-bowel lesions may lead to clinical and x-ray changes of obstruction. A malabsorption syndrome is common. Amyloidosis (AA or secondary) may also develop in association with other entities involving the gastrointestinal tract, especially tuberculosis (Chap. 150), granulomatous enteritis (Chap. 276), lymphoma (Chap. 97), and Whipple's disease (Chap. 275); differentiation of these conditions, which give rise to secondary amyloidosis, from diffuse primary amyloidosis of the small bowel may be difficult. Similarly, amyloidosis of the stomach may closely mimic gastric carcinoma, with obstruction, achlorhydria, and the radiologic appearance of tumor masses.

Nervous System   Neurologic manifestations, especially prominent in the heredofamilial amyloidoses, may include peripheral neuropathy, postural hypotension, inability to sweat, Adies's pupil, hoarseness, and sphincter incompetence (Chaps. 22 and 364). The cranial nerves are generally spared, except in the Finnish hereditary amyloidosis (AGel). Carpal tunnel syndrome may be caused by several amyloidoses, especially primary (AL) and chronic hemodialysis ($A\beta_2M$) amyloid. Peripheral neuropathy is frequent in the former type. $A\beta$ amyloid occurs in the central nervous system as a component of senile plaques and in blood vessels ("congophilic angiopathy") (Chap. 351). The protein concentration in the cerebrospinal fluid may be increased. Infiltrates of the cornea or vitreous body may be present in hereditary amyloid syndromes and give rise to a bilateral scalloping appearance of the pupil.

Endocrine   Amyloid may infiltrate the thyroid or other endocrine glands but rarely causes endocrine dysfunction. Local amyloid deposits almost invariably accompany medullary carcinoma of the thyroid (Chap. 320). Amyloid is often found in the adrenal gland, pituitary gland, and pancreas. Pancreatic islet amyloid as a complication of type 2 diabetes is especially prominent and is caused by the islet amyloid polypeptide (IAPP, amylin). Clinical dysfunction is present when there is significant replacement of the gland by amyloid (Chap. 323).

Joints and Muscles   Amyloid can directly, although rarely, involve articular structures by its presence in the synovial membrane and synovial fluid or in the articular cartilage. In these cases it is almost always of the AL type and associated with multiple myeloma (Chap. 98). Amyloid arthritis can mimic a number of the rheumatic diseases because it can present as a symmetric arthritis of small joints with nodules, morning stiffness, and fatigue (Chap. 311). The synovial fluid usually has a low white blood cell count, a good to fair mucin clot, a predominance of mononuclear cells, and no crystals. Studies of surgical specimens suggest a significant incidence of amyloid in cartilage, capsule, and synovium in osteoarthritis (Chap. 312). Amyloid infiltration of muscle may lead to a pseudomyopathy. Shoulder muscle infiltration can produce the "shoulder pad" sign. Amyloid is

TABLE 310-3   Diagnosis of Amyloidosis

BIOPSY

Common sites	Rare sites
Subcutaneous abdominal fat aspirate	Kidney
	Liver
Rectum	Bone marrow
Skin	Synovium
Gingiva	Spleen
Occasional sites	
Small intestine	
Muscle	
Nerve	

APPROPRIATE STAIN

Congo red, viewed by polarization microscopy
Thioflavin (less specific)
Potassium permanganate pretreatment, then Congo red stain
Other:
 Cotton dyes (comparable with Congo red)
 Crystal violet (less sensitive)

PROTEIN OR DNA STUDIES

Mutant protein identification
Immunocytochemistry: immunofluorescent or immunoperoxidase stains with specific antisera

found in muscle inclusion body disease, where $A\beta$ and/or PrP have been identified.

Deposition of β_2-microglobulin as amyloid fibrils in the musculoskeletal systems is a serious complication of long-term hemodialysis. $A\beta_2M$ presents as the carpal tunnel syndrome, cystic bone lesions, and even destructive spondyloarthropathy. Carpal tunnel syndrome is also associated with AL and ATTR (Chap. 262).

Respiratory System   The nasal sinuses, larynx, and trachea may be involved by accumulation of AL amyloid, which blocks the ducts, in the case of the sinuses, or the air passages. Amyloidosis of the lung

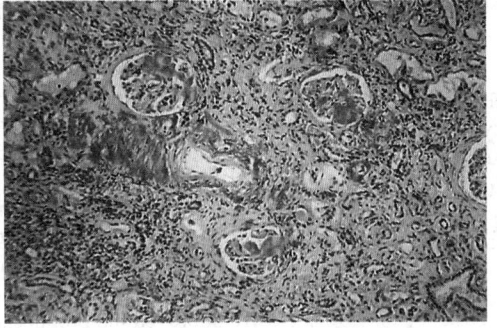
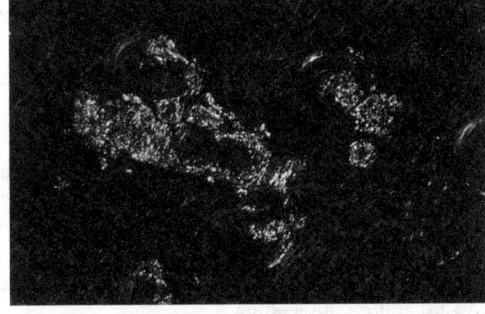
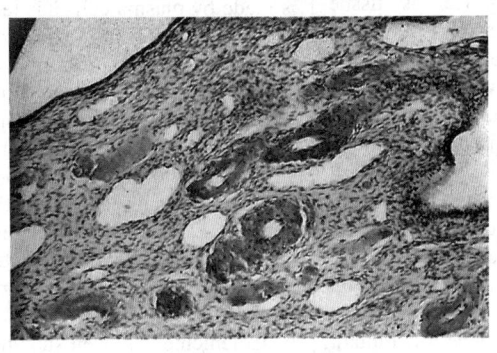
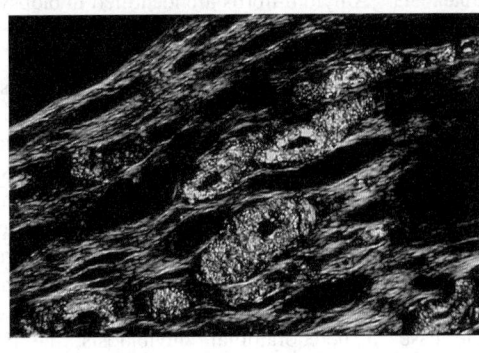

A   B   C   D

FIGURE 310-1   Microscopic tissue appearance of amyloid. *A.* Congo red–stained section of amyloidotic kidney. *B.* Polarization microscopy of section *A* showing green birefringence of glomeruli and blood vessels. *C.* Congo red–stained section of uterus. *D.* Polarization microscopy of section *C* showing the vascular amyloid as well as amyloid in the muscle wall.

TABLE 310-4 *Symptoms, Diagnosis, and Treatment of Systemic Amyloidosis*

AL (Primary)	AA (Secondary)	Familial Amyloidosis
SYMPTOMS		
Unexplained nephropathy, cardiomyopathy, neuropathy Hepatomegaly syndrome Macroglossia Malabsorption or unexplained diarrhea or constipation Any of the above *plus* monoclonal immunoglobulin in urine	Proteinuria Hepatomegaly and/or splenomegaly *plus* Chronic infection (osteomyelitis, tuberculosis) or chronic inflammation (rheumatoid arthritis, granulomatous ileitis)	Family history of peripheral neuropathy, nephropathy *plus* any of following: Carpal tunnel syndrome Vitreous opacities Renal disease Autonomic nervous system symptoms Cardiovascular disease Gastrointestinal disease Sensorimotor disassociation
LABORATORY DIAGNOSIS		
Serum, urine immunofixation electrophoresis Bone marrow biopsy with kappa and lambda light chain immunohistochemistry	Elevated serum amyloid A (SAA) Positive immunohistochemical staining for AA protein in tissue specimen	Identification of protein variant in serum DNA-based test for mutant gene
TREATMENT OPTIONS		

Depending upon cardiac involvement or stage of disease
  Cyclic oral melphalan and prednisolone
  High dose IV melphalan with stem cell rescue
	Aggressive treatment underlying inflammatory condition (monitor SAA)
	Surgical excision infection (bone resection, cholecystectomy)
	Colchicine for prevention and treatment of AA amyloidosis in FMF
		Organ transplantation (liver) (ATTR)

Note: FMF, familial Mediterranean fever.

involves the bronchi and alveolar septa diffusely. The lower respiratory tract is affected most frequently in primary (AL) amyloidosis and in the disease associated with dysproteinemia. Pulmonary symptoms attributable to amyloid are present in about 30% of cases. Amyloid may be localized in the bronchi or pulmonary parenchyma and may resemble a neoplasm. In these cases, local excision should be attempted and, when successful, may be followed by prolonged remissions.

Hematopoietic System Hematologic changes may include fibrinogenopenia, increased fibrinolysis, and selective deficiency of clotting factors (Chap. 53). Deficient factor X seems to be due to nonspecific calcium-dependent binding to the polyanionic amyloid fibrils. Splenectomy in the patient with such a factor X deficiency can relieve the deficiency and the associated bleeding disorder, since factor X has been shown to bind to the large masses of splenic amyloid. Endothelial damage together with the clotting abnormalities lead to a propensity toward abnormal bleeding.

DIAGNOSIS Amyloid fibrils are identified in biopsy or necropsy tissue sections (Table 310-3). The systemic amyloidoses offer a choice of biopsy sites; abdominal fat aspirates or renal or rectal biopsies are often performed. Microscopically, amyloid deposits stain pink with the hematoxylin-eosin stain and show metachromasia with crystal violet. The widely used and useful Congo red stain imparts a unique green birefringence when stained tissue sections are viewed using the polarizing microscope (Fig. 310-1). Fluorescent dyes such as thioflavin are sensitive screening stains for amyloid deposits in brain and other tissues; however, specificity should be confirmed. After amyloid has been identified by staining, it should be chemically classified by genomic DNA and protein studies and by immunohistochemistry. In the case of heredofamilial amyloidosis, the presence of mutant TTR (or gelsolin, Apo AI, etc.) establishes the specific diagnosis of the disease. Isoelectric focusing is used as a simple screening test for variant transthyretins associated with familial TTR amyloidosis. In order to establish the relationship of immunoglobulin-related amyloid

to multiple myeloma, electrophoretic and immunoelectrophoretic studies on serum and urine should be performed when the biopsy reveals amyloid deposition. Most of these patients will have only relatively small paraprotein components, and only a few will have frank multiple myeloma. If AL and familial amyloidosis have been ruled out, AA amyloidosis should be suspected in patients with renal amyloid and a chronic inflammatory condition (Table 310-4).

PROGNOSIS Generalized amyloidosis is usually a slowly progressive disease that leads to death if untreated. The average survival in most large series of AL amyloid is ~12 months and in familial amyloidosis is ~7 to 15 years. A number of individuals with amyloid have been followed 5 to 10 years and longer. The course of amyloidosis is difficult to document, because dating the time of origin of the disease is rarely possible. When amyloidosis deops in patients with rheumatoid arthritis, it seldom becomes evident when the arthritis is of less than 2 years' duration. When amyloidosis develops in patients with multiple myeloma, manifestations leading to initial hospitalization are more apt to be related to amyloid disease than to myeloma. In these cases, prognosis is very poor, and life expectancy is usually less than 6 months.

℞ TREATMENT

Rational therapy should be directed at (1) reducing precursor production, (2) inhibiting the extracellular deposition of amyloid fibrils, and (3) promoting lysis or mobilization of existing amyloid deposits. There are new specific therapies for the various amyloidoses. In certain of the heredofamilial amyloidoses, genetic counseling is an important aspect of treatment, and the removal of the site of synthesis of the mutant protein by liver transplantation has proven remarkably successful. Liver transplantation has been carried out since 1990 for ATTR patients in Sweden, the United States, Portugal, Spain, and other countries. It appears that disease progression is halted and that there is some improvement in autonomic nervous system function. The utilization of chronic hemodialysis and of kidney transplantation has clearly improved the prognosis of renal amyloid.

In the case of AL amyloid, the fact that immunoglobulin light chain is made by plasma cells has led to the use of alkylating agents. However, these agents are toxic and not very effective. The most effective form of treatment currently is stem cell transplantation and immunosuppressive drugs (melphalan). Several long-term remissions have been reported, but serious complications, even death, can occur. A novel anthracycline, iododoxorubicin (IDOX), has been shown to bind to AL amyloid (similar to Congo red) in vivo and promote amyloid resorption. A subset of AL patients responds transiently to this experimental agent; and it is thought that IDOX may prove useful in combination with other forms of treatment. Cardiac tranplantation in selected cases of AL or heredofamilial amyloidosis has its advocates and has been successful.

Colchicine has been shown to be effective in preventing acute attacks and amyloidosis in patients with FMF (Chap. 279). Several clinical trials are in progress for AD.

The major causes of death are heart disease and renal failure. Sudden death, presumably due to arrhythmias, is common. Occasionally, gastrointestinal hemorrhage, respiratory failure, intractable heart failure, and superimposed infections are the terminal events.

FURTHER READING

BENSON MD: Amyloidosis, in *The Metabolic and Molecular Bases of Inherited Disease*, 8th ed, CR Scriver et al (eds). New York, McGraw-Hill, 2000, pp 5345–5378.

COHEN AS, SIPE JD: Amyloidosis, in *Clinical Immunology*, 2d ed, RR Rich et al (eds). St. Louis, Mosby Year Book, 2001, Chap. 71, pp 1–8

FALK RH et al: The systemic amyloidoses. N Engl J Med 337:898, 1997

PICKEN MM: The changing concepts of amyloid. Arch Pathol Lab Med 125: 38, 2001

ROCKEN C, SHAKESPEARE A: Pathology, diagnosis and pathogenesis of AA amyloidosis. Virchows Archiv 440:111, 2002

SIPE JD: Amyloidosis. Crit Rev Clin Lab Sci 31:325, 1994

Section 3   Disorders of the Joints and Adjacent Tissues

311   APPROACH TO ARTICULAR AND MUSCULOSKELETAL DISORDERS
John J. Cush, Peter E. Lipsky

Musculoskeletal complaints account for more than 315 million outpatient visits per year. Recent surveys by the Centers for Disease Control and Prevention suggest that 33% (69.9 million) of the U.S. population is affected by arthritis or joint disorders. Many of these are self-limited conditions requiring minimal evaluation and only symptomatic therapy and reassurance. However, in some patients, musculoskeletal symptoms may herald a more serious condition that requires further evaluation or additional laboratory testing to confirm the suspected diagnosis or document the extent and nature of the pathologic process. The initial goal of the clinician is to formulate a differential diagnosis that leads to an accurate diagnosis and timely therapy, while avoiding excessive diagnostic testing and unnecessary treatment (Table 311-1). There are several urgent conditions that must be diagnosed promptly to avoid significant morbid or mortal sequelae. These "red flag" diagnoses include septic arthritis, acute crystal-induced arthritis (e.g., gout), and fracture. Each of these may be suspected by an acute onset with a monoarticular or focal presenting complaint (see below).

Individuals with musculoskeletal complaints should be evaluated in a uniform, logical manner with a thorough history, a comprehensive physical examination, and, if appropriate, laboratory testing. The goals of the initial encounter are to determine whether the musculoskeletal complaint is (1) *articular* or *nonarticular* in origin, (2) *inflammatory* or *noninflammatory* in nature, (3) *acute* or *chronic* in duration, and (4) *localized* or *widespread* (*systemic*) in distribution.

With such an approach and an understanding of the pathophysiologic processes that underlie musculoskeletal complaints, an adequate diagnosis can be made in the vast majority of individuals. However, some patients will not fit immediately into an established diagnostic category. Many musculoskeletal disorders resemble each other at the outset, and some may take weeks or months to evolve into a readily recognizable diagnostic entity. This consideration should temper the desire to establish a definitive diagnosis at the first encounter.

ARTICULAR VERSUS NONARTICULAR   The musculoskeletal evaluation must discriminate the anatomic site(s) of origin of the patient's complaint. For example, ankle pain can result from a variety of pathologic conditions involving disparate anatomic structures, including gonococcal arthritis, calcaneal fracture, Achilles tendinitis, cellulitis, and peripheral neuropathy. Distinguishing between articular and nonarticular conditions requires a careful and detailed examination. Articular structures include the synovium, synovial fluid, articular cartilage, intraarticular ligaments, joint capsule, and juxtaarticular bone. Nonarticular (or periarticular) structures, such as supportive extraarticular ligaments, tendons, bursae, muscle, fascia, bone, nerve, and overlying skin, may be involved in the pathologic process. Articular disorders may be characterized by deep or diffuse pain, limited range of motion on active and passive movement, swelling (caused by synovial proliferation, effusion, or bony enlargement), crepitation, instability, "locking," or deformity. By contrast, nonarticular disorders tend to be painful on active but not passive range of motion, demonstrate point or focal tenderness in regions distinct from articular structures, and have physical findings remote from the joint capsule. Moreover, nonarticular disorders seldom demonstrate crepitus, instability, or deformity.

INFLAMMATORY VERSUS NONINFLAMMATORY DISORDERS   In the course of a musculoskeletal evaluation, the examiner should elicit symptoms and signs that will narrow or establish the diagnosis. A primary objective is to identify the nature of the underlying pathologic process. Musculoskeletal disorders are generally classified as inflammatory or noninflammatory. Inflammatory disorders may be infectious (infection with *Neisseria gonorrhoea* or *Mycobacterium tuberculosis*), crystal-induced (gout, pseudogout), immune-related [rheumatoid arthritis (RA), systemic lupus erythematosus (SLE)], reactive (rheumatic fever, Reiter's syndrome), or idiopathic. Inflammatory disorders may be identified by the presence of all or some of the four cardinal signs of inflammation (erythema, warmth, pain, or swelling), systemic symptoms (prolonged morning stiffness, fatigue, fever, weight loss), or laboratory evidence of inflammation [elevated erythrocyte sedimentation rate (ESR) or C-reactive protein, thrombocytosis, anemia of chronic disease, or hypoalbuminemia]. Articular stiffness commonly accompanies chronic musculoskeletal disorders. However, the chronology and magnitude of stiffness may be diagnostically important. Morning stiffness related to inflammatory disorders (such as RA) is precipitated by prolonged rest, is often several hours in duration, and may improve with activity and anti-inflammatory medications. By contrast, intermittent stiffness associated with noninflammatory conditions (such as osteoarthritis) is precipitated by brief periods of rest, usually lasts <60 min, and is exacerbated by activity. Fatigue may accompany inflammation (as seen in RA and polymyalgia rheumatica) and can also be a feature of fibromyalgia (a noninflammatory disorder), anemia, cardiac failure, endocrinopathy, poor nutrition, poor sleep, or psychiatric disorders. Noninflammatory disorders may related to trauma (rotator cuff tear), ineffective repair (osteoarthritis), neoplasm (pigmented villonodular synovitis), or pain amplification (fibromyalgia). Noninflammatory disorders are often characterized by pain without swelling or

TABLE 311-1   *Evaluation of Patients with Musculoskeletal Complaints*

Goals
   Accurate diagnosis
   Timely provision of therapy
   Avoidance of unnecessary diagnostic testing
Approach
   Anatomic localization of complaint (articular vs. nonarticular)
   Determination of the nature of the pathologic process (inflammatory vs. noninflammatory)
   Determination of the extent of involvement (monarticular, polyarticular, focal, widespread)
   Determination of chronology (acute vs. chronic)
   Formulation of a differential diagnosis

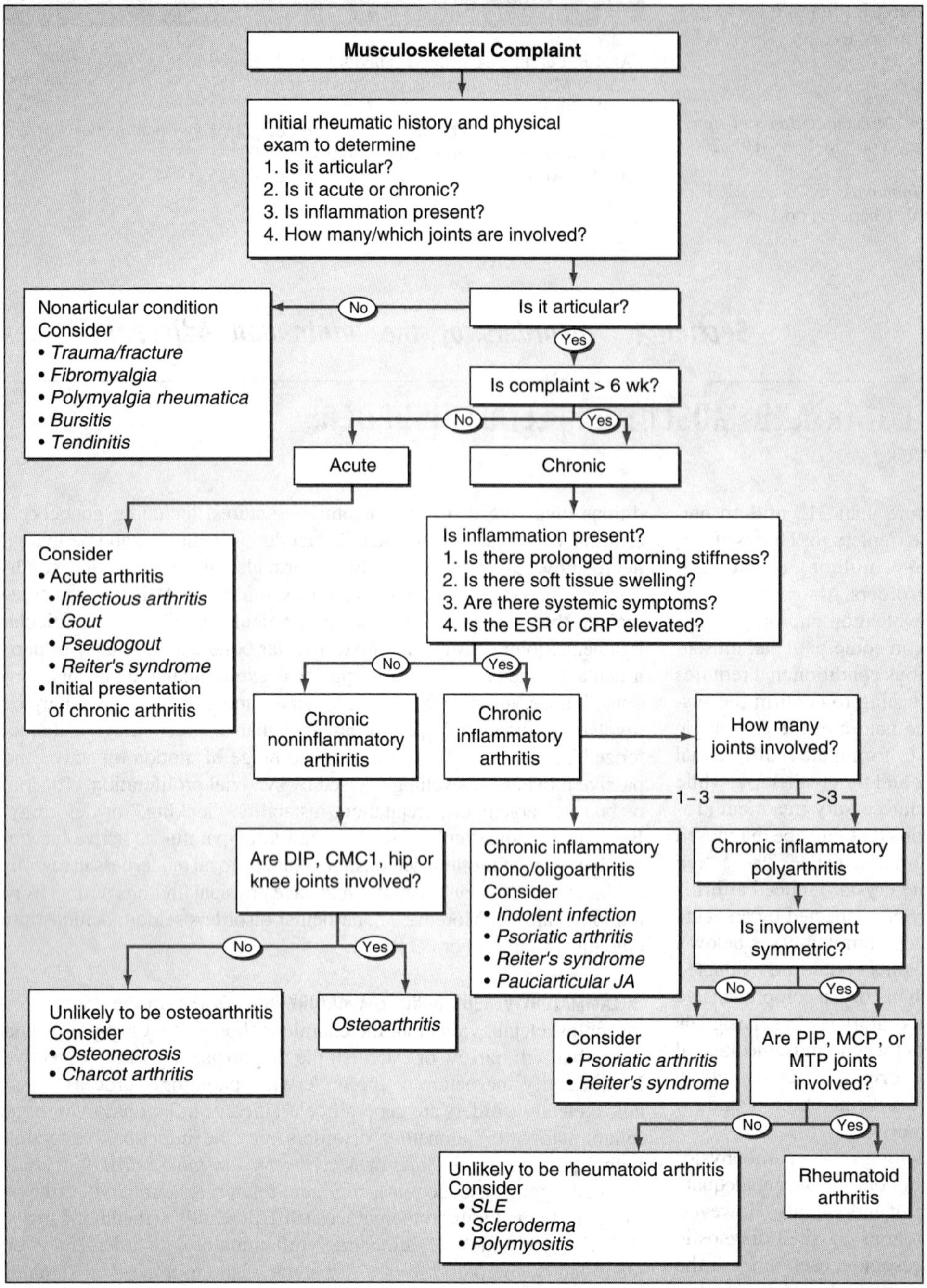

Musculoskeletal Complaint
Initial rheumatic history and physical exam to determine
1. Is it articular?
2. Is it acute or chronic?
3. Is inflammation present?
4. How many/which joints are involved?
Is it articular?
No
Yes
Nonarticular condition
Consider
• Trauma/fracture
• Fibromyalgia
• Polymyalgia rheumatica
• Bursitis
• Tendinitis
Is complaint > 6 wk?
No
Yes
Acute
Chronic
Consider
• Acute arthritis
• Infectious arthritis
• Gout
• Pseudogout
• Reiter's syndrome
• Initial presentation of chronic arthritis
Is inflammation present?
1. Is there prolonged morning stiffness?
2. Is there soft tissue swelling?
3. Are there systemic symptoms?
4. Is the ESR or CRP elevated?
No
Yes
Chronic noninflammatory arthiritis
Chronic inflammatory arthritis
How many joints involved?
1–3
>3
Are DIP, CMC1, hip or knee joints involved?
Chronic inflammatory mono/oligoarthritis
Consider
• Indolent infection
• Psoriatic arthritis
• Reiter's syndrome
• Pauciarticular JA
Chronic inflammatory polyarthritis
Is involvement symmetric?
No
Yes
Unlikely to be osteoarthritis
Consider
• Osteonecrosis
• Charcot arthritis
Osteoarthritis
No
Yes
Consider
• Psoriatic arthritis
• Reiter's syndrome
Are PIP, MCP, or MTP joints involved?
No
Yes
Unlikely to be rheumatoid arthritis
Consider
• SLE
• Scleroderma
• Polymyositis
Rheumatoid arthritis

FIGURE 311-1 Algorithm for the diagnosis of musculoskeletal complaints. An approach to formulating a differential diagnosis (shown in italics). (ESR, erythrocyte sedimentation rate; CRP, C-reactive protein; DIP, distal interphalangeal; CMC, carpometacarpal; PIP, proximal interphalangeal; MCP, metacarpophalangeal; MTP, metatarsophalangeal; PMR, polymyalgia rheumatica; SLE, systemic lupus erythematosus; JA, juvenile arthritis.)

warmth, absence of inflammatory or systemic features, minimal or absent morning stiffness, and normal (for age) or negative laboratory investigations.

Identification of the nature of the underlying process and the site of the complaint will enable the examiner to narrow the diagnostic considerations and to assess the need for immediate diagnostic or therapeutic intervention, or for continued observation. Figure 311-1 presents a logical approach to the evaluation of patients with musculoskeletal complaints.

CLINICAL HISTORY Additional historic features may be helpful in establishing the nature and extent of the pathologic process and may provide important clues to the diagnosis. Aspects of the patient profile, including age, sex, race, and family history, can provide important information. Certain diagnoses are more frequent in different *age* groups (Fig. 311-2). SLE, rheumatic fever, and Reiter's syndrome occur more frequently in the young, whereas fibromyalgia is most frequent in middle age and osteoarthritis and polymyalgia rheumatica are more prevalent among the elderly. Diagnostic clustering is also evident when *sex* and *race* are considered. Gout and the spondyloarthropathies (e.g., ankylosing spondylitis, Reiter's syndrome) are more common in men, whereas RA and fibromyalgia are more frequent in women. *Racial predilections* are noted with certain disorders. Thus, polymyalgia rheumatica, giant cell arteritis, and Wegener's granulomatosis commonly affect whites, whereas sarcoidosis and SLE more commonly affects African Americans. *Familial aggregation* may be seen in disorders such as ankylosing spondylitis, gout, RA, and Heberden's nodes of osteoarthritis.

The chronology of the complaint is an important diagnostic feature and can be divided into the *onset*, *evolution*, and *duration*. The onset of disorders such as septic arthritis or gout tends to be abrupt, whereas osteoarthritis, RA, and fibromyalgia may have more indolent presentations. The evolution of patients' complaints may also provide useful information. Disorders should be classified as either chronic (osteoarthritis), intermittent (gout), migratory (rheumatic fever, gonococcal or viral arthritis), or additive (RA, Reiter's syndrome). Musculoskeletal disorders are typically classified as acute or chronic based upon a disease duration that is either less than or greater than 6 weeks, respectively. Acute arthropathies tend to be infectious, crystal-induced, or reactive. Chronic arthritides often include noninflammatory and immunologic disorders such as osteoarthritis or RA, respectively. The duration of patients' complaints may alter the diagnostic considerations. For example, the musculoskeletal signs and symptoms of hepatitis B virus infection may be identical with those of early RA at the onset but rarely persist beyond 3 weeks.

The *number* and *distribution* of involved articulations should be noted. Articular disorders are classified based on the number of joints involved, as either *monarticular* (one joint), *oligoarticular* or *pauciarticular* (two to four joints), or *polyarticular* (more than 4 joints). Nonarticular disorders may be classified as either focal or widespread. Complaints secondary to trauma and gout are typically focal or monarticular, whereas others, such as polymyositis, RA, and fibromyalgia, are more diffuse or polyarticular in their presentation. Joint involvement in RA tends to be symmetric, whereas the spondyloarthropathies and gout are often asymmetric. The upper extremities are frequently involved in RA, whereas lower extremity arthritis is characteristic of Reiter's syndrome and gout at their onset. Involvement of the axial skeleton is common in osteoarthritis and ankylosing spondylitis but is infrequent in RA, with the notable exception of the cervical spine.

The clinical history should also identify *precipitating events*, such

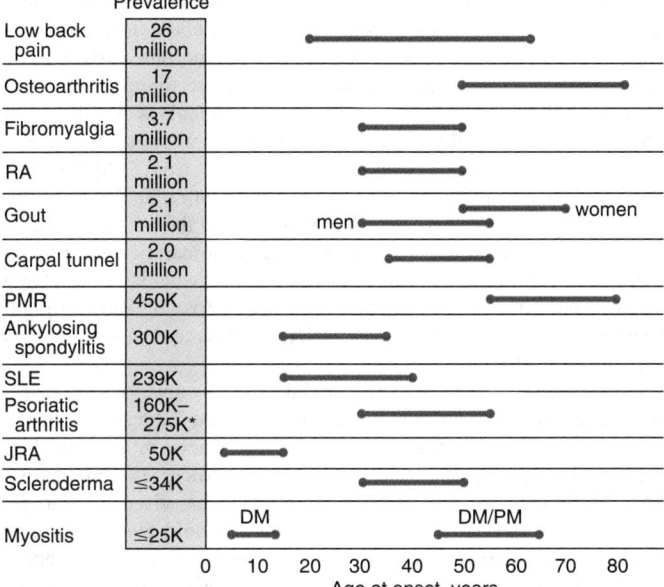

FIGURE 311-2   Age at onset for common rheumatic conditions; ranked by prevalance estimates in the United States in 1998. *Estimates vary. (RA, rheumatoid arthritis; PMR, polymyalgia rheumatica; SLE, systemic lupus erythematosus; JRA, juvenile rheumatoid arthritis; DM, dermatomyositis; PM, polymyositis.)

as trauma, drug administration (Table 311-2), or antecedent or intercurrent illnesses, that may have contributed to the patient's complaint. Lastly, a thorough *rheumatic review of systems* may disclose associated features outside the musculoskeletal system and provide useful diagnostic information. A variety of musculoskeletal disorders may be associated with systemic features such as fever (SLE, infection), rash (SLE, Reiter's syndrome, dermatomyositis), myalgias, weakness (polymyositis, polymyalgia rheumatica), or morning stiffness (inflammatory arthritis). In addition, some conditions are associated with involvement of other organ systems including the eyes (Behçet's disease, sarcoidosis, Reiter's syndrome), gastrointestinal tract (scleroderma, inflammatory bowel disease), genitourinary tract (Reiter's syndrome, gonococcemia), or the nervous system (Lyme disease, vasculitis).

PHYSICAL EXAMINATION   The goal of the physical examination is to ascertain the structures involved, the nature of the underlying pathology,

the extent and functional consequences of the process, and the presence of systemic or extraarticular manifestations. A knowledge of topographic anatomy is necessary to identify the primary site(s) of involvement and differentiate articular from nonarticular disorders. The musculoskeletal examination depends largely on careful inspection, palpation, and a variety of specific physical maneuvers to elicit diagnostic signs (Table 311-3). Although most articulations of the appendicular skeleton can be examined in this manner, adequate inspection and palpation are not possible for many axial (e.g., zygapophyseal) and inaccessible (e.g., sacroiliac or hip) joints. For such joints, there is a greater reliance upon specific maneuvers and imaging for assessment.

Examination of involved and uninvolved joints will determine whether *pain*, *warmth*, *erythema*, or *swelling* is present. The locale and level of pain elicited by palpation or movement should be quantified. For example, the number of tender joints on palpation or the patients' report of pain intensity (on a scale of 1 to 10) may be noted. The examination should distinguish true articular swelling caused by synovial effusion or synovial proliferation from nonarticular or periarticular involvement, which usually extends beyond the normal joint margins or full extent of the synovial space. Synovial effusion can be distinguished from synovial hypertrophy or bony hypertrophy by palpation or specific maneuvers. For example, small to moderate knee effusions may be identified by the "bulge sign" or "ballottement of the patellae." Bursal effusions (e.g., effusions of the olecranon or prepatellar bursa) overlie bony prominences and are fluctuant with sharply defined borders. Joint *stability* can be assessed by palpation and by the application of manual stress. *Subluxation* or *dislocation*, which may be secondary to traumatic, mechanical, or inflammatory causes, can be assessed by inspection and palpation. Joint *volume* can be assessed by palpation. Distention of the articular capsule usually causes pain. The patient will attempt to minimize the pain by maintaining the joint in the position of least intraarticular pressure and greatest volume, usually partial flexion. For this reason, inflammatory effusions may give rise to flexion contractures. Clinically, this may be detected as obvious swelling, voluntary or fixed flexion deformities, or diminished range of motion—especially on extension, when joint volumes are decreased. Active and passive *range of motion* should be assessed in all planes, with contralateral comparison. Serial evaluations of joint

TABLE 311-2   *Drug-Induced Musculoskeletal Conditions*

Arthralgias
  Quinidine, amphotericin B, cimetidine, quinolones, chronic acyclovir, interferon, IL-2, nicardipine, vaccines, rifabutin
Myalgias/myopathy
  Glucocorticoids, penicillamine, hydroxychloroquine, AZT, lovastatin, simvastatin, pravastatin, clofibrate, interferon, IL-2, alcohol, cocaine, taxol, docetaxel, colchicine, quinolones
Gout
  Diuretics, aspirin, cytotoxics, cyclosporine, alcohol, moonshine, ethambutol
Drug-induced lupus
  Hydralazine, procainamide, quinidine, phenytoin, methyldopa, isoniazid, chlorpromazine, lithium, penicillamine, tetracycline, infliximab
Osteonecrosis
  Glucocorticoids, alcohol, radiation
Osteopenia
  Glucocorticoids, chronic heparin, phenytoin, methotrexate
Scleroderma
  Vinyl chloride, bleomycin, pentazocine, organic solvents, carbidopa, tryptophan, rapeseed oil
Vasculitis
  Allopurinol, amphetamines, cocaine, thiazides, penicillamine, propylthiouracil

Note: IL-2, interleukin 2.

TABLE 311-3   *Glossary of Musculoskeletal Terms*

Crepitus
  A palpable (less commonly audible) vibratory or crackling sensation elicited with joint motion; fine joint crepitus is common and often insignificant in large joints; coarse joint crepitus indicates advanced cartilaginous and degenerative changes (as in osteoarthritis).
Subluxation
  Alteration of joint alignment such that articulating surfaces incompletely approximate each other
Dislocation
  Abnormal displacement of articulating surfaces such that the surfaces are not in contact
Range of motion
  For diarthrodial joints, the arc of measurable movement through which the joint moves in a single plane
Contracture
  Loss of full movement resulting from a fixed resistance due either to tonic spasm of muscle (reversible) or to fibrosis of periarticular structures (permanent)
Deformity
  Abnormal shape or size of a structure; may result from bony hypertrophy, malalignment of articulating structures, or damage to periarticular supportive structures
Enthesitis
  Inflammation of the entheses (tendinous or ligamentous insertions on bone)
Epicondylitis
  Infection or inflammation involving an epicondyle

motion may be recorded with a goniometer to quantify the arc of movement. Each joint should be passively manipulated through its full range of motion (including, as appropriate, flexion, extension, rotation, abduction, adduction, lateral bending, inversion, eversion, supination, pronation, and medial or lateral deviation, or bending). Limitation of motion is frequently caused by effusion, pain, deformity, or contracture. If passive motion exceeds active motion, a periarticular process (e.g., tendon rupture or myopathy) should be considered. *Contractures* may reflect antecedent synovial inflammation or trauma. Joint *crepitus* may be felt during palpation or maneuvers and may be prominent or coarse in osteoarthritis. Joint *deformity* usually indicates a long-standing or aggressive pathologic process. Deformities may result from ligamentous destruction, soft tissue contracture, bony enlargement, ankylosis, erosive disease, or subluxation. Examination of the musculature will document strength, atrophy, pain, or spasm. Muscle weakness should be characterized as proximal or distal. Muscle strength is graded on a 5-point scale: 0 for no movement; 1 for trace movement or twitch; 2 for movement with gravity eliminated; 3 for movement against gravity only; 4 for movement against gravity and resistance; and 5 for normal strength. The examiner should assess carefully for nonarticular or periarticular involvement, especially when articular complaints are not supported by objective findings referable to the joint capsule. The identification of musculoskeletal pain of soft tissue origin (nonarticular pain) will prevent unwarranted and often expensive additional evaluations. Specific maneuvers may reveal nonarticular abnormalities, such as a carpal tunnel syndrome (which can be identified by Tinel's or Phalen's sign). Other examples of soft tissue abnormalities include olecranon bursitis, epicondylitis (e.g., tennis elbow), enthesitis (e.g., Achilles tendinitis), and trigger points associated with fibromyalgia.

LABORATORY INVESTIGATIONS The vast majority of musculoskeletal disorders can be easily diagnosed by a complete history and physical examination. An additional objective of the initial encounter is to determine whether additional investigations or immediate therapy are required. A number of features indicate the need for additional evaluation. Monarticular conditions require additional evaluation, as do traumatic or inflammatory conditions and conditions accompanied by neurologic changes or systemic manifestations of serious disease. Finally, individuals with chronic symptoms (>6 weeks), especially when there has been a lack of response to symptomatic measures, are candidates for additional evaluation. The extent and nature of the additional investigation should be dictated by the clinical features and suspected pathologic process. Laboratory tests should be used to confirm a specific clinical diagnosis and not be used as a tool to screen or evaluate patients with vague rheumatic complaints. Indiscriminate use of broad batteries of diagnostic tests and radiographic procedures is rarely useful or cost-effective means to establish a diagnosis.

Besides a complete blood count, including a white blood cell (WBC) and differential count, the routine evaluation should include a determination of an acute-phase reactant such as the ESR or C-reactive protein, which can be useful in discriminating inflammatory from noninflammatory musculoskeletal disorders. Both are inexpensive and easily obtained and may be elevated with infections, inflammatory arthritis, autoimmune disorders, neoplasia, pregnancy, and advanced age. Serum uric acid determinations are useful only when gout has been diagnosed and therapy contemplated.

Serologic tests for rheumatoid factor, antinuclear antibodies (ANA), complement levels, Lyme and antineutrophil cytoplasmic antibodies, or antistreptolysin O titer should be carried out only when there is clinical evidence to suggest a relevant associated diagnosis, as these have poor predictive value when used for screening, especially when the pretest probability is low. Although, 4 to 5% of a healthy population will have positive tests for rheumatoid factor and ANA, only 1% and 0.4% of the population will have RA or SLE, respectively. IgM rheumatoid factor (autoantibodies against the Fc portion

of IgG) is found in 80% of patients with RA and may also be seen in low titers in patients with chronic infections (*tuberculosis*, leprosy); other autoimmune diseases (SLE, Sjögren's syndrome); and chronic pulmonary, hepatic, or renal diseases. ANAs are found in nearly all patients with SLE and may also be seen in patients with other autoimmune diseases (polymyositis, scleroderma, antiphospholipid syndrome), drug-induced lupus (resulting from hydralazine, procainamide, or quinidine), chronic hepatitic, or renal disorders. The interpretation of a positive ANA may depend on the magnitude of the titer and the pattern observed under immunofluorescence microscopy. Diffuse and speckled patterns are least specific, whereas a peripheral, or rim, pattern is highly specific and suggestive of autoantibodies against double-stranded (native) DNA. This pattern is seen only in patients with SLE.

Aspiration and analysis of synovial fluid are always indicated in acute monarthritis or when an infectious or crystal-induced arthropathy is suspected. Synovial fluid analysis may be crucial in distinguishing between noninflammatory and inflammatory processes. This distinction can be made on the basis of the appearance, viscosity, and cell count of the synovial fluid. Tests for synovial fluid glucose, protein, lactate dehydrogenase, lactic acid, or autoantibodies are not recommended as they are insensitive or have little discriminatory value. Normal synovial fluid is clear or a pale straw color and is viscous, primarily because of the high levels of hyaluronate. Noninflammatory synovial fluid is clear, viscous, and amber-colored, with a white blood cell count of $<2000/\mu$L and a predominance of mononuclear cells. The viscosity of synovial fluid is assessed by expressing fluid from the syringe one drop at a time. Normally there is a stringing effect, with a long tail behind each synovial drop. Effusions caused by osteoarthritis or trauma usually have normal viscosity. Inflammatory fluid is turbid and yellow, with an increased white cell count (2000 to 50,000/μL) and a polymorphonuclear leukocyte predominance. Inflammatory fluid has reduced viscosity, diminished hyaluronate, and little or no tail following each drop of synovial fluid. Such effusions are found in RA, gout, other inflammatory arthritides, and septic arthritis. Infectious fluid is opaque, and purulent, with a white cell count usually $>50,000/\mu$L, a predominance of polymorphonuclear leukocytes ($>75\%$), and low viscosity. Such effusions are typical of septic arthritis, but they occur rarely with sterile inflammatory arthritides such as RA or gout. In addition, hemorrhagic synovial fluid may be seen with trauma, hemarthrosis, or neuropathic arthritis. An algorithm for synovial fluid aspiration and analysis is shown in Fig. 311-3. Synovial fluid should be analyzed immediately for appearance, viscosity, and cell count. Cellularity and the presence of crystals may be assessed by either light or polarizing microscopy. Monosodium urate crystals, seen in gouty effusions, are long, needle-shaped, negatively birefringent, and usually intracellular, whereas calcium pyrophosphate dihydrate crystals, found in chondrocalcinosis and pseudogout, are usually short, rhomboid-shaped, positively birefringent crystals. Whenever infection is suspected, synovial fluid should be Gram-stained and cultured appropriately. If gonococcal arthritis is suspected, immediate plating of the fluid on appropriate culture medium is indicated. Synovial fluid from patients with chronic monarthritis should also be cultured for *M. tuberculosis* and fungi. Last, it should be noted that crystal-induced arthritis and infection occasionally occur together in the same joint.

DIAGNOSTIC IMAGING IN JOINT DISEASES Conventional radiography has been a valuable tool in the diagnosis and staging of articular disorders. Plain x-rays are most appropriate when there is a history of trauma, suspected chronic infection, progressive disability, or monarticular involvement; when therapeutic alterations are considered; or when a baseline assessment is desired for what appears to be a chronic process. However, in most inflammatory disorders, early radiography is rarely helpful in establishing a diagnosis and may only reveal soft tissue swelling or juxtaarticular demineralization. As the disease progresses, calcification (of soft tissues, cartilage, or bone), joint space narrowing, erosions, bony ankylosis, new bone formation (sclerosis, osteophytes,

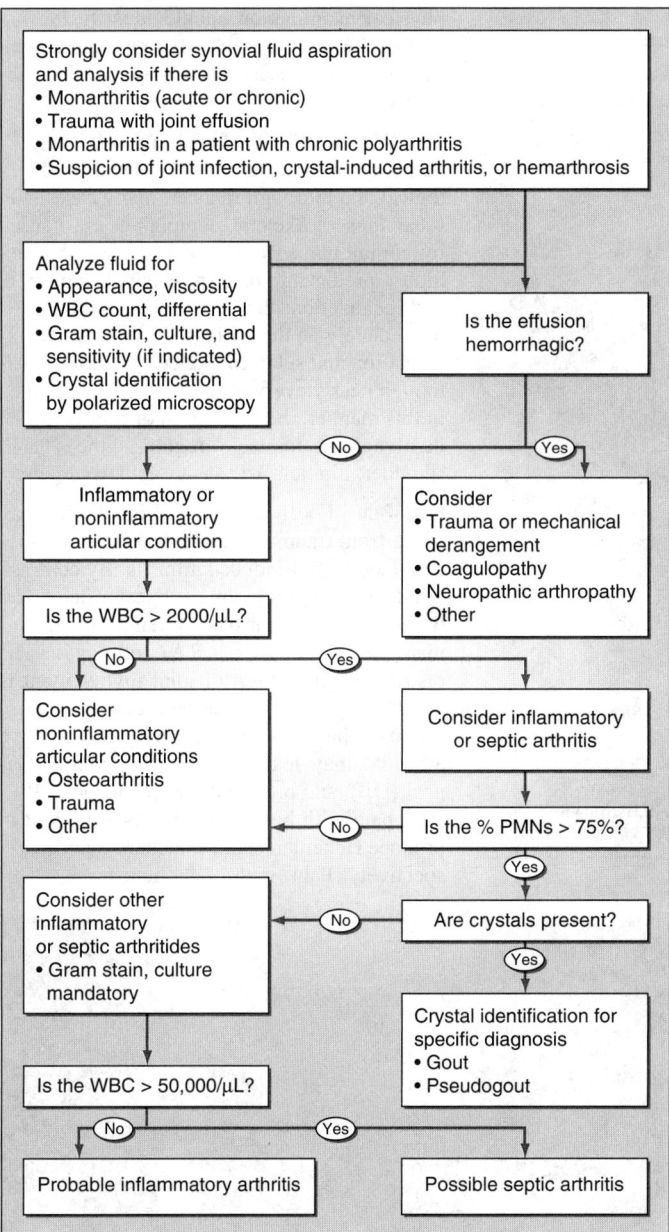

FIGURE 311-3 Algorithmic approach to the use and interpretation of synovial fluid aspiration and analysis. [WBC, white blood cell (count); PMNs, polymorphonuclear (leukocytes).]

or periostitis), or subchondral cysts may develop and suggest specific clinical entities. Consultation with a radiologist will help define proper imaging modality, technique, and positioning and prevent the need for further studies.

Additional imaging techniques may possess greater diagnostic sensitivity and facilitate early diagnosis in a limited number of articular disorders and in selected circumstances and are indicated when conventional radiography is not adequate (Table 311-4). *Ultrasonography* is useful in the detection of soft tissue abnormalities that cannot be fully appreciated by clinical examination. Although inexpensive and easily performed, in only a limited number of circumstances is it the preferred method of evaluation. The foremost application of ultrasound is in the diagnosis of synovial (Baker's) cysts, although rotator cuff tears and various tendon injuries may be evaluated with ultrasound by an experienced operator. *Radionuclide scintigraphy* provides useful information regarding the metabolic status of bone and, along with radiography, is well suited for total-body assessment of the extent and distribution of musculoskeletal involvement. Radionuclide imaging is a very sensitive, but poorly specific, means of detecting inflammatory

or metabolic alterations in bone or periarticular soft tissue structures. The limited tissue contrast resolution of scintigraphy may obscure the distinction between a bony or periarticular process and may necessitate the additional use of other imaging modalities. Scintigraphy, using ^{99m}Tc, ^{67}Ga, or ^{111}In-labeled WBCs has been applied to a variety of articular disorders with variable success (Table 311-4). [^{99m}Tc] pertechnate or diphosphate scintigraphy may be useful in identifying infection, neoplasia, inflammation, increased blood flow, bone remodeling, heterotopic bone formation, or avascular necrosis (Fig. 311-4). The poor specificity of ^{99m}Tc scanning has limited its use to investigational and serial assessments of joint or bone involvement, inflammatory or infectious processes, and surveys for bone metastases. ^{67}Ga binds to serum and cellular transferrin and lactoferrin and is preferentially taken up by neutrophils, macrophages, bacteria, and tumor tissue (e.g., lymphoma) and is useful in the identification of infection and malignancies. Scanning with ^{111}In-labeled WBCs has been used to detect both infectious and inflammatory arthritis. Although both have been used with success, ^{111}In-labeled WBC scanning is superior to ^{67}Ga in the early diagnosis of osteomyelitis and infected prosthetic joints. Prior treatment with antibiotics may reduce the diagnostic sensitivity of both ^{67}Ga and ^{111}In-labeled WBC scintigraphy.

Computed tomography (CT) provides rapid reconstruction of sagittal, coronal, and axial images and spatial relationships among anatomic structures. It has proved to be most useful in the assessment of the axial skeleton because of its ability to visualize in the axial plane. Articulations previously considered difficult to visualize using conventional radiography, such as the zygapophyseal, sacroiliac, sternoclavicular, and hip joints, can be effectively evaluated using CT. CT has been demonstrated to be useful in the diagnosis of low back pain syndromes, sacroiliitis, osteoid osteoma, tarsal coalition, osteomyelitis, intraarticular osteochondral fragments, and advanced osteonecrosis. Helical or spiral CT (with or without contrast angiography) is a novel technique that is rapid, cost effective, and sensitive in diagnosing pulmonary embolism or obscure fractures, often in the setting of initially equivocal findings. High-resolution CT can be advocated in the evaluation of suspected or established infiltrative lung disease (e.g., scleroderma or rheumatoid lung).

Magnetic resonance imaging (MRI) has significantly advanced the ability to image musculoskeletal structures. MRI has the advantages of providing multiplanar images with fine anatomic detail and contrast resolution (Fig. 311-5). Other advantages are the lack of ionizing radiation and adverse effects and the superior ability to visualize bone marrow and soft tissue periarticular structures, which have led to the increased use of this modality. The advantages of MRI are counterbalanced by high cost and long procedural time, factors that have limited its use in the evaluation of musculoskeletal disorders. MRI should be used only when it will provide necessary information that cannot be obtained by less expensive and noninvasive means.

MRI can image fascia, vessels, nerve, muscle, cartilage, ligaments, tendons, pannus, synovial effusions, and bone marrow. Visualization of particular structures can be enhanced by altering the pulse sequence to produce either T1- or T2-weighted spin echo, gradient echo, or inversion recovery [including short tau inversion recovery (STIR)] images. Because of its sensitivity to changes in marrow fat, MRI is a sensitive but nonspecific means of detecting osteonecrosis and osteomyelitis (Fig. 311-5). Because of its enhanced soft tissue resolution, MRI is more sensitive than arthrography or CT in the diagnosis of soft tissue injuries (e.g., meniscal and rotator cuff tears); intraarticular derangements; and spinal cord damage, subluxation, or synovitis.

RHEUMATOLOGIC EVALUATION OF THE ELDERLY The incidence of rheumatic diseases rises with age, and so ~58% of those >65 will have joint complaints. Musculoskeletal disorders in elderly patients are often not diagnosed because the signs and symptoms may be insidious, chronic, or overshadowed by comorbidities. These difficulties are compounded by the diminished reliability of laboratory testing in the elderly, who

Method	Imaging Time, h	Cost[a]	Current Indications
Ultrasound[b]	<1	+	Synovial cysts Rotator cuff tears Tendon injury
Radionuclide scintigraphy			
^{99m}Tc	1–4	++	Metastatic bone survey Evaluation of Paget's disease Quantitative joint assessment Acute infection Acute and chronic osteomyelitis
^{111}In-WBC	24	+++	Acute infection Prosthetic infection Acute osteomyelitis
^{67}Ga	24–48	++++	Acute and chronic infection Acute osteomyelitis
Computed tomography	<1	+++	Herniated intervertebral disk Sacroiliitis Spinal stenosis Spinal trauma Osteoid osteoma Tarsal coalition
Magnetic resonance imaging	1/2–2	+++++	Avascular necrosis Osteomyelitis Intraarticular derangement and soft tissue injury Derangements of axial skeleton and spinal cord Herniated intervertebral disk Pigmented villonodular synovitis Inflammatory and metabolic muscle pathology

[a] Relative cost for imaging study. [b] Results depend on operator.

often manifest nonpathologic abnormal results. For example, the ESR may be misleadingly elevated, and low-titer positive tests for rheumatoid factor and ANAs may be seen in up to 15% of elderly patients. Although nearly all rheumatic disorders afflict the elderly, certain diseases and drug-induced disorders (Table 311-2) are more common in this age group. The elderly should be approached in the same manner as other patients with musculoskeletal complaints, but with additional inquiries to exclude common geriatric musculoskeletal disorders. An emphasis on identifying the rheumatic consequences of intercurrent medical conditions and therapies is extremely important. Osteoarthritis, osteoporosis, gout, pseudogout, polymyalgia rheumatica, vasculitis, drug-induced lupus erythematosus, and chronic salicylate toxicity are all more common in the elderly than in other individuals. The

physical examination should identify the nature of the musculoskeletal complaint as well as coexisting diseases that may influence diagnosis and choice of treatment.

APPROACH TO REGIONAL RHEUMATIC COMPLAINTS

Although all patients should be evaluated in a logical and thorough manner, many cases with focal musculoskeletal complaints are caused by commonly encountered disorders that exhibit a predictable pattern of onset, evolution, and localization; they can often be diagnosed immediately on the basis of limited historic information and selected maneuvers or tests. Although nearly every joint could be approached in this manner, the evaluation of four common involved anatomical regions—the hand, shoulder, hip, and knee—are reviewed here.

Hand Pain Focal or unilateral hand pain may result from trauma, overuse, infection, or a reactive or crystal-induced arthritis. By contrast, bilateral hand complaints suggest a degenerative (e.g., osteoarthritis), systemic, or inflammatory/immune (e.g., RA) etiology. The distribution or pattern of joint involvement is highly suggestive of certain disorders (Fig. 311-6). Thus, osteoarthritis (or degenerative arthritis) may manifest as distal interphalangeal (DIP) and proximal interphalangeal (PIP) joint pain with bony hypertrophy sufficient to produce Heberden's and Bouchard's nodes, respectively. Pain, with or without bony swell-

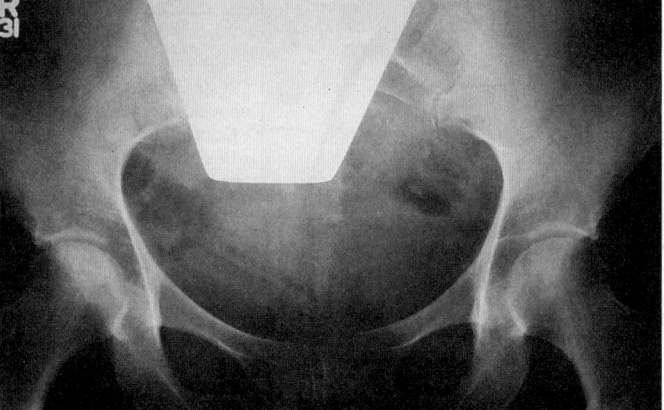
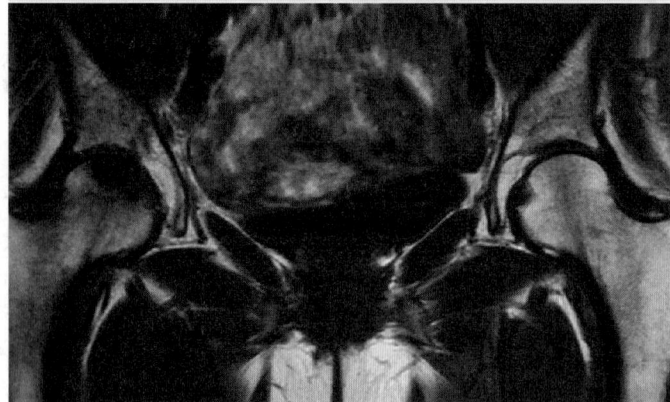

FIGURE 311-5 Superior sensitivity of magnetic resonance imaging in the diagnosis of osteonecrosis of the femoral head. A 45-year-old woman receiving high-dose glucocorticoids developed right hip pain. Conventional x-rays (*top*) demonstrated only mild sclerosis of the right femoral head. T1-weighted MRI (*bottom*) demonstrated low-density signal in the right femoral head, diagnostic of osteonecrosis.

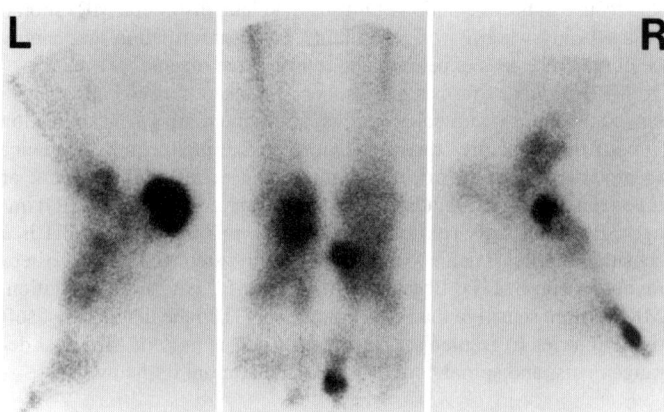

FIGURE 311-4 [^{99m}Tc]diphosphonate scintigraphy of the feet of a 33-year-old black male with Reiter's syndrome, manifested by sacroiliitis, urethritis, uveitis, asymmetric oligoarthritis, and enthesitis. This bone scan demonstrates increased uptake indicative of enthesitis involving the insertions of the left Achilles tendon, plantar aponeurosis, and right tibialis posterior tendon as well as arthritis of the right first interphalangeal joint.

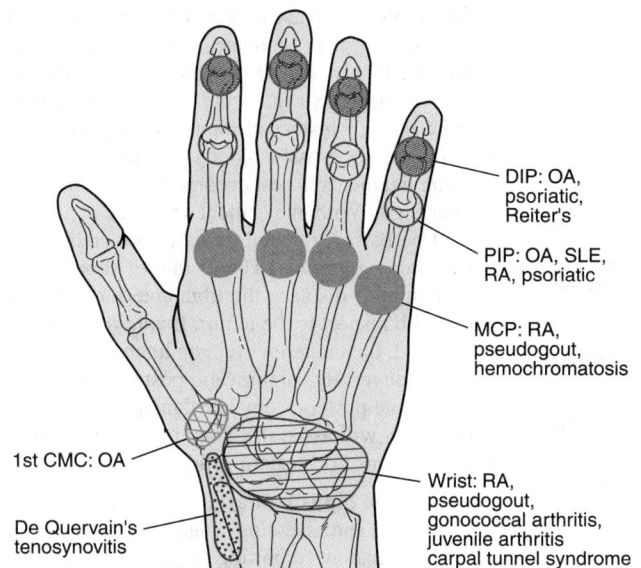

DIP: OA, psoriatic, Reiter's

PIP: OA, SLE, RA, psoriatic

MCP: RA, pseudogout, hemochromatosis

1st CMC: OA

De Quervain's tenosynovitis

Wrist: RA, pseudogout, gonococcal arthritis, juvenile arthritis carpal tunnel syndrome

FIGURE 311-6 Sites of hand or wrist involvement and their potential disease associations. (DIP, distal interphalangeal; OA, osteoarthritis; PIP, proximal interphalangeal; SLE, systemic lupus erythematosus; RA, rheumatoid arthritis; MCP, metacarpophalangeal; CMC, carpometacarpal.) *(From JJ Cush, AF Kavanaugh: Rheumatology: Diagnosis and Therapeutics. Baltimore, Lippincott Williams & Wilkins, 1999; with permission.)*

ing, involving the base of the thumb (first carpometacarpal joint) is also highly suggestive of osteoarthritis. By contrast, RA tends to involve the PIP, metacarpophalangeal, intercarpal, and carpometacarpal joints (wrist) with pain, prolonged stiffness, and palpable synovial tissue hypertrophy. Psoriatic arthritis may also involve the DIP and PIP joints and the carpus with inflammatory pain, stiffness, and synovitis. Moreover, the diagnosis of psoriatic arthritis can be suggested by nail pitting or onycholysis. Soft tissue swelling may also be noted over the dorsum of the hand and wrist and may suggest an inflammatory extensor tendon tenosynovitis possibly caused by gonococcal infection, gout, or inflammatory arthritis. The diagnosis of tenosynovitis may be suggested by local warmth and edema and is confirmed when pain is induced by maintaining the wrist in a fixed, neutral position and flexing the digits distal to the metacarpophalangeal joints to stretch the extensor tendon sheaths.

Focal wrist pain localized to the radial aspect may be caused by DeQuervains tenosynovitis resulting from inflammation of the tendon sheath(s) involving the abductor pollicis longus or extensor pollicis brevis (Fig. 311-6). This commonly results from overuse or follows pregnancy and may be diagnosed with Finkelstein's test. A positive result is present when local wrist pain is induced after the thumb is flexed across the palm and placed inside a clenched fist and the patient actively deviates the hand downward with ulnar deviation at the wrist. Carpal tunnel syndrome is another common disorder of the upper extremity and results from compression of the median nerve within the carpal tunnel. Manifestations include paresthesia in the thumb, second, third, and radial half of the fourth finger and, at times, atrophy of thenar musculature. Carpal tunnel syndrome is commonly associated with pregnancy, edema, trauma, osteoarthritis, inflammatory arthritis, and infiltrative disorders (e.g., amyloidosis). The diagnosis is suggested by a positive Tinel's or Phalen's sign. With each test, paresthesia in a median nerve distribution is induced or increased by either "thumping" the volar aspect of the wrist (Tinel's sign) or pressing the extensor surfaces of both flexed wrists against each other (Phalen's sign).

Shoulder Pain During the evaluation of shoulder disorders, the examiner should carefully note any history of trauma, infection, inflammatory disease, occupational hazards, or previous cervical disease. In addition, the patient should be questioned as to the activities or movement(s) that elicit shoulder pain. Shoulder pain is frequently referred from the cervical spine but may also be referred from intrathoracic

lesions (e.g., a Pancoast tumor) or from gall bladder, hepatic, or diaphragmatic disease. The shoulder should be put through its full range of motion both actively and passively (with examiner assistance): forward flexion, extension, abduction, adduction, and rotation. Manual inspection of the periarticular structures will often provide important diagnostic information. The examiner should apply direct manual pressure over the subacromial bursa that lies lateral to and immediately beneath the acromion. Subacromial bursitis is a frequent cause of shoulder pain. Anterior to the subacromial bursa, the bicipital tendon traverses the bicipital groove. This tendon is best identified by palpating it in its groove as the patient rotates the humerus internally and externally. Direct pressure over the tendon may reveal pain indicative of bicipital tendinitis. Palpation of the acromioclavicular joint may disclose local pain, bony hypertrophy, or, uncommonly, synovial swelling. Whereas osteoarthritis and RA commonly affect the acromioclavicular joint, osteoarthritis seldom involves the glenohumeral joint, unless there is a traumatic or occupational cause. The glenohumeral joint is best palpated anteriorly by placing the thumb over the humeral head (just medial and inferior to the coracoid process) and having the patient rotate the humerus internally and externally. Pain localized to this region is indicative of glenohumeral pathology. Synovial effusion or tissue is seldom palpable but, if present, may suggest infection, RA, or an acute tear of the rotator cuff.

Rotator cuff tendinitis or tear is a very common cause of shoulder pain. The rotator cuff is formed by the tendons of the supraspinatus, infraspinatus, teres minor, and subscapularis muscles. Rotator cuff tendinitis is suggested by pain on active abduction (but not passive abduction), pain over the lateral deltoid muscle, night pain, and evidence of the impingement sign. This maneuver is performed by the examiner raising the patient's arm into forced flexion while stabilizing and preventing rotation of the scapula. A positive sign is present if pain develops before 180° of forward flexion. A complete tear of the rotator cuff is more common in the elderly and often results from trauma; it may manifest in the same manner as tendinitis but is less common. The diagnosis is also suggested by the drop arm test in which the patient is unable to maintain his or her arm outstretched once it is passively abducted. If the patient is unable to hold the arm up once 90° of abduction is reached, the test is positive. Tendinitis or tear of the rotator cuff can be confirmed by MRI or arthrography.

Knee Pain A careful history should delineate the chronology of the knee complaint and whether there are predisposing conditions, trauma, or medications that might underlie the complaint. For example, patellofemoral disease (e.g., osteoarthritis) may cause anterior knee pain that worsens with climbing stairs. Observation of the patient's gait is also important. The knee should be carefully inspected in the upright (weight-bearing) and prone positions for swelling, erythema, contusion, laceration, or malalignment. The most common form of malalignment in the knee is *genu varum* (bowlegs) and *genu valgum* (knock knees). Bony swelling of the knee joint commonly results from hypertrophic osseous changes seen with disorders such as osteoarthritis and neuropathic arthropathy. Swelling caused by hypertrophy of intrasynovial structures (i.e., synovium or synovial effusion) may manifest as a fluctuant, ballotable, or soft tissue enlargement in the suprapatellar pouch (superior reflection of the synovial cavity) or lateral and medial to the patella. Synovial effusions may also be detected by balloting the patella downward toward the femoral groove or by eliciting a "bulge sign." With the the knee extended the examiner should manually compress, or "milk," synovial fluid down from the suprapatellar pouch and lateral to the patellae. The application of manual pressure lateral to the patella may cause an observable shift in synovial fluid (bulge) to the medial aspect. The examiner should note that this maneuver is only effective in detecting small to moderate effusions (<100 mL). Inflammatory disorders such as RA, gout, and Reiter's syndrome may involve the knee joint and produce significant pain, stiffness, swelling, or warmth. A popliteal or *Baker's cyst* is best palpated with

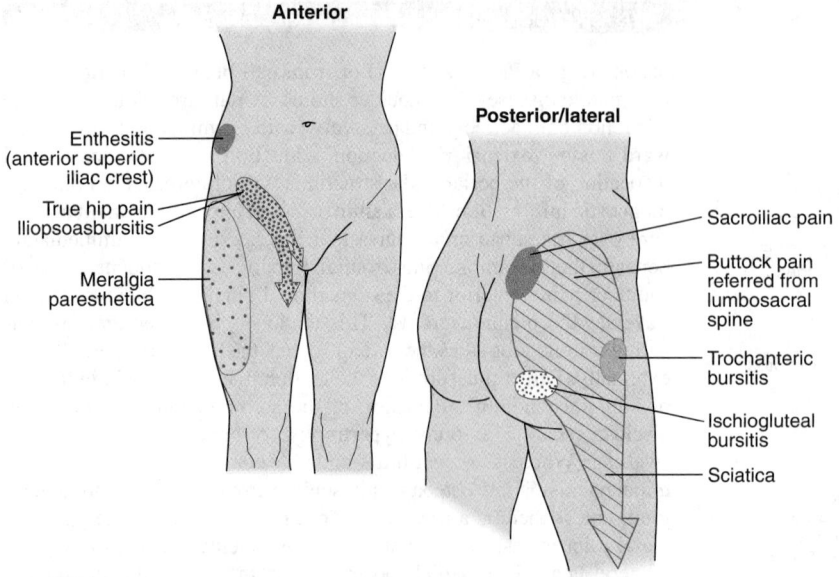

FIGURE 311-7 Origins of hip pain. *(From JJ Cush, AF Kavanaugh: Rheumatology: Diagnosis and Thera-peutics. Baltimore, Lippincott Williams & Wilkins, 1999; with permission.)*

the knee partially flexed and is best seen with the patient standing and knees fully extended to visualize popliteal swelling or fullness from a posterior view.

Anserine bursitis is an often missed periarticular cause of knee pain in adults. The pes anserine bursa underlies the semimembranosus tendon and may become inflamed and painful following trauma, overuse, or inflammation. It is often tender in patients with fibromyalgia. Anserine bursitis manifests primarily as point tenderness inferior and medial to the patella and overlies the medial tibial plateau. Swelling and erythema may not be present. Other forms of bursitis may also present as knee pain. The prepatellar bursa is superficial and is located over the inferior portion of the patella. The infrapatellar bursa is deeper and lies beneath the patellar ligament before its insertion on the tibial tubercle.

Internal derangement of the knee may result from trauma or degenerative processes. Damage to the meniscal cartilage (medial or lateral) frequently presents as chronic or intermittent knee pain. Such an injury should be suspected when there is a history of trauma or athletic activity and when the patient relates symptoms of "locking," clicking, or "giving way" of the joint. Pain may be detected during direct palpation over the medial or lateral joint line. The diagnosis may also be suggested by ipsilateral joint line pain when the knee is stressed laterally or medially. A positive McMurray test may indicated a meniscal tear. To perform this test, the knee is first flexed at 90°, and the leg is then extended while simultaneously the lower extremity is torqued medially or laterally. A painful click during inward rotation may in-

dicate a lateral meniscus tear, and pain during outward rotation may indicate a tear in the medial meniscus. Lastly, damage to the cruciate ligaments should be suspected with acute onset of pain, possibly with swelling, a history of trauma, or a synovial fluid aspirate that is grossly bloody. Examination of the cruciate ligaments is best accomplished by eliciting a drawer sign. With the patient recumbent, the knee should be partially flexed and the foot stabilized on the examining surface. The examiner should manually attempt to displace the tibia anteriorly or posteriorly with respect to the femur. If anterior movement is detected, then anterior cruciate ligament damage is likely. Conversely, significant posterior movement may indicate posterior cruciate damage. Contralateral comparison will assist the examiner in detecting significant anterior or posterior movement.

Hip Pain The hip is best evaluated by observing the patient's gait and assessing range of motion. The vast majority of patients reporting "hip pain" localize their pain unilaterally to the posterior or gluteal musculature (Fig. 311-7). Such pain may or may not be associated with low back pain and tends to radiate down the posterolateral aspect of the thigh. This presentation frequently results from degenerative arthritis of the lumbosacral spine and commonly follows a dermatomal distribution with involvement of nerve roots between L5 and S1. Some individuals instead localize their "hip pain" laterally to the area overlying the trochanteric bursa. Because of the depth of this bursa, swelling and warmth are usually absent. Diagnosis of trochanteric bursitis can be confirmed by inducing point tenderness over the trochanteric bursa. Range of movement may be limited by pain. Pain in the hip joint is less common and tends to be located anteriorly, over the inguinal ligament; it may radiate medially to the groin or along the anteromedial thigh. Uncommonly, iliopsoas bursitis may mimic true hip joint pain. Diagnosis of iliopsoas bursitis may be suggested by a history of trauma or inflammatory arthritis. Pain associated with an iliopsoas bursitis is localized to the groin or anterior thigh and tends to worsen with hyperextension of the hip; many patients prefer to flex and externally rotate the hip to reduce the pain from a distended bursa.

FURTHER READING

BROWER AC: Imaging techniques and modalities, in *Arthritis in Black and White*, AC Brower (ed). Philadelphia, Saunders, 1998, p 1

KAVANAUGH A: The utility of immunologic laboratory tests in patients with rheumatic diseases. Arthritis Rheum 44:2221, 2001

SCHUMACHER HR JR: Arthritis of recent onset: A guide to evaluation and initial therapy for primary care physicians. Postgrad Med 97:52, 1995

SHMERLING RH et al: Synovial fluid tests: What should be ordered? JAMA 264:1009, 1990

312 | OSTEOARTHRITIS
Kenneth D. Brandt

Osteoarthritis (OA), also erroneously called degenerative joint disease, represents failure of the diarthrodial (movable, synovial-lined) joint. In idiopathic (primary) OA, the most common form of the disease, no predisposing factor is apparent. Secondary OA is pathologically indistinguishable from idiopathic OA but is attributable to an underlying cause (Table 312-1).

EPIDEMIOLOGY AND RISK FACTORS OA is the most common joint disease of humans. Among the elderly, knee OA is the leading cause of chronic disability in developed countries; some 100,000 people in the United

States are unable to walk independently from bed to bathroom because of OA of the knee or hip.

In those <55 years, the joint distribution of OA in men and women is similar; in older individuals, hip OA is more common in men, while OA of interphalangeal joints and the thumb base is more common in women. Similarly, radiographic evidence of knee OA, and especially of *symptomatic* knee OA, is more common in women than in men (Table 312-2).

Racial differences exist in both the prevalence of OA and the pattern of joint involvement. The Chinese in Hong Kong have a lower incidence of hip OA than whites; OA is more frequent in Native Americans than in whites. Interphalangeal joint OA and especially hip OA are much less common in South African blacks than in whites in the same population. Whether these differences are genetic or due to

TABLE 312-1 Classification of Osteoarthritis

I. Idiopathic
  A. Localized OA
    1. Hands: Heberden's and Bouchard's nodes (nodal), erosive interphalangeal arthritis (nonnodal), 1st carpometacarpal joint
    2. Feet: hallux valgus, hallux rigidus, contracted toes (hammer/cock-up toes), talonavicular
    3. Knee:
      a. Medial compartment
      b. Lateral compartment
      c. Patellofemoral compartment
    4. Hip:
      a. Eccentric (superior)
      b. Concentric (axial, medial)
      c. Diffuse (coxae senilis)
    5. Spine:
      a. Apophyseal joints
      b. Intervertebral joints (disks)
      c. Spondylosis (osteophytes)
      d. Ligamentous (hyperostosis, Forestier's disease, diffuse idiopathic skeletal hyperstosis)
    6. Other single sites, e.g., glenohumoral, acromioclavicular, tibiotalar, sacroiliac, temporomandibular
  B. Generalized includes 3 or more of the areas listed above (Kellgren-Moore)
II. Secondary
  A. Trauma
    1. Acute
    2. Chronic (occupational, sports)
  B. Congenital or developmental
    1. Localized diseases: Legg-Calvé-Perthes, congenital hip dislocation, slipped epiphysis
    2. Mechanical factors: unequal lower extremity length, valgus/varus deformity, hypermobility syndromes
    3. Bone dysplasias: epiphyseal dysplasia, spondyloepiphyseal dysplasia, osteonychondystrophy
  C. Metabolic
    1. Ochronosis (alkaptonuria)
    2. Hemochromatosis
    3. Wilson's disease
    4. Gaucher's disease
  D. Endocrine
    1. Acromegaly
    2. Hyperparathyroidism
    3. Diabetes mellitus
    4. Obesity
    5. Hypothyroidism
  E. Calcium deposition diseases
    1. Calcium pyrophosphate dihydrate deposition
    2. Apatite arthropathy
  F. Other bone and joint diseases
    1. Localized: fracture, avascular necrosis, infection, gout
    2. Diffuse: rheumatoid (inflammatory) arthritis, Paget's disease, osteopetrosis, osteochondritis
  G. Neuropathic (Charcot joints)
  H. Endemic
    1. Kashin-Beck
    2. Mseleni
  I. Miscellaneous
    1. Frostbite
    2. Caisson's disease
    3. Hemoglobinopathies

Source: From HJ Mankin et al: J Rheumatol 13:1127, 1986, with permission.

differences in joint usage related to life-style or occupation is unknown.

In some cases, the relation of heredity to OA is less ambiguous. Thus, the mother and sister of a woman with distal interphalangeal (DIP) joint OA (Heberden's nodes) are, respectively, two to three times as likely to exhibit OA in these joints as the mother and sister of an unaffected woman. Association analyses have identified several candidate genes encoding structural proteins of the extracellular matrix of cartilage and bone and implicated in regulation of bone density. However, no mutation has been identified in the common primary (i.e.,

idiopathic) form of OA. Most of the mutations identified are associated with relatively rare syndromes, a feature of which can be classified as secondary OA. Mutations in COL2A1 genes, for example, have been associated with clinical phenotypes ranging from mild spondyloepiphyseal dysplasia to severe generalized OA, with onset at an early age. It is likely that classifications of "common OA" will eventually be developed based on causative gene defect rather than on variable clinical phenotypes. This could permit the development of tests permitting the diagnosis of molecular defects and, ideally, prophylactic therapy.

Age is the most powerful risk factor for OA. In a radiographic survey of women <45 years, only 2% had OA; between the ages of 45 and 64 years, however, the prevalence was 30%, and for those >65 years it was 68%. In males, the figures were similar, but somewhat lower, in the older age groups.

Major trauma and repetitive joint use are also important risk factors for OA. Anterior cruciate ligament insufficiency or meniscus damage (and meniscectomy) may lead to knee OA. Although damage to the articular cartilage may occur at the time of injury or subsequently, with use of the affected joint, even normal cartilage will degenerate if the joint is unstable. A person with a trimalleolar fracture will almost certainly develop ankle OA. The pattern of joint involvement in OA is influenced by prior vocational or avocational overload. Thus, although ankle OA is common in ballet dancers, elbow OA in baseball pitchers, and metacarpophalangeal joint OA in prize fighters, OA is not very common at any of these sites in the general population.

Given the growing participation of the population of the United States in cardiovascular fitness programs, it is important to note that, if major trauma is excluded, there are no convincing data to support an association between specific nonprofessional athletic activities and arthritis. Neither long-distance running nor jogging has been shown to cause OA. This apparent lack of association may, however, be due to the lack of good long-term studies, the difficulty in retrospective assessment of activities, and selection bias, i.e., early discontinuation of the activity by those incurring joint damage. In contrast, vocational activities, such as those performed by jackhammer operators, cotton mill and shipyard workers, and coal miners, may lead to OA in the joints exposed to repetitive occupational use. Men whose jobs required knee bending and at least moderate physical demands had a higher rate of radiographic evidence of knee OA, and more severe radiographic changes, than men whose jobs required neither.

Obesity is a risk factor for both knee and hand OA. For those in the highest quintile for body mass index at baseline examination, the relative risk for developing knee OA in the ensuing 36 years was 1.5 for men and 2.1 for women. For *severe* knee OA, the relative risk rose to 1.9 for men and 3.2 for women, suggesting that obesity plays an even larger role in the etiology of the most serious cases of knee OA. Obese subjects who have not yet developed OA can reduce their risk: A weight loss of only 5 kg was associated with a 50% reduction in the odds of developing symptomatic knee OA.

The correlation between the pathologic severity of OA and symptoms is poor. Many people with radiographic changes of advanced OA have no symptoms. The risk factors for *pain and disability* in affected individuals are poorly understood. Disability in subjects with knee OA is more strongly associated with quadriceps muscle weakness than with joint pain or radiographic severity. For the same degree of path-

TABLE 312-2 Risk Factors for OA

Age	Repetitive stress, e.g., vocational[a]
Female sex	Obesity[a]
Race	Congenital/developmental defects[a]
Genetic factors	Prior inflammatory joint disease
Major joint trauma[a]	Metabolic/endocrine disorders

[a] Potentially modifiable.
Source: Adapted from M Hochberg: J Rheumatol 18:1438, 1991, with permission.

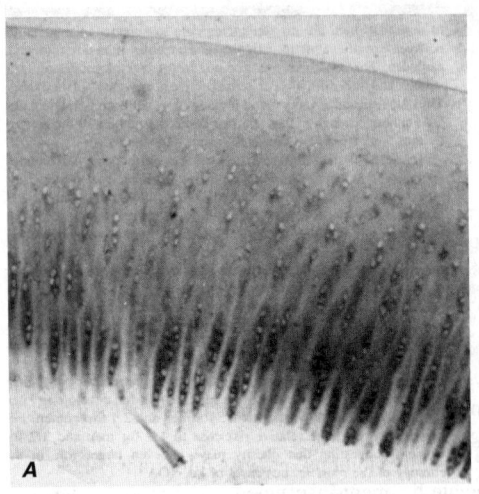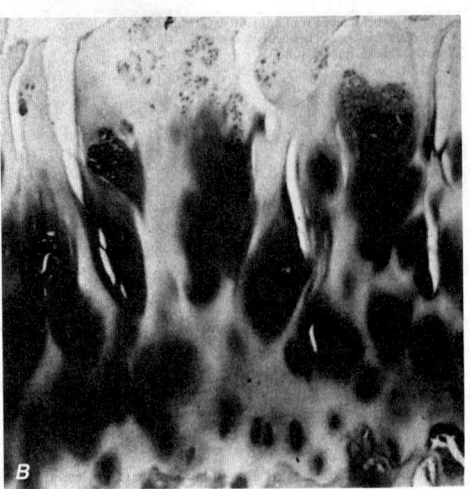

FIGURE 312-1 *A.* Normal articular cartilage. Note the intact surface and even distribution of chondrocytes. Mitotic figures are not present in normal adult articular cartilage. *B.* Osteoarthritic cartilage. Note the disruption of surface integrity, with vertical fissures (fibrillation) and irregular distribution of cells. Many of the chondrocytes have replicated and exist in clusters. Stained with safranin-O, which binds to the sulfated glycosaminoglycan chains of proteoglycans. Note patchy areas of diminished staining (pale extracellular matrix) due to proteoglycan depletion.

ologic severity, women are more likely to be symptomatic than men, those on welfare more likely than those who are working, and those who are divorced more likely than those who are married. For patients who had poor social support, periodic phone calls from a trained lay interviewer were as effective as a nonsteroidal anti-inflammatory drug (NSAID) in reducing joint pain, emphasizing the importance of psychosocial factors as determinants of pain.

PATHOLOGY Although the cardinal pathologic feature of OA is a progressive loss of articular cartilage, OA is not a disease of only the cartilage but a disease of an *organ*, the synovial joint, in which all of the tissues are affected: subchondral bone, synovium, meniscus, ligaments, and supporting neuromuscular apparatus as well as the cartilage.

The most striking morphologic changes in OA are usually seen in load-bearing areas of the articular cartilage. In the early stages the cartilage is thicker than normal, but with progression of OA the joint surface thins, the cartilage softens, the integrity of the surface is breached, and vertical clefts develop (fibrillation) (Fig. 312-1). Deep cartilage ulcers, extending to bone, may appear. Areas of fibrocartilaginous repair may develop, but these are inferior to pristine hyaline articular cartilage in their ability to withstand mechanical stress. All of the cartilage is metabolically active and the chondrocytes replicate, forming clusters (clones). Later, however, the cartilage becomes hypocellular.

Remodeling and hypertrophy of bone are major features of OA. Appositional bone growth occurs in the subchondral region, leading to the bony "sclerosis" seen radiographically. The abraded bone under a cartilage ulcer may take on the appearance of ivory (eburnation). Growth of cartilage and bone at the joint margins leads to osteophytes (spurs), which alter the contour of the joint and may restrict movement. A patchy chronic synovitis and thickening of the joint capsule may further restrict movement. Periarticular muscle wasting is common and may play a major role in symptoms and, as indicated above, in disability.

PATHOGENESIS The main load on articular cartilage—the major target tissue in OA—is generated by the contraction of the muscles that stabilize or move the joint. Although cartilage is an excellent shock absorber in terms of its bulk properties, at most sites it is only 1 to 2 mm thick—too thin to serve as the sole shock-absorbing structure in the joint. Additional protective mechanisms are provided by the subchondral bone and periarticular muscles.

Articular cartilage serves two essential functions within the joint, both of which are mechanical. First, it provides a remarkably smooth bearing surface, so that the bones glide effortlessly over each other with joint movement. With synovial fluid as lubricant, the coefficient of friction for cartilage rubbed against cartilage, even under physiologic loading, is 15 times lower than that of two ice cubes passed across each other! Second, articular cartilage prevents the concentration of stresses so the bones do not shatter when the joint is loaded.

OA develops in either of two settings: (1) the biomaterial properties of the articular cartilage and subchondral bone are normal, but excessive loading of the joint causes the tissues to fail; or (2) the applied load is reasonable, but the material properties of the cartilage or bone are inferior.

Although articular cartilage is highly resistant to wear under conditions of repeated oscillation, repetitive impact loading soon leads to joint failure. This fact accounts for the high prevalence of OA at specific sites related to vocational or avocational overloading. In general, the earliest changes occur at the sites in the joint that are subject to the greatest compressive loads. Some cases of so-called idiopathic OA of the hip may be due to subtle congenital or developmental defects, such as congenital subluxation/dislocation, acetabular dysplasia, Legg-Calvé-Perthes disease, or slipped capital femoral epiphysis, which increase joint congruity and concentrate the dynamic load.

Clinical conditions that reduce the ability of the cartilage or subchondral bone to deform are associated with development of OA. In ochronosis, for example, accumulation of homogentisic acid polymers leads to stiffening of the cartilage; in osteopetrosis, stiffness of the subchondral trabeculae occurs. In both conditions, severe generalized OA is usually apparent by the age of 40 years. If the subchondral bone is stiffened experimentally, repetitive impact loading soon leads to breakdown of the overlying cartilage. Conversely, osteoporosis, in which the bone is abnormally soft, may protect against OA.

The Extracellular Matrix of Normal Articular Cartilage Articular cartilage is composed of two major macromolecular species: proteoglycans (PGs), which are responsible for the compressive stiffness of the tissue and its ability to withstand load, and collagen, which provides tensile strength and resistance to shear. Although lysomal proteases (cathepsins) have been demonstrated within the cells and matrix of normal articular cartilage, their low pH optimum makes it likely that the proteoglycanase activity of these enzymes will be confined to intracellular sites or the immediate pericellular area. However, cartilage also contains a family of matrix metalloproteinases (MMPs), including stromelysin, collagenase, and gelatinase, which can degrade all the components of the extracellular matrix at neutral pH. Each is secreted by the chondrocyte as a latent proenzyme that must be activated by proteolytic cleavage of its N-terminal sequence. The level of MMP activity in the cartilage at any given time represents the balance between activation of the proenzyme and inhibition of the active enzyme by tissue inhibitors. Much of the total tissue pool of aggrecan, the major PG in articular cartilage, is degraded by a proteinase, which cleaves the protein core of the molecule at a site distinct from the cleavage site of the MMP. The enzyme responsible for this cleavage is referred to as *aggrecanase*.

The turnover of normal cartilage is affected through a degradative cascade; the driving force appears to be interleukin (IL) 1, a cytokine produced by mononuclear cells (including synovial lining cells) and synthesized by chondrocytes. IL-1 stimulates the synthesis and secretion of the latent MMPs and of tissue plasminogen activator. Plasminogen, the substrate for the latter enzyme, may be synthesized by the chondrocyte or may enter the cartilage from the synovial fluid. Both plasminogen and stromelysin may play a role in activation of the latent MMPs. In addition to its catabolic effect on cartilage, IL-1 suppresses PG synthesis by the chondrocyte, inhibiting matrix repair (see below). The major proteinases involved in degradation of matrix of human articular cartilage appear to be collagenase-3 (MMP-13) and aggrecanase-1 (ADAMTS4). Control of MMP-13 activity appears to be exerted via transcriptional activation by cytokines and activation of the pro-form at the cell surface. The transcriptional activity is mediated primarily through the p38 mitogen-activated protein kinase pathway, but also involves nuclear factor kappa B. Interest currently exists in the inhibition of cartilage matrix degradation by therapeutic agents that block the p38-dependant transcriptional activity of MMP-13 expression or control extracellular activation of the secreted form of ADAMTS4.

The balance of the system lies with inhibitors of matrix degrading enzymes, e.g., tissue inhibitor of metalloproteinase (TIMP) and plasminogen activator inhibitor-1 (PAI-1), which are synthesized by the chondrocyte and limit the degradative activity of MMPs and plasminogen activator, respectively. If TIMP or PAI-1 is destroyed or present in concentrations that are insufficient relative to those of active enzymes, stromelysin and plasmin are free to act on matrix substrates. Stromelysin can degrade the protein core of the PG and activate latent collagenase. Conversion of latent stromelysin to an active, highly destructive protease by plasmin provides a second mechanism for matrix degradation.

Polypeptide mediators, e.g., insulin-like growth factor-1 (IGF-1) and transforming growth factor β (TGF-β), stimulate biosynthesis of PGs. They regulate matrix metabolism in normal cartilage and may play a role in matrix repair in OA. These growth factors modulate catabolic as well as anabolic pathways of chondrocyte metabolism; by down-regulating chondrocyte receptors for IL-1, they may decrease PG degradation. In addition to its responsiveness to cytokines and a variety of other biologic mediators, chondrocyte metabolism in normal cartilage can be modulated directly by mechanical loading. Whereas static loading inhibits synthesis of PGs and protein, loads of relatively brief duration may stimulate matrix biosynthesis.

Pathophysiology of Cartilage Changes in OA Most investigators feel that the primary changes in OA begin in the cartilage. A change in the arrangement and size of the collagen fibers is apparent. Biochemical data are consistent with the presence of a defect in the collagen network of the matrix, perhaps due to disruption of the "glue" that binds adjacent fibers. This is among the earliest matrix changes observed and appears to be irreversible.

Although "wear" may be a factor in the loss of cartilage, strong evidence supports the concept that MMPs account for much of the loss of cartilage matrix in OA. Whether their synthesis and secretion are stimulated by IL-1 or by other factors (e.g., mechanical stimuli), MMPs, plasmin, and cathepsins all appear to be involved in the breakdown of articular cartilage in OA. TIMP and PAI-1 may work to stabilize the system, at least temporarily, while growth factors such as IGF-1 and TGF-β are implicated in repair processes that may heal the lesion or, at least, stabilize the process. A stoichiometric imbalance exists between the levels of active enzyme and the level of TIMP, which may be only modestly increased.

Nitric oxide (NO) may play a significant role in articular cartilage damage in OA insofar as NO stimulates synthesis of MMPs by chondrocytes. Chondrocytes are a major source of NO, the synthesis of which is stimulated by IL-1 and tumor necrosis factor and by shear stress. In an experimental model of OA, treatment with a selective inhibitor of inducible NO synthase reduced the severity of cartilage damage.

The chondrocytes in OA cartilage undergo active cell division and are very active metabolically, producing increased quantities of DNA, RNA collagen, PG, and noncollagenous proteins. For this reason, it is inaccurate to call OA *degenerative* joint disease. Prior to cartilage loss and PG depletion, this marked biosynthetic activity may lead to an increase in PG concentration, which may be associated with thickening

of the cartilage and a stage of homeostasis referred to as *compensated OA*. These mechanisms may maintain the joint in a reasonably functional state for years. The repair tissue, however, often does not hold up as well under mechanical stresses as does normal hyaline cartilage and eventually, at least in some cases, the rate of PG synthesis falls and "end-stage" OA develops, with full-thickness loss of cartilage.

Traumatic joint injury is a risk factor for secondary OA (Table 312-1). Mechanical injury to articular cartilage in vitro results in swelling, alteration in biomechanical properties, cell death, changes in biosynthesis of matrix macromolecules, loss of PGs, degradation of collagen, and an increase in MMP gene expression.

The extent to which the above changes are due to direct mechanical damage versus cell-mediated degradation is unclear. Injury may result in increased responsiveness of the chondrocyte to stimulation by cytokines. On the other hand, it may facilitate diffusion of cytokines into the matrix. In contrast to knee cartilage, glycosaminoglycan loss from ankle cartilage is not increased after mechanical injury of the tissue and exposure to cytokines. Chondrocytes in articular cartilage from some joints may react differently to cytokines, mechanical forces, and growth factors than to those in other joints, perhaps accounting for the lower incidence of OA in some joints than in others, e.g., ankle vs. knee.

CLINICAL FEATURES The joint pain of OA is often described as a deep ache localized to the involved joint. Typically, it is aggravated by joint use and relieved by rest but, as the disease progresses, it may become persistent. Nocturnal pain, interfering with sleep, is seen particularly in advanced OA of the hip and may be enervating. Stiffness of the involved joint after a period of inactivity (e.g., a night's sleep or automobile ride) may be prominent but usually lasts <20 min. Systemic manifestations are not a feature of primary OA.

Because articular cartilage is aneural, the joint pain in OA must arise from other structures (Table 312-3). In some cases it may be due to stretching of nerve endings in the periosteum covering osteophytes; in others, to microfractures in subchondral bone or medullary hypertension caused by distortion of blood flow by thickened subchondral trabeculae. Joint instability, leading to stretching of the joint capsule, and muscle spasm may also be sources of pain.

In some patients with OA, joint pain may be due to synovitis. In advanced OA, histologic evidence of synovial inflammation may be as marked as that in synovium of a patient with rheumatoid arthritis (Chap. 301). Synovitis in OA may be due to phagocytosis of shards of cartilage and bone from the abraded joint surface (wear particles), release from the cartilage of soluble matrix macromolecules, or crystals of calcium pyrophosphate or hydroxyapatite. In other cases, immune complexes, containing antigens derived from cartilage matrix, may be sequestered in collagenous tissues of the joint, leading to low-grade chronic synovitis. In contrast, in the earlier stages of OA, synovial inflammation may be absent, suggesting that the joint pain is due to one of the other factors mentioned above.

Physical examination of the OA joint may reveal localized tenderness and bony or soft tissue swelling. Bony crepitus (the sensation of bone rubbing against bone, evoked by joint movement) is characteristic. Synovial effusions, if present, are usually not large. Palpation may reveal some warmth over the joint. Periarticular muscle atrophy may be due to disuse or reflex inhibition of muscle contraction. In the

TABLE 312-3 *Causes of Joint Pain and Patients with OA*

Source	Mechanism
Synovium	Inflammation
Subchondral bone	Medullary hypertension, microfractures
Osteophyte	Stretching of periosteal nerve endings
Ligaments	Stretch
Capsule	Inflammation, distention
Muscle	Spasm

advanced stages of OA, there may be gross deformity, bony hypertrophy, subluxation, and marked loss of joint motion. The notion that OA is inexorably progressive, however, is incorrect. In many patients, the disease stabilizes; in some, regression of joint pain and even of radiographic changes occur.

Although the diagnosis of OA is often straightforward, because of the high prevalence of radiographic changes of OA in asymptomatic individuals, it is important to ensure that joint pain in a patient with radiographic evidence of OA is not due to some other cause, such as soft tissue rheumatism (e.g., anserine bursitis at the knee, trochanteric bursitis at the hip), radiculopathy, referral of pain from another joint (25% of patients with hip disease have pain referred to the knee), entrapment neuropathy, vascular disease (claudication), or some other type of arthritis (e.g., crystal-induced synovitis, septic arthritis). It is usually not difficult to differentiate OA from a systemic rheumatic disease, such as rheumatoid arthritis, because joint involvement in the latter disease is usually symmetric and polyarticular, with arthritis in wrists and metacarpophalangeal joints (sites not usually involved in OA), and constitutional features, such as prolonged morning stiffness, fatigue, weight loss, or fever, may be seen.

LABORATORY AND RADIOGRAPHIC FINDINGS The diagnosis of OA is usually based on clinical and radiographic features. In the early stages, the radiograph may be normal but joint space narrowing becomes evident as articular cartilage is lost. Other characteristic findings include subchondral bone sclerosis, subchondral cysts, and osteophytosis. A change in the contour of the joint, due to bony remodeling, and subluxation may be seen. Although tibiofemoral joint space narrowing has been considered to be a radiographic surrogate for articular cartilage thinning, joint space narrowing alone does not accurately indicate the status of the articular cartilage in patients with early OA who do not have radiographic evidence of bony changes (e.g., subchondral sclerosis or cysts, osteophytes). Similarly, osteophytosis alone, in the absence of other radiographic features of OA, may be due to aging rather than OA. As indicated above, there is often great disparity between the severity of radiographic findings, severity of symptoms, and functional ability in OA; while >90% of persons over age 40 have some radiographic changes of OA in weight-bearing joints, only 30% are symptomatic.

No laboratory studies are diagnostic for OA, but laboratory testing may help identify an underlying causes of secondary OA. Because primary OA is not systemic, the erythrocyte sedimentation rate, serum chemistry determinations, blood counts, and urinalysis are normal. Synovial fluid analysis reveals mild leukocytosis (<2000 white blood cells per microliter), with a predominance of mononuclear cells. Synovial fluid analysis is of particular value in excluding other conditions, such as calcium pyrophosphate dihydrate deposition disease (Chap. 313), gout (Chap. 313) or septic arthritis (Chap. 314).

Prior to the appearance of radiographic changes, the ability to clinically diagnose OA without an invasive procedure (e.g., arthroscopy) is limited. Magnetic resonance imaging and ultrasonography have not been sufficiently validated to justify their routine clinical use for diagnosis of OA or monitoring disease progression.

OA AT SPECIFIC JOINT SITES ■ **Interphalangeal Joints** Heberden's nodes (bony enlargement of the DIP joint) are the most common form of idiopathic OA (Fig. 312-2). A similar process at the proximal interphalangeal joints leads to Bouchard's nodes. Often, these nodes develop gradually, with little or no discomfort, and usually do not interfere significantly with function. However, they may present acutely with pain, redness, and swelling, sometimes triggered by minor trauma. Gelatinous dorsal cysts may develop at the insertion of the digital extensor tendon into the base of the distal phalanx.

EROSIVE OA In erosive OA, DIP and/or proximal interphalangeal joints of the hand are most prominently affected. Erosive OA is more destructive than typical nodal OA; x-ray evidence of collapse of the subchondral plate is characteristic, and bony ankylosis may occur. De-

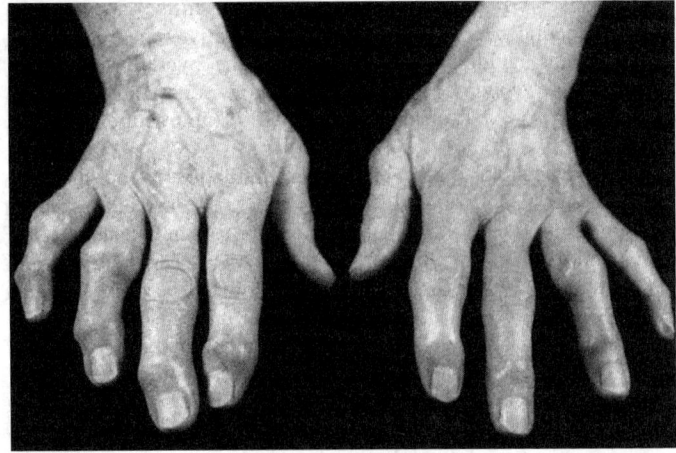

FIGURE 312-2 Nodal osteoarthritis. Note bony enlargement of distal and proximal interphalangeal joints (Heberden's nodes and Bouchard's nodes, respectively). (*Reprinted from the Clinical Slide Collection on the Rheumatic Diseases, 1991, 1995. Reproduced with permission of the American College of Rheumatology.*)

formity and functional impairment may be severe. The synovium is much more extensively infiltrated with mononuclear cells than in other forms of OA.

GENERALIZED OA Generalized OA is characterized by involvement of three or more joints or groups of joints (DIP and proximal interphalangeal joints are counted as one group each). Heberden's and Bouchard's nodes are prominent. "Flare-ups" of inflammation may be marked by soft tissue swelling, redness, and warmth. The erthryocyte sedimentation rate may be elevated, but serum rheumatoid factor tests are negative.

Thumb Base The second most frequent area of involvement in OA is the thumb base. Swelling, tenderness, and crepitus on movement of the joint and loss of motion and strength are common. Osteophytes may lead to a "squared" appearance (Fig. 312-3). Pain with pinch leads to adduction of the thumb and contracture of the first web space, often resulting in compensatory hyperextension of the first metacarpophalangeal joint and swan-neck deformity of the thumb.

Hip Congenital or developmental defects of the hip (e.g., acetabular dysplasia, Legg-Calvé-Perthes disease, slipped capital epiphysis) can lead to OA. Pain from hip OA is generally referred to the inguinal area but may be referred to the buttock or proximal thigh. Less commonly, hip OA presents as knee pain. Pain can be evoked by putting the involved hip through its range of motion. Flexion may be painless initially, but internal rotation will exacerbate pain. Loss of internal rotation occurs early, followed by loss of extension, adduction, and flexion due to capsular fibrosis and/or buttressing osteophytes.

Knee OA of the knee may involve the medial or lateral femorotibial compartment and/or the patellofemoral compartment. Palpation may

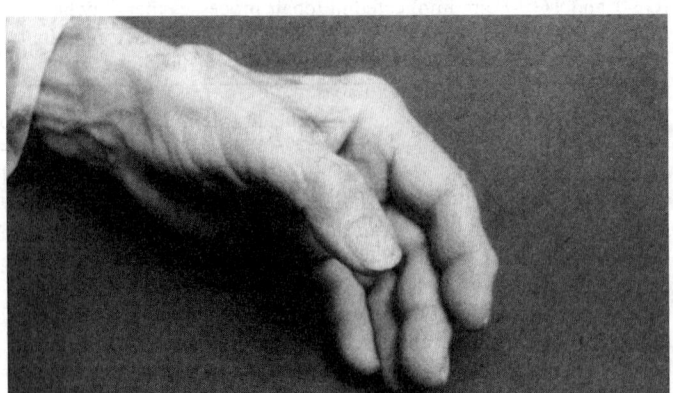

FIGURE 312-3 Osteoarthritis of the first carpometacarpal joint. Note the squared appearance of the thumb base, due to bony enlargement and remodeling of the joint.

reveal bony hypertrophy (osteophytes) and tenderness. Effusions, if present, are generally small. Joint movement commonly elicits bony crepitus. OA in the medial compartment may result in a varus (bow-leg) deformity; OA in the lateral compartment may produce a valgus (knock-knee) deformity. A positive "shrug" sign (pain with manual compression of the patella against the femur during quadriceps contraction) may be a sign of patellofemoral OA.

Chondromalacia patellae, which is also characterized by anterior knee pain and a positive shrug sign, is a syndrome of patellofemoral pain in teenagers and young adults. It is more common in females. It may be caused by a variety of factors (e.g., abnormal quadriceps angle, patella alta, trauma). Although exploration of the knee may reveal softening and fibrillation of cartilage on the posterior aspect of the patella, this change is usually not progressive; chondromalacia patellae is usually not a precursor of OA. In most cases, analgesics or NSAIDs and physical therapy are effective; in some, pain may be relieved by surgical correction of patellar malalignment.

Spine   OA of the spine can involve the apophyseal joints, intervertebral disks, and paraspinous ligaments. *Spondylosis* refers to degenerative disk disease. The diagnosis of spinal OA should be reserved for patients with involvement of the apophyseal joints, and not only disk degeneration. Symptoms of spinal OA include localized pain and stiffness. Nerve root compression by an osteophyte blocking a neural foramen, prolapse of a degenerated disk, or subluxation of an apophyseal joint may cause radicular pain and motor weakness.

Marked calcification and ossification of paraspinous ligaments occur in diffuse idiopathic skeletal hyperostosis (DISH), which must be distinguished from OA. Although DISH is often categorized as a variant of OA, the diarthrodial joints are not involved. In radiographs, ligamentous calcification and ossification in the anterior spinal ligaments give the appearance of "flowing wax" on the anterior vertebral bodies. However, a radiolucency may be seen between the newly deposited bone and the vertebral body, differentiating DISH from the marginal osteophytes in spondylosis. Intervertebral disk spaces are preserved, and sacroiliac and apophyseal joints appear normal, helping to differentiate DISH from spondylosis and from ankylosing spondylitis, respectively. DISH occurs in the middle-aged and elderly and is more common in men than in women. Patients are frequently asymptomatic but may have musculoskeletal stiffness. The radiographic changes are generally much more severe than might be predicted from the mild symptoms.

℞ TREATMENT

Treatment of OA is aimed at reducing pain, maintaining mobility, and minimizing disability. The vigor of the therapeutic intervention should be dictated by the severity of the condition in the individual patient. For those with only mild disease, reassurance, instruction in joint protection, and an occasional analgesic may be all that is required; for those with more severe OA, especially of knee or hip, a comprehensive program comprising a spectrum of nonpharmacologic measures supplemented by an analgesic and/or NSAID is appropriate.

Nonpharmacologic Measures ■ *REDUCTION OF JOINT LOADING*   OA may be caused or aggravated by poor body mechanics. Correction of poor posture and a support for excessive lumbar lordosis can be helpful. Excessive loading of the involved joint should be avoided. Patients with knee or hip OA should avoid prolonged standing, kneeling, and squatting. Obese patients should be counseled to lose weight. In patients with medial compartment knee OA, a wedged insole may decrease joint pain.

Rest periods during the day may be of benefit, but complete immobilization of the painful joint is rarely indicated, except in cases of hand OA. For DIP joint OA that is so painful that it interferes with hand function, a custom-molded thermoplastic splint that blocks flexion can reduce pain, improve overall hand function, and reduce muscle spasm. Splinting can also be very effective for trapeziometacarpal joint and pantrapezial OA. Rigid immobilization is not an acceptable long-term option for pain in the proximal interphalangeal joints, however,

because it limits hand function and can result in shortening of the collateral ligaments. In patients with unilateral OA of the hip or knee, a cane, held in the contralateral hand, may reduce joint pain by reducing the joint contact forces. Bilateral disease may necessitate use of crutches or a walker.

PATELLAR TAPING   OA of the patellofemoral compartment can cause severe pain, especially with kneeling, squatting, or climbing stairs. Medial taping of the patella can significantly reduce pain in such cases. The taping procedure is simple and inexpensive and patients can learn to apply their own tape after minimal instruction. The prompt relief of symptoms that may be achieved by taping may be maintained by isometric exercises to strengthen the vastus medialis obliquus component of the quadriceps muscle, facilitating realignment of the patella on a long-term basis.

WEDGED INSOLES/ORTHOSES   In patients with medial compartment knee OA, pain severity has been shown to be related to the magnitude of the external adduction moment (a measure of the varus torque on the knee during gait). Wedged insoles may be useful in conservative treatment of OA of the medial tibial femoral compartment. Their use may change the spatial position of the lower limb so that the mechanical axis becomes more nearly vertical and the calcaneal axis is shifted to a valgus position with respect to the tibiotalar joint, reducing excessive loading on the medial compartment of the knee and strain on the lateral collateral ligament. Use of lateral wedged insoles may result in a significant decrease in NSAID consumption by patients with knee OA. A polypropylene mesh insole is practical, inexpensive, and washable and may last about 2 years, i.e., approximately twice as long as a leather insole.

THERMAL MODALITIES   Application of heat to the OA joint may reduce pain and stiffness. A variety of modalities are available; often, the least expensive and most convenient is a hot shower or bath. Occasionally, better analgesia may be obtained with ice than with heat.

EXERCISE   Those who exercise regularly live longer and are healthier than those who are sedentary. Because OA of weight-bearing joints limits physical activity and the amount of exercise that an individual can perform, persons with this condition are at increased risk for hypertension, obesity, diabetes, and cardiovascular disease, i.e., diseases related to their inactivity. Only 24% of individuals with arthritis report a level of physical activity sufficient to achieve health; 75% do nothing or are not sufficiently active. Arthritis is *the* major reason that elderly individuals are not active or limit their activity and is a greater factor in limiting activity than heart disease, hypertension, blindness, or diabetes. Studies of cardiovascular health have shown that the aerobic capacity (cardiovascular fitness) of men with severe knee OA is >30% lower than that of controls who do not have OA. Even at slow speed, individuals with knee OA expend more energy (measured as oxygen consumption) in walking than age- and sex-matched controls.

Disability in patients with OA may have more to do with their ability to remain active and physically fit and maintain normal body weight than with pathologic changes in the OA joint. Even if we cannot cure OA, we can cure inactivity. Men in their forties who were not performing sufficient physical activity and had low scores on a treadmill test were found to have remarkably higher death rates than those who were fit. However, among those who were not fit at the outset but who *became* fit, the risk of mortality decreased by 44%.

The amount of *aerobic conditioning* (e.g., walking, cycling, aquatic exercise) necessary for cardiovascular fitness is not so great that it cannot be achieved by people with OA. Patients with OA of lower extremity joints who are able to perform moderate to vigorous exercise at least 3 days per week (i.e., 70 to 85% of maximal heart rate)—an intensity that permits an individual to talk while exercising continuously for 20 to 60 min—improve their fitness and health without exacerbating their joint pain or increasing their need for analgesic drugs. Persons with OA who exercise consistently at this level report decreases in joint pain and disability while improving their cardiovascular muscular fitness (strength and endurance). They also report improvement in function and quality of life and exhibit improved gait and walking speed. Patients with hip or knee OA can participate safely in conditioning exercises to improve fitness and health without increasing their joint pain or need for analgesics or NSAIDs.

Disuse of the OA joint because of pain will lead to muscle atrophy. Because periarticular muscles play a major role in protecting the articular cartilage from stress, strengthening exercises are important. In patients with knee OA, strengthening of the periarticular muscles may result, within weeks, in a decrease in joint pain as great as that seen with NSAIDs. Most of the information available about the benefits of *therapeutic exercise* relates to strength training. However, the benefits of therapeutic exercise go far beyond muscle strengthening. In studies that employed 4 to 10 instructional sessions followed by self-directed home exercise in which patients initially exercised up to 5 days per week, with recommendations to decrease the frequency over the next 6 months to 2 days per week, compliance was excellent. The results showed that pain, anxiety, and depression decreased, while lower extremity strength, endurance, proprioception, and functional status improved and disability was reduced. With fairly minimal intervention and self-directed exercise, patients with OA can achieve and maintain important gains.

PATIENT EDUCATION For effective management of many patients with OA, encouragement, reassurance, advice about exercise, and recommendation of measures to unload the arthritic joint (such as a cane and proper footwear) may be all that is required. Patient education programs offer benefits beyond those that can be achieved with an NSAID in symptomatic treatment of patients with OA. Patient education interventions provide an additive benefit 20 to 30% as great as that of NSAID treatment alone. Relevant education for the patient with OA is not education about joint anatomy or the definition of an osteophyte but is education in *self-management* that emphasizes the central role of the patient in managing the disease; furthermore, it teaches the skills required to permit patients to manage medically and emotionally and to maintain their role in society.

A variety of self-management programs have been developed for patients with OA, such as the Arthritis Self-Management Program that is sponsored in the United States by the Arthritis Foundation. Participation in a structured community-based education intervention, led by trained lay leaders, can result in significant decreases in pain, disability, and depression. Patients who participate in such programs report greater performance of self-management behaviors, e.g., taking their medication properly, communicating with their healthcare providers. Furthermore, the benefits may endure for years, even with no reinforcement of the intervention.

TIDAL IRRIGATION OF THE KNEE Copious irrigation of the OA knee through a large-bore needle, flushing out fibrin, cartilage shards, and other debris, has been reported to provide months of comfort for some patient whose joint pain has been refractory to analgesics, NSAIDs, and intraarticular glucocorticoid injections. However, results of a randomized controlled trial of patients with knee OA that included a sham-irrigation procedure led to the conclusion that the bulk of the benefit from this procedure is attributable to the placebo effect.

ARTHROSCOPIC DEBRIDEMENT AND LAVAGE Arthroscopic surgery can be helpful in alleviating knee pain and improving function in the subgroup of patients with knee OA in whom loose bodies, flaps of cartilage, or disruption of the meniscus (e.g., a bucket handle tear) cause mechanical symptoms, such as locking, giving way of the limb, or catching. Although arthroscopic debridement, e.g., smoothing of the surface of fibrillated articular cartilage or meniscus, trimming of osteophytes, and removal of inflamed synovium, is employed widely in patients with symptomatic knee OA who do not have mechanical symptoms, but who have not benefited from pharmacologic therapy,

this therapeutic modality appears to be of no greater symptomatic benefit than placebo in such patients.

Pharmacologic Therapy ■ *NSAIDs AND ACETAMINOPHEN (N-ACETYL-p-AMINOPHENOL, APAP)* Drug therapy for OA today is palliative; no pharmacologic agent has been shown to prevent, delay the progression of, or reverse the pathologic changes of OA in humans. Although claims have been made that some NSAIDs slow the rate of cartilage damage, adequately controlled clinical trials in humans with OA to support this view are lacking.

In management of OA pain, pharmacologic agents should be used as adjuncts to nonpharmacologic measures, such as those described above. The latter are the *keystone* of OA treatment. Although NSAIDs often decrease joint pain and improve mobility in OA, the magnitude of improvement is generally modest—on average, about 30% reduction in pain and 15% improvement in function. Many patients taking a full therapeutic dose of NSAIDs continue to experience a significant level of residual joint pain. On the other hand, low (i.e., analgesic) doses of NSAIDs may be as effective as anti-inflammatory doses; 30 to 40% of patients with OA may find APAP—an analgesic recommended for treatment of mild-moderate pain—as effective as an NSAID. Even in patients with clinical signs of joint inflammation (synovial effusion, tenderness), relief of joint pain by APAP may be as effective as that achieved with an NSAID. Nonetheless, if simple analgesics are inadequate, it is reasonable to prescribe an NSAID for the patient with OA.

However, concern over the use of NSAIDs in OA has grown in recent years because of the adverse effects of these agents, especially those related to the gastrointestinal tract. Those at greatest risk for OA, i.e., the elderly, appear to be at greater risk than younger individuals for gastrointestinal symptoms, ulceration, hemorrhage, and death as a result of NSAID use. The annual rate of hospitalization for peptic ulcer disease among elderly current NSAID users was 16 per 1000, i.e., four times greater than that for persons not taking an NSAID. Among people age ≥65, as many as 30% of all hospitalizations and deaths related to peptic ulcer disease have been attributed to NSAID use. Risk factors for hemorrhage and other ulcer complications associated with NSAID use include, in addition to age, a history of peptic ulcer disease or of upper gastrointestinal bleeding, concomitant use of glucocorticoids or anticoagulants, and, possibly, smoking and alcohol consumption (Table 312-4).

SELECTIVE COX-2 INHIBITORS In patients who carry risk factors for an NSAID-associated gastrointestinal catastrophe, a cyclooxygenase (COX)-2 selective NSAID may be preferable to even a low dose of a nonselective COX inhibitor. In contrast to the nonselective NSAIDs, all of which inhibit COX-1 as well as COX-2, selective COX-2 inhibitors, e.g., celecoxib, rofecoxib, valdecoxib, are now available. These exhibit no greater efficacy than nonselective NSAIDs, but endoscopic studies show that they are associated with a lower incidence of gastroduodenal ulcer than nonselective NSAIDs. Of additional advantage with respect to the issue of upper gastrointestinal bleeding, selective COX-2 inhibitors do not have a clinically significant effect on platelet aggregation or bleeding time.

Results of two large-size gastrointestinal safety studies, the CLASS trial and VIGOR study, have been published (Table 312-5). Both were designed to ascertain whether treatment with celecoxib or rofecoxib, respectively, resulted in a lower incidence of clinically important NSAID-associated ulcers and ulcer complications than that seen with

---

TABLE 312-4 *Risk Factors for Upper Gastrointestinal Adverse Events in Patients Taking NSAIDs*

Increasing age	History of upper gastrointestinal
Comorbidity (poor or fair general	bleeding
health)	Anticoagulation
Oral glucocorticoids	Combination NSAID therapy
History of peptic ulcer	Increasing NSAID dose

Note: NSAID, nonsteroidal anti-inflammatory drug.

nonselective NSAIDs. In the VIGOR trial, a clear reduction in the incidence of upper gastrointestinal events was apparent in the rofecoxib treatment arm, in comparison with the naproxen arm. The risk of all clinical upper gastrointestinal events was reduced by some 54% ($p < .01$), of complicated upper gastrointestinal events by 57% ($p = .005$), and of any gastrointestinal bleeding by 62% ($p < .01$). In the CLASS study, the annualized incidence rates of ulcer complications (the primary outcome measure) with celecoxib was not significantly different from that and with the comparator nonselective NSAIDs after 6 months of treatment, although the difference for ulcer complications combined with symptomatic ulcers was significant (2.08% vs 3.54%, respectively, $p = .02$). Although a significant reduction in ulcer complications was seen with celecoxib, use of low-dose aspirin for cardiovascular prophylaxis appeared to mitigate the gastroprotective effect of celecoxib. (Although only 22% of subjects in the CLASS study were taking low-dose aspirin, as many as 60% of patients with OA >60 years old may do so in clinical practice.) Furthermore, the superiority of celecoxib observed among nonaspirin users during the first 6 months was not sustained in patients treated for 12 months.

Unexpectedly, the incidence of myocardial infarction (MI) in the VIGOR study was fourfold greater among patients treated with rofecoxib than with naproxen. Although (1) the absolute number of MIs was small; (2) the study was not powered to compare the effects of the two treatments on MI; (3) the comparability of the treatment groups with respect to the prevalence of risk factors for MI (e.g., obesity, smoking, hypercholesterolemia, diabetes mellitus) was unknown; (4) the dose of rofecoxib was two to four times greater than that used for treatment of OA; and (5) the trial was conducted in patients with rheumatoid arthritis, in which the incidence of MI is about twice as great as that in OA. The rofecoxib label contains a caveat about use of this drug in patients predisposed to ischemic heart disease.

GLUCOCORTICOID INJECTION Systemic glucocorticoids have no place in the treatment of OA. However, intra- or periarticular injection of a depot glucocorticoid preparation may provide marked symptomatic relief for weeks to months. Because studies in animal models have suggested that glucocorticoids may produce cartilage damage, and frequent injections of large amounts of steroids have been associated with joint breakdown in humans, the injection should generally not be repeated in a given joint more often than every 4 to 6 months.

INTRAARTICULAR INJECTION OF HYALURONAN Intraarticular injection of hyaluronan has been approved for treatment of patients with knee OA who have failed a program of nonpharmacologic therapy and simple analgesics. Because the duration of benefit following treatment may exceed by many months the synovial half-life of exogenous hyaluronan, the mechanism of action is unclear. However, the placebo response to intraarticular injection of hyaluronan is often large and sustained. For example, the pivotal clinical trial of Hyalgan failed to demonstrate superiority of oral naproxen, 500 mg bid, over intraarticular injections of saline. Furthermore, intraarticular injection of a preparation of the high-molecular-weight hylan (Synvisc) which had been denatured to eliminate its viscoelasticity, was no less efficacious than injection of the intact hylan or non-cross-linked lower molecular weight hyaluronan. Consistent with this observation, no difference in efficacy was observed in a randomized placebo-controlled trial of Synvisc, a lower molecular weight hyaluronan formulation, and placebo.

OPIOIDS Health professionals and patients hold concerns about tolerance and physical and psychological dependence, and many physicians

TABLE 312-5 *Comparison of Study Designs for Rofecoxib (VIGOR) and Celecoxib (CLASS) Gastrointestinal (GI)*

Parameter	Trial	
	VIGOR	CLASS
Number of subjects	8076	7982
Mean age	~58 years	~60 years; ~38% >65 years
Underlying disease	Rheumatoid arthritis	Osteoarthritis 73%, rheumatoid arthritis 27%
Duration of follow-up	Median, 9 months	Median, 9 months
	Maximum, 13 months	Maximum, 13 months
Type of analysis	Intention to treat (includes events within 14 days of last dose of study drug)	Excludes events on day 0–2 and >6 months
Dose of Coxib	Rofecoxib, 50 mg/d	Celecoxib, 400 mg/d
Comparator NSAID	Naproxen, 1000 mg/d	Ibuprofen, 2400 mg/d or diclofenac, 150 mg/d
Low-dose aspirin	Not permitted	22%
Concurrent steroid use	56%	30%
Primary end point	Clinical upper GI events	Complicated ulcers
Secondary end point	Complicated upper GI events	Symptomatic + complicated ulcers

Note: NSAID, nonsteroidal anti-inflammatory drug.
Source: Derived from VIGOR: Bombardier C et al: N Engl J Med 343:1520, 2000, with permission; CLASS: Silverstein F et al: JAMA 284:1247, 2000.

hesitate to prescribe opioids for patients with nonmalignant chronic pain because of concerns about legal action by governmental regulatory authorities. However, the prevalence of narcotic abuse among older people is low: <1% of patients attending methadone maintenance programs are ≥60 years.

For acute flares of OA pain, when APAP or an NSAID does not provide adequate pain relief or is not well tolerated, a weak opioid, e.g., oral codeine, deserves consideration. Because codeine, when taken alone in a dose of 60 mg, is no more effective than 650 mg of aspirin or APAP, it is used in combination with these drugs to treat moderate or moderately severe OA pain.

Opioids may also be useful for chronic OA pain. The major problem associated with the use of chronic opioid therapy for OA pain is the side effects of these agents, e.g., nausea, vomiting, constipation, urinary retention, mental confusion, drowsiness, and respiratory depression. In the elderly, the central nervous system effects of opioids (e.g., dizziness) may have particularly serious consequences. Prescription of either codeine or propoxyphene may increase the risk of hip fracture by 60%. Concurrent use of these opioids and a psychotropic drug (e.g., sedative, antidepressant, antipsychotic) carries a fracture risk 2.6 times as high as that in nonusers of either drug class.

Tramadol hydrochloride is a centrally acting analgesic with a dual mechanism of action: the molecule is a μ-opioid agonist and also inhibits reuptake of norepinephrine and serotonin. Although the affinity of binding to the μ-opioid regimen is some 6000 times lower than that of morphine, the opioid and nonopioid activities are synergistic. In contrast to NSAIDs, tramadol does not inhibit prostaglandin synthesis and has no adverse effects on the gastric mucosa, kidney, or platelet. It is a useful adjunct in patients with OA in whom APAP or a low dose of NSAID is ineffective or contraindications exist to the use of an NSAID. Improvement with tramadol, 200 to 400 mg/d, is comparable to that with ibuprofen, 1200 to 2400 mg/d, in patients with chronic joint pain. Because development of tolerance or dependence appears to be uncommon with long-term administration, tramadol has not been scheduled as a controlled substance. In general, its efficacy and adverse event profile are comparable to those of APAP/codeine. The latter, however, is considerably less expensive.

The frequency and severity of side effects of tramadol may be reduced considerably if treatment is initiated at a very low dose (e.g., 25 mg/d), which can then be increased gradually every few days. However, this "start low, go slow" approach limits the usefulness of the drug in management of acute pain. Because it inhibits the reuptake of serotonin and norepinephrine, tramadol should not generally be given to patients receiving a tricyclic antidepressant, selective serotonin reuptake inhibitor, or monoamine oxidase inhibitor. These combinations have been reported to cause convulsions. Even in the absence of concomitant therapy with the above agents, however, seizures may occasionally occur in some patients taking tramadol.

A combination of tramadol and APAP in a 37.5 mg/325 mg tablet (ULTRACET) has recently become available. It has a more rapid onset of action than tramadol alone and longer duration of action than APAP alone. In subjects with an acute flare of hip or knee OA, who received 1 or 2 tablets of tramadol/APAP qid for 10 days in addition to their usual NSAID therapy, tramadol/APAP was significantly superior to placebo with respect to improvement in joint pain and global assessment by subjects and physicians. However, treatment-related adverse events (e.g., nausea, dizziness, vomiting) were reported in nearly 25% of the tramadol/APAP group, but in only 8% of the placebo group. Furthermore, the above figures may understate the true incidence of adverse events with this formulation, because subjects were excluded from the study if they had previously failed tramadol therapy or had discontinued tramadol because of an adverse event.

RUBEFACIENTS/CAPSAICIN Because use of systemic analgesics and NSAIDs is often accompanied by adverse effects and older individuals with OA often require medication for comorbid conditions (e.g., hypertension, heart disease, diabetes mellitus) and are at increased the risk of serious drug interactions with NSAIDs, topical therapy for management of OA has appeal.

Application of topical irritants to painful joints and muscles and the local heat provided by rubefacients may be beneficial. However, although topical medications are widely used in the United States as over-the-counter preparations, they are not often prescribed for OA in this country, chiefly because evidence of their efficacy is limited. Except for formulations of salicylate, topical NSAIDs have not been approved for use in the United States. It is unclear whether the benefit attributed to their use is mediated through a pharmacologic action, placebo effect, or their action as a rubefacient. Capsaicin cream, which depletes local sensory nerve endings of substance P, may reduce joint pain and tenderness when applied topically by patients with hand or knee OA, even when used as monotherapy, i.e., without NSAIDs or systemic analgesics.

Glucosamine, Chondroitin Sulfate Glucosamine and chondroitin sulfate have recently enjoyed striking popularity for treatment of OA. They are sold widely in pharmacies, supermarkets, and health food stores but are not approved for use in OA by the U.S. Food and Drug Administration. Several studies have shown glucosamine to be superior to placebo and comparable to NSAIDs with respect to efficacy in patients with knee OA, and to have a better safety profile than NSAIDs. However, the efficacy of neither glucosamine nor chondroitin sulfate has been examined in large, well-designed placebo-controlled trials. In a meta-analysis of randomized, double-blind, placebo-controlled studies of glucosamine and chondroitin sulfate, moderate symptomatic benefit was demonstrated for both agents, relative to placebo. In studies of chondroitin sulfate, symptomatic improvement was apparent as long as 12 months after the onset of treatment. However, when only high-quality or large-size trials were considered, the effect sizes for glucosamine and chondroitin sulfate were diminished, i.e., the better the study design, the smaller the therapeutic benefit. In three recent randomized, double-blind trials in which the manufacturer did not have access to the raw data and was not involved in data analysis, glucosamine was no more effective than placebo.

The question arises whether glucosamine is "chondroprotective." Results of two recent randomized clinical trials have led to the suggestion that glucosamine not only improves joint pain in patients with knee OA, but protects against articular cartilage damage, based upon analyses of changes in joint space width in the standing anteroposterior (AP) knee radiograph. However, concern has been expressed about the interpretation of the results of these studies because of limitations of the radiographic methods employed. A multicenter study supported by the National Institutes of Health, the Glucosamine Chondroitin Ar-

thritis Intervention Trial (GAIT), is in progress which is comparing glucosamine, chondroitin sulfate, the combination, and celecoxib with placebo in patients with knee OA. Although the primary outcome measure is joint pain after 6 months of treatment, approximately 50% of the subjects will be maintained on treatment for 2 years and radiographs obtained at baseline will be compared with those obtained after 1 year and 2 years of treatment.

Orthopedic Surgery Joint replacement surgery should be reserved for patients with advanced OA in whom aggressive medical management has failed. In such cases total joint arthroplasty may be remarkably effective in relieving pain and increasing mobility. Osteotomy, which is surgically more conservative than arthroplasty, can eliminate the concentration of peak dynamic loads and may provide effective pain relief in patients with hip or knee OA. It is of greatest benefit when the disease is only moderately advanced.

Cartilage Regeneration Chondroplasty (abrasion arthroplasty) has enjoyed some popularity as treatment for OA, but well-controlled studies of its efficacy are lacking and the fibrocartilage that resurfaces the abraded bone is inferior to normal hyaline cartilage in its ability to withstand mechanical loads. In one study, knee pain and function were not related to the extent of cartilage regeneration 2 years later in patients who had undergone tibial osteotomy for medial compartment knee OA. Autologous chondrocyte transplantation and attempts at cartilage repair using mesenchymal stem cells and autologous osteochondral plugs are currently being used experimentally for repair of focal chondral defects, but have not been proved to be effective in treatment of OA.

A Rational Approach to the Nonsurgical Management of OA Nonpharmacologic management, as described above, is the foundation of treatment of OA pain and is as important, or more important, than drug treatment, which plays an adjunctive or complementary role in management of this disease. Figure 312-4 provides an algorithm that might be applied to treatment of a newly diagnosed patient with knee OA. The progressive levels of treatment are associated with increasing cost, decreasing convenience for the patient, and increasing risk of side effects. The scheme should not be interpreted dogmatically as a fixed progression of steps. Treatment of OA must be individualized, and the treatment program flexible. For example, in some patients it may be reasonable to institute patellar taping or to prescribe a wedged insole on the initial visit, or an intraarticular glucocorticoid injection on a later visit. Maintaining regular contact with the patient, e.g., via periodic telephone calls, may reduce joint pain to a level beyond that which can be achieved with an NSAID alone and this, or some surrogate measure, warrants incorporation into the treatment program.

It is reasonable to prescribe APAP initially, in a dose up to 4000 mg/d, because of its low cost, excellent safety profile, and the fact that it is as efficacious as NSAIDs in many patients with OA when an analgesic is required for treatment of OA pain. If this does not control joint symptoms within a reasonable period of time, a *low dose* of NSAID (e.g., ibuprofen, 1200 mg/d; naproxen, 500 mg/d) may be substituted for, or added to, the APAP. In patients with significant risk factors for a serious upper gastrointestinal adverse event, if a nonselective NSAID is used, even in a low dose, it is reasonable to recommend coadministration of a gastroprotective agent, such as misoprostol or a proton pump inhibitor, which have been shown by endoscopy to be effective in treating and preventing NSAID gastropathy. Because the risk of an NSAID-associated gastrointestinal catastrophe is dose-dependent, the lowest effective dose of NSAID should be employed. Salsalate and other nonacetylated salicylates, which have only minimal effect on prostaglandin synthase, are as effective as other NSAIDs and have a lower rate of serious gastrointestinal side effects. However, ototoxicity and central nervous system toxicity may limit their use.

When NSAIDs are required, they may be prescribed on an "as needed" basis, rather than in a fixed daily dose; pain control has been shown to be comparable and the risk of toxicity will be reduced. Once treatment with an NSAID or simple analgesic is initiated, the need for

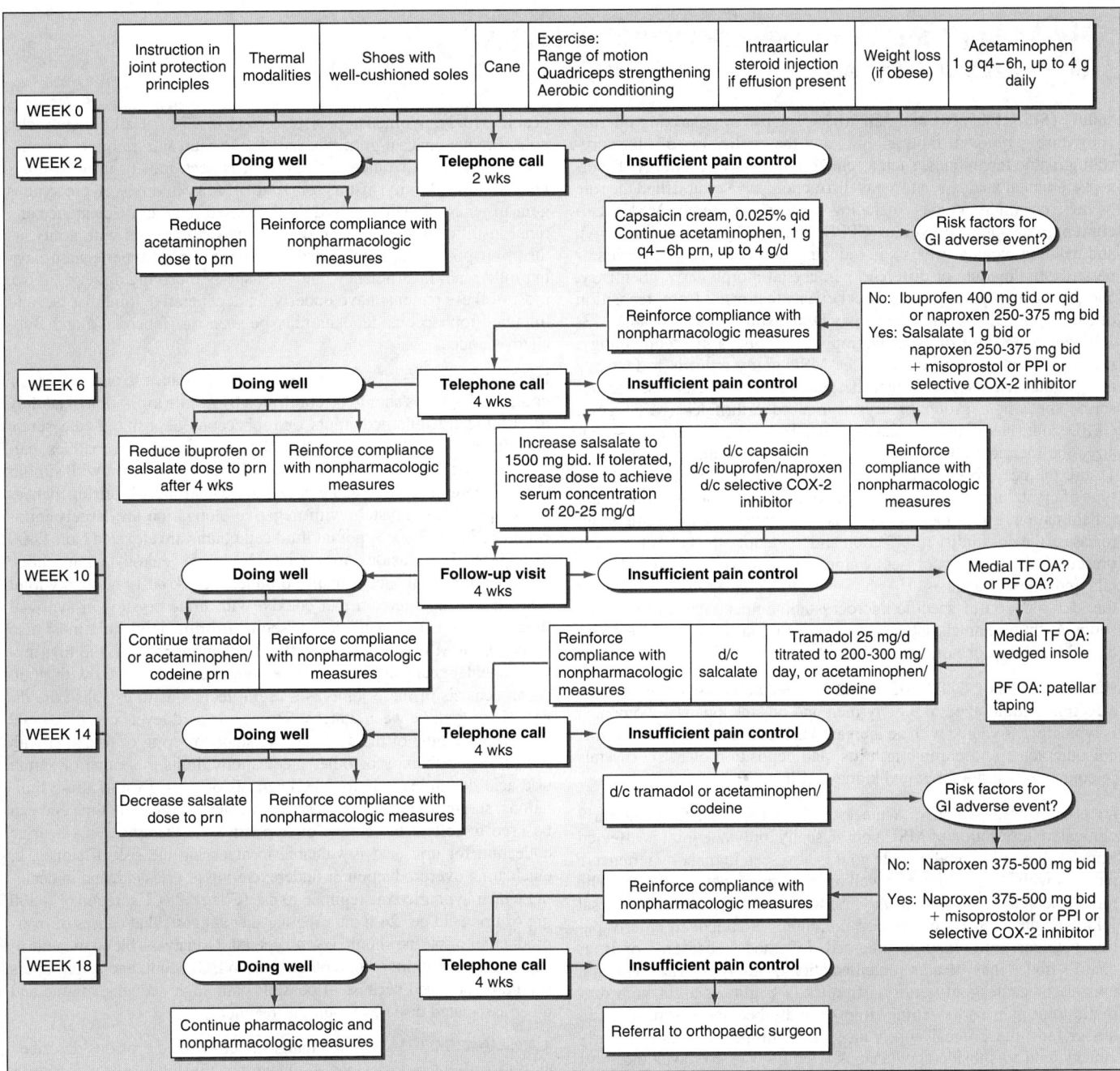

FIGURE 312-4 Algorithm for management of a newly diagnosed patient with knee OA. TF, tibiofemoral; PF, patellofemoral; PPI, proton pump inhibitor; d/c, discontinue.

(Modified from KD Brandt: Diagnosis and Nonsurgical Management of Osteoarthritis, 2d ed, Professional Communications, Inc., Caddo, OK, 2000, pp 1–304)

continuation of that treatment requires ongoing assessment. For many patients with OA, it will be possible eventually to reduce the dose of drug or to use the agent only intermittently during exacerbations of joint pain.

FURTHER READING

BOMBARDIER C et al: Comparison of upper gastrointestinal toxicity of rofecoxib and naproxen in patients with rheumatoid arthritis. N Engl J Med 343:1520, 2000

BRANDT KD, BRADLEY JD: Should the initial drug used to treat osteoarthritis pain be a nonsteroidal antiinflammatory drug? J Rheumatol 28:467, 2001

FELSON DT: Epidemiology of osteoarthritis, in *Osteoarthritis*, 2nd ed, KD Brandt et al (eds). Oxford, Oxford University Press, 2003, pp 9–16

JÜNI P et al: Are selective COX-2 inhibitors superior to traditional nonsteroidal anti-inflammatory drugs? Adequate analysis of the CLASS trial indicates that this may not be the case. BMJ 324:1287, 2002

MCALINDON T: An evaluation of glucosamine for the treatment of OA, in KD Brandt et al (eds): Proceedings of Symposium: Controversies and Practical Issues in the Management of Osteoarthritis. J Clin Rheum, 95(Suppl):S27, 2003

MINOR MA. The utility and importance of non-pharmacologic therapy for the patient with OA, in KD Brandt et al (eds): Proceedings of Symposium: Controversies and Practical Issues in the Management of Osteoarthritis. J Clin Rheum, 9(Suppl):S19, 2003

MOSELEY JB et al: A controlled trial of arthroscopic surgery for osteoarthritis of the knee. N Engl J Med 347:81, 2002

SILVERSTEIN FE et al: Gastrointestinal toxicity with celecoxib vs nonsteroidal anti-inflammatory drugs for osteoarthritis and rheumatoid arthritis. The CLASS Study: A randomized controlled trial. JAMA 284:1247, 2000

"GOUT" CRYSTALLOGRAPHY AND ARTHRITIS The use of polarizing microscopy during synovial fluid analysis and the application of other crystallographic techniques, such as electron microscopy, energy-dispersive elemental analysis, and x-ray diffraction, have established the role of different microcrystals, including monosodium urate (MSU), calcium pyrophosphate dihydrate (CPPD), calcium hydroxyapatite (HA), and calcium oxalate (CaOx), in inducing acute or chronic arthritis or periarthritis. In spite of differences in crystal morphology, chemistry, and physical properties, the clinical events that result from deposition of MSU, CPPD, HA, and CaOx may be indistinguishable (Table 313-1). Prior to the use of crystallographic techniques in rheumatology, much of what was considered to be MSU gouty arthritis in fact was not. Simkin has suggested that the generic term *gout* be used to describe the whole group of crystal-induced arthritides (MSU gout, CPPD gout, HA gout, and CaOx gout). This concept further emphasizes the identical clinical presentations of these entities (Table 313-1) and the need to perform synovial fluid analysis to distinguish the type of crystal involved. In the setting of acute articular or periarticular inflammation, aspiration and analysis of effusions are most important to assess the possibility of infection and to identify the type of crystals present. Polarization microscopy alone can identify most typical crystals and allow diagnosis. HA, however, is an exception. Apart from the identification of specific microcrystalline materials or organisms, synovial fluid characteristics are nonspecific, and synovial fluid can be inflammatory or noninflammatory.

MONOSODIUM URATE GOUT MSU gout is a metabolic disease most often affecting middle-aged to elderly men and postmenopausal women. It is typically associated with an increased uric acid pool, hyperuricemia, episodic acute and chronic arthritis, and deposition of MSU crystals in connective tissue tophi and kidneys (Chap. 338).

Acute and Chronic Arthritis Acute arthritis is the most frequent early clinical manifestation of MSU gout. Usually, only one joint is affected initially, but polyarticular acute gout is also seen in male hypertensive patients with ethanol abuse as well as in postmenopausal women. The metatarsophalangeal joint of the first toe is often involved, but tarsal joints, ankles, and knees are also commonly affected. In elderly patients, finger joints may be inflamed. Inflamed Heberden's or Bouchard's nodes may be a first manifestation of gouty arthritis. The first episode of acute gouty arthritis frequently begins at night with dramatic joint pain and swelling. Joints rapidly become warm, red, and tender, and the clinical appearance often mimics a cellulitis. Early attacks tend to subside spontaneously within 3 to 10 days, and most of the patients do not have residual symptoms until the next episode. Several events may precipitate acute gouty arthritis: dietary excess, trauma, surgery, excessive ethanol ingestion, adrenocorticotropic hormone (ACTH) and glucocorticoid withdrawal, hypouricemic therapy, and serious medical illnesses such as myocardial infarction and stroke.

After many acute mono- or oligoarticular attacks, a proportion of gouty patients may present with a chronic nonsymmetric synovitis, causing potential confusion with rheumatoid arthritis (Chap. 301). Less commonly, chronic gouty arthritis will be the only manifestation and, more rarely, the disease will manifest as inflamed or noninflamed periarticular tophaceous deposits in the absence of chronic synovitis.

TABLE 313-1 *Musculoskeletal Manifestations of Crystal-Induced Arthritis*

Acute mono- or polyarthritis	Destructive arthropathies
Bursitis	Pseudo-rheumatoid arthritis
Tendinitis	Pseudo-ankylosing spondylitis
Enthesitis	Spinal stenosis
Tophaceous deposits	Crown dens syndrome
Peculiar type of osteoarthritis	Carpal tunnel syndrome
Synovial osteochondromatosis	Tendon rupture

(Table 313-1). Women represent only 5 to 17% of all patients with gout. Premenopausal gout is a rare occurrence and accounts for only about 17% of all women with gout; it is seen mostly in individuals with a strong family history of gout. A few kindreds of precocious gout in young females caused by decreased renal urate clearance and renal insufficiency have been described. Most women with gouty arthritis are postmenopausal and elderly, have arterial hypertension causing mild renal insufficiency, and are usually receiving diuretics. Also, most of these patients have underlying degenerative joint disease, and inflamed tophaceous deposits may be seen on Heberden's and Bouchard's nodes.

LABORATORY DIAGNOSIS Even if the clinical appearance strongly suggests gout, the diagnosis should be confirmed by needle aspiration of acutely or chronically inflamed joints or tophaceous deposits. Acute septic arthritis, several of the other crystalline-associated arthropathies, palindromic rheumatism, and psoriatic arthritis may present with similar clinical features. During acute gouty attacks, strongly birefringent needle-shaped MSU crystals with negative elongation are largely intracellular (Fig. 313-1). Synovial fluid cell counts are elevated from 2000 to $60,000/\mu L$. Effusions appear cloudy due to leukocytes, and large amounts of crystals occasionally produce a thick pasty or chalky joint fluid. Bacterial infection can coexist with urate crystals in synovial fluid; if there is any suspicion of septic arthritis, joint fluid must also be cultured. MSU crystals can often be demonstrated in the first metatarsophalangeal joint and in knees not acutely involved with gout. Arthrocentesis of these joints is a useful technique to establish the diagnosis of gout between attacks. Serum uric acid levels can be normal or low at the time of the acute attack, since lowering of uric acid with hypouricemic therapy or other medications limits the value of serum uric acid determinations for the diagnosis of gout. Despite these limitations, serum uric acid is almost always elevated at some time and can be used to follow the course of hypouricemic therapy. A 24-h urine collection for uric acid is valuable in assessing the risk of stones, in elucidating overproduction or underexcretion of uric acid, and in deciding which hypouricemic regimen to use (Chap. 338). Excretion of >800 mg of uric acid per 24 h on a regular diet suggests that causes of overproduction of purine should be considered. Urinalysis, blood urea nitrogen, serum creatinine, white blood cell (WBC) count, and serum lipids should be obtained because of possible pathologic sequelae of gout and other associated diseases requiring treatment.

RADIOGRAPHIC FEATURES Cystic changes, well-defined erosions described as punched-out lytic lesions with overhanging bony edges [Martel's sign, or G sign (G for gout)], associated with soft tissue calcified masses are characteristic radiographic features of chronic tophaceous gout. However, similar radiographic signs can also be observed in erosive osteoarthritis, destructive apatite arthropathies, and rheumatoid arthritis.

℞ TREATMENT

Acute Gouty Arthritis The mainstay of treatment during an acute attack is the administration of an anti-inflammatory drug such as colchicine, nonsteroidal anti-inflammatory drugs (NSAIDs), or glucocorticoids depending on the age of the patient and comorbid conditions. Both colchicine and NSAIDs may be quite toxic in the elderly, particularly in the presence of renal insufficiency and gastrointestinal disorders. In elderly patients, one may favor the use of intraarticular glucocorticoid injections for attacks involving one or two larger joints or ice pack applications along with lower oral doses of colchicine for gouty synovitis affecting small joints. Colchicine given orally is a traditional and effective treatment, if used early in the attack, in at least 85% of patients. One tablet (0.6 mg) is given every hour until relief of symptoms or gastrointestinal toxicity occurs, or a total of four to eight tablets may be given in accordance with the age of the patient. The drug must be stopped promptly at the first sign of loose stools, and symptomatic treatment must be given for the diarrhea. Intravenous colchicine is sometimes used and can reduce, though not eliminate, the gastrointestinal side effects. Intravenous colchicine is most reliable for pre- or postoperative prophylaxis in 1- to 2-mg doses when patients cannot take medications orally. Life-threatening colchicine toxicity and sudden death have been described with the administration of >4 mg/d intravenously. The intravenous dose for acute gouty arthritis is 1 to 2 mg given slowly through an established venous line over 10 min in a soluset, and two additional doses of 1 mg each may be given at 6-h intervals, but the total dose should never exceed 4 mg. NSAIDs are affective in ~90% of patients, and the resolution of signs and symptoms usually occurs in 5 to 7 days. The most effective drugs are those with a short half-life and include indomethacin, 25 to 50 mg tid, ibuprofen, 800 mg tid, or diclofenac, 50 mg tid. Cyclooxigenase-2 highly selective inhibitors are probably equally effective but with less short-term gastrointestinal toxicity. Oral glucocorticoids such as prednisone, 30 to 50 mg/d as the initial dose and tapered over 5 to 7 days, a single intravenous dose of methylprednisolone, 7 mg of betametasone, or 20 to 40 mg of intraarticular triamcinolone acetonide have been equally effective. ACTH as an intramuscular injection of 40 to 80 IU in a single dose or every 12 h for 1 to 2 days is effective in patients with acute polyarticular refractory gout or with a contraindication for using colchicine or NSAIDs.

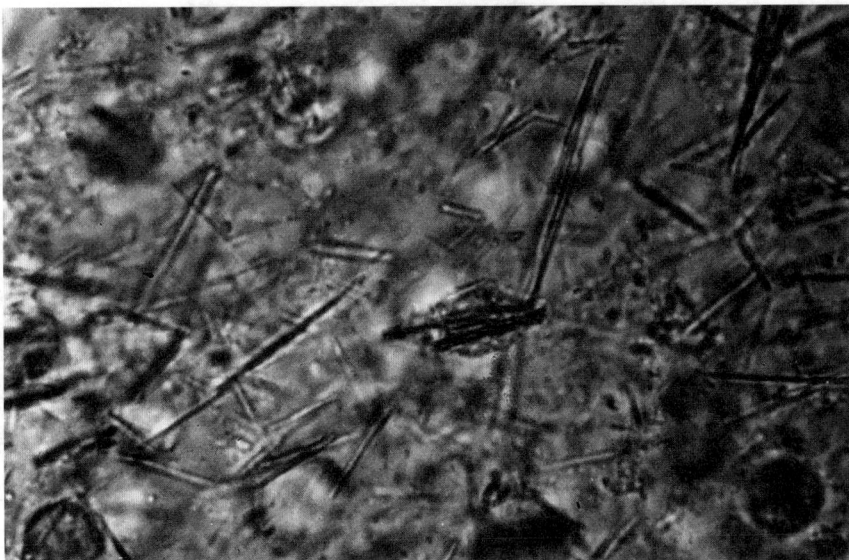

FIGURE 313-1 Extracellular and intracellular monosodium urate crystals, as seen in a fresh preparation of synovial fluid, illustrate needle- and rod-shaped strongly negative birefringent crystals (compensated polarized light microscopy; 400×).

Hypouricemic Therapy Attempts to normalize serum uric acid to <300 μmol/L (5.0 mg/dL) to prevent recurrent gouty attacks and eliminate tophaceous deposits entail a commitment to long-term hypouricemic regimens and medications that generally are required for life. Hypouricemic therapy should be considered when the hyperuricemia cannot be corrected by simple means (control of body weight, low-purine diet, increase in liquid ingestion, limitation of ethanol intake, and avoidance of diuretic use). The decision to initiate hypouricemic therapy is usually made taking into consideration the number of acute attacks, family history of gout, presence of MSU tophaceous deposits, uric acid excretion >800 mg per 24 hours, presence of uric acid stones, and risk for acute uric acid nephropathy during chemotherapy for myeloproliferative disorders. Uricosuric agents, such as probenecid, can be used in patients with good renal function who underexcrete uric acid, with <600 mg in a 24-hour urine sample. Urine volume must be maintained by ingestion of 1500 mL of water every day. Probenecid can be started at a dosage of 200 mg twice daily and increased gradually as needed up to 2 g in order to maintain a serum uric acid level <300 μmol/L (5 mg/dL). Probenecid is the drug of choice to treat elderly patients with hypertension and thiazide dependence; however, probenecid is not effective with a renal creatinine clearance <1 mL/s. These patients may require allopurinol or benzbromarone (not available in the United States), which is another uricosuric drug that is effective in patients with renal failure and who are receiving diuretics. Allopurinol is the best drug to lower serum urate in overproducers, stone formers, and patients with advanced renal failure. It can be given in a single morning dose, 300 mg initially and increasing up to 800 mg if needed. In most patients, it is not necessary to start at a lower dose; however, in patients with renal failure, the dosage should be adjusted depending on the serum creatinine concentration in order to minimize side effects. Patients with frequent acute attacks may require lower initial doses to prevent exacerbations. Toxicity of allopurinol has been recognized increasingly in patients with renal failure who use thiazide diuretics and in those patients allergic to penicillin and ampicillin. The most serious side effects include skin rash with progression to life-threatening toxic epidermal necrolysis, systemic vasculitis, bone marrow suppression, granulomatous hepatitis, and renal failure. Urate-lowering drugs should not be initiated during acute attacks. This is especially important in patients who have refractory acute arthritis or who had a flare-up previously with hypouricemic drugs. Colchicine prophylaxis in doses of 0.6 mg one to two times daily is usually continued, along with hypouricemic therapy, until the patient is normouricemic and without gouty attacks for 3 months. However, prophylactic colchicine treatment may be necessary as long as tophi are present. Recombinant urate oxidase uricase can be used in the short-term prophylaxis and treatment of chemotherapy-associated hyperuricemia in patients with lymphoproliferative and myeloproliferative disorders.

CPPD DEPOSITION DISEASE ■ Pathogenesis The deposition of CPPD crystals in articular tissues is most common in the elderly, affecting 10 to 15% of persons 65 to 75 years old and 30 to 60% of those >85 years old. In most cases this process is asymptomatic, and the cause of CPPD deposition is uncertain. Because >80% of patients are more than 60 years old and 70% have preexisting joint damage from other conditions, it is likely that biochemical changes in aging cartilage favor crystal nucleation. Examples of such chemical alterations include the following. There is an increased production of inorganic pyrophosphate and decreased levels of pyrophosphatases in cartilage extracts from patients with CPPD arthritis. This condition, which increases inorganic pyrophosphate and promotes CPPD crystal formation, may also inhibit hydroxyapatite formation. The increase in pyrophosphate production appears to be related to enhanced activity of ATP pyrophosphohydrolase and 5′-nucleotidase, which catalyze the reaction of ATP to adenosine and pyrophosphate. This pyrophosphate could combine with calcium to form CPPD crystals in matrix vesicles or on collagen fibers. There is a diminution in the levels of cartilage glycosaminoglycans that normally inhibit and regulate crystal nucleation. These deficiencies may lead to increased crystal deposition. In vitro studies have demonstrated that transforming growth factor β1 and epidermal growth factor both stimulate the production of pyrophosphate by articular cartilage and thus may contribute to the deposition of CPPD crystals. The release of CPPD crystals into the joint space is followed by the phagocytosis of these crystals by neutrophils, which respond by releasing inflammatory substances. In addition, neutrophils release a glycopeptide that is chemotactic for other neutrophils, thus augmenting the inflammatory events. The same substance is present in MSU gout.

A minority of patients with CPPD arthropathy have metabolic abnormalities or hereditary CPPD disease (Table 313-2). These associations suggest that a variety of different metabolic products may enhance CPPD deposition. Included among these conditions are the

TABLE 313-2 *Conditions Associated with Calcium Pyrophosphate Dihydrate Disease*

Aging
Disease-associated
  Primary hyperparathyroidism
  Hemochromatosis
  Hypophosphatasia
  Hypomagnesemia
  Chronic tophaceous gout
  Postmeniscectomy
Epiphyseal dysplasias
Hereditary: Slovakian-Hungarian, Spanish, Spanish-American (Argentinian,[a] Colombian, and Chilean), French,[a] Swedish, Dutch, Canadian, Mexican-American, Italian-American,[a] German-American, Japanese, Tunisian, Jewish, English[a]

[a] Mutations in the ANKH gene.

"four H's" of hyperparathyroidism, hemochromatosis, hypophosphatasia, and hypomagnesemia. Hemochromatosis and hyperparathyroidism are good examples. Ferrous ions and hypercalcemia may either directly alter cartilage or inhibit inorganic pyrophosphatases, leading to enhanced susceptibility to CPPD deposition. The presence of CPPD arthritis in individuals <50 years old should lead to consideration of these metabolic disorders and inherited forms of disease, including those identified in a variety of ethnic groups (Table 313-2). Genomic DNA studies performed on five different kindreds have shown a possible location of the genetic defects on chromosome 8q in one, and on chromosome 5p in the other four in a region that expresses the gene of a membrane pyrophosphate channel (*ANK* gene). A defective gene described in the *ank/ank* mice causes elevation of the intracellular pyrophosphate and reduction of the extracellular pyrophosphate and promotes apatite deposition. Mutations described in the human *ANK* gene in four kindreds with CPPD arthritis might increase extracellular pyrophosphate and induce CPPD crystal formation (Fig. 313-2). Identification of these genes will help elucidate the pathogenesis of both the familial and the more common sporadic form of the disease. Investigation should include inquiry for evidence of familial aggregation and evaluation of serum calcium, phosphorus, alkaline phosphatase, magnesium, serum ferritin, and transferritin saturation.

Clinical Manifestations CPPD arthropathy may be asymptomatic, acute, subacute, or chronic or cause acute synovitis superimposed on chronically involved joints. Acute CPPD arthritis was originally termed *pseudogout* by McCarty and coworkers because of its striking similarity to MSU gout. Other clinical manifestations of CPPD deposition include (1) induction or enhancement of peculiar forms of osteoarthritis; (2) induction of severe destructive disease that may radiographically mimic neuropathic arthritis; (3) production of symmetric proliferative synovitis, clinically similar to rheumatoid arthritis and frequently seen in familial forms with early onset; (4) intervertebral disk and ligament calcification with restriction of spine mobility, mimicking ankylosing spondylitis (also seen in hereditary forms); and (5) rarely spinal stenosis (most commonly seen in the elderly) (Table 313-1).

The knee is the joint most frequently affected in CPPD arthropathy.

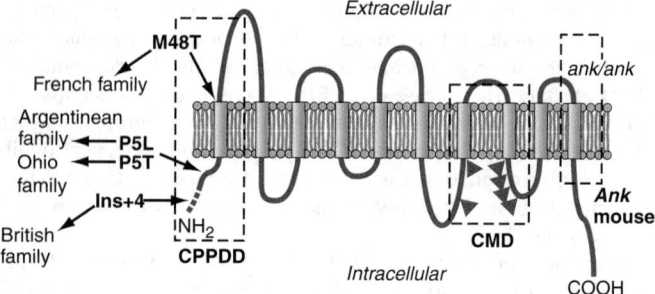

FIGURE 313-2 Mutations in *ANKH* gene associated with familial CPPD gout. CMD, cranial metaphyseal dysplasia.

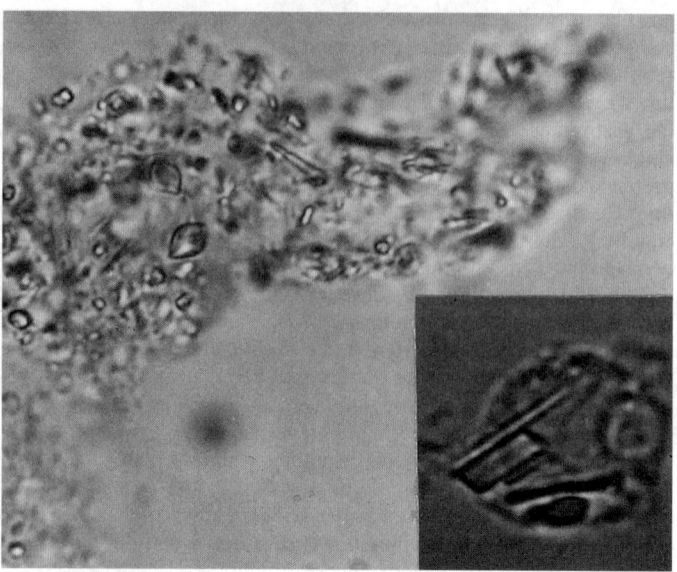

FIGURE 313-3 Intracellular and extracellular calcium pyrophosphate dihydrate crystals, as seen in a fresh preparation of synovial fluid, illustrate rectangular, rod-shaped, and rhomboid weakly positive birefringent crystals (compensated polarized light microscopy; 400×).

Other sites include the wrist, shoulder, ankle, elbow, and hands. Rarely, the temporomandibular joint and ligamentum flavum of the spinal canal are involved. Clinical and radiographic evidence indicates that CPPD deposition is polyarticular in at least two-thirds of patients. When the clinical picture resembles that of slowly progressive osteoarthritis, diagnosis may be more difficult. Joint distribution may provide important clues suggesting CPPD disease. For example, primary osteoarthritis rarely involves a metacarpophalangeal, wrist, elbow, shoulder, or ankle joint. If radiographs reveal punctate and/or linear radiodense deposits in fibrocartilaginous joint menisci or articular hyaline cartilage (chondrocalcinosis), the diagnostic certainty of CPPD is further enhanced. *Definitive diagnosis* requires demonstration of typical crystals in synovial fluid or articular tissue (Fig. 313-3). In the absence of joint effusion or indications to obtain a synovial biopsy, chondrocalcinosis is presumptive of CPPD deposition. One exception is chondrocalcinosis due to CaOx in some patients with chronic renal failure.

Acute attacks of CPPD arthritis may be precipitated by trauma, arthroscopy, or hyaluronate injections. Rapid diminution of serum calcium concentration, as may occur in severe medical illness or after surgery (especially parathyroidectomy), can also lead to pseudogout attacks.

In as many as 50% of cases, CPPD gout is associated with low-grade fever and, on occasion, temperatures as high as 40°C. Whether or not radiographic proof of chondrocalcinosis is evident in the involved joint(s), synovial analysis with microbial cultures is essential to rule out the possibility of infection. In fact, infection in a joint with any microcrystalline deposition process can lead to crystal shedding and subsequent synovitis from both crystals and microorganisms. Synovial fluid in acute CPPD gout has inflammatory qualities. The WBC count can range from several thousand cells to 100,000 cells/μL, the mean being about 24,000 cells/μL and the predominant cell being the neutrophil. Polarization microscopy usually reveals rhomboid crystals with weak positive birefringence inside fibrin clots and in neutrophils (Fig. 313-3).

℞ TREATMENT

Untreated acute attacks may last a few days to as long as a month. Treatment by joint aspiration and NSAIDs, or colchicine, or intraarticular glucocorticoid injection may result in return to prior status in ≤10 days. For patients with frequent recurrent attacks of CPPD gout, daily prophylactic treatment with low doses of colchicine may be helpful in decreasing the frequency of the attacks. Severe polyarticular attacks usually require short courses of glucocorticoids. Unfortunately, there is no effective way to remove CPPD deposits from cartilage and synovium. Uncontrolled studies suggest that radioactive synovectomy (with yttrium 90) or the administration of antimalarial agents may be helpful in controlling persistent synovitis. Patients with progressive destructive large-joint arthropathy usually require joint replacement.

CALCIUM HYDROXYAPATITE DEPOSITION DISEASE ■ Pathogenesis

HA is the primary mineral of bone and teeth. Abnormal accumulation can occur in areas of tissue damage (dystrophic calcification), in hypercalcemic or hyperparathyroid states (metastatic calcification), and in certain conditions of unknown cause (Table 313-3). In chronic renal failure, hyperphosphatemia enhances HA deposition both in and around joints. Familial aggregation is rarely seen, but no association with human *ANK* mutations have been described thus far.

HA may be released from exposed bone and cause the acute synovitis occasionally seen in chronic stable osteoarthritis (e.g., "hot" Heberden's nodes). HA deposition is also an important factor in an extremely destructive chronic arthropathy of the elderly that occurs most often in knees and shoulders (Milwaukee shoulder). Joint destruction is associated with attenuation or rupture of supporting structures, leading to instability and deformity. Progression tends to be indolent, and synovial fluid WBC counts are usually <2000/μL. Symptoms range from minimal to severe pain and disability that may lead to joint replacement surgery. Whether severely affected patients merely represent an extreme synovial tissue response to the HA crystals that are so common in osteoarthritis is uncertain. Synovial membrane tissue cultures exposed to HA (or CPPD) crystals markedly increased the release of collagenases and neutral proteases, underscoring the destructive potential of abnormally stimulated synovial lining cells.

Clinical Manifestations Periarticular and articular deposits may coexist and be associated with acute and/or chronic damage to the joint capsule, tendons, bursa, or articular surfaces. The most common sites of HA deposition include bursae and tendons in and/or around the knees, shoulders, hips, and fingers. Clinical manifestations include asymptomatic radiographic abnormalities, acute synovitis, bursitis, tendinitis,

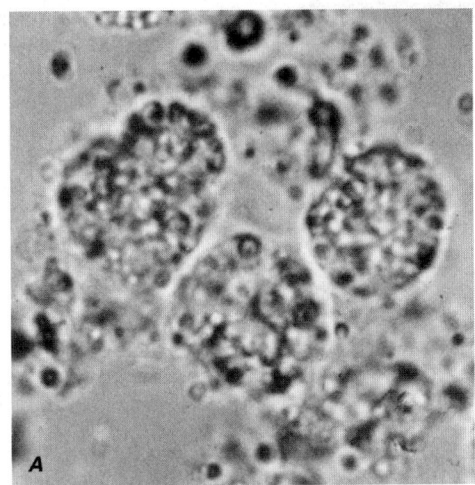 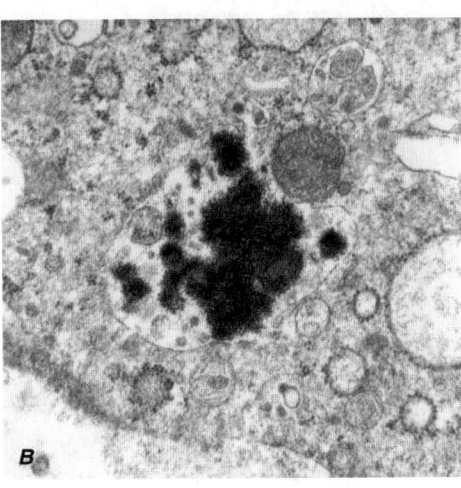

FIGURE 313-4 *A.* Cytoplasmic round inclusions inside synovial fluid cells represent aggregates of apatite crystals (fresh preparation, ordinary light microscopy; 288×). *B.* An electron micrograph demonstrates a cluster of dark apatite crystals within a synovial fluid mononuclear cell (21,600×).

and chronic destructive arthropathy. Most patients with HA arthropathy are elderly. Although the true incidence of HA arthritis is not known, 30 to 50% of patients with osteoarthritis have HA microcrystals in their synovial fluid. Such crystals can frequently be identified in clinically stable osteoarthritic joints, but they are more likely to come to attention in persons experiencing acute or subacute worsening of joint pain and swelling. The synovial fluid WBC count in HA arthritis is usually low (<2000/μL) but may at times have as many as 50,000/μL. Most synovial fluid analyses reveal a predominance of mononuclear cells. Occasionally, neutrophils may dominate.

Diagnosis Radiographic findings in HA arthropathy are not diagnostic. Intra- and/or periarticular calcifications with or without erosive, destructive, or hypertrophic changes may be present.

Definitive diagnosis of HA arthropathy depends on identification of crystals from synovial fluid or tissue (Fig. 313-4). Individual crystals are very small, nonbirefringent, and can only be seen by electron microscopy. Clumps of crystals may appear as 1- to 20-μm shiny intra- or extracellular globules that stain purplish with Wright's stain and bright red with alizarin red S. Absolute identification depends on electron microscopy with energy-dispersive elemental analysis, x-ray diffraction, or infrared spectroscopy.

℞ TREATMENT

Treatment of HA arthritis is nonspecific. Acute attacks of bursitis or synovitis may be self-limiting, resolving in from days to several weeks. Aspiration of effusions and the use of either NSAIDs or oral colchicine for 2 weeks or intra- or periarticular injection of glucocorticoid salts appears to shorten the duration and intensity of symptoms. In patients with underlying severe destructive articular changes, response to medical therapy is usually less rewarding.

CaOx DEPOSITION DISEASE ■ Pathogenesis

Primary oxalosis is a rare hereditary metabolic disorder (Chap. 343). Enhanced production of oxalic acid may result from at least two different enzyme defects, leading to hyperoxalemia and deposition of calcium oxalate crystals in tissues. Nephrocalcinosis, renal failure, and death usually occur before age 20. Acute and/or chronic CaOx arthritis and periarthritis may complicate primary oxalosis during later years of illness.

Secondary oxalosis is more common than the primary disorder. It is one of the many metabolic abnormalities that complicate end-stage renal disease (ESRD). In ESRD, calcium oxalate deposits have long been recognized in visceral organs, blood vessels, bones, and even cartilage. However, it was not until 1982 that such deposits were demonstrated to be one of the causes of arthritis in chronic renal failure. Thus far, reported patients have been dependent on long-term hemodialysis or peritoneal dialysis (Chap. 262), and many had received

---

TABLE 313-3 *Conditions Associated with Hydroxyapatite Deposition Disease*

Aging
Osteoarthritis
Hemorrhagic shoulder effusions in the elderly (Milwaukee shoulder)
Destructive arthropathy
Tendinitis, bursitis
Tumoral calcinosis (sporadic cases)
Disease-associated
  Hyperparathyroidism
  Milk-alkali syndrome
  Renal failure/long-term dialysis
  Connective tissue diseases (e.g., progressive systemic sclerosis, CREST syndrome, idiopathic myositis, SLE)
  Heterotopic calcification following neurologic catastrophes (e.g., stroke, spinal cord injury)
Hereditary
  Bursitis, arthritis
  Tumoral calcinosis
  Fibrodysplasia ossificans progressiva

Note: CREST, calcinosis cutis, Raynaud's phenomenon, esophageal dysmotility, sclerodactyly, telangiectasia; SLE, systemic lupus erythematosus.

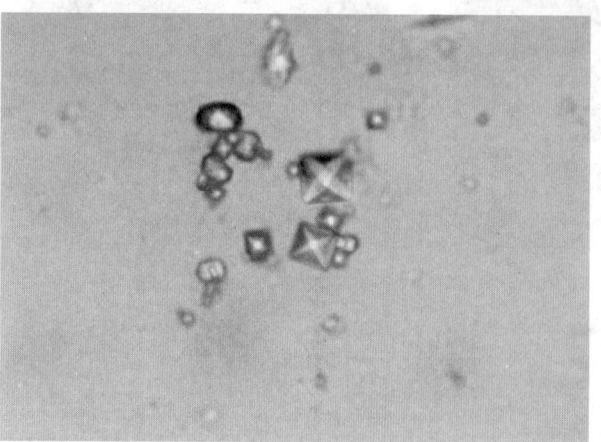

FIGURE 313-5 Bipyramidal and small polymorphic calcium oxalate crystals (ordinary light microscopy; 400×).

ascorbic acid supplements. Ascorbic acid is metabolized to oxalate, which is inadequately cleared in uremia and by dialysis. Such supplements are now usually avoided in dialysis programs because of the risk of enhancing hyperoxalosis and its sequelae.

Clinical Manifestations and Diagnosis   As was noted for the other calcium salts, CaOx aggregates can be found in bone, articular cartilage, synovium, and periarticular tissues. From these sites, crystals may be shed, causing acute synovitis. Persistent aggregates of CaOx may, like HA and CPPD, stimulate synovial proliferation and enzyme release, resulting in progressive articular destruction. Deposits have been documented in fingers, wrists, elbows, knees, ankles, and feet.

Each of the known microcrystalline arthropathies may be a complication of ESRD, and rare patients have more than one type of crystal present in a joint effusion. The advent of crystallographic techniques has made it clear that most arthritic problems in ESRD are not, as was once believed, due to MSU gout. Clinical features of acute CaOx arthritis may not be distinguishable from those due to sodium urate, CPPD, or HA. Radiographs may reveal chondrocalcinosis, a feature of either CPPD or CaOx deposition. CaOx-induced synovial effusions are usually noninflammatory, with <2000 leukocytes/μL. Neutrophils or mononuclear cells have predominated. CaOx crystals have a variable shape and variable birefringence to polarized light. The most easily recognized forms are bipyramidal and have strong positive birefringence (Fig. 313-5).

℞ TREATMENT

Treatment of CaOx arthropathy with NSAIDs, colchicine, intraarticular glucocorticoids, and/or an increased frequency of dialysis has produced only slight improvement. In primary oxalosis, liver transplantation has induced a significant reduction in crystal deposits (Chap. 343).

FURTHER READING

FAM AG: Difficult gout and new approaches for control of hyperuricemia in the allopurinol-allergic patient. Curr Rheumatol Rep 3:29, 2001

MALDONADO I et al: Familial calcium crystal diseases: What have we learned? Curr Opin Rheumatol 13:225, 2001

REGINATO AJ et al: Familial and clinical aspects of calcium pyrophosphate deposition disease. Curr Rheumatol Rep 1:112, 1999

SCHLESINGER N, SCHUMACHER HR JR: Gout: Can management be improved? Curr Opin Rheumatol 13:240, 2001

SCHUMACHER HR JR et al: Randomized double-blind trial of etoricoxib and indomethacin in treatment of acute gouty arthritis. BMJ 324:458, 2002

314 INFECTIOUS ARTHRITIS
Lawrence C. Madoff, Scott J. Thaler, James H. Maguire

INTRODUCTION AND APPROACH TO THE PATIENT   Although *Staphylococcus aureus*, *Neisseria gonorrhoeae*, and other bacteria are the most common causes of infectious arthritis, various mycobacteria, spirochetes, fungi, and viruses also infect joints. Since acute bacterial infection can rapidly destroy articular cartilage, all inflamed joints must be evaluated without delay to exclude noninfectious processes and to determine appropriate antimicrobial therapy and drainage procedures. For more detailed information on infectious arthritis due to specific organisms, the reader is referred to the chapters on those organisms.

Acute bacterial infection typically involves a single joint or a few joints. Subacute or chronic monarthritis or oligoarthritis suggests mycobacterial or fungal infection; episodic inflammation is seen in syphilis, Lyme disease, and the reactive arthritis that follows enteric infections and chlamydial urethritis (Table 314-1). Acute polyarticular inflammation occurs as an immunologic reaction during the course of endocarditis, rheumatic fever, disseminated neisserial infection, and acute hepatitis B. Bacteria and viruses occasionally infect multiple joints, the former most commonly in persons with rheumatoid arthritis.

Aspiration of synovial fluid—an essential element in the evaluation of potentially infected joints—can be performed without difficulty in most cases by the insertion of a large-bore needle into the site of maximal fluctuation or tenderness or by the route of easiest access. Ultrasonography or fluoroscopy may be used to guide aspiration of difficult-to-localize effusions of the hip and, occasionally, the shoulder and other joints. Normal synovial fluid contains <180 cells (predominantly mononuclear cells) per microliter. Synovial cell counts averaging 100,000/μL (range, 25,000 to 250,000/μL), with >90% neutro-

phils, are characteristic of acute bacterial infections. Crystal-induced, rheumatoid, and other noninfectious inflammatory arthritides are usually associated with <30,000 to 50,000 cells/μL; cell counts of 10,000 to 30,000/μL, with 50 to 70% neutrophils and the remainder lymphocytes, are common in mycobacterial and fungal infections. Definitive diagnosis of an infectious process relies on identification of the pathogen in stained smears of synovial fluid, isolation of the pathogen from cultures of synovial fluid and blood, or detection of microbial nucleic acids and proteins by polymerase chain reaction (PCR)–based assays and immunologic techniques.

ACUTE BACTERIAL ARTHRITIS ■ Pathogenesis   Bacteria enter the joint from the bloodstream; from a contiguous site of infection in bone or soft tissue; or by direct inoculation during surgery, injection, or trauma. In hematogenous infection, bacteria escape from synovial capillaries, which have no limiting basement membrane, and within hours provoke neutrophilic infiltration of the synovium. Neutrophils and bacteria enter the joint space; later, bacteria adhere to articular cartilage. Degradation of cartilage begins within 48 h as a result of increased intraarticular pressure, release of proteases and cytokines from chondrocytes and synovial macrophages, and invasion of the cartilage by bacteria and inflammatory cells. Histologic studies reveal bacteria lining the synovium and cartilage as well as abscesses extending into the synovium, cartilage, and—in severe cases—subchondral bone. Synovial proliferation results in the formation of a pannus over the cartilage, and thrombosis of inflamed synovial vessels develops. Bacterial factors that appear important in the pathogenesis of infective arthritis include various surface-associated adhesins in *S. aureus* that permit adherence to cartilage and endotoxins that promote chondrocyte-mediated breakdown of cartilage.

Microbiology   The hematogenous route of infection is the most common route in all age groups, and nearly every bacterial pathogen is capable of causing septic arthritis. In infants, group B streptococci, gram-negative enteric bacilli, and *S. aureus* are the usual pathogens. Since the advent of the *Haemophilus influenzae* vaccine, *S. aureus*, *Streptococcus pyogenes* (group A *Streptococcus*), and (in some centers) *Kingella kingae* have predominated among children <5 years of age. Among young adults and adolescents, *N. gonorrhoeae* is the most commonly implicated organism. *S. aureus* accounts for most nongonococcal isolates in adults of all ages; gram-negative bacilli, pneumococci, and β-hemolytic streptococci—particularly groups A and B, but also groups C, G, and F—are involved in up to one-third of cases in older adults, especially those with underlying comorbid illnesses.

Infections following surgical procedures or penetrating injuries are due most often to *S. aureus* and occasionally to other gram-positive bacteria or gram-negative bacilli. Infections with coagulase-negative staphylococci are unusual except after the implantation of prosthetic joints or arthroscopy. Anaerobic organisms, often in association with aerobic or facultative bacteria, are found after human bites and when decubitus ulcers or intraabdominal abscesses spread into adjacent joints. Polymicrobial infections complicate traumatic injuries with extensive contamination. Bites and scratches from cats and other animals may introduce *Pasteurella multocida* into joints.

Nongonococcal Bacterial Arthritis ■ *EPIDEMIOLOGY* Although hematogenous infections with virulent organisms such as *S. aureus*, *H. influenzae*, and pyogenic streptococci occur in healthy persons, there is an underlying host predisposition in many cases of septic arthritis. Patients with rheumatoid arthritis have the highest incidence of infective arthritis (most often secondary to *S. aureus*) because of chronically inflamed joints; glucocorticoid therapy; and frequent breakdown of rheumatoid nodules, vasculitic ulcers, and skin overlying deformed joints. Diabetes mellitus, glucocorticoid therapy, hemodialysis, and malignancy all carry an increased risk of infection with *S. aureus* and gram-negative bacilli. Tumor necrosis factor (TNF) inhibitors (etanercept and infliximab), increasingly used for the treatment of rheumatoid arthritis, predispose to mycobacterial infections and possibly to other pyogenic bacterial infections and could be associated with septic arthritis in this population. Pneumococcal infections complicate alcoholism, deficiencies of humoral immunity, and hemoglobinopathies. Pneumococci, *Salmonella*, and *H. influenzae* cause septic arthritis in persons infected with HIV. Persons with primary immunoglobulin deficiency are at risk for mycoplasmal arthritis, which results in permanent joint damage if treatment with tetracycline and intravenous (IV) immunoglobulin replacement is not administered promptly. Intravenous drug users acquire staphylococcal and streptococcal infections from their own flora and acquire pseudomonal and other gram-negative infections from drugs and injection paraphernalia.

CLINICAL MANIFESTATIONS Some 90% of patients present with involvement of a single joint—most commonly the knee, less frequently the hip, and still less often the shoulder, wrist, or elbow. Small joints of the hands and feet are more likely to be affected after direct inoculation or a bite. Among IV drug users, infections of the spine, sacroiliac joints, or sternoclavicular joints are more common than infections of the appendicular skeleton. Polyarticular infection is most common among patients with rheumatoid arthritis and may resemble a flare of the underlying disease.

The usual presentation consists of moderate to severe pain that is uniform around the joint, effusion, muscle spasm, and decreased range of motion. Fever in the range of 38.3° to 38.9°C (101° to 102°F) and sometimes higher is common but may be lacking, especially in persons with rheumatoid arthritis, renal or hepatic insufficiency, or conditions

TABLE 314-1 Differential Diagnosis of Arthritis Syndromes		
Acute Monarticular Arthritis	Chronic Monarticular Arthritis	Polyarticular Arthritis
Staphylococcus aureus	*Mycobacterium*	*Neisseria meningitidis*
Streptococcus pneumoniae	*tuberculosis*	*N. gonorrhoeae*
β-Hemolytic streptococci	Nontuberculous	Nongonococcal bacterial arthritis
Gram-negative bacilli	mycobacteria	Bacterial endocarditis
Neisseria gonorrhoeae	*Borrelia burgdorferi*	*Candida* species
Candida species	*Treponema pallidum*	Poncet's disease (tuberculous rheumatism)
Crystal-induced arthritis	*Candida* species	Hepatitis B virus
Fracture	*Sporothrix schenckii*	Parvovirus B19
Hemarthrosis	*Coccidioides immitis*	HIV
Foreign body	*Blastomyces dermatitidis*	Human T-lymphotropic virus type I
Osteoarthritis	*Aspergillus* species	Rubella virus
Ischemic necrosis	*Cryptococcus neoformans*	Arthropod-borne viruses
Monarticular rheumatoid	*Nocardia* species	Sickle cell disease flare
arthritis	*Brucella* species	Reactive arthritis
	Legg-Calvé-Perthes	Serum sickness
	disease	Acute rheumatic fever
	Osteoarthritis	Inflammatory bowel disease
		Systemic lupus erythematosus
		Rheumatoid arthritis/Still's disease
		Other vasculitides
		Sarcoidosis

requiring immunosuppressive therapy. The inflamed, swollen joint is usually evident on examination except in the case of a deeply situated joint, such as the hip, shoulder, or sacroiliac joint. Cellulitis, bursitis, and acute osteomyelitis, which may produce a similar clinical picture, should be distinguished from septic arthritis by their greater range of motion and less-than-circumferential swelling. A focus of extraarticular infection, such as a boil or pneumonia, should be sought. Peripheral-blood leukocytosis with a left shift and elevation of the erythrocyte sedimentation rate or C-reactive protein level are common.

Plain radiographs show evidence of soft tissue swelling, joint-space widening, and displacement of tissue planes by the distended capsule. Narrowing of the joint space and bony erosions indicate advanced infection and a poor prognosis. Ultrasound is useful for detecting effusions in the hip, and computed tomography or magnetic resonance imaging can demonstrate infections of the sacroiliac joint, the sternoclavicular joint, and the spine very well.

LABORATORY FINDINGS Specimens of peripheral blood and synovial fluid should be obtained before antibiotics are administered. Blood cultures are positive in up to 50% of *S. aureus* infections but are less frequently positive in infections due to other organisms. The synovial fluid is turbid, serosanguineous, or frankly purulent. Gram-stained smears confirm the presence of large numbers of neutrophils. Levels of total protein and lactate dehydrogenase in synovial fluid are elevated, and the glucose level is depressed; however, these findings are not specific for infection, and measurement of these levels is not necessary to make the diagnosis. The synovial fluid should be examined for crystals, because gout and pseudogout can resemble septic arthritis clinically, and infection and crystal-induced disease occasionally occur together. Organisms are seen on synovial fluid smears in nearly three-quarters of infections with *S. aureus* and streptococci and in 30 to 50% of infections due to gram-negative and other bacteria. Cultures of synovial fluid are positive in >90% of cases. Inoculation of synovial fluid into bottles containing liquid media for blood cultures increases the yield of culture, especially if the pathogen is a fastidious organism or the patient is taking an antibiotic. Although not yet widely available, PCR-based assays for bacterial DNA will also be useful for the diagnosis of partially treated or culture-negative bacterial arthritis.

℞ TREATMENT

Prompt administration of systemic antibiotics and drainage of the involved joint can prevent destruction of cartilage, postinfectious degenerative arthritis, joint instability, or deformity. Once samples of blood and synovial fluid have been obtained for culture, empirical antibiotics should be given that are directed against bacteria visualized on smears or against the pathogens that are likely, given the patient's age and risk factors. Initial therapy should consist of the IV administration of bactericidal agents; direct instillation of antibiotics into the joint is not necessary to achieve adequate levels in synovial fluid and tissue. An IV third-generation cephalosporin such as cefotaxime (1 g every 8 h) or ceftriaxone (1 to 2 g every 24 h) provides adequate empirical coverage for most community-acquired infections in adults when smears show no organisms. Either oxacillin or nafcillin (2 g every 4 h) is used if there are gram-positive cocci on the smear. If methicillin-resistant *S. aureus* is a possible pathogen (e.g., in hospitalized patients), IV vancomycin (1 g every 12 h) should be given. In addition, an aminoglycoside or third-generation cephalosporin should be given to IV drug users or other patients in whom *Pseudomonas aeruginosa* may be the responsible agent.

Definitive therapy is based on the identity and antibiotic susceptibility of the bacteria isolated in culture. Infections due to staphylococci are treated with oxacillin, nafcillin, or vancomycin for 4 weeks. Pneumococcal and streptococcal infections due to penicillin-susceptible organisms respond to 2 weeks of therapy with penicillin G (2 million units IV every 4 h); infections caused by *H. influenzae* and by strains of *S. pneumoniae* that are resistant to penicillin are treated with cefotaxime or ceftriaxone for 2 weeks. Most enteric gram-negative infections can be cured in 3 to 4 weeks by a second- or third-generation cephalosporin given intravenously or by a fluoroquinolone, such as levofloxacin (500 mg IV or orally every 24 h). *P. aeruginosa* infection should be treated for at least 2 weeks with a combination regimen of an aminoglycoside plus either an extended-spectrum penicillin, such as mezlocillin (3 g IV every 4 h), or an antipseudomonal cephalosporin, such as ceftazidime (1 g IV every 8 h). If tolerated, this regimen is continued for an additional 2 weeks; alternatively, a fluoroquinolone, such as ciprofloxacin (750 mg orally bid), is given by itself or with the penicillin or cephalosporin in place of the aminoglycoside.

Timely drainage of pus and necrotic debris from the infected joint is required for a favorable outcome. Needle aspiration of readily accessible joints such as the knee may be adequate if loculations or particulate matter in the joint does not prevent its thorough decompression. Arthroscopic drainage and lavage may be employed initially or within several days if repeated needle aspiration fails to relieve symptoms, decrease the volume of the effusion and the synovial white cell count, and clear bacteria from smears and cultures. In some cases, arthrotomy is necessary to remove loculations and debride infected synovium, cartilage, or bone. Septic arthritis of the hip is best managed with arthrotomy, particularly in young children, in whom infection threatens the viability of the femoral head. Septic joints do not require immobilization except for pain control before symptoms are alleviated by treatment. Weight bearing should be avoided until signs of inflammation have subsided, but frequent passive motion of the joint is indicated to maintain full mobility. While addition of glucocorticoids to antibiotic treatment improves the outcome of *S. aureus* arthritis in experimental animals, no clinical trials have yet evaluated this approach in humans.

Gonococcal Arthritis ■ *EPIDEMIOLOGY* Although its incidence has declined in recent years, gonococcal arthritis (Chap. 128) has accounted for up to 70% of episodes of infectious arthritis in persons <40 years of age in the United States. Arthritis due to *N. gonorrhoeae* is a consequence of bacteremia arising from gonococcal infection or, more frequently, from asymptomatic gonococcal mucosal colonization of the urethra, cervix, or pharynx. Women are at greatest risk during menses and during pregnancy and overall are two to three times more likely than men to develop disseminated gonococcal infection (DGI) and arthritis. Persons with complement deficiencies, especially of the terminal components, are prone to recurrent episodes of gonococcemia. Strains of gonococci that are most likely to cause DGI include those

that produce transparent colonies in culture, have the type IA outer-membrane protein, or are of the AUH-auxotroph type.

CLINICAL MANIFESTATIONS AND LABORATORY FINDINGS The most common manifestation of DGI is a syndrome of fever, chills, rash, and articular symptoms. Small numbers of papules that progress to hemorrhagic pustules develop on the trunk and the extensor surfaces of the distal extremities. Migratory arthritis and tenosynovitis of the knees, hands, wrists, feet, and ankles are prominent. The cutaneous lesions and articular findings are believed to be the consequence of an immune reaction to circulating gonococci and immune-complex deposition in tissues. Thus, cultures of synovial fluid are consistently negative, and blood cultures are positive in <45% of patients. Synovial fluid may be difficult to obtain from inflamed joints and usually contains only 10,000 to 20,000 leukocytes/μL.

True gonococcal septic arthritis is less common than the DGI syndrome and always follows DGI, which is unrecognized in one-third of patients. A single joint, such as the hip, knee, ankle, or wrist, is usually involved. Synovial fluid, which contains >50,000 leukocytes/μL, can be obtained with ease; the gonococcus is only occasionally evident in gram-stained smears, and cultures of synovial fluid are positive in <40% of cases. Blood cultures are almost always negative.

Because it is difficult to isolate gonococci from synovial fluid and blood, specimens for culture should be obtained from potentially infected mucosal sites. Cultures and gram-stained smears of skin lesions are occasionally positive. All specimens for culture should be plated onto Thayer-Martin agar directly or in special transport media at the bedside and transferred promptly to the microbiology laboratory in an atmosphere of 5% CO_2, as generated in a candle jar. PCR-based assays are extremely sensitive in detecting gonococcal DNA in synovial fluid. A dramatic alleviation of symptoms within 12 to 24 h after the initiation of appropriate antibiotic therapy supports a clinical diagnosis of the DGI syndrome if cultures are negative.

℞ TREATMENT

Initial treatment consists of ceftriaxone (1 g IV or intramuscularly every 24 h) to cover possible penicillin-resistant organisms. Once local and systemic signs are clearly resolving and if the sensitivity of the isolate permits, the 7-day course of therapy can be completed with an oral agent such as ciprofloxacin (500 mg twice daily). Ciprofloxacin (500 mg orally/400 mg IV twice daily) may also be used as initial therapy in areas where resistance has not become prevalent; if penicillin-susceptible organisms are isolated, amoxicillin (500 mg three times daily) may be used. Suppurative arthritis usually responds to needle aspiration of involved joints and 7 to 14 days of antibiotic treatment. Arthroscopic lavage or arthrotomy is rarely required. Patients with disseminated gonococcal infection should be treated for *Chlamydia trachomatis* infection unless this infection is ruled out by appropriate testing.

It is noteworthy that arthritis symptoms similar to those seen in DGI occur in meningococcemia. A dermatitis-arthritis syndrome, purulent monarthritis, and reactive polyarthritis have been described. All respond to treatment with IV penicillin.

SPIROCHETAL ARTHRITIS ■ **Lyme Disease** Lyme disease (Chap. 157) due to infection with the spirochete *Borrelia burgdorferi* causes arthritis in up to 70% of persons who are not treated. Intermittent arthralgias and myalgias—but not arthritis—occur within days or weeks of inoculation of the spirochete by the *Ixodes* tick. Later, there are three patterns of joint disease: (1) Fifty percent of untreated persons experience intermittent episodes of monarthritis or oligoarthritis involving the knee and/or other large joints. The symptoms wax and wane without treatment over months, and each year 10 to 20% of patients report loss of joint symptoms. (2) Twenty percent of untreated persons develop a pattern of waxing and waning arthralgias. (3) Ten percent of untreated patients develop chronic inflammatory synovitis resulting in erosive lesions and destruction of the joint. Serologic tests for IgG antibodies to *B. burgdorferi* are positive in >90% of persons with Lyme arthritis, and a PCR-based assay detects *Borrelia* DNA in 85%.

℞ TREATMENT

Lyme arthritis generally responds well to therapy. A regimen of oral doxycycline (100 mg twice daily for 30 days), oral amoxicillin (500 mg four times daily for 30 days), or parenteral ceftriaxone (2 g/d for 2 to 4 weeks) is recommended. Patients who do not respond to a total of 2 months of oral therapy or 1 month of parenteral therapy are unlikely to benefit from additional antibiotic therapy and are treated with anti-inflammatory agents or synovectomy. Failure of therapy is associated with host features such as the HLA-DR4 genotype, persistent reactivity to OspA (outer-surface protein A), and the presence of hLFA-1 (human leukocyte function–associated antigen 1), which cross-reacts with OspA.

Syphilitic Arthritis Articular manifestations occur in different stages of syphilis (Chap. 153). In early congenital syphilis, periarticular swelling and immobilization of the involved limbs (Parrot's pseudoparalysis) complicate osteochondritis of long bones. Clutton's joint, a late manifestation of congenital syphilis that typically develops between the ages of 8 and 15 years, is caused by chronic painless synovitis with effusions of large joints, particularly the knees and elbows. Secondary syphilis may be associated with arthralgias; with symmetric arthritis of the knees and ankles and occasionally of the shoulders and wrists; and with sacroiliitis. The arthritis follows a subacute to chronic course with a mixed mononuclear and neutrophilic synovial-fluid pleocytosis (typical cell counts, 5000 to 15,000/μL). Immunologic mechanisms may contribute to the arthritis, and symptoms usually improve rapidly with penicillin therapy. In tertiary syphilis, Charcot's joint is a result of sensory loss due to tabes dorsalis. Penicillin is not helpful in this setting.

MYCOBACTERIAL ARTHRITIS Tuberculous arthritis (Chap. 150) accounts for ~1% of all cases of tuberculosis and for 10% of extrapulmonary cases. The most common presentation is chronic granulomatous monarthritis. An unusual syndrome, Poncet's disease, is a reactive symmetric form of polyarthritis that affects persons with visceral or disseminated tuberculosis. No mycobacteria are found in the joints, and symptoms resolve with antituberculous therapy.

Unlike tuberculous osteomyelitis (Chap. 111), which typically involves the thoracic and lumbar spine (50% of cases), tuberculous arthritis primarily involves the large weight-bearing joints, in particular the hips, knees, and ankles, and only occasionally involves smaller non-weight-bearing joints. Progressive monarticular swelling and pain develop over months to years, and systemic symptoms are seen in only half of all cases. Tuberculous arthritis occurs as part of a disseminated primary infection or through late reactivation, often in persons with HIV infection or other immunocompromised hosts. Coexistent active pulmonary tuberculosis is unusual.

Aspiration of the involved joint yields fluid with an average cell count of 20,000/μL, with ~50% neutrophils. Acid-fast staining of the fluid yields positive results in fewer than one-third of cases, and cultures are positive in 80%. Culture of synovial tissue taken at biopsy is positive in ~90% of cases and shows granulomatous inflammation in most. DNA amplification methods such as PCR can shorten the time to diagnosis to 1 or 2 days. Radiographs reveal peripheral erosions at the points of synovial attachment, periarticular osteopenia, and eventually joint-space narrowing. Therapy for tuberculous arthritis is the same as that for tuberculous pulmonary disease, requiring the administration of multiple agents for 6 to 9 months. Therapy is more prolonged in immunosuppressed individuals, such as those infected with HIV.

Various atypical mycobacteria (Chap. 152) found in water and soil may cause chronic indolent arthritis. Such disease results from trauma and direct inoculation associated with farming, gardening, or aquatic activities. Smaller joints, such as the digits, wrists, and knees, are usually involved. Involvement of tendon sheaths and bursae is typical. The mycobacterial species involved include *Mycobacterium marinum*, *M. avium-intracellulare*, *M. terrae*, *M. kansasii*, *M. fortuitum*, and *M. chelonae*. In persons who have HIV infection or are receiving immunosuppressive therapy, hematogenous spread to the joints has been reported for *M. kansasii*, *M. avium-intracellulare*, and *M. haemophilum*. Diagnosis usually requires biopsy and culture, and therapy is based on antimicrobial susceptibility patterns.

FUNGAL ARTHRITIS Fungi are an unusual cause of chronic monarticular arthritis. Granulomatous articular infection with the endemic dimorphic fungi *Coccidioides immitis*, *Blastomyces dermatitidis*, and (less commonly) *Histoplasma capsulatum* results from hematogenous seeding or direct extension from bony lesions in persons with disseminated disease. Joint involvement is an unusual complication of sporotrichosis (infection with *Sporothrix schenckii*) among gardeners and other persons who work with soil or sphagnum moss. Articular sporotrichosis is six times more common among men than among women, and alcoholics and other debilitated hosts are at risk for polyarticular infection.

Candida infection involving a single joint—usually the knee, hip, or shoulder—results from surgical procedures, intraarticular injections, or (among critically ill patients with debilitating illnesses, such as diabetes mellitus or hepatic or renal insufficiency, and patients receiving immunosuppressive therapy) hematogenous spread. *Candida* infections in IV drug users typically involve the spine, sacroiliac joints, or other fibrocartilaginous joints. Unusual cases of arthritis due to *Aspergillus* species, *Cryptococcus neoformans*, *Pseudallescheria boydii*, and the dematiaceous fungi have also resulted from direct inoculation or disseminated hematogenous infection in immunocompromised persons.

The synovial fluid in fungal arthritis usually contains 10,000 to 40,000 cells/μL, with ~70% neutrophils. Stained specimens and cultures of synovial tissue often confirm the diagnosis of fungal arthritis when studies of synovial fluid give negative results. Treatment consists of drainage and lavage of the joint and systemic administration of an antifungal agent directed at a specific pathogen. The doses and duration of therapy are the same as for disseminated disease (see Part VI, Section 16). Intraarticular instillation of amphotericin B has been used in addition to IV therapy.

VIRAL ARTHRITIS Viruses produce arthritis by infecting synovial tissue during systemic infection or by provoking an immunologic reaction that involves joints. As many as 50% of women report persistent arthralgias and 10% report frank arthritis within 3 days of the rash that follows natural infection with rubella virus and within 2 to 6 weeks after receipt of live-virus vaccine. Episodes of symmetric inflammation of fingers, wrists, and knees uncommonly recur for >1 year, but a syndrome of chronic fatigue, low-grade fever, headaches, and myalgias can persist for months or years. Intravenous immunoglobulin has been helpful in selected cases. Self-limited monarticular or migratory polyarthritis may develop within 2 weeks of the parotitis of mumps; this sequela is more common among men than among women. Approximately 10% of children and 60% of women develop arthritis after infection with parvovirus B19. In adults, arthropathy sometimes occurs without fever or rash. Pain and stiffness, with less prominent swelling (primarily of the hands but also of the knees, wrists, and ankles), usually resolve within weeks, although a small proportion of patients develop chronic arthropathy.

About 2 weeks before the onset of jaundice, up to 10% of persons with acute hepatitis B develop an immune complex–mediated, serum sickness–like reaction with maculopapular rash, urticaria, fever, and arthralgias. Less common developments include symmetric arthritis involving the hands, wrists, elbows, or ankles and morning stiffness that resembles a flare of rheumatoid arthritis. Symptoms resolve at the time jaundice develops. Many persons with chronic hepatitis C infection report persistent arthralgia or arthritis, both in the presence and in the absence of cryoglobulinemia. Painful arthritis involving larger joints often accompanies the fever and rash of several arthropod-borne viral infections, including those caused by chikungunya, O'nyong-nyong, Ross River, Mayaro, and Barmah Forest viruses. Symmetric arthritis involving the hands and wrists may occur during the convalescent phase of infection with lymphocytic choriomeningitis virus. Patients infected with an enterovirus frequently report arthralgias, and echovirus has been isolated from patients with acute polyarthritis.

Several arthritis syndromes are associated with HIV infection. Reiter's syndrome with painful lower-extremity oligoarthritis often follows an episode of urethritis in HIV-infected persons. HIV-associated Reiter's syndrome appears to be extremely common among persons with the HLA-B27 haplotype, but sacroiliac joint disease is unusual and is seen mostly in the absence of HLA-B27. Up to one-third of HIV-infected persons with psoriasis develop psoriatic arthritis. Painless monarthropathy and persistent symmetric polyarthropathy occasionally complicate HIV infection. Chronic persistent oligoarthritis of the shoulders, wrists, hands, and knees occurs in women infected with human T-cell lymphotropic virus type I. Synovial thickening, destruction of articular cartilage, and leukemic-appearing atypical lymphocytes in synovial fluid are characteristic, but progression to T cell leukemia is unusual.

PARASITIC ARTHRITIS Arthritis due to parasitic infection is rare. The guinea worm *Dracunculus medinensis* may cause destructive joint lesions in the lower extremities as migrating gravid female worms invade joints or cause ulcers in adjacent soft tissues that become secondarily infected. Hydatid cysts infect bones in 1 to 2% of cases of infection with *Echinococcus granulosus*. The expanding destructive cystic lesions may spread to and destroy adjacent joints, particularly the hip and pelvis. In rare cases, chronic synovitis has been associated with the presence of schistosomal eggs in synovial biopsies. Monarticular arthritis in children with lymphatic filariasis appears to respond to therapy with diethylcarbamazine, even in the absence of microfilariae in synovial fluid. Reactive arthritis has been attributed to hookworm, *Strongyloides*, *Cryptosporidium*, and *Giardia* infection in case reports, but confirmation is required.

POSTINFECTIOUS OR REACTIVE ARTHRITIS Reiter's syndrome, a reactive polyarthritis, develops several weeks after ~1% of cases of nongonococcal urethritis and 2% of enteric infections, particularly those due to *Yersinia enterocolitica*, *Shigella flexneri*, *Campylobacter jejuni*, and *Salmonella* species. Only a minority of these patients have the other findings of classic Reiter's syndrome, including urethritis, conjunctivitis, uveitis, oral ulcers, and rash. Studies have identified microbial DNA or antigen in synovial fluid or blood, but the pathogenesis of this condition is poorly understood.

Reiter's syndrome is most common among young men (except after *Yersinia* infection) and has been linked to the HLA-B27 locus as a potential genetic predisposing factor. Patients report painful, asymmetric oligoarthritis affecting mainly the knees, ankles, and feet. Low-back pain is common, and radiographic evidence of sacroiliitis is found in patients with long-standing disease. Most patients recover within 6 months, but prolonged recurrent disease is more common in cases following chlamydial urethritis. Anti-inflammatory agents help to relieve symptoms, but the role of prolonged antibiotic therapy in eliminating microbial antigen from the synovium is controversial.

Migratory polyarthritis and fever constitute the usual presentation of acute rheumatic fever in adults (Chap. 302). This presentation is distinct from that of poststreptococcal reactive arthritis, which also follows infections with group A *Streptococcus* but is not migratory, lasts beyond the typical 3-week maximum of acute rheumatic fever, and responds poorly to aspirin.

INFECTIONS IN PROSTHETIC JOINTS Infection complicates 1 to 4% of total joint replacements. The majority of infections are acquired intraoperatively or immediately postoperatively as a result of wound breakdown

or infection; less commonly, these joint infections develop later after joint replacement and are the result of hematogenous spread or direct inoculation. The presentation may be acute, with fever, pain, and local signs of inflammation, especially in infections due to *S. aureus*, pyogenic streptococci, and enteric bacilli. Alternatively, infection may persist for months or years without causing constitutional symptoms when less virulent organisms, such as coagulase-negative staphylococci or diphtheroids, are involved. Such indolent infections are usually acquired during joint implantation and are discovered during evaluation of chronic unexplained pain or after a radiograph shows loosening of the prosthesis; the erythrocyte sedimentation rate and C-reactive protein level are usually elevated in such cases.

The diagnosis is best made by needle aspiration of the joint; accidental introduction of organisms during aspiration must be meticulously avoided. Synovial fluid pleocytosis with a predominance of polymorphonuclear leukocytes is highly suggestive of infection, since other inflammatory processes uncommonly affect prosthetic joints. Culture and Gram's stain usually yield the responsible pathogen. Use of special media for unusual pathogens such as fungi, atypical mycobacteria, and *Mycoplasma* may be necessary if routine and anaerobic cultures are negative.

℞ TREATMENT

Treatment includes surgery and high doses of parenteral antibiotics, which are given for 4 to 6 weeks because bone is usually involved. In most cases, the prosthesis must be replaced to cure the infection. Implantation of a new prosthesis is best delayed for several weeks or months because relapses of infection occur most commonly within this time frame. In some cases, reimplantation is not possible, and the patient must manage without a joint, with a fused joint, or even with amputation. Cure of infection without removal of the prosthesis is occasionally possible in cases that are due to streptococci or pneumococci and that lack radiologic evidence of loosening of the prosthesis. In these cases, antibiotic therapy must be initiated within several days of the onset of infection, and the joint should be drained vigorously either by open arthrotomy or arthroscopically. In selected patients who prefer to avoid the high morbidity associated with joint removal and reimplantation, suppression of the infection with antibiotics may be a reasonable goal. A high cure rate with retention of the prosthesis has been reported when the combination of oral rifampin and ciprofloxacin is given for 3 to 6 months to persons with staphylococcal prosthetic joint infection of short duration. This approach, which is based on the ability of rifampin to kill organisms adherent to foreign material and in the stationary growth phase, requires confirmation in prospective trials.

Prevention To avoid the disastrous consequences of infection, candidates for joint replacement should be selected with care. Rates of infection are particularly high among patients with rheumatoid arthritis, persons who have undergone previous surgery on the joint, and persons with medical conditions requiring immunosuppressive therapy. Perioperative antibiotic prophylaxis, usually with cefazolin, and measures to decrease intraoperative contamination, such as laminar flow, have lowered the rates of perioperative infection to <1% in many centers. After implantation, measures should be taken to prevent or rapidly treat extraarticular infections that might give rise to hematogenous spread to the prosthesis. The effectiveness of prophylactic antibiotics for the prevention of hematogenous infection following dental procedures has not been demonstrated; in fact, viridans streptococci and other components of the oral flora are extremely unusual causes of prosthetic joint infection. Accordingly, the American Dental Association and the American Academy of Orthopaedic Surgeons do not recommend antibiotic prophylaxis for most dental patients with total joint replacements. They do, however, recommend prophylaxis for patients who may be at high risk of hematogenous infection, including those with inflammatory arthropathies, immunosuppression, type 1 diabetes mellitus, joint replacement within 2 years, previous prosthetic joint infection, malnourishment, or hemophilia. The recommended regimen is amoxicillin (2 g orally) 1 h before dental procedures associated with a high incidence of bacteremia. Clindamycin (600 mg orally) is suggested for patients allergic to penicillin.

FURTHER READING

BARDIN T: Gonococcal arthritis. Best Pract Res Clin Rheumatol 17:201, 2003

DONATTO KC: Orthopedic management of septic arthritis. Rheum Dis Clin North Am 24:275, 1998

GOLDENBERG DL: Septic arthritis. Lancet 351:197, 1998

HARRINGTON JT: Mycobacterial and fungal arthritis. Curr Opin Rheumatol 10:335, 1998

MEDINA RODRIGUEZ F: Rheumatic manifestations of human immunodeficiency virus infection. Rheum Dis Clin North Am 29:145, 2003

MEEHAN AM et al: Outcome of penicillin-susceptible streptococcal prosthetic joint infection treated with debridement and retention of the prosthesis. Clin Infect Dis 36:845, 2003

STENGEL D et al: Systematic review and meta-analysis of antibiotic therapy for bone and joint infections. Lancet Infect Dis 1:175, 2001

YTTERBERG SR: Viral arthritis. Curr Opin Rheumatol 11:275, 1999

315 FIBROMYALGIA, ARTHRITIS ASSOCIATED WITH SYSTEMIC DISEASE, AND OTHER ARTHRITIDES
Bruce C. Gilliland

FIBROMYALGIA

Fibromyalgia is a commonly encountered disorder characterized by chronic widespread musculoskeletal pain, stiffness, paresthesia, disturbed sleep, and easy fatigability along with multiple painful tender points, which are widely and symmetrically distributed. Fibromyalgia affects predominantly women in a ratio of 9 to 1 compared to men. This disorder is found in most countries, in most ethnic groups, and in all types of climates. The prevalence of fibromyalgia in the general population of a community in the United States using the 1990 American College of Rheumatology (ACR) classification criteria (see below) was reported to be 3.4% in women and 0.5% in men. Contrary to some previous reports, fibromyalgia was not found to be present mainly in young women but, rather, to be most prevalent in women ≥50 years. The prevalence increased with age, being 7.4% in women between the ages of 70 and 79. Although not common, fibromyalgia also occurs in children. The reported prevalence of fibromyalgia in some rheumatology clinics has been as high as 20%. Most patients present with fibromyalgia between the ages of 30 to 50 years.

Pathogenesis Several causative mechanisms for fibromyalgia have been postulated to explain abnormal pain perception. Several abnormalities of the central nervous system have been suggested. Disturbed sleep has been implicated as a factor in the pathogenesis. Nonrestorative sleep or awakening unrefreshed has been observed in most patients with fibromyalgia. Sleep electroencephalographic studies in patients with fibromyalgia have shown disruption of normal stage 4 sleep [non–rapid eye movement (NREM) sleep] by many repeated α-wave intrusions. The idea that stage 4 sleep deprivation has a role in causing this disorder was supported by the observation that symptoms of fibromyalgia developed in normal subjects whose stage 4 sleep was disrupted artificially by induced α-wave intrusions. This sleep disturbance, however, has been demonstrated in healthy individuals; in emotionally distressed individuals; and in patients with sleep apnea, fever, osteoarthritis, or rheumatoid arthritis. Low levels of serotonin metabolites have been reported in the cerebrospinal fluid (CSF) of patients with fibromyalgia, suggesting that a deficiency of serotonin, a neurotransmitter that regulates pain and NREM sleep, might also be involved in the pathogenesis of fibromyalgia. Drugs that affect serotonin metabolism have not had a dramatic effect on fibromyalgia, however. Fibromyalgia patients as a group have been reported by some investigators to have reduced levels of growth hormone, which is important for muscle repair and strength. Growth hormone is secreted normally during stage 4 sleep, which is disturbed in patients with fibromyalgia. The reduction of growth hormone may explain the extended periods of muscle pain following exertion in these patients. The level of the neurotransmitter substance P has been reported to be increased in the CSF of fibromyalgia patients and may play a role in spreading muscle pain. Patients with fibromyalgia have a decreased cortisol response to stress. Low urinary free cortisol and a diminished cortisol response to corticotropin-releasing hormone suggest an abnormal hypothalamic-pituitary-adrenal axis. Autonomic dysfunction has also been suggested to play a role in the pathogenesis of fibromyalgia. Some patients experience orthostatic hypotension on tilt table testing and may have increased resting supine heart rates. Disturbances of the autonomic and peripheral nervous system may also account for the dry eyes and mouth and the cold sensitivity and Raynaud's-like symptoms seen in patients with fibromyalgia. Single photon emission computed tomography (SPECT) imaging has demonstrated reduced blood flow to the thalamus, caudate nucleus, and pontine tectum, which are areas in the brain involved in the signaling, integration, and modulation of pain. Patients with fibromyalgia have been shown to perceive stimuli such as heat or pressue as painful with less degree of stimulation than normal individuals. The actual threshold for detecting stimuli appears to be similar in both patients and normal subjects.

Many patients with fibromyalgia have psychological abnormalities; there has been disagreement as to whether some of these abnormalities represent reactions to the chronic pain or whether the symptoms of fibromyalgia are a reflection of psychiatric disturbance. Approximately 30% of patients fit a psychiatric diagnosis, the most common being depression, anxiety, somatization, and hypochondriases. Studies have also shown a high prevalence of sexual and physical abuse and eating disorders. However, fibromyalgia also occurs in patients without significant psychiatric problems.

Since patients experience pain from muscle and musculotendinous sites, many studies have been done to examine muscle, both structurally and physiologically. Inflammation or diagnostic muscle abnormalities have not been found. Evidence indicates deconditioning of muscles, and patients experience a greater degree of postexertional pain than do unaffected persons. A better understanding of fibromyalgia awaits further studies.

Clinical Manifestations Symptoms are generalized musculoskeletal aching and stiffness and fatigue. Patients may complain of low back pain, which may radiate into the buttocks and legs. Others complain of pain and tightness in the neck and across the upper posterior shoulders. Patients complain of muscle pain after even mild exertion and some degree of pain is always present. The pain has been described as a burning or gnawing pain or as soreness, stiffness, or aching. Pain may begin in one region, such as the shoulders, neck, or lower back (see "Myofascial Pain Syndrome," below) before it eventually becomes widespread. Patients may complain of joint pain and perceive that their joints are swollen; however, joint examination yields normal findings. Stiffness is usually present on arising in the morning; usually it improves during the day, but in some patients it lasts all day. Patients may complain of numbness of their hands and feet. They may also feel colder overall than others in the home, and some may experience Raynaud's-like phenomena or actual Raynaud's phenomenon. Patients complain of feeling fatigued and exhausted and wake up tired. They also awaken frequently at night and have trouble falling back to sleep.

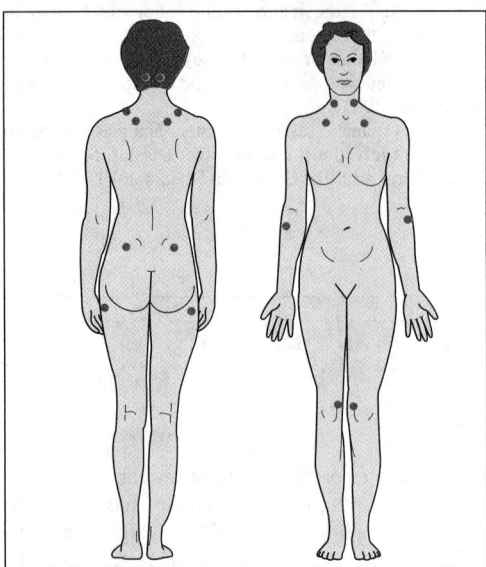

FIGURE 315-1 Tender points in fibromyalgia. Suboccipital muscle insertion at base of skull; anterior aspect of intertransverse process spaces at C5–7; midpoint of upper border of trapezius muscle; above scapular spine near medial border of scapula; second costochondral junction; lateral epicondyle; upper outer quadrant of buttocks; posterior aspect of trochanteric prominence; medial fat pad of knee (all bilateral). *(From the brochure "Fibromyalgia," Arthritis Information, Advise and Guidance, Disease Series. Used by permission of the Arthritis Foundation.)*

Patients may experience cognitive impairment with difficulty thinking and loss of short-term memory. Headaches, including migraine type, are also common symptons. Others experience episodes of light-headedness, dizziness, anxiety, or depression. Symptoms are made worse by stress or anxiety, cold, damp weather, and overexertion. Patients often feel better during warmer weather and vacations.

The characteristic feature on physical examination is the demonstration of specific sites or points, which are more tender or painful than the same sites in normal individuals. The ACR Criteria for Fibromyalgia defines 18 tender points (Fig. 315-1). These points of tenderness are remarkably constant in location. A moderate and consistent degree of pressure should be used in digital palpation of these tender points. As a guideline to reduce variability in the interpretation of point tenderness, the amount of force applied should be 4 kg (~9 lb), which is the degree of force required to just blanch the examiner's thumbnail. This amount of pressure does not produce significant tenderness or pain in normal subjects. Some workers recommend that the tender site be palpated using a rolling motion, which may be more effective in eliciting the tenderness. The tender sites can also be examined using a dolorimeter, which is a spring-loaded pressure gauge; however, digital palpation appears to be as effective and accurate. Some investigators have quantitated the degree of tenderness or pain, but the number of tender point sites is more diagnostic. Some patients are tender all over although still more tender or painful at the specific tender point sites.

Skinfold tenderness may be present, particularly over the upper scapular region. Subcutaneous nodules may be felt at sites of tenderness. Nodules in similar locations are present in normal persons but are not tender.

Fibromyalgia may be triggered by emotional stress, infections and other medical illness, surgery, hypothyroidism, and trauma. It has appeared in some patients with hepatitis C infection, HIV infection, parvovirus B19 infection, or Lyme disease. In the latter situation, fibromyalgia may persist despite adequate antibiotic treatment for Lyme disease, and especially anxious patients may believe that they still have Lyme disease. Disorders commonly associated with fibromyalgia include irritable bowel syndrome, irritable bladder, headaches (including migraine headaches), dysmenorrhea, premenstrual syn-

drome, restless leg syndrome, temporomandibular joint pain, non-cardiac chest pain, Raynaud's phenomenon, and sicca syndrome.

The course of fibromyalgia is variable. Symptoms wax and wane in some patients, while in others pain and fatigue are persistent regardless of therapy. Studies from tertiary medical centers indicate a poor prognosis for most patients. The prognosis may be better in community-treated patients. In a community-based study reported after 2 years of treatment, 24% of patients were in remission, and 47% no longer fulfilled the ACR criteria for fibromyalgia.

Diagnosis Fibromyalgia is diagnosed by a history of widespread musculoskeletal pain present for at least 3 months and the demonstration of significant tenderness or pain in at least 11 of the 18 tender point sites on digital palpation (Fig. 315-1). The ACR criteria are useful for standardizing the diagnosis; however, not all patients with fibromyalgia meet these criteria (Table 315-1). Some patients have fewer tender sites and more regional pain and may be considered to have fibromyalgia.

The musculoskeletal and neurologic examinations are normal in fibromyalgia patients, and there are no laboratory abnormalities. Fibromyalgia may occur in patients with rheumatoid arthritis, systemic lupus erythematosus (SLE), other connective tissue diseases, or other medical illness. A distinction is no longer made between primary and secondary fibromyalgia (concomitant with other disease), as the signs and symptoms are similar. Fibromyalgia and chronic fatigue syndrome have many similarities (Chap. 370). Both are associated with fatigue, abnormal sleep, musculoskeletal pain, impaired memory and concentration, and psychiatric conditions such as less severe forms of depression and anxiety. Patients with chronic fatigue syndrome, however, are more likely to have symptoms suggesting a viral illness. These include mild fever, sore throat, and pain in the axillary and anterior and posterior cervical lymph nodes. The onset of chronic fatigue syndrome is usually sudden; patients are usually able to date the onset. While many patients with chronic fatigue syndrome have tender or painful points, the diagnosis does not require their presence. Patients with fibromyalgia may be misdiagnosed with SLE or Sjögren's syndrome as these disorders have in common symptoms of musculoskeletal pain, dry eyes, cold hands, and fatigue. The antinuclear antibody (ANA) test may also be positive. The frequency of a positive ANA

TABLE 315-1 *The American College of Rheumatology 1990 Criteria for the Classification of Fibromyalgia[a]*

1. History of widespread pain. Pain is considered widespread when all of the following are present:
   a. Pain in the left side of the body
   b. Pain in the right side of the body
   c. Pain above the waist
   d. Pain below the waist
   e. Axial skeletal pain (cervical spine or anterior chest or thoracic spine or low back)
2. Pain on digital palpation in at least 11 of the following 18 tender point sites (see Fig. 315-1):
   a. Occiput: bilateral, at the suboccipital muscle insertion
   b. Low cervical: bilateral, at the anterior aspect of the intertransverse spaces at C5–7
   c. Trapezius: bilateral, at the midpoint of the upper border
   d. Supraspinatus: bilateral, at the origin, above the scapular spine near the medial border
   e. Second rib: bilateral, at the second costochondral junction, just lateral to the junction on the upper surface
   f. Lateral epicondyle: bilateral, 2 cm distal to the epicondyle
   g. Gluteal: bilateral, in the upper outer quadrant of the buttock
   h. Greater trochanter: bilateral, posterior to the trochanteric prominence
   i. Knee: bilateral, at the medial fat pad proximal to the joint line

Digital palpation should be performed with a moderate degree of pressure. For a tender point to be considered positive, the subject must state that the palpation was painful. "Tender" is not to be considered painful.

[a] For purposes of classification, patients will be said to have fibromyalgia if both criteria are satisfied. Widespread pain must have been present for at least 3 months. The presence of a second clinical disorder does not exclude the diagnosis of fibromyalgia.
Source: Modified from F Wolfe et al: Arthritis Rheum 33:171, 1990.

test in fibromyalgia patients, however, is the same as sex- and aged-matched normal controls. The predictive value of a positive ANA test in patients without characteristic symptoms and objective features of a connective tissue disease is quite low. Discretion is advised before ordering an ANA test. Patients with fibromyalgia may complain of muscle weakness, but on muscle strength testing, they have "give-away" weakness secondary to pain. Proximal muscle weakness and elevated muscle enzymes distinguish patients with polymyositis. Polymyalgia rheumatica is distinguished from fibromyalgia in an elderly patient by the presence of more proximal muscle stiffness and pain and an elevated erythrocyte sedimentation rate. Patients should be evaluated for hypothyroidism, which may have symptoms similar to fibromyalgia or may accompany fibromyalgia. Disturbed sleep, musculoskeletal pain, and fatigue occur in patients with sleep apnea and restless leg syndrome. A distinguishing feature of sleep apnea is the presence of significant daytime somnolence. These patients should be referred to a sleep laboratory for evaluation and treatment. Myofascial pain syndrome, which involves an area such as the shoulder or neck, may represent a localized form of fibromyalgia (see "Myofascial Pain Syndrome" below). Some patients with this syndrome progress to fibromyalgia.

The diagnosis of fibromyalgia has taken on a more complex significance in regard to labor and industry issues. This has become a significant issue since it has been reported that 10 to 25% of patients are not able to work in any capacity, while others require modification of their work. Disability evaluation in fibromyalgia is controversial. The diagnosis of fibromyalgia is not accepted by all. It is hard to evaluate patients' perceptions of their inability to function. The determination of tender points can also be subjective, on the part of both the physician and the patient, particularly when issues of compensation are pending. Patients also encounter difficulty in having their illness recognized as a disability. Physicians have been placed in the inappropriate role of assessing the patient's disability. Physicians are not in a position to quantitate disability at the workplace; that is better done by a work evaluation specialist. Better instruments are clearly needed for measuring disability, particularly in patients with fibromyalgia.

℞ TREATMENT

Patients should be informed that they have a condition that is not crippling, deforming, or degenerative, and that treatment is available. The initial step in treatment is to improve the quality of sleep. The use of tricyclics such as amitriptyline (10 to 50 mg), nortriptyline (10 to 75 mg), and doxepin (10 to 25 mg) or a pharmacologically similar drug, cyclobenzaprine (10 to 40 mg), 1 to 2 h before bedtime will give the patient restorative sleep (stage 4 sleep), resulting in clinical improvement. Patients should be started on a low dose, which is increased gradually as needed. Side effects of these tricyclics and cyclobenzoprine limit their use; these include constipation, dry mouth, weight gain, drowsiness, and difficulty thinking. Trazodone or zolpidem also improves sleep quality. In patients with restless leg syndrome, clonazepam may be effective. Depression and anxiety should next be treated with appropriate drugs and, when indicated, with psychiatric counseling. Fluoxetine, sertraline, paroxetine, citalopram, or other newer selective serotonin reuptake inhibitors can be used as antidepressants. Other useful antidepressants are trazodone and venlafaxine. Alprazolam and lorazepam are effective for anxiety. Patients may also benefit by regular aerobic exercises, which are started after patients begin to have improved sleep and less pain and fatigue. Exercise should be of a low-impact type and begun at a low level. Eventually, the patient should be exercising 20 to 30 min 3 to 4 days a week. Regular stretching exercises are also very important. Salicylates or other nonsteroidal anti-inflammatory drugs (NSAIDs) only partially improve symptoms. Glucocorticoids have been of little benefit and should not be used in these patients. Opiate analgesics should be avoided. For pain, acetaminophen or tramadol may be useful. Also gabapentin (300 to 1200 mg/d in divided doses) may reduce pain. Local measures such as heat, massage, injection of tender sites with steroids or lidocaine, and acupuncture provide only temporary relief of symptoms. Other therapies that may help to varying degrees including biofeedback, behavioral modification, hypnotherapy, and stress management and relaxation response training. Life stresses should be identified and discussed with the patient, and the patient should be provided with help on how to cope with these stresses. Patients may benefit from a multidisciplinary team approach involving a mental health professional, a physical therapist, and a physical medicine and rehabilitation specialist. Group therapy may be beneficial. Patients should be well educated about their disorder and taught the importance of self help. There are patient support groups in many communities. While treatment of fibromyalgia is effective in some patients, others continue to have chronic disease, which is relieved only partially if at all.

ARTHRITIS ASSOCIATED WITH SYSTEMIC DISEASE

ARTHROPATHY OF ACROMEGALY Acromegaly is the result of excessive production of growth hormone by an adenoma in the anterior pituitary gland (Chap. 318). Middle-aged persons are most often affected. The excessive secretion of growth hormone along with insulin-like growth factor I stimulates proliferation of cartilage, periarticular connective tissue, and bone, resulting in several musculoskeletal abnormalities, including osteoarthritis, back pain, muscle weakness, and carpal tunnel syndrome.

An arthropathy resembling osteoarthritis is a common feature, affecting most often the knees, shoulders, hips, and hands. Single or multiple joints may be affected. The overgrowth of cartilage initially produces widening of the joint space. The newly synthesized cartilage is not developed in an organized manner, making it susceptible to fissuring, ulceration, and destruction. Ligamental laxity of the joint resulting from the growth of connective tissue also contributes to the development of osteoarthritis. With breakdown and loss of cartilage, the joint space narrows, and subchondral sclerosis and osteophytes appear on radiographs. Joint examination reveals marked crepitus and hypermobility. Joint fluid is noninflammatory. Calcium pyrophosphate dihydrate crystals are found in the cartilage in some cases of acromegaly arthropathy and, when shed into the joint, can produce attacks of pseudogout. Chondrocalcinosis may also be observed radiographically. Approximately half of the patients with acromegaly experience back pain, which is predominantly lumbosacral. Hypermobility of the spine may be a contributing factor in back pain. Radiograph of the spine shows normal or increased intervertebral disk spaces, hypertrophic anterior osteophytes, and ligamental calcification. These changes are similar to those observed in patients with diffuse idiopathic skeletal hyperostosis. Dorsal kyphosis in conjunction with elongation of the ribs contributes to the development of the barrel chest seen in acromegalic patients. The hands and feet become enlarged owing to soft tissue proliferation. The fingers are thickened and have spadelike distal tufts. One-third of patients have a thickened heel pad. Approximately 25% of patients have Raynaud's phenomenon.

Carpal tunnel syndrome occurs in about half of patients. The median nerve is compressed by the excessive growth of connective tissue in the carpal tunnel. The median nerve also becomes enlarged. Patients with acromegaly also develop proximal muscle weakness, which is thought to be caused by the effect of growth hormone on muscle. Results of muscle enzyme assays and electromyography are normal. Muscle biopsy specimens show muscle fibers of varying size and no inflammatory changes.

ARTHROPATHY OF HEMOCHROMATOSIS Hemochromatosis is a disorder of iron storage. Excessive amounts of iron are absorbed from the intestine, leading to iron deposition in parenchymal cells, which results in tissue damage and impairment of organ function (Chap. 336). Symptoms of hemochromatosis usually begin between the ages of 40 and 60 but can occur earlier. Arthritis, which occurs in 20 to 40% of patients, usually begins after the age of 50 and may be the first clinical feature of hemochromatosis. The arthropathy is an osteoarthritis-like disorder affecting the small joints of the hands, followed later by larger joints such as knees, ankles, shoulders, and hips. The second and third metacarpophalangeal joints of both hands are often the first joints affected; they can provide an important clue to the possibility of hemochromatosis. Patients experience stiffness and pain. Morning stiffness usually lasts less than half an hour. The affected joints are enlarged and mildly tender. Synovial tissue is not appreciatively increased. Radiographs show irregular narrowing of the joint space, subchondral sclerosis, and subchondral cysts. There is juxtaarticular proliferation of bone, with frequent hooklike osteophytes. The synovial fluid is noninflammatory. The synovium shows mild to moderate proliferation of lining cells, fibrosis, and a low number of inflammatory cells, which are mononuclear. In approximately half of patients, there is evidence of calcium pyrophosphate deposition disease (CPDD), and patients may experience episodes of pseudogout. Iron can be demonstrated in the lining cells of the synovium and also in chondrocytes.

Iron may damage the articular cartilage in several ways. Iron catalyzes superoxide-dependent lipid peroxidation, which may play a role in joint damage. In animal models, ferric iron has been shown to interfere with collagen formation. Iron has also been shown to increase the release of lysosomal enzymes from cells in the synovial membrane. Iron may also play a role in the development of chondrocalcinosis. Iron inhibits synovial tissue pyrophosphatase in vitro and, therefore, may inhibit pyrophosphatase in vivo, resulting in chondrocalcinosis. Iron in synovial cells may also inhibit the clearance of calcium pyrophosphate from the joint.

℞ TREATMENT

The treatment of hemochromatosis is repeated phlebotomy. Unfortunately, this treatment has little effect on the arthritis, which, along with chondrocalcinosis, usually continues to progress. Treatment of the arthritis consists of administration of acetaminophen and NSAIDs. Acute pseudogout attacks are treated with higher doses of an NSAID or a short cause of glucocorticoids. Placement of a hip or knee prosthesis has been successful in advanced disease.

HEMOPHILIC ARTHROPATHY Hemophilia is a sex-linked recessive genetic disorder characterized by the absence or deficiency of factor VIII (hemophilia A, or classic hemophilia) or factor IX (hemophilia B, or Christmas disease) (Chap. 102). Hemophilia A is by far the more common type, constituting 85% of cases. Spontaneous hemarthrosis is a common problem with both types of hemophilia and can lead to a chronic deforming arthritis. The frequency and severity of hemarthrosis are related to the degree of clotting factor deficiency. Hemarthrosis is not common in other inherited disorders of coagulation, such as von Willebrand's disease or factor V deficiency.

Hemarthrosis becomes evident after 1 year of age, when the child begins to walk and run. In order of frequency, the joints most commonly affected are the knees, ankles, elbows, shoulders, and hips. Small joints of the hands and feet are occasionally involved.

In the initial stage of arthropathy, hemarthrosis produces a warm, tensely swollen, and painful joint. The patient holds the affected joint in flexion and guards against any movement. Blood in the joint remains liquid because of the absence of intrinsic clotting factors and the absence of tissue thromboplastin in the synovium. The blood in the joint space is resorbed over a period of a week or longer, depending on the size of the hemarthrosis. Joint function usually returns to normal or baseline in about 2 weeks.

Recurrent hemarthrosis leads to the development of a chronic arthritis. The involved joints remain swollen, and flexion deformities develop. In the later stages of arthropathy, joint motion is restricted and function is severely limited. Joint ankylosis, subluxation, and laxity are features of end-stage disease.

Bleeding into muscle and soft tissue also causes musculoskeletal

disorders. When bleeding into the iliopsoas muscle occurs, the hip is held in flexion because of the pain, resulting in a hip flexion contracture. Rotation of the hip is preserved, which distinguishes this problem from intraarticular hemorrhage. Expansion of the hematoma may place pressure on the femoral nerve, resulting in a femoral neuropathy. Another problem is shortening of the heel cord secondary to bleeding into the gastrocnemius. Hemorrhage into a closed compartment space, such as the volar compartment in the forearm, can result in muscle necrosis, neuropathy and flexion deformities of the wrist and fingers. When bleeding involves periosteum or bone, a pseudotumor forms. These occur distal to the elbows or knees in children and improve with treatment of the hemophilia. Surgical removal is indicated if the pseudotumor continues to enlarge. In adults, they occur in the femur and pelvis and are usually refractory to treatment. When bleeding occurs in muscle, cysts may develop within the muscle. Needle aspiration of a cyst is contraindicated because it can induce bleeding.

Septic arthritis can occur in hemophilia and is difficult at times to distinguish from acute hemarthrosis on physical examination. Whenever there is suspicion of an infected joint, the joint should be aspirated immediately, the fluid cultured, and the patient started on antibiotics that provide broad coverage until the results of the culture are known. The patient should be infused with the deficient clotting factor before the joint is tapped to decrease the risk of further bleeding.

Radiographs of joints reflect the stage of disease. In early stages there is only capsule distention; later, juxtaarticular osteopenia, marginal erosions, and subchondral cysts develop. In late disease, the joint space is narrowed and there is bony overgrowth. The changes are similar to those observed in osteoarthritis. Unique features of hemophilic arthropathy are widening of the femoral intercondylar notch, enlargement of the proximal radius, and squaring of the distal end of the patella.

Recurrent hemarthrosis produces synovial hyperplasia and hypertrophy. A pannus covers the cartilage. Cartilage is damaged by collagenase and other degradative enzymes released by mononuclear cells in the overlying synovium. Hemosiderin is found in synovial lining cells, the subsynovium, and chondrocytes and may also play a role in cartilage destruction.

℞ TREATMENT

The treatment of hemarthrosis is initiated with the immediate infusion of factor VIII or IX at the first sign of joint or muscle hemorrhage. The patient is placed at bed rest, with the involved joint in as much extension as the patient can tolerate. Analgesic doses of an NSAID and local icing may help with the pain. NSAIDs can be given safely for short periods even though they have a stabilizing effect on platelets. Studies have shown no significant abnormalities in platelet function or bleeding time in hemophiliacs receiving ibuprofen. The cyclooxygenase-2 inhibitors celecoxib, rofecoxib, and kaldecoxib do not interfere with platelet function and can be safely given for pain. Synovectomy, open or arthroscopic, may be indicated in patients with chronic synovial proliferation and recurrent hemarthrosis. Hypertrophied synovium is very vascular and subject to bleeding. Both types of synovectomy reduce the number of hemarthroses and slow the roentgenographic progression of hemophilic arthropathy. Open surgical synovectomy, however, is associated with some loss of range of motion. Radiosynovectomy with either yttrium 90 silicate or phosphorus 31 colloid has also been effective and may be a useful alternative when surgical synovectomy is not practical. Total joint replacement is indicated for severe joint destruction and incapacitating pain. Because of the young age of hemophilic patients, total-joint prostheses may need to be replaced more than once during their lives.

ARTHROPATHIES ASSOCIATED WITH HEMOGLOBINOPATHIES ■ **Sickle Cell Disease** Sickle cell disease (Chap. 91) is associated with several musculoskeletal abnormalities (Table 315-2). Children under the age of 5 may develop diffuse swelling, tenderness, and warmth of the hands and feet lasting from 1 to 3 weeks. The condition, referred to as *sickle cell dactylitis* or *hand-foot syndrome*, has also been observed in sickle cell

TABLE 315-2 *Musculoskeletal Abnormalities in Sickle Cell Disease*

Sickle cell dactylitis	Avascular necrosis
Joint effusions in sickle cell crises	Bone changes secondary to marrow
Osteomyelitis	hyperplasia
Infarction of bone	Septic arthritis
Infarction of bone marrow	Gouty arthritis

disease and sickle cell thalassemia. Dactylitis is believed to result from infarction of the bone marrow and cortical bone leading to periostitis and soft tissue swelling. Radiographs show periosteal elevation, subperiosteal new bone formation, and areas of radiolucency and increased density involving the metacarpals, metatarsals, and proximal phalanges. These bone changes disappear after several months. The syndrome leaves little or no residual damage. Because hematopoiesis ceases in the small bones of hands and feet with age, the syndrome is rarely seen after age 4 or 5 and does not occur in adults.

Sickle cell crisis is often associated with periarticular pain and joint effusions. The joint and periarticular area are warm and tender. Knees and elbows are most often affected, but other joints can be involved. Joint effusions are noninflammatory, with white cell counts <1000/μL; mononuclear cells predominate. There have been a few reports of sterile inflammatory effusion with high cell counts consisting of mostly polymorphonuclear white cells. Synovial biopsies have shown mild lining cell proliferation and microvascular thrombosis. Scintigraphic studies have shown decreased marrow uptake adjacent to the involved joint. The joint effusion and periarticular pain are considered to be the result of ischemia and infarction of the synovium and adjacent bone and bone marrow. The treatment is that for sickle cell crisis (Chap. 91).

Patients with sickle cell disease may also develop osteomyelitis, which commonly involves the long tubular bones (Chap. 111). These patients are particularly susceptible to bacterial infections, especially *Salmonella* infections, which are found in more than half of cases. The most common isolate is *S. typhimurium* (Chap. 137). Radiographs of the involved site show periosteal elevation initially, followed by disruption of the cortex. Treatment of the infection results in healing of the bone lesion. Sickle cell disease is also associated with bone infarction resulting from thrombosis secondary to the sickling of red cells. Bone infarction also occurs in hemoglobin S-C disease and sickle cell thalassemia (Chap. 91). The bone pain in sickle cell crisis is due to bone and bone marrow infarction. In children, infarction of the epiphyseal growth plate interferes with normal growth of the affected extremity. Radiographically, infarction of the bone cortex results in periosteal elevation and irregular thickening of the bone cortex. Infarction in the bone marrow leads to lysis, fibrosis, and new bone formation.

Avascular necrosis of the head of the femur is seen in ~5% of patients. It also occurs in the humeral head and less commonly in the distal femur, tibial condyles, distal radius, vertebral bodies, and other juxtaarticular sites. The mechanism for avascular necrosis is most likely the same as for bone infarction. Subchondral hemorrhage may play a role in the deterioration of articular cartilage. Irregularity of the femoral head or of other bone surfaces affected by avascular necrosis eventually results in degenerative joint disease. Radiograph of the affected joint may show patchy radiolucency and density followed by flattening of the bone. Magnetic resonance imaging (MRI) is a sensitive technique for detecting early avascular necrosis as well as bone infarction elsewhere. Total hip replacement and placement of prostheses in other joints may improve function and relieve pain in those patients with severe joint destruction.

Septic arthritis is occasionally encountered in sickle cell disease (Chap. 314). Multiple joints may be infected. Joint infection may result from hematogenous spread or from spread of contiguous osteomyelitis. Microorganisms identified include *Staphylococcus aureus*, *Streptococcus*, *Escherichia coli*, and *Salmonella*. The latter is not seen as frequently in septic arthritis as it is in osteomyelitis. Acute gouty arthritis is uncommon in sickle cell disease, even though 40% of patients

are hyperuremic. Hyperuricemia is due to overproduction of uric acid secondary to increased red cell turnover. Attacks may be polyarticular.

The bone marrow hyperplasia in sickle cell disease results in widening of the medullary cavities, thinning of the cortices, and coarse trabeculations and central cupping of the vertebral bodies. These changes are also seen to a lesser degree in hemoglobin S-C disease and sickle cell thalassemia. In normal individuals, red marrow is located mostly in the axial skeletal, but in sickle cell disease, red marrow is found in the bones of the extremities and even in the tarsal and carpal bones. Vertebral compression may lead to dorsal kyphosis, and softening of the bone in the acetabulum may result in protrusio acetabuli.

Thalassemia β-Thalassemia is a congenital disorder of hemoglobin synthesis characterized by impaired production of β chains (Chap. 91). Bone and joint abnormalities occur in β-thalassemia, being most common in the major and intermedia groups. In one study, ~50% of patients with β-thalassemia had evidence of symmetric ankle arthropathy, characterized by a dull aching pain aggravated by weight bearing. The onset was most often in the second or third decade of life. The degree of ankle pain in these patients varied. Some patients experienced self-limited ankle pain, which occurred only after strenuous physical activity and lasted several days to weeks. Other patients had chronic ankle pain, which became worse with walking. Symptoms eventually abated in a few patients. Compression of the ankle, calcaneus, or forefoot was painful in some patients. Synovial fluid from two patients was noninflammatory. Radiographs of ankle showed osteopenia, widened medullary spaces, thin cortices, and coarse trabeculations. These findings were largely the result of bone marrow expansion. The joint space was preserved. Specimens of bone from three patients revealed osteomalacia, osteopenia, and microfractures. Increased osteoblasts as well as increased foci of bone resorption were present on the bone surface. Iron staining was found in the bone trabeculae, in osteoid, and in the cement line. Synovium showed hyperplasia of lining cells, which contained deposits of hemosiderin. This arthropathy was considered to be related to the underlying bone pathology. The role of iron overload or abnormal bone metabolism in the pathogenesis of this arthropathy is not known. The arthropathy was treated with analgesics and splints. Patients were also transfused to decrease hematopoiesis and bone marrow expansion.

Patients with β-thalassemia major and intermedia also have involvement of other joints, including the knees, hips, and shoulders. Acquired hemochromatosis with arthropathy has been described in a patient with thalassemia. Gouty arthritis and septic arthritis can occur. Avascular necrosis is not a feature of thalassemia because there is no sickling of red cells leading to thrombosis and infarction.

β-Thalassemia minor (trait) is also associated with joint manifestations. Chronic seronegative oligoarthritis affecting predominantly ankles, wrists, and elbows has been described. These patients had mild persistent synovitis without large effusions. Joint erosions were not seen. Recurrent episodes of an acute asymmetric arthritis have also been reported; episodes last less than a week and may affect knees, ankles, shoulders, elbows, wrists, and metacarpal phalangeal joints. The mechanism for this arthropathy is unknown. Treatment with nonsteroidal drugs was not particularly effective.

MUSCULOSKELETAL DISORDERS ASSOCIATED WITH HYPERLIPIDEMIA (See also Chap. 335) Musculoskeletal manifestations may be the first indication of a hereditary disorder of lipoprotein metabolism. Patients with familial hypercholesterolemia (previously referred to as type II hyperlipoproteinemia) may have recurrent migratory polyarthritis involving knees and other large peripheral joints and, to a lesser degree, peripheral small joints. In a few patients, the arthritis is monarticular. Fever may accompany the arthritis. Pain ranges from moderate to very severe to incapacitating. The involved joints can be warm, erythematous, swollen, and tender. Arthritis usually has a sudden onset, lasts from a few days to 2 weeks, and does not cause joint damage. Episodes may suggest acute gout attacks. Several attacks occur a year. Synovial fluid from involved joints is not inflammatory and contains few white cells and no crystals. Joint involvement may actually represent inflammatory periarthritis or peritendinitis and not intraarticular disease. The recurrent, transient nature of the arthritis may suggest rheumatic fever, especially since patients with hyperlipoproteinemia have an elevated erythrocyte sedimentation rate and a falsely elevated antistreptolysin O titer. Patients may also experience Achilles tendinitis, which can be very painful. Attacks of tendinitis come on gradually and last only a few days. Fever is not present. Patients may be asymptomatic between attacks. During an attack the Achilles tendon is warm, erythematous, swollen, and tender to palpation. Achilles tendinitis and other joint manifestations often precede the appearance of xanthomas and may be the first clinical indication of hyperlipoproteinemia. Attacks of tendinitis may occur following treatment with a lipid-lowering drug. Patients also have tendinous xanthomas in the Achilles, patellar, and extensor tendons of the hands over the knuckles and feet. Xanthomas have also been reported in the peroneal tendon, the plantar aponeurosis, and the periosteum overlying the distal tibia. These xanthomas are located within tendon fibers. Tuberous xanthomas are soft subcutaneous masses located over the extensor surfaces of the elbows, knees, and hands, as well as on the buttocks. They appear in childhood in homozygous patients and after the age of 30 in heterozygous patients. Patients with elevated plasma levels of very low density lipoprotein (VLDL) and triglyceride (previously referred to as type IV hyperlipoproteinemia) may also have a mild inflammatory arthritis affecting large and small peripheral joints, usually in an asymmetric pattern with only a few joints involved at a time. The onset of arthritis is usually in middle age. Arthritis may be persistent or recurrent, with episodes lasting a few days to weeks. Joint pain is severe in some patients. Patients may experience morning stiffness. Joint tenderness and periarticular hyperesthesia may also be present, as may synovial thickening. Joint fluid is usually noninflammatory and without crystals but may have increased white blood cell counts with predominantly mononuclear cells. The fluid is occasionally lactescent. Radiographs may show juxtaarticular osteopenia and cystic lesions. Large bone cysts have been noted in a few patients. Xanthoma and bone cysts are also observed in other lipoprotein disorders. The pathogenesis of arthritis in patients with familial hypercholesterolemia or with elevated levels of VLDL and triglyceride is not well understood. Salicylates, other NSAIDs, or analgesics usually provide relief of symptoms. Clinical improvement may also occur in patients treated with lipid-lowering agents; however, patients treated with a HMG CoA reductase agent may experience myalgias, and a few patients may develop polymyositis or even rhabdomyolysis. Myositis has also been reported with the use of niacin (Chap. 370).

OTHER ARTHRITIDES

NEUROPATHIC JOINT DISEASE
Neuropathic joint disease (Charcot's joint) is a progressive destructive arthritis associated with loss of pain sensation, proprioception, or both. In addition, normal muscular reflexes that modulate joint movement are decreased. Without these protective mechanisms, joints are subjected to repeated trauma, resulting in progressive cartilage and bone damage. Neuropathic arthropathy was first described by Jean-Martin Charcot in 1868 in patients with tabes dorsalis. The term *Charcot joint* is commonly used interchangeably with *neuropathic joint*. Today, diabetes mellitus is the most frequent cause of neuropathic joint disease. A variety of other disorders are associated with neuropathic arthritis including leprosy, yaws, syringomyelia, meningomyelocoele, congenital indifference to pain, peroneal muscular atrophy (Charcot-Marie-Tooth disease), and amyloidosis. An arthritis resembling neuropathic joint disease is seen in patients who have received frequent intraarticular glucocorticoid injections into a weight-bearing joint and in patients with CPDD. The distribution of joint involvement depends on the underlying neurologic disorder (Table 315-3). In tabes dorsalis, knees, hips, and ankles are most com-

TABLE 315-3 *Disorders Associated with Neuropathic Joint Disease*

Diabetes mellitus	Amyloidosis
Tabes dorsalis	Leprosy
Meningomyelocele	Congenital indifference to pain
Syringomyelia	Peroneal muscular atrophy

monly affected; in syringomyelia, the glenohumeral joint, elbow, and wrist; and in diabetes mellitus, the tarsal and tarsometatarsal joints.

Pathology and Pathophysiology The pathologic changes in the neuropathic joint are similar to those found in the severe osteoarthritic joint. There is fragmentation and eventual loss of articular cartilage with eburnation of the underlying bone. Osteophytes are found at the joint margins. With more advanced disease, erosions are present on the joint surface. Fractures, devitalized bone, and intraarticular loose bodies may be present. Microscopic fragments of cartilage and bone are seen in the synovial tissue.

At least two underlying mechanisms are believed to be involved in the pathogenesis of neuropathic arthritis. An abnormal autonomic nervous system is thought to be responsible for the increased blood flow to the joint and subsequent resorption of bone. Loss of bone, particularly in the diabetic foot, may be the initial manifestation. With the loss of deep pain, proprioception, and protective neuromuscular reflexes, the joint is subjected to repeated injuries including ligamental tears and bone fractures. The mechanism of injury that occurs following frequent intraarticular glucocorticoid injections is thought to be due to the analgesic effect of glucocorticoids leading to overuse of an already damaged joint, which results in accelerated cartilage damage. It is not understood why only a few patients with neuropathies develop neuropathic arthritis.

Clinical Manifestations Neuropathic joint disease usually begins in a single joint and then progresses to involve other joints, depending on the underlying neurologic disorder. The involved joint progressively becomes enlarged from bony overgrowth and synovial effusion. Loose bodies may be palpated in the joint cavity. Joint instability, subluxation, and crepitus occur as the disease progresses. Neuropathic joints may develop rapidly, and a totally disorganized joint with multiple bony fragments may evolve in a patient within weeks or months. The amount of pain experienced by the patient is less than would be anticipated based on the degree of joint involvement. Patients may experience sudden joint pain from intraarticular fractures of osteophytes or condyles.

Neuropathic arthritis is encountered most often in patients with diabetes mellitus, with the incidence estimated in the range of 0.5%. The usual age of onset is ≥50 years following several years of diabetes, but exceptions occur. The tarsal and tarsometatarsal joints are most often affected, followed by the metatarsophalangeal and talotibial joints. The knees and spine are occasionally involved. In about 20%, neuropathic arthritis may be present in both feet. Patients often attribute the onset of foot pain to antecedent trauma such as twisting their foot. Neuropathic changes may develop rapidly following a foot fracture or dislocation. Swelling of the foot and ankle are often present. Downward collapse of the tarsal bones leads to convexity of the sole, referred to as a "rocker foot." Large osteophytes may protrude from the top of the foot. Calluses frequently form over the metatarsal heads and may lead to infected ulcers and osteomyelitis. Radiographs may show resorption and tapering of the distal metatarsal bones. The term *Lisfranc fracture-dislocation* is sometimes used to describe the destructive changes at the tarsometatarsal joints.

Diagnosis The diagnosis of neuropathic arthritis is based on the clinical features and characteristic radiographic findings in a patient with an underlying sensory neuropathy. The differential diagnosis of neuropathic arthritis includes osteomyelitis, osteonecrosis, advanced osteoarthritis, stress fractures, and CPDD. Radiographs in neuropathic arthritis initially show changes of osteoarthritis with joint space narrowing, subchondral bone sclerosis, osteophytes, and joint effusions followed later by marked destructive and hypertrophic changes. Soft tissue swelling, bone resorption, fractures, large osteophytes, extraarticular bone fragments, and subluxation are present with advanced arthropathy. The radiographic findings of neuropathic arthritis may be difficult to differentiate from those of osteomyelitis, especially in the diabetic foot. The joint margins in a neuropathic joint tend to be distinct, while in osteomyelitis, they are blurred. Imaging studies and cultures of fluid and tissue from the joint are often required to exclude osteomyelitis. MRI is helpful in differentiating these disorders. Another useful study is a bone scan using indium 111–labeled white blood cells or indium 111–labeled immunoglobulin G, which will show an increased uptake in osteomyelitis but not in a neuropathic joint. A technetium bone scan will not distinguish osteomyelitis from neuropathic arthritis as increased uptake is observed in both. The joint fluid in neuropathic arthritis is noninflammatory; may be xanthochromic or even bloody; and may contain fragments of synovium, cartilage, and bone. The finding of calcium pyrophosphate dihydrate crystals suggests the diagnosis of a crystal-associated neuropathic-like arthropathy. In the absence of such crystals, the presence of increased number of leukocytes may indicate osteomyelitis.

℞ TREATMENT

The primary focus of treatment is to provide stabilization of the joint. Treatment of the underlying disorder, even if successful, does not usually alter the joint disease. Braces and splints are helpful. Their use requires close surveillance, since patients may be unable to appreciate pressure from a poorly adjusted brace. In the diabetic patient, early recognition and treatment of a Charcot's foot by prohibiting weight bearing of the foot for at least 8 weeks may possibly prevent severe disease from developing. Fusion of a very unstable joint may improve function, but nonunion is frequent, especially when immobilization of the joint is inadequate.

HYPERTROPHIC OSTEOARTHROPATHY AND CLUBBING Hypertrophic osteoarthropathy (HOA) is characterized by clubbing of digits and, in more advanced stages, by periosteal new bone formation and synovial effusions. HOA occurs in primary or familial form and usually begins in childhood. The secondary form of HOA is associated with intrathoracic malignancies, suppurative lung disease, congenital heart disease, and a variety of other disorders and is more common in adults. Clubbing is almost always a feature of HOA but can occur as an isolated manifestation (Fig. 315-2). The presence of clubbing in isolation is generally considered to represent either an early stage or an element in the spectrum of HOA. The presence of only clubbing in a patient usually has the same clinical significance as HOA.

Pathology and Pathophysiology In HOA, the bone changes in the distal extremities begin as periostitis followed by new bone formation. At this stage, a radiolucent area may be observed between the new periosteal bone and subjacent cortex. As the process progresses, multiple

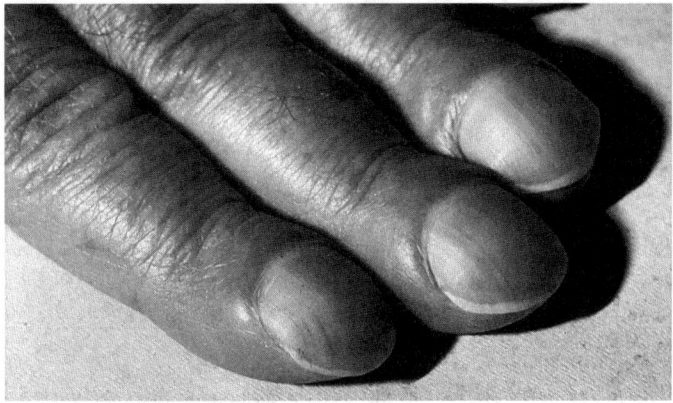

FIGURE 315-2 Clubbing of fingers. (*Reprinted from the Clinical Slide Collection on the Rheumatic Diseases, Copyright 1991, 1995. Used by permission of the American College of Rheumatology.*)

layers of new bone are deposited, which become contiguous with the cortex and result in cortical thickening. The outer portion of bone is laminated in appearance, with an irregular surface. Initially, the process of periosteal new bone formation involves the proximal and distal diaphyses of the tibia, fibula, radius, and ulna and, less frequently, the femur, humerus, metacarpals, metatarsals, and phalanges. Occasionally, scapulae, clavicles, ribs, and pelvic bones are also affected. In long-standing disease, these changes extend to involve metaphyses and musculotendinous insertions. The adjacent interosseous membranes may become ossified. The distribution of the bone manifestations is usually bilateral and symmetric. The soft tissue overlying the distal third of the arms and legs may be thickened. Mononuclear cell infiltration may be present in the adjacent soft tissue. Proliferation of connective tissue occurs in the nail bed and volar pad of digits, giving the distal phalanges a clubbed appearance. Small blood vessels in the clubbed digits are dilated and have thickened walls. In addition, the number of arteriovenous anastomoses is increased. The synovia of involved joints show edema, varying degrees of synovial cell proliferation, thickening of the subsynovium, vascular congestion, vascular obliteration with thrombi, and small numbers of lymphocyte infiltrates.

Several theories have been suggested for the pathogenesis of HOA. Most have either been disproved or have not explained the development in all clinical disorders associated with HOA. Previously proposed neurogenic and humoral theories are no longer considered likely explanations for HOA. The neurogenic theory was based on the observation that vagotomy resulted in symptomatic improvement in a small number of patients with lung tumors and HOA. It was postulated that vagal stimuli from the tumor site led via a neural reflex to efferent nerve impulses to the distal extremities, resulting in HOA. This theory, however, did not explain HOA in conditions where vagal stimulation did not occur, as in cyanotic congenital heart disease or arterial aneurysms. The humoral theory postulated that soluble substances that are normally inactivated or removed during passage through the lung reached the systemic circulation in an active form and stimulated the changes of HOA. Substances proposed included prostaglandins, ferritin, bradykinin, estrogen, and growth hormone. These substances seemed unlikely candidates, since their blood levels in HOA patients overlapped those in individuals without HOA. Furthermore, these substances did not explain the development of localized HOA associated with arterial aneurysms or infected arterial grafts.

Recent studies have suggested a role for platelets in the development of HOA. It has been observed that megakaryocytes and large platelet particles, present in venous circulation, were fragmented in their passage through normal lung. In patients with cyanotic congenital heart disease and in other disorders associated with right-to-left shunts, these large platelet particles bypass the lung and reach the distal extremities, where they can interact with endothelial cells. Platelet clumps have been demonstrated to form on an infected heart valve in bacterial endocarditis, in the wall of arterial aneurysms, and on infected arterial grafts. These platelet particles may also reach the distal extremities and interact with endothelial cells. Platelet-endothelial activation in the distal portion of extremities would then result in the release of platelet-derived growth factor (PDGF) and other factors leading to the proliferation of connective tissue and periosteum. Stimulation of fibroblasts by PDGF and transforming growth factor β results in cell growth and collagen synthesis. Elevated plasma levels of von Willebrand factor antigen have been found in patients with both primary and secondary forms of HOA, indicating endothelial activation or damage. Abnormalities of collagen synthesis have been demonstrated in the involved skin of patients with primary HOA. Fibroblasts from affected skin were shown to have increased collagen synthesis, increased $\alpha 1(I)$ procollagen mRNA, and evidence for upregulation of collagen transcription. Other factors are undoubtedly involved in the pathogenesis of HOA, and further studies are needed to better understand this disorder.

Clinical Manifestations Primary or familial HOA, also referred to as *pachydermoperiostitis* or *Touraine-Solente-Golé syndrome*, usually begins insidiously at puberty. In a smaller number of patients, the onset is in the first year of life. The disorder is inherited as an autosomal dominant trait with variable expression and is nine times more common in boys than in girls. Approximately one-third of patients have a family history of primary HOA.

Primary HOA is characterized by clubbing, periostitis, and unusual skin features. A small number of patients with this syndrome do not express clubbing. The skin changes and periostitis are prominent features of this syndrome. The skin becomes thickened and coarse. Deep nasolabial folds develop, and the forehead may become furrowed. Patients may have heavy-appearing eyelids and ptosis. The skin is often greasy, and there may be excessive sweating of the hands and feet. Patients may also experience acne vulgaris, seborrhea, and folliculitis. In a few patients, the skin over the scalp becomes very thick and corrugated, a feature that has been descriptively termed *cutis verticis gyrata*. The distal extremities, particularly the legs, become thickened owing to proliferation of new bone and soft tissue; when the process is extensive, the distal lower extremities resemble those of an elephant. The periostitis is usually not painful, as it may be in secondary HOA. Clubbing of the fingers may be extensive, producing large, bulbous deformities and clumsiness. Clubbing also affects the toes. Patients may experience articular and periarticular pain, especially in the ankles and knees, and joint motion may be mildly restricted owing to periarticular bone overgrowth. Noninflammatory effusions occur in the wrists, knees, and ankles. Synovial hypertrophy is not found. Associated abnormalities observed in patients with primary HOA include hypertrophic gastropathy, bone marrow failure, female escutcheon, gynecomastia, and cranial suture defects. In patients with primary HOA, the symptoms disappear when adulthood is reached.

HOA secondary to an underlying disease occurs more frequently than primary HOA. It accompanies a variety of disorders and may precede clinical features of the associated disorder by months. Clubbing is more frequent than the full syndrome of HOA in patients with associated illnesses. Because clubbing evolves over months and is usually asymptomatic, it is often recognized first by the physician and not the patient. Patients may experience a burning sensation in their fingertips. Clubbing is characterized by widening of the fingertips, enlargement of the distal volar pad, convexity of the nail contour, and the loss of the normal 15° angle between the proximal nail and cuticle. The thickness of the digit at the base of the nail is greater than the thickness at the distal interphalangeal joint. An objective measurement of finger clubbing can be made by determining the diameter at the base of the nail and at the distal interphalangeal joint of all 10 digits. Clubbing is present when the sum of the individual digit ratios is >10. At the bedside, clubbing can be appreciated by having the patient place the dorsal surface of the distal phalanges of the fourth fingers together with the nails of the fourth fingers opposing each other. Normally, an open area is visible between the bases of the opposing fingernails; when clubbing is present, this open space is no longer visible. The base of the nail feels spongy when compressed, and the nail can be easily rocked on its bed. Marked periungual erythema is usually present. When clubbing is advanced, the finger may have a drumstick appearance, and the distal interphalangeal joint can be hyperextended. Periosteal involvement in the distal extremities may produce a burning or deep-seated aching pain. The pain can be quite incapacitating and is aggravated by dependency and relieved by elevation of the affected limbs. The overlying soft tissue may be swollen, and the skin slightly erythematous. Pressure applied over the distal forearms and legs may be quite painful.

Patients may also experience joint pain, most often in the ankles, wrists, and knees. Joint effusions may be present; usually they are small and noninflammatory. The small joints of the hands are rarely affected. Severe joint or bone pain may be the presenting symptom of an underlying lung malignancy and may precede the appearance of

TABLE 315-4 *Disorders Associated with Hypertrophic Osteoarthropathy*

Pulmonary	Cardiovascular
Bronchogenic carcinoma and other neoplasms	Cyanotic congenital heart disease
Lung abscesses, empyema, bronchiectasis	Subacute bacterial endocarditis
Chronic interstitial pneumonitis	Infected arterial grafts[a]
Cystic fibrosis	Aortic aneurysm[b]
Chronic obstructive lung disease	Aneurysm of major extremity artery[a]
Sarcoidosis	Patent ductus arteriosus[b]
Gastrointestinal	Arteriovenous fistula of major extremity vessel[a]
Inflammatory bowel disease	Thyroid (thyroid acropachy)
Sprue	Hyperthyroidism (Graves' disease)
Neoplasms: esophagus, liver, bowel	

[a] Unilateral involvement.
[b] Bilateral lower extremity involvement.

clubbing. In addition, the progression of HOA tends to be more rapid when associated with malignancies, most notably bronchogenic carcinoma. Unlike primary HOA, excessive sweating and oiliness of the skin and thickening of the facial skin are uncommon in secondary HOA.

HOA occurs in 5 to 10% of patients with intrathoracic malignancies, the most common being bronchogenic carcinoma and pleural tumors (Table 315-4). Lung metastases infrequently cause HOA. HOA is also seen in patients with intrathoracic infections, including lung abscesses, empyema, bronchiectasis, chronic obstructive lung disease, and, uncommonly, pulmonary tuberculosis. HOA may also accompany chronic interstitial pneumonitis, sarcoidosis, and cystic fibrosis. In the latter, clubbing is more common than the full syndrome of HOA. Other causes of clubbing include congenital heart disease with right-to-left shunts, bacterial endocarditis, Crohn's disease, ulcerative colitis, sprue, and neoplasms of the esophagus, liver, and small and large bowel. In patients with congenital heart disease with right-to-left shunts, clubbing alone occurs more often than the full syndrome of HOA.

Unilateral clubbing has been found in association with aneurysms of major extremity arteries, infected arterial grafts, and with arteriovenous fistulas of brachial vessels. Clubbing of the toes but not fingers has been associated with an infected abdominal aortic aneurysm and patent ductus arteriosus. Clubbing of a single digit may follow trauma and has been reported in tophaceous gout and sarcoidosis. While clubbing occurs more commonly than the full syndrome in most diseases, periostitis in the absence of clubbing has been observed in the affected limb of patients with infected arterial grafts.

Hyperthyroidism (Graves' disease), treated or untreated, is occasionally associated with clubbing and periostitis of the bones of the hands and feet. This condition is referred to as *thyroid acropachy*. Periostitis is asymptomatic and occurs in the midshaft and diaphyseal portion of the metacarpal and phalangeal bones. The long bones of the extremities are seldom affected. Elevated levels of long-acting thyroid stimulator are found in the serum of these patients.

Laboratory Findings The laboratory abnormalities reflect the underlying disorder. The synovial fluid of involved joints has <500 white cells per microliter, and the cells are predominantly mononuclear. Radiographs show a faint radiolucent line beneath the new periosteal bone along the shaft of long bones at their distal end. These changes are observed most frequently at the ankles, wrists, and knees. The ends of the distal phalanges may show osseous resorption. Radionuclide studies show pericortical linear uptake along the cortical margins of long bones that may be present before any radiographic changes.

℞ TREATMENT

The treatment of HOA is to identify the associated disorder and treat it appropriately. The symptoms and signs of HOA may disappear completely with removal or effective chemotherapy of a tumor or with antibiotic therapy and drainage of a chronic pulmonary infection. Vagotomy or percutaneous block of the vagus nerve leads to symptomatic relief in some patients. Aspirin, other nonsteroidal anti-inflammatory drugs (NSAIDs), or analgesics may help control symptoms of HOA.

REFLEX SYMPATHETIC DYSTROPHY SYNDROME The reflex sympathetic dystrophy syndrome is now referred to as *complex regional pain syndrome, type 1*, by the new Classification of the International Association for the Study of Pain. It is characterized by pain and swelling, usually of a distal extremity, accompanied by vasomotor instability, trophic skin changes, and the rapid development of bony demineralization. →*Reflex sympathetic dystrophy syndrome, including its treatment, is covered in greater detail in Chap. 355.*

TIETZE'S SYNDROME AND COSTOCHONDRITIS Tietze's syndrome is manifested by painful swelling of one or more costochondral articulations. The age of onset is usually before 40, and both sexes are affected equally. In most patients only one joint is involved, usually the second or third costochondral joint. The onset of anterior chest pain may be sudden or gradual. The pain may radiate to the arms or shoulders and is aggravated by sneezing, coughing, deep inspirations, or twisting motions of the chest. The term *costochondritis* is often used interchangeably with *Tietze's syndrome*, but some workers restrict the former term to pain of the costochondral articulations without swelling. Costochondritis is observed in patients over age 40; tends to affect the third, fourth, and fifth costochondral joints; and occurs more often in women. Both syndromes may mimic cardiac or upper abdominal causes of pain. Rheumatoid arthritis, ankylosing spondylitis, and Reiter's syndrome may involve costochondral joints but are distinguished easily by their other clinical features. Other skeletal causes of anterior chest wall pain are xiphoidalgia and the slipping rib syndrome, which usually involves the tenth rib. Malignancies such as breast cancer, prostate cancer, plasma cell cytoma, and sarcoma can invade the ribs, thoracic spine, or chest wall and produce symptoms suggesting Tietze's syndrome. They should be easily distinguishable by radiographs and biopsy. Analgesics, anti-inflammatory drugs, and local glucocorticoid injections usually relieve symptoms.

MYOFASCIAL PAIN SYNDROME

Myofascial pain syndrome is characterized by localized musculoskeletal pain and tenderness in association with trigger points. The pain is deep and aching and may be accompanied by a burning sensation. Myofascial pain may follow trauma, overuse, or prolonged static contraction of a muscle or muscle group, which may occur when reading or writing at a desk or working at a computer. In addition, this syndrome may be associated with underlying osteoarthritis of the neck or low back. Trigger points are a diagnostic feature of this syndrome. Pain is referred from trigger points to defined areas distant from the original tender points. Palpation of the trigger point reproduces or accentuates the pain. The trigger points are usually located in the center of a muscle belly, but they can occur at other sites, such as costosternal junctions, the xyphoid process, ligamentous and tendinous insertions, fascia, and fatty areas. Trigger point sites in muscle have been described as feeling indurated and taut, and palpation may cause the muscle to twitch. These findings, however, have been shown not to be unique for myofascial pain syndrome, since in a controlled study they were also present in fibromyalgia patients and normal subjects. Myofascial pain most often involves the posterior neck, low back, shoulders, and chest. Chronic pain in the muscles of the posterior neck may involve referral of pain from the trigger point in the erector neck muscle or upper trapezius to the head, leading to persistent headaches, which may last for days. Trigger points in the paraspinal muscles of the low back may refer pain to the buttock. Pain may be referred down the leg from a trigger point in the gluteus medius and can mimic sciatica. A trigger point in the infraspinatus muscle may produce local and referred pain over the lateral deltoid and down the outside of the arm into the hand. Injection of a local anesthetic such as 1% lidocaine into the trigger point site often results in pain relief. Another useful technique is first to spray from the trigger point toward the area of referred pain with an agent such as ethyl chloride and then to stretch

the muscle. This maneuver may need to be repeated several times. Massage and application of ultrasound to the affected area may also be beneficial. Patients should be instructed in methods to prevent muscle stresses related to work and recreation. Posture and resting positions are important in preventing muscle tension. The prognosis in most patients is good. In some patients, myofascial pain syndrome may evolve into fibromyalgia. Patients at risk for developing fibromyalgia are thought to be those with anxiety, depression, nonrestorative sleep, and fatigue.

TUMORS OF JOINTS Primary tumors and tumor-like disorders of synovium are uncommon but should be considered in the differential diagnosis of monarticular joint disease. In addition, metastases to bone and primary bone tumors adjacent to a joint may produce joint symptoms. →*For further discussion, see Chap. 84.*

Pigmented villonodular synovitis is characterized by the slowly progressive, exuberant, benign proliferation of synovial tissue, usually involving a single joint. The most common age of onset is in the third decade, and women are affected slightly more often than men. The cause of this disorder is unknown.

The synovium has a brownish color and numerous large, finger-like villi that fuse to form pedunculated nodules. There is marked hyperplasia of synovial cells in the stroma of the villi. Hemosiderin granules and lipids are found in the cytoplasm of macrophages and in the interstitial tissue. Multinucleated giant cells may be present. The proliferative synovium grows into the subsynovial tissue and invades adjacent cartilage and bone.

The clinical picture of pigmented villonodular synovitis is characterized by the insidious onset of swelling and pain in one joint, most commonly the knee. Other joints affected include the hips, ankles, calcaneocuboid joints, elbows, and small joints of the fingers or toes. The disease may also involve the common flexor sheath of the hands or fingers. Less commonly, tendon sheaths in the wrist, ankle, or foot may be involved. Symptoms may be mild and intermittent and may be present for years before the patient seeks medical attention. Radiographs may show joint space narrowing, erosions, and subchondral cysts. The joint fluid contains blood and is dark red or almost black in color. Lipid-containing macrophages may be present in the fluid. The joint fluid may be clear if hemorrhages have not occurred.

The treatment of pigmented villonodular synovitis is complete synovectomy. With incomplete synovectomy, the villonodular synovitis recurs, and the rate of tissue growth may be faster than originally. Irradiation of the involved joint has been successful in some patients.

Synovial chondromatosis is a disorder characterized by multiple focal metaplastic growths of normal-appearing cartilage in the synovium or tendon sheath. Segments of cartilage break loose and continue to grow as loose bodies. When calcification and ossification of loose bodies occur, the disorder is referred to as *synovial osteochondromatosis*. The disorder is usually monarticular and affects young to middle-aged individuals. The knee is most often involved, followed by hip, elbow, and shoulder. Symptoms are pain, swelling, and decreased motion of the joint. Radiographs may show several rounded calcifications within the joint cavity. Treatment is synovectomy; however, the tumor may recur.

Hemangiomas occur in synovium and in tendon sheaths. The knee is affected most commonly. Recurrent episodes of joint swelling and pain usually begin in childhood. The joint fluid is bloody. Treatment is excision of the lesion. *Lipomas* occur most often in the knee, originating in the subsynovial fat on either side of the patellar tendon. Lipomas also appear in tendon sheaths of the hands, wrists, feet, and ankles. In some instances, surgical removal is necessary.

Synovial sarcoma is a malignant neoplasm often found near a large joint of both upper and lower extremities, being more common in the lower extremity. It seldom arises within the joint itself. Synovial sarcomas comprise 10% of soft tissue sarcomas. The tumor is believed to arise from primitive mesenchymal tissue that differentiates into epithelial cells and/or spindle cells. Small foci of calcification may be present in the tumor mass. It occurs most often in young adults and is more common in men. The tumor presents as a slowly growing deep seated mass near a joint, without much pain. The area of the knee is the most common site, followed by the foot, ankle, elbow, and shoulder. Other primary sites include the buttocks, abdominal wall, retroperitoneum, and mediastinum. The tumor spreads along tissue planes. The most common site of visceral metastasis is lung. The diagnosis is made by biopsy. Treatment is wide resection of the tumor including adjacent muscle and regional lymph nodes, followed by chemotherapy and radiation therapy. Currently used chemotherapeutic agents are doxorubicin, ifosfamide, and cisplatin. Amputation of the involved distal extremity may be required. Chemotherapy may be beneficial in some patients with metastatic disease. Isolated pulmonary metastasis can be surgically removed. The 5-year survival with treatment is variable depending on the staging of the tumor ranging from approximately 25 to 60% or higher. Synovial sarcomas tend to recur locally and eventually metastasize to regional lymph nodes, lungs, and skeleton.

FURTHER READING

ALTMAN RD, TENENBAUM J: Hypertrophic osteoarthropathy, in *Kelley's Textbook of Rheumatology*, 6th ed, S Ruddy et al (eds). Philadelphia, Saunders, 2001, pp 1589–1594

CRONIN ME: Rheumatic aspects of endocrinopathies, in *Arthritis and Allied Conditions,* 14th ed, WJ Koopman (ed). Philadelphia, Lippincott Williams & Wilkins, 2001, pp 2530–2547

GOLDENBERG DL: Fibromyalgia syndrome a decade later: What have we learned? Arch Intern Med 159:777, 1999

HECK LW JR: Arthritis associated with hematologic disorders, storage diseases, disorders of lipid metabolism, and dysproteinemias, in *Arthritis and Allied Conditions*, 14th ed, WJ Koopman (ed). Philadelphia, Lippincott Williams & Wilkins, 2001, pp 1903–1924

WOLFE F et al: The prevalence and characteristics of fibromyalgia in the general population. Arthritis Rheum 38:19, 1995

316 | PERIARTICULAR DISORDERS OF THE EXTREMITIES
Bruce C. Gilliland

A number of periarticular disorders have become increasingly common over the past two to three decades, due in part to greater participation in recreational sports by individuals of a wide range of ages. This chapter discusses some of the more common periarticular disorders of the extremities.

BURSITIS Bursitis is inflammation of a bursa, which is a thin-walled sac lined with synovial tissue. The function of the bursa is to facilitate movement of tendons and muscles over bony prominences. Excessive frictional forces from overuse, trauma, systemic disease (e.g., rheumatoid arthritis, gout), or infection may cause bursitis. *Subacromial bursitis* (subdeltoid bursitis) is the most common form of bursitis. The subacromial bursa, which is contiguous with the subdeltoid bursa, is located between the undersurface of the acromion and the humeral head, and is covered by the deltoid muscle. Bursitis is caused by repetitive overhead motion and often accompanies rotator cuff tendinitis. Another frequently encountered form is *trochanteric bursitis*, which involves the bursa around the insertion of the gluteus medius onto the greater trochanter of the femur. Patients experience pain over the lateral aspect of the hip and upper thigh and have tenderness over the posterior aspect of the greater trochanter. External rotation and resisted abduction of the hip elicit pain. *Olecranon bursitis* occurs over the posterior elbow, and when the area is acutely inflamed, infection or gout should be excluded by aspirating the bursa and performing a Gram stain and culture on the fluid as well as examining the fluid for urate crystals. *Achilles bursitis* involves the bursa located above the insertion of the tendon to the calcaneus and results from overuse and wearing tight shoes. *Retrocalcaneal bursitis* involves the bursa that is located between the calcaneus and posterior surface of the Achilles tendon. The pain is experienced at the back of the heel, and swelling appears on the medial and/or lateral side of the tendon. It occurs in association with spondyloarthropathies, rheumatoid arthritis, gout, or trauma. *Ischial bursitis* (weaver's bottom) affects the bursa separating the gluteus medius from the ischial tuberosity and develops from prolonged sitting and pivoting on hard surfaces. *Iliopsoas bursitis* affects the bursa that lies between the iliopsoas muscle and hip joint and is lateral to the femoral vessels. Pain is experienced over this area and is made worse by hip extension and flexion. *Anserine bursitis* is an inflammation of the sartorius bursa located over the medial side of the tibia just below the knee and under the conjoint tendon and is manifested by pain on climbing stairs. Tenderness is present over the insertion of the conjoint tendon of the sartorius, gracilis, and semitendinosus. *Prepatellar bursitis* (housemaid's knee) occurs in the bursa situated between the patella and overlying skin and is caused by kneeling on hard surfaces. Gout or infection may also occur at this site. Treatment of bursitis consists of prevention of the aggravating situation, rest of the involved part, administration of a nonsteroidal anti-inflammatory drug (NSAID), or local glucocorticoid injection.

ROTATOR CUFF TENDINITIS AND IMPINGEMENT SYNDROME Tendinitis of the rotator cuff is the major cause of a painful shoulder and is currently thought to be caused by inflammation of the tendon(s). The rotator cuff consists of the tendons of the supraspinatus, infraspinatus, subscapularis, and teres minor muscles, and inserts on the humeral tuberosities. Of the tendons forming the rotator cuff, the supraspinatus tendon is the most often affected, probably because of its repeated impingement (impingement syndrome) between the humeral head and the undersurface of the anterior third of the acromion and coracoacromial ligament above as well as the reduction in its blood supply that occurs with abduction of the arm (Fig. 316-1). The tendon of the infraspinatus and that of the long head of the biceps are less commonly involved. The process begins with edema and hemorrhage of the rotator cuff, which evolves to fibrotic thickening and eventually to rotator cuff degeneration with tendon tears and bone spurs. Subacromial bursitis also accompanies this syndrome. Symptoms usually appear

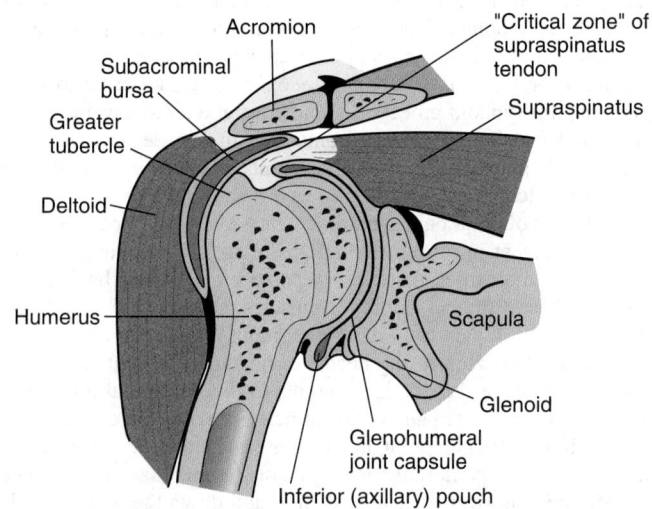

FIGURE 316-1 Coronal section of the shoulder illustrating the relationships of the glenohumeral joint, the joint capsule, the subacromial bursa, and the rotator cuff (supraspinatus tendon). [*From F Kozin, in WJ Koopman (ed): Arthritis and Allied Conditions, 13th ed. Baltimore, Williams & Wilkins, 1997, with permission.*]

after injury or overuse, especially with activities involving elevation of the arm with some degree of forward flexion. Impingement syndrome occurs in persons participating in baseball, tennis, swimming, or occupations that require repeated elevation of the arm. Those over age 40 are particularly susceptible. Patients complain of a dull aching in the shoulder, which may interfere with sleep. Severe pain is experienced when the arm is actively abducted into an overhead position. The arc between 60 and 120° is especially painful. Tenderness is present over the lateral aspect of the humeral head just below the acromion. NSAIDs, local glucocorticoid injection, and physical therapy may relieve symptoms. Surgical decompression of the subacromial space may be necessary in patients refractory to conservative treatment.

Patients may tear the supraspinatus tendon acutely by falling on an outstretched arm or lifting a heavy object. Symptoms are pain, along with weakness of abduction and external rotation of the shoulder. Atrophy of the supraspinatus muscles develops. The diagnosis is established by arthrogram, ultrasound or magnetic resonance imaging. Surgical repair may be necessary in patients who fail to respond to conservative measures. In patients with moderate to severe tears and functional loss, surgery is indicated.

CALCIFIC TENDINITIS This condition is characterized by deposition of calcium salts, primarily hydroxyapatite, within a tendon. The exact mechanism of calcification is not known but may be initiated by ischemia or degeneration of the tendon. The supraspinatus tendon is most often affected because it is frequently impinged on and has a reduced blood supply when the arm is abducted. The condition usually develops after age 40. Calcification within the tendon may evoke acute inflammation, producing sudden and severe pain in the shoulder. However, it may be asymptomatic or not related to the patient's symptoms.

BICIPITAL TENDINITIS AND RUPTURE Bicipital tendinitis, or tenosynovitis, is produced by friction on the tendon of the long head of the biceps as it passes through the bicipital groove. When the inflammation is acute, patients experience anterior shoulder pain that radiates down the biceps into the forearm. Abduction and external rotation of the arm are painful and limited. The bicipital groove is very tender to palpation. Pain may be elicited along the course of the tendon by resisting supination of the forearm with the elbow at 90° (Yergason's supination sign). Acute rupture of the tendon may occur with vigorous exercise of the arm and is often painful. In a young patient, it should be repaired surgically. Rupture of the tendon in an older person may be associated with little or no pain and is recognized by the presence of persistent swelling of the biceps ("Popeye" muscle) produced by the retraction of the long head of the biceps. Surgery is usually not necessary in this setting.

DE QUERVAINS' TENOSYNOVITIS In this condition, inflammation involves the abductor pollicis longus and the extensor pollicis brevis as these tendons pass through a fibrous sheath at the radial styloid process. The usual cause is repetitive twisting motion of the wrist. It may occur in pregnancy, and it also occurs in mothers from holding their babies with the thumb outstretched. Patients experience pain on grasping with their thumb such as with pinching. Swelling and tenderness are often present over the radial styloid process. The Finkelstein sign is positive, which is elicited by having the patient place the thumb in the palm and close the fingers over it. The wrist is then ulnarly deviated resulting in pain over the involved tendon sheath in the area of the radial styloid. Treatment consists initially of splinting the wrist and an NSAID. When severe or refractory to conservative treatment, glucocorticoid injections can be very effective.

PATELLAR TENDINITIS (JUMPER'S KNEE) Tendinitis involves the patellar tendon at its attachment to the lower pole of the patella. Patients may experience pain when jumping during basketball or volleyball, going up stairs, or when doing deep knee squats. Tenderness is noted on examination over the lower pole of the patella. Treatment consists of rest, icing, and NSAIDS, followed by strengthening and increasing flexibility.

ADHESIVE CAPSULITIS Often referred to as "frozen shoulder," adhesive capsulitis is characterized by pain and restricted movement of the shoulder, usually in the absence of intrinsic shoulder disease. Night pain is often present in the affected shoulder. Adhesive capsulitis, however, may follow bursitis or tendinitis of the shoulder or be associated with systemic disorders such as chronic pulmonary disease, myocardial infarction, and diabetes mellitus. Prolonged immobility of the arm contributes to the development of adhesive capsulitis, and reflex sympathetic dystrophy is thought to be a pathogenic factor. The capsule of the shoulder is thickened, and a mild chronic inflammatory infiltrate and fibrosis may be present.

Adhesive capsulitis occurs more commonly in women after age 50. Pain and stiffness usually develop gradually over several months to a year but progress rapidly in some patients. Pain may interfere with sleep. The shoulder is tender to palpation, and both active and passive movement are restricted. Radiographs of the shoulder show osteopenia. The diagnosis is confirmed by arthrography, in that only a limited amount of contrast material, usually <15 mL, can be injected under pressure into the shoulder joint.

In most patients, the condition improves spontaneously 1 to 3 years after onset. While pain usually improves, most patients are left with some limitation of shoulder motion. Early mobilization of the arm following an injury to the shoulder may prevent the development of this disease. Slow but forceful injection of contrast material into the joint may lyse adhesions and stretch the capsule, resulting in improvement of shoulder motion. Manipulation under anesthesia may be helpful in some patients. Once the disease is established, therapy may have little effect on its natural course. Local injections of glucocorticoids, NSAIDs, and physical therapy may provide relief of symptoms.

LATERAL EPICONDYLITIS (TENNIS ELBOW) Lateral epicondylitis, or tennis elbow, is a painful condition involving the soft tissue over the lateral aspect of the elbow. The pain originates at or near the site of attachment of the common extensors to the lateral epicondyle and may radiate into the forearm and dorsum of the wrist. This painful condition is thought to be caused by small tears of the extensor aponeurosis resulting from repeated resisted contractions of the extensor muscles. The pain usually appears after work or recreational activities involving repeated motions of wrist extension and supination against resistance. Most patients with this disorder injure themselves in activities other than tennis, such as pulling weeds, carrying suitcases or briefcases, or using a screwdriver. The injury in tennis usually occurs when hitting a backhand with the elbow flexed. Shaking hands and opening doors can reproduce the pain. Striking the lateral elbow against a solid object may also induce pain.

The treatment is usually rest along with administration of an NSAID. Ultrasound, icing, and friction massage may also help relieve pain. When pain is severe, the elbow is placed in a sling or splinted at 90° of flexion. When the pain is acute and well localized, injection of a glucocorticoid using a small-gauge needle may be effective. Following injection, the patient should be advised to rest the arm for at least 1 month and avoid activities that would aggravate the elbow. Once symptoms have subsided, the patient should begin rehabilitation to strengthen and increase flexibility of the extensor muscles before resuming physical activity involving the arm. A forearm band placed 2.5 to 5.0 cm (1 to 2 in.) below the elbow may help to reduce tension on the extensor muscles at their attachment to the lateral epicondyle. The patient should be advised to restrict activities requiring forcible extension and supination of the wrist. Improvement may take several months. The patient may continue to experience mild pain but, with care, can usually avoid the return of debilitating pain. In an occasional patient, surgical release of the extensor aponeurosis may be necessary.

MEDIAL EPICONDYLITIS Medial epicondylitis is an overuse syndrome resulting in pain over the medial side of the elbow with radiation into the forearm. The cause of this syndrome is considered to be repetitive resisted motions of wrist flexion and pronation, which lead to microtears and granulation tissue at the origin of the pronator teres and forearm flexors, particularly the flexor carpi radialis. This overuse syndrome is usually seen in patients >35 years and is much less common than lateral epicondylitis. It occurs most often in work-related repetitive activities but also occurs with recreational activities such as swinging a golf club (golfer's elbow) or throwing a baseball. On physical examination, there is tenderness just distal to the medial epicondyle over the origin of the forearm flexors. Pain can be reproduced by resisting wrist flexion and pronation with the elbow extended. Radiographs are usually normal. The differential diagnosis of patients with medial elbow symptoms include tears of the pronator teres, acute medial collateral ligament tear, and medial collateral ligament instability. Ulnar neuritis has been found in 25 to 50% of patients with medial epicondylitis and is associated with tenderness over the ulnar nerve at the elbow as well as hypesthesia and paresthesia on the ulnar side of the hand.

The initial treatment of medial epicondylitis is conservative, involving rest, NSAIDs, friction massage, ultrasound, and icing. Some patients may require splinting. Injections of glucocorticoids at the painful site may also be effective. Patients should be instructed to rest at least 1 month. Also, patients should be started on physical therapy once the pain has subsided. In patients with chronic debilitating medial epicondylitis that remains unresponsive after at least a year of treatment, surgical release of the flexor muscle at its origin may be necessary and is often successful.

FURTHER READING

GISPEN JG: Painful shoulder and the reflex sympathetic dystrophy syndrome, in *Arthritis and Allied Conditions*, 14th ed, WJ Koopman (ed). Philadelphia, Lippincott Williams & Wilkins, 2001, pp 2095–2142

LINTNER SA et al: Sports medicine, in *Kelley's Textbook of Rheumatology*, 6th ed, S Ruddy et al (eds). Philadelphia, Saunders, 2001, pp 439–456

MATSEN FA III, ARNTZ CT: Subacromial impingement, in *The Shoulder*, CA Rockwood Jr (ed). Philadelphia, Saunders, 1990, pp 623–646

NEER CS II: Impingement lesions. Clin Orthop 173:70, 1983

317 | PRINCIPLES OF ENDOCRINOLOGY
J. Larry Jameson

The management of endocrine disorders requires an understanding of such disparate areas as intermediary metabolism, reproductive physiology, bone metabolism, and growth. Accordingly, the practice of endocrinology is intimately linked to a conceptual framework for understanding hormone secretion, hormone action, and principles of feedback control systems. The endocrine system is evaluated primarily by measuring hormone concentrations, thereby arming the clinician with valuable diagnostic information. Most disorders of the endocrine system are amenable to effective treatment, once the correct diagnosis is determined. Endocrine deficiency disorders are treated with physiologic hormone replacement; hormone excess conditions, usually due to benign glandular adenomas, are managed by removing tumors surgically or by reducing hormone levels medically.

SCOPE OF ENDOCRINOLOGY

The specialty of endocrinology encompasses the study of glands and the hormones they produce. The term *endocrine* was coined by Starling to contrast the actions of hormones secreted internally (endocrine) with those secreted externally (*exocrine*) or into a lumen, such as the gastrointestinal tract. The term *hormone*, derived from a Greek phrase meaning "to set in motion," aptly describes the dynamic actions of hormones as they elicit cellular responses and regulate physiologic processes through feedback mechanisms.

Unlike many other specialties in medicine, it is not possible to define endocrinology strictly along anatomic lines. The classic endocrine glands—pituitary, thyroid, parathyroid, pancreatic islets, adrenal, and gonads—communicate broadly with other organs through the nervous system, hormones, cytokines, and growth factors. In addition to its traditional synaptic functions, the brain produces a vast array of peptide hormones, spawning the discipline of neuroendocrinology. Through the production of hypothalamic releasing factors, the central nervous system exerts a major regulatory influence over pituitary hormone secretion (Chap. 318). The peripheral nervous system modulates adrenal medulla and pancreatic islet hormone production. The immune and endocrine systems are also intimately intertwined. The adrenal glucocorticoid, cortisol, is a powerful immunosuppressant. Cytokines and interleukins (ILs) have profound effects on the functions of the pituitary, adrenal, thyroid, and gonads. Common endocrine diseases, such as autoimmune thyroid disease and type 1 diabetes mellitus, are caused by dysregulation of immune surveillance and tolerance. Less common diseases such as polyglandular failure, Addison's disease, and lymphocytic hypophysitis also have an immunologic basis.

The interdigitation of endocrinology with physiologic processes in other specialties sometimes blurs the role of hormones. For example, hormones play an important role in maintenance of blood pressure, intravascular volume, and peripheral resistance in the cardiovascular system. Vasoactive substances such as catecholamines, angiotensin II, endothelin, and nitric oxide are involved in dynamic changes of vascular tone, in addition to their multiple roles in other tissues. The heart is the principal source of atrial natriuretic peptide, which acts in classic endocrine fashion to induce natriuresis at a distant target organ (the kidney). Erythropoietin, a traditional circulating hormone, is made in the kidney and stimulates erythropoiesis in the bone marrow (Chap. 52). The kidney is also integrally involved in the renin-angiotensin axis (Chap. 321) and is a primary target of several hormones including parathyroid hormone (PTH), mineralocorticoids, and vasopressin. The gastrointestinal tract produces a surprising number of peptide hormones such as cholecystokinin, ghrelin, gastrin, secretin, and vasoactive intestinal peptide, among many others. Carcinoid and islet tumors can secrete excessive amounts of these hormones, leading to specific clinical syndromes (Chap. 329). Many of these gastrointestinal hormones are also produced in the central nervous system, where their functions remain poorly understood. As new hormones such as inhibin, ghrelin, and leptin are discovered, they become integrated into the science and practice of medicine on the basis of their functional roles rather than their tissues of origin or their structures or mechanisms of action.

Characterization of hormone receptors frequently reveals unexpected relationships to factors in nonendocrine disciplines. The growth hormone (GH) receptor, for example, is a member of the cytokine receptor family. The G protein–coupled receptors (GPCRs), which mediate the actions of many peptide hormones, are used in numerous physiologic processes including vision, smell, and neurotransmission.

It is apparent that hormones and growth factors play an important functional role in all organ systems. Though endocrinologists are not usually involved in the administration of the hormones or growth factors used to treat diseases in other specialties (e.g., cardiology, hematology), the principles of endocrinology can be applied in these cases, thus emphasizing the impact of endocrinology across multiple disciplines.

NATURE OF HORMONES

Hormones can be divided into five major classes: (1) *amino acid derivatives* such as dopamine, catecholamines, and thyroid hormone; (2) *small neuropeptides* such as gonadotropin-releasing hormone (GnRH), thyrotropin-releasing hormone (TRH), somatostatin, and vasopressin; (3) *large proteins* such as insulin, luteinizing hormone (LH), and PTH produced by classic endocrine glands; (4) *steroid hormones* such as cortisol and estrogen that are synthesized from cholesterol-based precursors; and (5) *vitamin derivatives* such as retinoids (vitamin A) and vitamin D. A variety of *peptide growth factors*, most of which act locally, share actions with hormones. As a rule, amino acid derivatives and peptide hormones interact with cell-surface membrane receptors. Steroids, thyroid hormones, vitamin D, and retinoids are lipid-soluble and interact with intracellular nuclear receptors.

HORMONE AND RECEPTOR FAMILIES

Many hormones and receptors can be grouped into families, reflecting their structural similarities (Table 317-1). The evolution of these families generates diverse but highly selective pathways of hormone action. Recognizing these relationships allows extrapolation of information gleaned from one hormone or receptor to other family members.

The glycoprotein hormone family, consisting of thyroid-stimulating hormone (TSH), follicle-stimulating hormone (FSH), LH, and human chorionic gonadotropin (hCG), illustrates many features of related hormones. The glycoprotein hormones are heterodimers that share the α subunit in common; the β subunits are distinct and confer specific biologic actions. The overall three-dimensional architecture of the β subunits is similar, reflecting the locations of conserved disulfide bonds that restrain protein conformation. The cloning of the β-subunit genes from multiple species suggests that this family arose from a common ancestral gene, probably by gene duplication and subsequent divergence to evolve new biologic functions.

As the hormone families enlarge and diverge, their receptors must co-evolve, if new biologic functions are to be derived. Related GPCRs, for example, have evolved for each of the glycoprotein hormones.

TABLE 317-1 *Membrane Receptor Families and Signaling Pathways*

Receptors	Effectors	Signaling Pathways
G protein–coupled seven-transmembrane (GPCR)		
β-Adrenergic	$G_s\alpha$, adenylate cyclase	Stimulation of cyclic AMP
LH, FSH, TSH	Ca^{2+} channels	production, protein kinase
Glucagon		A
PTH, PTHrP		Calmodulin, Ca^{2+}-dependent
ACTH, MSH		kinases
GHRH, CRH		
α-Adrenergic	$G_i\alpha$	Inhibition of cyclic AMP
		production
Somatostatin		Activation of K^+, Ca^{2+}
		channels
TRH, GnRH	G_q, G_{11}	Phospholipase C,
		diacylglycerol, IP_3, protein
		kinase C, voltage-
		dependent Ca^{2+} channels
Receptor tyrosine kinase		
Insulin, IGF-I	Tyrosine kinases, IRS-1 to IRS-4	MAP kinases, PI 3-kinase, RSK
EGF, NGF	Tyrosine kinases, ras	Raf, MAP kinases, RSK
Cytokine receptor–linked kinase		
GH, PRL	JAK, tyrosine kinases	STAT, MAP kinase, PI 3-kinase, IRS-1, IRS-2
Serine Kinase		
Activin, TGF-β, MIS	Serine kinase	Smads

Note: IP_3, inositol triphosphate; IRS, insulin receptor substrates; MAP, mitogen-activated protein; MSH, melanocyte-stimulating hormone; NGF, nerve growth factor; PI, phosphatylinositol; RSK, ribosomal S6 kinase; TGF-β, transforming growth factor β. For all other abbreviations, see text.

These receptors are structurally similar, and each is coupled to the $G_s\alpha$ signaling pathway. However, there is minimal overlap of hormone binding. For example, TSH binds with high specificity to the TSH receptor but interacts minimally with the LH or the FSH receptor. Nonetheless, there can be subtle physiologic consequences of hormone cross-reactivity with other receptors. Very high levels of hCG during pregnancy stimulate the TSH receptor and increase thyroid hormone levels.

Insulin, insulin-like growth factor (IGF) I, and IGF-II share structural similarities that are most apparent when precursor forms of the proteins are compared. In contrast to the high degree of specificity seen with the glycoprotein hormones, there is moderate cross-talk among the members of the insulin/IGF family. High concentrations of an IGF-II precursor produced by certain tumors (e.g., sarcomas) can cause hypoglycemia, partly because of binding to insulin and IGF-I receptors (Chap. 86). High concentrations of insulin also bind to the IGF-I receptor, perhaps accounting for some of the clinical manifestations seen in severe insulin resistance.

Another important example of receptor cross-talk is seen with PTH and parathyroid hormone–related peptide (PTHrP) (Chap. 332). PTH is produced by the parathyroid glands, whereas PTHrP is expressed at high levels during development and by a variety of tumors (Chap. 86). These hormones share amino acid sequence similarity, particularly in their amino-terminal regions. Both hormones bind to a single PTH receptor that is expressed in bone and kidney. Hypercalcemia and hypophosphatemia may therefore result from excessive production of either hormone, making it difficult to distinguish hyperparathyroidism from hypercalcemia of malignancy solely on the basis of serum chemistries. However, sensitive and specific assays for PTH and PTHrP now allow these disorders to be separated more readily.

Based on their specificities for DNA binding sites, the nuclear receptor family can be subdivided into type 1 receptors (GR, MR, AR, ER, PR) that bind steroids and type 2 receptors (TR, VDR, RAR, PPAR) that bind thyroid hormone, vitamin D, retinoic acid, or lipid derivatives. Certain functional domains in nuclear receptors, such as the zinc finger DNA-binding domains, are highly conserved. However,

selective amino acid differences within this domain confer DNA sequence specificity. The hormone-binding domains are more variable, providing great diversity in the array of small molecules that can bind to different nuclear receptors. With few exceptions, hormone binding is highly specific for a single type of nuclear receptor. One exception involves the highly related glucocorticoid and mineralocorticoid receptors. Because the mineralocorticoid receptor also binds glucocorticoids with high affinity, an enzyme (11β-hydroxysteroid dehydrogenase) located in renal tubular cells inactivates glucocorticoids, allowing selective responses to mineralocorticoids such as aldosterone. However, when very high glucocorticoid concentrations occur, as in Cushing's syndrome, the glucocorticoid degradation pathway becomes saturated, allowing excessive cortisol levels to exert mineralocorticoid effects (sodium retention, potassium wasting). This phenomenon is particularly pronounced in ectopic adrenocorticotropic hormone (ACTH) syndromes (Chap. 321). Another example of relaxed nuclear receptor specificity involves the estrogen receptor, which can bind an array of compounds, some of which share little structural similarity to the high-affinity ligand estradiol. This feature of the estrogen receptor makes it susceptible to activation by "environmental estrogens" such as resveratrol, octylphenol, and many other aromatic hydrocarbons. On the other hand, this lack of specificity provides an opportunity to synthesize a remarkable series of clinically useful antagonists (e.g., tamoxifen) and selective estrogen response modulators (SERMs), such as raloxifene. These compounds generate distinct conformations that alter receptor interactions with components of the transcription machinery (see below), thereby conferring their unique actions.

HORMONE SYNTHESIS AND PROCESSING

The synthesis of peptide hormones and their receptors occurs through a classic pathway of gene expression: transcription → mRNA → protein → posttranslational protein processing → intracellular sorting, membrane integration, or secretion (Chap. 56). Though endocrine genes contain regulatory DNA elements similar to those found in many other genes, their exquisite control by other hormones also necessitates the presence of specific hormone response elements. For example, the TSH genes are repressed directly by thyroid hormones acting through the thyroid hormone receptor, a member of the nuclear receptor family. Steroidogenic enzyme gene expression requires specific transcription factors such as steroidogenic factor-1 (SF-1), acting in conjunction with signals transmitted by trophic hormones (e.g., ACTH or LH). For some hormones, substantial regulation occurs at the level of translational efficiency. Insulin biosynthesis, while requiring ongoing gene transcription, is regulated primarily at the translational level in response to elevated levels of glucose or amino acids.

Many hormones are embedded within larger precursor polypeptides that are proteolytically processed to yield the biologically active hormone. Examples include: proopiomelanocortin (POMC) → ACTH; proglucagon → glucagon; proinsulin → insulin; pro-PTH → PTH, among others. In many cases, such as POMC and proglucagon, these precursors generate multiple biologically active peptides. It is provocative that hormone precursors are typically inactive, presumably adding an additional level of regulatory control. This is true not only for peptide hormones but also for certain steroids (testosterone → dihydrotestosterone) and thyroid hormone (T_4 → T_3).

Hormone precursor processing is intimately linked to intracellular sorting pathways that transport proteins to appropriate vesicles and enzymes, resulting in specific cleavage steps, followed by protein folding and translocation to secretory vesicles. Hormones destined for secretion are translocated across the endoplasmic reticulum under the guidance of an amino-terminal signal sequence that is subsequently cleaved. Cell-surface receptors are inserted into the membrane via short segments of hydrophobic amino acids that remain embedded within the lipid bilayer. During translocation through the Golgi and endoplasmic reticulum, hormones and receptors are also subject to a variety of posttranslational modifications, such as glycosylation and phosphorylation, which can alter protein conformation, modify circulating half-life, and alter biologic activity.

Synthesis of most steroid hormones is based on modifications of the precursor, cholesterol. Multiple regulated enzymatic steps are required for the synthesis of testosterone (Chap. 325), estradiol (Chap. 326), cortisol (Chap. 321), and vitamin D (Chap. 331). This large number of synthetic steps predisposes to multiple genetic and acquired disorders of steroidogenesis.

HORMONE SECRETION, TRANSPORT, AND DEGRADATION

The circulating level of a hormone is determined by its rate of secretion and its circulating half-life. After protein processing, peptide hormones (GnRH, insulin, GH) are stored in secretory granules. As these granules mature, they are poised beneath the plasma membrane for imminent release into the circulation. In most instances, the stimulus for hormone secretion is a releasing factor or neural signal that induces rapid changes in intracellular calcium concentrations, leading to secretory granule fusion with the plasma membrane and release of its contents into the extracellular environment and bloodstream. Steroid hormones, in contrast, diffuse into the circulation as they are synthesized. Thus, their secretory rates are closely aligned with rates of synthesis. For example, ACTH and LH induce steroidogenesis by stimulating the activity of *s*teroidogenic *a*cute *r*egulatory (StAR) protein (transports cholesterol into the mitochondrion) along with other rate-limiting steps (e.g., cholesterol side-chain cleavage enzyme, CYP11A1) in the steroidogenic pathway.

Hormone transport and degradation dictate the rapidity with which a hormonal signal decays. Some hormonal signals are evanescent (e.g., somatostatin), whereas others are longer lived (e.g., TSH). Because somatostatin exerts effects in virtually every tissue, a short half-life allows its concentrations and actions to be controlled locally. Structural modifications that impair somatostatin degradation have been useful for generating long-acting therapeutic analogues, such as octreotide (Chap. 318). On the other hand, the actions of TSH are highly specific for the thyroid gland. Its prolonged half-life accounts for relatively constant serum levels, even though TSH is secreted in discrete pulses.

An understanding of circulating hormone half-life is important for achieving physiologic hormone replacement, as the frequency of dosing and the time required to reach steady state are intimately linked to rates of hormone decay. T_4, for example, has a circulating half-life of 7 days. Consequently, >1 month is required to reach a new steady state, but single daily doses are sufficient to achieve constant hormone levels. T_3, in contrast, has a half-life of 1 day. Its administration is associated with more dynamic serum levels and it must be administered two to three times per day. Similarly, synthetic glucocorticoids vary widely in their half-lives; those with longer half-lives (e.g., dexamethasone) are associated with greater suppression of the hypothalamic-pituitary-adrenal (HPA) axis. Most protein hormones [e.g., ACTH, GH, prolactin (PRL); PTH, LH] have relatively short half-lives (<20 min), leading to sharp peaks of secretion and decay. The only accurate way to profile the pulse frequency and amplitude of these hormones is to measure levels in frequently sampled blood (every 10 min) over long durations (8 to 24 h). Because this is not practical in

a clinical setting, an alternative strategy is to pool three to four samples drawn at about 30-min intervals, recognizing that pulsatile secretion makes it difficult to establish a narrow normal range. Rapid hormone decay is useful in certain clinical settings. For example, the short half-life of PTH allows the use of intraoperative PTH determinations to confirm successful removal of an adenoma. This is particularly valuable diagnostically when there is a possibility of multicentric disease or parathyroid hyperplasia, as occurs with multiple endocrine neoplasia (MEN) or renal insufficiency.

Many hormones circulate in association with serum-binding proteins. Examples include: (1) T_4 and T_3 binding to thyroxine-binding globulin (TBG), albumin, and thyroxine-binding prealbumin (TBPA); (2) cortisol binding to cortisol-binding globulin (CBG); (3) androgen and estrogen binding to sex hormone–binding globulin (SHBG) (also called testosterone-binding globulin, TeBG); (4) IGF-I and -II binding to multiple IGF-binding proteins (IGFBPs); (5) GH interactions with GH-binding protein (GHBP), a circulating fragment of the GH receptor extracellular domain; and (6) activin binding to follistatin. These interactions provide a hormonal reservoir, prevent otherwise rapid degradation of unbound hormones, restrict hormone access to certain sites (e.g., IGFBPs), and modulate the unbound, or "free," hormone concentrations. Although a variety of binding protein abnormalities have been identified, most have little clinical consequence, aside from creating diagnostic problems. For example, TBG deficiency can greatly reduce total thyroid hormone levels, but the free concentrations of T_4 and T_3 remain normal. Liver disease and certain medications can also influence binding protein levels (e.g., estrogen increases TBG) or cause displacement of hormones from binding proteins (e.g., salsalate displaces T_4 from TBG). Only unbound hormone is available to interact with receptors and thereby elicit a biologic response. Short-term perturbations in binding proteins change the free hormone concentration, which in turn induces compensatory adaptations through feedback loops. SHBG changes in women are an exception to this self-correcting mechanism. When SHBG decreases because of insulin resistance or androgen excess, the unbound testosterone concentration is increased, potentially leading to hirsutism (Chap. 44). The increased unbound testosterone level does not result in an adequate compensatory feedback correction because estrogen, and not testosterone, is the primary regulator of the reproductive axis.

HORMONE ACTION THROUGH RECEPTORS

Receptors for hormones are divided into two major classes—membrane and nuclear. *Membrane receptors* primarily bind peptide hormones and catecholamines. *Nuclear receptors* bind small molecules that can diffuse across the cell membrane, such as thyroid hormone, steroids, and vitamin D. Certain general principles apply to hormone-receptor interactions, regardless of the class of receptor. Hormones bind to receptors with specificity and a high affinity that generally coincides with the dynamic range of circulating hormone concentrations. Low concentrations of free hormone (usually 10^{-12} to 10^{-9} M) rapidly associate and dissociate from receptors in a bimolecular reaction, such that the occupancy of the receptor at any given moment is a function of hormone concentration and the receptor's affinity for the hormone. Receptor numbers vary greatly in different target tissues, providing one of the major determinants of specific cellular responses to circulating hormones. For example, ACTH receptors are located almost exclusively in the adrenal cortex, and FSH receptors are found only in the gonads. In contrast, insulin and thyroid hormone receptors are widely distributed, reflecting the need for metabolic responses in all tissues.

MEMBRANE RECEPTORS

Membrane receptors for hormones can be divided into several major groups: (1) seven transmembrane GPCRs, (2) tyrosine kinase receptors, (3) cytokine receptors, and (4) serine kinase receptors (Fig. 317-

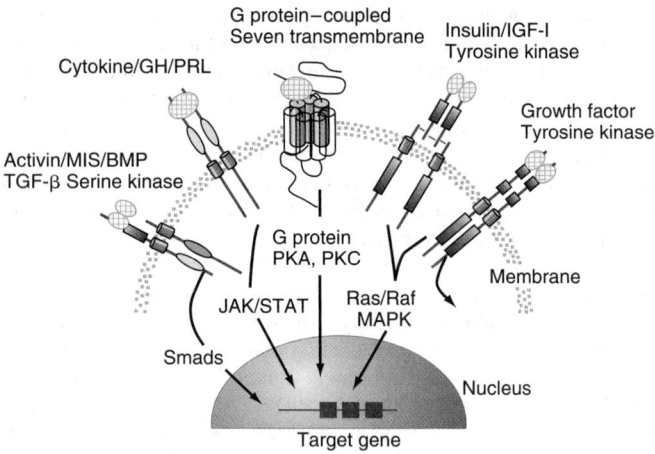

FIGURE 317-1   Membrane receptor signaling. MAPK, mitogen-activated protein kinase; PKA, -C, protein kinase A, C; TGF, transforming growth factor. For other abbreviations, see text.

1). The *seven transmembrane GPCR family* binds a remarkable array of hormones including large proteins (e.g., LH, PTH), small peptides (e.g., TRH, somatostatin), catecholamines (epinephrine, dopamine), and even minerals (e.g., calcium). The extracellular domains of GPCRs vary widely in size and are the major binding site for large hormones. The transmembrane-spanning regions are composed of hydrophobic α-helical domains that traverse the lipid bilayer. Like some channels, these domains are thought to circularize and form a hydrophobic pocket into which certain small ligands fit. Hormone binding induces conformational changes in these domains, transducing structural changes to the intracellular domain, which is a docking site for G proteins.

The large family of *G proteins*, so named because they bind guanine nucleotides (GTP, GDP), provides great diversity for coupling signaling pathways to different receptors. G proteins form a heterotrimeric complex that is composed of various α and $\beta\gamma$ subunits. The α subunit contains the guanine nucleotide–binding site and hydrolyzes GTP → GDP. The $\beta\gamma$ subunits are tightly associated and modulate the activity of the α subunit, as well as mediating their own effector signaling pathways. G protein activity is regulated by a cycle that

involves GTP hydrolysis and dynamic interactions between the α and $\beta\gamma$ subunits. Hormone binding to the receptor induces GDP dissociation, allowing Gα to bind GTP and dissociate from the $\beta\gamma$ complex. Under these conditions, the Gα subunit is activated and mediates signal transduction through various enzymes such as adenylate cyclase or phospholipase C. GTP hydrolysis to GDP allows reassociation with the $\beta\gamma$ subunits and restores the inactive state. As described below, a variety of endocrinopathies result from G protein mutations or from mutations in receptors that modify their interactions with G proteins.

There are more than a dozen isoforms of the Gα subunit. G$_s\alpha$ stimulates, whereas G$_i\alpha$ inhibits adenylate cyclase, an enzyme that generates the second messenger, cyclic AMP, leading to activation of protein kinase A (Table 317-1). G$_q$ subunits couple to phospholipase C, generating diacylglycerol and inositol triphosphate, leading to activation of protein kinase C and the release of intracellular calcium.

The *tyrosine kinase receptors* transduce signals for insulin and a variety of growth factors, such as IGF-I, epidermal growth factor (EGF), nerve growth factor, platelet-derived growth factor, and fibroblast growth factor. The cysteine-rich extracellular ligand-binding domains contain growth factor binding sites. After ligand binding, this class of receptors undergoes autophosphorylation, inducing interactions with intracellular adaptor proteins such as Shc and insulin receptor substrates 1 to 4. In the case of the insulin receptor, multiple kinases are activated including the Raf-Ras-MAPK and the Akt/protein kinase B pathways. The tyrosine kinase receptors play a prominent role in cell growth and differentiation as well as in intermediary metabolism.

The GH and PRL receptors belong to the *cytokine receptor* family (Chap. 295). Analogous to the tyrosine kinase receptors, ligand binding induces receptor interaction with intracellular kinases—the Janus kinases (JAKs), which phosphorylate members of the signal transduction and activators of transcription (STAT) family—as well as other signaling pathways (Ras, PI3-K, MAPK). The activated STAT proteins translocate to the nucleus and stimulate expression of target genes (Chap. 318).

The *serine kinase receptors* mediate the actions of activins, transforming growth factor β, müllerian-inhibiting substance (MIS, also known as anti-müllerian hormone, AMH), and bone morphogenic proteins (BMPs). This family of receptors (consisting of type I and II subunits) signal through proteins termed *smads* (fusion of terms for *Caenorhabditis elegans* sma + mammalian mad). Like the STAT proteins, the smads serve a dual role of transducing the receptor signal and acting as transcription factors. The pleomorphic actions of these growth factors dictate that they act primarily in a local (paracrine or autocrine) manner. Binding proteins, such as follistatin (which binds activin and other members of this family), function to inactivate the growth factors and restrict their distribution.

NUCLEAR RECEPTORS

The family of nuclear receptors has grown to nearly 100 members, many of which are still classified as orphan receptors because their ligands, if they exist, remain to be identified (Fig. 317-2). Otherwise, most nuclear receptors are classified based on the nature of their ligands. Though all nuclear receptors ultimately act to increase or decrease gene transcription, some (e.g., glucocorticoid receptor) reside primarily in the cytoplasm, whereas others (e.g., thyroid hormone receptor) are always located in the nucleus. After ligand binding, the cytoplasmically localized receptors translocate to the nucleus. There is growing evidence that certain nuclear receptors

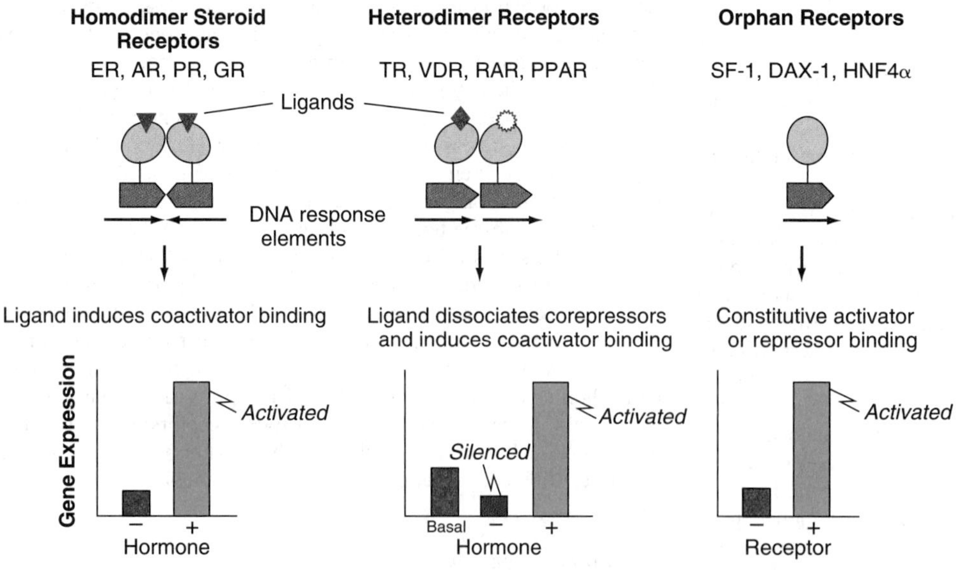

Homodimer Steroid Receptors
ER, AR, PR, GR

Heterodimer Receptors
TR, VDR, RAR, PPAR

Orphan Receptors
SF-1, DAX-1, HNF4α

Ligands — DNA response elements

Ligand induces coactivator binding — Ligand dissociates corepressors and induces coactivator binding — Constitutive activator or repressor binding

Gene Expression

Activated / Silenced / Activated / Activated

Basal − +   − +   − +
Hormone   Hormone   Receptor

FIGURE 317-2   Nuclear receptor signaling. ER, estrogen receptor; AR, androgen receptor; PR, progesterone receptor; GR, glucocorticoid receptor; TR, thyroid hormone receptor; VDR, vitamin D receptor; RAR, retinoic acid receptor; PPAR, peroxisome proliferator activated receptor; SF-1, steroidogenic factor-1; DAX, *dosage sensitive sex-reversal, adrenal hypoplasia congenita, X-chromosome*; HNF4α, hepatic nuclear factor 4α.

(e.g., glucocorticoid, estrogen) can also activate or repress signal transduction pathways, providing a mechanism for cross-talk between membrane and nuclear receptors.

The structures of nuclear receptors have been extensively studied, including by x-ray crystallography. The DNA binding domain, consisting of two zinc fingers, contacts specific DNA recognition sequences in target genes. Most nuclear receptors bind to DNA as dimers. Consequently, each monomer recognizes an individual DNA motif, referred to as a "half-site." The steroid receptors, including the glucocorticoid, estrogen, progesterone, and androgen receptors, bind to DNA as homodimers. Consistent with this twofold symmetry, their DNA recognition half-sites are palindromic. The thyroid, retinoid, peroxisome proliferator activated, and vitamin D receptors bind to DNA preferentially as heterodimers in combination with retinoid X receptors (RXRs). Their DNA half-sites are arranged as direct repeats. Receptor specificity for DNA sequences is determined by (1) the sequence of the half-site, (2) the orientation of the half-sites (palindromic, direct repeat), and (3) the spacing between the half-sites. For example, vitamin D, thyroid, and retinoid receptors recognize similar tandemly repeated half-sites (TAAGTCA), but these DNA repeats are spaced by three, four, and five nucleotides, respectively.

The carboxy-terminal hormone-binding domain mediates transcriptional control. For type II receptors, such as thyroid hormone receptor (TR) and retinoic acid receptor (RAR), co-repressor proteins bind to the receptor in the absence of ligand and silence gene transcription. Hormone binding induces conformational changes, triggering the release of co-repressors and inducing the recruitment of coactivators that stimulate transcription. Thus, these receptors are capable of mediating dramatic changes in the level of gene activity. Certain disease states are associated with defective regulation of these events. For example, mutations in the TR prevent co-repressor dissociation, resulting in a dominant form of hormone resistance (Chap. 320). In promyelocytic leukemia, fusion of RARα to other nuclear proteins causes aberrant gene silencing and prevents normal cellular differentiation. Treatment with retinoic acid reverses this repression and allows cellular differentiation and apoptosis to occur (Chap. 96). Most type 1 steroid receptors do not interact with co-repressors, but ligand binding still mediates interactions with an array of coactivators. X-ray crystallography shows that various SERMs induce distinct receptor conformations. The tissue-specific responses caused by these agents in breast, bone, and uterus appear to reflect distinct interactions with coactivators. The receptor-coactivator complex stimulates gene transcription by several pathways including (1) recruitment of enzymes (histone acetyl transferases) that modify chromatin structure, (2) interactions with additional transcription factors on the target gene, and (3) direct interactions with components of the general transcription apparatus to enhance the rate of RNA polymerase II–mediated transcription.

FUNCTIONS OF HORMONES

The functions of individual hormones are described in detail in subsequent chapters. Nevertheless, it is useful to illustrate how most biologic responses require integration of several different hormonal pathways. The physiologic functions of hormones can be divided into three general areas: (1) growth and differentiation, (2) maintenance of homeostasis, and (3) reproduction.

GROWTH

Multiple hormones and nutritional factors mediate the complex phenomenon of growth (Chap. 318). Short stature may be caused by GH deficiency, hypothyroidism, Cushing's syndrome, precocious puberty, malnutrition or chronic illness, or genetic abnormalities that affect the epiphyseal growth plates (e.g., *FGFR3* or *SHOX* mutations). Many factors (GH, IGF-I, thyroid hormone) stimulate growth, whereas others (sex steroids) lead to epiphyseal closure. Understanding these hormonal interactions is important in the diagnosis and management of growth disorders. For example, delaying exposure to high levels of sex steroids may enhance the efficacy of GH treatment.

MAINTENANCE OF HOMEOSTASIS

Though virtually all hormones affect homeostasis, the most important among these are the following:

1. Thyroid hormone—controls about 25% of basal metabolism in most tissues
2. Cortisol—exerts a permissive action for many hormones in addition to its own direct effects
3. PTH—regulates calcium and phosphorus levels
4. Vasopressin—regulates serum osmolality by controlling renal free water clearance
5. Mineralocorticoids—control vascular volume and serum electrolyte (Na^+, K^+) concentrations
6. Insulin—maintains euglycemia in the fed and fasted states

The defense against hypoglycemia is an impressive example of integrated hormone action (Chap. 324). In response to the fasted state and falling blood glucose, insulin secretion is suppressed, resulting in decreased glucose uptake and enhanced glycogenolysis, lipolysis, proteolysis, and gluconeogenesis to mobilize fuel sources. If hypoglycemia develops (usually from insulin administration or sulfonylureas), an orchestrated counterregulatory response occurs—glucagon and epinephrine rapidly stimulate glycogenolysis and gluconeogenesis, whereas GH and cortisol act over several hours to raise glucose levels and antagonize insulin action.

Although free water clearance is primarily controlled by vasopressin, cortisol and thyroid hormone are also important for facilitating renal tubular responses to vasopressin (Chap. 319). PTH and vitamin D function in an interdependent manner to control calcium metabolism (Chap. 331). PTH stimulates renal synthesis of 1,25 dihydroxyvitamin D, which increases calcium absorption in the gastrointestinal tract and enhances PTH action in bone. Increased calcium, along with vitamin D, feeds back to suppress PTH, thereby maintaining calcium balance.

Depending on the severity of a given stress and whether it is acute or chronic, multiple endocrine and cytokine pathways are activated to mount an appropriate physiologic response (Chap. 318). In severe acute stress such as trauma or shock, the sympathetic nervous system is activated and catecholamines are released, leading to increased cardiac output and a primed musculoskeletal system. Catecholamines also increase mean blood pressure and stimulate glucose production. Multiple stress-induced pathways converge on the hypothalamus, stimulating several hormones including vasopressin and corticotropin-releasing hormone (CRH). These hormones, in addition to cytokines (tumor necrosis factor α, IL-2, IL-6), increase ACTH and GH production. ACTH stimulates the adrenal gland, increasing cortisol, which in turn helps to sustain blood pressure and dampen the inflammatory response. Increased vasopressin acts to conserve free water.

REPRODUCTION

The stages of reproduction include: (1) sex determination during fetal development (Chap. 328); (2) sexual maturation during puberty (Chaps. 325 and 326); (3) conception, pregnancy, lactation, and child-rearing (Chap. 326); and (4) cessation of reproductive capability at menopause (Chap. 327). Each of these stages involves an orchestrated interplay of multiple hormones, a phenomenon well illustrated by the dynamic hormonal changes that occur during each 28-day menstrual cycle. In the early follicular phase, pulsatile secretion of LH and FSH stimulates the progressive maturation of the ovarian follicle. This results in gradually increasing estrogen and progesterone levels, leading to enhanced pituitary sensitivity to GnRH, which, when combined with accelerated GnRH secretion, triggers the LH surge and rupture of the mature follicle. Inhibin, a protein produced by the granulosa cells, enhances follicular growth and feeds back to the pituitary to selectively suppress FSH, without affecting LH. Growth factors such as EGF and IGF-I modulate follicular responsiveness to gonadotropins. Vascular endothelial growth factor and prostaglandins play a role in follicle vascularization and rupture.

During pregnancy, the increased production of prolactin, in combination with placentally derived steroids (e.g., estrogen and progesterone), prepares the breast for lactation. Estrogens induce the production of progesterone receptors, allowing for increased responsiveness to progesterone. In addition to these and other hormones involved in lactation, the nervous system and oxytocin mediate the suckling response and milk release.

HORMONAL FEEDBACK REGULATORY SYSTEMS

Feedback control, both negative and positive, is a fundamental feature of endocrine systems. Each of the major hypothalamic-pituitary-hormone axes is governed by negative feedback, a process that maintains hormone levels within a relatively narrow range (Chap. 318). Examples of hypothalamic-pituitary negative feedback include (1) thyroid hormones on the TRH-TSH axis, (2) cortisol on the CRH-ACTH axis, (3) gonadal steroids on the GnRH-LH/FSH axis, and (4) IGF-I on the growth hormone–releasing hormone (GHRH)-GH axis (Fig. 317-3). These regulatory loops include both positive (e.g., TRH, TSH) and negative components (e.g., T_4, T_3), allowing for exquisite control of hormone levels. As an example, a small reduction of thyroid hormone triggers a rapid increase of TRH and TSH secretion, resulting in thyroid gland stimulation and increased thyroid hormone production. When the thyroid hormone reaches a normal level, it feeds back to suppress TRH and TSH, and a new steady state is attained. Feedback regulation also occurs for endocrine systems that do not involve the pituitary gland, such as calcium feedback on PTH, glucose inhibition of insulin secretion, and leptin feedback on the hypothalamus. An understanding of feedback regulation provides important insights into endocrine testing paradigms (see below).

Positive feedback control also occurs but is not well understood. The primary example is estrogen-mediated stimulation of the midcycle LH surge. Though chronic low levels of estrogen are inhibitory, gradually rising estrogen levels stimulate LH secretion. This effect, which is illustrative of an endocrine rhythm (see below), involves activation of the hypothalamic GnRH pulse generator. In addition, estrogen-primed gonadotropes are extraordinarily sensitive to GnRH, leading to a 10- to 20-fold amplification of LH release.

PARACRINE AND AUTOCRINE CONTROL

The aforementioned examples of feedback control involve classic endocrine pathways in which hormones are released by one gland and act on a distant target gland. However, local regulatory systems, often involving growth factors, are increasingly recognized. *Paracrine regulation* refers to factors released by one cell that act on an adjacent cell in the same tissue. For example, somatostatin secretion by pancreatic islet δ cells inhibits insulin secretion from nearby β cells. *Autocrine regulation* describes the action of a factor on the same cell from which it is produced. IGF-I acts on many cells that produce it, including chondrocytes, breast epithelium, and gonadal cells. Unlike endocrine actions, paracrine and autocrine control are difficult to document because local growth factor concentrations cannot be readily measured.

Anatomic relationships of glandular systems also greatly influence hormonal exposure—the physical organization of islet cells enhances their intercellular communication; the portal vasculature of the hypothalamic-pituitary system exposes the pituitary to high concentrations of hypothalamic releasing factors; testicular seminiferous tubules gain exposure to high testosterone levels produced by the interdigitated Leydig cells; the pancreas receives nutrient information from the gastrointestinal tract; and the liver is the proximal target of insulin action because of portal drainage from the pancreas.

HORMONAL RHYTHMS

The feedback regulatory systems described above are superimposed on hormonal rhythms that are used for adaptation to the environment. Seasonal changes, the daily occurrence of the light-dark cycle, sleep, meals, and stress are examples of the many environmental events that affect hormonal rhythms. The *menstrual cycle* is repeated on average every 28 days, reflecting the time required to follicular maturation and ovulation (Chap. 326). Essentially all pituitary hormone rhythms are entrained to sleep and the *circadian cycle*, generating reproducible patterns that are repeated approximately every 24 h. The HPA axis, for example, exhibits characteristic peaks of ACTH and cortisol production in the early morning, with a nadir during the night. Recognition of these rhythms is important for endocrine testing and treatment. Patients with Cushing's syndrome characteristically exhibit increased midnight cortisol levels when compared to normal individuals (Chap. 321). In contrast, morning cortisol levels are similar in these groups, as cortisol is normally high at this time of day in normal individuals. The HPA axis is more susceptible to suppression by glucocorticoids administered at night as they blunt the early morning rise of ACTH. Understanding these rhythms allows glucocorticoid replacement that mimics diurnal production by administering larger doses in the morning than in the afternoon (Chap. 321). Disrupted sleep rhythms can alter hormonal regulation. For example, sleep deprivation causes mild insulin resistance and hypertension, which are reversible at least in the short term.

Other endocrine rhythms occur on a more rapid time scale. Many peptide hormones are secreted in discrete bursts every few hours. LH and FSH secretion are exquisitely sensitive to GnRH pulse frequency. Intermittent pulses of GnRH are required to maintain pituitary sensitivity, whereas continuous exposure to GnRH causes pituitary gonadotrope desensitization. This feature of the hypothalamic-pituitary-gonadotrope (HPG) axis forms the basis for using long-acting GnRH agonists to treat central precocious puberty or to decrease testosterone levels in the management of prostate cancer.

It is important to be aware of the pulsatile nature of hormone secretion and the rhythmic patterns of hormone production when relating serum hormone measurements to normal values. For some hormones, integrated markers have been developed to circumvent hormonal fluctuations. Examples include 24-h urine collections for cortisol, IGF-I as a biologic marker of GH action, and HbA1c as an index of long-term (weeks to months) blood glucose control.

Often, one must interpret endocrine data only in the context of other hormonal results. For example, PTH levels are typically assessed in combination with serum calcium concentrations. A high serum calcium level in association with elevated PTH is suggestive of hyperparathyroidism, whereas a suppressed PTH in this situation is more likely to be caused by hypercalcemia of malignancy or other causes of hypercalcemia. Similarly, TSH should be elevated when T_4 and T_3

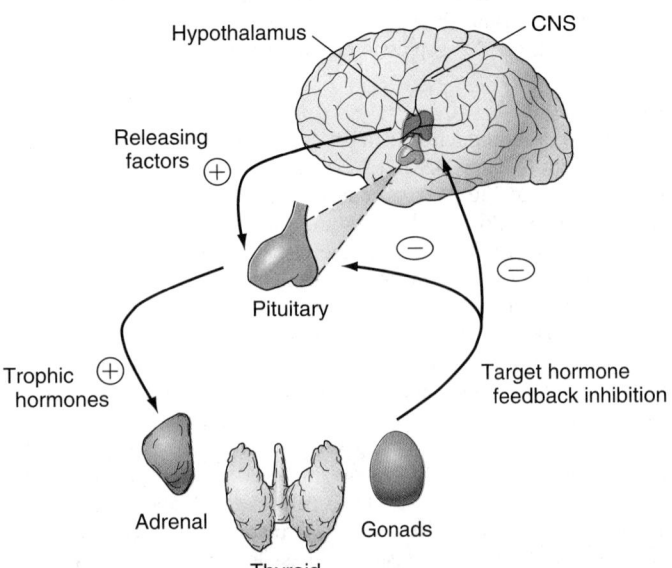

FIGURE 317-3   Feedback regulation of endocrine axes. CNS, central nervous system.

concentrations are low, reflecting reduced feedback inhibition. When this is not the case, it is important to consider other abnormalities in the hormonal axis, such as secondary hypothyroidism, which is caused by a defect at the level of the pituitary.

PATHOLOGIC MECHANISMS OF ENDOCRINE DISEASE

Endocrine diseases can be divided into three major types of conditions: (1) hormone excess, (2) hormone deficiency, and (3) hormone resistance (Table 317-2).

CAUSES OF HORMONE EXCESS

Syndromes of hormone excess can be caused by neoplastic growth of endocrine cells, autoimmune disorders, and excess hormone administration. Benign endocrine tumors, including parathyroid, pituitary, and adrenal adenomas, often retain the capacity to produce hormones, perhaps reflecting the fact that they are relatively well differentiated. Many endocrine tumors exhibit subtle defects in their "set points" for feedback regulation. For example, in Cushing's disease, impaired feedback inhibition of ACTH secretion is associated with autonomous function. However, the tumor cells are not completely resistant to feedback, as evidenced by ACTH suppression by higher doses of dexamethasone (e.g., high-dose dexamethasone test) (Chap. 321). Similar

set point defects are also typical of parathyroid adenomas and autonomously functioning thyroid nodules.

The molecular basis of some endocrine tumors, such as the MEN syndromes (MEN 1, 2A, 2B), have provided important insights into tumorigenesis (Chap. 330). MEN 1 is characterized primarily by the triad of parathyroid, pancreatic islet, and pituitary tumors. MEN 2 predisposes to medullary thyroid carcinoma, pheochromocytoma, and hyperparathyroidism. The *MEN1* gene, located on chromosome 11q13, encodes a putative tumor-suppressor gene, menin. Analogous to the paradigm first described for retinoblastoma, the affected individual inherits a mutant copy of the *MEN1* gene, and tumorigenesis ensues after a somatic "second hit" leads to loss of function of the normal *MEN1* gene (through deletion or point mutations).

In contrast to inactivation of a tumor-suppressor gene, as occurs in MEN 1 and most other inherited cancer syndromes, MEN 2 is caused by activating mutations in a single allele. In this case, activating mutations of the *RET* proto-oncogene, which encodes a receptor tyrosine kinase, leads to thyroid C-cell hyperplasia in childhood before the development of medullary thyroid carcinoma. Elucidation of the pathogenic mechanism has allowed early genetic screening for *RET* mutations in individuals at risk for MEN 2, permitting identification of those who may benefit from prophylactic thyroidectomy and biochemical screening for pheochromocytoma and hyperparathyroidism.

Mutations that activate hormone receptor signaling have been identified in several GPCRs. For example, activating mutations of the LH receptor cause a dominantly transmitted form of male-limited precocious puberty, reflecting premature stimulation of testosterone synthesis in Leydig cells (Chap. 325). Activating mutations in these GPCRs are predominantly located in the transmembrane domains and induce receptor coupling to $G_s\alpha$, even in the absence of hormone. Consequently, adenylate cyclase is activated and cyclic AMP levels increase in a manner that mimics hormone action. A similar phenomenon results from activating mutations in $G_s\alpha$. When these occur early in development, they cause McCune-Albright syndrome. When they occur only in somatotropes, the activating $G_s\alpha$ mutations cause GH-secreting tumors and acromegaly (Chap. 318).

In autoimmune Graves' disease, antibody interactions with the TSH receptor mimic TSH action, leading to hormone overproduction (Chap. 320). Analogous to the effects of activating mutations of the TSH receptor, these stimulating autoantibodies induce conformational changes that release the receptor from a constrained state, thereby triggering receptor coupling to G proteins.

CAUSES OF HORMONE DEFICIENCY

Most examples of hormone deficiency states can be attributed to glandular destruction caused by autoimmunity, surgery, infection, inflammation, infarction, hemorrhage, or tumor infiltration (Table 317-2). Autoimmune damage to the thyroid gland (Hashimoto's thyroiditis) and pancreatic islet β cells (type 1 diabetes mellitus) is a prevalent cause of endocrine disease. Mutations in a number of hormones, hormone receptors, transcription factors, enzymes, and channels can also lead to hormone deficiencies.

HORMONE RESISTANCE

Most severe hormone resistance syndromes are due to inherited defects in membrane receptors, nuclear receptors, or in the pathways that transduce receptor signals. These disorders are characterized by defective hormone action, despite the presence of increased hormone levels. In complete androgen resistance, for example, mutations in the androgen receptor cause genetic (XY) males to have a female phenotypic appearance, even though LH and testosterone levels are increased (Chap. 328). In addition to these relatively rare genetic disorders, more common acquired forms of functional hormone resistance include insulin resistance in type 2 diabetes mellitus, leptin resistance in obesity, and GH resistance in catabolic states. The pathogenesis of functional resistance involves receptor downregulation and

---

TABLE 317-2 *Causes of Endocrine Dysfunction*

Type of Endocrine Disorder	Examples
Hyperfunction	
Neoplastic	
Benign	Pituitary adenomas, hyperparathyroidism, autonomous thyroid or adrenal nodules, pheochromocytoma
Malignant	Adrenal cancer, medullary thyroid cancer, carcinoid
Ectopic	Ectopic ACTH, SIADH secretion
Multiple endocrine neoplasia	MEN1, MEN2
Autoimmune	Graves' disease
Iatrogenic	Cushing's syndrome, hypoglycemia
Infectious/inflammatory	Subacute thyroiditis
Activating receptor mutations	LH, TSH, Ca^{2+} and PTH receptors, $G_s\alpha$
Hypofunction	
Autoimmune	Hashimoto's thyroiditis, type 1 diabetes mellitus, Addison's disease, polyglandular failure
Iatrogenic	Radiation-induced hypopituitarism, hypothyroidism, surgical
Infectious/inflammatory	Adrenal insufficiency, hypothalamic sarcoidosis
Hormone mutations	GH, LHβ, FSHβ, vasopressin
Enzyme defects	21-Hydroxylase deficiency
Developmental defects	Kallmann syndrome, Turner syndrome, transcription factors
Nutritional/vitamin deficiency	Vitamin D deficiency, iodine deficiency
Hemorrhage/infarction	Sheehan's syndrome, adrenal insufficiency
Hormone resistance	
Receptor mutations	
Membrane	GH, vasopressin, LH, FSH, ACTH, GnRH, GHRH, PTH, leptin, Ca^{2+}
Nuclear	AR, TR, VDR, ER, GR, PPAR$_\gamma$
Signaling pathway mutations	Albright's hereditary osteodystrophy
Postreceptor	Type 2 diabetes mellitus, leptin resistance

Note: AR, androgen receptor; ER, estrogen receptor; GR, glucocorticoid receptor; PPAR, peroxisome proliferator activated receptor; SIADH, syndrome of inappropriate antidiuretic hormone; TR, thyroid hormone receptor; VDR, vitamin D receptor. For all other abbreviations, see text.

Disorder	Approx. Prevalence in Adults[a]	Screening/Testing Recommendations[b]	Specific Guidelines	Chapter
Obesity	23% BMI > 30 50% BMI > 25	Calculate BMI Measure waist circumference Exclude secondary causes Consider comorbid complications	NHLBI Clinical Guidelines on the Identification, Evaluation, and Treatment of Overweight and Obesity	64
Type 2 diabetes mellitus	>6%	Test every 3 years or more often in high-risk groups: Fasting plasma glucose (FPG) > 126 mg/dL Random plasma glucose > 200 mg/dL An elevated HbA1c Consider comorbid complications	Expert Committee on the Diagnosis and Classification of Diabetes Mellitus	323
Hyperlipidemia	15–20%	Cholesterol screening at least every 5 years; more often in high-risk groups Lipoprotein analysis (LDL, HDL) for increased cholesterol, CAD, diabetes Consider secondary causes	Expert Panel of the National Cholesterol Education Program (NCEP)	335
Hypothyroidism	5–10%, women 0.5–2%, men	TSH; confirm with free T_4 Screen women after age 35 and every 5 years thereafter	American Thyroid Association	320
Graves' disease	1–3%, women 0.1%, men	TSH, free T_4		320
Thyroid nodules and neoplasia	5%	Physical examination of thyroid Fine-needle aspiration biopsy	American Thyroid Association	320
Osteoporosis	5%, women 1%, men	Bone mineral density measurements in women >65 years or in postmenopausal women or men at risk Exclude secondary causes	World Health Organization National Osteoporosis Foundation	333
Hyperparathyroidism	0.1–0.5%, women > men	Serum calcium PTH, if calcium is elevated Assess comorbid conditions	NIH Consensus Conference on Diagnosis and Management of Asymptomatic Primary Hyperparathyroidism	332
Infertility	10%, couples	Investigate both members of couple Semen analysis in male Assess ovulatory cycles in female Specific tests as indicated		45
Polycystic ovarian syndrome	4–7% women	Free testosterone, DHEAS Consider comorbid conditions		326
Hirsutism	Variable	Free testosterone, DHEAS Exclude secondary causes Additional tests as indicated		44
Menopause	Median age, 51	FSH		327
Hyperprolactinemia	Common in women with amenorrhea or galactorrhea	PRL level MRI, if not medication-related		318
Erectile dysfunction	10–15%	PRL, testosterone Consider secondary causes (e.g., diabetes)		43
Gynecomastia	Common in older men	Often, no tests are indicated Consider Klinefelter syndrome Consider medications, hypogonadism, liver disease		325
Klinefelter syndrome	0.2%, men	Karyotype Testosterone		328
Turner syndrome	0.03%, women	Karyotype Consider comorbid conditions		328

[a] The prevalence of most disorders varies among ethnic groups and with aging.
[b] See individual chapters for additional information on evaluation and treatment. Early testing is indicated in patients with signs and symptoms of disease or in those at increased risk.

Note: BMI, body mass index; CAD, coronary artery disease; DHEAS, dehydroepiandrosterone; HDL, high-density lipoprotein; LDL, low-density lipoprotein. For other abbreviations, see text.

postreceptor desensitization of signaling pathways; functional forms of resistance are generally reversible.

APPROACH TO THE PATIENT

Because endocrinology interfaces with numerous physiologic systems, there is no standard endocrine history and examination. Moreover, because most glands are relatively inaccessible, the examination usually focuses on the manifestations of hormone excess or deficiency, as well as direct examination of palpable glands, such as the thyroid and gonads. For these reasons, it is important to evaluate patients in the context of their presenting symptoms, review of systems, family and social history, and exposure to medications that may affect the endocrine system. Astute clinical skills are required to detect subtle symptoms and signs suggestive of underlying endocrine disease. For example, a patient with Cushing's syndrome may manifest specific findings, such as central fat redistribution, striae, and proximal muscle weakness, in addition to features seen commonly in the general population, such as obesity, plethora, hypertension, and glucose intolerance. Similarly, the insidious onset of hypothyroidism—with mental slowing, fatigue, dry skin, and other features—can be difficult to distinguish from similar, nonspecific findings in the general population. Clinical judgment, based on knowledge of disease prevalence and pathophysiology, is required to decide when to embark on more extensive evaluation of these disorders. Laboratory testing plays an essential role in endocrinology by allowing quantitative assessment of hormone levels and dynamics. Radiologic imaging tests, such as computed tomography (CT) scan, magnetic resonance imaging (MRI), thyroid scan, and ultrasound, are also used for the diagnosis of endocrine disorders. However, these tests are generally employed only after a hormonal abnormality has been established by biochemical testing.

HORMONE MEASUREMENTS AND ENDOCRINE TESTING Radioimmunoassays are the most important diagnostic tool in endocrinology, as they allow sensitive, specific, and quantitative determination of steady-state and dynamic changes in hormone concentrations. Radioimmunoassays use antibodies to detect specific hormones. For many peptide hormones, these measurements are now configured as immunoradiometric assays (IRMAs), which use two different antibodies to increase binding affinity and specificity. There are many variations of these assays—a common format involves using one antibody to capture the antigen (hormone) onto an immobilized surface and a second antibody, labeled with a fluorescent or radioactive tag, to detect the antigen. These assays are sensitive enough to detect plasma hormone concentrations in the picomolar to nanomolar range, and they can readily distinguish structurally related proteins, such as PTH from PTHrP. A variety of other techniques are used to measure specific hormones, including mass spectroscopy, various forms of chromatography, and enzymatic methods; bioassays are now rarely used.

Most hormone measurements are based on plasma or serum samples. However, urinary hormone determinations remain useful for the evaluation of some conditions. Urinary collections over 24 h provide an integrated assessment of the production of a hormone or metabolite, many of which vary during the day. It is important to assure complete collections of 24-h urine samples; simultaneous measurement of creatinine provides an internal control for the adequacy of collection and can be used to normalize some hormone measurements. A 24-h urine free cortisol measurement largely reflects the amount of unbound cortisol, thus providing a reasonable index of biologically available hormone. Other commonly used urine determinations include: 17-hydroxycorticosteroids, 17-ketosteroids, vanillylmandelic acid (VMA), metanephrine, catecholamines, 5-hydroxyindoleacetic acid (5-HIAA), and calcium.

The value of quantitative hormone measurements lies in their correct interpretation in a clinical context. The normal range for most hormones is relatively broad, often varying by a factor of two- to tenfold. The normal ranges for many hormones are gender- and age-specific. Thus, using the correct normative database is an essential part of interpreting hormone tests. The pulsatile nature of hormones, and factors that can affect their secretion such as sleep, meals, and medications, must also be considered. Cortisol values increase fivefold between midnight and dawn; reproductive hormone levels vary dramatically during the female menstrual cycle.

For many endocrine systems, much information can be gained from basal hormone testing, particularly when different components of an endocrine axis are assessed simultaneously. For example, low testosterone and elevated LH levels suggest a primary gonadal problem, whereas a hypothalamic-pituitary disorder is likely if both LH and testosterone are low. Because TSH is a sensitive indicator of thyroid function, it is generally recommended as a first-line test for thyroid disorders. An elevated TSH level is almost always the result of primary hypothyroidism, whereas a low TSH is most often caused by thyrotoxicosis. These predictions can be confirmed by determining the free thyroxine level. Elevated calcium and PTH levels suggest hyperparathyroidism, whereas PTH is suppressed in hypercalcemia caused by malignancy or granulomatous diseases. A suppressed ACTH in the setting of hypercortisolemia, or increased urine free cortisol, is seen with hyperfunctioning adrenal adenomas.

It is not uncommon, however, for baseline hormone levels associated with pathologic endocrine conditions to overlap with the normal range. In this circumstance, dynamic testing is useful to further separate the two groups. There are a multitude of dynamic endocrine tests, but all are based on principles of feedback regulation, and most responses can be remembered based on the pathways that govern endocrine axes. *Suppression tests* are used in the setting of suspected endocrine hyperfunction. An example is the dexamethasone suppression test used to evaluate Cushing's syndrome (Chaps. 318 and 321). *Stimulation tests* are generally used to assess endocrine hypofunction. The ACTH stimulation test, for example, is used to assess the adrenal gland response in patients with suspected adrenal insufficiency. Other stimulation tests use hypothalamic-releasing factors such as TRH, GnRH, CRH, and GHRH to evaluate pituitary hormone reserve (Chap. 318). Insulin-induced hypoglycemia evokes pituitary ACTH and GH responses. Stimulation tests based on reduction or inhibition of endogenous hormones are now used infrequently. Examples include metyrapone inhibition of cortisol synthesis and clomiphene inhibition of estrogen feedback.

SCREENING AND ASSESSMENT OF COMMON ENDOCRINE DISORDERS Because many endocrine disorders are prevalent in the adult population (Table 317-3), most are diagnosed and managed by general internists, family practitioners, or other primary health care providers. The high prevalence and clinical impact of certain endocrine diseases justifies vigilance for features of these disorders during routine physical examinations; laboratory screening is indicated in selected high-risk populations.

FURTHER READING

LEO CP et al: Hormonal genomics. Endocr Rev 23:369, 2002

MCDONNELL DP et al: Definition of the molecular and cellular mechanisms underlying the tissue-selective agonist/antagonist activities of selective estrogen receptor modulators. Recent Prog Horm Res 57:295, 2002

MCKENNA NJ, O'MALLEY BW: Combinatorial control of gene expression by nuclear receptors and coregulators. Cell 108:465, 2002

NAKAE J et al: Distinct and overlapping functions of insulin and IGF-I receptors. Endocr Rev 22:818, 2001

WEINSTEIN LS et al: Endocrine manifestations of stimulatory G protein alpha-subunit mutations and the role of genomic imprinting. Endocr Rev 22:675, 2001

The anterior pituitary is often referred to as the "master gland" because, together with the hypothalamus, it orchestrates the complex regulatory functions of multiple other endocrine glands. The anterior pituitary gland produces six major hormones: (1) prolactin (PRL), (2) growth hormone (GH), (3) adrenocorticotropin hormone (ACTH), (4) luteinizing hormone (LH), (5) follicle-stimulating hormone (FSH), and (6) thyroid-stimulating hormone (TSH) (Table 318-1). Pituitary hormones are secreted in a pulsatile manner, reflecting stimulation by an array of specific hypothalamic releasing factors. Each of these pituitary hormones elicits specific responses in peripheral target tissues. The hormonal products of these peripheral glands, in turn, exert feedback control at the level of the hypothalamus and pituitary to modulate pituitary function (Fig. 318-1). Pituitary tumors cause characteristic hormone excess syndromes. Hormone deficiency may be inherited or acquired. Fortunately, efficacious treatments exist for the various pituitary hormone excess and deficiency syndromes. Nonetheless, these diagnoses are often elusive, emphasizing the importance of recognizing subtle clinical manifestations and performing the correct laboratory diagnostic tests. →*For discussion of disorders of the posterior pituitary, or neurohypophysis, see Chap. 319.*

ANATOMY AND DEVELOPMENT

ANATOMY The pituitary gland weighs ~600 mg and is located within the sella turcica ventral to the diaphragma sella; it comprises anatomically and functionally distinct anterior and posterior lobes. The sella is contiguous to vascular and neurologic structures, including the cavernous sinuses, cranial nerves, and optic chiasm. Thus, expanding intrasellar pathologic processes may have significant central mass effects in addition to their endocrinologic impact.

Hypothalamic neural cells synthesize specific releasing and inhibiting hormones that are secreted directly into the portal vessels of the pituitary stalk. Blood supply of the pituitary gland is derived from the superior and inferior hypophyseal arteries (Fig. 318-2). The hypothalamic-pituitary portal plexus provides the major blood source for the anterior pituitary, allowing reliable transmission of hypothalamic peptide pulses without significant systemic dilution; consequently, pituitary cells are exposed to sharp spikes of releasing factors and in turn release their hormones as discrete pulses (Fig. 318-3).

The posterior pituitary is supplied by the inferior hypophyseal arteries. In contrast to the anterior pituitary, the posterior lobe is directly innervated by hypothalamic neurons (supraopticohypophyseal and tuberohypophyseal nerve tracts) via the pituitary stalk (Chap. 319). Thus, posterior pituitary production of vasopressin (antidiuretic hormone; ADH) and oxytocin is particularly sensitive to neuronal damage by lesions that affect the pituitary stalk or hypothalamus.

PITUITARY DEVELOPMENT The embryonic differentiation and maturation of anterior pituitary cells have been elucidated in considerable detail. Pituitary development from Rathke's pouch involves a complex interplay of lineage-specific transcription factors expressed in pluripotential stem cells and gradients of locally produced growth factors (Table 318-1). The transcription factor Pit-1 determines cell-specific expression of GH, PRL, and TSH in somatotropes, lactotropes, and thyrotropes. Expression of high levels of estrogen receptors in cells that contain Pit-1 favors PRL expression, whereas thyrotrope embronic factor (TEF) induces TSH expression. Pit-1 binds to GH, PRL, and TSH gene regulatory elements, as well as to recognition sites on its own promoter, providing a mechanism for perpetuating selective pituitary phenotypic stability. The transcription factor Prop-1 induces the pituitary development of Pit-1-specific lineages, as well as gonadotropes. Gonadotrope cell development is further defined by the cell-specific expression of the nuclear receptors, steroidogenic factor (SF-1) and DAX-1. Development of corticotrope cells, which express the proopiomelanocortin (POMC) gene, requires corticotropin upstream transcription element (CUTE) and the PTX-1 transcription factor. Abnormalities of pituitary development caused by mutations of Pit-1, Prop-1, SF-1, and DAX-1 result in a series of rare, selective or combined, pituitary hormone deficits.

TABLE 318-1 *Anterior Pituitary Hormone Expression and Regulation*

Cell	Corticotrope	Somatotrope	Lactotrope	Thyrotrope	Gonadotrope
Tissue-specific transcription factor	PTX-1, CUTE	Prop-1, Pit-1	Prop-1, Pit-1	Prop-1, Pit-1, TEF	SF-1, DAX-1
Fetal appearance	6 weeks	8 weeks	12 weeks	12 weeks	12 weeks
Hormone	POMC	GH	PRL	TSH	FSH LH
Chromosomal locus	2p	17q	6	α -6q; β-1p	β-11p; β-19q
Protein	Polypeptide	Polypeptide	Polypeptide	Glycoprotein α, β subunits	Glycoprotein α, β subunits
Amino acids	266 (ACTH 1–39)	191	199	211	210 204
Stimulators	CRH, AVP, gp-130 cytokines	GHRH, GHRP	Estrogen, TRH, VIP	TRH	GnRH, activins, estrogen
Inhibitors	Glucocorticoids	Somatostatin, IGF-I	Dopamine	T_3, T_4, dopamine, somatostatin, glucocorticoids	Sex steroids, inhibin
Target gland	Adrenal	Liver, other tissues	Breast, other tissues	Thyroid	Ovary, testis
Trophic effect	Steroid production	IGF-I production, growth induction, insulin antagonism	Milk production	T_4 synthesis and secretion	Sex steroid production, follicle growth, germ cell maturation
Normal range	ACTH, 4–22 pg/L	<0.5 μg/L[a]	M < 15; F <20 μg/L	0.1–5 mU/L	M, 5–20 IU/L, F (basal), 5–20 IU/L

[a] Hormone secretion integrated over 24 h.

Note: M, male; F, female. For other abbreviations, see text.

Source: Adapted from I Shimon, S Melmed, in P Conn, S Melmed (eds): *Endocrinology: Basic and Clinical Principles.* Totowa, NJ, Humana, 1996.

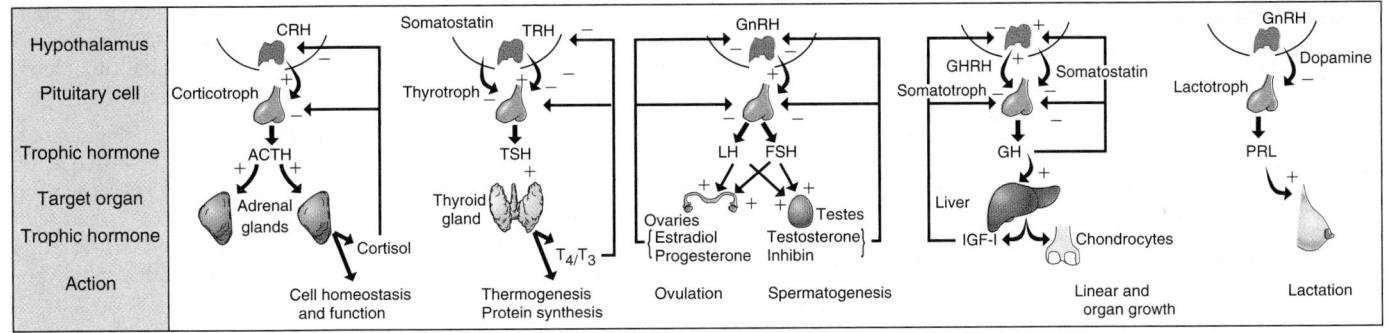

FIGURE 318-1 Diagram of pituitary axes. Hypothalamic hormones regulate anterior pituitary trophic hormones that, in turn, determine target gland secretion. Peripheral hormones feed back to regulate hypothalamic and pituitary hormones. For abbreviations, see text.

HYPOTHALAMIC AND ANTERIOR PITUITARY INSUFFICIENCY

Hypopituitarism results from impaired production of one or more of the anterior pituitary trophic hormones. Reduced pituitary function can result from inherited disorders; more commonly, it is acquired and reflects the mass effects of tumors or the consequences of inflammation or vascular damage. These processes may also impair synthesis or secretion of hypothalamic hormones, with resultant pituitary failure (Table 318-2).

DEVELOPMENTAL AND GENETIC CAUSES OF HYPOPITUITARISM ■ Pituitary Dysplasia
Pituitary dysplasia may result in aplastic, hypoplastic, or ectopic pituitary gland development. Because pituitary development requires midline cell migration from the nasopharyngeal Rathke's pouch, midline craniofacial disorders may be associated with pituitary dysplasia. Acquired pituitary failure in the newborn can also be caused by birth trauma, including cranial hemorrhage, asphyxia, and breech delivery.

SEPTO-OPTIC DYSPLASIA Hypothalamic dysfunction and hypopituitarism may result from dysgenesis of the septum pellucidum or corpus callosum. Affected children have mutations in the *HESX1* gene, which is involved in early development of the ventral prosencephalon. These children exhibit variable combinations of cleft palate, syndactyly, ear deformities, hypertelorism, optic atrophy, micropenis, and anosmia. Pituitary dysfunction leads to diabetes insipidus, GH deficiency and short stature and, occasionally, TSH deficiency.

Tissue-Specific Factor Mutations
Several pituitary cell–specific transcription factors, such as Pit-1 and Prop-1, are critical for determining the development and function of specific anterior pituitary cell lineages. Autosomal dominant or recessive Pit-1 mutations cause combined GH, PRL, and TSH deficiencies. These patients present with growth failure and varying degrees of hypothyroidism. The pituitary may appear hypoplastic on magnetic resonance imaging (MRI).

Prop-1 is expressed early in pituitary development and appears to be required for Pit-1 function. Familial and sporadic *PROP1* mutations result in combined GH, PRL, TSH, and gonadotropin deficiency, with preservation of ACTH. Over 80% of these patients have growth retardation and, by adulthood, all are deficient in TSH and gonadotropins. Because of gonadotropin deficiency, they do not enter puberty spontaneously. In some cases, the pituitary gland is enlarged.

Developmental Hypothalamic Dysfunction ■ *KALLMANN SYNDROME*
This syndrome results from defective hypothalamic gonadotropin-releasing hormone (GnRH) synthesis and is associated with anosmia or hyposmia due to olfactory bulb agenesis or hypoplasia (Chap. 325). The syndrome may also be associated with color blindness, optic atrophy, nerve deafness, cleft palate, renal abnormalities, cryptorchidism, and neurologic abnormalities such as mirror movements. Defects in the *KAL* gene, which maps to chromosome Xp22.3, prevent embryonic migration of GnRH neurons from the hypothalamic olfactory placode to the hypothalamus. Genetic abnormalities, in addition to *KAL* mutations, can also cause isolated GnRH deficiency, as autosomal recessive and dominant modes of transmission have been described. GnRH deficiency prevents progression through puberty. Males present with delayed puberty and pronounced hypogonadal features, including micropenis, probably the result of low testosterone levels during infancy. Female patients present with primary amenorrhea and failure of secondary sexual development.

Kallmann syndrome and other causes of congenital GnRH deficiency are characterized by low LH and FSH levels and low concentrations of sex steroids (testosterone or estradiol). In sporadic cases of isolated gonadotropin deficiency, the diagnosis is often one of exclusion after eliminating other causes of hypothalamic-pituitary dysfunction. Repetitive GnRH administration restores normal pituitary gonadotropin responses, pointing to a hypothalamic defect.

Long-term treatment of males with human chorionic gonadotropin

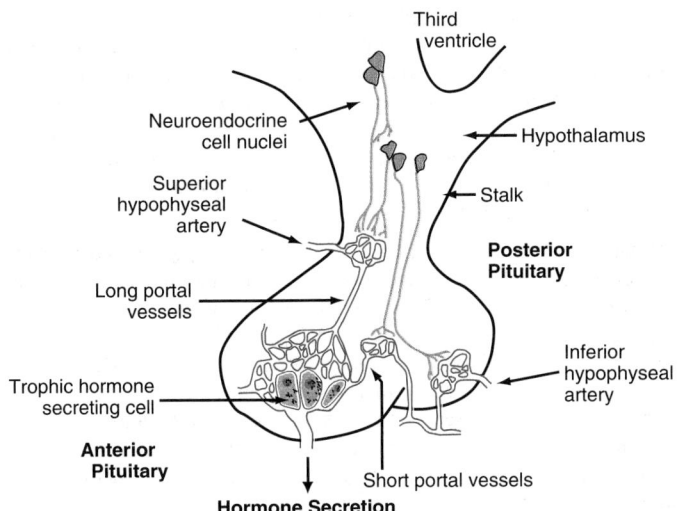

FIGURE 318-2 Diagram of hypothalamic-pituitary vasculature: The hypothalamic nuclei produce hormones that traverse the portal system and impinge on anterior pituitary cells to regulate pituitary hormone secretion. Posterior pituitary hormones are derived from direct neural extensions.

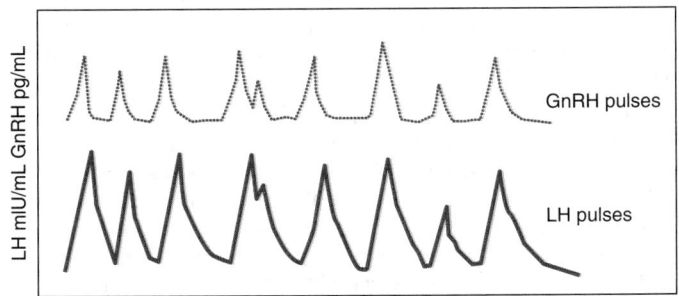

FIGURE 318-3 Hypothalamic gonadotropin-releasing hormone (GnRH) pulses induce secretory pulses of luteinizing hormone (LH).

TABLE 318-2 Etiology of Hypopituitarism*

Development/structural
   Transcription factor defect
   Pituitary dysplasia/aplasia
   Congenital CNS mass, encephalocele
   Primary empty sella
   Congenital hypothalamic disorders (septo-optic dysplasia, Prader-Willi
     syndrome, Laurence-Moon-Biedl syndrome, Kallmann syndrome)
Traumatic
   Surgical resection
   Radiation damage
   Head injuries
Neoplastic
   Pituitary adenoma
   Parasellar mass (meningioma, germinoma, ependymoma, glioma)
   Rathke's cyst
   Craniopharyngioma
   Hypothalamic hamartoma, gangliocytoma
   Pituitary metastases (breast, lung, colon carcinoma)
   Lymphoma and leukemia
   Meningioma
Infiltrative/inflammatory
   Hemochromatosis
   Lymphocytic hypophysitis
   Sarcoidosis
   Histiocytosis X
   Granulomatous hypophysitis
Vascular
   Pituitary apoplexy
   Pregnancy-related (infarction with diabetes; postpartum necrosis)
   Sickle cell disease
   Arteritis
Infections
   Fungal (histoplasmosis)
   Parasitic (toxoplasmosis)
   Tuberculosis
   Pneumocystis carinii

ª Trophic hormone failure associated with pituitary compression or destruction usually occurs sequentially GH > FSH > LH > TSH > ACTH. During childhood, growth retardation is often the presenting feature, and in adults hypogonadism is the earliest symptom.

(hCG) or testosterone restores pubertal development and secondary sex characteristics; females can be treated with cyclic estrogen and progestin. Fertility may also be restored by the administration of gonadotropins or by using a portable infusion pump to deliver subcutaneous, pulsatile GnRH.

LAURENCE-MOON-BARDET-BIEDL SYNDROME This rare autosomal recessive disorder is characterized by mental retardation; obesity; and hexadactyly, brachydactyly, or syndactyly. Central diabetes insipidus may or may not be associated. GnRH deficiency occurs in 75% of males and half of affected females. Retinal degeneration begins in early childhood, and most patients are blind by age 30.

FRÖHLICH SYNDROME (ADIPOSE GENITAL DYSTROPHY) A broad spectrum of hypothalamic lesions may be associated with hyperphagia, obesity, and central hypogonadism. Decreased GnRH production in these patients results in attenuated pituitary FSH and LH synthesis and release. Deficiencies of leptin, or its receptor, cause these clinical features (Chap. 64).

Prader-Willi Syndrome Chromosome 15q deletions are associated with hypogonadotropic hypogonadism, hyperphagia-obesity, chronic muscle hypotonia, mental retardation, and adult-onset diabetes mellitus (Chap. 57). Multiple somatic defects also involve the skull, eyes, ears, hands, and feet. Diminished hypothalamic oxytocin- and vasopressin-producing nuclei have been reported. Deficient GnRH synthesis is suggested by the observation that chronic GnRH treatment restores pituitary LH and FSH release.

ACQUIRED HYPOPITUITARISM Hypopituitarism may be caused by accidental or neurosurgical trauma; vascular events such as apoplexy;

pituitary or hypothalamic neoplasms such as pituitary adenomas, craniopharyngiomas, or metastatic tumors; inflammatory disease such as lymphocytic hypophysitis; infiltrative disorders such as sarcoidosis, hemochromatosis (Chap. 336), and tuberculosis; or irradiation.

Hypothalamic Infiltration Disorders These disorders—including sarcoidosis, histiocytosis X, amyloidosis, and hemochromatosis—frequently involve both hypothalamic and pituitary neuronal and neurochemical tracts. Consequently, diabetes insipidus occurs in half of patients with these disorders. Growth retardation is seen if attenuated GH secretion occurs before pubertal epiphyseal closure. Hypogonadotropic hypogonadism and hyperprolactinemia are also common.

Inflammatory Lesions Pituitary damage and subsequent dysfunction can be seen with chronic infections such as tuberculosis, opportunistic fungal infections associated with AIDS, and in tertiary syphilis. Other inflammatory processes, such as granulomas or sarcoidosis, may mimic a pituitary adenoma. These lesions may cause extensive hypothalamic and pituitary damage, leading to trophic hormone deficiencies.

Cranial Irradiation Cranial irradiation may result in long-term hypothalamic and pituitary dysfunction, especially in children and adolescents, as they are more susceptible to damage following whole-brain or head and neck therapeutic irradiation. The development of hormonal abnormalities correlates strongly with irradiation dosage and the time interval after completion of radiotherapy. Up to two-thirds of patients ultimately develop hormone insufficiency afer a median dose of 50 Gy (5000 rad) directed at the skull base. The development of hypopituitarism occurs over 5 to 15 years and usually reflects hypothalamic damage rather than absolute destruction of pituitary cells. Though the pattern of hormone loss is variable, GH deficiency is most common, followed by gonadotropin and ACTH deficiency. When deficiency of one or more hormones is documented, the possibility of diminished reserve of other hormones is likely. Accordingly, anterior pituitary function should be evaluated over the long term in previously irradiated patients, and replacement therapy instituted when appropriate (see below).

Lymphocytic Hypophysitis This occurs mainly in pregnant or post-partum women; it usually presents with hyperprolactinemia and MRI evidence of a prominent pituitary mass resembling an adenoma, with mildly elevated PRL levels. Pituitary failure caused by diffuse lymphocytic infiltration may be transient or permanent but requires immediate evaluation and treatment. Rarely, isolated pituitary hormone deficiencies have been described, suggesting a selective autoimmune process targeted to specific cell types. Most patients manifest symptoms of progressive mass effects with headache and visual disturbance. The erythrocyte sedimentation rate is often elevated. As the MRI image may be indistinguishable from that of a pituitary adenoma, hypophysitis should be considered in a post-partum woman with a newly diagnosed pituitary mass before embarking on unnecessary surgical intervention. The inflammatory process often resolves after several months of glucocorticoid treatment, and pituitary function may be restored, depending on the extent of damage.

Pituitary Apoplexy Acute intrapituitary hemorrhagic vascular events can cause substantial damage to the pituitary and surrounding sellar structures. Pituitary apoplexy may occur spontaneously in a preexisting adenoma (usually nonfunctioning); postpartum (Sheehan's syndrome); or in association with diabetes, hypertension, sickle cell anemia, or acute shock. The hyperplastic enlargement of the pituitary during pregnancy increases the risk for hemorrhage and infarction. Apoplexy is an endocrine emergency that may result in severe hypoglycemia, hypotension, central nervous system (CNS) hemorrhage, and death. Acute symptoms may include severe headache with signs of meningeal irritation, bilateral visual changes, ophthalmoplegia, and, in severe cases, cardiovascular collapse and loss of consciousness. Pituitary computed tomography (CT) or MRI may reveal signs of intratumoral or sellar hemorrhage, with deviation of the pituitary stalk and compression of pituitary tissue.

Patients with no evident visual loss or impaired consciousness can be observed and managed conservatively with high-dose glucocorticoids. Those with significant or progressive visual loss or loss of consciousness require urgent surgical decompression. Visual recovery after surgery is inversely correlated with the length of time after the acute event. Therefore, severe ophthalmoplegia or visual deficits are indications for early surgery. Hypopituitarism is very common after apoplexy.

Empty Sella A partial or apparently totally empty sella is often an incidental MRI finding. These patients usually have normal pituitary function, implying that the surrounding rim of pituitary tissue is fully functional. Hypopituitarism, however, may develop insidiously. Pituitary masses may undergo clinically silent infarction with development of a partial or totally empty sella by cerebrospinal fluid (CSF) filling the dural herniation. Rarely, functional pituitary adenomas may arise within the rim of pituitary tissue, and these are not always visible on MRI.

PRESENTATION AND DIAGNOSIS The clinical manifestations of hypopituitarism depend on which hormones are lost and the extent of the hormone deficiency. GH deficiency causes growth disorders in children and leads to abnormal body composition in adults (see below). Gonadotropin deficiency causes menstrual disorders and infertility in women and decreased sexual function, infertility, and loss of secondary sexual characteristics in men. TSH and ACTH deficiency usually develop later in the course of pituitary failure. TSH deficiency causes growth retardation in children and features of hypothyroidism in children and in adults. The secondary form of adrenal insufficiency caused by ACTH deficiency leads to hypocortisolism with relative preservation of mineralocorticoid production. PRL deficiency causes failure of lactation. When lesions involve the posterior pituitary, polyuria and polydipsia reflect loss of vasopressin secretion. Epidemiologic studies have documented an increased mortality rate in patients with long-standing pituitary damage, primarily from increased cardiovascular and cerebrovascular disease.

LABORATORY INVESTIGATION Biochemical diagnosis of pituitary insufficiency is made by demonstrating low levels of trophic hormones in the setting of low target hormone levels. For example, low free thyroxine in the setting of a low or inappropriately normal TSH level suggests secondary hypothyroidism. Similarly, a low testosterone level without elevation of gonadotropins suggests hypogonadotropic hypogonadism. Provocative tests may be required to assess pituitary reserve (Table 318-3). GH responses to insulin-induced hypoglycemia, arginine, L-dopa, growth hormone–releasing hormone (GHRH), or growth hormone–releasing peptides (GHRPs) can be used to assess GH reserve. PRL and TSH responses to thyrotropin-releasing hormone (TRH) reflect lactotrope and thyrotrope function. Corticotropin-

TABLE 318-3 *Tests of Pituitary Insufficiency*

Hormone	Test	Blood Samples	Interpretation
Growth hormone	Insulin tolerance test: Regular insulin (0.05–0.15 U/kg IV)	−30, 0, 30, 60, 120 min for glucose and GH	Glucose < 40 mg/dL; GH should be >3 μg/L
	GHRH test: 1 μg/kg IV	0, 15, 30, 45, 60, 120 min for GH	Normal response is GH >3 μg/L
	L-Arginine test: 30 g IV over 30 min	0, 30, 60, 120 min for GH	Normal response is GH >3 μg/L
	L-dopa test: 500 mg PO	0, 30, 60, 120 min for GH	Normal response is GH >3 μg/L
Prolactin	TRH test: 200–500 μg IV	0, 20, and 60 min for TSH and PRL	Normal prolactin is >2 μg/L and increase >200% of baseline
ACTH	Insulin tolerance test: Regular insulin (0.05–0.15 U/kg IV)	−30, 0, 30, 60, 90 min for glucose and cortisol	Glucose <40 mg/dL Cortisol should increase by >7 μg/dL or to >20 μg/dL
	CRH test: 1 μg/kg ovine CRH IV at 0800 h	0, 15, 30, 60, 90, 120 min for ACTH and cortisol	Basal ACTH increases 2- to 4-fold and peaks at 20–100 pg/mL Cortisol levels >20–25 μg/dL
	Metyrapone test: Metyrapone (30 mg/kg) at midnight	Plasma 11-deoxycortisol and cortisol at 8 A.M.; ACTH can also be measured	Plasma cortisol should be <4 μg/dL to assure an adequate response Normal response is 11-deoxycortisol >7.5 μg/dL or ACTH >75 pg/mL
	Standard ACTH stimulation test: ACTH 1-24 (Cosyntropin), 0.25 mg IM or IV	0, 30, 60 min for cortisol and aldosterone	Normal response is cortisol >21 μg/dL and aldosterone response of >4 ng/dL above baseline
	Low-dose ACTH test: ACTH 1-24 (Cosyntropin), 1 μg IV	0, 30, 60 min for cortisol	Cortisol should be >21 μg/dL
	3-day ACTH stimulation test consists of 0.25 mg ACTH 1-24 given IV over 8 h each day		Cortisol >21 μg/dL
TSH	Basal thyroid function tests: T₄, T₃, TSH	Basal tests	Low free thyroid hormone levels in the setting of TSH levels that are not appropriately increased
	TRH test: 200–500 μg IV	0, 20, 60 min for TSH and PRL	TSH should increase by >5 mU/L unless thyroid hormone levels are increased
LH, FSH	LH, FSH, testosterone, estrogen	Basal tests	Basal LH and FSH should be increased in postmenopausal women Low testosterone levels in the setting of low LH and FSH
	GnRH test: GnRH (100 μg) IV	0, 30, 60 min for LH and FSH	In most adults, LH should increase by 10 IU/L and FSH by 2 IU/L Normal responses are variable
Multiple hormones	Combined anterior pituitary test: GHRH (1 μg/kg), CRH (1 μg/kg), GnRH (100 μg), TRH (200 μg) are given IV	−30, 0, 15, 30, 60, 90, 120 min for GH, ACTH, cortisol, LH, FSH, and TSH	Combined or individual releasing hormone responses must be elevated in the context of basal target gland hormone values and may not be diagnostic (see text)

Note: For abbreviations, see text.

TABLE 318-4 *Hormone Replacement Therapy for Adult Hypopituitarism*[a]

Trophic Hormone Deficit	Hormone Replacement
ACTH	Hydrocortisone (10–20 mg A.M.; 10 mg P.M.)
	Cortisone acetate (25 mg A.M.; 12.5 mg P.M.)
	Prednisone (5 mg A.M.; 2.5 mg P.M.)
TSH	L-Thyroxine (0.075–0.15 mg daily)
FSH/LH	Males
	Testosterone enanthate (200 mg IM every 2 weeks)
	Testosterone skin patch (5 mg/d)
	Females
	Conjugated estrogen (0.65–1.25 mg qd for 25 days)
	Progesterone (5–10 mg qd) on days 16–25
	Estradiol skin patch (0.5 mg, every other day)
	For fertility: Menopausal gonadotropins, human chorionic gonadotropins
GH	Adults: Somatotropin (0.3–1.0 mg SC qd)
	Children: Somatotropin [0.02–0.05 (mg/kg per day)]
Vasopressin	Intranasal desmopressin (5–20 μg twice daily)
	Oral 300–600 μg qd

[a] All doses shown should be individualized for specific patients and should be reassessed during stress, surgery, or pregnancy. Male and female fertility requirements should be managed as discussed in Chap. 45.

Note: For abbreviations, see text.

releasing hormone (CRH) administration induces ACTH release, and administration of synthetic ACTH (cortrosyn) evokes adrenal cortisol release as an indirect indicator of pituitary ACTH reserve (Chap. 321). ACTH reserve is most reliably assessed during insulin-induced hypoglycemia. However, this test should be performed cautiously in patients with suspected adrenal insufficiency because of increased risk of hypoglycemia and hypotension. Insulin-induced hypoglycemia is contraindicated in patients with coronary heart disease or seizure disorders.

℞ TREATMENT

Hormone replacement therapy, including glucocorticoids, thyroid hormone, sex steroids, growth hormone, and vasopressin, is usually free of complications. Treatment regimens that mimic physiologic hormone production allow for maintenance of satisfactory clinical homeostasis. Effective dosage schedules are outlined in Table 318-4. Patients in need of glucocorticoid replacement require careful dose adjustments during stressful events such as acute illness, dental procedures, trauma, and acute hospitalization (Chap. 321).

HYPOTHALAMIC, PITUITARY, AND OTHER SELLAR MASSES

PITUITARY TUMORS Pituitary adenomas are the most common cause of pituitary hormone hypersecretion and hyposecretion syndromes in adults. They account for ~10% of all intracranial neoplasms. At autopsy, up to a quarter of all pituitary glands harbor an unsuspected microadenoma (<10 mm diameter). Similarly, pituitary imaging detects small pituitary lesions in at least 10% of normal individuals.

Pathogenesis Pituitary adenomas are benign neoplasms that arise from one of the five anterior pituitary cell types. The clinical and biochemical phenotype of pituitary adenomas depend on the cell type from which they are derived. Thus, tumors arising from lactotrope (PRL), somatotrope (GH), corticotrope (ACTH), thyrotrope (TSH), or gonadotrope (LH, FSH) cells hypersecrete their respective hormones (Table 318-5). Plurihormonal tumors that express combinations of GH, PRL, TSH, ACTH, and the glycoprotein hormone α subunit may be diagnosed by careful immunocytochemistry or may manifest as clinical syndromes that combine features of these hormonal hypersecretory syndromes. Morphologically, these tumors may arise from a single polysecreting cell type or consist of cells with mixed function within the same tumor.

Hormonally active tumors are characterized by autonomous hormone secretion with diminished responsiveness to the normal physiologic pathways of inhibition. Hormone production does not always correlate with tumor size. Small hormone-secreting adenomas may cause significant clinical perturbations, whereas larger adenomas that produce less hormone may be clinically silent and remain undiagnosed (if no central compressive effects occur). About one-third of all adenomas are clinically nonfunctioning and produce no distinct clinical hypersecretory syndrome. Most of these arise from gonadotrope cells and may secrete small amounts of α- and β-glycoprotein hormone subunits or, very rarely, intact circulating gonadotropins. True pituitary carcinomas with documented extracranial metastases are exceedingly rare.

Almost all pituitary adenomas are monoclonal in origin, implying the acquisition of one or more somatic mutations that confer a selective growth advantage. In addition to direct studies of oncogene mutations, this idea is supported by X-chromosomal inactivation analyses of tumors in female patients heterozygous for X-linked genes. Consistent with their clonal origin, complete surgical resection of small pituitary adenomas usually cures hormone hypersecretion. Nevertheless, hypothalamic hormones, such as GHRH or CRH, also enhance the mitotic activity of their respective pituitary target cells, in addition to their role in pituitary hormone regulation. Thus, patients harboring rare abdominal or chest tumors elaborating ectopic GHRH or CRH may present with somatotrope or corticotrope hyperplasia.

Several etiologic genetic events have been implicated in the development of pituitary tumors. The pathogenesis of sporadic forms of acromegaly has been particularly informative as a model of tumorigenesis. GHRH, after binding to its G protein–coupled somatotrope receptor, utilizes cyclic AMP as a second messenger to stimulate GH secretion and somatotrope proliferation. A subset (~35%) of GH-secreting pituitary tumors contain sporadic mutations in Gsα (Arg 201 → Cys or His; Gln 227 → Arg). These mutations inhibit intrinsic GTPase activity, resulting in constitutive elevation of cyclic AMP, Pit-1 induction, and activation of cyclic AMP response element binding protein (CREB), thereby promoting somatotrope cell proliferation.

TABLE 318-5 *Classification of Pituitary Adenomas*[a]

Adenoma Cell Origin	Hormone Product	Clinical Syndrome
Lactotrope	PRL	Hypogonadism, galactorrhea
Gonadotrope	FSH, LH, subunits	Silent or hypogonadism
Somatotrope	GH	Acromegaly/gigantism
Corticotrope	ACTH	Cushing's disease
Mixed growth hormone and prolactin cell	GH, PRL	Acromegaly, hypogonadism, galactorrhea
Other plurihormonal cell	Any	Mixed
Acidophil stem cell	PRL, GH	Hypogonadism, galactorrhea, acromegaly
Mammosomatotrope	PRL, GH	Hypogonadism, galactorrhea, acromegaly
Thyrotrope	TSH	Thyrotoxicosis
Null cell	None	Pituitary failure
Oncocytoma	None	Pituitary failure

[a] Hormone-secreting tumors are listed in decreasing order of frequency. All tumors may cause local pressure effects, including visual disturbances, cranial nerve palsy, and headache.

Note: For abbreviations, see text.

Source: Adapted from S Melmed, in JL Jameson (ed): *Principles of Molecular Medicine*, Totowa, Humana Press, 1998.

Characteristic loss of heterozygosity (LOH) in various chromosomes has been documented in large or invasive macroadenomas, suggesting the presence of putative tumor suppressor genes at these loci. LOH of chromosome region on 11q13, 13, and 9 is present in up to 20% of sporadic pituitary tumors including GH-, PRL-, and ACTH-producing adenomas and in some nonfunctioning tumors.

Compelling evidence also favors growth factor promotion of pituitary tumor proliferation. Basic fibroblast growth factor (bFGF) is abundant in the pituitary and has been shown to stimulate pituitary cell mitogenesis. Other factors involved in initiation and promotion of pituitary tumors include loss of negative-feedback inhibition (as seen with primary hypothyroidism or hypogonadism) and estrogen-mediated or paracrine angiogenesis. Growth characteristics and neoplastic behavior may also be influenced by several activated oncogenes, including *RAS* and pituitary tumor transforming gene (*PTTG*).

Genetic Syndromes Associated with Pituitary Tumors   Several familial syndromes are associated with pituitary tumors, and the genetic mechanisms for some of these have been unraveled.

Multiple endocrine neoplasia (MEN) 1 is an autosomal dominant syndrome characterized primarily by a genetic predisposition to parathyroid, pancreatic islet, and pituitary adenomas (Chap. 330). MEN1 is caused by inactivating germline mutations in *MENIN*, a constitutively expressed tumor-suppressor gene located on chromosome 11q13. Loss of heterozygosity, or a somatic mutation of the remaining normal *MENIN* allele, leads to tumorigenesis. About half of affected patients develop prolactinomas; acromegaly and Cushing's syndrome are less commonly encountered.

Carney syndrome is characterized by spotty skin pigmentation, myxomas, and endocrine tumors including testicular, adrenal, and pituitary adenomas. Acromegaly occurs in about 20% of patients. A subset of patients have mutations in the R1α regulatory subunit of protein kinase A (*PRKAR1A*).

McCune-Albright syndrome consists of polyostotic fibrous dysplasia, pigmented skin patches, and a variety of endocrine disorders, including GH-secreting pituitary tumors, adrenal adenomas, and autonomous ovarian function (Chap. 326). Hormonal hypersecretion is due to constitutive cyclic AMP production caused by inactivation of the GTPase activity of Gsα. The Gsα mutations occur postzygotically, leading to a mosaic pattern of mutant expression.

Familial acromegaly is a rare disorder in which family members may manifest either acromegaly or gigantism. The disorder is associated with LOH at a chromosome 11q13 locus distinct from that of *MENIN*.

OTHER SELLAR MASSES   *Craniopharyngiomas* are derived from Rathke's pouch. They arise near the pituitary stalk and commonly extend into the suprasellar cistern. These tumors are often large, cystic, and locally invasive. Many are partially calcified, providing a characteristic appearance on skull x-ray and CT images. More than half of all patients present before age 20, usually with signs of increased intracranial pressure, including headache, vomiting, papilledema, and hydrocephalus. Associated symptoms include visual field abnormalities, personality changes and cognitive deterioration, cranial nerve damage, sleep difficulties, and weight gain. Anterior pituitary dysfunction and diabetes insipidus are common. About half of affected children present with growth retardation.

Treatment usually involves transcranial or transsphenoidal surgical resection followed by postoperative radiation of residual tumor. This approach can result in long-term survival and ultimate cure, but most patients require lifelong pituitary hormone replacement. If the pituitary stalk is uninvolved and can be preserved at the time of surgery, the incidence of subsequent anterior pituitary dysfunction is significantly diminished.

Developmental failure of Rathke's pouch obliteration may lead to *Rathke's cysts*, which are small (<5 mm) cysts entrapped by squamous epithelium; these cysts are found in about 20% of individuals at autopsy. Although Rathke's cleft cysts do not usually grow and are often diagnosed incidentally, about a third present in adulthood with compressive symptoms, diabetes insipidus, and hyperprolactinemia due to stalk compression. Rarely, internal hydrocephalus develops. The diagnosis is suggested preoperatively by visualizing the cyst wall on MRI, which distinguishes these lesions from craniopharyngiomas. Cyst contents range from CSF-like fluid to mucoid material. *Arachnoid cysts* are rare and generate an MRI image isointense with cerebrospinal fluid.

Sella chordomas usually present with bony clival erosion, local invasiveness, and, on occasion, calcification. Normal pituitary tissue may be visible on MRI, distinguishing chordomas from aggressive pituitary adenomas. Mucinous material may be obtained by fine-needle aspiration.

Meningiomas arising in the sellar region may be difficult to distinguish from nonfunctioning pituitary adenomas. Meningiomas typically enhance on MRI and may show evidence of calcification or bony erosion. Meningiomas may cause compressive symptoms.

Histiocytosis X comprises a variety of syndromes associated with foci of eosinophilic granulomas. Diabetes insipidus, exophthalmos, and punched-out lytic bone lesions (*Hand-Schüller-Christian disease*) are associated with granulomatous lesions visible on MRI, as well as a characteristic axillary skin rash. Rarely, the pituitary stalk may be involved.

Pituitary metastases occur in ~3% of cancer patients. Blood-borne metastatic deposits are found almost exclusively in the posterior pituitary. Accordingly, diabetes insipidus can be a presenting feature of lung, gastrointestinal, breast, and other pituitary metastases. About half of pituitary metastases originate from breast cancer; about 25% of patients with breast cancer have such deposits. Rarely, pituitary stalk involvement results in anterior pituitary insufficiency. The MRI diagnosis of a metastatic lesion may be difficult to distinguish from an aggressive pituitary adenoma; the diagnosis may require histologic examination of excised tumor tissue. Primary or metastatic lymphoma, leukemias, and plasmacytomas also occur within the sella.

Hypothalamic hamartomas and *gangliocytomas* may arise from astrocytes, oligodendrocytes, and neurons with varying degrees of differentiation. These tumors may overexpress hypothalamic neuropeptides including GnRH, GHRH, or CRH. In GnRH-producing tumors, children present with precocious puberty, psychomotor delay, and laughing-associated seizures. Medical treatment of GnRH-producing hamartomas with long-acting GnRH analogues effectively suppresses gonadotropin secretion and controls premature pubertal development. Rarely, hamartomas are also associated with craniofacial abnormalities; imperforate anus; cardiac, renal, and lung disorders; and pituitary failure (*Pallister-Hall syndrome*). Hypothalamic hamartomas are often contiguous with the pituitary, and preoperative MRI diagnosis may not be possible. Histologic evidence of hypothalamic neurons in tissue resected at transsphenoidal surgery may be the first indication of a primary hypothalamic lesion.

Hypothalamic gliomas and *optic gliomas* occur mainly in childhood and usually present with visual loss. Adults have more aggressive tumors; about a third are associated with neurofibromatosis.

Brain germ-cell tumors may arise within the sellar region. These include *dysgerminomas*, which are frequently associated with diabetes insipidus and visual loss. They rarely metastasize. *Germinomas*, *embryonal carcinomas*, *teratomas*, and *choriocarcinomas* may arise in the parasellar region and produce hCG. These germ-cell tumors present with precocious puberty, diabetes insipidus, visual field defects, and thirst disorders. Many patients are GH-deficient with short stature.

METABOLIC EFFECTS OF HYPOTHALAMIC LESIONS   Lesions involving the anterior and preoptic hypothalamic regions cause paradoxical vasoconstriction, tachycardia, and hyperthermia. Acute hyperthermia is usually due to a hemorrhagic insult, but poikilothermia may also occur. Central disorders of thermoregulation result from posterior hypothalamic damage. The *periodic hypothermia syndrome* comprises episodic attacks of rectal temperatures <30°C, sweating, vasodilation, vomiting, and bradycardia (Chap. 19). Damage to the ventromedial nuclei by craniopharyngiomas, hypothalamic trauma, or inflammatory disorders may be associated with *hyperphagia* and *obesity*. This region appears to contain an energy-satiety center where melanocortin receptors are influenced by leptin, insulin, POMC products, and gastrointestinal peptides (Chap. 64). Hypothalamic gliomas in early childhood may be associated with a diencephalic syndrome characterized by progressive severe emaciation and growth failure. Polydipsia and hypodipsia are associated with damage to central osmo-receptors located in preoptic nuclei (Chap. 319). Slow-growing hypothalamic lesions can cause increased somnolence and disturbed sleep cycles as well as obesity, hypothermia, and emotional outbursts. Lesions of the central hypothalamus may stimulate sympathetic neurons, leading to elevated serum catecholamine and cortisol levels. These patients are predisposed to cardiac arrhythmias, hypertension, and gastric erosions.

EVALUATION ■ **Local Mass Effects** Clinical manifestations of sellar lesions vary, depending on the anatomic location of the mass and direction of its extension (Table 318-6). The dorsal roof of the sella presents the least resistance to soft tissue expansion from within the confines of the sella; consequently, pituitary adenomas frequently extend in a suprasellar direction. Bony invasion may ultimately occur as well.

Headaches are common features of small intrasellar tumors, even with no demonstrable suprasellar extension. Because of the confined nature of the pituitary, small changes in intrasellar pressure stretch the dural plate; however, the severity of the headache correlates poorly with adenoma size or extension.

Suprasellar extension can lead to visual loss by several mechanisms, the most common being compression of the optic chiasm, but direct invasion of the optic nerves or obstruction of CSF flow leading to secondary visual disturbances also occurs. Pituitary stalk compression by a hormonally active or inactive intrasellar mass may compress the portal vessels, disrupting pituitary access to the hypothalamic hormones and dopamine; this results in hyperprolactinemia and concurrent loss of other pituitary hormones. This "stalk section" phenomenon may also be caused by trauma, whiplash injury with posterior clinoid stalk compression, or skull base fractures. Lateral mass invasion may impinge on the cavernous sinus and compress its neural contents, leading to cranial nerve III, IV, and VI palsies as well as effects on the ophthalmic and maxillary branches of the fifth cranial nerve (Chap. 355). Patients may present with diplopia, ptosis, ophthalmoplegia, and decreased facial sensation, depending on the extent of neural damage. Extension into the sphenoid sinus indicates that the pituitary mass has eroded through the sellar floor. Aggressive tumors rarely invade the palate roof and cause nasopharyngeal obstruction, infection, and CSF leakage. Both temporal and frontal lobes may be invaded, leading to uncinate seizures, personality disorders, and anosmia. Direct hypothalamic encroachment by an invasive pituitary mass may cause important metabolic sequelae, precocious puberty or hypogonadism, diabetes insipidus, sleep disturbances, dysthermia, and appetite disorders.

MRI Sagittal and coronal T1-weighted spin-echo MRI imaging, before and after administration of gadolinium, allow precise visualization of the pituitary gland with clear delineation of the hypothalamus, pituitary stalk, pituitary tissue and surrounding suprasellar cisterns, cavernous sinuses, sphenoid sinus, and optic chiasm. Pituitary gland height ranges from 6 mm in children to 8 mm in adults; during pregnancy and puberty, the height may reach 10 to 12 mm. The upper aspect of the adult pituitary is flat or slightly concave, but in adolescent and pregnant individuals, this surface may be convex, reflecting physiologic pituitary enlargement. The stalk should be vertical. CT scan is indicated to define the extent of bony erosion or the presence of calcification.

The soft tissue consistency of the pituitary gland is slightly heterogeneous on MRI. Anterior pituitary signal intensity resembles that of brain matter on T1-imaging (Fig. 318-4). Adenoma density is usually lower than that of surrounding normal tissue on T1-weighted imaging, and the signal intensity increases with T2-weighted images. The high phospholipid content of the posterior pituitary results in a "pituitary bright spot."

Sellar masses are commonly encountered as incidental findings on MRI, and most of these are pituitary adenomas (incidentalomas). In the absence of hormone hypersecretion, these small lesions can be safely monitored by MRI, which is performed annually and then less often if there is no evidence of growth. Resection should be considered for incidentally discovered macroadenomas, as about one-third become invasive or cause local pressure effects. If hormone hypersecretion is evident, specific therapies are indicated. When larger masses (>1 cm) are encountered, they should also be distinguished from nonadenomatous lesions. Meningiomas are often associated with bony hyperostosis; craniopharyngiomas may be calcified and are usually hypodense, whereas gliomas are hyperdense on T2-weighted images.

TABLE 318-6	Features of Sellar Mass Lesions[a]
Impacted Structure	**Clinical Impact**
Pituitary	Hypogonadism
	Hypothyroidism
	Growth failure and adult hyposomatotropism
	Hypoadrenalism
Optic chiasm	Loss of red perception
	Bitemporal hemianopia
	Superior or bitemporal field defect
	Scotoma
	Blindness
Hypothalamus	Temperature dysregulation
	Appetite and thirst disorders
	Obesity
	Diabetes insipidus
	Sleep disorders
	Behavioral dysfunction
	Autonomic dysfunction
Cavernous sinus	Opthalmoplegia ± ptosis or diplopia
	Facial numbness
Frontal lobe	Personality disorder
	Anosmia
Brain	Headache
	Hydrocephalus
	Psychosis
	Dementia
	Laughing seizures

[a] As the intrasellar mass expands, it first compresses intrasellar pituitary tissue, then usually invades dorsally through the dura to lift the optic chiasm or laterally to the cavernous sinuses. Bony erosion is rare, as is direct brain compression. Microadenomas may present with headache.

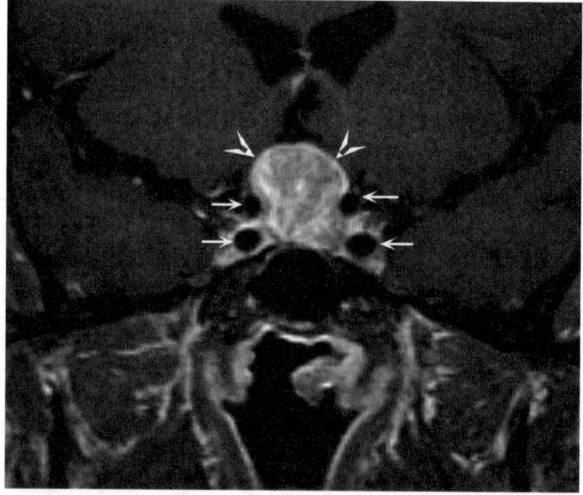

FIGURE 318-4 Pituitary adenoma. Coronal T1-weighted postcontrast MR image shows a homogeneously enhancing mass (*arrowheads*) in the sella turcica and suprasellar region compatible with a pituitary adenoma; the small arrows outline the carotid arteries.

Ophthalmologic Evaluation Because optic tracts may be contiguous to an expanding pituitary mass, reproducible visual field assessment that uses perimetry techniques should be performed on all patients with sellar mass lesions that abut the optic chiasm (Chap. 25). Bitemporal hemianopia or superior bitemporal defects are classically observed, reflecting the location of these tracts within the inferior and posterior part of the chiasm. Homonymous cuts are postchiasmal and monocular field cuts are prechiasmal. Loss of red perception is an early sign of optic tract pressure. Early diagnosis reduces the risk of blindness, scotomas, or other visual disturbances.

Laboratory Investigation The presenting clinical features of functional pituitary adenomas (e.g., acromegaly, prolactinomas, or Cushing's disease) should guide the laboratory studies (Table 318-7). However, for a sellar mass with no obvious clinical features of hormone excess, laboratory studies are geared towards determining the nature of the tumor and assessing the possible presence of hypopituitarism. When a pituitary adenoma is suspected based on MRI, initial hormonal evaluation usually includes: (1) basal PRL; (2) insulin-like growth factor (IGF) I; (3) 24-h urinary free cortisol (UFC) and/or overnight oral dexamethasone (1 mg) suppression test; (4) α-subunit, FSH, and LH levels; and (5) thyroid function tests. Additional hormonal evaluation may be indicated based on the results of these tests. Pending more detailed assessment of hypopituitarism, a menstrual history, testosterone level, 8 A.M. cortisol, and thyroid function tests usually identify patients with pituitary hormone deficiencies that require hormone replacement before further testing or surgery.

Histologic Evaluation Immunohistochemical staining of pituitary tumor specimens obtained at transsphenoidal surgery confirms clinical and laboratory studies and provides a histologic diagnosis when hormone studies are equivocal and in cases of clinically nonfunctioning tumors. Occasionally, ultrastructural assessment by electron microscopy is required for diagnosis.

℞ TREATMENT

OVERVIEW Successful management of sellar masses requires accurate diagnosis as well as selection of optimal therapeutic modalities. Most pituitary tumors are benign and slow-growing. Clinical features result from local mass effects and hormonal hypo- or hypersecretion syndromes caused directly by the adenoma or as a consequence of treatment. Thus, lifelong management and follow-up are necessary for these patients.

MRI technology with gadolinium enhancement for pituitary visualization, new advances in transsphenoidal surgery and in stereotactic

TABLE 318-7 *Screening Tests for Functional Pituitary Adenomas*

	Test	Comments
Acromegaly	Serum IGF-I	Interpret IGF-I relative to age- and gender-matched controls
	Oral glucose tolerance test with GH obtained at 0, 30, and 60 min	Normal subjects should suppress growth hormone to <1 μg/L
Prolactinoma	Exclude medications	MRI of the sella should be ordered if prolactin is elevated
Cushing's disease	24-h urinary free cortisol	Ensure urine collection is total and accurate
	Dexamethasone (1 mg) at 11 P.M. and fasting plasma cortisol measured at 8 A.M.	Normal subjects suppress to <5 μg/dL
	ACTH assay	Distinguishes adrenal adenoma (ACTH suppressed) from ectopic ACTH or Cushing's disease (ACTH normal or elevated)

Note: For abbreviations, see text.

radiotherapy (including gamma-knife radiotherapy), and novel therapeutic agents have improved pituitary tumor management. The goals of pituitary tumor treatment include normalization of excess pituitary secretion, amelioration of symptoms and signs of hormonal hypersecretion syndromes, and shrinkage or ablation of large tumor masses with relief of adjacent structure compression. Residual anterior pituitary function should be preserved and can sometimes be restored by removing tumor mass. Ideally, adenoma recurrence should be prevented.

TRANSSPHENOIDAL SURGERY Transsphenoidal rather than transfrontal resection is the desired surgical approach for pituitary tumors, except for the rare invasive suprasellar mass surrounding the frontal or middle fossa, the optic nerves, or invading posteriorly behind the clivus. Intraoperative microscopy facilitates visual distinction between adenomatous and normal pituitary tissue, as well as microdissection of small tumors that may not be visible by MRI (Fig. 318-5). Transsphenoidal surgery also avoids the cranial invasion and manipulation of brain tissue required by subfrontal surgical approaches. Endoscopic techniques with three-dimensional intraoperative localization have improved visualization and access to tumor tissue. The endoscopic approach is also less traumatic, as the technique is endonasal and does not require a transsphenoidal retractor.

In addition to correction of hormonal hypersecretion, pituitary surgery is indicated for mass lesions that impinge on surrounding structures. Surgical decompression and resection are required for an expanding pituitary mass accompanied by persistent headache, progressive visual field defects, cranial nerve palsies, internal hydrocephalus, and, occasionally, intrapituitary hemorrhage and apoplexy. Transsphenoidal surgery is sometimes used for pituitary tissue biopsy and histologic diagnosis.

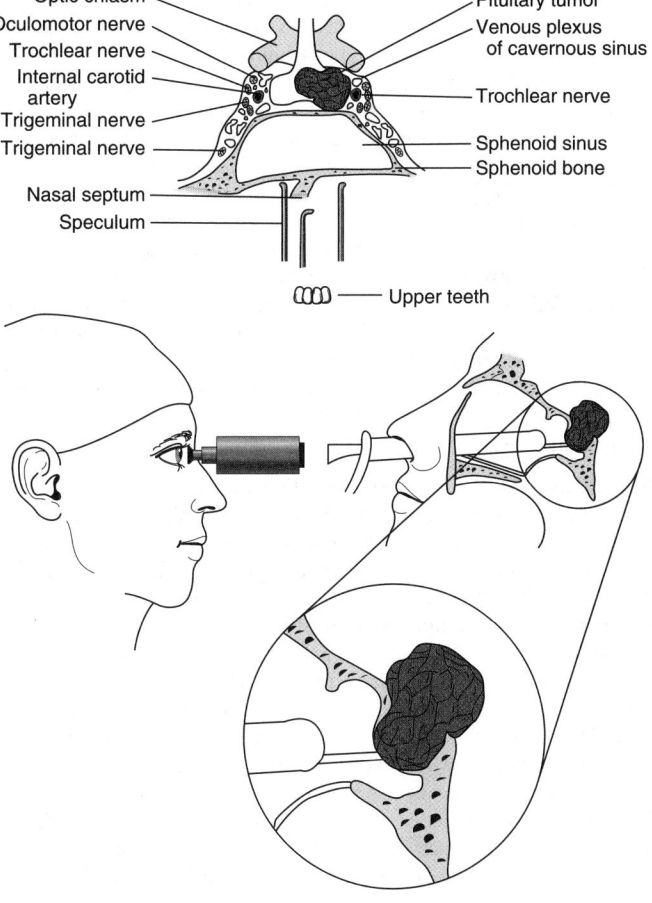

FIGURE 318-5 Transsphenoidal resection of pituitary mass via the endonasal approach. (*Adapted from Fahlbusch R: Endocrinol Metab Clin 21:669, 1992.*)

Whenever possible, the pituitary mass lesion should be selectively excised; normal tissue should be manipulated or resected only when critical for effective dissection. Nonselective hemihypophysectomy or total hypophysectomy may be indicated if no mass lesion is clearly discernible, multifocal lesions are present, or the remaining nontumorous pituitary tissue is obviously necrotic. This strategy increases the likelihood of hypopituitarism and the need for lifelong hormonal replacement.

Preoperative local compression signs, including visual field defects or compromised pituitary function, may be reversed by surgery, particularly when these deficits are not long-standing. For large and invasive tumors, it is necessary to determine the optimal balance between maximal tumor resection and preservation of anterior pituitary function, especially for preserving growth and reproductive function in younger patients. Similarly, tumor invasion outside of the sella is rarely amenable to surgical cure; the surgeon must judge the risk: benefit ratio of extensive tumor resection.

Side Effects   Tumor size and the degree of invasiveness largely determine the incidence of surgical complications. Operative mortality is about 1%. Transient diabetes insipidus and hypopituitarism occur in up to 20% of patients. Permanent diabetes insipidus, cranial nerve damage, nasal septal perforation, or visual disturbances may be encountered in up to 10% of patients. CSF leaks occur in 4% of patients. Less common complications include carotid artery injury, loss of vision, hypothalamic damage, and meningitis. Permanent side effects are rarely encountered after surgery for microadenomas.

RADIATION   Radiation is used either as a primary therapy for pituitary or parasellar masses or, more commonly, as an adjunct to surgery or medical therapy. Focused megavoltage irradiation is achieved by precise MRI localization, using a high-voltage linear accelerator and accurate isocentric rotational arcing. A major determinant of accurate irradiation is to reproduce the patient's head position during multiple visits and to maintain absolute head immobility. A total of <50 Gy (5000 rad) is given as 180-cGy (180 rad) fractions split over about 6 weeks. Stereotactic radiosurgery delivers a large single high-energy dose from a cobalt 60 source (gamma knife), linear accelerator, or cyclotron. Long-term effects of gamma-knife surgery are as yet unknown.

The role of radiation therapy in pituitary tumor management depends on multiple factors including the nature of the tumor, age of the patient, and the availability of surgical and radiation expertise. Because of its relatively slow onset of action, radiation therapy is usually reserved for postsurgical management. As an adjuvant to surgery, radiation is used to treat residual tumor and in an attempt to prevent regrowth. Irradiation offers the only effective means for ablating significant residual tumor tissue derived from nonfunctioning tumors. PRL-, GH-, and ACTH-secreting tumor tissues are also amenable to medical therapy.

Side Effects   In the short term, radiation may cause transient nausea and weakness. Alopecia and loss of taste and smell may be more longlasting. Failure of pituitary hormone synthesis is common in patients who have undergone head and neck or pituitary-directed irradiation. More than 50% of patients develop failure of GH, ACTH, TSH, and/or gonadotropin secretion within 10 years, usually due to hypothalamic damage. Lifelong follow-up with testing of anterior pituitary hormone reserve is therefore necessary after radiation treatment. Optic nerve damage with impaired vision due to optic neuritis is reported in about 2% of patients who undergo pituitary irradiation. Cranial nerve damage is uncommon now that radiation doses are ≤ 2 Gy (200 rad) at any one treatment session and the maximum dose is <50 Gy (5000 rad). The advent of stereotactic radiotherapy may reduce damage to adjacent structures. The cumulative risk of developing a secondary tumor after conventional radiation is 1.3% after 10 years and 1.9% after 20 years.

MEDICAL   Medical therapy for pituitary tumors is highly specific and depends on tumor type. For prolactinomas, dopamine agonists are the treatment of choice. For acromegaly and TSH-secreting tumors, somatostatin analogues and, occasionally, dopamine agonists are indicated. ACTH-secreting tumors and nonfunctioning tumors are generally not responsive to medication and require surgery and/or irradiation.

PROLACTIN

SYNTHESIS   PRL consists of 198 amino acids and has a molecular mass of 21,500 kDa; it is weakly homologous to GH and human placental lactogen (hPL), reflecting the duplication and divergence of a common GH-PRL-hPL precursor gene on chromosome 6. PRL is synthesized in lactotropes, which comprise about 20% of anterior pituitary cells. Lactotropes and somatotropes are derived from a common precursor cell that may give rise to a tumor secreting both PRL and GH. Marked lactotrope cell hyperplasia develops during the last two trimesters of pregnancy and the first few months of lactation. These transient adaptive changes in the lactotrope population are induced by estrogen.

SECRETION   Normal adult serum PRL levels are about 10 to 25 μg/L in women and 10 to 20 μg/L in men. PRL secretion is pulsatile, with the highest secretory peaks occurring during rapid eye movement sleep. Peak serum PRL levels (up to 30 μg/L) occur between 4:00 and 6:00 A.M. The circulating half-life of PRL is about 50 min.

PRL is unique among the pituitary hormones in that the predominant central control mechanism is inhibitory, reflecting dopamine-mediated suppression of PRL release. This regulatory pathway accounts for the spontaneous PRL hypersecretion that occurs after pituitary stalk section, often a consequence of mass lesions at the skull base. Pituitary, dopamine type 2 (D_2) receptors mediate PRL inhibition. Targeted disruption (gene knockout) of the murine D_2 receptor results in hyperprolactinemia and lactotrope proliferation. As discussed below, dopamine agonists play a central role in the management of hyperprolactinemic disorders.

TRH (pyro Glu-His-Pro-NH2) is a hypothalamic tripeptide that releases prolactin within 15 to 30 min after intravenous injection. The physiologic relevance of TRH for PRL regulation is unclear, as it appears primarily to regulate TSH (Chap. 320). *Vasoactive intestinal peptide* (VIP) also induces PRL release, whereas glucocorticoids and thyroid hormone weakly suppress PRL secretion.

Serum PRL levels rise after exercise, meals, sexual intercourse, minor surgical procedures, general anesthesia, acute myocardial infarction, and other forms of acute stress. PRL levels also increase significantly ($\sim$tenfold) during pregnancy and decline rapidly within 2 weeks of parturition. If breastfeeding is initiated, basal PRL levels remain elevated; suckling stimulates reflex increases in PRL levels that last for about 30 to 45 min. Breast suckling activates neural afferent pathways in the hypothalamus that induce PRL release. With time, the suckling-induced responses diminish and interfeeding PRL levels return to normal.

ACTION   The PRL receptor is a member of the type I cytokine receptor family that also includes GH and interleukin (IL) 6 receptors. Ligand binding leads to receptor dimerization followed by intracellular signaling mediated by Janus kinase (JAK) and components of the signal transduction and activators of transcription (STAT) family that translocate to the nucleus, where they act as transcription factors on target genes. In the breast, the lobuloalveolar epithelium proliferates in response to PRL, placental lactogens, estrogen, progesterone, and local paracrine growth factors.

PRL acts to induce and maintain lactation, decrease reproductive function, and suppress sexual drive. These functions are geared towards ensuring that maternal lactation is sustained and not interrupted by pregnancy. PRL inhibits reproductive function by suppressing hypothalamic GnRH and pituitary gonadotropin secretion and by impairing gonadal steroidogenesis in both female and male subjects. In the ovary, PRL blocks folliculogenesis and inhibits granulosa cell aromatase activity, leading to hypoestrogenism and anovulation. PRL also has a luteolytic effect, generating a shortened, or inadequate, luteal phase of the menstrual cycle. In males, attenuated LH secretion leads to low testosterone levels and decreased spermatogenesis. These hormonal changes decrease libido and reduce fertility in patients with hyperprolactinemia.

HYPERPROLACTINEMIA ■ **Etiology** Hyperprolactinemia is the most common pituitary hormone hypersecretion syndrome in both males and females. PRL-secreting pituitary adenomas (prolactinomas) are the most common cause of PRL levels >100 μg/L (see below). Less pronounced PRL elevation can also be seen with microprolactinomas but is more commonly caused by drugs, pituitary stalk compression, hypothyroidism, or renal failure (Table 318-8).

Pregnancy and lactation are the important physiologic causes of hyperprolactinemia. Sleep-associated hyperprolactinemia reverts to normal within an hour of awakening. Nipple stimulation and sexual orgasm may also cause acute PRL increases. Chest wall stimulation or trauma (including chest surgery and herpes zoster) invoke the reflex suckling arc with resultant hyperprolactinemia. Chronic renal failure elevates PRL by decreasing peripheral PRL clearance. Primary hypothyroidism is associated with mild hyperprolactinemia, probably because of enhanced TRH secretion.

Lesions of the hypothalamic-pituitary region that disrupt hypothalamic dopamine synthesis, portal vessel delivery, or lactotrope responses are associated with hyperprolactinemia. Thus, hypothalamic tumors, cysts, infiltrative disorders, and radiation-induced damage cause elevated PRL levels, usually in the range of 30 to 100 μg/L. Plurihormonal adenomas (including GH and ACTH tumors) may directly hypersecrete PRL. Clinically nonfunctioning pituitary tumors commonly compress the pituitary stalk to cause hyperprolactinemia.

Drug-induced inhibition or disruption of dopaminergic receptor function is a common cause of hyperprolactinemia (Table 318-8). Thus, many antipsychotics and antidepressants cause hyperprolactinemia. Methyldopa inhibits dopamine synthesis and verapamil blocks dopamine release, also leading to hyperprolactinemia. Hormonal agents that induce PRL include estrogens, antiandrogens, and TRH.

Presentation and Diagnosis Amenorrhea, galactorrhea, and infertility are the hallmarks of hyperprolactinemia in women. If hyperprolactinemia develops prior to the menarche, primary amenorrhea results. More commonly, hyperprolactinemia develops later in life and leads to oligomenorrhea and, ultimately, to amenorrhea. If hyperprolactinemia is sustained, vertebral bone mineral density can be reduced compared to age-matched controls, particularly when associated with pronounced hypoestrogenemia. Galactorrhea is present in up to 80% of hyperprolactinemic women. Though usually bilateral and spontaneous, it may be unilateral or only expressed manually. Patients may also complain of decreased libido, weight gain, and mild hirsutism.

In men with hyperprolactinemia, diminished libido or visual loss (from optic nerve compression) are the usual presenting symptoms. Gonadotropin suppression leads to reduced testosterone, impotence, and oligospermia. True galactorrhea is uncommon in men with hyperprolactinemia. If the disorder is longstanding, secondary effects of hypogonadism are evident, including osteopenia, reduced muscle mass, and decreased beard growth.

The diagnosis of idiopathic hyperprolactinemia is made by exclusion of known causes of hyperprolactinemia in the setting of a normal pituitary MRI. Some of these patients may have small microadenomas below MRI sensitivity (~2 mm).

Laboratory Investigation Basal, fasting morning PRL levels (normally <20 μg/L) should be measured to assess hypersecretion. Because hormone secretion is pulsatile and levels vary widely in some individuals with hyperprolactinemia, it may be necessary to measure levels on several different occasions when clinical suspicion is high. Both false-positive and false-negative results may be encountered. In patients with markedly elevated PRL levels (>1000 μg/L), results may be falsely lowered because of assay artifacts; sample dilution is required to measure these high values accurately. Falsely elevated values may be caused by aggregated forms of circulating PRL, which are biologically inactive (macroprolactinemia). Hypothyroidism should be excluded by measuring TSH and T_4 levels.

℞ TREATMENT

Treatment of hyperprolactinemia depends on the cause of elevated PRL levels. Regardless of the etiology, however, treatment should be aimed at normalizing PRL levels to alleviate suppressive effects on gonadal function, halt galactorrhea, and preserve bone mineral density. Dopamine agonists are effective for many different causes of hyperprolactinemia (see "Treatment" for "Prolactinoma," below).

If the patient is taking a medication known to cause hyperprolactinemia, the drug should be withdrawn, if possible. For psychiatric patients who require neuroleptic agents, dose titration or the addition of a dopamine agonist can help restore normoprolactinemia and alleviate reproductive symptoms. However, dopamine agonists sometimes worsen the underlying psychiatric condition, especially at high doses. Hyperprolactinemia usually resolves after adequate thyroid hormone replacement in hypothyroid patients or after renal transplantation in patients receiving dialysis. Resection of hypothalamic or sellar mass lesions can reverse hyperprolactinemia caused by reduced dopamine tone. Granulomatous infiltrates occasionally respond to glucocorticoid administration. In patients with irreversible hypothalamic damage, no treatment may be warranted. In up to 30% of patients with hyperprolactinemia—with or without a visible pituitary microadenoma—the condition resolves spontaneously.

GALACTORRHEA *Galactorrhea*, the inappropriate discharge of milk-containing fluid from the breast, is considered abnormal if it persists for longer than 6 months after childbirth or discontinuation of breast-feeding. Post-partum galactorrhea associated with amenorrhea is a self-limiting disorder usually associated with moderately elevated PRL levels. Galactorrhea may occur spontaneously, or be elicited by nipple pressure. In both males and females, galactorrhea may vary in color and consistency (transparent, milky, or bloody) and arise either unilaterally or bilaterally. Mammography or ultrasound is indicated for

---

TABLE 318-8 *Etiology of Hyperprolactinemia*

I. Physiologic hypersecretion
A. Pregnancy
B. Lactation
C. Chest wall stimulation
D. Sleep
E. Stress
II. Hypothalamic–pituitary stalk damage
A. Tumors
1. Craniopharyngioma
2. Suprasellar pituitary mass extension
3. Meningioma
4. Dysgerminoma
5. Metastases
B. Empty sella
C. Lymphocytic hypophysitis
D. Adenoma with stalk compression
E. Granulomas
F. Rathke's cyst
G. Irradiation
H. Trauma
1. Pituitary stalk section
2. Suprasellar surgery
III. Pituitary hypersecretion
A. Prolactinoma
B. Acromegaly
IV. Systemic disorders
A. Chronic renal failure
B. Hypothyroidism
C. Cirrhosis
D. Pseudocyesis
E. Epileptic seizures
V. Drug-induced hypersecretion
A. Dopamine receptor blockers
1. Phenothiazines: chlorpromazine, perphenazine
2. Butyrophenones: haloperidol
3. Thioxanthenes
4. Metoclopramide
B. Dopamine synthesis inhibitors
1. α-Methyldopa
C. Catecholamine depletors
1. Reserpine
D. Opiates
E. H_2 antagonists
1. Cimetidine, ranitidine
F. Imipramines
1. Amitriptyline, amoxapine
G. Serotonin-reuptake inhibitors
1. Fluoxetine
H. Calcium channel blockers
1. Verapamil
I. Hormones
1. Estrogens
2. Antiandrogens

Note: Hyperprolactinemia >100 μg/L almost invariably is indicative of a prolactin-secreting pituitary adenoma. Physiologic causes, hypothyroidism, and drug-induced hyperprolactinemia should be excluded before extensive evaluation.

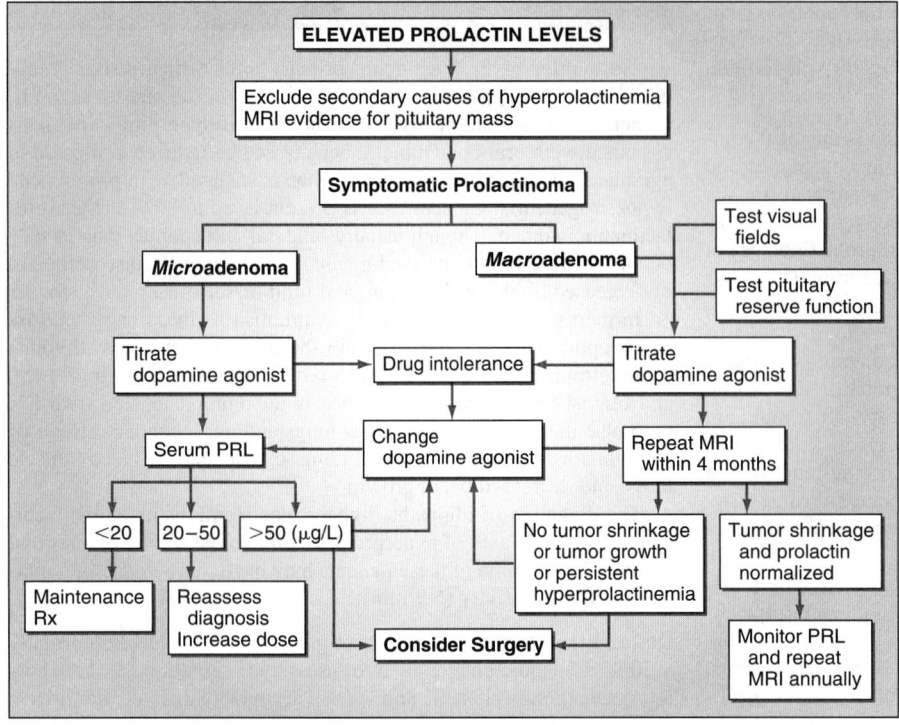

FIGURE 318-6 Management of prolactinoma. (MRI, magnetic resonance imaging; PRL, prolactin.)

bloody discharges (particularly from a single duct), which may be caused by breast cancer. Galactorrhea is commonly associated with hyperprolactinemia caused by any of the conditions listed in Table 318-8. Acromegaly is associated with galactorrhea in about one-third of patients. Treatment of galactorrhea usually involves managing the underlying disorder (e.g., replacing T_4 for hypothyroidism; discontinuing a medication; treating prolactinoma).

PROLACTINOMA ■ Etiology and Prevalence Tumors arising from lactotrope cells account for about half of all functioning pituitary tumors, with an annual incidence of ~3/100,000 population. Mixed tumors secreting combinations of GH and PRL, ACTH and PRL, and rarely TSH and PRL, are also seen. These plurihormonal tumors are usually recognized by immunohistochemistry, without apparent clinical manifestations from the production of additional hormones. Microadenomas are classified as <1 cm in diameter and do not usually invade the parasellar region. Macroadenomas are >1 cm in diameter and may be locally invasive and impinge on adjacent structures. The female:male ratio for microprolactinomas is 20:1, whereas the gender ratio is near 1:1 for macroadenomas. Tumor size generally correlates directly with PRL concentrations; values >100 μg/L are usually associated with macroadenomas. Males tend to present with larger tumors than females, possibly because the features of hypogonadism are less readily evident. PRL levels remain stable in most patients, reflecting the slow growth of these tumors. About 5% of microadenomas progress in the long term to macroadenomas. Hyperprolactinemia resolves spontaneously in about 30% of microadenomas.

Presentation and Diagnosis Women usually present with amenorrhea, infertility, and galactorrhea. If the tumor extends outside of the sella, visual field defects or other mass effects may be seen. Men often present with impotence, loss of libido, infertility, or signs of central CNS compression including headaches and visual defects. Assuming that known physiologic and medication-induced causes of hyperprolactinemia are excluded (Table 318-8), the diagnosis of prolactinoma is likely with a PRL level >100 μg/L. PRL levels <100 μg/L may be caused by microadenomas, other sellar lesions that decrease dopamine inhibition, or nonneoplastic causes of hyperprolactinemia. For this reason, an MRI should be performed in all patients with hyperprolactinemia. It is important to remember that hyperprolactinemia caused by

the mass effects of nonlactotrope lesions is also corrected by treatment with dopamine agonists. Consequently, PRL suppression by dopamine agonists does not necessarily indicate that the lesion is a prolactinoma.

℞ TREATMENT

As microadenomas rarely progress to become macroadenomas, no treatment may be needed if fertility is not desired. Estrogen replacement is indicated to prevent bone loss and other consequences of hypoestrogenemia and does not appear to increase the risk of tumor enlargement. These patients should be monitored by regular serial PRL and MRI measurements.

For symptomatic microadenomas, therapeutic goals include control of hyperprolactinemia, reduction of tumor size, restoration of menses and fertility, and improvement of galactorrhea. Dopamine agonists should be titrated to achieve maximal PRL suppression and restoration of reproductive function (Fig. 318-6). A normalized PRL level does not assure reduced tumor size. However, tumor shrinkage is not usually seen in those who do not respond with lowered PRL levels. For macroadenomas, formal visual field testing should be performed before initiating dopamine agonists. MRI and visual fields should be assessed at 6- to 12-month intervals until the mass shrinks and annually thereafter until maximum size reduction has occurred.

MEDICAL Oral dopamine agonists (cabergoline or bromocriptine) are the mainstay of therapy for patients with micro- or macroprolactinomas. Dopamine agonists suppress PRL secretion and synthesis as well as lactotrope cell proliferation. About 20% of patients are resistant to dopaminergic treatment; they may have decreased D_2 dopamine receptor numbers or a postreceptor defect. D_2 receptor gene mutations in the pituitary have not been reported.

Cabergoline An ergoline derivative, cabergoline is a long-acting dopamine agonist with high D_2 receptor affinity. The drug effectively suppresses PRL for >14 days after a single oral dose and induces prolactinoma shrinkage in most patients. Cabergoline (0.5 to 1.0 mg twice weekly) achieves normoprolactinemia and resumption of normal gonadal function in ~80% of patients with microadenomas; galactorrhea improves or resolves in 90% of patients. Cabergoline normalizes PRL and shrinks ~70% of macroprolactinomas. Mass effect symptoms, including headaches and visual disorders, usually improve dramatically within days after cabergoline initiation; improvement of sexual function requires several weeks of treatment but may occur before complete normalization of prolactin levels. Drug withdrawal usually results in recurrent hyperprolactinemia and tumor reexpansion, with the risk of visual compromise. After initial control of PRL levels has been achieved, cabergoline should be reduced to the lowest effective maintenance dose. In ~5% of treated patients, hyperprolactinemia may resolve and not recur when dopamine agonists are discontinued after long-term treatment. Cabergoline may also be effective in patients resistant to bromocriptine. Adverse effects and drug intolerance are encountered less commonly than with bromocriptine.

Bromocriptine The ergot alkaloid bromocriptine mesylate is a dopamine receptor agonist that suppresses prolactin secretion. Because it is short-acting, the drug is preferred when pregnancy is desired. In microadenomas the drug rapidly lowers serum prolactin levels to normal in up to 70% of patients, decreases tumor size, and restores gonadal function. In patients with macroadenomas, prolactin levels are also normalized in 70% of patients and tumor mass shrinkage (≥50%) is achieved in up to 40% of patients.

Therapy is initiated by administering a low bromocriptine dose (0.625 to 1.25 mg) at bedtime with a snack, followed by gradually increasing the dose. Most patients are successfully controlled with a daily dose of ≤7.5 mg (2.5 mg tid).

Nausea, vomiting, and postural hypotension with faintness may occur in ~25% of patients after the initial dose. These symptoms may persist in some patients.

Other Dopamine Agonists These include *pergolide mesylate*, an ergot derivative with dopaminergic properties; *lisuride*, an ergot derivative; and *quinagolide* (CV 205-502, Norprolac), a nonergot oral dopamine agonist with specific D_2 receptor activity.

Side Effects Side effects of dopamine agonists include constipation, nasal stuffiness, dry mouth, nightmares, insomnia, and vertigo; decreasing the dose usually alleviates these problems. For the approximately 15% of patients who are intolerant of oral bromocriptine, dostinex may be better tolerated. Intravaginal administration of bromocriptine is often efficacious. Auditory hallucinations, delusions, and mood swings have been reported in up to 5% of patients and may be due to the dopamine agonist properties or to the lysergic acid derivative of the compounds. Rare reports of leukopenia, thrombocytopenia, pleural fibrosis, cardiac arrhythmias, and hepatitis have been described with bromocriptine.

Surgery Indications for surgical debulking include dopamine resistance or intolerance or the presence of an invasive macroadenoma with compromised vision that fails to improve rapidly after drug treatment. Initial PRL normalization is achieved in about 70% of microprolactinomas after surgical resection, but only 30% of macroadenomas can be successfully resected. Follow-up studies have shown that recurrence of hyperprolactinemia occurs in up to 20% of patients within the first year after surgery; long-term recurrence rates exceed 50% for macroadenomas. Radiotherapy for prolactinomas is reserved for patients with aggressive tumors that do not respond to maximally tolerated dopamine agonists and/or surgery.

PREGNANCY The pituitary increases in size during pregnancy, reflecting the stimulatory effects of estrogen and perhaps other growth factors. About 5% of microadenomas significantly increase in size, but 15 to 30% of macroadenomas grow during pregnancy. Bromocriptine has been used for over 25 years to restore fertility in women with hyperprolactinemia, without evidence of untoward teratogenic effects. Nonetheless, most authorities recommend strategies to minimize fetal exposure to the drug. For women taking bromocriptine who desire pregnancy, mechanical contraception should be used through three regular menstrual cycles to allow for conception timing. When pregnancy is confirmed, bromocriptine should be discontinued and PRL levels followed serially, especially if headaches or visual symptoms occur. For women harboring macroadenomas, regular visual field testing is recommended, and the drug should be reinstituted if tumor growth is apparent. Although pituitary MRI may be safe during pregnancy, this procedure should be reserved for symptomatic patients with severe headache and/or visual field defects. Alternatively, surgical decompression may be indicated if vision is threatened. Though comprehensive data support the efficacy and relative safety of bromocriptine-facilitated fertility, patients should be advised of potential unknown deleterious effects and the risk of tumor growth during pregnancy. As cabergoline is long-acting with a high D_2-receptor affinity, it is not approved for routine use when fertility is desired.

GROWTH HORMONE

SYNTHESIS GH is the most abundant anterior pituitary hormone, and GH-secreting somatotrope cells constitute up to 50% of the total anterior pituitary cell population. Mammosomatotrope cells, which coexpress PRL with GH, can be identified using double immunostaining techniques. Somatotrope development and GH transcription are determined by expression of the cell-specific Pit-1 nuclear transcription factor. Five distinct genes on chromosome 17q22 encode GH and re-

lated proteins. The pituitary GH gene (*hGH-N*) produces two alternatively spliced products that give rise to 22-kDa GH (191 amino acids) and a less abundant, 20-kDa GH molecule, with similar biologic activity. Placental syncytiotrophoblast cells express a GH variant (*hGH-V*) gene; the related hormone human chorionic somatotropin (HCS) is expressed by distinct members of the gene cluster.

SECRETION GH secretion is controlled by complex hypothalamic and peripheral factors. *GHRH* is a 44 amino acid hypothalamic peptide that stimulates GH synthesis and release. Ghrelin, or octonoylated gastric-derived peptide, as well as synthetic agonists of the *GHRP* receptor stimulate GHRH and also directly stimulate GH release. *Somatostatin* [somatotropin-release inhibiting factor (SRIF)] is synthesized in the medial preoptic area of the hypothalamus and inhibits GH secretion. GHRH is secreted as discrete spikes that elicit GH pulses, whereas SRIF sets basal GH tone. SRIF is also expressed in many extrahypothalamic tissues, including the CNS, gastrointestinal tract, and pancreas, where it also acts to inhibit islet hormone secretion. *IGF-I*, the peripheral target hormone for GH, feeds back to inhibit GH; estrogen induces GH, whereas glucocorticoid excess suppresses GH release.

Surface receptors on the somatotrope regulate GH synthesis and secretion. The GHRH receptor is a G protein–coupled receptor (GPCR) that signals through the intracellular cyclic AMP pathway. Activation of this receptor stimulates somatotrope cell proliferation as well as hormone production. Inactivating mutations of the GHRH receptor cause profound dwarfism (see below). A distinct surface receptor for ghrelin, a gastric-derived GH secretagogue, is expressed in the hypothalamus and pituitary. Somatostatin binds to five distinct receptor subtypes (SSTR1 to SSTR5); SSTR2 and SSTR5 subtypes preferentially suppress GH (and TSH) secretion.

GH secretion is pulsatile, with greatest levels at night, generally correlating with the onset of sleep. GH secretory rates decline markedly with age so that hormone production in middle age is about 15% of production during puberty. These changes are paralleled by an age-related decline in lean muscle mass. GH secretion is also reduced in obese individuals, though IGF-I levels are usually preserved, suggesting a change in the setpoint for feedback control. Elevated GH levels occur within an hour of deep sleep onset as well as after exercise, physical stress, trauma, and during sepsis. Integrated 24-h GH secretion is higher in women and is also enhanced by estrogen replacement. Using standard assays, random GH measurements are undetectable in ~50% of daytime samples obtained from healthy subjects and are undetectable in most obese and elderly subjects. Thus, single random GH measurements do not distinguish patients with adult GH deficiency from normal persons.

GH secretion is profoundly influenced by nutritional factors. Using newer ultrasensitive chemiluminescence-based GH assays with a sensitivity of 0.002 μg/L, a glucose load can be shown to suppress GH to <0.7 μg/L in female and to <0.07 μg/L in male subjects. Increased GH pulse frequency and peak amplitudes occur with chronic malnutrition or prolonged fasting. GH is stimulated by high-protein meals and by L-arginine. GH secretion is induced by dopamine and apomorphine (a dopamine receptor agonist), as well as by α-adrenergic pathways. β-Adrenergic blockage induces basal GH and enhances GHRH- and insulin-evoked GH release.

ACTION The pattern of GH secretion may affect tissue responses. The higher GH pulsatility observed in males, as compared to the relatively continuous GH secretion in females, may be an important biologic determinant of linear growth patterns and liver enzyme induction.

The 70-kDa peripheral GH receptor protein shares structural homology with the cytokine/hematopoietic superfamily. A fragment of the receptor extracellular domain generates a soluble GH binding protein (GHBP) that interacts with GH in the circulation. The liver contains the greatest number of GH receptors. GH binding induces receptor dimerization, followed by signaling through the JAK/STAT pathway. The activated STAT proteins translocate to the nucleus, where they modulate expression of GH-regulated target genes. GH analogues that bind to the receptor, but are incapable of mediating receptor dimerization, are potent antagonists of GH action and are being investigated for potential use in the treatment of acromegaly and diabetic microangiopathy.

GH induces protein synthesis and nitrogen retention and impairs glucose tolerance by antagonizing insulin action. GH also stimulates lipolysis, leading to increased circulating fatty acid levels, reduced omental fat mass, and enhanced lean body mass. GH promotes sodium, potassium, and water retention and elevates serum levels of inorganic phosphate. Linear bone growth occurs as a result of complex hormonal and growth factor actions, including those of IGF-I. GH stimulates epiphyseal prechondrocyte differentiation. These precursor cells produce IGF-I locally and are also responsive to the growth factor.

INSULIN-LIKE GROWTH FACTORS   Though GH exerts direct effects in target tissues, many of its physiologic effects are mediated indirectly through IGF-I, a potent growth and differentiation factor. The major source of circulating IGF-I is hepatic in origin. Peripheral tissue IGF-I exerts local paracrine actions that appear to be both dependent and independent of GH. Thus, GH administration induces circulating IGF-I as well as stimulating IGF-I expression in multiple tissues.

Both IGF-I and -II are bound to high-affinity circulating IGF-binding proteins (IGFBPs) that regulate IGF bioactivity. Levels of IGFBP3 are GH-dependent, and it serves as the major carrier protein for circulating IGF-I. GH deficiency and malnutrition are associated with low IGFBP3 levels. IGFBP1 and -2 regulate local tissue IGF action but do not bind appreciable amounts of circulating IGF-I.

Serum IGF-I concentrations are profoundly affected by various physiologic factors. Levels increase during puberty, peak at 16 years, and subsequently decline by >80% during the aging process. IGF-I concentrations are higher in females than in males. Because GH is the major determinant of hepatic IGF-I synthesis, abnormalities of GH synthesis or action (e.g., pituitary failure, GHRH receptor defect, or GH receptor defect) reduce IGF-I levels. Hypocaloric states are associated with GH resistance; IGF-I levels are therefore low with cachexia, malnutrition, and sepsis. In acromegaly, IGF-I levels are invariably high and reflect a log-linear relationship with GH concentrations.

IGF-I Physiology   Though IGF-I is not an approved drug, investigational studies provide insight into its physiologic effects. Injected IGF-I (100 μg/kg) induces hypoglycemia, and lower doses improve insulin sensitivity in patients with severe insulin resistance and diabetes. In cachectic subjects, IGF-I infusion (12 μg/kg per hour) enhances nitrogen retention and lowers cholesterol levels. Longer-term subcutaneous IGF-I injections exert a marked anabolic effect with enhanced protein synthesis. Although bone formation markers are induced, bone turnover may also be stimulated by IGF-I.

IGF-I side effects are dose-dependent, and overdose may result in hypoglycemia, hypotension, fluid retention, temporomandibular jaw pain, and increased intracranial pressure, all of which are reversible. Avascular femoral head necrosis has been reported. Chronic excess IGF-I would presumably result in features of acromegaly.

DISORDERS OF GROWTH AND DEVELOPMENT ■ Skeletal Maturation and Somatic Growth   The growth plate is dependent on a variety of hormonal stimuli including GH, IGF-I, sex steroids, thyroid hormones, paracrine growth factors, and cytokines. The growth-promoting process also requires caloric energy, amino acids, vitamins, and trace metals and consumes about 10% of normal energy production. Malnutrition impairs chondrocyte activity and reduces circulating IGF-I and IGFBP3 levels.

Bone age is delayed in patients with all forms of true GH deficiency or GH receptor defects that result in attenuated GH action. Rarely, GH excess accelerates growth, particularly in the setting of delayed bone

age from concomitant hypogonadism. Bone age is delayed by thyroid hormone deficiency. Consequently, congenital or acquired hypothyroidism is associated with stunted growth, which is partially reversed by thyroid hormone replacement (Chap. 320). Elevated pubertal sex steroid levels (especially estrogen) induce the GHRH-GH-IGF-I axis and also directly stimulate epiphyseal growth. High doses of estrogen lead to epiphyseal closure. A mutation of the estrogen receptor α prevented epiphyseal closure, confirming the important role of this pathway in bone maturation. Several pathologic conditions accompanied by increased levels of sex steroids, including precocious puberty, androgen exposure (exogenous or endogenous), congenital adrenal hyperplasia, and obesity, are associated with accelerated bone maturation. Thus, children with these conditions have accelerated early growth, but end up with reduced final height. In contrast to sex steroids, glucocorticoid excess inhibits linear growth.

Linear bone growth rates are very high in infancy and are pituitary-dependent. Mean growth velocity is ~6 cm/year in later childhood and is usually maintained within a given range on a standardized percentile chart. Peak growth rates occur during midpuberty when bone age is 12 (girls) or 13 (boys). Secondary sexual development is associated with elevated sex steroids that cause progressive epiphyseal growth plate closure.

Short stature may occur as a result of constitutive intrinsic growth defects or because of acquired extrinsic factors that impair growth. In general, delayed bone age in a child with short stature is suggestive of a hormonal or systemic disorder, whereas normal bone age in a short child is more likely to be caused by a genetic cartilage dysplasia or growth plate disorder (Chap. 342).

GH Deficiency in Children ■ *GH DEFICIENCY*   Isolated GH deficiency is characterized by short stature, micropenis, increased fat, high-pitched voice, and a propensity to hypoglycemia. Familial modes of inheritance are seen in one-third of these individuals and may be autosomal dominant, recessive, or X-linked. About 10% of children with GH deficiency have mutations in the *GH-N* gene, including gene deletions and a wide range of point mutations. Mutations in transcription factors Pit-1 and Prop-1, which control somatotrope development, cause GH deficiency in combination with other pituitary hormone deficiencies, which may only become manifest in adulthood. The diagnosis of *idiopathic GH deficiency* (IGHD) should be made only after known molecular defects have been excluded.

GHRH RECEPTOR MUTATIONS   Recessive mutations of the GHRH receptor gene in subjects with severe proportionate dwarfism are associated with low basal GH levels that cannot be stimulated by exogenous GHRH, GHRP, or insulin-induced hypoglycemia. The syndrome exemplifies the importance of the GHRH receptor for somatotrope cell proliferation and hormonal responsiveness.

GROWTH HORMONE INSENSITIVITY   This is caused by defects of GH receptor structure or signaling. Homozygous or heterozygous mutations of the GH receptor are associated with partial or complete GH insensitivity and growth failure (*Laron syndrome*). The diagnosis is based on normal or high GH levels, with decreased circulating GHBP, and low IGF-I levels. Very rarely, defective IGF-I, IGF-I receptor, or IGF-I signaling defects are also encountered.

NUTRITIONAL SHORT STATURE   Caloric deprivation and malnutrition, uncontrolled diabetes, and chronic renal failure represent secondary causes of abrogated GH receptor function. These conditions also stimulate production of proinflammatory cytokines, which can block GH-mediated signal transduction. Children with these conditions typically exhibit features of acquired short stature with elevated GH and low IGF-I levels. Circulating GH receptor antibodies may rarely cause peripheral GH insensitivity.

PSYCHOSOCIAL SHORT STATURE   Emotional and social deprivation lead to growth retardation accompanied by delayed speech, discordant hyperphagia, and attenuated response to administered GH. A nurturing environment restores growth rates.

Presentation and Diagnosis Short stature is commonly encountered in clinical practice, and the decision to evaluate these children requires clinical judgement in association with auxologic data and family history. Short stature should be comprehensively evaluated if a patient's height is >3 SD below the mean for age or if the growth rate has decelerated. Skeletal maturation is best evaluated by measuring a radiologic bone age, which is based mainly on the degree of growth plate fusion. Final height can be predicted using standardized scales (Bayley-Pinneau or Tanner-Whitehouse) or estimated by adding 6.5 cm (boys) or subtracting 6.5 cm (girls) from the midparental height.

Laboratory Investigation Because GH secretion is pulsatile, GH deficiency is best assessed by examining the response to provocative stimuli including exercise, insulin-induced hypoglycemia, and other pharmacologic tests which normally increase GH to >7 μg/L in children. Random GH measurements do not distinguish normal children from those with true GH deficiency. Adequate adrenal and thyroid hormone replacement should be assured before testing. Age- and gender-matched IGF-I levels are not sufficiently sensitive or specific to make the diagnosis but can be useful to confirm GH deficiency. Pituitary MRI may reveal pituitary mass lesions or structural defects.

℞ TREATMENT

Replacement therapy with recombinant GH (0.02 to 0.05 mg/kg per day subcutaneously) restores growth velocity in GH-deficient children to ~10 cm/year. If pituitary insufficiency is documented, other associated hormone deficits should be corrected—especially adrenal steroids. GH treatment is also moderately effective for accelerating growth rates in children with Turner syndrome and chronic renal failure.

In patients with GH insensitivity and growth retardation due to mutations of the GH receptor, treatment with IGF-I bypasses the dysfunctional GH receptor. Growth rates have been maintained for several years, and this therapy now portends improved final adult stature in this group of patients.

ADULT GH DEFICIENCY (AGHD) This disorder is usually caused by hypothalamic or pituitary somatotrope damage. Acquired pituitary hormone deficiency follows a typical sequential pattern whereby loss of adequate GH reserve foreshadows subsequent hormone deficits. The sequential order of hormone loss is usually GH → FSH/LH → TSH → ACTH.

Presentation and Diagnosis The clinical features of AGHD include changes in body composition, lipid metabolism, and quality of life and cardiovascular dysfunction (Table 318-9). Body composition changes are common and include reduced lean body mass, increased fat mass

TABLE 318-9 *Features of Adult Growth Hormone Deficiency*

Clinical	Imaging
Impaired quality of life	Pituitary: Mass or structural damage
Decreased energy and drive	Bone: Reduced bone mineral density
Poor concentration	Abdomen: Excess omental adiposity
Low self-esteem	**Laboratory**
Social isolation	Evoked GH <3 ng/mL
Body composition changes	IGF-I and IGFBP3 low or normal
Increased body fat mass	Increased LDL-cholesterol
Central fat deposition	Concomitant gonadotropin, TSH,
Increased waist-hip ratio	and/or ACTH reserve deficits may
Decreased lean body mass	be present
Reduced exercise capacity	
Reduced maximum O$_2$ uptake	
Impaired cardiac function	
Reduced muscle mass	
Cardiovascular risk factors	
Impaired cardiac structure and	
function	
Abnormal lipid profile	
Decreased fibrinolytic activity	
Atherosclerosis	
Omental obesity	

Note: LDL, low-density lipoprotein; for other abbreviations, see text.

with selective deposition of intraabdominal visceral fat, and increased waist-to-hip ratio. Hyperlipidemia, left ventricular dysfunction, hypertension, and increased plasma fibrinogen levels may also be present. Bone mineral content is reduced, with resultant increased fracture rates. Patients may experience social isolation, depression, and difficulty in maintaining gainful employment. Adult hypopituitarism is associated with a threefold increased cardiovascular mortality rate in comparison to age- and sex-matched controls, and this may be due to GH deficiency.

Laboratory Investigation AGHD is rare, and in light of the nonspecific nature of associated clinical symptoms, patients appropriate for testing should be carefully selected on the basis of well-defined criteria. With few exceptions, testing should be restricted to patients with the following predisposing factors: (1) pituitary surgery, (2) pituitary or hypothalamic tumor or granulomas, (3) cranial irradiation, (4) radiologic evidence of a pituitary lesion, (5) childhood requirement for GH replacement therapy, or, rarely, (6) unexplained low age- and sex-matched IGF-I level. The transition of the GH-deficient adolescent to adulthood requires retesting to document adult GH deficiency. Up to 20% of patients treated for childhood-onset GH deficiency are found to be GH-sufficient on repeat testing as adults.

A significant proportion (~25%) of truly GH-deficient adults have low-normal IGF-I levels. Thus, as in the evaluation of GH deficiency in children, valid age- and gender-matched IGF-I measurements provide a useful index of therapeutic responses but are not sufficiently sensitive for diagnostic purposes. The most validated test to distinguish pituitary-sufficient patients from those with AGHD is insulin-induced (0.05 to 0.1 U/kg) hypoglycemia. After glucose reduction to ~40 mg/dL, most individuals experience neuroglycopenic symptoms (Chap. 324), and peak GH release occurs at 60 min and remains elevated for up to 2 h. About 90% of healthy adults exhibit GH responses >5 μg/L; AGHD is defined by a peak GH response to hypoglycemia of <3 μg/L. Although insulin-induced hypoglycemia is safe when performed under appropriate supervision, it is contraindicated in patients with diabetes, ischemic heart disease, cerebrovascular disease, or epilepsy, and in elderly patients. Alternative stimulatory tests include intravenous arginine (30 g), GHRH (1 μg/kg), and GHRP-6 (90 μg). Combinations of these tests may evoke GH secretion in subjects not responsive to a single test.

℞ TREATMENT

Once the diagnosis of AGHD is unequivocally established, replacement of GH may be indicated. Contraindications to therapy include the presence of an active neoplasm, intracranial hypertension, or uncontrolled diabetes and retinopathy. The starting dose of 0.15 to 0.3 mg/d should be titrated (up to a maximum of 1.25 mg/d) to maintain IGF-I levels in the mid-normal range for age- and gender-matched controls (Fig. 318-7). Women require higher doses than men, and elderly patients require less GH. Long-term GH maintenance sustains normal IGF-I levels and is associated with persistent body composition changes (e.g., enhanced lean body mass and lower body fat). High-density lipoprotein cholesterol increases, but total cholesterol and insulin levels do not change significantly. Lumbar spine bone mineral density increases, but this response is gradual (>1 year). Many patients note significant improvement in quality of life when evaluated by standardized questionnaires. The effect of GH replacement on mortality rates in GH-deficient patients is currently the subject of long-term prospective investigation.

About 30% of patients exhibit reversible dose-related fluid retention, joint pain, and carpal tunnel syndrome, and up to 40% exhibit myalgias and paresthesia. Patients receiving insulin require careful monitoring for dosing adjustments, as GH is a potent counterregulatory hormone for insulin action. Patients with type 2 diabetes mellitus initially develop further insulin resistance. However, glycemic control improves with the sustained loss of abdominal fat associated with

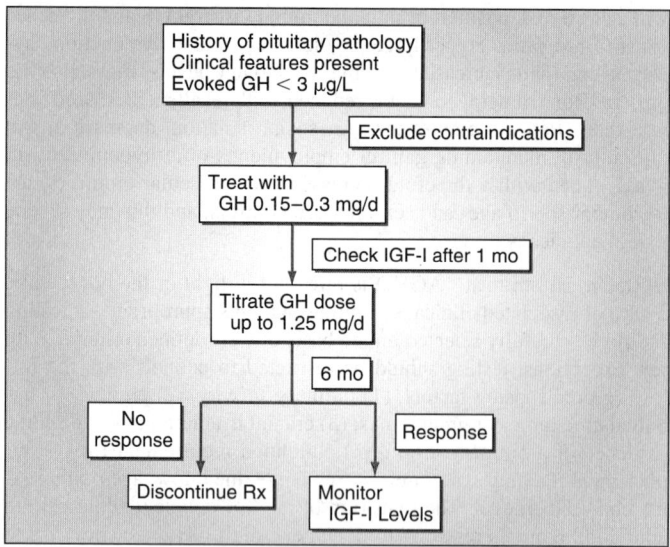

FIGURE 318-7   Management of adult growth hormone (GH) deficiency. (IGF, insulin-like growth factor.)

long-term GH replacement. Headache, increased intracranial pressure, hypertension, atrial fibrillation, and tinnitus occur rarely. Prevalence of pituitary tumor regrowth and potential progression of skin lesions are currently being assessed in long-term surveillance programs. To date, development of these potential side effects does not appear significant.

ACROMEGALY ■ **Etiology**   GH hypersecretion is usually the result of somatotrope adenomas but is also rarely caused by extrapituitary lesions (Table 318-10). In addition to typical GH-secreting somatotrope adenomas, mixed mammosomatotrope tumors and acidophilic stem-cell adenomas can secrete both GH and PRL. In patients with acidophilic stem-cell adenomas, features of hyperprolactinemia (hypogonadism and galactorrhea) predominate over the less clinically evident signs of acromegaly. Occasionally, mixed plurihormonal tumors are encountered that secrete ACTH, the glycoprotein hormone α subunit, or TSH, in addition to GH. Patients with partially empty sella may present with GH hypersecretion due to a small GH-secreting adenoma within the compressed rim of pituitary tissue; some of these may reflect the spon-

TABLE 318-10 *Causes of Acromegaly*

	Prevalence, %
Excess growth hormone secretion	
Pituitary	98
Densely or sparsely granulated GH cell adenoma	60
Mixed GH cell and PRL cell adenoma	25
Mammosomatrope cell adenoma	10
Plurihormonal adenoma	
GH cell carcinoma or metastases	
Multiple endocrine neoplasia-1 (GH cell adenoma)	
McCune-Albright syndrome	
Ectopic sphenoid or parapharyngeal sinus pituitary adenoma	
Extrapituitary tumor	
Pancreatic islet cell tumor	<1
Excess growth hormone–releasing hormone secretion	
Central	<1
Hypothalamic hamartoma, choristoma, ganglioneuroma	<1
Peripheral	<1
Bronchial carcinoid, pancreatic islet cell tumor, small cell lung cancer, adrenal adenoma, medullary thyroid carcinoma, pheochromocytoma	

Source: Adapted from S Melmed: N Engl J Med 322:966, 1990. Copyright © 1990, Massachusetts Medical Society. All rights reserved.

taneous necrosis of tumors that were previously larger. GH-secreting tumors rarely arise from ectopic pituitary tissue remnants in the nasopharynx or midline sinuses.

There are case reports of ectopic GH secretion by tumors of pancreatic, ovarian, or lung origin. Excess GHRH production may cause acromegaly because of chronic stimulation of somatotropes. These patients present with classic features of acromegaly, elevated GH levels, pituitary enlargement on MRI, and pathologic characteristics of pituitary hyperplasia. The most common cause of GHRH-mediated acromegaly is a chest or abdominal carcinoid tumor. Although these tumors usually express positive GHRH immunoreactivity, clinical features of acromegaly are evident in only a minority of patients with carcinoid disease. Excessive GHRH may also be elaborated by hypothalamic tumors, usually choristomas or neuromas.

Presentation and Diagnosis   Protean manifestations of GH and IGF-I hypersecretion are indolent and often are not clinically diagnosed for 10 years or more. Acral bony overgrowth results in frontal bossing, increased hand and foot size, mandibular enlargement with prognathism, and widened space between the lower incisor teeth. In children and adolescents, initiation of GH hypersecretion prior to epiphyseal long bone closure is associated with the development of pituitary gigantism (Fig. 318-8). Soft tissue swelling results in increased heel pad thickness, increased shoe or glove size, ring tightening, characteristic coarse facial features, and a large fleshy nose. Other commonly encountered clinical features include hyperhidrosis, deep and hollow-sounding voice, oily skin, arthropathy, kyphosis, carpal tunnel syndrome, proximal muscle weakness and fatigue, acanthosis nigricans, and skin tags. Generalized visceromegaly occurs, including cardiomegaly, macroglossia, and thyroid gland enlargement.

The most significant clinical impact of GH excess occurs with respect to the cardiovascular system. Coronary heart disease, cardiomyopathy with arrhythmias, left ventricular hypertrophy, decreased diastolic function, and hypertension occur in about 30% of patients. Upper airway obstruction with sleep apnea occurs in about 60% of patients and is associated with both soft tissue laryngeal airway obstruction and central sleep dysfunction. Diabetes mellitus develops in 25% of patients with acromegaly, and most patients are intolerant of a glucose load (as GH counteracts the action of insulin). Acromegaly is associated with an increased risk of colon polyps and colonic malignancy; polyps are diagnosed in up to one-third of acromegalic patients. Overall mortality is increased about threefold and is due primarily to cardiovascular and cerebrovascular disorders, malignancy, and respiratory disease. Unless GH levels are controlled, survival is reduced by an average of 10 years compared with an age-matched control population.

Laboratory Investigation   Age- and gender-matched serum IGF-I levels are elevated in acromegaly. Consequently, an IGF-I level provides a useful laboratory screening measure when clinical features raise the possibility of acromegaly. Due to the pulsatility of GH secretion, measurement of a single random GH level is not useful for the diagnosis or exclusion of acromegaly and does not correlate with disease severity. The diagnosis of acromegaly is confirmed by demonstrating the failure of GH suppression to < 1 μg/L within 1 to 2 h of an oral glucose load (75 g). About 20% of patients exhibit a paradoxical GH rise after glucose. About 60% of patients with GH-secreting tumors may exhibit paradoxical GH responses to TRH administration. PRL should be measured as it is elevated in ~25% of patients with acromegaly. Thyroid function, gonadotropins, and sex steroids may be attenuated because of tumor mass effects. Because most patients will undergo surgery with glucocorticoid coverage, tests of ACTH reserve in asymptomatic patients are more efficiently deferred until after surgery.

Rx TREATMENT

Surgical resection of GH-secreting adenomas is the initial treatment for most patients (Fig. 318-9). Somatostatin analogues are used as adjuvant treatment for preoperative shrinkage of large invasive macroadenomas, immediate relief of debilitating symptoms, and reduction of GH hypersecretion, in elderly patients experiencing morbidity, in patients who decline surgery, or, when surgery fails, to achieve biochemical control. Irradiation or repeat surgery may be required for patients who cannot tolerate or do not respond to adjunctive medical therapy. The high rate of late hypopituitarism and the slow rate (5 to 15 years) of biochemical response are the main disadvantages of radiotherapy. Irradiation is relatively ineffective in normalizing IGF-I levels. Stereotactic ablation of GH-secreting adenomas by gammaknife radiotherapy is promising, but long-term results are not available and the side effects have not been clearly delineated. Somatostatin analogues may be given while awaiting the full effect of radiotherapy. Systemic sequelae of acromegaly, including cardiovascular disease, diabetes, and arthritis, should also be managed aggressively. Maxillofacial surgery for mandibular repair may also be indicated.

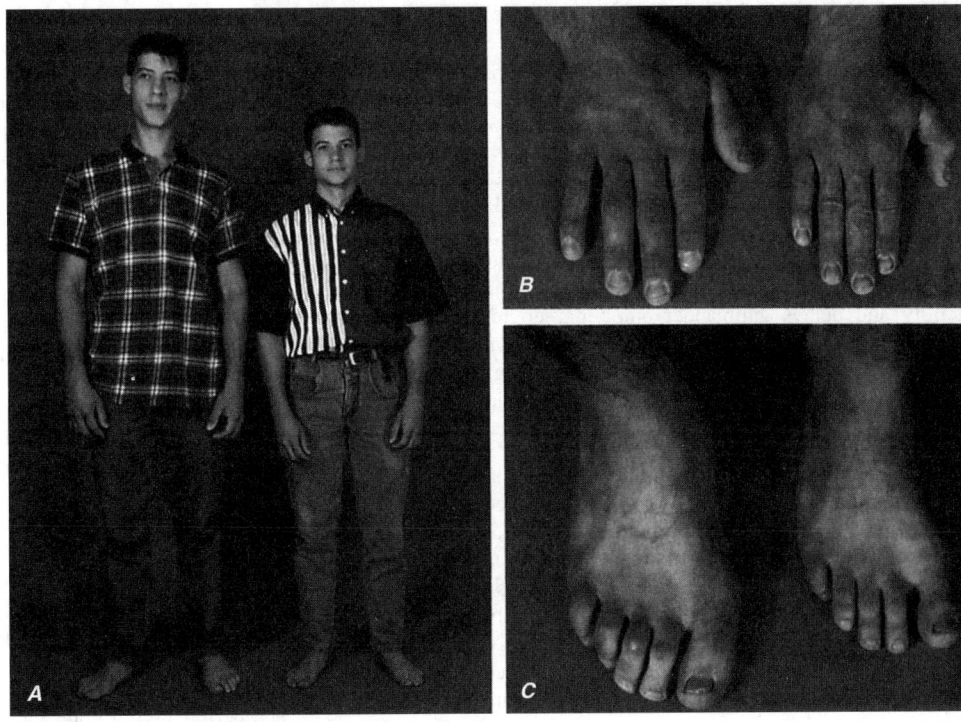

FIGURE 318-8 Features of acromegaly/gigantism. A 22-year-old man with gigantism due to excess growth hormone is shown to the left of his identical twin. The increased height and prognathism (*A*) and enlarged hand (*B*) and foot (*C*) of the affected twin are apparent. Their clinical features began to diverge at the age of approximately 13 years. (*Reproduced from R Gagel, IE McCutcheon: N Engl J Med 324:524, 1999, with permission.*)

SURGERY Transsphenoidal surgical resection by an experienced surgeon is the preferred primary treatment for both microadenomas (cure rate ~70%) and macroadenomas (<50% cured). Soft tissue swelling improves immediately after tumor resection. GH levels return to normal within an hour, and IGF-I levels are normalized within 3 to 4 days. In ~10% of patients, acromegaly may recur several years after apparently successful surgery; hypopituitarism develops in up to 15% of patients.

SOMATOSTATIN ANALOGUES Somatostatin analogues exert their therapeutic effects through SSTR2 and -5 receptors, both of which are expressed by GH-secreting tumors. Octreotide acetate is an 8-amino-acid synthetic somatostatin analogue. In contrast to native somatostatin, the analogue is relatively resistant to plasma degradation. It has a 2-h serum half-life and possesses 40-fold greater potency than native somatostatin to suppress GH. Octreotide is administered by subcutaneous injection, beginning with 50 μg tid; the dose can be gradually increased up to 1500 μg/d. Fewer than 10% of patients do not respond to the analogue. Octreotide suppresses integrated GH levels to <5 μg/L in ~70% of patients and to <2 μg/L in up to 60% of patients. It normalizes IGF-I levels in ~75% of treated patients. Prolonged use of the analogue is not associated with desensitization, even after ≥10 years of treatment. Rapid relief of headache and soft tissue swelling occurs in ~75% of patients within days to weeks of treatment initiation. Subjective clinical benefits of octreotide therapy occur more frequently than biochemical remission, and most patients report symptomatic improvement, including amelioration of headache, perspiration, obstructive apnea, and cardiac failure. Modest pituitary tumor size reduction occurs in about 40% of patients, but this effect is reversed when treatment is stopped.

Two long-acting somatostatin depot formulations, octreotide and lanreotide, are becoming the preferred medical treatment for acromegalic patients. *Sando-*

statin-LAR is a sustained-release, long-acting formulation of octreotide incorporated into microspheres that sustain drug levels for several weeks after intramuscular injection. GH suppression occurs for as long as 6 weeks after a 30-mg injection; long-term monthly treatment sustains GH and IGF-I suppression and reduction of pituitary tumor size. *Lanreotide,* a slow-release depot somatostatin preparation, is a cyclic somatostatin octapeptide analogue that suppresses GH and IGF-I hypersecretion for 10 to 14 days after a 30-mg intramuscular injection. Long-term administration controls GH hypersecretion in two-thirds of

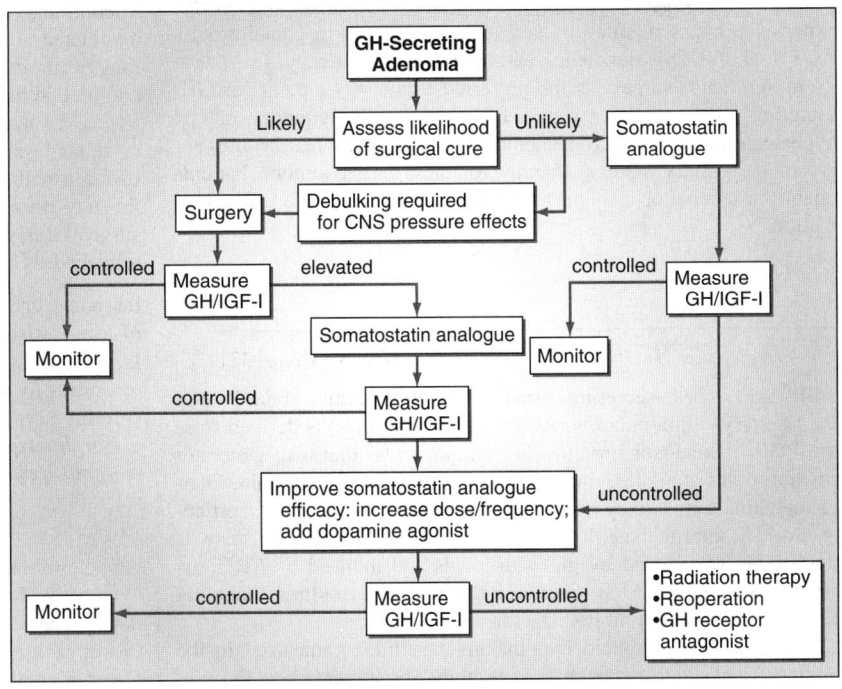

FIGURE 318-9 Management of acromegaly. (GH, growth hormone; CNS, central nervous system; IGF, insulin-like growth factor.) (*Adapted from S. Melmed et al: J Clin Endocrinol Metab 83:2646, 1998; © The Endocrine Society.*)

treated patients and improves patient compliance because of the long interval required between drug injections.

Side Effects Somatostatin analogues are well tolerated in most patients. Adverse effects are short-lived and mostly relate to drug-induced suppression of gastrointestinal motility and secretion. Nausea, abdominal discomfort, fat malabsorption, diarrhea, and flatulence occur in one-third of patients, though these symptoms usually remit within 2 weeks. Octreotide suppresses postprandial gallbladder contractility and delays gallbladder emptying; up to 30% of patients treated long-term develop echogenic sludge or asymptomatic cholesterol gallstones. Other side effects include mild glucose intolerance due to transient insulin suppression, asymptomatic bradycardia, hypothyroxinemia, and local pain at the injection site.

DOPAMINE AGONISTS Bromocriptine may suppress GH secretion in some acromegalic patients, particularly those with cosecretion of PRL. High doses (≥20 mg/d), administered as three to four daily doses, are usually required to lower GH, and therapeutic efficacy is modest. GH levels are suppressed to <5 µg/L in ~20% of patients, and IGF-I levels are normalized in only 10% of patients. Cabergoline also suppresses GH and decreases adenoma size when given at a relatively high dose of 0.5 mg/d. Combined treatment with octreotide and bromocriptine induces additive biochemical control compared to either drug alone.

GH ANTAGONISTS GH analogues (e.g., pegvisomant) antagonize endogenous GH action by blocking peripheral GH binding to its receptor. Consequently, serum IGF-I levels are suppressed, potentially reducing the deleterious effects of excess endogenous GH.

RADIATION External radiation therapy or high-energy stereotactic techniques are used as adjuvant therapy for acromegaly. An advantage of radiation is that patient compliance with long-term treatment is not required. Tumor mass is reduced, and GH levels are attenuated over time. However, 50% of patients require at least 8 years for GH levels to be suppressed to <5 µg/L; this level of GH reduction is achieved in about 90% of patients after 18 years but represents suboptimal GH suppression. Patients may require interim medical therapy for several years prior to attaining maximal radiation benefits. Most patients also experience hypothalamic-pituitary damage, leading to gonadotropin, ACTH, and/or TSH deficiency within 10 years of therapy.

In summary, surgery is the preferred primary treatment for GH-secreting microadenomas (Fig. 318-9). The high frequency of GH hypersecretion after macroadenoma resection usually necessitates adjuvant or primary medical therapy for these larger tumors. Patients unable to receive or respond to medical treatment can be offered radiation.

ADRENOCORTICOTROPIN HORMONE (See also Chap. 321)

SYNTHESIS ACTH-secreting corticotrope cells constitute about 20% of the pituitary cell population. ACTH (39 amino acids) is derived from the POMC precursor protein (266 amino acids) that also generates several other peptides, including β-lipotropin, β-endorphin, met-enkephalin, α melanocyte-stimulating hormone (MSH), and corticotropin-like intermediate lobe protein (CLIP). The POMC gene is powerfully suppressed by glucocorticoids and induced by CRH, arginine vasopressin (AVP), and proinflammatory cytokines, including IL-6, and leukemia inhibitory factor.

CRH, a 41-amino-acid hypothalamic peptide synthesized in the paraventricular nucleus as well as in higher brain centers, is the predominant stimulator of ACTH synthesis and release. The CRH receptor is a GPCR that is expressed on the corticotrope and induces POMC transcription.

SECRETION ACTH secretion is pulsatile and exhibits a characteristic circadian rhythm, peaking at 6 A.M. and reaching a nadir about midnight. Adrenal glucocorticoid secretion, which is driven by ACTH, follows a parallel diurnal pattern. ACTH circadian rhymicity is determined by variations in secretory pulse amplitude rather than changes in pulse frequency. Superimposed on this endogenous rhythm, ACTH levels are increased by AVP, physical stress, exercise, acute illness, and insulin-induced hypoglycemia.

Loss of cortisol feedback inhibition, as occurs in primary adrenal failure, results in extremely high ACTH levels. Glucocorticoid-mediated negative regulation of the hypothalamo-pituitary-adrenal (HPA) axis occurs as a consequence of both hypothalamic CRH suppression and direct attenuation of pituitary POMC gene expression and ACTH release.

Acute inflammatory or septic insults activate the HPA axis through the integrated actions of proinflammatory cytokines, bacterial toxins, and neural signals. The overlapping cascade of ACTH-inducing cytokines [tumor necrosis factor (TNF); IL-1, -2, and -6; and leukemia inhibitory factor] activates hypothalamic CRH and AVP secretion, pituitary POMC gene expression, and local paracrine pituitary cytokine networks. The resulting cortisol elevation restrains the inflammatory response and provides host protection. Concomitantly, cytokine-mediated central glucocorticoid receptor resistance impairs glucocorticoid suppression of the HPA. Thus, the neuroendocrine stress response reflects the net result of highly integrated hypothalamic, intrapituitary, and peripheral hormone and cytokine signals.

ACTION The major function of the HPA axis is to maintain metabolic homeostasis and to mediate the neuroendocrine stress response. ACTH induces cortical steroidogenesis by maintaining adrenal cell proliferation and function. The receptor for ACTH, designated *melanocortin-2 receptor*, is a GPCR that induces steroidogenesis by stimulating a cascade of steroidogenic enzymes (Chap. 321).

ACTH DEFICIENCY ■ **Presentation and Diagnosis** Secondary adrenal insufficiency occurs as a result of pituitary ACTH deficiency. It is characterized by fatigue, weakness, anorexia, nausea, vomiting, and, occasionally, hypoglycemia (due to diminished insulin counterregulation). In contrast to primary adrenal failure, hypocortisolism associated with pituitary failure is not usually accompanied by pigmentation changes or mineralocorticoid deficiency. ACTH deficiency is commonly due to glucocorticoid withdrawal following treatment-associated suppression of the HPA axis. Isolated ACTH deficiency may occur after surgical resection of an ACTH-secreting pituitary adenoma that has suppressed the HPA axis; this phenomenon is suggestive of a surgical cure. The mass effects of other pituitary adenomas or sellar lesions may lead to ACTH deficiency, but usually in combination with other pituitary hormone deficiencies. Partial ACTH deficiency may be unmasked in the presence of an acute medical or surgical illness, when clinically significant hypocortisolism reflects diminished ACTH reserve.

Laboratory Diagnosis Inappropriately low ACTH levels in the setting of low cortisol levels are characteristic of diminished ACTH reserve. Low basal serum cortisol levels are associated with blunted cortisol responses to ACTH stimulation and impaired cortisol response to insulin-induced hypoglycemia, or testing with metyrapone or CRH. →*For description of provocative ACTH tests, see "Tests of Pituitary-Adrenal Responsiveness" in Chap. 321.*

℞ **TREATMENT**

Glucocorticoid replacement therapy improves most features of ACTH deficiency. The total daily dose of hydrocortisone replacement should not exceed 30 mg daily, divided into two or three doses. Prednisone (5 mg each morning; 2.5 mg each evening) is longer acting and has fewer mineralocorticoid effects than hydrocortisone. Some authorities advocate lower maintenance doses in an effort to avoid cushingoid side effects. Doses should be increased several-fold during periods of acute illness or stress.

CUSHING'S DISEASE (ACTH-PRODUCING ADENOMA) (See also Chap. 321)

■ **Etiology and Prevalence** Pituitary corticotrope adenomas account for 70% of patients with endogenous causes of Cushing's syndrome. However, it should be recalled that iatrogenic hypercortisolism is the most common cause of cushingoid features. Ectopic tumor ACTH production, cortisol-producing adrenal adenomas, carcinoma, and hyperplasia account for the other causes; rarely, ectopic tumor CRH production is encountered.

ACTH-producing adenomas account for about 10 to 15% of all pituitary tumors. Because the clinical features of Cushing's syndrome often lead to early diagnosis, most ACTH-producing pituitary tumors are relatively small microadenomas. However, macroadenomas are also seen, and some ACTH-secreting adenomas are clinically silent. Cushing's disease is 5 to 10 times more common in women than in men. These pituitary adenomas exhibit unrestrained ACTH secretion, with resultant hypercortisolemia. However, they retain partial suppressibility in the presence of high doses of administered glucocorticoids, providing the basis for dynamic testing to distinguish pituitary and nonpituitary causes of Cushing's syndrome.

Presentation and Diagnosis The diagnosis of Cushing's syndrome presents two great challenges: (1) to distinguish patients with pathologic cortisol excess from those with physiologic or other disturbances of cortisol production; and (2) to determine the etiology of cortisol excess.

Typical features of chronic cortisol excess include thin, brittle skin, central obesity, hypertension, plethoric moon facies, purple striae and easy bruisability, glucose intolerance or diabetes mellitus, gonadal dysfunction, osteoporosis, proximal muscle weakness, signs of hyperandrogenism (acne, hirsutism), and psychologic disturbances (depression, mania, and psychoses) (Table 318-11). Hematopoietic features of hypercortisolism include leukocytosis, lymphopenia, and eosinopenia. Immune suppression includes delayed hypersensitivity. The protean manifestations of hypercortisolism make it challenging to decide which patients mandate formal laboratory evaluation. Certain features make pathologic causes of hypercortisolism more likely—these include characteristic central redistribution of fat, thin skin with striae and bruising, and proximal muscle weakness. In children and in young females, early osteoporosis may be particularly prominent. The primary cause of death is cardiovascular disease, but infections and risk of suicide are also increased.

Rapid development of features of hypercortisolism associated with skin hyperpigmentation and severe myopathy suggests the possibility

of ectopic sources of ACTH. Hypertension, hypokalemic alkalosis, glucose intolerance, and edema are also more pronounced in these patients. Serum potassium levels <3.3 mmol/L are evident in ~70% of patients with ectopic ACTH secretion but are seen in <10% of patients with pituitary-dependent Cushing's disease.

Laboratory Investigation The diagnosis of Cushing's syndrome is based on laboratory documentation of endogenous hypercortisolism. Measurements of 24-h urine free cortisol (UFC) is a precise and cost-effective screening test. Alternatively, the failure to suppress plasma cortisol after an overnight 1-mg dexamethasone suppression test can be used to identify patients with hypercortisolism. As nadir levels of cortisol occur at night, elevated midnight samples of cortisol are suggestive of Cushing's syndrome. Basal plasma ACTH levels often distinguish patients with ACTH-independent (adrenal or exogenous glucocorticoid) from those with ACTH-dependent (pituitary, ectopic ACTH) Cushing's disease. Mean basal ACTH levels are about eight-fold higher in patients with ectopic ACTH secretion compared to those with pituitary ACTH-secreting adenomas. However, extensive overlap of ACTH levels in these two disorders precludes using ACTH to make the distinction. Instead, dynamic testing, based on differential sensitivity to glucocorticoid feedback, or ACTH stimulation in response to CRH or cortisol reduction is used to discriminate ectopic versus pituitary sources of excess ACTH (Table 318-12). Very rarely, circulating CRH levels are elevated, reflecting ectopic tumor-derived secretion of CRH and often ACTH. →*For discussion of dynamic testing for Cushing's syndrome, see Chap. 321.*

Most ACTH-secreting pituitary tumors are <5 mm in diameter, and about half are undetectable by sensitive MRI. The high prevalence of incidental pituitary microadenomas diminishes the ability to distinguish ACTH-secreting pituitary tumors accurately by MRI.

TABLE 318-12 *Differential Diagnosis of ACTH-Dependent Cushing's Syndrome[a]*

	ACTH-Secreting Pituitary Tumor	Ectopic ACTH Secretion
Etiology	Pituitary corticotrope adenoma	Bronchial, abdominal carcinoid
	Plurihormonal adenoma	Small cell lung cancer Thymoma
Gender	F > M	M > F
Clinical features	Slow onset	Rapid onset Pigmentation Severe myopathy
Serum potassium <3.3 μg/L	<10%	75%
24-h urinary free cortisol (UFC)	High	High
Basal ACTH level	Inappropriately high	Very high
Dexamethasone suppression 1 mg overnight		
Low dose (0.5 mg q6h)	Cortisol >5 μg/dL	Cortisol >5 μg/dL
High dose (2 mg q6h)	Cortisol >5 μg/dL	Cortisol >5 μg/dL
UFC > 80% suppressed	Microadenomas: 90% Macroadenomas: 50%	10%
Inferior petrosal sinus sampling (IPSS) Basal		
IPSS: peripheral	>2	<2
CRH-induced		
IPSS: peripheral	>3	<3

[a] ACTH-independent causes of Cushing's syndrome are diagnosed by suppressed ACTH levels and an adrenal mass in the setting of hypercortisolism. Iatrogenic Cushing's syndrome is excluded by history.

Note: ACTH, adrenocorticotropin hormone; F, female; M, male; CRH, corticotropin-releasing hormone.

TABLE 318-11 *Clinical Features of Cushing's Syndrome (All Ages)*

Symptoms/Signs	Frequency, %
Obesity or weight gain (>115% ideal body weight)	80
Thin skin	80
Moon facies	75
Hypertension	75
Purple skin striae	65
Hirsutism	65
Abnormal glucose tolerance	55
Impotence	55
Menstrual disorders (usually amenorrhea)	60
Plethora	60
Proximal muscle weakness	50
Truncal obesity	50
Acne	45
Bruising	45
Mental changes	45
Osteoporosis	40
Edema of lower extremities	30
Hyperpigmentation	20
Hypokalemic alkalosis	15
Diabetes mellitus	15

Source: Adapted from MA Magiokou et al, in ME Wierman (ed), *Diseases of the Pituitary.* Totowa, NJ, Humana, 1997.

Inferior Petrosal Venous Sampling   Because pituitary MRI with gadolinium enhancement is insufficiently sensitive to detect small (<2 mm) pituitary ACTH-secreting adenomas, bilateral inferior petrosal sinus ACTH sampling before and after CRH administration may be required to distinguish these lesions from ectopic ACTH-secreting tumors that may have similar clinical and biochemical characteristics. Simultaneous assessment of ACTH concentrations in each inferior petrosal vein and in the peripheral circulation provides a strategy for confirming and localizing pituitary ACTH production. Sampling is performed at baseline and 2, 5, and 10 min after intravenous ovine CRH (1 μg/kg) injection. An increased ratio (>2) of inferior petrosal: peripheral vein ACTH confirms pituitary Cushing's disease. After CRH injection, peak petrosal:peripheral ACTH ratios of ≥3 confirm the presence of a pituitary ACTH-secreting tumor. The sensitivity of this test is >95%, with very rare false-positive results. False-negative results may be encountered in patients with aberrant venous anatomic drainage. Petrosal sinus catheterizations are technically difficult, and about 0.05% of patients develop neurovascular complications. The procedure should not be performed in patients with hypertension or in the presence of a well-visualized pituitary adenoma on MRI.

℞ TREATMENT

Selective transsphenoidal resection is the treatment of choice for Cushing's disease (Fig. 318-10). The remission rate for this procedure is ~80% for microadenomas but <50% for macroadenomas. After successful tumor resection, most patients experience a postoperative period of adrenal insufficiency that lasts for up to 12 months. This usually requires low-dose cortisol replacement, as patients experience steroid withdrawal symptoms as well as having a suppressed HPA axis. Biochemical recurrence occurs in approximately 5% of patients in whom surgery was initially successful.

When initial surgery is unsuccessful, repeat surgery is sometimes indicated, particularly when a pituitary source for ACTH is well documented. In older patients when growth and fertility are no longer important, hemi- or total hypophysectomy may be necessary if an adenoma is not recognized. Pituitary irradiation may be used after unsuccessful surgery, but it cures only about 15% of patients. Because radiation is slow and only partially effective in adults, steroidogenic

inhibitors are used in combination with pituitary irradiation to block the adrenal effects of persistently high ACTH levels.

Ketoconazole, an imidazole derivative antimycotic agent, inhibits several P450 enzymes and effectively lowers cortisol in most patients with Cushing's disease when administered twice daily (600 to 1200 mg/d). Elevated hepatic transaminases, gynecomastia, impotence, gastrointestinal upset, and edema are common side effects. *Metyrapone* (2 to 4 g/d) inhibits 11β-hydroxylase activity and normalizes plasma cortisol in up to 75% of patients. Side effects include nausea and vomiting, rash, and exacerbation of acne or hirsutism. *Mitotane* (o, p'-DDD; 3 to 6 g/d orally in four divided doses) suppresses cortisol hypersecretion by inhibiting 11β-hydroxylase and cholesterol side-chain cleavage enzymes and by destroying adrenocortical cells. Side effects of mitotane include gastrointestinal symptoms, dizziness, gynecomastia, hyperlipidemia, skin rash, and hepatic enzyme elevation. It may also lead to hypoaldosteronism. Other agents include *aminoglutethimide* (250 mg tid), *trilostane* (200 to 1000 mg/d), *cyproheptadine* (24 mg/d), and IV *etomidate* (0.3 mg/kg per hour). Glucocorticoid insufficiency is a potential side effect of agents used to block steroidogenesis.

The use of steroidogenic inhibitors has decreased the need for bilateral adrenalectomy. Removal of both adrenal glands corrects hypercortisolism but may be associated with significant morbidity and necessitates permanent glucocorticoid and mineralocorticoid replacement. Adrenalectomy in the setting of residual corticotrope adenoma tissue predisposes to the development of *Nelson's syndrome*, a disorder characterized by rapid pituitary tumor enlargement and increased pigmentation secondary to high ACTH levels. Radiation therapy may be indicated to prevent the development of Nelson's syndrome after adrenalectomy.

GONADOTROPINS: FSH AND LH

SYNTHESIS AND SECRETION   Gonadotrope cells comprise about 10% of anterior pituitary cells and produce two gonadotropins—LH and FSH. Like TSH and hCG, LH and FSH are glycoprotein hormones consisting of α and β subunits. The α subunit is common to these glycoprotein hormones; specificity is conferred by the β subunits, which are expressed by separate genes.

Gonadotropin synthesis and release are dynamically regulated. This is particularly true in females, in whom the rapidly fluctuating gonadal steroid levels vary throughout the menstrual cycle. Hypothalamic GnRH, a 10-amino-acid peptide, regulates the synthesis and secretion of both LH and FSH. GnRH is secreted in discrete pulses every 60 to 120 min, which in turn elicit LH and FSH pulses (Fig. 318-3). The pulsatile mode of GnRH input is essential to its action; pulses prime gonadotrope responsiveness, whereas continuous GnRH exposure induces desensitization. Based on this phenomenon, long-acting GnRH agonists are used to suppress gonadotropin levels in children with precocious puberty and in men with prostate cancer (Chap. 81) and are used in some ovulation-induction protocols to reduce endogenous gonadotropins (Chap. 45). Estrogens act at the hypothalamic and pituitary levels to control gonadotropin secretion. Chronic estrogen exposure is inhibitory, whereas rising estrogen levels, as occurs during the preovulatory surge, exert positive feedback to increase gonadotropin pulse frequency and amplitude. Progesterone slows GnRH pulse frequency but enhances gonadotropin responses to GnRH. Testosterone feedback in males also occurs at the hypothalamic and pituitary levels and partially reflects its conversion to estrogens.

Though GnRH is the main regulator of LH and FSH secretion, FSH synthesis is also under separate control by the gonadal peptides inhibin and activin, which are members of the transforming growth factor β (TGF-β) family. Inhibin selectively suppresses FSH, whereas activin stimulates FSH synthesis (Chap. 326).

ACTION   The gonadotropin hormones interact with their respective GPCRs expressed in the ovary and testis, evoking germ-cell development and maturation and steroid hormone biosynthesis. In women, FSH regulates ovarian follicle development and stimulates ovarian estrogen production. LH mediates ovulation and maintenance of the cor-

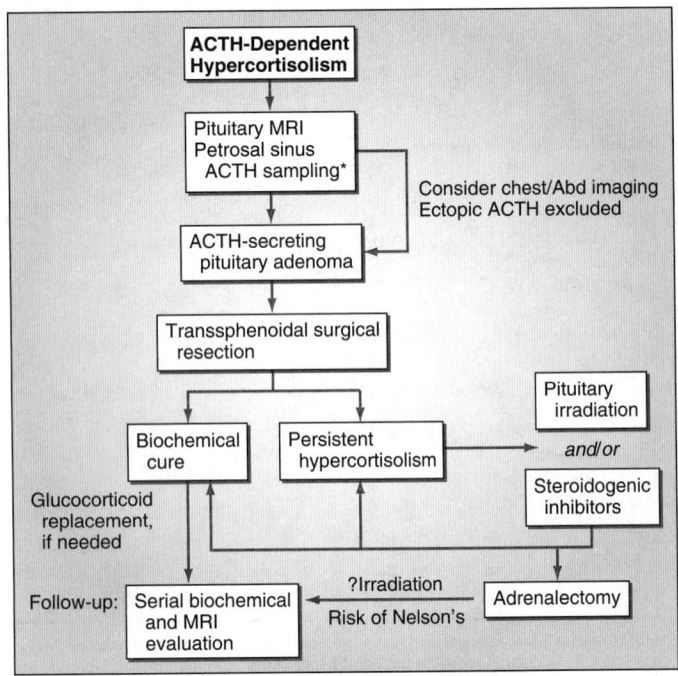

FIGURE 318-10   Management of Cushing's disease. (ACTH, adrenocorticotropin hormone; MRI, magnetic resonance imaging.) *, Not usually required.

pus luteum. In men, LH induces Leydig cell testosterone synthesis and secretion and FSH stimulates seminiferous tubule development and regulates spermatogenesis.

GONADOTROPIN DEFICIENCY Hypogonadism is the most common presenting feature of adult hypopituitarism, even when other pituitary hormones are also deficient. It is often a harbinger of hypothalamic or pituitary diseases that impair GnRH production or delivery through the pituitary stalk. As noted above, hypogonadotropic hypogonadism is a common presenting feature of hyperprolactinemia.

A variety of inherited and acquired disorders are associated with *isolated hypogonadotropic hypogonadism* (IHH) (Chap. 325). Hypothalamic defects associated with GnRH deficiency include two X-linked disorders, Kallmann syndrome (see above) and mutations in the *DAX1* gene. GnRH receptor mutations and inactivating mutations of the LH β and FSH β subunit genes are rare causes of selective gonadotropin deficiency. Acquired forms of GnRH deficiency leading to hypogonadotropism are seen in association with anorexia nervosa (Chap. 65), stress, starvation, and extreme exercise, but may also be idiopathic. Hypogonadotropic hypogonadism in these disorders is reversed by removal of the stressful stimulus.

Presentation and Diagnosis In premenopausal women, hypogonadotropic hypogonadism presents as diminished ovarian function leading to oligomenorrhea or amenorrhea, infertility, decreased vaginal secretions, decreased libido, and breast atrophy. In hypogonadal adult males, secondary testicular failure is associated with decreased libido and potency, infertility, decreased muscle mass with weakness, reduced beard and body hair growth, soft testes, and characteristic fine facial wrinkles. Osteoporosis occurs in both untreated hypogonadal females and males.

Laboratory Investigation Central hypogonadism is associated with low or inappropriately normal serum gonadotropin levels in the setting of low sex hormone concentrations (testosterone in males, estradiol in females). Three pooled serum samples drawn 20 min apart are used for accurate measurement of serum LH and FSH levels, thus allowing for the effects of hormone secretory pulses. Male patients have abnormal semen analysis.

Intravenous GnRH (100 μg) stimulates gonadotropes to secrete LH (which peaks within 30 min) and FSH (which plateaus during the ensuing 60 min). Normal responses vary according to menstrual cycle stage, age, and sex of the patient. Generally, LH levels increase about threefold, whereas FSH responses are less pronounced. In the setting of gonadotropin deficiency, a normal gonadotropin response to GnRH indicates intact gonadotrope function and suggests a hypothalamic abnormality. An absent response, however, cannot reliably distinguish pituitary from hypothalamic causes of hypogonadism. For this reason, GnRH testing usually adds little to the information gained from baseline evaluation of the hypothalamic-pituitary-gonadotrope axis, except in cases of isolated GnRH deficiency (e.g., Kallmann syndrome).

MRI examination of the sellar region and assessment of other pituitary functions are usually indicated in patients with documented central hypogonadism.

℞ TREATMENT

In males, testosterone replacement is necessary to achieve and maintain normal growth and development of the external genitalia, secondary sex characteristics, male sexual behavior, and androgenic anabolic effects including maintenance of muscle function and bone mass. Testosterone may be administered by intramuscular injections every 1 to 4 weeks or using patches that are replaced daily (Chap. 325). Testosterone creams are also available. Gonadotropin injections [hCG or human menopausal gonadotropin (hMG)] over 12 to 18 months are used to restore fertility. Pulsatile GnRH therapy (25 to 150 ng/kg every 2 h), administered by a subcutaneous infusion pump, is also effective for treatment of hypothalamic hypogonadism when fertility is desired.

In premenopausal women, cyclical replacement of estrogen and progesterone maintains secondary sexual characteristics and genitourinary tract integrity and prevents premature osteoporosis (Chap.

326). Gonadotropin therapy is used for ovulation induction. Follicular growth and maturation are initiated using hMG or recombinant FSH; hCG is subsequently injected to induce ovulation. As in men, pulsatile GnRH therapy can be used to treat hypothalamic causes of gonadotropin deficiency.

NONFUNCTIONING AND GONADOTROPIN-PRODUCING PITUITARY ADENOMAS ∎
Etiology and Prevalence Nonfunctioning pituitary adenomas include those that secrete little or no pituitary hormones, as well as tumors that produce too little hormone to result in recognizable clinical features. They are the most common type of pituitary adenoma and are usually macroadenomas at the time of diagnosis because clinical features are inapparent until tumor mass effects occur. Based on immunohistochemistry, most clinically nonfunctioning adenomas can be shown to originate from gonadotrope cells. These tumors typically produce small amounts of intact gonadotropins (usually FSH) as well as uncombined α and LH β and FSH β subunits. Tumor secretion may lead to elevated α and FSH β subunits and, rarely, to increased LH β subunit levels. Some adenomas express α subunits without FSH or LH. TRH administration often induces an atypical increase of tumor-derived gonadotropins or subunits.

Presentation and Diagnosis Clinically nonfunctioning tumors may present with optic chiasm pressure and other symptoms of local expansion or be incidentally discovered on an MRI performed for another indication. Menstrual disturbances or ovarian hyperstimulation rarely occur in women with large tumors that produce FSH and LH. More commonly, adenoma compression of the pituitary stalk or surrounding pituitary tissue leads to attenuated LH and features of hypogonadism. PRL levels are usually slightly increased, also because of stalk compression. It is important to distinguish this circumstance from true prolactinomas, as most nonfunctioning tumors respond poorly to treatment with dopamine agonists.

Laboratory Investigation The goal of laboratory testing in clinically nonfunctioning tumors is to classify the type of the tumor, to identify hormonal markers of tumor activity, and to detect possible hypopituitarism. Free α subunit levels may be elevated in 10 to 15% of patients with nonfunctioning tumors. In female patients, peri- or postmenopausal basal FSH concentrations are difficult to distinguish from tumor-derived FSH elevation. Premenopausal women have cycling FSH levels, also preventing clear-cut diagnostic distinction from tumor-derived FSH. In men, gonadotropin-secreting tumors may be diagnosed because of slightly increased gonadotropins (FSH > LH) in the setting of a pituitary mass. Testosterone levels are usually low, despite the normal or increased LH level, perhaps reflecting reduced LH bioactivity or the loss of normal LH pulsatility. Because this pattern of hormone tests is also seen in primary gonadal failure and, to some extent, with aging (Chap. 325), the increased gonadotropins alone are insufficient for the diagnosis of a gonadotropin-secreting tumor. In the majority of patients with gonadotrope adenomas, TRH administration stimulates LH β subunit secretion; this response is not seen in normal individuals. GnRH testing is not helpful for making the diagnosis. For nonfunctioning and gonadotropin-secreting tumors, the diagnosis usually rests on immunohistochemical analyses of resected tumor tissue, as the mass effects of these tumors usually necessitate resection.

Although acromegaly or Cushing's syndrome usually presents with unique clinical features, clinically inapparent somatotrope or corticotrope adenomas can be excluded by a normal IGF-I value and normal 24-h urinary free cortisol levels. If PRL levels are <100 μg/L in a patient harboring a pituitary mass, a nonfunctioning adenoma causing pituitary stalk compression should be considered.

℞ TREATMENT

Asymptomatic small nonfunctioning adenomas with no threat to vision may be followed with regular MRI and visual field testing without immediate intervention. However, for larger macroadenomas, trans-

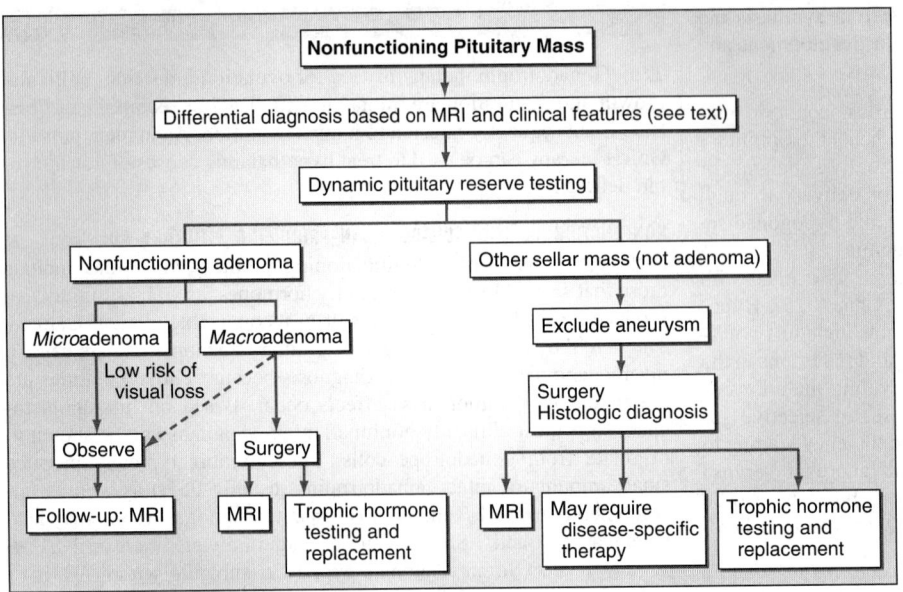

FIGURE 318-11 Management of a nonfunctioning pituitary mass.

sphenoidal surgery is the only effective way to reduce tumor size and relieve mass effects (Fig. 318-11). Although it is not usually possible to remove all adenoma tissue surgically, vision improves in 70% of patients with preoperative visual field defects. Preexisting hypopituitarism that results from tumor mass effects commonly improves or may resolve completely. Beginning about 6 months postoperatively, MRI scans should be performed yearly to detect tumor regrowth. Within 5 to 6 years following successful surgical resection, ~15% of nonfunctioning tumors recur. When substantial tumor remains after transsphenoidal surgery, adjuvant radiotherapy may be indicated to prevent tumor growth. Radiotherapy may be deferred if no postoperative residual mass is evident.

Nonfunctioning pituitary tumors respond poorly to dopamine agonist treatment, with modest tumor shrinkage occurring in <10% of patients. Although SSTR subtypes 2 and 5 have been identified on nonfunctioning pituitary adenomas, octreotide does not shrink these tumors and only modestly suppresses gonadotropin and α subunit levels. Visual improvement sometimes occurs without evident reduction of tumor size by MRI, presumably reflecting relief of pressure on the optic tracts. The selective GnRH antagonist, Nal-Glu GnRH, suppresses FSH hypersecretion but has no effect on adenoma size.

THYROID-STIMULATING HORMONE

SYNTHESIS AND SECRETION TSH-secreting thyrotrope cells comprise 5% of the anterior pituitary cell population. TSH is structurally related to LH and FSH. It shares a common α subunit with these hormones but contains a specific TSH β subunit. TRH is a hypothalamic tripeptide (pyroglutamyl histidylprolinamide) that acts through a GPCR to stimulate TSH synthesis and secretion; it also stimulates the lactotrope cell to secrete PRL. TSH secretion is stimulated by TRH, whereas thyroid hormones, dopamine, SRIF, and glucocorticoids suppress TSH by overriding TRH induction.

The thyrotrope is stimulated by a release from the negative feedback inhibition by thyroid hormones. Thus, thyroid damage, (including surgical thyroidectomy), radiation-induced hypothyroidism, chronic thyroiditis, or prolonged goitrogen exposure are associated with increased TSH. Long-standing untreated hypothyroidism can lead to thyrotrope hyperplasia and pituitary enlargement, which may be evident on MRI.

ACTION TSH is secreted in pulses, though the excursions are modest in comparison to other pituitary hormones because of the relatively low amplitude of the pulses and the relatively long half-life of TSH. Consequently, single determinations of TSH suffice to assess its circulating levels. TSH binds to a GPCR on thyroid follicular cells to stimulate thyroid hormone synthesis and release (Chap. 320).

TSH DEFICIENCY Features of central hypothyroidism, due to TSH deficiency, mimic those seen with primary hypothyroidism but are generally less severe. Pituitary hypothyroidism is characterized by low basal TSH levels in the setting of low free thyroid hormone. In contrast, patients with hypothyroidism of hypothalamic origin (presumably due to a lack of endogenous TRH) may exhibit normal or even slightly elevated TSH levels. There is evidence that the TSH produced in this circumstance has reduced biologic activity because of altered glycosylation.

TRH (200 μg) injected intravenously causes a two- to threefold increase in TSH (and PRL) levels within 30 min. Although TRH testing can be used to assess TSH reserve, abnormalities of the thyroid axis can usually be detected based on basal free T_4 and TSH levels, without the need for TRH testing.

Thyroid-replacement therapy should be initiated after establishing adequate adrenal function. Dose adjustment is based on thyroid hormone levels and clinical parameters rather than the TSH level.

TSH-SECRETING ADENOMAS TSH-producing macroadenomas are rare but are often large and locally invasive when they occur. Patients usually present with thyroid goiter and hyperthyroidism, reflecting overproduction of TSH. Diagnosis is based on demonstrating elevated serum free T_4 levels, inappropriately normal or high TSH secretion, and MRI evidence of a pituitary adenoma.

It is important to exclude other causes of inappropriate TSH secretion, such as resistance to thyroid hormone, an autosomal dominant disorder caused by mutations in the thyroid hormone β receptor (Chap. 320). The presence of a pituitary mass and elevated α subunit levels are suggestive of a TSH-secreting tumor. Dysalbuminemic hyperthyroxinemia syndromes, caused by various mutations in serum thyroid hormone binding proteins, are also characterized by elevated thyroid hormone levels, but with normal rather than suppressed TSH levels. Moreover, free thyroid hormone levels are normal in these disorders, most of which are familial.

℞ TREATMENT

The initial therapeutic approach is to remove or debulk the tumor mass surgically, using either a transsphenoidal or subfrontal approach. Total resection is not often achieved as most of these adenomas are large and locally invasive. Normal circulating thyroid hormone levels are achieved in about two-thirds of patients after surgery. Thyroid ablation or antithyroid drugs (methimazole or propylthiouracil) can be used to reduce thyroid hormone levels. Dopamine agonists are rarely effective for suppressing TSH secretion from these tumors. However, somatostatin analogue treatment effectively normalizes TSH and α subunit hypersecretion, shrinks the tumor mass in 50% of patients, and improves visual fields in 75% of patients; euthyroidism is restored in most patients. In some patients, octreotide markedly suppresses TSH, causing biochemical hypothyroidism that requires concomitant thyroid hormone replacement. Lanreotide (30 mg intramuscularly), a long-acting somatostatin analogue (see above), effectively suppresses TSH and thyroid hormone in patients treated every 14 days.

DIABETES INSIPIDUS

→*See Chap. 319 for diagnosis and treatment of diabetes insipidus.*

FURTHER READING

ATTANUSIO AF et al: Human growth hormone replacement in adult hypopituitary patients. J Clin Endocrinol Metab 87:1600, 2002

MELMED S et al: Consensus. Guidelines for acromegaly management. J Clin Endocrinol Metab 87:4054, 2002

MOLITCH ME: Diagnosis and treatment of prolactinomas. Adv Intern Med 44: 117, 1999

NEWELL-PRICE J et al: The diagnosis and differential diagnosis of Cushing's syndrome and pseudo-Cushing's states. Endocr Rev 19:647, 1998

OLSON LE, ROSENFELD MG: Perspective: Genetic and genomic approaches in elucidating mechanisms of pituitary development. Endocrinology 143: 2007, 2002

319 DISORDERS OF THE NEUROHYPOPHYSIS
Gary L. Robertson

The neurohypophysis, or posterior pituitary gland, is formed by axons that originate in large cell bodies in the supraoptic and paraventricular nuclei of the hypothalamus. It produces two hormones: (1) arginine vasopressin (AVP), also known as antidiuretic hormone; and (2) oxytocin. AVP acts on the renal tubules to reduce water loss by concentrating the urine. Oxytocin stimulates postpartum milk letdown in response to suckling. AVP deficiency causes diabetes insipidus (DI), characterized by the production of large amounts of dilute urine. Excessive or inappropriate AVP production predisposes to hyponatremia if water intake is not reduced in parallel with urine output.

VASOPRESSIN

ACTION AVP is a nonapeptide composed of a six-membered disulfide ring and a tripeptide tail (Fig. 319-1). The most important, if not the only, physiologic action of AVP is to reduce water excretion by promoting concentration of urine. This antidiuretic effect is achieved by increasing the hydroosmotic permeability of cells that line the distal tubule and medullary collecting ducts of the kidney (Fig. 319-2). In the absence of AVP, these cells are impermeable to water and reabsorb little, if any, of the relatively large volume of dilute filtrate that enters from the proximal nephron. This results in the excretion of very large volumes (as much as 0.2 mL/kg per min) of maximally dilute urine (specific gravity and osmolarity ~1.000 and 50 mosmol/L, respectively), a condition known as a *water diuresis*. In the presence of AVP, these cells become selectively permeable to water, allowing it to diffuse back down the osmotic gradient created by the hypertonic renal medulla. As a result, the dilute fluid passing through the tubules is concentrated and the rate of urine flow decreases. The magnitude of this effect varies in direct proportion to the plasma AVP concentration and, at maximum levels, approximates a urine flow rate as low as 0.35 mL/min and a urine osmolarity as high as 1200 mosmol/L. AVP action is mediated via binding to G protein–coupled V_2 receptors on the serosal surface of the cell, activation of adenyl cyclase, and insertion into the luminal surface of water channels composed of a protein known as *aquaporin 2*.

At high concentrations, AVP also causes contraction of smooth muscle in blood vessels and in the gastrointestinal tract, induces glycogenolysis in the liver, and potentiates adrenocorticotropic hormone (ACTH) release by corticotropin-releasing factor. These effects are mediated by V_{1a} or V_{1b} receptors that are coupled to phospholipase C. Their role, if any, in human physiology/pathophysiology is still uncertain.

SYNTHESIS AND SECRETION AVP secretion is synthesized via a polypeptide precursor that includes AVP, neurophysin, and copeptin. After preliminary processing and folding, the precursor is packaged in neurosecretory vesicles where it is transported down the axon, further processed to AVP, and stored until the hormone and other components are released by exocytosis into peripheral blood.

AVP secretion is regulated primarily by the "effective" osmotic pressure of body fluids. This control is mediated by specialized hypothalamic cells, known as *osmoreceptors*, which are extremely sensitive to small changes in the plasma concentration of sodium and certain other solutes but are insensitive to other solutes such as urea or glucose. The osmoreceptors appear to include inhibitory as well as stimulatory components that function in concert to form a threshold, or set point, control system for AVP release. Below this threshold, plasma AVP is suppressed to levels that permit the development of a maximum water diuresis. Above it, plasma AVP rises steeply in direct proportion to plasma osmolarity, quickly reaching levels sufficient to effect a maximum antidiuresis. The absolute levels of plasma osmolarity/sodium at which minimally and maximally effective levels of plasma AVP occur vary appreciably from person to person, owing apparently to genetic influences on the set and sensitivity of the system. However, the average threshold, or set point, for AVP release corresponds to a plasma osmolarity or sodium of about 280 mosmol/L or 135 meq/L, respectively; levels only 2 to 4% higher normally result in maximum antidiuresis. Though relatively stable in a healthy adult, the set of the osmoregulatory system can also be lowered by pregnancy, the menstrual cycle, and relatively large, acute reductions in blood pressure or volume.

The effects of acute changes in blood volume or pressure are mediated largely by neuronal afferents that originate in transmural pressure receptors of the heart and large arteries and project via the vagus and glossopharyngeal nerves to the brain stem, from whence postsynaptic projections ascend to the hypothalmus. These pathways maintain a tonic inhibitory tone that decreases when blood volume or pressure falls by >10 to 20%. This baroregulatory system is probably of minor importance in the physiology of AVP secretion because the hemodynamic changes required to affect it do not usually occur during normal activities. However, the baroregulatory system undoubtedly plays an important role in AVP secretion in patients with large, acute disturbances of hemodynamic function.

AVP secretion can also be stimulated by nausea, acute hypoglycemia, glucocorticoid deficiency, smoking, and, possibly, hyperangiotensinemia. The emetic stimuli are extremely potent since they typically elicit immediate, 50- to 100-fold increases in plasma AVP, even when the nausea is transient and unassociated with vomiting or other symptoms. They appear to act via the emetic center in the medulla and can be completely blocked by treatment with antiemetics such as fluphenazine. There is no evidence that pain or other noxious stresses have any affect on AVP unless they elicit a vasovagal reaction with its associated nausea and hypotension.

METABOLISM AVP distributes rapidly into a space roughly equal to the extracellular fluid volume. It is cleared irreversibly with a $t_{1/2}$ of 10 to 30 min. Most AVP clearance is due to degradation in the liver and kidneys. During pregnancy, the metabolic clearance of AVP is increased three- to fourfold due to placental production of an N-terminal peptidase.

THIRST Because AVP cannot reduce water loss below a certain minimum level obligated by urinary solute load and evaporation from skin

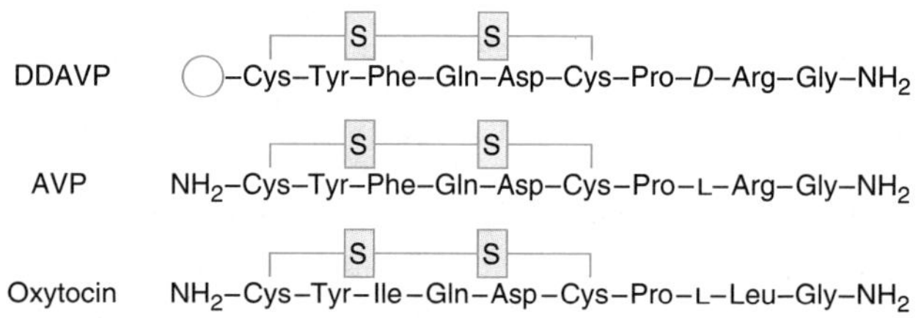

DDAVP ◯–Cys–Tyr–Phe–Gln–Asp–Cys–Pro–D-Arg–Gly–NH_2

AVP NH_2–Cys–Tyr–Phe–Gln–Asp–Cys–Pro–L-Arg–Gly–NH_2

Oxytocin NH_2–Cys–Tyr–Ile–Gln–Asp–Cys–Pro–L-Leu–Gly–NH_2

FIGURE 319-1 Primary structures of arginine vasopressin (AVP), oxytocin, and DDAVP.

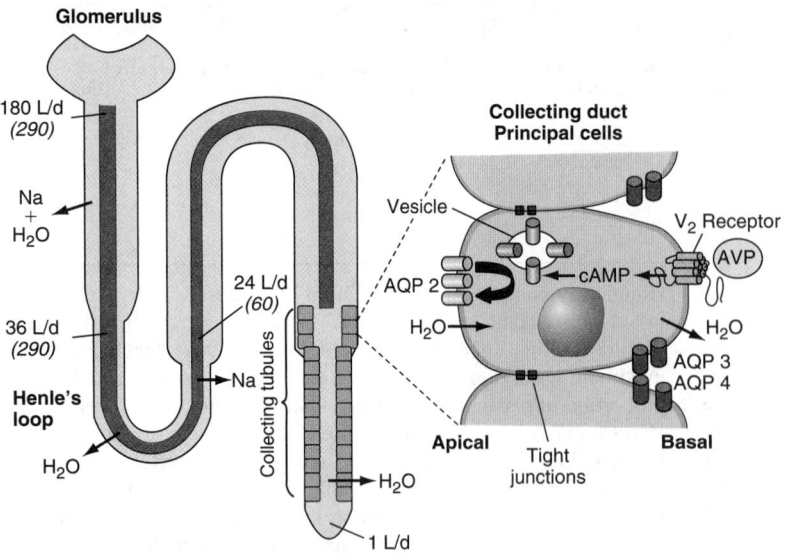

FIGURE 319-2 Antidiuretic effect of arginine vasopressin (AVP) in the regulation of urine volume. In a typical 70-kg adult, the kidney filters about 180 L/d of plasma. Of this, approximately 144 L (80%) is reabsorbed isosmotically in the proximal tubule and another 8 L (4 to 5%) is reabsorbed without solute in the descending limb of Henle's loop. The remainder is diluted to an osmolarity of about 60 mmol/kg by selective reabsorption of sodium and chloride in the ascending limb. In the absence of AVP, the urine issuing from the loop passes largely unmodified through the distal tubules and collecting ducts, resulting in a maximum water diuresis. In the presence of AVP, solute-free water is reabsorbed osmotically through the principal cells of the collecting ducts, resulting in the excretion of a much smaller volume of concentrated urine. This antidiuretic effect is mediated via a G protein–coupled V_2 receptor that increases intracellular cyclic AMP, thereby inducing translocation of aquaporin 2 (AQP 2) water channels into the apical membrane. The resultant increase in permeability permits an influx of water that diffuses out of the cell through AQP 3 and AQP 4 water channels on the basal-lateral surface. The net rate of flux across the cell is determined by the number of AQP 2 water channels in the apical membrane and the strength of the osmotic gradient between tubular fluid and the renal medulla. Tight junctions on the lateral surface of the cells serve to prevent unregulated water flow.

and lungs, a mechanism for ensuring adequate intake is essential for preventing dehydration. This vital function is performed by the thirst mechanism. Like AVP, thirst is regulated primarily by an osmostat that is located in the anteromedial hypothalamus and is able to detect very small changes in the plasma concentration of sodium and certain other effective solutes. The thirst osmostat appears to be "set" about 5% higher than the AVP osmostat. This arrangement ensures that thirst, polydipsia, and dilution of body fluids do not occur until plasma osmolarity/sodium start to exceed the defensive capacity of the antidiuretic mechanism.

OXYTOCIN

Oxytocin is also a nonapeptide and differs from AVP only at positions 3 and 8 (Fig. 319-1). However, it has relatively little antidiuretic effect and seems to act mainly on mammary ducts to facilitate milk letdown during nursing. It may also help to initiate or facilitate labor by stimulating contraction of uterine smooth muscle, but it is not yet clear if this action is physiologic or necessary for normal delivery.

DEFICIENCIES OF VASOPRESSIN SECRETION AND ACTION

DIABETES INSIPIDUS ■ **Clinical Characteristics** Decreased secretion or action of AVP usually manifests as DI, a syndrome characterized by the production of abnormally large volumes of dilute urine. The 24-h urine volume is >50 mL/kg body weight and the osmolarity is <300 mosmol/L. The polyuria produces symptoms of urinary frequency, enuresis, and/or nocturia, which may disturb sleep and cause mild daytime fatigue or somnolence. It is also associated with thirst and a commensurate increase in fluid intake (polydipsia). Clinical signs of dehydration are uncommon unless fluid intake is impaired.

Etiology Deficient secretion of AVP can be primary or secondary. The primary form usually results from agenesis or irreversible destruction of the neurohypophysis and is variously referred to as *neurohypophyseal DI*, *pituitary DI*, or *central DI*. It can be caused by a variety of

congenital, acquired, or genetic disorders but almost half the time it is idiopathic (Table 319-1). The genetic form of neurohypophyseal DI is usually transmitted in an autosomal dominant mode and is caused by diverse mutations in the coding region of the AVP–neurophysin II (or AVP-NPII) gene. In this type, the AVP deficiency and DI begin several months to several years after birth and appear to be a result of selective degeneration of AVP-producing magnocellular neurons. An autosomal recessive form, due to inactivating mutations in the AVP gene, and an X-linked recessive form, due to an unidentified gene on Xq28, have also been described. A primary deficiency of plasma AVP can also result from increased metabolism by an N-terminal aminopeptidase produced by the placenta. It is referred to as *gestational DI* since the signs and symptoms manifest during pregnancy and usually remit several weeks after delivery. However, a subclinical deficiency in AVP secretion can often be demonstrated in the nonpregnant state, indicating that damage to the neurohypophysis may also contribute to the AVP deficiency. Finally, a primary deficiency of AVP can also result from malformation or destruction of the neurohypophysis by a variety of diseases or toxins (Table 319-1).

Secondary deficiencies of AVP result from inhibition of secretion by excessive intake of fluids. They are referred to as *primary polydipsia* and can be divided into three subcategories. One of them, called *dipsogenic DI*, is characterized by an inappropriate increase in thirst caused by a reduction in the "set" of the osmoregulatory mechanism. It sometimes occurs in association with multifocal diseases of the brain such as neurosarcoid, tuberculous meningitis, or multiple sclerosis but is often idiopathic. The second subtype, called *psychogenic polydipsia*, is not associated with thirst, and the polydipsia seems to be a feature of psychosis. The third subtype, which may be referred to as *iatrogenic polydipsia*, results from recommendations of health professionals or the popular media to increase fluid intake for its presumed preventive or therapeutic benefits for other disorders.

Primary deficiencies in the antidiuretic action of AVP result in *nephrogenic DI* (Table 319-1). It can be genetic, acquired, or caused by exposure to various drugs. The genetic form is usually transmitted in an X-linked mode and is caused by mutations in the coding region of the V_2 receptor gene. Autosomal recessive or dominant forms result from mutations in the gene encoding the aquaporin protein that forms the water channels in the distal nephron.

Secondary deficiencies in the antidiuretic response to AVP result from polyuria per se. They are caused by washout of the medullary concentration gradient and/or suppression of aquaporin function. They usually resolve 24 to 48 h after the polyuria is corrected but often complicate interpretation of tests commonly used for differential diagnosis.

Pathophysiology When the secretion or action of AVP is reduced to <80 to 85% of normal, urine concentration ceases and the rate of output increases to symptomatic levels. If the defect is primary (e.g., the patient has pituitary, gestational, or nephrogenic DI), the polyuria results in a small (1 to 2%) decrease in body water and a commensurate increase in plasma osmolarity and sodium concentration that stimulate thirst and a compensatory increase in water intake. As a result, *overt physical or laboratory signs of dehydration do not develop unless the patient also has a defect in thirst (see below) or fails to drink for some other reason.*

The severity of the antidiuretic defect varies markedly among patients with pituitary, gestational, or nephrogenic DI. In some, the deficiencies in AVP secretion or action are so severe that basal urine output approximates the maximum (10 to 15 mL/min); even an intense stimulus such as nausea or severe dehydration does not raise plasma AVP enough to concentrate the urine. In others, however, the deficiency in AVP secretion or action is incomplete, and a modest stimulus such as a few hours of fluid deprivation, smoking, or a vasovagal reaction increases plasma AVP sufficiently to produce a profound antidiuresis. The maximum urine osmolarity achieved in these patients is usually less than normal, largely because their maximal concentrating capacity is temporarily impaired by chronic polyuria. However, in a few patients with partial pituitary or nephrogenic DI, it can reach levels as high as 800 mosmol/L.

In primary polydipsia, the pathogenesis of the polydipsia and polyuria is the reverse of that in pituitary, nephrogenic, and gestational DI. Thus, the excessive intake of fluids slightly increases body water, thereby reducing plasma osmolarity, AVP secretion, and urinary concentration. The latter results in a compensatory increase in urinary free-water excretion that varies in direct proportion to intake. Therefore, clinically appreciable overhydration is uncommon unless the compensatory water diuresis is impaired by a drug or disease that stimulates or mimics endogenous AVP.

In the dipsogenic form of primary polydipsia, fluid intake is excessive because the osmotic threshold for thirst appears to be reset to the left, often well below that for AVP release. When deprived of fluids or subjected to some other acute osmotic or nonosmotic stimulus, these individuals invariably increase plasma AVP normally, but the resultant increase in urine concentration is usually subnormal because their renal capacity to concentrate the urine is also blunted by chronic polyuria. Thus, their antidiuretic response to these stimuli may be indistinguishable from that in patients with partial pituitary, partial gestational, or partial nephrogenic DI. Patients with psychogenic or iatrogenic polydipsia respond similarly to fluid restriction but do not complain of thirst and usually offer other explanations for their high fluid intake.

TABLE 319-1 Causes of Diabetes Insipidus

Pituitary diabetes insipidus	Nephrogenic diabetes insipidus
Acquired	Acquired
Head trauma (closed and penetrating)	Drugs
Neoplasms	Lithium
Primary	Demeclocycline
Craniopharyngioma	Methoxyflurane
Pituitary adenoma (suprasellar)	Amphotericin B
Dysgerminoma	Aminoglycosides
Meningioma	Cisplatin
Metastatic (lung, breast)	Rifampin
Hematologic (lymphoma, leukemia)	Foscarnet
Granulomas	Metabolic
Neurosarcoid	Hypercalcemia, hypercalciuria
Histiocytosis	Hypokalemia
Xanthoma disseminatum	Obstruction (ureter or urethra)
Infectious	Vascular
Chronic meningitis	Sickle cell disease and trait
Viral encephalitis	Ischemia (acute tubular necrosis)
Toxoplasmosis	Granulomas
Inflammatory	Neurosarcoid
Lymphocytic infundibuloneurohypophysitis	Neoplasms
Wegener's granulomatosis	Sarcoma
Lupus erythematosus	Infiltration
Scleroderma	Amyloidosis
Chemical toxins	Pregnancy
Tetrodotoxin	Idiopathic
Snake venom	Genetic
Vascular	X-linked recessive (AVP receptor-2 gene)
Sheehan's syndrome	Autosomal recessive (aquaporin-2 gene)
Aneurysm (internal carotid)	Autosomal dominant (aquaporin-2 gene)
Aortocoronary bypass	**Primary polydipsia**
Hypoxic encephalopathy	Acquired
Pregnancy (vasopressinase)	Psychogenic
Idiopathic	Schizophrenia
Congenital malformations	Obsessive-compulsive disorder
Septooptic dysplasia	Dipsogenic (abnormal thirst)
Midline craniofacial defects	Granulomas
Holoprosencephaly	Neurosarcoid
Hypogenesis, ectopia of pituitary	Infectious
Genetic	Tuberculous meningitis
Autosomal dominant (AVP-neurophysin gene)	Head trauma (closed and penetrating)
Autosomal recessive (AVP-neurophysin gene)	Demyelination
Autosomal recessive-Wolfram-(4p − WFS 1 gene)	Multiple sclerosis
X-linked recessive (Xq28)	Drugs
Deletion chromosome 7q	Lithium
	Carbamazepine
	Idiopathic
	Iatrogenic

Differential Diagnosis When symptoms of urinary frequency, enuresis, nocturia, and/or persistent thirst are present, the presence of polyuria should be verified by documenting a 24-h urine output > 50 mL/kg per day (>3500 mL in a 70-kg man). If the osmolarity of the 24-h urine is >300 mosmol/L, the polyuria is due to a solute diuresis and the patient should be evaluated for uncontrolled diabetes mellitus or other less common causes of excessive solute excretion. However, if the 24-h urine osmolarity is <300 mosmol/L, the patient has a water diuresis and should be evaluated further to determine which type of DI is present.

In differentiating between the various types of DI, the history, physical examination, and routine laboratory tests may be helpful but are rarely sufficient because few, if any, of the findings are pathognomonic. Except in the rare patient who is clearly dehydrated under basal conditions of *ad libitum* fluid intake, this evaluation should begin with a *fluid deprivation test*. To minimize patient discomfort, avoid excessive dehydration, and maximize the information obtained, the test should be started in the morning and water balance should be monitored closely with hourly measurements of body weight, plasma osmolarity and/or sodium concentration, and urine volume and osmolarity.

If fluid deprivation does not result in urine concentration (osmolarity >300 mosmol/L, specific gravity >1.010) before body weight decreases by 5% or plasma osmolarity/sodium exceed the upper limit of normal, primary polydipsia or a partial defect in AVP secretion or action are largely excluded. In these patients, severe pituitary or nephrogenic DI are the only remaining possibilities, and they can usually be distinguished by administering desmopressin (DDAVP, 0.03 μg/kg subcutaneously or intravenously) and repeating the measurement of urine osmolarity 1 to 2 h later. An increase of >50% indicates severe pituitary DI, whereas a smaller or absent response is strongly suggestive of nephrogenic DI.

However, in patients who concentrate their urine during fluid deprivation, the change in urine osmolarity after administration of desmopressin is not useful for differential diagnosis because the values vary widely and over the same range in primary polydipsia, partial pituitary DI, and partial nephrogenic DI. The best way to differentiate these three conditions is to measure plasma or urine AVP before and during the fluid deprivation test and analyze the result in relation to the concurrent plasma or urine osmolarity (Fig. 319-3). This approach invariably differentiates partial nephrogenic DI from partial pituitary DI and primary polydipsia. It also differentiates pituitary DI from primary polydipsia if the hormone is measured when plasma osmolarity or sodium is clearly above the normal range. However, the requisite level of hypertonic dehydration is difficult to produce by fluid deprivation alone when urine concentration occurs. Therefore, it is usually

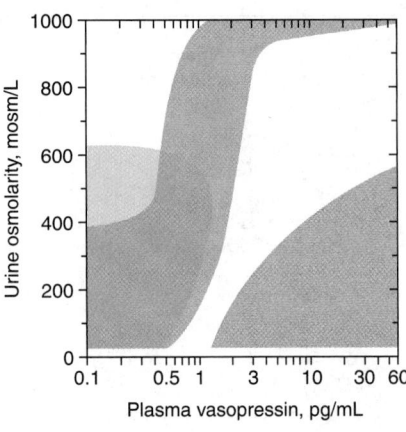
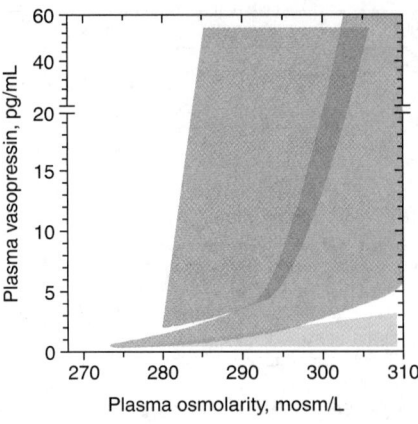

FIGURE 319-3 Relationship of plasma AVP to urine osmolarity (*left*) and plasma osmolarity (*right*) before and during fluid deprivation–hypertonic saline infusion test in patients who are normal or have primary polydipsia (■), pituitary diabetes insipidus (■), or nephrogenic diabetes insipidus (■).

necessary to add an infusion of hypertonic (3%) saline and repeat the AVP measurements when plasma osmolarity rises to >300 mosmol/L (Na^+ > 145 mmol/L). This endpoint is usually reached within 30 to 120 min if the hypertonic saline is infused at a rate of 0.1 mL/kg per min and the fluid deprivation is maintained.

The differential diagnosis of DI may also be facilitated by magnetic resonance imaging (MRI) of the pituitary and hypothalamus. In most healthy adults and children, the posterior pituitary emits a hyperintense signal in T1 weighted mid-saggital images. This "bright spot" is almost invariably absent or abnormally small in patients with pituitary DI but is present in 80 to 90% of patients with primary polydipsia. Thus, the presence of a normal bright spot virtually excludes pituitary DI, whereas its absence supports but does not prove this diagnosis. Therefore, the MRI findings must be interpreted with caution and only in conjunction with other diagnostic studies based on assays of AVP or the differential responses to treatment.

℞ TREATMENT

The signs and symptoms of uncomplicated pituitary DI can be eliminated completely by treatment with DDAVP (Fig. 319-4). It is a synthetic analogue of AVP (Fig. 319-1) that acts selectively at V_2 receptors to increase urine concentration and decrease urine flow in a dose-dependent manner. It is also more resistant to degradation than AVP and has a three- to fourfold longer duration of action. DDAVP can be given by intravenous or subcutaneous injection, nasal inhalation, or oral tablet. The doses required to completely control pituitary DI vary widely, depending on the patient and the route of administration. However, they usually range from 1 to 2 μg qd or bid by injection, 10 to 20 μg bid or tid by nasal spray, or 100 to 400 μg bid or tid orally. The onset of action is rapid, ranging from as little as 15 min after injection to 60 min after oral administration. When given in doses sufficient to completely normalize urinary osmolarity and flow, desmopressin produces a slight (1 to 3%) increase in total-body water and a commensurate decrease in plasma osmolarity and sodium concentration that rapidly eliminate thirst and polydipsia. Consequently, water balance is maintained and hyponatremia does not develop unless the patient has an associated abnormality in the osmoregulation of thirst or ingests/receives excessive amounts of fluid for some other reason. Fortunately, abnormal thirst occurs in <10% of patients with pituitary DI, and the other causes of excessive intake can usually be eliminated by educating the patient about the risks of drinking for reasons other than thirst. Therefore, most patients with pituitary DI can take DDAVP in doses sufficient to maintain a normal urine output continuously and do not need to endure the inconvenience and discomfort of allowing intermittent escape to prevent water intoxication.

Pituitary DI can also be treated with chlorpropamide (Diabinese). The mechanism of its antidiuretic action is uncertain but may involve potentiation of the effect of small amounts of AVP or direct activation of the V_2 receptor. In patients with severe or partial pituitary DI, doses of chlorpropamide similar to those used in the treatment of diabetes mellitus (125 to 500 mg once daily) increase urine concentration and decrease urine flow, thirst, and polydipsia in a manner similar to desmopressin. The antidiuresis is almost always sufficient to reduce urine output by 30 to 70%. Moreover, its antidiuretic effect can be enhanced appreciably by cotreatment with a thiazide diuretic. Side effects of chlorpropamide include hypoglycemia, which can be precipitated by severe reductions in caloric intake or heavy exercise, and it may cause a disulfiram (Antabuse)-like reaction to ethanol. Chlorpropamide is contraindicated in the treatment of gestational DI because its teratogenicity is unknown.

Primary polydipsia cannot be treated with desmopressin because a sustained inhibition of the compensatory water diuresis almost invariably results in the development of water intoxication within 24 to 48 h. Iatrogenic polydipsia can often be corrected by patient counseling; however, there is no effective treatment for either psychogenic or dipsogenic DI. In the latter, nocturia or nocturnal enuresis can often be controlled safely by administering a single small dose of desmopressin at bedtime. If the dose is adjusted carefully to provide no more than 8 to 10 h of antidiuresis, it will not result in water intoxication, because patients with dipsogenic, as well as other forms of DI, tend to drink less fluid at night than during the day.

The symptoms and signs of nephrogenic DI are not affected by treatment with DDAVP or chlorpropamide but may be reduced by treatment with a thiazide diuretic and/or amiloride in conjunction with a low-sodium diet. Inhibitors of prostaglandin synthesis (e.g., indomethacin) are also effective in some patients.

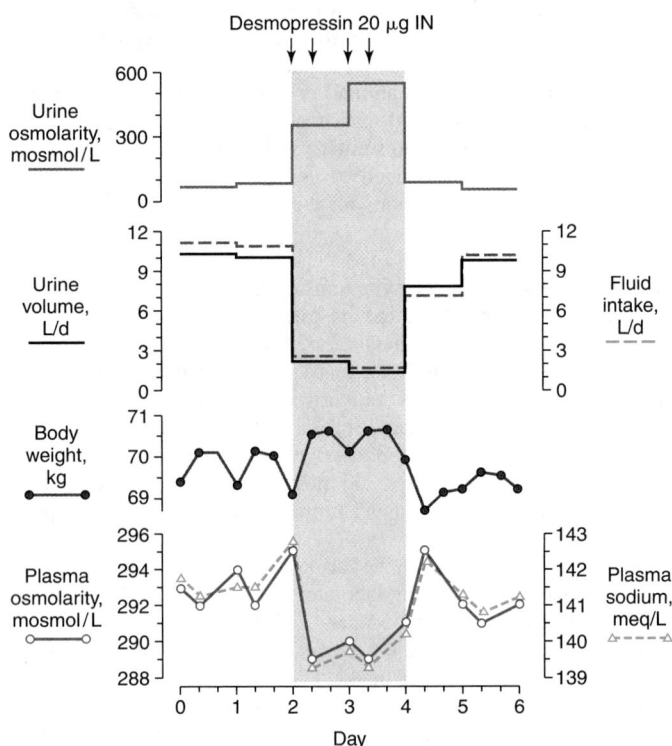

FIGURE 319-4 Effect of desmopressin therapy on water balance in patient with uncomplicated pituitary diabetes insipidus. Note that treatment rapidly reduces thirst and fluid intake as well as urine output to normal, with only a slight increase in body water (weight) and decrease in plasma osmolarity/sodium. [*From Endocrinology and Metabolism, 4th ed, P Felig, L Frohman (eds). New York, McGraw-Hill, 2001, with permission.*]

ADIPSIC HYPERNATREMIA ■ Clinical Characteristics
Adipsic hypernatremia is characterized by chronic or recurrent hypertonic dehydration and a deficient AVP response to osmotic stimulation. Despite hypertonic dehydration, these patients have little or no thirst and may even resist efforts to increase their oral intake of fluids. The hypernatremia varies in severity and usually is associated with commensurate signs of hypovolemia such as tachycardia, postural hypotension, azotemia, hyperuricemia, and hypokalemia. Muscle weakness, pain, rhabdomyolysis, hyperglycemia, hyperlipidemia, and acute renal failure may also occur.

Pathophysiology Adipsic hypernatremia is caused by agenesis or destruction of the hypothalamic osmoreceptors that normally regulate thirst and AVP secretion (Fig. 319-5). Lack of thirst and failure to drink enough water to replenish renal and extrarenal losses decrease total-body water and increase plasma osmolarity/sodium. Plasma renin activity and aldosterone secretion also increase, and plasma potassium falls due to increased urinary excretion. The osmoreceptor deficiency can usually be traced to an identifiable congenital or acquired disease in the hypothalamus but is sometimes idiopathic (Table 319-2). An MRI typically shows a normal posterior pituitary bright spot, and the AVP response to nonosmotic stimuli is also normal. Occasionally, the neurohypophysis is also affected, resulting in a combined defect in water balance that is particularly severe and difficult to manage.

Differential Diagnosis Adipsic hypernatremia should be distinguished from the hypernatremia that results from various other causes. These

TABLE 319-2 *Causes of Adipsic Hypernatremia*

Acquired
  Vascular: Occlusion anterior communicating artery
  Tumors
    Primary
      Craniopharyngioma
      Pinealoma, germinoma
      Meningioma
      Glioma
    Metastatic (lung, breast)
  Granulomas: Neurosarcoid
          Histiocytosis
  Trauma: Closed
        Penetrating (pituitary-hypothalamic surgery)
  Psychogenic: Psychotic depression
  Other: Hydrocephalus
      Neurodegenerative
      AIDS, cytomegalovirus encephalitis
  Idiopathic
Congenital
  Midline malformation (septum and corpus callosum)
  Microcephaly
  Genetic: Autosomal recessive (Schinzel-Giedion syndrome)

distinctions can usually be made from the history, physical examination, and routine laboratory tests. If a conscious patient denies thirst and/or does not drink vigorously in the presence of significant hypernatremia, the diagnosis of hypodipsia or adipsia can be made with confidence. This diagnosis is supported by physical laboratory evidence of hypovolemia (postural hypotension, azotemia, hypokalemia, hyperuricemia, hyperreninemia) and a relative deficiency of plasma AVP. During rehydration, patients may develop either DI or the syndrome of inappropriate antidiuretic hormone (SIADH) depending on whether they have partial or total deficiency of the osmoregulation of AVP (Fig. 319-5). If the patient is obtunded or otherwise unable to answer questions or drink at the time of presentation, the possibility of adipsic hypernatremia can be evaluated after rehydration by assessing the thirst and plasma AVP response to a controlled fluid deprivation–hypertonic saline infusion test similar to that described for evaluation of DI.

℞ TREATMENT

Adipsic hypernatremia should be treated by administering water by mouth, if the patient is alert, or 0.45% saline intravenously, if the patient is obtunded or uncooperative. The number of liters of free water that will be required to correct the deficit (ΔFW) can be estimated from body weight in kg (BW) and the serum sodium concentration in mmol/L (S_{Na}) by the formula $\Delta FW = 0.5BW \times [(S_{Na} - 140)/140]$. If serum glucose ($S_{Glu}$) is elevated, the measured S_{Na} should be corrected ($S_{Na}*$) by the formula $S_{Na}* = S_{Na} + [(S_{Glu} - 90)/36]$. This amount plus an allowance for continuing insensible and urinary losses should be given over a 24- to 48-h period. If DI is present or develops before rehydration is complete, desmopressin should also be given in standard doses to minimize urinary losses. If hyperglycemia and/or hypokalemia are present, insulin and/or potassium supplements should be given with the expectation that both can be discontinued after rehydration is complete. These variables plus urine output and plasma urea/creatinine should be monitored closely during treatment for signs of emerging DI, SIADH, or acute renal failure.

Once the acute fluid and electrolyte imbalances are corrected, an MRI of the brain and tests of anterior pituitary function should be performed. A long-term management plan to prevent or minimize recurrence of the fluid and electrolyte imbalance should also be developed. This should include a practical method that the patient can use to regulate fluid intake in accordance with day-to-day variations in water balance. The most effective way to accomplish these objectives is to prescribe desmopressin or chlorpropamide to completely control

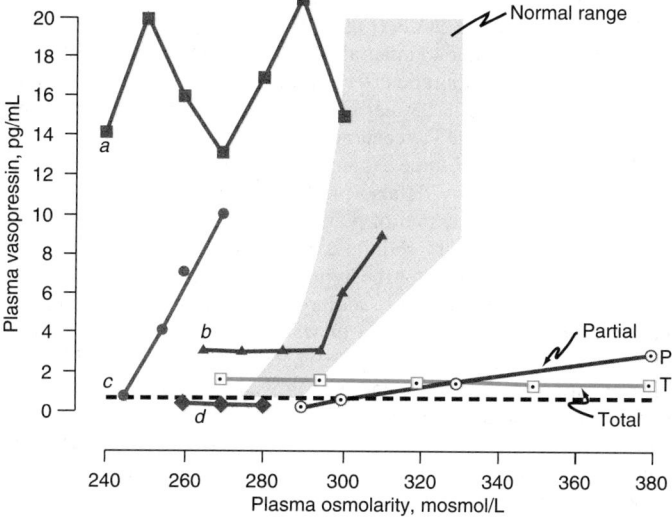

FIGURE 319-5 Heterogeneity of osmoregulatory dysfunction in adipsic hypernatremia (AH) and the syndrome of inappropriate antidiuretic hormone (SIADH). Each line depicts schematically the relationship of plasma arginine vasopressin (AVP) to plasma osmolarity during water loading and/or infusion of 3% saline in a patient with either AH (open symbols) or SIADH (closed symbols). The shaded area indicates the normal range of the relationship. The horizontal broken line indicates the plasma AVP level below which the hormone is undetectable and urinary concentration usually does not occur. Lines P and T represent patients with a selective deficiency in the osmoregulation of thirst and AVP that is either partial (O) or total (□). In the latter, plasma AVP does not change in response to increases or decreases in plasma osmolarity but remains within a range sufficient to concentrate the urine even if overhydration produces hypotonic hyponatremia. In contrast, if the osmoregulatory deficiency is partial (O), rehydration of the patient suppresses plasma AVP to levels that result in urinary dilution and polyuria before plasma osmolarity and sodium are reduced to normal. Lines a–d represent different defects in the osmoregulation of plasma AVP observed in patients with SIADH. In a (■), plasma AVP is markedly elevated and fluctuates widely without relation to changes in plasma osmolarity, indicating complete loss of osmoregulation. In b (▲), plasma AVP remains fixed at a slightly elevated level until plasma osmolarity reaches the normal range at which point it begins to rise appropriately, indicating a selective defect in the inhibitory component of the osmoregulatory mechanism. In c (●), plasma AVP rises in close correlation with plasma osmolarity before the latter reaches the normal range, indicating downward resetting of the osmostat. In d (♦), plasma AVP appears to be osmoregulated normally, suggesting that the inappropriate antidiuresis is caused by some other abnormality.

DI, if it is present, and teach the patient how to use day-to-day changes in body weight as a guide for adjusting fluid intake. Prescribing a constant fluid intake is less satisfactory because it does not take into account the large, uncontrolled variations in insensible loss that inevitably occur.

EXCESS VASOPRESSIN SECRETION AND ACTION

HYPONATREMIA (See also Chap. 41) ■ **Clinical Characteristics** Excessive secretion or action of AVP results in the production of decreased volumes of more highly concentrated urine. If not accompanied by a commensurate reduction in fluid intake, the reduced suppressibility of AVP results in water retention and a decrease in plasma osmolarity/sodium. If the hyponatremia develops gradually or has been present for more than a few days, it may be asymptomatic. However, if it develops acutely, it is almost always accompanied by symptoms and signs of water intoxication that may include mild headache, confusion, anorexia, nausea, vomiting, coma, and convulsions. Severe hyponatremia may be lethal. Depending on the cause of the antidiuresis, osmotically inappropriate thirst and/or fluid intake and other disturbances of fluid and electrolyte balance may also be present.

Etiology Osmotically inappropriate antidiuresis can be caused by a primary defect in AVP secretion or action or can be secondary to a recognized nonosmotic stimulus such as hypovolemia, hypotension, or glucocorticoid deficiency. The primary forms are generally referred to as SIADH or euvolemic (type III) hyponatremia. They have many different causes, including ectopic production of AVP by lung cancer or other neoplasms, eutopic release by various diseases or drugs, and exogenous administration of AVP, desmopressin, or large doses of oxytocin (Table 319-3). The ectopic forms result from abnormal expression of the AVP-NPII gene by primary or metastatic malignancies. They do not usually remit unless the ectopic source is eliminated. The eutopic forms manifest most often in patients with acute infections or strokes, but the mechanisms by which these diseases disrupt osmoregulation are not known. A form of acute or chronic euvolemic hyponatremia very similar to SIADH can also result from stimulation of AVP secretion by protracted nausea or isolated glucocorticoid defi-

ciency. In these patients the excess AVP secretion can be corrected quickly and completely by specific treatments (antiemetics or glucocorticoids) that are not useful in other forms of SIADH.

The secondary forms of osmotically inappropriate antidiuresis are usually divided into two groups: type I (hypervolemic) and type II (hypovolemic) hyponatremia. Type I occurs in sodium-retaining, edema-forming states such as congestive heart failure, cirrhosis, or nephrosis and is thought to be due to a reduction in "effective" blood volume. Type II occurs in sodium-depleted states such as severe gastroenteritis, diuretic abuse, or mineralocorticoid deficiency and is probably a result of reduction in extracellular volume as well as blood volume and/or pressure.

Pathophysiology In SIADH, interference with the osmotic suppression of AVP release results in significant expansion and dilution of body fluids only if water intake exceeds the rate of insensible and urinary output. The excess water intake often results from an associated defect in the osmoregulation of thirst but can also be due to psychogenic or iatrogenic factors, including the administration of intravenous fluids.

In SIADH, the abnormal osmoregulation of antidiuretic function can take any of four distinct forms (Fig. 319-5). For example, AVP secretion remains fully responsive to changes in plasma osmolarity/sodium, but the threshold, or set point, of the osmoregulatory system is abnormally low. Patients with this type of downward resetting of the osmostat differ from those with the other types of osmoregulatory defect in that they are able to maximally suppress plasma AVP and dilute their urine if their fluid intake is high enough to reduce their plasma osmolarity/sodium to the new set point. Another, smaller subgroup (about 10% of the total) does not have a demonstrable defect in the osmoregulation of AVP (Fig. 319-5). Thus, their inappropriate antidiuresis may be due to other abnormalities such as enhanced renal sensitivity to the antidiuretic effect of normally low levels of AVP or activation of aquaporin 2 water channels by a mechanism that is independent of AVP and V_2 receptors.

The extracellular volume expansion that results from excessive retention of water in SIADH also produces an increase in atrial natriuretic hormone, suppression of plasma renin activity, and a compensatory increase in urinary sodium excretion that serves to reduce the hypervolemia but aggravates the hyponatremia. Thus, hyponatremia is due to a decrease in total-body sodium as well as an increase in total-body water. The acute retention of water and fall in plasma sodium also increase intracellular volume. The resultant brain swelling increases intracranial pressure and probably causes the acute symptoms of water intoxication. After several days, this intracellular volume expansion may be reduced by inactivation or elimination of intracellular solutes, resulting in the remission of symptoms that often occur with hyponatremia of longer duration.

In type I (edematous) or type II (hypovolemic) hyponatremia, the osmotic inhibition of AVP and urine concentration is counteracted by a hemodynamic stimulus that results from a substantial reduction in effective or absolute blood volume. In both cases, the reduced suppression of AVP appears to be due to downward resetting of the osmostat. The resultant antidiuresis is usually enhanced by decreased distal delivery of filtrate that results from increased reabsorption of sodium in proximal nephrons secondary to the hypovolemia. If it is not associated with a commensurate reduction in water intake, the marked reduction in urine output that ensues also leads to expansion and dilution of body fluids with symptoms of hyponatremia. This attenuates, but does not completely eliminate, the antidiuresis because the amount of water retained is usually insufficient to fully correct the effective or absolute hypovolemia. Unlike in SIADH, therefore, plasma renin activity is elevated, causing secondary hyperaldosteronism and hypokalemia. The disturbance in salt and water balance that underlies the hyponatremia also differs from SIADH in that total-body sodium and water are increased in type I but decreased in type II.

Differential Diagnosis SIADH is a diagnosis of exclusion that can usually be accomplished with routine historic, physical, and laboratory information. In a patient with hyponatremia, the possibility of simple

TABLE 319-3 Causes of Syndrome of Inappropriate Antidiuretic Hormone (SIADH)	
Neoplasms	Neurologic
Carcinomas	Guillain-Barré syndrome
Lung	Multiple sclerosis
Duodenum	Delirium tremens
Pancreas	Amyotrophic lateral sclerosis
Ovary	Hydrocephalus
Bladder, ureter	Psychosis
Other neoplasms	Peripheral neuropathy
Thymoma	Congenital malformations
Mesothelioma	Agenesis corpus callosum
Bronchial adenoma	Cleft lip/palate
Carcinoid	Other midline defects
Gangliocytoma	Metabolic
Ewing's sarcoma	Acute intermittent porphyria
Head trauma (closed and penetrating)	Pulmonary
Infections	Asthma
Pneumonia, bacterial or viral	Pneumothorax
Abscess, lung or brain	Positive-pressure respiration
Cavitation (aspergillosis)	Drugs
Tuberculosis, lung or brain	Vasopressin or desmopressin
Meningitis, bacterial or viral	Chlorpropamide
Encephalitis	Oxytocin, high dose
AIDS	Vincristine
Vascular	Carbamazepine
Cerebrovascular occlusions,	Nicotine
hemorrhage	Phenothiazines
Cavernous sinus thrombosis	Cyclophosphamide
	Tricyclic antidepressants
	Monoamine oxidase inhibitors
	Serotonin reuptake inhibitors

dilution caused by an osmotically driven shift of water from the intracellular to the extracellular space should be excluded by measuring plasma glucose and/or plasma osmolarity. If the glucose is not elevated enough to account for the hyponatremia [serum sodium decreases ~1 meq/L for each rise in glucose 2.0 mmol/L (36 mg/dL)] and/or plasma osmolarity is reduced in proportion to sodium (each decrease in serum sodium of 1 meq/L should reduce plasma osmolarity by about 2 mosmol/L), the hyponatremia is "true" and can be typed or classified by standard clinical indicators of the extracellular fluid volume (Table 319-4). If these findings are ambiguous or contradictory, measuring the rate of urinary sodium excretion or plasma renin activity may be helpful. These measurements can be misleading, however, if SIADH is stable or resolving or if the patient has type II hyponatremia due to a primary defect in renal conservation of sodium, surreptitious diuretic abuse, or hyporeninemic hypoaldosteronism. The latter may be suspected if serum potassium is elevated instead of low as is usually seen in types I and II hyponatremia. Measurements of plasma AVP are currently of no diagnostic value since they exhibit the same wide variation in abnormalities in all three types of hyponatremia. In patients who fulfill the clinical criteria for type III (euvolemic) hyponatremia, plasma cortisol should also be measured to rule out unsuspected secondary adrenal insufficiency. If this is normal and there is no other obvious cause for SIADH, a careful search for occult lung cancer should also be undertaken.

TABLE 319-4 *Differential Diagnosis of Hyponatremia Based on Clinical Assessment of Extracellular Fluid Volume (ECFV)*

Clinical Findings	Type I, Hypervolemic	Type II, Hypovolemic	Type IIIA, Euvolemic	Type IIIB, Euvolemic (SIADH)
History				
CHF, cirrhosis, or nephrosis	Yes	No	No	No
Salt and water loss	No	Yes	No	No
ACTH–cortisol deficiency and/or nausea and vomiting	No	No	Yes	No
Physical examination				
Generalized edema, ascites	Yes	No	No	No
Postural hypotension	Maybe	Maybe	Maybe[a]	No
Laboratory				
BUN, creatinine	High-normal	High-normal	Low-normal	Low-normal
Uric acid	High-normal	High-normal	Low-normal	Low-normal
Serum potassium	Low-normal	Low-normal[b]	Normal[c]	Normal
Serum albumin	Low-normal	High-normal	Normal	Normal
Serum cortisol	Normal-high	Normal-high[d]	Low[e]	Normal
Plasma renin activity	High	High	Low[f]	Low
Urinary sodium (meq unit of time)[g]	Low	Low[h]	High[i]	High[i]

[a] Postural hypotension may occur in secondary (ACTH-dependent) adrenal insufficiency even though ECFV and aldosterone are usually normal.
[b] Serum potassium may be high if hypovolemia is due to aldosterone deficiency.
[c] Serum potassium may be low if vomiting causes alkalosis.
[d] Serum cortisol is low if hypovolemia is due to primary adrenal insufficiency (Addison's disease).
[e] Serum cortisol will be normal or high if the cause is nausea and vomiting rather than secondary (ACTH-dependent) adrenal insufficiency.
[f] Plasma renin activity may be high if the cause is secondary (ACTH) adrenal insufficiency.
[g] Urinary sodium should be expressed as the *rate of excretion* rather than the concentration. In a hyponatremic adult, an excretion rate > 25 meq/day (or 25 µeq/mg of creatinine) could be considered high.
[h] The rate of urinary sodium excretion may be high if the hypovolemia is due to diuretic abuse, primary adrenal insufficiency, or other causes of renal sodium wasting.
[i] The rate of urinary sodium excretion may be low if intake is curtailed by symptoms or treatment.
Note: SIADH, syndrome of inappropriate antidiuretic hormone; CHF, congestive heart failure; ACTH, adrenocorticotropic hormone; BUN, blood urea nitrogen.

℞ TREATMENT

In acute SIADH, the keystone to treatment of hyponatremia is to restrict total fluid intake to less than the sum of insensible losses and urinary output. Total intake should include the water derived from food (300 to 500 mL/d). Because insensible losses in adults usually approximate 500 mL/d, total discretionary intake (all water in liquid form) should be at least 500 mL less than urinary output. If achieved, this deficit usually reduces body water and increases serum sodium by about 1 to 2% per day. If more rapid correction of the hyponatremia is desired to eliminate severe symptoms or signs, the fluid restriction can be supplemented by intravenous infusion of hypertonic (3%) saline. This treatment has the advantage of correcting the sodium deficiency that is partly responsible for the hyponatremia as well as producing a solute diuresis that serves to remove some of the excess water. However, if the hyponatremia has been present for more than 24 to 48 h, correction that is too rapid has the potential to produce central pontine myelinolysis, an acute, potentially fatal neurologic syndrome characterized by quadriparesis, ataxia, and abnormal extraocular movements. The following guidelines appear to minimize, if not eliminate, the risk of this complication: the 3% saline should be infused at a rate ≤0.05 mL/kg body weight per min; the effect should be monitored continuously by STAT measurements of serum sodium at least once every 2 h; and the infusion should be stopped as soon as serum sodium increases by 12 mmol/L or to 130 mmol/L, whichever comes first. Urinary output should also be monitored continuously since spontaneous remission of the SIADH can occur at any time and can result in an acute water diuresis that greatly accelerates the rate of rise in serum sodium produced by fluid restriction and 3% saline infusion.

In chronic SIADH, the hyponatremia can be corrected by treatment with demeclocycline, 150 to 300 mg orally three or four times a day, or fludrocortisone, 0.05 to 0.2 mg orally twice a day. The effect of the demeclocycline manifests in 7 to 14 days and is due to production of a reversible form of nephrogenic DI. Potential side effects include phototoxicity and azotemia. The effect of fludrocortisone also requires 1 to 2 weeks and is partly due to increased retention of sodium and possibly inhibition of thirst. It also increases urinary potassium excretion, which may require replacement through dietary adjustments or supplements. Fludrocortisone may induce hypertension, occasionally necessitating discontinuation of the treatment.

One or more nonpeptide AVP antagonists that block the antidiuretic effect of AVP may soon be approved for use in the United States. Preliminary studies with these antagonists in acute or chronic SIADH indicate that they produce a dose-dependent increase in urinary free-water excretion, which, if combined with a modest restriction of fluid intake, gradually reduces body water and corrects the hyponatremia without any recognized adverse effect. Thus, they may become the treatment of choice for those forms of SIADH in which there is inappropriate secretion of AVP that cannot be corrected by other, more specific therapy such as antiemetics or glucocorticoids.

When an SIADH-like syndrome is due to protracted nausea and vomiting or isolated glucocorticoid deficiency, all abnormalities can be corrected quickly and completely by giving an antiemetic or hydrocortisone. As with other treatments, care must be taken to ensure that serum sodium does not rise too quickly or too far.

In type I hyponatremia, the only treatment currently available is severe fluid restriction, administration of urea or mannitol to produce a solute diuresis, and/or administration of cardiotonics or serum albumin to correct the effective hypovolemia. None of these treatments is particularly effective, and some (e.g., administration of mannitol or albumin) carry significant risks. Infusion of hypertonic saline is contraindicated because it worsens the sodium retention and edema and may precipitate cardiovascular decompensation. However, preliminary studies indicate that the AVP antagonists may be almost as effective and safe in type I hyponatremia as they are in SIADH. Thus, they may become the treatment of choice for this form of hyponatremia also.

In type II hyponatremia, the defect in AVP secretion and water balance can usually be corrected easily and quickly by stopping the loss of sodium and water and/or replacing the deficits by mouth or intravenous infusion of normal or hypertonic saline. As with the treatment of other forms of hyponatremia, care must be taken to ensure that plasma sodium does not increase too rapidly. Fluid restriction or administration of AVP antagonists is contraindicated as they would only aggravate the underlying volume depletion and could result in cardiovascular decompensation.

FURTHER READING

ADROGUE HJ, MADIAS NE: Hyponatremia. N Engl J Med 342:1581, 2000

HANSEN LK et al: The genetic basis of familial neurohypophyseal diabetes insipidus. Trends Endocrinol Metab 8:363, 1997

ROBERTSON GL: Antidiuretic hormone: Normal and disordered function. Endocrinol Metab Clin North Am 30:671, 2001

VERBALIS JG: Vasopressin V$_2$ receptor antagonists. J Mol Endocrinol 29:1, 2002

WONG LL, VERBALIS JG: Systemic disease associated with disorders of water homeostasis. Endocrinol Metab Clin North Am 31:121, 2002

320 DISORDERS OF THE THYROID GLAND
J. Larry Jameson, Anthony P. Weetman

The thyroid gland produces two related hormones, thyroxine (T$_4$) and triiodothyronine (T$_3$) (Fig. 320-1). Acting through nuclear receptors, these hormones play a critical role in cell differentiation during development and help maintain thermogenic and metabolic homeostasis in the adult. Disorders of the thyroid gland result primarily from autoimmune processes that either stimulate the overproduction of thyroid hormones (*thyrotoxicosis*) or cause glandular destruction and hormone deficiency (*hypothyroidism*). In addition, benign nodules and various forms of thyroid cancer are relatively common and amenable to detection by physical examination.

ANATOMY AND DEVELOPMENT

The thyroid gland is located in the neck, anterior to the trachea, between the cricoid cartilage and the suprasternal notch. The thyroid (Greek *thyreos*, shield, plus *eidos*, form) consists of two lobes that are connected by an isthmus. It is normally 12 to 20 g in size, highly vascular, and soft in consistency. Four parathyroid glands, which produce parathyroid hormone (Chap. 332), are located in the posterior region of each pole of the thyroid. The recurrent laryngeal nerves traverse the lateral borders of the thyroid gland and must be identified during thyroid surgery to avoid vocal cord paralysis.

The thyroid gland develops from the floor of the primitive pharynx during the third week of gestation. The gland migrates from the foramen cecum, at the base of the tongue, along the thyroglossal duct to reach its final location in the neck. This feature accounts for the rare ectopic location of thyroid tissue at the base of the tongue (lingual thyroid), as well as for the presence of thyroglossal duct cysts along this developmental tract. Thyroid hormone synthesis normally begins at about 11 weeks' gestation.

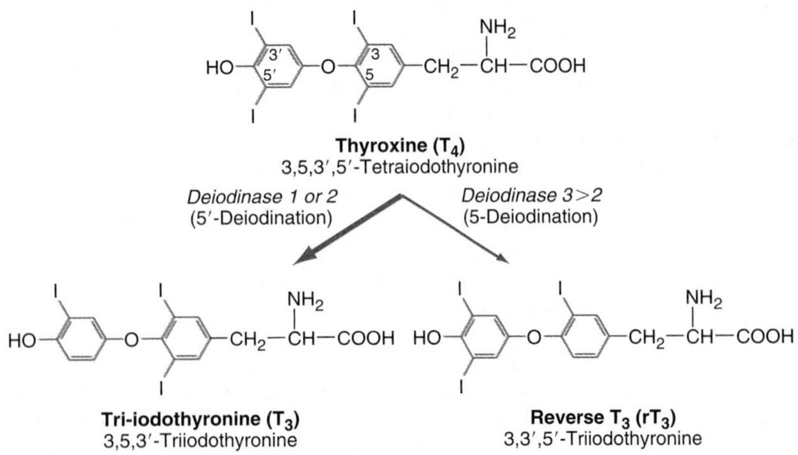

The parathyroid glands migrate from the third (inferior glands) and fourth (superior glands) pharyngeal pouches and become embedded in the thyroid gland. Neural crest derivatives from the ultimobranchial body give rise to thyroid medullary C cells that produce calcitonin, a calcium-lowering hormone. The C cells are interspersed throughout the thyroid gland, although their density is greatest in the juncture of the upper one-third and lower two-thirds of the gland.

Thyroid gland development is controlled by a series of developmental transcription factors. Thyroid transcription factor (TTF) 1 (also known as NKX2A), TTF-2 (also known as FKHL15), and paired homeobox-8 (PAX-8) are expressed selectively, but not exclusively, in the thyroid gland. In combination, they orchestrate thyroid cell development and the induction of thyroid-specific genes such as thyroglobulin (Tg), thyroid peroxidase (TPO), the sodium iodide symporter (NIS), and the thyroid-stimulating hormone receptor (TSH-R). Mutations in these developmental transcription factors or their downstream target genes are rare causes of thyroid agenesis or dyshormonogenesis and can cause congenital hypothyroidism (Table 320-1). Congenital hypothyroidism is common enough (approximately 1 in 4000 newborns) that neonatal screening is performed in most industrialized countries (see below). Though the underlying causes of most cases of congenital hypothyroidism are unknown, early treatment with thyroid hormone replacement precludes potentially severe developmental abnormalities.

The mature thyroid gland contains numerous spherical follicles composed of thyroid follicular cells that surround secreted colloid, a proteinaceous fluid that contains large amounts of thyroglobulin, the protein precursor of thyroid hormones (Fig. 320-2). The thyroid follicular cells are polarized—the basolateral surface is apposed to the bloodstream and an apical surface faces the follicular lumen. Increased demand for thyroid hormone, usually signaled by thyroid-stimulating hormone (TSH) binding to its receptor on the basolateral surface of the follicular cells, leads to Tg reabsorption from the follicular lumen and proteolysis within the cell to yield thyroid hormones for secretion into the bloodstream.

REGULATION OF THE THYROID AXIS

TSH, secreted by the thyrotrope cells of the anterior pituitary, plays a pivotal role in control of the thyroid axis and serves as the most useful physiologic marker of thyroid hormone action. TSH is a 31-kDa hormone composed of α and β subunits; the α subunit is common to the other glycoprotein hormones [luteinizing hormone, follicle-stimulating hormone, human chorionic gonadotropin (hCG)], whereas the TSH β subunit is unique to TSH. The extent and nature of carbohydrate modification are modulated by thyrotropin-releasing hormone (TRH) stimulation and influence the biologic activity of the hormone.

The thyroid axis is a classic example of an endocrine feedback loop. Hypothalamic TRH stimulates pituitary production of TSH, which, in turn, stimulates thyroid hor-

FIGURE 320-1   Structures of thyroid hormones. Thyroxine (T$_4$) contains four iodine atoms. Deiodination leads to production of the potent hormone, triiodothyronine (T$_3$), or the inactive hormone, reverse T$_3$.

mone synthesis and secretion. Thyroid hormones feed back negatively to inhibit TRH and TSH production (Fig. 320-2). The "set-point" in this axis is established by TSH. TRH is the major positive regulator of TSH synthesis and secretion. Peak TSH secretion occurs ~15 min after administration of exogenous TRH. Dopamine, glucocorticoids, and somatostatin suppress TSH but are not of major physiologic importance except when these agents are administered in pharmacologic doses. Reduced levels of thyroid hormone increase basal TSH production and enhance TRH-mediated stimulation of TSH. High thyroid hormone levels rapidly and directly suppress TSH and inhibit TRH-mediated stimulation of TSH, indicating that thyroid hormones are the dominant regulator of TSH production. Like other pituitary hormones, TSH is released in a pulsatile manner and exhibits a diurnal rhythm; its highest levels occur at night. However, these TSH excursions are modest in comparison to those of other pituitary hormones, in part because TSH has a relatively long plasma half-life (50 min). Consequently, single measurements of TSH are adequate for assessing its circulating level. TSH is measured using immunoradiometric assays that are highly sensitive and specific. These assays readily distinguish between normal and suppressed TSH values; thus, TSH can be used for the diagnosis of hyperthyroidism (low TSH) as well as hypothyroidism (high TSH).

TABLE 320-1 *Genetic Causes of Congenital Hypothyroidism*

Defective Gene Protein	Inheritance	Consequences
PROP-1	Autosomal recessive	Combined pituitary hormone deficiencies with preservation of adrenocorticotropic hormone
PIT-1	Autosomal recessive Autosomal dominant	Combined deficiencies of growth hormone, prolactin, thyroid-stimulating hormone (TSH)
TSHβ	Autosomal recessive	TSH deficiency
TTF-1	Autosomal dominant	Variable thyroid hypoplasia, choreoathetosis, pulmonary problems
TTF-2	Autosomal recessive	Thyroid agenesis, choanal atresia, spiky hair
PAX-8	Autosomal dominant	Thyroid dysgenesis
TSH-receptor	Autosomal recessive	Resistance to TSH
G$_{s\alpha}$ (Albright hereditary osteodystrophy)	Autosomal dominant	Resistance to TSH
Na$^+$/I$^-$ symporter	Autosomal recessive	Inability to transport iodide
THOX2	Autosomal dominant	Organification defect
Thyroid peroxidase	Autosomal recessive	Defective organification of iodide
Thyroglobulin	Autosomal recessive	Defective synthesis of thyroid hormone
Pendrin	Autosomal recessive	Pendred's syndrome: sensorineural deafness and partial organification defect in thyroid
Dehalogenase	Autosomal recessive	Loss of iodide reutilization

THYROID HORMONE SYNTHESIS, METABOLISM, AND ACTION

THYROID HORMONE SYNTHESIS Thyroid hormones are derived from Tg, a large iodinated glycoprotein. After secretion into the thyroid follicle, Tg is iodinated on selected tyrosine residues that are subsequently coupled via an ether linkage. Reuptake of Tg into the thyroid follicular cell initiates proteolysis and the release of newly synthesized T$_4$ and T$_3$.

Iodine Metabolism and Transport Iodide uptake is a critical first step in thyroid hormone synthesis. Ingested iodine is bound to serum proteins, particularly albumin. Unbound iodine is excreted in the urine. The thyroid gland extracts iodine from the circulation in a highly efficient manner. For example, 10 to 25% of radioactive tracer (e.g., ^{123}I) is taken up by the normal thyroid gland over 24 h; this value can rise to 70 to 90% in Graves' disease. Iodide uptake is mediated by the Na$^+$/I$^-$ symporter (NIS), which is expressed at the basolateral membrane of thyroid follicular cells. NIS is most highly expressed in the thyroid gland but low levels are present in the salivary glands, lactating breast, and placenta. The iodide transport mechanism is highly regulated, allowing adaptation to variations in dietary supply. Low iodine levels increase the amount of NIS and stimulate uptake, whereas high iodine levels suppress NIS expression and uptake. The selective expression of the NIS in the thyroid allows isotopic scanning, treatment of hyperthyroidism, and ablation of thyroid cancer with radioisotopes of iodine, without significant effects on other organs. Mutation of the *NIS* gene is a rare cause of congenital hypothyroidism, underscoring its importance in thyroid hormone synthesis. Another iodine transporter, pendrin, is located on the apical surface of thyroid cells and mediates iodine efflux into the lumen. Mutation of the *PENDRIN* gene causes *Pendred syndrome*, a disorder characterized by defective organification of iodine, goiter, and sensorineural deafness.

Iodine deficiency is prevalent in many mountainous regions and in central Africa, central South America, and northern Asia. In areas of relative iodine deficiency, there is an increased prevalence of goiter and, when deficiency is severe, hypothyroidism and cretinism. *Cretin-*

ism is characterized by mental and growth retardation and occurs when children who live in iodine-deficient regions are not treated with iodine or thyroid hormone to restore normal thyroid hormone levels during early childhood. These children are often born to mothers with iodine deficiency, and it is likely that maternal thyroid hormone deficiency worsens the condition. Concomitant selenium deficiency may also contribute to the neurologic manifestations of cretinism. Iodine supplementation of salt, bread, and other food substances has markedly reduced the prevalence of cretinism. Unfortunately, however, iodine deficiency remains the most common cause of preventable mental deficiency, often because of resistance to the use of food additives or the cost of supplementation. In addition to overt cretinism, mild iodine deficiency can lead to subtle reduction of IQ. Oversupply of iodine,

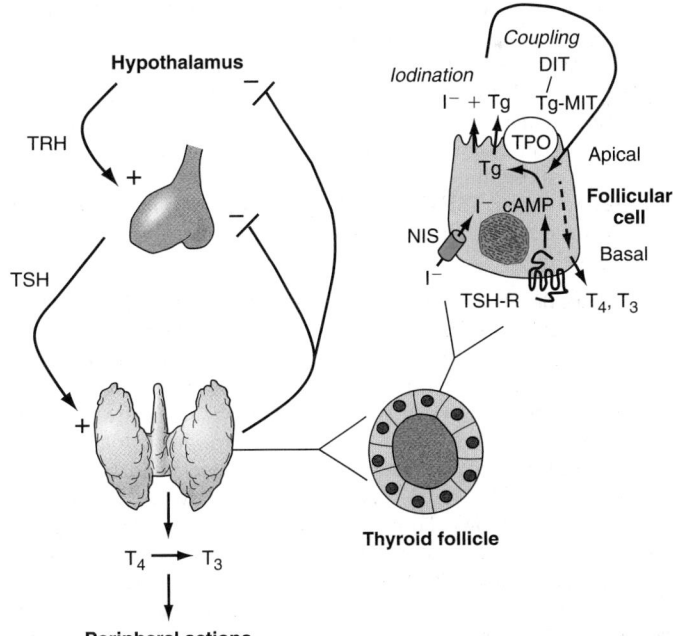

FIGURE 320-2 Regulation of thyroid hormone synthesis. *Left.* Thyroid hormones T$_4$ and T$_3$ feed back to inhibit hypothalamic production of thyrotropin-releasing hormone (TRH) and pituitary production of thyroid-stimulating hormone (TSH). TSH stimulates thyroid gland production of T$_4$ and T$_3$. *Right.* Thyroid follicles are formed by thyroid epithelial cells surrounding proteinaceous colloid, which contains thyroglobulin. Follicular cells, which are polarized, synthesize thyroglobulin and carry out thyroid hormone biosynthesis (see text for details). TSH-R, thyroid-stimulating hormone receptor; Tg, thyroglobulin; NIS, sodium-iodide symporter; TPO, thyroid peroxidase; DIT, di-iodotyrosine; MIT, monoiodotyrosine.

through supplements or foods enriched in iodine (e.g., shellfish, kelp), is associated with an increased incidence of autoimmune thyroid disease. The recommended average daily intake of iodine is 150 μg/d for adults, 90 to 120 μg/d for children, and 200 μg/d for pregnant women. Urinary iodine is >10 μg/dL in iodine-sufficient populations.

Organification, Coupling, Storage, Release   After iodide enters the thyroid, it is trapped and transported to the apical membrane of thyroid follicular cells where it is oxidized in an organification reaction that involves TPO and hydrogen peroxide. The reactive iodine atom is added to selected tyrosyl residues within Tg, a large (660 kDa) dimeric protein that consists of 2769 amino acids. The iodotyrosines in Tg are then coupled via an ether linkage in a reaction that is also catalyzed by TPO. Either T_4 or T_3 can be produced by this reaction, depending on the number of iodine atoms present in the iodotyrosines. After coupling, Tg is taken back into the thyroid cell where it is processed in lysosomes to release T_4 and T_3. Uncoupled mono- and diiodotyrosines (MIT, DIT) are deiodinated by the enzyme dehalogenase, thereby recycling any iodide that is not converted into thyroid hormones.

Disorders of thyroid hormone synthesis are rare causes of congenital hypothyroidism. The vast majority of these disorders are due to recessive mutations in TPO or Tg, but defects have also been identified in the TSH-R, NIS, pendrin, hydrogen peroxide generation, and in dehalogenase. Because of the biosynthetic defect, the gland is incapable of synthesizing adequate amounts of hormone, leading to increased TSH and a large goiter.

TSH Action   TSH regulates thyroid gland function through the TSH-R, a seven-transmembrane G protein–coupled receptor (GPCR). The TSH-R is coupled to the α subunit of stimulatory G protein ($G_{s\alpha}$), which activates adenylyl cyclase, leading to increased production of cyclic AMP. TSH also stimulates phosphatidylinositol turnover by activating phospholipase C. The functional roles of the TSH-R are exemplified by the consequences of naturally occurring mutations. Recessive loss-of-function mutations are a rare cause of thyroid hypoplasia and congenital hypothyroidism. Dominant gain-of-function mutations cause sporadic or familial nonautoimmune hyperthyroidism that is characterized by goiter, thyroid cell hyperplasia, and autonomous function. Most of these activating mutations occur in the transmembrane domain of the receptor. They are thought to mimic conformational changes similar to those induced by TSH binding or the interactions of thyroid-stimulating immunoglobulins (TSI) in Graves' disease. Activating TSH-R mutations also occur as somatic events and lead to clonal selection and expansion of the affected thyroid follicular cell (see below).

Other Factors that Influence Hormone Synthesis and Release   Although TSH is the dominant hormonal regulator of thyroid gland growth and function, a variety of growth factors, most produced locally in the thyroid gland, also influence thyroid hormone synthesis. These include insulin-like growth factor I (IGF-I), epidermal growth factor, transforming growth factor β (TGF-β), endothelins, and various cytokines. The quantitative roles of these factors are not well understood, but they are important in selected disease states. In acromegaly, for example, increased levels of growth hormone and IGF-I are associated with goiter and predisposition to multinodular goiter. Certain cytokines and interleukins (ILs) produced in association with autoimmune thyroid disease induce thyroid growth, whereas others lead to apoptosis. Iodine deficiency increases thyroid blood flow and upregulates the NIS, stimulating more efficient uptake. Excess iodide transiently inhibits thyroid iodide organification, a phenomenon known as the *Wolff-Chaikoff effect*. In individuals with a normal thyroid, the gland escapes from this inhibitory effect and iodide organification resumes; the suppressive action of high iodide may persist, however, in patients with underlying autoimmune thyroid disease.

THYROID HORMONE TRANSPORT AND METABOLISM ■ Serum Binding Proteins T_4 is secreted from the thyroid gland in at least 20-fold excess over

T_3 (Table 320-2). Both hormones are bound to plasma proteins, including thyroxine-binding globulin (TBG), transthyretin (TTR), formerly known as thyroxine-binding prealbumin, or TBPA), and albumin. The plasma-binding proteins increase the pool of circulating hormone, delay hormone clearance, and may modulate hormone delivery to selected tissue sites. The concentration of TBG is relatively low (1 to 2 mg/dL), but because of its high affinity for thyroid hormones ($T_4 > T_3$), it carries about 80% of the bound hormones. Albumin has relatively low affinity for thyroid hormones but has a high plasma concentration ($\sim$3.5 g/dL), and it binds up to 10% of T_4 and 30% of T_3. TTR carries about 10% of T_4 but little T_3.

When the effects of the various binding proteins are combined, approximately 99.98% of T_4 and 99.7% of T_3 are protein-bound. Because T_3 is less tightly bound than T_4, the amount of unbound T_3 is greater than unbound T_4, even though there is less total T_3 in the circulation. The unbound, or free, concentrations of the hormones are $\sim$2 × 10^{-11} M for T_4 and $\sim$6 × 10^{-12} M for T_3, which roughly correspond to the thyroid hormone receptor binding constants for these hormones (see below). Only the unbound hormone is biologically available to tissues. Therefore, homeostatic mechanisms that regulate the thyroid axis are directed towards maintenance of normal concentrations of unbound hormones.

Dysalbuminemic Hyperthyroxinemia   A number of inherited and acquired abnormalities affect thyroid hormone binding proteins. X-linked TBG deficiency is associated with very low levels of total T_4 and T_3. However, because unbound hormone levels are normal, patients are euthyroid and TSH levels are normal. The importance of recognizing this disorder is to avoid efforts to normalize total T_4 levels, as this leads to thyrotoxicosis and is futile because of rapid hormone clearance in the absence of TBG. TBG levels are elevated by estrogen, which increases sialylation and delays TBG clearance. Consequently, in women who are pregnant or taking estrogen-containing contraceptives, elevated TBG increases total T_4 and T_3 levels; however, unbound T_4 and T_3 levels are normal. Mutations in TBG, TTR, and albumin that increase binding affinity for T_4 and/or T_3 cause disorders known as *euthyroid hyperthyroxinemia* or *familial dysalbuminemic hyperthyroxinemia* (FDH) (Table 320-3). These disorders result in increased total T_4 and/or T_3, but unbound hormone levels are normal. The familial nature of the disorders, and the fact that TSH levels are normal rather than suppressed, suggest this diagnosis. Unbound hormone levels (ideally measured by dialysis) are normal in FDH. The diagnosis can be confirmed by using tests that measure the affinities of radiolabeled hormone binding to specific transport proteins or by performing DNA sequence analyses of the abnormal transport protein genes.

Certain medications, such as salicylates and salsalate, can displace thyroid hormones from circulating binding proteins. Although these drugs transiently perturb the thyroid axis by increasing free thyroid hormone levels, TSH is suppressed until a new steady state is reached, thereby restoring euthyroidism. Circulating factors associated with acute illness may also displace thyroid hormone from binding proteins (see "Sick Euthyroid Syndrome," below).

TABLE 320-2 *Characteristics of Circulating T_4 and T_3*

Hormone Property	T_4	T_3
Serum concentrations		
Total hormone	8 μg/dL	0.14 μg/dL
Fraction of total hormone in the free form	0.02%	0.3%
Free (unbound) hormone	21 × 10^{-12} M	6 × 10^{-12} M
Serum half-life	7 d	0.75 d
Fraction directly from the thyroid	100%	20%
Production rate, including peripheral conversion	90 μg/d	32 μg/d
Intracellular hormone fraction	$\sim$20%	$\sim$70%
Relative metabolic potency	0.3	1
Receptor binding	10^{-10} M	10^{-11} M

Deiodinases T_4 may be thought of as a precursor for the more potent T_3. T_4 is converted to T_3 by the deiodinase enzymes (Fig. 320-1). Type I deiodinase, which is located primarily in thyroid, liver, and kidney, has a relatively low affinity for T_4. Type II deiodinase has a higher affinity for T_4 and is found primarily in the pituitary gland, brain, brown fat, and thyroid gland. The presence of type II deiodinase allows it to regulate T_3 concentrations locally, a property that may be important in the context of levothyroxine (T_4) replacement. Type II deiodinase is also regulated by thyroid hormone—hypothyroidism induces the enzyme, resulting in enhanced $T_4 \rightarrow T_3$ conversion in tissues such as brain and pituitary. $T_4 \rightarrow T_3$ conversion is impaired by fasting, systemic illness or acute trauma, oral contrast agents, and a variety of medications (e.g., propylthiouracil, propranolol, amiodarone, glucocorticoids). Type III deiodinase inactivates T_4 and T_3 and is the most important source of reverse T_3 (rT_3). Massive hemangiomas that express type III deiodinase are a rare cause of hypothyroidism in infants.

THYROID HORMONE ACTION ■ Nuclear Thyroid Hormone Receptors

Thyroid hormones act by binding to nuclear *thyroid hormone receptors* (TRs) α and β. Both TRα and TRβ are expressed in most tissues, but their relative levels of expression vary among organs; TRα is particularly abundant in brain, kidney, gonads, muscle, and heart, whereas TRβ expression is relatively high in the pituitary and liver. Both receptors are variably spliced to form unique isoforms. The TRβ2 isoform, which has a unique amino terminus, is selectively expressed in the hypothalamus and pituitary, where it plays a role in feedback control of the thyroid axis. The TRα2 isoform contains a unique carboxy terminus that prevents thyroid hormone binding; it may function to block the action of other TR isoforms.

The TRs contain a central DNA-binding domain and a C-terminal ligand-binding domain. They bind to specific DNA sequences, termed *thyroid response elements* (TREs), in the promoter regions of target genes (Fig. 320-3). The receptors bind as homodimers or as heterodimers with retinoic acid X receptors (RXRs) (Chap. 317). The activated receptor can either stimulate gene transcription (e.g., myosin heavy chain α) or inhibit transcription (e.g., TSH β-subunit gene), depending on the nature of the regulatory elements in the target gene.

Thyroid hormones bind with similar affinities to TRα and TRβ. However, T_3 is bound with 10 to 15 times greater affinity than T_4, which explains its increased hormonal potency. Though T_4 is produced in excess of T_3, receptors are occupied mainly by T_3, reflecting $T_4 \rightarrow T_3$ conversion by peripheral tissues, greater T_3 bioavailability in the plasma, and receptors' greater affinity for T_3. After binding to TRs, thyroid hormone induces conformational changes in the receptors that modify its interactions with accessory transcription factors. In the absence of thyroid hormone binding, the aporeceptors bind to co-repressor proteins that inhibit gene transcription. Hormone binding dissociates the co-repressors and allows the recruitment of coactivators that enhance transcription. The discovery of TR interactions with co-repressors explains the fact that TR silences gene expression in the absence of hormone binding. Consequently, hormone deficiency has a profound effect on gene expression because it causes gene repression as well as loss of hormone-induced stimulation. This concept has been corroborated by the finding that targeted deletion of the TR genes in mice has a less pronounced phenotypic effect than hormone deficiency.

Thyroid Hormone Resistance

Resistance to thyroid hormone (RTH) is an autosomal dominant disorder characterized by elevated thyroid hormone levels and inappropriately normal or elevated TSH. Individuals with RTH do not, in general, exhibit signs and symptoms that are typical of hypothyroidism because hormone resistance is partial and is compensated by increased levels of thyroid hormone. The clinical features of RTH can include goiter, attention deficit disorder, mild reduction in IQ, delayed skeletal maturation, tachycardia, and impaired metabolic responses to thyroid hormone.

The disorder is caused by mutations in the TRβ receptor gene. These mutations, located in restricted regions of the ligand-binding domain, cause loss of receptor function. However, because the mutant receptors retain the capacity to dimerize with RXRs, bind to DNA, and recruit co-repressor proteins, they function as antagonists of the remaining, normal TRβ and TRα receptors. This property, referred to

---

TABLE 320-3 *Conditions Associated with Euthyroid Hyperthyroxinemia*

Disorder	Cause	Transmission	Characteristics
Familial dysalbuminemic hyperthyroxinemia (FDH)	Albumin mutations, usually R218H	AD	Increased T_4 Normal unbound T_4 Rarely increased T_3
TBG Familial excess	Increased TBG production	XL	Increased total T_4, T_3 Normal unbound T_4, T_3
Acquired excess	Medications (estrogen), pregnancy, cirrhosis, hepatitis	Acquired	Increased total T_4, T_3 Normal unbound T_4, T_3
Transthyretin[a] Excess	Islet tumors	Acquired	Usually normal T_4, T_3
Mutations	Increased affinity for T_4 or T_3	AD	Increased total T_4, T_3 Normal unbound T_4, T_3
Medications: propranolol, ipodate, iopanoic acid, amiodarone	Decreased $T_4 \rightarrow T_3$ conversion	Acquired	Increased T_4 Decreased T_3 Normal or increased TSH
Sick-euthyroid syndrome	Acute illness, especially psychiatric disorders	Acquired	Transiently increased unbound T_4 Decreased TSH T_4 and T_3 may also be decreased (see text)
Resistance to thyroid hormone (RTH)	Thyroid hormone receptor β mutations	AD	Increased unbound T_4, T_3 Normal or increased TSH Some patients clinically thyrotoxic

[a] Also known as thyroxine-binding prealbumin, TBPA.

Note: AD, autosomal dominant; TBG, thyroxine-binding globulin; TSH, thyroid-stimulating hormone; XL, X-linked.

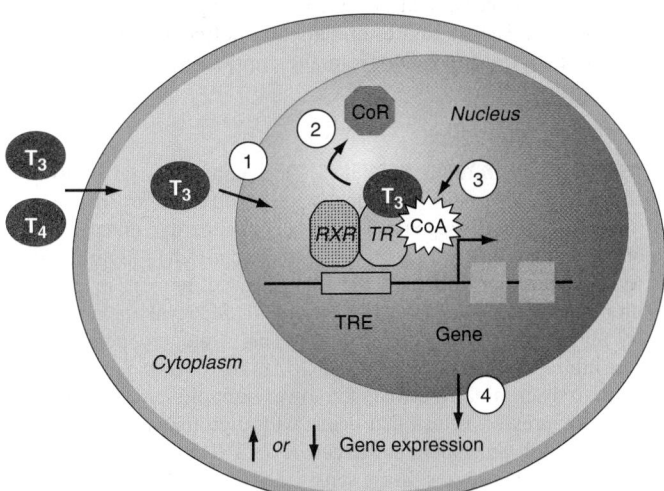

FIGURE 320-3 Mechanism of thyroid hormone receptor action. The thyroid hormone receptor (TR) and retinoid X receptor (RXR) form heterodimers that bind specifically to thyroid hormone response elements (TRE) in the promoter regions of target genes. In the absence of hormone, TR binds co-repressor (CoR) proteins that silence gene expression. The numbers refer to a series of ordered reactions that occur in response to thyroid hormone: (1) T_4 or T_3 enters the nucleus; (2) T_3 binding dissociates CoR from TR; (3) Coactivators (CoA) are recruited to the T_3-bound receptor; (4) gene expression is altered.

as "dominant negative" activity, explains the autosomal dominant mode of transmission. The diagnosis is suspected when unbound thyroid hormone levels are increased without suppression of TSH. Similar hormonal abnormalities are found in other affected family members, although the TRβ mutation arises de novo in about 20% of patients. DNA sequence analysis of the TRβ gene provides a definitive diagnosis. RTH must be distinguished from other causes of euthyroid hyperthyroxinemia (e.g., FDH) and inappropriate secretion of TSH by TSH-secreting pituitary adenomas (Chap. 318). In most patients, no treatment is indicated; the importance of making the diagnosis is to avoid inappropriate treatment of mistaken hyperthyroidism and to provide genetic counseling.

PHYSICAL EXAMINATION

In addition to the examination of the thyroid itself, the physical examination should include a search for signs of abnormal thyroid function and the extrathyroidal features of ophthalmopathy and dermopathy (see below). Examination of the neck begins by inspecting the seated patient from the front and side, and noting any surgical scars, obvious masses, or distended veins. The thyroid can be palpated with both hands from behind or while facing the patient, using the thumbs to palpate each lobe. It is best to use a combination of these methods, especially when the nodules are small. The patient's neck should be slightly flexed to relax the neck muscles. After locating the cricoid cartilage, the isthmus can be identified and followed laterally to locate either lobe (normally the right lobe is slightly larger than the left). By asking the patient to swallow sips of water, thyroid consistency can be better appreciated as the gland moves beneath the examiner's fingers.

Features to be noted include thyroid size, consistency, nodularity, and any tenderness or fixation. An estimate of thyroid size (normally 12 to 20 g) should be made, and a drawing is often the best way to record findings. However, ultrasound is the method of choice when it is important to determine thyroid size accurately. The size, location, and consistency of any nodules should also be defined. A bruit over the gland indicates increased vascularity, as occurs in hyperthyroidism. If the lower borders of the thyroid lobes are not clearly felt, a goiter may be retrosternal. Large retrosternal goiters can cause venous distention over the neck and difficulty breathing, especially when the arms are raised (Pemberton's sign). With any central mass above the thyroid, the tongue should be extended, as thyroglossal cysts then move upward. The thyroid examination is not complete without assessment for lymphadenopathy in the supraclavicular and cervical regions of the neck.

LABORATORY EVALUATION

MEASUREMENT OF THYROID HORMONES   The enhanced sensitivity and specificity of *TSH assays* have greatly improved laboratory assessment of thyroid function. Because TSH levels change dynamically in response to alterations of T_4 and T_3, a logical approach to thyroid testing is to first determine whether TSH is suppressed, normal, or elevated. With rare exceptions (see below), a normal TSH level excludes a primary abnormality of thyroid function. This strategy depends on the use of immunoradiometric assays (IRMAs) for TSH that are sensitive enough to discriminate between the lower limit of the reference range and the suppressed values that occur with thyrotoxicosis. Extremely sensitive (fourth generation) assays can detect TSH levels ≤0.004 mU/L, but for practical purposes assays sensitive to ≤0.1 mU/L are sufficient. The widespread availability of the TSH IRMA has rendered the TRH stimulation test obsolete, as the failure of TSH to rise after an intravenous bolus of 200 to 400 μg TRH has the same implications as a suppressed basal TSH measured by IRMA.

The finding of an abnormal TSH level must be followed by measurements of circulating thyroid hormone levels to confirm the diagnosis of hyperthyroidism (suppressed TSH) or hypothyroidism (elevated TSH). Radioimmunoassays are widely available for serum *total*

T_4 and *total* T_3. T_4 and T_3 are highly protein-bound, and numerous factors (illness, medications, genetic factors) can influence protein binding. It is useful, therefore, to measure the free, or unbound, hormone levels, which correspond to the biologically available hormone pool. Two direct methods are used to measure *unbound thyroid hormones*: (1) unbound thyroid hormone competition with radiolabeled T_4 (or an analogue) for binding to a solid-phase antibody, and (2) physical separation of the unbound hormone fraction by ultracentrifugation or equilibrium dialysis. Though early unbound hormone immunoassays suffered from artifacts, newer assays correlate well with the results of the more technically demanding and expensive physical separation methods. An indirect method to estimate unbound thyroid hormone levels is to calculate the free T_3 or free T_4 index from the total T_4 or T_3 concentration and the *thyroid hormone binding ratio* (THBR). The latter is derived from the T_3-resin uptake test, which determines the distribution of radiolabeled T_3 between an absorbent resin and the unoccupied thyroid hormone binding proteins in the sample. The binding of the labeled T_3 to the resin is increased when there is reduced unoccupied protein binding sites (e.g., TBG deficiency) or increased total thyroid hormone in the sample; it is decreased under the opposite circumstances. The product of THBR and total T_3 or T_4 provides the *free T_3 or T_4 index*. In effect, the index corrects for anomalous total hormone values caused by abnormalities in hormone-protein binding.

Total thyroid hormone levels are *elevated* when TBG is increased due to estrogens (pregnancy, oral contraceptives, hormone replacement therapy, tamoxifen), and *decreased* when TBG binding is reduced (androgens, the nephrotic syndrome). Genetic disorders and acute illness can also cause abnormalities in thyroid hormone binding proteins, and various drugs (phenytoin, carbamazepine, salicylates, and nonsteroidal anti-inflammatory drugs) can interfere with thyroid hormone binding. Because unbound thyroid hormone levels are normal and the patient is euthyroid in all of these circumstances, assays that measure unbound hormone are preferable to those for total thyroid hormones.

For most purposes, the unbound T_4 level is sufficient to confirm thyrotoxicosis, but 2 to 5% of patients have only an elevated T_3 level (T_3 toxicosis). Thus, unbound T_3 levels should be measured in patients with a suppressed TSH but normal unbound T_4 levels.

There are several clinical conditions in which the use of TSH as a screening test may be misleading, particularly without simultaneous unbound T_4 determinations. Any severe nonthyroidal illness can cause abnormal TSH levels (see below). Although hypothyroidism is the most common cause of an elevated TSH level, rare causes include a TSH-secreting pituitary tumor (Chap. 318), thyroid hormone resistance, and assay artifact. Conversely, a suppressed TSH level, particularly <0.1 mU/L, usually indicates thyrotoxicosis but may also be seen during the first trimester of pregnancy (due to hCG secretion), after treatment of hyperthyroidism (because TSH remains suppressed for several weeks), and in response to certain medications (e.g., high doses of glucocorticoids or dopamine). Importantly, secondary hypothyroidism, caused by hypothalamic-pituitary disease, is associated with a variable (low to high-normal) TSH level, which is inappropriate for the low T_4 level. Thus, *TSH should not be used to assess thyroid function in patients with suspected or known pituitary disease.*

Tests for the end-organ effects of thyroid hormone excess or depletion, such as estimation of basal metabolic rate, tendon reflex relaxation rates, or serum cholesterol, are not useful as clinical determinants of thyroid function.

TESTS TO DETERMINE THE ETIOLOGY OF THYROID DYSFUNCTION   Autoimmune thyroid disease is detected most easily by measuring circulating antibodies against TPO and Tg. As antibodies to Tg alone are uncommon, it is reasonable to measure only TPO antibodies. About 5 to 15% of euthyroid women and up to 2% of euthyroid men have thyroid antibodies; such individuals are at increased risk of developing thyroid dysfunction. Almost all patients with autoimmune hypothyroidism, and up to 80% of those with Graves' disease, have TPO antibodies, usually at high levels.

TSI are antibodies that stimulate the TSH-R in Graves' disease. They can be measured in bioassays or indirectly in assays that detect antibody binding to the receptor. The main use of these assays is to predict neonatal thyrotoxicosis caused by high maternal levels of TSI in the last trimester of pregnancy.

Serum Tg levels are increased in all types of thyrotoxicosis except *thyrotoxicosis factitia* caused by self-administration of thyroid hormone. The main role for Tg measurement, however, is in the follow-up of thyroid cancer patients. After total thyroidectomy and radioablation, Tg levels should be undetectable; measurable levels (>1 to 2 ng/mL) suggest incomplete ablation or recurrent cancer.

RADIOIODINE UPTAKE AND THYROID SCANNING The thyroid gland selectively transports radioisotopes of iodine (^{123}I, ^{125}I, ^{131}I) and ^{99m}Tc pertechnetate, allowing thyroid imaging and quantitation of radioactive tracer fractional uptake.

Nuclear imaging of Graves' disease is characterized by an enlarged gland and increased tracer uptake that is distributed homogeneously. Toxic adenomas appear as focal areas of increased uptake, with suppressed tracer uptake in the remainder of the gland. In toxic multinodular goiter, the gland is enlarged—often with distorted architecture—and there are multiple areas of relatively increased or decreased tracer uptake. Subacute thyroiditis is associated with very low uptake because of follicular cell damage and TSH suppression. Thyrotoxicosis factitia is also associated with low uptake.

Although the use of fine-needle aspiration (FNA) biopsy has diminished the use of thyroid scans in the evaluation of solitary thyroid nodules, the functional features of thyroid nodules have some prognostic significance. So-called cold nodules, which have diminished tracer uptake, are usually benign. However, these nodules are more likely to be malignant (~5 to 10%) than so-called hot nodules, which are almost never malignant.

Thyroid scanning is also used in the follow-up of thyroid cancer. After thyroidectomy and ablation using ^{131}I, there is diminished radioiodine uptake in the thyroid bed, allowing the detection of metastatic thyroid cancer deposits that retain the ability to transport iodine. Whole-body scans using 111 to 185 MBq (3 to 5 mCi) ^{131}I are typically performed after thyroid hormone withdrawal to raise the TSH level or after the administration of recombinant human TSH.

THYROID ULTRASOUND Ultrasonography is used increasingly to assist in the diagnosis of nodular thyroid disease, a reflection of the limitations of the physical examination and improvements in ultrasound technology. Using 10-MHz instruments, spatial resolution and image quality are excellent, allowing the detection of nodules and cysts >3 mm. In addition to detecting thyroid nodules, ultrasound is useful for monitoring nodule size, for guiding FNA biopsies, and for the aspiration of cystic lesions. Ultrasound is also used in the evaluation of recurrent thyroid cancer, including possible spread to cervical lymph nodes.

HYPOTHYROIDISM

Iodine deficiency remains the most common cause of hypothyroidism worldwide. In areas of iodine sufficiency, autoimmune disease (Hashimoto's thyroiditis) and iatrogenic causes (treatment of hyperthyroidism) are most common (Table 320-4).

CONGENITAL HYPOTHYROIDISM ■ **Prevalence** Hypothyroidism occurs in about 1 in 4000 newborns. It may be transient, especially if the mother has TSH-R blocking antibodies or has received antithyroid drugs, but permanent hypothyroidism occurs in the majority. Neonatal hypothyroidism is due to thyroid gland dysgenesis in 80 to 85%, inborn errors of thyroid hormone synthesis in 10 to 15%, and is TSH-R antibody-

TABLE 320-4 Causes of Hypothyroidism

Primary
  Autoimmune hypothyroidism: Hashimoto's thyroiditis, atrophic thyroiditis
  Iatrogenic: ^{131}I treatment, subtotal or total thyroidectomy, external irradiation of neck for lymphoma or cancer
  Drugs: iodine excess (including iodine-containing contrast media and amiodarone), lithium, antithyroid drugs, p-aminosalicyclic acid, interferon-α and other cytokines, aminoglutethimide
  Congenital hypothyroidism: absent or ectopic thyroid gland, dyshormonogenesis, TSH-R mutation
  Iodine deficiency
  Infiltrative disorders: amyloidosis, sarcoidosis, hemochromatosis, scleroderma, cystinosis, Riedel's thyroiditis
  Overexpression of type 3 deoiodinase in infantile hemangioma
Transient
  Silent thyroiditis, including postpartum thyroiditis
  Subacute thyroiditis
  Withdrawal of thyroxine treatment in individuals with an intact thyroid
  After ^{131}I treatment or subtotal thyroidectomy for Graves' disease
Secondary
  Hypopituitarism: tumors, pituitary surgery or irradiation, infiltrative disorders, Sheehan's syndrome, trauma, genetic forms of combined pituitary hormone deficiencies
  Isolated TSH deficiency or inactivity
  Bexarotene treatment
  Hypothalamic disease: tumors, trauma, infiltrative disorders, idiopathic

Note: TSH, thyroid-stimulating hormone; TSH-R, TSH receptor.

mediated in 5% of affected newborns. The developmental abnormalities are twice as common in girls. Mutations that cause congenital hypothyroidism are being increasingly recognized, but the vast majority remain idiopathic (Table 320-1).

Clinical Manifestations The majority of infants appear normal at birth, and <10% are diagnosed based on clinical features, which include prolonged jaundice, feeding problems, hypotonia, enlarged tongue, delayed bone maturation, and umbilical hernia. Importantly, permanent neurologic damage results if treatment is delayed. Typical features of adult hypothyroidism may also be present (Table 320-5). Other congenital malformations, especially cardiac, are four times more common in congenital hypothyroidism.

Diagnosis and Treatment Because of the severe neurologic consequences of untreated congenital hypothyroidism, neonatal screening programs have been established in developed countries. These are generally based on measurement of TSH or T$_4$ levels in heel-prick blood specimens. When the diagnosis is confirmed, T$_4$ is instituted at a dose of 10 to 15 μg/kg per day and the dosage is adjusted by close monitoring of TSH levels. T$_4$ requirements are relatively great during the first year of life, and a high circulating T$_4$ level is usually needed to normalize TSH. Early treatment with T$_4$ results in normal IQ levels, but subtle neurodevelopmental abnormalities may occur in those with the most severe hypothyroidism at diagnosis or when treatment is suboptimal.

TABLE 320-5 Signs and Symptoms of Hypothyroidism (Descending Order of Frequency)

Symptoms	Signs
Tiredness, weakness	Dry coarse skin; cool peripheral extremities
Dry skin	
Feeling cold	Puffy face, hands, and feet (myxedema)
Hair loss	
Difficulty concentrating and poor memory	Diffuse alopecia
Constipation	Bradycardia
Weight gain with poor appetite	Peripheral edema
Dyspnea	Delayed tendon reflex relaxation
Hoarse voice	Carpal tunnel syndrome
Menorrhagia (later oligomenorrhea or amenorrhea)	Serous cavity effusions
Paresthesia	
Impaired hearing	

AUTOIMMUNE HYPOTHYROIDISM ■ **Classification** Autoimmune hypothyroidism may be associated with a goiter (Hashimoto's, or *goitrous thyroiditis*) or, at the later stages of the disease, minimal residual thyroid tissue (*atrophic thyroiditis*). Because the autoimmune process gradually reduces thyroid function, there is a phase of compensation when normal thyroid hormone levels are maintained by a rise in TSH. Though some patients may have minor symptoms, this state is called *subclinical hypothyroidism* or *mild hypothyroidism*. Later, free T_4 levels fall and TSH levels rise further; symptoms become more readily apparent at this stage (usually TSH > 10 mU/L), which is referred to as *clinical hypothyroidism* or *overt hypothyroidism*.

Prevalence The mean annual incidence rate of autoimmune hypothyroidism is up to 4 per 1000 women and 1 per 1000 men. It is more common in certain populations, such as the Japanese, probably because of genetic factors and chronic exposure to a high-iodine diet. The mean age at diagnosis is 60 years, and the prevalence of overt hypothyroidism increases with age. Subclinical hypothyroidism is found in 6 to 8% of women (10% over the age of 60) and 3% of men. The annual risk of developing clinical hypothyroidism is about 4% when subclinical hypothyroidism is associated with positive TPO antibodies.

Pathogenesis In Hashimoto's thyroiditis, there is a marked lymphocytic infiltration of the thyroid with germinal center formation, atrophy of the thyroid follicles accompanied by oxyphil metaplasia, absence of colloid, and mild to moderate fibrosis. In atrophic thyroiditis, the fibrosis is much more extensive, lymphocyte infiltration is less pronounced, and thyroid follicles are almost completely absent. Atrophic thyroiditis likely represents the end stage of Hashimoto's thyroiditis rather than a distinct disorder.

As with most autoimmune disorders, susceptibility to autoimmune hypothyroidism is determined by a combination of genetic and environmental factors, and the risk of either autoimmune hypothyroidism or Graves' disease is increased among siblings. HLA-DR polymorphisms are the best documented genetic risk factors for autoimmune hypothyroidism, especially HLA-DR3, -DR4, and -DR5 in Caucasians. A weak association also exists between polymorphisms in *CTLA-4*, a T cell–regulating gene, and autoimmune hypothyroidism. Both of these genetic associations are shared by other autoimmune diseases, which may explain the relationship between autoimmune hypothyroidism and other autoimmune diseases, especially type 1 diabetes mellitus, Addison disease, pernicious anemia, and vitiligo (Chap. 330). HLA-DR and *CTLA*-4 polymorphisms account for approximately half of the genetic susceptibility to autoimmune hypothyroidism. The other contributory loci remain to be identified. A gene on chromosome 21 may be responsible for the association between autoimmune hypothyroidism and Down syndrome. The female preponderance of thyroid autoimmunity is most likely due to the effects of sex steroids on the immune response, but an X chromosome–related genetic factor is also possible, which may account for the high frequency of autoimmune hypothyroidism in Turner syndrome. Environmental susceptibility factors are also poorly defined at present. A high iodine intake may increase the risk of autoimmune hypothyroidism by immunologic effects or direct thyroid toxicity. There is no convincing evidence for a role of infection, except for the congenital rubella syndrome, in which there is a high frequency of autoimmune hypothyroidism. Viral thyroiditis does not induce subsequent autoimmune thyroid disease.

The thyroid lymphocytic infiltrate in autoimmune hypothyroidism is composed of activated CD4+ and CD8+ T cells, as well as B cells. Thyroid cell destruction is believed to be primarily mediated by the CD8+ cytotoxic T cells, which destroy their targets by either perforin-induced cell necrosis or granzyme B–induced apoptosis. In addition, local T cell production of cytokines, such as tumor necrosis factor (TNF), IL-1, and interferon (IFN) γ, may render thyroid cells more susceptible to apoptosis mediated by death receptors, such as Fas, which are activated by their respective ligands on T cells. These cytokines also impair thyroid cell function directly, and induce the expression of other proinflammatory molecules by the thyroid cells themselves, such as cytokines, HLA class I and class II molecules, adhesion molecules, CD40, and nitric oxide. Administration of high concentrations of cytokines for therapeutic purposes (especially IFN-α) is associated with increased autoimmune thyroid disease, possibly through mechanisms similar to those in sporadic disease.

Antibodies to Tg and TPO are clinically useful markers of thyroid autoimmunity, but any pathogenic effect is restricted to a secondary role in amplifying an ongoing autoimmune response. TPO antibodies fix complement, and complement membrane attack complexes are present in the thyroid in autoimmune hypothyroidism. However, transplacental passage of Tg or TPO antibodies has no effect on the fetal thyroid, which suggests that T cell–mediated injury is required to initiate autoimmune damage to the thyroid. Up to 20% of patients with autoimmune hypothyroidism have antibodies against the TSH-R, which, in contrast to TSI, do not stimulate the receptor but prevent the binding of TSH. These TSH-R-blocking antibodies therefore cause hypothyroidism and, especially in Asian patients, thyroid atrophy. Their transplacental passage may induce transient neonatal hypothyroidism. Rarely, patients have a mixture of TSI- and TSH-R-blocking antibodies, and thyroid function can oscillate between hyperthyroidism and hypothyroidism as one or the other antibody becomes dominant. Predicting the course of disease in such individuals is difficult, and they require close monitoring of thyroid function. Bioassays can be used to document that TSH-R-blocking antibodies reduce the cyclic AMP–inducing effect of TSH on cultured TSH-R-expressing cells, but these assays are difficult to perform. Assays that measure the binding of antibodies to the receptor by competition with radiolabeled TSH [TSH-binding inhibiting immunoglobulins (TBII)] do not distinguish between TSI- and TSH-R-blocking antibodies, but a positive result in a patient with spontaneous hypothyroidism is strong evidence for the presence of blocking antibodies. The use of these assays does not generally alter clinical management, although they may be useful to confirm the cause of transient neonatal hypothyroidism.

Clinical Manifestations The main clinical features of hypothyroidism are summarized in Table 320-5. The onset is usually insidious, and the patient may become aware of symptoms only when euthyroidism is restored. Patients with Hashimoto's thyroiditis may present because of goiter rather than symptoms of hypothyroidism. The goiter may not be large but is usually irregular and firm in consistency. It is often possible to palpate a pyramidal lobe, normally a vestigial remnant of the thyroglossal duct. Rarely, uncomplicated Hashimoto's thyroiditis is associated with pain.

Patients with atrophic thyroiditis, or the late stage of Hashimoto's thyroiditis, present with symptoms and signs of hypothyroidism. The skin is dry, and there is decreased sweating, thinning of the epidermis, and hyperkeratosis of the stratum corneum. Increased dermal glycosaminoglycan content traps water, giving rise to skin thickening without pitting (*myxedema*). Typical features include a puffy face with edematous eyelids and nonpitting pretibial edema (Fig. 320-4). There is pallor, often with a yellow tinge to the skin due to carotene accumulation. Nail growth is retarded, and hair is dry, brittle, difficult to manage, and falls out easily. In addition to diffuse alopecia, there is thinning of the outer third of the eyebrows, although this is not a specific sign of hypothyroidism.

Other common features include constipation and weight gain (despite a poor appetite). In contrast to popular perception, the weight gain is usually modest and due mainly to fluid retention in the myxedematous tissues. Libido is decreased in both sexes, and there may be oligomenorrhea or amenorrhea in long-standing disease, but menorrhagia is also common. Fertility is reduced and the incidence of miscarriage is increased. Prolactin levels are often modestly increased (Chap. 318) and may contribute to alterations in libido and fertility and cause galactorrhea.

Myocardial contractility and pulse rate are reduced, leading to a

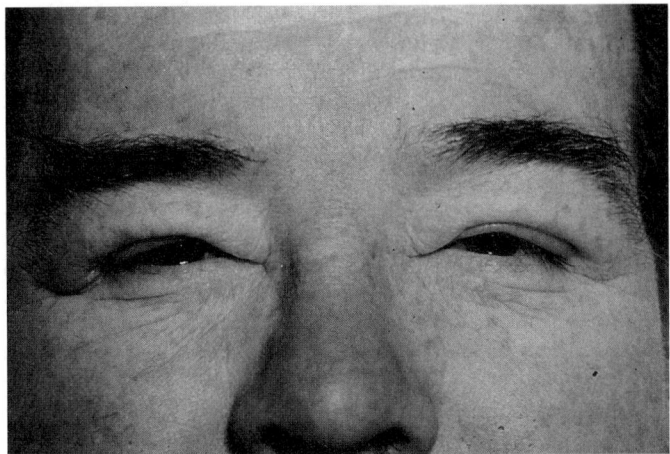

FIGURE 320-4 Facial appearance in hypothyroidism. Note puffy eyes and thickened, pale skin.

reduced stroke volume and bradycardia. Increased peripheral resistance may be accompanied by hypertension, particularly diastolic. Blood flow is diverted from the skin, producing the cool extremities. Pericardial effusions occur in up to 30% of patients but rarely compromise cardiac function. Though alterations in myosin heavy chain isoform expression have been documented, cardiomyopathy is unusual. Fluid may also accumulate in other serous cavities and in the middle ear, giving rise to conductive deafness. Pulmonary function is generally normal, but dyspnea may be caused by pleural effusion, impaired respiratory muscle function, diminished ventilatory drive, or sleep apnea.

Carpal tunnel and other entrapment syndromes are common, as is impairment of muscle function with stiffness, cramps, and pain. On examination, there may be slow relaxation of tendon reflexes and pseudomyotonia. Memory and concentration are impaired. Rare neurologic problems include reversible cerebellar ataxia, dementia, psychosis, and myxedema coma. *Hashimoto's encephalopathy* is a rare and distinctive syndrome associated with myoclonus and slow-wave activity on electroencephalography, which can progress to confusion, coma, and death. It is steroid-responsive and may occur in the presence of autoimmune thyroiditis, without hypothyroidism. The hoarse voice and occasionally clumsy speech of hypothyroidism reflect fluid accumulation in the vocal cords and tongue.

The features described above are the consequence of thyroid hormone deficiency. However, autoimmune hypothyroidism may be associated with signs or symptoms of other autoimmune diseases, particularly vitiligo, pernicious anemia, Addison disease, alopecia areata, and type 1 diabetes mellitus. Less common associations include celiac disease, dermatitis herpetiformis, chronic active hepatitis, rheumatoid arthritis, systemic lupus erythematosus (SLE), and Sjögren's syndrome. Thyroid-associated ophthalmopathy, which usually occurs in Graves' disease (see below), occurs in about 5% of patients with autoimmune hypothyroidism.

Autoimmune hypothyroidism is uncommon in children and usually presents with slow growth and delayed facial maturation. The appearance of permanent teeth is also delayed. Myopathy, with muscle swelling, is more common in children than in adults. In most cases, puberty is delayed, but precocious puberty sometimes occurs. There may be intellectual impairment if the onset is before 3 years and the hormone deficiency is severe.

Laboratory Evaluation A summary of the investigations used to determine the existence and cause of hypothyroidism is provided in Fig. 320-5. A normal TSH level excludes primary (but not secondary) hypothyroidism. If the TSH is elevated, an unbound T_4 level is needed to confirm the presence of clinical hypothyroidism, but T_4 is inferior to TSH when used as a screening test, as it will not detect subclinical or mild hypothyroidism. Circulating unbound T_3 levels are normal in about 25% of patients, reflecting adaptive responses to hypothyroidism. T_3 measurements are therefore not indicated.

Once clinical or subclinical hypothyroidism is confirmed, the etiology is usually easily established by demonstrating the presence of TPO antibodies, which are present in 90 to 95% of patients with autoimmune hypothyroidism. TBII can be found in 10 to 20% of patients, but these determinations are not needed routinely. If there is any doubt about the cause of a goiter associated with hypothyroidism, FNA biopsy can be used to confirm the presence of autoimmune thyroiditis. Other abnormal laboratory findings in hypothyroidism may include increased creatine phosphokinase, elevated cholesterol and triglycerides, and anemia (usually normocytic or macrocytic). Except when accompanied by iron deficiency, the anemia and other abnormalities gradually resolve with thyroxine replacement.

Differential Diagnosis An asymmetric goiter in Hashimoto's thyroiditis may be confused with a multinodular goiter or thyroid carcinoma, in which thyroid antibodies may also be present. Ultrasound can be used to show the presence of a solitary lesion or a multinodular goiter, rather than the heterogeneous thyroid enlargement typical of Hashimoto's thyroiditis. FNA biopsy is useful in the investigation of focal nodules. Other causes of hypothyroidism are discussed below but rarely cause diagnostic confusion (Table 320-4).

OTHER CAUSES OF HYPOTHYROIDISM *Iatrogenic hypothyroidism* is a common cause of hypothyroidism and can often be detected by screening before symptoms develop. In the first 3 to 4 months after radioiodine treatment, transient hypothyroidism may occur due to reversible radiation damage rather than to cellular destruction. Low-dose thyroxine treatment can be withdrawn if recovery occurs. Because TSH levels are suppressed by hyperthyroidism, unbound T_4 levels are a better measure of thyroid function than TSH in the months following ra-

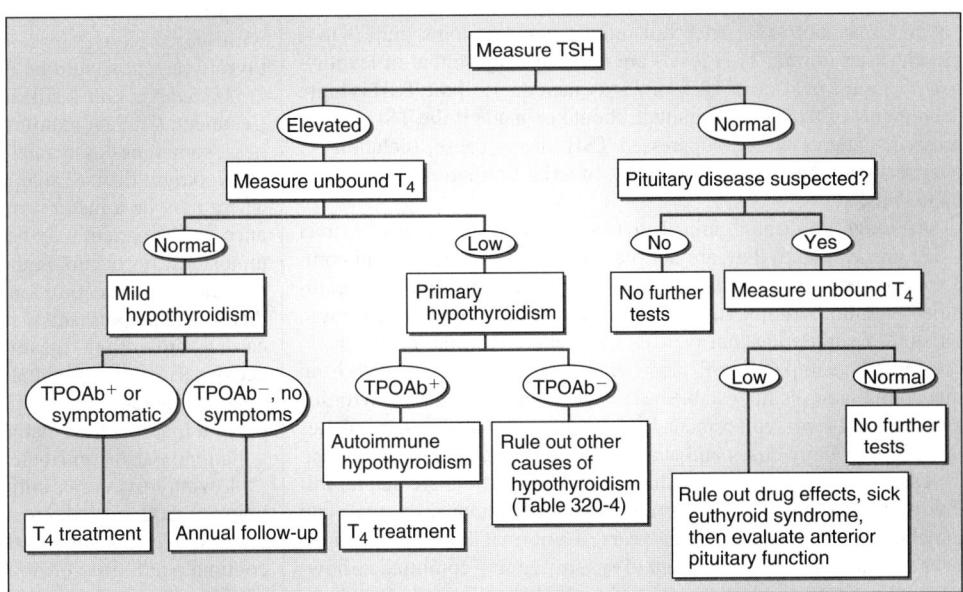

FIGURE 320-5 Evaluation of hypothyroidism. TPOAb+, thyroid peroxidase antibodies present; TPOAb−, thyroid peroxidase antibodies not present. TSH, thyroid-stimulating hormone.

dioiodine treatment. Mild hypothyroidism after subtotal thyroidectomy may also resolve after several months, as the gland remnant is stimulated by increased TSH levels.

Iodine deficiency is responsible for endemic goiter and cretinism but is an uncommon cause of adult hypothyroidism unless the iodine intake is very low or there are complicating factors, such as the consumption of thiocyanates in cassava or selenium deficiency. Though hypothyroidism due to iodine deficiency can be treated with thyroxine, public health measures to improve iodine intake should be advocated to eliminate this problem. Iodized salt or bread or a single bolus of oral or intramuscular iodized oil have all been used successfully.

Paradoxically, chronic iodine excess can also induce goiter and hypothyroidism. The intracellular events that account for this effect are unclear, but individuals with autoimmune thyroiditis are especially susceptible. Iodine excess is responsible for the hypothyroidism that occurs in up to 13% of patients treated with amiodarone (see below). Other drugs, particularly lithium, may also cause hypothyroidism. Transient hypothyroidism caused by thyroiditis is discussed below.

Secondary hypothyroidism is usually diagnosed in the context of other anterior pituitary hormone deficiencies; isolated TSH deficiency is very rare (Chap. 318). TSH levels may be low, normal, or even slightly increased in secondary hypothyroidism; the latter is due to secretion of immunoactive but bioinactive forms of TSH. The diagnosis is confirmed by detecting a low unbound T_4 level. The goal of treatment is to maintain unbound T_4 levels in the upper half of the reference range, as TSH levels cannot be used to monitor therapy.

℞ TREATMENT

Clinical Hypothyroidism   If there is no residual thyroid function, the daily replacement dose of levothyroxine is usually 1.6 μg/kg body weight (typically 100 to 150 μg). In many patients, however, lower doses suffice until residual thyroid tissue is destroyed. In patients who develop hypothyroidism after the treatment of Graves' disease, there is often underlying autonomous function, necessitating lower replacement doses (typically 75 to 125 μg/d).

Adult patients under 60 without evidence of heart disease may be started on 50 to 100 μg levothyroxine (T_4) daily. The dose is adjusted on the basis of TSH levels, with the goal of treatment being a normal TSH, ideally in the lower half of the reference range. TSH responses are gradual and should be measured about 2 months after instituting treatment or after any subsequent change in levothyroxine dosage. The clinical effects of levothyroxine replacement are often slow to appear. Patients may not experience full relief from symptoms until 3 to 6 months after normal TSH levels are restored. Adjustment of levothyroxine dosage is made in 12.5- or 25-μg increments if the TSH is high; decrements of the same magnitude should be made if the TSH is suppressed. Patients with a suppressed TSH of any cause, including T_4 overtreatment, have an increased risk of atrial fibrillation and reduced bone density.

Although dessicated animal thyroid preparations (thyroid extract USP) are available, they are not recommended as potency and composition vary between batches. Interest in using levothyroxine combined with liothyronine (triiodothyronine, T_3) has been revived, based on studies suggesting that patients feel better when taking the T_4/T_3 combination compared to T_4 alone. However, a long-term benefit from this combination is not established. There is no place for liothyronine alone as long-term replacement, because the short half-life necessitates three or four daily doses and is associated with fluctuating T_3 levels.

Once full replacement is achieved and TSH levels are stable, follow-up measurement of TSH is recommended at annual intervals and may be extended to every 2 to 3 years, if a normal TSH is maintained over several years. It is important to ensure ongoing compliance, however, as patients do not feel any difference after missing a few doses of levothyroxine, this sometimes leads to self-discontinuation.

In patients of normal body weight who are taking ≥200 μg of levothyroxine per day, an elevated TSH level is often a sign of poor compliance. This is also the likely explanation for fluctuating TSH levels, despite a constant levothyroxine dosage. Such patients often have normal or high unbound T_4 levels, despite an elevated TSH, because they remember to take medication for a few days before testing; this is sufficient to normalize T_4, but not TSH, levels. It is important to consider variable compliance, as this pattern of thyroid function tests is otherwise suggestive of disorders associated with inappropriate TSH secretion (Table 320-3). Because T_4 has a long half-life (7 days), patients who miss doses can be advised to take up to three doses of the skipped tablets at once. Other causes of increased levothyroxine requirements must be excluded, particularly malabsorption (e.g., celiac disease, small-bowel surgery), estrogen therapy, and drugs that interfere with T_4 absorption or clearance such as cholestyramine, ferrous sulfate, calcium supplements, lovastatin, aluminum hydroxide, rifampicin, amiodarone, carbamazepine, and phenytoin.

Mild Hypothyroidism   By definition, subclinical or mild hypothyroidism refers to biochemical evidence of thyroid hormone deficiency in patients who have few or no apparent clinical features of hypothyroidism. There are no universally accepted guidelines for the treatment of mild hypothyroidism. As long as excessive treatment is avoided, there is little risk in correcting a slightly increased TSH, and some patients likely derive modest clinical benefit from treatment. Moreover, there is some risk that patients will progress to overt hypothyroidism, particularly when the TSH level is >6 mU/L and TPO antibodies are present. Treatment is administered by starting with a low dose of levothyroxine (25 to 50 μg/d) with the goal of normalizing TSH. If thyroxine is not given, thyroid function should be evaluated annually.

Special Treatment Considerations   Rarely, levothyroxine replacement is associated with pseudotumor cerebri in *children*. Presentation appears to be idiosyncratic and occurs months after treatment has begun. Women with a history or high risk of hypothyroidism should ensure that they are euthyroid prior to conception and during early pregnancy as maternal hypothyroidism may adversely affect fetal neural development. Thyroid function should be evaluated once pregnancy is confirmed and at the beginning of the second and third trimesters. The dose of levothyroxine may need to be increased by ≥50% during pregnancy and returned to previous levels after delivery. *Elderly* patients may require up to 20% less thyroxine than younger patients. In the elderly, especially patients with known coronary artery disease, the starting dose of levothyroxine is 12.5 to 25 μg/d with similar increments every 2 to 3 months until TSH is normalized. In some patients it may be impossible to achieve full replacement, despite optimal antianginal treatment. *Emergency surgery* is generally safe in patients with untreated hypothyroidism, although routine surgery in a hypothyroid patient should be deferred until euthyroidism is achieved.

Myxedema coma still has a high mortality rate, despite intensive treatment. Clinical manifestations include reduced level of consciousness, sometimes associated with seizures, as well as the other features of hypothyroidism (Table 320-5). Hypothermia can reach 23°C (74°F). There may be a history of treated hypothyroidism with poor compliance, or the patient may be previously undiagnosed. Myxedema coma almost always occurs in the elderly and is usually precipitated by factors that impair respiration, such as drugs (especially sedatives, anesthetics, antidepressants), pneumonia, congestive heart failure, myocardial infarction, gastrointestinal bleeding, or cerebrovascular accidents. Sepsis should also be suspected. Exposure to cold may also be a risk factor. Hypoventilation, leading to hypoxia and hypercapnia, plays a major role in pathogenesis; hypoglycemia and dilutional hyponatremia also contribute to the development of myxedema coma.

Levothyroxine can initially be administered as a single intravenous bolus of 500 μg, which serves as a loading dose. Although further levothyroxine is not strictly necessary for several days, it is usually continued at a dose of 50 to 100 μg/d. If suitable intravenous preparation is not available, the same initial dose of levothyroxine can be given by nasogastric tube (though absorption may be impaired in myxedema). An alternative is to give liothyronine (T_3) intravenously or via nasogastric tube, in doses ranging from 10 to 25 μg every 8 to 12 h. This treatment has been advocated because $T_4 \rightarrow T_3$ conversion is impaired in myxedema coma. However, excess liothyronine has the potential to provoke arrhythmias. Another option is to combine levothyroxine (200 μg) and liothyronine (25 μg) as a single, initial intravenous bolus followed by daily treatment with levothyroxine (50 to 100 μg/d) and liothyronine (10 μg every 8 h).

Supportive therapy should be provided to correct any associated metabolic disturbances. External warming is indicated only if the temperature is <30°C, as it can result in cardiovascular collapse (Chap. 16). Space blankets should be used to prevent further heat loss. Parenteral hydrocortisone (50 mg every 6 h) should be administered, as there is impaired adrenal reserve in profound hypothyroidism. Any precipitating factors should be treated, including the early use of broad-spectrum antibiotics, pending the exclusion of infection. Ventilatory support with regular blood gas analysis is usually needed during the first 48 h. Hypertonic saline or intravenous glucose may be needed if there is hyponatremia or hypoglycemia; hypotonic intravenous fluids should be avoided because they may exacerbate water retention secondary to reduced renal perfusion and inappropriate vasopressin secretion. The metabolism of most medications is impaired, and sedatives should be avoided if possible or used in reduced doses. Medication blood levels should be monitored, when available, to guide dosage.

THYROTOXICOSIS

Thyrotoxicosis is defined as the state of thyroid hormone excess and is not synonymous with *hyperthyroidism*, which is the result of excessive thyroid function. However, the major etiologies of thyrotoxicosis are hyperthyroidism caused by Graves' disease, toxic multinodular goiter, and toxic adenomas. Other causes are listed in Table 320-6.

GRAVES' DISEASE ■ **Epidemiology** Graves' disease accounts for 60 to 80% of thyrotoxicosis, but the prevalence varies among populations, depending mainly on iodine intake (high iodine intake is associated with an increased prevalence of Graves' disease). Graves' disease occurs in up to 2% of women but is one-tenth as frequent in men. The disorder rarely begins before adolescence and typically occurs between 20 and 50 years of age, but it also occurs in the elderly.

PATHOGENESIS As in autoimmune hypothyroidism, a combination of genetic factors, including HLA-DR and *CTLA-4* polymorphisms, and environmental factors contribute to Graves' disease susceptibility. The concordance for Graves' disease in monozygotic twins is 20 to 30%,

compared to <5% in dizygotic twins. Indirect evidence suggests that stress is an important environmental factor, presumably operating through neuroendocrine effects on the immune system. Smoking is a minor risk factor for Graves' disease and a major risk factor for the development of ophthalmopathy. Sudden increases in iodine intake may precipitate Graves' disease, and there is a threefold increase in the occurrence of Graves' disease in the postpartum period.

The hyperthyroidism of Graves' disease is caused by TSI that are synthesized in the thyroid gland as well as in bone marrow and lymph nodes. Such antibodies can be detected by bioassays or using the more widely available TBII assays. The presence of TBII in a patient with thyrotoxicosis is strong indirect evidence for the existence of TSI, and these assays are useful in monitoring pregnant Graves' patients in whom high levels of TSI can cross the placenta and cause neonatal thyrotoxicosis. Other thyroid autoimmune responses, similar to those in autoimmune hypothyroidism (see above), occur concurrently in patients with Graves' disease. In particular, TPO antibodies occur in up to 80% of cases and serve as a readily measurable marker of autoimmunity. Because T cell–mediated cytotoxicity can also affect thyroid function, there is no direct correlation between the level of TSI and thyroid hormone levels. In the long term, spontaneous autoimmune hypothyroidism may develop in up to 15% of Graves' patients.

Cytokines appear to play a major role in thyroid-associated ophthalmopathy. There is infiltration of the extraocular muscles by activated T cells; the release of cytokines such as IFN-γ, TNF, and IL-1 results in fibroblast activation and increased synthesis of glycosaminoglycans that trap water, thereby leading to characteristic muscle swelling. Late in the disease, there is fibrosis and only then do the muscle cells show evidence of injury. Orbital fibroblasts may be uniquely sensitive to cytokines, perhaps explaining the anatomic localization of the immune response. Though the pathogenesis of thyroid-associated ophthalmopathy remains unclear, there is mounting evidence that expression of the TSH-R may provide an important orbital autoantigen. In support of this idea, injection of TSH-R into certain strains of mice induces autoimmune hyperthyroidism, as well as features of ophthalmopathy. A variety of autoantibodies against orbital muscle and fibroblast antigens have been detected in patients with ophthalmopathy, but these antibodies most likely arise as a secondary phenomenon, dependent on T cell–mediated autoimmune responses. Similar mechanisms are involved in dermopathy.

Clinical Manifestations Signs and symptoms include features that are common to any cause of thyrotoxicosis (Table 320-7) as well as those specific for Graves' disease. The clinical presentation depends on the severity of thyrotoxicosis, the duration of disease, individual susceptibility to excess thyroid hormone, and the patient's age. In the elderly, features of thyrotoxicosis may be subtle or masked, and patients may present mainly with fatigue and weight loss, leading to *apathetic hyperthyroidism*.

Thyrotoxicosis may cause unexplained weight loss, despite an enhanced appetite, due to the increased metabolic rate. Weight gain occurs in 5% of patients, however, because of increased food intake.

TABLE 320-6 *Causes of Thyrotoxicosis*

Primary hyperthyroidism
  Graves' disease
  Toxic multinodular goiter
  Toxic adenoma
  Functioning thyroid carcinoma metastases
  Activating mutation of the TSH receptor
  Activating mutation of $G_{s\alpha}$ (McCune-Albright syndrome)
  Struma ovarii
  Drugs: iodine excess (Jod-Basedow phenomenon)
Thyrotoxicosis without hyperthyroidism
  Subacute thyroiditis
  Silent thyroiditis
  Other causes of thyroid destruction: amiodarone, radiation, infarction of adenoma
  Ingestion of excess thyroid hormone (thyrotoxicosis factitia) or thyroid tissue
Secondary hyperthyroidism
  TSH-secreting pituitary adenoma
  Thyroid hormone resistance syndrome: occasional patients may have features of thyrotoxicosis
  Chorionic gonadotropin-secreting tumors[a]
  Gestational thyrotoxicosis[a]

[a] Circulating TSH levels are low in these forms of secondary hyperthyroidism.
Note: TSH, thyroid-stimulating hormone.

TABLE 320-7 *Signs and Symptoms of Thyrotoxicosis (Descending Order of Frequency)*

Symptoms	Signs[a]
Hyperactivity, irritability, dysphoria	Tachycardia; atrial fibrillation in the elderly
Heat intolerance and sweating	Tremor
Palpitations	Goiter
Fatigue and weakness	Warm, moist skin
Weight loss with increased appetite	Muscle weakness, proximal myopathy
Diarrhea	Lid retraction or lag
Polyuria	Gynecomastia
Oligomenorrhea, loss of libido	

[a] Excludes the signs of ophthalmopathy and dermopathy specific for Graves' disease.

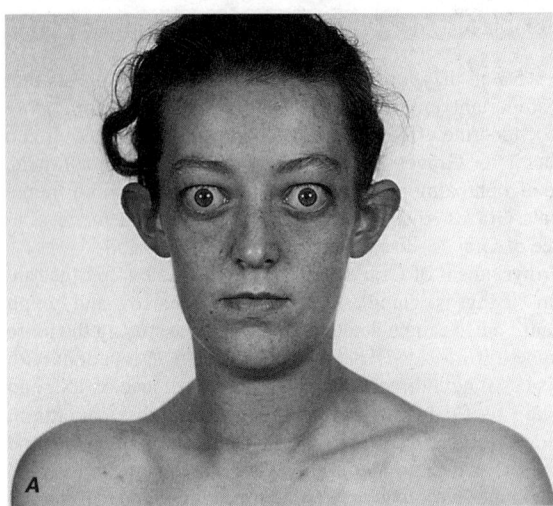

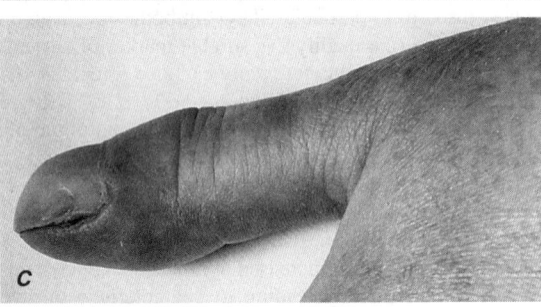

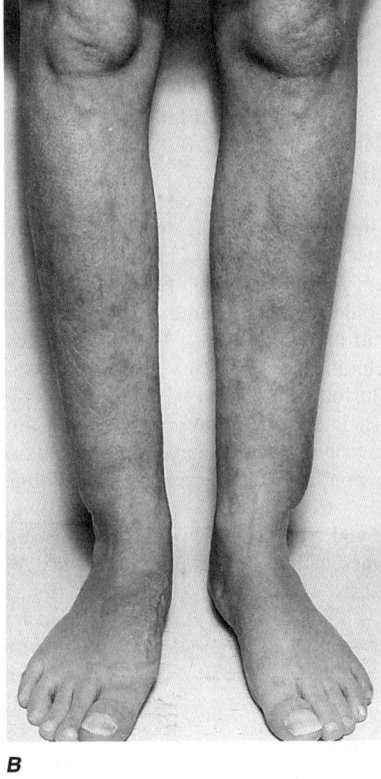

FIGURE 320-6 Features of Graves' disease. *A.* Facial appearance in Graves' disease; lid retraction, periorbital edema, and proptosis are marked. *B.* Thyroid dermopathy over the lateral aspects of the shins. *C.* Thyroid acropachy.

Other prominent features include hyperactivity, nervousness, and irritability, ultimately leading to a sense of easy fatiguability in some patients. Insomnia and impaired concentration are common; apathetic thyrotoxicosis may be mistaken for depression in the elderly. Fine tremor is a frequent finding, best elicited by having patients stretch out their fingers and feeling the fingertips with the palm. Common neurologic manifestations include hyperreflexia, muscle wasting, and proximal myopathy without fasciculation. Chorea is a rare feature. Thyrotoxicosis is sometimes associated with a form of hypokalemic periodic paralysis; this disorder is particularly common in Asian males with thyrotoxicosis.

The most common cardiovascular manifestation is sinus tachycardia, often associated with palpitations, occasionally caused by supraventricular tachycardia. The high cardiac output produces a bounding pulse, widened pulse pressure, and an aortic systolic murmur and can lead to worsening of angina or heart failure in the elderly or those with preexisting heart disease. Atrial fibrillation is more common in patients >50 years. Treatment of the thyrotoxic state alone reverts atrial fibrillation to normal sinus rhythm in fewer than half of patients, suggesting the existence of an underlying cardiac problem in the remainder.

The skin is usually warm and moist, and the patient may complain of sweating and heat intolerance, particularly during warm weather. Palmar erythema; onycholysis; and, less commonly, pruritus, urticaria, and diffuse hyperpigmentation may be evident. Hair texture may become fine, and a diffuse alopecia occurs in up to 40% of patients, persisting for months after restoration of euthyroidism. Gastrointestinal transit time is decreased, leading to increased stool frequency, often with diarrhea and occasionally mild steatorrhea. Women frequently experience oligomenorrhea or amenorrhea; in men there may be impaired sexual function and, rarely, gynecomastia. The direct effect of thyroid hormones on bone resorption leads to osteopenia in long-standing thyrotoxicosis; mild hypercalcemia occurs in up to 20% of patients, but hypercalciuria is more common. There is a small increase in fracture rate in patients with a previous history of thyrotoxicosis.

In Graves' disease the thyroid is usually diffusely enlarged to two to three times its normal size. The consistency is firm, but less so than in multinodular goiter. There may be a thrill or bruit due to the increased vascularity of the gland and the hyperdynamic circulation.

Lid retraction, causing a staring appearance, can occur in any form of thyrotoxicosis and is the result of sympathetic overactivity. However, Graves' disease is associated with specific eye signs that comprise *Graves' ophthalmopathy* (Fig. 320-6*A*). This condition is also called *thyroid-associated ophthalmopathy*, as it occurs in the absence of Graves' disease in 10% of patients. Most of these individuals have autoimmune hypothyroidism or thyroid antibodies. The onset of Graves' ophthalmopathy occurs within the year before or after the diagnosis of thyrotoxicosis in 75% of patients but can sometimes precede or follow thyrotoxicosis by several years, accounting for some cases of euthyroid ophthalmopathy.

Many patients with Graves' disease have little clinical evidence of ophthalmopathy. However, the enlarged extraocular muscles typical of the disease, and other subtle features, can be detected in almost all patients when investigated by ultrasound or computed tomography (CT) imaging of the orbits. Unilateral signs are found in up to 10% of patients. The earliest manifestations of ophthalmopathy are usually a sensation of grittiness, eye discomfort, and excess tearing. About a third of patients have proptosis, best detected by visualization of the sclera between the lower border of the iris and the lower eyelid, with the eyes in the primary position. Proptosis can be measured using an exophthalmometer. In severe cases, proptosis may cause corneal exposure and damage, especially if the lids fail to close during sleep. Periorbital edema, scleral injection, and chemosis are also frequent. In 5 to 10% of patients, the muscle swelling is so severe that diplopia results, typically but not exclusively when the patient looks up and laterally. The most serious manifestation is compression of the optic nerve at the apex of the orbit, leading to papilledema, peripheral field defects, and, if left untreated, permanent loss of vision.

Many scoring systems have been used to gauge the extent and activity of the orbital changes in Graves' disease. The "NO SPECS" scheme is an acronym derived from the following classes of eye change:

0 = No signs or symptoms
1 = Only signs (lid retraction or lag), no symptoms
2 = Soft tissue involvement (periorbital edema)
3 = Proptosis (>22 mm)
4 = Extraocular muscle involvement (diplopia)
5 = Corneal involvement
6 = Sight loss

Although useful as a mnemonic, the NO SPECS scheme is inadequate to describe the eye disease fully, and patients do not necessarily progress from one class to another. When Graves' eye disease is active and severe, referral to an ophthalmologist is indicated and objective measurements are needed, such as lid fissure width; corneal staining with fluorescein; and evaluation of extraocular muscle function (e.g., Hess chart), intraocular pressure and visual fields, acuity, and color vision.

Thyroid dermopathy occurs in <5% of patients with Graves' disease (Fig. 320-6*B*), almost always in the presence of moderate or severe ophthalmopathy. Although most frequent over the anterior and lateral aspects of the lower leg (hence the term *pretibial myxedema*), skin changes can occur at other sites, particularly after trauma. The typical lesion is a noninflamed, indurated plaque with a deep pink or purple color and an "orange-skin" appearance. Nodular involvement can occur, and the condition can rarely extend over the whole lower leg and foot, mimicking elephantiasis. *Thyroid acropachy* refers to a form of clubbing found in <1% of patients with Graves' disease (Fig. 320-6*C*). It is so strongly associated with thyroid dermopathy that an alternative cause of clubbing should be sought in a Graves' patient without coincident skin and orbital involvement.

Laboratory Evaluation Investigations used to determine the existence and cause of thyrotoxicosis are summarized in Fig. 320-7. In Graves' disease, the TSH level is suppressed and total and unbound thyroid hormone levels are increased. In 2 to 5% of patients (and more in areas of borderline iodine intake), only T_3 is increased (T_3 toxicosis). The converse state of T_4 toxicosis, with elevated total and unbound T_4 and normal T_3 levels, is occasionally seen when hyperthyroidism is induced by excess iodine, providing surplus substrate for thyroid hormone synthesis. Measurement of TPO antibodies is useful in differential diagnosis. Measurement of TBII or TSI will confirm the diagnosis but is not needed routinely. Associated abnormalities that may cause diagnostic confusion in thyrotoxicosis include elevation of bilirubin, liver enzymes, and ferritin. Microcytic anemia and thrombocytopenia may occur.

Differential Diagnosis Diagnosis of Graves' disease is straightforward in a patient with biochemically confirmed thyrotoxicosis, diffuse goiter on palpation, ophthalmopathy, positive TPO antibodies, and often a personal or family history of autoimmune disorders. For patients with thyrotoxicosis who lack these features, the most reliable diagnostic method is a radionuclide (^{99m}Tc, ^{123}I, or ^{131}I) scan of the thyroid, which will distinguish the diffuse, high uptake of Graves' disease from nodular thyroid disease, destructive thyroiditis, ectopic thyroid tissue, and factitious thyrotoxicosis. In secondary hyperthyroidism due to a TSH-secreting pituitary tumor, there is also a diffuse goiter. The presence of a nonsuppressed TSH level and the finding of a pituitary tumor on CT or magnetic resonance imaging (MRI) scan readily identify such patients.

Clinical features of thyrotoxicosis can mimic certain aspects of other disorders including panic attacks, mania, pheochromocytoma, and the weight loss associated with malignancy. The diagnosis of thyrotoxicosis can be easily excluded if the TSH and T_3 levels are normal. A normal TSH also excludes Graves' disease as a cause of diffuse goiter.

Clinical Course Clinical features generally worsen without treatment; mortality was 10 to 30% before the introduction of satisfactory therapy. Some patients with mild Graves' disease experience spontaneous relapses and remissions. Rarely, there may be fluctuation between hypo- and hyperthyroidism due to changes in the functional activity of TSH-R antibodies. About 15% of patients who enter remission after treatment with antithyroid drugs develop hypothyroidism 10 to 15 years later as a result of the destructive autoimmune process. The

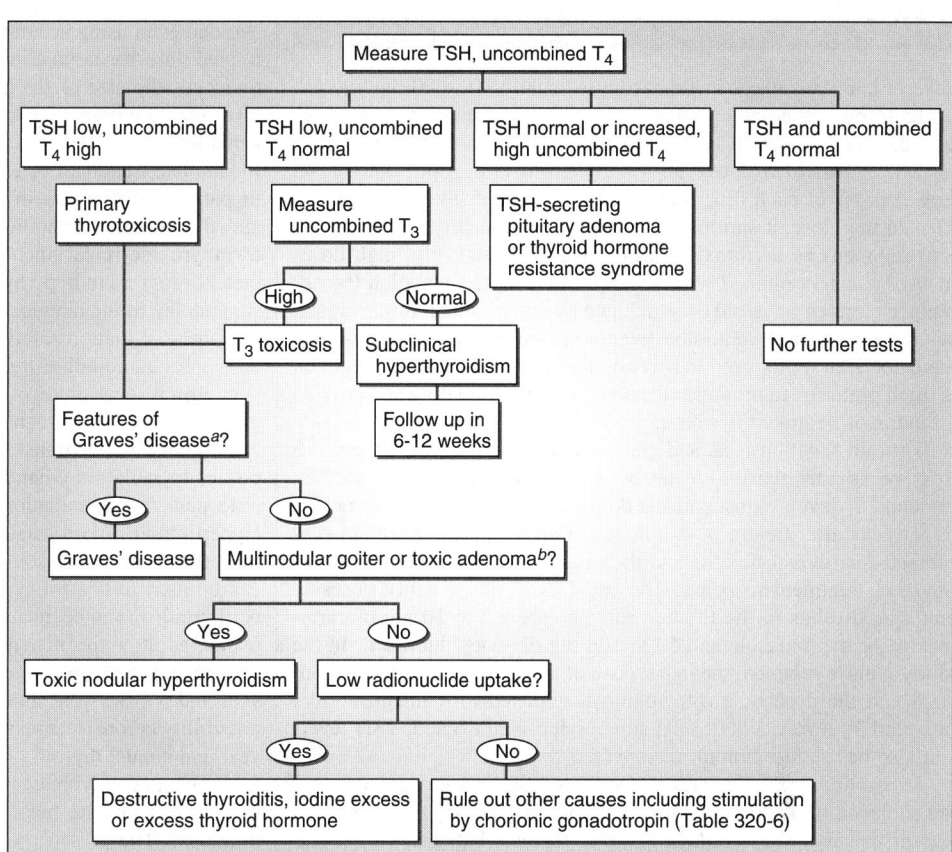

FIGURE 320-7 Evaluation of thyrotoxicosis. [a]Diffuse goiter, positive TPO antibodies, ophthalmopathy, dermopathy; [b]can be confirmed by radionuclide scan. TSH, thyroid-stimulating hormone.

clinical course of ophthalmopathy does not follow that of the thyroid disease. Ophthalmopathy typically worsens over the initial 3 to 6 months, followed by a plateau phase over the next 12 to 18 months, with spontaneous improvement, particularly in the soft tissue changes. However, the course is more fulminant in up to 5% of patients, requiring intervention in the acute phase if there is optic nerve compression or corneal ulceration. Diplopia may appear late in the disease due to fibrosis of the extraocular muscles. Some studies suggest that radioiodine treatment for hyperthyroidism worsens the eye disease in a small proportion of patients (especially smokers). Antithyroid drugs or surgery have no adverse effects on the clinical course of ophthalmopathy. Thyroid dermopathy, when it occurs, usually appears 1 to 2 years after the development of Graves' hyperthyroidism; it may improve spontaneously.

TREATMENT

The *hyperthyroidism* of Graves' disease is treated by reducing thyroid hormone synthesis, using antithyroid drugs, or by reducing the amount of thyroid tissue with radioiodine (^{131}I) treatment or by subtotal thyroidectomy. Antithyroid drugs are the predominant therapy in many centers in Europe and Japan, whereas radioiodine is more often the first line of treatment in North America. These differences reflect the fact that no single approach is optimal and that patients may require multiple treatments to achieve remission.

The main *antithyroid drugs* are the thionamides, such as propylthiouracil, carbimazole, and the active metabolite of the latter, methimazole. All inhibit the function of TPO, reducing oxidation and organification of iodide. These drugs also reduce thyroid antibody levels by mechanisms that remain unclear, and they appear to enhance rates of remission. Propylthiouracil inhibits deiodination of $T_4 \rightarrow T_3$. However, this effect is of minor benefit, except in the most severe thyrotoxicosis, and is offset by the much shorter half-life of this drug (90 min) compared to methimazole (6 h).

There are many variations of antithyroid drug regimens. The initial dose of carbimazole or methimazole is usually 10 to 20 mg every 8 or 12 h, but once-daily dosing is possible after euthyroidism is restored. Propylthiouracil is given at a dose of 100 to 200 mg every 6 to 8 h, and divided doses are usually given throughout the course. Lower doses of each drug may suffice in areas of low iodine intake. The starting dose of antithyroid drugs can be gradually reduced (titration regimen) as thyrotoxicosis improves. Alternatively, high doses may be given combined with levothyroxine supplementation (block-replace regimen) to avoid drug-induced hypothyroidism. Initial reports suggesting superior remission rates with the block-replace regimen have not been reproduced in several other trials. The titration regimen is often preferred to minimize the dose of antithyroid drug and provide an index of treatment response.

Thyroid function tests and clinical manifestations are reviewed 3 to 4 weeks after starting treatment, and the dose is titrated based on unbound T_4 levels. Most patients do not achieve euthyroidism until 6 to 8 weeks after treatment is initiated. TSH levels often remain suppressed for several months and therefore do not provide a sensitive index of treatment response. The usual daily maintenance doses of antithyroid drugs in the titration regimen are 2.5 to 10 mg of carbimazole or methimazole and 50 to 100 mg of propylthiouracil. In the block-replace regimen, the initial dose of antithyroid drug is held constant and the dose of levothyroxine is adjusted to maintain normal unbound T_4 levels. When TSH suppression is alleviated, TSH levels can also be used to monitor therapy.

Maximum remission rates (up to 30 to 50% in some populations) are achieved by 18 to 24 months. For unclear reasons, remission rates appear to vary in different geographic regions. Patients with severe hyperthyroidism and large goiters are most likely to relapse when treatment stops, but outcome is difficult to predict. All patients should be followed closely for relapse during the first year after treatment and at least annually thereafter.

The common side effects of antithyroid drugs are rash, urticaria, fever, and arthralgia (1 to 5% of patients). These may resolve spontaneously or after substituting an alternative antithyroid drug. Rare but major side effects include hepatitis, an SLE-like syndrome, and, most importantly, agranulocytosis (<1%). It is essential that antithyroid drugs are stopped and not restarted if a patient develops major side effects. Written instructions should be provided regarding the symptoms of possible agranulocytosis (e.g., sore throat, fever, mouth ulcers) and the need to stop treatment pending a complete blood count to confirm that agranulocytosis is not present. Management of agranulocytosis is described in Chap. 94. It is not useful to monitor blood counts prospectively, as the onset of agranulocytosis is idiosyncratic and abrupt.

Propranolol (20 to 40 mg every 6 h) or longer acting beta blockers, such as atenolol, may be helpful to control adrenergic symptoms, especially in the early stages before antithyroid drugs take effect. The need for anticoagulation with warfarin should be considered in all patients with atrial fibrillation. If digoxin is used, increased doses are often needed in the thyrotoxic state.

Radioiodine causes progressive destruction of thyroid cells and can be used as initial treatment or for relapses after a trial of antithyroid drugs. There is a small risk of thyrotoxic crisis (see below) after radioiodine, which can be minimized by pretreatment with antithyroid drugs for at least a month before treatment. Antecedent treatment with antithyroid drugs should be considered for all elderly patients or for those with cardiac problems, to deplete thyroid hormone stores before administration of radioiodine. Antithyroid drugs must be stopped at least 3 days before radioiodine administration to achieve optimum iodine uptake.

Efforts to calculate an optimal dose of radioiodine that achieves euthyroidism, without a high incidence of relapse or progression to hypothyroidism, have not been successful. Some patients inevitably relapse after a single dose because the biologic effects of radiation vary between individuals, and hypothyroidism cannot be uniformly avoided even using accurate dosimetry. A practical strategy is to give a fixed dose based on clinical features, such as the severity of thyrotoxicosis, the size of the goiter (increases the dose needed), and the level of radioiodine uptake (decreases the dose needed). ^{131}I dosage generally ranges between 185 MBq (5 mCi) to 555 MBq (15 mCi). Incomplete treatment or early relapse is more common in males and in patients <40 years of age. Many authorities favor an approach aimed at thyroid ablation (as opposed to euthyroidism), given that levothyroxine replacement is straightforward and most patients ultimately progress to hypothyroidism over 5 to 10 years, frequently with some delay in the diagnosis of hypothyroidism.

Certain radiation safety precautions are necessary in the first few days after radioiodine treatment, but the exact guidelines vary depending on local protocols. In general, patients need to avoid close, prolonged contact with children and pregnant women for several days because of possible transmission of residual isotope and excessive exposure to radiation emanating from the gland. Rarely there may be mild pain due to radiation thyroiditis 1 to 2 weeks after treatment. Hyperthyroidism can persist for 2 to 3 months before radioiodine takes full effect. For this reason, β-adrenergic blockers or antithyroid drugs can be used to control symptoms during this interval. Persistent hyperthyroidism can be treated with a second dose of radioiodine, usually 6 months after the first dose. The risk of hypothyroidism after radioiodine depends on the dosage but is at least 10 to 20% in the first year and 5% per year thereafter. Patients should be informed of this possibility before treatment and require close follow-up during the first year and annual thyroid function testing.

Pregnancy and breast feeding are absolute contraindications to radioiodine treatment, but patients can conceive safely 6 months after treatment. The presence of severe ophthalmopathy requires caution, and some authorities advocate the use of prednisone, 40 mg/d, at the time of radioiodine treatment, tapered over 2 to 3 months to prevent exacerbation of ophthalmopathy. The overall risk of cancer after radioiodine treatment in adults is not increased, but many physicians avoid radioiodine in children and adolescents because of the theoretical risks of malignancy.

Subtotal thyroidectomy is an option for patients who relapse after antithyroid drugs and prefer this treatment to radioiodine. Some experts recommend surgery in young individuals, particularly when the goiter is very large. Careful control of thyrotoxicosis with antithyroid drugs, followed by potassium iodide (3 drops SSKI orally tid), is needed prior to surgery to avoid thyrotoxic crisis and to reduce the vascularity of the gland. The major complications of surgery—i.e., bleeding, laryngeal edema, hypoparathyroidism, and damage to the recurrent laryngeal nerves—are unusual when the procedure is performed by highly experienced surgeons. Recurrence rates in the best series are <2%, but the rate of hypothyroidism is only slightly less than that following radioiodine treatment.

The titration regimen of antithyroid drugs should be used to manage Graves' disease in *pregnancy*, as blocking doses of these drugs produce fetal hypothyroidism. Propylthiouracil is usually used because of relatively low transplacental transfer and its ability to block $T_4 \rightarrow T_3$ conversion. Also, carbimazole and methimazole have been associated with rare cases of fetal *aplasia cutis* and other defects, such as choanal atresia. The lowest effective dose of propylthiouracil should be given, and it is often possible to stop treatment in the last trimester since TSH-R antibodies tend to decline in pregnancy. Nonetheless, the transplacental transfer of these antibodies rarely causes *fetal thyrotoxicosis* or *neonatal thyrotoxicosis*. Poor intrauterine growth, a fetal heart rate of >160 beats/min, and high levels of maternal TSH-R antibodies in the last trimester may herald this complication. Antithyroid drugs given to the mother can be used to treat the fetus and may be needed for 1 to 3 months after delivery, until the maternal antibodies disappear from the baby's circulation. The postpartum period is a time of major risk for relapse of Graves' disease. Breast feeding is safe with low doses of antithyroid drugs. Graves' disease in *children* is best managed with antithyroid drugs, often given as a prolonged course of the titration regimen. Surgery may be indicated for severe disease. Radioiodine can also be used in children, although most experts defer this treatment until adolescence or later.

Thyrotoxic crisis, or *thyroid storm*, is rare and presents as a life-threatening exacerbation of hyperthyroidism, accompanied by fever, delirium, seizures, coma, vomiting, diarrhea, and jaundice. The mortality rate due to cardiac failure, arrhythmia, or hyperthermia is as high as 30%, even with treatment. Thyrotoxic crisis is usually precipitated by acute illness (e.g., stroke, infection, trauma, diabetic ketoacidosis), surgery (especially on the thyroid), or radioiodine treatment of a patient with partially treated or untreated hyperthyroidism. Management requires intensive monitoring and supportive care, identification and treatment of the precipitating cause, and measures that reduce thyroid hormone synthesis. Large doses of propylthiouracil (600-mg loading dose and 200 to 300 mg every 6 h) should be given orally or by nasogastric tube or per rectum; the drug's inhibitory action on $T_4 \rightarrow T_3$ conversion makes it the antithyroid drug of choice. One hour after the first dose of propylthiouracil, stable iodide is given to block thyroid hormone synthesis via the Wolff-Chaikoff effect (the delay allows the antithyroid drug to prevent the excess iodine from being incorporated into new hormone). A saturated solution of potassium iodide (5 drops SSKI every 6 h), or ipodate or iopanoic acid (0.5 mg every 12 h), may be given orally. (Sodium iodide, 0.25 g intravenously every 6 h is an alternative but is not generally available.) Propranolol should also be given to reduce tachycardia and other adrenergic manifestations (40 to 60 mg orally every 4 h; or 2 mg intravenously every 4 h). Although other β-adrenergic blockers can be used, high doses of propranolol decrease $T_4 \rightarrow T_3$ conversion, and the doses can be easily adjusted. Caution is needed to avoid acute negative inotropic effects, but controlling the heart rate is important, as some patients develop a form of high-output heart failure. Additional therapeutic measures include glucocorticoids (e.g., dexamethasone, 2 mg every 6 h), antibiotics if infection is present, cooling, oxygen, and intravenous fluids.

Ophthalmopathy requires no active treatment when it is mild or moderate, as there is usually spontaneous improvement. General measures include meticulous control of thyroid hormone levels, advice about cessation of smoking, and an explanation of the natural history of ophthalmopathy. Discomfort can be relieved with artificial tears (e.g., 1% methylcellulose) and the use of dark glasses with side frames. Periorbital edema may respond to a more upright sleeping position or a diuretic. Corneal exposure during sleep can be avoided by taping the eyelids shut. Minor degrees of diplopia improve with prisms fitted to spectacles. Severe ophthalmopathy, with optic nerve involvement or chemosis resulting in corneal damage, is an emergency requiring joint management with an ophthalmologist. Short-term benefit can be gained in about two-thirds of patients by the use of high-dose glucocorticoids (e.g., prednisone, 40 to 80 mg daily), sometimes combined with cyclosporine. Glucocorticoid doses are tapered by 5 mg every 1 to 2 weeks, but the taper often results in reemergence of congestive symptoms. Pulse therapy with intravenous methylprednisolone (1 g of methylprednisolone in 250 mL of saline infused over 2 h daily for 1 week) followed by an oral regimen is also used. Once the eye disease has stabilized, surgery may be indicated for relief of diplopia and correction of the appearance of the eyes. Orbital decompression can be achieved by removing bone from any wall of the orbit, thereby allowing displacement of fat and swollen extraocular muscles. The transantral route is used most often, as it requires no external incision. Proptosis recedes an average of 5 mm, but there may be residual or even worsened diplopia. Alternatively, retrobulbar tissue can be decompressed without the removal of bony tissue. External beam radiotherapy of the orbits has been used for many years, especially for ophthalmopathy of recent onset, but the objective evidence that this therapy is beneficial remains equivocal.

Thyroid dermopathy does not usually require treatment but can cause cosmetic problems or interfere with the fit of shoes. Surgical removal is not indicated. If necessary, treatment consists of topical, high-potency glucocorticoid ointment under an occlusive dressing. Octreotide may be beneficial.

OTHER CAUSES OF THYROTOXICOSIS Destructive thyroiditis (subacute or silent thyroiditis) typically presents with a short thyrotoxic phase due to the release of preformed thyroid hormones and catabolism of Tg (see "Subacute Thyroiditis," below). True hyperthyroidism is absent, as demonstrated by a low radionuclide uptake. Circulating Tg and IL-6 levels are usually increased. Other causes of thyrotoxicosis with low or absent thyroid radionuclide uptake include *thyrotoxicosis factitia*; iodine excess and, rarely, ectopic thyroid tissue, particularly teratomas of the ovary (*struma ovarii*); and functional metastatic follicular carcinoma. Whole-body radionuclide studies can demonstrate ectopic thyroid tissue, and thyrotoxicosis factitia can be distinguished from destructive thyroiditis by the clinical features and low levels of Tg. Amiodarone treatment is associated with thyrotoxicosis in up to 10% of patients, particularly in areas of low iodine intake.

TSH-secreting pituitary adenoma is a rare causes of thyrotoxicosis. It can be identified by the presence of an inappropriately normal or increased TSH level in a patient with hyperthyroidism, diffuse goiter, and elevated T_4 and T_3 levels (Chap. 318). Elevated levels of the α subunit of TSH, released by the TSH-secreting adenoma, support this diagnosis, which can be confirmed by demonstrating the pituitary tumor on CT or MRI scan. A combination of transsphenoidal surgery, sella irradiation, and octreotide may be required to normalize TSH, as many of these tumors are large and locally invasive at the time of diagnosis. Radioiodine or antithyroid drugs can be used to control thyrotoxicosis.

Thyrotoxicosis caused by *toxic multinodular goiter* and *hyperfunctioning solitary nodules* is discussed below.

THYROIDITIS

A clinically useful classification of thyroiditis is based on the onset and duration of disease (Table 320-8).

ACUTE THYROIDITIS Acute thyroiditis is rare and due to suppurative infection of the thyroid. In children and young adults, the most common cause is the presence of a piriform sinus, a remnant of the fourth branchial pouch that connects the oropharynx with the thyroid. Such sinuses are predominantly left sided. A long-standing goiter and degeneration in a thyroid malignancy are risk factors in the elderly. The patient presents with thyroid pain, often referred to the throat or ears, and a small, tender goiter that may be asymmetric. Fever, dysphagia, and erythema over the thyroid are common, as are systemic symptoms of a febrile illness and lymphadenopathy.

The differential diagnosis of *thyroid pain* includes subacute or, rarely, chronic thyroiditis, hemorrhage into a cyst, malignancy including lymphoma, and, rarely, amiodarone-induced thyroiditis or amyloidosis. However, the abrupt presentation and clinical features of acute thyroiditis rarely cause confusion. The erythrocyte sedimentation rate (ESR) and white cell count are usually increased, but thyroid

TABLE 320-8 *Causes of Thyroiditis*

Acute
   Bacterial infection: especially *Staphylcoccus*, *Streptococcus*, and *Enterobacter*
   Fungal infection: *Aspergillus*, *Candida*, *Coccidioides*, *Histoplasma*, and *Pneumocystis*
   Radiation thyroiditis after ^{131}I treatment
   Amiodarone (may also be subacute or chronic)
Subacute
   Viral (or granulomatous) thyroiditis
   Silent thyroiditis (including postpartum thyroiditis)
   Mycobacterial infection
Chronic
   Autoimmunity: focal thyroiditis, Hashimoto's thyroiditis, atrophic thyroiditis
   Riedel's thyroiditis
   Parasitic thyroiditis: echinococcosis, strongyloidiasis, cysticercosis
   Traumatic: after palpation

function is normal. FNA biopsy shows infiltration by polymorpho-nuclear leukocytes; culture of the sample can identify the organism. Caution is needed in immunocompromised patients as fungal, myco-bacterial, or *Pneumocystis* thyroiditis can occur in this setting. Anti-biotic treatment is guided initially by Gram stain and subsequently by cultures of the FNA biopsy. Surgery may be needed to drain an ab-scess, which can be localized by CT scan or ultrasound. Tracheal ob-struction, septicemia, retropharyngeal abscess, mediastinitis, and jug-ular venous thrombosis may complicate acute thyroiditis but are uncommon with prompt use of antibiotics.

SUBACUTE THYROIDITIS   This is also termed *de Quervain's thyroiditis*, *granulomatous thyroiditis*, or *viral thyroiditis*. Many viruses have been implicated, including mumps, coxsackie, influenza, adenoviruses, and echoviruses, but attempts to identify the virus in an individual patient are often unsuccessful and do not influence management. The diag-nosis of subacute thyroiditis is often overlooked because the symptoms can mimic pharyngitis. The peak incidence occurs at 30 to 50 years, and women are affected three times more frequently than men.

Pathophysiology   The thyroid shows a characteristic patchy inflamma-tory infiltrate with disruption of the thyroid follicles and multinucle-ated giant cells within some follicles. The follicular changes progress to granulomas accompanied by fibrosis. Finally, the thyroid returns to normal, usually several months after onset. During the initial phase of follicular destruction, there is release of Tg and thyroid hormones, leading to increased circulating T_4 and T_3 and suppression of TSH (Fig. 320-8). During this destructive phase, radioactive iodine uptake is low or undetectable. After several weeks, the thyroid is depleted of stored thyroid hormone and a phase of hypothyroidism typically oc-curs, with low unbound T_4 (and sometimes T_3) and moderately in-creased TSH levels. Radioactive iodine uptake returns to normal or is even increased as a result of the rise in TSH. Finally, thyroid hormone and TSH levels return to normal as the disease subsides.

Clinical Manifestations   The patient usually presents with a painful and enlarged thyroid, sometimes accompanied by fever. There may be fea-tures of thyrotoxicosis or hypothyroidism, depending on the phase of the illness. Malaise and symptoms of an upper respiratory tract infec-tion may precede the thyroid-related features by several weeks. In other patients, the onset is acute, severe, and without obvious ante-cedent. The patient typically complains of a sore throat, and exami-nation reveals a small goiter that is exquisitely tender. Pain is often referred to the jaw or ear. Complete resolution is the usual outcome, but permanent hypothyroidism can occur, particularly in those with coincidental thyroid autoimmunity. A prolonged course over many months, with one or more relapses, occurs in a small percentage of patients.

Laboratory Evaluation   As depicted in Fig. 320-8, thyroid function tests characteristically evolve through three distinct phases over about 6 months: (1) thyrotoxic phase, (2) hypothyroid phase, and (3) recovery phase. In the thyrotoxic phase, T_4 and T_3 levels are increased, reflecting their discharge from the damaged thyroid cells, and TSH is suppressed. The T_4/T_3 ratio is greater than in Graves' disease or thyroid autonomy, in which T_3 is often disproportionately increased. The diagnosis is confirmed by a high ESR and low radioiodine uptake. Serum IL-6 levels increase during the thyrotoxic phase. The white blood cell count may be increased, and thyroid antibodies are negative. If the diagnosis is in doubt, FNA biopsy may be useful, particularly to distinguish unilateral involvement from bleeding into a cyst or neoplasm.

℞ **TREATMENT**

Relatively large doses of aspirin (e.g., 600 mg every 4 to 6 h) or nonsteroidal anti-inflammatory drugs are sufficient to control symp-toms in most cases. If this treatment is inadequate, or if the patient has marked local or systemic symptoms, glucocorticoids should be given. The usual starting dose is 40 to 60 mg prednisone, depending on se-verity. The dose is gradually tapered over 6 to 8 weeks, in response to improvement in symptoms and the ESR. If a relapse occurs during glucocorticoid withdrawal, treatment should be started again and with-drawn more gradually. In these patients, it is useful to wait until the radioactive iodine uptake normalizes before stopping treatment. Thy-roid function should be monitored every 2 to 4 weeks using TSH and unbound T_4 levels. Symptoms of thyrotoxicosis improve spontane-ously but may be ameliorated by β-adrenergic blockers; antithyroid drugs play no role in treatment of the thyrotoxic phase. Levothyroxine replacement may be needed if the hypothyroid phase is prolonged, but doses should be low enough (50 to 100 μg daily) to allow TSH-me-diated recovery.

SILENT THYROIDITIS   *Painless thyroiditis*, or *"silent" thyroiditis*, occurs in patients with underlying autoimmune thyroid disease. It has a clin-ical course similar to that of subacute thyroiditis, except that there is little or no thyroid tenderness. The condition occurs in up to 5% of women 3 to 6 months after pregnancy and is then termed *postpartum thyroiditis*. Typically, patients have a brief phase of thyrotoxicosis, lasting 2 to 4 weeks, followed by hypothyroidism for 4 to 12 weeks, and then resolution; often, however, only one phase is apparent. The condition is associated with the presence of TPO antibodies antepar-tum, and is three times more common in women with type 1 diabetes mellitus. As in subacute thyroiditis, the radioactive iodine uptake is initially suppressed. In addition to the painless goiter, silent thyroiditis can be distinguished from subacute thyroiditis by the normal ESR and the presence of TPO antibodies. Glucocorticoid treatment is not in-dicated for silent thyroiditis. Severe thyrotoxic symptoms can be man-aged with a brief course of propranolol, 20 to 40 mg three or four times daily. Thyroxine replacement may be needed for the hypothyroid phase but should be withdrawn after 6 to 9 months, as recovery is the rule. Annual follow-up thereafter is recommended, as a proportion of these individuals develop permanent hypothyroidism.

DRUG-INDUCED THYROIDITIS   Patients receiving IFN-α, IL-2, or amio-darone may develop painless thyroiditis. IFN-α, which is used to treat chronic hepatitis B or C, causes thyroid dysfunction in up to 5% of treated patients. It has been associated with painless thyroiditis, hy-pothyroidism, and Graves' disease. IL-2, which has been used to treat various malignancies, has also been associated with thyroiditis and hypothyroidism, though fewer patients have been studied. For discus-sion of amiodarone, see "Amiodarone Effects on Thyroid Function," below.

CHRONIC THYROIDITIS   Focal thyroiditis is present in 20 to 40% of eu-thyroid autopsy cases and is associated with serologic evidence of

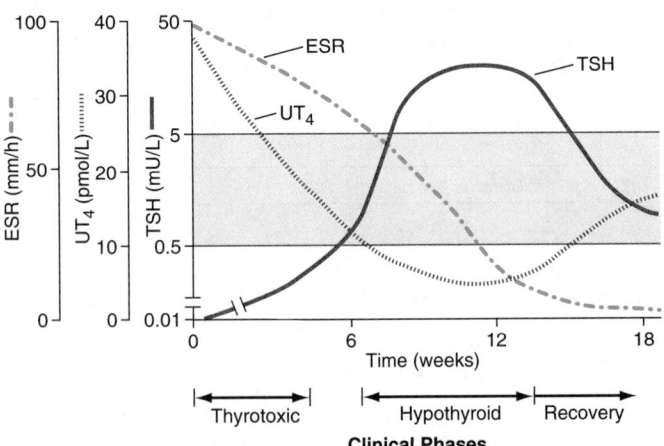

FIGURE 320-8 Clinical course of subacute thyroiditis. The release of thyroid hor-mones is initially associated with a thyrotoxic phase and suppressed thyroid-stimulating hormone (TSH). A hypothyroid phase then ensues, with low T_4 and TSH levels that are initially low but gradually increase. During the recovery phase, increased TSH levels combined with resolution of thyroid follicular injury leads to normalization of thyroid function, often several months after the beginning of the illness. ESR, erythrocyte sedimentation rate; UT_4, unbound T_4.

autoimmunity, particularly the presence of TPO antibodies. These antibodies are 4 to 10 times more common in otherwise healthy women than men. The most common clinically apparent cause of chronic thyroiditis is *Hashimoto's thyroiditis*, an autoimmune disorder that often presents as a firm or hard goiter of variable size (see above). *Riedel's thyroiditis* is a rare disorder that typically occurs in middle-aged women. It presents with an insidious, painless goiter with local symptoms due to compression of the esophagus, trachea, neck veins, or recurrent laryngeal nerves. Dense fibrosis disrupts normal gland architecture and can extend outside the thyroid capsule. Despite these extensive histologic changes, thyroid dysfunction is uncommon. The goiter is hard, nontender, often asymmetric and fixed, leading to suspicion of a malignancy. Diagnosis requires open biopsy as FNA biopsy is usually inadequate. Treatment is directed to surgical relief of compressive symptoms. Tamoxifen may also be beneficial. There is an association between Riedel's thyroiditis and idiopathic fibrosis at other sites (retroperitoneum, mediastinum, biliary tree, lung, and orbit).

SICK EUTHYROID SYNDROME

Any acute, severe illness can cause abnormalities of circulating TSH or thyroid hormone levels in the absence of underlying thyroid disease, making these measurements potentially misleading. The major cause of these hormonal changes is the release of cytokines. Unless a thyroid disorder is strongly suspected, the routine testing of thyroid function should be avoided in acutely ill patients.

The most common hormone pattern in sick euthyroid syndrome (SES) is a decrease in total and unbound T_3 levels (low T_3 syndrome) with normal levels of T_4 and TSH. The magnitude of the fall in T_3 correlates with the severity of the illness. T_4 conversion to T_3 via peripheral deiodination is impaired, leading to increased reverse T_3 (rT_3). Despite this effect, decreased clearance rather than increased production is the major basis for increased rT_3. Also, T_4 is alternately metabolized to the hormonally inactive T_3 sulfate. It is generally assumed that this low T_3 state is adaptive, as it can be induced in normal individuals by fasting. Teleologically, the fall in T_3 may limit catabolism in starved or ill patients.

Very sick patients may exhibit a dramatic fall in total T_4 and T_3 levels (low T_4 syndrome). This state has a poor prognosis. A key factor in the fall in T_4 levels is altered binding to TBG. T_4 assays usually demonstrate a normal unbound T_4 level in such patients, depending on the assay method used. Fluctuation in TSH levels also creates challenges in the interpretation of thyroid function in sick patients. TSH levels may range from <0.1 to >20 mU/L; these alterations reverse after recovery, confirming the absence of underlying thyroid disease. A rise in cortisol or administration of glucocorticoids may provide a partial explanation for decreased TSH levels. However, the exact mechanisms underlying the subnormal TSH seen in 10% of sick patients and the increased TSH seen in 5% remain unclear.

Any severe illness can induce changes in thyroid hormone levels, but certain disorders exhibit a distinctive pattern of abnormalities. Acute liver disease is associated with an initial rise in total (but not unbound) T_3 and T_4 levels, due to TBG release; these levels become subnormal with progression to liver failure. A transient increase in total and unbound T_4 levels, usually with a normal T_3 level, is seen in 5 to 30% of acutely ill psychiatric patients. TSH values may be transiently low, normal, or high in these patients. In the early stage of HIV infection, T_3 and T_4 levels rise, even if there is weight loss. T_3 levels fall with progression to AIDS, but TSH usually remains normal. Renal disease is often accompanied by low T_3 concentrations, but with normal rather than increased rT_3 levels, due to an unknown factor that increases uptake of rT_3 into the liver.

The diagnosis of SES is challenging. Historic information may be limited, and patients often have multiple metabolic derangements. Useful features to consider include previous history of thyroid disease and thyroid function tests, evaluation of the severity and time course of the patient's acute illness, documentation of medications that may affect thyroid function or thyroid hormone levels, and measurements

of rT_3 together with unbound thyroid hormones and TSH. The diagnosis of SES is frequently presumptive, given the clinical context and pattern of laboratory values; only resolution of the test results with clinical recovery can clearly establish this disorder. Treatment of SES with thyroid hormone (T_4 and/or T_3) is controversial, but most authorities recommend monitoring the patient's thyroid function tests during recovery, without administering thyroid hormone, unless there is historic or clinical evidence suggestive of hypothyroidism. Sufficiently large randomized controlled trials using thyroid hormone are unlikely to resolve this therapeutic controversy in the near future, because clinical presentations and outcomes are highly variable.

AMIODARONE EFFECTS ON THYROID FUNCTION

Amiodarone is a commonly used type III antiarrhythmic agent (Chap. 214). It is structurally related to thyroid hormone and contains 39% iodine by weight. Thus, typical doses of amiodarone (200 mg/d) are associated with very high iodine intake, leading to >40-fold increases in plasma and urinary iodine levels. Moreover, because amiodarone is stored in adipose tissue, high iodine levels persist for >6 months after discontinuation of the drug. Amiodarone inhibits deiodinase activity, and its metabolites function as weak antagonists of thyroid hormone action. Amiodarone has the following effects on thyroid function: (1) acute, transient suppression of thyroid function; (2) hypothyroidism in patients susceptible to the inhibitory effects of a high iodine load; and (3) thyrotoxicosis that may be caused by at least three mechanisms—a Jod-Basedow effect from the iodine load in the setting of multinodular goiter, a thyroiditis-like condition, and possibly induction of autoimmune Graves' disease.

The initiation of amiodarone treatment is associated with a transient decrease of T_4 levels, reflecting the inhibitory effect of iodine on T_4 release. Soon thereafter, most individuals escape from iodide-dependent suppression of the thyroid (Wolff-Chaikoff effect), and the inhibitory effects on deiodinase activity and thyroid hormone receptor action become predominant. These events lead to the following pattern of thyroid function tests: increased T_4, decreased T_3, increased rT_3, and a transient increase of TSH (up to 20 mU/L). TSH levels normalize or are slightly suppressed by 1 to 3 months.

The incidence of hypothyroidism from amiodarone varies geographically, apparently correlating with iodine intake. Hypothyroidism occurs in up to 13% of amiodarone-treated patients in iodine-replete countries, such as the United States, but is less common (<6% incidence) in areas of lower iodine intake, such as Italy or Spain. The pathogenesis appears to involve an inability of the thyroid to escape from the high iodine load. Consequently, amiodarone-associated hypothyroidism is more common in women and individuals with positive TPO antibodies. It is usually unnecessary to discontinue amiodarone for this side effect, as levothyroxine can be used to normalize thyroid function. TSH levels should be monitored, because T_4 levels are often increased for the reasons described above.

The management of amiodarone-induced thyrotoxicosis (AIT) is complicated by the fact that there are several causes of thyrotoxicosis and because the increased thyroid hormone levels exacerbate underlying arrhythmias and coronary artery disease. Amiodarone treatment causes thyrotoxicosis in 10% of patients living in areas of low iodine intake and in 2% of patients in regions of high iodine intake. There are two major forms of AIT, although some patients have features of both. Type 1 AIT is associated with an underlying thyroid abnormality (preclinical Graves' disease or nodular goiter). Thyroid hormone synthesis becomes excessive as a result of increased iodine exposure (Jod-Basedow phenomenon). Type 2 AIT occurs in individuals with no intrinsic thyroid abnormalities and is the result of drug-induced lysosomal activation leading to destructive thyroiditis with histiocyte accumulation in the thyroid. Mild forms of type 2 AIT can resolve spontaneously or can occasionally lead to hypothyroidism. Color-flow doppler thyroid scanning shows increased vascularity in type 1 AIT but decreased vascularity in type 2 AIT. Thyroid scans are difficult to interpret in this setting, because the high endogenous iodine levels diminish tracer uptake. However, the presence of normal or increased uptake favors type 1 AIT.

In AIT the drug should be stopped, if possible, although this is often impractical because of the underlying cardiac disorder. Discontinuation of amiodarone will not have an acute effect because of its storage and prolonged half-life. High doses of antithyroid drugs can be used in type 1 AIT but are often ineffective. In type 2 AIT, oral contrast agents, such as sodium ipodate (500 mg/d) or sodium tyropanoate (500 mg, 1 to 2 doses/d), rapidly reduce T_4 and T_3 levels, decrease $T_4 \rightarrow T_3$ conversion, and may block tissue uptake of thyroid hormones. Potassium perchlorate, 200 mg every 6 h, has been used to reduce thyroidal iodide content. Perchlorate treatment has been associated with agranulocytosis, though the risk appears relatively low with short-term use. Glucocorticoids, administered as for subacute thyroiditis, are of variable benefit in type 2 AIT. Lithium blocks thyroid hormone release and can provide modest benefit. Near-total thyroidectomy rapidly decreases thyroid hormone levels and may be the most effective long-term solution, if the patient can undergo the procedure safely.

THYROID FUNCTION IN PREGNANCY

Four factors alter thyroid function in pregnancy: (1) the transient increase in hCG during the first trimester, which stimulates the TSH-R; (2) the estrogen-induced rise in TBG during the first trimester, which is sustained during pregnancy; (3) alterations in the immune system, leading to the onset, exacerbation, or amelioration of an underlying autoimmune thyroid disease (see above); and (4) increased urinary iodide excretion, which can cause impaired thyroid hormone production in areas of marginal iodine sufficiency. Women with a precarious iodine intake (<50 μg/d) are most at risk of developing a goiter during pregnancy, and iodine supplementation should be considered to prevent maternal and fetal hypothyroidism and the development of neonatal goiter.

The rise in circulating hCG levels during the first trimester is accompanied by a reciprocal fall in TSH that persists into the middle of pregnancy. This appears to reflect weak binding of hCG, which is present at very high levels, to the TSH-R. Rare individuals have been described with variant TSH-R sequences that enhance hCG binding and TSH-R activation. hCG-induced changes in thyroid function can result in transient gestational hyperthyroidism and/or *hyperemesis gravidarum*, a condition characterized by severe nausea and vomiting and risk of volume depletion. Antithyroid drugs are rarely needed, and parenteral fluid replacement usually suffices until the condition resolves.

Maternal hypothyroidism occurs in 2 to 3% of women of childbearing age and is associated with increased risk of developmental delay in the offspring. Thyroid hormone requirements are increased by 25 to 50 μg/d during pregnancy.

GOITER AND NODULAR THYROID DISEASE

Goiter refers to an enlarged thyroid gland. Biosynthetic defects, iodine deficiency, autoimmune disease, and nodular diseases can each lead to goiter, though by different mechanisms. Biosynthetic defects and iodine deficiency are associated with reduced efficiency of thyroid hormone synthesis, leading to increased TSH, which stimulates thyroid growth as a compensatory mechanism to overcome the block in hormone synthesis. Graves' disease and Hashimoto's thyroiditis are also associated with goiter. In Graves' disease, the goiter results mainly from the TSH-R-mediated effects of TSI. The goitrous form of Hashimoto's thyroiditis occurs because of acquired defects in hormone synthesis, leading to elevated levels of TSH and its consequent growth effects. Lymphocytic infiltration and immune system–induced growth factors also contribute to thyroid enlargement in Hashimoto's

thyroiditis. Nodular disease is characterized by the disordered growth of thyroid cells, often combined with the gradual development of fibrosis. Because the management of goiter depends on the etiology, the detection of thyroid enlargement on physical examination should prompt further evaluation to identify its cause.

Nodular thyroid disease is common, occurring in about 3 to 7% of adults when assessed by physical examination. Using more sensitive techniques, such as ultrasound, it is present in >25% of adults. Thyroid nodules may be solitary or multiple, and they may be functional or nonfunctional.

DIFFUSE NONTOXIC (SIMPLE) GOITER ■ Etiology and Pathogenesis When diffuse enlargement of the thyroid occurs in the absence of nodules and hyperthyroidism, it is referred to as a *diffuse nontoxic goiter*. This is sometimes called *simple goiter*, because of the absence of nodules, or *colloid goiter*, because of the presence of uniform follicles that are filled with colloid. Worldwide, diffuse goiter is most commonly caused by iodine deficiency and is termed *endemic goiter* when it affects >5% of the population. In nonendemic regions, *sporadic goiter* occurs, and the cause is usually unknown. Thyroid enlargement in teenagers is sometimes referred to as *juvenile goiter*. In general, goiter is more common in women than men, probably because of the greater prevalence of underlying autoimmune disease and the increased iodine demands associated with pregnancy.

In *iodine-deficient areas*, thyroid enlargement reflects a compensatory effort to trap iodide and produce sufficient hormone under conditions in which hormone synthesis is relatively inefficient. Somewhat surprisingly, TSH levels are usually normal or only slightly increased, suggesting increased sensitivity to TSH or activation of other pathways that lead to thyroid growth. Iodide appears to have direct actions on thyroid vasculature and may indirectly affect growth through vasoactive substances such as endothelins and nitric oxide. Endemic goiter is also caused by exposure to environmental *goitrogens* such as cassava root, which contains a thiocyanate, vegetables of the Cruciferae family (e.g., brussels sprouts, cabbage, and cauliflower), and milk from regions where goitrogens are present in grass. Though relatively rare, inherited defects in thyroid hormone synthesis lead to a diffuse nontoxic goiter. Abnormalities at each step in hormone synthesis, including iodide transport (NIS), Tg synthesis, organification and coupling (TPO), and the regeneration of iodide (dehalogenase), have been described.

CLINICAL MANIFESTATIONS AND DIAGNOSIS If thyroid function is preserved, most goiters are asymptomatic. Spontaneous hemorrhage into a cyst or nodule may cause the sudden onset of localized pain and swelling. Examination of a diffuse goiter reveals a symmetrically enlarged, nontender, generally soft gland without palpable nodules. Goiter is defined, somewhat arbitrarily, as a lateral lobe with a volume greater than the thumb of the individual being examined. If the thyroid is markedly enlarged, it can cause tracheal or esophageal compression. These features are unusual, however, in the absence of nodular disease and fibrosis. *Substernal goiter* may obstruct the thoracic inlet. *Pemberton's sign* refers to symptoms of faintness with evidence of facial congestion and external jugular venous obstruction when the arms are raised above the head, a maneuver that draws the thyroid into the thoracic inlet. Respiratory flow measurements and CT or MRI should be used to evaluate substernal goiter in patients with obstructive signs or symptoms.

Thyroid function tests should be performed in all patients with goiter to exclude thyrotoxicosis or hypothyroidism. It is not unusual, particularly in iodine deficiency, to find a low total T_4, with normal T_3 and TSH, reflecting enhanced $T_4 \rightarrow T_3$ conversion. A low TSH, particularly in older patients, suggests the possibility of thyroid autonomy or undiagnosed Graves' disease, causing subclinical thyrotoxicosis. TPO antibodies may be useful to identify patients at increased risk of autoimmune thyroid disease. Low urinary iodine levels (<10 μg/dL) support a diagnosis of iodine deficiency. Thyroid scanning is not generally necessary but will reveal increased uptake in iodine deficiency and most cases of dyshormonogenesis. Ultrasound is not generally indicated in the evaluation of diffuse goiter, unless a nodule is palpable on physical examination.

 TREATMENT

Iodine or thyroid hormone replacement induces variable regression of goiter in iodine deficiency, depending on how long it has been present and the degree of fibrosis that has developed. Because of the possibility of underlying thyroid autonomy, caution should be exercised when instituting suppressive thyroxine therapy in other causes of diffuse nontoxic goiter, particularly if the baseline TSH is in the low-normal range. In younger patients, the dose of levothyroxine can be started at 100 μg/d and adjusted to suppress the TSH into the low-normal but detectable range. Treatment of elderly patients should be initiated at 50 μg/d. The efficacy of suppressive treatment is greater in younger patients and for those with soft goiters. Significant regression is usually seen within 3 to 6 months of treatment; after this time it is unlikely to occur. In older patients, and in those with some degree of nodular disease or fibrosis, fewer than one-third demonstrate significant shrinkage of the goiter. Surgery is rarely indicated for diffuse goiter. Exceptions include documented evidence of tracheal compression or obstruction of the thoracic inlet, which are more likely to be associated with substernal multinodular goiters (see below). Subtotal or near-total thyroidectomy for these or cosmetic reasons should be performed by an experienced surgeon to minimize complication rates, which occur in up to 10% of cases. Surgery should be followed by mild suppressive treatment with levothyroxine to prevent regrowth of the goiter. Radioiodine reduces goiter size by about 50% in the majority of patients. It is rarely associated with transient acute swelling of the thyroid, which is usually inconsequential unless there is severe tracheal narrowing. If not treated with levothyroxine, patients should be followed after radioiodine treatment for the possible development of hypothyroidism.

NONTOXIC MULTINODULAR GOITER ■ Etiology and Pathogenesis Depending on the population studied, multinodular goiter (MNG) occurs in up to 12% of adults. MNG is more common in women than men and increases in prevalence with age. It is more common in iodine-deficient regions but also occurs in regions of iodine sufficiency, reflecting multiple genetic, autoimmune, and environmental influences on the pathogenesis.

There is typically wide variation in nodule size. Histology reveals a spectrum of morphologies ranging from hypercellular regions to cystic areas filled with colloid. Fibrosis is often extensive, and areas of hemorrhage or lymphocytic infiltration may be seen. Using molecular techniques, most nodules within a MNG are polyclonal in origin, suggesting a hyperplastic response to locally produced growth factors and cytokines. TSH, which is usually not elevated, may play a permissive or contributory role. Monoclonal lesions also occur within a MNG, reflecting mutations in genes that confer a selective growth advantage to the progenitor cell.

Clinical Manifestations Most patients with nontoxic MNG are asymptomic and, by definition, euthyroid. MNG typically develops over many years and is detected on routine physical examination or when an individual notices an enlargement in the neck. If the goiter is large enough, it can ultimately lead to compressive symptoms including difficulty swallowing, respiratory distress (tracheal compression), or plethora (venous congestion), but these symptoms are uncommon. Symptomatic MNGs are usually extraordinarily large and/or develop fibrotic areas that cause compression. Sudden pain in a MNG is usually caused by hemorrhage into a nodule but should raise the possibility of invasive malignancy. Hoarseness, reflecting laryngeal nerve involvement, also suggests malignancy.

Diagnosis On examination, thyroid architecture is distorted and multiple nodules of varying size can be appreciated. Because many nodules are deeply embedded in thyroid tissue or reside in posterior or substernal locations, it is not possible to palpate all nodules. A TSH level should be measured to exclude subclinical hyper- or hypothy-

roidism, but thyroid function is usually normal. Tracheal deviation is common, but compression must usually exceed 70% of the tracheal diameter before there is significant airway compromise. Pulmonary function testing can be used to assess the functional effects of compression and to detect tracheomalacia, which characteristically causes inspiratory stridor. CT or MRI can be used to evaluate the anatomy of the goiter and the extent of substernal extension, which is often much greater than is apparent on physical examination. A barium swallow may reveal the extent of esophageal compression. MNG does not appear to predispose to thyroid carcinoma or to more aggressive carcinoma. For this reason, and because it is not possible to biopsy all nodular lesions, thyroid biopsies should be performed only if malignancy is suspected because of a dominant or enlarging nodule.

 TREATMENT

Most nontoxic MNGs can be managed conservatively. T$_4$ suppression is rarely effective for reducing goiter size and introduces the risk of thyrotoxicosis, particularly if there is underlying autonomy or if it develops during treatment. If levothyroxine is used, it should be started at low doses (50 μg) and advanced gradually while monitoring the TSH level to avoid excessive suppression. Contrast agents and other iodine-containing substances should be avoided because of the risk of inducing the *Jod-Basedow effect*, characterized by enhanced thyroid hormone production by autonomous nodules. Radioiodine is being used with increasing frequency because it often decreases goiter size and may selectively ablate regions of autonomy. Dosage of ^{131}I depends on the size of the goiter and radioiodine uptake but is usually about 3.7 MBq (0.1 mCi) per gram of tissue, corrected for uptake [typical dose, 370 to 1070 Mbq (10 to 29 mCi)]. Repeat treatment may be needed. It is possible to achieve a 40 to 50% reduction in goiter size in most patients. Earlier concerns about radiation-induced thyroid swelling and tracheal compression have diminished as recent studies have shown this complication to be rare. When acute compression occurs, glucocorticoid treatment or surgery may be needed. Radiation-induced hypothyroidism is less common than after treatment for Graves' disease. However, posttreatment autoimmune thyrotoxicosis may occur in up to 5% of patients treated for nontoxic MNG. Surgery remains highly effective but is not without risk, particularly in older patients with underlying cardiopulmonary disease.

TOXIC MULTINODULAR GOITER The pathogenesis of toxic MNG appears to be similar to that of nontoxic MNG; the major difference is the presence of functional autonomy in toxic MNG. The molecular basis for autonomy in toxic MNG remains unknown. As in nontoxic goiters, many nodules are polyclonal, while others are monoclonal and vary in their clonal origins. Genetic abnormalities known to confer functional autonomy, such as activating TSH-R or G$_{s\alpha}$ mutations (see below), are not usually found in the autonomous regions of toxic MNG goiter.

In addition to features of goiter, the clinical presentation of toxic MNG includes subclinical hyperthyroidism or mild thyrotoxicosis. The patient is usually elderly and may present with atrial fibrillation or palpitations, tachycardia, nervousness, tremor, or weight loss. Recent exposure to iodine, from contrast dyes or other sources, may precipitate or exacerbate thyrotoxicosis. The TSH level is low. The T$_4$ level may be normal or minimally increased; T$_3$ is often elevated to a greater degree than T$_4$. Thyroid scan shows heterogeneous uptake with multiple regions of increased and decreased uptake; 24-h uptake of radioiodine may not be increased.

 TREATMENT

The management of toxic MNG is challenging. Antithyroid drugs, often in combination with beta blockers, can normalize thyroid function and address clinical features of thyrotoxicosis. This treatment, however, often stimulates the growth of the goiter, and, unlike in

Graves' disease, spontaneous remission does not occur. Radioiodine can be used to treat areas of autonomy, as well as to decrease the mass of the goiter. Usually, however, some degree of autonomy remains, presumably because multiple autonomous regions emerge as soon as others are treated. Nonetheless, a trial of radioiodine should be considered before subjecting patients, many of whom are elderly, to surgery. Surgery provides definitive treatment of underlying thyrotoxicosis as well as goiter. Patients should be rendered euthyroid using antithyroid drugs before operation.

HYPERFUNCTIONING SOLITARY NODULE   A solitary, autonomously functioning thyroid nodule is referred to as *toxic adenoma*. The pathogenesis of this disorder has been unraveled by demonstrating the functional effects of mutations that stimulate the TSH-R signaling pathway. Most patients with solitary hyperfunctioning nodules have acquired somatic, activating mutations in the TSH-R (Fig. 320-9). These mutations, located primarily in the receptor transmembrane domain, induce constitutive receptor coupling to $G_{s\alpha}$, increasing cyclic AMP levels and leading to enhanced thyroid follicular cell proliferation and function. Less commonly, somatic mutations are identified in $G_{s\alpha}$. These mutations, which are similar to those seen in McCune-Albright syndrome (Chap. 326) or in a subset of somatotrope adenomas (Chap. 318), impair GTP hydrolysis, also causing constitutive activation of the cyclic AMP signaling pathway. In most series, activating mutations in either the TSH-R or the $G_{s\alpha}$ subunit genes are identified in >90% of patients with solitary hyperfunctioning nodules.

Thyrotoxicosis is usually mild. The disorder is suggested by the presence of the thyroid nodule, which is generally large enough to be palpable, and by the absence of clinical features suggestive of Graves' disease or other causes of thyrotoxicosis. A thyroid scan provides a definitive diagnostic test, demonstrating focal uptake in the hyperfunctioning nodule and diminished uptake in the remainder of the gland, as activity of the normal thyroid is suppressed.

℞ TREATMENT

Radioiodine ablation is usually the treatment of choice. Because normal thyroid function is suppressed, ^{131}I is concentrated in the hyperfunctioning nodule with minimal uptake and damage to normal thyroid tissue. Relatively large radioiodine doses [e.g., 370 to 1110 MBq (10 to 29.9 mCi)^{131}I] have been shown to correct thyrotoxicosis in about 75% of patients within 3 months. Hypothyroidism occurs in <10% of patients over the next 5 years. Surgical resection is also effective and is usually limited to enucleation of the adenoma or lobectomy, thereby preserving thyroid function and minimizing risk of hypoparathyroidism or damage to the recurrent laryngeal nerves. Medical therapy using antithyroid drugs and beta blockers can normalize thyroid function but is not an optimal long-term treatment. Ethanol injection under ultrasound guidance has been used successfully in some centers to ablate hyperfunctioning nodules. Repeated injections (often more than 5 sessions) are required to reduce nodule size. Normal thyroid function can be achieved in most patients using this technique.

BENIGN NEOPLASMS

The various types of benign thyroid nodules are listed in Table 320-9. These lesions are common (5 to 10% adults), particularly when assessed by sensitive techniques such as ultrasound. The risk of malignancy is very low for *macrofollicular adenomas* and *normofollicular adenomas*. *Microfollicular, trabecular, and Hürthle cell variants* raise greater concern, and the histology is more difficult to interpret. About one-third of palpable nodules are *thyroid cysts*. These may be recognized by their ultrasound appearance or based on aspiration of large amounts of pink or straw-colored fluid (colloid). Many are mixed cystic/solid lesions, in which case it is desirable to aspirate cellular components under ultrasound or harvest cells after cytospin of cyst fluid. Cysts frequently recur, even after repeated aspiration, and

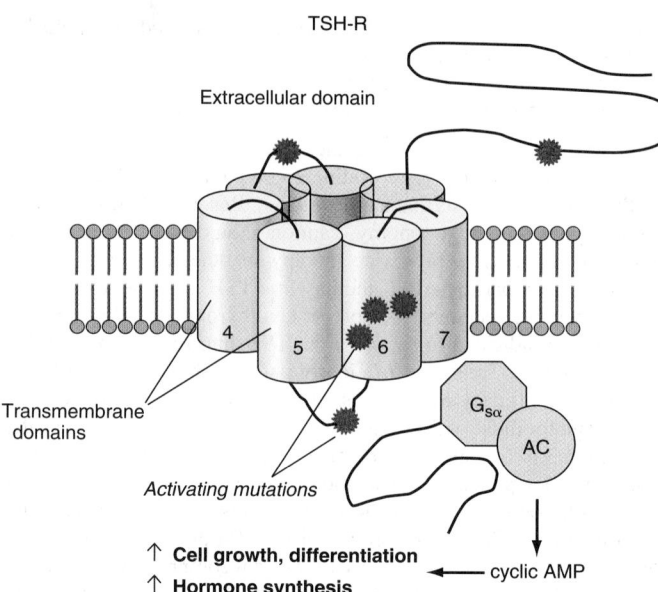

FIGURE 320-9   Activating mutations of the TSH-R. Mutations (*) that activate the thyroid-stimulating hormone receptor (TSH-R) reside mainly in transmembrane 5 and intracellular loop 3, though mutations have occurred in a variety of different locations. The effect of these mutations is to induce conformational changes that mimic TSH binding, thereby leading to coupling to stimulatory G protein ($G_{s\alpha}$) and activation of adenylate cyclase (AC), an enzyme that generates cyclic AMP.

may require surgical excision if they are large or if the cytology is suspicious. Sclerosis has been used with variable success but is often painful and may be complicated by infiltration of the sclerosing agent.

The treatment approach for benign nodules is similar to that for MNG. TSH suppression with levothyroxine decreases the size of about 30% of nodules and may prevent further growth. The TSH level should

TABLE 320-9   Classification of Thyroid Neoplasms

BENIGN	
Follicular epithelial cell adenomas	
Macrofollicular (colloid)	
Normofollicular (simple)	
Microfollicular (fetal)	
Trabecular (embryonal)	
Hürtle cell variant (oncocytic)	

MALIGNANT	**APPROXIMATE PREVALENCE, %**
Follicular epithelial cell	
Well-differentiated carcinomas	
Papillary carcinomas	80–90
Pure papillary	
Follicular variant	
Diffuse sclerosing variant	
Tall cell, columnar cell variants	
Follicular carcinomas	5–10
Minimally invasive	
Widely invasive	
Hürthle cell carcinoma (oncocytic)	
Insular carcinoma	
Undifferentiated (anaplastic) carcinomas	
C cell (calcitonin-producing)	
Medullary thyroid cancer	10
Sporadic	
Familial	
MEN 2	
Other malignancies	
Lymphomas	1–2
Sarcomas	
Metastases	
Others	

Note: MEN, multiple endocrine neoplasia.

be suppressed into the low-normal range, assuming there are no contraindications; alternatively, nodule size can be monitored without suppression. If a nodule has not decreased in size after 6 to 12 months of suppressive therapy, treatment should be discontinued as little benefit is likely to accrue from long-term treatment.

THYROID CANCER

Thyroid carcinoma is the most common malignancy of the endocrine system. Malignant tumors derived from the follicular epithelium are classified according to histologic features. Differentiated tumors, such as papillary thyroid cancer (PTC) or follicular thyroid cancer (FTC), are often curable, and the prognosis is good for patients identified with early-stage disease. In contrast, anaplastic thyroid cancer (ATC) is aggressive, responds poorly to treatment, and is associated with a bleak prognosis.

The incidence of thyroid cancer (~9/100,000 per year) increases with age, plateauing after about age 50 (Fig. 320-10). Age is also an important prognostic factor—thyroid cancer at a young age (<20) or in older persons (>65) is associated with a worse prognosis. Thyroid cancer is twice as common in women as men, but male sex is associated with a worse prognosis. Additional important risk factors include a history of childhood head or neck irradiation, large nodule size (≥4 cm), evidence for local tumor fixation or invasion into lymph nodes, and the presence of metastases (Table 320-10).

Several unique features of thyroid cancer facilitate its management: (1) thyroid nodules are readily palpable, allowing early detection and biopsy by FNA; (2) iodine radioisotopes can be used to diagnose (^{123}I) and treat (^{131}I) differentiated thyroid cancer, reflecting the unique uptake of this anion by the thyroid gland; and (3) serum markers allow the detection of residual or recurrent disease, including the use of Tg levels for PTC and FTC and calcitonin for medullary thyroid cancer (MTC).

CLASSIFICATION Thyroid neoplasms can arise in each of the cell types that populate the gland, including thyroid follicular cells, calcitonin-producing C cells, lymphocytes, and stromal and vascular elements, as well as metastases from other sites (Table 320-9). The American Joint Committee on Cancer (AJCC) has designated a staging system using the TNM classification (Table 320-11). Several other classification and staging systems are also widely used, some of which place greater emphasis on histologic features or risk factors such as age or gender.

PATHOGENESIS AND GENETIC BASIS ■ **Radiation** Early studies of the pathogenesis of thyroid cancer focused on the role of external radiation, which predisposes to chromosomal breaks, presumably leading to genetic rearrangements and loss of tumor-suppressor genes. External radiation of the mediastinum, face, head, and neck region was administered in the past to treat an array of conditions including acne and enlargement of the thymus, tonsils, and adenoids. Radiation exposure increases the risk of benign and malignant thyroid nodules, is associated with multicentric cancers, and shifts the incidence of thyroid cancer to an earlier age group. Radiation from nuclear fallout also increases the risk of thyroid cancer. Children seem more predisposed to the effects of radiation than adults. Of note, radiation derived from ^{131}I therapy appears to contribute little, if any, increased risk of thyroid cancer.

TSH and Growth Factors Thyroid growth is regulated primarily by TSH but also by a variety of growth factors and cytokines. Many differentiated thyroid cancers express TSH receptors and, therefore, remain responsive to TSH. This observation provides the rationale for T_4 suppression of TSH in patients with thyroid cancer. Residual expression of TSH receptors also allows TSH-stimulated uptake of ^{131}I therapy (see below).

Oncogenes and Tumor-Suppressor Genes Thyroid cancers are monoclonal in origin, consistent with the idea that they originate as a consequence of mutations that confer a growth advantage to a single cell. In addition to increased rates of proliferation, some thyroid cancers exhibit impaired apoptosis and features that enhance invasion, angiogenesis, and metastasis. By analogy with the model of multistep carcinogenesis proposed for colon cancer (Chap. 68), thyroid neoplasms have been analyzed for a variety of genetic alterations, but without clear evidence of an ordered acquisition of somatic mutations as they progress from the benign to the malignant state. On the other hand, certain mutations are relatively specific for thyroid neoplasia, some of which correlate with histologic classification (Table 320-12). For example, activating mutations of the TSH-R and the $G_{s\alpha}$ subunit are associated with autonomously functioning nodules. Though these mutations induce thyroid cell growth, this type of nodule is almost always benign. A variety of rearrangements involving the *RET* gene on chromosome 10 bring this receptor tyrosine kinase under the control of other promoters, leading to receptor overexpression. *RET* rearrangements occur in 20 to

TABLE 320-10 *Risk Factors for Thyroid Carcinoma in Patients with Thyroid Nodule*

History of head and neck irradiation	Family history of thyroid cancer or MEN 2
Age <20 or >70 years	Vocal cord paralysis, hoarse voice
Increased nodule size (>4 cm)	Nodule fixed to adjacent structures
New or enlarging neck mass	Suspected lymph node involvement
Male gender	Iodine deficiency (follicular cancer)

Note: MEN, multiple endocrine neoplasia.

TABLE 320-11 *American Joint Committee on Cancer Staging System for Thyroid Cancers Using the TNM Classification[a]*

Papillary or follicular thyroid cancers		
	<45 years	>45 years
Stage I	Any T, any N, M0	T1, N0, M0
Stage II	Any T, any N, M1	T2 or T3, N0, M0
Stage III	—	T4, N0, M0
		Any T, N1, M0
Stage IV	—	Any T, any N, M1
Anaplastic thyroid cancer		
Stage IV	All cases are stage IV	
Medullary thyroid cancer		
Stage I	T1, N0, M0	
Stage II	T2–T4, N0, M0	
Stage III	Any T, N1, M0	
Stage IV	Any T, any N, M1	

[a] Criteria include: T, the size and extent of the primary tumor (T1 ≤ 1 cm; 1 cm < T2 ≤ 4 cm; T3 > 4 cm; T4 direct invasion through the thyroid capsule); N, the absence (N0) or presence (N1) of regional node involvement; M, the absence (M0) or presence (M1) of metastases.

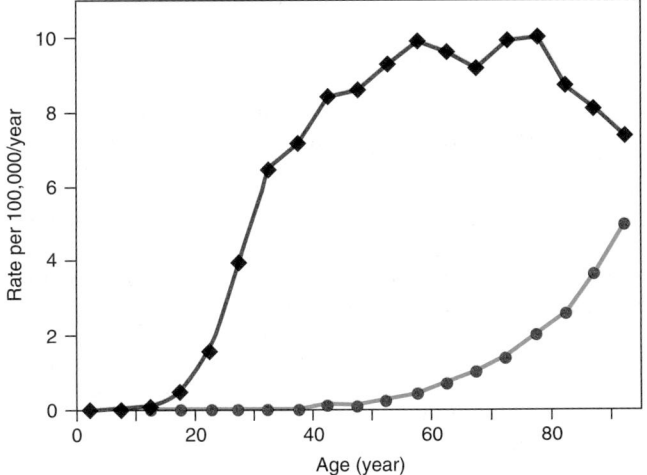

FIGURE 320-10 Age-associated incidence (—♦—) and mortality (—●—) rates for invasive thyroid cancer. [*Adapted from LAG Ries et al (eds): SEER Cancer Statistics Review, 1973–1996, Bethesda, National Cancer Institute, 1999.*]

TABLE 320-12 *Genetic Alterations in Thyroid Neoplasia*

Gene/Protein	Type of Gene	Chromosomal Location	Genetic Abnormality	Tumor
TSH receptor	GPCR receptor	14q31	Point mutations	Toxic adenoma, differentiated carcinomas
$G_{s\alpha}$	G protein	20q13.2	Point mutations	Toxic adenoma, differentiated carcinomas
RET/PTC	Receptor tyrosine kinase	10q11.2	Rearrangements PTC1: (inv(10)q11.2q21) PTC2: (t(10;17)(q11.2;q23)) PTC3: ELE1/TK	PTC
RET	Receptor tyrosine kinase	10q11.2	Point mutations	MEN 2, medullary thyroid cancer
TRK	Receptor tyrosine kinase	1q23-24	Rearrangements	Multinodular goiter, papillary thyroid cancer
RAS	Signal transducing p21	Hras 11p15.5 Kras 12p12.1; Nras 1p13.2	Point mutations	Differentiated thyroid carcinoma, adenomas
p53	Tumor suppressor, cell cycle control, apoptosis	17p13	Point mutations Deletion, insertion	Anaplastic cancer
APC	Tumor suppressor, adenomatous polyposis coli gene	5q21-q22	Point mutations	Anaplastic cancer, also associated with familial polyposis coli
p16 (MTS1, CDKN2A)	Tumor suppressor, cell cycle control	9p21	Deletions	Differentiated carcinomas
p21/WAF	Tumor suppressor, cell cycle control	6p21.2	Overexpression	Anaplastic cancer
MET	Receptor tyrosine kinase	7q31	Overexpression	Follicular thyroid cancer
c-MYC	Receptor tyrosine kinase	8q24.12.-13	Overexpression	Differentiated carcinoma
PTEN	Phosphatase	10q23	Point mutations	PTC in Cowden's syndrome (multiple hamartomas, breast tumors, gastrointestinal polyps, thyroid tumors)
Loss of heterozygosity (LOH)	?Tumor suppressors	3p; 11q13 Other loci	Deletions	Differentiated thyroid carcinomas, anaplastic cancer
PAX8-PPARγl	Transcription factor Nuclear receptor fusion	t(2;3)(q13;p25)	Translocation	Follicular adenoma or carcinoma

Note: TSH, thyroid-stimulating hormone; G$_{s\alpha}$, G-protein stimulating α-subunit; RET, rearranged during transfection proto-oncogene; PTC, papillary thyroid cancer; TRK, tyrosine kinase receptor; RAS, rat sarcoma proto-oncogene; p53, p53 tumor suppressor gene; MET, met proto-oncogene (hepatocyte growth factor receptor); c-MYC, cellular homologue of myelocytomatosis virus proto-oncogene; PTEN, phosphatase and tensin homologue; APC, adenomatous polyposis coli; MTS, multiple tumor suppressor; CDKN2A, cyclin-depen-dent kinase inhibitor 2A; P21, p21 tumor suppressor; WAF, wild-type p53 activated fragment; GPCR, G protein-coupled receptor; ELE1/TK, ret-activating gene ele1/tyrosine kinase; MEN 2, multiple endocrine neoplasia-2; PAX8, Paired domain transcription factor; PPARγl, peroxisome-proliferator activated receptor γl.

Source: Adapted with permission from P Kopp, JL Jameson, in JL Jameson (ed): *Principles of Molecular Medicine*. Totowa, NJ, Humana Press, 1998.

40% of PTCs in different series and were observed with increased frequency in tumors developing after the Chernobyl radiation disaster. Rearrangements in PTC have also been observed for another tyrosine kinase gene, *TRK1*, which is located on chromosome 1. To date, the identification of PTC with *RET* or *TRK1* rearrangements has not proven useful for predicting prognosis or treatment responses. Another rearrangement, linking the thyroid developmental transcription factor PAX8 to the nuclear receptor PPARγ, has been identified in a significance fraction of follicular adenomas and FTCs. *RAS* mutations are found in about 20 to 30% of thyroid neoplasms, including adenomas as well as PTC and FTC, suggesting that these mutations do not strongly affect tumor phenotype. Loss of heterozygosity, consistent with deletions of tumor-suppressor genes, is particularly common in FTC, often involving chromosomes 3p or 11q. Mutations of the tumor suppressor, p53, play an important role in the development of ATC. Because p53 plays a role in cell cycle surveillance, DNA repair, and apoptosis, its loss may contribute to the rapid acquisition of genetic instability as well as poor treatment responses (Chap. 69). The role of other tumor-suppressor genes in thyroid cancer is under investigation (Table 320-12).

MTC, when associated with multiple endocrine neoplasia (MEN) type 2, harbors an inherited mutation of the *RET* gene. Unlike the rearrangements of *RET* seen in PTC, the mutations in MEN2 are point mutations that induce constitutive activity of the tyrosine kinase (Chap. 330). MTC is preceded by hyperplasia of the C cells, raising the likelihood that as-yet-unidentified "second hits" lead to cellular transformation. A subset of sporadic MTC contain somatic mutations that activate *RET*.

WELL-DIFFERENTIATED THYROID CANCER ■ Papillary PTC is the most common type of thyroid cancer, accounting for 70 to 90% of well-differentiated thyroid malignancies. Microscopic PTC is present in up to 25% of thyroid glands at autopsy, but most of these lesions are very small (several millimeters) and are not clinically significant. Characteristic cytologic features of PTC help make the diagnosis by FNA or after surgical resection; these include psammoma bodies, cleaved nuclei with an "orphan-Annie" appearance caused by large nucleoli, and the formation of papillary structures.

PTC tends to be multifocal and to invade locally within the thyroid gland as well as through the thyroid capsule and into adjacent structures in the neck. It has a propensity to spread via the lymphatic system but can metastasize hematogenously as well, particularly to bone and lung. Because of the relatively slow growth of the tumor, a significant burden of pulmonary metastases may accumulate, sometimes with remarkably few symptoms. The prognostic implication of lymph node spread is debated. Lymph node involvement by thyroid cancer can be remarkably well tolerated but probably increases the risk of recurrence and mortality, particularly in older patients. The staging of PTC by the TNM system is outlined in Table 320-11. Most papillary cancers are identified in the early stages (>80% stages I or II) and have an excellent prognosis, with survival curves similar to expected survival (Fig. 320-11A). Mortality is markedly increased in stage IV disease (distant metastases), but this group comprises only about 1% of patients. The treatment of PTC is described below.

Follicular The incidence of FTC varies widely in different parts of the world; it is more common in iodine-deficient regions. FTC is difficult

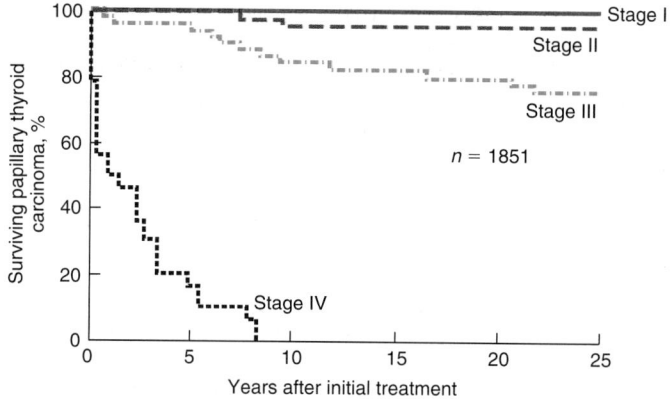

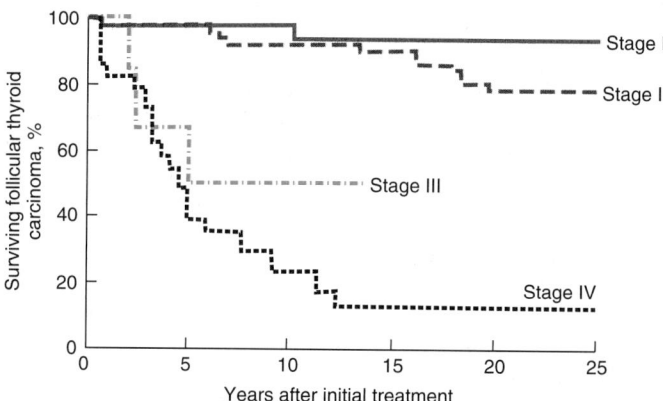

FIGURE 320-11   Survival rates in patients with differentiated thyroid cancer. *A.* Papillary cancer, cohort of 1851 patients. I, 1107 (60%), II, 408 (22%), III, 312 (17%), IV, 24 (1%); *n* = 1185. *B.* Follicular cancer, cohort of 153 patients. I, 42 (27%), II, 82 (54%), III, 6 (4%); IV, 23 (15%); *n* = 153. [*Adapted from PR Larsen et al: William's Textbook of Endocrinology, 9th ed, JD Wilson et al (eds). Philadelphia, Saunders, 1998, pp 389–575; with permission.*]

to diagnose by FNA because the distinction between benign and malignant follicular neoplasms rests largely on evidence of invasion into vessels, nerves, or adjacent structures. FTC tends to spread by hematogenous routes leading to bone, lung, and central nervous system metastases. Mortality rates associated with FTC are less favorable than for PTC, in part because a larger proportion of patients present with stage IV disease (Fig. 320-11*B*). Poor prognostic features include distant metastases, age >50 years, primary tumor size >4 cm, Hürthle cell histology, and the presence of marked vascular invasion.

℞ TREATMENT

Surgery   All well-differentiated thyroid cancers should be surgically excised. In addition to removing the primary lesion, surgery allows accurate histologic diagnosis and staging, and multicentric disease is commonly found in the contralateral thyroid lobe. Lymph node spread can also be assessed at the time of surgery, and involved nodes can be removed. Recommendations about the extent of surgery vary for stage I disease, as survival rates are similar for lobectomy and near-total thyroidectomy. Lobectomy is associated with a lower incidence of hypoparathyroidism and injury to the recurrent laryngeal nerves. However, it is not possible to monitor Tg levels or to perform whole-body ^{131}I scans in the presence of the residual lobe. Moreover, if final staging or subsequent follow-up indicates the need for radioiodine scanning or treatment, repeat surgery is necessary to remove the remaining thyroid tissue. Therefore, near-total thyroidectomy is preferable in almost all patients; complication rates are acceptably low if the surgeon is highly experienced in the procedure. This approach, in combination with postsurgical radioablation of the remnant thyroid tissue, facilitates the use of radioiodine scanning and Tg determinations to assess disease recurrence.

TSH Suppression Therapy   As most tumors are still TSH-responsive, levothyroxine suppression of TSH is a mainstay of thyroid cancer treatment. Though TSH suppression clearly provides therapeutic benefit, there are no prospective studies that identify the optimal level of TSH suppression. A reasonable goal is to suppress TSH as much as possible without subjecting the patient to unnecessary side effects from excess thyroid hormone, such as atrial fibrillation, osteopenia, anxiety, and other manifestations of thyrotoxicosis. For patients at low risk of recurrence, TSH should be suppressed into the low but detectable range (0.1 to 0.5 IU/L). For patients at high risk of recurrence, or with known metastatic disease, complete TSH suppression is indicated, if there are no strong contraindications to mild thyrotoxicosis. In this instance, unbound T$_4$ must also be monitored to avoid excessive treatment.

Radioiodine Treatment   Well-differentiated thyroid cancer still incorporates radioiodine, though less efficiently than normal thyroid follicular cells. Radioiodine uptake is determined primarily by expression of the NIS and is stimulated by TSH, requiring expression of the TSH-R. The retention time for radioactivity is influenced by the extent to which the tumor retains differentiated functions such as iodide trapping and organification. After near-total thyroidectomy, substantial thyroid tissue remains, particularly in the thyroid bed and surrounding the parathyroid glands. Consequently, ^{131}I ablation is necessary to eliminate remaining normal thyroid tissue and to treat residual tumor cells.

INDICATIONS   The use of therapeutic doses of radioiodine remains an area of controversy in thyroid cancer management. Postoperative thyroid ablation and radiodine treatment of known residual PTC or FTC reduce recurrence rates. For tumors that take up iodine, ^{131}I treatment can reduce or eliminate residual disease with relatively little associated toxicity. However, it is not clear that prophylactic radioiodine treatment reduces mortality for patients at relatively low risk. Most patients with stage 1 PTC with primary tumors <1.5 cm in size can be managed safely with thyroxine suppression, without radiation treatment, as the risk of recurrence and mortality is very low. For patients with larger papillary tumors, spread to the adjacent lymph nodes, FTC, or evidence of metastases, thyroid ablation and radioiodine treatment are generally indicated.

^{131}I THYROID ABLATION AND TREATMENT   As noted above, the decision to use ^{131}I for thyroid ablation should be coordinated with the surgical approach, as radioablation is much more effective when there is minimal remaining normal thyroid tissue. A typical strategy is to treat the patient for several weeks postoperatively with liothyronine (25 μg bid or tid), followed by thyroid hormone withdrawal. Ideally, the TSH level should increase to >50 IU/L over 3 to 4 weeks. The level to which TSH rises is dictated largely by the amount of normal thyroid tissue remaining postoperatively. A scanning dose of ^{131}I [usually 148 to 185 MBq (4 to 5 mCi)] will reveal the amount of residual tissue and provides guidance about the dose needed to accomplish ablation. A maximum outpatient ^{131}I dose is 1110 MBq (29.9 mCi) in the United States, though ablation is often more complete using greater doses [1850 to 2775 MBq (50 to 75 mCi)]. In patients with known residual cancer, the larger doses ensure thyroid ablation and may destroy remaining tumor cells. A whole-body scan following the high-dose radioiodine treatment is useful to identify possible metastatic disease.

FOLLOW-UP WHOLE-BODY THYROID SCANNING AND THYROGLOBULIN DETERMINATIONS   An initial whole-body scan should be performed about 6 months after surgery and thyroid ablation. The strategy for follow-up management of thyroid cancer has been altered by the availability of recombinant human TSH (rhTSH) to stimulate ^{131}I uptake and by the improved sensitivity of Tg assays to detect residual or recurrent disease. A scheme for using either rhTSH or thyroid hormone withdrawal for thyroid scanning is summarized in Fig. 320-12. After thyroid ablation, rhTSH can be used to stimulate ^{131}I uptake without subjecting patients to thyroid hormone withdrawal and its associated symptoms of hypothyroidism and the risk of prolonged TSH-stimulated tumor growth.

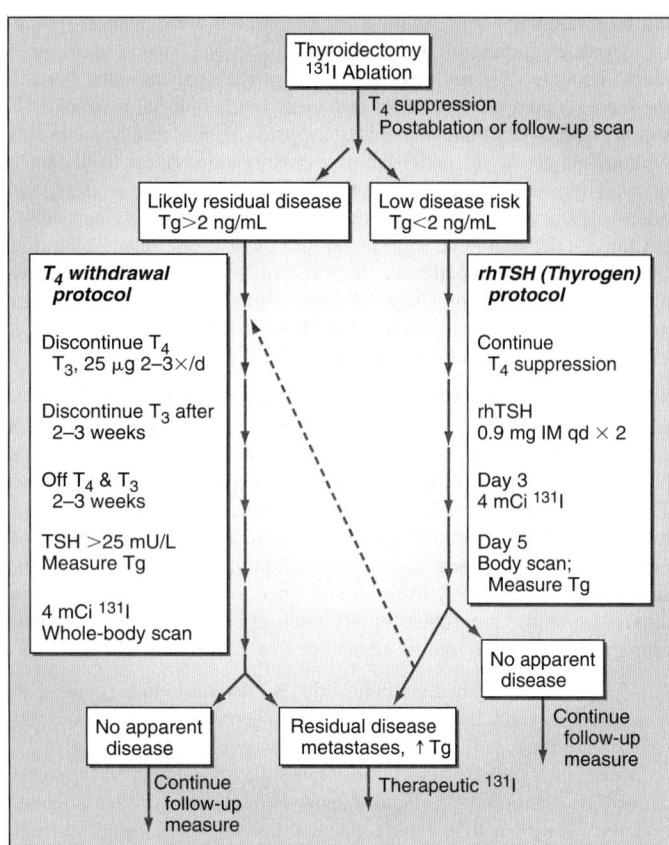

FIGURE 320-12 Use of recombinant thyroid-stimulating hormone (TSH) in the follow-up of patients with thyroid cancer. Tg, thyroglobulin; rhTSH, recombinant human TSH.

This approach is recommended for patients predicted to be at low risk of disease recurrence, since rhTSH is not currently approved for use in conjunction with therapeutic doses of ^{131}I. Alternatively, in patients who are likely to require ^{131}I treatment, the traditional approach of thyroid hormone withdrawal can be used to increase TSH. This involves switching patients from levothyroxine (T_4) to the more rapidly cleared hormone, liothyronine (T_3), thereby allowing TSH to increase more quickly. If residual disease is detected on the initial whole-body scan [148 to 185 MBq (4 to 5 mCi)], a larger treatment dose, usually between 2775 and 5550 MBq (75 and 150 mCi), can be administered depending on the degree of residual uptake and assessment of cancer risk. Because TSH stimulates Tg levels, Tg measurements should be obtained after administration of rhTSH or when TSH levels have risen after thyroid hormone withdrawal. Investigational protocols are measuring Tg levels after rhTSH stimulation but without radioiodine scanning. If the initial whole-body scan is negative and Tg levels are low, a repeat scan should be performed 1 year later. If still negative, the patient can be managed with suppressive therapy and measurements of Tg every 6 to 12 months. If a second follow-up scan is negative, no further scanning may be necessary if the patient is at low risk and there is no clinical or laboratory evidence of recurrence. Many authorities advocate radioiodine treatment for scan-negative, Tg-positive (Tg >5 to 10 ng/mL) patients, as many derive therapeutic benefit from a large dose of ^{131}I.

In addition to radioiodine, external beam radiotherapy is also used to treat specific metastatic lesions, particularly when they cause bone pain or threaten neurologic injury (e.g., vertebral metastases).

ANAPLASTIC AND OTHER FORMS OF THYROID CANCER ■ Anaplastic Thyroid Cancer

As noted above, ATC is a poorly differentiated and aggressive cancer. The prognosis is poor, and most patients die within 6 months of diagnosis. Because of the undifferentiated state of these tumors, the up-take of radioiodine is usually negligible, but it can be used therapeutically if there is residual uptake. Chemotherapy has been attempted with multiple agents, including anthracyclines and paclitaxel, but is usually ineffective. External radiation therapy can be attempted and continued if tumors are responsive.

Thyroid Lymphoma Lymphoma in the thyroid gland often arises in the background of Hashimoto's thyroiditis. A rapidly expanding thyroid mass suggests the possibility of this diagnosis. Diffuse large cell lymphoma is the most common type in the thyroid. Biopsies reveal sheets of lymphoid cells that can be difficult to distinguish from small cell lung cancer or ATC. These tumors are often highly sensitive to external radiation. Surgical resection should be avoided as initial therapy because it may spread disease that is otherwise localized to the thyroid. If staging indicates disease outside of the thyroid, treatment should follow guidelines used for other forms of lymphoma (Chap. 97).

MEDULLARY THYROID CARCINOMA MTC can be sporadic or familial and accounts for about 5 to 10% of thyroid cancers. There are three familial forms of MTC: MEN 2A, MEN 2B, and familial MTC without other features of MEN (Chap. 330). In general, MTC is more aggressive in MEN 2B than in MEN 2A, and familial MTC is more aggressive than sporadic MTC. Elevated serum calcitonin provides a marker of residual or recurrent disease. It is reasonable to test all patients with MTC for *RET* mutations, as genetic counseling and testing of family members can be offered to those individuals who test positive for mutations.

The management of MTC is primarily surgical. Unlike tumors derived from thyroid follicular cells, these tumors do not take up radioiodine. External radiation treatment and chemotherapy may provide palliation in patients with advanced disease (Chap. 330).

APPROACH TO THE PATIENT

Patient with a Thyroid Nodule Palpable thyroid nodules are found in about 5% of adults, but the prevalence varies considerably worldwide. Given this high prevalence rate, it is common for the practitioner to identify thyroid nodules. The main goal of this evaluation is to identify, in a cost-effective manner, the small subgroup of individuals with malignant lesions.

As described above, nodules are more common in iodine-deficient areas, in women, and with aging. Most palpable nodules are >1 cm in diameter, but the ability to feel a nodule is influenced by its location within the gland (superficial versus deeply embedded), the anatomy of the patient's neck, and the experience of the examiner. More sensitive methods of detection, such as thyroid ultrasound and pathologic studies, reveal thyroid nodules in >20% of glands. These findings have led to much debate about how to detect nodules and which nodules to investigate further. Most authorities still rely on physical examination to detect thyroid nodules, reserving ultrasound for monitoring nodule size or as an aid in thyroid biopsy.

It is important to distinguish whether a patient presents with a solitary thyroid nodule or a prominent nodule in the context of a MNG, as the incidence of malignancy is greater in solitary nodules. An approach to the evaluation of a solitary nodule is outlined in Fig. 320-13. Most patients with thyroid nodules have normal thyroid function tests. Nonetheless, thyroid function should be assessed by measuring a TSH level, which may be suppressed by one or more autonomously functioning nodules. If the TSH is suppressed, a radionuclide scan is indicated to determine if the identified nodule is "hot," as lesions with increased uptake are almost never malignant and FNA is unnecessary. Otherwise, FNA biopsy should be the first step in the evaluation of a thyroid nodule. FNA has good sensitivity and specificity when performed by physicians familiar with the procedure and when the results are interpreted by experienced cytopathologists. The technique is particularly accurate for detecting PTC. The distinction of benign and malignant follicular lesions is often not possible using cytology alone.

In several large studies, FNA biopsies yielded the following findings: 70% benign, 10% malignant or suspicious for malignancy, and 20% nondiagnostic or yielding insufficient material for diagnosis. Characteristic features of malignancy mandate surgery. A diagnosis of follicular neoplasm also warrants surgery, as benign and malignant lesions cannot be distinguished based on cytopathology or frozen section. The management of patients with benign lesions is more variable. Many authorities advocate TSH suppression, whereas others monitor nodule size without suppression. With either approach, thyroid nodule size should be monitored, either by palpation or ultrasound. Repeat FNA is indicated if a nodule enlarges, and a second biopsy should be performed within 2 to 5 years to confirm the benign status of the nodule.

Nondiagnostic biopsies occur for many reasons, including a fibrotic reaction with relatively few cells available for aspiration, a cystic lesion in which cellular components reside along the cyst margin, or a nodule that may be too small for accurate aspiration. For these reasons, ultrasound-guided FNA is useful when the FNA is repeated. Ultrasound is also increasingly used for initial biopsies in an effort to enhance nodule localization and the accuracy of sampling.

The evaluation of a thyroid nodule is stressful for most patients. They are concerned about the possibility of thyroid cancer, whether verbalized or not. It is constructive, therefore, to review the diagnostic approach and to reassure patients when malignancy is not found. When a suspicious lesion or thyroid cancer is identified, an explanation of the generally favorable prognosis and available treatment options should be provided.

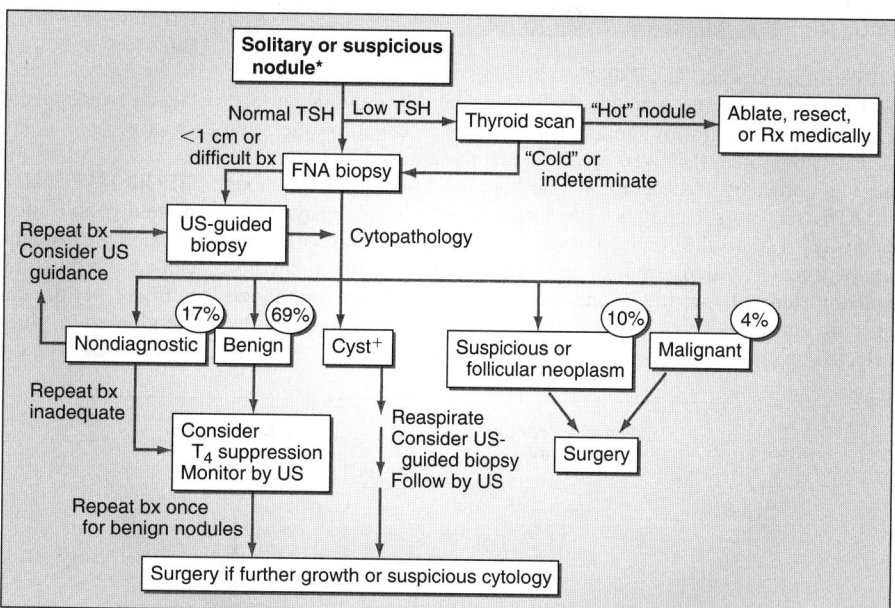

FIGURE 320-13 Approach to the patient with a thyroid nodule. *There are many exceptions to the suggested options. See text and references for details. †About one-third of nodules are cystic or mixed solid-cystic. US, ultrasound; TSH, thyroid-stimulating hormone; FNA, fine-needle aspiration.

FURTHER READING

DELANGE F et al: Iodine deficiency in the world: Where do we stand at the turn of the century? Thyroid 11:5, 2001

KOPP P: Perspective: Genetic defects in the etiology of congenital hypothyroidism. Endocrinology 143:2019, 2002

LADENSON PW et al: American Thyroid Association guidelines for detection of thyroid dysfunction. Arch Intern Med 160:1573, 2000

MAZZAFERRI EL et al: A concensus report of the role of serum thyroglobulin as a monitoring method for low-risk patients with papillary thyroid carcinoma. J Clin Endocrinol Metab 88:1433, 2003

WEETMAN AP: Graves' disease. N Engl J Med 343:1236, 2000

321 DISORDERS OF THE ADRENAL CORTEX
Gordon H. Williams, Robert G. Dluhy

BIOCHEMISTRY AND PHYSIOLOGY

The adrenal cortex produces three major classes of steroids: (1) glucocorticoids, (2) mineralocorticoids, and (3) adrenal androgens. Consequently, normal adrenal function is important for modulating intermediary metabolism and immune responses through glucocorticoids; blood pressure, vascular volume, and electrolytes through mineralocorticoids; and secondary sexual characteristics (in females) through androgens. The adrenal axis plays an important role in the stress response by rapidly increasing cortisol levels. Adrenal disorders include hyperfunction (Cushing's syndrome) and hypofunction (adrenal insufficiency), as well as a variety of genetic abnormalities of steroidogenesis.

STEROID NOMENCLATURE The basic structure of steroids is built upon a five-ring nucleus (Fig. 321-1). The carbon atoms are numbered in a sequence beginning with ring A. Adrenal steroids contain either 19 or 21 carbon atoms. The C_{19} steroids have methyl groups at C-18 and C-19. C_{19} steroids with a ketone group at C-17 are termed *17-ketosteroids*; C_{19} steroids have predominantly androgenic activity. The C_{21} steroids have a 2-carbon side chain (C-20 and C-21) attached at position 17 and methyl groups at C-18 and C-19; C_{21} steroids with a hydroxyl group at position 17 are termed *17-hydroxycorticosteroids*. The C_{21} steroids have either glucocorticoid or mineralocorticoid properties.

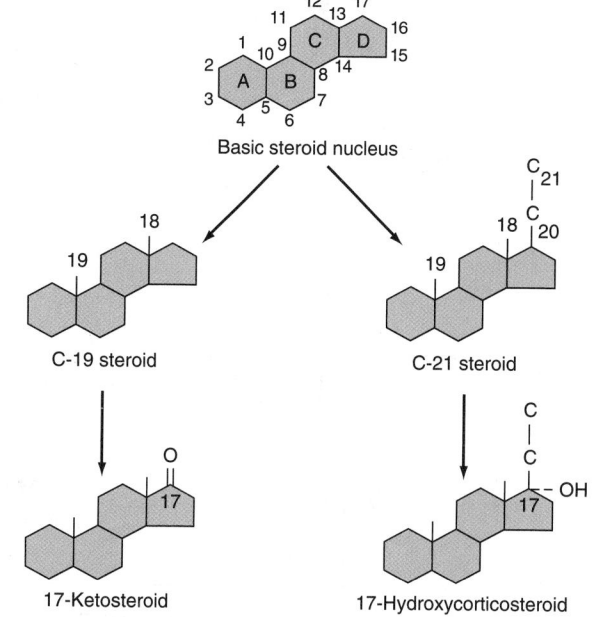

FIGURE 321-1 Basic steroid structure and nomenclature.

BIOSYNTHESIS OF ADRENAL STEROIDS   Cholesterol, derived from the diet and from endogenous synthesis, is the substrate for steroidogenesis. Uptake of cholesterol by the adrenal cortex is mediated by the low-density lipoprotein (LDL) receptor. With long-term stimulation of the adrenal cortex by adrenocorticotropic hormone (ACTH), the number of LDL receptors increases. The three major adrenal biosynthetic pathways lead to the production of glucocorticoids (cortisol), mineralocorticoids (aldosterone), and adrenal androgens (dehydroepiandrosterone). Separate zones of the adrenal cortex synthesize specific hormones (Fig. 321-2). This zonation is accompanied by the selective expression of the genes encoding the enzymes unique to the

formation of each type of steroid: aldosterone synthase is normally expressed only in the outer (glomerulosa) cell layer, whereas 21- and 17-hydroxylase are expressed in the (inner) faciculata-reticularis cell layers, which are the sites of cortisol and androgen biosynthesis, respectively.

STEROID TRANSPORT   Cortisol circulates in the plasma as free cortisol, protein-bound cortisol, and cortisol metabolites. *Free cortisol* is a physiologically active hormone that is not protein-bound and therefore can act directly on tissue sites. Normally, <5% of circulating cortisol is free. Only the unbound cortisol and its metabolites are filterable at the glomerulus. Increased quantities of free steroid are excreted in the urine in states characterized by hypersecretion of cortisol, because the

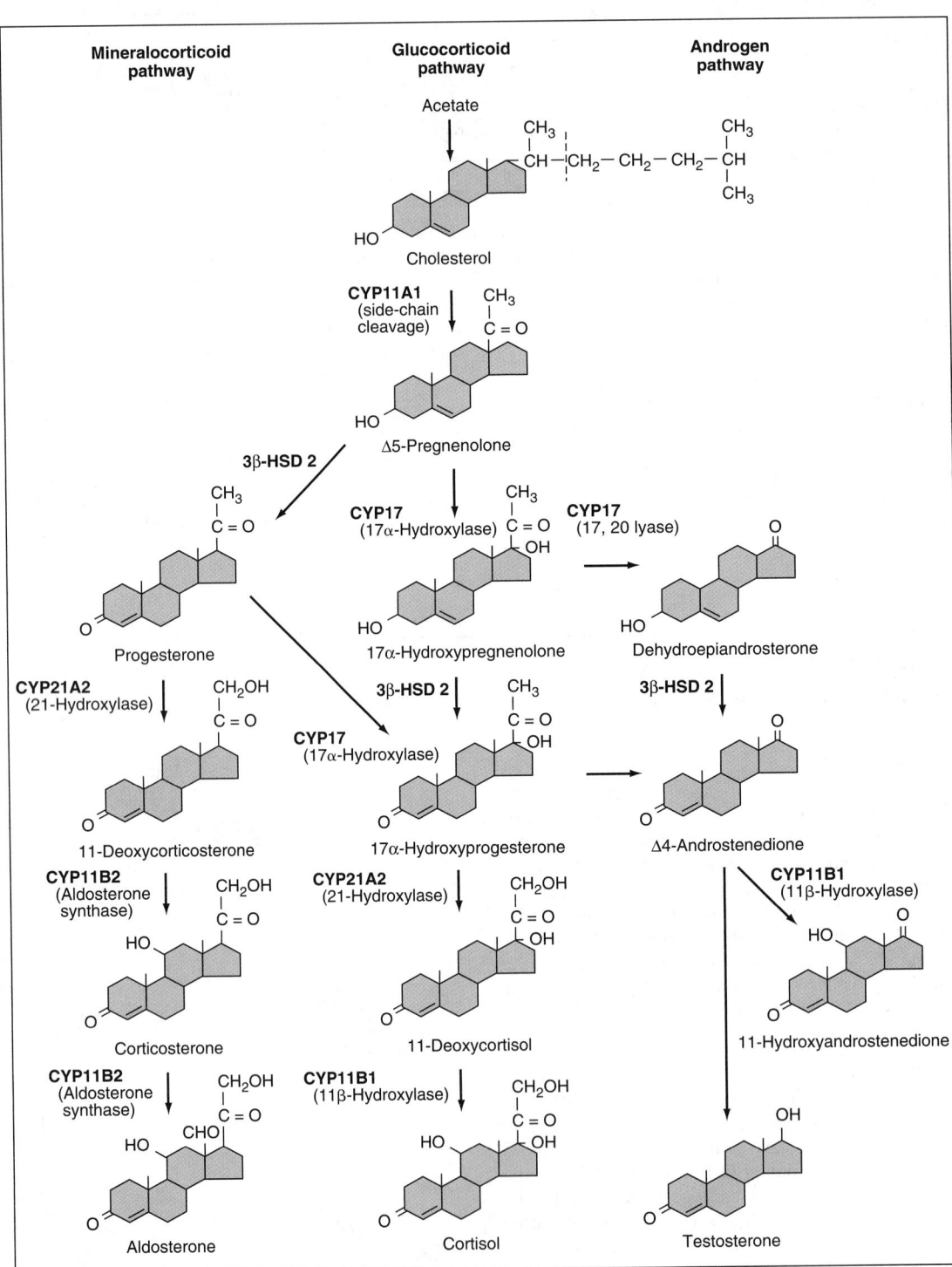

FIGURE 321-2   Biosynthetic pathways for adrenal steroid production; major pathways to mineralocorticoids, glucocorticoids, and androgens. 3β-HSD, 3β-hydroxysteroid dehydrogenase.

unbound fraction of plasma cortisol rises. Plasma has two cortisol-binding systems. One is a high-affinity, low-capacity α_2-globulin termed *transcortin* or *cortisol-binding globulin* (CBG), and the other is a low-affinity, high-capacity protein, *albumin*. Cortisol binding to CBG is reduced in areas of inflammation, thus increasing the local concentration of free cortisol. When the concentration of cortisol is >700 nmol/L (25 μg/dL), part of the excess binds to albumin, and a greater proportion than usual circulates unbound. CBG is increased in high-estrogen states (e.g., pregnancy, oral contraceptive administration). The rise in CBG is accompanied by a parallel rise in *protein-bound cortisol*, with the result that the total plasma cortisol concentration is elevated. However, the free cortisol level probably remains normal, and manifestations of glucocorticoid excess are absent. Most synthetic glucocorticoid analogues bind less efficiently to CBG (~70% binding). This may explain the propensity of some synthetic analogues to produce cushingoid effects at low doses. *Cortisol metabolites* are biologically inactive and bind only weakly to circulating plasma proteins.

Aldosterone is bound to proteins to a smaller extent than cortisol, and an ultrafiltrate of plasma contains as much as 50% of circulating aldosterone.

STEROID METABOLISM AND EXCRETION ■ Glucocorticoids
The daily secretion of cortisol ranges between 40 and 80 μmol (15 and 30 mg; 8–10 mg/m²), with a pronounced circadian cycle. The plasma concentration of cortisol is determined by the rate of secretion, the rate of inactivation, and the rate of excretion of free cortisol. The liver is the major organ responsible for steroid inactivation. A major enzyme regulating cortisol metabolism is 11β-hydroxysteroid dehydrogenase (11β-HSD). There are two isoforms: 11β-HSD I is primarily expressed in the liver and acts as a reductase, converting the inactive cortisone to the active glucocorticoid, cortisol; the 11β-HSD II isoform is expressed in a number of tissues and converts cortisol to the inactive metabolite, cortisone. Mutations in the *11BHSD1* gene are associated with rapid cortisol turnover, leading to activation of the hypothalamic-pituitary-adrenal (HPA) axis and excessive adrenal androgen production in women. In animal models, excess omental expression of 11β-HSD I increases local glucocorticoid production and is associated with central obesity and insulin resistance. The oxidative reaction of 11β-HSD I is increased in hyperthyroidism. Mutations in the *11BHSD2* gene cause the syndrome of *apparent mineralocorticoid excess*, reflecting insufficient inactivation of cortisol in the kidney, allowing inappropriate cortisol activation of the mineralocorticoid receptor (see below).

Mineralocorticoids
In individuals with normal salt intake, the average daily secretion of aldosterone ranges between 0.1 and 0.7 μmol (50 and 250 μg). During a single passage through the liver, >75% of circulating aldosterone is normally inactivated by conjugation with glucuronic acid. However, under certain conditions, such as congestive failure, this rate of inactivation is reduced.

Adrenal Androgens
The major androgen secreted by the adrenal is dehydroepiandrosterone (DHEA) and its sulfuric acid ester (DHEAS). Approximately 15 to 30 mg of these compounds is secreted daily. Smaller amounts of androstenedione, 11β-hydroxyandrostenedione, and testosterone are secreted. DHEA is the major precursor of the urinary 17-ketosteroids. Two-thirds of the urine 17-ketosteroids in the male are derived from adrenal metabolites, and the remaining one-third comes from testicular androgens. In the female, almost all urine 17-ketosteroids are derived from the adrenal.

Steroids diffuse passively through the cell membrane and bind to intracellular receptors (Chap. 317). Glucocorticoids and mineralocorticoids bind with nearly equal affinity to the mineralocorticoid receptor (MR). However, only glucocorticoids bind to the glucocorticoid receptor (GR). After the steroid binds to the receptor, the steroid-receptor complex is transported to the nucleus, where it binds to specific sites on steroid-regulated genes, altering levels of transcription. Some actions of glucocorticoids (e.g., anti-inflammatory effects) are mediated by GR-mediated inhibition of other transcription factors, such as ac-

tivating protein-1 (AP-1) or nuclear factor kappa B (NFκB), which normally stimulate the activity of various cytokine genes. Because cortisol binds to the MR with the same affinity as aldosterone, mineralocorticoid specificity is achieved by local metabolism of cortisol to the inactive compound cortisone by 11β-HSD II. The glucocorticoid effects of other steroids, such as high-dose progesterone, correlate with their relative binding affinities for the GR. Inherited defects in the GR cause glucocorticoid resistance states. Individuals with GR defects have high levels of cortisol but do not have manifestations of hypercortisolism.

ACTH PHYSIOLOGY ACTH and a number of other peptides (lipotropins, endorphins, and melanocyte-stimulating hormones) are processed from a larger precursor molecule of 31,000 mol wt—proopiomelanocortin (POMC) (Chap. 318). POMC is made in a variety of tissues, including brain, anterior and posterior pituitary, and lymphocytes. The constellation of POMC-derived peptides secreted depends on the tissue. ACTH, a 39-amino-acid peptide, is synthesized and stored in basophilic cells of the anterior pituitary. The N-terminal 18-amino-acid fragment of ACTH has full biologic potency, and shorter N-terminal fragments have partial biologic activity. Release of ACTH and related peptides from the anterior pituitary gland is stimulated by corticotropin-releasing hormone (CRH), a 41-amino-acid peptide produced in the median eminence of the hypothalamus (Fig. 321-3). Urocortin, a neuropeptide related to CRH, mimics many of the central effects of CRH (e.g., appetite suppression, anxiety), but its role in ACTH reg-

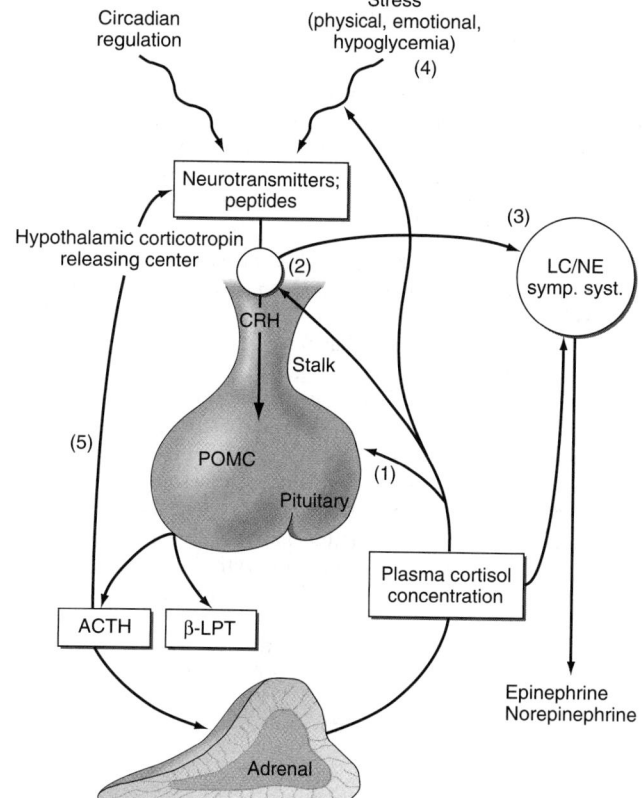

FIGURE 321-3 The hypothalamic-pituitary-adrenal axis. The main sites for feedback control by plasma cortisol are the pituitary gland (1) and the hypothalamic corticotropin-releasing center (2). Feedback control by plasma cortisol also occurs at the locus coeruleus/sympathetic system (3) and may involve higher nerve centers (4) as well. There may also be a short feedback loop involving inhibition of corticotropin-releasing hormone (CRH) by adrenocorticotropic hormone (ACTH) (5). Hypothalamic neurotransmitters influence CRH release; serotoninergic and cholinergic systems stimulate the secretion of CRH and ACTH; α-adrenergic agonists and γ-aminobutyric acid (GABA) probably inhibit CRH release. The opioid peptides β-endorphin and enkephalin inhibit, and vasopressin and angiotensin II augment, the secretion of CRH and ACTH. β-LPT, β-lipotropin; POMC, pro-opiomelanocortin; LC, locus coeruleus; NE, norepinephrine.

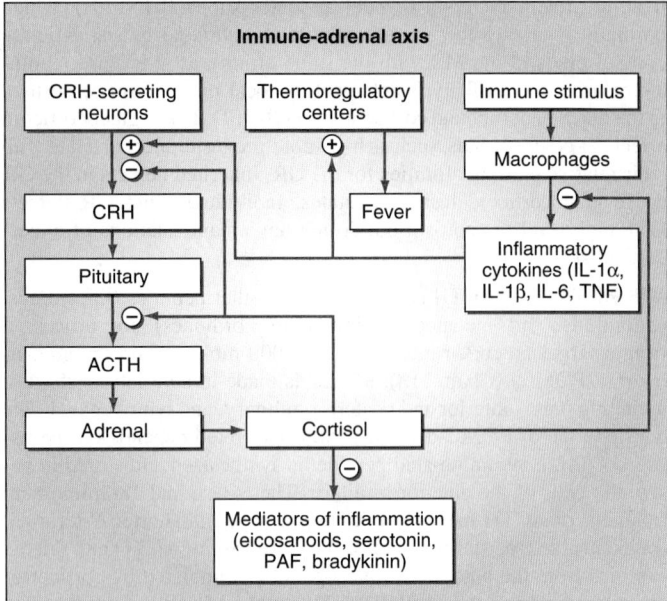

FIGURE 321-4 The immune-adrenal axis. Cortisol has anti-inflammatory properties that include effects on the microvasculature, cellular actions, and the suppression of inflammatory cytokines (the so-called immune-adrenal axis). A stress such as sepsis increases adrenal secretion, and cortisol in turn suppresses the immune response via this system. −, suppression; +, stimulation; CRH, corticotropin-releasing hormone; ACTH, adrenocorticotropic hormone; IL, interleukin; TNF, tumor necrosis factor; PAF, platelet activating factor.

ulation is unclear. Some related peptides such as β-lipotropin (β-LPT) are released in equimolar concentrations with ACTH, suggesting that they are cleaved enzymatically from the parent POMC before or during the secretory process. However, β-endorphin levels may or may not correlate with circulating levels of ACTH, depending on the nature of the stimulus.

The major factors controlling ACTH release include CRH, the free cortisol concentration in plasma, stress, and the sleep-wake cycle (Fig. 321-3). Plasma ACTH varies during the day as a result of its pulsatile secretion, and follows a circadian pattern with a peak just prior to waking and a nadir before sleeping. If a new sleep-wake cycle is adopted, the pattern changes over several days to conform to it. ACTH and cortisol levels also increase in response to eating. Stress (e.g., pyrogens, surgery, hypoglycemia, exercise, and severe emotional trauma) causes the release of CRH and arginine vasopressin (AVP) and activation of the sympathetic nervous system. These changes in turn enhance ACTH release, acting individually or in concert. For example, AVP release acts synergistically with CRH to amplify ACTH secretion; CRH also stimulates the locus coeruleus/sympathetic sys-

tem. Stress-related secretion of ACTH abolishes the circadian periodicity of ACTH levels but is, in turn, suppressed by prior high-dose glucocorticoid administration. The normal pulsatile, circadian pattern of ACTH release is regulated by CRH; this mechanism is the so-called open feedback loop. CRH secretion, in turn, is influenced by hypothalamic neurotransmitters including the serotoninergic and cholinergic pathways. The immune system also influences the HPA axis (Fig. 321-4). For example, inflammatory cytokines [tumor necrosis factor (TNF)-α, interleukin (IL) 1α, IL-1β, and IL-6] produced by monocytes increase ACTH release by stimulating secretion of CRH and/or AVP. Finally, ACTH release is regulated by the level of free cortisol in plasma. Cortisol decreases the responsiveness of pituitary corticotropic cells to CRH; the response of the POMC mRNA to CRH is also inhibited by glucocorticoids. In addition, glucocorticoids inhibit the locus coeruleus/sympathetic system and CRH release. The latter servomechanism establishes the primacy of cortisol in the control of ACTH secretion. The suppression of ACTH secretion that results in adrenal atrophy following *prolonged* glucocorticoid therapy is caused primarily by suppression of hypothalamic CRH release, as exogenous CRH administration in this circumstance produces a rise in plasma ACTH. Cortisol also exerts feedback effects on higher brain centers (hippocampus, reticular system, and septum) and perhaps on the adrenal cortex (Fig. 321-4).

The biologic half-life of ACTH in the circulation is <10 min. The action of ACTH is also rapid; within minutes of its release, the concentration of steroids in the adrenal venous blood increases. ACTH stimulates steroidogenesis via activation of adenyl cyclase. Adenosine-3′,5′-monophosphate (cyclic AMP), in turn, stimulates the synthesis of protein kinase enzymes, thereby resulting in the phosphorylation of proteins that activate steroid biosynthesis.

RENIN-ANGIOTENSIN PHYSIOLOGY Renin is a proteolytic enzyme that is produced and stored in the granules of the juxtaglomerular cells surrounding the afferent arterioles of glomeruli in the kidney. Renin acts on the basic substrate angiotensinogen (a circulating α₂-globulin made in the liver) to form the decapeptide angiotensin I (Fig. 321-5). Angiotensin I is then enzymatically transformed by angiotensin-converting enzyme (ACE), which is present in many tissues (particularly the pulmonary vascular endothelium), to the octapeptide angiotensin II by the removal of the two C-terminal amino acids. Angiotensin II is a potent pressor agent and exerts its action by a direct effect on arteriolar smooth muscle. In addition, angiotensin II stimulates production of aldosterone by the zona glomerulosa of the adrenal cortex; the heptapeptide angiotensin III may also stimulate aldosterone production. The two major classes of angiotensin receptors are termed *AT1* and *AT2*; AT1 may exist as two subtypes α and β. Most of the effects of angiotensins II and III are mediated by the AT1 receptor. Angiotensinases rapidly destroy angiotensin II (half-life, ~1 min), while the half-life of renin is more prolonged (10 to 20 min). In addition to circulating renin-angiotensin, many tissues have a local renin-angiotensin system and the ability to produce angiotensin II. These tissues include the uterus, placenta, vascular tissue, heart, brain, and, particularly, the adrenal cortex and kidney. Although the role of locally generated angiotensin II is not established, it may modulate the growth and function of the adrenal cortex and vascular smooth muscle.

The amount of renin released reflects the combined effects of four interdependent factors. The *juxtaglomerular cells*, which are specialized myoepithelial cells that cuff the afferent arterioles, act as miniature pressure transducers, sensing renal perfusion pressure and corresponding changes in afferent arteriolar perfusion pressures. For example, a reduction in circulating blood volume leads to a corresponding reduction in renal perfusion pressure and

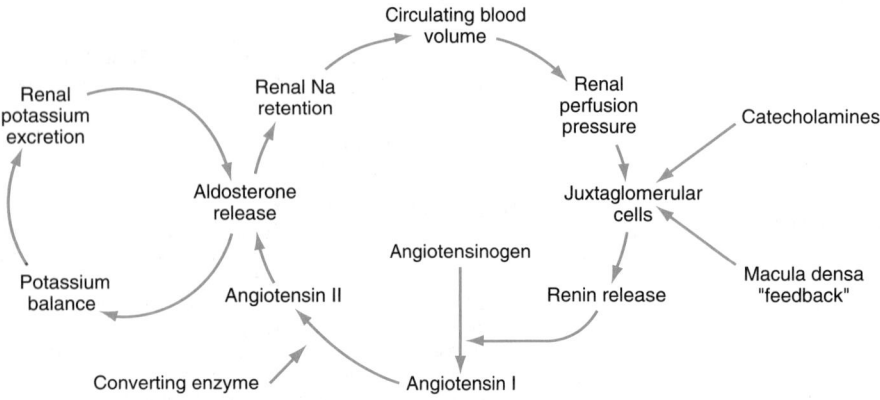

FIGURE 321-5 The interrelationship of the volume and potassium feedback loops on aldosterone secretion. Integration of signals from each loop determines the level of aldosterone secretion.

afferent arteriolar pressure (Fig. 321-5). This change is perceived by the juxtaglomerular cells as a decreased stretch exerted on the afferent arteriolar walls, and the juxtaglomerular cells release more renin into the renal circulation. This results in the formation of angiotensin I, which is converted in the kidney and peripherally to angiotensin II by ACE. Angiotensin II influences sodium homeostasis via two major mechanisms: it changes renal blood flow so as to maintain a constant glomerular filtration rate, thereby changing the filtration fraction of sodium, and it stimulates the adrenal cortex to release aldosterone. Increasing plasma levels of aldosterone enhance renal sodium retention and thus result in expansion of the extracellular fluid volume, which, in turn, dampens the stimulus for renin release. In this context, the renin-angiotensin-aldosterone system regulates volume by modifying renal hemodynamics and tubular sodium transport.

A second control mechanism for renin release is centered in the *macula densa cells*, a group of distal convoluted tubular epithelial cells directly opposed to the juxtaglomerular cells. They may function as chemoreceptors, monitoring the sodium (or chloride) load presented to the distal tubule. Under conditions of increased delivery of filtered sodium to the macula densa, a signal is conveyed to decrease juxtaglomerular cell release of renin, thereby modulating the glomerular filtration rate and the filtered load of sodium.

The *sympathetic nervous system* regulates the release of renin in response to assumption of the upright posture. The mechanism is either a direct effect on the juxtaglomerular cell to increase adenyl cyclase activity or an indirect effect on either the juxtaglomerular or the macula densa cells via vasoconstriction of the afferent arteriole.

Finally, circulating factors influence renin release. Increased dietary intake of potassium decreases renin release, whereas decreased potassium intake increases it. The significance of these effects is unclear. *Angiotensin II* exerts negative feedback control on renin release that is independent of alterations in renal blood flow, blood pressure, or aldosterone secretion. *Atrial natriuretic peptides* also inhibit renin release. Thus, the control of renin release involves both *intrarenal* (pressor receptor and macula densa) and *extrarenal* (sympathetic nervous system, potassium, angiotensin, etc.) mechanisms. Steady-state renin levels reflect all these factors, with the intrarenal mechanism predominating.

GLUCOCORTICOID PHYSIOLOGY The division of adrenal steroids into glucocorticoids and mineralocorticoids is arbitrary in that most glucocorticoids have some mineralocorticoid-like properties. The descriptive term *glucocorticoid* is used for adrenal steroids whose predominant action is on intermediary metabolism. Their overall actions are directed at enhancing the production of the high-energy fuel, glucose, and reducing all other metabolic activity not directly involved in that process. Sustained activation, however, results in a pathophysiologic state, e.g., Cushing's syndrome. The principal glucocorticoid is cortisol (hydrocortisone). The effect of glucocorticoids on intermediary metabolism is mediated by the GR. Physiologic effects of glucocorticoids include the regulation of protein, carbohydrate, lipid, and nucleic acid metabolism. Glucocorticoids raise the blood glucose level by antagonizing the secretion and actions of insulin, thereby inhibiting peripheral glucose uptake, which promotes hepatic glucose synthesis (gluconeogenesis) and hepatic glycogen content. The actions on protein metabolism are mainly catabolic, resulting in an increase in protein breakdown and nitrogen excretion. In large part, these actions reflect a mobilization of glycogenic amino acid precursors from peripheral supporting structures, such as bone, skin, muscle, and connective tissue, due to protein breakdown and inhibition of protein synthesis and amino acid uptake. Hyperaminoacidemia also facilitates gluconeogenesis by stimulating glucagon secretion. Glucocorticoids act directly on the liver to stimulate the synthesis of certain enzymes, such as tyrosine aminotransferase and tryptophan pyrrolase. Glucocorticoids regulate fatty acid mobilization by enhancing the activation of cellular lipase by lipid-mobilizing hormones (e.g., catecholamines and pituitary peptides).

The actions of cortisol on protein and adipose tissue vary in dif-

ferent parts of the body. For example, pharmacologic doses of cortisol can deplete the protein matrix of the vertebral column (trabecular bone), whereas long bones (which are primarily compact bone) are affected only minimally; similarly, peripheral adipose tissue mass decreases, whereas abdominal and interscapular fat expand.

Glucocorticoids have anti-inflammatory properties, which are probably related to effects on the microvasculature and to suppression of inflammatory cytokines. In this sense, glucocorticoids modulate the immune response via the so-called immune-adrenal axis (Fig. 321-4). This "loop" is one mechanism by which a stress, such as sepsis, increases adrenal hormone secretion, and the elevated cortisol level in turn suppresses the immune response. For example, cortisol maintains vascular responsiveness to circulating vasoconstrictors and opposes the increase in capillary permeability during acute inflammation. Glucocorticoids cause a leukocytosis that reflects release from the bone marrow of mature cells as well as inhibition of their egress through the capillary wall. Glucocorticoids produce a depletion of circulating eosinophils and lymphoid tissue, specifically T cells, by causing a redistribution from the circulation into other compartments. Thus, cortisol impairs cell-mediated immunity. Glucocorticoids also inhibit the production and action of the mediators of inflammation, such as the lymphokines and prostaglandins. Glucocorticoids inhibit the production and action of interferon by T lymphocytes and the production of IL-1 and IL-6 by macrophages. The antipyretic action of glucocorticoids may be explained by an effect on IL-1, which appears to be an endogenous pyrogen (Chap. 16). Glucocorticoids also inhibit the production of T cell growth factor (IL-2) by T lymphocytes. Glucocorticoids reverse macrophage activation and antagonize the action of migration-inhibiting factor (MIF), leading to reduced adherence of macrophages to vascular endothelium. Glucocorticoids reduce prostaglandin and leukotriene production by inhibiting the activity of phospholipase A_2, thus blocking release of arachidonic acid from phospholipids. Finally, glucocorticoids inhibit the production and inflammatory effects of bradykinin, platelet-activating factor, and serotonin. It is probably only at pharmacologic dosages that antibody production is reduced and lysosomal membranes are stabilized, the latter effect suppressing the release of acid hydrolases.

Cortisol levels respond within minutes to stress, whether physical (trauma, surgery, exercise), psychological (anxiety, depression), or physiologic (hypoglycemia, fever). The reasons why elevated glucocorticoid levels protect the organism under stress are not understood, but in conditions of glucocorticoid deficiency, such stresses may cause hypotension, shock, and death. Consequently, in individuals with adrenal insufficiency, glucocorticoid administration should be increased during stress.

Cortisol has major effects on body water. It helps regulate the extracellular fluid volume by retarding the migration of water into cells and by promoting renal water excretion, the latter effect mediated by suppression of vasopressin secretion, by an increase in the rate of glomerular filtration, and by a direct action on the renal tubule. The consequence is to prevent water intoxication by increasing solute-free water clearance. Glucocorticoids also have weak mineralocorticoid-like properties, and high doses promote renal tubular sodium reabsorption and increased urine potassium excretion. Glucocorticoids can also influence behavior; emotional disorders may occur with either an excess or a deficit of cortisol. Finally, cortisol suppresses the secretion of pituitary POMC and its derivative peptides (ACTH, β-endorphin, and β-LPT) and the secretion of hypothalamic CRH and vasopressin.

MINERALOCORTICOID PHYSIOLOGY Mineralocorticoids modify function in two classes of cells—epithelial and nonepithelial.

Effects on Epithelia Classically, mineralocorticoids are considered major regulators of extracellular fluid volume and are the major determinants of potassium metabolism. These effects are mediated by the binding of aldosterone to the MR in epithelial cells, primarily the principal cells in the renal cortical collecting duct. Because of its electrochemical gradient, sodium passively enters these cells from the urine via epithelial sodium channels located on the luminal membrane and is actively extruded from the cell via the Na/K-activated ATPase ("sodium pump") located on the basolateral membrane. The sodium pump also provides the driving force of potassium loss into the urine through potassium-selective luminal channels, again assisted by the electrochemical gradient for potassium in these cells. Aldosterone stimulates all three of these processes by increasing gene expression directly (for the sodium pump and the potassium channels) or via a complex process (for epithelial sodium channels) to increase both the number and activity of the sodium channels. Water passively follows the transported sodium, thus expanding intra- and extravascular volume.

Because the concentration of hydrogen ion is greater in the lumen than in the cell, hydrogen ion is also actively secreted. Mineralocorticoids also act on the epithelium of the salivary ducts, sweat glands, and gastrointestinal tract to cause reabsorption of sodium in exchange for potassium.

When normal individuals are given aldosterone, an initial period of sodium retention is followed by natriuresis, and sodium balance is reestablished after 3 to 5 days. As a result, edema does not develop. This process is referred to as the *escape phenomenon*, signifying an "escape" by the renal tubules from the sodium-retaining action of aldosterone. While renal hemodynamic factors may play a role in the escape, the level of atrial natriuretic peptide also increases. However, it is important to realize that there is no escape from the potassium-losing effects of mineralocorticoids.

Effect on Nonepithelial Cells   The MR has been identified in a number of nonepithelial cells, e.g., neurons in the brain, myocytes, endothelial cells, and vascular smooth-muscle cells. In these cells, the actions of aldosterone differ from those in epithelial cells in several ways:

1. They do not modify sodium-potassium homeostasis.
2. The groups of regulated genes differ, although only a few are known; for example, in nonepithelial cells, aldosterone modifies the expression of several collagen genes and/or genes controlling tissue growth factors, e.g., transforming growth factor (TGF) β and plasminogen activator inhibitor, type 1 (PAI-1).
3. In some of these tissues (e.g., myocardium and brain), the MR is not protected by the 11β-HSD II enzyme. Thus, cortisol rather than aldosterone may be activating the MR. In other tissues (e.g., the vasculature), 11β-HSD II is expressed in a manner similar to that of the kidney. Therefore, aldosterone is activating the MR.
4. Some effects on nonepithelial cells may be via nongenomic mechanisms. These actions are too rapid—occurring within 1 to 2 min and peaking within 5 to 10 min—to be considered genomic, suggesting that they are secondary to activation of a cell-surface receptor. However, no cell-surface MR has been identified, raising the possibility that the same MR is mediating both genomic and nongenomic effects. Rapid, nongenomic effects have also been described for other steroids including estradiol, progesterone, thyroxine, and vitamin D.
5. Some of these tissues—the myocardium and vasculature—may also produce aldosterone, although this theory is controversial.

Regulation of Aldosterone Secretion   Three primary mechanisms control adrenal aldosterone secretion: the renin-angiotensin system, potassium, and ACTH (Table 321-1). Whether these are also the primary regulatory mechanisms modifying nonadrenal production is uncertain. The renin-angiotensin system controls extracellular fluid volume via regulation of aldosterone secretion (Fig. 321-5). In effect, the renin-angiotensin system maintains the circulating blood volume constant by causing aldosterone-induced sodium retention during volume deficiency and by decreasing aldosterone-dependent sodium retention when volume is ample. There is an increasing body of evidence indicating that some tissues, in addition to the kidney, produce angiotensin II and may participate in the regulation of aldosterone secretion either from the adrenal or extraadrenal sources. Intriguingly, the ad-

TABLE 321-1   *Factors Regulating Aldosterone Biosynthesis*

Factor	Effect
Renin-angiotensin system	Stimulation
Sodium ion	Inhibition (?physiologic)
Potassium ion	Stimulation
Neurotransmitters	
Dopamine	Inhibition
Serotonin	Stimulation
Pituitary hormones	
ACTH	Stimulation
Non-ACTH pituitary hormones (e.g., growth hormone)	Permissive (for optimal response to sodium restriction)
β-Endorphin	Stimulation
γ-Melanocyte-stimulating hormone	Permissive
Atrial natriuretic peptide	Inhibition
Ouabain-like factors	Inhibition
Endothelin	Stimulation

Note: ACTH, adrenocorticotropic hormone.

renal itself is capable of synthesizing angiotensin II. What role(s) the extrarenal production of angiotensin II plays in normal physiology is still largely unknown. However, the tissue renin-angiotensin system is activated in utero in response to growth and development and/or later in life in response to injury.

Potassium ion directly stimulates aldosterone secretion, independent of the circulating renin-angiotensin system, which it suppresses (Fig. 321-5). In addition to a direct effect, potassium also modifies aldosterone secretion indirectly by activating the local renin-angiotensin system in the zona glomerulosa. This effect can be blocked by the administration of ACE inhibitors that reduce the local production of angiotensin II and thereby reduce the acute aldosterone response to potassium. An increase in serum potassium of as little as 0.1 mmol/L increases plasma aldosterone levels under certain circumstances. Oral potassium loading therefore increases aldosterone secretion, plasma levels, and excretion.

Physiologic amounts of ACTH stimulate aldosterone secretion acutely, but this action is not sustained unless ACTH is administered in a pulsatile fashion. Most studies relegate ACTH to a minor role in the control of aldosterone. For example, subjects receiving high-dose glucocorticoid therapy, and with presumed complete suppression of ACTH, have normal aldosterone secretion in response to sodium restriction.

Prior dietary intake of both potassium and sodium can alter the magnitude of the aldosterone response to acute stimulation. This effect results from a change in the expression and activity of aldosterone synthase. Increasing potassium intake or decreasing sodium intake sensitizes the response of the glomerulosa cells to acute stimulation by ACTH, angiotensin II, and/or potassium.

Neurotransmitters (dopamine and serotonin) and some peptides, such as atrial natriuretic peptide, γ-melanocyte-stimulating hormone (γ-MSH), and β-endorphin, also participate in the regulation of aldosterone secretion (Table 321-1). Thus, the control of aldosterone secretion involves both stimulatory and inhibitory factors.

ANDROGEN PHYSIOLOGY   Androgens regulate male secondary sexual characteristics and can cause virilizing symptoms in women (Chap. 44). Adrenal androgens have a minimal effect in males whose sexual characteristics are predominately determined by gonadal steroids (testosterone). In females, however, several androgen-like effects, e.g., sexual hair, are largely mediated by adrenal androgens. The principal adrenal androgens are DHEA, androstenedione, and 11-hydroxyandrostenedione. DHEA and androstenedione are weak androgens and exert their effects via conversion to the potent androgen testosterone in extraglandular tissues. DHEA also has poorly understood effects on the immune and cardiovascular systems. Adrenal androgen formation is regulated by ACTH, not by gonadotropins. Adrenal androgens are suppressed by exogenous glucocorticoid administration.

A basic assumption is that measurements of the plasma or urinary level of a given steroid reflect the rate of adrenal *secretion* of that steroid. However, urine *excretion* values may not truly reflect the secretion rate because of improper collection or altered metabolism. Plasma levels reflect the level of secretion only at the time of measurement. The plasma level (*PL*) depends on two factors: the secretion rate (*SR*) of the hormone and the rate at which it is metabolized, i.e., its metabolic clearance rate (*MCR*). These three factors can be related as follows:

$$PL = \frac{SR}{MCR} \quad or \quad SR = MCR \times PL$$

BLOOD LEVELS ■ Peptides The plasma levels of ACTH and angiotensin II can be measured by immunoassay techniques. Basal ACTH secretion shows a circadian rhythm, with lower levels in the early evening than in the morning. However, ACTH is secreted in a pulsatile manner, leading to rapid fluctuations superimposed on this circadian rhythm. Angiotensin II levels also vary diurnally and are influenced by dietary sodium and potassium intakes and posture. Both upright posture and sodium restriction elevate angiotensin II levels.

Most clinical determinations of the renin-angiotensin system, however, involve measurements of peripheral *plasma renin activity* (PRA) in which the renin activity is gauged by the generation of angiotensin I during a standardized incubation period. This method depends on the presence of sufficient angiotensinogen in the plasma as substrate. The generated angiotensin I is measured by radioimmunoassay. The PRA depends on the dietary sodium intake and on whether the patient is ambulatory. In normal humans, the PRA shows a diurnal rhythm characterized by peak values in the morning and a nadir in the afternoon. An alternative approach is to measure plasma active renin, which is easier and not dependent on endogenous substrate concentration. PRA and active renin correlate very well on low-sodium diets but less well on high-sodium diets.

Steroids Cortisol and aldosterone are both secreted episodically, and levels vary during the day, with peak values in the morning and low levels in the evening. In addition, the plasma level of aldosterone, but not of cortisol, is increased by dietary potassium loading, by sodium restriction, or by assumption of the upright posture. Measurement of the sulfate conjugate of DHEA may be a useful index of adrenal androgen secretion, as little DHEA sulfate is formed in the gonads and because the half-life of DHEA sulfate is 7 to 9 h. However, DHEA sulfate levels reflect both DHEA production and sulfatase activity.

URINE LEVELS For the assessment of glucocorticoid secretion, the urine 17-hydroxycorticosteroid assay has been replaced by measurement of urinary free cortisol. Elevated levels of urinary free cortisol correlate with states of hypercortisolism, reflecting changes in the levels of unbound, physiologically active circulating cortisol. Normally, the rate of excretion is higher in the daytime (7 A.M. to 7 P.M.) than at night (7 P.M. to 7 A.M.).

Urinary 17-ketosteroids originate in either the adrenal gland or the gonad. In normal women, 90% of urinary 17-ketosteroids is derived from the adrenal, and in men 60 to 70% is of adrenal origin. Urine 17-ketosteroid values are highest in young adults and decline with age.

A carefully timed urine collection is a prerequisite for all excretory determinations. Urinary creatinine should be measured simultaneously to determine the accuracy and adequacy of the collection procedure.

STIMULATION TESTS Stimulation tests are useful in the diagnosis of hormone deficiency states.

Tests of Glucocorticoid Reserve Within minutes after administration of ACTH, cortisol levels increase. This responsiveness can be used as an index of the functional reserve of the adrenal gland for production of cortisol. Under maximal ACTH stimulation, cortisol secretion increases tenfold, to 800 μmol/d (300 mg/d), but maximal stimulation can be achieved only with prolonged ACTH infusions.

A screening test (the so-called rapid ACTH stimulation test) involves the administration of 25 units (0.25 mg) of cosyntropin intra-venously or intramuscularly and measurement of plasma cortisol levels before administration and 30 and 60 min after administration, the test can be performed at any time of the day. The most clear-cut criterion for a normal response is a stimulated cortisol level of >500 nmol/L (>18 μg/dL), and the minimal stimulated normal increment of cortisol is >200 nmol/L (>7 μg/dL) above baseline. Severely ill patients with elevated basal cortisol levels may show no further increases following acute ACTH administration.

Tests of Mineralocorticoid Reserve and Stimulation of the Renin-Angiotensin System Stimulation tests use protocols designed to create a programmed volume depletion, such as sodium restriction, diuretic administration, or upright posture. A simple, potent test consists of severe sodium restriction and upright posture. After 3 to 5 days of a 10-mmol/d sodium intake, rates of aldosterone secretion or excretion should increase two- to threefold over the control values. Supine morning plasma aldosterone levels are usually increased three- to sixfold, and they increase a further two- to fourfold in response to 2 to 3 h of upright posture.

When the dietary sodium intake is normal, stimulation testing requires the administration of a potent diuretic, such as 40 to 80 mg furosemide, followed by 2 to 3 h of upright posture. The normal response is a two- to fourfold rise in plasma aldosterone levels.

SUPPRESSION TESTS Suppression tests to document hypersecretion of adrenal hormones involve measurement of the target hormone response after standardized suppression of its tropic hormone.

Tests of Pituitary-Adrenal Suppressibility The ACTH release mechanism is sensitive to the circulating glucocorticoid level. When blood levels of glucocorticoid are increased in normal individuals, less ACTH is released from the anterior pituitary and less steroid is produced by the adrenal gland. The integrity of this feedback mechanism can be tested clinically by giving a glucocorticoid and judging the suppression of ACTH secretion by analysis of urine steroid levels and/or plasma cortisol and ACTH levels. A potent glucocorticoid such as dexamethasone is used, so that the agent can be given in an amount small enough not to contribute significantly to the pool of steroids to be analyzed.

The best *screening* procedure is the overnight dexamethasone suppression test. This involves the measurement of plasma cortisol levels at 8 A.M. following the oral administration of 1 mg dexamethasone the previous midnight. The 8 A.M. value for plasma cortisol in normal individuals should be <140 nmol/L (5 μg/dL).

The definitive test of adrenal suppressibility involves administering 0.5 mg dexamethasone every 6 h for two successive days while collecting urine over a 24-h period for determination of creatinine and free cortisol and/or measuring plasma cortisol levels. In a patient with a normal hypothalamic-pituitary ACTH release mechanism, a fall in the urine free cortisol to <25 nmol/d (10 μg/d) or of plasma cortisol to <140 nmol/L (5 μg/dL) is seen on the second day of administration.

A normal response to either suppression test implies that the glucocorticoid regulation of ACTH and its control of the adrenal glands is physiologically normal. However, an isolated abnormal result, particularly to the overnight suppression test, does not in itself demonstrate pituitary and/or adrenal disease.

Tests of Mineralocorticoid Suppressibility These tests rely on an expansion of extracellular fluid volume, which should decrease circulating plasma renin activity and decrease the secretion and/or excretion of aldosterone. Various tests differ in the rate at which extracellular fluid volume is expanded. One convenient suppression test involves the intravenous infusion of 500 mL/h of normal saline solution for 4 h, which normally suppresses plasma aldosterone levels to <220 pmol/L (<8 ng/dL) from a sodium-restricted diet or to <140 pmol/L (<5 ng/dL) from a normal sodium intake. Alternatively, a high-sodium diet can be administered for 3 days with 0.2 mg fludrocortisone twice daily. Aldosterone excretion is measured on the third day and should be <28 nmol/d (10 μg/d). These tests should not be performed in potassium-depleted individuals since they carry a risk of precipitating hypokalemia.

TESTS OF PITUITARY-ADRENAL RESPONSIVENESS   Stimuli such as insulin-induced hypoglycemia, AVP, and pyrogens induce the release of ACTH from the pituitary by an action on higher neural centers or on the pituitary itself. Insulin-induced hypoglycemia is particularly useful, because it stimulates the release of both growth hormone and ACTH. In this test, regular insulin (0.05 to 0.1 U/kg body weight) is given intravenously as a bolus to reduce the fasting glucose level to at least 50% below basal. The normal cortisol response is a rise to >500 nmol/L (18 μg/dL). Glucose levels must be monitored during insulin-induced hypoglycemia, and it should be terminated by feeding or intravenous glucose, if subjects develop symptoms of hypoglycemia. This test is contraindicated in individuals with coronary artery disease or a seizure disorder.

Metyrapone inhibits 11β-hydroxylase in the adrenal. As a result, the conversion of 11-deoxycortisol (compound S) to cortisol is impaired, causing 11-deoxycortisol to accumulate in the blood and the blood level of cortisol to decrease (Fig. 321-2). The hypothalamic-pituitary axis responds to the declining cortisol blood levels by releasing more ACTH. Note that assessment of the response depends on both an intact hypothalamic-pituitary axis and an intact adrenal gland.

Although modifications of the original metyrapone test have been described, a commonly used protocol involves administering 750 mg of the drug by mouth every 4 h over a 24-h period and comparing the control and postmetyrapone plasma levels of 11-deoxycortisol, cortisol, and ACTH. In normal individuals, plasma 11-deoxycortisol levels should exceed 210 nmol/L (7 μg/dL) and ACTH levels should exceed 17 pmol/L (75 pg/mL) following metyrapone administration. The metyrapone test does not accurately reflect ACTH reserve if subjects are ingesting exogenous glucocorticoids or drugs that accelerate the metabolism of metyrapone (e.g., phenytoin).

A direct and selective test of the pituitary corticotrophs can be achieved with CRH. The bolus injection of ovine CRH (corticorelin ovine triflutate; 1 μg/kg body weight) stimulates secretion of ACTH and β-LPT in normal human subjects within 15 to 60 min. In normal individuals, the mean increment in ACTH is 9 pmol/L (40 pg/mL). However, the magnitude of the ACTH response is less than that produced by insulin-induced hypoglycemia, implying that additional factors (such as vasopressin) augment stress-induced increases in ACTH secretion.

The rapid ACTH test can often distinguish between primary and secondary adrenal insufficiency, because aldosterone secretion is preserved in secondary adrenal failure by the renin-angiotensin system and potassium. Cosyntropin (25 units) is given intravenously or intramuscularly, and plasma cortisol and aldosterone levels are measured before and at 30 and 60 min after administration. The cortisol response is abnormal in both groups, but patients with secondary insufficiency show an increase in aldosterone levels of at least 140 pmol/L (5 ng/dL). No aldosterone response is seen in patients in whom the adrenal cortex is destroyed. Alternatively, ACTH at a physiologic dose (1 μg), the so-called low-dose ACTH test, may be used to detect secondary adrenal insufficiency. An abnormal response is similar to that in the rapid ACTH test. However, levels need to be measured at 30 min, and the ACTH needs to be directly injected intravenously because it can be absorbed by plastic tubing. Because the use of a bolus of exogenous ACTH does not invariably exclude a diagnosis of secondary adrenocortical insufficiency, direct tests of pituitary ACTH reserve (metyrapone test, insulin-induced hypoglycemia) may be required in the appropriate clinical setting.

HYPERFUNCTION OF THE ADRENAL CORTEX

Excess cortisol is associated with Cushing's syndrome; excess aldosterone causes aldosteronism; and excess adrenal androgens cause adrenal virilism. These syndromes do not always occur in the "pure" form but may have overlapping features.

CUSHING'S SYNDROME ■ Etiology   Cushing described a syndrome characterized by truncal obesity, hypertension, fatigability and weakness, amenorrhea, hirsutism, purplish abdominal striae, edema, glucosuria, osteoporosis, and a basophilic tumor of the pituitary. As awareness of this syndrome has increased, the diagnosis of Cushing's syndrome has been broadened into the classification shown in Table 321-2. Regardless of etiology, all cases of endogenous Cushing's syndrome are due to increased production of cortisol by the adrenal. In most cases the cause is *bilateral adrenal hyperplasia* due to hypersecretion of pituitary ACTH or ectopic production of ACTH by a nonpituitary source. The incidence of pituitary-dependent adrenal hyperplasia is three times greater in women than in men, and the most frequent age of onset is the third or fourth decade. Most evidence indicates that the primary defect is the de novo development of a pituitary adenoma, as tumors are found in >90% of patients with pituitary-dependent adrenal hyperplasia. Alternatively, the defect may occasionally reside in the hypothalamus or in higher neural centers, leading to release of CRH inappropriate to the level of circulating cortisol. This primary defect leads to hyperstimulation of the pituitary, resulting in hyperplasia or tumor formation. In surgical series, most individuals with hypersecretion of pituitary ACTH are found to have a microadenoma (<10 mm in diameter; 50% are ≤5 mm in diameter), but a pituitary macroadenoma (>10 mm) or diffuse hyperplasia of the corticotrope cells may be found. Traditionally, only an individual who has an ACTH-producing pituitary tumor is defined as having *Cushing's disease*, whereas Cushing's syndrome refers to all causes of excess cortisol: exogenous ACTH tumor, adrenal tumor, pituitary ACTH-secreting tumor, or excessive glucocorticoid treatment.

The *ectopic ACTH syndrome* is caused by nonpituitary tumors that secrete either ACTH and/or CRH and cause bilateral adrenal hyperplasia (Chap. 86). The ectopic production of CRH results in clinical, biochemical, and radiologic features indistinguishable from those caused by hypersecretion of pituitary ACTH. The typical signs and symptoms of Cushing's syndrome may be absent or minimal with ectopic ACTH production, and hypokalemic alkalosis is a prominent manifestation. Most of these cases are associated with the primitive small cell (oat cell) type of bronchogenic carcinoma or with carcinoid tumors of the thymus, pancreas, or ovary; medullary carcinoma of the thyroid; or bronchial adenomas. The onset of Cushing's syndrome may be sudden, particularly in patients with carcinoma of the lung, and this feature accounts in part for the failure of these patients to exhibit the classic manifestations. On the other hand, patients with carcinoid tumors or pheochromocytomas have longer clinical courses and usually exhibit the typical cushingoid features. The ectopic secretion of ACTH is also accompanied by the accumulation of ACTH fragments in plasma and by elevated plasma levels of ACTH precursor molecules.

TABLE 321-2   *Causes of Cushing's Syndrome*

Adrenal hyperplasia
  Secondary to pituitary ACTH overproduction
    Pituitary-hypothalamic dysfunction
    Pituitary ACTH-producing micro- or macroadenomas
  Secondary to ACTH or CRH-producing nonendocrine tumors
    (bronchogenic carcinoma, carcinoid of the thymus, pancreatic
    carcinoma, bronchial adenoma)
Adrenal macronodular hyperplasia (including ectopic expression of GIP
  receptors in the adrenal cortex)
Adrenal micronodular dysplasia
  Sporadic
  Familial (Carney's syndrome)
Adrenal neoplasia
  Adenoma
  Carcinoma
Exogenous, iatrogenic causes
  Prolonged use of glucocorticoids
  Prolonged use of ACTH

Note: ACTH, adrenocorticotropic hormone; CRH, corticotropin-releasing hormone; GIP, gastric inhibitory peptide.

Because such tumors may produce large amounts of ACTH, baseline steroid values are usually very high and increased skin pigmentation may be present.

Approximately 20 to 25% of patients with Cushing's syndrome have an adrenal neoplasm. These tumors are usually unilateral, and about half are malignant. Occasionally, patients have biochemical features both of pituitary ACTH excess and of an adrenal adenoma. These individuals may have *nodular hyperplasia* of both adrenal glands, often the result of prolonged ACTH stimulation in the absence of a pituitary adenoma. Two additional entities cause nodular hyperplasia: a familial disorder in children or young adults (so-called pigmented micronodular dysplasia; see below) and an abnormal cortisol response to gastric inhibitory polypeptide or luteinizing hormone, secondary to ectopic expression of receptors for these hormones in the adrenal cortex.

The most common cause of Cushing's syndrome is *iatrogenic* administration of steroids for a variety of reasons. Although the clinical features bear some resemblance to those seen with adrenal tumors, these patients are usually distinguishable on the basis of history and laboratory studies.

Clinical Signs, Symptoms, and Laboratory Findings Many of the signs and symptoms of Cushing's syndrome follow logically from the known action of glucocorticoids (Table 321-3). Catabolic responses in peripheral supportive tissue causes muscle weakness and fatigability, osteoporosis, broad violaceous cutaneous striae, and easy bruisability. The latter signs are secondary to weakening and rupture of collagen fibers in the dermis. Osteoporosis may cause collapse of vertebral bodies and pathologic fractures of other bones. Decreased bone mineralization is particularly pronounced in children. Increased hepatic gluconeogenesis and insulin resistance can cause impaired glucose tolerance. Overt diabetes mellitus occurs in <20% of patients, who probably are individuals with a predisposition to this disorder. Hypercortisolism promotes the deposition of adipose tissue in characteristic sites, notably the upper face (producing the typical "moon" facies), the interscapular area (producing the "buffalo hump"), supraclavicular fat pads, and the mesenteric bed (producing "truncal" obesity) (Fig. 321-6). Rarely, episternal fatty tumors and mediastinal widening secondary to fat accumulation occur. The reason for this peculiar distribution of adipose tissue is not known, but it is associated with insulin resistance and/or elevated insulin levels. The face appears plethoric, even in the absence of any increase in red blood cell concentration. Hypertension is common, and emotional changes may be profound, ranging from irritability and emotional lability to severe depression, confusion, or even frank psychosis. In women, increased levels of adrenal androgens can cause acne, hirsutism, and oligomenorrhea or amenorrhea. Some signs and symptoms in patients with hypercortisolism—i.e., obesity, hypertension, osteoporosis, and diabetes—are nonspecific and therefore are less helpful in diagnosing the condition. On the other hand, easy bruising, typical striae, myopathy, and virilizing signs (although less frequent) are, if present, more suggestive of Cushing's syndrome (Table 321-3).

Except in iatrogenic Cushing's syndrome, plasma and urine cortisol levels are elevated. Occasionally, hypokalemia, hypochloremia, and metabolic alkalosis are present, particularly with ectopic production of ACTH.

Diagnosis The diagnosis of Cushing's syndrome depends on the demonstration of increased cortisol production and failure to suppress cortisol secretion normally when dexamethasone is administered (Chap. 318). Once the diagnosis is established, further testing is designed to determine the etiology (Fig. 321-7 and Table 321-4).

For initial screening, the overnight dexamethasone suppression test is recommended (see above). In difficult cases (e.g., in obese or depressed patients), measurement of a 24-h urine free cortisol can also be used as a screening test. A level >140 nmol/d (50 μg/d) is suggestive of Cushing's syndrome. The definitive diagnosis is then established by failure of urinary cortisol to fall to less than <25 nmol/d (10 μg/d) or of plasma cortisol to fall to <140 nmol/L (5 μg/dL) after a

TABLE 321-3 *Frequency of Signs and Symptoms in Cushing's Syndrome*

Sign or Symptom	Percent of Patients
Typical habitus (centripetal obesity)[a]	97
Increased body weight	94
Fatigability and weakness	87
Hypertension (blood pressure >150/90)	82
Hirsutism[a]	80
Amenorrhea	77
Broad violaceous cutaneous striae[a]	67
Personality changes	66
Ecchymoses[a]	65
Proximal myopathy[a]	62
Edema	62
Polyuria, polydipsia	23
Hypertrophy of clitoris	19

[a] Features more specific for Cushing's syndrome.

standard low-dose dexamethasone suppression test (0.5 mg every 6 h for 48 h). Owing to circadian variability, plasma cortisol and, to a certain extent, ACTH determinations are not meaningful when performed in isolation, but the absence of the normal fall of plasma cortisol at midnight is consistent with Cushing's syndrome because there is loss of the diurnal cortisol rhythm.

The task of determining the etiology of Cushing's syndrome is complicated by the fact that all the available tests lack specificity and by the fact that the tumors producing this syndrome are prone to spontaneous and often dramatic changes in hormone secretion (periodic hormonogenesis). No test has a specificity >95%, and it may be necessary to use a combination of tests to arrive at the correct diagnosis.

Plasma ACTH levels can be useful in distinguishing the various causes of Cushing's syndrome, particularly in separating ACTH-dependent from ACTH-independent causes. In general, measurement of plasma ACTH is useful in the diagnosis of ACTH-independent etiologies of the syndrome, since most adrenal tumors cause low or undetectable ACTH levels [<2 pmol/L (10 pg/mL)]. Furthermore, ACTH-secreting pituitary macroadenomas and ACTH-producing nonendocrine tumors usually result in elevated ACTH levels. In the ectopic ACTH syndrome, ACTH levels may be elevated to >110 pmol/L (500 pg/mL), and in most patients the level is >40 pmol/L (200 pg/mL). In Cushing's syndrome as the result of a microadenoma or pituitary-hypothalamic dysfunction, ACTH levels range from 6 to 30 pmol/L (30 to 150 pg/mL) [normal, <14 pmol/L (<60 pg/mL)],

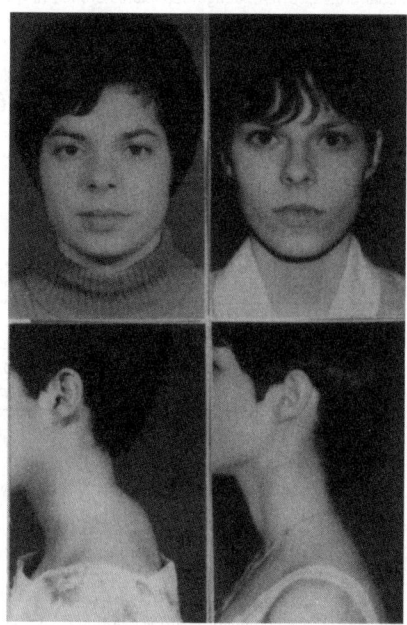

FIGURE 321-6 A woman with Cushing's syndrome due to a right adrenal cortical adenoma. *A.* One month prior to surgery, age 20. *B.* One year after surgery, age 21.

A   **B**

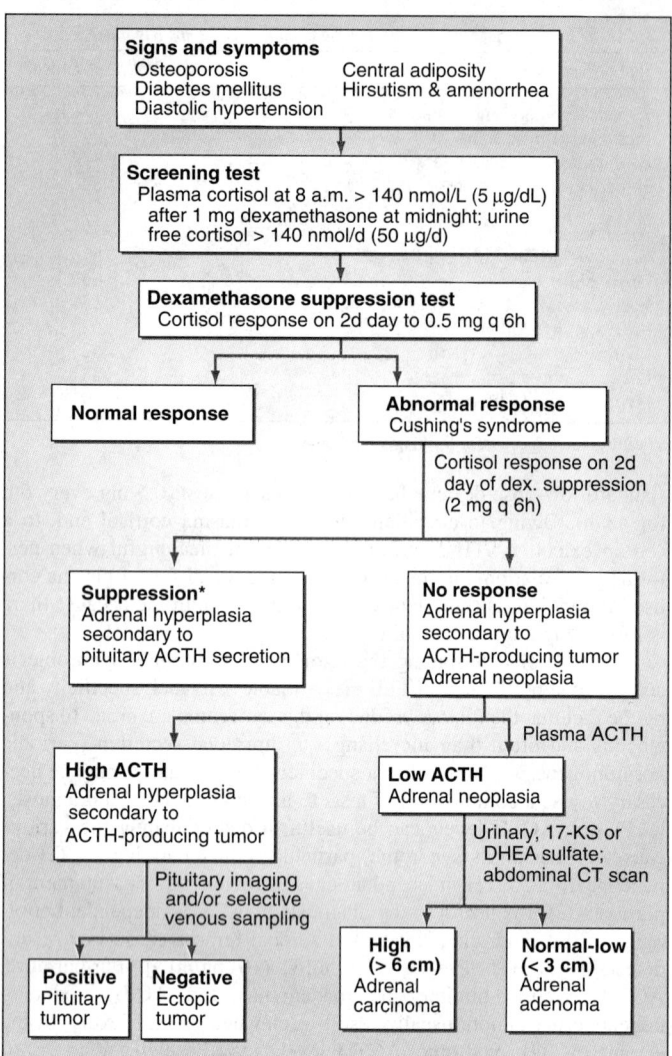

FIGURE 321-7 Diagnostic flowchart for evaluating patients suspected of having Cushing's syndrome. *This group probably includes some patients with pituitary-hypothalamic dysfunction and some with pituitary microadenomas. In some instances, a microadenoma may be visualized by pituitary magnetic resonance scanning. 17-KS, 17-ketosteroids; DHEA, dehydroepiandrosterone; ACTH, adrenocorticotropic hormone; CT, computed tomography.

with half of values falling in the normal range. However, the main problem with the use of ACTH levels in the differential diagnosis of Cushing's syndrome is that ACTH levels may be similar in individuals with hypothalamic-pituitary dysfunction, pituitary microadenomas, ectopic CRH production, and ectopic ACTH production (especially carcinoid tumors) (Table 321-4).

TABLE 321-4 *Diagnostic Tests to Determine the Type of Cushing's Syndrome*

Test	Pituitary Macroadenoma	Pituitary Microadenoma	Ectopic ACTH or CRH Production	Adrenal Tumor
Plasma ACTH level	↑ to ↑↑	N to ↑	↑ to ↑↑↑	↓
Percent who respond to high-dose dexamethasone	<10	95	<10	<10
Percent who respond to CRH	>90	>90	<10	<10

Note: ACTH, adrenocorticotropic hormone; CRH, corticotropin-releasing hormone; N, normal; ↑, elevated; ↓, decreased. See text for definition of a response.

A useful step to distinguish patients with an ACTH-secreting pituitary microadenoma or hypothalamic-pituitary dysfunction from those with other forms of Cushing's syndrome is to determine the response of cortisol output to administration of high-dose dexamethasone (2 mg every 6 h for 2 days). An alternative 8-mg, overnight high-dose dexamethasone test has been developed; however, this test has a lower sensitivity and specificity than the standard test. When the diagnosis of Cushing's syndrome is clear-cut on the basis of baseline urinary and plasma assays, the high-dose dexamethasone suppression test may be used without performing the preliminary low-dose suppression test. The high-dose suppression test provides close to 100% specificity if the criterion used is suppression of urinary free cortisol by >90%. Occasionally, in individuals with bilateral nodular hyperplasia and/or ectopic CRH production, steroid output is also suppressed. Failure of low- and high-dose dexamethasone administration to suppress cortisol production (Table 321-4) can occur in patients with adrenal hyperplasia secondary to an ACTH-secreting pituitary macroadenoma or an ACTH-producing tumor of nonendocrine origin and in those with adrenal neoplasms.

Because of these difficulties, several additional tests have been advocated, such as the metyrapone and CRH infusion tests. The rationale underlying these tests is that steroid hypersecretion by an adrenal tumor or the ectopic production of ACTH will suppress the hypothalamic-pituitary axis so that inhibition of pituitary ACTH release can be demonstrated by either test. Thus, most patients with pituitary-hypothalamic dysfunction and/or a microadenoma have an increase in steroid or ACTH secretion in response to metyrapone or CRH administration, whereas most patients with ectopic ACTH-producing tumors do not. Most pituitary macroadenomas also respond to CRH, but their response to metyrapone is variable. However, false-positive and false-negative CRH tests can occur in patients with ectopic ACTH and pituitary tumors.

The main diagnostic dilemma in Cushing's syndrome is to distinguish those instances due to microadenomas of the pituitary from those due to ectopic sources (e.g., carcinoids or pheochromocytoma) that produce CRH and/or ACTH. The clinical manifestations are similar unless the ectopic tumor produces other symptoms, such as diarrhea and flushing from a carcinoid tumor or episodic hypertension from a pheochromocytoma. Sometimes, one can distinguish between ectopic and pituitary ACTH production by using metyrapone or CRH tests, as noted above. In these situations, computed tomography (CT) of the pituitary gland is usually normal. Magnetic resonance imaging (MRI) with the enhancing agent gadolinium may be better than CT for this purpose but demonstrates pituitary microadenomas in only half of patients with Cushing's disease. Because microadenomas can be detected in up to 10 to 20% of individuals without known pituitary disease, a positive imaging study does not prove that the pituitary is the source of ACTH excess. In those with negative imaging studies, selective petrosal sinus venous sampling for ACTH is now used in many referral centers. ACTH levels are measured at baseline, 2, 5, and 10 min after ovine CRH (1 μ/kg IV) injections. Peak petrosal:peripheral ACTH ratios of >3 confirm the presence of a pituitary ACTH-secreting tumor. In centers where petrosal sinus sampling is performed frequently, it has proved highly sensitive for distinguishing pituitary and nonpituitary sources of ACTH excess. However, the catheterization procedure is technically difficult, and complications have occurred.

The diagnosis of a *cortisol-producing adrenal adenoma* is suggested by low ACTH and disproportionate elevations in baseline urine free cortisol levels with only modest changes in urinary 17-ketosteroids or plasma DHEA sulfate. Adrenal androgen secretion is usually reduced in these patients owing to the cortisol-induced suppression of ACTH and subsequent involution of the androgen-producing zona reticularis.

The diagnosis of *adrenal carcinoma* is suggested by a palpable abdominal mass and by markedly elevated baseline values of both urine 17-ketosteroids and plasma DHEA sulfate. Plasma and urine cortisol levels are variably elevated. Adrenal carcinoma is usually resistant to both ACTH stimulation and dexamethasone suppression. Elevated adrenal androgen secretion often leads to virilization in the female. Estrogen-producing adrenocortical carcinoma usually presents with gynecomastia in men and dysfunctional uterine bleeding in women. These adrenal tumors secrete increased amounts of androstenedione, which is converted peripherally to the estrogens estrone and estradiol. Adrenal carcinomas that produce Cushing's syndrome are often associated with elevated levels of the intermediates of steroid biosynthesis (especially 11-deoxycortisol), suggesting inefficient conversion of the intermediates to the final product. This feature also accounts for the characteristic increase in 17-ketosteroids. Approximately 20% of adrenal carcinomas are not associated with endocrine syndromes and are presumed to be nonfunctioning or to produce biologically inactive steroid precursors. In addition, the excessive production of steroids is not always clinically evident (e.g., androgens in adult men).

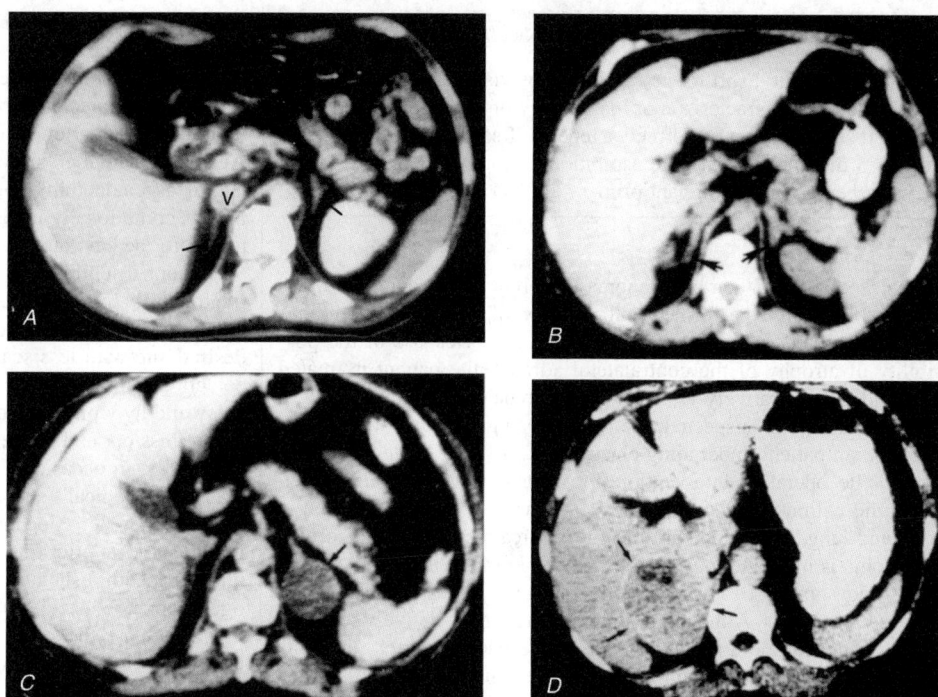

FIGURE 321-8 Computed tomography (CT) is the preferred method for visualizing the adrenal glands (*arrows*). *A.* The normal right adrenal gland is adjacent to the inferior vena cava (V) where it emerges from the liver. Approximately 90% of right adrenal glands appear as linear structures extending posteriorly from the inferior vena cava into the space between the right lobe of the liver and the crus of the diaphragm. The normal left adrenal gland is lateral to the left crus of the diaphragm and below the stomach. Most left adrenal glands are shaped like an inverted V or Y. *B.* Adrenal CT scan of a patient with ectopic ACTH production. Both adrenal glands (*arrows*) are enlarged (compare with *A*). In contrast, only 50% of patients with bilateral adrenal hyperplasia secondary to pituitary ACTH hypersecretion show enlargement of the adrenals when imaged by CT scan. *C.* CT scan of a patient with Cushing's syndrome with biochemical evidence only of cortisol overproduction. The left adrenal has been replaced by a racquet-shaped 2-cm tumor (*arrow*). Attenuation of the tumor is low because of its high lipid content. *D.* CT scan in a patient with Cushing's syndrome and biochemical evidence of an adrenal carcinoma. In contrast to the tumor in *C*, the right-sided mass in this patient is large and has a heterogeneous appearance—usual characteristics of an adrenal carcinoma.

Differential Diagnosis ■ *PSEUDO-CUSHING'S SYNDROME* Problems in diagnosis include patients with obesity, chronic alcoholism, depression, and acute illness of any type. Extreme *obesity* is uncommon in Cushing's syndrome; furthermore, with exogenous obesity, the adiposity is generalized, not truncal. On adrenocortical testing, abnormalities in patients with exogenous obesity are usually modest. Basal urine steroid excretion levels in obese patients are also either normal or slightly elevated, and the diurnal pattern in blood and urine levels is normal. Patients with *chronic alcoholism* and those with *depression* share similar abnormalities in steroid output: modestly elevated urine cortisol, blunted circadian rhythm of cortisol levels, and resistance to suppression using the overnight dexamethasone test. In contrast to alcoholic subjects, depressed patients do not have signs and symptoms of Cushing's syndrome. Following discontinuation of alcohol and/or improvement in the emotional status, results of steroid testing usually return to normal. One or more of three tests have been used to differentiate mild Cushing's syndrome and pseudo-Cushing's syndrome. The serum cortisol level following the standard 2-day low-dose dexamethasone test has very high sensitivity and specificity. Although the CRH test alone is less useful, in combination with the low-dose dexamethasone test, there is nearly complete discrimination between these two conditions. Finally, a midnight cortisol level obtained in awake patients may have similar predictive value as the low-dose dexamethasone test if a cut-off of 210 nmol/L (7.5 μg/dL) is used. Patients with *acute illness* often have abnormal results on laboratory tests and fail to exhibit pituitary-adrenal suppression in response to dexamethasone, since major stress (such as pain or fever) interrupts the normal regulation of ACTH secretion. *Iatrogenic Cushing's syndrome*, induced by the administration of glucocorticoids or other steroids such as megestrol that bind to the glucocorticoid receptor, is indistinguishable by physical findings from endogenous adrenocortical hyperfunction. The distinction can be made, however, by measuring blood or urine cortisol levels in a basal state; in the iatrogenic syndrome these levels are low secondary to suppression of the pituitary-adrenal axis. The severity of iatrogenic Cushing's syndrome is related to the total steroid dose, the biologic half-life of the steroid, and the duration of therapy. Also, individuals taking afternoon and evening doses of glucocorticoids develop Cushing's syndrome more readily and with a smaller total daily dose than do patients taking morning doses only.

Radiologic Evaluation for Cushing's Syndrome The preferred radiologic study for visualizing the adrenals is a CT scan of the abdomen (Fig. 321-8). CT is of value both for localizing adrenal tumors and for diagnosing bilateral hyperplasia. All patients believed to have hypersecretion of pituitary ACTH should have a pituitary MRI scan with gadolinium contrast. Even with this technique, small microadenomas may be undetectable; alternatively, false-positive masses due to cysts or nonsecretory lesions of the normal pituitary may be imaged. In patients with ectopic ACTH production, high-resolution chest CT is a useful first step.

Evaluation of Asymptomatic Adrenal Masses With abdominal CT scanning, many incidental adrenal masses (so-called incidentalomas) are discovered. This is not surprising, since 10 to 20% of subjects at autopsy have adrenocortical adenomas. The first step in evaluating such patients is to determine whether the tumor is functioning by means of appropriate screening tests, e.g., measurement of 24-h urine catecholamines and metabolites and serum potassium and assessment of adrenal cortical function by dexamethasone-suppression testing. However, 90% of incidentalomas are nonfunctioning. If an extraadrenal malignancy is present, there is a 30 to 50% chance that the adrenal tumor is a metastasis. If the primary tumor is being treated and there are no other metastases, it is prudent to obtain a fine-needle aspirate of the adrenal mass to establish the diagnosis. In the absence of a known malignancy the next step is unclear. The probability of adrenal carcinoma is <0.01%, the vast majority of adrenal masses being benign adenomas. Features suggestive of malignancy include large size (a size > 4 to 6 cm suggests carcinoma); irregular margins;

and inhomogeneity, soft tissue calcifications visible on CT (Fig. 321-8), and findings characteristic of malignancy on a chemical-shift MRI image. If surgery is not performed, a repeat CT scan should be obtained in 3 to 6 months. Fine-needle aspiration is not useful to distinguish between benign and malignant primary adrenal tumors.

Ŗ TREATMENT

Adrenal Neoplasm   When an adenoma or carcinoma is diagnosed, adrenal exploration is performed with excision of the tumor. Adenomas may be resected using laparoscopic techniques. Because of the possibility of atrophy of the contralateral adrenal, the patient is treated pre- and postoperatively as if for total adrenalectomy, even when a unilateral lesion is suspected, the routine being similar to that for an Addisonian patient undergoing elective surgery (see Table 321-8).

Despite operative intervention, most patients with adrenal carcinoma die within 3 years of diagnosis. Metastases occur most often to liver and lung. The principal drug for the treatment of adrenocortical carcinoma is mitotane (*o,p'*-DDD), an isomer of the insecticide DDT. This drug suppresses cortisol production and decreases plasma and urine steroid levels. Although its cytotoxic action is relatively selective for the glucocorticoid-secreting zone of the adrenal cortex, the zona glomerulosa may also be inhibited. Because mitotane also alters the extraadrenal metabolism of cortisol, plasma and urinary cortisol levels must be assessed to titrate the effect. The drug is usually given in divided doses three to four times a day, with the dose increased gradually to tolerability (usually <6 g daily). At higher doses, almost all patients experience side effects, which may be gastrointestinal (anorexia, diarrhea, vomiting) or neuromuscular (lethargy, somnolence, dizziness). All patients treated with mitotane should receive long-term glucocorticoid maintenance therapy, and, in some, mineralocorticoid replacement is appropriate. In approximately one-third of patients, both tumor and metastases regress, but long-term survival is not altered. In many patients, mitotane only inhibits steroidogenesis and does not cause regression of tumor metastases. Osseous metastases are usually refractory to the drug and should be treated with radiation therapy. Mitotane can also be given as adjunctive therapy after surgical resection of an adrenal carcinoma, although there is no evidence that this improves survival. Because of the absence of a long-term benefit with mitotane, alternative chemotherapeutic approaches based on platinum therapy have been used. However, there are no data presently available indicating a prolongation of life.

BILATERAL HYPERPLASIA   Patients with hyperplasia usually have a relative or absolute increase in ACTH levels. Since therapy would logically be directed at reducing ACTH levels, the ideal primary treatment for ACTH- or CRH-producing tumors, whether pituitary or ectopic, is surgical removal. Occasionally (particularly with ectopic ACTH production) surgical excision is not possible because the disease is far advanced. In this situation, "medical" or surgical adrenalectomy may correct the hypercortisolism.

Controversy exists as to the proper treatment for bilateral adrenal hyperplasia when the source of the ACTH overproduction is not apparent. In some centers, these patients (especially those who suppress after the administration of a high-dose dexamethasone test) undergo surgical exploration of the pituitary via a transsphenoidal approach in the expectation that a microadenoma will be found (Chap. 318). However, in most circumstances selective petrosal sinus venous sampling is recommended, and the patient is referred to an appropriate center if the procedure is not available locally. If a microadenoma is not found at the time of exploration, total hypophysectomy may be needed. Complications of transsphenoidal surgery include cerebrospinal fluid rhinorrhea, diabetes insipidus, panhypopituitarism, and optic or cranial nerve injuries.

In other centers, total adrenalectomy is the treatment of choice. The cure rate with this procedure is close to 100%. The adverse effects include the certain need for lifelong mineralocorticoid and glucocor-

ticoid replacement and a 10 to 20% probability of a pituitary tumor developing over the next 10 years (Nelson's syndrome; Chap. 318). It is uncertain whether these tumors arise de novo or if they were present prior to adrenalectomy but were too small to be detected. Periodic radiologic evaluation of the pituitary gland by MRI as well as serial ACTH measurements should be performed in all individuals after bilateral adrenalectomy for Cushing's disease. Such pituitary tumors may become locally invasive and impinge on the optic chiasm or extend into the cavernous or sphenoid sinuses.

Except in children, pituitary irradiation is rarely used as primary treatment, being reserved rather for postoperative tumor recurrences. In some centers, high levels of gamma radiation can be focused on the desired site with less scattering to surrounding tissues by using stereotactic techniques. Side effects of radiation include ocular motor palsy and hypopituitarism. There is a long lag time between treatment and remission, and the remission rate is usually <50%.

Finally, in occasional patients in whom a surgical approach is not feasible, "medical" adrenalectomy may be indicated (Table 321-5). Inhibition of steroidogenesis may also be indicated in severely cushingoid subjects prior to surgical intervention. Chemical adrenalectomy may be accomplished by the administration of the inhibitor of steroidogenesis ketoconazole (600 to 1200 mg/d). In addition, mitotane (2 or 3 g/d) and/or the blockers of steroid synthesis aminoglutethimide (1 g/d) and metyrapone (2 or 3 g/d) may be effective either alone or in combination. Mitotane is slow to take effect (weeks). Mifepristone, a competitive inhibitor of the binding of glucocorticoid to its receptor, may be a treatment option. Adrenal insufficiency is a risk with all these agents, and replacement steroids may be required.

ALDOSTERONISM   Aldosteronism is a syndrome associated with hypersecretion of the mineralocorticoid aldosterone. In *primary* aldosteronism the cause for the excessive aldosterone production resides within the adrenal gland; in *secondary* aldosteronism the stimulus is extraadrenal.

Primary Aldosteronism   In the original descriptions of excessive and inappropriate aldosterone production, the disease was the result of an *aldosterone-producing adrenal adenoma* (Conn's syndrome). Most cases involve a unilateral adenoma, which is usually small and may occur on either side. Rarely, primary aldosteronism is due to an adrenal carcinoma. Aldosteronism is twice as common in women as in men, usually occurs between the ages of 30 and 50, and is present in ~1% of unselected hypertensive patients. However, the prevalence may be as high as 5%, depending on the criteria and study population. In many patients with clinical and biochemical features of primary aldosteronism, a solitary adenoma is not found at surgery. Instead, these patients have *bilateral cortical nodular hyperplasia*. In the literature, this disease is also termed *idiopathic hyperaldosteronism*, and/or *nodular hyperplasia*. The cause is unknown.

SIGNS AND SYMPTOMS   Hypersecretion of aldosterone increases the renal distal tubular exchange of intratubular sodium for secreted potassium and hydrogen ions, with progressive depletion of body potassium and development of hypokalemia. Most patients have diastolic hypertension, which may be very severe, and headaches. The hypertension is probably due to the increased sodium reabsorption and extracellular volume expansion. *Potassium depletion* is responsible for the muscle

---

TABLE 321-5   Treatment Modalities for Patients with Adrenal Hyperplasia Secondary to Pituitary ACTH Hypersecretion

Treatments to reduce pituitary ACTH production
   Transsphenoidal resection of microadenoma
   Radiation therapy
Treatments to reduce or eliminate adrenocortical cortisol secretion
   Bilateral adrenalectomy
   Medical adrenalectomy (metyrapone, mitotane, aminoglutethimide, ketoconazole)[a]

[a] Not curative but effective as long as chronically administered in selected patients.
Note: ACTH, adrenocorticotropic hormone.

weakness and fatigue and is due to the effect of potassium depletion on the muscle cell membrane. The polyuria results from impairment of urinary concentrating ability and is often associated with polydipsia. However, some individuals with mild disease, particularly the bilateral hyperplasia type, may have normal potassium levels and therefore have no symptoms associated with hypokalemia.

Electrocardiographic and roentgenographic signs of left ventricular enlargement are, in part, secondary to the hypertension. However, the left ventricular hypertrophy is disproportionate to the level of blood pressure when compared to individuals with essential hypertension, and regression of the hypertrophy occurs even if blood pressure is not reduced after removal of an aldosteronoma. Electrocardiographic signs of potassium depletion include prominent U waves, cardiac arrhythmias, and premature contractions. In the absence of associated congestive heart failure, renal disease, or preexisting abnormalities (such as thrombophlebitis), edema is characteristically absent. However, structural damage to the cerebral circulation, retinal vasculature, and kidney occurs more frequently than would be predicted based on the level and duration of the hypertension. Proteinuria may occur in as many as 50% of patients with primary aldosteronism, and renal failure occurs in up to 15%. Thus, it is probable that excess aldosterone production induces cardiovascular damage independent of its effect on blood pressure.

LABORATORY FINDINGS   Laboratory findings depend on both the duration and the severity of potassium depletion. An overnight concentration test often reveals impaired ability to concentrate the urine, probably secondary to the hypokalemia. Urine pH is neutral to alkaline because of excessive secretion of ammonium and bicarbonate ions to compensate for the metabolic alkalosis.

Hypokalemia may be severe (<3 mmol/L) and reflects body potassium depletion, usually >300 mmol. In mild forms of primary aldosteronism, potassium levels may be normal. *Hypernatremia* is infrequent but may be caused by sodium retention, concomitant water loss from polyuria, and resetting of the osmostat. Metabolic alkalosis and elevation of serum bicarbonate are caused by hydrogen ion loss into the urine and migration into potassium-depleted cells. The alkalosis is perpetuated by potassium deficiency, which increases the capacity of the proximal convoluted tubule to reabsorb filtered bicarbonate. If hypokalemia is severe, serum magnesium levels are also reduced.

DIAGNOSIS   The diagnosis is suggested by persistent hypokalemia in a nonedematous patient with a normal sodium intake who is not receiving potassium-wasting diuretics (furosemide, ethacrynic acid, thiazides). If hypokalemia occurs in a hypertensive patient taking a potassium-wasting diuretic, the diuretic should be discontinued and the patient should be given potassium supplements. After 1 to 2 weeks, the potassium level should be remeasured, and if hypokalemia persists, the patient should be evaluated for a mineralocorticoid excess syndrome (Fig. 321-9).

The criteria for the diagnosis of primary aldosteronism are (1) diastolic hypertension without edema, (2) hyposecretion of renin (as judged by low plasma renin activity levels) that fails to increase appropriately during volume depletion (upright posture, sodium depletion), and (3) hypersecretion of aldosterone that does not suppress appropriately in response to volume expansion.

Patients with primary aldosteronism characteristically *do not have edema*, since they exhibit an "escape" phenomenon from the sodium-retaining aspects of mineralocorticoids. Rarely, pretibial edema is present in patients with associated nephropathy and azotemia.

The estimation of plasma renin activity is of limited value in separating patients with primary aldosteronism from those with hypertension of other causes. Although failure of plasma renin activity to rise normally during volume-depletion maneuvers is a criterion for a diagnosis of primary aldosteronism, suppressed renin activity also occurs in ~25% of patients with essential hypertension.

Although a renin measurement alone lacks specificity, the ratio of serum aldosterone to plasma renin activity is a very useful screening

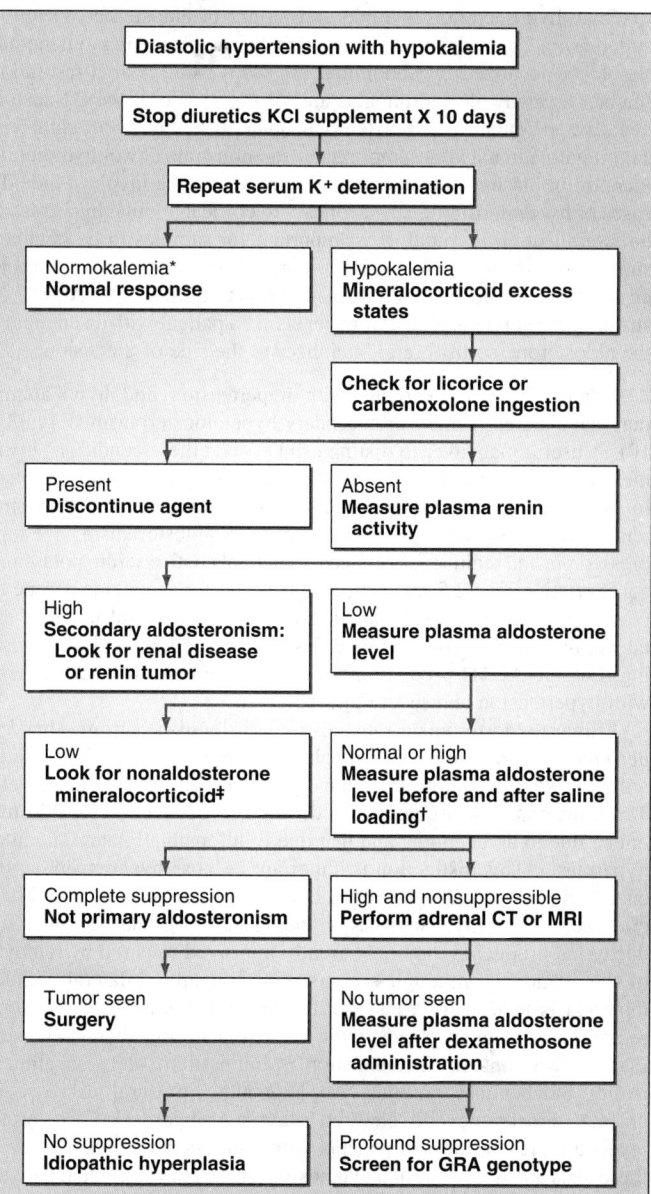

FIGURE 321-9 Diagnostic flowchart for evaluating patients with suspected primary aldosteronism. *Serum K⁺ may be normal in some patients with hyperaldosteronism who are taking potassium-sparing diuretics (spironolactone, triamterene) or who have a low sodium intake and a high potassium intake. †This step should not be taken if hypertension is severe (diastolic pressure > 115 mmHg) or if cardiac failure is present. Also, serum potassium levels should be corrected before the infusion of saline solution. Alternative methods that produce comparable suppression of aldosterone secretion include oral sodium loading (200 mmol/d) and the administration of fludrocortisone, 0.2 mg bid, for 3 days. ‡For example, Liddle's syndrome, apparent mineralocorticoid excess syndrome, or a deoxycorticosterone-secreting tumor. (GRA, glucocorticoid-remediable aldosteronism; CT, computed tomography; MRI, magnetic resonance imaging.)

test. A high ratio (>30), when aldosterone is expressed as ng/dL and plasma renin activity as ng/mL per hour, strongly suggests autonomy of aldosterone secretion. Aldosterone levels need to be >500 pmol/L (>15 ng/dL) when salt intake is not restricted. In some centers, the aldosterone/plasma renin activity ratio is used as a primary screen test in all normokalemic, difficult-to-control hypertensive patients, in addition to those with hypokalemia. Ultimately, it is necessary to demonstrate a lack of aldosterone suppression to diagnose primary aldosteronism (Fig. 321-9). The autonomy exhibited in these patients refers only to the resistance to suppression of secretion during volume expansion; aldosterone can and does respond in a normal or above-normal fashion to the stimulus of potassium loading or ACTH infusion.

Once hyposecretion of renin and failure of aldosterone secretion suppression are demonstrated, aldosterone-producing adenomas should be localized by abdominal CT scan, using a high-resolution scanner as many aldosteronomas are <1 cm in size. If the CT scan is negative, percutaneous transfemoral bilateral adrenal vein catheterization with adrenal vein sampling may demonstrate a two- to threefold increase in plasma aldosterone concentration on the involved side. In cases of hyperaldosteronism secondary to cortical nodular hyperplasia, no lateralization is found. It is important for samples to be obtained simultaneously if possible and for cortisol levels to be measured to ensure that false localization does not reflect dilution or an ACTH- or stress-induced rise in aldosterone levels. In a patient with an adenoma, the aldosterone/cortisol ratio lateralizes to the side of the lesion.

DIFFERENTIAL DIAGNOSIS Patients with hypertension and hypokalemia may have either primary or secondary hyperaldosteronism (Fig. 321-10). A useful maneuver to distinguish between these conditions is the measurement of plasma renin activity. Secondary hyperaldosteronism in patients with accelerated hypertension is due to elevated plasma renin levels; in contrast, patients with primary aldosteronism have suppressed plasma renin levels. Indeed, in patients with a serum potassium concentration of <2.5 mmol/L, a high ratio of plasma aldosterone to plasma renin activity in a random sample is usually sufficient to establish the diagnosis of primary aldosteronism without additional testing. Ectopic ACTH production should also be considered in patients with hypertension and severe hypokalemia.

Primary aldosteronism must also be distinguished from other *hypermineralocorticoid states*. Nonaldosterone mineralocorticoid states will have suppressed plasma renin activity but low aldosterone levels. The most common problem is to distinguish between hyperaldosteronism due to an adenoma and that due to idiopathic bilateral nodular hyperplasia. This distinction is important because hypertension associated with idiopathic hyperplasia does not usually benefit from bilateral adrenalectomy, whereas hypertension associated with aldosterone-producing tumors is usually improved or cured by removal of the adenoma. Although patients with idiopathic bilateral nodular hyperplasia tend to have less severe hypokalemia, lower aldosterone secretion, and higher plasma renin activity than do patients with primary aldosteronism, differentiation is impossible solely on clinical and/or biochemical grounds. An anomalous postural decrease in plasma aldosterone and elevated plasma 18-hydroxycorticosterone levels are present in most patients with a unilateral lesion. However, these tests are also of limited diagnostic value in the individual patient, because some adenoma patients have an increase in plasma aldosterone with upright posture, so-called renin-responsive aldosteronoma. A definitive diagnosis is best made by radiographic studies, including bilateral adrenal vein catheterization, as noted above.

In a few instances, hypertensive patients with hypokalemic alkalosis have adenomas that secrete deoxycorticosterone. Such patients have reduced plasma renin activity levels, but aldosterone levels are either normal or reduced, suggesting the diagnosis of mineralocorticoid excess due to a hormone other than aldosterone. Several inherited disorders have clinical features similar to those of primary aldosteronism (see below).

℞ TREATMENT

Primary aldosteronism due to an adenoma is usually treated by surgical excision of the adenoma. Where possible a laparoscopic approach is favored. However, dietary sodium restriction and the administration of an aldosterone antagonist—e.g., spironolactone—are effective in many cases. Hypertension and hypokalemia are usually controlled by doses of 25 to 100 mg spironolactone every 8 h. In some patients medical management has been successful for years, but chronic therapy in men is usually limited by side effects of spironolactone such as gynecomastia, decreased libido, and impotence.

When idiopathic bilateral hyperplasia is suspected, surgery is indicated only when significant, symptomatic hypokalemia cannot be controlled with medical therapy, i.e., by spironolactone, triamterene, or amiloride. Hypertension associated with idiopathic hyperplasia is usually not benefited by bilateral adrenalectomy.

Secondary Aldosteronism *Secondary aldosteronism* refers to an appropriately increased production of aldosterone in response to activation of the renin-angiotensin system (Fig. 321-10). The production rate of aldosterone is often higher in patients with secondary aldosteronism than in those with primary aldosteronism. Secondary aldosteronism usually occurs in association with the accelerated phase of hypertension or on the basis of an underlying edema disorder. Secondary aldosteronism in pregnancy is a normal physiologic response to estrogen-induced increases in circulating levels of renin substrate and plasma renin activity and to the anti-aldosterone actions of progestogens.

Secondary aldosteronism in hypertensive states is due either to a primary overproduction of renin (primary reninism) or to an overproduction of renin secondary to a decrease in renal blood flow and/or perfusion pressure (Fig. 321-10). Secondary hypersecretion of renin can be due to a narrowing of one or both of the major renal arteries by atherosclerosis or by fibromuscular hyperplasia. Overproduction of renin from both kidneys also occurs in severe arteriolar nephrosclerosis (malignant hypertension) or with profound renal vasoconstriction (the accelerated phase of hypertension). The secondary aldosteronism is characterized by hypokalemic alkalosis, moderate to severe increases in plasma renin activity, and moderate to marked increases in aldosterone levels.

Secondary aldosteronism with hypertension can also be caused by rare renin-producing tumors (primary reninism). In these patients, the biochemical characteristics are of renal vascular hypertension, but the primary defect is renin secretion by a juxtaglomerular cell tumor. The diagnosis can be made by demonstration of normal renal vasculature and/or demonstration of a space-occupying lesion in the kidney by radiographic techniques and documentation of a unilateral increase in renal vein renin activity. Rarely, these tumors arise in tissues such as the ovary.

Secondary aldosteronism is present in many forms of *edema*. The rate of aldosterone secretion is usually increased in patients with edema caused by either cirrhosis or the nephrotic syndrome. In congestive heart failure, elevated aldosterone secretion varies depending on the severity of cardiac failure. The stimulus for aldosterone release in these conditions appears to be *arterial hypovolemia* and/or hypotension. Thiazides and furosemide often exaggerate secondary aldosteronism via volume depletion; hypokalemia and, on occasion, alkalosis can then become prominent features. On occasion secondary hyperaldosteronism occurs without edema or hypertension (Bartter and Gitelman syndromes, see below).

Aldosterone and Cardiovascular Damage Although many studies have investigated the role of angiotensin II in mediating cardiovascular damage, additional evidence indicates that aldosterone has an important

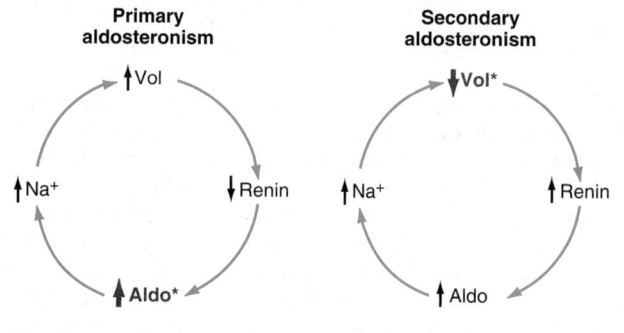

Primary aldosteronism

↑Vol

↑Na⁺   ↓Renin

↑Aldo*

Secondary aldosteronism

↓Vol*

↑Na⁺   ↑Renin

↑Aldo

*Initiating event

FIGURE 321-10 Responses of the renin-aldosterone volume control loop in primary versus secondary aldosteronism.

role that is independent of angiotensin II. Patients with primary aldosteronism (in which angiotensin II levels are usually very low) have a higher incidence of left ventricular hypertrophy (LVH), albuminuria, and stroke than do patients with essential hypertension. Experimental animal models mimicking secondary aldosteronism (angiotensin infusion) or primary aldosteronism (aldosterone infusion) reveal a common pathophysiologic sequence. Within the first few days there is activation of proinflammatory molecules with a histologic picture of perivascular macrophage infiltrate and inflammation, followed by cellular death, fibrosis, and ventricular hypertrophy. These events are prevented if an aldosterone receptor antagonist is used or if adrenalectomy is performed initially. The same pathophysiologic sequence is seen in animals with average aldosterone levels and cardiovascular damage, i.e., diabetes mellitus, or genetic hypertensive rats. Importantly, the level of sodium intake is a critical co-factor. If salt intake is severely restricted, no damage occurs even though the aldosterone levels are markedly elevated. Thus, it is not the level of aldosterone per se that is responsible for the damage, but its level relative to the volume or sodium status of the individual.

Four clinical studies support these experimental results. In the RALES trial, patients with class II/IV heart failure were randomized to standard care or a low dose of the mineralocorticoid receptor antagonist, spironolactone. There was a 30% reduction in all-cause mortality and cardiovascular mortality and hospitalizations after 36 months. Two studies in hypertensive subjects addressed the question of the relative importance of a reduction of angiotensin II formation versus blockade of the MR in mediating cardiovascular damage. Subjects were randomized to eplerenone (an MR antagonist), enalapril (an ACE inhibitor), or both agents. In the first study the subjects had LVH, with the end point being a reduction in LVH. In the second, the subjects had diabetes mellitus and proteinuria, with the end point being a reduction in proteinuria. In both studies all three treatment arms substantially reduced the primary end point; however, the most potent effect occurred in the combination arms of the studies. In the monotherapy LVH arms, the reduction in LVH was similar, while in the proteinuria study, eplerenone produced a greater reduction than did enalapril. The final study was the EPHESUS trial, where individuals who developed congestive heart failure after an acute myocardial infarction were randomized to standard-of-care treatment with or without a small dose of eplerenone. Eplerenone administration produced a significantly greater reduction in mortality (15 to 17%) and in cardiovascular-related hospitalizations than the placebo arm. Thus, these four clinical studies provide strong support to the hypothesis that MR blockade has a significant added advantage over standard-of-care therapy in reducing cardiovascular mortality and surrogate end points. However, regulatory approval is pending.

SYNDROMES OF ADRENAL ANDROGEN EXCESS   Adrenal androgen excess results from excess production of DHEA and androstenedione, which are converted to testosterone in extraglandular tissues; elevated testosterone levels account for most of the virilization. Adrenal androgen excess may be associated with the secretion of greater or smaller amounts of other adrenal hormones and may, therefore, present as "pure" syndromes of virilization or as "mixed" syndromes associated with excessive glucocorticoids and Cushing's syndrome. →*For further discussion of hirsutism and virilization, see Chap. 44.*

HYPOFUNCTION OF THE ADRENAL CORTEX

Cases of adrenal insufficiency can be divided into two general categories: (1) those associated with primary inability of the adrenal to elaborate sufficient quantities of hormone, and (2) those associated with a secondary failure due to inadequate ACTH formation or release (Table 321-6).

PRIMARY ADRENOCORTICAL DEFICIENCY (ADDISON'S DISEASE)   The original description of Addison's disease—"general languor and debility, feebleness of the heart's action, irritability of the stomach, and a peculiar change of the color of the skin"—summarizes the dominant clinical

TABLE 321-6   *Classification of Adrenal Insufficiency*

PRIMARY ADRENAL INSUFFICIENCY

Anatomic destruction of gland (chronic or acute)
  "Idiopathic" atrophy (autoimmune, adrenoleukodystrophy)
  Surgical removal
  Infection (tuberculous, fungal, viral—especially in AIDS patients)
  Hemorrhage
  Invasion: metastatic
Metabolic failure in hormone production
  Congenital adrenal hyperplasia
  Enzyme inhibitors (metyrapone, ketoconazole, aminoglutethimide)
  Cytotoxic agents (mitotane)
ACTH-blocking antibodies
Mutation in ACTH receptor gene
Adrenal hypoplasia congenita

SECONDARY ADRENAL INSUFFICIENCY

Hypopituitarism due to hypothalamic-pituitary disease
Suppression of hypothalamic-pituitary axis
  By exogenous steroid
  By endogenous steroid from tumor

Note: ACTH, adrenocorticotropic hormone.

features. Advanced cases are usually easy to diagnose, but recognition of the early phases can be a real challenge.

Incidence   Acquired forms of primary insufficiency are relatively rare, may occur at any age, and affect both sexes equally. Because of the common therapeutic use of steroids, secondary adrenal insufficiency is relatively common.

Etiology and Pathogenesis   Addison's disease results from progressive destruction of the adrenals, which must involve >90% of the glands before adrenal insufficiency appears. The adrenal is a frequent site for chronic granulomatous diseases, predominantly tuberculosis but also histoplasmosis, coccidioidomycosis, and cryptococcosis. In early series, tuberculosis was responsible for 70 to 90% of cases, but the most frequent cause now is *idiopathic* atrophy, and an autoimmune mechanism is probably responsible. Rarely, other lesions are encountered, such as adrenoleukodystrophy, bilateral hemorrhage, tumor metastases, HIV, cytomegalovirus (CMV), amyloidosis, adrenomyeloneuropathy, familial adrenal insufficiency, or sarcoidosis.

Although half of patients with idiopathic atrophy have circulating adrenal antibodies, autoimmune destruction is probably secondary to cytotoxic T lymphocytes. Specific adrenal antigens to which autoantibodies may be directed include 21-hydroxylase (CYP21A2) and side chain cleavage enzyme, but the significance of these antibodies in the pathogenesis of adrenal insufficiency is unknown. Some antibodies cause adrenal insufficiency by blocking the binding of ACTH to its receptors. Some patients also have antibodies to thyroid, parathyroid, and/or gonadal tissue (Chap. 330). There is also an increased incidence of chronic lymphocytic thyroiditis, premature ovarian failure, type 1 diabetes mellitus, and hypo- or hyperthyroidism. The presence of two or more of these autoimmune endocrine disorders in the same person defines the polyglandular autoimmune syndrome type II. Additional features include pernicious anemia, vitiligo, alopecia, nontropical sprue, and myasthenia gravis. Within families, multiple generations are affected by one or more of the above diseases. Type II polyglandular syndrome is the result of a mutant gene on chromosome 6 and is associated with the HLA alleles B8 and DR3.

The combination of parathyroid and adrenal insufficiency and chronic mucocutaneous candidiasis constitutes type I polyglandular autoimmune syndrome. Other autoimmune diseases in this disorder include pernicious anemia, chronic active hepatitis, alopecia, primary hypothyroidism, and premature gonadal failure. There is no HLA association; this syndrome is inherited as an autosomal recessive trait. It is caused by mutations in the *a*utoimmune *p*olyendocrinopathy *c*andidiasis *e*ctodermal *d*ystrophy (APECED) gene located on chromosome 21q22.3. The gene encodes a transcription factor thought to be involved in lymphocyte function. The type I syndrome usually presents during childhood, whereas the type II syndrome is usually manifested in adulthood.

Clinical suspicion of adrenal insufficiency should be high in patients with AIDS (Chap. 173). CMV regularly involves the adrenal glands (so-called CMV necrotizing adrenalitis), and involvement with *Mycobacterium avium-intracellulare*, *Cryptococcus*, and Kaposi's sarcoma has been reported. Adrenal insufficiency in AIDS patients may not be manifest, but tests of adrenal reserve frequently give abnormal results. When interpreting tests of adrenocortical function, it is important to remember that medications such as rifampin, phenytoin, ketoconazole, megestrol, and opiates may cause or potentiate adrenal insufficiency. Adrenal hemorrhage and infarction occur in patients on anticoagulants and in those with circulating anticoagulants and hypercoagulable states, such as the antiphospholipid syndrome.

There are several rare genetic causes of adrenal insufficiency that present primarily in infancy and childhood (see below).

Clinical Signs and Symptoms Adrenocortical insufficiency caused by gradual adrenal destruction is characterized by an insidious onset of fatigability, weakness, anorexia, nausea and vomiting, weight loss, cutaneous and mucosal pigmentation, hypotension, and occasionally hypoglycemia (Table 321-7). Depending on the duration and degree of adrenal hypofunction, the manifestations vary from mild chronic fatigue to fulminating shock associated with acute destruction of the glands, as described by Waterhouse and Friderichsen.

Asthenia is the cardinal symptom. Early it may be sporadic, usually most evident at times of stress; as adrenal function becomes more impaired, the patient is continuously fatigued, and bed rest is necessary.

Hyperpigmentation may be striking or absent. It commonly appears as a diffuse brown, tan, or bronze darkening of parts such as the elbows or creases of the hand and of areas that normally are pigmented such as the areolae about the nipples. Bluish-black patches may appear on the mucous membranes. Some patients develop dark freckles, and irregular areas of vitiligo may paradoxically be present. As an early sign, tanning following sun exposure may be persistent.

Arterial hypotension with postural accentuation is frequent, and blood pressure may be in the range of 80/50 or less.

Abnormalities of gastrointestinal function are often the presenting complaint. Symptoms vary from mild anorexia with weight loss to fulminating nausea, vomiting, diarrhea, and ill-defined abdominal pain, which may be so severe as to be confused with an acute abdomen. Patients may have personality changes, usually consisting of excessive irritability and restlessness. Enhancement of the sensory modalities of taste, olfaction, and hearing is reversible with therapy. Axillary and pubic hair may be decreased in women due to loss of adrenal androgens.

Laboratory Findings In the early phase of gradual adrenal destruction, there may be no demonstrable abnormalities in the routine laboratory

parameters, but adrenal reserve is decreased—that is, while basal steroid output may be normal, a subnormal increase occurs after stress. Adrenal stimulation with ACTH uncovers abnormalities in this stage of the disease, eliciting a subnormal increase of cortisol levels or no increase at all. In more advanced stages of adrenal destruction, serum sodium, chloride, and bicarbonate levels are reduced, and the serum potassium level is elevated. The hyponatremia is due both to loss of sodium into the urine (due to aldosterone deficiency) and to movement into the intracellular compartment. This extravascular sodium loss depletes extracellular fluid volume and accentuates hypotension. Elevated plasma vasopressin and angiotensin II levels may contribute to the hyponatremia by impairing free water clearance. Hyperkalemia is due to a combination of aldosterone deficiency, impaired glomerular filtration, and acidosis. Basal levels of cortisol and aldosterone are subnormal and fail to increase following ACTH administration. Mild to moderate hypercalcemia occurs in 10 to 20% of patients for unclear reasons. The electrocardiogram may show nonspecific changes, and the electroencephalogram exhibits a generalized reduction and slowing. There may be a normocytic anemia, a relative lymphocytosis, and a moderate eosinophilia.

Diagnosis The diagnosis of adrenal insufficiency should be made only with ACTH stimulation testing to assess adrenal reserve capacity for steroid production (see above for ACTH test protocols). In brief, the best screening test is the cortisol response 60 min after 250 μg of cosyntropin given intramuscularly or intravenously. Cortisol levels should exceed 495 nmol/L (18 μg/dL). If the response is abnormal, then primary and secondary adrenal insufficiency can be distinguished by measuring aldosterone levels from the same blood samples. In secondary, but not primary, adrenal insufficiency the aldosterone increment will be normal [≥150 pmol/l (5 ng/dL)]. Furthermore, in primary adrenal insufficiency, plasma ACTH and associated peptides (β-LPT) are elevated because of loss of the usual cortisol-hypothalamic-pituitary feedback relationship, whereas in secondary adrenal insufficiency, plasma ACTH values are low or "inappropriately" normal (Fig. 321-11).

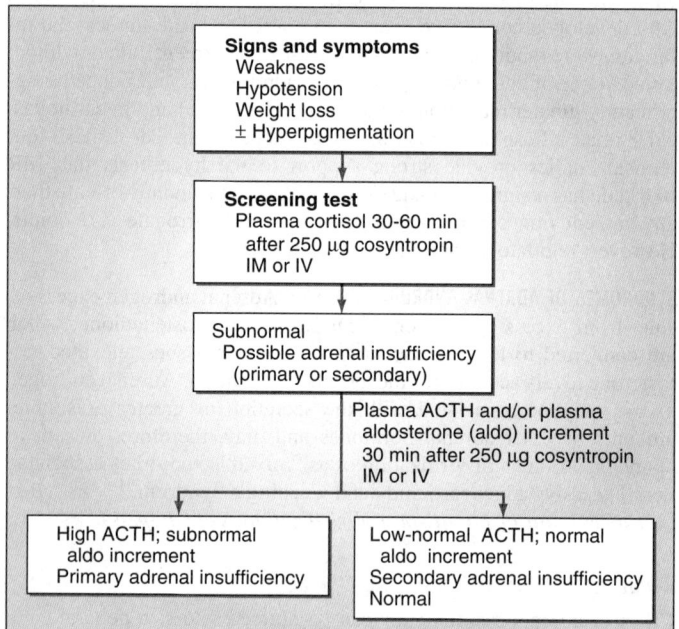

FIGURE 321-11 Diagnostic flowchart for evaluating patients with suspected adrenal insufficiency. Plasma adrenocorticotropic hormone (ACTH) levels are low in secondary adrenal insufficiency. In adrenal insufficiency secondary to pituitary tumors or idiopathic panhypopituitarism, other pituitary hormone deficiencies are present. On the other hand, ACTH deficiency may be isolated, as seen following prolonged use of exogenous glucocorticoids. Because the isolated blood levels obtained in these screening tests may not be definitive, the diagnosis may need to be confirmed by a continuous 24-h ACTH infusion. Normal subjects and patients with secondary adrenal insufficiency may be distinguished by insulin tolerance or metyrapone testing.

TABLE 321-7 *Frequency of Symptoms and Signs in Adrenal Insufficiency*

Sign or Symptom	Percent of Patients
Weakness	99
Pigmentation of skin	98
Weight loss	97
Anorexia, nausea, and vomiting	90
Hypotension (<110/70)	87
Pigmentation of mucous membranes	82
Abdominal pain	34
Salt craving	22
Diarrhea	20
Constipation	19
Syncope	16
Vitiligo	9

Differential Diagnosis Because weakness and fatigue are common, diagnosis of early adrenocortical insufficiency may be difficult. However, the combination of mild gastrointestinal distress, weight loss, anorexia, and a suggestion of increased pigmentation makes it mandatory to perform ACTH stimulation testing to rule out adrenal insufficiency, particularly before steroid treatment is begun. Weight loss is useful in evaluating the significance of weakness and malaise. Racial pigmentation may be a problem, but a *recent* and progressive *increase* in pigmentation is usually reported by the patient with gradual adrenal destruction. Hyperpigmentation is usually absent when adrenal destruction is rapid, as in bilateral adrenal hemorrhage. The fact that hyperpigmentation occurs with other diseases may also present a problem, but the appearance and distribution of pigment in adrenal insufficiency are usually characteristic. When doubt exists, measurement of ACTH levels and testing of adrenal reserve with the infusion of ACTH provide clear-cut differentiation.

TABLE 321-8 *Steroid Therapy Schedule for a Patient with Adrenal Insufficiency Undergoing Surgery*[a]

	Hydrocortisone Infusion, Continuous, mg/h		Hydrocortisone (Orally)		Fludrocortisone (Orally), 8 A.M.
			8 A.M.	4 P.M.	
Routine daily medication			20	10	0.1
Day before operation			20	10	0.1
Day of operation	10				
Day 1	5–7.5				
Day 2	2.5–5				
Day 3	2.5–5	*or*	40	20	0.1
Day 4	2.5–5	*or*	40	20	0.1
Day 5			40	20	0.1
Day 6			20	20	0.1
Day 7			20	10	0.1

[a] All steroid doses are given in milligrams. An alternative approach is to give 100 mg hydrocortisone as an intravenous bolus injection every 8 h on the day of the operation (see text).

TREATMENT

All patients with adrenal insufficiency should receive specific hormone replacement. These patients require careful education about the disease. Replacement therapy should correct both glucocorticoid and mineralocorticoid deficiencies. Hydrocortisone (cortisol) is the mainstay of treatment. The dose for most adults (depending on size) is 20 to 30 mg/d. Patients are advised to take glucocorticoids with meals or, if that is impractical, with milk or an antacid, because the drugs may increase gastric acidity and exert direct toxic effects on the gastric mucosa. To simulate the normal diurnal adrenal rhythm, two-thirds of the dose is taken in the morning, and the remaining one-third is taken in the late afternoon. Some patients exhibit insomnia, irritability, and mental excitement after initiation of therapy; in these, the dosage should be reduced. Other situations that may necessitate smaller doses are hypertension and diabetes mellitus. Obese individuals and those on anticonvulsive medications may require increased dosages. Measurements of plasma ACTH or cortisol or of urine cortisol levels do not appear to be useful in determining optimal glucocorticoid dosages.

Since the replacement dosage of hydrocortisone does not replace the mineralocorticoid component of the adrenal hormones, mineralocorticoid supplementation is usually needed. This is accomplished by the administration of 0.05 to 0.1 mg fludrocortisone per day by mouth. Patients should also be instructed to maintain an ample intake of sodium (3 to 4 g/d).

The adequacy of mineralocorticoid therapy can be assessed by measurement of blood pressure and serum electrolytes. Blood pressure should be normal and without postural changes; serum sodium, potassium, creatinine, and urea nitrogen levels should also be normal. Measurement of plasma renin levels may also be useful in titrating the dose.

In female patients with adrenal insufficiency, androgen levels are also low. Thus, some physicians believe that daily replacement with 25 to 50 mg of DHEA orally may improve quality of life and bone mineral density.

Complications of glucocorticoid therapy, with the exception of gastritis, are *rare* at the dosages recommended for treatment of adrenal insufficiency. Complications of mineralocorticoid therapy include hypokalemia, hypertension, cardiac enlargement, and even congestive heart failure due to sodium retention. Periodic measurements of body weight, serum potassium level, and blood pressure are useful. All patients with adrenal insufficiency should carry medical identification, should be instructed in the parenteral self-administration of steroids, and should be registered with a medical alerting system.

Special Therapeutic Problems During periods of intercurrent illness, especially in the setting of fever, the dose of hydrocortisone should be doubled. With severe illness it should be increased to 75 to 150 mg/d. When oral administration is not possible, parenteral routes should be employed. Likewise, before surgery or dental extractions, supplemental glucocorticoids should be administered. Patients should also be advised to increase the dose of fludrocortisone and to add salt to their otherwise normal diet during periods of strenuous exercise with sweating, during extremely hot weather, and with gastrointestinal upsets such as diarrhea. A simple strategy is to supplement the diet one to three times daily with salty broth (1 cup of beef or chicken bouillon contains 35 mmol of sodium). For a representative program of steroid therapy for the patient with adrenal insufficiency who is undergoing major surgery, see Table 321-8. This schedule is designed so that on the day of surgery it will mimic the output of cortisol in normal individuals undergoing prolonged major stress (10 mg/h, 250 to 300 mg/d). Thereafter, if the patient is improving and is afebrile, the dose of hydrocortisone is tapered by 20 to 30% daily. Mineralocorticoid administration is unnecessary at hydrocortisone doses >100 mg/d because of the mineralocorticoid effects of hydrocortisone at such dosages.

SECONDARY ADRENOCORTICAL INSUFFICIENCY ACTH deficiency causes *secondary* adrenocortical insufficiency; it may be a selective deficiency, as is seen following prolonged administration of excess glucocorticoids, or it may occur in association with deficiencies of multiple pituitary hormones (panhypopituitarism) (Chap. 318). Patients with secondary adrenocortical hypofunction have many symptoms and signs in common with those having primary disease but are *not hyperpigmented*, since ACTH and related peptide levels are low. In fact, plasma ACTH levels distinguish between primary and secondary adrenal insufficiency, since they are elevated in the former and decreased to absent in the latter. Patients with total pituitary insufficiency have manifestations of multiple hormone deficiencies. An additional feature distinguishing primary adrenocortical insufficiency is the *near-normal level of aldosterone secretion* seen in pituitary and/or isolated ACTH deficiencies (Fig. 321-11). Patients with pituitary insufficiency may have hyponatremia, which can be dilutional or secondary to a subnormal increase in aldosterone secretion in response to severe sodium restriction. However, severe *dehydration, hyponatremia,* and *hyperkalemia* are characteristic of severe mineralocorticoid insufficiency and favor a diagnosis of primary adrenocortical insufficiency.

Patients receiving long-term steroid therapy, despite physical findings of Cushing's syndrome, may develop adrenal insufficiency because of prolonged pituitary-hypothalamic suppression and adrenal atrophy secondary to the loss of endogenous ACTH. These patients have two deficits, a loss of adrenal responsiveness to ACTH and a failure of pituitary ACTH release. They are characterized by low blood cortisol and ACTH levels, a low baseline rate of steroid excretion, and abnormal ACTH and metyrapone responses. Most patients with steroid-induced adrenal insufficiency eventually recover normal HPA responsiveness, but recovery time varies from days to months. The rapid ACTH test provides a convenient assessment of recovery of HPA function. Because the plasma cortisol concentrations after injection of cosyntropin and during insulin-induced hypoglycemia are usually similar, the rapid ACTH test assesses the integrated HPA function (see "Tests of Pituitary-Adrenal Responsiveness," above). Some investigators suggest using the low-dose (1 μg) ACTH test for suspected secondary ACTH deficiency. Additional tests to assess pituitary ACTH reserve include the standard metyrapone and insulin-induced hypoglycemia tests.

Glucocorticoid therapy in patients with secondary adrenocortical insufficiency does not differ from that for the primary disorder. Mineralocorticoid therapy is usually not necessary, as aldosterone secretion is preserved.

ACUTE ADRENOCORTICAL INSUFFICIENCY   Acute adrenocortical insufficiency may result from several processes. On the one hand, *adrenal crisis* may be a rapid and overwhelming intensification of chronic adrenal insufficiency, usually precipitated by sepsis or surgical stress. Alternatively, acute hemorrhagic destruction of both adrenal glands can occur in previously well individuals. In children, this event is usually associated with septicemia with *Pseudomonas* or meningococcemia (Waterhouse-Friderichsen syndrome). In adults, anticoagulant therapy or a coagulation disorder may result in bilateral adrenal hemorrhage. Occasionally, bilateral adrenal hemorrhage in the newborn results from birth trauma. Hemorrhage has been observed during pregnancy, following idiopathic adrenal vein thrombosis, and as a complication of venography (e.g., infarction of an adenoma). The third and most frequent cause of acute insufficiency is the rapid withdrawal of steroids from patients with adrenal atrophy owing to chronic steroid administration. Acute adrenocortical insufficiency may also occur in patients with congenital adrenal hyperplasia or those with decreased adrenocortical reserve when they are given drugs capable of inhibiting steroid synthesis (mitotane, ketoconazole) or of increasing steroid metabolism (phenytoin, rifampin).

Adrenal Crisis   The long-term survival of patients with adrenocortical insufficiency depends largely on the prevention and treatment of adrenal crisis. Consequently, the occurrence of infection, trauma (including surgery), gastrointestinal upsets, or other stresses necessitates an immediate increase in hormone. In untreated patients, preexisting symptoms are intensified. Nausea, vomiting, and abdominal pain may become intractable. Fever may be severe or absent. Lethargy deepens into somnolence, and hypovolemic vascular collapse ensues. In contrast, patients previously maintained on chronic glucocorticoid therapy may not exhibit dehydration or hypotension until they are in a preterminal state, since mineralocorticoid secretion is usually preserved. In all patients in crisis, a precipitating cause should be sought.

℞ TREATMENT

Treatment is directed primarily toward repletion of circulating glucocorticoids and replacement of the sodium and water deficits. Hence an intravenous infusion of 5% glucose in normal saline solution should be started with a bolus intravenous infusion of 100 mg hydrocortisone followed by a continuous infusion of hydrocortisone at a rate of 10 mg/h. An alternative approach is to administer a 100-mg bolus of hydrocortisone intravenously every 6 h. However, only continuous infusion maintains the plasma cortisol constantly at stress levels [>830 nmol/L (30 μg/dL)]. Effective treatment of hypotension requires glucocorticoid replacement and repletion of sodium and water deficits. If the crisis was preceded by prolonged nausea, vomiting, and dehydration, several liters of saline solution may be required in the first few hours. Vasoconstrictive agents (such as dopamine) may be indicated in extreme conditions as adjuncts to volume replacement. With large doses of steroid, i.e., 100 to 200 mg hydrocortisone, the patient receives a maximal mineralocorticoid effect, and supplementary mineralocorticoid is superfluous. Following improvement, the steroid

dosage is tapered over the next few days to maintenance levels, and mineralocorticoid therapy is reinstituted if needed (Table 321-8).

ADRENAL CORTICOL INSUFFICIENCY IN ACUTELY ILL PATIENTS   The physiology of the HPA axis is dramatically altered during critical illnesses such as trauma, surgery, sepsis, and shock. In such situations cortisol levels rise four- to sixfold, diurnal variation is abolished, and the unbound fractions of cortisol rise in the circulation and in target tissues. Inadequate cortisol production during critical illness can result in hypotension, reduced systemic vascular resistance, shock, and death.

A major area of controversy in presumably normal individuals is the correlation of clinical outcomes with the cortisol levels measured during critical illness. Subnormal cortisol production during acute severe illness has been termed "functional" or "relative" adrenal insufficiency. Conceptually, the elevated cortisol levels that are observed are viewed as insufficient to control the inflammatory response and maintain blood pressure. If such patients can be identified, treatment with supplementary cortisol could be beneficial.

A level of cortisol in a critically ill patient below which replacement glucocorticoids may improve prognosis is not firmly established, although many have accepted a level of ≤441 nmol/L (15 μg/dL). On the other hand, a random cortisol >938 nmol/L (34 μg/dL) in the setting of critical illness is unlikely to be associated with relative adrenal insufficiency. In patients who have random cortisol levels between 441 and 938 nmol/L (15 and 34 μg/dL), a cosyntropin stimulation test may identify patients with diminished adrenal reserve [increment <255 nmol/L (9 μg/dL)] who may benefit from supplementary cortisol treatment. If the diagnosis of relative or functional adrenal insufficiency is considered in an acutely ill, hypotensive patient, treatment with supplementary cortisol should be initiated promptly following the measurement of a random cortisol level and/or performing a cosyntropin stimulation test. Supplemental cortisol may be particularly beneficial in patients with septic shock where glucocorticoids have been reported to reduce mortality and the duration of vasopressor therapy. Such patients should be treated with 50 to 75 mg of intravenous hydrocortisone every 6 h as bolus treatment or the same amount as a continuous infusion. Treatment can be terminated if the cortisol levels obtained at the outset are normal. On the other hand, those patients with abnormal testing should be treated for 1 week and then tapered. In surviving patients, adrenal function should be reevaluated after resolution of the critical illness.

HYPOALDOSTERONISM

Isolated aldosterone deficiency accompanied by normal cortisol production occurs in association with hyporeninism, as an inherited biosynthetic defect, postoperatively following removal of aldosterone-secreting adenomas, during protracted heparin administration, in pretectal disease of the nervous system, and in severe postural hypotension.

The feature common to all forms of hypoaldosteronism is the inability to increase aldosterone secretion appropriately in response to salt restriction. Most patients have unexplained hyperkalemia, which is often exacerbated by restriction of dietary sodium intake. In severe cases, urine sodium wastage occurs at a normal salt intake, whereas in milder forms, excessive loss of urine sodium occurs only with salt restriction.

Most cases of isolated hypoaldosteronism occur in patients with a deficiency in renin production (so-called hyporeninemic hypoaldosteronism), most commonly in adults with diabetes mellitus and mild renal failure and in whom hyperkalemia and metabolic acidosis are out of proportion to the degree of renal impairment. Plasma renin levels fail to rise normally following sodium restriction and postural changes. The pathogenesis is uncertain. Possibilities include renal disease (the most likely), autonomic neuropathy, extracellular fluid volume expansion, and defective conversion of renin precursors to active renin. Aldosterone levels also fail to rise normally after salt restriction and volume contraction; this effect is probably related to the hyporeninism, since biosynthetic defects in aldosterone secretion usually cannot be demonstrated. In these patients, aldosterone secretion increases promptly after ACTH stimulation, but it is uncertain whether the magnitude of the response is normal. On the other hand, the level of aldosterone appears to be subnormal in relationship to the hyperkalemia.

Hypoaldosteronism can also be associated with high renin levels and low or elevated levels of aldosterone (see below). Severely ill patients may also have hyperreninemic hypoaldosteronism; such patients have a high mortality rate (80%). Hyperkalemia is not present. Possible explanations for the hypoaldosteronism include adrenal necrosis (uncommon) or a shift in steroidogenesis from mineralocorticoids to glucocorticoids, possibly related to prolonged ACTH stimulation.

Before the diagnosis of isolated hypoaldosteronism is considered for a patient with hyperkalemia, "pseudohyperkalemia" (e.g., hemolysis, thrombocytosis) should be excluded by measuring the *plasma* potassium level. The next step is to demonstrate a normal cortisol response to ACTH stimulation. Then, the response of renin and aldosterone levels to stimulation (upright posture, sodium restriction) should be measured. Low renin and aldosterone levels establish the diagnosis of hyporeninemic hypoaldosteronism. A combination of high renin levels and low aldosterone levels is consistent with an aldosterone biosynthetic defect or a selective unresponsiveness to angiotensin II. Finally, there is a condition that clinically and biochemically mimics hypoaldosteronism with elevated renin levels. However, the aldosterone levels are not low but high—so-called pseudohypoaldosteronism. This inherited condition is caused by a mutation in the epithelial sodium channel (see below).

℞ TREATMENT

The treatment is to replace the mineralocorticoid deficiency. For practical purposes, the oral administration of 0.05 to 0.15 mg fludrocortisone daily should restore electrolyte balance if salt intake is adequate (e.g., 150 to 200 mmol/d). However, patients with hyporeninemic hypoaldosteronism may require higher doses of mineralocorticoid to correct hyperkalemia. This need poses a potential risk in patients with hypertension, mild renal insufficiency, or congestive heart failure. An alternative approach is to reduce salt intake and to administer furosemide, which can ameliorate acidosis and hyperkalemia. Occasionally, a combination of these two approaches is efficacious.

GENETIC CONSIDERATIONS   Glucocorticoid Diseases ■ *CONGENITAL ADRENAL HYPERPLASIA* Congenital adrenal hyperplasia (CAH) is the consequence of recessive mutations that cause one of several distinct enzymatic defects (see below). Because cortisol is the principal adrenal steroid regulating ACTH elaboration and because ACTH stimulates adrenal growth and function, a block in cortisol synthesis may result in the enhanced secretion of adrenal androgens and/or mineralocorticoids depending on the site of the enzyme block. In severe congenital virilizing hyperplasia, the adrenal output of cortisol may be so compromised as to cause adrenal deficiency despite adrenal hyperplasia.

CAH is the most common adrenal disorder of infancy and childhood (Chap. 328). Partial enzyme deficiencies can be expressed after adolescence, predominantly in women with hirsutism and oligomenorrhea but minimal virilization. Late-onset adrenal hyperplasia may account for 5 to 25% of cases of hirsutism and oligomenorrhea in women, depending on the population.

Etiology Enzymatic defects have been described in 21-hydroxylase (CYP21A2), 17α-hydroxylase/17,20-lyase (CYP17), 11β-hydroxylase (CYP11B1), and in (3β-HSD2) (Fig. 321-2). Although the genes encoding these enzymes have been cloned, the diagnosis of specific enzyme deficiencies with genetic techniques is not practical because of the large number of different deletions and missense mutations. CYP21A2 deficiency is closely linked to the HLA-B locus of chromosome 6 so that HLA typing and/or DNA polymorphism can be used to detect the heterozygous carriers and to diagnose affected individuals in some families (Chap. 296). The clinical expression in the different disorders is variable, ranging from virilization of the female (CYP2/A2) to feminization of the male (3β-HSD2) (Chap. 328).

Adrenal virilization in the female at birth is associated with ambiguous external genitalia (*female pseudohermaphroditism*). Virilization begins after the fifth month of intrauterine development. At birth there may be enlargement of the clitoris, partial or complete fusion of the labia, and sometimes a urogenital sinus in the female. If the labial fusion is nearly complete, the female infant has external genitalia resembling a penis with hypospadias. In the *postnatal* period, CAH is associated with virilization in the female and isosexual precocity in the male. The excessive androgen levels result in accelerated growth, so that bone age exceeds chronologic age. Because epiphyseal closure occurs early, growth stops, but truncal development continues, the characteristic appearance being a short child with a well-developed trunk.

The most common form of CAH (95% of cases) is a result of impairment of CYP21A2. In addition to cortisol deficiency, aldosterone secretion is decreased in approximately one-third of the patients. Thus, with CYP21A2 deficiency, adrenal virilization occurs with or without a salt-losing tendency due to aldosterone deficiency (Fig. 321-2).

CYP11B1 deficiency causes a "hypertensive" variant of CAH. Hypertension and hypokalemia occur because of the impaired conversion of 11-deoxycorticosterone to corticosterone, resulting in the accumulation of 11-deoxycorticosterone, a potent mineralocorticoid. The degree of hypertension is variable. Steroid precursors are shunted into the androgen pathway.

CYP17 deficiency is characterized by hypogonadism, hypokalemia, and hypertension. This rare disorder causes decreased production of cortisol and shunting of precursors into the mineralocorticoid pathway with hypokalemic alkalosis, hypertension, and suppressed plasma renin activity. Usually, 11-deoxycorticosterone production is elevated. Because CYP17 hydroxylation is required for biosynthesis of both adrenal androgens and gonadal testosterone and estrogen, this defect is associated with sexual immaturity, high urinary gonadotropin levels, and low urinary 17-ketosteroid excretion. Female patients have primary amenorrhea and lack of development of secondary sexual characteristics. Because of deficient androgen production, male patients have either ambiguous external genitalia or a female phenotype (*male pseudohermaphroditism*). Exogenous glucocorticoids can correct the hypertensive syndrome, and treatment with appropriate gonadal steroids results in sexual maturation.

With 3β-HSD2 deficiency, conversion of pregnenolone to progesterone is impaired, so that the synthesis of both cortisol and aldosterone is blocked, with shunting into the adrenal androgen pathway via 17α-hydroxypregnenolone and DHEA. Because DHEA is a weak androgen, and because this enzyme deficiency is also present in the gonad, the genitalia of the male fetus may be incompletely virilized or feminized. Conversely, in the female, overproduction of DHEA may produce partial virilization.

Diagnosis The diagnosis of CAH should be considered in infants having episodes of acute adrenal insufficiency or salt-wasting or hypertension. The diagnosis is further suggested by the finding of hypertrophy of the clitoris, fused labia, or a urogenital sinus in the female or of isosexual precocity in the male. In infants and children with a CYP21A2 defect, increased urine 17-ketosteroid excretion and increased plasma DHEA sulfate levels are typically associated with an increase in the blood levels of 17-hydroxyprogesterone and the excretion of its urinary metabolite pregnanetriol. Demonstration of elevated levels of 17-hydroxyprogesterone in amniotic fluid at 14 to 16 weeks of gestation allows prenatal detection of affected female infants.

The diagnosis of a *salt-losing form* of CAH due to defects in CYP21A2 is suggested by episodes of acute adrenal insufficiency with hyponatremia, hyperkalemia, dehydration, and vomiting. These infants and children often crave salt and have laboratory findings indicating deficits in both cortisol and aldosterone secretion.

With the *hypertensive form* of CAH due to CYP11B1 deficiency, 11-deoxycorticosterone and 11-deoxycortisol accumulate. The diagnosis is confirmed by demonstrating increased levels of 11-deoxycortisol in the blood or increased amounts of tetrahydro-11-deoxycortisol in the urine. Elevation of 17-hydroxyprogesterone levels does not imply a coexisting CYP21A2 deficiency.

Very high levels of urine DHEA with low levels of pregnanetriol and of cortisol metabolites in urine are characteristic of children with 3β-HSD2 deficiency. Marked salt-wasting may also occur.

Adults with *late-onset adrenal hyperplasia* (partial deficiency of CYP21A2, CYP11B1, or 3β-HSD2) are characterized by normal or moderately elevated levels of urinary 17-ketosteroids and plasma DHEA sulfate. A high basal level of a precursor of cortisol biosynthesis (such as 17-hydroxyprogesterone, 17-hydroxypregnenolone, or 11-deoxycortisol), or elevation of such a precursor after ACTH stimulation, confirms the diagnosis of a partial deficiency. Measurement of steroid precursors 60 min after bolus administration of ACTH is usually sufficient. Adrenal androgen output is easily suppressed by the standard low-dose (2 mg) dexamethasone test.

℞ TREATMENT

Therapy in CAH patients consists of daily administration of glucocorticoids to suppress pituitary ACTH secretion. Because of its low cost and intermediate half-life, prednisone is the drug of choice except in infants, in whom hydrocortisone is usually used. In adults with late-onset adrenal hyperplasia, the smallest single bedtime dose of a long- or intermediate-acting glucocorticoid that suppresses pituitary ACTH secretion should be administered. The amount of steroid required by children with CAH is approximately 1 to 1.5 times the normal cortisol production rate of 27 to 35 μmol (10 to 13 mg) of cortisol per square meter of body surface per day and is given in divided doses two or three times per day. The dosage schedule is governed by repetitive analysis of the urinary 17-ketosteroids, plasma DHEA sulfate, and/or precursors of cortisol biosynthesis. Skeletal growth and maturation must also be monitored closely, as overtreatment with glucocorticoid replacement therapy retards linear growth.

Receptor Mutations *Isolated glucocorticoid deficiency* is a rare autosomal recessive disease secondary to a mutation in the ACTH receptor. Usually mineralocorticoid function is normal. Adrenal insufficiency is manifest within the first 2 years of life as hyperpigmentation, convulsions, and/or frequent episodes of hypoglycemia. In some patients the adrenal insufficiency is associated with achalasia and alacrima—Allgrove's, or triple A, syndrome. However, in some triple A syndrome patients, no mutation in the ACTH receptor has been identified, suggesting that a distinct genetic abnormality causes this syndrome. *Adrenal hypoplasia congenita* is a rare X-linked disorder caused by a mutation in the *DAX1* gene. This gene encodes an orphan nuclear receptor that plays an important role in the development of the adrenal cortex and also the hypothalamic-pituitary-gonadal axis. Thus, patients present with signs and symptoms secondary to deficiencies of all three major adrenal steroids—cortisol, aldosterone, and adrenal androgens—as well as gonadotropin deficiency. Finally a rare cause of hypercortisolism without cushingoid stigmata is *primary cortisol resistance* due to mutations in the glucocorticoid receptor. The resistance is incomplete because patients do not exhibit signs of adrenal insufficiency.

Miscellaneous Conditions Adrenoleukodystrophy causes severe demyelination and early death in children, and adrenomyeloneuropathy is associated with a mixed motor and sensory neuropathy with spastic paraplegia in adults; both disorders are associated with elevated circulating levels of very long chain fatty acids and cause adrenal insufficiency. Autosomal recessive mutations in the *s*teroidogenic *a*cute *r*egulatory (STAR) protein gene cause congenital lipoid adrenal hyperplasia (Chap. 328), which is characterized by adrenal insufficiency and defective gonadal steroidogenesis. Because STAR mediates cholesterol transport into the mitochondrion, mutations in the protein cause massive lipid accumulation in steroidogenic cells, ultimately leading to cell toxicity.

MINERALOCORTICOID DISEASES Some forms of CAH have a mineralocorticoid component (see above). Others are caused by a mutation in other enzymes or ion channels important in mediating or mimicking aldosterone's action.

Hypermineralocorticoidism ■ *LOW PLASMA RENIN ACTIVITY* Rarely, hypermineralocorticoidism is due to a defect in cortisol biosynthesis, specifically 11- or 17-hydroxylation. ACTH levels are increased, with a resultant increase in the production of the mineralocorticoid 11-deoxycorticosterone. Hypertension and hypokalemia can be corrected by glucocorticoid administration. The definitive diagnosis is made by demonstrating an elevation of precursors of cortisol biosynthesis in the blood or urine or by direct demonstration of the genetic defect.

Glucocorticoid administration can also ameliorate hypertension or produce normotension even though a hydroxylase deficiency cannot be identified (Fig. 321-9). These patients have normal to slightly elevated aldosterone levels that do not suppress in response to saline but do suppress in response to 2 days of dexamethasone (2 mg/d). The condition is inherited as an autosomal dominant trait and is termed *glucocorticoid-remediable aldosteronism* (GRA). This entity is secondary to a chimeric gene duplication whereby the 11-β hydroxylase gene promoter (which is under the control of ACTH) is fused to the aldosterone synthase coding sequence. Thus, aldosterone synthase activity is ectopically expressed in the zona fasciculata and is regulated by ACTH, in a fashion similar to the regulation of cortisol secretion. Screening for this defect is best performed by assessing the presence or absence of the chimeric gene. Because the abnormal gene may be present in the absence of hypokalemia, its frequency as a cause of hypertension is unknown. Individuals with suppressed plasma renin levels and juvenile-onset hypertension or a history of early-onset hypertension in first-degree relatives should be screened for this disorder. Early hemorrhagic stroke also occurs in GRA-affected individuals.

GRA documented by genetic analysis may be treated with glucocorticoid administration or antimineralocorticoids, i.e., spironolactone, triamterene, or amiloride. Glucocorticoids should be used only in small doses to avoid inducing iatrogenic Cushing's syndrome. A combination approach is often necessary.

HIGH PLASMA RENIN ACTIVITY *Bartter syndrome* is characterized by severe hyperaldosteronism (hypokalemic alkalosis) with moderate to marked increases in renin activity and hypercalciuria, but normal blood pressure and no edema; this disorder usually begins in childhood. Renal biopsy shows juxtaglomerular hyperplasia. Bartter syndrome is caused by a mutation in the renal Na-K-2Cl co-transporter gene. The pathogenesis involves a defect in the renal conservation of sodium or chloride. The renal loss of sodium is thought to stimulate renin secretion and aldosterone production. Hyperaldosteronism produces potassium depletion, and hypokalemia further elevates prostaglandin production and plasma renin activity. In some cases, the hypokalemia may be potentiated by a defect in renal conservation of potassium.

Gitelman syndrome is an autosomal recessive trait characterized by renal salt wasting and as a result, as in Bartter syndrome, activation of the renin-angiotensin-aldosterone system. As a consequence affected individuals have low blood pressure, low serum potassium, low serum magnesium, and high serum bicarbonate. In contrast to Bartter syndrome, urinary calcium excretion is reduced. Gitelman syndrome results from loss-of-function mutations of the renal thiazide-sensitive Na-Cl co-transporter.

Increased Mineralocorticoid Action *Liddle syndrome* is a rare autosomal dominant disorder that mimicks hyperaldosteronism. The defect is in the genes encoding the β or η subunits of the epithelial sodium channel. Both renin and aldosterone levels are low, owing to the constitutively activated sodium channel and the resulting excess sodium reabsorption in the renal tubule.

TABLE 321-9 A Checklist for Use Prior to the Administration of Glucocorticoids in Pharmacologic Doses

Presence of tuberculosis or other chronic infection (chest x-ray, tuberculin test)
Evidence of glucose intolerance or history of gestational diabetes mellitus
Evidence of preexisting osteoporosis (bone density assessment in organ transplant recipients or postmenopausal patients)
History of peptic ulcer, gastritis, or esophagitis (stool guaiac test)
Evidence of hypertension or cardiovascular disease
History of psychological disorders

A rare autosomal recessive cause of hypokalemia and hypertension is 11β-HSD II deficiency, in which cortisol cannot be converted to cortisone and hence binds to the MR and acts as a mineralocorticoid. This condition, also termed *apparent mineralocorticoid excess syndrome*, is caused by a defect in the gene encoding the renal isoform of this enzyme, 11β-HSD II. Patients can be identified either by documenting an increased ratio of cortisol to cortisone in the urine or by genetic analysis. Patients with the 11β-HSD deficiency syndrome can be treated with small doses of dexamethasone, which suppresses ACTH and endogenous cortisol production but binds less well to the mineralocorticoid receptor than does cortisol.

The ingestion of candies or chewing tobacco containing certain forms of licorice produces a syndrome that mimics primary aldosteronism. The component of such agents that causes sodium retention is glycyrrhizinic acid, which inhibits 11β-HSD II and hence allows cortisol to act as a mineralocorticoid. The diagnosis is established or excluded by a careful history.

Decreased Mineralocorticoid Production or Action In patients with a deficiency in aldosterone biosynthesis, the transformation of corticosterone into aldosterone is impaired, owing to a mutation in the aldosterone synthase (CYP11B2) gene. These patients have low to absent aldosterone secretion, elevated plasma renin levels, and elevated levels of the intermediates of aldosterone biosynthesis (corticosterone and 18-hydroxycorticosterone).

Pseudohypoaldosteronism type I (PHA-I) is an autosomal recessive disorder that is seen in the neonatal period and is characterized by salt wasting, hypotension, hyperkalemia, and high renin and aldosterone levels. In contrast to the gain-of-function mutations in the epithelial sodium channel in Liddle syndrome, mutations in PHA-I result in loss of epithelial sodium channel function.

PHARMACOLOGIC CLINICAL USES OF ADRENAL STEROIDS

The widespread use of glucocorticoids emphasizes the need for a thorough understanding of the metabolic effects of these agents. Before adrenal hormone therapy is instituted, the expected gains should be weighed against undesirable effects. Several important questions should be addressed before initiating therapy. First, how serious is the disorder (the more serious, the greater the likelihood that the risk/benefit ratio will be positive)? Second, how long will therapy be required (the longer the therapy, the greater the risk of adverse side effects)? Third, does the individual have preexisting conditions that glucocorticoids may exacerbate (Table 321-9)? If so, then a careful risk/benefit assessment is required to ensure that the ratio is favorable given the increased likelihood of harm by steroids in these patients. Supplementary measures to minimize undesirable metabolic effects are shown in Table 321-10. Fourth, which preparation is best?

THERAPEUTIC CONSIDERATIONS The following considerations should be taken into account in deciding which steroid preparation to use:

1. *The biologic half-life.* The rationale behind alternate-day therapy is to decrease the metabolic effects of the steroids for a significant part of each 48 h period while still producing a pharmacologic effect durable enough to be effective. Too long a half-life would defeat the first purpose, and too short a half-life would defeat the second. In general, the more potent the steroid, the longer its biologic half-life.

TABLE 321-10 Supplementary Measures to Minimize Undesirable Metabolic Effects of Glucocorticoids

Monitor caloric intake to prevent weight gain.
Restrict sodium intake to prevent edema and minimize hypertension and potassium loss.
Provide supplementary potassium if necessary.
Provide antacid, H$_2$ receptor antagonist, and/or H$^+$,K$^+$-ATPase inhibitor therapy.
Institute alternate-day steroid schedule if possible. Patients receiving steroid therapy over a prolonged period should be protected by an appropriate increase in hormone level during periods of acute stress. A rule of thumb is to *double* the maintenance dose.
Minimize osteopenia by
  Administering gonadal hormone replacement therapy: 0.625–1.25 mg conjugated estrogens given cyclically with progesterone, unless the uterus is absent; testosterone replacement for hypogonadal men
Ensuring high calcium intake (should be approximately 1200 mg/d)
Administering supplemental vitamin D if blood levels of calciferol or 1,25(OH)$_2$ vitamin D are reduced
Administering bisphosphonate prophylactically, orally or parenterally, in high-risk patients

2. *The mineralocorticoid effects of the steroid.* Most synthetic steroids have less mineralocorticoid effect than hydrocortisone (Table 321-11).

3. *The biologically active form of the steroid.* Cortisone and prednisone have to be converted to biologically active metabolites before anti-inflammatory effects can occur. Because of this, in a condition for which steroids are known to be effective and when an adequate dose has been given without response, one should consider substituting hydrocortisone or prednisolone for cortisone or prednisone.

4. *The cost of the medication.* This is a serious consideration if chronic administration is planned. Prednisone is the least expensive of available steroid preparations.

5. *The type of formulation.* Topical steroids have the distinct advantage over oral steroids in reducing the likelihood of systemic side effects. In addition, some inhaled steroids have been designed to minimize side effects by increasing their hepatic inactivation if they are swallowed (Chap. 236). However, all topical steroids can be absorbed into the systemic circulation.

TABLE 321-11 Glucocorticoid Preparations

Commonly Used Name[a]	Estimated Potency[b]	
	Glucocorticoid	Mineralocorticoid
SHORT-ACTING		
Hydrocortisone	1	1
Cortisone	0.8	0.8
INTERMEDIATE-ACTING		
Prednisone	4	0.25
Prednisolone	4	0.25
Methylprednisolone	5	<0.01
Triamcinolone	5	<0.01
LONG-ACTING		
Paramethasone	10	<0.01
Betamethasone	25	<0.01
Dexamethasone	30–40	<0.01

[a] The steroids are divided into three groups according to the duration of biologic activity. Short-acting preparations have a biologic half-life <12 h; long-acting, >48 h; and intermediate, between 12 and 36 h. Triamcinolone has the longest half-life of the intermediate-acting preparations.

[b] Relative milligram comparisons with hydrocortisone, setting the glucocorticoid and mineralocorticoid properties of hydrocortisone as 1. Sodium retention is insignificant for commonly employed doses of methylprednisolone, triamcinolone, paramethasone, betamethasone, and dexamethasone.

ALTERNATE-DAY STEROID THERAPY   The most effective way to minimize the cushingoid effects of glucocorticoids is to administer the total 48-h dose as a *single dose* of *intermediate-acting steroid* in the morning, *every other day*. If symptoms of the underlying disorder can be controlled by this technique, it offers distinct advantages. Three considerations deserve mention: (1) The alternate-day schedule may be approached through transition schedules that allow the patient to adjust gradually; (2) supplementary nonsteroid medications may be needed on the "off" day to minimize symptoms of the underlying disorder; and (3) many symptoms that occur during the off day (e.g., fatigue, joint pain, muscle stiffness or tenderness, and fever) may represent relative adrenal insufficiency rather than exacerbation of the underlying disease.

The alternate-day approach capitalizes on the fact that cortisol secretion and plasma levels normally are highest in the early morning and lowest in the evening. The normal pattern is mimicked by administering an intermediate-acting steroid in the morning (7 to 8 A.M.) (Table 321-11).

Initially, the steroid regimen often requires daily or more frequent doses of steroid to achieve the desired anti-inflammatory or immunity-suppressing action. *Only after this desired effect is achieved is an attempt made to switch to an alternate-day program.* A number of schedules can be used for transferring from a daily to an alternate-day program. The key points to be considered are flexibility in arranging a program and the use of supportive measures on the off day. One may attempt a gradual transition to the alternate-day schedule rather than an abrupt changeover. One approach is to keep the steroid dose constant on one day and gradually reduce it on the alternate day. Alternatively, the steroid dose can be increased on one day and reduced on the alternate day. In any case, it is important to anticipate that some increase in pain or discomfort may occur in the 36 to 48 h following the last dose.

WITHDRAWAL OF GLUCOCORTICOIDS FOLLOWING LONG-TERM USE   It is possible to reduce a daily steroid dose gradually and eventually to discontinue it, but under most circumstances withdrawal of steroids should be initiated by first implementing an alternate-day schedule. Patients who have been on an alternate-day program for a month or more experience less difficulty during termination regimens. The dosage is gradually reduced and finally discontinued after a replacement dosage has been reached (e.g., 5 to 7.5 mg prednisone). Complications rarely ensue unless undue stress is experienced, and patients should understand that for ≥1 year after withdrawal from long-term high-dose steroid therapy, supplementary hormone should be given in the event of a serious infection, operation, or injury. A useful strategy in patients with symptoms of adrenal insufficiency on a tapering regimen is to measure plasma cortisol levels prior to the steroid dose. A level <140 nmol/L (5 μg/dL) indicates suppression of the pituitary-adrenal axis and implies that a more cautious tapering of steroids is indicated.

In patients on high-dose daily steroid therapy, it is advised to reduce dosage to ~20 mg prednisone daily as a single morning dose before beginning the transition to alternate-day therapy. If a patient cannot tolerate an alternate-day program, consideration should be given to the possibility that the patient has developed primary adrenal insufficiency.

FURTHER READING

BARZON L et al: Risk factors and long-term follow-up of adrenal incidentalomas. J Clin Endocrinol Metab 84:520, 1999

COOPER MS et al: Current concepts: Corticosteroid insufficiency in acutely ill patients. N Engl J Med 348: 727, 2003

NEWELL-PRICE J et al: Diagnosis and management of Cushing's syndrome. Lancet 353:2087, 1999

PITT B et al: Eplerenone, a selective aldosterone blocker, in patients with left ventricular dysfunction after myocardial infarction. N Engl J Med 348: 1309, 2003

YOUNG WF: Minireview: Primary aldosteronism—changing concepts in diagnosis and treatment. Endocrinology 144:2208, 2003

322 PHEOCHROMOCYTOMA
Lewis Landsberg, James B. Young

Pheochromocytomas produce, store, and secrete catecholamines. They are usually derived from the adrenal medulla but may develop from chromaffin cells in or about sympathetic ganglia (extraadrenal pheochromocytomas or paragangliomas). Related tumors that secrete catecholamines and produce similar clinical syndromes include chemodectomas derived from the carotid body and ganglioneuromas derived from the postganglionic sympathetic neurons.

The clinical features are due predominantly to the release of catecholamines and, to a lesser extent, to the secretion of other substances. Hypertension is the most common sign, and hypertensive paroxysms or crises, often spectacular and alarming, occur in over half the cases.

Pheochromocytoma occurs in approximately 0.1% of the hypertensive population but is, nevertheless, an important correctable cause of high blood pressure. Indeed, it is usually curable if diagnosed and treated, but it may be fatal if undiagnosed or mistreated. Postmortem series indicate that most pheochromocytomas are unsuspected clinically, even when the tumor is related to the fatal outcome.

PATHOLOGY ■ **Location and Morphology**   In adults, approximately 80% of pheochromocytomas are unilateral and solitary, 10% are bilateral, and 10% are extraadrenal. In children, a fourth of tumors are bilateral, and an additional fourth are extraadrenal. Solitary lesions inexplicably favor the right side. Although pheochromocytomas may grow to large size (>3 kg), most weigh <100 g and are <10 cm in diameter. Pheochromocytomas are highly vascular.

The tumors are made up of large, polyhedral, pleomorphic chromaffin cells. Fewer than 10% of these tumors are malignant. As with several other endocrine tumors, malignancy cannot be determined from the histologic appearance; tumors that contain large numbers of aneuploid or tetraploid cells, as determined by flow cytometry, are more likely to recur. Local invasion of surrounding tissues or distant metastases indicate malignancy.

EXTRAADRENAL PHEOCHROMOCYTOMAS   Extraadrenal pheochromocytomas usually weigh 20 to 40 g and are <5 cm in diameter. Most are located within the abdomen in association with the celiac, superior mesenteric, and inferior mesenteric ganglia. Approximately 10% are in the thorax, 1% are within the urinary bladder, and <3% are in the neck, usually in association with the sympathetic ganglia or the extracranial branches of the ninth or tenth cranial nerves.

Catecholamine Synthesis, Storage, and Release   Pheochromocytomas synthesize and store catecholamines by processes resembling those of the normal adrenal medulla. Little is known about the mechanisms of catecholamine release from pheochromocytomas, but changes in blood flow and necrosis within the tumor may be the cause in some instances. These tumors are not innervated, and catecholamine release does not result from neural stimulation. Pheochromocytomas also store and secrete a variety of peptides, including endogenous opioids, adrenomedullin, endothelin, erythropoietin, parathyroid hormone–related protein, neuropeptide Y, and chromagranin A. These peptides contribute to the clinical manifestations in selected cases, as noted below.

EPINEPHRINE, NOREPINEPHRINE, AND DOPAMINE   Most pheochromocytomas produce both norepinephrine and epinephrine, and the percentage of norepinephrine is usually greater than in the normal adrenal. Most extraadrenal pheochromocytomas secrete norepinephrine exclusively. Rarely, pheochromocytomas produce epinephrine alone, particularly in association with multiple endocrine neoplasia (MEN). Although epinephrine-producing tumors may cause a preponderance of metabolic and beta-receptor effects, in general the major catecholamine secreted cannot be predicted from the clinical presentation. Increased production of dopamine and homovanillic acid (HVA) is uncommon with benign lesions but may occur with malignant pheochromocytoma.

FAMILIAL PHEOCHROMOCYTOMA   Pheochromocytoma may be inherited as an autosomal dominant trait either alone or in combination with other abnormalities such as MEN type 2A (Sipple's syndrome) or type 2B (mucosal neuroma syndrome) (Chap. 330), von Hippel–Lindau's (VHL) retinal cerebellar hemangioblastomosis, or von Recklinghausen's neurofibromatosis (type 1) and in association with paragangliomas of the neck. Recent evidence suggests that 25% of patients with pheochromocytoma may have an inherited form of the disease. Features that suggest familial disease include bilaterality, multicentricity (within the adrenal and at diverse sites), and age of onset <30 years.

GENETIC CONSIDERATIONS   **MEN 2**   The MEN 2A and 2B syndromes are associated with abnormalities in the *RET* protooncogene located in pericentromeric region of chromosome 10 (Chap. 330). These mutations result in the constitutive activation of the receptor tyrosine kinase, causing adrenal medullary chromaffin cell and thyroid parafollicular C cell hyperplasia and rendering the cells susceptible to malignant transformation. The *RET* mutations are located in the extracellular domain in MEN 2A and in the intracellular portion of the receptor in families with the MEN 2B syndrome. Mutations at specific sites in the *RET* protooncogene are highly predictive of pheochromocytoma. Pheochromocytomas in MEN 2 are multicentric and bilateral but not extraadrenal. Individuals at risk for MEN 2A and 2B should be screened periodically for pheochromocytoma by assay of a 24-h urine sample for catecholamines, including measurement of epinephrine. Pheochromocytoma should be excluded or removed before thyroid or parathyroid surgery.

VHL   In the VHL syndrome, mutation of one copy of the VHL tumor-suppressor gene is associated with the development of tumors characteristic of the syndrome, including pheochromocytomas. Loss of function of the VHL tumor-suppressor gene promotes tumor formation by mechanisms that are incompletely understood but may involve alterations in mRNA transcript elongation. In the VHL syndrome, the frequency of pheochromocytoma varies considerably but may be as high as 60% in some kindreds. As in the MEN 2 syndromes, certain VHL mutations are highly associated with the development of pheochromocytoma. Of further interest is the recent finding that the VHL mutation has been identified in some kindreds with familial pheochromocytoma as the sole manifestation without other clinical evidence of the VHL syndrome. Missense mutations, as opposed to deletions, insertions, or nonsense mutations, appear to be more commonly associated with pheochromocytoma, which may be adrenal, extraadrenal, or multifocal. A high incidence of germ-line VHL mutations in patients with thoracic extraadrenal pheochromocytomas has also been reported.

Familial Paraganglioma Syndromes   Mutations in the genes encoding succinate dehydrogenase subunit B (SDHB) and subunit D (SDHD) may occur in kindreds with inherited paraganglioma, usually located in the head or neck (glomus tumors) or carotid body. Paraganglioma in these syndromes are distinct from extraadrenal pheochromocytomas, which are also commonly referred to as *paragangliomas*. Adrenal or extraadrenal pheochromocytomas are often inherited in association with these paragangliomas.

Neurofibromatosis Type I   Mutations in the *NF-I* gene predispose to the development of pheochromocytoma, although the association is not very common. It has been estimated that 1% of patients with pheochromocytoma have an *NF-I* mutation. Pheochromocytomas may occur in patients with minor clinical manifestations of neurofibromatosis such as a few café au lait spots, vertebral abnormalities, or kyphoscoliosis.

Nonsyndromic Familial Pheochromocytoma   Patients presenting with a solitary adrenal pheochromocytoma, negative family history, and no evidence of associated disease may still have an inherited form of the disease. This is most common with the *SDHB* and *SDHD* mutations but also occurs with alterations in the *VHL* gene.

Screening for Genetic Disease   Genetic screening for the *RET* mutation is available and of established utility in the evaluation of families for the MEN 2 syndromes. Genetic tests for the *SDH*, *NF-I*, and *VHL* mutations are not yet generally available. Screening in these kindreds therefore is dependent on a vigorous search for the associated diseases and a complete evaluation of family history.

CLINICAL FEATURES   Pheochromocytoma occurs at all ages but is most common in young to midadult life. Some series show a slight female preponderance. Most patients come to medical attention as a result of hypertensive crisis, paroxysmal symptoms suggestive of seizure disorder or anxiety attacks, or hypertension that responds poorly to conventional treatment. Less commonly, unexplained hypotension or shock in association with surgery or trauma will suggest the diagnosis. Aberrant reactions to medications such as opioids or tricyclic antidepressants may bring the patient to clinical attention. In most patients the hypertension is associated with other symptoms, such as headaches, excessive sweating, and/or palpitations.

Hypertension   Hypertension is the most common manifestation. In approximately 60% of cases the hypertension is sustained, although significant blood pressure lability is usually present, and half of patients with sustained hypertension have distinct crises or paroxysms. The other 40% have blood pressure elevations only during an attack. The hypertension is often severe, occasionally malignant, and may be resistant to treatment with standard antihypertensive drugs.

Paroxysms or Crises   The paroxysm or crisis occurs in over half of patients. In an individual patient, the symptoms are often similar with each attack. The paroxysms may be frequent or sporadic, occurring at intervals as long as weeks or months. With time, the paroxysms usually increase in frequency, duration, and severity.

The attack usually has a sudden onset. It may last from a few minutes to several hours or longer. Headache, profuse sweating, palpitations, and apprehension, often with a sense of impending doom, are common. Pain in the chest or abdomen may be associated with nausea and vomiting. Either pallor or flushing may occur during the attack. The blood pressure is elevated, often to alarming levels, and the elevation is usually accompanied by tachycardia.

The paroxysm may be precipitated by any activity that displaces the abdominal contents. In some cases a particular stimulus may induce an attack in a characteristic fashion, but in others no clearly defined precipitating event can be found. Although anxiety may accompany the attacks, mental or psychological stress does not usually provoke a crisis.

Other Distinctive Clinical Features   Symptoms and signs of an increased metabolic rate, such as profuse sweating and mild to moderate weight loss, are common. Orthostatic hypotension is a consequence of diminished plasma volume and blunted sympathetic reflexes. Both these factors predispose the patient with unsuspected pheochromocytoma to hypotension or shock during surgery or trauma. Secretion of the hypotensive peptide adrenomedullin may contribute to the hypotension in some patients.

CARDIAC MANIFESTATIONS   Sinus tachycardia, sinus bradycardia, supraventricular arrhythmias, and ventricular premature contractions have all been noted. Angina and acute myocardial infarction may occur even in the absence of coronary artery disease. A catecholamine-induced increase in myocardial oxygen consumption and, perhaps, coronary spasm may play a role in these ischemic events. Electrocardiographic changes, including nonspecific ST-T wave changes, prominent U waves, left ventricular strain patterns, and right and left bundle branch blocks may be present in the absence of demonstrable ischemia or infarction. Cardiomyopathy, either congestive with myocarditis and myocardial fibrosis or hypertrophic with concentric or asymmetric hypertrophy, may be associated with heart failure and cardiac arrhythmias. Multiorgan system failure with noncardiogenic pulmonary edema may be the presenting manifestation. Elevated levels of amylase originating from damaged pulmonary endothelium and abdominal pain may suggest acute pancreatitis, although serum lipase levels are normal.

CARBOHYDRATE INTOLERANCE   Over half of patients have impaired carbohydrate tolerance due to suppression of insulin and stimulation of hepatic glucose output. The impaired glucose tolerance may require treatment with insulin and disappears after removal of the tumor.

HEMATOCRIT   An elevated hematocrit may be secondary to diminished plasma volume. Rarely, production of erythropoietin by the tumor may cause a true erythrocytosis.

OTHER MANIFESTATIONS   Hypercalcemia has been attributed to the ectopic secretion of parathyroid hormone–related protein. Fever and an elevated erythrocyte sedimentation rate have been reported in association with the production of interleukin 6. Elevated temperature more commonly reflects catecholamine-mediated increases in metabolic rate and diminished heat dissipation secondary to vasoconstriction. Polyuria is an occasional finding, and rhabdomyolysis with myoglobinuric renal failure may result from extreme vasoconstriction with muscle ischemia. Ectopic production of adrenocorticotropic hormone and vasoactive intestinal peptide have been documented in association with the characteristic manifestations of inappropriate secretion of these hormones (Chap. 317).

PHEOCHROMOCYTOMA OF THE URINARY BLADDER   Pheochromocytoma in the wall of the urinary bladder may result in typical paroxysms in relation to micturition. The location in the bladder wall is responsible for the occurrence of symptoms while the tumors are quite small, and, consequently, catecholamine excretion may be normal or minimally elevated. Hematuria is present in over half of patients, and the tumor can often be visualized at cystoscopy.

Adverse Drug Interactions   Severe and occasionally fatal paroxysms have been induced by opiates, histamine, adrenocorticotropin, saralasin, and glucagon. These agents appear to release catecholamines directly from the tumor. Indirect-acting sympathomimetic amines, including methyldopa (when administered intravenously), may increase blood pressure by releasing catecholamines from the augmented stores within nerve endings. Drugs that block neuronal uptake of catecholamines, such as tricyclic antidepressants, may enhance the physiologic effects of circulating catecholamines. Indeed, all medications should be considered carefully and administered cautiously in patients with known or suspected pheochromocytoma.

DIAGNOSIS   The diagnosis is established by the demonstration of increased production of catecholamines or catecholamine metabolites. The diagnosis can usually be made by the analysis of a single 24-h urine sample, provided the patient is hypertensive or symptomatic at the time of collection.

Biochemical Tests   The assays employed include those for vanillylmandelic acid (VMA), the metanephrines, and unconjugated or "free" catecholamines. The VMA assay is both less sensitive and less specific than assays of metanephrines or catecholamines. Accuracy of diagnosis is improved when two of three determinations are employed. The following considerations apply to all the urinary tests: (1) Despite claims for the adequacy of determinations made on random urine samples, analysis of a full 24-h urine sample is preferable. Creatinine should also be determined to assess the adequacy of collection. (2) Where possible, the collection should be made when the patient is at rest, on no medication, and without recent exposure to radiographic

contrast media. When it is not practical to discontinue all medications, drugs known specifically to interfere with these assays (as noted below) should be avoided. (3) The urine should be acidified and refrigerated during and after collection. (4) With high-quality assays, dietary restrictions are minimal and should be specified by the laboratory performing the analyses. (5) Although most patients with pheochromocytoma excrete increased amounts of catecholamines and catecholamine metabolites at all times, the yield is increased in patients with paroxysmal hypertension if a 24-h urine collection is initiated during a crisis.

FREE CATECHOLAMINES   The upper limit of normal for total urinary catecholamines is between 590 and 885 nmol (100 and 150 μg) per 24 h. In most patients with pheochromocytoma, values >1480 nmol (250 μg) per day are obtained. Measurement of epinephrine is often of value, since increased epinephrine excretion [>275 nmol (50 μg) per 24 h] is usually due to an adrenal lesion and may be the only abnormality in cases associated with MEN 2. False-positive increases in catecholamine excretion result from exogenous catecholamines and related drugs such as methyldopa, levodopa, labetalol, and sympathomimetic amines, which may elevate catecholamine excretion for up to 2 weeks. Endogenous catecholamines from stimulation of the sympathoadrenal system may also increase urinary catecholamine excretion. Relevant clinical situations that cause such increases include hypoglycemia, strenuous exertion, central nervous system disease with increased intracranial pressure, severe hypoxia, and clonidine withdrawal.

METANEPHRINES AND VMA   In most laboratories, the upper limit of normal is 7 μmol (1.3 mg) of total metanephrines and 35 μmol (7.0 mg) of VMA excretion per 24 h. In most patients with pheochromocytoma, the increase in these urinary metabolites is considerable, often to more than three times the normal range. Metanephrine excretion is increased by exogenous and endogenous catecholamines and by treatment with monoamine oxidase inhibitors; propranolol may cause a spurious increase in metanephrine excretion, since a propranolol metabolite interferes in the commonly used spectrophotometric assay. VMA is less affected by endogenous and exogenous catecholamines but is spuriously increased by a variety of drugs, including carbidopa. VMA excretion is decreased by monoamine oxidase inhibitors.

PLASMA CATECHOLAMINES   Measurement of plasma catecholamines has a limited application. The care required in obtaining basal levels and the satisfactory results with urinary determinations make measurement of plasma catecholamines unnecessary in most cases. Plasma catecholamine levels are affected by the same drugs and physiologic perturbations that increase urinary catecholamine excretion. In addition, α- and β-adrenergic receptor blocking agents may elevate plasma catecholamines by impairing clearance.

When the clinical features suggest pheochromocytoma and the urinary assay results are borderline, measurement of plasma catecholamines may be worthwhile. Markedly elevated basal levels of total catecholamines support the diagnosis, although approximately one-third of patients with pheochromocytoma have normal or slightly elevated basal values. The usefulness of plasma catecholamine determinations may be increased by agents that suppress sympathetic nervous system activity. Clonidine and ganglionic blocking agents reduce plasma catecholamine levels in normal subjects and in patients with essential hypertension. These drugs have little effect on catecholamine levels in patients with pheochromocytoma. In patients with elevated or borderline basal catecholamine values, failure to suppress plasma or urinary levels with clonidine supports the diagnosis of pheochromocytoma.

PLASMA METANEPHRINES   Measurement of free (unconjugated) total plasma metanephrines, fractionated into normetanephrine and metanephrine, is a highly sensitive technique for the diagnosis of pheochromocytoma. Questions of specificity, particularly among the elderly, as well as the availability of high-quality assays need to be addressed before plasma metanephrines replace the 24-h urinary measurement of free catecholamines and metanephrines as the screening test of choice.

Pharmacologic Tests Reliable methods for the measurement of catecholamines and catecholamine metabolites in urine have rendered obsolete both the provocative and adrenolytic tests, which are nonspecific and entail considerable risk. A modified version of the adrenolytic test may be of some use, however, as a therapeutic trial in a patient in hypertensive crisis with features suggestive of pheochromocytoma. A positive response to phentolamine (5-mg bolus following a test dose of 0.5 mg) is a reduction in blood pressure of at least 35/25 mmHg after 2 min that persists for 10 to 15 min. The pharmacologic response is never diagnostic, and biochemical confirmation is essential. Provocative tests in normotensive patients are potentially dangerous and rarely indicated. However, a glucagon provocative test may be of use in patients with paroxysmal hypertension and nondiagnostic basal catecholamine levels. Glucagon has a negligible effect on blood pressure or plasma catecholamine levels in normal or hypertensive subjects. In patients with pheochromocytoma, on the other hand, glucagon may increase both blood pressure and circulating catecholamine levels. The elevation in plasma catecholamine concentration, moreover, may occur without a blood pressure response. It must be emphasized, however, that life-threatening pressor crises have occurred after administration of glucagon to patients with pheochromocytoma, so the test should never be performed casually. Careful continuous monitoring of the blood pressure is required, intravenous access must be adequate, and phentolamine must be at hand to terminate the test if a significant pressor reaction ensues.

Differential Diagnosis Since the manifestations of pheochromocytoma can be protean, the diagnosis must be considered and excluded in many patients with suggestive clinical features. In patients with essential hypertension and "hyperadrenergic" features such as tachycardia, sweating, and increased cardiac output, and in patients with anxiety attacks associated with blood pressure elevations, analysis of a 24-h urine collection is usually decisive in excluding the diagnosis. Repeated determinations on urine collected during attacks may be necessary, however, before the diagnosis can be excluded with certainty. Pressor crises associated with clonidine withdrawal and the use of cocaine or monoamine oxidase inhibitors may mimic the paroxysms of pheochromocytoma. Factitious crises may be produced by self-administration of sympathomimetic amines in psychiatrically disturbed patients.

Intracranial lesions, particularly posterior fossa tumors or subarachnoid hemorrhage, may cause hypertension and increased excretion of catecholamines or catecholamine metabolites. While this is most common in patients with an obvious neurologic catastrophe, the possibility of subarachnoid or intracranial hemorrhage secondary to pheochromocytoma should be considered. Diencephalic or autonomic epilepsy may be associated with paroxysmal spells, hypertension, and increased plasma catecholamine levels. This rare entity may be difficult to distinguish from pheochromocytoma, but an aura, an abnormal electroencephalogram, and a beneficial response to anticonvulsant medications will often suggest this diagnosis.

Rx **TREATMENT**

Preoperative Management The induction of stable α-adrenergic blockade provides the foundation for successful surgical treatment. Once the diagnosis is established, the patient should be placed on phenoxybenzamine to induce a long-lasting, noncompetitive α-receptor blockade. The usual initial dose is 10 mg every 12 h, with increments of 10 to 20 mg added every few days until the blood pressure is controlled and the paroxysms disappear. Because of the long duration of action, the therapeutic effects are cumulative, and the optimal dose must be achieved gradually with careful monitoring of supine and upright blood pressures. Most patients require between 40 and 80 mg phenoxybenzamine per day, although $\geq$200 mg may be necessary. Phenoxybenzamine should be administered for at least 10 to 14 days prior to surgery. Over this time, the combination of α-receptor block-

ade and a liberal salt intake will restore the contracted plasma volume to normal. Before adequate α-adrenergic blockade with phenoxybenzamine is achieved, paroxysms may be treated with oral prazosin or intravenous phentolamine. Selective α_1 antagonists have been employed for preoperative preparation, but their role in preparative management should be limited to the treatment of individual paroxysms. They may be useful as antihypertensive agents in patients with suspected pheochromocytoma while workup is in progress, since they are usually better tolerated than phenoxybenzamine and will prevent serious pressor crises if pheochromocytoma is present. Nitroprusside, calcium channel blocking agents, and possibly angiotensin-converting enzyme inhibitors reduce blood pressure in patients with pheochromocytoma. Nitroprusside may also be useful in the treatment of pressor crises.

β-Adrenergic receptor blocking agents should be given only after alpha blockade has been induced, since administration of such agents by themselves may cause a paradoxic increase in blood pressure by antagonizing beta-mediated vasodilation in skeletal muscle. Beta blockade is usually initiated when tachycardia develops during the induction of α-adrenergic blockade. Low doses often suffice, and a reasonable starting dose is 10 mg propranolol three to four times per day, increased as needed to control the pulse rate. Beta blockade is effective for catecholamine-induced arrhythmias, particularly those potentiated by anesthetic agents.

Preoperative Localization of the Tumor Once pheochromocytoma is diagnosed, localization should be undertaken while the patient is being prepared for surgery. Computed tomography (CT) or magnetic resonance imaging (MRI) of the adrenals is usually successful in identifying intraadrenal lesions. Extraadrenal tumors within the chest can frequently be identified by conventional chest films or CT. MRI or positron emission tomography (PET) scanning with ^{18}F dopa is useful in identifying extraadrenal tumors. Abdominal aortography (once α-adrenergic blockade is complete) or venous sampling at different levels of the inferior and superior vena cava in search of catecholamine gradients has been useful in the past but are rarely necessary now. An additional localization technique involves a radionuclide scintiscan after administration of the radiopharmaceutical [^{131}I]metaiodobenzylguanidine (MIBG). This agent is concentrated by the amine uptake process and produces an external scintigraphic image at the site of the tumor. This type of scanning may be useful in characterizing lesions discovered by CT when biochemical confirmation is indeterminate but is less useful at localizing extraadrenal pheochromocytomas than MRI or PET. Percutaneous fine-needle aspiration of chromaffin tumors is contraindicated; indeed, pheochromocytoma should be considered before adrenal lesions are aspirated.

Surgery Surgical treatment of pheochromocytoma is best performed in centers with experience in the preoperative, anesthetic, and intraoperative management of pheochromocytoma. Surgical mortality is <2 or 3%. Extensive experience with the laparoscopic approach over the past decade has demonstrated that in experienced hands pheochromocytoma can be safely and efficiently removed by this technique.

Monitoring during the surgical procedure should include continuous recording of arterial pressure and central venous pressure as well as electrocardiography; in the presence of cardiac disease or if congestive failure has been present, pulmonary capillary wedge pressure should be monitored. Adequate fluid replacement is crucial. Intraoperative hypotension responds better to volume replacement than to vasoconstrictors. Hypertension and cardiac arrhythmias are most likely during induction of anesthesia, intubation, and manipulation of the tumor. Intravenous phentolamine is usually sufficient to control the blood pressure, but nitroprusside may be required. Propranolol may be given in the treatment of tachycardia or ventricular ectopy.

PHEOCHROMOCYTOMA IN PREGNANCY Spontaneous labor and vaginal delivery in unprepared patients are usually disastrous for mother and fetus. In early pregnancy, the patient should be prepared with phenoxybenzamine, and the tumor should be removed as soon as the diagnosis is confirmed. The pregnancy need not be terminated, but the operative procedure itself may result in spontaneous abortion. In the third trimester, treatment with adrenergic blocking agents should be undertaken; when the fetus is of sufficient size, cesarean section may be followed by extirpation of the tumor. Although the safety of adrenergic blocking drugs in pregnancy is not established, these agents have been administered in several cases without obvious adverse effect. Antepartum diagnosis and treatment lowers the maternal death rate to that approaching nonpregnant pheochromocytoma patients; fetal death rate, however, remains elevated.

UNRESECTABLE AND MALIGNANT TUMORS   In cases of metastatic or locally invasive tumor in patients with intercurrent illness that precludes surgery, long-term medical management is required. When the manifestations cannot be adequately controlled by adrenergic blocking agents, the concomitant administration of metyrosine may be required. This agent inhibits tyrosine hydroxylase, diminishes catecholamine production by the tumor, and often simplifies chronic management. Malignant pheochromocytoma frequently recurs in the retroperitoneum, and it metastasizes most commonly to bone and lung. Although these malignant tumors are resistant to radiotherapy, combination chemotherapy is occasionally of some benefit. Use of ^{131}I-MIBG has had limited success in the treatment of malignant pheochromocytoma, due to poor uptake of the radioligand.

PROGNOSIS AND FOLLOW-UP   The 5-year survival rate after surgery is usually >95%, the recurrence rate is <10%. After successful surgery, catecholamine excretion returns to normal in about 2 weeks and should be measured to ensure complete tumor removal. Catecholamine excretion should be assessed at the reappearance of suggestive symptoms or yearly if the patient remains asymptomatic. For malignant pheochromocytoma, the 5-year survival rate is usually <50%, although long-term survival is occasionally noted.

Complete removal cures the hypertension in approximately three-fourths of patients. In the remainder, hypertension recurs but is usually well controlled by standard antihypertensive agents. In this group, either underlying essential hypertension or irreversible vascular damage induced by catecholamines may cause the persistence of the hypertension.

FURTHER READING

GILLAM MP, LANDSBERG L: Pheochromocytoma, in *Challenging Cases in Endocrinology*, M Molitch (ed). Humana Press 9:155–183, 2002

HARTMUT PH et al: Germ-line mutations in nonsyndromic pheochromocytoma. N Engl J Med 346:1459 2002

KERCHER KW et al: Laparoscopic adrenalectomy for pheochromocytoma. Surg Endosc 16:100, 2002

LENDERS JWM et al: Biochemical diagnosis of pheochromocytoma. JAMA 287:1427, 2002

SAWKA AM et al: A comparison of biochemical tests for pheochromocytoma: Measurement of fractionated plasma metanephrines compared with the combination of 24-h urinary metanephrines and catecholamines. J Clin Endocrinol Metab 88:553, 2003

323   DIABETES MELLITUS
Alvin C. Powers

Diabetes mellitus (DM) comprises a group of common metabolic disorders that share the phenotype of hyperglycemia. Several distinct types of DM exist and are caused by a complex interaction of genetics, environmental factors, and life-style choices. Depending on the etiology of the DM, factors contributing to hyperglycemia may include reduced insulin secretion, decreased glucose utilization, and increased glucose production. The metabolic dysregulation associated with DM causes secondary pathophysiologic changes in multiple organ systems that impose a tremendous burden on the individual with diabetes and on the health care system. In the United States, DM is the leading cause of end-stage renal disease (ESRD), nontraumatic lower extremity amputations, and adult blindness. With an increasing incidence worldwide, DM will be a leading cause of morbidity and mortality for the foreseeable future.

CLASSIFICATION

DM is classified on the basis of the pathogenic process that leads to hyperglycemia, as opposed to earlier criteria such as age of onset or type of therapy (Fig. 323-1). The two broad categories of DM are designated type 1 and type 2 (Table 323-1). Type 1A DM results from autoimmune beta cell destruction, which leads to insulin deficiency. Individuals with type 1B DM lack immunologic markers indicative of an autoimmune destructive process of the beta cells. However, they develop insulin deficiency by unknown mechanisms and are ketosis prone. Relatively few patients with type 1 DM are in the type 1B idiopathic category; many of these individuals are either African-American or Asian in heritage.

Type 2 DM is a heterogeneous group of disorders characterized by variable degrees of insulin resistance, impaired insulin secretion, and increased glucose production. Distinct genetic and metabolic defects

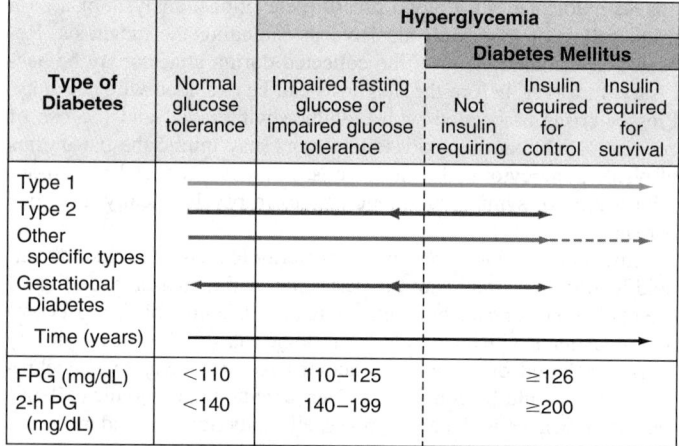

Type of Diabetes	Normal glucose tolerance	Hyperglycemia			
			Diabetes Mellitus		
		Impaired fasting glucose or impaired glucose tolerance	Not insulin requiring	Insulin required for control	Insulin required for survival
Type 1					
Type 2					
Other specific types					
Gestational Diabetes					
Time (years)					
FPG (mg/dL)	<110	110–125	≥126		
2-h PG (mg/dL)	<140	140–199	≥200		

FIGURE 323-1   Spectrum of glucose homeostasis and diabetes mellitus (DM). The spectrum from normal glucose tolerance to diabetes in type 1 DM, type 2 DM, other specific types of diabetes, and gestational DM is shown from left to right. In most types of DM, the individual traverses from normal glucose tolerance to impaired glucose tolerance to overt diabetes. Arrows indicate that changes in glucose tolerance may be bi-directional in some types of diabetes. For example, individuals with type 2 DM may return to the impaired glucose tolerance category with weight loss; in gestational DM diabetes may revert to impaired glucose tolerance or even normal glucose tolerance after delivery. The fasting plasma glucose (FPG) and 2-h plasma glucose (PG), after a glucose challenge for the different categories of glucose tolerance, are shown at the lower part of the figure. These values do not apply to the diagnosis of gestational DM. Some types of DM may or may not require insulin for survival, hence the dotted line. (Conventional units are used in the figure.) (*Adapted from American Diabetes Association, 2004.*)

in insulin action and/or secretion give rise to the common phenotype of hyperglycemia in type 2 DM (see below). Distinct pathogenic processes in type 2 DM have important potential therapeutic implications, as pharmacologic agents that target specific metabolic derangements

TABLE 323-1 *Etiologic Classification of Diabetes Mellitus*

I. Type 1 diabetes (β-cell destruction, usually leading to absolute insulin deficiency)
   A. Immune-mediated
   B. Idiopathic
II. Type 2 diabetes (may range from predominantly insulin resistance with relative insulin deficiency to a predominantly insulin secretory defect with insulin resistance)
III. Other specific types of diabetes
   A. Genetic defects of β-cell function characterized by mutations in:
      1. Hepatocyte nuclear transcription factor (HNF) 4α (MODY 1)
      2. Glucokinase (MODY 2)
      3. HNF-1α (MODY 3)
      4. Insulin promoter factor (IPF) 1 (MODY 4)
      5. HNF-1β (MODY 5)
      6. NeuroD1 (MODV6)
      7. Mitochondrial DNA
      8. Proinsulin or insulin conversion
   B. Genetic defects in insulin action
      1. Type A insulin resistance
      2. Leprechaunism
      3. Rabson-Mendenhall syndrome
      4. Lipodystrophy syndromes
   C. Diseases of the exocrine pancreas—pancreatitis, pancreatectomy, neoplasia, cystic fibrosis, hemochromatosis, fibrocalculous pancreatopathy
   D. Endocrinopathies—acromegaly, Cushing's syndrome, glucagonoma, pheochromocytoma, hyperthyroidism, somatostatinoma, aldosteronoma
   E. Drug- or chemical-induced—Vacor, pentamidine, nicotinic acid, glucocorticoids, thyroid hormone, diazoxide, β-adrenergic agonists, thiazides, phenytoin, α-interferon, protease inhibitors, clozapine, beta blockers
   F. Infections—congenital rubella, cytomegalovirus, coxsackie
   G. Uncommon forms of immune-mediated diabetes—"stiff-man" syndrome, anti-insulin receptor antibodies
   H. Other genetic syndromes sometimes associated with diabetes—Down's syndrome, Klinefelter's syndrome, Turner's syndrome, Wolfram's syndrome, Friedreich's ataxia, Huntington's chorea, Laurence-Moon-Biedl syndrome, myotonic dystrophy, porphyria, Prader-Willi syndrome
IV. Gestational diabetes mellitus (GDM)

Note: MODY, maturity onset of diabetes of the young.
Source: Adapted from American Diabetes Association, 2004.

have become available. Type 2 DM is preceded by a period of abnormal glucose homeostasis classified as impaired fasting glucose (IFG) or impaired glucose tolerance (IGT).

Two features of the current classification of DM diverge from previous classifications. First, the terms *insulin-dependent diabetes mellitus* (IDDM) and *noninsulin-dependent diabetes mellitus* (NIDDM) are obsolete. Since many individuals with type 2 DM eventually require insulin treatment for control of glycemia, the use of the term NIDDM generated considerable confusion. A second difference is that age is not a criterion in the classification system. Although type 1 DM most commonly develops before the age of 30, an autoimmune beta cell destructive process can develop at any age. It is estimated that between 5 and 10% of individuals who develop DM after age 30 have type 1A DM. Likewise, type 2 DM more typically develops with increasing age, but it also occurs in children, particularly in obese adolescents.

OTHER TYPES OF DM Other etiologies for DM include specific genetic defects in insulin secretion or action, metabolic abnormalities that impair insulin secretion, mitochondrial abnormalities, and a host of conditions that impair glucose tolerance (Table 323-1). *Maturity onset diabetes of the young* (MODY) is a subtype of DM characterized by autosomal dominant inheritance, early onset of hyperglycemia, and impairment in insulin secretion (discussed below). Mutations in the insulin receptor cause a group of rare disorders characterized by severe insulin resistance.

DM can result from pancreatic exocrine disease when the majority

of pancreatic islets (>80%) are destroyed. Hormones that antagonize the action of insulin can lead to DM. Thus, DM is often a feature of endocrinopathies, such as acromegaly and Cushing's disease. Viral infections have been implicated in pancreatic islet destruction, but are an extremely rare cause of DM. Congenital rubella greatly increases the risk for DM; however, most of these individuals also have immunologic markers indicative of autoimmune beta cell destruction.

GESTATIONAL DIABETES MELLITUS (GDM) Glucose intolerance may develop during pregnancy. Insulin resistance related to the metabolic changes of late pregnancy increases insulin requirements and may lead to IGT. GDM occurs in approximately 4% of pregnancies in the United States; most women revert to normal glucose tolerance post-partum but have a substantial risk (30 to 60%) of developing DM later in life.

EPIDEMIOLOGY

The worldwide prevalence of DM has risen dramatically over the past two decades. Likewise, prevalence rates of IFG are also increasing. Although the prevalence of both type 1 and type 2 DM is increasing worldwide, the prevalence of type 2 DM is expected to rise more rapidly in the future because of increasing obesity and reduced activity levels. DM increases with aging. In 2000, the prevalence of DM was estimated to be 0.19% in people <20 years old and 8.6% in people >20 years old. In individuals >65 years the prevalence of DM was 20.1%. The prevalence is similar in men and women throughout most age ranges but is slightly greater in men >60 years.

There is considerable geographic variation in the incidence of both type 1 and type 2 DM. Scandinavia has the highest incidence of type 1 DM (e.g., in Finland, the incidence is 35/100,000 per year). The Pacific Rim has a much lower rate (in Japan and China, the incidence is 1 to 3/100,000 per year) of type 1 DM; Northern Europe and the United States share an intermediate rate (8 to 17/100,000 per year). Much of the increased risk of type 1 DM is believed to reflect the frequency of high-risk HLA alleles among ethnic groups in different geographic locations. The prevalence of type 2 DM and its harbinger, IGT, is highest in certain Pacific islands, intermediate in countries such as India and the United States, and relatively low in Russia and China. This variability is likely due to genetic, behavioral, and environmental factors. DM prevalence also varies among different ethnic populations within a given country. In 2000, the prevalence of DM in the United States was 13% in African Americans, 10.2% in Hispanic Americans, 15.5% in Native Americans (American Indians and Alaska natives), and 7.8% in non-Hispanic whites. The onset of type 2 DM occurs, on average, at an earlier age in ethnic groups other than non-Hispanic whites.

DIAGNOSIS

The National Diabetes Data Group and World Health Organization have issued diagnostic criteria for DM (Table 323-2) based on the following premises: (1) the spectrum of fasting plasma glucose (FPG) and the response to an oral glucose load varies among normal indi-

TABLE 323-2 *Criteria for the Diagnosis of Diabetes Mellitus*

- Symptoms of diabetes plus random blood glucose concentration ≥ 11.1 mmol/L (200 mg/dL)[a]   *or*
- Fasting plasma glucose ≥ 7.0 mmol/L (126 mg/dL)[b]   *or*
- Two-hour plasma glucose ≥ 11.1 mmol/L (200 mg/dL) during an oral glucose tolerance test[c]

[a] Random is defined as without regard to time since the last meal.
[b] Fasting is defined as no caloric intake for at least 8 h.
[c] The test should be performed using a glucose load containing the equivalent of 75 g anhydrous glucose dissolved in water; not recommended for routine clinical use.
Note: In the absence of unequivocal hyperglycemia and acute metabolic decompensation, these criteria should be confirmed by repeat testing on a different day.
Source: Modified from American Diabetes Association, 2004.

viduals, and (2) DM is defined as the level of glycemia at which diabetes-specific complications occur rather than on deviations from a population-based mean. For example, the prevalence of retinopathy in Native Americans (Pima Indian population) begins to increase at a FPG > 6.4 mmol/L (116 mg/dL) (Fig. 323-2).

Glucose tolerance is classified into three categories based on the FPG: (1) FPG < 5.6 mmol/L (100 mg/dL) is considered normal; (2) FPG ≥ 5.6 mmol/L (100 mg/dL) but <7.0 mmol/L (126 mg/dL) is defined as IFG; and (3) FPG ≥ 7.0 mmol/L (126 mg/dL) warrants the diagnosis of DM. IFG is comparable to IGT, which is defined as plasma glucose levels between 7.8 and 11.1 mmol/L (140 and 200 mg/dL) 2 h after a 75-g oral glucose load (Table 323-2). Individuals with IFG or IGT are at substantial risk for developing type 2 DM (40% risk over the next 5 years) and cardiovascular disease.

The revised criteria for the diagnosis of DM emphasize the FPG as a reliable and convenient test for diagnosing DM in asymptomatic individuals. A random plasma glucose concentration ≥11.1 mmol/L (200 mg/dL) accompanied by classic symptoms of DM (polyuria, polydipsia, weight loss) is sufficient for the diagnosis of DM (Table 323-2). Oral glucose tolerance testing, although still a valid mechanism for diagnosing DM, is not recommended as part of routine care.

Some investigators have advocated the hemoglobin A1c (A1C) as a diagnostic test for DM. Though there is a strong correlation between elevations in the plasma glucose and the A1C (discussed below), the relationship between the FPG and the A1C in individuals with normal glucose tolerance or mild glucose intolerance is less clear and thus the use of the A1C is not currently recommended for the diagnosis of diabetes.

The diagnosis of DM has profound implications for an individual from both a medical and financial standpoint. Thus, these diagnostic criteria must be satisfied before assigning the diagnosis of DM. Abnormalities on screening tests for diabetes should be repeated before making a definitive diagnosis of DM, unless acute metabolic derangements or a markedly elevated plasma glucose are present (Table 323-2). The revised criteria also allow for the diagnosis of DM to be withdrawn in situations where the FPG reverts to normal.

SCREENING Widespread use of the FPG as a screening test for type 2 DM is recommended because: (1) a large number of individuals who meet the current criteria for DM are asymptomatic and unaware that they have the disorder, (2) epidemiologic studies suggest that type 2

DM may be present for up to a decade before diagnosis, (3) as many as 50% of individuals with type 2 DM have one or more diabetes-specific complications at the time of their diagnosis, and (4) treatment of type 2 DM may favorably alter the natural history of DM. The American Diabetes Association (ADA) recommends screening all individuals >45 years every 3 years and screening individuals with additional risk factors (Table 323-3) at an earlier age. In contrast to type 2 DM, a long asymptomatic period of hyperglycemia is rare prior to the diagnosis of type 1 DM. A number of immunologic markers for type 1 DM are becoming available (discussed below), but their routine use is discouraged pending the identification of clinically beneficial interventions for individuals at high risk for developing type 1 DM.

INSULIN BIOSYNTHESIS, SECRETION, AND ACTION

BIOSYNTHESIS Insulin is produced in the beta cells of the pancreatic islets. It is initially synthesized as a single-chain 86-amino-acid precursor polypeptide, preproinsulin. Subsequent proteolytic processing removes the aminoterminal signal peptide, giving rise to proinsulin. Proinsulin is structurally related to insulin-like growth factors I and II, which bind weakly to the insulin receptor (Chap. 317). Cleavage of an internal 31-residue fragment from proinsulin generates the C peptide and the A (21 amino acids) and B (30 amino acids) chains of insulin, which are connected by disulfide bonds. The mature insulin molecule and C peptide are stored together and cosecreted from secretory granules in the beta cells. Because the C peptide is less susceptible than insulin to hepatic degradation, it is a useful marker of insulin secretion and allows discrimination of endogenous and exogenous sources of insulin in the evaluation of hypoglycemia (Chap. 324). Human insulin is now produced by recombinant DNA technology; structural alterations at one or more residues are useful for modifying its physical and pharmacologic characteristics (see below).

SECRETION Glucose is the key regulator of insulin secretion by the pancreatic beta cell, although amino acids, ketones, various nutrients, gastrointestinal peptides, and neurotransmitters also influence insulin secretion. Glucose levels >3.9 mmol/L (70 mg/dL) stimulate insulin synthesis, primarily by enhancing protein translation and processing. Glucose stimulation of insulin secretion begins with its transport into the beta cell by the GLUT2 glucose transporter (Fig. 323-3). Glucose phosphorylation by glucokinase is the rate-limiting step that controls glucose-regulated insulin secretion. Further metabolism of glucose-6-phosphate via glycolysis generates ATP, which inhibits the activity of an ATP-sensitive K^+ channel. This channel consists of two separate proteins: one is the receptor for certain oral hypoglycemics (e.g., sulfonylureas, meglitinides); the other is an inwardly rectifying K^+ channel protein. Inhibition of this K^+ channel induces beta cell membrane depolarization, which opens voltage-dependent calcium channels (leading to an influx of calcium), and stimulates insulin secretion. Insulin secretory profiles reveal a pulsatile pattern of hormone release, with small secretory bursts occurring about every 10 min, superimposed upon greater amplitude oscillations of about 80 to 150 min. Meals or other major stimuli of insulin secretion induce large (four-

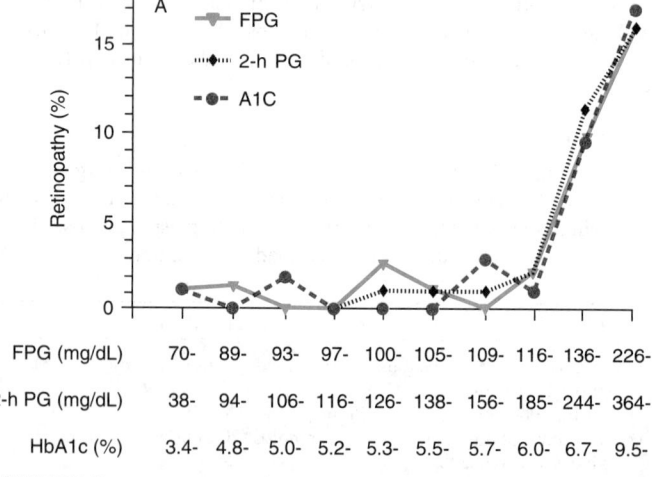

FPG (mg/dL)	70-	89-	93-	97-	100-	105-	109-	116-	136-	226-
2-h PG (mg/dL)	38-	94-	106-	116-	126-	138-	156-	185-	244-	364-
HbA1c (%)	3.4-	4.8-	5.0-	5.2-	5.3-	5.5-	5.7-	6.0-	6.7-	9.5-

FIGURE 323-2 Relationship of diabetes-specific complication and glucose tolerance. This figure shows the incidence of retinopathy in Pima Indians as a function of the fasting plasma glucose (FPG), the 2-h plasma glucose after a 75-g oral glucose challenge (2-h PG), or glycated hemoglobin (A1C). Note that the incidence of retinopathy greatly increases at a fasting plasma glucose >116 mg/dL, or a 2-h plasma glucose of 185 mg/dL, or a A1C >6.0%. (Conventional units for blood glucose are used in the figure.) *(Copyright 2002, American Diabetes Association. From Diabetes Care 25(Suppl 1): 55–520, 2002.)*

TABLE 323-3   Risk Factors for Type 2 Diabetes Mellitus

- Family history of diabetes (i.e., parent or sibling with type 2 diabetes)
- Obesity (BMI ≥ 25 kg/m²)
- Habitual physical inactivity
- Race/ethnicity (e.g., African American, Hispanic American, Native American, Asian American, Pacific Islander)
- Previously identified IFG or IGT
- History of GDM or delivery of baby >4 kg (>9 lb)
- Hypertension (blood pressure ≥ 140/90 mmHg)
- HDL cholesterol level ≤ 35 mg/dL (0.90 mmol/L) and/or a triglyceride level ≥250 mg/dL (2.82 mmol/L)
- Polycystic ovary syndrome or acanthosis nigracans
- History of vascular disease

Note: BMI, body mass index; IFG, impaired fasting glucose; IGT, impaired glucose tolerance; GDM, gestational diabetes mellitus; HDL, high-density lipoprotein.
Source: Adapted from American Diabetes Association, 2004.

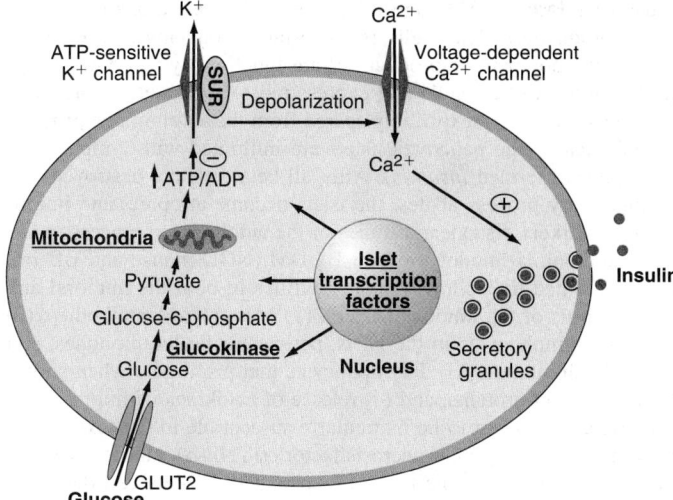

FIGURE 323-3 *Diabetes and abnormalities in glucose-stimulated insulin secretion. Glucose and other nutrients regulate insulin secretion by the pancreatic beta cell. Glucose is transported by the GLUT2 glucose transporter; subsequent glucose metabolism by the beta cell alters ion channel activity, leading to insulin secretion. The SUR receptor is the binding site for drugs that act as insulin secretagogues. Mutations in the events or proteins underlined are a cause of maturity onset diabetes of the young (MODY) or other forms of diabetes. SUR, sulfonylurea receptor; ATP, adenosine triphosphate; ADP, adenosine diphosphate. (Adapted from WL Lowe, in JL Jameson (ed): Principles of Molecular Medicine. Totowa, NJ, Humana, 1998.)*

to fivefold increase versus baseline) bursts of insulin secretion that usually last for 2 to 3 h before returning to baseline. Derangements in these normal secretory patterns are one of the earliest signs of beta cell dysfunction in DM.

ACTION Once insulin is secreted into the portal venous system, ~50% is degraded by the liver. Unextracted insulin enters the systemic circulation where it binds to receptors in target sites. Insulin binding to its receptor stimulates intrinsic tyrosine kinase activity, leading to receptor autophosphorylation and the recruitment of intracellular signaling molecules, such as insulin receptor substrates (IRS) (Fig. 323-4). These and other adaptor proteins initiate a complex cascade of phosphorylation and dephosphorylation reactions, resulting in the widespread metabolic and mitogenic effects of insulin. As an example, activation of the phosphatidylinositol-3'-kinase (PI-3-kinase) pathway stimulates translocation of glucose transporters (e.g., GLUT4) to the cell surface, an event that is crucial for glucose uptake by skeletal muscle and fat. Activation of other insulin receptor signaling pathways induces glycogen synthesis, protein synthesis, lipogenesis, and regulation of various genes in insulin-responsive cells.

Glucose homeostasis reflects a precise balance between hepatic glucose production and peripheral glucose uptake and utilization. Insulin is the most important regulator of this metabolic equilibrium, but neural input, metabolic signals, and hormones (e.g., glucagon) result in integrated control of glucose supply and utilization (Chap. 324; see Fig. 324-1). In the fasting state, low insulin levels increase glucose production by promoting hepatic gluconeogenesis

and glycogenolysis. Glucagon also stimulates glycogenolysis and gluconeogenesis by the liver and renal medulla. Low insulin levels decrease glycogen synthesis, reduce glucose uptake in insulin-sensitive tissues, and promote mobilization of stored precursors. Postprandially, the glucose load elicits a rise in insulin and fall in glucagon, leading to a reversal of these processes. The major portion of postprandial glucose is utilized by skeletal muscle, an effect of insulin-stimulated glucose uptake. Other tissues, most notably the brain, utilize glucose in an insulin-independent fashion.

PATHOGENESIS

TYPE 1 DM Type 1A DM develops as a result of the synergistic effects of genetic, environmental, and immunologic factors that ultimately destroy the pancreatic beta cells. The temporal development of type 1A DM is shown schematically as a function of beta cell mass in Fig. 323-5. Individuals with a genetic susceptibility have normal beta cell mass at birth but begin to lose beta cells secondary to autoimmune destruction that occurs over months to years. This autoimmune process is thought to be triggered by an infectious or environmental stimulus and to be sustained by a beta cell–specific molecule. In the majority of individuals, immunologic markers appear after the triggering event but before diabetes becomes clinically overt. Beta cell mass then begins to decline, and insulin secretion becomes progressively impaired, although normal glucose tolerance is maintained. The rate of decline in beta cell mass varies widely among individuals, with some patients progressing rapidly to clinical diabetes and others evolving more slowly. Features of diabetes do not become evident until a majority of beta cells are destroyed (~80%). At this point, residual functional beta cells still exist but are insufficient in number to maintain glucose tolerance. The events that trigger the transition from glucose intolerance to frank diabetes are often associated with increased insulin requirements, as might occur during infections or puberty. After the initial clinical presentation of type 1A DM, a "honeymoon" phase may ensue during which time glycemic control is achieved with modest doses of insulin or, rarely, insulin is not needed. However, this fleeting phase of endogenous insulin production from residual beta cells disappears

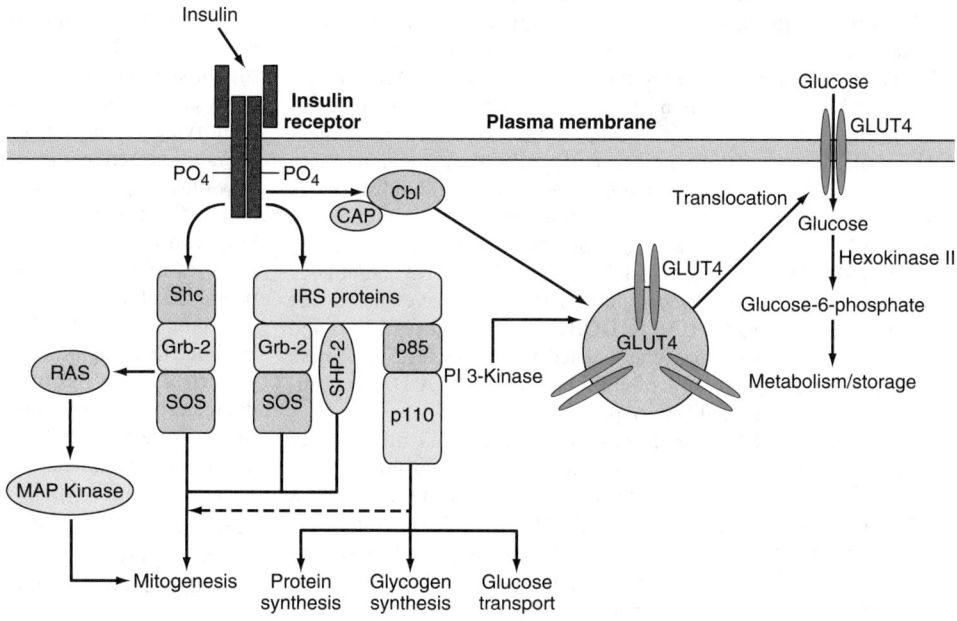

FIGURE 323-4 Insulin signal transduction pathway in skeletal muscle. The insulin receptor has intrinsic tyrosine kinase activity and interacts with insulin receptor substrates (IRS and Shc) proteins. A number of "docking" proteins bind to these cellular proteins and initiate the metabolic actions of insulin [GrB-2, SOS, SHP-2, p65, p110, and phosphatidylinositol-3'-kinase (PI-3-kinase)]. Insulin increases glucose transport through PI-3-kinase and the Cbl pathway, which promotes the translocation of intracellular vesicles containing GLUT4 glucose transporter to the plasma membrane. *(Adapted from WL Lowe, in Principles of Molecular Medicine, JL Jameson (ed). Totowa, NJ, Humana, 1998; A Virkamaki et al: J Clin Invest 103:931, 1999. For additional details see Saltiel and Kahn, 2001.)*

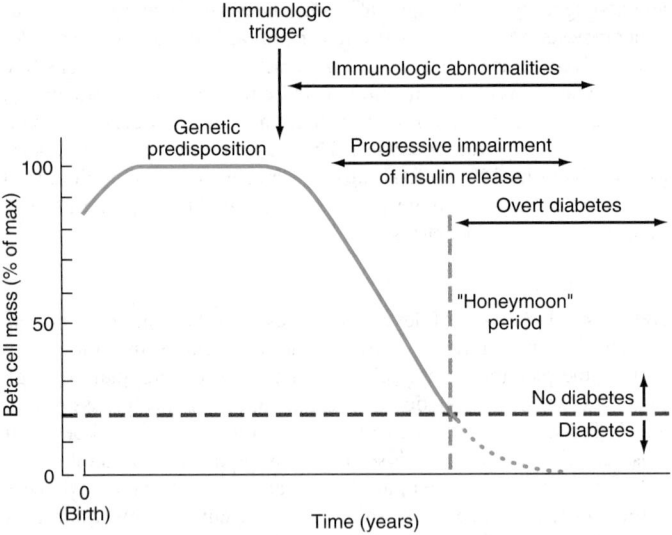

FIGURE 323-5 Temporal model for development of type 1 diabetes. Individuals with a genetic predisposition are exposed to an immunologic trigger that initiates an autoimmune process, resulting in a gradual decline in beta cell mass. The downward slope of the beta cell mass varies among individuals. This progressive impairment in insulin release results in diabetes when ~80% of the beta cell mass is destroyed. A "honeymoon" phase may be seen in the first 1 or 2 years after the onset of diabetes and is associated with reduced insulin requirements. *(Adapted from Medical Management of Type 1 Diabetes, 3d ed, JS Skyler (ed). Alexandria, VA, American Diabetes Association, 1998.)*

as the autoimmune process destroys the remaining beta cells, and the individual becomes completely insulin deficient.

GENETIC CONSIDERATIONS Genetic susceptibility to type 1A DM involves multiple genes. The concordance of type 1A DM in identical twins ranges between 30 and 70%, indicating that additional modifying factors must be involved in determining whether diabetes develops. The major susceptibility gene for type 1A DM is located in the HLA region on chromosome 6. Polymorphisms in the HLA complex account for 40 to 50% of the genetic risk of developing type 1A DM. This region contains genes that encode the class II MHC molecules, which present antigen to helper T cells and thus are involved in initiating the immune response (Chap. 296). The ability of class II MHC molecules to present antigen is dependent on the amino acid composition of their antigen-binding sites. Amino acid substitutions may influence the specificity of the immune response by altering the binding affinity of different antigens for class II molecules.

Most individuals with type 1A DM have the HLA DR3 and/or DR4 haplotype. Refinements in genotyping of HLA loci have shown that the haplotypes DQA1*0301, DQB1*0302, DQA1*501, and DQB1*0201 are most strongly associated with type 1A DM. These haplotypes are present in 40% of children with type 1A DM as compared to 2% of the normal U.S. population.

In addition to MHC class II associations, at least 17 different genetic loci contribute susceptibility to type 1A DM. For example, polymorphisms in the promoter region of the insulin gene account for ~10% of the predisposition to type 1A DM. Genes that confer protection against the development of the disease also exist. The haplotype DQA1*0102, DQB1*0602 is present in 20% of the U.S. population but is extremely rare in individuals with type 1A DM (<1%).

The risk of developing type 1A DM is increased tenfold in relatives of individuals with the disease. Nevertheless, most individuals with predisposing haplotypes do not develop diabetes. In addition, most individuals with type 1A DM do not have a first-degree relative with this disorder.

Autoimmune Factors Although other islet cell types [alpha cells (glucagon-producing), delta cells (somatostatin-producing), or PP cells (pancreatic polypeptide-producing)] are functionally and embryologically similar to beta cells and express most of the same proteins as beta cells, they are inexplicably spared from the autoimmune process. Pathologically, the pancreatic islets are infiltrated with lymphocytes (in a process termed *insulitis*). After all beta cells are destroyed, the inflammatory process abates, the islets become atrophic, and immunologic markers disappear. Studies of the autoimmune process in humans and animal models of type 1A DM (NOD mouse and BB rat) have identified the following abnormalities in both the humoral and cellular arms of the immune system: (1) islet cell autoantibodies; (2) activated lymphocytes in the islets, peripancreatic lymph nodes, and systemic circulation; (3) T lymphocytes that proliferate when stimulated with islet proteins; and (4) release of cytokines within the insulitis. Beta cells seem to be particularly susceptible to the toxic effect of some cytokines [tumor necrosis factor α (TNF-α), interferon γ, and interleukin-1 (IL-1)]. The precise mechanisms of beta cell death are not known but may involve formation of nitric oxide metabolites, apoptosis, and direct CD8+ T cell cytotoxicity. Islet autoantibodies are not thought to be involved in the destructive process, as these antibodies do not generally react with the cell surface of islet cells and are not capable of transferring diabetes mellitus to animals.

Pancreatic islet molecules targeted by the autoimmune process include insulin, glutamic acid decarboxylase (GAD, the biosynthetic enzyme for the neurotransmitter GABA), ICA-512/IA-2 (homology with tyrosine phosphatases), and phogrin (insulin secretory granule protein). Other less clearly defined autoantigens include an islet ganglioside and carboxypeptidase H. With the exception of insulin, none of the autoantigens are beta cell specific, which raises the question of how the beta cells are selectively destroyed. Current theories favor initiation of an autoimmune process directed at one beta cell molecule, which then spreads to other islet molecules as the immune process destroys beta cells and creates a series of secondary autoantigens. The beta cells of individuals who develop type 1A DM do not differ from beta cells of normal individuals, since transplanted islets are destroyed by a recurrence of the autoimmune process of type 1A DM.

Immunologic Markers Islet cell autoantibodies (ICAs) are a composite of several different antibodies directed at pancreatic islet molecules such as GAD, insulin, IA-2/ICA-512, and an islet ganglioside and serve as a marker of the autoimmune process of type 1A DM. Assays for autoantibodies to GAD-65 are commercially available. Testing for ICAs can be useful in classifying the type of DM as type IA and in identifying nondiabetic individuals at risk for developing type 1A DM. ICAs are present in the majority of individuals (>75%) diagnosed with new-onset type 1A DM, in a significant minority of individuals with newly diagnosed type 2 DM (5 to 10%), and occasionally in individuals with GDM (<5%). ICAs are present in 3 to 4% of first-degree relatives of individuals with type 1A DM. In combination with impaired insulin secretion after intravenous glucose tolerance testing, they predict a >50% risk of developing type 1A DM within 5 years. Without this impairment in insulin secretion, the presence of ICAs predicts a 5-year risk of <25%. Based on these data, the risk of a first-degree relative developing type 1A DM is relatively low. At present, the measurement of ICAs in nondiabetic individuals is a research tool because no treatments have been approved to prevent the occurrence or progression of type 1A DM.

Environmental Factors Numerous environmental events have been proposed to trigger the autoimmune process in genetically susceptible individuals; however, none have been conclusively linked to diabetes. Identification of an environmental trigger has been difficult because the event may precede the onset of DM by several years (Fig. 323-5). Putative environmental triggers include viruses (coxsackie and rubella most prominently), bovine milk proteins, and nitrosourea compounds.

Prevention of Type 1A DM A number of interventions have successfully delayed or prevented diabetes in animal models. Some interventions have targeted the immune system directly (immunosuppression, selective T cell subset deletion, induction of immunologic tolerance to islet proteins), whereas others have prevented islet cell death by blocking cytotoxic cytokines or increasing islet resistance to the destructive process. Though results in animal models are promising, these interventions have not been successful in preventing type 1A DM in humans. The Diabetes Prevention Trial—type 1 recently concluded that administering insulin to individuals at high risk for developing type 1A DM did not prevent type 1A DM.

TYPE 2 DM   Insulin resistance and abnormal insulin secretion are central to the development of type 2 DM. Although controversy remains regarding the primary defect, most studies support the view that insulin resistance precedes insulin secretory defects and that diabetes develops only if insulin secretion becomes inadequate.

GENETIC CONSIDERATIONS   Type 2 DM has a strong genetic component. Major genes that predispose to this disorder have yet to be identified, but it is clear that the disease is polygenic and multifactorial. Various genetic loci contribute to susceptibility, and environmental factors (such as nutrition and physical activity) further modulate phenotypic expression of the disease. The concordance of type 2 DM in identical twins is between 70 and 90%. Individuals with a parent with type 2 DM have an increased risk of diabetes; if both parents have type 2 DM, the risk approaches 40%. Insulin resistance, as demonstrated by reduced glucose utilization in skeletal muscle, is present in many nondiabetic, first-degree relatives of individuals with type 2 DM. However, definition of the genetic susceptibility remains a challenge because the genetic defect in insulin secretion or action may not manifest itself unless an environmental event or another genetic defect, such as obesity, is superimposed. Mutations in various molecules involved in insulin action (e.g., the insulin receptor and enzymes involved in glucose homeostasis) account for a very small fraction of type 2 DM. Likewise, genetic defects in proteins involved in insulin secretion have not been found in most individuals with type 2 DM. Genome-wide scanning for mutations or polymorphisms associated with type 2 DM is being used in an effort to identify genes associated with type 2 DM. The gene for the protease, calpain 10, is associated with type 2 DM in Hispanic and some other populations.

Pathophysiology   Type 2 DM is characterized by three pathophysiologic abnormalities: impaired insulin secretion, peripheral insulin resistance, and excessive hepatic glucose production. Obesity, particularly visceral or central (as evidenced by the hip-waist ratio), is very common in type 2 DM. Adipocytes secrete a number of biologic products (leptin, TNF-α, free fatty acids, resistin, and adiponectin) that modulate insulin secretion, insulin action, and body weight and may contribute to the insulin resistance. In the early stages of the disorder, glucose tolerance remains normal, despite insulin resistance, because the pancreatic beta cells compensate by increasing insulin output (Fig. 323-6). As insulin resistance and compensatory hyperinsulinemia progress, the pancreatic islets in certain individuals are unable to sustain the hyperinsulinemic state. IGT, characterized by elevations in postprandial glucose, then develops. A further decline in insulin secretion and an increase in hepatic glucose production lead to overt diabetes with fasting hyperglycemia. Ultimately, beta cell failure may ensue. Markers of inflammation such as IL-6 and C-reactive protein are often elevated in type 2 diabetes.

Metabolic Abnormalities ■ *INSULIN RESISTANCE*   The decreased ability of insulin to act effectively on peripheral target tissues (especially muscle and liver) is a prominent feature of type 2 DM and results from a combination of genetic susceptibility and obesity. Insulin resistance is relative, however, since supernormal levels of circulating insulin will normalize the plasma glucose. Insulin dose-response curves exhibit a rightward shift, indicating reduced sensitivity, and a reduced maximal response, indicating an overall decrease in maximum glucose utilization (30 to 60% lower than normal individuals). Insulin resistance impairs glucose utilization by insulin-sensitive tissues and increases hepatic glucose output; both effects contribute to the hyperglycemia.

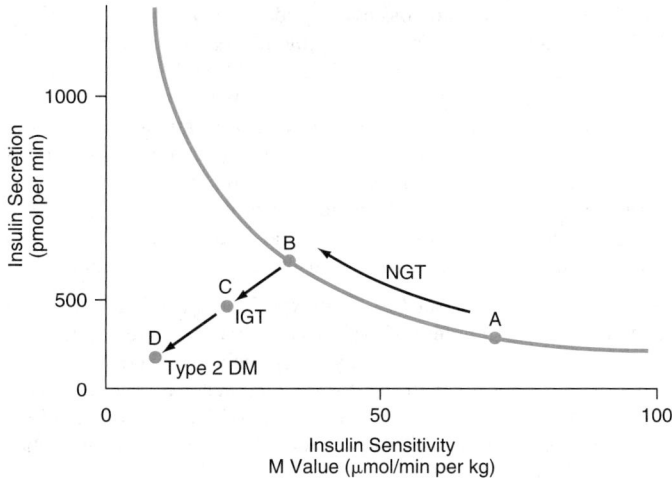

FIGURE 323-6   Metabolic changes during the development of type 2 diabetes mellitus (DM). Insulin secretion and insulin sensitivity are related, and as an individual becomes more insulin resistant (by moving from point A to point B), insulin secretion increases. A failure to compensate by increasing the insulin secretion results initially in impaired glucose tolerance (IGT; point C) and ultimately in type 2 DM (point D). *(Adapted from SE Kahn, J Clin Endocrinol Metab 86:4047, 2001; RN Bergman, M Ader, Trends Endocrinol Metab 11:351, 2000.)*

Increased hepatic glucose output predominantly accounts for increased FPG levels, whereas decreased peripheral glucose usage results in postprandial hyperglycemia. In skeletal muscle, there is a greater impairment in nonoxidative glucose usage (glycogen formation) than in oxidative glucose metabolism through glycolysis. Glucose metabolism in insulin-independent tissues is not altered in type 2 DM.

The precise molecular mechanism of insulin resistance in type 2 DM has not been elucidated. Insulin receptor levels and tyrosine kinase activity in skeletal muscle are reduced, but these alterations are most likely secondary to hyperinsulinemia and are not a primary defect. Therefore, postreceptor defects are believed to play the predominant role in insulin resistance (Fig. 323-4). Polymorphisms in IRS-1 may be associated with glucose intolerance, raising the possibility that polymorphisms in various postreceptor molecules may combine to create an insulin-resistant state. The pathogenesis of insulin resistance is currently focused on a PI-3-kinase signaling defect, which reduces translocation of GLUT4 to the plasma membrane, among other abnormalities. Of note, not all insulin signal transduction pathways are resistant to the effects of insulin [e.g., those controlling cell growth and differentiation and using the mitogen-activated protein (MAP) kinase pathway; Fig. 323-4]. Consequently, hyperinsulinemia may increase the insulin action through these pathways, potentially accelerating diabetes-related conditions such as atherosclerosis.

Another emerging theory proposes that elevated levels of free fatty acids, a common feature of obesity, may contribute to the pathogenesis of type 2 DM. Free fatty acids can impair glucose utilization in skeletal muscle, promote glucose production by the liver, and impair beta cell function.

IMPAIRED INSULIN SECRETION   Insulin secretion and sensitivity are interrelated (Fig. 323-6). In type 2 DM, insulin secretion initially increases in response to insulin resistance to maintain normal glucose tolerance. Initially, the insulin secretory defect is mild and selectively involves glucose-stimulated insulin secretion. The response to other nonglucose secretagogues, such as arginine, is preserved. Eventually, the insulin secretory defect progresses to a state of grossly inadequate insulin secretion.

The reason(s) for the decline in insulin secretory capacity in type 2 DM is unclear. Despite the assumption that a second genetic defect—superimposed upon insulin resistance—leads to beta cell failure, intense genetic investigation has so far excluded mutations in islet candidate genes. Islet amyloid polypeptide or amylin is cosecreted by the beta cell and likely forms the amyloid fibrillar deposit found in the islets of individuals with long-standing type 2 DM. Whether such islet amyloid deposits are a primary or secondary event is not known. The metabolic environment of diabetes may also negatively impact islet function. For example, chronic hyperglycemia paradoxically impairs islet function ("glucose toxicity") and leads to a worsening of hyperglycemia. Improvement in glycemic control is often associated with improved islet function. In addition, elevation of free fatty acid levels ("lipotoxicity") and dietary fat may also worsen islet function.

INCREASED HEPATIC GLUCOSE PRODUCTION In type 2 DM, insulin resistance in the liver reflects the failure of hyperinsulinemia to suppress gluconeogenesis, which results in fasting hyperglycemia and decreased glycogen storage by the liver in the postprandial state. Increased hepatic glucose production occurs early in the course of diabetes, though likely after the onset of insulin secretory abnormalities and insulin resistance in skeletal muscle.

Insulin Resistance Syndromes The insulin resistance condition comprises a spectrum of disorders, with hyperglycemia representing one of the most readily diagnosed features. The *metabolic syndrome*, the *insulin resistance syndrome*, or *syndrome X* are terms used to describe a constellation of metabolic derangements that includes insulin resistance, hypertension, dyslipidemia [low high-density lipoprotein (HDL) and elevated triglycerides], central or visceral obesity, type 2 diabetes or IGT/IFG, and accelerated cardiovascular disease. This syndrome is very common. The Centers for Disease Control and Prevention (CDC) estimates that 20% of U.S. adults have this syndrome. Epidemiologic evidence supports hyperinsulinemia as a marker for coronary artery disease risk, though an etiologic role has not been demonstrated.

A number of relatively rare forms of severe insulin resistance include features of type 2 DM or IGT (Table 323-1). *Acanthosis nigricans* and signs of hyperandrogenism (hirsutism, acne, and oligomenorrhea in women) are also common physical features. Two distinct syndromes of severe insulin resistance have been described in adults: (1) type A, which affects young women and is characterized by severe hyperinsulinemia, obesity, and features of hyperandrogenism; and (2) type B, which affects middle-aged women and is characterized by severe hyperinsulinemia, features of hyperandrogenism, and autoimmune disorders. Individuals with the type A insulin resistance syndrome have an undefined defect in the insulin-signaling pathway; individuals with the type B insulin resistance syndrome have autoantibodies directed at the insulin receptor. These receptor autoantibodies may block insulin binding or may stimulate the insulin receptor, leading to intermittent hypoglycemia.

Polycystic ovary syndrome (PCOS) is a common disorder that affects premenopausal women and is characterized by chronic anovulation and hyperandrogenism (Chap. 326). Insulin resistance is seen in a significant subset of women with PCOS, and the disorder substantially increases the risk for type 2 DM, independent of the effects of obesity. Both metformin and the thiazolidinediones attenuate hyperinsulinemia, ameliorate hyperandrogenism, induce ovulation, and improve plasma lipids, but they are not approved for this indication.

Prevention Type 2 DM is preceded by a period of IGT, and a number of life-style modifications and pharmacologic agents prevent or delay the onset of DM. The Diabetes Prevention Program (DPP) demonstrated that intensive changes in life-style (diet and exercise for 30 min/day five times/week) in individuals with IGT prevented or delayed the development of type 2 diabetes by 58% compared to placebo. This effect was seen in individuals regardless of age, sex, or ethnic group. In the same study, metformin prevented or delayed diabetes by 31% compared to placebo. The life-style intervention group lost 5 to 7% of their body weight during the 3 years of the study. Studies in Finnish and Chinese populations noted similar efficacy of diet and exercise in preventing or delaying type 2 DM; acarbose, metformin, and the thiazolidinediones prevent or delay type 2 DM, but are not approved for

this purpose. When administered to nondiabetic individuals for other reasons (cardiac, cholesterol lowering, etc.), two pharmacologic agents (ramipril, pravastatin) reduced the number of new cases of diabetes. Individuals with a strong family history, those at high risk for developing DM, or those with IFG or IGT should be strongly encouraged to maintain a normal body mass index (BMI) and engage in regular physical activity.

GENETICALLY DEFINED, MONOGENIC FORMS OF DIABETES MELLITUS

Several monogenic forms of DM have been identified. Five different variants of MODY, caused by mutations in genes encoding islet cell transcription factors or glucokinase (Fig. 323-3), have been identified so far, and all are transmitted as autosomal dominant disorders (Table 323-1). MODY 2 is the result of mutations in the glucokinase gene that lead to mild-to-moderate hyperglycemia. Glucokinase catalyzes the formation of glucose-6-phosphate from glucose, a reaction that is important for glucose sensing by the beta cells and for glucose utilization by the liver. As a result of glucokinase mutations, higher glucose levels are required to elicit insulin secretory responses, thus altering the set point for insulin secretion. Homozygous mutations in glucokinase cause severe, neonatal diabetes. MODY 1, MODY 3, and MODY 5 are caused by mutations in the hepatocyte nuclear transcription factors (HNF) 4α, HNF-1α, and HNF-1β, respectively. As their names imply, these transcription factors are expressed in the liver but also in other tissues, including the pancreatic islets and kidney (as a result, patients may also have renal absorption abnormalities and renal cysts). The mechanisms by which such mutations lead to DM is not well understood, but it is likely that these factors affect islet development or the transcription of genes that are important in stimulating insulin secretion. MODY 1 and 3 begin with mild hyperglycemia, but progressive impairment of insulin secretion requires treatment with oral agents or insulin. MODY 4 is a rare variant caused by mutations in the insulin promoter factor (IPF) 1, which is a transcription factor that regulates pancreatic development and insulin gene transcription. Homozygous inactivating mutations cause pancreatic agenesis, whereas heterozygous mutations result in DM. Studies of populations with type 2 DM suggest that mutations in the glucokinase gene and various islet cell transcription factors are very rare in ordinary type 2 DM.

ACUTE COMPLICATIONS OF DM

Diabetic ketoacidosis (DKA) and hyperglycemic hyperosmolar state (HHS) are acute complications of diabetes. DKA was formerly considered a hallmark of type 1 DM, but it also occurs in individuals who lack immunologic features of type 1A DM and who can subsequently be treated with oral glucose-lowering agents (these individuals with type 2 DM are often of Hispanic or African-American descent). HHS is primarily seen in individuals with type 2 DM. Both disorders are associated with absolute or relative insulin deficiency, volume depletion, and acid-base abnormalities. DKA and HHS exist along a continuum of hyperglycemia, with or without ketosis. The metabolic similarities and differences in DKA and HHS are highlighted in Table 323-4. Both disorders are associated with potentially serious complications if not promptly diagnosed and treated.

DIABETIC KETOACIDOSIS ■ **Clinical Features** The symptoms and physical signs of DKA are listed in Table 323-5 and usually develop over 24 hours. DKA may be the initial symptom complex that leads to a diagnosis of type 1 DM, but more frequently it occurs in individuals with established diabetes. Nausea and vomiting are often prominent, and their presence in an individual with diabetes warrants laboratory evaluation for DKA. Abdominal pain may be severe and can resemble acute pancreatitis or ruptured viscous. Hyperglycemia leads to glucosuria, volume depletion, and tachycardia. Hypotension can occur because of volume depletion in combination with peripheral vasodilation. Kussmaul respirations and a fruity odor on the patient's breath (secondary to metabolic acidosis and increased acetone) are classic signs of the disorder. Lethargy and central nervous system depression may evolve into coma with severe DKA but should also prompt evaluation for other reasons for altered mental status (infection, hypoxia, etc.). Cerebral edema, an extremely serious complication of DKA, is seen most frequently in children. Signs of infection, which may precipitate DKA, should be sought on physical examination, even in the absence of fever. Tissue ischemia (heart, brain) can also be a precipitating factor.

Pathophysiology DKA results from relative or absolute insulin deficiency combined with counterregulatory hormone excess (glucagon, catecholamines, cortisol, and growth hormone). Both insulin deficiency and glucagon excess, in particular, are necessary for DKA to develop. The decreased ratio of insulin to glucagon promotes gluconeogenesis, glycogenolysis, and ketone body formation in the liver, as well as increases in substrate delivery from fat and muscle (free fatty acids, amino acids) to the liver.

The combination of insulin deficiency and hyperglycemia reduces the hepatic level of fructose-2,6-phosphate, which alters the activity of phosphofructokinase and fructose-1,6-bisphosphatase. Glucagon excess decreases the activity of pyruvate kinase, whereas insulin deficiency increases the activity of phosphoenolpyruvate carboxykinase. These changes shift the handling of pyruvate toward glucose synthesis and away from glycolysis. The increased levels of glucagon and catecholamines in the face of low insulin levels promote glycogenolysis. Insulin deficiency also reduces levels of the GLUT4 glucose transporter, which impairs glucose uptake into skeletal muscle and fat and reduces intracellular glucose metabolism (Fig. 323-4).

Ketosis results from a marked increase in free fatty acid release from adipocytes, with a resulting shift toward ketone body synthesis in the liver. Reduced insulin levels, in combination with elevations in catecholamines and growth hormone, increase lipolysis and the release of free fatty acids. Normally, these free fatty acids are converted to triglycerides or very low density lipoproteins (VLDL) in the liver. However, in DKA, hyperglucagonemia alters hepatic metabolism to favor ketone body formation, through activation of the enzyme carnitine palmitoyltransferase I. This enzyme is crucial for regulating fatty acid transport into the mitochondria, where beta oxidation and conversion to ketone bodies occur. At physiologic pH, ketone bodies exist as ketoacids, which are neutralized by bicarbonate. As bicarbonate stores are depleted, metabolic acidosis ensues. Increased lactic acid production also contributes to the acidosis. The increased free fatty acids increase triglyceride and VLDL production. VLDL clearance is also reduced because the activity of insulin-sensitive lipoprotein lipase in muscle and fat is decreased. Hypertriglyceridemia may be severe enough to cause pancreatitis.

DKA is initiated by inadequate levels of plasma insulin (Table 323-5). Most commonly, DKA is precipitated by increased insulin requirements, as might occur during a concurrent illness. Failure to augment insulin therapy often compounds the problem. Occasionally, complete omission of insulin by the patient or health care team (in a hospitalized patient with type 1 DM) precipitates DKA. Patients using insulin infusion devices with short-acting insulin are at increased risk of DKA, since even a brief interruption in insulin delivery (e.g., mechanical malfunction) quickly leads to insulin deficiency.

Laboratory Abnormalities and Diagnosis The timely diagnosis of DKA is crucial and allows for prompt initiation of therapy. DKA is characterized by hyperglycemia, ketosis, and metabolic acidosis (increased anion gap) along with a number of secondary metabolic derangements (Table 323-4). Occasionally, the serum glucose is only minimally elevated. Serum bicarbonate is frequently <10 mmol/L, and arterial pH ranges between 6.8 and 7.3, depending on the severity of the acidosis. Despite a total-body potassium deficit, the serum potassium at presen-

tation may be mildly elevated, secondary to the acidosis. Total-body stores of sodium, chloride, phosphorous, and magnesium are also reduced in DKA but are not accurately reflected by their levels in the serum because of dehydration and hyperglycemia. Elevated blood urea nitrogen (BUN) and serum creatinine levels reflect intravascular volume depletion. Interference from acetoacetate may falsely elevate the serum creatinine measurement. Leukocytosis, hypertriglyceridemia, and hyperlipoproteinemia are commonly found as well. Hyperamylasemia may suggest a diagnosis of pancreatitis, especially when accompanied by abdominal pain. However, in DKA the amylase is usually of salivary origin and thus is not diagnostic of pancreatitis. Serum lipase should be obtained if pancreatitis is suspected.

The measured serum sodium is reduced as a consequence of the hyperglycemia [1.6 mmol/L (1.6 meq) reduction in serum sodium for each 5.6 mmol/L (100 mg/dL) rise in the serum glucose]. A normal serum sodium in the setting of DKA indicates a more profound water deficit. In "conventional" units, the calculated serum osmolality [2 × (serum sodium + serum potassium) + plasma glucose (mg/dL)/18 + BUN/2.8] is mildly to moderately elevated, though to a lesser degree than that found in HHS (see below).

In DKA, the ketone body, β-hydroxybutyrate, is synthesized at a threefold greater rate than acetoacetate; however, acetoacetate is preferentially detected by a commonly used ketosis detection reagent (nitroprusside). Serum ketones are present at significant levels (usually positive at serum dilution of 1:8 or greater). The nitroprusside tablet, or stick, is often used to detect urine ketones; certain medications such as captopril or penicillamine may cause false-positive reactions. Serum or plasma assays for β-hydroxybutyrate more accurately reflect the true ketone body level.

The metabolic derangements of DKA exist along a spectrum, beginning with mild acidosis with moderate hyperglycemia evolving into more severe findings. The degree of acidosis and hyperglycemia do not necessarily correlate closely since a variety of factors determine

TABLE 323-4 Laboratory Values in Diabetic Ketoacidosis (DKA) and Hyperglycemic Hyperosmolar State (HHS) (Representative Ranges at Presentation)

	DKA	HHS
Glucose,[a] mmol/L (mg/dL)	13.9–33.3 (250–600)	33.3–66.6 (600–1200)
Sodium, meq/L	125–135	135–145
Potassium,[a] meq/L	Normal to ↑[b]	Normal
Magnesium[a]	Normal[b]	Normal
Chloride[a]	Normal	Normal
Phosphate[a]	↓	Normal
Creatinine, μmol/L (mg/dL)	Slightly ↑	Moderately ↑
Osmolality (mOsm/mL)	300–320	330–380
Plasma ketones[a]	++++	+/−
Serum bicarbonate,[a] meq/L	<15 meq/L	Normal to slightly ↓
Arterial pH	6.8–7.3	>7.3
Arterial P_{CO_2},[a] mmHg	20–30	Normal
Anion gap[a] [Na − (Cl + HCO₃)], meq/L	↑	Normal to slightly ↑

[a] Large changes occur during treatment of DKA.
[b] Although plasma levels may be normal or high at presentation, total-body stores are usually depleted.

TABLE 323-5 Manifestations of Diabetic Ketoacidosis

Symptoms	Physical findings
Nausea/vomiting	Tachycardia
Thirst/polyuria	Dry mucous membranes/reduced
Abdominal pain	skin turgor
Shortness of breath	Dehydration / hypotension
Precipitating events	Tachypnea / Kussmaul
Inadequate insulin administration	respirations/respiratory distress
Infection (pneumonia/UTI/	Abdominal tenderness (may
gastroenteritis/sepsis)	resemble acute pancreatitis or
Infarction (cerebral, coronary,	surgical abdomen)
mesenteric, peripheral)	Lethargy /obtundation / cerebral
Drugs (cocaine)	edema / possibly coma
Pregnancy	

Note: UTI, urinary tract infection.

the level of hyperglycemia (oral intake, urinary glucose loss). Ketonemia is a consistent finding in DKA and distinguishes it from simple hyperglycemia. The differential diagnosis of DKA includes starvation ketosis, alcoholic ketoacidosis (bicarbonate >15 meq/L) and other increased anion gap acidosis (Chap. 42).

℞ TREATMENT

The management of DKA is outlined in Table 323-6. After initiating intravenous fluid replacement and insulin therapy, the agent or event that precipitated the episode of DKA should be sought and aggressively treated. If the patient is vomiting or has altered mental status, a nasogastric tube should be inserted to prevent aspiration of gastric contents. Central to successful treatment of DKA is careful monitoring and frequent reassessment to ensure that the patient and the metabolic derangements are improving. A comprehensive flow sheet should record chronologic changes in vital signs, fluid intake and output, and laboratory values as a function of insulin administered.

After the initial bolus of normal saline, replacement of the sodium and free water deficit is carried out over the next 24 h (fluid deficit is often 3 to 5 L). When hemodynamic stability and adequate urine output are achieved, intravenous fluids should be switched to 0.45% saline at a rate of 200 to 300 mL/h, depending on the calculated volume deficit. The change to 0.45% saline helps to reduce the trend toward hyperchloremia later in the course of DKA. Alternatively, initial use of lactated Ringer's intravenous solution may reduce the hyperchloremia that commonly occurs with normal saline.

A bolus of intravenous (0.15 units/kg) or intramuscular (0.4 units/kg) regular insulin should be administered immediately (Table 323-6), and subsequent treatment should provide continuous and adequate

---

TABLE 323-6 *Management of Diabetic Ketoacidosis*

1. Confirm diagnosis (↑ plasma glucose, positive serum ketones, metabolic acidosis).
2. Admit to hospital; intensive-care setting may be necessary for frequent monitoring or if pH < 7.00 or unconscious.
3. Assess: Serum electrolytes (K^+, Na^+, Mg^{2+}, Cl^-, bicarbonate, phosphate)
   Acid-base status—pH, HCO_3^-, P_{CO_2}, β-hydroxybutyrate
   Renal function (creatinine, urine output)
4. Replace fluids: 2–3 L of 0.9% saline over first 1–3 h (5–10 mL/kg per hour); subsequently, 0.45% saline at 150–300 mL/h; change to 5% glucose and 0.45% saline at 100–200 mL/h when plasma glucose reaches 250 mg/dL (14 mmol/L).
5. Administer regular insulin: IV (0.1 units/kg) or IM (0.4 units/kg), then 0.1 units/kg per hour by continuous IV infusion; increase 2- to 10-fold if no response by 2–4 h. If initial serum potassium is < 3.3 mmol/L (3.3 meq/L), do not administer insulin until the potassium is corrected to > 3.3 mmol/L (3.3.meq/L).
6. Assess patient: What precipitated the episode (noncompliance, infection, trauma, infarction, cocaine)? Initiate appropriate workup for precipitating event (cultures, CXR, ECG).
7. Measure capillary glucose every 1–2 h; measure electrolytes (especially K^+, bicarbonate, phosphate) and anion gap every 4 h for first 24 h.
8. Monitor blood pressure, pulse, respirations, mental status, fluid intake and output every 1–4 h.
9. Replace K^+: 10 meq/h when plasma K^+ < 5.5 meq/L, ECG normal, urine flow and normal creatinine documented; administer 40–80 meq/h when plasma K^+ <3.5 meq/L or if bicarbonate is given.
10. Continue above until patient is stable, glucose goal is 150–250 mg/dL, and acidosis is resolved. Insulin infusion may be decreased to 0.05–0.1 units/kg per hour.
11. Administer intermediate or long-acting insulin as soon as patient is eating. Allow for overlap in insulin infusion and subcutaneous insulin injection.

Note: CXR, chest x-ray; ECG, electrocardiogram.
Source: Adapted from M Sperling, in *Therapy for Diabetes Mellitus and Related Disorders*, American Diabetes Association, Alexandria, VA, 1998; and AE Kitabchi et al: Diabetes Care 24:131, 2001.

---

levels of circulating insulin. Intravenous administration is preferred (0.1 units/kg per hour), because it assures rapid distribution and allows adjustment of the infusion rate as the patient responds to therapy. Intravenous regular insulin should be continued until the acidosis resolves and the patient is metabolically stable. As the acidosis and insulin resistance associated with DKA resolve, the insulin infusion rate can be decreased (to 0.05 to 0.1 units/kg per hour). Intermediate or long-acting insulin, in combination with subcutaneous regular insulin, should be administered as soon as the patient resumes eating, as this facilitates transition to an outpatient insulin regimen and reduces length of hospital stay. It is crucial to continue the insulin infusion until adequate insulin levels are achieved by the subcutaneous route. Even relatively brief periods of inadequate insulin administration in this transition phase may result in DKA relapse.

Hyperglycemia usually improves at a rate of 4.2 to 5.6 mmol/L (75 to 100 mg/dL) per hour as a result of insulin-mediated glucose disposal, reduced hepatic glucose release, and rehydration. The latter reduces catecholamines, increases urinary glucose loss, and expands the intravascular volume. The decline in the plasma glucose within the first 1 to 2 h may be more rapid and is mostly related to volume expansion. When the plasma glucose reaches 13.9 mmol/L (250 mg/dL), glucose should be added to the 0.45% saline infusion to maintain the plasma glucose in the 11.1 to 13.9 mmol/L (200 to 250 mg/dL) range, and the insulin infusion should be continued. Ketoacidosis begins to resolve as insulin reduces lipolysis, increases peripheral ketone body use, suppresses hepatic ketone body formation, and promotes bicarbonate regeneration. However, the acidosis and ketosis resolve more slowly than hyperglycemia. As ketoacidosis improves, β-hydroxybutyrate is converted to acetoacetate. Ketone body levels may appear to increase if measured by laboratory assays that use the nitroprusside reaction, which only detects acetoacetate and acetone. The improvement in acidosis and anion gap, a result of bicarbonate regeneration and decline in ketone bodies, is reflected by a rise in the serum bicarbonate level and the arterial pH. Depending on the rise of serum chloride, the anion gap (but not bicarbonate) will normalize. A hyperchloremic acidosis [serum bicarbonate of 15 to 18 mmol/L (15 to 18 meq/L)] often follows successful treatment and gradually resolves as the kidneys regenerate bicarbonate and excretes chloride.

Potassium stores are depleted in DKA [estimated deficit 3 to 5 mmol/kg (3 to 5 meq/kg)]. During treatment with insulin and fluids, various factors contribute to the development of hypokalemia. These include insulin-mediated potassium transport into cells, resolution of the acidosis (which also promotes potassium entry into cells), and urinary loss of potassium salts of organic acids. Thus, potassium repletion should commence as soon as adequate urine output and a normal serum potassium are documented. If the initial serum potassium level is elevated, then potassium repletion should be delayed until the potassium falls into the normal range. Inclusion of 20 to 40 meq of potassium in each liter of intravenous fluid is reasonable, but additional potassium supplements may also be required. To reduce the amount of chloride administered, potassium phosphate or acetate can be substituted for the chloride salt. The goal is to maintain the serum potassium >3.5 mmol/L (3.5 meq/L). If the initial serum potassium is less than 3.3 mmol/L (3.3 meq/L), do not administer insulin until the potassium is supplemented to >3.3 mmol/L (3.3 meq/L).

Despite a bicarbonate deficit, bicarbonate replacement is not usually necessary. In fact, theoretical arguments suggest that bicarbonate administration and rapid reversal of acidosis may impair cardiac function, reduce tissue oxygenation, and promote hypokalemia. The results of most clinical trials do not support the routine use of bicarbonate replacement, and one study in children found that bicarbonate use was associated with an increased risk of cerebral edema. However, in the presence of severe acidosis (arterial pH < 7.0 after initial hydration), the ADA advises bicarbonate [50 mmol/L (meq/L) of sodium bicarbonate in 200 mL of 0.45% saline over 1 h if pH = 6.9 to 7.0; or 100 mmol/L (meq/L) of sodium bicarbonate in 400 mL of 0.45% saline over 2 h if pH 7 < 6.9]. Hypophosphatemia may result from increased glucose usage, but randomized clinical trials have not demonstrated that phosphate replacement is beneficial in DKA. If the serum phosphate is <0.32 mmol/L (1.0 mg/dL), then phosphate supplement should be considered and the serum calcium monitored. Hypomagnesemia may develop during DKA therapy and may also require supplementation.

With appropriate therapy, the mortality of DKA is low (<5%) and is related more to the underlying or precipitating event, such as infection or myocardial infarction. The major nonmetabolic complication of DKA therapy is cerebral edema, which most often develops in children as DKA is resolving. The etiology and optimal therapy for cerebral edema are not well established, but overreplacement of free water should be avoided. Venous thrombosis, upper gastrointestinal bleeding, and acute respiratory distress syndrome occasionally complicate DKA.

Following treatment, the physician and patient should review the sequence of events that led to DKA to prevent future recurrences. Foremost is patient education about the symptoms of DKA, its precipitating factors, and the management of diabetes during a concurrent illness. During illness or when oral intake is compromised, patients should: (1) frequently measure the capillary blood glucose; (2) measure urinary ketones when the serum glucose >16.5 mmol/L (300 mg/dL); (3) drink fluids to maintain hydration; (4) continue or increase insulin; and (5) seek medical attention if dehydration, persistent vomiting, or uncontrolled hyperglycemia develop. Using these strategies, early DKA can be prevented or detected and treated appropriately on an outpatient basis.

HYPERGLYCEMIC HYPEROSMOLAR STATE ■ Clinical Features   The prototypical patient with HHS is an elderly individual with type 2 DM, with a several week history of polyuria, weight loss, and diminished oral intake that culminates in mental confusion, lethargy, or coma. The physical examination reflects profound dehydration and hyperosmolality and reveals hypotension, tachycardia, and altered mental status. Notably absent are symptoms of nausea, vomiting, and abdominal pain and the Kussmaul respirations characteristic of DKA. HHS is often precipitated by a serious, concurrent illness such as myocardial infarction or stroke. Sepsis, pneumonia, and other serious infections are frequent precipitants and should be sought. In addition, a debilitating condition (prior stroke or dementia) or social situation that compromises water intake may contribute to the development of the disorder.

Pathophysiology   Relative insulin deficiency and inadequate fluid intake are the underlying causes of HHS. Insulin deficiency increases hepatic glucose production (through glycogenolysis and gluconeogenesis) and impairs glucose utilization in skeletal muscle (see above discussion of DKA). Hyperglycemia induces an osmotic diuresis that leads to intravascular volume depletion, which is exacerbated by inadequate fluid replacement. The absence of ketosis in HHS is not completely understood. Presumably, the insulin deficiency is only relative and less severe than in DKA. Lower levels of counterregulatory hormones and free fatty acids have been found in HHS than in DKA in some studies. It is also possible that the liver is less capable of ketone body synthesis or that the insulin/glucagon ratio does not favor ketogenesis.

Laboratory Abnormalities and Diagnosis   The laboratory features in HHS are summarized in Table 323-4. Most notable are the marked hyperglycemia [plasma glucose may be >55.5 mmol/L (1000 mg/dL)], hyperosmolality (>350 mosmol/L), and prerenal azotemia. The measured serum sodium may be normal or slightly low despite the marked hyperglycemia. The corrected serum sodium is usually increased [add 1.6 meq to measured sodium for each 5.6-mmol/L (100 mg/dL) rise in the serum glucose]. In contrast to DKA, acidosis and ketonemia are absent or mild. A small anion gap metabolic acidosis may be present secondary to increased lactic acid. Moderate ketonuria, if present, is secondary to starvation.

℞ TREATMENT

Volume depletion and hyperglycemia are prominent features of both HHS and DKA. Consequently, therapy of these disorders shares sev-

eral elements (Table 323-6). In both disorders, careful monitoring of the patient's fluid status, laboratory values, and insulin infusion rate is crucial. Underlying or precipitating problems should be aggressively sought and treated. In HHS, fluid losses and dehydration are usually more pronounced than in DKA due to the longer duration of the illness. The patient with HHS is usually older, more likely to have mental status changes, and more likely to have a life-threatening precipitating event with accompanying comorbidities. Even with proper treatment, HHS has a substantially higher mortality than DKA (up to 15% in some clinical series).

Fluid replacement should initially stabilize the hemodynamic status of the patient (1 to 3 L of 0.9% normal saline over the first 2 to 3 h). Because the fluid deficit in HHS is accumulated over a period of days to weeks, the rapidity of reversal of the hyperosmolar state must balance the need for free water repletion with the risk that too rapid a reversal may worsen neurologic function. If the serum sodium is >150 mmol/L (150 meq/L), 0.45% saline should be used. After hemodynamic stability is achieved, the intravenous fluid administration is directed at reversing the free water deficit using hypotonic fluids (0.45% saline initially then 5% dextrose in water, D_5W). The calculated free water deficit (which averages 9 to 10 L) should be reversed over the next 1 to 2 days (infusion rates of 200 to 300 mL/h of hypotonic solution). Potassium repletion is usually necessary and should be dictated by repeated measurements of the serum potassium. In patients taking diuretics, the potassium deficit can be quite large and may be accompanied by magnesium deficiency. Hypophosphatemia may occur during therapy and can be improved by using KPO_4 and beginning nutrition.

As in DKA, rehydration and volume expansion lower the plasma glucose initially, but insulin is also required. A reasonable regimen for HHS begins with an intravenous insulin bolus of 5 to 10 units followed by intravenous insulin at a constant infusion rate (3 to 7 units/h). As in DKA, glucose should be added to intravenous fluid when the plasma glucose falls to 13.9 mmol/L (250 mg/dL), and the insulin infusion rate should be decreased to 1 to 2 units/h. The insulin infusion should be continued until the patient has resumed eating and can be transferred to a subcutaneous insulin regimen. The patient should be discharged from the hospital on insulin, though some patients can later switch to oral glucose-lowering agents.

CHRONIC COMPLICATIONS OF DM

The chronic complications of DM affect many organ systems and are responsible for the majority of morbidity and mortality associated with the disease. Chronic complications can be divided into vascular and nonvascular complications (Table 323-7). The vascular complications

---

TABLE 323-7   *Chronic Complications of Diabetes Mellitus*

Microvascular
  Eye disease
    Retinopathy (nonproliferative/proliferative)
    Macular edema
  Neuropathy
    Sensory and motor (mono- and polyneuropathy)
    Autonomic
  Nephropathy
Macrovascular
  Coronary artery disease
  Peripheral vascular disease
  Cerebrovascular disease
Other
  Gastrointestinal (gastroparesis, diarrhea)
  Genitourinary (uropathy/sexual dysfunction)
  Dermatologic
  Infectious
  Cataracts
  Glaucoma

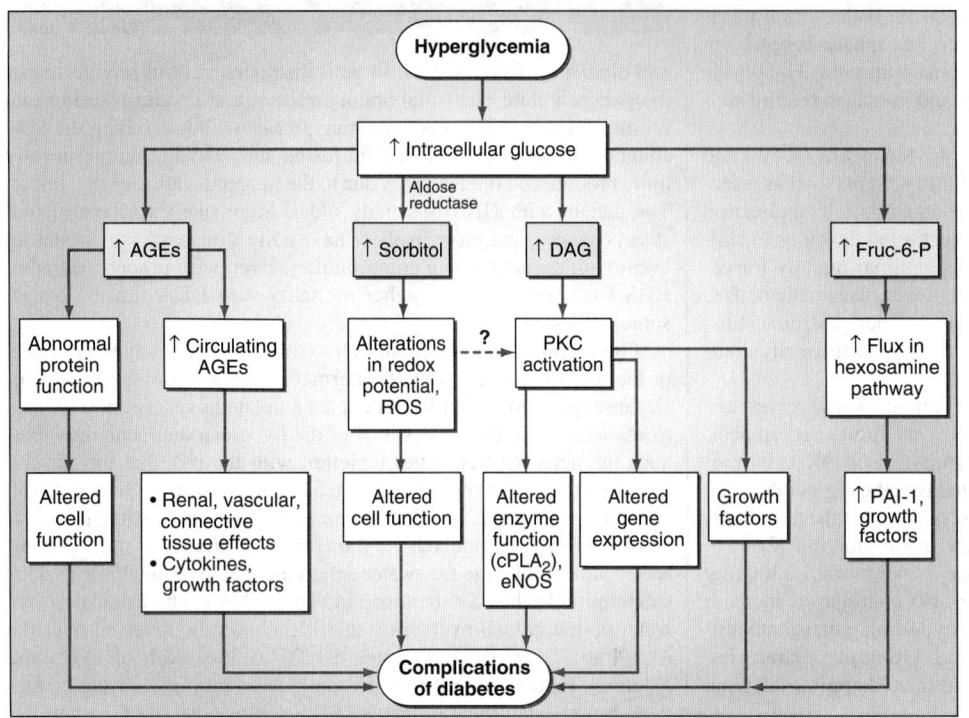

FIGURE 323-7 Possible molecular mechanisms of diabetes-related complications. AGEs, advanced glycation end products; PKC, protein kinase C; DAG, diacylglycerol; cPLA$_2$, phospholipase A$_2$; eNOS, endothelial nitric oxide synthase; ROS, reactive oxygen species; Fruc-6-P, fructose-6-phosphate; PAI-1, plasminogen activor inhibitor-1.

of DM are further subdivided into microvascular (retinopathy, neuropathy, nephropathy) and macrovascular complications (coronary artery disease, peripheral arterial disease, cerebrovascular disease). Nonvascular complications include problems such as gastroparesis, infections, and skin changes. The risk of chronic complications increases as a function of the duration of hyperglycemia; they usually become apparent in the second decade of hyperglycemia. Since type 2 DM often has a long asymptomatic period of hyperglycemia, many individuals with type 2 DM have complications at the time of diagnosis.

The microvascular complications of both type 1 and type 2 DM result from chronic hyperglycemia. Large, randomized clinical trials of individuals with type 1 or type 2 DM have conclusively demonstrated that a reduction in chronic hyperglycemia prevents or delays retinopathy, neuropathy, and nephropathy. Other incompletely defined factors may modulate the development of complications. For example, despite long-standing DM, some individuals never develop nephropathy or retinopathy. Many of these patients have glycemic control that is indistinguishable from those who develop microvascular complications, suggesting that there is a genetic susceptibility for developing particular complications.

Evidence implicating a causative role for chronic hyperglycemia in the development of macrovascular complications is less conclusive. However, coronary heart disease events and mortality are two to four times greater in patients with type 2 DM. These events correlate with fasting and postprandial plasma glucose levels as well as with the A1C. Other factors (dyslipidemia and hypertension) also play important roles in macrovascular complications.

MECHANISMS OF COMPLICATIONS Although chronic hyperglycemia is an important etiologic factor leading to complications of DM, the mechanism(s) by which it leads to such diverse cellular and organ dysfunction is unknown. Four prominent theories, which are not mutually exclusive, have been proposed to explain how hyperglycemia might lead to the chronic complications of DM (Fig. 323-7).

One theory is that increased intracellular glucose leads to the formation of advanced glycosylation end products (AGEs) via the nonenzymatic glycosylaton of intra- and extracellular proteins. Nonen-zymatic glycosylation results from the interaction of glucose with amino groups on proteins. AGEs have been shown to cross-link proteins (e.g., collagen, extracellular matrix proteins), accelerate atherosclerosis, promote glomerular dysfunction, reduce nitric oxide synthesis, induce endothelial dysfunction, and alter extracellular matrix composition and structure. The serum level of AGEs correlates with the level of glycemia, and these products accumulate as glomerular filtration rate declines.

A second theory is based on the observation that hyperglycemia increases glucose metabolism via the sorbitol pathway. Intracellular glucose is predominantly metabolized by phosphorylation and subsequent glycolysis, but when increased, some glucose is converted to sorbitol by the enzyme aldose reductase. Increased sorbitol concentration alters redox potential, increases cellular osmolality, generates reactive oxygen species, and likely leads to other types of cellular dysfunction. However, testing of this theory in humans, using aldose reductase inhibitors, has not demonstrated significant beneficial effects on clinical endpoints of retinopathy, neuropathy, or nephropathy.

A third hypothesis proposes that hyperglycemia increases the formation of diacylglycerol leading to activation of protein kinase C (PKC). Among other actions, PKC alters the transcription of genes for fibronectin, type IV collagen, contractile proteins, and extracellular matrix proteins in endothelial cells and neurons.

A fourth theory proposes that hyperglycemia increases the flux through the hexosamine pathway, which generates fructose-6-phosphate, a substrate for O-linked glycosylation and proteoglycan production. The hexosamine pathway may alter function by glycosylation of proteins such as endothelial nitric oxide synthase or by changes in gene expression of transforming growth factor β (TGF-β) or plasminogen activator inhibitor-1 (PAI-1).

Growth factors appear to play an important role in DM-related complications, and their production is increased by most of these proposed pathways. Vascular endothelial growth factor (VEGF) is increased locally in diabetic proliferative retinopathy and decreases after laser photocoagulation. TGF-β is increased in diabetic nephropathy and stimulates basement membrane production of collagen and fibronectin by mesangial cells. Other growth factors, such as platelet-derived growth factor, epidermal growth factor, insulin-like growth factor I, growth hormone, basic fibroblast growth factor, and even insulin, have been suggested to play a role in DM-related complications. A possible unifying mechanism is that hyperglycemia leads to increased production of reactive oxygen species or superoxide in the mitochondria; these compounds may activate all for of the pathways described above. Although hyperglycemia serves as the initial trigger for complications of diabetes, it is still unknown whether the same pathophysiologic processes are operative in all complications or whether some pathways predominate in certain organs.

GLYCEMIC CONTROL AND COMPLICATIONS The Diabetes Control and Complications Trial (DCCT) provided definitive proof that reduction in chronic hyperglycemia can prevent many of the early complications of type 1 DM. This large multicenter clinical trial randomized over 1400 individuals with type 1 DM to either intensive or conventional diabetes management, and prospectively evaluated the development of retinopathy, nephropathy, and neuropathy. Individuals in the intensive diabetes management group received multiple administrations of insulin each day along with extensive educational, psychological, and medical support. Individuals in the conventional diabetes management group received twice-daily insulin injections and quarterly nutritional, educational, and clinical evaluation. The goal in the former group was normoglycemia; the goal in the latter group was prevention of symptoms of diabetes. Individuals in the intensive diabetes management group achieved a substantially lower hemoglobin A1C (A1C; 7.3%) than individuals in the conventional diabetes management group (A1C; 9.1%).

The DCCT demonstrated that improvement of glycemic control reduced nonproliferative and proliferative retinopathy (47% reduction), microalbuminuria (39% reduction), clinical nephropathy (54% reduction), and neuropathy (60% reduction). Improved glycemic control also slowed the progression of early diabetic complications. There was a nonsignificant trend in reduction of macrovascular events. The results of the DCCT predicted that individuals in the intensive diabetes management group would gain 7.7 additional years of vision, 5.8 additional years free from ESRD, and 5.6 years free from lower extremity amputations. If all complications of DM were combined, individuals in the intensive diabetes management group would experience 15.3 more years of life without significant microvascular or neurologic complications of DM, compared to individuals who received standard therapy. This translates into an additional 5.1 years of life expectancy for individuals in the intensive diabetes management group. The benefit of the improved glycemic control during the DCCT persisted even after the study concluded and glycemic control worsened.

The benefits of an improvement in glycemic control occurred over the entire range of A1C values (Fig. 323-8), suggesting that at any A1C level, an improvement in glycemic control is beneficial. Therefore, there is no threshold beneath which the A1C can be reduced and the complications of DM prevented. The clinical implication of this finding is that the goal of therapy is to achieve an A1C level as close to normal as possible, without subjecting the patient to excessive risk of hypoglycemia.

The United Kingdom Prospective Diabetes Study (UKPDS) studied the course of >5000 individuals with type 2 DM for >10 years. This study utilized multiple treatment regimens and monitored the effect of intensive glycemic control and risk factor treatment on the development of diabetic complications. Newly diagnosed individuals with type 2 DM were randomized to (1) intensive management using various combinations of insulin, a sulfonylurea, or metformin; or (2) conventional therapy using dietary modification and pharmacotherapy with the goal of symptom prevention. In addition, individuals were randomly assigned to different antihypertensive regimens. Individuals in the intensive treatment arm achieved an A1C of 7.0%, compared to a 7.9% A1C in the standard treatment group. The UKPDS demonstrated that each percentage point reduction in A1C was associated with a 35% reduction in microvascular complications. As in the

DCCT, there was a continuous relationship between glycemic control and development of complications. Improved glycemic control did not conclusively reduce (nor worsen) cardiovascular mortality but was associated with improvement with lipoprotein risk profiles, such as reduced triglycerides and increased HDL.

One of the major findings of the UKPDS was that strict blood pressure control significantly reduced both macro- and microvascular complications. In fact, the beneficial effects of blood pressure control were greater than the beneficial effects of glycemic control. Lowering blood pressure to moderate goals (144/82 mmHg) reduced the risk of DM-related death, stroke, microvascular end points, retinopathy, and heart failure (risk reductions between 32 and 56%). Despite concerns that insulin therapy is associated with weight gain and may worsen underlying insulin resistance and hyperinsulinemia, most available data support strict glycemic control in individuals with type 2 DM.

Similar reductions in the risks of retinopathy and nephropathy were also seen in a small trial of lean Japanese individuals with type 2 DM randomized to either intensive glycemic control or standard therapy with insulin (Kumamoto study). These results demonstrate the effectiveness of improved glycemic control in individuals of different ethnicity, and, presumably a different etiology of DM (i.e., phenotypically different from those in the DCCT and UKPDS).

The findings of the DCCT, UKPDS, and Kumamoto study support the idea that chronic hyperglycemia plays a causative role in the pathogenesis of diabetic microvascular complications. These landmark studies prove the value of metabolic control and emphasize the importance of (1) intensive glycemic control in all forms of DM, and (2) early diagnosis and strict blood pressure control in type 2 DM.

OPHTHALMOLOGIC COMPLICATIONS OF DIABETES MELLITUS DM is the leading cause of blindness between the ages of 20 and 74 in the United States. The gravity of this problem is highlighted by the finding that individuals with DM are 25 times more likely to become legally blind than individuals without DM. Blindness is primarily the result of progressive diabetic retinopathy and clinically significant macular edema. Diabetic retinopathy is classified into two stages: nonproliferative and proliferative. *Nonproliferative diabetic retinopathy* usually appears late in the first decade or early in the second decade of the disease and is marked by retinal vascular microaneurysms, blot hemorrhages, and cotton wool spots (Fig. 323-9). Mild nonproliferative retinopathy progresses to more extensive disease, characterized by changes in venous vessel caliber, intraretinal microvascular abnormalities, and more numerous microaneurysms and hemorrhages. The pathophysiologic mechanisms invoked in nonproliferative retinopathy include loss of retinal pericytes, increased retinal vascular permeability, alterations in retinal blood flow, and abnormal retinal microvasculature, all of which lead to retinal ischemia.

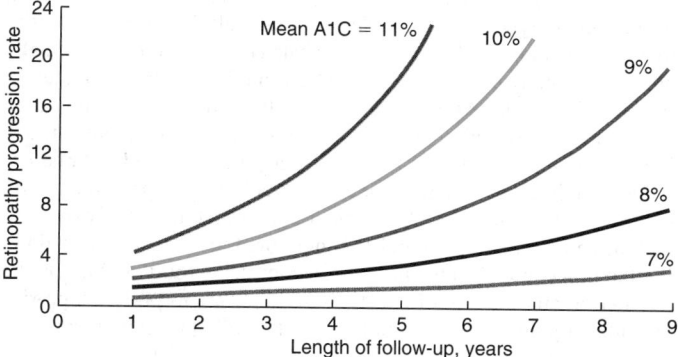

FIGURE 323-8 Relationship of glycemic control and diabetes duration to diabetic retinopathy. The progression of retinopathy in individuals in the Diabetes Control and Complications Trial is graphed as a function of the length of follow-up with different curves for different A1C values. (*Adapted from The Diabetes Control and Complications Trial Research Group, Diabetes 44:968, 1995.*)

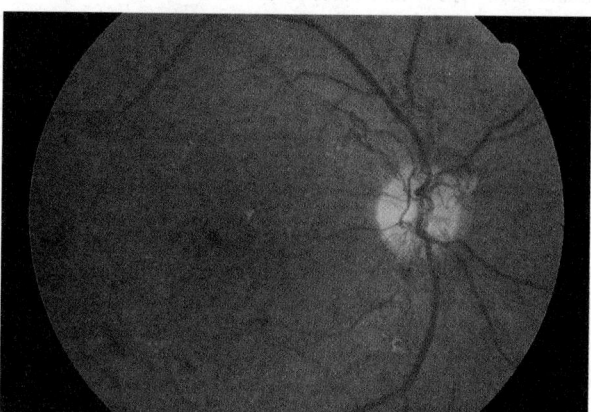

FIGURE 323-9 Diabetic retinopathy results in scattered hemorrhages and yellow exudates. This patient has neovascular vessels proliferating from the optic disc, requiring urgent pan retinal laser photocoagulation.

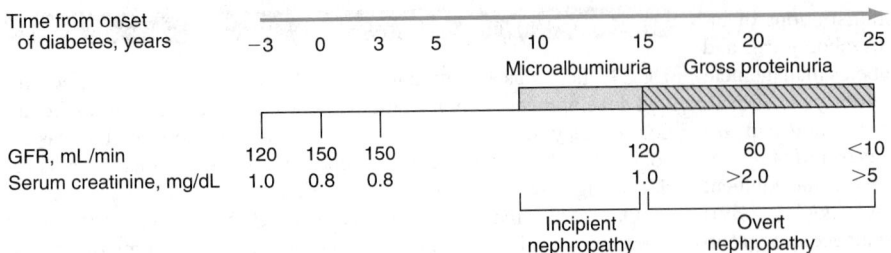

FIGURE 323-10 Time course of development of diabetic nephropathy. The relationship of time from onset of diabetes, the glomerular filtration rate (GFR), and the serum creatinine are shown. *(Adapted from RA DeFronzo, in Therapy for Diabetes Mellitus and Related Disorders, American Diabetes Association, Alexandria, VA, 1998.)*

The appearance of neovascularization in response to retinal hypoxia is the hallmark of *proliferative diabetic retinopathy*. These newly formed vessels appear near the optic nerve and/or macula and rupture easily, leading to vitreous hemorrhage, fibrosis, and ultimately retinal detachment. Not all individuals with nonproliferative retinopathy develop proliferative retinopathy, but the more severe the nonproliferative disease, the greater the chance of evolution to proliferative retinopathy within 5 years. This creates an important opportunity for early detection and treatment of diabetic retinopathy. *Clinically significant macular edema* can occur when only nonproliferative retinopathy is present. Fluorescein angiography is useful to detect macular edema, which is associated with a 25% chance of moderate visual loss over the next 3 years.

Duration of DM and degree of glycemic control are the best predictors of the development of retinopathy; hypertension is also a risk factor. Nonproliferative retinopathy is found in almost all individuals who have had DM for >20 years (25% incidence with 5 years, and 80% incidence with 15 years of type 1 DM). Although there is genetic susceptibility for retinopathy, it confers less influence than either the duration of DM or the degree of glycemic control.

℞ TREATMENT

The most effective therapy for diabetic retinopathy is prevention. Intensive glycemic and blood pressure control will delay the development or slow the progression of retinopathy in individuals with either type 1 or type 2 DM. Paradoxically, during the first 6 to 12 months of improved glycemic control, established diabetic retinopathy may transiently worsen. Fortunately, this progression is temporary, and in the long term, improved glycemic control is associated with less diabetic retinopathy. Individuals with known retinopathy are candidates for prophylactic photocoagulation when initiating intensive therapy. Once advanced retinopathy is present, improved glycemic control imparts less benefit, though adequate ophthalmologic care can prevent most blindness.

Regular, comprehensive eye examinations are essential for all individuals with DM. Most diabetic eye disease can be successfully treated if detected early. Routine, nondilated eye examinations by the primary care provider or diabetes specialist are *inadequate* to detect diabetic eye disease, which requires an ophthalmologist for optimal care of these disorders. Laser photocoagulation is very successful in preserving vision. Proliferative retinopathy is usually treated with panretinal laser photocoagulation, whereas macular edema is treated with focal laser photocoagulation. Although exercise has not been conclusively shown to worsen proliferative diabetic retinopathy, most ophthalmologists advise individuals with advanced diabetic eye disease to limit physical activities associated with repeated Valsalva maneuvers. Aspirin therapy (650 mg/d) does not appear to influence the natural history of diabetic retinopathy, but studies of other antiplatelet agents are under way.

RENAL COMPLICATIONS OF DIABETES MELLITUS Diabetic nephropathy is the leading cause of ESRD in the United States and a leading cause of DM-related morbidity and mortality. Proteinuria in individuals with DM is associated with markedly reduced survival and increased risk

of cardiovascular disease. Individuals with diabetic nephropathy almost always have diabetic retinopathy.

Like other microvascular complications, the pathogenesis of diabetic nephropathy is related to chronic hyperglycemia (Fig. 323-7). The mechanisms by which chronic hyperglycemia leads to ESRD, though incompletely defined, involve the effects of soluble factors (growth factors, angiotensin II, endothelin, AGEs), hemodynamic alterations in the renal microcirculation (glomerular hyperfiltration or hyperperfusion, increased glomerular capillary pressure), and structural changes in the glomerulus (increased extracellular matrix, basement membrane thickening, mesangial expansion, fibrosis). Some of these effects may be mediated through angiotensin II receptors. Smoking accelerates the decline in renal function.

The natural history of diabetic nephropathy is characterized by a fairly predictable sequence of events that was initially defined for individuals with type 1 DM but appears to be similar in type 2 DM (Fig. 323-10). Glomerular hyperperfusion and renal hypertrophy occur in the first years after the onset of DM and cause an increase of the glomerular filtration rate (GFR). During the first 5 years of DM, thickening of the glomerular basement membrane, glomerular hypertrophy, and mesangial volume expansion occur as the GFR returns to normal. After 5 to 10 years of type 1 DM, ~40% of individuals begin to excrete small amounts of albumin in the urine. *Microalbuminuria* is defined as 30 to 300 mg/d in a 24-h collection or 30 to 300 μg/mg creatinine in a spot collection (preferred method). The appearance of microalbuminuria (incipient nephropathy) in type 1 DM is an important predictor of progression to overt proteinuria (>300 mg/d) or overt nephropathy. Blood pressure may rise slightly at this point but usually remains in the normal range. Once overt proteinuria is present, there is a steady decline in GFR, and ~50% of individuals reach ESRD in 7 to 10 years. The early pathologic changes and albumin excretion abnormalities are reversible with normalization of plasma glucose. However, once overt nephropathy develops, the pathologic changes are likely irreversible.

The nephropathy that develops in type 2 DM differs from that of type 1 DM in the following respects: (1) microalbuminuria or overt nephropathy may be present when type 2 DM is diagnosed, reflecting its long asymptomatic period; (2) hypertension more commonly accompanies microalbuminuria or overt nephropathy in type 2 DM; and (3) microalbuminuria may be less predictive of diabetic nephropathy and progression to overt nephropathy in type 2 DM. Finally, it should be noted that albuminuria in type 2 DM may be secondary to factors unrelated to DM, such as hypertension, congestive heart failure, prostate disease, or infection. Diabetic nephropathy and ESRD secondary to this develop more commonly in African Americans, Native Americans, and Hispanic individuals than in Caucasians with type 2 DM.

Type IV renal tubular acidosis (hyporeninemic hypoaldosteronism) also occurs in type 1 or 2 DM. These individuals develop a propensity to hyperkalemia, which may be exacerbated by medications [especially angiotensin-converting enzyme (ACE) inhibitors and angiotensin receptor blockers (ARBs)]. Patients with DM are predisposed to radiocontrast-induced nephrotoxicity. Risk factors for radiocontrast-induced nephrotoxicity are preexisting nephropathy and volume depletion. Individuals with DM undergoing radiographic procedures with contrast dye should be well hydrated before and after dye exposure, and the serum creatinine should be monitored for several days following the procedure. Treatment with acetylcysteine (600 mg bid) on the day before and the day of the dye study appears to protect high-risk patients [creatinine, >212 μmol/L (>2.4 mg/dL)] from radiocontrast-induced nephrotoxicity.

℞ TREATMENT

The optimal therapy for diabetic nephropathy is prevention. As part of comprehensive diabetes care, microalbuminuria should be detected

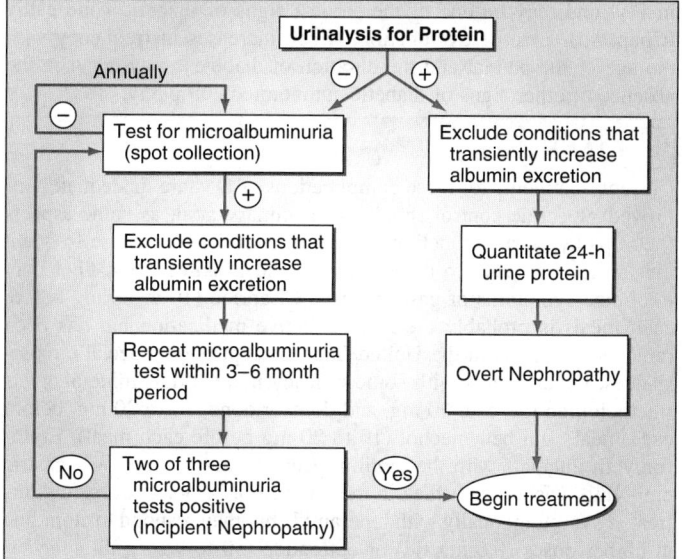

FIGURE 323-11 *Screening for microalbuminuria. (Adapted from RA DeFronzo, in Therapy for Diabetes Mellitus and Related Disorders, American Diabetes Association, Alexandria, VA, 1998.)*

at an early stage when effective therapies can be instituted. The recommended strategy for detecting microalbuminuria is outlined in Fig. 323-11. Interventions effective in slowing progression from microalbuminuria to overt nephropathy include: (1) near normalization of glycemia, (2) strict blood pressure control, and (3) administration of ACE inhibitors or ARBs, and (4) treatment of dyslipidemia.

Improved glycemic control reduces the rate at which microalbuminuria appears and progresses in type 1 and type 2 DM. However, once overt nephropathy exists, it is unclear whether improved glycemic control will slow progression of renal disease. During the phase of declining renal function, insulin requirements may fall as the kidney is a site of insulin degradation. Furthermore, glucose-lowering medications (sulfonylureas and metformin) are contraindicated in advanced renal insufficiency.

Many individuals with type 1 or type 2 DM develop hypertension. Numerous studies in both type 1 and type 2 DM demonstrate the effectiveness of strict blood pressure control in reducing albumin excretion and slowing the decline in renal function. Blood pressure should be maintained at <130/80 mmHg in diabetic individuals without proteinuria. A slightly lower blood pressure (125/75) should be considered for individuals with microalbuminuria or overt nephropathy (see "Hypertension," below).

ACE inhibitors and ARBs reduce the progression of overt nephropathy in individuals with type 1 or type 2 DM and should be prescribed in individuals with type 1 or type 2 DM and microalbuminuria. After 2 to 3 months of therapy, measurement of proteinuria should be repeated and the drug dose increased until either the albuminuria disappears or the maximum dose is reached. If an ACE inhibitor has an unacceptable side-effect profile (hyperkalemia, cough, and renal insufficiency), ARBs can be used as alternatives. If use of either of these types of agents is not possible, then calcium channel blockers (nondihydropyridine class) can be used. However, their efficacy in slowing the fall in the GFR is not proven. Blood pressure control with any agent is extremely important, but a drug-specific benefit in diabetic nephropathy, independent of blood pressure control, has been shown only for ACE inhibitors in type 1 DM and ARBs in type 2 DM.

A consensus panel of the ADA suggests modest restriction of protein intake in diabetic individuals with microalbuminuria (0.8 g/kg per day) or overt nephropathy (<0.8 g/kg per day, which is the adult Recommended Daily Allowance, or about 10% of the daily caloric intake). Conclusive proof of the efficacy of protein restriction is lacking.

Nephrology consultation should be considered after the diagnosis

of early incipient nephropathy. Once overt nephropathy ensues, the likelihood of ESRD is very high. As compared to nondiabetic individuals, hemodialysis in patients with DM is associated with more frequent complications, such as hypotension (due to autonomic neuropathy or loss of reflex tachycardia), more difficult vascular access, and accelerated progression of retinopathy. Survival after the onset of ESRD is shorter in the diabetic population compared to nondiabetics with similar clinical features. Atherosclerosis is the leading cause of death in diabetic individuals on dialysis, and hyperlipidemia should be treated aggressively. Renal transplantation from a living-related donor is the preferred therapy but requires chronic immunosuppression. Combined pancreas-kidney transplant offers the promise of normoglycemia but requires substantial expertise.

NEUROPATHY AND DIABETES MELLITUS Diabetic neuropathy occurs in approximately 50% of individuals with long-standing type 1 and type 2 DM. It may manifest as polyneuropathy, mononeuropathy, and/or autonomic neuropathy. As with other complications of DM, the development of neuropathy correlates with the duration of diabetes and glycemic control; both myelinated and unmyelinated nerve fibers are lost. Because the clinical features of diabetic neuropathy are similar to those of other neuropathies, the diagnosis of *diabetic neuropathy* should be made only after other possible etiologies are excluded (Chap. 363).

Polyneuropathy/Mononeuropathy The most common form of diabetic neuropathy is distal symmetric *polyneuropathy*. It most frequently presents with distal sensory loss. Hyperesthesia, paresthesia, and dysesthesia also occur. Any combination of these symptoms may develop as neuropathy progresses. Symptoms include a sensation of numbness, tingling, sharpness, or burning that begins in the feet and spreads proximally. Neuropathic pain develops in some of these individuals, occasionally preceded by improvement in their glycemic control. Pain typically involves the lower extremities, is usually present at rest, and worsens at night. Both an acute (lasting <12 months) and a chronic form of painful diabetic neuropathy have been described. As diabetic neuropathy progresses, the pain subsides and eventually disappears, but a sensory deficit in the lower extremities persists. Physical examination reveals sensory loss, loss of ankle reflexes, and abnormal position sense.

Diabetic polyradiculopathy is a syndrome characterized by severe disabling pain in the distribution of one or more nerve roots. It may be accompanied by motor weakness. Intercostal or truncal radiculopathy causes pain over the thorax or abdomen. Involvement of the lumbar plexus or femoral nerve may cause pain in the thigh or hip and may be associated with muscle weakness in the hip flexors or extensors (diabetic amyotrophy). Fortunately, diabetic polyradiculopathies are usually self-limited and resolve over 6 to 12 months.

Mononeuropathy (dysfunction of isolated cranial or peripheral nerves) is less common than polyneuropathy in DM and presents with pain and motor weakness in the distribution of a single nerve. A vascular etiology has been suggested, but the pathogenesis is unknown. Involvement of the third cranial nerve is most common and is heralded by diplopia. Physical examination reveals ptosis and opthalmoplegia with normal pupillary constriction to light. Sometimes cranial nerves IV, VI, or VII (Bell's palsy) are affected. Peripheral mononeuropathies or simultaneous involvement of more than one nerve (mononeuropathy multiplex) may also occur.

Autonomic Neuropathy Individuals with long-standing type 1 or 2 DM may develop signs of autonomic dysfunction involving the cholinergic, noradrenergic, and peptidergic (peptides such as pancreatic polypeptide, substance P, etc.) systems. DM-related autonomic neuropathy can involve multiple systems, including the cardiovascular, gastrointestinal, genitourinary, sudomotor, and metabolic systems. Autonomic neuropathies affecting the cardiovascular system cause a resting tachycardia and orthostatic hypotension. Reports of sudden death have also been attributed to autonomic neuropathy. Gastroparesis and bladder-emptying abnormalities are often caused by the autonomic neuropathy seen in DM (discussed below). Hyperhidrosis of the upper extremities and anhidrosis of the lower extremities result from sympathetic nervous system dysfunction. Anhidrosis of the feet can promote dry skin with cracking, which increases the risk of foot ulcers. Autonomic neuropathy may reduce counterregulatory hormone release, leading to an inability to sense hypoglycemia appropriately (*hypoglycemia unawareness*; Chap. 324), thereby subjecting the patient to the risk of severe hypoglycemia and complicating efforts to improve glycemic control.

TREATMENT

Treatment of diabetic neuropathy is less than satisfactory. Improved glycemic control should be pursued and will improve nerve conduction velocity, but the symptoms of diabetic neuropathy may not necessarily improve. Efforts to improve glycemic control may be confounded by autonomic neuropathy and hypoglycemia unawareness. Avoidance of neurotoxins (alcohol), supplementation with vitamins for possible deficiencies (B_{12}, B_6, folate; Chap. 61), and symptomatic treatment are the mainstays of therapy. Aldose reductase inhibitors do not offer significant symptomatic relief. Loss of sensation in the foot places the patient at risk for ulceration and its sequelae; consequently, prevention of such problems is of paramount importance. Since the pain of acute diabetic neuropathy may resolve over the first year, analgesics may be discontinued as progressive neuronal damage from DM occurs. Chronic, painful diabetic neuropathy is difficult to treat but may respond to tricyclic antidepressants (amitriptyline, desipramine, nortriptyline), gabapentin, nonsteroidal anti-inflammatory agents (avoid in renal dysfunction), and other agents (mexilitine, phenytoin, carbamazepine, capsaicin cream). Referral to a pain management center may be necessary.

Therapy of orthostatic hypotension secondary to autonomic neuropathy is challenging. A variety of agents have limited success (fludrocortisone, midodrine, clonidine, octreotide, and yohimbine) but each has significant side effects. Nonpharmacologic maneuvers (adequate salt intake, avoidance of dehydration and diuretics, and lower extremity support hose) may offer some benefit.

GASTROINTESTINAL/GENITOURINARY DYSFUNCTION Long-standing type 1 and 2 DM may affect the motility and function of gastrointestinal (GI) and genitourinary systems. The most prominent GI symptoms are delayed gastric emptying (gastroparesis) and altered small- and large-bowel motility (constipation or diarrhea). *Gastroparesis* may present with symptoms of anorexia, nausea, vomiting, early satiety, and abdominal bloating. Nuclear medicine scintigraphy after ingestion of a radiolabeled meal is the best study to document delayed gastric emptying, but noninvasive "breath tests" following ingestion of a radiolabeled meal are under development. Though parasympathetic dysfunction secondary to chronic hyperglycemia is important in the development of gastroparesis, hyperglycemia itself also impairs gastric emptying. Nocturnal diarrhea, alternating with constipation, is a common feature of DM-related GI autonomic neuropathy. In type 1 DM, these symptoms should also prompt evaluation for celiac sprue because of its increased frequency. Esophageal dysfunction in long-standing DM is common but usually asymptomatic.

Diabetic autonomic neuropathy may lead to genitourinary dysfunction including cystopathy, erectile dysfunction, and female sexual dysfunction (reduced sexual desire, dyspareunia, reduced vaginal lubrication). Symptoms of diabetic cystopathy begin with an inability to sense a full bladder and a failure to void completely. As bladder contractility worsens, bladder capacity and the post-void residual increase, leading to symptoms of urinary hesitancy, decreased voiding frequency, incontinence, and recurrent urinary tract infections. Diagnostic evaluation includes cystometry and urodynamic studies.

Erectile dysfunction and retrograde ejaculation are very common in DM and may be one of the earliest signs of diabetic neuropathy (Chap. 43). Erectile dysfunction, which increases in frequency with the age of the patient and the duration of diabetes, may occur in the absence of other signs of diabetic autonomic neuropathy.

TREATMENT

Current treatments for these complications of DM are inadequate. Improved glycemic control should be a primary goal, as some aspects (neuropathy, gastric function) may improve. Smaller, more frequent meals that are easier to digest (liquid) and low in fat and fiber may minimize symptoms of gastroparesis. Cisapride (10 to 20 mg before each meal) is probably the most effective medication but has been removed from use in the United States except under special circumstances. Other agents with some efficacy include dopamine agonists (metoclopramide, 5 to 10 mg, and domperidone, 10 to 20 mg, before each meal) and bethanechol (10 to 20 mg before each meal). Erythromycin interacts with the motilin receptor and may promote gastric emptying. Diabetic diarrhea in the absence of bacterial overgrowth is treated symptomatically with loperamide but may respond to clonidine at higher doses (0.6 mg tid) or octreotide (50 to 75 μg tid subcutaneously). Treatment of bacterial overgrowth with antibiotics is sometimes useful (Chap. 275).

Diabetic cystopathy should be treated with timed voiding or self-catherization. Medications (bethanechol) are inconsistently effective. The drug of choice for erectile dysfunction is sildenafil, but the efficacy in individuals with DM is slightly lower than in the nondiabetic population (Chap. 43). Sexual dysfunction in women may be improved with use of vaginal lubricants, treatment of vaginal infections, and systemic or local estrogen replacement.

CARDIOVASCULAR MORBIDITY AND MORTALITY Cardiovascular disease is increased in individuals with type 1 or type 2 DM. The Framingham Heart Study revealed a marked increase in peripheral arterial disease, congestive heart failure, coronary artery disease, myocardial infarction (MI), and sudden death (risk increase from one- to fivefold) in DM. The American Heart Association recently designated DM as a major risk factor for cardiovascular disease (same category as smoking, hypertension, and hyperlipidemia). Type 2 diabetes patients without a prior MI have a similar risk for coronary artery–related events as nondiabetic individuals who have had a prior myocardial infarction. Because of the extremely high prevalence of underlying cardiovascular disease in individuals with diabetes (especially in type 2 DM), evidence of atherosclerotic vascular disease should be sought in an individual with diabetes who has symptoms suggestive of cardiac ischemia, peripheral or carotid arterial disease, a resting electrocardiogram indicative of prior infarction, plans to initiate an exercise program, proteinuria, or two other cardiac risk factors (ADA recommendations). The absence of chest pain ("silent ischemia") is common in individuals with diabetes, and a thorough cardiac evaluation is indicated in individuals undergoing major surgical procedures. The prognosis for individuals with diabetes who have coronary artery disease or myocardial infarction is worse than for nondiabetics. Coronary artery disease is more likely to involve multiple vessels in individuals with DM.

The increase in cardiovascular morbidity and mortality appears to relate to the synergism of hyperglycemia with other cardiovascular risk factors. For example, after controlling for all known cardiovascular risk factors, type 2 DM increases the cardiovascular death rate twofold in men and fourfold in women. Risk factors for macrovascular disease in diabetic individuals include dyslipidemia, hypertension, obesity, reduced physical activity, and cigarette smoking. Additional risk factors specific to the diabetic population include microalbuminuria, gross proteinuria, an elevation of serum creatinine, and abnormal platelet function. Insulin resistance, as reflected by elevated serum insulin levels, is associated with an increased risk of cardiovascular complications in individuals with and without DM. Individuals with insulin resistance and type 2 DM have elevated levels of plasminogen activator inhibitors (especially PAI-1) and fibrinogen, which enhances the coagulation process and impairs fibrinolysis, thus favoring the development of thrombosis. Diabetes is also associated with endothelial, vascular smooth muscle, and platelet dysfunction.

Proof that improved glycemic control reduces cardiovascular complications in DM is lacking; in fact, it is possible that macrovascular complications may be unaffected or even worsened by such therapy. Concerns about the atherogenic potential of insulin remain, since in nondiabetic individuals, higher serum insulin levels (indicative of insulin resistance) are associated with a greater risk of cardiovascular morbidity and mortality. In the DCCT, the number of cardiovascular events did not differ between the standard and intensively treated groups. However, the duration of DM in these individuals was relatively short, and the total number of events was very low. An improvement in the lipid profile of individuals in the intensive group [lower total and low-density lipoprotein (LDL) cholesterol, lower triglycerides] suggested that intensive therapy may reduce the risk of cardiovascular morbidity and mortality associated with DM. In the UKPDS, improved glycemic control did not conclusively reduce cardiovascular mortality. Importantly, treatment with insulin and the sulfonylureas did not appear to increase the risk of cardiovascular disease in individuals with type 2 DM, refuting prior claims about the atherogenic potential of these agents.

In addition to coronary artery disease, cerebrovascular disease is increased in individuals with DM (threefold increase in stroke). Individuals with DM have an increased incidence of congestive heart failure (diabetic cardiomyopathy). The etiology of this abnormality is probably multifactorial and includes factors such as myocardial ischemia from atherosclerosis, hypertension, and myocardial cell dysfunction secondary to chronic hyperglycemia.

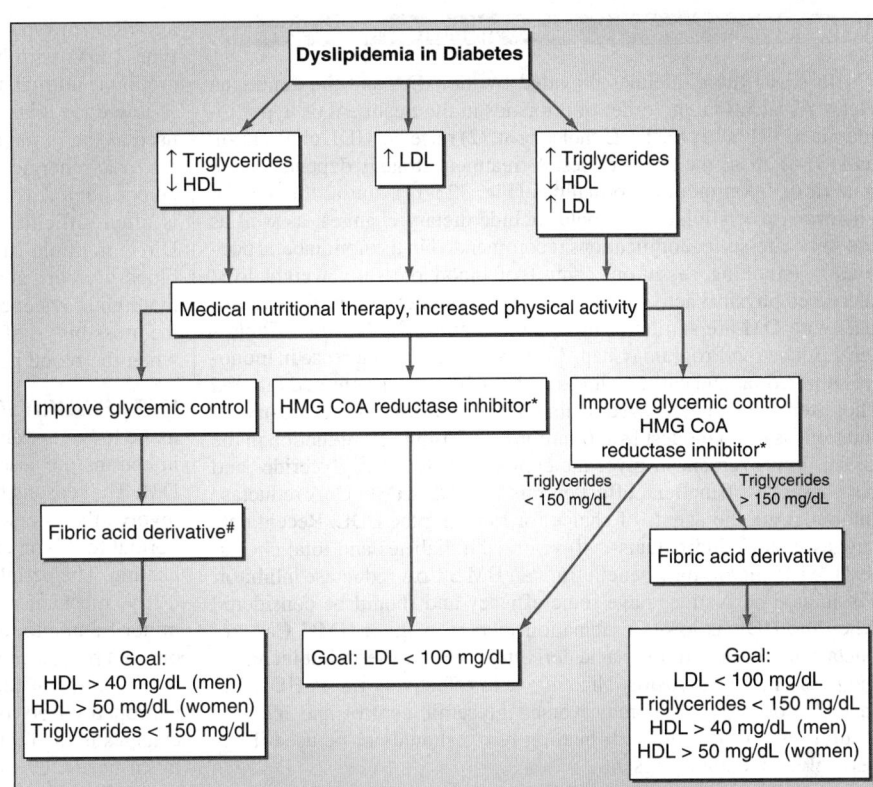

FIGURE 323-12 Dyslipidemia management in diabetes. *Second line treatment: fibric acid derivative or bile acid–binding resin. #Alternative treatment: high dose HMG CoA reductase inhibitor. The level of HDL in women should be 10 mg/dL higher. LDL, low-density lipoprotein; HDL, high-density lipoprotein.

RX TREATMENT

In general, the treatment of coronary disease is no different in the diabetic individual (Chap. 226). Revascularization procedures for coronary artery disease, including percutaneous coronary interventions (PCI) and coronary artery bypass grafting (CABG), are less efficacious in the diabetic individual. Initial success rates of PCI in diabetic individuals are similar to those in the nondiabetic population, but diabetic patients have higher rates of restenosis and lower long-term patency and survival rates. The use of stents and a GPIIb/IIIa platelet inhibitor has improved the outcome in diabetic patients. Perioperative mortality from CABG is not altered in DM, but both short- and long-term survival are reduced. Recent trials indicate that diabetic individuals with multivessel coronary artery disease or recent Q-wave MI have better long-term survival with CABG than PCI.

The ADA has emphasized the importance of glycemic control and aggressive cardiovascular risk modification in all individuals with DM. Past trepidation about using beta blockers in individuals who have diabetes should not prevent use of these agents since they clearly benefit diabetic patients after MI. ACE inhibitors may also be particularly beneficial and should be considered in individuals with type 2 DM and other risk factors (smoking, dyslipidemia, history of cardiovascular disease, microalbuminuria).

Antiplatelet therapy reduces cardiovascular events in individuals with DM who have coronary artery disease. Current recommendations by the ADA include the use of aspirin for secondary prevention of coronary events. Although data demonstrating efficacy in primary prevention of coronary events in DM are lacking, antiplatelet therapy should be strongly considered, especially in diabetic individuals with other coronary risk factors such as hypertension, smoking, or dysli-

pidemia. The aspirin dose (81 to 325 mg) is the same as that in nondiabetic individuals. Aspirin therapy does not have detrimental effects on renal function or hypertension, nor does it influence the course of diabetic retinopathy.

Cardiovascular Risk Factors ■ *DYSLIPIDEMIA* Individuals with DM may have several forms of dyslipidemia (Chap. 335). Because of the additive cardiovascular risk of hyperglycemia and hyperlipidemia, lipid abnormalities should be aggressively detected and treated as part of comprehensive diabetes care (Fig. 323-12). The most common pattern of dyslipidemia is hypertriglyceridemia and reduced HDL cholesterol levels. DM itself does not increase levels of LDL, but the small dense LDL particles found in type 2 DM are more atherogenic because they are more easily glycated and susceptible to oxidation. According to guidelines of the ADA and the American Heart Association, the target lipid values in diabetic individuals without cardiovascular disease should be: LDL < 2.6 mmol/L (100 mg/dL); HDL > 1.1 mmol/L (40 mg/dL) in men and >1.38 mmol/L (50 mg/dL) in women; and triglycerides < 1.7 mmol/L (150 mg/dL). The National Cholesterol Education Program Adult Treatment Panel III also recommends lowering the LDL to < 2.6 mmol/L (100 mg/dL) in diabetics. This is because the incidence of MI in type 2 DM is the same as that in patients without diabetes who have had a prior MI.

Almost all studies of diabetic dyslipidemia have been performed in individuals with type 2 DM because of the greater frequency of dyslipidemia in this form of diabetes. Interventional studies have shown that the beneficial effects of LDL reduction are similar in the diabetic and nondiabetic populations. Large prospective trials of primary and secondary intervention for coronary heart disease have included some individuals with type 2 DM, and subset analyses have consistently found that reductions in LDL reduce cardiovascular events and morbidity in individuals with DM. Most clinical trials used HMG CoA reductase inhibitors, although a fibric acid derivative has also shown to be beneficial. No prospective studies have addressed similar questions in individuals with type 1 DM.

Based on the guidelines provided by the ADA and the American Heart Association, the order of priorities in the treatment of hyperlipidemia is: (1) lower the LDL cholesterol, (2) raise the HDL cholesterol, and (3) decrease the triglycerides. A treatment strategy depends on the pattern of lipoprotein abnormalities (Fig. 323-11). Initial therapy for all forms of dyslipidemia should include dietary changes, as well as the same life-style modifications recommended in the nondiabetic population (smoking cessation, control of blood pressure, weight loss, increased physical activity). The dietary recommendations for individuals with DM are similar to those advocated by the National Cholesterol Education Program (Chap. 335) and include an increase in monounsaturated fat and carbohydrates and a reduction in saturated fats and cholesterol. Though viewed as important, the response to dietary alterations is often modest [<0.6-mmol/L (<25-mg/dL) reduction in the LDL]. Improvement in glycemic control will lower triglycerides and have a modest beneficial effect on raising HDL. HMG CoA reductase inhibitors are the agents of choice for lowering the LDL. Recent data suggest that all individuals >40 years with diabetes and total cholesterol >135 mg/dL may benefit from an HMG CoA reductase inhibitor. Fibric acid derivatives have some efficacy and should be considered when the HDL is low. Combination therapy with an HMG CoA reductase inhibitor and fibric acid derivative may be useful but increases the possibility of myositis. Nicotinic acid effectively raises HDL, but in high doses (>2 g/d) may worsen glycemic control and increase insulin resistance. Bile acid–binding resins should not be used if hypertriglyceridemia is present.

HYPERTENSION Hypertension can accelerate other complications of DM, particularly cardiovascular disease and nephropathy. Hypertension therapy should first emphasize life-style modifications such as weight loss, exercise, stress management, and sodium restriction. Antihypertensive agents should be selected based on the advantages and disadvantages of the therapeutic agent in the context of an individual patient's risk factor profile. DM-related considerations include the following:

1. ACE inhibitors are either glucose- and lipid-neutral or glucose- and lipid-beneficial and thus positively impact the cardiovascular risk profile. For example, captopril improves insulin resistance, reduces LDL slightly, and increases HDL slightly. α-Adrenergic blockers slightly improve insulin resistance and positively impact the lipid profile, whereas beta blockers and thiazide diuretics can increase insulin resistance and negatively impact the lipid profile. Calcium channel blockers, central adrenergic antagonists, and vasodilators are lipid- and glucose-neutral.

2. Beta blockers may slightly increase the risk of developing type 2 DM. Although often questioned because of the potential masking of hypoglycemic symptoms, beta blockers are safe in most patients with diabetes and reduce cardiovascular events. In one study of nondiabetic individuals, the ACE inhibitor ramipril reduced the risk of developing type 2 DM.

3. Sympathetic inhibitors and α-adrenergic blockers may worsen orthostatic hypotension in the diabetic individual with autonomic neuropathy.

4. Equivalent reduction in blood pressure by different classes of agents may not translate into equivalent protection from cardiovascular and renal endpoints. Thiazides, beta blockers, ACE inhibitors, and ARBs positively impact cardiovascular endpoints (MI or stroke). The cardiovascular protective effect of calcium channel blockers, central adrenergic antagonists, and α-adrenergic blockers is either controversial or not known. ACE inhibitors (in types 1 and 2 DM) and ARBs (in type 2 DM) slow the progression of diabetic renal disease; the effect of other classes of agents on diabetic nephropathy is not known.

5. Non-dihydropyridine calcium channel blockers (verapamil and diltiazem), rather than dihydropyridine agents (amlodipine and nifedipine), are preferred in diabetics.

If microalbuminuria or overt albuminuria is present, the optimal antihypertensive agent is an ACE inhibitor (in types 1 and 2 DM) or an ARB (in type 2 DM). Most prefer ARBs over ACE inhibitors in type 2 DM with hypertension and microalbuminuria. If albumin excretion is normal, then an ACE inhibitor is usually prescribed initially. A low-dose thiazide diuretic, beta blockers, or an ARB may also be used as the initial agent. Non-dihydropyridine calcium channel blockers, α-adrenergic blockers, and central adrenergic antagonists should be considered as additional or second-line agents. Since hypertension is often difficult to control with a single agent (especially in type 2 DM), multiple antihypertensive agents are usually required when blood pressure goals (<130/80 mmHg) are not achieved. Because of the high prevalence of atherosclerotic disease in individuals with DM, the possibility of renovascular hypertension should be considered when the blood pressure is not readily controlled.

LOWER EXTREMITY COMPLICATIONS DM is the leading cause of nontraumatic lower extremity amputation in the United States. Foot ulcers and infections are also a major source of morbidity in individuals with DM. The reasons for the increased incidence of these disorders in DM involve the interaction of several pathogenic factors: neuropathy, abnormal foot biomechanics, peripheral arterial disease, and poor wound healing. The peripheral sensory neuropathy interferes with normal protective mechanisms and allows the patient to sustain major or repeated minor trauma to the foot, often without knowledge of the injury. Disordered proprioception causes abnormal weight bearing while walking and subsequent formation of callus or ulceration. Motor and sensory neuropathy lead to abnormal foot muscle mechanics and to structural changes in the foot (hammer toe, claw toe deformity, prominent metatarsal heads, Charcot joint). Autonomic neuropathy results in anhidrosis and altered superficial blood flow in the foot, which promote drying of the skin and fissure formation. Peripheral arterial disease and poor wound healing impede resolution of minor breaks in the skin, allowing them to enlarge and to become infected.

Approximately 15% of individuals with DM develop a foot ulcer, and a significant subset will ultimately undergo amputation (14 to 24% risk with that ulcer or subsequent ulceration). Risk factors for foot ulcers or amputation include: male sex, diabetes >10 years' duration, peripheral neuropathy, abnormal structure of foot (bony abnormalities, callus, thickened nails), peripheral arterial disease, smoking, history of previous ulcer or amputation, and poor glycemic control.

℞ **TREATMENT**

The optimal therapy for foot ulcers and amputations is prevention through identification of high-risk patients, education of the patient, and institution of measures to prevent ulceration. High-risk patients should be identified during the routine foot examination performed on all patients with DM (see "Ongoing Aspects of Comprehensive Diabetes Care," below). Patient education should emphasize: (1) careful selection of footwear, (2) daily inspection of the feet to detect early signs of poor-fitting footwear or minor trauma, (3) daily foot hygiene to keep the skin clean and moist, (4) avoidance of self-treatment of foot abnormalities and high-risk behavior (e.g., walking barefoot), and (5) prompt consultation with a health care provider if an abnormality arises. Patients at high risk for ulceration or amputation may benefit from evaluation by a foot care specialist. Interventions directed at risk factor modification include orthotic shoes and devices, callus management, nail care, and prophylactic measures to reduce increased skin pressure from abnormal bony architecture. Attention to other risk factors for vascular disease (smoking, dyslipidemia, hypertension) and improved glycemic control are also important.

Despite preventive measures, foot ulceration and infection are common and represent a potentially serious problem. Due to the multifactorial pathogenesis of lower extremity ulcers, management of these lesions is multidisciplinary and often demands expertise in orthopedics, vascular surgery, endocrinology, podiatry, and infectious diseases. The plantar surface of the foot is the most common site of ulceration. Ulcers may be primarily neuropathic (no accompanying infection) or may have surrounding cellulitis or osteomyelitis. Cellulitis without ulceration is also frequent and should be treated with antibiotics that provide broad-spectrum coverage, including anaerobes (see below).

An infected ulcer is a clinical diagnosis, since superficial culture of any ulceration will likely find multiple possible bacterial pathogens. The infection surrounding the foot ulcer is often the result of multiple organisms (gram-positive and -negative organisms and anaerobes), and gas gangrene may develop in the absence of clostridial infection. Cultures taken from the debrided ulcer base or from purulent drainage are most helpful. Wound depth should be determined by inspection and probing with a blunt-tipped sterile instrument. Plain radiographs of the foot should be performed to assess the possibility of osteomyelitis in chronic ulcers that have not responded to therapy. Nuclear medicine bone scans may be helpful, but overlying subcutaneous infection is often difficult to distinguish from osteomyelitis. Indium-labeled white cell studies are more useful in determining if the infection involves bony structures or only soft tissue, but they are technically demanding. Magnetic resonance imaging of the foot may be the most specific modality, although distinguishing bony destruction due to osteomyelitis from destruction secondary to Charcot arthropathy is difficult. If surgical debridement is necessary, bone biopsy and culture may provide the answer.

Osteomyelitis is best treated by a combination of prolonged antibiotics (IV then oral) and possibly debridement of infected bone. The possible contribution of vascular insufficiency should be considered in all patients. Noninvasive blood-flow studies are often unreliable in DM, and angiography may be required, recognizing the risk of contrast-induced nephrotoxicity. Peripheral arterial bypass procedures are often effective in promoting wound healing and in decreasing the need for amputation of the ischemic limb.

A growing number of possible treatments for diabetic foot ulcers exist, but they have yet to demonstrate clear efficacy in prospective, controlled trials. A recent consensus statement from the ADA identified six interventions with demonstrated efficacy in diabetic foot wounds: (1) off-loading, (2) debridement, (3) wound dressings, (4) appropriate use of antibiotics, (5) revascularization, and (6) limited amputation. Off-loading is the complete avoidance of weight bearing on the ulcer, which removes the mechanical trauma that retards wound healing. Bed rest and a variety of orthotic devices or contact casting limit weight bearing on wounds or pressure points. Surgical debridement is important and effective, but clear efficacy of other modalities for wound cleaning (enzymes, soaking, whirlpools) is lacking. Dressings promote wound healing by creating a moist environment and protecting the wound. Antiseptic agents and topical antibiotics should be avoided. Referral for physical therapy, orthotic evaluation, and rehabilitation may be useful once the infection is controlled.

Mild or non-limb-threatening infections can be treated with oral antibiotics (cephalosporin, clindamycin, amoxicillin/clavulanate, and fluoroquinolones), surgical debridement of necrotic tissue, local wound care (avoidance of weight bearing over the ulcer), and close surveillance for progression of infection. More severe ulcers may require intravenous antibiotics as well as bed rest and local wound care. Urgent surgical debridement may be required. Intravenous antibiotics should provide broad-spectrum coverage directed toward *Staphylococcus aureus*, streptococci, gram-negative aerobes, and anaerobic bacteria. Initial antimicrobial regimens include cefotetan, ampicillin/sulbactam, or the combination of clindamycin and a fluoroquinolone. Severe infections, or infections that do not improve after 48 h of antibiotic therapy, require expansion of antimicrobial therapy to treat methicillin-resistant *S. aureus* (e.g., vancomycin) and *Pseudomonas aeruginosa*. If the infection surrounding the ulcer is not improving with intravenous antibiotics, reassessment of antibiotic coverage and reconsideration of the need for surgical debridement or revascularization are indicated. With clinical improvement, oral antibiotics and local wound care can be continued on an outpatient basis with close follow-up.

New information about wound biology has led to a number of new technologies (e.g., living skin equivalents and growth factors such as basic fibroblast growth factor) that may prove useful. Recombinant platelet-derived growth factor has some benefit and complement the therapies of off-loading, debridement, and antibiotics. Hyperbaric oxygen has been used, but rigorous proof of efficacy is lacking.

INFECTIONS Individuals with DM have a greater frequency and severity of infection. The reasons for this include incompletely defined abnormalities in cell-mediated immunity and phagocyte function associated with hyperglycemia, as well as diminished vascularization. Hyperglycemia aids the colonization and growth of a variety of organisms (*Candida* and other fungal species). Many common infections are more frequent and severe in the diabetic population, whereas several rare infections are seen almost exclusively in the diabetic population. Examples of this latter category includes rhinocerebral mucormycosis, emphysematous infections of the gall bladder and urinary tract, and "malignant" or invasive otitis externa. Invasive otitis externa is usually secondary to *P. aeruginosa* infection in the soft tissue surrounding the external auditory canal, usually begins with pain and discharge, and may rapidly progress to osteomyelitis and meningitis. These infections should be sought, in particular, in patients presenting with HHS.

Pneumonia, urinary tract infections, and skin and soft tissue infections are all more common in the diabetic population. In general, the organisms that cause pulmonary infections are similar to those found in the nondiabetic population; however, gram-negative organisms, *S. aureus*, and *Mycobacterium tuberculosis* are more frequent pathogens. Urinary tract infections (either lower tract or pyelonephritis) are the result of common bacterial agents such as *Escherichia coli*, though several yeast species (*Candida* and *Torulopsis glabrata*) are commonly observed. Complications of urinary tract infections include emphysematous pyelonephritis and emphysematous cystitis. Bacteriuria occurs frequently in individuals with diabetic cystopathy. Susceptibility to furunculosis, superficial candidal infections, and vulvovaginitis are increased. Poor glycemic control is a common denominator in individuals with these infections. Diabetic individuals have an increased rate of colonization of *S. aureus* in the skin folds and nares. Diabetic patients also have a greater risk of postoperative wound infections. Strict glycemic control reduces postoperative infections in diabetic individuals undergoing CABG and should be the goal in all diabetic patients with an infection.

DERMATOLOGIC MANIFESTATIONS The most common skin manifestations of DM are protracted wound healing and skin ulcerations. Diabetic dermopathy, sometimes termed *pigmented pretibial papules*, or "diabetic skin spots," begins as an erythematous area and evolves into an area of circular hyperpigmentation. These lesions result from minor mechanical trauma in the pretibial region and are more common in elderly men with DM. Bullous diseases (shallow ulcerations or erosions in the pretibial region) are also seen. *Necrobiosis lipoidica diabeticorum* is a rare disorder of DM that predominantly affects young women with type 1 DM, neuropathy, and retinopathy. It usually begins in the pretibial region as an erythematous plaque or papules that gradually enlarge, darken, and develop irregular margins, with atrophic centers and central ulceration. They may be painful. *Acanthosis nigricans* (hyperpigmented velvety plaques seen on the neck, axilla, or extensor surfaces) is sometimes a feature of severe insulin resistance and accompanying diabetes. Generalized or localized *granuloma annulare* (erythematous plaques on the extremities or trunk) and *scleredema* (areas of skin thickening on the back or neck at the site of previous superficial infections) are more common in the diabetic population. *Lipoatrophy* and *lipohypertrophy* can occur at insulin injection sites but are unusual with the use of human insulin. Xerosis and pruritus are common and are relieved by skin moisturizers.

APPROACH TO THE PATIENT

DM and its complications produce a wide range of symptoms and signs; those secondary to acute hyperglycemia may occur at any stage of the disease, whereas those related to chronic complications begin to appear during the second decade of hyperglycemia. Individuals with previously undetected type 2 DM may present with chronic complications of DM at the time of diagnosis. The history and physical examination should assess for symptoms or signs of acute hyperglycemia and should screen for the chronic complications and conditions associated with DM.

History A complete medical history should be obtained with special emphasis on DM-relevant aspects such as weight, family history of DM and its complications, risk factors for cardiovascular disease, exercise, smoking, and ethanol use. Symptoms of hyperglycemia include polyuria, polydipsia, weight loss, fatigue, weakness, blurry vision, frequent superficial infections (vaginitis, fungal skin infections), and slow healing of skin lesions after minor trauma. Metabolic derangements relate mostly to hyperglycemia (osmotic diuresis, reduced glucose entry into muscle) and to the catabolic state of the patient (urinary loss of glucose and calories, muscle breakdown due to protein degradation and decreased protein synthesis). Blurred vision results from changes in the water content of the lens and resolves as the hyperglycemia is controlled.

In a patient with established DM, the initial assessment should also include special emphasis on prior diabetes care, including the type of therapy, prior hemoglobin A1C levels, self-monitoring blood glucose results, frequency of hypoglycemia, presence of DM-specific complications, and assessment of the patient's knowledge about diabetes. The chronic complications may afflict several organ systems, and an individual patient may exhibit some, all, or none of the symptoms related to the complications of DM (see above). In addition, the presence of DM-related comorbidities should be sought (cardiovascular disease, hypertension, dyslipidemia).

Physical Examination In addition to a complete physical examination, special attention should be given to DM-relevant aspects such as weight or BMI, retinal examination, orthostatic blood pressure, foot examination, peripheral pulses, and insulin injection sites. Blood pressure > 130/80 mmHg is considered hypertension in individuals with diabetes. Careful examination of the lower extremities should seek evidence of peripheral neuropathy, calluses, superficial fungal infections, nail disease, and foot deformities (such as hammer or claw toes and Charcot foot) in order to identify sites of potential skin ulceration. Vibratory sensation (128-MHz tuning fork at the base of the great toe) and the ability to sense touch with a monofilament (5.07, 10-g monofilament) are useful to detect moderately advanced diabetic neuropathy. Since periodontal disease is more frequent in DM, the teeth and gums should also be examined.

Classification of DM in an Individual Patient The etiology of diabetes in an individual with new-onset disease can usually be assigned on the basis of clinical criteria. Individuals with type 1 DM tend to have the following characteristics: (1) onset of disease prior to age 30; (2) lean body habitus; (3) requirement of insulin as the initial therapy; (4) propensity to develop ketoacidosis; and (5) an increased risk of other autoimmune disorders such as autoimmune thyroid disease, adrenal insufficiency, pernicious anemia, and vitiligo. In contrast, individuals with type 2 DM often exhibit the following features: (1) develop diabetes after the age of 30; (2) are usually obese (80% are obese, but elderly individuals may be lean); (3) may not require insulin therapy initially; and (4) may have associated conditions such as insulin resistance, hypertension, cardiovascular disease, dyslipidemia, or PCOS. In type 2 DM, insulin resistance is often associated with abdominal obesity (as opposed to hip and thigh obesity) and hypertriglyceridemia. Although most individuals diagnosed with type 2 DM are older, the age of diagnosis is declining in some ethnic groups, and there is a marked increase among overweight children and adolescents. Some indi-

viduals with phenotypic type 2 DM present with DKA but lack autoimmune markers and may be later treated with oral glucose-lowering agents rather than insulin. On the other hand, some individuals (5–10%) with the phenotypic appearance of type 2 DM do not have absolute insulin deficiency but have autoimmune markers (ICA, GAD autoantibodies) suggestive of type 1A DM (termed *autoimmune diabetes not requiring insulin at diagnosis* or *latent autoimmune diabetes of the adult*). Such individuals are much more likely to require insulin treatment within 5 years. Thus, despite the revised classification of DM, it is remains difficult to categorize some patients unequivocally. Individuals who deviate from the clinical profile of type 1 and type 2 DM, or who have other associated defects such as deafness, pancreatic exocrine disease, and other endocrine disorders, should be classified accordingly (Table 323-1).

Laboratory Assessment The laboratory assessment should first determine whether the patient meets the diagnostic criteria for DM (Table 323-2) and then assess the degree of glycemic control (A1C, discussed below). In addition to the standard laboratory evaluation, the patient should be screened for DM-associated conditions (e.g., microalbuminuria, dyslipidemia, thyroid dysfunction). Individuals at high risk for cardiovascular disease should be screened for asymptomatic coronary artery disease by appropriate cardiac stress testing, when indicated.

The classification of the type of DM may be facilitated by laboratory assessments. Serum insulin or C-peptide measurements do not always distinguish type 1 from type 2 DM, but a low C-peptide level confirms a patient's need for insulin. Many individuals with new-onset type 1 DM retain some C-peptide production. Measurement of islet cell antibodies at the time of diabetes onset may be useful if the type of DM is not clear based on the characteristics described above.

LONG-TERM TREATMENT

OVERALL PRINCIPLES The goals of therapy for type 1 or type 2 DM are to: (1) eliminate symptoms related to hyperglycemia, (2) reduce or eliminate the long-term microvascular and macrovascular complications of DM, and (3) allow the patient to achieve as normal a life-style as possible. To reach these goals, the physician should identify a target level of glycemic control for each patient, provide the patient with the educational and pharmacologic resources necessary to reach this level, and monitor/treat DM-related complications. Symptoms of diabetes usually resolve when the plasma glucose is <11.1 mmol/L (200 mg/dL), and thus most DM treatment focuses on achieving the second and third goals.

The care of an individual with either type 1 or type 2 DM requires a multidisciplinary team. Central to the success of this team are the patient's participation, input, and enthusiasm, all of which are essential for optimal diabetes management. Members of the health care team include the primary care provider and/or the endocrinologist or diabetologist, a certified diabetes educator, and a nutritionist. In addition, when the complications of DM arise, subspecialists (including neurologists, nephrologists, vascular surgeons, cardiologists, ophthalmologists, and podiatrists) with experience in DM-related complications are essential.

A number of names are sometimes applied to different approaches to diabetes care, such as intensive insulin therapy, intensive glycemic control, and "tight control." The current chapter, however, will use the term *comprehensive diabetes care* to emphasize the fact that optimal diabetes therapy involves more than plasma glucose management. Though glycemic control is central to optimal diabetes therapy, comprehensive diabetes care of both type 1 and type 2 DM should also detect and manage DM-specific complications and modify risk factors for DM-associated diseases. In addition to the physical aspects of DM, social, family, financial, cultural, and employment-related issues may impact diabetes care.

PATIENT EDUCATION ABOUT DM, NUTRITION, AND EXERCISE

The patient with type 1 or type 2 DM should receive education about nutrition, exercise, care of diabetes during illness, and medications to lower the plasma glucose. Along with improved compliance, patient education allows individuals with DM to assume greater responsibility for their care. Patient education should be viewed as a continuing process with regular visits for reinforcement; it should *not* be a process that is completed after one or two visits to a nurse educator or nutritionist.

Diabetes Education The diabetes educator is a health care professional (nurse, dietician, or pharmacist) with specialized patient education skills who is certified in diabetes education (e.g., American Association of Diabetes Educators). Education topics important for optimal diabetes care include self-monitoring of blood glucose; urine ketone monitoring (type 1 DM); insulin administration; guidelines for diabetes management during illnesses; management of hypoglycemia; foot and skin care; diabetes management before, during, and after exercise; and risk factor–modifying activities.

Nutrition *Medical nutrition therapy* (MNT) is a term used by the ADA to describe the optimal coordination of caloric intake with other aspects of diabetes therapy (insulin, exercise, weight loss). Historically, nutrition education imposed restrictive, complicated regimens on the patient. Current practices have greatly changed, though many patients and health care providers still view the diabetic diet as monolithic and static. For example, MNT now includes foods with sucrose and seeks to modify other risk factors such as hyperlipidemia and hypertension rather than focusing exclusively on weight loss in individuals with type 2 DM. Like other aspects of DM therapy, MNT must be adjusted to meet the goals of the individual patient. Furthermore, MNT education is an important component of comprehensive diabetes care and should be reinforced by regular patient education. In general, the components of optimal MNT are similar for individuals with type 1 or type 2 DM (Table 323-8).

The goal of MNT in the individual with type 1 DM is to coordinate and match the caloric intake, both temporally and quantitatively, with the appropriate amount of insulin. MNT in type 1 DM and self-monitoring of blood glucose must be integrated to define the optimal insulin regimen. MNT must be flexible enough to allow for exercise, and the insulin regimen must allow for deviations in caloric intake. An important component of MNT in type 1 DM is to minimize the weight gain often associated with intensive diabetes management.

The goals of MNT in type 2 DM are slightly different and address the greatly increased prevalence of cardiovascular risk factors (hypertension, dyslipidemia, obesity) and disease in this population. The majority of these individuals are obese, and weight loss is strongly encouraged and should remain an important goal. Medical treatment of obesity is a rapidly evolving area and is discussed in Chap. 64. Hypocaloric diets and modest weight loss often result in rapid and dramatic glucose lowering in individuals with new-onset type 2 DM. Nevertheless, numerous studies document that long-term weight loss is uncommon. Current MNT for type 2 DM should emphasize modest caloric reduction, reduced fat intake, increased physical activity, and reduction of hyperlipidemia and hypertension. Increased consumption of soluble, dietary fiber may improve glycemic control in individuals with type 2 DM.

Exercise Exercise has multiple positive benefits including cardiovascular risk reduction, reduced blood pressure, maintenance of muscle mass, reduction in body fat, and weight loss. For individuals with type 1 or type 2 DM, exercise is also useful for lowering plasma glucose (during and following exercise) and increasing insulin sensitivity.

Despite its benefits, exercise presents challenges for individuals with DM because they lack the normal glucoregulatory mechanisms (insulin falls and glucagon rises during exercise). Skeletal muscle is a major site for metabolic fuel consumption in the resting state, and the increased muscle activity during vigorous, aerobic exercise greatly increases fuel requirements. Individuals with type 1 DM are prone to either hyperglycemia or hypoglycemia during exercise, depending on the preexercise plasma glucose, the circulating insulin level, and the level of exercise-induced catecholamines. If the insulin level is too low, the rise in catecholamines may increase the plasma glucose excessively, promote ketone body formation, and possibly lead to ketoacidosis. Conversely, if the circulating insulin level is excessive, this relative hyperinsulinemia may reduce hepatic glucose production (decreased glycogenolysis, decreased gluconeogenesis) and increase glucose entry into muscle, leading to hypoglycemia.

To avoid exercise-related hyper- or hypoglycemia, individuals with type 1 DM should: (1) monitor blood glucose before, during, and after exercise; (2) delay exercise if blood glucose is >14 mmol/L (250 mg/dL), <5.5 mmol/L (100 mg/dL), or if ketones are present; (3) monitor glucose during exercise and ingest carbohydrate to prevent hypoglycemia; (4) decrease insulin doses (based on previous experience) before exercise and inject insulin into a nonexercising area; and (5) learn individual glucose responses to different types of exercise and increase food intake for up to 24 h after exercise, depending on intensity and duration of exercise. In individuals with type 2 DM, exercise-related hypoglycemia is less common but can occur in individuals taking either insulin or sulfonylureas.

Because asymptomatic cardiovascular disease appears at a younger age in both type 1 and type 2 DM, formal exercise tolerance testing may be warranted in diabetic individuals with any of the following: age >35 years, diabetes duration >15 years (type 1 DM) or >10 years (type 2 DM), microvascular complications of DM (retinopathy, microalbuminuria, or nephropathy), peripheral arterial disease, other risk factors of coronary artery disease, or autonomic neuropathy. Untreated proliferative retinopathy is a relative contraindication to vigorous exercise, as this may lead to vitreous hemorrhage or retinal detachment.

MONITORING THE LEVEL OF GLYCEMIC CONTROL

Optimal monitoring of glycemic control involves plasma glucose measurements by the patient and an assessment of long-term control by the physician (measurement of hemoglobin A1C and review of the patient's self-measurements of plasma glucose). These measurements are complementary: the patient's measurements provide a picture of short-term glycemic control, whereas the A1C reflects average glycemic control over the previous 2 to 3 months.

Self-Monitoring of Blood Glucose Self-monitoring of blood glucose (SMBG) is the standard of care in diabetes management and allows the patient to monitor his or her blood glucose at any time. In SMBG, a small drop of blood and an easily detectable enzymatic reaction allow measurement of the capillary plasma glucose. A number of devices accurately measure glucose in blood obtained from the fingertip; al-

---

TABLE 323-8 *Nutritional Recommendations for All Persons with Diabetes*

- Protein to provide ~15–20% of kcal/d (~10% for those with nephropathy)
- Saturated fat to provide <10% of kcal/d (<7% for those with elevated LDL)
- Polyunsaturated fat to provide ~10% of kcal; avoid trans-unsaturated fatty acids
- 60–70% of calories to be divided between carbohydrate and monounsaturated fat, based on medical needs and personal tolerance; glycemic index of food not as important
- Use of caloric sweeteners, including sucrose, is acceptable.
- Fiber (20–35 g/d) and sodium (≤3000 mg/d) levels as recommended for the general healthy population
- Cholesterol intake ≤300 mg/d
- The same precautions regarding alcohol use in the general population also apply to individuals with diabetes. Alcohol may increase risk for hypoglycemia and therefore should be taken with food.

Note: LDL, low-density lipoprotein.
Source: Adapted from R Farkas-Hirsch, *Intensive Diabetes Management*, Alexandria, VA, American Diabetes Association, 1998; and American Diabetes Association: Diabetes Care 25:S1, 2002.

ternative testing sites (e.g., forearm) are less reliable. By combining glucose measurements with diet history, medication changes, and exercise history, the physician and patient can improve the treatment program.

The frequency of SMBG measurements must be individualized and adapted to address the goals of diabetes care. Individuals with type 1 DM should routinely measure their plasma glucose four to eight times per day to estimate and select mealtime boluses of short-acting insulin and to modify long-acting insulin doses. Most individuals with type 2 DM require less frequent monitoring, though the optimal frequency of SMBG has not been clearly defined. Individuals with type 2 DM who are on oral medications should utilize SMBG as a means of assessing the efficacy of their medication and the impact of diet. Since plasma glucose levels fluctuate less in these individuals, one to two SMBG measurements per day (or fewer) may be sufficient. Individuals with type 2 DM who are on insulin should utilize SMBG more frequently than those on oral agents. Urine glucose testing does not provide an accurate assessment of glycemic control.

Two devices for continuous blood glucose monitoring have been recently approved by the U.S. Food and Drug Administration (FDA). The Glucowatch uses iontophoresis to assess glucose in interstitial fluid, whereas the Minimed device uses an indwelling subcutaneous catheter to monitor interstitial fluid glucose. Both devices utilize immobilized glucose oxidase to generate electrons in response to changing glucose levels. Though clinical experience with these devices is limited, they perform well in clinical trials and appear to provide useful short-term information about the patterns of glucose changes as well as an enhanced ability to detect hypoglycemic episodes. These devices are not yet used routinely in diabetes management.

Ketones are an indicator of early diabetic ketoacidosis and should be measured in individuals with type 1 DM when the plasma glucose is consistently >16.7 mmol/L (300 mg/dL), during a concurrent illness; or with symptoms such as nausea, vomiting, or abdominal pain. Blood measurement of β-hydroxybutyrate is preferred over urine testing with nitroprusside-based assays that measure only acetoacetate and acetone.

Assessment of Long-Term Glycemic Control   Measurement of glycated hemoglobin is the standard method for assessing long-term glycemic control. When plasma glucose is consistently elevated, there is an increase in nonenzymatic glycation of hemoglobin; this alteration reflects the glycemic history over the previous 2 to 3 months, since erythrocytes have an average life span of 120 days. There are numerous laboratory methods for measuring the various forms of glycated hemoglobin, and these have significant interassay variations. Since glycated hemoglobin measurements are usually compared to prior measurements, it is essential for the assay results to be comparable. Depending on the assay methodology, hemoglobinopathies, anemias, and uremia may interfere with the A1C result.

Glycated hemoglobin or A1C should be measured in all individuals with DM during their initial evaluation and as part of their comprehensive diabetes care. As the primary predictor of long-term complications of DM, the A1C should mirror, to a certain extent, the short-term measurements of SMBG. These two measurements are complementary in that recent intercurrent illnesses may impact the SMBG measurements but not the A1C. Likewise, postprandial and nocturnal hyperglycemia may not be detected by the SMBG of fasting and preprandial capillary plasma glucose but will be reflected in the A1C. In standardized assays, the A1C approximates the following mean plasma glucose values: an A1C of 6% is 7.5 mmol/L (135 mg/dL), 7% is 9.5 mmol/L (170 mg/dL), 8% is 11.5 mmol/L (205 mg/dL), etc. [A 1% rise in the A1C translates into a 2.0-mmol/L (35 mg/dL) increase in the mean glucose.] In patients achieving their glycemic goal, the ADA recommends measurement of the A1C twice per year. More frequent testing (every 3 months) is warranted when glycemic control is inadequate, when therapy has changed, or in most patients

with type 1 DM. The degree of glycation of other proteins, such as albumin, has been used as an alternative indicator of glycemic control when the A1C is inaccurate (hemolytic anemia, hemoglobinopathies). The fructosamine assay (measuring glycated albumin) reflects the glycemic status over the prior 2 weeks. Current consensus statements do not favor the use of alternative assays of glycemic control, as there are no studies to indicate whether such assays accurately predict the complications of DM.

℞ TREATMENT

ESTABLISHMENT OF A TARGET LEVEL OF GLYCEMIC CONTROL   Because the complications of DM are related to glycemic control, normoglycemia or near normoglycemia is the desired, but often elusive, goal for most patients. However, normalization of the plasma glucose for long periods of time is extremely difficult, as demonstrated by the DCCT. Regardless of the level of hyperglycemia, improvement in glycemic control will lower the risk of diabetes complications (Fig. 323-8).

The target for glycemic control (as reflected by the A1C) must be individualized, and the goals of therapy should be developed in consultation with the patient after considering a number of medical, social, and life-style issues. Some important factors to consider include the patient's age, ability to understand and implement a complex treatment regimen, presence and severity of complications of diabetes, ability to recognize hypoglycemic symptoms, presence of other medical conditions or treatments that might alter the response to therapy, life-style and occupation (e.g., possible consequences of experiencing hypoglycemia on the job), and level of support available from family and friends.

The ADA has established suggested glycemic goals based on the premise that glycemic control predicts development of DM-related complications. In general, the target A1C should be <7.0% (Table 323-9). Other consensus groups (such as the Veterans Administration) have suggested A1C goals that take into account the patient's life expectancy at the time of diagnosis and the presence of microvascular complications. Such recommendations strive to balance the financial and personal costs of glycemic therapy with anticipated benefits (reduced health care costs, reduced morbidity). One limitation to this approach is that the onset of hyperglycemia in type 2 DM is difficult to ascertain and likely predates the diagnosis.

TYPE 1 DIABETES MELLITUS ■ General Aspects   The ADA recommendations for fasting and bedtime glycemic goals and A1C targets are summarized in Table 323-9. The goal is to design and implement insulin regimens that mimic physiologic insulin secretion. Because individuals with type 1 DM lack endogenous insulin production, administration of basal, exogenous insulin is essential for regulating glycogen breakdown, gluconeogenesis, lipolysis, and ketogenesis. Likewise, insulin replacement for meals should be appropriate for the carbohydrate intake and promote normal glucose utilization and storage.

Intensive Management   Intensive diabetes management has the goal of achieving euglycemia or near-normal glycemia. This approach requires multiple resources including thorough and continuing patient education, comprehensive recording of plasma glucose measurements and nutrition intake by the patient, and a variable insulin regimen that

TABLE 323-9   Ideal Goals for Glycemic Control[a]

Index	Goal
Preprandial plasma glucose, mmol/L (mg/dL)	5.0–7.2 (90–130)
Peak postprandial plasma glucose, mmol/L (mg/dL)	<10 (<180)
A1C, %	<7

[a] Plasma glucose values are 10–15% higher than whole blood values. The upper limit of the A1C reference range is 6.0% (mean 5.0%, with a standard deviation of 0.5%). These goals must be individualized for each patient and must consider the patient's age and other medical conditions.

Note: A1C, hemoglobin A1c.

Source: Adapted from American Diabetes Association, 2003.

TABLE 323-10 *Indications for Intensive Diabetes Management*

- Otherwise healthy adults with either type 1 or type 2 diabetes (selected adolescents and older children)
- Purposeful, therapeutic attempt to avoid or lessen microvascular complications
- All pregnant women with diabetes; all women with diabetes who are planning pregnancy
- Management of labile diabetes
- Availability of health care professionals with appropriate expertise
- Patients who have had kidney transplantation for diabetic nephropathy

Source: Adapted from R Farkas-Hirsch: *Intensive Diabetes Management*, Alexandria, VA American Diabetes Association, 1998.

matches glucose intake and insulin dose. Insulin regimens usually include multiple-component insulin regimens, multiple daily injections (MDI), or insulin infusion devices (each discussed below).

The benefits of intensive diabetes management and improved glycemic control include a reduction in the microvascular complications of DM and a possible delay or reduction in the macrovascular complications of DM. From a psychological standpoint, the patient experiences greater control over his or her diabetes and often notes an improved sense of well-being, greater flexibility in the timing and content of meals, and the capability to alter insulin dosing with exercise. In addition, intensive diabetes management in pregnancy reduces the risk of fetal malformations and morbidity. Intensive diabetes management is strongly encouraged in newly diagnosed patients with type 1 DM because it may prolong the period of C-peptide production, which may result in better glycemic control and a reduced risk of serious hypoglycemia.

Although intensive management confers impressive benefits, it is also accompanied by significant personal and financial costs and is therefore not appropriate for all individuals. Circumstances in which intensive diabetes management should be strongly considered are listed in Table 323-10.

Insulin Preparations Current insulin preparations are generated by recombinant DNA technology and consist of the amino acid sequence of human insulin or variations thereof. Animal insulin (beef or pork) is no longer used. Human insulin has been formulated with distinctive pharmacokinetics to mimic physiologic insulin secretion (Table 323-11). In the United States, all insulin is formulated as U-100 (100 units/mL), whereas in some other countries it is available in other units (e.g., U-40 = 40 units/mL). One short-acting insulin formulation, lispro, is an insulin analogue in which the 28th and 29th amino acids (lysine and proline) on the insulin B chain have been reversed by recombinant DNA technology. Insulin aspart is another genetically modified insulin analogue with very similar properties to lispro. These insulin analogues have full biologic activity but less tendency toward subcutaneous aggregation, resulting in more rapid absorption and onset of action and a shorter duration of action. These characteristics are particularly advantageous for allowing entrainment of insulin injection and action to rising plasma glucose levels following meals. The shorter duration of action also appears to be associated with a decreased number of hypoglycemic episodes, primarily because the decay of lispro action corresponds to the decline in plasma glucose after a meal. Insulin glargine is a long-acting biosynthetic human insulin that differs from normal insulin in that asparagine is replaced by glycine at amino acid 21, and two arginine residues are added to the C-terminus of the B chain. Compared to NPH insulin, the onset of insulin glargine action is later, the duration of action is longer (~24 h), and there is no pronounced

peak. A lower incidence of hypoglycemia, especially at night, has been reported with insulin glargine when compared to NPH insulin. Additional insulin analogues are currently under development.

Basal insulin requirements are provided by intermediate (NPH insulin or lente insulin) or long-acting (ultralente insulin or insulin glargine) insulin formulations. These are usually combined with short-acting insulin in an attempt to mimic physiologic insulin release with meals. Although mixing of intermediate and short-acting insulin formulations is common practice, this mixing may alter the insulin absorption profile (especially the short-acting insulins). For example, the absorption of regular insulin is delayed when mixed for even short periods of time (<5 min) with lente or ultralente insulin, but not when mixed with NPH insulin. Lispro absorption is delayed by mixing with NPH but not ultralente. Insulin glargine should not be mixed with other insulins and is not stable at room temperature. The miscibility of human regular and NPH insulin allows for the production of combination insulins that contain 70% NPH and 30% regular (70/30) or equal mixtures of NPH and regular (50/50). These combinations of insulin are more convenient for the patient but prevent adjustment of only one component of the insulin formulation. The alteration in insulin absorption when the patient mixes different insulin formulation should not discourage the patient from mixing insulin. However, the following guidelines should be followed: (1) mix the different insulin formulations in the syringe immediately before injection (inject within 2 min after mixing); (2) do not store insulin as a mixture; and (3) follow the same routine in terms of insulin mixing and administration to standardize the physiologic response to injected insulin. Several insulin formulations are available as insulin "pens," which may be more convenient for some patients.

Insulin Regimens Representations of the various insulin regimens that may be utilized in type 1 DM are illustrated in Fig. 323-13. Although the insulin profiles are depicted as "smooth," symmetric curves, there is considerable patient-to-patient variation in the peak and duration. In all regimens, intermediate- or long-acting insulins (NPH, lente, ultralente, or glargine insulin) supply basal insulin, whereas regular, insulin aspart, or lispro insulin provides prandial insulin. Lispro and insulin aspart should be injected just before or just after a meal; regular insulin is given 30 to 45 min prior to a meal.

A shortcoming of current insulin regimens is that injected insulin immediately enters the systemic circulation, whereas endogenous insulin is secreted into the portal venous system. Thus, exogenous insulin administration exposes the liver to subphysiologic insulin levels. No insulin regimen reproduces the precise insulin secretory pattern of

TABLE 323-11 *Pharmacokinetics of Insulin Preparations*

Preparation	Time of Action		
	Onset, h	Peak, h	Effective Duration, h
Short-acting			
Lispro	<0.25	0.5–1.5	3–4
Insulin aspart	<0.25	0.5–1.5	3–4
Regular	0.5–1.0	2–3	3–6
Intermediate-acting			
NPH	2–4	6–10	10–16
Lente	3–4	6–12	12–18
Long-acting			
Ultralente	6–10	10–16	18–20
Glargine	4	—[a]	24
Combinations			
75/25–75% protamine lispro, 25% lispro	0.5–1	Dual	10–14
70/30–70% NPH, 30% regular	0.5–1	Dual	10–16
50/50–50% NPH, 50% regular	0.5–1	Dual	10–16

[a] Glargine has minimal peak activity.
Source: Adapted from JS Skyler, *Therapy for Diabetes Mellitus and Related Disorders*, American Diabetes Association, Alexandria, VA, 1998.

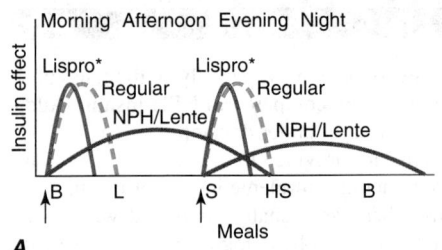
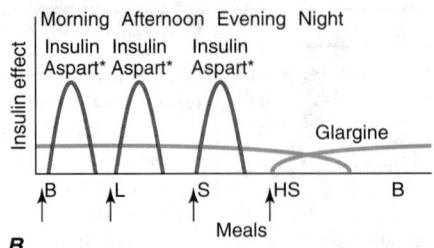
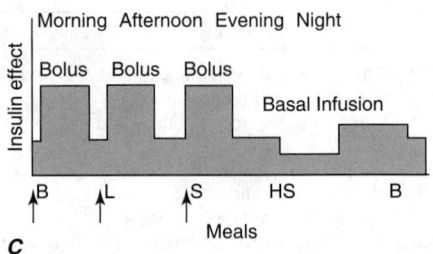

FIGURE 323-13   Representative insulin regimens for the treatment of diabetes. For each panel, the *y*-axis shows the amount of insulin effect and the *x*-axis shows the time of day. B, breakfast; L, lunch; S, supper; HS, bedtime; CSII, continuous subcutaneous insulin infusion. *either lispro or insulin aspart can be used. The time of insulin injection is shown with a vertical arrow. The type of insulin is noted above each insulin curve. *A.* The injection of two shots of intermediate-acting insulin (NPH or lente) and short-acting insulin (lispro, insulin aspart, or regular). Only one formulation of short-acting insulin is used. *B*: A multiple-component insulin regimen consisting of one shot of glargine at bedtime to provide basal insulin coverage and three shots of lispro or insulin aspart to provide glycemic coverage for each meal. *C*: Insulin administration by insulin infusion device is shown with the basal insulin and a bolus injection at each meal. The basal insulin rate is decreased during the evening and increased slightly prior to the patient awakening in the morning. (*Adapted from Intensive Diabetes Management, 2d ed, R. Farkas-Hirsch (ed). Alexandria, VA, American Diabetes Association, 1998.*)

the pancreatic islet. However, the most physiologic regimens entail more frequent insulin injections, greater reliance on short-acting insulin, and more frequent capillary plasma glucose measurements. In general, individuals with type 1 DM require 0.5 to 1.0 U/kg per day of insulin divided into multiple doses. Initial insulin-dosing regimens should be conservative; approximately 40 to 50% of the insulin should be given as basal insulin. A single daily injection of insulin is not appropriate therapy in type 1 DM.

One commonly used regimen consists of twice-daily injections of an intermediate insulin (NPH or lente) mixed with a short-acting insulin before the morning and evening meal (Fig. 323-13*A*). Such regimens usually prescribe two-thirds of the total daily insulin dose in the morning (with about two-thirds given as intermediate-acting insulin and one-third as short-acting) and one-third before the evening meal (with approximately one-half given as intermediate-acting insulin and one-half as short-acting). The drawback to such a regimen is that it enforces a rigid schedule on the patient, in terms of daily activity and the content and timing of meals. Although it is simple and effective at avoiding severe hyperglycemia, it does not generate near-normal glycemic control in most individuals with type 1 DM. Moreover, if the patient's meal pattern or content varies or if physical activity is increased, hyperglycemia or hypoglycemia may result. Moving the intermediate insulin from before the evening meal to bedtime may avoid nocturnal hypoglycemia and provide more insulin as glucose levels rise in the early morning (so-called dawn phenomenon). The insulin dose in such regimens should be adjusted based on SMBG results with the following general assumptions: (1) the fasting glucose is primarily determined by the prior evening intermediate-acting insulin; (2) the pre-lunch glucose is a function of the morning short-acting insulin; (3) the pre-supper glucose is a function of the morning intermediate-acting insulin; and (4) the bedtime glucose is a function of the pre-supper, short-acting insulin.

Multiple-component insulin regimens refer to the combination of basal insulin; preprandial short-acting insulin; and changes in short-acting insulin doses to accommodate the results of frequent SMBG, anticipated food intake, and physical activity. Also referred to as MDI, such regimens offer the patient more flexibility in terms of life-style and the best chance for achieving near normoglycemia. One such regimen, shown in Fig. 323-13*B*, consists of a basal insulin with glargine at bedtime and preprandial lispro or insulin aspart. The lispro or insulin aspart dose is based on individualized algorithms that integrate the preprandial glucose and the anticipated carbohydrate intake. An alternative regimen is two equal doses of ultralente (breakfast and evening; 10 to 12 h apart) and preprandial lispro or insulin aspart. Another alternative multiple-component insulin regimen consists of bedtime intermediate insulin, a small dose of intermediate insulin at breakfast (20 to 30 % of bedtime dose), and preprandial short-acting insulin. There are numerous variations of these regimens that can be optimized for individual patients. Frequent SMBG (four to eight times per day) is absolutely essential for these types of insulin regimens.

Continuous subcutaneous insulin infusion (CSII) is another mul-

tiple-component insulin regimen (Fig. 323-13*C*). Sophisticated insulin infusion devices can accurately deliver small doses of insulin (microliters per hour). For example, multiple basal infusion rates can be programmed to: (1) accommodate nocturnal versus daytime basal insulin requirement, (2) alter infusion rate during periods of exercise, or (3) select different waveforms of insulin infusion. A preprandial insulin ("bolus") is delivered by the insulin infusion device based on instructions from the patient, which follow individualized algorithms that account for preprandial plasma glucose and anticipated carbohydrate intake. These devices require a health professional with considerable experience with insulin infusion devices and very frequent patient interactions with the diabetes management team. Insulin infusion devices present unique challenges, such as infection at the infusion site, unexplained hyperglycemia because the infusion set becomes obstructed, or diabetic ketoacidosis if the pump becomes disconnected. Since most physicians use lispro or insulin aspart in CSII, the extremely short half-life of these insulins quickly lead to insulin deficiency if the delivery system is interrupted. Essential to the safe use of infusion devices is thorough patient education about pump function and frequent SMBG.

TYPE 2 DIABETES MELLITUS ■ **General Aspects**   The goals of therapy for type 2 DM are similar to those in type 1. While glycemic control tends to dominate the management of type 1 DM, the care of individuals with type 2 DM must also include attention to the treatment of conditions associated with type 2 DM (obesity, hypertension, dyslipidemia, cardiovascular disease) and detection/management of DM-related complications (Fig. 323-14). DM-specific complications may be present in up to 20 to 50% of individuals with newly diagnosed type 2 DM. Reduction in cardiovascular risk is of paramount importance as this is the leading cause of mortality in these individuals.

Diabetes management should begin with MNT (discussed above). An exercise regimen to increase insulin sensitivity and promote weight loss should also be instituted. After MNT and increased physical ac-

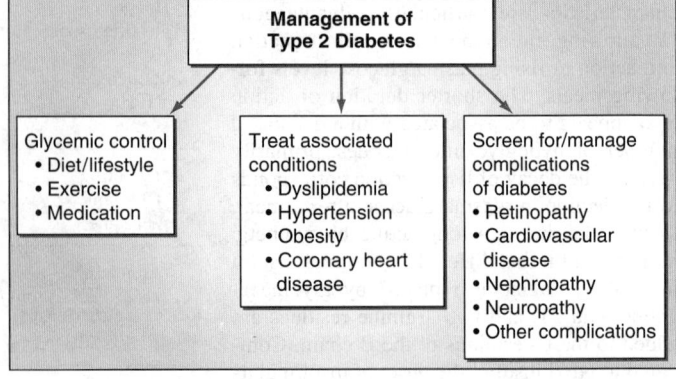

FIGURE 323-14   Essential elements in comprehensive diabetes care of type 2 diabetes.

tivity have been instituted, glycemic control should be reassessed; if the patient's glycemic target is not achieved after 3 to 4 weeks of MNT, pharmacologic therapy is indicated. Pharmacologic approaches to the management of type 2 DM include both oral glucose-lowering agents and insulin; most physicians and patients prefer oral glucose-lowering agents as the initial choice. Any therapy that improves glycemic control reduces "glucose toxicity" to the islet cells and improves endogenous insulin secretion. However, type 2 DM is a progressive disorder and ultimately requires multiple therapeutic agents and often insulin.

Glucose-Lowering Agents   Advances in the therapy of type 2 DM have generated considerable enthusiasm for oral glucose-lowering agents that target different pathophysiologic processes in type 2 DM. Based on their mechanisms of action, oral glucose-lowering agents are subdivided into agents that increase insulin secretion, reduce glucose production, or increase insulin sensitivity (Table 323-12). Oral glucose-lowering agents (with the exception of α-glucosidase inhibitors) are ineffective in type 1 DM and should not be used for glucose management of severely ill individuals with type 2 DM. Insulin is sometimes the initial glucose-lowering agent.

INSULIN SECRETAGOGUES   Insulin secretagogues stimulate insulin secretion by interacting with the ATP-sensitive potassium channel on the beta cell (Fig. 323-1). These drugs are most effective in individuals with type 2 DM of relatively recent onset (<5 years), who tend to be obese and have residual endogenous insulin production. At maximum doses, first-generation sulfonylureas are similar in potency to second-generation agents but have a longer half-life, a greater incidence of hypoglycemia, and more frequent drug interactions (Table 323-13). Thus, second-generation sulfonylureas are generally preferred. An advantage to a more rapid onset of action is better coverage of the postprandial glucose rise, but the shorter half-life of such agents requires more than once-a-day dosing. Sulfonylureas reduce both fasting and postprandial glucose and should be initiated at low doses and increased at 1- to 2-week intervals based on SMBG. In general, sulfonylureas increase

insulin acutely and thus should be taken shortly before a meal; with chronic therapy, though, the insulin release is more sustained. Repaglinide and nateglinide are not sulfonylureas but also interact with the ATP-sensitive potassium channel. Because of their short half-life, these agents are given with each meal or immediately before to reduce meal-related glucose excursions.

Insulin secretagogues are generally well tolerated. All of these agents, however, have the potential to cause profound and persistent hypoglycemia, especially in elderly individuals. Hypoglycemia is usually related to delayed meals, increased physical activity, alcohol intake, or renal insufficiency. Individuals who ingest an overdose of some agents develop prolonged and serious hypoglycemia and should be monitored closely in the hospital (Chap. 324). Most sulfonylureas are metabolized in the liver to compounds that are cleared by the kidney. Thus, their use in individuals with significant hepatic or renal dysfunction is not advisable. Weight gain, a common side effect of sulfonylurea therapy, results from the increased insulin levels and improvement in glycemic control. Some sulfonylureas have significant drug interactions with alcohol and some medications including warfarin, aspirin, ketoconazole, α-glucosidase inhibitors, and fluconazole. Despite prior concerns that use of sulfonylureas might increase cardiovascular risk, most recent trials have refuted this claim.

BIGUANIDES   Metformin is representative of this class of agents. It reduces hepatic glucose production through an undefined mechanism and improves peripheral glucose utilization slightly (Table 323-12). Metformin reduces fasting plasma glucose and insulin levels, improves the lipid profile, and promotes modest weight loss. The initial starting dose of 500 mg once or twice a day can be increased to 1000 mg bid. An extended-release form and a combination formulation with glyburide and glipizid are available. Because of its relatively slow onset of action and gastrointestinal symptoms with higher doses, the dose

TABLE 323-12 *Oral Glucose-Lowering Therapies in Type 2 Diabetes*

	Mechanism of Action	Examples	Anticipated Reduction in A1C, %	Agent-Specific Advantages	Agent-Specific Disadvantages	Contraindications
Insulin secretagogues	↑ Insulin		1–2			
Sulfonylureas		See Table 323-13		Lower fasting blood glucose	Hypoglycemia weight gain, hyperinsulinemia	Renal/liver disease
Nonsulfonylureas		See Table 323-13		Short onset of action, lower postprandial glucose	Hypoglycemia	Renal/liver disease
Biguanides	↓ Hepatic glucose production, weight loss, ↑ glucose utilization, ↓ insulin resistance	Metformin	1–2	Weight loss, improved lipid profile, no hypoglycemia	Lactic acidosis, diarrhea, nausea	Serum creatinine >1.5 mg/dL (men), >1.4 mg/dL (women), radiographic contrast studies, seriously ill patients, acidosis
α-Glucosidase inhibitors	↓ Glucose absorption	Acarbose, miglitol	0.5–1.0	No risk of hypoglycemia	GI flatulence, ↑ liver function tests	Renal/liver disease
Thiazolidinediones	↓ Insulin resistance, ↑ glucose utilization	Rosiglitazone, pioglitazone	1–2	↓ Insulin and sulfonylurea requirements, ↓ triglycerides	Frequent hepatic monitoring for idiosyncratic hepatocellular injury (see text)	Liver disease, congestive heart failure
Medical nutrition therapy and physical activity	↓ Insulin resistance	Low-calorie, low-fat diet, exercise	1–2	Other health benefits	Compliance difficult, long-term success low	

Note: A1C, hemoglobin A1c.

TABLE 323-13 *Characteristics of Agents that Increase Insulin Secretion*

Generic Name	Approved Daily Dosage Range, mg	Duration of Action, h	Clearance
Sulfonylurea—first generation			
Chlorpropamide	100–500	>48	Renal
Tolazamide	100–1000	12–24	Hepatic, renal
Tolbutamide	500–3000	6–12	Hepatic
Sulfonylurea—second generation			
Glimepiride	1–8	24	Hepatic, renal
Glipizide	2.5–40	12–18	Hepatic
Glipizide (extended release)	5–10	24	Hepatic
Glyburide	1.25–20	12–24	Hepatic, renal
Glyburide (micronized)	0.75–12	12–24	Hepatic, renal
Nonsulfonylureas			
Repaglinide	0.5–16	2–6	Hepatic
Nateglinide	180–360	2–4	Renal

Source: Adapted from BR Zimmerman (ed): *Medical Management of Type 2 Diabetes*, 4th ed. Alexandria, VA, American Diabetes Association, 1998.

should be escalated every 2 to 3 weeks based on SMBG measurements. The major toxicity of metformin, lactic acidosis, can be prevented by careful patient selection. Metformin should not be used in patients with renal insufficiency [serum creatinine >133 μmol/L (1.5 mg/dL) in men or >124 μmol/L (1.4 mg/dL) in women, with adjustments for age], any form of acidosis, congestive heart failure, liver disease, or severe hypoxia. Metformin should be discontinued in patients who are seriously ill, in patients who can take nothing orally, and in those receiving radiographic contrast material. Insulin should be used until metformin can be restarted. Though well tolerated in general, some individuals develop gastrointestinal side effects (diarrhea, anorexia, nausea, and metallic taste) that can be minimized by gradual dose escalation. Because the drug is metabolized in the liver, it should not be used in patients with liver disease or heavy ethanol intake.

α-GLUCOSIDASE INHIBITORS   α-Glucosidase inhibitors (acarbose and miglitol) reduce postprandial hyperglycemia by delaying glucose absorption; they do not affect glucose utilization or insulin secretion (Table 323-12). Postprandial hyperglycemia, secondary to impaired hepatic and peripheral glucose disposal, contributes significantly to the hyperglycemic state in type 2 DM. These drugs, taken just before each meal, reduce glucose absorption by inhibiting the enzyme that cleaves oligosaccharides into simple sugars in the intestinal lumen. Therapy should be initiated at a low dose (25 mg of acarbose or miglitol) with the evening meal and may be increased to a maximal dose over weeks to months (50 to 100 mg for acarbose or 50 mg for miglitol with each meal). The major side effects (diarrhea, flatulence, abdominal distention) are related to increased delivery of oligosaccharides to the large bowel and can be reduced somewhat by gradual upward dose titration. α-Glucosidase inhibitors may increase levels of sulfonylureas and increase the incidence of hypoglycemia. Simultaneous treatment with bile acid resins and antacids should be avoided. These agents should not be used in individuals with inflammatory bowel disease, gastroparesis, or a serum creatinine >177 μmol/L (2.0 mg/dL). This class of agents is not as potent as other oral agents in lowering the hemoglobin A1C but is unique because it reduces the postprandial glucose rise even in individuals with type 1 DM. If hypoglycemia occurs while taking these agents, the patient should consume glucose since the degradation and absorption of complex carbohydrates will be retarded.

THIAZOLIDINEDIONES   Thiazolidinediones reduce insulin resistance. These drugs bind to the PPAR-γ (peroxisome proliferator-activated receptor-γ) nuclear receptor. The PPAR-γ receptor is found at highest levels in adipocytes but is expressed at lower levels in many other tissues. Agonists of this receptor promote adipocyte differentiation and may re-

duce insulin resistance indirectly because of enhanced fatty acid uptake and storage (Table 323-12). Circulating insulin levels decrease with use of the thiazolidinediones, indicating a reduction in insulin resistance. Although direct comparisons are not available, the two currently available thiazolidinediones appear to have similar efficacy; the therapeutic range for pioglitazone is 15 to 45 mg/d in a single daily dose and for rosiglitazone the total daily dose is 2 to 8 mg/d administered either once daily or twice daily in divided doses. The ability of thiazolidinediones to influence other features of the insulin resistance syndrome is under investigation.

The prototype of this class of drugs, troglitazone, was withdrawn from the U.S. market after reports of hepatotoxicity and an association with an idiosyncratic liver reaction that sometimes led to hepatic failure. Although rosiglitazone and pioglitazone do not appear to induce the liver abnormalities seen with troglitazone, the FDA recommends measurement of liver function tests prior to initiating therapy with a thiazolidinedione and at regular intervals (every 2 months for the first year and then periodically). The thiazolidinediones raise LDL and HDL slightly and lower triglycerides by 10 to 15%, but the clinical significance of these changes is not known. Thiazolidinediones are associated with minor weight gain (1 to 2 kg), a small reduction in the hematocrit, and a mild increase in plasma volume. Cardiac function is not affected, but peripheral edema CHF may occur and is more common in individuals treated with insulin. They are contraindicated in patients with liver disease or congestive heart failure (class III or IV). Thiazolidinediones have been shown to induce ovulation in premenopausal women with PCOS. Women should be warned about the risk of pregnancy, since the safety of thiazolidinediones in pregnancy is not established.

INSULIN THERAPY IN TYPE 2 DM   Insulin should be considered as the initial therapy in type 2 DM, particularly in lean individuals or those with severe weight loss, in individuals with underlying renal or hepatic disease that precludes oral glucose-lowering agents, or in individuals who are hospitalized or acutely ill. Insulin therapy is ultimately required by a substantial number of individuals with type 2 DM because of the progressive nature of the disorder and the relative insulin deficiency that develops in patients with long-standing diabetes.

Because endogenous insulin secretion continues and is capable of providing some coverage of mealtime caloric intake, insulin is usually initiated in a single dose of intermediate- or long-acting insulin (0.3 to 0.4 U/kg per day), given either before breakfast (NPH, lente, or ultralente) or just before bedtime (NPH, lente, ultralente, or glargine). Since fasting hyperglycemia and increased hepatic glucose production are prominent features of type 2 DM, bedtime insulin is more effective in clinical trials than a single dose of morning insulin. Some physicians prefer a relatively low, fixed starting dose of intermediate-acting insulin (~15 to 20 units in the morning and 5 to 10 units at bedtime) to avoid hypoglycemia. The insulin dose may then be adjusted in 10% increments as dictated by SMBG results. Both morning and bedtime intermediate insulin may be used in combination with oral glucose-lowering agents (biguanides, α-glucosidase inhibitors, or thiazolidinediones).

CHOICE OF INITIAL GLUCOSE-LOWERING AGENT   The level of hyperglycemia should influence the initial choice of therapy. Assuming maximal benefit of MNT and increased physical activity has been realized, patients with mild to moderate hyperglycemia [fasting plasma glucose <11.1 to 13.9 mmol/L (200 to 250 mg/dL)] often respond well to a single oral glucose-lowering agent. Patients with more severe hyperglycemia [fasting plasma glucose >13.9 mmol/L (250 mg/dL)] may respond partially but are unlikely to achieve normoglycemia with oral monotherapy. A stepwise approach that starts with a single agent and adds a second agent to achieve the glycemic target can be used (see "Combination Therapy," below). Insulin can be used as initial therapy in individuals with severe hyperglycemia [fasting plasma glucose >13.9 to 16.7 mmol/L (250 to 300 mg/dL)]. This approach is based on the rationale that more rapid glycemic control will reduce "glucose toxicity" to the islet cells, improve endogenous insulin secretion, and possibly allow oral glucose-lowering agents to be more effective. If this occurs, the insulin may be discontinued.

Insulin secretagogues, biguanides, α-glucosidase inhibitors, thiazolidinediones, and insulin are approved for monotherapy of type 2 DM. Although each class of oral glucose-lowering agents has unique advantages and disadvantages, certain generalizations apply: (1) insulin secretagogues, biguanides, and thiazolidinediones improve glycemic control to a similar degree (1 to 2% reduction in A1C) and are more effective than α-glucosidase inhibitors; (2) assuming a similar degree of glycemic improvement, no clinical advantage to one class of drugs has been demonstrated, and any therapy that improves glycemic control is likely beneficial; (3) insulin secretagogues and α-glucosidase inhibitors begin to lower the plasma glucose immediately, whereas the glucose-lowering effects of the biguanides and thiazolidinediones are delayed by several weeks to months; (4) not all agents are effective in all individuals with type 2 DM (primary failure); (5) biguanides, α-glucosidase inhibitors, and thiazolidinediones do not directly cause hypoglycemia; and (6) most individuals will eventually require treatment with more than one class of oral glucose-lowering agents or insulin, reflecting the progressive nature of type 2 DM.

Considerable clinical experience exists with sulfonylureas and metformin because they have been available for several decades. It is assumed that the α-glucosidase inhibitors and thiazolidinediones, which are newer classes of oral glucose-lowering drugs, will reduce DM-related complications by improving glycemic control, although long-term data are not yet available. The thiazolidinediones are theoretically attractive because they target a fundamental abnormality in type 2 DM, namely insulin resistance. However, these agents are currently more costly than others and require liver function monitoring.

A reasonable treatment algorithm for initial therapy proposes either a sulfonylurea or metformin as initial therapy because of their efficacy, known side-effect profile, and relatively low cost (Fig. 323-14). Metformin has the advantage that it promotes mild weight loss, lowers insulin levels, improves the lipid profile slightly, and may have a lower secondary failure rate. Metformin is the initial choice of many physicians for the treatment of the obese, type 2 diabetic. However, there is no difference in response rate or degree of glycemic control when metformin and sulfonylureas are compared in randomized, prospective clinical trials. Based on SMBG results and the A1C, the dose of either the sulfonylurea or metformin should be increased until the glycemic target is achieved. Thiazolidinediones are alternative, initial agents, but are much more expensive; α-glucosidase inhibitors are the least potent agents and not as desirable for monotherapy (Fig. 323-15).

Approximately one-third of individuals will reach their target glycemic goal using either a sulfonylurea or metformin as monotherapy. Approximately 25% of individuals will not respond to sulfonylureas or metformin; under these circumstances, the drug usually should be discontinued. Some individuals respond to one agent but not the other. The remaining individuals treated with either sulfonylureas or metformin alone will exhibit some improvement in glycemic control but will not achieve their glycemic target and should be considered for combination therapy.

COMBINATION THERAPY WITH GLUCOSE-LOWERING AGENTS   A number of combinations of therapeutic agents are successful in type 2 DM, and the dosing of agents in combination is the same as when the agents are used alone. Because mechanisms of action of the first and second agents are different, the effect on glycemic control is usually additive. Commonly used regimens include: (1) insulin secretagogue with metformin or thiazolidinedione, (2) sulfonylurea with α-glucosidase inhibitor, and (3) insulin with metformin or thiazolidinedione. The combination of metformin and a thiazolidinedione is also effective and complementary. If adequate control is not achieved with two oral agents, bedtime insulin or a third oral agent may be added stepwise. However, long-term experience with any triple combination is lacking, and experience with two-drug combinations is relatively limited.

Insulin becomes required as type 2 DM enters the phase of relative insulin deficiency (as seen in long-standing DM) and is signaled by

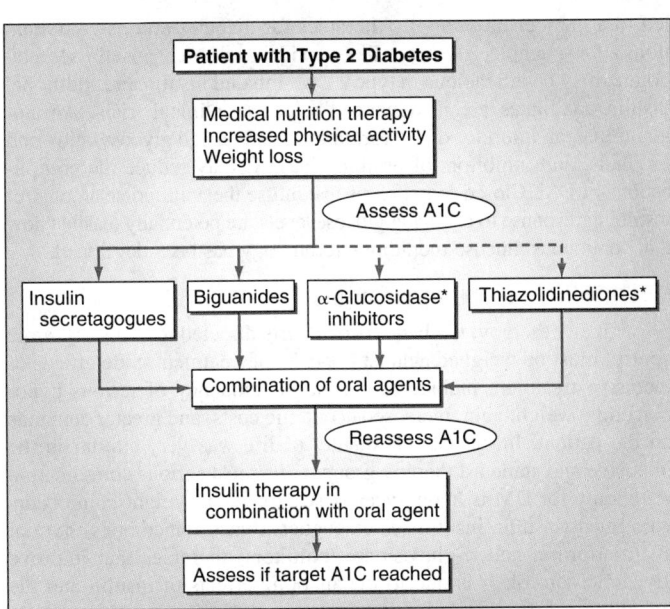

FIGURE 323-15   Glycemic management of type 2 diabetes. See text for discussion. *See text about use as monotherapy. The broken line indicates that biguanides or insulin secretagogues, but not α glucosidase inhibitors or thiazolidinediones, are preferred for initial therapy. A1C, hemoglobin A1c.

inadequate glycemic control with one or two oral glucose-lowering agents. Insulin can be used in combination with any of the oral agents in patients who fail to reach the glycemic target. For example, a single dose of intermediate- or long-acting insulin at bedtime is effective in combination with metformin. As endogenous insulin production falls further, multiple injections of intermediate-acting and short-acting insulin regimens are necessary to control postprandial glucose excursions. These combination regimens are identical to the intermediate-, long-acting, and short-acting combination regimens discussed above for type 1 DM. Since the hyperglycemia of type 2 DM tends to be more "stable," these regimens can be increased in 10% increments every 2 to 3 days using SMBG results. The daily insulin dose required can become quite large (1 to 2 units/kg per day) as endogenous insulin production falls and insulin resistance persists. Individuals who require >1 unit/kg per day of intermediate-acting insulin should be considered for combination therapy with metformin or a thiazolidinedione. The addition of metformin or a thiazolidinedione can reduce insulin requirements in some individuals with type 2 DM, while maintaining or even improving glycemic control.

Intensive diabetes management (Table 323-10) is a treatment option in type 2 patients who cannot achieve optimal glycemic control and are capable of implementing such regimens. A recent study from the Veterans Administration found that intensive diabetes management is not associated with a greater degree of side effects (hypoglycemia, weight gain) than standard insulin therapy. The effect of higher insulin levels associated with intensive diabetes management on the prognosis of diseases commonly associated with type 2 DM (cardiovascular disease, hypertension) is still debated. In selected patients with type 2 DM, insulin pumps improve glycemic control and are well tolerated.

EMERGING THERAPIES   Whole pancreas transplantation (conventionally performed concomitantly with a renal transplant) may normalize glucose tolerance and is an important therapeutic option in type 1 DM, though it requires substantial expertise and is associated with the side effects of immunosuppression. Pancreatic islet transplantation has been plagued by limitations in pancreatic islet isolation and graft survival, but recent advances in specific immunomodulation have greatly improved the results. Islet transplantation is an area of active clinical investigation.

New insights into normal mechanisms of glucose homeostasis have led to a number of emerging therapies for diabetes and its complications. For example, glucagon-like peptide 1, a potent insulin secretagogue, may be efficacious in type 2 DM. Inhaled insulin and additional insulin analogues are in advanced stages of clinical trials. Aminoguanidine, an inhibitor of the formation of advanced glycosylation end products, and inhibitors of protein kinase C may reduce the complications of DM. Closed-loop pumps that infuse the appropriate amount of insulin in response to changing glucose levels are potentially feasible now that continuous glucose-monitoring technology has been developed.

COMPLICATIONS OF THERAPY FOR DIABETES MELLITUS

As with any therapy, the benefits of efforts directed towards glycemic control must be weighed against the risks of treatment. Side effects of intensive treatment include an increased frequency of serious hypoglycemia, weight gain, increased economic costs, and greater demands on the patient. In the DCCT, quality of life was very similar in the intensive and standard therapy groups. The most serious complication of therapy for DM is hypoglycemia (Chap. 324). Weight gain occurs with most (insulin, insulin secretagogues, thiazolidinediones) but not all (metformin and α-glucosidase inhibitors) therapies that improve glycemic control. It is due to the anabolic effects of insulin and the reduction in glucosuria without a corresponding decrease in caloric intake. In the DCCT, individuals with the greatest weight gain exhibited increases in LDL cholesterol and triglycerides as well as increases in blood pressure (both systolic and diastolic) similar to those seen in individuals with type 2 DM and insulin resistance. These effects could increase the risk of cardiovascular disease in intensively managed patients. As discussed previously, transient worsening of diabetic retinopathy or neuropathy sometimes accompanies improved glycemic control.

ONGOING ASPECTS OF COMPREHENSIVE DIABETES CARE

The morbidity and mortality of DM-related complications can be greatly reduced by timely and consistent surveillance procedures (Table 323-14). These screening procedures are indicated for all individuals with DM, but numerous studies have documented that most individuals with diabetes do not receive comprehensive diabetes care. Screening for dyslipidemia and hypertension should be performed annually. In addition to routine health maintenance, individuals with diabetes should also receive the pneumococcal and tetanus vaccines (at recommended intervals) and the influenza vaccine (annually). As discussed above, aspirin therapy should be considered in many patients with diabetes.

An annual comprehensive eye examination should be performed by a qualified optometrist or ophthalmologist. If abnormalities are detected, further evaluation and treatment require an ophthalmologist skilled in diabetes-related eye disease. Because many individuals with type 2 DM have had asymptomatic diabetes for several years before diagnosis, the ADA recommends the following ophthalmologic examination schedule: (1) individuals with onset of DM at <29 years should have an initial eye examination within 3 to 5 years of diagnosis, (2) individuals with onset of DM at >30 years should have an initial eye examination at the time of diabetes diagnosis, and (3) women with

DM who are contemplating pregnancy should have an eye examination prior to conception and during the first trimester.

An annual foot examination should: (1) assess blood flow, sensation (monofilament testing), and nail care; (2) look for the presence of foot deformities such as hammer or claw toes and Charcot foot; and (3) identify sites of potential ulceration. Calluses and nail deformities should be treated by a podiatrist; the patient should be discouraged from self-care of even minor foot problems. The ADA advises a visual foot inspection for potential problems at each outpatient visit.

An annual microalbuminuria measurement (albumin-to-creatinine ratio in spot urine) is advised in individuals with type 1 or type 2 DM and no protein on a routine urinalysis (Fig. 323-10). If the urinalysis detects proteinuria, the amount of protein should be quantified by standard urine protein measurements. If the urinalysis was negative for protein in the past, microalbuminuria should be the annual screening examination. Routine urine protein measurements do not detect low levels of albumin excretion. Screening should commence 5 years after the onset of type 1 DM and at the time of onset of type 2 DM.

SPECIAL CONSIDERATIONS IN DIABETES MELLITUS

PSYCHOSOCIAL ASPECTS As with any chronic, debilitating disease, the individual with DM faces a series of challenges that affect all aspects of daily life. The individual with DM must accept that he or she may develop complications related to DM. Even with considerable effort, normoglycemia can be an elusive goal, and solutions to worsening glycemic control may not be easily identifiable. The patient should view him- or herself as an essential member of the diabetes care team and not as someone who is cared for by the diabetes team. Emotional stress may provoke a change in behavior so that individuals no longer adhere to a dietary, exercise, or therapeutic regimen. This can lead to the appearance of either hyper- or hypoglycemia. Depression and eating disorders, including binge eating disorders, bulimia, and anorexia nervosa, appear to occur more frequently individuals with type 1 or type 2 DM (Chap. 65).

MANAGEMENT IN THE HOSPITALIZED PATIENT Virtually all medical and surgical subspecialties may be involved in the care of hospitalized patients with diabetes. Hyperglycemia, whether in an individual with known diabetes or in one without diabetes, may be a predictor of poor outcome in hospitalized patients. General anesthesia, surgery, and concurrent illness raise the levels of counterregulatory hormones (cortisol, growth hormone, catecholamines, and glucagon), and infection may lead to transient insulin resistance and hyperglycemia. These factors increase insulin requirements by increasing glucose production and impairing glucose utilization and thus may worsen glycemic control. The concurrent illness or surgical procedure may lead to variable insulin absorption and also prevent the patient with DM from eating normally and may promote hypoglycemia. Glycemic control should be assessed (with A1C) and, if feasible, should be optimized prior to surgery. Electrolytes, renal function, and intravascular volume status should be assessed as well. The high prevalence of asymptomatic cardiovascular disease in individuals with DM (especially in type 2 DM) may require preoperative cardiovascular evaluation. Maintenance of a near normal glucose with insulin reduced the risk of postoperative infection after CABG, and in one study, reduced the morbidity and mortality in patients in a surgical intensive care unit.

The goals of diabetes management during hospitalization are avoidance of hypoglycemia, optimization of glycemic control and transition back to the outpatient diabetes treatment regimen. Optimal glycemic control in the hospitalized patient is <6.1 mmol/L (100 mg/dL, preprandial) and <10 mmol/L (180 mg/dL, postprandial). Attention to each stage in this process requires integrating information regarding the plasma glucose, diabetes treatment regimen, and clinical status of the patient. For example, some surgical procedures utilizing local anesthesia or epidural anesthesia may have minimal effects on glycemic control. If the patient is eating soon after the procedure and there is no disruption of the patient's regular meal plans, then glycemic control is usually maintained. A "consistent-carbohydrate diabetes meal plan" for hospital-

---

TABLE 323-14   *Guidelines for Ongoing Medical Care for Patients with Diabetes*

- Self-monitoring of blood glucose (individualized frequency)
- A1C testing (2–4 times/year)
- Patient education in diabetes management (annual)
- Medical nutrition therapy and education (annual)
- Eye examination (annual)
- Foot examination (1–2 times/year by physician; daily by patient)
- Screening for diabetic nephropathy (annual; see Fig. 323-11)
- Blood pressure measurement (quarterly)
- Lipid profile (annual)
- Influenza/pneumococcal immunizations
- Consider antiplatelet therapy (see text)

Note: A1C, hemoglobin A1c.

ized patients provides a similar amount of carbohydrate for a particular meal each day (but not necessarily the same amount for breakfast, lunch, and supper). The hospital diet should be determined by a nutritionist; terms such as "ADA diet" or "low sugar diet" are no longer used.

The physician caring for an individual with diabetes in the perioperative period, during times of infection or serious physical illness, or simply when fasting for a diagnostic procedure must monitor the plasma glucose vigilantly, adjust the diabetes treatment regimen, and provide glucose infusion as needed. Several different treatment regimens (intravenous or subcutaneous insulin regimens) can be employed successfully. Individuals with type 1 DM require continued insulin administration to maintain the levels of circulating insulin necessary to prevent DKA. Prolongation of a surgical procedure or delay in the recovery room is not uncommon and may result in periods of insulin deficiency. Even relatively brief periods without insulin may lead to mild DKA. Individuals with type 1 DM who are undergoing general anesthesia and surgery, or who are seriously ill, should receive continuous insulin, either through an intravenous insulin infusion or by subcutaneous administration of a reduced dose of long-acting insulin. Short-acting insulin alone is insufficient.

Perioperative Management Insulin infusions can effectively control plasma glucose in the perioperative period and when the patient is unable to take anything by mouth. The absorption of subcutaneous insulin may be variable in such situations because of changes in blood flow. The physician must consider carefully the clinical setting in which an insulin infusion will be utilized, including whether adequate ancillary personnel are available to monitor the plasma glucose frequently and whether they can adjust the insulin infusion rate, either based on an algorithm or in consultation with the physician. The initial rate for an insulin infusion may range from 0.5 to 5 units/h, depending on the degree of insulin resistance and the clinical situation. Based on hourly capillary glucose measurements, the insulin infusion rate is adjusted to maintain the plasma glucose within the optimal range. The insulin infusion can be temporarily discontinued if hypoglycemia occurs and may be resumed at a lower infusion rate once the plasma glucose exceeds 5.6 mmol/L (100 mg/dL).

Insulin infusion is the preferred method for managing patients with type 1 DM in the perioperative period or when serious concurrent illness is present (0.5 to 1.0 units/h of regular insulin). Insulin-infusion algorithms jointly developed and implemented by nursing and physician staff are advised. If the diagnostic or surgical procedure is brief and performed under local or regional anesthesia, a reduced dose of subcutaneous, long-acting insulin may suffice. This approach facilitates the transition back to the long-acting insulin after the procedure. The dose of long-acting insulin should be reduced by 30 to 40%, and short-acting insulin is either held or, likewise, reduced by 30 to 40%. Glucose may be infused to prevent hypoglycemia.

Individuals with type 2 DM can be managed with either regular insulin infusion 0.5 to 2 units/h or a reduced dose of subcutaneous intermediate- or long-acting insulin supplemented with short-acting insulin. Oral glucose-lowering agents are discontinued upon admission. Oral glucose-lowering agents are not useful in regulating the plasma glucose in clinical situations where the insulin requirements and glucose intake are changing rapidly. Moreover, these oral agents may be dangerous if the patient is fasting (e.g., hypoglycemia with sulfonylureas). Metformin should be withheld when radiographic contrast media will be given or if severe congestive heart failure, acidosis, or declining renal function is present.

Total Parenteral Nutrition (See also Chap. 63) Total parenteral nutrition (TPN) greatly increases insulin requirements. In addition, individuals not previously known to have DM may become hyperglycemic during TPN and require insulin treatment. Intravenous insulin infusion is the preferred treatment for hyperglycemia, and rapid titration to the required insulin dose is done most efficiently using a separate insulin infusion. After the total insulin dose has been determined, insulin may be added directly to the TPN solution or, preferably, given as a separate infusion. Often, individuals receiving either TPN or enteral nutrition

receive their caloric loads continuously and not at "meal times"; consequently, subcutaneous insulin regimens must be adjusted.

GLUCOCORTICOIDS Glucocorticoids increase insulin resistance, decrease glucose utilization, increase hepatic glucose production, and impair insulin secretion. These changes lead to a worsening of glycemic control in individuals with DM and may precipitate diabetes in other individuals ("steroid-induced diabetes"). The effects of glucocorticoids on glucose homeostasis are dose-related, usually reversible, and most pronounced in the postprandial period. If the fasting plasma glucose is near the normal range, oral diabetes agents (e.g., sulfonylureas, metformin) may be sufficient to reduce hyperglycemia. If the fasting plasma glucose >11.1 mmol/L (200 mg/dL), oral agents are usually not efficacious and insulin therapy is required. Short-acting insulin may be required to supplement long-acting insulin in order to control postprandial glucose excursions.

REPRODUCTIVE ISSUES Reproductive capacity in either men or women with DM appears to be normal. Menstrual cycles may be associated with alterations in glycemic control in women with DM. Pregnancy is associated with marked insulin resistance; the increased insulin requirements often precipitate DM and lead to the diagnosis of GDM. Glucose, which at high levels is a teratogen to the developing fetus, readily crosses the placenta, but insulin does not. Thus, hyperglycemia from the maternal circulation may stimulate insulin secretion in the fetus. The anabolic and growth effects of insulin may result in macrosomia. GDM complicates approximately 4% of pregnancies in the United States. The incidence of GDM is greatly increased in certain ethnic groups, including African Americans and Hispanic Americans, consistent with a similar increased risk of type 2 DM. Current recommendations advise screening for glucose intolerance between weeks 24 and 28 of pregnancy in women with high risk for GDM ($\geq$25 years; obesity; family history of DM; member of an ethnic group such as Hispanic American, Native American, Asian American, African American, or Pacific Islander). Therapy for GDM is similar to that for individuals with pregnancy-associated diabetes and involves MNT and insulin, if hyperglycemia persists. Oral glucose-lowering agents have not been approved for use during pregnancy. With current practices, the morbidity and mortality of the mother with GDM and the fetus are no different from those in the nondiabetic population. Individuals who develop GDM are at marked increased risk for developing type 2 DM in the future and should be screened periodically for DM. After delivery, glucose homeostasis should be reassessed in the mother. Most individuals with GDM revert to normal glucose tolerance, but some will continue to have overt diabetes or impairment of glucose tolerance. In addition, children of women with GDM appear to be at risk for obesity and glucose intolerance and have an increased risk of diabetes beginning in the later stages of adolescence.

Pregnancy in individuals with known DM requires meticulous planning and adherence to strict treatment regimens. Intensive diabetes management and normalization of the A1C are the standard of care for individuals with existing DM who are planning pregnancy. The most crucial period of glycemic control is soon after fertilization. The risk of fetal malformations is increased 4 to 10 times in individuals with uncontrolled DM at the time of conception and normal plasma glucose during the preconception period and throughout the periods of organ development in the fetus should be maintained.

LIPODYSTROPHIC DM Lipodystrophy, or the loss of subcutaneous fat tissue, may be generalized in certain genetic conditions such as leprechaunism. Generalized lipodystrophy is associated with severe insulin resistance and is often accompanied by acanthosis nigricans and dyslipidemia. Localized lipodystrophy associated with insulin injections has been reduced considerably by the use of human insulin.

Protease Inhibitors and Lipodystrophy Protease inhibitors used in the treatment of HIV disease (Chap. 173) have been associated with a centripetal accumulation of fat (visceral and abdominal area), accumulation of fat in the dorsocervical region, loss of extremity fat, decreased insulin sensitivity (elevations of the fasting insulin level and reduced glucose tolerance on intravenous glucose tolerance testing), and dyslipidemia. Although many aspects of the physical appearance of these individuals resemble Cushing's syndrome, increased cortisol levels do not account for this appearance. The possibility remains that this is related to HIV infection by some undefined mechanism, since some features of the syndrome were observed before the introduction of protease inhibitors. Therapy for HIV-related lipodystrophy is not well established.

FURTHER READING

AMERICAN DIABETES ASSOCIATION: Clinical practice recommendations 2002. Diabetes Care 27:51, 2004

CLEMENT S et al: Management of diabetes and hyperglycemia in hospitals. Diabetes Care 27:553, 2004

KIRPICHNIKOV D et al: Metformin: An update. Ann Intern Med 137:25, 2002

KNOWLER WC et al for the DIABETES PREVENTION PROGRAM RESEARCH GROUP: Reduction in the incidence of type 2 diabetes with lifestyle intervention or metformin. N Engl J Med 346:393, 2002

SALTIEL AR, KAHN CR: Insulin signalling and the regulation of glucose and lipid metabolism. Nature 414:799, 2001

THE WRITING TEAM FOR THE DIABETES CONTROL AND COMPLICATIONS TRIAL/EPIDEMIOLOGY OF THE DIABETES INTERVENTIONS AND COMPLICATIONS RESEARCH GROUP: Effect of intensive therapy on the microvascular complications of type 1 diabetes mellitus. JAMA 287:2563, 2002

UK PROSPECTIVE DIABETES STUDY GROUP: Intensive blood-glucose control with sulphonylureas or insulin compared with conventional treatment and risk of complications in patients with type 2 diabetes (UKPDS 33). Lancet 352:1998, 1998

324 HYPOGLYCEMIA
Philip E. Cryer

Hypoglycemia is most commonly the result of taking drugs used to treat diabetes mellitus or other drugs, including alcohol. However, a number of other disorders, including end-stage organ failure and sepsis, endocrine deficiencies, large mesenchymal tumors, insulinoma, and inherited metabolic disorders are also associated with hypoglycemia (Table 324-1). Hypoglycemia is sometimes defined as a plasma glucose level <2.5 to 2.8 mmol/L (<45 to 50 mg/dL). However, glucose thresholds for hypoglycemia-induced symptoms and physiologic responses vary widely, depending on the clinical setting. Therefore, an important framework for making the diagnosis of hypoglycemia is *Whipple's triad*: (1) symptoms consistent with hypoglycemia, (2) a low plasma glucose concentration, and (3) relief of symptoms after the plasma glucose level is raised. Hypoglycemia can cause significant morbidity and can be lethal, if severe and prolonged; it should be considered in any patient with confusion, altered level of consciousness, or seizures.

SYSTEMIC GLUCOSE BALANCE AND COUNTERREGULATION

Glucose is an obligate metabolic fuel for the brain under physiologic conditions. By contrast, other organs can use fatty acids, in addition to glucose, to generate energy. The brain cannot synthesize glucose and stores only a few minutes' supply as glycogen and therefore requires a continuous supply of glucose, which is delivered by facilitated diffusion from arterial blood. As the plasma glucose concentration falls below the physiologic range, blood-to-brain glucose transport becomes insufficient for adequate brain energy metabolism and functioning. Fortunately, redundant physiologic mechanisms prevent or rapidly correct hypoglycemia.

Plasma glucose levels are maintained within a narrow range, usually between 3.3 and 8.3 mmol/L (60 and 150 mg/dL), despite wide variation of food intake and activity level. This delicate balance requires dynamic regulation of glucose influx into the circulation as glucose utilization in various tissues can change rapidly. The diet is normally a major source of glucose. However, between meals or during fasting, plasma glucose levels are maintained primarily by the breakdown of glycogen and by gluconeogenesis (Fig. 324-1). In most persons, hepatic glycogen stores are sufficient to maintain plasma glucose levels for 8 to 12 h, but this time period can be shorter if glucose demand is increased by exercise or if glycogen stores are depleted by illness or starvation.

As glycogen stores are depleted, glucose is generated by gluconeogenesis, which occurs mainly in the liver but also in the kidneys. Gluconeogenesis requires a coordinated supply of precursors from

---

TABLE 324-1 Causes of Hypoglycemia

Drugs
  Especially insulin, sulfonylureas, ethanol
  Sometimes pentamidine, quinine
  Rarely salicylates, sulfonamides, and others
Critical illnesses
  Hepatic, renal, or cardiac failure
  Sepsis
  Starvation and inanition
Endocrine deficiencies
  Cortisol, growth hormone
  Glucagon and epinephrine (type 1 diabetes)
Non-β-cell tumors
  Fibrosarcoma, mesothelioma, rhabdomyosarcoma, liposarcoma, other sarcomas
  Hepatoma, adrenocortical tumors, carcinoid
  Leukemia, lymphoma, melanoma, teratoma
Endogenous hyperinsulinism
  Insulinoma
  Other β cell disorders
  Secretagogue (sulfonylurea)
  Autoimmune (autoantibodies to insulin, insulin receptor, β cell?)
  Ectopic insulin secretion
Disorders of infancy or childhood
  Transient intolerance of fasting
  Infants of diabetic mothers (hyperinsulinism)
  Congenital hyperinsulinism
  Inherited enzyme defects
Postprandial
  Reactive (after gastric surgery)
  Ethanol-induced
  Autonomic symptoms without true hypoglycemia
Factitious
  Insulin, sulfonylureas

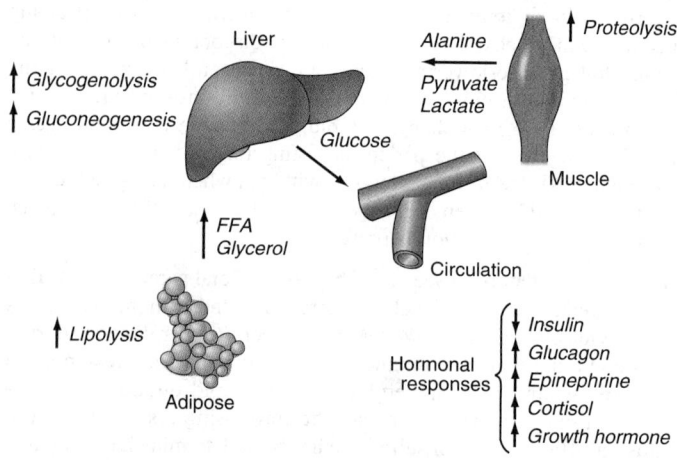

FIGURE 324-1 Overview of glucose metabolism and pathways of counterregulatory responses to fasting and hypoglycemia.

liver, muscle, and adipose tissue. Muscle provides lactate, pyruvate, alanine, and other amino acids. Triglycerides in adipose tissue are broken down into glycerol, which is a precursor for gluconeogenesis. Free fatty acids generate acetyl CoA for gluconeogenesis and provide an alternative fuel source to tissues other than the brain.

The balance of glucose production and its uptake and utilization in peripheral tissues are exquisitely regulated by a network of hormones, neural pathways, and metabolic signals (Chap. 323). Among the factors that control glucose production and utilization, insulin plays a dominant and pivotal role. In the fasting state, insulin is suppressed, allowing increased gluconeogenesis in the liver and the kidneys and enhancing glucose generation by the breakdown of liver glycogen. Low insulin levels also reduce glucose uptake and utilization in peripheral tissues and allow lipolysis and proteolysis to occur, which leads to the release of precursors for gluconeogenesis and provides alternative energy sources. In the fed state, insulin release from the pancreatic β cells reverses this process. Glycogenolysis and gluconeogenesis are inhibited, thereby reducing hepatic and renal glucose output; peripheral glucose uptake and utilization are enhanced; lipolysis and proteolysis are restrained; and energy storage is promoted by the conversion of substrates into glycogen, triglycerides, and proteins. Other hormones, such as glucagon, epinephrine, growth hormone, and cortisol, play less important roles in the control of glucose flux during normal physiologic circumstances. However, these hormones are critically important in the response to hypoglycemia.

As glucose levels approach, and ultimately enter, the hypoglycemic range, a characteristic sequence of *counterregulatory hormone responses* occurs. Glucagon is the first and most important of these responses. It promotes glycogenolysis and gluconeogenesis. Epinephrine can also play an important role in the acute response to hypoglycemia, particularly when glucagon is insufficient. It, too, stimulates glycogenolysis and gluconeogenesis and limits glucose utilization by insulin-sensitive tissues. When hypoglycemia is prolonged, growth hormone and cortisol also reduce glucose utilization and support its production.

The glucose thresholds at which various counterregulatory hormone responses occur are quite similar in healthy subjects (Table 324-2). Nevertheless, these thresholds are dynamic and can be influenced by recent metabolic events. A person with poorly controlled diabetes can have symptoms of hypoglycemia at higher-than-normal glucose levels. Recurrent hypoglycemia, which may occur in individuals with diabetes or an insulinoma, shifts thresholds for symptoms and counterregulatory responses to lower glucose levels.

CLINICAL MANIFESTATIONS

Symptoms of hypoglycemia can be divided into two categories, neuroglycopenic and neurogenic (or autonomic) responses. Neuroglycopenic symptoms are a direct result of central nervous system neuronal glucose deprivation. Symptoms include behavioral changes, confusion, fatigue, seizure, loss of consciousness, and, if hypoglycemia is severe and prolonged, death. Hypoglycemia-induced autonomic responses include adrenergic symptoms such as palpitations, tremor, and anxiety as well as cholinergic symptoms such as sweating, hunger, and paresthesia. Adrenergic symptoms are mediated by norepinephrine released from sympathetic postganglionic neurons and the release of epinephrine from the adrenal medullae. Increased sweating is mediated by cholinergic sympathetic nerve fibers. Patients with diabetes mellitus learn to recognize the characteristic symptoms of hypoglycemia, but

these are less familiar to individuals with other causes of hypoglycemia. Symptoms may be less pronounced with repeated hypoglycemic episodes (see below).

Common signs of hypoglycemia include pallor and diaphoresis. Heart rate and the systolic blood pressure are typically raised, but these findings may not be prominent. The neuroglycopenic manifestations are valuable, albeit nonspecific, signs. Transient focal neurologic deficits occur occasionally.

CAUSES

Hypoglycemia is traditionally classified as *postprandial* or *fasting*. However, in the clinical setting, hypoglycemia is most commonly a result of diabetes treatment. This topic is therefore addressed before considering the other causes of hypoglycemia.

HYPOGLYCEMIA IN DIABETES

FREQUENCY AND IMPACT Were it not for hypoglycemia, diabetes would be rather easy to treat by administering enough insulin (or any effective drug) to lower plasma glucose concentrations to, or below, the normal range. But because current insulin-replacement regimens are imperfect, individuals with type 1 diabetes are at ongoing risk for periods of relative hyperinsulinemia with resultant hypoglycemia. Those attempting to achieve near-normal glycemic control may experience several episodes of asymptomatic or symptomatic hypoglycemia each week. Plasma glucose levels may be <2.8 mmol/L (<50 mg/dL) as often as 10% of the time. Such patients suffer an average of one episode of severe, temporarily disabling hypoglycemia, often with seizure or coma, in a given year. Although seemingly complete recovery from the latter is the rule, the possibility of persistent cognitive deficits has been raised, but permanent neurologic defects are rare. About 2 to 4% of deaths associated with type 1 diabetes are estimated to be a result of hypoglycemia. Fear of hypoglycemia can also lead to disabling psychosocial morbidity.

Hypoglycemia is a less frequent problem in type 2 diabetes but still occurs in those treated with insulin or sulfonylureas. Transient, mild hypoglycemia may be seen with the shorter-acting sulfonylureas and repaglinide or nateglinide, which also act by enhancing insulin secretion. Patients who take the long-acting sulfonylureas, chlorpropamide and glyburide, may experience episodes of severe hypoglycemia that last between 24 and 36 h.

CONVENTIONAL RISK FACTORS Insulin excess is the primary determinant of risk from iatrogenic hypoglycemia. Relative or absolute insulin excess occurs when: (1) insulin (or oral agent) doses are excessive, ill timed, or of the wrong type; (2) the influx of exogenous glucose is reduced (e.g., during an overnight fast or following missed meals or snacks); (3) insulin-independent glucose utilization is increased (e.g., during exercise); (4) insulin sensitivity is increased (e.g., with effective

TABLE 324-2 Physiologic Responses to Decreasing Plasma Glucose Concentrations

Response	Glycemic Threshold, mmol/L (mg/dL)	Physiologic Effects	Role in the Prevention or Correction of Hypoglycemia (Glucose Counterregulation)
↓ Insulin	4.4–4.7 (80–85)	↑ R_a (↓R_d)	Primary glucose regulatory factor/first defense against hypoglycemia
↑ Glucagon	3.6–3.9 (65–70)	↑ R_a	Primary glucose counterregulatory factor
↑ Epinephrine	3.6–3.9 (65–70)	↑ R_a, ↓ R_d	Involved, critical when glucagon is deficient
↑ Cortisol and growth hormone	3.6–3.9 (65–70)	↑ R_a, ↓ R_d	Involved, not critical
Symptoms	2.8–3.1 (50–55)	↑ Exogenous glucose	Prompt behavioral defense (food ingestion)
↓ Cognition	< 2.8 (< 50)	—	(Compromises behavioral defense)

Note: R_a, rate of glucose appearance, glucose production by the liver and kidneys; R_d, rate of glucose disappearance, glucose utilization by insulin-sensitive tissues such as skeletal muscle. (R_d includes glucose utilization by the central nervous system, but the glucoregulatory hormones have no direct effects on that.)

intensive therapy, in the middle of the night, late after exercise, or with increased fitness or weight loss); (5) endogenous glucose production is reduced (e.g., following alcohol ingestion); and (6) insulin clearance is reduced (e.g., in renal failure). However, analyses of the Diabetes Control and Complications Trial (DCCT) indicate that these conventional risk factors explain only a minority of episodes of severe iatrogenic hypoglycemia; other causes are involved in the majority of episodes.

HYPOGLYCEMIA-ASSOCIATED AUTONOMIC FAILURE It is now clear that inadequate physiologic counterregulatory and behavioral responses greatly compound the problem of hypoglycemia caused by insulin excess. Hypoglycemia-associated autonomic failure has two main components: (1) reduced counterregulatory hormone responses, which result in impaired glucose generation; and (2) hypoglycemia unawareness, which precludes appropriate behavioral responses, such as eating.

Defective Glucose Counterregulation The counterregulatory hormone response is fundamentally altered in patients with established (e.g., absent C peptide) type 1 diabetes. As insulin deficiency progresses over the first few months or years of the disease, circulating insulin levels are no longer tightly coordinated with glucose levels and are a passive function of administered insulin. Thus, insulin levels do not decline as glucose levels fall; the first defense against hypoglycemia is lost. Over the same time frame, the glucagon response to falling glucose levels diminishes, and the second defense against hypoglycemia is lost. The cause of defective glucagon production by the pancreatic islet α cells is unknown, but it is tightly linked to the loss of insulin production by the β cells. It is a functional abnormality rather than an absolute deficiency of glucagon, as responses to stimuli other than hypoglycemia are intact. The third defense against hypoglycemia is compromised when the epinephrine response to hypoglycemia is reduced. In contrast to the absent glucagon response, epinephrine deficiency is a threshold abnormality; an epinephrine response can still be elicited, but a lower plasma glucose concentration is required. This threshold shift is largely a result of recent antecedent hypoglycemia, although an additional anatomic component may also be present in patients affected by classic diabetic autonomic neuropathy. The development of a reduced epinephrine response is a critical pathophysiologic event. Prospective studies have shown that patients with combined deficiencies of glucagon and epinephrine suffer severe hypoglycemia at rates 25-fold or greater than individuals with absent glucagon but intact epinephrine responses.

Hypoglycemia Unawareness *Hypoglycemia unawareness* refers to a loss of the warning symptoms that alert individuals to the presence of hypoglycemia and prompt them to eat and abort the episode. Under these circumstances, the first manifestation of hypoglycemia is neuroglycopenia, when it is often too late for patients to treat themselves. Like defective counterregulation, the presence of hypoglycemia unawareness has been shown in prospective studies to be associated with a high frequency of severe hypoglycemia.

The interplay of factors involved in hypoglycemia-associated autonomic failure in type 1 diabetes, and consequent hypoglycemia unawareness, is summarized in Fig. 324-2. Periods of relative or absolute therapeutic insulin excess, in the setting of absent glucagon responses, lead to episodes of iatrogenic hypoglycemia. These episodes, in turn, cause reduced autonomic (including adrenomedullary) responses to falling glucose concentrations. These impaired autonomic responses result in reduced symptoms of impending hypoglycemia (e.g., hypoglycemia unawareness) because epinephrine responses are reduced in the setting of absent glucagon responses. Thus, a vicious cycle of recurrent hypoglycemia is created and perpetuated. The syndrome of hypoglycemia unawareness and the reduced epinephrine component of defective glucose counterregulation are reversible but require >2 weeks of scrupulous avoidance of hypoglycemia. This involves a shift of glycemic thresholds back to higher plasma glucose concentrations.

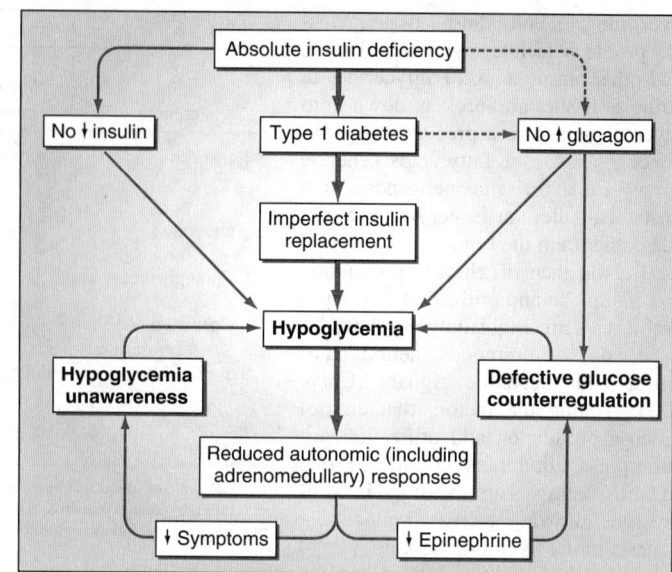

FIGURE 324-2 Hypoglycemia-associated autonomic failure and hypoglycemia unawareness in type 1 diabetes. (*PE Cryer: Diabetes 41:255, 1992.*)

HYPOGLYCEMIA RISK FACTOR REDUCTION A diagnosis of hypoglycemia unawareness can usually be made from the history. One should note that hypoglycemia unawareness implies that previous episodes of hypoglycemia have occurred, whether these are documented or not. If low glucose levels are not apparent from the patient's self-monitoring log, one should suspect hypoglycemia during the night. The presence of clinical hypoglycemia unawareness makes defective glucose counterregulation likely. It is possible to minimize the risk of hypoglycemia by applying the principles of modern therapy—patient education and empowerment, frequent self-monitoring of blood glucose, flexible insulin (and other drug) regimens, rational glycemic goals, and ongoing professional guidance and support. If hypoglycemia is a recognized problem, first consider each of the conventional risk factors summarized earlier and recommend the appropriate adjustments of medications, diet, and life-style. Nonselective beta blockers may attenuate the recognition of hypoglycemia and they impair glycogenolysis; a relatively selective β_1-antagonist (e.g., metoprolol or atenolol) is preferable when a beta blocker is indicated.

REACTIVE HYPOGLYCEMIA

Postprandial (reactive) hypoglycemia occurs only after meals and is self-limited. Postprandial hypoglycemia occurs in children with certain rare enzymatic defects in carbohydrate metabolism such as hereditary fructose intolerance and galactosemia (Chap. 341). Reactive hypoglycemia also occurs in some individuals who have undergone gastric surgery, which allows the rapid passage of food from the stomach to the small intestine. This type of *alimentary hypoglycemia* causes a rapid postprandial rise in plasma glucose levels and the release of gut incretins, which induce an exuberant insulin response and subsequent hypoglycemia. Administration of an α-glucosidase inhibitor, which delays carbohydrate digestion and thus glucose absorption from the intestine, can be considered for treatment of reactive hypoglycemia, although its efficacy remains to be established in controlled trials.

If postprandial symptoms occur as an idiopathic disorder, caution should be exercised before labeling a person with a diagnosis of hypoglycemia. Indeed, a self-diagnosis of hypoglycemia has often been reinforced by the finding of a "low" venous glucose concentration late after glucose ingestion. An oral glucose tolerance test should not be used in this setting. Plasma glucose falls as low as 2.4 mmol/L (43 mg/dL) after a 100-g glucose load in 5% of normal asymptomatic individuals, making it difficult to identify hypoglycemia based on the results of this test. The diagnosis of postprandial hypoglycemia requires documentation of Whipple's triad after a typical mixed meal. The cause of repetitive postprandial symptoms in certain individuals is unknown, but they may be particularly sensitive to the normal autonomic responses that follow ingestion of a meal.

FASTING HYPOGLYCEMIA

There are many causes of fasting hypoglycemia (Table 324-1). In addition to insulin and sulfonylureas used in the treatment of diabetes, ethanol use is a relatively common cause of hypoglycemia. Sepsis and renal failure are often complicated by hypoglycemia. Endocrine deficiencies, non-β-cell tumors, and endogenous hyperinsulinemia (including that caused by an insulinoma) are rare causes of hypoglycemia. Enzymatic metabolic errors that cause hypoglycemia are also rare but are being recognized more frequently in infants and children (Chaps. 341 and 343).

DRUGS In contrast to the sulfonylureas and rapid-acting insulin secretagogues (e.g., repaglinide, nateglinide), other oral hypoglycemic agents—biguanides (e.g., metformin), α-glucosidase inhibitors (e.g., acarbose, miglitol), and thiazolidinediones (e.g., rosiglitazone, pioglitazone)—do not act by stimulating insulin secretion. Therefore, with these agents, insulin levels usually decrease appropriately as plasma glucose levels fall. However, these drugs can contribute to hypoglycemia in other ways. Treatment with an α-glucosidase inhibitor alters the management of hypoglycemia; pure glucose should be used rather than ingestion of complex carbohydrates. Thiazolidinediones, as well as metformin, can predispose patients to hypoglycemia if they are receiving combined treatment with insulin or an insulin secretagogue.

Ethanol blocks gluconeogenesis but not glycogenolysis. Thus, alcohol-induced hypoglycemia typically occurs after a several-day ethanol binge during which the person eats little food, thereby causing glycogen depletion. Hypoglycemia in this setting can be profound, with mortality rates as high as 10%. Blood ethanol levels correlate poorly with plasma glucose concentrations at the time of diagnosis, as hypoglycemia occurs late in the sequence and often precludes further alcohol consumption.

Pentamidine, which is used to treat *Pneumocystis* pneumonia and other parasitic infections, is toxic to the pancreatic β cell. It causes insulin release initially, with hypoglycemia in about 10% of treated patients, and predisposes to the development of diabetes mellitus later. Quinine also stimulates insulin secretion. However, the relative contribution of hyperinsulinemia to the pathogenesis of hypoglycemia in quinine-treated patients who are critically ill with malaria is debated. Salicylates and sulfonamides can cause hypoglycemia, but do so rarely. There are reports of hypoglycemia attributed to nonselective β-adrenergic antagonists (e.g., propranolol) and a variety of other drugs.

CRITICAL ILLNESS Rapid and extensive hepatic destruction (e.g., severe toxic hepatitis) causes fasting hypoglycemia because the liver is the major site of endogenous glucose production. The mechanism of hypoglycemia reported in patients with cardiac failure is unknown but likely involves hepatic congestion. Although the kidneys are a source of glucose production, it is perhaps too simplistic to attribute hypoglycemia in persons with renal failure to this mechanism alone. The clearance of insulin is reduced substantially in renal failure, and reduced mobilization of gluconeogenic precursors has been reported.

Sepsis is sometimes complicated by hypoglycemia, which is multifactorial in origin. There is impaired endogenous glucose production, perhaps a result of hepatic hypoperfusion, and increased glucose utilization, which is induced by cytokines in macrophage-rich tissues such as the liver, spleen, and ileum and in muscle. Nutrition is also often inadequate in the setting of sepsis. Hypoglycemia can be seen with prolonged starvation, perhaps because of a loss of whole-body fat stores and the subsequent depletion of gluconeogenic precursors (e.g., amino acids), which necessitate increased glucose utilization.

ENDOCRINE DEFICIENCIES Neither cortisol nor growth hormone is critical to the prevention of acute hypoglycemia, at least in adults. However, hypoglycemia can occur with prolonged fasting in patients with untreated primary adrenocortical failure (Addison's disease) or hypopituitarism. Anorexia and weight loss are typical features of chronic

cortisol deficiency and likely result in glycogen depletion with increased reliance on gluconeogenesis. Cortisol deficiency is associated with low levels of gluconeogenic precursors, suggesting that substrate-limited gluconeogenesis, in the setting of glycogen depletion, is the cause of the impaired ability to tolerate fasting in cortisol-deficient individuals. Growth hormone deficiency can cause hypoglycemia in young children. In addition to extended fasting, high rates of glucose utilization (e.g., during exercise, pregnancy) or low rates of glucose production (e.g., following alcohol ingestion) can precipitate hypoglycemia in adults with hypopituitarism. Cortisol and growth hormone secretion should be evaluated in patients with fasting hypoglycemia when the history suggests pituitary or adrenal disease and when other causes of hypoglycemia are not apparent.

Hypoglycemia is not a feature of the epinephrine-deficient state that results from bilateral adrenalectomy when glucocorticoid replacement is adequate, nor does it occur during pharmacologic adrenergic blockage when other glucoregulatory systems are intact. There are case reports of fasting hypoglycemia attributed to isolated glucagon or epinephrine deficiency, although hyperinsulinemia was not excluded convincingly in neonatal cases and other counterregulatory defects may have contributed in the adults. Thus, the regular assessment of glucagon and epinephrine secretion is not warranted.

NON-β-CELL TUMORS Fasting hypoglycemia, often termed *non-islet cell tumor hypoglycemia*, occurs in some patients with large mesenchymal or other tumors (e.g., hepatoma, adrenocortical tumors, carcinoids; Chap. 86. The glucose kinetic patterns resemble those of hyperinsulinism, but insulin secretion is suppressed appropriately during hypoglycemia. In most instances, hypoglycemia is due to overproduction of an incompletely processed form of insulin-like growth factor (IGF) II. Although total IGF-II levels are not consistently elevated, circulating free IGF-II levels are high. Hypoglycemia results from IGF-II actions through the insulin or IGF-I receptors.

ENDOGENOUS HYPERINSULINISM Hypoglycemia due to excessive endogenous insulin secretion can be caused by: (1) a primary pancreatic islet β cell disorder, typically a β cell tumor (insulinoma), sometimes multiple insulinomas, or, especially in infants or young children, a functional β cell disorder without an anatomic correlate; (2) a β cell secretagogue, often a sulfonylurea, and, theoretically, a β cell–stimulating autoantibody; (3) an autoantibody to insulin; or (4) ectopic insulin secretion. None of these disorders is common. Endogenous hyperinsulinism is more likely to occur in an overtly healthy individual without other apparent causes of hypoglycemia such as a relevant drug history, critical illness, endocrine deficiencies, or a non-β-cell tumor. Accidental, surreptitious, or even malicious administration of a sulfonylurea or insulin should also be considered in such individuals.

The fundamental pathophysiologic feature of endogenous hyperinsulinism is the failure of insulin secretion to fall to very low rates during hypoglycemia. This is assessed by measuring insulin, proinsulin, and C peptide, which is derived from the processing of proinsulin. Critical diagnostic findings are a plasma insulin concentration ≥ 36 pmol/L (≥ 6 μU/mL) and a plasma C-peptide concentration ≥ 0.2 mmol/L (≥ 0.6 ng/mL) when the plasma glucose concentration is ≤ 2.5 mmol/L (≤ 45 mg/dL) in the fasting state with symptoms of hypoglycemia. Insulin and C-peptide levels do not need to be absolutely increased (e.g., relative to euglycemic normal values) but only inappropriately increased in the setting of fasting hypoglycemia. Plasma proinsulin concentrations are also inappropriately elevated, particularly in patients with an insulinoma. Sulfonylureas, because they stimulate insulin secretion, result in a pattern of glucose, insulin, and C-peptide levels that is indistinguishable from that produced by a primary β cell disorder. The measurement of sulfonylureas in plasma or urine distinguishes these conditions. Antibodies to insulin produce *autoimmune hypoglycemia* following the transition from the postprandial to the postabsorptive state, as insulin slowly dissociates from the antibodies. Total and free plasma insulin concentrations are inappropri-

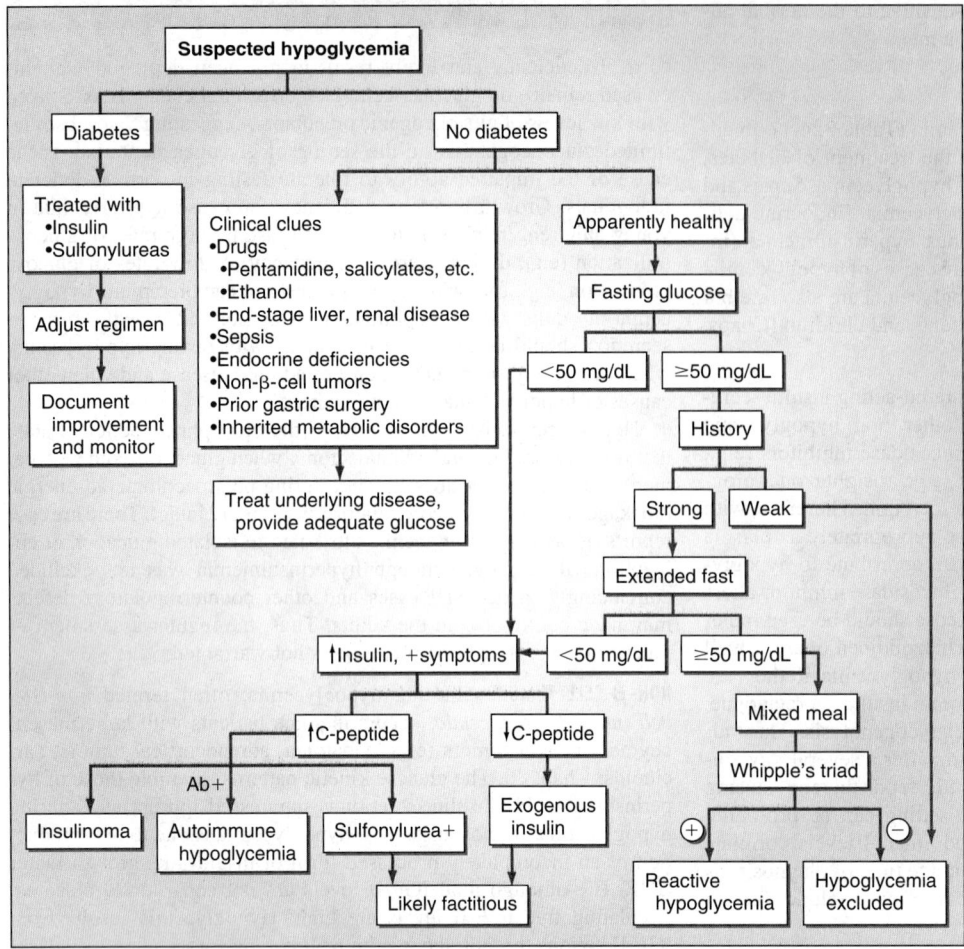

FIGURE 324-3 Diagnostic approach to a patient with suspected hypoglycemia based on a history of symptoms, a low plasma glucose concentration, or both.

phy has high sensitivity and may localize tumors not identified by palpation. Surgical resection of a solitary insulinoma is generally curative. Diazoxide, which inhibits insulin secretion, and the somatostatin analogue, octreotide, can be used to treat hypoglycemia in patients with unresectable insulinomas.

FACTITIOUS HYPOGLYCEMIA *Factitious hypoglycemia*, caused by malicious or self-administration of insulin or ingestion of a sulfonylurea, shares many clinical and laboratory features with insulinoma. It is most common among health care workers, patients with diabetes or their relatives, and people with a history of other factitious illnesses. When this diagnosis is suspected, it is useful to seek previous medical records, which may reveal admissions for similar episodes. In individuals taking exogenous insulin, factitious hypoglycemia can be distinguished from insulinoma by the presence of high insulin levels without a concomitant increase in the C-peptide level, which is suppressed by the exogenous insulin. As noted above, sulfonylureas stimulate endogenous insulin and can therefore be detected only by measuring drug levels in plasma or urine. Factitious or surreptitious hypoglycemia should be considered in every patient requiring a fasting test for hypoglycemia. In addition to laboratory tests, observing the patient's behavior may help make this diagnosis.

ately high. The distinguishing feature is the presence of circulating antibodies to insulin, but the need to measure these routinely is debated, since autoimmune hypoglycemia is rare. Autoantibodies to the insulin receptor are another rare cause of hypoglycemia and usually occur in the context of other autoimmune diseases. A few cases of ectopic insulin secretion (from a non-β-cell tumor) have been reported.

Insulinoma and Other Primary β Cell Disorders Insulinomas are uncommon, but because approximately 90% are benign, they are a treatable cause of potentially fatal hypoglycemia. The yearly incidence is estimated to be 1 in 250,000. About 60% of cases occur in women. The median age at presentation is 50 years in sporadic cases, but it usually presents in the third decade when associated with multiple endocrine neoplasia type 1 (Chap. 330). Insulinomas arise within the substance of the pancreas in >99% of cases and are usually small (1 to 2 cm). About 5 to 10% of insulinomas are malignant, as evidenced by the presence of metastases.

Insulinomas are almost always recognized because of hypoglycemia rather than mass effects. Unusually low plasma glucose concentrations may be required to produce symptoms and signs of hypoglycemia because recurrent hypoglycemia shifts the glycemic thresholds. Although symptomatic hypoglycemia can occur after an overnight fast, it often follows exercise. Rarely, symptomatic hypoglycemia occurs following meals, but most such patients have evidence of fasting hypoglycemia as well.

Octreotide scans localize approximately half of insulinomas. Arteriography has been used extensively in the past, but false-negative and false-positive results occur, and it is generally preferable to use less invasive computed tomography (CT) or magnetic resonance imaging (MRI) scans, which detect 45 to 75% of tumors. Preoperative ultrasound is valuable for some patients. Intraoperative ultrasonogra-

---

APPROACH TO THE PATIENT

In addition to recognition and documentation of hypoglycemia, and often urgent treatment, diagnosis of the hypoglycemic mechanism is critical for choosing a treatment that prevents, or at least minimizes, recurrent hypoglycemia. A diagnostic algorithm is shown in Fig. 324-3.

RECOGNITION AND DOCUMENTATION

Urgent treatment is often necessary in patients with suspected hypoglycemia. Blood should be drawn, whenever possible, before the administration of glucose to allow documentation of the plasma glucose level. Convincing documentation of hypoglycemia requires the fulfillment of Whipple's triad. Thus, *the ideal time to test the plasma glucose is during an episode associated with hypoglycemic symptoms*. A normal plasma glucose concentration measured when the patient is free of symptoms does not exclude hypoglycemia at the time of earlier symptoms. When the cause of hypoglycemia is obscure, additional assays should include glucose, insulin, C peptide, sulfonylurea levels, cortisol, and ethanol.

Hypoglycemia is sometimes detected serendipitously. A distinctly low plasma glucose measurement in a person without a history of corresponding symptoms raises the possibility of a laboratory error caused by ongoing metabolism of glucose by the formed elements of the blood after the sample is drawn. This type of artifactually low glucose level is particularly likely when leukocyte, erythrocyte, or platelet counts are abnormally high, but also if separation of the plasma or serum from the formed elements is delayed.

DIAGNOSIS OF THE HYPOGLYCEMIC MECHANISM

In an adult patient with documented hypoglycemia, a plausible hypoglycemic mechanism and further diagnostic evaluation can be guided by the history, physical examination, and available laboratory data (Fig. 324-3). In the absence of documented spontaneous hypoglycemia, overnight fasting, or food deprivation during observation in the outpatient setting, will sometimes elicit hypoglycemia and allow diagnostic evaluation. If there is a high degree of clinical suspicion, an extended fast lasting 48 to 72 h is often required to make the diagnosis. This procedure should be performed in the hospital with careful supervision and should be terminated if the plasma glucose drops to <2.5 mmol/L (<45 mg/dL) and the patient has symptoms. It is essential to draw blood samples for appropriate tests before administering glucose or allowing the patient to eat.

URGENT TREATMENT

Oral treatment with glucose tablets or glucose-containing fluids, candy, or food is appropriate if the patient is able and willing to take these. A reasonable initial dose is 20 g of glucose. If neuroglycopenia precludes oral feedings, parenteral therapy is necessary. Intravenous glucose (25 g) should be given using a 50% solution followed by a constant infusion of 5 or 10% dextrose. If intravenous therapy is not practical, subcutaneous or intramuscular glucagon can be used, particularly in patients with type 1 diabetes mellitus. Because it acts primarily by stimulating glycogenolysis, glucagon is ineffective in glycogen-depleted individuals (e.g., those with alcohol-induced hypoglycemia). It also stimulates insulin secretion and is therefore less useful in type 2 diabetes mellitus. These treatments raise plasma glucose concentrations only transiently, and patients should be encouraged to eat as soon as practical to replete glycogen stores.

PREVENTION OF RECURRENT HYPOGLYCEMIA

Prevention of recurrent hypoglycemia requires an understanding of the hypoglycemic mechanism. Offending drugs can be discontinued or their doses reduced. It should be remembered that hypoglycemia caused by sulfonylureas may recur after a period of several hours or days. Underlying critical illnesses can often be treated. Cortisol and growth hormone can be replaced if deficient. Surgical, radiotherapeutic, or chemotherapeutic reduction of a non-β-cell tumor can alleviate hypoglycemia, even if the tumor cannot be cured; glucocorticoid or growth hormone administration may also reduce hypoglycemic episodes in such patients. Surgical resection of an insulinoma is often curative; medical therapy with diazoxide or octreotide can be used if resection is not possible and in patients with a nontumor primary β cell disorder. The treatment of autoimmune hypoglycemia (e.g., with a glucocorticoid) is more problematic, but this disorder is often self-limited. Failing these treatments, frequent feedings and avoidance of fasting may be required. Uncooked cornstarch at bedtime or an overnight infusion of intragastric glucose may be necessary in some patients.

FURTHER READING

CRYER PE: *Hypoglycemia: Pathophysiology, Diagnosis and Treatment.* New York, Oxford Univ Press, 1997
———, CHILDS BP: Negotiating the barrier of hypoglycemia in diabetes. Diabetes Spectrum 15:20, 2001
SERVICE FJ: Hypoglycemic disorders. Endocrinol Metab Clin North Am 28: 467, 1999

---

325 | DISORDERS OF THE TESTES AND MALE REPRODUCTIVE SYSTEM
Shalendar Bhasin, J. Larry Jameson

The male reproductive system regulates sexual differentiation, virilization, and the hormonal changes that accompany puberty, ultimately leading to spermatogenesis and fertility. Under the control of the pituitary hormones—luteinizing hormone (LH) and follicle-stimulating hormone (FSH)—the Leydig cells of the testes produce testosterone and germ cells are nurtured by Sertoli cells to divide, differentiate, and mature into sperm. During embryonic development, testosterone and dihydrotestosterone (DHT) induce the wolffian duct and virilization of the external genitalia. During puberty, testosterone promotes somatic growth and the development of secondary sexual characteristics. In the adult, testosterone is necessary for spermatogenesis and stimulation of libido and normal sexual function. This chapter focuses on the physiology of the testes and disorders associated with decreased androgen production, which may be caused by gonadotropin deficiency or by primary testis dysfunction. A variety of testosterone formulations now allow more physiologic androgen replacement. Infertility occurs in ~5% of men and is increasingly amenable to treatment by hormone replacement or by using sperm transfer techniques (Chap. 45). →*For further discussion of sexual dysfunction, disorders of the prostate, and testicular cancer, see Chaps. 43, 81, 82, respectively.*

DEVELOPMENT AND STRUCTURE OF THE TESTIS

The fetal testis develops from the undifferentiated gonad after expression of a genetic cascade that is initiated by the SRY (Sex-related gene on the Y chromosome) (Chap. 328). SRY induces differentiation of Sertoli cells, which surround germ cells, and together with peritubular myoid cells form testis cords that will later develop into seminiferous tubules. Fetal Leydig cells and endothelial cells migrate into the gonad from the adjacent mesonephros but may also arise from interstitial cells

that reside between testis cords. Leydig cells produce testosterone, which supports the growth and differentiation of wolffian duct structures that develop into the epididymis, vas deferens, and seminal vesicles. Testosterone is also converted to DHT (see below), which induces formation of the prostate and the external male genitalia including the penis, urethra, and scrotum. Testicular descent through the inguinal canal is controlled in part by Leydig cell production of insulin-like factor 3 (INSL3), which acts via a receptor termed *Great* (*G* protein–coupled *re*ceptor *a*ffecting *t*estis descent). Sertoli cells produce müllerian inhibiting substance (MIS), which causes regression of the müllerian structures including the fallopian tube, uterus, and upper segment of the vagina.

NORMAL MALE PUBERTAL DEVELOPMENT

Although puberty commonly refers to the maturation of the reproductive axis and the development of secondary sex characteristics, it involves a coordinated response of multiple hormonal systems including the adrenal gland and the growth hormone (GH) axis (Fig. 325-1). The development of secondary sexual characteristics is initiated by *adrenarche*, which usually occurs between 6 and 8 years of age when the adrenal gland begins to produce greater amounts of androgens from the zona reticularis, the principal site of dehydroepiandrosterone (DHEA) production. The sexual maturation process is greatly accelerated by the activation of the hypothalamic-pituitary axis and the production of gonadotropin-releasing hormone (GnRH). The so-called GnRH pulse generator in the hypothalamus is active during fetal life and early infancy but is quiescent until the early stages of puberty, when the sensitivity to steroid inhibition is gradually lost, causing reactivation of GnRH secretion. Leptin, a hormone produced by adi-

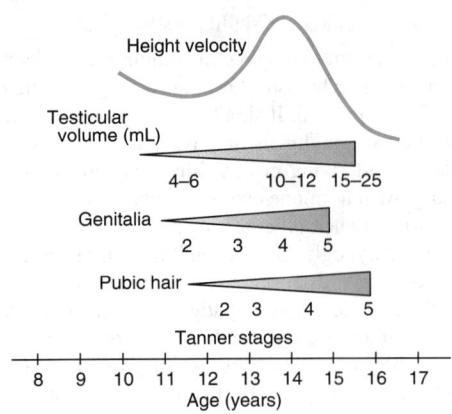

FIGURE 325-1   Pubertal events in males. Sexual maturity ratings for genitalia and pubic hair and divided into five stages. (*From WA Marshall, JM Tanner: Variations in the pattern of pubertal changes in boys. Arch Dis Child 45:13, 1970.*)

pose cells, may play a permissive role in this process, as leptin-deficient individuals fail to enter puberty (Chap. 64). Early puberty is characterized by nocturnal surges of LH and FSH. Growth of the testes is usually the first sign of puberty, reflecting an increase in seminiferous tubule volume. Increasing levels of testosterone deepen the voice and increase muscle growth. Conversion of testosterone to DHT leads to growth of the external genitalia and pubic hair. DHT also stimulates prostate and facial hair growth and initiates recession of the temporal hairline. The growth spurt occurs at a testicular volume of about 10 to 12 mL. GH increases early in puberty and is stimulated in part by the rise in gonadal steroids. GH increases the level of insulin-like growth factor 1 (IGF-1), which enhances linear bone growth. The prolonged pubertal exposure to gonadal steroids (mainly estradiol) ultimately causes epiphyseal closure and limits further bone growth.

REGULATION OF TESTICULAR FUNCTION

REGULATION OF THE HYPOTHALAMIC-PITUITARY-TESTIS AXIS IN ADULT MAN

Hypothalamic GnRH regulates the production of the pituitary gonadotropins, LH and FSH (Fig. 325-2). GnRH is released in discrete pulses approximately every 2 h, resulting in corresponding pulses of LH and FSH. These dynamic hormone pulses account in part for the wide variations in LH and testosterone, even within the same individual. LH acts primarily on the Leydig cell to stimulate testosterone synthesis. The regulatory control of androgen synthesis is mediated by testosterone and estrogen feedback on both the hypothalamus and the pituitary. FSH acts on the Sertoli cell to regulate spermatogenesis and the production of Sertoli products such as inhibin B, which acts to selectively suppress pituitary FSH. Despite these somewhat distinct Leydig and Sertoli cell–regulated pathways, testis function is integrated at several levels: GnRH regulates both gonadotropins; spermatogenesis requires high levels of testosterone; there are numerous paracrine interactions between Leydig and Sertoli cells that are necessary for normal testis function.

THE LEYDIG CELL: ANDROGEN SYNTHESIS

LH binds to its seven transmembrane, G protein–coupled receptor to activate the cyclic AMP pathway. Stimulation of the LH receptor induces *s*teroid *a*cute *r*egulatory (StAR) protein, along with several steroidogenic enzymes involved in androgen synthesis. LH receptor mutations cause Leydig cell hypoplasia or agenesis, underscoring the importance of this pathway for Leydig cell development and function. The rate-limiting process in testosterone synthesis is the delivery of cholesterol by the StAR protein to the inner mitochondrial membrane. Peripheral benzodiazepine receptor, a mitochondrial cholesterol-binding protein, is also an acute regulator of Leydig cell steroidogenesis. The five major enzymatic steps involved in testosterone synthesis are summarized in Fig. 325-3. After cholesterol transport into the mitochondrion, side chain cleavage by CYP11A1 to form pregnenolone is a limiting enzymatic step.

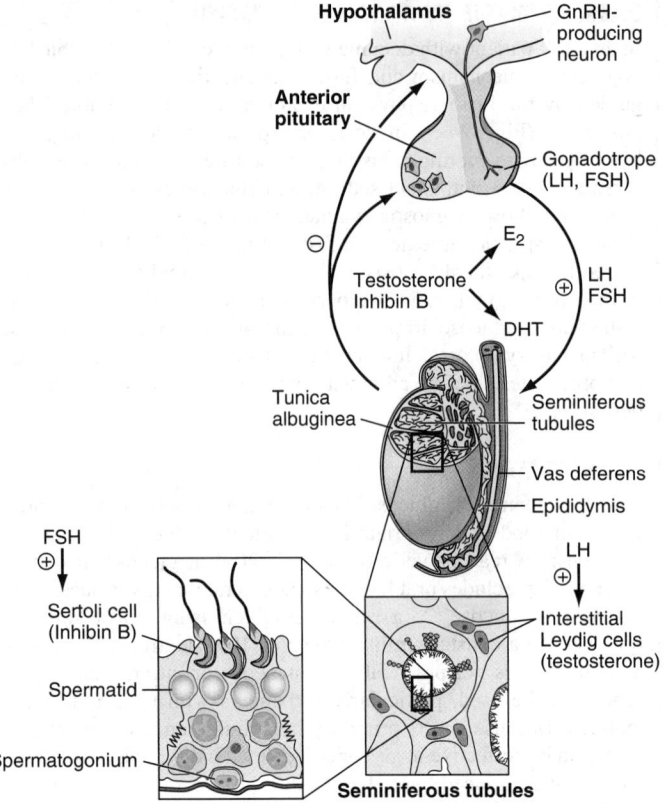

FIGURE 325-2   Human pituitary gonadotropin axis, structure of testis, seminiferous tubule. E_2, 17β estradiol; DHT, dihydrotestosterone.

The 17α-hydroxylase and the 17,20-lyase reactions are catalyzed by a single enzyme, CYP17; posttranslational modification (phosphorylation) of this enzyme and the presence of specific enzyme cofactors confer 17,20-lyase activity selectively in the testis and zona reticularis of the adrenal gland. Testosterone can be converted to the more potent DHT by 5α-reductase, or it can be aromatized to estradiol by CYP19 (aromatase).

Testosterone Transport and Metabolism   In males, 95% of circulating testosterone is derived from testicular secretion (3 to 10 mg/d). Direct secretion of testosterone by the adrenal and the peripheral conversion of androstenedione to testosterone collectively account for another 0.5 mg/d of testosterone. Only a small amount of DHT (70 μg/d) is secreted directly by the testis; most circulating DHT is derived from peripheral conversion of testosterone.

Circulating testosterone is bound to two plasma proteins: sex hormone–binding globulin (SHBG) and albumin (Fig. 325-4). SHBG binds testosterone with much greater affinity than albumin. Only 0.5 to 3% of testosterone is unbound. According to the "free hormone" hypothesis, only the unbound fraction is biologically active; however, albumin-bound hormone dissociates readily in the capillaries and may be bioavailable. SHBG concentrations are decreased by androgens, obesity, insulin, and nephrotic syndrome. Conversely, estrogen administration, hyperthyroidism, many chronic inflammatory illnesses, and aging are associated with high SHBG concentrations.

Testosterone is metabolized predominantly in the liver, although some degradation occurs in peripheral tissues, particularly the prostate and the skin. In the liver, testosterone is converted by a series of enzymatic steps into androsterone, etiocholanolone, DHT, and 3-α-androstanediol. These compounds undergo glucuronidation or sulfation before being excreted by the kidneys.

Mechanism of Androgen Action   The androgen receptor (AR) is homologous to other nuclear receptor proteins including the receptors for estrogen, glucocorticoids, and progesterone (Chap. 317). The AR is encoded by a gene on the long arm of the X chromosome and has a molecular mass of about 110 kDa. A polymorphic region in the amino

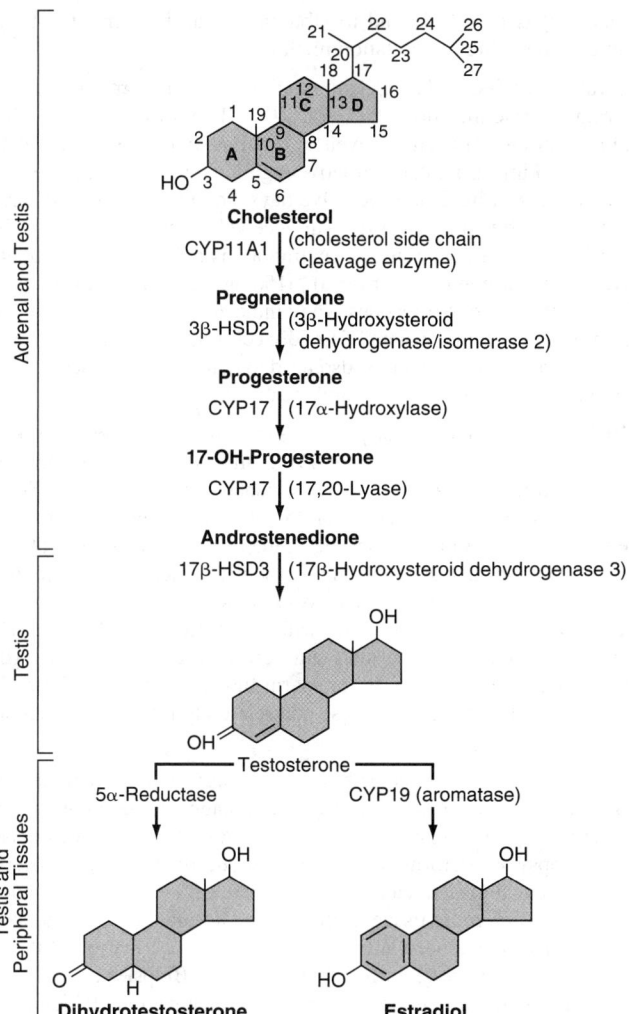

FIGURE 325-3 The biochemical pathway in the conversion of 27-carbon sterol cholesterol to androgens and estrogens.

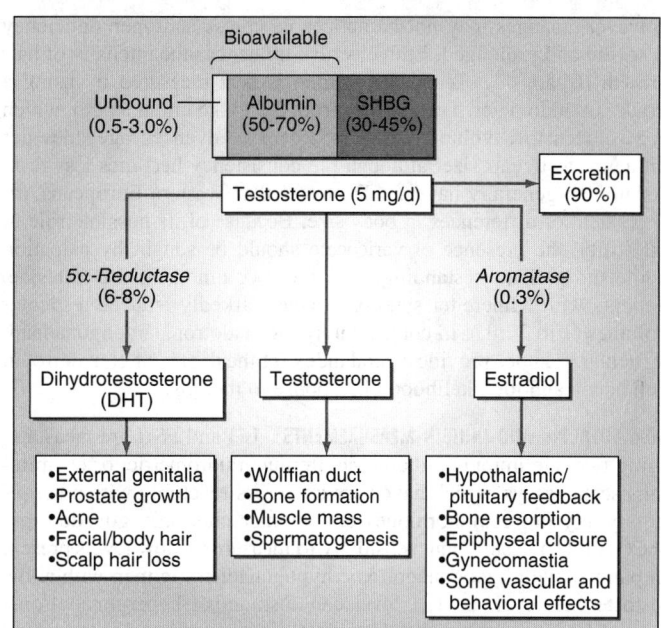

FIGURE 325-4 Androgen metabolism and actions. SHBG, sex hormone–binding globulin.

terminus of the receptor, which contains a variable number of glutamine repeats, modifies the transcriptional activity of the receptor. The AR protein is distributed in both the cytoplasm and the nucleus. Androgen binding to the AR causes it to translocate into the nucleus where it binds to DNA or other transcription factors already bound to DNA. The ligand also induces conformational changes that allow the recruitment and assembly of tissue-specific cofactors. Thus, the AR is a ligand-regulated transcription factor. Some androgen effects may be mediated by nongenomic AR signal transduction pathways. Testosterone binds to AR with half the affinity of DHT. The DHT-AR complex also has greater thermostability, and a slower dissociation rate, than the testosterone-AR complex. However, the molecular basis for selective testosterone versus DHT actions remains incompletely explained.

THE SEMINIFEROUS TUBULES: SPERMATOGENESIS The seminiferous tubules are convoluted, closed loops with both ends emptying into the rete testis, a network of progressively larger efferent ducts that ultimately form the epididymis (Fig. 325-2). The seminiferous tubules total about 600 m in length and comprise about two-thirds of testis volume. The walls of the tubules are formed by polarized Sertoli cells that are apposed to peritubular myoid cells. Tight junctions between Sertoli cells create a blood-testis barrier. Germ cells comprise the majority of the seminiferous epithelium (~60%) and are intimately embedded within the cytoplasmic extensions of the Sertoli cells, which function as "nurse cells." Germ cells progress through characteristic morphologic stages of spermiogenesis, requiring ~24 days. A pool of type A spermatogonia serve as stem cells capable of self-renewal. Primary sper-

matocytes are derived from type B spermatogonia and undergo meiosis before progressing to spermatids that mature and are ultimately released from Sertoli cells as mature spermatozoa. Peristaltic-type action by peritubular myoid cells transports sperm into the efferent ducts. The normal adult testes produce >100 million sperm per day.

Naturally occurring mutations in the *FSHβ* gene and in the FSH receptor confirm an important, but not essential, role for this pathway in spermatogenesis. Females with these mutations are hypogonadal and infertile because ovarian follicles do not mature; males exhibit variable degrees of reduced spermatogenesis, presumably because of impaired Sertoli cell function. Because Sertoli cells produce inhibin B, an inhibitor of FSH, seminiferous tubule damage (e.g., by radiation) causes a selective increase of FSH. Androgens reach very high concentrations locally in the testis and are essential for spermatogenesis. Several cytokines and growth factors are also involved in the regulation of spermatogenesis by paracrine and autocrine mechanisms. A number of knockout mouse models exhibit impaired germ cell development or spermatogenesis, presaging possible mutations associated with male infertility. In humans, microdeletions of several Y chromosome azoospermia factor (*AZF*) genes (e.g., RNA-binding motif, *RBM*; deleted in azoospermia, *DAZ*) are associated with oligospermia or azoospermia.

CLINICAL AND LABORATORY EVALUATION OF MALE REPRODUCTIVE FUNCTION

HISTORY AND PHYSICAL EXAMINATION The history should focus on developmental stages such as puberty and growth spurts, as well as androgen-dependent events such as early morning erections, frequency and intensity of sexual thoughts, and frequency of masturbation or intercourse. Although libido and the overall frequency of sexual acts is decreased in androgen-deficient men, young hypogonadal men may achieve erections in response to visual erotic stimuli. Men with acquired androgen deficiency often report decreased energy and increased irritability.

The physical examination should focus on secondary sex characteristics such as hair growth, possible gynecomastia, testicular volume, prostate, and height and body proportions. Eunuchoidal proportions are defined as an arm span >2 cm greater than height and suggest that androgen deficiency occurred before epiphyseal fusion. Hair growth in the face, axilla, chest, and pubic regions is androgen-dependent;

however, changes may not be noticeable unless androgen deficiency is severe and prolonged. Ethnicity also influences the intensity of hair growth (Chap. 44). Testicular volume is best measured by using a Prader orchidometer. Testes range from 3.5 to 5.5 cm in length, which corresponds to a volume of 12 to 25 mL. Advanced age does not influence testicular size, although the consistency becomes less firm. Asian men generally have smaller testes than western Europeans, independent of differences in body size. Because of its possible role in infertility, the presence of varicocele should be sought by palpation while the patient is standing; it is more common on the left side. Patients with Klinefelter syndrome have markedly reduced testicular volumes (1 to 2 mL). In congenital hypogonadotropic hypogonadism, testicular volumes provide a good index for the degree of gonadotropin deficiency and the likelihood of response to therapy.

GONADOTROPIN AND INHIBIN MEASUREMENTS LH and FSH are measured using two-site immunoradiometric, immunofluorometric, or chemiluminescent assays, which have very low cross-reactivity with other pituitary glycoprotein hormones and human chorionic gonadotropin (hCG) and have sufficient sensitivity to measure the low levels present in patients with hypogonadotropic hypogonadism. In men with a low testosterone level, an LH level can distinguish hypergonadotropic (high LH) versus hypogonadotropic (low or inappropriately normal LH) hypogonadism. An elevated LH level indicates a primary defect at the testicular level, whereas a low or inappropriately normal LH level suggests a defect at the hypothalamic-pituitary level. LH pulses occur about every 1 to 3 h in normal men. Thus, gonadotropin levels fluctuate, and samples should be pooled or repeated when results are equivocal. FSH is less pulsatile than LH because it has a longer half-life. Increased FSH suggests damage to the seminiferous tubules. Inhibin B, a Sertoli cell product that suppresses FSH, is reduced with seminiferous tubule damage. Inhibin B is a dimer with α-β_B subunits and is measured by two-site immunoassays.

GnRH Stimulation Testing The GnRH test is performed by measuring LH and FSH concentrations at baseline and at 30 and 60 min after intravenous administration of 100 μg of GnRH. A minimally acceptable response is a twofold LH increase and a 50% FSH increase. In the prepubertal period or with severe GnRH deficiency, the gonadotrope may not respond to a single bolus of GnRH because it has not been primed by endogenous hypothalamic GnRH; in these patients, GnRH responsiveness may be restored by chronic, pulsatile GnRH administration. With the availability of sensitive and specific LH assays, GnRH stimulation testing is used rarely except to evaluate gonadotrope function in patients who have undergone pituitary surgery or have a space-occupying lesion in the hypothalamic-pituitary region.

TESTOSTERONE ASSAYS ■ Total Testosterone Total testosterone includes both unbound and protein-bound testosterone and is measured by radioimmunoassays or immunometric assays. A single random sample provides a good approximation of the average testosterone concentration with the realization that testosterone levels fluctuate in response to pulsatile LH. Testosterone is generally lower in the late afternoon and is reduced by acute illness. The testosterone concentration in healthy young men ranges from 300 to 1000 ng/dL in most laboratories. Alterations in SHBG levels due to aging, obesity, some types of medications, chronic illness, or on a congenital basis can affect total testosterone levels.

Measurement of Free Testosterone Levels Most circulating testosterone is bound to SHBG and to albumin; only 0.5 to 3% of circulating testosterone is unbound or "free." Free testosterone concentrations can be calculated based on algorithms based on total testosterone and SHBG concentrations. The free fraction is best measured by equilibrium dialysis. Tracer analogue methods are relatively inexpensive and convenient but they are less reliable because changes in SHBG affect the results. Bioavailable testosterone refers to unbound testosterone plus testos-

terone that is loosely bound to albumin; it can be estimated by the ammonium sulfate precipitation method.

hCG Stimulation Test The hCG stimulation test is performed by administering a single injection of 1500 to 4000 IU of hCG intramuscularly and measuring testosterone levels at baseline and 24, 48, 72, and 120 h after hCG injection. An alternative regimen involves three injections of 1500 units of hCG on successive days, and measuring testosterone levels 24 h after the last dose. An acceptable response to hCG is a doubling of the testosterone concentration in adult men. In prepubertal boys, an increase in testosterone to >150 ng/dL indicates the presence of testicular tissue. No response may indicate an absence of testicular tissue or marked impairment of Leydig cell function. Measurement of MIS, a Sertoli cell product, is also used to detect the presence of testes in prepubertal boys with cryptorchidism.

SEMEN ANALYSIS Semen analysis is the most important step in the evaluation of male infertility (Chap. 45). Samples are collected by masturbation following a period of abstinence for 2 to 3 days. Semen volumes and sperm concentrations vary considerably among fertile men, and several samples may be needed before concluding that the results are abnormal. Analysis should be performed within an hour of collection. The normal ejaculate volume is 2 to 6 mL and contains sperm counts of >20 million/mL, with a motility of >50% and >15% normal morphology. Some men with low sperm counts are nevertheless fertile. A variety of tests for sperm function can be performed in specialized laboratories, but these add relatively little to the treatment options.

TESTICULAR BIOPSY Testicular biopsy is useful in some patients with oligospermia or azoospermia, as an aid in diagnosis and indication for the feasibility of treatment. Using local anesthesia, fine-needle aspiration biopsy is performed to aspirate tissue for histology. Alternatively, open biopsies can be performed under local or general anesthesia when more tissue is required. A normal biopsy in an azoospermic man with a normal FSH level suggests obstruction of the vas deferens, which may be correctable surgically. Biopsies are also used to harvest sperm for intracytoplasmic sperm injection (ICSI) and to classify disorders such as hypospermatogenesis (all stages present but in reduced numbers), germ cell arrest (usually at primary spermatocyte stage), and Sertoli cell–only syndrome (absent germ cells) or hyalinization (sclerosis with absent cellular elements).

DISORDERS OF SEXUAL DIFFERENTIATION

See Chap. 328

DISORDERS OF PUBERTY

PRECOCIOUS PUBERTY Puberty in boys before age 9 is considered precocious. *Isosexual precocity* refers to premature sexual development consistent with phenotypic sex and includes features such as the development of facial hair and phallic growth. Isosexual precocity is divided into gonadotropin-dependent and gonadotropin-independent causes of androgen excess (Table 325-1). *Heterosexual precocity* refers to the premature development of feminizing features in boys, such as breast development.

Gonadotropin-Dependent Precocious Puberty This disorder is also called *central precocious puberty* (CPP) and it is less common in boys than in girls. It is caused by premature activation of the GnRH pulse generator, sometimes because of central nervous system (CNS) lesions such as hypothalamic hamartomas, but it is often idiopathic. CPP is characterized by gonadotropin levels that are inappropriately elevated for age. Because pituitary priming has occurred, GnRH elicits LH and FSH responses typical of those seen in puberty or in adults. Magnetic resonance imaging (MRI) should be performed to exclude a mass, structural defect, or infectious or inflammatory process.

Gonadotropin-Independent Precocious Puberty This group of disorders includes hCG-secreting tumors; congenital adrenal hyperplasia; sex steroid–producing tumors of the testis, adrenal, and ovary; accidental or deliberate exogenous sex steroid administration; hypothyroidism; and

TABLE 325-1 *Causes of Precocious or Delayed Puberty in Boys*

I. Precocious puberty
  A. Gonadotropin-dependent
    1. Idiopathic
    2. Hypothalamic hamartoma or other lesions
    3. CNS tumor or inflammatory state
  B. Gonadotropin-independent
    1. Congenital adrenal hyperplasia
    2. hCG-secreting tumor
    3. McCune-Albright syndrome
    4. Activating LH receptor mutation
    5. Exogenous androgens
II. Delayed puberty
  A. Constitutional delay of growth and puberty
  B. Systemic disorders
    1. Chronic disease
    2. Malnutrition
    3. Anorexia nervosa
  C. CNS tumors and their treatment (radiotherapy and surgery)
  D. Hypothalamic-pituitary causes of pubertal failure (low gonadotropins)
    1. Congenital disorders (Table 325-2)
      a. Hypothalamic syndromes (e.g., Prader-Willi)
      b. Idiopathic hypogonadotropic hypogonadism
      c. Kallmann syndrome
      d. GnRH receptor mutations
      e. Adrenal hypoplasia congenita
      f. *PROP1* mutations
      g. Other mutations affecting pituitary development/function
    2. Acquired disorders
      a. Pituitary tumors
      b. Hyperprolactinemia
  E. Gonadal causes of pubertal failure (elevated gonadotropins)
    1. Klinefelter syndrome
    2. Bilateral undescended testes or anorchia
    3. Orchitis
    4. Chemotherapy or radiotherapy
  F. Androgen insensitivity

Note: CNS, central nervous system; hCG, human chronic gonadotropin; LH, luteinizing hormone; GnRH, gonadotropin-releasing hormone.

activating mutations of the LH receptor or $G_s\alpha$ subunit. In these cases, androgens from the testis or the adrenal are increased but gonadotropins are low.

FAMILIAL MALE-LIMITED PRECOCIOUS PUBERTY This is transmitted in an autosomal dominant manner. It is caused by activating mutations in the LH receptor, leading to constitutive stimulation of the cyclic AMP pathway and testosterone production. The disorder is also called *testotoxicosis*. Clinical features include premature virilization in boys, growth acceleration in early childhood, and advanced bone age followed by premature epiphyseal fusion. Testosterone is elevated and LH is suppressed. Treatment options include inhibitors of testosterone synthesis (e.g., ketoconazole), androgen receptor antagonists (e.g., flutamide), and aromatase inhibitors (e.g., anastrazole).

McCUNE-ALBRIGHT SYNDROME This is a sporadic disorder caused by somatic (postzygotic) activating mutations in the $G_s\alpha$ subunit that links G protein–coupled receptors to intracellular signaling pathways (Chap. 334). The mutations impair the guanosine triphosphatase activity of the $G_s\alpha$ protein, leading to constitutive activation of adenylyl cyclase. Like activating LH receptor mutations, this stimulates testosterone production and causes gonadotropin-independent precocious puberty. In addition to sexual precocity, affected individuals may have autonomy in the adrenals, pituitary, and thyroid glands. Café au lait spots are characteristic skin lesions that reflect the onset of the somatic mutations in melanocytes during embryonic development. Polyostotic fibrous dysplasia is caused by activation of the parathyroid hormone receptor pathway in bone. Treatment is similar to that in patients with activating LH receptor mutations. Bisphosphonates have been used to treat bone lesions.

CONGENITAL ADRENAL HYPERPLASIA Boys with congenital adrenal hyperplasia (CAH) who are not well controlled with glucocorticoid suppression

of adrenocorticotropic hormone (ACTH) can develop premature virilization because of excessive androgen production by the adrenal gland (Chaps. 321 and 328). LH is low and the testes are small. Rarely, adrenal rests may develop within the testis because of chronic ACTH stimulation.

Heterosexual Sexual Precocity Breast enlargement in prepubertal boys can result from familial aromatase excess, estrogen-producing tumors in the adrenal gland, Sertoli cell tumors in the testis, marijuana smoking, or estrogen use. Occasionally, germ cell tumors that secrete hCG can be associated with breast enlargement due to excessive stimulation of estrogen production (see "Gynecomastia," below).

APPROACH TO THE PATIENT

After verification of precocious development, serum LH and FSH levels should be measured to determine whether gonadotropins are increased in relation to chronologic age (gonadotropin-dependent) or whether sex steroid secretion is occurring independent of LH and FSH (gonadotropin-independent). In children with gonadotropin-dependent precocious puberty, CNS lesions should be excluded by history, neurologic examination, and MRI scan of the head. If organic causes are not found, one is left with the diagnosis of idiopathic central precocity. Patients with high testosterone but suppressed LH concentrations have gonadotropin-independent sexual precocity; in these patients; DHEA sulfate (DHEAS) and 17α-hydroxyprogesterone should be measured. High levels of testosterone and 17α-hydroxyprogesterone suggest the possibility of CAH due to 21α-hydroxylase or 11β-hydroxylase deficiency. If testosterone and DHEAS are elevated, adrenal tumors should be excluded by obtaining a computed tomography (CT) scan of the adrenal glands. Patients with elevated testosterone but without increased 17α-hydroxyprogesterone or DHEAS should undergo careful evaluation of the testis by palpation and ultrasound to exclude a Leydig cell neoplasm. Activating mutations of the LH receptor should be considered in children with gonadotropin-independent precocious puberty in whom CAH, androgen abuse, and adrenal and testicular neoplasms have been excluded.

$\underset{X}{R}$ TREATMENT

In patients with a known cause (e.g., a CNS lesion or a testicular tumor), therapy should be directed towards the underlying disorder. In patients with idiopathic CPP, long-acting GnRH analogues can be used to suppress gonadotropins and decrease testosterone, halt early pubertal development, delay accelerated bone maturation, and prevent early epiphyseal closure. The treatment is most effective for increasing final adult height if it is initiated before age 6. Puberty resumes after discontinuation of the GnRH analogue. Counseling is an important aspect of the overall treatment strategy. In children with gonadotropin-independent precocious puberty, inhibitors of steroidogenesis, such as ketoconazole, and AR antagonists have been used empirically without data from clinical trials.

DELAYED PUBERTY Puberty is delayed in boys if it has not ensued by age 14, an age that is 2 to 2.5 standard deviations above the mean for healthy children. Delayed puberty is more common in boys than in girls. There are four main categories of delayed puberty: (1) Constitutional delay of growth and puberty (~60% of cases); (2) functional hypogonadotropic hypogonadism caused by systemic illness or malnutrition (~20% of cases); (3) hypogonadotropic hypogonadism caused by genetic or acquired defects in the hypothalamic-pituitary region (~10% of cases); and (4) hypergonadotropic hypogonadism secondary to primary gonadal failure (~15% of cases) (Table 325-1). Functional hypogonadotropic hypogonadism is more common in girls than in boys. Permanent causes of hypogonadotropic or hypergonadotropic hypogonadism are identified in <25% of boys with delayed puberty.

Any history of systemic illness, eating disorders, excessive exercise, social and psychological problems, and abnormal patterns of linear growth during childhood should be verified. Boys with pubertal delay may have accompanying emotional and physical immaturity relative to their peers, which can be a source of anxiety. Physical examination should focus on height; arm span; weight; visual fields; and secondary sex characteristics including hair growth, testicular volume, phallic size, and scrotal reddening and thinning. Testicular size >2.5 cm generally indicates that the child has entered puberty.

The main diagnostic challenge is to distinguish those with constitutional delay, who will progress through puberty at a later age, from those with an underlying pathologic process. Constitutional delay should be suspected when there is a family history and when there are delayed bone age and short stature. Pituitary priming by pulsatile GnRH is required before LH and FSH are synthesized and secreted normally. Thus, blunted responses to exogenous GnRH can be seen in patients with constitutional delay, GnRH deficiency, or pituitary disorders (see "GnRH Stimulation Testing," above). On the other hand, low-normal basal gonadotropin levels or a normal response to exogenous GnRH is consistent with an early stage of puberty, which is often heralded by nocturnal GnRH secretion. Thus, constitutional delay is a diagnosis of exclusion that requires ongoing evaluation until the onset of puberty and the growth spurt.

TREATMENT

If therapy is considered appropriate, it can begin with 25 to 50 mg testosterone enanthate or testosterone cypionate every 2 weeks, or by using a 2.5-mg testosterone patch or 25-mg testosterone gel. Because aromatization of testosterone to estrogen is obligatory for mediating androgen effects on epiphyseal fusion, concomitant treatment with aromatase inhibitors may allow attainment of greater final adult height. Testosterone treatment should be interrupted after 6 months to determine if endogenous LH and FSH secretion have ensued. Other causes of delayed puberty should be considered when there are associated clinical features or when boys do not enter puberty spontaneously after a year of observation or treatment.

Reassurance without hormonal treatment is appropriate for many individuals with presumed constitutional delay of puberty. However, the impact of delayed growth and pubertal progression on a child's social relationships and school performance is often underappreciated.

DISORDERS OF THE MALE REPRODUCTIVE AXIS DURING ADULTHOOD

HYPOGONADOTROPIC HYPOGONADISM Because LH and FSH are trophic hormones for the testes, impaired secretion of these pituitary gonadotropins results in secondary hypogonadism, which is characterized by low testosterone in the setting of low LH and FSH. Those with the most severe deficiency have complete absence of pubertal development, sexual infantilism and, in some cases, hypospadias and undescended testes. Patients with partial gonadotropin deficiency have delayed or arrested sexual development. The 24-h LH secretory profiles are heterogeneous in patients with hypogonadotropic hypogonadism, reflecting variable abnormalities of LH pulse frequency or amplitude. In severe cases, basal LH is low and there are no LH pulses. A smaller subset of patients has low-amplitude LH pulses or markedly reduced pulse frequency. Occasionally, only sleep-entrained LH pulses occur, reminiscent of the pattern seen in the early stages of puberty. Hypogonadotropic hypogonadism can be classified into congenital and acquired disorders. Congenital disorders most commonly involve GnRH deficiency, which leads to gonadotropin deficiency. Acquired disorders are much more common than congenital disorders and may result from a variety of sellar mass lesions or infiltrative diseases of the hypothalamus or pituitary.

Congenital Disorders Associated with Gonadotropin Deficiency Most cases of congenital hypogonadotropic hypogonadism are idiopathic, despite extensive endocrine testing and imaging studies of the sellar region. Among known causes, familial hypogonadotropic hypogonadism can be transmitted as an X-linked (20%), autosomal recessive (30%), or autosomal dominant (50%) trait. Some individuals with idiopathic hypogonadotropic hypogonadism (IHH) have sporadic mutations in the same genes that cause inherited forms of the disorder. *Kallmann syndrome* is an X-linked disorder caused by mutations in the *KAL1* gene, which encodes anosmin, a protein that mediates the migration of neural progenitors of the olfactory bulb and GnRH-producing neurons. These individuals have GnRH deficiency and variable combinations of anosmia or hyposmia, renal defects, and neurologic abnormalities including mirror movements. Gonadotropin secretion and fertility can be restored by administration of pulsatile GnRH or by gonadotropin replacement. Mutations in the *FGFR1* gene cause an autosomal dominant form of hypogonadotropic hypogonadism that clinically resembles Kallmann syndrome. The *FGFR1* gene product may be the receptor for the *KAL1* gene product, anosmin, thereby explaining the similarity in clinical features. Other autosomal dominant causes remain unexplained. X-linked hypogonadotropic hypogonadism also occurs in adrenal hypoplasia congenita, a disorder caused by mutations in the *DAX1* gene, which encodes a nuclear receptor in the adrenal gland and reproductive axis. *Adrenal hypoplasia congenita* is characterized by absent development of the adult zone of the adrenal cortex, leading to neonatal adrenal insufficiency. Puberty usually does not occur or is arrested, reflecting variable degrees of gonadotropin deficiency. Although sexual differentiation is normal, some patients have testicular dysgenesis and impaired spermatogenesis despite gonadotropin replacement. *GnRH receptor mutations* account for ~40% of autosomal recessive and 10% of sporadic cases of hypogonadotropic hypogonadism. These patients have decreased LH response to exogenous GnRH. Some receptor mutations alter GnRH binding affinity, allowing apparently normal responses to pharmacologic doses of exogenous GnRH. Mutations in the G protein–coupled receptor, GPR54, cause gonadotropin deficiency without anosmia. Patients retain responsiveness to exogenous GnRA, suggesting an abnormality in the neural pathways controlling GnRH release. Rarely, recessive mutations in the *LHβ* or *FSHβ* genes have been described in patients with selective deficiencies of these gonadotropins. Deletions or mutations of the *GnRH* gene have not been found in patients with hypogonadotropic hypogonadism.

A number of homeodomain transcription factors are involved in the development and differentiation of the specialized hormone-producing cells within the pituitary gland (Table 325-2). Patients with mutations of *PROP1* have combined pituitary hormone deficiency that includes GH, prolactin (PRL) thyroid-stimulating hormone (TSH), LH, and FSH, but not ACTH. *LHX3* mutations cause combined pituitary hormone deficiency in association with cervical spine rigidity. *HESX1* mutations cause septooptic dysplasia and combined pituitary hormone deficiency.

Prader-Willi syndrome is characterized by obesity, hypotonic musculature, mental retardation, hypogonadism, short stature, and small hands and feet. Prader-Willi syndrome is a genomic imprinting disorder caused by deletions of the proximal portion of paternally derived chromosome 15q or by uniparental disomy of the maternal alleles (Chap. 57). *Laurence-Moon syndrome* is an autosomal recessive disorder characterized by obesity, hypogonadism, mental retardation, polydactyly, and retinitis pigmentosa. Recessive mutations of leptin, or its receptor, cause severe obesity and pubertal arrest, apparently because of hypothalmic GnRH deficiency (Chap. 64).

Acquired Hypogonadotropic Disorders ■ *SEVERE ILLNESS, STRESS, MALNUTRITION, AND EXERCISE* These may cause reversible gonadotropin deficiency. Although gonadotropin deficiency and reproductive dysfunction are well documented in these conditions in women, men exhibit similar but less pronounced responses. Unlike women, most male runners and other endurance athletes have normal gonadotropin and sex steroid

TABLE 325-2 *Causes of Congenital Hypogonadotropic Hypogonadism*

Gene	Locus	Inheritance	Associated Features
KAL1	Xp22	X-linked	Anosmia, renal agenesis, synkinesia, cleft lip/palate, oculomotor/visuospatial defects, gut malrotations
FGFR1	8p11–p12	AD	Anosmia, cleft lip/palate, synkinesia, syndactyly
LEP	7q31	AR	Obesity
LEPR	1p31	AR	Obesity
PC1	5q15-21	AR	Obesity, diabetes mellitus, ACTH deficiency
HESX1	3p21	AR	Septooptic dysplasia, CPHD
		AD	Isolated GH insufficiency
LHX3	9q34	AR	CPHD (ACTH spared), cervical spine rigidity
PROP1	5q35	AR	CPHD (ACTH usually spared)
GPR54	19p13	AR	None
GNRHR	4q21	AR	None
FSHβ	11p13	AR	↑ LH
LHβ	19q13	AR	↑ FSH
SF1 (NR5A1)	9p33	AD/AR	Primary adrenal failure, XY sex reversal
DAX1 (NR0B1)	Xp21	X-linked	Primary adrenal failure, impaired spermatogenesis

Abbreviations: ACTH, adrenocorticotropic hormone; AD, autosomal dominant; AR, autosomal recessive; CPHD, combined pituitary hormone deficiency; KAL1, Interval-1 gene; FGFR1, fibroblast growth factor receptor 1; LEP, leptin; LEPR, leptin receptor; PC1, prohormone convertase 1; HESX1, homeo box gene expressed in embryonic stem cells 1; LHX3, LIM homeobox gene 3; PROP1, Prophet of Pit 1; GPR54, G protein–coupled receptor 54; GNRHR, gonadotropin-releasing hormone receptor; FSHβ, follicle-stimulating hormone β-subunit; LHβ, luteinizing hormone β-subunit; SF1, steroidogenic factor 1; DAX1, *d*osage-sensitive sex-reversal, *a*drenal hypoplasia congenita, *X*-chromosome.

levels, despite low body fat and frequent intensive exercise. Testosterone levels fall at the onset of illness and recover during recuperation. The magnitude of gonadotropin suppression generally correlates with the severity of illness. Although hypogonadotropic hypogonadism is the most common cause of androgen deficiency in patients with acute illness, some have elevated levels of LH and FSH, which suggest primary gonadal dysfunction. The pathophysiology of reproductive dysfunction during acute illness is unknown but likely involves a combination of cytokine and/or glucocorticoid effects. There is a high frequency of low testosterone levels in patients with chronic illnesses such as HIV infection, end-stage renal disease, chronic obstructive lung disease, and many types of cancer and in patients receiving glucocorticoids. Some 20% of HIV-infected men with low testosterone levels have elevated LH and FSH levels; these patients presumably have primary testicular dysfunction. The remaining 80% have either normal or low LH and FSH levels; these men have a central hypothalamic-pituitary defect or a dual defect involving both the testis and the hypothalamic-pituitary centers. Muscle wasting is common in chronic diseases associated with hypogonadism, which also leads to debility, poor quality of life, and adverse outcome of disease. There is great interest in exploring strategies that can reverse androgen deficiency or attenuate the sarcopenia associated with chronic illness.

Men who are heavy users of marijuana have decreased testosterone secretion and sperm production. The mechanism of marijuana-induced hypogonadism is decreased GnRH secretion. Gynecomastia observed in marijuana users can also be caused by plant estrogens in crude preparations.

OBESITY In men with mild to moderate obesity, SHBG levels decrease in proportion to the degree of obesity, resulting in lower total testosterone levels. However, free testosterone levels usually remain within the normal range. The decrease in SHBG levels is caused by increased circulating insulin, which inhibits SHBG production. Estradiol levels are higher in obese men compared to healthy, non-obese controls, because of aromatization of testosterone to estradiol in adipose tissue. Weight loss is associated with reversal of these abnormalities including an increase in total and free testosterone levels and a decrease in

estradiol levels. A subset of massively obese men may have a defect in the hypothalamic-pituitary axis as suggested by low free testosterone in the absence of elevated gonadotropins.

HYPERPROLACTINEMIA (See also Chap. 318) Elevated PRL levels are associated with hypogonadotropic hypogonadism. PRL inhibits hypothalamic GnRH secretion either directly or through modulation of tuberoinfundibular dopaminergic pathways. A PRL-secreting tumor may also destroy the surrounding gonadotropes by invasion or compression of the pituitary stalk. Treatment with dopamine agonists reverses gonadotropin deficiency, although there may be a delay relative to PRL suppression.

SELLAR MASS LESIONS Neoplastic and nonneoplastic lesions in the hypothalamus or pituitary can directly or indirectly affect gonadotrope function. In adults, pituitary adenomas constitute the largest category of space-occupying lesions affecting gonadotropin and other pituitary hormone production. Pituitary adenomas that extend into the suprasellar region can impair GnRH secretion and mildly increase PRL secretion (usually <50 µg/L) because of impaired tonic inhibition by dopaminergic pathways. These tumors should be distinguished from prolactinomas, which typically secrete higher PRL levels. The presence of diabetes insipidus suggests the possibility of a craniopharyngioma, infiltrative disorder, or other hypothalamic lesions (Chap. 319).

HEMOCHROMATOSIS (See also Chap. 336) Both the pituitary and testis can be affected by excessive iron deposition. However, the pituitary defect is the predominant lesion in most patients with hemochromatosis and hypogonadism. The diagnosis of hemochromatosis is suggested by the association of characteristic skin pigmentation, hepatic enlargement or dysfunction, diabetes mellitus, arthritis, cardiac conduction defects, and hypogonadism.

PRIMARY TESTICULAR CAUSES OF HYPOGONADISM Common causes of primary testicular dysfunction include Klinefelter syndrome, uncorrected cryptorchidism, cancer chemotherapy, radiation to the testes, trauma, torsion, infectious orchitis, HIV infection, anorchia syndrome, and myotonic dystrophy. Primary testicular disorders may be associated with impaired spermatogenesis, decreased androgen production, or both. →*See Chap. 328 for disorders of testis development, androgen synthesis, and androgen action.*

Klinefelter Syndrome (See also Chap. 328) Klinefelter syndrome is the most common chromosomal disorder associated with testicular dysfunction and male infertility. It occurs in about 1 in 1000 live-born males. Azoospermia is the rule in men with Klinefelter syndrome who have the 47,XXY karyotype; however, men with mosaicism may have germ cells, especially at a younger age. Testicular histology shows hyalinization of seminiferous tubules and absence of spermatogenesis. Although their function is impaired, the number of Leydig cells appears to increase. Testosterone is decreased and estradiol is increased, leading to clinical features of undervirilization and gynecomastia.

Cryptorchidism Cryptorchidism occurs when there is incomplete descent of the testis from the abdominal cavity into the scrotum. About 3% of full-term and 30% of premature male infants have at least one cryptorchid testis at birth, but descent is usually complete by the first few weeks of life. The incidence of cryptorchidism is <1% by 9 months of age. Cryptorchidism is associated with increased risk of malignancy and infertility. Unilateral cryptorchidism, even when corrected before puberty, is associated with decreased sperm counts, possibly reflecting unrecognized damage to the fully descended testis.

Acquired Testicular Defects *Viral orchitis* may be caused by the mumps virus, echovirus, lymphocytic choriomeningitis virus, and group B arboviruses. Orchitis occurs in as many as one-fourth of adult men with mumps; the orchitis is unilateral in about two-thirds, and bilateral in the remainder. Orchitis usually develops a few days after the onset of parotitis but may precede it. The testis may return to normal size and function or undergo atrophy. Semen analysis returns to normal for three-fourths of men with unilateral involvement but normal for only one-third of men with bilateral orchitis. *Trauma*, including testicular torsion, can also cause secondary atrophy of the testes. The exposed position of the testes in the scrotum renders them susceptible to both thermal and physical trauma, particularly in men with hazardous occupations.

The testes are sensitive to *radiation damage*. Doses >200 mGy (20 rad) are associated with increased FSH and LH levels and damage to the spermatogonia. After ~800 mGy (80 rad), oligospermia or azoospermia develops, and higher doses may obliterate the germinal epithelium. Permanent androgen deficiency in adult men is uncommon after therapeutic radiation; however, most boys given direct testicular radiation therapy for acute lymphoblastic leukemia have permanently low testosterone levels. Sperm banking should be considered before patients undergo radiation treatment or chemotherapy.

Drugs interfere with testicular function by several mechanisms including inhibition of testosterone synthesis (e.g., ketoconazole), blockade of androgen action (e.g., spironolactone), increased estrogen (e.g., marijuana), or direct inhibition of spermatogenesis (e.g., chemotherapy). Cyclophosphamide causes azoospermia or extreme oligospermia within a few weeks after the initiation of therapy. In about half of patients, spermatogenesis returns within 3 years after cessation of therapy. Combination chemotherapy for acute leukemia, Hodgkin disease, and other malignancies may impair Leydig cell function. Alcohol, when consumed in excess for prolonged periods, decreases testosterone, independent of liver disease or malnutrition. Elevated estradiol and decreased testosterone levels may occur in men taking digitalis.

The occupational and recreational history should be carefully evaluated in all men with infertility because of the toxic effects of many *chemical agents* on spermatogenesis. Known environmental hazards include microwaves and ultrasound and chemicals such as nematocide dibromochloropropane, cadmium, and lead. In some populations, sperm density is said to have declined by as much as 40% in the past 50 years. Environmental estrogens or antiandrogens may be partly responsible.

Testicular failure also occurs as a part of *polyglandular autoimmune insufficiency* (Chap. 330). Sperm antibodies can cause isolated male infertility. In some instances, these antibodies are secondary phenomena resulting from duct obstruction or vasectomy. Granulomatous diseases can affect the testes, and testicular atrophy occurs in 10 to 20% of men with lepromatous leprosy because of direct tissue invasion by the mycobacteria. The tubules are involved initially, followed by endarteritis and destruction of Leydig cells.

Systemic disease can cause primary testis dysfunction in addition to suppressing gonadotropin production. In cirrhosis, a combined testicular and pituitary abnormality leads to decreased testosterone production independent of the direct toxic effects of ethanol. Impaired hepatic extraction of adrenal androstenedione leads to extraglandular conversion to estrone and estradiol, which partially suppresses LH. Testicular atrophy and gynecomastia are present in approximately one-half of men with cirrhosis. In chronic renal failure, androgen synthesis and sperm production decrease despite elevated gonadotropins. The elevated LH level is due to reduced clearance, but it does not restore normal testosterone production. About one-fourth of men with renal failure have hyperprolactinemia. Improvement in testosterone production with hemodialysis is incomplete, but successful renal transplantation may return testicular function to normal. Testicular atrophy is present in one-third of men with sickle cell anemia. The defect may be at either the testicular or the hypothalamic-pituitary level. Sperm density can decrease temporarily after acute febrile illness in the absence of a change in testosterone production. Infertility in men with celiac disease is associated with a hormonal pattern typical of androgen resistance, namely elevated testosterone and LH levels.

Neurologic diseases associated with altered testicular function include myotonic dystrophy, spinobulbar muscular atrophy, and paraplegia. In myotonic dystrophy, small testes may be associated with impairment of both spermatogenesis and Leydig cell function. Spinobulbar muscular atrophy is caused by an expansion of the glutamine repeat sequences in the amino-terminal region of the AR; this expansion impairs function of the AR, but it is unclear how the alteration is related to the neurologic manifestations. Men with spinobulbar muscular atrophy often have undervirilization and infertility as a late manifestation. Spinal cord lesions that cause paraplegia can lead to a temporary decrease in testosterone levels and may cause persistent defects in spermatogenesis; some patients retain the capacity for penile erection and ejaculation.

ANDROGEN INSENSITIVITY SYNDROMES Mutations in the AR cause resistance to the action of testosterone and DHT. These X-linked mutations are associated with variable degrees of defective male phenotypic development and undervirilization (Chap. 328). Although not technically hormone insensitivity syndromes, two genetic disorders impair testosterone conversion to active sex steroids. Mutations in the *SRD5A2* gene, which encodes 5α-reductase type 2, prevent the conversion of testosterone to DHT, which is necessary for the normal development of the male external genitalia. Mutations in the *CYP19* gene, which encodes aromatase, prevent testosterone conversion to estradiol. Males with *CYP19* mutations have delayed epiphyseal fusion, tall stature, eunuchoidal proportions, and osteoporosis, consistent with evidence from an estrogen receptor–deficient individual that these testosterone actions are mediated indirectly via estrogen.

GYNECOMASTIA

Gynecomastia refers to enlargement of the male breast. It is caused by excess estrogen action and is usually the result of an increased estrogen/androgen ratio. True gynecomastia is associated with glandular breast tissue that is >4 cm in diameter and is often tender. Glandular tissue enlargement should be distinguished from excess adipose tissue; glandular tissue is firmer and contains fibrous-like cords. Gynecomastia occurs as a normal physiologic phenomenon in the newborn, during puberty, and with aging, but it can also result from pathologic conditions associated with androgen deficiency or estrogen excess. The prevalence of gynecomastia increases with age and body mass index (BMI), likely because of increased aromatase activity in adipose tissue. Medications that alter androgen metabolism or action may also cause gynecomastia. The relative risk of breast cancer is increased in men with gynecomastia, although the absolute risk is relatively small.

PATHOLOGIC GYNECOMASTIA Any cause of *androgen deficiency* can lead to gynecomastia, reflecting an increased estrogen/androgen ratio, as estrogen synthesis still occurs by aromatization of residual adrenal and gonadal androgens. Gynecomastia is a characteristic feature of Klinefelter syndrome (Chap. 328). *Androgen insensitivity* disorders also cause gynecomastia. *Excess estrogen production* may be caused by tumors, including Sertoli cell tumors in isolation or in association with Peutz-Jegher syndrome or Carney complex. Tumors that produce hCG, including some testicular tumors, stimulate Leydig cell estrogen synthesis. *Increased conversion of androgens to estrogens* can be a result of increased availability of substrate (androstenedione) for extraglandular estrogen formation (CAH, hyperthyroidism, and most feminizing adrenal tumors) or to diminished catabolism of androstenedione (liver disease) so that estrogen precursors are shunted to aromatase in peripheral sites. Obesity is associated with increased aromatization of androgen precursors to estrogens. Extraglandular aromatase activity can also be increased in tumors of the liver or adrenal gland or rarely as an inherited disorder. Several families with *increased peripheral aromatase activity* inherited as an autosomal or as an X-linked disorder have been described. *Drugs* can cause gynecomastia by acting directly as estrogenic substances (e.g., oral contraceptives, phytoestrogens, digitalis), inhibiting androgen synthesis (e.g., ketoconazole), or action (e.g., spironolactone).

It is challenging to determine when to evaluate gynecomastia, since up to two-thirds of pubertal boys and half of hospitalized men have palpable glandular tissue (Fig. 325-5). In addition to the extent of gynecomastia, recent onset, rapid growth, tender tissue, and occur-

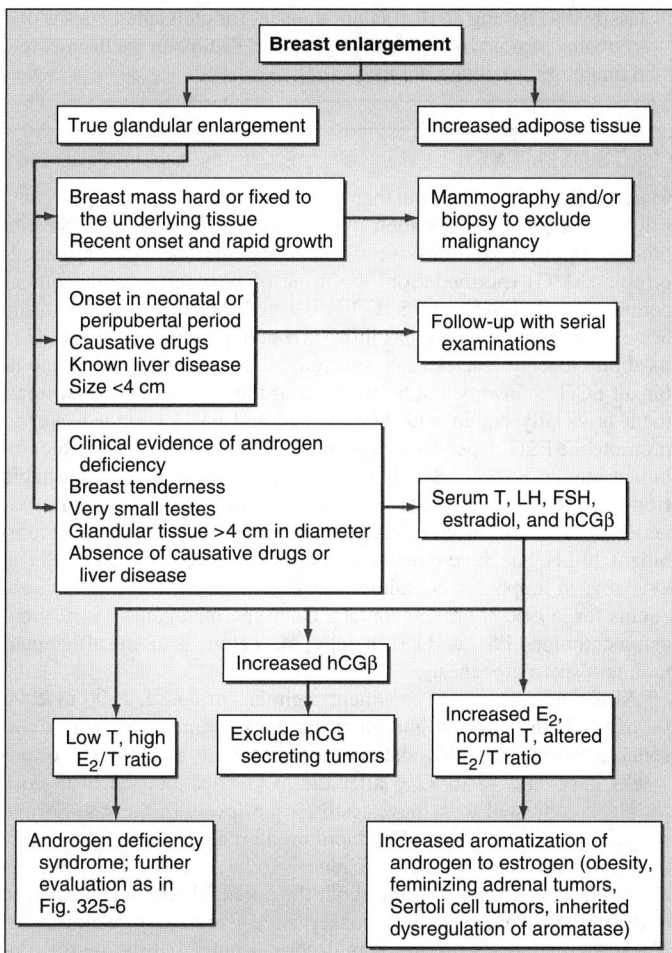

FIGURE 325-5 Evaluation of gynecomastia. T, testosterone; LH, luteinizing hormone; FSH, follicle-stimulating hormones; hCGβ, human chorionic gonadoltopin β; E₂, 17β-estradiol.

rence in a lean subject should prompt more extensive evaluation. This should include a careful drug history, measurement and examination of the testes, assessment of virilization, evaluation of liver function, and hormonal measurements including testosterone, estradiol, and androstenedione, LH, and hCG. If testes are small, a karyotype should be obtained to exclude Klinefelter syndrome. Despite this evaluation, the diagnosis is established in fewer than one-half of patients, probably because of subtle alterations of the estrogen/androgen ratio.

℞ TREATMENT

When the primary cause can be identified and corrected, breast enlargement usually subsides over several months. However, if gynecomastia is of long duration, surgery is the most effective therapy. Indications for surgery include severe psychologic and/or cosmetic problems, continued growth or tenderness, or suspected malignancy. In patients who have painful gynecomastia and who are not candidates for other therapy, treatment with antiestrogens such as tamoxifen (20 mg/d) reduces pain and breast tissue size in about two-thirds of patients. Aromatase inhibitors can be effective in the early proliferative phase of the disorder, although the experience is largely based on the use of testolactone, a relatively weak aromatase inhibitor; placebo-controlled trials with more potent aromatase inhibitors such as anastrazole, fadrozole, letrozole, or fromestane are needed.

AGING-RELATED CHANGES IN MALE REPRODUCTIVE FUNCTION

A number of cross-sectional and longitudinal studies (e.g., The Baltimore Longitudinal Study of Aging and the Massachusetts Male Aging Study) have established that testosterone concentrations decrease

with advancing age. This age-related decline starts in the third decade of life and progresses slowly; the rate of decline in testosterone concentrations is greater for men with chronic illness and for those taking medications than in healthy older men. Because SHBG concentrations are higher in older men than in younger men, free or bioavailable testosterone concentrations decline with aging to a greater extent than total testosterone concentrations. The age-related decline in testosterone is due to defects at all levels of the hypothalamic-pituitary-testicular axis: pulsatile GnRH secretion is attenuated, LH response to GnRH is reduced, and testicular response to LH is impaired. However, the gradual rise of LH with aging suggests that testis dysfunction is the main cause of declining androgen levels. The term *andropause* has been used to denote age-related decline in testosterone concentrations; this term is a misnomer because there is no discrete time when testosterone concentrations decline abruptly.

It is speculated that age-related decline in testosterone concentrations contributes to sexual dysfunction, loss of muscle mass and function, frailty, gain in fat mass, cognitive impairment, and loss of body hair. Initial studies of testosterone supplementation in older men with low or low normal testosterone levels have demonstrated a modest increase of fat-free mass and grip strength; a decrease in fat mass; an improved sense of well being, energy, visuo-spatial orientation, and verbal memory; and a modest increment in bone mineral density. However, the long-term risks of testosterone supplementation in older men remain largely unknown. In particular, physiologic testosterone replacement might increase the risk of prostate cancer or exacerbate cardiovascular disease. Population screening of all older men for low testosterone levels is not recommended, and testing should be restricted to men who have symptoms or physical features attributable to androgen deficiency. In men with documented androgen deficiency, testosterone replacement may be considered on an individualized basis and should be instituted after careful discussion of the risks and benefits (see "Testosterone Replacement," below).

Testicular morphology, semen production, and fertility are maintained up to a very old age in men. Although concern has been expressed about age-related increases in germ cell mutations and impairment of DNA repair mechanisms, the frequency of chromosomal aneuploidy or structural abnormalities does not increase in the sperm of older men. However, the incidence of autosomal dominant diseases, such as achondroplasia, polyposis coli, Marfan syndrome, and Apert syndrome, increases in the offspring of men who are advanced in age, consistent with transmission of sporadic missense mutations.

APPROACH TO THE PATIENT

Hypogonadism is often heralded by decreased sex drive, reduced frequency of sexual intercourse or inability to maintain erections, reduced beard growth, loss of muscle mass, decreased testicular size, and gynecomastia. Less than 10% of patients with erectile dysfunction alone have testosterone deficiency. Thus, it is useful to look for a constellation of symptoms and signs suggestive of androgen deficiency. Except when extreme, these clinical features may be difficult to distinguish from changes that occur with normal aging. Moreover, androgen deficiency may develop gradually. Population studies, such as the Massachusetts Male Aging Study, suggest that about 4% of men between the ages of 40 and 70 have testosterone levels <150 ng/dL. Thus, androgen deficiency is not uncommon. The changes for the clinician are (1) to decide when to evaluate a man for possible androgen deficiency, (2) to assess when there is laboratory evidence for androgen deficiency and determine its cause, and (3) to decide when and how to treat patients with androgen deficiency.

When symptoms or clinical features suggest possible androgen deficiency, the laboratory evaluation is initiated by the measurement of total testosterone, preferably in the morning (Fig. 325-6). A total testosterone level <200 ng/dL, in association with symp-

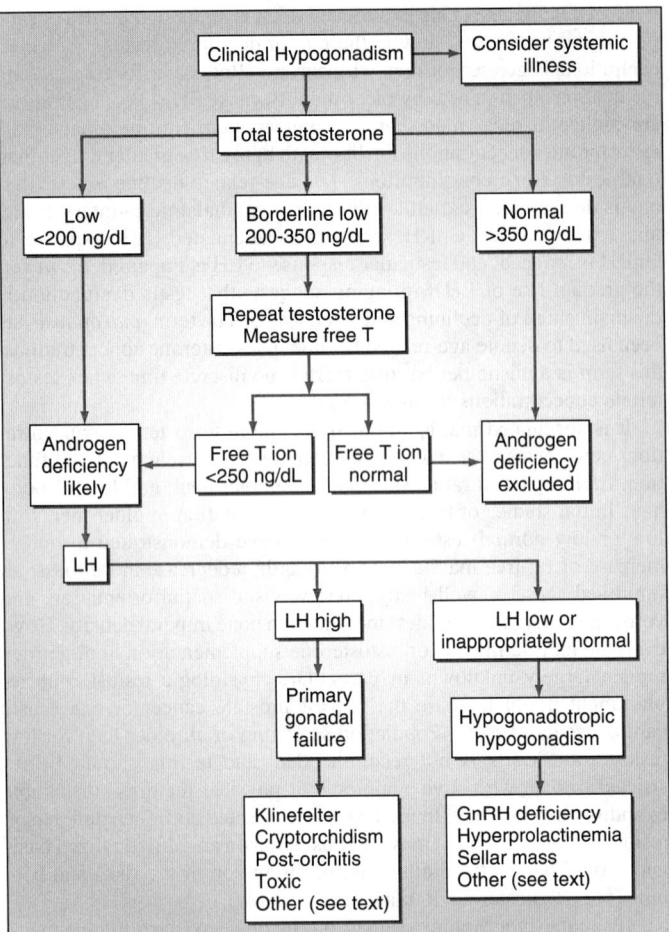

FIGURE 325-6   Evaluation of hypogonadism. T, testosterone; LH, luteinizing hormone; GnRH, gonadotropin-releasing hormone.

toms, is evidence of testosterone deficiency. An early-morning testosterone level >350 ng/dL makes the diagnosis of androgen deficiency unlikely. In men with testosterone levels between 200 and 350 ng/dL, the total testosterone level should be repeated and a free testosterone level should be measured. In older men and in patients with other clinical states that are associated with alterations in SHBG levels, a direct measurement of free testosterone level by equilibrium dialysis can be useful in unmasking testosterone deficiency.

When androgen deficiency has been confirmed by low testosterone concentrations, LH should be measured to classify the patient as having hypergonadotropic (high LH) or hypogonadotropic (low or inappropriately normal LH) hypogonadism. An elevated LH level indicates that the defect is at the testicular level. Common causes of primary testicular failure include Klinefelter syndrome, HIV infection, uncorrected cryptorchidism, cancer chemotherapeutic agents, radiation, surgical orchiectomy, or prior infectious orchitis. Unless causes of primary testicular failure are known, a karyotype should be performed in men with low testosterone and elevated LH to exclude Klinefelter syndrome. Men who have a low testosterone but "inappropriately normal" or low LH levels have hypogonadotropic hypogonadism; their defect resides at the hypothalamic-pituitary level. Common causes of acquired hypogonadotropic hypogonadism include space-occupying lesions of the sella, hyperprolactinemia, chronic illness, hemochromatosis, excessive exercise, and substance abuse. Measurement of PRL and MRI scan of the hypothalamic-pituitary region can help exclude the presence of a space-occupying lesion. Patients in whom known causes of hypogonadotropic hypogonadism have been excluded are

classified as having IHH. It is not unusual for congenital causes of hypogonadotropic hypogonadism, such as Kallmann syndrome, to be diagnosed in young adults.

Ṙ TREATMENT

Gonadotropins   Gonadotropin therapy is used to establish or restore fertility in patients with gonadotropin deficiency of any cause. Several gonadotropin preparations are available. Human menopausal gonadotropin (hMG) (purified from the urine of postmenopausal women) contains 75 IU FSH and 75 IU LH per vial. hCG (purified from the urine of pregnant women) has little FSH activity and resembles LH in its ability to stimulate testosterone production by Leydig cells. Recombinant hCG is now available. Because of the expense of hMG, treatment is usually begun with hCG alone, and hMG is added later to promote the FSH-dependent stages of spermatid development. Recombinant human FSH (hFSH) is now available and is indistinguishable from purified urinary hFSH in its biologic activity and pharmacokinetics in vitro and in vivo, although the mature β subunit of recombinant hFSH has seven fewer amino acids. Recombinant hFSH is available in ampoules containing 75 IU (~7.5 μg FSH), which accounts for >99% of protein content. Once spermatogenesis is restored using combined FSH and LH therapy, hCG alone is often sufficient to maintain spermatogenesis.

Although a variety of treatment regimens are used, 1500 to 2000 IU of hCG administered intramuscularly three times weekly is a reasonable starting dose. Testosterone levels should be measured 6 to 8 weeks later, and 48 to 72 h after the hCG injection; the hCG dose should be adjusted to achieve testosterone levels in the mid-normal range. Sperm counts should be monitored on a monthly basis. It may take several months for spermatogenesis to be restored; therefore, it is important to forewarn patients about the potential length and expense of the treatment and to provide conservative estimates of success rates. If testosterone levels are in the mid-normal range but the sperm concentrations are low after 6 months of therapy with hCG alone, FSH should be added. This can be done by using hMG, highly purified urinary hFSH, or recombinant hFSH. The selection of FSH dose is empirical. A common practice is to start with the addition of 75 IU FSH three times each week in conjunction with the hCG injections. If sperm densities are still low after 3 months of combined treatment, the FSH dose should be increased to 150 IU. Occasionally, it may take ≥18 to 24 months for spermatogenesis to be restored.

The two best predictors of success using gonadotropin therapy in hypogonadotropic men are testicular volume at presentation and time of onset. In general, men with testicular volumes >8 mL have better response rates than those who have testicular volumes <4 mL. Patients who became hypogonadotropic after puberty experience higher success rates than those who have never undergone pubertal changes. Spermatogenesis can usually be reinitiated by hCG alone, with high rates of success for men with postpubertal onset of hypogonadotropism. The presence of a primary testicular abnormality, such as cryptorchidism, will attenuate testicular response to gonadotropin therapy. Prior androgen therapy does not affect subsequent response to gonadotropin therapy.

GnRH   In patients with documented GnRH deficiency, both pubertal development and spermatogenesis can be successfully induced by pulsatile administration of low doses of GnRH. This response requires normal pituitary and testicular function. Therapy usually begins with an initial dose of 25 ng/kg per pulse administered subcutaneously every 2 h by a portable infusion pump. Testosterone, LH, and FSH levels should be monitored. The dose of GnRH is increased until testosterone levels reach the mid-normal range. Doses ranging from 25 to 200 ng/kg may be required to induce virilization. Once pubertal changes have been initiated, the dose of GnRH can often be reduced. Increased sperm counts and testicular volume have been reported in >70% of treated men, and improvements in sexual function and virilization can be induced in >90% of patients. Cutaneous infections occur but are infrequent and minor. Carrying a portable infusion device can be cumbersome, and follow-up of these patients requires physician supervision and laboratory monitoring. Some patients with IHH have cryptorchidism; men with this additional testicular defect may not respond to GnRH or gonadotropin therapy.

Comparative studies of gonadotropin therapy and pulsatile GnRH administration demonstrate that these two therapies are similar in terms of the time to first appearance of sperm or pregnancy rates; both approaches are equally effective in inducing spermatogenesis in men with hypogonadotropic hypogonadism caused by GnRH deficiency. However, most patients find intermittent gonadotropin injections preferable to wearing a continuous infusion pump.

Testosterone Replacement Androgen therapy is indicated to restore testosterone levels to normal to correct features of androgen deficiency. Testosterone replacement improves libido and overall sexual activity, increases energy, lean muscle mass, and bone density and provides the patient a better sense of well-being. The benefits of testosterone replacement therapy have only been proven in men who have documented androgen deficiency, as demonstrated by testosterone levels that are well below the lower limit of normal (<250 ng/dL).

Testosterone is available in a variety of formulations with distinct pharmacokinetics (Table 325-3). Testosterone serves as a prohormone and is converted to 17β-estradiol by aromatase and to 5α-dihydrotes-terone by 5α-reductase. Therefore, when evaluating testosterone formulations, it is important to consider whether the formulation being used can achieve physiologic estradiol and DHT concentrations, in addition to normal testosterone concentrations. Although testosterone concentrations at the lower end of the normal male range can restore sexual function, it is not clear whether low-normal testosterone levels can maintain bone mineral density and muscle mass. The current recommendation is to restore testosterone levels to the mid-normal range.

ORAL DERIVATIVES OF TESTOSTERONE Testosterone is well-absorbed after oral administration but quickly degrades during the first pass through the liver. Therefore, it is not possible to achieve sustained blood levels of testosterone after oral administration of crystalline testosterone. 17α-alkylated derivatives of testosterone (e.g., 17α-methyl testosterone, oxandrolone, fluoxymesterone) are relatively resistant to hepatic degradation and can be administered orally; however, because of the potential for hepatotoxicity, including cholestatic jaundice, peliosis, and hepatoma, these formulations should not be used for testosterone replacement. Hereditary angioedema due to C1 esterase deficiency is the only exception to this general recommendation; in this condition, oral 17α-alkylated androgens are useful because they stimulate hepatic synthesis of the C1 esterase inhibitor.

TABLE 325-3 *Clinical Pharmacology of Testosterone Formulations*

Formulation	Regimen	Pharmacokinetics	DHT and Estradiol	Advantages	Disadvantages
Testosterone enanthate or cypionate	100 mg IM weekly or 200 mg IM every 2 weeks	After a single IM injection, testosterone levels rise into the supraphysiologic range and then decline gradually into the hypogonadal range by the end of the dosing interval	DHT and estradiol levels rise in proportion to the increase in testosterone levels; T:DHT and T:E₂ ratios do not change	Corrects symptoms of androgen deficiency Relatively inexpensive, if self-administered Flexibility of dosing	Requires IM injection Peaks and valleys in testosterone levels
Scrotal testosterone patch	One scrotal patch designed to deliver 6 mg over 24 h applied daily	Normalizes testosterone levels in many but not all androgen-deficient men	Estradiol levels are in the physiologic male range, but DHT levels rise into the supraphysiologic range	Corrects symptoms of androgen deficiency	To promote optimum adherence of the patch, scrotal skin needs to be shaved High DHT levels
Nongenital transdermal system	One or two patches, designed to deliver 5–10 mg testosterone over 24 h applied daily on nonpressure areas	Restores testosterone, DHT, and estradiol levels into the physiologic male range	T:DHT and T:estradiol levels are in the physiologic male range	Ease of application, corrects symptoms of androgen deficiency, and mimics the normal diurnal rhythm of testosterone secretion. Lesser increase in hemoglobin than injectable esters	Testosterone levels in some androgen-deficient men may be in the low-normal range; these men may need application of two patches daily Skin irritation at the application site in some patients
Testosterone gel	Testosterone gel containing 50 to 100 mg testosterone should be applied daily	Restores testosterone and estradiol levels into the physiologic male range	DHT levels and T:DHT ratios are lower in hypogonadal men treated with the testosterone gel than in healthy eugonadal men	Corrects symptoms of androgen deficiency, provides flexibility of dosing, ease of application, good skin tolerability	Potential of transfer to a female partner or child by direct skin-to-skin contact; moderately high DHT levels
17α-methyl testosterone	Orally active, 17α-alkylated compound that should not be used because of potential for liver toxicity	Orally active			Clinical responses variable; potential for liver toxicity; should not be used for treatment of androgen deficiency
Buccal adhesive testosterone	An adhesive, 10-mg tablet applied to buccal mucosa twice daily	Absorbed through buccal mucosa	Serum T and DHT in the normal male range	Ease of application	Limited experience, no evidence of liver toxicity, effects of food and brushing unclear

Note: DHT, dihydrotestosterone; T, testosterone, E₂, 17β-estradiol.

Source: Adapted from: American College of Physicians/American Society of Internal Medicine Disease Management Module on Male Hypogonadism.

INJECTABLE FORMS OF TESTOSTERONE   The esterification of testosterone at the 17β-hydroxy position makes the molecule hydrophobic and extends its duration of action. The slow release of testosterone ester from an oily depot in the muscle accounts for its extended duration of action. The longer the side chain, the greater the hydrophobicity of the ester and longer the duration of action. Thus, testosterone enanthate and cypionate with longer side chains have longer duration of action than testosterone propionate. Within 24 h after intramuscular administration of 200 mg testosterone enanthate or cypionate, testosterone levels rise into the high-normal or supraphysiologic range and then gradually decline into the hypogonadal range over the next 2 weeks. A bimonthly regimen of testosterone enanthate or cypionate therefore results in peaks and troughs in testosterone levels that are accompanied by changes in a patient's mood, sexual desire, and energy level. The kinetics of testosterone enanthate and cypionate are similar. Estradiol and DHT levels are normal if testosterone replacement is physiologic.

TRANSDERMAL TESTOSTERONE   Three transdermal testosterone patches are commercially available: a scrotal testosterone patch (Testoderm) and two nongenital patches (Androderm and Testoderm TTS). The scrotal transdermal testosterone patch, when applied daily to the scrotal skin, produces mid-normal testosterone levels in hypogonadal men 4 to 8 h after application followed by a gradual decrease in testosterone levels over the next 24 h. Estradiol levels are normal but DHT levels are increased due to the conversion of testosterone to DHT by the high amounts of 5α-reductase in scrotal skin. There was initial concern that exposure to high DHT levels might have deleterious effects on the prostate; however, long-term follow-up of men treated with the scrotal patch has not revealed an unexpected increase in prostate problems.

With nongenital testosterone patches, testosterone, DHT, and estradiol levels are in the mid-normal range 4 to 12 h after application. Sexual function and a sense of well-being are restored in androgen-deficient men treated with the nongenital patch. One 5-mg patch may not be sufficient to increase testosterone into the mid-normal male range in all hypogonadal men; some patients may need daily administration of two 5-mg patches to achieve the targeted testosterone concentrations. The transdermal systems are more expensive than testosterone esters. The use of nongenital patches may be associated with skin irritation in some individuals.

TESTOSTERONE GEL   Two testosterone gels (Androgel) and Testim are available in 2.5- and 5-g unit doses that nominally deliver 25 and 50 mg of testosterone to the application site. Initial pharmacokinetic studies have demonstrated that 50-, 75-, and 100-mg doses applied daily to the skin can maintain total and free testosterone concentrations in the mid- to high-normal range in hypogonadal men. Total and free testosterone concentrations are uniform throughout the 24-h period. The current recommendations are to begin with a 50-mg dose and adjust the dose based on testosterone levels. The advantages of the testosterone gel are in its ease of application, its invisibility after application, and its flexibility of dosing. A major concern is the potential for inadvertent transfer of the gel to a sexual partner or to children who may come in close contact with the patient. The ratio of DHT to testosterone concentrations is higher in men treated with the testosterone gel.

A buccal adhesive testosterone tablet, which adheres to the buccal mucosa and releases testosterone as it is slowly dissolved, has been approved. After twice daily application of 10 to 20 mg tablets, serum testosterone levels are maintained within the normal male range in a majority of treated hypogonadal men. The adverse effects include buccal ulceration in a few subjects. The clinical experience with this formulation is limited, and the effects of food and brushing on absorption have not been studied in detail.

TESTOSTERONE FORMULATIONS NOT AVAILABLE IN THE UNITED STATES   Testosterone undecanoate, when administered orally in oleic acid, is absorbed preferentially through the lymphatics into the systemic circulation and is spared the first-pass degradation in the liver. Doses of 40 to 80 mg orally, two or three times daily, are typically used. However, the clinical responses are variable and suboptimal. DHT-to-testosterone ratios are higher in hypogonadal men treated with oral testosterone undecanoate, as compared to eugonadal men.

Implants of crystalline testosterone can be inserted in the subcutaneous tissue by means of a trocar through a small skin incision. Testosterone is released by surface erosion of the implant and absorbed into the systemic circulation. Four to six 200-mg implants can maintain testosterone in the mid- to high-normal range for up to 6 months. Potential drawbacks include incising the skin for insertion and removal, and spontaneous extrusions and fibrosis at the site of the implant.

NOVEL ANDROGEN FORMULATIONS   A number of androgen formulations with better pharmacokinetics or more selective activity profiles are under development. A biodegradable testosterone microsphere formulation provides physiologic testosterone levels for 10 to 11 weeks. Two long-acting esters, testosterone buciclate and testosterone undecanoate, when injected intramuscularly, can maintain circulating testosterone concentrations in the male range for 7 to 12 weeks. Initial clinical trials have demonstrated the feasibility of administering testosterone by the sublingual or buccal routes. 7α-methyl-19-nortestosterone is an androgen that cannot be 5α-reduced; therefore, compared to testosterone, it has relatively greater agonist activity in muscle and gonadotropin suppression but lesser activity on the prostate.

Analogous to the selective estrogen receptor modulators, such as raloxifene, it may be possible to develop selective androgen receptor modulators (SARMs) that exert the desired physiologic effects on muscle, bone, or sexual function but without adversely affecting the prostate and the cardiovascular system.

PHARMACOLOGIC USES OF ANDROGENS   In addition to hypogonadism, androgens have been used to treat a variety of disorders with the hope that anabolic actions of the agents (such as increase in nitrogen retention and muscle mass, increased hemoglobin) would outweigh any deleterious (e.g., virilization) actions of the drugs. The most common non-replacement uses of androgen have been attempts to improve nitrogen balance in catabolic states (e.g., AIDS), self-administration by athletes to increase muscle mass and/or athletic performance, attempts to enhance erythropoiesis in refractory anemias (including the anemia of renal failure), treatment of hereditary angioedema and endometriosis, and management of growth retardation of various etiologies. Most of the expected benefits in these disorders have not been realized. The modest pharmacologic doses of androgens have little physiologic effect in men when superimposed on normal testicular androgen; in women, the virilizing side effects of androgens are formidable.

The most pervasive form of androgen abuse is by male athletes with the expectation that it will improve muscle development and athletic performance. In controlled studies using modest pharmacologic doses (two to four times the usual replacement doses), these agents do not consistently improve performance. However, at the doses frequently taken by athletes (which sometimes exceed 10 times the replacement dose), androgens enhance nitrogen balance and muscle mass; since the drugs have multiple side effects at high doses, these benefits do not outweigh the risks associated with androgen abuse in men, while androgen use by female athletes is associated with disfiguring virilization. The only established indications for androgen therapy aside from male hypogonadism are in selected patients with anemia due to bone marrow failure (an indication largely supplanted by erythropoietin) or for hereditary angioedema.

RECOMMENDED REGIMENS FOR ANDROGEN REPLACEMENT   Testosterone esters are administered weekly at doses of 75 to 100 mg intramuscularly, or 150 to 200 mg every 2 weeks. One 6-mg scrotal patch should be applied daily after shaving the scrotal skin. One or two 5-mg nongenital testosterone patches can be applied daily over the skin of the back, thigh, or upper arm away from pressure areas. Testosterone gel is typically applied over a covered area of skin at a dose of 50 to 100 mg daily; patients should wash their hands after gel application.

ESTABLISHING EFFICACY OF TESTOSTERONE REPLACEMENT THERAPY Because a clinically useful marker of androgen action is not available, restoration of testosterone levels into the mid-normal range remains the goal of therapy. Measurements of LH and FSH are not useful in assessing the adequacy of testosterone replacement. Testosterone should be measured 3 months after initiating therapy to assess adequacy of therapy. In patients who are treated with testosterone enanthate or cypionate, testosterone levels should be 350 to 600 ng/dL 1 week after the injection. If testosterone levels are outside this range, adjustments should be made to either the dose or the interval between injections. In men on transdermal patch or gel therapy, testosterone levels should be in the mid-normal range (500 to 800 ng/dL) 4 to 12 h after application. If testosterone levels are outside this range, the dose should be adjusted.

Restoration of sexual function, secondary sex characteristics, and energy level and one's sense of well being are important objectives of testosterone replacement therapy. The patient should also be asked about sexual desire and activity, the presence of early morning erections, and whether he is able to achieve and maintain erections that are adequate for sexual intercourse. Some hypogonadal men continue to complain about sexual dysfunction even after testosterone replacement has been instituted; these patients may benefit from counseling. The hair growth in response to androgen replacement is variable and depends on ethnicity. Hypogonadal men with prepubertal onset of androgen deficiency who begin testosterone therapy in their late 20s or 30s may find it difficult to adjust to their newly found sexuality and may benefit from counseling. If the patient has a sexual partner, the partner should be included in counseling because of the dramatic physical and sexual changes that occur with androgen treatment.

CONTRAINDICATIONS FOR ANDROGEN ADMINISTRATION Testosterone administration is contraindicated in men with a history of prostate cancer because androgens can promote tumor growth (Table 325-4). Testosterone should not be prescribed to men with severe symptoms of benign prostatic hypertrophy (AUA symptom score > 22), because even small increases in prostate volume may exacerbate obstructive symptoms. Testosterone replacement should not be administered to men with baseline hematocrit ≥52%. Testosterone can induce and exacerbate sleep apnea because of its neuromuscular effects on the upper airway.

MONITORING POTENTIAL ADVERSE EXPERIENCES The clinical effectiveness and safety of testosterone replacement therapy should be performed 3 and 6 months after initiating testosterone therapy and annually thereafter.

Hemoglobin Levels Administration of testosterone to androgen-deficient men is typically associated with a 3 to 5% increase in hemoglobin levels. Clinically significant erythrocytosis is uncommon in young hypogonadal men but can occur in men who have sleep apnea, a significant smoking history, chronic obstructive lung disease, or who are older in age. The magnitude of hemoglobin increase during testosterone therapy appears related to the peak testosterone levels. Transdermal testosterone replacement may produce a smaller hemoglobin increase than testosterone esters.

Digital Examination of the Prostate and Serum PSA Levels Testosterone replacement therapy increases prostate volume to the size seen in age-matched controls but should not increase prostate volume beyond that expected for age. There is no evidence that testosterone replacement causes prostate cancer. However, androgen administration can exacerbate preexisting prostate cancer. Many older men harbor microscopic foci of cancer in their prostates. It is not known whether long-term testosterone administration will induce these microscopic foci to grow into clinically significant cancers.

Prostate-specific antigen (PSA) levels are lower in testosterone-deficient men and are restored to normal after testosterone replacement. There is considerable test-retest variability in PSA measurements; the average interassay coefficient of variation of PSA assays is 15%. The 95% confidence interval for the change in PSA values, measured 3 to 6 months apart, is 1.4 ng/mL. Increments in PSA levels after testosterone supplementation in androgen-deficient men are generally <0.5 ng/mL, and increments >1.0 ng/mL over a 3 to 6-month period are unusual. Nevertheless, administration of testosterone to men with baseline PSA levels between 2.5 and 4.0 ng/mL will cause PSA levels to exceed 4.0 ng/mL for some, and many of these men may undergo prostate biopsies. PSA velocity criterion can be used for patients who have sequential PSA measurements for >2 years; a change of >0.40 ng/mL per year merits closer urologic follow-up.

Cardiovascular Risk Assessment The long-term effects of testosterone supplementation on cardiovascular risk are unknown. Testosterone effects on lipids depend on the dose (physiologic or supraphysiologic), the route of administration (oral or parenteral), and the formulation (whether aromatizable or not). Physiologic testosterone replacement by an aromatizable androgen has a modest effect on high-density lipoprotein (HDL) or no effect at all. In middle-aged men with low testosterone levels, physiologic testosterone replacement has been shown to improve insulin sensitivity and reduce visceral obesity. In epidemiologic studies, testosterone concentrations are inversely related to waist-to-hip ratio and directly correlated with HDL cholesterol levels. These data suggest that physiologic testosterone concentrations is correlated with factors associated with reduced cardiovascular risk. However, no prospective studies have examined the effect on testosterone replacement on cardiovascular risk.

MALE SEXUAL DYSFUNCTION

See Chap. 43.

MALE INFERTILITY

See Chap. 45.

BENIGN AND MALIGNANT PROSTATE DISORDERS

See Chap. 81.

TESTICULAR NEOPLASMS

See Chap. 82.

ACKNOWLEDGMENT
We are grateful to James E. Griffin and Jean D. Wilson, authors of Disorders of the Testes in the 15th edition of Harrison's, for contributions to this chapter.

FURTHER READING

ACHERMANN JC et al: Inherited disorders of the gonadotropin hormones. Mol Cell Endocrinol 179:89, 2001

BHASIN S, BUCKWALTER JG: Testosterone supplementation of older men: A rational idea whose time has not yet come. J Androl 122:718, 2001

FELDMAN HA et al: Age trends in the level of serum testosterone and other hormones in middle-aged men: Longitudinal results from the Massachusetts male aging study. J Clin Endocrinol Metab 87:589, 2002

LIU PY et al: Androgens and cardiovascular disease. Endocr Rev 24:313, 2003

SEDLMEYER IL, PALMERT MR: Delayed puberty: Analysis of a large case series from an academic center. J Clin Endocrinol Metab 87:1613, 2002

TABLE 325-4 *Contraindications for Androgen Replacement*

- The presence or history of prostate cancer
- Baseline PSA ≥ 4 ng/mL or a palpable abnormality of the prostate without urologic evaluation to rule out prostate cancer
- Severe symptoms of lower urinary tract obstruction as indicated by IPSS or AUA symptom score of ≥22
- Baseline hematocrit > 52%
- Severe sleep apnea
- Class IV congestive heart failure

Note: PSA, prostate-specific antigen, IPSS, International Prostate Symptom Score; AUA, American Urological Association.

Normal female reproduction requires the integrated action of the central nervous system, the pituitary gland, and the ovary to orchestrate the monthly cycle of ovarian follicle development and the release of ova. The hormonal changes associated with the menstrual cycle prepare the uterus for implantation if fertilization occurs. After menopause, these cycles cease, and there is a marked reduction in sex steroid levels, leading to physiologic changes. Disorders of the female reproductive system may be developmental, structural, or hormonal in etiology. The reproductive tract is also susceptible to sexually transmitted diseases, which may cause active or chronic infections and predispose to infertility and neoplasia. Gynecologic malignancies, particularly of the ovary, uterus, and cervix, are relatively common. Although many women receive specialized care from obstetrician-gynecologists, a good understanding of the female reproductive system and its disorders is essential for comprehensive healthcare by internists and family practitioners.

DEVELOPMENT, STRUCTURE, AND FUNCTION OF THE OVARY

EMBRYOLOGY

The primordial germ cells migrate to the genital ridge adjacent to the mesonephric kidney by the fifth week of gestation and undergo mitotic division. The gonads exist in an undifferentiated state until the seventh week of fetal life, at which time the primitive ovary can be distinguished from the testis (Chap. 328). From the fifth month of fetal life, the primordial follicle consists of the primary oocyte arrested in meiosis, a single surrounding layer of granulosa cells, and a basement membrane that separates the primordial follicle from surrounding stromal (interstitial) tissues. The ovary contains a finite number of germ cells, the number peaking at about 7 million oogonia by the fifth to sixth month of gestation. Subsequently, the germ cells decrease in number through a process of atresia so that approximately 1 million remain at birth, 400,000 are present at menarche, and only a few remain at menopause.

PUBERTAL MATURATION

The final maturation of ovarian follicles commences during puberty. The two major hormones that regulate follicular development are the pituitary gonadotropins—follicle-stimulating hormone (FSH) and luteinizing hormone (LH) (Fig. 326-1). In the neonate, concomitant with the decrease in estrogen and progesterone levels caused by separation from the placenta, there is a rebound increase in gonadotropin secretion for the first few months of life. With continued maturation of the hypothalamic-pituitary system, the hypothalamic-pituitary axis (the so-called gonadostat) becomes exquisitely sensitive to negative feedback by low levels of circulating steroid hormones, and plasma gonadotropins again decrease. As the time of puberty nears, a decrease in the sensitivity of the gonadostat allows for increased secretion of FSH and LH, possibly secondary to increased episodic or pulsatile

secretion of gonadotropin-releasing hormone (GnRH) by the hypothalamus (Chap. 318). The increase in estrogen secretion exerts a positive feedback, which leads to an exaggeration of the pulsatile release of LH and eventually to menarche and ovulation, after which plasma gonadotropin concentrations reach adult values but vary across the menstrual cycle. After the menopause, plasma gonadotropin levels rise, then plateau 5 to 10 years after menopause and remain fairly constant until the eighth to ninth decade of life, when the levels may fall. Although ovarian function is regulated primarily by LH and FSH, the ovary is a source of protein hormones and growth factors such as inhibin and activin that play an important role in ovarian function and regulation. The production of inhibin by the mature ovary accounts, in part, for the selective reduction in FSH that is seen during the reproductive years (Fig. 326-1).

At age 10 to 11, the first secondary sexual characteristics begin to appear in girls, namely, development of the breast buds (*thelarche*), followed by the development of pubic hair (*pubarche*), and later by the development of axillary hair (*adrenarche*). The growth of pubic and axillary hair is believed to be initiated by adrenal androgens, the levels of which begin to rise at approximately 6 to 8 years of age. A growth spurt ensues, and peak growth rate is attained by age 12.

The culmination of puberty is the onset of predictable, cyclic menses. The average time between the beginning of breast development and the onset of menses (*menarche*) is 2 years. During the first few years after menarche, menstrual cycles are often irregular and unpredictable due to anovulation. The age of menarche is variable and is influenced by socioeconomic and genetic factors and by general health. In the United States, the mean age of menarche is believed to have decreased at a rate of 3 to 4 months per decade over the past 100 years and is now approximately 12 years of age, a change believed to be due to improved nutrition. Leptin levels have been correlated with the onset of the pubertal process. A critical combination of total body weight and percent body fat is associated with development of hypothalamic insensitivity to feedback by steroids that leads to increased secretion of gonadotropins and finally to menarche. Obese girls have earlier menarche than girls with normal body weight. In contrast, active participation in sports or ballet, malnutrition, and chronic debilitating disease can delay menarche.

MATURE OVARY

MORPHOLOGY The anatomic components and function of the adult ovary are illustrated schematically in Fig. 326-2. Under the influence of gonadotropins, a group of primary follicles are recruited, and by day 6 to 8 of the menstrual cycle, one follicle becomes mature or "dominant," a process characterized by accelerated growth of granulosa cells and enlargement of the fluid-filled antrum. The follicles not destined to ovulate undergo degeneration, similar to the atresia that occurs during embryogenesis. Just prior to ovulation, meiosis resumes in the ovum of the dominant follicle, and the first meiotic division results in formation of the first polar body. The antrum rapidly enlarges (up to 10 to 25 mm in size), follicular fluid increases in amount, and the follicular surface thins and forms a conical stigma. Ovulation from the dominant follicle occurs 16 to 23 h after the LH peak and 24 to 38 h after the onset of the LH surge when the follicular wall ruptures in the area of the stigma. The ovum is then expelled together with a mass of surrounding granulosa cells called *cumulus cells*. The rupture is believed to result from the action of hydrolytic enzymes on the surface of the follicle, possibly under the control of prostaglandins. The second meiotic division occurs after the egg is fertilized by a sperm, and the second polar body is then extruded. The formation of the *corpus luteum* begins in the retained remnant of the

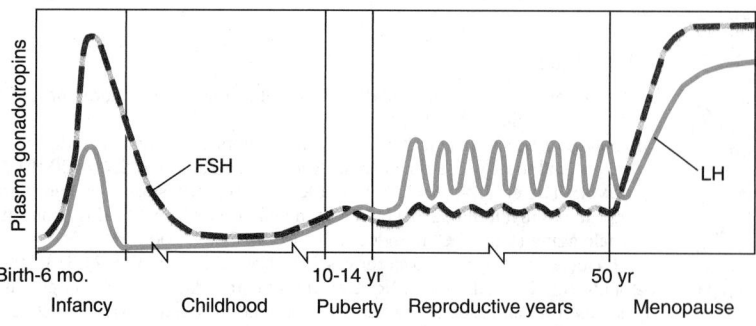

FIGURE 326-1 Pattern of gonadotropin secretion during different stages of life in women. FSH, follicle-stimulating hormone; LH, luteinizing hormone.

2198

ovulated follicle; the remaining granulosa and theca cells increase in size and accumulate lipids and a yellow pigment, lutein, to become "luteinized." After a period of 14 ± 2 days (the functional life of the corpus luteum), the corpus luteum begins to atrophy, to be replaced in time by a fibrous scar, the *corpus albicans*. The factors that limit the life span of the human corpus luteum are not known, but if pregnancy occurs, the corpus luteum persists under the influence of placental chorionic gonadotropin, and progesterone is produced by the corpus luteum for the support of pregnancy.

HORMONE FORMATION ■ Steroid Hormones

Like other steroid hormones, ovarian steroids are derived from cholesterol (Fig. 326-3). The ovary can synthesize cholesterol de novo and can also utilize cholesterol obtained from circulating lipoproteins as substrate for steroid hormone formation. Virtually all ovarian cells are believed to possess the complete complement of enzymes required for the synthesis of estradiol from cholesterol (Fig. 326-3); however, different cell types in the ovary contain different amounts of these enzymes so that the main steroids produced vary in different compartments. For example, the corpus luteum forms mainly progesterone and 17-hydroxyprogesterone, whereas theca and stromal cells convert cholesterol to androstenedione and testosterone. Granulosa cells are particularly rich in the aromatase enzyme responsible for estrogen synthesis and utilize as substrates for this process androgens synthesized in the adjacent theca cells.

LH acts primarily to regulate the early steps in steroid hormone biosynthesis, namely, the transport of cholesterol into the mitochondria by steroidogenic acute regulatory (StAR) protein and its conversion to pregnenolone. FSH acts mainly to regulate the final process by which androgens are aromatized to estrogens. As a consequence, LH enhances substrate flow and the formation of androgens and/or progesterone in the absence of FSH, whereas FSH action is impeded in the absence of LH because of diminished substrate for aromatization.

ESTROGENS The principal estrogen secreted by the ovary and the most potent estrogen is estradiol. Estrone is also produced by the ovary, but most estrone is formed by extraglandular conversion of androstenedione in peripheral tissues. Estriol (16-hydroxyestradiol), the main estrogen in urine, arises from the 16-hydroxylation of estrone and estradiol. Catechol estrogens are formed by hydroxylation of estrogens at the C-2 or C-4 position and may act as the intracellular mediators of some estrogen action. Estrogens promote development of the secondary sexual characteristics in women and cause uterine growth, thickening of the vaginal mucosa, thinning of the cervical mucus, and development of the ductule system of the breasts. Estrogens also alter lipid profiles and exert effects on the vascular endothelium. The classic mechanism of estrogen action in target tissues is similar to that for other steroid hormones and involves binding to a nuclear steroid receptor—either estrogen receptor (ER)α or ERβ—and enhancement of the transcription of various target genes (Chap. 317). There is growing evidence that ERs also act through nonclassic mechanisms to alter signal transduction, independent of receptor binding to DNA. ERs have specific tissue site expression and bind various estrogens with different affinities, thereby conferring selective actions. The relatively promiscuous binding of synthetic and environmental estrogens by the ER has allowed the development of selective estrogen receptor modulators (SERMs), such as tamoxifen and raloxifene.

PROGESTERONE Progesterone is the principal hormone secreted by the corpus luteum and is responsible for progestational effects, i.e., in-

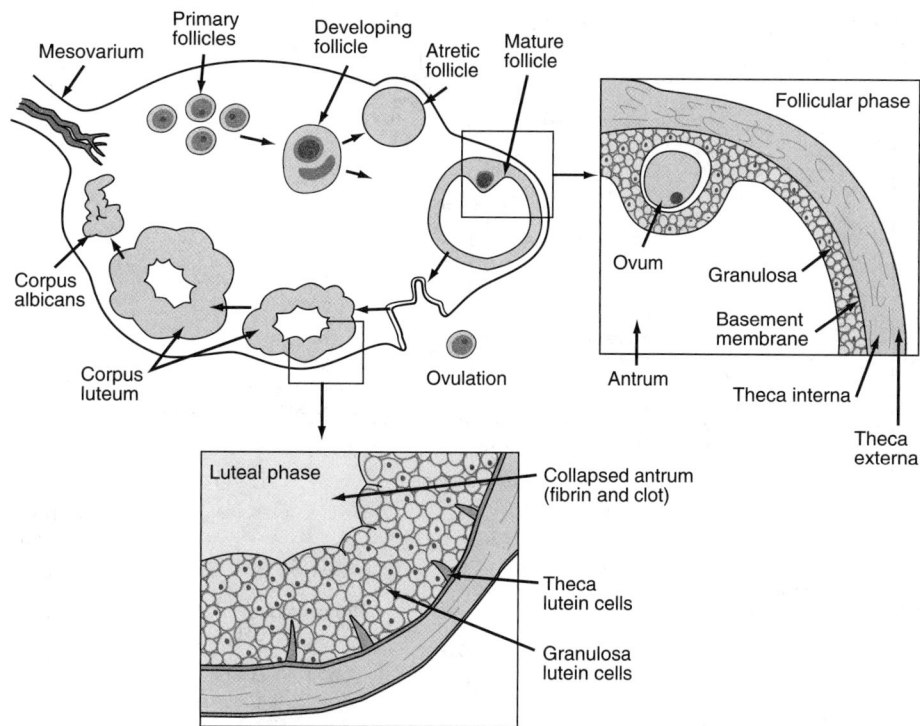

FIGURE 326-2 Developmental changes in the adult ovary during a complete 28-day cycle.

duction of secretory activity in the endometrium of the estrogen-primed uterus in preparation for implantation of the fertilized egg. Progesterone also induces a decidual reaction in endometrium. Other effects include inhibition of uterine contractions, an increase in the viscosity of cervical mucus, glandular development of the breasts, and an increase in basal body temperature (thermogenic effect).

ANDROGENS The ovary synthesizes a variety of 19-carbon steroids, including dehydroepiandrosterone, androstenedione, testosterone, and dihydrotestosterone, principally in stromal and thecal cells. The major ovarian 19-carbon steroid is androstenedione (Fig. 326-3), part of which is secreted into the plasma and part of which is converted to estrogen in granulosa cells or to testosterone in the interstitium. Androstenedione can also be converted to testosterone and estrogens in peripheral tissues. Only testosterone and dihydrotestosterone are true androgens that interact with the androgen receptor and induce virilizing signs in women (Chap. 44).

Other Hormones *Inhibin* is secreted in two forms (A and B) by the follicle and inhibits the release of FSH by the hypothalamic-pituitary unit. *Activin* is also secreted by the follicle and may enhance FSH secretion as well as having local effects on ovarian steroidogenesis. *Follistatin* is an activin-binding protein that attenuates the actions of activin and other members of the transforming growth factor (TGF)β family.

Some ovarian hormones play an uncertain role in human physiology. *Relaxin*, a polypeptide hormone produced by the human corpus luteum and by the decidua, causes softening of the cervix and loosening of the symphysis pubis in preparation for parturition in animals. *Oxytocin, vasopressin,* and other hypothalamic and pituitary hormones are also present in granulosa and/or luteal cells, but their function in these cells is unknown. Granulosa cells secrete *oocyte maturation inhibitor* (OMI), a factor that prevents premature ovulation. In addition, in the gonads of both sexes a *meiosis-inducing substance* triggers the onset of meiosis, an event that occurs earlier in ovarian than in testicular development. Local growth factors [including insulin-like growth factors (IGFs) 1 and 2 and TGFα and -β] may also influence steroid secretion by the ovary.

THE NORMAL MENSTRUAL CYCLE The menstrual cycle is divided into a follicular or proliferative phase and a luteal, or secretory, phase (Fig.

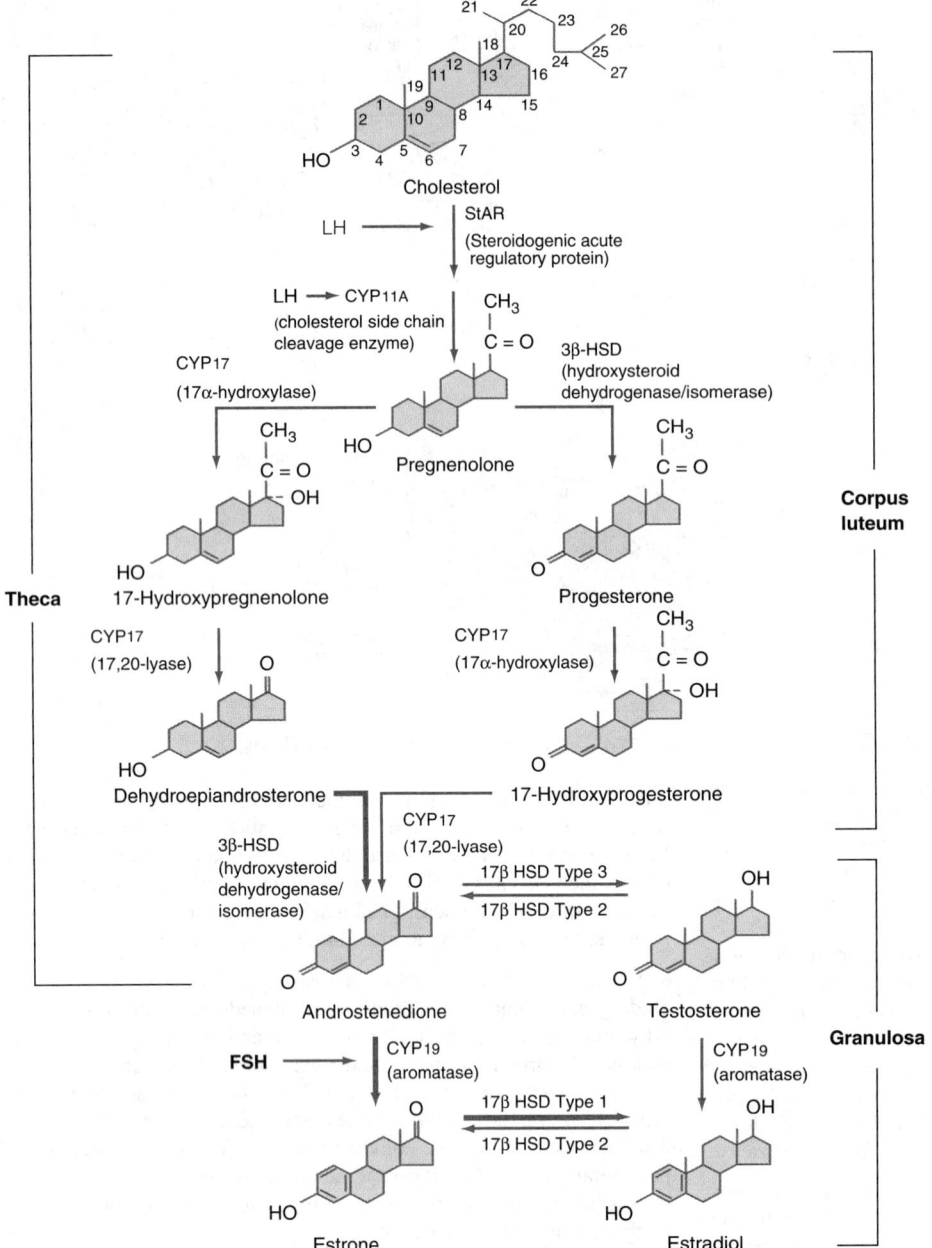

FIGURE 326-3 The principal pathway of steroid hormone biosynthesis in the ovary. The major enzyme complements for the corpus luteum, stroma, and granulosa cells are shown by the brackets; as a consequence, these cells produce predominantly progesterone and 17-OH progesterone, androgen, and estrogen, respectively. The major sites of action of luteinizing hormone (LH) and follicle-stimulating hormone (FSH) in mediating this pathway are shown in the horizontal arrows. The thin arrow emphasizes that the metabolism of 17-hydroxyprogesterone is limited in the human ovary. 17β HSD, 17β-hydroxysteroid dehydrogenase.

acterized by anovulation) occur at menarche and near the onset of menopause. At the end of a cycle, plasma levels of estrogen and progesterone fall and circulating levels of FSH increase. Under the influence of FSH, follicular recruitment results in development of the follicle that will be dominant during the next cycle.

After the onset of menses, follicular development continues, but FSH levels decrease. Approximately 8 to 10 days prior to the midcycle LH surge, plasma estradiol levels begin to rise as the result of estradiol formation by the granulosa cells of the dominant follicle. During the second half of the follicular phase, LH levels also begin to rise (owing to positive feedback). Just before ovulation, estradiol secretion reaches a peak and then falls. Immediately thereafter, a further rise in the plasma level of LH mediates the final maturation of the follicle, followed by follicular rupture and ovulation 16 to 23 h after the LH peak. The rise in LH is accompanied by a smaller increase in the level of plasma FSH, the physiologic significance of which is unclear. The plasma progesterone level also begins to rise just prior to midcycle and facilitates the positive feedback action of estradiol on LH secretion.

At the onset of the luteal phase, plasma gonadotropins decrease and plasma progesterone increases. A secondary rise in estrogens causes further gonadotropin suppression. Near the end of the luteal phase, progesterone and estrogen levels fall, and FSH levels begin to rise to initiate the development of the next follicle (usually in the contralateral ovary) and the next menstrual cycle. Inhibin A levels are low in the follicular phase but reach a peak in the luteal phase. Inhibin B levels, in contrast, are increased in the follicular phase and low in the luteal phase.

The endometrium lining the uterine cavity undergoes marked alterations in response to the changing plasma levels of ovarian hormones (Fig. 326-4). Concurrent with the decrease in plasma estrogen and progesterone and the decline of corpus luteum function in the late luteal phase, intense vasospasm occurs in the spiral arterioles supplying blood to the endometrium,

326-4). The secretion of FSH and LH is fundamentally under negative feedback control by ovarian steroids (particularly estradiol) and by inhibin (which selectively suppresses FSH), but the response of gonadotropins to different levels of estradiol varies. FSH secretion is inhibited progressively as estrogen levels increase—typical negative feedback. In contrast, LH secretion is suppressed maximally by sustained low levels of estrogen and is enhanced by a rising level of estradiol—positive feedback. Feedback of estrogen involves both the hypothalamus and pituitary. Negative feedback suppresses GnRH and inhibits gonadotropin production. Positive feedback is associated with an increased frequency of GnRH secretion and enhanced pituitary sensitivity to GnRH.

The length of the menstrual cycle is defined as the time from the onset of one menstrual bleeding episode to onset of the next. In women of reproductive age, the cycle averages 28 ± 3 days and the mean duration of flow is 4 ± 2 days. Longer menstrual cycles (usually char-

causing ischemic necrosis, endometrial desquamation, and bleeding. This vasospasm is caused by locally synthesized prostaglandins. The onset of bleeding marks the first day of the menstrual cycle. By the fourth to fifth day, the endometrium is thin. During the proliferative phase, glandular growth of the endometrium is mediated by estrogen. After ovulation, increased progesterone levels lead to further thickening of the endometrium, but the rapid growth slows. The endometrium then enters the secretory phase, characterized by tortuosity of the glands, curling of the spiral arterioles, and glandular secretion. As corpus luteum function begins to wane in the absence of conception, the sequence of events leading to menstruation is again set into action.

Biphasic changes in basal body temperature are characteristic of the ovulatory cycle and are mediated by alterations in progesterone levels (Fig. 326-4). An increase in basal body temperature by 0.3 to 0.5°C begins after ovulation, persists during the luteal phase, and returns to the normal baseline (36.2 to 36.4°C) after the onset of the subsequent menses.

MENOPAUSE

The *menopause* is defined as the final episode of menstrual bleeding in women. Menopause is the consequence of exhaustion of ovarian follicles, a process that begins during fetal development. The median age of women at the time of cessation of menstrual bleeding is 50 to 51 years. Preceding the menopause, the pattern of menstrual cycles is variable, but the interval between menses usually becomes shorter, as follicular recruitment is hastened by increases in FSH. Day 3 FSH and 17β-estradiol (E_2) levels are often elevated. Ovulatory cycles continue for some period of time, then anovulation becomes common.

The ovaries of postmenopausal women are small and wrinkled, and the residual cells are predominantly stromal. Estrogen and androgen levels in plasma are reduced but not absent. Before the menopause, plasma androstenedione is derived almost equally from the adrenals and the ovaries; after menopause, the ovarian contribution ceases so that the plasma levels of androstenedione fall by 50%. However, the menopausal ovary continues to secrete testosterone, presumably formed in stromal cells. After menopause, extraglandular estrogen formation is the major pathway for estrogen synthesis. Because adipose tissue is a major site of extraglandular estrogen production, peripheral estrogen formation may actually be enhanced in obese postmenopausal women. The predominant estrogen formed is estrone rather than estradiol. →*For discussion of the management of menopause, see Chap. 327.*

LABORATORY AND CLINICAL ASSESSMENT OF HORMONAL STATUS

The hormonal status of women can usually be assessed by history and physical examination. In general, the presence of secondary sexual characteristics such as normal female breast development indicates adequate estrogen secretion in the past, and the presence of regular, predictable, cyclic menses implies that ovulation and the production of gonadotropins, estrogen, progesterone, and androgens are adequate and that the outflow tract is intact. Such a history may be more valuable than laboratory tests in evaluating ovarian hormone status. However, laboratory tests provide valuable ancillary information in the evaluation of women with endocrine dysfunction or infertility (Chap. 45).

PITUITARY GONADOTROPINS

Plasma gonadotropins are assessed by immunoassay. Because both FSH and LH are secreted in a pulsatile manner, the results obtained from a single serum sample may be difficult to interpret. Moreover, the values vary widely during the menstrual cycle, particularly at the time of the midcycle gonadotropin surge. Consequently, plasma gonadotropin measurements are of greatest use in evaluating women with suspected ovarian failure and in supporting the diagnosis of polycystic ovarian syndrome (PCOS) or hypogonadotropic hypogonadism. FSH levels that are persistently >40 IU/L are diagnostic of ovarian failure, and an LH value <0.8 IU/L suggests hypogonadotropic hypogonadism. In practice, however, gonadotropin values may be equivocal and must be interpreted in the context of other historic, physical, and laboratory findings.

OVARIAN HORMONES

ESTROGEN The presence of normal secondary sexual characteristics implies that estrogen production was adequate in the past. The current estrogen status can be estimated by pelvic examination. The presence of a moist, rugated vagina with copious, clear, thin cervical mucus that

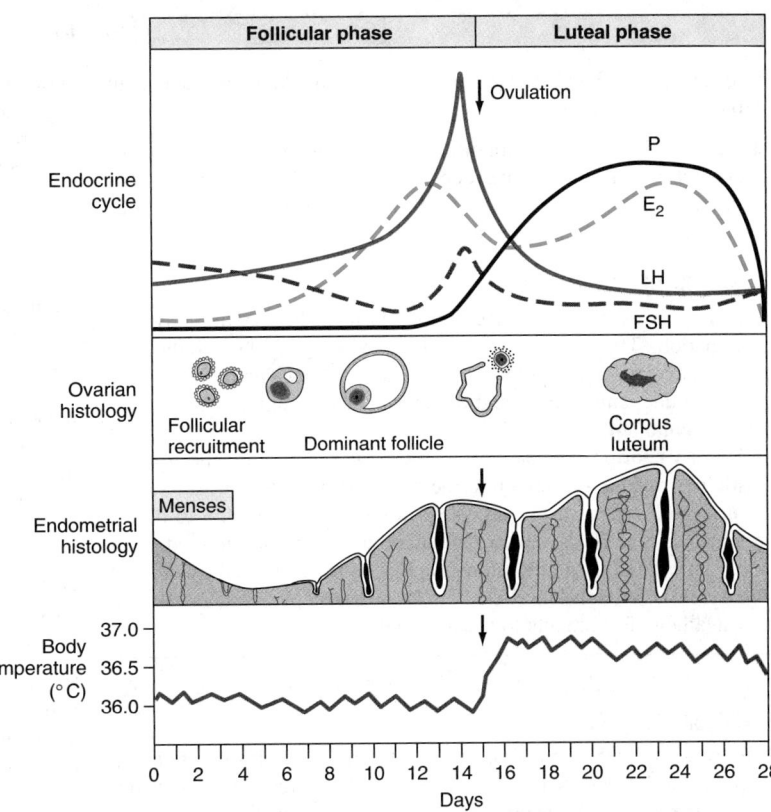

FIGURE 326-4 The hormonal, ovarian, endometrial, and basal body temperature changes and relationships throughout the normal menstrual cycle.

can be stretched and that exhibits arborization or ferning when spread on a slide is strong evidence of adequate estrogen production. Cytologic demonstration of mature vaginal epithelial cells and abundant cornified squamous epithelial cells with pyknotic nuclei confirms the presence of adequate estrogen levels.

The progesterone-withdrawal test provides a functional assessment of the endometrium, outflow tract, and estrogen status. If menses appear within a week to 10 days after the end of a trial of medroxyprogesterone acetate (10 mg by mouth once or twice a day for 5 days) or after a single intramuscular injection of progesterone (100 mg), then prior estrogen priming was adequate to allow withdrawal bleeding.

Owing to its variable level in plasma during the normal cycle and the difficulty of estimating the day of the cycle in women with abnormal cycles, the measurement of estrogen levels in plasma or urine is of little use in the routine assessment of estrogen status. Measurement of plasma estradiol is useful during attempts to induce ovulation with gonadotropins to prevent the development of the ovarian hyperstimulation syndrome and is used along with ultrasound assessment to monitor follicular growth in women during in vitro fertilization.

PROGESTERONE Cyclic, predictable menses also imply that adequate progesterone is secreted during the luteal phase of the menstrual cycle. Assessment of progesterone is useful to detect ovulation and to evaluate the adequacy of the luteal phase in infertile women. Several functional assays of progesterone can be used. The least expensive and most useful is the daily measurement of basal body temperature throughout a cycle. Owing to the thermogenic properties of progesterone, a normal biphasic monthly curve showing a temperature elevation lasting for approximately 2 weeks after ovulation is a valid indication of progesterone secretion during the luteal phase (Fig. 326-4). The presence of viscous cervical mucus that does not stretch or fern and of predominantly intermediate cells on vaginal cytology or demonstration of a secretory epithelium in an endometrial biopsy during the luteal phase on days 20 to 22 of the cycle provides additional assessment of progesterone secretion. In addition, plasma progesterone can be measured to assess the function of the corpus luteum; a level

$> 10 \mu$mol/L (> 3 ng/mL) suggests successful ovulation and adequate corpus luteum function.

ANDROGEN Under normal conditions, the ovary secretes androstenedione, testosterone, and dehydroepiandrosterone. In conditions of androgen excess, hirsutism and/or virilization are common. The evaluation of androgen excess is discussed in Chap. 44.

DIAGNOSIS OF PREGNANCY

Pregnancy is usually recognized on the basis of history and physical examination. That is, a woman with previously cyclic, predictable menses develops amenorrhea accompanied by breast tenderness, malaise, lassitude, and nausea, and on physical examination the uterus is soft and enlarged.

Human chorionic gonadotropin (hCG) is secreted by the trophoblastic cells of the placenta into the maternal plasma and excreted in the urine. Plasma or urine assays of hCG make it possible to detect pregnancies 8 to 10 days after ovulation, before the first missed menstrual period and long before pregnancy can be diagnosed by clinical assessments. Sensitive and specific hCG-based pregnancy tests are now available for patients to use at home.

DISORDERS OF OVARIAN FUNCTION

PREPUBERTAL YEARS

Puberty is said to be *precocious* if breast budding begins before age 8 or if menarche occurs before age 9. Those disorders in which the developing sexual characteristics are appropriate for the genetic and gonadal sex—i.e., feminization in girls or virilization in boys—are termed *isosexual precocity*, whereas *heterosexual precocity* occurs when sexual characteristics are not in accord with the genetic sex, namely, virilization in girls or feminization in boys. Pubertal disorders of boys are described in Chap. 325.

ISOSEXUAL PRECOCIOUS PUBERTY Isosexual precocious puberty in girls can be divided into three major categories (Table 326-1).

True Precocious Puberty True precocious puberty (gonadotropin-dependent) is characterized by an early but otherwise normal sequence of pubertal development, including increased secretion of gonadotropins and ovulatory menstrual cycles. Constitutional or idiopathic precocious puberty accounts for 90% of cases. The disorder is more common in girls than boys. No cause for the premature maturation of the central nervous system—hypothalamic-pituitary axis can be identified, and the diagnosis is confirmed by finding an adult pattern of LH and FSH release on a GnRH stimulation test. Premature appearance of secondary sexual characteristics and of ovulatory cycles with the accompa-

TABLE 326-1 *Differential Diagnosis of Sexual Precocity*

I. Isosexual precocity
  A. True precocious puberty
    1. Constitutional
    2. Organic brain disease
    3. Congenital adrenal hyperplasia
  B. Precocious pseudopuberty
    1. Ovarian tumors
    2. Adrenal tumors
    3. McCune-Albright syndrome
    4. Hypothyroidism
    5. Russell-Silver syndrome
    6. Estrogen-containing medications
  C. Incomplete sexual precocity
    1. Premature thelarche
    2. Premature adrenarche
    3. Premature pubarche
II. Heterosexual precocity
  A. Ovarian tumors
  B. Adrenal tumors
  C. Congenital adrenal hyperplasia

nying risk of fertility may cause significant emotional disturbance. Therefore, prompt initiation of therapy is imperative. GnRH analogues suppress gonadotropins and inhibit estrogen synthesis, thereby blocking precocious puberty; they may also prevent premature closure of the epiphyses and the resulting short stature.

About 10% of cases are due to organic brain diseases, including brain tumors (hypothalamic gliomas, astrocytomas, ependymomas, germinomas, and hamartomas), encephalitis, meningitis, hydrocephalus, head injury, tuberous sclerosis, and neurofibromatosis. It is essential to distinguish this group of patients from those with the idiopathic disorder, and patients whose disorder is designated as idiopathic occasionally prove to have such tumors. Most patients with organic lesions serious enough to cause precocious puberty have obvious neurologic signs and symptoms. Evaluation of all patients with precocious puberty should include, at a minimum, computed tomography (CT) or magnetic resonance imaging (MRI) of the brain. The success of treatment depends on the nature of the lesion, but surgical and radiation treatment of well-localized tumors is occasionally successful.

A rare cause of isosexual precocity is congenital adrenal hyperplasia due to 21-hydroxylase deficiency in girls when treatment has been delayed until 4 to 8 years of age (Chap. 321). After initiation of glucocorticoid replacement, such individuals may undergo isosexual precocious puberty.

Precocious Pseudopuberty Precocious pseudopuberty (gonadotropin-independent) occurs when girls undergo feminization as a consequence of enhanced estrogen formation but do not ovulate or develop cyclic menses. Ovarian cysts or tumors that secrete estrogen (granulosa-theca cell tumors) are the most frequent cause of precocious pseudopuberty. Granulosa-theca cell tumors associated with intestinal polyps and pigmentation of the mucous membranes occur in the Peutz-Jeghers syndrome. Other ovarian tumors that secrete estrogens (or androgens that can be converted to estrogens at extraglandular sites) include dysgerminomas, teratomas, cystadenomas, and ovarian carcinomas (Chap. 83). Ovarian tumors can usually be detected by rectoabdominal examination or by ultrasound, CT, MRI, and/or laparoscopy. Ovarian teratomas and choriocarcinomas and other carcinomas that secrete hCG do not cause precocious puberty in girls unless they also secrete estrogen (hCG or LH in the absence of FSH does not induce ovarian estrogen production). Rarely, feminizing tumors of the adrenal cause isosexual precocious puberty by direct formation of estrogens or by secretion of weak androgens, which are converted to estrogens in extraglandular tissues. The *McCune-Albright syndrome* (polyostotic fibrous dysplasia) is due to an activating mutation in the G protein, $G_{s\alpha}$, that occurs during embryogenesis, leading to a mosaic pattern of expression in various tissues. It is characterized by café au lait spots, cystic fibrous dysplasia of bones, and sexual precocity. In the ovary, the $G_{s\alpha}$ mutation mimics the action of FSH, leading to autonomous follicle development and estrogen formation. Occasionally, this disorder leads to true precocious puberty. *Primary hypothyroidism* is occasionally associated with enhanced secretion of FSH, inducing ovarian estrogen secretion. High levels of thyroid-stimulating hormone (TSH) caused by hypothyroidism may also stimulate the FSH receptor. The *Russell-Silver syndrome*, or congenital asymmetry, is associated with short stature and precocious feminization. *Estrogen-containing medications*, including use of estrogen-containing creams for diaper rash or the ingestion of meat from estrogen-treated animals or poultry or of any estrogen by mouth, can cause this disorder.

Incomplete Isosexual Precocity This term is used to describe the premature development of a single pubertal event and encompasses several entities. Breast budding before age 7 (*premature thelarche*) without other evidence of estrogen secretion and without premature bone maturation is believed to be due to a transient increase in estrogen secretion or to increased sensitivity to the small amounts of circulating estrogens formed before puberty. Usually, the disorder is self-limited and resolves spontaneously. Occasionally, axillary hair and/or pubic hair (*premature adrenarche* and *premature pubarche*) appear without any other secondary sexual development. The phenomenon is associated with adrenal androgen secretion in the range of normal puberty and can be distinguished from syndromes of virilization by the absence of clitoromegaly. It requires no treatment, and patients enter puberty at about the average time.

HETEROSEXUAL PRECOCITY Virilization in a prepubertal female is usually due to congenital adrenal hyperplasia or to androgen secretion by an ovarian or adrenal tumor. The manifestations of virilization are described in Chap. 44. Virilization in girls with congenital adrenal hyperplasia usually occurs in a background of variable sexual ambiguity (Chap. 328).

EVALUATION OF SEXUAL PRECOCITY The evaluation of sexual precocity involves a careful history and physical examination, including rectoabdominal examination, abdominal sonography, determination of bone age, and GnRH stimulation test, and measurement of thyroid hormones, TSH, and gonadotropins (and androgen or estrogen levels when appropriate). MRI and/or CT scans should be obtained if a neurologic disorder is suspected and no evidence of an ovarian or adrenal tumor is found.

REPRODUCTIVE YEARS

DISORDERS OF THE MENSTRUAL CYCLE ■ Abnormal Uterine Bleeding Between menarche and the menopause, almost every woman experiences one or more episodes of abnormal uterine bleeding, here defined as any bleeding pattern that differs in frequency, duration, or amount from the pattern observed during a normal menstrual cycle. In normal women, the average menstrual cycle is 28 ± 3 days, the mean duration of menstrual flow is 4 ± 2 days, and the average blood loss is 35 to 80 mL. A variety of descriptive terms (such as *menorrhagia, metrorrhagia,* and *menometrorrhagia*) have been used to characterize patterns of abnormal uterine bleeding. A more logical approach is to divide abnormal uterine bleeding into those patterns associated with ovulatory cycles and those associated with anovulatory cycles.

Ovulatory Cycles Normal menstrual bleeding with ovulatory cycles is spontaneous, regular, cyclic, and predictable and is frequently associated with discomfort (*dysmenorrhea*). Deviations from this pattern associated with cycles that are still regular and predictable are most often due to organic disease of the outflow tract. For example, regular but prolonged and excessive bleeding episodes unassociated with bleeding dyscrasias (hypermenorrhea or menorrhagia) can result from abnormalities of the uterus such as submucous leiomyomas, adenomyosis, or endometrial polyps. Regular, cyclic, predictable menstruation characterized by spotting or light bleeding is termed *hypomenorrhea* and is due to obstruction of the outflow tract as from intrauterine synechiae or scarring of the cervix. Intermenstrual bleeding between episodes of regular, ovulatory menstruation is also often due to cervical or endometrial lesions. An exception to the association between organic disease and abnormal uterine bleeding is the occurrence of regular menstruation more frequently than 21 days apart (*polymenorrhea*). Such cycles may be a normal variant.

Anovulatory Cycles Dysfunctional uterine bleeding refers to bleeding that is unpredictable with respect to amount, onset, and duration and is usually painless. This disorder is not due to abnormalities of the uterus but rather to chronic anovulation and occurs when there is interruption of the normal sequence of follicular and luteal phases under the influence of a dominant follicle and its resulting corpus luteum. As discussed above, uterine bleeding in ovulatory cycles occurs because of progesterone withdrawal and requires that the endometrium first be primed with estrogen. (When castrates or postmenopausal women are given progesterone, withdrawal bleeding usually does not occur.)

Dysfunctional uterine bleeding can occur in women who have a transient disruption of the synchronous hypothalamic-pituitary-ovarian patterns necessary for ovulatory cycles, most often at the extremes of the reproductive life—in the early menarche and in the perimenopausal period—but also after temporary stress or intercurrent illness.

Primary dysfunctional uterine bleeding can result from three disorders.

1. *Estrogen withdrawal bleeding* occurs when estrogen is given to a castrated or postmenopausal woman and then withdrawn. As in other types of dysfunctional uterine bleeding, this form of menstrual bleeding is usually painless.
2. *Estrogen breakthrough bleeding* occurs when there is continuous estrogen stimulation of the endometrium not interrupted by cyclic progesterone secretion and withdrawal. This is the most common type of dysfunctional uterine bleeding and is usually due to anovulation associated with chronic acyclic estrogen production, as in women with PCOS. Such women may have histories of irregular, unpredictable menses; oligomenorrhea; or amenorrhea (see below). Alternatively, estrogen breakthrough bleeding can occur in hypogonadal women given estrogens chronically rather than intermittently and in women with estrogen-secreting tumors of the ovary. Estrogen breakthrough bleeding may be profuse and is unpredictable with respect to duration, amount of flow, and time of occurrence. The endometrium is typically thin because its repair between episodes of bleeding is incomplete.
3. *Progesterone breakthrough bleeding* occurs in the presence of abnormally high ratios of progesterone to estrogen, i.e., in women using continuous low-dose oral contraceptives.

The approach to a patient with dysfunctional uterine bleeding begins with a careful history of menstrual patterns and prior hormonal therapy. Since not all urogenital tract bleeding is from the uterus, rectal, bladder, and vaginal or cervical sources must be excluded by physical examination. If the bleeding is from the uterus, a pregnancy-related disorder such as abortion or ectopic pregnancy must be ruled out.

℞ TREATMENT

Once the diagnosis of dysfunctional uterine bleeding is established, a rational approach to management is as follows: During a first episode of dysfunctional bleeding, it is reasonable to observe the patient without intervention, provided the bleeding is not copious and no evidence of bleeding dyscrasia is present. If bleeding is moderately severe, control can be achieved with relatively high dose estrogen oral contraceptives for 3 weeks. Alternatively, a regimen of three or four low-dose oral contraceptive pills per day for 1 week followed by tapering to the usual dosage for up to 3 weeks is also effective. If uterine bleeding is more severe, hospitalization, bed rest, and intramuscular injections of estradiol valerate (10 mg) and hydroxyprogesterone caproate (500 mg) or intravenous or intramuscular conjugated estrogens (25 mg) usually control the bleeding. After initial treatment, iron replacement should be instituted, and recurrence can be prevented by cyclic oral contraceptives for 2 to 3 months (or more if pregnancy is not desired). Alternatively, menses can be induced every 2 to 3 months with medroxyprogesterone acetate, 10 mg taken orally once or twice a day for 10 days. If hormone therapy fails to control uterine bleeding, an endometrial biopsy, hysteroscopy, or dilatation and curettage may be required for diagnosis and therapy. Indeed, uterine sampling should be performed prior to hormone therapy in women at risk for endometrial cancer (e.g., in women who are approaching the age of menopause or who are massively obese); endometrial cancer is rare in ovulatory women of reproductive age.

Amenorrhea An acceptable definition of amenorrhea is failure of menarche by age 15, irrespective of the presence or absence of secondary sexual characteristics, or the absence of menstruation for 6 months in a woman with previous periodic menses. However, women who do not fulfill these criteria should be evaluated if (1) the patient and/or her family are greatly concerned, (2) no breast development has occurred by age 13, or (3) any sexual ambiguity or virilization is present. Amenorrhea is commonly categorized as either primary (the woman has never menstruated) or secondary (when menstruation has been present for a variable period of time in the past and has ceased). How-ever, some disorders can cause either primary or secondary amenor-rhea. For example, most women with gonadal dysgenesis have primary amenorrhea, but some have a few follicles and ovulate for short periods so that pregnancy occurs rarely. Furthermore, patients with chronic anovulation (PCOS) usually have secondary amenorrhea but on oc-casion have primary amenorrhea. For these reasons, categorization of amenorrhea into primary and secondary types is less helpful than a classification based on the underlying physiologic derangements: (1) anatomic defects, (2) ovarian failure, and (3) chronic anovulation with or without estrogen present.

ANATOMIC DEFECTS Anatomic or structural defects of the genital tract can preclude menstrual bleeding. Starting from the caudal end of the fe-male genital tract, labial fusion is often associated with disorders of sexual development, particularly female pseudohermaphroditism (con-genital adrenal hyperplasia or exposure to maternal androgens in utero; Chap. 328). Congenital defects of the vagina, imperforate hymen, and transverse vaginal septae can also cause amenorrhea. These women frequently have accumulation of menstrual blood behind the obstruc-tion and may have cyclic, predictable episodes of abdominal pain.

More severe müllerian anomalies include müllerian agenesis (the Mayer-Rokitansky-Küster-Hauser syndrome), second in frequency only to gonadal dysgenesis as a cause of primary amenorrhea. It can be caused by mutations in the genes encoding anti-müllerian hormone (AMH) or its receptor (AMHR). Women with this syndrome have a 46,XX karyotype, female secondary sex characteristics, and normal ovarian function, including cyclic ovulation, but have absence or hy-poplasia of the vagina. The uterus usually consists of only rudimentary bicornuate cords, but if the uterus contains endometrium, cyclic ab-dominal pain and accumulation of blood may occur, as in other forms of outlet obstruction. One-third of women with this syndrome have abnormalities of the urogenital tract, and one-tenth have skeletal anom-alies, usually involving the spine. The major diagnostic problem is distinguishing müllerian agenesis from complete androgen insensitiv-ity syndrome, in which 46,XY genetic males with testes differentiate as phenotypic women but with a blind vaginal pouch and no uterus (Chap. 328). Androgen insensitivity can be diagnosed by demonstrat-ing a male level of serum testosterone and a 46,XY karyotype, whereas demonstration of a 46,XX karyotype, the biphasic basal body temper-ature curve characteristic of ovulation, and elevated levels of proges-terone during the luteal phase establish the diagnosis of müllerian agenesis.

Other abnormalities of the uterus that cause amenorrhea include obstruction due to scarring or stenosis of the cervix, often as a result of surgery, electrocautery, laser therapy, or cryosurgery. Such destruc-tion of the endometrium (Asherman's syndrome) usually follows vig-orous curettage for postpartum hemorrhage or after therapeutic abor-tion complicated by infection. This diagnosis is confirmed by hysterosalpingography or by direct visual examination of the endo-metrial scarring or synechiae using a hysteroscope.

Treatment of disorders of the outflow tract is surgical.

OVARIAN FAILURE Primary ovarian failure is associated with elevated plasma gonadotropin levels and can result from several causes. The most frequent cause is *gonadal dysgenesis*, in which the germ cells are absent and the ovary is replaced by a fibrous streak (Chap. 328). A 45,X karyotype is found in about half of women with this disorder, and most have somatic defects, including short stature, webbed neck, shield chest, and cardiovascular defects, collectively termed the *Turner phenotype*. The remainder of women with X chromosome abnormal-ities have chromosomal mosaicism with or without associated struc-tural abnormalities of the X. Approximately 90% of women with go-nadal dysgenesis due to partial or complete deletion of the X never have menstrual bleeding, and the remaining 10% have sufficient fol-licles to experience menses and, rarely, fertility; the menstrual and reproductive lives of such individuals are invariably brief.

One-tenth of individuals identified as having bilateral streak gonads have a normal 46,XX or 46,XY karyotype and are said to have *pure gonadal dysgenesis*. These individuals have either normal or above-average stature, owing to failure of estrogen-mediated epiphyseal clo-sure in the presence of a normal chromosomal constitution. Pure go-nadal dysgenesis does not constitute a phenotypic or chromosomally homogeneous disorder.

Other causes of ovarian failure and amenorrhea include deficiency of the *CYP17* gene that encodes 17α-hydroxylase and 17,20-lyase ac-tivities, premature ovarian failure, the resistant-ovary syndrome, and ovarian failure secondary to chemotherapy or radiation therapy for malignancy. *17α-Hydroxylase deficiency* is a rare, autosomal recessive disorder characterized by primary amenorrhea, sexual infantilism, and hypertension, the latter due to increased production of desoxycorti-costerone (DOC); women with *17,20-lyase deficiency* have primary amenorrhea and sexual infantilism with normal blood pressure. The diagnosis of *premature ovarian failure* or *premature menopause* ap-plies to women who cease menstruating before age 40. The ovaries in such women are similar to those of postmenopausal women, contain-ing few or no follicles as the result of accelerated follicular atresia. Premature ovarian failure due to ovarian antibodies may be one com-ponent of polyglandular failure, together with adrenal insufficiency, hypothyroidism, and other autoimmune disorders (Chap. 330). A rare form of ovarian failure is the *resistant-ovary syndrome*, in which the ovaries contain many follicles that are arrested in development prior to the antral stage, possibly because of resistance to the action of FSH in the ovary. A subset of these individuals have mutations in FSH or its receptor. To differentiate this disorder from the 46,XX variety of pure gonadal dysgenesis, which is also associated with sexual imma-turity, it is necessary to perform ovarian biopsy or genetic testing. Women with ovarian failure who desire pregnancy have been treated with hormone replacement and transfer of donor embryos to the uterine cavity or fallopian tubes.

℞ TREATMENT

In women with decreased estrogen production, whether due to ovarian dysfunction or to hypogonadotropic hypogonadism, treatment with cyclic estrogens should be instituted to induce the development and maintenance of female secondary sexual characteristics and to prevent osteoporosis. The most commonly used medications are conjugated estrogens (0.625 to 1.25 mg/d by mouth) together with medroxypro-gesterone acetate (2.5 mg/d or 5 to 10 mg during the last several days of monthly estrogen treatment to prevent development of endometrial hyperplasia). Alternatively, oral contraceptives may be given to pre-menopausal-age women (Chap. 45). Abnormal bleeding in women re-ceiving estrogen replacement mandates histologic evaluation of the endometrium.

Chronic Anovulation At least 80% or more of gynecologic endocrine disorders result from chronic anovulation. Women with chronic ano-vulation fail to ovulate spontaneously but may ovulate with appropri-ate therapy. The ovaries of such women do not secrete estrogen in a normal cyclic pattern. It is clinically useful to differentiate those women who produce enough estrogen to have withdrawal bleeding after progestogen therapy from those who do not; the latter often have hypothalamic-pituitary dysfunction.

CHRONIC ANOVULATION WITH ESTROGEN PRESENT This disorder is most com-monly caused by *polycystic ovarian syndrome*, which is characterized by infertility, hirsutism, obesity, insulin resistance, and amenorrhea or oligomenorrhea. When spontaneous uterine bleeding occurs in women with PCOS, it is unpredictable as to time of onset, duration, and amount; on occasion the bleeding can be severe.

PCOS, as originally described by Stein and Leventhal, was char-acterized by enlarged, polycystic ovaries, but it is now known to be associated with a variety of pathologic findings in the ovaries, only some of which result in enlargement and none of which are pathog-nomonic. The most common finding is a white, smooth, sclerotic ovary with a thickened capsule, multiple follicular cysts in various stages of atresia, a hyperplastic theca and stroma, and rare or absent corpora albicans. Other ovaries have hyperthecosis in which the ovarian stroma is hyperplastic and may contain lipid-laden luteal cells. Thus, the diagnosis of PCOS is a clinical one, based on the coexistence of chronic anovulation and varying degrees of androgen excess. The fundamental defect that causes PCOS is unknown, and it is likely to have several distinct causes.

In most women with PCOS, menarche occurs at the expected time, but oligomenorrhea ensues after a variable period. Signs of androgen excess (hirsutism) usually become evident soon after menarche. One scenario suggests that this disorder originates as an exaggerated adrenarche in obese girls (Fig. 326-5). The combination of elevated levels of adrenal androgens and obesity leads to increased formation of extraglandular estrogen. This estrogen exerts a positive feedback on LH secretion and negative feedback on FSH secretion, resulting in a ratio of LH to FSH levels in plasma that is characteristically greater than 2. The increased LH levels can then lead to hyperplasia of the ovarian stroma and theca cells and increased androgen production, which in turn provides more substrate for peripheral aromatization and perpetuates the chronic anovulation. In the advanced stage of the disorder, the ovary is the major site of androgen production, but the adrenal may continue to secrete excess androgen as well. Ovarian follicles from women with PCOS have low aromatase activity, but normal aromatase can be induced by treatment with FSH. An association exists between PCOS/hyperthecosis, virilization, acanthosis nigricans, and insulin resistance; in the ovary, insulin may interact via the insulin-like growth factor receptors to enhance androgen synthesis in insulin-resistant states. Women with PCOS have an increased incidence of impaired glucose tolerance and type 2 diabetes mellitus.

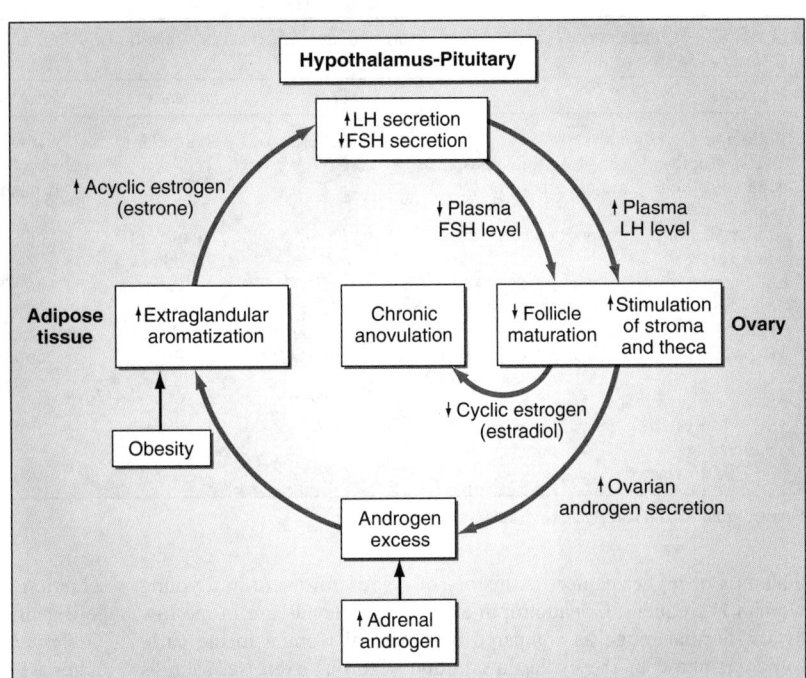

FIGURE 326-5 Proposed mechanism for the initiation and perpetuation of chronic anovulation in polycystic ovarian syndrome (PCOS). This cycle may be entered or initiated via adrenal androgen excess or obesity, both of which result in enhanced extraglandular formation of estrogens. The therapy of PCOS involves interruption of the cycle at any of several steps. *[From SSC Yen et al (eds), Reproductive Endocrinology. Philadelphia, Saunders, 1999; and from U Goebelmann, in Reproductive Endocrinology, Infertility, and Contraception, 2d ed, DR Mishell Jr, V Davajan (eds), Philadelphia, Davis, 1986.]*

℞ TREATMENT

Treatment of PCOS is directed toward interrupting the self-perpetuating cycle and can be accomplished in several ways, such as by decreasing ovarian androgen secretion (by wedge resection or the use of oral contraceptive agents), decreasing peripheral estrogen formation (by weight reduction), or enhancing FSH secretion [by administration of clomiphene, human menopausal gonadotropin (hMG), GnRH (gonadorelin) by portable infusion pump, or purified FSH (urofollitropin)]. The choice of therapy depends on the clinical findings and the needs of the patient. An attempt at weight reduction is appropriate in all who are obese. If the woman is not hirsute and does not desire pregnancy, periodic withdrawal menses can be induced with medroxyprogesterone acetate 10 days per month; such treatment prevents the development of endometrial hyperplasia. If the woman is hirsute and does not desire pregnancy, the ovarian (and possibly the adrenal) component of androgen production can be suppressed with combined estrogen-progestogen oral contraceptive agents. Combined oral contraceptives are also indicated if prolonged or excessive menstrual bleeding is present. Once androgen excess is controlled, treatment of previously existing hair growth by shaving, depilatories, or electrolysis may be indicated (Chap. 44). If pregnancy is desired, ovulation must be induced. Insulin-sensitizing drugs, such as metformin and the thiazolidinediones, improve fertility in women with PCOS. Clomiphene promotes ovulation in three-fourths of cases, or ovulation can be induced with hMG, urofollitropin, or gonadorelin (Chap. 45). Pretreatment with GnRH analogues prior to use of hMG, urofollitropin, or gonadorelin may improve the rates of ovulation and pregnancy. Women with PCOS are at increased risk of ovarian hyperstimulation after treatment with gonadotropins. They also experience increased rates of spontaneous abortion. An alternative therapy is ovarian drilling by laser or cautery performed at laparoscopy when hormonal therapy is not effective; however, the procedure is associated with a high incidence of ovarian adhesions.

Chronic anovulation with estrogen present may also occur with tumors of the ovary. These include granulosa-theca cell tumors, Brenner tumors, cystic teratomas, mucous cystadenomas, and Krukenberg tumors (Chap. 83). Such tumors can either secrete excess estrogen themselves or produce androgens that are aromatized in extraglandular sites. Chronic anovulation and the clinical features of PCOS result. Occasionally, areas of the ovary not involved with tumors show the characteristic histologic changes of PCOS. Other causes of chronic anovulation with estrogen present include adrenal production of excess androgen (usually adult-onset adrenal hyperplasia due to partial 21-hydroxylase deficiency) and hypothyroidism.

CHRONIC ANOVULATION WITH ESTROGEN ABSENT Women with chronic anovulation who have low or absent estrogen production and do not experience withdrawal bleeding after progestogen treatment usually have hypogonadotropic hypogonadism due to disease of either the pituitary or the central nervous system.

Isolated hypogonadotropic hypogonadism associated with defects of smell (olfactory bulb defects) is known as the *Kallmann syndrome* (Chap. 318), which is due to a single gene defect in the X-linked *KAL* gene. Affected women are sexually infantile and have a defect in the synthesis and/or release of GnRH. Hypothalamic lesions that impair GnRH production and cause hypogonadotropic hypogonadism include craniopharyngioma, germinoma (pinealoma), glioma, Hand-Schüller-Christian disease, teratomas, endodermal-sinus tumors, tuberculosis, sarcoidosis, and metastatic tumors that cause suppression or destruction of the hypothalamus. Central nervous system trauma and irradiation can also cause hypothalamic amenorrhea and deficiencies in secretion of growth hormone, adrenocorticotropic hormone (ACTH), vasopressin, and thyroid hormone. Rare, autosomal recessive defects in the GnRH receptor have also been described.

More commonly, gonadotropin deficiency leading to chronic anovulation is believed to arise from functional disorders of the hypo-

TABLE 326-2 *Incidence and Mode of Transmission of Single-Gene Mutations Associated with Reproductive Dysfunction in Women*

Phenotype	Gene	Incidence	Mode of Transmission
Kallmann's syndrome	KAL	1 in 50,000	X-linked
Gonadotropin-releasing hormone resistance	GNRHR	Rare	Autosomal recessive
Isolated follicle-stimulating hormone deficiency	FSHB	Rare	Autosomal recessive
Hypergonadotropic hypogonadal ovarian failure	FSHR	1 in 8300 (Finland)	Autosomal recessive
Luteinizing hormone resistance	LHR	Rare	Autosomal recessive
Congenital lipoid adrenal hyperplasia	STAR	Rare	Autosomal recessive
Galactosemia	GALT	1 in 187,000	Autosomal recessive
McCune-Albright syndrome	GNASI	Rare	Dominant postzygotic mutation
Aromatase deficiency	CYP19	Rare	Autosomal recessive
3β-Hydroxysteroid dehydrogenase type II deficiency	HSD3B2	Rare	Autosomal recessive
17α-Hydroxylase deficiency	CYP17	Rare	Autosomal recessive

Source: From Adashi and Hennebold, 1999, with permission.

thalamus or higher centers. A history of a stressful event in a young woman is frequent. Gonadotropin and estrogen levels are in the low to low-normal range as compared with normal women in the early follicular phase of the cycle. In addition, rigorous exercise, such as jogging or ballet, and diets that result in excessive weight loss may lead to chronic anovulation, particularly in girls with a history of prior menstrual irregularity. The amenorrhea in these women does not appear to be a result of weight loss alone but a combination of a decrease in body fat and chronic stress. An extreme form of weight loss with chronic anovulation occurs in anorexia nervosa (Chap. 65). In anorexia nervosa amenorrhea can precede, follow, or coincide with weight loss.

In addition, chronic debilitating diseases such as end-stage kidney disease, malignancy, inflammatory bowel disease, and malabsorption can lead to hypogonadotropic hypogonadism via a hypothalamic mechanism.

Treatment of chronic anovulation due to hypothalamic disorders includes ameliorating the stressful situation, decreasing exercise, and correcting weight loss, as appropriate. These women are susceptible to the development of osteoporosis; estrogen replacement therapy is recommended to induce and maintain normal secondary sexual characteristics and prevent bone loss in those who do not desire pregnancy, and gonadotropin or gonadorelin therapy is indicated when pregnancy is desired. When appropriate, therapy is directed at the primary disease of the hypothalamus.

Disorders of the pituitary can lead to the estrogen-deficient form of chronic anovulation by at least two mechanisms—direct interference with gonadotropin secretion by lesions that either obliterate or interfere with the gonadotrope cells (chromophobe adenomas, Sheehan's syndrome) or inhibition of gonadotropin secretion in association with excess prolactin (prolactinoma). *Pituitary tumors* may secrete no hormone, one hormone, or more than one hormone (Chap. 318). Prolactin levels are elevated in 50 to 70% of patients with pituitary tumors, either because of prolactin secretion by the tumor itself (in the case of prolactinomas) or because the tumor mass interferes with the normal hypothalamic inhibition of prolactin secretion.

Prolactin excess associated with low levels of LH and FSH constitutes a specific subtype of hypogonadotropic hypogonadism. One-tenth or more of amenorrheic women have increased levels of prolactin, and more than half of women with both galactorrhea and amenorrhea have elevated prolactin levels. The amenorrhea is most often associated with decreased or absent estrogen production, but prolactin-secreting tumors on occasion are associated with normal ovulatory menses or chronic anovulation with estrogen present. In the latter half of pregnancy, prolactin-secreting pituitary tumors may expand, leading to headaches, compression of the optic chiasm, bitemporal hemianopia, and blindness. Therefore, before inducing ovulation for the purposes of achieving pregnancy, it is mandatory to exclude the presence of a pituitary tumor. →*The evaluation, differential diagnosis, and management of hyperprolactinemia are described in Chap. 318.*

Large pituitary tumors such as null cell adenomas—whether or not hyperprolactinemia is present—are likely to be associated with deficiency of hormones in addition to gonadotropins (Chap. 318).

Craniopharyngiomas, which are thought to arise from remnants of Rathke's pouch, occur most frequently in the second decade of life and often extend into the suprasellar region. Many of these tumors calcify and can be diagnosed by conventional skull film or CT. Patients often present with sexual infantilism, delayed puberty, and amenorrhea due to gonadotropin deficiency; secretion of TSH, ACTH, growth hormone, and vasopressin may also be impaired.

Panhypopituitarism can be caused by mutations in transcription factors (Pit-1; Prop-1) involved in pituitary gland development, result from surgical or radiation treatment of pituitary adenomas, or develop after postpartum hemorrhage (Sheehan's syndrome) (Chap. 318). Table 326-2 outlines the incidence and mode of single gene mutations associated with reproductive dysfunction in women.

Evaluation of Amenorrhea A general scheme for the evaluation of women with amenorrhea is given in Fig. 326-6. On physical examination, attention should be given to three features: (1) the degree of maturation of the breasts, pubic and axillary hair, and external genitalia; (2) the current estrogen status; and (3) the presence or absence of a uterus. Pregnancy should be excluded in all women with amenorrhea; it is prudent to perform a suitable pregnancy screening test even when the history and physical examination are not suggestive. Once that is done, the cause of amenorrhea can frequently be diagnosed clinically. For example, Asherman's syndrome is suggested by a history of curettage in a woman who previously menstruated; in women with primary amenorrhea and sexual infantilism, the essential differential diagnosis is between gonadal dysgenesis and hypopituitarism; and the diagnosis of gonadal dysgenesis (Turner's syndrome) or of anatomic defects of the outflow tract (müllerian agenesis, testicular feminization, and cervical stenosis) is frequently suggested on the basis of physical findings. When a specific cause is suspected, it is appropriate to proceed directly to confirm the diagnosis (obtaining a chromosomal karyotype or measurement of plasma gonadotropins). It is also useful to measure serum prolactin and FSH levels during the initial evaluation.

Estrogen status is evaluated by determining if the vaginal mucosa is moist and rugated and if the cervical mucus can be stretched and shown to fern upon drying. If these criteria are indeterminate, a progestational challenge is indicated, most often the administration of 10 mg medroxyprogesterone acetate by mouth once or twice daily for 5 days or 100 mg progesterone in oil intramuscularly. (It should be emphasized that progestogen should never be administered until pregnancy is excluded.) If estrogen levels are adequate (and the outflow tract is intact), menstrual bleeding should occur within 1 week of ending the progestogen treatment. If withdrawal bleeding occurs, the diagnosis is chronic anovulation with estrogen present, usually caused by PCOS.

If no withdrawal bleeding or only minimal vaginal spotting occurs, the nature of the subsequent workup depends on the results of the initial prolactin assay. If plasma prolactin is elevated, or if galactorrhea is present, radiography of the pituitary should be undertaken. When the plasma prolactin level is normal in an anovulatory woman with estrogen absent and with elevated FSH levels, the diagnosis is ovarian failure. If the gonadotropins are in the low or normal range, the diagnosis is either hypothalamic-pituitary disorder or an anatomic defect of the outflow tract. As indicated previously, the diagnosis of outflow tract disorder is usually suspected or established on the basis of history and physical findings. When the physical findings are not clear-cut, it is useful to administer cyclic estrogen plus progestogen (1.25 mg oral conjugated estrogens per day for 3 weeks, with 10 mg medroxyprogesterone acetate added for the last 7 to 10 days of estrogen treatment), followed by 10 days of observation. If no bleeding occurs, the diagnosis of Asherman's syndrome or another anatomic defect of the outflow tract is confirmed by hysterosalpingography or hysteroscopy. If withdrawal bleeding occurs following the estrogen-progestogen combination, the diagnosis of chronic anovulation with estrogen absent (functional hypothalamic amenorrhea) is suggested. Radiologic evaluations of the pituitary-hypothalamic areas may be indicated in the latter cases—irrespective of the prolactin level—because of the risk of overlooking a pituitary-hypothalamic tumor and because the diagnosis of functional hypothalamic amenorrhea is one of exclusion.

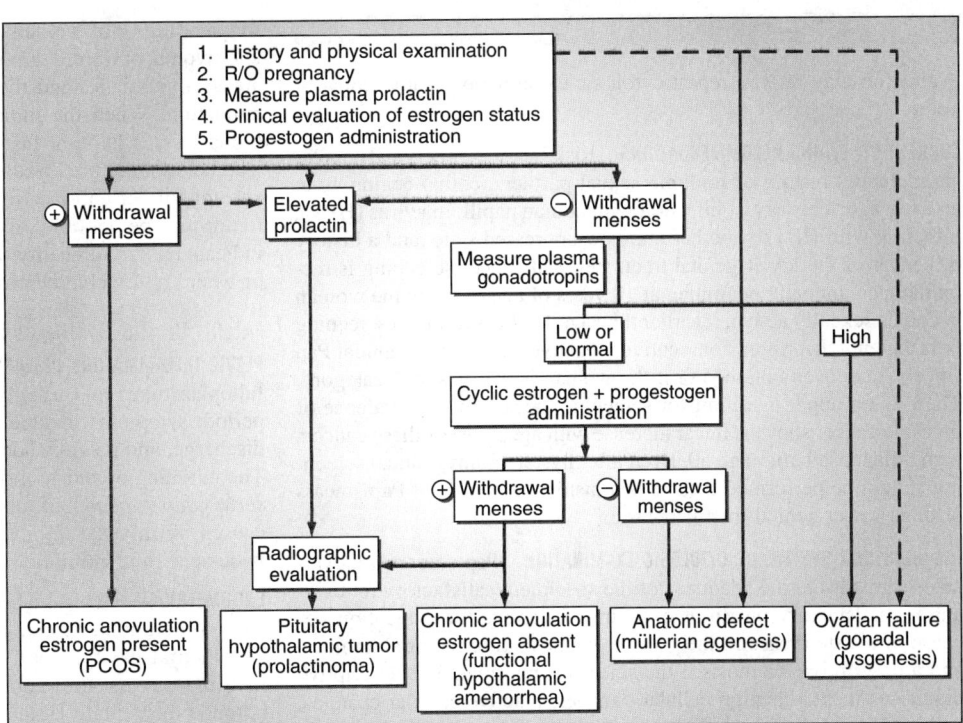

FIGURE 326-6 Flow diagram for the evaluation of women with amenorrhea. The most common diagnosis for each category is shown in parentheses. The dotted lines indicate that in some instances a correct diagnosis can be reached on the basis of history and physical examination alone. PCOS, polycystic ovarian syndrome.

INFERTILITY Infertility, the failure to become pregnant after 1 year of unprotected intercourse, affects approximately 10 to 15% of couples and is a common reason for seeking gynecologic assistance. Male factors account for at least 25% of infertility problems (Chap. 325). In women, failure of ovulation accounts for 40% of cases; pelvic factors, such as tubal disease or endometriosis, account for half. In 10 to 20% of infertile women no etiology is found. →*The evaluation and management of infertility are discussed in Chap. 45.*

PREGNANCY (See also Chap. 6) The possibility of pregnancy should be considered in all women of reproductive age who are evaluated for medical illness or considered for surgery. Procedures such as x-ray exposure, drugs, and anesthetics may be harmful to the developing fetus, and a variety of medical problems may worsen during pregnancy, including hypertension; diseases of the heart, lungs, kidney, and liver; and metabolic and endocrine disorders. Abnormal vaginal bleeding or amenorrhea during the reproductive years should prompt consideration of a complication of pregnancy, such as incomplete abortion, ectopic pregnancy, or trophoblastic disease (hydatidiform mole or choriocarcinoma). Women who present with these complications of pregnancy often have histories of abdominal pain and vaginal bleeding and may have evidence of intraabdominal hemorrhage.

Choriocarcinoma is a particular problem because of its protean manifestations. Half these malignancies follow pregnancies complicated by hydatidiform mole, and the remainder occur after spontaneous abortion, ectopic pregnancy, or normal deliveries. Patients may present with intraabdominal bleeding due to rupture of the uterus, liver, or ovary, with pulmonary manifestations (cough, hemoptysis, pleuritic pain, dyspnea, and respiratory failure) or gastrointestinal symptoms, usually chronic blood loss or melena. In addition, patients can present with cerebral metastases or renal involvement. The diagnosis can be established by demonstrating an elevated level of the β subunit of hCG in plasma. Treatment and cure are possible with chemotherapeutic agents (dactinomycin and/or methotrexate). →*The manifestations of choriocarcinoma in men are discussed in Chap. 82.*

OTHER DISORDERS OF THE FEMALE REPRODUCTIVE TRACT

VULVA

Most disorders of the vulva are a result of sexually transmitted diseases, most commonly syphilis (painless chancre), condylomata acuminata (venereal warts), and herpes vulvitis (painful ulcers; Chap. 115). All other lesions of the vulva, particularly in older women, must be biopsied. Early biopsy of cancer of the vulva is mandatory, because when it becomes symptomatic (pruritus and bleeding), it has often progressed to an advanced stage.

VAGINA

Infections of the vagina usually present as vaginal discharge and pruritus. The most frequent organisms are *Trichomonas*, *Candida albicans*, and *Gardnerella vaginalis* (Chap. 115). The diagnosis is made by microscopic examination of the discharge, and appropriate therapy can be instituted using vaginal or oral antibiotics.

Abnormalities of the vagina and cervix in female offspring of women given diethylstilbestrol during pregnancy include adenosis of the vagina and structural abnormalities of the vagina, cervix, and uterus; the risk of developing a rare vaginal cancer (adenocarcinoma, clear cell type) is increased (2 per 10,000 exposed women). Periodic examination of women at risk should begin at age 12 to 14, and reexamination should be done after any episode of abnormal bleeding.

CERVIX

Preinvasive lesions of the cervix (also known as *cervical intraepithelial neoplasia*) and invasive carcinoma of the cervix can be detected reliably by obtaining a Papanicolaou (Pap) smear.

EVALUATION OF THE PAP SMEAR The incidence of invasive cervical cancer has declined as a result of Pap smear screening. In the United States, approximately 2 to 3 million abnormal Pap smears are found each year. Most represent low-grade lesions but require appropriate follow-up. The follow-up of abnormal Pap smears requires an understanding of the Bethesda system for evaluating such smears (see below) and of the limitations of cytologic screening systems. Further evaluation may require repeat cytologic examination, colposcopy, or both.

CURRENT SCREENING RECOMMENDATIONS   Risk factors for cervical neoplasia include a history of multiple sexual partners, coitus beginning at an early age, a history of infection with human papilloma virus (HPV), infection with HIV or another immunosuppressed state, and a history of cancer of the lower genital tract. Cervical cancer screening is recommended annually beginning at 18 years of age or when the woman becomes sexually active, if earlier than age 18. Less frequent screening is sufficient when three consecutive, negative, satisfactory annual Pap smears have been obtained or if the woman is in a low-risk category. There is no upper age limit for screening, because the prevalence of invasive cancer shows a linear increase with age, most of these cancers being diagnosed after age 50. Even after hysterectomy, annual screening should be performed if there is a history of abnormal Pap smears or other lower genital tract neoplasia.

THE BETHESDA SYSTEM OF CYTOLOGIC EXAMINATION   Pap smears are evaluated in regard to the adequacy of the specimen (satisfactory for evaluation, satisfactory but limited, or unsatisfactory for evaluation because of a stated reason), the general diagnosis (normal or abnormal), and a descriptive diagnosis if the smear is abnormal. The descriptive diagnoses include benign cellular changes, reactive cellular changes, and epithelial cell abnormalities, the latter including (1) atypical squamous cells of undetermined significance (ASCUS); (2) low-grade squamous intraepithelial lesion (LSIL), which is further categorized to include HPV infection, cervical intraepithelial neoplasia (CIN 1), and high-grade squamous intraepithelial lesion (HSIL), which is itself subdivided into CIN 2 and CIN 3); and (3) squamous cell carcinoma.

GUIDELINES FOR THE MANAGEMENT OF WOMEN WITH ABNORMAL PAP SMEARS
For ASCUS smears that are unqualified or suggest a reactive process, a repeat smear should be obtained every 4 to 6 months for 2 years until three consecutive negative smears have been obtained. For ASCUS smears that are unqualified but have severe inflammation, any specific cause should be treated, and the smear should be repeated in 2 to 3 months; because invasive carcinoma can be obscured by severe inflammation, clinical evaluation is mandatory. For postmenopausal women not using hormone replacement, a course of topical estrogen should be applied before the test is repeated. For LSIL smears, the Pap test is repeated every 4 to 6 months for 2 years until three consecutive negative smears have been obtained; treatment of HPV is of no established benefit, and there is a high rate of regression of LSIL, so that in compliant, low-risk individuals, the outcome is usually favorable. If LSIL is persistent, colposcopy with directed biopsy is performed, and endocervical curettage is undertaken if a specific diagnosis is made by biopsy. Cervical cone biopsy or loop electrosurgical excision procedures are performed for higher-grade lesions such as HSIL. If cervical cancer is diagnosed by biopsy, clinical staging is performed, and the patient is treated with radiation therapy or surgery.

UTERUS

Only 40% of cases of endometrial adenocarcinoma are detected by Pap smear. In women at high risk for endometrial carcinoma (because of obesity, a history of chronic anovulatory cycles, diabetes mellitus, hypertension, or unopposed estrogen treatment), yearly endometrial sampling should be performed. Measurement of endometrial thickness by sonography can indicate which patients are at risk for endometrial pathology. Endometrial thickness <5 mm is rarely associated with either hyperplasia or cancer. Low-dose oral estrogen therapy rarely causes breakthrough or withdrawal bleeding in postmenopausal women. Therefore, irrespective of whether the patient is using estrogen therapy, the occurrence of postmenopausal bleeding makes it mandatory to obtain a tissue diagnosis by either endometrial sampling or curettage to exclude endometrial cancer.

One of the most common disorders of the uterus and the most frequent tumor of women (one of four women affected) is the uterine leiomyoma, or fibroid tumor. Three-fourths of women with leiomyoma are asymptomatic, and the diagnosis is made on routine pelvic examination. When the tumor is associated with excessive menstrual blood loss, is large or fast-growing, or causes significant pelvic pain (see below), the preferred treatment is hysterectomy if there is no desire for further childbearing. Embolism of the vascular supply to the tumor may be possible. In young women, myomectomy is sometimes indicated when infertility or repeated fetal wastage is a manifestation or where future childbearing is desired.

FALLOPIAN TUBES AND OVARIES

PELVIC INFLAMMATORY DISEASE (PID)   This is a common disorder of the fallopian tubes and usually becomes symptomatic after a menstrual period; symptoms include fever, chills, abdominal pain, and vaginal discharge, and pelvic tenderness on physical examination is common. The initiating organism most often is *Chlamydia trachomatis* or *Neisseria gonorrhoeae*, but tuboovarian abscess and sterility are probably caused by mixed aerobic and anaerobic superinfections and require wide-spectrum antibiotic treatment (Chap. 115).

ENDOMETRIOSIS   This is a benign disorder characterized by the presence and proliferation of endometrial tissue (stroma and glands) outside the endometrial cavity. The clinical manifestations are variable. Endometriosis occurs most commonly between the ages of 30 and 40 and is found incidentally at the time of surgery in approximately one-fifth of all gynecologic operations. The fertility rate is reduced in affected women. The disorder usually involves the posterior cul-de-sac or the ovaries and it occasionally involves distant sites (lung, umbilicus). The major symptom is pelvic pain, characteristically dysmenorrhea (see below). However, the frequency and severity of symptoms correlate poorly with the extent of disease. Other manifestations include dyspareunia, pain with defecation, and infertility. The characteristic physical findings are multiple tender nodules palpable along the uterosacral ligament at the time of rectal-vaginal examination, a posteriorly fixed uterus, or enlarged, cystic ovaries. The diagnosis can be confirmed only by direct visualization, usually at diagnostic laparoscopy. Treatment depends on the degree of involvement and the desires of the patient and includes observation for mild disease with no associated infertility or pain, hormonal suppressive therapy, conservative surgery by laparoscopy or laparotomy if fertility is desired, or removal of the uterus, tubes, and ovaries in severe disease. Endometriosis is rare after the menopause.

Any adnexal mass that persists for more than 6 weeks or is larger than 6 cm must be evaluated. Although ovarian cysts and neoplasms are the most common pelvic adnexal masses, tumors of the fallopian tubes, uterus, gastrointestinal tract, or urinary tract should also be considered. Sonography or radiographic evaluation is often helpful in identifying the nature of the adnexal mass prior to surgical exploration. →*For a discussion of ovarian tumors, see Chap. 83.*

EVALUATION OF PELVIC PAIN

The evaluation of pelvic pain requires a careful history and pelvic examination. This often leads to the correct diagnosis and institution of appropriate treatment. Pelvic pain may originate in the pelvis or be referred from another region of the body. A pelvic source is suggested by the history (e.g., dysmenorrhea and dyspareunia) and physical findings, but a high index of suspicion must be entertained for extrapelvic disorders that refer to the pelvis, such as appendicitis, diverticulitis, cholecystitis, intestinal obstruction, and urinary tract infections. If the pain is severe and the diagnosis is unclear, the workup should follow that outlined for the acute abdomen (Chap. 13).

"PHYSIOLOGIC" PELVIC PAIN

PAIN ASSOCIATED WITH OVULATION ("MITTELSCHMERZ")   Many women experience low abdominal discomfort with ovulation, typically a dull aching pain at midcycle in one lower quadrant lasting from minutes to hours. It is rarely severe or incapacitating. The pain may result from peritoneal irritation by follicular fluid released into the peritoneal cavity at ovulation. The onset of discomfort at midcycle, and short duration of pain, suggest this diagnosis.

PREMENSTRUAL OR MENSTRUAL PAIN   In normal ovulatory women, somatic symptoms during the few days prior to menses may be insignificant or disabling. Such symptoms include edema, breast engorgement, and abdominal bloating or discomfort. A symptom complex of cyclic irritability, depression, and lethargy is known as *premenstrual syndrome*, which appears to be caused by changes in gonadal steroid levels. Although there is no consensus about therapy, randomized, controlled trials suggest improvement in some women with the daily use of serotonin-reuptake inhibitors.

Severe or incapacitating uterine cramping during ovulatory menses and in the absence of demonstrable disorders of the pelvis is termed *primary dysmenorrhea*. Primary dysmenorrhea is caused by prostaglandin-induced uterine ischemia and is treated with nonsteroidal anti-inflammatory drugs and/or oral contraceptive agents.

PELVIC PAIN DUE TO ORGANIC CAUSES

Severe dysmenorrhea associated with disease of the pelvis is termed *secondary dysmenorrhea*. Organic causes of pelvic pain can be classified as (1) uterine, (2) adnexal, (3) vulvar or vaginal, and (4) pregnancy-associated.

UTERINE PAIN   Pain of uterine etiology is often chronic and continuous and increases in intensity during menstruation and intercourse. Causes include leiomyomas of the uterus (particularly submucous and degenerating leiomyomas), adenomyosis, and cervical stenosis. Infections of the uterus associated with intrauterine manipulation following dilatation and curettage or with the insertion of intrauterine devices can also cause pelvic pain. Pelvic pain due to endometrial or cervical cancer is usually a late manifestation.

ADNEXAL PAIN   The most common cause of pain in the adnexae (fallopian tubes and ovaries) is infection (Chap. 115). Acute salpingo-oophoritis presents as low abdominal pain, fever, and chills and begins a few days after a menstrual period. Chronic PID results from either a single episode or multiple episodes of infection and may present as infertility associated with chronic pelvic pain that increases in intensity with menses and intercourse. On physical examination, cervical motion tenderness, adnexal tenderness, and adnexal thickening and/or masses may be present. PID may become a surgical emergency if peritonitis results from rupture of a tuboovarian abscess. Ovarian cysts or neoplasms may cause pelvic pain that becomes more severe with torsion or rupture of the mass, and ectopic pregnancy must be considered in the differential diagnosis. If there is a question of an adnexal mass or if the patient is so obese as to preclude a thorough pelvic examination, abdominal or vaginal ultrasound may be useful. Endometriosis involving fallopian tubes, ovaries, or peritoneum may cause both chronic low abdominal pain and infertility; the magnitude of tissue involvement does not always correlate with the severity of symptoms. Endometriosis pain typically increases with menstruation and, if the posterior ligaments of the uterus are involved, with intercourse.

VULVAR OR VAGINAL PAIN   Pain in these areas is most often due to infectious vaginitis and is characteristically associated with vaginal discharge and pruritus. Herpetic vulvitis, other dermatologic conditions of the vulva, condyloma acumination, and cysts or abscesses of Bartholin's glands may also cause vulvar pain.

PREGNANCY-ASSOCIATED DISORDERS   Pregnancy must be considered in the differential diagnosis of pelvic pain during the reproductive years. Threatened abortion or incomplete abortion often presents with uterine cramping, bleeding, or passage of tissue following a period of amenorrhea. Ectopic pregnancy may be insidious in presentation or result in abrupt intraperitoneal hemorrhage and maternal death. A culdocentesis may be indicated if a ruptured ectopic pregnancy is suspected. Serial hCG measurements may help in establishing a diagnosis of tubal pregnancy and are useful in determining if an intrauterine pregnancy is viable.

FURTHER READING

ADASHI EY, HENNEBOLD JD: Single-gene mutations resulting in reproductive dysfunction in women. N Engl J Med 340:709, 1999

BRADLEY LD et al: Radiographic imaging techniques for the diagnosis of abnormal uterine bleeding. Obstet Gynecol Clin North Am 27:245, 2000

HEWITT GD: Acute and chronic pelvic pain in female adolescents. Med Clin North Am 84:1009, 2000

HUTCHINS FL et al: Embolotherapy for myoma-induced menorrhagia. Obstet Gynecol Clin North Am 27:397, 2000

MCGEE EA, HSUEH AWJ: Initial and cyclic recruitment of ovarian follicles. Endocr Rev 21:200, 2000

SHANG Y et al: Cofactor dynamics and sufficiency in estrogen receptor–regulated transcription. Cell 103: 843, 2000

---

327 THE MENOPAUSE TRANSITION AND POSTMENOPAUSAL HORMONE THERAPY
JoAnn E. Manson, Shari S. Bassuk

Menopause is the permanent cessation of menstruation due to loss of ovarian follicular function. It is diagnosed retrospectively after 12 months of amenorrhea. The average age at menopause is 51 years among U.S. women. *Perimenopause* refers to the time period preceding menopause, when fertility wanes and menstrual cycle irregularity increases, until the first year after cessation of menses. The onset of perimenopause precedes the final menses by 2 to 8 years, with a mean duration of 4 years. Smoking accelerates the menopausal transition by 2 years.

Although the peri- and postmenopausal periods share many symptoms, the physiology and clinical management of the two periods differ. Low-dose oral contraceptives have become a therapeutic mainstay in perimenopause, whereas postmenopausal hormone therapy (HT) has been a common method of symptom alleviation after menstruation ceases.

PERIMENOPAUSE

PHYSIOLOGY   Ovarian mass and fertility decline sharply after age 35 and even more precipitously during perimenopause; depletion of primary follicles, a process that begins before birth, occurs steadily until menopause (Chap. 326). In perimenopause, intermenstrual intervals shorten significantly (typically by 3 days) due to an accelerated follicular phase. Follicle-stimulating hormone (FSH) levels rise, due to altered folliculogenesis and reduced inhibin secretion. In contrast to the consistently high FSH and low estradiol levels seen in menopause, perimenopause is characterized by "irregularly irregular" hormone levels. The propensity for anovulatory cycles can produce a hyperestrogenic, hypoprogestagenic environment that may account for the increased incidence of endometrial hyperplasia or carcinoma, uterine polyps, and leiomyoma observed among women of perimenopausal age. Mean serum levels of selected ovarian and pituitary hormones during the menopausal transition are shown in Fig. 327-1. With transition into menopause, estradiol levels fall markedly, whereas estrone levels are relatively preserved, reflecting peripheral aromatization of adrenal and ovarian androgens. FSH levels increase more than those of luteinizing hormone (LH), presumably because of the loss of inhibin, as well as estrogen feedback.

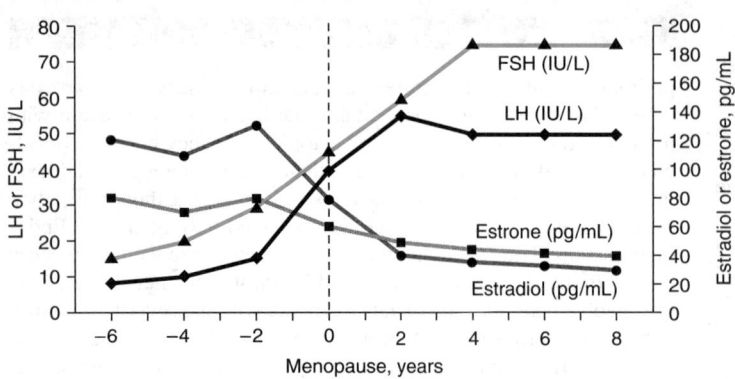

FIGURE 327-1 Mean serum levels of ovarian and pituitary hormones during the menopausal transition. FSH, follicle-stimulating hormone; LH, luteinizing hormone. *(From JL Shifren, Schiff: The aging ovary. J Women's Health Gend-Based Med 9:5–3, 2000, with permission.)*

DIAGNOSTIC TESTS Because of their extreme intraindividual variability, FSH and estradiol levels are imperfect diagnostic indicators of perimenopause in menstruating women. However, a low FSH in the early follicular phase (days 2 to 5) of the menstrual cycle is inconsistent with a diagnosis of perimenopause. FSH measurement can also aid in assessing fertility; levels of <20 mIU/mL, 20 to <30 mIU/mL, and ≥30 mIU/mL measured on day 3 of the cycle indicate a good, fair, and poor likelihood of achieving pregnancy, respectively.

SYMPTOMS Anovulatory cycles may be associated with irregular bleeding. Some perimenopausal women experience classic postmenopausal symptoms such as hot flashes and night sweats, insomnia, vaginal dryness, mood swings, or depression. In one U.S. study, nearly 60% of women reported hot flashes in the 2 years before their final menses. Symptom intensity, duration, and frequency are highly variable.

℞ TREATMENT

For women with irregular or heavy menses or hormonally related symptoms that impair quality of life, low-dose combined oral contraceptives are a staple of therapy. Static doses of estrogen and progestin (e.g., 20 μg of ethinyl estradiol and 1 mg of norethindrone acetate daily for 21 days each month) can eliminate vasomotor symptoms and restore regular cyclicity. Oral contraceptives provide other benefits, including protection against ovarian and endometrial cancers and increased bone density, although it is not clear whether use during perimenopause decreases fracture risk later in life. Moreover, the contraceptive benefit is important, given that the unintentional pregnancy rate among women in their forties rivals that of adolescents. Contraindications to oral contraceptive use include cigarette smoking, liver disease, a history of thromboembolism or cardiovascular disease, breast cancer, or unexplained vaginal bleeding. Progestin-only formulations (e.g., 0.35 mg norethindrone daily) or medroxyprogesterone (Depo-Provera) injections (e.g., 150 mg intramuscularly every 3 months) may provide an alternative for the treatment of perimenopausal menorrhagia in women who smoke or have cardiovascular risk factors. Although progestins neither regularize cycles nor reduce the number of bleeding days, they reduce the volume of menstrual flow.

Nonhormonal strategies to reduce menstrual flow include use of nonsteroidal anti-inflammatory agents such as mefenamic acid (initial dose of 500 mg at start of menses, then 250 mg qid for 2 to 3 days) or, when medical approaches fail, endometrial ablation. It should be noted that menorrhagia requires an evaluation to rule out uterine disorders. Transvaginal ultrasound with saline enhancement is useful for detecting leiomyomata or polyps, and endometrial aspiration can identify hyperplastic changes.

TRANSITION TO MENOPAUSE For sexually active women using contraceptive hormones to alleviate perimenopausal symptoms, the question of when and if to switch to HT must be individualized. Estrogen and

progestin doses in HT are lower than those in oral contraceptives and have not been documented to prevent pregnancy. Though a 1-year absence of spontaneous menses reliably indicates ovulation cessation, it is not possible to assess the natural menstrual pattern while a woman is taking an oral contraceptive. Women willing to switch to a barrier method of contraception should do so; if menses occur spontaneously, oral contraceptive use can be resumed. The average age of final menses among relatives can serve as a guide for when to initiate this process, which can be repeated yearly until menopause has occurred.

MENOPAUSE AND POSTMENOPAUSAL HORMONE THERAPY

One of the most complex health care decisions facing women is whether or not to use postmenopausal hormone therapy. HT, once prescribed primarily to relieve vasomotor symptoms, has been promoted as a strategy to forestall various disorders that accelerate after menopause, including osteoporosis and cardiovascular disease. More than 30% of postmenopausal women in the United States currently use HT. This widespread use is unwarranted given the paucity of conclusive data, until very recently, on the health consequences of such therapy. Although many women rely on their health care providers for a definitive answer to the question of whether to use postmenopausal hormones, balancing the benefits and risks for an individual patient is challenging.

Although observational studies suggest that HT prevents cardiovascular and other chronic diseases, the apparent benefits may result at least in part from differences between women who opt to take postmenopausal hormones and women who do not. Those choosing HT tend to be healthier, have greater access to medical care, are more compliant with prescribed treatments, and maintain a more health-promoting life-style. Randomized trials, which eliminate these confounding factors, have not consistently confirmed the benefits found in observational studies. Indeed, one arm of the largest trial of HT to date, the Women's Health Initiative (WHI), which examined more than 16,000 postmenopausal women for an average of 5.2 years, was stopped early because of an overall unfavorable risk-benefit ratio associated with estrogen-progestin therapy.

The following summary offers a decision-making guide based on a synthesis of currently available evidence. The decision is divided into one of short- (<5 years) or long-term (≥5 years) use of HT. Prevention of cardiovascular disease is eliminated from the equation due to lack of evidence for such benefits in recent randomized clinical trials.

BENEFITS AND RISKS OF POSTMENOPAUSAL HORMONE THERAPY (Table 327-1)

DEFINITE BENEFITS ■ **Symptoms of Menopause** Compelling evidence, including data from randomized clinical trials, indicates that estrogen therapy is highly effective for controlling vasomotor and genitourinary symptoms. Alternative approaches, including the use of antidepressants (such as venlafaxine, 75 to 150 mg/d), clonidine (0.1 to 0.2 mg/d), or vitamin E (400 to 800 IU/d) or the consumption of soy-based products or other phytoestrogens, may also alleviate vasomotor symptoms, although they are less effective than HT. For genitourinary symptoms, the efficacy of vaginal estrogen is similar to that of oral or transdermal estrogen.

Osteoporosis (see also Chap 333) ■ *BONE DENSITY* By reducing bone turnover and resorption rates, estrogen slows the aging-related bone loss experienced by most postmenopausal women. More than 50 randomized trials have demonstrated that postmenopausal estrogen therapy, with or without a progestin, rapidly increases bone mineral density at the spine by 4 to 6% and at the hip by 2 to 3%, and maintains those increases during treatment.

FRACTURES Data from observational studies indicate a 50 to 80% lower risk of vertebral fracture and a 25 to 30% lower risk of hip, wrist, and other peripheral fractures among current estrogen users; addition of a

Variable	Effect	Benefit or Risk		Sources of Evidence
		Relative	Absolute	
DEFINITE BENEFITS				
Symptoms of menopause (vasomotor, genitourinary)	Definite improvement	>70 to 80% decrease		Observational studies and randomized trials
Osteoporosis	Definite increase in bone mineral density and decrease in fracture risk	2–5% increase in bone density; 25–50% decrease in risk of fractures	WHI: 50 fewer hip fractures (100 vs. 150) per 100,000 woman-years	Observational studies and randomized trials, including WHI
DEFINITE RISKS				
Endometrial cancer	Definite increase in risk with use of unopposed[a] estrogen; no increase with use of estrogen plus progestin	8- to 10-fold increased risk with use of unopposed estrogen for ≥10 yr; no excess risk with estrogen-progestin therapy	46 excess cases (52 vs. 6) per 100,000 woman-years of unopposed estrogen use (≥10 years of use); no excess with estrogen-progestin therapy	Observational studies and randomized trials
Venous thromboembolism	Definite increase in risk	≥2-fold increase	Secondary prevention: 390 excess cases per 100,000 woman-years	Randomized trial (HERS)
			Primary prevention: 180 excess cases per 100,000 woman-years	Observational studies and randomized trial (WHI)
Breast cancer	Increase in risk with long-term use (≥5 yr)	1.35-fold overall increase with HT use ≥5 yr	10–30 excess cases per 10,000 women using HT for 5 yr; 30–90 excess cases after 10 yr of use; 50–200 excess cases after 15 yr of use	Observational data (meta-analysis of 51 studies)
		25–30% increase with 5.2 yr of estrogen-progestin therapy; no increase with estrogen-only	WHI: 80 excess cases (300 vs. 380) per 100,000 woman-years of estrogen-progestin therapy	Randomized trials (WHI, HERS)
PROBABLE OR UNCERTAIN RISKS AND BENEFITS				
Cardiovascular disease				
Primary prevention	Probable increase in risk	WHI: 29% increase in CHD with estrogen-progestin; no apparent increase or decrease with estrogen-only	WHI: 70 excess cases (370 vs. 300) of CHD per 100,000 woman-years with estrogen-progestin	Observational studies suggest a 35–50% decrease in risk, while randomized trials show no effect or a harmful effect; most studies have assessed conjugated equine estrogen alone or in combination with medroxyprogesterone acetate
		40% increase in stroke with either estrogen-progestin or estrogen-only	80 excess cases (290 vs. 210) of stroke per 100,000 woman-years	
Secondary prevention	Probable early increase in risk	HERS: 50% increase in CHD in year 1; no overall effect over 4 years	Equal number of CHD cases over 4 years	Observational studies and randomized secondary prevention trials
Gallbladder disease	Probable increase in risk	1.4-fold increase	360 excess cases per 100,000 woman-years	Randomized trials (HERS)
Colorectal cancer	Probable decrease in risk	20–37% decrease with estrogen-progestin	24–60 fewer cases per 100,000 woman-years	Observational data, randomized trial (WHI)
Cognitive dysfunction	Unproven decrease in risk	Apparent increase in dementia after age 65	Uncertain	Inconsistent data from observational studies and randomized trials

[a] "Unopposed estrogen" refers to the use of estrogen without progestin.
Note: WHI, Women's Health Initiative; HERS, Heart and Estrogen/progestin Replacement Study; CHD, coronary heart disease.

progestin does not appear to modify this benefit. Discontinuation of estrogen therapy leads to a diminution of protection. In the WHI, 5 to 6 years of either combined estrogen-progestin or estrogen-only was associated with a 30 to 40% reduction in hip fracture and 20 to 30% fewer total fractures among a population unselected for osteoporosis. Bisphosphonates (such as alendronate, 10 mg/d or 70 mg once per week or residronate, 5 mg/d or 35 mg once a week) and raloxifene (60 mg/d), a selective estrogen receptor modulator, have each been shown in randomized trials to increase bone mass density and decrease fracture rates. These agents, unlike estrogen, do not appear to have adverse effects on the endometrium or breast. Increased physical activity and adequate calcium (1000 to 1500 mg/d in two to three divided doses) and vitamin D (400 to 800 IU/d) intakes may also reduce the risk of osteoporosis-related fractures.

DEFINITE RISKS ■ Endometrial Cancer A combined analysis of 30 observational studies found a tripling of risk of endometrial cancer among short-term (1 to 5 years) users of unopposed estrogen and a nearly tenfold increased risk among users for 10 or more years. These findings are supported by results from the randomized Postmenopausal Estrogen/Progestin Interventions (PEPI) trial, in which 24% of women assigned to unopposed estrogen for 3 years developed atypical endometrial hyperplasia, a premalignant lesion, compared to only 1% of women assigned to placebo. Use of a progestin, which opposes the effects of estrogen on the endometrium, eliminates these risks.

Venous Thromboembolism A recent meta-analysis of 12 studies—8 case-control, 1 cohort, and 3 randomized trials—found that current estrogen use was associated with a doubling of risk for venous thromboembolism in postmenopausal women. Relative risks of thromboembolic events were even greater (2.7 to 5.1) in the three trials included in the meta-analysis. Results from the WHI indicate a twofold increase in risk of venous and pulmonary thromboembolism.

Breast Cancer An increased risk of breast cancer has been found among current or recent estrogen users in observational studies; this risk is directly related to duration of use. In a meta-analysis of 51 case-control and cohort studies, short-term use (<5 years) of postmenopausal hormone therapy did not appreciably elevate breast cancer incidence, whereas long-term use (≥5 years) was associated with a 35% increase in risk. In contrast to findings for endometrial cancer, combined estrogen-progestin regimens appear to increase breast cancer risk more than estrogen alone. Data from randomized trials also indicate that HT raises breast cancer risk. In the WHI, women assigned to receive combination therapy for an average of 5.2 years were 26% more likely to develop breast cancer than women assigned to placebo but estrogen-only did not increase risk. In the Heart and Estrogen/progestin Replacement Study (HERS), 4 years of combination therapy was associated with a 27% increase in breast cancer risk. Although the latter finding was not statistically significant, the totality of evidence strongly implicates estrogen-progestin therapy in breast carcinogenesis.

PROBABLE OR UNCERTAIN RISKS AND BENEFITS ■ Coronary Heart Disease/ Stroke Until recently, HT had been enthusiastically recommended as a possible cardioprotective agent. In the past three decades, multiple observational studies suggested, in the aggregate, that estrogen use leads to a 35 to 50% reduction in coronary heart disease incidence among postmenopausal women. The biologic plausibility of such an association is supported by data from randomized trials demonstrating that exogenous estrogen lowers plasma low-density lipoprotein (LDL) cholesterol and raises high-density lipoprotein (HDL) cholesterol levels by 10 to 15%. Administration of estrogen also favorably affects lipoprotein(a) levels, LDL oxidation, endothelial vascular function, and fibrinogen and plasminogen activator inhibitor-1. However, estrogen therapy also has unfavorable effects on other biomarkers of cardiovascular risk; it boosts triglyceride levels; promotes coagulation via factor VII, prothrombin fragments 1 and 2, and fibrinopeptide A elevations; and raises levels of the inflammatory marker C-reactive protein.

Randomized trials of estrogen or combined estrogen-progestin in women with preexisting cardiovascular disease have not confirmed the benefits reported in observational studies. In HERS, a secondary prevention trial designed to test the efficacy and safety of estrogen-progestin therapy on clinical cardiovascular outcomes, the 4-year incidence of coronary mortality and nonfatal myocardial infarction was similar in the active treatment and placebo groups, and a 50% increase in risk of coronary events was noted during the first year of the study among participants assigned to the active treatment group. Although it is possible that progestin may mitigate estrogen's benefits, the Estrogen Replacement and Atherosclerosis (ERA) trial indicated that angiographically determined progression of coronary atherosclerosis was unaffected by either opposed or unopposed estrogen treatment. Moreover, the Papworth Hormone Replacement Therapy Atherosclerosis

Study, a trial of transdermal estradiol with and without norethindone, the Women's Estrogen for Stroke Trial (WEST), a trial of oral 17β-estradiol, and the EStrogen in the Prevention of ReInfarction Trial (ESPRIT), a trial of oral estradiol valerate, found no cardiovascular benefits of the regimens studied. Thus, in clinical trials, HT has not proved effective for the secondary prevention of cardiovascular disease in postmenopausal women.

Primary prevention trials also suggest an early increase in cardiovascular risk and absence of cardioprotection with postmenopausal HT. Results from the large-scale WHI suggest a deleterious cardiovascular effect of hormone therapy. Women assigned to 5 years of estrogen-progestin therapy were 29% more likely to develop coronary heart disease and 41% more likely to suffer a stroke than those assigned to placebo. In the estrogen-only arm of the WHI, a similar increase in stroke and no effect on CHD were observed. Further research is needed on clinical characteristics as well as on biomarkers that predict increases or decreases in cardiovascular risk associated with exogenous hormone therapy. Whether different doses, formulations, or routes of administration of hormone therapy will produce different cardiovascular effects remains uncertain.

Gallbladder Disease Several large observational studies report a two- to threefold increased risk of gallstones or cholecystectomy among postmenopausal women taking estrogen. In HERS, women randomized to 4 years of estrogen-progestin therapy had a 38% greater risk of developing gallbladder disease than those assigned to placebo, a risk that climbed to 48% after 2.7 additional years of observational follow-up.

Colorectal Cancer Observational studies have suggested that HT reduces risks of colon and rectal cancer, although the estimated magnitudes of the relative benefits ranged from 8 to 33% in various meta-analyses. In the WHI, the only trial to examine the issue, estrogen-progestin therapy was associated with a significant 37% reduction in colorectal cancer over a 5-year period; no benefit was seen with estrogen-only.

Cognitive Decline and Dementia A meta-analysis of 10 case-control and 2 cohort studies suggested that postmenopausal HT is associated with a 33% decreased risk of dementia. Subsequent randomized trials, however, failed to demonstrate any benefit of estrogen therapy on the progression of mild to moderate Alzheimer's disease and indicated a potential adverse effect of estrogen-progestin therapy on the incidence of dementia.

Ovarian Cancer and Other Disorders On the basis of limited observational and randomized data, it has been hypothesized that HT increases the risk of ovarian cancer and reduces the risk of type 2 diabetes mellitus. These hypotheses require confirmation in additional clinical trials.

APPROACH TO THE PATIENT

The rational use of postmenopausal hormone therapy requires balancing the potential benefits and risks. Figure 327-2 provides one approach to decision making. The clinician should first determine whether the patient has an indication for initiating HT. Relief of menopausal symptoms and prevention of osteoporosis are the most valid reasons. The benefits and risks of such therapy should then be reviewed with the patient, giving more emphasis to absolute than to relative measures of effect, and pointing out uncertainties in clinical knowledge where relevant. Potential side effects—especially vaginal bleeding that may result from use of combined estrogen-progestin formulations recommended for women with an intact uterus—should be noted. The patient's own preference regarding therapy should be elicited and factored into the decision. Contraindications to HT should be assessed routinely and include unexplained vaginal bleeding, active liver disease, venous thromboembolism, or history of endometrial cancer (except stage 1 without deep invasion) or breast cancer. Relative contraindications include hypertriglyceridemia (>400 mg/dL) and active gallbladder disease (in such cases, transdermal estrogen is an option). Neither primary nor secondary prevention of heart disease should be viewed as an expected benefit of HT, and an increase in stroke and a small early increase in coronary artery disease risk should be considered. Nevertheless, such therapy may be appropriate, if the noncoronary benefits of treatment clearly outweigh risks. A woman who suffers an acute coronary event or stroke while on HT should stop therapy immediately.

Short-term use (<5 years) of HT is appropriate for relief of menopausal symptoms among women without contraindications to such use. However, such therapy should be avoided or considered only as a secondary option among women with preexisting heart disease or stroke due to their elevated baseline risk of future cardiovascular events. Women who have contraindications, or are opposed to HT, may derive benefit from the use of selective antidepressants, clonidine, or soy, and, for genitourinary symptoms, intravaginal estrogen creams or devices.

Long-term use (≥5 years) of HT is more problematic because a heightened risk of breast cancer must be factored into the decision. Reasonable candidates for such use include a small percentage of postmenopausal women and comprise those who have persistent severe vasomotor symptoms and/or have an increased risk of osteoporosis (e.g., those with osteopenia, a personal or family history of nontraumatic fracture, or a body mass index <22 kg/m²), who also have no personal or family history of breast cancer in a first-degree relative or other contraindications, and who have a strong personal preference for therapy. Poor candidates are women with cardiovascular disease, those at low risk of osteoporosis, and those at increased risk of breast cancer (e.g., women who have a first-degree relative with breast cancer, susceptibility genes such as *BRCA1* or *BRCA2*, or a personal history of cellular atypia detected by breast biopsy). Even in reasonable candidates, strategies to minimize dose and duration of use should be employed. For example, women using hormone replacement to relieve intense vasomotor symptoms in early postmenopause should consider discontinuing therapy before 5 years, resuming it only if vasomotor symptoms persist and/or an increased risk of osteoporosis is evident. In the latter situation, alternative therapies such as bisphosphonates or selective estrogen receptor modulators (SERMs) should be considered. Research on androgen-containing preparations has been limited, particularly in terms of long-term safety.

In addition to HT, control of symptoms and prevention of chronic disease can be accomplished by life-style choices, including smoking abstention, adequate physical activity, and a healthy diet. An expanding array of pharmacologic options—e.g., bisphosphonates or SERMs for osteoporosis, and cholesterol-lowering or antihypertensive agents for cardiovascular disease—should also reduce the widespread reliance on hormone use. However, short-term HT may still benefit some women.

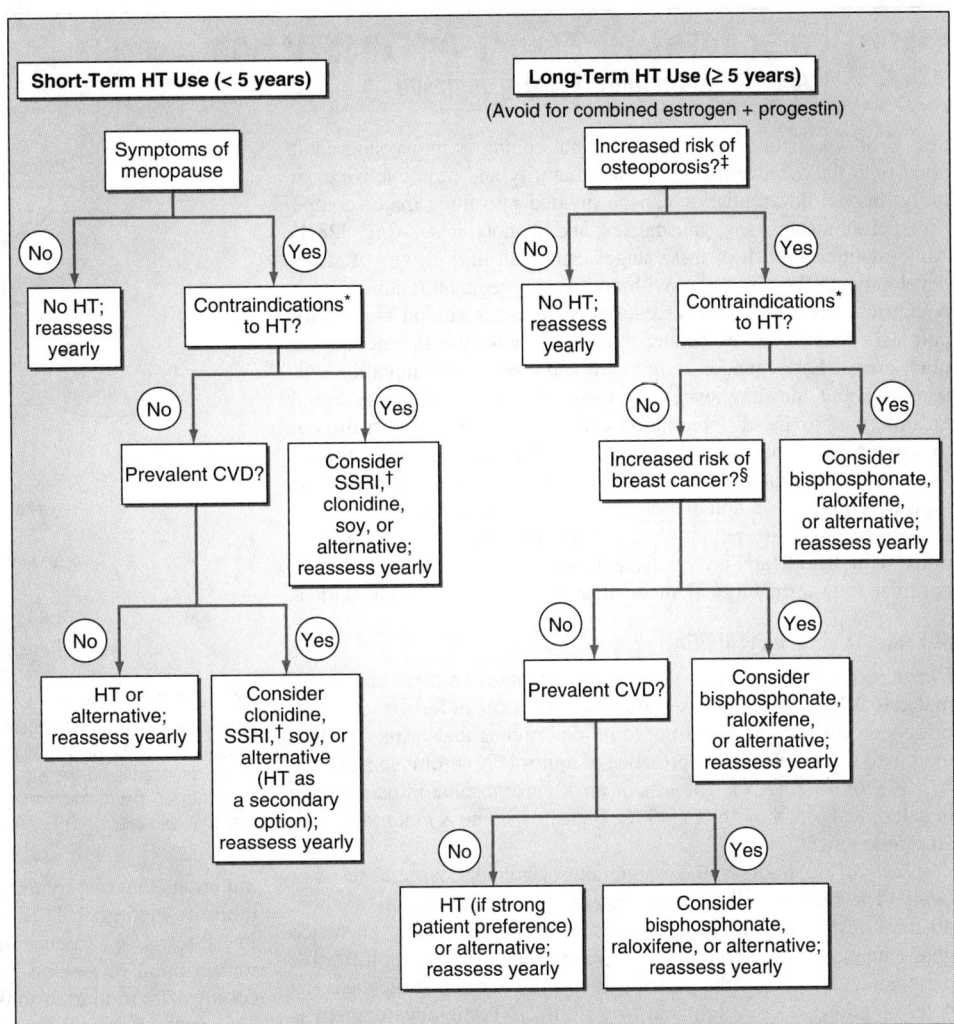

FIGURE 327-2 Flowchart for identifying appropriate candidates for short-term and long-term use of postmenopausal hormone therapy (HT). *Contraindications include unexplained vaginal bleeding, active liver disease, venous thromboembolism, or history of endometrial cancer (except stage 1 without deep invasion) or breast cancer. Relative contraindications include hypertriglyceridemia (>400 mg/dL) and active gallbladder disease (in such cases, transdermal estrogen is an option). †SSRI denotes selective serotonin reuptake inhibitor. ‡Increased risk of osteoporosis: documented osteopenia or osteoporosis, personal or family history of nontraumatic fracture, current smoking, or a body mass index <22 kg/m². §Increased risk of breast cancer: one or more first-degree relatives with breast cancer; susceptibility genes such as *BRCA1* or *BRCA2*; or a personal history of breast biopsy demonstrating atypia. CVD, cardiovascular disease. (*Adapted from Manson and Martin; with permission. Copyright © 2001 Massachusetts Medical Society. All rights reserved.*)

FURTHER READING

HULLEY S et al: Randomized trial of estrogen plus progestin for secondary prevention of coronary heart disease in postmenopausal women. Heart and Estrogen/progestin Replacement Study (HERS) Research Group. JAMA 280:605, 1998

MANSON JE, MARTIN KA: Clinical practice: Postmenopausal hormone-replacement therapy. N Engl J Med 345:34, 2001

NELSON HD et al: Postmenopausal hormone replacement therapy: Scientific review. JAMA 288:872, 2002

STEERING COMMITTEE FOR THE WOMEN'S HEALTH INITIATIVE: Effects of conjugated equine estrogen in postmenopausal women with hysterectomy: Principal results from the Women's Health Initiative randomized controlled trial. JAMA 2004, in press

WRITING GROUP FOR THE PEPI TRIAL: Effects of estrogen or estrogen/progestin regimens on heart disease risk factors in postmenopausal women. The Postmenopausal Estrogen/Progestin Interventions (PEPI) Trial. JAMA 273:199, 1995

WRITING GROUP FOR THE WOMEN'S HEALTH INITIATIVE INVESTIGATORS: Risks and benefits of estrogen plus progestin in healthy postmenopausal women. Principal results from the Women's Health Initiative randomized controlled trial. JAMA 288:321, 2002

Sexual differentiation begins in utero, but continues into young adulthood with the achievement of sexual maturity and reproductive capability. Sexual differentiation can be divided into three major components: chromosomal sex, gonadal sex, and phenotypic sex (Fig. 328-1). Abnormalities at each of these stages can result in disorders of sexual development. The child born with ambiguous genitalia requires urgent pediatric assessment, as some causes, such as congenital adrenal hyperplasia (CAH), are associated with potentially life-threatening adrenal crises. Early gender assignment and clear communication with parents about the diagnosis, prognosis, and treatment are essential. Disorders of sexual differentiation can also manifest later in life due to subtler forms of gonadal dysfunction [e.g., Klinefelter syndrome (KS)] and are often diagnosed by internists. There are many psychological, reproductive, and metabolic consequences associated with disorders of sexual differentiation; some of these patients avoid interactions with healthcare providers, and special effort is necessary to optimize long-term surgical, medical, and psychological management.

NORMAL SEXUAL DIFFERENTIATION

Chromosomal sex describes the sex chromosome complement (46,XY male; 46,XX female) that is established at the time of fertilization. The presence of a normal Y chromosome determines that testis development will occur, even in the presence of multiple X chromosomes (e.g., 47,XXY or 48,XXXY). The loss of an X chromosome impairs gonad development (45,X or 46,XY/45,X). Fetuses with no X material (45,Y) are not viable.

Gonadal sex refers to the assignment of gonadal tissue as testis or ovary. The embryonic gonad is bipotential, and can develop (at about 40 days gestation) into either a testis or ovary, depending on which genes are expressed. Ovarian development appears to be a constitutive pathway and occurs in the absence of specific genes that dictate testis determination and development (Fig. 328-2). Testis development is initiated by expression of the Y chromosome gene *SRY* (sex-determining region on the Y chromosome), which encodes an HMG box transcription factor. *SRY* is transiently expressed in cells destined to become Sertoli cells and serves as a pivotal switch to establish the testis lineage. Mutation of *SRY* prevents testis development in chromosomal 46,XY males, whereas translocation of *SRY* in 46,XX females is sufficient to induce testis development and a male phenotype. Other genes are necessary to continue testis development. *SOX9* (SRY-related HMG-box gene 9) is strikingly upregulated in the developing male gonad but is turned off in the female gonad. Transgenic expression of *SOX9* is sufficient to initiate testis formation in mice, and

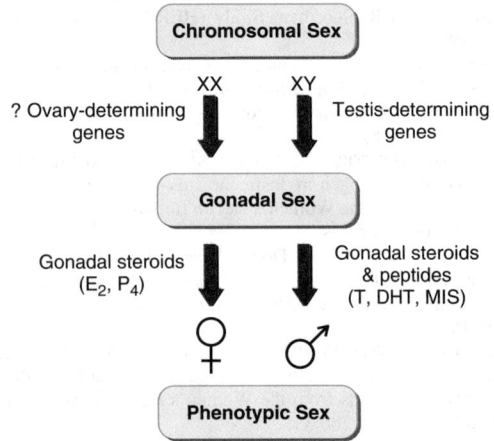

FIGURE 328-1 Sexual differentiation can be divided into three major components: chromosomal sex, gonadal sex, and phenotypic sex. T, testosterone; DHT, dihydrotestosterone; MIS, müllerian-inhibiting substance; E_2, estradiol; P_4, progesterone.

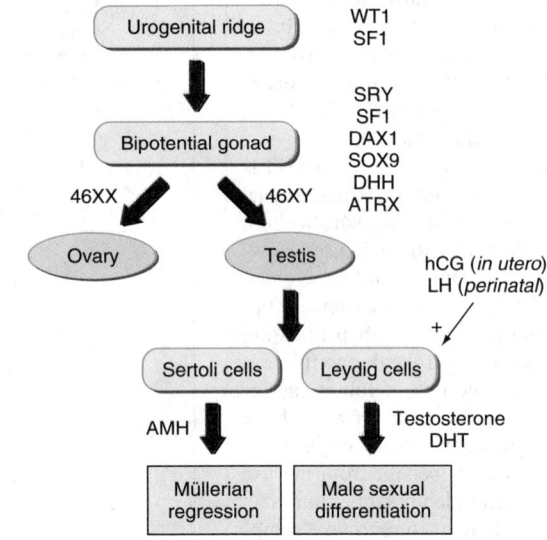

FIGURE 328-2 The genetic regulation of testis development. *WT1*, Wilms' tumor-related gene 1; *SF1*, steroidogenic factor 1; *SRY*, sex-related gene on the Y chromosome; *SOX9*, SRY-related HMG-box gene 9; *DHH*, desert hedgehog; *ATRX*, (α-thalassemia, mental retardation on the X); *DAX1*, dosage sensitive sex-reversal, adrenal hypoplasia congenita on the X chromosome, gene 1; *AMH*, anti-müllerian hormone (müllerian-inhibiting substance); DHT, dihydrotestosterone.

mutations that disrupt *SOX9* impair testis development. *WT1* (Wilms' tumor-related gene 1) is involved in renal and gonadal development. In the testis, *WT1* acts early in the genetic pathway and regulates the transcription of several genes including *SF1*, *DAX1*, and *AMH* (encoding *MIS*, müllerian-inhibiting substance). *SF1* (steroidogenic factor 1) encodes a nuclear receptor and is required for adrenal and gonadal development (both testis and ovary). It functions in cooperation with other transcription factors to regulate a large array of adrenal and gonadal genes, including many genes involved in steroidogenesis. The early expression pattern of *SF1* in the gonad parallels that of another orphan nuclear receptor, *DAX1* (dosage sensitive sex-reversal, adrenal hypoplasia congenita on the X chromosome, gene 1). In contrast to *SOX9*, *DAX1* is downregulated as the testis develops. Duplication of *DAX1* impairs testis development, possibly by antagonizing the function of SRY and SF1. Deletions or mutations of *DAX1*, on the other hand, lead to disordered formation of testis cords, revealing the exquisite sensitivity of the male sex-determining pathway to gene dosage effects. In addition to those mentioned above, human and murine mutations indicate that at least 10 other genes are also involved in gonadal differentiation and development as well as final positioning of the gonads.

It is unclear whether analogous "ovarian-determining genes" exist, or whether ovarian development only requires the absence of testis-determining genes. However, germ cells play a key role in supporting ovarian development and produce factors that inhibit the formation of testicular elements. This contrasts with the testis, which develops and undergoes steroidogenesis in the absence of germ cells. Once the ovary has formed, expression of a variety of specific genes is required for normal follicular development [e.g., follicle stimulating hormone (FSH) receptor, *GDF9*]. Steroidogenesis in the ovary requires the development of follicles containing granulosa cells and theca cells surrounding the oocytes (Chap. 326). Thus, there is minimal ovarian steroidogenesis until gonadotropins are produced at puberty.

Phenotypic sex refers to the structures of the external and internal genitalia, and secondary sex characteristics. The male phenotype requires the secretion of anti-müllerian hormone (AMH, müllerian-inhibiting substance) from Sertoli cells and testosterone from testicular

Leydig cells. AMH is a member of the TGF-β growth factor family and acts through specific receptors to cause regression of the müllerian structures (52 to 70 days gestation). At approximately 60 to 140 days gestation, testosterone supports the development of wolffian structures, including the epididymides, vasa deferentia, and seminal vesicles. Testosterone is also the precursor for dihydrotestosterone (DHT), a potent androgen that promotes development of the external genitalia, including the penis and scrotum (65–100 days, and beyond) (Fig. 328-3). The urogenital sinus develops into the prostate and prostatic urethra in the male and into the urethra and lower portion of the vagina in the female. The genital tubercle becomes the glans penis in the male and the clitoris in the female. The urogenital swellings form the scrotum or the labia majora, and the urethral folds fuse to form the shaft of the penis and the male urethra or the labia minora. In the female, wolffian ducts regress and the müllerian ducts form the fallopian tubes, uterus, and upper segment of the vagina. A normal female phenotype will develop in the absence of the gonad, but estrogen is needed for maturation of the uterus and breast at puberty.

DISORDERS OF CHROMOSOMAL SEX

Disorders of chromosomal sex result from abnormalities in the number or structure of the X or Y chromosomes (Table 328-1).

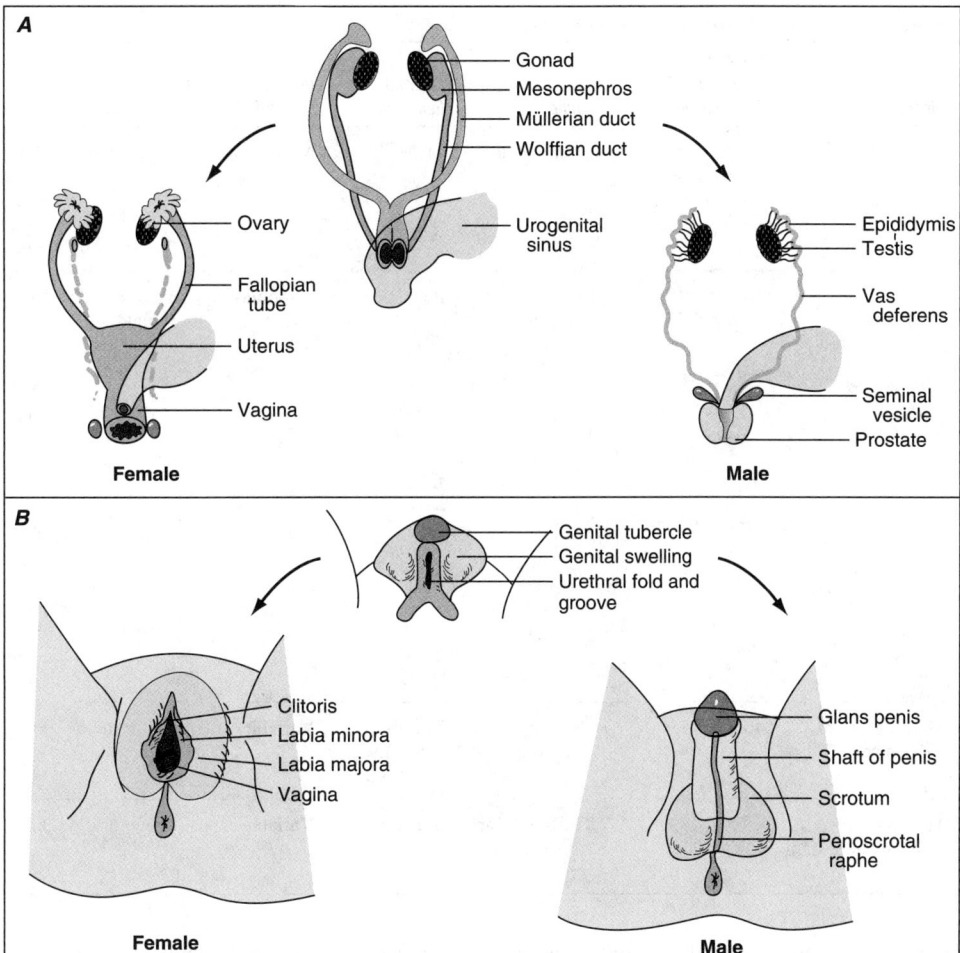

FIGURE 328-3   Normal sexual differentiation. *A.* Internal urogenital tract. *B.* External genitalia. [After JD Wilson, JE Griffin, in E Braunwald et al (eds): *Harrison's Principles of Internal Medicine*, 15th ed. New York, McGraw-Hill, 2001.]

KLINEFELTER SYNDROME (47,XXY AND MOSAIC VARIANTS) ■ Pathophysiology

The classic form of Klinefelter syndrome (KS) (47,XXY) occurs following meiotic nondisjunction of the sex chromosomes during gametogenesis (40% during spermatogenesis, 60% during oogenesis) (Chap. 57). Mosaic forms of KS (46,XY/47,XXY) are thought to result from chromosomal mitotic nondisjunction within the zygote, and occur in at least 10% of individuals with this condition. Other chromosomal variants of KS (e.g., 48,XXYY; 48,XXXY) have been reported but are less common.

Clinical Features   KS is characterized by small testes, infertility, gynecomastia, eunuchoid proportions, and poor virilization in phenotypic males. It has an incidence of 1 in 500 to 1000 men. In severe cases, individuals present prepubertally with small testes, or with impaired androgenization and gynecomastia at the time of puberty. Developmental delay and learning disabilities may be a feature. Later in life, eunuchoid features or infertility lead to the diagnosis. Testes are small and firm [median length 2.5 cm (4 mL volume); almost always <3.5 cm (12 mL)], and typically seem inappropriately small for the degree of androgenization. Biopsies are not usually necessary but reveal seminiferous tubule hyalinization and azoospermia. Other clinical features of KS are listed in Table 328-1. Plasma concentrations of follicle stimulating hormone (FSH) and luteinizing hormone (LH) are increased in most patients with 47,XXY (90 and 80%, respectively) and plasma testosterone is decreased (50–75%), reflecting primary gonadal failure. Estradiol is often increased because of chronic Leydig cell stimulation by LH and because of aromatization of androstenedione by adipose tissue; the increased ratio of estradiol/testosterone results in gynecomastia. Patients with mosaic forms of KS have less severe clinical features, larger testes, and sometimes achieve fertility.

℞ TREATMENT

Disfiguring gynecomastia should be treated by surgical reduction. Androgen supplementation (Chap. 325) improves virilization, libido, energy, and bone mineralization in underandrogenized men, but may worsen gynecomastia. Fertility has been achieved using in vitro fertilization in men with oligospermia, or with intracytoplasmic sperm injection when spermatids can be recovered from testicular biopsy. However, the risk of transmission of this chromosomal abnormality needs to be considered, and preimplantation screening may be desired.

TURNER SYNDROME (GONADAL DYSGENESIS) (45,X AND MOSAIC VARIANTS) ■

Pathophysiology   Approximately one-half of individuals with Turner syndrome (TS) have a 45,X karyotype, one-fourth have 46,XX/45,X mosaicism, and the remainder have structural abnormalities of the X chromosome such as X fragments, isochromosomes, or rings. The clinical features of TS result from haploinsufficiency of multiple X chromosomal genes (e.g., Short Stature Homeobox, *SHOX*). However, imprinted genes may also be affected when the inherited X has different parental origins.

Clinical Features   TS is characterized by bilateral streak gonads, primary amenorrhea, short stature, and multiple congenital anomalies in phenotypic females. It affects approximately 1 in 2500 women and is diagnosed at different ages depending on the dominant clinical features (Table 328-1). Prenatally, a diagnosis of TS is usually made incidentally after chorionic villous sampling or amniocentesis for unrelated reasons, such as advanced maternal age. Prenatal ultrasound findings include increased nuchal translucency and reduced fetal growth. The postnatal diagnosis of TS should be considered in female neonates or

TABLE 328-1 *Clinical Features of the Disorders of Chromosomal Sex*

Disorder	Common Chromosomal Complement	Gonad	External Genitalia	Internal Genitalia	Breast Development	Clinical Features
Klinefelter syndrome	47,XXY or 46,XY/47,XXY	Hyalinized testes	Male	Male	Gynecomastia	Small testes, azoospermia, decreased facial and axillary hair, decreased libido, tall stature & increased leg length, decreased penile length, increased risk of breast tumors, learning difficulties, obesity, varicose veins
Turner syndrome	45,X or 46,XX/45,X	Streak gonad or immature ovary	Female	Hypoplastic female	Immature female	Infancy: lymphedema, web neck, shield chest, low set hair line, cardiac defects and coarctation of the aorta, urinary tract malformations & horseshoe kidney Childhood: short stature, cubitus valgus, short neck, short 4th metacarpals, hypoplastic nails, micrognathia, scoliosis, otitis media & sensori-neural hearing loss, ptosis & amblyopia, multiple nevi & keloid formation, autoimmune thyroid disease, visuo-spatial learning difficulties Adulthood: pubertal failure & primary amenorrhea, hypertension, obesity, dyslipidemia, impaired glucose tolerance & insulin resistance, cardiovascular disease, aortic root dilatation, osteoporosis, inflammatory bowel disease, chronic hepatic dysfunction, increased risk of colon cancer, hearing loss
Mixed gonadal dysgenesis	46,XY/45,X	Testis or streak gonad	Variable— usually ambiguous	Variable	Usually male	Short stature, increased risk of gonadal tumors, some Turner syndrome features
True hermaphroditism	46,XY/46,XX	Testis & ovary or ovotestis	Variable— usually ambiguous	Variable	Gynecomastia	Increased risk of gonadal tumors

infants with lymphedema, nuchal folds, low hairline, or left-sided cardiac defects, and in girls with unexplained growth failure or pubertal delay. Although limited spontaneous pubertal development occurs in up to 30% of girls with TS (10%, 45,X; 30–40%, 45,X/46,XY), and approximately 2% reach menarche, the vast majority of women with TS develop complete ovarian failure. This diagnosis should be considered, therefore, in all women who present with primary or secondary amenorrhea and elevated gonadotropin levels.

℞ TREATMENT

The management of girls and women with TS requires a multidisciplinary approach because of the number of potentially involved organ systems. Detailed cardiac and renal evaluation should be performed at the time of diagnosis. Individuals with congenital heart defects (CHD) (30%) (bicuspid aortic valve, 30 to 50%; coarctation of the aorta, 30%; aortic root dilatation, 5%) require long-term follow-up by an experienced cardiologist, antibiotic prophylaxis for dental or surgical procedures, and serial imaging of aortic root dimensions, as progressive aortic root dilatation can occur. Individuals found to have congenital renal and urinary tract malformations (30%) are at risk for urinary tract infections, hypertension, and nephrocalcinosis. Hypertension can occur independent of cardiac and renal malformations, and should be monitored and treated as in other patients with essential hypertension. Clitoral enlargement or other evidence of virilization suggests the presence of covert, translocated Y chromosomal material and is associated with increased risk of gonadoblastoma, apparently the consequence of Y chromosomal genes distinct from *SRY*. Regular assessment of thyroid function, weight, dentition, hearing, speech, vision, and educational issues should be performed during childhood, and counseling about long-term growth and fertility issues should be provided. Patient support groups are active throughout the world.

The treatment of short stature in children with TS remains a challenge, as untreated final height rarely exceeds 150 cm. High-dose recombinant growth hormone stimulates growth rate in children with TS

and may be used alone or in combination with low doses of the non-aromatizable anabolic steroid oxandrolone (up to 0.05 mg/kg per d) in the older child (>8 years). However, final height increments are often modest (5–10 cm), and individualization of treatment regimens to response may be beneficial. Girls with evidence of gonadal failure require estrogen replacement to induce breast and uterine development, to support growth, and to maintain bone mineralization. Low-dose estrogen therapy (approximately one-sixth of the adult dose, 2 to 5 μg/d ethinylestradiol) is initiated between 12 to 14 years of age and increased gradually to induce feminization over a 2 to 3 year period. Progestins are later added to regulate withdrawal bleeds, and some women with TS have now achieved successful pregnancy after ovum donation and in vitro fertilization. Long-term follow-up of women with

TABLE 328-2 *Disorders Causing Undervirilization in Karyotypic Males (46,XY)*

Disorders of testis development
  True hermaphroditism (46,XY)
  Gonadal dysgenesis
  Absent testis syndrome
Disorders of androgen synthesis
  LH receptor mutations
  Smith-Lemli-Opitz syndrome
  Steroidogenic acute regulatory protein mutations
  Cholesterol side chain cleavage (*CYP11A1*) deficiency
  3β-Hydroxysteroid dehydrogenase 2 (*HSD3B2*) deficiency
  17α-Hydroxylase/17,20-lyase (*CYP17*) deficiency
  17β-Hydroxysteroid dehydrogenase 3 (*HSD17B3*) deficiency
  5α-Reductase 2 deficiency (*SRD5A2*)
  Aromatase overexpression
Disorders of androgen action
  Androgen Insensitivity Syndrome
  Androgen receptor cofactor defects
Other disorders of male reproductive tract
  Persistent müllerian duct syndrome
  Isolated hypospadias
  Cryptorchidism

TS involves careful surveillance of sex hormone replacement and reproductive function, bone mineralization, cardiac function and aortic root dimensions, blood pressure, weight and glucose tolerance, hepatic and lipid profiles, thyroid function, and hearing.

MIXED GONADAL DYSGENESIS (46,XY/45,X) Mixed gonadal dysgenesis typically results from 46,XY/45,X mosaicism. The phenotype of patients with this condition varies considerably, depending on the proportion and distribution of 46,XY cells. Although some patients have a predominantly female phenotype with somatic features of TS, streak gonads, and müllerian structures, other 46,XY/45,X individuals have a male phenotype and testes, and the diagnosis is made incidentally after amniocentesis or during investigation of infertility. In practice, most children who present to clinicians have ambiguous genitalia and variable somatic features. A female sex-of-rearing is often chosen (60%) if phallic development is poor, uterine structures are present, and if height potential is limited. However, gonadectomy is indicated to prevent further androgen secretion and to prevent development of gonadoblastoma (up to 25%). Individuals raised as males may require reconstructive surgery for hypospadias and removal of streak gonads. Scrotal testes can be preserved, but need regular examination for tumor development. Biopsy for carcinoma in situ is recommended in adolescence and testosterone supplementation may be required for virilization in puberty.

TRUE HERMAPHRODITISM (46,XY/46,XX) True hermaphroditism (TH) occurs when both an ovary and testis, or when an ovotestis, are found in one individual. For unclear reasons, gonadal asymmetry most often occurs with a testis on the right and an ovary on the left. True hermaphroditism due to 46,XY/46,XX mosaicism is rare and has a variable phenotype depending on the proportion of each cell line.

DISORDERS OF GONADAL AND PHENOTYPIC SEX

The clinical features of patients with disorders of gonadal and phenotypic sex are divided into the undervirilization of 46,XY males or inappropriate virilization of 46,XX females. These disorders comprise a spectrum of phenotypes ranging from complete "sex-reversal" (e.g., 46,XY phenotypic females or 46,XX males) to ambiguous genitalia.

UNDERVIRILIZED MALES (46,XY) (MALE PSEUDOHERMAPHRODITISM) Undervirilization of the male (46,XY) reflects defects in androgen production or action. It can result from disorders of testis development, defects of androgen synthesis, or resistance to testosterone and DHT (Table 328-2).

Disorders of Testis Development ■ *TESTICULAR DYSGENESIS* Patients with *pure gonadal dysgenesis* have streak gonads, müllerian structures (due to insufficient MIS secretion) and a complete absence of virilization.

TABLE 328-3 *Genetic Causes of Undervirilization of Karyotypic Males (46,XY)*

Gene	Inheritance	Gonad	Uterus	External Genitalia	Associated Features
DISORDERS OF TESTIS DEVELOPMENT					
WT1	AD	Dysgenetic testis	+/−	Female or ambiguous	Wilms' tumor, renal abnormalities, gonadal tumors (WAGR, Denys-Drash & Frasier syndromes)
SF1	AR/AD	Dysgenetic testis	+	Female or ambiguous	Primary adrenal failure
SRY	Y	Dysgenetic testis or ovary	+/−	Female or ambiguous	
SOX9	AD	Dysgenetic testis or ovary	+/−	Female or ambiguous	Campomelic dysplasia
DHH	AR	Testis/streak	+	Female	Minifascicular neuropathy
ATRX	X	Dysgenetic testis	−	Female or ambiguous	α-Thalassemia, developmental delay
ARX	X	Dysgenetic testis	−	Male or ambiguous	Mental retardation; X-linked lissencephaly
DAX1	dupXp21	Dysgenetic testis or ovary	+/−	Female or ambiguous	
WNT4	dup1p35	Dysgenetic testis	+	Ambiguous	
DISORDERS OF ANDROGEN SYNTHESIS					
LHR	AR	Testis	−	Female, ambiguous or micropenis	Leydig cell hypoplasia
DHCR7	AR	Testis	−	Variable	Smith-Lemli-Opitz syndrome: coarse facies, second-third toe syndactyly, failure to thrive, developmental delay, cardiac & visceral abnormalities
STAR	AR	Testis	−	Female	Congenital lipoid adrenal hyperplasia (primary adrenal failure)
CYP11A1	AR	Testis	−	Ambiguous	Congenital lipoid adrenal hyperplasia (primary adrenal failure)
HSD3B2	AR	Testis	−	Ambiguous	CAH, primary adrenal failure, partial virilization due to ↑ DHEA
CYP17	AR	Testis	−	Female or ambiguous	CAH, hypertension due to ↑ corticosterone & 11-deoxycorticosterone
HSD17B3	AR	Testis	−	Female or ambiguous	Partial virilization at puberty, ↑ androstenedione:testosterone ratio
SRD5A2	AR	Testis	−	Ambiguous	Partial virilization at puberty, ↑ testosterone:dihydrotestosterone ratio.
DISORDERS OF ANDROGEN ACTION					
Androgen receptor	X	Testis	−	Female, ambiguous, micropenis or normal male	Phenotypic spectrum from complete androgen insensitivity syndrome (female external genitalia) and partial androgen insensitivity (ambiguous) to normal male genitalia and infertility

Note: AR, autosomal recessive; AD, autosomal dominant; *WT1*, Wilms' tumor-related gene 1; WAGR, Wilms' tumor, aniridia, genitourinary anomalies, and mental retardation; *SF1*, steroidogenic factor 1; *SRY*, sex-related gene on the Y chromosome; *SOX9*, SRY-related HMG-box gene 9; *DHH*, desert hedgehog; *ATRX*, (α-thalassemia, mental retardation on the X); *ARX*, aristaless related homeobox, X-linked; *DAX1*, dosage sensitive sex-reversal, adrenal hypoplasia congenita on the X chromosome, gene 1; *WNT4*, wingless-type mouse mammary tumor virus integration site, 4; *LHR*, LH receptor; *DHCR7*, sterol 7δ reductase; *STAR*, steroidogenic acute regulatory protein; *CYP11A1*, P450 cholesterol side-chain cleavage; *HSD3B2*, 3β-hydroxysteroid dehydrogenase type 2; *CYP17*, 17α-hydroxylase and 17,20-lyase; *HSD17B3*, 17β-hydroxysteroid dehydrogenase type 3; *CYP19*, aromatase; *SRD5A2*, 5α-reductase type 2.

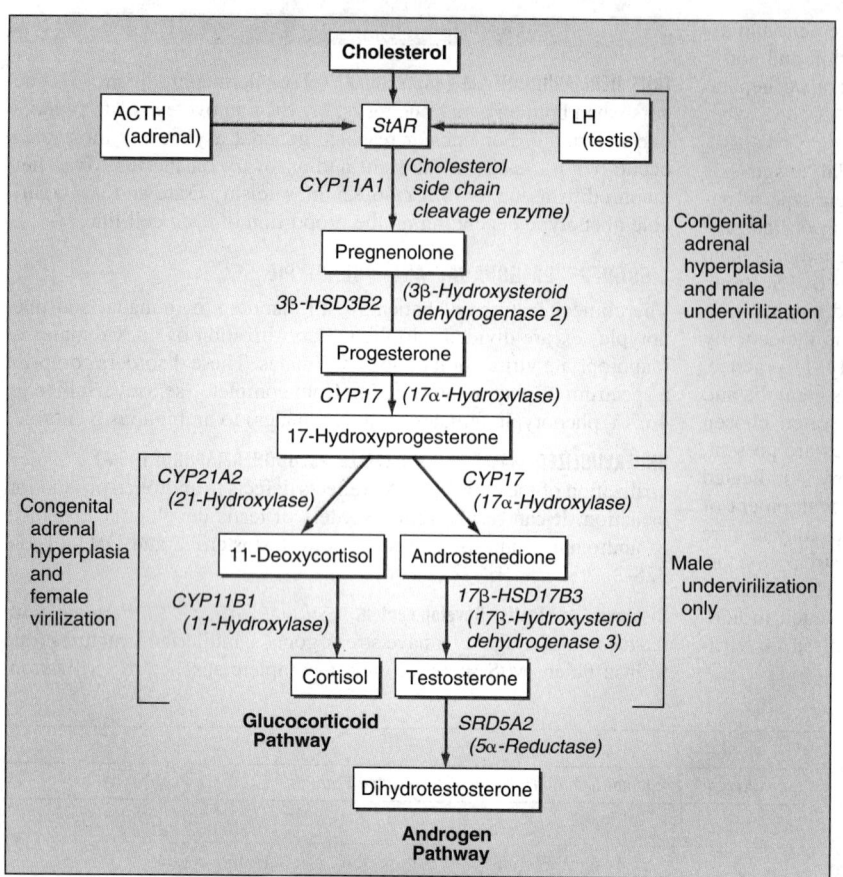

FIGURE 328-4 Pathways of glucocorticoid and androgen synthesis. Defects in *CYP21A2* and *CYP11B1* shunt steroid precursors into the androgen pathway and cause virilization of 46,XX females. Testosterone and dihydrotestosterone are synthesized in the testicular Leydig cells. Defects in enzymes involved in androgen synthesis result in undervirilization of 46,XY males. StAR, steroidogenic acute regulatory protein. [After JD Wilson, JE Griffin, in E Braunwald et al (eds): *Harrison's Principles of Internal Medicine*, 15th ed. New York, McGraw-Hill, 2001.]

Patients with *dysgenetic testes* produce enough MIS to regress the uterus and, sometimes, sufficient testosterone for partial virilization. Gonadal dysgenesis can result from mutations or deletions of testis-promoting genes (*WT1, SF1, SRY, SOX9, DAX1, DHH, ATRX, ARX*; also *DMRT*, and *SOX8* loci) or overexpression of factors that impair testis development when excessive (*WNT4, DAX1*) (Table 328-3). Associated clinical features may be present, reflecting additional functional roles for these genes. For example, renal dysfunction occurs in patients with specific *WT1* mutations (Denys-Drash and Frasier syndromes), primary adrenal failure occurs with *SF1* mutations, and severe cartilage abnormalities (campomelic dysplasia) are the predominant clinical feature of *SOX9* mutations. Dysgenetic testes should be removed to prevent malignancy, and estrogens can be used to induce secondary sex characteristics in 46,XY individuals raised as females. *Absent (vanishing) testis syndrome* reflects regression of the testis during development. The etiology is unknown but the absence of müllerian structures indicates adequate secretion of MIS in utero. Early testicular regression causes impaired virilization. Individuals raised as female should receive estrogen replacement at puberty. More frequently, late regression results in an otherwise normal male with anorchia. These individuals can be offered testicular prostheses and should receive androgen replacement in adolescence.

Disorders of Androgen Synthesis Defects in the pathway that regulates androgen synthesis (Fig. 328-4) cause undervirilization of the male fetus (Table 328-3). Müllerian regression is unaffected because Sertoli cell function is preserved.

LH RECEPTOR Mutations in the LH receptor cause Leydig cell hypoplasia and androgen deficiency. Defects of LH receptor synthesis or function preclude hCG (human chorionic gonadotropin) stimulation of

Leydig cells in utero, as well as LH stimulation of Leydig cells late in gestation and during the neonatal period. As a result, testosterone and DHT synthesis are insufficient for normal virilization of the internal and external genitalia, causing a spectrum of phenotypes that range from complete undervirilization to micropenis, depending on the severity of the mutation.

CONGENITAL ADRENAL HYPERPLASIA (CAH) Mutations in the genes that regulate cholesterol uptake and modification [*steroidogenic acute regulatory protein (StAR)*, *CYP11a*] affect both adrenal and gonadal steroidogenesis, and result in *congenital lipoid adrenal hyperplasia* (Chap. 321). Defects in *3β-hydroxysteroid dehydrogenase type 2 (HSD3B2)* also cause adrenal insufficiency, but the accumulation of dehydroepiandrosterone (DHEA) has a mild virilizing effect. Patients with congenital adrenal hyperplasia due to *17α-hydroxylase (CYP17) deficiency* have variable undervirilization and develop hypertension due to the potent salt-retaining effects of corticosterone and 11-deoxycorticosterone. Some mutations in *CYP17* selectively impair 17,20 lyase activity, without altering 17α-hydroxylase activity, leading to undervirilization without mineralocorticoid excess and hypertension.

SEX-STEROID PATHWAY ENZYMES Defects in *17β-hydroxysteroid dehydrogenase type 3 (HSD17B3)* and *5α-reductase type 2 (SRD5A2)* interfere with the synthesis of testosterone and DHT, respectively (Fig. 328-4). These conditions are characterized by minimal masculinization in childhood, but some phallic development can occur during adolescence due to the action of other enzyme isoforms. Individuals with *5α-reductase type 2* deficiency have normal wolffian structures and do not develop breast tissue. In some cultures, these individuals change gender role behavior from female to male at puberty, because the increase in testosterone induces muscle mass and other virilizing features. DHT cream can improve prepubertal phallic growth in patients raised as male. Individuals raised as female require gonadectomy, cosmetic surgery, and estrogen replacement.

Disorders of Androgen Action ■ *ANDROGEN INSENSITIVITY SYNDROME* Mutations in the androgen receptor (AR) cause resistance to androgen (testosterone, DHT) action or the *androgen insensitivity syndrome (AIS)*. AIS is a spectrum of disorders that affects at least 1 in 100,000 chromosomal males. Because the androgen receptor is X-linked, only males are affected and maternal carriers are phenotypically normal. XY individuals with *complete AIS (testicular feminization syndrome)* have a female phenotype, normal breast development, a short vagina but no uterus (because MIS production is normal), scanty pubic and axillary hair, and female psychosexual orientation. Gonadotropins and testosterone levels can be low, normal, or elevated, depending on the degree of androgen resistance and the contribution of estradiol to feedback inhibition of the hypothalamic-pituitary gonadal axis. Most patients present with inguinal herniae (containing testes) in childhood or with primary amenorrhea in adulthood. Gonadectomy is usually performed, as there is a low risk of malignancy, and estrogen replacement is prescribed. Surgical reconstruction or mechanical dilatation of the vagina permits sexual intercourse. *Partial AIS (Reifenstein syndrome)* results from less severe AR mutations. Patients present in infancy with perineoscrotal hypospadias, small cryptorchid testes, and with gynecomastia at the time of puberty. Those individuals raised as males require hypospadias repair in childhood and breast reduction in adolescence. Supplemental androgens rarely improve virilization significantly, as endogenous androgens are already increased. More severely undervirilized patients present with clitoral enlargement and labial fusion, and may be raised as females. The surgical and psychosexual management of both these groups of patients is complex and requires

TABLE 328-4 Disorders Causing Virilization in Karyotypic Females (46,XX)

Ovarian transdifferentiation
  True hermaphroditism (46,XX)
  XX male
Increased androgen synthesis
  3β-Hydroxysteroid dehydrogenase 2 (HSD3B2) deficiency
  21-Hydroxylase (CYP21A2) deficiency
  11β-Hydroxylase (CYP11B1) deficiency
  Aromatase (CYP19) deficiency
  Glucocorticoid receptor mutations
Increased androgen exposure
  Maternal virilizing tumors (e.g., luteomas of pregnancy)
Androgenic drugs
Nonvirilizing disorders of the female reproductive tract
  Ovarian dysgenesis
  Müllerian agenesis
  Vaginal agenesis

active involvement of the parents and the patient during the appropriate stages of development. *Azoospermia* and male-factor infertility has also been described in association with mild loss of function mutations in the androgen receptor. Trinucleotide (CAG) repeat expansion, from a mean of 22 repeats to greater than 40 repeats, within a highly polymorphic region of the androgen receptor is associated with spinal and bulbar muscular atrophy (also known as Kennedy disease). These patients may show evidence of partial androgen insensitivity in adolescence or adulthood (e.g., gynecomastia).

OTHER DISORDERS AFFECTING MALES (46,XY) *Persistent Müllerian Duct syndrome* is the presence of a uterus in an otherwise normal male. This condition can result from mutations in AMH or its receptor (AMHR2). The uterus may be removed, but damage to vasa deferentia must be avoided. *Isolated hypospadias* occurs in approximately 1 in 200 males and is treated by surgical repair. Most cases are idiopathic, although evidence of penoscrotal hypospadias and bilateral cryptorchidism require investigation for an underlying genetic disorder (e.g., defect in testosterone action). *Cryptorchidism* (unilateral) affects up to 3% of boys at birth. Orchidopexy should be considered if the testis has not descended by early childhood. Bilateral cryptorchidism occurs less frequently, and should raise suspicion of gonadotropin deficiency or disorders of sexual development. A subset of patients with cryptorchidism have mutations in the insulin-like 3 (INSL3) gene or its receptor LGR8 (also known as GREAT), which mediates normal testicular descent.

VIRILIZED FEMALES (46,XX) (FEMALE PSEUDOHERMAPHRODITISM) Inappropriate virilization of females can occur when the gonad (ovary) con-

tains androgen-secreting testicular material, or after increased androgen exposure (Table 328-4).

Gonadal Transdifferentiation Testicular tissue can develop in 46,XX true hermaphrodites, and in 46,XX males with a translocation of *SRY* or duplication of *SOX9* (Table 328-5).

Increased Androgen Exposure ■ *21-HYDROXYLASE DEFICIENCY* The *classic form* of 21-hydroxylase deficiency has an incidence of between 1 in 5000 and 15,000 and is the most frequent cause of virilization in chromosomal 46,XX females (Table 328-5; Chap. 321). Affected individuals are homozygous or compound heterozygous for severe mutations in the enzyme 21-hydroxylase (CYP21A2). This mutation causes a block in adrenal glucocorticoid and mineralocorticoid synthesis, increasing 17-hydroxyprogesterone, and shunting steroid precursors into the androgen synthesis pathway (Fig. 328-4). Glucocorticoid insufficiency causes a compensatory elevation of adrenocorticotropin (ACTH), resulting in adrenal hyperplasia and additional synthesis of steroid precursors proximal to the enzymatic block. Increased androgen synthesis *in utero* causes virilization of the female fetus. Ambiguous genitalia are seen at birth, with varying degrees of clitoral enlargement and labial fusion. Infants with the *salt-wasting* form of 21-hydroxylase deficiency develop primary adrenal failure in the first few weeks of life. Thus, a diagnosis of 21-hydroxylase deficiency should be considered in any baby with ambiguous genitalia; a salt-wasting crisis is a potentially life-threatening event. Males with this syndrome have no genital abnormalities at birth but are equally susceptible to adrenal insufficiency and salt-losing crises. If untreated, males undergo premature virilization (pseudopuberty) because of increased androgen levels during childhood. Females with the *classic simple virilizing* form of this disorder also present with genital ambiguity, but do not develop salt loss.

The diagnosis of classic 21-hydroxylase deficiency is made by neonatal screening tests for increased 17-hydroxyprogesterone in some centers. In most cases, 17-hydroxyprogesterone is markedly increased. In adults, ACTH stimulation (0.25 mg cosyntropin IV) with assays for 17-hydroxyprogesterone at 0 and 30 min can be useful for detecting nonclassic 21-hydroxylase deficiency and heterozygotes (Chap. 321).

℞ **TREATMENT**

Glucocorticoids must be given to correct the cortisol insufficiency and to suppress ACTH stimulation, thereby preventing further virilization, rapid skeletal maturation, and the development of polycystic ovaries. Typically, hydrocortisone (10 to 20 mg/m² per d in divided doses) is used with a goal of suppressing 17-hydroxyprogesterone to <1000 ng/

TABLE 328-5 Genetic Causes of Virilization of Karyotypic Females (46,XX)

Gene	Inheritance	Gonad	Uterus	External Genitalia	Associated Features
OVARIAN TRANSDIFFERENTIATION					
SRY	translocation	Testis or ovotestis	−	Male or ambiguous	
SOX9	dup17q24	Unknown	−	Male or ambiguous	
INCREASED ANDROGEN SYNTHESIS					
HSD3B2	AR	Ovary	+	Ambiguous	CAH, primary adrenal failure, partial virilization due to ↑ DHEA
CYP21A2	AR	Ovary	+	Ambiguous	CAH, phenotypic spectrum from severe salt-losing forms associated with adrenal failure to simple virilizing forms with compensated adrenal function, ↑ 17-hydroxyprogesterone
CYP11B1	AR	Ovary	+	Ambiguous	CAH, hypertension due to ↑ 11-deoxycortisol & 11-deoxycorticosterone
CYP19	AR	Ovary	+	Ambiguous	Maternal virilization during pregnancy, absent breast development at puberty
Glucocorticoid receptor	AR	Ovary	+	Ambiguous	↑ ACTH, 17-hydroxyprogesterone and cortisol; failure of dexamethasone suppression

Note: AR, autosomal recessive; *SRY*, sex-related gene on the Y chromosome; *SOX9*, SRY-related HMG-box gene 9; CAH, congenital adrenal hyperplasia; *HSD3B2*, 3β-hydroxy-steroid dehydrogenase type 2; *CYP21A2*, 21-hydroxylase; *CYP11B1*, 11β-hydroxylase; *CYP19*, aromatase; ACTH, adrenocorticotropin.

dL. It is difficult, however, to fully suppress androgen production without using excessive glucocorticoid treatment, which can impair growth and predispose to obesity. Older adolescents and adults are often treated with dexamethasone at night to provide more complete ACTH suppression. In very severe cases, adrenalectomy has been advocated but incurs the risks of major surgery and total adrenal insufficiency. Salt-wasting conditions are treated with mineralocorticoid replacement. Infants usually need salt supplements up to the first year of life. Plasma renin activity and electrolytes are used to monitor mineralocorticoid replacement. Newer therapeutic approaches, such as anti-androgens and aromatase inhibitors (to block premature epiphyseal closure) are under evaluation. Parents and patients should be aware of the need for increased doses of steroids during sickness and patients should carry medic alert systems.

Girls with significant virilization usually undergo clitoral reduction (maintaining the glans and nerve supply) and vaginal reconstruction, but the optimal timing of these procedures is the subject of debate. Surgical revision or regular vaginal dilatation may be needed in adolescence or adulthood, and long-term psychological support and psychosexual counseling may be appropriate.

Prenatal treatment of 21-hydroxylase deficiency by the administration of dexamethasone to mothers has been shown to reduce the degree of virilization in affected female fetuses. However, treatment on the mother and child must be started before 9 weeks gestation and ideally before 6–7 weeks; long-term effects are still under evaluation.

OTHER CAUSES Increased androgen synthesis can also occur in CAH due to defects in *11β-hydroxylase (CYP11B1)* and *3β-hydroxysteroid dehydrogenase type 2 (HSD3B2)*, and with mutations in the genes encoding *aromatase (CYP19)* and the glucocorticoid receptor. Increased androgen exposure *in utero* can occur with maternal virilizing tumors and with ingestion of androgenic compounds.

OTHER DISORDERS AFFECTING FEMALES (46,XX) *Congenital absence of the vagina* occurs in association with *müllerian agenesis* or *hypoplasia* as part of the Mayer-Rokitansky-Kuster-Hauser syndrome. This diagnosis should be considered in otherwise phenotypically normal females with primary amenorrhea. Rarer associated features include renal (agenesis) and cervical spinal abnormalities.

ACKNOWLEDGMENT
We are grateful to JD Wilson and JE Griffin, the authors of Disorders of Sexual Differentiation *in the 15th edition of* Harrison's, *for contributions to this chapter.*

FURTHER READING

ACHERMANN JC et al: Genetic causes of human reproductive disease. J Clin Endocrinol Metab 87:2447, 2002

AHMED SF, HUGHES IA: The genetics of male undermasculinization. Clin Endocrinol 56:1, 2002

ELSHEIKH M et al: Turner's syndrome in adulthood. Endocr Rev 23:120, 2002

KOOPMAN P: The genetics and biology of vertebrate sex determination. Cell 105:843, 2001

TILMANN C, CAPEL B: Cellular and molecular pathways regulating mammalian sex determination. Recent Prog Horm Res 57:1, 2002

329 | ENDOCRINE TUMORS OF THE GASTROINTESTINAL TRACT AND PANCREAS
Robert T. Jensen

Gastrointestinal neuroendocrine tumors (NETs) are tumors derived from the diffuse neuroendocrine system of the gastrointestinal (GI) tract, which is composed of amine- and acid-producing cells with different hormonal profiles, depending on the site of origin. The tumors they produce can be generally divided into carcinoid tumors and pancreatic endocrine tumors (PETs). These tumors were originally classified as APUDomas (for *a*mine *p*recursor *u*ptake and *d*ecarboxylation), as were pheochromocytomas, melanomas, and medullary thyroid carcinomas because they share certain cytochemical features as well as various pathologic, biologic, and molecular features (Table 329-1). APUDomas were thought to have a similar embryonic origin from neural crest cells, but the peptide-secreting cells are not of neuroectodermal origin.

CLASSIFICATION/PATHOLOGY/TUMOR BIOLOGY OF NETS

NETs are composed of monotonous sheets of small round cells with uniform nuclei; mitoses are uncommon. They can be tentatively identified on routine histology; however, these tumors are principally recognized by their histologic staining patterns due to shared cellular proteins. Historically, silver staining was used and tumors were classified as showing an argentaffin reaction if they took up and reduced silver or as being argyrophilic if they did not reduce it. Immunocytochemical localization of chromogranins (A, B, C), neuron-specific enolase, or synaptophysin, which are all neuroendocrine cell markers, are now used (Table 329-1). Chromogranin A is the most widely used.

Ultrastructurally, these tumors possess electron-dense neurosecretory granules and frequently contain small clear vesicles that correspond to synaptic vesicles of neurons. NETs synthesize numerous peptides, growth factors, and bioactive amines that may be ectopically secreted, giving rise to a specific clinical syndrome (Table 329-2). The diagnosis of the specific syndrome requires the clinical features of the disease and cannot be made from the immunocytochemistry results only. The presence or absence of a specific clinical syndrome cannot be predicted from the immunocytochemistry (Table 329-1). Further-

more, pathologists cannot distinguish between benign and malignant NETs unless metastases or invasion are present.

Carcinoid tumors are frequently classified according to their anatomic area of origin (i.e., foregut, midgut, hindgut), because tumors with similar areas of origin share functional manifestations, histochemistry, and secretory products (Table 329-3). Foregut tumors generally have a low serotonin (5HT) content, are argentaffin-negative but argyrophilic, occasionally secrete adrenocorticotropic hormone (ACTH) or 5-hydroxytryptophan (5HTP) causing an atypical carcinoid syndrome (Fig. 329-1), are often multihormonal, and may metastasize to bone. They uncommonly produce a clinical syndrome due to secreted products. Midgut carcinoids are argentaffin-positive, have a high serotonin content, most frequently cause the typical carcinoid syndrome when they metastasize (Table 329-3, Fig. 329-1), release serotonin and tachykinins (substance P, neuropeptide K, substance K), rarely secrete 5HTP or ACTH, and uncommonly metastasize to bone. Hindgut carcinoids (rectum, transverse and descending colon) are argentaffin-negative, often argyrophilic, rarely contain serotonin or cause the carcinoid syndrome (Fig. 329-1, Table 329-3), rarely secrete 5HTP or ACTH, contain numerous peptides, and may metastasize to bone.

PETs can be classified into nine well-established specific functional syndromes, two possible specific functional syndromes (PETs secreting calcitonin or renin), and nonfunctional PETs [pancreatic polypeptide (PP)-secreting tumors; PPomas] (Table 329-2). Each of the functional syndromes is associated with symptoms due to the specific hormone released. In contrast, nonfunctional PETs release no products that cause a specific clinical syndrome. "Nonfunctional" is a misnomer in the strict sense because they frequently secrete a number of peptides (PP, chromogranin A, ghrelin, neurotensin); however, they cause no specific clinical syndrome. The symptoms caused by nonfunctional PETs are entirely due to the tumor per se.

Carcinoid tumors can occur in almost any GI tissue; however, at present most (70%) originate from one of three sites: bronchus, jejuno-

TABLE 329-1 *General Characteristics of GI Neuroendocrine Tumors [Carcinoids, Pancreatic Endocrine Tumors (PETs)]*

I. Share general neuroendocrine cell markers
   A. Chromogranins (A, B, C) are acidic monomeric soluble proteins found in the large secretory granules; chromogranin A is most widely used
   B. Neuron-specific enolase (NSE) is the γ-γ dimer of the enzyme enolase and is a cytosolic marker of neuroendocrine differentiation
   C. Synaptophysin is an integral membrane glycoprotein of 38,000 molecular weight found in small vesicles of neurons and neuroendocrine tumors
II. Pathologic similarities
   A. All are APUDomas showing *amine precursor uptake and decarboxylation*
   B. Ultrastructurally they have dense-core secretory granules (>80 nm)
   C. Histologically appear similar with few mitoses and uniform nuclei
   D. Frequently synthesize multiple peptides/amines, which can be detected immunocytochemically but may not be secreted
   E. Presence or absence of clinical syndrome or type cannot be predicted by immunocytochemical studies
   F. Histologic classifications do not predict biologic behavior; only invasion or metastases establishes malignancy
III. Similarities of biologic behavior
   A. Generally slow growing, but a proportion are aggressive
   B. Secrete biologically active peptides/amines, which can cause clinical symptoms
   C. Generally have high densities of somatostatin receptors, which are used for both localization and treatment.
IV. Similarities/differences in molecular abnormalities
   A. Similarities
      1. Uncommon—alterations in common oncogenes (*ras, jun, fos,* etc)
      2. Uncommon—alterations in common tumor-suppressor genes (p53, retinoblastoma).
      3. Alterations at MEN-1 gene locus (11q13) and p16^{INK4a} (9p21) occur in a proportion (10–30%).
   B. Differences
      1. PETs—loss of 3p (8–47%), 3q (8–41%), 11q (21–62%), 6q (18–68%); gains at 17q (10–55%), 7q (16–68%).
      2. Carcinoids—loss of 18q (38–67%) >18p (33–43%) >9p (21%); gains at 17q, 19p (57%).

Note: MEN, multiple endocrine neoplasia; PETs, pancreatic endocrine tumors.

ileum, or colon/rectum (Table 329-3). In the past, carcinoid tumors most frequently occurred in the appendix (i.e., 40%); however, the bronchus/lung and small intestine are now the most common sites. Overall, GI carcinoids are the most common site for these tumors, comprising 64%, with the respiratory tract a distant second at 28%.

The term *pancreatic endocrine tumor*, although widely used and therefore retained here, is also a misnomer because these tumors can occur either almost entirely in the pancreas (insulinomas, glucagonomas, nonfunctional PETs, PETs causing hypercalcemia) or at both pancreatic and extrapancreatic sites [gastrinomas, VIPomas (VIP, vasoactive intestinal peptide), somatostatinomas, GRFomas (GRF, growth hormone–releasing factor)]. PETs are also called *islet cell tumors*; however, this term is discouraged because many do not originate from the islets and they can occur at extrapancreatic sites.

The exact incidence of carcinoid tumors or PETs varies according to whether only symptomatic or all tumors are considered. The incidence of clinically significant carcinoids is 7 to 13 cases per million population per year, whereas any malignant carcinoids at autopsy are reported in 21 to 84 cases per million population per year. Clinically significant PETs have a prevalence of 10 cases per million population, with insulinomas, gastrinomas, and nonfunctional PETs having an incidence of 0.5 to 2 cases per million population per year (Table 329-2). VIPomas are 2- to 8-fold less common, glucagonomas are 17- to 30-fold less common, and somatostatinomas the least common. In autopsy studies 0.5 to 1.5% of all cases have a PET; however, in <1 in 1000 cases was a functional tumor present.

Both carcinoid tumors and PETs commonly show malignant behavior (Tables 329-2, 329-3). Except for insulinomas, in which <10% are malignant, 50 to 100% of PETs are malignant. The fraction of

carcinoid tumors showing malignant behavior varies in different locations. For the three most common sites of occurrence the incidence of metastases varies greatly: jejuno-ileum (58%) > lung/bronchus (6%) > rectum (4%). A number of factors influence survival and the aggressiveness of the tumor (Table 329-4). The presence of liver metastases is the single most important prognostic factor for both carcinoid tumors and PETs. Particularly important in the development of liver metastases is the size of the primary tumor. For small-intestinal carcinoids, the most frequent cause of the carcinoid syndrome due to metastatic disease in the liver, metastases occur in 15 to 25% if the tumor diameter is <1 cm, 58 to 80% if it is 1 to 2 cm, and >75% if >2 cm. Similar data exist for gastrinomas and other PETs. The presence of lymph node metastases, the depth of invasion, various histologic features (differentiation, mitotic rates, growth indices), and the presence of aneuploidy are all important prognostic factors for the development of metastatic disease (Table 329-4). For patients with carcinoid tumors, additional poor prognosis factors include the development of the carcinoid syndrome, older age, male gender, the presence of a symptomatic tumor, or increases in a number of tumor markers [5-hydroxyindolactic acid (5-HIAA), neuropeptide K, chromogranin A]. With PETs or gastrinomas, the best studied PET, a worse prognosis is associated with female gender, overexpression of the *Ha-Ras* oncogene or p53, the absence of multiple endocrine neoplasia (MEN) type 1, and higher levels of various tumor markers (i.e., chromogranin A, gastrin).

A number of genetic disorders are associated with an increased incidence of NETs (Table 329-5). Each is caused by a loss of a putative tumor-suppressor gene. The most important is MEN-1, which is an autosomal dominant disorder due to a defect in a 10-exon gene on 11q13 that encodes for a 610-amino-acid nuclear protein, menin (Chap. 330). In patients with MEN-1, 95 to 100% develop hyperparathyroidism due to parathyroid hyperplasia, 80 to 100% develop PETs, 54 to 80% develop pituitary adenomas, and bronchial carcinoids develop in 8%, thymic carcinoids in 8%, and gastric carcinoids in 13 to 30% of the patients with Zollinger-Ellison syndrome (ZES). In patients with MEN-1, 80 to 100% develop nonfunctional PETs; functional PETs occur in 80%, with 54% developing ZES, 21% insulinomas, 3% glucagonomas, and 1% VIPomas. MEN-1 is present in 20 to 25% of all patients with ZES, in 4% with insulinomas, and in a low percentage (<5%) of the other PETs.

Three phacomatoses associated with NETs are von Hippel–Lindau disease, von Recklinghausen's disease [neurofibromatosis (NF) type 1], and tuberous sclerosis (Bourneville's disease). Von Hippel–Lindau disease is an autosomal dominant disorder due to defects on chromosome 3p25, which encodes for a 213-amino-acid protein that interacts with the elongin family of proteins as a transcriptional regulator (Chap. 358). In addition to cerebellar hemangioblastomas, renal cancer, and pheochromocytomas, 10 to 17% of these patients develop a PET. Most are nonfunctional, although insulinomas and VIPomas are reported. Patients with NF-1 have defects in a gene on chromosome 17q11.2 encoding for a 2845-amino-acid protein, neurofibromin, which functions in normal cells as a suppressor of the ras signaling cascade (Chap. 358). Up to 12% of these patients develop an upper GI carcinoid tumor, characteristically in the periampullary region (54%). Many are classified as somatostatinomas because they contain somatostatin immunocytochemically; however, they uncommonly secrete somatostatin or produce a clinical somatostatinoma syndrome. NF-1 has rarely been associated with insulinomas and ZES. Tuberous sclerosis is caused by mutations that alter either the 1164-amino-acid protein, hamartin (TSC1), or the 1807-amino-acid protein, tuberin (TSC2) (Chap. 358). Both hamartin and tuberin interact in a pathway related to cytosolic G protein regulation. A few cases including nonfunctional and functional PETs (insulinomas and gastrinomas) have been reported in these patients.

In contrast to most common nonendocrine tumors such as carcinoma of the breast, colon, lung or stomach, PETs and carcinoid tumors

TABLE 329-2 GI Neuroendocrine Tumor Syndromes

Name	Biologically Active Peptide(s) Secreted	Incidence New Cases/10⁶ Population/Year	Tumor Location	Malignant, %	Associated with MEN-1, %	Main Symptoms/Signs
I. ESTABLISHED SPECIFIC FUNCTIONAL SYNDROME						
Carcinoid tumor						
Carcinoid syndrome	Serotonin, possibly tachykinins, motilin, prostaglandins	0.5–2	Midgut (75–87%) Foregut (2–33%) Hindgut (1–8%) Unknown (2–15%)	95–100	Rare	Diarrhea (32–84%) Flushing (63–75%) Pain (10–34%) Asthma (4–18%) Heart disease (11–41%)
Pancreatic endocrine tumor						
Zollinger-Ellison syndrome	Gastrin	0.5–1.5	Duodenum (70%) Pancreas (25%) Other sites (5%)	60–90	20–25	Pain (79–100%) Diarrhea (30–75%) Esophageal symptoms (31–56%)
Insulinoma	Insulin	1–2	Pancreas (>99%)	<10	4–5	Hypoglycemic symptoms (100%)
VIPoma (Verner-Morrison syndrome, pancreatic cholera, WDHA)	Vasoactive intestinal peptide	0.05–0.2	Pancreas (90%, adult) Other (10%, neural, adrenal, periganglionic)	40–70	6	Diarrhea (90–100%) Hypokalemia (80–100%) Dehydration (83%)
Glucagonoma	Glucagon	0.01–0.1	Pancreas (100%)	50–80	1–20	Rash (67–90%) Glucose intolerance (38–87%) Weight loss (66–96%)
Somatostatinoma	Somatostatin	Rare	Pancreas (55%) Duodenum-jejunum (44%)	>70	45	Diabetes mellitus (63–90%) Cholelithiasis (65–90%) Diarrhea (35–90%)
GRFoma	Growth hormone–releasing hormone	Unknown	Pancreas (30%) Lung (54%) Jejunum (7%) Other (13%)	>60	16	Acromegaly (100%)
ACTHoma	ACTH	Rare	Pancreas (4–16%, all ectopic Cushing's)	>95	Rare	Cushing's syndrome (100%)
PET causing carcinoid syndrome	Serotonin, ? tachykinins	Rare (43 cases)	Pancreas (<1% all carcinoids)	60–88	Rare	Same as carcinoid syndrome above
PET causing hypercalcemia	PTHrP, others unknown	Rare	Pancreas (rare cause of hypercalcemia)	84	Rare	Abdominal pain due to hepatic metastases
II. POSSIBLE SPECIFIC FUNCTIONAL SYNDROME						
PET secreting calcitonin	Calcitonin	Rare	Pancreas (rare cause of hypercalcitonemia)	>80	16	Diarrhea (50%)
PET secreting renin	Renin	Rare	Pancreas	Unknown	No	Hypertension
III. NO FUNCTIONAL SYNDROME						
PPoma/nonfunctional	None	1–2	Pancreas (100%)	>60	18–44	Weight loss (30–90%) Abdominal mass (10–30%) Pain (30–95%)

Note: MEN, multiple endocrine neoplasia; VIPoma, tumor-secreting vasoactive intestinal peptide; WDHA, watery diarrhea, hypokalemia, and achlorhydria syndrome; ACTH, adrenocorticotrophic hormone; PET, pancreatic endocrine tumor; PTHrP, parathyroid hormone–related peptide; PPoma, tumor secreting pancreatic polypeptide.

do not have alterations in common oncogenes (ras, myc, fos, src, jun) or common tumor-suppressor genes (p53, retinoblastoma susceptibility gene) (Table 329-1). Alterations that may be important in their pathogenesis including changes in the *MEN-1* gene, p16/MTS1 tumor-suppressor gene, and DPC 4/*Smad* 4 gene, amplification of the HER-2/*neu* protooncogene and growth factors and their receptors, and deletions of unknown tumor-suppressor genes as well as gains in other unknown genes. Comparative genomic hybridization and genome-wide allelotyping studies have shown genetic differences between PETs and carcinoids (Table 329-1), some of which have prognostic significance (Table 329-4). Mutations in the *MEN-1* gene are particularly important. Loss of heterozygosity at the MEN-1 locus on chromosome 11q13 occurs in 46% of sporadic PETs (those without MEN-1) and in 26 to 75% of sporadic carcinoid tumors. Mutations in the *MEN-1* gene are reported in 31 to 34% of sporadic gastrinomas. The presence of a number of these molecular alterations correlates with tumor growth, tumor size, and disease extent or invasiveness and may have prognostic significance.

CARCINOID TUMORS AND CARCINOID SYNDROME

GENERAL TUMOR CHARACTERISTICS OF THE MOST COMMON GI CARCINOID TUMORS ■ Appendiceal Carcinoids
These occur in 1 in every 200 to 300 appendectomies, usually in the appendiceal tip. Most are <1 cm in diameter without metastases; however, up to 35% have metastases (Table 329-3). Among 1570 appendiceal carcinoids, 62% were localized and 27% had regional and 8% had distant metastases. Of tumors 1 to 2 cm in diameter, half metastasized to lymph nodes. The percentage of larger carcinoids has decreased from 43.9% (1950 to 1969) to 2.4% (1992 to 1999).

Small Intestinal Carcinoids
These are frequently multiple; 70 to 80% are present in the ileum and 70% are within 60 cm (24 in.) of the ileocecal valve. Some 40% are <1 cm in diameter, 32% are 1 to 2 cm, and 29% are >2 cm. Between 35 and 70% are associated with metastases (Table 329-3). They characteristically cause a marked fibrotic reaction that can lead to intestinal obstruction. Distant metastases occur to liver in 36 to 60% of patients, to bone in 3%, and to lung in 4%. Even small carcinoid tumors of the small intestine (<1 cm) have metastases in 15 to 25%; the incidence increases to 58 to 100% for tumors 1 to 2 cm in diameter. Carcinoids also occur in the duodenum, with 31% having metastases. No duodenal tumor <1 cm metastasized, whereas 33% of those >2 cm had metastases. Small-intestinal carcinoids are the most common cause (60 to 87%) of the carcinoid syndrome (Table 329-6).

TABLE 329-3 *Carcinoid Tumor Location, Frequency of Metastases, and Association with the Carcinoid Syndrome*

	Location (% of Total)	Incidence of Metastases	Incidence of Carcinoid Syndrome
Foregut			
Esophagus	<0.1	—	—
Stomach	4.6	10	9.5
Duodenum	2.0	—	3.4
Pancreas	0.7	71.9	20
Gallbladder	0.3	17.8	5
Bronchus, lung, trachea	27.9	5.7	13
Midgut			
Jejunum	1.8	} 58.4	9
Ileum	14.9		9
Meckel's diverticulum	0.5	—	13
Appendix	4.8	38.8	<1
Colon	8.6	51	5
Liver	0.4	32.2	—
Ovary	1.0	32	50
Testis	<0.1	—	50
Hindgut			
Rectum	13.6	3.9	—

Source: Location is from the PAN-SEER data (1973–1999), and incidence of metastases from the SEER data (1992–1999), reported by IM Modlin et al: Cancer 97:934, 2003. Incidence of carcinoid syndrome is from 4349 cases studied from 1950–1971, reported by JD Godwin: Cancer 36:560, 1975.

Rectal Carcinoids   Rectal carcinoids are found in 1 of every 2500 proctoscopies. Nearly all occur 4 to 13 cm above the dentate line. Most are small, with 66 to 80% being <1 cm in diameter; 5% metastasize. Tumors between 1 and 2 cm can metastasize in 5 to 30% of patients, and tumors >2 cm, which are uncommon, in >70%.

Bronchial Carcinoids   Bronchial carcinoids are not related to smoking. A number of different classifications have been proposed. In some

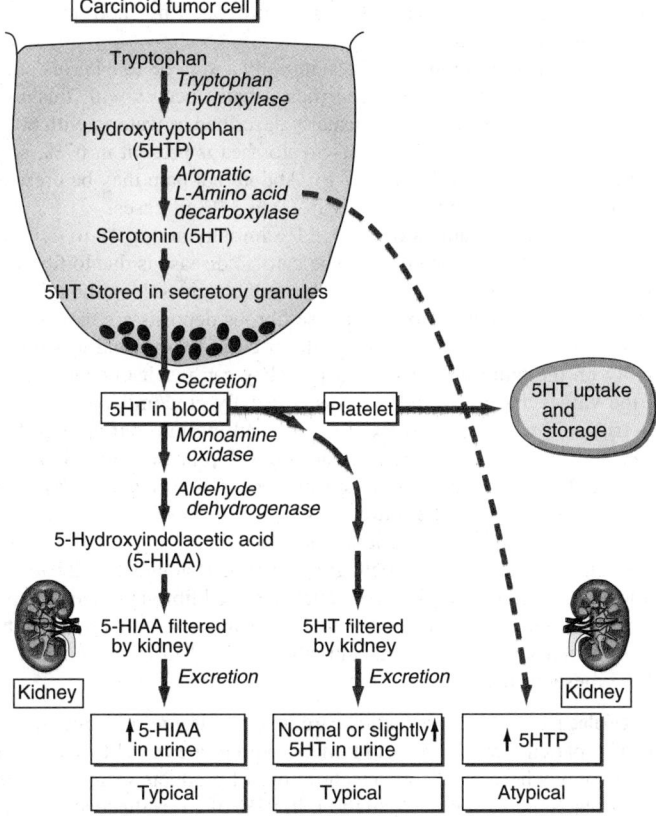

FIGURE 329-1   Synthesis, secretion, and metabolism of serotonin (5HT) in patients with typical and atypical carcinoid syndromes. Abbreviations: 5-HIAA, 5-hydroxyindolacetic acid.

TABLE 329-4 *Prognostic Factors in Neuroendocrine Tumors*

Both carcinoid tumors and PETs
  Presence of liver metastases ($p < .001$)
  Extent of liver metastases ($p < .001$)
  Presence of lymph node metastases ($p < .001$)
  Depth of invasion ($p < .001$)
  Primary tumor site ($p < .001$)
  Primary tumor size ($p < .005$)
  Various histologic features
    Tumor differentiation ($p < .001$)
    High growth indices (high Ki-67 index, PCNA expression)
    High mitotic counts ($p < .001$)
    Vascular or perineural invasion
    Flow cytometric features (i.e., aneuploidy)
Carcinoid tumors
  Presence of carcinoid syndrome
  Laboratory results [urinary 5-HIAA level ($p < .01$), plasma neuropeptide K ($p < .05$), serum chromogranin A ($p < .01$)]
  Presence of a secondary malignancy
  Male gender ($p < .001$)
  Older age ($p < .01$)
  Mode of discovery (incidental > symptomatic)
  Molecular findings [TGF-α expression ($p < .05$), chr 16q LOH or gain chr 4p ($p < .05$)]
PETs
  Ha-Ras oncogene or p53 overexpression
  Female gender
  MEN-1 syndrome absent
  Laboratory findings (increased chromogranin A in some studies; gastrinomas—increased gastrin level)
  Molecular findings [increased HER2/*neu* expression ($p = .032$), chr 1q, 3p,3q, or 6q LOH ($p = .0004$), EGF receptor overexpression ($p = .034$), gains in chr 7q, 17q, 17p, 20q]

Note: PET, pancreatic endocrine tumor; Ki-67, proliferation-associated nuclear antigen recognized by Ki-67 monoclonal antibody; PCNA, proliferating cell nuclear antigen; 5-HIAA, 5-hydroxy indolacetic acid; TGF-α, transforming growth factor α; chr, chromosome; LOH, loss of heterozygosity; MEN, multiple endocrine neoplasia; EGF, epidermal growth factor.

studies lung NETs are classified into four categories: typical carcinoid [also called bronchial carcinoid tumor, Kulchitsky cell carcinoma (KCC)-I]; atypical carcinoid (also called well-differentiated neuroendocrine carcinoma, KCC-II); intermediate small cell neuroendocrine carcinoma; and small cell neuroendocarcinoma (KCC-III). Another proposed classification includes three categories: benign or low-grade malignant (typical carcinoid); low-grade malignant (atypical carcinoid), and high-grade malignant (poorly differentiated carcinoma of the large cell or small cell type). These different categories of lung NETs have different prognoses varying from excellent for typical carcinoid to poor for small cell neuroendocrine carcinomas.

Gastric Carcinoids   These account for 3 of every 1000 gastric neoplasms. Three different subtypes of gastric carcinoids are observed. Each originates from gastric enterochromaffin-like (ECL) cells in the gastric mucosa. Two subtypes are associated with hypergastrinemic states: (1) chronic atrophic gastritis (type I) (80% of all gastric carcinoids), or (2) ZES, almost always as part of the MEN-1 syndrome (type II) (6% of all cases). These tumors generally pursue a benign course, with 9 to 30% associated with metastases. They are usually multiple and small and infiltrate only to the submucosa. The third subtype of gastric carcinoid (type III) (sporadic) occurs without hypergastrinemia (14% of all carcinoids) and pursues an aggressive course, with 54 to 66% developing metastases. Sporadic carcinoids are usually single, large tumors, 50% have atypical histology, and they can be a cause of the carcinoid syndrome. Gastric carcinoids as a percentage of all carcinoids are increasing in frequency [1.96% (1969 to 1971), 3.6% (1973 to 1991), 5.8% (1991 to 1999)].

CARCINOID TUMORS WITHOUT THE CARCINOID SYNDROME   The age of patients at diagnosis ranges from 10 to 93 years, with a mean age of 63 years for small intestine and 66 years for the rectum. The presentation

Syndrome	Location of Gene Mutation and Gene Product	NETs Seen/Frequency
Multiple endocrine neoplasia type 1 (MEN-1)	11q13 (encodes 610-amino-acid protein, menin)	80–100% develop PETs: (nonfunctional > gastrinoma > insulinoma) Carcinoids: gastric (13–30%), bronchial/thymic (8%)
von Hippel–Lindau disease	3q25 (encodes 213-amino-acid-protein)	12–17% develop PETs (almost always nonfunctional)
von Recklinghausen's disease [neurofibromatosis1 (NF-1)]	17q11.2 (encodes 2485-amino-acid protein, neurofibromin)	Duodenal somatostatinomas (usually nonfunctional) Rarely insulinoma, gastrinoma
Tuberous sclerosis	9q34 (TSCI) (encodes 1164-amino-acid protein, hamartin) 16p13 (TSC2) (encodes 1807-amino-acid protein, tuberin)	Uncommonly develop PETs [nonfunctional and functional (insulinoma, gastrinoma)]

is diverse and related to the site of origin and extent of malignant spread. In the appendix, carcinoid tumors are usually found incidentally during surgery for suspected appendicitis. Small-intestinal carcinoids in the jejunoileum present with periodic abdominal pain (51%), intestinal obstruction with ileus/invagination (31%), an abdominal tumor (17%), or GI bleeding (11%). Because of the vagueness of the symptoms the diagnosis is usually delayed about 2 years from onset of the symptoms, with a range up to 20 years. Duodenal, gastric, and rectal carcinoids are most frequently found by chance at endoscopy. The most common symptoms of rectal carcinoids are melena/bleeding (39%), constipation (17%), and diarrhea (12%). Bronchial carcinoids are frequently discovered as a lesion on a chest radiograph, and 31% of the patients are asymptomatic. Thymic carcinoids present as anterior mediastinal masses, usually on chest radiograph or computed tomography (CT) scan. Ovarian and testicular carcinoids usually present as masses discovered on physical examination or ultrasound. Metastatic carcinoid tumor in the liver frequently presents as hepatomegaly in a patient who may have minimal symptoms and near-normal liver function tests.

CARCINOID TUMORS WITH SYSTEMIC SYMPTOMS DUE TO SECRETED PRODUCTS

Carcinoid tumors immunocytochemically can contain numerous GI peptides: gastrin, insulin, somatostatin, motilin, neurotensin, tachykinins (substance K, substance P, neuropeptide K), glucagon, gastrin-releasing peptide, VIP, PP, other biologically active peptides (ACTH, calcitonin, growth hormone), prostaglandins, and bioactive amines (serotonin). These substances may or may not be released in sufficient

amounts to cause symptoms. In patients with carcinoid tumors, elevated serum levels of PP were found in 43%, motilin in 14%, gastrin in 15%, and VIP in 6%. Foregut carcinoids are more likely to produce various GI peptides than midgut carcinoids. Ectopic ACTH production causing Cushing's syndrome is increasingly seen with foregut carcinoids (respiratory tract primarily) and in some series was the most common cause of the ectopic ACTH syndrome, accounting for 64% of all cases. Acromegaly due to GRF release occurs with foregut carcinoids; the somatostatinoma syndrome with duodenal carcinoids. The most common systemic syndrome with carcinoid tumors is the carcinoid syndrome.

CARCINOID SYNDROME ■ Clinical Features
The cardinal features at presentation and during the disease course are shown in Table 329-6. Flushing and diarrhea are the two most common symptoms, occurring in up to 73% initially and in up to 89% during the course of the disease. The characteristic flush is of sudden onset; it is a deep red or violaceous erythema of the upper body (especially the neck and face), often associated with a feeling of warmth, and occasionally associated with pruritus, lacrimation, diarrhea, or facial edema. Flushes may be precipitated by stress, alcohol, exercise, or certain foods such as cheese or by certain agents such as catecholamines, pentagastrin, and serotonin reuptake inhibitors. Flushing episodes may be brief, lasting 2 to 5 min, especially initially, or may last hours, especially later in the disease course. Flushing is usually seen with midgut carcinoids but can also occur with foregut carcinoids. With bronchial carcinoids the flushes are frequently prolonged for hours to days, reddish in color, and associated with salivation, lacrimation, diaphoresis, diarrhea, and hypotension. The flush associated with gastric carcinoids is also reddish in color but patchy in distribution over the face and neck. It may be provoked by food and have accompanying pruritus.

Diarrhea is present in 32 to 73% initially and in 68 to 84% at some time in their disease course. Diarrhea usually occurs with flushing (85% of cases). The diarrhea is usually described as watery, with 60% having <1 L per day of diarrhea. Steatorrhea is present in 67%, and in 46% it is >15 g/d (normal <7 g). Abdominal pain may be present with the diarrhea or independently in 10 to 34% of cases.

Cardiac manifestations occur in 11% initially and in 14 to 41% at some time in the disease course. The cardiac disease is due to fibrosis involving the endocardium, primarily on the right side, although left side lesions can occur also. The dense fibrous deposits are most commonly on the ventricular aspect of the tricuspid valve and less commonly on the pulmonary valve cusps. They can result in constriction of the valves and pulmonic stenosis is usually predominant, whereas the tricuspid valve is often fixed open, resulting in regurgitation. Up to 80% of patients with cardiac lesions develop heart failure. Lesions on the left side are much less extensive, occur in 30% at autopsy, and most frequently affect the mitral valve.

Other clinical manifestations include wheezing or asthma-like symptoms (8 to 18%) and pellagra-like skin lesions (2 to 25%). A variety of noncardiac problems due to increased fibrous tissue may be seen including retroperitoneal fibrosis causing urethral obstruction, Peyronie's disease of the penis, intraabdominal fibrosis, and occlusion of the mesenteric arteries or veins.

Pathobiology   In different studies carcinoid syndrome occurred in 8% of 8876 patients with carcinoid tumors, with a rate of 1.4 to 18.4%. It occurs only when sufficient concentrations of products secreted by the tumor reach the systemic circulation. In 91% of cases this occurs after distant metastases to the liver. Rarely primary gut carcinoids with nodal metastases with extensive retroperitoneal invasion, pancreatic carcinoids with retroperitoneal lymph nodes, or carcinoids of the lung

	At Presentation	During Course of Disease
Symptoms/signs		
Diarrhea	32–73%	68–84%
Flushing	23–65%	63–74%
Pain	10%	34%
Asthma/wheezing	4–8%	3–18%
Pellagra	2%	5%
None	12%	22%
Carcinoid heart disease present	11%	14–41%
Demographics		
Male	46–59%	46–61%
Age		
Mean	57 yrs	52–54 yrs
Range	25–79 yrs	9–91 yrs
Tumor location		
Foregut	5–9%	2–33%
Midgut	78–87%	60–87%
Hindgut	1–5%	1–8%
Unknown	2–11%	2–15%

or ovary with direct access to the systemic circulation can cause the carcinoid syndrome without hepatic metastases. All carcinoid tumors do not have the same propensity to metastasize and cause the carcinoid syndrome (Table 329-3). Midgut carcinoids account for 60 to 67% of the cases of carcinoid syndrome, foregut tumors for 2 to 33%, hindgut for 1 to 8%, and an unknown primary location for 2 to 15% (Tables 329-2, 329-3).

One of the main secretory products of carcinoid tumors involved in the carcinoid syndrome is serotonin (Fig. 329-1), which is synthesized from tryptophan. Up to 50% of dietary tryptophan can be used in this synthetic pathway by tumor cells, which can result in inadequate supplies for conversion to niacin; thus, some patients (2.5%) develop pellagra-like lesions. Serotonin has numerous biologic effects including stimulating intestinal secretion, inhibition of absorption, increasing intestinal motility, and stimulating fibrogenesis. Serotonin overproduction is found in 56 to 88% of all carcinoid tumors; however, 12 to 26% of patients do not have the carcinoid syndrome. In 90 to 100% of patients with the carcinoid syndrome serotonin is overproduced. Through its effects on gut motility and intestinal secretion, serotonin is thought to be predominantly responsible for the diarrhea. Serotonin receptor antagonists (especially $5HT_3$ antagonists) relieve the diarrhea in most patients. However, prostaglandin E_2 and tachykinins may be important mediators of the diarrhea in some patients. Serotonin does not appear to be involved in the flushing, because flushing is not relieved by serotonin receptor antagonists. In patients with gastric carcinoids the red, patchy pruritic flush is likely due to histamine release, because it can be prevented by H_1 and H_2 receptor antagonists. Numerous studies show tachykinins are stored in carcinoid tumors and released during flushing. However, octreotide can relieve the flushing induced by pentagastrin in these patients without altering the stimulated increase in plasma substance P, suggesting other mediators must be involved in the flushing. Both histamine and serotonin may be responsible for the wheezing as well as the fibrotic reactions involving the heart, Peyronie's disease, and intraabdominal fibrosis. The exact mechanism of the heart disease is unclear. The valvular heart disease caused by the appetite-suppressant drug dexfenfluramine is histologically indistinguishable from that observed in carcinoid disease or after long exposure to $5HT_2$-preferring ergot drugs. Metabolites of fenfluramine have high affinity for $5HT_2$ receptors whose activation is known to cause fibroblast mitogenesis. High levels of $5HT_{2B}$ and $5HT_{2C}$ receptor transcripts are known to occur in heart valves. Studies on sheep aortic valve interstitial cells demonstrate serotonin interacts primarily with $5HT_{2A/2B}$ receptors and stimulates transforming growth factor-β and collagen biosynthesis. Thus, serotonin overproduction is important for the valvular changes, possibly by activating $5HT_2$ receptors in the endocardium. Both the magnitude of serotonin overproduction and prior chemotherapy are important predictors of progression of the heart disease. Atrial natriuretic peptide overproduction is also reported in patients with cardiac disease, but its role in the pathogenesis is unknown.

Patients may develop either a typical or atypical carcinoid syndrome (Fig. 329-1). In patients with the typical form, characteristically caused by a midgut carcinoid tumor, the conversion of tryptophan to 5HTP is the rate-limiting step. Once 5HTP is formed it is rapidly converted to 5HT and stored in secretory granules of the tumor or in platelets. A small amount remains in plasma and is converted to 5-HIAA, which appears in large amounts in the urine. These patients have an expanded serotonin pool size, increased blood and platelet serotonin, and increased urinary 5-HIAA. Some carcinoid tumors cause an atypical carcinoid syndrome thought due to a deficiency in the enzyme dopa decarboxylase in which 5HTP cannot be converted to 5HT (serotonin), and 5HTP is secreted into the bloodstream. In these patients plasma serotonin levels are normal but urinary levels may be increased because some 5HTP is converted to 5HT in the kidney. Characteristically, urinary 5HTP and 5HT are increased, but urinary 5-HIAA levels are only slightly elevated. Foregut carcinoids are the most likely to cause an atypical carcinoid syndrome.

One of the most life-threatening complications of the carcinoid syndrome is the development of a carcinoid crisis. This is more fre-

quent in patients who have intense symptoms from foregut tumors or have greatly increased urinary 5-HIAA levels (i.e., >200 mg/d). The crises may occur spontaneously or be provoked by stress, anesthesia, chemotherapy, or a biopsy. Patients develop intense flushing, diarrhea, abdominal pain, and cardiac abnormalities including tachycardia, hypertension, or hypotension. If not adequately treated it can be fatal.

Diagnosis of the Carcinoid Syndrome and Carcinoid Tumors The diagnosis of carcinoid syndrome relies on measurement of urinary or plasma serotonin or its metabolites in the urine. The measurement of 5-HIAA is most frequently used. False-positive elevations may occur if the patient is eating serotonin-rich foods, such as bananas, pineapple, walnuts, pecans, avocados, or hickory nuts, or taking certain medications (cough syrup containing guaifenesin, acetaminophen, salicylates, or L-dopa). The normal range in daily urinary 5-HIAA excretion is between 2 and 8 mg/d. 5-HIAA has 73% sensitivity and 100% specificity for carcinoid syndrome.

Most physicians use only the urinary 5-HIAA excretion rate; however, plasma and platelet serotonin levels, if available, may give additional information. Platelet serotonin levels are more sensitive than urinary 5-HIAA but are not generally available. Patients with foregut carcinoids may produce an atypical carcinoid syndrome. If this syndrome is suspected and the urinary 5-HIAA is minimally elevated or normal, other urinary metabolites of tryptophan such as 5HTP or 5HT should be measured (Fig. 329-1).

Flushing occurs in a number of other diseases including systemic mastocytosis or chronic myeloid leukemia with increased histamine release; in menopause; as a reaction to alcohol or glutamate; or as side effects of chlorpropamide, calcium channel blockers, and nicotinic acid. None of these conditions cause an increase in urinary 5-HIAA.

The diagnosis of carcinoid tumor can be suggested by the carcinoid syndrome, by recurrent abdominal symptoms in a healthy-appearing individual, or by discovering hepatomegaly or hepatic metastases associated with minimal symptoms. Ileal carcinoids, which make up 25% of all clinically detected carcinoids, should be suspected in patients with bowel obstruction, abdominal pain, flushing, or diarrhea.

Serum chromogranin A levels are elevated in 56 to 100% of patients with carcinoid tumors, and the level correlates with tumor bulk. Serum chromogranin A levels are not specific for carcinoid tumors because they are also elevated in patients with PETs and other NETs. Plasma neuron-specific enolase levels are also used as a marker of carcinoid tumors but are less sensitive than chromogranin A, being increased in only 17 to 47% of patients.

R̲x̲ TREATMENT

Carcinoid Syndrome Treatment includes avoiding conditions that precipitate flushing, dietary supplementation with nicotinamide, treatment of heart failure with diuretics, treatment of wheezing with oral bronchodilators, and controlling the diarrhea with antidiarrheal agents such as loperamide or diphenoxylate. If patients still have symptoms, serotonin receptor antagonists or somatostatin analogues (Fig. 329-2) are the drugs of choice.

There are 14 subclasses of serotonin (5HT) receptors; antagonists for most are not available. The $5HT_1$ and $5HT_2$ receptor antagonists methysergide, cyproheptadine, and ketanserin have all been used to control diarrhea but usually do not decrease flushing. The use of methysergide is limited because it can cause or enhance retroperitoneal fibrosis. Ketanserin diminishes diarrhea in 30 to 100% of patients. $5HT_3$ receptor antagonists (ondansetron, tropisetron, alosetron) can control diarrhea and nausea in up to 100% of patients and occasionally ameliorate the flushing. A combination of histamine H_1 and H_2 receptor antagonists (i.e., diphenhydramine and cimetidine or ranitidine) may control flushing in patients with foregut carcinoids.

Synthetic analogues of somatostatin (octreotide, lanreotide) are now the most widely used agents to control the symptoms of patients with carcinoid syndrome (Fig. 329-2). These drugs are effective at

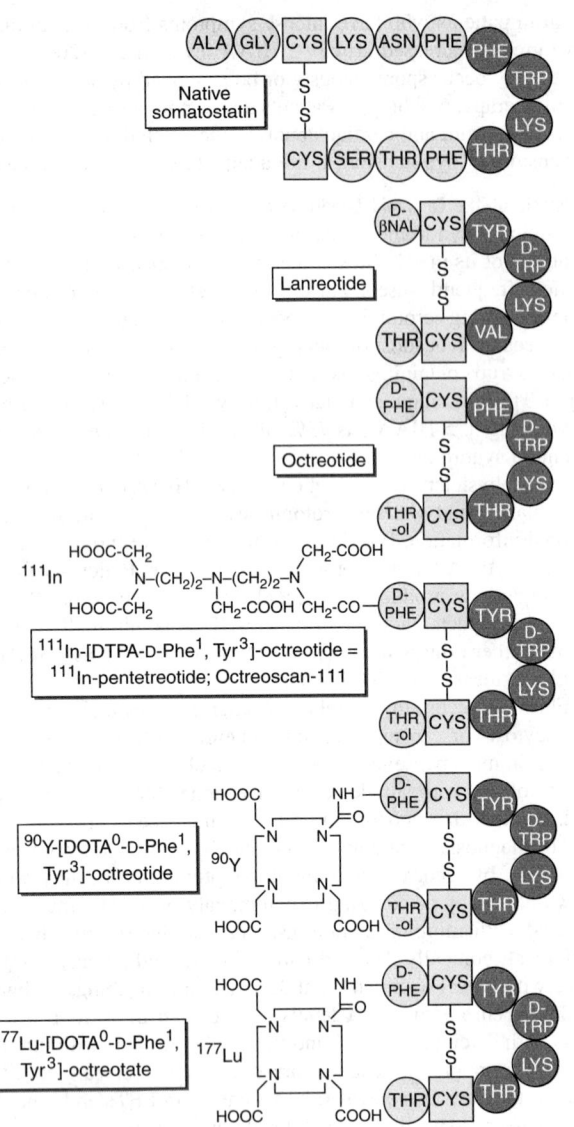

FIGURE 329-2   Structure of somatostatin and synthetic analogues used for diagnostic or therapeutic indications.

trolling the symptoms of the carcinoid syndrome (61 to 85% of patients).

Short-term side effects occur in 40 to 60% of patients receiving subcutaneous somatostatin analogues. Pain at the injection site and side effects related to the GI tract (59% discomfort, 15% nausea, diarrhea) are the most common. They are usually short-lived and do not interrupt treatment. Important long-term side effects include gallstone formation, steatorrhea, and deterioration in glucose tolerance. The overall incidence of gallstones/biliary sludge is 52%, with 7% having symptomatic disease requiring surgical treatment.

Interferon-α controls symptoms of the carcinoid syndrome either alone or combined with hepatic artery embolization. The response rate to interferon-α alone is 42%, and when combined with hepatic artery embolization, diarrhea was controlled for 1 year in 43% and flushing in 86%.

Hepatic artery embolization alone or with chemotherapy (chemoembolization) has been used to control the symptoms of carcinoid syndrome. Embolization alone is reported to control symptoms in up to 76% of patients, and chemoembolization (5-fluorouracil, adriamycin, cisplatin, mitomycin) in 60 to 75% of patients. Hepatic artery embolization can have major side effects including nausea, vomiting, pain, and fever. The mortality rate is 5 to 7%.

Other drugs have been used successfully in small numbers of patients to control the symptoms of carcinoid syndrome. Parachlorophenylanine can inhibit tryptophan hydroxylase and therefore the conversion of tryptophan to 5HTP (Fig. 329-1). However, its severe side effects, including psychiatric disturbances, make it intolerable for long-term use. α-Methyldopa inhibits the conversion of 5HTP to 5HT; however, its effects are only partial.

Carcinoid Tumors (Nonmetastatic)   Surgery is the only potentially curative therapy. Because the probability of metastatic disease increases with increasing primary tumor size, the extent of surgical resection is determined accordingly. With appendiceal carcinoids, simple appendectomy was curative in 103 patients followed for up to 35 years. With rectal carcinoids <1 cm, local resection is curative. With small-intestinal carcinoids <1 cm, consensus has not been reached. Because 15 to 69% of small-intestinal carcinoids this size have metastases in different studies, some recommend a wide resection with en bloc resection of the adjacent lymph-bearing mesentery. If the carcinoid tumor is >2 cm in rectal, appendiceal, or small-intestinal sites, a full cancer operation should be done. This includes a right hemicolectomy for appendiceal carcinoid, an abdominoperineal resection or low anterior resection for rectal carcinoids, and an en bloc resection of adjacent lymph nodes for small-intestinal carcinoids. For carcinoids 1 to 2 cm in the appendix, a simple appendectomy is proposed by some, whereas others favor a formal right hemicolectomy. For rectal carcinoids of 1 to 2 cm, a wide local full-thickness excision is recommended.

With type I or II gastric carcinoids, which are usually <1 cm, endoscopic removal is recommended. For type I or II gastric carcinoids >2 cm or locally invasive, some recommend total gastrectomy; others recommend antrectomy in type 1. For types I and III gastric carcinoids of 1 to 2 cm, some recommend endoscopic treatment, others surgical treatment. With type III gastric carcinoids >2 cm, excision and regional lymph node clearance are recommended. Most tumors <1 cm are treated endoscopically.

Resection of isolated or limited hepatic metastases may be beneficial (see below).

PANCREATIC ENDOCRINE TUMORS

Functional PETs usually present with symptoms due to hormone excess. Only late in the course of the disease does the tumor per se cause prominent symptoms such as abdominal pain. In contrast, all of the symptoms due to nonfunctional PETs are due to the tumor per se. The overall result is that some functional PETs may present with severe symptoms with a small or undetectable primary tumor, whereas nonfunctional tumors almost always present late in their disease course with large tumors that are usually metastatic. The mean delay between

relieving symptoms and decreasing urinary 5-HIAA levels in patients with carcinoid syndrome. Octreotide controls symptoms in >80% of patients, including the diarrhea and flushing, and produces a >50% decrease in urinary 5-HIAA excretion in 70% of patients. Patients with mild to moderate symptoms should initially be treated with 100 μg subcutaneously every 8 h. Individual responses vary; doses as high as 3000 μg/d have been given. About 40% of patients escape control after a median 4 months, and the dose may need to be increased. Similar results are reported with lanreotide.

In patients with carcinoid crises, somatostatin analogues are effective at both treating the condition as well as preventing its development during known precipitating events such as surgery, anesthesia, chemotherapy, or stress. Octreotide, 150 to 250 μg subcutaneously every 6 to 8 h, should be used 24 to 48 h before anesthesia and then continued throughout the procedure.

Sustained-release preparations of both octreotide [octreotide-LAR, (long-acting release)] and lanreotide [lanreotide-PR (prolonged release)] have been developed. Octreotide-LAR (30 mg/month) gives a plasma level ≥ 1 ng/mL for 25 days, whereas the non-sustained-release form would need to be injected three to six times a day to achieve this level. Lanreotide-PR is given intramuscularly every 10 to 14 days. Both sustained-release forms are highly effective at con-

onset of continuous symptoms and diagnosis of a functional PET syndrome is 4 to 7 years. Therefore, the diagnoses are frequently missed for extended periods of time.

Treatment of PETs requires two different strategies. Treatment must be directed at the hormone excess state such as the gastric acid hypersecretion in gastrinomas or hypoglycemia in insulinomas. Ectopic hormone secretion usually causes the presenting symptoms and can cause life-threatening complications. Second, with all of the tumors except insulinomas, >50% are malignant (Table 329-2); therefore, treatment must also be directed against the tumor per se. Because these tumors are not frequently surgically curable due to the extent of disease, in many cases surgical resection for cure, which addresses both treatment aspects, is not possible.

GASTRINOMA (ZOLLINGER-ELLISON SYNDROME)
A gastrinoma is a NET that secretes gastrin. The chronic hypergastrinemia results in marked gastric acid hypersecretion (ZES) and growth of the gastric mucosa, with increased numbers of parietal cells and proliferation of gastric ECL cells. The gastric acid hypersecretion characteristically causes peptic ulcer disease (PUD), often refractory and severe, as well as diarrhea. The most common presenting symptoms are abdominal pain (70 to 100%), diarrhea (37 to 73%), and gastroesophageal reflux disease (GERD) (30 to 35%), though 10 to 20% have diarrhea only. Although peptic ulcers may occur in unusual locations, most patients have a typical duodenal ulcer. Important observations that should suggest this diagnosis include PUD with diarrhea; PUD in an unusual location or with multiple lesions; and PUD that is refractory to treatment or persistent, associated with prominent gastric folds, associated with findings suggestive of MEN-1 (endocrinopathy, family history of ulcer or endocrinopathy, nephrolithiasis), or without *Helicobacter pylori* present. *H. pylori* is present in >90% of idiopathic peptic ulcers but is present in <50% of patients with gastrinomas. Chronic unexplained diarrhea should also suggest gastrinoma.

About 20 to 25% of patients have MEN-1, and in most cases the hyperparathyroidism is present before the gastrinoma. These patients are treated differently from those without MEN-1; therefore, MEN-1 should be sought in all patients by family history, by measuring plasma ionized calcium and prolactin levels and plasma hormone levels (parathormone, growth hormone).

Most gastrinomas (50 to 70%) are present in the duodenum, followed by the pancreas (20 to 40%) and other intraabdominal sites (mesentery, lymph nodes, biliary tract, liver, stomach, ovary). Rare cases may originate outside the abdominal cavity. In MEN-1 the gastrinomas are also usually in the duodenum (70 to 90%) or the pancreas (10 to 30%), and they are almost always multiple. Between 60 and 90% of gastrinomas are malignant (Table 329-2), with metastatic spread to lymph nodes and liver. Distant metastases to bone occur in 12 to 30% of patients with liver metastases.

Diagnosis The diagnosis of gastrinoma requires the demonstration of fasting hypergastrinemia and an increased basal gastric acid output (BAO) (hyperchlorhydria). Nearly all patients with gastrinomas have fasting hypergastrinemia, although in 40 to 60% the level may be elevated by less than a factor of 10. Therefore, when the diagnosis is suspected a fasting gastrin level should be determined first. Potent gastric acid–suppressant drugs such as proton pump inhibitors (omeprazole, pantoprazole, lansoprazole, rabeprazole) can suppress acid secretion sufficiently to cause hypergastrinemia; because of their prolonged duration of action, these drugs need to be discontinued for a week before the gastrin determination. If the gastrin level is elevated, gastric pH should be measured. If gastric pH < 2.0, the hypergastrinemia is not a physiologic response to achlorhydria (atrophic gastritis, pernicious anemia), another common cause of hypergastrinemia. If the fasting gastrin > 1000 μg/L (10 times increased) and the pH < 2.0, which occurs in 40 to 60% of patients with gastrinoma, the diagnosis is established after ruling out the possibility of retained antrum syndrome by history. In patients with hypergastrinemia with fasting gastrin < 1000 μg/L and gastric pH < 2.0, other conditions such as *H. pylori* infections, antral G cell hyperplasia/hyperfunction, gastric outlet

obstruction, or, rarely, renal failure can masquerade as a gastrinoma. To establish the diagnosis in this group, a determination of BAO and a secretin provocative test should be done. In patients with gastrinomas, BAO is usually (>80%) elevated (i.e., >15 meq/h) and the secretin provocative test is positive (i.e., >200 μg/L increase in serum gastrin level) (Chap. 274).

℞ TREATMENT

The gastric acid hypersecretion in patients with gastrinomas can be controlled in almost every case by oral gastric antisecretory drugs. Because of their long duration of action and potency, allowing once or twice a day dosing, the proton pump inhibitors (H$^+$, K$^+$-ATPase inhibitors) are the drugs of choice. Histamine H$_2$-receptor antagonists are also effective, although more frequent (every 4 to 8 h) and high doses are usually required. In patients with MEN-1 with hyperparathyroidism, correction of the hyperparathyroidism increases the sensitivity to gastric antisecretory drugs and decreases the BAO.

Although gastric acid secretion can be controlled, more than half the patients who are not cured (>60%) will die from tumor-related causes. Careful imaging studies are essential to localize the extent of the tumor (see below). About one-third of patients present with hepatic metastases; in <15% of those with hepatic metastases, the disease is limited so that surgical resection may be possible. Surgical cure is possible in 30 to 60% of all patients without MEN-1 or liver metastases (40% of all patients). In patients with MEN-1, surgical cure is rare because the tumors are multiple, frequently with lymph node metastases.

INSULINOMAS
An insulinoma is an endocrine tumor of the pancreas derived from β cells that ectopically secrete insulin, which results in hypoglycemia. The average age of occurrence is in persons 40 to 50 years old. The most common clinical symptoms are due to the effect of the hypoglycemia on the central nervous system (neuroglycemic symptoms) and include confusion, headache, disorientation, visual difficulties, irrational behavior, or even coma. Also, most patients have symptoms due to excess catecholamine release secondary to the hypoglycemia including sweating, tremor, and palpitations. Characteristically these attacks are associated with fasting.

Insulinomas are generally small (>90% are <2 cm), usually not multiple (90%), and only 5 to 15% are malignant. They almost invariably occur only in the pancreas, distributed equally in the pancreatic head, body, and tail. Insulinomas should be suspected in all patients with hypoglycemia, especially those with attacks provoked by fasting or with a family history of MEN-1. Insulin is synthesized as proinsulin which consists of a 21-amino-acid α chain and a 30-amino-acid β chain connected by a 33-amino-acid connecting peptide (C peptide). In insulinomas, in addition to elevated plasma insulin levels, elevated plasma proinsulin levels are found and C-peptide levels can be elevated.

Diagnosis The diagnosis of insulinoma requires the demonstration of an elevated plasma insulin level at the time of hypoglycemia. Other causes of fasting hypoglycemia include the inadvertent or surreptitious use of insulin or oral hypoglycemic agents, severe liver disease, alcoholism, poor nutrition, or other extrapancreatic tumors. The most reliable test to diagnose insulinoma is a fast up to 72 h with serum glucose, C-peptide, and insulin measurements every 4 to 8 h. If at any point the patient becomes symptomatic or glucose levels are persistently <2.2 mmol/L (<40 mg/dL), the test should be terminated and repeat samples for the above studies obtained before glucose is given. Between 70 and 80% of patients with insulinoma will develop hypoglycemia during the first 24 h and 98% by 48 h. In nonobese normal subjects serum insulin levels should decrease to <43 pmol/L (<6 μU/mL) when blood glucose decreases to ≤2.2 mmol/L (<40 mg/dL) and the ratio of insulin to glucose is <0.3 (in mg/dL). In addition to having an insulin level > 6 μU/mL when blood glucose ≤ 40 mg/dL, some investigators also require an elevated C-peptide and serum proinsulin level and/or insulin:glucose ratio >0.3 for the diagnosis of insulinoma. Surreptitious use of insulin or hypoglycemic agents may be difficult to distinguish from the symptoms of insulinomas. The combination of proinsulin levels (normal in exogenous insulin/hypoglycemic agent users), C-peptide levels (low in exogenous insulin users), antibodies to insulin (positive in exogenous insulin users), and sulfonylurea levels in serum or plasma will allow the correct diagnosis to be made.

℞ TREATMENT

Only 5 to 15% of insulinomas are malignant; therefore, after appropriate imaging (see below), surgery should be performed. Some 75 to 95% of patients are cured by surgery. Before surgery, the hypoglycemia can be controlled by frequent small meals and the use of diazoxide (150 to 800 mg/d). Diazoxide is a benzothiadiazide whose hyperglycemic effect is attributed to inhibition of insulin release; 50 to 60% of patients respond to diazoxide. Its side effects are sodium retention and GI symptoms such as nausea. Other agents effective in some patients include verapamil and diphenylhydantoin. Long-acting somatostatin analogues such as octreotide are acutely effective in 40% of patients. However, octreotide needs to be used with care because it inhibits growth hormone secretion and can alter plasma glucagon levels and so worsen the hypoglycemia in some patients.

For the 5 to 15% of patients with malignant insulinomas, the above drugs or somatostatin analogues are used initially. If they are not effective, various antitumor treatments such as hepatic arterial embolization, chemoembolization, or chemotherapy have been used. These will be discussed below.

GLUCAGONOMAS A glucagonoma is an endocrine tumor of the pancreas that secretes excessive amounts of glucagon, which causes a distinct syndrome characterized by dermatitis, glucose intolerance or diabetes, and weight loss. Glucagonomas occur in persons between 45 and 70 years of age and are clinically heralded by a characteristic dermatitis (migratory necrolytic erythema) (67 to 90%), accompanied by glucose intolerance (40 to 90%), weight loss (66 to 96%), anemia (33 to 85%), diarrhea (15 to 29%), and thromboembolism (11 to 24%). The characteristic rash usually starts as an annular erythema at intertriginous and periorificial sites, especially in the groin or buttock. It subsequently becomes raised, and bullae form and leave erosions when the bullae rupture. The lesions can wax and wane. A characteristic laboratory finding is hypoaminoacidemia, which occurs in 26 to 100% of patients.

Glucagonomas are generally large tumors at diagnosis, with average size of 5 to 10 cm. From 50 to 80% occur in the pancreatic tail, and from 50 to 82% have metastatic spread at presentation, usually to the liver. Glucagonomas are rarely extrapancreatic and usually occur singly.

Diagnosis The diagnosis is confirmed by demonstrating an increased plasma glucagon level (normal is <150 μg/L). Plasma glucagon levels are >1000 μg/mL in 90%, are between 500 and 1000 μg/mL in 7%, and <500 μg/mL in 3%. A plasma glucagon level > 1000 μg/L is considered diagnostic of glucagonoma. Other diseases causing increased plasma glucagon levels include renal insufficiency, acute pancreatitis, hypercorticism, hepatic insufficiency, prolonged fasting, or familial hyperglucagonomia. These disorders do not increase plasma glucagon to >500 μg/L except cirrhosis.

℞ TREATMENT

In 50 to 80% of patients metastases are present at presentation, so curative surgical resection is not possible. Surgical debulking in patients with advanced disease or other antitumor treatments may be beneficial and will be discussed below. Long-acting somatostatin analogues such as octreotide or lanreotide improve the skin rash in 75%

of patients and may improve the weight loss, pain, and diarrhea, but usually do not improve the glucose intolerance.

SOMATOSTATINOMA SYNDROME The somatostatinoma syndrome is due to a NET that secretes excessive amounts of somatostatin, which causes a distinct syndrome characterized by diabetes mellitus, gallbladder disease, diarrhea, and steatorrhea. Usually no distinction is made between a tumor that contains somatostatin-like immunoreactivity (somatostatinoma) and that does or does not produce a clinical syndrome (somatostatinoma syndrome) by secreting somatostatin (11 to 45% and 55 to 89%, respectively). In one review of 173 cases of somatostatinomas, only 11% were associated with the somatostatinoma syndrome. The mean age of patients is 51 years. Somatostatinomas occur primarily in the pancreas and small intestine, and the frequency of the symptoms differs in each. Each of the usual symptoms is more frequent in pancreatic than intestinal somatostatinomas: diabetes mellitus (95% vs. 21%), gallbladder disease (94% vs. 43%), diarrhea (92% vs. 38%), steatorrhea (83% vs. 12%), hypochlorhydria (86% vs. 12%), and weight loss (90% vs. 69%). Somatostatinomas occur in the pancreas in 56 to 74% of cases, with the primary location being in the pancreatic head. The tumors are usually solitary (90%) and large, with a mean size of 4.5 cm. Liver metastases are frequent (69 to 84% of patients).

Somatostatin is a tetradecapeptide (Fig. 329-2) that is widely distributed in the central nervous system and gastrointestinal tract, where it functions as a neurotransmitter or has paracrine and autocrine actions. It is a potent inhibitor of many processes, including release of almost all hormones, acid secretion, intestinal and pancreatic secretion, and intestinal absorption. Most of the clinical manifestations are directly related to these inhibitory actions.

Diagnosis In most cases somatostatinomas have been found by accident either at the time of cholecystectomy or during endoscopy. The presence of psammoma bodies in a duodenal tumor should particularly raise suspicion. Duodenal somatostatin-containing tumors are increasingly associated with von Recklinghausen's disease. Most of these do not cause the somatostatinoma syndrome. The diagnosis of the somatostatinoma syndrome requires elevated plasma somatostatin levels.

℞ TREATMENT

Pancreatic tumors are frequently metastatic at presentation (70 to 92%), whereas 30 to 69% of small-intestinal somatostatinomas have metastases. Surgery is the treatment of choice for those without widespread hepatic metastases. Symptoms in patients with the somatostatinoma syndrome are also improved by octreotide treatment.

VIPOMAS VIPomas are endocrine tumors that secrete excessive amounts of VIP, which causes a distinct syndrome characterized by large-volume watery diarrhea, hypokalemia, and dehydration. This syndrome is also called Verner-Morrison syndrome, pancreatic cholera, or WDHA syndrome for *w*atery *d*iarrhea, *h*ypokalemia, and *a*chlorhydria, which some patients develop. The mean age of patients is 49 years; however, it can occur in children, and when it does is usually caused by a ganglioneuroma or ganglioneuroblastoma.

The principal symptoms are large-volume diarrhea (100%) severe enough to cause hypokalemia (80 to 100%), dehydration (83%), hypochlorhydria (54 to 76%), and flushing (20%). The diarrhea is secretory in nature, persists during fasting, and is almost always >1 L/d and >3 L/d in 70%. Most patients do not have accompanying steatorrhea (16%), and the increased stool volume is due to increased excretion of sodium and potassium, which, with the anions, account for the osmolality of the stool. Patients frequently have hyperglycemia (25 to 50%) and hypercalcemia (25 to 50%).

VIP is a 28-amino-acid peptide that is an important neurotransmitter ubiquitously present in the central nervous system and GI tract. Its known actions include stimulation of small-intestinal chloride secretion and effects on smooth-muscle contractility, inhibition of acid secretion, and vasodilatory effects which explain most features of the clinical syndrome.

In adults 80 to 90% of VIPomas are pancreatic in location, with the rest due to VIP-secreting pheochromocytomas, intestinal carcinoids, and rarely ganglioneuromas. These tumors are usually not multiple, 50 to 75% are in the pancreatic tail, and 37 to 68% have hepatic metastases at diagnosis. In children <10 years, the syndrome is usually due to ganglioneuromas or ganglioblastomas, which are less malignant and account for 10% of VIPomas in adults.

Diagnosis The diagnosis requires the demonstration of an elevated plasma VIP level and the presence of large-volume diarrhea. A stool volume of <700 mL/d excludes the diagnosis of VIPoma. By fasting the patient, a number of causes can be excluded that can cause marked diarrhea. Other diseases that can give a secretory large-volume diarrhea include gastrinomas, chronic laxative abuse, carcinoid syndrome, systemic mastocytosis, rarely medullary thyroid cancer, diabetic diarrhea, and AIDS. Of these conditions, only VIPomas caused a marked increase in plasma VIP.

TREATMENT

The most important initial treatment is to correct their dehydration, hypokalemia, and electrolyte losses with fluid and electrolyte replacement. These patients may require 5 L/d of fluid and >350 meq/d of potassium. Because 37 to 68% of adults with VIPomas have metastatic disease in the liver at presentation, a significant number of patients cannot be cured surgically. In these patients, long-acting somatostatin analogues such as octreotide or lanreotide are the drugs of choice.

Octreotide will control the diarrhea in 87% of patients. In nonresponsive patients, the combination of glucocorticoids and octreotide has proved helpful in a small number of patients. Other drugs reported to be helpful in small numbers of patients include prednisone (60 to 100 mg/d), clonidine, indomethacin, phenothiazines, loperamide, lidamidine, lithium, propranolol, and metochlorpramide.

Treatment of advanced disease with embolization, chemoembolization, and chemotherapy may also be helpful (see below).

NONFUNCTIONAL PANCREATIC ENDOCRINE TUMORS Nonfunctional PETs are endocrine tumors that originate in the pancreas and either secrete no products or their secreted products do not cause a specific clinical syndrome. The symptoms are due entirely to the tumor per se. Nonfunctional PETs almost always secrete chromogranin A (90 to 100%), chromogranin B (90 to 100%), PP (58%), α-human chorionic gonadotropin (hCG) (40%), and β-hCG (20%), but none cause a specific syndrome. Because the symptoms are due to the tumor per se, patients with nonfunctional PETs usually present late in their disease course with invasive tumors and hepatic metastases (64 to 92%), and the tumors are usually large (72% are >5 cm). These tumors are usually solitary except in patients with MEN-1, where they are multiple, and occur primarily in the pancreatic head. Even though these tumors do not cause a functional syndrome, immunocytochemical studies show that they synthesize numerous peptides and cannot be distinguished from functional tumors by immunocytochemistry.

The most common symptoms are abdominal pain (30 to 80%); jaundice (20 to 35%); and weight loss, fatigue, or bleeding; 10 to 15% are found incidentally. The average time from the beginning of symptoms to diagnosis is 5 years.

Diagnosis The diagnosis is established by histologic confirmation in a patient with a PET without either clinical symptoms or elevated plasma hormone levels of one of the established syndromes. Even though chromogranin A levels are elevated in almost every patient, this is not specific for this disease as it can be found in functional PETs, carcinoids, and other neuroendocrine disorders. Plasma PP is increased in 22 to 71% of patients and should strongly suggest the diagnosis in a patient with a pancreatic mass because it is usually normal in patients with pancreatic adenocarcinomas. Elevated plasma PP is not diagnostic of this tumor because it is elevated in a number of other conditions such as chronic renal failure, old age, inflammatory conditions, and diabetes.

TREATMENT

Unfortunately, surgical curative resection can be considered only in the minority of patients because of the high frequency of metastatic disease. Treatment needs to be directed against the tumor per se (see below).

GRFOMAS GRFomas are endocrine tumors that secrete excessive amounts of GRF, which causes acromegaly. The true frequency of this syndrome is not known. GRF is a 44-amino-acid peptide, and 25 to 44% of PETs have GRF immunoreactivity, although it is uncommonly secreted. GRFomas are lung tumors in 47 to 54% of cases, PETs in 29 to 30%, and small-intestinal carcinoids in 8 to 10%, and up to 12% occur at other sites. Patients have a mean age of 38 years, and the symptoms are usually due to either acromegaly or the tumor per se. The acromegaly caused by GRFomas is indistinguishable from classic acromegaly. The pancreatic tumors are usually large (>6 cm) and liver metastases are present in 39%. They should be suspected in any patient with acromegaly and an abdominal tumor, in a patient with MEN-1 with acromegaly, or in a patient without a pituitary adenoma with acromegaly or associated with hyperprolactinemia, which occurs in 70% of GRFomas. GRFomas are an uncommon cause of acromegaly. The diagnosis is established by performing plasma assays for GRF and growth hormone. The normal level for GRF is <5 μg/L in men and <10 μg/L in women. Most GRFomas have a plasma GRF level ≥300 μg/L. Patients with GRFomas also have increased plasma insulin-like growth factor 1 levels similar to those in classic acromegaly. Surgery is the treatment of choice if diffuse metastases are not present. Long-acting somatostatin analogues such as octreotide or lanreotide are the agents of choice, with 75 to 100% of patients responding.

OTHER RARE PANCREATIC ENDOCRINE TUMOR SYNDROMES Cushing's (ACTHoma) due to a PET occurs in 4 to 16% of all ectopic Cushing's syndrome cases. It occurs in 5% of cases of sporadic gastrinomas, almost invariably in patients with hepatic metastases, and is an independent, poor prognostic factor. Paraneoplastic hypercalcemia due to PETs releasing parathyroid hormone–related peptide (PTHrP), a parathyroid hormone–like material, or unknown factor is rarely reported. The tumors are usually large, and liver metastases are usually present. Most (88%) appear to be due to release of PTHrP. PETs can occasionally cause the carcinoid syndrome. PETs secreting calcitonin appear to have a specific clinical syndrome. Half the patients have diarrhea, which disappears with resection of the tumor. That this could be a discrete syndrome is supported by finding that 25 to 42% of patients with medullary thyroid cancer with hypercalcitonemia develop diarrhea, likely secondary to a motility disorder. This is classified in Table 329-2 as a possible specific disorder because so few cases have been described. A renin-producing PET has been described in a patient presenting with hypertension (Table 329-2). Ghrelin is a 28-amino-acid peptide with growth hormone–releasing effect and a strong influence on appetite, among other functions. Even though it is detectable immunohistochemically in most PETs, only 1 in 24 patients (4%) with a PET had elevated plasma ghrelin levels and the patient was asymptomatic, suggesting that no specific syndrome is associated with release of ghrelin by a PET.

TUMOR LOCALIZATION

Localization of the primary tumor and determination of the extent of disease are essential to the proper management of all carcinoids and PETs. Without proper localization studies it is not possible (1) to determine whether the patient is a candidate for curative resection or cytoreductive surgery or requires antitumor treatment (2) or to predict the patient's prognosis.

Numerous tumor localization methods are used in both types of NETs including conventional imaging studies [CT scanning, magnetic resonance imaging (MRI), transabdominal ultrasound, selective angiography] and somatostatin receptor scintigraphy (SRS). In PETs, endoscopic ultrasound (EUS) and functional localization by measuring venous hormonal gradients are also useful. Bronchial carcinoids are usually detected by a standard chest radiograph and assessed by CT. Rectal, duodenal, colonic, and gastric carcinoids are usually detected by GI endoscopy.

PETs and carcinoid tumors frequently overexpress high-affinity somatostatin receptors in both their primary and their metastatic tumors. Of the five types of somatostatin receptors (sst_{1-5}), radiolabeled octreotide binds with high affinity to sst_2 and sst_5, lower for sst_3, and has a very low affinity for sst_1 and sst_4. Nearly all carcinoid tumors and PETs express sst_2, and many also have the other four sst subtypes. Interaction with these receptors can be used to localize NETs using [^{111}In-DTPA-D-Phe^1]octreotide (Fig. 329-2) and radionuclide scanning (SRS) as well as for treatment of the hormone excess state with octreotide or lanreotide. Because of its sensitivity and ability to localize tumor throughout the body at one time, SRS is now the initial imaging modality of choice for localizing both primary NETs and metastases. SRS localizes tumor in 73 to 89% of patients with carcinoids and in 56 to 100% of patients with PETs, except for insulinomas. Insulinomas are usually small and have low densities of sst receptors, resulting in SRS being positive in only 12 to 50% of insulinomas. SRS has greater sensitivity than conventional imaging studies in localizing both the primary tumor and metastases. Figure 329-3 shows an example of the increased sensitivity of SRS in a patient with a gastrinoma. The CT scan (Fig. 329-3, *top*) did not show any disease after resection of the primary tumor; however, hypergastrinemia remained and the SRS demonstrated a metastasis in the liver (Fig. 329-3, *bottom*). Occasional

false-positive responses with SRS can occur (12% in one study) because numerous other normal tissues and diseases can have high densities of sst receptors including granulomas (sarcoid, tuberculosis, etc.), thyroid diseases (goiter, thyroiditis), and activated lymphocytes (lymphomas, wound infections). For PETs located in the pancreas, EUS is highly sensitive localizing 77 to 93% of insulinomas, which occur almost exclusively within the pancreas. EUS is less sensitive for extrapancreatic tumors. If liver metastases are identified by SRS, either a CT scan or MRI is then recommended to assess the size and exact location of the metastases because SRS does not give information on tumor size. Functional localization measuring hormone gradients after intraarterial calcium injections in insulinomas (insulin) or gastrin gradients after secretin injections in gastrinoma is a sensitive method, being positive in 80 to 100% of patients. However, this method gives only regional localization and is reserved for cases where the other imaging modalities are negative.

℞ TREATMENT

Advanced Disease (Diffuse Metastatic Disease)   The single most important prognostic factor for survival is the presence of liver metastases (Fig. 329-4). For patients with foregut carcinoids without hepatic metastases, the 5-year survival is 95% and with distant metastases is 20% (Fig. 329-4, *bottom*). With gastrinomas the 5-year survival without liver metastases is 98%, with limited metastases in one hepatic lobe it is 78%, and with diffuse metastases it is 16% (Fig. 329-4, *top*). Therefore, treatment for advanced metastatic disease is important. A number of different modalities are effective, including cytoreductive surgery

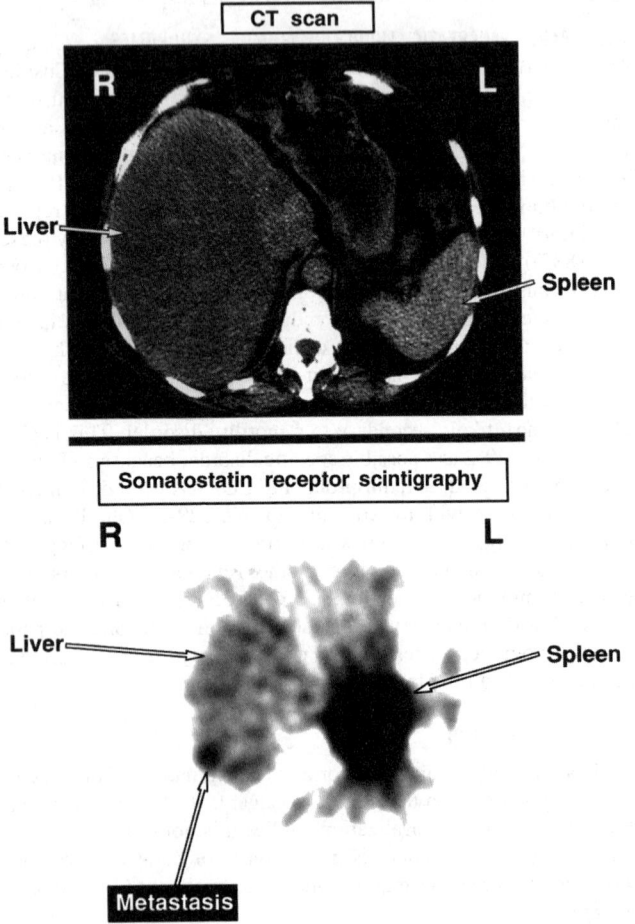

FIGURE 329-3   Ability of computed tomography (*top*) or somatostatin receptor scintigraphy (*bottom*) to localize metastatic gastrinoma in the liver in a patient with Zollinger-Ellison syndrome.

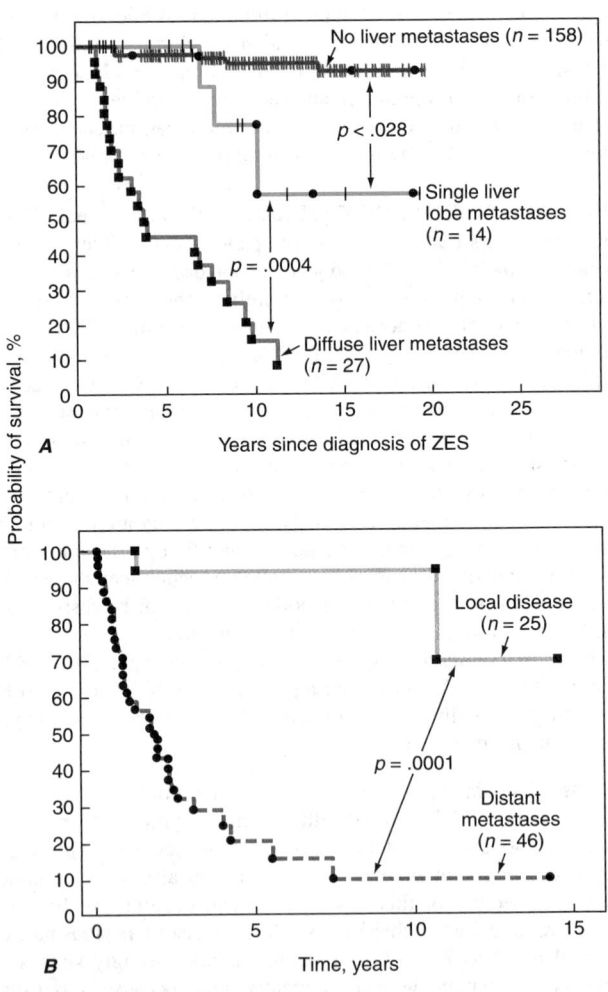

FIGURE 329-4   Effect of the presence and extent of liver metastases on survival in patients with gastrinomas (*top*) or carcinoid tumors (*bottom*). (*Top panel is drawn from data from 199 patients with gastrinomas modified from F Yu et al: J Clin Oncol 17:615, 1999. Bottom panel is drawn from data from 71 patients with foregut carcinoid tumors from EW McDermott et al: Br J Surg 81:1007, 1994; with permission.*)

(removal of all visible tumor), treatment with chemotherapy, somatostatin analogues, interferon α, hepatic embolization alone or with chemotherapy (chemoembolization), radiotherapy, and liver transplantation.

Specific Antitumor Treatments   Cytoreductive surgery, unfortunately, is only possible in 9 to 22% of patients who present with limited hepatic metastases. Although no randomized studies have proven it extends life, results from a number of studies suggest it likely increases survival, and therefore it is recommended if possible.

Chemotherapy for metastatic carcinoid tumors has generally been disappointing, with response rates of 0 to 40% with various two- or three-drug combinations. Chemotherapy for PETs has been more successful with tumor shrinkage reported in 30 to 70% of patients. The current regimen of choice is streptozocin and doxorubicin.

Long-acting somatostatin analogues, such as octreotide and lanreotide, and interferon α rarely decrease tumor size (i.e., 0 to 17%); however, these drugs have tumoristic effects, stopping additional growth in 26 to 95% of patients with NETs. How long tumor stabilization lasts or whether it prolongs survival has not been established. Somatostatin analogues can induce apoptosis in carcinoid tumors.

Hepatic embolization and chemoembolization (with dacarbazine, cisplatin, doxorubicin, 5-fluorouracil, or streptozocin) may decrease tumor bulk and help control the symptoms of the hormone-excess state. These modalities are generally reserved for cases in which treatment with somatostatin analogues, interferon (carcinoids), or chemotherapy (PETs) fails. Embolization, when combined with treatment with octreotide and interferon α, significantly reduces tumor progression compared to treatment with embolization and octreotide alone in patients with advanced midgut carcinoids.

Radiotherapy with radiolabeled somatostatin analogues (Fig. 329-2) that are internalized by the tumors is an approach being investigated.

Three different radionuclides are being used. High doses of [^{111}In-DTPA-D-Phe^1]octreotide (emits γ rays, internal conversion, and Auger electrons) and yttrium-90 (emits high energy β-particles) coupled by a DOTA-chelating group (Fig. 329-2) to octreotide or octreotate are being used as well as ^{177}Lu-coupled analogues (emit β- and γ-rays). In one study, treatment with the ^{111}In or ^{177}Lu compounds caused tumor stabilization in 41% and 40%, respectively, and a decrease in tumor size in 30% and 38%, respectively, in patients with advanced metastatic NETs. Hormone-directed radiation therapy may be helpful in patients with advanced, widespread metastatic disease.

The use of liver transplantation has been abandoned for treatment of most metastatic tumors to the liver. However, for metastatic NETs it is still a consideration. In a recent review of 103 cases of malignant NETs (48 PETs, 43 carcinoids) the 2- and 5-year survival rates were 60% and 47%, respectively. However, recurrence-free survival was low (<24%). For younger patients with metastatic NETs limited to the liver, liver transplantation may be justified.

FURTHER READING

CAPLIN ME et al: Carcinoid tumour. Lancet 352:799, 1998.

CORLETO VD et al: Molecular insights into gastrointestinal neuroendocrine tumors: Importance and recent advances. Dig Liver Dis 34:668, 2002

KULKE MH, MAYER RJ: Carcinoid tumors. N Engl J Med 340:858, 1999

KWEKKEBOOM D et al: Peptide receptor imaging and therapy. J Nucl Med 41: 1704, 2000

METZ DC, JENSEN RT: Endocrine tumors of the gastrointestinal tract, in AK Rustgi, JM Crawford (eds): *Gastrointestinal Cancers*. Edinburgh, Saunders, 2003, pp 681–720

MODLIN IM et al: A 5-decade analysis of 13,715 carcinoid tumors. Cancer 97: 934, 2003

330 DISORDERS AFFECTING MULTIPLE ENDOCRINE SYSTEMS
Steven I. Sherman, Robert F. Gagel

NEOPLASTIC DISORDERS AFFECTING MULTIPLE ENDOCRINE ORGANS

Several distinct genetic disorders predispose to endocrine gland neoplasia and cause hormone excess syndromes (Table 330-1). DNA-based genetic testing is now available for these disorders, but effective management requires an understanding of endocrine neoplasia and the range of clinical features that may be manifest in an individual patient.

MULTIPLE ENDOCRINE NEOPLASIA (MEN) TYPE 1 ■ Clinical Manifestations

MEN1, or Wermer's syndrome, is an autosomal dominant genetic syndrome characterized by neoplasia of parathyroid, pituitary, pancreatic islet, and other neuroendocrine cell types (Table 330-1). Each child born to an affected parent has a 50% probability of inheriting the gene. The variable penetrance of the several neoplastic components can make the differential diagnosis challenging.

Hyperparathyroidism is the most common manifestation of MEN1. Hypercalcemia may develop during the teenage years, and most individuals are affected by age 40 (Fig. 330-1). The neoplastic changes in hyperparathyroidism exemplify one of the cardinal features of endocrine tumors in MEN1—multicentricity. The neoplastic changes inevitably affect multiple parathyroid glands, making surgical cure difficult. Screening for hyperparathyroidism involves measurement of either an albumin-adjusted or ionized serum calcium level. The diagnosis is established by demonstrating elevated levels of serum calcium and inappropriately normal or high intact parathyroid hormone. Manifestations of hyperparathyroidism in MEN1 do not differ substantially from those in sporadic hyperparathyroidism and include calcium-containing kidney stones, bone abnormalities, and gastrointestinal and musculoskeletal complaints (Chap. 332).

Other familial disorders associated with hypercalcemia include familial isolated hyperparathyroidism, a broad categorization that includes at least two types, HRPT1 and HRPT2. The first type, HRPT1, includes familial parathyroid hyperplasia and adenomatosis. The second type, HRPT2, is associated with multiple cystic parathyroid ade-

TABLE 330-1 *Disease Associations in the Multiple Endocrine Neoplasia (MEN) Syndromes*

MEN1	MEN2	Mixed Syndromes
Parathyroid hyperplasia or adenoma	MEN2A MTC Pheochromocytoma Parathyroid hyperplasia or adenoma	von Hippel–Lindau syndrome, pheochromocytoma, islet cell tumor, renal cell carcinoma, hemangioblastoma of central nervous system, retinal angiomas
Islet cell hyperplasia, adenoma, or carcinoma		
Pituitary hyperplasia or adenoma	Cutaneous lichen amyloidosis	Neurofibromatosis with features of MEN1 or 2
Other less common manifestations: foregut carcinoid, pheochromocytoma, subcutaneous or visceral lipomas	Hirschsprung disease Familial MTC MEN2B MTC Pheochromocytoma Mucosal and gastro-intestinal neuromas Marfanoid features	Carney complex Myxomas of heart, skin, and breast Spotty cutaneous pigmentation Testicular, adrenal, and GH-producing pituitary tumors Peripheral nerve schwannomas

Note: MTC, medullary thyroid carcinoma.

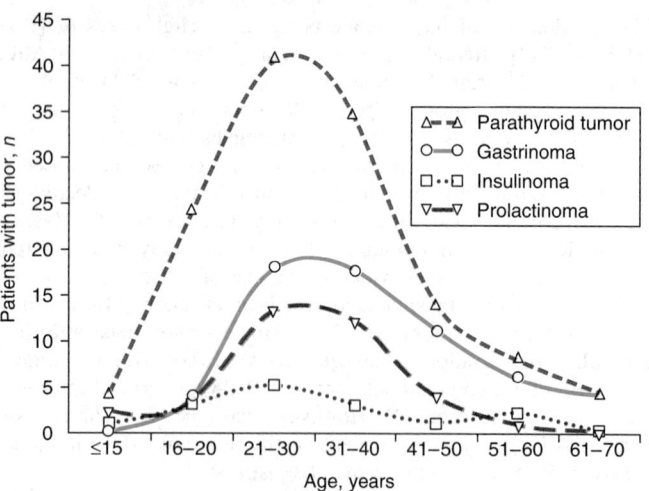

FIGURE 330-1 Age at onset of endocrine tumor expression in multiple endocrine neoplasia type 1 (MEN1). Data derived from retrospective analysis for each endocrine organ hyperfunction in 130 cases of MEN1. Age at onset is the age at first symptom or, with tumors not causing symptoms, age at the time of the first abnormal finding on a screening test. The rate of diagnosis of hyperparathyroidism increased sharply between ages 16 and 20 years. (*Reprinted with permission from S Marx et al: Ann Intern Med 129:484, 1998.*)

nomas and ossifying jaw fibromas. Inactivating mutations of the gene that encodes parafibromin were recently identified in nearly all families with HRPT2. Subsequent analysis of this gene in families with HRPT1 indicates that some patients with HRPT1 have mutations of the HRPT2 gene. Inactivating mutations of HRPT2 are also found commonly in sporadic parathyroid cancers. MEN2 (to be discussed below) should also be considered in the differential diagnosis. Another cause of familial hypercalcemia is familial hypercalcemic hypocalciuria (FHH), an autosomal dominant form of hypercalcemia caused by inactivating mutations of the calcium sensor, a transmembrane G protein–coupled receptor found in parathyroid tissue and kidney (Chap. 332). Hypercalcemia associated with MEN1, MEN2, HRPT1, and HRPT2 is characterized by increased urine calcium excretion (calcium/creatinine clearance ratio > 0.01) whereas in FHH it is associated with low urine calcium excretion (calcium/creatinine clearance ratio < 0.01). Another distinguishing feature is that the serum calcium level is rarely elevated at birth in patients with MEN1 but is frequently elevated in newborns with FHH.

Differentiation of hyperparathyroidism of MEN1 from other forms of familial primary hyperparathyroidism is usually based on family history, histologic features of resected parathyroid tissue, and, sometimes, long-term observation to determine whether other manifestations of MEN1 develop. Parathyroid hyperplasia is the most common cause of hyperparathyroidism in MEN1, although single and multiple adenomas have been described. Hyperplasia of one or more parathyroid glands is common in younger patients; adenomas are usually found in older patients or those with long-standing disease.

Neoplasia of the pancreatic islets is the second most common manifestation of MEN1 and tends to occur in parallel with hyperparathyroidism (Fig. 330-1). Increased pancreatic islet cell hormones include pancreatic polypeptide (75 to 85%), gastrin [60%; Zollinger-Ellison syndrome (ZES)], insulin (25 to 35%), vasoactive intestinal peptide (VIP) (3 to 5%; Verner-Morrison, or watery diarrhea, syndrome), glucagon (5 to 10%), and somatostatin (1 to 5%). The tumors rarely produce adrenocorticotropin (ACTH), corticotropin-releasing hormone (CRH), growth hormone–releasing hormone (GHRH), calcitonin gene products, neurotensin, gastric inhibitory peptide, and others. Many of the tumors produce more than one peptide. The pancreatic neoplasms differ from the other components of MEN1 in that approximately one-third of the tumors display malignant features, including hepatic metastases (Chap. 329).

Pancreatic islet cell tumors are diagnosed by identification of a characteristic clinical syndrome, hormonal assays with or without provocative stimuli, or radiographic techniques. One approach involves annual screening of individuals at risk with measurement of basal and meal-stimulated levels of pancreatic polypeptide to identify the tumors as early as possible; the rationale of this screening strategy is that surgical removal of islet cell tumors at an early stage will be curative. Other approaches to screening include measurement of serum gastrin and pancreatic polypeptide levels every 2 to 3 years, with the rationale that pancreatic neoplasms will be detected at a later stage but can be managed medically, if possible, or by surgery. High-resolution, early-phase computed tomography (CT) scanning or endoscopic ultrasound provides the best preoperative technique for identification of these tumors; intraoperative ultrasonography is the most sensitive method for detection of small tumors.

ZES is caused by excessive gastrin production and occurs in more than half of MEN1 patients with pancreatic islet cell tumors or small carcinoid-like tumors in the duodenal wall (Fig. 330-1) (Chap. 329). Approximately one-fourth of all ZES occurs in the context of MEN1. Clinical features include increased gastric acid production, recurrent peptic ulcers, diarrhea, and esophagitis. The ulcer diathesis is refractory to conservative therapy such as antacids. The diagnosis is made by finding increased gastric acid secretion, elevated basal gastrin levels in serum [generally >115 pmol/L (200 pg/mL)], and an exaggerated response of serum gastrin to either secretin or calcium. Other causes of elevated serum gastrin levels, such as achlorhydria, treatment with H_2 receptor antagonists or omeprazole, retained gastric antrum, small-bowel resection, gastric outlet obstruction, and hypercalcemia, should be excluded.

Insulinoma causes hypoglycemia in about one-third of MEN1 patients with pancreatic islet cell tumors (Fig. 330-1). The tumors may be benign or malignant (25%). The diagnosis can be established by documenting hypoglycemia during a short fast with simultaneous inappropriate elevation of serum insulin and C-peptide levels. More commonly, it is necessary to subject the patient to a supervised 12- to 72-h fast to provoke hypoglycemia (Chap. 324). Large insulinomas may be identified by CT scanning; small tumors not detected by radiographic techniques may be localized by selective arteriographic injection of calcium into each of the arteries that supply the pancreas and timed sampling of the hepatic vein for insulin to determine the anatomic region containing the tumor. Intraoperative ultrasonography can also be used to localize these tumors, but preoperative calcium injection data are helpful in guiding the appropriate pancreatic surgical procedure if multiple or no abnormalities are detected by intraoperative ultrasonography.

Glucagonoma in occasional MEN1 patients causes a syndrome of hyperglycemia, skin rash (necrolytic migratory erythema), anorexia, glossitis, anemia, depression, diarrhea, and venous thrombosis. In about half of these patients the plasma glucagon level is high, leading to its designation as the *glucagonoma syndrome*, although elevation of plasma glucagon level in MEN1 patients is not necessarily associated with these symptoms. Some patients with this syndrome also have elevated plasma ghrelin levels. The glucagonoma syndrome may represent a complex interaction between glucagon and ghrelin overproduction and the nutritional status of the patient.

The *Verner-Morrison syndrome*, or *watery diarrhea syndrome*, consists of watery diarrhea, hypokalemia, hypochlorhydria, and metabolic acidosis. The diarrhea can be voluminous and is almost always found in association with an islet cell tumor, prompting use of the term *pancreatic cholera*. However, the syndrome is not restricted to pancreatic islet tumors and has been observed with carcinoids or other tumors. This syndrome is believed to be due to overproduction of VIP, although plasma VIP levels are not always elevated. Hypercalcemia may be induced by the effects of VIP on bone as well as by hyperparathyroidism. The differential diagnosis includes other causes of chronic diarrhea, infectious or parasitic diseases, inflammatory bowel disease, or sprue or other endocrine causes such as ZES, carcinoid syndrome, or medullary thyroid carcinoma.

Pituitary tumors occur in more than half of patients with MEN1 and tend to be multicentric, making them difficult to resect (Chap. 318). Prolactinomas are most common (Fig. 330-1) and are diagnosed by finding serum prolactin levels >200 μg/L, with or without a pituitary mass evident by magnetic resonance imaging (MRI). Values <200 μg/L may be due to a prolactin-secreting neoplasm or to compression of the pituitary stalk by a different type of pituitary tumor. Acromegaly due to excessive growth hormone (GH) production is the second most common syndrome caused by pituitary tumors in MEN1 (Chap. 318) but is rarely caused by production of GHRH by an islet cell tumor (see above). Cushing's disease can be caused by ACTH-producing pituitary tumors or by ectopic production of ACTH or CRH by other components of MEN1 syndrome including islet cell or carcinoid tumors. Diagnosis of pituitary Cushing's disease is generally best accomplished by a high-dose dexamethasone suppression test or by petrosal venous sinus sampling for ACTH after intravenous injection of CRH (Chap. 318). Differentiation of a primary pituitary tumor from an ectopic CRH-producing tumor may be difficult because the pituitary is the source of ACTH in both disorders; documentation of CRH production by a pancreatic islet or carcinoid tumor may be the only method of proving ectopic CRH production. Adrenal cortical tumors are found in almost one-half of gene carriers but are rarely functional; malignancy in the cortical adenomas is uncommon.

Carcinoid tumors in MEN1 are of the foregut type and are derived from thymus, lung, stomach, or duodenum; they may metastasize or be locally invasive. These tumors usually produce serotonin, calcitonin, or CRH. The typical carcinoid syndrome with flushing, diarrhea, and bronchospasm is rare (Chap. 329). Mediastinal carcinoid tumors (an upper mediastinal mass) are more common in men; bronchial carcinoid tumors are more common in women. Carcinoid tumors are a late manifestation of MEN1; screening regularly for mediastinal carcinoid tumors by chest CT scans has been recommended because of the high rate of malignant transformation.

UNUSUAL MANIFESTATIONS OF MEN1 Subcutaneous or visceral lipomas and cutaneous leiomyomas may also be present but rarely undergo malignant transformation. Skin angiofibromas or collagenomas are seen in most patients with MEN1 when carefully sought.

GENETIC CONSIDERATIONS MEN1 is transmitted as an autosomal dominant trait, reflecting the fact that the gene that causes MEN1, located on chromosome 11q13, encodes a tumor-suppressor protein termed *menin* (Fig. 330-2). Affected individuals typically harbor a germline mutation in *MEN1* and acquire a "second hit" in the normal gene as a result of another mutation or, more commonly, loss of the portion of chromosome 11 that contains the MEN1 locus (Chap. 68). Though the function of menin is not well understood, it is a nuclear protein that interacts with at least two transcriptional factors, SMAD 3 and Jun D, suggesting a regulatory role in cell growth.

MEN1 gene mutations are found in >90% of families with the syndrome (Fig. 330-2). Genetic testing can be performed in individuals at risk for the development of MEN1 and is now commercially available in the United States and Europe. The major value of genetic testing in a kindred with an identifiable mutation is the assignment or exclusion of gene carrier status. In those identified as carrying the mutant gene, routine screening for individual manifestations of MEN1 should be performed as outlined above. Those with negative genetic test results (in a kindred with an identified mutation) can be excluded from further screening for MEN1. A significant percentage of sporadic

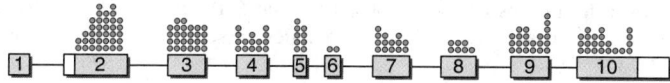

FIGURE 330-2 Schematic depiction of the MEN1 gene and the distribution of mutations. The shaded areas show coding sequence. The closed circles show the relative distribution of mutations, mostly inactivating, in each exon. Mutation data are derived from the Human Gene Mutation Database from which more detailed information can be obtained (*www.uwcm.ac.uk/uwcm/mg/hgmd0.html*). (*From M Krawczak, DN Cooper: Trends Genet 13:1321, 1998, with permission.*)

parathyroid, islet cell, and carcinoid tumors also have loss or mutation of *MEN1*. It is presumed that these mutations are somatic and occur in a single cell, leading to subsequent transformation.

℞ TREATMENT

Almost everyone who inherits a mutant *MEN1* gene develops at least one clinical manifestation of the syndrome. Most develop hyperparathyroidism, 80% develop pancreatic islet cell tumors, and more than half develop pituitary tumors. For most of these tumors, initial surgery is not curative and patients frequently require multiple surgical procedures on two or more endocrine glands during a lifetime. For this reason, it is essential to establish clear goals for management of these patients rather than to recommend surgery casually each time a tumor is discovered. Ranges for acceptable management are discussed below.

Hyperparathyroidism Individuals with serum calcium levels >3.0 mmol/L (12 mg/dL), evidence of calcium nephrolithiasis or renal dysfunction, neuropathic or muscular symptoms, or bone involvement (including osteopenia) should undergo parathyroid exploration. There is less agreement regarding the necessity for parathyroid exploration in individuals who do not meet these criteria, and observation may be appropriate in the MEN1 patient with asymptomatic hyperparathyroidism.

When parathyroid surgery is indicated in MEN1, all parathyroid tissue should be identified and removed at the time of primary operation, and parathyroid tissue should be implanted in the nondominant forearm. Thymectomy should also be performed because of the potential for later development of malignant carcinoid tumors. If reoperation for hyperparathyroidism is necessary at a later date, transplanted parathyroid tissue can be resected from the forearm under local anesthesia with titration of tissue removal to lower the intact parathyroid hormone (PTH) to <50% of basal.

A less desirable approach is to remove 3 to 3.5 parathyroid glands from the neck (leaving ~50 mg of parathyroid tissue), carefully marking the location of residual tissue so that the remaining tissue can be located easily during subsequent surgery. If this approach is utilized, intraoperative PTH measurements should be utilized to monitor adequacy of removal of parathyroid tissue with a goal of reducing postoperative serum intact PTH to ≤50% of basal values.

Pancreatic Islet Tumors (See Chap. 329 for discussion of pancreatic islet tumors not associated with MEN1.) Two features of pancreatic islet cell tumors in MEN1 complicate the management. First, the pancreatic islet cell tumors are multicentric, malignant about a third of the time, and cause death in 10 to 20% of patients. Second, removal of all pancreatic islets to prevent malignancy causes diabetes mellitus, a disease with significant long-term complications that include neuropathy, retinopathy, and nephropathy. These features make it difficult to formulate clear-cut guidelines, but some general concepts appear to be valid. First, islet cell tumors producing insulin, glucagon, VIP, GHRH, or CRH should be resected because medical therapy for the hormonal effects of these tumors is generally ineffective. Second, gastrin-producing islet cell tumors that cause ZES are frequently multicentric. Recent experience suggests that a high percentage of ZES in MEN1 is caused by duodenal wall tumors and that resection of these tumors improves the cure rate. Treatment with H₂ receptor antagonists (cimetidine or ranitidine) and the H⁺,K⁺-ATPase inhibitors (omeprazole or lansoprazole) provides an alternative, and some think preferable, therapy to surgery for control of ulcer disease in patients with multicentric tumors or with hepatic metastases. Third, total pancreatectomy at an early age may be justified to prevent malignancy for families who have a high incidence of malignant cell tumors that cause death.

Management of metastatic islet cell carcinoma is unsatisfactory. Hormonal abnormalities can sometimes be controlled. For example, ZES can be treated with H₂ receptor antagonists or H⁺,K⁺-ATPase inhibitors; the somatostatin analogues, octreotide or lanreotide, are useful in the management of carcinoid and the watery diarrhea syndrome. Bilateral adrenalectomy may be required for ectopic ACTH syndrome if medical therapy is ineffective (Chap. 321). Islet cell carcinomas frequently metastasize to the liver but may grow slowly. Hepatic artery embolization or chemotherapy (5-fluorouracil, streptozocin, chlorozotocin, doxorubicin, or dacarbazine) may reduce tumor mass, control symptoms of hormone excess, and prolong life; however, these treatments are never curative.

Pituitary Tumors   Treatment of prolactinomas with dopamine agonists (bromocriptine, cabergoline, or quinagolide) usually returns the serum prolactin level to normal and prevents further tumor growth (Chap. 318). Surgical resection of a prolactinoma is rarely curative but may relieve mass effects. Transsphenoidal resection is appropriate for neoplasms that secrete ACTH, GH, or the α-subunit of the pituitary glycoprotein hormones. Octreotide reduces tumor mass in one-third of GH-secreting tumors and reduces GH and insulin-like growth factor I levels in >75% of patients. Pegvisomant, a GH receptor antagonist, rapidly lowers insulin-like growth factor levels 1/(IGF-1) and is now approved for treatment of acromegaly. Radiation therapy may be useful for large or recurrent tumors.

Advances in the management of MEN1, particularly islet cell and pituitary tumors, have improved outcome in these patients substantially. As a result, other neoplastic manifestations that develop later in the course of this disorder, such as carcinoid syndrome, are now seen with increased frequency.

MULTIPLE ENDOCRINE NEOPLASIA TYPE 2 ■ **Clinical Manifestations**   Medullary thyroid carcinoma (MTC) and pheochromocytoma are associated in two major syndromes: MEN type 2A and MEN type 2B (Table 330-1). MEN2A is the combination of MTC, hyperparathyroidism, and pheochromocytoma. Three subvariants of MEN2A are familial medullary thyroid carcinoma (FMTC), MEN2A with cutaneous lichen amyloidosis, and MEN2A with Hirschsprung disease. MEN2B is the combination of MTC, pheochromocytoma, mucosal neuromas, intestinal ganglioneuromatosis, and marfanoid features.

MULTIPLE ENDOCRINE NEOPLASIA TYPE 2A   MTC is the most common manifestation. This tumor usually develops in childhood, beginning as hyperplasia of the calcitonin-producing cells (C cells) of the thyroid. MTC is typically located at the junction of the upper one-third and lower two-thirds of each lobe of the thyroid, reflecting the high density of C cells in this location; tumors >1 cm in size are frequently associated with local or distant metastases. Measurement of the serum calcitonin level after calcium or pentagastrin injection makes it possible to diagnose this disorder at an early stage in its development (see below).

Pheochromocytoma occurs in ~50% of patients with MEN2A and causes hypertension with palpitations, nervousness, headaches, and sometimes sweating (Chap. 322). About half the tumors are bilateral. After unilateral adrenalectomy, >50% of patients develop a pheochromocytoma in the contralateral gland within a decade. A second feature of these tumors is a disproportionate increase in the secretion of epinephrine relative to norepinephrine. This characteristic differentiates the MEN2 pheochromocytomas from sporadic pheochromocytoma and those associated with von Hippel–Lindau (VHL) syndrome, hereditary paraganglioma, or neurofibromatosis. Capsular invasion is common, but metastasis is uncommon. Finally, the pheochromocytomas are almost always found in the adrenal gland, differentiating the pheochromocytomas in MEN2 from the extraadrenal tumors found in hereditary paraganglioma syndromes.

Hyperparathyroidism occurs in 15 to 20% of patients, with the peak incidence in the third or fourth decade. The manifestations of hyperparathyroidism do not differ from those in other forms of primary hyperparathyroidism (Chap. 332). Diagnosis is established by finding hypercalcemia, hypophosphatemia, hypercalciuria, and an inappropriately high serum level of intact PTH. Multiglandular parathyroid hyperplasia is the most common histologic finding, although with long-standing disease, adenomatous changes may be superimposed on hyperplasia.

The most common subvariant of MEN2A is familial MTC, an autosomal dominant syndrome in which MTC is the only manifestation (Table 330-1). The clinical diagnosis of FMTC is established by the identification of MTC in multiple generations without a pheochromocytoma. Since the penetrance of pheochromocytoma is 50% in MEN2A, it is possible that MEN2A could masquerade as FMTC in small kindreds. It is important to consider this possibility carefully before classifying a kindred as having FMTC; failure to do so could lead to death or serious morbidity from pheochromocytoma in an affected kindred member.

MULTIPLE ENDOCRINE NEOPLASIA TYPE 2B   The association of MTC, pheochromocytoma, mucosal neuromas, and a marfanoid habitus is designated MEN2B. MTC in MEN2B develops earlier and is more aggressive than in MEN2A. Metastatic disease has been described prior to 1 year of age, and death commonly occurs in the second or third decade of life. However, the prognosis is not invariably bad even in patients with metastatic disease, as evidenced by a number of multigenerational families with this disease.

Pheochromocytoma occurs in more than half of MEN2B patients and does not differ from that in MEN2A. Hypercalcemia is rare in MEN2B, and there are no well-documented examples of hyperparathyroidism.

The mucosal neuromas and marfanoid body habitus are the most distinctive features and are recognizable in childhood. Neuromas are present on the tip of the tongue, under the eyelids, and throughout the gastrointestinal tract and are true neuromas, distinct from neurofibromas. The most common presentation in children relates to gastrointestinal symptomatology, including intermittent colic, pseudoobstruction, and diarrhea.

⧖ **GENETIC CONSIDERATIONS**   Mutations of the *RET* proto-oncogene have been identified in most patients with MEN2 (Fig. 330-3). *RET* encodes a tyrosine kinase receptor that, in combination with a co-receptor, GDNF family-receptor alpha (GFRα), is normally activated by glial cell–derived neurotropic factor or other members of this transforming growth factor–like family of peptides including artemin, persephin, and neurturin. In the C cell there is evidence that persephin normally activates the RET/GFRα-4 receptor complex and is partially responsible for migration of the C cells into the thyroid gland, whereas in the gastrointestinal tract, glial cell–derived neurotrophic factor activates a RET/GFRα-1 complex. *RET* mutations induce constitutive activity of the receptor, explaining the autosomal dominant transmission of the disorder.

Naturally occurring mutations localize to two regions of the RET tyrosine kinase receptor. The first is a cysteine-rich extracellular domain; point mutations in the coding sequence for one of six cysteines (codons 609, 611, 618, 620, 630, or 634) cause amino acid substitutions that induce receptor dimerization and activation in the absence of its ligand. Codon 634 mutations occur in 80% of MEN2A kindreds and are most commonly associated with classic MEN2A features (Figs. 330-3 and 330-2); an arginine substitution at this codon accounts for half of all MEN2A mutations. All reported families with MEN2A and cutaneous lichen amyloidosis have a codon 634 mutation. Mutations of codons 609, 611, 618, or 620 occur in 10 to 15% of MEN2A kindreds and are more commonly associated with FMTC (Fig. 330-3). Mutations in codons 609, 618, and 620 have also been identified in a variant of MEN2A that includes Hirschsprung disease (Fig. 330-3).

The second region of the RET tyrosine kinase that is mutated in MEN2 is in the substrate recognition pocket at codon 918 (Fig. 330-3). This activating mutation is present in ~95% of patients with MEN2B and accounts for 5% of all *RET* proto-oncogene mutations in MEN2. Mutations of codons 883 and 922 have also been identified in a few patients with MEN2B.

Uncommon mutations (initially <5% of the total) include those of codons 533 (exon 8), 768, 790, 791, 804, 891, and 912. Mutations associated with only FMTC include codons 533, 768, V804M, and 912. A cautionary note is that rare mutations that were once associated with FMTC only (791, V804L, and 891) have been found in families with MEN2A as there are occasional reports of pheochromocytoma. At present it is reasonable to conclude that only kindreds with codon 533, 768, V804M, or 912 mutations are consistently associated with FMTC; in kindreds with all other *RET* mutations, pheochromocytoma is a possibility. Germline mutations occur in at least 6% of patients with apparently sporadic MTC, leading to the recommendation that all patients with MTC should be screened for these mutations. These findings mirror results in other malignancies where germline mutations of cancer-causing genes contribute to a greater percentage of apparently sporadic cancer than previously considered. The recognition of new mutations of *RET* almost 10 years following the initial discovery of *RET* mutations suggests that more will be identified in the future.

Somatic mutations (found only in the tumor and not transmitted in the germline) of the *RET* proto-oncogene have been identified in sporadic MTC; 25 to 35% of sporadic tumors have codon 918 mutations, and somatic mutations in codons 630, 768, and 804 have also been identified (Fig. 330-3).

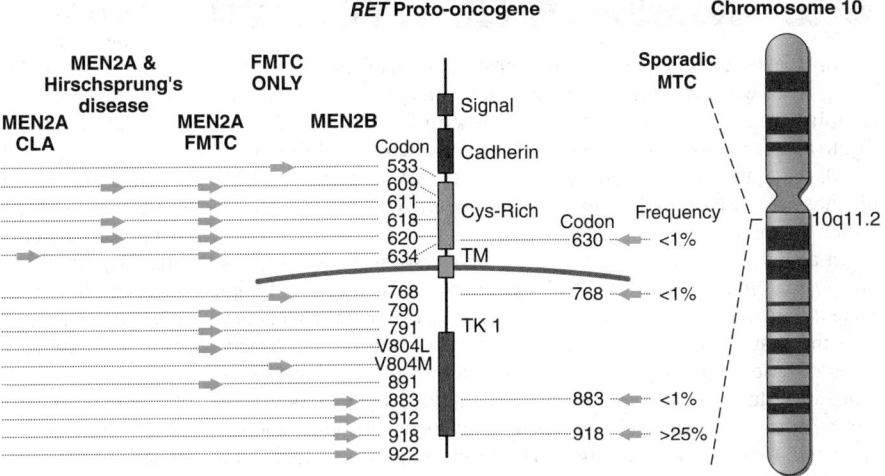

FIGURE 330-3 Schematic diagram of the *RET* proto-oncogene showing mutations found in MEN type 2 and sporadic medullary thyroid carcinoma (MTC). The *RET* proto-oncogene is located on the proximal arm of chromosome 10q (10q11.2). Activating mutations of two functional domains of the RET tyrosine kinase receptor have been identified. The first affects a cysteine-rich (Cys-Rich) region in the extracellular portion of the receptor. Each germline mutation changes a cysteine at codons 609, 611, 618, 620, or 634 to another amino acid. The second region is the intracellular tyrosine kinase (TK) domain. Codon 634 mutations account for ~80% of all germline mutations. Mutations of codons 630, 768, 883, and 918 have been identified as somatic (nongermline) mutations that occur in a single parafollicular or C cell within the thyroid gland in sporadic MTC. A codon 918 mutation is the most common somatic mutation. Abbreviations: MEN2, multiple endocrine neoplasia type 2; CLA cutaneous lichen amyloidosis; FMTC, familial medullary thyroid carcinoma; Signal, the signal peptide; Cadherin, a cadherin-like region in the extracellular domain; TM, transmembrane domain; TK, tyrosine kinase domain.

Rx TREATMENT

Screening for Multiple Endocrine Neoplasia Type 2 Death from MTC can be prevented by early thyroidectomy. The identification of *RET* proto-oncogene mutations and the application of DNA-based molecular diagnostic techniques to identify these mutations has simplified the screening process. During the initial evaluation of a kindred, a *RET* proto-oncogene analysis should be performed on an individual with proven MEN2A. Establishment of the specific germline mutation facilitates the subsequent analysis of other family members. Each family member at risk should be tested twice for the presence of the specific mutation; the second analysis should be performed on a new DNA sample and, ideally, in a second laboratory to exclude sample mix-up or technical error (see *www.genetests.org* for an up-to-date list of laboratory testing sites). Both false-positive and false-negative analyses have been described; a false-negative test result is of the greatest concern because calcitonin testing is now rarely performed as a diagnostic backup study; if there is a genetic test error, a child may present in the second or third decade with metastatic MTC. Individuals in a kindred with a known mutation who have two normal analyses can be excluded from further screening.

There is general consensus that children with codon 883, 918, and 922 mutations, those associated with MEN2B, should have a total thyroidectomy and central lymph node dissection (level VI) performed during the first months of life or soon after identification of the syndrome. If local metastasis is discovered, a more extensive lymph node dissection (levels II to V) is generally indicated. In children with codon 611, 618, 620, 630, 634, and 891 mutations, thyroidectomy should be performed before age 6 because of reports of local metastatic disease in children this age. Finally, there are kindreds with codon 609, 768, 790, 791, 804, and 912 mutations where the phenotype of MTC appears to be less aggressive. In kindreds with these mutations, two management approaches have been suggested: (1) perform a total thyroidectomy, with or without central node dissection, at some arbitrary age (perhaps 6 to 10 years of age); or (2) continue annual or biannual

calcitonin provocative testing with performance of total thyroidectomy, with or without central neck dissection, when the test becomes abnormal. The pentagastrin test involves measurement of serum calcitonin basally and at 2, 5, 10, and 15 min after a bolus injection of 5 μg pentagastrin per kilogram body weight. Before injection, patients should be warned of epigastric tightness, nausea, warmth, and tingling of extremities and reassured that the symptoms will last ~2 min. The recent unavailability of pentagastrin in the United States has led to use of a short calcium infusion, performed by obtaining a baseline serum calcitonin and then infusing 150 mg calcium salt intravenously over 10 min with measurement of serum calcium and calcitonin at 5, 10, 15, and 30 min after initiation of the infusion.

The *RET* proto-oncogene analysis should be performed in patients with suspected MEN2B to detect codon 883, 918, and 922 mutations, especially in newborn children where the diagnosis is suspected but the clinical phenotype is not fully developed. Other family members at risk for MEN2B should also be tested because the mucosal neuromas can be subtle and not always identified. Most MEN2B mutations represent de novo germline mutations derived from the paternal allele. In the rare families with proven germline transmission of MTC but no identifiable *RET* proto-oncogene mutation, annual pentagastrin or calcium-pentagastrin testing should be performed on members at risk.

Annual screening for pheochromocytoma in subjects with germline *RET* mutations should be performed by measuring basal plasma or 24-h urine catecholamines and metanephrines. The goal is to identify a pheochromocytoma before it causes significant symptoms or is likely to cause sudden death, an event most commonly associated with large tumors. Radiographic studies, such as MRI or CT scans, are generally reserved for individuals with abnormal screening tests or with symptoms suggestive of pheochromocytoma (Chap. 322). Women should be tested during pregnancy because undetected pheochromocytoma can cause maternal death during childbirth.

Measurement of serum calcium and parathyroid hormone levels every 2 to 3 years provides an adequate screen for hyperparathyroidism, except in those families in which hyperparathyroidism is a prominent component.

Medullary Thyroid Carcinoma Hereditary MTC is a multicentric disorder. Total thyroidectomy with a central lymph node dissection should be performed in children who carry the mutant gene. Incomplete thyroidectomy leaves the possibility of later transformation of residual C cells. The goal of early therapy is to cure, and a strategy that does not accomplish this goal is short-sighted. Long-term follow-up studies indicate an excellent outcome with ~90% of children free of disease 15 to 20 years after surgery. In contrast, 15 to 25% of patients whose diagnosis is based on a palpable thyroid nodule die from the disease within 15 to 20 years.

In adults with MTC >1 cm in size, metastases to regional lymph nodes are common (>75%). Total thyroidectomy with central lymph node dissection and selective dissection of other regional chains provide the best chance for cure. In patients with extensive local metastatic disease in the neck, external radiation may prevent local recurrence or reduce tumor mass but is not curative. Chemotherapy with combinations of adriamycin, vincristine, cyclophosphamide, and dacarbazine may provide palliation. The recent success of gleevec for treatment of chronic myelogenous leukemia and gastrointestinal stromal tumors has prompted efforts to develop inhibitors that target the RET tyrosine kinase. Preliminary in vitro studies have identified several promising agents, and human trials are forthcoming.

Pheochromocytoma The long-term goal for management of pheochromocytoma is to prevent death and cardiovascular complications. Improvements in radiographic imaging of the adrenals make direct examination of the apparently normal contralateral gland during surgery less important, and the rapid evolution of laparoscopic surgery has simplified management of early pheochromocytoma. The major question is whether to remove both adrenal glands or to remove only the affected adrenal at the time of primary surgery. Issues to be considered in this decision include the possibility of malignancy (<15 reported cases), the high probability of developing pheochromocytoma in the apparently unaffected gland over an 8- to 10-year period, and the risks of adrenal insufficiency caused by removal of both glands (at least two deaths related to adrenal insufficiency in MEN2 patients). Most clinicians recommend removing only the affected gland. If both adrenals are removed, glucocorticoid and mineralocorticoid replacement are mandatory. An alternative approach is to perform a cortical-sparing adrenalectomy, removing the pheochromocytoma and adrenal medulla, leaving the adrenal cortex behind. This approach is usually successful and eliminates the necessity for steroid hormone replacement in most patients, although the pheochromocytoma recurs in a small percentage.

Hyperparathyroidism Hyperparathyroidism has been managed by one of two approaches. Removal of 3.5 glands with maintenance of the remaining half gland in the neck is the usual procedure. In families in whom hyperparathyroidism is a prominent manifestation (almost always associated with a codon 634 *RET* mutation) and recurrence is common, total parathyroidectomy with transplantation of parathyroid tissue into the nondominant forearm is preferred. This approach is discussed above in the context of hyperparathyroidism associated with MEN1.

OTHER GENETIC ENDOCRINE TUMOR SYNDROMES

A number of mixed syndromes exist in which the neoplastic associations differ from those in MEN1 or 2 (Table 330-1).

The cause of VHL syndrome, the association of central nervous system tumors, renal cell carcinoma, pheochromocytoma, and islet cell neoplasms, is a mutation in the *VHL* tumor-suppressor gene. Germline-inactivating mutations of the *VHL* gene cause tumor formation when there is additional loss or somatic mutation of the normal *VHL* allele in brain, kidney, pancreatic islet, or adrenal medullary cells. Missense mutations have been identified in >40% of VHL families with pheochromocytoma, suggesting that families with this type of mutation should be surveyed routinely for pheochromocytoma. A point that may be useful in differentiating VHL from MEN1 (overlapping features include islet cell tumor and rare pheochromocytoma) or MEN2 (overlapping feature is pheochromocytoma) is that hyperparathyroidism rarely occurs in VHL.

The molecular defect in type 1 neurofibromatosis inactivates neurofibromin, a cell membrane–associated protein that normally activates a GTPase. Inactivation of this protein impairs GTPase and causes continuous activation of p21 Ras and its downstream tyrosine kinase pathway. Endocrine tumors also form in less common neoplastic genetic syndromes. These include Cowden's disease, Carney complex, familial acromegaly, and familial carcinoid syndrome. Carney complex comprises myxomas of the heart, skin, and breast; peripheral nerve schwannomas; spotty skin pigmentation; and testicular, adrenal, and GH-secreting pituitary tumors. Linkage analysis has identified two loci: chromosome 2p in half of families and 17q in the others. The 17q gene has been identified as the regulatory subunit (type IA) of protein kinase A (PRKA1A).

IMMUNOLOGIC SYNDROMES AFFECTING MULTIPLE ENDOCRINE ORGANS

When immune dysfunction affects two or more endocrine glands and other nonendocrine immune disorders are present, the polyglandular autoimmune (PGA) syndromes should be considered. The PGA syndromes are classified as two main types: the type I syndrome starts in childhood and is characterized by mucocutaneous candidiasis, hypoparathyroidism, and adrenal insufficiency; the type II, or Schmidt syndrome, is more likely to present in adults and most commonly comprises adrenal insufficiency, thyroiditis, and type 1 diabetes mellitus (Table 330-2).

POLYGLANDULAR AUTOIMMUNE SYNDROME TYPE I PGA type I is usually recognized in the first decade of life and requires two of three components for diagnosis: mucocutaneous candidiasis, hypoparathyroidism, and adrenal insufficiency. Mineralocorticoids and glucocorticoids may be lost simultaneously or sequentially. This disorder is also called *autoimmune polyendocrinopathy-candidiasis-ectodermal dystrophy* (APECED). Other endocrine defects can include gonadal failure, hypothyroidism, anterior hypophysitis, and, less commonly, destruction of the β cells of the pancreatic islets and development of insulin-dependent (type 1) diabetes mellitus. Additional features include hypoplasia of the dental enamel, ungual dystrophy, tympanic membrane sclerosis, vitiligo, keratopathy, and gastric parietal cell dysfunction resulting in pernicious anemia. Some patients develop autoimmune hepatitis, malabsorption (variably attributed to intestinal lymphangiectasia, IgA deficiency, bacterial overgrowth, or hypoparathyroidism), asplenism, achalasia, and cholelithiasis (Table 330-2). At the outset, only one organ may be involved, but the number increases with time so that patients eventually manifest two to five components of the syndrome.

Most patients initially present with oral candidiasis in childhood; it is poorly responsive to treatment and relapses frequently. Chronic hypoparathyroidism usually occurs before adrenal insufficiency de-

TABLE 330-2 *Features of Polyglandular Autoimmune (PGA) Syndromes*

PGA I	PGA II
EPIDEMIOLOGY	
Autosomal recessive	Polygenic inheritance
Mutations in APECED gene	HLA-DR3 and HLA-DR4 associated
Childhood onset	Adult onset
Equal male:female ratio	Female predominance
DISEASE ASSOCIATIONS	
Mucocutaneous candidiasis	Adrenal insufficiency
Hypoparathyroidism	Hypothyroidism
Adrenal insufficiency	Graves' disease
Hypogonadism	Type 1 diabetes
Alopecia	Hypogonadism
Hypothyroidism	Hypophysitis
Dental enamel hypoplasia	Myasthenia gravis
Malabsorption	Vitiligo
Chronic active hepatitis	Alopecia
Vitiligo	Pernicious anemia
Pernicious anemia	Celiac disease

Note: APECED, autoimmune polyendocrinopathy-candidiasis-ectodermal dystrophy.

velops. More than 60% of postpubertal women develop premature hypogonadism. The endocrine components, including adrenal insufficiency and hypoparathyroidism, may not develop until the fourth decade, making continued surveillance necessary.

Type I PGA syndrome is usually inherited as an autosomal recessive trait. The responsible gene, designated as either *APECED* or *AIRE*, encodes a transcription factor that is expressed in thymus and lymph nodes; a variety of different mutations have been reported.

POLYGLANDULAR AUTOIMMUNE SYNDROME TYPE II PGA type II is characterized by two or more of the endocrinopathies listed in Table 330-2. Most often these include primary adrenal insufficiency, Graves' disease or autoimmune hypothyroidism, type 1 diabetes mellitus, and primary hypogonadism. Because adrenal insufficiency is relatively rare, it is frequently used to define the presence of the syndrome. Among patients with adrenal insufficiency, type 1 diabetes mellitus coexists in 52% and autoimmune thyroid disease occurs in 69%. However, many patients with antimicrosomal and antithyroglobulin antibodies never develop abnormalities of thyroid function. Thus, increased antibody titers alone are poor predictors of future disease. Other associated conditions include hypophysitis, celiac disease, atrophic gastritis, and pernicious anemia. Vitiligo, caused by antibodies against the melanocyte (see Fig. 46-12), and alopecia are less common than in the type I syndrome. Mucocutaneous candidiasis does not occur. A few patients develop a late-onset, usually transient hypoparathyroidism caused by antibodies that compete with parathyroid hormone for binding to the PTH receptor. Up to 25% of patients with myasthenia gravis, and an even higher percentage who have myasthenia and a thymoma, have PGA type II (Chap. 366).

The type II syndrome is familial in nature, often transmitted as an autosomal dominant trait with incomplete penetrance. Like many of the individual autoimmune endocrinopathies, certain HLA-DR3 and HLA-DR4 alleles increase disease susceptibility; several different genes probably contribute to the expression of this syndrome.

A variety of autoantibodies are seen in PGA type II, including antibodies directed against: (1) thyroid antigens such as thyroid peroxidase, thyroglobulin, or the thyroid-stimulating hormone (TSH) receptor; (2) adrenal side chain cleavage enzyme, steroid 21-hydroxylase, or ACTH receptor; and (3) pancreatic islet glutamic acid decarboxylase or the insulin receptor, among others.

DIAGNOSIS The clinical manifestations of adrenal insufficiency often develop slowly, may be difficult to detect, and can be fatal if not diagnosed and treated appropriately. Thus, prospective screening should be performed routinely in all patients and family members at risk for PGA types I and II. The most effective screening test for adrenal disease is a cosyntropin stimulation test (Chap. 321). A fasting blood glucose level can be obtained to screen for hyperglycemia. Additional screening tests should include measurements of TSH, luteinizing hormone, follicle-stimulating hormone, and, in men, testosterone levels. In families with suspected type I PGA syndrome, calcium and phosphorus levels should be measured. These screening studies should be performed every 1 to 2 years up to about age 50 in families with PGA type II syndrome and until about age 40 in patients with type I syndrome. Screening measurements of autoantibodies against potentially affected endocrine organs are of uncertain prognostic value. The differential diagnosis of PGA syndrome should include the DiGeorge syndrome (hypoparathyroidism due to glandular agenesis and mucocutaneous candidiasis), Kearns-Sayre syndrome (hypoparathyroidism, primary hypogonadism, type 1 diabetes mellitus, and panhypopituitarism), Wolfram's syndrome (congenital diabetes insipidus and diabetes mellitus), IPEX syndrome (*immunodysregulation, polyendocrinopathy, and enteropathy, X-linked*), and congenital rubella (type 1 diabetes mellitus and hypothyroidism).

Rx **TREATMENT**

With the exception of Graves' disease, the management of each of the endocrine components of the disease involves hormone replacement and is covered in detail in the chapters on adrenal, thyroid, gonadal,

and parathyroid disease (Chaps. 320, 321, 325, 326, and 332). One aspect of therapy deserves special emphasis. Namely, primary hypothyroidism can mask adrenal insufficiency by prolonging the half-life of cortisol; consequently, administration of thyroid hormone to a patient with unsuspected adrenal insufficiency can precipitate adrenal crisis. Thus, all patients with hypothyroidism in the context of PGA syndrome should be screened for adrenal disease and, if it is present, be treated with glucocorticoids prior to or concurrently with thyroid hormone therapy.

OTHER AUTOIMMUNE ENDOCRINE SYNDROMES ■ **Insulin Receptor Antibodies**
Rare insulin-resistance syndromes occur in patients who develop antibodies that block the interaction of insulin with its receptor. Conversely, other classes of anti-insulin receptor antibodies can activate the receptor and can cause hypoglycemia; this disorder should be considered in the differential diagnosis of fasting hypoglycemia (Chap. 324).

Patients with insulin receptor antibodies and acanthosis nigricans are often middle-aged women who acquire insulin resistance in association with other autoimmune disorders such as systemic lupus erythematosus or Sjögren's syndrome. Vitiligo, alopecia, Raynaud's phenomenon, and arthritis may also be seen. Other autoimmune endocrine disorders, including thyrotoxicosis, hypothyroidism, and hypogonadism, occur rarely. Acanthosis nigricans, a velvety, hyperpigmented, thickened skin lesion, is prominent on the dorsum of the neck and other skin fold areas in the axillae or groin and often heralds the diagnosis in these patients. However, acanthosis nigricans also occurs in patients with obesity or polycystic ovarian syndrome, in which insulin resistance appears to be due to a postreceptor defect; thus acanthosis nigricans itself is not diagnostic of the immunologic form of insulin resistance.

Ataxia telangiectasia is an autosomal recessive disorder caused by mutations in *ATM*, a gene involved in cellular responses to ionizing radiation and oxidative damage (Chap. 352). This disorder is characterized by ataxia, telangiectasia, immune abnormalities, and an increased incidence of malignancies. Insulin-resistant diabetes mellitus occurs and is associated with anti-insulin antibodies.

Autoimmune Insulin Syndrome with Hypoglycemia This disorder typically occurs in patients with other autoimmune disorders and is caused by polyclonal insulin-binding autoantibodies that bind to endogenously synthesized insulin. If the insulin dissociates from the antibodies several hours or more after a meal, hypoglycemia can result. Most cases of the syndrome have been described in Japan, and there may be a genetic component. In plasma cell dyscrasias such as multiple myeloma, the plasma cells may produce monoclonal antibodies against insulin and cause hypoglycemia by a similar mechanism.

Antithyroxine Antibodies and Hypothyroidism Circulating autoantibodies against thyroid hormones in patients with both immune thyroid disease and plasma cell dyscrasias such as Waldenström's macroglobulinemia can bind thyroid hormones, decrease their biologic activity, and result in primary hypothyroidism. In other patients the antibodies simply interfere with thyroid hormone immunoassays and cause false elevations or decreases in measured hormone levels.

Crow-Fukase Syndrome The features of this syndrome are highlighted by an acronym that emphasizes its important features: *p*olyneuropathy, *o*rganomegaly, *e*ndocrinopathy, *M*-proteins, and *s*kin changes (POEMS). The most important feature is a severe, progressive sensorimotor polyneuropathy associated with a plasma cell dyscrasia. Localized collections of plasma cells (plasmacytomas) can cause sclerotic bone lesions and produce monoclonal IgG or IgA proteins. Endocrine manifestations include amenorrhea in women and impotence and gynecomastia in men, hypogonadism, hyperprolactinemia, type 2 diabetes mellitus, primary hypothyroidism, adrenal insufficiency, and hyperparathyroidism. Skin changes include hyperpigmentation, thickening of the dermis, hirsutism, and hyperhidrosis. Hepatomegaly and lymphadenopathy occur in about two-thirds of patients, and spleno-megaly is seen in about one-third. Other manifestations include increased cerebrospinal fluid pressure with papilledema, peripheral edema, ascites, pleural effusions, glomerulonephritis, and fever. Median survival may be >10 years, though shorter in patients with extravascular volume overload or clubbing.

The systemic nature of the disorder may cause confusion with other connective tissue diseases. The endocrine manifestations suggest an autoimmune basis of the disorder, but circulating antibodies against endocrine cells have not been demonstrated. Increased serum and tissue levels of interleukin 6, interleukin 1β, vascular endothelial growth factor, matrix metalloproteins, and tumor necrosis factor α are present, but the pathophysiologic basis for the POEMS syndrome is uncertain. Therapy directed against the plasma cell dyscrasia such as local radi-ation of bony lesions, chemotherapy, thalidomide, plasmapheresis, bone marrow or stem cell transplantation, and treatment with all-*trans* retinoic acid may result in endocrine improvement.

FURTHER READING

BETTERLE C et al: Autoimmune adrenal insufficiency and autoimmune poly-endocrine syndromes: Autoantibodies, autoantigens, and their applicability in diagnosis and disease prediction. Endocr Rev 23:327, 2002
DISPENZIERI A et al: POEMS syndrome: Definitions and long-term outcome. Blood First Edition Paper, prepublished online November 27, 2002; DOI 10.1182/blood-2002-07-2299
HEINO M et al: Mutation analyses of North American APS-1 patients. Hum Mutat 13:69, 1999
MACHENS A et al: Early malignant progression of hereditary medullary thyroid carcinoma. N Engl J Med 349: 1517, 2003
PERHEENTUPA J: APS-1/APECED: The clinical disease and therapy. Endo-crinol Metab Clin North Am 31:295, 2002

Section 2   Disorders of Bone and Mineral Metabolism

331 | BONE AND MINERAL METABOLISM IN HEALTH AND DISEASE
F. Richard Bringhurst, Marie B. Demay, Stephen M. Krane, Henry M. Kronenberg

BONE STRUCTURE AND METABOLISM

Bone is a dynamic tissue that is remodeled constantly throughout life. The arrangement of compact and cancellous bone provides a strength and density suitable for mobility and protection. In addition, bone provides a reservoir for calcium, magnesium, phosphorus, sodium, and other ions necessary for homeostatic functions. The skeleton is highly vascular and receives about 10% of the cardiac output. Remodeling of bone is accomplished by two distinct cell types: osteoblasts produce bone matrix and osteoclasts resorb the matrix.

The extracellular components of bone consist of a solid mineral phase in close association with an organic matrix, of which 90 to 95% is type I collagen (Chap. 342). The noncollagenous portion of the organic matrix is heterogeneous and contains serum proteins, such as albumin, as well as many locally produced proteins, whose functions are incompletely understood. These proteins include cell attachment/signaling proteins, such as thrombospondin, osteopontin, and fibro-nectin; calcium-binding proteins such as matrix gla protein and osteo-calcin; and proteoglycans such as biglycan and decorin. Some of these proteins organize collagen fibrils; others initiate mineralization and binding of the mineral phase to the matrix.

The mineral phase is made up of calcium and phosphate and is best characterized as a poorly crystalline hydroxyapatite. The mineral phase of bone is deposited initially in intimate relation to the collagen fibrils and is found in specific locations in the "holes" between the collagen fibrils. This architectural arrangement of mineral and matrix results in a two-phase material well suited to withstand mechanical stresses. The organization of collagen influences the amount and type of mineral phase formed in bone. Although the primary structures of type I collagen in skin and bone tissues are similar, there are differences in posttranslational modifications and distribution of intermolecular cross-links. The holes in the packing structure of the collagen are larger in mineralized collagen of bone and dentin than in unmineralized collagens such as tendon. Single amino-acid substitutions in the helical portion of either the α1 (*COL1A1*) or α2 (*COL1A2*) chains of type I collagen disrupt the organization of bone in osteogenesis imperfecta. The severe skeletal fragility associated with these disorders highlights the importance of the fibrillar matrix in the structure of bone (Chap. 342).

Osteoblasts synthesize and secrete the organic matrix. They are derived from cells of mesenchymal origin (Fig. 331-1A). Active osteoblasts are found on the surface of newly forming bone. As an osteoblast secretes matrix, which is then mineralized, the cell becomes an *osteocyte*, still connected with its blood supply through a series of canaliculi. Osteocytes represent the vast majority of the cells in bone. They are thought to be the mechanosensors in bone that communicate signals to surface osteo-

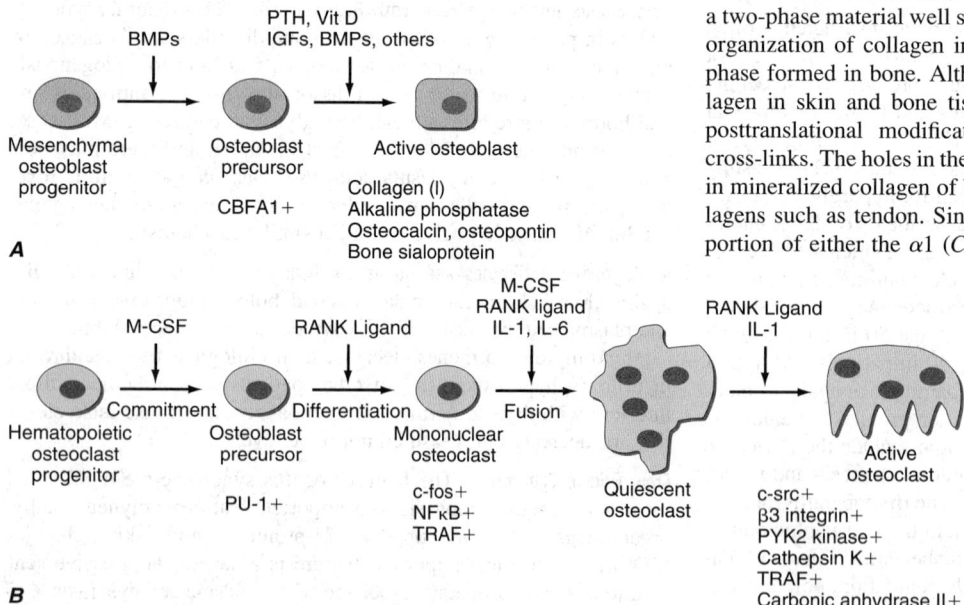

FIGURE 331-1 Pathways regulating development of (A) osteoblasts and (B) osteoclasts. Hormones, cytokines, and growth factors that control cell proliferation and differentiation are shown above the arrows. Transcription factors and other markers specific for various stages of development are depicted below the arrows. BMPs, bone morphogenic proteins; PTH, parathyroid hormone; Vit D, vitamin D; IGFs, insulin-like growth factors; CBFA1, core binding factor A1; M-CSF, macrophage colony-stimulating factor; PU-1, a monocyte- and B lymphocyte–specific ets family transcription factor; NFκB, nuclear factor κB; TRAF, tumor necrosis factor receptor–associated factors; RANK ligand, receptor activator of NFκB ligand; IL-1, interleukin-1; IL-6, interleukin-6. (*Modified from Suda et al, with permission.*)

blasts and their progenitors through the canalicular network. Mineralization of the matrix, both in trabecular bone and in osteones of compact cortical bone (*haversian systems*), begins soon after the matrix is secreted (primary mineralization) but is not completed for several weeks or even longer (secondary mineralization). While this mineralization takes advantage of the high concentrations of calcium and phosphate already near saturation in serum, mineralization is a carefully regulated process dependent on the activity of osteoblast-derived alkaline phosphatase, which probably works by hydrolyzing inhibitors of mineralization.

Genetic studies in humans and mice have identified several key genes that control osteoblast development. Core-binding factor A1 (*CBFA1*, also called *RUNX2*), is a transcription factor expressed specifically in chondrocyte (cartilage cells) and osteoblast progenitors, as well as in mature osteoblasts. *CBFA1* regulates the expression of several important osteoblast proteins including osterix (another transcription factor needed for osteoblast maturation), osteopontin, bone sialoprotein, type I collagen, osteocalcin, and receptor-activator of NFκB (RANK) ligand. *CBFA1* expression is regulated, in part, by bone morphogenic proteins (BMPs). *CBFA1*-deficient mice are devoid of osteoblasts, whereas mice with a deletion of only one allele (*CBFA1* +/−) exhibit a delay in formation of the clavicles and some cranial bones. The latter abnormalities are similar to those in the human disorder *cleidocranial dysplasia*, which is also caused by heterozygous inactivating mutations in *CBFA1*.

The paracrine signaling molecule, Indian hedgehog (Ihh), also plays a critical role in osteoblast development, as evidenced by Ihh-deficient mice that lack osteoblasts in bone formed on a cartilage mold (endochondral ossification). Signals originating from members of the wnt (wingless-type mouse mammary tumor virus integration site) family of paracrine factors are also important. Humans and mice missing a wnt-family co-receptor, LRP5 (lipoprotein receptor–related protein 5), have osteoporosis. Remarkably, humans with an overactive form of LPR5 have increased bone mass. Numerous other growth-regulatory factors affect osteoblast function, including the three closely related transforming growth factor βs, fibroblast growth factors (FGFs) 2 and 18, platelet-derived growth factor, and insulin-like growth factors (IGFs) I and II. Hormones, such as parathyroid hormone (PTH) and 1,25-dihydroxyvitamin D [1,25(OH)$_2$D] activate receptors expressed by osteoblasts to assure mineral homeostasis and to influence a variety of bone cell functions.

Resorption of bone is carried out mainly by *osteoclasts*, multinucleated cells that are formed by fusion of cells derived from the common precursor of macrophages and osteoclasts. Multiple factors regulating osteoclast development have been identified (Fig. 331-1*B*). Factors produced by osteoblasts or marrow stromal cells allow osteoblasts to control osteoclast development and activity. Macrophage colony-stimulating factor (M-CSF) plays a critical role during several steps in the pathway and ultimately leads to fusion of osteoclast progenitor cells to form multinucleated, active osteoclasts. RANK ligand, a member of the tumor necrosis factor (TNF) family, is expressed on the surface of osteoblast progenitors and stromal fibroblasts. In a process involving cell-cell interactions, RANK ligand binds to the RANK receptor on osteoclast progenitors, stimulating osteoclast differentiation and activation. Alternatively, a soluble decoy receptor, referred to as osteoprotegerin, can bind RANK ligand and inhibit osteoclast differentiation. Several growth factors and cytokines (including interleukins 1, 6, and 11; TNF; and interferon γ) modulate osteoclast differentiation and function. Most hormones that influence osteoclast function do not directly target this cell but instead influence M-CSF and RANK ligand signaling by osteoblasts. Both PTH and 1,25(OH)$_2$D increase osteoclast number and activity, whereas estrogen decreases osteoclast number and activity by this indirect mechanism. Calcitonin, in contrast, binds to its receptor on the basal surface of osteoclasts and directly inhibits osteoclast function.

Osteoclast-mediated resorption of bone takes place in scalloped spaces (*Howship's lacunae*) where the osteoclasts are attached through a specific $\alpha_v\beta_3$ integrin to components of the bone matrix such as

osteopontin. The osteoclast forms a tight seal to the underlying matrix and secretes protons, chloride, and proteinases into a confined space likened to an extracellular lysosome. The active osteoclast surface forms a ruffled border that contains a specialized proton-pump ATPase, which secretes acid and solubilizes the mineral phase. Carbonic anhydrase (type II isoenzyme) within the osteoclast generates the needed protons. The bone matrix is resorbed in the acid environment adjacent to the ruffled border by proteases that act at low pH, such as cathepsin K.

In the embryo and in the growing child, bone develops by remodeling and replacing previously calcified cartilage (endochondral bone formation) or is formed without a cartilage matrix (intramembranous bone formation). Chondrocytes proliferate, secrete and mineralize a matrix, enlarge (hypertrophy), and then die, thereby enlarging bone and providing the matrix and factors that stimulate endochondral bone formation. This program is regulated by both local factors, such as IGF-I and -II, parathyroid hormone–related peptide (PTHrP), and FGFs, and by systemic hormones such as growth hormone, glucocorticoids, and estrogen.

New bone, whether formed in infants or in adults during repair, has a relatively high ratio of cells to matrix and is characterized by coarse fiber bundles of collagen that are interlaced and randomly dispersed (woven bone). In adults, the more mature bone is organized with fiber bundles regularly arranged in parallel or concentric sheets (lamellar bone). In long bones, deposition of lamellar bone in a concentric arrangement around blood vessels forms the haversian systems. Growth in length of bones is dependent on proliferation of cartilage cells and on the endochondral sequence at the growth plate. Growth in width and thickness is accomplished by formation of bone at the periosteal surface and by resorption at the endosteal surface, with the rate of formation exceeding that of resorption. In adults, after the growth plates close, growth in length and endochondral bone formation cease, except for some activity in the cartilage cells beneath the articular surface. Even in adults, however, remodeling of bone (within haversian systems as well as trabecular bone) continues throughout life. In adults, ~4% of the surface of trabecular bone (such as iliac crest) is involved in active resorption, whereas 10 to 15% of trabecular surfaces is covered with osteoid. Radioisotope studies indicate that as much as 18% of the total skeletal calcium is deposited and removed each year. Thus, bone is an active metabolizing tissue that requires an intact blood supply. The cycle of bone resorption and formation is a highly orchestrated process carried out by the basic multicellular unit, composed of a group of osteoclasts and osteoblasts (Fig. 331-2).

The response of bone to fractures, infection, and interruption of blood supply and to expanding lesions is relatively limited. Dead bone must be resorbed, and new bone must be formed, a process carried out in association with growth of new blood vessels into the involved area. In injuries that disrupt the organization of the tissue, such as a fracture in which apposition of fragments is poor or when motion exists at the fracture site, the progenitor stromal cells differentiate into cells with functional capacities different from those of osteoblasts, and varying amounts of fibrous tissue and cartilage are formed. When there is good apposition with fixation and little motion at the fracture site, repair occurs predominantly by formation of new bone without other scar tissue.

Remodeling of bone occurs along lines of force generated by mechanical stress. The signals from these mechanical stresses are sensed by osteocytes, which transmit signals to osteoclasts or osteoblasts, or their precursors. A bowing deformity increases new bone formation at the concave surface and resorption at the convex surface, seemingly designed to produce the strongest mechanical structure. Expanding lesions in bone, such as tumors, induce resorption at the surface in contact with the tumor, by producing ligands, such as PTHrP, that stimulate osteoclast differentiation and function. Even in a disorder as architecturally disruptive as Paget's disease, remodeling is dictated by mechanical forces. Thus, bone plasticity reflects the interaction of cells with each other and with the environment.

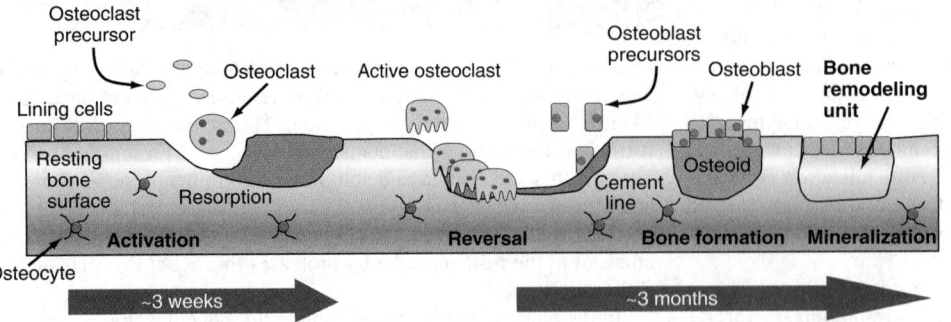

FIGURE 331-2 Schematic representation of bone remodeling. The cycle of bone remodeling is carried out by the basic multicellular unit (BMU), comprising a group of osteoclasts and osteoblasts. In cortical bone, the BMUs tunnel through the tissue, whereas in cancellous bone, they move across the trabecular surface. The process of bone remodeling is initiated by contraction of the lining cells and the recruitment of osteoclast precursors. These precursors fuse to form multinucleated, active osteoclasts that mediate bone resorption. Osteoclasts adhere to bone and subsequently remove it by acidification and proteolytic digestion. As the BMU advances, osteoclasts leave the resorption site and osteoblasts move in to cover the excavated area and begin the process of new bone formation by secreting osteoid, which is eventually mineralized into new bone. After osteoid mineralization, osteoblasts flatten and form a layer of lining cells over new bone.

The products of osteoblast and osteoclast activity can assist in the diagnosis and management of bone diseases. Osteoblast activity can be assessed by measuring serum bone-specific alkaline phosphatase. Similarly, osteocalcin, a protein secreted from osteoblasts, is made virtually only by osteoblasts. Osteoclast activity can be assessed by measurement of products of collagen degradation. Collagen molecules are covalently linked to each other in the extracellular matrix through the formation of hydroxypyridinium crosslinks (Chap. 342). These cross-linked peptides can be measured both in urine and in blood.

CALCIUM METABOLISM

Over 99% of the 1 to 2 kg of calcium present normally in the adult human body resides in the skeleton, where it provides mechanical stability and serves as a reservoir sometimes needed to maintain extracellular fluid (ECF) calcium concentration (Fig. 331-3). Skeletal calcium accretion first becomes significant during the third trimester of fetal life, accelerates throughout childhood and adolescence, reaches a peak in early adulthood, and gradually declines thereafter at rates that rarely exceed 1 to 2% per year. These slow changes in total skeletal calcium content contrast with relatively high daily rates of closely matched fluxes of calcium into and out of bone (approximately 250 to 500 mg each), a process mediated by coupled osteoblastic and osteoclastic activity. Another 0.5 to 1% of skeletal calcium is freely exchangeable (e.g., in chemical equilibrium) with that in the ECF.

The concentration of ionized calcium in the ECF must be maintained within a narrow range because of the critical role it plays in a

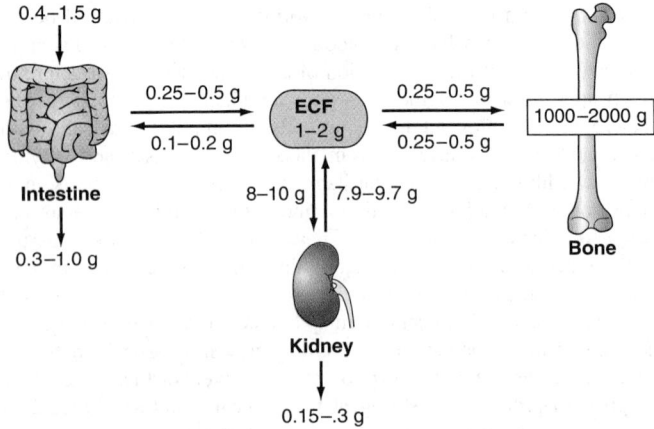

FIGURE 331-3 Calcium homeostasis. Schematic illustration of calcium content of extracellular fluid (ECF) and bone as well as of diet and feces; magnitude of calcium flux per day as calculated by various methods is shown at sites of transport in intestine, kidney, and bone. Ranges of values shown are approximate and chosen to illustrate certain points discussed in text. In conditions of calcium balance, rates of calcium release from and uptake into bone are equal.

wide array of cellular functions, especially those involved in neuromuscular activity, secretion, and signal transduction. Intracellular cytosolic free calcium levels are approximately 100 nmol/L and are 10,000-fold lower than ionized calcium concentration in the blood and ECF (1.1 to 1.3 mmol/L). This steep chemical gradient promotes rapid calcium influx through various membrane calcium channels that can be activated by hormones, metabolites, or neurotransmitters, swiftly changing cellular function. In blood, total calcium concentration is normally 2.2 to 2.6 mM (8.5 to 10.5 mg/dL), of which approximately 50% is ionized. The remainder is bound ionically to negatively charged proteins (predominantly albumin and immunoglobulins) or loosely complexed with phosphate, citrate, sulfate, or other anions. Alterations in serum protein concentrations directly affect the total blood calcium concentration, even if the ionized calcium concentration remains normal. An algorithm to correct for protein changes adjusts the total serum calcium (in mg/dL) upward by 0.8 times the deficit in serum albumin (g/dL) or by 0.5 times the deficit in serum immunoglobulin (in g/dL). Such corrections provide only rough approximations of actual free calcium concentrations, however, and may be misleading. Acidosis also alters ionized calcium by reducing its association with proteins. The best practice is to measure blood ionized calcium directly by a method that employs calcium-selective electrodes.

Control of the ionized calcium concentration in the ECF ordinarily is accomplished by adjusting the rates of calcium movement across intestinal and renal epithelia. These adjustments are mediated mainly via changes in blood levels of the hormones PTH and $1,25(OH)_2D$. Blood ionized calcium directly suppresses PTH secretion by activating parathyroid calcium-sensing receptors (CaSRs). Also, ionized calcium indirectly affects PTH secretion via effects on $1,25(OH)_2D$ production. This active vitamin D metabolite inhibits PTH production by an incompletely understood mechanism of negative feedback (Chap. 332).

Normal dietary calcium intake in the United States varies widely, ranging from 10 to 37 mmol/d (400 to 1500 mg/d). Many individuals, in an effort to prevent osteoporosis, routinely supplement this further with oral calcium salts to a total intake of 37 to 50 mmol/d (1500 to 2000 mg/d). Intestinal absorption of ingested calcium involves both active (transcellular) and passive (paracellular) mechanisms. Passive calcium absorption is nonsaturable and approximates 5% of daily calcium intake, whereas the active mechanism, controlled principally by $1,25(OH)_2D$, normally ranges from 20 to 70%. Active calcium transport occurs mainly in the proximal small bowel (duodenum and proximal jejunum), although some active calcium absorption occurs in most segments of the small intestine. Optimal rates of calcium absorption require gastric acid. This is especially true for weakly dissociable calcium supplements such as calcium carbonate. In fact, large boluses of calcium carbonate are poorly absorbed because of their neutralizing effect upon gastric acid. In achlorhydric subjects or for those taking drugs that inhibit gastric acid secretion, supplements should be taken with meals to optimize their absorption. Use of calcium citrate may be preferable in these circumstances. Calcium absorption may also be blunted in disease states such as pancreatic or biliary insufficiency, where ingested calcium remains bound to unabsorbed fatty acids or other food constituents. At high levels of calcium intake, synthesis of $1,25(OH)_2D$ is reduced, which decreases the rate of active intestinal calcium absorption. The opposite occurs with dietary calcium restriction. Some calcium, approximately 2.5 to 5.0 mmol/d (100 to 200 mg/d), is excreted as an obligate component of intestinal secretions and is not regulated by calciotropic hormones.

The feedback-controlled hormonal regulation of intestinal absorptive efficiency results in a relatively constant daily net calcium absorption of approximately 5 to 7.5 mmol/d (200 to 400 mg/d), despite large changes in daily dietary calcium intake. This daily load of absorbed calcium is excreted by the kidneys in a manner that is also tightly regulated by the concentration of ionized calcium in the blood. Approximately 8 to 10 g/d of calcium are filtered by the glomeruli, of which only 2 to 3% appears in the urine. Most filtered calcium (65%) is reabsorbed in the proximal tubules via a passive, paracellular route that is coupled to concomitant NaCl reabsorption and not specifically regulated. The cortical thick ascending limb of Henle's loop (cTAL) reabsorbs roughly another 20% of filtered calcium, also via a paracellular mechanism. Calcium reabsorption in the cTAL requires a tight-junctional protein called paracellin-1 and is inhibited by increased blood concentrations of calcium or magnesium, acting via the CaSR, which is highly expressed on basolateral membranes in this nephron segment. Operation of the renal CaSR provides a mechanism, independent of those engaged directly by PTH or 1,25(OH)$_2$D, whereby serum ionized calcium can control renal calcium reabsorption. Finally, ~10% of filtered calcium is reabsorbed in the distal convoluted tubules (DCT) by a transcellular mechanism. Calcium enters the luminal surface of the cell through specific apical calcium channels, whose number is regulated. It then moves across the cell in association with a specific calcium-binding protein (calbindin-D28k) that buffers cytosolic calcium concentrations from the large mass of transported calcium. Ca^{2+}-ATPases and Na/ Ca^{2+} exchangers actively extrude calcium across the basolateral surface and thereby maintain the transcellular calcium gradient. All of these steps are increased, directly or indirectly, by PTH. The DCT is also the site of action of thiazide diuretics, which lower urinary calcium excretion by blocking a NaCl transporter expressed on the apical surface of these cells. Conversely, dietary sodium loads, or increased distal sodium delivery caused by loop diuretics or saline infusion, reduce DCT calcium reabsorption by an action opposite to that of thiazides.

The homeostatic mechanisms that normally maintain a constant serum ionized calcium concentration may fail at extremes of calcium intake or when the hormonal systems or organs involved are compromised. Thus, even with maximal activity of the vitamin D–dependent intestinal active transport system, sustained calcium intakes <5 mmol/d (<200 mg/d) cannot provide enough net calcium absorption to replace obligate losses via the intestine, kidney, sweat, or other secretions. In this case, increased blood levels of PTH and 1,25(OH)$_2$D activate osteoclastic bone resorption to obtain needed calcium from bone, which leads to progressive bone loss and negative calcium balance. Increased PTH and 1,25(OH)$_2$D also enhance renal calcium reabsorption, and 1,25(OH)$_2$D enhances calcium absorption in the gut. At very high calcium intakes [> 100 mmol/d; > 4 g/d], passive intestinal absorption continues to deliver calcium into the ECF, despite maximally down-regulated intestinal active transport and renal tubular calcium reabsorption. This can cause severe hypercalciuria, nephrocalcinosis, progressive renal failure, and hypercalcemia (e.g., "milk alkali syndrome"). Deficiency or excess of PTH or vitamin D, intestinal disease, and renal failure represent other commonly encountered challenges to normal calcium homeostasis (Chap. 332).

PHOSPHORUS METABOLISM

Although 85% of the ~600 g of body phosphorus is present in bone mineral, phosphorus is also a major intracellular constituent, both as the free anion(s) and as a component of numerous organophosphate compounds including structural proteins, enzymes, transcription factors, carbohydrate and lipid intermediates, high-energy stores (ATP, creatine phosphate), and nucleic acids. Unlike calcium, phosphorus exists intracellularly at concentrations close to those present in ECF (e.g., 1 to 2 mmol/L). In cells and in the ECF, phosphorus exists in several forms, predominantly as H$_2$PO$_4$$^-$ or NaHPO$_4$$^-$, with perhaps 10% as HPO$_4$$^{2-}$. This mixture of anions will be referred to here as "phosphate." In serum, about 12% of phosphorus is bound to proteins. Concentrations of phosphates in blood and ECF are generally expressed in terms of elemental phosphorus, the normal range in adults

being 0.75 to 1.45 mmol/L (2.5 to 4.5 mg/dL). Because the volume of the intracellular fluid compartment is twice that of the ECF, measurements of ECF phosphate may not accurately reflect phosphate availability within cells that follows even modest shifts of phosphate from one compartment to the other.

Phosphate is widely available in foods and is efficiently absorbed (65%) by the small intestine, even in the absence of vitamin D. On the other hand, phosphate absorptive efficiency may be further enhanced (to 85 to 90%) via active transport mechanisms that are stimulated by 1,25(OH)$_2$D. These involve activation of Na$^+$/PO$_4$$^{2-}$ co-transporters that move phosphate into intestinal cells against an unfavorable electrochemical gradient. Daily net intestinal phosphate absorption varies widely according to the composition of the diet but is generally in the range of 500 to 1000 mg/d. Phosphate absorption can be inhibited by large doses of calcium salts or by sevelamer hydrochloride (Renagel), strategies commonly used to control levels of serum phosphate in renal failure. Aluminum hydroxide antacids also reduce phosphate absorption but are less commonly used because of the potential for aluminum toxicity. Low serum phosphate directly stimulates renal proximal tubular synthesis of 1,25(OH)$_2$D.

Serum phosphate levels vary by as much as 50% on a normal day. This reflects the effect of food intake but also an underlying circadian rhythm that produces a nadir between 7 and 10 A.M. Carbohydrate administration, especially as intravenous dextrose solutions in fasting subjects, can decrease serum phosphate by >0.7 mmol/L (2 mg/dL) due to rapid uptake into, and utilization by, cells. A similar response is observed in the treatment of diabetic ketoacidosis and during metabolic or respiratory alkalosis. Because of this wide variation in serum phosphate, it is best to perform measurements in the basal, fasting state.

Control of serum phosphate is determined mainly by the rate of renal tubular reabsorption of the filtered load, which approximates 4 to 6 g/d. Because intestinal phosphate absorption is highly efficient, urinary excretion is not constant but varies directly with dietary intake. The fractional excretion of phosphate (ratio of phosphate to creatinine clearance) is generally in the range of 10 to 15%. The proximal tubule is the principal site at which renal phosphate reabsorption is regulated. This is accomplished by changes in the apical expression and activity of a specific Na$^+$/PO$_4$$^{2-}$ co-transporter (NaPi-2) in the proximal tubule. Apical expression of NaPi-2 is rapidly reduced by PTH, the major known hormonal regulator of renal phosphate excretion. FGF23 can dramatically impair phosphate reabsorption. Activating *FGF23* mutations cause the rare disorder autosomal dominant hypophosphatemic rickets. In contrast to PTH, this molecule also leads to reduced synthesis of 1,25(OH)$_2$D, which may worsen the resulting hypophosphatemia by lowering intestinal phosphate absorption. Renal reabsorption of phosphate is responsive to changes in dietary intake, such that experimental dietary phosphate restriction leads to a dramatic lowering of urinary phosphate within hours, preceding any decline in serum phosphate (e.g., filtered load). This physiologic renal adaptation to changes in dietary phosphate availability occurs independently of PTH. Findings in *FGF23*-knockout mice suggest that FGF23 normally acts to lower blood phosphate and 1,25(OH)$_2$D levels.

Renal phosphate reabsorption is impaired by hypocalcemia, hypomagnesemia, and severe hypophosphatemia. Phosphate clearance is enhanced by ECF volume expansion and impaired by dehydration. Phosphate retention is an important pathophysiologic feature of renal insufficiency (Chap. 261).

HYPOPHOSPHATEMIA ■ **Causes** Hypophosphatemia can occur by one or more of three primary mechanisms: (1) inadequate intestinal phosphate absorption, (2) excessive renal phosphate excretion, or (3) rapid redistribution of phosphate from the ECF into bone or soft tissue (Table 331-1). Because phosphate is so abundant in foods, inadequate intestinal absorption is almost never observed now that aluminum hydroxide antacids, which bind phosphate in the gut, are no longer commonly

TABLE 331-1 *Causes of Hypophosphatemia*

  I. Reduced renal tubular phosphate reabsorption
   A. PTH/PTHrP-dependent
     1. Primary hyperparathyroidism
     2. Secondary hyperparathyroidism
       a. Vitamin D deficiency/resistance
       b. Calcium starvation/malabsorption
       c. Bartter syndrome
       d. Autosomal recessive renal hypercalciuria with hypomagnesemia
     3. PTHrP-dependent hypercalcemia of malignancy
     4. Familial hypocalciuric hypercalcemia
   B. PTH/PTHrP-independent
     1. Genetic hypophosphatemia
       a. X-linked hypophosphatemic rickets
       b. Dent disease
       c. Autosomal dominant hypophosphatemic rickets
       d. Fanconi syndrome(s)
       e. Cystinosis
       f. Wilson disease
       g. McCune-Albright syndrome (fibrous dysplasia)
       h. Idiopathic hypercalciuria (absorptive subtype)
       i. Hereditary hypophosphatemia with hypercalciuria (Bedouins)
     2. Tumor-induced osteomalacia
     3. Other systemic disorders
       a. Poorly controlled diabetes mellitus
       b. Alcoholism
       c. Hyperaldosteronism
       d. Hypomagnesemia
       e. Amyloidosis
       f. Hemolytic uremic syndrome
       g. Renal transplantation or partial liver resection
       h. Rewarming or induced hyperthermia
     4. Drugs or toxins
       a. Ethanol
       b. Acetazolamide, other diuretics
       c. High-dose estrogens or glucocorticoids
       d. Heavy metals (lead, cadmium)
       e. Toluene, *N*-methyl formamide
       f. Cisplatin, ifosfamide, foscarnet, rapamycin
       g. Calcitonin, pamidronate
 II. Impaired intestinal phosphate absorption
   A. Aluminum-containing antacids
   B. Sevalamer
III. Shifts of extracellular phosphate into cells
   A. Intravenous glucose
   B. Insulin therapy of prolonged hyperglycemia or diabetic ketoacidosis
   C. Catecholamines (epinephrine, dopamine, albuterol)
   D. Acute respiratory alkalosis
   E. Gram-negative sepsis, toxic shock syndrome
   F. Recovery from starvation or acidosis
   G. Rapid cellular proliferation
     1. Leukemic blast crisis
     2. Intensive erythropoetin, other CSF therapy
IV. Accelerated net bone formation
   A. Following parathyroidectomy
   B. Treatment of vitamin D deficiency, Paget disease
   C. Osteoblastic metastases

Note: CSF, cerebrospinal fluid.

amples of genetic disorders in this category (Chap. 332). Several genetic diseases cause PTH/PTHrP-independent tubular phosphate wasting, with associated rickets and osteomalacia. The most common of these is X-linked hypophosphatemic rickets (XLHR), which results from inactivating mutations in an endopeptidase termed *PHEX* (*p*hosphate-regulating gene with *h*omologies to *e*ndopeptidases on the *X* chromosome) that is most abundantly expressed on the surface of mature osteoblasts. It is believed that PHEX normally inactivates a phosphaturic hormone (phosphatonin) that impairs both renal tubular phosphate reabsorption and $1,25(OH)_2D$ synthesis in the proximal renal tubules. Disorders likely to share a related pathophysiology with XLHR are autosomal dominant hypophosphatemic rickets (ADHR) and tumor-induced osteomalacia (TIO). All of these manifest severe hypophosphatemia; renal phosphate wasting, sometimes accompanied by aminoaciduria; low blood levels of $1,25(OH)_2D$; low or low-normal serum levels of calcium; and evidence of impaired cartilage or bone mineralization. ADHR results from activating mutations in the gene encoding FGF23, which is phosphaturic when administered to mice. TIO is an acquired disorder in which tumors, usually of mesenchymal origin and generally histologically benign, secrete a phosphatonin-like molecule (Chap. 87). The hypophosphatemic syndrome resolves completely within hours to days following successful resection of the responsible tumor. Such tumors express large amounts of FGF23 mRNA, raising the possibility that FGF23 may be a phosphatonin. It is not yet clear if FGF23 is a physiologic substrate for PHEX, however. Dent's disease is an X-linked recessive disorder caused by inactivating mutations in CLCN5, a chloride transporter expressed in endosomes of the proximal tubule; features include hypercalciuria, hypophosphatemia, and recurrent kidney stones. Renal phosphate wasting is common among poorly controlled diabetics and alcoholics, who therefore are at risk for iatrogenic hypophosphatemia when treated with insulin or intravenous glucose, respectively. Diuretics and certain other drugs and toxins can cause defective renal tubular phosphate reabsorption (Table 331-1).

In hospitalized patients, hypophosphatemia is often attributable to massive redistribution of phosphate from the ECF into cells. Insulin therapy of diabetic ketoacidosis is a paradigm for this phenomenon, in which the severity of the hypophosphatemia is related to the extent of antecedent depletion of phosphate and other electrolytes (Chap. 323). The hypophosphatemia is usually greatest at a point many hours after initiation of insulin therapy and is difficult to predict from baseline measurements of serum phosphate at the time of presentation, when prerenal azotemia can obscure significant phosphate depletion. Other factors that may contribute to such acute redistributive hypophosphatemia include antecedent starvation or malnutrition, administration of intravenous glucose without other nutrients, elevated blood catecholamines (endogenous or exogenous), respiratory alkalosis, and recovery from metabolic acidosis.

Hypophosphatemia can also occur transiently (over weeks to months) during the phase of accelerated net bone formation following parathyroidectomy for severe primary hyperparathyroidism or during treatment of vitamin D deficiency or lytic Paget's disease. This is usually most prominent in patients who preoperatively have evidence of high bone turnover (e.g., high serum levels of alkaline phosphatase). Osteoblastic metastases can also lead to this syndrome.

Clinical and Laboratory Findings The clinical manifestations of severe hypophosphatemia reflect a generalized defect in cellular energy metabolism because of ATP depletion, a shift from oxidative phosphorylation toward glycolysis, and associated tissue or organ dysfunction. Acute, severe hypophosphatemia occurs mainly or exclusively in hospitalized patients with underlying serious medical or surgical illness and preexisting phosphate depletion due to excessive urinary losses, severe malabsorption, or malnutrition. Chronic hypophosphatemia tends to be less severe, with a clinical presentation dominated by musculoskeletal complaints such as bone pain, pseudofractures, and proximal muscle weakness or, in children, rickets and short stature.

Neuromuscular manifestations of severe hypophosphatemia are

used. Fasting or starvation, however, may result in depletion of body phosphate and predispose to subsequent hypophosphatemia during refeeding, especially if this is accomplished with intravenous glucose alone.

Chronic hypophosphatemia usually signifies a persistent renal tubular phosphate-wasting disorder. Excessive activation of PTH/PTHrP receptors in the proximal tubule, because of primary or secondary hyperparathyroidism or because of the PTHrP-mediated hypercalcemia syndrome in malignancy (Chap. 332), is among the more common causes of renal hypophosphatemia, especially because of the high prevalence of vitamin D deficiency in older Americans. Familial hypocalciuric hypercalcemia and Jansen's chondrodystrophy are rare ex-variable but may include muscle weakness, lethargy, confusion, disorientation, hallucinations, dysarthria, dysphagia, oculomotor palsies, anisocoria, nystagmus, ataxia, cerebellar tremor, ballismus, hyporeflexia, impaired sphincter control, distal sensory deficits, paresthesia, hyperesthesia, generalized or Guillain Barré–like ascending paralysis, seizures, coma, and death. Serious sequelae such as paralysis, confusion, and seizures are likely only at phosphate concentrations <0.25 mmol/L (< 0.8 mg/dL). Rhabdomyolysis may develop during rapidly progressive hypophosphatemia. The diagnosis of hypophosphatemia-induced rhabdomyolysis may be overlooked, as up to 30% of patients with acute hypophosphatemia (< 0.7 mM) have creatine phosphokinase elevations that peak 1 to 2 days after the nadir in serum phosphate, when the release of phosphate from injured myocytes may have led to a near-normalization of circulating levels of phosphate.

Respiratory failure and cardiac dysfunction, reversible with phosphate treatment, may occur at serum phosphate levels of 0.5 to 0.8 mmol/L (1.5 to 2.5 mg/dL). Renal tubular defects, including tubular acidosis, glycosuria, and impaired reabsorption of sodium and calcium, may occur. Hematologic abnormalities correlate with reductions in intracellular ATP and 2,3-diphosphoglycerate and may include erythrocyte microspherocytosis and hemolysis; impaired oxyhemoglobin dissociation; defective leukocyte chemotaxis, phagocytosis, and bacterial killing; and platelet dysfunction with spontaneous gastrointestinal hemorrhage.

℞ TREATMENT

Severe hypophosphatemia [< 0.75 mmol/L (< 2 mg/dL)], particularly in the setting of underlying phosphate depletion, constitutes a dangerous electrolyte abnormality that should be corrected promptly. Unfortunately, the cumulative deficit in body phosphate cannot be easily predicted from knowledge of the circulating level of phosphate, and therapy must be approached empirically. The threshold for intravenous phosphate therapy and the dose administered should reflect consideration of renal function, the likely severity and duration of the underlying phosphate depletion, and the presence and severity of symptoms consistent with those of hypophosphatemia. In adults, phosphate may be safely administered intravenously as neutral mixtures of sodium and potassium phosphate salts at initial doses of 0.2 to 0.8 mmol/kg of elemental phosphorus over 6 h (e.g., 10 to 50 mmol over 6 h), with doses >20 mmol/6 h reserved for those who have serum levels <0.5 mmol/L (1.5 mg/dL) and normal renal function. A suggested approach is presented in Table 331-2. Serum levels of phosphate and calcium must be monitored closely (every 6 to 12 h) throughout treatment. It is necessary to avoid a serum calcium-phosphorus product >50 to reduce the risk of heterotopic calcification. Hypocalcemia, if present,

TABLE 331-2 Intravenous Therapy of Hypophosphatemia

Consider
Likely severity of underlying phosphate depletion
Concurrent parenteral glucose administration
Presence of neuromuscular, cardiopulmonary, or hematologic complications of hypophosphatemia
Renal function [reduce dose by 50% if serum creatinine >220 μmol/L (>2.5 mg/dL)]
Serum calcium level (correct hypocalcemia first; reduce dose by 50% in hypercalcemia)

Guidelines

Serum Phosphorus, mM(mg/dL)	Rate of Infusion, mmol/h	Duration, h	Total Administered, mmol
<0.8 (<2.5)	2.0	6	12
<0.5 (<1.5)	4.0	6	24
<0.3 (<1.0)	8.0	6	48

Rates shown are calculated for a 70-kg person; levels of serum calcium and phosphorus must be measured every 6 to 12 h during therapy; infusions can be repeated to achieve stable serum phosphorus levels > 0.8 mmol/L (>2.5 mg/dL); most formulations available in the United States provide 3 mmol/mL of sodium or potassium phosphate.

should be corrected before administering intravenous phosphate. Less severe hypophosphatemia, in the range of 0.5 to 0.8 mmol/L (1.5 to 2.5 mg/dL), can usually be treated with oral phosphate in divided doses of 750 to 2000 mg/d, as elemental phosphorus; higher doses can cause bloating and diarrhea.

Management of chronic hypophosphatemia requires knowing the cause(s) of the disorder. Hypophosphatemia related to the secondary hyperparathyroidism of vitamin D deficiency usually responds to treatment with vitamin D and calcium alone. XLHR, ADHR, TIO, and related renal tubular disorders are usually managed with divided oral doses of phosphate, often with calcium and 1,25(OH)$_2$D supplements to bypass the block in renal 1,25(OH)$_2$D synthesis and prevent secondary hyperparathyroidism caused by suppression of ECF calcium levels. Thiazide diuretics may be used to prevent nephrocalcinosis in patients who are managed this way. Complete normalization of hypophosphatemia is generally not possible in these conditions. Optimal therapy of TIO is extirpation of the responsible tumor, which may be localized by radiographic skeletal survey or bone scan (many are located in bone) or by radionuclide scanning using sestamibi or labeled octreotide. Successful treatment of TIO-induced hypophosphatemia with octreotide has been reported in a small number of patients.

HYPERPHOSPHATEMIA ■ **Causes**   When the filtered load of phosphate and glomerular filtration rate (GFR) are normal, control of serum phosphate levels is achieved by adjusting the rate at which phosphate is reabsorbed by the proximal tubular NaPi-2 co-transporter. The principal hormonal regulator of NaPi-2 activity is PTH. Hyperphosphatemia, defined in adults as a fasting serum phosphate concentration >1.8 mmol/L (5.5 mg/dL), usually results from impaired glomerular filtration, hypoparathyroidism, excessive delivery of phosphate into the ECF (from bone, gut, or parenteral phosphate therapy), or some combination of these factors (Table 331-3). The upper limit of normal serum phosphate concentrations is higher in children and neonates [2.4 mmol/L (7 mg/dL)]. It is useful to distinguish hyperphosphatemia caused by impaired renal phosphate excretion from that which results from excessive delivery of phosphate into the ECF (Table 331-3).

TABLE 331-3 Causes of Hyperphosphatemia

I. Impaired renal phosphate excretion
  A. Renal insufficiency
  B. Hypoparathyroidism
    1. Developmental
    2. Autoimmune
    3. After neck surgery or radiation
    4. Activating mutations of the calcium-sensing receptor
  C. Parathyroid suppression
    1. Parathyroid-independent hypercalcemia
      a. Vitamin D or vitamin A intoxication
      b. Sarcoidosis, other granulomatous diseases
      c. Immobilization, osteolytic metastases
      d. Milk-alkali syndrome
    2. Severe hypermagnesemia or hypomagnesemia
  D. Pseudohypoparathyroidism
  E. Acromegaly
  F. Tumoral calcinosis
  G. Heparin therapy
II. Massive extracellular fluid phosphate loads
  A. Rapid administration of exogenous phosphate (intravenous, oral, rectal)
  B. Extensive cellular injury or necrosis
    1. Crush injuries
    2. Rhabdomyolysis
    3. Hyperthermia
    4. Fulminant hepatitis
    5. Cytotoxic therapy
    6. Severe hemolytic anemia
  C. Transcellular phosphate shifts
    1. Metabolic acidosis
    2. Respiratory acidosis

In chronic renal insufficiency, reduced GFR leads to phosphate retention. Hyperphosphatemia, in turn, further impairs renal synthesis of $1,25(OH)_2D$ and stimulates PTH secretion and hypertrophy, both directly and indirectly (by lowering blood ionized calcium levels). Thus, hyperphosphatemia is a major cause of the secondary hyperparathyroidism of renal failure and must be addressed early in the course of the disease (Chaps. 261 and 332).

Hypoparathyroidism leads to hyperphosphatemia via increased expression of NaPi-2 co-transporters in the proximal tubule. Hypoparathyroidism, or parathyroid suppression, has multiple potential causes including autoimmune disease; developmental, surgical, or radiation-induced absence of functional parathyroid tissue; vitamin D intoxication or other causes of PTH-independent hypercalcemia; cellular PTH resistance (pseudohypoparathyroidism or hypomagnesemia); infiltrative disorders such as Wilson disease and hemochromatosis; and impaired PTH secretion caused by hypermagnesemia, severe hypomagnesemia, or activating mutations in the CaSR. Hypocalcemia may also contribute directly to impaired phosphate clearance, as calcium infusion can induce hyperphosphaturia in hypoparathyroid subjects. Increased tubular phosphate reabsorption also occurs in acromegaly, during heparin administration, and in tumoral calcinosis. Tumoral calcinosis is a rare genetic disorder in which elevated serum $1,25(OH)_2D$, parathyroid suppression, increased intestinal calcium absorption, and focal hyperostosis with large, lobulated periarticular heterotopic ossifications (especially at shoulders or hips) are accompanied by hyperphosphatemia. In some forms of tumoral calcinosis serum phosphorus levels are normal.

When large amounts of phosphate are rapidly delivered into the ECF, hyperphosphatemia can occur despite normal renal function. Examples include overzealous intravenous phosphate therapy, oral or rectal administration of large amounts of phosphate-containing laxatives or enemas (especially in children), extensive soft tissue injury or necrosis (crush injuries, rhabdomyolysis, hyperthermia, fulminant hepatitis, cytotoxic chemotherapy), extensive hemolytic anemia, or transcellular phosphate shifts induced by severe metabolic or respiratory acidosis.

Clinical Findings   The clinical consequences of acute, severe hyperphosphatemia are due mainly to the formation of widespread calcium phosphate precipitates and resulting hypocalcemia. Thus, tetany, seizures, accelerated nephrocalcinosis (with renal failure, hyperkalemia, hyperuricemia, and metabolic acidosis), and pulmonary or cardiac calcifications (including development of acute heart block) may occur. The severity of these complications relates to the elevation of serum phosphate levels, which can reach concentrations as high as 7 mmol/L (20 mg/dL) in instances of massive soft tissue injury or tumor lysis syndrome.

℞ TREATMENT

Therapeutic options for management of severe hyperphosphatemia are limited. Volume expansion may enhance renal phosphate clearance. Aluminum hydroxide antacids or sevalamer may be helpful in chelating and limiting absorption of offending phosphate salts present in the intestine. Hemodialysis is the most effective therapeutic strategy and should be considered early in the course of severe hyperphosphatemia, especially in the setting of renal failure and symptomatic hypocalcemia.

MAGNESIUM METABOLISM

Magnesium is the major intracellular divalent cation. Normal concentrations of extracellular magnesium and calcium are crucial for normal neuromuscular activity. Intracellular magnesium forms a key complex with ATP and is an important cofactor for a wide range of enzymes, transporters, and nucleic acids required for normal cellular function, replication, and energy metabolism. The concentration of magnesium in serum is closely regulated within the range of 0.7 to 1.0 mmol/L (1.5 to 2.0 meq/L; 1.7 to 2.4 mg/dL), of which 30% is protein-bound and another 15% is loosely complexed to phosphate and other anions. Half of the 25 g (1000 mmol) of total body magnesium is located in bone, only half of which is insoluble in the mineral phase. Almost all extraskeletal magnesium is present within cells, where the total concentration is 5 mM, 95% of which is bound to proteins and other macromolecules. Because only 1% of body magnesium resides in the ECF, measurements of serum magnesium levels may not accurately reflect the level of total body magnesium stores.

Dietary magnesium content normally ranges from 6 to 15 mmol/d (140 to 360 mg/d), of which 30 to 40% is absorbed, mainly in the jejunum and ileum. Intestinal magnesium absorptive efficiency is stimulated by $1,25(OH)_2D$ and can reach 70% during magnesium deprivation. Urinary magnesium excretion normally matches net intestinal absorption and is approximately 4 mmol/d (100 mg/d). Regulation of serum magnesium concentrations is achieved mainly by control of renal magnesium reabsorption. Only 20% of filtered magnesium is reabsorbed in the proximal tubule, whereas 60% is reclaimed in the cTAL and another 5 to 10% in the DCT. Magnesium reabsorption in the cTAL occurs via a paracellular route that requires both a lumen-negative potential, created by NaCl reabsorption, and the tight-junction protein, paracellin-1. Magnesium reabsorption in the cTAL is increased by PTH but inhibited by hypercalcemia or hypermagnesemia, both of which activate the CaSR in this nephron segment.

HYPOMAGNESIA ■ Causes   Hypomagnesemia usually signifies substantial depletion of body magnesium stores (0.5 to 1 mmol/kg). Hypomagnesemia can result from intestinal malabsorption; protracted vomiting, diarrhea, or intestinal drainage; defective renal tubular magnesium reabsorption; or rapid shifts of magnesium from the ECF into cells, bone, or third spaces (Table 331-4). Dietary magnesium deficiency is unlikely except possibly in the setting of alcoholism. A rare genetic disorder causing selective intestinal magnesium malabsorption has been described (primary infantile hypomagnesemia). Mal-

TABLE 331-4   Causes of Hypomagnesemia

I. Impaired intestinal absorption
  A. Primary infantile hypomagnesemia
  B. Malabsorption syndromes
  C. Vitamin D deficiency
II. Increased intestinal losses
  A. Protracted vomiting/diarrhea
  B. Intestinal drainage, fistulae
III. Impaired renal tubular reabsorption
  A. Genetic magnesium-wasting syndromes
    1. Gitelman syndrome
    2. Bartter syndrome
    3. Paracellin-1 mutations
    4. Na-K-ATPase g-subunit mutations (FXYD2)
    5. Autosomal dominant, with low bone mass
  B. Acquired renal disease
    1. Tubulointerstitial disease
    2. Postobstruction, ATN (diuretic phase)
    3. Renal transplantation
  C. Drugs and toxins
    1. Ethanol
    2. Diuretics (loop, thiazide, osmotic)
    3. Cisplatin
    4. Pentamidine, foscarnet
    5. Cyclosporine
    6. Aminoglycosides, amphotericin B
  D. Other
	IV. Extracellular fluid volume expansion
	  A. Hyperaldosteronism
	  B. SIADH
	  C. Diabetes mellitus
	  D. Hypercalcemia
	  E. Phosphate depletion
	  F. Metabolic acidosis
	  G. Hyperthyroidism
	V. Rapid shifts from extracellular fluid
	  A. Intracellular redistribution
	    1. Recovery from diabetic ketoacidosis
	    2. Refeeding syndrome
	    3. Correction of respiratory acidosis
	    4. Catecholamines
	  B. Accelerated bone formation
	    1. Post parathyroidectomy
	    2. Treatment of vitamin D deficiency
	    3. Osteoblastic metastases
	  C. Other
	    1. Pancreatitis, burns, excessive sweating
	    2. Pregnancy (3rd trimester) and lactation

Note: ATN, acute tubular necrosis; SIADH, syndrome of inappropriate anti-diuretic hormone.

absorptive states, often compounded by vitamin D deficiency, can critically limit magnesium absorption and produce hypomagnesemia, despite the compensatory effects of secondary hyperparathyroidism and of hypocalcemia and hypomagnesemia to enhance cTAL magnesium reabsorption. Diarrhea or surgical drainage fluid may contain ≥5 mmol/L of magnesium.

Several genetic magnesium-wasting syndromes are described, including inactivating mutations of genes encoding the DCT NaCl cotransporter (Gitelman syndrome), proteins required for cTAL Na-K-Cl_2 transport (Bartter syndrome), paracellin-1 (autosomal recessive renal hypomagnesemia with hypercalciuria), and a DCT Na-K-ATPase γ-subunit (autosomal dominant renal hypomagnesemia with hypocalciuria). ECF expansion, hypercalcemia, and severe phosphate depletion may impair magnesium reabsorption, as can various forms of renal injury, including those caused by drugs such as cisplatin, cyclosporine, aminoglycosides, and pentamidine (Table 331-4). A rising blood concentration of ethanol directly impairs tubular magnesium reabsorption, and persistent glycosuria with osmotic diuresis leads to magnesium wasting and likely contributes to the high frequency of hypomagnesemia in poorly controlled diabetics. Magnesium depletion is aggravated by metabolic acidosis, which causes intracellular losses as well.

Hypomagnesemia due to rapid shifts of magnesium from ECF into the intracellular compartment can occur during recovery from diabetic ketoacidosis, from starvation, or from respiratory acidosis. Less acute shifts may be seen during rapid bone formation after parathyroidectomy, with treatment of vitamin D deficiency, or with osteoblastic metastases. Large amounts of magnesium may be lost with acute pancreatitis, extensive burns, protracted and severe sweating, and during pregnancy and lactation.

Clinical and Laboratory Findings Hypomagnesemia may cause generalized alterations in neuromuscular function, including tetany, tremor, seizures, muscle weakness, ataxia, nystagmus, vertigo, apathy, depression, irritability, delirium, and psychosis. Patients are usually asymptomatic when serum magnesium concentrations are >0.5 mmol/L (1 meq/L; 1.2 mg/dL), although the severity of symptoms may not correlate with serum magnesium levels. Cardiac arrhythmias may occur, including sinus tachycardia, other supraventricular tachycardias, and ventricular arrhythmias. Electrocardiographic abnormalities may include prolonged PR or QT intervals, T-wave flattening or inversion, and ST straightening. Sensitivity to digitalis toxicity may be enhanced.

Other electrolyte abnormalities often seen with hypomagnesemia, including hypocalcemia (with hypocalciuria) and hypokalemia, may not be easily corrected unless magnesium is administered as well. The hypocalcemia may be a result of concurrent vitamin D deficiency, although hypomagnesemia can cause impaired synthesis of 1,25(OH)$_2$D, cellular resistance to PTH and, at very low serum magnesium [< 0.4 mmol/L (<0.8 meq/L; < 1 mg/dL)], a defect in PTH secretion; these abnormalities are reversible with therapy.

℞ TREATMENT

Mild, asymptomatic hypomagnesemia may be treated with oral magnesium salts [MgCl$_2$, MgO, Mg(OH)$_2$] in divided doses totaling 20 to 30 mmol/d (40 to 60 meq/d). Diarrhea may occur with larger doses. More severe hypomagnesemia should be treated parenterally, preferably with intravenous MgCl$_2$, which can be administered safely as a continuous infusion of 50 mmol/d (100 meq Mg^{2+}/d) if renal function is normal. If GFR is reduced, the infusion rate should be lowered by 50 to 75%. Use of intramuscular MgSO$_4$ is discouraged; the injections are painful and provide relatively little magnesium (2 mL of 50% MgSO$_4$ supplies only 4 mmol). MgSO$_4$ may be given intravenously instead of MgCl$_2$, although the sulfate anions may bind calcium in serum and urine and aggravate hypocalcemia. Serum magnesium should be monitored at intervals of 12 to 24 h during therapy, which may continue for several days because of impaired renal conservation of magnesium (only 50 to 70% of the daily intravenous magnesium dose is retained) and delayed repletion of intracellular deficits, which may be as high as 1 to 1.5 mmol/kg (2 to 3 meq/kg).

It is important to consider the need for calcium, potassium, and phosphate supplementation in patients with hypomagnesemia. Vitamin D deficiency frequently coexists and should be treated with oral or parenteral vitamin D or 25(OH)D [but not 1,25(OH)$_2$D, which may impair tubular magnesium reabsorption, possibly via PTH suppression]. In severely hypomagnesemic patients with concomitant hypocalcemia and hypophosphatemia, administration of intravenous magnesium alone may worsen hypophosphatemia, provoking neuromuscular symptoms or rhabdomyolysis, due to rapid stimulation of PTH secretion. This is avoided by administering both calcium and magnesium.

HYPERMAGNESEMIA ■ **Causes** Hypermagnesemia is rarely seen in the absence of renal insufficiency, as normal kidneys can excrete large amounts (250 mmol/d) of magnesium. Mild hypermagnesemia due to excessive reabsorption in the cTAL occurs with calcium-sensing receptor mutations in familial hypocalciuric hypercalcemia and has been described in some patients with adrenal insufficiency, hypothyroidism, or hypothermia. Massive exogenous magnesium exposures, usually via the gastrointestinal tract, can overwhelm renal excretory capacity and cause life-threatening hypermagnesemia (Table 331-5). A notable example of this is prolonged retention of even normal amounts of magnesium-containing cathartics in patients with intestinal ileus, obstruction, or perforation. Extensive soft tissue injury or necrosis can also deliver large amounts of magnesium into the ECF in patients who have suffered trauma, shock, sepsis, cardiac arrest, or severe burns.

Clinical and Laboratory Findings The most prominent clinical manifestations of hypermagnesemia are vasodilation and neuromuscular blockade, which may appear at serum magnesium concentrations >2 mmol/L (> 4 meq/L; > 4.8 mg/dL). Hypotension, refractory to vasopressors or volume expansion, may be an early sign. Nausea, lethargy, and weakness may progress to respiratory failure, paralysis, and coma, with hypoactive tendon reflexes, at serum magnesium levels >4 mmol/L. Other findings may include gastrointestinal hypomotility or ileus; facial flushing; pupillary dilation; paradoxical bradycardia; prolongation of PR, QRS, and QT intervals, heart block; and, at serum magnesium levels approaching 10 mmol/L, asystole.

Hypermagnesemia, acting via the CaSR, causes hypocalcemia and hypercalciuria due to both parathyroid suppression and impaired cTAL calcium reabsorption.

℞ TREATMENT

Successful treatment of hypermagnesemia generally involves identifying and interrupting the source of magnesium and employing measures to increase magnesium clearance from the ECF. Use of magnesium-free cathartics or enemas may be helpful in clearing ingested magnesium from the gastrointestinal tract. Vigorous intravenous hydration should be attempted, if appropriate. Hemodialysis is effective and may be required in patients with significant renal insufficiency. Calcium, administered intravenously in doses of 100 to 200 mg over 1 to 2 h, has been reported to provide temporary improvement in signs and symptoms of hypermagnesemia.

TABLE 331-5 Causes of Hypermagnesemia

Impaired Mg excretion	Rapid Mg mobilization from
Renal failure	soft tissues
Familial hypocalciuric	Trauma
hypercalcemia	Extensive burns
Excessive Mg intake	Shock, sepsis
Cathartics	Post cardiac arrest
Intestinal obstruction/perforation	Other disorders
following magnesium ingestion	Adrenal insufficiency
Parenteral magnesium administration	Hypothyroidism
Magnesium-rich urologic irrigants	Hypothermia

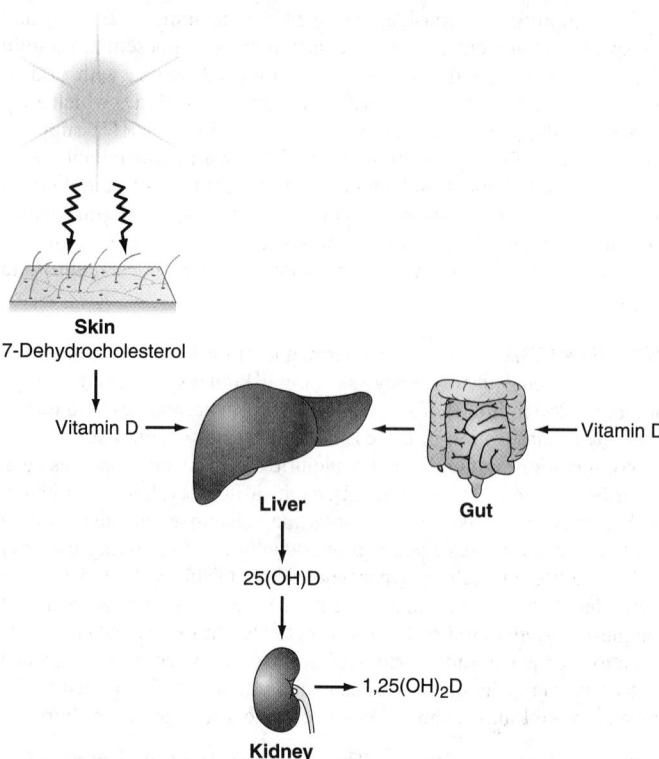

FIGURE 331-4 Vitamin D synthesis and activation. Vitamin D is synthesized in the skin in response to ultraviolet radiation and is also absorbed from the diet. It is then transported to the liver, where it undergoes 25-hydroxylation. This metabolite is the major circulating form of vitamin D. The final step in hormone activation, 1α-hydroxylation, occurs in the kidney.

VITAMIN D

SYNTHESIS AND METABOLISM 1,25-dihydroxyvitamin D [1,25(OH)$_2$D] is the major steroid hormone involved in mineral ion homeostasis regulation. Vitamin D and its metabolites are hormones and hormone precursors rather than vitamins, since in the proper biologic setting, they can be synthesized endogenously (Fig. 331-4). In response to ultraviolet radiation of the skin, a photochemical cleavage results in the formation of vitamin D from 7-dehydrocholesterol. Cutaneous production of vitamin D is decreased by melanin and high solar protection factor sunblocks, which effectively impair skin penetration of ultraviolet light. The increased use of sunblocks in North America and Western Europe and a reduction in the magnitude of solar exposure of the general population over the past several decades has led to an increased reliance on dietary sources of vitamin D. In the United States and Canada, these sources largely consist of fortified cereals and dairy products, in addition to fish oils and egg yolks. Vitamin D from plant sources is in the form of vitamin D$_2$, whereas that from animal sources is vitamin D$_3$. These two forms have equivalent biologic activity and are activated equally well by the vitamin D hydroxylases in humans. Vitamin D enters the circulation, whether absorbed from the intestine or synthesized cutaneously, bound to vitamin D–binding protein, an α-globulin synthesized in the liver. Vitamin D is subsequently 25-hydroxylated in the liver by cytochrome P450–like enzymes in the mitochondria and microsomes. The activity of this hydroxylase is not tightly regulated, and the resultant metabolite, 25-hydroxyvitamin D [25(OH)D], is the major circulating and storage form of vitamin D. Approximately 88% of 25(OH)D circulates bound to the vitamin D–binding protein, 0.03% is free, and the rest circulates bound to albumin. The half-life of 25(OH)D is approximately 2 to 3 weeks; however, it is dramatically shortened when vitamin D–binding protein levels are reduced, as can occur with increased urinary losses in the nephrotic syndrome.

The final hydroxylation required for mature hormone formation occurs in the kidney (Fig. 331-5). The 25(OH)D-1α-hydroxylase is a tightly regulated cytochrome P450–like mixed function oxidase expressed in proximal convoluted tubule cells. PTH stimulates this microsomal enzyme, whereas calcium and the product of the enzyme's action, 1,25(OH)$_2$D, repress it. The 25(OH)D-1α-hydroxylase is also present in epidermal keratinocytes, but keratinocyte production of 1,25(OH)$_2$D is not thought to contribute to circulating levels of this hormone. The 1α-hydroxylase is present in the trophoblastic layer of the placenta and is produced in the granulomas of sarcoidosis, tuberculosis, and berylliosis as well as in lymphomas. In these latter pathologic states, the activity of the enzyme is induced by interferon γ and TNF but is not regulated by calcium or 1,25(OH)$_2$D; therefore, hypercalcemia may occur because of elevated levels of 1,25(OH)$_2$D. Treatment of sarcoidosis-associated hypercalcemia with glucocorticoids, ketoconazole, or chloroquine has been shown to lower serum 1,25(OH)$_2$D levels.

The major pathway for inactivation of vitamin D metabolites is an additional hydroxylation step by vitamin D–24-hydroxylase, an enzyme that is expressed in most tissues. 1,25(OH)$_2$D, the major inducer of vitamin D–24-hydroxylase, thus promotes its own inactivation, thereby limiting its biologic effects. Polar metabolites of 1,25(OH)$_2$D are secreted into the bile and reabsorbed via the enterohepatic circulation. Impairment of this circulation, seen with diseases of the terminal ileum, leads to accelerated losses of vitamin D metabolites.

ACTIONS OF 1,25(OH)$_2$D 1,25(OH)$_2$D mediates its biologic effects by binding to a member of the nuclear receptor superfamily, the vitamin D receptor (VDR). This receptor belongs to the subfamily that includes the thyroid hormone receptors, the retinoid receptors, and the peroxisome proliferator–activated receptors (Chap. 317). In contrast to the

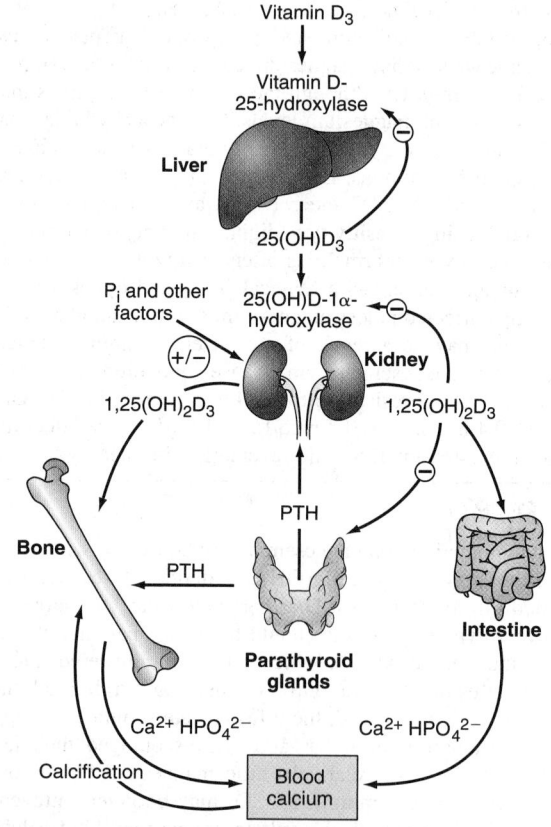

FIGURE 331-5 Schematic representation of the hormonal control loop for vitamin D metabolism and function. A reduction in the serum calcium below approximately 2.2 mmol/L (8.8 mg/dL) prompts a proportional increase in the secretion of parathyroid hormone (PTH) and so mobilizes additional calcium from the bone. PTH promotes the synthesis of 1,25(OH)$_2$D in the kidney, which, in turn, stimulates the mobilization of calcium from bone and intestine and regulates the synthesis of PTH by negative feedback.

other members of this subfamily, however, only one VDR isoform has been isolated. The VDR binds to target DNA sequences as a heterodimer with the retinoid X receptor, recruiting a series of coactivators that result in the induction of target gene expression. When the VDR causes repression of target gene expression, it either interferes with the action of activating transcription factors or recruits novel proteins to the VDR complex that cause transcriptional repression.

The affinity of the VDR for 1,25(OH)$_2$D is approximately three orders of magnitude higher than for the other vitamin D metabolites. Under normal physiologic circumstances, these other metabolites do not stimulate receptor-dependent actions. However, in states of vitamin D toxicity, the markedly elevated levels of 25(OH)D may lead to hypercalcemia by interacting directly with the VDR and by displacing 1,25(OH)$_2$D from serum vitamin D–binding protein, resulting in increased bioavailability of the active hormone.

The VDR is expressed in a wide range of cells and tissues. The molecular actions of 1,25(OH)$_2$D have been most extensively studied in tissues involved in the regulation of mineral ion homeostasis. This hormone is a major inducer of calbindin 9K, a calcium-binding protein expressed in the intestine, which is thought to play an important role in the active transport of calcium across the enterocyte. The two major calcium transporters expressed by intestinal epithelia, ECaC and ICaC, are also vitamin D responsive. By inducing the expression of these and other genes in the small intestine, 1,25(OH)$_2$D increases the efficiency of intestinal calcium absorption.

The VDR regulates the expression of several genes in osteoblasts. Target genes include the bone matrix proteins, osteocalcin and osteopontin, which are upregulated by 1,25(OH)$_2$D, in addition to type I collagen, which is transcriptionally repressed by 1,25(OH)$_2$D. 1,25(OH)$_2$D, as well as PTH, induces the expression of RANK ligand, which promotes osteoclast differentiation and increases osteoclast activity.

In the parathyroid gland, the VDR exerts antiproliferative effects on parathyroid cells and suppresses the transcription of the PTH gene. These effects of 1,25(OH)$_2$D on the parathyroid gland provide part of the rationale for current therapies directed at preventing and treating hyperparathyroidism associated with renal insufficiency.

The VDR is also expressed in tissues and organs that do not play a role in mineral ion homeostasis. Notable in this respect is the observation that 1,25(OH)$_2$D has an antiproliferative effect on several cell types, including keratinocytes, breast cancer cells, and prostate cancer cells. Alopecia is seen in humans and mice with mutant VDRs, but alopecia is not a feature of vitamin D deficiency, suggesting hormone-independent effects of the receptor.

VITAMIN D DEFICIENCY The mounting concern about the relationship between solar exposure and the development of skin cancer has led to increased reliance on dietary sources of vitamin D. Although the prevalence of vitamin D deficiency varies, the third National Health and Nutrition Examination Survey (NHANES III) revealed that vitamin D deficiency is common throughout the United States. The clinical syndrome of vitamin D deficiency can result from deficient production of vitamin D in the skin, lack of dietary intake, accelerated losses of vitamin D, impaired vitamin D activation, or resistance to the biologic effects of 1,25(OH)$_2$D (Table 331-6). The elderly and nursing home residents are particularly at risk for vitamin D deficiency, since both the efficiency of vitamin D synthesis in the skin and the absorption of vitamin D from the intestine decline with age.

Intestinal malabsorption of dietary fats can also lead to vitamin D deficiency. This is further exacerbated in the presence of terminal ileal disease, which results in impaired enterohepatic circulation of vitamin D metabolites. In addition to intestinal diseases, accelerated inactivation of vitamin D metabolites can be seen with drugs such as barbiturates, phenytoin, and rifampin, which induce hepatic cytochrome P450 mixed function oxidases. Impaired 25-hydroxylation, associated with severe liver disease or isoniazid, is an infrequent cause of vitamin D deficiency. Impaired 1α-hydroxylation is prevalent in the population with profound renal dysfunction, and therapeutic interventions should be considered in patients whose creatinine clearance is <0.5 mL/s (30 mL/min).

Mutations in the renal 1α-hydroxylase are the basis for the genetic disorder, pseudo-vitamin D–deficiency rickets. This autosomal recessive disorder presents with the syndrome of vitamin D deficiency in the first year of life. Affected children manifest growth retardation, rickets, and hypocalcemic seizures. Serum 1,25(OH)$_2$D levels are low, despite normal 25(OH)D levels and elevated PTH levels. Treatment with vitamin D metabolites that do not require 1α-hydroxylation corrects this disorder and must be continued throughout life. A second autosomal recessive disorder, hereditary vitamin D–resistant rickets, is caused by VDR mutations. Affected children present in a similar fashion during the first year of life, but alopecia often accompanies the disorder, demonstrating a functional role of the VDR in postnatal hair regeneration. Serum levels of 1,25(OH)$_2$D are dramatically elevated in these individuals, both because of increased production due to stimulation of 1α-hydroxylase activity as a consequence of secondary hyperparathyroidism and because of impaired inactivation, since induction of the 24-hydroxylase by 1,25(OH)$_2$D requires an intact VDR. Since the receptor mutation results in hormone resistance, daily calcium and phosphorus infusions may be required to bypass the defect in intestinal mineral ion absorption.

Regardless of the cause, the clinical manifestations of vitamin D deficiency are largely a consequence of impaired intestinal calcium absorption. Mild to moderate vitamin D deficiency is asymptomatic, whereas long-standing vitamin D deficiency results in hypocalcemia accompanied by secondary hyperparathyroidism, impaired mineralization of the skeleton (osteopenia on x-ray or decreased bone mineral density), and proximal myopathy. In the absence of an intercurrent illness, the hypocalcemia associated with long-standing vitamin D deficiency rarely presents with acute symptoms of hypocalcemia, such as numbness, tingling, or seizures. The concurrent development of hypomagnesemia, however, which impairs parathyroid gland function, or the administration of potent bisphosphonates, which impairs bone resorption, can lead to acute symptomatic hypocalcemia in vitamin D–deficient individuals.

RICKETS AND OSTEOMALACIA In children, prior to epiphyseal fusion, vitamin D deficiency results in growth retardation associated with an expansion of the growth plate known as *rickets*. Three layers of chondrocytes are present in the normal growth plate: the reserve zone, the proliferating zone, and the hypertrophic zone. Rickets, associated with impaired vitamin D action, is characterized by expansion of the hypertrophic chondrocyte layer. The expansion of the growth plate is thought to be a result of impaired apoptosis of the late hypertrophic chondrocytes, an event that precedes replacement of these cells by osteoblasts during endochondral bone formation. Investigations in mice lacking the VDR have demonstrated that maintenance of normal mineral ion homeostasis prevents the development of rickets. The observation that phosphate promotes chondrocyte apoptosis, combined with the presence of rickets in syndromes associated with renal phosphate wasting, suggests that hypophosphatemia, which in vitamin D deficiency is a consequence of secondary hyperparathyroidism, is a key etiologic factor in the development of the rachitic growth plate.

TABLE 331-6   *Causes of Impaired Vitamin D Action*

Vitamin D deficiency	Impaired 1α-hydroxylation
Impaired cutaneous production	Hypoparathyroidism
Dietary absence	Renal failure
Malabsorption	Ketoconazole
Accelerated loss of vitamin D	1α-hydroxylase mutation
Increased metabolism (barbiturates,	Oncogenic osteomalacia
phenytoin, rifampin)	X-linked hypophosphatemic
Impaired enterohepatic circulation	rickets
Impaired 25-hydroxylation	Target organ resistance
Liver disease	Vitamin D receptor mutation
Isoniazid	Phenytoin

The hypocalcemia and hypophosphatemia that accompany vitamin D deficiency result in impaired mineralization of bone matrix, a condition known as *osteomalacia*. Osteomalacia is also a feature of long-standing hypophosphatemia, which may be a consequence of renal phosphate wasting or chronic use of etidronate or phosphate-binding antacids. This hypomineralized matrix is biomechanically inferior to normal bone and, as a result, patients with vitamin D deficiency are prone to bowing of weight-bearing extremities because of abnormal remodeling and to skeletal fractures. Vitamin D and calcium supplementation have been shown to decrease the incidence of hip fracture among ambulatory nursing home residents in France, suggesting that undermineralization of bone contributes significantly to morbidity in the elderly. Proximal myopathy is a striking feature of severe vitamin D deficiency, both in children and in adults. Rapid resolution of the myopathy is observed after vitamin D repletion.

Though vitamin D deficiency is the most common cause of rickets and osteomalacia, many disorders lead to inadequate mineralization of the growth plate and bone. Calcium deficiency without vitamin D deficiency, the disorders of vitamin D metabolism previously discussed, and hypophosphatemia can all lead to inefficient mineralization. Even in the presence of normal calcium and phosphate levels, chronic acidosis and drugs such as bisphosphonates can lead to osteomalacia. The inorganic calcium/phosphate mineral phase of bone cannot form at low pH, and bisphosphonates bind to and prevent mineral crystal growth. Since alkaline phosphatase is necessary for normal mineral deposition, probably because the enzyme can hydrolyze inhibitors of mineralization such as inorganic pyrophosphate, genetic inactivation of the alkaline phosphatase gene (hereditary hypophosphatasia) can also lead to rickets and osteomalacia in the setting of normal calcium and phosphate levels.

DIAGNOSIS OF VITAMIN D DEFICIENCY, RICKETS, AND OSTEOMALACIA The most specific screening test for vitamin D deficiency in otherwise healthy individuals is a serum 25(OH)D level. While the normal ranges vary, levels of 25(OH)D <37 nmol/L (<15 ng/mL) are associated with increasing PTH levels and lower bone density, suggesting the need to revise normative values. Vitamin D deficiency leads to impaired intestinal absorption of calcium, resulting in decreased serum total and ionized calcium levels. Hypocalcemia results in secondary hyperparathyroidism, a homeostatic response that initially maintains serum calcium levels at the expense of the skeleton. Alkaline phosphatase levels are often increased because of the PTH-induced increase in bone turnover. In addition to increasing bone resorption, PTH decreases urinary calcium excretion, while promoting phosphaturia. This results in hypophosphatemia, which exacerbates the mineralization defect in the skeleton. With prolonged vitamin D deficiency resulting in osteomalacia, calcium stores in the skeleton become relatively inaccessible, since osteoclasts cannot resorb unmineralized osteoid, and frank hypocalcemia ensues. Since PTH is a major stimulus for the renal 1α-hydroxylase, there is increased synthesis of the active hormone, $1,25(OH)_2D$. Paradoxically, levels of this hormone may be normal in vitamin D deficiency. Measurements of $1,25(OH)_2D$, therefore, do not provide an accurate index of vitamin D stores and should not be used to diagnose vitamin D deficiency in patients with normal renal function.

Radiologic features of vitamin D deficiency in children include a widened, expanded growth plate, characteristic of rickets. These findings are apparent not only in the long bones, but also at the costochondral junctions, where the expansion of the growth plate leads to swellings known as "rachitic rosaries." Impairment of intramembranous bone mineralization leads to delayed fusion of the calvarial sutures and a decrease in the radio-opacity of cortical bone in the long bones. If vitamin D deficiency occurs after epiphyseal fusion, the main radiologic finding is a decrease in cortical thickness and relative radiolucency of the skeleton. A specific radiologic feature of osteomalacia,

whether associated with phosphate wasting or vitamin D deficiency, is pseudofractures or Looser's zones (Fig. 331-6). These are radiolucent lines that occur where large arteries are in contact with the underlying skeletal elements; it is believed that the arterial pulsations lead to the radiolucencies. As a result, these pseudofractures are usually a few millimeters wide, several centimeters long, and are seen particularly in the scapula, the pelvis, and the femoral neck.

℞ TREATMENT

Daily intake of a multivitamin preparation that contains 400 IU of vitamin D is often insufficient to prevent vitamin D deficiency. Based on the observation that 800 IU of vitamin D, with calcium supplementation, decreases the risk of hip fractures in elderly women, 800 IU is considered to be a more appropriate daily dosage for prevention of vitamin D deficiency. The safety margin for vitamin D is large, and vitamin D toxicity is usually observed only in patients taking doses >40,000 IU daily. Treatment of vitamin D deficiency should be directed at the underlying disorder, if possible, and tailored to the severity of the condition. Vitamin D should always be repleted in conjunction with calcium supplementation since most, if not all, of the consequences of vitamin D deficiency are a result of impaired mineral ion homeostasis.

In patients whose 1α-hydroxylation is impaired, vitamin D analogues not requiring this activation step are preferred. These include dihydrotachysterol (DHT, 0.2 to 1.0 mg daily), $1,25(OH)_2D_3$ [calcitriol (Rocaltrol), 0.25 to 0.5 μg daily], and 1α-hydroxyvitamin D_2 [doxercalciferol (Hectorol), 2.5 to 5 μg daily]. If the pathway required for activation of vitamin D is intact, severe vitamin D deficiency can be treated with pharmacologic repletion initially (50,000 IU weekly for 3 to 12 weeks), followed by maintenance therapy (800 IU daily). Pharmacologic doses may be required for maintenance therapy in patients who are taking drugs such as barbiturates or phenytoin that accelerate the metabolism of, or cause resistance to, 1,25-dihydroxyvitamin D. If intestinal malabsorption is a contributing factor, up to tenfold higher doses of vitamin D may be needed, or repletion can be performed with intramuscular vitamin D (250,000 IU biannually). Calcium supplementation should include 1.5 to 2.0 g of elemental calcium daily. Normocalcemia is usually observed within 1 week of institution of therapy, although increases in PTH and alkaline phosphatase levels may persist for 3 to 6 months.

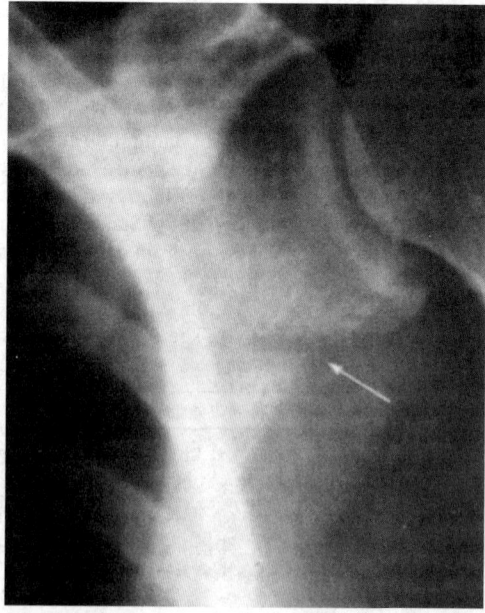

FIGURE 331-6 Radiograph of the scapula of a 58-year-old woman with phosphaturia as a cause of osteomalacia. The presence of a pseudofracture or Looser's zone is indicated by an arrow.

The most efficacious methods to monitor treatment and resolution of vitamin D deficiency are serum and urinary calcium measurements. For patients who are vitamin D replete and are taking adequate calcium supplementation, the 24-h urinary calcium excretion should be in the range of 100 to 250 mg/24 h. Lower levels suggest problems with adhering to the treatment regimen or with absorption of calcium or vitamin D supplements. The 25(OH)D level can be remeasured to address the latter, although the half-life of this metabolite is long (3 weeks) and levels may continue to increase for many months on a stable regimen. Urinary calcium excretion >250 mg/24 h predisposes to nephrolithiasis and should prompt a reduction in vitamin D dosage and/or calcium supplementation.

FURTHER READING

MANOLAGAS SC: Birth and death of bone cells: Basic regulatory mechanisms and implications for the pathogenesis and treatment of osteoporosis. Endocr Rev 21:115, 2000

SHIMADA T et al: Cloning and characterization of FGF23 as a causative factor of tumor-induced osteomalacia. Proc Natl Acad Sci USA 98:6500, 2001

SUDA T et al: Modulation of osteoclast differentiation and function by the new members of the tumor necrosis factor receptor and ligand families. Endocr Rev 20:345, 1999

THOMAS MK, DEMAY MB: Vitamin D deficiency and disorders of vitamin D metabolism. Endocrinol Metab Clin North Am 29:611, 2000

WAGNER EF, KARSENTY G: Genetic control of skeletal development. Curr Opin Genet Dev 11:527, 2001

332 DISEASES OF THE PARATHYROID GLAND AND OTHER HYPER- AND HYPOCALCEMIC DISORDERS
John T. Potts, Jr

The four parathyroid glands are located posterior to the thyroid gland. They produce parathyroid hormone (PTH), which is the primary regulator of calcium physiology. PTH acts directly on bone, where it induces calcium resorption, and on the kidney, where it stimulates calcium reabsorption and synthesis of 1,25-dihydroxyvitamin D [$1,25(OH)_2D$], a hormone that stimulates gastrointestinal calcium absorption. Serum PTH levels are tightly regulated by a negative feedback loop. Calcium, acting through the calcium-sensing receptor, and vitamin D, acting through its nuclear receptor, inhibit PTH release and synthesis. Understanding the hormone pathways that regulate calcium levels and bone metabolism is essential for effective diagnosis and management of a wide array of hyper- and hypocalcemic disorders.

Hyperparathyroidism, characterized by excess production of PTH, is a common cause of hypercalcemia and is usually the result of autonomously functioning adenomas or hyperplasia. Surgery for this disorder is highly effective and has been shown to reverse some of the deleterious effects of long-standing PTH excess on bone density. Hypercalcemia of malignancy is also common and is usually due to the overproduction of parathyroid hormone–related peptide (PTHrP) by cancer cells. The similarities in the biochemical characteristics of hyperparathyroidism and hypercalcemia of malignancy, first noted by Albright in 1941, are now known to reflect the actions of PTH and PTHrP through the same G protein–coupled PTH/PTHrP receptor.

The genetic basis of multiple endocrine neoplasia (MEN) types 1 and 2, familial hypocalciuric hypercalcemia (FHH), the different forms of pseudohypoparathyroidism (PHP), Jansen's syndrome, disorders of vitamin D synthesis and action, and the molecular events associated with parathyroid gland neoplasia have provided new insights into calcium metabolism. The advent of new drugs, including bisphosphonates and selective estrogen receptor modulators (SERMs), offers new avenues for the treatment and prevention of metabolic bone disease. PTH analogues are promising therapeutic agents for the treatment of postmenopausal or senile osteoporosis, and calcimimetic agents, which act through the calcium-sensing receptor, may provide new approaches for PTH suppression.

PARATHYROID HORMONE

PHYSIOLOGY The primary function of PTH is to maintain the extracellular fluid (ECF) calcium concentration within a narrow normal range. The hormone acts directly on bone and kidney and indirectly on intestine through its effects on synthesis of $1,25(OH)_2D$ to increase serum calcium concentrations; in turn, PTH production is closely regulated by the concentration of serum ionized calcium. This feedback system is the critical homeostatic mechanism for maintenance of ECF calcium. Any tendency toward hypocalcemia, as might be induced by calcium-deficient diets, is counteracted by an increased secretion of PTH. This in turn (1) increases the rate of dissolution of bone mineral, thereby increasing the flow of calcium from bone into blood; (2) reduces the renal clearance of calcium, returning more of the calcium filtered at the glomerulus into ECF; and (3) increases the efficiency of calcium absorption in the intestine by stimulating the production of $1,25(OH)_2D$. Immediate control of blood calcium is due to PTH effects on bone and, to a lesser extent, on renal calcium clearance. Maintenance of steady-state calcium balance, on the other hand, probably results from the effects of $1,25(OH)_2D$ on calcium absorption (Chap. 331). The renal actions of the hormone are exerted at multiple sites and include inhibition of phosphate transport (proximal tubule), increased reabsorption of calcium (distal tubule), and stimulation of the renal 25(OH)D-1α-hydroxylase. As much as 12 mmol (500 mg) calcium is transferred between the ECF and bone each day (a large amount in relation to the total ECF calcium pool), and PTH has a major effect on this transfer. The homeostatic role of the hormone can preserve calcium concentration in blood at the cost of bone destruction.

PTH has multiple actions on bone, some direct and some indirect. PTH-mediated changes in bone calcium release can be seen within minutes. The chronic effects of PTH are to increase the number of bone cells, both osteoblasts and osteoclasts, and to increase the remodeling of bone; these effects are apparent within hours after the hormone is given and persist for hours after PTH is withdrawn. Continuous exposure to elevated PTH (as in hyperparathyroidism or long-term infusions in animals) leads to increased osteoclast-mediated bone resorption. However, the intermittent administration of PTH, elevating hormone levels for 1 to 2 h each day, leads to a net stimulation of bone formation rather than bone breakdown. Striking increases, especially in trabecular bone in the spine and hip, have been reported with the use of PTH in combination with estrogen. PTH as monotherapy caused a highly significant reduction in fracture incidence in a worldwide placebo-controlled trial.

Osteoblasts (or stromal cell precursors), which have PTH receptors, are crucial to this bone-forming effect of PTH; osteoclasts, which mediate bone breakdown, lack PTH receptors. PTH-mediated stimulation of osteoclasts is believed to be indirect, acting in part through cytokines released from osteoblasts to activate osteoclasts; in experimental studies of bone resorption in vitro, osteoblasts must be present for PTH to activate osteoclasts to resorb bone (Chap. 331).

STRUCTURE PTH is an 84-amino-acid single-chain peptide. The amino acid portion, PTH(1–34), is highly conserved and is critical for the biologic actions of the molecule. Modified synthetic fragments of the amino-terminal sequence as small as PTH(1–11) are sufficient to activate the major receptor (see below). The carboxyl-terminal region of

PTH binds to a separate receptor (cPTH-R), but it has not yet been cloned. Fragments shortened at the amino terminus bind to cPTH-R and inhibit the actions of the full-length PTH(1–84) or the PTH(1–34) active fragments.

BIOSYNTHESIS, SECRETION, AND METABOLISM ■ Synthesis

Parathyroid cells have multiple methods of adapting to increased needs for PTH production. Most rapid (within minutes) is secretion of preformed hormone in response to hypocalcemia. Second, within hours, PTH mRNA expression is induced by sustained hypocalcemia. Finally, protracted challenge leads within days to cellular replication to increase gland mass.

PTH is initially synthesized as a larger molecule (preproparathyroid hormone, consisting of 115 amino acids), which is then reduced in size by a second cleavage (proparathyroid hormone, 90 amino acids) before secretion as the 84-amino-acid peptide. In one kindred with hypoparathyroidism, a mutation in the preprotein region of the gene interferes with hormone transport and secretion.

Transcriptional suppression of the PTH gene by calcium is nearly maximal at physiologic calcium concentrations. Hypocalcemia increases transcriptional activity within hours. $1,25(OH)_2D_3$ strongly suppresses PTH gene transcription. In patients with renal failure, intravenous administration of supraphysiologic levels of $1,25(OH)_2D_3$ or analogues of the active metabolite can dramatically suppress PTH overproduction, which is sometimes difficult to control due to severe secondary hyperparathyroidism. Regulation of proteolytic destruction of preformed hormone (posttranslational regulation of hormone production) is an important mechanism for mediating rapid (minutes) changes in hormone availability. High calcium increases and low calcium inhibits the proteolytic destruction of hormone stores.

Regulation of PTH Secretion

PTH secretion increases steeply to a maximum value of five times the basal rate of secretion as calcium concentration falls from normal to the range of 1.9 to 2.0 mmol/L (7.5 to 8.0 mg/dL) (measured as total calcium). The ionized fraction of blood calcium is the important determinant of hormone secretion. Severe intracellular magnesium deficiency impairs PTH secretion (see below).

ECF calcium controls PTH secretion by interaction with a calcium sensor, a G protein–coupled receptor (GPCR) for which Ca^{2+} ions act as the ligand (see below). This receptor is a member of a distinctive subfamily of the GPCR superfamily that is characterized by a large extracellular domain suitable for "clamping" the small-molecule ligand. Stimulation of the receptor by high calcium levels suppresses PTH secretion. The receptor is present in parathyroid glands and the calcitonin-secreting cells (C cells) of the thyroid, as well as in other sites such as brain and kidney. Genetic evidence has revealed a key biologic role for the calcium-sensing receptor in parathyroid gland responsiveness to calcium and in renal calcium clearance. Point mutations associated with loss of function cause a syndrome FHH resembling hyperparathyroidism but with hypocalciuria. On the other hand, gain-of-function mutations cause a form of hypocalcemia resembling hypoparathyroidism (see below).

Metabolism

The secreted form of PTH is indistinguishable by immunologic criteria and by molecular size from the 84-amino-acid peptide (PTH 1–84) extracted from glands. However, much of the immunoreactive material found in the circulation is smaller than the extracted or secreted hormone. The principal circulating fragments of immunoreactive hormone lack a portion of the critical amino-terminal sequence required for biologic activity and, hence, are biologically inactive fragments (so-called middle- and carboxyl-terminal fragments). Much of the proteolysis of hormone occurs in the liver and kidney. Peripheral metabolism of PTH does not appear to be regulated by physiologic states (high versus low calcium, etc.); hence peripheral metabolism of hormone, although responsible for rapid clearance of secreted hormone, appears to be a high-capacity, metabolically invariant catabolic process.

The rate of clearance of the secreted 84-amino-acid peptide from blood is more rapid than the rate of clearance of the biologically inactive fragment(s) corresponding to the middle- and carboxyl-terminal regions of PTH. Consequently, the interpretation of PTH immunoassays is influenced by the nature of the peptide fragments detected by the antibodies.

Although the problems inherent in PTH measurements have been largely circumvented by use of double-antibody assays that detect only the intact molecule, new evidence has revealed the existence of a hitherto unappreciated larger PTH fragment that may affect the interpretation of most currently available double-antibody assays. A large amino-terminally truncated form of PTH, possibly PTH(7–84), is present in normal and uremic individuals in addition to PTH(1–84). The concentration of the putative (7–84) fragment relative to that of intact PTH(1–84) is higher with induced hypercalcemia than in eucalcemic or hypocalcemic conditions and is higher in patients with renal failure. Growing evidence suggests that the PTH(7–84)-like amino-terminally truncated fragments can act as an inhibitor of PTH action and may be of clinical significance, particularly in renal failure. Efforts to prevent secondary hyperparathyroidism by a variety of measures (vitamin D analogues, higher calcium intake, and phosphate-lowering strategies) may have led to oversuppression of biologically active intact PTH since the amino-terminally truncated PTH reacts in many first-generation double-antibody PTH assays. The role, if any, of excessive PTH suppression due to inaccurate measurement of PTH in adynamic bone disease in renal failure (see below) is unknown. Newer assays with extreme amino-terminal epitopes that detect only full-length PTH(1–84) are being studied intensively.

PARATHYROID HORMONE–RELATED PROTEIN

The paracrine factor termed *PTHrP* is responsible for most instances of hypercalcemia of malignancy (Chap. 86), a syndrome that resembles hyperparathyroidism. Many different cell types produce PTHrP, including brain, pancreas, heart, lung, mammary tissue, placenta, endothelial cells, and smooth muscle. In fetal animals, PTHrP directs transplacental calcium transfer, and high concentrations of PTHrP are produced in mammary tissue and secreted into milk. Human and bovine milk contain very high concentrations of the hormone, the biologic significance of which is unknown. PTHrP may also play a role in uterine contraction and other biologic functions.

PTH and PTHrP, although distinctive products of different genes, exhibit considerable functional and structural homology (Fig. 332-1) and may have evolved from a shared ancestral gene. The structure of the gene for human PTHrP, however, is more complex than that of PTH, containing multiple exons and multiple sites for alternate splicing patterns during formation of the mature mRNA. Protein products of 141, 139, and 173 amino acids are produced, and other molecular forms may result from tissue-specific degradation at accessible internal cleavage sites. The biologic roles of these various molecular species and the nature of the circulating forms of PTHrP are unclear. It is uncertain whether PTHrP circulates at any significant level in adults; as a paracrine factor, PTHrP may be produced, act, and be destroyed locally within tissues. In adults PTHrP appears to have little influence on calcium homeostasis, except in disease states, when large tumors, especially of the squamous cell type, lead to massive overproduction of the hormone.

PTH AND PTHrP HORMONE ACTION

Both PTH and PTHrP bind to and activate the PTH/PTHrP receptor. The 500-amino-acid PTH/PTHrP receptor (also known as the PTH-1 receptor, PTH1R) belongs to a subfamily of GPCRs that includes those for glucagon, secretin, and vasoactive intestinal peptide. The extracellular regions are involved in hormone binding, and the intracellular domains, after hormone activation, bind G protein subunits to transduce hormone signaling into cellular responses through stimulation of second messengers. A second receptor that binds PTH, termed the *PTH-2 receptor* (PTH2R), is expressed in brain, pancreas, and several other tissues. PTH1R responds equivalently to PTH and PTHrP, whereas PTH2R responds only to PTH. The endogenous ligand of this receptor is now believed to be a

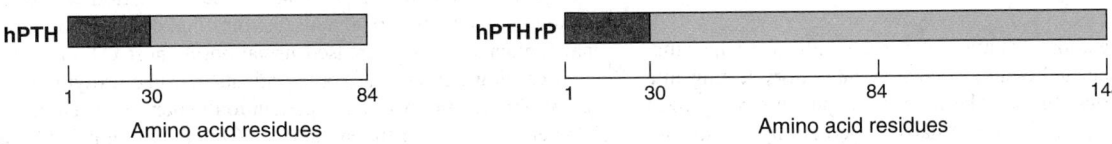

	1		5		10		15		20		25		30

hPTH H-ALA VAL SER GLU ILE GLN LEU MET HIS ASN LEU GLY LYS HIS LEU –ASN SER MET GLU ARG VAL GLU TRP LEU ARG LYS LYS LEU GLN ASP

hPTHrp –   –   –   – HIS –   – LEU – ASP LYS –   – SER ILE GLN   LEU ARG   ARG PHE PHE   HIS HIS LEU ILE ALA GLU

hPTH | **hPTHrP**

Amino acid residues: 1 30 84 (hPTH); 1 30 84 144 (hPTHrP)

FIGURE 332-1 Schematic diagram to illustrate similarities and differences in structure of human parathyroid hormone (PTH) and human PTH-related peptide (PTHrP). Close structural (and functional) homology exists between the first 30 amino acids of hPTH and hPTHrP. The PTHrP sequence may be ≥144 amino acid residues in length. PTH is only 84 residues long; after residue 30, there is little structural homology between the two. Dashed lines in the PTHrP sequence indicate identity; underlined residues, although different from those of PTH, still represent conservative changes (charge or polarity preserved). Eleven amino acids are identical, and a total of 21 of 30 are homologues.

peptide distinct from PTH, a 39-amino-acid hypothalamic peptide (*tubular infundibular peptide*, TIP-39). PTH1R and PTH2R can be traced backward in evolutionary time to fish. Zebrafish PTH1R and PTH2R exhibit the same selective responses to PTH and PTHrP as do human PTH1R and PTH2R. The evolutionary conservation of structure and function suggests unique biologic roles for these receptors.

Studies using cloned PTH1R confirm that it can be coupled to more than one G protein and second-messenger kinase pathway, apparently explaining the multiplicity of pathways stimulated by PTH. Stimulation of protein kinases (A and C) and calcium transport channels is associated with a variety of hormone-specific tissue responses. These responses include inhibition of phosphate and bicarbonate transport, stimulation of calcium transport, and activation of renal 1α-hydroxylase in the kidney. The responses in bone include effects on collagen synthesis; increased alkaline phosphatase, ornithine decarboxylase, citrate decarboxylase, and glucose-6-phosphate dehydrogenase activities; DNA, protein, and phospholipid synthesis; and calcium and phosphate transport. Ultimately, these biochemical events lead to an integrated hormonal response in bone turnover and calcium homeostasis. PTH also activates Na^+/Ca^{2+} exchanges in renal distal tubular sites and stimulates translocation of preformed calcium transport channels, moving them from the interior to the apical surface to mediate increased tubular uptake of calcium. PTH-dependent stimulation of phosphate excretion (blocking reabsorption—the opposite effect from actions on calcium in the kidney) involves the sodium-dependent phosphate cotransporter, NPT-2, lowering its apical membrane content (and therefore function). Similar shifts may be involved in other renal tubular transport effects of PTH.

PTHrP exerts important developmental influences on fetal bone development and in adult physiology. A homozygous knockout of the PTHrP gene (or the gene for the PTH receptor) in mice causes a lethal deformity in which animals are born with severe skeletal deformities resembling chondrodysplasia (Fig. 332-2).

CALCITONIN (See also Chap. 330)

Calcitonin is a hypocalcemic peptide hormone that in several mammalian species acts as an antagonist to PTH. Calcitonin seems to be of limited physiologic significance in humans, however, at least in calcium homeostasis. It is of medical significance because of its role as a tumor marker in sporadic and hereditary cases of medullary carcinoma and its medical use as an adjunctive treatment in severe hypercalcemia and in Paget's disease of bone.

The hypocalcemic activity of calcitonin is accounted for primarily by inhibition of osteoclast-mediated bone resorption and secondarily by stimulation of renal calcium clearance. These effects are mediated by receptors on osteoclasts and renal tubular cells. Calcitonin exerts additional effects through receptors present in brain, gastrointestinal tract, and the immune system. The hormone, for example, exerts analgesic effects directly on cells in the hypothalamus and related structures, possibly by interacting with receptors for related peptide hormones, such as calcitonin gene–related peptide (CGRP) or amylin. The latter ligands have specific high-affinity receptors and can also

bind to and trigger calcitonin receptors. The calcitonin receptors are homologous in structure to PTH1R.

The thyroid is the major source of the hormone, and the cells involved in calcitonin synthesis arise from neural crest tissue. During embryogenesis, these cells migrate into the ultimobranchial body, derived from the last branchial pouch. In submammalian vertebrates, the ultimobranchial body constitutes a discrete organ, anatomically separate from the thyroid gland; in mammals, the ultimobranchial gland fuses with and is incorporated into the thyroid gland.

The naturally occurring calcitonins consist of a peptide chain of 32 amino acids. There is considerable sequence variability among species. Calcitonin from salmon, which is used therapeutically, is 10 to 100 times more potent than mammalian forms in lowering serum calcium.

There are two calcitonin genes, α and β; the transcriptional control of these genes is complex. Two different mRNA molecules are transcribed from the α gene; one is translated into the precursor for calcitonin, and the other message is translated into an alternative product, CGRP. CGRP is synthesized wherever the calcitonin mRNA is expressed, e.g., in medullary carcinoma of the thyroid. The β, or CGRP-2, gene is transcribed into the mRNA for CGRP in the central nervous system (CNS); this gene does not produce calcitonin, however. CGRP has cardiovascular actions and may serve as a neurotransmitter or play a developmental role in the CNS.

The circulating level of calcitonin in humans is lower than that in many other species. In humans, even extreme variations in calcitonin production do not change calcium and phosphate metabolism; no definite effects are attributable to calcitonin deficiency (totally thyroidectomized patients receiving only replacement thyroxine) or excess (patients with medullary carcinoma of the thyroid, a calcitonin-secreting tumor) (Chap. 330). Calcitonin has been a useful pharmacologic agent to suppress bone resorption in Paget's disease (Chap. 334) and osteoporosis (Chap. 333) and in the treatment of hypercalcemia

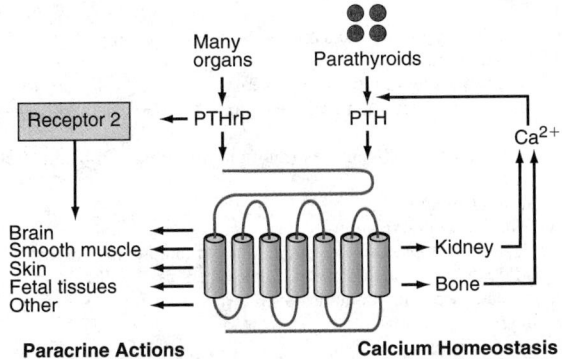

FIGURE 332-2 Dual role for the actions of the PTH/PTHrP receptor (PTH1R). Parathyroid hormone (PTH; endocrine-calcium homeostasis) and PTH-related peptide (PTHrP; paracrine—multiple tissue actions including growth plate cartilage in developing bone) use the single receptor for their disparate functions mediated by the amino-terminal 30 residues of either peptide. Other regions of both ligands interact with other receptors (not shown).

of malignancy (see below). However, the physiologic role, if any, of calcitonin in humans is uncertain.

HYPERCALCEMIA

Hypercalcemia can be a manifestation of a serious illness such as malignancy or can be detected coincidentally by laboratory testing in a patient with no obvious illness. The number of patients recognized with asymptomatic hypercalcemia, usually hyperparathyroidism, increased in the late twentieth century but is now declining somewhat, perhaps due to decreased use of routine blood calcium measurements or for other unknown reasons.

Whenever hypercalcemia is confirmed, a definitive diagnosis must be established. Although hyperparathyroidism, a frequent cause of asymptomatic hypercalcemia, is a chronic disorder in which manifestations, if any, may be expressed only after months or years, hypercalcemia can also be the earliest manifestation of malignancy, the second most common cause of hypercalcemia in the adult. The causes of hypercalcemia are numerous (Table 332-1), but hyperparathyroidism and cancer account for 90% of cases.

Before undertaking a diagnostic workup, it is essential to be sure that true hypercalcemia, not a false-positive laboratory test, is present. A false-positive diagnosis of hypercalcemia is usually the result of inadvertent hemoconcentration during blood collection or elevation in serum proteins such as albumin. Hypercalcemia is a chronic problem, and it is cost-effective to obtain several serum calcium measurements; these tests need not be in the fasting state.

Clinical features are helpful in differential diagnosis. Hypercalcemia in an adult who is asymptomatic is usually due to primary hyperparathyroidism. In malignancy-associated hypercalcemia the disease is usually not occult; rather, symptoms of malignancy bring the patient to the physician, and hypercalcemia is discovered during the evaluation. In such patients the interval between detection of hypercalcemia and death is often <6 months. Accordingly, if an asymptomatic individual has had hypercalcemia or some manifestation of hypercalcemia, such as kidney stones, for >1 or 2 years, it is unlikely that malignancy is the cause. Nevertheless, differentiating primary hyperparathyroidism from *occult* malignancy can occasionally be difficult, and careful evaluation is required, particularly when the duration of the hypercalcemia is unknown. Hypercalcemia not due to hyperparathyroidism or malignancy can result from excessive vitamin D action, high bone turnover from any of several causes, or from renal

---

TABLE 332-1   Classification of Causes of Hypercalcemia

I. Parathyroid-related
   A. Primary hyperparathyroidism
      1. Solitary adenomas
      2. Multiple endocrine neoplasia
   B. Lithium therapy
   C. Familial hypocalciuric hypercalcemia
II. Malignancy-related
   A. Solid tumor with metastases (breast)
   B. Solid tumor with humoral mediation of hypercalcemia (lung, kidney)
   C. Hematologic malignancies (multiple myeloma, lymphoma, leukemia)
III. Vitamin D–related
   A. Vitamin D intoxication
   B. ↑ 1,25(OH)$_2$D; sarcoidosis and other granulomatous diseases
   C. Idiopathic hypercalcemia of infancy
IV. Associated with high bone turnover
   A. Hyperthyroidism
   B. Immobilization
   C. Thiazides
   D. Vitamin A intoxication
V. Associated with renal failure
   A. Severe secondary hyperparathyroidism
   B. Aluminum intoxication
   C. Milk-alkali syndrome

---

failure (Table 332-1). Dietary history and a history of ingestion of vitamins or drugs are often helpful in diagnosing some of the less frequent causes. PTH immunoassays based on double-antibody methods serve as the principal laboratory test in differential diagnosis.

Hypercalcemia from any cause can result in fatigue, depression, mental confusion, anorexia, nausea, vomiting, constipation, reversible renal tubular defects, increased urination, a short QT interval in the electrocardiogram, and, in some patients, cardiac arrhythmias. There is a variable relation from one patient to the next between the severity of hypercalcemia and the symptoms. Generally, symptoms are more common at calcium levels >2.9 to 3 mmol/L (11.5 to 12.0 mg/dL), but some patients, even at this level, are asymptomatic. When the calcium level is >3.2 mmol/L (13 mg/dL), calcification in kidneys, skin, vessels, lungs, heart, and stomach occurs and renal insufficiency may develop, particularly if blood phosphate levels are normal or elevated due to impaired renal function. Severe hypercalcemia, usually defined as ≥3.7 to 4.5 mmol/L (15 to 18 mg/dL), can be a medical emergency; coma and cardiac arrest can occur.

Acute management of the hypercalcemia is usually successful. The type of treatment is based on the severity of the hypercalcemia and the nature of associated symptoms, as outlined below.

PRIMARY HYPERPARATHYROIDISM ■ Natural History and Incidence Primary hyperparathyroidism is a generalized disorder of calcium, phosphate, and bone metabolism due to an increased secretion of PTH. The elevation of circulating hormone usually leads to hypercalcemia and hypophosphatemia. There is great variation in the manifestations. Patients may present with multiple signs and symptoms, including recurrent nephrolithiasis, peptic ulcers, mental changes, and, less frequently, extensive bone resorption. However, with greater awareness of the disease and wider use of multiphasic screening tests, including measurements of blood calcium, the diagnosis is frequently made in patients who have no symptoms and minimal, if any, signs of the disease other than hypercalcemia and elevated levels of PTH. The manifestations may be subtle, and the disease may have a benign course for many years or a lifetime. This milder form of the disease is usually termed *asymptomatic hyperparathyroidism*. Rarely, hyperparathyroidism develops or worsens abruptly and causes severe complications, such as marked dehydration and coma, so-called hypercalcemic parathyroid crisis.

The annual incidence of the disease is calculated to be as high as 0.2% in patients >60, with an estimated prevalence, including undiscovered asymptomatic patients, of ≥1%; some reports suggest the incidence may be declining, perhaps reflecting earlier overestimates. The disease has a peak incidence between the third and fifth decades but occurs in young children and in the elderly.

Etiology ■ SOLITARY ADENOMAS The cause of hyperparathyroidism is one or more hyperfunctioning glands. A single abnormal gland is the cause in ~80% of patients; the abnormality in the gland is usually a benign neoplasm or adenoma and rarely a parathyroid carcinoma. Some surgeons and pathologists report that the enlargement of multiple glands is common; double adenomas are reported. In ~15% of patients, all glands are hyperfunctioning; *chief cell parathyroid hyperplasia* is usually hereditary and frequently associated with other endocrine abnormalities.

MULTIPLE ENDOCRINE NEOPLASIA Hereditary hyperparathyroidism can occur without other endocrine abnormalities but is usually part of a *multiple endocrine neoplasia* syndrome (Chap. 330). MEN 1 (Wermer's syndrome) consists of hyperparathyroidism and tumors of the pituitary and pancreas, often associated with gastric hypersecretion and peptic ulcer disease (Zollinger-Ellison syndrome). MEN 2A is characterized by pheochromocytoma and medullary carcinoma of the thyroid, as well as hyperparathyroidism; MEN 2B has additional associated features such as multiple neuromas but usually lacks hyperparathyroidism. Each of these MEN syndromes is transmitted in an apparent autosomal dominant manner, although, as noted below, the genetic basis does not always involve a dominant allele.

Pathology　Adenomas are most often located in the inferior parathyroid glands, but in 6 to 10% of patients, parathyroid adenomas may be located in the thymus, the thyroid, the pericardium, or behind the esophagus. Adenomas are usually 0.5 to 5 g in size but may be as large as 10 to 20 g (normal glands weigh 25 mg on average). Chief cells are predominant in both hyperplasia and adenoma. With chief cell hyperplasia, the enlargement may be so asymmetric that some involved glands appear grossly normal. If generalized hyperplasia is present, however, histologic examination reveals a uniform pattern of chief cells and disappearance of fat even in the absence of an increase in gland weight. Thus, microscopic examination of biopsy specimens of several glands is essential to interpret findings at surgery.

Parathyroid carcinoma is usually not aggressive. Long-term survival without recurrence is common if at initial surgery the entire gland is removed without rupture of the capsule. Recurrent parathyroid carcinoma is usually slow-growing with local spread in the neck, and surgical correction of recurrent disease may be feasible. Occasionally, however, parathyroid carcinoma is more aggressive, with distant metastases (lung, liver, and bone) found at the time of initial operation. It may be difficult to appreciate initially that a primary tumor is carcinoma; increased numbers of mitotic figures and increased fibrosis of the gland stroma may precede invasion. The diagnosis of carcinoma is often made in retrospect. Hyperparathyroidism from a parathyroid carcinoma may be indistinguishable from other forms of primary hyperparathyroidism; a potential clue to the diagnosis, however, is provided by the degree of calcium elevation. Calcium values of 3.5 to 3.7 mmol/L (14 to 15 mg/dL) are frequent with carcinoma and may alert the surgeon to remove the abnormal gland with care to avoid capsular rupture.

GENETIC CONSIDERATIONS　**Defects Associated with Hyperparathyroidism**　As in many other types of neoplasia, two fundamental types of genetic defects have been identified in parathyroid gland tumors: (1) overactivity of protooncogenes, and (2) loss of function of tumor-suppressor genes. The former, by definition, can lead to uncontrolled cellular growth and function by activation (gain-of-function

mutation) of a single allele of the responsible gene, whereas the latter requires loss of function of both allelic copies.

Mutations in the *MENIN* gene locus on chromosome 11q13 are responsible for causing MEN 1; the normal allele of this gene fits the definition of a tumor-suppressor gene. A mutation of one allele is inherited; loss of the other allele via somatic cell mutation leads to monoclonal expansion and tumor development. In ~20% of sporadic parathyroid adenomas, the *MENIN* locus on chromosome 11 is deleted, implying that the same defect responsible for MEN 1 can also cause the sporadic disease (Fig. 332-3*A*). Consistent with the Knudson hypothesis for two-step neoplasia in certain inherited cancer syndromes (Chap. 68), the earlier onset of hyperparathyroidism in the hereditary syndromes reflects the need for only one mutational event to trigger the monoclonal outgrowth. In sporadic adenomas, typically occurring later in life, two different somatic events must occur before the *MENIN* gene is silenced.

Other presumptive antioncogenes involved in hyperparathyroidism include a gene mapped to chromosome 1p seen in 40% of sporadic parathyroid adenomas and a gene mapped to chromosome Xp11 in patients with secondary hyperparathyroidism and renal failure, who progressed to "tertiary" hyperparathyroidism, now known to reflect monoclonal outgrowths within previously hyperplastic glands.

The *Rb* gene, a tumor-suppressor gene located on chromosome 13q14, was initially associated with retinoblastomas but has since been implicated in many other forms of neoplasia including parathyroid carcinoma. Allelic deletion (with a presumed point mutation in the second allele) has been identified in all parathyroid carcinomas examined; there is also an abnormal staining pattern of the protein product of the gene. Allelic deletion is also seen in 10% of parathyroid adenomas, although the abnormal staining pattern of the Rb protein is not seen. Other gene loci on chromosome 13 may be involved in addition to the *Rb* locus.

There are two rare syndromes associated with hyperparathyroidism that involve one or more genes located on chromosome 1q. The he-

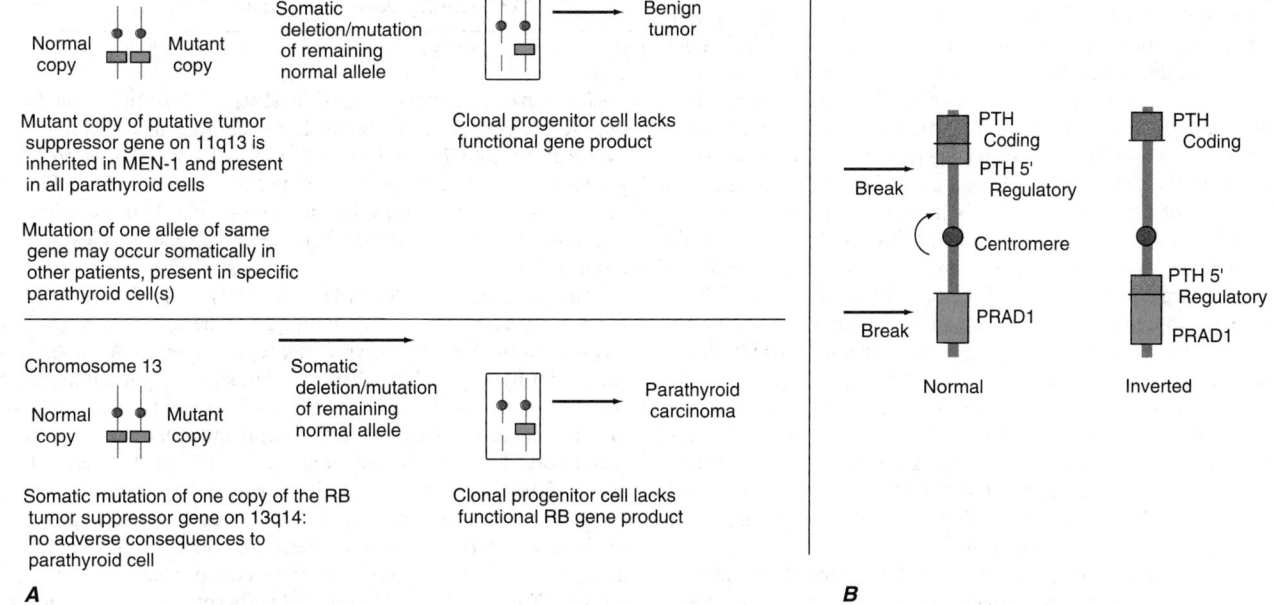

FIGURE 332-3　*A*. Schematic diagram indicating concept of autosomal recessive rather than autosomal dominant inheritance of tumor susceptibility. The patient with the hereditary abnormality (multiple endocrine neoplasia, or MEN) is envisioned as having one defective gene inherited from the affected parent on chromosome 11, but one copy of the normal gene is present from the other parent. In the monoclonal tumor (benign tumor), a somatic event, here partial chromosomal deletion, removes the remaining normal gene from a cell. In nonhereditary tumors, two successive somatic mutations must occur, a process that takes a longer time. By either pathway, the cell, deprived of growth-regulating influence from this gene, has unregulated growth and becomes a tumor. A different genetic locus also involving loss of a tumor-suppressor gene on chromosome 13 is involved in the pathogenesis of parathyroid carcinoma. *B*. Schematic illustration of the mechanism and consequences of gene rearrangement and overexpression of the PRAD 1 protooncogene (pericentromeric inversion of chromosome 11) in parathryoid adenomas. The excessive expression of PRAD 1 (a cell cycle control protein, cyclin D_1) by the highly active PTH gene promoter in the parathyroid cell contributes to excess cellular proliferation. [*From J Habener et al, in L DeGroot, JL Jameson (eds): Endocrinology, 4th ed. Philadelphia, Saunders, 2001, with permission.*]

reditary *hyperparathyroidism jaw tumor* (HPT-JT) syndrome shows an autosomal dominant inheritance pattern; the jaw tumors are benign, but the parathyroid pathology may involve carcinoma as well as adenoma. Parathyroid carcinoma may also appear in the other syndrome, *familial isolated primary hyperparathyroidism* (FIPH). Both syndromes have been mapped through linkage studies to the chromosome 1q21-q31 region. Certain findings have led to speculation that this chromosome region might contain a protooncogene rather than a tumor-suppressor gene.

In some parathyroid adenomas, activation of a protooncogene has been identified (Fig. 332-3*B*). A reciprocal translocation involving chromosome 11 has been identified that juxtaposes the PTH gene promoter upstream of a gene product termed *PRAD-1*, a cyclin D protein that plays a key role in normal cell division. This translocation is found in as many as 15% of parathyroid adenomas, usually in larger tumors. Targeted overexpression of cyclin D_1 in the parathyroid glands of transgenic mice causes the development of hyperparathyroidism, consistent with the role of this cell cycle control protein in parathyroid neoplasia.

A mutated protooncogene, *RET*, is involved in each of the clinical variants of MEN 2 (Chap. 330). *RET* encodes a tyrosine kinase–type receptor; specific mutations lead to constitutive activity of the receptor, thereby explaining the autosomal dominant mode of transmission and the relatively early onset of neoplasia.

Signs and Symptoms　Half or more of patients with hyperparathyroidism are asymptomatic. In series in which patients are followed without operation, as many as 80% are classified as without symptoms. Manifestations of hyperparathyroidism involve primarily the kidneys and the skeletal system. Kidney involvement, due either to deposition of calcium in the renal parenchyma or to recurrent nephrolithiasis, was present in 60 to 70% of patients prior to 1970. With earlier detection, renal complications occur in <20% of patients in many large series. Renal stones are usually composed of either calcium oxalate or calcium phosphate. In occasional patients, repeated episodes of nephrolithiasis or the formation of large calculi may lead to urinary tract obstruction, infection, and loss of renal function. Nephrocalcinosis may also cause decreased renal function and phosphate retention.

The distinctive bone manifestation of hyperparathyroidism is *osteitis fibrosa cystica*, which occurred in 10 to 25% of patients in series reported 50 years ago. Histologically, the pathognomonic features are an increase in the giant multinucleated osteoclasts in scalloped areas on the surface of the bone (Howship's lacunae) and a replacement of the normal cellular and marrow elements by fibrous tissue. X-ray changes include resorption of the phalangeal tufts and replacement of the usually sharp cortical outline of the bone in the digits by an irregular outline (subperiosteal resorption). In recent years, osteitis fibrosa cystica is very rare in primary hyperparathyroidism, probably due to the earlier detection of the disease.

With the use of multiple markers of bone turnover, such as formation indices (bone-specific alkaline phosphatase, osteocalcin, and type I procollagen peptides) and bone resorption indices (including hydroxypyridinium collagen cross-links and telopeptides of type I collagen), increased skeletal turnover is detected in essentially all patients with established hyperparathyroidism.

Computed tomography (CT) scan and dual-energy x-ray absorptiometry (DEXA) of the spine provide reproducible quantitative estimates (within a few percent) of spinal bone density (Chap. 333). Similarly, bone density in the extremities can be quantified by densitometry of the hip or of the distal radius at a site chosen to be primarily cortical. Cortical bone density is reduced while cancellous bone density, especially in the spine, is relatively preserved. Serial studies in patients who choose to be followed without surgery have indicated that in the majority there is little further change over a number of years, consistent with laboratory data indicating relatively unchanged blood

calcium and PTH levels. After an initial loss of bone mass in patients with mild asymptomatic hyperparathyroidism, a new equilibrium may be reached, with bone density and biochemical manifestations of the disease remaining relatively unchanged.

In symptomatic patients, dysfunctions of the CNS, peripheral nerve and muscle, gastrointestinal tract, and joints also occur. It has been reported that severe neuropsychiatric manifestations may be reversed by parathyroidectomy; it remains unclear, in the absence of controlled studies, whether this improvement has a defined cause-and-effect relationship. Generally, the fact that hyperparathyroidism is common in elderly patients, in whom there are often other problems, suggests the possibility that such coexisting problems as hypertension, renal deterioration, and depression may not be parathyroid-related and suggests caution in recommending parathyroid surgery as a cure for these manifestations.

When present, neuromuscular manifestations may include proximal muscle weakness, easy fatigability, and atrophy of muscles and may be so striking as to suggest a primary neuromuscular disorder. The distinguishing feature is the complete regression of neuromuscular disease after surgical correction of the hyperparathyroidism.

Gastrointestinal manifestations are sometimes subtle and include vague abdominal complaints and disorders of the stomach and pancreas. Again, cause and effect are unclear. In MEN 1 patients with hyperparathyroidism, duodenal ulcer may be the result of associated pancreatic tumors that secrete excessive quantities of gastrin (Zollinger-Ellison syndrome). Pancreatitis has been reported in association with hyperparathyroidism, but the incidence and the mechanism are not established.

DIAGNOSIS　The diagnosis is typically made by detecting an elevated immunoreactive PTH level in a patient with asymptomatic hypercalcemia (see "Differential Diagnosis: Special Tests," below). Serum phosphate is usually low but may be normal, especially if renal failure has developed.

Many tests based on renal responses to excess PTH (renal calcium and phosphate clearance; blood phosphate, chloride, magnesium; urinary or nephrogenous cyclic AMP) were used in earlier decades. These tests have low specificity for hyperparathyroidism and are therefore not cost-effective; they have been replaced by PTH immunoassays.

℞ TREATMENT

Medical Surveillance versus Surgical Treatment　The critical management question is whether the disease should be treated surgically. If severe hypercalcemia [3.7 to 4.5 mmol/L (15 to 18 mg/dL)] is present, surgery is mandatory as soon as the diagnosis can be confirmed by a PTH immunoassay. However, in most patients with hyperparathyroidism, hypercalcemia is mild and does not require urgent surgical or medical treatment.

The National Institutes of Health (NIH) held a Consensus Conference on Management of Asymptomatic Hyperparathyroidism in 1990. *Asymptomatic hyperparathyroidism* was defined as documented (presumptive) hyperparathyroidism without signs or symptoms attributable to the disease. The consensus was that patients <50 should undergo surgery, given the long surveillance that would be required. Other considerations that favored surgery included concern that consistent follow-up would be unlikely or that coexistent illness would complicate management. Patients >50 were deemed appropriate for medical monitoring if certain criteria were met, the patients wished to avoid surgery, or the guidelines for recommending surgery were not present (Table 332-2). Careful evaluation of patients over the subsequent dozen years has both provided reassurance that in some patients medical monitoring rather than surgery is still prudent yet has promoted new questions about the natural history of the disease with or without surgery.

Data developed since the Consensus Conference indicated that a subgroup of patients had selective vertebral osteopenia out of proportion to bone loss at other sites and responded to surgery with striking restoration of bone mass (average >20%). In addition, as much as a

5% increase in bone mineral density in the spine and hip have been reported with alendronate use in asymptomatic hyperparathyroid patients. In light of this new information, the NIH convened a Workshop on Asymptomatic Hyperparathyroidism in 2002, and an independent (non-NIH) panel offered a revised set of recommendations. The changes reflect both practical considerations (such as the difficulty in creatinine clearance measurements and therefore substituting calculations based on serum creatinine) and concerns regarding potential deleterious skeletal effects in untreated patients (Tables 332-2 and 332-3). Accordingly, indication for surgical intervention was lowered (i.e., stricter serum calcium and bone density criteria). Asymptomatic patients should be monitored regularly. Surgical correction of hyperparathyroidism can always be undertaken when indicated, since the success rate is high (>90%), mortality is low, and morbidity is minimal. The goals of monitoring are early detection of worsening hypercalcemia, deteriorating bone or renal status, or other complications of hyperparathyroidism. No specific recommendations about medical therapy were made, but the promise of the newer agents was stressed, with the prediction that they would be used in clinical practice to increase bone mass in patients not electing surgery as further experience is gained. Neither panel recommended estrogen use in patients for whom surgery was not elected because there was insufficient cumulative experience with such therapy to balance theoretical risks (breast and endometrial cancer) versus benefits. Raloxifene (Evista), the first of the SERMS, has been shown to have many of the bone-protective effects of estrogen in osteoporotic subjects yet at the same time lowers the incidence of breast cancer; preliminary use of this agent in a small series of hyperparathyroid patients led to increased bone density. Experience with calcimimetics, drugs that selectively stimulate the calcium sensor and suppress PTH secretion, indicates that these agents decrease calcium levels to normal and lower PTH levels by at least 50% for >1 year of continuous use.

Surgical Treatment Parathyroid exploration is challenging and should be undertaken by an experienced surgeon. Certain features help in predicting the pathology (e.g., multiple abnormal glands in familial cases). However, some critical decisions regarding management can be made only during the operation.

As discussed above, there are many unresolved issues to consider in surgery for this disease. One surgical strategy is based on the view that typically only one gland (the adenoma) is abnormal. If an enlarged gland is found, a normal gland should be sought. In this view, if a biopsy of a normal-sized second gland confirms its histologic (and presumed functional) normality, no further exploration, biopsy, or excision is needed. At the other extreme is the minority viewpoint that all four glands be sought and that most of the total parathyroid tissue mass should be removed. The concern with the former approach is that the recurrence rate of hyperparathyroidism may be high if a second abnormal gland is missed; the latter approach could involve unnecessary surgery and an unacceptable rate of hypoparathyroidism. The majority viewpoint favors conservative surgery, i.e., removal of what is usually only one enlarged gland but only after four-gland exploration to eliminate the possibility that more than one gland is abnormal. When normal glands are found in association with one enlarged gland, excision of the single adenoma usually leads to cure or at least years free of symptoms. Long-term follow-up studies are limited to establish true rates of recurrence.

Recently, there has been growing experience with new surgical strategies that feature a minimally invasive approach guided by improved preoperative localization and intraoperative monitoring by PTH assays. Preoperative ^{99m}Tc sestamibi scans with positron emission computed tomography (SPECT) are used to predict the location of an abnormal gland and intraoperative sampling of PTH before and at 5-min intervals after removal of a suspected adenoma to confirm a rapid fall (>50%) to normal levels of PTH. In several centers, a combination of preoperative sestamibi imaging, cervical block anesthesia, minimal surgical incision, and intraoperative PTH measurements has allowed successful outpatient surgical management with a clear-cut cost benefit compared to general anesthesia and more extensive neck surgery. The use of these minimally invasive approaches requires clinical judgment to select patients unlikely to have multiple gland disease (e.g., MEN or secondary hyperparathyroidism). The growing acceptance of the technique and its relative ease for the patient has lowered the threshold for surgery.

When parathyroid carcinoma is encountered, the tissue should be widely excised; care must be taken to avoid rupture of the capsule to prevent local seeding of tumor cells.

Multiple gland hyperplasia, as predicted in familial cases, poses more difficult questions of surgical management. Once a diagnosis of hyperplasia is established, all the glands must be identified. Two schemes have been proposed for surgical management. One is to totally remove three glands with partial excision of the fourth gland; care is taken to leave a good blood supply for the remaining gland. Other surgeons advocate total parathyroidectomy with immediate transplantation of a portion of a removed, minced parathyroid gland into the muscles of the forearm, with the view that surgical excision is easier from the ectopic site in the arm if there is recurrent hyperfunction.

In a minority of cases, if no abnormal parathyroid glands are found in the neck, the issue of further exploration must be decided. There are documented cases of five or six parathyroid glands and of unusual locations for adenomas, such as in the mediastinum.

When a second parathyroid exploration is indicated, the minimally invasive techniques such as ultrasound, CT scan, and isotope scanning may be combined with venous sampling and/or selective digital arteriography in one of the centers specializing in these techniques. Intraoperative monitoring of PTH levels by rapid PTH immunoassays may be useful in guiding the surgery, especially in patients who are reexplored after an initial unsuccessful operation. At one center, long-term cures have been achieved with selective embolization or injection of large amounts of contrast material into the end-arterial circulation feeding the parathyroid tumor.

A decline in serum calcium occurs within 24 h after successful surgery; usually blood calcium falls to low-normal values for 3 to 5

TABLE 332-2 *Guidelines for Parathyroid Surgery in Asymptomatic Primary Hyperparathyroidism[a]*

Measurement	Guidelines, 1990	Guidelines, 2002
Serum calcium (above upper limit of normal)	0.3–0.4 mmol/L (1–6 mg/dL)	0.3 mmol/L (1.0 mg/dL)
24-h urinary calcium	>400 mg	>400 mg
Creatinine clearance	Reduced by 30%	Reduced by 30%
Bone mineral density	Z-score < −2.0 (forearm)	T-score < −2.5 at any site
Age	<50	<50

[a] Surgery is also indicated in patients for whom medical surveillance is neither desired nor possible.
Source: From JP Bilezikian et al: J Clin Endocrinol Metab 87:5353, 2002.

TABLE 332-3 *Management Guidelines for Patients with Asymptomatic Primary Hyperparathyroidism Who Do Not Undergo Parathyroid Surgery*

Measurement	Older Guidelines	New Guidelines
Serum calcium	Biannually	Biannually
24-h urinary calcium	Annually	Not recommended[a]
Creatinine clearance	Annually	Not recommended[a]
Serum creatinine	Annually	Annually[b]
Bone density	Annually (forearm)	Annually (lumbar spine, hip, forearm)
Abdominal x-ray (+/− ultrasound)	Annually	Not recommended[a]

[a] Except at the time of initial evaluation.
[b] If the serum creatinine concentration suggests a change in the creatinine clearance when the Cockroft-Gault equation is applied, further, more direct assessments of the creatinine clearance are recommended.
Source: From JP Bilezikian et al: J Clin Endocrinol Metab 87:5353, 2002.

days until the remaining parathyroid tissue resumes hormone secretion. Severe postoperative hypocalcemia is likely only if osteitis fibrosa cystica is present or if injury to all the normal parathyroid glands occurs during surgery. In general, patients with uncomplicated disease such as a single adenoma (the clear majority) who do not have symptomatic bone disease or a large deficit in bone mineral and who have good renal and gastrointestinal function have few problems with postoperative hypocalcemia. The extent of postoperative hypocalcemia varies with the surgical approach. If all glands are biopsied, hypocalcemia may be transiently symptomatic and more prolonged. Hypocalcemia is more likely to be symptomatic after second parathyroid explorations, particularly when normal parathyroid tissue was removed at the initial operation and when the manipulation and/or biopsy of the remaining normal glands is more extensive in the search for the missing adenoma.

Patients with hyperparathyroidism have efficient intestinal calcium absorption due to the increased levels of $1,25(OH)_2D$ stimulated by PTH excess. Once hypocalcemia signifies successful surgery, patients can be put on a high-calcium intake or be given oral calcium supplements. Despite mild hypocalcemia, most patients do not require parenteral therapy. If the serum calcium falls to <2 mmol/L (8 mg/dL), *and if the phosphate level rises simultaneously*, the possibility that surgery has caused hypoparathyroidism must be considered. With unexpected hypocalcemia, coexistent hypomagnesemia should be considered, as it interferes with PTH secretion and causes functional hypoparathyroidism (see below). Signs of hypocalcemia include symptoms such as muscle twitching, a general sense of anxiety, and positive Chvostek and Trousseau signs coupled with serum calcium consistently <2 mmol/L (8 mg/dL). Parenteral calcium replacement at a low level should be instituted when hypocalcemia is symptomatic. The rate and duration of intravenous therapy are determined by the severity of the symptoms and the response of the serum calcium to treatment. An infusion of 0.5 to 2 (mg/kg)/h or 30 to 100 mL/h of a 1-mg/mL solution usually suffices to relieve symptoms. Usually, parenteral therapy is required for only a few days. If symptoms worsen or if parenteral calcium is needed for >2 to 3 days, therapy with a vitamin D analogue and/or oral calcium (2 to 4 g/d) should be started (see below). It is cost-effective to use calcitriol (doses of 0.5 to 1.0 μg/d) because of the rapidity of onset of effect and prompt cessation of action when stopped, in comparison to other forms of vitamin D (see below). A rise in blood calcium after several months of vitamin D replacement may indicate restoration of parathyroid function to normal. It is also appropriate to monitor serum PTH serially to estimate gland function in such patients.

Magnesium deficiency may also complicate the postoperative course. Magnesium deficiency impairs the secretion of PTH, and so hypomagnesemia should be corrected whenever detected. Magnesium chloride is effective by mouth, but this compound is not widely available. Repletion is usually parenteral. Because the depressant effect of magnesium on central and peripheral nerve functions does not occur at levels <2 mmol/L (normal range 0.8 to 1.2 mmol/L), parenteral replacement can be given rapidly. A cumulative dose as great as 0.5 to 1 mmol/kg of body weight can be administered if severe hypomagnesemia is present; often, however, total doses of 20 to 40 mmol are sufficient. The magnesium is given either as an intravenous infusion over 8 to 12 h or in divided doses intramuscularly (magnesium sulfate, USP).

OTHER PARATHYROID-RELATED CAUSES OF HYPERCALCEMIA ■ Lithium Therapy

Lithium, used in the management of bipolar depression and other psychiatric disorders, causes hypercalcemia in ~10% of treated patients. The hypercalcemia is dependent on continued lithium treatment, remitting and recurring when lithium is stopped and restarted. The parathyroid adenomas reported in some hypercalcemic patients with lithium therapy may reflect the presence of an independently occurring parathyroid tumor; a permanent effect of lithium on parathyroid gland growth need not be implicated as most patients have complete reversal of hypercalcemia when lithium is stopped. However, long-standing stimulation of parathyroid cell replication by lithium may predispose to development of adenomas (as is documented in secondary hyperparathyroidism and renal failure).

At the levels achieved in blood in treated patients, lithium can be shown in vitro to shift the PTH secretion curve to the right in response to calcium; i.e., higher calcium levels are required to lower PTH secretion, probably acting at the calcium sensor (see below); this effect can cause elevated PTH levels and consequent hypercalcemia in otherwise normal individuals. Fortunately, there are alternative medications for the underlying psychiatric illness. Parathyroid surgery should not be recommended unless hypercalcemia and elevated PTH levels persist after lithium is discontinued.

GENETIC DISORDERS CAUSING HYPERPARATHYROID-LIKE SYNDROMES ■ Familial Hypocalciuric Hypercalcemia

FHH (also called *familial benign hypercalcemia*) is inherited as an autosomal dominant trait. Affected individuals are discovered because of asymptomatic hypercalcemia. This disorder and Jansen's disease (discussed below) are variants of hyperparathyroidism. FHH involves excessive secretion of PTH, whereas Jansen's disease is caused by excessive biologic activity of the PTH receptor in target tissues. Neither disorder, however, involves a primary growth disorder of the parathyroids.

The pathophysiology of FHH is now understood. The primary defect is abnormal sensing of the blood calcium by the parathyroid gland and renal tubule, causing inappropriate secretion of PTH and excessive renal reabsorption of calcium. The calcium sensor is a member of the third family of GPCRs (type C, or III). The receptor responds to the ECF calcium concentration, suppressing PTH secretion through second messenger signaling, thereby providing negative-feedback regulation of PTH secretion. Many different mutations in the calcium-sensing receptor have been identified in patients with FHH (Fig. 332-4). These mutations lower the capacity of the sensor to bind calcium, and the mutant receptors function as though blood calcium levels were low; excessive secretion of PTH occurs from an otherwise normal gland. Approximately two-thirds of patients with FHH have mutations within the protein-coding region of the gene. The remaining one-third of kindreds may have mutations in the gene promoter or may involve still unknown mechanisms in other regions of the genome identified through mapping studies (e.g., chromosome 19).

Even before elucidation of the pathophysiology of FHH, abundant clinical evidence served to separate the disorder from primary hyperparathyroidism. Patients with primary hyperparathyroidism have <99% renal calcium reabsorption, whereas most patients with FHH have >99% reabsorption. The hypercalcemia in FHH is often detectable in affected members of the kindreds in the first decade of life, whereas hypercalcemia rarely occurs in patients with primary hyperparathyroidism or the MEN syndromes who are <10. PTH may be elevated in FHH, but the values are usually normal or lower for the same degree of calcium elevation than in patients with primary hyperparathyroidism. Parathyroid surgery in a few patients with FHH led to permanent hypoparathyroidism, but hypocalciuria persisted nevertheless, establishing that hypocalciuria, therefore, is not PTH-dependent (now known to be due to the abnormal calcium sensor in the kidney).

Few clinical signs or symptoms are present in patients with FHH, and other endocrine abnormalities are not present. Most patients are detected as a result of family screening after hypercalcemia is detected in a proband. In those patients inadvertently operated upon, the parathyroids appeared normal or moderately hyperplastic. Parathyroid surgery is not appropriate, nor, in view of the lack of symptoms, does medical treatment seem needed to lower the calcium. Calcimimetic agents that bind to the calcium sensor and elevate the set point are under investigation.

One striking exception to the rule against parathyroid surgery in this syndrome is the occurrence, usually in consanguineous marriages (due to the rarity of the gene mutation), of a homozygous or compound heterozygote state, resulting in complete loss of the calcium sensor function. In this condition, neonatal severe hypercalcemia, total parathyroidectomy is mandatory.

Jansen's Disease Mutations in the PTH1R have been identified as responsible for this rare autosomal dominant syndrome (Fig. 332-4). Because the mutations lead to constitutive receptor function, one abnormal copy of the mutant receptor is sufficient to cause the disease, thereby accounting for its dominant mode of transmission. The disorder leads to short-limbed dwarfism due to abnormal regulation of the bone growth plate. In adult life, there are numerous abnormalities in bone, including multiple cystic resorptive areas resembling those seen in severe hyperparathyroidism. Hypercalcemia and hypophosphatemia with undetectable or low PTH levels are typically seen. The pathogenesis of the disease has been confirmed by transgenic experiments in which targeted expression of the mutant receptor to the growth plate emulated several features of the disorder.

MALIGNANCY-RELATED HYPERCALCEMIA ■ **Clinical Syndromes and Mechanisms of Hypercalcemia** Hypercalcemia due to malignancy is common (occurring with 10 to 15% of certain types of tumor, such as lung carcinoma), often severe and difficult to manage, and occasionally difficult to distinguish from primary hyperparathyroidism. Although malignancy is often clinically obvious or readily detectable by medical history, hypercalcemia can occasionally be due to an occult tumor. Previously, hypercalcemia associated with malignancy was thought to be due to local invasion and destruction of bone by tumor cells; many cases are now known to result from the elaboration by the malignant cells of humoral mediators of hypercalcemia. PTHrP is the responsible humoral agent in most solid tumors that cause hypercalcemia.

The histologic character of the tumor is more important than the extent of skeletal metastases in predicting hypercalcemia. Small-cell carcinoma (oat cell) and adenocarcinoma of the lung, although the most common lung tumors associated with skeletal metastases, rarely cause hypercalcemia. By contrast, as many as 10% of patients with squamous cell carcinoma of the lung develop hypercalcemia. Histologic studies of bone in patients with squamous cell or epidermoid carcinoma of the lung, in sites invaded by tumor as well as areas remote from tumor invasion, reveal increased bone remodeling, including osteoclastic and osteoblastic activity.

Two main mechanisms of hypercalcemia are operative in cancer hypercalcemia. Many solid tumors associated with hypercalcemia, particularly squamous cell and renal tumors, produce and secrete PTHrP that causes increased bone resorption and mediate the hypercalcemia through systemic actions on the skeleton. Alternatively, direct bone marrow invasion occurs with hematologic malignancies such as leukemia, lymphoma, and multiple myeloma. Lymphokines and cytokines produced by cells involved in the marrow response to the tumors promote resorption of bone through local destruction. Several hormones, hormone analogues, cytokines, and growth factors have been implicated as the result of clinical assays, in vitro tests, or chemical isolation. The etiologic factor produced by activated normal lymphocytes and by myeloma and lymphoma cells, termed *osteoclast activation factor*, now appears to represent the biologic action of several different cytokines, probably interleukin 1 and lymphotoxin or tumor necrosis factor. In some lymphomas, typically B cell lymphomas, there is a third mechanism, caused by an increased blood level of $1,25(OH)_2D$, which is probably produced by lymphocytes.

The more common mechanism, usually termed *humoral hypercalcemia of malignancy*, solid tumors (cancers of the lung and kidney, in particular), in which bone metastases are absent, minimal, or not de-

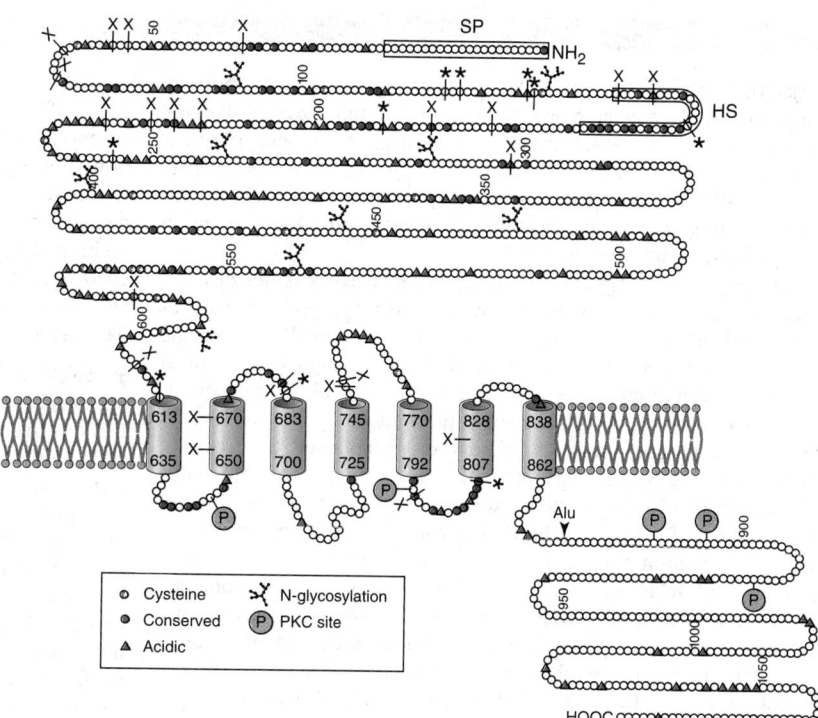

FIGURE 332-4 Mutations in the calcium sensor receptor. The extracellular domain binds calcium, leading to conformational changes that stimulate Gq-coupled activation of the phospholipase C and suppression of PTH. The identified sequence alterations (X) cause loss of function and lead to inadequate suppression of parathyroid hormone release and, therefore, mild hypercalcemia (FHH); *, a gain-of-function mutation that causes hypocalcemia; •, conserved residues; ▲, acidic residues. (*From EM Brown et al: J Nutr 125:1965S, 1995, with permission.*)

tectable clinically, secrete PTHrP measurable by immunoassay. Secretion by the tumors of the PTH-like factor, PTHrP, activates the PTH1R, resulting in a pathophysiology closely resembling hyperparathyroidism. The clinical picture resembles primary hyperparathyroidism (hypophosphatemia accompanies hypercalcemia), and elimination or regression of the primary tumor leads to disappearance of the hypercalcemia.

As in hyperparathyroidism, patients with the humoral hypercalcemia of malignancy have elevated urinary nephrogenous cyclic AMP excretion, hypophosphatemia, and increased urinary phosphate clearance. However, in humoral hypercalcemia of malignancy, immunoreactive PTH is undetectable or suppressed, making the differential diagnosis easier. Other features of the disorder differ from those of true hyperparathyroidism. Patients may have high, rather than low, renal calcium clearance (relative to serum calcium when compared to true hyperparathyroidism, unlike the expected elevation) and low to normal levels of $1,25(OH)_2D$. The reason that the humoral syndrome differs from hyperparathyroidism in these parameters is unclear since the biologic actions of PTH and PTHrP are presumably exerted through the same receptor. Other cytokines elaborated by the malignancy may be responsible for these variations from hyperparathyroidism. In some patients with the humoral hypercalcemia of malignancy, osteoclastic resorption is unaccompanied by an osteoblastic or bone-forming response, implying inhibition of the normal coupling of bone formation and resorption. Thus the interaction of more than one substance may determine whether hypercalcemia develops in a particular patient.

Several different assays (single- or double-antibody, different epitopes) have been developed to detect PTHrP. Most data indicate that circulating PTHrP levels are undetectable (or low) in normal individuals, elevated in most cancer patients with the humoral syndrome, and high in human milk. The etiologic mechanisms in cancer hypercalcemia may be multiple in the same patient. For example, in breast carcinoma (metastatic to bone) and in a distinctive type of T cell lymphoma/leukemia initiated by human T cell lymphotropic virus I, hypercalcemia is caused by direct local lysis of bone as well as by a humoral mechanism involving excess production of PTHrP.

Diagnostic Issues Levels of PTH measured by the double-antibody technique are undetectable or extremely low in tumor hypercalcemia, as would be expected with the mediation of the hypercalcemia by a factor other than PTH (the hypercalcemia suppresses the normal parathyroid glands). In a patient with minimal symptoms referred for hypercalcemia, low or undetectable PTH levels would focus attention on a possible occult malignancy.

Ordinarily, the diagnosis of cancer hypercalcemia is not difficult because tumor symptoms are prominent when hypercalcemia is detected. Indeed, hypercalcemia may be noted incidentally during the workup of a patient with known or suspected malignancy. Clinical suspicion that malignancy is the cause of the hypercalcemia is heightened when there are other paraneoplastic signs or symptoms, such as weight loss, fatigue, muscle weakness, or unexplained skin rash, or when symptoms specific for a particular tumor are present. Squamous cell tumors are most frequently associated with hypercalcemia, particularly tumors of the lung, kidney, head and neck, and urogenital tract. Radiologic examinations can focus on these areas when clinical evidence is unclear. Bone scans with technetium-labeled bisphosphonate are useful for detection of osteolytic metastases; the sensitivity is high, but specificity is low; results must be confirmed by conventional x-rays to be certain that areas of increased uptake are due to osteolytic metastases per se. Bone marrow biopsies are helpful in patients with anemia or abnormal peripheral blood smears.

℞ TREATMENT

Treatment of the hypercalcemia of malignancy is first directed to control of tumor; reduction of tumor mass usually corrects hypercalcemia. If a patient has severe hypercalcemia yet has a good chance for effective tumor therapy, treatment of the hypercalcemia should be vigorous while awaiting the results of definitive therapy. If hypercalcemia occurs in the late stages of a tumor that is resistant to anti-tumor therapy, the treatment of the hypercalcemia should be judicious as high calcium levels can have a mild sedating effect. Standard therapies for hypercalcemia (discussed below) are applicable to patients with malignancy.

VITAMIN D–RELATED HYPERCALCEMIA Hypercalcemia caused by vitamin D can be due to excessive ingestion or abnormal metabolism of the vitamin. Abnormal metabolism of the vitamin is usually acquired in association with a widespread granulomatous disorder. Vitamin D metabolism is carefully regulated, particularly the activity of renal 1α-hydroxylase, the enzyme responsible for the production of $1,25(OH)_2D$ (Chap. 331). The regulation of 1α-hydroxylase and the normal feedback suppression by $1,25(OH)_2D$ seem to work less well in infants than in adults and to operate poorly, if at all, in sites other than the renal tubule; these phenomena explain the occurrence of hypercalcemia secondary to excessive $1,25(OH)_2D_3$ production in infants with Williams' syndrome (see below) and in adults with sarcoidosis or lymphoma.

Vitamin D Intoxication Chronic ingestion of 50 to 100 times the normal physiologic requirement of vitamin D (amounts >50,000 to 100,000 U/d) is usually required to produce significant hypercalcemia in normal individuals. An upper limit of dietary intake of 2000 U/d (50 μg/d) in adults is now recommended because of concerns about potential toxic effects of cumulative supraphysiologic doses. Vitamin D excess increases intestinal calcium absorption and, if severe, also increases bone resorption.

Hypercalcemia in vitamin D intoxication is due to an excessive biologic action of the vitamin, perhaps the consequence of increased levels of 25(OH)D rather than merely increased levels of the active metabolite $1,25(OH)_2D$ (the latter may not be elevated in vitamin D intoxication). 25(OH)D has definite, if low, biologic activity in intestine and bone. The production of 25(OH)D is less tightly regulated than is the production of $1,25(OH)_2D$. Hence concentrations of 25(OH)D are elevated several-fold in patients with excess vitamin D intake.

The diagnosis is substantiated by documenting elevated levels of 25(OH)D >100 ng/mL. Hypercalcemia is usually controlled by restriction of dietary calcium intake and appropriate attention to hydration. These measures, plus discontinuation of vitamin D, usually lead to resolution of hypercalcemia. However, vitamin D stores in fat may be substantial, and vitamin D intoxication may persist for weeks after vitamin D ingestion is terminated. Such patients are responsive to glucocorticoids, which in doses of 100 mg/d of hydrocortisone or its equivalent, usually return serum calcium levels to normal over several days; severe intoxication may require intensive therapy.

Sarcoidosis and Other Granulomatous Diseases In patients with sarcoidosis and other granulomatous diseases, such as tuberculosis and fungal infections, excess $1,25(OH)_2D$ is synthesized in macrophages or other cells in the granulomas. Indeed, increased $1,25(OH)_2D$ levels have been reported in anephric patients with sarcoidosis and hypercalcemia. Macrophages obtained from granulomatous tissue convert 25(OH)D to $1,25(OH)_2D$ at an increased rate. There is a positive correlation in patients with sarcoidosis between 25(OH)D levels (reflecting vitamin D intake) and the circulating concentrations of $1,25(OH)_2D$, whereas normally there is no increase in $1,25(OH)_2D$ with increasing 25(OH)D levels due to multiple feedback controls on renal 1α-hydroxylase (Chap. 331). The usual regulation of active metabolite production by calcium or PTH does not operate in these patients; hypercalcemia does not lead to a reduction in the blood levels of $1,25(OH)_2D$ in patients with sarcoidosis. Clearance of $1,25(OH)_2D$ from blood may be decreased in sarcoidosis as well. PTH levels are usually low and $1,25(OH)_2D$ levels are elevated, but primary hyperparathyroidism and sarcoidosis may coexist in some patients.

Management of the hypercalcemia can often be accomplished by avoiding excessive sunlight exposure and limiting vitamin D and calcium intake. Presumably, however, the abnormal sensitivity to vitamin D and abnormal regulation of $1,25(OH)_2D$ synthesis will persist as long as the disease is active. Alternatively, glucocorticoids in the equivalent of ≤100 mg/d of hydrocortisone control hypercalcemia. Glucocorticoids appear to act by blocking excessive production of $1,25(OH)_2D$ as well as the response to it in target organs.

Idiopathic Hypercalcemia of Infancy This rare disorder, usually referred to as *Williams' syndrome*, is an autosomal dominant disorder characterized by multiple congenital development defects, including supravalvular aortic stenosis, mental retardation, and an elfin facies, in association with hypercalcemia due to abnormal sensitivity to vitamin D. The syndrome was first recognized in England after the fortification of milk with vitamin D. Levels of $1,25(OH)_2D$ are elevated, ranging from 46 to 120 nmol/L (150 to 500 pg/mL). The mechanism of the abnormal sensitivity to vitamin D and of the increased circulating levels of $1,25(OH)_2D$ is still unclear. Studies suggest that mutations involving the elastin locus and perhaps other genes on chromosome 7 may play a role in the pathogenesis.

HYPERCALCEMIA ASSOCIATED WITH HIGH BONE TURNOVER ▪ **Hyperthyroidism** As many as 20% of hyperthyroid patients have high-normal or mildly elevated serum calcium concentrations; hypercalciuria is even more common. The hypercalcemia is due to increased bone turnover, with bone resorption exceeding bone formation. Severe calcium elevations are not typical, and the presence of such suggests a concomitant disease such as hyperparathyroidism. Usually, the diagnosis is obvious, but signs of hyperthyroidism may occasionally be occult, particularly in the elderly (Chap. 320). Hypercalcemia is managed by treatment of the hyperthyroidism.

Immobilization Immobilization is a rare cause of hypercalcemia in adults in the absence of an associated disease but may cause hypercalcemia in children and adolescents, particularly after spinal cord injury and paraplegia or quadriplegia. With resumption of ambulation, the hypercalcemia in children usually returns to normal.

The mechanism appears to involve a disproportion between bone formation and bone resorption. Hypercalciuria and increased mobilization of skeletal calcium can develop in normal volunteers subjected to extensive bed rest, although hypercalcemia is unusual. Immobilization of an adult with a disease associated with high bone turnover, however, such as Paget's disease, may cause hypercalcemia.

Thiazides Administration of benzothiadiazines (thiazides) can cause hypercalcemia in patients with high rates of bone turnover, such as patients with hypoparathyroidism treated with high doses of vitamin D. Traditionally, thiazides are associated with aggravation of hypercalcemia in primary hyperparathyroidism, but this effect can be seen in other high-bone-turnover states as well. The mechanism of thiazide action is complex. Chronic thiazide administration leads to reduction in urinary calcium; the hypocalciuric effect appears to reflect the enhancement of proximal tubular resorption of sodium and calcium in response to sodium depletion. Some of this renal effect is due to augmentation of PTH action and is more pronounced in individuals with intact PTH secretion. However, thiazides cause hypocalciuria in hypoparathyroid patients on high-dose vitamin D and oral calcium replacement if sodium intake is restricted. This finding is the rationale for the use of thiazides as an adjunct to therapy in hypoparathyroid patients, as discussed below. Thiazide administration to normal individuals causes a transient increase in blood calcium (usually within the high-normal range) that reverts to preexisting levels after a week or more of continued administration. If hormonal function and calcium and bone metabolism are normal, homeostatic controls are reset to counteract the calcium-elevating effect of the thiazides. In the presence of hyperparathyroidism or increased bone turnover from another cause, homeostatic mechanisms are ineffective. The abnormal effects of the thiazide on calcium metabolism disappear within days of cessation of the drug.

Vitamin A Intoxication Vitamin A intoxication is a rare cause of hypercalcemia and is most commonly a side effect of dietary faddism (Chap. 61). Calcium levels can be elevated into the 3 to 3.5 mmol/L (12 to 14 mg/dL) range after the ingestion of 50,000 to 100,000 units of vitamin A daily (10 to 20 times the minimum daily requirement). Typical features of severe hypercalcemia include fatigue, anorexia, and, in some, severe muscle and bone pain. Excess vitamin A intake is presumed to increase bone resorption.

The diagnosis can be established by history and by measurement of vitamin A levels in serum. Occasionally, skeletal x-rays reveal periosteal calcifications, particularly in the hands. Withdrawal of the vitamin is usually associated with prompt disappearance of the hypercalcemia and reversal of the skeletal changes. As in vitamin D intoxication, administration of 100 mg/d hydrocortisone or its equivalent leads to a rapid return of the serum calcium to normal.

HYPERCALCEMIA ASSOCIATED WITH RENAL FAILURE ▪ **Severe Secondary Hyperparathyroidism** Secondary hyperparathyroidism occurs when partial resistance to the metabolic actions of PTH leads to excessive production of the hormone. Parathyroid gland hyperplasia occurs because resistance to the normal level of PTH leads to hypocalcemia, which, in turn, is a stimulus to parathyroid gland enlargement.

Secondary hyperparathyroidism occurs not only in patients with renal failure but also in those with osteomalacia due to multiple causes (Chap. 331), including deficiency of vitamin D action, and PHP (deficient response to PTH at the level of the receptor). Hypocalcemia seems to be the common denominator in initiating secondary hyperparathyroidism. Primary and secondary hyperparathyroidism can be distinguished conceptually by the autonomous growth of the parathyroid glands in primary hyperparathyroidism (presumably irreversible) and the adaptive response of the parathyroids in secondary hyperparathyroidism (typically reversible). In fact, reversal over weeks from an abnormal pattern of secretion, presumably accompanied by involution of parathyroid gland mass to normal, occurs in patients who have been treated effectively to reverse the resistance to PTH (such as with calcium and vitamin D in osteomalacia).

Patients with secondary hyperparathyroidism may develop bone pain, ectopic calcification, and pruritus. The bone disease seen in patients with secondary hyperparathyroidism and renal failure is termed *renal osteodystrophy*. Osteomalacia (predominantly due to vitamin D and calcium deficiency) and/or osteitis fibrosa cystica (excessive PTH action on bone) may occur.

Two other skeletal disorders are associated with long-term dialysis in patients with renal failure. Aluminum deposition (see below) is associated with an osteomalacia-like picture. The other entity is a low-bone-turnover state termed "aplastic" or "adynamic" bone disease; PTH levels are lower than in typical secondary hyperparathyroidism. It is believed that the condition is caused, at least in part, by excessive PTH suppression, which may be even greater than previously appreciated in light of evidence that some of the immunoreactive PTH detected by most commercially available PTH assays is not the full-length biologically active molecule (as discussed above).

℞ TREATMENT

Medical therapy to reverse secondary hyperparathyroidism includes reduction of excessive blood phosphate by restriction of dietary phosphate, the use of nonabsorbable antacids, and careful, selective addition of calcitriol (0.25 to 2.0 μg/d); calcium carbonate is preferred over aluminum-containing antacids to prevent aluminum toxicity. Intravenous calcitriol, administered as several pulses each week, helps control secondary hyperparathyroidism. Aggressive but carefully administered medical therapy can often, but not always, reverse hyperparathyroidism and its symptoms and manifestations.

Occasional patients develop severe manifestations of secondary hyperparathyroidism, including hypercalcemia, pruritus, extraskeletal calcifications, and painful bones, despite aggressive medical efforts to suppress the hyperparathyroidism. PTH hypersecretion no longer responsive to medical therapy, a state of severe hyperparathyroidism in patients with renal failure that requires surgery, has been referred to as *tertiary hyperparathyroidism*. Parathyroid surgery is necessary to control this condition. Based on genetic evidence from examination of tumor samples in these patients, the emergence of autonomous parathyroid function is due to a monoclonal outgrowth of one or more previously hyperplastic parathyroid glands. The adaptive response has become an independent contributor to disease; this finding seems to emphasize the importance of optimal medical management to reduce the proliferative response of the parathyroid cells that enables the irreversible genetic change.

Aluminum Intoxication Aluminum intoxication (and often hypercalcemia as a complication of medical treatment) may occur in patients on chronic dialysis; manifestations include acute dementia and unresponsive and severe osteomalacia. Bone pain, multiple nonhealing fractures, particularly of the ribs and pelvis, and a proximal myopathy may occur. Hypercalcemia develops when these patients are treated with vitamin D or calcitriol because of impaired skeletal responsiveness. Aluminum is present at the site of osteoid mineralization, osteoblastic activity is minimal, and calcium incorporation into the skeleton is impaired. Prevention is accomplished by avoidance of aluminum excess in the dialysis regimen; treatment of established disease involves mobilizing aluminum through the use of the chelating agent deferoxamine (Chap. 339).

Milk-Alkali Syndrome The milk-alkali syndrome is due to excessive ingestion of calcium and absorbable antacids such as milk or calcium carbonate. It is much less frequent since nonabsorbable antacids and other treatments became available for peptic ulcer disease. However, the increased use of calcium carbonate in the management of osteoporosis has led to reappearance of the syndrome. Several clinical presentations—acute, subacute, and chronic—have been described, all of which feature hypercalcemia, alkalosis, and renal failure. The chronic form of the disease, termed *Burnett's syndrome*, is associated with irreversible renal damage. The acute syndromes reverse if the excess calcium and absorbable alkali are stopped.

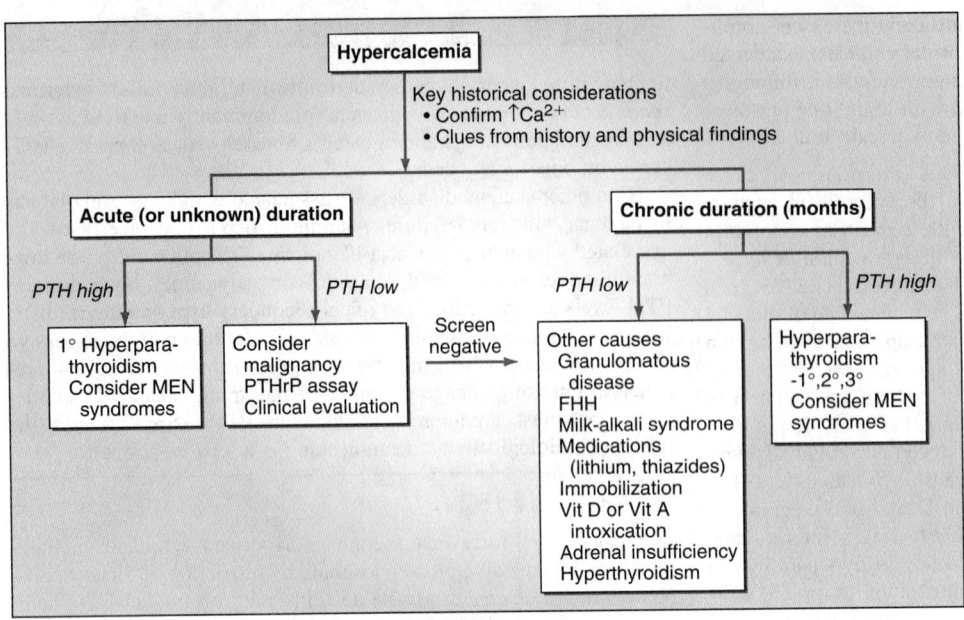

FIGURE 332-5   Algorithm for the evaluation of patients with hypercalcemia. See text for details. FHH, familial hypocalciuric hypercalcemia; MEN, multiple endocrine neoplasia; PTH, parathyroid hormone; PTHrP, parathyroid hormone–related peptide.

Individual susceptibility is important in the pathogenesis, as many patients are treated with calcium carbonate alkali regimens without developing the syndrome. One variable is the fractional calcium absorption as a function of calcium intake. Some individuals absorb a high fraction of calcium, even with intakes as high as 2 g or more of elemental calcium per day, instead of reducing calcium absorption with high intake, as occurs in most normal individuals. Resultant mild hypercalcemia after meals in such patients is postulated to contribute to the generation of alkalosis. Development of hypercalcemia causes increased sodium excretion and some depletion of total-body water. These phenomena and perhaps some suppression of endogenous PTH secretion due to mild hypercalcemia lead to increased bicarbonate resorption and to alkalosis in the face of continued calcium carbonate ingestion. Alkalosis per se selectively enhances calcium resorption in the distal nephron, thus aggravating the hypercalcemia. The cycle of mild hypercalcemia → bicarbonate retention → alkalosis → renal calcium retention → severe hypercalcemia perpetuates and aggravates hypercalcemia and alkalosis as long as calcium and absorbable alkali are ingested.

DIFFERENTIAL DIAGNOSIS: SPECIAL TESTS   Differential diagnosis of hypercalcemia is best achieved by using clinical criteria, but the immunoassay for PTH is especially useful in distinguishing among major causes (Fig. 332-5). The clinical features that deserve emphasis are the presence or absence of symptoms or signs of disease and evidence of chronicity. If one discounts fatigue or depression, >90% of patients with primary hyperparathyroidism have *asymptomatic hypercalcemia*; symptoms of malignancy are usually present in cancer-associated hypercalcemia. Disorders other than hyperparathyroidism and malignancy cause <10% of cases of hypercalcemia, and some of the nonparathyroid causes are associated with clear-cut manifestations such as renal failure.

Hyperparathyroidism is the likely diagnosis in patients with *chronic hypercalcemia*. If hypercalcemia has been manifest for >1 year, malignancy can usually be excluded as the cause. A striking feature of malignancy-associated hypercalcemia is the rapidity of the course, whereby signs and symptoms of the underlying malignancy are evident within months of the detection of hypercalcemia. Although clinical considerations are helpful in arriving at the correct diagnosis of the cause of hypercalcemia, appropriate laboratory testing is essential for definitive diagnosis. The immunoassay for PTH should separate hyperparathyroidism from all other causes of hypercalcemia. Patients with hyperparathyroidism have elevated PTH levels despite hypercal-

cemia, whereas patients with malignancy and the other causes of hypercalcemia (except for disorders mediated by PTH such as lithium-induced hypercalcemia) have levels of hormone below normal or undetectable. Assays based on the double-antibody method for PTH exhibit very high sensitivity (especially if serum calcium is simultaneously evaluated) and specificity for the diagnosis of primary hyperparathyroidism (Fig. 332-6).

In summary, PTH values are elevated in >90% of parathyroid-related causes of hypercalcemia, undetectable or low in malignancy-related hypercalcemia, and undetectable or normal in vitamin D–related and high-bone-turnover causes of hypercalcemia. In view of the specificity of the PTH immunoassay and the high frequency of hyperparathyroidism in hypercalcemic patients, it is cost-effective to measure the PTH level in all hypercalcemic patients unless malignancy or a specific nonparathyroid disease is obvious. False-positive PTH assay results are rare. There are very rare reports of ectopic production of excess PTH by nonparathyroid tumors. Immunoassays for PTHrP are helpful in diagnosing certain types of malignancy-associated hypercalcemia. Although FHH is parathyroid-related, the disease should be managed distinctively from hyperparathyroidism. Clinical features and the low urinary calcium excretion can help make the distinction. Because the

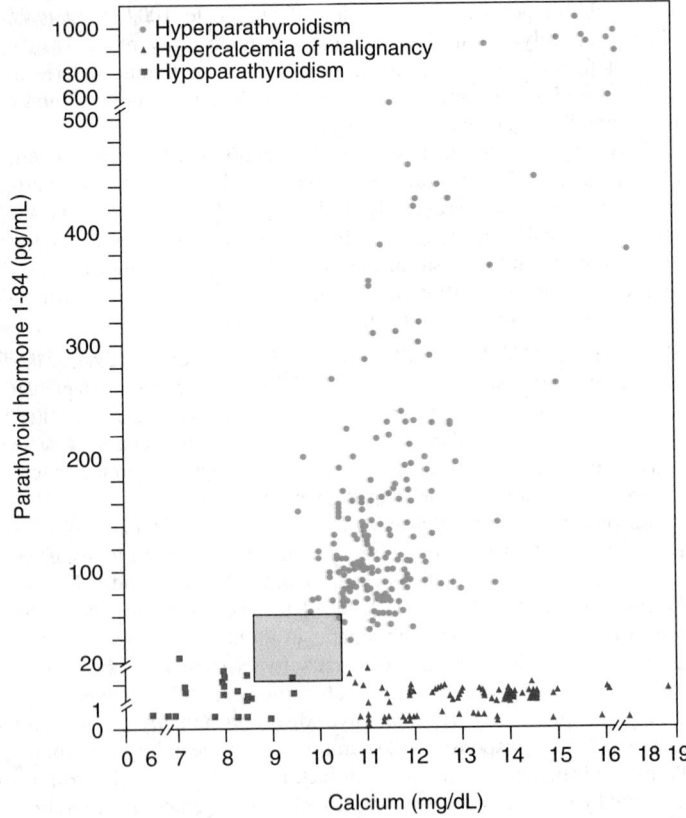

FIGURE 332-6   Levels of immunoreactive parathyroid hormone (PTH) detected in patients with primary hyperparathyroidism, hypercalcemia of malignancy, and hypoparathyroidism. Boxed area represents the upper and normal limits of blood calcium and/or immunoreactive PTH. [*From SR Nussbaum, JT Potts, Jr, in L DeGroot, JL Jameson (eds): Endocrinology, 4th ed. Philadelphia, Saunders, 2001, with permission.*]

incidence of malignancy and hyperparathyroidism both increase with age, they can coexist as two independent causes of hypercalcemia.

1,25$(OH)_2$D levels are elevated in many (but not all) patients with primary hyperparathyroidism. In other disorders associated with hypercalcemia, concentrations of 1,25$(OH)_2$D are low or, at the most, normal. However, this test is of low specificity and is not cost-effective, as not all patients with hyperparathyroidism have elevated 1,25$(OH)_2$D levels, and not all nonparathyroid hypercalcemic patients have suppressed 1,25$(OH)_2$D. Measurement of 1,25$(OH)_2$D is, however, critically valuable in establishing the cause of hypercalcemia in sarcoidosis and certain B cell lymphomas.

A useful general approach is outlined in Fig. 332-5. If the patient is *asymptomatic* and there is evidence of *chronicity* to the hypercalcemia, hyperparathyroidism is almost certainly the cause. If PTH levels (usually measured at least twice) are elevated, the clinical impression is confirmed and little additional evaluation is necessary. If there is only a short history or no data as to the duration of the hypercalcemia, *occult malignancy* must be considered; if the PTH levels are not elevated, then a thorough workup must be undertaken for malignancy, including chest x-ray, CT of chest and abdomen, and bone scan. Immunoassays for PTHrP may be especially useful in such situations. Attention should also be paid to clues for underlying hematologic disorders such as anemia, increased plasma globulin, and abnormal serum immunoelectrophoresis; bone scans can be negative in some patients with metastases, such as in multiple myeloma. Finally, if a patient with chronic hypercalcemia is asymptomatic and malignancy therefore seems unlikely on clinical grounds, but PTH values are not elevated, it is useful to search for other chronic causes of hypercalcemia, such as occult sarcoidosis. A careful history of dietary supplements and drug use may suggest intoxication with vitamin D or vitamin A or the use of thiazides.

℞ TREATMENT

Hypercalcemic States   The approach to medical treatment of hypercalcemia varies with its severity (Table 332-4). Mild hypercalcemia, <3.0 mmol/L (12 mg/dL), can be managed by hydration. More severe hypercalcemia [levels of 3.2 to 3.7 mmol/L (13 to 15 mg/dL)] must be managed aggressively; above that level, hypercalcemia can be life-threatening and requires emergency measures. By using a combination of approaches in severe hypercalcemia, the serum calcium concentration can be decreased by 0.7 to 2.2 mmol/L (3 to 9 mg/dL) within 24 to 48 h in most patients, enough to relieve acute symptoms, prevent death from hypercalcemic crisis, and permit diagnostic evaluation. Therapy can then be directed at the underlying disorder—the second priority.

Hypercalcemia develops because of excessive skeletal calcium release, increased intestinal calcium absorption, or inadequate renal calcium excretion. Understanding the particular pathogenesis helps guide therapy. For example, hypercalcemia in patients with malignancy is primarily due to excessive skeletal calcium release and is, therefore, minimally improved by restriction of dietary calcium. On the other hand, patients with vitamin D hypersensitivity or vitamin D intoxication have excessive intestinal calcium absorption, and restriction of dietary calcium is beneficial. Decreased renal function or ECF depletion decreases urinary calcium excretion. In such situations, rehydration may rapidly reduce or reverse the hypercalcemia, even though increased bone resorption persists. As outlined below, the more severe the hypercalcemia, the greater the number of combined therapies that should be used. Rapid acting (hours) approaches—rehydration, forced diuresis, and calcitonin—can be used with the most effective antiresorptive agents, such as bisphosphonates (since severe hypercalcemia usually involves excessive bone resorption).

HYDRATION, INCREASED SALT INTAKE, MILD AND FORCED DIURESIS   The first principle of treatment is to restore normal hydration. Many hypercalcemic patients are dehydrated because of vomiting, inanition, and/or hypercalcemia-induced defects in urinary concentrating ability. The resultant drop in glomerular filtration rate is accompanied by an additional decrease in renal tubular sodium and calcium clearance. Restoring a normal ECF volume corrects these abnormalities and increases urine calcium excretion by 2.5 to 7.5 mmol/d (100 to 300

TABLE 332-4	Therapies for Severe Hypercalcemia			
Treatment	Onset of Action	Duration of Action	Advantages	Disadvantages
MOST USEFUL THERAPIES				
Hydration with saline	Hours	During infusion	Rehydration invariably needed	Volume overload, cardiac decompensation, intensive monitoring, electrolyte disturbance, inconvenience
Forced diuresis; saline plus loop diuretic	Hours	During treatment	Rapid action	
Bisphosphonates 1st generation: etidronate	1–2 days	5–7 days in doses used	First available bisphosphonate; intermediate onset of action	Less effective than other bisphosphonates
2d generation: pamidronate	1–2 days	10–14 days to weeks	High potency; intermediate onset of action	Fever in 20% hypophosphatemia, hypocalcemia, hypomagnesemia
3d generation: zolendronate	1–2 days	>3 weeks	High potency; rapid infusion; prolonged duration of action	Minor; fever, rarely hypocalcemia or hypophosphatemia
Calcitonin	Hours	1–2 days	Rapid onset of action; useful as adjunct in severe hypercalcemia	Rapid tachyphylaxis
SPECIAL USE THERAPIES				
Phosphate Oral	24 h	During use	Chronic management (with hypophosphatemia); low toxicity if P < 4 mg/dL	Limited use except as adjuvant or chronic therapy
Intravenous	Hours	During use and 24–48 h afterward	Rapid action, highly potent but *rarely used* except with severe hypercalcemia and cardiac and renal decompensation present	Ectopic calcification; renal damage, fatal hypocalcemia
Glucocorticoids	Days	Days, weeks	Oral therapy, antitumor agent	Active only in certain malignancies; glucocorticoid side effects
Dialysis	Hours	During use and 24–48 h afterward	Useful in renal failure; onset of effect in hours; can immediately reverse life-threatening hypercalcemia	Complex procedure, reserved for extreme or special circumstances

mg/d). Increasing urinary sodium excretion to 400 to 500 mmol/d increases urinary calcium excretion even further than simple rehydration. After rehydration has been achieved, saline can be administered or furosemide or ethacrynic acid can be given twice daily to depress the tubular reabsorptive mechanism for calcium (care must be taken to prevent dehydration). The combined use of these therapies can increase urinary calcium excretion to ≥12.5 mmol/d (500 mg/d) in most hypercalcemic patients. Since this is a substantial percentage of the exchangeable calcium pool, the serum calcium concentration usually falls 0.25 to 0.75 mmol/L (1 to 3 mg/dL) within 24 h. Precautions should be taken to prevent potassium and magnesium depletion; calcium-containing renal calculi are a potential complication.

Under life-threatening circumstances, the preceding approach can be pursued more aggressively, giving as much as 6 L isotonic saline (900 mmol sodium) daily plus furosemide or equivalent in doses up to 100 mg every 1 to 2 h or ethacrynic acid in doses to 40 mg every 1 to 2 h. Urinary calcium excretion may exceed 25 mmol/d (1000 mg/d), and the serum calcium may decrease by ≥1 mmol/L (4 mg/dL) within 24 h. Depletion of potassium and magnesium is inevitable unless replacements are given; pulmonary edema can be precipitated. The potential complications can be reduced by careful monitoring of central venous pressure and plasma or urine electrolytes; catheterization of the bladder may be necessary. This treatment approach should be supplemented with agents to block bone resorption. Though these agents do not become effective for several days, forced diuresis is difficult to sustain even in patients with good cardiopulmonary and renal function.

BISPHOSPHONATES The bisphosphonates are analogues of pyrophosphate, with high affinity for bone, especially in areas of increased bone turnover, where they are powerful inhibitors of bone resorption. These bone-seeking compounds are stable in vivo because phosphatase enzymes cannot hydrolyze the central carbon-phosphorus-carbon bond. The bisphosphonates are concentrated in areas of high bone turnover and are taken up by and inhibit osteoclast action; the mechanism of action is complex. Bisphosphonates alter osteoclast proton pump function or impair the release of acid hydrolases into the extracellular lysosomes contiguous with mineralized bone. They may also inhibit the differentiation of monocyte-macrophage precursors into osteoclasts and possibly have effects on osteoblasts as well. The bisphosphonate molecules that contain amino groups in the side chain structure (see below) interfere with prenylation of proteins and can lead to cellular apoptosis. The highly active non-amino group–containing bisphosphonates are also metabolized to cytotoxic products.

The initial bisphosphonate widely used in clinical practice, etidronate, was effective but had several disadvantages, including the capacity to inhibit bone formation as well as blocking resorption. Subsequently, a number of second-generation compounds have become the mainstays of antiresorptive therapy for treatment of hypercalcemia and osteoporosis. The newer bisphosphonates have a highly favorable ratio of blocking resorption versus inhibiting bone formation; they inhibit osteoclast-mediated skeletal resorption yet do not cause mineralization defects at ordinary doses. Though the bisphosphonates have similar structures, the routes of administration, efficacy, toxicity, and side effects vary. The potency of the compounds for inhibition of bone resorption varies a thousandfold, increasing in the order of etidronate, tiludronate, pamidronate, alendronate, and risedronate. Oral alendronate and risedronate are approved for the therapy of osteoporosis in the United States, but in Europe only for the chronic treatment of hypercalcemia. Only the intravenous use of pamidronate is approved for the treatment of hypercalcemia in the United States; between 30 and 90 mg pamidronate, given as a single intravenous dose over a few hours, returns serum calcium to normal within 24 to 48 h with an effect that lasts for weeks in 80 to 100% of patients.

Even more potent third-generation bisphosphonates have been recently introduced into clinical practice. Zolendronate, said to be sev-

eralfold more potent than second-generation compounds, is reported in preliminary trials to be superior in treatment of hypercalcemia, normalizing calcium faster and for longer periods of time after infusion. Doses of 1 to 4 mg can be given over a few minutes intravenously.

CALCITONIN Calcitonin acts within a few hours of its administration, through receptors on osteoclasts, to block bone resorption and, in addition, to increase urinary calcium excretion by inhibition of renal tubular calcium reabsorption. Results with calcitonin, particularly after 24 h of use, are variable, with minimal lowering of calcium. Tachyphylaxis, a known phenomenon with this drug, may explain the results. However, in life-threatening hypercalcemia, calcitonin can be used effectively within the first 24 h in combination with rehydration and saline diuresis while waiting for more sustained effects from a simultaneously administered bisphosphonate such as pamidronate. Usual doses of calcitonin are 2 to 8 U/kg of body weight intravenously, subcutaneously, or intramuscularly every 6 to 12 h.

OTHER THERAPIES Plicamycin (formerly mithramycin), which inhibits bone resorption, has been a useful therapeutic agent but is now seldom used because of its toxicity and the effectiveness of bisphosphonates. Plicamycin must be given intravenously, either as a bolus or by slow infusion; the usual dose is 25 μg/kg body weight. Gallium nitrate exerts a hypocalcemic action by inhibiting bone resorption and altering the structure of bone crystals. It is not often used now because of superior alternatives.

Glucocorticoids have utility, especially in hypercalcemia complicating certain malignancies. They increase urinary calcium excretion and decrease intestinal calcium absorption when given in pharmacologic doses, but they also cause negative skeletal calcium balance. In normal individuals and in patients with primary hyperparathyroidism, glucocorticoids neither increase nor decrease the serum calcium concentration. In patients with hypercalcemia due to certain osteolytic malignancies, however, glucocorticoids may be effective as a result of antitumor effects. The malignancies in which hypercalcemia responds to glucocorticoids include multiple myeloma, leukemia, Hodgkin's disease, other lymphomas, and carcinoma of the breast, at least early in the course of the disease. Glucocorticoids are also effective in treating hypercalcemia due to vitamin D intoxication and sarcoidosis. In all the preceding situations, the hypocalcemic effect develops over several days, and the usual glucocorticoid dosage is 40 to 100 mg prednisone (or its equivalent) daily in four divided doses. The side effects of chronic glucocorticoid therapy may be acceptable in some circumstances.

Dialysis is often the treatment of choice for severe hypercalcemia complicated by renal failure, which is difficult to manage medically. Peritoneal dialysis with calcium-free dialysis fluid can remove 5 to 12.5 mmol (200 to 500 mg) of calcium in 24 to 48 h and lower the serum calcium concentration by 0.7 to 3 mmol/L (3 to 12 mg/dL). Large quantities of phosphate are lost during dialysis, and serum inorganic phosphate concentrations usually fall, thus aggravating hypercalcemia. Therefore, the serum inorganic phosphate concentration should be measured after dialysis, and phosphate supplements should be added to the diet or to dialysis fluids if necessary.

Phosphate therapy, oral or intravenous, has a limited role in certain circumstances. Correcting hypophosphatemia lowers the serum calcium concentration by several mechanisms, including bone/calcium exchange. The usual oral treatment is 1 to 1.5 g phosphorus per day for several days, given in divided doses. It is generally believed, but not established, that toxicity does not occur if therapy is limited to restoring serum inorganic phosphate concentrations to normal.

Raising the serum inorganic phosphate concentration above normal decreases serum calcium levels, sometimes strikingly. Intravenous phosphate is one of the most dramatically effective treatments available for severe hypercalcemia but is toxic and even dangerous (fatal hypocalcemia). For these reasons, it is used rarely and only in severely hypercalcemic patients with cardiac or renal failure. A phosphate phosphorus dose of ≥1500 mg intravenously over 6 to 8 h leads to a prompt decrease in serum calcium of as much as 1.2 to 2.5 mmol/L (5 to 10 mg/dL) in patients with initially normal serum inorganic phosphate concentrations. This therapy should be employed only in extreme emergencies. Inorganic phosphate is commercially available for oral use in liquid, powder, and capsule form and as a liquid for intravenous use. If used, it is important to calculate doses in terms of phosphate phosphorus.

Summary The various therapies for hypercalcemia are listed in Table 332-4. The choice depends on the underlying disease, the severity of the hypercalcemia, the serum inorganic phosphate level, and the renal, hepatic, and bone marrow function. Mild hypercalcemia [≤3 mmol/L (12 mg/dL)] can usually be managed by hydration. Severe hypercalcemia [≥3.7 mmol/L (15 mg/dL)] requires rapid correction. Calcitonin should be given for its rapid, albeit short-lived, blockade of bone resorption, and intravenous pamidronate or zolendronate should be administered, although its onset of action is delayed for 1 to 2 days. In addition, for the first 24 to 48 h, aggressive sodium-calcium diuresis with intravenous saline and large doses of furosemide or ethacrynic acid following initial hydration should be initiated, but only if appropriate monitoring is available and cardiac and renal function are adequate. Otherwise, dialysis may be necessary. Intermediate degrees of hypercalcemia between 3.0 and 3.7 mmol/L (12 and 15 mg/dL) should be approached with vigorous hydration and then the most appropriate selection for the patient of the combinations used with severe hypercalcemia.

HYPOCALCEMIA

PATHOPHYSIOLOGY OF HYPOCALCEMIA: CLASSIFICATION BASED ON MECHANISM
Chronic hypocalcemia is less common than hypercalcemia; causes include chronic renal failure, hereditary and acquired hypoparathyroidism, vitamin D deficiency, PHP, and hypomagnesemia.

Acute rather than chronic hypocalcemia is seen in critically ill patients or as a consequence of certain medications and often does not require specific treatment. Transient hypocalcemia is seen with severe sepsis, burns, acute renal failure, and extensive transfusions with citrated blood. Although as many as half of patients in an intensive care setting are reported to have calcium concentrations <2.1 mmol/L (8.5 mg/dL), most do not have a reduction in ionized calcium. Patients with severe sepsis may have a decrease in ionized calcium (true hypocalcemia), but in other severely ill individuals, hypoalbuminemia is the primary cause of the reduced total calcium concentration. Alkalosis increases calcium binding to proteins, and in this setting direct measurements of ionized calcium should be made.

Medications such as protamine, heparin, and glucagon may cause transient hypocalcemia. These forms of hypocalcemia are usually not associated with tetany and resolve with improvement in the overall medical condition. The hypocalcemia after repeated transfusions of citrated blood usually resolves quickly.

Patients with *acute pancreatitis* have hypocalcemia that persists during the acute inflammation and varies in degree with the severity of the pancreatitis. The cause of hypocalcemia remains unclear. PTH values are reported to be low, normal, or elevated, and both resistance to PTH and impaired PTH secretion have been postulated. Occasionally, a chronic low total calcium and low ionized calcium concentration are detected in an elderly patient without obvious cause and with a paucity of symptoms; the pathogenesis is unclear.

Chronic hypocalcemia, however, is usually symptomatic and requires treatment. Neuromuscular and neurologic manifestations of chronic hypocalcemia include muscle spasms, carpopedal spasm, facial grimacing, and, in extreme cases, laryngeal spasm and convulsions. Respiratory arrest may occur. Increased intracranial pressure occurs in some patients with long-standing hypocalcemia, often in association with papilledema. Mental changes include irritability, depression, and psychosis. The QT interval on the electrocardiogram is prolonged, in contrast to its shortening with hypercalcemia. Arrhythmias occur, and digitalis effectiveness may be reduced. Intestinal cramps and chronic malabsorption may occur. Chvostek's or Trousseau's sign can be used to confirm latent tetany.

The classification of hypocalcemia shown in Table 332-5 is based on an organizationally useful premise that PTH is responsible for minute-to-minute regulation of plasma calcium concentration and, therefore, that the occurrence of hypocalcemia must mean a failure of the homeostatic action of PTH. Failure of the PTH response can occur if there is hereditary or acquired parathyroid gland failure, if PTH is ineffective in target organs, or if the action of the hormone is overwhelmed by the loss of calcium from the ECF at a rate faster than it can be replaced.

PTH ABSENT Whether hereditary or acquired, hypoparathyroidism has a number of common components. Symptoms of untreated hypocalcemia are shared by both types of hypoparathyroidism, although the onset of hereditary hypoparathyroidism is more gradual and is often associated with other developmental defects. Basal ganglia calcification and extrapyramidal syndromes are more common and earlier in onset in hereditary hypoparathyroidism. In earlier decades, acquired hypoparathyroidism secondary to surgery in the neck was more common than hereditary hypoparathyroidism, but the frequency of surgically induced parathyroid failure has diminished as a result of improved surgical techniques that spare the parathyroid glands and increased use of nonsurgical therapy for hyperthyroidism. PHP, an example of ineffective PTH action rather than a failure of parathyroid gland production, may share several features with hypoparathyroidism, including extraosseous calcification and extrapyramidal manifestations such as choreoathetotic movements and dystonia.

Papilledema and raised intracranial pressure may occur in both hereditary and acquired hypoparathyroidism, as do chronic changes in fingernails and hair and lenticular cataracts, the latter usually reversible with treatment of hypocalcemia. Certain skin manifestations, including alopecia and candidiasis, are characteristic of hereditary hypoparathyroidism associated with autoimmune polyglandular failure (Chap. 330).

Hypocalcemia associated with hypomagnesemia is associated with both deficient PTH release and impaired responsiveness to the hormone. Patients with hypocalcemia secondary to hypomagnesemia have absent or low levels of circulating PTH, indicative of diminished hormone release despite maximum physiologic stimulus by hypocalcemia. Plasma PTH levels return to normal with correction of the hypomagnesemia. Thus hypoparathyroidism with low levels of PTH in blood can be due to hereditary gland failure, acquired gland failure, or acute but reversible gland dysfunction (hypomagnesemia).

Genetic Abnormalities and Hereditary Hypoparathyroidism Hereditary hypoparathyroidism can occur as an isolated entity without other endocrine or dermatologic manifestations (idiopathic hypoparathyroidism).

TABLE 332-5 *Functional Classification of Hypocalcemia (Excluding Neonatal Conditions)*

PTH ABSENT	
Hereditary hypoparathyroidism Acquired hypoparathyroidism	Hypomagnesemia

PTH INEFFECTIVE	

Chronic renal failure
Active vitamin D lacking
  ↓ Dietary intake or sunlight
Defective metabolism:
  Anticonvulsant therapy
  Vitamin D–dependent
  rickets type I
	Active vitamin D ineffective
	Intestinal malabsorption
	Vitamin D–dependent rickets
	  type II
	Pseudohypoparathyroidism

PTH OVERWHELMED	

Severe, acute hyperphosphatemia
  Tumor lysis
  Acute renal failure
  Rhabdomyolysis
	Osteitis fibrosa after
	  parathyroidectomy

Note: PTH, parathyroid hormone.

More typically, it occurs in association with other abnormalities such as defective development of the thymus or failure of other endocrine organs such as the adrenal, thyroid, or ovary (Chap. 330). Idiopathic and hereditary hypoparathyroidism are often manifest within the first decade but may appear later.

A rare form of hypoparathyroidism associated with defective development of both the thymus and the parathyroid glands is termed the *DiGeorge syndrome*, or the *velocardiofacial syndrome*. Congenital cardiovascular, facial, and other developmental defects are present, and most patients die in early childhood with severe infections, hypocalcemia and seizures, or cardiovascular complications. Some survive into adulthood, and milder, incomplete forms occur. Most cases are sporadic, but an autosomal dominant form involving microdeletions of chromosome 22q11.2 has been described. Smaller deletions in this region are seen in incomplete forms of the DiGeorge syndrome, appearing in childhood or adolescence, that are manifest primarily by parathyroid gland failure.

Hypoparathyroidism can occur in association with a complex hereditary autoimmune syndrome involving failure of the adrenals, the ovaries, the immune system, and the parathyroids in association with recurrent mucocutaneous candidiasis, alopecia, vitiligo, and pernicious anemia (Chap. 330). The responsible gene on chromosome 21q22.3 has been identified. The protein product, which resembles a transcription factor, has been termed the *autoimmune regulator*, or AIRE. A stop codon mutation occurs in many Finnish families with the disorder, commonly referred to as *polyglandular autoimmune type 1 deficiency*.

Gain-of-function mutations in the calcium-sensing receptor cause *autosomal dominant hypocalcemia*. These mutations induce constitutive receptor functions that lead to features that are the inverse of FHH. The activated receptor suppresses PTH secretion, leading to hypocalcemia; receptor activation in the kidney results in excessive renal calcium excretion. Recognition of the syndrome is important because efforts to treat the hypocalcemia of these patients with vitamin D analogues and increased oral calcium exacerbate the already excessive urinary calcium secretion (several grams or more per 24 h), leading to irreversible renal damage from stones and ectopic calcification.

Hypoparathyroidism is seen in two disorders associated with mitochondrial dysfunction and myopathy, one termed the *Kearns-Sayre syndrome* (KSS), with ophthalmplegia and pigmentary retinopathy, and the other termed the *MELAS syndrome*, *m*itochondrial *e*ncephalopathy, *l*actic *a*cidosis, and *s*troke-like episodes. Mutations or deletions in mitochondrial genes have been identified.

The two other rare forms of hypoparathyroidism with other multisystem developmental abnormalities follow either an autosomal dominant pattern, with deafness and/or renal dysplasia, or an autosomal recessive pattern, with growth retardation and dysmorphic features.

Hereditary hypoparathyroidism occurs also as an isolated entity without any other defects. The pattern of inheritance varies and includes autosomal dominant, autosomal recessive, and X-linked inheritance patterns. In one family in which the disorder is transmitted as an autosomal dominant trait, a structural abnormality in the PTH gene has been identified. A defect in the signal sequence needed for processing of the hormone impairs PTH secretion. In another kindred with autosomal recessive inheritance, the mutant allele in the first intron of the PTH gene causes a splicing defect in mRNA production. An X-linked recessive form of hypoparathyroidism has been described in males and the defect has been localized to chromosome Xq26-q27.

Acquired Hypoparathyroidism *Acquired chronic hypoparathyroidism* is usually the result of inadvertent surgical removal of all the parathyroid glands; in some instances, not all the tissue is removed, but the remainder undergoes vascular supply compromise secondary to fibrotic changes in the neck after surgery. In the past, the most frequent cause of acquired hypoparathyroidism was surgery for hyperthyroidism. Hypoparathyroidism now usually occurs after surgery for hyperparathy-

roidism when the surgeon, facing the dilemma of removing too little tissue and thus not curing the hyperparathyroidism, removes too much. Parathyroid function may not be totally absent in all patients with postoperative hypoparathyroidism.

Even rarer causes of acquired chronic hypoparathyroidism include radiation-induced damage subsequent to radioiodine therapy of hyperthyroidism and glandular damage in patients with hemochromatosis or hemosiderosis after repeated blood transfusions. Infection may involve one or more of the parathyroids but usually does not cause hypoparathyroidism because all four glands are rarely involved.

Transient hypoparathyroidism is frequent following surgery for hyperparathyroidism. After a variable period of hypoparathyroidism, normal parathyroid function may return due to hyperplasia or recovery of remaining tissue. Occasionally, recovery occurs months after surgery.

℞ TREATMENT

Treatment of acquired and hereditary hypoparathyroidism involves replacement with vitamin D or $1,25(OH)_2D_3$ (calcitriol) combined with a high oral calcium intake. In most patients, blood calcium and phosphate levels are satisfactorily regulated, but some patients show resistance and a brittleness, with a tendency to alternate between hypocalcemia and hypercalcemia. For many patients, vitamin D in doses of 40,000 to 120,000 U/d (1 to 3 mg/d) combined with ≥ 1 g elemental calcium is satisfactory. The wide dosage range reflects the variation encountered from patient to patient; precise regulation of each patient is required. Compared to typical daily requirements in euparathyroid patients of 200 U/d, the high dose of vitamin D reflects the reduced conversion of vitamin D to $1,25(OH)_2D$. Many physicians now use 0.5 to 1.0 μg of calcitriol in management of such patients, especially if they are difficult to control. Because of its storage in fat, when vitamin D is withdrawn, weeks are required for the disappearance of the biologic effects, compared with a few days for calcitriol, which has a rapid turnover.

Oral calcium and vitamin D restore the overall calcium-phosphate balance but do not reverse the lowered urinary calcium reabsorption typical of hypoparathyroidism. Therefore, care must be taken to avoid excessive urinary calcium excretion after vitamin D and calcium replacement therapy; otherwise, kidney stones can develop. Thiazide diuretics lower urine calcium by as much as 100 mg/d in hypoparathyroid patients on vitamin D, provided they are maintained on a low-sodium diet. Use of thiazides seems to be of benefit in mitigating hypercalciuria and easing the daily management of these patients.

Hypomagnesemia Severe hypomagnesemia (<0.4 mmol/L; <0.8 meq/L) is associated with hypocalcemia (Chap. 331). Restoration of the total-body magnesium deficit leads to rapid reversal of hypocalcemia. There are at least two causes of the hypocalcemia—impaired PTH secretion and reduced responsiveness to PTH. →*For discussion of causes and treatment of hypomagnesemia, see Chap. 331.*

The effects of magnesium on PTH secretion are similar to those of calcium; hypermagnesemia suppresses and hypomagnesemia stimulates PTH secretion. The effects of magnesium on PTH secretion are normally of little significance, however, because the calcium effects dominate. Greater change in magnesium than in calcium is needed to influence hormone secretion. Nonetheless, hypomagnesemia might be expected to increase hormone secretion. It is therefore surprising to find that severe hypomagnesemia is associated with blunted secretion of PTH. The explanation for the paradox is that severe, chronic hypomagnesemia leads to intracellular magnesium deficiency, which interferes with secretion and peripheral responses to PTH. The mechanism of the cellular abnormalities caused by hypomagnesemia is unknown, although effects on adenylate cyclase (for which magnesium is a cofactor) have been proposed.

PTH levels are undetectable or inappropriately low in severe hypomagnesemia despite the stimulus of severe hypocalcemia, and acute repletion of magnesium leads to a rapid increase in PTH level. Serum phosphate levels are often not elevated, in contrast to the situation with acquired or idiopathic hypoparathyroidism, probably because phosphate deficiency is a frequent accompaniment of hypomagnesemia.

Diminished peripheral responsiveness to PTH also occurs in some patients, as documented by subnormal response in urinary phosphorus and urinary cyclic AMP excretion after administration of exogenous PTH to patients who are hypocalcemic and hypomagnesemic. Both blunted PTH secretion and lack of renal response to administered PTH can occur in the same patient. When acute magnesium repletion is undertaken, the restoration of PTH levels to normal or supranormal may precede restoration of normal serum calcium by several days.

℞ TREATMENT

Repletion of magnesium cures the condition. Repletion should be parenteral. Attention must be given to restoring the intracellular deficit, which may be considerable. After intravenous magnesium administration, serum magnesium may return transiently to the normal range, but unless replacement therapy is adequate serum magnesium will again fall. If the cause of the hypomagnesemia is renal magnesium wasting, magnesium may have to be given chronically to prevent recurrence (Chap. 331).

PTH INEFFECTIVE PTH is ineffective when the hormone receptor–guanyl nucleotide–binding protein complex is defective (PHP, discussed below), when PTH action to promote calcium absorption from the diet is impaired because of vitamin D deficiency or because vitamin D is ineffective (receptor or synthesis defects), or in chronic renal failure in which the calcium-elevating action of PTH is impaired.

Typically, hypophosphatemia is more severe than hypocalcemia in vitamin D deficiency states because of the increased secretion of PTH, which, although only partly effective in elevating blood calcium, is capable of promoting phosphaturia.

PHP, on the other hand, has a pathophysiology different from the other disorders of ineffective PTH action. PHP resembles hypoparathyroidism (in which PTH synthesis is deficient) and is manifested by hypocalcemia and hyperphosphatemia. The cause of the disorder is defective hormone activation of guanyl nucleotide–binding proteins, resulting in failure of PTH to increase intracellular cyclic AMP (see below).

Chronic Renal Failure Improved medical management of chronic renal failure now allows many patients to survive for years and hence time enough to develop features of renal osteodystrophy, which must be controlled to avoid its morbidity. Phosphate retention and impaired production of $1,25(OH)_2D$ are the principal factors that cause calcium deficiency, secondary hyperparathyroidism, and bone disease. Low levels of $1,25(OH)_2D$ due to hyperphosphatemia and destruction of renal tissue are critical in the development of hypocalcemia. The uremic state also causes impairment of intestinal absorption by mechanisms other than defects in vitamin D metabolism. Nonetheless, treatment with supraphysiologic amounts of vitamin D or calcitriol corrects the impaired calcium absorption.

Hyperphosphatemia in renal failure lowers blood calcium levels by several mechanisms, including extraosseous deposition of calcium and phosphate, impairment of the bone-resorbing action of PTH, and reduction in $1,25(OH)_2D$ production by remaining renal tissue.

℞ TREATMENT

Therapy of chronic renal failure (Chap. 261) involves appropriate management of patients prior to dialysis and adjustment of regimens once dialysis is initiated. Attention should be paid to restriction of phosphate in the diet; avoidance of aluminum-containing phosphate-binding antacids to prevent the problem of aluminum intoxication; provision of an adequate calcium intake by mouth, usually 1 to 2 g/d; and supplementation with 0.25 to 1.0 μg/d calcitriol. Each patient must be monitored closely. The aim of therapy is to restore normal calcium balance to prevent osteomalacia and secondary hyperparathyroidism and, in light of evidence of genetic changes and monoclonal outgrowths of parathyroid glands in renal failure patients, to prevent sec-

ondary from becoming autonomous hyperparathyroidism. Reduction of hyperphosphatemia and restoration of normal intestinal calcium absorption by calcitriol can improve blood calcium levels and reduce the manifestations of secondary hyperparathyroidism. Since adynamic bone disease can occur in association with low PTH levels, it is important to avoid excessive suppression of the parathyroid glands while recognizing the beneficial effects of controlling the secondary hyperparathyroidism. These patients should probably be closely monitored with PTH assays that detect only the full-length PTH(1–84) to ensure that biologically active PTH and not inactive, inhibitory PTH fragments are measured.

Vitamin D Deficiency Due to Inadequate Diet and/or Sunlight Vitamin D deficiency due to inadequate intake of dairy products enriched with vitamin D, lack of vitamin supplementation, and reduced sunlight exposure in the elderly, particularly during winter in northern latitudes, is more common in the United States than previously recognized. Biopsies of bone in elderly patients with hip fracture (documenting osteomalacia) and abnormal levels of vitamin D metabolites, PTH, calcium, and phosphate indicate that vitamin D deficiency may occur in as many as 25% of elderly patients, particularly in northern latitudes in the United States. Concentrations of 25(OH)D are low or low-normal in these patients. Quantitative histomorphometry of bone biopsy specimens reveals widened osteoid seams consistent with osteomalacia (Chap. 331). PTH hypersecretion compensates for the tendency for the blood calcium to fall but also induces renal phosphate wasting and results in osteomalacia.

Treatment involves adequate replacement with vitamin D and calcium until the deficiencies are corrected. Severe hypocalcemia rarely occurs in moderately severe vitamin D deficiency of the elderly, but vitamin D deficiency must be considered in the differential diagnosis of mild hypocalcemia.

Defective Vitamin D Metabolism ■ *ANTICONVULSANT THERAPY* Anticonvulsant therapy with any of several agents induces acquired vitamin D deficiency by increasing the conversion of vitamin D to inactive compounds. The more marginal the vitamin D intake in the diet, the more likely that anticonvulsant therapy will lead to abnormal mineral and bone metabolism →***For discussion of treatment, see Chap. 331.***

VITAMIN D–DEPENDENT RICKETS TYPE I Rickets can be due to *resistance to the action* of vitamin D as well as to vitamin D deficiency. Vitamin D–dependent rickets type I, previously termed *pseudo-vitamin D–resistant rickets*, differs from true vitamin D–resistant rickets (vitamin D-dependent rickets type II, see below) in that it is less severe and the biochemical and radiographic abnormalities can be reversed with appropriate doses of the vitamin or the active metabolite, $1,25(OH)_2D_3$. Physiologic amounts of calcitriol cure the disease (Chap. 331). This finding fits with the pathophysiology of the disorder, which is autosomal recessive, and is now known to be caused by mutations in the gene encoding 25(OH)D-1α-hydroxylase. Both alleles are inactivated in all patients, and compound heterozygotes, harboring distinct mutations, are common.

Clinical features include hypocalcemia, often with tetany or convulsions, hypophosphatemia, secondary hyperparathyroidism, and osteomalacia, often associated with skeletal deformities and increased alkaline phosphatase. Treatment involves physiologic replacement doses of $1,25(OH)_2D_3$ (Chap. 331).

Vitamin D Ineffective ■ *INTESTINAL MALABSORPTION* Mild hypocalcemia, secondary hyperparathyroidism, severe hypophosphatemia, and a variety of nutritional deficiencies occur with gastrointestinal diseases. Hepatocellular dysfunction can lead to reduction in 25(OH)D levels, as in portal or biliary cirrhosis of the liver, and malabsorption of vitamin D and its metabolites, including $1,25(OH)_2D$, may occur in a variety of bowel diseases, hereditary or acquired. Hypocalcemia itself can lead to steatorrhea, due to deficient production of pancreatic enzymes and bile salts. Depending on the disorder, vitamin D or its

TABLE 332-6 *Classification of Pseudohypoparathyroidism (PHP) and Pseudopseudohypoparathyroidism (PPHP)*

Type	Hypocalcemia, Hyperphosphatemia	Response of Urinary cAMP to PTH	Serum PTH	$G_{s}\alpha$ Subunit Deficiency	AHO	Resistance to Hormones in Addition to PTH
PHP-Ia	Yes	↓	↑	Yes	Yes	Yes
PHP-Ib	Yes	↓	↑	No	No	No
PHP-II	Yes	Normal	↑	No	No	No
PPHP	No	Normal	Normal	Yes	Yes	±

Note: ↓, decreased; ↑, increased; AHO, Albright's hereditary osteodystrophy; PTH, parathyroid hormone.

metabolites can be given parenterally, guaranteeing adequate blood levels of active metabolites.

VITAMIN D–DEPENDENT RICKETS TYPE II Vitamin D–dependent rickets type II results from end-organ resistance to the active metabolite $1,25(OH)_2D_3$. The clinical features resemble those of the type I disorder and include hypocalcemia, hypophosphatemia, secondary hyperparathyroidism, and rickets but also partial or total alopecia. Plasma levels of $1,25(OH)_2D$ are at least three times normal, in keeping with the refractoriness of the end organs. All of the genetically characterized phenotypes have mutations in the gene for the vitamin D receptor. Treatment is difficult, given the receptor defect (Chap. 331).

Pseudohypoparathyroidism PHP is a hereditary disorder characterized by symptoms and signs of hypoparathyroidism, typically in association with distinctive skeletal and developmental defects. The hypoparathyroidism is due to a deficient end-organ response to PTH. Hyperplasia of the parathyroids, a response to hormone resistance, causes elevation of PTH levels. Studies, both clinical and basic, have clarified some aspects of this syndrome, including the variable clinical spectrum, the pathophysiology, the genetic defects, and the inheritance.

A working classification of the various forms of PHP is given in Table 332-6. The classification scheme is based on the signs of ineffective PTH action (low calcium and high phosphate), urinary cyclic AMP response to exogenous PTH, the presence or absence of *Albright's hereditary osteodystrophy* (AHO), and assays of the concentration of the $G_{s}\alpha$ subunit of the adenylate cyclase enzyme. Using these criteria, there are four types: PHP type I, subdivided into a and b categories; PHP-II; and pseudopseudohypoparathyroidism (PPHP).

PHP-IA AND PHP-IB Individuals with PHP-I, the most common of the disorders, show a deficient urinary cyclic AMP response to administration of exogenous PTH. Patients with PHP-I are divided into type a, who have reduced amounts of $G_{s}\alpha$ in vitro assays with erythrocytes, and type b, with normal amounts of $G_{s}\alpha$ in erythrocytes. There is a third type (PHP-Ic, reported in a few patients) that differs from PHP-Ia only in having normal erythroycte levels of $G_{s}\alpha$ despite having AHO, hypocalcemia, and decreased urinary cyclic AMP responses to PTH (presumably with a post-$G_{s}\alpha$ defect in adenyl cyclase stimulation).

Most patients show characteristic features of AHO, consisting of short stature, round face, skeletal anomalies (brachydactyly), and heterotopic calcification. Patients have low calcium and high phosphate levels, as with true hypoparathyroidism. PTH levels, however, are elevated, reflecting resistance to hormone action.

Amorphous deposits of calcium and phosphate are found in the basal ganglia in about half of patients. The defects in metacarpal and metatarsal bones are sometimes accompanied by short phalanges as well, possibly reflecting premature closing of the epiphyses. The typical findings are short fourth and fifth metacarpals and metatarsals. The defects are usually bilateral. Exostoses and radius curvus are frequent. Impairments in olfaction and taste and unusual dermatoglyphic abnormalities have been reported.

PPHP Multiple defects have now been identified in the *GNAS-1* gene in PHP-Ia and PPHP patients. This gene, which is located on chromosome 20q13, encodes the stimulatory G protein subunit $G_{s}\alpha$, among other products (see below). Mutations include abnormalities in splice junctions associated with deficient mRNA production and point mu-

tations that result in a protein with defective function as well as a 50% reduction in $G_{s}\alpha$ levels in erythrocytes.

Detailed analyses of disease transmission in affected kindreds have clarified many features of PHP-Ia, PPHP, and PHP-Ib (Fig. 332-7). The former two entities, traced through multiple kindreds, have an inheritance pattern consistent with gene imprinting—only females, not males, can transmit the full disease with hypocalcemia—and PHP and PPHP do not coexist in the same generation. The phenomenon of gene imprinting involves selective inactivation of either the maternal or the paternal allele (Chap. 56). In the case of the $G_{s}\alpha$ gene, it is paternally imprinted (silenced) so that the disease PHP-Ia is never inherited from the father carrying the defective allele but only from the mother. On the other hand, the defective allele is not imprinted or silenced in all tissues. It seems possible, therefore, that the AHO phenotype recognized in PPHP as well as PHP-Ia reflects haplotype insufficiency during embryonic development. In the renal cortex, however, it is postulated that only the maternal allele is normally active, such that lack of activity from a defective paternal allele is not of consequence. This explains the occurrence in PHP-Ia of hypocalcemia, hyperphosphatemia, and other stigmata such as variable resistance to other hormones (if similar tissue-specific imprinting occurs in other organs). Strong evidence favoring this overall hypothesis comes from gene knockout studies in the mouse (ablating exon 2 of the gene). Mice inheriting the mutant allele from the female had undetectable $G_{s}\alpha$ protein in renal cortex and were hypocalcemic and resistant to renal actions of PTH. Offspring inheriting the mutant allele from the male showed no evidence of PTH resistance or hypercalcemia.

The complex mechanisms that control the *GNAS-1* gene also contribute to challenges involved in unraveling the pathogenesis of these disorders. Alternative splicing patterns produce three different transcripts that encode distinct proteins. In addition to $G_{s}\alpha$, this gene encodes a second protein product with a unique NH_2-terminus (the XL exon); $XL_{\alpha}s$ includes exons 2–13. It is unknown whether this protein can function as a stimulatory G protein, but the mRNA encoding it is

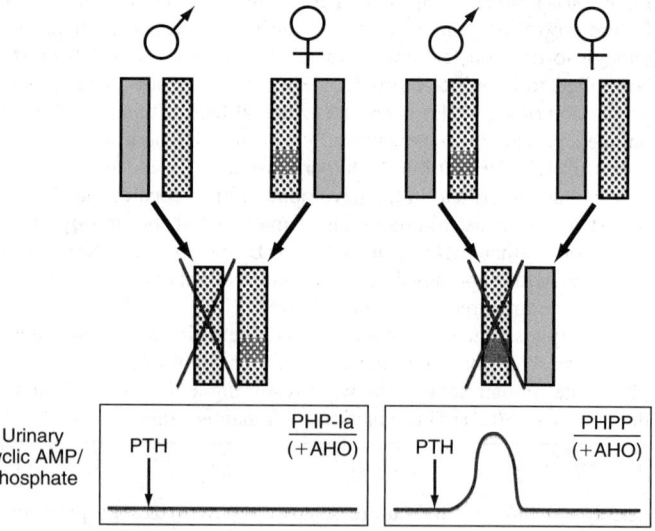

FIGURE 332-7 Paternal imprinting of renal parathyroid hormone (PTH) resistance (*GNAS-1* gene for $G_{s}\alpha$ subunit) in pseudohypoparathyroidism (PHP). An impaired excretion of urinary cyclic AMP and phosphate is observed in patients with PHP. In the renal cortex, there is selective silencing of the paternal $G_{s}\alpha$ gene mRNA. The disease becomes manifest only in patients who inherit the defective gene from an obligate female carrier (*left*). If the genetic defect is inherited from an obligate male gene carrier, there is no biochemical abnormality; administration of PTH causes an appropriate increase in the urinary cyclic AMP and phosphate concentration [pseudo-PHP (PPHP)]; *right*]. Both patterns of inheritance lead to Albright's hereditary osteodystrophy (AHO), perhaps because of haplotype insufficiency—i.e., both copies of $G_{s}\alpha$ must be active in the fetus for normal bone development.

expressed in numerous endocrine tissues and is transcribed from only the paternal allele. A third transcript is transcribed from only the maternal allele and encodes the protein product, NESP55, which contains no homology with $XL_\alpha s$ or $G_s\alpha$.

PHP-Ib, lacking the AHO phenotype, shares with PHP-Ia the resistance to PTH action and a blunted urinary cyclic AMP response to administered PTH, a standard test for hormone resistance (Table 332-6). PHP-Ib patients, however, show normal levels of $G_s\alpha$ in erythrocytes. Bone responsiveness may be excessive rather than blunted in PHP-Ib compared to PHP-Ia patients, based on case reports that have emphasized an osteitis fibrosa–like pattern in some PHP patients who lack the AHO phenotype. The inheritance patterns in PHP-Ib kindreds are clearly consistent with paternal imprinting and lack male transmission of symptomatic disease; gene cloning studies have narrowed the responsible region to chromosome 20, close to—if not within—the *GNAS-1* gene locus. Elucidation of the responsible genetic and pathogenetic mechanisms in this disorder may further illuminate the function of the complex *GNAS-1* gene and the role of its products in hormonal signaling.

PHP-II refers to patients with hypocalcemia and hyperphosphatemia who have a normal urinary cyclic AMP response to PTH. These patients are assumed to have a defect in the response to PTH at a locus distal to cyclic AMP production, although at least some patients may instead have occult vitamin D deficiency.

The diagnosis of these hormone-resistant states can usually be made without difficulty when there is a positive family history for developmental defects and/or the presence of developmental anomalies, including brachydactyly, in association with the signs and symptoms of hypoparathyroidism. In all categories—PHP-Ia, -Ib, and -II—serum PTH levels are elevated, particularly when patients are hypocalcemic. However, patients with PHP-Ib or PHP-II do not have phenotypic abnormalities, only hypocalcemia with high PTH levels, confirming hormone resistance. In PHP-Ib, the response of urinary cyclic AMP to the administration of exogenous PTH is blunted. Levels of $G_s\alpha$ subunits in erythrocyte membranes are, however, normal in those with PHP-Ib. The diagnosis of PHP-II is more complex, in that cyclic AMP responses in urine are, by definition, normal. Since vitamin D deficiency itself can dissociate phosphaturic and urinary cyclic AMP responses to exogenous PTH, vitamin D deficiency must be excluded before the diagnosis of PHP-II can be entertained.

℞ TREATMENT

Treatment of PHP is similar to that of hypoparathyroidism, except that the doses of vitamin D and calcium are usually lower than those required in true hypoparathyroidism, presumably because the defect in PHP is only partial because of imprinting in specific tissues (renal cortex vs. renal medulla). Variability in response makes it necessary to establish the optimal regimen for each patient, based on maintaining the appropriate blood calcium level and urinary calcium excretion.

PTH Overwhelmed Occasionally, loss of calcium from the ECF is so severe that PTH cannot compensate. Such situations include acute pancreatitis and severe, acute hyperphosphatemia, often in association with renal failure, conditions in which there is rapid efflux of calcium from the ECF. Severe hypocalcemia can occur quickly; PTH rises in response to hypocalcemia but does not return blood calcium to normal.

Severe, Acute Hyperphosphatemia Severe hyperphosphatemia is associated with extensive tissue damage or cell destruction (Chap. 331). The combination of increased release of phosphate from muscle and impaired ability to excrete phosphorus because of renal failure causes moderate to severe hyperphosphatemia, the latter causing calcium loss from the blood and mild to moderate hypocalcemia. Hypocalcemia is usually reversed with tissue repair and restoration of renal function as phosphorus and creatinine values return to normal. There may even be a mild hypercalcemic period in the oliguric phase of renal function recovery. This sequence, severe hypocalcemia followed by mild hypercalcemia, reflects widespread deposition of calcium in muscle and

subsequent redistribution of some of the calcium to the ECF after phosphate levels return to normal.

Other causes of hyperphosphatemia include hypothermia, massive hepatic failure, and hematologic malignancies, either because of high cell turnover of malignancy or because of cell destruction by chemotherapy.

℞ TREATMENT

Treatment is directed toward lowering of blood phosphate by the administration of phosphate-binding antacids or dialysis, often needed for the management of renal failure. Although calcium replacement may be necessary if hypocalcemia is severe and symptomatic, calcium administration during the hyperphosphatemic period tends to increase extraosseous calcium deposition and aggravate tissue damage. The levels of $1,25(OH)_2D$ may be low during the hyperphosphatemic phase and return to normal during the oliguric phase of recovery.

Osteitis Fibrosis after Parathyroidectomy Severe hypocalcemia after parathyroid surgery is rare now that osteitis fibrosa cystica is an infrequent manifestation of hyperparathyroidism. When osteitis fibrosa cystica is severe, however, bone mineral deficits can be large. After parathyroidectomy, hypocalcemia can persist for days if calcium replacement is inadequate. Treatment may require parenteral administration of calcium; addition of calcitriol and oral calcium supplementation is sometimes needed for weeks to a month or two until bone defects are filled (which, of course, is of therapeutic benefit in the skeleton), making it possible to discontinue parenteral calcium and/or reduce the amount.

DIFFERENTIAL DIAGNOSIS OF HYPOCALCEMIA Care must be taken to ensure that true hypocalcemia is present; in addition, acute transient hypocalcemia can be a manifestation of a variety of severe, acute illnesses, as discussed above. *Chronic hypocalcemia*, however, can usually be ascribed to a few disorders associated with absent or ineffective PTH. Important clinical criteria include the duration of the illness, signs or symptoms of associated disorders, and the presence of features that suggest a hereditary abnormality. A nutritional history can be helpful in recognizing a low intake of vitamin D and calcium in the elderly, and a history of excessive alcohol intake may suggest magnesium deficiency.

Hypoparathyroidism and PHP are typically lifelong illnesses, usually (but not always) appearing by adolescence; hence a recent onset of hypocalcemia in an adult is more likely due to nutritional deficiencies, renal failure, or intestinal disorders that result in deficient or ineffective vitamin D. Neck surgery, even long past, however, can be associated with a delayed onset of postoperative hypoparathyroidism. A history of seizure disorder raises the issue of anticonvulsive medication. Developmental defects may point to the diagnosis of PHP. Rickets and a variety of neuromuscular syndromes and deformities may indicate ineffective vitamin D action, either due to defects in vitamin D metabolism or to vitamin D deficiency.

A pattern of *low calcium with high phosphorus* in the absence of renal failure or massive tissue destruction almost invariably means hypoparathyroidism or PHP. A *low calcium and low phosphorus* points to absent or ineffective vitamin D, thereby impairing the action of PTH on calcium metabolism (but not phosphate clearance). The relative ineffectiveness of PTH in calcium homeostasis in vitamin D deficiency, anticonvulsant therapy, gastrointestinal disorders, and hereditary defects in vitamin D metabolism leads to secondary hyperparathyroidism as a compensation. The excess PTH on renal tubule phosphate transport accounts for renal phosphate wasting and hypophosphatemia.

Exceptions to these patterns may occur. Most forms of hypomagnesemia are due to long-standing nutritional deficiency as seen in chronic alcoholics. Despite the fact that the hypocalcemia is principally due to an acute absence of PTH, phosphate levels are usually low, rather than elevated as in hypoparathyroidism. Chronic renal failure is often associated with hypocalcemia and hyperphosphatemia, despite secondary hyperparathyroidism.

Diagnosis is usually established by application of the PTH immunoassay, tests for vitamin D metabolites, and measurements of the urinary cyclic AMP response to exogenous PTH. In hereditary and acquired hypoparathyroidism and in severe hypomagnesemia, PTH is either undetectable or in the normal range. This finding in a hypocalcemic patient is supportive of hypoparathyroidism, as distinct from ineffective PTH action, in which even mild hypocalcemia is associated with elevated PTH levels. Hence a failure to detect elevated PTH levels establishes the diagnosis of hypoparathyroidism; elevated levels suggest the presence of secondary hyperparathyroidism, as found in many of the situations in which the hormone is ineffective due to associated abnormalities in vitamin D action. Assays for 25(OH)D and 1,25(OH)$_2$D can be helpful. Low or low normal 25(OH)D indicates vitamin D deficiency due to lack of sunlight, inadequate vitamin D intake, or intestinal malabsorption. A low level of 1,25(OH)$_2$D in the presence of elevated concentrations of PTH suggests ineffective PTH action in disorders such as chronic renal failure, severe vitamin D deficiency, vitamin D–dependent rickets type I, and PHP. Recognition that mild hypocalcemia, rickets, and hypophosphatemia are due to anticonvulsant therapy is made by history.

℞ TREATMENT

Hypocalcemic States   The management of hypoparathyroidism, PHP, chronic renal failure, and hereditary defects in vitamin D metabolism involves the use of vitamin D or vitamin D metabolites and calcium supplementation. Vitamin D itself is the least expensive form of vitamin D replacement and is frequently used in the management of uncomplicated hypoparathyroidism and some disorders associated with ineffective vitamin D action. When vitamin D is used prophylactically, as in the elderly or in those with chronic anticonvulsant therapy, there is a wider margin of safety than with the more potent

metabolites. However, most of the conditions in which vitamin D is administered chronically for hypocalcemia require amounts 50 to 100 times the daily replacement dose because the formation of 1,25(OH)$_2$D is deficient. In such situations, vitamin D is no safer than the active metabolite because intoxication can occur with high-dose therapy (because of storage in fat). Calcitriol is more rapid in onset of action and also has a short biologic half-life.

Vitamin D [200 U (5 μg/d)] or calcifediol and lower doses of calcitriol (0.25 to 1.0 μg/d) are required to prevent rickets in normal individuals. In contrast, 40,000 to 12,000 U (1 to 3 mg) of vitamin D$_2$ or D$_3$ is typically required in hypoparathyroidism; doses of calcifediol are also high (several hundred micrograms per day). The dose of calcitriol is unchanged in hypoparathyroidism, since the defect is in hydroxylation by the 25(OH)D-1α-hydroxylase.

Patients with hypoparathyroidism should be given 2 to 3 g elemental calcium by mouth each day. The two agents, vitamin D or calcitriol and oral calcium, can be varied independently. If hypocalcemia alternates with episodes of hypercalcemia in more brittle patients with hypoparathyroidism, administration of calcitriol and use of thiazides, as discussed above, may make management easier.

FURTHER READING

BASTEPE M, JÜPPNER H: Pseudohypoparathyroidism: New insights into an old disease. Endocrinol Metab Clin North Am 29:569, 2000

BILEZIKIAN JP, POTTS JT JR: Asymptomatic primary hyperparathyroidism: New issues and new questions—bridging the past with the future. J Bone Min Res 17(Suppl 2):N57, 2002

CHEN H et al: Outpatient minimally invasive parathyroidectomy: A combination of sestamibi-SPECT localization, cervical block anesthesia, and intraoperative parathyroid hormone assay. Surgery 126:1021, 1999

REID R et al: Intravenous zoledronic acid in postmenopausal women with low bone mineral density. N Engl J Med 346:653, 2002

SILVERBERG SJ et al: Primary hyperparathyroidism: 10-year course with or without parathyroid surgery. N Engl J Med 332:1249, 1999

THAKKER RV: Molecular genetics of parathyroid disease. Curr Opin Endocrinol Diab 3:521, 1996

333   OSTEOPOROSIS
Robert Lindsay, Felicia Cosman

Osteoporosis, a condition characterized by decreased bone strength, is prevalent among postmenopausal women but also occurs in men and women with underlying conditions or major risk factors associated with bone demineralization. Its chief clinical manifestations are vertebral and hip fractures, although fractures can occur at any skeletal site. Osteoporosis affects >10 million individuals in the United States, but only a small proportion are diagnosed and treated.

DEFINITION   *Osteoporosis* is defined as a reduction of bone mass (or density) or the presence of a fragility fracture. Loss of bone tissue causes deterioration in the architecture of the skeleton, the combination leading to a markedly increased risk of fracture. Based on recommendation of a WHO committee, osteoporosis is defined operationally as a bone density that falls 2.5 standard deviations (SD) below the mean for young healthy adults of the same race and gender—also referred to as a *T-score* of −2.5. Those who fall at the lower end of the young normal range (a T-score of >1 SD below the mean) are defined as having low bone density and are considered to be at increased risk of osteoporosis.

EPIDEMIOLOGY   In the United States, as many as 8 million women and 2 million men have osteoporosis (T-score < −2.5), and an additional 18 million individuals have bone mass levels that put them at increased risk of developing osteoporosis (e.g., bone mass T-score < −1.0). Osteoporosis occurs more frequently with increasing age as bone tissue is progressively lost. In women, the loss of ovarian function at

menopause (typically about age 50) precipitates rapid bone loss such that most women meet the diagnostic criteria for osteoporosis by age 70 to 80.

The epidemiology of fractures follows similar trends as bone density loss. Fractures of the distal radius increase in frequency before age 50 and plateau by age 60, with only a modest age-related increase thereafter. In contrast, incidence rates for hip fractures double every 5 years after age 70 (Fig. 333-1). This distinct epidemiology may be related to the way people fall as they age, with fewer falls on an outstretched hand and more directly on the hip. At least 1.5 million fractures occur each year in the United States as a consequence of osteoporosis. As the population continues to age, the total number of fractures will continue to escalate.

About 300,000 hip fractures occur each year in the United States, most of which require hospital admission and surgical intervention. The probability that a 50-year-old white individual will have a hip fracture during his or her lifetime is 14% for women and 5% for men; the risk for African Americans is lower (about half these rates). Hip fractures are associated with a high incidence of deep vein thrombosis and pulmonary embolism (20 to 50%) and a mortality rate between 5 and 20% during the year after surgery.

There are about 700,000 vertebral crush fractures per year in the United States. Only a fraction of these are recognized clinically, since many are relatively asymptomatic and are identified incidentally during radiography for other purposes (Fig. 333-2). Vertebral fractures rarely require hospitalization but are associated with long-term morbidity and a slight increase in mortality. Multiple fractures lead to height loss (often of several inches), kyphosis, and secondary pain and discomfort related to altered biomechanics of the back. Thoracic frac-

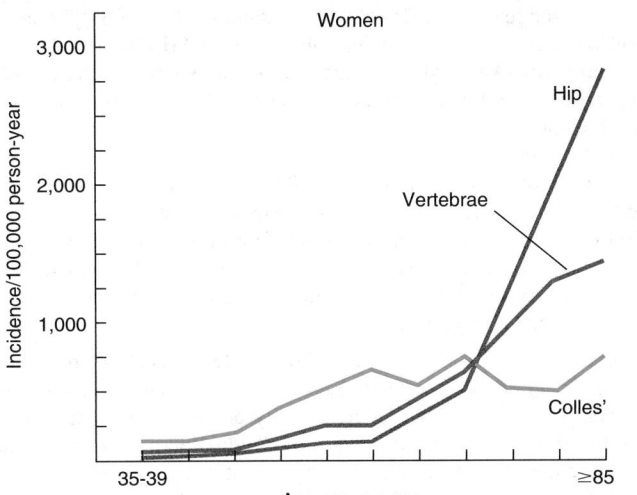

FIGURE 333-1 Epidemiology of vertebral, hip, and Colles' fractures with age. [Adapted from LJ Melton III, in BL Riggs, LJ Melton II (eds): Osteoporosis: Etiology, Diagnosis and Management, 2d ed. Rochester, MN, Mayo Foundation, 1995.]

tures can be associated with restrictive lung disease, whereas lumbar fractures are associated with abdominal symptoms including distention, early satiety, and constipation.

Approximately 250,000 wrist fractures occur in the United States each year. Fractures of other bones (estimated to be about 300,000 per year) also occur with osteoporosis, which is not surprising given that bone loss is a systemic phenomenon. Fractures of the pelvis and proximal humerus are clearly associated with osteoporosis. Although some fractures are the result of major trauma, the threshold for fracture is reduced for an osteoporotic bone (Fig. 333-3). A list of common risk factors for osteoporotic fractures is summarized in Table 333-1. Prior fractures, a family history of osteoporotic fractures, and low body weight are each independent predictors of fracture. Chronic diseases that increase the risk of falling or frailty, including dementia, Parkinson's disease, and multiple sclerosis, also increase fracture risk.

In the United States and Europe, osteoporosis-related fractures are more common among women than men, presumably due to a lower peak bone mass as well as postmenopausal bone loss in women. However, this gender difference in bone density and age-related increase in hip fractures is not as apparent in some other cultures, possibly due to genetics, physical activity level, or diet.

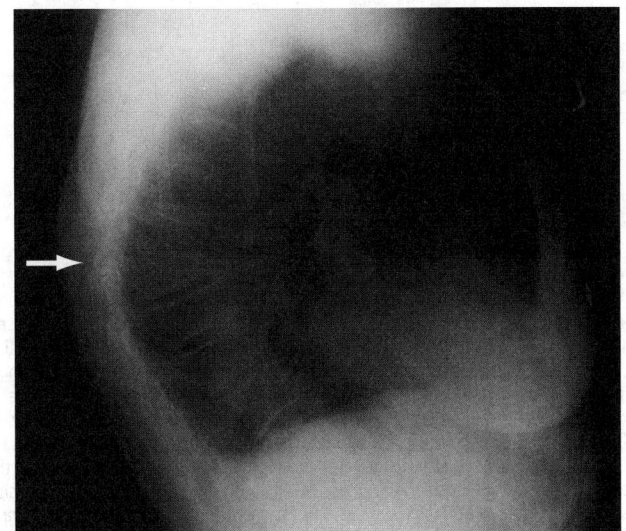

FIGURE 333-2 Lateral spine x-ray showing severe osteopenia and a severe wedge-type deformity (severe anterior compression).

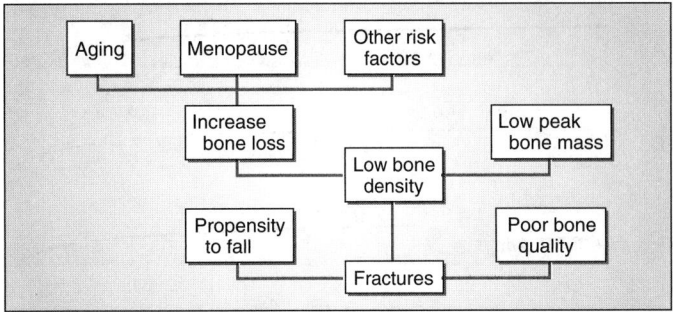

FIGURE 333-3 Factors leading to osteoporotic fractures.

PATHOPHYSIOLOGY ■ Bone Remodeling Osteoporosis results from bone loss due to normal age-related changes in bone remodeling as well as extrinsic and intrinsic factors that exaggerate this process. These changes may be superimposed on a low peak bone mass. Consequently, understanding the bone remodeling process is fundamental to understanding the pathophysiology of osteoporosis (Chap. 331). The skeleton increases in size by linear growth and by apposition of new bone tissue on the outer surfaces of the cortex (Fig. 333-4). This latter process is called *modeling*, a process that also allows the long bones to adapt in shape to the stresses placed upon them. Increased sex hormone production at puberty is required for skeletal maturation, which reaches maximum mass and density in early adulthood. Nutrition and life-style also play an important role in growth, though genetic factors are the major determinants of peak skeletal mass and density. Numerous genes control skeletal growth, peak bone mass, and body size, but it is likely that separate genes control skeletal structure and density. Heritability estimates of 50 to 80% for bone density and size have been derived based on twin studies. Though peak bone mass is often lower among individuals with a family history of osteoporosis, association studies of candidate genes [vitamin D receptor; type I collagen, the estrogen receptor (ER), interleukin (IL) 6; and insulin-like growth factor (IGF) I] and bone mass, bone turnover, and fracture prevalence have been inconsistent. Linkage studies suggest that a genetic locus on chromosome 11 is associated with high bone mass. Recently, a family with extremely high bone mass was identified with a point mutation in LRP 5, a low-density lipoprotein receptor–related protein.

Bone remodeling has two primary functions: (1) to repair microdamage within the skeleton to maintain skeletal strength, and (2) to supply calcium from the skeleton to maintain serum calcium. Remodeling may be activated by microdamage to bone as a result of excessive or accumulated stress. Acute demands for calcium involve osteoclast-mediated resorption as well as calcium transport by osteocytes.

Bone remodeling is also regulated by several circulating hormones, including estrogens, androgens, vitamin D, and parathyroid hormone (PTH), as well as locally produced growth factors such as IGF-I and -II, transforming growth factor (TGF) β, parathyroid hormone–related peptide (PTHrP), ILs, prostaglandins, and tumor necrosis factor

TABLE 333-1 Risk Factors for Osteoporosis Fracture	
Nonmodifiable	Estrogen deficiency
Personal history of fracture as an adult	Early menopause (<45 years) or bilateral ovariectomy
History of fracture in first-degree relative	Prolonged premenstrual amenorrhea (>1 year)
Female sex	Low calcium intake
Advanced age	Alcoholism
Caucasian race	Impaired eyesight despite adequate correction
Dementia	Recurrent falls
Potentially modifiable	Inadequate physical activity
Current cigarette smoking	Poor health/frailty
Low body weight [<58 kg (127 lb)]	

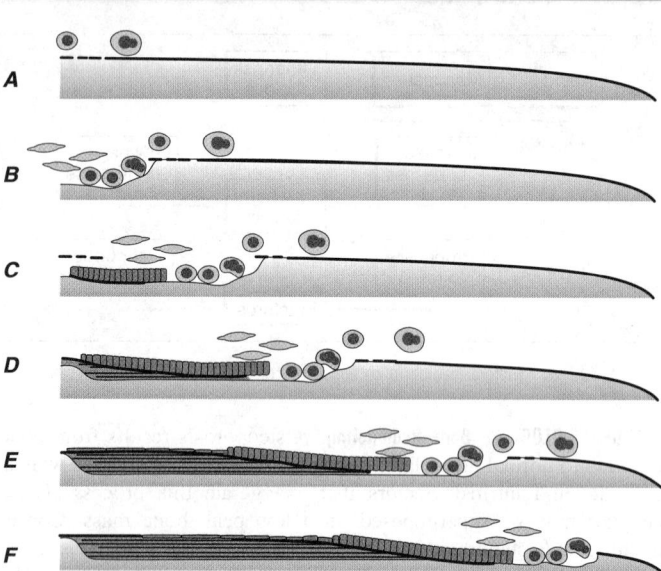

FIGURE 333-4 *Mechanism of bone remodeling. The basic molecular unit (BMU) moves along the trabecular surface at a rate of about 10 μm/d. The figure depicts remodeling over ~120 days. A. Origination of BMU-lining cells contract to expose collagen and attract preosteoclasts. B. Osteoclasts fuse into multinucleated cells that resorb a cavity. Mononuclear cells continue resorption and preosteoblasts are stimulated to proliferate. C. Osteoblasts align at bottom of cavity and start forming osteoid (black). D. Osteoblasts continue formation and mineralization. Previous osteoid starts to mineralize (horizontal lines). E. Osteoblasts begin to flatten. F. Osteoblasts turn into lining cells; bone remodeling at initial surface (left of drawing) is now complete, but BMU is still advancing (to the right). [Adapted from: SM Ott, in JP Bilezikian et al (eds): Principles of Bone Biology, vol. 18. San Diego, Academic Press, 1996, pp 231–241.]*

(TNF). The cytokine responsible for communication between the osteoblast and osteoclast has been identified as RANK or osteoprotegerin ligand (Chap. 331). The osteoclast receptor for this protein is referred to as RANK. A humoral decoy for RANK ligand is referred to as osteoprotegerin (Fig. 333-5). Modulation of osteoclast recruitment and activity appears to be related to the interplay among these three factors.

Additional influences include nutrition (particularly calcium intake) and physical activity level. The end result of this remodeling process is that the resorbed bone is replaced by an equal amount of new bone tissue. Thus, the mass of the skeleton remains constant after peak bone mass is achieved in adulthood. After age 30 to 45, however, the resorption and formation processes become imbalanced, and resorption exceeds formation. This imbalance may begin at different ages and varies at different skeletal sites; it becomes exaggerated in women after menopause. Excessive bone loss can be due to an increase in osteoclastic activity and/or a decrease in osteoblastic activity. In addition, an increase in remodeling activation frequency can magnify the small imbalance seen at each remodeling unit.

In trabecular bone, if the osteoclasts penetrate trabeculae, they leave no template for new bone formation to occur and, consequently, may cause rapid bone loss. In cortical bone, increased activation of remodeling creates more porous bone. The effect of this increased porosity on cortical bone strength may be modest if the overall diameter of the bone is not changed. However, decreased apposition of new bone on the periosteal surface coupled with increased endocortical resorption of bone decreases the biomechanical strength of long bones. Even a slight exaggeration in normal bone loss increases the risk of osteoporotic fracture.

Calcium Nutrition Peak bone mass may be impaired by inadequate calcium intake during growth among other nutritional factors (calories, protein, and other minerals), thereby leading to increased risk of osteoporosis later in life. During the adult phase of life, insufficient calcium intake induces secondary hyperparathyroidism and an increase in the rate of remodeling to maintain normal serum calcium levels. PTH stimulates the hydroxylation of vitamin D in the kidney, leading

to increased levels of 1,25-dihydroxyvitamin D [1,25(OH)$_2$D] and enhanced gastrointestinal calcium absorption. PTH also reduces renal calcium loss. Although these are appropriate short-term homeostatic responses for adjusting calcium economy, the long-term effects are detrimental to the skeleton because of the ongoing imbalance at remodeling sites.

Total daily calcium intakes of <400 mg are likely to be detrimental to the skeleton, but there are fewer data about intakes in the 600- to 800-mg range, which is the average intake among adults in the United States. The recommended daily required intake of 1000 to 1200 mg for adults accommodates population heterogeneity in controlling calcium balance (Chap. 60).

Vitamin D (See also Chap. 331) Severe vitamin D deficiency causes rickets in children or osteomalacia in adults. There is accumulating evidence that vitamin D deficiency may be more prevalent than previously thought, particularly among individuals at increased risk, such as the elderly; those living in northern latitudes; and in individuals with poor nutrition, malabsorption, or chronic liver or renal disease. Modest vitamin D deficiency [25-hydroxyvitamin D levels ≤50 nmol/L (20 ng/mL)] leads to compensatory secondary hyperparathyroidism and is an important risk factor for osteoporosis and fractures. Some studies have shown that >50% of inpatients on a general medical service exhibit biochemical features of vitamin D deficiency, including increased levels of PTH and alkaline phosphatase and lower levels of ionized calcium. In women living in northern latitudes, it has been shown that vitamin D levels decline during the winter months. This is associated with a striking seasonal bone loss, reflecting increased bone turnover. Even among healthy ambulatory individuals, mild vitamin D deficiency is increasing in prevalence. Treatment with vitamin D can return vitamin D levels to normal [>50 μmol/L (20 ng/mL)] and prevent the associated increase in bone remodeling, bone loss, and fractures. Reduced fracture rates have also been documented among individuals in northern latitudes who have greater vitamin D intake and have higher 25-hydroxyvitamin D [25(OH)D] levels (see below).

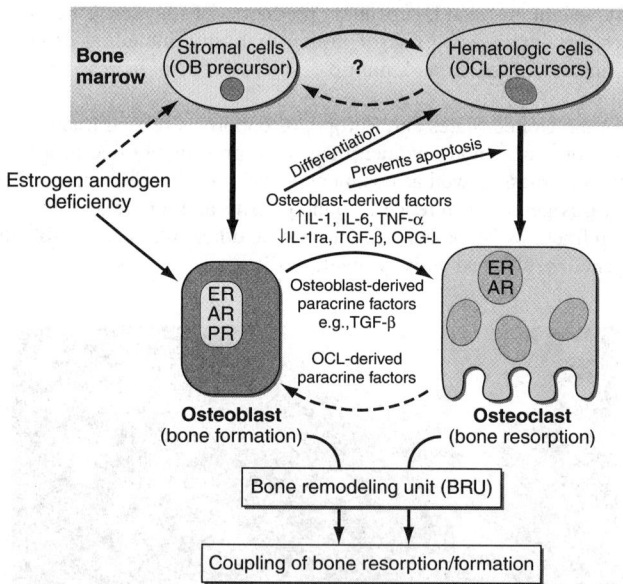

FIGURE 333-5 *Steroid actions and interactions with growth factors/cytokines in bone cells at bone resorption and formation sites. Estrogen inhibits osteoclasts (OCL), cells that mediate bone resorption; estrogen stimulates osteoblasts (OB), cells that mediate bone formation. OBs produce many growth factors and cytokines that mediate estrogen action, some of which regulate the OCL indirectly. Estrogen deficiency stimulates OB production of IL-1, IL-6, and TNF-α (and inhibits apoptosis and extends the life span of OCLs). Estrogen deficiency decreases IL-1ra leading to enhanced OCL sensitivity to IL-1. Estrogen deficiency also decreases production of TGF-β and OPG-L, factors that mediate osteoclast apoptosis. Solid lines indicate well-documented pathways. Dashed lines indicate less well defined pathways. ER, estrogen receptor; AR, androgen receptor; OPG, osteoprotegerin; OPG-L, osteoprotegerin-ligand; IL, interleukin; IL-1ra, interleukin 1 receptor antagonist; TGF-β, transforming growth factor β; TNF-α, tumor necrosis factor α. (Adapted from TC Spelsberg et al: Mol Endocrinol 13:819, 1999.)*

Estrogen Status Estrogen deficiency probably causes bone loss by two distinct but interrelated mechanisms: (1) activation of new bone remodeling sites, and (2) exaggeration of the imbalance between bone formation and resorption. The change in activation frequency causes a transient bone loss until a new steady state between resorption and formation is achieved. The remodeling imbalance, however, results in a permanent decrement in mass that can only be corrected by a remodeling event during which bone formation exceeds resorption. In addition, the very presence of more remodeling sites in the skeleton increases the probability that trabeculae will be penetrated, thereby eliminating the template upon which new bone can be formed and accelerating the loss of bony tissue.

The most frequent estrogen-deficient state is the cessation of ovarian function at the time of menopause, which occurs on average at the age of 51. Thus, with current life expectancy, an average woman will spend about 30 years without ovarian supply of estrogen. The mechanism by which estrogen deficiency causes bone loss is summarized in Fig. 333-5. Marrow cells (macrophages, monocytes, osteoclast precursors, mast cells) as well as bone cells (osteoblasts, osteocytes, osteoclasts) express ERs α and β. The net effect of estrogen deficiency is increased osteoclast recruitment and perhaps activity. Estrogen may also play an important role in determining the life span of bone cells by controlling the rate of apoptosis. Thus, in situations of estrogen deprivation, the life span of osteoblasts may be decreased whereas the longevity of osteoclasts is increased.

Since remodeling is initiated at the surface of bone, it follows that trabecular bone—which has a considerably larger surface area (80% of the total) than cortical bone—will be preferentially affected by estrogen deficiency. Fractures occur earliest at sites where trabecular bone contributes most to bone strength; consequently, vertebral fractures are the most common early consequence of estrogen deficiency.

Physical Activity Inactivity, such as prolonged bed rest or paralysis, results in significant bone loss. Concordantly, athletes have higher bone mass than the general population. These changes in skeletal mass are most marked when the stimulus begins during growth and before the age of puberty. Adults are less capable than children of increasing bone mass following restoration of physical activity. Epidemiologic data support the beneficial effects on the skeleton of chronic high levels of physical activity. Fracture risk is lower in rural communities and in countries where physical activity is maintained into old age. However, when exercise is initiated during adult life, the effects of moderate exercise are modest, with a bone mass increase of 1 to 2% in short-term studies of <2 years duration. It is argued that more active individuals are less likely to fall and are more capable of protecting themselves upon falling, thereby reducing fracture risk.

Chronic Disease Various genetic and acquired diseases are associated with an increase in the risk of osteoporosis (Table 333-2). Mechanisms that contribute to bone loss are unique for each disease and typically result from multiple factors including nutrition, reduced physical activity levels, and factors that affect bone-remodeling rates.

Medications A large number of medications used in clinical practice have potentially detrimental effects on the skeleton (Table 333-3). *Glucocorticoids* are the most common cause of medication-induced osteoporosis. It is often not possible to determine the extent to which osteoporosis is related to the glucocorticoid or to other factors, as treatment is superimposed on the effects of the primary disease, which may in itself be associated with bone loss (e.g., rheumatoid arthritis). Excessive doses of thyroid hormone can accelerate bone remodeling and result in bone loss.

Other medications have less detrimental effects upon the skeleton than pharmacologic doses of glucocorticoids. *Anticonvulsants* are thought to increase the risk of osteoporosis, although many affected individuals have concomitant vitamin D insufficiency, as some anticonvulsants induce the cytochrome P450 system and vitamin D metabolism. Patients undergoing transplantation are at high risk for rapid bone loss and fracture not only from glucocorticoids but also from treatment with other *immunosuppressants*, such as cyclosporine and

TABLE 333-2 *Diseases Associated with an Increased Risk of Generalized Osteoporosis in Adults*

Hypogonadal states	Hematologic disorders/malignancy
Turner syndrome	Multiple myeloma
Klinefelter syndrome	Lymphoma and leukemia
Anorexia nervosa	Malignancy-associated parathyroid
Hypothalamic amenorrhea	hormone (PTHrP) production
Hyperprolactinemia	Mastocytosis
Other primary or secondary	Hemophilia
hypogonadal states	Thalassemia
Endocrine disorders	Selected inherited disorders
Cushing's syndrome	Osteogenesis imperfecta
Hyperparathyroidism	Marfan syndrome
Thyrotoxicosis	Hemochromatosis
Type 1 diabetes mellitus	Hypophosphatasia
Acromegaly	Glycogen storage diseases
Adrenal insufficiency	Homocystinuria
Nutritional and gastrointestinal	Ehlers-Danlos syndrome
disorders	Porphyria
Malnutrition	Menkes' syndrome
Parenteral nutrition	Epidermolysis bullosa
Malabsorption syndromes	Other disorders
Gastrectomy	Immobilization
Severe liver disease, espe-	Chronic obstructive pulmonary
cially biliary cirrhosis	disease
Pernicious anemia	Pregnancy and lactation
Rheumatologic disorders	Scoliosis
Rheumatoid arthritis	Multiple sclerosis
Ankylosing spondylitis	Sarcoidosis
	Amyloidosis

tacrolimus (FK506). In addition, these patients often have underlying metabolic abnormalities, such as hepatic or renal failure, that predispose to bone loss.

Cigarette Consumption The use of cigarettes over a long period has detrimental effects on bone mass. These effects may be mediated directly, by toxic effects on osteoblasts, or indirectly by modifying estrogen metabolism. On average, cigarette smokers reach menopause 1 to 2 years earlier than the general population. Cigarette smoking also produces secondary effects that can modulate skeletal status, including intercurrent respiratory and other illnesses, frailty, decreased exercise, poor nutrition, and the need for additional medications (e.g., glucocorticoids for lung disease).

MEASUREMENT OF BONE MASS Several noninvasive techniques are now available for estimating skeletal mass or density. These include dual-energy x-ray absorptiometry (DXA), single-energy x-ray absorptiometry (SXA), quantitative computed tomography (CT), and ultrasound.

DXA is a highly accurate x-ray technique that has become the standard for measuring bone density in most centers. Though it can be used for measurements of any skeletal site, clinical determinations are usually made of the lumbar spine and hip. Portable DXA machines have been developed that measure the heel (calcaneus), forearm (radius and ulna), or finger (phalanges). DXA can also be used to measure body composition. In the DXA technique, two x-ray energies are used to estimate the area of mineralized tissue, and the mineral content is divided by the area, which partially corrects for body size. However, this correction is only partial since DXA is a two-dimensional scanning technique and cannot estimate the depths or posteroanterior length of the bone. Thus, small people tend to have lower-than-average bone

TABLE 333-3 *Drugs Associated with an Increased Risk of Generalized Osteoporosis in Adults*

Glucocorticoids	Excessive thyroxine
Cyclosporine	Aluminum
Cytotoxic drugs	Gonadotropin-releasing hormone agonists
Anticonvulsants	Heparin
Excessive alcohol	Lithium

mineral density (BMD). Bone spurs, which are frequent in osteoarthritis, tend to falsely increase bone density of the spine. Because DXA instrumentation is provided by several different manufacturers, the output varies in absolute terms. Consequently, it has become standard practice to relate the results to "normal" values using T-scores, which compare individual results to those in a young population that is matched for race and gender. Z-scores compare individual results to those of an age-matched population that is also matched for race and gender. Thus, a 60-year-old woman with a Z-score of −1 (1 SD below mean for age) has a T-score of −2.5 (2.5 SD below mean for a young control group) (Fig. 333-6).

CT is used primarily to measure the spine, and peripheral CT is used to measure bone in the forearm or tibia. Research into the use of CT for measurement of the hip is ongoing. The results obtained from CT are different from all others currently available since this technique specifically analyzes trabecular bone in vertebrae, eliminating posterior cortical elements of the spine, and can provide a true density (mass of bone per unit volume) measurement. However, CT remains expensive, involves greater radiation exposure, and is less reproducible.

Ultrasound is used to measure bone mass by calculating the attenuation of the signal as it passes through bone or the speed with which it traverses the bone. It is unclear whether ultrasound assesses bone quality, but this may be an advantage of the technique. Because of its relatively low cost and mobility, ultrasound is amenable for use as a screening procedure.

All of these techniques for measuring BMD have been approved by the U.S. Food and Drug Administration (FDA) based upon their capacity to predict fracture risk. The hip is the preferred site of measurement in most individuals, since it predicts the risk of hip fracture, the most important consequence of osteoporosis, better than any other bone density measurement site. When hip measurements are performed by DXA, the spine can be measured at the same time. In younger individuals, such as perimenopausal or early postmenopausal women, spine measurements may be the most sensitive indicator of bone loss.

When to Measure Bone Mass   Clinical guidelines developed by the National Osteoporosis Foundation recommend bone mass measurements in postmenopausal women, assuming they have risk factors for osteoporosis in addition to age, gender, and estrogen deficiency. The guidelines further recommend that bone mass measurement be considered in *all* women by age 65, a position ratified by the U.S. Preventive Health Services Task Force. Criteria approved for Medicare reimbursement of BMD are summarized in Table 333-4.

When to Treat Based Upon Bone Mass Results   Several guidelines suggest that patients be considered for treatment when BMD is >2.5 SD below the mean value for young adults (T-score ≤ −2.5). Treatment should also be considered in postmenopausal women with risk factors if BMD of the hip is <−2.0. Because the fracture risk increases continuously as T-scores decline, there is no critical threshold and treatment deci-

TABLE 333-4   FDA-Approved Indications for BMD Tests[a]

Estrogen-deficient women at clinical risk of osteoporosis
Vertebral abnormalities on x-ray suggestive of osteoporosis (osteopenia, vertebral fracture)
Glucocorticoid treatment equivalent to ≥7.5 mg of prednisone, or duration of therapy >3 months
Primary hyperparathyroidism
Monitoring response to an FDA-approved medication for osteoporosis
Repeat BMD evaluations at >23-month intervals, or more frequently, if medically justified

[a] Criteria adapted from the 1998 Bone Mass Measurement Act.
Note: FDA, U.S. Food and Drug Administration; BMD, bone mineral density.

sions must be individualized. Clearly clinical status must be evaluated carefully, considering age, prior fracture history, weight, and family history of osteoporosis. Moreover, high bone turnover, particularly in older individuals, should be considered an independent risk factor for fracture and should prompt treatment at a higher BMD level.

APPROACH TO THE PATIENT

The perimenopausal transition is a good opportunity to initiate discussion about risk factors for osteoporosis and to consider indications for a BMD test. A careful history and physical examination should be performed to identify risk factors for osteoporosis. A low Z-score increases the suspicion of a secondary disease. Height loss >2.5 to 3.8 cm (>1 to 1.5 in.) is an indication for radiography to rule out asymptomatic vertebral fractures, as is the presence of significant kyphosis or back pain, particularly if it began after menopause. For patients who present with fractures, it is important to ensure that the fractures are not caused by an underlying malignancy. Usually this is clear on routine radiography, but on occasion, CT, magnetic resonance imaging, or radionuclide scans may be necessary.

Routine Laboratory Evaluation   There is no established algorithm for the evaluation of women presenting with osteoporosis. A general evaluation that includes complete blood count, serum calcium, and perhaps urine calcium is helpful for identifying selected secondary causes of low bone mass, particularly for women with fractures or very low Z-scores. An elevated serum calcium level suggests hyperparathyroidism or malignancy, whereas a reduced serum calcium level may reflect malnutrition and osteomalacia. In the presence of hypercalcemia, a serum PTH level differentiates between hyperparathyroidism (PTH↑) and malignancy (PTH↓), and a high PTHrP level can help document the presence of humoral hypercalcemia of malignancy (Chap. 332). A low urine calcium (<50 mg/24 h) suggests osteomalacia, malnutrition, or malabsorption; a high urine calcium (>300 mg/24 h) is indicative of hypercalciuria and must be investigated further. Hypercalciuria occurs primarily in three situations: (1) a renal calcium leak, which is more frequent in males with osteoporosis; (2) absorptive hypercalciuria, which can be idiopathic or associated with increased $1,25(OH)_2D$ in granulomatous disease; or (3) hematologic malignancies or conditions associated with excessive bone turnover such as Paget's disease, hyperparathyroidism, and hyperthyroidism.

Possible hyperthyroidism can be evaluated by measuring thyroid-stimulating hormone (TSH). When there is clinical suspicion of Cushing's syndrome, urinary free cortisol levels or a fasting serum cortisol should be measured after overnight dexamethasone. When bowel disease, malabsorption, or malnutrition is suspected, serum albumin, cholesterol, and a complete blood count should be checked. Asymptomatic malabsorption might be heralded by anemia (macrocytic-vitamin B_{12} or folate deficiency; or microcytic-iron deficiency) or low serum cholesterol or urinary calcium levels. If these or other features suggest malabsorption, further evaluation is required. Asymptomatic celiac disease with selective malabsorption is being found with increasing prevalence; the diagnosis can be made by testing for antigliadin, antiendomysial, or transglutam-

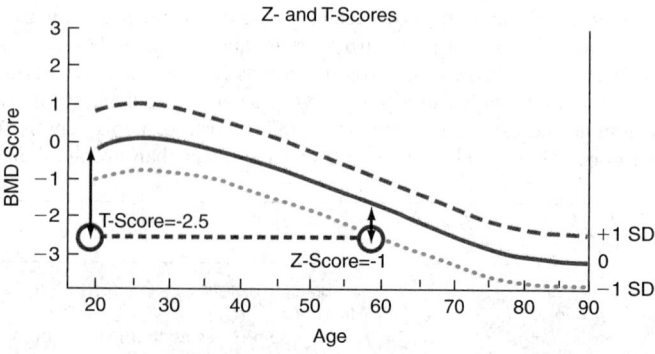

FIGURE 333-6   Relationship between Z-scores and T-scores in a 60-year-old woman (BMD, bone mineral density; SD, standard deviation).

TABLE 333-5 *Biochemical Markers of Bone Metabolism in Clinical Use*

Bone formation
   Serum bone-specific alkaline phosphatase
   Serum osteocalcin
   Serum propeptide of type I procollagen
Bone resorption
   Urine and serum cross-linked N-telopeptide
   Urine and serum cross-linked C-telopeptide
   Urine total free deoxypyridinoline
   Urine hydroxyproline
   Serum tartrate-resistant acid phosphatase
   Serum bone sialoprotein
   Urine hydroxylysine glycosides

inase antibodies but may require endoscopic biopsy. A trial of a gluten-free diet can be confirmatory (Chap. 275). When osteoporosis is found associated with symptoms of rash, multiple allergies, diarrhea, or flushing, mastocytosis should be excluded using 24-h urine histamine collection or serum tryptase.

Myeloma can masquerade as generalized osteoporosis, although it more commonly presents with bone pain and characteristic "punched-out" lesions on radiography. Serum and urine electrophoresis and evaluation for light chains in urine are required to exclude this diagnosis. A bone marrow biopsy may be required to rule out myeloma (in patients with equivocal electrophoretic results) and can also be used to exclude mastocytosis, leukemia, and other marrow infiltrative disorders, such as Gaucher's disease.

Bone Biopsy Tetracycline labeling of the skeleton allows determination of the rate of remodeling as well as evaluation for other metabolic bone diseases. The current use of BMD tests, in combination with hormonal evaluation and biochemical markers of bone remodeling, has largely replaced bone biopsy.

Biochemical Markers Several biochemical tests are now available that provide an index of the overall rate of bone remodeling (Table 333-5). Biochemical markers are usually characterized as those related primarily to *bone formation* or *bone resorption*. These tests measure the overall state of bone remodeling at a single point in time. Clinical use of these tests has been hampered by biologic variability (in part related to circadian rhythm) as well as to analytical variability.

For the most part, remodeling markers do not predict rates of bone loss well enough to use this information clinically. However, markers of bone resorption may help in the prediction of fracture risk, particularly in older individuals. In women ≥65 years, when bone density results are greater than the usual treatment thresholds noted above, a high level of bone resorption should prompt consideration of treatment. The primary use of biochemical markers is for monitoring the response to treatment. With the introduction of antiresorptive therapeutic agents, bone remodeling declines rapidly, with the fall in resorption occurring earlier than the fall in formation. Inhibition of bone resorption is maximal within 3 to 6 months. Thus, measurement of bone resorption prior to initiating therapy and 4 to 6 months after starting therapy provides an earlier estimate of patient response than does bone densitometry. A decline in resorptive markers can be ascertained after treatment with bisphosphonates or estrogen; this effect is less marked after treatment with either raloxifene or intranasal calcitonin. A biochemical marker response to therapy is particularly useful for asymptomatic patients and might help to ensure long-term compliance. Bone turnover markers are also useful in monitoring the effects of PTH, or teriparatide, which rapidly increases bone formation and later bone resorption.

℞ **TREATMENT**

Management of Osteoporotic Fractures Treatment of the patient with osteoporosis frequently involves management of acute fractures as well

as treatment of the underlying disease. Hip fractures almost always require surgical repair if the patient is to become ambulatory again. Depending on the location and severity of the fracture, condition of the neighboring joint, and general status of the patient, procedures may include open reduction and internal fixation with pins and plates, hemiarthroplasties, and total arthroplasties. These surgical procedures are followed by intense rehabilitation in an attempt to return patients to their prefracture functional level. Long bone fractures often require either external or internal fixation. Other fractures (e.g., vertebral, rib, and pelvic fractures) are usually managed with only supportive care, requiring no specific orthopedic treatment.

Only ~25 to 30% of vertebral compression fractures present with sudden-onset back pain. For acutely symptomatic fractures, treatment with analgesics is required, including nonsteroidal anti-inflammatory agents and/or acetaminophen, sometimes with the addition of a narcotic agent (codeine or oxycodone). A few small, randomized clinical trials suggest that calcitonin may reduce pain related to acute vertebral compression fracture. A recently developed technique involves percutaneous injection of artificial cement (polymethylmethacrylate) into the vertebral body (vertebroplasty or kyphoplasty); this has been reported to offer significant immediate pain relief in the majority of patients. Long-term effects are unknown, and conclusions are based on observational studies in patients with severe persistent back pain from acute or subacute vertebral fractures. There have been no randomized controlled trials of either vertebroplasty or kyphoplasty to date. Short periods of bed rest may be helpful for pain management, but, in general, early mobilization is recommended as it helps prevent further bone loss associated with immobilization. Occasionally, use of a soft elastic-style brace may facilitate earlier mobilization. Muscle spasms often occur with acute compression fractures and can be treated with muscle relaxants and heat treatments.

Severe pain usually resolves within 6 to 10 weeks. Chronic pain is probably not bony in origin; instead, it is related to abnormal strain on muscles, ligaments, and tendons and to secondary facet-joint arthritis associated with alterations in thoracic and/or abdominal shape. Chronic pain is difficult to treat effectively and may require analgesics, sometimes including narcotic analgesics. Frequent intermittent rest in a supine or semireclining position is often required to allow the soft tissues, which are under tension, to relax. Back-strengthening exercises (paraspinal) may be beneficial. Heat treatments help relax muscles and reduce the muscular component of discomfort. Various physical modalities, such as ultrasound and transcutaneous nerve stimulation, may be beneficial in some patients. Pain also occurs in the neck region, not as a result of compression fractures (which almost never occur in the cervical spine as a result of osteoporosis) but because of chronic strain associated from trying to elevate the head in a person with a severe thoracic kyphosis.

Multiple vertebral fractures are often associated with psychological symptoms, not always commonly appreciated. The changes in body configuration and back pain can lead to marked loss of self-image and a secondary depression. Altered balance, precipitated by the kyphosis and the anterior movement of the body's center of gravity, leads to a fear of falling, a consequent tendency to remain indoors, and the onset of social isolation. These symptoms can sometimes be alleviated by family support and/or psychotherapy. Medication may be necessary when depressive features are present.

Management of the Underlying Disease ■ *RISK FACTOR REDUCTION* Patients should be thoroughly educated to reduce the likelihood of risk factors associated with bone loss and falling. Medications should be reviewed to ensure that any glucocorticoid medication is truly indicated and is being given in doses as low as possible. For those on thyroid hormone replacement, TSH testing should be performed to determine that an excessive dose is not being used, as thyrotoxicosis can be associated with increased bone loss. In patients who smoke, efforts should be made to facilitate smoking cessation. Reducing risk factors for falling also includes alcohol abuse treatment and a review of the medical regimen for any drugs that might be associated with orthostatic hypotension and/or sedation, including hypnotics and anxiolytics. If nocturia occurs, the frequency should be reduced, if possible (e.g., by decreasing or modifying diuretic use), as arising in the middle of sleep is a common precipitant of a fall. Patients should be instructed about environmental safety with regard to eliminating exposed wires, curtain strings, slippery rugs, and mobile tables. Avoiding stocking feet on wood floors, checking carpet condition (particularly on stairs), and providing good light in paths to bathrooms and outside the home are important preventive measures. Treatment for impaired vision is recommended, particularly a problem with depth perception, which is specifically associated with increased falling risk. Elderly patients with neurologic impairment (e.g., stroke, Parkinson's disease, Alzheimer's disease) are particularly at risk of falling and require specialized supervision and care.

NUTRITIONAL RECOMMENDATIONS ■ Calcium   A large body of data indicates that optimal calcium intake reduces bone loss and suppresses bone turnover. Recommended intakes from a recent report from the Institute of Medicine are shown in Table 333-6. The National Health and Nutritional Evaluation Studies (NHANES) have consistently documented that average calcium intakes fall considerably short of these recommendations. The preferred source of calcium is from dairy products and other foods, but many patients require calcium supplementation. Food sources of calcium are dairy products (milk, yogurt, and cheese) and fortified foods such as certain cereals, waffles, snacks, juices, and crackers. Some of these fortified foods contain as much calcium per serving as milk.

If a calcium supplement is required, it should be taken in doses ≤600 mg at a time, as the calcium absorption fraction decreases at higher doses. Calcium supplements should be calculated based on the elemental calcium content of the supplement, not the weight of the calcium salt (Table 333-7). Calcium supplements containing carbonate are best taken with food since they require acid for solubility. Calcium citrate supplements can be taken at any time.

Several controlled clinical trials of calcium plus vitamin D have confirmed reductions in clinical fractures, including fractures of the hip (~20 to 30% risk reduction). All recent studies of pharmacologic agents have been conducted in the context of calcium replacement (± vitamin D). Thus, it is standard practice to ensure an adequate calcium and vitamin D intake in patients with osteoporosis, whether they are receiving additional pharmacologic therapy or not.

Although side effects from supplemental calcium are minimal, individuals with a history of kidney stones should have a 24-h urine calcium determination before starting increased calcium to avoid hypercalciuria.

Vitamin D   Vitamin D is synthesized in skin under the influence of heat and ultraviolet light (Chap. 331). However, large segments of the population do not obtain sufficient vitamin D to maintain what is now considered an adequate supply [serum 25(OH)D consistently >50 μmol/L (20 ng/mL)]. Since vitamin D supplementation at doses that

TABLE 333-6   Adequate Calcium Intake

Life Stage Group	Estimated Adequate Daily Calcium Intake, mg/d
Young children (1–3 years)	500
Older children (4–8 years)	800
Adolescents and young adults (9–18 years)	1300
Men and women (19–50 years)	1000
Men and women (51 and older)	1200

Note: Pregnancy and lactation needs are the same as for nonpregnant women (e.g., 1300 mg/d for adolescents/young adult and 1000 mg/d for ≥19 years.)
Source: Adapted from the Standing Committee on the Scientific Evaluation of Dietary Reference Intakes. Food and Nutrition Board. Institute of Medicine. Washington, DC, 1997. National Academy Press.

TABLE 333-7   Elemental Calcium Content of Various Oral Calcium Preparations

Calcium Preparation	Elemental Calcium Content
Calcium citrate	60 mg/300 mg
Calcium lactate	80 mg/600 mg
Calcium gluconate	40 mg/500 mg
Calcium carbonate	400 mg/g
Calcium carbonate + 5 μg vitamin D$_2$ (OsCal 250)	250 mg/tablet
Calcium carbonate (Tums 500)	500 mg/tablet

Source: Adapted from SM Krane and MF Holick, Chap. 355 in HPIM, 14 ed, 1998.

would achieve these serum levels is safe and inexpensive, the Institute of Medicine recommends daily intakes of 200 IU for adults <50 years of age, 400 IU for those from 50 to 70 years, and 600 IU for those >70 years. Multivitamin tablets usually contain 400 IU, and many calcium supplements also contain vitamin D. Some data suggest that higher doses may be required in the elderly and chronically ill.

Other Nutrients   Other nutrients such as salt and caffeine may have modest effects on calcium excretion or absorption. Adequate vitamin K status is required for optimal carboxylation of osteocalcin. States in which vitamin K nutrition or metabolism is impaired, such as with long-term warfarin therapy, have been associated with reduced bone mass.

Magnesium is abundant in foods, and magnesium deficiency is quite rare in the absence of a serious chronic disease. Magnesium supplementation may be warranted in patients with inflammatory bowel disease, celiac disease, chemotherapy, severe diarrhea, malnutrition, or alcoholism. Dietary phytoestrogens, which are derived primarily from soy products and legumes (e.g., garbanzo beans, chickpeas, and lentils), exert some estrogenic activity but are insufficiently potent to justify their use in place of a pharmacologic agent in the treatment of osteoporosis.

Patients with hip fracture are often frail and relatively malnourished. Some data suggest an improved outcome in such patients when they are provided calorie and protein supplementation. Excessive protein intake can increase renal calcium excretion but this can be corrected by an adequate calcium intake.

EXERCISE   Exercise in young individuals increases the likelihood that they will attain the maximal genetically determined peak bone mass. Meta-analyses of studies performed in postmenopausal women indicate that weight-bearing exercise prevents bone loss but does not appear to result in substantial gain of bone mass. This beneficial effect wanes if exercise is discontinued. Exercise also has beneficial effects on neuromuscular function, and it improves coordination, balance, and strength, thereby reducing the risk of falling. A walking program is a practical way to start. Other activities such as dancing, racquet sports, cross-country skiing, and use of gym equipment are also recommended, depending on the patient's personal preference. Even women who cannot walk benefit from swimming or water exercises, not so much for the effects on bone, which are quite minimal, but because of effects on muscle. Exercise habits should be consistent, optimally at least three times a week.

Pharmacologic Therapies   Until fairly recently, estrogen treatment, either by itself or in concert with a progestin, was the primary therapeutic agent for prevention or treatment of osteoporosis. Over the past 10 years, a number of new drugs have appeared, and more are expected in the near future. Some are agents that specifically treat osteoporosis (bisphosphonates, calcitonin, PTH); others, such as selective estrogen response modulators (SERMs), have broader effects. The availability of these drugs allows therapy to be tailored to the needs of an individual patient.

ESTROGENS   A large body of clinical trial data indicates that various types of estrogens (conjugated equine estrogens, estradiol, estrone, esterified estrogens, ethinyl estradiol, and mestranol) reduce bone turnover, prevent bone loss, and induce small increases in bone mass of the spine, hip, and total body. The effects of estrogen are seen in women with natural or surgical menopause and in late postmenopausal women with or without established osteoporosis. Estrogens are efficacious when administered orally or transdermally. For both oral and transdermal routes of administration, combined estrogen/progestin preparations are now available in many countries, obviating the problem of taking two tablets or using a patch and oral progestin. One large study, referred to as PEPI (Postmenopausal Estrogen/Progestin Intervention Trial), indicated that C-21 progestins alone do not augment the effect of standard estrogen doses on bone mass (Fig. 333-7).

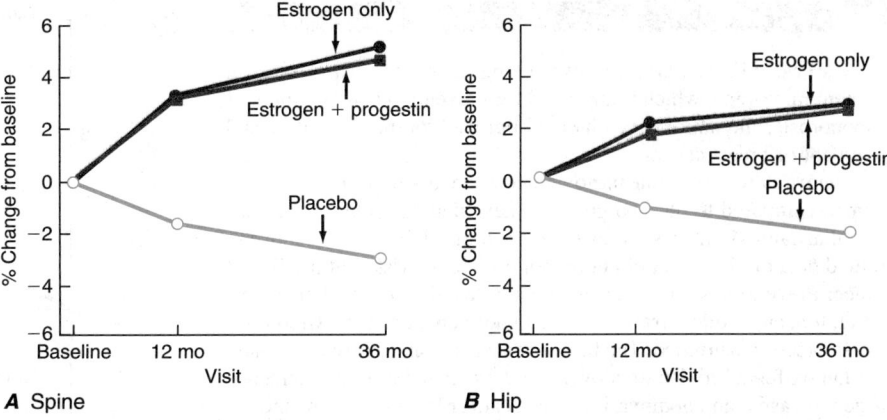

A Spine   **B** Hip

FIGURE 333-7   Results of hormone therapy regimens on bone mineral density (BMD) of the spine (*A*) and hip (*B*). Unadjusted mean percent change in BMD in the hip by treatment assignment and visit: adherent PEPI participants only. Results From the Postmenopausal Estrogen/Progestin Interventions (PEPI) Trial. Estrogen, conjugated equine estrogen 0.625 mg/d; progestin, medroxyprogesterone acetate 10 mg/d. (*Adapted from TL Bush et al: JAMA 276: 1389, 1996.*)

Dose of Estrogen   For oral estrogens, the standard recommended doses are 0.3 mg/d for esterified estrogens, 0.625 mg/d for conjugated equine estrogens, and 5μg/d for ethinyl estradiol. For transdermal estrogen, the commonly used dose supplies 50 μg estradiol per day, but a lower dose may be appropriate for some individuals. Dose response data for conjugated equine estrogens indicate that lower doses are effective.

Fracture Data   Epidemiologic databases indicate that women who take estrogen replacement have a 50% reduction, on average, of osteoporotic fractures, including hip fractures. The beneficial effect of estrogen is greatest among those who start replacement early and continue the treatment; the benefit declines after discontinuation such that there is no residual protective effect against fracture by 10 years after discontinuation. The first clinical trial evaluating fractures as secondary outcomes, the Heart and Estrogen-Progestin Replacement Study (HERS) trial, showed no effect of hormone therapy against hip or other clinical fractures in women with established coronary artery disease. These data made the results of the Women's Health Initiative (WHI) exceedingly important (Chap. 327). The estrogen-progestin arm of the WHI in >16,000 postmenopausal healthy women indicated that hormone therapy reduces the risk of hip fracture by 34% and all clinical fractures by 24%.

A few clinical trials have evaluated spine fracture occurrence as an outcome with estrogen therapy. One that used high doses of estrogen (2.5 mg/d conjugated equine estrogen) indicated marked vertebral fracture reduction in estrogen-treated women. Several other small studies, using lower estrogen doses, have consistently shown that estrogen treatment reduces the incidence of vertebral compression fracture.

The WHI has now provided a vast amount of data on the multisystemic effects of hormone therapy. Although earlier observational studies suggested that estrogen replacement might reduce heart disease, the WHI showed that combined estrogen-progestin treatment increased risk of fatal and nonfatal myocardial infarction by about 29%, confirming data from the HERS study. Other important relative risks included a 40% increase in stroke, 100% increase in venous thromboembolic disease, and a 26% increase in risk of breast cancer. Subsequent analyses have confirmed the increased risk of stroke and shown a twofold increase in dementia. Benefits other than the fracture reductions noted above included a 37% reduction in risk of colon cancer. These relative risks have to be interpreted in light of absolute risk (Fig. 333-8). For example, out of 10,000 women treated with estrogen-progestin for 1 year, there will be 8 excess heart attacks, 8 excess breast cancers, 18 excess venous thromboembolic events, 5 fewer hip fractures, 44 fewer clinical fractures, and 6 fewer colorectal cancers. These numbers must be multiplied by years of hormone treatment. There was no effect of hormone treatment on risk of uterine cancer or total mortality.

It is important to note that the WHI findings apply specifically to hormone treatment in the form of conjugated equine estrogen plus medroxyprogesterone acetate. Furthermore the relative benefits and

risks of unopposed estrogen in women who had hysterectomy are still being evaluated in the estrogen-only arm of the WHI.

Mode of Action   Two subtypes of ERs, α and β, have been identified in bone and other tissues. Cells of monocyte lineage express both ERα and -β, as do osteoblasts. Estrogen-mediated effects vary depending on the receptor type. Using ER knockout mouse models, elimination of ERα produces a modest reduction in bone mass, whereas mutation of ERβ has less effect on bone. A male patient with a homozygous mutation of ERα had markedly decreased bone density as well as abnormalities in epiphyseal closure, confirming the important role of ERα in bone biology. The mechanism of estrogen action in bone is an area of active investigation (Fig. 333-5). Although data are conflicting, estrogens may inhibit osteoclasts directly. However, the majority of estrogen (and androgen) effects on bone resorption are mediated indirectly through paracrine factors produced by osteoblasts. These actions include: (1) increasing IGF-I and TGF-β, and (2) suppressing IL-1 (α and β), IL-6, TNF-α, and osteocalcin synthesis. The indirect estrogen actions primarily decrease bone resorption.

PROGESTINS   In women with a uterus, daily progestin or cyclical progestins at least 12 days per month are prescribed in combination with estrogens to reduce the risk of uterine cancer. Medroxyprogesterone acetate and norethindrone acetate blunt the high-density lipoprotein response to estrogen, but micronized progesterone does not. Neither medroxyprogesterone acetate nor micronized progesterone appears to have an independent effect on bone; at lower doses, norethindrone acetate might have an additive benefit. On breast tissue, progestins may increase the risk of breast cancer.

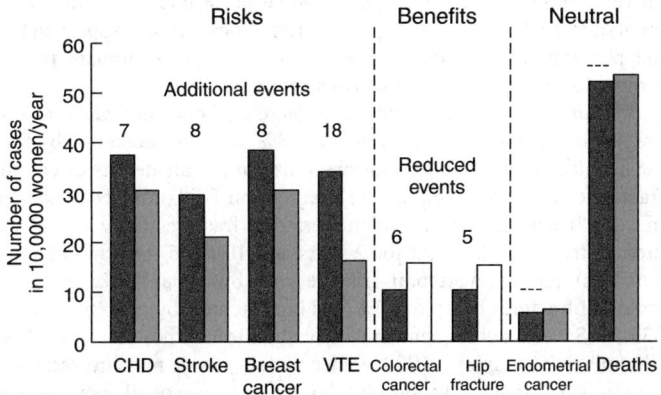

FIGURE 333-8   Effects of hormone therapy on event rates (CHD, coronary heart disease; VTE, venous thromboembolic events). (*Adapted from: Women's Health Initiative. WHI HRT Update. Available at http://www.nhlbi.nih.gov/whi/hrtupd/upd20002.htm.2002.*)

SERMS Two SERMs are currently being used in postmenopausal women: raloxifene, which is approved for prevention and treatment of osteoporosis, and tamoxifen, which is approved for the prevention and treatment of breast cancer.

Tamoxifen reduces bone turnover and bone loss in postmenopausal women compared to placebo groups. These findings support the concept that tamoxifen acts as an estrogenic agent in bone. There are limited data on the effect of tamoxifen on fracture risk, but the Breast Cancer Prevention study indicated a possible reduction in clinical vertebral, hip, and Colles' fractures. The major benefit of tamoxifen is on breast cancer occurrence. The breast cancer prevention trial indicated that tamoxifen administration over 4 to 5 years reduced the incidence of new invasive and noninvasive breast cancer by ~45% in women at increased risk of breast cancer. The incidence of ER-positive breast cancers was reduced by 65%.

Raloxifene (60 mg/d) has effects on bone turnover and bone mass that are very similar to those of tamoxifen, indicating that this agent is also estrogenic on the skeleton. The effect of raloxifene on bone density (+1.4 to 2.8% versus placebo in the spine, hip, and total body) is somewhat less than that seen with standard doses of estrogens. Raloxifene reduces the occurrence of vertebral fracture by 30 to 50%, depending on the subpopulation; however, there are no data confirming that raloxifene can reduce the risk of nonvertebral fractures.

Raloxifene, like tamoxifen and estrogen, has effects in other organ systems. The most beneficial effect appears to be a reduction in invasive breast cancer (mainly decreased ER-positive) occurrence of about 65% in women who take raloxifene compared to placebo. In contrast to tamoxifen, raloxifene is not associated with an increase in the risk of uterine cancer or benign uterine disease. Raloxifene increases the occurrence of hot flashes but reduces serum total and low-density lipoprotein cholesterol, lipoprotein(a), and fibrinogen. In women at high risk of heart disease, preliminary data suggest that raloxifene may reduce the occurrence of heart disease and stroke outcomes by about 40%. A large ongoing pivotal study, called Raloxifene Use for the Heart (RUTH), will further evaluate vascular disease and breast cancer outcomes.

Mode of Action of SERMs All SERMs bind to the ER, but each agent produces a unique receptor conformation. As a result, specific coactivator or co-repressor proteins are bound to the receptor (Chap. 317), resulting in differential effects on gene transcription that vary depending on other transcription factors present in the cell. Another aspect of selectivity is the affinity of each SERM for the different ERα and -β subtypes, which are expressed differentially in various tissues. These tissue-selective effects of SERMs offer the possibility of tailoring estrogen therapy to best meet the needs and risk factor profile of an individual patient.

BISPHOSPHONATES Both alendronate and risedronate are approved for the prevention and treatment of postmenopausal osteoporosis and treatment of steroid-induced osteoporosis. Risedronate is also approved for the prevention of steroid-induced osteoporosis. Alendronate is approved for treatment of osteoporosis in men.

Alendronate has been shown to decrease bone turnover and increase bone mass in the spine by up to 8% versus placebo and by 6% versus placebo in the hip. Multiple trials have evaluated its effect on fracture occurrence. The Fracture Intervention Trial provided evidence in >2000 women with prevalent vertebral fractures that daily alendronate treatment (5 mg/d for 2 years and 10 mg/d for 9 months afterwards) reduces vertebral fracture risk by about 50%, multiple vertebral fractures by up to 90%, and hip fractures by up to 50% (Fig. 333-9). Several subsequent trials have confirmed these findings. For example, in a study of >1900 women with low bone mass treated with alendronate (10 mg/d) versus placebo, the incidence of all nonvertebral fractures was reduced by ~47% after only 1 year.

Trials comparing once-weekly alendronate, 70 mg, with daily 10-mg dosing have shown equivalence with regard to bone mass and bone

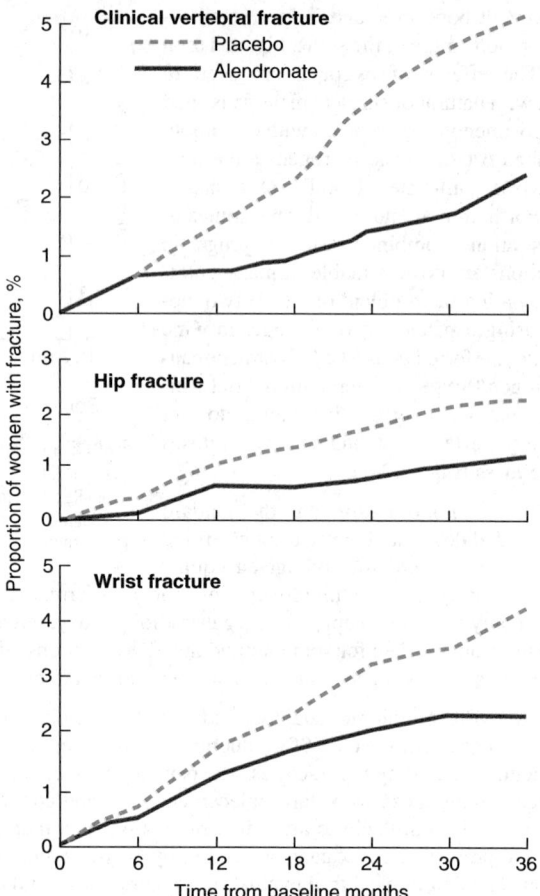

FIGURE 333-9 Cumulative proportions of women with osteoporosis who suffered clinical vertebral, hip, or wrist fracture during 3 years of treatment with alendronate or placebo (FIT 1). (*From DM Black et al: Lancet 348:1535, 1996.*)

turnover responses. Consequently, once-weekly therapy is generally preferred because of low incidence of gastrointestinal side effects and ease of administration. Alendronate should be given with a full glass of water before breakfast, as bisphosphonates are poorly absorbed. Because of the potential for esophageal irritation, alendronate is contraindicated in patients who have stricture or inadequate emptying of the esophagus. It is recommended that patients remain upright for at least 30 min after taking the medication to avoid esophageal irritation. Cases of esophagitis, esophageal ulcer, and esophageal stricture have been described, but the incidence appears to be low. In clinical trials, overall gastrointestinal symptomatology was no different with alendronate compared to placebo.

Risedronate also reduces bone turnover and increases bone mass. Controlled clinical trials have demonstrated 40 to 50% reduction in vertebral fracture risk over 3 years, accompanied by a 40% reduction in clinical nonspine fractures. The only clinical trial specifically designed to evaluate hip fracture outcome (HIP) indicated that risedronate reduced hip fracture risk in women in their 70s with confirmed osteoporosis by 40%. In contrast, risedronate was not effective at reducing hip fracture occurrence in older women without proven osteoporosis. Studies have shown that 35 mg of risedronate administered once weekly is therapeutically equivalent to 5 mg/d. Patients should take risedronate with a full glass of plain water [0.18 to 0.25 L (6 to 8 oz)], to facilitate delivery to the stomach, and should not lie down for 30 min after taking the drug. The incidence of gastrointestinal side effects in trials with risedronate was similar to that of placebo.

Etidronate was the first bisphosphonate to be approved, initially for use in Paget's disease and hypercalcemia. This agent has also been used in osteoporosis trials of smaller magnitude than those performed for alendronate and risedronate but is not approved by the FDA for treatment of osteoporosis. Etidronate probably has some efficacy against vertebral fracture when given as an intermittent cyclical regimen (2 weeks on, 2 1/2 months off). There has not been any study of its effectiveness against nonvertebral fractures.

Zoledronate and ibandronate are potent bisphosphonates with unique administration regimens (once yearly intravenously, once monthly orally) and are currently in clinical development.

Mode of Action Bisphosphonates are structurally related to pyrophosphates, compounds that are incorporated into bone matrix. Bisphosphonates specifically impair osteoclast function and reduce osteoclast number, in part by the induction of apoptosis. Recent evidence suggests that the nitrogen-containing bisphosphonates also inhibit protein prenylation, one of the end products in the mevalonic acid pathway. This effect disrupts intracellular protein trafficking and may ultimately lead to apoptosis. Some bisphosphonates have very long retention in the skeleton and may exert long-term effects.

CALCITONIN Calcitonin is a polypeptide hormone produced by the thyroid gland (Chap. 332). Its physiologic role is unclear as no skeletal disease has been described in association with calcitonin deficiency or calcitonin excess. Calcitonin preparations are approved by the FDA for Paget's disease, hypercalcemia, and osteoporosis in women >5 years past menopause.

Injectable calcitonin produces small increments in bone mass of the lumbar spine. However, difficulty of administration and frequent reactions, including nausea and facial flushing, make general use limited. In 1995, a nasal spray containing calcitonin (200 IU/d) was approved for treatment of osteoporosis in postmenopausal women. One study suggests that nasal calcitonin produces small increments in bone mass and a small reduction in new vertebral fractures in calcitonin-treated patients versus those on calcium alone. There has been no proven effectiveness against nonvertebral fractures.

Calcitonin is not indicated for prevention of osteoporosis and is not sufficiently potent to prevent bone loss in early postmenopausal women. As mentioned above, calcitonin might have an analgesic effect on bone pain, both in the subcutaneous and possibly the nasal form.

Mode of Action Calcitonin suppresses osteoclast activity by direct action on the osteoclast calcitonin receptor. Osteoclasts exposed to calcitonin cannot maintain their active ruffled border, which normally maintains close contact with underlying bone.

PARATHYROID HORMONE Endogenous PTH is an 84-amino-acid peptide that is largely responsible for calcium homeostasis (Chap. 332). Although chronic elevation of PTH, as occurs in hyperparathyroidism, is associated with bone loss (particularly cortical bone), PTH can also exert anabolic effects on bone. Consistent with this, some observational studies have indicated that mild elevations in PTH are associated with maintenance of trabecular bone mass. On the basis of these findings, preclinical and early clinical studies have been performed using an exogenous PTH analogue (1-34 PTH). The first randomized controlled trial in postmenopausal women showed that PTH, when superimposed on ongoing estrogen therapy, produced substantial increments in bone mass (13% over a 3-year period compared to estrogen alone) and reduced the risk of vertebral compression deformity. In one study (median 19 months' duration), 20 μg PTH(1-34) reduced vertebral fractures by 65% and nonvertebral fractures by 45% (Fig. 333-10). PTH(1-34) has now been approved by the FDA for treatment of patients with osteoporosis (both women and men) at high risk of fracture. Treatment is administered as a single daily injection given for a maximum of 2 years. Although there are no randomized controlled studies to confirm the need for an antiresorptive agent after PTH withdrawal, based on observational data and animal studies, it is likely that antiresorptive agents will be required to maintain PTH-induced benefits on bone mass and fracture. In contrast to combination

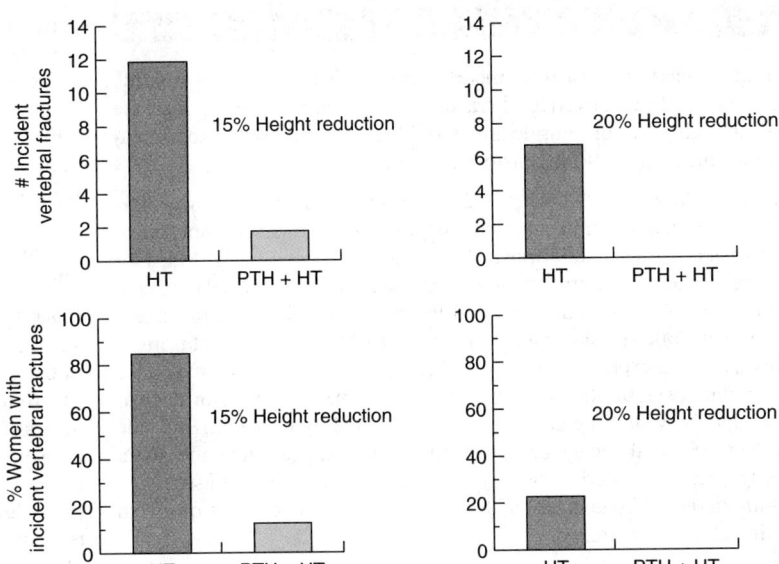

FIGURE 333-10 Number of incident vertebral deformities (15% and 20% reductions) in women with osteoporosis on hormone therapy (HT), compared to HT + PTH over 3 years. (HT, hormone therapy; PTH, parathyroid hormone.) (*From Cosman et al.*)

treatment with estrogen, there are no published data on use of PTH in combination with bisphosphonates or SERMs.

Side effects are generally mild and can include muscle pains, weakness, dizziness, headache, and nausea. Rodents given prolonged treatment with PTH in relatively high doses developed osteogenic sarcomas. It is not believed that this finding has any relevance to humans.

PTH use may be limited by its mode of administration; alternative modes of delivery are being investigated. The optimal frequency of administration also remains to be established, and it is possible that PTH might also be effective when used intermittently. Cost may also be a limiting factor.

Mode of Action Exogenously administered PTH appears to have direct actions on osteoblast activity, with biochemical and histomorphometric evidence of de novo bone formation early in response to PTH, prior to activation of bone resorption. Subsequently, PTH activates bone remodeling but still appears to favor bone formation over bone resorption. PTH stimulates IGF-I and collagen production and appears to increase osteoblast number by stimulating replication, enhancing osteoblast recruitment, and inhibiting apoptosis. Unlike all other treatments, PTH produces a true increase in bone tissue and an apparent restoration of bone microarchitecture (Fig. 333-11).

FLUORIDE Fluoride has been available for many years and is a potent stimulator of osteoprogenitor cells when studied in vitro. It has been used in multiple osteoporosis studies with conflicting results, in part related to use of varying doses and preparations. Despite increments

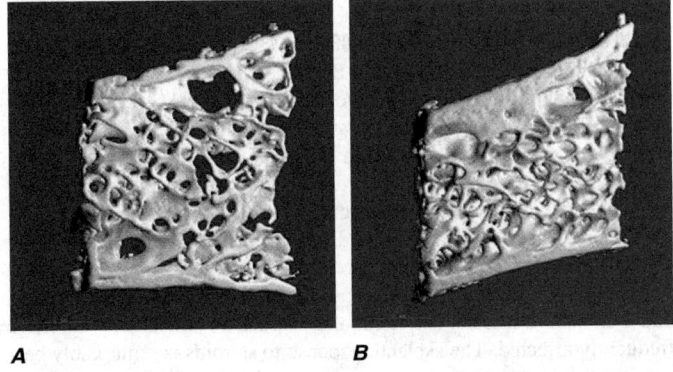

FIGURE 333-11 Effect of parathyroid hormone (PTH) treatment on bone microarchitecture. Paired biopsy specimens from a 64-year-old woman before (*A*) and after (*B*) treatment with PTH. (*From DW Dempster et al: J Bone Miner Res 16:1846, 2001.*)

in bone mass of up to 10%, there are no consistent effects of fluoride on vertebral or nonvertebral fracture, which might actually increase when high doses of fluoride are used. Fluoride remains an experimental agent, despite its long history and multiple studies.

OTHER POTENTIAL ANABOLIC AGENTS   Several small studies of growth hormone (GH), alone or in combination with other agents, have not shown consistent or substantial positive effects on skeletal mass. Many of these studies are relatively short-term, and the effects of GH, growth hormone–releasing hormone, and the IGFs are still under investigation. Anabolic steroids, mostly derivatives of testosterone, act primarily as antiresorptive agents to reduce bone turnover but may also stimulate osteoblastic activity. Effects on bone mass remain unclear but appear weak, in general, and use is limited by masculinizing side effects. Several recent observational studies suggest that the statin drugs, currently used to treat hypercholesterolemia, may be associated with increased bone mass and reduced fractures, but conclusions from clinical trials are mixed.

Nonpharmacologic Approaches   Protective pads worn around the outer thigh, which cover the trochanteric region of the hip can prevent hip fractures in elderly residents in nursing homes. The use of hip protectors is limited largely by compliance and comfort, but new devices are being developed that may circumvent these problems and provide adjunctive treatments.

Kyphoplasty and *vertebroplasty* are also useful nonpharmacologic approaches for the treatment of painful vertebral fractures. However, no long-term data are available.

Treatment Monitoring   There are currently no well-accepted guidelines for monitoring treatment of osteoporosis. Because most osteoporosis treatments produce small or moderate bone mass increments on average, it is reasonable to consider BMD as a monitoring tool. Changes must exceed ~4% in the spine and 6% in the hip to be considered significant in any individual. The hip is the preferred site due to larger surface area and greater reproducibility. Medication-induced increments may require several years to produce changes of this magnitude (if they do at all). Consequently, it can be argued that BMD should not be repeated at intervals <2 years. Only significant BMD reductions should prompt a change in medical regimen, as it is expected that many individuals will not show responses greater than the detection limits of the current measurement techniques.

Biochemical markers of bone turnover may prove useful for treatment monitoring, but there is currently little hard evidence to support this concept; it remains unclear which endpoint is most useful. If bone turnover markers are used, a determination should be made before starting therapy and repeated ≥4 months after therapy is initiated. In general, a change in bone turnover markers must be 30 to 40% lower than the baseline to be significant because of the biologic and technical variability in these tests. A positive change in biochemical markers and/or bone density can be useful to help patients adhere to treatment regimens.

GLUCOCORTICOID-INDUCED OSTEOPOROSIS   Osteoporotic fractures are a well-characterized consequence of the hypercortisolism associated with Cushing's syndrome. However, the therapeutic use of glucocorticoids is by far the most common form of glucocorticoid-induced osteoporosis. Glucocorticoids are widely used in the treatment of a variety of disorders, including chronic lung disorders, rheumatoid arthritis and other connective tissue diseases, inflammatory bowel disease, and posttransplantation. Osteoporosis and related fractures are serious side effects of chronic glucocorticoid therapy. Because the effects of glucocorticoids on the skeleton are often superimposed upon the consequences of aging and menopause, it is not surprising that women and the elderly are most frequently affected. The skeletal response to steroids is remarkably heterogeneous, however, and even young, growing individuals treated with glucocorticoids can present with fractures.

The risk of fractures depends on the dose and duration of gluco-

corticoid therapy, although recent data suggest that there may be no completely safe dose. Bone loss is more rapid during the early months of treatment, and trabecular bone is more severely affected than cortical bone. As a result, fractures have been shown to increase within 3 months of steroid treatment. There is an increase in fracture risk in both the axial and appendicular skeleton, including risk of hip fracture. Bone loss can occur with any route of steroid administration including high-dose inhaled glucocorticoids and intraarticular injections. Alternate-day delivery does not appear to ameliorate the skeletal effects of glucocorticoids.

Pathophysiology   Glucocorticoids increase bone loss by multiple mechanisms including: (1) inhibition of osteoblast function and an increase in osteoblast apoptosis, resulting in impaired synthesis of new bone; (2) stimulation of bone resorption, probably as a secondary effect; (3) impairment of the absorption of calcium across the intestine, probably by a vitamin D–independent effect; (4) increase of urinary calcium loss and induction of some degree of secondary hyperparathyroidism; (5) reduction of adrenal androgens and suppression of ovarian and testicular secretion of estrogens and androgens; and (6) induction of glucocorticoid myopathy, which may exacerbate effects on skeletal and calcium homeostasis as well as increase the risk of falls.

Evaluation of the Patient   Because of the prevalence of glucocorticoid-induced bone loss, it is important to evaluate the status of the skeleton in all patients starting or already receiving long-term glucocorticoid therapy. Modifiable risk factors should be identified, including those for falls. Examination should include height and muscle strength testing. Laboratory evaluation should include an assessment of 24-h urinary calcium. A task force of the American College of Rheumatology recommends that all patients on long-term (>6 months) glucocorticoids have measurement of bone mass at both the spine and hip using DXA. If only one skeletal site can be measured, it is best to assess the spine in individuals <60 years and the hip for those >60 years.

Prevention   Bone loss caused by glucocorticoids can be prevented, and the risk of fractures significantly reduced. Strategies must include using the lowest dose of glucocorticoid for disease management. Topical and inhaled routes of administration are preferred, where appropriate. Risk factor reduction is important, including smoking cessation, limitation of alcohol consumption, and participation in weight-bearing exercise, when appropriate. All patients should receive an adequate calcium and vitamin D intake from the diet or from supplements.

℞ TREATMENT

Only bisphosphonates have been demonstrated in large clinical trials to reduce the risk of fractures in patients being treated with glucocorticoids. Risedronate prevents bone loss and reduces vertebral fracture risk by about 70%. Similar beneficial effects are observed in studies of alendronate and etidronate. Controlled trials of hormone therapy have shown bone-sparing effects, and calcitonin also has some protective effect in the spine. Thiazides reduce urine calcium loss, but their role in prevention of fractures is unclear. PTH has also been studied in a small group of women with glucocorticoid-induced osteoporosis. Bone mass increased substantially, but no fracture data are available.

FURTHER READING

COSMAN F, LINDSAY R: Selective estrogen receptors modulators: Clinical spectrum. Endocr Rev 20:418, 1999

——— et al: Parathyroid hormone added to established hormone therapy: Effects on vertebral fracture and maintenance of bone mass after parathyroid hormone withdrawal. J Bone Miner Res 16:925, 2001

GUYATT G et al: Meta-analyses of therapies for postmenopausal osteoporosis. Endocr Rev 23:495, 2002

NEER RM et al: Effect of parathyroid hormone (1-34) on fractures and bone mineral density in postmenopausal women with osteoporosis. N Engl J Med 344:1434, 2001

WRITING GROUP FOR THE WOMEN'S HEALTH INITIATIVE INVESTIGATORS: Risks and benefits of estrogen plus progestin in healthy postmenopausal women: Principal results from the Women's Health Initiative randomized controlled trial. JAMA 288:321, 2002

PAGET DISEASE OF BONE

Paget disease is a localized bone disorder that often affects widespread areas of the skeleton through increased bone remodeling. The pathologic process is initiated by overactive osteoclastic bone resorption followed by a compensatory increase in osteoblastic new bone formation. New pagetic bone is structurally disorganized and more susceptible to deformities and fractures. Although most patients are asymptomatic, a variety of symptoms and complications may result directly from bony involvement or secondarily from the expansion of bone and subsequent compression of surrounding neural tissue.

EPIDEMIOLOGY There is a marked geographic variation in the frequency of Paget disease, with high prevalence in Western Europe (Great Britain, France, and Germany but not Switzerland or Scandinavia) and among those who have immigrated to Australia, New Zealand, South Africa, and North and South America. The disease is rare in native populations of the Americas, Africa, Asia, and the Middle East. The prevalence is greater in males and increases with age. Autopsy series reveal Paget disease in about 3% of those over age 40. Prevalence of positive skeletal radiographs in patients over age 55 is 2.5% for men and 1.6% for women. Elevated alkaline phosphatase (ALP) levels in asymptomatic patients has an age-adjusted incidence of 12.7 and 7 per 100,000 person-years in men and women, respectively. The frequency of diagnosis by either radiographic or biochemical criteria has decreased during the past 20 years.

ETIOLOGY The etiology of Paget disease of bone remains unknown, but evidence supports both genetic and viral etiologies. A positive family history is found in 5 to 25% of patients and, when present, raises the prevalence of the disease seven- to tenfold among first-degree relatives. Familial patterns of disease in several large kindred are consistent with an autosomal dominant pattern of inheritance with variable penetrance. A susceptibility locus for Paget disease has been mapped to chromosome 18q21-22, a region that contains the gene responsible for a rare Paget disease–like skeletal disorder known as familial expansile osteolysis. The gene encodes the receptor activator of nuclear factor-κB (RANK), a member of the tumor necrosis factor superfamily critical for osteoclast differentiation (Fig. 334-1). In other families, susceptibility loci have been mapped to loci on chromosomes 18q23, 6p21.3, 5q31, and 5q35. A homozygous deletion of the *TNFRSF11B* gene, which encodes osteoprotegrin (Fig. 334-1), causes juvenile Paget disease, a disorder characterized by uncontrolled osteoclastic differentiation and resorption. Thus, it is likely that Paget disease is genetically heterogeneous with divergent pathogenetic mechanisms in sporadic and familial forms.

Several lines of evidence suggest a viral etiology of Paget disease, including (1) the presence of cytoplasmic and nuclear inclusions resembling paramyxoviruses (measles and respiratory syncytial virus) in pagetic osteoclasts, and (2) viral mRNA in precursor and mature osteoclasts. The viral etiology is further supported by conversion of osteoclast precursors to pagetic-like osteoclasts by vectors containing the measles virus nucleocapsid or matrix genes. However, the viral etiology has been questioned by the inability to culture a live virus from pagetic bone and by failure to clone the full-length viral genes from material obtained from patients with Paget disease.

PATHOPHYSIOLOGY The principal abnormality in Paget disease is the increased number and activity of osteoclasts. Pagetic osteoclasts are large, increased 10- to 100-fold in number, and have a greater number of nuclei (as many as 100 compared to 3 to 5 nuclei in the normal osteoclast). The overactive osteoclasts create a sevenfold increase in resorptive surfaces and an erosion rate of 9 μg/d (normal is 1 μg/d). Several causes for the increased number and activity of pagetic osteoclasts have been identified: (1) osteoclastic precursors are hypersen-

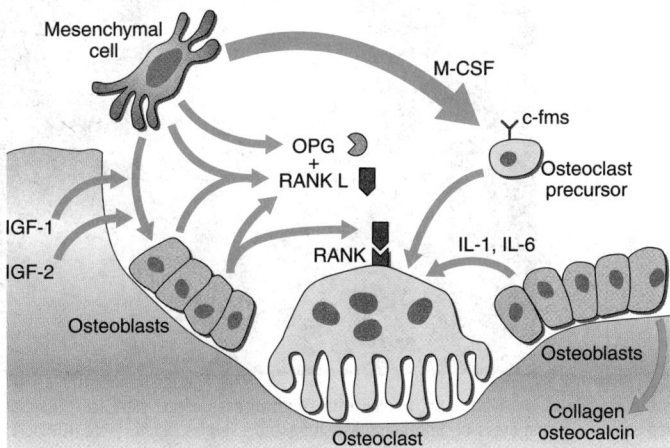

FIGURE 334-1 Diagram illustrating factors that promote differentiation and function of osteoclasts and osteoblasts and the role of the RANK pathway. Stromal bone marrow (mesenchymal) cells and differentiated osteoblasts produce multiple growth factors and cytokines, including macrophage colony-stimulating factor (M-CSF), to modulate osteoclastogenesis. RANKL (receptor activator of NFκB ligand) is produced by osteoblast progenitors and mature osteoblasts and can bind to a soluble decoy receptor known as OPG (osteoprotegrin) to inhibit RANKL action. Alternatively, a cell-cell interaction between osteoblast and osteoclast progenitors allows RANKL to bind to its membrane-bound receptor, RANK, thereby stimulating osteoclast differentiation and function. RANK binds intracellular proteins called TRAFS (tumor necrosis factor receptor-associated factors) that mediate receptor signaling through transcription factors such as NFκB. M-CSF binds to its receptor, c-fms, which is the cellular homologue of the *fms* oncogene. See text for the potential role of these pathways in disorders of osteoclast function such as Paget disease and osteopetrosis.

sitive to 1,25(OH)$_2$D$_3$; (2) osteoclasts are hyperresponsive to RANK ligand (RANKL), the osteoclast stimulatory factor that mediates the effects of most osteotropic factors on osteoclast formation; (3) marrow stromal cells from pagetic lesions have increased RANKL expression; (4) osteoclast precursor recruitment is increased by interleukin (IL) 6, which is increased in the blood of patients with active Paget disease and is overexpressed in pagetic osteoclasts; (5) expression of the proto-oncogene c-*fos*, which increases osteoclastic activity, is increased; and (6) the antiapoptotic oncogene *Bcl*-2 in pagetic bone is overexpressed. Numerous osteoblasts are recruited to active resorption sites and produce large amounts of new bone matrix. As a result, bone turnover is high and bone mass is normal or increased, not reduced.

The characteristic feature of Paget disease is increased bone resorption accompanied by accelerated bone formation. An initial osteolytic phase involves prominent bone resorption and marked hypervascularization. Radiographically, this manifests as an advancing lytic wedge, or "blade of grass" lesion. The second phase is a period of very active bone formation and resorption that replaces normal lamellar bone with haphazard (woven) bone. The mosaic pattern of woven bone is structurally inferior and can bow and fracture more readily. At the same time, fibrous connective tissue may replace normal bone marrow. In the final sclerotic phase, bone resorption declines progressively and leads to a hard, dense, less vascular pagetic or mosaic bone, which represents the so-called burned-out phase of Paget disease. All three phases may be present at the same time at different skeletal sites.

CLINICAL MANIFESTATIONS Asymptomatic patients are often diagnosed by discovery of an elevated ALP level on routine blood chemistry testing or from an abnormality on a skeletal radiograph obtained for another indication. The skeletal sites most commonly involved are the pelvis, vertebral bodies, skull, femur, and tibia. Numerous active sites of skeletal involvement are more common in familial cases with an early presentation.

Pain is the most common presenting symptom. It results from in-

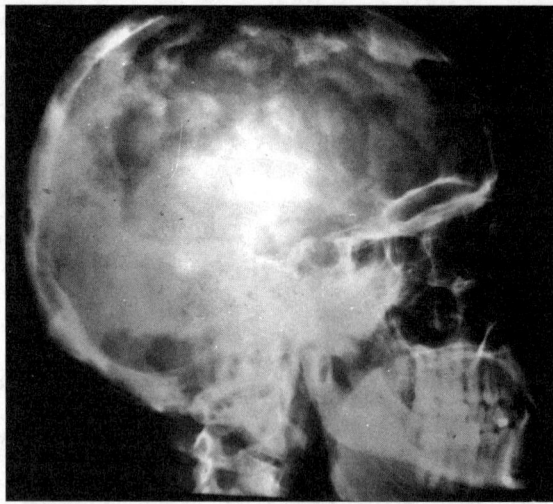

FIGURE 334-2   A 48-year-old woman with Paget disease of the skull. *Left.* Lateral radiograph showing areas of both bone resorption and sclerosis. *Right.* ^{99m}Tc HDP bone scan with anterior, posterior, and lateral views of the skull showing diffuse isotope uptake by the frontal, parietal, occipital, and petrous bones.

creased bony vascularity, expanding lytic lesions, fractures, bowing, or other deformities of the extremities. Bowing of the femur or tibia causes gait abnormalities and abnormal mechanical stresses with secondary osteoarthritis of the hip or knee joints. Long bone bowing also causes extremity pain by stretching the muscles attached to the bone softened by the pagetic process. Back pain results from enlarged pagetic vertebrae, vertebral compression fractures, spinal stenosis, degenerative changes of the joints, and altered body mechanics with kyphosis and forward tilt of the upper back. Rarely, spinal cord compression may result from bone enlargement or from the vascular steal syndrome. Skull involvement may cause headaches, symmetric or asymmetric enlargement of the parietal or frontal bones (frontal bossing), and increased head size. Cranial expansion may narrow cranial foramina and cause neurologic complications including hearing loss from cochlear nerve damage from temporal bone involvement, cranial nerve palsies, and softening of the base of the skull (*platybasia*) and the risk of brainstem compression. Pagetic involvement of the facial bones may cause facial deformity, loss of teeth and other dental conditions, and rarely, airway compression.

Fractures are serious complications of Paget disease and usually occur in long bones at areas of active or advancing lytic lesions. Common fracture sites are the femoral shaft and subtrochanteric regions. Neoplasms arising from pagetic bone are rare. The incidence of sarcoma appears to be decreasing, possibly because of earlier, more effective treatment with potent antiresorptive agents. The majority of tumors are osteosarcomas, which usually present with new pain in a long-standing pagetic lesion. Osteoclast-rich benign giant cell tumors may arise in areas adjacent to pagetic bone and respond to glucocorticoid therapy.

Cardiovascular complications may occur in patients with involvement of large (15 to 35%) portions of the skeleton and a high degree of disease activity (ALP four times above normal). The extensive arteriovenous shunting and marked increases in blood flow through the vascular pagetic bone lead to a high-output state and cardiac enlargement. However, high-output heart failure is relatively rare and usually develops in patients with concomitant cardiac pathology. In addition, calcific aortic stenosis and diffuse vascular calcifications have been associated with Paget disease.

DIAGNOSIS   The diagnosis may be suggested on clinical examination by the presence of enlarged skull with frontal bossing, bowing of an extremity, or short stature with simian posturing. An extremity with an area of warmth and tenderness to palpation may suggest an underlying pagetic lesion. Other findings include bony deformity of the pelvis, skull, spine and extremities; arthritic involvement of the joints adjacent to lesions; and leg length discrepancy resulting from deformities of the long bones.

2280

Paget disease is usually diagnosed from radiologic and biochemical abnormalities. Radiographic findings typical of Paget disease include enlargement or expansion of an entire bone or area of a long bone, cortical thickening, coarsening of trabecular markings, and typical lytic and sclerotic changes. Skull radiographs (Fig. 334-2) reveal regions of "cotton wool," or osteoporosis circumscripta; thickening of diploic areas; and enlargement and sclerosis of a portion or all of one or more skull bones. Vertebral cortical thickening of the superior and inferior end plates creates a "picture frame" vertebra. Diffuse radiodense enlargement of a vertebra is referred to as "ivory vertebra." Pelvic radiographs may demonstrate disruption or fusion of the sacroiliac joints; porotic and radiodense lesions of the ilium with whorls of coarse trabeculation; thickened and sclerotic ileopectinal line (Brim sign); and softening with protrusio acetabuli, with axial migration of the hips and functional flexion contracture. Radiographs of long bones reveal bowing deformity and typical pagetic changes of cortical thickening and expansion and areas of lucency and sclerosis (Fig. 334-3). Radionuclide ^{99m}Tc bone scans are less specific but are more sensitive than standard radiographs for identifying sites of active skeletal lesions. Suspected areas of malignant transformation are best distinguished from pagetic bone by computed tomography (CT) or magnetic

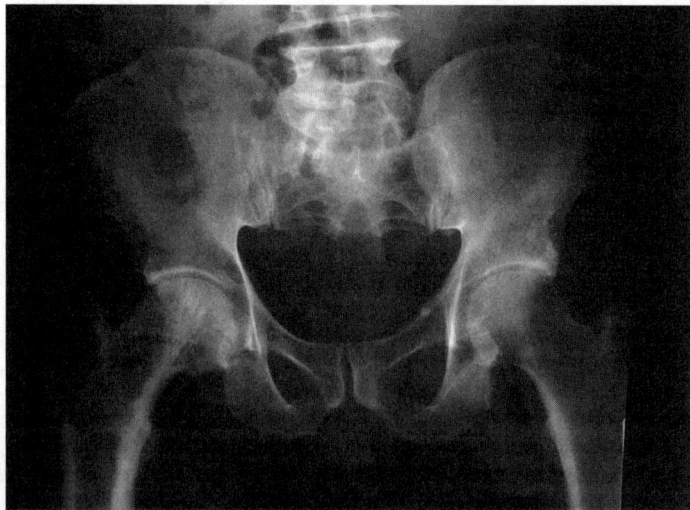

FIGURE 334-3   Radiograph of a 73-year-old man with Paget disease of the right proximal femur. Note the coarsening of the trabecular pattern with marked cortical thickening and narrowing of the joint space consistent with osteoarthritis secondary to pagetic deformity of the right femur.

resonance imaging (MRI). Definitive diagnosis of malignancy requires bone biopsy.

Biochemical evaluation is useful in the diagnosis and management of Paget disease. The marked increase in bone turnover can be monitored using biochemical markers of bone formation and resorption. The parallel rise in serum ALP and urinary hydroxyproline levels, markers of bone formation and resorption, respectively, confirm the coupling of bone formation and resorption in Paget disease. The degree of bone marker elevation reflects the extent and severity of the disease. Patients with the highest elevation of ALP (10 times the upper limit of normal) typically have involvement of the skull and at least one other skeletal site. Lower values suggest less extensive involvement or a quiescent phase of the disease. For most patients, serum total ALP remains the test of choice both for diagnosis and assessing response to therapy. Occasionally, a symptomatic patient with evidence of progression at a single site may have a normal total ALP level but increased bone-specific ALP. Serum osteocalcin, a marker of bone formation, is not always elevated in patients with active Paget disease and is not recommended for use in diagnosis or management.

Urinary and serum deoxypyridinoline, N-telopeptide, and C-telopeptide levels are products of type I collagen degradation and are more specific for bone resorption than hydroxyproline. These newer bone resorption markers have distinct advantages over measurement of 24-h or second-morning void hydroxyproline/creatinine ratio, which requires control of dietary gelatin intake and precise urine collection and analysis. The new resorption markers decrease more rapidly in response to therapy than does ALP.

Serum calcium and phosphate levels are normal in Paget disease. Immobilization of a patient with active Paget disease may rarely cause hypercalcemia and hypercalciuria and increase the risk for nephrolithiasis. However, the discovery of hypercalcemia, even in the presence of immobilization, should prompt a search for another cause of hypercalcemia. In contrast, hypocalcemia or mild secondary hyperparathyroidism may develop in Paget patients with very active bone formation and insufficient dietary calcium intake. Hypocalcemia can occur during bisphosphonate therapy when bone resorption is rapidly suppressed and active bone formation continues. Hypocalcemia may be prevented by adequate calcium and vitamin D intake.

Rx TREATMENT

The development of effective and potent pharmacologic agents (Table 334-1) has changed the treatment philosophy from treating only symptomatic patients to treating asymptomatic patients who are at risk for complications. Pharmacologic therapy is indicated in the following circumstances: to control symptoms caused by metabolically active Paget disease such as bone pain, fracture, headache, pain from pagetic radiculopathy or arthropathy, or neurologic complications; to decrease local blood flow and minimize operative blood loss in patients undergoing surgery at an active pagetic site; to reduce hypercalciuria that may occur during immobilization; and to decrease the risk of complications when disease activity is high (elevated ALP) and when the site of involvement involves weight-bearing bones, areas adjacent to major joints, vertebral bodies, and skull. Whether early therapy prevents late complications remains to be determined. However, the restoration of normal bone architecture following suppression of pagetic activity suggests that treatment may prevent further deformities and complications.

Agents approved for treatment of Paget disease suppress the very high rates of bone resorption and secondarily decrease the high rates of bone formation (Table 334-1). As a result of decreasing bone turnover, pagetic structural patterns, including areas of poorly mineralized

TABLE 334-1 *Pharmacologic Agents Approved for Treatment of Paget Disease*

Name (Brand)	Potency[a]	Dose	Mode of Administration[b]
Etidronate (Didronel)	1	400 mg/d for 6 mos	Fasting with 6 oz tap water 2 h before or after a meal
Tiludronate (Skelid)	10	400 mg/d for 3 mos	Fasting with 6 oz tap water and wait 45 min before food, liquids are taken
Pamidronte (Aredia)	100	30 mg IV daily for 3 days or 60 to 90 mg IV at various intervals as determined by disease	
Alendronate (Fosamax)	700	40 mg/d for 6 mos	Fasting with 6 oz tap water and wait 45 min before food, liquids are taken
Risedronate (Actonel)	1000	30 mg/d for 2 mos	Fasting with 6 oz tap water and wait 45 min before food, liquids are taken
Calcitonin (Miacalcin)	NA	100 U sc daily	Dose may be reduced to 50 U qod for 6–18 mos

[a] Potency is relative to etidronate. For each tablet, etidronate strength is 400 mg; tiludronate is 200 mg; alendronate is 40 mg; and risedronate is 30 mg. Miacalcin nasal spray is not approved for use in Paget disease.
[b] 6 oz is 175 mL.

woven bone, are replaced by more normal cancellous or lamellar bone. The improvement in skeletal structure can be demonstrated on standard radiographs and ^{99m}Tc bone scans, which show decreased isotope accumulation in pagetic sites. Reduced bone turnover can be documented by a decline in urine or serum resorption markers (pyridinoline, deoxypyridinoline, N-telopeptide, C-telopeptide) and serum markers of bone formation (ALP, osteocalcin).

The potencies of various bisphosphonates are expressed relative to that of etidronate, the first clinically useful agent in this class. Etidronate use is now limited as the doses required to suppress bone resorption may impair mineralization. Thus, etidronate is administered in 6-month treatment cycles followed by a 6-month drug-free period. Failure to adhere to the cyclic regimen can produce osteomalacia manifested by bone pain and fractures. Etidronate should not be used in patients with advanced lytic lesions in weight-bearing bones. The major advantage of etidronate is that it is relatively well tolerated and only occasionally causes transient diarrhea or bone pain.

The second-generation oral bisphosphonates tiludronate, alendronate, and risedronate are more potent than etidronate in controlling bone turnover and thus induce a longer remission at a lower dose. The lower doses reduce the risks of impaired mineralization and osteomalacia. Oral bisphosphonates are poorly absorbed and have a potential to produce esophageal ulceration, reflux, and rarely, perforation. They should be taken first thing in the morning on an empty stomach, followed by maintenance of upright posture with no food or drink for 30 to 60 min. Other medications, liquids, and food should be delayed for at least 30 to 60 min after taking bisphosphonates to optimize absorption. Tiludronate daily for 3 months normalizes ALP in 24 to 35% of moderately affected patients. In patients with moderate to severe disease, alendronate for 6 months normalizes ALP in >67% of patients, with an overall fall in ALP of 79% compared to 44% with etidronate. In patients with moderately active disease, risedronate daily for 2 to 3 months reduces serum ALP by 80% and normalizes indices of bone turnover in 73% of patients compared to 15% of those receiving etidronate.

Pamidronate is the only bisphosphonate currently approved for intravenous use in Paget disease. The recommended dose is 30 mg dissolved in 500 mL of normal saline or dextrose intravenously over 4 h on three consecutive days. The dose can be adjusted to each patient's requirements. A single 60-mg dose of pamidronate intravenously may normalize bone turnover in patients with mild disease. In contrast, patients with moderate to severe disease (elevation of ALP of three to four times normal) may require two to four doses of pamidronate, 60 to 90 mg intravenously, every 1 to 2 weeks. Patients with very severe disease may require a total dose of pamidronate of 300 to 500 mg given weekly over several weeks. Although suppression of urinary bone markers occurs after a few days to weeks, normalization of serum ALP levels often requires at least 3 months. Consequently, the effects of pamidronate are best evaluated 3 months after the initial dose. Pamidronate is generally well tolerated; however, a small number of patients experience a flulike syndrome that may begin 24 h after the first infusion. In patients with high bone turnover, vitamin D (400 to 800 IU daily) and calcium (500 mg three times daily) should be provided to prevent hypocalcemia and secondary hyperparathyroidism. Indications for intravenous therapy include mild disease and normalization of bone turnover after a single infusion, previous prevention of disease progression, refractoriness to oral therapy, need for rapid response such for those with neurologic symptoms or with severe bone pain due to a lytic lesion, risk of an impending fracture, and as pretreatment prior to elective surgery in an area of active disease. Remission following pamidronate therapy may persist for as long as 1 year. Other bisphosphonate agents are in development.

The subcutaneous injectable form of salmon calcitonin is approved for the treatment of Paget disease. Intranasal calcitonin spray is approved for osteoporosis at a dose of 200 U/d; however, the efficacy of this dose in Paget disease has not been thoroughly studied. The usual starting dose of injectable calcitonin (100 U/d) reduces ALP by 50% and may relieve skeletal symptoms. The dose may be reduced to 50 U/day three times weekly after an initial favorable response to 100 U daily; however, the lower dose may require long-term use to sustain efficacy. The common side effects of calcitonin therapy are nausea and facial flushing. Secondary resistance after prolonged use may be due to either the formation of anti-calcitonin antibodies or downregulation of osteoclastic cell-surface calcitonin receptors. The lower potency and injectable mode of delivery make this agent a less attractive treatment option that should be reserved for patients who either do not tolerate or do not respond to bisphosphonates.

SCLEROSING BONE DISORDERS

OSTEOPETROSIS   *Osteopetrosis* refers to a group of disorders caused by severe impairment of osteoclast-mediated bone resorption. Other terms that are often used include marble bone disease, which captures the solid x-ray appearance of the involved skeleton, and Albers-Schonberg disease, which refers to the milder, adult form of osteopetrosis also known as autosomal dominant osteopetrosis type II. The major types of osteopetrosis include malignant (severe, infantile, autosomal recessive) osteopetrosis and benign (adult, autosomal dominant) osteopetrosis types I and II. A rare autosomal recessive intermediate form has a more benign prognosis. Autosomal recessive carbonic anhydrase (CA) II deficiency produces osteopetrosis of intermediate severity associated with renal tubular acidosis and cerebral calcification.

Etiology and Genetics   Naturally occurring and gene knockout animal models with phenotypes similar to those of the human disorders have been used to explore the genetic basis of osteopetrosis. The primary defect in osteopetrosis is the loss of osteoclastic bone resorption and preservation of normal osteoblastic bone formation. Osteoprotegerin (OPG) is a soluble decoy receptor that binds osteoblast-derived RANK ligand, which mediates osteoclast differentiation and activation (Fig. 334-1). Transgenic mice that overexpress OPG develop osteopetrosis, presumably by blocking RANK ligand. Mice deficient in RANK lack osteoclasts and develop severe osteopetrosis.

Recessive mutations of CA II prevent osteoclasts from generating an acid environment in the clear zone between its ruffled border and the adjacent mineral surface. Absence of CA II, therefore, impairs osteoclastic bone resorption. Other forms of human disease have less clear genetic defects. About one-half of the patients with malignant infantile osteopetrosis have a mutation in the *TCIRG1* gene encoding the osteoclast-specific subunit of the vacuolar proton pump, which mediates the acidification of the interface between bone mineral and the osteoclast ruffled border. Mutations in the *CICN7* chloride channel gene cause autosomal dominant osteopetrosis type II.

Clinical Presentation   The incidence of autosomal recessive severe (malignant) osteopetrosis ranges from 1 in 200,000 to 1 in 500,000 live births. As bone and cartilage fail to undergo modeling, paralysis of one or more cranial nerves may occur due to narrowing of the cranial foramina. Failure of skeletal modeling also results in inadequate marrow space, leading to extramedullary hematopoiesis with hypersplenism and pancytopenia. Hypocalcemia due to lack of osteoclastic bone resorption may occur in infants and young children. The untreated infantile disease is fatal, often before age 5.

Adult (benign) osteopetrosis is an autosomal dominant disease that is usually diagnosed by the discovery of typical skeletal changes in young adults who undergo radiologic evaluation of a fracture. The prevalence is 1 in 100,000 to 1 in 500,000 adults. The course is not always benign, as fractures may be accompanied by loss of vision, deafness, psychomotor delay, mandibular osteomyelitis, and other complications usually associated with the juvenile form. In some kindred, nonpenetrance results in skip generations, while in other families severely affected children are born into families with benign disease. The milder form of the disease does not usually require treatment.

Radiography   Typically, there are generalized symmetric increases in bone mass with thickening of both cortical and trabecular bone. Diaphyses and metaphyses are broadened, and alternating sclerotic and lucent bands may be seen in the iliac crests, at the ends of long bones, and in vertebral bodies. The cranium is usually thickened, particularly at the base of the skull, and the paranasal and mastoid sinuses are underpneumatized.

Laboratory Findings   The only significant laboratory findings are elevated serum levels of osteoclast-derived tartrate-resistant acid phosphatase (TRAP) and the brain isoenzyme of creatine kinase. Serum calcium may be low in severe disease, and parathyroid hormone and 1,25-dihydroxyvitamin D levels may be elevated in response to hypocalcemia.

℞ TREATMENT

Allogenic HLA-identical bone marrow transplantation has been successful in some children. Following transplantation, the marrow contains progenitor cells and normally functioning osteoclasts. A cure is most likely when children are transplanted before age 4. Marrow transplantation from nonidentical HLA-matched donors has a much higher failure rate. Limited studies in small numbers of patients have suggested variable benefits following treatment with interferon gamma-1b, 1,25-dihydroxyvitamin D (which stimulates osteoclasts directly), methylprednisolone, and a low calcium/high-phosphate diet.

Surgical intervention is indicated to decompress optic or auditory nerve compression. Orthopedic management is required for the surgical treatment of fractures and their complications including malunion and post-fracture deformity.

PYKNODYSOSTOSIS   This is an autosomal recessive form of osteosclerosis that is believed to have affected the French impressionist painter Henri de Toulouse-Lautrec. The molecular basis involves mutations in the gene that encodes cathepsin K, a lysosomal metalloproteinase highly expressed in osteoclasts and important for bone matrix degradation. Osteoclasts are present but do not function normally. Pyknodysostosis is a form of short-limb dwarfism that presents with frequent fractures but usually normal life span. Clinical features include short stature; kyphoscoliosis and deformities of the chest; high arched palate; proptosis; blue sclerae; dysmorphic features including small face and chin, frontooccipital prominence, pointed beaked nose, large cranium, and obtuse mandibular angle; and small square hands with hypoplastic nails. Radiographs demonstrate a generalized increase in bone density, but in contrast to osteopetrosis, the long bones are normally shaped. Separated cranial sutures, including the persistent patency of the anterior fontanel, are characteristic of the disorder. There may also be hypoplasia of the sinuses, mandible, distal clavicles, and terminal phalanges. Persistence of deciduous teeth and sclerosis of the calvarium and base of the skull are also common. Histologic evaluation shows normal cortical bone architecture with decreased osteoblastic and osteoclastic activities. Serum chemistries are normal, and unlike osteopetrosis, there is no anemia. There is no known treatment for this condition, and no reports of attempted bone marrow transplant.

PROGRESSIVE DIAPHYSEAL DYSPLASIA Also known as Camurati-Engelman disease, progressive diaphyseal dysplasia is an autosomal dominant disorder that is characterized radiographically by diaphyseal hyperostosis and a symmetric thickening and increased diameter of the endosteal and periosteal surfaces of the diaphyses of the long bones, particularly the femur and tibia, and, less often, the fibula, radius, and ulna. The genetic defect responsible for the disease has been localized to the area of chromosome 19q13.2 encoding tumor growth factor (TGF)-β1. The mutation promotes activation of TGF-β1. The clinical severity is variable. The most common presenting symptoms are pain and tenderness of the involved areas, fatigue, muscle wasting, and gait disturbance. The weakness may be mistaken for muscular dystrophy. Characteristic body habitus includes thin limbs with little muscle mass yet prominent and palpable bones and, when the skull is involved, large head with prominent forehead and proptosis. Patients may also display signs of cranial nerve palsies, hydrocephalus, central hypogonadism, and Raynaud phenomenon. Radiographically, patchy progressive endosteal and periosteal new bone formation is observed along the diaphyses of the long bones. Bone scintigraphy shows increased radiotracer uptake in involved areas.

Treatment with low-dose glucocorticoids relieves bone pain and may reverse the abnormal bone formation. Intermittent bisphosphonate therapy has produced clinical improvement in a limited number of patients.

HYPEROSTOSIS CORTICALIS GENERALISATA This is also known as Van Buchem disease; it is an autosomal recessive disorder characterized by endosteal hyperostosis in which osteosclerosis involves the skull, mandible, clavicles, and ribs. The major manifestations are due to narrowed cranial foramina with neural compressions that may result in optic atrophy, facial paralysis, and deafness. Adults may have an enlarged mandible. Serum ALP levels may be elevated, which reflects the uncoupled bone remodeling with high osteoblastic formation rates and low osteoclastic resorption. As a result, there is increased accumulation of normal bone. Endosteal hyperostosis with syndactyly, known as *sclerosteosis*, is a more severe form. The genetic defects for both sclerosteosis and van Buchem disease have been assigned to the same region of the chromosome 17q12-q21. It is possible that both conditions may have deactivating mutations in the *BEER* (bone-expressed equilibrium regulator) gene.

MELORHEOSTOSIS Melorheostosis (Greek, "flowing hyperostosis") may occur sporadically or follow a pattern consistent with an autosomal recessive disorder. The major manifestation is progressive linear hyperostosis in one or more bones of one limb, usually a lower extremity. The name comes from the radiographic appearance of the involved bone, which resembles melted wax that has dripped down a candle. Symptoms appear during childhood as pain or stiffness in the area of sclerotic bone. There may be associated ectopic soft tissue masses, composed of cartilage or osseous tissue, and skin changes overlying the involved bone, consisting of scleroderma-like areas and hypertrichosis. The disease does not progress in adults, but pain and stiffness may persist. Laboratory tests are unremarkable. No specific etiology is known. There is no specific treatment. Surgical interventions to correct contractures are often unsuccessful.

OSTEOPOIKILOSIS The literal translation of osteopoikilosis is "spotted bones"; it is a benign autosomal dominant condition in which numerous small, variably shaped (usually round or oval) foci of bony sclerosis are seen in the epiphyses and adjacent metaphyses. The lesions may involve any bone except the skull, ribs, and vertebrae. They may be misidentified as metastatic lesions. The main differentiating points are that bony lesions of osteopoikilosis are stable over time and do not accumulate radionucleotide on bone scanning. In some kindred, osteopoikilosis is associated with connective tissue nevi known as

dermatofibrosis lenticularis disseminata, also known as *Buschke-Ollendorf syndrome*. Histologic inspection reveals thickened but otherwise normal trabeculae and islands of normal cortical bone. No treatment is indicated.

DISORDERS ASSOCIATED WITH DEFECTIVE MINERALIZATION

HYPOPHOSPHATASIA This is a rare inherited disorder that presents as rickets in infants and children or osteomalacia in adults with paradoxically low serum levels of ALP. The frequency of the severe neonatal and infantile forms is about 1 in 100,000 live births in Canada, where the disease is most common because of its high prevalence among Mennonites and Hutterites. It is rare in African Americans. The severity of the disease is remarkably variable, ranging from intrauterine death associated with profound skeletal hypomineralization at one extreme, to premature tooth loss as the only manifestation in some adults. Severe cases are inherited in an autosomal recessive manner, but the genetic patterns are less clear for the milder forms. The disease is caused by a deficiency of tissue nonspecific (bone/liver/kidney) ALP (*TNSALP*), which, although ubiquitous, results only in bone abnormalities. Protein levels and functions of the other ALP isozymes (germ cell, intestinal, placental) are normal. Defective ALP permits accumulation of its major naturally occurring substrates including phosphoethanolamine (PEA), inorganic pyrophosphate (PPi), and pyridoxal 5′-phosphate (PLP). The accumulation of PPi interferes with mineralization through its action as a potent inhibitor of hydroxyapatite crystal growth.

Perinatal hypophosphatasia becomes manifest during pregnancy and is often complicated by polyhydroamnios and intrauterine death. The infantile form becomes clinically apparent before age 6 months with failure to thrive, rachitic deformities, functional craniosynostosis despite widely open fontanels (which are actually hypomineralized areas of the calvarium), raised intracranial pressure, and flail chest and predisposition to pneumonia. Hypercalcemia and hypercalciuria are common. This form has a mortality rate of about 50%. Prognosis seems to improve for the children who survive infancy. Childhood hypophosphatasia has variable clinical presentation. Premature loss of deciduous teeth (before age 5 years) is the hallmark of the disease. Rickets causes delayed walking with waddling gait, short stature, and dolichocephalic skull with frontal bossing. The disease often improves during puberty but may recur in adult life. Adult hypophosphatasia presents during middle age with painful, poorly healing metatarsal stress fractures or thigh pain due to femoral pseudofractures.

Laboratory investigation reveals low ALP levels and normal or elevated levels of serum calcium and phosphorus despite clinical and radiologic evidence of rickets or osteomalacia. Serum parathyroid hormone, 25-hydroxyvitamin D, and 1,25-dihydroxyvitamin D levels are normal. The elevation of PLP is specific for the disease and may even be present in asymptomatic parents of severely affected children. As vitamin B$_6$ increases PLP levels, vitamin B$_6$ supplements should be discontinued 1 week before testing.

There is no established medical therapy. In contrast to other forms of rickets and osteomalacia, calcium and vitamin D supplementation should be avoided as they may aggravate hypercalcemia and hypercalciuria. A low-calcium diet, glucocorticoids, and calcitonin have been used in a small number of patients with variable responses. Because fracture healing is poor, placement of intramedullary rods is best for acute fracture repair and for prophylactic prevention of fractures.

AXIAL OSTEOMALACIA This is a rare disorder characterized by defective skeletal mineralization despite normal serum calcium and phosphate levels. Clinically, the disorder presents in middle-aged or elderly men with chronic axial skeletal discomfort. Cervical spine pain may also be present. Radiographic findings are mainly osteosclerosis due to coarsened trabecular patterns typical of osteomalacias. Spine, pelvis, and ribs are most commonly affected. Histologic changes show defective mineralization and flat, inactive osteoblasts. The primary defect appears to be an acquired defect in osteoblast function. The course is benign and there is no established treatment. Calcium and vitamin D therapies are not effective.

FIBROGENESIS IMPERFECTA OSSIUM   The is a rare condition of unknown etiology. It presents in both sexes, in middle age or later, with progressive, intractable skeletal pain and fractures, worsening immobilization, and a debilitating course. Radiographic evaluation reveals generalized osteomalacia, osteopenia, and occasional pseudofractures. Histologic features include a tangled pattern of collagen fibrils with abundant osteoblasts and osteoclasts. There is no effective treatment. Spontaneous remission has been reported in a small number of patients. Calcium and vitamin D have not been beneficial.

FIBROUS DYSPLASIA AND McCUNE ALBRIGHT SYNDROME

Fibrous dysplasia is a sporadic disorder characterized by the presence of one (monoostotic) or more (polyostotic) expanding fibrous skeletal lesions composed of bone-forming mesenchyme. The association of the polyostotic form with café-au-lait spots and hyperfunction of an endocrine system such as pseudo-precocious puberty of ovarian origin is known as *McCune-Albright syndrome* (MAS). A spectrum of the phenotypes is caused by activating mutations in the *GNAS1* gene, which encodes the α subunit of the stimulatory G protein ($G_s\alpha$). As the postzygotic mutations occur at different stages of early development, the extent and type of tissue affected are variable and explain the mosaic pattern of skin and bone changes. GTP binding activates the $G_s\alpha$ regulatory protein and mutations in regions of $G_s\alpha$ that selectively inhibit GTPase activity, which results in constitutive stimulation of the cyclic AMP–protein kinase A signal transduction pathway. Such mutations of the $G_s\alpha$ protein–coupled receptor may cause autonomous function in bone (parathyroid hormone receptor); skin (melanocyte-stimulating hormone receptor); and various endocrine glands including ovary (follicle-stimulating hormone receptor), thyroid (thyroid-stimulating hormone receptor), adrenal (adrenocorticotropic hormone receptor), and pituitary (growth hormone–releasing hormone receptor). The skeletal lesions are composed largely of mesenchymal cells that do not differentiate into osteoblasts, resulting in the formation of imperfect bone. In some areas of bone, fibroblast-like cells develop features of osteoblasts in that they produce extracellular matrix that organizes into woven bone. Calcification may occur in some areas. In other areas, cells have features of chondrocytes and produce cartilage-like extracellular matrix.

CLINICAL PRESENTATION   Fibrous dysplasia occurs with equal frequency in both sexes, whereas MAS with precocious puberty is more common (10:1) in girls. The monoostotic form is the most common and is usually diagnosed in patients between 20 and 30 years of age without associated skin lesions. The polyostotic form typically manifests in children <10 years of age and may progress with age. Early-onset disease is generally more severe. Lesions may become quiescent in puberty and progress during pregnancy or with estrogen therapy. In polyostotic fibrous dysplasia, the lesions most commonly involve the maxilla and other craniofacial bones, ribs, and metaphyseal or diaphyseal portions of the proximal femur or tibia. Expanding bone lesions may cause pain, deformity, fractures, and nerve entrapment. Sarcomatous degeneration involving the facial bones or femur is infrequent (<1%). The risk of malignant transformation is increased by radiation, which has proven to be ineffective treatment. In rare patients with widespread lesions, renal phosphate wasting and hypophosphatemia may cause rickets or osteomalacia. Hypophosphatemia may be due to production of a phosphaturic factor by the abnormal fibrous tissue.

MAS patients may have café-au-lait spots, which are flat, hyperpigmented skin lesions that have rough borders ("coast of Maine") in contrast to the café-au-lait lesions of neurofibromatosis that have smooth borders ("coast of California"). The most common endocrinopathy is isosexual pseudo-precocious puberty in girls. Other less

common endocrine disorders include thyrotoxicosis, Cushing syndrome, acromegaly, hyperparathyroidism, hyperprolactinemia, and pseudo-precocious puberty in boys.

RADIOGRAPHIC FINDINGS   In long bones, the fibrous dysplastic lesions are typically well-defined, radiolucent areas with thin cortices and a ground-glass appearance. Lesions may be lobulated with trabeculated areas of radiolucency (Fig. 334-4). Involvement of facial bones usually presents as radiodense lesions, which may create a leonine appearance (leontiasis osea). Expansile cranial lesions may narrow foramina and cause optic lesions, reduce hearing, and create other manifestations of cranial nerve compression.

LABORATORY RESULTS   Serum ALP is occasionally elevated but calcium, parathyroid hormone, 25-hydroxyvitamin D, and 1,25-dihydroxyvitamin D levels are normal. Patients with extensive polyostotic lesions may have hypophosphatemia, hyperphosphaturia, and osteomalacia. Biochemical markers of bone turnover may be elevated.

℞ TREATMENT

Spontaneous healing of the lesions does not occur, and there is no established effective treatment. Improvement in bone pain and partial or complete resolution of radiographic lesions have been reported after intravenous bisphosphonate therapy. Surgical stabilization is used to prevent pathologic fracture or destruction of a major joint space, and to relieve nerve root or cranial nerve compression or sinus obstruction.

OTHER DYSPLASIAS OF BONE AND CARTILAGE

PACHYDERMOPERIOSTOSIS   Pachydermoperiostosis, or hypertrophic osteoarthropathy (primary or idiopathic), is an autosomal dominant disorder characterized by periosteal new bone formation that involves the distal extremities. The lesions present as clubbing of the digits and hyperhydrosis and thickening of the skin, primarily of the face and forehead. The changes usually appear during adolescence, progress over the next decade, and then become quiescent. During the active phase, progressive enlargement of the hands and feet produces a paw-like appearance, which may be mistaken for acromegaly. Arthralgias, pseudogout, and limited mobility may also occur. The disorder must be differentiated from secondary hypertrophic osteopathy that develops during the course of serious pulmonary disorders. The two con-

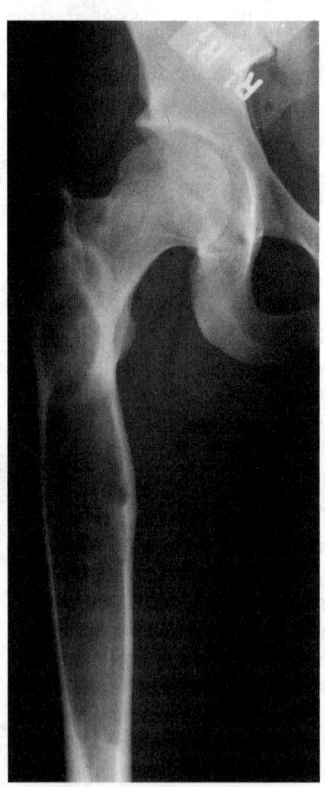

FIGURE 334-4   Radiograph of a 16-year-old male with fibrous dysplasia of the right proximal femur. Note the multiple cystic lesions, including the large lucent lesion in the proximal mid-shaft with scalloping of the interior surface. The femoral neck contains two lucent cystic lesions.

ditions can be differentiated by standard radiography of the digits in which secondary pachydermoperiostosis has exuberant periosteal new bone formation and a smooth and undulating surface. In contrast, primary hypertrophic osteopathy has an irregular periosteal surface.

There are no diagnostic blood or urine tests. Synovial fluid does not have an inflammatory profile. There is no specific therapy, although a limited experience with colchicine suggests some benefit in controlling the arthralgias.

OSTEOCHONDRODYSPLASIAS These include several hundred heritable disorders of connective tissue. These primary abnormalities of cartilage manifest as disturbances in cartilage and bone growth. Selected growth plate chondrodysplasias are described here. →*For discussion of chondrodysplasias, see Chap. 342.*

Achondrodysplasia This is a relatively common form of short-limb dwarfism that occurs in 1 in 15,000 to 1 in 40,000 live births. The disease is caused by a mutation of the fibroblast growth factor receptor 3 (*FGFR3*) gene that results in a gain-of-function state. Most cases are sporadic mutations. However, when the disorder appears in families, the inheritance pattern is consistent with an autosomal dominant disorder. The primary defect is abnormal chondrocyte proliferation at the growth plate that causes development of short but proportionately thick long bones. Other regions of the long bones may be relatively unaffected. The disorder is manifest by the presence of short limbs (particularly the proximal portions), normal trunk, large head, saddle nose, and an exaggerated lumbar lordosis. Severe spinal deformity may lead to cord compression. The homozygous disorder is more serious than the sporadic form and may cause neonatal death. Pseudo-achondroplasia clinically resembles achondroplasia but has no skull abnormalities.

Enchondromatosis This is also called dyschondroplasia, or Ollier disease; it is also a disorder of the growth plate in which the primary cartilage is not resorbed. Cartilage ossification proceeds normally but it is not resorbed normally, leading to cartilage accumulation. The changes are most marked at the ends of long bones where the highest growth rates occur. Chondrosarcoma develops infrequently. The association of enchondromatosis and cavernous hemangiomas of the skin and soft tissues is known as *Maffucci syndrome*. Both Ollier disease and Maffucci syndrome are associated with various malignancies, including granulosa cell tumor of the ovary and cerebral glioma.

Multiple Exostoses This is also called diaphyseal aclasis, or osteochondromatosis; it is a genetic disorder that follows an autosomal dominant pattern of inheritance. In this condition, areas of growth plates become displaced, presumably by growing through a defect in the perichondrium. The lesion begins with vascular invasion of the growth plate cartilage, resulting in a characteristic radiographic finding of a mass that is in direct communication with the marrow cavity of the parent bone. The underlying cortex is resorbed. The disease is caused by inactivating mutations of the *EXT1* and *EXT2* genes, whose products normally regulate processing of chondrocyte cytoskeletal proteins. The products of the *EXT* gene likely function as tumor suppressors, with the loss-of-function mutation resulting in abnormal proliferation of growth plate cartilage. Solitary or multiple lesions are located in the metaphyses of long bones. Although usually asymptomatic, the lesions may interfere with joint or tendon function or compress peripheral nerves. The lesions stop growing when growth ceases but may recur during pregnancy. There is a small risk for malignant transformation into chondrosarcoma.

EXTRASKELETAL (ECTOPIC) CALCIFICATION AND OSSIFICATION

Deposition of calcium phosphate crystals (*calcification*) or formation of true bone (*ossification*) in nonosseous soft tissue may occur by one of three mechanisms: (1) metastatic calcification due to a supranormal calcium x phosphate concentration product in extracellular fluid; (2) dystrophic calcification due to mineral deposition into metabolically impaired or dead tissue despite normal serum levels of calcium and phosphate; and (3) ectopic ossification, or true bone formation. Dis-

orders that may cause extraskeletal calcification or ossification are listed in Table 334-2.

METASTATIC CALCIFICATION Soft tissue calcification may complicate diseases associated with significant hypercalcemia, hyperphosphatemia, or both. In addition, vitamin D and phosphate treatments or calcium administration in the presence of mild hyperphosphatemia, such as during hemodialysis, may induce ectopic calcification. Calcium phosphate precipitation may complicate any disorder when the serum calcium $\times$ phosphate concentration product >75. The initial calcium phosphate deposition is in the form of small, poorly organized crystals, which subsequently organize into hydroxyapatite crystals. Calcifications that occur in hypercalcemic states with normal or low phosphate have a predilection for kidney, lungs, and gastric mucosa. Hyperphosphatemia with normal or low serum calcium may promote soft tissue calcification with predilection for the kidney and arteries. The disturbances of calcium and phosphate in renal failure and hemodialysis are common causes of soft tissue (metastatic) calcification.

TUMORAL CALCINOSIS This is a rare genetic disorder characterized by masses of metastatic calcifications in soft tissues around major joints, most often shoulders, hips, and ankles. Tumoral calcinosis differs from other disorders in that the periarticular masses contain hydroxyapatite crystals or amorphous calcium phosphate complexes, while in fibrodysplasia ossificans progressiva (below), true bone is formed in soft tissues. About one-third of tumoral calcinosis cases are familial, with both autosomal recessive and autosomal dominant modes of inheritance reported. The disease is also associated with a variably expressed abnormality of dentition marked by short bulbous roots, pulp calcification, and radicular dentin deposited in swirls. The primary defect responsible for the metastatic calcification appears to be hyperphosphatemia resulting from the increased capacity of the renal tubule to reabsorb filtered phosphate. Spontaneous soft tissue calcification is related to the elevated serum phosphate, which along with normal serum calcium exceeds the concentration product of 75.

All of the North American patients reported have been African-American. The disease usually presents in childhood and continues lifelong. The calcific masses are typically painless and grow at variable rates, sometimes becoming large and bulky. The masses are often located near major joints but remain extracapsular. Joint range of motion is not usually restricted unless the tumors are very large. Complications include compression of neural structures and ulceration of the overlying skin with drainage of chalky fluid and risk of secondary infection. Small deposits not detected by standard radiographs may be detected by ^{99m}Tc bone scanning. The most common laboratory findings are hyperphosphatemia and elevated serum 1,25-dihydroxyvitamin D levels. Serum calcium, parathyroid hormone, and ALP levels are usually normal. Renal function is also usually normal. Urine cal-

TABLE 334-2 Diseases and Conditions Associated with Ectopic Calcification and Ossification

Metastatic calcification	Dystrophic calcification
Hypercalcemic states	Inflammatory disorders
Primary hyperparathyroidism	Scleroderma
Sarcoidosis	Dermatomyositis
Vitamin D intoxication	Systemic lupus
Milk-alkali syndrome	erythematosus
Renal failure	Trauma-induced
Hyperphosphatemia	Ectopic ossification
Tumoral calcinosis	Myositis ossificans
Secondary hyperparathyroidism	Post surgery
Pseudohypoparathyroidism	Burns
Renal failure	Neurologic injury
Hemodialysis	Other trauma
Cell lysis following chemotherapy	Fibrodysplasia ossificans
Therapy with vitamin D and	progressiva
phosphate	

cium and phosphate excretions are low, and calcium and phosphate balances are positive.

An acquired form of the disease may occur with other causes of hyperphosphatemia, such as secondary hyperparathyroidism associated with hemodialysis, hypoparathyroidism, pseudohypoparathyroidism, and massive cell lysis following chemotherapy for leukemia. Tissue trauma from joint movement may contribute to the periarticular calcifications. Metastatic calcifications are also seen in conditions associated with hypercalcemia, such as in sarcoidosis, vitamin D intoxication, milk-alkali syndrome, and primary hyperparathyroidism. In these conditions, however, mineral deposits are more likely to occur in proton-transporting organs such as kidney, lungs, and gastric mucosa in which an alkaline milieu is generated by the proton pumps.

Rx TREATMENT

Therapeutic successes have been achieved with surgical removal of subcutaneous calcified masses, which tend not to recur if all calcification is removed from the site. Reduction of serum phosphate by chronic phosphorus restriction may be accomplished using low dietary phosphorus intake alone or in combination with oral phosphate binders. The addition of the phosphaturic agent acetazolamide may be useful. Limited experience using the phosphaturic action of calcitonin deserves further testing.

DYSTROPHIC CALCIFICATION Posttraumatic calcification may occur with normal serum calcium and phosphate levels and normal ion solubility product. The deposited mineral is either in the form of amorphous calcium phosphate or hydroxyapatite crystals. Soft tissue calcification complicating connective tissue disorders such as scleroderma, dermatomyositis, and systemic lupus erythematosus may involve localized areas of the skin or deeper subcutaneous tissue and is referred to as *calcinosis circumscripta*. Mineral deposition at sites of deeper tissue injury including periarticular sites is called *calcinosis universalis*.

ECTOPIC OSSIFICATION True extraskeletal bone formation that begins in areas of fasciitis following surgery, trauma, burns, or neurologic injury is referred to as *myositis ossificans*. The bone formed is organized as lamellar or trabecular, with normal osteoblasts and osteoclasts conducting active remodeling. Well-developed haversian systems and marrow elements may be present. A second cause of ectopic bone formation occurs in an inherited disorder, *fibrodysplasia ossificans progressiva*.

FIBRODYSPLASIA OSSIFICANS PROGRESSIVA This is also called *myositis ossificans progressiva*; it is a rare autosomal dominant disorder characterized by congenital deformities of the hands and feet and episodic soft tissue swellings that ossify. Ectopic bone formation occurs in fascia, tendons, ligaments, and connective tissue within voluntary muscles. Tender, rubbery induration, sometimes precipitated by trauma, develops in the soft tissue and gradually calcifies. Eventually, heterotopic bone forms at these sites of soft tissue trauma. Morbidity results from heterotopic bone interfering with normal movement and function of muscle and other soft tissues. Mortality is usually related to restrictive lung disease caused by an inability of the chest to expand. Laboratory tests are unremarkable.

There is no effective medical therapy. Bisphosphonates, glucocorticoids, and a low-calcium diet have largely been ineffective in halting progression of the ossification. Surgical removal of ectopic bone is not recommended, as the trauma of surgery may precipitate formation of new areas of heterotopic bone. Dental complications including frozen jaw may occur following injection of local anesthetics. Thus, CT imaging of the mandible should be undertaken to detect early sites of soft tissue ossification before they are appreciated by standard radiography.

ACKNOWLEDGMENT
The authors wish to acknowledge the contributions of Dr. Stephen M. Krane to this chapter in previous editions of Harrison's.

FURTHER READING

HOCKING LJ et al: Domain-specific mutations in sequestosome 1 (SQSTM1) cause familial and sporadic Paget disease. Hum Mol Genet 11:2735, 2002

HOFBAUER LC, HEUFELDER AE: Role of receptor activator of nuclear factor-kappa B ligand and osteoprotegerin in bone cell biology. J Mol Med 79: 243, 2001

SOBACCHI C et al: The mutational spectrum of human malignant autosomal recessive osteopetrosis. Hum Mol Genet 10:1767, 2001

WEINSTEIN LS et al: Endocrine manifestations of stimulatory G protein alpha-subunit mutations and the role of genomic imprinting. Endocrine Rev 22: 675, 2001

WHYTE MP et al: Osteoprotegrin deficiency and juvenile Paget disease. N Engl J Med 347:175, 2002

Section 3   Disorders of Intermediary Metabolism

335 DISORDERS OF LIPOPROTEIN METABOLISM
Daniel J. Rader, Helen H. Hobbs

Lipoproteins are complexes of lipids and proteins that are essential for the transport of cholesterol, triglycerides, and fat-soluble vitamins. Until recently, lipoprotein disorders were the purview of lipidologists, but the demonstration that lipid-lowering therapy significantly reduces the clinical complications of atherosclerotic cardiovascular disease (ASCVD) has brought the diagnosis and treatment of these disorders into the domain of the general internist. The metabolic consequences associated with changes in diet and lifestyle have increased the number of hyperlipidemic individuals who could benefit from lipid-lowering therapy. The development of safe, effective, and well-tolerated pharmacologic agents has greatly expanded the therapeutic armamentarium available to the physician to treat disorders of lipid metabolism. Therefore, the appropriate diagnosis and management of lipid disorders is critically important to the practice of medicine. This chapter reviews normal lipoprotein physiology, the pathophysiology of the known single-gene disorders of lipoprotein metabolism, the environmental factors that influence lipoprotein metabolism, and the practical approaches to their diagnosis and management.

LIPOPROTEIN METABOLISM

LIPOPROTEIN CLASSIFICATION AND COMPOSITION Lipoproteins are large, mostly spherical complexes that transport lipids (primarily triglycerides, cholesteryl esters, and fat-soluble vitamins) through body fluids (plasma, interstitial fluid, and lymph) to and from tissues. Lipoproteins play an essential role in the absorption of dietary cholesterol, long-chain fatty acids, and fat-soluble vitamins; the transport of triglycerides, cholesterol, and fat-soluble vitamins from the liver to peripheral tissues; and the transport of cholesterol from peripheral tissues to the liver.

Lipoproteins contain a core of hydrophobic lipids (triglycerides and cholesteryl esters) surrounded by hydrophilic lipids (phospholipids, unesterified cholesterol) and proteins that interact with body fluids.

The plasma lipoproteins are divided into five major classes based on their relative densities (Fig. 335-1 and Table 335-1): chylomicrons, very low density lipoproteins (VLDL), intermediate-density lipoproteins (IDL), low-density lipoproteins (LDL), and high-density lipoproteins (HDL). Each lipoprotein class comprises a family of particles that vary slightly in density, size, migration during electrophoresis, and protein composition. The density of a lipoprotein is determined by the amount of lipid and protein per particle. HDL is the smallest and most dense lipoprotein, whereas chylomicrons and VLDL are the largest and least dense lipoprotein particles. Most triglyceride is transported in chylomicrons or VLDL, and most cholesterol is carried as cholesteryl esters in LDL and HDL.

TABLE 335-1 *Major Lipoprotein Classes^a*

Lipoprotein	Density, g/mL^b	Size nm^c	Electrophoretic Mobility^d	Apolipoproteins Major	Apolipoproteins Other	Other Constituents
Chylomicrons	0.930	75–1200	Origin	ApoB-48	A-I, A-IV, C-I, C-II, C-III	Retinyl esters
Chylomicron remnants	0.930–1.006	30–80	Slow pre-β	ApoB-48	E, A-I, A-IV, C-I, C-II, C-III	Retinyl esters
VLDL	0.930–1.006	30–80	Pre-β	ApoB-100	E, A-I, A-II, A-V, C-I, C-II, C-III	Vitamin E
IDL	1.006–1.019	25–35	Slow pre-β	ApoB-100	E, C-I, C-II, C-III	Vitamin E
LDL	1.019–1.063	18–25	β	ApoB-100		Vitamin E
HDL	1.063–1.210	5–12	Alpha	ApoA-I	A-II, A-IV, E, C-III	LCAT, CETP paroxonase
Lp(a)	1.050–1.120	25	Pre-β	ApoB-100	Apo(a)	

^{a} All of the lipoprotein classes contain phospholipids, esterified and unesterified cholesterol, and triglycerides to varying degrees.
^{b} The density of the particle is determined by ultracentrifugation.
^{c} The size of the particle is measured using gel electrophoresis.
^{d} The electrophoretic mobility of the particle on agarose gel electrophoresis reflects the size and surface charge of the particle, with β being the position of LDL and α the position of HDL.
Note: VLDL, very low density lipoprotein; IDL, intermediate-density lipoprotein; LDL, low-density lipoprotein; HDL, high-density lipoprotein; Lp(a), lipoprotein A; LCAT, lecithin-cholesterol acyltransferase; CETP, cholesteryl ester transfer protein.

The apolipoproteins are required for the assembly and structure of lipoproteins (Table 335-2). Apolipoproteins also serve to activate enzymes important in lipoprotein metabolism and to mediate the binding of lipoproteins to cell-surface receptors. ApoA-I, which is synthesized in the liver and intestine, is found on virtually all HDL particles. ApoA-II is the second most abundant HDL apolipoprotein and is found on approximately two-thirds of all HDL particles. ApoB is the major structural protein of chylomicrons, VLDL, IDL, and LDL; one molecule of apoB, either apoB-48 (chylomicrons) or apoB-100 (VLDL, IDL, or LDL), is present on each lipoprotein particle. The human liver makes only apoB-100, and the intestine makes apoB-48, which is derived from the same gene by mRNA editing. ApoE is present in multiple copies on chylomicrons, VLDL, and IDL and plays a critical role in the metabolism and clearance of triglyceride-rich particles. Three apolipoproteins of the C-series (apoC-I, -II, and -III) also participate in the metabolism of triglyceride-rich lipoproteins. The other apolipoproteins are listed in Table 335-2.

TRANSPORT OF DIETARY LIPIDS (EXOGENOUS PATHWAY) The exogenous pathway of lipoprotein metabolism permits efficient transport of dietary lipids (Fig. 335-2). Dietary triglycerides are hydrolyzed by pancreatic lipases within the intestinal lumen and are emulsified with bile acids to form micelles. Dietary cholesterol and retinol are esterified (by the addition of a fatty acid) in the enterocyte to form cholesteryl esters and retinyl esters, respectively. Longer-chain fatty acids (>12 carbons) are incorporated into triglycerides and packaged with apoB-48, cholesteryl esters, retinyl esters, phospholipids, and cholesterol to form chylomicrons. Nascent chylomicrons are secreted into the intestinal lymph and delivered directly to the systemic circulation, where they are extensively processed by peripheral tissues before reaching the liver. The particles encounter lipoprotein lipase (LPL), which is anchored to proteoglycans that decorate the capillary endothelial surfaces of adipose tissue, heart, and skeletal muscle (Fig. 335-2). The triglycerides of chylomicrons are hydrolyzed by LPL, and free fatty acids are released; apoC-II, which is transferred to circulating chylomicrons, acts as a cofactor for LPL in this reaction. The released free fatty acids are taken up by adjacent myocytes or adipocytes and either oxidized or reesterified and stored as triglyceride. Some free fatty acids bind albumin and are transported to other tissues, especially the liver. The chylomicron particle progressively shrinks in size as the hydrophobic core is hydrolyzed and the hydrophilic lipids (cholesterol and phospholipids) on the particle surface are transferred to HDL. The resultant smaller, more cholesterol ester–rich particles are referred to as *chylomicron remnants*. The remnant particles are rapidly removed from the circulation by the liver in a process that requires apoE. Consequently, few, if any, chylomicrons are present in the blood after a 12-h fast, except in individuals with disorders of chylomicron metabolism.

TRANSPORT OF HEPATIC LIPIDS (ENDOGENOUS PATHWAY) The *endogenous pathway of lipoprotein metabolism* refers to the hepatic secretion and metabolism of VLDL to IDL and LDL (Fig. 335-2). VLDL particles resemble chylomicrons in protein composition but contain apoB-100 rather than apoB-48 and have a higher ratio of cholesterol to triglyceride (~1 mg of cholesterol for every 5 mg of triglyceride). The triglycerides of VLDL are derived predominantly from the esterification of long-chain fatty acids. The packaging of hepatic triglycerides with the other major components of the nascent VLDL particle (apoB-100, cholesteryl esters, phospholipids, and vitamin E) requires the action of the enzyme microsomal transfer protein (MTP). After secretion into the plasma, VLDL acquires multiple copies of apoE and apolipoproteins of the C series. The triglycerides of VLDL are hydrolyzed by LPL, especially in muscle and adipose tissue. As VLDL remnants undergo further hydrolysis, they continue to shrink in size and become *IDL*, which contain similar amounts of cholesterol and triglyceride. The liver removes approximately 40 to 60% of VLDL remnants and IDL by LDL receptor–mediated endocytosis via binding to apoE. The remainder of IDL is remodeled by hepatic lipase (HL) to form LDL; during this process, most of the triglyceride in the particle is hydrolyzed and all apolipoproteins except apoB-100 are transferred to other lipoproteins. The cholesterol in LDL accounts for ~70% of the plasma cholesterol in most individuals. Approximately 70% of circulating LDLs are cleared by LDL receptor–mediated endocytosis in the liver.

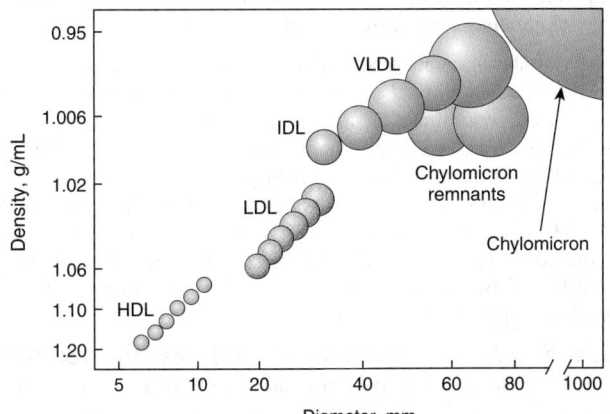

FIGURE 335-1 The density and size-distribution of the major classes of lipoprotein particles. Lipoproteins are classified by density and size, which are inversely related. VLDL, very low density lipoproteins; IDL, intermediate-density lipoproteins; LDL, low-density lipoproteins; HDL, high-density lipoproteins.

TABLE 335-2 *Major Apolipoproteins*

Apolipoprotein	Primary Source	Lipoprotein Association	Function
ApoA-I	Intestine, liver	HDL, chylomicrons	Structural protein for HDL; activates LCAT
ApoA-II	Liver	HDL, chylomicrons	Structural protein for HDL
ApoA-IV	Intestine	HDL, chylomicrons	Unknown
ApoA-V	Liver	VLDL	Unknown
ApoB-48	Intestine	Chylomicrons	Structural protein for chylomicrons
ApoB-100	Liver	VLDL, IDL, LDL, Lp(a)	Structural protein for VLDL, LDL, IDL, Lp(a); ligand for binding to LDL receptor
ApoC-I	Liver	Chylomicrons, VLDL, HDL	Unknown
ApoC-II	Liver	Chylomicrons, VLDL, HDL	Cofactor for LPL
ApoC-III	Liver	Chylomicrons, VLDL, HDL	Inhibits lipoprotein binding to receptors
ApoD	Spleen, brain, testes, adrenals	HDL	Unknown
ApoE	Liver	Chylomicron remnants, IDL, HDL	Ligand for binding to LDL receptor
ApoH	Liver	Chylomicrons, VLDL, LDL, HDL	B_2 glycoprotein I
ApoJ	Liver	HDL	Unknown
ApoL	Unknown	HDL	Unknown
Apo(a)	Liver	Lp(a)	Unknown

Note: HDL, high-density lipoprotein; LCAT, lecithin-cholesterol acyltransferase; VLDL, very low density lipoprotein; IDL, intermediate-density lipoprotein; LDL, low-density lipoprotein; Lp(a), lipoprotein A; LPL, lipoprotein lipase.

Lipoprotein(a) [Lp(a)] is a lipoprotein similar to LDL in lipid and protein composition, but it contains an additional protein called apolipoprotein(a) [apo(a)]. Apo(a) is synthesized in the liver and is attached to apoB-100 by a disulfide linkage. The mechanism by which Lp(a) is removed from the circulation is not known.

HDL METABOLISM AND REVERSE CHOLESTEROL TRANSPORT All nucleated cells synthesize cholesterol but only hepatocytes can efficiently metabolize and excrete cholesterol from the body. The predominant route of cholesterol elimination is by excretion into the bile, either directly or after conversion to bile acids. Cholesterol in peripheral cells is transported from the plasma membranes of peripheral cells to the liver by an HDL-mediated process termed *reverse cholesterol transport* (Fig. 335-3).

Nascent HDL particles are synthesized by the intestine and the liver. The newly formed discoidal HDL particles contain apoA-I and phospholipids (mainly lecithin) but rapidly acquire unesterified cholesterol and additional phospholipids from peripheral tissues via transport by the membrane protein ATP-binding cassette protein A1 (ABCA1). Once incorporated in the HDL particle, cholesterol is esterified by lecithin-cholesterol acyltransferase (LCAT), a plasma enzyme associated with HDL. As HDL acquires more cholesteryl ester it becomes spherical, and additional apolipoproteins and lipids are transferred to the particles from the surfaces of chylomicrons and VLDL during lipolysis.

HDL cholesterol is transported to hepatoctyes by both an indirect and a direct pathway. HDL cholesteryl esters are transferred to apoB-containing lipoproteins in exchange for triglyceride by the cholesteryl ester transfer protein (CETP). The cholesteryl esters are then removed from the circulation by LDL receptor–mediated endocytosis. HDL cholesterol can also be taken up directly by hepatocytes via the scavenger receptor class BI (SR-BI), a cell-surface receptor that mediates the selective transfer of lipids to cells.

HDL particles undergo extensive remodeling within the plasma compartment as they transfer lipids and proteins to lipoproteins and cells. For example, after CETP-mediated lipid exchange, the triglyceride-enriched HDL becomes a substrate for HL, which hydrolyzes the triglycerides and phospholipids to generate smaller HDL particles.

DISORDERS OF LIPOPROTEIN METABOLISM

The identification and characterization of genes responsible for the genetic forms of hyperlipidemia have provided important molecular

insight into the critical roles of apolipoproteins, enzymes, and receptors in lipid metabolism.

PRIMARY DISORDERS OF ApoB-CONTAINING LIPOPROTEIN BIOSYNTHESIS CAUSING LOW PLASMA CHOLESTEROL LEVELS (KNOWN ETIOLOGY) The synthesis and secretion of apoB-containing lipoproteins in the enterocytes of the proximal small bowel and in the hepatocytes of the liver involve a complex series of events that coordinate the coupling of various lipids with apoB-48 and apoB-100, respectively.

Abetalipoproteinemia Abetalipoproteinemia is a rare autosomal recessive disease caused by mutations in the gene encoding MTP, which transfers lipids to nascent chylomicrons and VLDL in the intestine and liver, respectively. Plasma cholesterol and triglyceride levels are extremely low in this disorder, and no chylomicrons, VLDL, LDL, or apoB are detectable. The parents of patients with abetalipoproteinemia (who are obligate heterozygotes) have normal plasma lipid and apoB levels. Abetalipoproteinemia usually presents in early childhood with diarrhea and failure to thrive and is characterized clinically by fat malabsorption, spinocerebellar degeneration, pigmented retinopathy, and acanthocytosis. The initial neurologic manifestations are loss of deep-tendon reflexes, followed by decreased distal lower extremity vibratory and proprioceptive sense, dysmetria, ataxia, and the development of a spastic gait, often by the third or fourth decade. Patients with abetalipoproteinemia also develop a progressive pigmented retinopathy presenting with decreased night and color vision, followed by reductions in daytime visual acuity and ultimately progressing to near blindness. The presence of spinocerebellar degeneration and pigmented retinopathy in this disease has resulted in misdiagnosis of Friedreich's ataxia. Rarely, patients with abetalipoproteinemia develop a cardiomyopathy with associated life-threatening arrhythmias.

Most clinical manifestations of abetalipoproteinemia result from defects in the absorption and transport of fat-soluble vitamins. Vitamin E and retinyl esters are normally transported from enterocytes to the liver by chylomicrons, and vitamin E is dependent on VLDL for transport out of the liver and into the circulation. Patients with abetalipoproteinemia are markedly deficient in vitamin E and are also mildly to moderately deficient in vitamin A and vitamin K. Treatment of abetalipoproteinemia consists of a low-fat, high-caloric, vitamin-enriched diet accompanied by large supplemental doses of vitamin E. It is imperative for treatment to be initiated as soon as possible to obviate the development of neurologic sequelae.

Familial Hypobetalipoproteinemia Familial homozygous hypobetalipoproteinemia has a clinical picture similar to abetalipoproteinemia but is autosomal codominant in inheritance pattern. The disease can be differentiated from abetalipoproteinemia since the parents of the probands with this disorder have levels of plasma LDL-C and apoB that are less than half of the normal levels. Mutations in the gene encoding apoB-100 that interfere with protein synthesis are common causes of this disorder. These patients, like those with abetalipoproteinemia, should be referred to specialized centers for confirmation of the diagnosis and appropriate therapy.

PRIMARY DISORDERS OF ApoB-CONTAINING LIPOPROTEIN CATABOLISM CAUSING ELEVATED PLASMA CHOLESTEROL LEVELS (KNOWN ETIOLOGY) Single-gene defects can result in the accumulation of specific classes of lipoprotein particles. Mutations in genes encoding key proteins in the metabolism and clearance of apoB-containing lipoproteins cause type I (chylomicronemia), type II (elevations in LDL) and type III (elevations in IDL) hyperlipoproteinemias (Table 335-3).

Lipoprotein Lipase and ApoC-II Deficiency (Familial Chylomicronemia Syndrome; Type I Hyperlipoproteinemia)

LPL is required for the hydrolysis of triglycerides in chylomicrons and VLDL. ApoC-II is a cofactor for LPL (Fig. 335-2). Genetic deficiency of either LPL or apoC-II results in impaired lipolysis and profound elevations in plasma chylomicrons. These patients also have elevations in plasma VLDL, but chylomicronemia predominates. Normally chylomicrons are delipidated and removed from the circulation within 12 h of the last meal, but in LPL-deficient patients, the triglyceride-rich chylomicrons persist in the circulation for days. The fasting plasma is turbid, and if left at 4°C for a few hours, the chylomicrons float to the top and form a creamy supernatant. In these disorders, called *familial chylomicronemia syndromes*, fasting triglyceride levels are almost invariably >11.3 μmol/L (1000 mg/dL). Fasting cholesterol levels are also usually elevated, but to a much less severe degree.

LPL deficiency is autosomal recessive and has a population frequency of approximately one in a million. ApoC-II deficiency is also recessive in inheritance pattern and is even less common than LPL deficiency. Multiple mutations in the LPL and apoC-II genes cause these diseases. Obligate LPL heterozygotes have normal or mild to moderate elevations in plasma triglyceride levels, whereas individuals heterozygous for mutation in apoC-II are not hypertriglyceridemic.

Both LPL and apoC-II deficiency usually present in childhood with recurrent episodes of severe abdominal pain caused by acute pancreatitis. On fundoscopic examination the retinal blood vessels are opalescent (*lipemia retinalis*). Eruptive xanthomas, which are small yellowish-white papules, often appear in clusters on the back, buttocks, and extensor surfaces of the arms and legs. These typically painless skin lesions may become pruritic as they regress. Hepatosplenomegaly results from the uptake of circulating chylomicrons by reticuloendothelial cells in the liver and spleen. For reasons unknown, some patients with persistent and pronounced chylomicronemia never develop pancreatitis, eruptive xanthomas, or hepatosplenomegaly. Premature ASCVD has not been consistently demonstrated to be a feature of familial chylomicronemia syndromes.

The diagnoses of LPL and apoC-II deficiency are established enzymatically by assaying triglyceride lipolytic activity in post-heparin plasma. Blood is sampled after an intravenous heparin injection to release the endothelial-bound lipases. LPL activity is profoundly reduced in both LPL and apoC-II deficiency; in patients with apoC-II deficiency, the addition of normal pre-heparin plasma (a source of apoC-II) normalizes LPL activity, but this correction does not occur in patients with LPL deficiency.

The major therapeutic intervention in familial chylomicronemia syndromes is dietary fat restriction (to as little as 15 g/d) with fat-

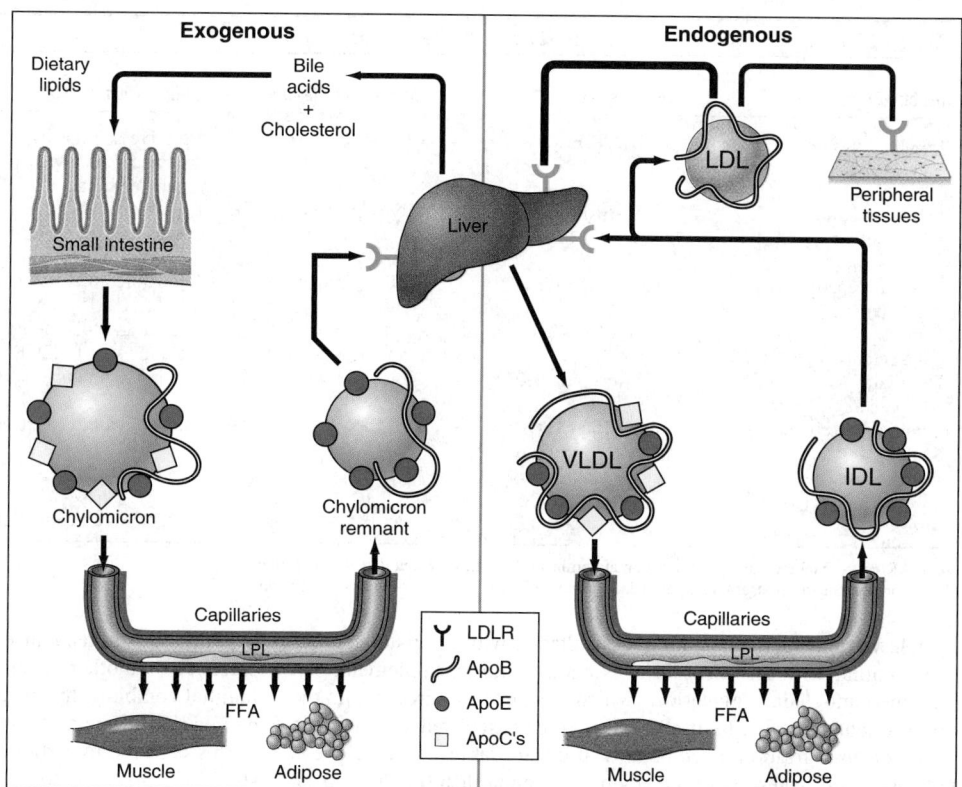

FIGURE 335-2 The exogenous and endogenous lipoprotein metabolic pathways. The exogenous pathway transports dietary lipids to the periphery and the liver. The endogenous pathway transports hepatic lipids to the periphery. LPL, lipoprotein lipase; FFA, free fatty acids; VLDL, very low density lipoproteins; IDL, intermediate-density lipoproteins; LDL, low-density lipoproteins; LDLR, low-density lipoprotein receptor.

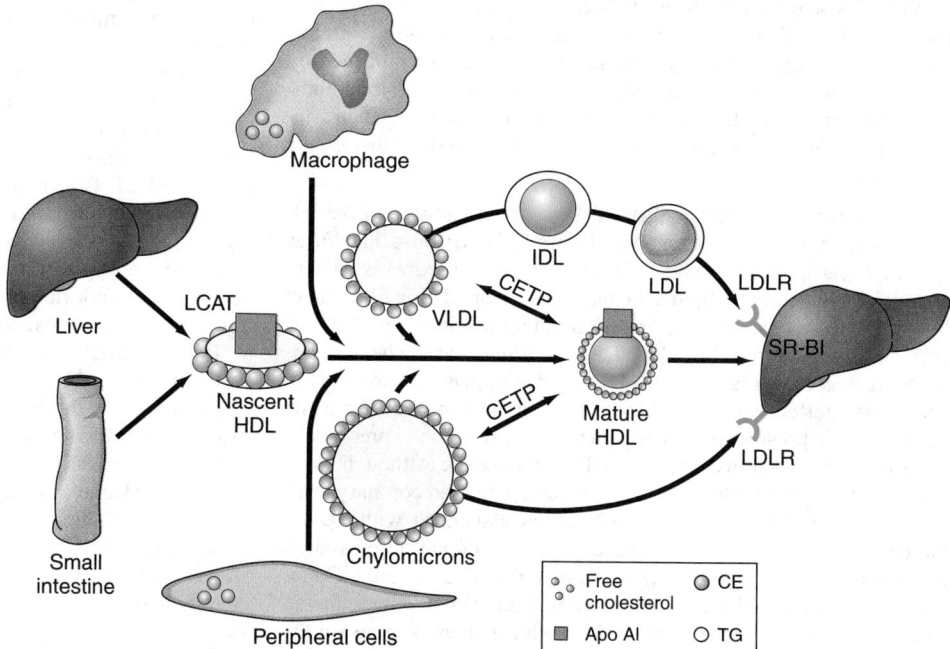

FIGURE 335-3 HDL metabolism and reverse cholesterol transport. This pathway transports excess cholesterol from the periphery back to the liver for excretion in the bile. The liver and the intestine produce nascent HDL. Free cholesterol is acquired from macrophages and other peripheral cells and esterfied by LCAT, forming mature HDL. HDL cholesterol can be selectively taken up by the liver via SR-BI. Alternatively, HDL cholesteryl ester can be transferred by CETP from HDL to VLDL and chylomicrons, which can then be taken up by the liver. LCAT, lecithin-cholesterol acyltransferase; CETP, cholesteryl ester transfer protein; VLDL, very low density lipoproteins; IDL, intermediate-density lipoproteins; LDL, low-density lipoproteins; HDL, high-density lipoproteins; LDLR, low-density lipoprotein receptor; TG, triglycerides.

Genetic Disorder	Gene Defect	Lipoproteins Elevated	Clinical Findings	Genetic Transmission	Estimated Incidence
Lipoprotein lipase deficiency	LPL (*LPL*)	Chylomicrons	Eruptive xanthomas, hepatosplenomegaly pancreatitis	AR	1/1,000,000
Familial apolipoprotein C-II deficiency	ApoC-II (*APOC2*)	Chylomicrons	Eruptive xanthomas, hepatosplenomegaly pancreatitis	AR	<1/1,000,000
Familial hepatic lipase deficiency	Hepatic lipase (*LIPC*)	VLDL remnants	Premature atherosclerosis	AR	<1/1,000,000
Familial dysbetalipoproteinemia	ApoE (*APOE*)	Chylomicron and VLDL remnants	Palmar and tuberoeruptive xanthomas, CHD, PVD	AR AD	1/10,000
Familial hypercholesterolemia	LDL receptor (*LDLR*)	LDL	Tendon xanthomas, CHD	AD	1/500
Familial defective apoB-100	ApoB-100 (*APOB*) (Arg$_{3500}$ → Gln)	LDL	Tendon xanthomas, CHD	AD	1/1000
Autosomal recessive hypercholesterolemia	ARH (*ARH*)	LDL	Tendon xanthomas, CHD	AR	<1/1,000,000
Sitosterolemia	*ABCG5* or *ABCG8*	LDL	Tendon xanthomas, CHD	AR	<1/1,000,000

Note: AR, autosomal recessive; AD, autosomal dominant; VLDL, very low density lipoprotein; CHD, coronary heart disease; PVD, peripheral vascular disease; LDL, low-density lipoprotein.

soluble vitamin supplementation. Consultation with a registered dietician familiar with this disorder is essential. Caloric supplementation with medium-chain triglycerides, which are absorbed directly into the portal circulation, can be useful but may be associated with hepatic fibrosis if used for prolonged periods. If dietary fat restriction alone is not successful in resolving the chylomicronemia, fish oils have been effective in some patients. In patients with apoC-II deficiency, apoC-II can be provided by infusing fresh-frozen plasma to resolve the chylomicronemia. Management of patients with familial chylomicronemia syndrome is particularly challenging during pregnancy when VLDL production is increased. Plasmapheresis may be required if pancreatitis develops and the chylomicronemia is not responsive to diet therapy.

Hepatic Lipase Deficiency HL is a member of the same gene family as LPL and hydrolyzes triglycerides and phospholipids in remnant lipoproteins and HDL. HL deficiency is a very rare autosomal recessive disorder characterized by elevated plasma cholesterol and triglycerides (mixed hyperlipidemia) due to the accumulation of lipoprotein remnants. HDL-C is normal or elevated. The diagnosis is confirmed by measuring HL activity in post-heparin plasma. Due to the small number of patients with HL deficiency, the association of this genetic defect with ASCVD is not known, but lipid-lowering therapy is recommended.

Familial Dysbetalipoproteinemia (Type III Hyperlipoproteinemia) Like HL deficiency, familial dysbetalipoproteinemia (FDBL) (also known as *type III hyperlipoproteinemia* or *familial broad β disease*) is characterized by a mixed hyperlipidemia due to the accumulation of remnant lipoprotein particles. ApoE is present in multiple copies on chylomicron and VLDL remnants and mediates their removal via hepatic lipoprotein receptors (Fig. 335-2). FDBL is due to genetic variations in apoE that interfere with its ability to bind lipoprotein receptors. The *APOE* gene is polymorphic in sequence resulting in the expression of three common isoforms: apoE3, apoE2, and apoE4. Although associated with slightly higher LDL-C levels and increased coronary heart disease (CHD) risk, the apoE4 allele is not associated with FDBL. Patients with apoE4 have an increased incidence of late-onset Alzheimer disease. ApoE2 has a lower affinity for the LDL receptor. Therefore, chylomicron and VLDL remnants containing apoE2 are removed from plasma at a slower rate. Individuals who are homozygous for the E2 allele (the E2/E2 genotype) comprise the most common subset of patients with FDBL.

Approximately 1% of the general population are apoE2/E2 homozygotes but only a small minority of these individuals develop FDBL. In most cases an additional, identifiable factor precipitates the development of hyperlipoproteinemia. The most common precipitating factors are a high-caloric, high-fat diet, diabetes mellitus, obesity,

hypothyroidism, renal disease, estrogen deficiency, alcohol use, or the presence of another genetic form of hyperlipidemia, most commonly familial combined hyperlipidemia (FCHL) or familial hypercholesterolemia (FH). Rare mutations in apoE cause dominant forms of FDBL; in this case the hyperlipidemia is fully manifest in the heterozygous state.

Patients with FDBL usually present in adulthood with xanthomas and premature coronary and peripheral vascular disease. The disease seldom presents in women before menopause. Two distinctive types of xanthomas are seen in FDBL patients: tuberoeruptive and palmar xanthomas. *Tuberoeruptive xanthomas* begin as clusters of small papules on the elbows, knees, or buttocks and can grow to the size of small grapes. *Palmar xanthoma* (alternatively called *xanthomata striata palmaris*) are orange-yellow discolorations of the creases in the palms. In FDBL, the plasma cholesterol and triglyceride are elevated to a relatively similar degree until the triglyceride levels reach ~5.6 mol/L (~500 mg/dL), and then the triglycerides tends to be greater than cholesterol.

The traditional approach to diagnose this disorder is to use lipoprotein electrophoresis; in FDBL, the remnant lipoproteins accumulate in a broad β band. The preferred method to confirm the diagnosis of FDBL is to measure VLDL-C by ultracentrifugation and determine the ratio of VLDL-C to total plasma triglyceride; a ratio >0.30 is consistent with the diagnosis of FDBL. Protein methods (apoE phenotyping) or DNA-based methods (apoE genotyping) can be performed to confirm homozygosity for apoE2. However, absence of the apoE2/2 genotype does not rule out the diagnosis of FDBL, since other mutations in apoE can cause this condition.

Because FDBL is associated with increased risk of premature ASCVD, it should be treated aggressively. Other metabolic conditions that can worsen the hyperlipidemia (see above) should be actively treated. Patients with FDBL are typically very diet responsive and can respond dramatically to weight reduction and to low-cholesterol, low-fat diets. Alcohol intake should be curtailed. In postmenopausal women with FDBL, the dyslipidemia responds to estrogen-replacement therapy. HMG-CoA reductase inhibitors, fibrates, and niacin are all generally effective in the treatment of FDBL, and combination drug therapy is sometimes required.

Familial Hypercholesterolemia FH is an autosomal codominant disorder characterized by elevated plasma LDL-C with normal triglycerides, tendon xanthomas, and premature coronary atherosclerosis. FH is caused by >750 mutations in the LDL receptor gene and has a higher incidence in certain populations, such as Afrikaners, Christian Lebanese, and French Canadians, due to the founder effect. The elevated levels of LDL-C in FH are due to delayed catabolism of LDL and its precursor particles from the blood, resulting in increased rates of LDL production. There is a major gene dose effect, in that individuals with two mutated LDL receptor alleles (FH homozygotes) are much more affected than those with one mutant allele (FH heterozygotes).

Homozygous FH occurs in approximately 1 in 1 million persons world-wide. Patients with homozygous FH can be classified into one of two groups based on the amount of LDL receptor activity measured in their skin fibroblasts: those patients with <2% of normal LDL receptor activity (receptor negative) and those patients with 2 to 25% of normal LDL receptor activity (receptor defective). Most patients with homozygous FH present in childhood with cutaneous xanthomas on the hands, wrists, elbows, knees, heels, or buttocks. Arcus cornea is usually present and some patients have xanthelasmas. Total cholesterol levels are usually >12.93 mmol/L (500 mg/dL) and can be >25.86 mmol/L (1000 mg/dL). Accelerated atherosclerosis is a devastating complication of homozygous FH and can result in disability and death in childhood. Atherosclerosis often develops first in the aortic root and can cause aortic valvular or supravalvular stenosis and typically extends into the coronary ostia. Children with homozygous FH often develop symptomatic vascular disease before puberty, when symptoms can be atypical and sudden death is common. Untreated, receptor-negative patients with homozygous FH rarely survive beyond the second decade; patients with receptor-defective LDL receptor defects have a better prognosis but almost invariably develop clinically apparent atherosclerotic vascular disease by age 30, and often much sooner. Carotid and femoral disease develop later in life and are usually not clinically significant.

A careful family history should be taken, and plasma lipid levels should be measured in the parents and other first-degree relatives of patients with homozygous FH. The diagnosis can be confirmed by obtaining a skin biopsy and measuring LDL receptor activity in cultured skin fibroblasts or by quantifying the number of LDL receptors on the surfaces of lymphocytes using cell-sorting technology.

Combination therapy with an HMG-CoA reductase inhibitor and a bile acid sequestrant sometimes results in modest reductions in plasma LDL-C in the FH homozygote. Patients with homozygous FH invariably require additional lipid-lowering therapy. Since the liver is quantitatively the most important tissue for removing circulating LDL via the LDL receptor, liver transplantation is effective in decreasing plasma LDL-C levels in this disorder. Liver transplantation is, however, associated with substantial risks, including the requirement for long-term immunosuppression. The current treatment of choice for homozygous FH is LDL apheresis (a process where the LDL particles are selectively removed from the circulation), which can promote regression of xanthomas and may slow the progression of atherosclerosis. Initiation of LDL apheresis should be delayed until approximately 5 years of age except when evidence of atherosclerotic vascular disease is present.

Heterozygous FH is caused by the inheritance of one mutant LDL receptor allele and occurs in approximately 1 in 500 persons worldwide, making it one of the most common single gene disorders. It is characterized by elevated plasma LDL-C [usually 5.17 to 10.34 μmol/L (200 to 400 mg/dL)] and normal triglyceride levels. Patients with heterozygous FH have hypercholesterolemia from birth, although the disease is often not detected until adulthood, usually due to the detection of hypercholesterolemia on routine screening, the appearance of tendon xanthomas, or the premature development of symptomatic coronary atherosclerotic disease. Since the disease is codominant in inheritance and has a high penetrance (>90%), one parent and ~50% of the patient's siblings are usually hypercholesterolemic. The family history is frequently positive for premature ASCVD on one side of the family, particularly among male relatives. Corneal arcus is common, and tendon xanthomas involving the dorsum of the hands, elbows, knees, and especially the Achilles tendons are present in ~75% of patients. The age of onset of ASCVD is highly variable and depends in part on the molecular defect in the LDL receptor gene and other coexisting cardiac risk factors. FH heterozygotes with elevated plasma Lp(a) appear to be at greater risk for cardiovascular complications.

Untreated men with heterozygous FH have an ~50% chance of having a myocardial infarction before age 60. Although the age of onset of atherosclerotic heart disease is later in women with FH, coronary disease is significantly more common in women with FH than in the general female population.

No definitive diagnostic test for heterozygous FH is available. Although FH heterozygotes tend to have reduced levels of LDL receptor function in skin fibroblasts, there is significant overlap with the levels in normal fibroblasts. The clinical diagnosis is usually not problematic, but it is critical that hypothyroidism, nephrotic syndrome, and obstructive liver disease be excluded before initiating therapy.

FH patients should be treated aggressively to lower plasma levels of LDL-C. Initiation of a low-cholesterol, low-fat diet is recommended, but heterozygous FH patients inevitably require lipid-lowering drug therapy. HMG-CoA reductase inhibitors are especially effective in heterozygous FH, inducing upregulation of the normal LDL receptor allele in the liver. Many heterozygous FH patients can achieve desired LDL-C levels with HMG-CoA reductase inhibitor therapy alone, but combination drug therapy with the addition of a bile acid sequestrant or nicotinic acid is frequently required. Heterozygous FH patients who cannot be adequately controlled on combination drug therapy are candidates for LDL apheresis.

Familial Defective ApoB-100 Familial defective apoB-100 (FDB) is a dominantly inherited disorder that clinically resembles heterozygous FH. FDB occurs with a frequency of ~1 in 1000 in western populations. The disease is characterized by elevated plasma LDL-C levels with normal triglycerides, tendon xanthomas, and an increased incidence of premature ASCVD. FDB is caused by mutations in the LDL receptor–binding domain of apoB-100. Almost all patients with FDB have a substitution of glutamine for arginine at position 3500 in apoB-100, although other rarer mutations have been reported to cause this disease. As a consequence of the mutation in apoB-100, LDL binds the LDL receptor with reduced affinity and LDL is removed from the circulation at a reduced rate. Patients with FDB cannot be clinically distinguished from patients with heterozygous FH, although patients with FDB tend to have lower plasma LDL-C than FH heterozygotes. The apoB-100 gene mutation can be detected directly, but currently genetic diagnosis is not encouraged since the recommended management of FDB and heterozygous FH is identical.

Autosomal Recessive Hypercholesterolemia Autosomal recessive hypercholesterolemia (ARH) is a rare disorder (except in Sardinia) due to mutations in a protein (ARH) involved in LDL receptor–mediated endocytosis in the liver. ARH clinically resembles homozygous FH and is characterized by hypercholesterolemia, tendon xanthomas, and premature coronary artery disease. The hypercholesterolemia tends to be intermediate between the levels seen in FH homozygotes and FH heterozygotes. LDL receptor function in cultured fibroblasts is normal or only modestly reduced in ARH, whereas LDL receptor function in lymphocytes and the liver is negligible. Unlike FH homozygotes, the hyperlipidemia responds partially to treatment with HMG-CoA reductase inhibitors, but these patients usually require LDL apheresis to lower plasma LDL-C to recommended levels.

Wolman Disease and Cholesteryl Ester Storage Disease Wolman disease is an autosomal recessive disorder caused by complete deficiency of lysosomal acid lipase. After LDL is taken up from the cell surface by LDL receptor–mediated endocytosis, it is delivered from endosomes to lysosomes. In the acidic environment of the endosome, the particle dissociates from the receptor, which recycles to the cell surface. In the lysosome, apoB-100 is degraded and the cholesteryl esters and triglycerides of LDL are hydrolyzed by lysosomal acid lipase. Patients with Wolman disease fail to hydrolyze the neutral lipids, resulting in their accumulation within cells. The disease presents within the first weeks of life with hepatosplenomegaly, steatorrhea, adrenal calcification, and failure to thrive. The disease is usually fatal within the first year of life and can be diagnosed by measuring acid lipase activity in fibroblasts or liver tissue biopsy specimens. Cholesteryl ester storage disease is a less severe form of the same genetic disorder in which there is low, but detectable, acid lipase activity. Patients with this disorder sometimes present in childhood with hepatomegaly and a mixed hyperlipidemia, due to elevations in the levels of plasma LDL and VLDL. Other patients present later in life with hepatic fibrosis, portal hypertension, or with premature atherosclerosis.

Sitosterolemia Sitosterolemia is a rare autosomal recessive disease caused by mutations in one of two members of the adenosine triphosphate (ATP)-binding cassette transporter family, ABCG5 and ABCG8. These genes are expressed in the intestine and liver, where they form a functional complex to limit intestinal absorption and promote biliary excretion of plant- and animal-derived neutral sterols. In normal individuals, <5% of dietary plant sterols, of which sitosterol is the most plentiful, are absorbed by the proximal small intestine and delivered to the liver. Plant sterols in the liver are preferentially secreted into the bile, and plasma plant sterol levels are normally very low. In sitosterolemia, the intestinal absorption of plant sterols is increased and biliary excretion of the sterols is reduced, resulting in increased plasma levels of sitosterol and other plant sterols. The trafficking of cholesterol is also impaired. Patients with sitosterolemia can have either normal or elevated plasma levels of cholesterol. Irrespective of the plasma cholesterol level, these patients develop cutaneous and tendon xanthomas as well as premature atherosclerosis. Episodes of hemolysis, presumably secondary to the incorporation of plant sterols into the red blood cell membrane, are a distinctive clinical feature of this disease. The hypercholesterolemia in patients with sitosterolemia is unusually responsive to reductions in dietary cholesterol content. Sitosterolemia should be suspected when the plasma cholesterol level falls by >40% on a low-cholesterol diet (without associated weight loss).

Sitosterolemia is confirmed by demonstrating an elevated plasma sitosterol level. The hypercholesterolemia does not respond to HMG-CoA reductase inhibitors, but bile acid sequestrants and cholesterol-absorption inhibitors, such as ezetimibe, are effective in reducing plasma sterol levels in these patients.

PRIMARY DISORDERS OF ApoB-CONTAINING LIPOPROTEIN METABOLISM (UNKNOWN ETIOLOGY) A large proportion of patients with elevated levels of apoB-containing lipoproteins have disorders in which the molecular defect has not been defined, largely because multiple other genetic and nongenetic factors contribute to the hyperlipidemia.

Familial Hypertriglyceridemia Familial hypertriglyceridemia (FHTG) is a relatively common (1 in 500) autosomal dominant disorder of unknown etiology characterized by moderately elevated plasma triglycerides accompanied by more modest elevations in cholesterol. VLDL is the major class of lipoproteins elevated in this disorder, which is

often referred to as type IV hyperlipoproteinemia (Frederickson classification, Table 335-4). The elevated plasma VLDL is due to increased VLDL production, impaired VLDL catabolism, or a combination of the two. Some patients with FHTG have a more severe form of hyperlipidemia in which both VLDL and chylomicrons are elevated (type V hyperlipidemia), as these two classes of lipoproteins compete for the same lipolytic pathway. Increased intake of simple carbohydrates, obesity, insulin resistance, alcohol use, or estrogen treatment, all of which increase VLDL synthesis, can precipitate the development of chylomicronemia. FHTG does not appear to be associated with increased risk of ASCVD in many families.

The diagnosis of FHTG is suggested by the triad of elevated plasma triglycerides [2.8 to 11.3 mmol/L (250 to 1000 mg/dL)], normal or only mildly increased cholesterol levels [<6.5 mmol/L (<250 mg/dL)], and reduced plasma HDL-C. Plasma LDL-C is generally not increased and is often reduced due to defective metabolism of the triglyceride-rich particles. The identification of other first-degree relatives with hypertriglyceridemia is useful in making the diagnosis. FDBL and FCHL should also be ruled out as these two conditions are associated with a significantly increased risk of ASCVD. The plasma apoB levels and the ratio of plasma cholesterol to triglyceride tend to be lower in FHTG than in either FDBL or FCHL.

It is important to exclude secondary causes of the hypertriglyceridemia before making the diagnosis of FHTG. Lipid-lowering drug therapy can frequently be avoided with appropriate dietary and lifestyle changes. Patients with plasma triglyceride levels >4.5 to 6.8 mmol/L (>400 to 600 mg/dL), after a trial of diet and exercise, should be considered for drug therapy to avoid the development of chylomicronemia and pancreatitis. A fibrate is a reasonable first line drug for FHTG, and niacin can also be considered in this condition.

Familial Combined Hyperlipidemia The molecular etiology of FCHL is unknown but is likely to involve defects in several different genes. FCHL is the most common primary lipid disorder, occurring in approximately 1 in 200 persons. Approximately 20% of patients who develop CHD before age 60 have FCHL.

FCHL is characterized by moderate elevation of plasma triglycerides and cholesterol and reduced plasma HDL-C. The disease is autosomal dominant, and affected family members typically have one of three possible phenotypes: (1) elevated plasma LDL-C, (2) elevated plasma triglycerides and VLDL-C, or (3) elevated plasma LDL-C and VLDL-C. A classic feature of FCHL is that the lipoprotein phenotype can switch among these phenotypes. FCHL can manifest in childhood but is sometimes not fully expressed until adulthood. Visceral obesity, glucose intolerance, insulin resistance, hypertension, and hyperuricemia are often present. These patients do not develop xanthomas.

Patients with FCHL almost always have significantly elevated plasma apoB. The levels of apoB are disproportionately high relative to plasma LDL-C due to the presence of small dense LDL particles,

TABLE 335-4 *Frederickson Classification of Hyperlipoproteinemias*

Phenotype	I	IIa	IIb	III	IV	V
Lipoprotein elevated	Chylomicrons	LDL	LDL and VLDL	Chylomicron and VLDL remnants	VLDL	Chylomicrons and VLDL
Triglycerides	++++	−−	++	++ to +++	++	++++
Cholesterol	+ to ++	+++	++ to +++	++ to +++	−− to +	++ to +++
LDL-cholesterol	↓	↑	↑	↓	↓	↓
HDL-cholesterol	↓↓↓	↓	↓	—	↓↓	↓↓↓
Plasma appearance	Lactescent	Clear	Clear	Turbid	Turbid	Lactescent
Xanthomas	Eruptive	Tendon, tuberous	None	Palmar, tuberoeruptive	None	Eruptive
Pancreatitis	+++	0	0	0	0	+++
Coronary atherosclerosis	0	+++	+++	+++	+/−	+/−
Peripheral atherosclerosis	0	+	+	++	+/−	+/−
Molecular defects	LPL and apoC-II	LDL receptor and apoB-100	Unknown	ApoE	Unknown	Unknown
Genetic nomenclature	FCS	FH, FDB	FCHL	FDBL	FHTG	FHTG

Note: LPL, lipoprotein lipase; apo, apolipoprotein; FCS, familial chylomicronemia syndrome; FH, familial hypercholesterolemia; FDB, familiar defective apoB; FCHL, familial combined hyperlipidemia; FDBL, familial dysbetalipoproteinemia; FHTG, familial hypertriglyceridemia.

which are characteristic of this syndrome and are highly atherogenic. *Hyperapobetalipoproteinemia* has been used as a term to describe the coupling of elevated plasma apoB with normal plasma cholesterol, and is probably a form of FCHL.

A mixed dyslipidemia [plasma triglyceride levels between 2.3 and 9.0 mmol/L (200 and 800 mg/dL), cholesterol levels between 5.2 and 10.3 mmol/L (200 and 400 mg/dL), and HDL-C levels <10.3 mmol/L (<40 mg/dL)] and a family history of hyperlipidemia and/or premature CHD suggests the diagnosis of FCHL. An elevated plasma apoB level or an increased number of small dense LDL particles in the plasma supports this diagnosis. FDBL should be considered and ruled out by beta-quantification in suspected patients with a mixed hyperlipidemia.

Individuals with FCHL should be treated aggressively due to significantly increased risk of premature CHD. Decreased dietary intake of saturated fat and simple carbohydrates, aerobic exercise, and weight loss have beneficial effects on the lipid profile. Patients with diabetes should be aggressively treated to maintain good glucose control. Most patients with FCHL require lipid-lowering drug therapy to reduce lipoprotein levels to the recommended range. HMG-CoA reductase inhibitors are very effective in lowering plasma levels of LDL-C and can also significantly reduce VLDL-C. Nicotinic acid decreases both LDL-C and VLDL-C, while raising plasma HDL-C, and is frequently effective for this condition when used in combination with HMG-CoA reductase inhibitors.

Polygenic Hypercholesterolemia Polygenic hypercholesterolemia is characterized by hypercholesterolemia with a normal plasma triglyceride in the absence of secondary causes of hypercholesterolemia. Plasma LDL-C levels are not as elevated as they are in FH and FDB. Family studies are useful to differentiate polygenic hypercholesterolemia from the single-gene disorders described above; half of the first-degree relatives of patients with FH and FDB are hypercholesterolemic, whereas <10% of first-degree relatives of patients with polygenic hypercholesterolemia are hypercholesterolemic. Treatment of polygenic hypercholesterolemia is identical to that of other forms of hypercholesterolemia.

GENETIC DISORDERS OF HDL METABOLISM (KNOWN ETIOLOGY) Mutations in certain genes encoding critical proteins in HDL synthesis and catabolism cause marked variations in plasma HDL-C levels. Unlike the genetic forms of hypercholesterolemia, which are invariably associated with premature coronary atherosclerosis, genetic forms of hypoalphalipoproteinemia (low HDL-C) are not always associated with accelerated atherosclerosis. Whereas high plasma LDL-C is invariably associated with increased atherosclerosis, the risk associated with low plasma levels of HDL-C depends on the underlying mechanism. Analysis of the genetic disorders of HDL metabolism has provided insights into the less well understood etiologic relationship between plasma HDL-C levels and atherosclerosis.

ApoA-I Deficiency and ApoA-I Mutations Complete genetic deficiency of apoA-I due to mutations in the apoA-I gene result in the virtual absence of HDL from the plasma. The genes encoding apoA-I, apoC-III, apoA-IV, and apoA-V are clustered together on chromosome 11, and some patients with complete absence of apoA-I have deletions that include more than one of these genes. Because apoA-I is required for LCAT function, plasma and tissue levels of free cholesterol are increased, resulting in the development of corneal opacities and planar xanthomas. Clinically apparent coronary atherosclerosis typically appears between the fourth and seventh decade in the apoA-I-deficient patient.

Although missense mutations in the apoA-I gene have been identified in selected patients with low plasma HDL [usually 0.39 to 0.78 mmol/L (15 to 30 mg/dL)], they are very rare causes of low HDL-C levels in the general population. Patients with apoA-I$_{Milano}$ have very low plasma levels of HDL due to the rapid catabolism of the apolipoprotein, but these patients do not have an increased risk of premature CHD. Other than corneal opacities, most individuals with low plasma HDL-C levels due to missense mutations in apoA-I have no clinical sequelae. A few specific mutations in apoA-I cause systemic amyloi-

dosis, and the mutant apoA-I has been found as a component of the amyloid plaque.

Tangier Disease Tangier disease is a rare autosomal codominant form of low plasma HDL-C caused by mutations in the gene encoding ABCA1, a cellular transporter that facilitates efflux of unesterified cholesterol and phospholipids from cells to apoA-I (Fig. 335-3). ABCA1 plays a critical role in the generation and stabilization of the mature HDL particle. In its absence, HDL is rapidly cleared from the circulation. Patients with Tangier disease have plasma HDL-C levels <0.13 mmol/L (<5 mg/dL) and extremely low circulating levels of apoA-I. The disease is associated with cholesterol accumulation in the reticuloendothelial system, resulting in hepatosplenomegaly and pathognomonic enlarged, grayish yellow or orange tonsils. An intermittent peripheral neuropathy (mononeuritis multiplex) or a sphingomyelia-like neurologic disorder can also be seen in this disorder. Tangier disease is associated with premature atherosclerotic disease, but the risk is not as high as might be anticipated given the markedly decreased plasma HDL-C and apoA-I. Plasma LDL-C is also low and this may attenuate the atherosclerotic risk. Obligate heterozygotes for ABCA1 mutations have moderately reduced plasma HDL-C levels and are also at increased risk of premature CHD.

LCAT Deficiency LCAT deficiency is a rare disorder caused by mutations in lecithin:cholesterol acyltransferase (Fig. 335-3). LCAT is synthesized in the liver and secreted into the plasma, where it circulates associated with lipoproteins. Because the enzyme mediates the esterification of cholesterol, the proportion of free cholesterol in circulating lipoproteins is greatly increased (from ~25% to >70% of total plasma cholesterol). Lack of normal cholesterol esterification impairs the formation of mature HDL particles and leads to rapid catabolism of circulating apoA-I. Two genetic forms of LCAT deficiency have been described in humans—complete deficiency (also called *classic LCAT deficiency*) and partial deficiency (also called *fish-eye disease*). Progressive corneal opacification due to the deposition of free cholesterol in the lens, very low plasma HDL-C [usually <0.26 mmol/L (<10 mg/dL)], and variable hypertriglyceridemia are characteristic of both types. In partial LCAT deficiency, there are no other known clinical sequelae. In contrast, complete LCAT deficiency is characterized by a hemolytic anemia and progressive renal insufficiency that eventually leads to end-stage renal disease (ESRD). Despite the extremely low plasma levels of HDL-C and apoA-I, premature ASCVD is not a feature of either complete or partial LCAT deficiency, once again exemplifying the complex relationship between low plasma levels of HDL-C and the development of ASCVD. The diagnosis can be confirmed by assaying LCAT activity in the plasma.

CETP Deficiency Mutations in the gene encoding cholesteryl ester transfer protein (CETP) cause a high HDL-C condition called *CETP deficiency*. CETP facilitates the transfer of cholesteryl esters among lipoproteins, especially from HDL to apoB-containing lipoproteins in exchange for triglycerides (Fig. 335-3). Homozygous deficiency of CETP, which occurs predominantly in Japan, results in very high plasma HDL-C [>3.88 mmol/L (>150 mg/dL)] due to accumulation of large, cholesterol-rich HDL particles. Heterozygotes for CETP deficiency have only modestly elevated HDL-C. The relationship of CETP deficiency to risk of ASCVD remains a matter of debate.

PRIMARY DISORDERS OF HDL METABOLISM (UNKNOWN ETIOLOGY) The gene defect in other individuals with either very high or very low plasma HDL-C is not known.

Primary Hypoalphalipoproteinemia The most common inherited cause of low plasma HDL-C is termed *primary or familial hypoalphalipoproteinemia*. Hypoalphalipoproteinemia is defined as a plasma HDL-C level below the 10th percentile in the setting of relatively normal cholesterol and triglyceride levels, no apparent secondary causes of low plasma HDL-C, and no clinical signs of LCAT deficiency or Tangier disease. This syndrome is often referred to as "isolated low HDL." A family history of low HDL-C facilitates the diagnosis of an inherited condition, which usually follows an autosomal dominant pattern. The metabolic etiology of this disease appears to be primarily accelerated catabolism of HDL and its apolipoproteins. Several kindreds with primary hypoalphalipoproteinemia have been described in association with an increased incidence of premature ASCVD.

Familial Hyperalphalipoproteinemia Familial hyperalphalipoproteinemia has a dominant inheritance pattern. Plasma HDL-C is usually >2.07 mmol/L (80 mg/dL) in affected women and >1.81 mmol/L (70 mg/dL) in affected men. The genetic basis of primary hyperalphalipoproteinemia is not known, and the condition may be associated with decreased risk of CHD and increased longevity in some cases.

SECONDARY DISORDERS OF LIPOPROTEIN METABOLISM Significant changes in plasma levels of lipoproteins are seen in a variety of diseases. It is critical that secondary causes of hyperlipidemias (Table 335-5) are considered prior to initiation of lipid-lowering therapy.

Obesity Obesity is frequently, though not invariably, accompanied by hyperlipidemia. The increase in adipocyte mass and accompanying decrease in insulin sensitivity associated with obesity have multiple effects on lipid metabolism. More free fatty acids are delivered from the expanded adipose tissue to the liver where they are re-esterified in hepatocytes to form triglycerides, which are packaged into VLDL for secretion into the circulation. High dietary intake of simple carbohydrates also drives hepatic production of VLDL, leading to increases in VLDL and/or LDL in some obese individuals. Plasma HDL-C tends to be low in obesity. Weight loss is often associated with a reduction of plasma apoB-containing lipoproteins and an increase of plasma HDL-C.

Diabetes Mellitus Patients with type 1 diabetes mellitus are generally not hyperlipidemic if they are under good glycemic control. Diabetic ketoacidosis is frequently accompanied by hypertriglyceridemia due to increased hepatic influx of free fatty acids from adipose tissue. The hypertriglyceridemia responds dramatically to administration of insulin in the insulinopenic diabetic.

Patients with type 2 diabetes mellitus are usually dyslipidemic, even if under relatively good glycemic control. The high levels of insulin and insulin resistance associated with type 2 diabetes have multiple effects on fat metabolism: (1) a decrease in LPL activity resulting in reduced catabolism of chylomicrons and VLDL, (2) an increase in the release of free fatty acid from the adipose tissue, (3) an increase in fatty acid synthesis in the liver, and (4) an increase in hepatic VLDL production. Patients with type 2 diabetes mellitus have several lipid abnormalities, including elevated plasma triglycerides (due to increased VLDL and lipoprotein remnants), elevated dense LDL, and decreased HDL-C. In some diabetic patients, especially those with a genetic defect in lipid metabolism, the triglycerides can be extremely elevated. Elevated plasma LDL-C levels are usually not a feature of diabetes mellitus and suggest the presence of an underlying lipoprotein abnormality or may indicate the development of diabetic nephropathy. Patients with lipodystrophy, who have profound insulin resistance, have markedly elevated VLDL and chylomicrons.

Thyroid Disease Hypothyroidism is associated with elevated plasma LDL-C due primarily to a reduction in hepatic LDL receptor function and delayed clearance of LDL. Conversely, plasma LDL-C is often reduced in the hyperthyroid patient. Hypothyroid patients may have increased circulating IDL, and some are mildly hypertriglyceridemic [<3.34 μmol/L (<300 mg/dL)]. Because hypothyroidism is easily overlooked, all patients presenting with elevated plasma LDL-C or IDL should be screened for hypothyroidism. Thyroid replacement therapy usually ameliorates the hypercholesterolemia.

Renal Disorders Nephrotic syndrome is associated with hyperlipoproteinemia, which is usually mixed but can manifest as hypercholesterolemia or hypertriglyceridemia alone. The hyperlipidemia of nephrotic syndrome appears to be due to a combination of increased hepatic production and decreased clearance of VLDL, with increased LDL production. Effective treatment of the underlying renal disease normalizes the lipid profile, but most patients with chronic nephrotic syndrome require lipid-lowering drug therapy.

ESRD is often associated with mild hypertriglyceridemia [<3.34 μmol/L (<300 mg/dL)] due to the accumulation of VLDL and remnant lipoproteins in the circulation. Triglyceride lipolysis and remnant clearance are both reduced in patients with renal failure. Because the risk of ASCVD is increased in hyperlipidemic patients with ESRD, they should be treated aggressively with lipid-lowering agents.

Patients with renal transplants are usually hyperlipidemic due to immunosuppression drugs (cyclosporine and glucocorticoids); they present a difficult management problem as HMG-CoA reductase inhibitors must be used cautiously in these patients.

Liver Disorders Because the liver is the principal site of formation and clearance of lipoproteins, it is not surprising that liver diseases can

---

TABLE 335-5 *Secondary Forms of Hyperlipidemia*

LDL Elevated	LDL Reduced	HDL Elevated	HDL Reduced	VLDL Elevated	IDL Elevated	Chylomicrons Elevated	Lp(a) Elevated
Hypothyroidism	Severe liver disease	Alcohol	Smoking	Obesity	Multiple myeloma	Autoimmune disease	Renal insufficiency
Nephrotic syndrome	Malabsorption	Exercise	DM type 2	DM type 2	Monoclonal gammopathy	Drugs: Isotretinoin	Inflammation
Cholestasis	Malnutrition	Exposure to chlorinated hydrocarbons	Obesity	Glycogen storage disease	Autoimmune disease		Menopause
Acute intermittent porphyria	Gaucher disease	Drugs: estrogen	Malnutrition	Hepatitis	Hypothyroidism		Orchidectomy
Anorexia nervosa	Chronic infectious disease		Gaucher disease	Alcohol			Hypothyroidism
Hepatoma	Hyperthyroidism		Drugs: anabolic steroids, beta blockers	Renal failure			Acromegaly
Drugs: thiazides, cyclosporine, tegretol	Drugs: niacin toxicity			Sepsis			Nephrosis
				Stress			Drugs: growth hormone
				Cushing syndrome			
				Pregnancy			
				Acromegaly			
				Lipodystrophy			
				Drugs: estrogen, beta blockers, furosemide, glucocorticoids, bile acid–binding resins, retinoic acid, HIV protease inhibitors			

Note: LDL, low-density lipoprotein; HDL, high-density lipoprotein; VLDL, very low density lipoprotein; IDL, intermediate-density lipoprotein; Lp(a), lipoprotein A; DM, diabetes mellitus.

profoundly affect plasma lipid levels in a variety of ways. Hepatitis due to infection, drugs, or alcohol is often associated with increased VLDL synthesis and mild to moderate hypertriglyceridemia. Severe hepatitis and liver failure are associated with dramatic reductions in plasma cholesterol and triglycerides due to reduced lipoprotein biosynthetic capacity. Cholestasis is associated with hypercholesterolemia, which sometimes can be very severe. The major pathway by which cholesterol is excreted is via secretion into bile, either directly or after conversion to bile acids. Cholestasis blocks this critical excretory pathway. In cholestasis, free cholesterol coupled with phospholipids are secreted into the plasma as constituents of a lamellar particle called *Lp(X)*. These particles can deposit in skin folds, producing lesions resembling those seen in patients with FDBL (xanthomata strata palmaris). Planar and eruptive xanthomas can also be seen in patients with cholestasis.

Alcohol Regular alcohol consumption has a variable effect on plasma lipid levels. The most common effect of alcohol is to increase plasma triglyceride levels. Alcohol consumption stimulates hepatic secretion of VLDL, possibly by inhibiting the hepatic oxidation of free fatty acids, which then promote hepatic triglyceride synthesis and VLDL secretion. The usual lipoprotein pattern seen with alcohol consumption is type IV (increased VLDL), but persons with an underlying primary lipid disorder may develop severe hypertriglyceridemia (type V) if they drink alcohol. Regular alcohol use is also associated with a mild to moderate increase in plasma levels of HDL-C.

Estrogen Estrogen administration is associated with increased VLDL and HDL synthesis resulting in elevated plasma triglycerides and HDL-C. This lipoprotein pattern is distinctive since the levels of plasma triglyceride and HDL-C are typically inversely related. Estrogen treatment may convert a person with type IV to type V hyperlipidemia. Plasma triglyceride levels should be monitored when birth control pills or estrogen replacement therapy is initiated. Use of low-dose estrogen preparations or the estrogen patch can minimize the effect of exogenous estrogen on lipids.

Glycogen Storage Diseases Other rarer causes of secondary hyperlipidemias include glycogen storage diseases such as *von Gierke's disease*, which is caused by mutations in glucose-6-phosphatase. The inability to mobilize hepatic glucose during fasting results in hypoinsulinemia and increased release of free fatty acids from adipose tissue. Hepatic fatty acids synthesis is also increased, resulting in fat accumulation in the liver and increased VLDL secretion. The hyperlipidemia associated with this disease can be very severe but responds well to treatment of the underlying disorder.

Cushing Syndrome Glucocorticoid excess is associated with increased VLDL synthesis and hypertriglyceridemia. Patients with Cushing syndrome can also have mild elevations in plasma LDL-C.

Drugs Many drugs have a significant impact on lipid metabolism and can result in significant alterations in the lipoprotein profile (Table 335-5).

SCREENING Guidelines for the screening and management of lipid disorders have been provided by an expert Adult Treatment Panel (ATP) convened by the National Cholesterol Education Program (NCEP) of the National Heart Lung and Blood Institute. The NCEP ATPIII guidelines published in 2001 recommend that all adults over age 20 have plasma levels of cholesterol, triglyceride, LDL-C, and HDL-C measured after a 12-h overnight fast. In most clinical laboratories, the total cholesterol and triglycerides in the plasma are measured enzymatically and then the cholesterol in the supernatant is measured after precipitation of apoB-containing lipoproteins to determine the HDL-C. The LDL-C is estimated using the following equation:

$$\text{LDL-C} = \text{total cholesterol} - (\text{triglycerides}/5) - \text{HDL-C}$$

The VLDL-C is estimated by dividing the plasma triglyceride by 5, reflecting the ratio of cholesterol to triglyceride in VLDL particles. This formula is reasonably accurate if test results are obtained on fasting plasma and if the triglyceride level $<\sim4.0$ μmol/L (350 mg/dL).

The accurate determination of LDL-C levels in patients with triglyceride levels greater than this requires application of ultracentrifugation techniques (beta quantification), although direct assays for LDL-C are also available in some laboratories. →*For further discussion about screening, see Chap. 225.*

℞ TREATMENT

Multiple epidemiologic studies have demonstrated a strong relationship between serum cholesterol and CHD. Randomized controlled clinical trials have unequivocally documented that lowering plasma cholesterol reduces the risk of clinical events due to atherosclerosis (Chaps. 224 and 225). Although the proportional benefit accrued from reducing plasma LDL-C is similar over the entire range of LDL-C values, the absolute risk reduction depends on the baseline LDL-C, the presence of established CHD, and other cardiovascular risk factors.

Elevated plasma triglyceride levels are also associated with increased risk of CHD, but this relationship weakens considerably when statistical corrections are made for the plasma levels of LDL-C and HDL-C. Plasma levels of HDL-C are strongly and consistently inversely related to the prevalence and incidence of CHD, and yet no clinical trial data are available demonstrating that increasing plasma levels of HDL-C reduces the frequency of cardiovascular events. No pharmacologic agents are available that exclusively either lower plasma triglyceride levels or increase plasma HDL-C levels, contributing to the dearth of clinical trial data addressing the role of treatment of these lipid abnormalities in CHD prevention. Since both hypertriglyceridemia and low plasma levels of HDL-C confer higher ASCVD risk, the NCEP ATPIII recommends more aggressive therapy to lower the plasma LDL-C in patients with these dyslipidemias.

Nonpharmacologic Treatment ■ *DIET* Dietary modification is an important component in the management of hyperlipidemia. In the hypercholesterolemic patient, dietary saturated fat and cholesterol should be restricted. For patients who are hypertriglyceridemic, the intake of simple sugars should also be curtailed. For severe hypertriglyceridemia [>11.3 mmol/L (>1000 mg/dL)], restriction of total fat intake is critical. The most widely used diet to lower the LDL-C level is the "Step 1 diet" developed by the American Heart Association. Most patients have a relatively modest ($<10\%$) decrease in plasma levels of LDL-C on a step I diet in the absence of any associated weight loss. Almost all persons experience a decrease in plasma HDL-C levels with a reduction in the amount of total and saturated fat in their diet.

FOODS AND ADDITIVES Certain foods and dietary additives are associated with modest reductions in plasma cholesterol levels. Plant stanol and sterol esters are available in a variety of foods such as spreads, salad dressings, and snack bars. They interfere with cholesterol absorption and reduce plasma LDL-C levels by ~10 to 15% when taken three times per day. The addition to the diet of psyllium, soy protein, or Chinese red yeast rice (which contains lovastatin) can have modest cholesterol-lowering effects. Other herbal approaches such as guggulipid require further study to assess their effectiveness.

WEIGHT LOSS AND EXERCISE The treatment of obesity, if present, can have a favorable impact on plasma lipid levels and should be actively encouraged. Plasma triglyceride and LDL-C levels tend to fall and HDL-C levels tend to increase in obese persons who lose weight. Aerobic exercise has a very modest elevating effect on plasma levels of HDL-C in most individuals but has cardiovascular benefits that extend beyond the effects on plasma lipid levels.

Pharmalogic Treatment The decision to use drug therapy depends on the cardiovascular risk (Chap. 225). An effective way to estimate absolute risk of a cardiovascular event over 10 years is to use a scoring system based on the Framingham Heart Study database. Patients with a 10-year absolute CHD risk of $>20\%$ are considered "CHD risk equivalents." Current NCEP ATPIII guidelines call for drug therapy to reduce LDL-C to <2.6 mmol/L (<100 mg/dL) in patients with established

CHD, other ASCVD (aortic aneurysm, peripheral vascular disease, or cerebrovascular disease), diabetes mellitus, or CHD risk equivalents. Based on these guidelines, most CHD and CHD risk–equivalent patients require cholesterol-lowering drug therapy. Moderate risk patients with two or more risk factors and a 10-year absolute risk of 10 to 20% should be treated to a goal LDL-C of <3.4 mmol/L (<130 mg/dL). All other individuals have a goal of LDL-C <4.1 mmol/L (<160 mg/dL), but not all persons are candidates for drug therapy to achieve this goal.

Persons with markedly elevated plasma LDL-C levels [>4.9 mmol/L (>190 mg/dL)] should be considered for drug therapy even if their 10-year absolute CHD risk is not particularly elevated. The decision to initiate drug treatment in individuals with plasma LDL-C levels between 3.4 and 4.9 mmol/L (130 and 190 mg/dL) can be difficult. Although it is desirable to avoid drug treatment in patients who are unlikely to develop CHD, a very high proportion of patients who eventually develop CHD have plasma LDL-C levels that are in this range. Other clinical information can assist in the decision-making process. For example, a low plasma HDL-C [<1.0 mmol/L (<40 mg/dL) supports a decision in favor of more aggressive therapy. The diagnosis of the metabolic syndrome (Chap. 225) also identifies a higher risk individual who should be targeted for therapeutic life-style changes and might be a candidate for more aggressive drug therapy. Other laboratory tests, such as an elevated plasma Lp(a) or high-sensitivity C-reactive protein, may help to identify additional high-risk individuals. In persons at low risk, the emphasis should primarily be on dietary and life-style modification.

Drug treatment is also indicated in patients with triglycerides >11.3 mmol/L (>1000 mg/dL) who have been screened and treated for secondary causes of chylomicronemia. The goal is to reduce plasma triglycerides to <4.5 mmol/L (400 mg/dL) to prevent the risk of acute pancreatitis. Most major clinical end-point trials with statins have excluded persons with triglyceride levels >3.9 to 5.1 mmol/L (>350 to 450 mg/dL), and therefore there are few data regarding the effectiveness of statins in reducing cardiovascular risk in persons with triglycerides higher than this threshold. Combination therapy is often required for optimal control of mixed dyslipidemia.

HMG-COA REDUCTASE INHIBITORS   3-Hydroxy-3-methylglutaryl coenzyme A (HMG-CoA reductase) is the rate-limiting step in cholesterol bio-synthesis, and inhibition of this enzyme decreases cholesterol synthesis. By inhibiting cholesterol biosynthesis, HMG-CoA reductase inhibitors (statins) lead to increased hepatic LDL receptor activity and accelerated clearance of circulating LDL, resulting in a dose-dependent reduction in plasma LDL-C. There is wide interindividual variation in the initial response to a statin, but once a patient is on the medication, the doubling of the dose produces a 6% further reduction of plasma LDL-C. The HMG-CoA reductase inhibitors currently available differ in their LDL-C reducing effects (Table 335-6). HMG-CoA reductase inhibitors also reduce plasma triglycerides in a dose-dependent fashion, which is proportional to their LDL-C lowering effects [if the triglycerides are <3.9 mmol/L (<350 mg/dL)]. HMG-CoA reductase inhibitors have a modest HDL-raising effect (5 to 10%), and this effect is not dose-dependent.

HMG-CoA reductase inhibitors are well tolerated and can be taken in tablet form once a day. Potential side effects include dyspepsia, headaches, fatigue, and muscle or joint pains. Severe myopathy and even rhabdomyolysis occurs rarely. The risk of myopathy is increased by the presence of renal insufficiency and by coadministration of drugs that interfere with the metabolism of HMG-CoA reductase inhibitors, such as erythromycin and related antibiotics, antifungal agents, immunosuppressive drugs, and fibric acid derivatives. Severe myopathy can usually be avoided by careful patient selection, avoidance of interacting drugs, and by instructing the patient to contact the physician immediately in the event of unexplained muscle pain. In the event of muscle symptoms, the plasma creatine phosphokinase (CPK) level should be obtained to document the myopathy, but serum CPK levels do not need to be monitored on a routine basis as an elevated CPK in the absence of symptoms does not predict the development of myopathy and does not necessarily suggest the need for discontinuing the drug.

Another side effect of HMG-CoA reductase inhibitor therapy is hepatitis. Liver transaminases (ALT and AST) should be checked before starting therapy, at 8 weeks, and then every 6 months. Substantial (>3 × upper limit of normal) elevation in transaminases is relatively rare, and mild to moderate (1 to 3 × normal) elevation in transaminases in the absence of symptoms need not mandate discontinuing the medication. Severe clinical hepatitis associated with HMG-CoA reductase inhibitors is exceedingly rare, and the trend is toward less frequent monitoring of transaminases in patients taking HMG-CoA reductase inhibitors. The HMG-CoA reductase inhibitor–associated elevation in liver enzymes resolves after discontinuation of the medication.

TABLE 335-6   *Summary of the Major Drugs Used for the Treatment of Hyperlipidemia*

Drug	Major Indications	Starting Dose	Maximal Dose	Mechanism	Common Side Effects
HMG-CoA reductase inhibitors (statins)	Elevated LDL			↓ Cholesterol synthesis, ↓ hepatic LDL receptors, ↓ VLDL production	Myalgias, arthralgias, elevated transaminases, dyspepsia
Lovastatin		20 mg daily	80 mg daily		
Pravastatin		40 mg qhs	80 mg qhs		
Simvastatin		20 mg qhs	80 mg qhs		
Fluvastatin		20 mg qhs	80 mg qhs		
Atorvastatin		10 mg qhs	80 mg qhs		
Rosuvastatin		10 mg qhs	40 mg qhs		
Bile acid sequestrants	Elevated LDL			↑ Bile acid excretion and ↑ LDL receptors	Bloating, constipation, elevated triglycerides
Cholestyramine		4 g daily	32 g daily		
Colestipol		5 g daily	40 g daily		
Colesevelam		3750 mg daily	4375 mg daily		
Nicotinic acid	Elevated LDL, low HDL, elevated TG			↓ VLDL hepatic synthesis	Cutaneous flushing; GI upset; elevated glucose, uric acid, and liver function tests
Immediate-release		100 mg tid	2 g tid		
Sustained-release		250 mg bid	1.5 g bid		
Extended-release		500 mg qhs	2 g qhs		
Fibric acid derivatives	Elevated TG, elevated remnants			↑ LPL, ↓ VLDL synthesis	Dyspepsia, myalgia, gallstones, elevated transaminases
Gemfibrozil		600 mg bid	600 mg bid		
Fenofibrate		160 mg qd	160 mg qd		
Fish oils	Severely elevated TG	3 g daily	12 g daily	↓ Chylomicron and VLDL production	Dyspepsia, diarrhea, fishy odor to breath
Cholesterol absorption inhibitors				↓ Intestinal cholesterol absorption	Elevated transaminases
Ezetimibe	Elevated LDL	10 mg daily	10 mg daily		

Note: LDL, low-density lipoprotein; VLDL, very low density lipoprotein; HDL, high-density lipoprotein; TG, triglycerides; LPL, lipoprotein lipase.

Overall, HMG-CoA reductase inhibitors appear to be remarkably safe. Over 50,000 patients have been treated with HMG-CoA reductase inhibitors for over 5 to 6 years as a part of large randomized controlled clinical trials and no increase in any major noncardiac diseases have been seen in these individuals. HMG-CoA reductase inhibitors are the drug class of choice for LDL-C reduction and are by far the most widely used class of lipid-lowering drugs.

BILE ACID SEQUESTRANTS (RESINS) Bile acid sequestrants bind bile acids in the intestine and promote their excretion in the stool. In order to maintain an adequate bile acid pool, the liver diverts cholesterol to bile acid synthesis. The decreased hepatic intracellular cholesterol content upregulates the LDL receptor and enhances LDL clearance from the plasma. Bile acid sequestrants, including cholestyramine, colestipol, and colesevelam (Table 335-6), primarily reduce plasma LDL-C levels but can increase plasma triglycerides. Therefore, patients with hypertriglyceridemia should not be treated with bile acid–binding resins.

Cholestyramine and colestipol are insoluble resins that must be mixed with liquids. Colestipol is also available in large tablets but multiple tablets must be taken to achieve significant lowering of plasma LDL-C levels. The newest bile acid sequestrant, colesevelam, has greater bile acid–binding capacity than traditional resins. The colesevelam tablets are smaller, and fewer tablets per day are required. Most side effects of resins are limited to the gastrointestinal tract and include bloating and constipation. Bile acid sequestrants may bind other drugs (e.g., digoxin, warfarin) and interfere with their absorption. Therefore, all other medications should be taken either 1 h before or 4 h after the bile acid sequestrants.

Bile acid sequestrants are not systemically absorbed and are very safe. They are the cholesterol-lowering drug of choice in children and in women of childbearing age who are lactating, pregnant, or could become pregnant. These drugs can also be useful in young, well-motivated patients with moderate hypercholesterolemia who wish to avoid systemic drug therapy. This class of drugs is also useful in combination with HMG-CoA reductase inhibitors in patients who are unable to reach their LDL-C goal on HMG-CoA reductase inhibitor monotherapy and have relatively normal triglyceride levels.

NICOTINIC ACID (NIACIN) Nicotinic acid, or niacin, is a B-complex vitamin that reduces plasma triglyceride and LDL-C levels and raises the plasma HDL-C (Table 335-6) in high doses. Niacin is the only currently available lipid-lowering drug that significantly reduces plasma levels of Lp(a). If properly prescribed and monitored, niacin is a safe and effective lipid-lowering agent.

The cheapest form of niacin is immediate-release crystalline niacin. Niacin should be started at a low dose (100 mg three times a day) and taken with meals to delay absorption. The dose of niacin should be increased every 4 to 7 days by 100 mg until a dose of 500 mg tid is obtained. After 1 month on this dose, lipids and pertinent chemistries (glucose, uric acid, liver transaminases) should be measured. The dose can be further increased as needed up to a total dose of 6 g/d. The most frequent side effect is cutaneous flushing, but this improves with continued administration. In many patients, taking an aspirin 30 min prior to the niacin prevents flushing. Over-the-counter sustained-release forms of niacin are generally administered twice a day and are associated with less flushing, but some have been associated with rare cases of severe hepatitis. A clue to the development of niacin-induced hepatitis is a sudden, precipitous drop in the plasma lipid levels. A prescription form of extended-release niacin that is administered once daily at bedtime has not been associated with severe hepatic toxicity. Mild elevations in transaminases occur in up to 15% of patients treated with any form of niacin, but these elevations rarely require discontinuation of the medication. Niacin potentiates the effect of warfarin, and these two drugs should be prescribed together with caution. Acanthosis nigricans and maculopathy are infrequent side effects of niacin. Niacin is contraindicated in patients with peptic ulcer disease and can exacerbate the symptoms of esophageal reflux. Niacin can raise plasma levels of uric acid and precipitate gouty attacks in susceptible patients.

Niacin can raise fasting plasma glucose levels, but concerns regarding the use of niacin in diabetic patients have been allayed by the results of two studies. In one study, short-acting niacin treatment of dyslipidemia was associated with only a slight increase in fasting glucose and no significant change from baseline in the HbA1c. In the other, low-dose niacin was found to reduce triglycerides effectively and raise HDL-C in diabetics without adversely impacting glycemic control.

Successful therapy with niacin requires careful education and motivation of the patient. Its advantages are its low cost and long-term safety. It is the most effective drug currently available for raising HDL-C levels. It is particularly useful in patients with combined hyperlipidemia and low plasma levels of HDL-C and is effective in combination with statins.

FIBRIC ACID DERIVATIVES (FIBRATES) Fibric acid derivatives, or fibrates, are agonists of PPARα, a nuclear receptor involved in the regulation of carbohydrate and lipid metabolism. Fibrates stimulate LPL activity (enhancing triglyceride hydrolysis), reduce apoC-III synthesis (enhancing lipoprotein remnant clearance), and may reduce VLDL production. Fibrates are the most effective drugs available for reducing triglyceride levels, and they also raise HDL-C levels (Table 335-6). Fibrates have variable effects on LDL-C, and in hypertriglyceridemic patients can sometimes be associated with increases in plasma LDL-C levels.

Fibrates are generally very well tolerated. The most common side effect is dyspepsia. Myopathy and hepatitis occur rarely in the absence of other lipid-lowering agents. Fibrates promote cholesterol secretion into bile and are associated with an increased risk of gallstones. Importantly, fibrates can potentiate the effect of warfarin and certain oral hypoglycemic agents; the anticoagulation status and plasma glucose levels should be closely monitored in patients on these agents.

Fibrates are the drug class of choice in patients with severe hypertriglyceridemia [11.3 mmol/L (>1000 mg/dL)] and are a reasonable consideration in patients with moderate hypertriglyceridemia [4.5 to 11.3 mmol/L (400 to 1000 mg/dL)]. The Veterans Affairs High-Density Lipoprotein Intervention Trial study also suggests that they may have a role in high-risk patients with well-controlled LDL-C levels but elevated plasma triglyceride levels and low plasma levels of HDL-C. The relative indications of fibrates vs. statins and the role of combined therapy will be determined by ongoing and future trials.

Omega-3 Fatty Acids (Fish Oils) N-3 polyunsaturated fatty acids (PUFAs) are present in high concentration in fish and in flax seeds. The most widely used n-3 PUFAs for the treatment of hyperlipidemias are the two active molecules in fish oil, eicosapentanoic acid (EPA) and decohexanoic acid (DHA). N-3 PUFAs have been concentrated into tablets and in doses of 3 to 6 g/d decrease fasting and postprandial triglycerides. At least 6 g/d is usually required for a substantial triglyceride-lowering effect, and many patients require 9 to 12 g/d. Fish oil treatment of hypertriglyceridemia can be associated with a significant increase in plasma LDL-C levels. Fish oil supplements can be used in combination with fibrates, niacin, or statins to treat hypertriglyceridemia. In general, fish oils are well tolerated and appear to be safe, at least at doses up to 3 g. The large number of capsules required for a therapeutic effect, the associated dyspepsia, and fishy aftertaste have limited the clinical use of these agents. Although fish oil administration is associated with a prolongation in the bleeding time, no increase in bleeding has been seen in clinical trials.

CHOLESTEROL ABSORPTION INHIBITORS A new mechanism of cholesterol-lowering is the inhibition of intestinal cholesterol absorption. Ezetimibe (Table 335-6) inhibits the absorption of dietary and biliary cholesterol from the intestinal lumen. It reduces LDL-C cholesterol levels by ~18% as monotherapy or in combination with a statin. Cholesterol absorption inhibitors are particularly useful in combination with a statin in patients unable to reach their LDL-C goal on statin monotherapy.

COMBINATION DRUG THERAPY Combination drug therapy is frequently used in the following situations: (1) patients unable to reach their LDL-C goal on a single drug, (2) patients with combined hypertriglyceridemia and hypercholesterolemia that cannot be adequately controlled with a single drug, and (3) patients with elevated LDL-C and low HDL-C levels. Inability to achieve LDL-C goal is not uncommon on statin monotherapy. If the patient has a normal plasma triglyceride level, a bile acid sequestrant can be added. A cholesterol absorption inhibitor can also be used in this setting. Combination of niacin with a statin is an attractive option for high-risk patients who do not attain their target LDL-C level on statin monotherapy and who have an HDL-C <10.3 mmol/L (<40 mg/dL). One product currently available offers the combination of lovastatin and extended-release niacin in a single tablet.

Patients with combined hyperlipidemia frequently have persistent hypertriglyceridemia on statin monotherapy. Addition of niacin or a fibrate can reduce the plasma triglyceride level in these patients. Conversely, hypertriglyceridemic patients treated with a fibrate often fail to reach their LDL-C goal and are therefore candidates for the addition of a statin. Coadministration of statins and fibrates has obvious appeal in patients with combined hyperlipidemia, but no clinical trials have assessed the effectiveness of a statin-fibrate combination compared with either a statin or a fibrate alone in reducing cardiovascular events and the long-term safety of this combination is not known. Statin-fibrate combinations are known to be associated with an increased incidence of severe myopathy (up to 2.5%) and rhabdomyolysis, and patients treated with these two drugs must be carefully counseled and monitored. This combination of drugs should be used cautiously in patients with underlying renal or hepatic insufficiency; in the elderly, frail, and chronically ill; and in those on multiple medications.

Other Approaches Occasionally, patients cannot tolerate any of the existing lipid-lowering drugs at doses required for adequate control of their lipid levels. Some patients, mostly those with genetic lipid disorders, remain significantly hypercholesterolemic despite combination drug therapy. These patients are at high risk for development or progression of CHD and clinical CHD events.

LDL APHERESIS The preferred option for management of patients with refractory or drug-resistant hypercholesterolemia is LDL apheresis. In this process, the patient's plasma is passed over a column that selectively removes the LDL, and the LDL-depleted plasma is returned to the patient. Patients on maximally tolerated combination drug therapy who have CHD and a plasma LDL-C level >5.2 mmol/L (>200 mg/dL) or no CHD and a plasma LDL-C level >7.8 mmol/L (>300 mg/dL), are candidates for every-other-week LDL apheresis.

PARTIAL ILEAL BYPASS Partial ileal bypass interrupts the enterohepatic circulation of bile acids, resulting in upregulation of the hepatic LDL receptor and reduction in plasma LDL-C levels. Diarrhea is a common side effect, and the incidence of kidney stones, gallstones, and intestinal obstruction is increased after ileal bypass surgery. The clinical utility of partial ileal bypass at this time is limited to severely hypercholesterolemic patients with normal triglycerides who cannot tolerate existing lipid-lowering medications and do not have access to LDL apheresis. Partial ileal bypass has not been proven effective in patients with severe hypercholesterolemia who have not responded adequately to statins.

Management of Low HDL-C Severely reduced plasma HDL-C [<0.5 mmol/L (<20 mg/dL)] accompanied by triglycerides <4.5 mmol/L (<400 mg/dL) usually indicates the presence of a genetic disorder, such as a mutation in apoA-I, LCAT deficiency, or Tangier disease. HDL-C levels <0.5 mmol/L (<20 mg/dL) are common in the setting of severe hypertriglyceridemia, in which case the primary focus should be on the management of the triglycerides. Secondary causes of more moderate reductions in plasma HDL [0.5 to 10.3 mmol/L (20 to 40 mg/dL)] should be considered (Table 335-5). Smoking should be discontinued, obese persons should be encouraged to lose weight, sedentary persons should be encouraged to exercise, and diabetes should be optimally controlled. When possible, medications associated with reduced plasma levels of HDL-C should be discontinued. The presence of an isolated low plasma HDL-C level in a patient with a borderline plasma LDL-C should prompt consideration of LDL-lowering drug therapy in high-risk individuals. Statins increase plasma levels of HDL-C only modestly (~5 to 10%). Fibrates also have a modest effect on plasma HDL-C levels (increasing levels ~5 to 15%) except in patients with coexisting hypertriglyceridemia, where they can be more effective. Niacin is the most effective therapeutic agent and can increase plasma HDL-C levels by up to ~30%.

The issue of whether pharmacologic intervention should be used to specifically raise HDL-C levels has not been adequately addressed in clinical trials. Pending these studies, it may be reasonable to initiate therapy (with a fibrate or niacin) directed specifically at reducing plasma triglyceride levels and raising the plasma HDL-C level in persons with established CHD and low HDL-C levels whose plasma LDL-C levels are at or below the goal.

FURTHER READING

Executive Summary of the Third Report of the National Cholesterol Education Program (NCEP) expert panel on detection, evaluation, and treatment of high blood cholesterol in adults (Adult Treatment Panel III). JAMA 285: 2486, 2001

GOLDSTEIN JL et al: Familial hypercholesterolemia, in *The Metabolic and Molecular Bases of Inherited Disease*, 8th ed, CR Scriver et al (ed). New York, McGraw-Hill, 2001, pp 2863–2913

GRUNDY SM (ed): *Cholesterol-Lowering Therapy: Evaluation of Clinical Trial Evidence*. New York, Marcel Dekker, 2000

HEART PROTECTION STUDY COLLABORATIVE GROUP: MRC/BHF Heart Protection Study of cholesterol lowering with simvastatin in 20,536 high-risk individuals: A randomised placebo-controlled trial. Lancet 360:7, 2002

MULDOON MF et al: Cholesterol reduction and non-illness mortality: Meta-analysis of randomised clinical trials. BMJ 322:11, 2001

WILSON PWF et al: Prediction of coronary heart disease using risk factor categories. Circulation 97:1837, 1998

336 | HEMOCHROMATOSIS
Lawrie W. Powell

DEFINITION

Hemochromatosis is a common disorder of iron storage in which an inappropriate increase in intestinal iron absorption results in deposition of excessive amounts of iron in parenchymal cells with eventual tissue damage and impaired function of organs. The iron-storage pigment in tissues was called *hemosiderin* because it was believed to be derived from the blood. The term *hemosiderosis* is used to describe the presence of stainable iron in tissues, but tissue iron must be quantified to assess body iron status accurately (see below and Chap. 90). *Hemo-chromatosis* implies potentially severe progressive iron overload leading to fibrosis and organ failure. Cirrhosis of the liver, diabetes mellitus, arthritis, cardiomyopathy, and hypogonadotrophic hypogonadism are common manifestations.

Although there is debate about definitions, it seems logical to use the following terminology:

1. *Hereditary hemochromatosis* or *genetic hemochromatosis*: This disorder is most often caused by inheritance of a mutant gene, termed *HFE*, which is tightly linked to the HLA-A locus on chromosome 6p (see below). Rarer forms of non-*HFE* hemochromatosis due to mutation in other key genes involved in iron metabolism have recently been described (Table 336-1). The disease can be recognized during its early stages when iron overload and organ damage are min-

TABLE 336-1	Classification of Iron Overload States

HEREDITARY HEMOCHROMATOSIS

Hemochromatosis, *HFE*-related (type 1)
  C282Y homozygosity
  C282Y/H63D compound heterozygosity
Hemochromatosis non-*HFE*-related
  Juvenile hemochromatosis (type 2)
  Mutated transferrin receptor 2 *TFR2* (type 3)
  Mutated ferroportin 1 (Ireg1) gene, *SLC11A3* (type 4)
  Mutated H Ferritin IRE (type 5)
  Solomon Island hemochromatosis (?defect) (type 6)

ACQUIRED IRON OVERLOAD

Iron-loading anemias	Chronic liver disease
Thalassemia major	Hepatitis C
Sideroblastic anemia	Alcoholic cirrhosis, especially
Chronic hemolytic	when advanced
anemia	Nonalcoholic steatohepatitis
Transfusional and	Porphyria cutanea tarda
parenteral iron	Dysmetabolic iron overload
overload	syndrome
Dietary iron overload	Post portacaval shunting

MISCELLANEOUS

Iron overload in sub-Sahara Africa
Neonatal iron overload
Aceruloplasminemia
Congenital atransferrinemia

imal. At this stage the disease is best referred to as *early hemochromatosis* or *precirrhotic hemochromatosis*.

2. *Secondary iron overload*: Tissue injury usually occurs secondary to an iron-loading anemia such as thalassemia or sideroblastic anemia, in which increased erythropoiesis is ineffective. In the acquired iron-loading disorders, massive iron deposits in parenchymal tissues can lead to the same clinical and pathologic features as in hemochromatosis.

PREVALENCE

HFE-associated hemochromatosis is one of the most common genetic diseases, although its prevalence varies in different ethnic groups. It is most common in populations of northern European extraction in whom approximately 1 in 10 persons are heterozygous carriers and 0.3 to 0.5% are homozygotes. However, expression of the disease is modified by several factors, especially alcohol consumption and dietary iron intake, blood loss associated with menstruation and pregnancy, and blood donation. The clinical expression of the disease is 5 to 10 times more frequent in men than in women. Nearly 70% of affected patients develop the first symptoms between ages 40 and 60. The disease is rarely evident before age 20, although with family screening (see below) and periodic health examinations, asymptomatic subjects with iron overload can be identified, including young menstruating women. Recent studies in European non-blood bank populations have revealed that 30% or more of homozygous individuals do not have evidence of iron overload. Thus, the penetrance of the mutation is variable.

GENETIC BASIS AND MODE OF INHERITANCE

The *HFE* gene involved in the most common form of hemochromatosis was cloned in 1996. A homozygous G → A mutation resulting in a cysteine to tyrosine substitution at position 282 (C282Y) is the most common mutation. It is identified in 85 to 100% of patients with hereditary hemochromatosis in populations of northern European descent but is found in only 60% of cases from Mediterranean populations (e.g., southern Italy). A second, relatively common *HFE* mutation has also been identified. This results in an amino acid substitution of histidine to aspartic acid at position 63 (H63D). Homozygosity for H63D is not associated with clinically significant iron overload. Some compound heterozygotes (e.g., one copy each of C282Y and H63D) have mild to moderately increased body iron stores. Thus, *HFE*-

associated hemochromatosis is inherited as an autosomal recessive trait; heterozygotes have no, or minimal, increase in iron stores. However, in some cases this slight increase in hepatic iron acts as a cofactor that aggravates other diseases such as porphyria cutanea tarda (PCT) and nonalcoholic steatohepatitis.

Mutations in other genes are responsible for non-*HFE* associated hemochromatosis, including juvenile hemochromatosis, which affects persons in the second and third decade of life (Table 336-1).

PATHOGENESIS

Normally, the body iron content of 3 to 4 g is maintained such that intestinal mucosal absorption of iron is equal to iron loss. This amount is approximately 1 mg/d in men and 1.5 mg/d in menstruating women. In hemochromatosis, mucosal absorption is inappropriate to body needs and amounts to 4 mg/d or more. The progressive accumulation of iron causes an early elevation in plasma iron, an increased saturation of transferrin, and progressive elevation of plasma ferritin level (Fig. 336-1). A liver protein, hepcidin, is proposed to increase *HFE*-mediated reticuloendothelial cell iron retention and to decrease intestinal iron uptake, thereby linking body stores with intestinal iron absorption.

The *HFE* gene encodes a 343-amino-acid protein that is structurally related to MHC class I proteins. The basic defect in hemochromatosis is a lack of cell surface expression of HFE (due to the C282Y mutation). The normal (wild type) HFE protein forms a complex with β_2-microglobulin and transferrin, and the C282Y mutation completely abrogates this interaction. As a result, the mutant HFE protein remains trapped intracellularly, reducing transferrin receptor–mediated iron uptake by the intestinal crypt cell. This is postulated to upregulate the divalent metal transporter (DMT-1) on the brush border of the villus cells, leading to inappropriately increased intestinal iron absorption (Fig. 336-2). In advanced disease, the body may contain 20 g or more of iron that is deposited mainly in parenchymal cells of the liver, pancreas, and heart. Iron may be increased 50- to 100-fold in the liver and pancreas and 5- to 25-fold in the heart. Iron deposition in the pituitary causes hypogonadotropic hypogonadism in both men and women. Tis-

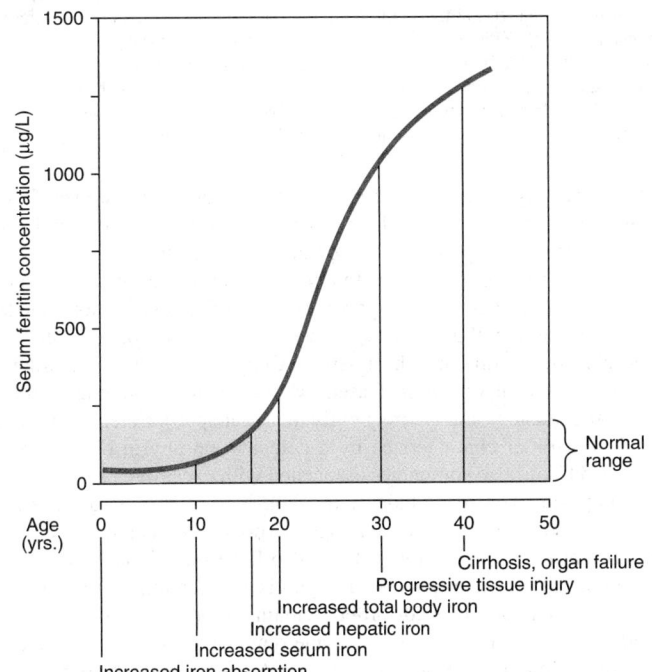

FIGURE 336-1 Sequence of events in genetic hemochromatosis and their correlation with the serum ferritin concentration. Increased iron absorption is present throughout life. Overt, symptomatic disease usually develops between ages 40 and 60, but latent disease can be detected long before this.

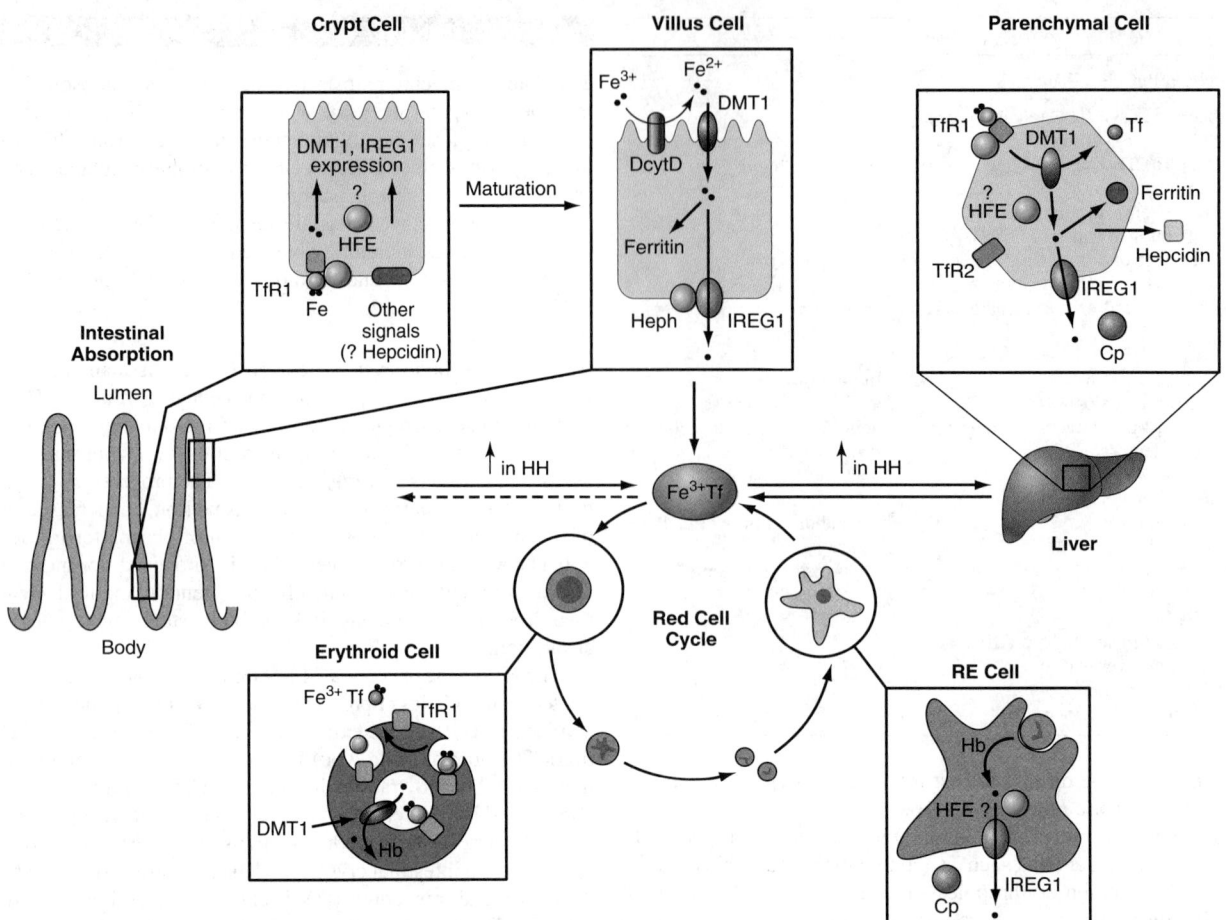

FIGURE 336-2 *Pathways of normal iron homeostasis.* Iron is absorbed in the proximal intestine after conversion from the ferric (Fe^{3+}) to the ferrous (Fe^{2+}) state by duodenal cytochrome D (DcytD), a ferrireductase. At the apical membrane of the mature villus cell, iron is imported by the divalent metal transporter (DMT1). Iron may be stored within the cell as ferritin or transferred across the basolateral membrane by the transporter, IREG1 (ferroportin-1), and is reoxidized by hephaestin (Heph) before binding to the transport protein, transferrin (Tf). Circulating iron is acquired by the liver primarily through the classic transferrin receptor-1 (TfR1) and by the related transferrin receptor-2 (TfR2). Reticuloendothelial macrophages acquire iron mainly by phagocytosis of senescent erythrocytes, and the iron is released via the iron export protein, IREG1. The released iron is oxidized to the ferric state by ceruloplasmin (Cp) before binding to transferrin. In response to increased iron, the liver produces hepcidin, which appears to communicate the level of iron stores to intestinal cells and reticuloendothelial (RE) cells. Hepcidin deficiency mimics hemochromatosis, as it is associated with increased intestinal iron absorption and decreased iron uptake in reticuloendothelial cells. HFE is a MHC class 1 molecule that forms a complex with β_2 microglobulin (β_2-M) and binds to TfR1.

Patients with hereditary hemochromatosis (HH) caused by *HFE* mutations fail to express a functional β_2-M:HFE:TfR complex. In addition, they have decreased hepatic expression of hepcidin. Although the pathogenesis of HH is incompletely understood, decreased expression of HFE in the intestine is thought to result in low iron levels in the crypt cells, leading to inappropriate upregulation of DMT1 and IREG1. This causes increased intestinal iron absorption, leading to increased tissue iron stores, with paradoxical sparing of iron loading in the RE system, perhaps because iron is efficiently exported by IREG1. Hb, hemoglobin. Also, a decreased expression of HPE in the liver may result in decreased hepcidin synthesis and upregulation of iron absorption.

sue injury may result from disruption of iron-laden lysosomes, from lipid peroxidation of subcellular organelles by excess iron, or from stimulation of collagen synthesis by activated stellate cells.

Secondary iron overload with deposition in parenchymal cells occurs in chronic disorders of erythropoiesis, particularly in those due to defects in hemoglobin synthesis or ineffective erythropoiesis such as sideroblastic anemia and thalassemia (Chap. 91). In these disorders, the absorption of iron is increased. Moreover, these patients require blood transfusions and are frequently treated inappropriately with iron. PCT, a disorder characterized by a defect in porphyrin biosynthesis (Chap. 337), is also sometimes associated with excessive parenchymal iron deposits. The magnitude of the iron load in PCT is usually insufficient to produce tissue damage. However, recent reports have found that many patients with PCT also have mutations in the *HFE* gene, and some have associated hepatitis C infection. Although the relationship among these disorders remains to be clarified, iron overload accentuates the inherited enzyme deficiency in PCT and should be avoided along with other agents (alcohol, estrogens, haloaromatic compounds) that may exacerbate PCT. Another cause of hepatic parenchymal iron overload is hereditary aceruloplasminemia. In this disorder, impairment of iron mobilization due to deficiency of ceruloplasmin (a ferroxidase) causes iron overload in hepatocytes. End-stage liver disease may also be associated with iron overload of the degree seen in hemochromatosis. The mechanism is uncertain, although hemolysis plays a role. Hemochromatosis in a heavy drinker can be distinguished from alcoholic liver disease by the presence of the C282Y mutation.

Excessive iron ingestion over many years rarely results in hemochromatosis. An important exception has been reported in South Africa among groups who brew fermented beverages in vessels made of iron. Hemochromatosis has been described in apparently normal persons who have taken medicinal iron over many years, but such individuals probably had a genetic disorder.

The common denominator in all patients with hemochromatosis is *excessive amounts of iron in parenchymal tissues.* Parenteral administration of iron in the form of blood transfusions or iron preparations results predominantly in reticuloendothelial cell iron overload. This appears to lead to less tissue damage than iron loading of parenchymal cells.

PATHOLOGY

At autopsy, the enlarged nodular liver and pancreas are rusty in color. Histologically, iron is increased in many organs, particularly in the liver, heart, and pancreas, and to a lesser extent in the endocrine glands.

The epidermis of the skin is thin, and melanin is increased in the cells of the basal layer. Deposits of iron are present around the synovial lining cells of the joints.

In the liver of patients with hemochromatosis, parenchymal iron is in the form of ferritin and hemosiderin. In the early stages these deposits are seen in the periportal parenchymal cells, especially within lysosomes in the pericanalicular cytoplasm of the hepatocytes. This stage progresses to perilobular fibrosis and eventually to deposition of iron in bile duct epithelium, Kupffer cells, and fibrous septa due to activation of stellate cells. In the advanced stage, a macronodular or mixed macro- and micronodular cirrhosis develops.

CLINICAL MANIFESTATIONS

Initial symptoms include weakness, lassitude, change in skin color, abdominal pain, loss of libido, and symptoms of diabetes mellitus. Hepatomegaly, increased pigmentation, spider angiomas, splenomegaly, arthropathy, ascites, cardiac arrhythmias, congestive heart failure, loss of body hair, testicular atrophy, and jaundice are prominent in advanced disease.

The *liver* is usually the first organ to be affected, and hepatomegaly is present in more than 95% of symptomatic patients. Hepatic enlargement may exist in the absence of symptoms or of abnormal liver function tests. Indeed, over half of patients with symptomatic hemochromatosis have little laboratory evidence of functional impairment of the liver, in spite of hepatomegaly and fibrosis. Loss of body hair, palmar erythema, testicular atrophy, and gynecomastia are common. Manifestations of portal hypertension and esophageal varices occur less commonly than in cirrhosis from other causes. Hepatocellular carcinoma develops in about 30% of patients with cirrhosis, and it is the most common cause of death in treated patients; hence the importance of early diagnosis and therapy. Its incidence increases with age, is more common in men, and occurs almost exclusively in cirrhotic patients. Splenomegaly occurs in approximately half of symptomatic cases.

Excessive skin pigmentation is present in over 90% of symptomatic patients at the time of diagnosis. The characteristic metallic or slate gray hue is sometimes referred to as bronzing and results from increased melanin and iron in the dermis. Pigmentation usually is diffuse and generalized, but it may be more pronounced on the face, neck, extensor aspects of the lower forearms, dorsa of the hands, lower legs, genital regions, and in scars.

Diabetes mellitus occurs in about 65% of patients and is more likely to develop in those with a family history of diabetes, suggesting that direct damage to the pancreatic islets by iron deposition occurs in combination with a genetic predisposition. The management is similar to that of other forms of diabetes, although pronounced insulin resistance is more common in association with hemochromatosis. Late complications are the same as seen in other causes of diabetes mellitus.

Arthropathy develops in 25 to 50% of patients. It usually occurs after age 50, but may occur as a first manifestation, or long after therapy. The joints of the hands, especially the second and third metacarpophalangeal joints, are usually the first joints involved, a feature that helps to distinguish the chondrocalcinosis associated with hemochromatosis from the idiopathic form (Chap. 313). A progressive polyarthritis involving wrists, hips, ankles, and knees may also ensue. Acute brief attacks of synovitis may be associated with deposition of calcium pyrophosphate (chondrocalcinosis or pseudogout), mainly in the knees. Radiologic manifestations include cystic changes of the subchondral bones, loss of articular cartilage with narrowing of the joint space, diffuse demineralization, hypertrophic bone proliferation, and calcification of the synovium. The arthropathy tends to progress despite removal of iron by phlebotomy. Although the relation of these abnormalities to iron metabolism is not known, the fact that similar changes occur in other forms of iron overload suggests that iron is directly involved.

Cardiac involvement is the presenting manifestation in about 15% of patients. The most common manifestation is congestive heart fail-

ure, which occurs in about 10% of young adults with the disease, especially those with juvenile hemochromatosis. Symptoms of congestive failure may develop suddenly, with rapid progression to death if untreated. The heart is diffusely enlarged and may be misdiagnosed as idiopathic cardiomyopathy if other overt manifestations are absent. Cardiac arrhythmias include premature supraventricular beats, paroxysmal tachyarrhythmias, atrial flutter, atrial fibrillation, and varying degrees of atrioventricular block.

Hypogonadism occurs in both sexes and may antedate other clinical features. Manifestations include loss of libido, impotence, amenorrhea, testicular atrophy, gynecomastia, and sparse body hair. These changes are primarily the result of decreased production of gonadotropins due to impairment of hypothalamic-pituitary function by iron deposition; however, primary testicular dysfunction may be seen in some cases. Adrenal insufficiency, hypothyroidism, and hypoparathyroidism may also occur.

DIAGNOSIS

The association of (1) hepatomegaly, (2) skin pigmentation, (3) diabetes mellitus, (4) heart disease, (5) arthritis, and (6) hypogonadism should suggest the diagnosis. However, a parenchymal iron overload of comparatively short duration or modest degree may exist with none or only some of these manifestations [e.g., in young patients (Fig. 336-1)]. Therefore, a high index of suspicion is needed to make the diagnosis early. Treatment before there is permanent organ damage can reverse the iron toxicity and restore life expectancy to normal.

The history should be particularly detailed in regard to disease in other family members, alcohol ingestion, iron intake, and ingestion of large doses of ascorbic acid, which promotes iron absorption (Chap. 61). Appropriate tests should be performed to exclude iron deposition due to hematologic disease. The presence of liver, pancreatic, cardiac, and joint disease should be confirmed by physical examination, roentgenography, and standard function tests of these organs. The degree of increase in total-body iron stores should be assessed with particular attention to an increase in parenchymal iron concentration, with or without tissue damage.

The methods available for assessing parenchymal iron stores include (1) measurement of serum iron and the percent saturation of transferrin (or the unsaturated iron-binding capacity); (2) measurement of serum ferritin concentration; (3) liver biopsy with measurement of the iron concentration and calculation of the hepatic iron index (Table 336-2), (4) estimation of chelatable iron stores following the administration of deferoxamine; and (5) computed tomography (CT) and/or magnetic resonance imaging (MRI) of the liver. Each has its advantages and limitations. The serum iron level and percent saturation of transferrin are elevated early in the course, but their specificity is reduced by significant false-positive and false-negative rates. For example, serum iron concentration may be increased in patients with alcoholic liver disease without iron overload; in this situation, however, the hepatic iron index is usually not increased as in hemochromatosis (Table 336-1). In otherwise healthy persons, a fasting serum transferrin saturation greater than 50% is abnormal and suggests homozygosity for hemochromatosis.

The serum ferritin concentration is usually a good index of body iron stores, whether decreased or increased. In fact, an increase of 1 μg/L in serum ferritin level reflects an increase of about 65 mg in body stores. In most untreated patients with hemochromatosis, the serum ferritin level is greatly increased (Fig. 336-1 and Table 336-1). However, in patients with inflammation and hepatocellular necrosis, serum ferritin levels may be elevated out of proportion to body iron stores due to increased release from tissues. A repeat determination of serum ferritin should therefore be carried out after acute hepatocellular damage has subsided, e.g., in alcoholic liver disease. Ordinarily, the combined measurements of the percent transferrin saturation and serum ferritin level provide a simple and reliable screening test for hemochromatosis, including the precirrhotic phase of the disease. If ei-

Determination	Normal	Symptomatic Hemochromatosis	Homozygotes with Early, Asymptomatic Hemochromatosis	Heterozygotes	Alcoholic Liver Disease
Plasma iron, μmol/L (μg/dL)	9–27 (50–150)	32–54 (180–300)	Usually elevated	Elevated or normal	Often elevated
Total iron-binding capacity, μmol/L (μg/dL)	45–66 (250–370)	36–54 (200–300)	36–54 (200–300)	Elevated or normal	45–66 (250–370)
Transferrin saturation, percent	22–46	50–100	50–100	Normal or elevated	27–60
Serum ferritin, μg/L	10–200	900–6000	200–500	Usually <500	10–500
Urinary iron,[a] mg/24 h	0–2	9–23	2–5	2–5	Usually <5
Liver iron, μg/g dry wt	300–1400	6000–18,000	2000–4000	300–3000	300–2000
Hepatic iron index (μg/g dry wt) $\dfrac{}{56 \times age}$	<1.0	>2	Usually >2	<2	<2

[a] After intramuscular administration of 0.5 g deferoxamine.

ther of these tests is abnormal, genetic testing for hemochromatosis should be performed (Fig. 336-3).

The role of liver biopsy in the diagnosis and management of hemochromatosis has been reassessed as a result of the widespread availability of genetic testing for the C282Y mutation. The absence of severe fibrosis can be accurately predicted in most patients using clinical and biochemical variables. Thus, there is virtually no risk of severe fibrosis in a C282Y homozygous subject with: (1) serum ferritin level less than 1000 μg/L; (2) normal serum alanine amino transaminase values; (3) no hepatomegaly; and (4) no excess alcohol intake. However, it should be emphasized that liver biopsy is the only reliable method for establishing or excluding the presence of hepatic cirrhosis, which is the critical factor determining prognosis and the risk of developing hepatocellular carcinoma. Biopsy also permits histochemical estimation of tissue iron and measurement of hepatic iron concentration. Increased density of the liver due to iron deposition can be demonstrated by CT or MRI. A retrospective assessment of body iron storage is also provided by performing weekly phlebotomy and calculating the amount of iron removed before iron stores are exhausted (1 mL blood = approximately 0.5 mg iron).

SCREENING FOR HEMOCHROMATOSIS

When the diagnosis of hemochromatosis is established, it is important to counsel and screen other family members (Chap. 58). Asymptomatic as well as symptomatic family members with the disease usually have an increased saturation of transferrin and an increased serum ferritin concentration. These changes occur even before the iron stores are greatly increased (Fig. 336-1). All first-degree relatives of patients with hemochromatosis should be tested for the C282Y and H63D mutations and advised appropriately. In affected individuals, it is important to confirm or exclude the presence of cirrhosis and begin therapy as early as possible. When children of a proband are affected, a homozygote-heterozygote mating is most likely.

The role of population screening for hemochromatosis is controversial. Hemochromatosis fulfills the criteria established by the World Health Organization for population screening, and DNA testing could, in principle, be performed along with other neonatal tests. However, because iron overload does not develop until the second, third, or fourth decades, and the degree of penetrance is still uncertain, screening for phenotypic expression in adults is more practical at present (Fig. 336-3).

℞ TREATMENT

The therapy of hemochromatosis involves removal of the excess body iron and supportive treatment of damaged organs. Iron removal is best begun by weekly or twice-weekly phlebotomy of 500 mL. Although there is an initial modest decline in the volume of packed red blood cells to about 35 mL/dL, the level stabilizes after several weeks. The plasma transferrin saturation remains increased until the available iron stores are depleted. In contrast, the plasma ferritin concentration falls progressively, reflecting the gradual decrease in body iron stores. Since one 500-mL unit of blood contains 200 to 250 mg iron and about 25 g iron should be removed, weekly phlebotomy may be required for 1 or 2 years. When the transferrin saturation and ferritin level become normal, phlebotomies are performed at appropriate intervals to maintain levels within the normal range. The measurements promptly become abnormal with iron reaccumulation. Usually one phlebotomy every 3 months will suffice.

Chelating agents such as deferoxamine, when given parenterally, remove 10 to 20 mg iron per day, which is much less than that mobilized by once-weekly phlebotomy. Phlebotomy is also less expensive, more convenient, and safer for most patients. However, chelating agents are indicated when anemia or hypoproteinemia is severe enough to preclude phlebotomy. Subcutaneous infusion of deferoxamine using a portable pump is the most effective means of administration.

Alcohol consumption should be severely curtailed or eliminated as it increases the risk of cirrhosis in hereditary hemochromatosis nearly tenfold. The management of hepatic failure, cardiac failure, and diabetes mellitus is similar to conventional therapy for these conditions. Loss of libido and change in secondary sex characteristics are partially

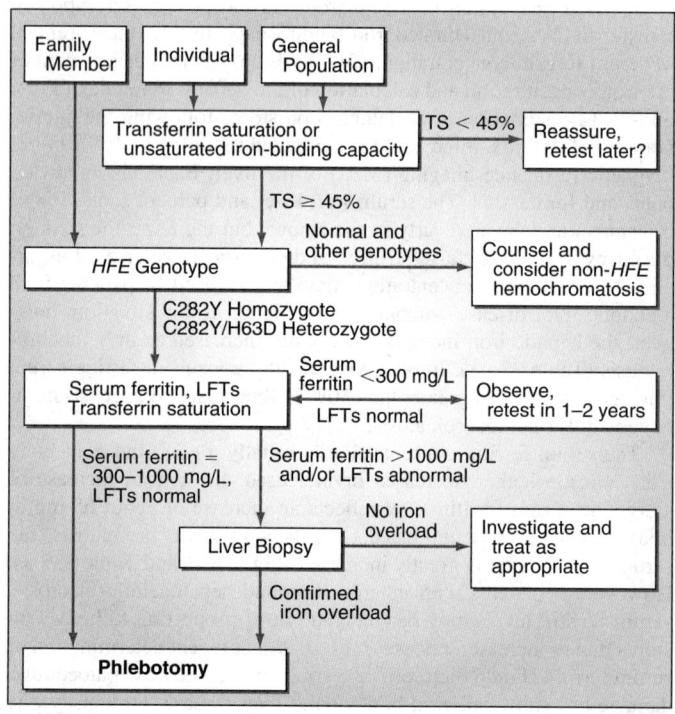

FIGURE 336-3 Algorithm for screening for *HFE*-associated hemochromatosis. LFT, liver function tests; TS, transferrin saturation. (*With permission from The Canadian Journal of Gastroenterology.*)

relieved by parenteral testosterone or gonadotropin therapy (Chap. 325).

PROGNOSIS

The principal causes of death are cardiac failure (30%), hepatocellular failure or portal hypertension (25%), and hepatocellular carcinoma (30%).

Life expectancy is improved by removal of the excessive stores of iron and maintenance of these stores at near-normal levels. The 5-year survival rate with therapy increases from 33 to 89%. With repeated phlebotomy, the liver and spleen decrease in size, liver function improves, pigmentation of skin decreases, and cardiac failure may be reversed. Diabetes improves in about 40%, but removal of excess iron has little effect on hypogonadism or arthropathy. Hepatic fibrosis may decrease, but cirrhosis is irreversible. End-stage liver disease can be treated with orthotopic liver transplantation, but the results are suboptimal unless excess iron stores are first corrected. Hepatocellular carcinoma usually occurs as a late sequela in patients who are cirrhotic at presentation. The apparent increase in its incidence in treated patients is probably related to their increased life span. Hepatocellular carcinoma does not appear to develop if the disease is treated in the precirrhotic stage. Indeed, the life expectancy of homozygotes treated before the development of cirrhosis is normal.

The importance of family screening and early therapy cannot be emphasized too strongly. Asymptomatic individuals detected by family studies should have phlebotomy therapy if iron stores are moderately to severely increased. Assessment of iron stores at appropriate intervals is also important. With this management approach, most manifestations of the disease can be prevented.

ACKNOWLEDGMENT
The author acknowledges the contribution of Dr. Kurt J. Isselbacher to this chapter in previous editions of Harrison's.

FURTHER READING

BEUTLER E et al: Penetrance of 845G → A (C282Y) *HFE* hereditary haemochromatosis mutation in the USA. Lancet 359:211, 2002

BRIDLE KR et al: Disrupted hepcidin regulation in HFE-associated haemochromatosis and the liver as a regulator of body iron homeostasis. Lancet 361:669, 2003

EDWARDS CQ et al: Prevalence of hemochromatosis among 11,065 presumably healthy blood donors. N Engl J Med 318:1355, 1988

FLEMING RE, SLY WS: Mechanisms of iron accumulation in hereditary hemochromatosis. Annu Rev Physiol 64:663, 2002

NICOLAS G et al: Lack of hepcidin expression and severe tissue iron overload in upstream stimulatory factor 2 (USF2) knockout mice. Proc Natl Acad Sci USA 98:8780, 2001

OLYNYK JK et al: A population based study of the clinical expression of the hemochromatosis gene. N Engl J Med 341:718, 1999

337 THE PORPHYRIAS
Robert J. Desnick

The porphyrias are inherited disorders, each involving a specific enzyme in the heme biosynthetic pathway (Fig. 337-1). These disorders are classified as either *hepatic* or *erythropoietic* depending on the primary site of overproduction and accumulation of the porphyrin precursor or porphyrin (Tables 337-1 and 337-2), although some have overlapping features. The major manifestations of the hepatic porphyrias are neurologic, including neuropathic abdominal pain, neuropathy, and mental disturbances, whereas the erythropoietic porphyrias characteristically cause cutaneous photosensitivity. The reason for neurologic involvement in the hepatic porphyrias is poorly understood. Cutaneous sensitivity to sunlight is due to long-wave ultraviolet light excitation of excess porphyrins in the skin, leading to cell damage, scarring, and deformation. Steroid hormones, drugs, and nutrition influence the production of porphyrin precursors and porphyrins, thereby precipitating or increasing the severity of some porphyrias. Thus, the porphyrias are ecogenetic disorders in which environmental, physiologic, and genetic factors interact to cause disease.

Because many symptoms of the porphyrias are nonspecific, diagnosis is often delayed. Laboratory testing is required to confirm or exclude the various types of porphyria (Table 337-2). Urinary δ-aminolevulinic acid (ALA) and porphobilinogen (PBG) are easily quantitated by chemical methods; the urinary porphyrin isomers can be separated and quantitated by high-performance liquid chromatography. The diagnostic profile of accumulated precursors and/or porphyrins in each disorder can also be defined by extraction and thin-layer chromatography of fecal porphyrins. However, a definite diagnosis requires demonstration of the specific enzyme deficiency or gene defect. The isolation and characterization of the cDNAs encoding the heme biosynthetic enzymes have permitted identification of the genetic basis of each porphyria. Molecular genetic analyses now make it possible to provide precise heterozygote identification and prenatal diagnoses in families with known mutations.

HEME BIOSYNTHESIS The first and last three enzymes in the heme biosynthetic pathway are located in the mitochondrion, whereas the other four are cytosolic (Fig. 337-1). The first enzyme, δ-aminolevulinate synthase (ALA-synthase), catalyzes the condensation of glycine, activated by pyridoxal phosphate and succinyl coenzyme A, to form ALA. In the liver, this rate-limiting enzyme can be induced by a variety of drugs, steroids, and other chemicals. Distinct erythroid-specific and nonerythroid (e.g., housekeeping) forms of ALA-synthase are encoded by separate genes; defects in the erythroid form cause X-linked sideroblastic anemia (XLSA).

The second enzyme, δ-aminolevulinate dehydratase (ALA-dehydratase), catalyzes the condensation of two molecules of ALA to form PBG. Four molecules of PBG condense to form the tetrapyrrole uroporphyrinogen (URO) III by a two-step process catalyzed by hydroxymethylbilane (HMB) synthase (also known as PBG-deaminase or URO I synthase) and URO III synthase. HMB-synthase catalyzes the head-to-tail condensation of four PBG molecules by a series of deaminations to form the linear tetrapyrrole, HMB. URO-synthase catalyzes the rearrangement and rapid cyclization of HMB to form the asymmetric, physiologic, octacarboxylate porphyrinogen URO III isomer.

The fifth enzyme in the pathway, URO-decarboxylase, catalyzes the sequential removal of the four carboxyl groups from the acetic acid side chains of URO III to form coproporphyrinogen (COPRO) III, a tetracarboxylate porphyrinogen. This compound then enters the mitochondrion, where COPRO-oxidase, the sixth enzyme, catalyzes the decarboxylation of two of the four propionic acid groups to form the two vinyl groups of protoporphyrinogen (PROTO) IX, a dicarboxylate porphyrinogen. Next, PROTO-oxidase oxidizes PROTO IX to protoporphyrin IX by the removal of six hydrogen atoms. The product of the reaction is a porphyrin (oxidized form), in contrast to the preceding tetrapyrrole intermediates, which are porphyrinogens (reduced forms). Finally, ferrous iron is inserted into protoporphyrin IX to form heme, a reaction catalyzed by the eighth enzyme in the pathway, ferrochelatase (also known as heme synthetase or protoheme ferrolyase).

Mutations causing their respective porphyria have been identified in each of these genes. Thus, molecular diagnosis is now available for each porphyria, which is important in many cases where the diagnosis by other methods may be difficult.

REGULATION OF HEME BIOSYNTHESIS About 85% of the heme produced in the body is synthesized in erythroid cells to provide heme for hemoglobin; most of the remainder is produced in the liver, where the

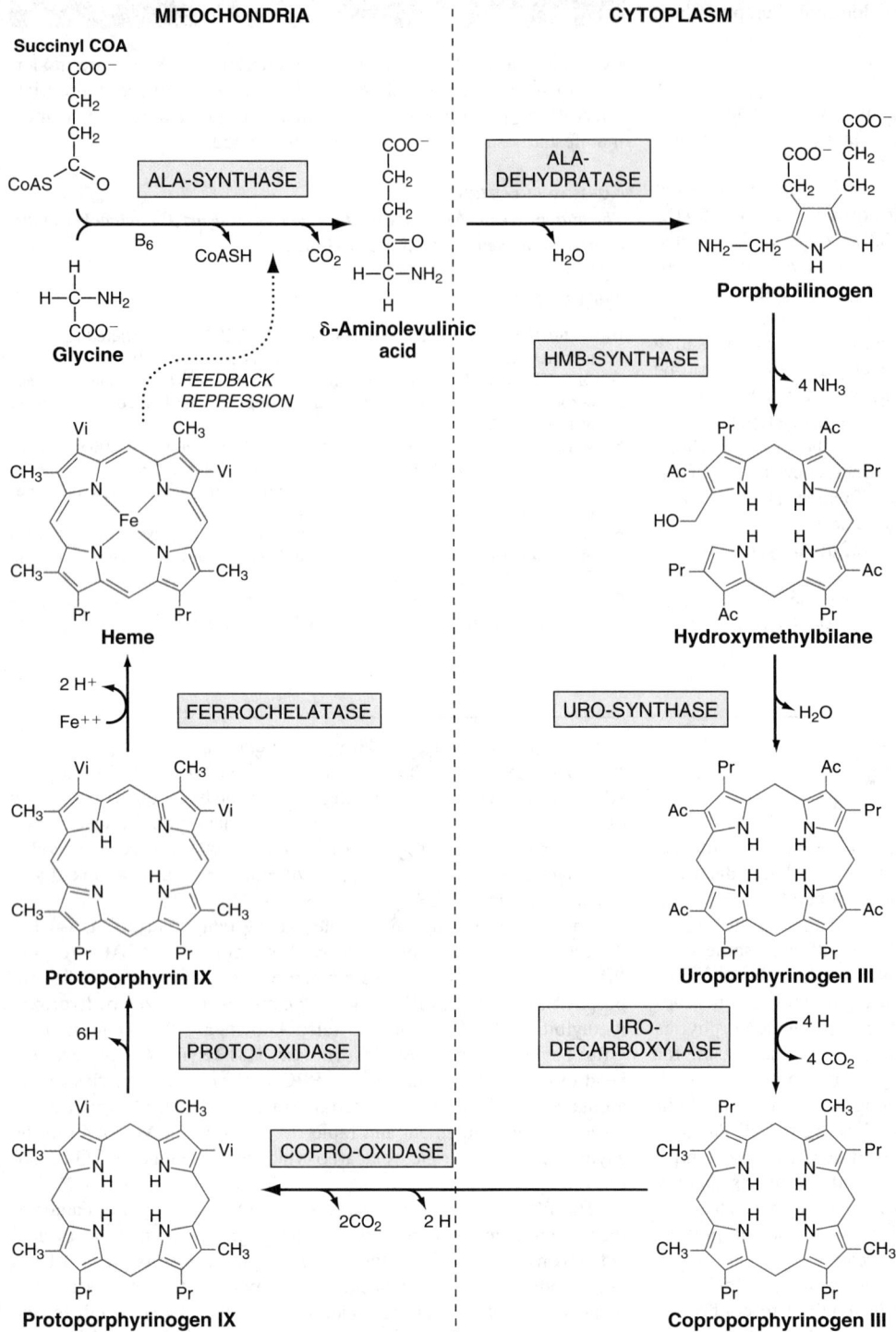

MITOCHONDRIA   **CYTOPLASM**

Succinyl COA

ALA-SYNTHASE

Glycine

FEEDBACK REPRESSION

δ-Aminolevulinic acid

ALA-DEHYDRATASE

Porphobilinogen

Heme

FERROCHELATASE

HMB-SYNTHASE

Hydroxymethylbilane

Protoporphyrin IX

URO-SYNTHASE

Uroporphyrinogen III

PROTO-OXIDASE

URO-DECARBOXYLASE

Protoporphyrinogen IX

COPRO-OXIDASE

Coproporphyrinogen III

FIGURE 337-1   The human heme biosynthetic pathway.

biosynthetic pathway is under negative feedback control. "Free" heme in the liver regulates the synthesis and mitochondrial translocation of the housekeeping form of ALA-synthase. Heme represses the synthesis of the ALA-synthase mRNA and interferes with the transport of the enzyme from the cytosol into mitochondria. ALA-synthase is increased by many of the same chemicals that induce the cytochrome P450 enzymes in the endoplasmic reticulum of the liver. Because most of the heme in the liver is used for the synthesis of cytochrome P450 enzymes, hepatic ALA-synthase and the cytochrome P450s are regulated in a coordinated fashion.

Different regulatory mechanisms control the production of heme for hemoglobin. The erythroid-specific ALA-synthase is encoded on the X-chromosome and it is expressed at higher levels than the hepatic

enzyme. An erythroid-specific control mechanism regulates iron transport into erythroid cells. During erythroid differentiation, the activities of the heme biosynthetic enzymes are increased.

THE HEPATIC PORPHYRIAS

The acute hepatic porphyrias are characterized by the rapid onset of neurologic manifestations. During the acute attack, individuals have markedly elevated plasma and urinary concentrations of the porphyrin precursors ALA and PBG, which originate from the liver.

ALA-DEHYDRATASE–DEFICIENT PORPHYRIA This is a rare autosomal recessive disorder that has been described in only a few patients. Onset and severity of the disease are variable, presumably depending on the amount of residual ALA-dehydratase activity. Clinical features include abdominal pain and neuropathy, resembling acute intermittent porphyria (AIP; see below). Patients have increased urinary levels of ALA and coproporphyrin. ALA-dehydratase activity in erythrocytes is <5% of normal. Lead intoxication and hereditary tyrosinemia (fumarylacetoacetase deficiency) should be considered in the differential diagnosis of ALA-dehydratase–deficient porphyria, as they can inhibit ALA-dehydratase. DNA analyses reveal a variety of missense mutations that result in the amino acid substitutions in ALA-dehydratase. Heterozygotes are clinically asymptomatic and do not excrete increased levels of ALA, but they can be detected by demonstration of intermediate levels of erythrocyte ALA-dehydratase activity or by demonstrating a specific mutation in the *ALA-dehydratase* gene. Prenatal diagnosis of this disorder has not been achieved but should be possible by determination of the ALA-dehydratase activity and/or gene mutation in cultured chorionic villi or amniocytes. Treatment and prevention of the neurologic complications are the same as for other acute porphyrias (see below).

ACUTE INTERMITTENT PORPHYRIA This hepatic porphyria is an autosomal dominant condition resulting from the half-normal level of HMB-synthase activity. The disease is widespread but is especially common in Scandinavia and Great Britain. The enzyme deficiency can be demonstrated in most heterozygous individuals, but clinical expression is highly variable. Activation of the disease is related to environmental or hormonal factors, such as drugs, diet, and steroid hormones, which can precipitate the manifestations. Attacks can be prevented by avoiding known precipitating factors.

Clinical Features Most heterozygotes remain clinically asymptomatic (latent) unless exposed to factors that increase the production of porphyrins. Endogenous and exogenous gonadal steroids, porphyrinogenic drugs, alcohol ingestion, and low-calorie diets, usually instituted for weight loss, are common precipitating factors. Table 337-3 provides a partial list of the major drugs that are harmful in AIP [and also in hereditary coproporphyria (HCP) and variegate porphyria (VP)] and some drugs and anesthetic agents known to be safe. More extensive lists of drugs considered harmful or safe are available (Anderson et al., 2001), but information is incomplete for many of them. Attacks also can be provoked by infections and surgery.

Because the neurovisceral symptoms rarely occur before puberty and are often nonspecific, a high index of suspicion is required to make the diagnosis. The disease can be disabling but is rarely fatal. Abdominal pain, the most common symptom, is usually steady and poorly localized but may be due to cramps. Ileus, abdominal distention, and decreased bowel sounds are common. However, increased bowel sounds and diarrhea may occur. Abdominal tenderness, fever, and leukocytosis are usually absent or mild because the symptoms are neurologic rather than inflammatory. Nausea, vomiting, constipation, tachycardia, hypertension, mental symptoms, pain in the limbs, head, neck, or chest, muscle weakness, sensory loss, dysuria, and urinary retention are characteristic. Tachycardia, hypertension, restlessness, tremors, and excess sweating are due to sympathetic overactivity.

The peripheral neuropathy is due to axonal degeneration (rather than demyelinization) and primarily affects motor neurons. Significant neuropathy does not occur with all acute attacks; abdominal symptoms are usually more prominent. Motor neuropathy affects the proximal muscles initially, more often in the shoulders and arms. The course and degree of involvement are variable. Deep tendon reflexes may be normal or hyperactive but are usually decreased or absent with advanced neuropathy. Motor weakness can be asymmetric and focal and may involve cranial nerves. Sensory changes such as paresthesia and loss of sensation are less prominent. Progressive muscle weakness can lead to respiratory and bulbar paralysis and death when diagnosis and treatment are delayed. Sudden death may result from sympathetic overactivity and cardiac arrhythmia.

Mental symptoms such as anxiety, insomnia, depression, disorientation, hallucinations, and paranoia can occur in acute attacks. Seizures can be due to neurologic effects or to hyponatremia. Treatment of seizures is difficult because virtually all antiseizure drugs (except bromides) may exacerbate AIP (clonazepam may be safer than phenytoin or barbiturates). Hyponatremia results from hypothalamic involvement and inappropriate vasopressin secretion or from electrolyte depletion due to vomiting, diarrhea, poor intake, or excess renal sodium loss. Persistent hypertension and impaired renal function may occur. When an attack resolves, abdominal pain may disappear within hours, and paresis begins to improve within days and may continue to improve over several years.

TABLE 337-1 *Classification of the Human Porphyrias*

Type/Porphyria	Deficient Enzyme	Inheritance[a]	Photosensitivity	Neurovisceral Symptoms
HEPATIC PORPHYRIAS				
ALA-dehydratase deficiency (ADP)	ALA-dehydratase	AR	−	+
Acute intermittent porphyria (AIP)	HMB-synthase	AD	−	+
Porphyria cutanea tarda (PCT)	URO-decarboxylase	AD	+++	−
Hereditary coproporphyria (HCP)	COPRO-oxidase	AD	+	+
Variegate porphyria (VP)	PROTO-oxidase	AD	+	+
ERYTHROPOIETIC PORPHYRIAS				
X-linked sideroblastic anemia (XLSA)	ALA-synthase	XLR	−	−
Congenital erythropoietic porphyria (CEP)	URO-synthase	AR	+++	−
Erythropoietic protoporphyria (EPP)	Ferrochelatase	AD	+	−

[a] AR, autosomal recessive; AD, autosomal dominant; XLR, X-linked recessive.
Note: ALA, δ-aminolevulinic acid; HMB, hydroxymethylbilane; URO, uroporphyrinogen; COPRO, coproporphyrinogen; PROTO, protoporphyrinogen.

Diagnosis ALA and PBG levels are increased in plasma and urine during acute attacks. Urinary PBG excretion is usually 220 to 880 μmol/d (50 to 200 mg/d) [normal, 0 to 18 μmol/d (0 to 4 mg/d)], and urinary ALA excretion is 150 to 760 μmol/d (20 to 100 mg/d) [normal, 8 to 53 μmol/d (1 to 7 mg/d)]. The excretion of these compounds generally decreases with clinical improvement, particularly after hematin infusions (see below). A normal urinary PBG level effectively excludes AIP as a cause for current symptoms. Fecal porphyrins are usually normal or minimally increased in AIP, in contrast to HCP and VP. Most asymptomatic ("latent") heterozygotes with HMB-synthase deficiency have normal urinary excretion of ALA and PBG. Therefore, measurement of HMB-synthase in erythrocytes, or better, the detection of the family's HMB-synthase mutation, will diagnose asymptomatic family members.

The enzyme deficiency is detectable in erythrocytes from most AIP heterozygotes (*classic AIP*). Note that the activity is higher in young erythrocytes and may increase into the normal range in AIP when erythropoiesis is increased due to a concurrent condition. However, patients with the rare erythroid form of AIP (*erythroid, or variant, AIP*) have normal enzyme levels in erythrocytes and deficient activity in nonerythroid tissues (see below). The erythroid and housekeeping forms of HMB-synthase are encoded by a single gene, which has two promoters: one promoter generates the ubiquitously expressed housekeeping mRNA; the other promoter transcribes the erythroid-specific mRNA. Several deletions and >175 different mutations have been

TABLE 337-2 *The Major Metabolites Accumulated in the Human Porphyrias*

Type/Porphyria	Increased Erythrocyte Porphyrins	Porphyrin Excretion	
		Urine	Stool
HEPATIC PORPHYRIAS			
ALA-dehydratase deficiency (ADP)	Zn-protoporphyrins	ALA, Coproporphyrin III	—
Acute intermittent porphyria (AIP)	—	ALA, PBG	—
Porphyria cutanea tarda (PCT)	—	Uroporphyrin I, 7-Carboxylate Porphyrin	Isocoproporphyrin
Hereditary coproporphyria (HCP)	—	ALA, PBG, Coproporphyrin III	Coproporphyrin III
Variegate porphyria (VP)	—	ALA, PBG Coproporphyrin III	Protoporphyrin IX 5-Carboxylate Porphyrin
ERYTHROPOIETIC PORPHYRIAS			
X-linked sideroblastic anemia (XLSA)	—	—	—
Congenital erythropoietic porphyria (CEP)	Uroporphyrin I	Uroporphyrin I	Coproporphyrin I, Uroporphyrin I
Erythropoietic protoporphyria (EPP)	Protoporphyrin IX	—	Protoporphyrin IX

Note: ALA, δ-aminolevulinic acid; PBG, porphobilinogen

TABLE 337-3 *Categories of Unsafe and Safe Drugs in AIP, HCP, and VP*

Unsafe	Safe
Barbiturates	Narcotic analgesics
Sulfonamide antibiotics	Aspirin
Meprobamate	Acetaminophen
Glutethimide	Phenothiazines
Methyprylon	Penicillin and derivatives
Ethchlorvynol	Streptomycin
Mephenytoin	Glucocorticoids
Succinimides	Bromides
Carbamazepine	Insulin
Valproic acid	Atropine
Pyrazolones	
Griseofulvin	
Ergots	
Synthetic estrogens and progestogens	
Danazol	
Alcohol	

found in the coding region of the gene in unrelated AIP families. These mutations alter the kinetic properties and/or stability of the mutant enzymes or create premature termination codons. Mutations that cause erythroid AIP variants with half-normal enzyme in nonerythroid tissues, but normal activity in erythrocytes, include point mutations in the initiation methionine codon (which prevent translation) and in the 5' donor splice site of intron 1 (which cause abnormal splicing of the HMB-synthase transcript) and a mutation in the housekeeping promoter. The prenatal diagnosis of a fetus at risk can be made with cultured amniotic cells or chorionic villi.

℞ TREATMENT

During acute attacks, narcotic analgesics may be required for abdominal pain, and phenothiazines are useful for nausea, vomiting, anxiety, and restlessness. Chloral hydrate can be given for insomnia, and benzodiazepines are probably safe in low doses, if a minor tranquilizer is required. Although intravenous glucose (at least 300 g/d) can be effective in acute attacks of porphyria, a more complete parenteral nutritional regimen may be beneficial if oral feeding is not possible for a prolonged period. However, intravenous heme is more effective than glucose in reducing porphyrin precursor excretion and probably leads to more rapid recovery. The response to heme therapy is reduced if delayed. Therefore, 3 to 4 mg of heme, in the form of hematin (Abbott Laboratories), heme albumin, or heme arginate (Leiras Oy, Turku, Finland), may be infused daily for 4 days beginning as soon as possible after onset of an attack. Heme arginate and heme albumin are chemically stable and are less likely than hematin to produce phlebitis or an anticoagulant effect. The rate of recovery from an acute attack depends on the degree of neuronal damage and may be rapid (1 to 2 days) with prompt therapy. Recovery from severe motor neuropathy may require months or years. Identification and avoidance of inciting factors can hasten recovery from an attack and prevent future attacks. Multiple inciting factors may contribute to a symptomatic episode. Frequent clear-cut cyclical attacks occur in some women and can be prevented with a long-acting gonadotropin-releasing hormone analogue (this indication is not approved by the U.S. Food and Drug Administration).

PORPHYRIA CUTANEA TARDA Porphyria cutanea tarda (PCT), the most common of the porphyrias, can be sporadic (type I) or familial (types II and III) and can also develop after exposure to halogenated aromatic hydrocarbons. Hepatic URO-decarboxylase is deficient in all types of PCT; however, in types I and III PCT, URO-decarboxylase activity is normal in erythrocytes. In type II PCT, an autosomal dominant disorder, the enzyme is deficient in erythrocytes and other tissues. In type III PCT, deficiency of the enzyme is limited to the liver. Deficient hepatic URO-decarboxylase and a porphyrin pattern resembling PCT

can be produced by exposure of normal individuals to a number of halogenated aromatic hydrocarbons. Hepatoerythropoietic porphyria (HEP) is an autosomal recessive form of porphyria that results from marked systemic deficiency of URO-decarboxylase activity.

Clinical Features Cutaneous photosensitivity is the major clinical feature. Neurologic manifestations are not observed. Fluid-filled vesicles and bullae develop on sun-exposed areas such as the face, the dorsa of the hands and feet, the forearms, and the legs. The skin in these areas is friable, and minor trauma may lead to the formation of bullae. The appearance of small white plaques, termed *milia*, may precede or follow vesicle formation. Bullae and denuded skin heal slowly and are subject to infection. Other features include hypertrichosis and hyperpigmentation, especially of the face, and thickening, scarring, and calcification resembling the cutaneous changes of systemic sclerosis.

A number of factors contribute to the development of hepatic URO-decarboxylase deficiency, including excess alcohol, iron, and estrogens. The importance of excess hepatic iron as a precipitating factor is underscored by the finding that the incidence of the common hemochromatosis-causing mutations, *HFE* C282Y and H63D, are increased in patients with types I and II PCT (Chap. 336). Various chemicals can also induce PCT; an epidemic of PCT occurred in eastern Turkey in the 1950s as a consequence of wheat contaminated with the fungicide hexachlorobenzene. PCT also occurs after exposure to other chemicals, including di- and trichlorophenols and 2,3,7,8-tetrachlorodibenzo-(*p*)-dioxin (TCDD, dioxin). Patients with PCT characteristically have liver damage and are at risk for hepatocellular carcinoma. These carcinomas do not produce porphyrins.

HEP resembles congenital erythropoietic porphyria (CEP) and usually presents with blistering skin lesions, hypertrichosis, scarring, and red urine in infancy or childhood.

Diagnosis Porphyrins are increased in the liver, plasma, urine, and stool. The urinary ALA level may be slightly increased, but the PBG level is normal. Urinary porphyrins consist mostly of uroporphyrin and 7-carboxylate porphyrin, with lesser amounts of coproporphyrin and 5- and 6-carboxylate porphyrins. Plasma porphyrins are also increased in a pattern that resembles that in urine. Isocoproporphyrins are increased in feces and sometimes in plasma and urine. The finding of increased isocoproporphyrins is diagnostic for hepatic URO-decarboxylase deficiency.

Type II PCT and HEP can be distinguished from types I and III by finding decreased URO-decarboxylase in erythrocytes. URO-decarboxylase activity in liver, erythrocytes, and cultured skin fibroblasts in type II PCT is approximately 50% of normal in affected individuals and in family members with latent disease. In HEP, the URO-decarboxylase activity is markedly deficient, with typical levels of 3 to 10% of normal. Over 50 mutations have been identified in the coding region of the *URO-decarboxylase* gene from unrelated type II PCT and HEP patients. Excess hepatic iron contributes to development of sporadic and familial forms of PCT. As noted above, coinheritance of *HFE* mutations that cause hemochromatosis increases susceptibility to PCT-precipitating factors. In the familial forms (types II and III), iron inhibits the residual normal enzyme, so that enzymatic activity in liver is <50% of normal. In type I PCT the decreased hepatic URO-decarboxylase activity is not accompanied by a decrease in the amount of enzyme protein, suggesting that the enzyme is present in an inactive form; hepatic URO-decarboxylase activity gradually increases after a remission is induced by phlebotomy.

℞ TREATMENT

Alcohol, estrogens, iron supplements, and, if possible, any drugs that may exacerbate the disease should be discontinued, but this step does not always lead to improvement. A complete response can almost always be achieved by repeated phlebotomy to reduce hepatic iron. A unit (450 mL) of blood can be removed every 1 to 2 weeks. Because iron overload is not marked in most cases, remission may occur after only five or six phlebotomies. Hemoglobin levels and serum ferritin should be followed closely to prevent development of iron deficiency and anemia. After remission, continued phlebotomy may not be needed even if ferritin levels return to normal. Relapses are treated by additional phlebotomy.

PCT can also be treated with chloroquine or hydroxychloroquine, both of which form a complex with the excess porphyrins and promote their excretion. Small doses (e.g., 125 mg chloroquine phosphate twice weekly) should be given, because standard doses can induce transient, sometimes marked increases in photosensitivity and hepatocellular damage. Hepatic imaging can diagnose or exclude complicating hepatocellular carcinoma. Treatment of PCT in patients with end-stage renal disease is facilitated by administration of erythropoietin.

HEREDITARY COPROPORPHYRIA HCP is an autosomal dominant form of hepatic porphyria that results from half-normal levels of COPRO-oxidase activity. Photosensitivity may occur. A few cases of homozygous HCP have been reported.

Clinical Features HCP is influenced by the same factors that cause attacks in AIP. The disease is latent before puberty, and symptoms are more common in women. Neurovisceral symptoms and other manifestations are virtually identical to those of AIP. Photosensitivity may resemble that in PCT and VP. Cutaneous lesions may begin in childhood in rare homozygous cases.

Diagnosis Coproporphyrin is markedly increased in the urine and feces in symptomatic disease and sometimes when there are no symptoms. Urinary ALA and PBG levels are increased during acute attacks but may return to normal when symptoms resolve. Although the diagnosis can be confirmed by measuring COPRO-oxidase activity, these assays are not widely available and require cells other than erythrocytes. Since the *COPRO-oxidase* gene has been cloned and >30 mutations, two-thirds of which are missense, have been identified in unrelated patients, DNA diagnosis of suspected patients is also available.

℞ TREATMENT

Neurologic symptoms are treated as in AIP (see above). Phlebotomy and chloroquine are ineffective when cutaneous lesions are present.

VARIEGATE PORPHYRIA VP, a hepatic porphyria that results from the deficient activity of PROTO-oxidase, is transmitted in an autosomal dominant manner and can present with neurologic symptoms, photosensitivity, or both.

Clinical Features Neurovisceral signs and symptoms develop after puberty and are similar to those of AIP or HCP (see above). Attacks are provoked by the same drugs, steroids, and nutritional factors that are detrimental in AIP. Skin manifestations are more common than in HCP but usually occur apart from the neurovisceral symptoms. Because the skin lesions in VP, HCP, and PCT are not distinguishable by clinical examination or biopsy, these conditions are diagnosed by assay of porphyrins and porphyrin precursors in blood, urine, and feces.

VP is particularly common in South Africa, where 3 of every 1000 whites have the disorder. Most are descendants of a couple who emigrated from Holland to South Africa in 1688. Homozygous VP is associated with photosensitivity, neurologic symptoms, and developmental disturbances, including growth retardation in infancy or childhood; all cases had increased erythrocyte levels of zinc protoporphyrin, a characteristic finding in all homozygous porphyrias so far described.

Dual porphyria, the simultaneous occurrence of VP and familial PCT, has been documented in several kindreds. *Chester porphyria* was described in a large British family in which individuals had acute porphyric attacks and deficiency of both PROTO-oxidase and HMB-synthase. Photosensitivity was not observed. It is unclear whether Chester porphyria is a variant of VP or AIP.

Diagnosis When VP is symptomatic, levels of fecal protoporphyrin and coproporphyrin and of urinary coproporphyrin are increased. Urinary ALA and PBG levels are increased during acute attacks. Plasma levels of porphyrins are increased, particularly when there are cutaneous lesions. VP can be distinguished rapidly from all other porphyrias by examining the fluorescence emission spectrum of porphyrins in plasma at neutral pH. This test is particularly useful for differentiating VP from PCT.

Assays of PROTO-oxidase activity in cultured fibroblasts or lymphocytes are not widely available. Some latent cases of VP can be diagnosed by measurement of fecal porphyrins in relatives of VP patients. Over 90 mutations have been found in the *PROTO-oxidase* gene; 52% are missense mutations and 30% are small deletions or insertions.

℞ TREATMENT

Acute attacks are treated with hematin as in AIP. Other than avoiding sun exposure, there are few effective measures for treating the skin lesions. β-Carotene, phlebotomy, and chloroquine are not helpful.

THE ERYTHROPOIETIC PORPHYRIAS

In the erythropoietic porphyrias, porphyrins from bone marrow erythrocytes and plasma are deposited in the skin and lead to cutaneous photosensitivity.

X-LINKED SIDEROBLASTIC ANEMIA XLSA results from the deficient activity of the erythroid form of ALA-synthase and is associated with ineffective erythropoiesis, weakness, and pallor.

Clinical Features Typically, males with XLSA develop refractory hemolytic anemia, pallor, and weakness during infancy. They have secondary hypersplenism, become iron overloaded, and can develop hemosiderosis. The severity depends on the level of residual erythroid ALA-synthase activity and on the responsiveness of the specific mutation to pyridoxal 5'-phosphate supplementation (see below). Peripheral blood smears reveal a hypochromic, microcytic anemia with striking anisocytosis, poikilocytosis, and polychromasia; the leukocytes and platelets appear normal. Hemoglobin content is reduced, and the mean corpuscular volume and mean corpuscular hemoglobin concentration are decreased. Patients with milder, late-onset disease have been reported.

Diagnosis Bone marrow examination reveals hypercellularity with a left shift and megaloblastic erythropoiesis with abnormal maturation. A variety of Prussian blue–staining sideroblasts are observed. Levels of urinary porphyrin precursors and of both urinary and fecal porphyrins are normal. The level of erythroid ALA-synthase is decreased in bone marrow, but this enzyme is difficult to measure in the presence of the normal ALA-synthase housekeeping enzyme. Definitive diagnosis requires the demonstration of mutations in the *erythroid ALA-synthase* gene.

℞ TREATMENT

The severe anemia may respond to pyridoxine supplementation. This cofactor is essential for ALA-synthase activity, and mutations in the pyridoxine-binding site of the enzyme have been found in several responsive patients. Cofactor supplementation may make it possible to eliminate or reduce the frequency of transfusion. Unresponsive patients may be transfusion-dependent and require chelation therapy.

CONGENITAL ERYTHROPOIETIC PORPHYRIA CEP (also known as *Gunther's disease*) is an autosomal recessive disorder due to markedly deficient activity of URO-synthase; it is associated with hemolytic anemia and cutaneous lesions. CEP is characterized by accumulation of uroporphyrin I and coproporphyrin I isomers.

Clinical Features Severe cutaneous photosensitivity begins in early infancy. The skin over sun-exposed areas is friable, and bullae and vesicles are prone to rupture and infection. Skin thickening, focal hypo- and hyperpigmentation, and hypertrichosis of the face and extremities are characteristic. Secondary infection of the cutaneous lesions can lead to disfigurement of the face and hands. Porphyrins are deposited in teeth and in bones. As a result, the teeth are reddish-brown and fluoresce on exposure to long-wave ultraviolet light. Hemolysis is probably due to the marked increase in erythrocyte porphyrins and leads to splenomegaly. Adults with a milder form of the disease have been described.

Diagnosis   Uroporphyrin and coproporphyrin (mostly type I isomers) accumulate in the bone marrow, erythrocytes, plasma, urine, and feces. The diagnosis should be confirmed by demonstration of markedly deficient URO-synthase activity. The disease can be detected in utero by measuring porphyrins in amniotic fluid and URO-synthase activity in cultured amniotic cells or chorionic villi. Molecular analyses of the mutant alleles have revealed multiple different mutations, including four mutations in the recently discovered erythroid-specific promoter of the *URO-synthase* gene.

℞ TREATMENT

The transfusion of sufficient blood to suppress erythropoiesis is effective but results in iron overload. Splenectomy may reduce hemolysis and decrease transfusion requirements. Protection from sunlight and minor skin trauma is important. β-Carotene may be of some value. Complicating bacterial infections should be treated promptly. Recently, bone marrow transplantation has proven effective in several transfusion-dependent children, providing the rationale for stem-cell gene therapy.

ERYTHROPOIETIC PROTOPORPHYRIA   Erythropoietic protoporphyria (EPP) is an autosomal dominant disorder due to the partial deficiency of ferrochelatase activity. Protoporphyrin accumulates in erythroid cells and plasma and is excreted in bile and feces. EPP is the most common erythropoietic porphyria and, after PCT, the second most common porphyria.

Clinical Features   Skin photosensitivity usually begins in childhood. The skin manifestations differ from those of other porphyrias. Vesicular lesions are uncommon. Redness, swelling, burning, and itching can develop within minutes of sun exposure and resemble angioedema. Symptoms may seem out of proportion to the visible skin lesions. Sparse vesicles and bullae occur in 10% of cases. Chronic skin changes may include lichenification, leathery pseudovesicles, labial grooving, and nail changes. Severe scarring is rare, as are pigment changes, friability, and hirsutism.

The primary source of excess protoporphyrin is the bone marrow reticulocyte. Erythrocyte protoporphyrin is free (not complexed with zinc) and is mostly bound to hemoglobin. In plasma, protoporphyrin is bound to albumin. Hemolysis and anemia are usually absent or mild.

Liver function is usually normal, but in some patients accumulation of protoporphyrin causes chronic liver disease that can progress to liver failure and death. The hepatic complications are often preceded by increasing levels of erythrocyte and plasma protoporphyrin and probably result, in part, from protoporphyrin accumulation in the liver. Protoporphyrin is insoluble, forms crystalline structures in liver cells, and can decrease hepatic bile flow. Gallstones composed at least in part of protoporphyrin occur in some patients.

Some obligate heterozygotes are asymptomatic and have little or no increase in erythrocyte protoporphyrin. Thus there is phenotypic variation in this disease.

Diagnosis   Protoporphyrin levels are increased in bone marrow, circulating erythrocytes, plasma, bile, and feces. Urinary levels of porphyrin and porphyrin precursors are normal. Ferrochelatase activity in cultured lymphocytes or fibroblasts is decreased. DNA diagnosis by mutation analysis is possible, and multiple missense and nonsense mutations have been identified in the *ferrochelatase* gene.

℞ TREATMENT

Oral β-carotene (120 to 180 mg/d) improves tolerance to sunlight in many patients. The dosage may need to be adjusted to maintain serum carotene levels in the recommended range of 10 to 15 μmol/L (600 to 800 μg/dL). Mild skin discoloration due to carotenemia is the only significant side effect. The beneficial effects of β-carotene may involve quenching of singlet oxygen or free radicals. Unfortunately, this drug is less effective in other forms of porphyria associated with photosensitivity.

Treatment of hepatic complications is difficult. However, cholestyramine and other porphyrin absorbents such as activated charcoal may interrupt the enterohepatic circulation of protoporphyrin and promote its fecal excretion, leading to some improvement. Splenectomy may be helpful when the disease is accompanied by hemolysis and significant splenomegaly. Caloric restriction and drugs or hormones that may induce the heme pathway or impair hepatic excretory function should be avoided. Iron deficiency should be prevented or treated. Transfusions or intravenous heme therapy may suppress erythroid and hepatic protoporphyrin production and are sometimes beneficial. Liver transplantation has been carried out in some patients with severe liver complications.

FURTHER READING

ANDERSON KE et al: Disorders of heme biosynthesis: X-linked sideroblastic anemia and the porphyrias, in *The Metabolic and Molecular Bases of Inherited Disease*, 8th ed, CR Scriver et al (eds). New York, McGraw-Hill, 2001, p 2991

DESNICK RJ, ASTRIN KH: Congenital erythropoietic porphyria: Advances in pathogenesis and treatment. Br J Hematol 117:779, 2002

GROSS U et al: Erythropoietic and hepatic porphyria. J Inherit Metab Dis 23:641, 2002

LAMBRECT RW, BONKOVSKY HL: Hemachromatosis and porphyria. Semin Gastrointest Dis 13:109, 2002

SARKANY RPE: The management of porphyria cutanea tarda. Clin Exp Dermatol 26:225, 2001

338 DISORDERS OF PURINE AND PYRIMIDINE METABOLISM
Robert L. Wortmann

Purines (adenine and guanine) and pyrimidines (cytosine, thymine, uracil) serve fundamental roles in the replication of genetic material, gene transcription, protein synthesis, and cellular metabolism. Disorders that involve abnormalities of nucleotide metabolism range from relatively common diseases such as hyperuricemia and gout, in which there is increased production or impaired excretion of a metabolic end product of purine metabolism (uric acid), to rare enzyme deficiencies that affect purine and pyrimidine synthesis or degradation. Understanding these biochemical pathways has led, in some instances, to the development of specific forms of treatment, such as the use of allopurinol to reduce uric acid production.

URIC ACID METABOLISM

Uric acid is the final breakdown product of purine degradation in humans. It is a weak acid with pK_as of 5.75 and 10.3. Urates, the ionized forms of uric acid, predominate in plasma extracellular fluid and synovial fluid, with approximately 98% existing as monosodium urate at pH 7.4. Monosodium urate is easily dialyzed from plasma. Binding of urate to plasma proteins has little physiologic significance.

Plasma is saturated with monosodium urate at a concentration of 415 μmol/L (6.8 mg/dL) at 37°C. At higher concentrations, plasma is therefore supersaturated, creating the potential for urate crystal precipitation. However, precipitation sometimes does not occur even at plasma urate concentrations as high as 4800 μmol/L (80 mg/dL), perhaps because of the presence of solubilizing substances in plasma.

Uric acid is more soluble in urine than in water, possibly because of the presence of urea, proteins, and mucopolysaccharides. The pH of urine greatly influences its solubility. At pH 5.0, urine is saturated with uric acid at concentrations ranging from 360 to 900 μmol/L (6 to 15 mg/dL). At pH 7.0, saturation is reached at concentrations between 9480 and 12,000 μmol/L (158 and 200 mg/dL). Ionized forms of uric acid in urine include mono- and disodium, potassium, ammonium, and calcium urates.

Although purine nucleotides are synthesized and degraded in all tissues, urate is produced only in tissues that contain xanthine oxidase, primarily the liver and small intestine. Urate production varies with the purine content of the diet and the rates of purine biosynthesis, degradation, and salvage (Fig. 338-1). Normally, two-thirds to three-fourths of urate is excreted by the kidneys, and most of the remainder is eliminated through the intestines. A four-component model describes the renal handling of uric acid in humans: (1) glomerular filtration, (2) tubular reabsorption, (3) secretion, and (4) postsecretory reabsorption (Fig. 338-2). Approximately 8 to 12% of urate filtered by the glomeruli is excreted in the urine as uric acid. After filtration, 98 to 100% of the urate is reabsorbed; about half of the reabsorbed urate is secreted back into the proximal tubule, and about 40% of that is again reabsorbed.

Serum urate levels vary with age and sex. Most children have serum urate concentrations of 180 to 240 μmol/L (3.0 to 4.0 mg/dL). Levels begin to rise in males during puberty but remain low in females until menopause. Mean serum urate values of adult men and premenopausal women are 415 and 360 μmol/L (6.8 and 6.0 mg/dL), respectively. After menopause, values for women increase to approximate those of men. In adulthood, concentrations rise steadily over time and vary with height, body weight, blood pressure, renal function, and alcohol intake.

HYPERURICEMIA

Hyperuricemia can result from increased production or decreased excretion of uric acid or from a combination of the two processes. Sustained hyperuricemia predisposes some individuals to develop clinical manifestations including gouty arthritis (Chap. 313), urolithiasis, and renal dysfunction (see below).

Hyperuricemia is defined as a plasma (or serum) urate concentration >420 μmol/L (7.0 mg/dL). The risk of developing gouty arthritis or urolithiasis increases with higher urate levels and escalates in proportion to the degree of elevation. Hyperuricemia is present in between

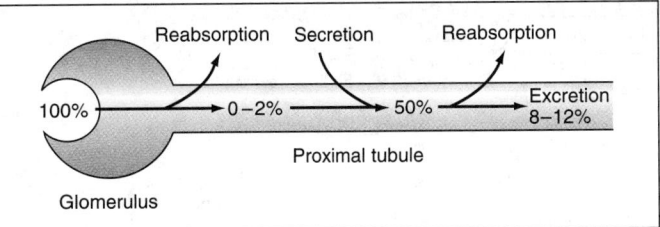

FIGURE 338-2   Schematic for handling of uric acid by the kidney. Components are illustrated with the percentage of filtered urate.

2.0 and 13.2% of ambulatory adults and is even more frequent in hospitalized individuals.

CAUSES OF HYPERURICEMIA   Hyperuricemia may be classified as primary or secondary depending on whether the cause is innate or is the result of an acquired disorder. However, it is more useful to classify hyperuricemia in relation to the underlying pathophysiology, i.e., whether it results from increased production, decreased excretion, or a combination of the two (Fig. 338-1, Table 338-1).

Increased Urate Production   Diet contributes to the serum urate in proportion to its purine content. Strict restriction of purine intake reduces the mean serum urate level by about 60 μmol/L (1.0 mg/dL) and urinary uric acid excretion by approximately 1.2 mmol/d (200 mg/d). Foods high in nucleic acid content include liver, "sweetbreads" (i.e., thymus and pancreas), kidney, and anchovy.

Endogenous sources of purine production also influence the serum urate level (Fig. 338-3). De novo purine biosynthesis is an 11-step process that forms inosine monophosphate (IMP). The rates of purine biosynthesis and urate production are determined, for the most part, by amidophosphoribosyltransferase (amidoPRT), which combines phosphoribosylpyrophosphate (PRPP) and glutamine. AmidoPRT is regulated by the substrate PRPP, which drives the reaction forward, and by the end products of biosynthesis (IMP and other ribonucleotides), which provide feedback inhibition. A secondary regulatory pathway is the salvage of purine bases by hypoxanthine phosphoribosyltransferase (HPRT). HPRT catalyzes the combination of the purine bases hypoxanthine and guanine with PRPP to form the respective ribonucleotides IMP and guanosine monophosphate (GMP). Increased

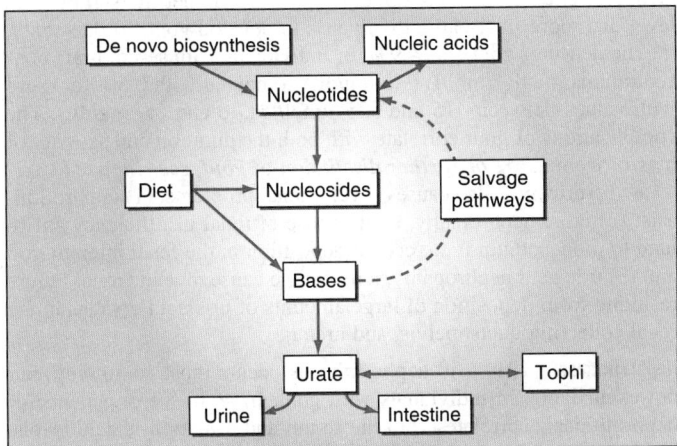

FIGURE 338-1   The total-body urate pool is the net result between urate production and excretion. Urate production is influenced by dietary intake of purines and the rates of de novo biosynthesis of purines from nonpurine precursors, nucleic acid turnover, and salvage by phosphoribosyltransferase activities. The formed urate is normally excreted by urinary and intestinal routes. Hyperuricemia can result from increased production, decreased excretion, or a combination of both mechanisms. When hyperuricemia exists, urate can precipitate and deposit in tissues as tophi.

TABLE 338-1   *Classification of Hyperuricemia by Pathophysiology*

URATE OVERPRODUCTION

Primary idiopathic	Myeloproliferative	Rhabdomyolysis
HPRT deficiency	diseases	Exercise
PRPP synthetase	Polycythemia vera	Alcohol
overactivity	Psoriasis	Obesity
Hemolytic processes	Paget's disease	Purine-rich diet
Lymphoproliferative	Glycogenosis III, V,	
diseases	and VII	

DECREASED URIC ACID EXCRETION

Primary idiopathic	Starvation ketosis	Drug ingestion
Renal insufficiency	Berylliosis	Salicylates (>2 g/d)
Polycystic kidney	Sarcoidosis	Diuretics
disease	Lead intoxication	Alcohol
Diabetes insipidus	Hyperparathyroidism	Levodopa
Hypertension	Hypothyroidism	Ethambutol
Acidosis	Toxemia of pregnancy	Pyrazinamide
Lactic acidosis	Bartter's syndrome	Nicotinic acid
Diabetic	Down syndrome	Cyclosporine
ketoacidosis		

COMBINED MECHANISM

Glucose-6-phosphatase	Fructose-1-phosphate	Alcohol
deficiency	aldolase deficiency	Shock

Note: HPRT, hypoxanthine phosphoribosyltransferase; PRPP, phosphoribosylpyrophosphate.

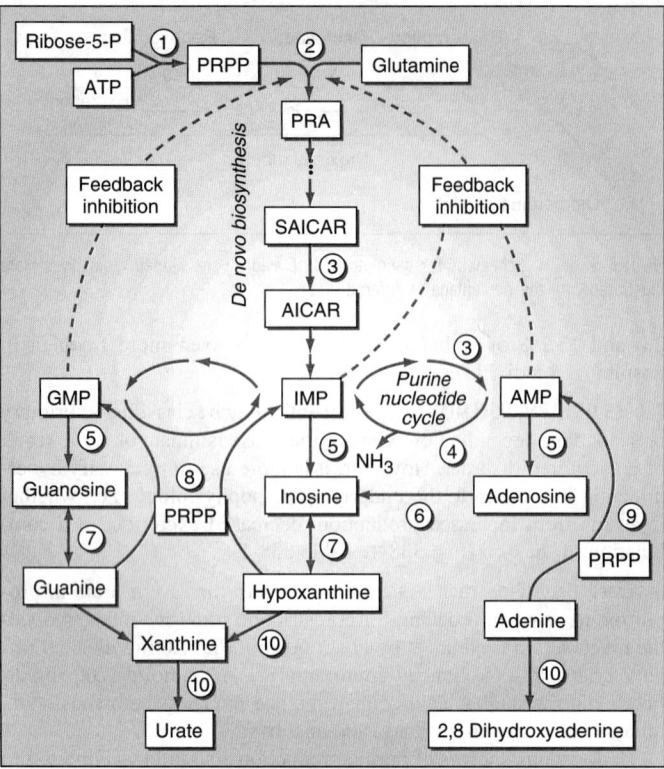

FIGURE 338-3 Abbreviated scheme of purine metabolism. (1) Phosphoribosylpyro-phosphate (PRPP) synthetase, (2) amidophosphoribosyltransferase (amidoPRT), (3) ad-enylosuccinate lyase, (4) adenylate (AMP) deaminase, (5) 5'-nucleotidase, (6) adenosine deaminase, (7) purine nucleoside phosphorylase, (8) hypoxanthine phos-phoribosyltransferase (HPRT), (9) adenine phosphoribosyltransferase (APRT), and (10) xanthine oxidase. PRA, phosphoribosylamine; SAICAR, succinylaminoimidazole carbox-amide ribotide; AICAR, aminoimidazole carboxamide ribotide; GMP, guanylate; IMP, inosine monophosphate.

salvage activity thus retards de novo synthesis by reducing PRPP levels and increasing concentrations of inhibitory ribonucleotides.

Serum urate levels are closely coupled to the rates of de novo purine biosynthesis, which is driven in part by the level of PRPP, as evidenced by two X-linked inborn errors of purine metabolism. Both increased PRPP synthetase activity and HPRT deficiency are associated with overproduction of purines, hyperuricemia, and hyperuricaciduria (see below for clinical descriptions).

Accelerated purine nucleotide degradation can also cause hyper-uricemia, i.e., with conditions of rapid cell turnover, proliferation, or cell death, as in leukemic blast crises, cytotoxic therapy for malig-nancy, hemolysis, or rhabdomyolysis. Hyperuricemia can result from excessive degradation of skeletal muscle ATP after strenuous physical exercise or status epilepticus and in glycogen storage diseases types III, V, and VII (Chap. 341). The hyperuricemia of myocardial infarc-tion, smoke inhalation, and acute respiratory failure may also be re-lated to accelerated breakdown of ATP.

Decreased Uric Acid Excretion Over 90% of individuals with sustained hyperuricemia have a defect in the renal handling of uric acid. Gouty individuals excrete approximately 40% less uric acid than nongouty individuals for any given plasma urate concentration. Uric acid excre-tion increases in gouty and nongouty individuals when plasma urate levels are raised by purine ingestion or infusion, but in those with gout, plasma urate concentrations must be 60 to 120 μmol/L (1 to 2 mg/dL) higher than normal to achieve equivalent uric acid excretion rates.

Altered uric acid excretion could theoretically result from de-creased glomerular filtration, decreased tubular secretion, or enhanced

tubular reabsorption. Decreased urate filtration does not appear to cause primary hyperuricemia but does contribute to the hyperuricemia of renal insufficiency. Although hyperuricemia is invariably present in chronic renal disease, the correlation between serum creatinine, urea nitrogen, and urate concentration is poor. Uric acid excretion per unit of glomerular filtration rate increases progressively with chronic renal insufficiency, but tubular secretory capacity tends to be preserved, tu-bular reabsorptive capacity is reduced, and extrarenal clearance of uric acid increases as renal damage becomes more severe.

Decreased tubular secretion of urate causes the secondary hyper-uricemia of acidosis. Diabetic ketoacidosis, starvation, ethanol intox-ication, lactic acidosis, and salicylate intoxication are accompanied by accumulations of organic acids (β-hydroxybutyrate, acetoacetate, lac-tate, or salicylates) that compete with urate for tubular secretion. Hy-peruricemia may be due to enhanced reabsorption of uric acid distal to the site of secretion. This mechanism is known to be responsible for the hyperuricemia of extracellular volume depletion that occurs with diabetes insipidus or diuretic therapy.

Alcohol promotes hyperuricemia because of increased urate pro-duction and decreased uric acid excretion. Excessive alcohol con-sumption accelerates hepatic breakdown of ATP to increase urate pro-duction. Alcohol consumption can also induce hyperlacticacidemia, which blocks uric acid secretion. The higher purine content in some alcoholic beverages such as beer may also be a factor.

EVALUATION OF HYPERURICEMIA Hyperuricemia does not necessarily rep-resent a disease, nor is it a specific indication for therapy. The decision to treat depends on the cause and the potential consequences of the hyperuricemia in each individual.

Quantification of uric acid excretion can be used to determine whether hyperuricemia is caused by overproduction or decreased ex-cretion. On a purine-free diet, men with normal renal function excrete <3.6 mmol/d (600 mg/d). Thus, the hyperuricemia of individuals who excrete uric acid above this level while on a purine-free diet is due to purine overproduction; for those who excrete lower amounts on the purine-free diet, it is due to decreased excretion. If the assessment is performed while the patient is on a regular diet, the level of 4.2 mmol/d (800 mg/d) can be used as the discriminating value.

Pyrazinamide, which has a suppressive action on tubular secretion, can be used to investigate presecretory reabsorption of uric acid. Pro-benecid, an agent that inhibits postsecretory reabsorption, can be used to evaluate tubular secretion and postsecretory reabsorption.

COMPLICATIONS OF HYPERURICEMIA The most recognized complication of hyperuricemia is *gouty arthritis*. In the general population the prev-alence of hyperuricemia ranges between 2.0 and 13.2%, and the prev-alence of gout is between 1.3 and 3.7%. The higher the serum urate level, the more likely an individual is to develop gout. In one study, the incidence of gout was 4.9% for individuals with serum urate con-centrations >540 μmol/L (9.0 mg/dL) compared with 0.5% for those with values between 415 and 535 μmol/L (7.0 and 8.9 mg/dL). The complications of gout correlate with both the duration and severity of hyperuricemia. →*For further discussion of gout, see Chap. 313.*

Hyperuricemia also causes several renal problems: (1) nephrolithi-asis; (2) urate nephropathy, a rare cause of renal insufficiency attrib-uted to monosodium urate crystal deposition in the renal interstitium; and (3) uric acid nephropathy, a reversible cause of acute renal failure resulting from deposition of large amounts of uric acid crystals in the renal collecting ducts, pelvis, and ureters.

Nephrolithiasis Uric acid nephrolithiasis occurs most commonly, but not exclusively, in individuals with gout. In gout, the prevalence of nephrolithiasis correlates with the serum and urinary uric acid levels, reaching approximately 50% with serum urate levels of 770 μmol/L (13 mg/dL) or urinary uric acid excretion >6.5 mmol/d (1100 mg/d).

Uric acid stones can develop in individuals with no evidence of arthritis, only 20% of whom are hyperuricemic. Uric acid can also play a role in other types of kidney stones. Some nongouty individuals with calcium oxalate or calcium phosphate stones have hyperuricemia or hyperuricaciduria. Uric acid may act as a nidus on which calcium oxalate can precipitate or lower the formation product for calcium oxalate crystallization.

Urate Nephropathy Urate nephropathy, sometimes referred to as *urate nephrosis*, is a late manifestation of severe gout and is characterized histologically by deposits of monosodium urate crystals surrounded by a giant cell inflammatory reaction in the medullary interstitium and pyramids. The disorder is now rare and cannot be diagnosed in the absence of gouty arthritis. The lesions may be clinically silent or cause proteinuria, hypertension, and renal insufficiency.

Uric Acid Nephropathy This reversible cause of acute renal failure is due to precipitation of uric acid in renal tubules and collecting ducts that causes obstruction to urine flow. Uric acid nephropathy develops following sudden urate overproduction and marked hyperuricaciduria. Factors that favor uric acid crystal formation include dehydration and acidosis. This form of acute renal failure occurs most often during an aggressive "blastic" phase of leukemia or lymphoma prior to or coincident with cytolytic therapy but has also been observed in individuals with other neoplasms, following epileptic seizures, and after vigorous exercise with heat stress. Autopsy studies have demonstrated intraluminal precipitates of uric acid, dilated proximal tubules, and normal glomeruli. The initial pathogenic events are believed to include obstruction of collecting ducts with uric acid and obstruction of distal renal vasculature.

If recognized, uric acid nephropathy is potentially reversible. Appropriate therapy has reduced the mortality from about 50% to practically nil. Serum levels cannot be relied on for diagnosis because this condition has developed in the presence of urate concentrations varying from 720 to 4800 μmol/L (12 to 80 mg/dL). The distinctive feature is the urinary uric acid concentration. In most forms of acute renal failure with decreased urine output, urinary uric acid content is either normal or reduced, and the ratio of uric acid to creatinine is <1. In acute uric acid nephropathy the ratio of uric acid to creatinine in a random urine sample or 24-h specimen is >1, and a value that high is essentially diagnostic.

HYPERURICEMIA AND SYNDROME X Syndrome X is characterized by abdominal obesity with visceral adiposity, impaired glucose tolerance due to insulin resistance with hyperinsulinemia, hypertriglyceridemia, increased low-density lipoprotein cholesterol, decreased high-density lipoprotein cholesterol, and hyperuricemia. Hyperinsulinemia reduces the renal excretion of uric acid and sodium. Not surprisingly, hyperuricemia resulting from euglycemic hyperinsulinemia may precede the onset of type 2 diabetes, hypertension, coronary artery disease, and gout in individuals with syndrome X.

R℞ TREATMENT

ASYMPTOMATIC HYPERURICEMIA Hyperuricemia is present in approximately 5% of the population and in up to 25% of hospitalized individuals. The vast majority are at no clinical risk. Hyperuricemia does not appear to have a causal role in the development of coronary heart disease or death from cardiovascular disease. In the past, the association of hyperuricemia with cardiovascular disease and renal failure led to the use of urate-lowering agents for people with asymptomatic hyperuricemia. This practice is no longer recommended except for individuals receiving cytolytic therapy for neoplastic disease, in which treatment is given in an effort to prevent uric acid nephropathy. Because hyperuricemia can be a component of syndrome X, its presence is an indication to screen for and aggressively treat any accompanying obesity, hyperlipidemia, diabetes mellitus, or hypertension.

Hyperuricemic individuals are at risk to develop gouty arthritis, especially those with higher serum urate levels. However, most hyperuricemic persons never develop gout and prophylactic treatment is not indicated. Furthermore, neither structural kidney damage nor tophi are identifiable before the first attack. Reduced renal function cannot be attributed to asymptomatic hyperuricemia, and treatment of asymp-

tomatic hyperuricemia does not alter the progression of renal dysfunction in patients with renal disease. Increased risk of stone formation in people with asymptomatic hyperuricemia is not established.

Thus, because treatment with antihyperuricemic agents entails inconvenience, cost, and potential toxicity, routine treatment of asymptomatic hyperuricemia cannot be justified other than for prevention of acute uric acid nephropathy. In addition, routine screening for asymptomatic hyperuricemia is not recommended. If hyperuricemia is diagnosed, however, the cause should be determined. Causal factors should be corrected if the condition is secondary, and associated problems such as hypertension, hypercholesterolemia, diabetes mellitus, and obesity should be treated.

Symptomatic Hyperuricemia ■ *NEPHROLITHIASIS* (See Chap. 313 for treatment of gout.) Antihyperuricemic therapy is recommended for the individual who has both gouty arthritis and either uric acid– or calcium-containing stones, both of which may occur in association with hyperuricaciduria. Regardless of the nature of the calculi, fluid ingestion should be sufficient to produce a daily urine volume >2 L. Alkalinization of the urine with sodium bicarbonate or acetazolamide may be justified to increase the solubility of uric acid. Specific treatment of uric acid calculi requires reducing the urine uric acid concentration with allopurinol. Allopurinol administration decreases the serum urate concentration and the urinary excretion of uric acid in the first 24 h, with a maximum reduction occurring within 2 weeks. The average effective dose of allopurinol is 300 mg/d. Allopurinol can be given once a day because of the long half-life (18 h) of its active metabolite oxypurinol. The drug is effective in patients with renal insufficiency, but the dose should be reduced. Allopurinol is also useful in reducing the recurrence of calcium oxalate stones in gouty patients and in nongouty individuals with hyperuricemia or hyperuricaciduria. Potassium citrate (30 to 80 mmol/d orally in divided doses) is an alternative therapy for patients with uric acid stones alone or mixed calcium/uric acid stones. Allopurinol is also indicated for the treatment of 2,8-dihydroxyadenine kidney stones.

URIC ACID NEPHROPATHY Uric acid nephropathy is often preventable, and immediate, appropriate therapy has greatly reduced the mortality rate. Vigorous intravenous hydration and diuresis with furosemide dilute the uric acid in the tubules and promote urine flow to ≥100 mL/h. The administration of acetazolamide, 240 to 500 mg every 6 to 8 h, and sodium bicarbonate, 89 mmol/L, intravenously enhances urine alkalinity and thereby solubilizes more uric acid. It is important to ensure that the urine pH remains >7.0 and to watch for circulatory overload. In addition, antihyperuricemic therapy in the form of allopurinol in a single dose of 8 mg/kg is administered to reduce the amount of urate that reaches the kidney. If renal insufficiency persists, subsequent daily doses should be reduced to 100 to 200 mg because oxypurinol, the active metabolite of allopurinol, accumulates in renal failure. Despite these measures, hemodialysis may be required.

TABLE 338-2 *Medications with Uricosuric Activity*	
Acetohexamide	Glyceryl guaiacolate
ACTH	Glycopyrrolate
Ascorbic acid	Halofenate
Azauridine	Meclofenamate
Benzbromarone	Phenolsulfonphthalein
Calcitonin	Phenylbutazone
Chlorprothixene	Probenecid
Citrate	Radiographic contrast agents
Dicumarol	Salicylates (>2 g/2d)
Diflunisal	Sulfinpyrazone
Estrogens	Tetracycline that is outdated
Glucocorticoids	Zoxazolamine

TABLE 338-3 *Inborn Errors of Purine Metabolism*

Enzyme	Activity	Inheritance	Clinical Features
Hypoxanthine phosphoribosyl-transferase	Complete deficiency	X-linked	Self-mutilation, choreoathetosis, hyperuricemia, gout, and uric acid lithiasis
	Partial deficiency	X-linked	Hyperuricemia, gout, and uric acid lithiasis
Phosphoribosyl-pyrophosphate synthetase	Overactivity	X-linked	Hyperuricemia, gout, uric acid lithiasis, and deafness
Adenine phosphoribosyl-transferase	Deficiency	Autosomal recessive	2,8-Dihydroxyadenine lithiasis
Xanthine oxidase	Deficiency	Autosomal recessive	Xanthinuria and xanthine lithiasis
Adenylosuccinate lyase	Deficiency	Autosomal recessive	Autism and psychomotor retardation
Myoadenylate deaminase	Deficiency	Autosomal recessive	Myopathy with exercise intolerance or asymptomatic
Adenosine deaminase	Deficiency	Autosomal recessive	Severe combined immunodeficiency disease and chrondro-osseous dysplasia
Purine nucleoside phosphorylase	Deficiency	Autosomal recessive	T cell–mediated immunodeficiency

HYPOURICEMIA

Hypouricemia, defined as a serum urate concentration <120 μmol/L (2.0 mg/dL) can result from decreased production of urate, increased excretion of uric acid, or a combination of both mechanisms. It occurs in <0.2% of the general population and <0.8% of hospitalized individuals. Hypouricemia causes no symptoms or pathology and therefore requires no therapy.

Most hypouricemia results from increased renal uric acid excretion. The finding of normal amounts of uric acid in a 24-h urine collection in an individual with hypouricemia is evidence for a renal cause. Medications with uricosuric properties (Table 338-2) include aspirin (at doses >2.0 g/d), x-ray contrast materials, and glycerylguaiacholate. Total parenteral hyperalimentation can also cause hypouricemia, possibly a result of the high glycine content of the infusion formula. Other causes of increased urate clearance include conditions such as neo-plastic disease, hepatic cirrhosis, diabetes mellitus, and inappropriate secretion of vasopressin; defects in renal tubular transport such as primary Fanconi syndrome and Fanconi syndromes caused by Wilson's disease, cystinosis, multiple myeloma, and heavy metal toxicity; and isolated congenital defects in the bidirectional transport of uric acid. Hypouricemia can also be caused by inherited forms of decreased urate production.

SELECTED INBORN ERRORS OF PURINE METABOLISM

(See also Table 338-3, Fig. 338-3)

HPRT DEFICIENCY The HPRT gene is located on the X chromosome. Affected males are hemizygous for the mutant gene; carrier females are asymptomatic. A complete deficiency of HPRT, the Lesch-Nyhan syndrome, is characterized by hyperuricemia, self-mutilative behavior, choreoathetosis, spasticity, and mental retardation. A partial deficiency of HPRT, the Kelley-Seegmiller syndrome, is associated with hyperuricemia but no central nervous system manifestations. In both disorders, the hyperuricemia results from urate overproduction and can cause uric acid crystalluria, nephrolithiasis, obstructive uropathy, and gouty arthritis. Early diagnosis and appropriate therapy with allopurinol can prevent or eliminate all the problems attributable to hyperuricemia but have no effect on the behavioral or neurologic abnormalities.

INCREASED PRPP SYNTHETASE ACTIVITY Like the HPRT deficiency states, PRPP synthetase overactivity is X-linked and results in gouty arthritis and uric acid nephrolithiasis. Nerve deafness occurs in some families.

ADENINE PHOSPHORIBOSYLTRANSFERASE (APRT) DEFICIENCY APRT deficiency is inherited as an autosomal recessive trait. Affected individuals develop kidney stones composed of 2,8-dihydroxyadenine. Caucasians with the disorder have a complete deficiency (type I), whereas Japanese subjects have some measurable enzyme activity (type II). Expression of the defect is similar in the two populations, as is the frequency of the heterozygous state (0.4 to 1.1 per 100). Allopurinol treatment prevents stone formation.

HEREDITARY XANTHINURIA A deficiency of xanthine oxidase causes all purine in the urine to occur in the form of hypoxanthine and xanthine. About two-thirds of deficient individuals are asymptomatic. The remainder develop kidney stones composed of xanthine.

MYOADENYLATE DEAMINASE DEFICIENCY Primary (inherited) and secondary (acquired) forms of myoadenylate deaminase deficiency have been described. The primary form is inherited as an autosomal recessive trait. Clinically, some may have relatively mild myopathic symptoms with exercise or other triggers, but most individuals with this defect are asymptomatic. Therefore, another explanation for the myopathy should be sought in symptomatic patients with this deficiency. The acquired deficiency occurs in association with a wide variety of neuromuscular disease, including muscular dystrophies, neuropathies, inflammatory myopathies, and collagen vascular diseases.

ADENYLOSUCCINATE LYASE DEFICIENCY Deficiency of this enzyme is due to an autosomal recessive trait and

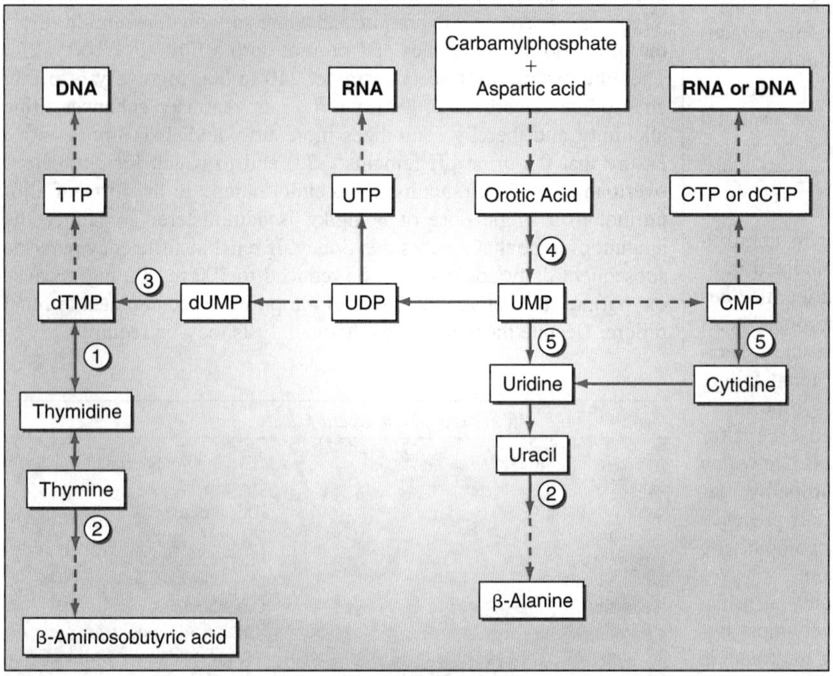

FIGURE 338-4 Abbreviated scheme of pyrimidine metabolism. (1) thymidine kinase, (2) dihydropyrimidine dehydrogenase, (3) thymidylate synthase, (4) UMP synthase, (5) 5'-nucleotidase. CMP, cytidine-5'-monophosphate; UMP, uridine-5'-monophosphate; UDP, uridine-5'-diphosphate; dUMP, deoxyuridine-5'-monophosphate; dTMP, deoxythymidine-5'monophosphate.

causes profound psychomotor retardation, seizures, and other movement disorders. All individuals with this deficiency are mentally retarded, and most are autistic.

ADENOSINE DEAMINASE DEFICIENCY AND PURINE NUCLEOSIDE PHOSPHORYLASE DEFICIENCY See Chap. 297.

PYRIMIDINE DISORDERS

The pyrimidine, cytidine, is found in both DNA and RNA; it is a complementary base pair for guanine. Thymidine is found only in DNA where it is paired with adenine. Uridine is found only in RNA and can pair with either adenine or guanine in RNA secondary structures. Pyrimidines can be synthesized by a de novo pathway (Fig. 338-4) or reused in a salvage pathway. Although more than 25 different enzymes are involved in pyrimidine metabolism, disorders of these pathways are rare. Seven disorders of pyrimidine metabolism have been discovered (Table 338-4), three of which are discussed below.

OROTIC ACIDURIA Hereditary orotic aciduria is caused by mutations in a bifunctional enzyme, uridine-5'-monophosphate (UMP) synthase, which converts orotic acid to UMP in the de novo synthesis pathway (Fig. 338-4). The disorder is characterized by hypochromic megaloblastic anemia that is unresponsive to vitamin B_{12} and folic acid, growth retardation, and neurologic abnormalities. Increased excretion of orotic acid causes crystalluria and obstructive uropathy. Replacement of uridine (100 to 200 mg/kg per day) corrects the anemia, reduces orotic acid excretion, and improves the other sequelae of the disorder.

PYRIMIDINE 5'-NUCLEOTIDASE DEFICIENCY Pyrimidine 5'-nucleotidase catalyzes the removal of the phosphate group from pyrimidine ribonucleoside monophosphates (cytidine-5'-monophosphate or UMP) (Fig. 338-4). An inherited deficiency of this enzyme causes hemolytic anemia with prominent basophilic stippling of erythrocytes. The accumulation of pyrimidines or cytidine diphosphate choline (CDPC) is thought to induce hemolysis. There is no specific treatment. Acquired pyrimidine 5'nucleotidase deficiency has been reported in lead poisoning and in thalassemia.

DIHYDROPYRIMIDINE DEHYDROGENASE DEFICIENCY Dihydropyrimidine dehydrogenase (DPD) is the rate-limiting enzyme in the pathway of uracil and thymine degradation (Fig. 338-4). Deficiency of this enzyme causes excessive urinary excretion of uracil and thymine. DPD deficiency causes nonspecific cerebral dysfunction with convulsive disorders, motor retardation, and mental retardation. No specific treatment is available.

TABLE 338-4 *Inborn Errors of Pyrimidine Metabolism*

Enzyme	Activity	Inheritance	Clinical Features
Uridine-5'-monophosphate synthetase	Deficiency	Autosomal recessive	Aortic acid crystalluria; obstructive uropathy, hypochromic megaloblastic anemia
Pyrimidine 5'-nucleotidase	Deficiency	Autosomal recessive	Hemolytic anemia
Pyrimidine 5'-nucleotidase	Superactivity	Uncertain	Developmental delay, seizures, ataxia, language deficit
Thymidine phosphorylase	Deficiency	Autosomal recessive	Mitochondrial neurogastrointestinal encephalopathy
Dihydropyrimidine dehydrogenase	Deficiency	Autosomal recessive	Seizures, motor and mental retardation
Dihydropyrimidinase	Deficiency	Uncertain	Seizures, mental retardation
Ureidopropionase	Deficiency	Uncertain	Hypotonia, dystonia, developmental delay

MEDICATION EFFECTS ON PYRIMIDINE METABOLISM A variety of medications can influence pyrimidine metabolism. The anticancer agents fluorodeoxyuridine and 5-fluorouracil (5-FU) and the antimicrobial agent fluorocytosine cause cytotoxicity when converted to fluorodeoxyuridylate (FdUMP), a specific suicide inhibitor of thymidylate synthase. Fluorocytosine must be converted to 5-FU to be effective. This conversion is catalyzed by cytosine deaminase activity. Fluorocytosine's action is selective because cytosine deaminase is present in bacteria and fungi but not in human cells.

DPD is involved in the degradation of 5-FU. Consequently, deficiency of this enzyme is associated with 5-FU neurotoxicity.

Leflunomide, which is used to treat rheumatoid arthritis, inhibits de novo pyrimidine synthesis by inhibiting dihydroorotate dehydrogenase, resulting in an antiproliferative effect on T cells. Allopurinol, which is used to block xanthine oxidase and purine synthesis, also inhibits orotidine-5'-phosphate decarboxylase, a step in UMP synthesis. Consequently, allopurinol use is associated with increased excretion of orotidine and orotic acid; there are no known clinical effects of this inhibition.

FURTHER READING

BECKER MA: Hyperuricemia and gout, in *The Metabolic and Molecular Bases of Inherited Disease*, 8th ed, CR Scriver et al (eds). New York, McGraw-Hill, 2001, pp 2513–2535

CULLETON BF et al: Serum uric acid risk for cardiovascular disease and death: The Framingham heart study. Ann Intern Med 131:7, 1999

FAM AG: Gout, diet, and the insulin resistance syndrome. J Rheumatol 29: 1350, 2002

WEBSTER DR et al: Hereditary orotic aciduria and other disorders of pyrimidine metabolism, in *The Metabolic and Molecular Bases of Inherited Disease*, 8th ed, CR Scriver et al (eds). New York, McGraw-Hill, 2001, pp 2663–2702

WORTMANN RL, KELLEY WN: Gout and hyperuricemia, in *Kelly's Textbook of Rheumatology*, 6th ed, ED Harris, Jr, S Ruddy, CB Sledge (eds). Philadelphia, Saunders, 2001, pp 1339–1376

339 WILSON DISEASE
George J. Brewer

Wilson disease is an autosomal recessive disorder caused by mutations in the *ATP7B* gene, a membrane-bound copper-transporting ATPase. Clinical manifestations are caused by copper toxicity and primarily involve the liver and the brain. Because effective treatment is available, it is important to make this diagnosis early.

GENETIC CONSIDERATIONS The frequency of Wilson disease in most populations is about 1 in 40,000, and the frequency of carriers of *ATP7B* mutations is about 1%. Based on these gene frequencies, the risk of Wilson disease in the children of an affected patient

is about 1 in 200. Because a large number of inactivating mutations have been reported in the *ATP7B* gene, mutation screening is not practical, but DNA haplotype analysis can be used to genotype siblings of an affected patient.

PATHOGENESIS ATP7B protein deficiency impairs biliary copper excretion, resulting in positive copper balance, hepatic copper accumulation, and copper toxicity from oxidant damage. Excess hepatic copper is initially bound to metallothionein, but as this storage capacity is exceeded, liver damage begins as early as 3 years of age. Defective copper incorporation into apoceruloplasmin leads to excess catabolism and low blood levels of ceruloplasmin. Serum copper levels are usually lower than normal because of low blood ceruloplasmin, which normally binds >90% of serum copper. As the disease progresses, non-

TABLE 339-1 Useful Diagnosis Tests for Wilson Disease

Test	Usefulness[a]	Normal Value	Heterozygous Carriers	Wilson Disease
Serum ceruloplasmin	+	180–350 mg/L (18–35 mg/dL)	Low in 20%	Low in 85%
KF rings	++	Absent	Absent	Present in 99% + if neurologic or psychiatric symptoms present
				Present in 30–50% in hepatic presentation and presymptomatic state
24-h urine Cu	+++	0.3–0.8 μmol (20–50 μg)	Normal to 1.3 μmol (80 μg)	>1.6 μmol (>100 μg) in symptomatic patients
				0.9 to >1.6 μmol (60 to >100 μg) in presymptomatic patients
Liver Cu	++++	0.3–0.8 μmol/g (20–50 μg) tissue	Normal to 2.0 μmol (125 μg)	>3.1 μmol (200 μg) (obstructive liver disease can cause false-positive results)
Haplotype analysis	++++ (Siblings only)	0 Matches	1 Match	2 Matches

[a] Usefulness: +, somewhat useful, to ++++, very useful.
Abbreviations: KF, Kayser-Fleischer; Cu, copper.

ceruloplasmin serum copper ("free") levels increase, resulting in copper buildup in other parts of the body, such as the brain, leading to neurologic and psychiatric disease.

CLINICAL PRESENTATION ■ **Hepatic** Wilson disease may present as hepatitis, cirrhosis, or as hepatic decompensation, typically in the mid- to late-teenage years in western countries, although the age of presentation is quite broad and extends into the fourth decade of life. In India and countries in the Far East, the hepatic presentation may occur much earlier, often in children only five or six years of age.

An episode of hepatitis may occur, with elevated blood transaminase enzymes, with or without jaundice, and then spontaneously regress. Hepatitis often reoccurs, and most of these patients eventually develop cirrhosis.

Hepatic decompensation is associated with elevated serum bilirubin, reduced serum albumin and coagulation factors, ascites, peripheral edema, and hepatic encephalopathy. In severe hepatic failure, hemolytic anemia may occur because large amounts of copper are released into the bloodstream. The association of hemolysis and liver disease makes Wilson disease a likely diagnosis.

Neurologic The neurologic manifestations of Wilson disease typically occur in patients in their early twenties, although the age of onset extends from the second to the fifth decades of life. Magnetic resonance imaging and computed tomography scans reveal damage in the basal ganglia and occasionally in the pons, medulla, thalamus, cerebellum, and subcortical areas. The three main neurologic problems are of a movement disorder type: dystonia, incoordination, and tremor. Dysarthria and dysphagia are common. In some patients, the clinical picture closely resembles that of Parkinson's disease. Dystonia can involve any part of the body and eventually leads to grotesque positions of the limbs, neck, and trunk. Tremor, which is common, can be of any type. Autonomic disturbances may include orthostatic hypotension and sweating abnormalities as well as bowel, bladder, and sexual dysfunction. Memory loss, migraine-type headaches, and seizures may occur. Patients have difficulties focusing on tasks, but cognition is not usually grossly impaired. Sensory abnormalities and muscular weakness are not features of the disease.

Psychiatric A history of behavioral disturbances, with onset in the five years before diagnosis, is present in half of patients with neurologic disease. The features are diverse and may include loss of emotional control (temper tantrums, crying bouts), depression, hyperactivity, or loss of sexual inhibition.

Other Manifestations Some female patients have repeated spontaneous abortions, and most become amenorrheic prior to diagnosis. Cholelithiasis and nephrolithiasis occur with increased frequencies. Some patients may have osteoarthritis, particularly of the knee. Microscopic hematuria is common, and increased urinary excretion of phosphates, amino acids, glucose, or urates may occur; however, a full-blown Fanconi syndrome is rare. Sunflower cataracts and Kayser-Fleischer rings (copper deposits in the outer rim of the cornea) may be seen. Electrocardiographic and other cardiac abnormalities have been reported but are not common.

DIAGNOSIS Diagnostic tests for Wilson disease are listed in Table 339-1. Serum ceruloplasmin levels should be used only to affect the index of suspicion, because they are not always low in affected patients and are reduced in 20% of carriers. Kayser-Fleischer rings can only be diagnosed definitively by an ophthalmologist using a slit lamp. They are present in >99% of patients with neurologic/psychiatric forms of the disease and have been described very rarely in the absence of Wilson disease. Kayser-Fleischer rings are present in only about 30 to 50% of patients diagnosed in the hepatic or presymptomatic state; thus, the absence of rings does not exclude the diagnosis.

Symptomatic patients invariably have urine copper levels > 1.6 μmol (>100 μg) per 24 h. Heterozygotes never have values >1.6 μmol (>100 μg) per 24 h. About half of presymptomatic patients who are ultimately diagnosed as affected have urine copper values in an intermediate range between 0.9 and 1.6 μmol (60 and 100 μg) per 24 h. Because heterozygotes may have values up to 1.3 μmol (80 μg) per 24 h, patients in this range may require a liver biopsy for definitive diagnosis.

The "gold standard" for diagnosis remains liver biopsy with quantitative copper assays. Affected patients have values >3.1 μmol/g

TABLE 339-2 Recommended Anticopper Treatments for Wilson Disease

Disease Status	First Choice	Second Choice
Initial hepatic		
Hepatitis or cirrhosis without decompensation	Zinc[a]	Trientine
Hepatic decompensation		
Mild	Trientine[b] and zinc	Penicillamine[b] and zinc
Moderate	Trientine and zinc	Hepatic transplantation
Severe	Hepatic transplantation	Trientine and zinc
Initial neurologic/ psychiatric	Tetrathiomolybdate[c] and zinc	Trientine and zinc
Maintenance	Zinc	Trientine
Presymptomatic	Zinc	Trientine
Pediatric	Zinc	Trientine
Pregnant	Zinc	Trientine

[a] Zinc acetate is supplied as Galzin. Recommended adult dose for all the above indications is 50 mg of elemental zinc three times daily, each dose separated from food and beverages other than water by at least 1 h, and separated from trientine or penicillamine doses by at least 1 h.
[b] Trientine is supplied as Syprine and penicillamine as Cuprimine. Recommended adult dosage for both drugs is 500 mg twice daily, each dose at least ½ h before or 2 h after meals.
[c] Tetrathiomolybdate is not yet commercially available but is expected to be marketed in the near future.

(>200 μg/g) dry weight of liver. Copper stains are not reliable. False-positive results can occur with long-standing obstructive liver disease, which can elevate hepatic and urine copper and rarely causes Kayser-Fleischer rings.

TABLE 339-3 *Prognostic Index of Nazer*

Laboratory Measurement	Normal Value	Score (in Points)				
		0	1	2	3	4
Serum bilirubin*	0.2–1.2 mg/dl	<5.8	5.8–8.8	8.8–11.7	11.7–17.5	>17.5
Serum aspartate transferase (AST)	10–35 IU/L	<100	100–150	151–200	201–300	>300
Prolongation of prothrombin time (seconds)	—	<4	4–8	9–12	13–20	>20

* If hemolysis is present, the serum bilirubin cannot be used as a measure of liver function until the hemolysis subsides.
Source: Modified with permission from Nazer H et al: Wilson's disease: Clinical presentation and use of prognostic index. *Gut* 1986; 27:1377–81, with permission from BMJ Publishing Group.

℞ TREATMENT

Recommended anticopper treatments are listed in Table 339-2. Penicillamine was previously the primary anticopper treatment but now plays a minor role because of its toxicity and because it worsens existing neurologic disease if used as initial therapy. If penicillamine is given, it should always be accompanied by 25 mg/d of pyridoxine. Trientine is a less toxic chelator and has largely supplanted penicillamine.

For patients with hepatitis or cirrhosis, without evidence of hepatic decompensation other than a mildly elevated bilirubin level and without neurologic or psychiatric symptoms from Wilson disease, zinc is the therapy of choice, although some advocate therapy with trientene. Zinc has proven efficacy in Wilson disease and is essentially nontoxic. It produces a negative copper balance by blocking intestinal absorption of copper, and it induces hepatic metallothionein synthesis, which sequesters additional toxic copper. All presymptomatic patients should be treated prophylactically, since the disease is close to 100% penetrant.

The first step in evaluating patients presenting with hepatic decompensation is to establish disease severity, which can be estimated using the Nazer prognostic index (Table 339-3). Patients with scores ≤6 can usually be managed with medical therapy. Patients with scores ≥10 should be considered immediately for liver transplantation, and those with scores between 7 and 9 require clinical judgment as to whether to recommend transplantation or medical therapy. A combination of trientine and zinc has been used to treat patients with Nazer scores as high as 9, but such patients should be watched carefully for indications of hepatic deterioration, which mandates transplantation.

For initial medical therapy of patients with hepatic decompensation, a chelator (trientine is preferred) plus zinc is recommended (Table 339-2). Zinc should not, however, be ingested simultaneously with trientine, as it will chelate zinc and form therapeutically ineffective complexes; the two drugs should be separated by at least 1 h. Hepatic transplantation is necessary for patients with severe hepatic decompensation.

For initial neurologic therapy, tetrathiomolybdate is emerging as the drug of choice because of its rapid action, preservation of neurologic function, and low toxicity. However, until tetrathiomolybdate is commercially available, trientine and zinc are recommended for 8 weeks, at which time the trientine can be stopped, and zinc continued for maintenance therapy. Although hepatic transplantation may improve neurologic symptoms, it does so only by removing copper, which can be done more safely and inexpensively with anticopper drugs.

Anticopper therapy must be lifelong. With treatment, liver function usually recovers after about a year, although residual liver damage is usually present. Neurologic and psychiatric symptoms usually improve between 6 and 24 months of treatment.

Monitoring Anticopper Therapy When first using trientine or penicillamine, it is necessary to monitor for drug toxicity, particularly bone marrow suppression and proteinuria. Complete blood counts, standard biochemical profiles, and a urinalysis should be performed at weekly intervals for a month, then at 2-weekly intervals for 2 to 3 months, then at monthly intervals for 3 or 4 months, and at 4- to 6-monthly intervals thereafter.

The anticopper effects of trientine and penicillamine can be monitored by following 24-h "free" serum copper. Changes in urine copper are more difficult to interpret because excretion reflects the effect of the drug, as well as body loading with copper. Free serum copper is calculated by subtracting the ceruloplasmin copper from the total serum copper. Each 10 mg/L (mg/dL) of ceruloplasmin contributes 0.5 μmol/L (3.0 μg/dL) of serum copper. The normal free copper value is 1.6 to 2.4 μmol/L (10 to 15 μg/dL), and it often is as high as 7.9 μmol/L (50 μg/dL) in untreated Wilson disease. With treatment, free copper should be <3.9 μmol/L (<25 μg/dL).

Zinc treatment does not require blood or urine monitoring for toxicity. Its only significant side effect is gastric burning or nausea in about 10% of patients, usually with the first morning dose. This can be mitigated by taking the first dose an hour after breakfast or taking the zinc with a small amount of protein. Because zinc mainly affects stool copper, 24-h urine copper can be used to reflect body loading. The typical value in untreated symptomatic patients is >3.1 μmol (>200 μg) per 24 h. This level should decrease during the first 1 to 2 years of therapy to <2.0 μmol (<125 μg) per 24 h. A normal value [0.3 to 0.8 μmol (20 to 50 μg)] is rarely reached during the first decade of therapy and should raise concern about overtreatment (copper deficiency), the first sign of which is anemia and/or leukopenia.

FURTHER READING

BREWER GJ: Recognition, diagnosis and management of Wilson's disease. Proc Soc Ex Biol Med 223:39, 2000

BREWER GJ et al: Treatment of Wilson disease with ammonium tetrathiomolybdate: III. Initial therapy in 55 neurologically affected patients and follow-up with zinc therapy. Arch Neurol 60:379, 2003

———: Treatment of Wilson's disease with zinc: XV. Long-term follow-up studies. J Lab Clin Med 132:264, 1998

BULL PC et al: The Wilson disease gene is a putative copper transporting P-type ATPase similar to the Menkes gene. Nature Genet 5:327, 1993

COX DW, ROBERTS EA: Wilson Disease. GeneClinics, University of Washington, Seattle. Online. Available at *http://www.geneclinics.org/profiles/wilson/details.html*

SCHILSKY ML et al: Liver transplantation for Wilson's disease: Indications and outcome. Hepatology 19:583, 1994

340 LYSOSOMAL STORAGE DISEASES
Robert J. Hopkin, Gregory A. Grabowski

Lysosomes are heterogeneous subcellular organelles containing specific hydrolyases that allow targeted processing or degradation of proteins, nucleic acids, carbohydrates, and lipids. There are >30 different lysosomal storage diseases and these are classified based on the nature of the stored material (Table 340-1). The most prevalent among these disorders in adults will be reviewed here, including Fabry disease, Gaucher disease, and Niemann-Pick disease. Lysosomal storage diseases should be considered in the differential diagnosis of patients with neurologic, renal, or muscular degeneration and unexplained hepatomegaly, splenomegaly, cardiomyopathy, or skeletal dysplasias and deformations. Physical findings are disease-specific, and definitive diagnosis is made by enzyme assays.

TABLE 340-1   Selected Lysosomal Storage Diseases

Disorder[a]	Enzyme Deficiency	Stored Material	Clinical Types (Onset)	Inheritance	Neurologic
MUCOPOLYSACCHARIDOSES (MPS)					
MPS I H, Hurler (136)	α-L-Iduronidase	Dermatan sulfate Heparan sulfate	Infantile	AR	Mental retardation
MPS I H/S, Hurler/Scheie			Intermediate		Mental retardation
MPS I S, Scheie			Adult		None
MPS II, Hunter (136)	Iduronate sulfatase	Dermatan sulfate Heparan sulfate	Severe infantile Mild juvenile	X-linked	Mental retardation, less in mild form
MPS III A, Sanfilippo A (136)	Heparan-N-sulfatase	Heparan sulfate	Late infantile	AR	Severe mental retardation
MPS III B, Sanfilippo B	N-Acetyl-α-glucosaminidase	Heparan sulfate	Late infantile	AR	Severe mental retardation
MPS III C, Sanfilippo C	Acetyl-CoA: α-glucosaminide N-acetyltransferase	Heparan sulfate	Late infantile	AR	Severe mental retardation
MPS III D, Sanfilippo D	N-Acetylglucosamine-6-sulfate sulfatase	Heparan sulfate	Late infantile	AR	Severe mental retardation
MPS IV A, Morquio (136)	N-Acetylgalactosamine-6-sulfate sulfatase	Keratan sulfate Chondroitin-6 sulfate	Childhood	AR	None
MPS VI B, Morquio (136)	β-Galactosidase		Childhood	AR	None
MPS VI, Maroteaux-Lamy (136)	Arylsulfatase B	Dermatan sulfate	Late infantile	AR	None
MPS VII (136)	β-Glucuronidase	Dermatan sulfate Heparan sulfate	Neonatal Infantile Adult	AR	Mental retardation, absent in some adults
GM₂ GANGLIOSIDOSES					
Tay-Sachs' disease (153)	β-Hexosaminidase A	GM_2 gangliosides	Infantile Juvenile	AR	Mental retardation, seizures, later juvenile form
Sandhoff's disease (153)	β-Hexosaminidases A and B	GM_2 gangliosides	Infantile	AR	Mental retardation, seizures
NEUTRAL GLYCOSPHINGOLIPIDOSES					
Fabry disease (150)	α-Galactosidase A	Globotriaosylceramide	Childhood	X-linked	Painful acroparesthesias
Gaucher disease (146)	Acid β-glucosidase	Glucosylceramide	Type 1 Type 2 Type 3	AR	None ++++ ++
Niemann-Pick disease (144) A and B	Sphingomyelinase	Sphingomyelin	Neuronopathic, type A Nonneuronopathic, type B	AR	Mental retardation and seizures
GLYCOPROTEINOSES					
Fucosidosis (140)	α-Fucosidase	Glycopeptides, oligosaccharides	Infantile Juvenile	AR	Mental retardation
α-Mannosidosis (140)	α-Mannosidase	Oligosaccharides	Infantile Milder variant	AR	Mental retardation
β-Mannosidosis (140)	β-Mannosidase	Oligosaccharides		AR	Seizures, mental retardation
Aspartylglucosaminuria (140)	Aspartylglucosaminidase	Aspartylglucosamine, glycopeptides	Young adult onset	AR	Mental retardation
Sialidosis (140)	Neuraminidase	Sialyloligosaccharides	Type I, congenital Type II, infantile and juvenile forms	AR	Myoclonus, mental retardation
MUCOLIPIDOSES (ML)					
ML-II, I-cell disease (138)	UDP-N-Acetylglucosamine-1-phosphotransferase	Glycoprotein, glyco-lipids	Infantile	AR	Mental retardation
ML-III, pseudo-Hurler polydystrophy (138)	UDP-N-Acetylglucosamine-1-phosphotransferase	Glycoprotein, glyco-lipids	Late infantile	AR	Mild mental retardation
LEUKODYSTROPHIES					
Krabbe's disease (147)	Galactosylceramidase	Galactosylceramide, Galactosyl sphingosine	Infantile	AR	Mental retardation
Metachromatic leukodystrophy (148)	Arylsulfatase A	Cerebroside sulfate	Infantile Juvenile Adult	AR	Mental retardation, dementia, and psychosis in adult
Multiple sulfatase deficiency (149)	Active site cysteine to C_α-formylglycine-converting enzyme	Sulfatides, mucopolysaccharides	Late infantile	AR	Mental retardation
DISORDERS OF NEUTRAL LIPIDS					
Wolman disease (142)	Acid lysosomal lipase	Cholesterol esters, triglycerides	Infantile	AR	Mild mental retardation
Cholesteryl ester storage disease (142)	Acid lysosomal lipase	Cholesteryl esters	Childhood	AR	None
Farber disease (142)	Acid ceramidase	Ceramide	Infantile Juvenile	AR	Occasional mental retardation

[a] Numbers in parentheses refer to the chapters in Scriver et al, 8th edition, for detailed reviews.   *Note:* AR, autosomal recessive.

Liver Spleen Enlargement	Skeletal Disease	Ophthalmologic	Hematologic	Unique Features
		Clinical Features		
+++	++++	Corneal clouding	Vacuolated lymphocytes	Coarse facies, cardiovascular involvement, joint stiffness
+++	++++	Retinal degeneration, no corneal clouding	Granulated lymphocytes	Coarse facies, cardiovascular, joint stiffness, distinctive pebbly skin lesions
+	+	None	Granulated lymphocytes	Mild coarse facies
+	+	None	Granulated lymphocytes	Mild coarse facies
+	+	None	Granulated lymphocytes	Mild coarse facies
+	+	None	Granulated lymphocytes	Mild coarse facies
+	++++	Corneal clouding	Granulated neutrophils	Distinctive skeletal deformity, odontoid hypoplasia, aortic valve disease
±	++++			
++	++++	Corneal clouding	Granulated neutrophils and lymphocytes	Coarse facies, valvular heart disease
+++	+++	Corneal clouding	Granulated neutrophils	Coarse facies, vascular involvement, hydrops fetalis in neonatal form
None	None	Cherry red spot in infantile form	None	Macrocephaly, hyperacusis in infantile form
++	±	Cherry red spot	None	Macrocephaly, hyperacusis
None	None	Corneal dystrophy, vascular lesions	None	Cutaneous angiokeratomas, hypohydrosis
++++	++++	None	Gaucher cells in bone marrow, cytopenias	Adult form highly variable
+++	+	Eye movements		
++++	++++	Eye movements		
++++	None	Macular degeneration	Foam cells in bone marrow	Pulmonary infiltrates
	Osteoporosis			Lung failure
++	++	None	Vacuolated lymphocytes, foam cells	Coarse facies, angiokeratomas in juvenile form
+++	++	Cataracts, corneal clouding	Vacuolated lymphocytes, granulated neutrophils	Coarse facies, enlarged tongue
	++	None	Vacuolated lymphocytes, foam cells	Angiokeratomas
±	++	None	Vacuolated lymphocytes, foam cells	Coarse facies
++, less in type I	++ less in type I	Cherry red spot	Vacuolated lymphocytes	MPS phenotype in type II
±	++++	Corneal clouding	Vacuolated and granulated neutrophils	Coarse facies, absence of mucopolysacchariduria, gingival hypoplasia
None	+++	Corneal clouding, mild retinopathy, hyperopic astigmatism		Coarse facies, stiffness of hands and shoulders
None	None	None	None	White matter globoid cells
None	None	Optic atrophy	None	Gait abnormalities in late infantile form
+	++	Retinal degeneration	Vacuolated and granulated cells	Absent activity of all known cellular sulfatases
+++	None	None	None	Adrenal calcification
Hepatomegaly	None	None	None	Cirrhosis
+/−	None	Macular degeneration	None	Arthropathy, subcutaneous nodules

2317

PATHOGENESIS OF LYSOSOMAL STORAGE DISEASES

Lysosomal biogenesis involves ongoing synthesis of lysosomal hydrolases, membrane constitutive proteins, and new membranes. Lysosomes originate from the fusion of *trans*-Golgi network (TGN) vesicles with late endosomes. Progressive vesicular acidification accompanies the maturation of TGN vesicles, and this gradient facilitates the pH-dependent dissociation of receptors and ligands, as well as activating lysosomal hydrolases.

Abnormalities at any biosynthetic step can impair enzyme activation and lead to a lysosomal storage disorder. Following leader sequence clipping, complex oligosaccharide modifications occur during transit through the Golgi, including the mannose-6-phosphate modification of high-mannose oligosaccharide chains of many soluble lysosomal hydrolases. Lysosomal integral or associated membrane proteins are sorted to the membrane or interior of the lysosome by several different signals. Phosphorylation, sulfation, additional proteolytic processing, and macromolecular assembly of heteromers occur concurrently. These are critical to enzyme function, and defects can result in multiple enzyme/protein deficiencies.

The final common pathway for lysosomal storage diseases is the accumulation of specific macromolecules within tissues and cells that normally have a high flux of these substrates. The majority of lysosomal enzyme deficiencies result from point mutations or genetic rearrangements at a locus that encodes a single lysosomal hydrolase. However, some mutations cause deficiencies of several different lysosomal hydrolases by altering the enzymes/proteins involved in targeting, active site modifications, or macromolecular association or trafficking. All are inherited as autosomal recessive disorders, except Hunter (mucopolysaccharidosis, type II) and Fabry diseases, which are X-linked. Substrate accumulation leads to lysosomal distortion, which has significant pathologic consequences. In addition, abnormal amounts of metabolites may also have pharmacologic effects important to disease pathophysiology.

For many lysosomal diseases, the accumulated substrates are endogenously synthesized within particular tissue sites of pathology. Other diseases have greater exogenous substrate supplies, For example, they are delivered by low-density lipoprotein receptor–mediated uptake in Fabry and cholesteryl ester storage diseases or by phagocytosis in Gaucher disease type 1. The *threshold hypothesis* refers to a level of enzyme activity below which disease develops. Consequently, small changes in enzyme activity near the threshold can lead to or prevent disease. A critical element of this model is that enzymatic activity can be challenged by changes in substrate flux based on genetic background, cell turnover, recycling, or metabolic demands. Thus, a set level of residual enzyme may be adequate for substrate in some tissues or cells, but not in others.

SELECTED DISORDERS

TAY-SACHS DISEASE About 1 in 30 Ashkenazi Jews is a carrier for Tay-Sachs disease, which is caused by total hexosaminidase A (Hex A) deficiency. The infantile form is a fatal neurodegenerative disease with macrocephaly, loss of motor skills, increased startle reaction, and a macular cherry red spot. The juvenile-onset form presents with ataxia and dementia, with death by age 10 to 15 years. The adult-onset disorder is characterized by clumsiness in childhood; progressive motor weakness in adolescence; and additional spinocerebellar, lower motor neuron symptoms, and dysarthria in adulthood. Intelligence declines slowly, and psychosis is common. Screening for Tay-Sachs disease carriers is recommended in the Ashkenazi Jewish population. *Sandhoff disease* is nearly identical to Tay-Sachs disease, but hepatosplenomegaly and bony dysplasias are also present.

FABRY DISEASE Fabry disease is an X-linked disorder that results from mutations in the α-galactosidase gene. The estimated prevalence of hemizygous males is 1/40,000. Clinically, the disease manifests with angiokeratomas (telangiectatic skin lesions); hypohidrosis; corneal and lenticular opacities; acroparesthesia; and small-vessel disease of the kidney, heart, and brain.

The angiokeratomas and acroparesthesia may appear in childhood and lead to early diagnosis, if suspected. Angiokeratomas are punctate, dark red to blue-black, flat or slightly raised, usually symmetric, and do not blanch with pressure. They range from barely visible to several millimeters in diameter and have a tendency to increase in size and number with age. They usually are most dense between the umbilicus and knees—"the bathing suit area"—but may occur anywhere, including the mucosal surfaces. Angiokeratomas also occur in Fordyce scrotal angiokeratoma and several other lysosomal storage diseases. Corneal and lenticular lesions, detectable on slit-lamp examination, may help in establishing a diagnosis. Debilitating episodic burning pain of the hands, feet, and proximal extremities, acroparesthesia, can last from minutes to days and can be precipitated by changes in temperature, exercise, fatigue, or fever. Abdominal pain can resemble that from appendicitis or renal colic. Proteinuria, isosthenuria, and progressive renal dysfunction occur in the second to fourth decades. Hypertension, left ventricular hypertrophy, anginal chest pain with or without myocardial ischemia or infarction, and congestive heart failure can occur in the third to fourth decades. Leg lymphedema without hypoproteinemia and episodic diarrhea also occur. Death is due to renal failure or cardiovascular or cerebrovascular disease in untreated patients. Variants with residual α-galactosidase activity may have late-onset manifestations limited to the cardiovascular system that resemble hypertrophic cardiomyopathy. Up to 70% of heterozygous females may exhibit clinical manifestations, including central nervous system (CNS) and cardiac disease, but usually do not develop renal failure.

Phenytoin and carbamazepine diminish the chronic and episodic acroparesthesia. Chronic hemodialysis or kidney transplantation can be lifesaving in patients with renal failure. Enzyme therapy clears stored lipids from a variety of cells, particularly those of the renal, cardiac, and skin vascular endothelium. Renal insufficiency appears irreversible. Early institution of enzyme therapy likely will prevent or slow the progression of the life-threatening complications.

GAUCHER DISEASE Gaucher disease is an autosomal recessive disorder that results from defective activity of acid β-glucosidase; >175 mutations have been described. Disease variants are classified based on the absence or presence and severity of neuronopathic involvement.

Type 1 Gaucher disease is a nonneuronopathic disease that can present in childhood to adulthood with slowly to rapidly progressive visceral disease. The average age at diagnosis is ~20 years in Caucasian populations and somewhat younger in other groups. This pattern of presentation is distinctly bimodal, with peaks at <10 to 15 years and at ~25 years. Younger patients tend to have a greater degree of hepatosplenomegaly and accompanying blood cytopenias. In contrast, the older group has a greater tendency for chronic bone disease. Hepatosplenomegaly occurs in virtually all symptomatic patients and can be minor or massive. Accompanying anemia and thrombocytopenia are variable and are not linearly related to liver or spleen volume. Severe liver dysfunction is unusual. Splenic infarctions can resemble an acute abdomen. Pulmonary hypertension and alveolar Gaucher cell accumulation are uncommon, but life-threatening, and can occur at any age.

All patients with Gaucher disease have nonuniform infiltration of bone marrow by lipid-laden macrophages, termed *Gaucher cells*. This can lead to marrow packing with subsequent infarction, ischemia, necrosis, and cortical bone destruction. Bone marrow involvement spreads from proximal to distal in the limbs and can involve the axial skeleton extensively, causing vertebral collapse. In addition to bone marrow involvement, bone remodeling is defective, with loss of total bone calcium leading to osteopenia, osteonecrosis, avascular infarction, and vertebral compression fractures and spinal cord involvement. Aseptic necrosis of the femoral head is common, as is fracture of the femoral neck. The mechanism by which diseased bone marrow macrophages interact with osteoclasts and/or osteoblasts to cause bone disease is not well understood. Chronic, ill-defined bone pain can be debilitating and poorly correlated with radiographic findings. "Bone crises" are associated with localized, excruciating pain, and, on occasion, local erythema, fever, and leukocytosis. Some patients have frequent crises, whereas other patients experience only one. These crises represent acute infarctions of bone, as evidenced in nuclear scans by localized absent uptake of pyrophosphate agents. Osteomyelitis should be excluded by appropriate cultures.

Decreased acid β-glucosidase activity (0 to 20% of normal) in nucleated cells makes the diagnosis. The enzyme is not present in bodily fluids. The sensitivity of enzyme testing is poor for heterozygote detection; molecular testing is preferred when the mutations are known. The disease frequency varies from about 1 in 1000 in Ashkenazi Jews to <1 in 100,000 in other populations. About 1 in 12 to 15 Ashkenazi Jews carries a Gaucher disease allele. Four common mutations account for ~90 to 95% of the mutations in affected patients: N370S (1226G), 84GG (a G insertion at cDNA position 84), L444P (1448C), and IVS-2 (an intron 2 splice junction mutation).

Genotype/phenotype studies indicate a significant correlation, though not absolute, between disease type and severity and the acid β-glucosidase genotype. The most common mutation in the Ashkenazi Jewish population (N370S) shares a 100% association with nonneuronopathic type 1 Gaucher disease. The N370S/N370S and N370S/other mutant allele genotypes are associated with later onset/less severe and with earlier onset/severe disease, respectively. As many as 50 to 60% of patients with the N370S/N370S genotype are discovered as asymptomatic family members. The other alleles are L444P (very low activity), 84GG (null), or IVS-2 (null), and rare/private or uncharacterized alleles. The L444P/L444P patients almost always have life-threatening to very severe/early-onset disease, and many, though not all, develop CNS involvement in the first two decades of life.

Symptomatic management of the blood cytopenias and joint replacement surgeries continue to have important roles in management. However, enzyme therapy is currently the treatment of choice in significantly affected patients and is highly efficacious and safe in diminishing the hepatosplenomegaly and improving bone marrow involvement and hematologic findings. The bone disease is decreased but not eliminated by enzyme replacement therapy. Adult patients may benefit from adjunctive treatment with bisphosphonates, which improves bone mineralization.

Type 2 Gaucher disease is a rare, severe CNS disease that leads to death by 2 years of age. *Type 3 Gaucher disease* has highly variable manifestations in the CNS and viscera. It can present in early childhood with rapidly progressive, massive visceral disease and slowly progressive to static CNS involvement; in adolescence with dementia; or in early adulthood with rapidly progressive, uncontrollable myoclonic seizures and mild visceral disease. Visceral disease in type 3 is nearly identical to that in type 1 but is generally more severe. Early CNS findings may be limited to defects in lateral gaze tracking, which may remain static for decades. Mental retardation can be slowly progressive or static. This variant is most frequent among individuals of Swedish descent.

NIEMANN-PICK DISEASE This is an autosomal recessive disorder that results from defects in acid sphingomyelinase. Types A and B are distinguished by an early age of onset and progressive CNS disease in type A. Type A typically has onset in the first 6 months, with rapidly progressive CNS deterioration, spasticity, failure to thrive, and massive hepatosplenomegaly. In contrast, B has a later, more variable onset and progression of hepatosplenomegaly, with eventual development of cirrhosis and hepatic replacement by foam cells. Affected patients develop progressive pulmonary disease with dyspnea, hypoxemia, and a reticular infiltrative pattern on chest x-ray. Foam cells are present in alveoli, lymphatic vessels, and pulmonary arteries. Progressive hepatic or lung disease lead to demise in adolescence to early adulthood.

The diagnosis is established by markedly decreased (1 to 10% of normal) sphingomyelinase activity in nucleated cells. There is no specific treatment for Neimann-Pick disease. The efficacy of hepatic or bone marrow transplantation has not been proven. Clinical trials using enzyme therapy are anticipated in the near future.

FURTHER READING

RISCH N: *Molecular epidemiology of Tay-Sachs disease.* Adv Genet 44:233, 2001

SCHIFFMANN R, BRADY RO: *New prospects for the treatment of lysosomal storage diseases.* Drugs 62:733, 2002

SCRIVER CR et al (eds): *The Metabolic and Molecular Bases of Inherited Diseases*, 8th ed. New York, McGraw-Hill, 2001

ZHAO H, GRABOWSKI GA: *Gaucher disease: Perspectives on a prototype lysosomal disease.* Cell Mol Life Sci 59:694, 2002

341 | GLYCOGEN STORAGE DISEASES AND OTHER INHERITED DISORDERS OF CARBOHYDRATE METABOLISM
Yuan-Tsong Chen

Carbohydrate metabolism plays a vital role in cellular function by providing the energy required for most metabolic processes. The relevant biochemical pathways involved in the metabolism of these carbohydrates are shown in Fig. 341-1. Glucose is the principle substrate of energy metabolism in humans. Metabolism of glucose generates ATP via glycolysis and mitochondrial oxidative phosphorylation. Dietary sources of glucose are obtained by ingesting polysaccharides, primarily starch, and disaccharides including lactose, maltose, and sucrose. Galactose and fructose are two other monosaccharides that provide fuel for cellular metabolism; however, their role as fuel sources is much less significant than that of glucose. Galactose is derived from lactose (galactose + glucose), which is found in milk products, and is an important component for certain glycolipids, glycoproteins, and glycosaminoglycans. The two dietary sources of fructose are sucrose (fructose + glucose), a commonly used sweetener, and fructose itself, which is found in fruits, vegetables, and honey.

Glycogen, the storage form of glucose in animal cells, is composed of glucose residues joined in straight chains by α1-4 linkages and branched at intervals of 4 to 10 residues by α1-6 linkages. Glycogen forms a treelike molecule and can have a molecular weight of many millions; it may aggregate to form structures recognizable by electron microscopy. Defects in glycogen metabolism typically cause an accumulation of glycogen in the tissues; hence, the name *glycogen storage diseases*. The defects in gluconeogenesis or glycolytic pathways, including galactose and fructose metabolism, do not usually result in glycogen accumulation.

Clinical manifestations of the various disorders of carbohydrate metabolism differ markedly. The symptoms range from harmless to lethal. Unlike disorders of lipid metabolism, mucopolysaccharidoses, or other storage diseases, dietary therapy has been effective in many of the carbohydrate disorders. All of the genes responsible for the inherited defects of carbohydrate metabolism have been cloned, and mutations have been identified. Advances in our understanding of the molecular basis of these diseases are being used to improve diagnosis and management, and some of these disorders are candidates for enzyme replacement and early trials of gene therapy.

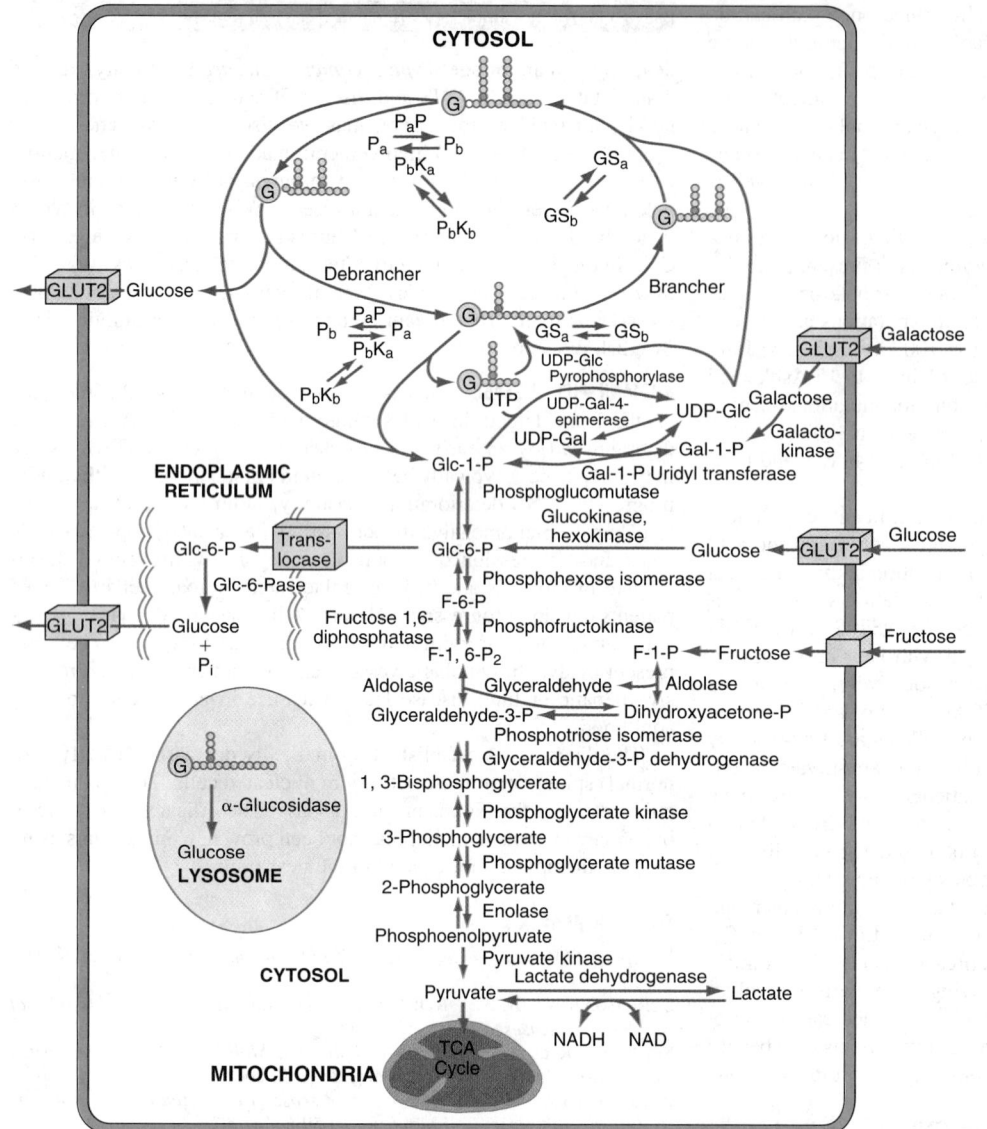

FIGURE 341-1 Metabolic pathways related to glycogen storage diseases and galactose and fructose disorders. Nonstandard abbreviations are as follows: GS$_a$, active glycogen synthase; GS$_b$, inactive glycogen synthase; P$_a$, active phosphorylase; P$_b$, inactive phosphorylase; P$_a$P, phosphorylase a phosphatase; P$_b$K$_a$, active phosphorylase b kinase; P$_b$K$_b$, inactive phosphorylase b kinase; G, glycogenin, the primer protein for glycogen synthesis. [*Modified from AR Beaudet, in KJ Isselbacher et al (eds): Harrison's Principles of Internal Medicine, 13th ed. New York, McGraw-Hill, 1994, p 1855.*]

Historically, the glycogen storage diseases were categorized numerically in the order in which the enzymatic defects were identified. They are also classified by the organs involved and clinical manifestations, the system followed in this chapter (Table 341-1). The overall frequency of all forms of glycogen storage disease is approximately 1 in 20,000 live births; most are inherited as autosomal recessive traits, but phosphoglycerate kinase deficiency and one form of phosphorylase kinase deficiency are X-linked disorders. The most common childhood disorders are glucose-6-phosphatase deficiency (type I), lysosomal acid α-glucosidase deficiency (type II), debrancher deficiency (type III), and liver phosphorylase kinase deficiency (type IX). The most common adult disorder is myophosphorylase deficiency (type V, or McArdle disease).

SELECTED LIVER GLYCOGENOSES

DISORDERS WITH HEPATOMEGALY AND HYPOGLYCEMIA ■ Type I Glycogen Storage Disease (Glucose-6-Phosphatase or Translocase Deficiency, von Gierke Disease) Type I glycogen storage disease is an autosomal recessive disorder that causes glucose-6-phosphatase deficiency in liver, kidney, and intestinal mucosa. It can be divided into two subtypes: type Ia, in which the glucose-6-phosphatase enzyme is defective, and type Ib,

which is due to a defect in the translocase that transports glucose-6-phosphate across the microsomal membrane. The defects in both subtypes lead to inadequate conversion in the liver of glucose-6-phosphate to glucose and thus make affected individuals susceptible to fasting hypoglycemia.

CLINICAL AND LABORATORY FINDINGS Persons with type I disease may develop hypoglycemia and lactic acidosis during the neonatal period, but, more commonly, they present at 3 to 4 months of age with hepatomegaly. Hypoglycemia and lactic acidosis can develop after a short fast. These children often have doll-like faces with fat cheeks, relatively thin extremities, short stature, and a protuberant abdomen that is due to massive hepatomegaly; the kidneys are enlarged, but the spleen and heart are of normal size. The hepatocytes are distended by glycogen and fat with large and prominent lipid vacuoles. Despite hepatomegaly, liver enzymes are usually normal or near normal. Easy bruising and epistaxis are associated with a prolonged bleeding time as a result of impaired platelet aggregation/adhesion. Hyperuricemia is present. Hyperlipidemia includes elevation of triglycerides, cholesterol, and phospholipids.

LONG-TERM COMPLICATIONS Gout usually becomes symptomatic around puberty as a result of the long-term hyperuricemia. Puberty is often delayed. Virtually all females have ultrasound findings consistent with polycystic ovaries; however, the other clinical features of polycystic ovary syndrome, such as acne and hirsutism, are not seen. Secondary to the lipid abnormalities, there is an increased risk of pancreatitis. The dyslipidemia together with elevated erythrocyte aggregation predispose these patients to atherosclerosis. Frequent fractures and radiographic evidence of osteopenia are not uncommon in adult patients, and radial bone mineral content is significantly reduced in prepubertal patients. By the second or third decade of life, most patients with type I glycogen storage disease develop hepatic adenomas that can hemorrhage and, in some cases, become malignant. Renal disease is a serious late complication. Almost all patients older than 20 years have proteinuria and many have hypertension, kidney stones, nephrocalcinosis, and altered creatinine clearance. In some patients, renal function deteriorates and progresses to failure, requiring dialysis or transplantation.

DIAGNOSIS The diagnosis of type I disease can be suspected on the basis of clinical presentation and abnormal plasma lactate and lipid values. Before the glucose-6-phosphatase and glucose-6-phosphate translocase genes were cloned, a definitive diagnosis required a liver biopsy to demonstrate a deficiency. Gene-based mutation analysis now provides a noninvasive way of diagnosis for most patients with types Ia and Ib disease.

Rx TREATMENT

Treatment is designed to maintain normal blood glucose levels and is achieved by continuous nasogastric infusion of glucose or oral admin-

Type/Common Name	Basic Defect	Clinical Features	Comments
LIVER GLYCOGENOSES			
Disorders with hepatomegaly and hypoglycemia			
Ia/von Gierke	Glucose-6-phosphatase	Growth retardation, enlarged liver and kidney, hypoglycemia, elevated blood lactate, cholesterol, triglycerides, and uric acid	Common, severe hypoglycemia Late complications in adulthood
Ib	Glucose-6-phosphate translocase	As for Ia, with additional findings of neutropenia and neutrophil dysfunction	~10% of type I
IIIa/Cori or Forbes	Liver and muscle debranching enzyme	Childhood: Hepatomegaly, growth retardation, muscle weakness, hypoglycemia, hyperlipidemia, elevated liver transaminases; liver symptoms improve with age Adulthood: muscle atrophy and weakness; onset: third to fourth decades; variable cardiomyopathy	Common, intermediate severity of hypoglycemia Liver cirrhosis can occur
IIIb	Liver debranching enzyme (normal muscle debrancher activity)	Liver symptoms same as in type IIIa; no muscle symptoms	~15% of type III
VI/Hers	Liver phosphorylase	Hepatomegaly, mild hypoglycemia, hyperlipidemia and ketosis; symptoms improve with age	Rare, "benign" glycogenosis
IX/phosphorylase kinase deficiency	Liver phosphorylase kinase α subunit	As for VI	Common, "benign glycogenosis," X-linked
0/glycogen synthase deficiency	Glycogen synthase	Fasting hypoglycemia and ketosis, elevated lactic acid and hyperglycemia after glucose load	Decreased glycogen stores
XI/Fanconi-Bickel	Glucose transporter-2	Failure to thrive, rickets, hepatomegaly, proximal renal tubular dysfunction, impaired glucose and galactose utilization	Rare, consanguinity in 70%
Disorders with liver cirrhosis			
IV/Andersen	Branching enzyme	Failure to thrive, hypotonia, hepatomegaly, splenomegaly, progressive liver cirrhosis and failure (death usually before fifth year); some without progression	One of the rarer glycogenoses; other neuromuscular variants exist
MUSCLE GLYCOGENOSES			
Disorders with muscle-energy impairment			
V/McArdle	Muscle phosphorylase	Exercise intolerance, muscle cramps, myoglobinuria on strenuous exercise, increased CK	Common, male predominance
VII/Tarui	Phosphofructokinase—M subunit	As for type V, with additional findings of a compensated hemolysis	Prevalent in Ashkenazi Jews and Japanese
Phosphoglycerate kinase deficiency	Phosphoglycerate kinase	As for type V, with additional findings of a hemolytic anemia and CNS dysfunction	Rare, X-linked
Phosphoglycerate mutase deficiency	Phosphoglycerate mutase—M subunit	As for type V	Rare; most patients are African American
Lactate dehydrogenase deficiency	Lactic acid dehydrogenase—M subunit	As for type V, with additional findings of erythematous skin eruption and uterine stiffness resulting in childbirth difficulty in female	Rare
Fructose 1,6-bisphosphate aldolase A deficiency	Fructose 1,6-bisphosphate aldolase A	As for type V, with additional finding of hemolytic anemia	Rare
Pyruvate kinase deficiency	Pyruvate kinase—muscle isozyme	Muscle cramps and/or fixed muscle weakness	Rare
Muscle phosphorylase kinase deficiency	Muscle-specific phosphorylase kinase	As for type V, some patients may have muscle weakness and atrophy	Rare, autosomal recessive
β-enolase deficiency	Muscle β-enolase	Exercise intolerance	Rare
Disorders with progressive skeletal myopathy and/or cardiomyopathy			
II/Pompe	Lysosomal acid α-glucosidase	Infantile: hypotonia, muscle weakness, cardiac enlargement and failure, fatal early Juvenile and adult: progressive skeletal muscle weakness and atrophy, proximal muscle and respiratory muscle are seriously affected	Common, undetectable, or very low level of enzyme activity in infantile form; residual enzyme activity in late-onset
Cardiac phosphorylase kinase deficiency	Cardiac-specific phosphorylase kinase	Severe cardiomyopathy and early heart failure	Very rare
GALACTOSE DISORDERS			
Galactosemia with uridyl transferase deficiency	Galactose 1-phosphate uridyl transferase	Vomiting, hepatomegaly, jaundice, cataracts, amino aciduria, failure to thrive	Long-term complications exist despite early diagnosis and treatment
Galactokinase deficiency	Galactokinase	Cataracts	Benign
Uridine diphosphate galactose 4-epimerase deficiency	Uridine diphosphate galactose 4-epimerase	Similar to transferase deficiency with additional findings of hypotonia and nerve deafness	Benign variant exists
FRUCTOSE DISORDERS			
Essential fructosuria	Fructokinase	Asymptomatic, positive urine reducing substance	Benign
Hereditary fructose intolerance	Fructose 1-phosphate aldolase B	Vomiting, lethargy, failure to thrive, hepatic failure	Prognosis good with early diagnosis and fructose restriction
Fructose 1,6-diphosphatase deficiency	Fructose 1,6-diphosphatase	Episodic hypoglycemia and lactic acidosis	Avoid fasting, good prognosis

Note: CK, creatine kinase; M, muscle; CNS, central nervous system.

istration of uncooked cornstarch. Uncooked cornstarch acts as a slow-release form of glucose and can be given at a dose of 1.6 g/kg every 4 h for infants younger than 2 years. As the child grows older, the cornstarch regimen can be changed to every 6 h, and can be given by mouth as a liquid (1:2, weight:volume) at a dose of 1.75 to 2.5 g/kg of body weight. Because fructose and galactose cannot be converted to free glucose, their dietary intake should be restricted. Dietary supplements of multivitamins and calcium are required. Allopurinol is given to lower uric acid levels. The hyperlipidemia can be reduced with lipid-lowering drugs such as HMG-CoA reductase inhibitors and fibric acids. Preliminary studies of treating microalbuminuria, an early indicator of renal dysfunction in these patients, have also shown angiotensin-converting enzyme (ACE) inhibitors to be beneficial. Citrate supplement may be beneficial in preventing or ameliorating nephrocalcinosis and development of urinary calculi.

Type III Glycogen Storage Disease (Debrancher Deficiency, Limit Dextrinosis)

Type III glycogenoses are autosomal recessive disorders caused by a deficiency of glycogen debranching enzyme. Debranching enzyme and phosphorylase are responsible for complete degradation of glycogen; when debranching enzyme is defective, glycogen breakdown is incomplete and an abnormal glycogen accumulates that has short outer chains and resembles limit dextrin.

CLINICAL AND LABORATORY FINDINGS   Deficiency of glycogen debranching enzyme causes hepatomegaly, hypoglycemia, short stature, variable skeletal myopathy, and cardiomyopathy. The disorder usually involves both liver and muscle and is termed *type IIIa glycogen storage disease*. However, in about 15% of patients, the disease appears to involve only the liver and is classified as *type IIIb*. Remarkably, hepatomegaly and hepatic symptoms in most patients with type III disease improve with age and usually disappear after puberty.

Hypoglycemia, hyperlipidemia, and elevated liver transaminases occur in children. In contrast to type I disease, fasting ketosis is prominent, and blood lactate and uric acid concentrations are usually normal. Serum creatine kinase levels can sometimes be used to identify patients with muscle involvement, but normal levels do not rule out muscle enzyme deficiency.

DIAGNOSIS   In type IIIa glycogen storage disease, deficient debranching enzyme activity can be demonstrated in liver, skeletal muscle, and heart. In contrast, patients with type IIIb have debranching enzyme deficiency in the liver but not in muscle. In the past, definitive assignment of subtype required enzyme assays in both liver and muscle. DNA-based analyses now provide a noninvasive way of subtyping these disorders in most patients.

℞ TREATMENT

Dietary management of type III disease is less demanding than that of type I. If hypoglycemia is present, frequent high-carbohydrate meals with cornstarch supplements or nocturnal gastric drip feedings are usually effective. A high-protein diet during the day plus overnight protein enteral infusion may be tried in patients with myopathy, but it is not established whether such a regimen is effective.

Type VI Glycogen Storage Disease [Liver Phosphorylase Deficiency (Hers Disease)]

These patients present with hepatomegaly and growth retardation early in childhood. Hypoglycemia, hyperlipidemia, and hyperketosis are usually mild, if present. Plasma lactic acid and uric acid levels are normal. The heart and skeletal muscles are not involved. The hepatomegaly and growth retardation improve with age and usually disappear at puberty. Treatment is symptomatic. A high-carbohydrate diet and frequent feeding are effective in preventing hypoglycemia, but most patients require no specific treatment.

Type IX Glycogen Storage Disease (Liver Phosphorylase Kinase Deficiency)

Defects of phosphorylase kinase cause a heterogeneous group of glycogenoses. The phosphorylase kinase enzyme complex consists of four subunits (α, β, γ, and δ), each encoded by different genes (X chromosome as well as autosomes) that are differentially expressed in various tissues. Phosphorylase kinase deficiency can be divided into several subtypes on the basis of the gene/subunit involved, the tissues that are primarily affected, and the mode of inheritance. The most common subtype is X-linked liver phosphorylase kinase deficiency, which is also one of the most common liver glycogenoses. Phosphorylase kinase activity may also be deficient in erythrocytes and leukocytes but is normal in muscle. Typically, a child between the ages of 1 and 5 presents with growth retardation and hepatomegaly. Levels of cholesterol, triglycerides, and liver enzymes are mildly elevated. Ketosis may occur after fasting. Lactic and uric acid levels are normal. Hypoglycemia is mild, if present. Hepatomegaly and abnormal blood chemistries gradually return to normal with age. Most adults achieve a normal final height and are practically asymptomatic, despite a persistent phosphorylase kinase deficiency.

Treatment is symptomatic. A high-carbohydrate diet and frequent feedings are effective in preventing hypoglycemia; some patients require no specific treatment. Prognosis is usually good; adult patients have normal stature and minimal hepatomegaly.

Other subtypes of Type IX include an autosomal recessive form of liver and muscle phosphorylase kinase deficiency, an autosomal recessive form of liver phosphorylase kinase deficiency that often develops into liver cirrhosis, a muscle-specific phosphorylase kinase deficiency that causes cramps and myoglobinuria with exercise, and a cardiac-specific phosphorylase kinase deficiency that is lethal during infancy because of massive glycogen deposition in the myocardium.

Other Liver Glycogenoses with Hepatomegaly and Hypoglycemia

These disorders include glycogen synthase deficiency (type 0) and hepatic glycogenosis with renal Fanconi syndrome (type XI). The latter is caused by defects in the facilitative glucose transporter 2 (GLUT-2), which transports glucose in and out of hepatocytes, pancreatic cells, and the basolateral membranes of intestinal and renal epithelial cells. The disease is characterized by proximal renal tubular dysfunction, impaired glucose and galactose utilization, and accumulation of glycogen in liver and kidney.

SELECTED MUSCLE GLYCOGENOSES

DISORDERS WITH MUSCLE-ENERGY IMPAIRMENT ■ Type V Glycogen Storage Disease (Muscle Phosphorylase Deficiency, McArdle Disease)

Type V glycogen storage disease is an autosomal recessive disorder caused by deficiency of muscle phosphorylase. McArdle disease is a prototypical muscle energy disorder as the enzyme deficiency limits ATP generation by glycogenolysis and results in glycogen accumulation.

CLINICAL AND LABORATORY FINDINGS   Symptoms usually develop first in adulthood and are characterized by exercise intolerance with muscle cramps. Two types of activity tend to cause symptoms: (1) brief exercise of great intensity, such as sprinting or carrying heavy loads; and (2) less intense but sustained activity, such as climbing stairs or walking uphill. Moderate exercise, such as walking on level ground, can be performed by most patients for long periods. About half of patients report burgundy-colored urine after exercise, the consequence of myoglobinuria secondary to rhabdomyolysis. Intense myoglobinuria after vigorous exercise may cause renal failure. In rare cases, electromyography (EMG) findings may suggest an inflammatory myopathy, and the diagnosis can be confused with polymyositis.

The level of serum creatine kinase is usually elevated at rest and increases after exercise. Exercise also increases the levels of blood ammonia, inosine, hypoxanthine, and uric acid. The latter abnormalities are attributed to accelerated recycling of muscle purine nucleotides in the face of insufficient ATP production.

DIAGNOSIS   Lack of an increase in blood lactate and exaggerated blood ammonia elevations after an ischemic exercise test are indicative of muscle glycogenosis and suggest a defect in the conversion of glycogen or glucose to lactate. The abnormal exercise response, however, is not limited to type V disease and can occur with other defects in glycogenolysis or glycolysis, such as deficiencies of muscle phosphofructokinase or debranching enzyme (when the test is done after fasting). Definitive diagnosis is made by enzymatic assay in muscle tissue or by mutation analysis of the myophosphorylase gene.

 TREATMENT

In general, avoidance of strenuous exercise can prevent major episodes of rhabdomyolysis; however, regular and moderate exercise is recommended to improve exercise capacity. A high-protein diet may increase exercise endurance, and creatine supplement has been shown to improve muscle function in some patients. In general, longevity does not appear to be affected.

DISORDERS WITH PROGRESSIVE SKELETAL MUSCLE MYOPATHY AND/OR CARDIOMYOPATHY ■ Type II Glycogen Storage Disease (Acid α-1,4 Glucosidase Deficiency, Pompe Disease)

Type II disease is an autosomal recessive disorder caused by a deficiency of lysosomal acid α-1,4 glucosidase (acid maltase), an enzyme responsible for the degradation of glycogen in lysosomal vacuoles. It is characterized by the accumulation of glycogen in lysosomes as opposed to its accumulation in cytoplasm as in the other glycogenoses.

CLINICAL AND LABORATORY FINDINGS   The disorder encompasses a range of phenotypes, each including myopathy but differing in age of onset, organ involvement, and clinical severity. The most severe is the infantile-onset disease with cardiomegaly, hypotonia, and death before age 1. Infants appear normal at birth but soon develop generalized muscle weakness with feeding difficulties, macroglossia, hepatomegaly, and congestive heart failure due to a hypertrophic cardiomyopathy.

The juvenile, or late-childhood, form is characterized by skeletal muscle manifestations, usually without cardiac involvement, and a slowly progressive course. The juvenile form typically presents as delayed motor milestones (if age of onset is early enough) and difficulty in walking. These manifestations are followed by swallowing difficulties, proximal muscle weakness, and respiratory muscle involvement. Death may occur before the end of the second decade.

An adult form of type II disease presents as a slowly progressive myopathy without cardiac involvement and has its onset between the second and seventh decades. The clinical picture is dominated by slowly progressive proximal muscle weakness with truncal involvement. The pelvic girdle, paraspinal muscles, and the diaphragm are most seriously affected. The initial symptoms may be respiratory insufficiency manifested by somnolence, morning headache, orthopnea, and exertional dyspnea.

Laboratory findings include elevated levels of serum creatine kinase, aspartate transaminase, and lactate dehydrogenase, particularly in infants. Muscle biopsy shows the presence of vacuoles that stain positively for glycogen, and muscle acid phosphatase is increased, presumably from a compensatory increase of lysosomal enzymes. EMG reveals myopathic features with irritability of muscle fibers and pseudomyotonic discharges. Serum creatine kinase is not always elevated in adults and, depending on the muscle biopsied or tested, muscle histology or EMG may not be abnormal. It is prudent to examine affected muscle.

DIAGNOSIS   Diagnosis can be established by demonstration of the absence or reduced levels of acid α-glucosidase activity in muscle or cultured skin fibroblasts. Deficiency is usually more severe in the infantile form than in the juvenile and adult disorders.

 TREATMENT

Definitive therapy is not currently available; a high-protein diet may be useful for the juvenile and adult forms. Nocturnal ventilatory support in late-onset patients improves the quality of life and is beneficial during a period of respiratory decompensation. Clinical trials of enzyme replacement therapy have begun. Preliminary data have shown that recombinant acid α-glucosidase is capable of improving cardiac and skeletal muscle function in these patients.

SELECTED DISORDERS OF GALACTOSE METABOLISM

"Classic" *galactosemia* is due to galactose 1-phosphate uridyl transferase deficiency. It is a serious disease with an early onset of symptoms; the incidence is 1 in 60,000. The newborn infant normally receives up to 20% of caloric intake as lactose, which consists of glucose and galactose. Without the transferase, the infant is unable to metabolize galactose 1-phosphate (Fig. 341-1), the accumulation of which results in injury to parenchymal cells of the kidney, liver, and brain.

Widespread newborn screening for galactosemia has identified these infants early and allowed them to be placed on dietary restriction. Elimination of galactose from the diet reverses growth failure and renal and hepatic dysfunction and improves the prognosis. However, on long-term follow-up, these patients still have ovarian failure manifest as primary or secondary amenorrhea, as well as developmental delay and learning disabilities, which increase in severity with age. In addition, most patients have speech disorders, and a smaller number demonstrate poor growth and impaired motor function and balance (with or without overt ataxia). The treatment of galactosemia to prevent long-term complications remains a challenge.

Deficiency of *galactokinase* (Fig. 341-1) causes cataracts. Deficiency of *uridine diphosphate galactose 4-epimerase* can be benign when the enzyme deficiency is limited to blood cells but can be as severe as "classic" galactosemia when the enzyme deficiency is generalized.

SELECTED DISORDERS OF FRUCTOSE METABOLISM

Fructokinase deficiency (Fig. 341-1) causes a benign condition that is usually an incidental finding made through the detection of fructose as a reducing substance in the urine.

Deficiency of *fructose 1,6-bisphosphate aldolase* (aldolase B, hereditary fructose intolerance) is a serious disease of infants because of a defect in gluconeogenesis. These patients are healthy and asymptomatic until fructose or sucrose (table sugar) is ingested (usually from fruit, fruit juice, or sweetened cereal). Clinical manifestations may include jaundice, hepatomegaly, vomiting, lethargy, irritability, and convulsions. Laboratory findings include prolonged clotting time, hypoalbuminemia, elevation of bilirubin and transaminases, and proximal renal tubular dysfunction. If the disease is not diagnosed and intake of the noxious sugar persists, hypoglycemic episodes recur, and liver and kidney failure progress, eventually leading to death. Treatment consists of the complete elimination of all sources of sucrose, fructose, and sorbitol from the diet. With this treatment, liver and kidney dysfunction improve, and catch-up growth is common. Intellectual development is usually unimpaired. As the patient matures, symptoms become milder, even after fructose ingestion, and the long-term prognosis is good.

Fructose 1,6-diphosphatase deficiency is characterized by childhood life-threatening episodes of acidosis, hypoglycemia, hyperventilation, convulsions, and coma. These episodes are triggered by febrile infections and gastroenteritis when oral food intake decreases. Laboratory findings include low blood glucose, high lactate and uric acid levels, and metabolic acidosis. In contrast to hereditary fructose intolerance, there is usually no aversion to sweets, and renal tubular and liver functions are normal. Treatment of acute attacks consists of correction of hypoglycemia and acidosis by intravenous infusion. Later, avoidance of fasting and elimination of fructose and sucrose from the diet prevent further episodes. For long-term prevention of hypoglycemia, a slowly released carbohydrate such as cornstarch is useful. Prognosis is good as patients who survive childhood develop normally.

FURTHER READING

AMALFITANO A et al: Recombinant human acid-α-glucosidase enzyme therapy for infantile glycogen storage disease type II: Results of a phase I/II clinical trial. Genet Med 3:132, 2001

DIMAURO S, LAMPERTI C: Muscle glycogenoses. Muscle Nerve 24:984, 2001

SCRIVER CR et al (Eds): *The Metabolic and Molecular Bases of Inherited Disease*, 8th ed, New York, McGraw-Hill, 2001

SHEN J-J, CHEN Y-T: Molecular characterization of glycogen storage disease type III. Curr Mol Med 2:167, 2002

Heritable disorders that involve the major connective tissues of the body such as bone, skin, cartilage, blood vessels, and basement membranes are among the most common genetic diseases in human beings. Here we will focus primarily on those disorders that can have severe manifestations, are relatively common, and are sufficiently understood at the molecular level to provide useful paradigms: osteogenesis imperfecta (OI), the Ehlers-Danlos syndrome (EDS), chondrodysplasias (CDs), the Marfan syndrome (MFS), epidermolysis bullosa (EB), and the Alport syndrome (AS).

THE CHALLENGE OF CLASSIFYING THE DISEASES The original classification of connective tissue diseases was based on the pattern of inheritance, the cluster of signs and symptoms, the histologic changes in tissues, and limited information about the molecular defects involved. This classification included about a dozen types and subtypes for OI, about the same number for the EDS, and over 150 for the CDs. Several limitations in these original classifications are now apparent. One is that the same mutation does not always produce the same disease phenotype in terms of severity of the condition or its clinical course. Such phenotypic variation occurs in many genetic diseases, including the connective tissue disorders, in which some members of a family are severely affected, whereas others with the same mutation have a mild disorder.

Most patients with classic features of a severe connective tissue disease have a mutation in a gene, or genes, coding for a single protein.

For example, the majority of patients with OI have a mutation in one of the two genes coding for type I procollagen. Similarly, most patients with MFS have mutations in a gene for fibrillin. For other disease categories, the situation is more complex. In EDS, for example, the type IV variant is usually caused by mutations in the gene for type III procollagen, the type VI variant by defects in the gene for lysyl hydroxylase, and the type VII variant by defects in a gene required for processing type I procollagen to type I collagen.

Classifications of these disorders also tend to overemphasize the etiologic differences between severe genetic diseases that are apparent in infants and the more common diseases that appear much later in life. Single-gene defects can cause subsets of late-onset diseases such as osteoporosis, aneurysms, and osteoarthritis. For example, a small subset of patients with postmenopausal osteoporosis have mutations in the genes for procollagen I similar to the mutations in the same genes that produce lethal variants of OI. Likewise, a subset of patients with familial aortic aneurysms have mutations in the gene for procollagen III similar to the mutations in the same gene that cause lethal variants of type IV EDS, and occasional patients with osteoarthritis have mutations in the gene for procollagen II similar to the mutations in the same gene that cause lethal CDs.

DEFINITION AND COMPOSITION OF CONNECTIVE TISSUES The distinguishing feature of connective tissues is that it consists of complex macromolecules that are assembled into an insoluble extracellular matrix (Table 342-1). The macromolecules include at least 25 different types of collagens, the related fibrous proteins known as *elastin* and *fibrillin*, a series of proteoglycans, and other components whose structure and function are only partially defined. Differences in the connective tissues of bone, skin, and cartilage are partially explained by differences in the content of specific components (Table 342-1). For example, tendons and ligaments consist primarily of type I collagen fibrils and small amounts of other components that help organize the type I fibrils into thick fibers and fiber bundles. Cartilage consists primarily of fibrils of type II collagen in the form of arcades that are distended by highly charged proteoglycans. The extracellular matrix of the aorta contains collagens that provide tensile strength and elastin that provides elasticity. Differences among the connective tissues also depend on the three-dimensional organization of the molecular components. The type I collagen fibrils in tendon are packed into thick, parallel bundles of fibers, whereas type I collagen fibrils in skin are randomly oriented. In cortical bone, type I collagen fibrils form helical arrays around haversian canals.

BIOSYNTHESIS OF CONNECTIVE TISSUE Connective tissues form primarily by a process of self-assembly, in which a molecule of the correct size, shape, and surface property binds to other molecules with the same or similar structure in a spontaneous and precisely ordered manner. The molecular mechanisms and driving forces are similar to those involved in crystal formation.

Collagen Synthesis Collagens have a triple-helical conformation, because each of the three α chains has a simple, repetitive amino acid se-

TABLE 342-1	Constituents of Connective Tissues in Various Tissues		
Connective Tissue	**Major Constituents**	**Approximate Amounts, % dry wt**	**Characteristics or Functions**
Dermis, ligaments, tendons	Type I collagen	80	Bundles of fibrils
	Type III collagen	5–15	Thin fibrils
	Type IV collagen, laminin, nidogen	<5	In basal laminae under epithelium and endothelium
	Types V, VI, and VII collagens	<5	VII forms anchoring fibrils; others unknown
	Elastin, fibrillin	<5	Provides elasticity
	Fibronectin	<5	Associated with collagen fibers and cell surfaces
	Proteoglycans,[a] hyaluronate	0.5	Provide resiliency
Bone (demineralized)	Type I collagen	90	Complex fibril network
	Type VI collagen	1–2	Function unclear
	Proteoglycans[a]	1	Function unclear
	Osteonectin, osteopontin, osteocalcin, α2-glycoprotein, sialoproteins	1–5	May regulate mineralization
Aorta	Type I collagen	20–40	Fibril network
	Type III collagen	20–40	Thin fibrils
	Elastin, fibrillin	20–40	Provide elasticity
	Type IV collagen, laminin, nidogen	<5	Form basal lamina
	Types V and VI collagens	<2	Functions unclear
	Proteoglycans[a]	<3	Provide resiliency
Cartilage	Type II collagen	40–50	Arcades of thin fibrils
	Type IX collagen	5–10	Links type II fibrils
	Type X collagen	5–10	Surrounds hypertrophic cells
	Type XI collagen	<10	Function unclear
	Proteoglycans,[a] hyaluronate	15–50	Provides resiliency

[a] As discussed in text, >30 proteoglycans have now been identified. They differ in the structures of their core proteins and their contents of glycosaminoglycan side chains of chondroitin-4-sulfate, chondroitin-6-sulfate, dermatan sulfate, and keratin sulfate. Basal lamina contain a proteoglycan with a side chain of heparan sulfate that resembles heparin.

quence of about 1000 amino acids in which glycine (Gly) appears as every third amino acid. Therefore, the sequence of each α chain can be designated as (-Gly-X-Y-)$_{333}$, where X and Y represent amino acids other than glycine. To fold into a triple helix, every third amino acid in an α chain must be glycine, the smallest amino acid, since this residue must fit in a sterically restricted space where the three chains of the triple helix come together. Many of the X- and Y-position amino acids are proline and hydroxyproline, which, because of their ring structure, provide rigidity to the triple helix.

Twenty-five different collagens have been identified. Many are minor constituents that probably have highly specialized functions. The fibrillar collagens are abundant proteins that are found in tissues as long, highly ordered fibrils with a characteristic banding pattern revealed by electron microscopy. Type I collagen, the most abundant, is composed of two identical α chains called α1(I) and a third called α2(I). Type II collagen, the fibrillar collagen of cartilage, is composed of three identical α chains called α1(II). Type III collagen is found in small amounts in many tissues that contain type I collagen and in large amounts in large blood vessels; it is composed of three identical chains called α1(III). Type IV collagen in basement membranes self-assembles into a complex three-dimensional network that provides a diffusion barrier in the renal glomerulus, pulmonary alveolus, and other tissues.

Collagens are first synthesized as larger and more soluble precursors called *procollagens* that are composed of proα chains. As the proα chains of procollagen are synthesized on ribosomes, the free ends move into the cisternae of the rough endoplasmic reticulum (Fig. 342-1). Hydrophobic signal peptides at the N termini are cleaved, and additional posttranslational reactions begin. Proline residues in the Y position of the repeating -Gly-X-Y- sequences are converted to hydroxyproline by prolyl hydroxylase. The requirement for ascorbic acid as cofactor in the hydroxylation of prolyl residues explains why wounds fail to heal in scurvy (Chap. 61). If sufficient proline residues are not converted to hydroxyproline, collagen cannot fold into a triple helix that is stable at body temperature. The abnormal protein accumulates in the cisternae of the rough endoplasmic reticulum and is slowly degraded. Lysine residues in the Y position are similarly hydroxylated to hydroxylysine by lysyl hydroxylase. Many of the hydroxylysine residues are glycosylated with galactose or with galactose and glucose. A large mannose-rich oligosaccharide is assembled on the C-terminal propeptide of each chain.

After secretion, procollagen is processed to collagen by cleavage of the N-propeptides by procollagen N-proteinase and of the C-propeptides by procollagen C-proteinase. The processing converts the precursor to type I collagen and thereby decreases the solubility of the protein about 1000-fold. The entropic energy that is released drives the spontaneous self-assembly of the collagen into fibrils. Self-assembled collagen fibers have considerable tensile strength, which is increased by cross-linking reactions that form covalent bonds between α chains in one molecule and α chains in adjacent molecules. The first step in cross-linking is oxidation by lysyl oxidase of amino groups on a few lysine or hydroxylysine residues to form aldehydes that interact to form stable covalent bonds.

During growth and development, the collagen fibrils in all tissues undergo repeated synthesis, degradation, and resynthesis. The degradation of collagen fibers in tissues is initiated by specific collagenases. Collagen fibers in most tissues of normal adults undergo very little metabolic turnover. One exception to this is the collagen fibrils that are degraded and resynthesized as part of the continual remodeling of bone. Also, although the collagen in many adult tissues is metabolically stable, the rate of turnover increases under some circumstances. In starvation, a large fraction of the collagen in skin and other con-

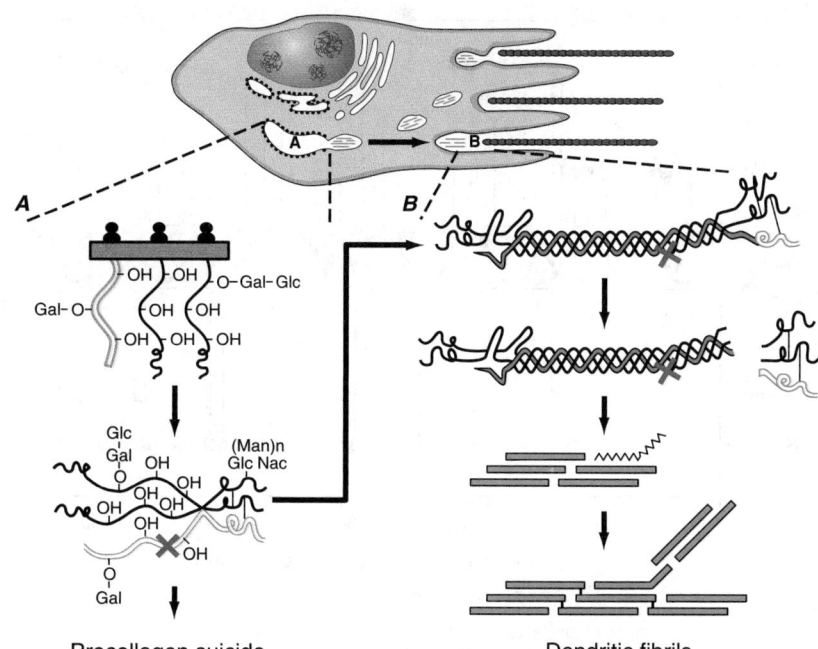

FIGURE 342-1 Schematic representation of synthesis of a type I collagen fibril by a fibroblast. *A.* Intracellular steps in the assembly of the procollagen molecule. Hydroxylations and glycosylations of the proα chains begin soon after the amino termini pass into the cisternae of the rough endoplasmic reticulum and continue after the three chains associate through their carboxy-terminal propeptides and become disulfide linked. *B.* Cleavage of procollagen to collagen, self-assembly of the collagen molecule into quarter-staggered fibrils, and cross-linking of the molecules in the fibrils. Cleavage of the propeptides may occur within crypts of the fibroblast, as shown here, or some distance from the cell. Mutations (depicted by X) cause the synthesis of structurally abnormal proα1(I) or proα2(I) chains of type I procollagen by interfering either with protein assembly (procollagen suicide) *(A)* or with processing to normal collagen fibrils *(B)*. *(From DJ Prockop et al, Am J Med Genet 34:60, 1989, with permission.)*

nective tissues is degraded, thus providing amino acids for gluconeogenesis. Large losses of collagen also occur in most connective tissues during immobilization or prolonged periods of low-gravitational stress. In rheumatoid arthritis, pannus invasion causes a rapid degradation of collagen in the articular cartilage. Glucocorticoids decrease the collagen content of most connective tissues, including bone, by decreasing the rate of collagen synthesis. Decreases in collagen weaken tissues. In many pathologic states, however, collagen is deposited in excess. With injury to tissue, inflammation is usually followed by increased deposition primarily of type I collagen fibrils in the form of fibrotic tissue and scars. The deposition of collagen fibrils during the repair process is largely irreversible and is a major feature of the pathologic changes in hepatic cirrhosis, pulmonary fibrosis, atherosclerosis, and nephrosclerosis and in the scarring of skin and ligaments after surgery or trauma.

Elastin Synthesis Elastin assembly appears to be closely related to that of collagen, since a few of the prolines in the protein are hydroxylated to hydroxyproline by prolyl hydroxylase. The elastin monomer, however, is a single polypeptide that does not fold into a defined three-dimensional structure and is not synthesized as a larger precursor molecule. Instead, it is slowly secreted from cells into extracellular compartments, where it forms amorphous deposits around previously deposited microfibrils. The elastin deposits then become covalently cross-linked through oxidation of lysine residues to aldehydes by the same lysyl oxidase that initiates the cross-linking of collagen. The microfibrils in elastin deposits are largely composed of fibrillin, a large protein that forms beadlike strands.

Proteoglycan Synthesis The synthesis of proteoglycans begins in the cisternae of the rough endoplasmic reticulum with assembly of a core protein that then undergoes sequential additions of sugars to generate large side chains of glycosaminoglycans. At least 30 proteoglycans have been identified by differences in the structures of their core proteins and their side chains. The major proteoglycan of cartilage, called

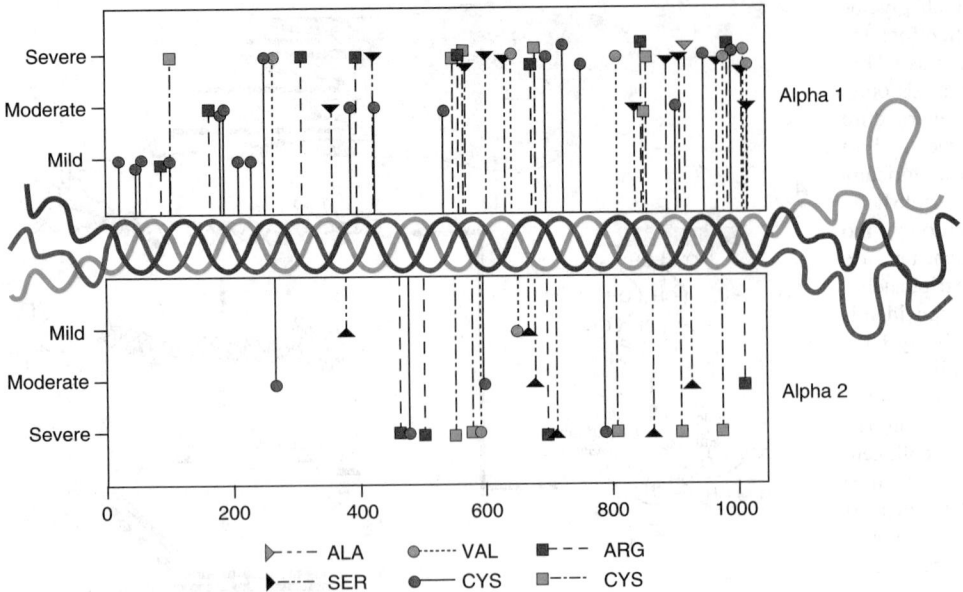

FIGURE 342-2 Examples of single-base mutations found in type I procollagen in patients with osteogenesis imperfecta (OI) and osteoporosis. Mild refers to type I OI, severe to type II OI, and moderate to type III or type IV OI.

aggrecan, has a core protein of about 2000 amino acids, which are bound multiple side chains of chondroitin sulfate and keratin sulfate, polysaccharides consisting of highly charged and repetitive disaccharide sequences. The highly charged proteoglycan aggregate binds water and small ions that distend the collagen network and thereby make the tissue resilient to pressure.

MUTATIONS THAT PRODUCE DISEASES OF CONNECTIVE TISSUES The most complete data on mutations causing heritable disorders of connective tissue are available on OI. Most patients with OI have mutations in either the gene for the proα1(I) chain or the gene for the proα2(I) chain of type I procollagen (the COL1A1 and COL1A2 genes). Most of the mutations in patients with severe OI cause synthesis of a structurally abnormal but partially functional proα chain. They include partial gene deletions, partial gene duplications, and RNA splicing mutations. The most common mutations, however, cause the substitution of single amino acids with bulky side chains for the glycine residues that appear as every third amino acid in the triple-helical domain of a proα chain (Fig. 342-2). The structurally abnormal proα chains exert their effects primarily through one of three mechanisms (Fig. 342-1). First, the presence of an abnormal proα chain in a procollagen molecule containing two normal proα chains can prevent folding of the protein into a triple-helical conformation and lead to degradation of the whole molecule in a process called *procollagen suicide*. Similar dominant negative mutations are seen with other multisubunit proteins. The net result of procollagen suicide is accumulation of the unfolded protein in the rough endoplasmic reticulum of cells and a reduction in the amount of collagen available for fibril assembly. Second, the presence of one abnormal proα chain in a procollagen molecule can interfere with cleavage of the N-propeptide from the protein. The persistence of the N-propeptide on a fraction of the molecules interferes with the self-assembly of normal collagen so that thin and irregular collagen fibrils are formed. Third, the substitution of a bulkier amino acid for glycine can produce a change in the conformation of the mol-

ecule and result in the assembly of collagen fibrils that are abnormally branched or abnormally thick and short.

Over 500 mutations in the two genes for type I procollagen have been found in patients with OI (Fig. 342-2). The data on mutations in type I procollagen that cause OI have been used as a paradigm for defining other mutations in other collagen and procollagen genes that cause other disorders of connective tissue.

Several generalizations can be made about mutations in collagen genes. One is that unrelated patients rarely have the same mutation in the same gene. Another is that mutations that cause the most severe disease are usually new mutations in one allele that occur either during the generation of the germline in one of the parents or during meiosis in the fertilized egg (Chap. 56). Another general trend is that similar mutations in different regions of the same gene can produce different disease syndromes in both severity and the major tissues involved. One reason for heterogeneity in pathologic manifestations is that different regions of a large molecule may be more important for its function in some connective tissues than in others. For example, some regions of the type I collagen molecule may be essential for the binding of mineralizing proteins in bone so that mutations in these regions cause fragile bones but do not impair function in skin and other nonmineralizing tissues. It is more difficult, however, to explain how the same mutation can produce a severe phenotype in some and a mild phenotype in other members of the same family. Such phenotypic variation appears to be characteristic of OI, where some subjects are short and have multiple fractures from minor trauma, whereas others in the same family can be of normal stature and free of fractures. In the past, such phenotypic variation was explained by undefined variations in the genetic background of different family members. Studies in transgenic mice, however, demonstrated similar phenotypic variation with expression of a mutated collagen gene in an inbred strain of mice whose genetic background was uniform. Therefore, the phenotypic variation is probably caused by undefined stochastic or chance events during embryonic and fetal development. Although dramatic phenotypic variations are relatively rare in OI and related disorders, it is important to consider in counseling families about the consequences of inherited mutations.

SPECIFIC DISORDERS

OSTEOGENESIS IMPERFECTA OI causes a generalized decrease in bone mass (osteopenia) and makes the bones brittle. The disorder is frequently associated with blue sclerae, dental abnormalities (dentinogenesis imperfecta), progressive hearing loss, and a positive family history. The most severe forms cause death in utero, at birth, or shortly thereafter. The course of mild and moderate forms is more variable. Some patients appear normal at birth and become progressively worse. Some have multiple fractures in infancy and childhood, improve after puberty, and fracture more frequently later in life. Women are particularly prone to fracture during pregnancy and after menopause. A few women from families with mild variants of OI do not develop fractures until after menopause, and their disease may be difficult to distinguish from postmenopausal osteoporosis.

Classification The most common classification for OI was developed by Sillence (Table 342-2). Type I, the mildest form, is inherited as an

Type	Bone Fragility	Blue Sclerae	Abnormal Dentition	Hearing Loss	Inheritance[a]
I	Mild	Present	Present in some	Present in most	AD
II	Extreme	Present	Present in some	Unknown	S, rarely AR
III	Severe	Bluish at birth	Present in some	High incidence	AD, rarely AR
IV	Variable	Absent	Absent in IVA, present in IVB	High incidence	AD

TABLE 342-2 Classification of Osteogenesis Imperfecta (OI)

[a] AD, autosomal dominant; AR, autosomal recessive; S, sporadic.

autosomal dominant trait. Most patients have distinctly blue sclerae. Type II is lethal in utero or shortly after birth. Types III and IV are intermediate in severity between types I and II. They differ from type I because they are greater in severity and because blue sclerae are absent or only slightly bluish in infancy and white in adulthood. Type III differs from type IV because it tends to become more severe with age. The distinction between type IV and type III OI may not be helpful. Therefore, it may be sufficient to classify patients simply as mild (type I), lethal (type II), and moderately severe (type III).

Incidence Type I OI has a frequency of about 1 in 30,000. Type II OI has a reported incidence at birth of about 1 in 60,000, but the combined incidence of the three severe forms that are recognizable at birth (types II, III, and IV) may be much higher.

Skeletal Changes In type I OI, the fragility of bones may be severe enough to limit physical activity or so mild that individuals are unaware of any disability. Radiographs of the skull in patients with mild disease may show a mottled appearance because of small islands of irregular ossification. In type II OI, bones and other connective tissues are so fragile that massive injuries can occur in utero or during delivery. Ossification of many bones is frequently incomplete. Continuously beaded or broken ribs and crumpled long bones (accordina femora) may be present. For unclear reasons, the long bones may be either thick or thin. In types III and IV, multiple fractures from minor physical stress can produce severe deformities. Kyphoscoliosis can impair respiration, cause cor pulmonale, and predispose to pulmonary infections. On radiographs the appearance of "popcorn-like" deposits of mineral on the ends of long bones is an ominous sign. Progressive neurologic symptoms may result from basilar compression and communicating hydrocephalus.

In all forms of OI, bone mineral density in unfractured bone is decreased. However, the degree of osteopenia may be difficult to evaluate because recurrent fractures limit exercise and thereby worsen the decrease in bone mass. Surprisingly, fractures appear to heal normally.

Ocular Changes The sclerae can be normal, slightly bluish, or bright blue. The color is probably caused by a thinness of the collagen layers of the sclerae that allows the choroid layers to be seen. Blue sclerae, however, are an inherited trait in some families who do not have increased bone fragility.

Dentinogenesis Imperfecta The teeth may be normal, moderately discolored, or grossly abnormal. The enamel generally appears normal, but the teeth may have a characteristic amber, yellowish brown, or translucent bluish gray color because of improper deposition or deficiency of dentin. The deciduous teeth are usually smaller than normal, whereas permanent teeth are frequently bell-shaped and restricted at the base. In some patients, the teeth readily fracture and need to be extracted. The defect in dentin is directly attributable to the fact that normal dentin is rich in type I collagen. Similar tooth defects, however, can be inherited without any evidence of OI.

Hearing Loss Hearing loss usually begins during the second decade of life and occurs in more than 50% of individuals over age 30. The loss can be conductive, sensorineural, or mixed and varies in severity. The middle ear usually exhibits maldevelopment, deficient ossification, persistence of cartilage in areas that are normally ossified, and abnormal calcium deposits.

Associated Features Changes in other connective tissues can include thin skin that scars extensively, joint laxity with permanent dislocations indistinguishable from those of EDS, and, occasionally, cardiovascular manifestations such as aortic regurgitation, floppy mitral valves, mitral incompetence, and fragility of large blood vessels. For reasons unknown, some patients develop a hypermetabolic state with elevated serum thyroxine levels, hyperthermia, and excessive sweating.

Molecular Defects Most patients with OI have mutations in one of the two genes that encode type I procollagen. Over 90% of patients with type I OI and blue sclerae have mutations in the proα1(I) gene that

decrease the steady-state levels of the mRNA for proα1(I) chains and decrease the rates of synthesis of proα1(I) chains relative to those for proα2(I) chains. In more severe forms (types II, III, and IV), the effects of mutations that cause synthesis of abnormal proα chains are amplified by the three mechanisms discussed above (Fig. 342-1). Mutations that change the structure of the protein near the N-proteinase cleavage site cause accumulation of a partially processed procollagen and produce lax joints similar to those in type VII EDS that is caused by mutations in the gene for the N-proteinase. Mutations that change the structure in the middle or near the C terminus of the molecule tend to cause severe or lethal variants of OI. It is difficult, however, to correlate the site or nature of the mutation with the clinical phenotype (Fig. 342-2). Most patients are heterozygotes with mutations in a single allele, but rare patients are homozygotes with two mutated alleles for proα1(I) or proα2(I) chains.

Mosaicism in Germ-Line Cells and in Somatic Cells Most lethal OI is the result of new autosomal dominant mutations. The frequency of a second child with lethal OI in the same family, however, is about 7% because of germ-line mosaicism in one of the parents. The presence of germ-line mosaicism has been indicated in several fathers of patients with type II OI by demonstrating the mutated gene in a fraction of their sperm. Because of the possibility for germ-line mosaicism, asymptomatic parents of a child with severe OI should be counseled that recurrence can occur.

Diagnosis Diagnosis is usually made on the basis of clinical criteria. The presence of fractures together with blue sclerae, dentinogenesis imperfecta, or family history of the disease is usually sufficient to make the diagnosis. Other causes of pathologic fractures must be excluded, including the battered child syndrome, nutritional deficiencies, malignancies, and other inherited disorders such as CDs and hypophosphatasia. The absence of superficial bruises can be helpful in distinguishing OI from battered child syndrome. X-rays usually reveal a decrease in bone density that can be verified by photon or x-ray absorptiometry. There is no consensus, however, as to whether the diagnosis can be made by microscopy of bone. A molecular defect in type I procollagen can be demonstrated in at least half of patients by incubating skin fibroblasts with radioactive amino acids and then analyzing the proα chains by polyacrylamide gel electrophoresis. The analysis detects decreases in the rate of synthesis of proα1(I) chains relative to proα2(I) chains, abnormally long proα chains, abnormally short proα chains, and proα chains with excessive posttranslational modification because of an amino acid substitution that impairs folding of the triple helix. The mutations themselves can be defined in most patients by the sequencing of genomic DNA. Because each proband and family usually has a "private" mutation, extensive analysis of about 10,000 bases in each of the two genes is required to identify the exact mutation. After a mutation in a type I procollagen gene is identified, a simple test based on the polymerase chain reaction can be used to screen family members at risk and for prenatal diagnosis.

℞ TREATMENT

Many patients with OI have successful careers despite severe deformities. Those with mild disorder may need little treatment when fractures decrease after puberty, but women require special attention during pregnancy and after menopause, when fractures again increase. More severely affected children require a comprehensive program of physical therapy, surgical management of fractures and skeletal deformities, and vocational education.

Many of the fractures are only slightly displaced and have little soft tissue swelling. Therefore, they can be treated with minimal support or traction for a week or two followed by a light cast. If fractures are relatively painless, physical therapy can be initiated early. A judicious amount of exercise prevents loss of bone mass secondary to physical inactivity. Some physicians advocate insertion of steel rods into long bones to correct limb deformities; the risk/benefits and cost/

benefits of such procedures are difficult to evaluate. Aggressive conventional intervention is usually warranted for pneumonia and cor pulmonale. For severe hearing loss, stapedectomy or replacement of the stapes with a prosthesis may be successful. Moderately to severely affected patients should be evaluated periodically to anticipate possible neurologic problems. About half of children have a substantial increase in growth when given growth hormone. Treatment with bisphosphonates to decrease bone loss has been introduced on an experimental basis. Initial results are promising, but the long-term effects of decreasing bone resorption are unknown. Also, a clinical trial has been initiated to use stromal cells from bone marrow that can differentiate into osteoblasts after systemic infusion. In the first phase of the trial, four children with severe OI (type III) showed clinical improvement after marrow ablation and transplantation of whole bone marrow from an HLA-compatible sibling.

Counseling and emotional support are important for patients and their parents; and lay organizations in some countries provide help in these areas. Prenatal ultrasonography will detect severely affected fetuses at about 16 weeks of pregnancy. Diagnosis by demonstrating synthesis of abnormal proα chains or by DNA sequencing can be carried out in chorionic villa biopsies at 8 to 12 weeks of pregnancy.

EHLERS-DANLOS SYNDROME EDS is characterized by hyperelasticity of the skin and hypermobile joints.

Classification Nine types of EDS were initially defined primarily based on the extent to which the skin, joints, and other tissues are involved. Type I is the classic, severe form of the disease, with both severe joint hypermobility and skin that is velvety in texture, hyperextensible, and easily scarred. Type II is similar to type I but milder. In type III, joint hypermobility is more prominent than skin changes. In type IV, the skin changes are more prominent than joint changes. However, type IV patients are predisposed to sudden death from rupture of large blood vessels or other hollow organs. Type V is similar to type II but is inherited as an X-linked trait. Type VI is characterized by scoliosis, ocular fragility, and a cone-shaped deformity of the cornea (keratoconus). Type VII is characterized by marked joint hypermobility that is difficult to distinguish from type III except by the specific molecular defects in the processing of type I procollagen to collagen. Type VIII is distinguished by prominent periodontal changes. Types IX, X, and XI were defined on the basis of preliminary biochemical and clinical data, but these classifications have not proven to be useful. Because of overlapping signs and symptoms, many patients and families with some of the features of EDS cannot be assigned to any of the defined types.

Incidence The incidence of EDS is difficult to establish, largely because patients with mild skin or joint symptoms rarely seek medical attention. It is also difficult to define the normal range of variation for joint mobility or skin elasticity. The incidence may be about 1 in 5000 births, although a higher value has been reported for blacks. Types I, II, and III account for most diagnoses.

Skin The changes vary from thin and velvety skin to skin that is either dramatically hyperextensible ("rubber man" syndrome) or easily torn or scarred. Type I patients develop characteristic "cigarette-paper" scars. In type IV extensive scars and hyperpigmentation develop over bony prominences, and the skin may be so thin that subcutaneous blood vessels are visible. In type VIII the skin is more fragile than hyperextensible, and it heals with atrophic, pigmented scars. Easy bruisability occurs in several types of EDS.

Ligament and Joint Changes Laxity and hypermobility of joints vary from mild to unreducible dislocations of hips and other large joints. In mild forms, patients learn to reduce dislocations by limiting physical activity. In more severe forms, surgical repair may be required. Some patients have progressive difficulty with age, but severe joint laxity is compatible with a normal life span.

Associated Changes Mitral valve prolapse and hernias occur, particularly with type I. Pes planus and mild to moderate scoliosis are common. Extreme joint laxity and repeated dislocations may lead to degenerative arthritis. In type VI, the eye may rupture with minimal trauma, and kyphoscoliosis can cause respiratory impairment. Also, sclerae may be blue.

Molecular Defects Mutations in two of the three genes for type V collagen have been found in patients with types I and II EDS. Mutations in both the α1(V) and α2(V) chain are found in patients with type I EDS, but to date only mutations in the α1(V) chain have been found in patients with type II EDS.

Most patients with type IV EDS have a defect either in the synthesis or structure of type III procollagen, a finding consistent with the fact that these patients are prone to spontaneous rupture of the aorta and intestines, tissues rich in type III collagen. The thinness and scarring of skin are more difficult to explain, since type III constitutes a small fraction of the collagen in skin (Table 342-1). Most of the 500 or more mutations in the type III procollagen gene lead to synthesis of abnormal but partially functional proα1(III) chains that produce procollagen suicide or alter fibril formation by the same mechanisms that amplify the effects of mutations in the genes for type I procollagen. Similar mutations in type III procollagen can cause aortic aneurysms in some individuals without other evidence of EDS type IV, MFS, or other inherited disorders of connective tissue.

Type VI EDS is caused by mutations in the gene that encodes lysyl hydroxylase. In one series, all the patients were homozygous or compound heterozygotes for the mutated genes, and all the mutations caused profound deficiency of lysyl hydroxylase, a decrease in the hydroxylysine content of collagen, and a decrease in the cross-links in collagen fibers. The decrease in cross-links is explained by the observation that some cross-links are less stable if formed from lysine instead of hydroxylysine.

Type VII EDS occurs because of a defect in the conversion of procollagen to collagen caused either by mutations that make type I procollagen resistant to cleavage by procollagen N-proteinase or by mutations that decrease the activity of the enzyme. The type VIIA mutations alter the cleavage site in the proα1(I) chain, and the type VIIB mutations alter the cleavage site in the proα2(I) chain. Both types are dominantly inherited. Type VIIC is caused by mutations that decrease the activity of procollagen N-proteinase and is inherited as an autosomal recessive trait. In all three forms of type VII EDS, the persistence of the N-propeptide causes the formation of collagen fibrils that are thin and irregular. Since most patients do not have clinical osteopenia, the thin and irregular fibrils apparently suffice for the structural integrity of bone but do not provide the necessary tensile strength for ligaments and joint capsules. However, some patients fracture easily, and their disorder is difficult to distinguish from variants of OI.

The cause of type VIII EDS is unknown. Type IX is a disorder of copper transport. The syndrome, also referred to as *Menkes' syndrome*, is due to an X-linked defect and is associated with cutis laxa, hypopigmentation, unusual hair ("kinky"), vascular aneurysms, neurologic degeneration, and mental retardation. Mutations in a gene coding for a copper-transporting ATPase cause the disease (Chaps. 339 and 344). Type X EDS may be caused by defects in fibronectin, but no specific mutations have been defined.

Diagnosis The diagnosis is based on clinical criteria. Biochemical assays and gene analyses for known molecular defects in EDS are difficult and time-consuming, but specific diagnostic tests should be available in the future for families in whom the genes at fault have been defined.

Rx **TREATMENT**

There is no specific therapy. Surgical repair and tightening of joint ligaments require careful evaluation of individual patients, as the ligaments frequently do not hold sutures. Patients with easy bruisability should be evaluated for other bleeding disorders. Patients with type IV EDS and members of their families should probably be evaluated at regular intervals by sonography and related techniques for early detection of aneurysms. Surgical repair of aneurysms may be difficult because of increased friability of tissues, and there is limited experience with elective surgery in such patients. Also, women with type IV EDS should be counseled about the increased risk of uterine rupture, bleeding, and other complications of pregnancy.

CHONDRODYSPLASIAS (See also Chap. 334.)   The CDs are inherited skeletal disorders that cause dwarfism and abnormal body proportions. The category also includes some individuals with normal stature and body proportions who have features such as ocular changes or cleft palate that are common in more severe CDs. Many patients develop degenerative joint changes, and mild CD in adults may be difficult to differentiate from primary generalized osteoarthritis. Some authors refer to the disorders as "skeletal dysplasias," but CD is a more widely used term.

Classification   Over 150 distinct types and subtypes have been defined based on criteria such as "bringing death" (thanatophoric), causing "twisted" bones (diastrophic), affecting metaphyses (metaphyseal), affecting epiphyses (epiphyseal), and producing histologic changes such as an apparent increase in the fibrous material in the epiphyses (fibrochondrogenesis). Also, a number of eponyms are based on the first or most comprehensive case reports. Severe forms of the diseases produce gross distortions of most cartilaginous structures and of the eye. Mild forms are more difficult to classify. Among the features are cataracts, degeneration of the vitreous and retinal detachment, high forehead, hypoplastic facies, cleft palate, short extremities, and gross distortions of the epiphyses, metaphyses, and joint surfaces.

Incidence   Data on the frequency of most CDs are not available, but the incidence of the Stickler syndrome may be as high as 1 in 10,000. Therefore, the diseases are probably among the more common heritable disorders of connective tissue.

Molecular Defects   The first mutations shown to cause CDs were in the COL2A1 gene for type II collagen, the most abundant protein in cartilage. A number of mutations in this gene have now been reported in variants of CD ranging from mild to lethal. A large fraction of patients with lethal CDs, a smaller number of patients with moderately severe CDs, and about 2% of families with early-onset generalized osteoarthritis have mutations in the same gene. However, similar phenotypes can also be caused by mutations in other genes, including genes for three other collagens, additional components of the cartilage matrix, growth factors, growth factor receptors, and transcription factors. The number of mutated genes reported does not necessarily reflect the incidence of such mutations in the diseases themselves but rather the complexity of the genes and the technical difficulties in searching the complete gene for mutations. Also, it reflects the availability of large families for DNA linkage analysis and the vigor with which investigators have pursued their interest in a given gene. It is likely that mutations in additional genes will be found.

Mutations in the COL2A1 gene were first found in patients with severe CDs characterized by gross deformities of bones and cartilage such as spondyloepiphyseal dysplasia congenita, hypochondrogenesis/achondrogenesis II, and the Kniest syndrome. However, mutations in the COL2A1 gene have been found in a few families where few if any symptoms are present in childhood, but joint stiffness, joint pain, and degenerative changes of osteoarthritis develop in midlife. The mutations in the COL2A1 gene are similar to the mutations in the genes for types I and III procollagens, and the correlations between genotype and the severity of the phenotype are equally difficult. Stickler syndrome and related syndromes are caused by mutations in three different genes: the COL2AI gene for type II collagen and the COL11A1 and COL11A2 genes for type XI collagen. A series of mutations that introduce premature terminal signals in the COL2A1 gene lead to classic Stickler syndrome. However, some patients with classic Stickler syndrome have glycine substitutions in COL11A1. RNA splicing mutations in the COL11A1 gene are found in patients with the Marshall

syndrome, which is similar to classic Stickler syndrome but with milder eye changes and more severe hearing loss.

Many individuals with the Schmid metaphyseal CD, characterized by short stature, *coxa vara*, flaring metaphyses, and waddling gait, have mutations in the gene for the type X collagen, a short, network-forming collagen found primarily in the hypertrophic zone of endochondral cartilage.

Mutations in the receptor for fibroblast growth factor (FGFR3) are present in most patients with achondroplasia, the most common cause of short-limbed dwarfism accompanied by macrocephaly and dysplasias of the metaphyses of long bones. The same single-base mutation in the gene that converts glycine to arginine at position 380 is present in >90% of patients. Most patients represent sporadic new mutations, and this nucleotide change must be one of the most common recurring mutations in the human genome. The mutation causes unregulated signal transduction through the receptor and inappropriate development of cartilage. Mutations that alter other domains of FGFRE3 have been found in patients with the more severe disorders hypochondroplasia and thanatophoric dysplasia and in a few families with a variant of craniosynostosis. However, most patients with craniosynostosis appear to have mutations in the related *FGFR2 gene.*

Mutations in the gene for the cartilage oligomeric matrix protein (COMP) have been found in patients with multiple epiphyseal dysplasia or pseudoachondroplasia and in related syndromes characterized by short limbs and degenerative arthritis. However, some families with multiple epiphyseal dysplasia had a mutation in the gene for the $\alpha1(IX)$, $\alpha2(IX)$, or $\alpha3(IX)$ chain of type IX collagen (COL9A1, COL9A2, and COL9A3), or matrilin-3. All the known mutations in these two type IX collagen genes in patients with multiple epiphyseal dysplasia cause splicing out of the codons in the same domain. One predisposing mutation in COL9A2 and one predisposing mutation in COL9A3 were found in Finnish patients with the common condition of sciatica and herniations of vertebral discs.

Diagnosis   The diagnosis of severe forms of CD is made on the basis of the physical appearance, x-ray findings, histologic changes, and clinical course.

℞ TREATMENT

No definitive therapy is available. Symptomatic treatment is directed to secondary features such as degenerative arthritis. Many patients require joint replacement surgery and corrective surgery for cleft palate. The eyes should be monitored carefully for the development of cataracts and the need for laser therapy to prevent retinal detachment. Patients should probably be advised to avoid obesity and contact sports. Counseling for the psychological problems of short stature is critical, and support groups have formed in many countries. Ultrasonography is sometimes successful for prenatal diagnosis but is less successful than for OI. Specific DNA tests are available for the CDs caused by mutations in most of the genes identified to date.

MARFAN SYNDROME   MFS is characterized by a triad of features: (1) long, thin extremities frequently associated with other skeletal changes, such as loose joints and arachnodactyly; (2) reduced vision as the result of dislocations of the lenses (ectopia lentis); and (3) aortic aneurysms that typically begin at the base of the aorta.

Classification   The clinical diagnosis is frequently problematic because some affected members of families with MFS present with only one or two features of the typical clinical triad. Also, many patients present with one or two of the features of MFS without a family history, apparently because they represent sporadic mutations. Therefore, it is frequently difficult to determine whether a patient with ectopia lentis or the characteristic body habitus of MFS is at risk for developing a life-threatening aortic aneurysm on the basis of clinical data alone. The new DNA diagnostic tests for mutations in the fibrillin-1 and fibrillin-2 genes can probably resolve most, but not all, of these problems. Most patients who are prone to develop an aortic aneurysm as a component of MFS can be identified by detection of mutations in the fibrillin-1 gene. Some of these patients develop aortic aneurysms because of a mutation in the fibrillin-1 gene without the skeletal or ocular changes characteristic of MFS. Patients with the rarer form of MFS, which is characterized by contractural arachnodactyly instead of loose joints, can usually be identified by detection of a mutation in the fibrillin-2 gene that is similar in structure to the gene for fibrillin-1. Preliminary data suggest that patients with mutations in the fibrillin-2 gene are not prone to develop aneurysms. However, affected members of some rare families with a mutation in the fibrillin-1 gene also do not develop aortic aneurysms, even though they may show the skeletal or ocular changes. Therefore, the DNA tests are most helpful if: (1) a mutation is detected in either of the two genes, and (2) informative data are available on the clinical symptoms that the same mutation produces in the patient's family or in other families with similar clinical features.

Incidence and Inheritance   MFS has an incidence of about 1 in 10,000 in most racial and ethnic groups. The disorder is inherited as an autosomal dominant trait; at least one-fourth of patients do not have an affected parent, and therefore probably represent new mutations.

Skeletal Changes   Patients have long limbs and are usually tall compared to other members of the same family. The ratio of the upper segment (top of the head to the top of the pubic ramus) to the lower segment (top of the pubic ramus to the floor) is usually 2 SDs below mean for age, race, and sex. The fingers and hands are long and slender and have a spider-like appearance (arachnodactyly). Many patients have severe chest deformities, including depression (pectus excavatum), protrusion (pectus carinatum), or asymmetry. Scoliosis is frequent and usually accompanied by kyphosis. High-arched palate and high pedal arches or pes planus are common. A few patients have severe joint hypermobility similar to EDS.

Cardiovascular Changes   Cardiovascular abnormalities are the major source of morbidity and mortality (Chap. 231). Mitral valve prolapse develops early in life and in about one-quarter of patients progresses to mitral valve regurgitation of increasing severity because of redundancy of the leaflets, stretching of the chordae tendineae, and dilatation of the valvulae annulus. Dilatation of the root of the aorta and the sinuses of Valsalva are characteristic and ominous features of the disease that can develop at any age and in rare instances may be detected by echocardiography in utero. The rate of dilatation is unpredictable, but it can lead to aortic regurgitation, dissection of the aorta, and rupture. Dilatation is probably accelerated by physical and emotional stress, as well as by pregnancy.

Ocular Changes   Dislocations of the lens may be readily apparent, but diagnosis usually requires pupillary dilatation and slit-lamp examination. The displacement is usually not progressive but may contribute to the formation of cataracts. The ocular globe is frequently elongated; most patients are myopic, and some develop retinal detachment. A few patients have lattice degeneration and retinal tears; most have adequate vision.

Associated Changes   Striae may occur over the shoulders and buttocks. Otherwise the skin is normal. A number of patients develop spontaneous pneumothorax. Inguinal and incisional hernias are common. Marked dilatation of the dural sac is seen frequently in computed tomography scans, but the condition is usually asymptomatic. Patients are typically thin with little subcutaneous fat, but adults may develop centripetal obesity.

Molecular Defects   Most patients with the classic features of MFS are heterozygotes for mutations in a gene on chromosome 15 that encodes fibrillin-1, a glycoprotein of 350 kDa that is a major component of elastin-associated microfibrils. These microfibrils are abundant in large blood vessels and the suspensory ligaments of the lens. Mutations in the fibrillin-1 gene include missense, nonsense, in-frame deletions, and RNA splicing mutations. Many of the mutations are single amino acid substitutions in the epidermal growth factor-like domains of the molecule that may be involved in calcium binding. Mutations in the fibrillin-2 gene that cause the MFS variant characterized by contractures appear to follow a similar pattern. As with most genetic diseases, the nature and location of mutations in the genes are only an approximate guide to the severity of the phenotype unless the same mutation has been seen in other members of the same family or in similar unrelated patients. However, there is a clustering of mutations in the middle portion of the molecule of fibrillin-1 encoded by exons 23 to 32 that causes the most severe phenotype, referred to as *neonatal MFS*. The function of fibrillin has not been defined, but the data suggest that fibrillin self-assembles into a fibrillar structure and that the conformation and surface properties of the entire molecule are critical for normal assembly. Therefore, the functional consequences of mutations that change the amino acid sequence of fibrillin may be similar to the effects of mutations that change the conformation of a fibrillar collagen.

Diagnosis   The diagnosis is easily established if the patient and other members of the family have dislocated lenses, aortic dilatation, and long and thin extremities together with kyphoscoliosis or other chest deformities. The diagnosis is frequently made if ectopia lentis and an aneurysm of the ascending aorta occur in the absence of a Marfan habitus or a positive family history. All patients with suspected diagnosis should have a slit-lamp examination and an echocardiogram. Also, homocystinuria should be ruled out by a negative cyanide-nitroprusside test for disulfides in the urine (Chap. 343). A few patients with types I, II, and III EDS have ectopia lentis but lack the Marfan habitus and instead have characteristic skin changes not present in MFS. Patients with familial aortic aneurysms tend to develop aneurysms at the base of the abdominal aorta. The location of the aneurysms, however, is somewhat variable, and the high incidence of aortic aneurysms in the general population (1 in 100) makes the differential diagnosis difficult unless other features of MFS are clearly present. A few families with familial aortic aneurysms have mutations in the gene for type III procollagen.

℞ TREATMENT

There is no established treatment, but several investigators have recommended use of propranolol or other β-adrenergic blocking agents to lower blood pressure and thereby delay or prevent aortic dilatation. Surgical correction of the aorta, aortic valve, and mitral valve has been successful in some patients; all patients should be followed carefully with echocardiography and other techniques for evaluation of cardiovascular changes (Chap. 231). Patients should probably be advised of the risks of severe physical and emotional stress and of pregnancy.

The scoliosis tends to be progressive and should be treated by mechanical bracing and physical therapy if >20° or by surgery if it progresses to >45°. Dislocated lenses rarely require surgical removal, but patients should be followed closely for retinal detachment.

Diagnostic tests based on detection of fibrillin defects in cultured skin fibroblasts or DNA analysis of the gene are now available from several laboratories.

DISEASES RELATED TO ELASTIN   As may be expected from the role of elastin in maintaining the elasticity of skin, mutations in the elastin gene cause *cutis laxa*, a rare and heterogeneous group of disorders characterized by skin that is both lax and inelastic.

EPIDERMOLYSIS BULLOSA   EB consists of a group of similar disorders in which the skin and related epithelial tissues break and blister as the result of minor trauma. As with most heritable disorders of connective tissues, the clinical manifestations range from lethal to mild.

Classification   Four types of EB are defined on the basis of the level at which blistering occurs: EB simplex for blistering in the epidermis, EB hemidesmosomal for fissures between keratinocytes and the basal lamina, EB junctional for blistering in the dermal-epidermal junction, and EB dystrophica for blistering in the dermis.

Incidence The incidence of EB in the United States is estimated to be 1 in 50,000.

Molecular Defects The molecular basis of several specific variants of EB has been defined. A series of patients with EB simplex were found to have mutations in either keratin 14 or keratin 5, two of the major keratins in basal epithelial cells. Patients with the related syndrome, epidermolytic icthyosis, have mutations in keratin 1 and keratin 10. The new disease phenotype of hemidesmosomal EB has three clinical variants that are caused by mutations in one of four genes: (1) A generalized atrophic and benign form of EB is caused by mutations in the COL17A1 gene for type XVII collagen; (2) a variant with EB associated with pyloric atresia and other intestinal abnormalities is caused by mutations in either the gene for the α6 integrin (ITG A6) or the gene for the β4 integrin (ITG B4); and (3) another variant characterized by relatively mild blistering at birth but associated with late-onset muscular dystrophy is caused by mutations in the gene for plectin (PLEC-1). Junctional EB is caused by mutations in any one of three genes for laminin (LAMA-3, LAMB-3, LAMC-2). The most severe dystrophic form of EB is caused by mutations in the gene for type VII collagen (COL7A1) that forms the anchoring fibers binding the epidermis to the dermis.

Diagnosis The diagnosis is based on skin that readily breaks and forms blisters. Also, DNA diagnostic tests are available. EB simplex and EB hemidesmosomal are generally milder than EB junctional or EB dystrophica. EB dystrophica variants usually cause large and prominent scars. Precise classification within subtypes usually requires electron microscopy. The treatment is symptomatic.

ALPORT SYNDROME AS is an inherited disorder characterized by hematuria. Four forms of the disease are now recognized: (1) classic AS, which is inherited as an X-linked disorder with hematuria, sensorineural deafness, and conical deformation of the anterior surface of the lens (lenticonus); (2) a subtype of the X-linked form associated with diffuse leiomyomatosis; (3) an autosomal recessive form; and (4) an autosomal dominant form. The two autosomal forms can cause renal disease without deafness or lenticonus.

Incidence The incidence of AS is about 1 in 10,000 in the general population and as high as 1 in 5000 in some ethnic groups. About 80% of AS patients have the X-linked variant.

Molecular Defects Electron microscopy of kidneys from patients with classic AS demonstrates that the glomerular basement membrane is up to five times thicker than normal and the lamina densa is distorted and split. The X-linked and autosomal recessive forms are caused primarily by mutations in genes for the α3(IV), α4(IV), α5(IV), or α6(IV) chains of type IV collagen, a major component of basement membranes. The genes for the proteins are arranged in tandem pairs on different chromosomes in a head-to-head orientation and with overlapping promoters, i.e., the α1(IV) and α2(IV) genes are head-to-head on chromosome 13q34, the α3(IV) and α4(IV) genes are on chromosome 2q35-37, and the α5(IV) and α6(IV) genes are on chromosome Xq22. An X-linked variant is caused by mutations in the COL4A5 gene, and the X-linked variant associated with leiomyomatosis is caused by deletions that involve both the COL4A5 gene and the nearby COL4A6 gene. The autosomal recessive variants are caused by mutations in either the COL4A3 or COL4A4 genes. The mutations responsible for the autosomal dominant variants are still unknown, but they have been mapped to the same locus as the COL4A3 and COL4A4 genes.

Diagnosis The diagnosis of classic AS is based on X-linked inheritance of hematuria, sensorineural deafness, and lenticonus. Because of the X-linked transmission, women are generally underdiagnosed and are usually less severely affected than men. The hematuria progresses to nephritis and may cause renal failure in late adolescence in affected males and at older ages in some women. The sensorineural deafness is primarily in the high-tone range. It can frequently be detected only by an audiogram and is usually not progressive. The lenticonus can occur without nephritis but is generally considered to be pathognomonic of classic ASR. Renal transplantation is usually successful.

ACKNOWLEDGMENT
The authors acknowledge the contributions of Helena Kuivaniemi and Gerard Tromp to this chapter in previous editions of Harrison's.

FURTHER READING

INTERNATIONAL WORKING GROUP ON CONSTITUTIONAL DISEASES OF BONE: International nomenclature and classification of the osteochondrodysplasias (1997). Am J Med Genet 79:376, 1998

KUIVANIEMI H et al: Mutations in the fibrillar collagens (types I, II, III, IX and XI), and fibril-associated collagen, and the network-forming collagen (type X) cause a spectrum of diseases of bone, cartilage and blood vessels. Hum Mutat 9:300, 1997

MARINI JC: Osteogenesis imperfecta. Comprehensive management. Adv Pediatr 35:391, 1988

PEPIN M et al: Clinical and genetic features of Ehlers-Danlos syndrome type IV, the vascular type. N Engl J Med 342:673, 2000

RAMIREZ F et al: Marfan syndrome: New clues to genotype-phenotype correlations. Ann Med 31:202, 1999

343 | INHERITED DISORDERS OF AMINO ACID METABOLISM PRESENTING IN ADULTS
Nicola Longo

Amino acids are not only the building blocks of proteins but also serve as neurotransmitters (glycine, glutamate, γ-aminobutyric acid) or as precursors of hormones, coenzymes, pigments, purines, or pyrimidines. Eight amino acids, referred to as *essential*, cannot be synthesized by humans and must be obtained from dietary sources. The others are formed endogenously. Each amino acid has a unique degradative pathway by which its nitrogen and carbon components are used for the synthesis of other amino acids, carbohydrates, and lipids. Disorders of amino acid metabolism and transport (Chap. 344) are individually rare—the incidences range from 1 in 10,000 for cystinuria or phenylketonuria to 1 in 200,000 for homocystinuria or alkaptonuria—but collectively they affect perhaps 1 in 1000 newborns. Almost all are transmitted as autosomal recessive traits.

The features of inherited disorders of amino acid catabolism are summarized in Table 343-1. In general, these disorders are named for the compound that accumulates to highest concentration in blood

(-*emias*) or urine (-*urias*). For many conditions (often called *aminoacidopathies*), the parent amino acid is found in excess; for others, generally referred to as *organic acidemias*, products in the catabolic pathway accumulate. Which compound(s) accumulates depends, of course, on the site of the enzymatic block, the reversibility of the reactions proximal to the lesion, and the availability of alternative pathways of metabolic "runoff." Biochemical and genetic heterogeneity are common. Five distinct forms of hyperphenylalaninemia, seven forms of homocystinuria, and seven types of methylmalonic acidemia are recognized. Such heterogeneity reflects the presence of an even larger array of molecular defects.

The manifestations of these conditions differ widely (Table 343-1). Some, such as sarcosinemia, produce no clinical consequences. At the other extreme, complete deficiency of ornithine transcarbamylase is lethal in the untreated neonate. Central nervous system (CNS) dysfunction, in the form of developmental retardation, seizures, alterations

TABLE 343-1 Inherited Disorders of Amino Acid Metabolism

Aminoacid(s)	Condition	Enzyme Defect	Clinical Findings	Inheritance[a]
Phenylalanine	Phenylketonuria type I	Phenylalanine hydroxylase	Mental retardation, microcephaly, hypopigmented skin and hairs, eczema, "mousy" odor	AR
	Phenylketonuria type II	Dihydropteridine reductase	Mental retardation, hypotonia, spasticity, myoclonus	AR
	Phenylketonuria type III	6-Pyruvoyl-tetrahydropterin synthase	Dystonia, neurologic deterioration, seizures, mental retardation	AR
	GTP cyclohydrolase I deficiency	GTP cyclohydrolase I	Mental retardation, seizures, dystonia, temperature instability	AR
	Carbinolamine dehydratase deficiency	Pterin-4α-carbinolamine dehydratase	Transient hyperphenylalaninemia (benign)	AR
Tyrosine	Tyrosinemia type I (hepatorenal)	Fumarylacetoacetate hydrolase	Liver failure, cirrhosis, rickets, failure to thrive, peripheral neuropathy, "boiled cabbage" odor	AR
	Tyrosinemia type II (oculocutaneous)	Tyrosine transaminase	Palmoplantar keratosis, painful corneal erosions with photophobia, mental retardation (?)	AR
	Tyrosinemia type III	4-Hydroxyphenylpyruvate dioxygenase	Hypertyrosinemia with normal liver function, occasional mental delay	AR
	Hawkinsinuria	4-Hydroxyphenylpyruvate dioxygenase	Transient failure to thrive, metabolic acidosis in infancy	AD
	Alkaptonuria	Homogentisic acid oxidase	Ochronosis, arthritis, cardiac valve involvement, coronary artery calcification	AR
	Albinism (oculocutaneous)	Tyrosinase	Hypopigmentation of hair, skin, and optic fundus; visual loss; photophobia	AR
	Albinism (ocular)	Different enzymes or transporters	Hypopigmentation of optic fundus, visual loss	AR, XL
	DOPA-responsive dystonia	Tyrosine hydroxylase	Rigidity, truncal hypotonia, tremor, mental retardation	AR
GABA	4-Hydroxybutyric aciduria	Succinic semialdehyde dehydrogenase	Seizures, mental retardation, ataxia	AR
Tryptophan	Tryptophanuria	Unknown	Mental retardation, ataxia, skin photosensitivity	AR
	Hydroxykinureninuria	Kynureninase	Mental retardation, spasticity	AR
Histidine	Histidinemia	Histidine-ammonia lyase	Benign	AR
	Urocanic aciduria	Urocanase	Benign	AR
	Formiminoglutamic aciduria	Formiminotransferase	Occasional mental retardation	AR
Glycine	Glycine encephalopathy	Glycine cleavage (4 enzymes)	Infantile seizures, lethargy, apnea, profound mental retardation	AR
	Sarcosinemia	Sarcosine dehydrogenase	Benign	AR
	Hyperoxaluria type I	Alanine:glyoxylate aminotransferase	Calcium oxalate nephrolithiasis, renal failure	AR
	Hyperoxaluria type II	D-Glyceric acid dehydrogenase/glyoxylate reductase	Calcium oxalate nephrolithiasis, renal failure	AR
Serine	Phosphoglycerate dehydrogenase deficiency	Phosphoglycerate dehydrogenase	Seizures, microcephaly, mental retardation	AR
Proline	Hyperprolinemia type I	Proline oxidase	Benign	AR
	Hyperprolinemia type II	Δ^1-Pyrroline-5-carboxylate dehydrogenase	Febrile seizures, mental retardation	AR
	Hyperhydroxyprolinemia	Hydroxyproline oxidase	Benign	AR
	Prolidase deficiency	Prolidase	Mild mental retardation, chronic dermatitis	AR
Methionine	Hypermethioninemia	Methionine adenosyltransferase	Usually benign	AR
Homocystine	Homocystinuria	Cystathionine β-synthase	Lens dislocation, thrombotic vascular disease, mental retardation, osteoporosis	AR
	Homocystinuria	5,10-Methylene-tetrahydrofolate reductase	Mental retardation, gait and psychiatric abnormalities, recurrent strokes	AR
	Homocystinuria	Methionine synthase (CblE, -G)	Mental retardation, hypotonia, seizures, megaloblastic anemia	AR
	Homocystinuria and methylmalonic acidemia	Vitamin B$_{12}$ lysosomal efflux and metabolism (CblC, -D, -F)	Mental retardation, lethargy, failure to thrive, hypotonia, seizures, megaloblastic anemia	AR
Cystathionine	Cystathioninuria	γ-Cystathioninase	Benign	AR
Cystine	Cystinosis	Cystinosin CTNS (lysosomal efflux)	Renal Fanconi syndrome, rickets, photophobia, hypotonia, renal failure	AR
S-Sulfo-L-cysteine	Sulfocysteinuria	Sulfate oxidase or molibdenum cofactor deficiency	Seizures, mental retardation, dislocated lenses	AR
Lysine	Hyperlysinemia, saccharopinuria	α-Aminoadipic semialdehyde synthase	Benign	AR
Lysine, tryptophan	α-Ketoadipic acidemia	α-Ketoadipic acid dehydrogenase	Benign	?
	Glutaric acidemia type I	Glutaryl-CoA dehydrogenase	Progressive severe dystonia and athetosis, mild mental retardation	AR
	Glutaric acidemia type II	Electron transfer flavoprotein, ETF ubiquinone oxidoreductase	Hypoglycemia, metabolic acidosis, "sweaty feet" odor, hypotonia, cardiomyopathy	AR

(continued)

TABLE 343-1—(Continued)

Aminoacid(s)	Condition	Enzyme Defect	Clinical Findings	Inheritance[a]
Ornithine	Gyrate atrophy of the choroid and retina	Ornithine-δ-aminotransferase	Myopia, night blindness, loss of peripheral vision, cataracts, chorioretinal degeneration	AR
Urea cycle	Carbamylphosphate synthase deficiency	Carbamylphosphate synthase I	Lethargy progressing to coma, protein aversion, mental retardation, hyperammonemia	AR
	N-Acetylglutamate synthase deficiency	N-Acetylglutamate synthase	Lethargy progressing to coma, protein aversion, mental retardation, hyperammonemia	AR
	Ornithine transcarbamylase deficiency	Ornithine transcarbamylase	Lethargy progressing to coma, protein aversion, mental retardation, hyperammonemia	XL
	Citrullinemia type I	Argininosuccinate synthase	Lethargy progressing to coma, protein aversion, mental retardation, hyperammonemia	AR
	Argininosuccinic acidemia	Argininosuccinate lyase	Lethargy progressing to coma, protein aversion, mental retardation, hyperammonemia	AR
	Arginase deficiency	Arginase	Spastic tetraparesis, mental retardation, mild hyperammonemia	AR
	Hyperornithinemia, hyperammonemia, homocitrullinuria	Mitochondrial ornithine carrier ORNT1	Vomiting, lethargy, failure to thrive, mental retardation, episodic confusion, hyperammonemia, protein intolerance	AR
	Citrullinemia type II	Mitochondrial aspartate/glutamate carrier CTLN2	Neonatal intrahepatic cholestasis, adult presentation with sudden behavioral changes and stupor, coma, hyperammonemia	AR
Valine	Hypervalinemia	Valine aminotransferase	Vomiting, fever, failure to thrive, hypotonia	AR
Leucine, isoleucine	Hyperleucine-isoleucinemia	Leucine-isoleucine aminotransferase	Seizures, failure to thrive, mental retardation	?
Valine, leucine, isoleucine	Maple syrup urine disease (defective E1α, E1β, E2, E3)	Branched-chain ketoacid dehydrogenase	Lethargy, vomiting, encephalopathy, seizures, mental retardation, "maple syrup" odor, protein intolerance	AR
Leucine	Isovaleric acidemia	Isovaleryl-CoA dehydrogenase	Acidosis, ketosis, vomiting, coma, hyperammonemia, "sweaty feet" odor, protein intolerance	AR
	3-Methylcrotonyl glycinuria	3-Methylcrotonyl-CoA carboxylase	Stress-induced metabolic acidosis, hypotonia, hypoglycemia, "cat's urine" odor	AR
	3-Methylglutaconic aciduria type I	3-Methylglutaconyl-CoA hydratase deficiency	Stress-induced acidosis, mental retardation, hypotonia, hepatomegaly	AR
	3-Hydroxy-3-methylglutaric aciduria	3-Hydroxy-3-methylglutaryl-CoA lyase	Stress-induced hypoketotic hypoglycemia and acidosis, encephalopathy, hyperammonemia	AR
Isoleucine	3-Oxothiolase deficiency	3-Oxothiolase	Fasting-induced acidosis and ketosis, vomiting, lethargy	AR
Valine, isoleucine, methionine, threonine	Propionic acidemia (pccA, -B,-C)	Propionyl-CoA carboxylase (pcc)	Metabolic ketoacidosis, hyperammonemia, hypotonia, lethargy, coma, protein intolerance, mental retardation, hyperglycinemia	AR
	Multiple carboxylase/biotinidase deficiency	Holocarboxylase synthase or biotinidase	Metabolic ketoacidosis, diffuse rash, alopecia, seizures, mental retardation	AR
	Methylmalonic acidemia (mutase, CblA, -B)	Methylmalonyl-CoA mutase or cobalamin reductase/adenosyltransferase	Metabolic ketoacidosis, hyperammonemia, hypertonia, lethargy, coma, protein intolerance, mental retardation, hyperglycinemia	AR

[a] AR, autosomal recessive; XL, X-linked, AD, autosomal dominant.

Note: GTP, guanosine 5′-triphosphate; DOPA, dihydroxyphenylalanine; GABA, γ-aminobutyric acid; Cbl, cobalamin.

in sensorium, or behavioral disturbances, is present in more than half the disorders. Protein-induced vomiting, neurologic dysfunction, and hyperammonemia occur in many disorders of urea cycle intermediates. Metabolic ketoacidosis, often accompanied by hyperammonemia, is a frequent presenting finding in disorders of branched-chain amino acid metabolism. Some disorders produce focal tissue or organ involvement such as liver disease, renal failure, cutaneous abnormalities, or ocular lesions.

The analysis of plasma amino acids (by ion-exchange chromatography) and urine organic acids (by gas chromatography/mass spectrometry) is commonly used to diagnose and monitor most of these disorders. The diagnosis is confirmed by enzyme assay on cells or tissues from the patients or by DNA testing. The clinical manifestations in many of these conditions can be prevented or mitigated if a diagnosis is achieved early and appropriate treatment (i.e., dietary protein or amino acid restriction or vitamin supplementation) is instituted promptly. For this reason, several of these disorders are routinely screened for in newborns. Selected disorders that illustrate the principles, properties, and problems presented by the disorders of amino acid metabolism are discussed in this chapter.

THE HYPERPHENYLALANINEMIAS

The hyperphenylalaninemias (Table 343-1) result from impaired conversion of phenylalanine to tyrosine. The most common and clinically important is *phenylketonuria* (frequency 1:10,000), which is an autosomal recessive disorder characterized by an increased concentration of phenylalanine and its by-products in body fluids and by severe mental retardation if untreated in infancy. It results from reduced activity of phenylalanine hydroxylase (phenylketonuria type I). The accumulation of phenylalanine inhibits the transport of other amino acids required for protein or neurotransmitter synthesis, reduces synthesis and increases degradation of myelin, and leads to inadequate formation of norepinephrine and serotonin. Phenylalanine is a competitive inhibitor of tyrosinase, a key enzyme in the pathway of melanin synthesis, and accounts for the hypopigmentation of hair and skin. Untreated children with classic phenylketonuria are normal at birth, but fail to attain early developmental milestones, develop microcephaly, and demonstrate progressive impairment of cerebral function. Hyperactivity, seizures, and severe mental retardation are major clinical problems later in life. Electroencephalographic abnormalities; "mousy" odor of skin, hair, and urine (due to phenylacetate accumulation); and a ten dency to hypopigmentation and eczema complete the devastating clinical picture. In contrast, affected children who are detected and treated at birth show none of these abnormalities. To prevent mental retardation, diagnosis and initiation of dietary treatment of classic phenylketonuria must occur before the child is 3 weeks of age. For this reason, most newborns in North America and Europe are screened by determinations of blood phenylalanine levels. Abnormal values are confirmed using quantitative analysis of plasma amino acids. Dietary phenylalanine restriction is usually instituted if blood phenylalanine levels are >250 μmol/L (4 mg/dL). Treatment consists in a special diet low in phenylalanine and supplemented with tyrosine, since tyrosine becomes an essential amino acid in phenylalanine hydroxylase deficiency. With therapy, plasma phenylalanine concentrations should be maintained between 120 and 360 μmol/L (2 and 6 mg/dL). Dietary restriction should be continued and monitored indefinitely. Some patients with milder forms of phenylketonuria (phenylalanine <1200 μm at presentation) show increased tolerance to dietary proteins and improved metabolic control when treated with tetrahydrobiopterin (20 mg/kg per day), an essential cofactor of phenylalanine hydroxylase.

A number of women with phenylketonuria who have been treated since infancy will have reached adulthood and become pregnant. If maternal phenylalanine levels are not strictly controlled before and during pregnancy, their offspring are at increased risk for congenital defects and microcephaly (*maternal phenylketonuria*). After birth, these children have severe mental and growth retardation. Pregnancy risks can be minimized by continuing lifelong phenylalanine-restricted diets and assuring strict phenylalanine restriction 2 months prior to conception and throughout gestation.

THE HOMOCYSTINURIAS (HYPERHOMOCYSTEINEMIAS)

The homocystinurias are seven biochemically and clinically distinct disorders (Table 343-1) characterized by increased concentration of the sulfur-containing amino acid homocystine in blood and urine.

Classic homocystinuria, the most common (frequency 1:200,000), results from reduced activity of cystathionine β-synthase, the pyridoxal phosphate–dependent enzyme that condenses homocysteine with serine to form cystathionine. Most patients present between 3 and 5 years of age with dislocated optic lenses and mental retardation (in about half of cases). Some patients develop a marfanoid habitus and radiologic evidence of osteoporosis. Life-threatening vascular complications (affecting coronary, renal, and cerebral arteries) can occur during the first decade of life and are the major cause of morbidity and mortality. Classic homocystinuria can be diagnosed with analysis of plasma amino acids, showing elevated methionine and presence of free homocystine. Total plasma homocysteine is also extremely elevated (usually >100 μM). Treatment consists in a special diet restricted in protein and methionine and supplemented with cystine. In approximately half of patients, oral pyridoxine (25 to 500 mg/d) produces a fall in plasma methionine and homocystine concentration in body fluids. Folate deficiency should be prevented by adequate supplementation. Betaine is also effective in reducing homocystine levels in pyridoxine-unresponsive patients.

The other forms of homocystinuria are the result of impaired remethylation of homocysteine to methionine. This can be caused by defective methionine synthase or reduced availability of two essential cofactors, 5-methyltetrahydrofolate and methylcobalamin (methylvitamin B_{12}).

Hyperhomocysteinemia refers to increased total plasma concentration of homocysteine with or without an increase in free homocystine (disulfide form). Hyperhomocysteinemia, in the absence of significant homocystinuria, is found in some heterozygotes for the genetic defects noted above or in homozygotes for milder variants. Changes of homocysteine levels are also observed with increasing age; in postmenopausal women; in patients with renal failure, hypothyroidism, leukemias, or psoriasis; and during therapy with drugs such as methotrexate, nitrous oxide, isoniazid, and some antiepileptic agents. Homocysteine acts as an atherogenic and thrombophilic agent. An increase in total plasma homocysteine represents an independent risk factor for coronary, cerebrovascular, and peripheral arterial disease as well as for deep-vein thrombosis (Chap. 224). Homocysteine is synergistic with hypertension and smoking, and it is additive with other risk factors that predispose to peripheral arterial disease. In addition, hyperhomocysteinemia and folate and vitamin B_{12} deficiency have been associated with an increased risk of neural tube defects in pregnant women. Vitamin supplements are effective in reducing plasma homocysteine levels in these cases.

ALKAPTONURIA

Alkaptonuria is a rare (frequency 1:200,000) disorder of tyrosine catabolism in which deficiency of homogentisate 1,2-dioxygenase (also known as *homogentisic acid oxidase*) leads to excretion of large amounts of homogentisic acid in urine and accumulation of oxidized homogentisic acid pigment in connective tissues (*ochronosis*). Alkaptonuria may go unrecognized until middle life when degenerative joint disease develops. Prior to this time, about half of the patients might be diagnosed for the presence of dark urine. Foci of gray-brown scleral pigment and generalized darkening of the concha, anthelix, and, finally, helix of the ear usually develop after age 30. Low back pain usually starts between 30 and 40 years of age. *Ochronotic arthritis* is heralded by pain, stiffness, and some limitation of motion of the hips, knees, and shoulders. Acute arthritis may resemble rheumatoid arthritis, but small joints are usually spared. Pigmentation of heart valves, larynx, tympanic membranes, and skin occurs, and occasional patients develop pigmented renal or prostatic calculi. Degenerative cardiovascular disease is increased in older patients. The diagnosis should be suspected in a patient whose urine darkens to blackness. Homogentistic acid in urine is identified by urine organic acid analysis or by a specific colorimetric test. Ochronotic arthritis is treated symptomatically (Chap. 312). Ascorbic acid and protein restriction are not effective in reducing homogentisic acid production. By contrast, nitisone [2-(2-nitro-4-trifluoromethylbenzoyl)-1,3-cyclohexanedione], a drug used in tyrosinemia type I, reduces urinary excretion of homogentisic acid and, in conjunction with a low-protein diet, might prevent the long-term complications of alkaptonuria.

FURTHER READING

MONTAU AC et al: Tetrahydrobiopterin as an alternative treatment for mild phenylketonuria. N Engl J Med 347:2122, 2002

MUDD SH et al: Disorders of transulfuration, in *The Molecular & Metabolic Bases of Inherited Disease*, 8th ed., CR Scriver et al (eds). New York, McGraw-Hill, 2001, pp 2007–2056

NYHAN WL, OZAND PT: *Atlas of Metabolic Diseases*. London, Chapman & Hall Medical, 1998

PHORNPHUTKUL C et al: One hundred years later: Alkaptonuria in the twenty-first century. N Engl J Med, 347:2111, 2002

Specific membrane transporters mediate the passage of a wide variety of substances across cellular membranes. Classes of substrates include amino acids, sugars, cations, anions, vitamins, and water. The number of inherited disorders of membrane transport continues to increase with the identification of new transporters and the clarification of the molecular basis of diseases with previously unknown pathophysiology. The first transport disorders identified affected the gut or the kidney, but transport processes are now proving essential for the normal function of every organ. Mutations in transporter molecules demonstrate in disorders of the heart, muscle, brain, and endocrine and sensory organs (Table 344-1). Inherited defects impairing the transport of selected amino acids that can present in adults are discussed here as examples of the abnormalities encountered; others are considered elsewhere in this text.

CYSTINURIA Cystinuria (frequency of 1 in 10,000 to 1 in 15,000) is an autosomal recessive disorder caused by defective transporters in the apical brush border of proximal renal tubule and small intestinal cells. It is characterized by impaired reabsorption and excessive urinary excretion of the dibasic amino acids lysine, arginine, ornithine, and cystine. Because cystine is poorly soluble, its overexcretion predisposes to the formation of renal, ureteral, and bladder stones. Such stones are responsible for the signs and symptoms of the disorder.

There are two variants of cystinuria. Homozygotes for both variants have high urinary excretion of cystine, lysine, arginine, and ornithine. Type I heterozygotes have normal urinary amino, whereas non-type I (formerly type II and type III) heterozygotes have moderately increased urinary excretion of each of the four amino acids. The gene for type I cystinuria (*SLC3A1*, chromosome 2p16.3) encodes a membrane glycoprotein. Non-type I cystinuria is caused by mutations in *SLC7A9* (chromosome 19q13) that encodes the $b^{0,+}$ amino acid transporter. The glycoprotein encoded by *SLC3A1* favors the correct processing of the $b^{0,+}$ membrane transporter, and explains why mutations in two different genes cause a similar disease.

Cystine stones account for 1 to 2% of all urinary tract calculi but are the most common cause of stones in children. Cystinuria homozygotes regularly excrete 2400 to 7200 μmol (600 to 1800 mg) of cystine daily. Since the maximum solubility of cystine in the physiologic urinary pH range of 4.5 to 7.0 is about 1200 μmol/L (300 mg/L), cystine needs to be diluted to 2.5 to 7 L of water to prevent crystalluria. Stone formation usually manifests in the second or third decade but may occur in the first year of life. Symptoms and signs are those typical of urolithiasis: hematuria, flank pain, renal colic, obstructive uropathy, and infection (Chap. 268). Recurrent urolithiasis may lead to progressive renal insufficiency.

Cystinuria is suspected after observing typical hexagonal crystals in the sediment of acidified, concentrated, chilled urine or after performing a urinary nitroprusside test. Quantitative urine amino acid analysis confirms the diagnosis of cystinuria by showing selective overexcretion of cystine, lysine, arginine, and ornithine. Quantitation is important for differentiating heterozygotes from homozygotes and for following free cystine excretion during therapy.

Management is aimed at preventing cystine crystal formation by increasing urinary volume and by maintaining an alkaline urine pH. Fluid ingestion in excess of 4 L/d is essential, and 5 to 7 L/d is optimal. Urinary cystine concentration should be <1000 μmol/L (250 mg/L). The daily fluid ingestion necessary to maintain this dilution of excreted cystine should be spaced over 24 h, with one-third of the total volume ingested between bedtime and 3 A.M. Cystine solubility rises sharply above pH 7.5, and urinary alkalinization (with bicarbonate or polycitrates) can be therapeutic. Penicillamine (1 to 3 g/d) and tiopronin (α-mercaptopropionylglycine, 800 to 1200 mg/d in four divided doses) undergo sulfhydryl-disulfide exchange with cystine to form mixed disulfides. Since these disulfides are much more soluble than cystine,

pharmacologic therapy can prevent and promote dissolution of calculi. Penicillamine can have significant side effects and should be reserved for patients who fail to respond to hydration alone or who are in a high-risk category (one remaining kidney, renal insufficiency). When medical management fails, urologic surgery is required but should be a last resort as cystine stones reform more easily in scarred epithelium. Occasional patients progress to renal failure and require kidney transplantation.

DIBASIC AMINOACIDURIA This disorder is characterized by a defect in renal tubular reabsorption of the three dibasic amino acids lysine, arginine, and ornithine but *not* cystine. There are two variants, transmitted as autosomal recessive traits. In the common form of dibasic aminoaciduria (type II), also known as *lysinuric protein intolerance*, homozygotes show defective intestinal transport of dibasic amino acids as well as exaggerated renal losses. It is most common in Finland (1 in 60,000) and is rare elsewhere. The transport defect affects basolateral rather than luminal membrane transport and is associated with impairment of the urea cycle. The defective gene (*SLC7A7*, chromosome 14q11.2) encodes a unique membrane transporter, y+LAT, which associates with the cell-surface glycoprotein 4F2 heavy chain to form the complete sodium-independent transporter y+L.

Manifestations are related to the losses of ornithine, arginine, and lysine. Affected patients present in childhood with hepatosplenomegaly, protein intolerance, and episodic ammonia intoxication. Older patients may present with severe osteoporosis, impairment of kidney function, or interstitial changes in the lungs. Plasma concentrations of lysine, arginine, and ornithine are reduced, whereas urinary excretion of lysine and orotic acid are increased. Hyperammonemia may develop after the ingestion of protein loads or with infections, probably because of insufficient amounts of arginine and ornithine to maintain proper function of the urea cycle. The clinical features have been attributed to the hyperammonemia, to insufficient amounts of lysine to support protein synthesis during growth, and to decreased production of nitric oxide caused by arginine deficiency.

Therapy consists of dietary protein restriction and supplementation of citrulline (2 to 8 g/d), a neutral amino acid that fuels the urea cycle when metabolized to arginine and ornithine. Pulmonary disease responds to glycocorticoids or bronchoalveolar lavage in some patients.

HARTNUP DISEASE Hartnup disease (frequency 1 in 24,000) is an autosomal recessive disorder characterized by pellagra-like skin lesions, variable neurologic manifestations, and neutral and aromatic aminoaciduria. Alanine, serine, threonine, valine, leucine, isoleucine, phenylalanine, tyrosine, tryptophan, glutamine, asparagine, and histidine are excreted in urine in quantities 5 to 10 times normal, and intestinal transport of these same amino acids is defective. The clinical manifestations result from nutritional deficiency of the essential amino acid tryptophan, caused by its intestinal and renal malabsorption, and of niacin, which derives in part from tryptophan metabolism. Only a small fraction of patients with the chemical findings of this disorder develop a pellagra-like syndrome, implying that manifestations depend on other factors in addition to the transport defect. The diagnosis of Hartnup disease should be suspected in any patient with clinical features of pellagra who does not have a history of dietary niacin deficiency (Chap. 61). The neurologic and psychiatric manifestations range from attacks of cerebellar ataxia to mild emotional lability to frank delirium and are usually accompanied by exacerbations of the erythematous, eczematoid skin rash. Fever, sunlight, stress, and sulfonamide therapy provoke clinical relapses. Diagnosis is made by detection of the neutral aminoaciduria, which does not occur in dietary niacin deficiency. Treatment is directed at niacin repletion and includes a high-protein diet and daily nicotinamide supplementation (50 to 250 mg).

TABLE 344-1 *Genetic Disorders of Membrane Transport (Selected Examples)*

Class of Substance and Disorder	Individual Substrates	Tissues Manifesting Transport Defect	Proposed Molecular Basis of Defect	Major Clinical Manifestations	Inheritance
AMINO ACIDS					
Classic cystinuria	Cystine, lysine, arginine, ornithine	Proximal renal tubule, jejunal mucosa	Shared dibasic-cystine transport protein SLC3A1, SLC7A9	Cystine nephrolithiasis	AR
Dibasic amino-aciduria	Lysine, arginine, ornithine	Proximal renal tubule, jejunal mucosa	Dibasic transport protein SLC7A7	Type I: Benign Type II: Protein intolerance, hyperammonemia, retardation	AR
Hypercystinuria	Cystine	Proximal renal tubule	Cystine transport protein	Some risk of cystine nephrolithiasis	AR
Lysinuria	Lysine	Proximal renal tubule, jejunal mucosa	Lysine transport protein	Seizures, physical and mental retardation	Probable AR
Hartnup disease	Neutral amino acids	Proximal renal tubule, jejunal mucosa	Shared neutral amino acid transport protein	Constant neutral aminoaciduria, intermittent symptoms of pellagra	AR
Tryptophan malabsorption	Tryptophan	Jejunal mucosa	Tryptophan transport protein	Indoluria, ?hypercalcemia, ?nephrocalcinosis	Probable AR
Methionine malabsorption	Methionine	Jejunal mucosa	Methionine transport protein	White hair, mental retardation, convulsions, hyperpneic attacks, edema	Probable AR
Histidinuria	Histidine	Proximal renal tubule, jejunal mucosa	Histidine transport protein	Mental retardation	AR
Iminoglycinuria	Glycine, proline, hydroxyproline	Proximal renal tubule, jejunal mucosa	Shared glycine–imino acid transport protein	None	AR
Dicarboxylic-aminoaciduria	Glutamic acid, aspartic acid	Proximal renal tubule, jejunal mucosa	Shared dicarboxylic amino acid transport protein	None	Probable AR
Cystinosis	Cystine	Lysosomal membranes	Cystine transport protein	Renal failure, hypothyroidism, blindness	AR
HEXOSES					
Glucose-galactose malabsorption	D-Glucose D-Galactose	Jejunal mucosa, proximal renal tubule	Shared Na$^+$-dependent glucose-galactose transport protein SGLT1	Watery diarrhea on feeding glucose, lactose, sucrose, or galactose	AR
Glucose-transport defect	D-Glucose	Ubiquitous	Facilitative glucose transporter GLUT1	Seizures, mental retardation	AD
Fanconi-Bickel syndrome	D-Glucose	Liver, kidney, pancreas, intestine	Facilitative glucose transporter GLUT2	Growth retardation, rickets, hepatorenal glycogenosis, hypo- and hyperglycemia	AR
URATE					
Hypouricemia	Uric acid	Proximal renal tubule	Urate transport protein SLC22A12	Hypouricemia, hyperuricosuria, ?hypercalciuria	AR
ANIONS					
Congenital chloridorrhea	Chloride, sulfate	Ileal and colonic mucosa	Cl$^-$/HCO$_3^-$ exchange pump carrier protein (DRA)	Hydramnios, watery diarrhea, elevated fecal chloride, metabolic alkalosis with volume depletion, hyperaldosteronism	AR
Dent disease, X-linked recessive hypophosphatemic rickets and nephrocalcinosis	Chloride, phosphate	Proximal renal tubule	Voltage-gated Cl$^-$ channel CLCN5	Proteinuria, hypercalciuria, nephrocalcinosis, nephrolithiasis, rickets	XL
CATIONS					
Nesidioblastosis of pancreas	Potassium	Pancreatic β cell	Sulfonylurea receptor SUR1, K$^+$ channel KCNJ11	Neonatal hypoglycemia, hyperinsulinemia	AR
Benign familial neonatal epilepsy	Potassium	Brain	Voltage-gated K$^+$ channels KCNQ2, KCNQ3	Neonatal convulsions, normal development	AD

(continued)

TABLE 344-1 — *(Continued)*

Class of Substance and Disorder	Individual Substrates	Tissues Manifesting Transport Defect	Proposed Molecular Basis of Defect	Major Clinical Manifestations	Inheritance
WATER					
Nephrogenic diabetes insipidus	Water	Collecting tubule	Aquaporin 2 (water channel)	Polyuria, dehydration, hyposthenuria	AR, AD
VITAMINS					
Rogers' syndrome	Thiamine	Ubiquitous	Thiamine transporter SLC19A2	Megaloblastic anemia, diabetes, deafness	AR
OTHER					
Carnitine deficiency	Carnitine	Muscle, kidney, fibroblasts	High-affinity carnitine transporter OCTN2	Hypoketotic hypoglycemia, cardiomyopathy, hypotonia	AR
Benign recurrent and progressive familial intrahepatic cholestasis	Bile salts	Liver	Phosphatidylcholine transporter MDR3, phospholipid transporter ATP8B1, bile salt export pump BSEP	Cholestasis, hepatomegaly, cirrhosis, liver failure	AR

Note: AR, autosomal recessive; AD, autosomal dominant; XL, X-linked recessive.

FURTHER READING

BROER S, WAGNER CA: *Membrane Transporter Diseases. Molecular Bases of Inherited Transport Defects*. Kluver Academic/Plenum, New York, 2003, in press

LEVY HL: Hartnup disorder, in *The Molecular and Metabolic Bases of Inherited Disease*, 8th ed, CR Scriver et al (eds). New York, McGraw-Hill, 2001, pp 4957–4969

PALACIN M et al: Cystinuria, in *The Molecular and Metabolic Bases of Inherited Disease*, 8th ed, CR Scriver et al (eds). New York, McGraw-Hill, 2001, pp 4909–4932

———: The molecular bases of cystinuria and lysinuric protein intolerance. Curr Opin Genet Dev 11:328, 2001

345 NEUROBIOLOGY OF DISEASE
Stephen L. Hauser, M. Flint Beal

The human nervous system is the organ of consciousness, cognition, ethics, and behavior; as such, it is the most intricate structure known to exist. One-third of the 35,000 genes encoded in the human genome are expressed in the nervous system. Each mature brain is composed of 100 billion neurons, several million miles of axons and dendrites, and $>10^{15}$ synapses. Neurons exist within a dense parenchyma of multifunctional glial cells that synthesize myelin, preserve homeostasis, and regulate immune responses. Measured against this background of complexity, the achievements of molecular neuroscience have been extraordinary. Advances in cell biology and genetics have provided new tools to explore the pathophysiology of nervous system diseases, clarifying their underlying causes, revealing new unanticipated groupings, and raising realistic hope that novel therapies and prevention strategies will be possible. This chapter reviews selected themes in neurobiology that provide a context for understanding fundamental mechanisms underlying neurologic disorders.

ION CHANNELS AND CHANNELOPATHIES The resting potential of neurons and the action potentials responsible for impulse conduction are generated by ion currents and ion channels. Most ion channels are gated, meaning that they can transition between conformations that are open or closed to ion conductance. Individual ion channels are distinguished by the specific ions they conduct; by their kinetics; and by whether they directly sense voltage, are linked to receptors for neurotransmitters or other ligands such as neurotrophins, or are activated by second messengers. The diverse characteristics of different ion channels provide a means by which neuronal excitability can be exquisitely modulated at both the cellular and the subcellular levels. Mutations in ion channels—channelopathies—are responsible for a growing list of human neurologic disorders (Table 345-1). One example is epilepsy, a syndrome of diverse causes characterized by repetitive, synchronous firing of neuronal action potentials. Action potentials are normally generated by the opening of sodium channels and the inward movement of sodium ions down the intracellular concentration gradient. Depolarization of the neuronal membrane opens potassium channels, resulting in outward movement of potassium ions, repolarization, closure of the sodium channel, and hyperpolarization. Sodium or potassium channel subunit genes have long been considered candidate disease genes in inherited epilepsy syndromes, and recently such mutations have been identified (Chap. 348). These mutations appear to alter the normal gating function of these channels, increasing the inherent excitability of neuronal membranes in regions where the abnormal channels are expressed.

Whereas the specific clinical manifestations of channelopathies are quite variable, one common feature is that manifestations tend to be intermittent or paroxysmal, such as occurs in epilepsy, migraine, ataxia, myotonia, or periodic paralysis. Exceptions are clinically progressive channel disorders such as autosomal dominant hearing impairment. The neurologic channelopathies identified to date are all uncommon disorders caused by obvious mutations in channel genes. As the full repertoire of human ion channels and related proteins are identified, it is likely that additional channel-opathies will be discovered. In addition to rare disorders that result from obvious mutations, it is possible that subtle allelic variations in channel genes or in their pattern of expression might underlie susceptibility to some common forms of epilepsy, migraine, or other disorders.

NEUROTRANSMITTERS AND NEUROTRANSMITTER RECEPTORS Synaptic neurotransmission is the predominant means by which neurons communicate with each other. Classic neurotransmitters are synthesized in the presynaptic region of the nerve terminal; stored in vesicles; and released into the synaptic cleft, where they bind to receptors on the postsynaptic cell. Secreted neurotransmitters are eliminated by reuptake into the presynaptic neuron (or glia), by diffusion away from the synaptic cleft, and/or by specific inactivation. In addition to the classic neurotransmitters, many neuropeptides have been identified as definite or probable neurotransmitters; these include substance P, neurotensin, enkephalins, β-endorphin, histamine, vasoactive intestinal polypeptide, cholecystokinin, neuropeptide Y, and somatostatin. Peptide neurotransmitters are synthesized in the cell body rather than the nerve terminal and may colocalize with classic neurotransmitters in single neurons. Nitric oxide and carbon monoxide are gases that appear also to function as neurotransmitters, in part by signaling in a retrograde fashion from the postsynaptic to the presynaptic cell.

Neurotransmitters modulate the function of postsynaptic cells by binding to specific neurotransmitter receptors, of which there are two major types. *Ionotropic receptors* are direct ion channels that open after engagement by the neurotransmitter. *Metabotropic receptors* interact with G proteins, stimulating production of second messengers and activating protein kinases, which modulate a variety of cellular events. Ionotropic receptors are multiple subunit structures, whereas metabotropic receptors are composed of single subunits only. One important difference between ionotropic and metabotropic receptors is that the kinetics of ionotropic receptor effects are fast (generally <1 ms) because neurotransmitter binding directly alters the electrical properties of the postsynaptic cell, whereas metabotropic receptors function over longer time periods. These different properties contribute to the potential for selective and finely modulated signaling by neurotransmitters.

Neurotransmitter systems are perturbed in a large number of clinical disorders, examples of which are highlighted in Table 345-2. One example is the involvement of dopaminergic neurons originating in the substantia nigra of the midbrain and projecting to the striatum

TABLE 345-1 *Examples of Neurologic Channelopathies*

Category	Disorder	Channel Type	Gene	Chap. Ref.
Ataxias	Episodic ataxia-1	K	*KCNAI*	352
	Episodic ataxia-2	Ca	*CACNLIAd*	
	Spinocerebellar ataxia-6	Ca	*CACNLIAd*	
Migraine	Familial hemiplegic migraine	Ca	*CACNLIAd*	14
Epilepsy	Benign neonatal familial convulsions	K	*KCNQ2, KCNQ3*	348
	Generalized epilepsy with febrile convulsions plus	Na	*SCNIβ*	
Periodic paralysis	Hyperkalemic periodic paralysis	Na	*SCN4A*	368
	Hypokalemic periodic paralysis	Ca	*CACNLIA3*	
Myotonia	Myotonia congenita	Cl	*CLCNI*	368
	Paramyotonia congenita	Na	*SCN4A*	
Deafness	Jorvell and Lange-Nielsen syndrome (deafness, prolonged QT interval, and arrythmia)	K	*KCNQI, KCNEI*	26
	Autosomal dominant progressive deafness	K	*KCNQ4*	

(nigrostriatal pathway) in Parkinson's disease (Chap. 351) and in heroin addicts after the ingestion of the toxin MPTP (1-methyl-4-phenyl-1,2,5,6-tetrahydropyridine).

A second important dopaminergic system arising in the midbrain is the mediocorticolimbic pathway, which is implicated in the pathogenesis of addictive behaviors including drug reward. Its key components include the midbrain ventral tegmental area (VTA), median forebrain bundle, and nucleus accumbens (Fig. 345-1). *Addictive drugs share the property of increasing dopamine release in the nucleus accumbens.* Amphetamine increases intracellular release of dopamine from vesicles and reverses transport of dopamine through the dopamine transporters. Patients prone to addiction show increased activation of the nucleus accumbens following administration of amphetamine. Cocaine binds to dopamine transporters and inhibits dopamine reuptake. Ethanol inhibits inhibitory neurons in the VTA, leading to increased dopamine release in the nucleus accumbens. Opioids also disinhibit these dopaminergic neurons by binding to μ receptors expressed by GABA-containing interneurons in the VTA. Nicotine increases dopamine release by activating nicotinic acetylcholine receptors on cell bodies and nerve terminals of dopaminergic VTA neurons. Tetrahydrocannabinol, the active ingredient of cannabis, also increases dopamine levels in the nucleus accumbens. Blockade of dopamine in the nucleus accumbens can terminate the rewarding effects of addictive drugs.

Not all cell-to-cell communication in the nervous system occurs via neurotransmission. Gap junctions provide for direct neuron-neuron electrical conduction and also create openings for the diffusion of ions and metabolites between cells. In addition to neurons, gap junctions

TABLE 345-2 *Principal Classic Neurotransmitters*

Neurotransmitter	Anatomy	Clinical Aspects
Acetylcholine (ACh) $CH_3-\overset{\overset{O}{\|\|}}{C}-O-CH_2-CH_2-N-(CH_3)_3$	Motor neurons in spinal cord → neuromuscular junction	Acetylcholinesterases (nerve gases) Myasthenia gravis (antibodies to ACh receptor) Congenital myasthenic syndromes (mutations in ACh receptor subunits) Lambert-Eaton syndrome (antibodies to Ca channels impair ACh release) Botulism (toxin disrupts ACh release by exocytosis)
	Basal forebrain → widespread cortex	Alzheimer's disease (selective cell death) Autosomal dominant frontal lobe epilepsy (mutations in CNS ACh receptor)
	Interneurons in striatum Autonomic nervous system (preganglionic and postganglionic sympathetic)	Parkinson's disease (tremor)
Dopamine $HO\text{-}\underset{HO}{\bigcirc}-CH_2-CH_2-NH_3$	Substantia nigra → striatum (nigrostriatal pathway)	Parkinson's disease (selective cell death) MPTP parkinsonism (toxin transported into neurons)
	Substantia nigra → limbic system and widespread cortex	Addiction, behavioral disorders
	Arcuate nucleus of hypothalamus → anterior pituitary (via portal veins)	Inhibits prolactin secretion
Norepinephrine (NE) $HO\text{-}\underset{HO}{\bigcirc}-\underset{OH}{CH}-CH_2-NH_2$	Locus coeruleus (pons) → limbic system, hypothalamus, cortex Medulla → locus coeruleus, spinal cord Postganglionic neurons of sympathetic nervous system	Mood disorders (MAOA inhibitors and tricyclics increase NE and improve depression) Anxiety Orthostatic tachycardia syndrome (mutations in NE transporter)
Serotonin $HO\text{-indole ring}\text{-}CH_2-CH_2-NH_2$	Pontine raphe nuclei → widespread projections Medulla/pons → dorsal horn of spinal cord	Mood disorders (SSRIs improve depression) Migraine pain pathway Pain pathway
γ-Aminobutyric acid (GABA) $H_2N-CH_2-CH_2-CH_2-COOH$	Major inhibitory neurotransmitter in brain; widespread cortical interneurons and long projection pathways	Stiff person syndrome (antibodies to glutamic acid decarboxylase, the biosynthetic enzyme for GABA) Epilepsy (gabapentin and valproic acid increase GABA)
Glycine H_2N-CH_2-COOH	Major inhibitory neurotransmitter in spinal cord	Spasticity Hyperekplexia (myoclonic startle syndrome) due to mutations in glycine receptor
Glutamate $H_2N-\underset{COOH}{CH}-CH_2-CH_2-COOH$	Major excitatory neurotransmitter; located throughout CNS, including cortical pyramidal cells	Seizures due to ingestion of domoic acid (a glutamate analogue) Rasmussen's encephalitis (antibody against glutamate receptor 3) Excitotoxic cell death

Note: CNS, central nervous system; MPTP, 1-methyl-4-phenyl-1,2,3,6-tetrahydropyridine; MAOA, monoamine oxidase A; SSRI, selective serotonin reuptake inhibitor.

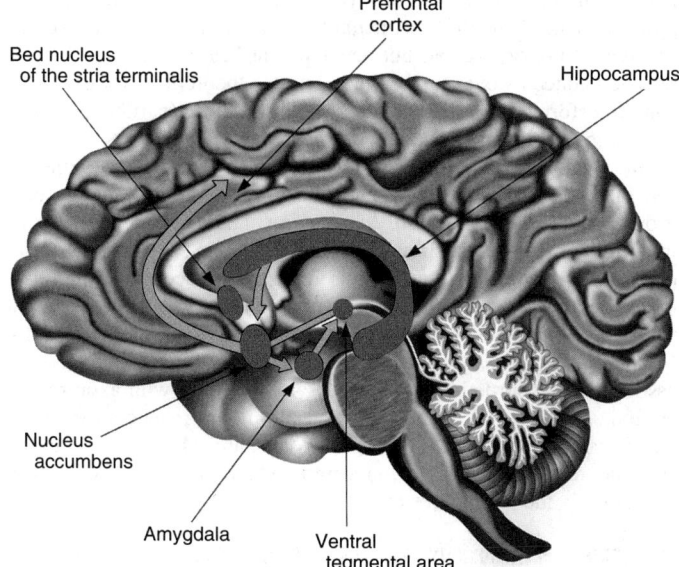

Prefrontal cortex

Bed nucleus of the stria terminalis

Hippocampus

Nucleus accumbens

Amygdala

Ventral tegmental area

FIGURE 345-1 Mid-sagittal section of the human brain demonstrating limbic structures involved in brain reward pathways.

are also widespread in glia, creating a syncytium that protects neurons by removing glutamate and potassium from the extracellular environment. Gap junctions consist of membrane-spanning proteins, termed *connexins*, that pair across adjacent cells. Mechanisms that involve gap junctions have been related to a variety of neurologic disorders. Mutations in connexin 32, a gap junction protein expressed by Schwann cells, are responsible for the X-linked form of Charcot-Marie-Tooth disease (Chap. 364). Mutations in either of two gap junction proteins expressed in the inner ear—connexin 26 and connexin 31—result in autosomal dominant progressive hearing loss (Chap. 26). Glial calcium waves mediated through gap junctions also appear to explain the phenomenon of spreading depression associated with migraine auras and the march of epileptic discharges. Spreading depression is a neural response that follows a variety of different stimuli and is characterized by a circumferentially expanding negative potential that propagates at a characteristic speed of 20 m/s and is associated with an increase in extracellular potassium.

SIGNALING PATHWAYS AND GENE TRANSCRIPTION

The fundamental issue of how memory, learning, and thinking are encoded in the nervous system is likely to be clarified by identifying the signaling pathways involved in neuronal differentiation, axon guidance, and synapse formation, and by understanding how these pathways are modulated by experience. Many families of transcription factors, each comprising multiple individual components, are expressed in the nervous system. Elucidation of these signaling pathways has already begun to provide insights into the cause of a variety of neurologic disorders, including inherited disorders of cognition such as X-linked mental retardation. This problem affects approximately 1 in 500 males, and linkage studies in different families suggest that as many as 60 different X-chromosome encoded genes may be responsible. Rett syndrome, a common cause of (dominant) X-linked progressive mental retardation in females, is due to a mutation in a gene (*MECP2*) encoding a DNA-

binding protein involved in transcriptional repression. As the X chromosome comprises only ~3% of germline DNA, then by extrapolation the number of genes that potentially contribute to clinical disorders affecting intelligence in humans must be potentially very large. As discussed below, there is increasing evidence that abnormal gene transcription may play a role in neurodegenerative diseases such as Huntington's disease in which proteins with polyglutamine expansions bind to and sequester transcription factors. A critical transcription factor for neuronal survival is CREB (cyclic adenosine monophosphate responsive element-binding) protein, which also plays an important role in memory in the hippocampus.

MYELIN Myelin is the multilayered insulating substance that surrounds axons and speeds impulse conduction by permitting action potentials to jump between naked regions of axons (nodes of Ranvier) and across myelinated segments. A single oligodendrocyte usually ensheaths multiple axons in the central nervous system (CNS), whereas in the peripheral nervous system (PNS) each Schwann cell typically myelinates a single axon. Myelin is a lipid-rich material formed by a spiraling process of the membrane of the myelinating cell around the axon, creating multiple membrane bilayers that are tightly apposed (compact myelin) by charged protein interactions. A number of clinically important neurologic disorders are caused by inherited mutations in myelin proteins of the CNS or PNS. Constituents of myelin also have a propensity to be targeted as autoantigens in autoimmune demyelinating disorders (Fig. 345-2).

NEUROTROPHIC FACTORS Neurotrophic factors (Table 345-3) are secreted proteins that modulate neuronal growth, differentiation, repair, and survival; some have additional functions, including roles in neurotransmission and in the synaptic reorganization involved in learning and memory. The neurotrophin (NT) family contains nerve growth factor (NGF), brain-derived neurotrophic factor (BDNF), NT3, and NT4/5. The neurotrophins act at TrK and p75 receptors to promote survival of neurons. Because of their survival-promoting and anti-

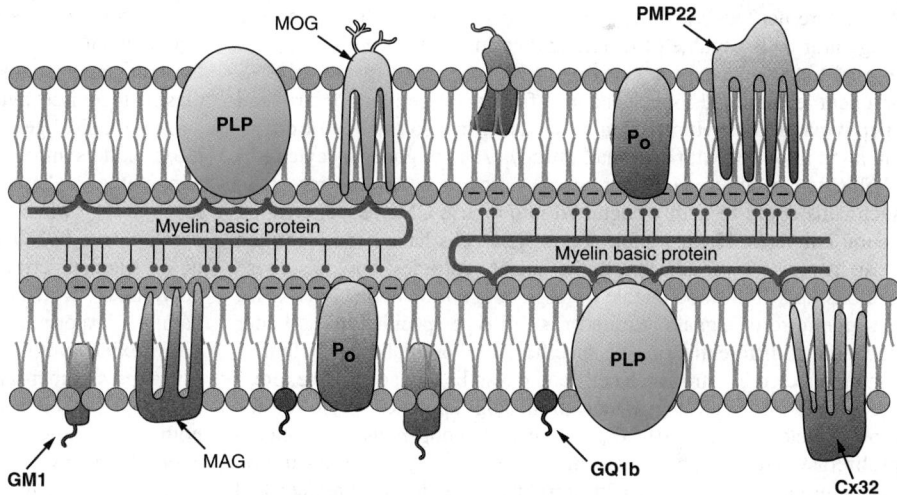

MOG PMP22 PLP P₀ Myelin basic protein Myelin basic protein P₀ PLP GM1 MAG GQ1b Cx32

FIGURE 345-2 The molecular architecture of the myelin sheath illustrating the most important disease-related proteins. The illustration represents a composite of CNS and PNS myelin. Proteins restricted to CNS myelin are shown in green, proteins of PNS myelin are lavender, and proteins present in both CNS and PNS are red. In the CNS, the X-linked allelic disorders, Pelizaeus Merzbacher disease and one variant of familial spastic paraplegia, are caused by mutations in the gene for proteolipid protein (PLP) that normally promotes extracellular compaction between adjacent myelin lamellae. The homologue of PLP in the PNS is the P₀ protein, mutations in which cause the neuropathy Charcot-Marie-Tooth disease (CMT) type 1B. The most common form of CMT is the 1A subtype caused by a duplication of the *PMP22* gene; deletions in *PMP22* are responsible for another inherited neuropathy termed hereditary liability to pressure palsies (Chap. 364).

In multiple sclerosis (MS), myelin basic protein (MBP) and the quantitatively minor CNS protein, myelin oligodendrocyte glycoprotein (MOG), are likely T cell and B cell antigens, respectively (Chap. 359). The location of MOG at the outermost lamella of the CNS myelin membrane may facilitate its targeting by autoantibodies. In the PNS, autoantibodies against myelin gangliosides are implicated in a variety of disorders, including GQ1b in the Fisher variant of Guillain-Barré syndrome, GM1 in multifocal motor neuropathy, and sulfatide constituents of myelin-associated glycoprotein (MAG) in peripheral neuropathies associated with monoclonal gammopathies (Chap. 365).

TABLE 345-3 *Neurotrophic Factors*

Neurotrophin family	Transforming growth factor β
Nerve growth factor	family
Brain-derived neurotrophic	Glial-derived neurotrophic family
factor	Neurturin
Neurotrophin-3	Persephin
Neurotrophin-4	Fibroblast growth factor family
Neurotrophin-6	Hepatocyte growth factor
Cytokine family	Insulin-like growth factor (IGF)
Ciliary neurotrophic factor	family
Leukemia inhibitory factor	IGF-1
Interleukin-6	IGF-2
Cardiotrophin-1	

apoptotic effects, neurotrophic factors are in theory outstanding candidates for therapy of disorders characterized by premature death of neurons such as occurs in amyotrophic lateral sclerosis (ALS) and other degenerative motor neuron disorders. Knockout mice lacking receptors for ciliary neurotrophic factor (CNTF) or BDNF show loss of motor neurons, and experimental motor neuron death can be rescued by treatment with various neurotrophic factors including CNTF and BDNF. However, in phase 3 clinical trials, growth factors were ineffective in human ALS. The growth factor glial-derived neurotrophic factor (GDNF) is important for survival of dopaminergic neurons. It has shown promising neurorestorative effects in experimental models of Parkinson's disease and in early stage human clinical trials.

STEM CELLS AND TRANSPLANTATION   The nervous system is traditionally considered to be a nonmitotic organ, in particular with respect to neurons. These concepts have been challenged by the finding that neural progenitor or stem cells exist in the adult CNS that are capable of differentiation, migration over long distances, and extensive axonal arborization and synapse formation with appropriate targets. These capabilities also indicate that the repertoire of factors required for growth, survival, differentiation, and migration of these cells exists in the mature nervous system. In rodents, neural stem cells, defined as progenitor cells capable of differentiating into mature cells of neural or glial lineage, have been experimentally propagated from fetal CNS and neuroectodermal tissues and also from adult germinal matrix and ependyma regions. Human fetal CNS tissue is also capable of differentiation into cells with neuronal, astrocyte, and oligodendrocyte morphology when cultured in the presence of growth factors. Impressively, such cells could be stably engrafted into mouse CNS tissue, creating neural chimeras. Human adult neural stem cells have been identified in an astrocyte layer adjacent to the lateral ventricles; however, these neurons appeared to be unable to migrate or form connections. Once the repertoire of signals required for cell type specification is better understood, differentiation into specific neural or glial subpopulations can be directed in vitro; such cells could also be engineered to express therapeutic molecules. Another promising approach is to utilize growth factors, such as BDNF, to stimulate endogenous stem cells to proliferate and migrate to areas of neuronal damage. Administration of epidermal growth factor with fibroblast growth factor replenished up to 50% of hippocampal CA1 neurons a month after global ischemia in rats. The new neurons made connections and improved performance in a memory task.

Experimental transplantation of human fetal dopaminergic neurons in patients with Parkinson's disease has shown that these transplanted cells can survive within the host striatum; however, some patients developed disabling dyskinesias and this approach is no longer in clinical development. Studies of transplantation for patients with Huntington's disease have also reported encouraging, although very preliminary, results. Oligodendrocyte precurser cells transplanted into mice with a dysmyelinating disorder effectively migrated in the new environment, interacted with axons, and mediated myelination; such experiments raise hope that similar transplantation strategies may be feasible in human disorders of myelin such as multiple sclerosis. The promise of stem cells for treatment of both neurodegenerative diseases and neural injury is great, but development has been slowed by unresolved concerns over safety (including the theoretical risk of malignant transformation of transplanted cells), ethics (particularly with respect to use of fetal tissue), and efficacy.

In developing brain, the extracellular matrix provides stimulatory and inhibitory signals that promote neuronal migration, neurite outgrowth, and axonal extension. After neuronal damage, reexpression of inhibitory molecules such as chondroitin sulfate proteoglycans may prevent tissue regeneration. Chondroitinase degraded these inhibitory molecules and enhanced axonal regeneration and motor recovery in a rat model of spinal cord injury. Several myelin proteins, specifically Nogo, oligodendrocyte myelin glycoprotein (OMGP), and myelin-associated glycoprotein (MAG), may also interfere with axon regeneration. Antibodies against Nogo promote regeneration after experimental focal ischemia. Nogo, OMGP, and MAG all bind to the same neural receptor, the Nogo receptor, which mediates its inhibitory function via the p75 neurotrophin receptor signaling.

CELL DEATH—EXCITOTOXICITY AND APOPTOSIS   *Excitotoxicity* refers to neuronal cell death caused by activation of excitatory amino acid receptors (Fig. 345-3). Compelling evidence for a role of excitotoxicity, especially in ischemic neuronal injury, is derived from experiments in animal models. Experimental models of stroke are associated with increased extracellular concentrations of the excitatory amino acid neurotransmitter glutamate, and neuronal damage is attenuated by denervation of glutamate-containing neurons or the administration of glutamate receptor antagonists. The distribution of cells sensitive to ischemia corresponds closely with that of *N*-methyl-D-aspartate (NMDA) receptors (except for cerebellar Purkinje cells, which are vulnerable to hypoxia-ischemia but lack NMDA receptors); and competitive and noncompetitive NMDA antagonists are effective in preventing focal ischemia. In global cerebral ischemia, non-NMDA receptors (kainic acid and AMPA) are activated, and antagonists to these receptors are protective. Experimental brain damage induced by hypoglycemia is also attenuated by NMDA antagonists.

Excitotoxicity is not a single event but rather a cascade of cell injury. Excitotoxicity causes influx of calcium into cells, and much of the calcium is sequestered in mitochondria rather than in the cytoplasm. Increased cytoplasmic calcium causes metabolic dysfunction and free radical generation; activates protein kinases, phospholipases, nitric oxide synthase, proteases, and endonucleases; and inhibits protein synthesis. Activation of nitric oxide synthase generates nitric oxide (NO$^\bullet$), which can react with superoxide (O$_2^\bullet$) to generate peroxynitrite (ONOO$^-$), which may play a direct role in neuronal injury. Another critical pathway is activation of poly-ADP-ribose polymerase, which occurs in response to free radical–mediated DNA damage. Experimentally, mice with knockout mutations of neuronal nitric oxide synthase or poly-ADP-ribose polymerase, or those that overexpress superoxide dismutase, are resistant to focal ischemia.

Apoptosis, or programmed cell death, plays an important role in both physiologic and pathologic conditions. During embryogenesis, apoptotic pathways operate to destroy neurons that fail to differentiate appropriately or reach their intended targets. There is mounting evidence for an increased rate of apoptotic cell death in a variety of acute and chronic neurologic diseases. Apoptosis is characterized by neuronal shrinkage, chromatin condensation, and DNA fragmentation, whereas necrotic cell death is associated with cytoplasmic and mitochondrial swelling followed by dissolution of the cell membrane. Apoptotic and necrotic cell death can coexist or be sequential events, depending on the severity of the initiating insult. Cellular energy reserves appear to have an important role in these two forms of cell death, with apoptosis favored under conditions in which ATP levels are preserved. Evidence of DNA fragmentation has been found in a number of degenerative neurologic disorders, including Alzheimer's disease, Huntington's disease, and ALS. The best characterized genetic neurologic disorder related to apoptosis is infantile spinal muscular atrophy (Werdnig-Hoffmann disease), in which two genes thought to be involved in the apoptosis pathways are causative.

Mitochondria are essential in controlling specific apoptosis pathways. The redistribution of cytochrome c, as well as apoptosis-inducing factor (AIF), from mitochondria during apoptosis leads to the activation of a cascade of intracellular proteases known as caspases. Caspase-independent apoptosis occurs after DNA damage, activation of poly-ADP-ribose polymerase, and translocation of AIF into the nucleus. Redistribution of cytochrome c is prevented by overproduction of the apoptotic protein BCL2 and is promoted by the proapoptotic protein BAX. These pathways may be triggered by activation of a large pore in the mitochondrial inner membrane known as the *permeability transition pore*, although in other circumstances they occur independently. Recent studies suggest that blocking the mitochondrial pore reduces both hypoglycemic and ischemic cell death.

PROTEIN AGGREGATION AND NEURODEGENERATION

The possibility that protein aggregation plays a role in the pathogenesis of neurodegenerative diseases is a major focus of current research. Protein aggregation is a major histopathologic hallmark of neurodegenerative diseases. Deposition of β-amyloid is strongly implicated in the pathogenesis of Alzheimer's disease. Genetic mutations in familial Alzheimer's disease produce increased amounts of β-amyloid with 42 amino acids, which has an increased propensity to aggregate, as compared to β-amyloid with 40 amino acids. Mutations in genes encoding the microtubule-associated protein tau lead to altered splicing of tau and the production of neurofibrillary tangles in frontotemporal dementia and progressive supranuclear palsy. Familial Parkinson's disease is associated with mutations in α-synuclein, parkin, and the ubiquitin carboxy-terminal hydrolase. Parkin, which causes autosomal recessive early-onset Parkinson's disease, is a ubiquitin ligase. The characteristic histopathologic feature of Parkinson's disease is the Lewy body, an eosinophilic cytoplasmic inclusion that contains both neurofilaments and α-synuclein. Huntington's disease and cerebellar degenerations are associated with expansions of polyglutamine repeats in proteins, which aggregate to produce neuronal intranuclear inclusions. Familial ALS is associated with superoxide dismutase mutations and cytoplasmic inclusions containing superoxide dismutase. In autosomal dominant neurohypophyseal diabetes insipidus, mutations in vasopressin result in abnormal protein processing, accumulation in the endoplasmic reticulum, and cell death (Chap. 319).

The current major scientific question is whether protein aggregates contribute to neuronal death or whether they are merely secondary bystanders. Protein aggregates are usually ubiquinated, which targets them for degradation by the 26S component of the proteosome. An inability to degrade protein aggregates could lead to cellular dysfunction, impaired axonal transport, and cell death by apoptotic mechanisms.

In experimental models of Huntington's disease and cerebellar degeneration, protein aggregates are not well correlated with neuronal death. A substantial body of evidence suggests that the mutant proteins

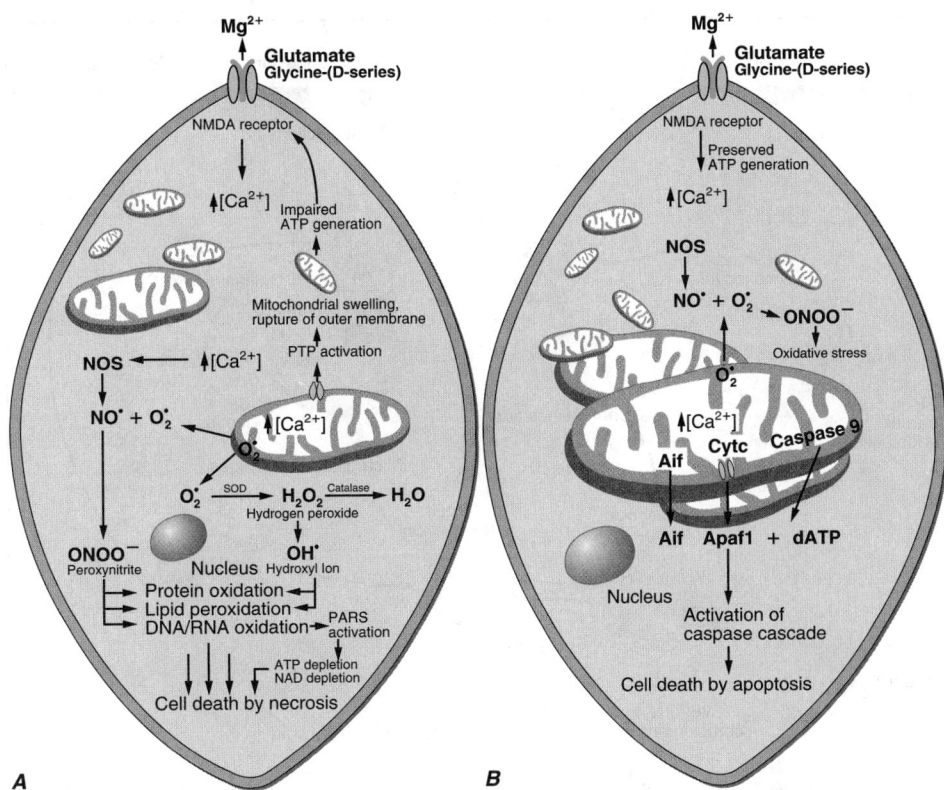

FIGURE 345-3 Involvement of mitochondria in cell death. A severe excitotoxic insult (*A*) results in cell death by necrosis, whereas a mild excitotoxic insult (*B*) results in apoptosis. After a severe insult (such as ischemia), there is a large increase in glutamate activation of NMDA receptors, an increase in intracellular Ca²⁺ concentrations, activation of nitric oxide synthase (NOS), and increased mitochondrial Ca²⁺ and superoxide generation followed by the formation of ONOO⁻. This sequence results in damage to cellular macromolecules including DNA, leading to activation of poly-ADP-ribose polymerase (PARS). Both mitochondrial accumulation of Ca²⁺ and oxidative damage lead to activation of the permeability transition pore (PTP) that is linked to excitotoxic cell death. A mild excitotoxic insult can occur due either to an abnormality in an excitotoxicity amino acid receptor, allowing more Ca²⁺ flux, or to impaired functioning of other ionic channels or of energy production, which may allow the voltage-dependent NMDA receptor to be activated by ambient concentrations of glutamate. This event can then lead to increased mitochondrial Ca²⁺ and free radical production, yet relatively preserved ATP generation. The mitochondria may then release cytochrome c (Cytc), caspase 9, apoptosis-inducing factor (Aif), and perhaps other mediators that lead to apoptosis. The precise role of the PTP in this mode of cell death is still being clarified, but there does appear to be involvement of the adenine nucleotide transporter that is a key component of the PTP.

with polyglutamine expansions in these diseases bind to transcription factors and that this contributes to disease pathogenesis. Agents that upregulate gene transcription are neuroprotective in animal models of these diseases. A number of compounds have been developed to block β-amyloid production and/or aggregation, and these agents are being studied in early clinical trials in humans.

NEUROIMMUNOLOGY

The nervous system is traditionally considered to be an immunologically privileged organ, a concept originally derived from observations that tissue grafts implanted in the brain were not rejected efficiently. In this context, immune privilege of the CNS may be maintained by a variety of mechanisms, including the lack of an efficient surveillance function by T cells; the absence of a traditional lymphoid system; limited expression of major histocompatibility complex (MHC) molecules required for T cell recognition of antigen; effects of regulatory cytokines secreted spontaneously or in response to mediators such as NGF, creating an immunosuppressive milieu; and also from expression of fas ligand that can induce apoptosis of fas-expressing immune cells that enter the brain. The blood-brain barrier (BBB) partially isolates the brain from the peripheral environment and contributes to immune privilege. Anatomically, the barrier is created by the presence of impermeable tight junctions between endothelial cells and by a relative absence of transendothelial conduits for the passive diffusion of soluble molecules. The BBB serves to preserve CNS homeostasis by excluding neuroactive substances present in the serum, such as neurotransmitters and neurotrophic factors. Because of the BBB, lipid-insoluble molecules must utilize either ion channels or

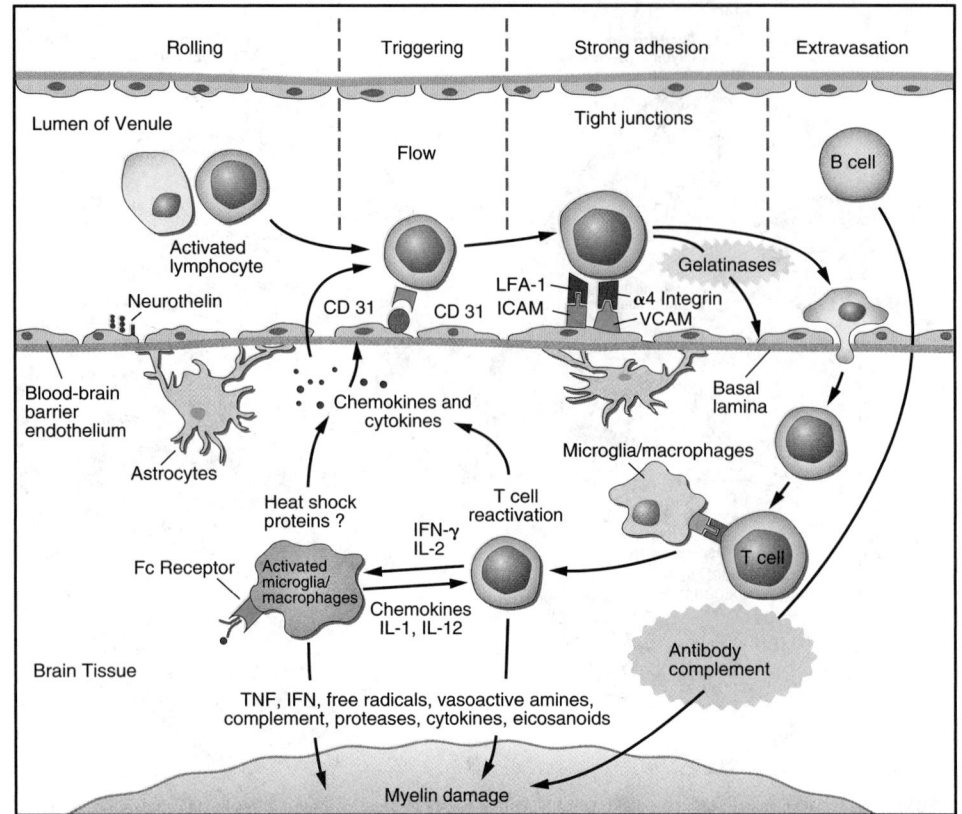

FIGURE 345-4 A model for experimental allergic encephalomyelitis (EAE). Crucial steps for disease initiation and progression include peripheral activation of preexisting autoreactive T cells; homing to the CNS and extravasation across the blood-brain barrier; reactivation of T cells by exposed autoantigens; secretion of cytokines; activation of microglia and astrocytes and recruitment of a secondary inflammatory wave; and immune-mediated myelin destruction. ICAM, intercellular adhesion molecule; LFA-1, leukocyte function-associated antigen-1; VCAM, vascular cell adhesion molecule; IFN, interferon; IL, interleukin; TNF, tumor necrosis factor.

demyelinating disorders multiple sclerosis and acute disseminated encephalomyelitis; the sequence of events in EAE is illustrated in Fig. 345-4.

Under normal circumstances the BBB is impermeable to antibodies. For autoantibodies to reach the CNS, the BBB must first be disrupted. In inflammatory conditions it is thought that this disruption most often occurs via actions of proinflammatory cytokines elaborated within the brain consequent to interactions between pathogenic T cells and antigen-presenting cells (APCs). In contrast to the BBB, in the PNS the blood-nerve barrier is incomplete. Endothelial tight junctions are lacking, and the capacity of charged molecules, including antibodies, to cross the barrier appears to be greatest in two regions of the PNS: proximally in the spinal roots and distally at neuromuscular junctions. This anatomic feature is likely to contribute to the propensity of antibody-mediated autoimmune disorders of the PNS to target proximal nerves (Guillain-Barré syndrome) or the neuromuscular junction (myasthenia gravis, Eaton-Lambert syndrome).

The major APCs in the CNS are microglial cells and macrophages; both cell types express MHC class 2 molecules as well as co-stimulatory molecules required for antigen presentation. Neurons do not express MHC class 2 molecules; however, some neurons express MHC class 1 proteins, which may be further increased in response to neuronal activity. Neuronal MHC class 1 molecules may function as retrograde postsynaptic signaling molecules that interact with presynaptic CD3 molecules to stabilize active synapses and transsynaptically modulate neuronal function. A role of microglial activation as a contributer to cell death in neurodegenerative and chronic neuroinflammatory diseases is likely and is being actively investigated.

FURTHER READING

DAWSON TM, DAWSON VL: Rare genetic mutations shed light on the pathogenesis of Parkinson's disease. J Clin Invest 111:145, 2003

GAGE FH: Neurogenesis in the adult brain. J Neurosci 22:612, 2002

SANAI N et al: Unique astrocyte ribbon in adult human brain contains neural stem cells but lacks chain migration. Nature 427:740, 2004

SOTO C: Unfolding the role of protein misfolding in neurodegenerative diseases. Nature Rev Neurosci 4:49, 2003

WATKINS TA, BARRES BA: Nerve regeneration: Regrowth stumped by shared receptor. Curr Biol 12:654, 2002

specific transport systems (for glucose or various amino acids) to gain entry to the CNS. Astrocyte foot processes that encircle the subendothelial basal surface of small blood vessels in the brain contribute to development and maintenance of the BBB.

The concept of immune privilege is at odds with clinical experience that vigorous immune reactions readily occur in the nervous system in response to infections and that autoimmune diseases of the nervous system are relatively common. Although primary (sensitizing) immune responses are not easily generated in the CNS for the reasons outlined above, this is not the case for secondary immune responses. When sensitization to nervous system antigens occurs *outside* the nervous system (e.g., in a regional lymph node), activated autoreactive T lymphocytes are easily generated, and these cells readily cross the BBB and induce immune-mediated injury. The paradigm for this mechanism of T cell–mediated CNS disease is experimental allergic encephalomyelitis (EAE), a laboratory model for the human autoimmune

346 APPROACH TO THE PATIENT WITH NEUROLOGIC DISEASE
Joseph B. Martin, Daniel H. Lowenstein, Stephen L. Hauser

Neurologic diseases are common and costly. According to one estimate, 180 million Americans suffer from a nervous system disorder, resulting in an annual cost of $634 billion (Table 346-1). Globally, these disorders are responsible for 28% of all years lived with a disability. Most patients with neurologic symptoms seek care from internists and other generalists rather than from neurologists, and this situation is likely to continue as primary care–based health care systems become increasingly prevalent. Because useful therapies now ex-

ist for these disorders, a skillfull approach to diagnosis is essential. Many errors result from an overreliance on costly neuroimaging procedures and laboratory tests, which, while useful, do not substitute for an adequate history and examination. The proper approach to the patient with a neurologic illness begins with the patient and focuses the clinical problem first in anatomic and then in pathophysiologic terms; only then should a specific diagnosis be entertained. The direct evaluation of the patient also informs the subsequent workup and ensures

TABLE 346-1 *Impact of Neurologic and Psychiatric Diseases in the U.S.*

Disorder	Patients, Millions	Cost, Billion $
Addiction	17.5	160
Alzheimer's disease	4	100
Blindness/vision loss	13	38.4
Deafness/hearing loss	28	56
Depression/manic depressive illness	17.5	47.3
Developmental disorders	8.6	30
Epilepsy	2.5	3.5
Head injury	2	25
Huntington's disease	0.03	—
Multiple sclerosis	0.3	2.5
Pain	80	100
Parkinson's disease	1	6
Schizophrenia	2	30
Spinal cord injury	0.25	5
Stroke	3	30
Total	**180**	**634**

Source: Modified from Dana Alliance for Brain Initiatives.

that technology is judiciously applied, a correct diagnosis is established in an efficient manner, and treatment is promptly initiated.

THE NEUROLOGIC METHOD ■ Locate the Lesion(s)   The first priority is to identify the region of the nervous system that is likely to be responsible for the symptoms. Can the disorder be mapped to one specific location, is it multifocal, or is a diffuse process present? Are the symptoms restricted to the nervous system, or do they arise in the context of a systemic illness? Is the problem in the central nervous system (CNS), the peripheral nervous system (PNS), or both? If in the CNS, is the cerebral cortex, basal ganglia, brainstem, cerebellum, or spinal cord responsible? Are the pain-sensitive meninges involved? If in the PNS, could the disorder be located in peripheral nerves and, if so, are motor or sensory nerves primarily affected, or is a lesion in the neuromuscular junction or muscle more likely?

The first clues to defining the anatomic area of involvement appear in the history, and the examination is then directed to confirm or rule out these impressions and to clarify uncertainties suggested by the history. A more detailed examination of a particular region of the CNS or PNS is often indicated. For example, the examination of a patient who presents with a history of ascending paresthesias and weakness should be directed toward deciding, among other things, if the location of the lesion is in the spinal cord or peripheral nerves. Focal back pain, a spinal cord sensory level, and incontinence suggest a spinal cord origin, whereas a stocking-glove pattern of sensory loss suggests peripheral nerve disease; areflexia usually indicates peripheral neuropathy but may also be present with spinal shock in acute spinal cord disorders.

Deciding "where the lesion is" accomplishes the task of limiting the possible etiologies to a manageable, finite number. In addition, this strategy safeguards against making tragic errors. Symptoms of recurrent vertigo, diplopia, and nystagmus should not trigger "multiple sclerosis" as an answer (etiology) but "brainstem" or "pons" (location); then a diagnosis of brainstem arteriovenous malformation will not be missed for lack of consideration. Similarly, the combination of optic neuritis and spastic ataxic paraparesis should initially suggest optic nerve and spinal cord disease; multiple sclerosis, CNS syphilis, and vitamin B_{12} deficiency are treatable disorders that can produce this syndrome. Once the question, "Where is the lesion?" is answered, then the question, "What is the lesion?" can be addressed.

Define the Pathophysiology   Clues to the pathophysiology of the disease process may also be present in the history. Primary neuronal (gray matter) disorders may present as early cognitive disturbances, movement disorders, or seizures, whereas white matter involvement produces predominantly "long tract" disorders of motor, sensory, visual, and cerebellar pathways. Progressive and symmetric symptoms often have a metabolic or degenerative origin; in such cases lesions are usu-

ally not sharply circumscribed. Thus, a patient with paraparesis and a clear spinal cord sensory level is unlikely to have vitamin B_{12} deficiency as the explanation. A Lhermitte symptom (electric shock–like sensations evoked by neck flexion) is due to ectopic impulse generation in white matter pathways and occurs with demyelination in the cervical spinal cord. Symptoms that worsen after exposure to heat or exercise may indicate conduction block in demyelinated axons, as occurs in multiple sclerosis. A patient with recurrent episodes of diplopia and dysarthria associated with exercise or fatigue may have a disorder of neuromuscular transmission such as myasthenia gravis. Slowly advancing visual scotoma with luminous edges, termed *fortification spectra*, indicates spreading cortical depression, typically with migraine.

THE NEUROLOGIC HISTORY   As in all other aspects of clinical medicine, attention to the description of the symptoms experienced by the patient and substantiated by family members and others often permits an accurate localization and determination of the probable cause of the complaints, even before the neurologic examination is performed. Furthermore, a careful analysis of the history is a necessary prerequisite for bringing a focus to the neurologic examination that follows. Each complaint should be pursued as far as possible to elucidate the location of the lesion, the likely underlying pathophysiology, and potential etiologies. For example, a patient complains of weakness of the right arm. What are the associated features? Does the patient have difficulty with brushing hair or reaching upward (proximal) or buttoning buttons or opening a twist-top bottle (distal)? Also, negative associations may also be crucial. A patient with a right hemiparesis without a language deficit likely has a lesion (internal capsule, brainstem, or spinal cord) different from that of a patient with a right hemiparesis and aphasia (left hemisphere). Additional features of the history include the following:

1. *Temporal course of the illness.* It is important to determine the precise time of appearance and rate of progression of the symptoms experienced by the patient. The rapid onset of a neurologic complaint, occurring within seconds or minutes, usually indicates a vascular event, a seizure, or migraine. The onset of sensory symptoms located in one extremity that spread over a few seconds to adjacent portions of that extremity and then to the other regions of the body suggests a seizure. A more gradual onset and less well localized symptoms point to the possibility of a transient ischemic attack (TIA). A similar but slower temporal march of symptoms accompanied by headache, nausea, or visual disturbance suggests migraine. The presence of "positive" sensory symptoms (e.g., tingling or sensations that are difficult to describe) or involuntary motor movements suggests a seizure; in contrast, transient loss of function (negative symptoms) suggests a TIA. A stuttering onset where symptoms appear, stabilize, and then progress over hours or days also suggests cerebrovascular disease; an additional history of transient remission or regression indicates that the process is more likely due to ischemia rather than hemorrhage. A gradual evolution of symptoms over hours or days suggests a toxic, metabolic, infectious, or inflammatory process. Progressing symptoms associated with the systemic manifestations of fever, stiff neck, and altered level of consciousness imply an infectious process. Relapsing and remitting symptoms involving different levels of the nervous system suggest multiple sclerosis or other inflammatory processes; these disorders can occasionally produce new symptoms that are rapidly progressive over hours. Slowly progressive symptoms without remissions are characteristic of neurodegenerative disorders, chronic infections, gradual intoxications, and neoplasms.

2. *Patients' descriptions of the complaint.* The same words often mean different things to different patients. "Dizziness" may imply impending syncope, a sense of disequilibrium, or true spinning vertigo. "Numbness" may mean a complete loss of feeling, a positive sensation such as tingling, or paralysis. "Blurred vision" may be used to describe unilateral visual loss, as in transient monocular blindness, or diplopia.

The interpretation of the true meaning of the words used by patients to describe symptoms becomes even more complex when there are differences in primary languages and cultures.

3. *Corroboration of the history by others.* It is almost always helpful to obtain additional information from family, friends, or other observers to corroborate or expand the patient's description. Memory loss, aphasia, loss of insight, intoxication, and other factors may impair the patient's capacity to communicate normally with the examiner or prevent openness about factors that have contributed to the illness. Episodes of loss of consciousness necessitate that details be sought from observers to ascertain precisely what has happened during the event.

4. *Family history.* Many neurologic disorders have an underlying genetic component. The presence of a Mendelian disorder, such as Huntington's disease or Charcot-Marie-Tooth neuropathy, is often obvious if family data are available. More detailed questions about family history are often necessary in polygenic disorders such as multiple sclerosis, migraine, and many types of epilepsy. It is important to elicit family history about all illnesses, in addition to neurologic and psychiatric disorders. A familial propensity to hypertension or heart disease is relevant in a patient who presents with a stroke. There are numerous inherited neurologic diseases that are associated with multisystem manifestations that may provide clues to the correct diagnosis (e.g., neurofibromatosis, Wilson's disease, neuro-ophthalmic syndromes).

5. *Medical illnesses.* Many neurologic diseases occur in the context of systemic disorders. Diabetes mellitus, hypertension, and abnormalities of blood lipids predispose to cerebrovascular disease. A solitary mass lesion in the brain may be an abscess in a patient with valvular heart disease, a primary hemorrhage in a patient with a coagulopathy, a lymphoma or toxoplasmosis in a patient with AIDS, or a metastasis in a patient with underlying cancer. Patients with malignancy may also present with a paraneoplastic syndrome (Chap. 87) or complications from chemotherapy or radiotherapy. Marfan's syndrome and related collagen disorders predispose to dissection of the cranial arteries and aneurysmal subarachnoid hemorrhage; the latter may also occur with polycystic kidney disease. A recent onset of asthma suggests the possibility of polyarteritis nodosa. Various neurologic disorders occur with dysthyroid states or other endocrinopathies. It is especially important to look for the presence of systemic diseases in patients with peripheral neuropathy. Most patients with coma in a hospital setting have a metabolic, toxic, or infectious cause.

6. *Drug use and abuse and toxin exposure.* It is essential to inquire about the history of drug use, both prescribed and illicit. Aminoglycoside antibiotics may exacerbate symptoms of weakness in patients with disorders of neuromuscular transmission, such as myasthenia gravis, and may cause dizziness secondary to ototoxicity. Vincristine and other antineoplastic drugs can cause peripheral neuropathy, and immunosuppressive agents such as cyclosporine can produce encephalopathy. Excessive vitamin ingestion can lead to disease; for example vitamin A and pseudotumor cerebri, or pyridoxine and peripheral neuropathy. Many patients are unaware that over-the-counter sleeping pills, cold preparations, and diet pills are actually drugs. Alcohol, the most prevalent neurotoxin, is often not recognized as such by patients, and other drugs of abuse such as cocaine and heroin can cause a wide range of neurologic abnormalities. A history of environmental or industrial exposure to neurotoxins may provide an essential clue; consultation with the patient's co-workers or employer may be required.

7. *Formulating an impression of the patient.* Use the opportunity while taking the history to form an impression of the patient. Is the information forthcoming, or does it take a circuitous course? Is there evidence of anxiety, depression, hypochondriasis? Are there any clues to defects in language, memory, insight, or inappropriate behavior? The neurologic assessment begins as soon as the patient comes into the room and the first introduction is made.

THE NEUROLOGIC EXAMINATION   The neurologic examination is challenging and complex; it has many components and includes a number of skills that can be mastered only through repeated use of the same techniques on a large number of individuals with and without neurologic disease. Mastery of the complete neurologic examination is usually important only for physicians in neurology and associated specialties. However, knowledge of the basics of the examination, especially those components that are effective in screening for neurologic dysfunction, is essential for all clinicians, especially generalists.

There is no single, universally accepted sequence of the examination that must be followed, but most clinicians begin with assessment of mental status followed by the cranial nerves, motor system, sensory system, coordination, and gait. Whether the examination is basic or comprehensive, it is essential that it be performed in an orderly and systematic fashion to avoid errors and serious omissions. Thus, the best way to learn and gain expertise in the examination is to choose one's own approach and practice it frequently and do it in the same exact sequence each time.

The detailed description of the neurologic examination that follows describes the more commonly used parts of the examination, with a particular emphasis on the components that are considered most helpful for the assessment of common neurologic problems. Each section also includes a brief description of the minimal examination necessary for adequate screening for abnormalities in a patient who has no symptoms suggesting neurologic dysfunction. A screening examination done in this way can be completed in 3 to 5 min.

Several additional points about the examination are worth noting. First, in recording observations, it is important to describe what is found rather than to apply a poorly defined medical term (e.g., "patient groans to sternal rub" rather than "obtunded"). Second, subtle CNS abnormalities are best detected by carefully comparing a patient's performance on tasks that require simultaneous activation of both cerebral hemispheres (e.g., eliciting a pronator drift of an outstretched arm with the eyes closed; extinction on one side of bilaterally applied light touch, also with eyes closed; or decreased arm swing or a slight asymmetry when walking). Third, if the patient's complaint is brought on by some activity, reproduce the activity in the office. If the complaint is of dizziness when the head is turned in one direction, have the patient do this and look for associated signs on examination (e.g., nystagmus or dysmetria). If pain occurs after walking two blocks, have the patient leave the office and walk this distance and immediately return, and repeat the relevant parts of the examination. Finally, the use of tests that are individually tailored to the patient's problem can be of value in assessing changes over time. Tests of walking a 7.5-m (25-ft) distance (normal, 5 to 6 s; note assistance, if any), repetitive finger or toe tapping (normal, 20 to 25 taps in 5 s), or handwriting are examples.

Mental Status Examination (See also Chaps. 23, 257, and 350)

- *The bare minimum: During the interview, look for difficulties with communication and determine whether the patient has recall and insight into recent and past events.*

The mental status examination is underway as soon as the physician begins observing and talking with the patient. If the history raises any concern for abnormalities of higher cortical function or if cognitive problems are observed during the interview, then detailed testing of the mental status is indicated. The patient's ability to understand the language used for the examination, cultural background, educational experience, sensory or motor problems, or co-morbid conditions need to be factored into the applicability of the tests and interpretation of results.

The Folstein mini-mental status examination (MMSE) (Table 350-4) is a standardized screening examination of cognitive function that is extremely easy to administer and takes <10 min to complete. Using age-adjusted values for defining normal performance, the test is ~85% sensitive and 85% specific for making the diagnosis of dementia that is moderate or severe, especially in educated patients. When there is sufficient time available, the MMSE is one of the best methods for documenting the current mental status of the patient, and this is especially useful as a baseline assessment to which future scores of the MMSE can be compared.

Individual elements of the mental status examination can be subdivided into level of consciousness, orientation, speech and language, memory, fund of information, insight and judgment, abstract thought, and calculations.

Level of consciousness is the patient's relative state of awareness of the self and the environment, and ranges from fully awake to comatose. When the patient is not fully awake, the examiner should describe the responses to the minimum stimulus necessary to elicit a reaction, ranging from verbal commands to a brief, painful stimulus such as a squeeze of the trapezius muscle. Responses that are directed toward the stimulus and signify some degree of intact cerebral function (e.g., opening the eyes and looking at the examiner or reaching to push away a painful stimulus) must be distinguished from reflex responses of a spinal origin (e.g., triple flexion response—flexion at the ankle, knee, and hip in response to a painful stimulus to the foot). *Orientation* is tested by asking the person to state his or her name, location, and time (day of the week and date); time is usually the first to be affected in a variety of conditions. *Speech* is assessed by observing articulation, rate, rhythm, and prosody (i.e., the changes in pitch and accentuation of syllable and words). *Language* is assessed by observing the content of the patient's verbal and written output, response to spoken commands, and ability to read. A typical testing sequence is to ask the patient to name successively more detailed components of clothing, a watch or a pen; repeat the phrase "No ifs, ands, or buts"; follow a three-step, verbal command; write a sentence; and read and respond to a written command. *Memory* should be analyzed according to three main time scales: (1) immediate memory can be tested by saying a list of three items and having the patient repeat the list immediately, (2) short-term memory is assessed by asking the patient to recall the same three items 5 and 15 min later, and (3) long-term memory is evaluated by determining how well the patient is able to provide a coherent chronologic history of his or her illness or personal events. *Fund of information* is assessed by asking questions about major historic or current events, with special attention to educational level and life experiences. Abnormalities of *insight and judgment* are usually detected during the patient interview; a more detailed assessment can be elicited by asking the patient to describe how he or she would respond to situations having a variety of potential outcomes (e.g., "What would you do if you found a wallet on the sidewalk?"). *Abstract thought* can be tested by asking the patient to describe similarities between various objects or concepts (e.g., apple and orange, desk and chair, poetry and sculpture) or to list items having the same attributes (e.g., a list of four-legged animals). *Calculation ability* is assessed by having the patient carry out a computation that is appropriate to the patient's age and education (e.g., serial subtraction of 7 from 100 or 3 from 20; or word problems involving simple arithmetic).

Cranial Nerve Examination (See also Chaps. 25, 26, and 355)

- *The bare minimum: Check the fundi, visual fields, pupil size and reactivity, extraocular movements, and facial movements.*

The cranial nerves (CN) are best examined in numerical order, except for grouping together CN III, IV, and VI because of their similar function.

CN I (OLFACTORY) Testing is usually omitted unless there is suspicion for inferior frontal lobe disease (e.g., meningioma). With eyes closed, ask the patient to sniff a mild stimulus such as toothpaste or coffee and identify the odorant.

CN II (OPTIC) Check visual acuity (with eyeglasses or contact lens correction) using a Snellen chart or similar tool. Test the visual fields by confrontation, i.e., by comparing the patient's visual fields to your own. As a screening test, it is usually sufficient to examine the visual fields of both eyes simultaneously; individual eye fields should be tested if there is any reason to suspect a problem of vision by the history or other elements of the examination, or if the screening test

reveals an abnormality. Face the patient at a distance of approximately 0.6 to 1.0 m (2 to 3 ft) and place your hands at the periphery of your visual fields in the plane that is equidistant between you and the patient. Instruct the patient to look directly at the center of your face and to indicate when and where he or she sees one of your fingers moving. Beginning with the two inferior quadrants and then the two superior quadrants, move your index finger of the right hand, left hand, or both hands simultaneously and observe whether the patient detects the movements. A single small-amplitude movement of the finger is sufficient for a normal response. Focal perimetry and tangent screen examinations should be used to map out visual field defects fully or to search for subtle abnormalities. Optic fundi should be examined with an ophthalmoscope, and the color, size, and degree of swelling or elevation of the optic disc noted, as well as the color and texture of the retina. The retinal vessels should be checked for size, regularity, arterial-venous nicking at crossing points, hemorrhage, exudates, etc.

CN III, IV, VI (OCULOMOTOR, TROCHLEAR, ABDUCENS) Describe the size and shape of pupils and reaction to light and accommodation (i.e., as the eyes converge while following your finger as it moves toward the bridge of the nose). To check extraocular movements, ask the patient to keep his or her head still while tracking the movement of the tip of your finger. Move the target slowly in the horizontal and vertical planes; observe any paresis, nystagmus, or abnormalities of smooth pursuit (saccades, oculomotor ataxia, etc.). If necessary, the relative position of the two eyes, both in primary and multidirectional gaze, can be assessed by comparing the reflections of a bright light off both pupils. However, in practice it is typically more useful to determine whether the patient describes diplopia in any direction of gaze; true diplopia should almost always resolve with one eye closed. Horizontal nystagmus is best assessed at 45° and not at extreme lateral gaze (which is uncomfortable for the patient); the target must often be held at the lateral position for at least a few seconds to detect an abnormality.

CN V (TRIGEMINAL) Examine sensation within the three territories of the branches of the trigeminal nerve (ophthalmic, maxillary, and mandibular) on each side of the face. As with other parts of the sensory examination, testing of two sensory modalities derived from different anatomic pathways (e.g., light touch and temperature) is sufficient for a screening examination. Testing of other modalities, the corneal reflex, and the motor component of CN V (jaw clench—masseter muscle) is indicated when suggested by the history.

CN VII (FACIAL) Look for facial asymmetry at rest and with spontaneous movements. Test eyebrow elevation, forehead wrinkling, eye closure, smiling, and cheek puff. Look in particular for differences in the lower versus upper facial muscles; weakness of the lower two-thirds of the face with preservation of the upper third suggests an upper motor neuron lesion, whereas weakness of an entire side suggests a lower motor neuron lesion.

CN VIII (VESTIBULOCOCHLEAR) Check the patient's ability to hear a finger rub or whispered voice with each ear. Further testing for air versus mastoid bone conduction (Rinne) and lateralization of a 512-Hz tuning fork placed at the center of the forehead (Weber) should be done if an abnormality is detected by history or examination. Any suspected problem should be followed up with formal audiometry. →*For further discussion of assessing vestibular nerve function in the setting of dizziness or coma, see Chaps. 20 and 257, respectively.*

CN IX, X Observe the position and symmetry of the palate and uvula at rest and with phonation ("aah"). The pharyngeal ("gag") reflex is evaluated by stimulating the posterior pharyngeal wall on each side with a sterile, blunt object (e.g., tongue blade), but the reflex is often absent in normal individuals.

CN XI Check shoulder shrug (trapezius muscle) and head rotation to each side (sternocleidomastoid) against resistance.

CN XII Inspect the tongue for atrophy or fasciculations, position with protrusion, and strength when extended against the inner surface of the cheeks on each side.

Motor Examination (See also Chap. 21)

- *The bare minimum: Look for muscle atrophy and check extremity tone. Assess upper extremity strength by checking for pronator drift and strength of wrist or finger extensors. Tap the biceps, patellar, and Achilles reflexes. Test for lower extremity strength by having the patient walk normally and on heels and toes.*

The motor examination includes observations of muscle appearance, tone, strength, and reflexes. Although gait is in part a test of motor function, it is usually evaluated separately at the end of the examination.

APPEARANCE Inspect and palpate muscle groups under good light and with the patient in a comfortable and symmetric position. Check for muscle fasciculations, tenderness, and atrophy or hypertrophy. Involuntary movements may be present at rest (e.g., tics, myoclonus, choreoathetosis), during maintained posture (pill-rolling tremor of Parkinson's disease), or with voluntary movements (intention tremor of cerebellar disease or familial tremor).

TONE Muscle tone is tested by measuring the resistance to passive movement of a relaxed limb. Patients often have difficulty relaxing during this procedure, so it is useful to distract the patient to minimize active movements. In the upper limbs, tone is assessed by rapid pronation and supination of the forearm and flexion and extension at the wrist. In the lower limbs, while the patient is supine the examiner's hands are placed behind the knees and rapidly raised; with normal tone the ankles drag along the table surface for a variable distance before rising, whereas increased tone results in an immediate lift of the heel off the surface. Decreased tone is most commonly due to lower motor neuron or peripheral nerve disorders. Increased tone may be evident as spasticity (resistance determined by the angle and velocity of motion; corticospinal tract disease), rigidity (similar resistance in all angles of motion; extrapyramidal disease), or paratonia (fluctuating changes in resistance; frontal lobe pathways or normal difficulty in relaxing). Cogwheel rigidity, in which passive motion elicits jerky interruptions in resistance, is seen in parkinsonism.

STRENGTH Testing for pronator drift is an extremely useful method for screening upper limb weakness. The patient is asked to hold both arms fully extended and parallel to the ground with eyes closed. This position should be maintained for ~10 s; any flexion at the elbow or fingers or pronation of the forearm, especially if asymmetric, is a sign of potential weakness. Muscle strength is further assessed by having the patient exert maximal effort for the particular muscle or muscle group being tested. It is important to isolate the muscles as much as possible, i.e., hold the limb so that only the muscles of interest are active. It is also helpful to palpate accessible muscles as they contract. Grading muscle strength and evaluating the patient's effort is an art that takes time and practice. Muscle strength is traditionally graded using the following scale:

> 0 = no movement
> 1 = flicker or trace of contraction but no associated movement at a joint
> 2 = movement with gravity eliminated
> 3 = movement against gravity but not against resistance
> 4− = movement against a mild degree of resistance
> 4 = movement against moderate resistance
> 4+ = movement against strong resistance
> 5 = full power

However, in many cases it is more practical to use the following terms:

> Paralysis = no movement
> Severe weakness = movement with gravity eliminated

> Moderate weakness = movement against gravity but not against mild resistance
> Mild weakness = movement against moderate resistance
> Full strength

Noting the pattern of weakness is as important as assessing the magnitude of weakness. Unilateral or bilateral weakness of the upper limb extensors and lower limb flexors ("pyramidal weakness") suggests a lesion of the pyramidal tract, bilateral proximal weakness suggests myopathy, and bilateral distal weakness suggests peripheral neuropathy.

REFLEXES ■ *Muscle Stretch Reflexes* Those that are typically assessed include the biceps (**C5**, C6), brachioradialis (C5, **C6**), and triceps (**C7**, C8) reflexes in the upper limbs and the patellar or quadriceps (**L3**, L4) and Achilles (**S1**, S2) reflexes in the lower limbs. The patient should be relaxed and the muscle positioned midway between full contraction and extension. Reflexes may be enhanced by asking the patient to voluntarily contract other, distant muscle groups (Jendrassik maneuver). For example, upper limb reflexes may be reinforced by voluntary teeth-clenching, and the Achilles reflex by hooking the flexed fingers of the two hands together and attempting to pull them apart. For each reflex tested, the two sides should be tested sequentially, and it is important to determine the smallest stimulus required to elicit a reflex rather than the maximum response. Reflexes are graded according to the following scale:

> 0 = absent   3 = exaggerated
> 1 = present but diminished   4 = clonus
> 2 = normoactive

Cutaneous Reflexes The plantar reflex is elicited by stroking, with a noxious stimulus such as a tongue blade, the lateral surface of the sole of the foot beginning near the heel and moving across the ball of the foot to the great toe. The normal reflex consists of plantar flexion of the toes. With upper motor neuron lesions above the S1 level of the spinal cord, a paradoxical extension of the toe is observed, associated with fanning and extension of the other toes (termed an *extensor plantar response*, or *Babinski sign*). Superficial abdominal reflexes are elicited by gently stroking the abdominal surface near the umbilicus in a diagonal fashion with a sharp object (e.g., the wooden end of a cotton-tipped swab) and observing the movement of the umbilicus. Normally, the umbilicus will pull toward the stimulated quadrant. With upper motor neuron lesions, these reflexes are absent. They are most helpful when there is preservation of the upper (spinal cord level T9) but not lower (T12) abdominal reflexes, indicating a spinal lesion between T9 and T12, or when the response is asymmetric. Other useful cutaneous reflexes include the cremasteric (ipsilateral elevation of the testicle following stroking of the medial thigh; mediated by L1 and L2) and anal (contraction of the anal sphincter when the perianal skin is scratched; mediated by S2, S3, S4) reflexes. It is particularly important to test for these reflexes in any patient with suspected injury to the spinal cord or lumbosacral roots.

Primitive Reflexes With disease of the frontal lobe pathways, several primitive reflexes not normally present in the adult may appear. The suck response is elicited by lightly touching the center of the lips, and the root response the corner of the lips, with a tongue blade; the patient will move the lips to suck or root in the direction of the stimulus. The grasp reflex is elicited by touching the palm between the thumb and index finger with the examiner's fingers; a positive response is a forced grasp of the examiner's hand. In many instances stroking the back of the hand will lead to its release. The palmomental response is contraction of the mentalis muscle (chin) ipsilateral to a scratch stimulus diagonally applied to the palm.

Sensory Examination (See also Chap. 22)

- *The bare minimum: Ask whether the patient can feel light touch and the temperature of a cool object in each distal extremity. Check double simultaneous stimulation using light touch on the hands.*

Evaluating sensation is usually the most unreliable part of the examination, because it is subjective and is difficult to quantify. In the compliant and discerning patient, the sensory examination can be extremely helpful for the precise localization of a lesion. With patients who are uncooperative or lack an understanding of the tests, it may be useless. The examination should be focused on the suspected lesion. For example, in spinal cord, spinal root, or peripheral nerve abnormalities, all major sensory modalities should be tested while looking for a pattern consistent with a spinal level and dermatomal or nerve distribution. In patients with lesions at or above the brainstem, screening the primary sensory modalities in the distal extremities along with tests of "cortical" sensation is usually sufficient.

The five primary sensory modalities—light touch, pain, temperature, vibration, and joint position—are tested in each limb. Light touch is assessed by stimulating the skin with single, very gentle touches of the examiner's finger or a wisp of cotton. Pain is tested using a new pin, and temperature is assessed using a metal object (e.g., tuning fork) that has been immersed in cold and warm water. Vibration is tested using a 128-Hz tuning fork applied to the distal phalynx of the great toe or index finger just below the nailbed. By placing a finger on the opposite side of the joint being tested, the examiner compares the patient's threshold of vibration perception with his or her own. For joint position testing, the examiner grasps the digit or limb laterally and distal to the joint being assessed; small 1- to 2-mm excursions can usually be sensed. The Romberg maneuver is primarily a test of proprioception. The patient is asked to stand with the feet as close together as necessary to maintain balance while the eyes are open, and the eyes are then closed. A loss of balance with the eyes closed is an abnormal response.

"Cortical" sensation is mediated by the parietal lobes and represents an integration of the primary sensory modalities; testing cortical sensation is only meaningful when primary sensation is intact. Double simultaneous stimulation is especially useful as a screening test for cortical function; with the patient's eyes closed, the examiner lightly touches one or both hands and asks the patient to identify the stimuli. With a parietal lobe lesion, the patient may be unable to identify the stimulus on the contralateral side when both hands are touched. Other modalities relying on the parietal cortex include the discrimination of two closely placed stimuli as separate (two-point discrimination), identification of an object by touch and manipulation alone (stereognosis), and the identification of numbers or letters written on the skin surface (graphesthesia).

Coordination Examination (See also Chap. 21)

- *The bare minimum: Test rapid alternating movements of the fingers and feet, and the finger-to-nose maneuver.*

Coordination refers to the orchestration and fluidity of movements. Even simple acts require cooperation of agonist and antagonist muscles, maintenance of posture, and complex servomechanisms to control the rate and range of movements. Part of this integration relies on normal function of the cerebellar and basal ganglia systems. However, coordination also requires intact muscle strength and kinesthetic and propioceptive information. Thus, if the examination has disclosed abnormalities of the motor or sensory systems, the patient's coordination should be assessed with these limitations in mind.

Rapid alternating movements in the upper limbs are tested separately on each side by having the patient make a fist, partially extend the index finger, and then tap the index finger on the distal thumb as quickly as possible. In the lower limb, the patient rapidly taps the foot against the floor or the examiner's hand. Finger-to-nose testing is primarily a test of cerebellar function; the patient is asked to touch his or her index finger repetitively to the nose and then to the examiner's outstretched finger, which moves with each repetition. A similar test in the lower extremity is to have the patient raise the leg and touch

the examiner's finger with the great toe. Another cerebellar test in the lower limbs is the heel-knee-shin maneuver; in the supine position the patient is asked to slide the heel of each foot from the knee down the shin of the other leg. For all these movements, the accuracy, speed, and rhythm are noted.

Gait Examination (See also Chap. 21)

- *The bare minimum: Observe the patient while walking normally, on the heels and toes, and along a straight line.*

Watching the patient walk is the most important part of the neurologic examination. Normal gait requires that multiple systems—including strength, sensation, and coordination—function in a highly integrated fashion. Unexpected abnormalities may be detected that prompt the examiner to return, in more detail, to other aspects of the examination. The patient should be observed while walking and turning normally, walking on the heels, walking on the toes, and walking heel-to-toe along a straight line. The examination may reveal decreased arm swing on one side (corticospinal tract disease), a stooped posture and short-stepped gait (parkinsonism), a broad-based unstable gait (ataxia), scissoring (spasticity), or a high-stepped, slapping gait (posterior column or peripheral nerve disease), or the patient may appear to be stuck in place (apraxia with frontal lobe disease).

NEUROLOGIC DIAGNOSIS The clinical data obtained from the history and the examination are interpreted in terms of neuroanatomy and neurophysiology and assembled into one of the known syndromes (see Table 346-2; online). From the syndrome the physician should be able to determine the anatomic localization that best explains the clinical findings, to narrow the list of diagnostic possibilities, and to select the laboratory tests most likely to be informative. The laboratory assessment may include (1) serum electrolytes; complete blood count; and renal, hepatic, endocrine, and immune studies; (2) cerebrospinal fluid examination; (3) focused neuroimaging studies (Chap. 347); or (4) electrophysiologic studies (Chaps. 348 and 363). The anatomic localization, mode of onset and course of illness, other medical data, and laboratory findings are then integrated to establish an etiologic diagnosis.

It should be emphasized that the neurologic examination may be normal even in patients with a serious neurologic disease, such as seizures, chronic meningitis, or a TIA. A comatose patient may arrive with no available history, and in such cases the approach is as described in Chap. 257. In other patients, an inadequate history may be overcome by a succession of examinations from which the course of the illness can be inferred. In perplexing cases it is useful to remember that uncommon presentations of common diseases are more likely than rare etiologies. Thus, even in tertiary care settings, multiple strokes are usually due to emboli and not vasculitis, and dementia with myoclonus is usually Alzheimer's disease and not a prionopathy or a paraneoplastic disorder. Finally, the most important task of a primary care physician faced with a patient who has a new neurologic complaint is to assess the urgency of referral to a specialist. Here, the imperative is to rapidly identify patients likely to have nervous system infections, acute strokes, and spinal cord compression or other treatable mass lesions and arrange for immediate care.

FURTHER READING

BLUMENTHAL H: *Neuroanatomy Through Clinical Cases*. Sinauer Associates, 2002

DANA ALLIANCE FOR BRAIN INITIATIVES: *Delivery Results: A Progress Report on Brain Research*. New York, Dana Press, 1996

VICTOR M et al: *Principles of Neurology*, 7th Ed. New York, McGraw-Hill, 2001

The clinician caring for patients with neurologic symptoms is faced with an expanding number of imaging options, including computed tomography (CT), CT angiography (CTA), perfusion CT (pCT), magnetic resonance imaging (MRI), MR angiography (MRA), functional MRI (fMRI), MR spectroscopy (MRS), MR neurography, and perfusion MRI (pMRI). In addition, an increasing number of interventional neuroradiologic techniques are available including angiography; embolization and stenting of vascular structures; and spine interventions such as discography, selective nerve root injection, and epidural injections. Recent developments, such as multidetector CT angiography and gadolinium-enhanced MRA, have narrowed the indications for conventional angiography, which is now reserved for patients in whom small-vessel detail is essential for diagnosis or for whom interventional therapies are planned (Table 347-1).

In general, MRI is more sensitive than CT for the detection of lesions affecting the central nervous system (CNS), particularly those of the spinal cord, cranial nerves, and posterior fossa structures. Diffusion MR, a sequence that detects reduction of microscopic motion of water, is the most sensitive technique for detecting acute ischemic stroke and is useful in the detection of encephalitis, abscesses, and prion diseases. CT, however, can be quickly obtained and is widely available, making it a pragmatic choice for the initial evaluation of patients with suspected acute stroke, hemorrhage, and intracranial or spinal trauma. CT is also more sensitive than MRI for visualizing fine osseous detail and is indicated in the initial evaluation of conductive hearing loss as well as lesions affecting the skull base and calvarium.

COMPUTED TOMOGRAPHY ■ **Technique** The CT image is a cross-sectional representation of anatomy created by a computer-generated analysis of the attenuation of x-ray beams passed through a section of the body. As the x-ray beam, collimated to the desired slice width, rotates around the patient, it passes through selected regions in the body. X-rays that are not attenuated by the body are detected by sensitive x-ray detectors aligned 180° from the x-ray tube. A computer calculates a "back projection" image from the 360° x-ray attenuation profile. Greater x-ray attenuation, e.g., as caused by bone, results in areas of high "density," while soft tissue structures, which have poor attenuation of x-rays, are lower in density. The resolution of an image depends on the radiation dose, the collimation (slice thickness), the field of view, and the matrix size of the display. A modern CT scanner is capable of obtaining sections as thin as 0.5 to 1 mm with submillimeter resolution at a speed of 0.5 to 1 s per section; complete studies of the brain can be completed in 20 to 60 s.

Helical CT is a type of scanner in which continuous CT information is obtained while the patient moves through the x-ray beam. In the helical scan mode, the table moves continuously through the rotating x-ray beam, generating a "helix" of information that can be reformatted into various slice thicknesses. Single or multiple (from 4 to 32) detectors positioned 180 degrees to the x-ray source may result in multiple slices per revolution of the beam around the patient. These "multidetector" scanners have further decreased the time per examination and permit rapid assessment of vascular anatomy as well as perfusion characteristics of brain parenchyma (Figs. 347-1 and 347-2). Advantages of multidetector scanning include shorter scan times, reduced patient and organ motion, and the ability to acquire images dynamically during the infusion of intravenous contrast that can be used to construct CT angiograms of vascular structures and CT perfusion images (Figs. 347-1B and 347-2). CTA images may be processed later for display in three dimensions to yield angiogram-like images (Figs. 347-1C and 349-12). CTA has proven useful in assessing the carotid bifurcation and intracranial arterial and venous anatomy.

Intravenous contrast is often administered prior to or during a CT study to identify vascular structures and to detect defects in the blood-brain barrier (BBB), which are associated with disorders such as tumors, infarcts, and infections. In the normal CNS, only vessels and structures lacking a BBB (e.g., the pituitary gland, choroid plexus, and dura) enhance after contrast administration. The use of iodinated contrast agents carries a risk of allergic reaction and adds additional expense and radiation dose. While helpful in characterizing mass lesions as well as essential for the acquisition of CTA studies, the decision to use contrast material should always be considered carefully.

Indications CT is the primary study of choice in the evaluation of acute trauma to the brain and spine, suspected subarachnoid hemorrhage, and conductive hearing loss (Table 347-1). CT is complementary to MR in the evaluation of the skull base, orbit, and osseous structures of the spine. In the spine, CT is useful in evaluating patients with osseous spinal stenosis and spondylosis, but MRI is often preferred in those with neurologic deficits. CT can also be obtained following intrathecal contrast injection to evaluate the intracranial cisterns (*CT cisternography*) for cerebrospinal fluid (CSF) fistula, as well as the spinal subarachnoid space (*CT myelography*).

Complications CT is safe, fast, and reliable. Radiation exposure is between 3 and 5 cGy per study. Care must be taken to reduce exposure when imaging children. The most frequent complications are associ-

TABLE 347-1 *Guidelines for the Use of CT , Ultrasound, and MRI*

Condition	Recommended Technique
Hemorrhage	
Acute parenchymal	CT > MR
Subacute/chronic	MRI
Subarachnoid hemorrhage	CT, CTA, lumbar puncture → angiography
Aneurysm	Angiography > CTA, MRA
Ischemic infarction	
Hemorrhagic infarction	CT
Bland infarction	MRI > CT
Carotid or vertebral dissection	MRI/MRA
Vertebral basilar insufficiency	CTA, MRI/MRA
Carotid stenosis	CTA > Doppler ultrasound, MRA
Suspected mass lesion	
Neoplasm, primary or metastatic	MRI + contrast
Infection/abscess	MRI + contrast
Immunosuppressed with focal findings	MRI + contrast
Vascular malformation	MRI +/− angiography
White matter disorders	MRI
Demyelinating disease	MRI +/− contrast
Dementia	MRI
Trauma	
Acute trauma	CT (noncontrast)
Shear injury/chronic hemorrhage	MRI
Headache/migraine	CT (noncontrast) / MRI
Seizure	
First time, no focal neurologic deficits	?CT as screen
Partial complex/refractory	MRI with coronal T2W imaging
Cranial neuropathy	MRI with contrast
Meningeal disease	MRI with contrast
SPINE	
Low back pain	
No neurologic deficits	MRI or CT after 4 weeks
With focal deficits	MRI > CT
Spinal stenosis	MRI or CT
Cervical spondylosis	MRI or CT myelography
Infection	MRI + contrast, CT
Myelopathy	MRI + contrast > myelography
Arteriovenous malformation	MRI, myelography/angiography

Note: CT, computed tomography; MRI, magnetic resonance imaging; MRA, MR angiography; CTA, CT angiography; T2W, T2-weighted.

ated with use of intravenous contrast agents. Two broad categories of contrast media, ionic and nonionic, are in use. Although ionic agents are relatively safe and inexpensive, they are associated with a higher incidence of reactions and side effects. As a result, ionic agents have been largely replaced by safer nonionic compounds (Table 347-2).

Contrast nephropathy may result from hemodynamic changes, renal tubular obstruction and cell damage, or immunologic reactions to contrast agents. A rise in serum creatinine of at least 85 μmol/L (1 mg/dL) within 48 h of contrast administration is often used as a definition of contrast nephropathy, although other causes of acute renal failure must be excluded. The prognosis is usually favorable, with serum creatinine levels returning to baseline within 1 to 2 weeks. Risk factors for contrast nephropathy include advanced age, preexisting renal disease, diabetes, dehydration, and high contrast dose. Patients with diabetes and those with mild renal failure should be well hydrated prior to the administration of contrast agents, although careful consideration should be given to alternative imaging techniques, such as MR imaging. Nonionic, low-osmolar media produce fewer abnormalities in renal blood flow and less endothelial cell damage but should still be used carefully in patients at risk (Table 347-3).

Other side effects are rare but include a sensation of warmth throughout the body and a metallic taste during intra-

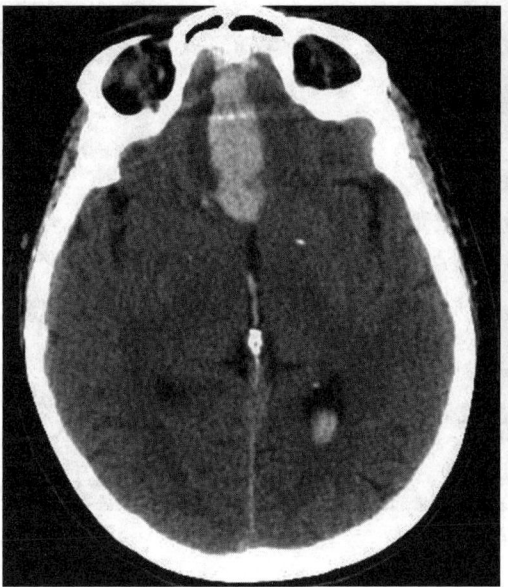

A

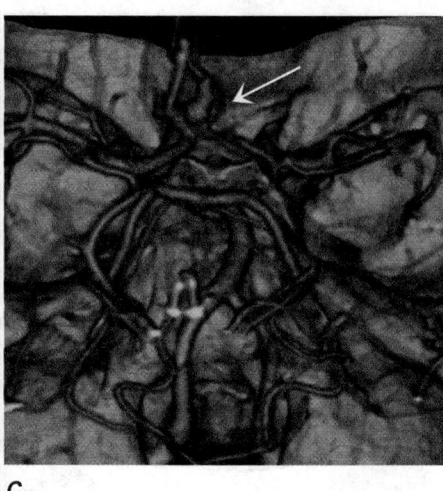

C

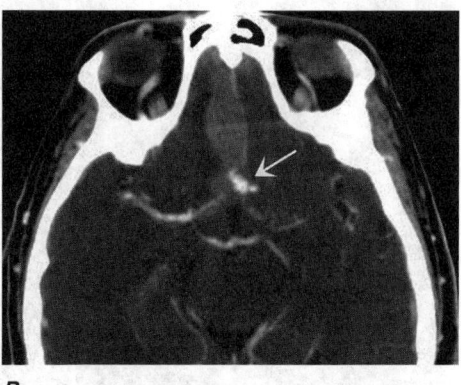

B

FIGURE 347-1 CT angiography (CTA) of ruptured anterior cerebral artery aneurysm. A 45-year-old man presents with acute headache. *A.* Noncontrast CT demonstrates intraventricular, subarachnoid, and frontal lobe hemorrhage. *B.* A partition from CT angiography demonstrates a suspicious enlargement of the anterior cerebral cerebral artery (*arrow*). *C.* 3D surface reconstruction using a workstation confirms the anterior cerebral aneurysm and demonstrates its orientation and relationship to nearby vessels (*arrow*). CTA image is produced by 1-mm helical CT scans performed during a rapid bolus infusion of intravenous contrast medium.

venous administration of iodinated contrast media. Anaphylactic reactions to intravenous contrast media, while rare, are the most serious side effects and range from mild hives to bronchospasm, acute anaphylaxis, and death. The pathogenesis of these allergic reactions is not fully understood, but it is thought to include the release of mediators such as histamine, antibody-antigen reactions, and complement activation. Severe allergic reactions occur in ~0.04% of patients receiving nonionic media, sixfold fewer than with ionic media. Risk factors include a history of prior contrast reaction, food allergies to shellfish, and atopy (asthma and hay fever). In such patients, a noncontrast CT or MRI procedure should be considered as an alternative to contrast administration. If iodinated contrast is absolutely required, a nonionic agent should be used in conjunction with pretreatment with glucocorticoids and antihistamines (Table 347-4). Patients with allergic reactions to iodinated contrast material do not usually react to gadolinium-based MR contrast material, although it would be wise to pretreat patients with a prior allergic history to MR contrast administration in a similar fashion.

MAGNETIC RESONANCE IMAGING ■ **Technique** Magnetic resonance is a complex interaction between hydrogen protons in biologic tissues, a static magnetic field (the magnet), and energy in the form of radiofrequency (Rf) waves of a specific frequency introduced by coils placed next to the body part of interest. Spatial localization is achieved by magnetic gradients surrounding the main magnet, which impart slight changes in magnetic field throughout the imaging volume. The energy state of the hydrogen protons is transiently excited by the Rf, which is administered at a frequency specific for the field strength of the magnet. The subsequent return to equilibrium energy state (*relaxation*) of the protons results in a release of Rf energy (the *echo*), which is detected by the coils that delivered the Rf pulses. The echo is trans-

formed by Fourier analysis into the information used to form an MR image. The MR image thus consists of a map of the distribution of hydrogen protons, with signal intensity imparted by both density of hydrogen protons as well as differences in the relaxation time (see below) of hydrogen protons on different molecules.

T1 AND T2 RELAXATION TIMES The rate of return to equilibrium of perturbed protons is called the *relaxation rate*. The relaxation rate varies among normal and pathologic tissues. The relaxation rate of a hydrogen proton in a tissue is influenced by local interactions with surrounding molecules and atomic neighbors. Two relaxation rates, T1 and T2, influence the signal intensity of the image. The T1 relaxation time is the time, measured in milliseconds, for 63% of the hydrogen protons to return to their normal equilibrium state, while the T2 relaxation is the time for 63% of the protons to become dephased owing to interactions among nearby protons. The intensity of the signal within various tissues and image contrast can be modulated by altering acquisition parameters, such as the interval between Rf pulses (TR) and the time between the Rf pulse and the signal reception (TE). So-called T1-weighted (T1W) images are produced by keeping the TR and TE relatively short. T2-weighted (T2W) images are produced by using longer TR and TE times. Fat and subacute hemorrhage have short T1 relaxation rates and a high signal intensity on T1W images. Structures containing more water, such as CSF and edema, have long T1 and T2 relaxation rates, a low signal intensity on T1W images, and a high signal intensity on T2W images (Table 347-5). Gray matter contains 10 to 15% more water than white matter, which accounts for much of its contrast on MRI (Fig. 347-3). T2W images are more sensitive than T1W images to edema, demyelination, infarction, and chronic hemorrhage, while T1-weighted imaging is more sensitive to subacute hemorrhage and fat-containing structures.

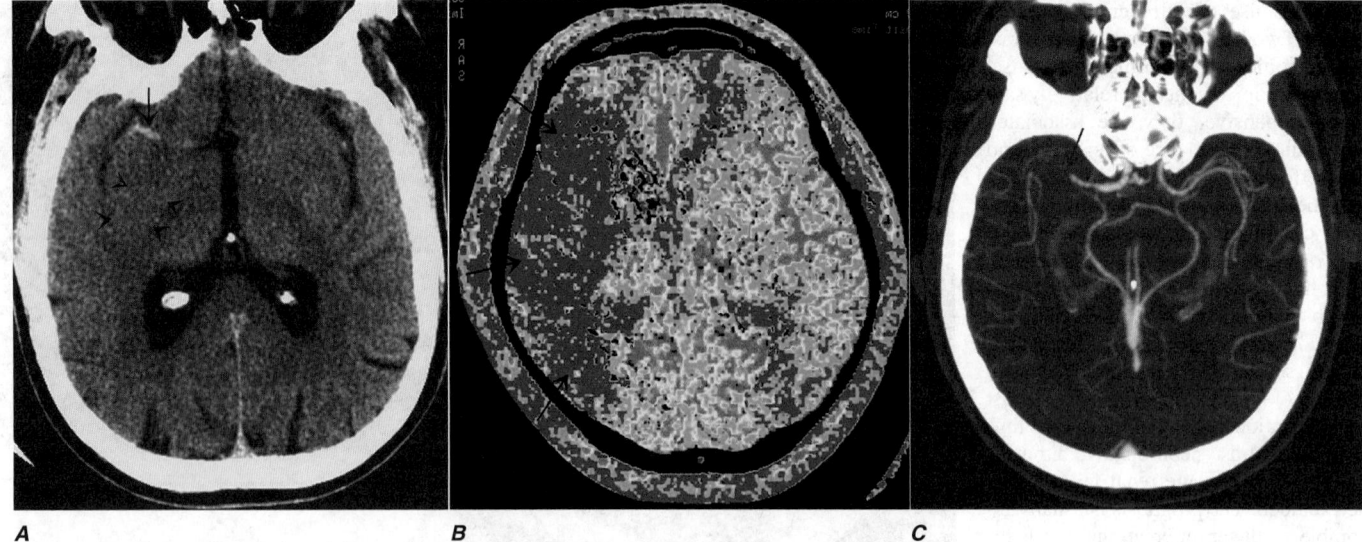

A   B   C

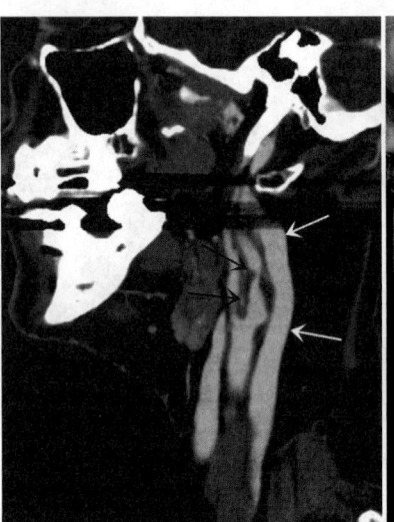
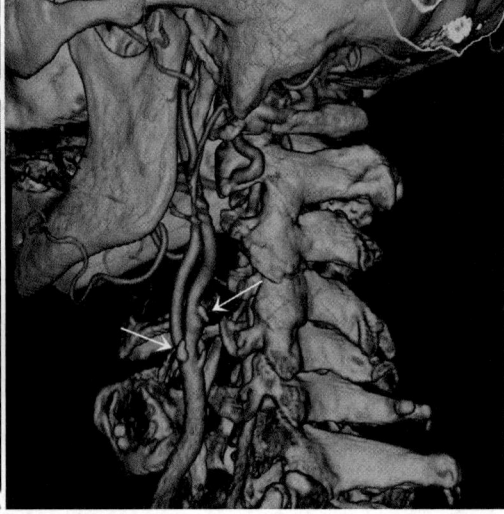

D   E

FIGURE 347-2 A 49-year-old man with acute neck pain and right hemiparesis. *A.* Axial noncontrast CT scan demonstrates high density within the right middle cerebral artery (*arrow*) associated with subtle low density involving the right putamen (*arrowheads*). *B.* Mean transit time map calculated from a CT perfusion study obtained with a 40-cc contrast injection during which 45 images were obtained at the same slice location. Prolongation of the mean transit time is visible throughout the right hemisphere (*arrows*). *C.* Axial maximum intensity projection from CTA study through the Circle of Willis demonstrates an abrupt occlusion of the proximal right middle cerebral artery (*arrow*). Reconstitution of flow via collaterals is seen distal to the occlusion, however, the patient sustained a right basal ganglia infarction. *D.* Sagittal reformation through the right internal carotid artery. Low-density lipid laden plaque (*arrows*) narrows the lumen of the internal carotid artery (*black arrows*). The internal jugular vein is shown (*white arrows*). *E.* 3D surface CTA images (different patient) demonstrate calcification and narrowing of the right internal carotid artery, consistent with atherosclerotic disease.

Many different MR pulse sequences exist, and each can be obtained in various planes (Figs. 347-3, 4, 5). The selection of a proper protocol that will best answer a clinical question depends on an accurate clinical history and indication for the examination. Fluid-attenuated inversion recovery (FLAIR) is a useful pulse sequence that produces T2W images in which the normally high signal intensity of CSF is suppressed

TABLE 347-3 *Indications for Use of Nonionic Contrast Media*

- Prior adverse reaction to contrast media, with the exception of heat, flushing, or an episode of nausea or vomiting
- Asthma or other serious lung disease
- History of atopic allergies (pretreatment with steroid/antihistamines recommended)
- Children under the age of 2 years
- Renal failure or creatinine >177 μmol/L (>2.0 mg/dL)
- Cardiac dysfunction, including recent or imminent cardiac decompensation, severe arrhythmias, unstable angina pectoris, recent myocardial infarction, and pulmonary hypertension
- Diabetes
- Severe debilitation

TABLE 347-2 *Guidelines for Use of Intravenous Contrast in Patients with Impaired Renal Function*

Serum Creatinine, μmol/L (mg/dL)[a]	Recommendation
<133 (<1.5)	Use either ionic or nonionic at 2 mL/kg to 150 mL total
133–177 (1.5–2.0)	Nonionic; hydrate diabetics 1 mL/kg per hour × 10 h
>177 (>2.0)	Consider noncontrast CT or MRI; nonionic contrast if required
177–221 (2.0–2.5)	Nonionic only if required (as above); contraindicated in diabetics
>265 (>3.0)	Nonionic IV contrast given only to patients undergoing dialysis within 24 h

[a] Risk is greatest in patients with rising creatinine levels.
Note: CT, computed tomography; MRI, magnetic resonance imaging.

TABLE 347-4 *Guidelines for Premedication of Patients with Prior Contrast Allergy*

12 h prior to examination:
 Prednisone, 40 mg PO *or* methylprednisolone, 32 mg PO
2 h prior to examination:
 Prednisone, 40 mg PO *or* methylprednisolone, 32 mg PO *and*
 Cimetidine, 300 mg PO *or* ranitidine, 150 mg PO
Immediately prior to examination:
 Benadryl, 50 mg IV (alternatively, can be given PO 2 h prior to exam)

TABLE 347-5   *Some Common Intensities on T1- and T2-Weighted MRI Sequences*

			Signal Intensity			
Image	TR	TE	CSF	Fat	Brain	Edema
T1W	Short	Short	Low	High	Low	Low
T2W	Long	Long	High	Low	High	High

Note: TR, interval between radiofrequency (Rf) pulses; TE, interval between Rf pulse and signal reception; CSF, cerebrospinal fluid; T1W and T2W, T1- and T2-weighted.

(Fig. 347-5*A*). FLAIR images are more sensitive than standard spine echo images for the detection of lesions within or adjacent to CSF. Gradient echo imaging is most sensitive to magnetic susceptibility as seen with blood, calcium, and air, and is indicated in patients with traumatic brain injury. MR images can be generated in sagittal, coronal, axial, or oblique planes without changing the patient's position. Each plane obtained requires a separate sequence lasting 1 to 10 min. Three-dimensional volumetric imaging is also possible with MRI, resulting in a volume of data that can be reformatted in any orientation on a workstation to highlight certain disease processes.

MR CONTRAST MATERIAL   The heavy-metal element gadolinium forms the basis of all currently approved intravenous MR contrast agents. Gadolinium is a paramagnetic substance, which means that it reduces the T1 and T2 relaxation times of nearby water protons, resulting in a high signal on T1W images and a low signal on T2W images (the latter requires a sufficient local concentration, usually in the form of a bolus). Unlike iodinated contrast agents, the effect of MR contrast agents depends on the presence of local hydrogen protons on which it must act to achieve the desired effect. Gadolinium is chelated to DTPA (diethylenetriaminepentaacetic acid), which allows safe renal excretion. Approximately 0.2 mL/kg body weight is administered intravenously; the cost is ~$60 per dose. Gadolinium-DTPA does not cross the intact BBB but will enhance lesions lacking a BBB (Fig. 347-4*A*) and areas of the brain that normally are devoid of the BBB. The agent is well tolerated, and severe allergic reactions to gadolinium are rare but have been reported. The adverse reaction rate in patients with a prior history of atopy or asthma is 3.7%; however, the reaction rate increases to 6.3% in those patients with a prior history of unspecified allergic reaction to iodinated contrast. These agents can be administered safely to children as well as adults. Renal failure does not occur.

Complications and Contraindications   From the patient's perspective, an MRI examination can be intimidating, and a higher level of cooperation is required than with CT. The patient lies on a table that is moved into a long, narrow gap within the magnet. Approximately 5% of the population experiences severe claustrophobia in the MR environment. This can be reduced by mild sedation but remains a problem for some. Unlike CT, movement of the patient during an MR sequence distorts all the images; therefore, uncooperative patients should either be sedated for the MR study or scanned with CT. Generally, children under the age of 10 years usually require conscious sedation in order to complete the MR examination without motion degradation.

MRI is considered safe for patients, even at very high field strengths (>3 to 4 T). Serious injuries have been caused, however, by attraction of ferromagnetic objects into the magnet, which act as missiles if brought too close to the magnet. Likewise, ferromagnetic implants, such as aneurysm clips, may torque within the magnet, causing damage to vessels and even death. Metallic foreign bodies in the eye have moved and caused intraocular hemorrhage; screening for ocular metallic fragments is indicated in those with a history of metal work or ocular metallic foreign bodies. Implanted cardiac pacemakers are a contraindication to MRI owing to the risk of induced arrhythmias. All health care personnel and patients must be screened and educated thoroughly to prevent such disasters as the magnet is always "on." Table 347-6 lists common contraindications for MRI.

MAGNETIC RESONANCE ANGIOGRAPHY   On routine spin echo MR sequences, moving protons (e.g., flowing blood, CSF) exhibit complex MR signals that range from high to low signal intensity relative to background stationary tissue. Fast-flowing blood returns no signal (flow void) on routine T1W or T2W spin echo MR images. Slower flowing blood, as occurs in veins or distal to arterial stenoses, may appear high in signal. However, using special pulse sequences called *gradient echo sequences*, it is possible to increase the signal intensity of moving protons in contrast to the low signal background intensity of stationary tissue. This creates angiography-like images, which can be manipulated in three dimensions to highlight vascular anatomy and relationships.

Two MRA techniques, time-of-flight (TOF) and phase-contrast, are routinely used. TOF, currently the technique used most frequently, relies on the suppression of nonmoving tissue to provide a low-intensity background for the high signal intensity of flowing blood entering the section; arterial or venous structures may be highlighted. A typical TOF angiography sequence results in a series of contiguous thin MR sections (0.9 mm thick), which can be viewed as a stack and manipulated to create an angiographic image data set that can be reformatted

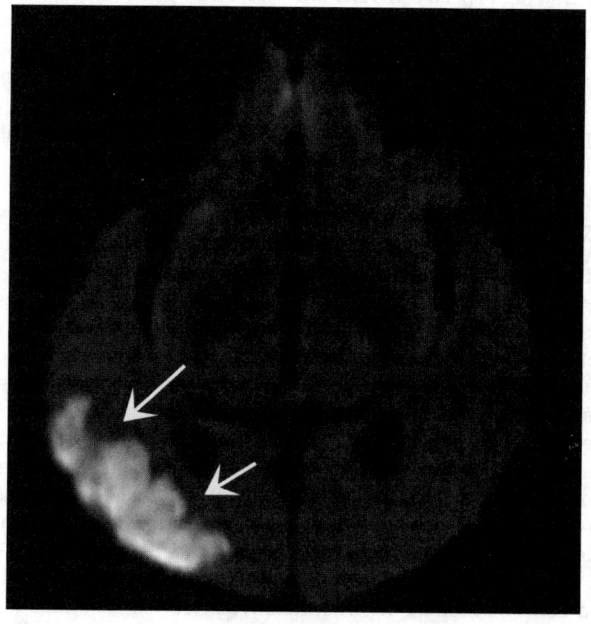

A

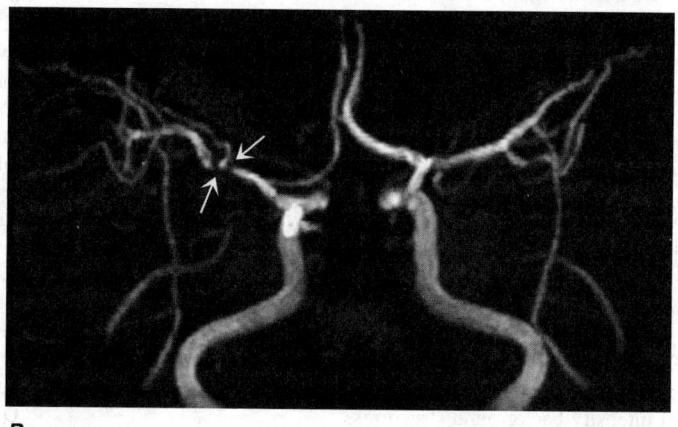

B

FIGURE 347-3   *A.* Axial echo-planar diffusion-weighted MR image demonstrates a large area of reduced diffusion consistent with acute cerebral ischemia (*arrows*) located in the right posterior frontotemporal lobe. Reduced diffusion is consistent with cytotoxic edema and is most commonly associated with acute cerebral infarction. *B.* Time-of-flight MR angiography through the circle of Willis demonstrates a high-grade stenosis at the left middle cerebral artery bifurcation (*arrows*).

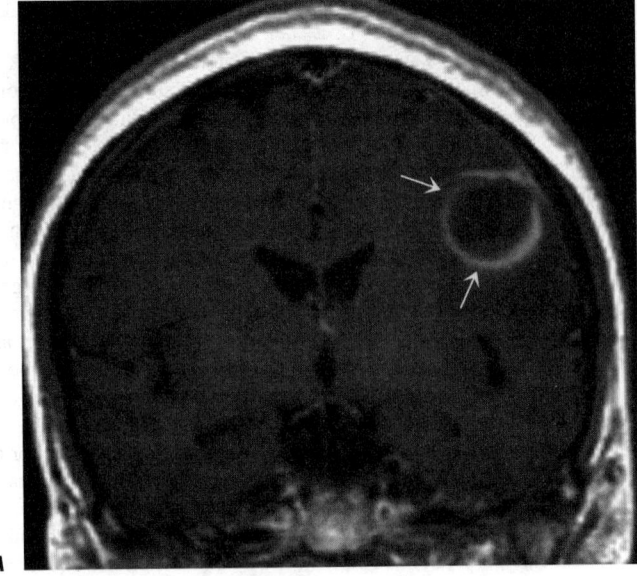

A

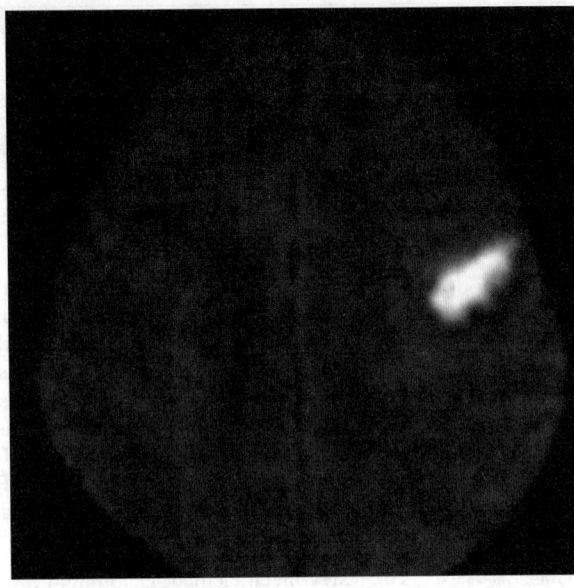

B

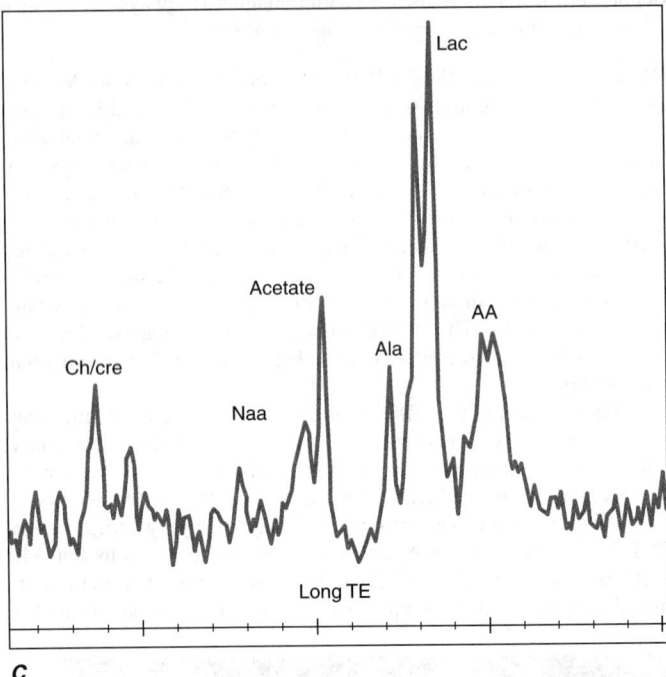

C

and viewed in various planes and angles, much like that seen with conventional angiography (Fig. 347-3*B*). Noncontrast enhanced MRA provides a vascular flow map rather than the anatomic map shown by conventional angiography.

Phase-contrast MRA has a longer acquisition time than TOF MRA, but in addition to providing anatomic information similar to that of TOF imaging, it can be used to reveal the velocity and direction of blood flow in a given vessel. Through the selection of different imaging parameters, differing blood velocities can be highlighted; selective venous and arterial MRA images can thus be obtained. One advantage of phase-contrast MRA is the excellent suppression of high signal intensity background structures.

MRA can also be acquired during infusion of contrast material. Recently, contrast-enhanced MRA has become the standard for extracranial vascular MRA. This technique entails rapid imaging using coronal three-dimensional TOF sequences during a bolus infusion of 15 to 20 mL of gadolinium-DTPA. Proper technique and timing of acquisition relative to bolus arrival are critical for success. Advantages include a reduction in the time of acquisition (1 to 2 min vs. 10 min) and flow-related artifacts.

MRA is lower in spatial resolution compared with conventional film-based angiography, and therefore the detection of small-vessel detail, such as is required in the workup of vasculitis, is problematic. MRA is also less sensitive to slowly flowing blood and thus may not reliably differentiate complete from near-complete occlusions. Motion, either by the patient or by anatomic structures, may distort the MRA images, creating artifacts. These limitations notwithstanding, MRA has proved useful in evaluation of the extracranial carotid and vertebral circulation as well as of larger-caliber intracranial arteries and dural sinuses. It has also proved useful in the noninvasive detection of intracranial aneurysms and vascular malformations.

ECHO-PLANAR MR IMAGING Recent improvements in gradients, software, and high-speed computer processors now permit extremely rapid MRI of the brain. With echo-planar MRI (EPI), fast gradients are switched on and off at high speeds to create the information used to form an image. In routine spin echo imaging, images of the brain can be obtained in 5 to 10 min. With EPI, all of the information required for processing an image is accumulated in 50 to 150 ms, and the information for the entire brain is obtained in 1 to 2 min, depending on the degree of resolution required or desired. Fast MRI reduces patient and organ motion, permitting diffusion imaging (Figs. 347-3, 4, 5 and Fig. 349-13), perfusion imaging during contrast infusion fMRI, and kinematic motion studies.

Perfusion and diffusion imaging are EPI techniques that are useful in early detection of ischemic injury of the brain and may be useful together to demonstrate infarcted tissue as well as ischemic but potentially viable tissue at risk of infarction (e.g., the ischemic penumbra). Diffusion-weighted imaging (DWI) assesses microscopic motion of water; restriction of motion appears as relative high signal intensity on diffusion-weighted images. DWI is the most sensitive technique for detection of acute cerebral infarction of <7 days' duration and is also sensitive to encephalitis and abscess formation, all of which demonstrate reduced diffusion or high signal.

Perfusion MRI involves the acquisition of EPI images during a rapid bolus of contrast material. Relative perfusion abnormalities can be identified. The relative cerebral blood volume, mean transit time,

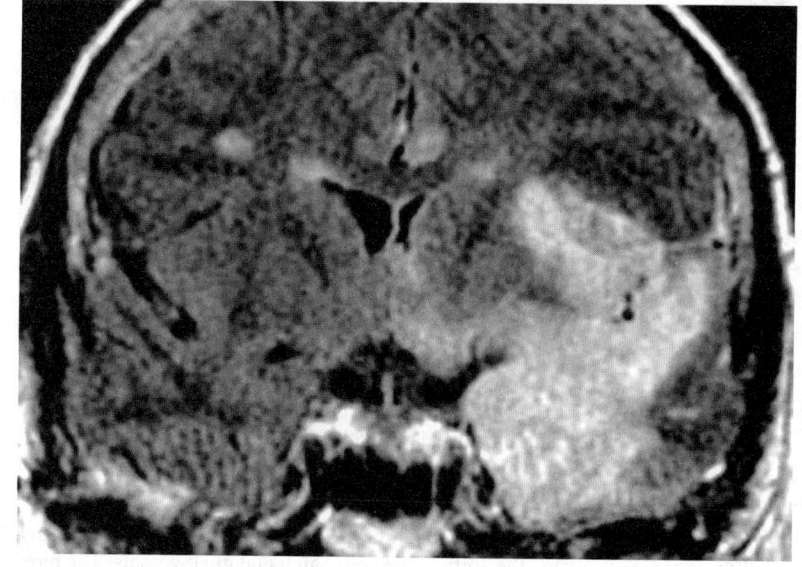

FIGURE 347-5 Herpes encephalitis. A 40-year-old man presents with altered mental status and fever. *A.* Coronal T2-weighted FLAIR image demonstrates expansion and high signal intensity involving the left medial temporal lobe, insular cortex, and left cingulate gyrus. *B.* Diffusion weighted image demonstrates high signal intensity indicative of restricted diffusion involving the left medial temporal lobe and hippocampus (*arrows*). This is most consistent with neuronal destruction and can be seen in acute infarction as well as infectious and inflammatory encephalitis. PCR evaluation of the CSF confirmed Herpes encephalitis. (*Case courtesy of Howard Rowley, MD, University of Wisconsin.*)

and cerebral blood flow throughout the image can be calculated within regions of interest. Delay in mean transit time and reduction in cerebral blood volume and cerebral blood flow are typically seen in infarction. Elevated or normal cerebral blood volume in a setting of reduced blood flow may indicate tissue that is at risk of infarction. pMRI imaging can also be used in the assessment of brain tumors where it has been shown to be helpful in differentiating intraaxial primary tumors from extraaxial tumors or metastasis.

Diffusion tract imaging (DTI) is a special diffusion technique that is capable of demonstrating white matter tracts and their relationship to lesions of the brain. Preferential microscopic motion of water along white matter tracts is detected by diffusion MR, which can also indicate the direction of white matter fiber tracts. This new technique has great potential in the assessment of brain maturation as well as disease entities that undermine the integrity of the white matter architecture.

fMRI of the brain is an EPI technique that localizes regions of activity in the brain following task activation. Neuronal activity elicits an increase in the delivery of oxygenated blood flow to a specific region of the brain, resulting in a slight alteration in the balance of oxyhemoglobin and deoxyhemoglobin, which yields a 2 to 3% increase in signal intensity within draining veins. Further work will determine whether these techniques are cost effective or clinically useful, but currently preoperative somatosensory and auditory cortex localization is possible. This technique has proved useful to neuroscientists interested in interrogating the localization of certain brain functions.

MAGNETIC RESONANCE NEUROGRAPHY MR neurography is an MR technique that shows promise in detecting increased signal in irritated, inflamed, or infiltrated nerves. These images are obtained with fat-suppressed fast spin echo imaging or short inversion recovery sequences, and they may indicate nerves that are responsible for pain syndromes more precisely. Irritated or infiltrated nerves will demonstrate high signal on T2W imaging.

POSITRON EMISSION TOMOGRAPHY (PET) PET relies on the detection of positrons emitted during the decay of a radionuclide that has been injected into a patient. The most frequently used moiety is 2-[^{18}F]fluoro-2-deoxy-D-glucose (FDG), which is an analogue of glucose and is taken up by cells competitively with 2-deoxyglucose. Multiple images of glucose uptake activity are formed after 45 to 60 min. Images reveal differences in regional glucose activity among normal and pathologic brain structures. A lower activity of FDG in the parietal lobes has been associated with Alzheimer's disease. FDG PET is used primarily for the detection of extracranial metastatic disease. PET is no longer used primarily for differentiation of tumor from radiation necrosis.

MYELOGRAPHY ▪ Technique Myelography involves the intrathecal instillation of specially formulated water-soluble iodinated contrast medium into the lumbar or cervical subarachnoid space. CT scanning is usually performed after myelography (*CT myelography*) to better demonstrate the spinal cord and roots, which appear as filling defects in the opacified subarachnoid space. *Low-dose CT myelography*, in which CT is performed after the subarachnoid injection of a small amount of relatively dilute contrast material, has replaced conventional myelography for many indications, thereby reducing exposure to radiation and contrast media. Newer multidetector scanners now obtain CT studies quickly so that reformations in sagittal and coronal planes, equivalent to traditional myelography projections, are now routine.

Indications Myelography has been largely replaced by CT myelography and MRI for diagnosis of diseases of the spinal canal and cord (Table 347-1). Remaining indications for conventional plain film myelography include the evaluation of suspected meningeal or arachnoid cysts and the localization of spinal dural arteriovenous or CSF fistulas. Conventional myelography and CT myelography provide the most precise information in patients with prior spinal fusion and spinal fixation hardware.

Contraindications Myelography is relatively safe; however, it should be performed with caution in any patient with elevated intracranial pressure or a history of allergic reaction to intrathecal contrast media. In patients with a suspected spinal block, MR is the preferred technique. If myelography is necessary, only a small amount of contrast medium should be instilled below the lesion in order to minimize the risk of neurologic deterioration. Lumbar puncture is to be avoided in patients with bleeding disorders, including patients receiving anticoagulant therapy, as well as in those with infections of the soft tissues.

Complications Headache, nausea, and vomiting are the most frequent complications of myelography, occurring in up to 38% of patients. These symptoms are thought to result from neurotoxic effects of the contrast agent, persistent leakage of CSF at the puncture site, or psy-

TABLE 347-6 *Common Contraindications to MR Imaging*

Cardiac pacemaker or permanent pacemaker leads	Omniphase penile implant
Internal defibrillatory device	Swan-Ganz catheter
Cochlear prostheses	Magnetic stoma plugs
Bone growth stimulators	Magnetic dental implants
Spinal cord stimulators	Magnetic sphincters
Electronic infusion devices	Ferromagnetic IVC filters, coils,
Intracranial aneurysm clips (some but not all)	stents—safe 6 weeks after implantation
Ocular implants (some) or ocular metallic foreign body	Tattooed eyeliner (contains ferromagnetic material and may irritate eyes)
McGee stapedectomy piston prosthesis	

chological reactions to the procedure. Vasovagal syncope may occur during lumbar puncture; it is accentuated by the upright position used during lumbar myelography. Adequate hydration before and after myelography will reduce the incidence of this complication. Postural headache (post–lumbar puncture headache) is generally due to leakage of CSF from the puncture site, resulting in CSF hypotension; management is discussed in Chap. 14. Hearing loss is a rare complication of myelography. It may result from a direct toxic effect of the contrast medium or from an alteration of the pressure equilibrium between CSF and perilymph in the inner ear. Puncture of the spinal cord is a rare but serious complication of cervical (C1-2) and high lumbar puncture. The risk of cord puncture is greatest in patients with spinal stenosis or conditions that reduce CSF volume. In these settings, a low-dose lumbar injection followed by thin-section CT or MRI is a safer alternative to cervical puncture. Intrathecal contrast reactions are rare, but aseptic meningitis and encephalopathy may occur. The latter is usually dose-related and associated with contrast entering the intracranial subarachnoid space. Seizures occur following myelography in 0.1 to 0.3% of patients. Risk factors include a preexisting seizure disorder and the use of a total iodine dose of >4500 mg. Other reported symptoms include hyperthermia, hallucinations, depression, and anxiety states. These side effects have been reduced by the development of nonionic, water-soluble contrast agents, as well as by head elevation and generous hydration following myelography.

SPINE INTERVENTIONS ■ **Discography** The evaluation of back pain and radiculopathy may require diagnostic procedures that attempt either to reproduce the patient's pain or relieve it, indicating its correct source. Discography is performed by fluoroscopic placement of a 22- to 25-gauge needle into the intervertebral disc and subsequent injection of 1 to 3 mL of contrast media. The intradiscal pressure is recorded, as is an assessment of the patient's response to the injection of contrast material. Typically little or no pain is felt during injection of a normal disc, which does not accept much more than 1 mL of contrast material, even at pressures as high as 415 to 690 kPa (60 to 100 lb/in²). CT and plain films are obtained following the procedure.

Selective Nerve Root and Epidural Spinal Injections Percutaneous selective nerve root and epidural blocks with glucocorticoid and anesthetic mixtures may be both therapeutic as well as diagnostic, especially if a patient's pain is relieved. Typically 1 to 2 mL of an equal mixture of a long-acting glucocorticoid such as betamethasone and a long-acting anesthetic such as bupivicain 0.75% is instilled under CT or fluoroscopic guidance in the intraspinal epidural space or adjacent to an existing nerve root.

ANGIOGRAPHY ■ **Technique** Catheter angiography is indicated in the evaluation of patients with vascular pathology, particularly of smaller intracranial vessels. However, it carries the greatest risk of morbidity of all diagnostic imaging procedures, owing to the necessity of inserting a catheter into a blood vessel, directing the catheter to the required location, injecting contrast material to visualize the vessel, and removing the catheter while maintaining hemostasis. Therapeutic

transcatheter procedures (see below) have become important options for the treatment of some cerebrovascular diseases. The decision to undertake a diagnostic or therapeutic angiographic procedure requires careful assessment of the goals of the investigation and its attendant risks.

To improve tolerance to contrast agents, patients undergoing angiography should be well hydrated before and after the procedure. Since the femoral route is used most commonly, the femoral artery must be compressed after the procedure to prevent a hematoma from developing. The puncture site and distal pulses should be evaluated carefully after the procedure; complications can include thigh hematoma or lower extremity emboli.

Indications Table 347-1 lists some of the indications for conventional angiography. Angiography has been replaced for many indications by CT/CTA or MRI/MRA; however, angiography is still used for evaluating intracranial small-vessel pathology (such as vasculitis), for assessing vascular malformations and aneurysms, and in endovascular therapeutic procedures.

Complications A common femoral arterial puncture provides retrograde access via the aorta to the aortic arch and great vessels. The most feared complication of cerebral angiography is stroke. Thrombus can form on or inside the tip of the catheter, and atherosclerotic thrombus or plaque can be dislodged by the catheter or guidewire or by the force of injection and can embolize distally in the cerebral circulation. Risk factors for ischemic complications include limited experience on the part of the angiographer, atherosclerosis, vasospasm, low cardiac output, decreased oxygen-carrying capacity, advanced age, and possibly migraine. The risk of a neurologic complication varies but is ~4% for transient ischemic attack and stroke, 1% for permanent deficit, and <0.1% for death.

Ionic contrast material injected into the cerebral vasculature can be neurotoxic if the BBB is breached, either by an underlying disease or by the injection of hyperosmolar contrast agent. Ionic contrast media are less well tolerated than nonionic media, probably because they can induce changes in cell membrane electrical potentials. Patients with dolichoectasia of the basilar artery can suffer reversible brainstem dysfunction and acute short-term memory loss during angiography, owing to the slow percolation of the contrast material and the consequent prolonged exposure of the brain. Rarely, an intracranial aneurysm ruptures during an angiographic contrast injection, causing subarachnoid hemorrhage, perhaps as a result of injection under high pressure.

Spinal Angiography Spinal angiography may be indicated to evaluate vascular malformations and tumors and to identify the artery of Adamkiewicz (Chap. 356) prior to aortic aneurysm repair. The procedure is lengthy and requires the use of relatively large volumes of contrast; the incidence of serious complications, including paraparesis, subjective visual blurring, and altered speech, is ~2%. Gadolinium-enhanced MRA has been used successfully in this setting and has promise for replacing diagnostic spinal angiography for some indications.

INTERVENTIONAL NEURORADIOLOGY This rapidly developing field is providing new therapeutic options for patients with difficult neurovascular problems. Available procedures include detachable coil therapy for aneurysms, particulate or liquid adhesive embolization of arteriovenous malformations, balloon angioplasty and stenting of arterial stenosis or vasospasm, transarterial or transvenous embolization of dural arteriovenous fistulas, balloon occlusion of carotid-cavernous and vertebral fistulas, endovascular treatment of vein-of-Galen malformations, preoperative embolization of tumors, and thrombolysis of acute arterial or venous thrombosis. Many of these disorders place the patient at high risk of cerebral hemorrhage, stroke, or death.

The highest complication rates are found with the therapies designed to treat the highest-risk diseases. In a large series of surgically difficult intracranial aneurysms treated with detachable balloons, Higashida and colleagues reported a 7.4% incidence of stroke and a 9.8% death rate. These figures must be considered in light of the high morbidity and mortality associated with untreated and surgically unapproachable aneurysms (Chap. 349). The advent of the electrolytically detachable coil has reduced these rates and ushered in a new era in the treatment of cerebral aneurysms. One recent double-blind trial (ISAT) found a 28% reduction of morbity and mortality at 1 year among those treated for anterior circulation aneurysm with detachable coils versus

neurosurgical clipping. It remains to be determined what the role of coils will be relative to surgical options, but in many centers, coiling of aneurysms has become standard therapy for many aneurysms.

Section 2 Diseases of the Central Nervous System

348 SEIZURES AND EPILEPSY
Daniel H. Lowenstein

A *seizure* (from the Latin *sacire*, "to take possession of") is a paroxysmal event due to abnormal, excessive, hypersynchronous discharges from an aggregate of central nervous system (CNS) neurons. Depending on the distribution of discharges, this abnormal CNS activity can have various manifestations, ranging from dramatic convulsive activity to experiential phenomena not readily discernible by an observer. Although a variety of factors influence the incidence and prevalence of seizures, ~5 to 10% of the population will have at least one seizure, with the highest incidence occurring in early childhood and late adulthood.

The meaning of the term seizure needs to be carefully distinguished from that of epilepsy. *Epilepsy* describes a condition in which a person has *recurrent* seizures due to a chronic, underlying process. This definition implies that a person with a single seizure, or recurrent seizures due to correctable or avoidable circumstances, does not necessarily have epilepsy. Epilepsy refers to a clinical phenomenon rather than a single disease entity, since there are many forms and causes of epilepsy. However, among the many causes of epilepsy there are various *epilepsy syndromes* in which the clinical and pathologic characteristics are distinctive and suggest a specific underlying etiology.

Using the definition of epilepsy as two or more unprovoked seizures, the incidence of epilepsy is ~0.3 to 0.5% in different populations throughout the world, and the prevalence of epilepsy has been estimated at 5 to 10 persons per 1000.

CLASSIFICATION OF SEIZURES

Determining the type of seizure that has occurred is essential for focusing the diagnostic approach on particular etiologies, selecting the appropriate therapy, and providing potentially vital information regarding prognosis. In 1981, the International League Against Epilepsy (ILAE) published a modified version of the International Classification of Epileptic Seizures that has continued to be a useful classification system (Table 348-1). This system is based on the clinical features of seizures and associated electroencephalographic findings. Other potentially distinctive features such as etiology or cellular substrate are not considered in this classification system, although this will un-

doubtedly change in the future as more is learned about the pathophysiologic mechanisms that underlie specific seizure types.

A fundamental principle is that seizures may be either partial (synonymous with focal) or generalized. *Partial seizures* are those in which the seizure activity is restricted to discrete areas of the cerebral cortex. *Generalized seizures* involve diffuse regions of the brain simultaneously. Partial seizures are usually associated with structural abnormalities of the brain. In contrast, generalized seizures may result from cellular, biochemical, or structural abnormalities that have a more widespread distribution.

PARTIAL SEIZURES Partial seizures occur within discrete regions of the brain. If consciousness is fully preserved during the seizure, the clinical manifestations are considered relatively simple and the seizure is termed a *simple partial seizure*. If consciousness is impaired, the symptomatology is more complex and the seizure is termed a *complex partial seizure*. An important additional subgroup comprises those seizures that begin as partial seizures and then spread diffusely throughout the cortex, i.e., *partial seizures with secondary generalization*.

Simple Partial Seizures Simple partial seizures cause motor, sensory, autonomic, or psychic symptoms without an obvious alteration in consciousness. For example, a patient having a partial motor seizure arising from the right primary motor cortex in the vicinity controlling hand movement will note the onset of involuntary movements of the contralateral, left hand. These movements are typically clonic (i.e., repetitive, flexion/extension movements) at a frequency of ~2 to 3 Hz; pure tonic posturing may be seen as well. Since the cortical region controlling hand movement is immediately adjacent to the region for facial expression, the seizure may also cause abnormal movements of the face synchronous with the movements of the hand. The electroencephalogram (EEG) recorded with scalp electrodes during the seizure (i.e., an ictal EEG) may show abnormal discharges in a very limited region over the appropriate area of cerebral cortex if the seizure focus involves the cerebral convexity. Seizure activity occurring within deeper brain structures is often not recorded by the standard EEG, however, and may require intracranial electrodes for its detection.

Three additional features of partial motor seizures are worth noting. First, in some patients the abnormal motor movements may begin in a very restricted region such as the fingers and gradually progress (over seconds to minutes) to include a larger portion of the extremity. This phenomenon, described by Hughlings Jackson and known as a "Jacksonian march," represents the spread of seizure activity over a progressively larger region of motor cortex. Second, patients may experience a localized paresis (Todd's paralysis) for minutes to many hours in the involved region following the seizure. Third, in rare instances the seizure may continue for hours or days. This condition, termed *epilepsia partialis continua*, is often refractory to medical therapy.

Simple partial seizures may also manifest as changes in somatic sensation (e.g., paresthesias), vision (flashing lights or formed hallucinations), equilibrium (sensation of falling or vertigo), or autonomic function (flushing, sweating, piloerection). Simple partial seizures arising from the temporal or frontal cortex may also cause alterations in hearing, olfaction, or higher cortical function (psychic symptoms). This includes the sensation of unusual, intense odors (e.g., burning rubber or kerosene) or sounds (crude or highly complex sounds), or an epigastric sensation that rises from the stomach or chest to the head. Some patients describe odd, internal feelings such as fear, a sense of

---

TABLE 348-1 *Classification of Seizures*

1. Partial seizures
   a. Simple partial seizures (with motor, sensory, autonomic, or psychic signs)
   b. Complex partial seizures
   c. Partial seizures with secondary generalization
2. Primarily generalized seizures
   a. Absence (petit mal)
   b. Tonic-clonic (grand mal)
   c. Tonic
   d. Atonic
   e. Myoclonic
3. Unclassified seizures
   a. Neonatal seizures
   b. Infantile spasms

impending change, detachment, depersonalization, déjà vu, or illusions that objects are growing smaller (micropsia) or larger (macropsia). When such symptoms precede a complex partial or secondarily generalized seizure, these simple partial seizures serve as a warning, or *aura*.

Complex Partial Seizures   Complex partial seizures are characterized by focal seizure activity accompanied by a transient impairment of the patient's ability to maintain normal contact with the environment. The patient is unable to respond appropriately to visual or verbal commands during the seizure and has impaired recollection or awareness of the ictal phase. The seizures frequently begin with an aura (i.e., a simple partial seizure) that is stereotypic for the patient. The start of the ictal phase is often a sudden behavioral arrest or motionless stare, which marks the onset of the period of amnesia. The behavioral arrest is usually accompanied by *automatisms*, which are involuntary, automatic behaviors that have a wide range of manifestations. Automatisms may consist of very basic behaviors such as chewing, lip smacking, swallowing, or "picking" movements of the hands, or more elaborate behaviors such as a display of emotion or running. The patient is typically confused following the seizure, and the transition to full recovery of consciousness may range from seconds up to an hour. Examination immediately following the seizure may show an anterograde amnesia or, in cases involving the dominant hemisphere, a postictal aphasia.

The routine, interictal (i.e., between seizures) EEG in patients with complex partial seizures is often normal or may show brief discharges termed *epileptiform spikes*, or *sharp waves*. Since complex partial seizures can arise from the medial temporal lobe or inferior frontal lobe, i.e., regions distant from the scalp, the EEG recorded during the seizure may be nonlocalizing. However, the seizure focus is often detected using sphenoidal or surgically placed intracranial electrodes.

The range of potential clinical behaviors linked to complex partial seizures is so broad that extreme caution is advised before concluding that stereotypic episodes of bizarre or atypical behavior are not due to seizure activity. In such cases additional, detailed EEG studies may be helpful.

Partial Seizures with Secondary Generalization   Partial seizures can spread to involve both cerebral hemispheres and produce a generalized seizure, usually of the tonic-clonic variety (discussed below). Secondary generalization is observed frequently following simple partial seizures, especially those with a focus in the frontal lobe, but may also be associated with partial seizures occurring elsewhere in the brain. A partial seizure with secondary generalization is often difficult to distinguish from a primarily generalized tonic-clonic seizure, since bystanders tend to emphasize the more dramatic, generalized convulsive phase of the seizure and overlook the more subtle, focal symptoms present at onset. In some cases, the focal onset of the seizure becomes apparent only when a careful history identifies a preceding aura (i.e., simple partial seizure). Often, however, the focal onset is not clinically evident and may be established only through careful EEG analysis. Nonetheless, distinguishing between these two entities is extremely important, as there may be substantial differences in the evaluation and treatment of partial versus generalized seizure disorders.

GENERALIZED SEIZURES   By definition, generalized seizures arise from both cerebral hemispheres simultaneously. However, it is currently impossible to exclude entirely the existence of a focal region of abnormal activity that initiates the seizure prior to rapid secondary generalization. For this reason, generalized seizures may be practically defined as bilateral clinical and electrographic events without any detectable focal onset. Fortunately, several types of generalized seizures have distinctive features that facilitate clinical diagnosis.

Absence Seizures (Petit Mal)   Absence seizures are characterized by sudden, brief lapses of consciousness without loss of postural control. The seizure typically lasts for only seconds, consciousness returns as sud-

denly as it was lost, and there is no postictal confusion. Although the brief loss of consciousness may be clinically inapparent or the sole manifestation of the seizure discharge, absence seizures are usually accompanied by subtle, bilateral motor signs such as rapid blinking of the eyelids, chewing movements, or small-amplitude, clonic movements of the hands.

Absence seizures usually begin in childhood (ages 4 to 8) or early adolescence and are the main seizure type in 15 to 20% of children with epilepsy. The seizures can occur hundreds of times per day, but the child may be unaware of or unable to convey their existence. The patient may be constantly piecing together experiences that have been interrupted by the seizures. Since the clinical signs of the seizures are subtle, especially to new parents, it is not surprising that the first clue to absence epilepsy is often unexplained "daydreaming" and a decline in school performance recognized by a teacher.

The electrophysiologic hallmark of typical absence seizures is a generalized, symmetric, 3-Hz spike-and-wave discharge that begins and ends suddenly, superimposed on a normal EEG background. Periods of spike-and-wave discharges lasting more than a few seconds usually correlate with clinical signs, but the EEG often shows many more brief bursts of abnormal cortical activity than were suspected clinically. Hyperventilation tends to provoke these electrographic discharges and even the seizures themselves and is routinely used when recording the EEG.

Typical absence seizures are often associated with generalized, tonic-clonic seizures, but patients usually have no other neurologic problems and respond well to treatment with specific anticonvulsants. Although estimates vary, ~60 to 70% of such patients will have a spontaneous remission during adolescence.

Atypical Absence Seizures   Atypical absence seizures have features that deviate both clinically and electrophysiologically from typical absence seizures. For example, the lapse of consciousness is usually of longer duration and less abrupt in onset and cessation, and the seizure is accompanied by more obvious motor signs that may include focal or lateralizing features. The EEG shows a generalized, slow spike-and-wave pattern with a frequency of $\leq2.5/s$, as well as other abnormal activity. Atypical absence seizures are usually associated with diffuse or multifocal structural abnormalities of the brain and therefore may accompany other signs of neurologic dysfunction such as mental retardation. Furthermore, the seizures are less responsive to anticonvulsants compared to typical absence seizures.

Generalized, Tonic-Clonic Seizures (Grand Mal)   Primarily generalized, tonic-clonic seizures are the main seizure type in ~10% of all persons with epilepsy. They are also the most common seizure type resulting from metabolic derangements and are therefore frequently encountered in many different clinical settings. The seizure usually begins abruptly without warning, although some patients describe vague premonitory symptoms in the hours leading up to the seizure. This prodrome is distinct from the stereotypic auras associated with focal seizures that secondarily generalize. The initial phase of the seizure is usually tonic contraction of muscles throughout the body, accounting for a number of the classic features of the event. Tonic contraction of the muscles of expiration and the larynx at the onset will produce a loud moan or "ictal cry." Respirations are impaired, secretions pool in the oropharynx, and cyanosis develops. Contraction of the jaw muscles may cause biting of the tongue. A marked enhancement of sympathetic tone leads to increases in heart rate, blood pressure, and pupillary size. After 10 to 20 s, the tonic phase of the seizure typically evolves into the clonic phase, produced by the superimposition of periods of muscle relaxation on the tonic muscle contraction. The periods of relaxation progressively increase until the end of the ictal phase, which usually lasts no more than 1 min. The postictal phase is characterized by unresponsiveness, muscular flaccidity, and excessive salivation that can cause stridorous breathing and partial airway obstruction. Bladder or bowel incontinence may occur at this point. Patients gradually regain consciousness over minutes to hours, and during this transition there is typically a period of postictal confusion. Patients subsequently complain of headache, fatigue, and muscle ache that can last for many hours. The duration of impaired consciousness in the postictal phase can be extremely long, i.e., many hours, in patients with prolonged seizures or underlying CNS diseases such as alcoholic cerebral atrophy.

The EEG during the tonic phase of the seizure shows a progressive increase in generalized low-voltage fast activity, followed by generalized high-amplitude, polyspike discharges. In the clonic phase, the high-amplitude activity is typically interrupted by slow waves to create a spike-and-wave pattern. The postictal EEG shows diffuse slowing that gradually recovers as the patient awakens.

There are many variants of the generalized tonic-clonic seizure, including pure tonic and pure clonic seizures. Brief tonic seizures lasting only a few seconds are especially noteworthy since they are usually associated with specific epileptic syndromes having mixed seizure phenotypes, such as the Lennox-Gastaut syndrome (discussed below).

Atonic Seizures Atonic seizures are characterized by sudden loss of postural muscle tone lasting 1 to 2 s. Consciousness is briefly impaired, but there is usually no postictal confusion. A very brief seizure may cause only a quick head drop or nodding movement, while a longer seizure will cause the patient to collapse. This can be extremely dangerous, since there is a substantial risk of direct head injury with the fall. The EEG shows brief, generalized spike-and-wave discharges followed immediately by diffuse slow waves that correlate with the loss of muscle tone. Similar to pure tonic seizures, atonic seizures are usually seen in association with known epileptic syndromes.

Myoclonic Seizures Myoclonus is a sudden and brief muscle contraction that may involve one part of the body or the entire body. A normal, common physiologic form of myoclonus is the sudden jerking movement observed while falling asleep. Pathologic myoclonus is most commonly seen in association with metabolic disorders, degenerative CNS diseases, or anoxic brain injury (Chap. 21). Although the distinction from other forms of myoclonus is imprecise, myoclonic seizures are considered to be true epileptic events since they are caused by cortical (versus subcortical or spinal) dysfunction. The EEG may show bilaterally synchronous spike-and-wave discharges synchronized with the myoclonus, although these can be obscured by movement artifact. Myoclonic seizures usually coexist with other forms of generalized seizure disorders but are the predominant feature of juvenile myoclonic epilepsy (discussed below).

UNCLASSIFIED SEIZURES Not all seizure types can be classified as partial or generalized. This appears to be especially true of seizures that occur in neonates and infants. The distinctive phenotypes of seizures at these early ages likely result, in part, from differences in neuronal function and connectivity in the immature versus mature CNS.

EPILEPSY SYNDROMES

Epilepsy syndromes are disorders in which epilepsy is a predominant feature, and there is sufficient evidence (e.g., through clinical, EEG, radiologic, or genetic observations) to suggest a common underlying mechanism. Three important epilepsy syndromes are listed below; additional examples with a known genetic basis are shown in Table 348-2.

JUVENILE MYOCLONIC EPILEPSY Juvenile myoclonic epilepsy (JME) is a generalized seizure disorder of unknown cause that appears in early adolescence and is usually characterized by bilateral myoclonic jerks that may be single or repetitive. The myoclonic seizures are most frequent in the morning after awakening and can be provoked by sleep deprivation. Consciousness is preserved unless the myoclonus is especially severe. Many patients also experience generalized tonic-clonic seizures, and up to one-third have absence seizures. The condition is otherwise benign, and although complete remission is uncommon, the seizures respond well to appropriate anticonvulsant medication. There is often a family history of epilepsy, and genetic linkage studies suggest a polygenic cause.

LENNOX-GASTAUT SYNDROME Lennox-Gastaut syndrome occurs in children and is defined by the following triad: (1) multiple seizure types (usually including generalized tonic-clonic, atonic, and atypical absence seizures); (2) an EEG showing slow (<3 Hz) spike-and-wave discharges and a variety of other abnormalities; and (3) impaired cognitive function in most but not all cases. Lennox-Gastaut syndrome is associated with CNS disease or dysfunction from a variety of causes, including developmental abnormalities, perinatal hypoxia/ischemia, trauma, infection, and other acquired lesions. The multifactorial nature of this syndrome suggests that it is a nonspecific response of the brain to diffuse neural injury. Unfortunately, many patients have a poor prognosis due to the underlying CNS disease and the physical and psychosocial consequences of severe, poorly controlled epilepsy.

MESIAL TEMPORAL LOBE EPILEPSY SYNDROME Mesial temporal lobe epilepsy (MTLE) is the most common syndrome associated with complex partial seizures and is an example of a symptomatic, partial epilepsy with distinctive clinical, electroencephalographic, and pathologic features (Table 348-3). High-resolution magnetic resonance imaging (MRI) can detect the characteristic hippocampal sclerosis that appears to be essential in the pathophysiology of MTLE for many patients (Fig. 348-1). Recognition of this syndrome is especially important because it tends to be refractory to treatment with anticonvulsants but responds extremely well to surgical intervention. Advances in the understanding of basic mechanisms of epilepsy have come through studies of experimental models of MTLE, discussed below.

THE CAUSES OF SEIZURES AND EPILEPSY

Seizures are a result of a shift in the normal balance of excitation and inhibition within the CNS. Given the numerous properties that control neuronal excitability, it is not surprising that there are many different ways to perturb this normal balance, and therefore many different causes of both seizures and epilepsy. Three clinical observations emphasize how a variety of factors determine why certain conditions may cause seizures or epilepsy in a given patient.

1. *The normal brain is capable of having a seizure under the appropriate circumstances, and there are differences between individuals in the susceptibility or threshold for seizures.* For example, seizures may be induced by high fevers in children who are otherwise normal and who never develop other neurologic problems, including epilepsy. However, febrile seizures occur only in a relatively small proportion of children. This implies there are various underlying, *endogenous factors* that influence the threshold for having a seizure. Some of these factors are clearly genetic, as it has been shown that a family history of epilepsy will influence the likelihood of seizures occurring in otherwise normal individuals. Normal development also plays an important role, since the brain appears to have different seizure thresholds at different maturational stages.

2. *There are a variety of conditions that have an extremely high likelihood of resulting in a chronic seizure disorder.* One of the best examples of this is severe, penetrating head trauma, which is associated with up to a 50% risk of subsequent epilepsy. The high propensity for severe traumatic brain injury to lead to epilepsy suggests that the injury results in a long-lasting, pathologic change in the CNS that transforms a presumably normal neural network into one that is abnormally hyperexcitable. This process is known as *epileptogenesis*, and the specific changes that result in a lowered seizure threshold can be considered *epileptogenic factors*. Other processes associated with epileptogenesis include stroke, infections, and abnormalities of CNS development. Likewise, the genetic abnormalities associated with epilepsy likely involve processes that trigger the appearance of specific sets of epileptogenic factors.

3. *Seizures are episodic.* Patients with epilepsy have seizures intermittently and, depending on the underlying cause, many patients are completely normal for months or even years between seizures. This implies there are important provocative or *precipitating factors* that

TABLE 348-2 *Examples of Genes Associated with Epilepsy Syndromes*[a]

Gene (Locus)	Function of Gene	Clinical Syndrome	Comments
CHRNA4 (20q13.2) CHRNB2 (1q21.3)	Nicotinic acetylcholine receptor subunit; mutations cause alterations in Ca^{2+} flux through the receptor; this may reduce amount of GABA release in presynaptic terminals	Autosomal dominant nocturnal frontal lobe epilepsy (ADNFLE); childhood onset; brief, nighttime seizures with prominent motor movements; often misdiagnosed as primary sleep disorder	Rare; first identified in a large Australian family; other families found to have mutations in CHRNA2 or CHRNB2, and some families appear to have mutations at other loci
KCNQ2 (20q13.3) KCNQ3 (8q24)	Voltage-gated potassium channel subunits; mutation in pore regions may cause a 20–40% reduction of potassium currents, which will lead to impaired repolarization	Benign familial neonatal convulsions (BFNC); autosomal dominant inheritance; onset in 1st week of life in infants who are otherwise normal; remission usually within weeks to months; long-term epilepsy in 10–15%	Rare; sequence and functional homology to KCNQ1, mutations of which cause long QT syndrome and a cardiac-auditory syndrome
SCN1B (19q12.1)	β-subunit of a voltage-gated sodium channel; mutation disrupts disulfide bridge that is crucial for structure of extracellular domain; mutated β-subunit leads to slower sodium channel inactivation	Generalized epilepsy with febrile seizures plus (GEFS+); autosomal dominant inheritance; presents with febrile seizures at median 1 year, which may persist >6 years, then variable seizure types not associated with fever	Incidence uncertain; GEFS+ identified in other families with mutations in other sodium channel subunits (SCN1A and SCN2A) and GABA$_A$ receptor subunit (GABRG2); significant phenotypic heterogeneity within same family, including members with febrile seizures only
LGI1 (10q24)	Leucine-rich glioma-inactivated gene; previous evidence for role in glial tumor progression; likely to be involved in nervous system development	Autosomal dominant partial epilepsy with auditory features (ADPEAF); temporal lobe epilepsy with wide range of auditory and other sensory symptoms as major manifestation; age of onset usually between 10 and 25 years	Rare; at least one family with similar syndrome has mutation(s) elsewhere; LGI1 mutation is the only known mutation identified in temporal lobe epilepsy and the only non-ion-channel gene mutation known in idiopathic epilepsy
CSTB (21q22.3)	Cystatin B, a noncaspase cysteine protease inhibitor; normal protein may block neuronal apoptosis by inhibiting caspases directly or indirectly (via cathepsins), or controlling proteolysis	Progressive myoclonus epilepsy (PME) (Unverricht-Lundborg disease); autosomal recessive inheritance; age of onset between 6–15 years, myoclonic seizures, ataxia, and progressive cognitive decline; brain shows neuronal degeneration	Overall rare, but relatively common in Finland and Western Mediterranean (>1 in 20,000); precise role of cystatin B in human disease unknown, although mice with null mutations of cystatin B have similar syndrome
EPM2A (6q24)	Laforin, a protein tyrosine phosphatase (PTP); may influence glycogen metabolism, which is known to be regulated by phosphatases	Progressive myoclonus epilepsy (Lafora's disease); autosomal recessive inheritance; onset age 6–19 years, death within 10 years; brain degeneration associated with polyglucosan intracellular inclusion bodies in numerous organs	Most common PME in Southern Europe, Middle East, Northern Africa, and Indian subcontinent; genetic heterogeneity; unknown whether seizure phenotype due to degeneration or direct effects of abnormal laforin expression.
Doublecortin (Xq21-24)	Doublecortin, expressed primarily in frontal lobes; function unknown; potentially an intracellular signalling molecule	Classic lissencephaly associated with severe mental retardation and seizures in males; subcortical band heterotopia with more subtle findings in females (presumably due to random X-inactivation); X-linked dominant	Relatively rare but of uncertain incidence, recent increased ascertainment due to improved imaging techniques; relationship between migration defect and seizure phenotype unknown

[a] The first four syndromes listed in the table (ADNFLE, BFNC, GEFS+, and ADPEAF) are examples of idiopathic generalized epilepsies associated with identified gene mutations. The last three syndromes are examples of the numerous Mendelian disorders in which seizures are one part of the phenotype.
Note: GABA, γ-aminobutyric acid.

induce seizures in patients with epilepsy. Similarly, precipitating factors are responsible for causing the single seizure in someone without epilepsy. Precipitants include those due to intrinsic physiologic processes, such as psychological or physical stress, sleep deprivation, or hormonal changes associated with the menstrual cycle. They also include exogenous factors such as exposure to toxic substances and certain medications.

These observations emphasize the concept that the many causes of seizures and epilepsy result from a dynamic interplay between endogenous factors, epileptogenic factors, and precipitating factors. The potential role of each needs to be carefully considered when determining the appropriate management of a patient with seizures. For example, the identification of predisposing factors (e.g., family history of epilepsy) in a patient with febrile seizures may increase the necessity for closer follow-up and a more aggressive diagnostic evaluation. Finding an epileptogenic lesion may help in the estimation of seizure recurrence and duration of therapy. Finally, removal or modification of a precipitating factor may be an effective and safer method for preventing further seizures than the prophylactic use of anticonvulsant drugs.

CAUSES ACCORDING TO AGE In practice, it is useful to consider the etiologies of seizures based on the age of the patient, as age is one of the most important factors determining both the incidence and likely causes of seizures or epilepsy (Table 348-4). During the *neonatal period and early infancy*, potential causes include hypoxic-ischemic encephalopathy, trauma, CNS infection, congenital CNS abnormalities, and metabolic disorders. Babies born to mothers using neurotoxic drugs such as cocaine, heroin, or ethanol are susceptible to drug-withdrawal seizures in the first few days after delivery. Hypoglycemia and hypocalcemia, which can occur as secondary complications of peri-

TABLE 348-3 *Characteristics of the Mesial Temporal Lobe Epilepsy Syndrome*

History
    History of febrile seizures
    Family history of epilepsy
    Early onset
    Rare secondarily generalized seizures
    Seizures may remit and reappear
    Seizures often intractable

Clinical observations
    Aura common
    Behavioral arrest/stare
    Complex automatisms
    Unilateral posturing
    Postictal disorientation, memory loss, dysphasia (with focus in dominant hemisphere)

Laboratory studies
    Unilateral or bilateral anterior temporal spikes on EEG
    Hypometabolism on interictal PET
    Hypoperfusion on interictal SPECT
    Material-specific memory deficits on intracranial amobarbital (Wada) test
    MRI findings
        Small hippocampus with increased signal on T2-weighted sequences
        Small temporal lobe
        Enlarged temporal horn
    Pathologic findings
        Highly selective loss of specific cell populations within hippocampus in most cases

Note: EEG, electroencephalogram; PET, positron emission tomography; SPECT, single photon emission computed tomography.

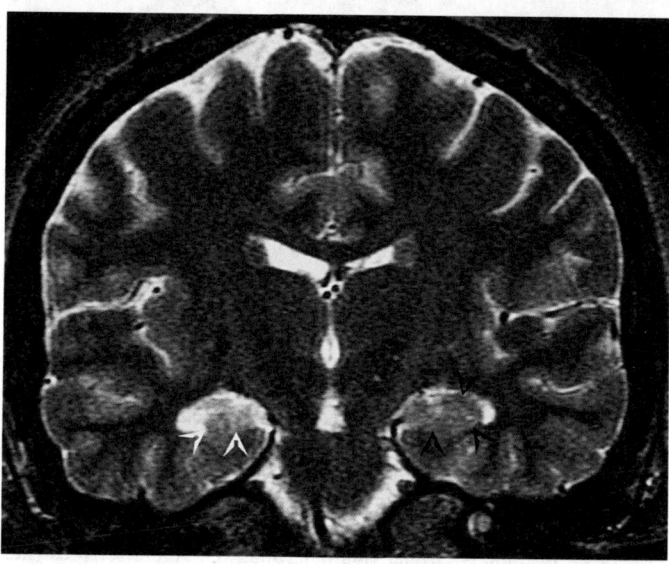

FIGURE 348-1 Mesial temporal lobe epilepsy. The EEG suggested a right temporal lobe focus. Coronal high-resolution T2-weighted fast spin echo magnetic resonance image obtained through the body of the hippocampus demonstrates abnormal high signal intensity in the right hippocampus (white arrows; compare with the normal hippocampus on the left, black arrows) consistent with mesial temporal sclerosis.

natal injury, are also causes of seizures early after delivery. Seizures due to inborn errors of metabolism usually present once regular feeding begins, typically 2 to 3 days after birth. Pyridoxine (vitamin B_6) deficiency, an important cause of neonatal seizures, can be effectively treated with pyridoxine replacement. The idiopathic or inherited forms of benign neonatal convulsions are also seen during this time period.

The most common seizures arising in *late infancy and early childhood* are febrile seizures, which are seizures associated with fevers but without evidence of CNS infection or other defined causes. The overall prevalence is 3 to 5% and even higher in some parts of the world, such as Asia. Patients often have a family history of febrile seizures or epilepsy. Febrile seizures usually occur between 3 months and 5 years of age and have a peak incidence between 18 and 24 months. The typical scenario is a child who has a generalized, tonic-clonic seizure during a febrile illness in the setting of a common childhood infection such as otitis media, respiratory infection, or gastroenteritis. The seizure is likely to occur during the rising phase of the temperature curve (i.e., during the first day) rather than well into the course of the illness. A *simple* febrile seizure is a single, isolated event, brief, and symmetric in appearance. *Complex* febrile seizures are characterized by repeated seizure activity, duration >15 min, or have focal features. Approximately one-third of patients with febrile seizures will have a recurrence, but <10% have three or more episodes. Recurrences are much more likely when the febrile seizure occurs in the first year of life. Simple febrile seizures are not associated with an increase in the risk of developing epilepsy, while complex febrile seizures have a risk of 2 to 5%; other risk factors include the presence of preexisting neurologic deficits and a family history of nonfebrile seizures.

Childhood marks the age at which many of the well-defined epilepsy syndromes present. Some children who are otherwise normal develop idiopathic, generalized tonic-clonic seizures without other features that fit into specific syndromes. Temporal lobe epilepsy usually presents in childhood and may be related to mesial temporal lobe sclerosis (as part of the MTLE syndrome) or other focal abnormalities such as cortical dysgenesis. Other types of partial seizures, including those with secondary generalization, may be the relatively late manifestation of a developmental disorder, an acquired lesion such as head trauma, CNS infection (especially viral encephalitis), or very rarely a CNS tumor.

The period of *adolescence and early adulthood* is one of transition during which the idiopathic or genetically based epilepsy syndromes, including JME and juvenile absence epilepsy, become less common, while epilepsies secondary to acquired CNS lesions begin to predominate. Seizures that begin in patients in this age range may be associated with head trauma, CNS infections (including parasitic infections such as cysticercosis), brain tumors, congenital CNS abnormalities, illicit drug use, or alcohol withdrawal.

TABLE 348-4 *Causes of Seizures*

Neonates (<1 month)	Perinatal hypoxia and ischemia
	Intracranial hemorrhage and trauma
	Acute CNS infection
	Metabolic disturbances (hypoglycemia, hypocalcemia, hypomagnesemia, pyridoxine deficiency)
	Drug withdrawal
	Developmental disorders
	Genetic disorders
Infants and children (>1 mo and <12 years)	Febrile seizures
	Genetic disorders (metabolic, degenerative, primary epilepsy syndromes)
	CNS infection
	Developmental disorders
	Trauma
	Idiopathic
Adolescents (12–18 years)	Trauma
	Genetic disorders
	Infection
	Brain tumor
	Illicit drug use
	Idiopathic
Young adults (18–35 years)	Trauma
	Alcohol withdrawal
	Illicit drug use
	Brain tumor
	Idiopathic
Older adults (>35 years)	Cerebrovascular disease
	Brain tumor
	Alcohol withdrawal
	Metabolic disorders (uremia, hepatic failure, electrolyte abnormalities, hypoglycemia)
	Alzheimer's disease and other degenerative CNS diseases
	Idiopathic

Note: CNS, central nervous system.

Head trauma is a common cause of epilepsy in adolescents and adults. The head injury can be caused by a variety of mechanisms, and the likelihood of developing epilepsy is strongly correlated with the severity of the injury. A patient with a penetrating head wound, depressed skull fracture, intracranial hemorrhage, or prolonged posttraumatic coma or amnesia has a 40 to 50% risk of developing epilepsy, while a patient with a closed head injury and cerebral contusion has a 5 to 25% risk. Recurrent seizures usually develop within 1 year after head trauma, although intervals of ≥10 years are well known. In controlled studies, mild head injury, defined as a concussion with amnesia or loss of consciousness of <30 min, was found to be associated with only a slightly increased likelihood of epilepsy. Nonetheless, most epileptologists know of patients who have partial seizures within hours or days of a mild head injury and subsequently develop chronic seizures of the same type; such cases may represent rare examples of chronic epilepsy resulting from mild head injury.

The causes of seizures in *older adults* include cerebrovascular disease, trauma (including subdural hematoma), CNS tumors, and degenerative diseases. Cerebrovascular disease may account for ~50% of new cases of epilepsy in patients older than 65. Acute seizures (i.e., occurring at the time of the stroke) are seen more often with embolic rather than hemorrhagic or thrombotic stroke. Chronic seizures typically appear months to years after the initial event and are associated with all forms of stroke.

Metabolic disturbances such as electrolyte imbalance, hypo- or hyperglycemia, renal failure, and hepatic failure may cause seizures at any age. Similarly, endocrine disorders, hematologic disorders, vasculitides, and many other systemic diseases may cause seizures over a broad age range. A wide variety of medications and abused substances are known to precipitate seizures as well (Table 348-5).

BASIC MECHANISMS

MECHANISMS OF SEIZURE INITIATION AND PROPAGATION Partial seizure activity can begin in a very discrete region of cortex and then spread to neighboring regions, i.e., there is a *seizure initiation* phase and a *seizure propagation* phase. The initiation phase is characterized by two concurrent events in an aggregate of neurons: (1) high-frequency bursts of action potentials, and (2) hypersynchronization. The bursting activity is caused by a relatively long-lasting depolarization of the neuronal membrane due to influx of extracellular calcium (Ca^{2+}), which leads to the opening of voltage-dependent sodium (Na^+) channels, influx of Na^+, and generation of repetitive action potentials. This is followed by a hyperpolarizing afterpotential mediated by γ-aminobutyric acid (GABA) receptors or potassium (K^+) channels, depending on the cell type. The synchronized bursts from a sufficient number of neurons result in a so-called spike discharge on the EEG.

Normally, the spread of bursting activity is prevented by intact

hyperpolarization and a region of surrounding inhibition created by inhibitory neurons. With sufficient activation there is a recruitment of surrounding neurons via a number of mechanisms. Repetitive discharges lead to the following: (1) an increase in extracellular K^+, which blunts hyperpolarization and depolarizes neighboring neurons; (2) accumulation of Ca^{2+} in presynaptic terminals, leading to enhanced neurotransmitter release; and (3) depolarization-induced activation of the N-methyl-D-aspartate (NMDA) subtype of the excitatory amino acid receptor, which causes Ca^{2+} influx and neuronal activation. The recruitment of a sufficient number of neurons leads to a loss of the surrounding inhibition and propagation of seizure activity into contiguous areas via local cortical connections, and to more distant areas via long commissural pathways such as the corpus callosum.

Many factors control neuronal excitability, and thus there are many potential mechanisms for altering a neuron's propensity to have bursting activity. Mechanisms *intrinsic* to the neuron include changes in the conductance of ion channels, response characteristics of membrane receptors, cytoplasmic buffering, second-messenger systems, and protein expression as determined by gene transcription, translation, and posttranslational modification. Mechanisms *extrinsic* to the neuron include changes in the amount or type of neurotransmitters present at the synapse, modulation of receptors by extracellular ions and other molecules, and temporal and spatial properties of synaptic and nonsynaptic input. Nonneural cells, such as astrocytes and oligodendrocytes, have an important role in many of these mechanisms as well.

Certain recognized causes of seizures are explained by these mechanisms. For example, accidental ingestion of domoic acid, which is an analogue of glutamate (the principal excitatory neurotransmitter in the brain), causes profound seizures via direct activation of excitatory amino acid receptors throughout the CNS. Penicillin, which can lower the seizure threshold in humans and is a potent convulsant in experimental models, reduces inhibition by antagonizing the effects of GABA at its receptor. The basic mechanisms of other precipitating factors of seizures, such as sleep deprivation, fever, alcohol withdrawal, hypoxia, and infection, are not as well understood but presumably involve analogous perturbations in neuronal excitability. Similarly, the endogenous factors that determine an individual's seizure threshold may relate to these properties as well.

Knowledge of the mechanisms responsible for initiation and propagation of most generalized seizures (including tonic-clonic, myoclonic, and atonic types) remains rudimentary and reflects the limited understanding of the connectivity of the brain at a systems level. Much more is understood about the origin of generalized spike-and-wave discharges in absence seizures. These appear to be related to oscillatory rhythms normally generated during sleep by circuits connecting the thalamus and cortex. This oscillatory behavior involves an interaction between $GABA_B$ receptors, T-type Ca^{2+} channels, and K^+ channels located within the thalamus. Pharmacologic studies indicate that modulation of these receptors and channels can induce absence seizures, and there is speculation that the genetic forms of absence epilepsy may be associated with mutations of components of this system.

MECHANISMS OF EPILEPTOGENESIS Epileptogenesis refers to the transformation of a normal neuronal network into one that is chronically hyperexcitable. There is often a delay of months to years between an initial CNS injury such as trauma, stroke, or infection and the first seizure. The injury appears to initiate a process that gradually lowers the seizure threshold in the affected region until a spontaneous seizure occurs. In many genetic and idiopathic forms of epilepsy, epileptogenesis is presumably determined by developmentally regulated events.

Pathologic studies of the hippocampus from patients with temporal lobe epilepsy have led to the suggestion that some forms of epileptogenesis are related to *structural changes in neuronal networks*. For example, many patients with MTLE have a highly selective loss of neurons that may contribute to inhibition of the main excitatory neurons within the dentate gyrus. There is also evidence that, in response to the loss of neurons, there is reorganization or "sprouting" of sur-

---

TABLE 348-5 *Drugs and Other Substances That Can Cause Seizures*

Antimicrobials/antivirals	Psychotropics
β-lactam and related compounds	Antidepressants
Quinolones	Antipsychotics
Acyclovir	Lithium
Isoniazid	Radiographic contrast agents
Ganciclovir	Theophylline
Anesthetics and analgesics	Sedative-hypnotic drug
Meperidine	withdrawal
Tramadol	Alcohol
Local anesthetics	Barbiturates
Immunomodulatory drugs	Benzodiazepines
Cyclosporine	Drugs of abuse
OKT3 (monoclonal antibodies to	Amphetamine
T cells)	Cocaine
Tacrolimus (FK-506)	Phencyclidine
Interferons	Methylphenidate
	Flumazenil[a]

[a] In benzodiazepine-dependent patients.

viving neurons in a way that affects the excitability of the network. Some of these changes can be seen in experimental models of prolonged electrical seizures or traumatic brain injury. Thus, an initial injury such as head injury may lead to a very focal, confined region of structural change that causes local hyperexcitability. The local hyperexcitability leads to further structural changes that evolve over time until the focal lesion produces clinically evident seizures. Similar models have also provided strong evidence for long-term alterations in *intrinsic, biochemical properties of cells* within the network, such as chronic changes in glutamate receptor function.

GENETIC CAUSES OF EPILEPSY The most important recent progress in epilepsy research has been the identification of genetic mutations associated with a variety of epilepsy syndromes (Table 348-2). Although all of the mutations identified to date cause rare forms of epilepsy, their discovery has led to extremely important conceptual advances. For example, it appears that many of the inherited, idiopathic epilepsies (i.e., the relatively "pure" forms of epilepsy in which seizures are the phenotypic abnormality and brain structure and function are otherwise normal) are due to mutations affecting ion channel function. These syndromes are therefore part of the larger group of channelopathies causing paroxysmal disorders such as cardiac arrhythmias, episodic ataxia, periodic weakness, and familial hemiplegic migraine. In contrast, gene mutations observed in symptomatic epilepsies (i.e., disorders in which other neurologic abnormalities, such as cognitive impairment, coexist with seizures) are proving to be associated with pathways influencing CNS development or neuronal homeostasis. A current challenge is to identify the multiple susceptibility genes that underlie the more common forms of idiopathic epilepsies.

MECHANISMS OF ACTION OF ANTIEPILEPTIC DRUGS Antiepileptic drugs appear to act primarily by blocking the initiation or spread of seizures. This occurs through a variety of mechanisms that modify the activity of ion channels or neurotransmitters, and in most cases the drugs have pleiotropic effects. The mechanisms include inhibition of Na^+-dependent action potentials in a frequency-dependent manner (e.g., phenytoin, carbamazepine, lamotrigine, topiramate, zonisamide), inhibition of voltage-gated Ca^{2+} channels (phenytoin), decrease of glutamate release (lamotrigine), potentiation of GABA receptor function (benzodiazepines and barbiturates), and increase in the availability of GABA (valproic acid, gabapentin, tiagabine). The two most effective drugs for absence seizures, ethosuximide and valproic acid, probably act by inhibiting T-type Ca^{2+} channels in thalamic neurons.

In contrast to the relatively large number of antiepileptic drugs that can attenuate seizure activity, there are currently no drugs known to prevent the formation of a seizure focus following CNS injury. The eventual development of such "antiepileptogenic" drugs will provide an important means of preventing the emergence of epilepsy following injuries such as head trauma, stroke, and CNS infection.

EVALUATION OF THE PATIENT WITH A SEIZURE

When a patient presents shortly after a seizure, the first priorities are attention to vital signs, respiratory and cardiovascular support, and treatment of seizures if they resume (see "Treatment"). Life-threatening conditions such as CNS infection, metabolic derangement, or drug toxicity must be recognized and managed appropriately.

When the patient is not acutely ill, the evaluation will initially focus on whether there is a history of earlier seizures (Fig. 348-2). If this is the first seizure, then the emphasis will be to (1) establish whether the reported episode was a seizure rather than another paroxysmal event, (2) determine the cause of the seizure by identifying risk factors and precipitating events, and (3) decide whether anticonvulsant therapy is required in addition to treatment for any underlying illness.

In the patient with prior seizures or a known history of epilepsy, the evaluation is directed toward (1) identification of the underlying cause and precipitating factors, and (2) determination of the adequacy of the patient's current therapy.

HISTORY AND EXAMINATION The first goal is to determine whether the event was truly a seizure. An in-depth history is essential, for *in many*

cases the diagnosis of a seizure is based solely on clinical grounds— the examination and laboratory studies are often normal. Questions should be focused on the symptoms before, during, and after the episode in order to discriminate a seizure from other paroxysmal events (see "Differential Diagnosis of Seizures"). Seizures frequently occur out-of-hospital, and the patient may be unaware of the ictal and immediate postictal phases; thus witnesses to the event should be interviewed carefully.

The history should also focus on risk factors and predisposing events. Clues for a predisposition to seizures include a history of febrile seizures, earlier auras or brief seizures not recognized as such, and a family history of seizures. Epileptogenic factors such as prior head trauma, stroke, tumor, or vascular malformation should be identified. In children, a careful assessment of developmental milestones may provide evidence for underlying CNS disease. Precipitating factors such as sleep deprivation, systemic diseases, electrolyte or metabolic derangements, acute infection, drugs that lower the seizure threshold (Table 348-5), or alcohol or illicit drug use should also be identified.

The general physical examination includes a search for signs of infection or systemic illness. Careful examination of the skin may reveal signs of neurocutaneous disorders, such as tuberous sclerosis or neurofibromatosis, or chronic liver or renal disease. A finding of organomegaly may indicate a metabolic storage disease, and limb asymmetry may provide a clue to brain injury early in development. Signs of head trauma and use of alcohol or illicit drugs should be sought. Auscultation of the heart and carotid arteries may identify an abnormality that predisposes to cerebrovascular disease.

All patients require a complete neurologic examination, with particular emphasis on eliciting signs of cerebral hemispheric disease (Chap. 346). Careful assessment of mental status (including memory, language function, and abstract thinking) may suggest lesions in the anterior frontal, parietal, or temporal lobes. Testing of visual fields will help screen for lesions in the optic pathways and occipital lobes. Screening tests of motor function such as pronator drift, deep tendon reflexes, gait, and coordination may suggest lesions in motor (frontal) cortex, and cortical sensory testing (e.g., double simultaneous stimulation) may detect lesions in the parietal cortex.

LABORATORY STUDIES Routine blood studies are indicated to identify the more common metabolic causes of seizures, such as abnormalities in electrolytes, glucose, calcium, or magnesium, and hepatic or renal disease. A screen for toxins in blood and urine should also be obtained from all patients in appropriate risk groups, especially when no clear precipitating factor has been identified. A lumbar puncture is indicated if there is any suspicion of meningitis or encephalitis and is mandatory in all patients infected with HIV, even in the absence of symptoms or signs suggesting infection.

Electroencephalography All patients who have a possible seizure disorder should be evaluated with an EEG as soon as possible. The EEG measures electrical activity of the brain by recording from electrodes placed on the scalp. The potential difference between pairs of electrodes is amplified and displayed on a computer monitor, oscilloscope, or paper. The characteristics of the normal EEG depend on the patient's age and level of arousal. The recorded activity represents the postsynaptic potentials of vertically oriented pyramidal cells in the cerebral cortex and is characterized by its frequency. In normal awake adults lying quietly with the eyes closed, an 8- to 13-Hz alpha rhythm is seen posteriorly in the EEG, intermixed with a variable amount of generalized faster beta activity (>13 Hz), and it is attenuated when the eyes are opened (Fig. 348-3). During drowsiness, the alpha rhythm is also attenuated; with light sleep, slower activity in the theta (4 to 7 Hz) and delta (<4 Hz) ranges becomes more apparent.

The EEG is best recorded from several different electrode arrangements (montages) in turn, and activating procedures are usually performed in an attempt to provoke abnormalities. Such procedures com-

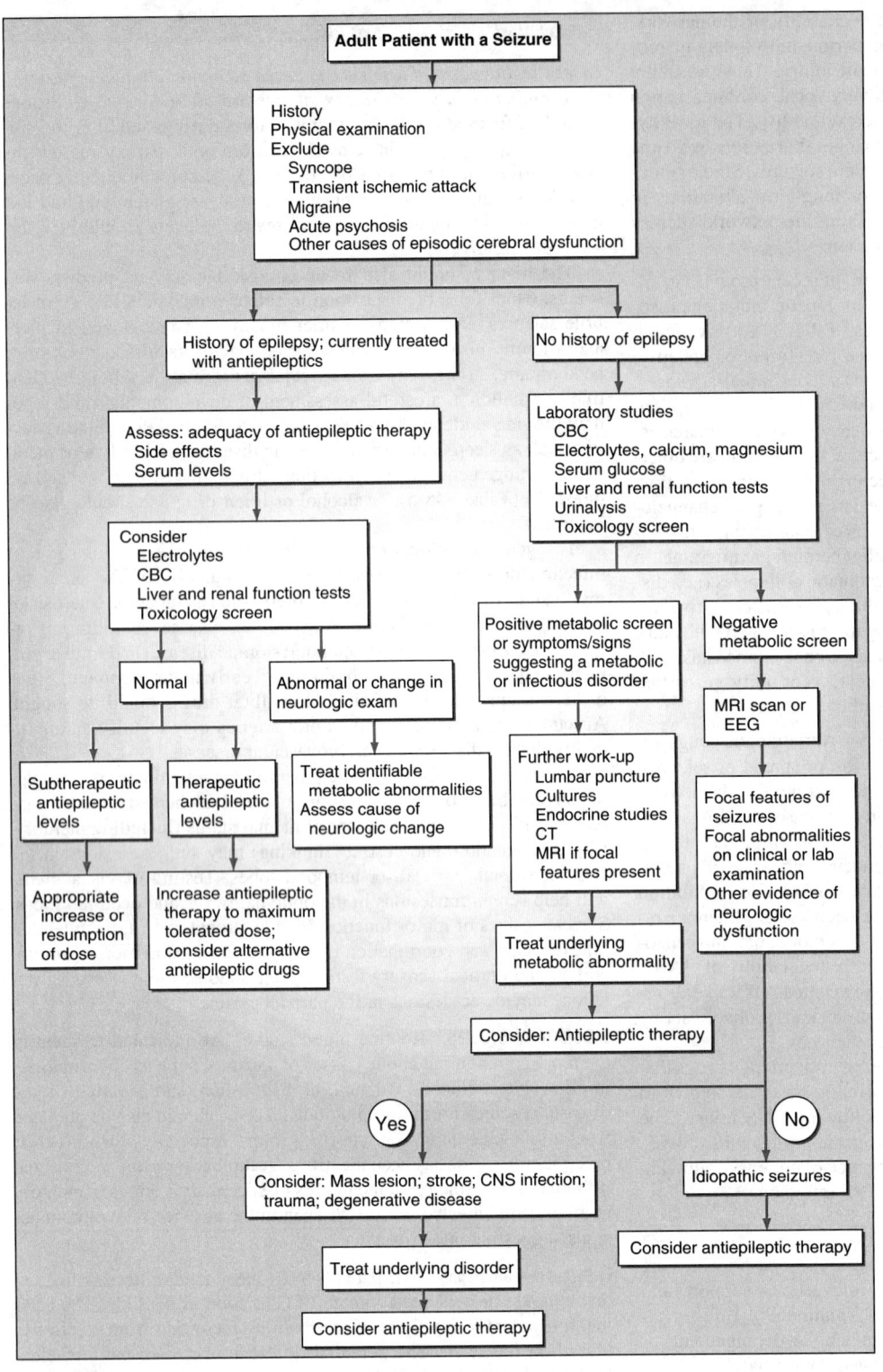

FIGURE 348-2 Evaluation of the adult patient with a seizure. CBC, complete blood count; CT, computed tomography; MRI, magnetic resonance imaging; EEG, electroencephalogram; CNS, central nervous system.

zures are typically infrequent and unpredictable, it is often not possible to obtain the EEG during a clinical event. Continuous monitoring for prolonged periods in video-EEG telemetry units for hospitalized patients or the use of portable equipment to record the EEG continuously on cassettes for ≥24 h in ambulatory patients has made it easier to capture the electrophysiologic accompaniments of clinical events.

The EEG may also be helpful in the interictal period by showing certain abnormalities that are highly supportive of the diagnosis of epilepsy. Such *epileptiform activity* consists of bursts of abnormal discharges containing spikes or sharp waves. The presence of epileptiform activity is not specific for epilepsy, but it has a much greater prevalence in patients with epilepsy than in normal individuals. However, even in an individual who is known to have epilepsy, the initial routine interictal EEG may be normal up to 60% of the time. Thus, the EEG cannot establish the diagnosis of epilepsy in many cases.

The EEG is also used for classifying seizure disorders and aiding in the selection of anticonvulsant medications. For example, episodic generalized spike-wave activity is usually seen in patients with typical absence epilepsy and may be seen with other generalized epilepsy syndromes. Focal interictal epileptiform discharges would support the diagnosis of a partial seizure disorder such as temporal lobe epilepsy or frontal lobe seizures, depending on the location of the discharges.

The routine scalp-recorded EEG may also be used to assess the prognosis of seizure disorders; in general, a normal EEG implies a better prognosis, whereas an abnormal background or profuse epileptiform activity suggests a poor outlook. Unfortunately, the EEG has not proved to be useful in predicting which patients with predisposing conditions, such as head injury or brain tumor, will go on to develop epilepsy, because in such circumstances epileptiform activity is commonly encountered regardless of whether seizures occur.

Brain Imaging Almost all patients with new-onset seizures should have a brain imaging study to determine whether there is an underlying structural abnormality that is responsible. The only potential exception to this rule is children who have an unambiguous history and examination suggestive of a benign, generalized seizure disorder such as absence epilepsy. MRI has been shown to be superior to computed tomography (CT) for the detection of cerebral lesions associated with epilepsy. In some cases MRI will identify lesions such as tumors, vascular malformations, or other pathologies that need immediate therapy. The use of newer MRI methods, such as fluid-attenuated inversion recovery (FLAIR), has increased the sensitivity for detection of abnormalities

monly include hyperventilation (for 3 or 4 min), photic stimulation, sleep, and sleep deprivation on the night prior to the recording.

In the evaluation of a patient with suspected epilepsy, the presence of *electrographic seizure activity* during the clinically evident event, i.e., of abnormal, repetitive, rhythmic activity having an abrupt onset and termination, clearly establishes the diagnosis. The absence of electrographic seizure activity does not exclude a seizure disorder, however, because simple or complex seizures may originate from a region of cortex that is not within range of the scalp electrodes. The EEG is always abnormal during generalized tonic-clonic seizures. Since sei-

of cortical architecture, including hippocampal atrophy associated with mesial temporal sclerosis, and abnormalities of cortical neuronal migration. In such cases the findings may not lead to immediate therapy, but they do provide an explanation for the patient's seizures and point to the need for chronic anticonvulsant therapy or possible surgical resection.

In the patient with a suspected CNS infection or mass lesion, CT scanning should be performed emergently when MRI is not immediately available. Otherwise, it is usually appropriate to obtain an MRI study within a few days of the initial evaluation. Functional imaging procedures such as positron emission tomography (PET) and single photon emission computed tomography (SPECT) are also used to evaluate certain patients with medically refractory seizures (discussed below).

DIFFERENTIAL DIAGNOSIS OF SEIZURES

Disorders that may mimic seizures are listed in Table 348-6. In most cases seizures can be distinguished from other conditions by meticulous attention to the history and relevant laboratory studies. On occasion, additional studies, such as video-EEG monitoring, sleep studies, tilt table analysis, or cardiac electrophysiology, may be required to reach a correct diagnosis. Two of the more common nonepileptic syndromes in the differential diagnosis are detailed below.

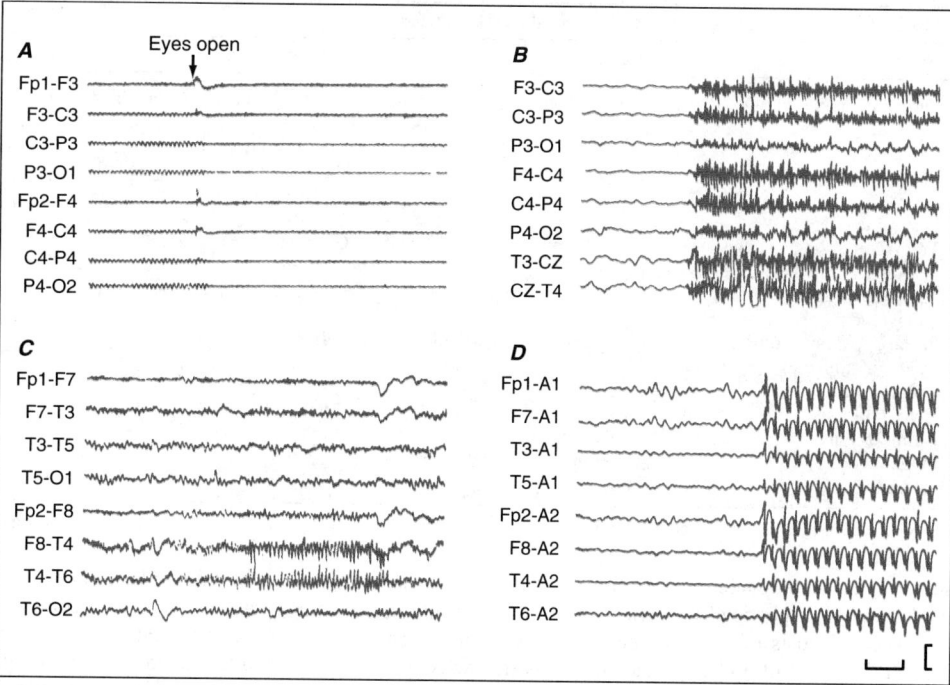

FIGURE 348-3 *A.* A normal EEG showing a posteriorly situated 9-Hz alpha rhythm that attenuates with eye opening. *B.* Onset of a tonic seizure showing generalized repetitive sharp activity with synchronous onset over both hemispheres. *C.* Burst of repetitive spikes in the right temporal region during a clinical spell suggestive of a complex partial seizure. *D.* Generalized 3-Hz spike-wave activity occurring synchronously over both hemispheres during an absence seizure. Horizontal calibration: 1s; vertical calibration: 200 μV in *A* and *C*, 400 μV in *B*, and 750 μV in *D*. Electrode placements are indicated at the left of each panel in accord with the international 10:20 system. A, earlobe; C, central; F, frontal; Fp, frontal polar; P, parietal; T, temporal; O, occipital. Right-sided placements are indicated by even numbers, left-sided placements by odd numbers, and midline placements by Z. [*From MJ Aminoff (ed): Electrodiagnosis in Clinical Neurology, 4th ed. New York, Churchill Livingstone, 1999.*]

Syncope (See also Chap. 20) The diagnostic dilemma encountered most frequently is the distinction between a generalized seizure and syncope. Observations by the patient and bystanders that can help discriminate between the two are listed in Table 348-7. Characteristics of a seizure include the presence of an aura, cyanosis, unconsciousness, motor manifestations lasting >30 s, postictal disorientation, muscle soreness, and sleepiness. In contrast, a syncopal episode is more likely if the event was provoked by acute pain or anxiety or occurred immediately after arising from the lying or sitting position. Patients with syncope often describe a stereotyped transition from consciousness to unconsciousness that includes tiredness, sweating, nausea, and tunneling of vision, and they experience a relatively brief loss of consciousness. Headache or incontinence usually suggests a seizure but may on occasion also occur with syncope. A brief period (i.e., 1 to 10 s) of convulsive motor activity is frequently seen immediately at the onset of a syncopal episode, especially if the patient remains in an upright posture after fainting (e.g., in a dentist's chair) and therefore has a sustained decrease in cerebral perfusion. Rarely, a syncopal episode can induce a full tonic-clonic seizure. In such cases the evaluation must focus on both the cause of the syncopal event as well as the possibility that the patient has a propensity for recurrent seizures.

Psychogenic Seizures Psychogenic seizures are nonepileptic behaviors that resemble seizures. They are often part of a conversion reaction precipitated by underlying psychological distress. Certain behaviors, such as side-to-side turning of the head, asymmetric and large-amplitude shaking movements of the limbs, twitching of all four extremities without loss of consciousness, and pelvic thrusting are more commonly associated with psychogenic rather than epileptic seizures. Psychogenic seizures often last longer than epileptic seizures and may wax and wane over minutes to hours. However, the distinction is sometimes difficult on clinical grounds alone, and there are many examples

of diagnostic errors made by experienced epileptologists. This is especially true for psychogenic seizures that resemble complex partial seizures, since the behavioral manifestations of complex partial seizures (especially of frontal lobe origin) can be extremely unusual, and in both cases the routine surface EEG may be normal. Video-EEG monitoring is often useful when historic features are nondiagnostic. Generalized tonic-clonic seizures always produce marked EEG abnormalities during and after the seizure. For suspected complex partial seizures of temporal lobe origin, the use of additional electrodes beyond the standard scalp locations (e.g., sphenoidal electrodes) may be required to localize a seizure focus. Measurement of serum prolactin levels may also help to discriminate between organic and psychogenic seizures, since most generalized seizures and many complex partial

TABLE 348-6 *Differential Diagnosis of Seizures*

Syncope	Transient ischemic attack (TIA)
Vasovagal syncope	Basilar artery TIA
Cardiac arrhythmia	Sleep disorders
Valvular heart disease	Narcolepsy/cataplexy
Cardiac failure	Benign sleep myoclonus
Orthostatic hypotension	Movement disorders
Psychological disorders	Tics
Psychogenic seizure	Nonepileptic myoclonus
Hyperventilation	Paroxysmal choreoathetosis
Panic attack	Special considerations in children
Metabolic disturbances	Breath-holding spells
Alcoholic blackouts	Migraine with recurrent
Delirium tremens	abdominal pain and cyclic
Hypoglycemia	vomiting
Hypoxia	Benign paroxysmal vertigo
Psychoactive drugs (e.g.,	Apnea
hallucinogens)	Night terrors
Migraine	Sleepwalking
Confusional migraine	
Basilar migraine	

TABLE 348-7 *Features That Distinguish Generalized Tonic-Clonic Seizure from Syncope*

Features	Seizure	Syncope
Immediate precipitating factors	Usually none	Emotional stress, Valsalva, orthostatic hypotension, cardiac etiologies
Premonitory symptoms	None or aura (e.g., odd odor)	Tiredness, nausea, diaphoresis, tunneling of vision
Posture at onset	Variable	Usually erect
Transition to unconsciousness	Often immediate	Gradual over seconds[a]
Duration of unconsciousness	Minutes	Seconds
Duration of tonic or clonic movements	30–60 s	Never more than 15 s
Facial appearance during event	Cyanosis, frothing at mouth	Pallor
Disorientation and sleepiness after event	Many minutes to hours	<5 min
Aching of muscles after event	Often	Sometimes
Biting of tongue	Sometimes	Rarely
Incontinence	Sometimes	Sometimes
Headache	Sometimes	Rarely

[a] May be sudden with certain cardiac arrhythmias.

seizures are accompanied by rises in serum prolactin (during the immediate 30-min postictal period), whereas psychogenic seizures are not. The diagnosis of psychogenic seizures does not exclude a concurrent diagnosis of epilepsy, since the two often coexist.

℞ TREATMENT

Therapy for a patient with a seizure disorder is almost always multimodal and includes treatment of underlying conditions that cause or contribute to the seizures, avoidance of precipitating factors, suppression of recurrent seizures by prophylactic therapy with antiepileptic medications or surgery, and addressing a variety of psychological and social issues. Treatment plans must be individualized, given the many different types and causes of seizures as well as the differences in efficacy and toxicity of antiepileptic medications for each patient. In almost all cases a neurologist with experience in the treatment of epilepsy should design and oversee implementation of the treatment strategy. Furthermore, patients with refractory epilepsy or those who require polypharmacy with antiepileptic drugs should remain under the regular care of a neurologist.

Treatment of Underlying Conditions If the sole cause of a seizure is a metabolic disturbance such as an abnormality of serum electrolytes or glucose, then treatment is aimed at reversing the metabolic problem and preventing its recurrence. Therapy with antiepileptic drugs is usually unnecessary unless the metabolic disorder cannot be corrected promptly and the patient is at risk of having further seizures. If the apparent cause of a seizure was a medication (e.g., theophylline) or illicit drug use (e.g., cocaine), then appropriate therapy is avoidance of the drug; there is usually no need for antiepileptic medications unless subsequent seizures occur in the absence of these precipitants.

Seizures caused by a structural CNS lesion such as a brain tumor, vascular malformation, or brain abscess may not recur after appropriate treatment of the underlying lesion. However, despite removal of the structural lesion, there is a risk that the seizure focus will remain in the surrounding tissue or develop de novo as a result of gliosis and other processes induced by surgery, radiation, or other therapies. Most patients are therefore maintained on an antiepileptic medication for at least 1 year, and an attempt is made to withdraw medications only if the patient has been completely seizure-free. If seizures are refractory to medication, the patient may benefit from surgical removal of the epileptic brain region (see below).

Avoidance of Precipitating Factors Unfortunately, little is known about the specific factors that determine precisely when a seizure will occur in a patient with epilepsy. Some patients can identify particular situations that appear to lower their seizure threshold; these situations should be avoided. For example, a patient who has seizures in the setting of sleep deprivation should obviously be advised to maintain a normal sleep schedule. Many patients note an association between alcohol intake and seizures, and they should be encouraged to modify their drinking habits accordingly. There are also relatively rare cases of patients with seizures that are induced by highly specific stimuli such as a video game monitor, music, or an individual's voice ("reflex epilepsy"). If there is an association between stress and seizures, stress reduction techniques such as physical exercise, meditation, or counseling may be helpful.

Antiepileptic Drug Therapy Antiepileptic drug therapy is the mainstay of treatment for most patients with epilepsy. The overall goal is to completely prevent seizures without causing any untoward side effects, preferably with a single medication and a dosing schedule that is easy for the patient to follow. Seizure classification is an important element in designing the treatment plan, since some antiepileptic drugs have different activities against various seizure types. However, there is considerable overlap between many antiepileptic drugs, such that the choice of therapy is often determined more by specific needs of the patient, especially the patient's assessment of side effects.

WHEN TO INITIATE ANTIEPILEPTIC DRUG THERAPY Antiepileptic drug therapy should be started in any patient with recurrent seizures of unknown etiology or a known cause that cannot be reversed. Whether to initiate therapy in a patient with a single seizure is controversial. Patients with a single seizure due to an identified lesion such as a CNS tumor, infection, or trauma, in which there is strong evidence that the lesion is epileptogenic, should be treated. The risk of seizure recurrence in a patient with an apparently unprovoked or idiopathic seizure is uncertain, with estimates ranging from 31 to 71% in the first 12 months after the initial seizure. This uncertainty arises from differences in the underlying seizure types and etiologies in various published epidemiologic studies. Generally accepted risk factors associated with recurrent seizures include the following: (1) an abnormal neurologic examination, (2) seizures presenting as status epilepticus, (3) postictal Todd's paralysis, (4) a strong family history of seizures, or (5) an abnormal EEG. Most patients with one or more of these risk factors should be treated. Issues such as employment or driving may influence the decision whether or not to start medications as well. For example, a patient with a single, idiopathic seizure whose job depends on driving may prefer taking antiepileptic drugs rather than risk a seizure recurrence and the potential loss of driving privileges.

SELECTION OF ANTIEPILEPTIC DRUGS Antiepileptic drugs available in the United States are shown in Table 348-8, and the main pharmacologic characteristics of commonly used drugs are listed in Table 348-9. Older medications such as phenytoin, valproic acid, carbamazepine, and ethosuximide are generally used as first-line therapy for most seizure disorders since, overall, they are as effective as recently marketed drugs and significantly less expensive. Most of the new drugs that have become available in the past decade are used as add-on or alternative therapy.

In addition to efficacy, factors influencing the choice of an initial medication include the convenience of dosing (e.g., once daily versus three or four times daily) and potential side effects. Almost all of the commonly used antiepileptic drugs can cause similar, dose-related side effects such as sedation, ataxia, and diplopia. Close follow-up is required to ensure these are promptly recognized and reversed. Most of the drugs can also cause idiosyncratic toxicity such as rash, bone marrow suppression, or hepatotoxicity. Although rare, these side effects should be considered during drug selection, and patients require laboratory tests (e.g., complete blood count and liver function tests) prior to the institution of a drug (to establish baseline values) and during initial dosing and titration of the agent.

Antiepileptic Drug Selection for Partial Seizures Carbamazepine, phenytoin, or lamotrigine is currently the initial drug of choice for the treatment of partial seizures, including those that secondarily generalize. Overall they have very similar efficacy, but differences in pharmacokinetics and toxicity are the main determinants for use in a given patient. Phenytoin has a relatively long half-life and offers the advantage of once or twice daily dosing compared to two or three times daily dosing for carbamazepine (although a more expensive, extended-release form of carbamazepine is now available) and lamotrigine. An advantage of carbamazepine is that its metabolism follows first-order pharmacokinetics, and the relationship between drug dose, serum levels, and toxicity is linear. By contrast, phenytoin shows properties of saturation kinetics, such that small increases in phenytoin doses above a standard maintenance dose can precipitate marked side effects. This is one of the main causes of acute phenytoin toxicity. Long-term use of phenytoin is associated with untoward cosmetic effects (e.g., hirsutism, coarsening of facial features, and gingival hypertrophy), and effects on bone metabolism, so it is often avoided in young patients who are likely to require the drug for many years. Carbamazepine can cause leukopenia, aplastic anemia, or hepatotoxicity and would therefore be contraindicated in patients with predispositions to these problems. A major concern with lamotrigine is the occurrence of skin rash during the initiation of therapy. This can be extremely severe and lead to Stevens-Johnson syndrome if unrecognized and if the medication is not discontinued immediately. This risk can be reduced by slow introduction and titration. Lamotrigine must be started slowly when used as add-on therapy with valproic acid, since valproic acid can inhibit its metabolism, thereby substantially prolonging its half-life.

Valproic acid is an effective alternative for some patients with partial seizures, especially when the seizures secondarily generalize. Gastrointestinal side effects are fewer when using the valproate semisodium formulation (Depakote). Valproic acid also rarely causes reversible bone marrow suppression and hepatotoxicity, and laboratory testing is required to monitor toxicity. This drug should generally be avoided in patients with preexisting bone marrow or liver disease. Irreversible, fatal hepatic failure appearing as an idiosyncratic rather than dose-related side effect is a relatively rare complication; its risk is highest in children <2 years old, especially those taking other antiepileptic drugs or with inborn errors of metabolism.

Topiramate, tiagabine, levetiracetam, zonisamide, gabapentin, and oxcarbazepine are additional drugs currently used for the treatment of partial seizures with or without secondary generalization. Until recently, phenobarbital and other barbiturate compounds were commonly used as first-line therapy for many forms of epilepsy. However, the barbiturates frequently cause sedation in adults, hyperactivity in children, and other more subtle cognitive changes; thus, their use should be limited to situations in which no other suitable treatment alternatives exist.

Antiepileptic Drug Selection for Generalized Seizures Valproic acid is currently considered the best initial choice for the treatment of primarily generalized, tonic-clonic seizures. Lamotrigine, followed by carbamazepine and phenytoin, are suitable alternatives. Valproic acid is also particularly effective in absence, myoclonic, and atonic seizures and is therefore the drug of choice in patients with generalized epilepsy syndromes having mixed seizure types. Importantly, both carbamazepine and phenytoin can worsen certain types of generalized seizures, including absence, myoclonic, tonic, and atonic seizures. Ethosuximide is a particularly effective drug for the treatment of uncomplicated absence seizures, but it is not useful for tonic-clonic or partial seizures. Ethosuximide rarely causes bone marrow suppression, so that periodic monitoring of blood cell counts is required. Although approved for

TABLE 348-8 *Selection of Antiepileptic Drugs*

	Primary Generalized Tonic-Clonic	Partial[a]	Absence	Atypical Absence, Myoclonic, Atonic
First-Line	Valproic acid Lamotrigine	Carbamazepine Phenytoin Lamotrigine Valproic acid	Valproic acid Ethosuximide	Valproic acid
Alternatives	Phenytoin Carbamazepine Topiramate[b] Zonisamide[b] Felbamate Primidone Phenobarbital	Topiramate[b] Levetiracetam[b] Tiagabine[b] Zonisamide[b] Gabapentin[b] Primidone Phenobarbital	Lamotrigine Clonazepam	Lamotrigine Topiramate[b] Clonazepam Felbamate

[a] Includes simple partial, complex partial, and secondarily generalized seizures.
[b] As adjunctive therapy.

use in partial seizure disorders, lamotrigine appears to be effective in epilepsy syndromes with mixed, generalized seizure types such as JME and Lennox-Gastaut syndrome. Topiramate, zonisamide, and felbamate may have similar broad efficacy. Clinical trials are underway to establish the usefulness of levetiracetam in generalized seizure syndromes.

INITIATION AND MONITORING OF THERAPY Because the response to any antiepileptic drug is unpredictable, patients should be carefully educated about the approach to therapy. The goal is to prevent seizures and minimize the side effects of therapy; determination of the optimal dose is often a matter of trial and error. This process may take months or longer if the baseline seizure frequency is low. Most anticonvulsant drugs need to be introduced relatively slowly to minimize side effects, and patients should expect that minor side effects such as mild sedation, slight changes in cognition, or imbalance will typically resolve within a few days. Starting doses are usually the lowest value listed under the dosage column in Table 348-9. Subsequent increases should be made only after achieving a steady state with the previous dose (i.e., after an interval of five or more half-lives).

Monitoring of serum antiepileptic drug levels can be very useful for establishing the initial dosing schedule. However, the published therapeutic ranges of serum drug concentrations are only an approximate guide for determining the proper dose for a given patient. The key determinants are the clinical measures of seizure frequency and presence of side effects, not the laboratory values. Conventional assays of serum drug levels measure the total drug (i.e., both free and protein-bound). However, it is the concentration of free drug that reflects extracellular levels in the brain and correlates best with efficacy. Thus, patients with decreased levels of serum proteins (e.g., decreased serum albumin due to impaired liver or renal function) may have an increased ratio of free to bound drug, yet the concentration of free drug may be adequate for seizure control. These patients may have a "subtherapeutic" drug level, but the dose should be changed only if seizures remain uncontrolled, not just to achieve a "therapeutic" level. It is also useful to monitor free drug levels in such patients. In practice, other than during the initiation or modification of therapy, monitoring of antiepileptic drug levels is most useful for documenting compliance.

If seizures continue despite gradual increases to the maximum tolerated dose and documented compliance, then it becomes necessary to switch to another antiepileptic drug. This is usually done by maintaining the patient on the first drug while a second drug is added. The dose of the second drug should be adjusted to decrease seizure frequency without causing toxicity. Once this is achieved, the first drug can be gradually withdrawn (usually over weeks unless there is significant toxicity). The dose of the second drug is then further optimized based on seizure response and side effects. Monotherapy should be the goal whenever possible.

WHEN TO DISCONTINUE THERAPY Overall, about 70% of children and 60% of adults who have their seizures completely controlled with antiepi-

Generic Name	Trade Name	Principal Uses	Typical Dose; Dose Interval	Half-Life	Therapeutic Range	Adverse Effects Neurologic	Adverse Effects Systemic	Drug Interactions
Phenytoin (diphenyl-hydantoin)	Dilantin	Tonic-clonic (grand mal) Focal-onset	300–400 mg/d (3–6 mg/kg, adult; 4–8 mg/kg, child); qd-bid	24 h (wide variation, dose-dependent)	10–20 μg/mL	Dizziness Diplopia Ataxia Incoordination Confusion	Gum hyperplasia Lymphade-nopathy Hirsutism Osteomalacia Facial coarsening Skin rash	Level increased by isoniazid, sulfonamides, fluoxetine Level decreased by enzyme-inducing drugs[a] Altered folate metabolism
Carbamaze-pine	Tegretol Carbatrol	Tonic-clonic Focal-onset	600–1800 mg/d (15–35 mg/kg, child); bid-qid	10–17 h	6–12 μg/mL	Ataxia Dizziness Diplopia Vertigo	Aplastic anemia Leukopenia Gastrointestinal irritation Hepatotoxicity Hyponatremia	Level decreased by enzyme-inducing drugs[a] Level increased by erythromy-cin, propoxy-phene, isonia-zid, cimetidine, fluoxetine
Valproic acid	Depakene Depakote	Tonic-clonic Absence Atypical absence Myoclonic Focal-onset	750–2000 mg/d (20–60 mg/kg); bid-qid	15 h	50–150 μg/mL	Ataxia Sedation Tremor	Hepatotoxicity Thrombocy-topenia Gastrointestinal irritation Weight gain Transient alopecia Hyperam-monemia	Level decreased by enzyme-inducing drugs[a]
Lamotrigine	Lamictal	Focal-onset Tonic-clonic Atypical absence Myoclonic Lennox-Gastaut syndrome	150–500 mg/d; bid	25 h 14 h (with enzyme-inducers) 59 h (with valproic acid)	Not established	Dizziness Diplopia Sedation Ataxia Headache	Skin rash Stevens-Johnson syndrome	Level decreased by enzyme-inducing drugs[a] Level increased by valproic acid
Ethosuxi-mide	Zarontin	Absence (petit mal)	750–1250 mg/d (20-40 mg/kg); qd-bid	60 h, adult 30 h, child	40–100 μg/mL	Ataxia Lethargy Headache	Gastrointestinal irritation Skin rash Bone marrow suppression	
Gabapentin	Neurontin	Focal-onset	900–2400 mg/d; tid-qid	5–9 h	Not established	Sedation Dizziness Ataxia Fatigue	Gastrointestinal irritation Weight gain Edema	No known significant interactions
Topiramate	Topamax	Focal-onset Tonic-clonic Lennox-Gastaut syndrome	200–400 mg/d; bid	20–30 h	Not established	Psychomotor slowing Sedation Speech or language problems Fatigue Paresthesias	Renal stones (avoid use with other carbonic anhydrase inhibitors) Weight loss	Level decreased by enzyme-inducing drugs[a]
Tiagabine	Gabitril	Focal-onset Tonic-clonic	32–56 mg/d; bid-qid	7–9 h	Not established	Confusion Sedation Depression Dizziness Speech or language problems Paresthesias Psychosis	Gastrointestinal irritation	Level decreased by enzyme-inducing drugs[a]

(continued)

TABLE 348-9—(Continued)

Generic Name	Trade Name	Principal Uses	Typical Dose; Dose Interval	Half-Life	Therapeutic Range	Adverse Effects		Drug Interactions
						Neurologic	Systemic	
Phenobarbital	Luminol	Tonic-clonic Focal-onset	60–180 mg/d (1–4 mg/kg, adult); (3–6 mg/kg, child); qd	90 h (70 h in children)	10–40 μg/mL	Sedation Ataxia Confusion Dizziness Decreased libido Depression	Skin rash	Level increased by valproic acid, phenytoin
Primidone	Mysoline	Tonic-clonic Focal-onset	750–1000 mg/d (10–25 mg/kg); bid-tid	Primidone, 8–15 h Phenobarbital, 90 h	Primidone, 4–12 μg/mL Phenobarbital, 10–40 μg/mL	Same as phenobarbital		
Clonazepam	Klonopin	Absence Atypical absence Myoclonic	1–12 mg/d (0.1–0.2 mg/kg); qd-tid	24–48 h	10–70 ng/mL	Ataxia Sedation Lethargy	Anorexia	Level decreased by enzyme-inducing drugs[a]
Felbamate	Felbatol	Focal-onset Lennox-Gastaut syndrome	2400–3600 mg/d, (45 mg/kg, child); tid-qid	16–22 h	Not established	Insomnia Dizziness Sedation Headache	Aplastic anemia Hepatic failure Weight loss Gastrointestinal irritation	Increases phenytoin, valproic acid, active carbamazepine metabolite
Levetiracetam	Keppra	Focal-onset	1000–3000 mg/d; bid	6–8 h	Not established	Sedation Fatigue Incoordination Psychosis	Anemia Leukopenia	None known
Zonisamide	Zonegran	Focal-onset	200–400 mg/d; qd-bid	50–68 h	Not established	Sedation Dizziness Confusion Headache Psychosis	Anorexia Renal stones	Level decreased by enzyme-inducing drugs[a]
Oxcarbazepine	Trileptal	Focal-onset	900–2400 mg/d (30–45 mg/kg, child); bid	10–17 h (for active metabolite)	Not established	Fatigue Ataxia Dizziness Diplopia Vertigo Headache	See carbamazepine	Level decreased by enzyme-inducing drugs[a] May increase phenytoin

[a] Phenytoin, carbamazepine, phenobarbital.

leptic drugs can eventually discontinue therapy. The following patient profile yields the greatest chance of remaining seizure-free after drug withdrawal: (1) complete medical control of seizures for 1 to 5 years; (2) single seizure type, either partial or generalized; (3) normal neurologic examination, including intelligence; and (4) normal EEG. The appropriate seizure-free interval is unknown and undoubtedly varies for different forms of epilepsy. However, it seems reasonable to attempt withdrawal of therapy after 2 years in a patient who meets all of the above criteria, is motivated to discontinue the medication, and clearly understands the potential risks and benefits. In most cases it is preferable to reduce the dose of the drug gradually over 2 to 3 months. Most recurrences occur in the first 3 months after discontinuing therapy, and patients should be advised to avoid potentially dangerous situations such as driving or swimming during this period.

TREATMENT OF REFRACTORY EPILEPSY Approximately one-third of patients with epilepsy do not respond to treatment with a single antiepileptic drug, and it becomes necessary to try a combination of drugs to control seizures. Patients who have focal epilepsy related to an underlying structural lesion or those with multiple seizure types and developmental delay are particularly likely to require multiple drugs. There are currently no clear guidelines for rational polypharmacy, although in theory a combination of drugs with different mechanisms of action

may be most useful. In most cases the initial combination therapy combines first-line drugs, i.e., carbamazepine, phenytoin, valproic acid, and lamotrigine. If these drugs are unsuccessful, then the addition of a newer drug such as topiramate or levetiracetam is indicated. Patients with myoclonic seizures resistant to valproic acid may benefit from the addition of clonazepam, and those with absence seizures may respond to a combination of valproic acid and ethosuximide. The same principles concerning the monitoring of therapeutic response, toxicity, and serum levels for monotherapy apply to polypharmacy, and potential drug interactions need to be recognized. If there is no improvement, a third drug can be added while the first two are maintained. If there is a response, the less effective or less well-tolerated of the first two drugs should be gradually withdrawn.

Surgical Treatment of Refractory Epilepsy Approximately 20% of patients with epilepsy are resistant to medical therapy despite efforts to find an effective combination of antiepileptic drugs. For some, surgery can be extremely effective in substantially reducing seizure frequency and even providing complete seizure control. Understanding the potential value of surgery is especially important when, at the time of diagnosis, a patient has an epilepsy syndrome that is considered likely to be drug-resistant. Rather than submitting the patient to years of unsuccessful medical therapy and the psychosocial trauma and increased mortality associated with ongoing seizures, the patient should have an efficient but relatively brief attempt at medical therapy and then be referred for surgical evaluation.

The most common surgical procedure for patients with temporal lobe epilepsy involves resection of the anteromedial temporal lobe (temporal lobectomy) or a more limited removal of the underlying hippocampus and amygdala (amygdalohippocampectomy). Focal seizures arising from extratemporal regions may be abolished by a focal neocortical resection with precise removal of an identified lesion (lesionectomy). When the cortical region cannot be removed, multiple subpial transection, which disrupts intracortical connections, is sometimes used to prevent seizure spread. Hemispherectomy or multilobar resection is useful for some patients with severe seizures due to hemispheric abnormalities such as hemimegaloencephaly or other dysplastic abnormalities, and corpus callosotomy has been shown to be effective for disabling tonic or atonic seizures, usually when they are part of a mixed-seizure syndrome (e.g., Lennox-Gastaut syndrome).

Presurgical evaluation is designed to identify the functional and structural basis of the patient's seizure disorder. Inpatient video-EEG monitoring is used to define the anatomic location of the seizure focus and to correlate the abnormal electrophysiologic activity with behavioral manifestations of the seizure. Routine scalp or scalp-sphenoidal recordings are usually sufficient for localization, and advances in neuroimaging have made the use of invasive electrophysiologic monitoring such as implanted depth electrodes or subdural electrodes less common. A high-resolution MRI scan is routinely used to identify structural lesions. Functional imaging studies such as SPECT and PET are adjunctive tests that may help verify the localization of an apparent epileptogenic region. Once the presumed location of the seizure onset is identified, additional studies, including neuropsychological testing and the intracarotid amobarbital test (Wada test) may be used to assess language and memory localization and to determine the possible functional consequences of surgical removal of the epileptogenic region. In some cases, the exact extent of the resection to be undertaken is determined by performing cortical mapping at the time of the surgical procedure, allowing for a tailored resection. This involves electrocorticographic recordings made with electrodes on the surface of the brain to identify the extent of epileptiform disturbances. If the region to be resected is within or near brain regions suspected of having sensorimotor or language function, electrical cortical stimulation mapping is performed in the awake patient to determine the function of cortical regions in question in order to avoid resection of so-called eloquent cortex, and thereby minimize postsurgical deficits.

Advances in presurgical evaluation and microsurgical techniques have led to a steady increase in the success of epilepsy surgery. Clinically significant complications of surgery are <5%, and the use of functional mapping procedures has markedly reduced the neurologic sequelae due to removal or sectioning of brain tissue. For example, about 70% of patients treated with temporal lobectomy will become seizure-free, and another 15 to 25% will have at least a 90% reduction in seizure frequency. Marked improvement is also usually seen in patients treated with hemispherectomy for catastrophic seizure disorders due to large hemispheric abnormalities. Postoperatively, patients generally need to remain on antiepileptic drug therapy, but the marked reduction of seizures following surgery can have a very beneficial effect on quality of life.

Vagus Nerve Stimulation (VNS)   VNS is a new treatment option for patients with medically refractory epilepsy who are not candidates for resective brain surgery. The procedure involves placement of a bipolar electrode on the midcervical portion of the left vagus nerve. The electrode is connected to a small, subcutaneous generator located in the infraclavicular region, and the generator is programmed to deliver intermittent electrical pulses to the vagus nerve. Unlike medications, there may be a delay between the initiation of VNS and the appearance of antiseizure effects. The precise mechanism of action of VNS is unknown, although experimental studies have shown that stimulation of vagal nuclei leads to widespread activation of cortical and subcortical pathways and an associated increased seizure threshold. In practice, the efficacy of VNS appears to be no greater than recently introduced anticonvulsant medications. Adverse effects of the surgery are rare, and stimulation-induced side effects, including transient hoarseness, cough, and dyspnea, are usually mild and well tolerated.

STATUS EPILEPTICUS   Status epilepticus refers to continuous seizures or repetitive, discrete seizures with impaired consciousness in the interictal period. The duration of seizure activity sufficient to meet the definition of status epilepticus has traditionally been specified as 15 to 30 min. However, a more practical definition is to consider status epilepticus as a situation in which the duration of seizures prompts the acute use of anticonvulsant therapy, typically when seizures last beyond 5 min.

Status epilepticus is an emergency and must be treated immediately, since cardiorespiratory dysfunction, hyperthermia, and metabolic derangements can develop as a consequence of prolonged seizures, and these can lead to irreversible neuronal injury. Furthermore, CNS injury can occur even when the patient is paralyzed with neuromuscular blockade but continues to have electrographic seizures. The most common causes of status epilepticus are anticonvulsant withdrawal or noncompliance, metabolic disturbances, drug toxicity, CNS infection, CNS tumors, refractory epilepsy, and head trauma.

Generalized status epilepticus is obvious when the patient is having overt convulsions. However, after 30 to 45 min of uninterrupted seizures, the signs may become increasingly subtle. Patients may have mild clonic movements of only the fingers, or fine, rapid movements of the eyes. There may be paroxysmal episodes of tachycardia, hypertension, and pupillary dilation. In such cases, the EEG may be the only method of establishing the diagnosis. Thus, if the patient stops having overt seizures, yet remains comatose, an EEG should be performed to rule out ongoing status epilepticus.

The first step in the management of a patient in status epilepticus is to attend to any acute cardiorespiratory problems or hyperthermia, perform a brief medical and neurologic examination, establish venous access, and send samples for laboratory studies to identify metabolic abnormalities. Anticonvulsant therapy should then begin without delay; a treatment approach is shown in Fig. 348-4.

BEYOND SEIZURES: OTHER MANAGEMENT ISSUES

Interictal Behavior   The adverse effects of epilepsy often go beyond the occurrence of clinical seizures, and the extent of these effects depends largely upon the etiology of the seizure disorder, the degree to which the seizures are controlled, and the presence of side effects from antiepileptic therapy. Many patients with epilepsy are completely normal between seizures and able to live highly successful and productive lives. In contrast, patients with seizures secondary to developmental abnormalities or acquired brain injury may have impaired cognitive function and other neurologic deficits. Frequent interictal EEG abnormalities have been shown to be associated with subtle dysfunction of memory and attention. Patients with many seizures, especially those emanating from the temporal lobe, often note an impairment of short-term memory that may progress over time.

Patients with epilepsy are at risk of developing a variety of psychiatric problems including depression, anxiety, and psychosis. This risk varies considerably depending on many factors, including the etiology, frequency, and severity of seizures and the patient's age and previous history. Depression occurs in ~20% of patients, and the incidence of suicide is higher in epileptic patients than in the general population. Depression should be treated through counseling or medication. The selective serotonin reuptake inhibitors typically have no effect on seizures, while the tricyclic antidepressants may lower the seizure threshold. Anxiety can appear as a manifestation of a seizure, and anxious or psychotic behavior can sometimes be observed as part of a postictal delirium. Postictal psychosis is a rare phenomenon that typically occurs after a period of increased seizure frequency. There is usually a brief lucid interval lasting up to a week, followed by days to weeks of agitated, psychotic behavior. The psychosis will usually resolve spontaneously but may require treatment with antipsychotic or anxiolytic medications.

There is ongoing controversy as to whether some patients with epilepsy (especially temporal lobe epilepsy) have a stereotypical "interictal personality." The predominant view is that the unusual or abnormal personality traits observed in such patients are, in most cases, not due to epilepsy but result from an underlying structural brain lesion, the effects of antiepileptic drugs, or psychosocial factors related to suffering from a chronic disease.

Mortality of Epilepsy Patients with epilepsy have a risk of death that is roughly two to three times greater than expected in a matched population without epilepsy. Most of the increased mortality is due to the underlying etiology of epilepsy, e.g., tumors or strokes in older adults. However, a significant number of patients die from accidents, status epilepticus, and a syndrome known as *sudden unexpected death in epileptic patients* (SUDEP), which usually affects young people with convulsive seizures and tends to occur at night. The cause of SUDEP is unknown; it may result from brainstem-mediated effects of seizures on cardiac rhythms or pulmonary function.

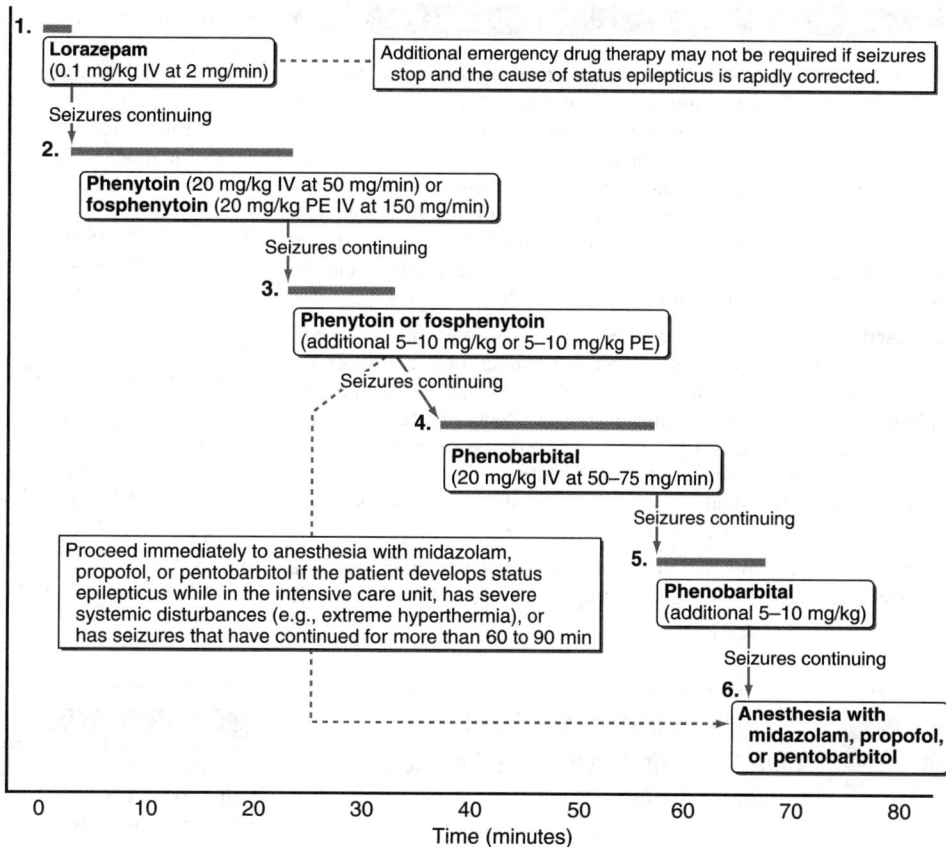

FIGURE 348-4 Pharmacologic treatment of generalized tonic-clonic status epilepticus in adults. IV, intravenous; PE, phenytoin equivalents. The horizontal bars indicate the approximate duration of drug infusions.

Psychosocial Issues There continues to be a cultural stigma about epilepsy, although it is slowly declining in societies with effective health education programs. Many patients with epilepsy harbor fears, such as the fear of becoming mentally retarded or dying during a seizure. These issues need to be carefully addressed by educating the patient about epilepsy and by ensuring that family members, teachers, fellow employees, and other associates are equally well informed. The Epilepsy Foundation of America (1-800-EFA-1000) is a patient advocacy organization and a useful source of educational material.

Employment and Driving Many patients with epilepsy face difficulty in obtaining or maintaining employment, even when their seizures are well controlled. Federal and state legislation is designed to prevent employers from discriminating against patients with epilepsy, and patients should be encouraged to understand and claim their legal rights. Patients in these circumstances also benefit greatly from the assistance of health providers who act as strong patient advocates.

Loss of driving privileges is one of the most disruptive social consequences of epilepsy. Physicians should be very clear about local regulations concerning driving and epilepsy, since the laws vary considerably among states and countries. In all cases, it is the physician's responsibility to warn patients of the danger imposed on themselves and others while driving if their seizures are uncontrolled (unless the seizures are not associated with impairment of consciousness or motor control). In general, most states allow patients to drive after a seizure-free interval (on or off medications) between 3 months and 2 years.

SPECIAL ISSUES RELATED TO WOMEN AND EPILEPSY

Catamenial Epilepsy Some women experience a marked increase in seizure frequency around the time of menses. This is thought to reflect either the effects of estrogen and progesterone on neuronal excitability or changes in antiepileptic drug levels due to altered protein binding. Acetazolamide (250 to 500 mg/d) may be effective as adjunctive therapy in some cases when started 7 to 10 days prior to the onset of menses and continued until bleeding stops. Some patients may benefit from increases in antiepileptic drug dosages during this time or from control of the menstrual cycle through the use of oral contraceptives. Natural progestins may be of benefit to a subset of women.

Pregnancy Most women with epilepsy who become pregnant will have an uncomplicated gestation and deliver a normal baby. However, epilepsy poses some important risks to a pregnancy. Seizure frequency during pregnancy will remain unchanged in ~50% of women, increase in 30%, and decrease in 20%. Changes in seizure frequency are attributed to endocrine effects on the CNS, variations in antiepileptic drug pharmacokinetics (such as acceleration of hepatic drug metabolism or effects on plasma protein binding), and changes in medication compliance. It is useful to see patients at frequent intervals during pregnancy and monitor serum antiepileptic drug levels. Measurement of the unbound drug concentrations may be useful if there is an increase in seizure frequency or worsening of side effects of antiepileptic drugs.

The overall incidence of fetal abnormalities in children born to mothers with epilepsy is 5 to 6%, compared to 2 to 3% in healthy women. Part of the higher incidence is due to teratogenic effects of antiepileptic drugs, and the risk increases with the number of medications used (e.g., 10% risk of malformations with three drugs). A syndrome comprising facial dysmorphism, cleft lip, cleft palate, cardiac defects, digital hypoplasia, and nail dysplasia was originally ascribed to phenytoin therapy, but it is now known to occur with other first-line antiepileptic drugs (i.e., valproic acid and carbamazepine) as well. Also, valproic acid and carbamazepine are associated with a 1 to 2% incidence of neural tube defects compared with a baseline of 0.5 to 1%. Little is currently known about the safety of newer drugs.

Since the potential harm of uncontrolled seizures on the mother and fetus is considered greater than the teratogenic effects of antiepileptic drugs, it is currently recommended that pregnant women be maintained on effective drug therapy. When possible, it seems prudent to have the patient on monotherapy at the lowest effective dose, especially during the first trimester. Patients should also take folate (1 to 4 mg/d), since the antifolate effects of anticonvulsants are thought to play a role in the development of neural tube defects, although the benefits of this treatment remain unproved in this setting.

Enzyme-inducing drugs such as phenytoin, phenobarbital, and primidone cause a transient and reversible deficiency of vitamin K–dependent clotting factors in ~50% of newborn infants. Although neonatal hemorrhage is uncommon, the mother should be treated with oral vitamin K (20 mg daily) in the last 2 weeks of pregnancy, and the infant should receive vitamin K (1 mg) at birth.

Contraception Special care should be taken when prescribing antiepileptic medications for women who are taking oral contraceptive agents. Drugs such as carbamazepine, phenytoin, phenobarbital, and topiramate can significantly antagonize the effects of oral contraceptives via enzyme induction and other mechanisms. Patients should be advised to consider alternative forms of contraception, or their contraceptive medications should be modified to offset the effects of the antiepileptic medications.

Breast Feeding Antiepileptic medications are excreted into breast milk to a variable degree. The ratio of drug concentration in breast milk relative to serum is ~80% for ethosuximide, 40 to 60% for phenobarbital, 40% for carbamazepine, 15% for phenytoin, and 5% for valproic acid. Given the overall benefits of breast feeding and the lack of evidence for long-term harm to the infant by being exposed to antiepileptic drugs, mothers with epilepsy can be encouraged to breast feed. This should be reconsidered, however, if there is any evidence of drug effects on the infant, such as lethargy or poor feeding.

ACKNOWLEDGMENT
The editors acknowledge the contributions of Michael J. Aminoff to this chapter in earlier editions of Harrison's.

FURTHER READING

CHANG B, LOWENSTEIN D: Mechanisms of disease: Epilepsy. N Engl J Med 349:1257, 2003

LOWENSTEIN DH, ALLDREDGE BK: Status epilepticus. N Engl J Med 338:970, 1998

NOEBELS J: Exploring new gene discoveries in idiopathic generalized epilepsy. Epilepsia 44(Suppl 2):16, 2003

PACK AM, MORRELL MJ: Treatment of women with epilepsy. Semin Neurol 22:289, 2002

WIEBE S et al: A randomized, controlled trial of surgery for temporal-lobe epilepsy. N Engl J Med 345:311, 2001

349 CEREBROVASCULAR DISEASES
Wade S. Smith, S. Claiborne Johnston, J. Donald Easton

Cerebrovascular diseases include some of the most common and devastating disorders: ischemic stroke, hemorrhagic stroke, and cerebrovascular anomalies such as intracranial aneurysms and arteriovenous malformations (AVMs). They cause ~200,000 deaths each year in the United States and are a major cause of disability. The incidence of cerebrovascular diseases increases with age, and the number of strokes is projected to increase as the elderly population grows, with a doubling in stroke deaths in the United States by 2030. Most cerebrovascular diseases are manifest by the abrupt onset of a focal neurologic deficit, as if the patient was "struck by the hand of God". A stroke, or cerebrovascular accident, is defined by this abrupt onset of a neurologic deficit that is attributable to a focal vascular cause. Thus, the definition of stroke is clinical, and laboratory studies including brain imaging are used to support the diagnosis. The clinical manifestations of stroke are highly variable because of the complex anatomy of the brain and its vasculature. *Cerebral ischemia* is caused by a reduction in blood flow that lasts longer than several seconds. Neurologic symptoms are manifest within seconds because neurons lack glycogen, so energy failure is rapid. When blood flow is quickly restored, brain tissue can recover fully and the patient's symptoms are only transient: this is called a *transient ischemic attack* (TIA). Typically the neurologic signs and symptoms of a TIA last for 5 to 15 min but, by definition, must last <24 h. If the cessation of flow lasts for more than a few minutes, *infarction* or death of brain tissue results. Stroke has occurred if the neurologic signs and symptoms last for >24 h. A generalized reduction in cerebral blood flow due to systemic hypotension (e.g., cardiac arrhythmia, myocardial infarction, or hemorrhagic shock) usually produces syncope (Chap. 20). If low cerebral blood flow persists for a longer duration, then infarction in the border zones between the major cerebral artery distributions may develop. In more severe instances, *global hypoxia-ischemia* causes widespread brain injury; the constellation of cognitive sequelae that ensue is called *hypoxic-ischemic encephalopathy* (Chap. 258). *Focal ischemia* or infarction, on the other hand, is usually caused by thrombosis of the cerebral vessels themselves or by emboli from a proximal arterial source or the heart. *Cerebral hemorrhage* produces neurologic symptoms by producing a mass effect on neural structures or from the toxic effects of blood itself.

APPROACH TO THE PATIENT

Patients with acute stroke often do not seek medical assistance on their own, both because they are rarely in pain, as well as because they may lose the appreciation that something is wrong (**anosagnosia**). It is often a family member or a bystander who calls for help. The rapid evaluation of patients is essential for use of time-sensitive treatments such as thrombolysis. Patients at risk for stroke should be counseled to call emergency medical services immediately if they experience the sudden onset of any of the following: loss of sensory and/or motor function on one side of the body (nearly 85% of ischemic stroke patients have hemiparesis); change in vision, gait, or ability to speak or understand; or if they experience a sudden, severe headache.

There are several common causes of sudden-onset neurologic symptoms that may mimic stroke. An adequate history from an observer that no convulsive activity occurred at the onset reasonably excludes seizure. Tumors may present with acute neurologic symptoms due to hemorrhage, seizure, or hydrocephalus. Surprisingly, migraine can mimic cerebral ischemia, even in patients without a significant migraine history. When it develops without head pain (*acephalgic migraine*), the diagnosis may remain elusive. Patients without any prior history of complicated migraine may develop acephalgic migraine even after age 65. A sensory disturbance is often prominent, and the sensory deficit, as well as any motor deficits, tends to migrate slowly across a limb over minutes. The diagnosis of migraine becomes more secure as the cortical disturbance begins to cross vascular boundaries or if typical visual symptoms are present, such as scintillating scotomata (Chap. 14). At times it may be difficult to make the diagnosis until multiple episodes have occurred leaving behind no residual stroke or magnetic resonance imaging (MRI) changes consistent with stroke. Classically, metabolic encephalopathies produce fluctuating mental status without focal neurologic findings. However, in the setting of prior stroke or brain injury, a patient with fever or sepsis may manifest hemiparesis, which clears rapidly when the infection is remedied. The metabolic process serves to "unmask" a prior deficit. Once the diagnosis of stroke is made, a brain imaging study is necessary to determine if the cause of stroke is ischemia or hemorrhage (Fig. 349-1). Computed tomography (CT) imaging of the brain is the standard imaging modality to detect the presence or absence of intracranial hemorrhage (see "Imaging Studies," below). If the stroke is ischemic, administration of tissue plasminogen activator

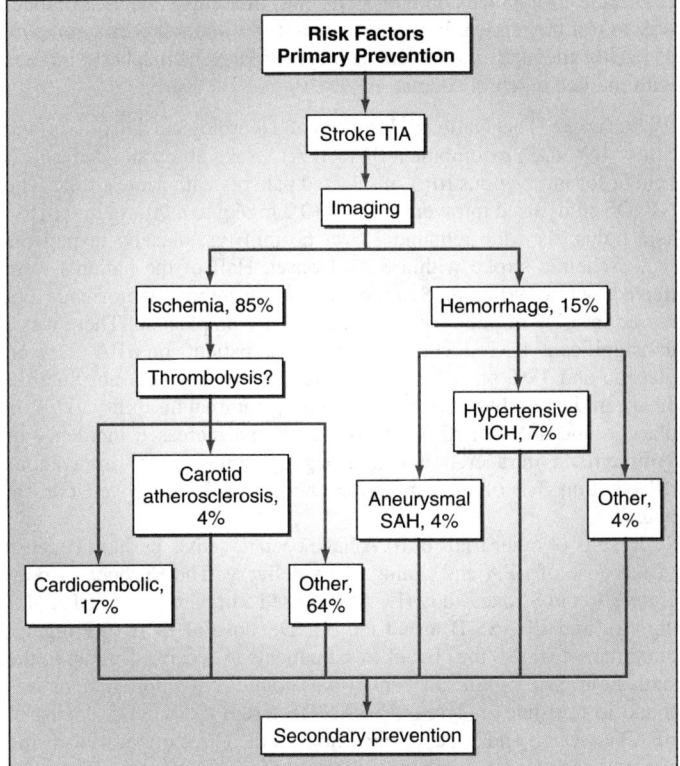

FIGURE 349-1 *Schematic approach to acute stroke. Numbers are percentage of all strokes. Abbreviations: TIA, transient ischemic attack; SAH, subarachnoid hemorrhage; ICH, intracerebral hemorrhage.*

(tPA) may be beneficial in restoring cerebral perfusion (see "Treatment" below). Medical management to reduce the risk of complications becomes the next priority, followed by plans for secondary prevention. For ischemic stroke, several strategies can reduce the risk of subsequent stroke in all patients, while other strategies are effective for patients with specific causes of stroke such as cardiac embolus and carotid atherosclerosis. For hemorrhagic stroke, aneurysmal subarachnoid hemorrhage (SAH) is the most important treatable condition followed by hypertensive intracranial hemorrhage.

ISCHEMIC STROKE

PATHOPHYSIOLOGY OF ISCHEMIC STROKE Acute occlusion of an intracranial vessel causes reduction in blood flow to the brain region it supplies. The magnitude of flow reduction is a function of collateral blood flow and this depends on individual vascular anatomy and the site of occlusion. A fall in cerebral blood flow to zero causes death of brain tissue within 4 to 10 min; values <16 to 18 mL/100 g tissue per min cause infarction within an hour; and values <20 mL/100 g tissue per min cause ischemia without infarction unless prolonged for several hours or days. If blood flow is restored prior to a significant amount of cell death, the patient may experience only transient symptoms, i.e., a TIA. Tissue surrounding the core region of infarction is ischemic but reversibly dysfunctional and is referred to as the *ischemic penumbra*. The penumbra may be imaged by using perfusion-diffusion imaging with MRI (see below and Fig. 349-13). The ischemic penumbra will eventually infarct if no change in flow occurs, and hence saving the ischemic penumbra

is the goal of thrombolytic therapy and newer therapies under investigation.

The complex processes that are involved in focal cerebral infarction are summarized in Fig. 349-2. Cellular death occurs via two distinct pathways: (1) a necrotic pathway in which cellular cytoskeletal breakdown is rapid, due principally to energy failure of the cell; and (2) an apoptotic pathway in which cells become programmed to die. Ischemia produces necrosis by starving neurons of glucose which in turn results in failure of mitochondria to produce ATP. Without ATP, membrane ion pumps stop functioning and neurons depolarize, allowing intracellular calcium to rise. Cellular depolarization also causes glutamate release from synaptic terminals; excess extracellular glutamate produces neurotoxicity by agonizing postsynaptic glutamate receptors that increase neuronal calcium influx. Free radicals are produced by membrane lipid degradation and mitochondrial dysfunction. Free radicals cause catalytic destruction of membranes and likely damage other vital functions of cells. Lesser degrees of ischemia, as are seen within the ischemic penumbra, favor apoptotic cellular death causing cells to die days to weeks later. There are no clinically proven strategies that alter these ischemic cascades despite extensive clinical study. It is clear, however, that fever dramatically worsens ischemia, as does hyperglycemia [glucose > 11.1 to 16.7 mmol/L (200 to 300 mg/dL)], so it is reasonable to suppress fever and prevent hyperglycemia as much as possible. Hypothermia and other neuroprotective strategies are subjects of continuing clinical research.

℞ TREATMENT

Acute Ischemic Stroke After the clinical diagnosis of stroke is made, an orderly process of evaluation and treatment should follow (Table 349-1). The first goal is to prevent or reverse brain injury. After initial stabilization, an emergency noncontrast head CT scan should be performed to differentiate ischemic from hemorrhagic stroke; there are no reliable clinical findings that conclusively separate ischemia from hemorrhage, although a more depressed level of consciousness and higher initial blood pressure favor hemorrhage, and a deficit that remits suggests ischemia. Treatments designed to reverse or lessen the amount of tissue infarction fall within five categories: (1) medical support, (2) thrombolysis, (3) anticoagulation, (4) antiplatelet agents, and (5) neuroprotection.

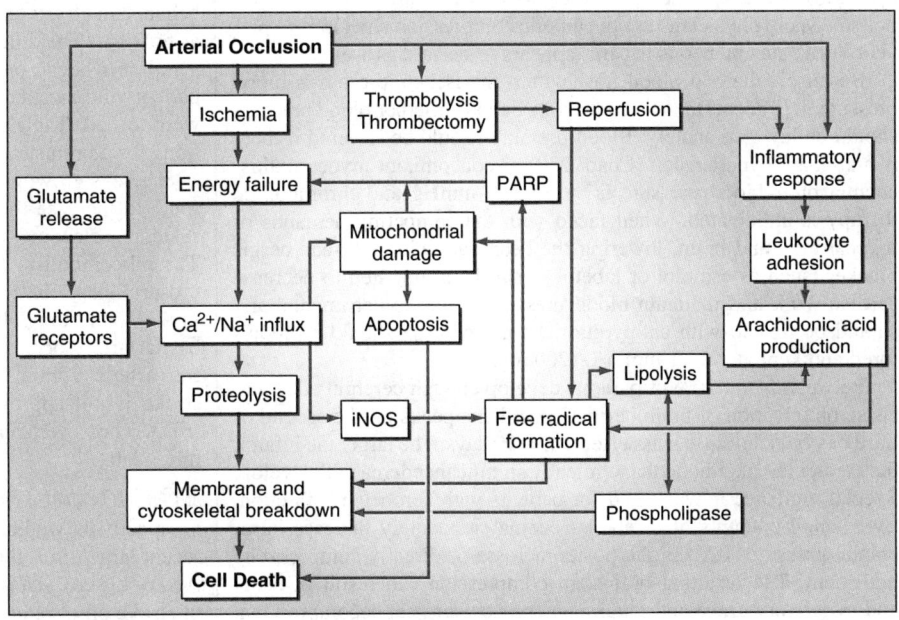

FIGURE 349-2 *Major steps in the cascade of cerebral ischemia. See text for details. Abbreviations: PARP, poly-A ribose polymerase; iNOS, inducible nitric oxide synthase.*

TABLE 349-1 *Clinical Management of Acute Stroke*

New onset of neurologic deficit: Stroke or TIA?	Differential diagnosis of new focal deficit 　Stroke or TIA 　Seizure with postictal Todd's paresis 　Tumor 　Migraine 　Metabolic encephalopathy 　　Fever/infection and old stroke 　　Hyperglycemia 　　Hypercalcemia 　　Hepatic encephalopathy
Initial assessment and management	ABCs, serum glucose Noncontrast head CT 　Hemorrhage 　　Medical and surgical management 　Tumor or other CNS process 　　Treat as indicated 　Normal or hypodense area consistent with acute ischemic stroke 　　Consider thrombolysis, aspirin 　　Maintain blood pressure and hydrate 　　Admit patient to appropriate level of care depending on concomitant medical problems and airway
Subsequent hospital management	Establish cause of stroke and risk factors Plan for secondary prophylaxis (drugs, risk factor modifications) Obtain physical, occupational, and speech therapy consultation and social work as appropriate Provide nutrition Plan for discharge, including prescriptions for risk factor reduction, including when to institute antihypertensive treatment, and antithrombotic medication prophylaxis

Note: ABCs, airway management, breathing, cardiac status; CNS, central nervous system; CT, computed tomography; TIA, transient ischemic attack.

MEDICAL SUPPORT When cerebral infarction occurs, the immediate goal is to optimize cerebral perfusion in the surrounding ischemic penumbra. Attention is also directed toward preventing the common complications of bedridden patients—infections (pneumonia, urinary tract, and skin) and deep venous thrombosis (DVT) with pulmonary embolism. Many physicians use pneumatic compression stockings to prevent DVT; subcutaneous heparin appears to be safe as well.

Because collateral blood flow within the ischemic brain is blood pressure dependent, there is controversy about whether blood pressure should be lowered acutely. Blood pressure should be lowered if there is malignant hypertension (Chap. 230) or concomitant myocardial ischemia or if blood pressure is >185/110 mmHg and thrombolytic therapy is anticipated. When faced with the competing demands of myocardium and brain, lowering the heart rate with a β_1-adrenergic blocker (such as esmolol or labetolol) can be a first step to decrease cardiac work and maintain blood pressure. Fever is detrimental and should be treated with antipyretics. Serum glucose should be monitored and kept at <11.1 mmol/L (200 mg/dL).

Between 5 and 10% of patients develop enough cerebral edema to cause obtundation or brain herniation. Edema peaks on the second or third day but can cause mass effect for ~10 days. The larger the infarct, the greater the likelihood that clinically significant edema will develop. Special vigilance is warranted for patients with cerebellar infarction. Even small amounts of cerebellar edema can acutely increase intracranial pressure (ICP) in the posterior fossa or directly compress the brainstem. The resulting brainstem compression can result in coma and respiratory arrest and require emergency surgical decompression. Water restriction and intravenous mannitol may be used to raise the serum osmolarity, but hypovolemia should be avoided as this may

contribute to hypotension and worsening infarction. Trials are under way to test the clinical benefits of craniotomy and temporary removal of part of the skull (hemicraniectomy) for large hemispheric infarcts with marked cerebral edema.

THROMBOLYSIS The National Institute of Neurological Disorders and Stroke (NINDS) recombinant tPA (rtPA) Stroke Study showed a clear benefit for intravenous rtPA in selected patients with acute stroke. The NINDS study used intravenous rtPA (0.9 mg/kg to a 90-mg max; 10% as a bolus, then the remainder over 60 min) vs. placebo in patients with ischemic stroke within 3 h of onset. Half of the patients were treated within 90 min. Symptomatic intracerebral hemorrhage occurred in 6.4% of patients on rtPA and 0.6% on placebo. There was a nonsignificant 4% reduction in mortality in patients on rtPA (21% on placebo and 17% on rtPA); there was a significant 12% absolute increase in the number of patients with only minimal disability (32% on placebo and 44% on rtPA.) Thus, despite an increased incidence of symptomatic intracerebral hemorrhage, treatment with intravenous rtPA within 3 h of the onset of ischemic stroke improved clinical outcome.

Results of other trials of rtPA have been negative, perhaps because of the dose of rtPA and timing of its delivery. The European Cooperative Acute Stroke Study (ECASS) I used a higher dose of rtPA (1.2 mg/kg), and ECASS-II tested the NINDS dose of rtPA (0.9 mg/kg; maximum dose, 90 mg) but allowed patients to receive drug up to the sixth hour. No significant benefit was found, but improvement was found in post hoc analyses. ATLANTIS tested the NINDS dosing of rtPA between 3 and 5 h and found no benefit. Three major trials using streptokinase reported increased mortality for patients receiving streptokinase. Early administration of the fibrinolytic agent ancrod appears to improve outcomes for patients with acute ischemic stroke; although the drug has not been approved for clinical use, its efficacy provides further evidence that thrombolytics should have a role in treatment of acute ischemic stroke.

Because of the marked differences in trial design, including drug and dose used, time to thrombolysis, and severity of stroke, the precise efficacy of intravenous thrombolytics for acute ischemic stroke remains unclear. The risk of intracranial hemorrhage appears to rise with larger strokes, longer times from onset of symptoms, and higher doses of rtPA administered. The established dose of 0.9 mg/kg administered intravenously within 3 h of stroke onset appears safe. Many hospitals have developed expert stroke teams to facilitate this treatment. The drug is now approved in the United States, Canada, and Europe for acute stroke when given within 3 h from the time the stroke symptoms began, and efforts should be made to give it as early in this 3-h window as possible. The time of stroke onset is defined as the time the patient's symptoms began or the time the patient was last seen as normal. A patient who awakens with stroke has the onset defined as when they went to bed. Table 349-2 summarizes eligibility criteria and instructions for administration of rtPA.

There is growing interest in using thrombolytics via an intraarterial route to increase the concentration of drug at the clot and minimize systemic bleeding complications. The Prolyse in Acute Cerebral Thromboembolism (PROACT) II trial found benefit for intraarterial pro-urokinase for acute middle cerebral artery (MCA) occlusions up to the sixth hour following onset of stroke. Intraarterial treatment of basilar artery occlusions may also be beneficial for selected patients. Intraarterial administration of a thrombolytic agent for acute ischemic stroke is not approved by the U.S. Food and Drug Administration (FDA); however, many stroke centers offer this treatment based on these data.

ANTIPLATELET AGENTS Aspirin is the only antiplatelet agent that has been prospectively studied for the treatment of acute ischemic stroke. The recent large trials, the International Stroke Trial (IST) and the Chinese Acute Stroke Trial (CAST), found that the use of aspirin within 48 h of stroke onset reduced both stroke recurrence risk and mortality minimally. Among 19,435 patients in IST, those allocated to aspirin, 300 mg/d, had slightly fewer deaths within 14 days (9.0 vs. 9.4%), signif-

TABLE 349-2 *Administration of Intravenous Recombinant Tissue Plasminogen Activator (rtPA) for Acute Ischemic Stroke*[a]

Indication	Contraindication
Clinical diagnosis of stroke	Sustained BP > 185/110 despite
Onset of symptoms to time of	treatment
drug administration ≤3 h	Platelets < 100,000;
CT scan showing no hemorrhage	HCT < 25%; glucose < 50
or edema of >⅓ of the MCA	or > 400 mg/dL
territory	Use of heparin within 48 h and
Age ≥18 years	prolonged PTT, or elevated INR
Consent by patient or surrogate	Rapidly improving symptoms
	Prior stroke or head injury within 3
	months; prior intracranial
	hemorrhage
	Major surgery in preceding 14 days
	Minor stroke symptoms
	Gastrointestinal bleeding in
	preceding 21 days
	Recent myocardial infarction
	Coma or stupor

Administration of rtPA

Intravenous access with two peripheral IV lines (avoid arterial or central line placement)

Review eligibility for rtPA

Administer 0.9 mg/kg intravenously (maximum 90 mg) IV as 10% of total dose by bolus, followed by remainder of total dose over 1 h

Frequent cuff blood pressure monitoring

No other antithrombotic treatment for 24 h

For decline in neurologic status or uncontrolled blood pressure, stop infusion, give cryoprecipitate, and reimage brain emergently

Avoid urethral catheterization for ≥2 h

[a] See Activase (tissue plasminogen activator) package insert for complete list of contraindications and dosing.

Note: BP, blood pressure; CT, computed tomography; HCT, hematocrit; INR, international normalized ratio; MCA, middle cerebral artery; PTT, partial thromboplastin time.

icantly fewer recurrent ischemic strokes (2.8 vs. 3.9%), no excess of hemorrhagic strokes (0.9 vs. 0.8%), and a trend towards a reduction in death or dependence at 6 months (61.2 vs. 63.5%). In CAST, 21,106 patients with ischemic stroke received 160 mg/d of aspirin or a placebo for up to 4 weeks. There were very small reductions in the aspirin group in early mortality (3.3 vs. 3.9%), recurrent ischemic strokes (1.6 vs. 2.1%), and dependency at discharge or death (30.5 vs. 31.6%). These trials demonstrate that the use of aspirin in the treatment of acute ischemic stroke is safe and produces a small net benefit. For every 1000 acute strokes treated with aspirin, about 9 deaths or nonfatal stroke recurrences will be prevented in the first few weeks and ~13 fewer patients will be dead or dependent at 6 months.

Agents that act at the glycoprotein IIb/IIIa receptor are undergoing clinical trials in acute stroke treatment. Early results show that intravenous abciximab can be used safely within 6 h of stroke onset and suggest that it may be effective.

Anticoagulation The role of anticoagulation in atherothrombotic cerebral ischemia is uncertain. Several trials have investigated antiplatelet versus anticoagulant medications given within 12 to 24 h of the initial event. The U.S. Trial of Organon 10172 in Acute Stroke Treatment (TOAST), an investigational low-molecular-weight heparin, failed to show any benefit over aspirin. Use of subcutaneous unfractionated heparin versus aspirin was tested in IST. Heparin given subcutaneously afforded no additional benefit over aspirin and increased bleeding rates. Several trials of low-molecular-weight heparins have also shown no consistent benefit in acute ischemic stroke. Therefore, trials do not support the use of heparin or other anticoagulants for patients with atherothrombotic stroke.

In spite of the absence of evidence, heparin is still used frequently to treat stroke and TIA, primarily based on beliefs about its impact on pathophysiology. Theoretically, heparin may prevent propagation of clot within a thrombosed vessel or may prevent more emboli from occurring. Heparin is widely used for crescendo TIAs (TIAs that increase in frequency), despite the absence of data from controlled studies regarding this indication. In ~20% of patients with acute stroke,

deficits will progress over several hours to 1 to 2 days. Some physicians heparinize all patients with recent mild ischemic stroke in order to prevent some of this worsening, but this practice is discouraged. The bleeding complication rate for 7 days of heparin is about 10%, with a serious bleed rate of ~2%. Clearly the value of this approach must be clarified. Heparinization is generally accomplished by beginning an infusion without bolus and is monitored to maintain the activated partial thromboplastin time (PTT) at approximately twice normal.

Neuroprotection Neuroprotection is the concept of providing a treatment that prolongs the brain's tolerance to ischemia. Hypothermia is a powerful neuroprotective treatment in patients with cardiac arrest, but it has not been adequately studied in patients with stroke. Drugs that block the excitatory amino acid pathways have been shown to protect neurons and glia in animals, but despite multiple clinical trials, they have not yet been proven to be beneficial in humans. Even so, interest in neuroprotection continues because of the potential for agents to have limited risk, even when administered in the pre-hospital setting or in conjunction with thrombolytic agents.

Stroke Centers and Rehabilitation Patient care in comprehensive stroke units followed by rehabilitation services improves neurologic outcomes and reduces mortality. Use of clinical pathways and staff dedicated to the stroke patient can improve care. Stroke teams that provide emergency 24-h evaluation of acute stroke patients for acute medical management and consideration of thrombolysis are important.

Proper rehabilitation of the stroke patient includes early physical, occupational, and speech therapy. It is directed toward educating the patient and family about the patient's neurologic deficit, preventing the complications of immobility (e.g., pneumonia, DVT and pulmonary embolism, pressure sores of the skin, and muscle contractures), and providing encouragement and instruction in overcoming the deficit. The goal of rehabilitation is to return the patient to home and to maximize recovery by providing a safe, progressive regimen suited to the individual patient. Additionally, the use of restraint therapy has been shown to improve hemiparesis following stroke, even years following the stroke, suggesting that physical therapy can recruit unused neural pathways. This finding suggests that the human nervous system is more adaptable than originally thought and has stimulated active research into physical and pharmacologic strategies that can enhance long-term neural recovery.

ETIOLOGY OF ISCHEMIC STROKE (Table 349-3) Although the initial management of acute ischemic stroke often does not depend on the etiology, establishing a cause is essential in reducing the risk of recurrence. The clinical presentation and examination findings often establish the cause of stroke or narrow the possibilities to a few. Judicious use of laboratory testing and imaging studies completes the initial evaluation. Nevertheless, nearly 30% of strokes remain unexplained despite extensive evaluation.

Clinical examination should be focused on the peripheral and cervical vascular system (carotid auscultation for bruits, blood pressure, and pressure comparison between arms), the heart (dysrhythmia, murmurs), extremities (peripheral emboli), and retina [effects of hypertension and cholesterol emboli (Hollenhorst plaques)]. A complete neurologic examination is performed to localize the site of stroke. An imaging study of the brain is nearly always performed and is required for patients being considered for thrombolysis. A chest x-ray, electrocardiogram (ECG), urinalysis, complete blood count, erythrocyte sedimentation rate, serum electrolytes, blood urea nitrogen, creatinine, blood sugar, serologic test for syphilis, serum lipid profile, prothrombin time, and PTT are often useful and should be considered in all patients. An ECG may demonstrate conduction abnormalities and arrhythmias or reveal evidence of recent myocardial infarction (MI).

Cardioembolic Stroke Cardioembolism is responsible for ~20% of all ischemic strokes. Stroke caused by heart disease is primarily due to embolism of thrombotic material forming on the atrial or ventricular

TABLE 349-3 *Causes of Ischemic Stroke*

Common Causes	Uncommon Causes
Thrombosis	Hypercoagulable disorders
Lacunar stroke (small	Protein C deficiency
vessel)	Protein S deficiency
Large vessel thrombosis	Antithrombin III deficiency
Dehydration	Antiphospholipid syndrome
Embolic occlusion	Factor V Leiden mutation[a]
Artery-to-artery	Prothrombin G20210 mutation[a]
Carotid bifurcation	Systemic malignancy
Aortic arch	Sickle cell anemia
Arterial dissection	β-Thalassemia
Cardioembolic	Polycythemia vera
Atrial fibrillation	Systemic lupus erythematosus
Mural thrombus	Homocysteinemia
Myocardial infarction	Thrombotic thrombocytopenic
Dilated cardiomyopathy	purpura
Valvular lesions	Disseminated intravascular
Mitral stenosis	coagulation
Mechanical valve	Dysproteinemias
Bacterial endocarditis	Nephrotic syndrome
Paradoxical embolus	Inflammatory bowel disease
Atrial septal defect	Oral contraceptives
Patent foramen ovale	Venous sinus thrombosis[b]
Atrial septal aneurysm	Fibromuscular dysplasia
Spontaneous echo	Vasculitis
contrast	Systemic vasculitis (PAN, Wegner's,
	Takayasu's, giant cell arteritis)
	Primary CNS vasculitis
	Meningitis (syphilis, tuberculosis,
	fungal, bacterial, zoster
	Cardiogenic
	Mitral valve calcification
	Atrial myxoma
	Intracardiac tumor
	Marantic endocarditis
	Libman-Sacks endocarditis
	Subarachnoid hemorrhage vasospasm
	Drugs: cocaine, amphetamine
	Moyamoya disease
	Eclampsia

[a] Chiefly cause venous sinus thrombosis.
[b] May be associated with any hypercoagulable disorder.
Note: CNS, central nervous system; PAN, polyarteritis nodosa.

wall or the left heart valves. These thrombi then detach and embolize into the arterial circulation. The thrombus may fragment or lyse quickly, producing only TIA. Alternatively, the arterial occlusion may last longer, producing stroke. Embolic strokes tend to be sudden in onset, with maximum neurologic deficit at once. With reperfusion following more prolonged ischemia, petechial hemorrhage can occur within the ischemic territory. This is usually of no clinical significance and should be distinguished from frank intracranial hemorrhage into a region of ischemic stroke where the mass effect from the hemorrhage can cause a decline in neurologic function.

Emboli from the heart most often lodge in the MCA, the posterior cerebral artery (PCA), or one of their branches; infrequently, the anterior cerebral artery (ACA) territory is involved. Emboli large enough to occlude the stem of the MCA (3 to 4 mm) lead to large infarcts that involve both deep gray and white matter and some portions of the cortical surface and its underlying white matter. A smaller embolus may occlude a small cortical or penetrating arterial branch. The location and size of an infarct within a vascular territory depend on the extent of the collateral circulation.

The most significant causes of cardioembolic stroke in most of the world are nonrheumatic (often called nonvalvular) atrial fibrillation, MI, prosthetic valves, rheumatic heart disease, and ischemic cardiomyopathy (Table 349-3). Cardiac disorders causing brain embolism are discussed in the respective chapters on heart diseases. A few pertinent aspects are highlighted here.

Nonrheumatic atrial fibrillation is the most common cause of cerebral embolism overall. The presumed stroke mechanism is thrombus formation in the fibrillating atrium or atrial appendage, with subsequent embolization. Patients with atrial fibrillation have an average annual risk of stroke of ~5%. The risk varies according to the presence of certain risk factors, including older age, hypertension, poor left ventricular function, prior cardioembolism, diabetes, and thyrotoxicosis. Patients younger than 60 with none of these risk factors have an annual risk for stroke of ~0.5%, while those with most of the factors have a rate of ~15% per year. Left atrial enlargement and congestive heart failure are additional risk factors for formation of atrial thrombi. Rheumatic heart disease usually causes ischemic stroke when there is prominent mitral stenosis or atrial fibrillation. Guidelines for the use of warfarin and aspirin for secondary prevention are based on risk factors (Table 349-4).

Recent MI may be a source of emboli, especially when transmural and involving the anteroapical ventricular wall, and prophylactic anticoagulation following MI has been shown to reduce stroke risk. Mitral valve prolapse is not usually a source of emboli unless the prolapse is severe.

Paradoxical embolization occurs when venous thrombi migrate to the arterial circulation, usually via a patent foramen ovale or atrial septal defect. Bubble-contrast echocardiography (intravenous injection of agitated saline coupled with either transthoracic or transesophageal echocardiography) can demonstrate a cardiac right-to-left shunt, revealing the conduit for paradoxical embolization. Alternatively, a right-to-left shunt is implied if immediately following intravenous injection of agitated saline, high-intensity transients are observed during transcranial Doppler insonation of the MCA. Both techniques are highly sensitive for detection of right-to-left shunts. Besides venous clot, fat and tumor emboli, bacterial endocarditis, intravenous air, and amniotic fluid emboli associated with delivery may occasionally be responsible for paradoxical embolization. The importance of right-to-left shunt as a cause of stroke is debated, particularly because such shunts occur in ~15% of the general population. Some studies have suggested that the risk is only elevated in the presence of a coexisting atrial septal aneurysm. The presence of a venous source of embolus, most commonly a deep venous thrombus, may provide confirmation of the importance of a right-to-left shunt in a particular case.

Bacterial endocarditis can cause valvular vegetations that can give rise to multiple septic emboli (Chap. 109). The appearance of multifocal symptoms and signs in a patient with stroke makes bacterial endocarditis more likely. Infarcts of microscopic size occur, and large septic infarcts may evolve into brain abscesses or cause hemorrhage into the infarct, which generally precludes use of anticoagulation or thrombolytics. Mycotic aneurysms caused by septic emboli give rise to SAH or intracerebral hemorrhage.

Artery-to-Artery Embolic Stroke Thrombus formation on atherosclerotic plaques may embolize to intracranial arteries producing an artery-to-artery embolic stroke. Alternatively, a diseased vessel may acutely thrombose; the resulting blockage causes stroke by producing ischemia within the region of brain it supplied. Unlike the myocardial vessels, artery-to-artery embolism appears to be the dominant vascular mech-

TABLE 349-4 *Consensus Recommendation for Antithrombotic Prophylaxis in Atrial Fibrillation*

Age	Risk Factors[a]	Recommendation
Age ≤65	≥1	Warfarin INR 2–3
	0	Aspirin or no treatment
Age 65–75	≥1	Warfarin INR 2–3
	0	Warfarin INR 2–3 or aspirin
Age >75		Warfarin INR 2–3

[a] Risk factors include previous transient ischemic attack or stroke, hypertension, heart failure, diabetes, clinical coronary artery disease, mitral stenosis, prosthetic heart valves, or thyrotoxicosis.
Source: Modified from GW Albers et al: Antithrombotic therapy in atrial fibrillation. Chest 119:194S, 2001; with permission.

anism causing ischemia rather than thrombosis. The most common source of embolism is the carotid bifurcation, but any diseased vessel may be a source, including the aortic arch and common carotid, internal carotid, vertebral, and basilar arteries. Carotid bifurcation atherosclerosis is the most common source of artery-to-artery embolus, and specific treatments have proven efficacy in reducing risk.

CAROTID ATHEROSCLEROSIS Atherosclerosis within the carotid artery occurs most frequently within the common carotid bifurcation and proximal internal carotid artery. Additionally, the carotid siphon (portion within the cavernous sinus) is also vulnerable to atherosclerosis. Male gender, older age, smoking,

TABLE 349-5 *Risk Factors for Stroke*

Risk Factor	Relative Risk	Relative Risk Reduction with Treatment	Number Needed to Treat[a]	
			Primary Prevention	Secondary Prevention
Hypertension	2–5	38%	100–300	50–100
Atrial fibrillation	1.8–2.9	68% warfarin, 21% aspirin	20–83	13
Diabetes	1.8–6	No proven effect		
Smoking	1.8	50% at 1 year, baseline risk at 5 years post cessation		
Hyperlipidemia	1.8–2.6	10–29%		—
Asymptomatic carotid stenosis	2.0	53%	85	N/A
Symptomatic carotid stenosis (70–99%)		65% at 2 years	N/A	12
Symptomatic carotid stenosis (50–69%)		29% at 5 years	N/A	77

[a] Number needed to treat to prevent one stroke annually. Prevention of other cardiovascular outcomes is not considered here.
Note: N/A, not applicable.

hypertension, diabetes, and hypercholesterolemia are risk factors for carotid disease, as they are for stroke in general (Table 349-5). Carotid atherosclerosis produces an estimated 5% of ischemic stroke, and the risk of stroke rises the higher the degree of carotid narrowing. →*For further discussion of the pathogenesis of atherosclerosis, see Chap. 224.*

Carotid disease can be classified by whether the stenosis is symptomatic or asymptomatic and by the degree of stenosis (percent narrowing of the narrowest segment compared to a more distal internal carotid segment). Symptomatic carotid disease implies that the patient has experienced a stroke or TIA within the vascular distribution of the artery, and it is associated with a greater risk of subsequent stroke than asymptomatic stenosis, in which the patient is symptom free and the stenosis is detected through screening. Greater degrees of arterial narrowing are generally associated with a greater risk of stroke.

℞ TREATMENT

Surgical Therapy Surgery for atherosclerotic occlusive disease is largely limited to *carotid endarterectomy* for plaques located at the origin of the internal carotid artery in the neck.

Symptomatic carotid stenosis was studied in the North American Symptomatic Carotid Endarterectomy Trial (NASCET) and the European Carotid Surgery Trial (ECST). Both showed a substantial benefit for surgery in patients with a stenosis of >70%. In NASCET, the average cumulative ipsilateral stroke risk at 2 years was 26% for patients treated medically and 9% for those receiving the same medical treatment plus a carotid endarterectomy. This 17% *absolute* reduction in the surgical group is a 65% *relative* risk reduction favoring surgery (Table 349-5). NASCET also showed a significant benefit for patients with 50 to 70% stenosis, although less robust. ECST found harm for patients with stenosis in the 0 to 30% range treated surgically.

A patient's risk of stroke and possible benefit from surgery are related to the presence of retinal versus hemispheric symptoms, degree of arterial stenosis, extent of associated medical conditions, institutional surgical morbidity and mortality, and other factors. A patient with multiple atherosclerosis risk factors, symptomatic hemispheric ischemia, high-grade stenosis in the appropriate internal carotid artery, and an institutional perioperative morbidity and mortality rate of ≤6% generally should undergo carotid endarterectomy. If the perioperative stroke rate is >6% for any particular surgeon, however, the benefits of carotid endarterectomy are questionable.

The indications for surgical treatment of *asymptomatic carotid disease* have been clarified by the results of the Asymptomatic Carotid Atherosclerosis Study (ACAS), which randomized patients with ≥60% stenosis to medical treatment with aspirin or the same medical treatment plus carotid endarterectomy. The surgical group had a risk over 5 years for ipsilateral stroke (and any perioperative stroke or death) of 5.1%, compared to a risk in the medical group of 11%. While

this demonstrates a 53% *relative* risk reduction, the *absolute* risk reduction is only 5.9% over 5 years, or 1.2% annually (Table 349-5). The perioperative complication rate was higher in women, so they received only a 17% relative risk reduction over 5 years. Nearly half of the strokes in the surgery group were caused by preoperative angiograms.

The natural history of asymptomatic stenosis is an ~2% per year stroke rate, while symptomatic patients experience a 13% per year risk of stroke. Whether to recommend carotid revascularization for an asymptomatic patient remains controversial and depends on many factors including patient preference, age, and comorbidities. Medical therapy for reduction of atherosclerosis risk factors, including statins and aspirin, is generally recommended for patients with asymptomatic carotid stenosis. As with atrial fibrillation, it is imperative to counsel the patient about TIAs so their therapy can be revised if they become symptomatic.

Balloon angioplasty coupled with stenting is being used with increasing frequency to open stenotic carotid arteries and maintain their patency. This method has not yet been compared prospectively with endarterectomy, except in high-risk patients where one small trial suggested less morbidity with stenting compared with endarterectomy. Concern exists about distal embolization of plaque during vessel dilation, and many new devices designed to prevent distal embolization are undergoing clinical trials. Extracranial to intracranial (EC-IC) bypass surgery has been proven ineffective for atherosclerotic stenoses that are inaccessible to conventional carotid endarterectomy. However, using more functional techniques [positron emission tomography (PET) imaging] to select patients who may benefit from EC-IC bypass is currently being studied.

OTHER CAUSES OF ARTERY-TO-ARTERY EMBOLIC STROKE *Intracranial atherosclerosis* produces stroke either by an embolic mechanism or by in-situ thrombosis of a diseased vessel and is more common in patients of Asian and African-American descent. It is estimated that following a stroke or TIA from intracranial atherosclerosis the risk of a second stroke is ~15% per year. There is no proven superior treatment for stroke prevention in this disorder. Warfarin sodium and aspirin are being compared in a U.S. based prospective trial. Many neurointerventional centers are using intracranial angioplasty coupled with intracranial stenting, but this has not been compared with antithrombotic strategies for stroke prevention.

Dissection of the internal carotid or vertebral arteries or even vessels beyond the circle of Willis is a common source of embolic stroke in young (age <60 years) patients. The dissection is usually painful and precedes the stroke by several hours or days. Extracranial dissections rarely cause hemorrhage because of the tough adventitia of these vessels. Intracranial dissections, on the other hand, may produce SAH because the adventitia of intracranial vessels is thin and pseudoaneurysms may form, requiring treatment to prevent rerupture. The cause of dissection is usually unknown and recurrence is rare. Ehlers-Danlos type IV, Marfan's disease, cystic medial necrosis, and fibromuscular dysplasia are associated with dissections. Trauma (usually a motor vehicle accident or a sports injury) can cause carotid and vertebral artery dissections. Spinal manipulative therapy is independently associated with vertebral artery dissection and stroke. Most dissections heal spontaneously, and stroke or TIA is uncommon beyond 2 weeks. Although there are no trials comparing anticoagulation to antiplatelet agents, many physicians treat with anticoagulants for 3 to 6 months then convert to antiplatelet therapy after demonstration of vascular recanalization.

Small-Vessel Stroke   The term *lacunar infarction* refers to infarction following atherothrombotic or lipohyalinotic occlusion of a small artery (30 to 300 μm) in the brain. The term *small-vessel stroke* denotes occlusion of such a small penetrating artery and is now the preferred term. Small-vessel strokes account for ~20% of all strokes.

PATHOPHYSIOLOGY   The MCA stem, the arteries comprising the circle of Willis (A1 segment, anterior and posterior communicating arteries, and P1 segment), and the basilar and vertebral arteries all give rise to 30- to 300-μm branches that penetrate the deep gray and white matter of the cerebrum or brainstem (Fig. 349-3). Each of these small branches can occlude either by atherothrombotic disease at its origin or by the development of lipohyalinotic thickening. Thrombosis of these vessels causes small infarcts that are referred to as *lacunes* (Latin for "lake" of fluid noted at autopsy). They range in size from 3 mm to 2 cm. Hypertension and age are the principal risk factors.

CLINICAL MANIFESTATIONS   The most common *lacunar syndromes* are the following: (1) Pure motor hemiparesis from an infarct in the posterior limb of the internal capsule or basis pontis; the face, arm, and leg are almost always involved; (2) pure sensory stroke from an infarct in the ventrolateral thalamus; (3) ataxic hemiparesis from an infarct in the base of the pons; (4) dysarthria and a clumsy hand or arm due to infarction in the base of the pons or in the genu of the internal capsule; and (5) pure motor hemiparesis with "motor (Broca's) aphasia" due to thrombotic occlusion of a lenticulostriate branch supplying the genu and anterior limb of the internal capsule and adjacent white matter of the corona radiata.

Transient symptoms (small vessel TIAs) may herald a small-vessel infarct; they may occur several times a day and last only a few minutes. Recovery from a small-vessel stroke often begins within hours or days, and over weeks or months may be nearly complete; in some cases, however, there is severe permanent disability. Often, institution of combined antithrombotic treatments does not prevent eventual stroke in "stuttering lacunes."

A large-vessel source (either thrombosis or embolism) may manifest initially as a lacunar syndrome with small-vessel infarction. Therefore, the search for embolic sources (carotid and heart) should not be completely abandoned in the evaluation of these patients. Secondary prevention of lacunar stroke involves risk factor modification, specifically reduction in blood pressure (see "Primary and Secondary Prevention," below).

LESS COMMON CAUSES OF STROKE (Table 349-3)   *Hypercoagulable disorders* (Chap. 53) primarily cause increased risk of venous thrombosis and therefore may cause venous sinus thrombosis. Protein S deficiency and homocysteinemia may cause arterial thromboses as well. Systemic lupus erythematosus with Liebman-Sacks endocarditis can be a cause of embolic stroke. These conditions overlap with the antiphospholipid syndrome, which probably requires long-term anticoagulation to prevent further stroke.

Venous sinus thrombosis of the lateral or sagittal sinus or of small cortical veins (cortical vein thrombosis) occurs as a complication of pregnancy and the postpartum period, sepsis, and intracranial infections (meningitis). It is also seen with increased incidence in patients with laboratory-confirmed thrombophilia (Table 349-3) including polycythemia, sickle cell anemia, proteins C and S deficiency, factor V Leiden mutation (resistance to activated protein C), antithrombin III deficiency, homocysteinemia, and the prothrombin G20210 mutation. Women who take oral contraceptives and have the prothrombin G20210 mutation may be at high risk for sinus thrombosis. Patients present with headache, focal neurologic signs (especially paraparesis), and seizures. Often, CT imaging is normal unless an intracranial venous hemorrhage has occurred, but the venous sinus occlusion is readily visualized using magnetic resonance (MR) venography or conventional x-ray angiography. With greater degrees of sinus thrombosis, the patient may develop signs of increased ICP and coma. Intravenous heparin, regardless of the presence of intracranial hemorrhage, has been shown to reduce morbidity and mortality, and the long-term outcome is generally good. Heparin prevents further thrombosis and reduces venous hypertension and ischemia. If an underlying hypercoagulable state is not found, many physicians treat with warfarin sodium for 3 to 6 months then convert to aspirin, depending on the degree of resolution of the venous sinus thrombus. Anticoagulation is often continued indefinitely if thrombophilia is diagnosed.

Fibromuscular dysplasia affects the cervical arteries and occurs mainly in women. The carotid or vertebral arteries show multiple rings of segmental narrowing alternating with dilatation. Occlusion is usually incomplete. The process is often asymptomatic but occasionally is associated with an audible bruit, TIAs, or stroke. The cause and natural history of fibromuscular dysplasia is unknown (Chap. 232). TIA or stroke generally occurs only when the artery is severely narrowed or dissects. Anticoagulation or antiplatelet therapy may be helpful.

Temporal (giant cell) arteritis (Chap. 306) is a relatively common affliction of elderly persons in which the external carotid system, particularly the temporal arteries, becomes the site of a subacute granu-

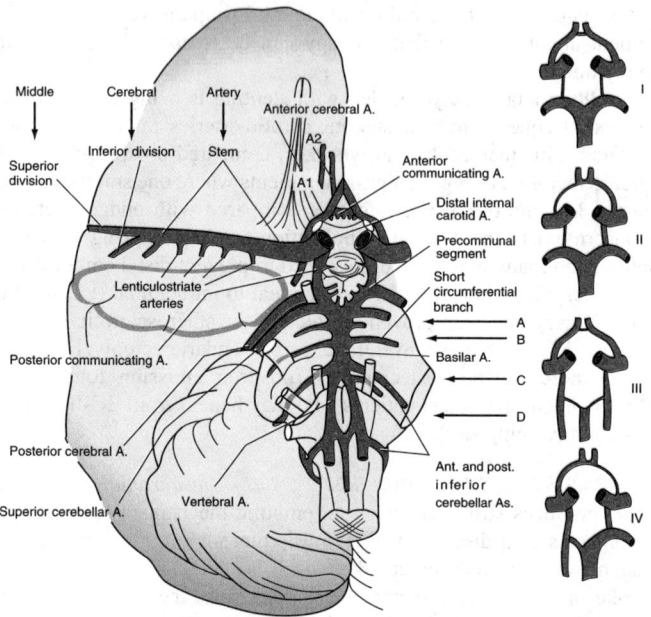

FIGURE 349-3   Diagram of the brainstem, cerebellum, inferior right frontal lobe, and transected temporal lobe. Principal branches of the vertebral basilar arterial system are pictured. The stem of the middle cerebral artery with its small, deep penetrating lenticulostriate arteries and the circle of Willis with its small, deep penetrating branches are shown. Roman numerals I, II, III, and IV represent some of the possible variations of the circle of Willis. *A, B, C,* and *D* arrows indicate the four levels of the brainstem diagrammed below (*A*, Fig. 349-11; *B*, Fig. 349-10; *C*, Fig. 349-9; *D*, Fig. 349-8). Although typical vascular syndromes of the pons and medulla have been designated by the shaded areas in Figs. 349-8 to 349-11, the shading is approximate only. Great variability in infarct size and location occurs when the basilar or vertebral arteries or one of their penetrating branches becomes occluded. This variability is because of variation in arterial anatomic location and available collateral circulation. Thus the stroke syndromes produced are often atypical, incomplete, or merge with one another. (*Courtesy of CM Fisher, MD.*)

lomatous inflammation with giant cells. Occlusion of posterior ciliary arteries derived from the ophthalmic artery results in blindness in one or both eyes and can be prevented with glucocorticoids. It rarely causes stroke as the internal carotid artery is usually not inflamed. Idiopathic giant cell arteritis involving the great vessels arising from the aortic arch (*Takayasu's arteritis*) may cause carotid or vertebral thrombosis; it is rare in the western hemisphere.

Necrotizing (or granulomatous) arteritis, occurring alone or in association with generalized polyarteritis nodosa or Wegener's granulomatosis, involves the distal small branches (<2 mm diameter) of the main intracranial arteries and produces small ischemic infarcts in the brain, optic nerve, and spinal cord. The cerebrospinal fluid often shows pleocytosis, and the protein level is elevated. *Primary central nervous system vasculitis* is rare; small or medium-sized vessels are usually affected. Brain biopsy or high-resolution conventional x-ray angiography is usually required to make the diagnosis. Patients with any form of vasculitis may present with insidious progression of combined white and gray matter infarctions, prominent headache, and cognitive decline. Aggressive immunosuppression with glucocorticoids, and often cyclophosphamide, is usually necessary to prevent progression. Depending upon the duration of the disease, many patients can make an excellent recovery.

Drugs, in particular amphetamines and perhaps cocaine, may cause stroke on the basis of acute hypertension and drug-induced vasculitis. Abstinence appears to be the best treatment, as no data exist on use of any treatment. Phenylpropanolamine has been linked with intracranial hemorrhage as has cocaine, perhaps related to a drug-induced vasculitis. Arteritis can also occur as a consequence of bacterial, tuberculous, and syphilitic meningitis.

Moyamoya disease is a poorly understood occlusive disease involving large intracranial arteries, especially the distal internal carotid artery and the stem of the middle and anterior cerebral arteries. Vascular inflammation is absent. The lenticulostriate arteries develop a rich collateral circulation around the occlusive lesion, which gives the impression of a "puff of smoke" (*moyamoya* in Japanese) on conventional x-ray angiography. Other collaterals include transdural anastomoses between the cortical surface branches of the meningeal and scalp arteries. The disease occurs mainly in Asian children or young adults, but the appearance may be identical in adults who have atherosclerosis. The etiology of the childhood form is unknown. Because of the occurrence of intracranial hemorrhage from rupture of the transdural and pial anastomotic channels, anticoagulation is risky. Breakdown of dilated lenticulostriate arteries may produce parenchymal hemorrhage, and progressive occlusion of large surface arteries can occur, producing large-artery distribution strokes. Bypass of extracranial carotid arteries to the dura or MCAs may prevent stroke and hemorrhage.

Reversible posterior leukoencephalopathy can occur in head injury, migraine, sympathomimetic drug use, eclampsia, and the postpartum period. The etiology is unclear but likely involves widespread cerebral segmental vasoconstriction. Patients complain of headache and manifest fluctuating neurologic symptoms and signs, especially visual symptoms. Sometimes cerebral infarction ensues. Conventional x-ray angiography is the only means of establishing the diagnosis, but because angiography itself can cause spasm of vessels, even the existence of this vascular entity is debated.

Binswanger's disease (chronic progressive subcortical encephalopathy) is a rare condition in which infarction of the subcortical white matter occurs subacutely. CT or MRI scans detect periventricular white matter infarcts and gliosis. There is lipohyalinosis in the small arteries of the deep white matter, as in hypertension. There are usually associated lacunar infarcts. Binswanger's disease may represent a type of border zone ischemic infarction in the deep white matter between the penetrating arteries of the circle of Willis and of the cortex. The pathophysiologic basis of the disease is unclear, but it typically occurs in older patients with severe long-standing hypertension.

CADASIL (cerebral autosomal dominant arteriopathy with subcortical infarcts and leukoencephalopathy) is an inherited disorder that presents as small-vessel strokes, progressive dementia, and extensive symmetric white matter changes visualized by MRI. Approximately 40% of patients have migraine with aura, often manifest as transient motor or sensory deficits. Onset is usually in the fourth or fifth decade of life. This autosomal dominant condition is caused by one of several mutations in Notch-3, a member of a highly conserved gene family characterized by epidermal growth factor repeats in its extracellular domain. CADASIL is the only monogenic ischemic stroke syndrome so far described. Genetic testing is available.

TRANSIENT ISCHEMIC ATTACKS TIAs are episodes of stroke symptoms that last only briefly; the current definition of duration is <24 h, but the average duration of a TIA is ~12 min. The causes of TIA are similar to all causes of stroke, but because TIAs may herald stroke they are an important risk factor that should be considered separately. TIAs may arise from emboli to the brain or from in situ thrombosis of an intracranial vessel. With a TIA, the occluded blood vessel reopens and neurologic function is restored. However, infarcts of the brain do occur in 15 to 40% of TIAs even though neurologic signs and symptoms are absent.

In addition to the stroke syndromes discussed below, there are a few specific TIA symptoms that should receive special notice. *Amaurosis fugax*, or transient monocular blindness, occurs from emboli to the central retinal artery of one eye. This may indicate carotid stenosis as the cause or local ophthalmic artery disease.

The risk of stroke after a TIA is ~10% in the first 3 months, with most events occurring in the first 2 days. Therefore, urgent evaluation and treatment are justified. Since etiologies for stroke and TIA are identical, evaluation for TIA should parallel that of stroke (Tables 349-1 and 349-3). The improvement characteristic of TIA is a contraindication to thrombolysis. Acute antiplatelet therapy has not been tested specifically after TIA but is likely to be effective and is recommended. No large-scale trial has evaluated acute anticoagulation after TIA, a setting in which the risk of hemorrhage may be lower.

RISK FACTORS FOR ISCHEMIC STROKE Identification and control of modifiable risk factors is the best strategy to reduce the burden of stroke, as the total number of strokes could be reduced substantially by these means (Table 349-5).

PRIMARY AND SECONDARY PREVENTION ■ **General Principles** A number of medical and surgical interventions, as well as life-style modifications, are available for preventing stroke. Some of these can be widely applied because of their low cost and minimal risk; others are expensive and carry substantial risk but may be valuable for selected high-risk patients.

Evaluation of a patient's *clinical risk profile* can help determine which preventive treatments to offer. In addition to known risk factors for ischemic stroke (above), certain clinical characteristics also contribute to an increased risk of stroke (Table 349-5). NASCET found that even in patients with the same degree of carotid artery stenosis, specifically 70 to 99%, nine prospectively selected risk factors predicted the risk of vascular outcomes in the medically treated patients. The overall risk of stroke was much greater in a high-risk group (those with more than six risk factors) than in a low-risk group (those with fewer than six risk factors). Fully 39% of patients in the high-risk group treated medically experienced an ipsilateral stroke within 2 years. The rate for the low-risk group was less than half that but was still 17%.

Atherosclerosis Risk Factors The relationship of various factors to the risk of atherosclerosis is described in Chap. 225. Older age, family history of thrombotic stroke, diabetes mellitus, hypertension, tobacco smoking, abnormal blood cholesterol [particularly, low high-density lipoprotein (HDL) and/or high low-density lipoprotein (LDL), and other factors are either proven or probable risk factors for ischemic stroke, largely by their link to atherosclerosis. Risk of second stroke is strongly influenced by prior stroke or TIA, depending on cause.

Many cardiac conditions predispose to stroke, including atrial fibrillation and recent MI. Oral contraceptives may increase stroke risk, and certain inherited and acquired hypercoagulable states predispose to stroke. Hypertension is the most significant of the risk factors; in general, all hypertension should be treated. The presence of known cerebrovascular disease is not a contraindication to treatment aimed at achieving normotension. Also, the value of treating systolic hypertension in older patients has been clearly established. Lowering blood pressure to levels below those traditionally defining hypertension appears to reduce the risk of stroke even further. Data are particularly strong in support of angiotensin-converting enzyme inhibitors and angiotensin receptor blockers.

Several trials have confirmed that statin drugs reduce the risk of stroke even in patients without elevated LDL or low HDL. Although studies specifically targeting prevention of second stroke are still underway, results for patients with cardiovascular risk factors or dyslipidemia have been compelling, with a 20 to 30% relative risk reduction for stroke. Therefore, a statin should be considered in all patients with prior ischemic stroke. Tobacco smoking should be discouraged in all patients (Chap. 375). Whether or not tight control of blood sugar in patients with diabetes lowers stroke risk is uncertain.

Antiplatelet Agents   *Platelet antiaggregation agents* can prevent atherothrombotic events, including TIA and stroke, by inhibiting the formation of intraarterial platelet aggregates. These can form on diseased arteries, induce thrombus formation, and occlude the artery or embolize into the distal circulation. Aspirin, clopidogrel, and the combination of aspirin plus extended-release dipyridamole are the antiplatelet agents most commonly used for this purpose. Ticlopidine has been largely abandoned because of its adverse effects.

Aspirin is the most widely studied antiplatelet agent. Aspirin acetylates platelet cyclooxygenase, which irreversibly inhibits the formation in platelets of thromboxane A_2, a platelet aggregating and vasoconstricting prostaglandin. This effect is permanent and lasts for the usual 8-day life of the platelet. Paradoxically, aspirin also inhibits the formation in endothelial cells of prostacyclin, an antiaggregating and vasodilating prostaglandin. This effect is transient. As soon as aspirin is cleared from the blood, the nucleated endothelial cells again produce prostacyclin. Aspirin in low doses given once daily inhibits the production of thromboxane A_2 in platelets without substantially inhibiting prostacyclin formation. The FDA recommends 50 to 325 mg of aspirin daily for stroke prevention.

Ticlopidine and clopidogrel block the ADP receptor on platelets and thus prevent the cascade resulting in activation of the glycoprotein IIb/IIIa receptor that leads to fibrinogen binding to the platelet and consequent platelet aggregation. Ticlopidine is more effective than aspirin; however, it has the disadvantage of causing diarrhea, skin rash, a low incidence of neutropenia, and thrombotic thrombocytopenic purpura. Clopidogrel is not associated with these important side effects. However, the CAPRIE (Clopidogrel versus Aspirin in Patients at Risk of Ischemic Events) trial, which led to FDA approval, found that it was only marginally more effective than aspirin in reducing risk of stroke. Studies of clopidogrel in combination with aspirin are in progress in both cerebrovascular and cardiovascular patients.

Dipyridamole is an antiplatelet agent that inhibits the uptake of adenosine by a variety of cells, including those of the vascular endothelium. The accumulated adenosine is an inhibitor of aggregation. At least in part through its effects on platelet and vessel wall phosphodiesterases, dipyridamole also potentiates the antiaggregatory effects of prostacyclin and nitric oxide produced by the endothelium and acts by inhibiting platelet phosphodiesterase, which is responsible for the breakdown of cyclic AMP. The resulting elevation in cyclic AMP inhibits aggregation of platelets. Dipyridamole has a controversial history in stroke prevention. The European Stroke Prevention Study-2 showed efficacy of both 50 mg daily of aspirin and extended-release dipyridamole in preventing stroke, and a significantly better risk re-

duction when the two agents were combined. A combination capsule of extended-release dipyridamole and aspirin is approved for prevention of stroke.

Many large clinical trials have demonstrated clearly that most antiplatelet agents reduce the risk of all important vascular atherothrombotic events (i.e., ischemic stroke, MI, and death due to all vascular causes) in patients at risk for these events. The overall *relative* reduction in risk of nonfatal stroke is about 25 to 30% and of all vascular events is about 25%. The *absolute* reduction varies considerably depending on the particular patient's risk. Individuals at very low risk for stroke seem to experience the same relative reduction, but their risk may be so low that the "benefit" is meaningless. On the other hand, individuals with a 10 to 15% risk of vascular events per year experience a reduction to about 7.5 to 11%.

Aspirin is inexpensive, can be given in low doses, and could be recommended for all adults to prevent both stroke and MI. However, it causes epigastric discomfort, gastric ulceration, and gastrointestinal hemorrhage, which may be asymptomatic or life-threatening. Consequently, not every 40- or 50-year-old should be advised to take aspirin regularly because the risk of atherothrombotic stroke is extremely low and is outweighed by the risk of adverse side effects. Conversely, every patient who has experienced an atherothrombotic stroke or TIA and has no contraindication should be taking an antiplatelet agent regularly because the average annual risk of another stroke is 8 to 10%; another few percent will experience a MI or vascular death. Clearly, the likelihood of benefit far outweighs the risks of treatment.

The choice of antiplatelet agent and dose must balance the risk of stroke, the expected benefit, and the risk and cost of treatment. However, there are no definitive data, and opinions vary. Many authorities believe low-dose (30 to 75 mg daily) and high-dose (650 to 1300 mg daily) aspirin are about equally effective. Some advocate very low doses to avoid adverse effects, and still others advocate very high doses to be sure the benefit is maximal. Most physicians in North America recommend 81 to 325 mg daily, while most Europeans recommend 50 to 100 mg. Similarly, the choice of aspirin, clopidogrel, or dipyridamole plus aspirin must balance the fact that the latter are more effective than aspirin but the cost is higher.

Anticoagulation Therapy and Noncardiogenic Stroke   There are few data to support the use of long-term warfarin for preventing atherothrombotic stroke, either intracranially or extracranially. The WARSS study found no benefit of warfarin sodium (INR, 2 to 3) over aspirin, 325 mg, for secondary prevention of stroke but did find a slightly higher bleeding rate in the warfarin group. A prospective trial is ongoing to study warfarin versus aspirin in secondary stroke prevention for intracranial atherosclerosis.

Anticoagulation Therapy and Embolic Stroke   Several trials have shown that anticoagulation (INR range, 2 to 3) in patients with chronic nonvalvular (nonrheumatic) atrial fibrillation prevents cerebral embolism and is safe. For primary prevention and for patients who have experienced stroke or TIA, anticoagulation with warfarin reduces the risk by about 67% which clearly outweighs the 1% risk per year of a major bleeding complication.

The decision to use anticoagulation for primary prevention is based primarily on risk factors (Table 349-4). The presence of any risk factor tips the balance in favor of anticoagulation.

Because of the high annual stroke risk in untreated rheumatic heart disease, primary prophylaxis against stroke has not been studied in a double-blind fashion. These patients generally receive long-term anticoagulation.

Anticoagulation also reduces the risk of embolism in acute MI. Most clinicians recommend a 3-month course of anticoagulation when there is anterior Q-wave infarction, substantial left ventricular dysfunction, congestive heart failure, mural thrombosis, or atrial fibrillation. Warfarin is recommended long-term if atrial fibrillation persists. Warfarin is currently being studied in patients with congestive heart failure.

Thromboembolism is one of the most serious complications of

prosthetic heart valve implantation. Anticoagulation has been proven effective for preventing strokes in this situation, while antiplatelet therapy alone has not. However, coupled with warfarin anticoagulation, aspirin adds substantial benefit. A greater degree of anticoagulation (INR of 3 to 4, depending on valve type) is recommended for some patients with prosthetic heart valves.

If the embolic source cannot be eliminated, anticoagulation should in most cases be continued indefinitely. Many neurologists recommend combining antiplatelet agents with anticoagulants for patients who "fail" one form of therapy (i.e., have another stroke or TIA). This empirical approach subjects the patient to an increased bleeding risk.

Other Causes of Stroke ◼ *CAROTID DISEASE* Surgical or endovascular repair of carotid atherosclerosis is preferred over medical therapy for symptomatic carotid artery disease (see section above). Anticoagulation has not been directly compared with antiplatelet therapy for carotid disease.

DURAL SINUS THROMBOSIS Limited evidence exists to support short-term usage of anticoagulants, regardless of the presence of intracranial hemorrhage for venous infarction following sinus thrombosis.

STROKE SYNDROMES A careful history and neurologic examination can often localize the region of brain dysfunction; if this region corresponds to a particular arterial distribution, the possible causes responsible for the syndrome can be narrowed. This is of particular importance when the patient presents with a TIA and a normal examination. For example, if a patient develops language loss and a right homonymous hemianopia, a search for causes of left middle cerebral emboli should be performed. A finding of an isolated stenosis of the right internal carotid artery in that patient, for example, suggests an asymptomatic carotid stenosis, and the search for other causes of stroke should continue. The following sections describe the clinical findings of cerebral ischemia associated with cerebral vascular territories depicted in Figs. 349-3 through 349-11. Stroke syndromes are divided into: (1) large-vessel stroke within the anterior circulation, (2) large-vessel stroke within the posterior circulation, and (3) small-vessel disease of either vascular bed.

Stroke Within the Anterior Circulation The internal carotid artery and its branches comprise the anterior circulation of the brain. These vessels can be occluded by intrinsic disease of the vessel (e.g., atherosclerosis or dissection) or by embolic occlusion from a proximal source as discussed above. Occlusion of each major intracranial vessel has distinct clinical manifestations.

MIDDLE CEREBRAL ARTERY Occlusion of the proximal MCA or one of its major branches is most often due to an embolus (artery-to-artery, cardiac, or of unknown source) rather than intracranial atherothrombosis. Atherosclerosis of the proximal MCA may cause distal emboli to the

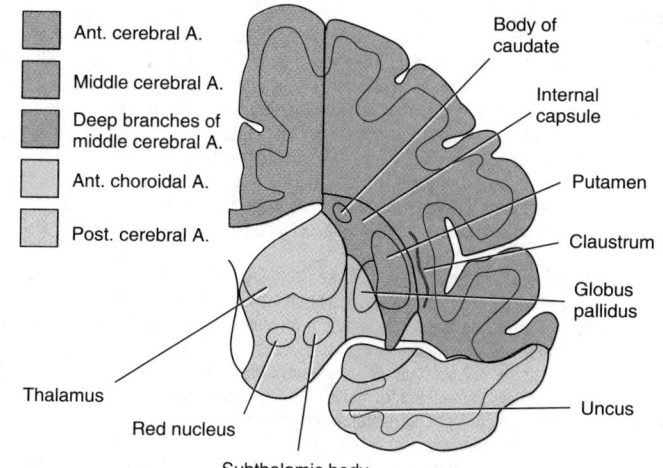

FIGURE 349-4 Diagram of a cerebral hemisphere in coronal section showing the territories of the major cerebral vessels. *(Courtesy of CM Fisher, MD.)*

Legend for Figure 349-4:
- Ant. cerebral A.
- Middle cerebral A.
- Deep branches of middle cerebral A.
- Ant. choroidal A.
- Post. cerebral A.

Labels: Body of caudate, Internal capsule, Putamen, Claustrum, Globus pallidus, Uncus, Thalamus, Red nucleus, Subthalamic body

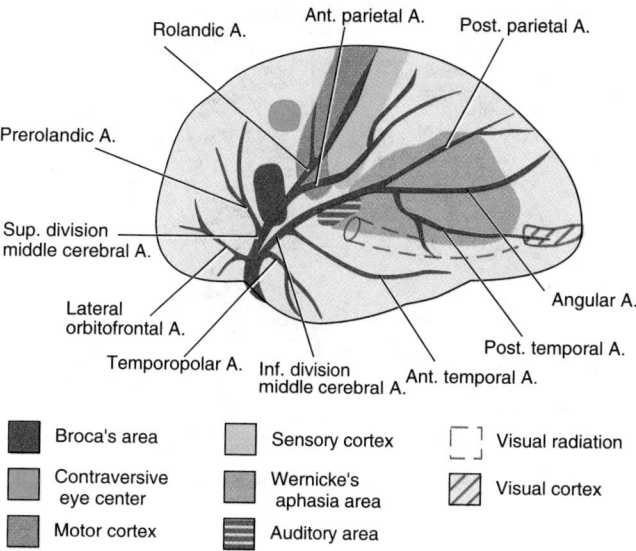

Legend for Figure 349-5:
- Broca's area
- Contraversive eye center
- Motor cortex
- Sensory cortex
- Wernicke's aphasia area
- Auditory area
- Visual radiation
- Visual cortex

Labels: Rolandic A., Ant. parietal A., Post. parietal A., Prerolandic A., Sup. division middle cerebral A., Lateral orbitofrontal A., Temporopolar A., Inf. division middle cerebral A., Ant. temporal A., Post. temporal A., Angular A.

FIGURE 349-5 Diagram of a cerebral hemisphere, lateral aspect, showing the branches and distribution of the middle cerebral artery and the principal regions of cerebral localization. Note the bifurcation of the middle cerebral artery into a superior and inferior division. *(Courtesy of CM Fisher, MD.)*

Signs and symptoms: *Structures involved*

Paralysis of the contralateral face, arm, and leg; sensory impairment over the same area (pinprick, cotton touch, vibration, position, two-point discrimination, stereognosis, tactile localization, barognosis, cutaneographia): *Somatic motor area for face and arm and the fibers descending from the leg area to enter the corona radiata and corresponding somatic sensory system*

Motor aphasia: *Motor speech area of the dominant hemisphere*

Central aphasia, word deafness, anomia, jargon speech, sensory agraphia, acalculia, alexia, finger agnosia, right-left confusion (the last four comprise the Gerstmann syndrome): *Central, suprasylvian speech area and parietooccipital cortex of the dominant hemisphere*

Conduction aphasia: *Central speech area (parietal operculum)*

Apractognosia of the nondominant hemisphere, anosognosia, hemiasomatognosia, unilateral neglect, agnosia for the left half of external space, dressing "apraxia," constructional "apraxia," distortion of visual coordinates, inaccurate localization in the half field, impaired ability to judge distance, upside-down reading, visual illusions (e.g., it may appear that another person walks through a table): *Nondominant parietal lobe (area corresponding to speech area in dominant hemisphere); loss of topographic memory is usually due to a nondominant lesion, occasionally to a dominant one*

Homonymous hemianopia (often homonymous inferior quadrantanopia): *Optic radiation deep to second temporal convolution*

Paralysis of conjugate gaze to the opposite side: *Frontal contraversive field or projecting fibers*

middle cerebral territory or, less commonly, may produce low-flow TIAs. Collateral formation via leptomeningeal vessels often prevents MCA stenosis from becoming symptomatic.

The cortical branches of the MCA supply the lateral surface of the hemisphere except for (1) the frontal pole and a strip along the superomedial border of the frontal and parietal lobes supplied by the ACA, and (2) the lower temporal and occipital pole convolutions supplied by the PCA (Figs. 349-4, 349-6, and 349-7).

The proximal MCA (M1 segment) gives rise to penetrating branches (termed *lenticulostriate arteries*) that supply the putamen, outer globus pallidus, posterior limb of the internal capsule, the adjacent corona radiata, and most of the caudate nucleus. In the sylvian fissure, the MCA in most patients divides into *superior* and *inferior* divisions (M2 branches). Branches of the inferior division supply the inferior parietal and temporal cortex, and those from the superior division supply the frontal and superior parietal cortex (Fig. 349-5).

If the entire MCA is occluded at its origin (blocking both its penetrating and cortical branches) and the distal collaterals are limited, the clinical findings are contralateral hemiplegia, hemianesthesia, homonymous hemianopia, and a day or two of gaze preference to the ipsilateral side. Dysarthria is common because of facial weakness.

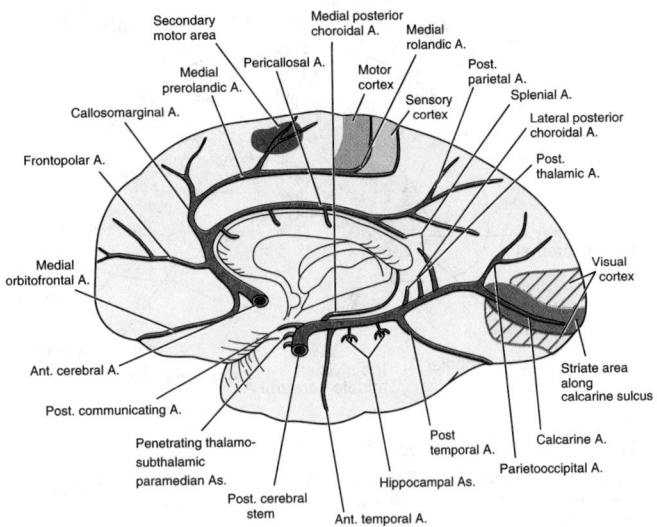

FIGURE 349-6 Diagram of a cerebral hemisphere, medial aspect, showing the branches and distribution of the anterior cerebral artery and the principal regions of cerebral localization. (*Courtesy of CM Fisher, MD.*)

Signs and symptoms: *Structures involved*

Paralysis of opposite foot and leg: *Motor leg area*

A lesser degree of paresis of opposite arm: *Arm area of cortex or fibers descending to corona radiata*

Cortical sensory loss over toes, foot, and leg: *Sensory area for foot and leg*

Urinary incontinence: *Sensorimotor area in paracentral lobule*

Contralateral grasp reflex, sucking reflex, gegenhalten (paratonic rigidity): *Medial surface of the posterior frontal lobe (?) supplemental motor area*

Abulia (akinetic mutism), slowness, delay, intermittent interruption, lack of spontaneity, whispering, reflex distraction to sights and sounds: *Uncertain localization—probably cingulate gyrus and medial inferior portion of frontal, parietal, and temporal lobes*

Impairment of gait and stance (gait apraxia): *Frontal cortex near leg motor area*

Dyspraxia of left limbs, tactile aphasia in left limbs: *Corpus callosum*

When the dominant hemisphere is involved, global aphasia is present also, and when the nondominant hemisphere is affected, anosognosia, constructional apraxia, and neglect are found (Chap. 23).

Complete MCA syndromes occur most often when an embolus occludes the stem of the artery. Cortical collateral blood flow and differing arterial configurations are probably responsible for the development of many partial syndromes. Partial syndromes may also be due to emboli that enter the proximal MCA without complete occlusion, occlude distal MCA branches, or fragment and move distally.

Partial syndromes due to embolic occlusion of a single branch include hand, or arm and hand, weakness alone (brachial syndrome) or facial weakness with nonfluent (Broca) aphasia (Chap. 23), with or without arm weakness (frontal opercular syndrome). A combination of sensory disturbance, motor weakness, and nonfluent aphasia suggests that an embolus has occluded the proximal superior division and infarcted large portions of the frontal and parietal cortices (Fig. 349-5). If a fluent (Wernicke's) aphasia occurs without weakness, the inferior division of the MCA supplying the posterior part (temporal cortex) of the dominant hemisphere is probably involved. Jargon speech and an inability to comprehend written and spoken language are prominent features, often accompanied by a contralateral, homonymous superior quadrantanopia. Hemineglect or spatial agnosia without weakness indicates that the inferior division of the MCA in the nondominant hemisphere is involved.

Occlusion of a lenticulostriate vessel produces small-vessel (lacunar) stroke within the internal capsule. This produces pure motor stroke or sensory-motor stroke contralateral to the lesion. Ischemia within the genu of the internal capsule causes primarily facial weakness followed by arm then leg weakness as the ischemia moves posterior within the capsule. Alternatively, the contralateral hand may become ataxic and dysarthria will be prominent (clumsy hand, dys-

arthria lacunar syndrome). Lacunar infarction affecting the globus pallidus and putamen often has few clinical signs, but parkinsonism and hemiballismus have been reported.

ANTERIOR CEREBRAL ARTERY The ACA is divided into two segments: the precommunal (A1) circle of Willis, or stem, which connects the internal carotid artery to the anterior communicating artery, and the postcommunal (A2) segment distal to the anterior communicating artery (Figs. 349-3 and 349-7). The A1 segment gives rise to several deep penetrating branches that supply the anterior limb of the internal capsule, the anterior perforate substance, amygdala, anterior hypothalamus, and the inferior part of the head of the caudate nucleus (Fig. 349-4).

Occlusion of the proximal ACA is usually well tolerated because of collateral flow through the anterior communicating artery and collaterals through the MCA and PCA. Occlusion of a single A2 segment results in the contralateral symptoms noted in Fig. 349-6. If both A2 segments arise from a single anterior cerebral stem (contralateral A1

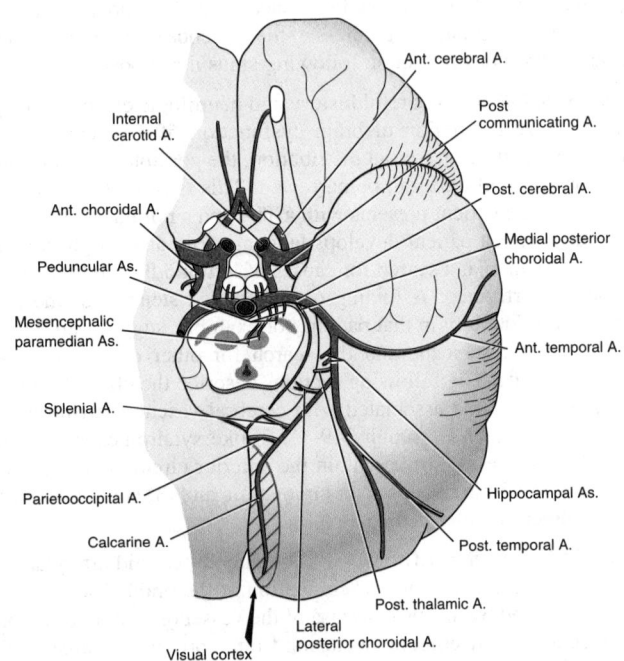

FIGURE 349-7 Inferior aspect of the brain with the branches and distribution of the posterior cerebral artery and the principal anatomic structures shown. (*Courtesy of CM Fisher, MD.*)

Signs and symptoms: *Structures involved*

Peripheral territory (see also Fig. 349-11). Homonymous hemianopia (often upper quadrantic): *Calcarine cortex or optic radiation nearby.* Bilateral homonymous hemianopia, cortical blindness, awareness or denial of blindness; tactile naming, achromatopia (color blindness), failure to see to-and-fro movements, inability to perceive objects not centrally located, apraxia of ocular movements, inability to count or enumerate objects, tendency to run into things that the patient sees and tries to avoid: *Bilateral occipital lobe with possibly the parietal lobe involved.* Verbal dyslexia without agraphia, color anomia: *Dominant calcarine lesion and posterior part of corpus callosum.* Memory defect: *Hippocampal lesion bilaterally or on the dominant side only.* Topographic disorientation and prosopagnosia: *Usually with lesions of nondominant, calcarine, and lingual gyrus.* Simultagnosia, hemivisual neglect: *Dominant visual cortex, contralateral hemisphere.* Unformed visual hallucinations, peduncular hallucinosis, metamorphopsia, teleopsia, illusory visual spread, palinopsia, distortion of outlines, central photophobia: *Calcarine cortex.* Complex hallucinations: *Usually nondominant hemisphere.*

Central territory. Thalamic syndrome: sensory loss (all modalities), spontaneous pain and dysesthesias, choreoathetosis, intention tremor, spasms of hand, mild hemiparesis: *Posteroventral nucleus of thalamus; involvement of the adjacent subthalamus body or its afferent tracts.* Thalamoperforate syndrome: crossed cerebellar ataxia with ipsilateral third nerve palsy (Claude's syndrome): *Dentatothalamic tract and issuing third nerve.* Weber's syndrome: third nerve palsy and contralateral hemiplegia: *Third nerve and cerebral peduncle.* Contralateral hemiplegia: *Cerebral peduncle.* Paralysis or paresis of vertical eye movement, skew deviation, sluggish pupillary responses to light, slight miosis and ptosis (retraction nystagmus and "tucking" of the eyelids may be associated): *Supranuclear fibers to third nerve, interstitial nucleus of Cajal, nucleus of Darkschewitsch, and posterior commissure.* Contralateral rhythmic, ataxic action tremor; rhythmic postural or "holding" tremor (rubral tremor): *Dentatothalamic tract (?).*

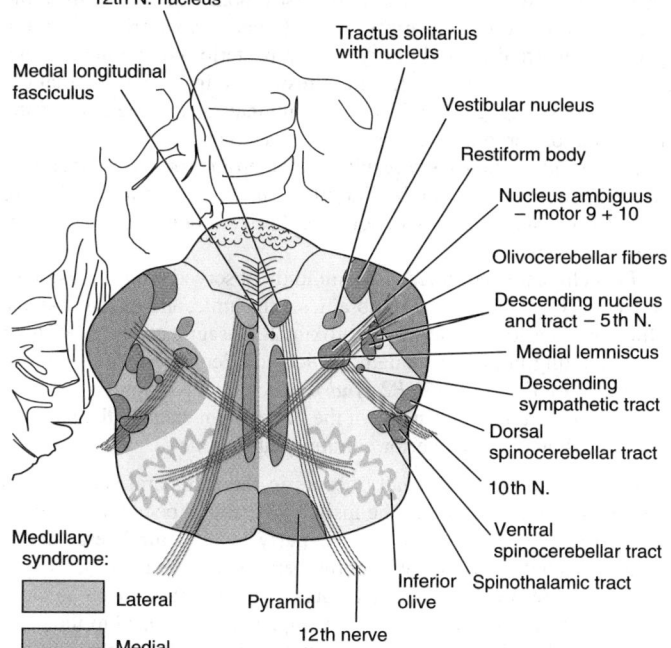

FIGURE 349-8 *(Courtesy of CM Fisher, MD.)*
Signs and symptoms: *Structures involved*

1. Medial medullary syndrome (occlusion of vertebral artery or of branch of vertebral or lower basilar artery)
    On side of lesion
    Paralysis with atrophy of half the tongue: *Ipsilateral twelfth nerve*
    On side opposite lesion
    Paralysis of arm and leg, sparing face; impaired tactile and proprioceptive sense over half the body: *Contralateral pyramidal tract and medial lemniscus*
2. Lateral medullary syndrome (occlusion of any of five vessels may be responsible—vertebral, posterior inferior cerebellar, superior, middle, or inferior lateral medullary arteries)
    On side of lesion
    Pain, numbness, impaired sensation over half the face: *Descending tract and nucleus fifth nerve*
    Ataxia of limbs, falling to side of lesion: *Uncertain—restiform body, cerebellar hemisphere, cerebellar fibers, spinocerebellar tract (?)*
    Nystagmus, diplopia, oscillopsia, vertigo, nausea, vomiting: *Vestibular nucleus*
    Horner's syndrome (miosis, ptosis, decreased sweating): *Descending sympathetic tract*
    Dysphagia, hoarseness, paralysis of palate, paralysis of vocal cord, diminished gag reflex: *Issuing fibers ninth and tenth nerves*
    Loss of taste: *Nucleus and tractus solitarius*
    Numbness of ipsilateral arm, trunk, or leg: *Cuneate and gracile nuclei*
    On side opposite lesion
    Impaired pain and thermal sense over half the body, sometimes face: *Spinothalamic tract*
3. Total unilateral medullary syndrome (occlusion of vertebral artery): Combination of medial and lateral syndromes
4. Lateral pontomedullary syndrome (occlusion of vertebral artery): Combination of lateral medullary and lateral inferior pontine syndrome
5. Basilar artery syndrome (the syndrome of the lone vertebral artery is equivalent): A combination of the various brainstem syndromes plus those arising in the posterior cerebral artery distribution.
    Bilateral long tract signs (sensory and motor; cerebellar and peripheral cranial nerve abnormalities): *Bilateral long tract; cerebellar and peripheral cranial nerves*
    Paralysis or weakness of all extremities, plus all bulbar musculature: *Corticobulbar and corticospinal tracts bilaterally*

segment atresia), the occlusion may affect both hemispheres. Profound abulia (a delay in verbal and motor response) and bilateral pyramidal signs with paraparesis and urinary incontinence result.

ANTERIOR CHOROIDAL ARTERY This artery arises from the internal carotid artery and supplies the posterior limb of the internal capsule and the white matter posterolateral to it, through which pass some of the geniculocalcarine fibers (Figs. 349-4 and 349-7). The complete syndrome of anterior choroidal artery occlusion consists of contralateral hemi-

plegia, hemianesthesia (hypesthesia), and homonymous hemianopia. However, because this territory is also supplied by penetrating vessels of the proximal MCA and the posterior communicating and posterior choroidal arteries, minimal deficits may occur, and patients frequently recover substantially. Anterior choroidal strokes are usually the result of in situ thrombosis of the vessel, and the vessel is particularly vulnerable to iatrogenic occlusion during surgical clipping of aneurysms arising from the internal carotid artery.

INTERNAL CAROTID ARTERY The clinical picture of internal carotid occlusion varies depending on whether the cause of ischemia is propagated thrombus, embolism, or low flow. The cortex supplied by the MCA territory is affected most often. With a competent circle of Willis, occlusion may go unnoticed. If the thrombus propagates up the internal carotid artery into the MCA or embolizes it, symptoms are identical to proximal MCA occlusion (see above). Sometimes there is massive infarction of the entire deep white matter and cortical surface. When the origins of both the ACA and MCA are occluded at the top of the carotid artery, abulia or stupor occurs with hemiplegia, hemianes-

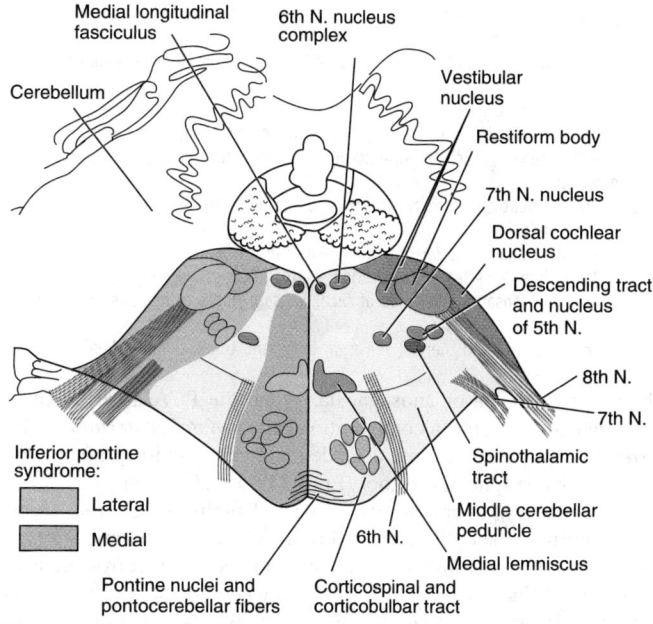

FIGURE 349-9 *(Courtesy of CM Fisher, MD.)*
Signs and symptoms: *Structures involved*

1. Medial inferior pontine syndrome (occlusion of paramedian branch of basilar artery)
    On side of lesion
    Paralysis of conjugate gaze to side of lesion (preservation of convergence): *Center for conjugate lateral gaze*
    Nystagmus: *Vestibular nucleus*
    Ataxia of limbs and gait: *Middle cerebellar peduncle (?)*
    Diplopia on lateral gaze: *Abducens nerve*
    On side opposite lesion
    Paralysis of face, arm, and leg: *Corticobulbar and corticospinal tract in lower pons*
    Impaired tactile and proprioceptive sense over half of the body: *Medial lemniscus*
2. Lateral inferior pontine syndrome (occlusion of anterior inferior cerebellar artery)
    On side of lesion
    Horizontal and vertical nystagmus, vertigo, nausea, vomiting, oscillopia: *Vestibular nerve or nucleus*
    Facial paralysis: *Seventh nerve*
    Paralysis of conjugate gaze to side of lesion: *Center for conjugate lateral gaze*
    Deafness, tinnitus: *Auditory nerve or cochlear nucleus*
    Ataxia: *Middle cerebellar peduncle and cerebellar hemisphere*
    Impaired sensation over face: *Descending tract and nucleus fifth nerve*
    On side opposite lesion
    Impaired pain and thermal sense over half the body (may include face): *Spinothalamic tract*

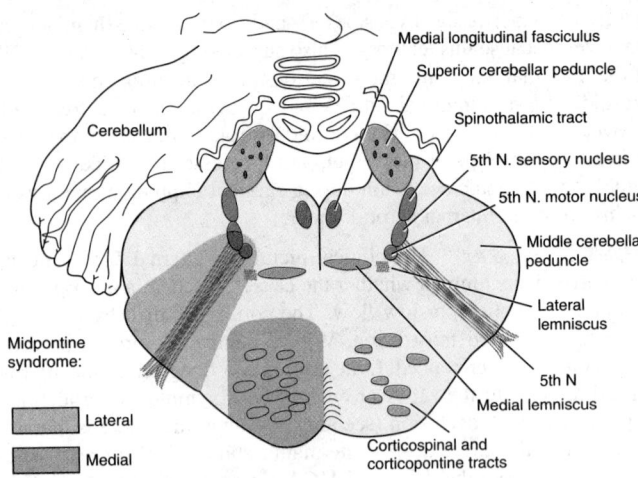

FIGURE 349-10   *(Courtesy of CM Fisher, MD.)*
Signs and symptoms: *Structures involved*

1. Medial midpontine syndrome (paramedian branch of midbasilar artery)
    On side of lesion
        Ataxia of limbs and gait (more prominent in bilateral involvement): *Pontine nuclei*
    On side opposite lesion
        Paralysis of face, arm, and leg: *Corticobulbar and corticospinal tract*
        Variable impaired touch and proprioception when lesion extends posteriorly: *Medial lemniscus*
2. Lateral midpontine syndrome (short circumferential artery)
    On side of lesion
        Ataxia of limbs: *Middle cerebellar peduncle*
        Paralysis of muscles of mastication: *Motor fibers or nucleus of fifth nerve*
        Impaired sensation over side of face: *Sensory fibers or nucleus of fifth nerve*
    On side opposite lesion
        Impaired pain and thermal sense on limbs and trunk: *Spinothalamic tract*

thesia, and aphasia or anosognosia. When the PCA arises from the internal carotid artery (a configuration called a *fetal posterior cerebral artery*), it may also become occluded and give rise to symptoms referable to its peripheral territory (Figs. 349-6 and 349-7).

In addition to supplying the ipsilateral brain, the internal carotid artery perfuses the optic nerve and retina via the ophthalmic artery. In about 25% of symptomatic internal carotid disease, recurrent transient monocular blindness (amaurosis fugax) warns of the lesion. Patients typically describe a horizontal shade that sweeps down or up across the field of vision. They may also complain that their vision was blurred in that eye or that the upper or lower half of vision disappeared. In most cases, these symptoms last only a few minutes. Rarely, ischemia or infarction of the ophthalmic artery or central retinal arteries occurs at the time of cerebral TIA or infarction.

A high-pitched prolonged carotid bruit fading into diastole is often associated with tightly stenotic lesions. As the stenosis grows tighter and flow distal to the stenosis becomes reduced, the bruit becomes fainter and may disappear when occlusion is imminent.

COMMON CAROTID ARTERY   All symptoms and signs of internal carotid occlusion may also be present with occlusion of the common carotid artery. Bilateral common carotid artery occlusions at their origin may occur in Takayasu's arteritis (Chap. 306).

Stroke Within the Posterior Circulation   The posterior circulation is composed of the paired vertebral arteries, the basilar artery, and the paired posterior cerebral arteries. The vertebral arteries join to form the basilar artery at the pontomedullary junction. The basilar artery divides into two posterior cerebral arteries in the interpeduncular fossa (Fig. 349-3). These major arteries give rise to long and short circumferential branches and to smaller deep penetrating branches that supply the cerebellum, medulla, pons, midbrain, subthalamus, thalamus, hippocampus, and medial temporal and occipital lobes. Occlusion of each vessel produces its own distinctive syndrome.

POSTERIOR CEREBRAL ARTERY   In 75% of cases, both PCAs arise from the bifurcation of the basilar artery; in 20%, one has its origin from the ipsilateral internal carotid artery via the posterior communicating artery; in 5%, both originate from the respective ipsilateral internal carotid arteries (Fig. 349-3). The precommunal, or P1, segment of the true posterior cerebral artery is atretic in such cases.

PCA syndromes usually result from atheroma formation or emboli that lodge at the top of the basilar artery; posterior circulation disease may also be caused by dissection of either vertebral artery and fibromuscular dysplasia.

Two clinical syndromes are commonly observed with occlusion of the PCA: (1) *P1 syndrome*: midbrain, subthalamic, and thalamic signs, which are due to disease of the proximal P1 segment of the PCA or its penetrating branches (thalamogeniculate, Percheron, and posterior choroidal arteries); and (2) *P2 syndrome*: cortical temporal and occipital lobe signs, due to occlusion of the P2 segment distal to the junction of the PCA with the posterior communicating artery.

P1 Syndromes   Infarction usually occurs in the ipsilateral subthalamus and medial thalamus and in the ipsilateral cerebral peduncle and midbrain (Fig. 349-7). A third nerve palsy with contralateral ataxia (Claude's syndrome) or with contralateral hemiplegia (Weber's syndrome) may result. The ataxia indicates involvement of the red nucleus or dentatorubrothalamic tract; the hemiplegia is localized to the cerebral peduncle. If the subthalamic nucleus is involved, contralateral

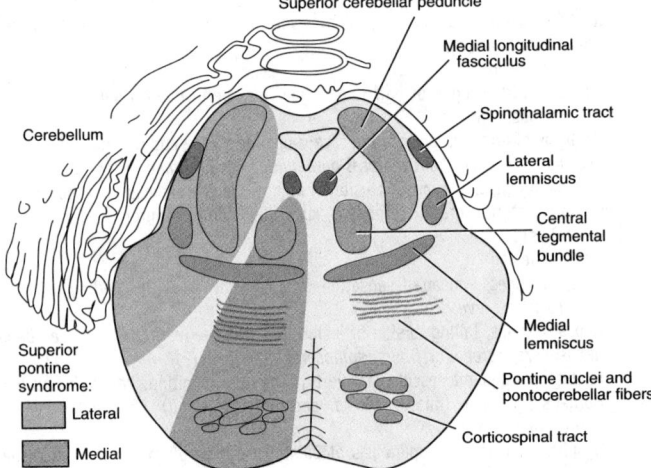

FIGURE 349-11   *(Courtesy of CM Fisher, MD.)*
Signs and symptoms: *Structures involved*

1. Medial superior pontine syndrome (paramedian branches of upper basilar artery)
    On side of lesion
        Cerebellar ataxia (probably): *Superior and/or middle cerebellar peduncle*
        Internuclear ophthalmoplegia: *Medial longitudinal fasciculus*
        Myoclonic syndrome, palate, pharynx, vocal cords, respiratory apparatus, face, oculomotor apparatus, etc.: *Localization uncertain—central tegmental bundle (?), dentate projection (?), inferior olivary nucleus (?)*
    On side opposite lesion
        Paralysis of face, arm, and leg: *Corticobulbar and corticospinal tract*
        Rarely touch, vibration, and position are affected: *Medial lemniscus*
2. Lateral superior pontine syndrome (syndrome of superior cerebellar artery)
    On side of lesion
        Ataxia of limbs and gait, falling to side of lesion: *Middle and superior cerebellar peduncles, superior surface of cerebellum, dentate nucleus*
        Dizziness, nausea, vomiting; horizontal nystagmus: *Vestibular nucleus*
        Paresis of conjugate gaze (ipsilateral): *Pontine contralateral gaze*
        Skew deviation: *Uncertain*
        Miosis, ptosis, decreased sweating over face (Horner's syndrome): *Descending sympathetic fibers*
        Tremor: *Dentate nucleus (?), superior cerebellar peduncle (?)*
    On side opposite lesion
        Impaired pain and thermal sense on face, limbs, and trunk: *Spinothalamic tract*
        Impaired touch, vibration, and position sense, more in leg than arm (there is a tendency to incongruity of pain and touch deficits): *Medial lemniscus (lateral portion)*

hemiballismus may occur. Occlusion of the artery of Percheron produces paresis of upward gaze and drowsiness, and often abulia. Extensive infarction in the midbrain and subthalamus occurring with bilateral proximal PCA occlusion presents as coma, unreactive pupils, bilateral pyramidal signs, and decerebrate rigidity.

Occlusion of the penetrating branches of thalamic and thalamogeniculate arteries produces less extensive thalamic and thalamocapsular lacunar syndromes. The *thalamic Déjerine-Roussy syndrome* consists of contralateral hemisensory loss followed later by an agonizing, searing or burning pain in the affected areas. It is persistent and responds poorly to analgesics. Anticonvulsants (carbamazepine or gabapentin) or tricyclic antidepressants may be beneficial.

P2 Syndromes (See also Fig. 349-7)   Occlusion of the distal PCA causes infarction of the medial temporal and occipital lobes. Contralateral homonymous hemianopia with macula sparing is the usual manifestation. Occasionally, only the upper quadrant of visual field is involved. If the visual association areas are spared and only the calcarine cortex is involved, the patient may be aware of visual defects. Medial temporal lobe and hippocampal involvement may cause an acute disturbance in memory, particularly if it occurs in the dominant hemisphere. The defect usually clears because memory has bilateral representation. If the dominant hemisphere is affected and the infarct extends to involve the splenium of the corpus callosum, the patient may demonstrate alexia without agraphia. Visual agnosia for faces, objects, mathematical symbols, and colors and anomia with paraphasic errors (amnestic aphasia) may also occur in this setting, even without callosal involvement. Occlusion of the posterior cerebral artery can produce *peduncular hallucinosis* (visual hallucinations of brightly colored scenes and objects).

Bilateral infarction in the distal PCAs produces cortical blindness (blindness with preserved pupillary light reaction). The patient is often unaware of the blindness or may even deny it (*Anton's syndrome*). Tiny islands of vision may persist, and the patient may report that vision fluctuates as images are captured in the preserved portions. Rarely, only peripheral vision is lost and central vision is spared, resulting in "gun-barrel" vision. Bilateral visual association area lesions may result in *Balint's syndrome*, a disorder of the orderly visual scanning of the environment (Chap. 23), usually resulting from infarctions secondary to low flow in the "watershed" between the distal posterior and middle cerebral artery territories, as occurs after cardiac arrest. Patients may experience persistence of a visual image for several minutes despite gazing at another scene (*palinopia*). Embolic occlusion of the top of the basilar artery can produce any or all of the central or peripheral territory symptoms. The hallmark is the sudden onset of bilateral signs, including ptosis, pupillary asymmetry or lack of reaction to light, and somnolence.

VERTEBRAL AND POSTERIOR INFERIOR CEREBELLAR ARTERIES   The vertebral artery, which arises from the innominate artery on the right and the subclavian artery on the left, consists of four segments. The first (V1) extends from its origin to its entrance into the sixth or fifth transverse vertebral foramen. The second segment (V2) traverses the vertebral foramina from C6 to C2. The third (V3) passes through the transverse foramen and circles around the arch of the atlas to pierce the dura at the foramen magnum. The fourth (V4) segment courses upward to join the other vertebral artery to form the basilar artery; only the fourth segment gives rise to branches that supply the brainstem and cerebellum. The posterior inferior cerebellar artery (PICA) in its proximal segment supplies the lateral medulla and, in its distal branches, the inferior surface of the cerebellum.

Atherothrombotic lesions have a predilection for V1 and V4 segments of the vertebral artery. The first segment may become diseased at the origin of the vessel and may produce posterior circulation emboli; collateral flow from the contralateral vertebral artery or the ascending cervical, thyrocervical, or occipital arteries is usually sufficient to prevent low-flow TIAs or stroke. When one vertebral artery is atretic and an atherothrombotic lesion threatens the origin of the other, the collateral circulation, which may also include retrograde

flow down the basilar artery, is often insufficient (Figs. 349-3 and 349-7). In this setting, low-flow TIAs may occur, consisting of syncope, vertigo, and alternating hemiplegia; this state also sets the stage for thrombosis. Disease of the distal fourth segment of the vertebral artery can promote thrombus formation manifest as embolism or with propagation as basilar artery thrombosis. Stenosis proximal to the origin of the posterior inferior cerebellar artery can threaten the lateral medulla and posterior inferior surface of the cerebellum.

If the subclavian artery is occluded proximal to the origin of the vertebral artery, there is a reversal in the direction of blood flow in the ipsilateral vertebral artery. Exercise of the ipsilateral arm may increase demand on vertebral flow, producing posterior circulation TIAs, or "subclavian steal."

Although atheromatous disease rarely narrows the second and third segments of the vertebral artery, this region is subject to dissection, fibromuscular dysplasia, and, rarely, encroachment by osteophytic spurs within the vertebral foramina.

Embolic occlusion or thrombosis of a V4 segment causes ischemia of the lateral medulla. The constellation of vertigo, numbness of the ipsilateral face and contralateral limbs, diplopia, hoarseness, dysarthria, dysphagia, and ipsilateral Horner's syndrome is called the lateral medullary (or Wallenberg's) syndrome (Fig. 349-8). Most cases result from ipsilateral vertebral artery occlusion; in the remainder, PICA occlusion is responsible. Occlusion of the medullary penetrating branches of the vertebral artery or PICA results in partial syndromes. *Hemiparesis is not a feature of vertebral artery occlusion.*

Rarely, a *medial medullary syndrome* occurs with infarction of the pyramid and contralateral hemiparesis of the arm and leg, sparing the face. If the medial lemniscus and emerging hypoglossal nerve fibers are involved, contralateral loss of joint position sense and ipsilateral tongue weakness occur.

Cerebellar infarction with edema can lead to *sudden respiratory arrest* due to raised ICP in the posterior fossa. Drowsiness, Babinski signs, dysarthria, and bifacial weakness may be absent, or present only briefly, before respiratory arrest ensues. Gait unsteadiness, headache, dizziness, nausea, and vomiting may be the only early symptoms and signs and should arouse suspicion of this impending complication, which may require neurosurgical decompression, often with an excellent outcome. Separating these symptoms from those of viral labrynthitis can be a challenge, but headache, neck stiffness, and unilateral dysmetria favor stroke.

BASILAR ARTERY   Branches of the basilar artery supply the base of the pons and superior cerebellum and fall into three groups: (1) paramedian, 7 to 10 in number, which supply a wedge of pons on either side of the midline; (2) short circumferential, 5 to 7 in number, which supply the lateral two-thirds of the pons and middle and superior cerebellar peduncles; and (3) bilateral long circumferential (superior cerebellar and anterior inferior cerebellar arteries), which course around the pons to supply the cerebellar hemispheres.

Atheromatous lesions can occur anywhere along the basilar trunk but are most frequent in the proximal basilar and distal vertebral segments. Typically, lesions occlude either the proximal basilar and one or both vertebral arteries. The clinical picture varies depending on the availability of retrograde collateral flow from the posterior communicating arteries. Rarely, dissection of a vertebral artery may involve the basilar artery and, depending on the location of true and false lumen, may produce multiple penetrating artery strokes.

Although atherothrombosis occasionally occludes the distal portion of the basilar artery, emboli from the heart or proximal vertebral or basilar segments are more commonly responsible for "top of the basilar" syndromes.

Because the brainstem contains many structures in close apposition, a diversity of clinical syndromes may emerge with ischemia, reflecting involvement of the corticospinal and corticobulbar tracts, ascending sensory tracts, and cranial nerve nuclei (Figs. 349-9, 349-10, and 349-11).

The symptoms of transient ischemia or infarction in the territory of the basilar artery often do not indicate whether the basilar artery itself or one of its branches is diseased, yet this distinction has important implications for therapy. *The picture of complete basilar occlusion, however, is easy to recognize as a constellation of bilateral long tract signs (sensory and motor) with signs of cranial nerve and cerebellar dysfunction.* A "locked-in" state of preserved consciousness with quadriplegia and cranial nerve signs suggests complete pontine and lower midbrain infarction. The therapeutic goal is to identify *impending* basilar occlusion before devastating infarction occurs. A series of TIAs and a slowly progressive, fluctuating stroke are extremely significant as they often herald an atherothrombotic occlusion of the distal vertebral or proximal basilar artery.

TIAs in the proximal basilar distribution may produce dizziness (often described by patients as "swimming," "swaying," "moving," "unsteadiness" or "light-headedness"). Other symptoms that warn of basilar thrombosis include diplopia, dysarthria, facial or circumoral numbness, and hemisensory symptoms. In general, symptoms of basilar branch TIAs affect one side of the brainstem, whereas symptoms of basilar artery TIAs usually affect both sides, though a "herald" hemiparesis has been emphasized as an initial symptom of basilar occlusion. Most often TIAs, whether due to impending occlusion of the basilar artery or a basilar branch, are short-lived (5 to 30 min) and repetitive, occurring several times a day. The pattern suggests intermittent reduction of flow. Many neurologists treat with heparin to prevent clot propagation.

Atherothrombotic occlusion of the basilar artery with infarction usually causes *bilateral* brainstem signs. A gaze paresis or internuclear ophthalmoplegia associated with ipsilateral hemiparesis may be the only manifestation of bilateral brainstem ischemia. More often, unequivocal signs of bilateral pontine disease are present. Complete basilar thrombosis carries a high mortality.

Occlusion of a branch of the basilar artery usually causes *unilateral* symptoms and signs involving motor, sensory, and cranial nerves. As long as symptoms remain unilateral, concern over pending basilar occlusion should be reduced.

Occlusion of the superior cerebellar artery results in severe ipsilateral cerebellar ataxia, nausea and vomiting, dysarthria, and contralateral loss of pain and temperature sensation over the extremities, body, and face (spino- and trigeminothalamic tract). Partial deafness, ataxic tremor of the ipsilateral upper extremity, Horner's syndrome, and palatal myoclonus may occur rarely. Partial syndromes occur frequently (Fig. 349-11). With large strokes, swelling and mass effects may compress the midbrain or produce hydrocephalus; these symptoms may evolve rapidly. Neurosurgical intervention may be lifesaving in such cases.

Occlusion of the anterior inferior cerebellar artery produces variable degrees of infarction because the size of this artery and the territory it supplies vary inversely with those of the PICA. The principal symptoms include: (1) ipsilateral deafness, facial weakness, vertigo, nausea and vomiting, nystagmus, tinnitus, cerebellar ataxia, Horner's syndrome, and paresis of conjugate lateral gaze; and (2) contralateral loss of pain and temperature sensation. An occlusion close to the origin of the artery may cause corticospinal tract signs (Fig. 349-9).

Occlusion of one of the short circumferential branches of the basilar artery affects the lateral two-thirds of the pons and middle or superior cerebellar peduncle, whereas occlusion of one of the paramedian branches affects a wedge-shaped area on either side of the medial pons (Figs. 349-9 through 349-11).

IMAGING STUDIES (See also Chap. 347) ■ **Computed Tomographic Scans** CT radiographic images identify or exclude hemorrhage as the cause of stroke, and they identify extraparenchymal hemorrhages, neoplasms, abscesses, and other conditions masquerading as stroke. Scans obtained in the first several hours after an infarction generally show

no abnormality, and the infarct may not be seen reliably for 24 to 48 h. CT may fail to show small ischemic strokes in the posterior fossa because of bone artifact; small infarcts on the cortical surface may also be missed.

Contrast-enhanced CT scans add specificity by showing contrast enhancement of subacute infarcts and allow visualization of venous structures. Coupled with newer generation scanners, CT angiography (CTA) can be performed with administration of intravenous iodinated contrast allowing visualization of the cervical and intracranial arteries. Carotid disease and intracranial vascular occlusions are readily identified with this method (Fig. 349-12). After an intravenous bolus of contrast, deficits in brain perfusion produced by vascular occlusion can also be demonstrated (Fig. 349-12 *C*). CT imaging is also sensitive for detecting subarachnoid hemorrhage, and CTA can readily identify intracranial aneurysms (see below). Because of its speed and wide availability, noncontrast head CT is the imaging modality of choice in patients with acute stroke (Fig. 349-1), and CTA and CT perfusion imaging may also be useful and convenient adjuncts.

Magnetic Resonance Imaging (MRI) MRI reliably documents the extent and location of infarction in all areas of the brain, including the posterior fossa and cortical surface. It also identifies intracranial hemorrhage and other abnormalities but is less sensitive than CT for detecting acute blood. MRI scanners with magnets of higher field strength produce more reliable and precise images. Diffusion-weighted imaging is more sensitive for early brain infarction than standard MR sequences (Fig. 349-13), as is FLAIR (fluid-attenuated inversion recovery) imaging (Chap. 347). Using intravenous administration of gadolinium contrast, MR perfusion studies can be performed. Brain regions showing poor perfusion but no abnormality on diffusion are considered equivalent to the ischemic penumbra (see "Pathophysiol-

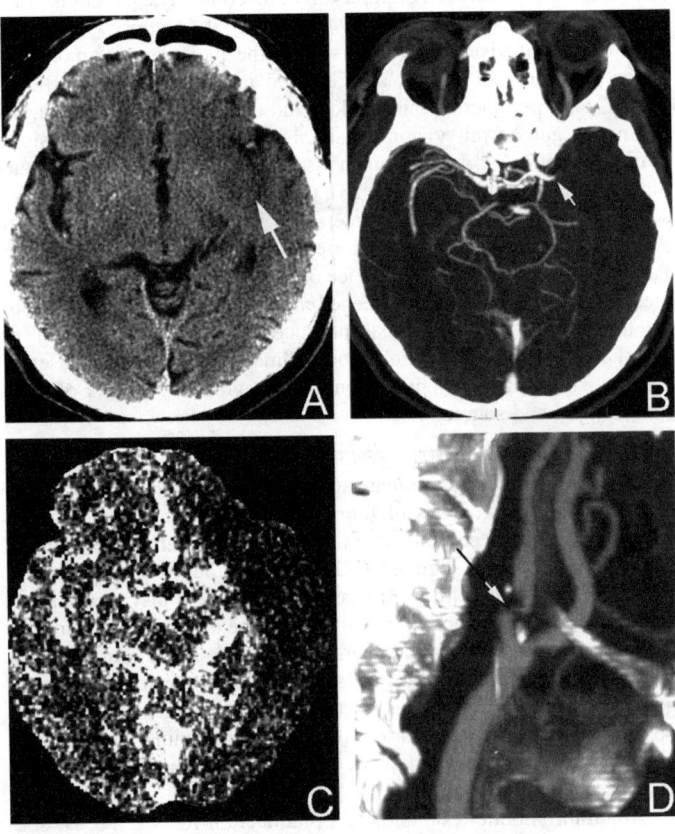

FIGURE 349-12 *A.* Computed tomography (CT) scan of the brain of a patient with a left middle cerebral artery (MCA) stroke of 3 h duration. As an earliest indicator of infarction, the "insular ribbon sign" is caused by edema (darker signal) within the left insular cortex and basal ganglia (*arrow*). *B.* Embolic occlusion of the MCA imaged with CT angiography during the acute stroke (*arrow*). *C.* Cerebral blood flow measured with CT perfusion; blood flow is reduced over a wider region of brain than appeared edematous in *A. D.* CT angiogram of a carotid artery showing high-grade stenosis (*arrow*) from atheroma in another patient.

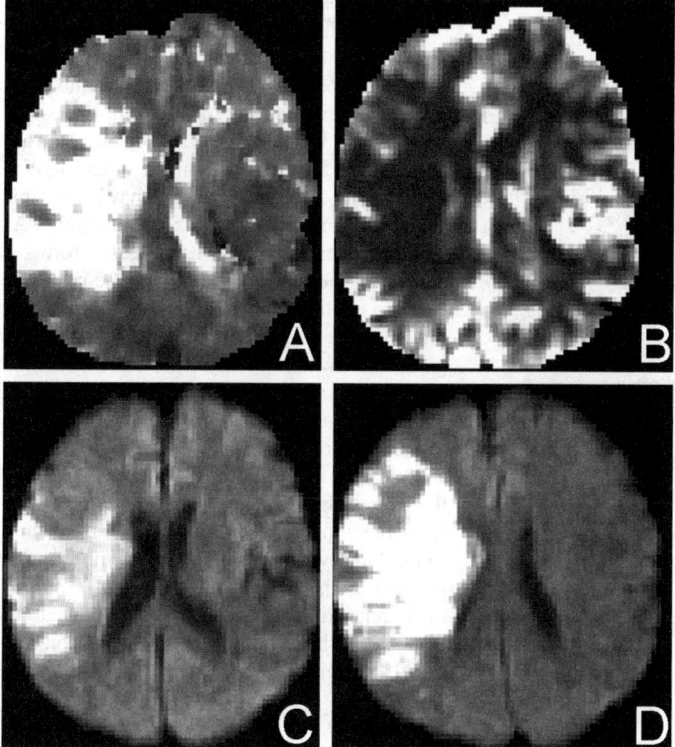

FIGURE 349-13 Magnetic resonance imaging of acute stroke. *A.* Perfusion defect within this right hemisphere (bright signal) imaged after administration of an intravenous bolus of gadolinium contrast. *B.* Cerebral blood flow measured at the same time as in *A*; darker signal reflects decreased blood flow. *C.* Diffusion-weighted image obtained 5 h after onset of a right middle cerebral artery stroke; bright signal indicates regions of restricted diffusion that will progress to infarction. The discrepancy between the region of poor perfusion shown in *A* and *B* and the diffusion deficit, is called *diffusion-perfusion mismatch* and is a measure of the ischemic penumbra. Without specific therapy the region of infarction expands to match the perfusion deficit, as shown in the diffusion weighted image in *D* obtained 5 days later. *(Courtesy of Gregory Albers and Vincent Thijs, MD, Stanford University)*

ogy of Ischemic Stroke," above), and patients showing large regions of mismatch may be better candidates for acute revascularization. MR angiography is highly sensitive for stenosis of extracranial internal carotid arteries and of large intracranial vessels. With higher degrees of stenosis, MR angiography tends to overestimate the degree of stenosis when compared to conventional x-ray angiography. MRI with fat saturation is an imaging sequence used to visualize extra- or intracranial arterial dissection. This sensitive technique images clotted blood within the dissected vessel wall.

MRI is less sensitive for acute blood products than CT and is more expensive and time consuming and less readily available. Claustrophobia also limits its application. Most acute stroke protocols use CT because of these limitations. However, MRI may be useful outside the acute period by more clearly defining the extent and possible source of a stroke.

Cerebral Angiography Conventional x-ray cerebral angiography is the "gold standard" for identifying and quantifying atherosclerotic stenoses of the cerebral arteries and for identifying and characterizing other pathologies, including aneurysm, vasospasm, intraluminal thrombi, fibromuscular dysplasia, arteriovenous fistula, vasculitis, and collateral channels of blood flow. Endovascular techniques, which are evolving rapidly, can be used to deploy stents within delicate intracranial vessels, to perform balloon angioplasty of stenotic lesions, and to treat intracranial aneurysms by embolization. Recent studies have documented that intraarterial delivery of thrombolytic agents to patients with acute MCA stroke can effectively recanalize vessels and improve clinical outcomes. Although its use is investigational in many centers, cerebral angiography coupled with endovascular techniques for cerebral revascularization may become routine in the near future. Conven-

tional angiography carries risks of arterial damage, groin hemorrhage, embolic stroke, and renal failure from contrast nephropathy, so it should be reserved for situations where less invasive means are inadequate.

Ultrasound Techniques Stenosis at the origin of the internal carotid artery can be identified and quantified reliably by ultrasonography that combines a B-mode ultrasound image with a Doppler ultrasound assessment of flow velocity ("duplex" ultrasound). Transcranial Doppler (TCD) assessment of middle, anterior, and posterior cerebral artery flow and of vertebrobasilar flow is also useful. This latter technique can detect stenotic lesions in the large intracranial arteries because such lesions increase systolic flow velocity. In many cases, MR angiography combined with carotid and transcranial ultrasound studies eliminates the need for conventional x-ray angiography in evaluating vascular stenosis. Alternatively, CT angiography of the entire head and neck can be performed during the initial imaging of acute stroke. Because this images the entire arterial system relevant to stroke, with the exception of the heart, much of the clinician's stroke workup can be completed with one imaging study.

Perfusion Techniques Both xenon techniques (principally xenon-CT) and PET can quantify cerebral blood flow. These tools are generally used for research (Chap. 347) but can be useful for determining the significance of arterial stenosis and planning for revascularization surgery. Single photon emission tomography (SPECT), CT perfusion, and MR perfusion techniques report relative cerebral blood flow. Since CT imaging is used as the initial imaging modality for acute stroke, many centers now combine both CT angiography and CT perfusion imaging together with the noncontrast CT scan. CT perfusion imaging increases the sensitivity and improves accuracy in imaging ischemic brain. Alternatively, MR perfusion can be combined with MR diffusion imaging to identify the ischemic penumbra as the mismatch between these two imaging sequences (Fig. 349-13). The ability to image the ischemic penumbra allows more judicious selection of patients who may or may not benefit from acute interventions such as thrombolysis or investigational neuroprotective strategies.

INTRACRANIAL HEMORRHAGE

Hemorrhages are classified by their location and the underlying vascular pathology. Bleeding into subdural and epidural spaces is principally produced by trauma (Chap. 357). Intraparenchymal, intraventricular, and subarachnoid hemorrhage will be considered here.

DIAGNOSIS Intracranial hemorrhage is often discovered on noncontrast CT imaging of the brain during the acute evaluation of stroke. Since CT is more sensitive than routine MRI for acute blood, CT imaging is the preferred method for acute stroke evaluation (Fig. 349-1). The location of the hemorrhage narrows the differential diagnosis to a few entities. Table 349-6 lists the causes and anatomic spaces involved in hemorrhages.

EMERGENCY MANAGEMENT Close attention should be paid to airway management since a reduction in the level of consciousness is common. The initial blood pressure should be maintained until the results of the CT scan are reviewed. Patients with acute SAH should have blood pressure lowered to a normal range with nonvasodilating agents such as nicardipine, labetalol, or esmolol. Patients with cerebellar hemorrhages or with depressed mental status and radiographic evidence of hydrocephalus should undergo urgent neurosurgical evaluation. Based on the clinical examination and CT findings, further imaging studies may be necessary, including MRI or conventional x-ray angiography. Stuporous or comatose patients generally are treated presumptively for elevated ICP, with tracheal intubation and hyperventilation, mannitol administration, and elevation of the head of the bed while surgical consultation is obtained (Chap. 258).

SUBARACHNOID HEMORRHAGE Excluding head trauma, the most common cause of SAH is rupture of a saccular aneurysm. Other causes

TABLE 349-6 *Causes of Intracranial Hemorrhage*

Cause	Location	Comments
Head trauma	Intraparenchymal: frontal lobes, anterior temporal lobes; subarachnoid	Coup and contracoup injury during brain deceleration
Hypertensive hemorrhage	Putamen, globus pallidus, thalamus, cerebellar hemisphere, pons	Chronic hypertension produces hemorrhage from small (~100 μm) vessels in these regions
Transformation of prior ischemic infarction	Basal ganglion, subcortical regions, lobar	Occurs in 1–6% of ischemic strokes with predilection for large hemispheric infarctions
Metastatic brain tumor	Lobar	Lung, choriocarcinoma, melanoma, renal cell carcinoma, thyroid, atrial myxoma
Coagulopathy	Any	Uncommon cause; often associated with prior stroke or underlying vascular anomaly
Drug	Lobar, subarachnoid	Cocaine, amphetamine, phenylpropranolamine
Arteriovenous malformation	Lobar, intraventricular, subarachnoid	Risk is ~2–4% per year for bleeding
Aneurysm	Subarachnoid, intraparenchymal, rarely subdural	Mycotic and nonmycotic forms of aneurysms
Amyloid angiopathy	Lobar	Degenerative disease of intracranial vessels; linkage to Alzheimer's disease, rare in patients <60
Cavernous angioma	Intraparenchymal	Multiple cavernous angiomas linked to chromosome 7q
Dural arteriovenous fistula	Lobar, rarely subarachnoid	Produces bleeding by venous hypertension
Capillary telangiectasias	Usually brainstem	Rare cause of hemorrhage

include bleeding from a vascular anomaly and extension into the subarachnoid space from a primary intracerebral hemorrhage. Some idiopathic SAHs are localized to the perimesencephalic cisterns and are benign; they probably have a venous or capillary source, and angiography is unrevealing.

Saccular ("Berry") Aneurysm Autopsy and angiography studies have found that about 2% of adults harbor intracranial aneurysms, for a prevalence of 4 million persons in the United States; the aneurysm will rupture, producing SAH, in 25,000 to 30,000 cases per year. For patients who arrive alive at hospital, the mortality rate over the next month is about 45%. Of those who survive, more than half are left with major neurologic deficits as a result of the initial hemorrhage, cerebral vasospasm with infarction, or hydrocephalus. If the patient survives but the aneurysm is not obliterated, the rate of rebleeding is about 20% in the first 2 weeks and about 3% per year afterwards. Given these alarming figures, the major therapeutic emphasis is on preventing the predictable early complications of the SAH.

Unruptured, asymptomatic aneurysms are much less dangerous than a recently ruptured aneurysm. The annual risk of rupture for aneurysms <10 mm in size is ~0.1%, and for aneurysms ≥10 mm in size is ~0.5 to 1%; the surgical morbidity far exceeds these percentages. As more data become available, a true risk-benefit analysis for treating these aneurysms will result.

Giant aneurysms, those >2.5 cm in diameter, occur at the same sites (see below) as small aneurysms and account for 5% of cases. The three most common locations are the terminal internal carotid artery, MCA bifurcation, and top of the basilar artery. Their risk of rupture is about 6% in the first year after identification and may remain high indefinitely. They often cause symptoms by compressing the adjacent brain or cranial nerves.

Mycotic aneurysms are usually located distal to the first bifurcation of major arteries of the circle of Willis. Most result from infected emboli due to bacterial endocarditis causing septic degeneration of arteries and subsequent dilatation and rupture. Whether these lesions should be sought and repaired prior to rupture, or left to heal spontaneously, is controversial.

PATHOPHYSIOLOGY Saccular aneurysms occur at the bifurcations of the large to medium-sized intracranial arteries; rupture is into the subarachnoid space in the basal cisterns and often into the parenchyma of the adjacent brain. Approximately 85% of aneurysms occur in the anterior circulation, mostly on the circle of Willis. About 20% of patients have multiple aneurysms, many at mirror sites bilaterally. As an aneurysm develops, it typically forms a neck with a dome. The length of the neck and the size of the dome vary greatly and are factors that are important in planning neurosurgical obliteration or endovascular embolization. The arterial internal elastic lamina disappears at the base of the neck. The media thins, and connective tissue replaces smooth-muscle cells. At the site of rupture (most often the dome) the wall thins, and the tear that allows bleeding is often no more than 0.5 mm long. Aneurysm size and site are important in predicting risk of rupture. Those >7 mm in diameter and those at the top of the basilar artery and at the origin of the posterior communicating artery are at greater risk of rupture.

CLINICAL MANIFESTATIONS Most unruptured intracranial aneurysms are completely asymptomatic. Symptoms are usually due to rupture and resultant SAH. At the moment of aneurysmal rupture with major SAH, the ICP suddenly rises. This may account for the sudden transient loss of consciousness that occurs in nearly half of patients. Sudden loss of consciousness may be preceded by a brief moment of excruciating headache, but most patients first complain of headache upon regaining consciousness. In 10% of cases, aneurysmal bleeding is severe enough to cause loss of consciousness for several days. In about 45% of cases, severe headache associated with exertion is the presenting complaint. The patient often calls the headache "the worst headache of my life." Occasionally these ruptures may present as headache of only moderate intensity or as a change in the patient's usual headache pattern. The headache is usually generalized, often with neck stiffness, and vomiting is common.

Although sudden headache in the absence of focal neurologic symptoms is the hallmark of aneurysmal rupture, focal neurologic deficits may occur. Anterior communicating artery or MCA bifurcation aneurysms may rupture into the adjacent brain or subdural space and form a hematoma large enough to produce mass effect. The common deficits that result include hemiparesis, aphasia, and abulia.

Occasionally, prodromal symptoms suggest the location of a progressively enlarging unruptured aneurysm. A third cranial nerve palsy, particularly when associated with pupillary dilatation, loss of ipsilateral (but retained contralateral) light reflex, and focal pain above or behind the eye, may occur with an expanding aneurysm at the junction of the posterior communicating artery and the internal carotid artery. A sixth nerve palsy may indicate an aneurysm in the cavernous sinus, and visual field defects can occur with an expanding supraclinoid carotid or anterior cerebral artery aneurysm. Occipital and posterior cervical pain may signal a posterior inferior cerebellar artery or anterior inferior cerebellar artery aneurysm. Pain in or behind the eye and in the low temple can occur with an expanding MCA aneurysm. Thunderclap headache is a variant of migraine that simulates a SAH. Before concluding that a patient with sudden, severe headache has thunderclap migraine, a definitive workup for aneurysm or other intracranial pathology is required.

Aneurysms can undergo small ruptures and leaks of blood into the subarachnoid space, so-called sentinel bleeds. Sudden unexplained headache at any location should raise suspicion of SAH and be investigated, because a major hemorrhage may be imminent.

DELAYED NEUROLOGIC DEFICITS   There are four major causes of delayed neurologic deficits: rerupture, hydrocephalus, vasospasm, and hyponatremia.

1. *Rerupture.* The incidence of rerupture of an untreated aneurysm in the first month following SAH is ~30%, with the peak in the first 7 days. Rerupture is associated with a 60% mortality and poor outcome. Early treatment eliminates this risk.

2. *Hydrocephalus.* Acute hydrocephalus can cause stupor and coma. More often, subacute hydrocephalus develops over a few days or weeks and causes progressive drowsiness or slowed mentation (abulia) with incontinence. Hydrocephalus is differentiated from cerebral vasospasm with a CT scan, TCD ultrasound, or conventional x-ray angiography. Hydrocephalus may clear spontaneously or require temporary ventricular drainage. Chronic hydrocephalus may develop weeks to months after SAH and manifest as gait difficulty, incontinence, or impaired mentation. Subtle signs may be a lack of initiative in conversation or a failure to recover independence.

3. *Vasospasm.* Narrowing of the arteries at the base of the brain following SAH causes symptomatic ischemia and infarction in ~30% of patients and is the major cause of delayed morbidity and death. Signs of ischemia appear 4 to 14 days after the hemorrhage, most often at 7 days. The severity and distribution of vasospasm determine whether infarction will occur.

Delayed vasospasm is believed to result from direct effects of clotted blood and its breakdown products on the artery. In general, the more blood that surrounds the arteries, the greater the chance of symptomatic vasospasm. Spasm of major arteries produces symptoms referable to the appropriate vascular territory (see "Stroke Syndromes," above). All of these focal symptoms may present abruptly, fluctuate, or develop over a few days. In most cases, focal spasm is preceded by a decline in mental status.

Vasospasm can be detected reliably with conventional x-ray angiography, but this invasive procedure is expensive and carries risk of stroke and other complications. TCD ultrasound is based on the principle that the velocity of blood flow within an artery will rise as the lumen diameter is narrowed. By directing the probe along the MCA and proximal ACA, carotid terminus, vertebral, and basilar arteries on a daily or every-other-day basis, vasospasm can be reliably detected and treatments initiated to prevent cerebral ischemia (see below). CT angiography is another method that can reliably detect vasospasm.

Severe cerebral edema in patients with infarction from vasospasm may increase the ICP enough to reduce cerebral perfusion pressure. Treatment is with mannitol and hyperventilation (Chap. 258).

4. *Hyponatremia.* Hyponatremia may be profound and develop quickly in the first 2 weeks following SAH. It usually results from inappropriate secretion of vasopressin (Chap. 319) and secretion of atrial and brain natriuretic factors, which produce a natriuresis. This "cerebral salt-wasting syndrome" clears over the course of 1 to 2 weeks and, in the setting of SAH, should not be treated with free-water restriction as this may increase the risk of stroke (see below).

LABORATORY EVALUATION AND IMAGING (Fig. 349-14)   The hallmark of aneurysmal rupture is blood in the cerebrospinal fluid (CSF). More than 95% of cases have enough blood to be visualized on a high-quality noncontrast CT scan obtained within 72 h. If the scan fails to establish the diagnosis of SAH and no mass lesion or obstructive hydrocephalus is found, a lumbar puncture should be performed to establish the presence of subarachnoid blood. Lysis of the red blood cells and subsequent conversion of hemoglobin to bilirubin stains the spinal fluid yellow within 6 to 12 h of SAH. This xanthochromic spinal fluid peaks in intensity at 48 h and lasts for 1 to 4 weeks, depending on the amount of subarachnoid blood.

The extent and location of subarachnoid blood on noncontrast CT scan help locate the underlying aneurysm, identify the cause of any neurologic deficit, and predict delayed vasospasm. A high incidence of symptomatic vasospasm in the MCA and ACA has been found when early CT scans show subarachnoid clots >5 × 3 mm in the basal cisterns or layers of blood >1 mm thick in the cerebral fissures. CT scans less reliably predict vasospasm in the vertebral, basilar, or posterior cerebral arteries.

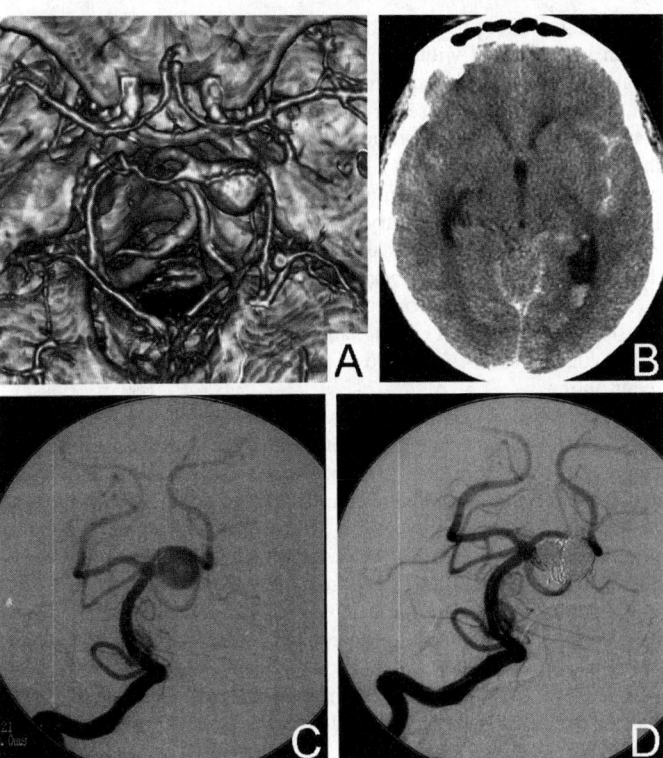

FIGURE 349-14   Subarachnoid hemorrhage. *A.* Computed tomography (CT) angiography revealing an aneurysm of the left superior cerebellar artery. *B.* Noncontrast CT scan at the level of the third ventricle revealing subarachnoid blood in the left sylvian fissure (bright) and within the left lateral ventricle. *C.* Conventional anteroposterior x-ray angiogram of the right vertebral and basilar artery showing the large aneurysm. *D.* Conventional angiogram following coil embolization of the aneurysm, whereby the aneurysm body is filled with platinum delivered through a microcatheter navigated from the femoral artery into the aneurysm neck.

Lumbar puncture prior to an imaging procedure is indicated only if a CT scan is not available at the time of the suspected SAH. Once the diagnosis of hemorrhage from a ruptured saccular aneurysm is suspected, four-vessel conventional x-ray angiography (both carotids and both vertebrals) is generally performed to localize and define the anatomic details of the aneurysm and to determine if other unruptured aneurysms exist (Fig. 349-14). CT angiography is an alternative method for locating the aneurysm and may be sufficient to plan definitive therapy. At some centers, the ruptured aneurysm can be treated using endovascular techniques at the time of the initial angiogram (see below).

The ECG frequently shows ST-segment and T-wave changes similar to those associated with cardiac ischemia. Prolonged QRS complex, increased QT interval, and prominent "peaked" or deeply inverted symmetric T waves are usually secondary to the intracranial hemorrhage. There is evidence that structural myocardial lesions produced by circulating catecholamines may occur after SAH, causing reversible cardiomyopathy sufficient to cause shock or congestive heart failure. Serious ventricular dysrhythmias are unusual.

Close monitoring (daily or twice daily) of electrolytes is important because hyponatremia can occur precipitously during the first 2 weeks following SAH (see above).

℞ TREATMENT

Early aneurysm repair prevents rerupture and allows the safe application of techniques to improve blood flow (e.g., induced hypertension and hypervolemia) should symptomatic vasospasm develop. An aneurysm can be "clipped" by a neurosurgeon or "coiled" by a neurointerventional radiologist. Surgical repair involves placing a metal clip across the aneurysm neck, thereby immediately eliminating the risk of rebleeding. This approach requires craniotomy and brain retraction, which is associated with neurologic morbidity. The newer endovascular technique involves placing platinum coils within the aneurysm via a catheter that is passed from the femoral artery. The aneurysm is packed tightly to enhance thrombosis and over time is walled-off from the circulation (Fig. 349-14). The only prospective randomized trial of surgery versus endovascular treatment for ruptured aneurysm, the International Study of Aneurysm Treatment (ISAT), was terminated early when 24% of patients treated with endovascular therapy were dead or dependent at 1 year compared to 31% treated with surgery, a 23% relative reduction. However, some aneurysms have a morphology that is not amenable to coiling, and only a few endovascular centers are available world-wide. Thus, surgery remains an important treatment option.

The medical management of SAH centers on protecting the airway, managing blood pressure before and after aneurysm treatment, preventing rebleeding prior to treatment, managing vasospasm, treating hydrocephalus, treating hyponatremia, and preventing pulmonary embolus.

Intracranial hypertension following aneurysmal rupture occurs secondary to subarachnoid blood, parenchymal hematoma, acute hydrocephalus, or loss of vascular autoregulation. Patients who are stuporous should undergo emergent ventriculostomy to prevent cerebral ischemia from high ICP. Medical therapies designed to combat raised ICP (e.g., mild hyperventilation, mannitol, and sedation) can also be used as needed (Chap. 258). High ICP refractory to treatment is a poor prognostic sign.

Prior to definitive treatment of the ruptured aneurysm, care is required to maintain adequate cerebral perfusion pressure while avoiding excessive elevation of arterial pressure. Occasionally an intracranial hematoma causing neurologic deterioration requires removal.

Because rebleeding is common, all patients who are not candidates for early aneurysm repair are put on bed rest in a quiet room and are given stool softeners to prevent straining. If headache or neck pain is severe, mild sedation and analgesia are prescribed. Extreme sedation is avoided because it can obscure changes in neurologic status. Adequate hydration is necessary to avoid a decrease in blood volume predisposing to brain ischemia.

Seizures are uncommon at the onset of aneurysmal rupture. The quivering, jerking, and extensor posturing that often accompany loss of consciousness are probably related to the sharp rise in ICP or, perhaps, acute generalized vasospasm. However, phenytoin is often given as prophylactic therapy since a seizure may promote rebleeding.

Glucocorticoids may help reduce the head and neck ache caused by the irritative effect of the subarachnoid blood. There is no good evidence that they reduce cerebral edema, are neuroprotective, or reduce vascular injury, and their routine use therefore is not recommended.

Antifibrinolytic agents are not routinely prescribed but may be considered in patients in whom aneurysm treatment cannot proceed immediately. They are associated with a reduced incidence of aneurysmal rerupture but are also associated with an increased incidence of delayed cerebral infarction and DVT.

Vasospasm remains the leading cause of morbidity and mortality following aneurysmal SAH and treatment of the aneurysm. Treatment with the calcium channel antagonist nimodipine (60 mg orally every 4 h) improves outcome, perhaps by preventing ischemic injury rather than reducing the risk of vasospasm. Nimodipine can cause significant hypotension in some patients, which may worsen cerebral ischemia in patients with vasospasm. Symptomatic cerebral vasospasm can also be treated by increasing the cerebral perfusion pressure by raising mean arterial pressure through plasma volume expansion and the judicious use of vasopressor agents, usually phenylephrine or dopamine. Raised perfusion pressure has been associated with clinical improvement in many patients, but high arterial pressure may promote rebleeding in unprotected aneurysms. Treatment with induced hypertension and hypervolemia generally requires monitoring of arterial and central venous pressures. Volume expansion helps prevent hypotension, augments cardiac output, and reduces blood viscosity by reducing the hematocrit. This method is called "triple-H" (hypertension, hemodilution, and hypervolemic) therapy.

If symptomatic vasospasm persists despite optimal medical therapy, intraarterial vasodilators and percutaneous transluminal angioplasty are considered. Vasodilatation following angioplasty appears to be permanent, allowing triple-H therapy to be tapered sooner. The pharmacologic vasodilators (verapamil and nicardipine) do not last more than 8 to 24 h, and therefore multiple treatments may be required until the subarachnoid blood is reabsorbed.

Acute hydrocephalus can cause stupor or coma. It may clear spontaneously or require temporary ventricular drainage. When chronic hydrocephalus develops, ventricular shunting is the treatment of choice.

Free-water restriction is contraindicated in patients with SAH at risk for vasospasm because hypovolemia and hypotension may occur and precipitate cerebral ischemia. Many patients continue to experience a decline in serum sodium despite receiving parenteral fluids containing normal saline. Frequently, supplemental oral salt coupled with normal saline will mitigate hyponatremia, but often patients also require hypertonic saline. Care must be taken not to correct serum sodium too quickly in patients with marked hyponatremia of several days' duration, as central pontine myelinolysis (Chap. 258) may occur.

All patients should have pneumatic compression stockings applied to prevent pulmonary embolism. Systemic heparin is contraindicated in patients with ruptured and untreated aneurysms; it is a relative contraindication following craniotomy, and it may delay thrombosis of a coiled aneurysm.

INTRAPARENCHYMAL HEMORRHAGE   Intraparenchymal hemorrhage is the most common type of intracranial hemorrhage. It accounts for about 10% of all strokes and is associated with a 50% case fatality rate. Incidence rates are particularly high in Asians and African Americans. Hypertension, trauma, and cerebral amyloid angiopathy cause the majority of these hemorrhages. Advanced age and heavy alcohol consumption increase the risk, and cocaine use is one of the most important causes in the young.

Hypertensive Intraparenchymal Hemorrhage ■ *PATHOPHYSIOLOGY* Hypertensive intraparenchymal hemorrhage (hypertensive hemorrhage or hypertensive intracerebral hemorrhage) usually results from spontaneous rupture of a small penetrating artery deep in the brain. The most common sites are the basal ganglia (putamen, thalamus, and adjacent deep white matter), deep cerebellum, and pons. When hemorrhages occur in other brain areas or in nonhypertensive patients, greater consideration should be given to hemorrhagic disorders, neoplasms, vascular malformations, and other causes. The small arteries in these areas seem most prone to hypertension-induced vascular injury. The hemorrhage may be small or a large clot may form and compress adjacent tissue, causing herniation and death. Blood may dissect into the ventricular space, which substantially increases morbidity and may cause hydrocephalus.

Most hypertensive intraparenchymal hemorrhages develop over 30 to 90 min, whereas those associated with anticoagulant therapy may evolve for as long as 24 to 48 h. Within 48 h macrophages begin to phagocytize the hemorrhage at its outer surface. After 1 to 6 months, the hemorrhage is generally resolved to a slitlike orange cavity lined with glial scar and hemosiderin-laden macrophages.

CLINICAL MANIFESTATIONS Although not particularly associated with exertion, intracerebral hemorrhages almost always occur while the patient is awake and sometimes when stressed. The hemorrhage generally presents as the abrupt onset of focal neurologic deficit. Seizures are uncommon. The focal deficit typically worsens steadily over 30 to 90 min and is associated with a diminishing level of consciousness and signs of increased ICP, such as headache and vomiting.

The putamen is the most common site for hypertensive hemorrhage, and the adjacent internal capsule is invariably damaged (Fig.

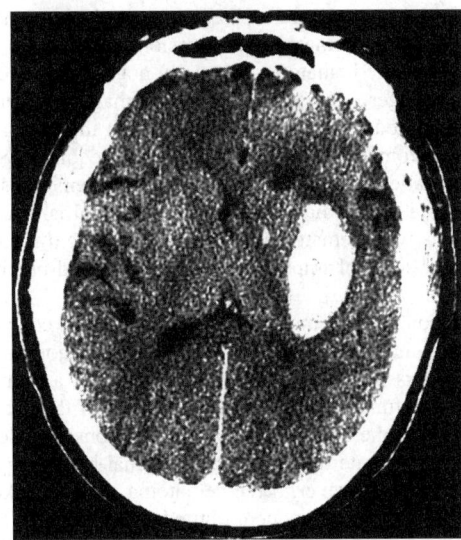

FIGURE 349-15　Transaxial noncontrast computed tomography scan through the region of the basal ganglia reveals a hematoma involving the left putamen in a patient with rapidly progressive onset of right hemiparesis. This is a typical hypertensive hemorrhage.

349-15). Contralateral hemiparesis is therefore the sentinel sign. When mild, the face sags on one side over 5 to 30 min, speech becomes slurred, the arm and leg gradually weaken, and the eyes deviate away from the side of the hemiparesis. The paralysis may worsen until the affected limbs become flaccid or extend rigidly. When hemorrhages are large, drowsiness gives way to stupor as signs of upper brainstem compression appear. Coma ensues, accompanied by deep, irregular, or intermittent respiration, a dilated and fixed ipsilateral pupil, and decerebrate rigidity. In milder cases, edema in adjacent brain tissue may cause progressive deterioration over 12 to 72 h.

Thalamic hemorrhages also produce a contralateral hemiplegia or hemiparesis from pressure on, or dissection into, the adjacent internal capsule. A prominent sensory deficit involving all modalities is usually present. Aphasia, often with preserved verbal repetition, may occur after hemorrhage into the dominant thalamus, and apractognosia or mutism occurs in some cases of nondominant hemorrhage. There may also be a homonymous visual field defect. Thalamic hemorrhages cause several typical ocular disturbances by virtue of extension medially into the upper midbrain. These include deviation of the eyes downward and inward so that they appear to be looking at the nose, unequal pupils with absence of light reaction, skew deviation with the eye opposite the hemorrhage displaced downward and medially, ipsilateral Horner's syndrome, absence of convergence, paralysis of vertical gaze, and retraction nystagmus. Patients may later develop a chronic, contralateral pain syndrome (Déjerine-Roussy syndrome).

In pontine hemorrhages, deep coma with quadriplegia usually occurs over a few minutes. There is often prominent decerebrate rigidity and "pin-point" (1 mm) pupils that react to light. There is impairment of reflex horizontal eye movements evoked by head turning (doll's-head or oculocephalic maneuver) or by irrigation of the ears with ice water (Chap. 257). Hyperpnea, severe hypertension, and hyperhidrosis are common. Death often occurs within a few hours, but small hemorrhages are compatible with survival.

Cerebellar hemorrhages usually develop over several hours and are characterized by occipital headache, repeated vomiting, and ataxia of gait. In mild cases there may be no other neurologic signs other than gait ataxia. Dizziness or vertigo may be prominent. There is often paresis of conjugate lateral gaze toward the side of the hemorrhage, forced deviation of the eyes to the opposite side, or an ipsilateral sixth nerve palsy. Less frequent ocular signs include blepharospasm, involuntary closure of one eye, ocular bobbing, and skew deviation. Dysarthria and dysphagia may occur. As the hours pass, the patient often becomes stuporous and then comatose from brainstem compression or

obstructive hydrocephalus; immediate surgical evacuation before brainstem compression occurs may be lifesaving. Hydrocephalus from fourth ventricle compression can be relieved by external ventricular drainage, but definitive hematoma evacuation is essential for survival. If the deep cerebellar nuclei are spared, full recovery is common.

Lobar Hemorrhage　Symptoms and signs appear over several minutes. Most lobar hemorrhages are small and cause a restricted clinical syndrome that simulates an embolus to an artery supplying one lobe. For example, the major neurologic deficit with an occipital hemorrhage is hemianopia; with a left temporal hemorrhage, aphasia and delirium; with a parietal hemorrhage, hemisensory loss; and with frontal hemorrhage, arm weakness. Large hemorrhages may be associated with stupor or coma if they compress the thalamus or midbrain. Most patients with lobar hemorrhages have focal headaches, and more than half vomit or are drowsy. Stiff neck and seizures are uncommon.

Other Causes of Intracerebral Hemorrhage　*Cerebral amyloid angiopathy* is a disease of the elderly in which arteriolar degeneration occurs and amyloid is deposited in the walls of the cerebral arteries. Amyloid angiopathy causes both single and recurrent lobar hemorrhages and is probably the most common cause of lobar hemorrhage in the elderly. It accounts for some intracranial hemorrhages associated with intravenous thrombolysis given for MI. This disorder can be suspected in patients who present with multiple hemorrhages (and infarcts) over several months or years, or in patients with "micro-bleeds" seen on brain MRI sequences sensitive for hemosiderin, but it is definitively diagnosed by demonstration of Congo red staining of amyloid in cerebral vessels. There is no specific therapy.

Cocaine is a frequent cause of stroke in young (age < 45) patients. Intracerebral hemorrhage, ischemic stroke, and SAH are all associated with cocaine use. Angiographic findings vary from completely normal arteries to large-vessel occlusion or stenosis, vasospasm, or changes consistent with vasculitis. The mechanism of cocaine-related stroke is not known, but cocaine enhances sympathetic activity causing acute, sometimes severe, hypertension, and this may lead to hemorrhage. Slightly more than half of cocaine-related intracranial hemorrhages are intracerebral, and the rest are subarachnoid. In cases of SAH, a saccular aneurysm is usually identified. Presumably, acute hypertension causes aneurysmal rupture.

Head injury often causes intracranial bleeding. The common sites are intracerebral (especially temporal and inferior frontal lobes) and into the subarachnoid, subdural, and epidural spaces. Trauma must be considered in any patient with an unexplained acute neurologic deficit (hemiparesis, stupor, or confusion), particularly if the deficit occurred in the context of a fall (Chap. 357).

Intracranial hemorrhages associated with *anticoagulant therapy* can occur at any location; they are often lobar or subdural. Anticoagulant-related intracerebral hemorrhages may evolve slowly, over 24 to 48 h. Coagulopathy should be reversed with fresh-frozen plasma or factor replacement and vitamin K to limit the volume of hemorrhage. When intracerebral hemorrhage is associated with thrombocytopenia (platelet count < $50,000/\mu L$), transfusion of fresh platelets is indicated. Intracerebral hemorrhage associated with *hematologic disorders* (leukemia, aplastic anemia, thrombocytopenic purpura) can occur at any site and may present as multiple intracerebral hemorrhages. Skin and mucous membrane bleeding is usually evident and offers a diagnostic clue.

Hemorrhage into a *brain tumor* may be the first manifestation of neoplasm. Choriocarcinoma, malignant melanoma, renal cell carcinoma, and bronchogenic carcinoma are among the most common metastatic tumors associated with intracerebral hemorrhage. Glioblastoma multiforme in adults and medulloblastoma in children may also have areas of intracerebral hemorrhage.

Hypertensive encephalopathy is a complication of malignant hypertension. In this acute syndrome, severe hypertension is associated with headache, nausea, vomiting, convulsions, confusion, stupor, and coma. Focal or lateralizing neurologic signs, either transitory or permanent, may occur but are infrequent and therefore suggest some other vascular disease (hemorrhage, embolism, or atherosclerotic thrombosis). There are retinal hemorrhages, exudates, papilledema (hypertensive retinopathy), and evidence of renal and cardiac disease. In most cases ICP and CSF protein levels are elevated. The hypertension may be essential or due to chronic renal disease, acute glomerulonephritis, acute toxemia of pregnancy, pheochromocytoma, or other causes. Lowering the blood pressure reverses the process, but stroke can occur, especially if blood pressure is lowered too rapidly. Neuropathologic examination reveals multifocal to diffuse cerebral edema and hemorrhages of various sizes from petechial to massive. Microscopically, there are necrosis of arterioles, minute cerebral infarcts, and hemorrhages. The term *hypertensive encephalopathy* should be reserved for this syndrome and not for chronic recurrent headaches, dizziness, recurrent TIAs, or small strokes that often occur in association with high blood pressure.

Primary intraventricular hemorrhage is rare. It usually begins within the substance of the brain and dissects into the ventricular system without leaving signs of intraparenchymal hemorrhage. Alternatively, bleeding can arise from periependymal veins. Vasculitis, usually polyarteritis nodosa or lupus erythematosus, can produce hemorrhage into any region of the central nervous system; most hemorrhages are associated with hypertension, but the arteritis itself may cause bleeding by disrupting the vessel wall. *Sepsis* can cause small petechial hemorrhages throughout the cerebral white matter. *Moyamoya disease*, mainly an occlusive arterial disease that causes ischemic symptoms, may on occasion produce intraparenchymal hemorrhage, particularly in the young. Hemorrhages into the spinal cord are usually the result of an AVM or metastatic tumor. *Epidural spinal hemorrhage* produces a rapidly evolving syndrome of spinal cord or nerve root compression (Chap. 356). Spinal hemorrhages usually present with sudden back pain and some manifestation of myelopathy.

Laboratory and Imaging Evaluation   The CT scan reliably detects acute focal hemorrhages in the supratentorial space. Small pontine hemorrhages may not be identified because of motion and bone-induced artifact that obscure structures in the posterior fossa. After the first 2 weeks, x-ray attenuation values of clotted blood diminish until they become isodense with surrounding brain. Mass effect and edema may remain. In some cases, a surrounding rim of contrast enhancement appears after 2 to 4 weeks and may persist for months. MRI, though more sensitive for delineating posterior fossa lesions, is generally not necessary in most instances. Images of flowing blood on MRI scan may identify AVMs as the cause of the hemorrhage. MRI, CT angiography, and conventional x-ray angiography are used when the cause of intracranial hemorrhage is uncertain, particularly if the patient is young or not hypertensive and the hematoma is not in one of the four usual sites for hypertensive hemorrhage. For example, hemorrhage into the temporal lobe suggests rupture of a MCA saccular aneurysm.

Since patients typically have focal neurologic signs and obtundation, and often show signs of increased ICP, a lumbar puncture should be avoided as it may induce cerebral herniation.

℞ TREATMENT

Acute Management   Nearly 50% of patients with a hypertensive intracerebral hemorrhage die, but others may have a good to complete recovery if they survive the initial hemorrhage. The volume and location of the hematoma determine the prognosis. In general, supratentorial hematomas with volumes <30 mL have a good prognosis; 30 to 60 mL, an intermediate prognosis; and >60 mL, a poor prognosis during initial hospitalization. Extension into the ventricular system worsens the prognosis. Except in patients who are on therapeutic anticoagulation or who have a bleeding disorder, little can be done about the hemorrhage itself. Hematomas may expand for several hours following the initial hemorrhage, so treating severe hypertension seems reasonable to prevent hematoma progression.

Evacuation of the hematoma is usually not helpful, except in cerebellar hemorrhages. For cerebellar hemorrhages, a neurosurgeon should be consulted immediately to assist with the evaluation; most cerebellar hematomas >3 cm in diameter will require surgical evacuation. If the patient is alert without focal brainstem signs and if the hematoma is <1 cm in diameter, surgical removal is usually unnecessary. Patients with hematomas between 1 and 3 cm require careful observation for signs of impaired consciousness and precipitous respiratory failure.

Tissue surrounding hematomas is displaced and compressed but not necessarily infarcted. Hence, in survivors, major improvement commonly occurs as the hematoma is reabsorbed and the adjacent tissue regains its function. Careful management of the patient during the acute phase of the hemorrhage can lead to considerable recovery.

Surprisingly, despite large intraparenchymal hemorrhages, ICP is often not elevated. However, if the hematoma causes marked midline shift of structures with consequent obtundation, coma, or hydrocephalus, osmotic agents coupled with induced hyperventilation can be instituted to lower ICP (Chap. 258). These maneuvers will provide enough time to place a ventriculostomy or ICP monitor. Once ICP is recorded, further hyperventilation and osmotic therapy can be tailored to the individual patient. For example, if ICP is found to be high, CSF can be drained from the ventricular space and osmotic therapy continued; persistent or progressive elevation in ICP may prompt surgical evacuation of the clot or withdrawal of support. Alternately, if ICP is normal or only mildly elevated, induced hyperventilation can be reversed and osmotic therapy tapered. Since hyperventilation may actually produce ischemia by cerebral vasoconstriction, induced hyperventilation should be limited to acute resuscitation of the patient with presumptive high ICP and eliminated once other treatments (osmotic therapy or surgical treatments) have been instituted. Glucocorticoids are not helpful for the edema from intracerebral hematoma.

Prevention   Hypertension is the leading cause of primary intracerebral hemorrhage. Prevention is aimed at reducing hypertension, excessive alcohol use, and use of illicit drugs such as cocaine and amphetamines.

VASCULAR ANOMALIES

Vascular anomalies can be divided into congenital vascular malformations and acquired vascular lesions.

CONGENITAL VASCULAR MALFORMATIONS   True *arteriovenous malformations*, venous anomalies, and capillary telangiectasias are lesions that usually remain clinically silent through life. Although most AVMs are congenital, cases of acquired lesions have been reported.

True AVMs are congenital shunts between the arterial and venous systems that may present as headache, seizures, and intracranial hemorrhage. AVMs consist of a tangle of abnormal vessels across the cortical surface or deep within the brain substance. AVMs vary in size from a small blemish a few millimeters in diameter to a large mass of tortuous channels composing an arteriovenous shunt of sufficient magnitude to raise cardiac output. The blood vessels forming the tangle interposed between arteries and veins are usually abnormally thin and do not have a normal structure. AVMs occur in all parts of the cerebral hemispheres, brainstem, and spinal cord, but the largest ones are most frequently in the posterior half of the hemispheres, commonly forming a wedge-shaped lesion extending from the cortex to the ventricle.

Although the lesion is present from birth, bleeding or other symptoms are most common between the ages of 10 and 30, occasionally as late as the fifties. AVMs are more frequent in men, and rare familial cases have been described.

Headache (without bleeding) may be hemicranial and throbbing, like migraine, or diffuse. Focal seizures, with or without generalization, occur in about 30% of cases. Half of AVMs become evident as intracerebral hemorrhages. In most, the hemorrhage is mainly intraparenchymal with extension into the subarachnoid space in some cases. Blood is usually not deposited in the basal cisterns, and symptomatic cerebral vasospasm is rare. The risk of rerupture is about 18% per year and is particular high in the first few weeks. Hemorrhages may be massive, leading to death, or may be as small as 1 cm in diameter, leading to minor focal symptoms or no deficit. The AVM may be large enough to steal blood away from adjacent normal brain tissue or to increase venous pressure significantly to produce venous ischemia locally and in remote areas of the brain. This is seen most often with large AVMs in the territory of the MCA.

Large AVMs of the anterior circulation may be associated with a systolic and diastolic bruit (sometimes self-audible) over the eye, forehead, or neck and a bounding carotid pulse. Headache at the onset of AVM rupture is not generally as explosive as with aneurysmal rupture. MRI is better than CT for diagnosis, although contrast CT scanning sometimes detects calcification of the AVM.

Surgical treatment of symptomatic AVMs, often with preoperative embolization to reduce operative bleeding, is usually indicated for accessible lesions. Stereotaxic radiation, an alternative to surgery, can produce a slow sclerosis of arterial channels over 2 to 3 years.

Patients with asymptomatic AVMs have about a 2% per year risk for hemorrhage. Several angiographic features of the AVM can be used to help predict future bleeding risk. Paradoxically, smaller lesions seem to have a higher hemorrhage rate. The mortality rate with each bleed is about 15%. Given this natural history, surgical treatment is probably indicated for most AVMs that can be treated with reasonable surgical risk.

Venous anomalies are the result of development of anomalous cerebral, cerebellar, or brainstem drainage. These structures, unlike AVMs, are functional venous channels. They are of little clinical significance and should be ignored if found incidentally on brain imaging studies. Surgical resection of these anomalies may result in venous infarction and hemorrhage. Venous anomalies may be associated with cavernous malformations (see below), which do carry some bleeding risk. If resection of a cavernous malformation is attempted, the venous anomaly should not be disturbed.

Capillary telangiectasias are true capillary malformations that often form extensive vascular networks through an otherwise normal brain structure. The pons and deep cerebral white matter are typical locations, and these capillary malformations can be seen in patients with hereditary hemorrhagic telangiectasia (Osler-Rendu-Weber) syndrome. If bleeding does occur, it rarely produces mass effect or significant symptoms. No treatment options exist.

ACQUIRED VASCULAR LESIONS   *Cavernous angiomas* are tufts of capillary sinusoids that form within the deep hemispheric white matter and brainstem with no normal intervening neural structures. The pathogenesis is unclear. Familial cavernous angiomas have been mapped to several different chromosomal loci; the gene responsible for the 7q-linked form encodes a protein that interacts with a member of the RAS family of GTPases. Cavernous angiomas are typically <1 cm in diameter and are often associated with a venous anomaly. Bleeding is usually of small volume, causing slight mass effect only. The bleeding risk for single cavernous malformations is 0.7 to 1.5% per year and may be higher for patients with prior clinical hemorrhage or multiple malformations. Seizures may occur if the malformation is located near the cerebral cortex. Surgical resection eliminates bleeding risk and may reduce seizure risk, but it is reserved for those malformations that form near the brain surface. Radiation treatment has not been shown to be of benefit.

Dural arteriovenous fistulas are acquired connections usually from a dural artery to a dural sinus. Patients may complain of a pulse-synchronous cephalic bruit ("pulsatile tinnitus") and headache. Depending on the magnitude of the shunt, venous pressures may rise high enough to cause cortical ischemia or venous hypertension and hemorrhage. Surgical and endovascular techniques are usually curative. These fistulas may form because of trauma, but most are idiopathic. There is an association between fistulas and dural sinus thrombosis. Fistulas have been observed to appear months to years following venous sinus thrombosis, suggesting that angiogenesis factors elaborated from the thrombotic process may cause these anomalous connections to form. Alternatively, dural arteriovenous fistulas can produce venous sinus occlusion over time, perhaps from the high pressure and high flow through a venous structure.

FURTHER READING

ADAMS HP et al: Guidelines for the early management of patients with ischemic stroke: A scientific statement from the Stroke Council of the American Stroke Association. Stroke 34:1056, 2003

JOHNSTON SC: Clinical practice. Transient ischemic attack. N Engl J Med 347:1687, 2002

———— et al: Recommendations for the endovascular treatment of intracranial aneurysms: A statement for healthcare professionals from the Committee on Cerebrovascular Imaging of the American Heart Association Council on Cardiovascular Radiology. Stroke. 33:2536, 2002

MAS JL et al: Recurrent cerebrovascular events associated with patent foramen ovale, atrial septal aneurysm, or both. N Engl J Med 345:1740, 2001

MOHR JP et al: A comparison of warfarin and aspirin for the prevention of recurrent ischemic stroke. N Engl J Med. 345:1444, 2001

MOLYNEUX A: International Subarachnoid Aneurysm Trial (ISAT) of neurosurgical clipping versus endovascular coiling in 2143 patients with ruptured intracranial aneurysms: A randomised trial. Lancet 360:1267, 2002

OGILVY CS et al: AHA Scientific Statement: Recommendations for the management of intracranial arteriovenous malformations: A statement for healthcare professionals from a special writing group of the Stroke Council, American Stroke Association. Stroke 32:1458, 2001

PROGRESS COLLABORATIVE GROUP: Randomised trial of a perindopril-based blood-pressure-lowering regimen among 6105 individuals with previous stroke or transient ischaemic attack. Lancet 358:1033, 2001

ROTHWELL PM et al: Analysis of pooled data from the randomised controlled trials of endarterectomy for symptomatic carotid stenosis. Lancet 361:107, 2003

STAESSEN JA et al: Hypertension prevalence and stroke mortality across populations. JAMA 289:2420, 2003

350   ALZHEIMER'S DISEASE AND OTHER DEMENTIAS
Thomas D. Bird, Bruce L. Miller

Dementia, a syndrome of many causes, affects >4 million Americans and results in a total health care cost of >$100 billion annually. It is defined as an acquired deterioration in cognitive abilities that impairs the successful performance of activities of daily living. Memory is the most common cognitive ability lost with dementia; 10% of persons over age 70 and 20 to 40% of individuals over age 85 have clinically identifiable memory loss. In addition to memory, other mental faculties are also affected in dementia, such as language, visuospatial ability, calculation, judgment, and problem solving. Neuropsychiatric and social deficits develop in many dementia syndromes resulting in depression, withdrawal, hallucinations, delusions, agitation, insomnia, and disinhibition. The common forms of dementia are progressive, but some dementing illnesses are static or fluctuate dramatically from day to day.

MEMORY

Memory is a complex function of the brain that uses several storage buffers of differing capacity and duration. It can be divided into three major types: working, episodic, and long-term, or remote, memory. Working memory lasts for <30 s and has a limited storage capacity. Normal individuals can hold seven (plus or minus two) bits of information in working memory where these bits can be manipulated and either discarded or retained as a more permanent memory store. Working memory is highly vulnerable to distraction, requiring attention and vigilance for its maintenance. It is tested by asking the patient to recall digits backwards. The reticular activating system and prefrontal and parietal lobe networks are activated during working memory tasks.

Episodic memory lasts for minutes to many months or even years and binds information about "what," "where," and "when." Normal individuals lay down multiple episodic memories throughout the day, which allow them to move through life connected to previous experiences. On entering this memory buffer, information undergoes a process of consolidation. Significant events are more likely to be consolidated as a more permanent trace. Episodic memory is commonly tested by asking a patient to recall three words after 3 to 5 min. Other simple ways to test episodic memory include determining whether patients can remember what they had for breakfast, how they got to the office, or who examined them earlier in the day. The hippocampal complex is critical for episodic memory, and physiologic changes in synapses in this brain region accompany new episodic memories. Eventually episodic memories become independent of the hippocampal complex and move to neocortex.

Remote, or long-term, memory stores information lasting weeks to a lifetime and contains most of our personal experiences and knowledge. Some information appears to be stored accurately for an indefinite time, whereas other items fade or become distorted. More permanent stores of words, dates, historic facts, or names require the left anterior temporal cortex. The specific localization of other types of long-term memories is unknown, although the neocortex appears to be particularly important. Animal experiments have shown that long-term memory requires new protein synthesis, and the stabilization process probably involves physical changes at neuronal synapses.

Memory function includes *registration* (encoding or acquisition), *retention* (storage or consolidation), *stabilization* (consolidation), and *retrieval* (decoding or recall). Registration and retrieval are conscious processes. The process of encoding is dependent upon the frontal lobes and hippocampal complex, while the process of retrieval requires the frontal lobes. The hippocampal complex is vulnerable to metabolic insults such as seizures, hypoglycemia, hypoxia, and neurodegenerative processes, which explains why episodic memory deficits are the most common cognitive deficits that follow these varied disorders.

Several additional terms for memory types are sometimes used. *Amnesia* is a term used to describe an impairment in memory function. *Semantic memory* contains unchanging facts, principles, associations, and rules (for example, the number of days in a week). Injury to the anterior temporal neocortex will lead to loss of semantic memory. *Declarative (explicit) memory* refers to facts about the world and past personal events that must be consciously retrieved to be remembered. Episodic memory is the prototypical declarative, or explicit, memory. *Procedural (implicit) memory* is involved in learning and retaining a skill or procedure such as riding a bicycle, getting dressed, or driving a car. Abilities stored in procedural memory become automatic and do not require conscious implementation.

Finally, the term *executive function* refers to mental activity involved in planning, initiating, and regulating behavior. It is considered the central organizing function of the brain that results in systematic, goal-directed activity and is highly dependent upon working memory. Executive functions are active in situations where reflex or automatic behavior is not adequate. Executive functions are presumed to involve the frontal lobes (Chap. 23). Deficits in executive function occur frequently in patients with dementia.

FUNCTIONAL ANATOMY OF THE DEMENTIAS

Dementia results from disorders of cerebral neuronal circuits and is a result of the total quantity of neuronal loss combined with the specific location of such loss (Chap. 23). Episodic memory requires the dorsomedial nucleus of the thalamus (damaged in Korsakoff's syndrome due to thiamine deficiency) and the medial temporal lobes. Unilateral

temporal lobe lesions produce mild to moderate amnesia for either verbal or nonverbal material, while bilateral lesions produce a severe anterograde learning disorder, i.e., an inability to store new memories, often with retained ability to recall old ones.

The components of the medial temporal lobe memory system include the hippocampus and adjacent cortex, including the entorhinal, perirhinal, and parahippocampal regions (Fig. 350-1). This includes a circular pathway of neurons from the entorhinal cortex to the dentate gyrus, CA3 and CA1 neurons of the hippocampus to the subiculum, and back to the entorhinal cortex; this pathway is heavily damaged in Alzheimer's disease (AD). This system is fast, has limited capacity, and performs a crucial function at the time of learning and establishing declarative memory and semantic associations. Its role continues after learning during a lengthy period of reorganization and consolidation, whereby memory stored in neocortex eventually becomes independent of the medial temporal lobe memory system. This process, by which the burden of long-term (permanent) memory storage is gradually assumed by neocortex, ensures that the medial temporal lobe system is constantly available for the acquisition of new information.

Functional imaging studies indicate that learning and memory involve many of the same regions of the cortex that process sensory information and control motor output. The forms of perceptual and motor learning that can occur without conscious recollections are mediated in part by contractions and expansions of representations in the sensory and motor cortex. One study, for example, has shown that the cortical representation of the fingers of the left hand of musical string players is larger than that in controls, suggesting that the representation of different parts of the body in the primary somatosensory cortex of humans depends on use and changes to conform to the current needs and experiences of the individual. Discrete cortical regions exist in the anterior temporal lobes in which object knowledge (such as words related to color, animals, tools, or action) is organized as a distributed system. Here the attributes of an object are stored close to the regions of the cortex that mediate perception of those attributes.

Procedural (implicit) memory appears to involve centers outside the hippocampus such as amygdala, basal ganglia, cerebellum, and sensory cortex. Different frontal regions are activated for different kinds of memory storage. Functional magnetic resonance imaging (MRI) studies show that the magnitude of focal activation in left prefrontal-temporal regions and right prefrontal-bilateral parahippocampal regions predicts how well verbal or visual stimuli, respectively, will be remembered.

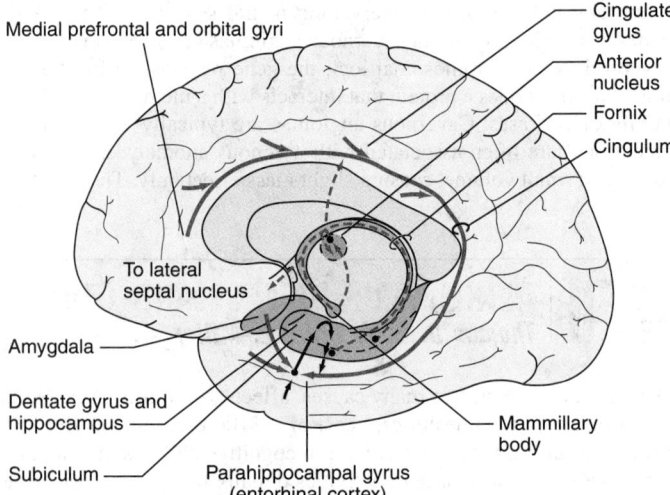

FIGURE 350-1 *The principal connections of the hippocampus. Afferent connections (red arrows) from the cingulate gyrus (cortical association fibers) and amygdala converge on the entorhinal cortex (part of the parahippocampal gyrus) and connect with the hippocampus via a polysynaptic circuit (black arrows) from dentate to CA3, CA1, and subiculum neurons with output back to the entorhinal cortex. Efferent connections (broken arrows) are principally via the fornix to the anterior nucleus of the thalamus, septal nucleus, and mammillary body.*

The cholinergic system plays an important role in memory, and anticholinergic agents such as atropine and scopolamine interfere with memory. Choline acetyltransferase (the enzyme catalyzing the formation of acetylcholine) and cholinergic receptors are known to be deficient in the cortex of patients with AD. The brains of AD patients show severe neuronal loss in the nucleus basalis of Meynert, the major source of cholinergic input to the cerebral cortex. These findings form the basis for the use of cholinesterase inhibitors in the treatment of AD, with benefits thought to arise from increased available levels of acetylcholine. Behavior and mood are modulated by noradrenergic, serotonergic, and dopaminergic pathways, and norepinephrine has been shown to be reduced in the brainstem locus coeruleus in AD. Neurotrophins (Chap. 345) are also postulated to play a role in memory in part by preserving cholinergic neurons.

Long-term potentiation (LTP), which refers to a long-lasting enhancement of synaptic transmission resulting from repetitive stimulation of excitatory synapses, is presumed to be involved in memory acquisition and storage. LTP occurs in the hippocampus and is mediated by N-methyl-D-aspartate (NMDA) receptors as well as cyclic AMP-responsive element-binding (CREB) protein. Dementias have anatomically specific patterns of neuronal degeneration, which dictate the clinical symptomatology. AD begins in the entorhinal cortex, spreads to the hippocampus, then moves to posterior temporal and parietal neocortex and eventually causes a relatively diffuse degeneration throughout the cerebral cortex. Multi-infarct dementia is associated with focal damage in a random patchwork of cortical regions. Diffuse white matter damage may disrupt intracerebral connections and cause dementia syndromes similar to those associated with leukodystrophies, multiple sclerosis, and Binswanger's disease (see below). Subcortical structures including the caudate, putamen, thalamus, and substantia nigra also modulate cognition and behavior in ways that are not yet well understood. AD primarily presents as memory loss and is often associated with aphasia or other disturbance of language. In contrast, patients with frontal lobe or subcortical dementias such as frontotemporal dementia (FTD) or Huntington's disease are less likely to begin with memory and language problems and more likely to have difficulties with attention, judgment, awareness, and behavior.

Lesions of specific cortical-subcortical pathways will have important effects on behavior (Chap. 23). The dorsolateral prefrontal cortex has connections with the dorsolateral caudate, globus pallidus, and thalamus. Lesions of these pathways result in poor organization and planning, decreased cognitive flexibility, and impaired judgment. The lateral orbital frontal cortex connects with the ventromedial caudate, globus pallidus, and thalamus. Lesions of these connections cause irritability, impulsiveness, and distractibility. The anterior cingulate cortex connects with the nucleus accumbens, globus pallidus, and thalamus. Interruption of these connections produces apathy and poverty of speech or even akinetic mutism.

THE CAUSES OF DEMENTIA

The many causes of dementia are listed in Table 350-1. The frequency of each condition depends on the age group under study, the access of the group to medical care, the country of origin, and perhaps racial or ethnic background. AD is the most common cause of dementia in western countries, representing more than half of demented patients. Vascular disease is the second most common cause of dementia in the United States, representing 10 to 20%. In populations with limited access to medical care, where vascular risk factors are undertreated, the prevalence of vascular dementia can be much higher. Dementia associated with Parkinson's disease is the next most common category, and in many instances these patients suffer from dementia with Lewy bodies (DLB). Chronic intoxications including those resulting from alcohol and prescription drugs are an important, often treatable cause of dementia. Other disorders listed in the table are uncommon but important because many are reversible. The classification of dementing illnesses into two broad groups of reversible and irreversible disorders is a useful approach to the differential diagnosis of dementia.

In a study of 1000 persons attending a memory disorders clinic, 19% had a potentially reversible cause of the cognitive impairment and 23% had a potentially reversible concomitant condition. The three most common potentially reversible diagnoses were depression, hydrocephalus, and alcohol dependence.

The single strongest risk factor for dementia is increasing age. The prevalence of disabling memory loss increases with each decade over age 50 and is associated most often with the microscopic changes of AD at autopsy. Slow accumulation of mutations in neuronal mitochondria is also hypothesized to contribute to the increasing prevalence of dementia with age. Nonetheless, some centenarians have

TABLE 350-1 *Differential Diagnosis of Dementia*

MOST COMMON CAUSES OF DEMENTIA

Alzheimer's disease	Alcoholism[a]
Vascular dementia	Parkinson's disease
Multi-infarct	Drug/medication intoxication[a]
Diffuse white matter disease (Binswanger's)	

LESS COMMON CAUSES OF DEMENTIA

Vitamin deficiencies	Toxic disorders
Thiamine (B₁): Wernicke's encephalopathy[a]	Drug, medication, and narcotic poisoning[a]
B₁₂ (pernicious anemia)[a]	Heavy metal intoxication[a]
Nicotinic acid (pellagra)[a]	Dialysis dementia (aluminum)
Endocrine and other organ failure	Organic toxins
Hypothyroidism[a]	Psychiatric
Adrenal insufficiency and Cushing's syndrome[a]	Depression (pseudodementia)[a]
Hypo- and hyperparathyroidism[a]	Schizophrenia[a]
Renal failure[a]	Conversion reaction[a]
Liver failure[a]	Degenerative disorders
Pulmonary failure[a]	Huntington's disease
Chronic infections	Pick's disease
HIV	Dementia with Lewy bodies
Neurosyphilis[a]	Progressive supranuclear palsy (Steel-Richardson syndrome)
Papovavirus (progressive multifocal leukoencephalopathy)	Multisystem degeneration (Shy-Drager syndrome)
Prion (Creutzfeldt-Jakob and Gerstmann-Sträussler-Scheinker diseases)	Hereditary ataxias (some forms)
Tuberculosis, fungal, and protozoal[a]	Motor neuron disease [amyotrophic lateral sclerosis (ALS); some forms]
Sarcoidosis[a]	Frontotemporal dementia
Whipple's disease[a]	Cortical basal degeneration
Head trauma and diffuse brain damage	Multiple sclerosis
Dementia pugilistica	Adult Down's syndrome with Alzheimer's
Chronic subdural hematoma[a]	ALS–Parkinson's–Dementia complex of Guam
Postanoxia	Miscellaneous
Postencephalitis	Vasculitis[a]
Normal-pressure hydrocephalus[a]	CADASIL
Neoplastic	Acute intermittent porphyria[a]
Primary brain tumor[a]	Recurrent nonconvulsive seizures[a]
Metastatic brain tumor[a]	Additional conditions in children or adolescents
Paraneoplastic limbic encephalitis	Hallervorden-Spatz disease
	Subacute sclerosing panencephalitis
	Metabolic disorders (e.g., Wilson's and Leigh's diseases, leukodystrophies, lipid storage diseases, mitochondrial mutations)

[a] Potentially reversible dementia.

TABLE 350-2 *Evaluation of the Patient with Dementia*

Routine Evaluation	Optional Focused Tests	Occasionally Helpful Tests
History	HIV	EEG
Physical examination	Chest x-ray	Parathyroid function
Laboratory tests	Lumbar puncture	Adrenal function
Thyroid function (TSH)	Liver function	Urine heavy metals
Vitamin B$_{12}$	Renal function	RBC sedimentation rate
Complete blood count	Urine toxin screen	Angiogram
Electrolytes	Psychometric testing	Brain biopsy
VDRL	Apolipoprotein E	SPECT
CT/MRI		

DIAGNOSTIC CATEGORIES

Reversible Causes	Irreversible/Degenerative Dementias	Psychiatric Disorders
Examples	Examples	Depression
Hypothyroidism	Alzheimer's	Schizophrenia
Thiamine deficiency	Frontotemporal dementia	Conversion reaction
Vitamin B$_{12}$ deficiency	Huntington's	
Normal-pressure	Dementia with Lewy bodies	
hydrocephalus	Multi-infarct	
Chronic infection	Leukoencephalopathies	
Brain tumor	Parkinson's	
Drug intoxication		

Associated Treatable Conditions

Depression	Agitation
Seizures	Caregiver "burnout"
Insomnia	Drug side effects

intact memory function and no evidence of clinically significant dementia. Whether dementia is an inevitable consequence of normal human aging remains controversial.

Subtle cumulative decline in episodic memory is a natural part of aging. This frustrating experience, often the source of jokes and humor, is referred to as *benign forgetfulness of the elderly*. Benign means that it is not so progressive or serious that it impairs reasonably successful and productive daily functioning, although the distinction between benign and more significant memory loss can be difficult to make. At age 85 years the average person is able to remember approximately one-half the number of words that he or she could at age 18. A mild cognitive problem that has subtly begun to interfere with daily activities is referred to as *mild cognitive impairment* (MCI). A sizeable proportion of persons with MCI will progress to frank dementia, usually caused by AD. The conversion rate from MCI to AD is ~12% per year. It remains unclear why some individuals show progression and others do not. Factors that predict progression from MCI to AD include a memory deficit >1.5 standard deviations from the norm, family history of dementia, the presence of an apolipoprotein ε4 (Apo ε4) allele, and small hippocampal volumes.

The major degenerative dementias include AD, FTD and related disorders, DLB, and prion disorders including Creutzfeldt-Jakob disease (CJD). These disorders are all associated with the abnormal aggregation of a specific protein: $A\beta_{42}$ in AD, tau in FTD, α-synuclein in DLB, and PrP in CJD.

APPROACH TO THE PATIENT

(Tables 350-1 and 350-2) Three major issues should be kept in the forefront: (1) What is the most accurate diagnosis? (2) Is there a treatable or reversible component to the dementia? (3) Can the physician help to alleviate the burden on caregivers? The major degenerative dementias can usually be distinguished by the initial symptoms; neuropsychological, neuropsychiatric, and neurologic findings; and neuroimaging features (Table 350-3).

History The history should focus on the onset, duration, and tempo of progression of the dementia. An acute or subacute onset of confusion may represent delirium and should trigger the search for intoxication, infection, or metabolic derangement. An elderly person with slowly progressive memory loss over several years is likely to suffer from AD. Nearly 75% of AD patients begin with memory symptoms, but other early symptoms include difficulty with managing money, driving, shopping, following instructions, finding words, or navigating. A change in personality, disinhibition, gain of weight, or food obsession suggests FTD, not AD. FTD is also suggested by the finding of apathy, loss of executive function, progressive abnormalities in speech, or by a relative sparing of memory or spatial abilities. The diagnosis of DLB is suggested by the early presence of visual hallucinations, parkinsonism, delirium, rapid-eye-movement (REM) sleep disorder (the merging of dream states into wakefulness), or *Capgras syndrome*, the delusion that a familiar person has been replaced by an impostor.

A history of sudden stroke with an irregular stepwise progression suggests multi-infarct dementia. Multi-infarct dementia is also commonly seen in the setting of hyper-

TABLE 350-3 *Clinical Differentiation of the Major Dementias*

Disease	Initial Symptom	Mental Status	Neuropsychiatry	Neurology	Imaging
AD	Memory loss	Episodic memory loss	Initially normal	Initially normal	Entorhinal and hippocampal atrophy
Vascular	Often sudden; variable initial symptoms; apathy, falls, focal weakness	Frontal/executive cognitive slowing; can spare memory	Apathy, delusions, anxiety	Usually motor slowing, spasticity; can be normal	Cortical and/or subcortical infarctions, confluent white matter disease
FTD	Apathy; reduced judgment/ insight/speech/ language; hyperorality	Frontal/executive, language; spares drawing	Apathy, disinhibition, hyperorality, euphoria, depression	Vertical gaze palsy, axial rigidity, dystonia, alien hand (due to PSP/CBD overlap)	Frontal and/or temporal atrophy; spares posterior parietal lobe
DLB	Visual hallucinations, REM-sleep disorder, delirium, Capgras syndrome, parkinsonism	Drawing and frontal/ executive; spares memory; delirium prone	Visual hallucinations, depression, sleep disorder, delusions	Parkinsonism	Posterior parietal; hippocampi larger than in AD
Prion	Dementia, mood changes, anxiety, movement disorder	Variable, frontal/ executive, focal cortical, memory	Depression, anxiety	Myoclonus, rigidity, parkinsonism	Cortical ribboning and basal ganglia hyperintensities on diffusion/flare MRI

Note: AD, Alzheimer's disease; FTD, frontotemporal dementia; PSP, progressive supranuclear palsy; CBD, cortical basal degeneration; DLB, dementia with Lewy bodies; MRI, magnetic resonance imaging.

tension, atrial fibrillation, peripheral vascular disease, and diabetes. In patients suffering from cerebrovascular disease it can be difficult to determine whether the dementia is due to AD, multi-infarct dementia, or a mixture of the two. Rapid progression of the dementia in association with motor rigidity and myoclonus suggests a prion disease. Seizures may indicate strokes or neoplasm. Gait disturbance is commonly seen with multi-infarct dementia, Parkinson's disease, or normal-pressure hydrocephalus. Multiple sex partners or intravenous drug use should trigger a search for a central nervous system (CNS) infection, especially in persons with HIV. A history of recurrent head trauma could indicate chronic subdural hematoma, dementia pugilistica, or normal-pressure hydrocephalus. Alcoholism may suggest malnutrition and thiamine deficiency. A remote history of gastric surgery may result in loss of intrinsic factor and vitamin B_{12} deficiency. Certain occupations such as working in a battery or chemical factory might indicate heavy metal intoxication. A careful review of medications, especially of sedatives and tranquilizers, may raise the issue of chronic drug intoxication. A family history of dementia is found in Huntington's disease, familial AD, or familial FTD. Depressive signs such as insomnia or weight loss are often seen with pseudodementia due to depression, which can also be caused by the recent death of a loved one.

Physical and Neurologic Examination   A thorough examination is essential to document the dementia, look for other signs of nervous system involvement, and search for clues of a systemic disease that might be responsible for the cognitive disorder. AD does not affect motor systems until late in the course. In contrast, FTD patients often develop axial rigidity, supranuclear gaze palsy, or features of amyotrophic lateral sclerosis (ALS). In DLB, initial symptoms may be the new onset of a parkinsonian syndrome (resting tremor, cogwheel rigidity, bradykinesia, and festinating gait) with the dementia following later, or vice-versa. Corticobasal degeneration (CBD) is associated with dystonia and alien hand (unilateral involuntary movements of the upper limb resembling purposeful actions) and with asymmetric motor deficits or myoclonus. A presentation with unexplained falls, axial rigidity, and gaze deficits suggests progressive supranuclear palsy (PSP). CJD is suggested by diffuse rigidity, an akinetic state, and myoclonus.

Hemiparesis or other focal neurologic deficits may occur in multi-infarct dementia or brain tumor. Dementia with a myelopathy and peripheral neuropathy suggests vitamin B_{12} deficiency. A peripheral neuropathy could also indicate an underlying vitamin deficiency or heavy metal intoxication. Dry cool skin, hair loss, and bradycardia suggest hypothyroidism. Confusion associated with repetitive stereotyped movements may indicate ongoing seizure activity. Hearing impairment or visual loss may produce confusion and disorientation misinterpreted as dementia. Such sensory deficits are common in the elderly.

Cognitive and Neuropsychiatric Examination   Brief screening tools such as the mini-mental status examination (MMSE) help to confirm the presence of cognitive impairment and to follow the progression of dementia (Table 350-4). The MMSE is an easily administered 30-point test of cognitive function and contains tests of orientation, working and episodic memory, language comprehension, naming, and copying. In most patients with MCI and some with clinically apparent AD, the MMSE may be normal and a more rigorous set of neuropsychological tests will be required. Additionally, when the etiology for the dementia syndrome remains in doubt, a specially tailored evaluation should be performed that includes tasks of working and episodic memory, frontal executive tasks, language, visuospatial function, and perception. In AD the deficits involve episodic memory, category generation ("name as many animals as you can in one minute"), and visuoconstructive ability. Deficits in verbal or visual episodic memory are often the first neuropsychological abnormalities seen with AD, and tasks that require the patient to recall a long list of words or pictures after a predetermined

TABLE 350-4   *The Mini-Mental Status Examination*

	Points
Orientation	
Name: season/date/day/month/year	5 (1 for each name)
Name: hospital/floor/town/state/country	5 (1 for each name)
Registration	
Identify three objects by name and ask patient to repeat	3 (1 for each object)
Attention and calculation	
Serial 7s; subtract from 100 (e.g., 93–86–79–72–65)	5 (1 for each subtraction)
Recall	
Recall the three objects presented earlier	3 (1 for each object)
Language	
Name pencil and watch	2 (1 for each object)
Repeat "No ifs, ands, or buts"	1
Follow a 3-step command (e.g., "Take this paper, fold it in half, and place it on the table")	3 (1 for each command)
Write "close your eyes" and ask patient to obey written command	1
Ask patient to write a sentence	1
Ask patient to copy a design (e.g., intersecting pentagons)	1
TOTAL	30

delay will demonstrate deficits in most AD patients. In FTD the earliest deficits often involve frontal executive function or language (speech or naming). DLB patients have more severe deficits in visuospatial function but do better on episodic memory tasks than do patients with AD. Patients with vascular dementia often demonstrate a mixture of frontal executive and visuospatial deficits. In delirium, deficits tend to occur in the areas of attention, working memory, and frontal tasks.

A functional assessment should also be performed. The physician should determine the day-to-day impact of the disorder on the patient's memory, community affairs, hobbies, judgment, dressing, and eating. Knowledge of the patient's day-to-day function will help to organize a therapeutic approach with the family.

Neuropsychiatric assessment is important for diagnosis, prognosis, and treatment. In the early stages of AD mild depressive features, social withdrawal, and denial of illness are the most prominent psychiatric changes. However, patients often maintain their social skills into the middle stages of the illness when delusions, agitation, and sleep disturbance become more common. In FTD dramatic personality change, apathy, overeating, repetitive compulsions, disinhibition, euphoria, and loss of empathy are common. DLB shows visual hallucinations, delusions related to personal identity, and day-to-day fluctuation. Vascular dementia can present with psychiatric symptoms such as depression, delusions, disinhibition, or apathy.

Laboratory Tests   The choice of laboratory tests in the evaluation of dementia is not straightforward. A reversible or treatable cause must not be missed, yet no single etiology is common; thus a screen must employ multiple tests, each of which has a low yield. Cost/benefit ratios are difficult to assess, and many laboratory screening algorithms for dementia discourage multiple tests. Nevertheless, even a test with only a 1 to 2% positive rate is probably worth undertaking if the alternative is missing a treatable cause of dementia. The algorithm in Table 350-2 lists most screening tests for dementia. Recently the American Academy of Neurology recommended the routine measurement of thyroid function tests, a vitamin B_{12} level, and a neuroimaging study [computed tomography (CT) or MRI].

Neuroimaging studies will identify primary and secondary neoplasms, locate areas of infarction, reveal subdural hematomas, and suggest normal-pressure hydrocephalus or diffuse white matter disease. They also lend support to the diagnosis of AD, especially if there is hippocampal atrophy in addition to diffuse cortical atrophy. Focal frontal and/or anterior temporal atrophy suggest FTD. There is no specific pattern yet determined for DLB, although these patients tend to have less hippocampal atrophy than is seen in AD. Diffusion-weighted MRI will detect abnormalities in the cortical-ribbon and basal ganglia in the vast majority of patients with CJD. Large white matter abnormalities correlate with a vascular etiology for dementia. The role of functional imaging in the diagnosis of dementia is still under study. Single photon emission computed tomography (SPECT) and positron emission tomography (PET) scanning reveal temporal-parietal hypoperfusion or hypometabolism in AD, and frontotemporal hypoperfusion or hypometabolism in FTD, but most of these changes reflect atrophy. Recently, amyloid imaging has shown promise for the diagnosis of AD. Similarly, MRI perfusion and brain activation studies using functional MRI are under study as diagnostic tools.

Lumbar puncture need not be done routinely in the evaluation of dementia but is indicated if CNS infection is a serious consideration. Cerebrospinal fluid (CSF) levels of tau protein are increased and $A\beta_{42}$ amyloid decreased in some AD patients; however, the sensitivity and specificity of these measures are not sufficiently high to warrant routine measurement. Formal psychometric testing is not necessary in every patient but helps to document the severity of dementia, suggest psychogenic causes, and provide a semiquantitative method for following the disease course. An electroencephalogram (EEG) is rarely helpful except to suggest CJD (repetitive bursts of diffuse high-voltage sharp waves) or an underlying nonconvulsive seizure disorder (epileptiform discharges). Brain biopsy (including meninges) is not advised except to diagnose vasculitis, potentially treatable neoplasms, unusual infections, or systemic disorders such as vasculitis or sarcoid or in young persons where the diagnosis is uncertain. Angiography should be considered when cerebral vasculitis is a possible cause of the dementia.

SPECIFIC DEMENTIAS

ALZHEIMER'S DISEASE   AD is the most common cause of dementia in western countries. Approximately 10% of all persons over the age of 70 have significant memory loss, and in more than half the cause is AD. AD can occur, however, in any decade of adulthood. The annual cost of caring for a single AD patient in an advanced stage of the disease is estimated at $50,000. The disease also exacts a heavy emotional toll on family members and caregivers. AD most often presents with subtle onset of memory loss followed by a slowly progressive dementia that has a course of several years. Pathologically there is diffuse atrophy of the cerebral cortex with secondary enlargement of the ventricular system. Microscopically there are neuritic plaques containing $A\beta$ amyloid, silver-staining neurofibrillary tangles (NFTs) in neuronal cytoplasm, and accumulation of $A\beta$ amyloid in arterial walls of cerebral blood vessels. The identification of four different susceptibility genes has provided a foundation for rapid progress in understanding the biologic basis of AD.

Clinical Manifestations   The cognitive changes with AD tend to follow a characteristic pattern, beginning with memory impairment and spreading to language and visuospatial deficits. However, ~20% of AD patients present with nonmemory complaints such as word-finding, organizational, or navigational difficulty. In the early stages of the disease, the memory loss may go unrecognized or may be ascribed to benign forgetfulness. Once the memory loss begins to affect day-to-day activities or falls to <1.5 standard deviations from normal on standardized memory tasks, the disease is defined as MCI. Slowly the cognitive problems begin to interfere with daily activities, such as

keeping track of finances, following instructions on the job, driving, shopping, and housekeeping. Some patients are unaware of these difficulties (*anosognosia*), while others have considerable insight. Change of environment may be bewildering, and the patient may become lost on walks or while driving an automobile. In the middle stages of AD, the patient is unable to work, is easily lost and confused, and requires daily supervision. Social graces, routine behavior, and superficial conversation may be surprisingly retained. Language becomes impaired: first naming, then comprehension, and finally fluency. In some patients, *aphasia* is an early and prominent feature. Word-finding difficulties and circumlocution may be a problem even when formal testing demonstrates intact naming and fluency. *Apraxia* emerges and patients have trouble carrying out sequential motor tasks. Visuospatial deficits begin to interfere with dressing, eating, solving simple puzzles, and copying geometric figures. Patients may be unable to perform simple calculations or tell time.

In the late stages of the disease, some persons remain ambulatory but wander aimlessly. Loss of judgment, reason, and cognitive abilities occurs. Delusions are common, usually simple in quality, involving delusions of theft, infidelity, or misidentification. Approximately 10% of AD patients develop the Capgras syndrome, believing that a caregiver has been replaced by an impostor. In contrast to DLB where the Capgras syndrome is an early feature, in AD this syndrome emerges later in the course of the illness. Loss of inhibitions and aggression may alternate with passivity and withdrawal. Sleep-wake patterns are prone to disruption, and nighttime wandering becomes disturbing to the household. Some patients develop a shuffling gait, with generalized muscle rigidity associated with slowness and awkwardness of movement. Patients often look parkinsonian (Chap. 351) but rarely have tremor. In end-stage AD, patients become rigid, mute, incontinent, and bedridden. Help may be needed with the simplest tasks, such as eating, dressing, and toilet function. Hyperactive tendon reflexes may be noted. Myoclonic jerks (sudden brief contractions of various muscles or the whole body) may occur spontaneously or in response to physical or auditory stimulation. Myoclonus raises the possibility of a prion disease (Chap. 362), but the course of AD is much more prolonged. Generalized seizures may also occur. Often, death results from malnutrition, secondary infections, pulmonary emboli, or heart disease. The typical duration of AD is 8 to 10 years, but the course can range from 1 to 25 years. For unknown reasons, some AD patients show a steady downhill decline in function, while others have prolonged plateaus without major deterioration.

Diagnosis   Early in the disease course, other etiologies of dementia should be excluded (see above). Neuroimaging studies (CT and MRI) do not show a single specific pattern with AD and may be normal early in the course of the disease. As AD progresses, diffuse cortical atrophy becomes apparent, and MRI scans show atrophy of the hippocampus (Fig. 350-2A, B). Functional imaging studies in AD reveal hypoperfusion or hypometabolism in the posterior temporal-parietal cortex (Fig. 350-2C, D). The EEG is normal or shows nonspecific slowing. Routine spinal fluid examination is also normal. The use of blood Apo ε genotyping is discussed under "Genetic Considerations" below.

Slowly progressive decline in memory and orientation, normal results on laboratory tests, and an MRI or CT scan showing only diffuse or posteriorly predominant cortical and hippocampal atrophy are highly suggestive of AD. A clinical diagnosis of AD, reached after careful evaluation, is confirmed at autopsy ~90% of the time, with misdiagnosed cases usually representing one of the other dementing disorders (Table 350-3).

Epidemiology   The most important risk factors for AD are old age and a positive family history. The frequency of AD increases with each decade of adult life, reaching 20 to 40% of the population over the age of 85. A positive family history of dementia suggests a genetic cause of AD. Female gender may also be a risk factor independent of the greater longevity of women. Some AD patients have a past history of head trauma with concussion, but this appears to be a relatively minor risk factor. AD is more common in groups with lower educational attainment, but education influences test-taking ability, and it is clear that AD can affect persons of all intellectual levels. One study found that the capacity to express complex written language in early adulthood correlated with a decreased risk for AD. Numerous environmental factors, including aluminum, mercury, and viruses, have been proposed as causes of AD, but none has been demonstrated to play a significant role. Several studies suggest that the use of nonsteroidal anti-inflammatory agents is associated with a decreased risk of AD, but this has not been confirmed in large prospective studies. Vascular disease does not seem to be a direct cause of AD, but amyloid angiopathy can lead to ischemic infarctions or hemorrhages. Elevated homocysteine and cholesterol levels, hypertension, and insufficient exercise are all being explored as potential risk factors for AD.

Pathology   The most severe pathology is usually found in the hippocampus, temporal cortex, and nucleus basalis of Meynert (lateral septum). The most important microscopic findings are neuritic "senile" plaques and NFTs. These lesions accumulate in small numbers during normal aging of the brain but occur in excess in AD. Neuritic plaques contain a central core that includes $A\beta$ amyloid, proteoglycans, Apo ε4, α_1 antichymotrypsin, and other proteins. $A\beta$ amyloid is a protein of 39 to 42 amino acids that is derived proteolytically from a larger transmembrane protein, amyloid precursor protein (APP), which has neurotrophic and neuroprotective activity. The normal function of $A\beta$ amyloid is unknown. Soluble amyloid fibrils may represent the initial pathologic event in AD leading to formation of neuritic plaques. The plaque core is surrounded by the debris of degenerating neurons, microglia, and macrophages. The accumulation of $A\beta$ amyloid in cerebral arterioles, termed *amyloid angiopathy*, may lead to cerebral lobar hemorrhages. NFTs are silver-staining, twisted neurofilaments in neuronal cytoplasm that represent abnormally phosphorylated tau protein and appear as paired helical filaments by electron microscopy. Tau is a microtubule-associated protein that may function to assemble and stabilize the microtubules that convey cell organelles, glycoproteins, and other important materials through the neuron.

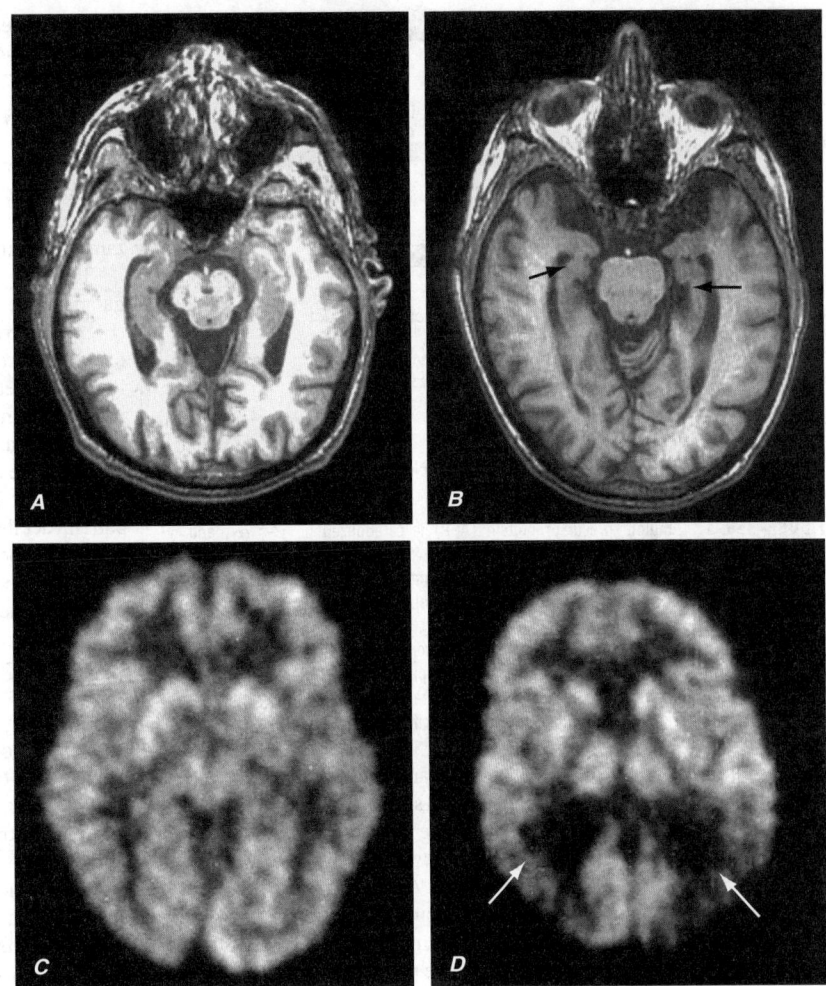

FIGURE 350-2   Alzheimer's disease. Axial T1-weighted MR images through the midbrain of a normal 86-year-old athletic individual (*A*) and a 77-year-old male (*B*) with Alzheimer's disease. Note that both individuals have prominent sulci and slight dilatation of the lateral ventricles. However, there is a reduction in the volume of the hippocampus of the patient with Alzheimer's disease (*arrows*) compared with that of the normal-for-age hippocampus of the older individual. Fluorodeoxyglucose positron emission tomographic scans of a normal control (*C*) and a patient with Alzheimer's disease (*D*). Note that the patient with Alzheimer's disease has decreased activity in the parietal lobes bilaterally (*arrows*), a typical finding in this condition. (*Images courtesy of TF Budinger, University of California.*)

A hyperphosphorylated state of tau impairs its capacity to bind to microtubules. AD is also associated with decreased levels of several proteins and neurotransmitters in the cerebral cortex, especially acetylcholine, its synthetic enzyme choline acetyltransferase, and nicotinic cholinergic receptors. Reduction of acetylcholine may result from degeneration of cholinergic neurons in the nucleus basalis of Meynert that project to many areas of the cortex. There is also reduction in norepinephrine levels in brainstem nuclei such as the locus coeruleus.

GENETIC CONSIDERATIONS   Several genes have been found to play important roles in the pathogenesis of at least some cases of AD. The first to be identified was the *APP* gene on chromosome 21. Point mutations in *APP* produce early-onset, autosomal dominant AD. APP is a membrane-spanning protein that is subsequently processed into smaller units, including $A\beta$ amyloid that is deposited in neuritic plaques. $A\beta$ peptide results from cleavage of APP by β- and γ-secretases (Fig. 350-3). Only very rare families with AD-producing *APP* mutations have been identified. However, adults with trisomy 21 (Down's syndrome) who survive beyond age 40 consistently develop a progressive dementia superimposed upon their baseline mental retardation and accompanied by typical neuropathologic changes of AD. Presumably the extra dose of the *APP* gene on chromosome 21 is the initiating cause of AD in adult Down's syndrome and results in an excess of cerebral amyloid.

Investigation of large families with multigenerational familial AD led to the discovery of two additional AD genes, termed the *presenilins*. Presenilin-1 (*PS-1*) is on chromosome 14 and encodes a protein called S182. Mutations in this gene cause an early-onset AD (onset before age 60 and often before age 50) transmitted in an autosomal dominant, highly penetrant fashion. More than 50 different mutations have been found in the *PS-1* gene in families from a wide range of ethnic backgrounds. Presenilin-2 (*PS-2*) is on chromosome 1 and encodes a protein called STM2. The two genes (*PS-1* and *PS-2*) are highly homologous and encode similar proteins that at first appeared to have seven transmembrane domains (hence the designation *STM*), but subsequent studies have suggested eight such domains with a ninth submembrane region. Both S182 and STM2 are cytoplasmic neuronal proteins that are widely expressed throughout the nervous system. They are homologous to a cell-trafficking protein, sel 12, found in the nematode *Coenorhabditis elegans*. Patients with mutations in these genes have elevated plasma levels of $A\beta_{42}$ amyloid, suggesting a possible link between the presenilins and APP. There is evidence that *PS-1* is involved in the cleavage of APP at the γ-secretase site, and mutations in either gene (*PS-1* or *PS-2*) may disturb this function. Mutations in *PS-1* have thus far proved to be the most common cause of early-onset familial AD, representing 40 to 70% of this relatively rare syndrome. Mutations in *PS-1* tend to produce AD with an earlier age of onset (mean onset, 45 years) and a shorter, more rapidly pro-

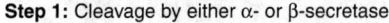

Step 1: Cleavage by either α- or β-secretase

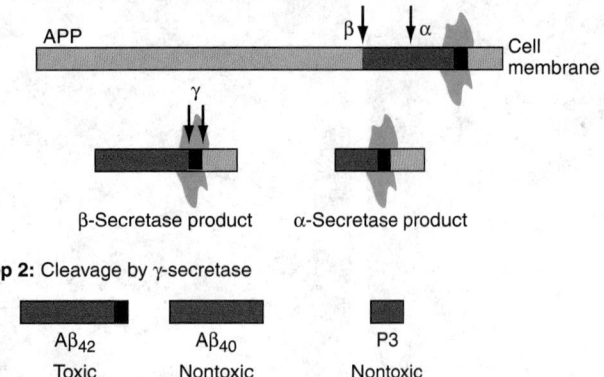

Step 2: Cleavage by γ-secretase

FIGURE 350-3 Amyloid precursor protein (APP) is catabolized by β-, α-, and γ-secretases. A key initial step is the digestion by either β-secretase (BASE) or α-secretase [(ADAM10 or ADAM17 (TACE))], producing smaller nontoxic products. Cleavage of the β-secretase product by γ-secretase (step 2) results in either the toxic Aβ42 or the nontoxic Aβ40 peptide; cleavage of the α-secretase product by γ-secretase produces the nontoxic P3 peptide. Excess production of Aβ42 is a key initiator of cellular damage in Alzheimer's disease. Current AD research is focused on developing therapies designed to reduce accumulation of Aβ42 by antagonizing β- or γ-secretases; promoting α-secretase; or clearing Aβ42 that has already formed by use of specific antibodies.

gressive course (mean duration 6 to 7 years) than the disease caused by mutations in *PS-2* (mean onset 53 years; duration 11 years). Some carriers of uncommon *PS-2* mutations have had onset of dementia after the age of 70. Mutations in the *presenilins* are rarely involved in the more common sporadic cases of late-onset AD occurring in the general population. DNA testing for these uncommon mutations is now possible on a research basis, and mutation analysis of *PS-1* is commercially available. Such testing is likely to be positive only in early-onset familial cases of AD. Any testing of asymptomatic at-risk individuals should be done only in the context of formal genetic counseling.

A discovery of great importance has implicated the *Apo ε* gene on chromosome 19 in the pathogenesis of late-onset familial and sporadic forms of AD. *Apo ε* is involved in cholesterol transport (Chap. 335) and has three alleles, designated 2, 3, and 4. The Apo ε4 allele has a strong association with AD in the general population, including sporadic and late-onset familial cases. Approximately 40 to 65% of AD patients, compared to 24 to 30% of the nondemented Caucasian population, has at least one ε4 allele. Many AD patients have no ε4 allele, however, and individuals with ε4 may never develop AD. Nevertheless, it is clear that the Apo ε4 allele, especially in the homozygous 4/4 state, is an important risk factor for AD. It appears to act as a dose-dependent modifier of age of onset, with the earliest onset associated with the ε4/4 homozygous state. Apo ε may be involved with the clearance of amyloid; clearance is least efficient with Apo ε4. Apo ε is present in the neuritic amyloid plaques of AD, and it may be involved in NFT formation, because it binds to tau. Apo ε4 decreases neurite outgrowth in cultures of dorsal root ganglion neurons, perhaps indicating a deleterious role in the brain's response to injury. Some cognitively normal ε4 heterozygotes and homozygotes have also been found by PET to have decreased cerebral cortical metabolic rates, suggesting possible presymptomatic abnormalities compatible with the earliest stage of AD. Finally, there is suggestive evidence that the ε2 allele may be "protective."

Apo ε testing is not indicated as a predictive test for AD in normal persons. In demented persons who meet clinical criteria for AD, the finding of an ε4 allele increases the reliability of diagnosis; however, its absence does not eliminate the diagnosis of AD. Furthermore, all patients with dementia, including those with an ε4 allele, require a search for reversible causes of their cognitive impairment. The ε4 allele is not associated with FTD, DLB, or CJD.

Additional genes are also likely to be involved in AD. Potential candidate genes have been described on chromosomes 12 (α2-macroglobulin) and 10.

℞ TREATMENT

AD cannot be cured, and no highly effective drug exists. The focus is on judicious use of cholinesterase inhibitor drugs; symptomatic management of behavioral problems; and building rapport with the patient, family members, and other caregivers.

Tacrine (tetrahydroaminoacridine), donepezil, rivastigmine, and galantamine are approved by the U.S. Food and Drug Administration (FDA) for treatment of AD. Their pharmacologic action is presumed to be inhibition of cholinesterase, with a resulting increase in cerebral levels of acetylcholine. Controlled studies indicate that cholinesterase inhibitors improve caregiver ratings of patients' functioning and decrease the rate of decline in cognitive test scores over periods of up to 3 years. The average patient on an anticholinesterase compound maintains his or her MMSE score at 1 year, whereas a placebo-treated patient declines two to three points over the same time period. Nevertheless, these compounds are only modestly efficacious and offer little or no benefit in the late stages of AD. Tacrine is expensive and may cause hepatotoxicity, thus it is rarely used. Donepezil avoids liver toxicity and can be administered once daily (5 to 10 mg), offering an advantage over the other cholinesterase inhibitors.

In a prospective observational study, the use of estrogen-replacement therapy appeared to protect—by ~50%—against development of AD in women. This study appeared to confirm the results of two earlier case-controlled studies. However, a prospective placebo-controlled study of a combined estrogen-progesterone therapy for asymptomatic postmenopausal women appeared to increase the prevalence of dementia. This study has markedly dampened enthusiasm for hormone treatments for the prevention of dementia. Additionally, no benefit has been found in the treatment of established AD with estrogen.

In patients with moderately advanced AD, a prospective trial of the antioxidants selegiline (Chap. 351), α-tocopherol (vitamin E), or both slowed institutionalization and progression to death. Because vitamin E has less potential for toxicity than selegiline and is inexpensive, the doses used in this study of 1000 IU twice daily are offered to many patients with AD. However, the beneficial effects of vitamin E are likely to be small.

A controlled trial of an extract of *Ginkgo biloba* found modest improvement in cognitive function in subjects with AD and vascular dementia. This study requires confirmation before *Ginkgo biloba* is considered an effective treatment for dementia because there was a high subject dropout rate and no improvement on a clinician's judgment scale.

One study of AD subjects in the mid-stages of disease showed a slowing of progression over a 28-week course in patients treated with memantine, an NMDA receptor antagonist.

There has been considerable enthusiasm for a strategy involving vaccination against the Aβ protein. This approach was highly effective in mouse models of AD; amyloid deposits were effectively cleared, and cognitive decline was arrested. The mechanism appears to involve generation of antibodies against Aβ, which cross the blood-brain barrier and eliminate neuritic plaques. Unfortunately, in human trials this approach led to life-threatening meningoencephalitis in some vaccinated individuals. Modifications of the vaccine approach are under development.

Several retrospective studies have suggested that nonsteroidal anti-inflammatory agents and statins (HMG-CoA reductase inhibitors) may protect against dementia. Controlled prospective studies are under way. Other prospective studies designed to lower serum homocysteine levels are in progress, based upon epidemiologic studies that revealed an association of elevated homocysteine levels with dementia progression.

Mild to moderate depression, common in the early stages of AD, may respond to antidepressant or cholinesterase inhibitors. Selective serotonin reuptake inhibitors (SSRIs) are commonly used due to their low anticholinergic side effects. Generalized seizures should be treated with an appropriate anticonvulsant, such as phenytoin or carbamazepine. For management of behavioral disturbances and suggestions for caregivers, see "General Symptomatic Treatment of the Patient with Dementia," below.

VASCULAR DEMENTIA Dementia associated with cerebrovascular disease can be divided into two general categories: multi-infarct dementia and diffuse white matter disease (also called subcortical arteriosclerotic encephalopathy, or Binswanger's disease). Cerebrovascular disease appears to be a more common cause of dementia in Asia than in Europe and North America. Individuals who have had several strokes may develop chronic cognitive deficits, commonly called *multi-infarct dementia*. The strokes may be large or small (sometimes lacunar) and usually involve several different brain regions. The occurrence of dementia appears to depend partly on the total volume of damaged cortex, but it is also more common in individuals with left-hemisphere lesions, independent of any language disturbance. Patients typically report a history of discrete episodes of sudden neurologic deterioration. Many multi-infarct dementia patients have a history of hypertension, diabetes, coronary artery disease, or other manifestations of widespread atherosclerosis. Physical examination usually shows focal neurologic deficits such as hemiparesis, a unilateral Babinski reflex, a visual field defect, or pseudobulbar palsy. The recurrent strokes result in a stepwise progression of disease. Neuroimaging studies show multiple areas of infarction. Thus, the history and neuroimaging findings differentiate this condition from AD. However, both AD and multiple infarctions are common and sometimes occur together. With normal aging, there is also an accumulation of amyloid in cerebral blood vessels, leading to a condition called *cerebral amyloid angiopathy of aging* (not associated with dementia), which predisposes older persons to hemorrhagic lobar stroke. AD patients with amyloid angiopathy may be at increased risk of cerebral infarction.

Some individuals with dementia are discovered on MRI to have bilateral subcortical white matter abnormalities, termed *diffuse white matter disease* (or leukoaraiosis), often occurring in association with lacunar infarctions (Fig. 350-4). The dementia may be insidious in onset and progress slowly, features that distinguish it from multi-infarct dementia, although other patients can show a stepwise deterioration more typical of multi-infarct dementia. Early symptoms are mild confusion, apathy, changes in personality, depression, psychosis, and

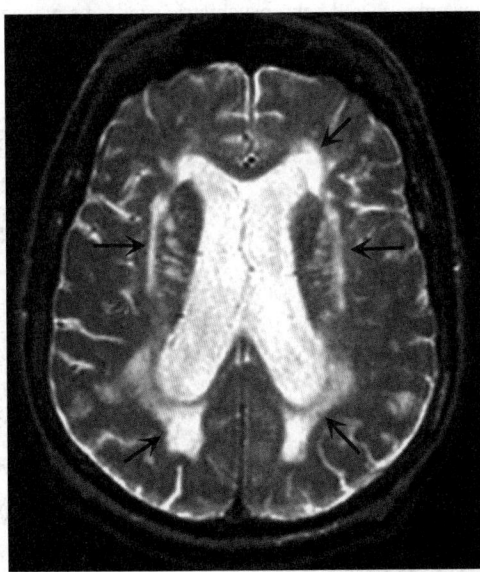

FIGURE 350-4 Diffuse white matter disease (Binswanger's disease). Axial T2-weighted MR image through the lateral ventricles reveals multiple areas of abnormal high signal intensity involving the periventricular white matter as well as the corona radiata and lentiform nuclei (*arrows*). While seen in some individuals with normal cognition, this appearance is more pronounced in patients with dementia of a vascular etiology.

memory or executive deficits. Marked difficulties in judgment and orientation and dependence on others for daily activities develop later. Euphoria, elation, depression, or aggressive behaviors are common. Both pyramidal and cerebellar signs may be present in the same patient. A gait disorder appears in at least half of affected patients. With advanced disease, urinary incontinence and dysarthria with or without other pseudobulbar features (e.g., dysphagia, emotional lability) are frequent. Seizures and myoclonic jerks appear in a minority of patients. This disorder is a microangiopathy due to occlusive disease of small penetrating cerebral arteries and arterioles. The patients usually, but not always, have a history of hypertension, but any disease causing stenosis of small cerebral vessels may be the critical underlying factor. The term *Binswanger's disease* should be used with caution, because it does not really identify a single entity.

A dominantly inherited form of diffuse white matter disease is known as *cerebral autosomal dominant arteriopathy with subcortical infarcts and leukoencephalopathy* (CADASIL). Clinically there is a progressive dementia developing in the fifth to seventh decades in multiple family members who may also have a history of migraine and recurrent stroke without hypertension. Skin biopsy may show characteristic dense bodies in the media of arterioles. The disease is caused by mutations in the notch 3 gene, and there is a commercially available genetic test. The frequency of this disorder is unknown, and there are no known treatments. Mitochondrial disorders can present with strokelike episodes and can selectively injure basal ganglia or cortex. Many such patients show other findings suggestive of a neurologic or systemic disorder such as ophthalmoplegia, retinal degeneration, deafness, myopathy, neuropathy, or diabetes. Diagnosis is difficult, but serum, and especially CSF, levels of lactate and pyruvate may be abnormal, and biopsy of affected tissue is often diagnostic.

Treatment of vascular dementia must be focused on the underlying causes, such as hypertension, atherosclerosis, and diabetes. Recovery of lost cognitive function is not likely to occur, although fluctuations with periods of improvement are common. Anticholinesterase compounds appear to be useful, as in AD (see above).

FRONTOTEMPORAL DEMENTIA AND RELATED DISORDERS ■ **Frontotemporal Dementia** FTD often begins between 50 and 70 years of age, and in this age group its prevalence may approach that of AD. Men and women are equally affected. Unlike AD, behavioral symptoms often predominate in the early stages of FTD. FTD can be sporadic or familial. The clinical heterogeneity is remarkable; patients demonstrate combinations of disinhibition, dementia, apraxia, parkinsonism, and motor neuron disease. In many families with an autosomal dominant pattern of inheritance, mutations in the tau gene on chromosome 17 have been found; in others, the dementia has been linked to 17 but does not involve tau. In still other families, chromosomes 3 and 9 have been linked to FTD.

Early symptoms are divided between cognitive, behavioral, and sometimes motor abnormalities, reflecting degeneration of the anterior frontal and temporal regions, basal ganglia, and motor neurons. Cognitive presentations typically spare memory and involve planning, judgment, or language. Poor business decisions, difficulty organizing work plans, and speech and language deficits emerge. Insight into the disorder is often severely impaired. Common behavioral deficits associated with FTD include apathy, disinhibition, weight gain, food fetishes, compulsions, and euphoria.

Findings at the bedside are dictated by the anatomic localization of the disorder. Asymmetric left frontal cases present with nonfluent aphasias, while left anterior temporal degeneration is characterized by loss of words and concepts related to language (semantic dementia). Nonfluent patients quickly progress to mutism, while those with semantic dementia develop features of visual agnosia, losing the ability to recognize faces, objects, and words (Chap. 23). Copying, calculating, and navigation often remain normal into later in the illness. These left hemisphere presentations of FTD have been called *primary pro-*

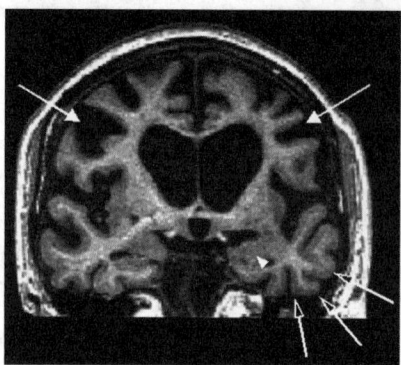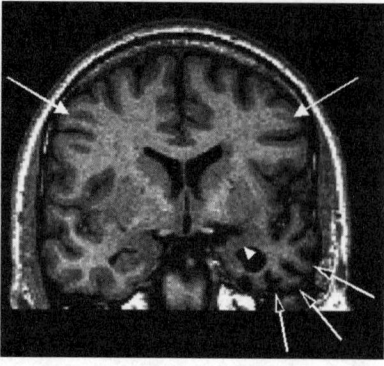

FIGURE 350-5 Frontotemporal dementia (FTD). Coronal MRI sections from one patient with frontally predominant FTD (*left*) and another with temporally predominant FTD (*right*). Prominent atrophy affecting the frontal gyri (*white arrows*) is present in frontally predominant FTD, particularly affecting the right frontal region; note also the thinning of the corpus callosum superior to the lateral ventricles. This patient presented with dysinhibition and antisocial behavior. In the temporally predominant patient, severe atrophy in the left temporal lobe (*open arrows*) and amygdala (*white arrowheads*) is present; this patient presented with progressive aphasia. (*Images courtesy of H Rosen and G Schauer, University of California at San Francisco.*)

gressive aphasia. In contrast, right frontal or temporal cases show profound alterations in social conduct with loss of empathy, disinhibition, and antisocial behaviors predominating. Memory and visuospatial skills are relatively spared in most FTD patients. There is a striking overlap between FTD and PSP, CBD, and motor neuron disease; ophthalmoplegia, dystonia, swallowing symptoms, and fasciculations are common at presentation of FTD or emerge during the course of the illness.

The anatomic hallmark of FTD is a marked atrophy of the temporal and/or frontal lobes, which can be visualized by neuroimaging studies (Figs. 350-5 and 350-6). The atrophy is sometimes remarkably asymmetric. A variety of pathologies have been associated with the clinical syndrome. The most consistent microscopic findings include gliosis and neuronal loss, and many cases show swollen or ballooned neurons containing cytoplasmic inclusions that in the majority of cases stain for tau. These aggregates sometimes resemble those found in PSP and CBD; tau is accepted as playing a major role in the pathogenesis of all three conditions. A toxic gain of function related to tau underlies the pathogenesis of many familial cases and is presumed to play a role in sporadic cases as well. Finally, many patients show no cellular inclusions, and the pathology remains bland with frontal and temporal gliosis, vacuolar changes, and neuronal loss the only evidence for disease. Nearly 80% of FTD patients show involvement of the basal ganglia at autopsy, and 15% go on to develop motor neuron disease, indicating the multisystem nature of this illness. Depletion of seratonergic and glutamatergic neurons is present in many patients. In contrast to AD, the cholinergic system is relatively spared in FTD.

Pick's disease was historically described as a progressive degenerative disorder of the anterior frontal and temporal neocortex accompanied by intracellular inclusions (*Pick's bodies*) that stain positive with silver (argyrophilic) and tau. Many of the τ-positive inclusions in FTD cases, however, are not labeled with silver stains. Although the nomenclature for these patients has remained controversial, the term *FTD* is increasingly used for all patients with frontotemporal degenerations, whereas Pick's disease is used to classify pathologically the subset of FTD cases that show Pick's bodies at autopsy.

The burden on caregivers of FTD patients is extremely high. Treatment is symptomatic, and there are currently no therapies known to slow progression or improve cognitive symptoms. Many of the behaviors that accompany FTD such as depression, hyperorality, compulsions, and irritability can be ameliorated with serotonin-modifying antidepressants. The co-association with motor disorders necessitates the careful use antipsychotics, which can exacerbate this problem.

Progressive Supranuclear Palsy PSP is a degenerative disease that usually begins with falls and a vertical supranuclear gaze paresis and progresses to symmetric rigidity and dementia. A stiff, unstable posture

with hyperextension of the neck and slow gait with frequent falls is characteristic. Early in the disease, patients have difficulty with downgaze and lose vertical opticokinetic nystagmus on downward movement of a target. Although patients have very limited voluntary eye movements, oculocephalic reflexes (doll's head maneuver) are retained; thus, the eye movement disorder is supranuclear. Frequent unexplained and sometimes spectacular falls are common secondary to a combination of axial rigidity, inability to look down, and bad judgment. The dementia is similar to FTD with apathy, frontal/executive dysfunction, poor judgment, slowed thought processes, impaired verbal fluency, and difficulty with sequential actions and with shifting from one task to another. These cognitive deficits are usually evident at the time of presentation and often precede the motor syndrome.

PSP is often confused with Parkinson's disease. Dementia does occur in ~20% of Parkinson's disease patients, often secondary to DLB. Furthermore, the behavioral syndromes seen with DLB differ from those of PSP (see below). The occurrence of dementia in Parkinson's disease is more likely with increasing age, increasing severity of extrapyramidal signs, a long duration of disease, and the presence of depression. Cortical atrophy is usually present on brain imaging studies. Neuropathologically, there may be Alzheimer changes in the cortex (amyloid plaques and NFTs), neuronal Lewy body inclusions in both the substantia nigra and the cortex, or no specific microscopic changes other than gliosis and neuronal loss. →*PSP and Parkinson's disease are discussed in detail in Chap. 351.*

Cortical Basal Degeneration CBD is a slowly progressive dementing illness that typically presents with a unilateral onset with rigidity, dystonia, and apraxia of one arm and hand, sometimes called the "alien hand." Eventually the condition becomes bilateral and includes dysarthria, slow gait, action tremor, and dementia. →*CBD is discussed in detail in Chap. 351.*

DEMENTIA WITH LEWY BODIES This syndrome is characterized by visual hallucinations, parkinsonism, fluctuating alertness, and falls. Dementia can precede or follow the appearance of parkinsonism. DLB may present in a patient with longstanding Parkinson's disease without cognitive impairment who slowly develops dementia associated with visual hallucinations, parkinsonism, and fluctuating alertness. In other patients the dementia and neuropsychiatric syndrome precede the parkinsonism. DLB patients are highly susceptible to metabolic perturbations, and in some the first manifestation of illness is a delirium,

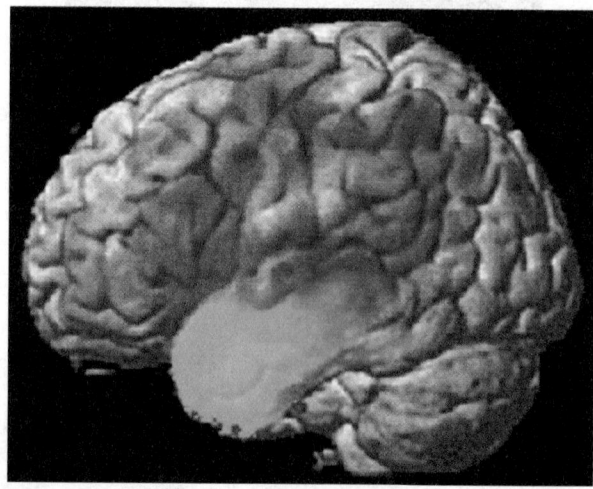

FIGURE 350-6 Voxel-based morphometry (VBM) analysis showing differing patterns of brain atrophy in the frontal variant of frontotemporal dementia (red), temporal variant of frontotemporal dementia (green), and Alzheimer's disease (blue). This technique allows comparison of MRI gray matter volumes between groups of subjects. (*Image courtesy of Marilu Gorno-Tempini, University of California at San Francisco.*)

often precipitated by an infection or other systemic disturbance. A delirium induced by L-dopa, prescribed for parkinsonian symptoms attributed to Parkinson's disease, may be the initial clue that the correct diagnosis is DLB. Even without an underlying precipitant, fluctuations can be marked in DLB patients, with the occurrence of episodic confusion admixed with lucid intervals. However, despite the fluctuating pattern, the clinical features persist over a long period of time, unlike delirium, which resolves following correction of the underlying precipitant. Cognitively, DLB patients tend to have relatively better memory, but more severe visuospatial deficits, than individuals with AD.

The key neuropathologic feature is the presence of Lewy bodies throughout the cortex, amygdala, cingulated cortex, and substantia nigra. Lewy bodies are intraneuronal cytoplasmic inclusions that stain with periodic acid–Schiff (PAS) and ubiquitin. They are composed of straight neurofilaments 7 to 20 nm long with surrounding amorphous material. They are recognized by antibodies against phosphorylated and nonphosphorylated neurofilament proteins, ubiquitin, and a presynaptic protein called α-synuclein. Lewy bodies are traditionally found in the substantia nigra of patients with idiopathic Parkinson's disease. A profound cholinergic deficit is present in many patients with DLB and may be a factor responsible for the fluctuations and visual hallucinations present in these patients. In patients without other pathologic features, the condition is referred to as *diffuse Lewy body disease*. In patients whose brains also contain excessive amounts of amyloid plaques and NFTs, the condition is called the *Lewy body variant of AD*. The quantity of Lewy bodies required to establish the diagnosis is not agreed on, but a definite diagnosis requires pathologic confirmation. At autopsy, 10 to 30% of demented patients show cortical Lewy bodies.

Due to the overlap with AD and the cholinergic deficit in DLB, anticholinesterase compounds may be helpful. Exercise programs are also helpful to maximize the motor function of these patients. Antidepressants are often necessary to treat depressive syndromes that accompany DLB. Atypical antipsychotics in low doses are sometimes needed to alleviate psychosis, although even low doses can increase extrapyramidal syndromes, which rarely may be life-threatening. As noted above, patients with DLB are extremely sensitive to dopaminergic medications, which must be carefully titrated; tolerability may be improved by concomitant use of cholinesterase inhibitors.

OTHER CAUSES OF DEMENTIA *Huntington's disease (HD)* (Chap. 351) is an autosomal dominant, degenerative brain disorder. A DNA repeat expansion (CAG repeat) of the gene encoding huntingtin on chromosome 4 forms the basis of a diagnostic blood test for the disease gene. The clinical hallmarks of the disease are chorea, behavioral disturbance, and a frontal/executive disorder. Onset is usually in the fourth or fifth decade, but there is a wide range in age of onset, from childhood to >70 years. Memory is frequently not impaired until late in the disease, but attention, judgment, awareness, and executive functions may be seriously deficient at an early stage. Depression, apathy, social withdrawal, irritability, and intermittent disinhibition are common. Delusions and obsessive-compulsive behavior may occur. The disease duration is typically about 15 years but is quite variable. There is no specific treatment, but the adventitious movements and behavioral changes may partially respond to phenothiazines, haloperidol, or benzodiazepines. Asymptomatic adult children at risk for HD should

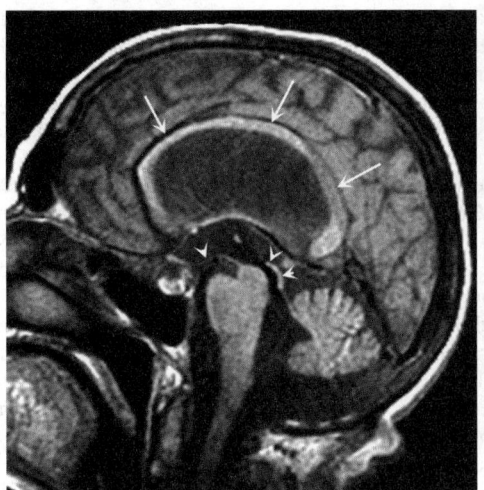 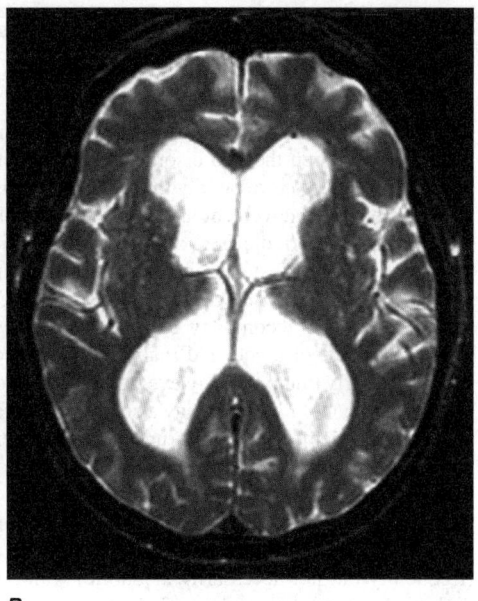

A   **B**

FIGURE 350-7 Normal pressure hydrocephalus. *A.* Sagittal T1-weighted MR image demonstrates dilatation of the lateral ventricle and stretching of the corpus callosum (*arrows*), depression of the floor of the third ventricle (*single arrowhead*), and enlargement of the aqueduct (*double arrowheads*). Note the diffuse dilatation of the lateral, third, and fourth ventricles with a patent aqueduct, typical of communicating hydrocephalus. *B.* Axial T2-weighted MR images demonstrate dilatation of the lateral ventricles without generalized cortical atrophy. This patient underwent successful ventriculoperitoneal shunting.

receive careful genetic counseling prior to DNA testing, because a positive result may have serious emotional and social consequences.

Normal-pressure hydrocephalus (NPH) is a relatively uncommon syndrome consisting of an abnormal gait (ataxic or apractic), dementia (usually mild to moderate), and urinary incontinence. Historically, many individuals who have been treated as having NPH have suffered from other dementias, particularly AD, multi-infarct dementia, and DLB. Neuroimaging findings in NPH are those of a communicating hydrocephalus with a patent aqueduct of Sylvius (Fig. 350-7). In many cases periventricular edema is present. Lumbar puncture findings include an opening pressure in the high-normal range and normal CSF protein, sugar concentrations, and cell count. NPH is presumed to be caused by obstruction to normal flow of CSF over the cerebral convexity and delayed absorption into the venous system. The indolent nature of the process results in enlarged lateral ventricles but relatively little increase in CSF pressure. There is presumably stretching and distortion of white matter tracts in the corona radiata, but the exact physiologic cause of the clinical syndrome is unclear. Some patients have a history of conditions producing scarring of the basilar meninges (blocking upward flow of CSF) such as previous meningitis, subarachnoid hemorrhage, or head trauma. Others with longstanding but asymptomatic congenital hydrocephalus may have an adult-onset deterioration in gait or memory that is confused with NPH; in these patients, the aqueduct of Sylvius is small, in contrast to patients with NPH. Unlike in AD, the NPH patient has an early and prominent gait disturbance and no evidence of cortical or hippocampal atrophy on neuroimaging studies. A number of attempts have been made to use various special studies to improve the diagnosis of NPH and predict the success of ventricular shunting. These include radionuclide cisternography (showing a delay in CSF absorption over the convexity) and various attempts to monitor and alter CSF flow dynamics. None has proved to be specific or consistently useful. There is sometimes a transient improvement in gait or cognition following lumbar puncture (or serial punctures) with removal of ≥30 mL of CSF, but this finding is not a reliable predictor of post-shunt improvement. Approximately 30 to 50% of patients identified by careful diagnosis as having NPH will show improvement with a ventricular shunting procedure. Gait may improve more than memory. Transient, short-lasting improvement is common. Patients should be carefully selected for this operation, because subdural hematoma and infection are known complications.

Prion diseases such as CJD are rapidly progressive disorders associated with dementia, focal cortical signs, rigidity, and myoclonus. The rapidity of progression seen with CJD is uncommon in AD so that distinction between the two disorders is usually straightforward. CBD and DLB progress more rapidly than AD and are associated with prominent disorders of movement and so are more likely to be mistaken for CJD. Abnormal periodic EEG discharges and cortical and basal ganglia abnormalities on diffusion-weighted MRI are unique diagnostic features of CJD. →*Prion diseases are discussed in detail in Chap. 362.*

Dementia can accompany *chronic alcoholism* (Chap. 372). This may be a result of associated malnutrition, especially of B vitamins and particularly thiamine. However, other as yet poorly defined aspects of chronic alcohol ingestion may also produce cerebral damage. A rare syndrome of dementia and seizures with degeneration of the corpus callosum has been reported primarily in male Italian drinkers of red wine (Marchiafava-Bignami disease).

Thiamine (vitamin B₁) deficiency causes Wernicke's encephalopathy (Chap. 258). The clinical presentation is a malnourished individual (frequently but not necessarily alcoholic) with confusion, ataxia, and diplopia from ophthalmoplegia. Thiamine deficiency damages the thalamus, mammillary bodies, midline cerebellum, periaqueductal gray matter of the midbrain, and peripheral nerves. Damage to the dorsomedial thalamic regions correlates most closely with memory loss. Prompt administration of parenteral thiamine may reverse the disease if given in the first few days of symptom onset. However, prolonged untreated thiamine deficiency can result in an irreversible dementia/amnestic syndrome known as *Korsakoff's syndrome*. Here, the patient is unable to recall new information despite normal immediate memory, attention span, and level of consciousness. Memory for new events is seriously impaired, whereas memory of knowledge prior to the illness is relatively intact. Patients are easily confused, disoriented, and incapable of recalling new information for more than a brief interval. Superficially, they may be conversant, entertaining, able to perform simple tasks, and follow immediate commands. Confabulation is common, although not always present, and may result in obviously erroneous statements and elaborations. There is no specific treatment because the previous thiamine deficiency has produced irreversible damage to the medial thalamic nuclei and mammillary bodies. Mammillary body atrophy may be visible on high-resolution MRI (Fig. 258-6).

Vitamin B₁₂ deficiency, as can occur in pernicious anemia, causes a macrocytic anemia and may also damage the nervous system (Chaps. 92 and 356). Neurologically it most commonly produces a spinal cord syndrome (myelopathy) affecting the posterior columns (loss of position and vibratory sense) and corticospinal tracts (hyperactive tendon reflexes with Babinski responses); it also damages peripheral nerves, resulting in sensory loss with depressed tendon reflexes. Damage to cerebral myelinated fibers may also cause dementia. The mechanism of neurologic damage is unclear but may be related to a deficiency of *S*-adenosylmethionine (required for methylation of myelin phospholipids) due to reduced methionine synthase activity or accumulation of methylmalonate, homocysteine, and propionate, providing abnormal substrates for fatty acid synthesis in myelin. The neurologic signs of vitamin B₁₂ deficiency are usually associated with macrocytic anemia, but on occasion may occur in its absence. Treatment with parenteral vitamin B₁₂ stops progression of the disease if instituted promptly, but reversal of advanced nervous system damage will not occur.

Deficiency of nicotinic acid (pellagra) is associated with sun-exposed skin rash, glossitis, and angular stomatitis (Chap. 61). Severe dietary deficiency of nicotinic acid along with other B vitamins such as pyridoxine may result in spastic paraparesis, peripheral neuropathy, fatigue, irritability, and dementia. This syndrome has been seen in prisoner-of-war and concentration camps. Low serum folate levels appear to be a rough index of malnutrition, but isolated folate deficiency has not been proved to be a specific cause of dementia.

Infections of the CNS usually cause delirium and other acute neurologic syndromes (Chap. 258). However, some chronic CNS infections, particularly those associated with chronic meningitis (Chap. 361), may produce a dementing illness. The possibility of chronic infectious meningitis should be suspected in patients presenting with a dementia or behavioral syndrome who also have headache, meningismus, cranial neuropathy, and/or radiculopathy. Between 20 and 30% of patients in the advanced stages of infection with HIV become demented (Chap. 173). Cardinal features include psychomotor retardation, apathy, and impaired memory. This may result from secondary opportunistic infections but can also be caused by direct infection of CNS neurons with HIV. Neurosyphilis (Chap. 153) was a common cause of dementia in the preantibiotic era; it is now uncommon but can still be encountered in patients with multiple sex partners. Characteristic CSF changes consist of pleocytosis, increased protein, and a positive Venereal Disease Research Laboratory (VDRL) test.

Primary and metastatic neoplasms of the CNS (Chap. 358) usually produce focal neurologic findings and seizures rather than dementia. However, if tumor growth begins in the frontal or temporal lobes, the initial manifestations may be memory loss or behavioral changes. A paraneoplastic syndrome of dementia associated with occult carcinoma (often small cell lung cancer) is termed *limbic encephalitis* (Chap. 87). In this syndrome, confusion, agitation, seizures, poor memory, movement disorders, and dementia occur in association with sensory neuropathy.

A *nonconvulsive seizure disorder* may underlie a syndrome of confusion, clouding of consciousness, and garbled speech. Psychiatric disease is often suspected, but an EEG demonstrates the seizure discharges. If recurrent or persistent, the condition may be termed *complex partial status epilepticus*. The cognitive disturbance often responds to anticonvulsant therapy. The etiology may be previous small strokes or head trauma; some cases are idiopathic.

It is important to recognize systemic diseases that indirectly affect the brain and produce chronic confusion or dementia. Such conditions include hypothyroidism; vasculitis; and hepatic, renal, or pulmonary disease. Hepatic encephalopathy may begin with irritability and confusion and slowly progress to agitation, lethargy, and coma (Chap. 258).

Isolated vasculitis of the CNS (CNS granulomatous vasculitis) (Chaps. 306 and 349) occasionally causes a chronic encephalopathy with confusion, disorientation, and clouding of consciousness. Headache is common, and strokes and cranial neuropathies may occur. Brain imaging studies may be normal or nonspecifically abnormal. CSF studies reveal a mild pleocytosis or elevation in the protein level. Cerebral angiography often shows multifocal stenosis and narrowing of vessels. A few patients have only small-vessel disease that is not revealed on angiography. The angiographic appearance is nonspecific and may be mimicked by atherosclerosis, infection, or other causes of vascular disease. Brain or meningeal biopsy demonstrates abnormal arteries with endothelial cell proliferation and infiltrates of mononuclear cells. The prognosis is often poor; however, the disorder may remit spontaneously. Some patients respond to glucocorticoids or chemotherapy.

Chronic metal exposure may produce a dementing syndrome. The key to diagnosis is to elicit a history of exposure at work, home, or even as a consequence of a medical procedure such as dialysis. Chronic lead poisoning may present as fatigue, depression, and confusion and may be associated with episodic abdominal pain and peripheral neuropathy. Inadequately fired glazed pottery has been reported as a cause. Gray lead lines appear in the gums. There is usually an anemia with basophilic stippling of red cells. The clinical presentation can resemble that of acute intermittent porphyria, including elevated levels of urine porphyrins as a result of the inhibition of δ-aminolevulinic acid dehydrase. The treatment is chelation therapy with agents such as ethylenediamine tetraacetic acid (EDTA). Chronic mercury poisoning produces dementia, peripheral neuropathy, ataxia, and tremulousness that may progress to choreoathetosis. Chronic arsenic intoxication can produce confusion and memory loss associated with nausea, weight loss, peripheral neuropathy, pigmentation and scaling of the skin, and transverse white lines of the fingernails (Mee's lines). Treatment is chelation therapy with dimercaprol (BAL). Aluminum poisoning has been best documented with the dialysis dementia syndrome in which water used during renal dialysis was contaminated with excessive amounts of aluminum. A progressive encephalopathy ensued, associated with confusion, aphasia, memory loss, agitation, and, later, lethargy and stupor. Speech arrest and myoclonic jerks were common and associated with severe and generalized EEG changes. The condition has been eliminated by the use of deionized water for dialysis.

Recurrent head trauma in professional boxers may lead to dementia, sometimes called the "punch drunk" syndrome or *dementia pugilistica*. The symptoms can be progressive, beginning late in a boxer's career or even long after retirement. The severity of the syndrome correlates with the length of the boxing career and number of bouts. Early on, a personality change associated with social instability and sometimes paranoia and delusions occurs. Later, memory loss progresses to full dementia, often associated with parkinsonian signs and ataxia or intention tremor. At autopsy, the cerebral cortex may show changes similar to those in AD, although NFTs are usually more prominent than amyloid plaques (which are usually diffuse rather than neuritic). There may also be loss of neurons in the substantia nigra. Chronic subdural hematoma (Chap. 357) is also occasionally associated with dementia, often in the context of underlying cortical atrophy from conditions such as AD or Huntington's disease. In these latter cases, evacuation of the subdural hematoma will not alter the underlying degenerative process.

Transient global amnesia (TGA) is characterized by the sudden onset of a severe episodic memory deficit, usually occurring in persons over age 50. Often, the memory loss occurs in the setting of an emotional stimulus or physical exertion. During the attack the individual is alert and communicative, general cognition seems intact, and there are no other neurologic signs or symptoms. The patient may seem confused and repeatedly ask about present events. The ability to form new memories returns after a period of hours, and the individual returns to normal with no recall for the period of the attack. Frequently no cause is determined, but cerebrovascular disease, epilepsy (7% in one study), migraine, or cardiac arrhythmia have all been implicated. A Mayo Clinic review of 277 patients with TGA found a past history of migraine in 14% and cerebrovascular disease in 11%, but these conditions were not temporally related to the TGA episodes. Approximately one-quarter of the patients had recurrent attacks, but they were not at increased risk for subsequent stroke. Rare instances of permanent memory loss after sudden onset have been reported, usually representing ischemic infarction of the hippocampi or medial thalamic nuclei bilaterally.

The ALS/parkinsonian/dementia complex of Guam is a rare degenerative disease that has occurred in the Chamorro natives on the island of Guam. Any combination of parkinsonian features, dementia, and motor neuron disease may occur. The most characteristic pathologic features are the presence of NFTs in degenerating neurons of the cortex and substantia nigra and loss of motor neurons in the spinal cord. Epidemiologic evidence supports a possible environmental cause, such as exposure to a neurotoxin with a long latency period. One interesting but unproven candidate neurotoxin occurs in the seed of the false palm tree, which Guamanians traditionally used to make flour. The ALS syndrome is decreasing in frequency on Guam, but a dementing illness with rigidity continues to be seen.

Rarely adult-onset leukodystrophies, neuronal storage diseases, and other genetic disorders can cause dementia late in life. Adult metachromatic leukodystrophy (arylsulfatase A deficiency) can present as a dementia associated with large frontal white matter lesions. Adult presentations of adrenaleukodystrophy have been reported, and in these cases involvement of the spinal cord and posterior white matter is common. This is diagnosed with measurement of medium- and long-chain fatty acids (Chap. 356). The neuronal cerebrolipofuscinoses are a genetically heterogeneous group of disorders associated with myoclonus, seizures, and progressive dementia. Diagnosis is made by finding curvilinear inclusions within white blood cells or neuronal tissue.

Psychogenic amnesia for personally important memories is common, although whether this results from deliberate avoidance of unpleasant memories or from unconscious repression is currently unknown. The event-specific amnesia is more likely to occur after violent crimes such as homicide of a close relative or friend or sexual abuse. It may also develop in association with drug or alcohol intoxication and sometimes with schizophrenia. More prolonged psychogenic amnesia occurs in fugue states that also commonly follow severe emotional stress. The patient with a fugue state suffers from a sudden loss of personal identity and may be found wandering far from home. In contrast to organic amnesia, fugue states are associated with amnesia for personal identity and events closely associated with the personal past. At the same time, memory for other recent events and the ability to learn and use new information are preserved. The episodes usually last hours or days and occasionally weeks or months while the patient takes on a new identity. On recovery, there is a residual amnesia for the period of the fugue. Very rarely, selective loss of autobiographical information represents a focal injury in the brain areas involved with these functions.

Psychiatric diseases may mimic dementia. Severely depressed individuals may appear demented, a phenomenon called *pseudodementia*. Memory and language are usually intact when carefully tested in depressed persons, and a significant memory disturbance usually suggests an underlying dementia, even if the patient is depressed. The patient with pseudodementia may feel confused and unable to accomplish routine tasks. Vegetative symptoms are common, such as insomnia, lack of energy, poor appetite, and concern with bowel function. The onset is often abrupt, and the psychosocial milieu may suggest prominent reasons for depression. Such patients respond to treatment of the depression. Schizophrenia is usually not difficult to distinguish from dementia, but occasionally the distinction can be problematic. Schizophrenia usually has a much earlier age of onset (second and third decades) than most dementing illnesses and is associated with intact memory. The delusions and hallucinations of schizophrenia are usually more complex and bizarre than those of dementia. Some chronic schizophrenics develop an unexplained progressive dementia late in life that is not related to AD. Conversely, FTD, HD, vascular dementia, DLB, AD, or leukoencephalopathy can begin with schizophrenia-like features, leading to the misdiagnosis of a psychiatric condition. The later age of onset, presence of significant deficits on cognitive testing, and neuroimaging findings point toward a degenerative condition. Memory loss may also be part of a conversion reaction. In this situation, patients commonly complain bitterly of memory loss, but careful cognitive testing either does not confirm the deficits or demonstrates inconsistent or unusual patterns of cognitive problems. The patient's behavior and "wrong" answers to questions often indicate that he or she understands the question and knows the correct answer.

Clouding of cognition by chronic drug or medication use, often prescribed by physicians, is an important cause of dementia. Sedatives, tranquilizers, and analgesics used to treat insomnia, pain, anxiety, or agitation may cause confusion, memory loss, and lethargy, especially in the elderly. Discontinuation of the offending medication often improves mentation.

GENERAL SYMPTOMATIC TREATMENT OF THE PATIENT WITH DEMENTIA

The major goals of management are to treat any correctable causes of the dementia and to provide comfort and support to the patient and caregivers. Removal of sedating or cognition-impairing drugs and medications is often beneficial. If the patient is depressed rather than demented, the depression should be vigorously treated. Patients with degenerative diseases may also be depressed, and that portion of their condition may respond to antidepressant therapy. Antidepressants that are low in cognitive side effects, such as SSRIs (Chap. 371), are advisable when treatment is necessary. Anticonvulsants are used to control seizures.

Agitation, hallucinations, delusions, and confusion are difficult to treat. These behavioral problems represent major causes for nursing home placement and institutionalization. Before treating these behaviors with medications, a thorough search for potentially modifiable environmental or metabolic factors should be sought. Hunger, lack of exercise, toothache, constipation, urinary tract infection, or drug toxicity all represent easily correctable factors that can be treated without psychoactive drugs. Medications that may calm agitation and insomnia without worsening dementia include low-dose haloperidol (0.5 to 2 mg), trazodone, buspirone, or propranolol. The new atypical antipsychotics including risperidone, olanzapine, and quetiapine are increasingly used for patients with difficult behaviors. When patients do not respond it is usually a mistake to advance to higher doses or to use anticholinergics or sedatives (such as barbiturates or benzodiazepines). The few controlled studies comparing drugs with behavioral intervention in the treatment of agitation suggest that both approaches are effective. However, careful, daily, nondrug behavior management is often not available, rendering medication necessary. Sometimes, apathy, visual hallucinations, and other psychiatric symptoms respond to the cholinesterase inhibitors, obviating the need for other therapies.

A proactive strategy has been shown to reduce the occurrence of delirium in hospitalized patients. This includes frequent orientation, cognitive activities, sleep-enhancement measures, vision and hearing aids, and correction of dehydration.

Nondrug behavior therapy has an important place in the management of dementia. The primary goal is to make the demented patient's life comfortable, uncomplicated, and safe. Memory aids such as notebooks, lists, and posted daily reminders are frequently helpful. It is also useful to stress familiar routines, short-term tasks, walks, and simple physical exercises. For many demented patients, the memory for facts is worse than that for routine activities, and they still may be able to take part in remembered physical activities such as walking, bowling, dancing, and golf. Demented patients usually object to losing control over familiar tasks such as driving, cooking, and handling finances. Attempts to help or take over may be greeted with complaints, depression, or anger. Hostile responses on the part of the caretaker are useless and sometimes harmful. Explanation, reassurance, distraction, and calm statements are more productive responses in this setting. Eventually, tasks such as finances and driving must be assumed by others, and the patient will conform and adjust. Safety is an important issue that includes not only driving but the environment of the kitchen, bathroom, and sleeping area. These areas need to be monitored, supervised, and made as safe as possible. A move to a retirement home, assisted-living center, or nursing home can initially increase confusion and agitation. Repeated reassurance, reorientation, and careful introduction to the new personnel will help to smooth the process. Provision of activities that are known to be enjoyable to the patient can be of considerable benefit. Attention should also be paid to frustration and depression in family members and caregivers. Caregiver guilt and burn-out are common, often resulting in nursing home placement of the patient. Family members often feel overwhelmed and helpless and may vent their frustrations on the patient, each other, and health care providers. Caregivers should be encouraged to take advantage of day-care facilities and respite breaks. Education and counseling about dementia are important. Local and national support groups, such as the Alzheimer's Disease and Related Disorders Association, can be of considerable help.

FURTHER READING

BOEVE BF et al: Current management of sleep disturbances in dementia: Curr Neurol Neurosci Rep 2:169, 2002

HEJI A et al: Potentially reversible conditions in 1000 consecutive memory clinic patients. J Neurol Neurosurg Psychiatry 73:390, 2002

REISBERG B et al: Memantine in moderate to severe Alzheimer's disease. N Engl J Med 348:1333, 2003

ROSEN HJ et al: Utility of clinical criteria in differentiating frontotemporal lobar degeneration (FTLD) from AD. Neurology 58:1608, 2002

SHUMAKER SA et al: Estrogen plus progestin and the incidence of dementia and mild cognitive impairment in postmenopausal women: The Women's Health Initiative Memory Study: A randomized controlled trial. JAMA 289: 2651, 2003

VERMEER SE et al: Silent brain infarcts and the risk of dementia and cognitive decline. N Engl J Med 348:1215, 2003

351 PARKINSON'S DISEASE AND OTHER MOVEMENT DISORDERS
Mahlon R. DeLong, Jorge L. Juncos

PARKINSON'S DISEASE

Parkinson's disease (PD) is the most common example of a family of neurodegenerative disorders characterized by a neuronal accumulation of the presynaptic protein α-synuclein and by variable degrees of *parkinsonism*, defined as a paucity and slowness of movement (*bradykinesia*), tremor at rest, rigidity, shuffling gait, and flexed posture. Nearly all forms of parkinsonism result from a reduction of dopaminergic transmission within the basal ganglia. Sporadic and idiopathic PD account for ~75% of all cases of parkinsonism; the remaining 25% result from genetically defined etiologies and other causes including other neurodegenerative disorders, cerebrovascular disease, and drugs.

Epidemiology PD afflicts >1 million individuals in the United States (~1% of those >55 years). Its peak age of onset is in the 60s (range is 35 to 85 years), and the course of the illness ranges between 10 and 25 years. Familial clusters of autosomal dominant and recessive forms of PD comprise ~5% of cases (Table 351-1). These are characterized by an earlier age of onset (typically before age 50 years) and a longer course than the more typical "sporadic" PD. Although most patients with PD appear to have no strong genetic determinant, epidemiologic evidence points to a complex interaction between genetic vulnerability and environmental factors (Fig. 351-1). Risk factors include a positive family history, male gender, head injury, exposure to pesticides, con-

TABLE 351-1 *Familial Parkinson's Disease*

Locus	Gene	Inheritance
PARK1	α-Synuclein	AD
PARK2	Parkin	AR
PARK4	α-Synuclein triplication	AD
PARK5	UCHL1	AD
PARK7	DJ-1	AR
PARK3,4,6,8,9	Unknown	AD and AR mutations
PARK10	Unknown	Late-onset susceptibility gene

sumption of well water, and rural living. Factors linked to a reduced incidence of PD include coffee drinking, smoking, use of nonsteroidal anti-inflammatory drugs, and estrogen replacement in postmenopausal women.

Clinical Features A diagnosis of PD can be made with some confidence in patients who present with at least two of the three cardinal signs—rest tremor, rigidity, and bradykinesia. Tremor is particularly important, as it is present in 85% of patients with true PD; a diagnosis of PD is particularly difficult when tremor is absent. A unilateral and gradual onset of symptoms further supports the diagnosis. Masked facies, decreased eye blinking, stooped posture, and decreased arm swing complete the early picture. The onset may also be heralded by vague feelings of weakness and fatigue, incoordination, aching, and discomfort.

Motor Features The most disabling feature of PD is bradykinesia, which interferes with all aspects of daily living such as walking, rising from a chair, turning in bed, dressing. Fine motor control is also impaired as evidenced by decreased manual dexterity and handwriting (*micrographia*). Soft speech (*hypophonia*) and sialorrhea are other troubling manifestations of (bulbar) bradykinesia. Rest tremor, at a frequency of 4 to 6 Hz, typically appears unilaterally, first distally, involving the digits and wrist where it may have a "pill-rolling" character. Tremor usually spreads proximally, ipsilaterally, and occasionally to the leg before crossing to the other side after a year or more. It may appear later in the lips, tongue, and jaw but spares the head. Rigidity is felt as a uniform resistance to passive movement about a joint throughout the full range of motion, giving rise to a characteristic "plastic" quality. Brief, regular interruptions of resistance during passive movement, corresponding to subclinical tremor, may give rise to a "cogwheeling" sensation. Dystonia involving the distal arm or leg may occur early in the disease, unrelated to treatment, especially in younger patients. It can also be provoked by antiparkinsonian drug therapy.

Gait disturbance with shuffling short steps and a tendency to turn en bloc is a prominent feature of PD. Festinating gait, a classic parkinsonian sign, results from the combination of flexed posture and loss of postural reflexes, which cause the patient to accelerate in an effort to "catch up" with the body's center of gravity. Freezing of gait, a feature of more advanced PD, occurs commonly at the onset of locomotion (start hesitation), when attempting to change direction or turn around, and upon entering a narrow space such as a doorway.

Abnormalities of balance and posture tend to increase in prominence as the disease progresses. Flexion of the head, stooping and tilting of the upper trunk, and a tendency to hold the arm in a flexed posture while walking are common, as are changes in the posture of the fingers and hands. Postural instability is one of the most disabling features of advanced PD, contributing to falls and injuries and leading to major morbidity and mortality. Significant postural instability and falls in the first years of the illness, however, strongly suggest a diagnosis other than PD.

Non-Motor Features Non-motor aspects of PD include depression and anxiety, cognitive impairment, sleep disturbances, sensory abnormalities and pain, loss of smell (*anosmia*), and disturbances of autonomic function. Together they may contribute as much to the burden of the disease as the more obvious motor abnormalities. Some of these (e.g., anosmia, depression, and sleep disorders) may be present long before the onset of motor signs. The physiologic basis of the non-motor signs and symptoms are explained in part by widespread involvement of brainstem, olfactory, thalamic, and cortical structures, as discussed below.

Sensory symptoms most often manifest as a distressing sensation of inner restlessness presumed to be a form of akathisia. Aching pain and discomfort in the extremities can be a prominent presenting symptom or develop when antiparkinson medications are wearing off. Other patients develop a subjective shortness of breath in the absence of any underlying cardiorespiratory pathology.

Sleep disorders are common in PD. Daytime drowsiness and frequent napping are typical signs of sleep disruption. Factors that disrupt sleep include nighttime reemergence of bradykinesia and rigidity, with difficulty turning in bed, as well as tremor and involuntary movements (e.g., myoclonic jerks or periodic leg movements). Restless legs and rapid eye movement–behavioral disorder (RBD) are present in considerable numbers of patients, often preceding the onset of PD. Vivid dreams and hallucinations related to dopaminomimetic therapy may

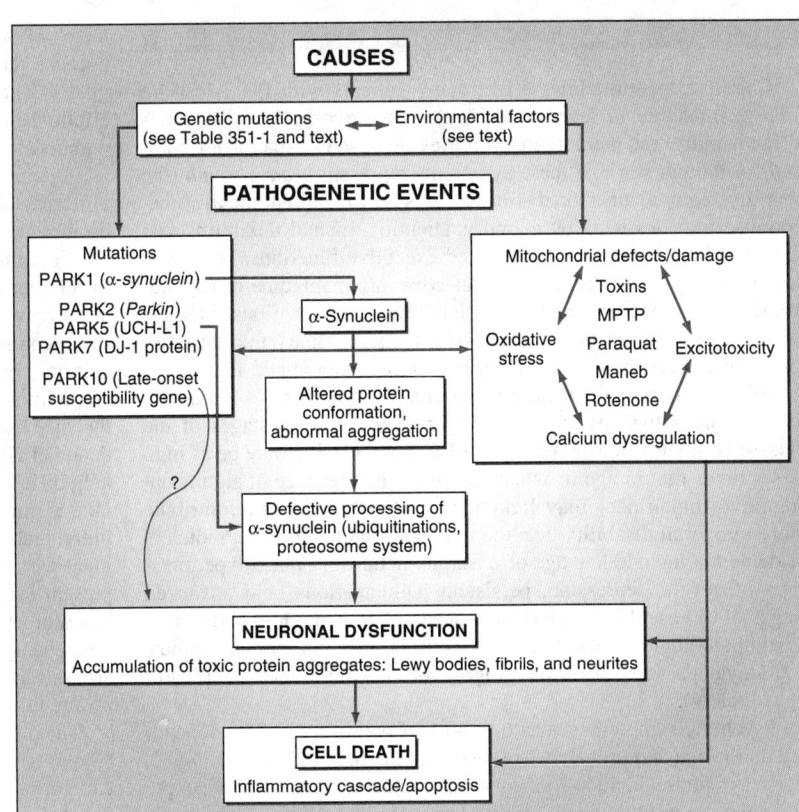

FIGURE 351-1 Possible cascade of pathogenic events leading to neuronal cell death in Parkinson's disease.

also contribute to sleep disruption. Finally, sleep apnea and other sleep disturbances can occur.

Autonomic dysfunction can produce diverse manifestations, including orthostatic hypotension, constipation, urinary urgency and frequency, excessive sweating, and seborrhea. Orthostatic hypotension is present in many patients resulting from sympathetic denervation of the heart or as a side effect of dopaminomimetic therapy. This rarely leads to syncope unless the patient has developed true autonomic failure or has an unrelated cardiac problem. Drenching sweats may occur in advanced PD, often related to wearing off of medication.

Neuropsychiatric Symptoms Changes in mood, cognition, and behavior are common accompaniments of the later stages of PD and may be the direct result of PD or its comorbid pathologies [e.g., Alzheimer's disease (AD), cortical dementia with Lewy bodies (DLB)], or occur as a side effect of its pharmacotherapy.

Depression affects approximately half of patients with PD and can occur at any phase of the illness. It is often difficult to diagnose due to the overlap between the somatic and vegetative symptoms of PD and depression. As a consequence, depression often goes unrecognized and untreated. There is compelling evidence that depression in PD is an intrinsic part of the illness and not simply a reaction to disability. Recognizing even mild depression is particularly important since it can account for otherwise unexplained worsening parkinsonian motor symptoms, new somatic symptoms, and sleep disruption. Depression can also be induced or aggravated iatrogenically by antiparkinsonian and psychotropic agents used to treat other symptoms. Finally, other causes for depressive symptoms and refractory depression should always be considered, including hypothyroidism, hypogonadism, and vitamin B$_{12}$ deficiency.

Anxiety disorders in PD can appear in isolation or as an accompaniment of depression or progressive cognitive impairment. They can also be due to an akathisia equivalent mediated by "dopamine hunger" due to undertreatment of motor symptoms. The development of drug-induced motor fluctuations can compound the problem by precipitating fluxes in anxiety during the off periods that mimic panic attacks.

Cognitive abnormalities affect many patients with PD. Most are mild to moderate in severity. Difficulties with complex tasks, long-term planning, and memorizing or retrieving new information are common. Although some of these symptoms represent *bradyphrenia* (the cognitive equivalent of bradykinesia), it is now clear that the dysfunction also includes working memory, attention, mental flexibility, visuospatial function, word fluency, and executive functions. Iatrogenic contributors include the indiscriminate use of amantadine or psychotropic, anticholinergic, and dopaminomimetic medications. Depression and intercurrent medical illnesses, such as urinary tract or other infections, are reversible causes of cognitive symptoms in PD.

Whether these nondementing abnormalities form a continuum with the dementias that affect a subset of patients in later stages of the disease is unknown. The incidence of dementia in PD may be as high as six times that in age-matched controls. The presence of significant cognitive impairment may limit therapeutic options and contribute more to overall disability than the motor symptoms in PD. Predictors of dementia include late age of onset, akinetic rigid phenotype, presence of severe depression, persistent hallucinations, and advanced stages of disease. In most instances accumulating amyloid and α-synuclein pathologies in the frontal lobes, basal forebrain, hippocampus, and amygdala account for the progression of symptoms (see "Pathology," below).

Psychotic symptoms affect 6 to 40% of patients with PD, depending on the age and prevalence of dementia in the population surveyed. Early symptoms include formed visual hallucinations (usually people and animals) with retained insight. Although depression and dementia are the most important risk factors for psychotic symptoms in PD, the symptoms are often triggered by drug therapy and are dose-dependent. Dopaminomimetics, anticholinergics, amantadine, and selegiline are the chief offenders. Delusions are more disturbing than hallucinations because they place an even heavier burden on the family and caregivers. The prodrome to these psychotic symptoms includes subtle erratic behaviors with temperamental and sometimes unreasonable outbursts.

Differential Diagnosis   The differential diagnosis of parkinsonian syndromes requires a careful history and physical examination (Table 351-2). Neuroimaging with magnetic resonance imaging (MRI) is useful to rule out disorders such as normal pressure hydrocephalus, vascular disease, or mass lesions. Positron emission tomography (PET) is helpful in confirming suspected atypical forms (see "Corticobasal Degeneration," below). Essential tremor (ET) is sometimes confused with rest tremor in PD, but the absence of other signs of parkinsonism and the bilaterality, higher frequency (8 to 10 Hz), and postural dependency of ET plus significant relief with even a small amount of alcohol help differentiate this from the rest tremor of PD. In individuals under 40 it is important to rule out Wilson's disease (Chap. 339). In younger individuals Huntington's disease (HD) sometimes presents with prominent parkinsonian features. Although parkinsonian features are often present in AD, they are greatly outweighed by the cognitive and behavioral disturbances. In DLB, the parkinsonian features are compounded by the early appearance of hallucinations and disturbances in arousal and behavior. Parkinsonism may also develop following exposure to certain neurotoxins such as carbon monoxide or manganese.

The differentiation of sporadic PD from atypical parkinsonism (see below) is the most difficult task, since early in their course these atypical forms often meet diagnostic criteria for PD. Accordingly, it is important not to settle on a definite diagnosis at the first visit. The development of early imbalance and falls suggests progressive supranuclear palsy (PSP); early urinary incontinence, orthostatic hypotension, and dysarthria suggest multiple system atrophy (MSA). The

TABLE 351-2   *Differential Diagnosis of Parkinsonism*

PRIMARY PARKINSONISM	SECONDARY PARKINSONISM

I. Familial ("primary") PD (rare; see Table 351-1)
II. Idiopathic ("sporadic") PD (most common form)
  Phenotype may be influenced by vulnerability genes and environmental factors
III. Other neurodegenerative disorders
  A. Disorders associated with α-synuclein pathology
    1. Multiple systems atrophies (glial and neuronal inclusions)
      a. Striatonigral degeneration
      b. Olivopontocerebellar atrophy
      c. Shy-Drager syndrome
      d. Motor neuron disease with PD features
    2. Dementia with Lewy bodies (cortical and brainstem neuronal inclusions)
  B. Disorders associated with primary tau pathology ("tauopathies")
    1. Progressive supranuclear palsy
    2. Corticobasal degeneration
    3. Frontotemporal dementia
  C. Disorders associated with primary amyloid pathology ("amyloidopathies")
    1. Alzheimer's disease with parkinsonism
IV. Genetically mediated disorders with occasional parkinsonian features
  A. Wilson's disease
  B. Hallervorden-Spatz disease
  C. Chédiak-Higashi disease
  D. SCA-3 spinocerebellar ataxia
  E. X-linked dystonia-parkinsonism (DYT3)
  F. Fragile X premutation associated ataxia-tremor-parkinsonism syndrome
  G. Huntington's disease (Westphalt variant)
  H. Prion disease
V. Miscellaneous acquired conditions
  A. Vascular parkinsonism
  B. Normal pressure hydrocephalus
  C. Catatonia
  D. Cerebral Palsy
	I. Repeated head trauma ("dementia pugilistica" with parkinsonian features)
	II. Infectious and postinfectious diseases
	  A. Postencephalitic PD
	  B. Neurosyphillis
	III. Metabolic conditions
	  A. Hypoparathyroidism or pseudohypoparathyroidism with basal ganglia calcifications
	  B. Non-Wilsonian hepatolenticular degeneration
	IV. Drugs
	  A. Neuroleptics (typical antipsychotics)
	  B. Selected atypical antipsychotics (see text)
	  C. Antiemetics (e.g., compazine, metoclopramide)
	  D. Dopamine-depleting agents (reserpine, tetrabenazine)
	  E. α-Methyldopa
	  F. Lithium carbonate
	  G. Valproic acid
	  H. Fluoxetine
	V. Toxins
	  A. 1-Methyl-1,2,4,6 tetrahydropyridine (MPTP)
	  B. Manganese
	  C. Cyanide
	  D. Methanol
	  E. Carbon monoxide
	  F. Carbon disulfide
	  G. *N*-hexane?

Note: PD, Parkinson's disease.

early appearance of drug-induced hallucinations strongly favors the diagnosis of DLB. As a rule the different forms of atypical parkinsonism can be reliably differentiated from sporadic PD within the first 3 to 4 years.

Pathology Gross pathologic examination of the brain in PD reveals mild frontal atrophy with loss of the normal dark melanin pigment of the midbrain. Microscopically there is degeneration of the dopaminergic cells with the presence of Lewy bodies (LBs) in the remaining neurons and processes of the substantia nigra pars compacta (SNpc), other brainstem nuclei, and regions such as the medial temporal, limbic, and frontal cortices. LBs have a high concentration of α-synuclein and are the pathologic hallmark of the disorder. Mutations in the α-synuclein gene can cause familial PD by promoting the formation of α-synuclein-positive filaments that aggregate into LBs and Lewy neurites (Fig. 351-2). This pathology may begin in the anterior olfactory nuclei and lower brainstem (glossopharyngeal and vagal nerve nuclei), with ascending brainstem involvement of the locus coeruleus, n. gigantocellularis, and the raphe, before extending to the magnocellular nuclei of the basal forebrain, the central nucleus of the amygdala, and the SNpc. Involvement of these nuclei may play a role in the non-motor (e.g., autonomic, sleep, emotional, and cognitive) and refractory motor aspects (e.g., postural instability, gait, and bulbar disturbances) of PD.

The biochemical consequence of dopaminergic cell loss in the SNpc is gradual denervation of the striatum, the main target projection for the SNpc neurons. Other target regions of these neurons include the intralaminar and parafascicular nuclei of the thalamus, the globus pallidus, and the subthalamic nucleus (STN). Dopamine denervation of the striatum leads to many of the motor symptoms of PD. Symptoms develop when striatal dopamine depletion reaches 50 to 70% of normal. Pharmacologic restoration of dopamine transmission is the basis for symptomatic drug treatment of PD.

GENETIC CONSIDERATIONS Although >90% of cases of idiopathic PD appear to be sporadic, increasing evidence indicates that genetic factors play an important role in many forms PD. Much of this evidence comes from studies of the concordance rates for PD among monozygotic and dizygotic twins. These studies suggest that heredity plays an important role in cases with age of onset <50 years and a less important role in older patients. Four genes have been clearly linked to familial forms of PD (Table 351-1), and a number of other candidate genes or genetic loci have been identified as possibly causative of PD. Among the former, PARK1 and PARK5 lead to an autosomal dominant form of PD with atypical features such as early age of onset and rapid progression of symptoms. PARK1 encodes α-synuclein, leading to its abnormal aggregation. PARK2 and PARK7 lead to autosomal recessive disorders also with atypical features, including juvenile forms of parkinsonism. PARK2 encodes *parkin*, an E3 ubiquitin protein ligase. Mutations in *parkin* appear to be the major cause of autosomal recessive PD. Remarkably, PARK5 codes for the ubiquitin carboxy-terminal hydroxylase L1 (UCH-L1), another component of the ubiquitin proteosomal system. Because ubiquitination of proteins targets them for degradation in the proteosome, these findings suggest that abnormal proteosomal processing is important in the pathogenesis of PD. Other mutations with yet-to-be identified genes include PARK10, a late-onset PD susceptibility gene. All these mutations are thought to affect α-synuclein or its biochemical processing, either directly or indirectly. The identification of these and other mutations are proving invaluable in refining the correlation between genotypes and phenotypes, in generating animal models to study pathogenesis, and in identifying target pathways for possible therapeutic intervention.

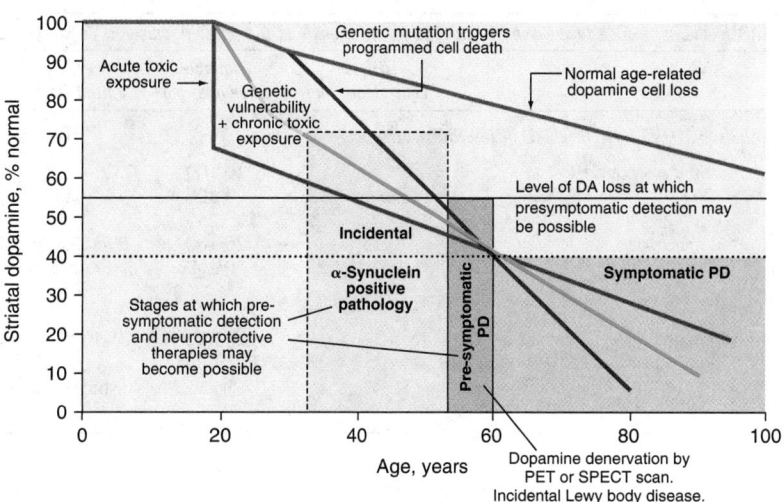

FIGURE 351-2 Proposed stages of Parkinson's disease (PD) based on extrapolations from epidemiologic field studies and on brain imaging data using PET and SPECT technology. At presymptomatic stages the patient would not meet criteria for the clinical diagnosis of PD but may instead exhibit striatal dopamine denervation on PET scan or, in familial cases, have a positive genetic test. This stage is thought to last about 5 years. The presence of incidental α-synuclein positive pathology (Lewy neurites or LBs) at autopsy may be the earliest recognizable stage of PD. PET, positron emission tomography using 18-F fluorodopa; SPECT, single proton emission computerized tomography using β-CIT, both presynaptic markers of presynaptic dopamine innervation.

Pathogenesis (Fig. 351-1) In PD dopaminergic and other cells die due to a combination of factors including: (1) genetic vulnerability, (2) oxidative stress, (3) proteosomal dysfunction, and (4) environmental factors, most of which have yet to be identified.

Oxidative stress appears to play an important role in the sporadic forms of PD. Endogenous sources of oxidative stress include the free-radicals produced by the metabolism of dopamine and melanin. Additional stress may come from defects in mitochondrial complex I of the oxidative phosphorylation chain in patients with PD. This defect has been detected in platelets and muscle and in postmortem tissue from the substantia nigra. Several toxins have been shown to cause oxidative toxicity and dopamine cell death in animal models of PD, further strengthening the above hypothesis. The most important of these are MPTP, a meperidine derivative, and rotenone, a commonly used insecticide. Both cause oxidative damage by inhibiting complex I. In vitro, oxidative stress can lead to aggregation of α-synuclein and proteosomal dysfunction. Proteosomal system abnormalities have also been described in the substantia nigra from sporadic cases of PD. The other factors of the selective dopamine neuron degeneration in PD are microglial activation, low-grade inflammation, and apoptosis, each a potential target for therapeutic intervention.

TREATMENT

General Considerations The goals of therapy in PD are to maintain function and quality of life and to avoid drug-induced complications. Bradykinesia, tremor, rigidity, and abnormal posture respond well to symptomatic therapy early in the course of the illness. In contrast, cognitive symptoms, hypophonia, autonomic dysfunction, and balance difficulties respond poorly. Primary motor disability in PD is often aggravated by secondary disability resulting from physical deconditioning following a sedentary life-style. Prevention of secondary disability requires a consistent program of physical activity, thus regular activity is strongly encouraged. Remaining mentally active is probably equally important.

A current priority is to move beyond symptom control to neuroprotective therapies. Unfortunately, no such therapy is yet available, although selegiline (deprenyl) may, in addition to a mild symptomatic effect, have a neuroprotective function. High doses of coenzyme Q_{10} and intrastriatal infusion of neurotrophic factors show promise in early clinical trials. Animal studies have shown that exercise can promote neuroprotection against neurotoxins.

CARBIDOPA/LEVODOPA (TYPICAL INITIAL STRENGTH)		LD Dose Equivalency, mg	Available Strengths, mg	Initial Dose	Other Considerations
Carbidopa/levodopa IR 25/100	→	100 (anchor dose)	10/100 25/100 25/250	25/100; 0.5 tab tid	Target dose = 3–6 25/100 tabs/d
Carbidopa/levodopa CR 50/200	→	150	25/100 50/200	50/200; one tab bid to tid	Increased bioavailability with food; splitting the tablet negates the CR property
Carbidopa/levodopa/entacapone 25/100/200	→	120	12.5/50/200 25/100/200 37.5/150/200	25/100/200; one tab bid to tid	Do not split tablets

	DA Equivalent to LD Anchor Dose Above, mg[a]	Available Strengths, mg	Approximate Target Doses			Other Considerations
			Initial Dose, mg	As Monotherapy, mg/d	As Adjuncts to LD, mg/d	
DOPAMINE AGONISTS						
Non-ergot alkaloids						
Ropinirole	5	0.25, 0.5, 1, 2, 3, 4, 5	0.25 tid	12–24	6–16	Hepatic metabolism; potential drug-drug interactions Occasionally associated with "sleep attacks"
Pramipexole	1	0.125, 0.25, 1, 1.5	0.125 tid	1.5–4.5	0.375–3.0	Renal metabolism; dose adjustments needed in renal insufficiency Occasionally associated with "sleep attacks"
Ergot alkaloids						
Pergolide	1	0.05, 0.25, 1.0	0.05 tid	1.5–6	0.3–3	Rare reports of valvular heart disease; fewer reports of sleep attacks compared to non-ergots
Bromocriptine	2	2.5, 5.0	1.25 bid to tid	7.5–15	3.75–7.5	Rare reports of pulmonary and retroperitoneal fibrosis Relative incidence of sleep attacks not well studied

[a] Equivalency doses are approximations based on clinical experience and may not correlate with the relative in vitro binding properties of these compounds.

Note: LD, levodopa (with carbidopa); IR, immediate release; CR, controlled release; DA, dopamine agonist. Carbidopa/levodopa/entacapone, Stalevo.

Initiation of Therapy From a practical standpoint, dopaminomimetic therapy should be initiated as soon as the patient's symptoms begin to interfere with quality of life. The ideal agent for initiation of symptomatic therapy depends on the age and cognitive status of the patient and, to a lesser extent, the patient's clinical type and finances. The choices consist of either a levodopa preparation or a dopamine agonist. Controlled studies support the view that, in early PD, dopamine agonist monotherapy is well tolerated and significantly reduces the risk of later treatment-related complications such as motor fluctuations and dyskinesias. *Motor fluctuations* are the exaggerated ebb and flow of parkinsonian signs experienced by many patients between doses of antiparkinsonian medications. *Dyskinesias* refer to choreiform and dystonic movements that can occur as a peak dose effect or at the beginning or end of the dose (diphasic dyskinesias). More than 50% of patients with PD treated over five years with levodopa will develop these complications.

Successful dopamine agonist monotherapy requires a higher dose of the agonist than is typically needed when the agonist is used to supplement levodopa (Table 351-3). In both cases titration has to be slow and cautious to avoid unnecessary side effects. Patients benefit greatly from education and support during this titration. Most patients will require the addition of levodopa or another agent within 1 to 3 years of initiating dopamine agonist monotherapy. Preclinical studies suggest that the advantages of dopamine agonist monotherapy can be maintained with agonist-dominant therapy. In this case dopamine agonists continue to provide the bulk of dopaminomimetic therapy, with levodopa playing a supplementary role.

Although dopamine agonist monotherapy is considered the initial treatment of choice for most patients with PD, the long-term benefits noted above must be balanced against a higher incidence of non-motor side effects and a slightly higher level of motor disability than with levodopa. These recommendations may need to be modified in patients with psychotic symptoms or severe daytime sleep disturbances. Older patients and those with akinetic rigid phenotypes of PD have a lower risk of motor complications and dyskinesias compared to the average PD patient and may be satisfactorily treated with levodopa.

Pharmacotherapy of Motor Symptoms The above advances in the initiation of therapy notwithstanding, levodopa remains the most effective treatment for PD. It significantly improves motor symptoms and increases quality of life and independence. The aim of all dopaminomimetic strategies is to restore dopamine transmission in the striatum. This is accomplished by stimulating postsynaptic receptors (directly with dopamine agonists), increasing dopamine precursor availability (levodopa), blocking the metabolism of levodopa in the periphery and in the brain, and blocking the catabolism of dopamine at the presynaptic terminal.

DOPAMINE AGONISTS Dopamine agonists readily cross the blood-brain barrier and act directly on postsynaptic dopamine receptors (primarily D_2 type). Compared to levodopa, they are longer acting and thus provide a more uniform stimulation of dopamine receptors. They are effective as monotherapeutic agents and as adjuncts to carbidopa/levodopa therapy. They can also be used in combination with anticholinergics and amantadine. Table 351-3 provides a guide to the doses and uses of these agents.

Available agents include two ergot alkaloids, pergolide and bromocriptine, and two non-ergot alkaloids, pramipexole and ropinirole. Apomorphine has been available for subcutaneous infusion and injection in Europe and Canada for many years and will soon become available in the United States as "rescue therapy" to help control motor fluctuations ("off" spells) in patients with moderate to advanced disease. These agents are particularly effective in treating bradykinesia and gait disturbances, but they are less effective in treating tremor. Side effects include nausea, postural hypotension, psychiatric symptoms, daytime sedation, and occasional sleep attacks. These can be managed using the above strategies and, in severe cases, through the introduction of peripheral dopamine blockers such as domperidone (not available in the United States) or short courses of trimethobenzamide or dronabinol until the symptoms subside. Patients need to be warned against the potential for sleep attacks, which can occur without warning and have resulted in traffic accidents. This phenomenon has been most often associated with agonists and less so with carbidopa/levodopa. Pergolide has recently been shown to be associated with valvular disease. When used as adjuncts to levodopa therapy these agents can aggravate dyskinesias if the doses of carbidopa/levodopa are not adjusted accordingly, and they are more expensive than carbidopa/levodopa, which is now available in generic form.

CARBIDOPA/LEVODOPA FORMULATIONS Carbidopa/levodopa is available in regular, immediate release (IR) formulations (Sinemet, Atamet and others; 10/100 mg, 25/100 mg, and 25/250 mg), controlled release (CR) formulations (Sinemet CR 25/100 mg, 50/200 mg), and more recently as Stalevo (Table 351-3). The latter combines IR carbidopa/levodopa with 200 mg of entacapone (see below). In most individuals, at least 75 mg/d of carbidopa is necessary to block peripheral levodopa decarboxylation into dopamine and thus symptoms of nausea and orthostasis often associated with the initiation of levodopa. Initial target doses of these medications are summarized in the table. Individualized and gradual escalation of these doses is recommended. Initiation of dosing at mealtimes will reduce the incidence and severity of nausea. As patients develop tolerance to nausea and other side effects, these medications can be administered on an empty stomach, which generally leads to a more brisk and predictable absorption.

LEVODOPA AUGMENTATION Selegiline is a selective and irreversible monoamine oxidase (MAO) B inhibitor with a weak symptomatic effect when used as monotherapy or as an adjunct to carbidopa/levodopa. Typically, selegiline is used as initial therapy or is added to alleviate tremor or levodopa-associated wearing-off. The usual dose is 5 mg with breakfast and lunch. At this dose there is no need for dietary restrictions, as is the case with non-selective and MAO-A inhibitors. A significant side-effect of selegiline is insomnia. Older individuals, and those with significant cardiac abnormalities, may benefit from doses as low as 2.5 mg/d. The potential role of selegiline (or desmethylselegiline) as neuroprotective therapy remains controversial.

The catechol *O*-methyltransferase (COMT) inhibitors entacapone and tolcapone offer yet another strategy to augment the effects of levodopa by blocking the enzymatic degradation of levodopa and dopamine. Entacapone is preferred to tolcapone because of the low but potentially serious incidence of hepatic and hematologic side effects of the latter. When used in conjunction with carbidopa/levodopa, these agents increase the area under the curve of plasma levodopa by >30%. They alleviate wearing-off symptoms and increase by 1 to 2 h the time a patient remains "on" (i.e., well medicated) during the day. The more common side effects are gastrointestinal and hyperdopaminergic, including increased dyskinesias that may require reductions in the dose of carbidopa/levodopa. The dose of entacapone is 200 mg coadministered with each dose of carbidopa/levodopa. The dose of tolcapone is 50 to 200 mg tid.

Anticholinergics and amantadine are appropriate adjuncts to dopaminomimetic therapy. Anticholinergics are particularly useful for controlling rest tremor and dystonia, and amantadine can reduce drug-induced dyskinesias by up to 70%. The mechanisms of action of amantadine are unknown, although there is evidence it has both anticholinergic and dopaminomimetic properties. Recently amantadine has been shown to have weak glutamate antagonist properties, a mechanism thought responsible for reducing drug-induced dyskinesias. The side-effects of amantadine are nausea, headaches, edema, erythema, and livedo reticularis. In older patients, it may aggravate confusion and psychosis. Doses need to be adjusted in patients with renal failure.

Therapy of Non-Motor Symptoms Patients with frequent nighttime awakenings due to nocturnal akinesia or tremor can be treated with supplemental doses of carbidopa/levodopa at night. A bedtime dose of dopamine agonists helps restless leg symptoms and urinary urgency. Treatment of other bladder symptoms will improve sleep for many elderly patients. Depression typically responds to antidepressants [e.g., tricyclics, selective serotonin reuptake inhibitors (SSRIs)]. The combination of SSRIs and selegiline carries an exceedingly low risk of a hyperserotonergic syndrome (delirium with myoclonus and hyperpyrexia). Electroconvulsive therapy (ECT) is highly effective in drug-refractory cases or in patients intolerant of oral antidepressants. There are several reports indicating that ECT, in addition, has short-term benefit for parkinsonian motor symptoms.

In patients with psychotic symptoms or confusion, anticholinergics and amantadine should be eliminated first. In severe cases not responding to the above approach, some dopaminomimetics may have to be reduced or eliminated. Further drug simplification and dose reductions should proceed in the following order: selegiline, nocturnal doses of dopamine agonists, Sinemet CR, daytime doses of dopamine agonists, and finally, daytime doses of carbidopa/levodopa. If the patient improves after only a modest reduction of antiparkinsonian therapy, the overall impact on the parkinsonian motor symptoms will be negligible. If in the process parkinsonian symptoms worsen, most specialists initiate treatment with an atypical antipsychotic with a low incidence of extrapyramidal side effects rather than continuing to lower dopaminomimetic therapy. Quetiapine is recommended first because, although not as well studied in PD as clozapine, it has proved to be effective in open-label studies and lacks the small risk of agranulocytosis associated with clozapine. Typical doses of quetiapine are 12.5 to 100 mg/d, and for clozapine 12.5 to 100 mg/d. Both are dosed at night to promote sleep and minimize daytime sedation and orthostasis. Other atypical antipsychotics, such as risperidone and olanzapine, are not well tolerated by most patients with PD because they are associated with dose-dependent parkinsonism. Early evidence suggests that the use of acetylcholinesterase inhibitors may be well tolerated and capable of treating hallucinations and delusions in patients with PD and dementia.

Given the complexity of the above polypharmacy, the management of non-motor symptoms is best carried out in an interdisciplinary setting, coordinated by a neurologist who specializes in PD together with a psychiatrist and the patient's primary care physician.

Neuroprotective Therapy Reducing the progression of PD through neuroprotective or restorative therapy is a major focus of research. Epidemiologic studies suggest that the chronic use of nonsteroidal anti-inflammatory agents or the use of estrogen replacement in postmenopausal women may delay or prevent the onset of PD through yet unclear mechanisms. From a pharmacologic standpoint, current strategies involve interrupting the cascade of biochemical events that leads to death of dopaminergic cells (Fig. 351-2). The first such clinical trial in PD was the large multicenter DATATOP study in which selegiline monotherapy delayed the need for levodopa therapy by 9 to 12 months in newly diagnosed patients. Most evidence indicates that this delay was due to a mild symptomatic effect of selegiline. Long-term follow-up of the DATATOP cohort revealed that patients who remained on selegiline for 7 years experienced slower motor decline compared to those who were changed to placebo after 5 years. The 7-year patient group was more likely to develop dyskinesias but less likely to develop freezing gait. Finally, the metabolite of selegiline, desmethylselegiline, has been shown in laboratory studies to have powerful neuroprotective effects, possibly through interactions of glyceraldehyde-3-phosphate dehydrogenase (GAPDH) and other cellular protective (antiapoptotic) factors. Clinical trials to test this agent are under way.

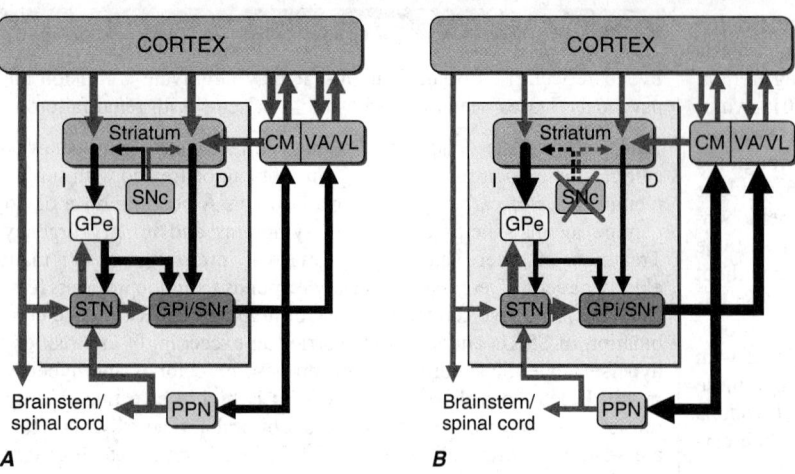

FIGURE 351-3 Schematic diagram of the basal ganglia–thalamocortical circuitry under normal conditions and in Parkinson's disease (PD). Inhibitory connections are shown as black arrows and excitatory connections as red arrows. Note that in PD, striatal dopamine denervation results in increased traffic in the indirect pathway and decreased traffic in the direct pathway. The downstream consequence of this is increased activity in striatal outflow stemming from the increased activity of STN and ultimately GPi/SNr neurons. Because striatal outflow is inhibitory to the thalamus (main neurotransmitter = γ-aminobutyric acid), there is a decrease in the ability of the thalamus to activate the frontal cortex leading to signs of parkinsonism. As discussed, changes in discharge pattern are also a major factor. D, direct pathway; I, indirect pathway; GPe, external segment of the globus pallidus; GPi, internal segment of the globus pallidus; SNr, substantia nigra, pars reticulata; SNc, substantia nigra, pars compacta; STN, subthalamic nucleus; VA/VL, ventral anterior and ventrolateral thalamus; CM, centromedian nucleus; PPN, pedunculopontine nucleus. *(Courtesy of T Wichmann, MD, Emory University School of Medicine.)*

In a recent trial, coenzyme Q_{10}, an antioxidant and a cofactor of complex I of the mitochondrial oxidative chain, appeared to delay progression of early disability in PD. Other potentially neuroprotective agents under investigation are acetyl-levo-carnitine and creatine monohydrate. A large controlled study of the antiglutamatergic agent riluzole (Chap. 353) was prematurely discontinued after a futility analysis revealed little effect on progression of symptoms. Dopamine agonists are also under investigation as putative agents to slow disease progression in PD, based on their possible antioxidant properties resulting in part from their ability in vitro to decrease dopamine turnover, scavenge free radicals, and interfere with proapoptotic cell signals. Other promising agents include nitric oxide synthetase inhibitors, antiapoptotic agents such as Jun N-terminal kinase inhibitors, and the antibiotic minocycline. Minocycline can inhibit microglial activation in vitro and interrupt apoptosis by inhibiting caspase 1 and 3, which are involved in the enzymatic processing of α-synuclein.

Surgical Treatments Over the past decade there has been a renaissance in the surgical treatment of PD and other movement disorders. Although both pallidotomy and thalmotomy were performed widely in the 1950s, the introduction of levodopa in the 1960s led to the virtual abandonment of surgery. The resurgence in the use of surgery has been motivated by the fact that after ≥5 years of treatment, many patients develop significant drug-induced motor fluctuations and dyskinesias. Second, advances in understanding of the functional organization of the basal ganglia and the pathophysiologic basis of parkinsonism have provided a clearer rationale for the effectiveness of these procedures and guidance for targeting specific structures (Fig. 351-3). The demonstration, in animal models of PD, that ablation of the STN (subthalamotomy) resulted in a dramatic reduction in all of the cardinal features of parkinsonism was a critical finding.

The selection of suitable patients for surgery is most important, since in general patients with atypical Parkinson's do not have a favorable response. The major indications for surgery are (1) a diagnosis of idiopathic PD, (2) a clear response to levodopa, (3) significant intractable symptoms of PD, and/or (4) drug-induced dyskinesias and wearing-off. Contraindications to surgery include atypical forms of PD, cognitive impairment, major psychiatric illness, substantial medical comorbidities, and advanced age (a relative factor). Signs and symptoms not responding to levodopa, such as postural instability and falling, hypophonia, micrographia, drooling, and autonomic dysfunction, are unlikely to benefit from surgery. As a rule of thumb, the benefits from surgery are unlikely to exceed the benefits of antiparkinson medication. In general, the decision for surgery should be made by a movement disorder neurologist who is part of a team including a neurosurgeon trained in functional neurosurgery, a psychiatrist, a neuropsychologist, and trained technicians.

ABLATION VERSUS DEEP BRAIN STIMULATION (DBS) The use of ablation (e.g., pallidotomy or thalamotomy) has decreased greatly since the introduction of DBS and is generally reserved for individuals who for medical or economic reasons cannot have DBS. Major advantages of DBS are that it is somewhat less invasive and more reversible than ablation, and in addition may be adjusted to best effect following implantation. Although the choice between the STN and the internal segment of the globus pallidus for DBS has shifted toward the STN, the data to support this are lacking. Several clinical trials are now under way to compare these two targets. The available evidence suggests that both are effective for all the cardinal features of PD as well as for dyskinesias and motor fluctuations. Unilateral stimulation is appropriate for patients with asymmetric disease, although bilateral surgery is generally necessary for patients with more advanced disease and for those with significant bilateral manifestations. Reductions in drug dosages appear to be easier with STN than globus pallidus procedures.

The mechanism of action of DBS remains controversial. Since clinically it appears that ablation and stimulation of a given target have a similar effect, it has been assumed that stimulation caused a functional blockade. It is likely, however, that multiple factors are involved. The basis for improvement may be the replacement of abnormal neural activity by a more tolerable pattern of activity. Following ablation or DBS, the remaining motor systems in the brainstem, thalamus, and cortex are able to compensate more effectively for the abnormal activity associated with the parkinsonian state. Whatever the mechanism, it is clear that these approaches can offer impressive results in properly selected patients.

NEUROTRANSPLANTATION AND OTHER SURGICAL APPROACHES Despite highly encouraging open-label pilot studies of fetal cell transplantation, this approach has suffered considerable disappointment with the recent publication of the results from two large, well-controlled clinical trials. The first, using sham surgery, showed only modest benefit in patients under 60 and no benefit in those over 60. An unexpected complication in a number of patients was the development of symptomatic dyskinesias, occurring off medication. The second study has shown similar findings with regard to benefit and the development of dyskinesias. A puzzling feature of these studies is the apparent successful grafting observed by PET and autopsy. Because of these disappointing results, the considerable obstacles to obtaining sufficient fetal tissue, and opposition to the use of fetal tissue on ethical grounds, this approach is now viewed as purely investigational. It is hoped that these issues can be addressed with the development of other strategies to enhance dopaminergic cell function (e.g., carotid body cells; stem cells; encapsulated and genetically engineered cells capable of producing levodopa, dopamine, and/or trophic factors). The favorable response from direct infusion of glial cell–derived neurotrophic factor (GDNF) to the putamen in a small number of patients with PD has raised hopes that this approach, or the use of gene-transfer of trophic factors such as GDNF, will succeed. Preliminary studies in primate models of PD have been encouraging in this regard.

DEMENTIA IN PARKINSON'S DISEASE As noted above, the incidence of dementia in PD may be as high as six times that in the general non-PD population. Approximately a quarter of patients will develop dementia of the Alzheimer type simply due to the overlap of these two common age-related disorders. Pathologically, the incidence of AD-type findings in postmortem tissue from patients dying with PD is as high as 40%. Conversely, 25% of AD patients have at least mild clinical parkinsonian features such as rigidity and bradykinesia, and ≥60% have coexistent α-synuclein pathology in the cortex. Patients with PD-dementia (PDD) typically have the akinetic/rigid form of the disorder where tremor is less prominent than in idiopathic PD. The course of PDD is more rapid and the management is more difficult than in PD due to the high incidence of cognitive side effects from antiparkinsonian therapy, particularly anticholinergics and amantadine. Central dopaminomimetic toxicity can present in many ways, ranging from sleep disruption with daytime sleepiness, personality changes, depression and mental dullness, episodic confusion, hallucinations, and disruptive behaviors.

DLB is an increasingly recognized form of dementia with prominent parkinsonian features. The dementia may precede or follow the parkinsonian syndrome. In patients presenting with parkinsonian features, the dementia is often heralded by levodopa-induced sedation, myoclonus, and hallucinations. Early on, the phenotype can be indistinguishable from PD. Features that help differentiate this entity from PD include the presence of an action rather than a rest tremor, a rapidly fading response to levodopa, and rapidly fluctuating, spontaneous, and drug-induced problems with arousal. Another feature of DLB is the higher incidence of neuropsychiatric symptoms than in idiopathic PD. These symptoms include apathy, personality changes, depression, fixed delusions, and hallucinations. Finally, patients with DLB exhibit a heightened sensitivity to drug-induced parkinsonism (DIP) when exposed to any dopamine blocker. The progression of symptoms in DLB is intermediate between the PD and PD/AD overlap. →*DLB is discussed in detail in Chap. 350.*

OTHER PARKINSONIAN DISORDERS

PARKINSONIAN DISORDERS ASSOCIATED WITH ABNORMAL METABOLISM OF α-SYNUCLEIN (α-SYNUCLEINOPATHIES) ■ Multiple System Atrophy   MSA represents a sporadic group of disorders characterized by varying degrees of parkinsonism and cerebellar, corticospinal, and autonomic dysfunction. The average age of onset is 50 years (earlier than in PD), and the median survival 6 to 9 years. The clinical presentation is highly varied and may begin with any of the above clinical signs. The unifying pathologic hallmark is the presence of α-synuclein-positive inclusions located in various brain regions.

CLINICAL PHENOTYPES   With disease progression, 90% percent of patients exhibit parkinsonian signs, 80% signs of autonomic failure, and a similarly high percentage exhibit upper motor neuron signs. Tremor is common but, unlike in PD, this and other parkinsonian signs are more likely to present symmetrically. Parkinsonian symptoms are typically poorly responsive to dopaminergic therapy, although some patients may respond favorably for years. Drug-induced dyskinesias typically involve the face and neck rather than the trunk and limbs, as is the case in PD. Corticospinal signs consist of spasticity, involving the legs more than the arms, and pseudobulbar palsy. This aspect of the illness may mimic primary lateral sclerosis with lower motor neurons being occasionally involved. A few patients develop myoclonus.

Signs of autonomic failure include orthostatic hypotension, leg swelling not due to drug therapy, changes in sweating patterns, and autonomic storms with diaphoresis and flushing. Orthostatic hypotension can present with dizziness, faintness, or syncope. Once patients are successfully treated for syncope, they often develop fatigue and lassitude. This is due in part to chronic tissue hypoperfusion caused by marginal blood pressures while sitting or standing. More aggressive management of the blood pressure is warranted but not always successful. Urinary symptoms include urgency, retention, and incontinence. In men impotence is one of the earliest and most prominent signs. The autonomic dysfunction can precede or follow the development of other neurologic signs by several years. Dementia may not be as frequent as in PD.

The clinical phenotype of MSA can fall into one of three broad categories, termed *striatonigral degeneration* (SND), *olivopontocerebellar atrophy* (OPCA), and *progressive autonomic failure* (PAF), either without parkinsonism or with parkinsonism (Shy-Drager syndrome). Patients presenting with a relatively pure form of akinetic rigid parkinsonism and a limited response to levodopa are designated as SND. The diagnosis is difficult. Individuals with other signs such as ataxia, upper motor neuron and corticobulbar involvement, myoclonus, oculomotor abnormalities, peripheral neuropathy, and deafness fit into the category of OPCA. This phenotype is notably heterogeneous, with sporadic and hereditary forms. The sporadic forms are more likely to form part of the spectrum referred to in this section, with the hereditary forms usually representing one of the spinocerebellar ataxias (Chap. 352). Finally, a diagnosis of Shy-Drager syndrome is justified when the parkinsonian features are associated with prominent signs of autonomic dysfunction. Although the above categories remain clinically useful, it should be noted that as disease progresses, there tends to be more clinical and pathologic overlap than separation between these entities.

The spectrum of disease in MSA is determined by the location and density of the LB pathology. For instance, in PD the LBs are confined to neurons in the brainstem, and in DLB to the brainstem, cortex, and hippocampus. In MSA these deposits take the form of glial α-synuclein-positive intracytoplasmic inclusions in the substantia nigra, putamen, inferior olives, pontine nuclei, pigmented nuclei of the brainstem, the intermediolateral nucleus of the spinal cord, and the cerebellum. In addition in MSA there are myelin degeneration and oligodendroglia containing argyrophilic glial cytoplasmic inclusions that are immunoreactive for ubiquitin and α-synuclein. Similar inclusions can be found in neuronal cell bodies and processes.

Several diagnostic tests help differentiate MSA from PD and other parkinsonian syndromes. In OPCA, brain MRI reveals prominent atrophy of the cerebellum, pons, and olivary eminence of the medulla. In SND, prominent volume loss and T2-weighted image hyperintensity in the putamen, globus pallidus, and white matter may be present. Electrodiagnostic studies may reveal rectal sphincter abnormalities with signs of degeneration with reinnervation due to anterior horn cell loss. Commercially available genetic tests are available for many of the spinocerebellar ataxias (Chap. 352) that present with features that overlap OPCA.

℞ TREATMENT

Early in the course of the illness parkinsonian features may respond to dopaminomimetic agents. These have to be used with caution due to their tendency to provoke orthostatic hypotension. →*Treatment of orthostatic hypotension and other autonomic symptoms is discussed in Chap. 354.*

PARKINSONIAN DISORDERS ASSOCIATED WITH ABNORMALITIES OF TAU METABOLISM (TAUOPATHIES)   As in the synucleopathies, the discovery that a group of familial and sporadic disorders with pathology involving the microtubule-associated protein tau has helped classify a group of disorders characterized by atypical parkinsonism and dementia. In the less common familial forms, mutations in the *tau* gene have been linked to rare forms of parkinsonism and to frontotemporal dementia, another tauopathy discussed in Chap. 350. This discussion will focus on two entities that typically present with movement disorders. The first, PSP, has not been linked to mutations in the *tau* gene but is associated with overrepresentation of the H1 *tau* gene haplotype. These and other findings support the view that abnormal processing of tau may be directly linked to the pathogenesis of sporadic and familial tauopathies.

Progressive Supranuclear Palsy   This is a sporadic neurodegenerative disorder of unknown etiology associated with tau pathology. It presents in the sixth to seventh decades and progresses faster than PD, with death in 5 to 10 years. Risk factors include head trauma, vascular disease, dietary exposure to benzyl-tetrahydroisoquinolines (TIQ, reticuline), and beta-carbolines (reports from the West Indies).

PSP is characterized by akinetic rigid parkinsonism, dizziness, unsteadiness, slowness, falls, and pseudobulbar dysarthria. Tremor is distinctly uncommon. Supranuclear eye movement abnormalities affecting downgaze occur first, followed by variable limitations of upward and horizontal eye movement. Because the vestibular ocular reflex ("doll's eyes" maneuver) and the Bell's reflex (elevation and abduction of eyes on attempted lid closure) are intact, these abnormalities are termed *supranuclear*. Neurologic examination often reveals prominent stare and furrowed brow, axial (especially nuchal) and proximal distal limb rigidity and dystonia, as well as upper motor neuron and occasional cerebellar signs. Virtually all patients develop frontal-type cognitive dysfunction (Chap. 350), and a significant number may develop dementia with distinct subcortical features (e.g., abulia, mental inflexibility, and defects in memory retrieval). Brain MRI reveals midbrain atrophy (superior colliculus), and PET studies show symmetric frontal and striatal hypometabolism. Although some response may occur to levodopa and other antiparkinson medications, especially early in the course, treatment is generally not highly effective. The diagnosis is made on clinical grounds.

Pathologically, PSP is characterized by deposition of neurofibrillary tangles histochemically positive for tau (mostly 4-repeat tau) and negative for amyloid or α-synuclein. The deposits are associated with varying degrees of degeneration in the brainstem, basal ganglia, and cerebellum. There is loss of dopamine and dopamine receptors due to intrinsic striatal damage. This is thought to account for the poor response to therapy.

Corticobasal Degeneration (CBD) CBD, another sporadic tauopathy, is less common and has a broader range of clinical presentations than PSP. As with most atypical forms of parkinsonism, it begins insidiously in the sixth to seventh decades with varying degrees of asymmetric progressive apraxia, rigidity, dystonia, bradykinesia, and myoclonic jerks with or without cortical sensory loss. Alien limb phenomena is a characteristic sign present in many cases. The disorder progresses to become bilateral over 2 to 5 years, leading to total incapacity with, ultimately, paraplegia in flexion. A significant number of cases present with frontotemporal dementia or progressive aphasia, followed by asymmetric cortical sensory signs, including abnormalities of graphesthesia and astereognosis (Chap. 350). Brain MRI reveals focal cortical loss in the contralateral superior frontal and parietal lobes with corresponding hypometabolic changes on PET scan, as well as hyperintense signal abnormalities in white matter and sometimes atrophy of the corpus callosum. Treatment is largely ineffective.

Grossly, CBD is a focal cortical degenerative process with asymmetric pathology and volume loss in the parietal and frontal regions. Most of the damage is in the dorsal peri-Rolandic, superior frontal, and superior parietal cortices, whereas cases with aphasia show abnormalities in the peri-Sylvian regions. Histologically, gliosis and swollen (ballooned) achromatic neurons and neuronal loss are present in these cortical regions as well as in the nigra, caudate, putamen, and thalamus. Recent clinicopathologic evidence indicates the syndrome can occur in the absence of basal ganglia or nigral degeneration.

SECONDARY PARKINSONISM ■ **Drug-Induced Parkinsonism** DIP closely resembles PD except for the tremor, which is generally (but not always) less prominent. It is commonly due to neuroleptics, some atypical antipsychotics, lithium carbonate, or antiemetic agents (especially metochlopramide). Less common causes include valproic acid and, more recently, fluoxetine. DIP can be induced as well by the chronic administration of antihypertensive agents such as reserpine and alpha-methyldopa. Exposure to manganese, carbon monoxide or disulfides, cyanide, and methanol can also lead to a parkinsonian state. The severity of the parkinsonian symptoms usually correlates with the dose or exposure to a medication or toxin. If due to medication, the symptoms tend to disappear within days to weeks after stopping the offending agent but may be permanent. Patients with permanent symptoms may have been in the process of developing parkinsonism. DIP may respond to anticholinergic agents, amantadine, and levodopa.

Vascular Parkinsonism The concept of vascular or atherosclerotic parkinsonism remains a topic of controversy. Generally, patients with vascular parkinsonism exhibit an akinetic-rigid syndrome with short mincing steps without tremor. Most have neurologic signs distinguishable from those associated with PD, including upper motor neuron signs, pseudobulbar palsy, or dementia. A poor response to levodopa therapy is characteristic. Imaging studies are heterogeneous and may reveal basal ganglia lacunes or multiple infarcts. The hypertensive and diabetic microangiopathy and diffuse white matter disease (Chap. 349) typically present with patchy, confluent or diffuse white matter in the centrum semiovale. Other causes of microangiopathy can also rarely be a cause. The premortem diagnosis of these disorders is difficult to make with certainty, given the absence of disease markers.

TREMOR

Tremor is defined as an "approximately rhythmic and roughly sinusoidal movement of variable amplitude and frequency" (Elble and Koller). Not all tremors are abnormal; most are involuntary with occasional voluntary tremors occurring in malingerers. Individuals with conversion disorders may show partial control over their tremor symptom. Physiologic tremor is a normal high-frequency, low-amplitude tremor notable only during hyperadrenergic states. Parkinsonian rest tremor is discussed above. Cerebellar kinetic tremor is discussed in Chaps. 21 and 352. Kinetic tremors can be postural, action, or both. Postural tremor is most prominent when the arms are held in front of the chest. Action or intention tremor is most notable when reaching to a target. Most tremor disorders have a predominant tremor type and a variable representation of other tremor types.

ESSENTIAL TREMOR ET is perhaps the most common movement disorder, affecting 5 to 10 million adults and a few children in the United States. It is characterized by a 6- to 12-Hz postural and kinetic tremor affecting the arms in almost all cases. In order of decreasing frequency, other body parts that can also be involved include the head (titubation), legs, the larynx (voice tremor), and the trunk. Diagnosis is made on clinical grounds. An autosomal dominant inheritance pattern is likely; thus a positive family history is very helpful, as is a history of partial response to alcohol consumption. Drugs that can aggravate any tremor include valproic acid, lithium, β-adrenergic agonists, methylxanthines, thyroxin, glucocorticoids, tricyclic antidepressants, and serotonin reuptake blockers. Withdrawal from drugs associated with tolerance, or medical conditions such as thyrotoxicosis and other enhanced adrenergic states, can amplify physiologic tremor, mimic pathologic tremors, or aggravate ET.

Compared to PD, symptoms of ET are generally bilateral from onset and the course slower. A small subset of patients has comorbid PD. ET can nonetheless be associated with significant disability, depending on amplitude of the tremor and the body region involved. Anxiety disorders are comorbid in a significant number of cases, and, as in all movement disorders, symptoms and signs worsen during emotional and physiologic stress. There is no consensus with respect to any pathology associated with ET, and diagnostic imaging of the brain is normal.

℞ **TREATMENT**

There is no cure for ET, but symptoms can be managed adequately with pharmacologic interventions in ~50% of cases and with surgical interventions in 80% of patients. Primidone and propranolol are the first-line treatments for ET; both have shown efficacy in double-blind, placebo-controlled studies. Primidone (50 to 750 mg/d) is often highly effective. The starting dose should be 25 mg (one-half of a 50-mg tab) at bedtime, with slowly increasing doses to minimize sedation. Propranolol (40 to 320 mg/d) is better tolerated but no more effective and is contraindicated in patients with asthma, bradycardia, and some cardiac conduction defects. Additional medications with potential efficacy (with or without the primary agents) include benzodiazepines, gabapentin, topiramate, and botulinum toxin injections to affected muscle groups. Approximately 80% of patients resistant or intolerant to pharmacotherapy respond to thalamotomy or to deep brain stimulation of the ventral intermediate nucleus of the thalamus.

HYPERKINETIC DISORDERS

Hyperkinetic movement disorders (Chap. 21) encompass a wide variety of involuntary movements, which may occur in isolation or in combination. Hyperkinesias have a wide spectrum of severity ranging from subtle restlessness to the violent movements of hemiballismus and the highly complex and emotionally laden vocal tics and coprolalia in Tourette syndrome.

HEMIBALLISMUS/HEMICHOREA Hemiballismus, a dramatic disorder, is typically acute in onset and ranges from mild chorea to the wild flinging movements of ballism. Hemiballismus may be viewed as a large-amplitude, violent form of chorea affecting the proximal more than the distal limbs. The most common cause is a lesion of the subthalamic nucleus, most often a hypertensive lacunar stroke (Fig. 351-4). Other cerebral lesions associated with hemiballismus and hemichorea include cortical, thalamic, and basal ganglia infarcts or lesions and demyelinating disease. Medical management of hemiballismus consists of supportive care to avoid injuries, exhaustion, and dehydration. The condition is difficult to treat pharmacologically but the drugs most consistently beneficial are tetrabenazine (not available in the United States), haloperidol, propranolol, phenytoin, clonazepam, and baclofen. Although hemiballismus was once thought to carry a poor prognosis, with proper treatment there is a high likelihood of survival and improvement over weeks to months. In intractable cases, pallidotomy or thalamotomy can be highly effective.

HUNTINGTON'S DISEASE HD is a fatal autosomal dominant disorder characterized by progressive motor, emotional, and cognitive dysfunction. Onset is typically between the ages of 35 and 45 years (range 3 to 70). HD occurs worldwide, with a prevalence of 10 cases per 100,000. It is caused by mutations in the Huntington's gene on the short arm of

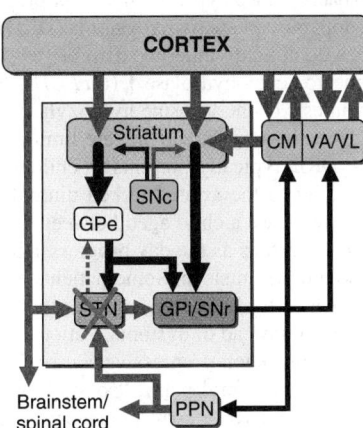

FIGURE 351-4 Schematic diagram of the basal ganglia–thalamocortical circuitry in hemiballismus, a surrogate in this case for other hyperkinetic movement disorders. As in Fig. 351-3, inhibitory connections are shown as black arrows and excitatory connections as red arrows. In hemiballismus the sudden loss of activity in STN neurons or their connections results in the loss of the normal thalamic inhibition by basal ganglia outflow, leading to poorly modulated and excessive thalamic activation of cortex. Clinically the patient exhibits abnormal contralateral choreiform movements. Dopamine antagonists help reduce the violence of the movements by decreasing neuronal activity in the direct pathway and increasing it in the indirect pathway, elevating neuronal activity in GPi/SNr. Parodoxically, surgical lesions of GPi/SNr are also beneficial, suggesting that abnormalities in neuronal discharge patterns are a major factor as well. D, direct pathway; I, indirect pathway; GPe, external segment of the globus pallidus; GPi, internal segment of the globus pallidus; SNr, substantia nigra, pars reticulata; SNc, substantia nigra, pars compacta; STN, subthalamic nucleus; VA/VL, ventral anterior and ventrolateral thalamus; CM, centromedian nucleus; PPN, pedunculopontine nucleus. (*Courtesy of T Wichmann, MD, Emory University School of Medicine.*)

chromosome 4, specifically an expanding and unstable polyglutamine repeat (CAG) in its coding sequence. The gene encodes the highly conserved cytoplasmic protein huntingtin, which is present in all neurons.

Clinical Features A clinical diagnosis of HD can be made readily in cases with a positive family history and an insidious onset of chorea with variable degrees of dementia and emotional symptoms. The term *chorea* ("dance") refers to arrhythmic involuntary movements that are typically sudden and brief and that seem to flow from one part of the body to another. When combined with slower writhing movements or dystonic posturing, the term *choreoathetosis* is often used. Examples of other involuntary movements that may be confused with chorea include myoclonus and tics. Myoclonic jerks are lightning fast but lack the rhythmic flow of activity seen in chorea. While patients with myoclonic jerks commonly lose motor control and drop objects, this rarely happens with chorea or tics. Unlike chorea and myoclonus, motor tics can be readily suppressed voluntarily.

The clinical course of HD can last 15 to 20 years. In the early stages the chorea is focal and segmental (i.e., increased blinking, grimacing) but progresses to involve multiple body parts. The chorea typically peaks within 10 years and is gradually replaced by bradykinesia, rigidity, and dystonia. In 6 to 10% of cases HD may present with a parkinsonian syndrome rather than with chorea (Westphalt variant). The latter cases typically have an early onset (e.g., < 20 years). The behavioral and cognitive disturbances characteristic of HD most often account for the brunt of the patient's disability and most of the hardship to the family. Approximately one-third develop dysthymia or an affective disorder; one-third an intermittent explosive disorder; and the remaining third substance-abuse problems, sexual dysfunction, antisocial personality traits, or schizophreniform symptoms. Depression with suicidal tendencies is not uncommon. Even the minority who may not manifest behavioral problems ultimately succumb to dementia.

The diagnosis of HD is confirmed with genetic testing, which is also helpful in the differential diagnosis of chorea of unknown etiology and in cases of atypical dementia or psychosis. Genetic testing is also used for genetic counseling in adults but is usually not necessary in symptomatic individuals if there is genetic or pathologic confirmation of HD in other family members. Other conditions important in the differential diagnosis of HD include so-called senile chorea occurring in older individuals, benign hereditary chorea in younger individuals, and neuroacanthocytosis, a progressive autosomal recessive degeneration of the basal ganglia associated with acanthocytosis of red cells in the peripheral smear and normal plasma lipoproteins. Ancillary diagnostic measures include MRI to determine if there is caudate atrophy. Other diagnostic measures may be helpful in atypical cases without a clear family history and in cases where the genetic testing results are indeterminate. These tests include PET, which typically reveals decreased striatal metabolic activity before atrophy is apparent, and neuropsychologic testing.

Pathology and Pathophysiology The neuropathology of HD consists of widespread cerebral atrophy with prominent involvement of the striatum and cerebral cortex. Neuronal loss and gliosis are maximal in the caudate initially, with lesser involvement of the cortex and other subcortical structures. Although the mechanism of cell death in HD remains unclear, there is now experimental evidence to support the hypothesis that abnormal glutamatergic transmission with excitotoxicity of striatal cells bearing glutamate receptors plays a role.

℞ TREATMENT

Treatment should involve a multidisciplinary team that can provide social, medical, neuropsychiatric, and genetic guidance to patients and families throughout the course of the illness. Although dopamine blockers are moderately effective for chorea, they may aggravate bradykinesia and dystonia. Atypical antipsychotics such as clozapine, risperidone, and olanzapine are better tolerated but may not be as effective. The indications for treating chorea include interference with activities of daily living and social embarrassment.

Depression responds to conventional antidepressant therapy. The therapy needs to be monitored carefully since it can produce mania or precipitate suicide, a particularly serious problem in HD. Anxiety responds to benzodiazepines as well as to effective treatment of depression. Long-acting benzodiazepines are favored over short-acting ones because of the lesser potential for abuse and paradoxical excitation.

Psychosis can be treated with atypical neuroleptics clozapine (50 to 600 mg/d), quetiapine (100 to 600 mg/d), and risperidone (2 to 8 mg/d). These medications control dyskinesias as well as traditional neuroleptics but have fewer extrapyramidal side effects. When these drugs cannot be tolerated, smaller doses combined with tetrabenazine can be tried. There is currently no adequate treatment for the motor and cognitive decline of HD.

DYSTONIA ■ Clinical Features

Dystonia is a syndrome consisting of involuntary muscular contractions that result in twisting and repetitive movements and/or abnormal postures. Dystonia comprises a large and heterogeneous group of disorders. Although dystonia is one of the more common movement disorders, it is also one of the most frequently under- and misdiagnosed due to its highly variable presentations. The prevalence is not certain because of underreporting but probably exceeds 300,000 cases in the United States, a prevalence equal to that of multiple sclerosis.

Co-contraction of agonist and antagonist muscles is a fundamental feature of dystonia, distinguishing it from chorea, tics, and other dyskinesias. Also, unlike other hyperkinetic movement disorders, dystonia is characteristically present during attempted voluntary movement (so-called action dystonia). It is also associated with "overflow," the abnormal spread of activation to muscles other than those required for the intended movement. As with most movement disorders, dystonia is exacerbated by stress and fatigue. A unique feature of dystonia is that it can often be attenuated by sensory (tactile or proprioceptive) input (so-called sensory tricks). For instance, in patients with torticollis, placing a finger on the chin or the hand on the neck may reduce the twisting movements or abnormal postures. Another common feature of primary dystonia is the presence of dystonic tremor, which may appear in a form resembling essential tremor or as a succession of rapid dystonic movements.

The dystonias can be classified according to: (1) age of onset (childhood vs. adult), (2) region of the body involved, and (3) etiology. Using an etiologic scheme, similar to that used for PD, the dystonias may be divided into primary, secondary, dystonia-plus syndromes, and hereditary degenerative disorders.

PRIMARY DYSTONIA

Primary dystonia includes syndromes in which dystonia is the only clinical manifestation of the disease (other than tremor), and no pathologic changes are evident. Primary dystonia is often inherited and a number of genes have been identified. The major childhood disorder in this group is idiopathic torsion dystonia (ITD), or Oppenheim's dystonia. Sporadic adult-onset focal dystonias are the most common forms of primary dystonia.

Oppenheim's Dystonia

ITD dystonia is an autosomal dominant hereditary disorder affecting primarily Ashkenazy Jewish families (up to 90% of all cases of dystonia) but also present in non-Jewish families. The gene is located on chromosome 9q34 and results in a loss of glutamic acid in the protein Torsin A. The penetrance is about 30%. Families with ITD dystonia may exhibit either generalized or focal dystonia. The age of onset is typically in childhood for generalized and later for focal dystonia. The first signs of dystonia generally occur in the foot during walking or in the arms during voluntary movement. Dystonia later occurs at rest, leading to postural abnormalities. It usually spreads to the arm on the same side before spreading to the other side of the body. The age of onset is typically later in cases in which the symptoms begin in the arm or neck. In late-onset ITD the dystonia

tends to remain focal, in contrast to early-onset forms that usually become generalized.

Focal Dystonias

The most common forms of dystonia are the focal dystonias, which present primarily in adults. These may affect (1) the eyelids, causing them to close involuntarily (*blepharospasm*); (2) the neck and shoulders (*cervical dystonia*), causing the neck to twist to the side (*torticollis*), forward (*anterocollis*), or backward (*retrocollis*); (3) the lower face and jaw or a syndrome causing the jaw to move incessantly (*oromandibular dystonia*); and (4) the larynx (*spasmodic dysphonia*), causing the voice to have a strained and discontinuous quality due to involuntary closing of the vocal cords with phonation. The combination of lower facial and jaw dystonia (*Meige's syndrome*) is not uncommon. Another type of task-specific focal dystonia affects the hand and forearm in specific activities such as handwriting (writer's cramp), typing, or playing a musical instrument (musician's cramp). Dystonia can, in fact, occur in almost any situation involving repetitive activities of the hand or other body parts. The focal dystonias are still often misdiagnosed as psychiatric or orthopedic problems.

The role of hereditary and environmental factors in adult-onset focal dystonia is not well understood. There is now mounting evidence that in some cases dystonia can develop from peripheral factors such as trauma to peripheral nerves. In addition to peripheral injury, discrete cerebral lesions, typically involving the basal ganglia but also the thalamus, cortex, or brainstem, can cause unilateral dystonia. The most frequent cause is a cerebral infarction but trauma, tumor, and other lesions may be accountable. In the case of infarction, the onset of dystonia is typically delayed by weeks to months as the associated hemiparesis clears.

SECONDARY DYSTONIAS

Secondary dystonias are largely due to drugs and other environmental factors. The drug-induced phenomena include levodopa-induced dystonia as well as acute and tardive dystonia associated with dopamine receptor blockers (see "Drug-Induced Movement Disorders," below). External factors producing dystonia include cerebral palsy (athetoid form), cerebral trauma, peripheral nerve injury, cerebral hypoxia, some infectious and postinfectious states, and toxic exposure to manganese, cyanide, and 3-nitro proprionic acid.

Dystonia-Plus Syndromes

Two types of dystonia-plus syndromes deserve mention—dopamine-responsive dystonia (DRD) and myoclonic dystonia. DRD is a dominantly inherited disorder associated with mutations in the gene for cyclohydrolase I (*GTPCH*), the rate-limiting enzyme in the synthesis of the tyrosine hydroxylase cofactor tetrahydrobiopterin. Tyrosine hydroxylase is the rate-limiting enzyme for dopamine synthesis. DRD typically presents in childhood beginning in the legs and spreading to the arms. Marked diurnal fluctuations are common. In the typical case a child aged between 4 and 8 develops a stiff-legged gait that worsens as the day progresses but improves dramatically on awakening from sleep. Some patients exhibit parkinsonism and signs of spasticity. In late-onset cases the presentation may consist of parkinsonism instead of dystonia. Patients have an excellent response to levodopa and a non-progressive course. DRD may be misdiagnosed as "athetoid" cerebral palsy, "spastic" paraplegia, or parkinsonism. Although rare, DRD is so responsive to levodopa that many feel that a trial of levodopa is warranted in all cases of dystonia.

The hereditary syndrome of myoclonic dystonia (also called hereditary dystonia with lightning jerks) is not always easily distinguished from primary dystonia or heredity essential myoclonus. It is distinguished not only by its character but also by its responsiveness to alcohol.

The hereditary degenerative diseases that may manifest dystonia typically present with more prominent parkinsonian features and include Wilson's disease, HD, PD, corticobasal degeneration (CBD), progressive supranuclear palsy (PSP), the Lubag form of dystonia-parkinsonism (DYT3), Leigh's disease, and other mitochondrial encephalopathies.

Pathophysiology

There is now considerable evidence for a loss of inhibition at multiple levels in the central nervous system (CNS), including the cortex, brainstem, and spinal cord, in patients with both generalized and focal dystonia. Dystonia appears to result primarily from dysfunction within the basal ganglia. As in PD, both ablation and DBS of the internal segment of the globus pallidus are effective in ameliorating the abnormal motor signs. Experimental studies in humans and animals have demonstrated a degradation of sensorimotor representation in the cortex, suggesting a disturbance of neuroplasticity.

℞ TREATMENT

Treatment for dystonia is for the most part symptomatic except in the rare instances such as Wilson's disease (Chap. 339) or DRD, where known mechanisms are present and specific therapies are available. The available treatments include physical and emotional support, physical therapy and neurorehabilitation, drugs, and surgery. The importance of education and supportive care must be recognized. Sensory retraining in humans with focal dystonias has resulted in a substantial recovery of function in some patients. Patients with generalized dystonia benefit from a team approach in a specialized center.

Pharmacotherapy Anticholinergic drugs are the most effective forms of treatment for generalized primary dystonia. Trihexyphenidyl is most commonly used. Doses ≥120 mg/d in children may be necessary, with a usual range of 20 to 50 mg/d. Adults can rarely tolerate these high doses. The limiting factors include constipation, dry mouth, blurred vision, and urinary retention as well as impaired short-term memory, confusion, and hallucinations. Benzodiazepines, including clonazepam or diazepam, are also effective for dystonia, alone or in combination with anticholinergics. Dosages are raised slowly until benefits are obtained or side effects, including sedation, ataxia, and confusion, prevent further escalation. Baclofen, a drug similar to the naturally occurring neurotransmitter γ-aminobutyric acid (GABA), is also effective for treating both focal and generalized dystonia. Relatively high doses are required (60 to 100 mg); however, side effects are often limiting. A baclofen pump for intrathecal infusion may be helpful for such cases. Dystonia involving the legs and trunk is most responsive to this form of therapy. Unfortunately, sustained benefits are not the rule and complications are not infrequent. Dopaminergic drugs are occasionally beneficial in both generalized and focal dystonias, but the most dramatic effects are seen in individuals with DRD, who experience a dramatic and sustained improvement with even a small dose of levodopa. Paradoxically, a fair percentage of patients with generalized dystonia (and craniocervical dystonia) respond to dopaminergic antagonists, such as haloperidol or pimozide. Sometimes the combination of tetrabenazine, pimozide, and trihexyphenidyl is effective.

Botulinum Toxin Although the focal dystonias are generally poorly responsive to drugs, they often respond dramatically to botulinum toxin injected into the affected muscle groups. Botulinum toxin can also be used in generalized dystonia for the occasional treatment of focal problems. Botulinum toxin acts by blocking the release of acetylcholine at the neuromuscular junction, resulting in dose-dependent weakness. Repeated injections are required every 2 to 5 months. Botulinum toxin serotypes A and B are now available, providing an alternative should resistance develop to either serotype.

Surgical Approaches Prior to the introduction of botulinum toxin, peripheral denervation procedures, such as dorsal or anterior cervical rhizotomy and selective peripheral denervation, were commonly performed, primarily for the treatment of cervical dystonia. These are now performed far less frequently, generally in patients with cervical dystonia who fail botulinum toxin injections. Stereotactic surgery is used primarily for severe generalized dystonia unresponsive to other treatments. In recent years following the success in PD, pallidotomy and DBS of the pallidum are being used with promising results. The best candidates for surgery appear to be individuals with primary (DYT1) dystonia. Patients with secondary forms of dystonia are less likely to benefit. Bilateral surgery is usually necessary to obtain control of axial dystonia.

TOURETTE SYNDROME

The most common disorder characterized by tics is Tourette syndrome (TS), a neurodevelopmental disorder with neurologic and behavioral manifestations. The true prevalence of TS disorders is unknown but has been estimated at 0.05%. In addition to tics, approximately half of patients develop comorbidities, specifically obsessive-compulsive disorder (OCD) and attention-deficit hyperactivity disorder (ADHD).

Clinical Features A *tic* is a brief, rapid, repetitive, and seemingly purposeless stereotyped action that may involve one or more muscle groups. Tics are divided into motor or vocal types, depending on the affected muscle group, and into simple and complex, depending on the number of muscle groups involved and the associated behaviors. They can range from the barely detectable and easily rationalized "nervous habits" such as blinking, twitching of the nose, and jerking of the neck, to the complex, emotionally laden, and sometimes offensive utterances of a minority of patients (*coprolalia*). Tics can be associated with brief focal sensory experiences termed *sensory tics* that commonly affect the face, head, and neck areas. Some tics may be difficult to distinguish from other fast "jerky" movements, such as chorea and myoclonus, but are unique in that they can be voluntarily inhibited for a brief period of time.

Developmentally, attentional problems develop before school and tics present during the first years of school. OCD symptoms develop later, just before or during adolescence. Tics and ADHD symptoms tend to stabilize with aging. The OCD symptoms have a more variable course.

The inheritance pattern of TS best fits the model of a major gene or genes with low penetrance, modifier genes, and a phenotype influenced by environmental factors. The risk of a family with one affected child of having another is 25%. No specific gene has been linked to TS, however. In PET studies using selective dopamine D_2-receptor ligands, alleles of this gene have been shown to modify symptom severity.

℞ TREATMENT

Tic symptoms have been ascribed to an overactivity of dopaminergic circuits. Accordingly dopamine blockers have consistently improved symptoms. Tics are not the most disabling feature of the illness, and treatment is generally indicated only when tics interfere with quality of life. The typical antipsychotics, Fluphenazine, haloperidol, and pimozide, thought to be very effective at treating tics, have been associated with extrapyramidal symptoms and school phobias. More recently, selected atypical antipsychotics have been shown to control tic symptoms and to have a lower incidence of these complications compared to typical antipsychotics. Drugs in this category include risperidone (0.5 to 4 mg/d), olanzapine (5 to 30 mg/d), and ziprasidone (80 to 200 mg/d). Other treatments for tics include clonidine (0.1 to 0.4 mg/d or the equivalent as transdermal patch), guanifencine (0.5 to 2 mg/d), and clonazepam (0.5 to 4.0 mg/d). Botulinum toxin injections can be effective in controlling focal tics involving small muscle groups. In general, symptoms of anxiety and OCD should be treated first since their control may preclude the need to treat the tics (Chap. 371).

DRUG-INDUCED HYPERKINETIC DISORDERS

This important group of iatrogenic and mostly reversible movement disorders is primarily associated with drugs that directly or indirectly affect central dopaminergic transmission. CNS stimulants, levodopa, dopamine agonists, and dopamine receptor blockers are the most common offending agents. The mechanism of acute and subacute movement disorders appears to result from idiosyncratic extensions of the intended action of the compound. By contrast, the mechanism of delayed or tardive dyskinesia (TD) syndromes remains more obscure.

DRUG-INDUCED MOVEMENT DISORDERS ■ Acute Reactions in this category include acute dystonia in response to dopamine antagonists, which appears most frequently in a generalized form in children and in a focal form (e.g., blepharospasm, torticollis, or oromandibular dystonia) in adults. These movements can be readily treated with the parenteral administration of anticholinergics (benztropine or diphenhydramine) or benzodiazepines (lorazepam or diazepam). Other acute movement disorders include dyskinesias, stereotypic behaviors, and tics after exposure to CNS stimulants such as methylphenidate, dextroamphetamine, and pemoline.

Subacute Probably the most common of these reactions is neuroleptic-induced akathisia, a state of motor restlessness with a feeling of restlessness and a need to move, which tends to alleviate the symptoms temporarily. Therapy consists of removing the offending agent(s). When this is not possible, symptoms can be ameliorated with benzodiazepines, anticholinergics, beta blockers, and, in some cases, dopamine agonists.

Tardive Tardive movement disorders such as TD are primarily due to chronic exposure to central dopamine blockers. The movements are most often choreatic, affecting first the mouth, lips, and tongue and later the trunk and limbs. In a fully developed case there can be head nodding, pelvic rocking, and fine movements of the fingers and toes. The diaphragm is affected rarely, producing respiratory distress. Other tardive syndromes include tardive dystonia, which generally presents with more axial than appendicular involvement; tardive akathisia; tardive tics; and even tardive tremor.

Approximately one-third of patients with TD remit within 3 months of stopping neuroleptic therapy, and in most patients the movements will gradually remit within 5 years. Patients at risk of permanent TD include the elderly, the edentulous, and those with underlying organic cerebral dysfunction. Patients with affective illnesses appear more likely to develop TD than patients with schizophrenia. Since treatment of TD is most often unsatisfactory and frustrating for both patient and physician, it is critical that typical antipsychotics be used judiciously and that, once started, their continued need be reassessed periodically. Abrupt drug cessation may result in "withdrawal dyskinesias," which presage the development of frank TD.

℞ TREATMENT

Atypical antipsychotics (clozapine, risperidone, olanzepine, quetiapine, ziprasidone, and aripiprazole) significantly lower the risk of TD compared to typical antipsychotics. Accordingly, if withdrawal of the offending antipsychotic is not possible, replacing traditional with atypical antipsychotics should be tried. Furthermore, it appears that atyp-

ical antipsychotics can successfully block the dyskinesias themselves. Elimination of stimulants and anticholinergics will also alleviate dyskinesias. In refractory cases, choreatic TD can be treated with the catecholamine depletors reserpine and tetrabenazine. Reserpine should be started at 0.125 mg/d and escalated slowly as needed up to 6 mg/d. Tetrabenazine should be started at 12.5 mg/d and gradually increased as necessary up to 200 mg/d. The elderly are less likely to tolerate the dose-dependent sedation and orthostatic hypotension associated with these drugs. Approximately 15% of patients on catecholamine depletors develop depression with chronic use of reserpine. Another strategy employs GABAergic medications such as baclofen (40 to 80 mg/d), clonazepam (1 to 8 mg/d), or valproic acid (750 to 3,000 mg/d). The latter strategy is particularly helpful in patients with tardive dystonia, which may also benefit from anticholinergic therapy and botulinum toxin injections.

Neuroleptic Malignant Syndrome (NMS) This serious complication of neuroleptic medications occurs in 1 to 2% of treated individuals; the mortality rate is as high as 20%. Muscle rigidity with myonecrosis; an altered mental status resembling catatonia; and autonomic dysfunction with hyperthermia, tachycardia, and a labile blood pressure constitute the principal manifestations. Symptoms typically evolve subacutely over several days and usually occur in the first few weeks following initial exposure to the drug, but can develop anytime. NMS can also be precipitated by the abrupt withdrawal of antiparkinson medications.

℞ TREATMENT

Treatment begins with immediate cessation of the offending antipsychotic drug as well as lithium and anticholinergic agents, which appear to increase the risk of NMS. Careful monitoring of body temperature, hydration, electrolytes (especially K^+), and blood pressure are essential. Specific pharmacologic agents include dopamine agonists or levodopa, amantadine, and benzodiazepines as well as dantrolene. Supportive measures include antipyretics, cooling blankets, fluids, and measures to maintain blood pressure.

FURTHER READING

AHLSKOG JE: Slowing Parkinson's disease progression: Recent dopamine agonist trials. Neurology 60:381, 2003
DAWSON TM, DAWSON VL: Molecular pathways of neurodegeneration in Parkinson's disease. Science 302:819, 2003
PAHWA R, LYONS K: Essential tremor: Differential diagnosis and current therapy. Am J Med 115:134, 2003
SIDEROWF A, STERN M: Update on Parkinson's disease. Ann Intern Med 138: 651, 2003

352 | ATAXIC DISORDERS
Roger N. Rosenberg

APPROACH TO THE PATIENT

Symptoms and signs of ataxia consist of gait impairment, unclear ("scanning") speech, visual blurring due to nystagmus, hand incoordination, and tremor with movement (Chap. 21). These result from the involvement of the cerebellum and its afferent and efferent pathways, including the spinocerebellar pathways, and the fronto-pontocerebellar pathway originating in the rostral frontal lobe. True cerebellar ataxia must be distinguished from ataxia associated with vestibular nerve or labyrinthine disease, as the latter results in a disorder of gait associated with a significant degree of dizziness, light-headedness, or the perception of movement (Chap. 20). True cerebellar ataxia is devoid of these vertiginous complaints and is clearly an unsteady gait due to imbalance. Sensory disturbances can also on occasion simulate the imbalance of cerebellar disease;

with sensory ataxia, imbalance dramatically worsens when visual input is removed (Romberg sign). Rarely, weakness of proximal leg muscles mimics cerebellar disease. In the patient who presents with ataxia, the rate and pattern of the development of cerebellar symptoms help to narrow the diagnostic possibilities (Table 352-1). A gradual and progressive increase in symptoms with bilateral and symmetric involvement suggests a biochemical, metabolic, immune, or toxic etiology. Conversely, focal, unilateral symptoms with headache and impaired level of consciousness accompanied by ipsilateral cranial nerve palsies and contralateral weakness imply a space-occupying cerebellar lesion.

Symmetric Ataxia Progressive and symmetric ataxia can be classified with respect to onset as acute (over hours or days), subacute (weeks or months), or chronic (months to years). Acute and reversible ataxias include those caused by intoxication with alcohol, phenytoin, lithium, barbiturates, and other drugs. Intoxication caused by toluene exposure, gasoline sniffing, glue sniffing, spray painting, or exposure to methyl mercury or bismuth are additional

TABLE 352-1 *Etiology of Cerebellar Ataxia*

Symmetric and Progressive Signs			Focal and Ipsilateral Cerebellar Signs		
Acute (Hours to Days)	*Subacute (Days to Weeks)*	*Chronic (Months to Years)*	*Acute (Hours to Days)*	*Subacute (Days to Weeks)*	*Chronic (Months to Years)*
Intoxication: alcohol, lithium, diphenylhydantoin, barbiturates (positive history and toxicology screen) Acute viral cerebellitis (CSF supportive of acute viral infection) Postinfection syndrome	Intoxication: mercury, solvents, gasoline, glue; cytotoxic chemotherapeutic drugs Alcoholic-nutritional (vitamin B$_1$ and B$_{12}$ deficiency) Lyme disease	Paraneoplastic syndrome Anti-gliadin antibody syndrome Hypothyroidism Inherited diseases Tabes dorsalis (tertiary syphilis) Phenytoin toxicity	Vascular: cerebellar infarction, hemorrhage, or subdural hematoma Infectious: cerebellar abscess (positive mass lesion on MRI/CT, positive history in support of lesion)	Neoplastic: cerebellar glioma or metastatic tumor (positive for neoplasm on MRI/CT) Demyelinating: multiple sclerosis (history, CSF, and MRI are consistent) AIDS-related multifocal leukoencephalopathy (positive HIV test and CD4+ cell count for AIDS)	Stable gliosis secondary to vascular lesion or demyelinating plaque (stable lesion on MRI/CT older than several months) Congenital lesion: Chiari or Dandy-Walker malformations (malformation noted on MRI/CT)

Abbreviations: CSF, cerebrospinal fluid; CT, computed tomography; MRI, magnetic resonance imaging.

causes of acute or subacute ataxia, as is treatment with cytotoxic chemotherapeutic drugs such as fluorouracil and paclitaxel. Patients with a postinfectious syndrome (especially after varicella) may develop gait ataxia and mild dysarthria, both of which are reversible (Chap. 359). Rare infectious causes of acquired ataxia include poliovirus, coxsackievirus, echovirus, Epstein-Barr virus, toxoplasmosis, *Legionella*, and Lyme disease.

The subacute development of ataxia of gait over weeks to months (degeneration of the cerebellar vermis) may be due to the combined effects of alcoholism and malnutrition, particularly with deficiencies of vitamins B$_1$ and B$_{12}$. Hyponatremia has also been associated with ataxia. Paraneoplastic cerebellar ataxia is associated with a number of different tumors (and autoantibodies) such as breast and ovarian cancers (anti-Yo), small-cell lung cancer (anti-PQ type voltage-gated calcium channel), and Hodgkin's disease (anti-Tr) (Chap. 87). Another paraneoplastic syndrome associated with myoclonus and opsoclonus occurs with breast (anti-Ri) and lung cancers and neuroblastoma. For all of these paraneoplastic ataxias, the neurologic syndrome may be the presenting symptom of the cancer. Another immune-mediated progressive ataxia is associated with anti-gliadin (and anti-endomysium) antibodies and the HLA DQB1*0201 haplotype; in some affected patients, biopsy of the small intestine reveals villous atrophy consistent with gluten-sensitive enteropathy (Chap. 275). Finally, subacute progressive ataxia may be caused by a prion disorder, especially when an infectious etiology, such as transmission from contaminated human growth hormone, is responsible (Chap. 362).

Chronic symmetric gait ataxia suggests an inherited ataxia (discussed below), a metabolic disorder, or a chronic infection. Hypothyroidism must always be considered as a readily treatable and reversible form of gait ataxia. Infectious diseases that can present with ataxia are meningovascular syphilis and tabes dorsalis due to degeneration of the posterior columns and spinocerebellar pathways in the spinal cord.

Focal Ataxia Acute focal ataxia commonly results from cerebrovascular disease, usually ischemic infarction, or cerebellar hemorrhage. These lesions typically produce cerebellar symptoms ipsilateral to the injured cerebellum and may be associated with an impaired level of consciousness due to brainstem compression and increased intracranial pressure; ipsilateral pontine signs, including sixth and seventh nerve palsies, may be present. Focal and worsening signs of acute ataxia should also prompt consideration of a posterior fossa subdural hematoma, bacterial abscess, or primary or metastatic cerebellar tumor. Computed tomography (CT) or magnetic resonance imaging (MRI) studies will reveal clinically significant processes of this type. Many of these lesions represent true neurologic emergencies, as sudden herniation, either rostrally through the tentorium or caudal herniation of cerebellar tonsils through the foramen magnum, can occur and is usually devastating. Acute surgical decompression may be required (Chap. 258). Lymphoma or progressive multifocal leukoencephalopathy (PML) in a patient with AIDS may present with an acute or subacute focal cerebellar syndrome. Chronic etiologies of progressive ataxia include multiple sclerosis (Chap. 359) and congenital lesions such as a Chiari malformation (Chap. 356) or a congenital cyst of the posterior fossa (Dandy-Walker syndrome).

THE INHERITED ATAXIAS

These may show autosomal dominant, autosomal recessive, or maternal (mitochondrial) modes of inheritance. A genomic classification (Table 352-2) has now largely superseded previous ones based on clinical expression alone.

Although the clinical manifestations and neuropathologic findings of cerebellar disease dominate the clinical picture, there may also be characteristic changes in the basal ganglia, brainstem, spinal cord, optic nerves, retina, and peripheral nerves. In large families with dominantly inherited ataxias, many gradations are observed from purely cerebellar manifestations to mixed cerebellar and brainstem disorders, cerebellar and basal ganglia syndromes, and spinal cord or peripheral nerve disease. Rarely, dementia is present as well. The clinical picture may be homogeneous within a family with dominantly inherited ataxia, but sometimes most affected family members show one characteristic syndrome, while one or several members have an entirely different phenotype.

AUTOSOMAL DOMINANT ATAXIAS The autosomal spinocerebellar ataxias (SCAs) include SCA type 1 through SCA22, dentatorubropallidoluysian atrophy (DRPLA), and episodic ataxia (EA) types 1 and 2 (Table 352-2). SCA1, SCA2, SCA3 [Machado-Joseph disease (MJD)], SCA6, SCA7, and SCA17 are caused by CAG triplet repeat expansions in different genes. SCA8 is due to an untranslated CTG repeat expansion, SCA12 is linked to an untranslated CAG repeat, and SCA10 is caused by an untranslated pentanucleotide repeat. The clinical phenotypes of these SCAs overlap. The genotype has become the "gold standard" for diagnosis and classification. CAG encodes glutamine, and these expanded CAG triplet repeat expansions result in expanded polyglutamine proteins, termed *ataxins*, that produce a toxic gain of function with autosomal dominant inheritance. Although the phenotype is variable for any given disease gene, a pattern of neuronal loss with gliosis is produced that is relatively unique for each ataxia. Immunohistochemical and biochemical studies have shown cytoplasmic (SCA2), neuronal (SCA1, MJD, SCA7), and nucleolar (SCA7) accumulation of the

TABLE 352-2 Genotype Classification of the Spinocerebellar Ataxias

Name	Locus	Phenotype
SCA1 (autosomal dominant type 1)	6p22-p23 with CAG repeats (exonic) Ataxin-1	Ataxia with ophthalmoparesis, pyramidal and extrapyramidal findings
SCA2 (autosomal dominant type 2)	12q23-q24.1 with CAG repeats (exonic) Ataxin-2	Ataxia with slow saccades and minimal pyramidal and extrapyramidal findings
Machado-Joseph disease/SCA3 (autosomal dominant type 3)	14q24.3-q32 with CAG repeats (exonic) MJD–ataxin-3	Ataxia with ophthalmoparesis and variable pyramidal, extrapyramidal, and amyotrophic signs
SCA4 (autosomal dominant type 4)	16q24-ter	Ataxia with normal eye movements, sensory axonal neuropathy, and pyramidal signs
SCA5 (autosomal dominant type 5)	Centromeric region of chromosome II	Ataxia and dysarthria
SCA6 (autosomal dominant type 6)	19p13.2 with CAG repeats in α_{1A}-voltage–dependent calcium channel gene (exonic)	Ataxia and dysarthria, nystagmus, mild proprioceptive sensory loss
SCA7 (autosomal dominant type 7)	3p14.1-p21.1 with CAG repeats (exonic) Ataxin-7	Ophthalmoparesis, visual loss, ataxia, dysarthria, extensor plantar response, pigmentary retinal degeneration
SCA8 (autosomal dominant type 8)	13q21 with CTG repeats; noncoding	Gait ataxia, dysarthria, nystagmus, leg spasticity, and reduced vibratory sensation
SCA10 (autosomal dominant type 10)	22q; ATTCT repeat; noncoding	Gait ataxia, dysarthria, nystagmus; partial complex and generalized motor seizures; polyneuropathy
SCA11 (autosomal dominant type 11)	15q14-q21.3 by linkage	Slowly progressive gait and extremity ataxia, dysarthria, vertical nystagmus, hyperreflexia
SCA12 (autosomal dominant type 12)	5q31-q33 by linkage; CAG repeat; protein phosphatase 2A	Tremor, decreased movement, increased reflexes, dystonia, ataxia, dysautonomia, dementia, dysarthria
SCA13 (autosomal dominant type 13)	19q13.3-q14.4	Mutation unknown
SCA14 (autosomal dominant type 14)	19q-13.4	Mutation unknown
SCA15 (autosomal dominant type 15)	Mutation unknown in 1 family; other known loci were excluded	Gait and extremity ataxia, dysarthria
SCA16 (autosomal dominant type 16)	8q22.1-24.1	Mutation unknown; pure cerebellar ataxia and head tremor, gait ataxia, and dysarthria; horizontal gaze–evoked nystagmus
SCA17 (autosomal dominant type 17)	6q27; CAG expansion in the TATA-binding protein (*TBP*) gene	Gait ataxia, dementia, parkinsonism, dystonia, chorea, seizures; MRI shows cerebral & cerebellar atrophy
SCA18 (autosomal dominant type 18)	7q22-q32	Ataxia motor/sensory neuropathy
SCA19 (autosomal dominant type 19)	1p21-q21	Ataxia, tremor, cognitive impairment, myoclonus
SCA20 (assigned but not yet published)	—	—
SCA21 (autosomal dominant type 21)	7p21.3-p15.1	Ataxia, extrapyramidal features of akinesia, rigidity, tremor, cognitive defect
SCA22 (assigned but not yet published)	—	
Dentatorubropallidoluysian atrophy (autosomal dominant)	12p12-ter with CAG repeats (exonic) Atrophin	Ataxia, choreoathetosis, dystonia, seizures, myoclonus, dementia
Friedreich's ataxia (autosomal recessive)	9q13-q21.1 with intronic GAA repeats Frataxin	Ataxia, areflexia, extensor plantar responses, position sense deficits, cardiomyopathy, diabetes mellitus, scoliosis, foot deformities; defective iron transport from mitochondria
Friedreich's ataxia (autosomal recessive)	8q13.1-q13.3; (α-TTP deficiency)	Same as phenotype that maps to 9q but associated with vitamin E deficiency
Autosomal recessive spastic ataxia of Charlevoix-Saguenay (ARSACS)	Chromosome 13; SACS gene; loss of Sacsin peptide activity	Childhood onset of ataxia, spasticity, dysarthria, distal muscle wasting, foot deformity, retinal striations, mitral valve prolapse
Kearns-Sayre syndrome (sporadic)	mtDNA deletion and duplication mutations	Ptosis, ophthalmoplegia, pigmentary retinal degeneration, cardiomyopathy, diabetes mellitus, deafness, heart block, increased CSF protein, ataxia
Myoclonic epilepsy and ragged red fiber syndrome (MERRF) (maternal inheritance)	Mutation in mtDNA of the $tRNA^{lys}$ at 8344; also mutation at 8356	Myoclonic epilepsy, ragged red fiber myopathy, ataxia
Mitochondrial encephalopathy, lactic acidosis, and stroke syndrome (MELAS) (maternal inheritance)	$tRNA^{leu}$ mutation at 3243; also at 3271 and 3252	Headache, stroke, lactic acidosis, ataxia
Leigh's disease; subacute necrotizing encephalopathy (maternal inheritance or autosomal recessive)	mtDNA complex V defect (ATPase gene at 8993) or mitochondrial protein synthesis defect (both maternally inherited); or complex IV defect (autosomal recessive)	Obtundation, hypotonia, cranial nerve defects, respiratory failure, hyperintense signals on T2-weighted MRI in basal ganglia, cerebellum, or brainstem; ataxia
Episodic ataxia, type 1 (EA-1) (autosomal dominant)	12p; potassium channel gene, *KCNA1*	Episodic ataxia for minutes; provoked by startle or exercise; with facial and hand myokymia; cerebellar signs are not progressive; responds to phenytoin
Episodic ataxia, type 2 (EA-2) (autosomal dominant)	19p-13(*CACNA1A*) (allelic with SCA6) (α_{1A}-voltage–dependent calcium channel subunit)	Episodic ataxia for days; provoked by stress, fatigue; with down-gaze nystagmus; cerebellar atrophy results; progressive cerebellar signs; responds to acetazolamide
Ataxia telangiectasia (autosomal recessive)	11q22-23; *ATM* gene for regulation of cell cycle; mitogenic signal transduction and meiotic recombination	Telangiectasia, ataxia, dysarthria, pulmonary infections, neoplasms of lymphatic system; IgA and IgG deficiencies; diabetes mellitus, breast cancer

(continued)

TABLE 352-2—(Continued)

Name	Locus	Phenotype
Infantile-onset spinocerebellar ataxia of Nikali et al (autosomal recessive)	10q23.3-q24.1	Infantile ataxia, sensory neuropathy; athetosis, hearing deficit, ophthalmoplegia, optic atrophy; primary hypogonadism in females
Hypoceruloplasminemia with ataxia and dysarthria (autosomal recessive)	Ceruloplasmin gene; 3q23-q25 (trp 858 ter)	Gait ataxia and dysarthria; hyperreflexia; cerebellar atrophy by MRI; iron deposition in cerebellum, basal ganglia, thalamus, and liver; onset in the 4th decade
Spinocerebellar ataxia with neuropathy (SCAN1) (autosomal recessive)	Tryosyl-DNA phosphodiesterase-1 (TDP-1) 14q31-q32	Onset in 2nd decade; gait ataxia, dysarthria, seizures, cerebellar vermis atrophy on MRI, dysmetria

Abbreviations: MRI, magnetic resonance imaging; CSF, cerebrospinal fluid.

specific mutant polyglutamine containing ataxin proteins. Expanded polyglutamine ataxins with more than ~40 glutamines are potentially toxic to neurons for a variety of reasons including the following: high levels of gene expression for the mutant polyglutamine ataxin in affected neurons; conformational change of the aggregated protein to a β-pleated structure; abnormal transport of the ataxin into the nucleus (SCA1, MJD, SCA7); binding to other polyglutamine proteins, including the TATA-binding transcription protein and the CREB-binding protein, impairing their functions; altering the efficiency of the ubiquitin-proteosome system of protein turnover; and inducing neuronal apoptosis. An earlier age of onset (anticipation) and more aggressive disease in subsequent generations are due to further expansion of the CAG triplet repeat and increased polyglutamine number in the mutant ataxin. The most common disorders are discussed below.

SCA1 SCA1 was previously referred to as *olivopontocerebellar atrophy*, but genomic data have shown that that entity represents several different genotypes with overlapping clinical features.

SYMPTOMS AND SIGNS SCA1 is characterized by the development in early or middle adult life of progressive cerebellar ataxia of the trunk and limbs, impairment of equilibrium and gait, slowness of voluntary movements, scanning speech, nystagmoid eye movements, and oscillatory tremor of the head and trunk. Dysarthria, dysphagia, and oculomotor and facial palsies may also occur. Extrapyramidal symptoms include rigidity, an immobile face, and parkinsonian tremor. The reflexes are usually normal, but knee and ankle jerks may be lost, and extensor plantar responses may occur. Dementia may be noted but is usually mild. Impairment of sphincter function is common, with urinary and sometimes fecal incontinence. Cerebellar and brainstem atrophy are evident on MRI (Fig. 352-1).

Marked shrinkage of the ventral half of the pons, disappearance of

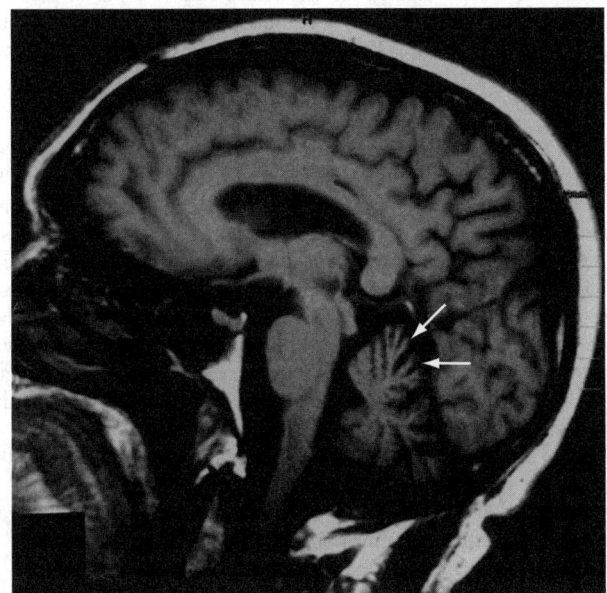

FIGURE 352-1 Sagittal MRI of the brain of a 60-year-old man with gait ataxia and dysarthria due to SCA1, illustrating cerebellar atrophy (*arrows*).

the olivary eminence on the ventral surface of the medulla, and atrophy of the cerebellum are evident on gross postmortem inspection of the brain. Variable loss of Purkinje cells, reduced numbers of cells in the molecular and granular layer, demyelination of the middle cerebellar peduncle and the cerebellar hemispheres, and severe loss of cells in the pontine nuclei and olives are found on histologic examination. Degenerative changes in the striatum, especially the putamen, and loss of the pigmented cells of the substantia nigra may be found in cases with extrapyramidal features. More widespread degeneration in the central nervous system (CNS), including involvement of the posterior columns and the spinocerebellar fibers, is often present.

GENETIC CONSIDERATIONS SCA1 encodes a gene product, called ataxin-1, which is a novel protein of unknown function. The mutant allele has 40 CAG repeats located within the coding region, whereas alleles from unaffected individuals have ≤36 repeats. A few patients with 38 to 40 CAG repeats have been described. There is a direct correlation between a larger number of repeats and a younger age of onset for SCA1. Juvenile patients have higher numbers of repeats, and anticipation is present in subsequent generations. Transgenic mice carrying SCA1 developed ataxia and Purkinje cell pathology. Nuclear localization, but not aggregation, of ataxin-1 appears to be required for cell death initiated by the mutant protein.

SCA2 ■ *SYMPTOMS AND SIGNS* Another clinical phenotype, SCA2, has been described in Cubans. These patients probably are descendants of a common ancestor, and the population may be the largest homogeneous group of patients with ataxia yet described. The age of onset ranges from 2 to 65 years, and there is considerable clinical variability within families. Although neuropathologic and clinical findings are compatible with a diagnosis of SCA1, including slow saccadic eye movements, ataxia, dysarthria, parkinsonian rigidity, optic disk pallor, mild spasticity, and retinal degeneration, SCA2 is a unique form of cerebellar degenerative disease.

GENETIC CONSIDERATIONS The gene in SCA2 families also contains CAG repeat expansions coding for a polyglutamine-containing protein, ataxin-2. Normal alleles contain 15 to 32 repeats; mutant alleles have 35 to 77 repeats.

Machado-Joseph Disease/SCA3 MJD was first described among the Portuguese and their descendants in New England and California. Subsequently, MJD has been found in families from Portugal, Australia, Brazil, Canada, China, England, France, India, Israel, Italy, Japan, Spain, Taiwan, and the United States. In most populations, it is the most common autosomal dominant ataxia.

SYMPTOMS AND SIGNS MJD has been classified into three clinical types. In type I MJD (amyotrophic lateral sclerosis–parkinsonism–dystonia type), neurologic deficits appear in the first two decades and involve weakness and spasticity of extremities, especially the legs, often with dystonia of the face, neck, trunk, and extremities. Patellar and ankle clonus are common, as are extensor plantar responses. The gait is slow and stiff, with a slightly broadened base and lurching from side to side; this gait results from spasticity, not true ataxia. There is no truncal titubation. Pharyngeal weakness and spasticity cause difficulty with speech and swallowing. Of note is the prominence of horizontal and vertical nystagmus, loss of fast saccadic eye movements, hypermetric and hypometric saccades, and impairment of upward vertical gaze. Facial fasciculations, facial myokymia, lingual fasciculations without atrophy, ophthalmoparesis, and ocular prominence are common early manifestations.

In type II MJD (ataxic type), true cerebellar deficits of dysarthria and gait and extremity ataxia begin in the second to fourth decades along with corticospinal and extrapyramidal deficits of spasticity, rigidity, and dystonia. Type II is the most common form of MJD. Ophthalmoparesis, upward vertical gaze deficits, and facial and lingual fasciculations are also present. Type II MJD can be distinguished from the clinically similar disorders SCA1 and SCA2.

Type III MJD (ataxic-amyotrophic type) presents in the fifth to the seventh decades with a pancerebellar disorder that includes dysarthria and gait and extremity ataxia. Distal sensory loss involving pain, touch, vibration, and position senses and distal atrophy are prominent, indicating the presence of peripheral neuropathy. The deep tendon reflexes are depressed to absent, and there are no corticospinal or extrapyramidal findings.

The mean age of onset of symptoms in MJD is 25 years. Neurologic deficits invariably progress and lead to death from debilitation within 15 years of onset, especially in patients with types I and II disease. Usually, patients retain full intellectual function.

The major pathologic findings are variable loss of neurons and glial replacement in the corpus striatum and severe loss of neurons in the pars compacta of the substantia nigra. A moderate loss of neurons occurs in the dentate nucleus of the cerebellum and in the red nucleus. Purkinje cell loss and granule cell loss occur in the cerebellar cortex. Cell loss also occurs in the dentate nucleus and in the cranial nerve motor nuclei. Sparing of the inferior olives distinguishes MJD from other dominantly inherited ataxias.

GENETIC CONSIDERATIONS The gene for MJD maps to 14q24.3-q32. Unstable CAG repeat expansions are present in the MJD gene coding for a polyglutamine-containing protein named ataxin-3, or MJD-ataxin. An earlier age of onset is associated with longer repeats. Alleles from normal individuals have between 12 and 37 CAG repeats, and MJD alleles have 60 to 84 CAG repeats. Polyglutamine-containing aggregates of ataxin-3 (MJD-ataxin) have been described in neuronal nuclei undergoing degeneration.

SCA6 Genomic screening for CAG repeats in other families with autosomal dominant ataxia and vibratory and proprioceptive sensory loss have yielded another locus. Of interest is that different mutations in the same gene for the α_{1A} voltage-dependent calcium channel subunit (CACNLIA4; also referred to as the *CACNA1A* gene) at 19p13 result in different clinical disorders. CAG repeat expansions (21 to 27 in patients; 4 to 16 triplets in normal individuals) result in late-onset progressive ataxia with cerebellar degeneration. Missense mutations in this gene result in familial hemiplegic migraine. Nonsense mutations resulting in termination of protein synthesis of the gene product yield hereditary paroxysmal cerebellar ataxia or EA. Some patients with familial hemiplegic migraine develop progressive ataxia and also have cerebellar atrophy.

SCA7 This disorder is distinguished from all other SCAs by the presence of retinal pigmentary degeneration. The visual abnormalities first appear as blue-yellow color blindness and proceed to frank visual loss with macular degeneration. In almost all other respects, SCA7 resembles several other SCAs in which ataxia is accompanied by various noncerebellar findings, including ophthalmoparesis and extensor plantar responses. The genetic defect is an expanded CAG repeat in the SCA7 gene. The expanded repeat size in SCA7 is highly variable. Consistent with this, the severity of clinical findings varies from essentially asymptomatic to mild late-onset symptoms to severe, aggressive disease in childhood with rapid progression. Marked anticipation has been recorded, especially with paternal transmission. The disease protein, ataxin-7, forms aggregates in nuclei of affected neurons, as has also been described for SCA1 and SCA3/MJD.

SCA8 This form of ataxia is caused by a CTG repeat expansion in an untranslated region of a gene on chromosome 13q21. There is marked maternal bias in transmission, perhaps reflecting contractions of the repeat during spermatogenesis. The mutation is not fully penetrant. Symptoms include slowly progressive dysarthria and gait ataxia beginning at ~40 years of age with a range between 20 and 65 years. Other features include nystagmus, leg spasticity, and reduced vibratory sensation. Severely affected individuals are nonambulatory by the fourth to sixth decades. MRI shows cerebellar atrophy. The mechanism of disease may involve a dominant "toxic" effect occurring at the RNA level, as occurs in myotonic dystrophy.

Dentatorubropallidoluysian Atrophy DRPLA has a variable presentation that may include progressive ataxia, choreoathetosis, dystonia, seizures, myoclonus, and dementia. DRPLA is due to unstable CAG triplet repeats in the open reading frame of a gene named *atrophin* located on chromosome 12p12-ter. Larger expansions are found in patients with earlier onset. The number of repeats is 49 in patients with DRPLA and ≤26 in normal individuals. Anticipation occurs in successive generations, with earlier onset of disease in association with an increasing CAG repeat number in children who inherit the disease from their father. One well-characterized family in North Carolina has a phenotypic variant known as the *Haw River syndrome*, now recognized to be due to the DRPLA mutation.

Episodic Ataxia EA types 1 and 2 are two rare dominantly inherited disorders that have been mapped to chromosomes 12p (a potassium channel gene) for type 1 and 19p for type 2. Patients with EA-1 have brief episodes of ataxia with myokymia and nystagmus that last only minutes. Startle, sudden change in posture, and exercise can induce episodes. Acetazolamide or anticonvulsants may be therapeutic. Patients with EA-2 have episodes of ataxia with nystagmus that can last for hours or days. Stress, exercise, or excessive fatigue may be precipitants. Acetazolamide may be therapeutic and can reverse the relative intracellular alkalosis detected by magnetic resonance spectroscopy. Stop codon, nonsense mutations causing EA-2 have been found in the *CACNA1A* gene, encoding the α_{1A} voltage-dependent calcium channel subunit (see "SCA6," above).

AUTOSOMAL RECESSIVE ATAXIAS ■ Friedreich's Ataxia This is the most common form of inherited ataxia, comprising one-half of all hereditary ataxias. It can occur in a classic form or in association with a genetically determined vitamin E deficiency syndrome; the two forms are clinically indistinguishable.

SYMPTOMS AND SIGNS Friedreich's ataxia presents before 25 years of age with progressive staggering gait, frequent falling, and titubation. The lower extremities are more severely involved than the upper ones. Dysarthria occasionally is the presenting symptom; rarely, progressive scoliosis, foot deformity, nystagmus, or cardiopathy is the initial sign.

The neurologic examination reveals nystagmus, loss of fast saccadic eye movements, truncal titubation, dysarthria, dysmetria, and ataxia of trunk and limb movements. Extensor plantar responses (with normal tone in trunk and extremities), absence of deep tendon reflexes, and weakness (greater distally than proximally) are usually found. Loss of vibratory and proprioceptive sensation occurs. The median age of death is 35 years. Women have a significantly better prognosis than men.

Cardiac involvement occurs in 90% of patients. Cardiomegaly, symmetric hypertrophy, murmurs, and conduction defects are reported. Moderate mental retardation or psychiatric syndromes are present in a small percentage of patients. A high incidence of diabetes mellitus (20%) is found and is associated with insulin resistance and pancreatic β-cell dysfunction. Musculoskeletal deformities are com-

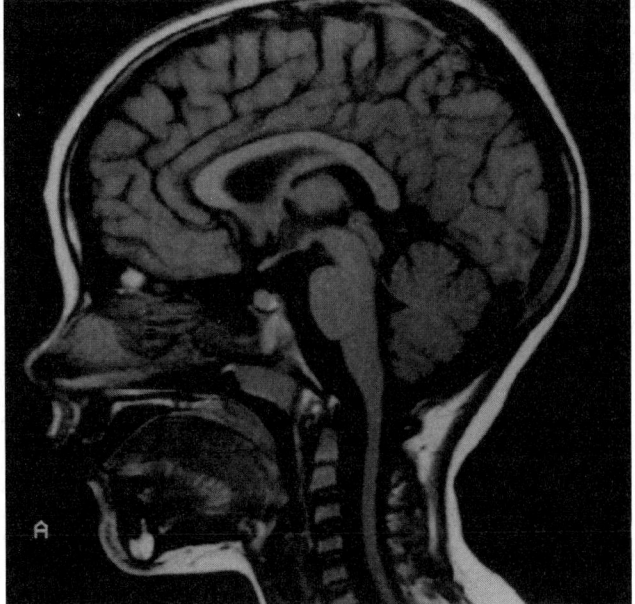

FIGURE 352-2 Sagittal MRI of the brain and spinal cord of a patient with Friedreich's ataxia, demonstrating spinal cord atrophy.

mon and include pes cavus, pes equinovarus, and scoliosis. MRI of the spinal cord shows atrophy (Fig. 352-2).

The primary sites of pathology are the spinal cord, dorsal root ganglion cells, and the peripheral nerves. Slight atrophy of the cerebellum and cerebral gyri may occur. Sclerosis and degeneration occur predominantly in the spinocerebellar tracts, lateral corticospinal tracts, and posterior columns. Degeneration of the glossopharyngeal, vagus, hypoglossal, and deep cerebellar nuclei is described. The cerebral cortex is histologically normal except for loss of Betz cells in the precentral gyri. The peripheral nerves are extensively involved, with a loss of large myelinated fibers. Cardiac pathology consists of myocytic hypertrophy and fibrosis, focal vascular fibromuscular dysplasia with subintimal or medial deposition of periodic acid–Schiff (PAS)–positive material, myocytopathy with unusual pleomorphic nuclei, and focal degeneration of nerves and cardiac ganglia.

GENETIC CONSIDERATIONS The classic form of Friedreich's ataxia has been mapped to 9q13-q21.1, and the mutant gene, *frataxin*, contains expanded GAA triplet repeats in the first intron. There is homozygosity for expanded GAA repeats in >95% of patients. Normal persons have 7 to 22 GAA repeats, and patients have 200 to 900 GAA repeats. A more varied clinical syndrome has been described in compound heterozygotes who have one copy of the GAA expansion and the other copy a point mutation in the *frataxin* gene. When the point mutation is located in the region of the gene that encodes the amino-terminal half of frataxin, the phenotype is milder, often consisting of a spastic gait, retained or exaggerated reflexes, no dysarthria, and mild or absent ataxia.

Patients with Friedreich's ataxia have undetectable or extremely low levels of *frataxin* mRNA, as compared with carriers and unrelated individuals; thus, disease appears to be caused by a loss of expression of the frataxin protein. Frataxin is a mitochondrial protein involved in iron homeostasis. Mitochondrial iron accumulation due to loss of the iron transporter coded by the mutant *frataxin* gene results in oxidized intramitochondrial iron. Excess oxidized iron results in turn in the oxidation of cellular components and irreversible cell injury.

Two forms of hereditary ataxia associated with abnormalities in the interactions of vitamin E (α-tocopherol) with very low density lipoprotein (VLDL) have been delineated. These are abetalipoproteinemia (Bassen-Kornzweig syndrome) and ataxia with vitamin E deficiency (AVED). Abetalipoproteinemia is caused by mutations in the gene coding for the larger subunit of the microsomal triglyceride transfer protein (MTP). Defects in MTP result in impairment of formation and secretion of VLDL in liver. This defect results in a deficiency of delivery of vitamin E to tissues, including the central and peripheral nervous system, as VLDL is the transport molecule for vitamin E and other fat-soluble substitutes. AVED is due to mutations in the gene for α-tocopherol transfer protein (α-TTP). These patients have an impaired ability to bind vitamin E into the VLDL produced and secreted by the liver, resulting in a deficiency of vitamin E in peripheral tissues. Hence, either absence of VLDL (abetalipoproteinemia) or impaired binding of vitamin E to VLDL (AVED) causes an ataxic syndrome. Once again, a genotype classification has proved to be essential in sorting out the various forms of the Friedreich's disease syndrome, which may be clinically indistinguishable.

Ataxia Telangiectasia ■ *SYMPTOMS AND SIGNS* Patients with ataxia telangiectasia (AT) present in the first decade of life with progressive telangiectatic lesions associated with deficits in cerebellar function and nystagmus. The neurologic manifestations correspond to those in Friedreich's disease, which should be included in the differential diagnosis. Truncal and limb ataxia, dysarthria, extensor plantar responses, myoclonic jerks, areflexia, and distal sensory deficits may develop. There is a high incidence of recurrent pulmonary infections and neoplasms of the lymphatic and reticuloendothelial system in patients with AT. Thymic hypoplasia with cellular and humoral (IgA and IgG2) immunodeficiencies, premature aging, and endocrine disorders such as type 1 diabetes mellitus are described. There is an increased incidence of lymphomas, Hodgkin's disease, acute leukemias of the T cell type, and breast cancer.

The most striking neuropathologic changes include loss of Purkinje, granule, and basket cells in the cerebellar cortex as well as of neurons in the deep cerebellar nuclei. The inferior olives of the medulla may also have neuronal loss. There is a loss of anterior horn neurons in the spinal cord and of dorsal root ganglion cells associated with posterior column spinal cord demyelination. A poorly developed or absent thymus gland is the most consistent defect of the lymphoid system.

GENETIC CONSIDERATIONS The gene for AT (the *ATM* gene) encodes a protein that is similar to several yeast and mammalian phosphatidylinositol-3'-kinases involved in mitogenic signal transduction, meiotic recombination, and cell cycle control. Defective DNA repair in AT fibroblasts exposed to ultraviolet light has been demonstrated. The discovery of *ATM* will make possible the identification of heterozygotes who are at risk for cancer (e.g., breast cancer) and permit early diagnosis.

Mitochondrial Ataxias Spinocerebellar syndromes have been identified with mutations in mitochondrial DNA (mtDNA). Thirty pathogenic mtDNA point mutations and 60 different types of mtDNA deletions are known, several of which cause or are associated with ataxia (Chap. 368).

℞ TREATMENT

The most important goal in management of patients with ataxia is to identify treatable disease entities. Mass lesions must be recognized promptly and treated appropriately. Paraneoplastic disorders can often be identified by the clinical patterns of disease that they produce, measurement of specific autoantibodies, and uncovering the primary cancer; these disorders are often refractory to therapy, but some patients improve following removal of the tumor or immunotherapy (Chap. 87). Ataxia with anti-gliadin antibodies and gluten-sensitive enteropathy may improve with a gluten-free diet. Malabsorption syndromes leading to vitamin E deficiency may lead to ataxia. The vitamin E deficiency form of Friedreich's ataxia must be considered, and serum vitamin E levels measured. Vitamin E therapy is indicated for these rare patients. Vitamin B_1 and B_{12} levels in serum should be measured, and the vitamins administered to patients having deficient levels. Hypothyroidism is easily treated. The cerebrospinal fluid should be tested for a syphilitic infection in patients with progressive ataxia and other features of tabes dorsalis. Similarly, antibody titers for Lyme disease and *Legionella* should be measured, and appropriate antibiotic therapy should be instituted in antibody-positive patients. Aminoacidopathies, leukodystrophies, urea-cycle abnormalities, and mitochondrial encephalomyopathies may produce ataxia, and some dietary or metabolic therapies are available for these disorders. The deleterious effects of diphenylhydantoin and alcohol on the cerebellum are well known and these exposures should be avoided in patients with ataxia of any cause.

There is no proven therapy for any of the autosomal dominant ataxias (SCA1 to 22). There is preliminary evidence that idebenone, a free-radical scavenger, can improve myocardial hypertrophy in pa-
tients with classic Friedreich ataxia; there is no current evidence, however, that it improves neurologic function. Iron chelators and antioxidant drugs are potentially harmful in Friedreich's patients as they may increase heart muscle injury. Acetazolamide can reduce the duration of symptoms of episodic ataxia. At present, identification of an at-risk person's genotype, together with appropriate family and genetic counseling, can reduce the incidence of these cerebellar syndromes in future generations (Chap. 58).

FURTHER READING

HADJIVASSILIOU M et al: Gluten ataxia in perspective: Epidemiology, genetic susceptibility and clinical characteristics. Brain 136:685, 2003

LYNCH DR et al: Friedrich ataxia: Effects of genetic understanding on clinical evaluation and therapy. Arch Neurol 59:743, 2002

ROSENBERG RN, PAULSON HL: The inherited ataxias, in *The Molecular and Genetic Basis of Neurologic and Psychiatric Disease*, 3rd ed, RN Rosenberg et al (eds). Philadelphia, Elsevier Science, and Boston, Butterworth-Heinemann, 2003

---

353   AMYOTROPHIC LATERAL SCLEROSIS AND OTHER MOTOR NEURON DISEASES
Robert H. Brown, Jr.

AMYOTROPHIC LATERAL SCLEROSIS   Amyotrophic lateral sclerosis (ALS) is the most common form of progressive motor neuron disease. It is a prime example of a neurodegenerative disease and is arguably the most devastating of the neurodegenerative disorders.

Pathology   The pathologic hallmark of motor neuron degenerative disorders is death of lower motor neurons (consisting of anterior horn cells in the spinal cord and their brainstem homologues innervating bulbar muscles) and upper, or corticospinal, motor neurons (originating in layer five of the motor cortex and descending via the pyramidal tract to synapse with lower motor neurons, either directly or indirectly via interneurons) (Chap. 21). Although at its onset ALS may involve selective loss of function of only upper or lower motor neurons, it ultimately causes progressive loss of both categories of motor neurons. Indeed, in the absence of clear involvement of both motor neuron types, the diagnosis of ALS is questionable.

Other motor neuron diseases involve only particular subsets of motor neurons (Tables 353-1 and 353-2). Thus, in bulbar palsy and spinal muscular atrophy (SMA; also called progressive muscular atrophy), the lower motor neurons of brainstem and spinal cord, respectively, are most severely involved. By contrast, pseudobulbar palsy, primary lateral sclerosis (PLS), and familial spastic paraplegia (FSP) affect only upper motor neurons innervating the brainstem and spinal cord.

In each of these diseases, the affected motor neurons undergo shrinkage, often with accumulation of the pigmented lipid (lipofuscin) that normally develops in these cells with advancing age. In ALS, the motor neuron cytoskeleton is typically affected early in the illness. Focal enlargements are frequent in proximal motor axons; ultrastructurally, these "spheroids" are composed of accumulations of neurofilaments. Also seen is proliferation of astroglia and microglia, the inevitable accompaniment of all degenerative processes in the central nervous system (CNS).

The death of the peripheral motor neurons in the brainstem and spinal cord leads to denervation and consequent atrophy of the corresponding muscle fibers. Histochemical and electrophysiologic evidence indicates that in the early phases of the illness denervated muscle can be reinnervated by sprouting of nearby distal motor nerve terminals, although reinnervation in this disease is considerably less extensive than in most other disorders affecting motor neurons (e.g., poliomyelitis, peripheral neuropathy). As denervation progresses, muscle atrophy is readily recognized in muscle biopsies and on clinical examination. This is the basis for the term *amyotrophy*. The loss of cortical motor neurons results in thinning of the corticospinal tracts that travel via the internal capsule (Fig. 353-1) and brainstem to the lateral and anterior white matter columns of the spinal cord. The loss
of fibers in the lateral columns and resulting fibrillary gliosis impart a particular firmness (*lateral sclerosis*). A remarkable feature of the disease is the selectivity of neuronal cell death. By light microscopy, the entire sensory apparatus, the regulatory mechanisms for the control and coordination of movement, and the components of the brain that are needed for cognitive processes, remain intact. However, immunostaining indicates that neurons bearing ubiquitin, a marker for degeneration, are also detected in nonmotor systems. Moreover, studies of glucose metabolism in the illness also indicate that there is neuronal dysfunction outside of the motor system. Within the motor system, there is some selectivity of involvement. Thus, motor neurons required for ocular motility remain unaffected, as do the parasympathetic neurons in the sacral spinal cord (the nucleus of Onufrowicz, or Onuf) that innervate the sphincters of the bowel and bladder.

Clinical Manifestations   The manifestations of ALS are somewhat variable depending on whether corticospinal neurons or lower motor neurons in the brainstem and spinal cord are more prominently involved. With lower motor neuron dysfunction and early denervation, typically the first evidence of the disease is insidiously developing asymmetric weakness, usually first evident distally in one of the limbs. A detailed history often discloses recent development of cramping with volitional movements, typically in the early hours of the morning (e.g., while stretching in bed). Weakness caused by denervation is associated with progressive wasting and atrophy of muscles and, particularly early in the illness, spontaneous twitching of motor units, or fasciculations. In the hands, a preponderance of extensor over flexor weakness is common. When the initial denervation involves bulbar rather than limb muscles, the problem at onset is difficulty with chewing, swallowing, and movements of the face and tongue. Early involvement of the muscles of respiration may lead to death before the disease is far advanced elsewhere. With prominent corticospinal involvement, there is hyperactivity of the muscle-stretch reflexes (tendon jerks) and, often, spastic resistance to passive movements of the affected limbs. Patients with significant reflex hyperactivity complain of muscle stiffness often out of proportion to weakness. Degeneration of the corticobulbar projections innervating the brainstem results in dysarthria and exaggeration of the motor expressions of emotion. The latter leads to involuntary excess in weeping or laughing (so-called pseudobulbar affect).

Virtually any muscle group may be the first to show signs of disease, but, as time passes, more and more muscles become involved until ultimately the disorder takes on a symmetric distribution in all regions. It is characteristic of ALS that, regardless of whether the initial disease involves upper or lower motor neurons, both will eventually be implicated. Even in the late stages of the illness, sensory, bowel

TABLE 353-1 *Etiology and Investigation of Motor Neuron Disorders*

Diagnostic Category	Investigations
Structural lesions	MRI scan of head (including
Parasagittal or foramen magnum	foramen magnum), cervical
tumors	spine[a]
Cervical spondylosis	
Chiari malformation or syrinx	
Spinal cord arteriovenous	
malformation	
Infections	CSF exam, culture[a]
Bacterial—tetanus, Lyme	Lyme antibody titer[a]
Viral—poliomyelitis, herpes	Antiviral antibody titers
zoster	
Retroviral myelopathy	HTLV-1 titers
Intoxications, physical agents	
Toxins—lead, aluminum, others	24-h urine for heavy metals[a]
Drugs—strychnine, phenytoin	Serum for lead level[a]
Electric shock, x-irradiation	
Immunologic mechanisms	Complete blood count[a]
Plasma cell dyscrasias	Sedimentation rate[a]
Autoimmune polyradiculoneu-	Protein immunoelectrophoresis[a]
ropathy	
Motor neuropathy with	Anti-GM1 antibodies[a]
conduction block	
Paraneoplastic	Anti-Hu antibody
Paracarcinomatous/lymphoma	MRI scan, bone marrow biopsy
Metabolic	
Hypoglycemia	Fasting blood sugar (FBS), routine
	chemistries including calcium[a]
Hyperparathyroidism	PTH, calcium, phosphate
Hyperthyroidism	Thyroid function[a]
Deficiency of folate, vitamin	Vitamin B_{12}, vitamin E, folate
B_{12}, vitamin E	levels[a]
Malabsorption	24-h stool fat, carotene,
	prothrombin time
Mitochondrial dysfunction	Fasting lactate, pyruvate, ammonia
	Consider mtDNA analysis
Hereditary biochemical disorders	
Superoxide dismutase 1 gene	White blood cell DNA analysis
mutation	
Androgen receptor defect	Abnormal CAG insert in androgen
(Kennedy's disease)	receptor gene
Hexosaminidase deficiency	Lysosomal enzyme screen
Infantile (α-glucosidase	
deficiency/Pompe's disease)	
Hyperlipidemia	Lipid electrophoresis
Hyperglycinuria	Urine and serum amino acids
Methylcrotonylglycinuria	CSF amino acids

[a] Denotes studies that should be obtained in all cases.
Note: CSF, cerebrospinal fluid; HTLV, human T cell lymphotropic virus; MRI, magnetic resonance imaging.

TABLE 353-2 *Sporadic Motor Neuron Diseases*

CHRONIC

Upper and lower motor neurons
  Amyotrophic lateral sclerosis
Predominantly upper motor neurons
  Primary lateral sclerosis
Predominantly lower motor neurons
  Multifocal motor neuropathy with conduction block
  Motor neuropathy with paraproteinemia or cancer
  Motor-predominant peripheral neuropathies
Other
  Associated with other degenerative disorders
  Secondary motor neuron disorders (see Table 353-1)

ACUTE

Poliomyelitis
Herpes zoster
Coxsackie virus

---

and bladder, and cognitive functions are preserved. Even when there is severe brainstem disease, ocular motility is spared until the very late stages of the illness. Dementia is not a component of sporadic ALS. In some families, ALS is co-inherited with frontotemporal dementia, characterized by early behavioral abnormalities with prominent behavioral features indicative of frontal lobe dysfunction.

A committee of the World Federation of Neurology has established diagnostic guidelines for ALS. Essential for the diagnosis is simultaneous upper and lower motor neuron involvement with progressive weakness, and the exclusion of all alternative diagnoses. The disorder is ranked as "definite" ALS when three or four of the following are involved: bulbar, cervical, thoracic, and lumbosacral motor neurons. When two sites are involved, the diagnosis is "probable," and when only one site is implicated, the diagnosis is "possible." An exception is made for those who have progressive upper and lower motor neuron signs at only one site and a mutation in the gene encoding superoxide dismutase (SOD1; below).

Epidemiology The illness is relentlessly progressive, leading to death from respiratory paralysis; the median survival is from 3 to 5 years. There are very rare reports of stabilization or even regression of ALS. In most societies there is an incidence of 1 to 3 per 100,000 and a prevalence of 3 to 5 per 100,000. Several endemic foci of higher prevalence exist in the western Pacific (e.g., in specific regions of Guam or Papua New Guinea). In the United States and Europe, males are somewhat more frequently affected than females. While ALS is overwhelmingly a sporadic disorder, some 5 to 10% of cases are inherited as an autosomal dominant trait.

Familial ALS Several forms of selective motor neuron disease are inheritable (Table 353-3). Two involve both corticospinal and lower motor neurons. The most common is familial ALS (FALS). Apart from its inheritance as an autosomal dominant trait, it is clinically indistinguishable from sporadic ALS. Genetic studies have identified mutations in the gene encoding the cytosolic, copper- and zinc-binding enzyme SOD1 as the cause of one form of FALS. However, this accounts for only 20% of inherited cases of ALS. Rare mutations in other genes are also clearly implicated in ALS-like diseases. Thus, a familial, predominantly lower motor neuron disease with bulbar predominance has been ascribed to mutations in the gene encoding the cellular motor protein dynactin. Another familial, adult-onset disorder that may mimic aspects of ALS is Kennedy's syndrome; as described below, this arises from distinctive mutations in the androgen receptor. Genetic

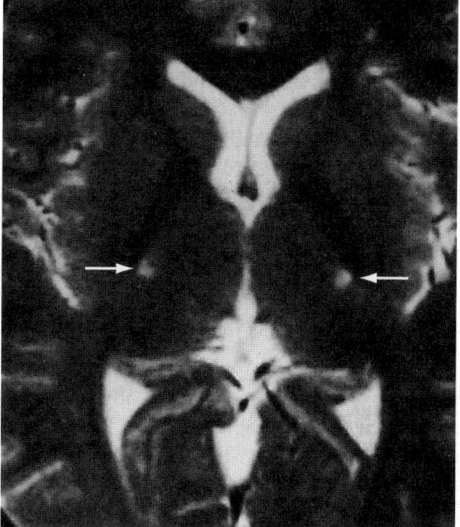

FIGURE 353-1 Amyotrophic lateral sclerosis. Axial T2-weighted MRI scan through the lateral ventricles of the brain reveals abnormal high signal intensity within the corticospinal tracts (*arrows*). This MRI feature represents an increase in water content in myelin tracts undergoing Wallerian degeneration secondary to cortical motor neuronal loss. This finding is commonly present in ALS, but can also be seen in AIDS-related encephalopathy, infarction, or other disease processes that produce corticospinal neuronal loss in a symmetric fashion.

TABLE 353-3   *Genetic Motor Neuron Diseases*

Disease	Locus	Gene
I. Upper and lower motor neurons (familial ALS)		
A. Autosomal dominant	2p	Dynactin
	21q	Superoxide dismutase
	22q	Neurofilament heavy subunit
	9q	Unknown
	16q	Unknown
	20p	Unknown
	X$_{cent}$	Unknown
B. Autosomal recessive (juvenile)	2q	Alsin
	15q	Unknown
C. Mitochondrial	mtDNA	Cytochrome c oxidase
II. Lower motor neurons		
A. Spinal muscular atrophies	5q	Survival motor neuron protein
B. X-linked spinobulbar muscular atrophy	Xq	Androgen receptor
C. G$_{M2}$ gangliosidosis		
1. Adult Tay-Sach's disease	15q	Hexosaminidase A
2. Sandhoff disease	5q	Hexosaminidase B
3. AB variant	5q	G$_{M2}$ activator protein
III. Upper motor neurons/selected FSPs		
A. Autosomal dominant	2p	Spastin
	2q	Mitochondrial heat shock protein
	12q	Kinesin heavy chain KIF5A
	14q	Unknown
B. Autosomal recessive	16q	Paraplegin
C. X-linked	Xq21	Proteolipid protein
	Xq28	L1 CAM
D. Adrenomyeloneuropathy	Xq21	Adrenoleukodystrophy protein
IV. ALS-plus syndromes		
A. ALS with frontotemporal dementia	9q	Unknown
B. Amyotrophy with behavioral disorder and parkinsonian features	17q	Tau protein

Note: ALS, amyotrophic lateral sclerosis; FSP, familial spastic paraplegia.

analyses are also beginning to illuminate the pathogenesis of some childhood-onset motor neuron diseases. For example, a slowly disabling degenerative, predominantly upper motor neuron disease that starts in the first decade is caused by mutations in a gene that expresses a novel signaling molecule with properties of a guanine-exchange factor, termed *alsin*. In other instances, chromosomal locations for motor neuron diseases, but not the causative genes themselves, have been identified. Typical FALS has been genetically mapped to chromosomes 16 and 20 in several families, and a juvenile-onset, dominantly inherited form of ALS has been mapped to the long-arm of chromosome 9.

Differential Diagnosis   Because ALS is currently untreatable, it is imperative that potentially remediable causes of motor neuron dysfunction be excluded (Table 353-1). This is particularly true in cases that are atypical by virtue of (1) restriction to either upper or lower motor neurons, (2) involvement of neurons other than motor neurons, and (3) evidence of motor neuronal conduction block on electrophysiologic testing. Compression of the cervical spinal cord or cervicomedullary junction from tumors in the cervical regions or at the foramen magnum or from cervical spondylosis with osteophytes projecting into the vertebral canal can produce weakness, wasting, and fasciculations in the upper limbs and spasticity in the legs, closely resembling ALS. The absence of cranial nerve involvement may be helpful in differentiation,

although some foramen magnum lesions may compress the twelfth cranial (hypoglossal) nerve, with resulting paralysis of the tongue. Absence of pain or of sensory changes, normal bowel and bladder function, normal roentgenographic studies of the spine, and normal cerebrospinal fluid (CSF) all favor ALS. Where doubt exists, magnetic resonance imaging (MRI) scans and contrast myelography should be performed to visualize the cervical spinal cord.

Another important entity in the differential diagnosis of ALS is *multifocal motor neuropathy with conduction block* (MMCB), discussed below. A diffuse, lower motor axonal neuropathy mimicking ALS sometimes evolves in association with hematopoietic disorders such as lymphoma. In this clinical setting, the presence of an M-component in serum should prompt consideration of a bone marrow biopsy. Lyme disease (Chap. 157) may also cause an axonal, lower motor neuropathy.

Other treatable disorders that occasionally mimic ALS are chronic lead poisoning and thyrotoxicosis. These disorders may be suggested by the patient's social or occupational history or by unusual clinical features. When the family history is positive, disorders involving the genes encoding cytosolic SOD1, hexosaminidase A, or α-glucosidase deficiency must be excluded (Chap. 340). These are readily identified by appropriate laboratory tests. Benign fasciculations are occasionally a source of concern because on inspection they resemble the fascicular twitchings that accompany motor neuron degeneration. The absence of weakness, atrophy, or denervation phenomena on electrophysiologic examination usually excludes ALS or other serious neurologic disease. Patients who have recovered from poliomyelitis may experience a delayed deterioration of motor neurons that presents clinically with progressive weakness, atrophy, and fasciculations. Its cause is unknown, but it is thought to reflect sublethal prior injury to motor neurons by poliovirus (Chap. 175).

Rarely, ALS develops concurrently with features indicative of more widespread neurodegeneration. Thus, one infrequently encounters otherwise typical ALS patients with a parkinsonian movement disorder or dementia. It remains unclear whether this reflects the unlikely simultaneous occurrence of two disorders or a primary defect triggering two forms of neurodegeneration. The latter is suggested by the observation that multisystem neurodegenerative diseases may be inherited. For example, prominent amyotrophy has been described as a dominantly inherited disorder in individuals with bizarre behavior and a movement disorder suggestive of parkinsonism; many such cases have now been ascribed to mutations that alter the expression of tau protein in brain (Chap. 350). In other cases, ALS develops simultaneously with a striking frontotemporal dementia. These disorders may be dominantly co-inherited; in some families, this trait is linked to a locus on chromosome 9q, although the underlying genetic defect is not established.

Pathogenesis   The cause of sporadic ALS is not well defined. Several mechanisms that impair motor neuron viability have been elucidated in mice and rats induced to develop motor neuron disease by SOD1 transgenes with ALS-associated mutations. It is evident that excitotoxic neurotransmitters such as glutamate participate in the death of motor neurons in ALS. This may be a consequence of diminished uptake of synaptic glutamate by an astroglial glutamate transporter, EAAT2. It is striking that one cellular defense against such excitotoxicity is the enzyme SOD1, which detoxifies the free radical superoxide anion (Chap. 345). Because SOD1 is mutated in some familial cases of ALS, it may be that glutamate excitotoxicity and ALS result from free radical accumulations in motor neurons. Precisely why the SOD1 mutations are toxic to motor nerves is not established, although it is clear the effect is not simply loss of normal scavenging of the superoxide anion. The mutant protein is conformationally unstable and prone to aberrant catalytic reactions. In turn, these features lead to aggregation of SOD1 protein, impairment of axonal transport, reduced production of ATP and other perturbations of mitochondrial function, activation of cyclo-oxygenase within the ALS spinal cord, and ultimately induction of cell death via pathways that are at least partially dependent on caspases. Recent studies have raised the hypothesis that genetic variants in the vascular endothelial growth factor gene (VEGF) that reduce VEGF expression increase the risk of ALS; whether this is a consequence of spinal cord hypoxia or diminished neurotrophic influence of VEGF remains to be established.

℞ TREATMENT

No treatment arrests the underlying pathologic process in ALS. The drug riluzole (100 mg/d) was approved for ALS because it produces a modest lengthening of survival. In one trial, the survival rate at 18 months with riluzole was similar to placebo at 15 months. The mechanism of this effect is not known with certainty; riluzole may reduce excitotoxicity by diminishing glutamate release. Riluzole is generally well tolerated; nausea, dizziness, weight loss, and elevated liver enzymes occur occasionally. Several agents have failed in clinical trials in human ALS including brain-derived neurotrophic factor, glial-derived neurotrophic factor, the anti-glutamate compound topiramate, and creatine. The latter was somewhat surprising as creatine was proven to be beneficial in transgenic ALS mice, perhaps by augmenting intracellular ATP stores. Insulin-like growth factor 1 (IGF-1) produced inconsistent results in ALS patients and is undergoing further clinical trials. The finding that cyclo-oxygenase activity is enhanced in the spinal cords of ALS mice led to a preclinical study of the COX-2 inhibitor, celecoxib, which significantly increased life span in that model. As a consequence, celecoxib is currently being tested in human ALS. Analogously, because minocycline produced a modest benefit in ALS mice, presumably by inhibiting late stages of the apoptotic cascade, it is now being tested in a multicenter ALS trial.

In the absence of a primary therapy for ALS, a variety of rehabilitative aids may substantially assist ALS patients. Foot-drop splints facilitate ambulation by obviating the need for excessive hip flexion and by preventing tripping on a floppy foot. Finger extension splints can potentiate grip. Respiratory support may be life-sustaining. For patients electing against long-term ventilation by tracheostomy, positive-pressure ventilation by mouth or nose provides transient (several weeks) relief from hypercarbia and hypoxia. Also extremely beneficial for some patients is a respiratory device (In-exsufflator or Cough Assist Device) that produces an artificial cough. This is highly effective in clearing airways and preventing aspiration pneumonia. When bulbar disease prevents normal chewing and swallowing, gastrostomy is uniformly helpful, restoring normal nutrition and hydration. Fortunately, an increasing variety of speech synthesizers are now available to augment speech when there is advanced bulbar palsy. These facilitate oral communication and may be effective for telephone use.

In contrast to ALS, several of the disorders (Tables 353-1 and 353-3) that bear some clinical resemblance to ALS are treatable. For this reason, a careful search for causes of secondary motor neuron disease is warranted.

SELECTED LOWER MOTOR NEURON DISORDERS In these motor neuron diseases, the peripheral motor neurons are affected without evidence of involvement of the corticospinal motor system (Tables 353-1 to 353-3).

X-Linked Spinobulbar Muscular Atrophy (Kennedy's Disease) This is an X-linked lower motor neuron disorder in which progressive weakness and wasting of limb and bulbar muscles begins in males in mid-adult life and is conjoined with androgen insensitivity manifested by gynecomastia and reduced fertility (Chap. 325). In addition to gynecomastia, which may be subtle, two findings distinguishing this disorder from ALS are the absence of signs of pyramidal tract disease (spasticity) and the presence of a subtle sensory neuropathy in some patients. The underlying molecular defect is an expanded trinucleotide repeat (-CAG-) in the first exon of the androgen receptor gene on the X chromosome. DNA testing is available. An inverse correlation appears to exist between the number of -CAG- repeats and the age of onset of the disease.

Adult Tay-Sach's Disease Several reports have described adult-onset, predominantly lower motor neuropathies arising from deficiency of the enzyme β-hexosaminidase (hex A). These tend to be distinguishable from ALS because they are very slowly progressive; dysarthria and radiographically evident cerebellar atrophy may be prominent. In rare cases, spasticity may also be present, although it is generally absent (Chap. 340).

Spinal Muscular Atrophy The SMAs are a family of selective lower motor neuron diseases of early onset. Despite some phenotypic variability (largely in age of onset), the defect in the majority of families with SMA maps to a locus on chromosome 5 encoding a putative motor neuron survival protein (SMN, for survival motor neuron) that is important in the formation and trafficking of RNA complexes across the nuclear membrane. Neuropathologically these disorders are characterized by extensive loss of large motor neurons; muscle biopsy reveals evidence of denervation atrophy. Several clinical forms exist.

Infantile SMA (SMA I, Werdnig-Hoffmann Disease) has the earliest onset and most rapidly fatal course. In some instances it is apparent even before birth, as indicated by decreased fetal movements late in the third trimester. Though alert, afflicted infants are weak and floppy (hypotonic) and lack muscle stretch reflexes. Death generally ensues within the first year of life. *Chronic childhood SMA* (SMA II) begins later in childhood and evolves with a more slowly progressive course. *Juvenile SMA* (SMA III, Kugelberg-Welander disease) manifests during late childhood and runs a slow, indolent course. Unlike most denervating diseases, in this chronic disorder weakness is greatest in the proximal muscles; indeed, the pattern of clinical weakness can suggest a primary myopathy such as limb-girdle dystrophy. Electrophysiologic and muscle biopsy evidence of denervation distinguish SMA III from the myopathic syndromes.

Multifocal Motor Neuropathy with Conduction Block In this disorder lower motor neuron function is regionally and chronically disrupted by remarkably focal blocks in conduction. Many cases have elevated serum titers of mono- and polyclonal antibodies to ganglioside GM1; it is hypothesized that the antibodies produce selective, focal, paranodal demyelination of motor neurons. MMCB is not typically associated with corticospinal signs. In contrast with ALS, MMCB may respond dramatically to therapy such as intravenous immunoglobulin or chemotherapy; it is thus imperative that MMCB be excluded when considering a diagnosis of ALS.

Other Forms of Lower Motor Neuron Disease In individual families, other syndromes characterized by selective lower motor neuron dysfunction in an SMA-like pattern have been described. There are rare X-linked and autosomal dominant forms of apparent SMA. There is an ALS variant of juvenile onset, the Fazio-Londe syndrome, that involves mainly the musculature innervated by the brainstem. A component of lower motor neuron dysfunction is also found in degenerative disorders such as Machado-Joseph disease and the related olivopontocerebellar degenerations (Chap. 352).

SELECTED DISORDERS OF THE UPPER MOTOR NEURON ■ Primary Lateral Sclerosis This exceedingly rare disorder arises sporadically in adults in mid- to late life. Clinically PLS is characterized by progressive spastic weakness of the limbs, preceded or followed by spastic dysarthria and dysphagia, indicating combined involvement of the corticospinal and corticobulbar tracts. Fasciculations, amyotrophy, and sensory changes are absent; neither electromyography nor muscle biopsy shows denervation. On neuropathologic examination there is selective loss of the large pyramidal cells in the precentral gyrus and degeneration of the corticospinal and corticobulbar projections. The peripheral motor neurons and other neuronal systems are spared. The course of PLS is variable; while long-term survival is documented, the course may be as aggressive as in ALS, with ~3-year survival from onset to death. Early in its course, PLS raises the question of multiple sclerosis or other demyelinating diseases such as adrenoleukodystrophy as diagnostic considerations (Chap. 359). A myelopathy suggestive of PLS is infrequently seen with infection with the retrovirus human T cell lymphotropic virus (HTLV-I) (Chap. 356). The clinical course and laboratory testing will distinguish these possibilities.

Familial Spastic Paraplegia   In its pure form, FSP is usually transmitted as an autosomal trait; most adult-onset cases are dominantly inherited. It arises in the third or fourth decade and is characterized by progressive spastic weakness beginning in the distal lower extremities. FSP typically has a long survival, presumably because respiratory function is spared. Late in the illness there may be urinary urgency and incontinence and sometimes fecal incontinence; sexual function tends to be preserved. In pure forms of FSP, ataxia, posterior column sensory loss, and amyotrophy are absent or minimal; however, in some patients, minor sensory changes (impaired vibration and position sense) may be observed in late stages. Some family members may have spasticity without clinical symptoms. Neuropathologically, in FSP there is degeneration of the corticospinal tracts, which appear nearly normal in the brainstem but show increasing atrophy at more caudal levels in the spinal cord. It is now apparent that defects at numerous loci underlie both dominantly and recessively inherited forms of FSP (Table 353-3). An infantile-onset form of X-linked, recessive FSP arises from mutations in the gene for myelin proteolipid protein (Chap. 345). This is an example of rather striking allelic variation, as most other mutations in the same gene cause not FSP but Pelizaeus-Merzbacher disease, a widespread disorder of CNS myelin. Defects in genes encoding the proteins spastin and paraplegin have been associated respectively with dominantly and recessively inherited FSP. The latter gene is of particular interest as it has homology to metalloproteases that are important in mitochondrial function in yeast. Defects in the gene *spartin*, a protein with homology to spastin, are associated with recessively inherited spasticity and distal weakness of early childhood onset. A kinesin heavy chain protein implicated in microtubule motor function was found to be defective in a family with dominantly inherited FSP of variable onset age.

Rarely, FSP may arise concomitantly with significant involvement of other regions of the nervous system. Thus, it has been described concurrently with amyotrophy, mental retardation, mental retardation with skin thickening, optic atrophy, and sensory neuropathy. In some cases there is loss of fibers in the ascending posterior columns and the spinocerebellar tracts, features reminiscent of Friedreich's ataxia (Chap. 352). These complicated forms of FSP emphasize the challenge inherent in classifying the neurodegenerative disorders; there may be considerable overlap of the clinical phenotypes in diseases otherwise classified as distinct. Fortunately, it is likely that increasingly available genetic testing will clarify these nosologic difficulties.

WEB SITES   Several web sites provide valuable information on ALS including those offered by the Muscular Dystrophy Association (www.mdausa.org), the Amyotrophic Lateral Sclerosis Association (www.alsa.org), and the World Federation of Neurology and the Neuromuscular Unit At Washington University in St. Louis (www.neuro.wustl.edu/neuromuscular).

FURTHER READING

CLEVELAND DW, ROTHSTEIN JD: From Charcot to Lou Gehrig: Deciphering selective motor neuron death in ALS. Nat Rev Neurosci 2:806, 2001

HADANO S et al: A gene encoding a putative GTPase regulator is mutated in familial amyotrophic lateral sclerosis. Nat Genet 29:166, 2001

LAMBRECHTS D et al: VEGF is a modifier of amyotrophic lateral sclerosis in mice and humans and protects motoneurons against ischemic death. Nat Genet 34(4):384, 2003

PULS I et al: Mutant dynactin in motor neuron disease. Nat Genet 33:455, 2003

YANG Y et al: The gene encoding alsin, a protein with three guanine-nucleotide exchange factor domains, is mutated in a form of recessive amyotrophic lateral sclerosis. Nat Genet 29:160, 2001

354 | DISORDERS OF THE AUTONOMIC NERVOUS SYSTEM
Phillip A. Low, John W. Engstrom

The autonomic nervous system (ANS) innervates the entire neuraxis and permeates all organ systems. It regulates blood pressure (BP), heart rate, sleep, and bladder and bowel function. It operates in the background, so that its full importance becomes recognized only when ANS function is compromised, resulting in dysautonomia. →*Hypothalamic disorders that cause disturbances in homeostasis are discussed in Chaps. 16 and 318.*

ANATOMIC ORGANIZATION   The activity of the autonomic nervous system is regulated by central neurons responsive to diverse afferent inputs. After central integration of afferent information, autonomic outflow is adjusted to permit the functioning of the major organ systems in accordance with the needs of the organism as a whole. Connections between the cerebral cortex and the autonomic centers in the brainstem coordinate autonomic outflow with higher mental functions.

The preganglionic neurons of the parasympathetic nervous system leave the central nervous system (CNS) in the third, seventh, ninth, and tenth cranial nerves as well as the second and third sacral nerves, while the preganglionic neurons of the sympathetic nervous system exit the spinal cord between the first thoracic and the second lumbar segments (Fig. 354-1). The postganglionic neurons, located in ganglia outside the CNS, give rise to the postganglionic autonomic nerves that innervate organs and tissues throughout the body. Responses to sympathetic and parasympathetic stimulation are frequently antagonistic (Table 354-1), reflecting highly coordinated interactions within the CNS; the resultant changes in parasympathetic and sympathetic activity provide more precise control of autonomic responses than could be achieved by the modulation of a single system.

Acetylcholine (ACh) is the preganglionic neurotransmitter for both divisions of the ANS as well as the postganglionic neurotransmitter of the parasympathetic neurons. Norepinephrine (NE) is the neurotransmitter of the postganglionic sympathetic neurons, except for cholinergic neurons innervating the eccrine sweat glands and perhaps some blood vessels supplying skeletal muscle.

CLINICAL EVALUATION ■ **Classification**   Disorders of the ANS may result from pathology of either the CNS or the peripheral nervous system (PNS) (Table 354-2). Signs and symptoms may result from interruption of the afferent limb, CNS processing centers, or efferent limb of reflex arcs controlling autonomic responses. For example, a lesion of the medulla produced by a posterior fossa tumor can impair BP responses to postural changes and result in orthostatic hypotension (OH). OH can also be caused by lesions of the spinal cord or peripheral vasomotor nerve fibers (e.g., diabetic autonomic neuropathy). The site of reflex interruption is usually established by the clinical context in which the dysautonomia arises, combined with judicious use of ANS testing and neuroimaging studies. Important elements of the clinical context include the presence or absence of CNS signs (pathophysiology and prognosis differ), association with sensory or motor polyneuropathy, family history, and pathologic findings. Some syndromes do not fit easily into any classification scheme.

Symptoms of Autonomic Dysfunction   Clinical manifestations result from a loss of function (e.g., impaired baroreflexes leading to OH), overactivity (e.g., hyperhidrosis, hypertension, tachycardia), or loss of regulation (e.g., autonomic storms, autonomic dysreflexia) of autonomic circuits. The disorder may be widespread or regional in distribution.

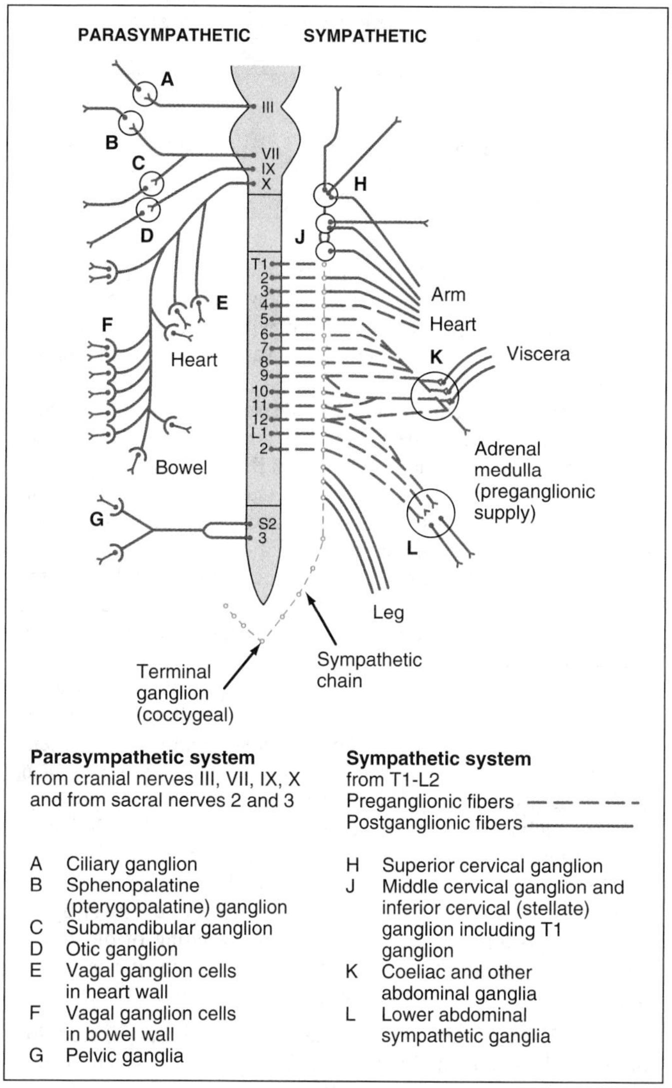
PARASYMPATHETIC
SYMPATHETIC
A
B
C
D
E
F
G
H
J
K
L
III
VII
IX
X
T1
2
3
4
5
6
7
8
9
10
11
12
L1
2
S2
3
Heart
Bowel
Arm
Heart
Viscera
Adrenal medulla (preganglionic supply)
Leg
Terminal ganglion (coccygeal)
Sympathetic chain
Parasympathetic system
from cranial nerves III, VII, IX, X and from sacral nerves 2 and 3
Sympathetic system
from T1-L2
Preganglionic fibers
Postganglionic fibers
A Ciliary ganglion
B Sphenopalatine (pterygopalatine) ganglion
C Submandibular ganglion
D Otic ganglion
E Vagal ganglion cells in heart wall
F Vagal ganglion cells in bowel wall
G Pelvic ganglia
H Superior cervical ganglion
J Middle cervical ganglion and inferior cervical (stellate) ganglion including T1 ganglion
K Coeliac and other abdominal ganglia
L Lower abdominal sympathetic ganglia

FIGURE 354-1 Schematic representation of the autonomic nervous system. (*From M Moskowitz: Clin Endocrinol Metab 6:77, 1977.*)

An autonomic history focuses on systemic functions (BP, heart rate, sleep, thermoregulation) and individual organ systems (pupils, bowel, bladder, sexual function). More formal assessment is possible using a standardized instrument such as the autonomic symptom profile. It is also important to recognize the modulating effects of age and gender. For instance, OH commonly results in lightheadedness in the young, whereas cognitive slowing is much more important in the elderly. Specific symptoms of orthostatic intolerance are quite diverse (Table 354-3). Autonomic symptoms may vary dramatically, reflecting the dynamic nature of autonomic control over homeostatic function. For example, OH might be manifest only in the early morning, following a

TABLE 354-1 *Functional Consequences of Normal ANS Activation*

	Sympathetic	*Parasympathetic*
Heart rate	Increased	Decreased
Blood pressure	Increased	Mildly decreased
Bladder	Increased sphincter tone	Voiding (decreased tone)
Bowel motility	Decreased motility	Increased
Lung	Bronchodilation	Bronchoconstriction
Sweat glands	Sweating	—
Pupils	Dilation	Constriction
Adrenal glands	Catecholamine release	—
Sexual function	Ejaculation, orgasm	Erection
Lacrimal glands	—	Tearing
Parotid glands	—	Salivation

TABLE 354-2 *Classification of Clinical Autonomic Disorders*

I. Autonomic disorders with brain involvement
  A. Associated with multisystem degeneration
    1. Multisystem degeneration: autonomic failure clinically prominent
      a. Multiple system atrophy (MSA)
      b. Parkinson's disease with autonomic failure
      c. Diffuse Lewy body disease (some cases)
    2. Multisystem degeneration: autonomic failure clinically not usually prominent
      a. Parkinson's disease
      b. Other extrapyramidal disorders (inherited spinocerebellar atrophies, progressive supranuclear palsy, corticobasal degeneration, Machado-Joseph disease)
  B. Unassociated with multisystem degeneration
    1. Disorders mainly due to cerebral cortex involvement
      a. Frontal cortex lesions causing urinary/bowel incontinence
      b. Partial complex seizures
    2. Disorders of the limbic and paralimbic circuits
      a. Shapiro's syndrome (agenesis of corpus callosum, hyperhidrosis, hypothermia)
      b. Autonomic seizures
    3. Disorders of the hypothalamus
      a. Wernicke-Korsakoff syndrome
      b. Diencephalic syndrome
      c. Neuroleptic malignant syndrome
      d. Serotonin syndrome
      e. Fatal familial insomnia
      f. Antidiuretic hormone (ADH) syndromes (diabetes insipidus, inappropriate ADH)
      g. Disturbances of temperature regulation (hyperthermia, hypothermia)
      h. Disturbances of sexual function
      i. Disturbances of appetite
      j. Disturbances of BP/HR and gastric function
      k. Horner's syndrome
    4. Disorders of the brainstem and cerebellum
      a. Posterior fossa tumors
      b. Syringobulbia and Arnold-Chiari malformation
      c. Disorders of BP control (hypertension, hypotension)
      d. Cardiac arrhythmias
      e. Central sleep apnea
      f. Baroreflex failure
      g. Horner's syndrome
II. Autonomic disorders with spinal cord involvement
  A. Traumatic tetraplegia
  B. Syringomyelia
  C. Subacute combined degeneration
  D. Multiple sclerosis
  E. Amyotrophic lateral sclerosis
  F. Tetanus
  G. Stiff-man syndrome
  H. Spinal cord tumors
III. Autonomic neuropathies
  A. Acute/subacute autonomic neuropathies
    1. Subacute autoimmune autonomic neuropathy (panautonomic neuropathy, pandysautonomia)
      a. Subacute paraneoplastic autonomic neuropathy
      b. Guillain-Barré syndrome
      c. Botulism
      d. Porphyria
      e. Drug induced autonomic neuropathies
      f. Toxic autonomic neuropathies
  B. Chronic peripheral autonomic neuropathies
    1. Distal small fiber neuropathy
    2. Combined sympathetic and parasympathetic failure
      a. Amyloid
      b. Diabetic autonomic neuropathy
      c. Autoimmune autonomic neuropathy (paraneoplastic and idiopathic)
      d. Sensory neuronopathy with autonomic failure
      e. Familial dysautonomia (Riley-Day syndrome)

Note: BP, blood pressure; HR, heart rate.

TABLE 354-3 Symptoms of Orthostatic Intolerance

Lightheadedness (dizziness)	88%
Weakness or tiredness	72%
Cognitive difficulty (thinking/concentrating)	47%
Blurred vision	47%
Tremulousness	38%
Vertigo	37%
Pallor	31%
Anxiety	29%
Palpitations	26%
Clammy feeling	19%
Nausea	18%

Source: From Low et al.

meal, or with exercise, depending upon the regional vascular bed affected by dysautonomia.

Early symptoms may be overlooked. Impotence, although not specific for autonomic failure, often heralds autonomic failure in men and may precede other symptoms by years (Chap. 43). A decrease in the frequency of spontaneous early morning erections may occur months before loss of nocturnal penile tumescence and development of total impotence. Bladder dysfunction may appear early in men and women, particularly in those with CNS involvement. Brain and spinal cord disease above the level of the lumbar spine results first in urinary frequency and small bladder volumes, and eventually in incontinence (upper motor neuron or spastic bladder). Disease of PNS autonomic nerve fibers to and from the bladder results in large bladder volumes, urinary frequency, and overflow incontinence (lower motor neuron bladder or flaccid bladder). Measurement of bladder volume (postvoid residual) is a useful bedside test for distinguishing between upper and lower motor neuron bladder dysfunction in the early stages of dysautonomia. Gastrointestinal autonomic dysfunction typically presents as severe constipation. Diarrhea occurs occasionally (as in diabetes mellitus) due to rapid transit of contents or uncoordinated small-bowel motor activity, or on an osmotic basis from bacterial overgrowth associated with small-bowel stasis. Impaired glandular secretory function may cause difficulty with food intake due to decreased salivation or with eye irritation due to decreased lacrimation. Occasionally, temperature elevation and vasodilation can result from anhidrosis because sweating is normally important for heat dissipation (Chap. 16).

OH (also called "postural hypotension") is perhaps the most disabling feature of autonomic dysfunction. The prevalence of OH is relatively high, especially when OH associated with aging is included (Table 354-4). OH can cause a variety of symptoms including dimming or loss of vision, lightheadedness, diaphoresis, diminished hearing, pallor, and weakness. Syncope results when the drop in BP impairs cerebral perfusion. Other manifestations of impaired baroreflexes are supine hypertension, a heart rate that is fixed regardless of posture, postprandial hypotension, and an excessively high nocturnal BP. Many patients with OH have a preceding diagnosis of hypertension, reflecting the great importance of baroreflexes in maintaining postural and supine normotension. The most common causes of OH are not neurologic in origin; these must be distinguished from the neurogenic causes. →*Neurocardiogenic and cardiac syncope are considered in Chap. 20.*

APPROACH TO THE PATIENT

The first step in the evaluation of symptomatic OH is the exclusion of treatable causes. The history should include a review of medications that may cause OH (e.g., diuretics, antihypertensives, antidepressants, phenothiazines, ethanol, narcotics, insulin, barbiturates, and calcium channel blocking agents). However, the precipitation of OH by medications may also be the first sign of an underlying autonomic disorder. The history may reveal an underlying cause for symptoms (e.g., diabetes, Parkinson's disease) or specific underlying mechanisms (e.g., cardiac pump failure, re-

TABLE 354-4 Prevalence of Orthostatic Hypotension in Different Disorders

Disorder	Prevalence
Aging	14–20%
Diabetic neuropathy	10%
Other autonomic neuropathies	10–50 per 100,000
Multiple system atrophy	5–15 per 100,000
Pure autonomic failure	10–30 per 100,000

duced intravascular volume). The relationship of symptoms to meals (splanchnic pooling), standing on awakening in the morning (intravascular volume depletion), ambient warming (vasodilation), or exercise (muscle arteriolar vasodilatation) should be sought.

Physical examination includes measurement of supine and standing pulse and BP. OH is defined as a sustained drop in systolic ($\geq$20 mmHg) or diastolic ($\geq$10 mmHg) BP within 3 min of standing up. In nonneurogenic causes of OH (such as hypovolemia), the BP drop is accompanied by a compensatory increase in heart rate of >15 beats/min. An important clinical clue that the patient has neurogenic OH is the aggravation or precipitation of OH by autonomic stressors (such as a meal, hot tub/hot bath, and exercise). Neurologic evaluation should include a mental status examination (to exclude neurodegenerative disorders), cranial nerve examination (impaired downgaze is found with progressive supranuclear palsy), abnormal pupils (Horner's or Adie's pupils), motor examination (Parkinson's disease and parkinsonian syndromes), and sensory examination (polyneuropathies). In patients without a clear initial diagnosis, follow-up neurologic examinations and repeat laboratory evaluations over 1 to 2 years may reveal an evolution of findings that enables a specific diagnosis to be made.

Disorders of autonomic function should be considered in patients with symptoms of altered sweating (hyperhidrosis or hypohidrosis), gastroparesis (bloating, nausea, vomiting of old food), constipation, impotence, or bladder dysfunction (urinary frequency, hesitancy, or incontinence).

Autonomic Testing Autonomic function tests (Table 354-5) are helpful when the history and physical examination findings are inconclusive, when detection of subclinical involvement is important to evaluate the extent and severity of abnormalities, or to follow the course of an autonomic disorder or its response to therapy.

HEART RATE VARIATION WITH DEEP BREATHING This is a test of parasympathetic influence on cardiovascular function. Results are influenced by the subject's posture, rate and depth of respiration [6 breaths per minute and a forced vital capacity (FVC) >1.5 L are optimal], age, medications, and hypocapnea. Interpretation of results requires comparison of test data with results from normal individuals collected under the same test conditions. For example, the lower limit of normal heart rate variation with deep breathing

TABLE 354-5 Neural Pathways Underlying Some Standardized Autonomic Tests

Test Evaluated	Procedure	Autonomic Function
HRBD	6 deep breaths/min	Cardiovagal function
Valsalva ratio	Expiratory pressure, 40 mmHg for 10–15 s	Cardiovagal function
QSART	Axon-reflex test 4 limb sites	Postganglionic sudomotor function
BP_BB to VM	BP_BB response to VM	Adrenergic function: baroreflex adrenergic control of vagal and vasomotor function
HUT	BP_BB and heart rate response to HUT	Adrenergic and cardiovagal responses to HUT

Note: HRDB, heart rate response to deep breathing; BP_BB, beat-to-beat blood pressure; QSART, quantitative sudomotor axon-reflex test; VM, Valsalva maneuver; HUT, head-up tilt.

in persons <20 years is >15 to 20 beats/min, but for persons over age 60 it is 5 to 8 beats/min. Heart rate variation with deep breathing (respiratory sinus arrhythmia) is abolished by the administration of atropine.

VALSALVA RESPONSE This response (Table 354-5) assesses integrity of the baroreflex control of heart rate (parasympathetic) and BP (adrenergic). The response is obtained with the subject supine. A constant expiratory pressure of 40 mmHg is maintained for 15 s while measuring changes in heart rate and beat-to-beat BP. There are four phases of BP and heart rate response to the Valsalva maneuver. Phases I and III are mechanical and related to changes in intrathoracic and intraabdominal pressure. In early phase II, reduced venous return results in a fall in stroke volume and BP, counteracted by a combination of reflex tachycardia and increased total peripheral resistance. Increased total peripheral resistance arrests the BP drop ~5 to 8 s after the onset of the maneuver. Late phase II begins with a progressive rise in BP to or above baseline. Venous return and cardiac output return to normal in phase IV. Persistent peripheral arteriolar vasoconstriction and increased cardiac adrenergic tone results in a temporary BP overshoot and phase IV bradycardia (mediated by the baroreceptor reflex).

Autonomic function during the Valsalva maneuver can be measured using beat-to-beat blood pressure or heart rate changes. The Valsalva ratio is defined as the maximum phase II tachycardia divided by the minimum phase IV bradycardia. The ratio reflects cardiovagal function.

SUDOMOTOR FUNCTION Sweating is induced by release of ACh from sympathetic postganglionic fibers. The quantitative sudomotor axon reflex test (QSART) is a measure of regional autonomic function mediated by ACh-induced sweating. A reduced or absent response indicates a lesion of the postganglionic sudomotor axon. For example, sweating may be reduced in the legs as a result of peripheral neuropathy (e.g., in diabetes) before other signs of autonomic dysfunction emerge. The thermoregulatory sweat test (TST) is a qualitative measure of regional sweat production in response to an elevation of body temperature. An indicator powder placed on the anterior body surface changes color with sweat production during temperature elevation. The pattern of color changes is a measure of regional sweat secretion. Combining TST and QSART results will determine the site of the lesion. A postganglionic lesion is present if both QSART and TST show absent sweating. In a preganglionic lesion, QSART is intact but TST shows anhidrosis. Measurement of galvanic skin responses in the limbs after an induced electrical potential is another qualitative test for detecting the presence or absence of sweating.

ORTHOSTATIC BP RECORDINGS Beat-to-beat BP measurements determined in supine, 70° tilt, and tilt-back positions are useful to quantitate orthostatic failure of BP control. It is important to allow a 20-min period of supine rest before assessing changes in BP during tilting. The BP change combined with heart rate monitoring can be useful for the evaluation of patients with suspected OH or unexplained syncope or to detect vagally mediated syncope.

PHARMACOLOGIC TESTS Pharmacologic assessments can help localize an autonomic defect to the CNS or the PNS. A useful method to evaluate the systemic adrenergic response is the measurement of plasma NE, first with the patient supine and then after standing for at least 5 min. Supine values are reduced in postganglionic disorders (such as autonomic neuropathy or pure autonomic failure) and may fail to increase in preganglionic or postganglionic disorders (e.g., multiple system atrophy).

Administration of tyramine (releases NE from postganglionic terminals) and phenylephrine (denervation supersensitivity—directly acting α_1-agonist) is often used to evaluate postganglionic adrenergic function. In a postganglionic lesion, the response to tyramine is reduced and there is an excessive response to subthreshold doses of phenylephrine. Other strategies include ganglionic

blockade with trimethaphan (greater fall in resulting BP with a preganglionic lesion) or administration of arginine vasopressin (to evaluate afferent central pathways).

SPECIFIC SYNDROMES OF ANS DYSFUNCTION ■ **Multiple System Atrophy**
Multiple system atrophy (MSA) is an uncommon entity that comprises autonomic failure (OH and/or a neurogenic bladder are required for diagnosis) combined with either striatonigral degeneration (Shy-Drager syndrome) or sporadic olivopontocerebellar atrophy (Chap. 351). The parkinsonism is usually unassociated with rest tremor and is not responsive to levodopa. Levodopa-induced dyskinesia is also uncommon. Autonomic function tests can usually differentiate MSA from Parkinson's disease in that the severity and distribution of autonomic failure is more severe and generalized in MSA. Cardiac postganglionic adrenergic innervation, measured as labeled metaiodobenzylguanidine (MIBG) uptake on single photon emission computed tomography or fluorodopamine on positron emission tomography (PET), is markedly impaired in the dysautonomia of Parkinson's disease but is normal in MSA.

MSA generally progresses relentlessly to death 7 to 10 years after onset. Neuropathologic changes include primary neuronal degeneration with loss of neurons and gliosis in many CNS regions, including the brainstem, the cerebellum, the striatum, and the intermediolateral cell column of the thoracolumbar spinal cord.

Spinal Cord Spinal cord lesions from any cause may result in focal autonomic deficits or autonomic hyperreflexia. Spinal cord transection or hemisection may be attended by autonomic hyperreflexia affecting bowel, bladder, sexual, temperature-regulation, or cardiovascular functions. Dangerous increases or decreases in body temperature may result from inability to experience the sensory accompaniments of heat or cold exposure below the level of the injury. Quadriparetic patients exhibit both supine hypertension and OH after upward tilting. Markedly increased autonomic discharge can be elicited by bladder pressure or stimulation of the skin or muscles; suprapubic palpation of the bladder, a distended bladder, catheter insertion, catheter obstruction, or urinary infection are common and correctable precipitants. This phenomenon, termed *autonomic dysreflexia*, affects 85% of patients with a traumatic spinal cord lesion above the C6 level. In patients with supine hypertension, BP can be lowered by tilting the head upward. Vasodilator drugs may be used to treat acute elevations in BP. Clonidine is used prophylactically to reduce the hypertension resulting from bladder stimulation. Sudden, dramatic increases in BP can lead to intracranial hemorrhage and death.

Peripheral Nerve and Neuromuscular Junction Disorders Peripheral neuropathies (Chap. 363) are the most common cause of chronic autonomic insufficiency. Neuropathies that affect small myelinated and unmyelinated fibers of the sympathetic and parasympathetic nerves occur in diabetes mellitus, amyloidosis, chronic alcoholism, porphyria, and Guillain-Barré syndrome. Neuromuscular junction disorders include botulism and Lambert-Eaton syndrome.

DIABETES MELLITUS Autonomic neuropathy typically begins ~10 years after the onset of diabetes (Chap. 323) and slowly progresses. The earliest autonomic abnormalities, typically asymptomatic, consist of vagal disturbances, which can be detected as reduced heart rate variation with deep breathing, and loss of distal sudomotor function, detected by QSART. Loss of small myelinated and unmyelinated nerve fibers in the splanchnic distribution, carotid sinus, and vagus nerves is characteristic. In advanced disease, widespread enteric neuropathy can cause profound disturbances in gut motility (*gastroparesis*), nausea and vomiting, malnutrition, achlorhydria, and bowel incontinence. Other symptoms can include impotence, urinary incontinence, pupillary abnormalities, and OH. Typical symptoms and signs of hypoglycemia may fail to appear because damage to the sympathetic innervation of the adrenal gland can result in a lack of epinephrine release. Insulin increases flow through arteriovenous shunts and may also aggravate OH. Autonomic dysfunction may lengthen the QT interval, increasing the risk of sudden death due to cardiac arrhythmia. There is postganglionic cardiac denervation with some proximal segments showing increased uptake of labeled hydroxyephedrine, indicative of hyperadrenergic innervation, on PET scanning. This finding is of interest in that these areas could be potentially arrhythmogenic. Hyperglycemia appears to be a direct risk factor for autonomic involvement in diabetes. Biochemical and pharmacologic studies in diabetic neuropathy are compatible with autonomic failure localized to the PNS. Supine plasma NE levels can be reduced, and a minority of patients experience a phase of hyperadrenegic autonomic function characterized by exaggerated orthostatic pressor responsiveness.

AMYLOIDOSIS   Autonomic neuropathy occurs in both sporadic and familial forms of amyloidosis (Chap. 310). The AL (immunoglobulin light chain) type is associated with primary amyloidosis or amyloidosis secondary to multiple myeloma. The ATTR type, with transthyretin as the primary protein component, is responsible for the most common form of inherited amyloidosis. Although patients usually present with a distal painful neuropathy accompanied by sensory loss, autonomic insufficiency can precede the development of the polyneuropathy or occur in isolation. Death is usually due to cardiac or renal impairment. Postmortem studies reveal amyloid deposition in many organs, including two sites that contribute to autonomic failure: intraneural blood vessels and autonomic ganglia. Pathologic examination reveals a loss of unmyelinated and myelinated nerve fibers.

ALCOHOLIC NEUROPATHY   Abnormalities in parasympathetic vagal and efferent sympathetic function are usually mild in individuals with alcoholic neuropathy. Pathologic changes can be demonstrated in the parasympathetic (vagus) and sympathetic fibers and in ganglia. OH is usually due to brainstem involvement. Impotence is a major problem, but concurrent gonadal hormone abnormalities may obscure the parasympathetic component. Clinical symptoms of autonomic failure generally appear when the polyneuropathy is severe and there is usually coexisting Wernicke's encephalopathy (Chap. 258). Autonomic involvement may contribute to the high mortality rates associated with alcoholism (Chap. 372).

PORPHYRIA   Although each of the porphyrias can cause autonomic dysfunction, the condition is most extensively documented in the acute intermittent type (Chap. 337). Autonomic symptoms include tachycardia, sweating, urinary retention, and hypertension, or, less commonly, hypotension. Other prominent symptoms include anxiety, abdominal pain, nausea, and vomiting. Abnormal autonomic function can occur both during acute attacks and during remissions. Elevated catecholamine levels during acute attacks correlate with the degree of tachycardia and hypertension that are present.

GUILLAIN-BARRÉ SYNDROME   BP fluctuations and arrhythmias can be severe (Chap. 365). It is estimated that 2 to 10% of patients seriously ill with Guillain-Barré syndrome suffer fatal cardiovascular collapse. Gastrointestinal autonomic involvement is common. Abnormal sweating, sphincter disturbance, and pupillary dysfunction also occur. Demyelination has been described in the vagus and glossopharyngeal nerves, the sympathetic chain, and the white rami communicantes. The presence of autonomic involvement is not clearly related to the severity of motor or sensory involvement.

AUTOIMMUNE AUTONOMIC NEUROPATHY   The development of serologic testing for the ganglionic ACh receptor (A_3 AChR) autoantibody, which is a putative effector of autoimmune dysautonomia, now allows definition of the entity of autoimmune autonomic neuropathy (AAN). This disorder presents as the subacute development of autonomic failure with OH, enteric neuropathy (gastroparesis, ileus, constipation/diarrhea), and cholinergic failure; the latter consists of loss of sweating, sicca complex, and a tonic pupil. In general, the antibody titer correlates with the severity of autonomic failure. Symptoms of cholinergic failure

are also predictive of a high antibody titer. Onset of the neuropathy follows a viral infection in approximately half of cases. Some patients appear to respond to immunotherapy. The spectrum of AAN is broader than originally thought, and some antibody-positive cases have an insidious onset and slow progression with a pure autonomic failure (see below) phenotype. An experimental autonomic neuropathy has recently been produced by immunization of rabbits with this receptor.

AAN can have a paraneoplastic basis (Chap. 87). The clinical features of the autonomic neuropathy may be indistinguishable from the nonparaneoplastic form, or a coexisting paraneoplastic syndrome, such as cerebellar involvement or dementia, may be present (Tables 87-2 and 87-3). The neoplasm may be truly occult, possibly suppressed by the autoantibody.

BOTULISM   Botulinum toxin binds presynaptically to cholinergic nerve terminals and, after uptake into the cytosol, blocks ACh release. Manifestations consist of motor paralysis and autonomic disturbances that include blurred vision, dry mouth, nausea, unreactive or sluggishly reactive pupils, constipation, and urinary retention (Chap. 125).

Pure Autonomic Failure (PAF)   This sporadic syndrome consists of postural hypotension, impotence, bladder dysfunction, and defective sweating. The disorder begins in the middle decades and occurs in women more often than men. The symptoms can be disabling, but the disease does not shorten life span. The clinical and pharmacologic characteristics suggest primary involvement of postganglionic sympathetic neurons. There is a severe reduction in the density of neurons within sympathetic ganglia that results in low supine plasma NE levels and noradrenergic supersensitivity. Recent studies have questioned the specificity of PAF as a distinct clinical entity. Some cases are ganglionic antibody–positive and thus represent a type of AAN. Between 10 and 15% of cases evolve into MSA.

Postural Orthostatic Tachycardia Syndrome (POTS)   This syndrome is characterized by symptomatic orthostatic intolerance (not OH) and by either an increase in heart rate to >120 beats/min or an increase of 30 beats/min with standing that subsides on sitting or lying down. Women are affected approximately five times more often than men, and most develop the syndrome between the ages of 15 and 50 years. Approximately half of affected patients report an antecedent viral infection. Syncopal symptoms (lightheadedness, weakness, blurred vision) combined with those of autonomic overactivity (palpitations, tremulousness, nausea) are common. Recurrent unexplained episodes of dysautonomia and fatigue also occur. The pathogenesis is unclear in most cases; hypovolemia, venous pooling, impaired brainstem regulation, or β-receptor supersensitivity may play a role. In one affected individual, a mutation in the NE transporter, which resulted in impaired NE clearance from synapses, was responsible. Some cases are due to an underlying limited autonomic neuropathy. Although ~80% of patients improve, only one-quarter eventually resume their usual daily activities (including exercise and sports). Expansion of fluid volume and postural training (see "Treatment") are initial approaches to treatment. When these approaches are inadequate, midodrine, fludrocortisone, phenobarbital, beta blockers, and clonidine have been used with some success.

Inherited Disorders   There are five known hereditary sensory and autonomic neuropathies (HSAN I–V). The most important ones are HSAN I and HSAN III (Riley-Day syndrome; familial dysautonomia). HSAN I is dominantly inherited and often presents as a distal small-fiber neuropathy (burning feet syndrome). The responsible gene, on chromosome 9q, is designated *SPTLC1*. SPTLC is an important enzyme in the regulation of ceramide. Cells from HSAN I patients affected by mutation of *SPTLC1* produce higher-than-normal levels of glucosyl ceramide, perhaps triggering apoptosis.

HSAN III, an autosomal recessive disorder of infants and children that occurs among Ashkenazi Jews, is much less prevalent than HSAN I. Decreased tearing, hyperhidrosis, reduced sensitivity to pain, areflexia, absent fungiform papillae on the tongue, and labile BP may be present. Episodic abdominal crises and fever are common. Pathologic examination of nerves reveals a loss of small myelinated and unmyelinated nerve fibers. The defective gene, named *IKBKAP*, is also located on the long arm of chromosome 9. Pathogenic mutations may prevent normal transcription of important molecules in neural development.

Primary Hyperhidrosis This syndrome presents with excess sweating of the palms of the hands and soles of the feet. The disorder affects 0.6 to 1.0% of the population; the etiology is unclear but there may be a genetic component. While not dangerous, the condition can be socially embarrassing (e.g., shaking hands) or disabling (e.g., inability to write without soiling the paper). Onset of symptoms is usually in adolescence; the condition tends to improve with age. Topical antiperspirants are occasionally helpful. More useful are potent anticholinergic drugs such as glycopyrrolate, 1 to 2 mg tid. T2 ganglionectomy or sympathectomy is successful in >90% of patients with palmar hyperhidrosis. The advent of endoscopic transaxillary T2 sympathectomy has lowered the complication rate of the procedure. The most common postoperative complication is compensatory hyperhidrosis, which improves spontaneously over months; other potential complications include recurrent hyperhidrosis (16%), Horner's syndrome (<2%), gustatory sweating, wound infection, hemothorax, and intercostal neuralgia. Local injection of botulinum toxin has also been used to block cholinergic, postganglionic sympathetic fibers to sweat glands in patients with palmar hyperhidrosis. This approach is limited by the need for repetitive injections (the effect usually lasts 4 months before waning), pain with injection, the high cost of botulinum toxin, and the possibility of temporary intrinsic hand muscle weakness. Tap water iontophoresis has been successful for some patients.

Miscellaneous Other conditions associated with autonomic failure include infections, poisoning (organophosphates), malignancy, and aging. Disorders of the hypothalamus can affect autonomic function and produce abnormalities in temperature control, satiety, sexual function, and circadian rhythms (Chap. 318).

Reflex Sympathetic Dystrophy and Causalgia The failure to identify a primary role of the ANS in the pathogenesis of these disorders has resulted in a change of nomenclature. Complex regional pain syndrome (CRPS) types I and II are now used in place of reflex sympathetic dystrophy (RSD) and causalgia, respectively.

CRPS type I is a regional pain syndrome that usually develops after tissue trauma. Examples of associated trauma include myocardial infarction, minor shoulder or limb injury, and stroke. *Allodynia* (the perception of a nonpainful stimulus as painful), *hyperpathia* (an exaggerated pain response to a painful stimulus), and spontaneous pain occur. The symptoms are unrelated to the severity of the initial trauma and are not confined to the distribution of a single peripheral nerve. CRPS type II is a regional pain syndrome that develops after injury to a peripheral nerve, usually a major nerve trunk. Spontaneous pain initially develops within the territory of the affected nerve but eventually may spread outside the nerve distribution.

Pain is the primary clinical feature of CRPS. Vasomotor dysfunction, sudomotor abnormalities, or focal edema may occur alone or in combination but must be present for diagnosis. Limb pain syndromes that do not meet these criteria are best classified as "limb pain—not otherwise specified." In CRPS, localized sweating (increased resting sweat output) and changes in blood flow may produce temperature differences between affected and unaffected limbs.

CRPS type I (RSD) has classically been divided into three clinical phases but is now considered to be more variable. Phase I consists of pain and swelling in the distal extremity occurring within weeks to 3 months after the precipitating event. The pain is diffuse, spontaneous, and either burning, throbbing, or aching in quality. The involved extremity is warm and edematous, and the joints are tender. Increased sweating and hair growth develop. In phase II (3 to 6 months after onset), thin, shiny, cool skin appears. After an additional 3 to 6 months (phase III), atrophy of the skin and subcutaneous tissue plus flexion contractures complete the clinical picture.

The natural history of typical CRPS may be more benign than reflected in the literature. A variety of surgical and medical treatments have been developed, with conflicting reports of efficacy. Clinical trials suggest that early mobilization with physical therapy or a brief course of glucocorticoids may be helpful for CRPS type I. Other medical treatments include the use of adrenergic blockers, nonsteroidal anti-inflammatory drugs (NSAIDs), calcium channel blockers, phenytoin, opioids, and calcitonin. Stellate ganglion blockade is a commonly used invasive therapeutic technique that often provides temporary pain relief, but the efficacy of repetitive blocks is uncertain.

Rx TREATMENT

Management of autonomic failure is aimed at specific treatment of the cause and alleviation of symptoms. Of particular importance is the removal of drugs or amelioration of underlying conditions that cause or aggravate the autonomic symptom. For instance, OH can be caused or aggravated by angiotensin-converting enzyme inhibitors, calcium channel blocking agents, tricyclic antidepressants, levodopa, alcohol, or insulin.

Patient Education OH can be asymptomatic or symptomatic. Neurogenic OH requires treatment, but only a minority of patients require pharmacologic treatment. All patients should be taught the mechanisms of postural normotension (volume status, resistance and capacitance bed, autoregulation) and the nature of orthostatic stressors (time of day and the influence of meals, heat, standing, and exercise). Patients should learn to recognize orthostatic symptoms early in their evolution (especially subtle cognitive symptoms, weakness, and fatigue) and to modify activities that provoke episodes. Other helpful measures may include keeping a BP log, dietary education (salt/fluids), monitoring urine volume and sodium excretion, or recognizing medications and situations to avoid. Learning physical countermaneuvers that reduce standing OH, practicing postural and resistance training, and learning to manage worsening OH in specific situations and at specific times are helpful measures.

Symptomatic Treatment Nonpharmacologic approaches are summarized in Table 354-6. Adequate intake of salt and fluids to produce a voiding volume between 1.5 to 2.5 L of urine (containing >170 meq of Na^+) each 24 h is essential. Sleeping with the head of the bed elevated will minimize the effects of supine nocturnal hypertension. Prolonged recumbency should be avoided when possible. Patients are advised to sit with legs dangling over the edge of the bed for several minutes before attempting to stand in the morning; other postural stresses should be similarly approached in a gradual manner. Physical countermaneuvers that can reduce OH include leg-crossing, with maintained contraction of leg muscles for 30 s. Such maneuvers compress leg veins and increase systemic resistance. Compressive garments such as compression stockings and abdominal binders may be helpful; some patients find these uncomfortable. Anemia should be corrected, if necessary, with erythropoietin, administered subcutaneously at doses of 25 to 75 U/kg three times per week. The hematocrit increases after 2 to 6 weeks. A weekly maintenance dose is usually necessary. The increased intravascular volume that accompanies the rise in hematocrit can exacerbate supine hypertension.

If these measures are not sufficient, drug treatment might be nec-

TABLE 354-6   Initial Treatment of Orthostatic Hypotension (OH)

Patient education: mechanisms and stressors of OH
High-salt diet (10–20 g/d)
High-fluid intake (2 L/D)
Elevate head of bed 10 cm (4 in.)
Maintain postural stimuli
Learn physical countermaneuvers
Compression garments
Correct anemia

essary. Midodrine is effective but can aggravate supine hypertension at higher doses. The drug is a directly acting α_1-agonist that does not cross the blood-brain barrier. It has a duration of action of 2 to 4 h. The usual dose is 5 to 10 mg orally tid, but some patients respond best to a decremental dose (e.g., 15 mg on awakening, 10 mg at noon, and 5 mg in the afternoon). Midodrine should not be taken after 6 P.M. Side effects include pruritus, uncomfortable piloerection, and supine hypertension. Pyridostigmine appears to improve OH without aggravating supine hypertension by enhancing ganglionic transmission (maximal when orthostatic, minimal supine). Fludrocortisone will reduce OH, but it aggravates supine hypertension. At doses between 0.1 mg/d and 0.3 mg bid orally, it enhances renal sodium conservation and increases the sensitivity of arterioles to NE. Susceptible patients may develop fluid overload, congestive heart failure, supine hypertension, or hypokalemia. Potassium supplements are often necessary with chronic administration of fludrocortisone. Sustained elevations of supine BP >180/110 mmHg should be avoided.

Postprandial OH may respond to several measures. Frequent, small, low-carbohydrate meals may diminish splanchnic shunting of blood after meals and reduce postprandial OH. Prostaglandin inhibitors (ibuprofen or indomethacin) taken with meals or midodrine (10 mg with the meal) can be helpful. The somatostatin analogue octreotide can be useful in the treatment of postprandial syncope by inhibiting the release of gastrointestinal peptides that have vasodilator and hypotensive

effects. The subcutaneous dose ranges from 25 μg bid to 100 to 200 μg tid.

The patient should be taught to self-treat transient worsening of OH. Drinking two 250-mL (8-oz) glasses of water can raise standing BP 20 to 30 mmHg for about 2 h, beginning ~20 min after the fluid load. The patient can increase intake of salt and fluids (bouillon treatment), increase use of physical countermaneuvers, temporarily resort to a full-body stocking (compression pressure 30 to 40 mmHg), or increase the dose of midodrine. Supine hypertension (>180/110 mmHg) can be self-treated by avoiding the supine position and reducing fludrocortisone. A daily glass of wine, if requested by the patient, can be taken shortly before bedtime. If these simple measures are not adequate, drugs to be considered include oral hydralazine (25 mg qhs), oral procardia (10 mg qhs), or a nitroglycerin patch.

ACKNOWLEDGMENT

In the previous edition, Lewis Landsberg and James B. Young contributed the section on the anatomic organization of the autonomic nervous system.

FURTHER READING

KLEIN CM et al: The spectrum of autoimmune autonomic neuropathies. Ann Neurol 53:752, 2003

LOW PA et al: Prospective evaluation of clinical characteristics of orthostatic hypotension. Mayo Clin Proc 70:617, 1995

SINGER W et al: Acetylcholinesterase inhibition—a novel approach in the treatment of neurogenic orthostatic hypotension. J Neurol Neurosurg Psychiatry 74:1294, 2003

355 | TRIGEMINAL NEURALGIA, BELL'S PALSY, AND OTHER CRANIAL NERVE DISORDERS
M. Flint Beal, Stephen L. Hauser

Symptoms and signs of cranial nerve pathology are common in internal medicine. They often develop in the context of a widespread neurologic disturbance, and in such situations cranial nerve involvement may represent the initial manifestation of the illness. In other disorders, involvement is largely restricted to one or several cranial nerves; these distinctive disorders are reviewed in this chapter. Disorders of ocular movement are discussed in Chap. 25; disorders of smell, taste, and hearing in Chap. 26; and vertigo and disorders of vestibular function in Chap. 20.

FACIAL PAIN OR NUMBNESS

ANATOMIC CONSIDERATIONS The trigeminal (fifth cranial) nerve supplies sensation to the skin of the face and anterior half of the head (Fig.

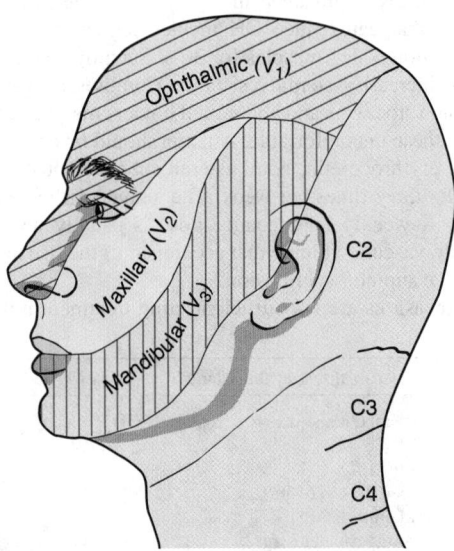

FIGURE 355-1 The three major sensory divisions of the trigeminal nerve consist of the ophthalmic, maxillary, and mandibular nerves.

355-1). Its motor part innervates the masseter and pterygoid masticatory muscles.

TRIGEMINAL NEURALGIA (TIC DOULOUREUX) ■ **Clinical Manifestations** Trigeminal neuralgia is characterized by excruciating paroxysms of pain in the lips, gums, cheek, or chin and, very rarely, in the distribution of the ophthalmic division of the fifth nerve. The pain seldom lasts more than a few seconds or a minute or two but may be so intense that the patient winces, hence the term *tic*. The paroxysms, experienced as single jabs or clusters, tend to recur frequently, both day and night, for several weeks at a time. They may occur spontaneously or with movements of affected areas evoked by speaking, chewing, or smiling. Another characteristic feature is the presence of trigger zones, typically on the face, lips, or tongue, that provoke attacks; patients may report that tactile stimuli—e.g. washing the face, brushing the teeth, or exposure to a draft of air—generate excruciating pain. *An essential feature of trigeminal neuralgia is that objective signs of sensory loss cannot be demonstrated on examination.*

Trigeminal neuralgia is relatively common, with an estimated annual incidence of 4.5 per 100,000 individuals. Middle-aged and elderly persons are affected primarily, and ~60% of cases occur in women. Onset is typically sudden, and bouts tend to persist for weeks or months before remitting spontaneously. Remissions may be longlasting, but in most patients the disorder ultimately recurs.

Pathophysiology Symptoms result from ectopic generation of action potentials in pain-sensitive afferent fibers of the fifth cranial nerve root just before it enters the lateral surface of the pons. Compression or other pathology in the nerve leads to demyelination of large myelinated fibers that do not themselves carry pain sensation but become hyperexcitable and electrically coupled with smaller unmyelinated or poorly myelinated pain fibers in close proximity; this may explain why tactile stimuli, conveyed via the large myelinated fibers, can stimulate paroxysms of pain. Compression of the trigeminal nerve root by a blood vessel, most often the superior cerebellar artery or on occasion a tortuous vein, is the source of trigeminal neuralgia in a substantial proportion of patients. In cases of vascular compression, age-related brain sagging and increased vascular thickness and tortuosity may explain the prevalence of trigeminal neuralgia in later life.

Differential Diagnosis Trigeminal neuralgia must be distinguished from other causes of face and head pain (Chap. 14) and from pain arising from diseases of the jaw, teeth, or sinuses. Pain from migraine or cluster headache tends to be deep seated and steady, unlike the superficial stabbing quality of trigeminal neuralgia; rarely, cluster headache is associated with trigeminal neuralgia, a syndrome known as *cluster-tic*. In temporal arteritis, superficial facial pain is present but is not typically shock-like, the patient frequently complains of myalgias and other systemic symptoms and an elevated erythrocyte sedimentation rate (ESR) is usually present (Chap. 306). When trigeminal neuralgia develops in a young adult or is bilateral, multiple sclerosis is a key consideration, and in such cases the cause is a demyelinating plaque at the root entry zone of the fifth nerve in the pons; often, evidence of facial sensory loss can be found on careful examination. Cases that are secondary to mass lesions—such as aneurysms, neurofibromas, or meningiomas—also usually produce objective signs of sensory loss in the trigeminal nerve distribution (trigeminal neuropathy, see below).

Laboratory Evaluation An ESR is indicated if temporal arteritis is suspected. In typical cases of trigeminal neuralgia, neuroimaging studies are not necessary.

℞ TREATMENT

Drug therapy with carbamazepine is effective in ~50 to 75% of patients. Carbamazepine should be started as a single daily dose of 100 mg taken with food, and increased gradually (by 100 mg daily every 1 to 2 days) until substantial (>50%) pain relief is achieved. Most patients require a maintenance dose of 200 mg qid. Doses >1200 mg daily provide no additional benefit. Dizziness, imbalance, sedation, and rare cases of agranulocytosis are the most important side effects of carbamazepine. If treatment is effective, it is usually continued for approximately 1 month and then tapered as tolerated. If carbamazepine is not well tolerated or is ineffective, phenytoin, 300 to 400 mg daily, can be tried. Baclofen may also be administered, either alone or in combination with carbamazepine or phenytoin. The initial dose is 5 to 10 mg tid, gradually increasing as needed to 20 mg qid.

If drug treatment fails, surgical therapy should be offered. The most widely applied procedure creates a heat lesion of the trigeminal (gasserian) ganglion or nerve, a method termed *radiofrequency thermal rhizotomy*. Injection of glycerol in Meckel's cave is a method preferred by some surgeons. Either procedure produces short-term relief in >95% of patients; however, long-term studies indicate that pain recurs in a substantial percentage of treated patients. Complications are infrequent in experienced hands. These procedures result in partial numbness of the face and carry a risk of corneal denervation with secondary keratitis when used for first-division trigeminal neuralgia.

A third treatment, microvascular decompression, requires a suboccipital craniotomy. This procedure has a >70% efficacy rate and a low rate of pain recurrence in responders; in a small number of cases, there is perioperative damage to the eighth or seventh nerve. High-resolution magnetic resonance angiography may be useful preoperatively to visualize the relationships between the fifth cranial nerve root and nearby blood vessels.

TRIGEMINAL NEUROPATHY A variety of diseases may affect the trigeminal nerve (Table 355-1). Most present with sensory loss on the face or with weakness of the jaw muscles. Deviation of the jaw on opening indicates weakness of the pterygoids on the side to which the jaw deviates. Some cases are due to Sjögren's syndrome or a collagen-vascular disease such as systemic lupus erythematosus, scleroderma, or mixed connective tissue disease. Among infectious causes, herpes zoster and leprosy should be considered. Tumors of the middle cranial fossa (meningiomas), of the trigeminal nerve (schwannomas), or of the base of the skull (metastatic tumors) may cause a combination of motor and sensory signs. Lesions in the cavernous sinus can affect the

TABLE 355-1 *Trigeminal Nerve Disorders*

Nuclear (brainstem) lesions	Peripheral nerve lesions
Multiple sclerosis	Nasopharyngeal carcinoma
Stroke	Trauma
Syringobulbia	Guillain-Barré syndrome
Glioma	Sjögren's syndrome
Lymphoma	Collagen-vascular diseases
Preganglionic lesions	Sarcoidosis
Acoustic neuroma	Leprosy
Meningioma	Drugs (stilbamidine, trichloroethylene)
Metastasis	Idiopathic trigeminal neuropathy
Chronic meningitis	
Cavernous carotid	
aneurysm	
Gasserian ganglion lesions	
Trigeminal neuroma	
Herpes zoster	
Infection (spread from	
otitis media or	
mastoiditis)	

first and second divisions of the trigeminal nerve, and lesions of the superior orbital fissure can affect the first (ophthalmic) division; the accompanying corneal anesthesia increases the risk of ulceration (neurokeratitis).

Loss of sensation over the chin (mental neuropathy) can be the only manifestation of systemic malignancy. Rarely, an idiopathic form of trigeminal neuropathy is observed. It is characterized by numbness and paresthesia, sometimes bilaterally, with loss of sensation in the territory of the trigeminal nerve but without weakness of the jaw. Gradual recovery is the rule. Tonic spasm of the masticatory muscles, known as *trismus*, is symptomatic of tetanus (Chap. 124) or may occur in patients treated with phenothiazine drugs.

FACIAL WEAKNESS

ANATOMIC CONSIDERATIONS (Fig. 355-2) The seventh cranial nerve supplies all the muscles concerned with facial expression. The sensory component is small (the nervus intermedius); it conveys taste sensation from the anterior two-thirds of the tongue and probably cutaneous impulses from the anterior wall of the external auditory canal. The motor nucleus of the seventh nerve lies anterior and lateral to the abducens nucleus. After leaving the pons, the seventh nerve enters the internal auditory meatus with the acoustic nerve. The nerve continues its course in its own bony channel, the facial canal, and exits from the

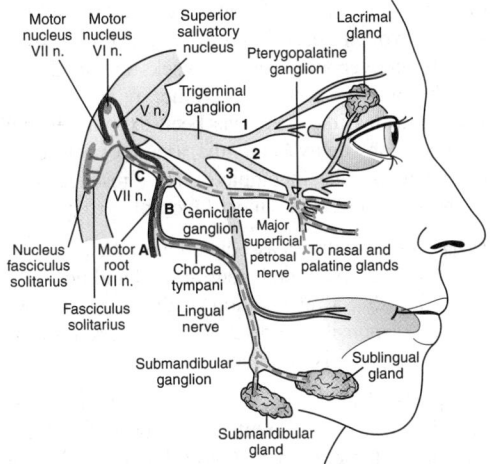

FIGURE 355-2 The facial nerve. A, B, and C denote lesions of the facial nerve at the stylomastoid foramen, distal and proximal to the geniculate ganglion, respectively. Green lines indicate the parasympathetic fibers, red line indicates motor fibers, and purple lines indicate visceral afferent fibers (taste). (*Adapted from Carpenter, 1978.*)

skull via the stylomastoid foramen. It then passes through the parotid gland and subdivides to supply the facial muscles.

A complete interruption of the facial nerve at the stylomastoid foramen paralyzes all muscles of facial expression. The corner of the mouth droops, the creases and skin folds are effaced, the forehead is unfurrowed, and the eyelids will not close. Upon attempted closure of the lids, the eye on the paralyzed side rolls upward (*Bell's phenomenon*). The lower lid sags and falls away from the conjunctiva, permitting tears to spill over the cheek. Food collects between the teeth and lips, and saliva may dribble from the corner of the mouth. The patient complains of a heaviness or numbness in the face, but sensory loss is rarely demonstrable and taste is intact.

If the lesion is in the middle ear portion, taste is lost over the anterior two-thirds of the tongue on the same side. If the nerve to the stapedius is interrupted, there is hyperacusis (sensitivity to loud sounds). Lesions in the internal auditory meatus may affect the adjacent auditory and vestibular nerves, causing deafness, tinnitus, or dizziness. Intrapontine lesions that paralyze the face usually affect the abducens nucleus as well, and often the corticospinal and sensory tracts.

If the peripheral facial paralysis has existed for some time and recovery of motor function is incomplete, a continuous diffuse contraction of facial muscles may appear. The palpebral fissure becomes narrowed, and the nasolabial fold deepens. Attempts to move one group of facial muscles may result in contraction of all (associated movements, or *synkinesis*). Facial spasms, initiated by movements of the face, may develop (*hemifacial spasm*). Anomalous regeneration of seventh nerve fibers may result in other troublesome phenomena. If fibers originally connected with the orbicularis oculi come to innervate the orbicularis oris, closure of the lids may cause a retraction of the mouth, or if fibers originally connected with muscles of the face later innervate the lacrimal gland, anomalous tearing ("crocodile tears") may occur with any activity of the facial muscles, such as eating. Another facial synkinesia is triggered by jaw opening, causing closure of the eyelids on the side of the facial palsy (jaw-winking).

BELL'S PALSY   The most common form of facial paralysis is *Bell's palsy*. The annual incidence of this idiopathic disorder is between 11 and 40 per 100,000 annually, or about 1 in 60 persons in a lifetime.

Clinical Manifestations   The onset of Bell's palsy is fairly abrupt, maximal weakness being attained by 48 h as a general rule. Pain behind the ear may precede the paralysis for a day or two. Taste sensation may be lost unilaterally, and hyperacusis may be present. In some cases there is mild cerebrospinal fluid lymphocytosis. Magnetic resonance imaging (MRI) may reveal swelling and uniform enhancement of the geniculate ganglion and facial nerve, and, in some cases, entrapment of the swollen nerve in the temporal bone. Approximately 80% of patients recover within a few weeks or months. Electromyography may be of some prognostic value; evidence of denervation after 10 days indicates that there has been axonal degeneration and that there will be a long delay (3 months, as a rule) before regeneration occurs and that it may be incomplete. The presence of incomplete paralysis in the first week is the most favorable prognostic sign.

Pathophysiology   Bell's palsy is associated with the presence of herpes simplex virus type 1 DNA in endoneurial fluid and posterior auricular muscle, suggesting that a reactivation of this virus in the geniculate ganglion may be responsible. However, a causal role for herpes simplex virus in Bell's palsy is unproven.

Differential Diagnosis   There are many other causes of facial palsy that must be considered in the differential diagnosis of Bell's palsy. Tumors that invade the temporal bone (carotid body, cholesteatoma, dermoid) may produce a facial palsy, but the onset is insidious and the course progressive. The *Ramsay Hunt syndrome*, presumably due to herpes zoster of the geniculate ganglion, consists of a severe facial palsy associated with a vesicular eruption in the pharynx, external auditory canal, and other parts of the cranial integument; often the eighth cranial nerve is affected as well. *Acoustic neuromas* frequently involve the facial nerve by local compression. Infarcts, demyelinating lesions of multiple sclerosis, and tumors are the common pontine lesions that interrupt the facial nerve fibers; other signs of brainstem involvement are usually present. Bilateral facial paralysis (facial diplegia) occurs in *Guillain-Barré syndrome* (Chap. 365) and also in a form of sarcoidosis known as *uveoparotid fever* (*Heerfordt syndrome*). Lyme disease is a frequent cause of facial palsies in endemic areas. The rare *Melkersson-Rosenthal syndrome* consists of a triad of recurrent facial paralysis, recurrent—and eventually permanent—facial (particularly labial) edema, and less constantly, plication of the tongue; its cause is unknown. Leprosy frequently involves the facial nerve, and facial neuropathy may also occur in diabetes mellitus.

All these forms of nuclear or peripheral facial palsy must be distinguished from the supranuclear type. In the latter, the frontalis and orbicularis oculi muscles are involved less than those of the lower part of the face, since the upper facial muscles are innervated by corticobulbar pathways from both motor cortices, whereas the lower facial muscles are innervated only by the opposite hemisphere. In supranuclear lesions there may be a dissociation of emotional and voluntary facial movements, and often some degree of paralysis of the arm and leg or an aphasia (in dominant hemisphere lesions) is conjoined.

Laboratory Evaluation   The diagnosis of Bell's palsy can usually be made clinically in patients with (1) a typical presentation, (2) no risk factors or preexisting symptoms for other causes of facial paralysis, (3) absence of cutaneous lesions of herpes zoster in the external ear canal, and (4) a normal neurologic examination with the exception of the facial nerve. Particular attention to the eighth cranial nerve, which courses near to the facial nerve in the pontomedullary junction and in the temporal bone, and to other cranial nerves is essential. In atypical or uncertain cases, an ESR, testing for diabetes mellitus, a Lyme titer, angiotensin-converting enzyme and chest x-ray for possible sarcoidosis, or MRI scanning may be indicated.

℞ TREATMENT

Symptomatic measures include (1) the use of paper tape to depress the upper eyelid during sleep and prevent corneal drying, and (2) massage of the weakened muscles. A course of glucocorticoids, given as prednisone 60 to 80 mg daily during the first 5 days and then tapered over the next 5 days, appears to shorten the recovery period and modestly improve the functional outcome. In one double-blind study, patients treated within 3 days of onset with both prednisone and acyclovir (400 mg five times daily for 10 days) had a better outcome than patients treated with prednisone alone.

OTHER MOTOR DISORDERS OF THE FACE   *Hemifacial spasm* consists of painless irregular involuntary contractions on one side of the face. Symptoms may develop as a sequela to Bell's palsy but may also be due to an irritative lesion of the facial nerve (e.g., an acoustic neuroma, an aberrant artery that compresses the nerve, or a basilar artery aneurysm). However, in the most common form of hemifacial spasm, the cause and pathology are unknown. Hemifacial spasm can be treated successfully with carbamazepine or, if this drug fails, with baclofen. Refractory cases due to vascular compression usually respond to surgical decompression of the facial nerve. *Blepharospasm* is an involuntary recurrent spasm of both eyelids that occurs in elderly persons as an isolated phenomenon or with varying degrees of spasm of other facial muscles. Severe, persistent cases of blepharospasm can be treated by local injection of botulinum toxin into the orbicularis oculi; the spasms are relieved for 3 to 4 months, and the injections can be repeated. *Facial myokymia* refers to a fine rippling activity of the facial muscles; it may be caused by multiple sclerosis or follow Guillain-Barré syndrome (Chap. 365).

Facial hemiatrophy occurs mainly in females and is characterized by a disappearance of fat in the dermal and subcutaneous tissues on one side of the face. It usually begins in adolescence or early adult years and is slowly progressive. In its advanced form, the affected side of the face is gaunt, and the skin is thin, wrinkled, and rather brown. The facial hair may turn white and fall out, and the sebaceous glands become atrophic. The muscles and bones are not involved as a rule. Sometimes the atrophy becomes bilateral. The condition is a form of lipodystrophy. Treatment is cosmetic, consisting of transplantation of skin and subcutaneous fat.

OTHER CRANIAL NERVE DISORDERS

GLOSSOPHARYNGEAL NEURALGIA This form of neuralgia involves the ninth (glossopharyngeal) and sometimes portions of the tenth (vagus) cranial nerves. It resembles trigeminal neuralgia in many respects but is much less common. The pain is intense and paroxysmal; it originates on one side of the throat, approximately in the tonsillar fossa. In some cases the pain is localized in the ear or may radiate from the throat to the ear because of involvement of the tympanic branch of the glossopharyngeal nerve. Spasms of pain may be initiated by swallowing or coughing. There is no demonstrable motor or sensory deficit; the glossopharyngeal nerve supplies taste sensation to the posterior third of the tongue and, together with the vagus nerve, sensation to the posterior pharynx. Cardiac symptoms—bradycardia, hypotension, and fainting—have been reported. Medical therapy is similar to that for trigeminal neuralgia, and carbamazepine is generally the first choice. If drug therapy is unsuccessful, surgical procedures, including microvascular decompression if vascular compression is evident, or rhizotomy of glossopharyngeal and vagal fibers in the jugular bulb is frequently successful.

Very rarely, herpes zoster involves the glossopharyngeal nerve. Glossopharyngeal neuropathy in conjunction with vagus and accessory nerve palsies may also occur with a tumor or aneurysm in the posterior fossa or in the jugular foramen. Hoarseness due to vocal cord paralysis, some difficulty in swallowing, deviation of the soft palate to the intact side, anesthesia of the posterior wall of the pharynx, and weakness of the upper part of the trapezius and sternocleidomastoid muscles make up the jugular foramen syndrome (Table 355-2).

DYSPHAGIA AND DYSPHONIA When the intracranial portion of one vagus (tenth cranial) nerve is interrupted, the soft palate droops ipsilaterally and does not rise in phonation. There is loss of the gag reflex on the

affected side, as well as of the "curtain movement" of the lateral wall of the pharynx, whereby the faucial pillars move medially as the palate rises in saying "ah." The voice is hoarse and slightly nasal, and the vocal cord lies immobile midway between abduction and adduction. Loss of sensation at the external auditory meatus and the posterior pinna may also be present.

The pharyngeal branches of both vagal nerves may be affected in diphtheria; the voice has a nasal quality, and regurgitation of liquids through the nose occurs during the act of swallowing.

The vagus nerve may be involved at the meningeal level by neoplastic and infectious processes and within the medulla by tumors, vascular lesions (e.g., the lateral medullary syndrome), and motor neuron disease. This nerve may be involved by infection with herpes zoster virus. Polymyositis and dermatomyositis, which cause hoarseness and dysphagia by direct involvement of laryngeal and pharyngeal muscles, may be confused with diseases of the vagus nerves. Also, dysphagia is a symptom in some patients with myotonic dystrophy. →*See Chap. 33 for discussion of nonneurologic forms of dysphagia.*

The recurrent laryngeal nerves, especially the left, are most often damaged as a result of intrathoracic disease. Aneurysm of the aortic arch, an enlarged left atrium, and tumors of the mediastinum and bronchi are much more frequent causes of an isolated vocal cord palsy than are intracranial disorders. However, a substantial number of cases of recurrent laryngeal palsy remain idiopathic.

When confronted with a case of laryngeal palsy, the physician must attempt to determine the site of the lesion. If it is intramedullary, there are usually other signs, such as ipsilateral cerebellar dysfunction, loss of pain and temperature sensation over the ipsilateral face and contralateral arm and leg, and an ipsilateral Horner syndrome. If the lesion is extramedullary, the glossopharyngeal and spinal accessory nerves are frequently involved (jugular foramen syndrome). If it is extracranial in the posterior laterocondylar or retroparotid space, there may be a combination of ninth, tenth, eleventh, and twelfth cranial nerve palsies and a Horner syndrome (Table 355-2). If there is no sensory loss over the palate and pharynx and no palatal weakness or dysphagia, the lesion is below the origin of the pharyngeal branches, which leave the vagus nerve high in the cervical region; the usual site of disease is then the mediastinum.

NECK WEAKNESS Isolated involvement of the accessory (eleventh cranial) nerve can occur anywhere along its route, resulting in partial or complete paralysis of the sternocleidomastoid and trapezius muscles. More commonly, involvement occurs in combination with deficits of the ninth and tenth cranial nerves in the jugular foramen or after exit from the skull (Table 355-2). An idiopathic form of accessory neuropathy, akin to Bell's palsy, has been described, and it may be recurrent in some cases. Most but not all patients recover.

TONGUE PARALYSIS The hypoglossal (twelfth cranial) nerve supplies the ipsilateral muscles of the tongue. The nucleus of the nerve or its fibers of exit may be involved by intramedullary lesions such as tumor, poliomyelitis, or most often motor neuron disease. Lesions of the basal meninges and the occipital bones (platybasia, invagination of occipital condyles, Paget's disease) may compress the nerve in its extramedullary course or in the hypoglossal canal. Isolated lesions of unknown cause can occur. Atrophy and fasciculation of the tongue develop weeks to months after interruption of the nerve.

MULTIPLE CRANIAL NERVE PALSIES

Several cranial nerves may be affected by the same disease process. In this situation, the main clinical problem is to determine whether the lesion lies within the brainstem or outside it. Lesions that lie on the surface of the brainstem are characterized by involvement of adjacent cranial nerves (often occurring in succession) and late and rather slight involvement of the long sensory and motor pathways and segmental structures lying within the brainstem. The opposite is true of primary lesions within the brainstem. The extramedullary lesion is more likely

TABLE 355-2 *Cranial Nerve Syndromes*

Site	Cranial Nerves	Usual Cause
Sphenoid fissure (superior orbital)	III, IV, first division V, VI	Invasive tumors of sphenoid bone; aneurysms
Lateral wall of cavernous sinus	III, IV, first division V, VI, often with proptosis	Infection, thrombosis, aneurysm, or fistula of cavernous sinus; invasive tumors from sinuses and sella turcica; benign granuloma responsive to glucocorticoids
Retrosphenoid space	II, III, IV, V, VI	Large tumors of middle cranial fossa
Apex of petrous bone	V, VI	Petrositis; tumors of petrous bone
Internal auditory meatus	VII, VIII	Tumors of petrous bone (dermoids, etc.); infectious processes; acoustic neuroma
Pontocerebellar angle	V, VII, VIII, and sometimes IX	Acoustic neuroma; meningioma
Jugular foramen	IX, X, XI	Tumors and aneurysms
Posterior laterocondylar space	IX, X, XI, XII	Tumors of parotid gland and carotid body and metastatic tumors
Posterior retroparotid space	IX, X, XI, XII and Horner syndrome	Tumors of parotid gland, carotid body, lymph nodes; metastatic tumor; tuberculous adenitis

to cause bone erosion or enlargement of the foramens of exit of cranial nerves. The intramedullary lesion involving cranial nerves often produces a crossed sensory or motor paralysis (cranial nerve signs on one side of the body and tract signs on the opposite side).

Involvement of multiple cranial nerves outside the brainstem is frequently the result of diabetes or trauma, localized infections such as herpes zoster, infectious and noninfectious (especially carcinomatous) causes of meningitis (Chap. 361), granulomatous diseases such as Wegener's granulomatosis, Behçet's disease, enlarging saccular aneurysms, or tumors. Among the tumors, nasopharyngeal cancers, lymphomas, neurofibromas, meningiomas, chordomas, cholesteatomas, carcinomas, and sarcomas have all been observed to involve a succession of lower cranial nerves. Owing to their anatomic relationships, the multiple cranial nerve palsies form a number of distinctive syndromes, listed in Table 355-2. Sarcoidosis is the cause of some cases of multiple cranial neuropathy, and chronic glandular tuberculosis the cause of a few others. Platybasia, basilar invagination of the skull, and the adult Chiari malformation are additional causes. A purely motor disorder without atrophy always raises the question of myasthenia gravis (Chap. 366). As noted above, Guillain-Barré syndrome commonly affects the facial nerves bilaterally. In the Fisher variant of the Guillain-Barré syndrome, oculomotor paresis occurs with ataxia and areflexia in the limbs (Chap. 365). Wernicke encephalopathy can cause a severe ophthalmoplegia combined with other brainstem signs.

The *cavernous sinus syndrome* (Fig. 355-3) is a distinctive and frequently life-threatening disorder. It often presents as orbital or facial pain; orbital swelling and chemosis due to occlusion of the ophthalmic veins; fever; oculomotor neuropathy affecting the third, fourth, and sixth cranial nerves; and trigeminal neuropathy affecting the ophthalmic (V_1) and occasionally the maxillary (V_2) divisions of the trigeminal nerve. Cavernous sinus thrombosis, often secondary to infection from orbital cellulitis (frequently *Staphylococcus aureus*), a cutaneous source on the face, or sinusitis (especially with mucormycosis in diabetic patients), is the most frequent cause; other etiologies include aneurysm of the carotid artery, a carotid-cavernous fistula (orbital bruit may be present), meningioma, nasopharyngeal carcinoma, other tumors, or an idiopathic granulomatous disorder (Tolosa-Hunt syndrome). The two cavernous sinuses directly communicate via intercavernous channels, thus involvement on one side may extend to become bilateral. Early diagnosis is essential, especially when due to infection, and treatment depends upon the underlying etiology. In infectious cases, prompt administration of broad-spectrum antibiotics, drainage of any abscess cavities, and identification of the offending organism is essential. Anticoagulant therapy may benefit cases of primary thrombosis. Repair or occlusion of the carotid artery may be

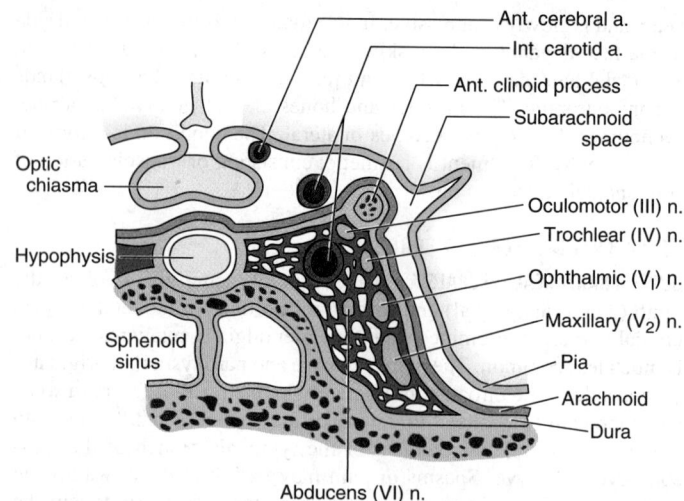

FIGURE 355-3 Anatomy of the cavernous sinus in coronal section, illustrating the location of the cranial nerves in relation to the vascular sinus, internal carotid artery (which loops anteriorly to the section), and surrounding structures.

required for treatment of fistulas or aneurysms. The Tolosa-Hunt syndrome generally responds to glucocorticoids.

An idiopathic form of multiple cranial nerve involvement on one or both sides of the face is occasionally seen. The syndrome consists of a subacute onset of boring facial pain, followed by paralysis of motor cranial nerves. The clinical features overlap those of the Tolosa-Hunt syndrome and appear to be due to idiopathic inflammation of the dura mater, which may be visualized by MRI. The syndrome is frequently responsive to glucocorticoids.

ACKNOWLEDGMENT
The authors acknowledge the contributions of Dr. Joseph B. Martin to this chapter in previous editions.

FURTHER READING

CARPENTER MB. *Core Text of Neuroanatomy*, 2d ed. Baltimore, Williams & Wilkins, 1978

GROGAN PM, GRONSETH GS: Practice parameter: Steroids, acyclovir, and surgery for Bell's palsy (an evidence-based review). Report of the Quality Standards Subcommittee of the American Academy of Neurology. Neurology 56:830, 2001

LOVE S, COAKHAM HB: Trigeminal neuralgia: Pathology and pathogenesis. Brain 124:2347, 2002

PATEL A et al: Microvascular decompression in the management of glossopharyngeal neuralgia: Analysis of 217 cases. Neurosurgery 50:705, 2002

SWEENEY CJ, GILDEN DH: Ramsay Hunt syndrome. J Neurol Neurosurg Psychiatry 71:149, 2001

356 DISEASES OF THE SPINAL CORD
Stephen L. Hauser, Allan H. Ropper

Diseases of the spinal cord are frequently devastating. They can produce quadriplegia, paraplegia, and sensory deficits far beyond the damage they would inflict elsewhere in the nervous system because the spinal cord contains, in a small cross-sectional area, almost the entire motor output and sensory input of the trunk and limbs. Many spinal cord diseases are reversible if recognized and treated at an early stage (Table 356-1); thus, they are among the most critical of neurologic emergencies. The efficient use of diagnostic procedures, guided by a knowledge of the anatomy and the clinical features of common spinal cord diseases, is required for a successful outcome.

APPROACH TO THE PATIENT

SPINAL CORD ANATOMY RELEVANT TO CLINICAL SIGNS The spinal cord is a thin, tubular extension of the central nervous system contained within the bony spinal canal. It originates at the medulla and continues caudally to the conus medullaris at the lumbar level; its fibrous extension, the filum terminale, terminates at the coccyx. The adult spinal cord is ~46 cm (18 in.) long, oval or round in shape, and enlarged in the cervical and lumbar regions, where neurons that innervate the upper and lower extremities, respectively, are located. The white matter tracts containing ascending sensory and descending motor pathways are located peripherally, whereas nerve cell bodies are clustered in an inner region shaped like a four-leaf clover that surrounds the central canal (anatomically an extension

TABLE 356-1 *Some Treatable Spinal Cord Disorders*

Compressive
    Epidural, intradural, or intramedullary neoplasm
    Epidural abscess
    Epidural hemorrhage
    Cervical spondylosis
    Herniated disc
    Posttraumatic compression by fractured or displaced vertebra or
        hemorrhage
Vascular
    Arteriovenous malformation
    Antiphospholipid syndrome and other hypercoagulable states
Inflammatory
    Multiple sclerosis including neuromyelitis optica
    Transverse myelitis
    Sarcoidosis
    Vasculitis
Infectious
    Viral: VZV, HSV-1 and -2, CMV, HIV, HTLV-I, others
    Bacterial and mycobacterial: *Borrelia*, *Listeria*, syphilis, others
    Mycoplasma pneumoniae
    Parasitic: schistosomiasis, toxoplasmosis
Developmental
    Syringomyelia
    Meningomyelocoele
    Tethered cord syndrome
Metabolic
    Vitamin B_{12} deficiency (subacute combined degeneration)
    Adrenomyeloneuropathy

Note: VZV, varicella-zoster virus; HSV, herpes simplex virus; CMV, cytomegalovirus; HTLV, human T cell lymphotropic virus.

of the fourth ventricle). The membranes that cover the spinal cord—the pia, arachnoid, and dura—are continuous with those of the brainstem and cerebral hemispheres.

The spinal cord has 31 segments, each defined by an exiting ventral motor root and entering dorsal sensory root. During embryologic development, growth of the cord lags behind that of the vertebral column, and in the adult the spinal cord (conus segments) ends at approximately the first lumbar vertebral body. The lower spinal nerves take an increasingly downward course to exit via intervertebral foramina. The first seven pairs of cervical spinal nerves exit above the same-numbered vertebral bodies, whereas all the subsequent nerves exit below the same-numbered vertebral bodies; this situation is due to the presence of eight cervical spinal cord segments but only seven cervical vertebrae. The relationship between spinal cord segments and the corresponding vertebral bodies is shown in Table 356-2. These relationships assume particular importance for localization of lesions that cause spinal cord compression; a T10 spinal cord level, for example, indicates involvement of the cord adjacent to the seventh or eighth thoracic vertebral body. In addition, at every level the main ascending and descending tracts are somatotopically organized with a laminated distribution that reflects the origin or destination of nerve fibers.

Level of the Lesion (Fig. 356-1)   The presence of a horizontally defined level below which sensory, motor, and/or autonomic function is impaired is a hallmark of spinal cord disease. A sensory level is sought by asking the patient to identify a pinprick or cold stimulus

TABLE 356-2 *Spinal Cord Levels Relative to the Vertebral Bodies*

Spinal Cord Level	Corresponding Vertebral Body
Upper cervical	Same as cord level
Lower cervical	1 level higher
Upper thoracic	2 levels higher
Lower thoracic	2 to 3 levels higher
Lumbar	T10-T12
Sacral	T12-L1
Coccygeal	L1

(i.e., a dry tuning fork after immersion in cold water) applied to the low back and sequentially moved up toward the neck on each side. The presence of a sensory level indicates damage to the spinothalamic tract, but the lesion is located one to two segments above the perceived level of a unilateral spinal cord lesion and at the level of the lesion when bilateral. That is the result of the ascent of second-order sensory fibers, which originate in the dorsal horn, proceed to cross anterior to the central canal, and join the opposite spinothalamic tract. Lesions that transect the descending corticospinal and other motor tracts cause paraplegia or quadriplegia, with increased muscle tone, exaggerated deep tendon reflexes, and extensor plantar signs (the upper motor neuron syndrome). Such lesions also typically produce autonomic disturbances consisting of disturbed sweating and bladder, bowel, and sexual dysfunction.

The uppermost level of a spinal cord lesion can also be localized by attention to the *segmental signs* corresponding to disturbed motor or sensory innervation by an individual cord segment. A band of altered sensation (hyperalgesia or hyperpathia) at the upper end of the sensory disturbance, fasciculations or atrophy in muscles innervated by one or several segments, or a diminished or absent deep tendon reflex may be noted. These signs also occur with focal root or peripheral nerve disorders; thus, segmental signs are most useful when they occur with signs of long tract damage. With severe and acute transverse lesions, the limbs initially may be flaccid rather than spastic. This state of "spinal shock" lasts for several days, rarely for weeks, and should not be mistaken for extensive damage to many segments of the cord or for a polyneuropathy.

The main features of transverse damage at each level of the spinal cord are summarized below.

CERVICAL CORD   Extensive lesions near the junction of the cervical cord and medulla are usually fatal owing to involvement of adjacent medullary vasomotor and respiratory centers. Upper cervical cord lesions produce quadriplegia and weakness of the diaphragm. Breathing is possible only by use of accessory muscles of respiration. Lesions at C4-C5 produce quadriplegia; at C5-C6, there is loss of power and reflexes in the biceps; at C7 weakness is found in finger and wrist extensors and triceps; and at C8, finger and wrist flexion are impaired. A Horner's syndrome (miosis, ptosis, and facial hypohidrosis) may accompany a cervical cord lesion at any level.

THORACIC CORD   Lesions here are localized by the sensory level on the trunk and midline back pain if it accompanies the syndrome. The sensory dermatomes of the body are shown in Fig. 22-2; useful markers are the nipples (T4) and umbilicus (T10). Leg weakness and disturbances of bladder and bowel function accompany the paralysis. Lesions at T9-T10 paralyze the lower, but not the upper, abdominal muscles, resulting in upward movement of the umbilicus when the abdominal wall contracts (Beevor's sign).

LUMBAR CORD   The lumbar and sacral cord segments are small and are situated behind the T12 to L1 vertebrae. Lesions at L2-L4 paralyze flexion and adduction of the thigh, weaken leg extension at the knee, and abolish the patellar reflex. Lesions at L5-S1 paralyze movements of the foot and ankle, flexion at the knee, and extension of the thigh, and abolish the ankle jerk (S1).

SACRAL CORD/CONUS MEDULLARIS   The conus medullaris is the tapered caudal termination of the spinal cord, comprising the lower sacral and single coccygeal segments. The conus syndrome is distinctive, consisting of bilateral saddle anesthesia (S3-S5), prominent bladder and bowel dysfunction (urinary retention and incontinence with lax anal tone), and impotence. The bulbocavernosus (S2-S4) and anal (S4-S5) reflexes are absent (Chap. 346). Muscle strength is largely preserved. Lesions of the conus must be distinguished from those

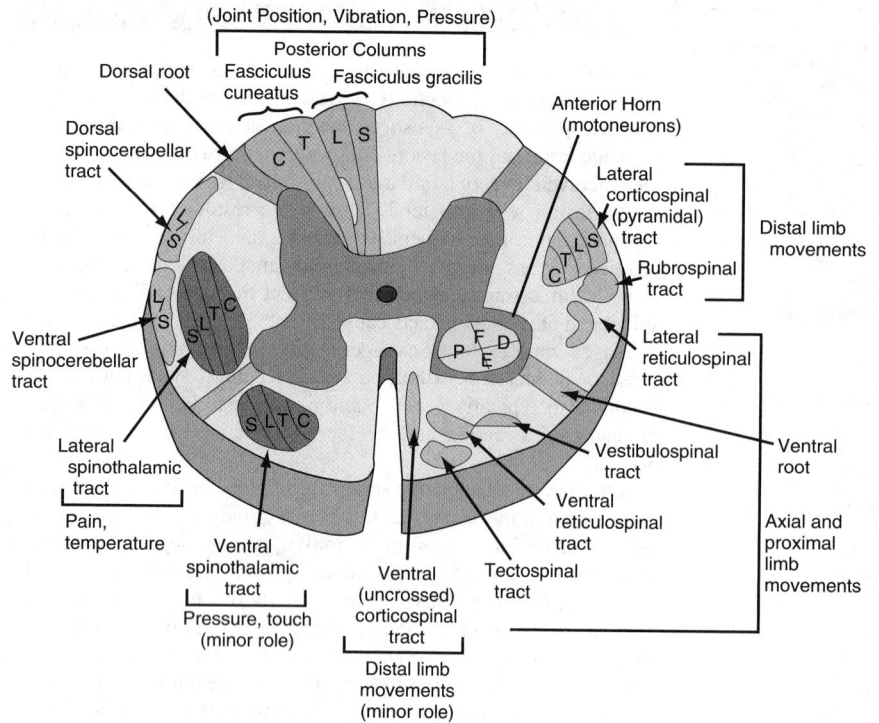

FIGURE 356-1 Transverse section through the spinal cord, composite representation, illustrating the principal ascending (*left*) and descending (*right*) pathways. The lateral and ventral spinothalamic tracts (*dark-brown*) ascend contralateral to the side of the body that is innervated. C, cervical; T, thoracic; L, lumbar; S, sacral; P, proximal; D, distal; F, flexors; E, extensors.

ANTERIOR SPINAL ARTERY SYNDROME Infarction of the cord is generally the result of occlusion or diminished flow in this artery. The result is extensive bilateral tissue destruction that spares the posterior columns. All spinal cord functions—motor, sensory, and autonomic—are lost below the level of the lesion, with the striking exception of retained vibration and position sensation.

LESIONS OF THE FORAMEN MAGNUM Partial lesions in this area interrupt decussating pyramidal tract fibers destined for the legs, which cross below those of the arms, resulting in a "crural paresis" of the lower limbs. Compressive lesions near the foramen magnum may produce weakness of the ipsilateral shoulder and arm followed by weakness of the ipsilateral leg, then the contralateral leg, and finally the contralateral arm (an "around the clock" pattern that may begin in any of the four limbs). There is typically suboccipital pain spreading to the neck and shoulders.

INTRAMEDULLARY AND EXTRAMEDULLARY SYNDROMES It is useful to differentiate intramedullary processes, arising within the substance of the cord, from extramedullary ones that compress the spinal cord or its vascular supply. The differentiating features are only relative and serve as rough guides to clinical decision making. With extramedullary lesions, radicular pain is often prominent, and there are early sacral sensory loss (lateral spinothalamic tract) and spastic weakness in the legs (corticospinal tract); this is due to the superficial location of the leg fibers in the corticospinal tract. Intramedullary lesions tend to produce poorly localized burning pain rather than radicular pain and spare sensation in the perineal and sacral areas ("sacral sparing") reflecting the laminated configuration of the spinothalamic tract with these fibers outermost; corticospinal tract signs appear later. Regarding extramedullary lesions, a further distinction is made between extradural and intradural masses, as the former are generally malignant and the latter benign (neurofibroma being the common cause); for this reason, a long duration of symptoms favors an intradural origin.

ACUTE AND SUBACUTE SPINAL CORD DISEASES

The initial symptom is often focal neck or back pain, followed by various combinations of paresthesias, sensory loss, motor weakness, and sphincter disturbance evolving over hours to several days. There may be mild sensory symptoms only or a devastating functional transection of the cord. Partial forms may selectively involve the posterior columns, anterior spinothalamic tracts, or one hemicord. Paresthesias or numbness may begin in the feet and ascend either symmetrically or asymmetrically, earlier in one leg than in the other; these symptoms may initially raise a question of Guillain-Barré syndrome, but involvement of the trunk with a sharply demarcated spinal cord level indicates the myelopathic nature of the process. In severe cases, areflexia indicating spinal shock may be present, but hyperreflexia soon supervenes; persistent areflexic paralysis indicates necrosis over multiple segments of the spinal cord.

APPROACH TO THE PATIENT

Distinguishing Compressive from Noncompressive Myelopathy The first priority is to identify a treatable mass lesion. The common causes in this category are tumor, epidural abscess or hematoma, herniated disc, or other vertebral pathology. Epidural compression due to malignancy or abscess often causes warning signs of neck or back pain, bladder disturbances, and sensory symptoms that precede the development of paralysis. Spinal subluxation, hemorrhage, and noncompressive etiologies such as infarction are more likely to produce myelopathy without antecedent symptoms. Magnetic res-

of the cauda equina, the cluster of nerve roots derived from the lower cord. Cauda equina lesions are characterized by low back or radicular pain, asymmetric leg weakness and sensory loss, variable areflexia in the lower extremities, and relative sparing of bowel and bladder function. Mass lesions in the lower spinal canal often produce a mixed clinical picture in which elements of both cauda equina and conus medullaris syndromes coexist; the typical cause is an ependymoma in that region. →*Cauda equina syndromes are discussed in Chap. 15.*

Special Patterns of Spinal Cord Disease The location of the major ascending and descending pathways of the spinal cord are shown in Fig. 356-1. Most fiber tracts—including the posterior columns and the spinocerebellar and pyramidal tracts—are situated on the side of the body they innervate. Afferent fibers mediating pain and temperature sensation ascend the spinothalamic tract contralateral to the side they supply. The anatomic relationships of these various fiber tracts produce characteristic clinical syndromes that provide clues to the underlying disease process.

BROWN-SEQUARD HEMICORD SYNDROME This consists of ipsilateral weakness (corticospinal tract) and loss of joint position and vibratory sense (posterior column), with contralateral loss of pain and temperature sense (spinothalamic tract) one or two levels below the lesion. Segmental signs, such as radicular pain, muscle atrophy, or loss of a deep tendon reflex, are unilateral. This classical syndrome is rare, and partial forms are more commonly encountered.

CENTRAL CORD SYNDROME The central cord syndrome results from damage to the gray matter nerve cells and crossing spinothalamic tracts near the central canal. In the cervical cord, the central cord syndrome produces arm weakness out of proportion to leg weakness and a "dissociated" sensory loss signifying a loss of pain and temperature sense in a cape distribution over the shoulders, lower neck, and upper trunk in contrast to intact light touch, joint position, and vibration sense in these regions. Trauma, syringomyelia, tumors, and anterior spinal artery ischemia are main causes.

onance imaging (MRI) with contrast of the clinically suspected level of pathology is the initial diagnostic procedure; in some cases it is appropriate to image the entire spine (cervical through sacral regions) to search for additional, clinically silent, lesions. Once compressive lesions have been excluded, noncompressive causes of acute myelopathy that are intrinsic to the cord are considered: primarily vascular, inflammatory, and infectious etiologies.

COMPRESSIVE MYELOPATHIES ■ Neoplastic Spinal Cord Compression In adults, most neoplasms are epidural in origin, resulting from metastases to the adjacent spinal bones. The propensity of solid tumors to metastasize to the vertebral column probably reflects the high percentage of bone marrow located in the axial skeleton. Almost any malignant tumor can metastasize to the spinal column, with breast, lung, prostate, kidney, lymphoma, and plasma cell dyscrasia being particularly frequent. The thoracic cord is most commonly involved; exceptions are metastases from prostate and ovarian cancer, which occur disproportionately in the sacral and lumbar vertebrae, perhaps resulting from spread through Batson's plexus, a network of veins along the anterior epidural space. Retroperitoneal neoplasms (especially lymphomas or sarcomas) enter the spinal canal through the intervertebral foramina; they produce radicular pain and other signs of root involvement prior to cord compression.

Pain is the initial symptom; it may be either aching and localized or sharp and radiating in quality. The pain typically worsens with movement, coughing, or sneezing and characteristically awakens patients at night. A recent onset of persistent back pain, particularly if in the thoracic spine (which is uncommonly involved by spondylosis), should prompt consideration of vertebral metastasis. Rarely, pain is mild or absent. Pain typically precedes signs of cord compression by weeks or even months. However, once cord compression occurs, it usually advances rapidly. Plain radiographs of the spine and radionuclide bone scans have only a limited role in diagnosis because they do not identify 15 to 20% of metastatic vertebral lesions and fail to detect paravertebral masses that reach the epidural space through the intervertebral foramina. MRI provides excellent anatomic resolution of the site and extent of spinal tumors (Fig. 356-2); MRI has largely replaced computed tomography (CT) and myelography in the diagnosis of epidural masses. MRI can often distinguish between malignant lesions and other masses—epidural abscess, tuberculoma, or epidural hemorrhage, among others—that present in a similar fashion. Vertebral metastases are usually hypointense relative to a normal bone marrow signal on T1-weighted MRI scans; after the administration of gadolinium, contrast enhancement may "normalize" the appearance of the tumor by increasing its intensity to that of normal bone marrow. Infections of the spinal column (osteomyelitis and related disorders) are distinctive in that, unlike tumor, they may cross the disk space.

It is important to convey to the radiologist an estimate of the urgency of the imaging procedure requested. If signs of spinal cord involvement are present, imaging should be obtained promptly. If there are radicular symptoms but no evidence of myelopathy, it is usually safe, if necessary, to defer imaging for 24 to 48 h. With back or neck pain only, imaging studies may be obtained within a few days. Up to 40% of patients who present with symptomatic disease at one level are found to have asymptomatic epidural disease elsewhere; thus, the length of the spine should be imaged when epidural malignancy is in question.

℞ TREATMENT

Management includes glucocorticoids to reduce cord edema, local radiotherapy (initiated as early as possible) to the symptomatic lesion, and specific therapy for the underlying tumor type. Glucocorticoids (dexamethasone, 40 mg daily) can be administered before the imaging study if the clinical suspicion is strong and continued at a lower dose (20 mg daily in divided doses) until radiotherapy (a total of 3000 cGy administered in 15 daily fractions) is completed. Radiotherapy appears to be as effective as surgery, even for classically radioresistant metastases. Biopsy of the epidural mass is unnecessary in patients with known preexisting cancer, but the procedure may be indicated if a history of underlying cancer is lacking. Surgery, either decompression or vertebral body resection, should be considered when signs of cord compression worsen despite radiotherapy, when the maximum tolerated dose of radiotherapy has been delivered previously to the site, or when a vertebral compression fracture contributes to cord compression. A good response to radiotherapy can be expected in individuals who are ambulatory at presentation; new weakness is prevented, and some recovery of motor function occurs in approximately half of treated patients. Fixed motor deficits—paraplegia or quadriplegia—once established for >12 h, do not usually improve, and beyond 48 h the prognosis for substantial motor recovery is poor.

In contrast to tumors of the epidural space, most intradural mass lesions are slow-growing and benign. Meningiomas and neurofibromas account for most of these lesions, with occasional cases representing chordoma, lipoma, dermoid, or sarcoma (Chap. 358). Meningiomas (Fig. 356-3) are often located posterior to the thoracic cord or near the foramen magnum, although they can arise from the meninges anywhere along the spinal canal. Neurofibromas are benign tumors of the nerve sheath that typically arise near the posterior root; when multiple, neurofibromatosis is the likely etiology. Symptoms usually begin with radicular sensory symptoms followed by an asymmetric, progressive spinal cord syndrome. Therapy is by surgical resection.

Primary intramedullary tumors of the spinal cord are uncommon. They typically present as central cord or hemicord syndromes, often in the cervical region; there may be poorly localized burning pain in the extremities and sparing of sacral sensation. In adults, most of these lesions are ependymomas, hemangioblastomas, or low-grade astrocytomas (Fig. 356-4). Complete resection of an intramedullary ependymoma is often possible with microsurgical techniques. Debulking of an intramedullary astrocytoma can also be helpful, as these are often slowly growing lesions; the value of adjunctive radiotherapy is uncertain. Secondary (metastatic) intramedullary tumors are seen on most oncology services (Chap. 358).

Spinal Epidural Abscess Spinal epidural abscess presents as a clinical triad of pain, fever, and rapidly progressive weakness. Prompt recognition of this distinctive and treatable process will in most cases prevent permanent sequelae. Aching pain is almost always present, either over the spine or in a radicular pattern. The duration of pain prior to presentation is generally ≤2 weeks but may on occasion be several

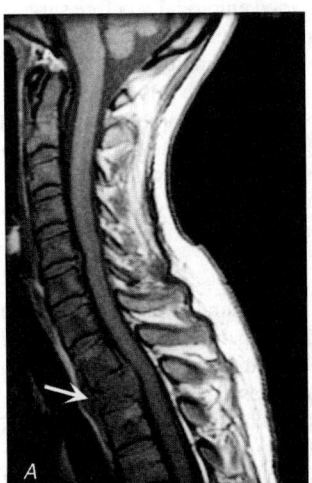
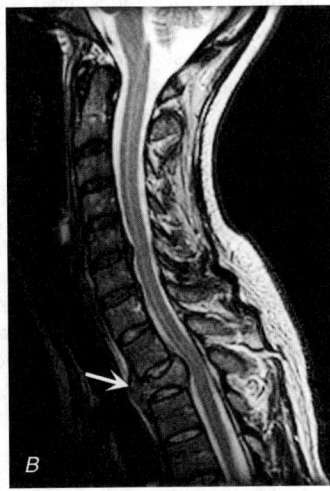

FIGURE 356-2 Epidural spinal cord compression due to breast carcinoma. Sagittal T1-weighted (*A*) and T2-weighted (*B*) MRI scans through the cervicothoracic junction reveal a compression fracture of the second thoracic vertebral body with posterior displacement and compression of the upper thoracic spinal cord. The low-intensity bone marrow signal in *A* signifies replacement by tumor.

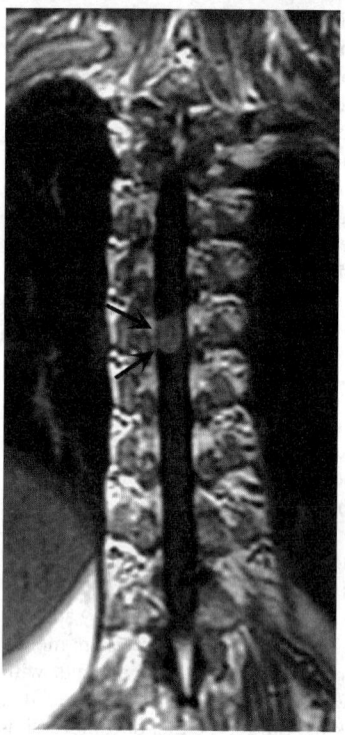

FIGURE 356-3   MRI of a thoracic meningioma. Coronal T1-weighted post-contrast image through the thoracic spinal cord demonstrates intense enhancement of a well-circumscribed extramedullary mass (*arrows*) which displaces the spinal cord to the left, widening the cistern adjacent to the mass.

months or longer. Fever is usual, accompanied by an elevated white blood cell count and sedimentation rate. As the abscess expands, further spinal cord damage results from venous congestion and thrombosis in the epidural space. Once weakness and other signs of myelopathy appear, progression may be rapid. A more chronic granulomatous form of abscess is also known.

Risk factors include an impaired immune status (diabetes mellitus, renal failure, alcoholism, malignancy), intravenous drug abuse, and infections of the skin or other tissues. Two-thirds of epidural infections result from hematogenous spread from the skin (furunculosis), soft tissue (pharyngeal or dental abscesses), or deep viscera (bacterial endocarditis). One-third result from direct extension of a local infection to the subdural space; examples of local predisposing conditions are vertebral osteomyelitis; decubitus ulcers; or iatrogenic complications of lumbar puncture, epidural anesthesia, or spinal surgery. Most cases are due to *Staphylococcus aureus*; gram-negative bacilli, *Streptococcus*, anaerobes, and fungi can also cause epidural abscesses. Tuber-

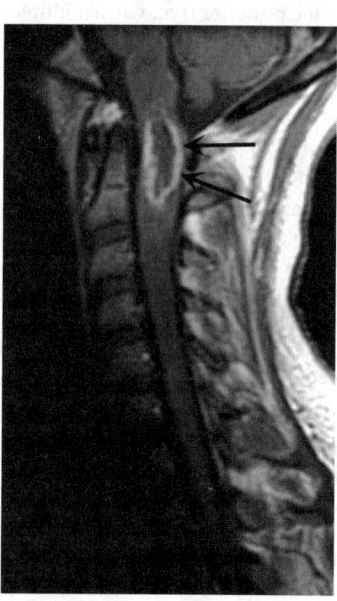

FIGURE 356-4   MRI of an intramedullary astrocytoma. Sagittal T1-weighted postcontrast image through the cervical spine demonstrates expansion of the upper cervical spine by a mass lesion emanating from within the spinal cord at the cervicomedullary junction. Irregular peripheral enhancement occurs within the mass (*arrows*).

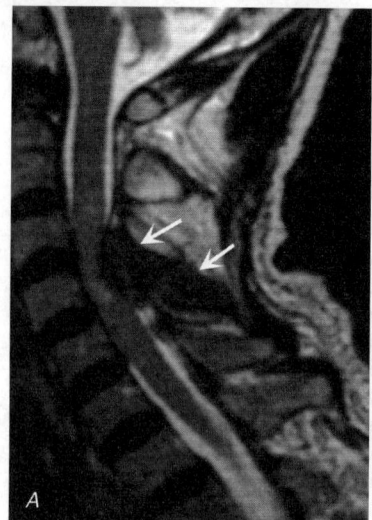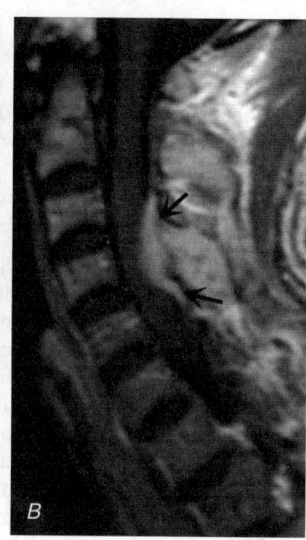

FIGURE 356-5   MRI of a spinal epidural abscess due to tuberculosis. *A.* Sagittal T2-weighted free spin-echo MR sequence. A hypointense mass replaces the posterior elements of C3 and extends epidurally to compress the spinal cord (*arrows*). *B.* Sagittal T1-weighted image after contrast administration reveals a diffuse enhancement of the epidural process (*arrows*) with extension into the epidural space.

culosis from an adjacent vertebral source remains an important cause in the underdeveloped world. MRI scans (Fig. 356-5) localize the abscess and exclude other causes of myelopathy. Lumbar puncture is not required but may be indicated if encephalopathy or other clinical signs raise the question of associated meningitis, a feature that is found in <25% of cases. In such situations, the level of the puncture should be planned to minimize the risk of inducing meningitis by passage of the needle through infected tissue, or herniation from decompression below an area of obstruction to the flow of cerebrospinal fluid (CSF). A high cervical tap is often the safest approach. CSF abnormalities in subdural abscess consist of pleocytosis with a preponderance of polymorphonuclear cells, an elevated protein level, and a reduced glucose level, but the responsible organism is not cultured unless there is an associated meningitis. Blood cultures are positive in <25% of cases.

℞ TREATMENT

Treatment is by decompressive laminectomy with debridement combined with long-term antibiotic treatment. Surgical evacuation prevents development of paralysis and may improve or reverse paralysis in evolution, but it is unlikely to improve deficits of more than several days duration. Antibiotics should be started empirically before surgery and then modified on the basis of culture results; medication is continued for at least 4 weeks. If surgery is contraindicated or if there is a fixed paraplegia or quadriplegia that is unlikely to improve following surgery, long-term administration of systemic and oral antibiotics can be used; in such cases, the choice of antibiotics may be guided by results of blood cultures. However, paralysis may develop or progress during antibiotic therapy; thus, initial surgical management remains the treatment of choice unless the abscess is very limited in size and causes no neurologic signs.

Epidural Hematoma   Hemorrhage into the epidural (or subdural) space causes an acute onset of focal or radicular pain followed by variable signs of a spinal cord or conus medullaris disorder. Therapeutic anticoagulation, trauma, tumor, or blood dyscrasias are predisposing conditions. Rare cases complicate lumbar puncture or epidural anesthesia, sometimes in association with use of low-molecular-weight heparin. MRI and CT confirm the clinical suspicion and can delineate the extent of the bleeding. Extrinsic spinal cord compression from any cause is an urgent condition, and appropriate treatment consists of prompt reversal of any underlying clotting disorder and surgical decompression. Surgery may be followed by substantial recovery, especially in patients with some preservation of motor function preoperatively. Because of the risk of hemorrhage, lumbar puncture should be avoided whenever possible in patients with thrombocytopenia or other coagulopathies.

Hematomyelia   Hemorrhage into the substance of the spinal cord is a rare result of trauma, intraparenchymal vascular malformation (see below), vasculitis due to polyarteritis nodosa or systemic lupus erythematosus (SLE), bleeding disorders, or a spinal cord neoplasm. Hematomyelia presents as an acute painful transverse myelopathy. With large lesions, extension into the subarachnoid space may occur, resulting in subarachnoid hemorrhage (Chap. 349). Diagnosis is made by MRI. Therapy is supportive, and surgical intervention is generally not useful. An exception is hematomyelia due to an underlying vascular malformation, in which selective spinal angiography may be indicated, followed by surgery to evacuate the clot and remove the underlying vascular lesion.

NONCOMPRESSIVE MYELOPATHIES   Acute transverse myelopathies (ATM) are rapidly progressive spinal cord syndromes with limb weakness, incontinence, and bilateral sensory loss accompanied by a sensory level and not due to cord compression. The time from onset to maximum symptoms is often hours or a few days, but some cases progress more slowly, over several weeks. Five general causes of ATM need to be considered: spinal cord infarction; systemic disorders including SLE and sarcoidosis; infectious (especially viral) causes; demyelinating diseases such as multiple sclerosis or neuromyelitis optica; and idiopathic transverse myelitis. The evaluation begins with a lumbar puncture and a search for systemic disease that may underlie the myelopathy (Table 356-3).

Spinal Cord Infarction   The cord is supplied by three arteries that course vertically over its surface: a single anterior spinal artery and paired posterior spinal arteries. At each segment, paired penetrating vessels branch from the anterior spinal artery to supply the anterior two-thirds of the spinal cord; the posterior spinal arteries, which often become less distinct below the midthoracic level, supply the posterior columns. Rostrally, the spinal arteries arise from the vertebral arteries. During embryogenesis, arterial feeders arise at each segmental level, but most involute before birth; generally, between three and eight major feeders remain, arising from the vertebral, subclavian, intercostal (from the aorta), iliac, and sacral arteries. In addition to the vertebral arteries, anterior spinal artery feeders arise at C6, at an upper thoracic level, and, most consistently, at T11-L2 (artery of Adamkiewicz).

Spinal cord ischemia can occur at any level; however, the presence of the artery of Adamkiewicz creates a watershed of marginal blood flow in the upper-thoracic segments. With systemic hypotension, cord infarction occurs at the level of greatest ischemic risk, often T3-T4, and also at boundary zones between the anterior and posterior spinal artery territories. The latter may result in an acute—or more commonly progressive—syndrome of weakness and spasticity with little sensory change, superficially resembling amyotrophic lateral sclerosis (ALS).

Acute infarction in the territory of the anterior spinal artery produces paraplegia or quadriplegia, dissociated sensory loss affecting pain and temperature sense but sparing vibration and position sense, and loss of sphincter control. Onset may be sudden and dramatic but more typically is progressive over minutes or a few hours, quite unlike stroke in the cerebral hemispheres. Sharp midline or radiating back pain localized to the area of ischemia is frequent. Partial infarction of one anterior hemicord (hemiplegia or monoplegia and crossed pain and temperature loss) may also occur. Areflexia due to spinal shock is often present initially; with time, hyperreflexia and spasticity appear. Infarction in the territory of the posterior spinal arteries, resulting in loss of posterior column function, also occurs and may be underrecognized as a cause of obscure loss of position and vibration sense.

Spinal cord infarction is associated with aortic atherosclerosis, dissecting aortic aneurysm (chest or back pain with diminished pulses in legs), or hypotension from any cause. Cardiogenic emboli; vasculitis related to collagen vascular disease, particularly SLE and the antiphospholipid antibody syndrome (see below); and surgical interruption of aortic aneurysms are other causative conditions. Occasional cases develop by an unknown mechanism that leads to embolism of nucleus pulposus material into spinal vessels. In a substantial number of cases, no cause can be found, and thromboembolism in arterial feeders is suspected. The MRI may not demonstrate limited infarctions of the cord but is more often abnormal at the affected level.

Therapy is directed at treatment of any predisposing condition. In cord infarction due to presumed thromboembolism, acute anticoagulation is probably not indicated, with the exception of the unusual transient ischemic attack or incomplete infarction with a stuttering or progressive course. The antiphospholipid antibody syndrome is treated with anticoagulation, as described in Chap. 300.

Immune-Mediated Diseases   ATM occurs in ~1% of patients with SLE (Chap. 300) and may appear as the presenting manifestation of SLE. In some patients the ATM may be preceded or followed by optic neuritis (neuromyelitis optica; Chap. 359). Antiphospholipid antibodies are present in nearly two-thirds of patients with SLE-associated ATM. CSF is usually normal or shows a lymphocytic pleocytosis; oligoclonal bands are generally negative. Possible responses to glucocorticoids and/or cyclophosphamide have been reported. Other immune-mediated disorders associated with ATM include Sjögren's syndrome (Chap. 304), mixed connective tissue disease (Chap. 303), Behçet's syndrome (Chap. 307), and vasculitis with perinuclear antineutrophilic cytoplasmic (p-ANCA) antibodies (Chap. 306).

Another important consideration is sarcoid myelopathy (Chap. 309), in which a large edematous swelling of the spinal cord may mimic tumor; there is almost always enhancement of the lesion and the adjacent surface of the cord. The CSF profile consists of variable lymphocytic pleocytosis, and oligoclonal bands are present in one-third of cases. The diagnosis of sarcoid affecting the spinal cord is particularly difficult when systemic manifestations of sarcoid are meager or absent (50% of cases) or when other neurologic manifestations of the disease—such as cranial neuropathy, hypothalamic involvement, or meningeal enhancement visualized by MRI—are lacking. Whenever neurosarcoid is considered, a careful slit-lamp examination of the eye to search for uveitis, chest x-ray and CT to assess pulmonary involvement and mediastinal lymphadenopathy, serum angiotensin-converting enzyme (positive in only one-quarter of cases), serum calcium, and a gallium scan may be indicated. Initial treatment is with

TABLE 356-3   Evaluation of Acute Transverse Myelopathy

1. MRI of spinal cord with and without contrast (exclude compressive causes).
2. CSF studies: Cell count, protein, glucose, IgG index/synthesis rate, oligoclonal bands, VDRL; Gram's stain, acid-fast bacilli, and India ink stains; PCR for VZV, HSV-2, HSV-1, EBV, CMV, HHV-6, enteroviruses, HIV; antibody for HTLV-I, *B. burgdorferi*, *M. pneumoniae*, and *Chlamydia pneumoniae*; viral, bacterial, mycobacterial, and fungal cultures.
3. Blood studies for infection: HIV; RPR; IgG and IgM enterovirus antibody; IgM mumps, measles, rubella, group B arbovirus, *Brucella melitensis*, *Chlamydia psittaci*, *Bartonella henselae*, schistosomal antibody; cultures for *B. melitensis*. Also consider nasal/pharyngeal/anal cultures for enteroviruses; stool O&P for *Schistosoma* ova.
4. Immune-mediated disorders: ESR; ANA; ENA; dsDNA; rheumatoid factor; anti-SSA; anti-SSB, complement levels; antiphospholipid and anticardiolipin antibodies; p-ANCA; antimicrosomal and antithyroglobulin antibodies; if Sjögren syndrome suspected, Schirmer test, salivary gland scintography, and salivary/lacrimal gland biopsy.
5. Sarcoidosis: Serum angiotensin-converting enzyme; serum Ca; 24 hour urine Ca; chest x-ray; chest CT; total body gallium scan; lymph node biopsy.
6. Demyelinating disease: Brain MRI scan, evoked potentials.
7. Vascular causes: CT myelogram; spinal angiogram.

Note: VDRL, Venereal Disease Research Laboratory; PCR, polymerase chain reaction; VZV, varicella-zoster virus; HHV, human herpes virus; RPR, rapid plasma reagin (test); O&P, ova and parasites; ESR, erythrocyte sedimentation rate; ANA, antinuclear antibodies; ENA, epithelial neutrophil-activity (protein).

oral glucocorticoids; immunosuppressent drugs are used for resistant cases.

Recurrent episodes of myelitis are usually due to an immune-mediated disease such as SLE or sarcoid, a demyelinating disease, or infection with herpes simplex virus (HSV) type 2 (below).

Infectious and Parainfectious Myelitis   Many viruses have been associated with an acute myelitis that is caused by direct infection of the spinal cord. Herpes zoster is the most common viral cause of acute myelitis; HSV types 1 and 2, Epstein-Barr virus (EBV), cytomegalovirus (CMV), and rabies virus are other well-described etiologies. HSV-2 can produce a distinctive syndrome of recurrent sacral myelitis in association with outbreaks of genital herpes which mimics multiple sclerosis (MS). Poliomyelitis is the prototypic virus that produces acute infection of the spinal cord. In some cases it may be appropriate to begin specific therapy based upon the suspicion that a particular viral agent might be responsible for myelitis, pending laboratory confirmation. Herpes zoster, HSV, and EBV myelitis are treated with acyclovir (10 mg/kg tid for 10 to 14 days); CMV with ganciclovir (5 mg/kg IV bid) plus foscarnet (60 mg/kg IV tid) or with cidofovir (5 mg/kg per week for 2 weeks).

Bacterial and mycobacterial etiologies are less common than viral causes. Almost any pathogenic species may be responsible, including *Listeria monocytogenes*, *Borrelia burgdorferi* (Lyme disease), and *Treponema pallidum* (syphilis). *Mycoplasma pneumoniae* may be underrecognized as a cause of ATM.

Schistosomiasis (Chap. 203) is an important cause of parasitic myelitis in endemic areas. The myelitis is intensely inflammatory and granulomatous in nature, caused by a local response to tissue-digesting enzymes from the ova of the parasite. Toxoplasmosis (Chap. 198) can occasionally cause a focal myelopathy, and this diagnosis should be considered, particularly in patients with AIDS.

Other cases of myelitis, termed *postinfectious myelitis*, or *postvaccinial myelitis*, follow an infection or vaccination. Many infectious agents have been implicated, including influenza, measles, varicella, rubeola, and mumps. As in the related disorder, acute disseminated encephalomyelitis (Chap. 359), postinfectious transverse myelitis often begins as the patient appears to be recovering from the infection, but an infectious agent cannot be isolated from the nervous system or spinal fluid. These features suggest that the myelitis represents an autoimmune disorder triggered by infection and is not due to direct infection of the spinal cord.

Demyelinating Diseases   Multiple sclerosis (Chap. 359) may present as ATM, particularly in individuals of Asian or African ancestry. In Caucasians, MS rarely causes ATM (e.g., transverse myelitis with acute bilateral signs) but is a common cause of acute partial myelopathy, Unlike infectious and parainfectious ATM, MS-associated ATM is usually not associated with fever, rash, or other manifestations of an antecedent infection. Neuromyelitis optica (Devic's disease; Chap. 359) is a demyelinating syndrome related to MS that presents as ATM associated with optic neuritis; the optic neuritis is often bilateral and may precede or follow the myelitis by weeks or months. A neuromyelitis optica syndrome is also associated with SLE (see above) and other immune-mediated diseases, and with the antiphospholipid syndrome.

MRI findings in MS-associated ATM consist of mild swelling and edema of the cord and diffuse or multifocal areas of abnormal signal on T2-weighted sequences, often extending over several cord segments. Contrast enhancement, indicating disruption in the blood-brain barrier associated with inflammation, is present in acute cases. A brain MRI should be obtained to assess the likelihood that the myelitis represents an initial attack of MS. A normal scan indicates that the risk of evolution to MS is low—~10% over 5 years; by contrast, the finding of multiple periventricular T2-bright lesions indicates a risk of >50%. The CSF may be normal, but more often there is a mild pleocytosis, occasionally up to several hundred mononuclear cells per microliter. CSF protein levels are normal or at most mildly elevated; oligoclonal banding is a variable finding but, when present, implicates MS.

There are no adequate trials of therapy for MS-associated ATM. Intravenous methylprednisolone (500 mg qd for 3 days) followed by oral prednisone (1 mg/kg per day for several weeks, then gradual taper) is the initial treatment of choice; a course of plasma exchange may be tried if glucocorticoids are ineffective.

Idiopathic Transverse Myelitis   In approximately one-quarter of cases of ATM, no underlying cause can be identified. Some will later manifest additional symptoms of a systemic immune-mediated disease such as SLE or a demyelinating disorder. In cases associated with inflammation (e.g., contrast enhancement of the lesion by spinal MRI or CSF pleocytosis) but not evidence of infection, glucocorticoids and plasma exchange are the first and second options, as for demyelinating causes (above).

CHRONIC MYELOPATHIES

SPONDYLITIC MYELOPATHY   Spondylitic myelopathy is one of the most common causes of gait difficulty in the elderly. Neck and shoulder pain with stiffness are early symptoms; impingement of bone and soft tissue overgrowth on nerve roots results in radicular arm pain, most often in a C5 or C6 distribution. Compression of the cervical cord produces a slowly progressive spastic paraparesis, at times asymmetric, and often accompanied by paresthesias in the feet and hands. Vibratory sense is diminished in the legs, and occasionally there is a sensory level for vibration on the upper thorax. In some cases coughing or straining produces leg weakness or radiating arm or shoulder pain. Dermatomal sensory loss in the arms, atrophy of intrinsic hand muscles, increased deep tendon reflexes in the legs, and extensor plantar responses are common. Urinary urgency or incontinence occurs in advanced cases. A tendon reflex in the arms is often diminished at some level; the biceps is most often affected (C5-C6). In individual cases, radicular, myelopathic, or combined signs may predominate. The diagnosis should be considered in cases of progressive cervical myelopathy, paresthesias of the feet and hands, or wasting of the hands.

Diagnosis is best made by MRI. Extrinsic cord compression is appreciated on axial views, and T2-weighted sequences may reveal areas of high signal intensity within the cord adjacent to the site of compression. Definitive therapy consists of surgical relief of the compression. Posterior laminectomy or an anterior approach with resection of the protruded disc material may be required. A cervical collar may be very helpful in milder cases. →*Cervical spondylosis and related degenerative diseases of the spine are discussed in Chap. 15.*

VASCULAR MALFORMATIONS   Although uncommon, vascular malformations of the cord are important lesions because they represent a treatable cause of progressive myelopathy. Arteriovenous malformations (AVMs) are most often located posteriorly, within the dura or along the surface of the cord, at or below the midthoracic level. The typical presentation is a middle-aged man with a progressive myelopathy. The myelopathy may worsen slowly or rapidly or may have periods of apparent remission with superimposed worsenings, resembling MS. Acute deterioration due to hemorrhage into the spinal cord or subarachnoid space may also occur. At presentation, most patients have sensory, motor, and bladder disturbances. The motor disorder may predominate and produce a mixture of upper and lower motor neuron signs, simulating amyotrophic lateral sclerosis (ALS). Pain, either dysesthesias or radicular pain, is also common. Other symptoms suggestive of AVM include intermittent claudication (symptoms that appear with exercise and are relieved by rest), or symptoms that change with posture, menses, or fever. A rare AVM syndrome presents as a progressive thoracic myelopathy with paraparesis developing over weeks or several months, associated with abnormally thick, hyalinized vessels (Foix-Alajouanine syndrome).

Spinal bruits are infrequent but should be sought at rest and after exercise. High-resolution MRI with contrast administration detects most AVMs (Fig. 356-6). A small number of AVMs not detected by

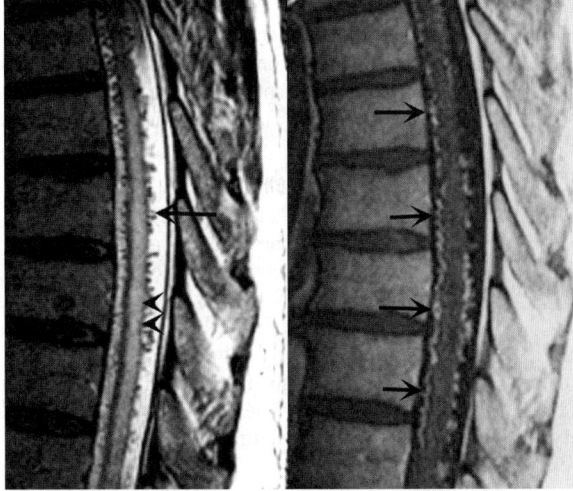

FIGURE 356-6 Arteriovenous malformation. Sagittal MR scans of the thoracic spinal cord: T2 fast spin-echo technique (*left*) and T1 post-contrast image (*right*). On the T2-weighted image (*left*), abnormally high signal intensity is noted in the central aspect of the spinal cord (*arrowheads*). Numerous punctate flow voids indent the dorsal and ventral spinal cord (*arrow*). These represent the abnormally dilated venous plexus supplied by a dural arteriovenous fistula. After contrast administration (*right*), multiple, serpentine, enhancing veins (*arrows*) on the ventral and dorsal aspect of the thoracic spinal cord are visualized, diagnostic of arteriovenous fistula. This patient was a 54-year-old man with a 4-year history of progressive paraparesis.

MRI may be visualized by CT myelography as enlarged vessels along the surface of the cord. Definitive diagnosis requires selective spinal angiography, which will also define the feeding vessels and the extent of the malformation. Spinal angiography should be considered when the clinical suspicion of an AVM is high, even when myelography is unrevealing. Embolization with occlusion of the major feeding vessels may stabilize a progressive neurologic deficit or produce a gradual recovery.

RETROVIRUS-ASSOCIATED MYELOPATHIES The myelopathy associated with the human T cell lymphotropic virus type I (HTLV-I), formerly called tropical spastic paraparesis, presents as a slowly progressive spastic paraparesis with variable sensory and bladder disturbance. The myelopathy typically implicates a thoracic level. Approximately half of patients have back or leg pain. The signs may be asymmetric, often lacking a well-defined sensory level; the only sign in the arms is hyperreflexia. The onset is generally insidious, and the tempo of progression is variable, but most patients are nonambulatory within 10 years of onset. This presentation may resemble primary progressive MS or a thoracic AVM. Diagnosis is made by demonstration of HTLV-I–specific antibody in serum by enzyme-linked immunosorbent assay (ELISA), confirmed by radioimmunoprecipitation or western blot analysis. There is no effective treatment, but symptomatic therapy for spasticity and bladder symptoms may be helpful. →*HTLV-I infections of the nervous system are discussed in Chap. 173.*

A progressive myelopathy may also occur in AIDS, characterized by vacuolar degeneration of the posterior and lateral tracts resembling subacute combined degeneration (see below).

SYRINGOMYELIA Syringomyelia is a developmental, slowly enlarging cavitary expansion of the cervical cord that produce progressive myelopathy. Symptoms begin insidiously in adolescence or early adulthood, progress irregularly, and may undergo spontaneous arrest for several years; most patients acquire a cervical-thoracic scoliosis. More than half of all cases are associated with Chiari type 1 malformations in which the cerebellar tonsils protrude through the foramen magnum and into the cervical spinal canal. The pathophysiology of the syrinx is controversial. Some interference with the normal flow of CSF seems likely. Acquired cavitations of the cord are also termed *syrinx cavities*; these may follow trauma, myelitis, chronic arachnoiditis due to tuberculosis and other etiologies, or necrotic spinal cord tumors.

The classic presentation is of a central cord syndrome with dissociated sensory loss and areflexic weakness in the upper limbs. The sensory deficit consists of loss of pain and temperature sensation with sparing of touch and vibration which is "suspended" over the nape of the neck, shoulders, and upper arms in a cape distribution or is in the hands. Most cases begin asymmetrically with unilateral sensory loss in the hands and unappreciated burns. Muscle wasting in the lower neck, shoulders, arms, and hands with asymmetric or absent reflexes reflects extension of the cavity to the anterior horns. As the lesion enlarges, spasticity and weakness of the legs, bladder and bowel dysfunction, and, in some cases, a Horner's syndrome appear. Thoracic kyphoscoliosis is a frequent additional finding. Some patients develop facial numbness and sensory loss from damage to the descending tract of the trigeminal nerve (C2 level or above). With Chiari malformations, cough headache, and neck, arm, or facial pain are common. Extension of the syrinx into the medulla, syringobulbia, may present as palatal or vocal cord paralysis, dysarthria, horizontal or vertical nystagmus, episodic dizziness, and/or tongue weakness.

MRI scans accurately identify developmental and acquired syrinx cavities and their associated spinal cord enlargement (Fig. 356-7). MRI scans of the brain and the entire spinal cord should be obtained to delineate the full longitudinal extent of the syrinx, assess posterior fossa structures, and determine whether hydrocephalus is present. If a Chiari malformation is not found, a contrast-enhanced MRI scan should be obtained to search for abnormal enhancement from an associated spinal cord tumor.

℞ TREATMENT

Treatment is generally unsatisfactory. Syringomyelia associated with tonsillar herniation is treated with posterior fossa decompression, generally consisting of suboccipital craniectomy, upper cervical laminectomy, and placement of a dural graft. If obstruction of fourth ventricular outflow is present, flow may be reestablished by enlargement of the opening. If the syrinx cavity is large, some surgeons recommend direct decompression of the fluid cavity, but the added benefit of this procedure is uncertain, and morbidity may occur. With Chiari malformations, shunting of hydrocephalus should generally precede any attempt to correct the syrinx. Surgery may stabilize the neurologic deficit; some patients have improvement postoperatively. Syringomyelia secondary to trauma or infection is treated with a decompression and drainage procedure in which a small shunt is inserted between the syrinx cavity and the subarachnoid space. Syringomyelia due to

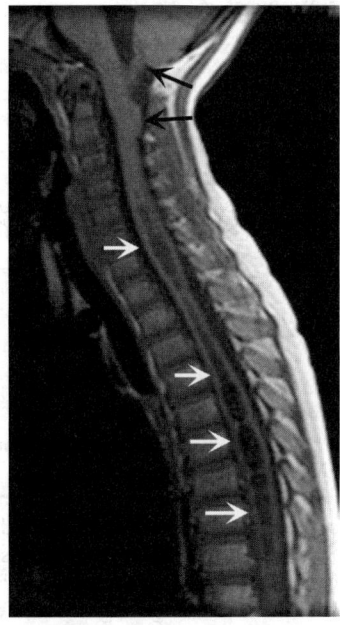

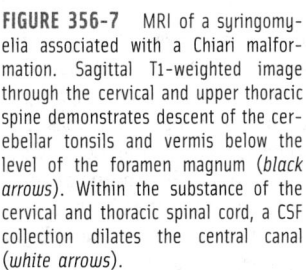

FIGURE 356-7 MRI of a syringomyelia associated with a Chiari malformation. Sagittal T1-weighted image through the cervical and upper thoracic spine demonstrates descent of the cerebellar tonsils and vermis below the level of the foramen magnum (*black arrows*). Within the substance of the cervical and thoracic spinal cord, a CSF collection dilates the central canal (*white arrows*).

TABLE 356-4 *Expected Neurologic Function Following Complete Cord Lesions*

Level	Self-Care	Transfers	Maximum Mobility
High quadriplegia (C1-C4)	Dependent on others; requires respiratory support	Dependent on others	Motorized wheelchair
Low quadriplegia (C5-C8)	Partially independent with adaptive equipment	May be dependent or independent	May use manual wheelchair, drive an automobile with adaptive equipment
Paraplegia (below T1)	Independent	Independent	Ambulates short distances with aids

Source: Adapted from JF Ditunno, CS Formal: Chronic spinal cord injury. N Engl J Med 330:550, 1994; with permission.

an intramedullary spinal cord tumor is managed by resection of the tumor, if feasible; decompression of the cyst cavity may produce temporary relief, but recurrence is common.

MULTIPLE SCLEROSIS Spinal cord involvement is common in MS. It may develop acutely as an exacerbation in a patient with known MS or appear as the presenting manifestation of the disease (see above). Chronic progressive myelopathy is the most frequent cause of disability in both primary progressive and secondary progressive forms of MS. Involvement is typically asymmetric, producing motor, sensory, and bladder/bowel disturbances. Diagnosis is facilitated by identification of earlier attacks that may not be initially recalled by the patient; by MRI, CSF and evoked response testing; and by exclusion of other conditions. The diagnosis may be particularly difficult to establish in patients with primary progressive MS. Therapy with interferon β or glatiramer acetate is indicated for patients with coexisting relapses of MS. →*MS is discussed in Chap. 359.*

SUBACUTE COMBINED DEGENERATION (VITAMIN B$_{12}$ DEFICIENCY) This treatable myelopathy presents with parasthesias in the hands and feet, early loss of vibration and position sensation, and a progressive spastic and ataxic weakness. Loss of reflexes due to a superimposed peripheral neuropathy, present in many patients, is an important diagnostic clue. Optic atrophy and irritability and other mental changes may be prominent in advanced cases and on occasion are the presenting symptoms (megaloblastic madness). The myelopathy of subacute combined degeneration tends to be diffuse rather than focal; signs are generally symmetric and reflect predominant involvement of the posterior and lateral tracts, including Romberg's sign. The diagnosis is confirmed by the finding of macrocytic red cells, a low serum B$_{12}$ concentration, elevated levels of homocysteine and methylmalonic acid in uncertain cases, and a positive Schilling test (Chap. 61).

TABES DORSALIS The classic syndromes of tabes dorsalis and meningovascular syphilis of the spinal cord are rare but must be considered in the differential diagnosis of spinal cord disorders. The most common symptoms of tabes are characteristic fleeting and repetitive lancinating pains, which occur primarily in the legs and less commonly in the back, thorax, abdomen, arms, and face. Ataxia of the legs and gait due to loss of position sense occurs in half of patients. Paresthesias, bladder disturbances, and acute abdominal pain with vomiting (visceral crisis) occur in 15 to 30% of patients. The cardinal signs of tabes are loss of reflexes in the legs, impaired position and vibratory sense, Romberg's sign, and bilateral Argyll Robertson pupils, which fail to constrict to light but react with accommodation. In the modern era, diabetic polyradiculopathy simulates tabes.

FAMILIAL SPASTIC PARAPLEGIA (Chap. 353) Some cases of progressive myelopathy are genetic in origin. More than 20 different loci have been identified, including autosomal dominant, autosomal recessive, and X-linked forms. Most patients present with progressive spasticity and weakness in the legs; the syndrome is usually but not always symmetric. Sensory symptoms and signs are usually absent or mild. Sphincter disturbances may be present. In some families in which the condition is referred to as "complicated" familial spastic paraplegia, additional neurologic signs, e.g., nystagmus, ataxia, or optic atrophy,

occur. Onset may be as early as the first year of life or as late as middle adulthood. The causative mutations responsible for several forms of familial spastic paraplegia are now known (Table 353-3). No therapies are currently available.

ADRENOMYELONEUROPATHY This X-linked disorder, a variant of adrenoleukodystrophy, most commonly presents as a progressive spastic paraparesis beginning in early adulthood; some patients also have a mild peripheral neuropathy. Affected males usually have a history of adrenal insufficiency beginning in childhood. Rare heterozygous females may also present with adult-onset myelopathy. Diagnosis is usually made by demonstration of elevated levels of very long chain fatty acids in plasma and in cultured fibroblasts. The responsible gene, located at Xq17-28, encodes a protein involved in peroxysomal transport. Steroid replacement is indicated if hypoadrenalism is present, and bone marrow transplantation has been attempted for this condition, although without clear evidence of efficacy.

OTHER CHRONIC MYELOPATHIES Primary lateral sclerosis (Chap. 353) is a degenerative disorder characterized by progressive spasticity with weakness, often accompanied by dysarthria and dysphonia. Sensory function is spared. The disorder resembles ALS, but there is no evidence of a lower motor neuron disturbance. Toxic causes of spastic myelopathy include (1) lathyrism due to ingestion of chick peas containing the excitotoxin β-N-oxalylaminoalanine (BOAA) and seen primarily in the undeveloped world, and (2) nitrous oxide inhalation producing a myelopathy identical to subacute combined degeneration. SLE (Chap. 300), Sjögren's syndrome (Chap. 304), and sarcoid (Chap. 309), as mentioned above, have all been associated with progressive myelopathy, which may involve the cord even without evidence of overt systemic disease. Cancer-related causes include chronic paraneoplastic myelopathy (Chap. 87) or radiation injury (Chap. 358); metastases to the cord are probably more common than either of these. Finally, as in ATM, in some patients the etiology of a chronic myelopathy may not be determined initially. A cause can often be identified through periodic reassessment. →*Traumatic spinal cord lesions are discussed in Chap. 357.*

MEDICAL REHABILITATION OF SPINAL CORD DISORDERS

The prospects for recovery from an acute spinal cord lesion fade after ~6 months. There are currently no effective means to promote repair of injured spinal cord tissue; promising experimental approaches include the use of factors that influence reinnervation by axons of the corticospinal tract, nerve graft bridges that promote reinnervation across spinal cord lesions, and the local injection of stem cells. The disability associated with irreversible spinal cord damage is determined primarily by the level of the lesion and by whether the disturbance in function is complete or incomplete (Table 356-4). Even a complete high cervical cord lesion may be compatible with a productive life. Development of a rehabilitation plan framed by realistic expectations, and attention to the neurologic, medical, and psychological complications that commonly arise, are primary goals of treatment.

Many of the usual symptoms associated with medical illnesses, especially somatic and visceral pain, may be lacking because of the destruction of afferent pain pathways. Unexplained fever, worsening of spasticity, or deterioration in neurologic function should prompt a search for infection, thrombophlebitis, or an intraabdominal pathology; these etiologies are far more likely to be responsible than primary neurologic events such as meningitis, secondary syringomyelia, or chronic arachnoiditis. The loss of normal thermoregulation and inability to maintain normal body temperature can produce recurrent fever (*quadriplegic fever*), although most episodes of fever are due to infection of the urinary tract, lung, skin, or bone.

Bladder dysfunction generally results from loss of supraspinal innervation of the detrusor muscle of the bladder wall and the sphincter musculature. Detrusor spasticity is treated with anticholinergic drugs (oxybutinin, 2.5 to 5 mg qid) or tricyclic antidepressants with anticholinergic properties (imipramine, 25 to 200 mg/d). Failure of the sphincter muscle to relax during bladder emptying (urinary dyssynergia) may be managed with the α-adrenergic blocking agent terazosin hydrochloride (1 to 2 mg tid or qid), with intermittent catheterization, or, if that is not feasible, by use of a condom catheter in men or a permanent indwelling catheter. Surgical options include the creation of an artificial bladder by isolating a segment of intestine that can be catheterized intermittently (enterocystoplasty) or can drain continuously to an external appliance (urinary conduit). Bladder areflexia due to acute spinal shock or conus lesions is best treated by catheterization.

Bladder paralysis predisposes the patient to urinary tract infection. Bacteriuria due to asymptomatic colonization is extremely common and is generally not treated. Prophylaxis with antiseptics or antibiotics is a controversial practice. Urinary tract infections may present only as foul-smelling urine or a change in voiding pattern; the development of high fever or other systemic signs often indicates pyelonephritis. Bowel regimens and disimpaction are necessary in most patients to ensure at least biweekly evacuation and avoid colonic distention or obstruction.

High cervical cord lesions cause various degrees of mechanical respiratory failure requiring artificial ventilation. In cases of incomplete respiratory failure, chest physical therapy is useful, and a negative-pressure cuirass may alleviate atelectasis, particularly if the major lesion is below C4. With severe respiratory failure, tracheal intubation, followed by tracheotomy, provides tracheal access for ventilation and suctioning. Phrenic nerve pacing may be an option in some patients with lesions at C5 or above.

Patients with acute cord injury are at high risk for venous thrombosis and pulmonary embolism. During the first 2 weeks, use of calf-compression devices and anticoagulation with heparin (5000 U subcutaneously every 12 h) or warfarin (INR, 2 to 3) are recommended. In cases of persistent paralysis, anticoagulation should probably be continued for 3 months.

Prophylaxis against decubitus ulcers should involve frequent changes in position in a chair or bed, the use of special mattresses, and cushioning of areas where pressure sores often develop, such as the sacral prominence and heels. Early treatment of ulcers with careful cleansing, surgical or enzyme debridement of necrotic tissue, and appropriate dressing and drainage may prevent infection of adjacent soft tissue or bone.

Spasticity (Chap. 21) is aided by stretching exercises to maintain mobility of joints. Drug treatment is effective but may result in reduced function, as some patients depend upon spasticity as an aid to stand, transfer, or walk. Baclofen (15 to 240 mg/d in divided doses) is the most effective drug; it acts by facilitating GABA-mediated inhibition of motor reflex arcs. Diazepam acts by a similar mechanism and is useful for leg spasms that interrupt sleep (2 to 4 mg at bedtime). For nonambulatory patients, the direct muscle inhibitor dantrolene (25 to 100 mg qid) may be used, but it is potentially hepatotoxic. In severe cases, intrathecal baclofen administered via an implanted pump, botulinum toxin injections, or dorsal rhizotomy may be required to control spasticity.

A dramatic paroxysmal autonomic hyperreflexia may occur following lesions above the major splanchnic sympathetic outflow at T6. Headache, flushing, and diaphoresis above the level of the lesion, and hypertension with bradycardia or tachycardia, are the major symptoms. The trigger is typically a noxious stimulus—for example, bladder or bowel distention, a urinary tract infection, or a decubitus ulcer—below the level of the cord lesion. Treatment consists of removal of offending stimuli; ganglionic blocking agents (mecamylamine, 2.5 to 5 mg) or other short-acting antihypertensive drugs are useful in some patients.

Attention to these details allows longevity and a productive life for patients with myelopathy.

FURTHER READING

DE SEZE J et al: Acute myelopathies: Clinical, laboratory and outcome profiles in 79 cases. Brain 124:1509, 2001

KALB RG: Getting the spinal cord to think for itself. Arch Neurol 60:805, 2003

TRANSVERSE MYELITIS CONSORTIUM WORKING GROUP: Proposed diagnostic criteria and nosology of acute transverse myelitis. Neurology 59:499, 2002

357 | CONCUSSION AND OTHER HEAD INJURIES
Allan H. Ropper

Almost 10 million head injuries occur annually in the United States, about 20% of which are serious enough to cause brain damage. Among men under 35 years, accidents, usually motor vehicle collisions, are the chief cause of death, and >70% of these involve head injury. Furthermore, minor head injuries are so common that almost all physicians will be called upon to provide immediate care or to see patients who are suffering from various sequelae.

Medical personnel caring for head injury patients should be aware that (1) spinal injury often accompanies head injury, and care must be taken to prevent compression of the spinal cord due to instability of the spinal column; (2) intoxication is an important accompaniment of traumatic brain injury and, when appropriate, testing should be carried out for drugs and alcohol; and (3) systemic injuries, including rupture of abdominal organs, may produce vascular collapse or respiratory compromise requiring immediate attention.

TYPES OF HEAD INJURIES

CONCUSSION This refers to an immediate but transient loss of consciousness that is associated with a short period of amnesia. Patients may appear dazed or report feeling "star struck." It typically occurs after a blunt forward impact that creates a sudden deceleration of the cranium and a movement of the brain within the skull. Severe concussion may precipitate a brief convulsion or autonomic signs such as facial pallor, bradycardia, faintness with mild hypotension, or sluggish pupillary reaction, but most patients are soon neurologically normal. The mechanism of loss of consciousness in concussion is believed to be a transient electrophysiologic dysfunction of the reticular activating system in the upper midbrain caused by rotation of the cerebral hemispheres on the relatively fixed brainstem (Chap. 257).

Gross and light-microscopic changes in the brain are usually absent following concussion, but biochemical and ultrastructural changes, such as mitochondrial ATP depletion and local disruption of the blood-brain barrier, suggest that transient abnormalities occur. CT and MRI scans are usually normal; however, approximately 3% of patients will be found to have an intracranial hemorrhage of some type.

The amnesia of concussion typically occurs in individuals who have experienced at least a few moments of unresponsiveness, but on rare occasions no loss of consciousness is reported. The memory loss spans the time of, and moments before, mild impact injuries but may encompass previous weeks (rarely months) in cases of more severe trauma. In most cases, the extent of retrograde amnesia correlates with the severity of injury. Any anterograde amnesia is usually brief and disappears rapidly in alert patients. Memory is regained in an orderly way from the most distant to recent memories, with islands of amnesia occasionally remaining in severe cases. The mechanism of peritraumatic amnesia is not known. Hysterical posttraumatic amnesia is not uncommon and should be suspected when inexplicable abnormalities of behavior occur, such as recounting events that cannot be recalled

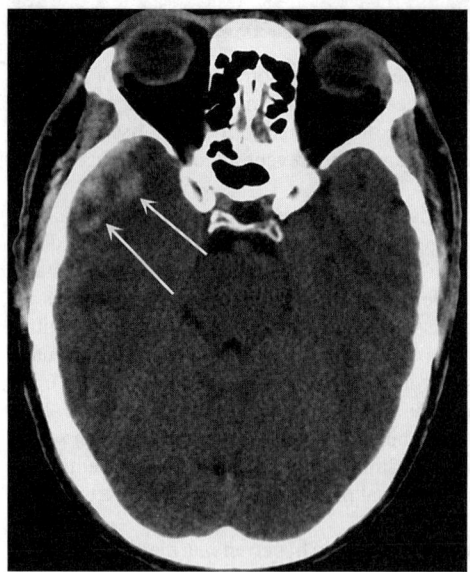

FIGURE 357-1 Traumatic cerebral contusion. Noncontrast CT scan demonstrating a hyperdense hemorrhagic region in the anterior temporal lobe.

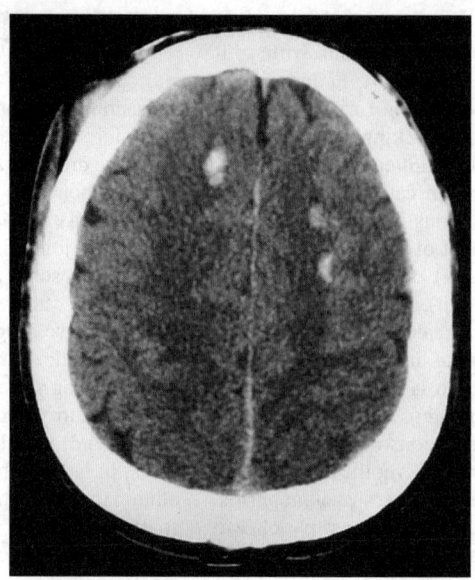

FIGURE 357-2 Multiple small areas of hemorrhage and tissue disruption in the white matter of the frontal lobes on noncontrast CT scan. These appear to reflect an extreme type of the diffuse axonal shearing lesions that occur with closed head injury.

diathesis or cerebrovascular amyloidosis in the elderly. For unexplained reasons, deep cerebral hemorrhages may not develop until several days after severe injury. Sudden neurologic deterioration in a comatose patient or a sudden rise in intracranial pressure (ICP) should therefore prompt investigation with a CT scan.

Another type of deep white matter lesion consists of widespread acute disruption, or shearing, of axons at the time of impact. Most characteristic are small areas of tissue disruption in the corpus callosum and dorsolateral pons. The presence of widespread axonal damage of both hemispheres, a state called *diffuse axonal injury*, explains persistent coma and the vegetative state, but small ischemic-hemorrhagic lesions in the midbrain and thalamus are as often the cause. Only severe shearing lesions that contain blood are visualized by CT, usually in the corpus callosum and centrum semiovale (Fig. 357-2); however, within days of the injury, MRI scan demonstrates such lesions throughout the white matter with the use of special imaging sequences.

on later testing, a bizarre affect, forgetting one's own name, or a persistent anterograde deficit that is excessive in comparison with the degree of injury. →*For further discussion of amnesia, see Chap. 23.*

A single, uncomplicated head injury only infrequently produces permanent neurobehavioral changes in patients who are free of preexisting psychiatric problems and substance abuse. These minor problems in memory and concentration may have an anatomic correlate in small shearing or other microscopic lesions (see below).

CONTUSION, BRAIN HEMORRHAGE, AND AXONAL SHEARING LESIONS
A surface bruise of the brain, or *contusion*, consists of varying degrees of petechial hemorrhage, edema, and tissue destruction. Contusions and deeper hemorrhages result from mechanical forces that displace the hemispheres forcefully relative to the skull by deceleration of the brain against the inner skull, either under a point of impact (coup lesion) or, as the brain swings back, in the antipolar area (contrecoup lesion). Trauma sufficient to cause prolonged unconsciousness usually produces some degree of contusion. Blunt impact, as from an automobile dashboard or from falling forward while drunk, typically causes contusions on the orbital surfaces of the frontal lobes and the anterior and basal portions of the temporal lobes. With lateral forces the contusions are situated on the lateral convexity of the hemispheres. In both instances there may be contrecoup contusions on the opposite side of the impact. The clinical signs are determined by the location and size of the contusion; a hemiparesis or gaze preference is fairly typical. Large bilateral contusions produce coma with extensor posturing. Contusions limited to the frontal lobes cause an abulic-taciturn state, and those in the temporal lobe may cause an aggressive, combative, or delirious syndrome, described below.

Contusions are visible on CT and MRI scans, appearing early as inhomogeneous hyperdensities on CT and as hyperintensities on MRI; the signal changes reflect small scattered areas of cortical and subcortical blood and localized brain edema (Fig. 357-1); there is also some degree of subarachnoid bleeding, which may be detected by scans or lumbar puncture. Subacutely, contusions acquire a surrounding contrast enhancement that may be mistaken for tumor or abscess. Glial and macrophage reactions may result in scarred, hemosiderin-stained depressions on the surface (*plaques jaunes*) that are the main source of posttraumatic epilepsy.

Torsion or shearing forces in the brain can cause basal ganglial and other deep hematomas independent of surface damage. Large single hemorrhages after minor trauma may be associated with a bleeding

SKULL FRACTURES
A blow to the skull causes a fracture if the elastic tolerance of the bone is exceeded. Intracranial lesions accompany two-thirds of skull fractures, and the presence of a skull fracture increases manyfold the chances of an underlying subdural or epidural hematoma. Consequently, fractures are primarily markers of the site and severity of injury. They provide pathways for entry of bacteria (meningitis) or air (pneumocephalus) to the cerebrospinal fluid (CSF) and for leakage of CSF out through the dura.

Linear fractures, which are most often associated with subdural or epidural hematomas, account for 80% of all skull fractures. They are usually oriented from the point of impact toward the base of the skull. Basilar skull fractures are often extensions of adjacent fractures over the convexity of the skull but may occur independently owing to stresses on the floor of the middle cranial fossa or occiput. They are located parallel to the petrous bone or along the sphenoid bone toward the sella turcica and ethmoidal groove. Although most are uncomplicated, basilar skull fractures can cause CSF leakage, pneumocephalus, and cavernous-carotid fistulas. Hemotympanum (blood behind the tympanic membrane), delayed ecchymosis over the mastoid process (Battle's sign), or periorbital ecchymosis ("racoon sign") all signify fracture of the base of the skull. Because routine x-ray examination may fail to disclose basilar fractures, they should be suspected if these clinical signs are present. CSF may leak through the cribriform plate or the adjacent sinus and manifest as a watery discharge from the nose (CSF rhinorrhea). Persistent rhinorrhea and recurrent meningitis are indications for surgical repair of torn dura underlying the fracture. The precise site of the leak is often difficult to determine, but useful diagnostic tests include the instillation of water-soluble contrast into the CSF followed by CT with the patient in various positions, and injection of radionuclide compounds or fluorescein into the CSF with an assessment of uptake of these compounds by absorptive nasal pledgets. The site of an intermittent leak is rarely delineated, and most resolve spontaneously. Sellar fractures, even ones associated with serious neuroendocrine dysfunction, are sometimes radiologically occult. Fractures of the dorsum sella may cause sixth or seventh nerve palsies or optic nerve damage. An air-fluid level in the sphenoid sinus suggests a fracture of the sellar floor.

Petrous bone fractures, especially those oriented along the long axis of the bone, may be associated with facial palsy, disruption of ear ossicles, and CSF otorrhea. Transverse petrous fractures are less common; they almost always damage the cochlea or labyrinths and often the facial nerve. External bleeding from the ear is usually from local abrasion of the external canal but can also result from petrous fracture.

Fractures of the frontal bone are often depressed, involving the frontal and paranasal sinuses and the orbits; permanent anosmia results if the olfactory filaments in the cribriform plate are disrupted. Depressed skull fractures are typically compound, but they are often neurologically asymptomatic because the impact energy is dissipated in breaking the bone; however, some are associated with brain contusions and focal neurologic signs caused by damage to the underlying cortical area. Prompt debridement and exploration of compound fractures are required in order to avoid infection.

CRANIAL NERVE INJURIES   The cranial nerves likely to be injured with head trauma include the olfactory, optic, oculomotor, and trochlear nerves; the first and second branches of the trigeminal nerve; and the facial and auditory nerves. Anosmia and an apparent loss of taste (actually a loss of perception of aromatic flavors, with elementary tastes retained) occur in ~10% of persons with serious head injuries, particularly after falls on the back of the head. This sequela results from displacement of the brain and shearing of the olfactory nerve filaments and may occur in the absence of a fracture. Recovery is the rule, leaving residual hyposmia, but if bilateral anosmia persists for several months, the prognosis is poor. Partial optic nerve injuries from closed trauma result in blurring of vision, central or paracentral scotomas, or sector defects. Direct orbital injury may cause short-lived blurred vision for close objects and pupillary paralysis because of reversible iridoplegia. Diplopia limited to downward gaze and corrected when the head is tilted away from the affected eye indicates trochlear nerve damage. It occurs as an isolated problem after minor injury and can develop after a delay of several days. Direct facial nerve injury by a basal fracture is present immediately in 3% of severe injuries; it may also be delayed 5 to 7 days. Fractures through the petrous bone, particularly the less common transverse type, are liable to produce this injury. Delayed facial palsy, the mechanism of which is unknown, has a good prognosis. Injury to the eighth cranial nerve from a fracture of the petrous bone causes loss of hearing, vertigo, and nystagmus immediately after injury. Deafness from nerve injury must be distinguished from that due to rupture of the eardrum, blood in the middle ear, or disruption of the ossicles from fracture through the middle ear. A high-tone hearing loss occurs with direct cochlear concussion.

SEIZURES   *Convulsions* are surprisingly uncommon immediately after a head injury, but a brief period of tonic extensor posturing or a few clonic movements of the limbs just after the moment of impact may occur. However, the superficial cortical scars that evolve from contusions are highly epileptogenic and may later manifest as seizures, even after many years (Chap. 348). The severity of injury determines the risk of future seizures. It has been estimated that 17% of individuals with brain contusion, subdural hematoma, or prolonged loss of consciousness will develop a seizure disorder and that this risk extends for an indefinite period of time, whereas the risk is only 2% after mild injury. The majority of convulsions in the latter group occur within 5 years of injury.

SUBDURAL AND EPIDURAL HEMATOMAS   Hemorrhages beneath the dura (subdural) or between the dura and skull (epidural) may be associated with contusions and other injuries, making it difficult to determine their relative contribution to the clinical state. However, subdural and epidural hematomas as often occur as the sole manifestation of injury, and each has characteristic clinical and radiologic features. Because the mass effect and the rise in ICP caused by these hemorrhages may be life threatening, it is imperative that hemorrhages be identified immediately by CT or MRI scan and evacuated when appropriate.

Acute Subdural Hematoma   These lesions become symptomatic minutes or hours after injury. Up to one-third of patients have a lucid interval before coma supervenes, but most are drowsy or comatose from the moment of injury. Direct cranial trauma is not required for acute subdural hemorrhage to occur; acceleration forces alone, as from whip-

lash, are adequate, especially in the elderly and those taking anticoagulant medications. A unilateral headache and slightly enlarged pupil on the same side are frequently but not invariably found. Stupor or coma, a hemiparesis, and unilateral pupillary enlargement are the signs of larger hematomas. In an acutely deteriorating patient with diminished alertness and with pupillary enlargement, burr (drainage) holes or an emergency craniotomy are appropriate. Small subdural hematomas may be asymptomatic and usually do not require evacuation. A subacute syndrome due to subdural hematoma occurs days to weeks after injury with drowsiness, headache, confusion, or mild hemiparesis; it is seen in alcoholics and in the elderly. Subdural hematomas appear as crescentic collections over the convexity of the hemisphere and are located over the frontotemporal region, less often in the inferior middle fossa or over the occipital poles (Fig. 357-3).

Interhemispheric, posterior fossa, or bilateral convexity hematomas are less common and are difficult to diagnose clinically, although drowsiness and the signs expected for each region can be detected (Chap. 23). Larger hematomas are primarily venous in origin, though additional arterial bleeding sites are often found; a few large hematomas, when explored surgically, have an exclusively arterial cause.

Epidural Hematoma (Fig. 357-4)   These evolve more rapidly than subdural hematomas and are therefore more treacherous. They occur in up to 10% of severe head injury cases and are less often associated with underlying cortical damage than are subdural hematomas. Most patients are unconscious when first seen. A "lucid interval" of several minutes to hours before coma supervenes is most characteristic of epidural hemorrhage, but it is still uncommon, and epidural hemorrhage by no means is the only cause of this temporal sequence of events.

Chronic Subdural Hematoma   A history of trauma may or may not be elicited; 20 to 30% of patients recall no head injury, particularly the elderly and those with bleeding diatheses. The causative injury may be trivial and is often forgotten because it was remote. Headache (common but not invariable), slowed thinking, change in personality, a seizure, or a mild hemiparesis emerges weeks or months afterwards. The headache may fluctuate in severity, sometimes with position changes. Many chronic subdural hematomas are bilateral and produce perplexing clinical syndromes. The initial clinical impression is of a stroke, brain tumor, drug intoxication, depression, or a dementing illness because drowsiness, inattentiveness, and incoherence of thought are more prominent than focal signs such as hemiparesis. Patients with undetected small bilateral subdural hematomas seem to have a low tolerance for surgery, anesthesia, and drugs that depress the nervous system, remaining drowsy or confused for long periods postoperatively. Occasionally a chronic hematoma causes brief episodes of hemiparesis or aphasia that are indistinguishable from transient ischemic attacks.

Skull x-rays are usually normal except for a shift of the calcified pineal body to one side or an occasional unexpected fracture. In longstanding cases the irregular calcification of membranes that surround the collection may be appreciated. CT performed soon after injury (without contrast infusion) shows a low-density mass over the convexity of the hemisphere (Fig. 357-5), but between 2 to 6 weeks after the initial bleeding the hemorrhage appears isodense compared to adjacent brain. Bilateral chronic hematomas may fail to be detected because of the absence of lateral tissue shifts; this circumstance is suggested by a "hypernormal" CT scan with fullness of the cortical sulci and small ventricles in an older patient. CT with contrast demonstrates the vascular fibrous capsule surrounding the hemorrhage. MRI reliably identifies either a subacute or chronic hematoma. Chronic subdural hematomas can expand gradually and clinically resemble tumors of the brain.

Clinical observation and serial imaging are reasonable in patients with few symptoms and small chronic subdural collections. Treatment with glucocorticoids alone is sufficient in some larger hematomas, but surgical evacuation is more often successful. The fibrous membranes

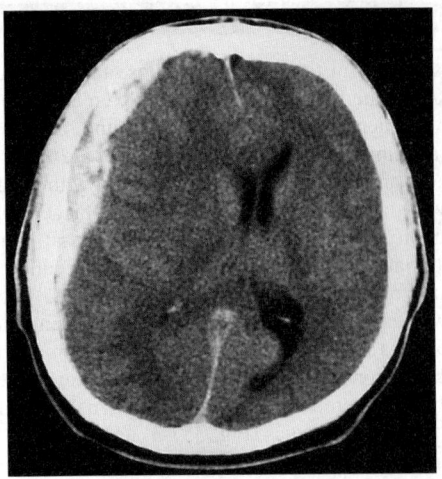

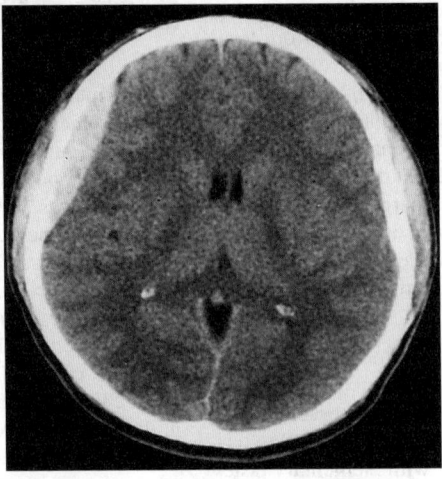

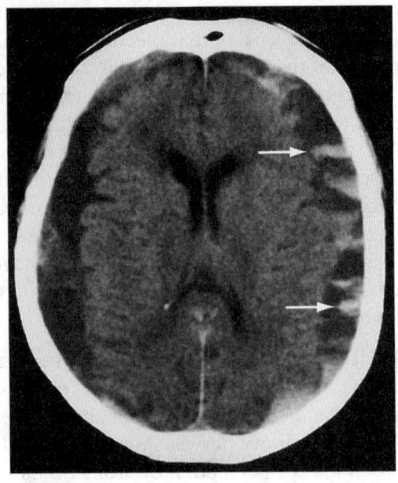

FIGURE 357-3 Acute subdural hematoma in a non-contrast CT scan. The hyperdense clot has an irregular border with the brain and causes more horizontal displacement (mass effect) than might be expected from its thickness. The disproportionate mass effect is the result of the large rostral-caudal extent of these hematomas. Compare to Fig. 357-4.

FIGURE 357-4 Acute epidural hematoma. The tightly attached dura is stripped from the inner table of the skull, producing a characteristic lenticular-shaped hemorrhage on CT scan. Epidural hematomas are usually caused by disruption of the middle meningeal artery following fracture of the temporal bone.

FIGURE 357-5 CT scan of chronic bilateral subdural hematomas of different ages. The collections began as acute hematomas and have become hypodense in comparison to the adjacent brain after a period during which they were isodense and difficult to appreciate. Some areas of resolving blood are contained on the more recently formed collection on the left (arrows).

that grow from the dura and encapsulate the region require surgical resection to prevent recurrent fluid accumulation. Small hematomas are largely resorbed, leaving only the organizing membranes.

CLINICAL SYNDROMES AND TREATMENT OF HEAD INJURY

MINOR INJURY The patient who is fully alert and attentive after head injury but who has one or more symptoms of headache, faintness, nausea, a single episode of emesis, difficulty with concentration, or slight blurring of vision has a good prognosis with little risk of subsequent deterioration. Such patients have usually sustained a concussion and are expected to have a brief amnestic period. Children and young adults are particularly prone to drowsiness, vomiting, and irritability, which is sometimes delayed for several hours after apparently minor injuries. Occasionally, vasovagal syncope follows several minutes to an hour after the injury and may cause undue concern. Constant generalized or frontal headache is common in the days following trauma; it may be migrainous (throbbing and hemicranial) in nature. After several hours of observation, patients with this category of injury may be accompanied home and observed by a family member or friend. Most patients with this syndrome do not have a skull fracture on x-ray or hemorrhage on CT. The decision to perform these tests therefore depends largely on clinical signs suggesting that the impact was severe (e.g., prolonged concussion, periorbital or mastoid hematoma, repeated vomiting, apparent fracture), on the seriousness of other bodily injuries, and on the degree of surveillance that can be anticipated at home. Persistent severe headache and repeated vomiting in the context of normal alertness and no focal neurologic signs are usually benign, but radiologic studies should be obtained and observation in the hospital is justified.

INJURY OF INTERMEDIATE SEVERITY Patients who are not comatose but who have persistent confusion, behavioral changes, subnormal alertness, extreme dizziness, or focal neurologic signs such as hemiparesis should be admitted to the hospital and soon thereafter have a CT scan. Usually a contusion or hematoma is found. The clinical syndromes most common in this group, in addition to postconcussive drowsiness, headache, dizziness, and vomiting, include (1) delirium with a disinclination to be examined or moved, expletive speech, and resistance if disturbed (anterior temporal lobe contusions); (2) a quiet, disinterested, slowed mental state (abulia) with dull facial appearance and irascibility (inferior frontal and frontopolar contusions); (3) a focal deficit such as aphasia or mild hemiparesis (due to subdural hematoma or convexity contusion, or, less often but frequently missed, carotid

artery dissection); (4) confusion with inattention, poor performance on simple mental tasks, and fluctuating or slightly erroneous orientation (associated with several types of injuries, including the first two described above as well as medial frontal contusions and interhemispheric subdural hematoma); (5) repetitive vomiting, nystagmus, drowsiness, and unsteadiness (usually from labyrinthine concussion, but occasionally due to a posterior fossa subdural hematoma or vertebral artery dissection); and (6) diabetes insipidus (damage to the median eminence or pituitary stalk). *It should be emphasized that intermediate-grade injuries are often complicated by drug or alcohol intoxication.*

Clinical observation is necessary to detect increasing drowsiness, change in respiratory pattern, or pupillary enlargement and to ensure restriction of free water (unless there is diabetes insipidus). Most patients in this category improve over several days. During the first week, the state of alertness, memory, and other cognitive functions often fluctuates, and irascibility or agitation is common. Behavioral changes are worse at night, as with many other encephalopathies, and may be treated with small doses of antipsychotic medications. Subtle abnormalities of attention, intellect, spontaneity, and memory tend to return to normal weeks or months after the injury, sometimes surprisingly abruptly; persistent problems in cognition are discussed below.

SEVERE INJURY Patients who are comatose from the onset require immediate neurologic attention and resuscitation. After intubation, with care taken to avoid deforming the cervical spine, the depth of coma, pupillary size and reactivity, limb movements, and Babinski responses are assessed. As soon as vital functions permit and cervical spine x-rays and a CT scan have been obtained, the patient should be transported to a critical care unit where ICP can be monitored, and where the systemic complications that follow severe brain injury can be treated. The finding of an epidural or subdural hematoma or large intracerebral hemorrhage is an indication for prompt surgery and intracranial decompression in otherwise salvageable patients. →*Management of raised ICP is discussed in Chap. 258.*

PROGNOSIS In severe head injury, eye opening, the best motor response of the limbs, and verbal output have been found to be roughly predictive of outcome; these are summarized using the "Glasgow Coma Scale" (Table 357-1). Over 85% of patients with aggregate scores of 3 or 4 die within 24 h. However, a number of patients with slightly higher scores and a poor initial prognosis, including a few without pupillary light responses, survive, suggesting that an initially

TABLE 357-1 *Glasgow Coma Scale for Head Injury*

Eye opening (E)		Verbal response (V)	
Spontaneous	4	Oriented	5
To loud voice	3	Confused, disoriented	4
To pain	2	Inappropriate words	3
Nil	1	Incomprehensible sounds	2
Best motor response (M)		Nil	1
Obeys	6		
Localizes	5		
Withdraws (flexion)	4		
Abnormal flexion posturing	3		
Extension posturing	2		
Nil	1		

Note: Coma score = E + M + V. Patients scoring 3 or 4 have an 85 percent chance of dying or remaining vegetative, while scores above 11 indicate only a 5 to 10 percent likelihood of death or vegetative state and 85 percent chance of moderate disability or good recovery. Intermediate scores correlate with proportional chances of recovery.

aggressive approach is justified in most patients. Patients <20 years, particularly children, may make remarkable recoveries after having grave early neurologic signs. In one large study of severe head injury, 55% of children had a good outcome at 1 year, compared with 21% of adults. Older age, increased ICP, hypoxia and hypotension, and CT scan evidence of compression of the cisterns surrounding the brainstem and shift of midline structures are all poor prognostic signs. Delayed evacuation of large intracerebral hemorrhages is associated with a poor prognosis. Carrier status for the apolipoprotein E-4 allele is also associated with poor recovery following traumatic brain injury.

POSTCONCUSSION SYNDROME

A structural basis has been sought for the posttraumatic nervous instability termed the *postconcussion syndrome*, which consists of fatigue, dizziness, headache, and difficulty in concentration after mild or moderate injury. Most instances are difficult to distinguish from asthenia and depression. Based largely on experimental models, some investigators believe that subtle axonal shearing lesions or yet undefined biochemical alterations account for the cognitive symptoms even when the findings are normal on brain imaging, evoked potentials, and electroencephalogram. In moderate and severe trauma, neuropsychological changes such as difficulty with attention, memory, and other cognitive deficits are undoubtedly present, sometimes severe, but many deficits identified in formal testing are not important for daily functioning. Test scores tend to improve rapidly during the first 6 months after injury, then more slowly for years.

Treatment of the various symptoms of the postconcussive syndrome first requires a symptomatic approach to identify and treat depression and loss of energy, sleeplessness, anxiety, persistent headache, and dizziness. Often, reassurance and treatment directed at anxious depression and sleep problems are all that are required. Care is taken to avoid prolonged use of drugs that produce dependence. Vestibular exercises (Chap. 26) and small doses of vestibular suppressants such as phenergan are helpful when dizziness is the main problem. Patients who after minor or moderate injury report difficulty with memory or with complex cognitive tasks at work may also be reassured that these problems usually improve over 6 to 12 months. It is helpful in this group to obtain focused, serial, and quantified neuropsychological testing in order to adjust the work environment to the patient's current abilities and to document improvement. Whether cognitive exercises are useful is uncertain, but patients certainly report them to be helpful. Previously energetic individuals are usually found to have the best recoveries. In patients with persistent symptoms, the possibility of malingering exists. Physicians should be aware that symptoms tend to persist when litigation regarding the injury is prolonged.

In the absence of adequate data, a common sense approach has been taken to deciding when an athlete who has suffered a concussion should resume athletic activities. Generally, it is advisable to avoid

TABLE 357-2 *Guidelines for Management of Concussion in Sports*

SEVERITY OF CONCUSSION

Grade 1: Transient confusion, no loss of consciousness (LOC), all symptoms resolve within 15 min.
Grade 2: Transient confusion, no LOC, but concussive symptoms or mental status abnormalities persist longer than 15 min.
Grade 3: Any LOC, either brief (seconds) or prolonged (minutes).

ON-SITE EVALUATION

1. Mental status testing
   a. Orientation—time, place, person, circumstances of injury
   b. Concentration—digits backward, months of year in reverse order
   c. Memory—names of teams, details of contest, recent events, recall of three words and objects at 0 and 5 min
2. Finger-nose-finger with eyes open and closed
3. Pupillary symmetry and reaction
4. Romberg and tandem gait
5. Provocative testing—40-yard sprint, 5 push ups, 5 sit ups, 5 knee bends (development of dizziness, headaches, or other symptoms is abnormal)

MANAGEMENT GUIDELINES

Grade 1: Remove from contest. Examine immediately and at 5 min intervals. May return to contest if exam clears within 15 min. A second grade 1 concussion eliminates player for 1 week, with return contingent upon normal neurologic assessment at rest and with exercise.
Grade 2: Remove from contest, cannot return for at least 1 week. Examine at frequent intervals on sideline. Formal neurologic exam the next day. If headache or other symptoms persist for 1 week or longer, CT or MRI scan is indicated. After 1 full asymptomatic week, repeat neurologic assessment at rest and with exercise before cleared to resume play. A second grade 2 concussion eliminates player for at least 2 weeks following complete resolution of symptoms.
Grade 3: Transport by ambulance to emergency department if still unconscious or worrisome signs are present; cervical spine stabilization may be indicated. Neurologic exam and, when indicated, CT or MRI scan will guide subsequent management. Hospital admission indicated when signs of pathology are present or if mental status remains abnormal. If findings are normal at the time of the initial medical evaluation, the athlete may be sent home, but daily exams as an outpatient are indicated. A brief (LOC for seconds) grade 3 concussion eliminates player for 1 week, and a prolonged (LOC for minutes) grade 3 concussion for 2 weeks, following complete resolution of symptoms. A second grade 3 concussion should eliminate player from sports for at least 1 month following resolution. Any abnormality on CT or MRI scans should result in termination of the season for the athlete, and return to play at any future time should be discouraged.

Note: CT, computed tomography; MRI, magnetic resonance imaging.
Source: Modified from Quality Standards Subcommittee of the American Academy of Neurology: *The American Academy of Neurology Practice Handbook*. The American Academy of Neurology, St. Paul, MN, 1997.

contact sports for several days at least, and for weeks after a second concussion or if there are protracted neurologic symptoms (Table 357-2). These guidelines are designed to avoid an extremely rare complication of recurrent head injury, termed the *second impact syndrome*, in which devastating cerebral swelling follows a minor head injury superimposed upon a recent concussion. There is some evidence that repeated concussions in football and soccer players are associated with mild but cumulative cognitive deficits.

FURTHER READING

LOVELL MR et al: Recovery from concussion in high school athletes. J Neurosurg 98:296, 2003

ROPPER AH (ed): *Neurological and Neurosurgical Intensive Care*, 4th ed. Philadelphia, Lippincott Williams & Wilkins, 2004

SAVOLA O, HILBLOM M: Early predictors of post-concussion symptoms in patients with mild head injury. Eur J Neurol 10:175, 2003

Malignant primary tumors of the central nervous system (CNS) occur in ~16,500 individuals and account for an estimated 13,000 deaths in the United States annually, a mortality rate of 6 per 100,000. An approximately equal number of benign tumors of the CNS are diagnosed, with a much lower mortality rate. Glial tumors account for 50 to 60% of primary brain tumors, meningiomas for 25%, schwannomas for 10%, and all other CNS tumors for the remainder.

Brain and vertebral metastases from systemic cancer are more prevalent than primary CNS tumors. About 15% of patients who die of cancer (80,000 individuals each year in the United States) have symptomatic brain metastases; an additional 5% suffer spinal cord involvement. Brain and spinal metastases therefore pose a major problem in the management of systemic cancer.

BRAIN TUMORS

APPROACH TO THE PATIENT

Clinical Features Brain tumors usually present with one of three syndromes: (1) subacute progression of a focal neurologic deficit; (2) seizure; or (3) nonfocal neurologic disorder such as headache, dementia, personality change, or gait disorder. The presence of systemic symptoms such as malaise, weight loss, anorexia, or fever suggests a metastatic rather than a primary brain tumor.

Progressive focal neurologic deficits result from compression of neurons and white matter tracts by expanding tumor and surrounding edema. Less commonly, a brain tumor presents with a sudden stroke-like onset of a focal neurologic deficit. Although this presentation may be caused by hemorrhage into the tumor, often no hemorrhage can be demonstrated and the mechanism is obscure. Tumors frequently associated with hemorrhage include high-grade gliomas and metastatic melanoma and choriocarcinoma.

Seizures may result from disruption of cortical circuits. Tumors that invade or compress the cerebral cortex, even small meningiomas, are more likely to be associated with seizures than subcortical neoplasms. Nonfocal neurologic dysfunction usually reflects increased intracranial pressure (ICP), hydrocephalus, or diffuse tumor spread. Tumors in some areas of the brain may produce behavioral disorders; for example, frontal lobe tumors may present with personality change, dementia, or depression.

Headache may result from focal irritation or displacement of pain-sensitive structures (Chap. 14) or from a generalized increase in ICP. A headache that worsens rather than abates with recumbency is suggestive of a mass lesion. Headaches from increased ICP are usually holocephalic and episodic, occurring more than once a day. They typically develop rapidly over several minutes, persist for 20 to 40 min, and subside quickly. They may awaken the patient from a sound sleep, generally 60 to 90 min after retiring, or may be precipitated by coughing, sneezing, or straining. Vomiting may occur with severe headaches. As elevated ICP becomes sustained, the headache becomes continuous but varying in intensity. Elevated ICP may cause papilledema (Chap. 25), although it is often not present in infants or patients >55 years.

The Karnofsky performance scale is useful in assessing and following patients with brain tumors (Chap. 66). A score ≥70 indicates that the patient is ambulatory and independent in self-care activities; it is often taken as a level of function justifying aggressive therapy.

Laboratory Examination Primary brain tumors typically do not produce serologic abnormalities such as an elevated sedimentation rate or tumor-specific antigens associated with systemic cancers. In contrast, metastases to the nervous system, depending on the type and extent of the primary tumor, may be associated with systemic signs of malignancy (Chap. 66). Lumbar puncture may precipitate brain herniation in patients with mass lesions and should be performed only in patients with suspected CNS infection or meningeal metastasis. Findings in the cerebrospinal fluid (CSF) of patients with primary and metastatic nervous system tumors may include raised opening pressure, elevated protein level, and a mild lymphocytic pleocytosis. The CSF rarely contains malignant cells, with the important exceptions of leptomeningeal metastases, primary CNS lymphoma, and primitive neuroectodermal tumors, including medulloblastoma.

Neuroimaging Computed tomography (CT) and magnetic resonance imaging (MRI) can reveal mass effect and contrast enhancement. Mass effect reflects the volume of neoplastic tissue as well as surrounding edema. Brain tumors typically produce a vasogenic pattern of edema, with accumulation of excess water in white matter. Contrast enhancement reflects a breakdown of the blood-brain barrier within the tumor, permitting leakage of contrast agent. Low-grade gliomas typically do not exhibit contrast enhancement.

Positron emission tomography (PET) and single-photon emission tomography (SPECT) have ancillary roles in the imaging of brain tumors, primarily in distinguishing tumor recurrence from tissue necrosis that can occur after irradiation (see below). Electroencephalography (EEG) has a role in the evaluation of patients with seizures. Functional imaging with PET, MRI, or magnetoencephalography may be of use in surgical or radiosurgical planning to define the anatomic relationship of the tumor to critical brain regions such as the primary motor or language cortex.

℞ TREATMENT

Symptomatic Glucocorticoids decrease the volume of edema surrounding brain tumors and improve neurologic function; dexamethasone (12 to 20 mg/d in divided doses orally or intravenously) is used because it has relatively little mineralocorticoid activity.

Tumors that involve the cerebral cortex or hippocampus may produce epilepsy. Anticonvulsants are therefore used therapeutically and prophylactically; phenytoin, carbamazepine, and valproic acid are equally effective (Chap. 348). If the tumor is subcortical in location, prophylactic anticonvulsants are unnecessary.

Gliomas and primary CNS lymphomas are associated with an increased risk for deep vein thrombosis and pulmonary embolism, probably because these tumors secrete procoagulant factors into the systemic circulation. Even though hemorrhage within gliomas is a frequent histopathologic finding, patients appear to be at no increased risk for symptomatic intracranial bleeding following treatment with an anticoagulant. Prophylaxis with low-dose subcutaneous heparin should be considered for patients with brain tumors who have lower limb immobility, which places them at risk for deep venous thrombosis.

PRIMARY BRAIN TUMORS

ETIOLOGY Exposure to ionizing radiation is the only well-documented environmental risk factor for the development of gliomas. A number of hereditary syndromes are associated with an increased risk of brain tumors (Table 358-1). Genes that contribute to the development of brain tumors, as well as other malignancies, fall into two general classes, *tumor-suppressor genes* and *proto-oncogenes* (Chap. 68). Whereas germ-line mutations of tumor-suppressor genes are rare, somatic mutations are almost invariably found in malignant tumors, including brain tumors. Likewise, the activation of proto-oncogenes occurs frequently in brain tumors. Moreover, cytogenetic analysis often reveals characteristic changes. In astrocytic tumors, DNA is commonly lost on chromosomes 10p, 17p, 13q, and 9. Oligodendrogliomas frequently have deletions of 1p and 19q. In meningiomas portions of 22q, which contains the gene for neurofibromatosis (NF) type 2, are often lost. In approximately one-third of glioblastomas, there is amplification of the *EGFR* gene.

The particular constellation of genetic alterations varies among individual gliomas, even those that are histologically indistinguishable. Moreover, gliomas are genetically unstable. Genetic abnormalities tend to accumulate with time, and these changes correspond with an increasingly malignant phenotype. There are at least two genetic routes for the development of malignant glioma (Fig. 358-1). One route involves the progression, generally over years, from a low-grade astrocytoma with deletions of chromosome 17 and inactivation of the *p53* gene to a malignant

TABLE 358-1	Hereditary Syndromes Associated with Brain Tumors		
Syndrome	**Gene (Locus)**	**Gene Product (Function)**	**Nervous System Neoplasms**
Neurofibromatosis type 1 (von Recklinghausen's Disease)[a]	*NF1* (17q)	Neurofibromin (GTPase activating protein)	Neuroma, schwannoma, meningioma, optic glioma
Neurofibromatosis type 2[a]	*NF2* (22q)	Merlin (cytoskeletal protein)	Schwannoma, glioma, ependymoma, meningioma
Tuberous sclerosis	*TSC1* (9q) *TSC2* (16p)	Hamartin (unknown function) Tuberin (GTPase activating protein)	Astrocytoma
von Hippel-Lindau[a]	*VHL* (3p)	pVHL (modulator of cellular hypoxic response)	Hemangioblastoma of retina, cerebellum and spinal cord; pheochromocytoma
Li-Fraumeni[a]	*p53* (17p)	TP53 (cell cycle and transcriptional regulator)	Malignant glioma
Retinoblastoma[a]	*RB1* (13q)	RB (cell cycle regulator)	Retinoblastoma, pineoblastoma, malignant glioma
Turcot	*APC* (5q) (adenomatous polyposis coli)	APC (cell adhesion)	Medulloblastoma, malignant glioma
Gorlin (basal cell nevus syndrome)	*PTCH* (9q) (patched)	PTH (developmental regulator)	Medulloblastoma
Multiple endocrine neoplasia 1 (Werner syndrome)[a]	*MEN1* (11q13)	Menin (cofactor for transcription)	Pituitary adenoma, malignant schwannoma

[a] Genetic testing possible.

glioma with additional chromosomal alterations. The second route is characterized by the de novo appearance of a malignant glioma with amplification of the *EGFR* gene and an intact *p53* gene. In both pathways, inactivation of the *PTEN* gene as a result of the loss of chromosome 10 occurs frequently.

ASTROCYTOMAS Tumors with astrocytic cytologic features are the most common primary intracranial neoplasms (Fig. 358-2). The most widely used histologic grading system is the World Health Organization four-tiered grading system. Grade I is reserved for special histologic variants of astrocytoma that have an excellent prognosis after surgical excision. These include *juvenile pilocytic astrocytoma*, *subependymal giant cell astrocytoma* (which occurs in patients with tuberous sclerosis), and *pleiomorphic xanthoastrocytoma*. At the other extreme is grade IV, *glioblastoma multiforme*, a clinically aggressive tumor. *Astrocytoma* (grade II) and *anaplastic astrocytoma* (grade III) are intermediate in their histologic and clinical manifestations. The histologic features associated with higher grade are hypercellularity, nuclear and cytoplasmic atypia, endothelial proliferation, mitotic activity, and necrosis. Endothelial proliferation and necrosis are predictors of aggressive behavior.

A limitation of all grading schemes, especially when applied to a single biopsy, is that astrocytic tumors are histologically variable from region to region, and their histopathology may change with time. It is common for low-grade astrocytomas to progress over time to a higher histopathologic grade and a more aggressive clinical course.

Quantitative measures of mitotic activity also correlate with prognosis. The proliferation index can be determined by immunohistochemical staining with antibodies to the proliferating cell nuclear antigen (PCNA) or with a monoclonal antibody termed *Ki-67*, which recognizes a histone protein expressed in proliferating but not quiescent cells. These measures provide estimates of DNA synthesis and correlate with malignant clinical behavior of the tumor.

The overall prognosis is poor. In a representative Finnish population, the median survival was 93.5 months for patients with grade I or II astrocytomas, 12.4 months for patients with grade III (anaplastic astrocytoma), and 5.1 months for patients with grade IV (glioblastoma) tumors. In the United States, the median survival of patients with high-grade brain tumors is ~12 months. Clinical features that correlate with poor prognosis include age >65 and a poor functional status, as defined by the Karnofsky performance scale.

Low-Grade Astrocytoma Low-grade astrocytomas are more common in children than adults. Pilocytic astrocytoma, named for its characteristic spindle-shaped cells, is the most common childhood brain tumor. It frequently occurs in the cerebellum. Typically, this tumor is cystic and well demarcated from adjacent brain. Complete surgical excision usually produces long-term, disease-free survival.

The optimal management of grade II astrocytomas, termed *fibril-

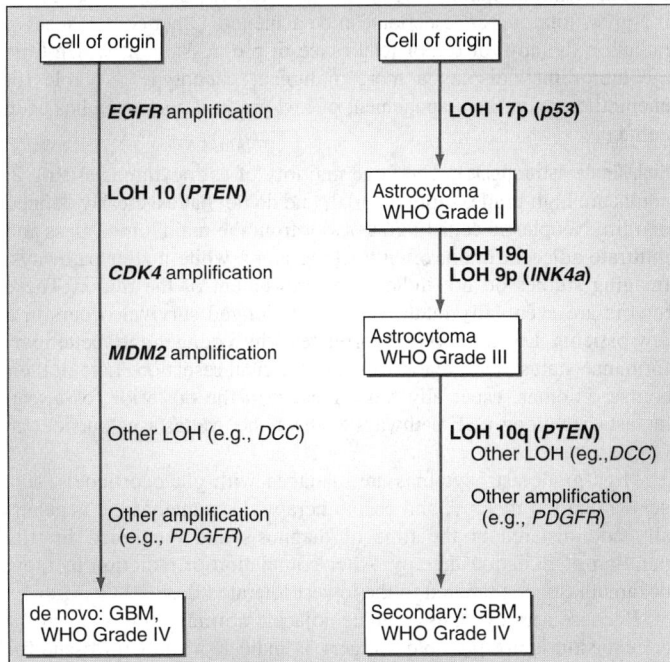

FIGURE 358-1 Model for the pathogenesis of human astrocytoma. Glioblastoma multiforme (GBM) typically presents without evidence of a precursor lesion, referred to as de novo GBM, frequently associated with amplification of the epidermal growth factor receptor (*EGFR*) gene. Less commonly, GBM arises in association with progressive genetic alterations after the diagnosis of a lower grade astrocytoma. These tumors are referred to as secondary GBM. The most widely described alterations are mutations of *p53* and *INK4a*. Other genes implicated in the development of these primary brain tumors include *CDK4*, *MDM2*, *DDC*, and *PDGFR*. LOH, loss of heterozygosity.

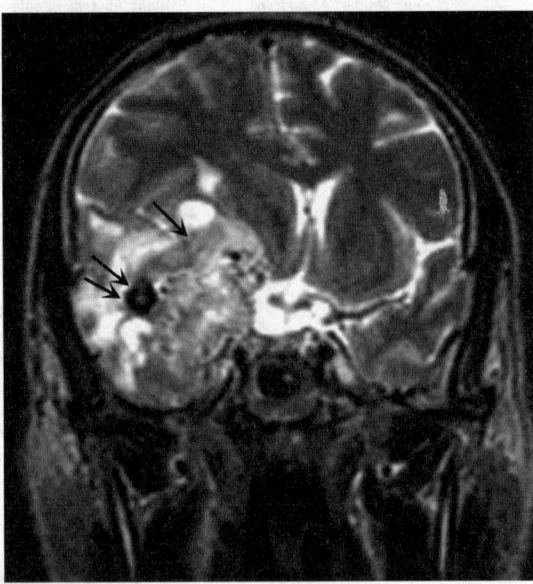

FIGURE 358-2 Malignant astrocytoma (glioblastoma). Coronal proton density–weighted MR scan through the temporal lobes demonstrates a heterogeneous right temporal lobe mass (*arrows*) compressing the third and lateral ventricles. The area of hypointense signal (*double arrows*) indicates either hemorrhage or calcification. Heterogeneous MR signal intensity is typical of glioblastoma.

lary astrocytomas, is controversial. For patients who are symptomatic from mass effect or poorly controlled epilepsy, surgical excision can relieve symptoms. For patients who are asymptomatic or minimally symptomatic at presentation, a diagnostic biopsy should be performed and, when surgically feasible, the tumor may be resected. The indications for postoperative radiation therapy are uncertain. In many centers, when only a biopsy or partial resection is possible, postoperative external beam radiation therapy is administered, whereas it is not used if a gross total tumor resection can be achieved. Other centers reserve radiation therapy for tumor recurrence or progression, at which time the tumor may display a more malignant phenotype. No role for chemotherapy in the management of low-grade astrocytoma has been defined.

High-Grade Astrocytoma   The large majority of astrocytomas arising in adults are high grade, supratentorial, and do not have a clearly defined margin. Neoplastic cells migrate away from the main tumor mass and infiltrate adjacent brain, often tracking along white matter pathways. Imaging studies do not indicate the full extent of the tumor. These tumors are eventually fatal, although prolonged survival occurs in a few patients. Longer survival correlates with younger age, better performance status, and greater extent of surgical resection. Late in their course, gliomas, especially those located in the posterior fossa, can metastasize along CSF pathways to the spine. Metastases outside the CNS are rare.

High-grade astrocytomas are managed with glucocorticoids, surgery, radiation therapy, and chemotherapy. Dexamethasone is generally administered at the time of diagnosis and continued for the duration of radiation therapy. After completion of radiation therapy, dexamethasone is tapered to the lowest tolerated dose.

Because astrocytomas infiltrate adjacent normal brain, total surgical excision is not possible. Surgery is indicated to obtain tissue for pathologic diagnosis and to control mass effect. Moreover, retrospective studies indicate that the extent of tumor resection correlates with survival, at least in younger patients. Therefore, accessible astrocytomas are resected aggressively in patients <65 years old who are in good general medical condition.

Postoperative radiation therapy prolongs survival and improves quality of life, although the duration of benefit is only a few months. Treated with dexamethasone alone following surgery, the mean sur-

vival of patients <65 years with glioblastoma is 7 to 9 months. Survival is prolonged to 11 to 13 months with radiation therapy. Focal brain irradiation is less toxic and is as effective as whole-brain radiation for primary glial tumors. Radiation is generally administered to the tumor mass, as defined by contrast enhancement on a CT or MRI scan, plus a 3- to 4-cm margin. A total dose of 5000 to 7000 cGy is administered in 25 to 35 equal fractions, 5 days per week.

The roles of stereotaxic radiosurgery and interstitial brachytherapy in glioma treatment are uncertain. *Stereotaxic radiosurgery* is the administration of a focused high dose of radiation to a precisely defined volume of tissue in a single treatment. Stereotaxic radiosurgery can potentially achieve tumor ablation within the treated volume. A major limitation of stereotaxic radiosurgery is that it can be used for only relatively small tumors, generally <4 cm in maximum diameter. *Interstitial brachytherapy*, the implantation of radioactive material into the tumor mass, is generally reserved for tumor recurrence because of its associated toxicity—in particular, necrosis of adjacent brain tissue.

Chemotherapy is marginally effective and is often used as an adjuvant therapy following surgery and radiation therapy. Nitrosoureas, including carmustine (BCNU) and lomustine (CCNU), are the most effective available agents. Since a typical glioma infiltrates normal brain where the blood-brain barrier is relatively intact, lipid-soluble agents such as the nitrosoureas, which cross the blood-brain barrier, may reach more malignant cells than water-soluble agents. Temozolomide is an orally administered alkylating agent, has activity against gliomas, and is generally better tolerated than the nitrosoureas. Experimental approaches include intraarterial infusion of chemotherapy, the implantation of chemotherapy-releasing wafers or injection of chemotherapeutic agents into the tumor resection cavity, and administration of chemotherapy after disruption of the blood-brain barrier.

Gliomatosis cerebri is a rare form of astrocytoma in which there is diffuse infiltration of the brain by malignant astrocytes without a focal enhancing mass. It generally presents as a multifocal CNS syndrome or a more generalized disorder including dementia, personality change, or seizures. Neuroimaging studies are often nonspecific, and biopsy is required to establish the diagnosis. Gliomatosis cerebri is treated with whole-brain radiation therapy and, in selected patients, with radiation to the entire neuroaxis and systemic chemotherapy.

OLIGODENDROGLIOMAS   Oligodendrogliomas, which comprise about 15% of gliomas in adults, have a more benign course and are more responsive to cytotoxic treatment than astrocytomas. Five-year survival is >50%, and 10-year survival is 25 to 34%.

Oligodendrogliomas occur chiefly in supratentorial locations; in adults, ~30% contain areas of calcification (Fig. 358-3). Many gliomas contain mixtures of cells with astrocytic and oligodendroglial features. If this mixed histology is prominent, the tumor is termed a *mixed glioma* or an *oligoastrocytoma*. The greater the oligodendroglial component, the more benign the clinical course. As a rule, oligodendrogliomas are less infiltrative than astrocytomas, permitting more complete surgical excision. Histologic features of mitoses, necrosis, and nuclear atypia are associated with a more aggressive clinical course. If these features are prominent, the tumor is termed an *anaplastic oligodendroglioma*.

Surgery, at minimum a stereotaxic biopsy, is necessary to establish a diagnosis. Many oligodendrogliomas are amenable to gross total surgical resection. In addition, oligodendrogliomas may respond dramatically to systemic combination chemotherapy with procarbazine, lomustine, and vincristine (PCV). Oligodendrogliomas with deletions of chromosome 1p always respond to PCV, but only ~25% of oligodendrogliomas lacking 1p deletion respond to chemotherapy. The simultaneous deletion of 1p and 19q predicts a durable response to chemotherapy (>31 months on average) and survival >10 years. Many centers therefore use 1p deletion as an indication for adjuvant or neo-adjuvant chemotherapy and reserve external beam irradiation for tumor recurrence.

EPENDYMOMAS   In adults ependymomas are typically located in the spinal canal, especially in the lumbosacral region. They typically arise from the filum terminale of the spinal cord and have a myxopapillary histology, with a papillary arrangement of cells and mucin production. In children, ependymomas occur within the ventricles, most often the fourth ventricle, and have a different histology, typically with ependymal rosettes. Ependymomas with histologic signs of malignancy, including cellular atypia, frequent mitotic figures, or a high labeling index virtually always recur after surgical resection. Imaging with CT or MRI scans reveals ependymomas as uniformly enhancing masses that are relatively well demarcated from adjacent neural tissue. Ependymomas may metastasize via CSF pathways: brain tumor metastases that spread to the spinal cord by this means are termed *drop metastases*.

Following the gross total excision of an ependymoma, the prognosis is excellent. The 5-year disease-free survival is >80%. However, many ependymomas cannot be totally excised, and postoperative focal external beam radiation or stereotaxic radiosurgery is used. Whether focal radiation is adequate or whether the entire neuraxis needs to be irradiated is not known.

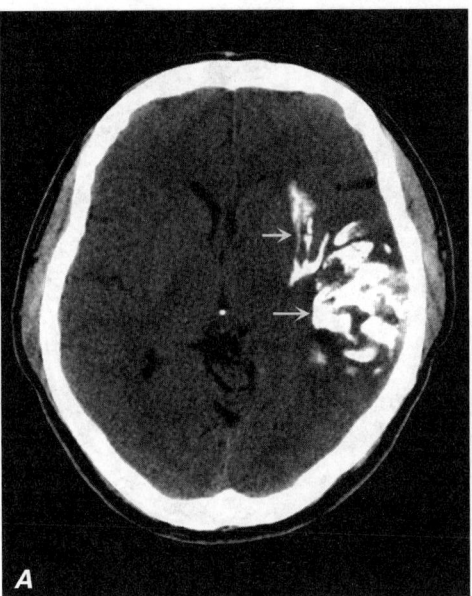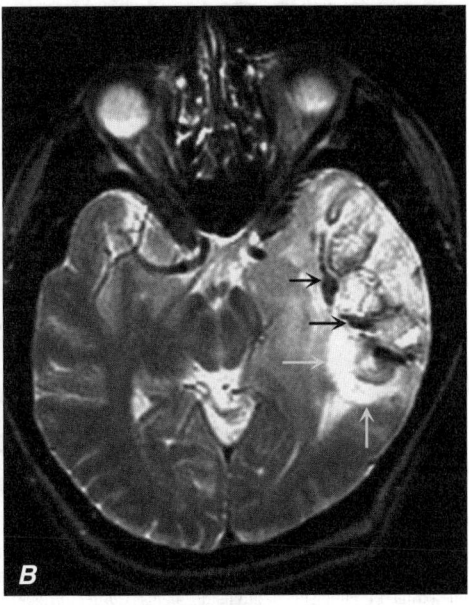

FIGURE 358-3 Oligodendroglioma. *A.* Noncontrast CT scan reveals a calcified mass involving the left temporal lobe (*arrows*) associated with mild mass effect but little edema. *B.* An MR T2-weighted image demonstrates a heterogeneous mass with hypointense signal (*black arrows*) surrounded by a zone of higher signal intensity (*white arrows*), consistent with a calcified temporal lobe mass. The tumor extends into the left medial temporal lobe and compresses the midbrain.

GERMINOMAS These tumors most commonly present during the second decade of life, generally at sites within or adjacent to the third ventricle, including the pineal region. Germinomas are the most frequent variety of *germ cell tumor*, a tumor type arising in midline structures and including *teratoma*, yolk sac tumor (*endodermal sinus tumor*), *embryonal carcinoma*, and *choriocarcinoma*. Germinomas of the CNS may be benign but are more often aggressive and invasive. Due to their location, patients frequently present with hypothalamic-pituitary dysfunction including diabetes insipidus, visual field deficits, disturbances of memory or mood, or hydrocephalus (Chap. 318). Neuroimaging demonstrates germinomas to be uniformly enhancing masses that may not have well-defined borders. The treatment of choice is complete surgical resection. For unresectable tumors, a stereotaxic biopsy is performed for diagnosis, and focal radiation is the primary therapy. When the extent of disease or very young age precludes radiotherapy as primary treatment, platinum-based chemotherapy may decrease tumor size and facilitate subsequent radiation therapy of residual disease or recurrent tumor. Prognosis depends on the histology and surgical resectability of the tumor. Germinomas are generally radiosensitive and chemosensitive. Five year survival is >85%.

MEDULLOBLASTOMAS AND PRIMITIVE NEUROECTODERMAL TUMORS (PNET)
These highly cellular malignant tumors are thought to arise from neural precursor cells. Medulloblastomas of the posterior fossa are the most frequent malignant brain tumor of children. PNET is a term applied to tumors histologically indistinguishable from medulloblastoma but occurring either in adults or supratentorially in children. In adults, >50% present in the posterior fossa. These tumors frequently disseminate along CSF pathways.

If possible, these tumors should be surgically excised, although outcome is not related to the extent of surgery. In adults, surgical excision of a PNET should be followed by chemotherapy and irradiation of the entire neuraxis, with a boost in radiation dose to the primary tumor. If the tumor is not disseminated at presentation, the prognosis is generally favorable. Aggressive treatment can result in prolonged survival, although half of adult patients relapse within 5 years of treatment.

CNS LYMPHOMA ■ **Primary CNS Lymphoma** These are high-grade B cell malignancies that present within the neuraxis without evidence of systemic lymphoma. They occur most frequently in immunocompromised individuals, specifically organ transplant recipients or patients with AIDS (Chap. 173). In immunocompromised patients, CNS lymphomas are invariably associated with Epstein-Barr virus infection of the tumor cells.

In immunocompetent patients, neuroimaging studies most often reveal a uniformly enhancing mass lesion. In immunocompromised patients, primary CNS lymphoma is likely to be multicentric and exhibit ring enhancement or to arise in the meninges (Fig. 358-4). Stereotaxic needle biopsy can be used to establish the diagnosis. Leptomeningeal involvement is present in ~15% of patients at presentation and in 50% at some time during the course of the illness. Moreover, the disease extends to the eyes in up to 15% of patients. Therefore, a slit-lamp examination and, if indicated, anterior chamber paracentesis or vitreous biopsy is necessary to define radiation ports.

The prognosis of primary CNS lymphoma is poor compared to histologically similar lymphoma occurring outside the CNS. Many patients experience a dramatic clinical and radiographic response to glucocorticoids; however, relapse almost invariably occurs within weeks. The mainstay of definitive therapy is chemotherapy including high-dose methotrexate. This is followed in patients <60 years with whole-brain irradiation. Whole-brain irradiation is postponed as long as possible in patients >60 because of the risk of dementia as a manifestation of late-delayed radiation toxicity. Consolidation therapy is with high-dose cytarabine. Intraarterial chemotherapy with or without blood-brain barrier disruption is an alternative. Intrathecal chemotherapy with methotrexate can be added if leptomeningeal disease is present. Despite aggressive therapy, >90% of patients develop recurrent CNS disease. Historically, the survival of immunocompetent patients with CNS lymphoma has been ~18 months but is now longer with the use of systemic chemotherapy. In organ transplant recipients, reversal of the immunosuppressed state can improve outcome. Survival with AIDS-related primary CNS lymphoma is very poor, generally ≤3 months; pretreatment performance status, the degree of immunosuppression, and the extent of CNS dissemination at diagnosis all appear to influence outcome.

Secondary CNS Lymphoma Secondary CNS lymphoma is a manifestation of systemic disease and almost always occurs in adults with progressive B cell lymphoma or B cell leukemia who have tumor involvement of bone, bone marrow, testes, or the cranial sinuses. Leptomeningeal lymphoma is usually detectable with contrast-enhanced CT or gado-

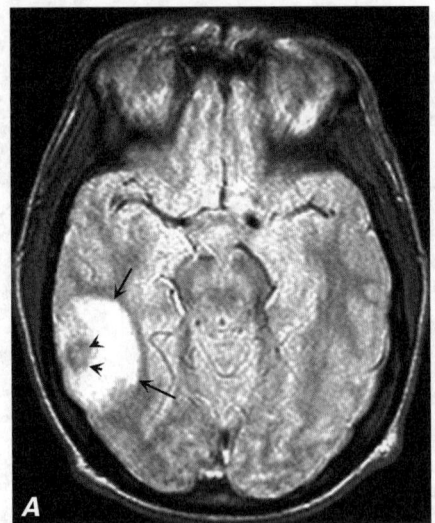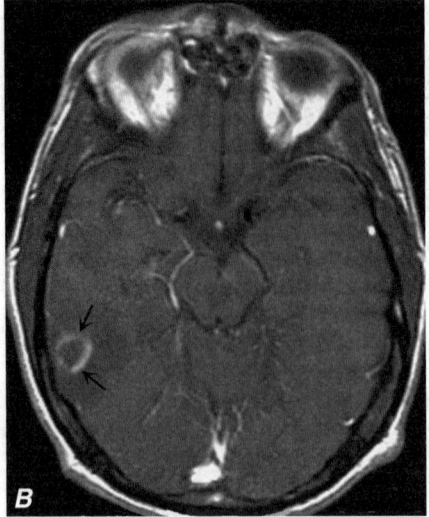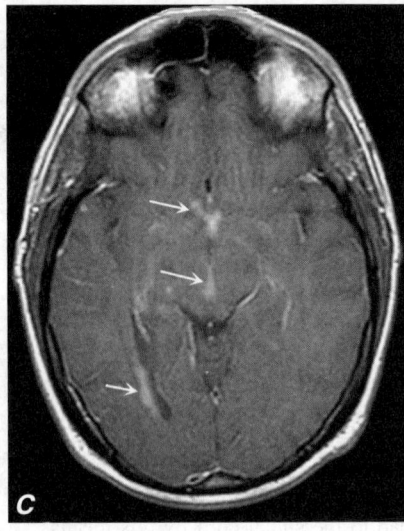

FIGURE 358-4 CNS lymphoma. *A.* Proton density–weighted MR image through the temporal lobe demonstrates a low signal intensity nodule (*small arrows*) surrounded by a ring of high signal intensity edema (*larger arrows*). *B.* T1-weighted contrast-enhanced axial MRI demonstrates ring enhancement surrounded by a nonenhanced rim of edema. In this patient with AIDS, a solitary lesion of this type is consistent with either lymphoma or toxoplasmosis; the presence of multiple lesions favors toxoplasmosis. *C.* In a different patient with lymphomatous meningitis, an axial postcontrast T1-weighted MRI through the midbrain demonstrates multiple areas of abnormal enhancement in periventricular and subependymal regions (*arrows*). Lymphoma tends to spread subependymally at interfaces of CSF and brain parenchyma.

linium-enhanced MRI of the brain and spine or by CSF examination. Treatment consists of systemic chemotherapy, intrathecal chemotherapy, and CNS irradiation. It is usually possible to suppress the leptomeningeal disease effectively, although the overall prognosis is determined by the course of the systemic lymphoma.

PITUITARY ADENOMAS See Chap. 318.

MENINGIOMAS Meningiomas are derived from mesoderm, probably from cells giving rise to the arachnoid granulations. These tumors are usually benign and attached to the dura. They may invade the skull but only infrequently invade the brain. Meningiomas most often occur along the sagittal sinus, over the cerebral convexities, in the cerebellar-pontine angle, and along the dorsum of the spinal cord. They are more frequent in women than men, with a peak incidence in middle age.

Meningiomas may be found incidentally on a CT or MRI scan or may present with a focal seizure, a slowly progressive neurologic deficit, or symptoms of raised ICP. The radiologic image of a dural-based, extraaxial mass with dense, uniform contrast enhancement is essentially diagnostic, although a dural metastasis must also be considered (Fig. 358-5). A meningioma may have a "dural tail," a streak of dural enhancement flanking the main tumor mass; however, this finding may also be present with other dural tumors.

Total surgical resection of benign meningiomas is curative. If a total resection cannot be achieved, local external beam radiotherapy or stereotaxic radiosurgery reduces the recurrence rate to <10%. For meningiomas that are not surgically accessible, targeted radiosurgery or heavy particle radiation should be considered. Small asymptomatic meningiomas incidentally discovered in older patients can safely be followed radiologically; these tumors grow at an average rate of ~0.24 cm in diameter per year and only rarely become symptomatic.

Rare meningiomas invade the brain or have histologic evidence of malignancy such as nuclear pleomorphism and cellular atypia. A high mitotic index is also predictive of aggressive behavior. *Hemangiopericytoma*, although not strictly a meningioma, is a meningeal tumor with an especially aggressive behavior. Meningiomas with features of aggressiveness and hemangiopericytomas, even if totally excised by gross inspection, frequently recur and should receive postoperative radiotherapy. Chemotherapy has no proven benefit.

SCHWANNOMAS These tumors are also called *neuromas, neurinomas,* or *neurolemmomas.* They arise from Schwann cells of nerve roots, most frequently in the eighth cranial nerve (*vestibular schwannoma,* formerly termed *acoustic schwannoma*). The fifth cranial nerve is the second most frequent site; however, schwannomas may arise from any cranial or spinal root except the optic and olfactory nerves, which are myelinated by oligodendroglia rather than Schwann cells. NF type 2 (see below) strongly predisposes to vestibular schwannoma. Schwannomas of spinal nerve roots also occur in patients with NF type 2 as well as patients with NF type 1.

Eighth nerve schwannomas typically arise from the vestibular division of the nerve. They are densely and uniformly enhancing neoplasms on MRI (Fig. 358-6). Vestibular schwannomas enlarge the internal auditory canal, an imaging feature that helps distinguish them from other cerebellopontine angle masses. Because the vestibular system adapts to slow destruction of the eighth nerve, vestibular schwannomas characteristically present as progressive unilateral hearing loss rather than with dizziness or other vestibular symptoms. Unexplained unilateral hearing loss merits evaluation with audiometry and either brainstem auditory evoked potentials or an MRI scan (Chap. 26). As

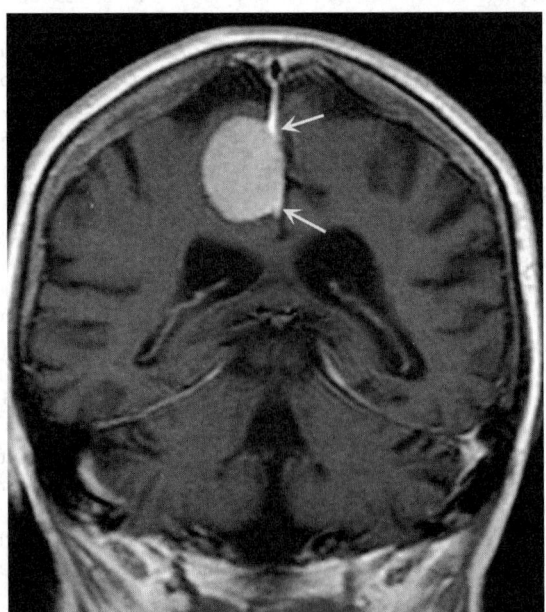

FIGURE 358-5 Meningioma. Coronal postcontrast T1-weighted MR image demonstrates an enhancing extraaxial mass arising from the falx cerebri (*arrows*). There is a "dural tail" of contrast enhancement extending superiorly along the intrahemispheric septum.

a vestibular schwannoma grows, it can compress the cerebellum, pons, or facial nerve. With rare exceptions schwannomas are histologically and clinically benign.

Whenever possible, schwannomas should be surgically excised. When the tumors are small, it is usually possible to preserve hearing in the involved ear. In the case of large tumors, the patient is usually deaf at presentation; nonetheless, surgery is indicated to prevent further compression of posterior fossa structures. Stereotaxic radiosurgery is also effective treatment for schwannoma and has a complication rate equivalent to that of surgery.

OTHER BENIGN BRAIN TUMORS *Epidermoid tumors* are cystic tumors with proliferative epidermal cells at the periphery and more mature epidermal cells towards the center of the cyst. The mature cells desquamate into the liquid center of the cyst. Epidermoid tumors are thought to arise from embryonic epidermal rests within the cranium. They occur extraaxially near the midline, in the middle cranial fossa, the suprasellar region, or the cerebellopontine angle. These well-demarcated lesions are amenable to complete surgical excision. Postoperative radiation therapy is unnecessary.

Dermoid cysts are thought to arise from embryonic rests of skin tissue trapped within the CNS during closure of the neural tube. The most frequent locations are in the midline supratentorially or at the cerebellopontine angle. Histologically, they are composed of all elements of the dermis, including epidermis, hair follicles, and sweat glands; they frequently calcify. Treatment is surgical excision.

Craniopharyngiomas are thought to arise from remnants of Rathke's pouch, the mesodermal structure from which the anterior pituitary gland is derived (Chap. 318). Craniopharyngiomas typically present as suprasellar masses. Histologically, craniopharyngiomas resemble epidermoid tumors; they are usually cystic, and in adults 80% are calcified. Because of their location, they may present as growth failure in children, endocrine dysfunction in adults, or visual loss in either age group. Treatment is surgical excision; postoperative external beam radiation or stereotaxic radiosurgery is added if total surgical removal cannot be achieved.

Colloid cysts are benign tumors of unknown cellular origin that occur within the third ventricle and can obstruct CSF flow. *Rare benign primary brain tumors* include neurocytomas, subependymomas, and pleomorphic xanthoastrocytomas. Surgical excision of these neoplasms is the primary treatment and can be curative.

NEUROCUTANEOUS SYNDROMES

This group of genetic disorders, also known as the *phakomatoses*, produces a variety of developmental abnormalities of skin along with an increased risk of nervous system tumors (Table 358-1). These disorders are inherited as autosomal dominant conditions with variable penetrance.

NEUROFIBROMATOSIS TYPE 1 (VON RECKLINGHAUSEN'S DISEASE) NF1 is characterized by cutaneous *neurofibromas*, pigmented lesions of the skin called *café au lait spots*, freckling in non-sun-exposed areas such as the axilla, hamartomas of the iris termed *Lisch nodules*, and pseudoarthrosis of the tibia. Neurofibromas are benign peripheral nerve tumors composed of proliferating Schwann cells and fibroblasts. They present as multiple, palpable, rubbery, cutaneous tumors. They are generally asymptomatic; however, if they grow in an enclosed space, e.g., the intervertebral foramen, they may produce a compressive radiculopathy or neuropathy. Aqueductal stenosis with hydrocephalus, scoliosis, short stature, hypertension, epilepsy, and mental retardation may also occur.

Patients with NF1 are at increased risk of developing nervous system neoplasms, including plexiform neurofibromas, optic pathway gliomas, ependymomas, meningiomas, astrocytomas, and pheochro-

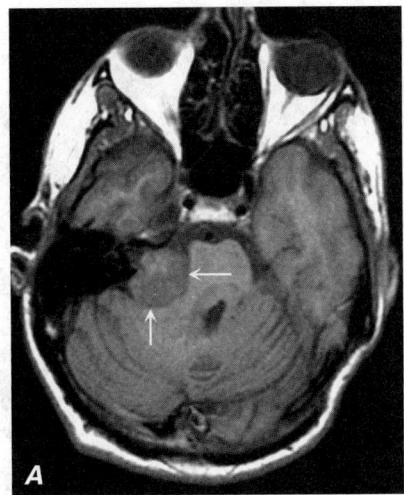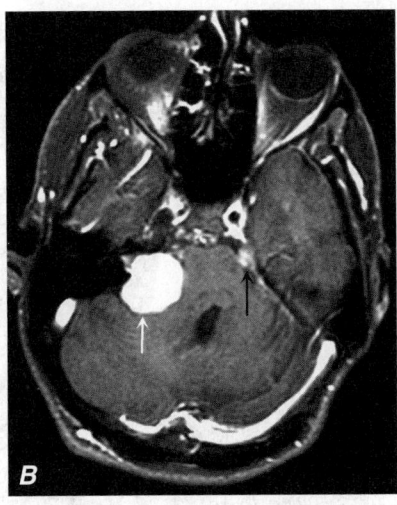

FIGURE 358-6 Vestibular schwannoma. *A.* Axial noncontrast MR scan through the cerebellopontine angle demonstrates an extraaxial mass that extends into a widened internal auditory canal, displacing the pons (*arrows*). *B.* Postcontrast T1-weighted image demonstrates intense enhancement of the vestibular schwannoma (*white arrow*). Abnormal enhancement of the left fifth nerve (*black arrow*) most likely represents another schwannoma in this patient with neurofibromatosis type 2.

mocytomas. Neurofibromas may undergo secondary malignant degeneration and become sarcomatous.

Mutation of the *NF1* gene on chromosome 17 causes von Recklinghausen's disease. The *NF1* gene is a tumor-suppressor gene; it encodes a protein, *neurofibromin*, which modulates signal transduction through the *ras* GTPase pathway.

NEUROFIBROMATOSIS TYPE 2 NF2 is characterized by the development of bilateral vestibular schwannomas in >90% of individuals who inherit the gene. Patients with NF2 also have a predisposition for the development of meningiomas, gliomas, and schwannomas of cranial and spinal nerves. In addition, a characteristic type of cataract, juvenile posterior subcapsular lenticular opacity, occurs in NF2. Multiple café au lait spots and peripheral neurofibromas occur rarely.

In patients with NF2, vestibular schwannomas usually present with progressive unilateral deafness early in the third decade of life. Bilateral vestibular schwannomas are generally detectable by MRI at that time (Fig. 358-6). Surgical management is designed to treat the underlying tumor and preserve hearing as long as possible.

This syndrome is caused by mutation of the *NF2* gene on chromosome 22q; *NF2* encodes a protein called *neurofibromin 2, schwannomin,* or *merlin,* with homology to a family of cytoskeletal proteins that includes moesin, ezrin, and radixin.

TUBEROUS SCLEROSIS (BOURNEVILLE'S DISEASE) Tuberous sclerosis is characterized by cutaneous lesions, seizures, and mental retardation. The cutaneous lesions include adenoma sebaceum (facial angiofibromas), ash leaf–shaped hypopigmented macules (best seen under ultraviolet illumination with a Wood's lamp), shagreen patches (yellowish thickenings of the skin over the lumbosacral region of the back), and depigmented nevi. On neuroimaging studies, the presence of subependymal nodules, which may be calcified, is characteristic. Patients inheriting the tuberous sclerosis gene are at increased risk of developing ependymomas and childhood astrocytomas, of which >90% are *subependymal giant cell astrocytomas.* These are benign neoplasms that may develop in the retina or along the border of the lateral ventricles. They may obstruct the foramen of Monro and produce hydrocephalus. Rhabdomyomas of the myocardium and angiomyomas of the kidney, liver, adrenals, and pancreas may also occur.

Treatment is symptomatic. Anticonvulsants for seizures, shunting for hydrocephalus, and behavioral and educational strategies for mental retardation are the mainstays of management. Severely affected individuals generally die before age 30.

Mutations at both 9q(*TSC-1*) and 16p(*TSC-2*) are associated with tuberous sclerosis. The mutated genes encode *tuberins*, proteins that modulate the GTPase activity of other cellular proteins.

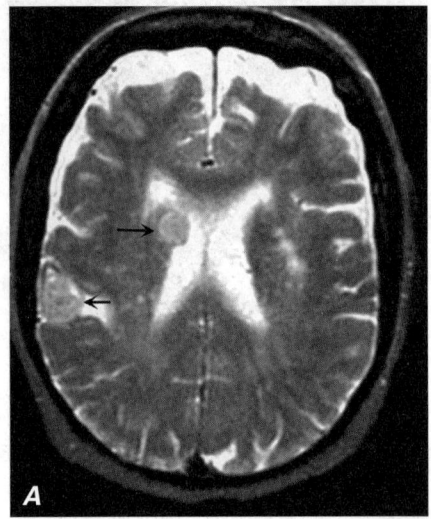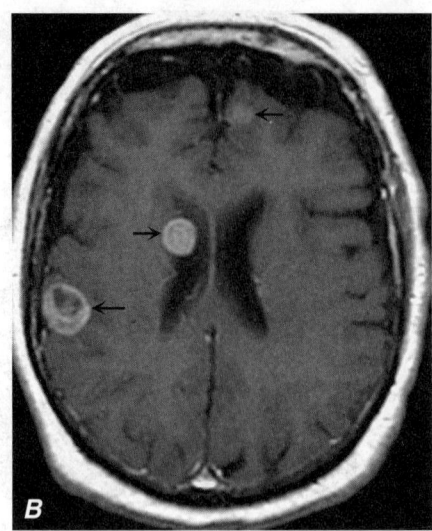

FIGURE 358-7 Brain metastasis. *A.* Axial T2-weighted MRI through the lateral ventricles reveals two isodense masses, one in the subependymal region and one near the cortex (*arrows*). *B.* T1-weighted postcontrast image at the same level as *A* reveals enhancement of the two masses seen on the T2-weighted image as well as a third mass in the left frontal lobe (*arrows*).

Small metastases often enhance uniformly. Larger metastases typically produce ring enhancement surrounding a central mass of nonenhancing necrotic tissue that develops as the metastasis outgrows its blood supply. Metastases are surrounded by variable amounts of edema. Blood products may also be seen, reflecting hemorrhage of abnormal tumor vessels.

The radiologic appearance of a brain metastasis is not specific. The differential diagnosis of ring-enhancement lesions includes brain abscess, radiation necrosis, toxoplasmosis, granulomas (tuberculosis, sarcoidosis), demyelinating lesions, primary brain tumors, primary CNS lymphoma, stroke, hemorrhage, and trauma. Contrast-enhanced CT scanning is less sensitive than MRI for the detection of brain metastases. Cytologic examination of the CSF is not indicated, since intraparenchymal brain metastases almost never shed cells into the CSF. Measuring CSF levels of tumor markers such as carcinoembryonic antigen (CEA) is rarely helpful in management.

VON HIPPEL–LINDAU SYNDROME This syndrome consists of retinal, cerebellar, and spinal hemangioblastomas, which are slowly growing cystic tumors. Hypernephroma, renal cell carcinoma, pheochromocytoma, and benign cysts of the kidneys, pancreas, epididymis, or liver may also occur. Erythropoietin production by hemangioblastomas may result in polycythemia. The von Hippel–Lindau (*VHL*) gene on chromosome 3p is a tumor suppressor that encodes a protein with multiple functions, including mediating signal transduction in response to cellular hypoxia.

TUMORS METASTATIC TO BRAIN

MECHANISMS OF BRAIN METASTASES The large majority of brain metastases disseminate by hematogenous spread. The anatomic distribution of brain metastases generally parallels regional cerebral blood flow, with a predilection for the gray matter–white matter junction and for the border zone between middle cerebral and posterior cerebral artery distributions. The lung is the most common origin of brain metastases; both primary lung cancer (adenocarcinoma and small cell lung cancer) and cancers metastatic to the lung can metastasize to the brain. Breast cancer (especially ductal carcinoma) has a propensity to metastasize to the cerebellum and the posterior pituitary gland. Moreover, breast cancer that metastasizes to bone tends not to metastasize to the brain. Other common origins of brain metastases are gastrointestinal malignancies, and melanoma (Table 358-2). Certain less common tumors have a special propensity to metastasize to brain, including germ cell tumors and thyroid cancer. By contrast, prostate cancer, ovarian cancer, and Hodgkin's disease rarely metastasize to the brain.

EVALUATION OF METASTASES FROM KNOWN CANCER On MRI scans brain metastases typically appear as well-demarcated, approximately spherical lesions that are hypointense or isointense relative to brain on T1-weighted images and bright on T2-weighted images. They invariably enhance with gadolinium, reflecting extravasation of gadolinium through tumor vessels that lack a blood-tumor barrier (Fig. 358-7).

BRAIN METASTASES WITHOUT A KNOWN PRIMARY TUMOR In general hospital populations, up to one-third of patients presenting with brain metastases do not have a known underlying cancer. These patients generally present with either a seizure or a progressive neurologic deficit. Neuroimaging studies demonstrate one or multiple ring-enhancement lesions. In individuals who are not immunocompromised and not at risk for brain abscesses, this radiologic pattern is most likely due to brain metastasis.

Diagnostic evaluation begins with a search for the primary tumor. Blood tests should include CEA and liver function tests. Examination of the skin for melanoma and the thyroid gland for masses should be carried out. A CT scan of the chest, abdomen, and pelvis should be obtained. If these are all negative, further imaging studies, including bone scan, other radionuclide scans, mammography, and upper and lower gastrointestinal barium studies, are unlikely to be productive. The search for a primary cancer most often discloses lung cancer, particularly small cell lung cancer, or melanoma. In 30% of patients no primary tumor can be identified, even after extensive evaluation.

A tissue diagnosis is essential. If a primary tumor is found, it will usually be more accessible to biopsy than a brain lesion. If a single brain lesion is found in a surgically accessible location, if a primary tumor is not found, or if the primary tumor is in a location difficult to biopsy, the brain metastasis should be biopsied or resected.

℞ TREATMENT

Once a systemic cancer metastasizes to the brain it is, with rare exception, incurable. Therapy is therefore palliative, designed to prevent disability and suffering and, if possible, to prolong life. Published outcome studies have focused on survival as the primary end point, leaving questions regarding quality of life unanswered. There is, however, widespread agreement that glucocorticoids, anticonvulsants, and radiation therapy improve the quality of life for many patients. The roles of surgery and chemotherapy are less well established.

General Measures Glucocorticoids frequently ameliorate symptoms of brain metastases. Improvement is often dramatic, occurs within 24 h, and is sustained with continued administration, although the toxicity of glucocorticoids is cumulative. Therefore, if possible, a more definitive therapy for metastases should be instituted to permit withdrawal of glucocorticoid therapy. One-third of patients with brain metastases have one or more seizures. Anticonvulsants are used empirically for seizure prophylaxis when supratentorial metastases are present.

Specific Measures ■ *RADIATION THERAPY* Radiation is the primary treatment for brain metastases. Since multiple microscopic deposits of tu-

TABLE 358-2	*Frequency of Nervous System Metastases by Common Primary Tumors*		
Site of Primary Tumor	Brain Metastases, %	Leptomeningeal Metastases, %	Spinal Cord Compression, %
Lung	40	24	18
Breast	19	41	24
Melanoma	10	12	4
Gastrointestinal tract	7	13	6
Genitourinary tract	7		18
Other	17	10	30

mor cells throughout the brain are likely to be present in addition to metastases visualized by neuroimaging studies, whole-brain irradiation is usually used. Its benefit has been established in controlled studies, but no clear dose response has been shown. Usually, 30 to 37.5 Gy is administered in 10 to 15 fractions; an additional dose ("boost") of focal irradiation to a single or large metastasis may also be administered. Stereotaxic radiosurgery is of benefit in patients with four or fewer metastases demonstrable by MRI.

SURGERY Up to 40% of patients with brain metastases have only a single tumor mass identified by CT. Accessible single metastases are usually surgically excised as a palliative measure. If the systemic disease is under control, total resection of a single brain lesion has been demonstrated to improve survival and minimize disability. Survival appears to be improved if surgery is followed by whole-brain irradiation.

CHEMOTHERAPY Brain metastases of certain tumors, including breast cancer, small cell lung cancer, and germ cell tumors, are often responsive to systemic chemotherapy. Although metastases frequently do not respond as well as the primary tumor, dramatic responses to systemic chemotherapy or hormonal therapy may occur in some cases. In patients who are neurologically stable, two to four cycles of systemic chemotherapy may be administered initially to reduce tumor mass and render the residual tumor more amenable to radiation therapy. Even if a complete radiologic remission is achieved from chemotherapy, whole-brain irradiation should then be administered.

EXPERIMENTAL THERAPIES These include gene therapy, immunotherapy, intraarterial chemotherapy, and chemotherapy administered following osmotic disruption of the blood-brain barrier.

LEPTOMENINGEAL METASTASES

Leptomeningeal metastases are also called *carcinomatous meningitis, meningeal carcinomatosis,* and, in the cases of specific tumors, *leukemic meningitis* or *lymphomatous meningitis.* Clinical evidence of leptomeningeal metastases is present in 8% of patients with metastatic solid tumors; at necropsy, the prevalence is as high as 19%. Among solid tumors, adenocarcinomas of the breast, lung, and gastrointestinal tract and melanoma are the most common cause of leptomeningeal metastases (Table 358-2). In one-quarter of patients the systemic cancer is under control; thus effective control of leptomeningeal disease can improve the quality and duration of life.

Cancer usually metastasizes to the meninges via the bloodstream. Alternatively, a superficially located parenchymal brain metastasis may shed cells directly into the subarachnoid space. Some tumors, including squamous cell carcinoma of the skin and some non-Hodgkin's lymphomas, have a propensity to grow along peripheral nerves and may seed the meninges by that route.

CLINICAL FEATURES Leptomeningeal metastases present with signs and symptoms at multiple levels of the nervous system, most often in a setting of known systemic malignancy. Encephalopathy is frequent, and cranial neuropathy or spinal radiculopathy from nodular nerve root compression is characteristic. Hydrocephalus results from obstruction of CSF outflow. Focal neurologic deficits from coexisting intraparenchymal metastases may occur.

LABORATORY EVALUATION Leptomeningeal metastases are diagnosed by cytologic demonstration of malignant cells in the CSF, by MRI demonstration of nodular tumor deposits in the meninges or diffuse meningeal enhancement (Fig. 358-8), or by meningeal biopsy. CSF findings are usually those of an inflammatory meningitis, consisting of lymphocytic pleocytosis, elevated protein levels, and normal or low CSF glucose. A complete MRI examination of the neuraxis may demonstrate hydrocephalus due to obstruction of CSF pathways and identify nodular meningeal metastases.

℞ TREATMENT

In selected patients, intrathecal chemotherapy or focal external beam radiotherapy to sites of nodular leptomeningeal disease is employed.

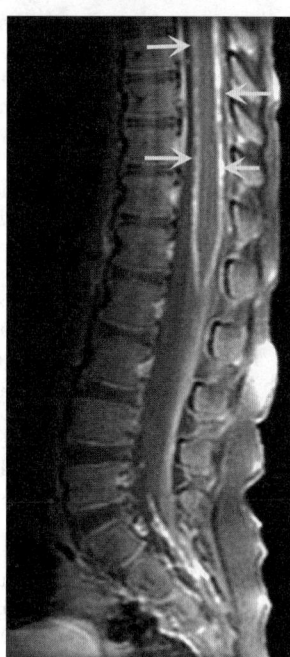

FIGURE 358-8 *Carcinomatous meningitis. Sagittal postcontrast MRI through the lower thoracic region demonstrates diffuse pial enhancement along the surface of the spinal cord (arrows), typical of CSF spread of neoplasm.*

Although the prognosis of leptomeningeal metastases is poor, ~20% of patients treated aggressively for leptomeningeal metastases can expect a response of ≥6 months. Intrathecal therapy exposes meningeal tumor implants to high concentrations of chemotherapy with minimal systemic toxicity. Methotrexate can be safely administered intrathecally and is effective against leptomeningeal metastases from a variety of solid tumors and lymphoma; cytarabine and thiotepa are alternative agents. Intrathecal chemotherapy may be administered either by repeated lumbar puncture or through an indwelling Ommaya reservoir, which consists of a catheter in one lateral ventricle attached to a reservoir implanted under the scalp. If there is a question of patency of CSF pathways, a radionuclide flow study through the reservoir may be performed.

Large, nodular deposits of tumor on the meninges or along nerve roots are unlikely to respond to intrathecal chemotherapy, as the barrier to diffusion is too great. Therefore, external beam radiation is employed. Hydrocephalus is treated with a ventriculoperitoneal shunt, although seeding of the peritoneum by tumor is a risk.

MALIGNANT SPINAL CORD COMPRESSION

Spinal cord compression from solid tumor metastases usually results from expansion of a vertebral metastasis into the epidural space. Primary tumors that frequently metastasize to bone include lung, breast, and prostate cancer. Back pain is usually the first symptom and is prominent at presentation in 90% of patients. The pain is typically dull, aching, and may be associated with localized tenderness. If a nerve root is compressed, radicular pain is also present. The thoracic cord is most often affected. Weakness, sensory loss, and autonomic dysfunction (urinary urgency and incontinence, fecal incontinence, and sexual impotence in men) are the hallmarks of spinal cord compression. Once signs of spinal cord compression appear, they tend to progress rapidly. It is thus essential to recognize and treat this serious complication of malignancy promptly in order to prevent irreversible neurologic deficits. →*Diagnosis and management are discussed in Chap. 356.*

METASTASES TO THE PERIPHERAL NERVOUS SYSTEM

Systemic cancer may compress or invade peripheral nerves. Compression of the brachial plexus may occur by direct extension of Pancoast's tumors (cancer of the apex of the lung) or by extension of local lymph node metastases of breast or lung cancer or lymphoma. The lumbosacral plexus may be compressed by the retroperitoneal spread of prostate or ovarian cancer or lymphoma. Skull metastases may compress cranial nerve branches as they pass through the skull, and pituitary metastases may extend into the cavernous sinus. The epineurium generally provides an effective barrier to invasion of the peripheral nerves by solid tumors, but certain tumors characteristically invade and spread along peripheral nerves. Squamous cell carcinoma of the skin may spread along the trigeminal nerve and extend intracranially. Non-Hodgkin's lymphoma may be neurotrophic and cause polyradiculopathy or a syndrome resembling mononeuropathy multiplex. Focal external beam radiation may reduce pain, prevent irreversible loss of peripheral nerve function, and possibly restore function.

In patients with cancer who have brachial or lumbosacral plexopathy, it may be difficult to distinguish tumor invasion from radiation injury. High radiation dose or the presence of myokymia (rippling contractions of muscle) suggests radiation injury, whereas pain suggests tumor. Radiographic imaging studies may be equivocal, and surgical exploration is sometimes required.

COMPLICATIONS OF THERAPY

RADIATION TOXICITY The nervous system is vulnerable to injury by therapeutic radiation. Histologically, there is demyelination, degeneration of small arterioles, and eventually brain infarction and necrosis.

Acute radiation injury occurs during or immediately after therapy. It is rarely seen with current protocols of external beam radiation but may occur after stereotaxic radiosurgery. Manifestations include headache, sleepiness, and worsening of preexisting neurologic deficits.

Early delayed radiation injury occurs within 4 months of therapy. It is associated with an increased white matter T2 signal on MRI scans. In children, the *somnolence syndrome* is a common form of early delayed radiation injury in which somnolence and ataxia develop after whole-brain irradiation. Irradiation of the cervical spine may cause Lhermitte's phenomenon, an electricity-like sensation evoked by neck flexion. Acute and early delayed radiation injury are self-limited and glucocorticoid-responsive disorders that do not appear to increase the risk of late radiation injury.

Late delayed radiation injury produces permanent damage to the nervous system. It occurs >4 months (generally 8 to 24 months) after completion of therapy; onset 15 years after therapy has been described. After whole-brain irradiation, progressive dementia can occur, sometimes accompanied by gait apraxia. White matter signal abnormalities are present on MRI studies (Fig. 358-9). Following focal brain irradiation, radiation necrosis occurs within the radiation field producing a contrast-enhancing (frequently ring-enhancing) mass. MRI or CT scans are often unable to distinguish radiation necrosis from recurrent tumor, but PET or SPECT scans may demonstrate that glucose metabolism is increased in tumor tissue but decreased in radiation necrosis. Magnetic resonance spectroscopy may demonstrate a high lactate concentration with relatively low choline concentration in areas of necrosis. Biopsy is frequently required to establish the correct diagnosis. Peripheral nerves, including the brachial and lumbosacral plexuses, may also develop late delayed radiation injury.

If untreated, radiation necrosis of the CNS may act as an expanding mass lesion, although it may resolve spontaneously or after treatment with glucocorticoids. Progressive radiation necrosis is best treated with surgical resection if the patient has a life expectancy of at least 6 months and a Karnofsky performance score >70. There are anecdotal reports that anticoagulation with heparin or warfarin may be beneficial. Radiation injury also accelerates the development of atherosclerosis in large arteries, but an increase in the risk of stroke becomes significant only years after radiation treatment.

Endocrine dysfunction frequently follows exposure of the hypothalamus or pituitary gland to therapeutic radiation. Growth hormone is the pituitary hormone most sensitive to radiation therapy, and thyroid-stimulating hormone is the least sensitive; ACTH, prolactin, and the gonadotropins have an intermediate sensitivity.

Development of a second neoplasm is another risk of therapeutic radiation that generally occurs many years after radiation exposure. Depending on the irradiated field, the risk of gliomas, meningiomas, sarcomas, and thyroid cancer is increased.

COMPLICATIONS OF CHEMOTHERAPY Chemotherapy regimens used to treat primary brain tumors have generally included a nitrosourea and are well tolerated. Infrequently, nitrosoureas and other drugs used to treat CNS neoplasms cause altered mental states (e.g., confusion, depression), ataxia, and seizures. Chemotherapy for systemic malignancy is a more frequent cause of nervous system toxicity. Cisplatin commonly produces tinnitus and high-frequency bilateral hearing loss, especially in younger patients. At cumulative doses, >450 mg/m^2, cisplatin can produce a symmetric, large-fiber axonal neuropathy that is predominantly sensory; paclitaxel (Taxol) produces a similar picture. Fluorouracil and high-dose cytarabine can cause cerebellar dysfunction that resolves after discontinuation of therapy. Vincristine, which is commonly used to treat lymphoma, may cause an acute ileus and is frequently associated with development of a progressive distal, symmetric sensory-motor neuropathy with foot drop and paresthesia.

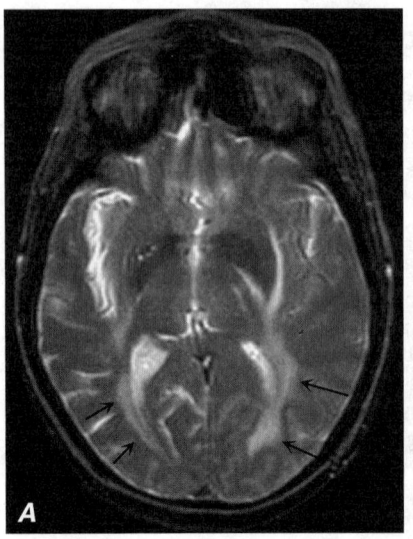 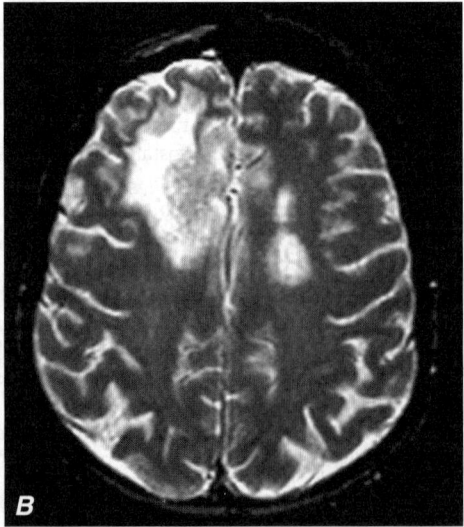 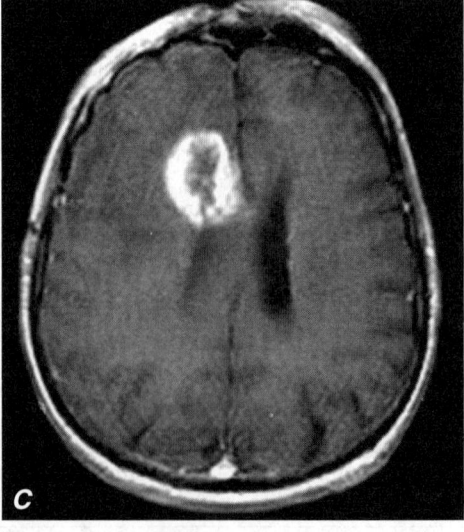

FIGURE 358-9 Radiation injury. *A.* Late-delayed radiation injury 1 year after whole-brain radiation (5500 cGy). T2-weighted MR image at the level of the temporal lobes reveals high signal intensity abnormality in periventricular white matter (*arrows*). *B* and *C.* Focal radiation necrosis 3 years after radiotherapy (7000 cGy) for carcinoma of the nasopharynx. Axial T2-weighted MRI (*B*) demonstrates a mass in the right frontal lobe with surrounding vasogenic edema. Abnormal signal changes are also present on the left. T1-weighted postcontrast MRI (*C*) reveals a heterogeneously enhancing mass in the right cingulate gyrus.

FURTHER READING

BEHIN A et al: Primary brain tumors in adults. Lancet 361:323, 2003

GLANTZ M et al: Temozolomide as an alternative to irradiation for elderly patients with newly diagnosed malignant gliomas. Cancer 97:2262, 2003

ZHU Y, PARADA LF: The molecular and genetic basis of neurological tumors. Nat Rev Cancer 2:616, 2002

359 MULTIPLE SCLEROSIS AND OTHER DEMYELINATING DISEASES
Stephen L. Hauser, Douglas S. Goodin

Demyelinating disorders are characterized by inflammation and selective destruction of central nervous system (CNS) myelin. The peripheral nervous system (PNS) is spared, and most patients have no evidence of an associated systemic illness.

MULTIPLE SCLEROSIS

Multiple sclerosis (MS) is characterized by a triad of inflammation, demyelination, and gliosis (scarring); the course can be relapsing-remitting or progressive. Lesions of MS are typically disseminated in time and location. MS affects ~350,000 Americans and 1.1 million individuals worldwide. In western societies, MS is second only to trauma as a cause of neurologic disability in early to middle adulthood. Manifestations of MS vary from a benign illness to a rapidly evolving and incapacitating disease requiring profound life-style adjustments.

PATHOGENESIS ■ Anatomy These lesions (plaques) vary in size from 1 or 2 mm to several centimeters. Acute MS lesions are characterized by perivenular cuffing with inflammatory mononuclear cells, predominantly T cells and macrophages, which also infiltrate the surrounding white matter. At sites of inflammation, the blood-brain barrier (BBB) is disrupted but, unlike vasculitis, the vessel wall is preserved. In more than half of cases, myelin-specific autoantibodies promote demyelination and stimulate macrophages and microglial cells (bone marrow–derived CNS phagocytes) that scavenge the myelin debris. As lesions evolve, astrocytes proliferate (gliosis). Surviving oligodendrocytes or those that differentiate from precursor cells may partially remyelinate the surviving naked axons, producing so-called shadow plaques. Ultrastructural studies of MS lesions suggest that fundamentally different underlying pathologies may exist in different patients. Heterogeneity has been observed in terms of: (1) whether the inflammatory cell infiltrate is associated with deposition of antibody and activation of complement, and (2) whether the target of the immunopathologic process is the myelin sheath itself or the cell body of the oligodendrocyte. Although sparing of axons is typical of MS, partial or total axonal destruction can also occur. Indirect evidence suggests that axonal loss is a major cause of irreversible neurologic disability in MS.

Physiology Nerve conduction in myelinated axons occurs in a saltatory manner, with the nerve impulse jumping from one node of Ranvier to the next without depolarization of the axonal membrane underlying the myelin sheath between nodes (Fig. 359-1). This produces considerably faster conduction velocities (~70 m/s) than the slow velocities (~1 m/s) produced by continuous propagation in unmyelinated nerves. Conduction block occurs when the nerve impulse is unable to traverse the demyelinated segment. This can happen when the resting axon membrane becomes hyperpolarized due to the exposure of voltage-dependent potassium channels that are normally buried underneath the myelin sheath. A temporary conduction block often follows a demyelinating event before the sodium channels (originally concentrated at the nodes) have had a chance to redistribute themselves along the naked axon (Fig. 359-1). This redistribution ultimately allows the continuous propagation of nerve action potentials through the demyelinated segment but, before this happens, the leakage currents are too large for the nerve impulse to jump the internode distance and conduction fails. On occasion, conduction block is incomplete, affecting, for example, high- but not low-frequency volleys of impulses. Variable conduction block can occur with raised body temperature or metabolic alterations and may explain clinical fluctuations (typical of MS) that

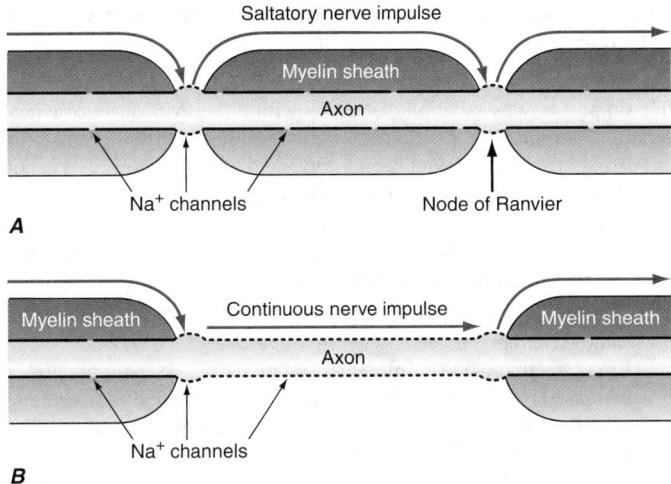

FIGURE 359-1 Nerve conduction in myelinated and demyelinated axons. *A.* Saltatory nerve conduction in myelinated axons occurs with the nerve impulse jumping from one node of Ranvier to the next. Sodium channels are concentrated at the nodes where axonal depolarization occurs. *B.* Following demyelination, the sodium channels are redistributed along the axon, thereby supporting continuous propagation of the nerve action potential in this region.

vary from hour to hour or in association with fever or exercise. Conduction slowing occurs when the demyelinated segments support only (slow) continuous nerve impulse propagation.

Epidemiology MS is approximately twice as common in women as in men. The age of onset is typically between 20 and 40 years (slightly later in men than in women). Rarely, it can begin as early as 2 years of age or as late as the eighth decade.

The highest known prevalence for MS (250 per 100,000) occurs in the Orkney islands, located north of Scotland, and similarly high rates are found throughout northern Europe, the northern United States, and Canada. By contrast, the prevalence is low in Japan (2 per 100,000), in other parts of Asia, in equatorial Africa, and in the Middle East. In general, prevalence increases with increasing distance from the equator, although certain exceptions are notable. Thus, the incidence of MS in the Eskimo population of Alaska is rare compared to the incidence in Caucasians living at similar latitudes. Similarly, native South Africans have a markedly lower prevalence compared to South Africans of European descent who live in the same geographic area. However, distinctive migration patterns of certain populations may artifactually suggest a relationship between MS and climate. Thus, when Scandanavians migrated to the United States or when the Scots migrated to New Zealand, they tended to migrate preferentially to places (e.g., the northern United States or southern New Zealand) with similar climates to their native lands. Such considerations point to potential genetic mechanisms (see below) rather than to an influence of temperate climate per se.

CHANGES IN INCIDENCE/PREVALENCE Studies from the United States, Europe, Australia, and the Middle East suggest that the prevalence of MS may be increasing, although improved methods of diagnosis may account for the apparent change. Other reports suggest that individuals who move from an area of high prevalence to one of low prevalence (or vice versa) before the age of 15 years adopt the risk of MS in their new environment, whereas if they move after this age, they retain the risk of their native land. The reliability of these observations is uncertain, although, if correct, they would suggest an environmental factor in the pathogenesis of MS.

REPORTED CLUSTERS Clusters of MS cases are occasionally reported. Often these apparent epidemics cannot be distinguished easily from chance occurrences, although some reports (e.g., the clustering of MS cases in the Faeroe Islands after British occupation during World War II) are more convincing than others. Such clustering, however, seems to be rare.

The Relationship of MS to Trauma and Stress The existing evidence does not support any association of trauma with either MS onset or exacerbation. Similarly, a relationship between stress and either onset or exacerbation of MS has not been established, although this area is not easily studied because of difficulties in quantifying stress.

 GENETIC CONSIDERATIONS A genetic susceptibility to MS exists, as evidenced by the following observations:

1. The prevalence of MS differs among ethnic groups residing in the same environment.
2. First-, second-, and third-degree relatives of MS patients are at increased risk for the disease. Siblings of affected individuals have a lifetime risk of 2 to 5%, whereas the risk to parents or children of affected individuals is somewhat lower.
3. Twin studies demonstrate concordance rates of 25 to 30% in monozygotic twins compared to only 2 to 5% in dizygotic twins (similar to the risk in nontwin siblings).

The inheritance of MS cannot be explained by a simple genetic model. Susceptibility is probably polygenic, with each gene contributing a relatively small amount to the overall risk. It is also likely that genetic heterogeneity (different susceptibilities among individuals) also exists. The major histocompatibility complex (MHC) on chromosome 6p21 (encoding proteins involved in presenting peptide antigens to T cells) is the most important MS susceptibility region identified to date. MS susceptibility is associated with the class II region of the MHC, specifically with the DR2 (DRB1*1501) allele and its corresponding haplotype. Other genetic regions implicated in MS susceptibility are located on chromosomal regions 19q35 and 17q13.

Immunology An autoimmune cause for MS is supported by the laboratory model of experimental allergic encephalomyelitis (EAE) and by studies of the immune system in MS patients.

AUTOREACTIVE T LYMPHOCYTES Myelin basic protein (MBP) is an important T cell antigen in EAE and probably also in human MS. Activated MBP-reactive T cells are often found in the blood or cerebrospinal fluid (CSF) of MS patients and, occasionally also, in MS lesions. Moreover, DR2 may influence the autoimmune response because it binds with high affinity to a fragment of MBP (spanning amino acids 89 to 96), stimulating T cell responses to this self-protein.

AUTOANTIBODIES Autoantibodies, directed against myelin antigens such as myelin oligodendrocyte glycoprotein (MOG), probably act in concert with a pathogenic T cell response to cause the demyelinating lesions in many patients. Recent evidence suggests that the presence of anti MOG antibodies in the serum of patients with a clinically isolated syndrome (CIS) is highly predictive of the development of MS in the future. Also, evidence of an abnormal humoral immune response is present in the CSF of MS patients. Membrane attack complexes (from complement-mediated antibody damage) can be detected in CSF, and elevated CSF immunoglobulin (synthesized locally) is characteristic of MS. Oligoclonal antibody (derived from expansion of a selected group of plasma cells) is present in most cases. Oligoclonal immunoglobulin is also detected in other chronic inflammatory conditions,

including infections, and thus is not specific to MS. The pattern of banding is unique to each individual, and attempts to identify the targets of these antibodies have been unsuccessful.

CYTOKINES (Chap. 295) The proinflammatory T_H1 cytokines such as interleukin (IL) 2, tumor necrosis factor (TNF) α, and interferon (IFN) γ are thought to be central to MS pathogenesis and some (e.g., TNF-α and IFN-γ) may directly injure oligodendrocytes or the myelin membranes. Nevertheless, the notion of an isolated T_H1 imbalance causing MS is probably simplistic. The presence of autoantibodies in MS suggests that regulatory T_H2 cytokines (including IL-4, -5, and -10) may also play a pathogenic role. Moreover, T_H1-based therapies have often proved to be unhelpful or, in the case of certain TNF-α inhibitors, harmful to patients.

TRIGGERS Magnetic resonance imaging (MRI) has demonstrated bursts of disease activity 7 to 10 times more frequently than is clinically apparent. This finding indicates that there is a large reservoir of subclinical disease activity in MS, especially during the early stages of the disease. The triggers causing these bursts are unknown, although the fact that patients may experience relapses after nonspecific upper respiratory infections suggests that either molecular mimicry between viruses and myelin antigens or viral superantigens activating pathogenic T cells may play a role in MS pathogenesis. (Chap. 299).

Microbiology As noted above, epidemiologic evidence supports the role of an environmental exposure in MS. MS risk also correlates with high socioeconomic status, which may reflect improved sanitation and delayed initial exposures to infectious agents. By analogy, some viral infections (e.g., poliomyelitis and measles viruses) produce neurologic sequelae more frequently when the age of initial infection is delayed. The best studied experimental model of virus-induced demyelinating disease is infection with Theiler virus, a murine coronavirus similar to measles, which produces a chronic oligodendrocyte infection with multifocal perivascular lymphocytic infiltration and demyelination, closely resembling lesions of MS.

High antibody titers against many viruses have been reported in serum and CSF of MS patients, including measles, herpes simplex, varicella, rubella, Epstein-Barr, and influenza C and some parainfluenza strains. Numerous viruses and bacteria (or their genomic sequences) have been recovered from MS tissues and fluids. Most recently human herpes virus type 6 (HHV-6) and *Chlamydia pneumoniae* have been implicated, although a causal role for any infectious agent in MS remains unproven.

CLINICAL MANIFESTATIONS The onset of MS may be abrupt or insidious. Symptoms may be severe or seem so trivial that a patient may not seek medical attention for months or years. Indeed, at autopsy some individuals who were asymptomatic during life will be found, unexpectedly, to have MS. In other cases an MRI scan obtained for an unrelated reason may show evidence of asymptomatic MS. Symptoms of MS are extremely varied and depend upon the location of lesions within the CNS (Table 359-1). Examination generally reveals evidence of neurologic dysfunction, often in asymptomatic locations. For example, a patient may present with symptoms in one leg and signs in both.

TABLE 359-1 *Initial Symptoms of MS*

Symptom	Percent of Cases	Symptom	Percent of Cases
Sensory loss	37	Lhermitte	3
Optic neuritis	36	Pain	3
Weakness	35	Dementia	2
Paresthesias	24	Visual loss	2
Diplopia	15	Facial palsy	1
Ataxia	11	Impotence	1
Vertigo	6	Myokymia	1
Paroxysmal attacks	4	Epilepsy	1
Bladder	4	Falling	1

Source: After WB Matthews et al, *McAlpine's Multiple Sclerosis,* New York, Churchill Livingstone, 1991.

Weakness of the limbs may manifest as loss of strength or dexterity, fatigue, or a disturbance of gait. Exercise-induced weakness is a characteristic symptom of MS. The weakness is of the upper motor neuron type (Chap. 20) and is frequently accompanied by other pyramidal signs such as spasticity, hyperreflexia and Babinski signs. Occasionally, a tendon reflex may be lost (simulating a lower motor neuron lesion) if an MS lesion disrupts the afferent reflex fibers in the spinal cord.

Spasticity (Chap. 21) is often associated with spontaneous and movement-induced muscle spasms. More than 30% of MS patients have moderate to severe spasticity, especially in the legs. It is often accompanied by painful spasms and can interfere with a patient's ability to ambulate or work or with self-care. Occasionally, spasticity may provide nonvolitional support for the body weight during ambulation. In these cases, treatment of spasticity may actually do more harm than good.

Optic neuritis (ON) generally presents as diminished visual acuity, dimness, or decreased color perception (desaturation) in the central field of vision. These symptoms may be mild or may progress to severe visual loss. Rarely, there is complete loss of light perception. Visual symptoms are generally monocular but may occur bilaterally. Periorbital pain (aggravated by eye movement) often precedes or accompanies the visual loss. An afferent pupillary defect (Chap. 25) may be found. Funduscopic examination may be normal or reveal optic disc swelling (papillitis). Pallor of the optic disc (optic atrophy) commonly follows ON. Uveitis is rare and should raise the possibility of alternative diagnoses. →*ON is discussed in detail in Chap. 25.*

Visual blurring in MS may result from ON or diplopia. Visual blurring that resolves when either eye is covered is due to diplopia.

Diplopia may result from internuclear ophthalmoplegia (INO) or from palsy of the sixth cranial nerve (rarely the third or fourth). An INO consists of impaired adduction of one eye due to a lesion in the ipsilateral medial longitudinal fasciculus (Chap. 25). Prominent nystagmus is often observed in the abducting eye, along with a small skew deviation. A bilateral INO is particularly suggestive of MS. Other common gaze disturbances in MS include: (1) a horizontal gaze palsy, (2) a "one and a half" syndrome (horizontal gaze palsy plus an INO), and (3) acquired pendular nystagmus.

Sensory symptoms are varied and include both paresthesias (e.g., tingling, prickling sensations, formications, "pins and needles," or painful burning) and hypesthesia (e.g., reduced sensation, numbness or a "dead" feeling). Unpleasant sensations (e.g., feelings that body parts are swollen, wet, raw, or tightly wrapped) are also common. Sensory impairment of the trunk and legs below a horizontal line on the torso (a sensory level) suggests that the spinal cord is the origin of the sensory disturbance. It is often accompanied by a bandlike sensation of tightness around the torso. Pain is a common symptom of MS, experienced by >50% of patients. Pain can occur anywhere on the body and can change locations over time.

Ataxia usually manifests as cerebellar tremors (Chap. 21). Ataxia may also involve the head and trunk or the voice, producing a characteristic cerebellar dysarthria (scanning speech). The true extent of cerebellar involvement may be difficult to determine in an individual patient, because motor and sensory deficits can affect coordination and weakness may interfere with coordination testing.

Bladder and bowel dysfunction arise from different causes and frequently different types of dysfunction coexist. During normal reflex voiding, relaxation of the bladder sphincter (α-adrenergic innervation) is coordinated with contraction of the detrusor muscle in the bladder wall (muscarinic cholinergic innervation). Stoppage of the urinary stream is accomplished with a coordinated sphincter contraction and detrusor relaxation. Bladder-stretch (during filling) activates this reflex, which is inhibited by supraspinal (voluntary) input. Symptoms of bladder dysfunction are present in >90% of MS patients and, in a third, dysfunction results in weekly or more frequent episodes of incontinence.

Detrusor hyperreflexia, due to impairment of suprasegmental inhibition, causes urinary frequency, urgency, nocturia, and uncontrolled bladder emptying. *Detrusor sphincter dyssynergia*, due to loss of synchronization between detrusor and sphincter muscles, causes difficulty in initiating and/or stopping the urinary stream, thereby producing hesitancy. It can also lead to urinary retention, large postvoid residual volumes, overflow incontinence, and recurrent infection.

Constipation occurs in >30% of patients. Fecal urgency or *bowel incontinence* is less common (15%) but can be socially debilitating.

Cognitive dysfunction can include memory loss, impaired attention, difficulties in problem-solving, slowed information processing, and problems shifting between cognitive tasks. Euphoria (elevated mood) was once thought to be characteristic of MS but is actually uncommon, occurring in <20% of patients. Cognitive dysfunction sufficient to impair activities of daily living also occurs but is rare.

Depression, experienced by 50 to 60% of patients, can be reactive, endogenous, or part of the illness itself and can contribute to fatigue. Suicide in MS patients is 7.5-fold more common than in age-matched controls.

Fatigue is experienced by 90% of patients and is moderate or severe in half. Symptoms include generalized motor weakness, limited ability to concentrate, extreme lassitude, loss of energy, decreased endurance, and an overwhelming sense of exhaustion that requires the patient to rest or fall asleep. Fatigue (either alone or with other symptoms) is the most common reason for work-related disability in MS. Fatigue can be exacerbated by elevated temperatures, by depression, by expending exceptional effort to accomplish basic activities of daily living, or by sleep disturbances (e.g., from frequent nocturnal awakenings to urinate). MS-related fatigue may be maximum during mid-afternoon or continuous throughout the day, and it is often difficult to treat.

Sexual dysfunction is common in MS. Men report impotence, less desire, impaired genital sensation, impaired ejaculation, and inability to achieve/maintain an erection. Women report genital numbness, diminished orgasmic response, decreased libido, unpleasant sensations during intercourse, and diminished vaginal lubrication. Adductor spasticity (in women) can also interfere with intercourse, and urinary incontinence (in either men or women) can be problematic.

Facial weakness due to a lesion in the intraparenchymal pathway of the seventh cranial nerve may resemble idiopathic Bell's palsy. However, unlike Bell's palsy, facial weakness in MS is generally not associated with ipsilateral loss of taste sensation or retroauricular pain (Chap. 355).

Vertigo may appear suddenly and resemble acute labyrinthitis. A brainstem rather than end-organ origin is suggested by the presence of coexisting trigeminal or facial nerve involvement; vertical nystagmus; or nystagmus that has no latency to onset, no direction reversal, and doesn't fatigue (Chap. 20). Hearing loss may also occur in MS but is uncommon.

Ancillary Symptoms *Heat sensitivity* refers to neurologic symptoms produced by an elevation of the body's core temperature. For example, transient unilateral visual blurring or loss may occur during a hot shower or with physical exercise (*Uhthoff's symptom*). It is common for MS symptoms to worsen transiently, sometimes dramatically, during febrile illnesses (see pseudoexacerbation, below). Such heat-related symptoms probably result from transient conduction block (see above).

Lhermitte's symptom is the electric shock–like sensation (evoked by neck flexion or other movement) that radiates down the back into the legs. Rarely, it radiates into the arms. It is generally self-limited but may persist for years. Lhermitte's symptom can also occur with other disorders of the cervical spine (e.g., cervical spondylosis).

Paroxysmal symptoms are distinguished by their brief duration (30 s to 2 min), high frequency (5 to 40 episodes per day), lack of any alteration of consciousness or change in background electroencephalogram during episodes, and a self-limited course (generally lasting weeks to months). They may be precipitated by hyperventilation or movement. These syndromes include Lhermitte's symptom; tonic contractions of a limb, face, or trunk (tonic seizures); paroxysmal dysarthria/ataxia; paroxysmal sensory disturbances; and several other less well characterized syndromes. Paroxysmal symptoms probably result from spontaneous discharges, arising at the edges of demyelinated plaques, and spreading ephaptically to adjacent white matter tracts.

Trigeminal neuralgia, hemifacial spasm, and glossopharyngeal neuralgia can occur when the demyelinating lesion involves the root entry (or exit) zone of the fifth, seventh, and ninth cranial nerve, respectively. *Trigeminal neuralgia* (tic douloureux) is a very brief lancinating facial pain often triggered by an afferent input from the face or teeth. Most cases of trigeminal neuralgia are not MS-related. However, the occurrence of atypical features (Chap. 355) such as the onset before age 50 years, bilateral symptoms, objective sensory loss, or nonparoxysmal pain should raise concerns that a symptomatic cause such as MS is responsible.

Facial myokymia consists of either persistent rapid flickering contractions of the facial musculature (especially the lower portion of the orbicularis oculus) or a contraction that slowly spreads across the face. It results from lesions of the corticobulbar tracts or brainstem course of the facial nerve.

DISEASE COURSE   Four clinical types of MS have been described (Fig. 359-2):

1. *Relapsing/remitting MS* (RRMS) accounts for 85% of MS cases at onset and is characterized by discrete attacks that generally evolve over days to weeks (rarely over hours). Often, but not invariably, there is complete recovery over the ensuing weeks to months (Fig. 359-2*A*). However, when ambulation is severely impaired during an attack, approximately half will fail to improve. Between attacks, patients are neurologically stable.

2. *Secondary progressive MS* (SPMS) always begins as RRMS (Fig. 359-2*B*). At some point, however, the RRMS clinical course changes so that the patient experiences a steady deterioration in function unassociated with acute attacks (which may continue or cease during the progressive phase). SPMS produces a greater amount of fixed neurologic disability than RRMS. Approximately 50% of patients with RRMS will have developed SPMS after 15 years, and longer follow-up points indicate that the great majority of RRMS ultimately evolves into SPMS. Thus, SPMS appears to represent a late-stage of the same underlying illness as RRMS.

3. *Primary progressive MS* (PPMS) accounts for ~15% of cases. These patients do not experience attacks but only a steady functional decline from disease onset (Fig. 359-2*C*). Compared to RRMS, the

sex distribution is more even, the disease begins later in life (mean age, ~40 years), and disability develops faster. Whether PPMS is an unusual phenotype of the same underlying illness as RRMS or whether these are distinct illnesses is unknown.

4. *Progressive/relapsing MS* (PRMS) overlaps PPMS and SPMS and accounts for ~5% of MS patients. Like patients with PPMS, these patients experience a steady deterioration in their condition from disease onset. However, like SPMS patients, they experience occasional attacks superimposed upon their progressive course (Fig. 359-2*D*). The early stages of RPMS are indistinguishable from those of PPMS (i.e., until the first clinical attack).

DIAGNOSIS   There is no definitive diagnostic test for MS. Diagnostic criteria for clinically definite MS require documentation of two or more episodes of symptoms and two or more signs that reflect pathology in anatomically noncontiguous white matter tracts of the CNS (Table 359-2). Symptoms must last for >24 h and occur as distinct episodes that are separated by a month or more. At least one of the two required signs must be present on neurologic examination. The second may be documented by certain abnormal paraclinical tests such as MRI or evoked potentials (EPs). In patients who experience gradual progression of disability for ≥6 months without superimposed relapses, documentation of intrathecal IgG and visual EP testing may be used to support the diagnosis.

DIAGNOSTIC TESTS ■ **Magnetic Resonance Imaging**   MRI has revolutionized the diagnosis and management of MS (Fig. 359-3); characteristic abnormalities are found in >95% of patients. An increase in vascular permeability from a breakdown of the BBB is detected by leakage of intravenous gadolinium (Gd) into the parenchyma. Such leakage occurs early in the development of an MS lesion and serves as a useful marker of inflammation. Gd-enhancement persists for up to 3 months, and the residual MS plaque remains visible indefinitely as a focal area of hyperintensity (a lesion) on spin-echo (T2-weighted) and proton-density images. Lesions are frequently oriented perpendicular to the

---

TABLE 359-2   Diagnostic Criteria for MS

1. Examination must reveal *objective* abnormalities of the CNS.
2. Involvement must reflect predominantly disease of white matter long tracts, usually including (a) pyramidal pathways, (b) cerebellar pathways, (c) medial longitudinal fasciculus, (d) optic nerve, and (e) posterior columns.
3. Examination or history must implicate involvement of two or more areas of the CNS.
    a. MRI may be used to document a second lesion when only one site of abnormality has been demonstrable on examination. A confirmatory MRI must have either four lesions involving the white matter or three lesions if one is periventricular in location. Acceptable lesions must be >3 mm in diameter. For patients older than 50 years, two of the following criteria must also be met: (a) lesion size >5 mm, (b) lesions adjacent to the bodies of the lateral ventricles, and (c) lesion(s) present in the posterior fossa.
    b. Evoked response testing may be used to document a second lesion not evident on clinical examination.
4. The clinical pattern must consist of (a) two or more separate episodes of worsening involving different sites of the CNS, each lasting at least 24 h and occurring at least 1 month apart, or (b) gradual or stepwise progression over at least 6 months if accompanied by increased IgG synthesis or two or more oligoclonal bands. MRI may be used to document dissemination in time if a new T2 lesion or a Gd-enhancing lesion is seen 3 or more months after a clinically isolated syndrome.
5. The patient's neurologic condition could not better be attributed to another disease.

DIAGNOSTIC CATEGORIES

1. *Definite MS:* All five criteria fulfilled.
2. *Probable MS:* All five criteria fulfilled except (a) only one objective abnormality despite two symptomatic episodes or (b) only one symptomatic episode despite two or more objective abnormalities.
3. *At risk for MS:* Criteria 1, 2, 3, and 5 fulfilled; patient has only one symptomatic episode and one objective abnormality.

Note: CNS, central nervous system; MRI, magnetic resonance imaging; Gd, gadolinium.

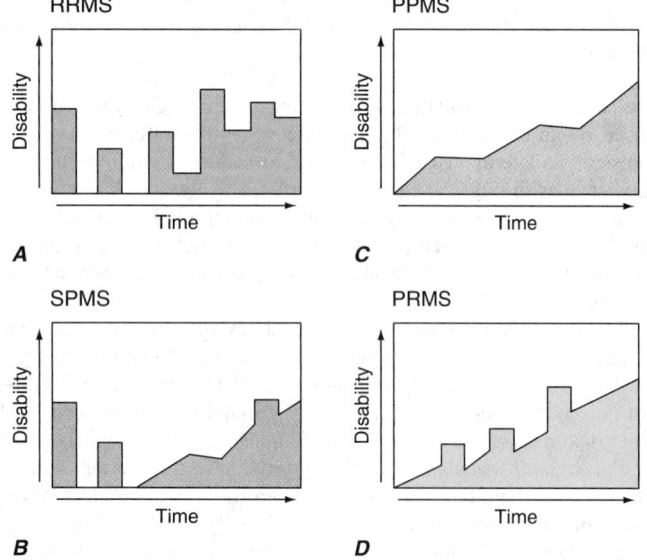

FIGURE 359-2   Clinical course of multiple sclerosis (MS). *A.* Relapsing/remitting MS. *B.* Secondary progressive MS. *C.* Primary progressive MS. *D.* Progressive/relapsing MS.

ventricular surface, corresponding to the pathologic pattern of perivenous demyelination (Dawson's fingers). Lesions are multifocal within the brain, brainstem, and spinal cord. Lesions in the anterior corpus callosum are helpful diagnostically because this site is usually spared in cerebrovascular disease. Different criteria for the use of MRI in the diagnosis of MS have been proposed (Table 359-2).

The total volume of T2-weighted signal abnormality (the "burden of disease") shows a significant (albeit weak) correlation with clinical disability. Approximately one-third of T2-weighted lesions appear as hypointense lesions (black holes) on T1-weighted imaging. Black holes may be a better marker of irreversible demyelination and axonal loss than T2 hyperintensities, although even this measure depends upon the timing of the image acquisition (e.g., most acute Gd-enhancing T2 lesions are T1 dark).

Newer MRI measures such as brain atrophy, magnetization transfer ratio (MTR) imaging and proton magnetic resonance spectroscopic imaging (MRSI) may ultimately serve as surrogate markers of clinical disability. For example, MRSI can quantitate molecules such as N-acetyl aspartate (NAA), which is a marker of axonal integrity, and MTR may be able to distinguish demyelination from edema.

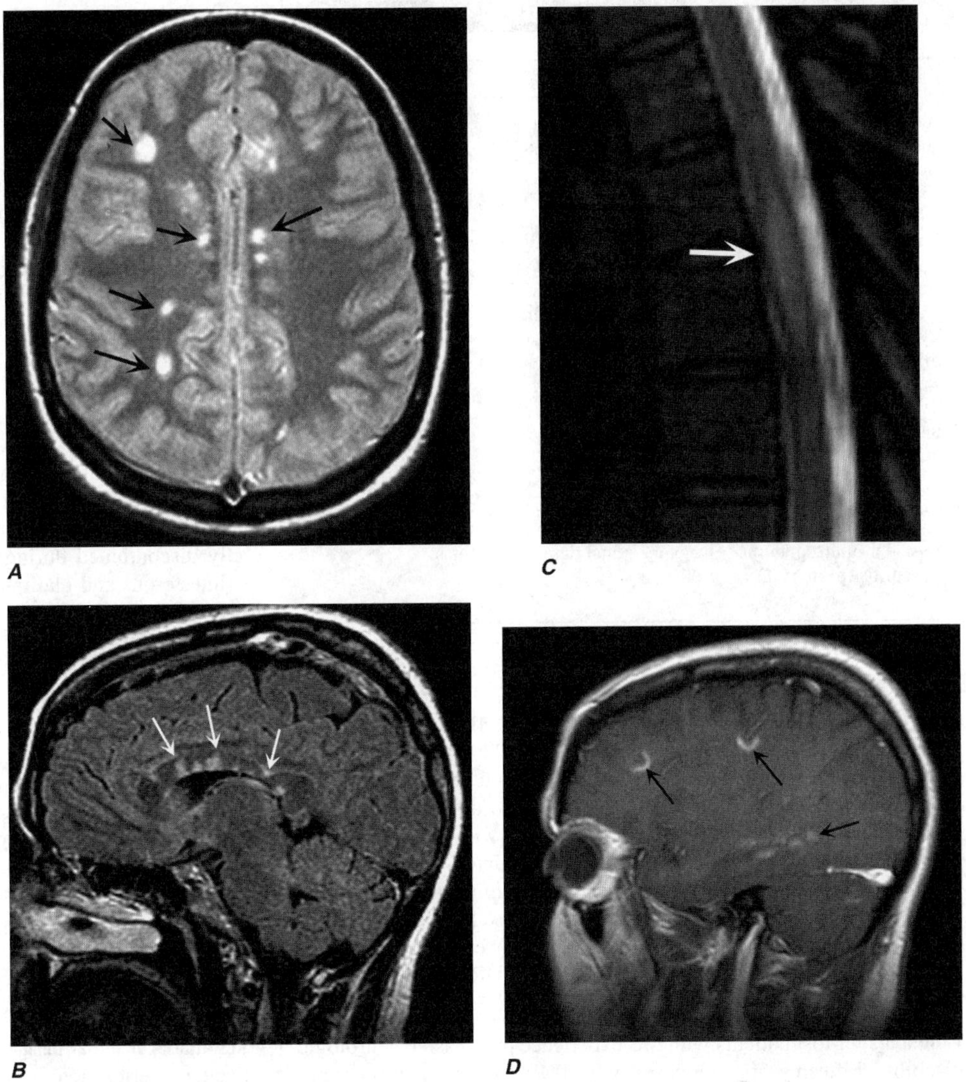

Evoked Potentials EP testing assesses function in afferent (visual, auditory, and somatosensory) or efferent (motor) CNS pathways. EPs use computer averaging to measure CNS electric potentials evoked by repetitive stimulation of selected peripheral nerves or of the brain. These tests provide the most information when the pathways studied are clinically uninvolved. For example, in a patient with a remitting and relapsing spinal cord syndrome with sensory deficits in the legs, an abnormal somatosensory EP following posterior tibial nerve stimulation provides little new information. By contrast, an abnormal visual EP in this circumstance would permit a diagnosis of clinically definite MS (Table 359-2). Abnormalities on one or more EP modalities occur in 80 to 90% of MS patients. EP abnormalities are not specific to MS, although a marked delay in the latency of a specific EP component (as opposed to a reduced amplitude) is suggestive of demyelination.

Cerebrospinal Fluid CSF abnormalities found in MS include a mononuclear cell pleocytosis and an increased level of intrathecally synthesized IgG. The total CSF protein is usually normal or slightly elevated. Various formulas distinguish intrathecally synthesized IgG from IgG that may have entered the CNS passively from the serum. One formula (the CSF IgG index) expresses the ratio of IgG to albumin in the CSF divided by the same ratio in the serum. A more complicated formula, the IgG synthesis rate, makes certain assumptions but uses the same serum and CSF IgG and albumin measurements to calculate the rate of CNS IgG synthesis. The measurement of oligoclonal banding (OCB) in the CSF also assesses intrathecal production of IgG. OCBs are detected by agarose gel electrophoresis. Two or more OCBs are

FIGURE 359-3 MRI findings in MS. *A.* Axial first-echo image from T2-weighted sequence demonstrates multiple bright signal abnormalities in white matter, typical for MS. *B.* Sagittal T2-weighted FLAIR (fluid attenuated inversion recovery) image in which the high signal of CSF has been suppressed. CSF appears dark, while areas of brain edema or demyelination appear high in signal as shown here in the corpus callosum (*arrows*). Lesions in the anterior corpus callosum are frequent in MS and rare in vascular disease. *C.* Sagittal T2-weighted fast spin echo image of the thoracic spine demonstrates a fusiform high signal intensity lesion in the mid thoracic spinal cord. *D.* Sagittal T1-weighted image obtained after the intravenous administration of gadolinium DTPA reveals focal areas of blood-brain barrier disruption, identified as high-signal-intensity regions (*arrows*).

found in 75 to 90% of patients with MS. OCBs may be absent at the onset of MS, and in individual patients the number of bands present may increase with time. It is important that paired serum samples be studied to exclude a peripheral (i.e., non-CNS) origin of any OCBs detected in the CSF.

A mild CSF pleocytosis ($>$5 cells/μL) is present in $\sim$25% of cases, usually in young patients with RRMS. A pleocytosis of $>$75 cells/μL, the presence of polymorphonuclear leukocytes, or a protein concentration of $>$1.0 g/L ($>$100 mg/dL) in CSF should raise concern that the patient may not have MS.

DIFFERENTIAL DIAGNOSIS No single clinical sign or test is diagnostic of MS. The diagnosis is readily made in a young adult with relapsing and remitting symptoms involving different areas of CNS white matter. The possibility of an alternative diagnosis should always be considered (Table 359-3), particularly when (1) symptoms are localized exclusively to the posterior fossa, craniocervical junction, or spinal cord; (2) the patient is $<$15 or $>$60 years of age; (3) the clinical course is progressive from onset; (4) the patient has never experienced visual, sensory, or bladder symptoms; or (5) laboratory findings (e.g., MRI, CSF, or EPs) are atypical. Similarly, uncommon or rare symptoms in

TABLE 359-3 *Disorders that Can Mimic MS*

Acute disseminated encephalomyelitis (ADEM)
Antiphospholipid antibody syndrome
Behçet's disease
Cerebral autosomal dominant arteriopathy, subcortical infarcts, and
  leukoencephalopathy (CADASIL)
Congenital leukodystrophies (e.g., adrenoleukodystrophy, metachromatic
  leukodystrophy)
Human immunodifficiency virus (HIV) infection
Ischemic optic neuropathy (arteritic and nonarteritic)
Lyme disease
Mitochondrial encephalopathy with lactic acidosis and stroke (MELAS)
Neoplasms (e.g., lymphoma, glioma, meningioma)
Sarcoid
Sjögren's syndrome
Stroke and ischemic cerebrovascular disease
Syphilis
Systemic lupus erythematosus and related collagen vascular disorders
Tropical spastic paraparesis (HTLV I/II infection)
Vascular malformations (especially spinal dural AV fistulas)
Vasculitis (primary CNS or other)
Vitamin B_{12} deficiency

Note: HTLV, human T cell leukemia/lymphoma virus; AV, arteriovenous; CNS, central nervous system.

MS (e.g., aphasia, parkinsonism, chorea, isolated dementia, severe muscular atrophy, peripheral neuropathy, episodic loss of consciousness, fever, headache, seizures, or coma) should increase concern about an alternative diagnosis. Diagnosis is also difficult in patients with a rapid or explosive (stroke-like) onset or with mild symptoms and a normal neurologic examination. Rarely, intense inflammation and swelling may produce a mass lesion that mimics a primary or metastatic tumor. The specific tests required to exclude alternative diagnoses will vary with each clinical situation; however, an erythrocyte sedimentation rate, serum B_{12} level, ANA, and VDRL should probably be obtained in all patients with suspected MS.

PROGNOSIS Most patients with MS experience progressive neurologic disability. Fifteen years after onset, only 20% of patients have no functional limitation; half will have progressed to SPMS and will require assistance with ambulation. Twenty-five years after onset, >80% of MS patients will have reached this level of disability. In 1998, it was estimated that the total annual economic burden of MS in the United States exceeded $6.8 billion.

However, even if the prognosis for disability is grave for the average patient, the prognosis in an individual is difficult to establish. Certain clinical features suggest a more favorable prognosis. Patients with ON or sensory symptoms at onset, patients who recover completely from early attacks, patients <40 years at onset (but not beginning in childhood), women, patients with RRMS, patients with fewer than two relapses in the first year of illness, and patients with minimal impairment after 5 years do better than patients without these clinical features. By contrast, patients with truncal ataxia, action tremor, pyramidal symptoms, or a progressive disease course are more likely to become disabled. A purely progressive disease course carries a graver outlook at all disease stages than does a disease course accompanied by occasional relapses.

Importantly, some MS patients have a benign variant of MS and never develop neurologic disability. The likelihood of having benign MS is thought to be <20%, although it may be underestimated by existing natural history studies. One recent study of patients with benign MS 15 years after onset reported that, although most patients had developed disability by 25 years, those patients with entirely normal neurologic examinations maintained their benign course.

In patients with their first demyelinating event (i.e., a clinically isolated syndrome), the brain MRI provides prognostic information. With three or more typical T2-weighted lesions, the risk of developing MS after 10 years is 70 to 80%. Conversely, with a normal brain MRI,

the likelihood of developing MS is <20%. Similarly, two or more Gd-enhancing lesions at baseline is highly predictive of future MS, as is the appearance of either new T2-weighted lesions or new Gd enhancement ≥3 months after the episode. Typical abnormalities on EP testing and CSF examination provide similar prognostic information, although these relationships are not as well characterized.

Mortality as a direct consequence of MS is uncommon, although it has been estimated that the 25-year survival is only 85% of expected. Death can occur during an acute MS attack, although this is distinctly rare. More commonly, death occurs as a complication of MS (e.g., pneumonia in a debilitated individual). Death also results from suicide.

Effect of Pregnancy Pregnant MS patients experience fewer attacks than expected during gestation (especially in the last trimester) but more attacks than expected in the first 3 months post-partum. When considering the pregnancy year as a whole (i.e., 9 months pregnancy plus 3 months post-partum), the overall disease course is unaffected. Decisions about childbearing should thus be made based upon (1) the mother's physical state, (2) her ability to care for the child, and (3) the availability of social support. Disease-modifying therapy is generally discontinued during pregnancy, although the actual risk from the interferons and glatiramer acetate (see below) appears to be quite low.

℞ TREATMENT

Current therapy for MS can be divided into several categories: (1) treatment of acute attacks as they occur; (2) treatment with disease-modifying agents that reduce the biological activity of MS, and (3) symptomatic therapy. Treatments that promote remyelination or neural repair do not currently exist but would be highly desirable.

The Kurtzke Expanded Disability Status Score (EDSS) is a measure of neurologic impairment in MS (Table 359-4). The EDSS provides a useful snapshot of the disease status of a patient at a given time and a composite picture of the disease course over time. Most patients with EDSS scores <3.5 have RRMS, walk normally, and are not disabled; by contrast, patients with EDSS scores >5.5 have progressive MS (SPMS or PPMS) and are gait-impaired and occupationally disabled.

Acute Attacks or Initial Demyelinating Episodes When patients experience an acute deterioration, it is important to consider whether this change reflects new disease activity or a "pseudoexacerbation" resulting from an increase in ambient temperature, fever, or an infection. In such instances, glucocorticoid treatment is inappropriate. Glucocorticoids are used to manage either first attacks or acute exacerbations. They provide short-term clinical benefit by reducing the severity and shortening the duration of attacks. Whether treatment provides any long-term benefit on the course of the illness is less clear. As a result, mild attacks are often not treated. Physical and occupational therapy can help with mobility and manual dexterity.

Glucocorticoid treatment is administered as intravenous methylprednisolone, 500 to 1000 mg/d for 3 to 5 days, either without a taper or followed by a course of oral prednisone beginning at a dose of 60 to 80 mg/d and gradually tapered over 2 weeks. Outpatient treatment is usually possible. If intravenous therapy is unavailable or inconvenient, oral glucocorticoids can be substituted.

Side effects of short-term glucocorticoid therapy include fluid retention, potassium loss, weight gain, gastric disturbances, acne, and emotional lability. Concurrent use of a low-salt, potassium-rich diet and avoidance of potassium-wasting diuretics is advisable. Lithium carbonate (300 mg orally bid) may help to manage emotional lability and insomnia associated with glucocorticoid therapy. Patients with a history of peptic ulcer disease may require cimetidine (400 mg bid) or ranitidine (150 mg bid).

Plasma exchange (7 exchanges: 54 mL/kg or 1.1 plasma volumes per exchange, every other day for 14 days) may benefit patients with fulminant attacks of demyelination (not only MS) that are unresponsive to glucocorticoids. However, because the cost is high, and the evidence of efficacy is preliminary, plasma exchange should be considered only in selected cases.

TABLE 359-4 *Scoring Systems for MS*

KURTZKE EXPANDED DISABILITY STATUS SCORE (EDSS)

0.0 = Normal neurologic exam [all grade 0 in functional status (FS)]	6.0 = Unilateral assistance required to walk about 100 m with or without resting
1.0 = No disability, minimal signs in one FS (i.e., grade 1)	6.5 = Constant bilateral assistance required to walk about 20 m without resting
1.5 = No disability, minimal signs in more than one FS (more than one grade 1)	7.0 = Unable to walk beyond about 5 m even with aid; essentially restricted to wheelchair; wheels self and transfers alone
2.0 = Minimal disability in one FS (one FS grade 2, others 0 or 1)	7.5 = Unable to take more than a few steps; restricted to wheelchair; may need aid to transfer
2.5 = Minimal disability in two FS (two FS grade 2, others 0 or 1)	8.0 = Essentially restricted to bed or chair or perambulated in wheelchair, but out of bed most of day; retains many self-care functions; generally has effective use of arms
3.0 = Moderate disability in one FS (one FS grade 3, others 0 or 1) or mild disability in three or four FS (three/four FS grade 2, others 0 or 1) though fully ambulatory	8.5 = Essentially restricted to bed much of the day; has some effective use of arm(s); retains some self-care functions
3.5 = Fully ambulatory but with moderate disability in one FS (one grade 3) and one or two FS grade 2; or two FS grade 3; or five FS grade 2 (others 0 or 1)	9.0 = Helpless bed patient; can communicate and eat
4.0 = Ambulatory without aid or rest for ≥ 500 m	9.5 = Totally helpless bed patient; unable to communicate or eat
4.5 = Ambulatory without aid or rest for ≥ 300 m	10.0 = Death due to MS
5.0 = Ambulatory without aid or rest for ≥ 200 m	
5.5 = Ambulatory without aid or rest for ≥ 100 m	

FUNCTIONAL STATUS (FS) SCORE

A. Pyramidal functions	5 = Loss (essentially) of sensation in 1 or 2 limbs or moderate decrease in touch or pain and/or loss of proprioception for most of the body below the head
0 = Normal	6 = Sensation essentially lost below the head
1 = Abnormal signs without disability	E. Bowel and bladder functions
2 = Minimal disability	0 = Normal
3 = Mild or moderate paraparesis or hemiparesis, or severe monoparesis	1 = Mild urinary hesitancy, urgency, or retention
4 = Marked paraparesis or hemiparesis, moderate quadriparesis, or monoplegia	2 = Moderate hesitancy, urgency, retention of bowel or bladder, or rare urinary incontinence
5 = Paraplegia, hemiplegia, or marked quadriparesis	3 = Frequent urinary incontinence
6 = Quadriplegia	4 = In need of almost constant catheterization
B. Cerebellar functions	5 = Loss of bladder function
0 = Normal	6 = Loss of bowel and bladder function
1 = Abnormal signs without disability	F. Visual (or optic) functions
2 = Mild ataxia	0 = Normal
3 = Moderate truncal or limb ataxia	1 = Scotoma with visual acuity (corrected) better than 20/30
4 = Severe ataxia all limbs	2 = Worse eye with scotoma with maximal visual acuity (corrected) of 20/30 to 20/59
5 = Unable to perform coordinated movements due to ataxia	3 = Worse eye with large scotoma, or moderate decrease in fields, but with maximal visual acuity (corrected) of 20/60 to 20/99
C. Brainstem functions	4 = Worse eye with marked decrease of fields and maximal acuity (corrected) of 20/100 to 20/200; grade 3 plus maximal acuity of better eye of 20/60 or less
0 = Normal	5 = Worse eye with maximal visual acuity (corrected) less than 20/200; grade 4 plus maximal acuity of better eye of 20/60 or less
1 = Signs only	6 = Grade 5 plus maximal visual acuity of better eye of 20/60 or less
2 = Moderate nystagmus or other mild disability	G. Cerebral (or mental) functions
3 = Severe nystagmus, marked extraocular weakness, or moderate disability of other cranial nerves	0 = Normal
4 = Marked dysarthria or other marked disability	1 = Mood alteration only (does not affect EDSS score)
5 = Inability to swallow or speak	2 = Mild decrease in mentation
D. Sensory functions	3 = Moderate decrease in mentation
0 = Normal	4 = Marked decrease in mentation
1 = Vibration or figure-writing decrease only, in 1 or 2 limbs	5 = Chronic brain syndrome—severe or incompetent
2 = Mild decrease in touch or pain or position sense, and/or moderate decrease in vibration in 1 or 2 limbs, or vibratory decrease alone in 3 or 4 limbs	
3 = Moderate decrease in touch or pain or position sense, and/or essentially lost vibration in 1 or 2 limbs, or mild decrease in touch or pain, and/or moderate decrease in all proprioceptive tests in 3 or 4 limbs	
4 = Marked decrease in touch or pain or loss of proprioception, alone or combined, in 1 or 2 limbs or moderate decrease in touch or pain and/or severe proprioceptive decrease in more than 2 limbs	

Source: After JF Kurtzke: Rating neurologic impairment in multiple sclerosis: An expanded disability status scale (EDSS). Neurology 33:1444, 1983.

Disease-Modifying Therapies for Relapsing Forms of MS (RRMS SPMS with Exacerbations) Four such agents are approved in the United States: (1) IFN-β1a (Avonex), (2) IFN-β1a (Rebif); (3) IFN-β1b (Betaseron); and (4) glatiramer acetate (Copaxone). Each of these treatments is also used in SPMS patients who still experience attacks, because SPMS can be difficult to distinguish from RRMS and the clinical trials suggest that such patients also derive therapeutic benefit. In Phase III clinical trials, recipients of IFNβ1b, IFNβ1a, and glatiramer acetate experienced ~30% fewer clinical exacerbations and fewer new MRI lesions compared to placebo recipients. Mitoxantrone (Novantrone), an immune suppressant, has also been approved in the United States, although, because of its potential toxicity, it is generally reserved for patients with progressive disability who have failed other treatments.

INTERFERON β AND GLATIRAMER ACETATE IFN-β is a class I interferon originally identified by its antiviral properties. Efficacy in MS, however,

probably results from immunomodulatory properties including: (1) downregulating expression of MHC molecules on antigen-presenting cells; (2) inhibiting proinflammatory and increasing regulatory cytokine levels; (3) inhibition of T cell proliferation; and (4) limiting the trafficking of inflammatory cells in the CNS. Glatiramer acetate is a synthetic, random polypeptide composed of four amino acids (L-glutamic acid, L-lysine, L-alanine, and L-tyrosine). Its mechanism of action may include: (1) induction of antigen-specific suppressor T cells; (2) binding to MHC molecules, thereby displacing bound MBP; or (3) altering the balance between proinflammatory and regulatory cytokines.

IFN-β reduces the attack rate (whether measured clinically or by MRI) in MS patients. It also improves disease severity measures such as EDSS progression and MRI-documented disease burden. The efficacy of IFN-β in SPMS patients is less convincing than the efficacy in RRMS patients. IFN-β should be considered in patients with either RRMS or SPMS with superimposed relapses. In patients with SPMS but without relapses, efficacy has not been established. Higher IFN-β doses appear to have slightly greater efficacy but are also more likely to induce neutralizing antibodies, which may reduce the clinical benefit (see below).

Glatiramer acetate also reduces the attack rate (whether measured clinically or by MRI) in RRMS. Glatiramer acetate may also benefit disease severity measures, although this is less well established than for the relapse rate. Therefore, glatiramer acetate should be considered in RRMS patients. However, its usefulness in progressive disease is entirely unknown.

The long-term efficacy of these treatments remains largely unknown. For the interferons, clear-cut beneficial effects in reducing the relapse rate and, more substantially, in reducing CNS inflammation inferred by MRI has not been matched by similar success in treating patients with progressive symptoms (see below). This discordance has led to a reconsideration of the MS disease process as having two separate phases: inflammatory and neurodegenerative. In this model, the former leads to attacks and the latter to progression. It is likely that a gradual loss of axons underlies progressive MS symptoms, and this process could hypothetically result from loss of trophic influences provided by intact myelin. If true, then an MS attack early in the course might lead to a progressive symptom many years later. Because of this possibility, many experts currently believe that very early treatment with a disease-modifying drug is appropriate for most MS patients. It is reasonable to delay initiating treatment in patients with (1) normal neurologic exams; (2) a single attack or a low attack frequency; and (3) a low burden of disease as assessed by brain MRI. Untreated patients need to be followed closely with periodic brain MRI scans; the

need for therapy is reassessed if the scans reveal evidence of ongoing, subclinical disease.

Most treated patients with relapsing forms of MS receive IFN-β as first-line therapy. Regardless of which agent is chosen first, treatment should probably be altered in patents who continue to have frequent attacks or progressive disability (Fig. 359-4). The value of combination therapy is unknown.

IFN-β1a (Avonex), 30 μg, is administered by intramuscular injection once every week. IFN-β1a (Rebif), 44 μg, is administered by subcutaneous injection three times per week. IFN-β1b (Betaseron), 250 μg, is administered by subcutaneous injection every other day. Glatiramer acetate, 20 mg, is administered by subcutaneous injection every day. Common side effects of IFN-β therapy include flulike symptoms (e.g., fevers, chills, and myalgias) and mild abnormalities on routine laboratory evaluation (e.g., elevated liver function tests or lymphopenia). Rarely, more severe hepatotoxicity may occur. Subcutaneous IFN-β also causes reactions at the injection site (e.g., pain, redness, induration, or, rarely, skin necrosis). Side effects can usually be managed with concomitant nonsteroidal anti-inflammatory medications and with the use of an auto-injector. Depression, increased spasticity, and cognitive changes have been reported, although these symptoms can also be due to the underlying disease. In any event, side effects to IFN-β therapy usually subside with time.

Approximately 2 to 10% of IFN-β1a (Avonex) recipients, 15 to 25% of IFN-β1a (Rebif) recipients, and 30 to 40% of IFN-β1b (Betaseron) recipients develop neutralizing antibodies to IFN-β, which may disappear over time. Some evidence suggests that neutralizing antibodies reduce efficacy, especially for MRI outcomes. The current clinical data, however, are quite conflicted. Moreover, there are few situations where measurement of antibodies is necessary. Thus, for a patient doing well on therapy, the presence of antibodies should not matter. Conversely, for a patient doing poorly on therapy, alternative

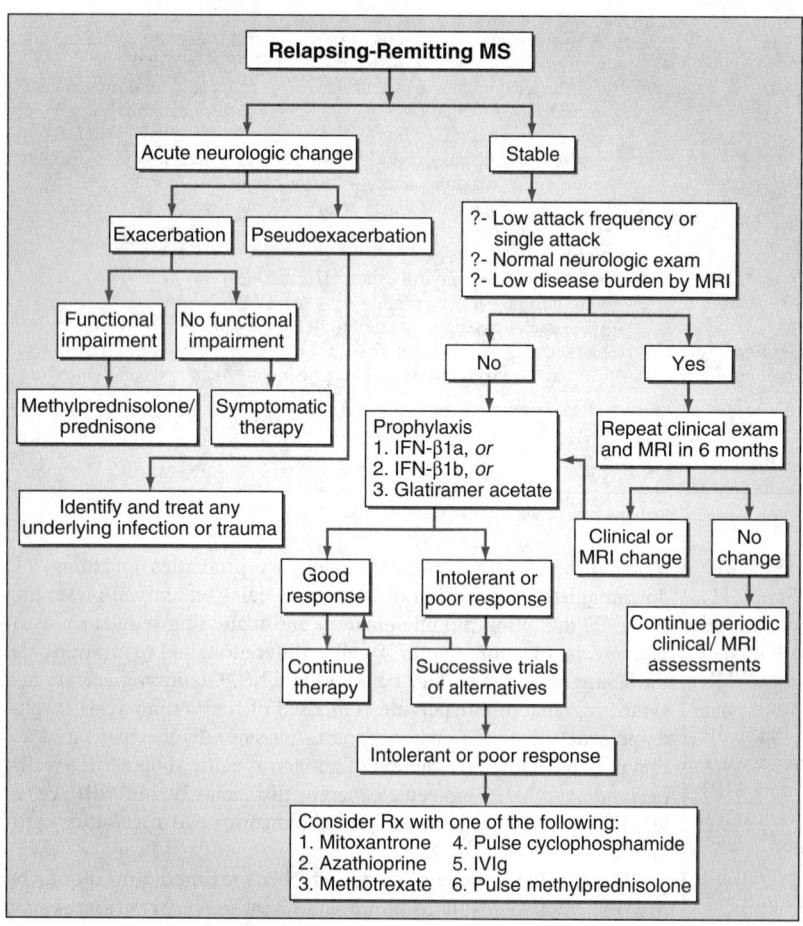

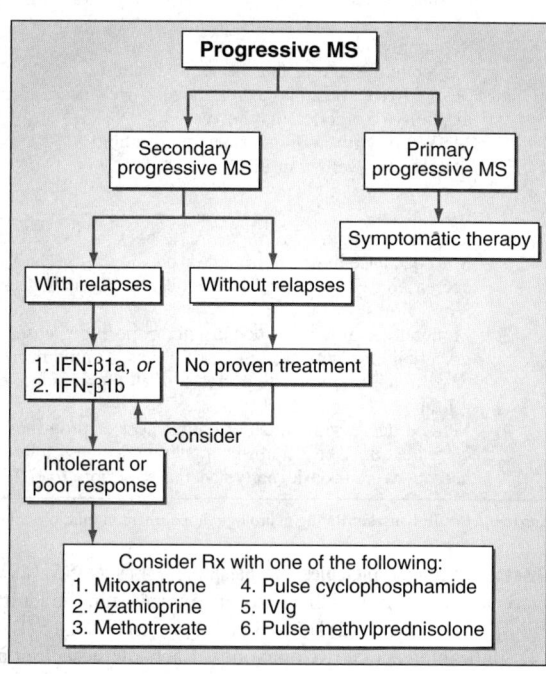

FIGURE 359-4   Therapeutic decision making for MS.

treatment should be considered, even if there are no detectable antibodies.

Injection site reactions also occur with glatiramer acetate but are less severe than with IFN-β1b. Approximately 15% of patients experience one or more episodes of flushing, chest tightness, dyspnea, palpitations, and anxiety after injection. This systemic reaction is unpredictable, brief (duration <1 h), and tends not to recur.

MITOXANTRONE HYDROCHLORIDE Mitoxantrone (Novantrone), an anthracenedione, exerts its antineoplastic action by (1) intercalating into DNA and producing both strand breaks and interstrand cross-links, (2) interfering with RNA synthesis and, (3) inhibiting topoisomerase II (involved in DNA repair). The U.S. Food and Drug Administration (FDA) approved mitoxantrone on the basis of a single (relatively small) phase III clinical trial in Europe, in addition to an even smaller phase II study completed earlier. Mitoxantrone received (from the FDA) the broadest indication of any current treatment for MS. Thus, mitoxantrone is indicated for use in SPMS, in PRMS, and in patients with worsening RRMS (defined as patients whose neurologic status remains significantly abnormal between MS attacks). Despite this broad indication, however, the data supporting its efficacy are weaker than for other approved therapies.

Mitoxantrone can produce cardiac problems (e.g., cardiomyopathy, reduced left ventricular ejection fraction, and irreversible congestive heart failure). As a result, a cumulative dose >140 mg/m^2 is not recommended. At currently approved doses (12 mg/m^2 every 3 months), the maximum duration of therapy can be only 2 to 3 years. Furthermore, >40% of women will experience amenorrhea, which may be permanent. Finally, there is risk of acute leukemia, and this complication has already been reported in several mitoxantrone-treated MS patients.

Given these risks, mitoxantrone should not be used as a first-line agent in either RRMS or relapsing SPMS. It is reasonable to consider mitoxantrone in selected patients with a progressive course who have failed other approved therapies.

Disease-Modifying Therapies for SPMS without Relapses

High-dose IFN-β probably has a beneficial effect in patients with SPMS who are still experiencing acute relapses. IFN-β is probably ineffective in patients with SPMS who are not having acute attacks.

Although mitoxantrone has been approved for patients with progressive MS, this is not the population studied in the pivotal trial. Therefore no evidence-based recommendation can be made with regard to its use in this setting.

PPMS

No currently available therapies have shown any promise for treating PPMS at this time. A phase III clinical trial of glatiramer acetate in PPMS was recently stopped because of an apparent lack of efficacy. A trial of mitoxantrone in PPMS is in progress.

Off-Label Treatment Options for RRMS and SPMS

Azathioprine (2 to 3 mg/kg body weight) has been used primarily in SPMS. Meta-analysis of published trials suggests that azathioprine is marginally effective at lowering relapse rates, although a benefit on disability progression has not been demonstrated.

Methotrexate (7.5 to 20 mg/wk) was shown in one study to slow the progression of upper extremity dysfunction in SPMS. Because of the possibility of developing irreversible liver damage, some experts recommend a blind liver biopsy after 2 years of therapy.

Cyclophosphamide (700 mg/m^2, every other month) may be helpful for treatment-refractory patients who are (1) otherwise in good health, (2) ambulatory, and (3) <40 years of age. Because cyclophosphamide can be used for periods in excess of 3 years, it may be preferable to mitoxantrone in these circumstances.

Intravenous immunoglobulin (IVIg), administered in monthly pulses (up to 1 g/kg) for up to 2 years, appears to reduce annual exacerbation rates. However, its use is limited because of its high cost, questions about optimal dose, and uncertainty about its effect on long-term disability outcome.

Methylprednisolone administered in one study as monthly high-dose intravenous pulses, reduced disability progression (see above).

Other Therapeutic Claims

Many purported treatments for MS have never been subjected to scientific scrutiny. These include dietary therapies (e.g., the Swank diet in addition to others), megadose vitamins, calcium orotate, bee stings, cow colostrum, hyperbaric oxygen, procarin (a combination of histamine and caffeine), chelation, acupuncture, acupressure, various Chinese herbal remedies, and removal of mercury amalgam tooth fillings, among many others. Patients should avoid costly or potentially hazardous unproven treatments. Many such treatments lack biologic plausibility. For example, no reliable case of mercury poisoning resembling typical MS has ever been described.

Although potential roles for human herpes virus 6 and/or chlamydia have been suggested for MS, these reports are unconfirmed, and treatment with antiviral agents or antibiotics is not currently appropriate.

Symptomatic Therapy

Potassium channel blockers (e.g., 4-aminopyridine, 10 to 40 mg/d; and 3,4-di-aminopyridine, 40 to 80 mg/d) may be helpful for *weakness*, especially for heat-sensitive symptoms. At high doses they may cause seizures. These agents are not FDA-approved but can be obtained from compounding pharmacies around the United States.

Ataxia/tremor is often intractable. Clonazepam, 1.5 to 20 mg/d; mysoline, 50 to 250 mg/d; propranolol, 40 to 200 mg/d; or ondansetron, 8 to 16 mg/d may help. Wrist-weights occasionally reduce tremor in the arm or hand. Thalamotomy or deep brain stimulation has been tried with mixed success.

Spasticity and *spasms* may improve with physical therapy, regular exercise, and stretching. Avoidance of triggers (e.g., infections, fecal impactions, bed sores) is extremely important. Effective medications include lioresal (20 to 120 mg/d), diazepam (2 to 40 mg/d), tizanidine (8 to 32 mg/d), dantroline (25 to 400 mg/d), and cyclobenzaprine hydrochloride (10 to 60 mg/d). For severe spasticity, a lioresal pump (delivering medication directly into the CSF) can provide substantial relief.

Pain is treated with anticonvulsants (carbamazepine, 100 to 1000 mg/d; phenytoin, 300 to 600 mg/d; or gabapentin, 300 to 3600 mg/d), antidepressants (amitriptyline, 25 to 150 mg/d; nortryptiline, 25 to 150 mg/d; desipramine, 100 to 300 mg/d; or venlafaxine, 75 to 225 mg/d), or antiarrhythmics (mexiletine, 300 to 900 mg/d). If these approaches fail, patients should be referred to a comprehensive pain management program.

Bladder dysfunction management is best guided by urodynamic testing. Evening fluid restriction or frequent voluntary voiding may help *detrusor hyperreflexia*. If these methods fail, propantheline bromide (10 to 15 mg/d), oxybutinin (5 to 15 mg/d), hycosamine sulfate (0.5 to 0.75 mg/d), or tolteridine tartrate (2 to 4 mg/d) may help. Coadministration of pseudoephedrine (30 to 60 mg) is sometimes beneficial.

Detrusor/sphyncter dyssynergia may respond to phenoxybenzamine (10 to 20 mg/d) or terazosin hydrochloride (1 to 20 mg/d). Loss of reflex bladder wall contraction may respond to bethanecol (30 to 150 mg/d). However, both conditions often require catheterization.

Urinary tract infections should be treated promptly. Patients with large postvoid residual urine volumes are predisposed to infections. Prevention by urine acidification (with cranberry juice or vitamin C) inhibits some bacteria. Prophylactic administration of antibiotics is sometimes necessary but may lead to colonization by resistant organisms. Intermittent catheterization may help to prevent recurrent infections.

Treatment of *constipation* includes high-fiber diets and fluids. Natural or other laxatives may help. *Fecal incontinence* may respond to a reduction in dietary fiber.

Depression should be treated. Useful drugs include the selective serotonin reuptake inhibitors (fluoxitine, 20 to 80 mg/d, or sertraline, 50 to 200 mg/d); the tricyclic antidepressants, (amitriptyline, 25 to 150 mg/d, nortryptiline, 25 to 150 mg/d, or desipramine, 100 to 300 mg/d); and the non-tricyclic antidepressants (venlafaxine, 75 to 225 mg/d).

Fatigue may improve with assistive devices, help in the home, or successful management of spasticity. Patients with frequent nocturia may benefit from anticholinergic medication at bedtime. Primary MS fatigue may respond to amantadine (200 mg/d), pemoline (37.5 to 75 mg/d), methylphenidate (5 to 25 mg/d), or modafinil (100 to 400 mg/d).

Cognitive problems may respond to the cholinesterase inhibitor donepezil hydrochloride (10 mg/d).

Paroxysmal symptoms respond dramatically to low-dose anticonvulsants (acetazolamide, 200 to 600 mg/d; carbamazepine, 50 to 400 mg/d; phenytoin, 50 to 300 mg/d; or gabapentin, 600 to 1800 mg/d).

Heat sensitivity may respond to heat-avoidance, air conditioning, or cooling garments.

Sexual dysfunction may be helped by lubricants to aid in genital stimulation and sexual arousal. Management of pain, spasticity, fatigue, and bladder/bowel dysfunction may also help. Sildenafil (50 to 100 mg) taken 1 to 2 h before sex is now the standard treatment for maintaining erections.

Promising Experimental Therapies   Numerous clinical trials are currently underway. These include: (1) combination therapies; (2) higher-dose IFN-β than currently prescribed; (3) monoclonal antibodies against α_4-integrin to prevent adhesion of lymphocytes to endothelial surfaces, against CD52 to induce global lymphocyte depletion, or against CD20 to deplete B cells selectively; (4) use of statins as immunomodulators; (5) estriol to induce a pregnancy-like state; (6) bone marrow transplants; and (7) schwann cell transplants.

CLINICAL VARIANTS OF MS   *Neuromyelitis optica* (NMO), or Devic's syndrome, consists of separate attacks of acute ON and myelitis. ON may be unilateral or bilateral and precede or follow an attack of myelitis by days, months, or years. In contrast to MS, patients with NMO do not experience brainstem, cerebellar, and cognitive involvement, and the brain MRI is typically normal. A focal enhancing region of swelling and cavitation, extending over three or more spinal cord segments, is typically seen on MRI. Histopathology of these lesions may reveal areas of necrosis and thickening of blood vessel walls. NMO, which is uncommon in Caucasians compared with Asians and Africans, is best understood as a syndrome with diverse causes. Some patients have a systemic autoimmune disorder, often systemic lupus erythematosus, Sjögren's syndrome, p-ANCA (perinuclear antineutrophil cytoplasmic antibody) associated vasculitis, or mixed connective tissue disease. In others, onset may be associated with acute infection with varicella-zoster virus or HIV. More frequently, however, NMO is idiopathic and probably represents an MS variant.

Occasional patients present with apparent NMO but have periventricular MRI changes indicating typical MS. Furthermore, in the MS disease model EAE, immunization with peptides of MOG can produce an NMO-like disorder. Disease-modifying therapies for MS have not been rigorously studied in NMO. Acute attacks are usually treated with high-dose glucocorticoids as for MS exacerbations (see above). Because of the possibility that NMO is antibody-mediated, plasma exchange has also been used empirically for acute episodes that fail to respond to glucocorticoids. Immunosuppressants or interferons are sometimes used in the hope that further relapses will be prevented.

Acute MS (Marburg's variant) is a fulminant demyelinating process that progresses to death within 1 to 2 years. Typically, there are no remissions. Diagnosis is established by biopsy or at autopsy, revealing widespread demyelination, axonal loss, edema, and macro-phage infiltration. Discrete plaques may also be seen. Recent evidence strongly supports an antibody-mediated process in the demyelinating lesions. Marburg's variant does not seem to follow infection or vaccination, and it is unclear whether this syndrome represents an extreme form of MS or another disease altogether. No controlled trials of therapy exist; high-dose glucocorticoids, plasma exchange, and cyclophosphamide have been tried, with uncertain benefit.

ACUTE DISSEMINATED ENCEPHALOMYELITIS (ADEM)

ADEM has a monophasic course and is frequently associated with antecedent immunization (postvaccinal encephalomyelitis) or infection (postinfectious encephalomyelitis). The hallmark of ADEM is the presence of widely scattered small foci of perivenular inflammation and demyelination. In its most explosive form, acute hemorrhagic leukoencephalitis of Weston Hurst, the lesions are vasculitic and hemorrhagic, and the clinical course is devastating.

Postvaccinal encephalomyelitis may follow the administration of smallpox and certain rabies vaccines. Postinfectious encephalomyelitis is most frequently associated with the viral exanthems of childhood. Infection with measles virus is the most common antecedent (1 in 1000 cases). Worldwide, measles encephalomyelitis is still common, although use of the live measles vaccine has dramatically reduced its incidence in developed countries. An ADEM-like illness rarely follows vaccination with live measles vaccine (1 to 2 in 10^6 immunizations). ADEM is now most frequently associated with varicella (chickenpox) infections (1 in 4000 to 10,000 cases). It may also follow infection with rubella, mumps, influenza, parainfluenza, and infectious mononucleosis viruses and with *Mycoplasma*. Some patients may have a nonspecific upper respiratory infection or no known antecedent illness.

An autoimmune response to MBP can be detected in the CSF from many patients with ADEM. This response has been most clearly established after rabies vaccination and infection with measles virus. With measles infection, the induction of immune responses to a variety of CNS antigens may occur, but only the response to MBP correlates with the development of ADEM. Many cases of postvaccinal encephalomyelitis may result from sensitization with brain material that contaminates the viral vaccines. Attempts to demonstrate direct viral invasion of the CNS have been unsuccessful.

CLINICAL MANIFESTATIONS   In severe cases, onset is abrupt, and progression rapid (hours to days). In postinfectious ADEM, the neurologic syndrome generally begins late in the course of the viral illness as the exanthem is fading. Fever reappears, and headache, meningismus, and lethargy progressing to coma may develop. Seizures are common. Signs of disseminated neurologic disease are consistently present (e.g., hemiparesis or quadriparesis, extensor plantar responses, lost or hyperactive tendon reflexes, sensory loss and brainstem involvement). In ADEM due to chickenpox, cerebellar involvement is often conspicuous. CSF protein is modestly elevated [0.5 to 1.5 g/L (50 to 150 mg/dL)]. Lymphocytic pleocytosis, generally 200 cells/μl, occurs in 80% of patients. Occasional patients have higher counts or a mixed polymorphonuclear-lymphocytic pattern during the initial days of the illness. Transient CSF oligoclonal banding has been reported. MRI may reveal extensive gadolinium enhancement of white matter in brain and spinal cord.

DIAGNOSIS   The diagnosis is easily established when there is a history of recent vaccination or exanthematous illness. In severe cases with predominantly cerebral involvement, acute encephalitis due to infection with herpes simplex or other viruses may be difficult to exclude. The simultaneous onset of disseminated symptoms and signs is common in ADEM and rare in MS. Similarly, meningismus, drowsiness or coma, or seizures suggest ADEM rather than MS. Unlike in MS, in ADEM optic nerve involvement is generally bilateral and transverse myelopathy complete. MRI findings that may support a diagnosis of ADEM include extensive and relatively symmetric white matter abnormalities and Gd enhancement of all abnormal areas, indicating active disease and a monophasic course.

℞ TREATMENT

Initial treatment is with high-dose glucocorticoids as for exacerbations of MS (see above). Patients who fail to respond may benefit from a course of plasma exchange or intravenous immunoglobulin. The prognosis reflects the severity of the underlying acute illness. Measles encephalomyelitis is associated with a mortality rate of 5 to 20%, and most survivors have permanent neurologic sequelae. Children who recover may have persistent seizures and behavioral and learning disorders.

FURTHER READING

BERGER T et al: Antimyelin antibodies as a predictor of clinically definite multiple sclerosis after a first demyelinating event. N Engl J Med 349:139, 2003
CREE BAC et al: Neuromyelitis optica. Semin Neurol 22:105, 2002
GOODIN DS et al: Disease modifying therapies in multiple sclerosis: Report of the Therapeutics and Technology Assessment Subcommittee of the American Academy of Neurology. Neurology 58:169, 2002
OKSENBERG J et al: Mapping multiple sclerosis susceptibility to the HLA-DR locus in African Americans. Am J Hum Genet 74:160, 2004

360 MENINGITIS, ENCEPHALITIS, BRAIN ABSCESS, AND EMPYEMA
Karen L. Roos, Kenneth L. Tyler

Acute infections of the nervous system are among the most important problems in medicine because early recognition, efficient decision-making, and rapid institution of therapy can be lifesaving. These distinct clinical syndromes include acute bacterial meningitis, viral meningitis, encephalitis, focal infections such as brain abscess and subdural empyema, and infectious thrombophlebitis. Each may present with a nonspecific prodrome of fever and headache, which in a previously healthy individual may initially be thought to be benign, until (with the exception of viral meningitis) altered consciousness, focal neurologic signs, or seizures appear. Key goals of early management are to emergently distinguish between these conditions, identify the responsible pathogen, and initiate appropriate antimicrobial therapy.

APPROACH TO THE PATIENT

(Fig. 360-1) The first task is to identify whether an infection predominantly involves the subarachnoid space ("meningitis") or whether there is evidence of either generalized or focal involvement of brain tissue in the cerebral hemispheres, cerebellum, or brainstem. When brain tissue is directly injured by a viral infection the disease is referred to as "encephalitis," whereas focal bacterial, fungal, or parasitic infections involving brain tissue are classified as either "cerebritis" or "abscess," depending on the presence or absence of a capsule.

Nuchal rigidity is the pathognomonic sign of meningeal irritation and is present when the neck resists passive flexion. Kernig's and Brudzinski's signs are also classic signs of meningeal irritation. *Kernig's sign* is elicited with the patient in the supine position. The thigh is flexed on the abdomen, with the knee flexed; attempts to passively extend the knee elicit pain when meningeal irritation is present. *Brudzinski's sign* is elicited with the patient in the supine position and is positive when passive flexion of the neck results in spontaneous flexion of the hips and knees. Although commonly tested on physical examinations, the sensitivity and specificity of Kernig's and Brudzinski's signs are uncertain. Both may be absent or reduced in very young or elderly patients, immunocompromised individuals, or patients with a severely depressed mental status. The high prevalence of cervical spine disease in older individuals may result in false-positive tests for nuchal rigidity.

Initial management can be guided by several considerations: (1) Empirical therapy should be initiated promptly whenever bacterial meningitis is a significant diagnostic consideration. (2) All patients who have had recent head trauma, are immunocompromised, have known malignant lesions or central nervous system (CNS) neoplasms, or have focal neurologic findings including papilledema or a depressed level of consciousness should undergo computed tomography (CT) or magnetic resonance imaging (MRI) of the brain prior to lumbar puncture (LP). In these cases empirical antibiotic therapy should not be delayed pending test results but should be administered prior to neuroimaging and LP. (3) A significantly depressed mental status (e.g., somnolence, coma), seizures, or focal neurologic deficits only rarely occur in viral ("aseptic") meningitis; patients with these symptoms should be hospitalized for further evaluation and treated empirically for bacterial and viral meningoencephalitis. (4) Immunocompetent patients with a normal level of consciousness, no prior antimicrobial treatment, and a cerebrospinal fluid (CSF) profile consistent with viral meningitis (lymphocytic pleocytosis and a normal glucose concentration) can often be treated as outpatients, if appropriate contact and monitoring can be ensured. Failure of a patient with suspected viral meningitis to improve within 48 h should prompt a reevaluation including follow-up neurologic and general medical examination and repeat imaging and laboratory studies, often including a second LP.

ACUTE BACTERIAL MENINGITIS

DEFINITION Bacterial meningitis is an acute purulent infection within the subarachnoid space. It is associated with a CNS inflammatory reaction that may result in decreased consciousness, seizures, raised intracranial pressure (ICP), and stroke. The meninges, the subarachnoid space, and the brain parenchyma are all frequently involved in the inflammatory reaction (*meningoencephalitis*).

EPIDEMIOLOGY Bacterial meningitis is the most common form of suppurative CNS infection, with an annual incidence in the United States of >2.5 cases/100,000 population. The epidemiology of bacterial meningitis has changed significantly in recent years, reflecting a dramatic decline in the incidence of meningitis due to *Haemophilus influenzae*, and a smaller decline in that due to *Neisseria meningitidis*, following the introduction and increasingly widespread use of vaccines for both these organisms. Currently, the organisms most commonly responsible for community-acquired bacterial meningitis are *Streptococcus pneumoniae* (~50%), *N. meningitidis* (~25%), group B streptococci (~15%), and *Listeria monocytogenes* (~10%). *H. influenzae* now accounts for <10% of cases of bacterial meningitis in most series.

ETIOLOGY *S. pneumoniae* (Chap. 121) is the most common cause of meningitis in adults >20 years of age, accounting for nearly half the reported cases (1.1 per 100,000 persons per year). There are a number of predisposing conditions that increase the risk of pneumococcal meningitis, the most important of which is pneumococcal pneumonia. Additional risk factors include coexisting acute or chronic pneumococcal sinusitis or otitis media, alcoholism, diabetes, splenectomy, hypogammaglobulinemia, complement deficiency, and head trauma with basilar skull fracture and CSF rhinorrhea. Mortality remains ~20% despite antibiotic therapy.

N. meningitidis (Chap. 127) accounts for 25% of all cases of bacterial meningitis (0.6 cases per 100,000 persons per year) and for up to 60% of cases in children and young adults between the ages of 2 and 20. The presence of petechial or purpuric skin lesions can provide an important clue to the diagnosis of meningococcal infection. In some patients the disease is fulminant, progressing to death within hours of symptom onset. Infection may be initiated by nasopharyngeal colo-

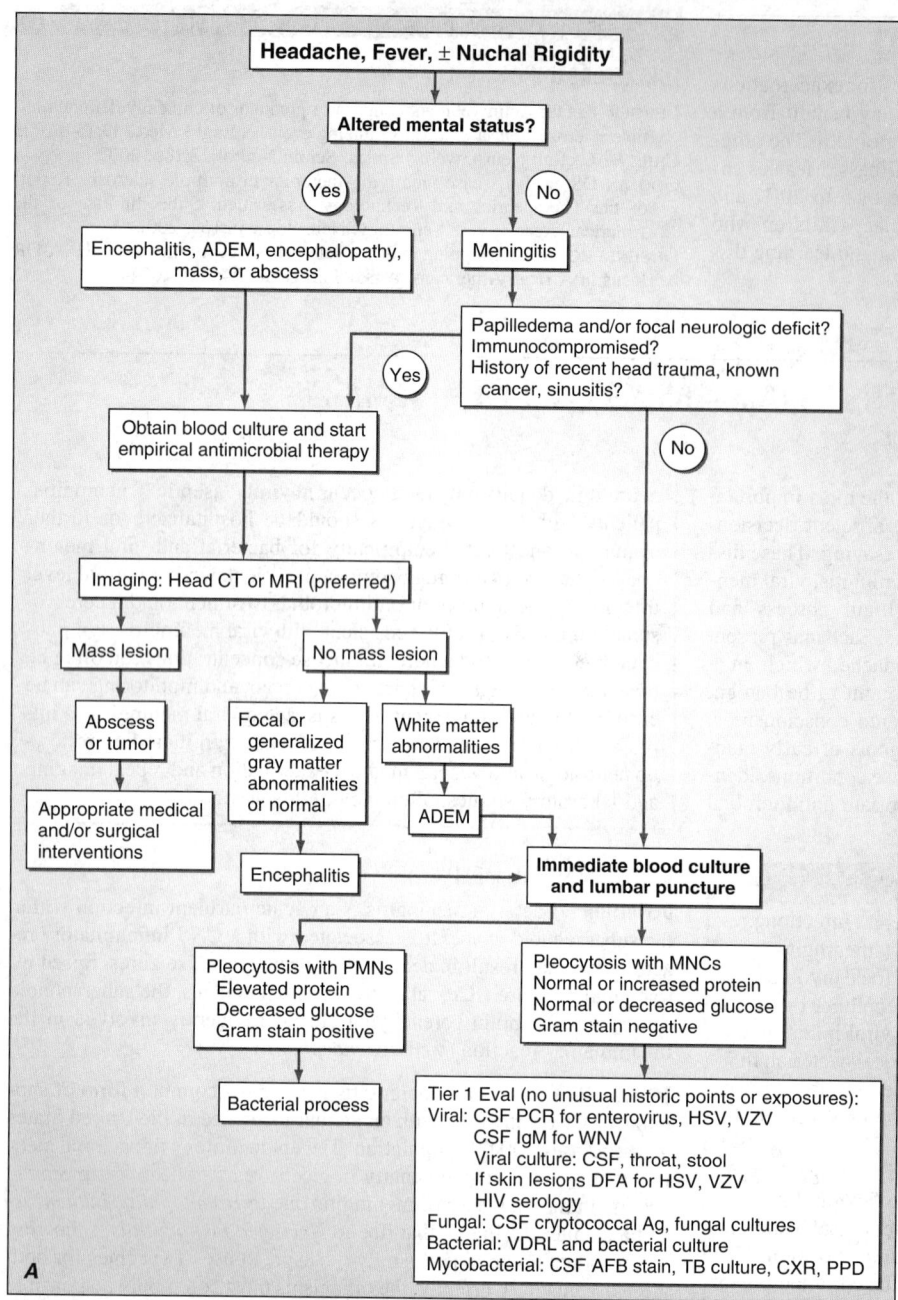

Headache, Fever, ± Nuchal Rigidity

Altered mental status?

Yes → **Encephalitis, ADEM, encephalopathy, mass, or abscess**

No → **Meningitis**

Papilledema and/or focal neurologic deficit? Immunocompromised? History of recent head trauma, known cancer, sinusitis?

Yes → **Obtain blood culture and start empirical antimicrobial therapy**

No →

Imaging: Head CT or MRI (preferred)

Mass lesion → **Abscess or tumor** → **Appropriate medical and/or surgical interventions**

No mass lesion →
- **Focal or generalized gray matter abnormalities or normal** → **Encephalitis**
- **White matter abnormalities** → **ADEM**

Immediate blood culture and lumbar puncture

Pleocytosis with PMNs Elevated protein Decreased glucose Gram stain positive → **Bacterial process**

Pleocytosis with MNCs Normal or increased protein Normal or decreased glucose Gram stain negative →

Tier 1 Eval (no unusual historic points or exposures):
Viral: CSF PCR for enterovirus, HSV, VZV
  CSF IgM for WNV
  Viral culture: CSF, throat, stool
  If skin lesions DFA for HSV, VZV
  HIV serology
Fungal: CSF cryptococcal Ag, fungal cultures
Bacterial: VDRL and bacterial culture
Mycobacterial: CSF AFB stain, TB culture, CXR, PPD

FIGURE 360-1 *A.* Algorithm for management of patients with suspected CNS infections. ADEM, acute disseminated encephalomyelitis; CT, computed tomography; MRI, magnetic resonance imaging; PMNs, polymorphonuclear leukocytes; MNCs, mononuclear cells; CSF, cerebrospinal fluid; PCR, polymerase chain reaction; HSV, herpes simplex virus; VZV, varicella-zoster virus; WNV, West Nile Virus; DFA, direct fluorescent antibody; Ag, antigen; VDRL, Venereal Disease Research Laboratory; AFB, acid-fast bacillus; TB, tuberculosis; CXR, chest x-ray; PPD, purified protein derivative; EBV, Epstein-Barr virus; CTFV, Colorado tick fever virus; HHV, human herpesvirus; LCMV, lymphocytic choriomeningitis virus.

Group B streptococcus, or *S. agalactiae*, was previously responsible for meningitis predominantly in neonates, but it has been reported with increasing frequency in individuals >50 years of age, particularly those with underlying diseases.

L. monocytogenes (Chap. 123) has become an increasingly important cause of meningitis in neonates (<1 month of age), pregnant women, individuals >60 years, and immunocompromised individuals of all ages. Infection is acquired by ingesting foods contaminated by *Listeria*. Foodborne human listerial infection has been reported from contaminated coleslaw, milk, soft cheeses, and several types of "ready-to-eat" foods including delicatessen meat and uncooked hotdogs.

The frequency of *H. influenzae* type b meningitis in children has declined dramatically since the introduction of the Hib conjugate vaccine, although rare cases of Hib meningitis in vaccinated children have been reported. More frequently, *H. influenzae* causes meningitis in unvaccinated children and adults.

Staphylococcus aureus and coagulase-negative staphylococci (Chap. 120) are important causes of meningitis that follows invasive neurosurgical procedures, particularly shunting procedures for hydrocephalus, or that occurs as a complication of the use of subcutaneous Ommaya reservoirs for administration of intrathecal chemotherapy.

PATHOPHYSIOLOGY The most common bacteria that cause meningitis, *S. pneumoniae* and *N. meningitidis*, initially colonize the nasopharynx by attaching to nasopharyngeal epithelial cells. Bacteria are transported across epithelial cells in membrane-bound vacuoles to the intravascular space or invade the intravascular space by creating separations in the apical tight junctions of columnar epithelial cells. Once in the bloodstream, bacteria are able to avoid phagocytosis by neutrophils and classic complement–mediated bactericidal activity because of the presence of a polysaccharide capsule. Bloodborne bacteria can reach the intraventricular choroid plexus, directly infect choroid plexus epithelial cells, and gain access to the CSF. Some bacteria, such as *S. pneumoniae*, can adhere to cerebral capillary endothelial cells and subsequently migrate through or between these cells to reach the CSF. Bacteria are able to multiply rapidly within CSF because of the absence of effective host immune defenses. Normal CSF contains few white blood cells (WBCs) and relatively small amounts of complement proteins and immunoglobulins. The paucity of the latter two prevents effective opsonization of bacteria, an essential prerequisite for bacterial phagocytosis by neutrophils. Phagocytosis of bacteria is further impaired by the fluid nature of CSF, which is less conducive to phagocytosis than a solid tissue substrate.

A critical event in the pathogenesis of bacterial meningitis is the inflammatory reaction induced by the invading bacteria. Many of the neurologic manifestations and complications of bacterial meningitis result from the immune response to the invading pathogen rather than from direct bacteria-induced tissue injury. As a result, neurologic injury can progress even after the CSF has been sterilized by antibiotic therapy.

nization, which can result in either an asymptomatic carrier state or invasive meningococcal disease. The risk of invasive disease following nasopharyngeal colonization depends on both bacterial virulence factors and host immune defense mechanisms, including the host's capacity to produce antimeningococcal antibodies and to lyse meningococci by both the classic and alternative complement pathways. Individuals with deficiencies of any of the complement components, including properdin, are highly susceptible to meningococcal infections.

Enteric gram-negative bacilli are an increasingly common cause of meningitis in individuals with chronic and debilitating diseases such as diabetes, cirrhosis, or alcoholism and in those with chronic urinary tract infections. Gram-negative meningitis can also complicate neurosurgical procedures, particularly craniotomy.

The lysis of bacteria with the subsequent release of cell-wall components into the subarachnoid space is the initial step in the induction of the inflammatory response and the formation of a purulent exudate in the subarachnoid space (Fig. 360-2). Bacterial cell-wall components, such as the lipopolysaccharide (LPS) molecules of gram-negative bacteria and teichoic acid and peptidoglycans of *S. pneumoniae*, induce meningeal inflammation by stimulating the production of inflammatory cytokines and chemokines by microglia, astrocytes, monocytes, microvascular endothelial cells, and CSF leukocytes. In experimental models of meningitis, cytokines including tumor necrosis factor (TNF) and interleukin (IL) 1 are present in CSF within 1 to 2 h of intracisternal inoculation of LPS. This cytokine response is quickly followed by an increase in CSF protein concentration and leukocytosis. Chemokines (cytokines that induce chemotactic migration in leukocytes) and a variety of other proinflammatory cytokines are also produced and secreted by leukocytes and tissue cells that are stimulated by IL-1 and TNF. In addition, bacteremia and the inflammatory cytokines induce the production of excitatory amino acids, reactive oxygen and nitrogen species (free oxygen radicals, nitric oxide, and peroxynitrite), and other mediators that can induce death of brain cells.

Much of the pathophysiology of bacterial meningitis is a direct consequence of elevated levels of CSF cytokines and chemokines. TNF and IL-1 act synergistically to increase the permeability of the blood-brain barrier, resulting in induction of vasogenic edema and the leakage of serum proteins into the subarachnoid space (Fig. 360-2). The subarachnoid exudate of proteinaceous material and leukocytes obstructs the flow of CSF through the ventricular system and diminishes the resorptive capacity of the arachnoid granulations in the dural sinuses, leading to obstructive and communicating hydrocephalus and concomitant interstitial edema.

Inflammatory cytokines upregulate the expression of selectins on cerebral capillary endothelial cells and leukocytes, promoting leukocyte adherence to vascular endothelial cells and subsequent migration into the CSF. The adherence of leukocytes to capillary endothelial cells increases the permeability of blood vessels, allowing for the leakage of plasma proteins into the CSF, which adds to the inflammatory exudate. Neutrophil degranulation results in the release of toxic metabolites that contribute to cytotoxic edema, cell injury, and death. Contrary to previous beliefs, CSF leukocytes probably do little to contribute to the clearance of CSF bacterial infection.

During the very early stages of meningitis there is an increase in cerebral blood flow, soon followed by a decrease in cerebral blood flow and a loss of cerebrovascular autoregulation (Chap. 258). Narrowing of the large arteries at the base of the brain due to encroachment by the purulent exudate in the subarachnoid space and infiltration of the arterial wall by inflammatory cells with intimal thickening (*vasculitis*) also occur and may result in ischemia and infarction, obstruction of branches of the middle cerebral artery by thrombosis, thrombosis of the major cerebral venous sinuses, and thrombophlebitis of the cerebral cortical veins. The combination of interstitial, vasogenic, and cytotoxic edema leads to raised ICP and coma. Cerebral herniation usually results from the effects of cerebral edema, either focal or generalized; hydrocephalus and dural sinus or cortical vein thrombosis may also play a role.

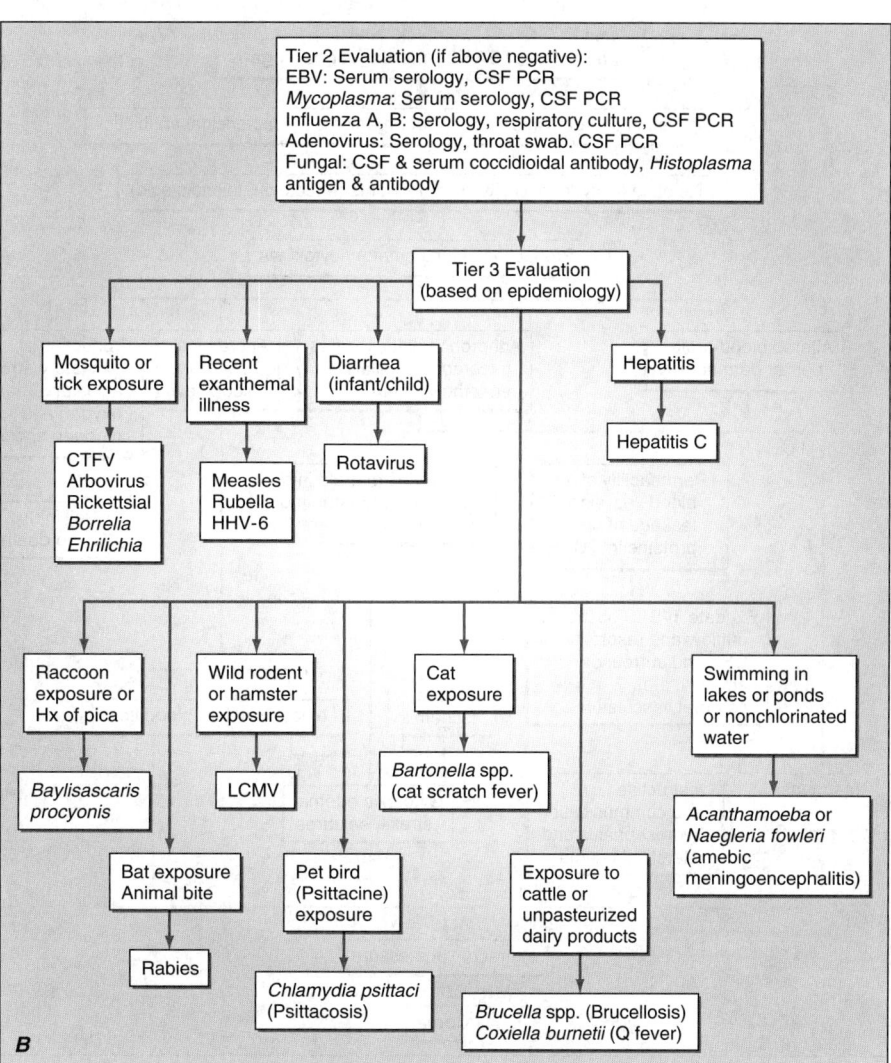

FIGURE 360-1B—*(Continued)*

CLINICAL PRESENTATION Meningitis can present as either an acute fulminant illness that progresses rapidly in a few hours or as a subacute infection that progressively worsens over several days. The classic clinical triad of meningitis is fever, headache, and nuchal rigidity ("stiff neck"). Each of these signs and symptoms occurs in >90% of cases. Alteration in mental status occurs in >75% of patients and can vary from lethargy to coma. Nausea, vomiting, and photophobia are also common complaints.

Seizures occur as part of the initial presentation of bacterial meningitis or during the course of the illness in 20 to 40% of patients. Focal seizures are usually due to focal arterial ischemia or infarction, cortical venous thrombosis with hemorrhage, or focal edema. Generalized seizure activity and status epilepticus may be due to hyponatremia, cerebral anoxia, or, less commonly, the toxic effects of antimicrobial agents such as high-dose penicillin.

Raised ICP is an expected complication of bacterial meningitis and is the major cause of obtundation and coma in this disease. More than 90% of patients will have a CSF opening pressure >180 mmH₂O, and 20% have opening pressures >400 mmH₂O. Signs of increased ICP include a deteriorating or reduced level of consciousness, papilledema, dilated poorly reactive pupils, sixth nerve palsies, decerebrate posturing, and the Cushing reflex (bradycardia, hypertension, and irregular respirations). The most disastrous complication of increased ICP is cerebral herniation. The incidence of herniation in patients with bacterial meningitis has been reported to occur in as few as 1% to as many as 8% of cases.

Specific clinical features may provide clues to the diagnosis of

2473

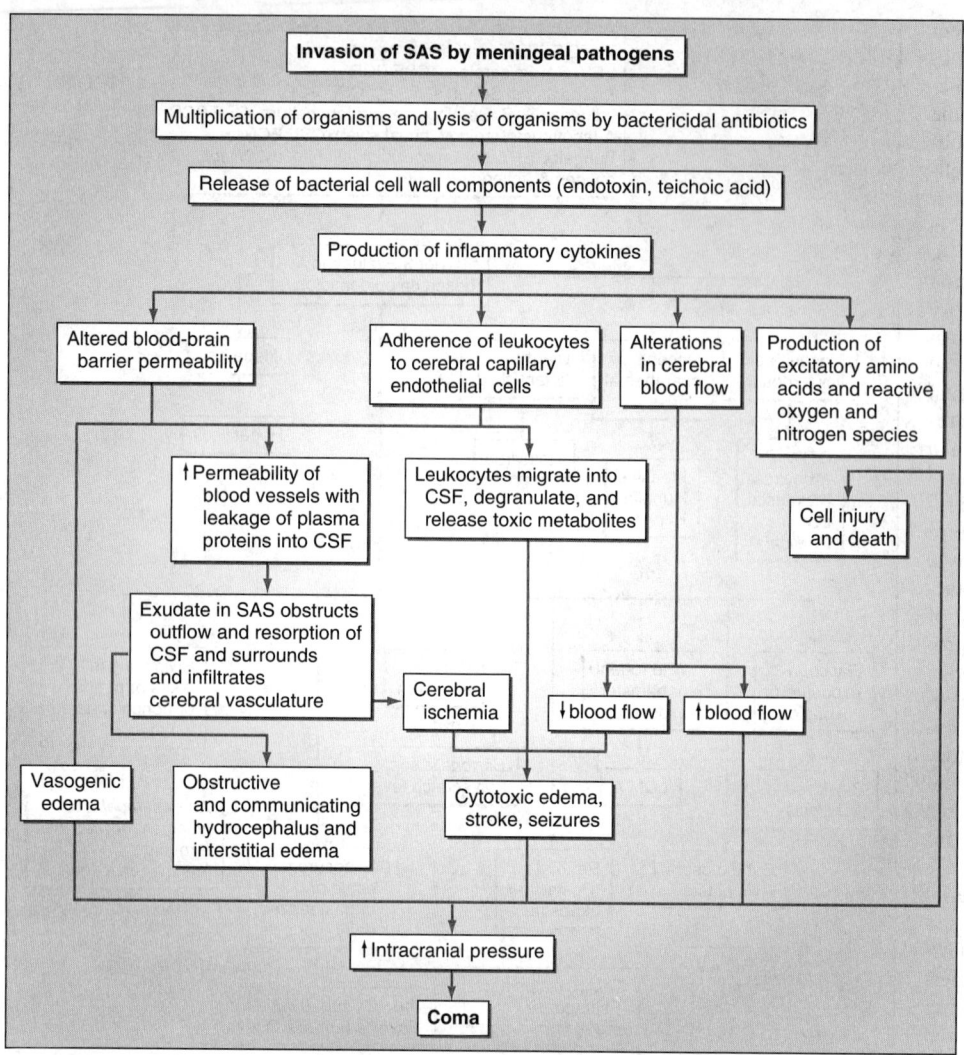

FIGURE 360-2 The pathophysiology of the neurologic complications of bacterial meningitis. SAS, subarachnoid space; CSF, cerebrospinal fluid.

individual organisms and are discussed in more detail in specific chapters devoted to individual pathogens. The most important of these clues is the rash of meningococcemia, which begins as a diffuse erythematous maculopapular rash resembling a viral exanthem, but the skin lesions of meningococcemia rapidly become petechial. Petechiae are found on the trunk and lower extremities, in the mucous membranes and conjunctiva, and occasionally on the palms and soles.

DIAGNOSIS When bacterial meningitis is suspected, blood cultures should be immediately obtained and empirical antimicrobial therapy initiated without delay. The diagnosis of bacterial meningitis is made by examination of the CSF (Table 360-1). The need to obtain neuroimaging studies (CT or MRI) prior to LP requires clinical judgment. In an immunocompetent patient with no known history of recent head trauma, a normal level of consciousness, and no evidence of papilledema or focal neurologic deficits, it is safe to perform LP without prior neuroimaging studies. If LP is delayed in order to obtain neuroimaging studies, empirical antibiotic therapy should be initiated after blood cultures are obtained. Antibiotic therapy initiated a few hours prior to LP will not significantly alter the CSF WBC count or glucose concentration, nor is it likely to prevent visualization of organisms by Gram's stain.

The classic CSF abnormalities in bacterial meningitis (Table 360-1) are (1) polymorphonuclear (PMN) leukocytosis (>100 cells/μL in 90%), (2) decreased glucose concentration [<2.2 mmol/L (<40 mg/dL) and/or CSF/serum glucose ratio of <0.4 in ~60%], (3) increased protein concentration [>0.45 g/L (>45 mg/dL) in 90%], and (4) increased opening pressure (>180 mmH$_2$O in 90%). CSF bacterial cul-

tures are positive in >80% of patients, and CSF Gram's stain demonstrates organisms in >60%.

CSF glucose concentrations <2.2 mmol/L (<40 mg/dL) are abnormal, and a CSF glucose concentration of zero can be seen in bacterial meningitis. Use of the CSF/serum glucose ratio corrects for hyperglycemia that may mask a relative decrease in the CSF glucose concentration. The CSF glucose concentration is low when the CSF/serum glucose ratio is <0.6. A CSF/serum glucose ratio <0.4 is highly suggestive of bacterial meningitis but may also be seen in other conditions, including fungal, tuberculous, and carcinomatous meningitis. It takes from 30 min to several hours for CSF glucose concentration to reach equilibrium with blood glucose concentrations; therefore, administration of 50 mL of 50% glucose (D50) prior to LP, as commonly occurs in emergency room settings, is unlikely to alter CSF glucose concentration significantly unless more than a few hours have elapsed between glucose administration and LP.

The latex agglutination (LA) test for the detection of bacterial antigens of *S. pneumoniae*, *N. meningitidis*, *H. influenzae* type b, group B streptococcus, and *Escherichia coli* K1 strains in the CSF is very useful for making a rapid diagnosis of bacterial meningitis, especially in patients who have been pretreated with antibiotics and in whom CSF Gram's stain and culture are negative. The CSF LA test has a *specificity* of 95 to 100% for *S. pneumoniae* and *N. meningitidis*, so a positive test is virtually diagnostic of bacterial meningitis caused by these organisms. However, the *sensitivity* of the CSF LA test is only 70 to 100% for detection of *S. pneumoniae* and 33 to 70% for detection of *N. meningitidis* antigens, so a negative test does not exclude infection by these organisms. The Limulus amebocyte lysate assay is a rapid diagnostic test for the detection of gram-negative endotoxin in CSF, and thus for making a diagnosis of gram-negative bacterial meningitis. The test has a specificity of 85 to 100% and a sensitivity approaching 100%. Thus, a positive Limulus amebocyte lysate assay occurs in virtually all patients with gram-negative bacterial meningitis, but false-positives may occur. CSF polymerase chain

TABLE 360-1 Cerebrospinal Fluid (CSF) Abnormalities in Bacterial Meningitis

Opening pressure	>180 mmH$_2$O
White blood cells	10/μL to 10,000/μL; neutrophils predominate
Red blood cells	Absent in nontraumatic tap
Glucose	<2.2 mmol/L (<40 mg/dL)
CSF/serum glucose	<0.4
Protein	>0.45 g/L (>45 mg/dL)
Gram's stain	Positive in >60%
Culture	Positive in >80%
Latex agglutination	May be positive in patients with meningitis due to *S. pneumoniae*, *N. meningitidis*, *H. influenzae* type b, *E. coli*, group B streptococci
Limulus lysates	Positive in cases of gram-negative meningitis
PCR for bacterial DNA	Research test

Note: PCR, polymerase chain reaction.

reaction (PCR) tests are not as useful in the diagnosis of bacterial meningitis as they are in the diagnosis of viral CNS infections. A CSF PCR test has been developed for detecting DNA from bacteria in CSF, but its sensitivity and specificity need to be better characterized before its role in diagnosis can be defined.

Almost all patients with bacterial meningitis will have neuroimaging studies performed during the course of their illness. MRI is preferred over CT because of its superiority in demonstrating areas of cerebral edema and ischemia. In patients with bacterial meningitis, diffuse meningeal enhancement is often seen after the administration of gadolinium. Meningeal enhancement is not diagnostic of meningitis but occurs in any CNS disease associated with increased blood-brain barrier permeability.

Petechial skin lesions, if present, should be biopsied. The rash of meningococcemia results from the dermal seeding of organisms with vascular endothelial damage, and biopsy may reveal the organism on Gram's stain.

DIFFERENTIAL DIAGNOSIS Viral meningoencephalitis, and particularly herpes simplex virus (HSV) encephalitis, can mimic the clinical presentation of bacterial meningitis (see "Encephalitis," below). HSV encephalitis typically presents with headache, fever, altered consciousness, focal neurologic deficits (e.g., dysphasia, hemiparesis), and focal or generalized seizures. The findings on CSF studies, neuroimaging, and electroencephalogram (EEG) distinguish HSV encephalitis from bacterial meningitis. The typical CSF profile with viral CNS infections is a lymphocytic pleocytosis with a normal glucose concentration, in contrast to PMN pleocytosis and hypoglycorrhachia characteristic of bacterial meningitis. MRI abnormalities (other than meningeal enhancement) are not seen in uncomplicated bacterial meningitis. By contrast, in HSV encephalitis parenchymal changes, especially in orbitofrontal and medial temporal lobes, are usually found. Some patients with HSV encephalitis have a distinctive periodic pattern on EEG (see below).

Rickettsial disease can resemble bacterial meningitis (Chap. 158). Rocky Mountain spotted fever (RMSF) is transmitted by a tick bite and caused by the bacteria *Rickettsia rickettsii*. The disease may present acutely with high fever, prostration, myalgia, headache, and nausea and vomiting. Most patients develop a characteristic rash within 96 h of the onset of symptoms. The rash is initially a diffuse erythematous maculopapular rash that may be difficult to distinguish from that of meningococcemia. It progresses to a petechial rash, then to a purpuric rash, and, if untreated, to skin necrosis or gangrene. The color of the lesions changes from bright red to very dark red, then yellowish-green to black. The rash typically begins in the wrist and ankles, and then spreads distally and proximally within a matter of a few hours and involves the palms and soles. Diagnosis is made by immunofluorescent staining of skin biopsy specimens.

Focal suppurative CNS infections (see below), including subdural and epidural empyema and brain abscess, should also be considered, especially when focal neurologic findings are present. MRI should be performed promptly in all patients with suspected meningitis who have focal features, both to detect the intracranial infection and to search for associated areas of infection in the sinuses or mastoid bones.

A number of noninfectious CNS disorders can mimic bacterial meningitis. Subarachnoid hemorrhage (SAH; Chap. 349) is generally the major consideration. Other possibilities include chemical meningitis due to rupture of tumor contents into the CSF (e.g., from a cystic glioma, craniopharyngioma epidermoid or dermoid cyst); drug-induced hypersensitivity meningitis; carcinomatous or lymphomatous meningitis; meningitis associated with inflammatory disorders such as sarcoid, systemic lupus erythematosus (SLE), and Behçet disease; pituitary apoplexy; and uveomeningitic syndromes (Vogt-Koyanagi-Harada syndrome).

Subacutely evolving meningitis (Chap. 361) may on occasion be considered in the differential diagnosis of acute meningitis. The principal causes include *Mycobacterium tuberculosis* (Chap. 150), *Cryptococcus neoformans* (Chap. 186), *Histoplasma capsulatum* (Chap.

183), *Coccidioides immitis* (Chap. 184), and *Treponema pallidum* (Chap. 153).

℞ TREATMENT

Empirical Antimicrobial Therapy (Table 360-2)   Bacterial meningitis is a medical emergency. The goal is to begin antibiotic therapy within 60 min of a patient's arrival in the emergency room. Empirical antimicrobial therapy is initiated in patients with suspected bacterial meningitis before the results of CSF Gram's stain and culture are known. *S. pneumoniae* (Chap. 119) and *N. meningitidis* (Chap. 127) are the most common etiologic organisms of community-acquired bacterial meningitis. Due to the emergence of penicillin- and cephalosporin-resistant *S. pneumoniae*, empirical therapy of community-acquired bacterial meningitis in children and adults should include a third-generation cephalosporin (e.g., ceftriaxone or cefotaxime) and vancomycin. Ceftriaxone or cefotaxime provide good coverage for susceptible *S. pneumoniae*, group B streptococci, and *H. influenzae* and adequate coverage for *N. meningitidis*. Cefepime is a broad-spectrum fourth-generation cephalosporin with in vitro activity similar to that of cefotaxime or ceftriaxone against *S. pneumoniae* and *N. meningitidis* and greater activity against *Enterobacter* spp. and *Pseudomonas aeruginosa*. In clinical trials, cefepime has been demonstrated to be equivalent to cefotaxime in the treatment of penicillin-sensitive pneumococcal and meningococcal meningitis, but its efficacy in bacterial meningitis caused by penicillin- and cephalosporin-resistant pneumococcal organisms, *Enterobacter* spp., and *P. aeruginosa* has not been established. Ampicillin should be added to the empirical regimen for coverage of *L. monocytogenes* in individuals <3 months of age, those >55, or those with suspected impaired cell-mediated immunity because of chronic illness, organ transplantation, pregnancy, malignancies, or immunosuppressive therapy. In hospital-acquired menin-

TABLE 360-2 *Antibiotics Used in Empirical Therapy of Bacterial Meningitis and Focal CNS Infections[a]*

Indication	Antibiotic
Preterm infants to infants <1 month	Ampicillin + cefotaxime
Infants 1–3 mos	Ampicillin + cefotaxime or ceftriaxone
Immunocompetent children > 3 mos and adults <55	Cefotaxime or ceftriaxone + vancomycin
Adults > 55 and adults of any age with alcoholism or other debilitating illnesses	Ampicillin + cefotaxime or ceftriaxone + vancomycin
Hospital-acquired meningitis, posttraumatic or postneurosurgery meningitis, neutropenic patients, or patients with impaired cell-mediated immunity	Ampicillin + ceftazidime + vancomycin

	Total Daily Dose and Dosing Interval	
Antimicrobial Agent	Child (>1 month)	Adult
Ampicillin	200 (mg/kg)/d, q4h	12 g/d, q4h
Cefepime	150 (mg/kg)/d, q8h	6 g/d, q8h
Cefotaxime	200 (mg/kg)/d, q6h	12 g/d, q4h
Ceftriaxone	100 (mg/kg)/d, q12h	4 g/d, q12h
Ceftazidime	150 (mg/kg)/d, q8h	6 g/d, q8h
Gentamicin	7.5 (mg/kg)/d, q8h[b]	7.5 (mg/kg)/d, q8h
Meropenem	120 (mg/kg)/d, q8h	3 g/d, q8h
Metronidazole	30 (mg/kg)/d, q6h	1500–2000 mg/d, q6h
Nafcillin	100–200 (mg/kg)/d, q6h	9–12 g/d, q4h
Penicillin G	400,000 (U/kg)/d, q4h	20–24 million U/d, q4h
Vancomycin	60 (mg/kg)/d, q6h	2 g/d, q12h[b]

[a] All antibiotics are administered intravenously; doses indicated assume normal renal and hepatic function.
[b] Doses should be adjusted based on serum peak and trough levels: gentamicin therapeutic level: peak: 5–8 μg/mL; trough:<2 μg/mL; vancomycin therapeutic level: peak: 25–40 μg/mL; trough:5–15 μg/mL.

gitis, and particularly meningitis following neurosurgical procedures, staphylococci and gram-negative organisms including *P. aeruginosa* are the most common etiologic organisms. In these patients, empirical therapy should include a combination of vancomycin and ceftazidime. Ceftazidime should be substituted for ceftriaxone or cefotaxime in neurosurgical patients and in neutropenic patients, as ceftazidime is the only cephalosporin with adequate activity against CNS infection with *P. aeruginosa*. Meropenem is a carbapenem antibiotic that is highly active in vitro against *L. monocytogenes*, has been demonstrated to be effective in cases of meningitis caused by *P. aeruginosa*, and shows good activity against penicillin-resistant pneumococci. In experimental pneumococcal meningitis, meropenem was comparable to ceftriaxone and inferior to vancomycin in sterilizing CSF cultures. The number of patients with bacterial meningitis enrolled in clinical trials of meropenem has not been sufficient to definitively assess the efficacy of this antibiotic.

Specific Antimicrobial Therapy (Table 360-3) ■ *MENINGOCOCCAL MENINGITIS* Although ceftriaxone and cefotaxime provide adequate empirical coverage for *N. meningitidis*, penicillin G remains the antibiotic of choice for meningococcal meningitis caused by susceptible strains. Isolates of *N. meningitidis* with moderate resistance to penicillin have been identified, but patients infected with these strains have still been successfully treated with penicillin. CSF isolates of *N. meningitidis* should be tested for penicillin and ampicillin susceptibility, and if resistance is found, cefotaxime or ceftriaxone should be substituted for penicillin. A 7-day course of intravenous antibiotic therapy is adequate for uncomplicated meningococcal meningitis. The index case and all close contacts should receive chemoprophylaxis with a 2-day regimen of rifampin (600 mg every 12 h for 2 days in adults and 10 mg/kg every 12 h for 2 days in children >1 year). Rifampin is not recommended in pregnant women. Alternatively, adults can be treated with one dose of ciprofloxacin (750 mg), one dose of azithromycin (500 mg), or one intramuscular dose of ceftriaxone (250 mg). Close contacts are defined as those individuals who have had contact with oropharyngeal secretions either through kissing or by sharing toys, beverages, or cigarettes.

PNEUMOCOCCAL MENINGITIS Antimicrobial therapy of pneumococcal meningitis is initiated with a cephalosporin (ceftriaxone, cefotaxime, or cefepime) and vancomycin. All CSF isolates of *S. pneumoniae* should be tested for sensitivity to penicillin and the cephalosporins. Once the results of antimicrobial susceptibility tests are known, therapy can be modified accordingly (Table 360-3). For *S. pneumoniae* meningitis, an isolate of *S. pneumoniae* is considered to be susceptible to penicillin with a minimal inhibitory concentration (MIC) < 0.06 μg/mL, to have

intermediate resistance when the MIC is 0.1 to 1.0 μg/mL, and to be highly resistant when the MIC > 1.0 μg/mL. Isolates of *S. pneumoniae* that have cephalosporin MICs ≤ 0.5 μg/mL are considered sensitive to the cephalosporins (cefotaxime, ceftriaxone, cefepime). Those with MICs of 1 μg/mL are considered to have intermediate resistance, and those with MICs ≥ 2 μg/mL are considered resistant. For meningitis due to pneumococci with cefotaxime or ceftriaxone MICs ≥ 0.5 μg/mL, treatment with cefotaxime or ceftriaxone is usually adequate. If the MIC > 1 μg/mL, vancomycin is the antibiotic of choice. Rifampin can be added to vancomycin for its synergistic effect but is inadequate as monotherapy because resistance develops rapidly when it is used alone.

Patients with *S. pneumoniae* meningitis should have a repeat LP performed 24 to 36 h after the initiation of antimicrobial therapy to document sterilization of the CSF. Failure to sterilize the CSF after 24 to 36 h of antibiotic therapy should be considered presumptive evidence of antibiotic resistance. Patients with penicillin- and cephalosporin-resistant strains of *S. pneumoniae* who do not respond to intravenous vancomycin alone may benefit from the addition of intraventricular vancomycin. The intraventricular route of administration is preferred over the intrathecal route because adequate concentrations of vancomycin in the cerebral ventricles are not always achieved with intrathecal administration. A 2-week course of intravenous antimicrobial therapy is recommended for pneumococcal meningitis.

L. MONOCYTOGENES MENINGITIS Meningitis due to this organism is treated with ampicillin for at least 3 weeks (Table 360-3). Gentamicin is often added (2 mg/kg loading dose, then 5.1 mg/kg per day given every 8 h and adjusted for serum levels and renal function). The combination of trimethoprim [10 to 20 (mg/kg)/d] and sulfamethoxazole [50 to 100 (mg/kg)/d] given every 6 h may provide an alternative in penicillin-allergic patients.

STAPHYLOCOCCAL MENINGITIS Meningitis due to susceptible strains of *S. aureus* or coagulase-negative staphylococci is treated with nafcillin (Table 360-3). Vancomycin is the drug of choice for methicillin-resistant staphylococci and for patients allergic to penicillin. In these patients, the CSF should be monitored during therapy. If the CSF is not sterilized after 48 h of intravenous vancomycin therapy, then either intrathecal or intraventricular vancomycin, 20 mg once daily, can be added.

GRAM-NEGATIVE BACILLARY MENINGITIS The third-generation cephalosporins, cefotaxime, ceftriaxone, and ceftazidime, are equally efficacious for the treatment of gram-negative bacillary meningitis, with the exception of meningitis due to *P. aeruginosa*, which should be treated with ceftazidime (Table 360-3). A 3-week course of intravenous antibiotic therapy is recommended for meningitis due to gram-negative bacilli.

Adjunctive Therapy The release of bacterial cell-wall components by bactericidal antibiotics leads to the production of the inflammatory cytokines IL-1 and TNF in the subarachnoid space. Dexamethasone exerts its beneficial effect by inhibiting the synthesis of IL-1 and TNF at the level of mRNA, decreasing CSF outflow resistance, and stabilizing the blood-brain barrier. The rationale for giving dexamethasone 20 min before antibiotic therapy is that dexamethasone inhibits the production of TNF by macrophages and microglia only if it is administered before these cells are activated by endotoxin. Dexamethasone does not alter TNF production once it has been induced. The results of clinical trials of dexamethasone therapy in children, predominantly with meningitis due to *H. influenzae* and *S. pneumoniae*, have demonstrated its efficacy in decreasing meningeal inflammation and neurologic sequelae such as the incidence of sensorineural hearing loss.

A prospective European trial of adjunctive therapy for acute bacterial meningitis in 301 adults found that dexamethasone reduced the number of unfavorable outcomes (15% vs. 25%, *p* = .03) including death (7% vs. 15%, *p* = .04). The benefits were most striking in patients with pneumococcal meningitis. Dexamethasone (10 mg intra-

TABLE 360-3 Antimicrobial Therapy of CNS Bacterial Infections Based on Pathogen[a]	
Organism	**Antibiotic**
Neisseria meningitides	
Penicillin-sensitive	Penicillin G or Ampicillin
Penicillin-resistant	Ceftriaxone or cefotaxime
Streptococcus pneumoniae	
Penicillin-sensitive	Penicillin G
Penicillin-intermediate	Ceftriaxone or cefotaxime
Penicillin-resistant	(Ceftriaxone or cefotaxime) + vancomycin
Gram-negative bacilli (except *Pseudomonas* spp.)	Ceftriaxone or cefotaxime
Pseudomonas aeruginosa	Ceftazidime
Staphylococci spp.	
Methicillin-sensitive	Nafcillin
Methicillin-resistant	Vancomycin
Listeria monocytogenes	Ampicillin + gentamicin
Haemophilus influenzae	Ceftriaxone or cefotaxime
Streptococcus agalactiae	Penicillin G or ampicillin
Bacteroides fragilis	Metronidazole
Fusobacterium spp.	Metronidazole

[a] Doses are as indicated in Table 360-2.

venously) was administered 15 to 20 min before the first dose of an antimicrobial agent, and the same dose was repeated every 6 h for 4 days. These results were confirmed in a second trial of dexamethasone in adults with pneumococcal meningitis. Therapy with dexamethasone should ideally be started 20 min before, or not later than concurrent with, the first dose of antibiotics. It is unlikely to be of significant benefit if started >6 h after antimicrobial therapy has been initiated. Dexamethasone may decrease the penetration of vancomycin into CSF, and it delays the sterilization of CSF in experimental models of *S. pneumoniae* meningitis. As a result, its potential benefit should be carefully weighed when vancomycin is the antibiotic of choice. Alternatively, vancomycin can be administered by the intraventricular route.

Increased Intracranial Pressure Emergency treatment of increased ICP includes elevation of the patient's head to 30 to 45°, intubation and hyperventilation (Pa_{CO_2} 25 to 30 mmHg), and mannitol. Patients with increased ICP should be managed in an intensive care unit; accurate ICP measurements are best obtained with an ICP monitoring device. →*Treatment of increased intracranial pressure is discussed in detail in Chap. 258.*

PROGNOSIS Mortality is 3 to 7% for meningitis caused by *H. influenzae*, *N. meningitidis*, or group B streptococci; 15% for that due to *L. monocytogenes*; and 20% for *S. pneumoniae*. In general, the risk of death from bacterial meningitis increases with (1) decreased level of consciousness on admission, (2) onset of seizures within 24 h of admission, (3) signs of increased ICP, (4) young age (infancy) and age >50, (5) the presence of comorbid conditions including shock and/or the need for mechanical ventilation, and (6) delay in the initiation of treatment. Decreased CSF glucose concentration [<2.2 mmol/L (<40 mg/dL)] and markedly increased CSF protein concentration [>3 g/L (>300 mg/dL)] have been predictive of increased mortality and poorer outcomes in some series. Moderate or severe sequelae occur in ~25% of survivors, although the exact incidence varies with the infecting organism. Common sequelae include decreased intellectual function, memory impairment, seizures, hearing loss and dizziness, and gait disturbances.

ACUTE VIRAL MENINGITIS

CLINICAL MANIFESTATIONS Viral meningitis presents as fever, headache, and meningeal irritation coupled with an inflammatory CSF profile (see below). Fever may be accompanied by malaise, myalgia, anorexia, nausea and vomiting, abdominal pain, and/or diarrhea. It is not uncommon to see a mild degree of lethargy or drowsiness. The presence of more profound alterations in consciousness, such as stupor, coma, or marked confusion, should prompt consideration of alternative diagnoses. Similarly, seizures or other focal neurologic signs or symptoms suggest involvement of the brain parenchyma and do not occur in uncomplicated viral meningitis. The headache associated with viral meningitis is usually frontal or retroorbital and often associated with photophobia and pain on moving the eyes. Nuchal rigidity is present in most cases but may be mild and present only near the limit of neck anteflexion. Evidence of severe meningeal irritation, such as Kernig's and Brudzinski's signs, is generally absent.

ETIOLOGY Enteroviruses account for 75 to 90% of aseptic meningitis cases in most series (Table 360-4). Viruses belonging to the *Enterovirus* genus are members of the family Picornaviridae and include the coxsackieviruses, echoviruses, polioviruses, and human enteroviruses 68 to 71. Using a variety of diagnostic techniques including CSF PCR tests, culture, and serology, a specific viral cause can be found in 75 to 90% of cases of viral meningitis. CSF cultures are positive in 30 to 70% of patients, the frequency of isolation depending on the specific viral agent. Approximately two-thirds of culture-negative cases of aseptic meningitis have a specific viral etiology identified by CSF PCR testing (see below).

EPIDEMIOLOGY The exact incidence of viral meningitis in the United States is impossible to determine since most cases go unreported to

TABLE 360-4 *Viruses Causing Acute Meningitis and Acute Encephalitis*

Common	Less Common	Rare
ACUTE MENINGITIS		
Enteroviruses	HSV-1	Adenoviruses
Arboviruses	LCMV	CMV
HIV	VZV	EBV
HSV-2		Influenza A, B, parainfluenza, mumps, rubella
ACUTE ENCEPHALITIS		
Arboviruses	CMV	Adenoviruses, CTFV, hepatitis C,
Enteroviruses	EBV	influenza A, LCMV, parainfluenza,
HSV-1	HIV	rabies, rotavirus, rubella
	Mumps	

Note: CMV, cytomegalovirus; CTFV, Colorado tick fever virus; EBV, Epstein-Barr virus; HSV, herpes simplex virus; LCMV, lymphocytic choriomeningitis virus; VZV, varicella-zoster virus.

public health authorities, although a reasonable estimate would be ~75,000 cases per year. In temperate climates, there is a substantial increase in cases during the summer and early fall months, reflecting the seasonal predominance of enterovirus and arthropod-borne encephalitis virus ("arbovirus") infections, with a peak monthly incidence of about 1 reported case per 100,000 population. The dramatic seasonal predilections of some viruses causing meningitis provide a valuable clue to diagnosis (Table 360-5).

LABORATORY DIAGNOSIS ■ CSF Examination The most important laboratory test in the diagnosis of viral meningitis is examination of the CSF. The typical profile is a lymphocytic pleocytosis (25 to 500 cells/μL) a normal or slightly elevated protein concentration [0.2 to 0.8 g/L (20 to 80 mg/dL)], a normal glucose concentration, and a normal or mildly elevated opening pressure (100 to 350 mmH$_2$O). Organisms are *not* seen on Gram's or acid-fast stained smears or india ink preparations of CSF. Rarely, PMNs may predominate in the first 48 h of illness, especially in patients with infections due to echovirus 9, West Nile virus or Eastern equine encephalitis virus, or mumps. Recent studies suggest that in some patients with West Nile virus infection, PMN pleocytosis can persist for up to a week before shifting to a lymphocytic pleocytosis. Despite these exceptions, the presence of a CSF PMN pleocytosis in a patient with suspected viral meningitis should always prompt consideration of an alternative diagnosis including bacterial meningitis or parameningeal infections. The total CSF cell count in viral meningitis is typically 25 to 500/μL, although cell counts of several thousand per microliter are occasionally seen, especially with infections due to lymphocytic choriomeningitis virus (LCMV) and mumps virus. The CSF glucose concentration is typically normal in viral infections, although it may be decreased in 10 to 30% of cases due to mumps as well as in cases due to LCMV. Rare instances of decreased CSF glucose concentration occur in cases of meningitis due to echoviruses and other enteroviruses, HSV type 2, and varicella-zoster virus (VZV). As a rule, a lymphocytic pleocytosis with a low glucose concentration should suggest fungal, listerial, or tuberculous meningitis or noninfectious disorders (e.g., sarcoid, neoplastic meningitis).

A number of tests measuring levels of various CSF proteins, enzymes, and mediators, including C-reactive protein, lactic acid, lactate dehydrogenase, neopterin, quinolinate, IL,-1β, IL-6, soluble IL-2 receptor, β_2-microglobulin, and TNF, have been proposed as potential

TABLE 360-5 *Seasonal Prevalence of Viruses Commonly Causing Meningitis*

Summer/Early Fall	Fall/Winter	Winter/Spring	Nonseasonal
Arboviruses	LCMV	Mumps	HSV
Enteroviruses			HIV

Note: Abbreviations are as in Table 360-4.

TABLE 360-6 *Features of Selected Arbovirus Encephalitides*

Feature	WNV	WEE	EEE	VEE	SLE	CE
Region	All	West, midwest	Atlantic and Gulf coasts	SW, W	All	East and NC
Age	Adults > 60	Infants, adults > 50	Children, adults > 60	Adults	Adults > 60	Children
Deaths	7%	3–15%	50–75%	1%	2–20%	<1%
Sequelae	?	Common	80%	Rare	20%	Rare
Vector	M	M	M	M	M	M
Animal reservoir	B	B	B	H, sm M	B	sm M

Note: WNV, West Nile virus; WEE, Western equine encephalitis (virus); EEE, Eastern equine encephalitis (virus); VEE, Venezuelan equine encephalitis (virus); SLE, St. Louis encephalitis; CE, California encephalitis (virus); B, bird; H, horse; M, mosquito; NC, north central United States; sm M, small mammal; SW, southwest; W, west.

discriminators between viral and bacterial meningitis or as markers of specific types of viral infection (e.g., infection with HIV), but remain of uncertain sensitivity and specificity and are not widely used for diagnostic purposes.

Polymerase Chain Reaction Amplification of Viral Nucleic Acid   Amplification of viral-specific DNA or RNA from CSF using PCR amplification has become the single most important method for diagnosing CNS viral infections. In both enteroviral and HSV infections of the CNS, PCR has become the diagnostic procedure of choice and is substantially more sensitive than viral cultures. HSV PCR is also an important diagnostic test in patients with recurrent episodes of "aseptic" meningitis, many of whom have amplifiable HSV DNA in CSF despite negative viral cultures. CSF PCR is also used routinely to diagnose CNS viral infections caused by cytomegalovirus (CMV), Epstein-Barr virus (EBV), and VZV.

CSF Culture   The overall results of CSF culture for the diagnosis of viral infection are disappointing, presumably because of the generally low concentration of infectious virus present and the need to customize isolation procedures for individual viruses. For viral isolation, 2 mL of CSF should be brought promptly to the microbiology laboratory, where it should be refrigerated and processed as speedily as possible. CSF specimens for viral isolation should never be stored in a −20°C freezer since viruses are often unstable at this temperature, and most freezers have "frostfree" warm-up cycles that are detrimental to viral stability. Storage for >24 h is probably best done in a −70°C freezer.

Other Sources for Viral Isolation   Viruses may also be isolated from sites and body fluids other than CSF, including throat, stool, blood, and urine. Enteroviruses and adenoviruses may be found in feces; arboviruses, some enteroviruses, and LCMV, in blood; mumps and CMV, in urine; and enteroviruses, mumps, and adenoviruses, in throat washings. During enteroviral infections, viral shedding in stool may persist for several weeks. The presence of enterovirus in stool is not diagnostic and may result from residual shedding from a previous enteroviral infection; it also occurs in some asymptomatic individuals during enteroviral epidemics.

Serologic Studies   For some viruses, including many arboviruses such as West Nile virus (WNV), serologic studies remain a crucial diagnostic tool. Serum serologic studies are less useful for viruses such as HSV, VZV, CMV, and EBV for which the prevalence of antibody seropositivity in the general population is high. Diagnosis of acute viral infection can be made by documenting seroconversion between acute-phase and convalescent sera (typically obtained after 2 to 4 weeks) or by demonstrating the presence of virus-specific IgM antibodies. Documentation of intrathecal synthesis of virus-specific antibodies, as shown by an increased IgG index or the presence of IgM antibodies in CSF, is often significantly more useful than serum serology alone and can provide presumptive evidence of CNS infection. Although serum and CSF IgM antibodies generally persist for only a few months after acute infection, there are exceptions to this rule. For example, WNV IgM has been shown to persist in some patients for >1 year following acute infection. Unfortunately, the delay between

onset of infection and the generation by the host of a virus-specific antibody response often means that serologic data are useful mainly for the retrospective establishment of a specific diagnosis, rather than in urgent diagnosis or management.

Agarose electrophoresis or isoelectric focusing of CSF γ-globulins may reveal the presence of oligoclonal bands. These bands have been found in association with a number of viral infections, including infections with HIV, human T cell lymphotropic virus (HTLV) type I, VZV, mumps, subacute sclerosing panencephalitis (SSPE), and progressive rubella panencephalitis. The associated antibodies are often directed against viral proteins. The finding of oligoclonal bands may be of some diagnostic utility, since typically they are not seen with arbovirus, enterovirus, or HSV infections. Oligoclonal bands are also encountered in certain noninfectious neurologic diseases (e.g., multiple sclerosis) and may be found in nonviral infections (e.g., syphilis, Lyme borreliosis).

Other Laboratory Studies   All patients with suspected viral meningitis should have a complete blood count and differential; liver function tests; and measurement of the erythrocyte sedimentation rate (ESR), blood urea nitrogen (BUN), and plasma levels of electrolytes, glucose, creatinine, creatine kinase, aldolase, amylase, and lipase. Abnormalities in specific test results may suggest particular etiologic diagnoses. MRI, CT, EEG, evoked response studies, electromyography (EMG), and nerve conduction studies are not necessary in most cases. They are best used selectively when atypical presentations or unusual features present diagnostic problems.

DIFFERENTIAL DIAGNOSIS   The most important issue in the differential diagnosis is the exclusion of nonviral causes that can mimic viral meningitis. The major categories of disease that should always be considered and excluded are (1) bacterial meningitis and other infectious meningidities (e.g., *Mycoplasma*, *Listeria*, *Brucella*, *Coxiella*, and *Rickettsia*); (2) parameningeal infections or partially treated bacterial meningitis; (3) nonviral infectious meningidities where cultures may be negative (e.g., fungal, tuberculous, parasitic, or syphilitic disease); (4) neoplastic meningitis; and (5) meningitis secondary to noninfectious inflammatory diseases such as sarcoid, Behçet's disease, and the uveomeningitic syndromes.

SPECIFIC VIRAL ETIOLOGIES   *Enteroviruses* (Chap. 175) are the most common cause of viral meningitis (>75% of cases in which a specific etiology can be identified) and should be considered the most likely cause of viral meningitis when a typical case occurs in the summer months, especially in a child (<15 years). However, despite their summer predominance, sporadic cases of enteroviral CNS infection are seen year-round. The physical examination should include a careful search for exanthemata, hand-foot-mouth disease, herpangina, pleurodynia, myopericarditis, and hemorrhagic conjunctivitis, which may be stigmata of enterovirus infections. PCR amplification of enteroviral RNA from CSF has become the diagnostic procedure of choice for these infections.

Arbovirus infections (Chap. 180) typically occur in the summer months, may have clear circumscribed geographic localization, and occur in both endemic and epidemic form, all factors reflecting the ecology of their transmission through infected insect vectors (Fig. 360-2; Tables 360-5 and 360-6). Arboviral meningitis should be considered when clusters of meningitis cases occur in a restricted geographic region during the summer or early fall. WNV infection should be suspected when bird deaths precede clusters of human cases of meningitis or encephalitis in an area known to harbor the virus. A history of tick exposure or travel or residence in the appropriate geographic area should suggest the possibility of Colorado tick fever virus or Powassan virus infection, although nonviral diseases producing meningitis (e.g.,

Lyme disease) or headache with meningismus (e.g., RMSF) may also present this way.

HSV-2 meningitis (Chap. 163) occurs in ~25% of women and 11% of men at the time of an initial (primary) episode of genital herpes. Of these patients, 20% go on to have recurrent attacks of meningitis. In some series, HSV-2 has been the most important cause of aseptic meningitis in adults, especially women, and overall it is probably second only to enteroviruses as a cause of viral meningitis. Although HSV-2 can be cultured from CSF during a first episode of meningitis, cultures are invariably negative during recurrent episodes of HSV-2 meningitis. Diagnosis depends on amplification of HSV-2 DNA from CSF by PCR. Almost all cases of recurrent HSV meningitis are due to HSV-2, although rare cases due to HSV-1 have been reported. Most cases of benign recurrent lymphocytic meningitis, including cases previously diagnosed as "Mollaret's meningitis," appear to be due to HSV. Genital lesions may not be present, and most patients give no history of genital herpes. CSF cultures are negative, although HSV DNA can be amplified from CSF by PCR during attacks of meningitis but not during symptom-free intervals.

VZV meningitis should be suspected in the presence of concurrent chickenpox or shingles. However, it is important to recognize that in some series up to 40% of VZV meningitis cases have been reported to occur in the absence of rash. The frequency of VZV as a cause of meningitis is extremely variable, ranging from as low as 3% to as high as 20% in different series. In addition to meningitis, encephalitis (see below), and shingles (see below), VZV can also produce acute cerebellar ataxia. This typically occurs in children and presents with the abrupt onset of limb and truncal ataxia. A similar syndrome occurs less commonly in association with EBV and enteroviral infection. PCR has rapidly become a major tool in the diagnosis of VZV CNS infections. In patients with negative CSF PCR results, the diagnosis of VZV CNS infection can be made by the demonstration of VZV-specific intrathecal antibody synthesis and/or the presence of VZV CSF IgM antibodies, or by positive CSF cultures.

EBV infections may also produce aseptic meningitis, with or without accompanying evidence of the infectious mononucleosis syndrome. The diagnosis may be suggested by the finding of atypical lymphocytes in the CSF or an atypical lymphocytosis in peripheral blood. The demonstration of IgM antibody to viral capsid antigen (VCA), or antibody to the diffuse (D) component of early antigen (EA) in the absence of or preceding detectable antibody to nuclear antigen (EBNA), are indicative of acute EBV infection. EBV is almost never cultured from CSF, but EBV DNA can be amplified from CSF in some patients with EBV-associated CNS infections. HIV-infected patients with primary CNS lymphoma may have a positive CSF PCR for EBV DNA even in the absence of meningoencephalitis.

HIV meningitis should be suspected in any patient with known or identified risk factors for HIV infection. Aseptic meningitis is a common manifestation of primary exposure to HIV and occurs in 5 to 10% of cases. In some patients, seroconversion may be delayed for several months; however, detection of the presence of HIV genome by PCR or p24 protein establishes the diagnosis. HIV can be cultured from CSF in some patients. Cranial nerve palsies, most commonly involving cranial nerves V, VII, or VIII, are more common in HIV meningitis than in other viral infections. →*For further discussion of HIV infection, see Chap. 173.*

Mumps (Chap. 178) should be considered when meningitis occurs in the late winter or early spring, especially in males (male/female ratio 3:1). With the widespread use of the live attenuated mumps vaccine in the United States since 1967, the incidence of mumps meningitis has fallen by >95%. Rare cases of mumps vaccine–associated meningitis have been reported, but they are not usually seen after vaccination with the attenuated Jeryl-Lynn strain of virus used in the United States. The presence of orchitis, oophoritis, parotitis, pancreatitis, or elevations in serum lipase and amylase are suggestive but can be found with other viruses, and their absence does not exclude the diagnosis. Clinical meningitis occurs in 5% of patients with parotitis, but only 50% of patients with meningitis have associated parotitis.

Mumps infection confers lifelong immunity, so a documented history of previous infection excludes this diagnosis. The presence of hypoglycorrhachia, found in 10 to 30% of patients, may be an additional diagnostic clue, once other causes have been excluded (see above). Up to 25% of patients may have a PMN-predominant CSF pleocytosis, and CSF abnormalities may persist for months. Diagnosis is typically made by isolation of virus from CSF and/or demonstration of seroconversion between acute-phase and convalescent sera.

LCMV infection (Chap. 180) should be considered when aseptic meningitis occurs in the late fall or winter, and in individuals with a history of exposure to house mice (*Mus musculus*), pet or laboratory rodents (e.g., hamsters), or their excreta. Some patients have an associated rash, pulmonary infiltrates, alopecia, parotitis, orchitis, or myopericarditis. Laboratory clues to the diagnosis of LCMV, in addition to the clinical findings noted above, may include the presence of leukopenia, thrombocytopenia, or abnormal liver function tests. Some cases present with a marked CSF pleocytosis (>1000 cells/μL) and hypoglycorrachia (<30%).

℞ TREATMENT

In the usual case of viral meningitis, treatment is symptomatic and hospitalization is not required. Exceptions include patients with deficient humoral immunity, neonates with overwhelming infection, and patients in whom the clinical or CSF profile suggests the possibility of a bacterial or other nonviral cause of infection. Patients with suspected bacterial meningitis should receive appropriate empirical therapy pending culture results (see above). Patients usually prefer to rest undisturbed in a quiet, darkened room. Analgesics can be used to relieve headache, which is often reduced by the initial diagnostic LP. Antipyretics may help to reduce fever, which rarely exceeds 40°C. Hyponatremia may develop as a result of inappropriate vasopressin secretion [syndrome of inappropriate secretion of antidiuretic hormone (SIADH)], so fluid and electrolyte status should be monitored. Repeat LP is indicated only in patients whose fever and symptoms fail to resolve after a few days, in patients with an initial PMN pleocytosis or hypoglycorhachia, or if there is doubt about the initial diagnosis.

Oral or intravenous acyclovir may be of benefit in patients with meningitis caused by HSV-1 or -2 and in cases of severe EBV or VZV infection. Data concerning treatment of HSV, EBV, and VZV meningitis are extremely limited. Seriously ill patients should probably receive intravenous acyclovir (30 mg/kg per day in three divided doses) for 7 days. Oral acyclovir (800 mg, five times daily), famciclovir (500 mg, tid), or valacyclovir (1000 mg, tid) for a week may be tried in less severely ill patients, although data on efficacy are lacking. Patients with HIV meningitis should receive highly active antiretroviral therapy (Chap. 173).

Patients with viral meningitis who are known to have deficient humoral immunity (e.g. X-linked agammaglobulinemia), and who are not already receiving either intramuscular γ-globulin or intravenous immunoglobulin (IVIg), should be treated with these agents. Intraventricular administration of immunoglobulin through an Ommaya reservoir has been tried in some patients with chronic enteroviral meningitis who have not responded to intramuscular or intravenous immunoglobulin.

An experimental drug, pleconaril (Viropharma Inc., VP 63843), has shown efficacy against a variety of enteroviral infections and has good oral bioavailability and excellent CNS penetration. Ongoing clinical trials in patients with enteroviral meningitis suggest that pleconaril decreases the duration of symptoms compared to placebo. Since most cases of enteroviral CNS infection are benign and self-limited, the indications for pleconaril therapy need to be better defined. Antiviral treatment might benefit patients with chronic CNS enteroviral infections in the setting of agammaglobulinemia or those who develop poliomyelitis as a complication of polio vaccine administration.

Vaccination is an effective method of preventing the development of meningitis and other neurologic complications associated with poliovirus, mumps, and measles infection. A live attenuated VZV vaccine (Varivax) is available in the United States. Clinical studies indicate an effectiveness rate of 70 to 90% for this vaccine, but a booster may be required to maintain immunity. An inactivated varicella vaccine is available for transplant recipients.

PROGNOSIS In adults, the prognosis for full recovery from viral meningitis is excellent. Rare patients complain of persisting headache, mild mental impairment, incoordination, or generalized asthenia for weeks to months. The outcome in infants and neonates (<1 year) is less certain; intellectual impairment, learning disabilities, hearing loss, and other lasting sequelae have been reported in some studies.

VIRAL ENCEPHALITIS

DEFINITION In contrast to viral meningitis, where the infectious process and associated inflammatory response are limited largely to the meninges, in encephalitis the brain parenchyma is also involved. Many patients with encephalitis also have evidence of associated meningitis (meningoencephalitis) and, in some cases, involvement of the spinal cord or nerve roots (encephalomyelitis, encephalomyeloradiculitis).

CLINICAL MANIFESTATIONS In addition to the acute febrile illness with evidence of meningeal involvement characteristic of meningitis, the patient with encephalitis commonly has confusion, behaviroral abnormalities, an altered level of consciousness, and evidence of either focal or diffuse neurologic signs and symptoms. Any degree of altered consciousness may occur, ranging from mild lethargy to deep coma. Patients with encephalitis may have hallucinations, agitation, personality change, behavioral disorders, and, at times, a frankly psychotic state. Focal or generalized seizures occur in many patients with severe encephalitis. Virtually every possible type of focal neurologic disturbance has been reported in viral encephalitis; the signs and symptoms reflect the sites of infection and inflammation. The most commonly encountered focal findings are aphasia, ataxia, hemiparesis (with hyperactive tendon reflexes and extensor plantar responses), involuntary movements (e.g., myoclonic jerks, tremor), and cranial nerve deficits (e.g., ocular palsies, facial weakness). Involvement of the hypothalamic-pituitary axis may result in temperature dysregulation, diabetes insipidus, or the development of SIADH. Despite the clear neuropathologic evidence that viruses differ in the regions of the CNS they injure, it is often impossible to distinguish reliably on clinical grounds alone one type of viral encephalitis (e.g., that caused by HSV) from others (see "Differential Diagnosis," below).

ETIOLOGY In the United States, there are ~20,000 reported cases of encephalitis per year; the actual number is likely to be significantly higher. Hundreds of viruses are capable of causing encephalitis, although only a limited subset is responsible for most cases in which a specific cause is identified (Table 360-4). The same organisms responsible for aseptic meningitis are also responsible for encephalitis, although their relative frequencies differ. The most important viruses causing sporadic cases of encephalitis in immunocompetent adults are HSV-1 (Fig. 360-3), VZV and, less commonly, enteroviruses. Epidemics of encephalitis are caused by arboviruses, which belong to several different viral taxonomic groups including *Alphaviruses* (e.g. Eastern equine encephalitis virus, Western equine encephalitis virus), *Flaviviruses* (e.g., WNV, St. Louis encephalitis virus, Powassan virus), and *Bunyaviruses* (e.g., California encephalitis virus serogroup, LaCrosse virus). Historically, the largest number of cases of arbovirus encephalitis in the United States has been due to St. Louis encephalitis virus and the California encephalitis virus serogroup. However, in 2002, WNV produced the largest epidemic of encephalitis ever recorded in the United States, with 4156 cases and 284 deaths. New causes of viral encephalitis are constantly appearing, as evidenced by the recent outbreak of 257 cases of encephalitis with a 40% mortality rate in Malaysia caused by Nipah virus, a new member of the Paramyxovirus family.

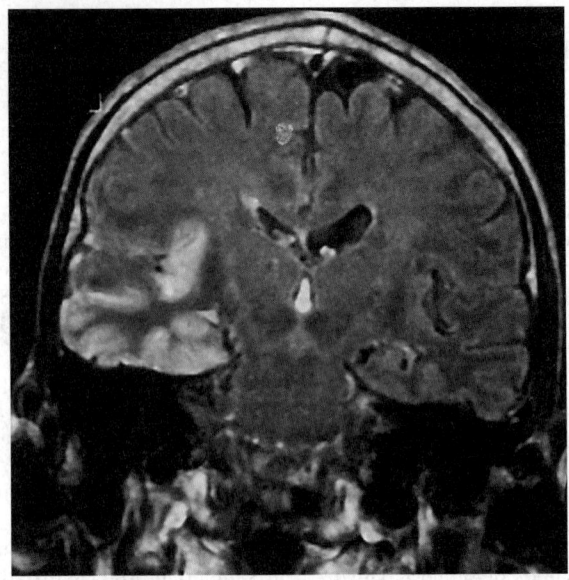

FIGURE 360-3 Coronal FLAIR magnetic resonance image from a patient with herpes simplex encephalitis. Note the area of increased signal in the temporal lobe (left) confined predominantly to the gray matter. This patient had predominantly unilateral disease; bilateral lesions are more common but may be quite asymmetric in their intensity.

LABORATORY DIAGNOSIS ■ CSF Examination CSF examination should be performed in all patients with suspected viral encephalitis unless contraindicated by the presence of severely increased ICP. The characteristic CSF profile is indistinguishable from that of viral meningitis and consists of a lymphocytic pleocytosis, a mildly elevated protein concentration, and a normal glucose concentration. A CSF pleocytosis (>5 cells/μL) occurs in >95% of patients with documented viral encephalitis. In rare cases, a pleocytosis may be absent on the initial LP but present on subsequent LPs. Patients who are severely immunocompromised by HIV infection, glucocorticoid or other immunosuppressant drugs, chemotherapy, or lymphoreticular malignancies may fail to mount a CSF inflammatory response. CSF cell counts exceed 500/μL in only about 10% of patients with encephalitis. Infections with certain arboviruses (e.g., Eastern equine encephalitis or California encephalitis viruses), mumps, and LCMV may occasionally result in cell counts >1000/μL, but this degree of pleocytosis should suggest the possibility of nonviral infections or other inflammatory processes. Atypical lymphocytes in the CSF may be seen in EBV infection and less commonly with other viruses, including CMV, HSV, and enteroviruses. The presence of substantial numbers of PMNs after the first 48 h should prompt consideration of bacterial infection, leptospirosis, amebic infection, and noninfectious processes such as acute hemorrhagic leukoencephalitis. PMN pleocytosis that can persist for up to a week has also been reported in cases of WNV encephalitis. Large numbers of CSF PMNs may be present in patients with viral encephalitis due to Eastern equine encephalitis virus, echovirus 9, and, more rarely, other enteroviruses. About 20% of patients with encephalitis will have a significant number of red blood cells (>500/μL) in the CSF in a nontraumatic tap. The pathologic correlate of this finding may be a hemorrhagic encephalitis of the type seen with HSV, Colorado tick fever virus, and occasionally California encephalitis virus. A decreased CSF glucose concentration is distinctly unusual in viral encephalitis and should suggest the possibility of bacterial, fungal, tuberculous, parasitic, leptospiral, syphilitic, sarcoid, or neoplastic meningitis. Rare patients with mumps, LCMV, or advanced HSV encephalitis may have low CSF glucose concentrations.

CSF PCR CSF PCR has become the primary diagnostic test for CNS infections caused by CMV, EBV, VZV and enteroviruses (see "Viral Meningitis," above). The sensitivity and specificity of CSF PCRs vary with the virus being tested. Recent studies with HSV encephalitis indicate that the sensitivity (~98%) and specificity (~94%) of CSF PCR equal or exceed those of brain biopsy. It is important to recognize that CSF HSV PCR results need to be interpreted after considering the likelihood of disease in the patient being tested, the timing of the test in relationship to onset of symptoms, and the prior use of antiviral therapy. A negative HSV CSF PCR test performed in a patient with a high likelihood of HSV encephalitis based on clinical and laboratory tests significantly reduces the likelihood of HSV encephalitis but does not exclude it. There have been several recent reports of initially negative CSF HSV PCR tests that were obtained early ($\leq$72 h) following symptom onset, that became positive when repeated 1 to 3 days later. The frequency of positive CSF HSV PCRs in patients with herpes encephalitis also decreases as a function of the duration of illness, with only ~20% of cases remaining positive after $\geq$14 days. PCR results are generally not affected by $\leq$1 week of antiviral therapy. In one study 98% of CSF specimens remained PCR-positive during the first week of initiation of antiviral therapy, but the numbers fell to ~50% by 8 to 14 days and to ~21% by >15 days after initiation of therapy.

The sensitivity and specificity of CSF PCR tests for viruses other than herpes simplex have not been definitively characterized. Enteroviral CSF PCR appears to have a sensitivity and specificity of >95%. The specificity of EBV CSF PCR has not been established, and apparent false-positive results can occur in patients with CNS lymphoma and in patients with inflammatory CSF specimens. In patients with CNS infection due to VZV, CSF antibody and PCR studies should be considered complementary, as several cases with positive serologies and negative PCR studies have been reported. In the case of WNV infection, CSF PCR is considerably less sensitive (~70% sensitivity) than detection of WNV specific CSF IgM in diagnosis of WNV encephalitis.

CSF Culture   Attempts to culture viruses from the CSF in cases of encephalitis are often disappointing. Cultures are invariably negative in cases of HSV-1 encephalitis.

Serologic Studies and Antigen Detection   The basic approach to the serodiagnosis of viral encephalitis is identical to that discussed earlier for viral meningitis. In patients with HSV encephalitis, both antibodies to HSV-1 glycoproteins and glycoprotein antigens have been detected in the CSF. Optimal detection of both HSV antibodies and antigen typically occurs after the first week of illness, limiting the utility of these tests in acute diagnosis. Nonetheless, CSF HSV antibody testing may be of value in selected patients whose illness is >1 week in duration and who are CSF PCR-negative for HSV. Demonstration of WNV IgM antibodies is diagnostic of WNV encephalitis, as IgM antibodies do not cross the blood-brain barrier and their presence in CSF is therefore indicative of intrathecal synthesis.

MRI, CT, EEG   Patients with suspected encephalitis almost invariably undergo neuroimaging studies and often EEG. These tests help identify or exclude alternative diagnoses and assist in the differentiation between a focal, as opposed to a diffuse, encephalitic process. Focal findings in a patient with encephalitis should always raise the possibility of HSV encephalitis. Examples of focal findings include: (1) areas of increased signal intensity in the frontotemporal, cingulate, or insular regions of the brain on T2-weighted, fluid-attenuated inversion recovery (FLAIR), or diffusion-weighted MRI images (Fig. 360-3); (2) temporoparietal areas of low absorption, mass effect, and contrast enhancement on CT; or (3) periodic focal temporal lobe spikes on a background of slow or low-amplitude ("flattened") activity on EEG. Approximately 10% of patients with PCR-documented HSV encephalitis will have a normal MRI, although nearly 90% will have abnormalities in the temporal lobe. CT is less sensitive than MRI and is normal in up to 33% of patients. The addition of FLAIR and diffusion-weighted images to the standard MRI sequences enhances sensitivity. EEG abnormalities occur in >90% of PCR-documented cases of HSV encephalitis; they typically involve the temporal lobes but are often nonspecific. Some patients with HSV encephalitis have a distinctive EEG pattern consisting of periodic, stereotyped, sharp-and-slow complexes originating in one or both temporal lobes and repeating at regular intervals of 2 to 3 s. The periodic complexes are typically noted between the second and the fifteenth day of the illness and are present in two-thirds of pathologically proven cases of HSV encephalitis.

Significant MRI abnormalities are found in only ~30% of patients with WNV encephalitis, a frequency significantly less than that of HSV encephalitis. When present, abnormalities often involve deep brain structures including the thalamus, basal ganglia, and brainstem rather than the cortex. Patients with VZV encephalitis may show areas of hemorrhagic infarction reflecting the tendency of this virus to produce a CNS vasculopathy rather than a true encephalitis.

Brain Biopsy   Brain biopsy is now generally reserved for patients in whom CSF PCR studies fail to lead to a specific diagnosis, who have focal abnormalities on MRI, and who continue to show progressive clinical deterioration despite treatment with acyclovir and supportive therapy. The isolation of HSV from brain tissue obtained at biopsy was once considered the "gold standard" for the diagnosis of HSV encephalitis, although with the advent of CSF PCR tests for HSV it is rarely necessary to perform brain biopsy for this purpose. The need for brain biopsy to diagnose other forms of viral encephalitis has also declined greatly with the widespread availability of CSF PCR diagnostic tests for EBV, CMV, VZV, and enteroviruses. When biopsy is performed, the tissue is cultured for virus and examined histopathologically and ultrastructurally. Tissue should be taken from a site that appears to be significantly involved on the basis of clinical and laboratory criteria. Although brain biopsy is not an innocuous procedure, the mortality rate is low (<0.2%) and serious complications occur in only 0.5 to 2.0% of cases. Potential morbidity, in addition to that related to general anesthesia, includes local bleeding and edema, the development of a seizure focus, and wound dehiscence or infection.

DIFFERENTIAL DIAGNOSIS   Some of the most common illnesses masquerading as viral encephalitis, as identified in multicenter clinical trials using brain biopsy as a diagnostic standard, were vascular diseases; abscess and empyema; fungal, parasitic, rickettsial, and tuberculous infections; tumors; Reye's syndrome; toxic encephalopathy; subdural hematoma; and SLE. Acute disseminated encephalomyelitis (ADEM), limbic encephalitis, prion diseases, and Hashimoto's encephalopathy are additional considerations. Of the nonviral infections, particular attention should be paid to *Listeria*, *Mycoplasma*, *Leptospira*, *Cryptococcus*, and *Mucor* infections, as well as to toxoplasmosis and tuberculosis.

Meningoencephalitis caused by ameba can also mimic viral encephalitis. Infection caused by *Naegleria fowleri* usually causes an acute syndrome (primary amebic meningoencephalitis), whereas that caused by *Acanthamoeba* and *Balamuthia* more typically produces subacute or chronic granulomatous amebic meningoencephalitis. *Naegleria* thrive in warm iron-rich pools of water including those found in drains, canals, and both natural and man-made outdoor pools. Infection has typically occurred in immunocompetent children with a history of swimming in potentially infected water. The presentation is of an acute encephalitis, with a CSF neutrophilic pleocytosis and hypoglycorrhachia identical to that seen in bacterial meningitis. Motile trophozoites can be seen in a wet mount of warm fresh CSF. No effective treatment has been identified, and mortality approaches 100%.

There have also been several recent reports of encephalitis caused by the raccoon pinworm *Baylisascaris procyonis*. Clues to the diagnosis include a history of raccoon exposure, and especially of playing in or eating dirt potentially contaminated with raccoon feces. Most patients are children, and many have an associated eosinophilia.

Infection with *Bartonella* species, the agents of cat scratch fever, can also produce a meningoencephalitis. In some recent surveys, *Bartonella* infection has been the most common bacterial infection mimicking viral encephalitis. Infection is transmitted by the bite or scratch of a cat, with an increased risk associated with kittens and feral cats. Patients often develop regional lymphadenopathy; 2 to 4% of infected patients develop encephalopathy, retinitis, or less commonly cranial or peripheral neuropathy. CSF shows a lymphocytic pleocytosis with normal glucose in about one-third of cases, the remainder having no abnormalities or only mild protein elevation. Neuroimaging results are nonspecific, and diagnosis is based on serology. Antibiotic therapy is of uncertain value in immunocompetent hosts, although doxycycline (200 mg daily for 3 months) is often tried in patients with CNS disease.

Once nonviral causes of encephalitis have been excluded, the major diagnostic challenge is to distinguish HSV from other viruses that cause encephalitis. This distinction is particularly important because in virtually every other instance the therapy is supportive, whereas specific and effective antiviral therapy is available for HSV, and its efficacy is enhanced when it is instituted early in the course of infection. HSV encephalitis should be considered when clinical features suggesting involvement of the inferomedial frontotemporal regions of the brain are present, including prominent olfactory or gustatory hallucinations, anosmia, unusual or bizarre behavior or personality alterations, or memory disturbance. HSV encephalitis should always be suspected in patients with focal findings on clinical examination, neuroimaging studies, or EEG. The diagnostic procedure of choice in these patients is CSF PCR analysis for HSV. A positive CSF PCR establishes the diagnosis, and a negative test dramatically reduces the likelihood of HSV encephalitis (see above).

The anatomic distribution of lesions may provide an additional clue to diagnosis. Patients with rapidly progressive encephalitis and prominent brainstem signs, symptoms or neuroimaging abnormalities may be infected by flaviviruses (WNV, Japanese encephalitis virus), HSV, rabies or *L. monocytogenes*. Significant involvement of deep gray matter structures including the basal ganglia and thalamus should also suggest possible flavivirus infection. These patients may present clinically with prominent movement disorders (tremor, myoclonus) or Parkinson's disease–like features. Patients with WNV infection can also present with acute poliomyelitis-like areflexic paralysis, as can patients infected with enterovirus 71 and less commonly other enteroviruses. Despite an aggressive World Health Organization poliovirus eradication initiative, cases of wild-type poliovirus-induced poliomyelitis continue to be reported in at least seven countries worldwide: Egypt, Somalia, Niger, Nigeria, India, Pakistan, and Afghanistan. Rare cases continue to occur in the United States in nonvaccinated individuals exposed to vaccine strains of virus that have reverted to virulence. A recent outbreak of poliomyelitis on Hispaniola (the Dominican Republic and Haiti) has been attributed to vaccine strain–derived viruses that have reverted to virulence after apparently recombining with other circulating enteroviruses. Acute ascending paralysis resembling Guillain-Barré syndrome but associated with CSF pleocytosis can occur with HIV infection, rabies, and WNV infection.

Epidemiologic factors may provide important clues. Particular attention should be paid to the season of the year (Table 360-5); the age of the patient (Table 360-6); the geographic location and travel history (Table 360-6); and possible exposure to animal bites or scratches, rodents, and ticks. Although transmission from the bite of an infected dog remains the most common cause of rabies worldwide, in the United States very few cases of dog rabies occur, and the most common risk factor is exposure to bats—although a clear history of a bite or scratch is often lacking. The classic clinical presentation of encephalitic (furious) rabies is of fever and autonomic hyperactivity with fluctuating mental status. Phobic spasms of the larynx, pharynx, neck muscles, and diaphragm can be triggered by attempts to swallow water (*hydrophobia*) or by inspiration (*aerophobia*). Patients may also present with paralytic (dumb) rabies characterized by acute ascending paralysis. Patients with rabies have a CSF lymphocytic pleocytosis and may show areas of increased T2 signal abnormality in the brainstem, hippocampus, and hypothalamus. Diagnosis can be made by finding rabies virus antigen in brain tissue or in the neural innervation of hair follicles at the nape of the neck. PCR amplification of viral nucleic acid from CSF and saliva or tears may also enable diagnosis. Serology is frequently negative in both serum and CSF in the first week after onset of infection, which limits its acute diagnostic utility.

No specific therapy is available, and cases are almost invariably fatal, with isolated survivors having devastating neurologic sequelae.

Morbidity and Mortality Weekly Reports provides regular information about the prevalence of particular viruses causing encephalitis by season and region of the country. State public health authorities provide another valuable resource concerning isolation of particular agents in individual regions. Deaths in crows and other corvid birds in the local area have preceded human infection by WNV during outbreaks in the United States. Details of the occurrence of WNV in mosquitoes, birds, horses, and humans can be found on the Centers for Disease Control and Prevention (CDC) and U.S. Geological Survey (USGS) websites (and http://westnilemaps.usgs.gov/).

℞ TREATMENT

Specific antiviral therapy should be initiated when appropriate. Vital functions, including respiration and blood pressure, should be monitored continuously and supported as required. In the initial stages of encephalitis, many patients will require care in an intensive care unit. Basic management and supportive therapy should include careful monitoring of ICP, fluid restriction and avoidance of hypotonic intravenous solutions, and suppression of fever. Seizures should be treated with standard anticonvulsant regimens, and prophylactic therapy should be considered in view of the high frequency of seizures in severe cases of encephalitis. As with all seriously ill, immobilized patients with altered levels of consciousness, encephalitis patients are at risk for aspiration pneumonia, stasis ulcers and decubiti, contractures, deep venous thrombosis and its complications, and infections of indwelling lines and catheters.

Acyclovir is of benefit in the treatment of HSV and should be started empirically in patients with suspected viral encephalitis while awaiting viral diagnostic studies. Treatment should be discontinued in patients found not to have HSV encephalitis, with the possible exception of patients with severe encephalitis due to VZV or EBV. HSV, VZV, and EBV all encode an enzyme, deoxypyrimidine (thymidine) kinase, that phosphorylates acyclovir to produce acyclovir-5′-monophosphate. Host cell enzymes then phosphorylate this compound to form a triphosphate derivative. It is the triphosphate that acts as an antiviral agent by inhibiting viral DNA polymerase and by causing premature termination of nascent viral DNA chains. The specificity of action depends on the fact that uninfected cells do not phosphorylate significant amounts of acyclovir to acyclovir-5′-monophosphate. A second level of specificity is provided by the fact that the acyclovir triphosphate is a more potent inhibitor of viral DNA polymerase than of the analogous host cell enzymes.

Adults should receive a dose of 10 mg/kg of acyclovir intravenously every 8 h (30 mg/kg per day total dose) for a minimum of 14 days. Although no studies directly addressing this issue are yet available, repeating the CSF PCR after completion of acyclovir therapy should be considered. Patients with a persisting positive CSF PCR for HSV after completing a standard course of acyclovir therapy should be treated for an additional 7 days, followed by a repeat CSF PCR test. Neonatal HSV CNS infection is less responsive to acyclovir therapy than HSV encephalitis in adults; it is recommended that neonates with HSV encephalitis receive 20 mg/kg of acyclovir every 8 h (60 mg/kg per day total dose) for a minimum of 21 days.

Prior to intravenous administration, acyclovir should be diluted to a concentration ≤7 mg/mL. (A 70-kg person would receive a dose of 700 mg, which would be diluted in a volume of 100 mL.) Each dose should be infused slowly over 1 h rather than by rapid or bolus infusion, to minimize the risk of renal dysfunction. Care should be taken to avoid extravasation or intramuscular or subcutaneous administration. The alkaline pH of acyclovir can cause local inflammation and phlebitis (9%). Dose adjustment is required in patients with impaired renal glomerular filtration. Penetration into CSF is excellent, with average drug levels ~50% of serum levels. Complications of therapy include elevations in BUN and creatinine levels (5%), thrombocytopenia (6%), gastrointestinal toxicity (nausea, vomiting, diarrhea) (7%), and neurotoxicity (lethargy or obtundation, disorientation, confusion, agitation, hallucinations, tremors, seizures) (1%). Acyclovir resistance may be mediated by changes in either the viral deoxypyrimidine kinase or DNA polymerase. To date, acyclovir-resistant isolates have not been a significant clinical problem in immunocompetent individuals. However, there have been reports of clinically virulent acyclovir-resistant HSV isolates from sites outside the CNS in immunocompromised individuals, including those with AIDS.

Oral antiviral drugs with efficacy against HSV, VZV, and EBV, including acyclovir, famciclovir, and valacyclovir, have not been evaluated in the treatment of encephalitis either as primary therapy or as supplemental therapy following completion of a course of parenteral acyclovir. An NIAID/NINDS-sponsored phase III trial of supplemental oral valacyclovir therapy (2 g, tid for 3 months) following the initial 14- to 21-day course of therapy with parenteral acyclovir has recently been initiated by the Collaborative Antiviral Study Group (CASG) in patients with HSV encephalitis (CASG 204); it may help clarify the role of extended oral antiviral therapy.

Both ganciclovir and foscarnet have been shown to be effective in the treatment of CMV-related CNS infections. These drugs are often used in combination. Cidofovir (see below) may provide an alternative in patients who fail to respond to ganciclovir and foscarnet, although data concerning its use in CMV CNS infections are extremely limited.

Ganciclovir is a synthetic nucleoside analogue of 2'-deoxyguanosine. The drug is preferentially phosphorylated by virus-induced cellular kinases. Ganciclovir triphosphate acts as a competitive inhibitor of the CMV DNA polymerase, and its incorporation into nascent viral DNA results in premature chain termination. Following intravenous administration, CSF concentrations of ganciclovir are 25 to 70% of coincident plasma levels. The usual dose for treatment of severe neurologic illnesses is 5 mg/kg every 12 h given intravenously at a constant rate over 1 h. Induction therapy is followed by maintenance therapy of 5 mg/kg every day for an indefinite period. Induction therapy should be continued until patients show a decline in CSF pleocytosis and a reduction in CSF CMV DNA copy number on quantitative PCR testing (where available). Doses should be adjusted in patients with renal insufficiency. Treatment is often limited by the development of granulocytopenia and thrombocytopenia (20 to 25%), which may require reduction in or discontinuation of therapy. Gastrointestinal side effects including nausea, vomiting, diarrhea, and abdominal pain occur in ~20% of patients. Some patients treated with ganciclovir for CMV retinitis have developed retinal detachment, but the causal relationship to ganciclovir treatment is unclear.

Foscarnet is a pyrophosphate analogue that inhibits viral DNA polymerases by binding to the pyrophosphate-binding site. Following intravenous infusion, CSF concentrations range from 15 to 100% of coincident plasma levels. The usual dose for serious CMV-related neurologic illness is 60 mg/kg every 8 h administered by constant infusion over 1 h. Induction therapy for 14 to 21 days is followed by maintenance therapy (60 to 120 mg/kg per day). Induction therapy may need to be extended in patients who fail to show a decline in CSF pleocytosis and a reduction in CSF CMV DNA copy number on quantitative PCR tests (where available). Approximately one-third of patients develop renal impairment during treatment, which is reversible following discontinuation of therapy in most, but not all, cases. This is often associated with elevations in serum creatinine and proteinuria and is less frequent in patients who are adequately hydrated. Many patients experience fatigue and nausea. Reduction in serum calcium, magnesium, and potassium occur in ~15% of patients and may be associated with tetany, cardiac rhythm disturbances, or seizures.

Cidofovir is a nucleotide analogue that is effective in treating CMV retinitis and equivalent or better than ganciclovir in some experimental models of murine CMV encephalitis, although data concerning its efficacy in human CMV CNS disease are limited. The usual dose is 5 mg/kg intravenously once weekly for 2 weeks, then biweekly for 2 or more additional doses, depending on clinical response. Patients must be prehydrated with normal saline (e.g., 1 L over 1 to 2 h) prior to each dose and treated with probenecid (e.g., 1 g 3 h before cidofovir

and 1 g 2 and 8 h after cidofovir). Nephrotoxicity is common; the dose should be reduced if renal function deteriorates.

Intravenous ribavarin (15 to 25 mg/kg per day in divided doses given every 8 h) has been reported to be of benefit in isolated cases of severe encephalitis due to California encephalitis (LaCrosse) virus. Ribavarin might be of benefit for the rare patients, typically infants or young children, with severe adenovirus or rotavirus encephalitis and in patients with encephalitis due to LCMV or other arenaviruses. However, clinical trials are lacking. Hemolysis, with resulting anemia, has been the major side effect limiting therapy.

No specific antiviral therapy of proven efficacy is currently available for treatment of WNV encephalitis. Small groups of patients have been treated with interferon α, ribavarin, and IVIg preparations of non-U.S. origin containing high titer anti-WNV antibody. Evidence is insufficient to establish efficacy of any of these therapies.

SEQUELAE There is considerable variation in the incidence and severity of sequelae in patients surviving viral encephalitis. In the case of Eastern equine encephalitis virus infection, nearly 80% of survivors have severe neurologic sequelae. At the other extreme are infections due to EBV, California encephalitis virus, and Venezuelan equine encephalitis virus, where severe sequelae are unusual. For example, ~5 to 15% of children infected with LaCrosse virus have a residual seizure disorder, and 1% have persistent hemiparesis. Detailed information about sequelae in patients with HSV encephalitis treated with acyclovir are available from the NIAID-CASG trials. Of 32 acyclovir-treated patients, 26 survived (81%). Of the 26 survivors, 12 (46%) had no or only minor sequelae, 3 (12%) were moderately impaired (gainfully employed but not functioning at their previous level), and 11 (42%) were severely impaired (requiring continuous supportive care). The incidence and severity of sequelae were directly related to the age of the patient and the level of consciousness at the time of initiation of therapy. Patients with severe neurologic impairment (Glasgow coma score 6) at initiation of therapy either died or survived with severe sequelae. Young patients (<30 years) with good neurologic function at initiation of therapy did substantially better (100% survival, 62% with no or mild sequelae) compared with their older counterparts (>30 years); (64% survival, 57% no or mild sequelae). Some recent studies using quantitative CSF PCR tests for HSV indicate that clinical outcome following treatment also correlates with the amount of HSV DNA present in CSF at the time of presentation. Many patients with WNV infection have acute sequelae including cognitive impairment; weakness; and hyper- or hypo-kinetic movement disorders including tremor, myoclonus, and parkinsonism. Improvement in these symptoms may occur over the subsequent 6 to 12 months, although detailed clinical studies of the duration and severity of WNV sequelae are still lacking.

SUBACUTE MENINGITIS

CLINICAL MANIFESTATIONS Patients with subacute meningitis typically have an unrelenting headache, stiff neck, low-grade fever, and lethargy for days to several weeks before they present for evaluation. Cranial nerve abnormalities and night sweats may be present. This syndrome overlaps that of chronic meningitis discussed in detail in Chap. 361.

ETIOLOGY Common causative organisms include *M. tuberculosis*, *C. neoformans*, *H. capsulatum*, *C. immitis*, and *T. pallidum*. Initial infection with *M. tuberculosis* is acquired by inhalation of aerosolized droplet nuclei. Tuberculous meningitis in adults does not develop acutely from hematogenous spread of tubercle bacilli to the meninges. Rather, millet seed–size (miliary) tubercles form in the parenchyma of the brain during hematogenous dissemination of tubercle bacilli in the course of primary infection. These tubercles enlarge and are usually caseating. The propensity for a caseous lesion to produce meningitis is determined by its proximity to the SAS and the rate at which fibrous encapsulation develops. Subependymal caseous foci cause meningitis via discharge of bacilli and tuberculous antigens into the SAS. Mycobacterial antigens produce an intense inflammatory reaction that leads to the production of a thick exudate that fills the basilar cisterns and surrounds the cranial nerves and major blood vessels at the base of the brain.

Fungal infections are typically acquired by the inhalation of airborne fungal spores. The initial pulmonary infection may be asymptomatic or present with fever, cough, sputum production, and chest pain. The pulmonary infection is often self-limited. A localized pulmonary fungal infection can then remain dormant in the lungs until there is an abnormality in cell-mediated immunity that allows the fungus to reactivate and disseminate to the CNS. The most common pathogen causing fungal meningitis is *C. neoformans*. This fungus is found worldwide in soil and bird excreta. *H. capsulatum* is endemic to the Ohio and Mississippi River valleys of the central United States and to parts of Central and South America. *C. immitis* is endemic to the desert areas of the southwest United States, northern Mexico, and Argentina.

Syphilis is a sexually transmitted disease that is manifest by the appearance of a painless chancre at the site of inoculation. *T. pallidum* invades the CNS early in the course of syphilis. Cranial nerves VII and VIII are most frequently involved.

LABORATORY DIAGNOSIS The classic CSF abnormalities in tuberculous meningitis are as follows: (1) elevated opening pressure, (2) lymphocytic pleocytosis (10 to 500 cells/μL), (3) elevated protein concentration in the range of 1 to 5 g/L (10 to 500 mg/dL), and (4) decreased glucose concentration in the range of 1.1 to 2.2 mmol/L (20 to 40 mg/dL). *The combination of unrelenting headache, stiff neck, fatigue, night sweats, and fever with a CSF lymphocytic pleocytosis and a mildly decreased glucose concentration is highly suspicious for tuberculous meningitis.* The last tube of fluid collected at LP is the best tube to send for a smear for acid-fast bacilli (AFB). If there is a pellicle in the CSF or a cobweb-like clot on the surface of the fluid, AFB can best be demonstrated in a smear of the clot or pellicle. Positive smears are typically reported in only 10 to 40% of cases of tuberculous meningitis in adults. Cultures of CSF take 4 to 8 weeks to identify the organism and are positive in ~50% of adults. Culture remains the "gold standard" to make the diagnosis of tuberculous meningitis. PCR for the detection of *M. tuberculosis* DNA has a sensitivity of 70 to 80% but at the present time is limited by a high rate of false-positive results.

The characteristic CSF abnormalities in fungal meningitis are a mononuclear or lymphocytic pleocytosis, an increased protein concentration, and a decreased glucose concentration. There may be eosinophils in the CSF in *C. immitis* meningitis. Large volumes of CSF are often required to demonstrate the organism on India ink smear or grow the organism in culture. If spinal fluid examined by LP on two separate occasions fails to yield an organism, CSF should be obtained by high-cervical or cisternal puncture.

The cryptococcal polysaccharide antigen test is a highly sensitive and specific test for cryptococcal meningitis. A reactive CSF cryptococcal antigen test establishes the diagnosis. The detection of the *histoplasma* polysaccharide antigen in CSF establishes the diagnosis of a fungal meningitis but is not specific for meningitis due to *H. capsulatum*. It may be falsely positive in coccidioidal meningitis. The CSF complement fixation antibody test is reported to have a specificity of 100% and a sensitivity of 75% for coccidioidal meningitis.

The diagnosis of syphilitic meningitis is made when a reactive serum treponemal test [fluorescent treponemal antibody, absorbed (FTA-ABS) or microhemagglutination-*T. pallidum* (MHA-TP)] is associated with a CSF lymphocytic or mononuclear pleocytosis and an elevated protein concentration, or when the CSF VDRL is positive. A reactive CSF-FTA-ABS is not definitive evidence of neurosyphilis. The CSF-FTA-ABS can be falsely positive from blood contamination. A negative CSF VDRL does not rule out neurosyphilis. A negative CSF FTA-ABS or MHA-TP rules out neurosyphilis.

℞ TREATMENT

Empirical therapy of tuberculous meningitis is often initiated on the basis of a high index of suspicion without adequate laboratory support. Initial therapy is a combination of isoniazid (300 mg/d), rifampin (10 mg/kg per day), pyrazinamide (30 mg/kg per day in divided doses), ethambutol (15 to 25 mg/kg per day in divided doses), and pyridoxine (50 mg/d). If the clinical response is good, pyrazinamide and ethambutol can be discontinued after 8 weeks and isoniazid and rifampin continued alone for the next 6 to 12 months. A 6-month course of therapy is acceptable, but therapy should be prolonged for 9 to 12 months in patients who have an inadequate resolution of symptoms of meningitis or who have positive mycobacterial cultures of CSF during the course of therapy. Dexamethasone therapy is recommended for patients who develop hydrocephalus.

Meningitis due to *C. neoformans* is treated with amphotericin B (0.7 mg/kg per day) and flucytosine (100 mg/kg per day in four divided doses) for 2 weeks, followed by an 8- to 10-week course of fluconazole (400 to 800 mg/d). If the CSF culture is sterile after 10 weeks of acute therapy, the dose of fluconazole is decreased to 200 mg/d for 6 months to a year. Patients with HIV infection may require indefinite maintenance therapy. Meningitis due to *H. capsulatum* is treated with amphotericin B (0.7 to 1.0 mg/kg per day) for 4 to 12 weeks followed by itraconazole (400 mg/d). Therapy with amphotericin B is not discontinued until fungal cultures are sterile. After completing a course of amphotericin B, maintenance therapy with itraconazole is initiated and continued for at least 6 months to a year. *C. immitis* meningitis is treated with intravenous amphotericin B (0.5 to 0.7 mg/kg per day) for ≥4 weeks until CSF fungal cultures are negative. Intrathecal amphotericin B may be required to eradicate the infection. Lifelong therapy with fluconazole is recommended to prevent relapse. Ambisome (4 mg/kg per day) or amphotericin B lipid complex (5 mg/kg per day) can be substituted for amphotericin B in patients who have or who develop significant renal dysfunction. The most common complication of fungal meningitis is hydrocephalus. Patients who develop hydrocephalus should receive a CSF diversion device. A ventriculostomy can be used until CSF fungal cultures are sterile, at which time the ventriculostomy is replaced by a ventriculoperitoneal shunt.

Syphilitic meningitis is treated with aqueous penicillin G in a dose of 3 to 4 million units intravenously every 4 h for 10 to 14 days. An alternative regimen is 2.4 million units of procaine penicillin G intramuscularly daily with 500 mg of oral probenecid four times daily for 10 to 14 days. Either regimen is followed with 2.4 million units of benzathine penicillin G intramuscularly once a week for 3 weeks. The standard criterion for treatment success is reexamination of the CSF. The CSF should be reexamined at 6-month intervals for 2 years. The cell count is expected to normalize within 12 months, and the VDRL titer to decrease by two dilutions or revert to nonreactive within 2 years of completion of therapy. Failure of the CSF pleocytosis to resolve or an increase in the CSF VDRL titer by two or more dilutions requires re-treatment.

CHRONIC ENCEPHALITIS

PROGRESSIVE MULTIFOCAL LEUKOENCEPHALOPATHY ▪ Clinical Features and Pathology Progressive multifocal leukoencephalopathy (PML) is a progressive disorder characterized pathologically by multifocal areas of demyelination of varying size distributed throughout the CNS. In addition to demyelination, there are characteristic cytologic alterations in both astrocytes and oligodendrocytes. Astrocytes are tremendously enlarged and contain hyperchromatic, deformed, and bizarre nuclei and frequent mitotic figures. Oligodendrocytes have enlarged, densely staining nuclei that contain viral inclusions formed by crystalline arrays of JC virus particles. Patients often present with visual deficits (45%), typically a homonymous hemianopia, and mental impairment (38%) (dementia, confusion, personality change). Motor weakness may not be present early but eventually occurs in 75% of cases.

Almost all patients have an underlying immunosuppressive disorder. Prior to the HIV epidemic, common associated diseases included lymphoproliferative disorders, immune deficiency states, myeloproliferative disease, and chronic infectious or granulomatous diseases. More than 60% of currently diagnosed PML cases occur in patients with AIDS. Conversely, it has been estimated that nearly 1% of AIDS patients will develop PML. The basic features of AIDS-associated and non-AIDS-associated PML are identical.

Diagnostic Studies   MRI reveals multifocal asymmetric, coalescing white matter lesions located periventricularly, in the centrum semiovale, in the parietal-occipital region, and in the cerebellum. These lesions have increased T2 and decreased T1 signal, are generally nonenhancing or show only minimal peripheral enhancement, and are not associated with edema or mass effect. CT scans, which are less sensitive than MRI for the diagnosis of PML, often show hypodense nonenhancing white matter lesions.

The CSF is typically normal, although mild elevation in protein and/or IgG may be found. Pleocytosis occurs in <25% of cases, is predominantly mononuclear, and rarely exceeds 25 cells/μL. PCR amplification of JC virus DNA from CSF has become an important diagnostic tool. CSF PCR for JC virus DNA has high specificity, but sensitivity has varied among studies. Rare cases of positive CSF PCR for JC virus DNA in the absence of clinical or radiographic evidence of PML have been described in HIV-infected patients. It remains to be established whether these results are false positives or indicate preclinical PML.

A positive CSF PCR for JC virus DNA in association with typical MRI lesions in the appropriate clinical setting is diagnostic of PML. Patients with negative CSF PCR studies may require brain biopsy for definitive diagnosis; JC virus antigen and nucleic acid can be detected by immunocytochemistry, in situ hybridization, or PCR amplification. Detection of JC virus antigen or genomic material should be considered diagnostic of PML only if accompanied by characteristic pathologic changes, since both antigen and genomic material have been found in the brains of normal patients.

℞ **TREATMENT**

No effective therapy is available. Recent trials in HIV-associated PML failed to show benefit from either cytarabine or cidofovir. Some patients with HIV-associated PML have shown dramatic clinical improvement associated with improvement in their immune status following institution of highly active antiretroviral therapy.

SUBACUTE SCLEROSING PANENCEPHALITIS   SSPE is a rare progressive demyelinating disease of the CNS associated with a chronic infection of brain tissue with measles virus. Most patients give a history of primary measles infection at an early age (2 years), which is followed after a latent interval of 6 to 8 years by the development of insidious intellectual decline and mood and personality changes. Typical signs of a CNS viral infection, including fever and headache, do not occur. Focal and/or generalized seizures, myoclonus, ataxia, and visual disturbances occur as the disease progresses. The EEG shows a characteristic periodic pattern with bursts every 3 to 8 s of high-voltage, sharp slow waves, followed by periods of attenuated ("flat") background. The CSF is acellular with a normal or mildly elevated protein level and a markedly elevated γ-globulin level (>20% of total CSF protein). CSF antimeasles antibody levels are invariably elevated, and oligoclonal antimeasles antibodies are often present. CT and MRI show evidence of multifocal white matter lesions and generalized atrophy. Measles virus can be cultured from brain tissue, and viral genome can be detected by in situ hybridization or PCR amplification. Treatment with isoprinosine (Inosiplex) (100 mg/kg per day), alone or in combination with intrathecal or intraventricular interferon, has been reported to prolong survival and produce clinical improvement in some patients but has never been subjected to a controlled clinical trial.

PROGRESSIVE RUBELLA PANENCEPHALITIS   This is an extremely rare disorder that primarily affects males with congenital rubella syndrome, although isolated cases have been reported following childhood rubella. After a latent period of 8 to 19 years, patients develop progres-

sive neurologic deterioration. The manifestations are similar to those seen in SSPE. CSF shows a mild lymphocytic pleocytosis, slightly elevated protein level, markedly increased γ-globulin, and rubella virus–specific oligoclonal bands. No therapy is available.

BRAIN ABSCESS

DEFINITION   A brain abscess is a focal, suppurative infection within the brain parenchyma, typically surrounded by a vascularized capsule. The term *cerebritis* is often employed to describe a nonencapsulated brain abscess.

EPIDEMIOLOGY   A bacterial brain abscess is a relatively uncommon intracranial infection, with an incidence of ~1 in 100,000 persons per year. Predisposing conditions include otitis media and mastoiditis, paranasal sinusitis, pyogenic infections in the chest or other body sites, penetrating head trauma or neurosurgical procedures, and dental infections. In most modern series, an increasing proportion of brain abscesses are not caused by classic pyogenic bacteria, but rather by fungi and parasites including *Toxoplasma gondii*, *Aspergillus* spp., *Nocardia* spp., *Mycobacteria* spp., and *C. neoformans*. These organisms are almost exclusively restricted to immunocompromised hosts with underlying HIV infection, organ transplantation, cancer, or immunosuppressive therapy. In Latin America and in immigrants from Latin America, the most common cause of brain abscess is *Taenia solium* (neurocysticercosis). In India and the Far East, mycobacterial infection (tuberculoma) remains a major cause of focal CNS mass lesions.

ETIOLOGY   A brain abscess may develop (1) by direct spread from a contiguous cranial site of infection, such as paranasal sinusitis, otitis media, mastoiditis, or dental infection; (2) following head trauma or a neurosurgical procedure; or (3) as a result of hematogenous spread from a remote site of infection. In up to 25% of cases no obvious primary source of infection is apparent (cryptogenic brain abscess).

Up to one-third of brain abscesses are associated with otitis media and mastoiditis, often with an associated cholesteatoma. Otogenic abscesses occur predominantly in the temporal lobe (55 to 75%) and cerebellum (20 to 30%). In some series up to 90% of cerebellar abscesses are otogenic. Common organisms include streptococci, *Bacteroides* spp., *P. aeruginosa*, and Enterobacteriaceae. Abscesses that develop as a result of direct spread of infection from the frontal, ethmoidal, or sphenoidal sinuses and those that occur due to dental infections are usually located in the frontal lobes. Approximately 10% of brain abscesses are associated with paranasal sinusitis, and this association is particularly strong in young males in their second and third decades of life. The most common pathogens in brain abscesses associated with paranasal sinusitis are streptococci (especially *S. milleri*), *Haemophilus* spp., *Bacteroides* spp., *Pseudomonas* spp., and *S. aureus*. Dental infections are associated with ~2% of brain abscesses, although it is often suggested that many "cryptogenic" abscesses are in fact due to dental infections. The most common pathogens in this setting are streptococci, staphylococci, and *Bacteroides* and *Fusobacterium* spp.

Hematogenous abscesses account for ~25% of brain abscesses. These abscesses show a predilection for the territory of the middle cerebral artery (i.e., posterior frontal or parietal lobes). Hematogenous abscesses are often located at the junction of the gray and white matter and are often poorly encapsulated. Not surprisingly, hematogenous abscesses are often multiple, and multiple abscesses often have a hematogenous origin. The microbiology of these hematogenous abscesses is dependent on the primary source of infection. For example, brain abscesses that develop as a complication of infective endocarditis are often due to viridans streptococci or *S. aureus*. Abscesses associated with pyogenic lung infections such as lung abscess or bronchiectasis are often due to Streptococci, staphylococci, or *Bacteroides* or *Fusobacterium* spp. Enterobacteriaceae and *P. aeruginosa* are important causes of abscesses associated with urinary sepsis. Abscesses that follow penetrating head trauma or neurosurgical procedures are frequently due to staphylococci, Enterobacteriaceae, and *Pseudomonas* species. Congenital cardiac malformations that produce a right-to-left shunt (congenital cyanotic heart disease), such as tetralogy of Fallot, patent ductus arteriosus, and atrial and ventricular septal defects, allow bloodborne bacteria to bypass the pulmonary capillary bed and reach the brain. Similar phenomena can occur with pulmonary arteriovenous malformations. The decreased arterial oxygenation and saturation from the right-to-left shunt and polycythemia may cause focal areas of cerebral ischemia, thus providing a nidus for microorganisms that bypassed the pulmonary circulation to multiply and form an abscess. Streptococci are the most common pathogens in this setting.

PATHOGENESIS AND HISTOPATHOLOGY   The intact brain parenchyma is relatively resistant to infection; preexisting brain ischemia, necrosis, or hypoxia appears to be a prerequisite for effective bacterial invasion. Once infection is established, brain abscess frequently evolves through a series of stages, influenced by the nature of the infecting organism and by the immunocompetence of the host. The early cerebritis stage (days 1 to 3) is characterized by a perivascular infiltration of inflammatory cells, which surround a central core of coagulative necrosis. Marked edema surrounds the lesion at this stage. In the late cerebritis stage (days 4 to 9), pus formation leads to enlargement of the necrotic center, which is surrounded at its border by an inflammatory infiltrate of macrophages and fibroblasts. A thin capsule of fibroblasts and reticular fibers gradually develops, and the surrounding area of cerebral edema becomes more distinct than in the previous stage. The third stage, early capsule formation (days 10 to 13), is characterized by the formation of a capsule that is better developed on the cortical than on the ventricular side of the lesion. This stage correlates with the appearance of a ring-enhancing capsule on neuroimaging studies. The final stage, late capsule formation (day 14 and beyond), is defined by a well-formed necrotic center surrounded by a dense collagenous capsule. The surrounding area of cerebral edema has regressed, but marked gliosis with large numbers of reactive astrocytes has developed outside the capsule. This gliotic process may contribute to the development of seizures as a sequelae of brain abscess.

CLINICAL PRESENTATION   A brain abscess typically presents as an expanding intracranial mass lesion, rather than as an infectious process. Although the evolution of signs and symptoms is extremely variable, ranging from hours to weeks or even months, most patients present to the hospital 11 to 12 days following onset of symptoms. The classic clinical triad of headache, fever, and a focal neurologic deficit is present in <50% of cases. The most common symptom in patients with a brain abscess is headache, occurring in >75% of patients. The headache is often characterized as a constant, dull, aching sensation, either hemicranial or generalized, and it becomes progressively more severe and refractory to therapy. Fever is present in only 50% of patients at the time of diagnosis, and its absence should not exclude the diagnosis. The new onset of focal or generalized seizure activity is a presenting sign in 15 to 35% of patients. Focal neurologic deficits

including hemiparesis, aphasia, or visual field defects are part of the initial presentation in >60% of patients.

The clinical presentation of a brain abscess depends on its location, the nature of the primary infection if present, and on the level of the ICP. Hemiparesis is the most common localizing sign of a frontal lobe abscess. A temporal lobe abscess may present with a disturbance of language (dysphasia) or an upper homonymous quadrantanopia. Nystagmus and ataxia are signs of a cerebellar abscess. Signs of raised ICP—papilledema, nausea and vomiting, and drowsiness or confusion—can be the dominant presentation of some abscesses, particularly those in the cerebellum. Meningismus is not present unless the abscess has ruptured into the ventricle or the infection has spread to the subarachnoid space.

DIAGNOSIS   Diagnosis is made by neuroimaging studies. MRI (Fig. 360-4) is better than CT for demonstrating abscesses in the early (cerebritis) stages and is superior to CT for identifying abscesses in the posterior fossa. A mature brain abscess appears on CT as a focal area of hypodensity surrounded by ring enhancement. The CT and MRI appearance, particularly of the capsule, may be altered by treatment with glucocorticoids. The distinction between a brain abscess and other focal lesions such as tumors may be facilitated with diffusion-weighted imaging (DWI) sequences in which brain abscesses typically show increased signal and low apparent diffusion coefficient.

Microbiologic diagnosis of the etiologic agent is most accurately determined by Gram's stain and culture of abscess material obtained by stereotactic needle aspiration. Up to 10% of patients will also have positive blood cultures. LP should not be performed in patients with known or suspected focal intracranial infections such as abscess or empyema; CSF analysis contributes nothing to diagnosis or therapy, and LP increases the risk of herniation.

Additional laboratory studies may provide clues to the diagnosis of brain abscess in patients with a CNS mass lesion. About 50% of patients have a peripheral leukocytosis, 60% an elevated ESR, and 80% an elevated C-reactive protein.

DIFFERENTIAL DIAGNOSIS   Conditions that can cause headache, fever, focal neurologic signs, and seizure activity include brain abscess, subdural empyema, bacterial meningitis, viral meningoencephalitis, superior sagittal sinus thrombosis, and acute disseminated encephalomyelitis. When fever is absent, primary and metastatic brain tumors become the major differential diagnosis. Less commonly, cerebral infarction or hematoma can have an MRI or CT appearance resembling brain abscess.

Rx TREATMENT

Optimal therapy of brain abscesses involves a combination of high-dose parenteral antibiotics and neurosurgical drainage. Empirical therapy of community-acquired brain abscess in an immunocompetent patient typically includes a third-generation cephalosporin (e.g., cefotaxime or ceftriaxone) and metronidazole (see Table 360-2 for antibiotic dosages). In patients with penetrating head trauma or recent neurosurgical procedures, treatment should include ceftazidime as the

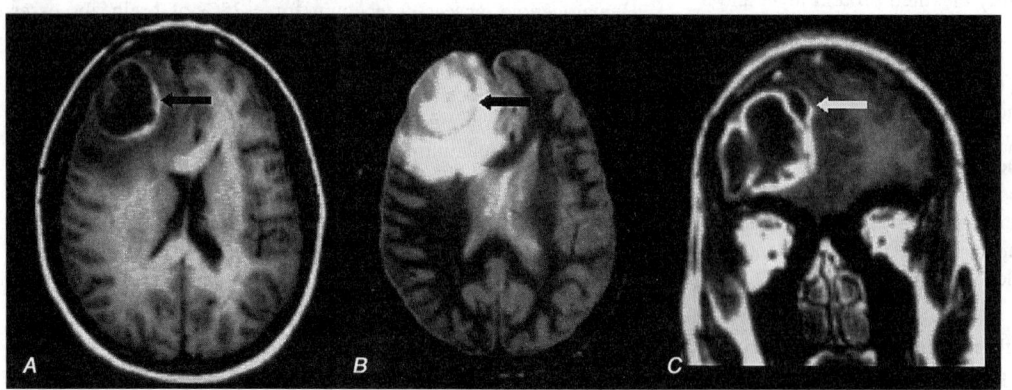

FIGURE 360-4 Pneumococcal brain abscess. Note that the abscess wall has hyperintense signal on the axial T1-weighted image (*A*, black arrow), hypointense signal on the axial proton density images (*B*, black arrow), and enhances prominently after gadolinium administration on the coronal T1-weighted image (*C*). The abscess is surrounded by a large amount of vasogenic edema and has a small "daughter" abscess (*C*, white arrow). (*Courtesy of Joseph Lurito, MD.*)

third-generation cephalosporin to enhance coverage of *Pseudomonas* spp. and vancomycin for coverage of staphylococci. Meropenem plus vancomycin also provides good coverage in this setting.

Aspiration and drainage of the abscess under stereotaxic guidance are beneficial for both diagnosis and therapy. Empirical antibiotic coverage should be modified based on the results of Gram's stain and culture of the abscess contents. Complete excision of a bacterial abscess via craniotomy or craniectomy is generally reserved for multiloculated abscesses or those in which stereotactic aspiration is unsuccessful.

Medical therapy alone is not optimal for treatment of brain abscess and should be reserved for patients whose abscesses are neurosurgically inaccessible, for patients with small nonencapsulated abscesses (cerebritis), and patients whose condition is too tenuous to allow performance of a neurosurgical procedure. All patients should receive a minimum of 6 to 8 weeks of parenteral antibiotic therapy. The role, if any, of supplemental oral antibiotic therapy following completion of a standard course of parenteral therapy has never been adequately studied.

Patients should also receive prophylactic anticonvulsant therapy because of the high risk of seizures. Anticonvulsant therapy is continued for at least 3 months after resolution of the abscess, and decisions regarding withdrawal are then based on the EEG. If the EEG is abnormal, anticonvulsant therapy should be continued. If the EEG is normal, anticonvulsant therapy can be slowly withdrawn, with close follow-up and repeat EEG after the medication has been discontinued.

Glucocorticoids should not be given routinely to patients with brain abscesses. Intravenous dexamethasone therapy (10 mg every 6 h) is usually reserved for patients with substantial periabscess edema and associated mass effect and increased ICP. Dexamethasone should be tapered as rapidly as possible to avoid delaying the natural process of encapsulation of the abscess.

Serial MRI or CT scans should be obtained on a monthly or twice-monthly basis to document resolution of the abscess. More frequent studies (e.g., weekly) are probably warranted in the subset of patients who are receiving antibiotic therapy alone. A small amount of enhancement may remain for months after the abscess has been successfully treated.

PROGNOSIS The mortality of brain abscess has declined in parallel with the development of enhanced neuroimaging techniques, improved neurosurgical procedures for stereotactic aspiration, and improved antibiotics. In modern series the mortality is typically <15%. Significant sequelae including seizures, persisting weakness, aphasia, or mental impairment occur in ≥20% of survivors.

NONBACTERIAL CAUSES OF INFECTIOUS FOCAL CNS LESIONS

ETIOLOGY Neurocysticercosis is the most common parasitic disease of the CNS worldwide. Humans acquire cysticercosis by the ingestion of food contaminated with the eggs of the parasite *T. solium*. Eggs are contained in undercooked pork or in drinking water or other foods contaminated with human feces. *T. gondii* is a parasite that is acquired from the ingestion of undercooked meat and from handling cat feces.

CLINICAL PRESENTATION The most common manifestation of neurocysticercosis is new-onset partial seizures with or without secondary generalization. Cysticerci may develop in the brain parenchyma and cause seizures or focal neurologic deficits. When present in the subarachnoid or ventricular spaces, cysticerci can produce increased ICP by interference with CSF flow. Spinal cysticerci can mimic the presentation of intraspinal tumors. When the cysticerci first lodge in the brain, they frequently cause little in the way of an inflammatory response. As the cysticercal cyst degenerates, it elicits an inflammatory response that may present clinically as a seizure. Eventually the cyst dies, a process that may take several years, and is typically associated with resolution of the inflammatory response and often abatement of seizures.

Primary *toxoplasma* infection is often asymptomatic. However, during this phase parasites may spread to the CNS, where they become latent. Reactivation of CNS infection is almost exclusively associated with immunocompromised hosts, particularly those with HIV infection. During this phase patients present with headache, fever, seizures, and focal neurologic deficits.

DIAGNOSIS The lesions of neurocysticercosis are readily visualized by MRI or CT scans. Parenchymal brain calcifications are the most common finding. The scolex can often be visualized on MRI. A very early sign of cyst death is hypointensity of the vesicular fluid on T2-weighted images when compared with CSF. MRI findings consist of multiple lesions in the deep white matter, the thalamus, and basal ganglia and at the gray-white junction in the cerebral hemispheres. With contrast administration, the majority of the lesions enhance in a ringed, nodular, or homogeneous pattern and are surrounded by edema. In the presence of the characteristic neuroimaging abnormalities of this parasitic infection, serum anti–*T. gondii* antibodies should be obtained; if positive, the patient should be treated.

℞ TREATMENT

Anticonvulsant therapy is initiated when the patient with neurocysticercosis presents with a seizure. There is controversy about whether or not antihelminthic therapy should be given to all patients. Such therapy does not necessarily reduce the risk of seizure recurrence, but the control of seizures is easier after treatment with cysticidal drugs than when the disease is untreated. Albendazole and praziquantel are used in the treatment of neurocysticercosis. Approximately 85% of parenchymal cysts are destroyed by a single course of albendazole and ~75% are destroyed by a single course of praziquantel. The dose of albendazole is 15 mg/kg per day in two doses for 8 days. The dose of praziquantel is 50 mg/kg per day for 15 days, although a number of other dosage regimens are also frequently cited. Antiepileptic therapy can be stopped once the follow-up CT scan shows resolution of the lesion. Long-term antiepileptic therapy is recommended when seizures occur after resolution of edema and resorption or calcification of the degenerating cyst.

CNS toxoplasmosis is treated with a combination of sulfadiazine, 1.5 to 2.0 g orally qid, plus pyrimethamine, 100 mg orally to load then 75 to 100 mg orally qd, plus folinic acid, 10 to 15 mg orally qd. Folinic acid is added to the regimen to prevent megaloblastic anemia. Therapy is continued until there is no evidence of active disease on neuroimaging studies, which typically takes at least 6 weeks, and then the dose of sulfadiazine is reduced to 2 to 4 g/d and pyrimethamine to 50 mg/d. Clindamycin plus pyrimethamine is an alternative therapy for patients who cannot tolerate sulfadiazine, but the combination of pyrimethamine and sulfadiazine is more effective.

SUBDURAL EMPYEMA

A subdural empyema (SDE) is a collection of pus between the dura and arachnoid membranes (Fig. 360-5).

EPIDEMIOLOGY SDE is a rare disorder that accounts for 15 to 25% of focal suppurative CNS infections. Sinusitis is the most common predisposing condition and typically involves the frontal sinuses, either alone or in combination with the ethmoid and maxillary sinuses. Sinusitis-associated empyema has a striking predilection for young males, possibly reflecting sex-related differences in sinus anatomy and development. It has been suggested that SDE may complicate 1 to 2% of cases of frontal sinusitis severe enough to require hospitalization. As a consequence of this epidemiology, SDE shows an ~3:1 male:female predominance, with 70% of cases occurring in the second and third decades of life. SDE may also develop as a complication of head trauma or neurosurgery. Secondary infection of a subdural effusion may also result in empyema, although secondary infection of hematomas, in the absence of a prior neurosurgical procedure, is rare.

ETIOLOGY Aerobic and anaerobic streptococci, staphylococci, Enterobacteriaceae, and anaerobic bacteria are the most common causative

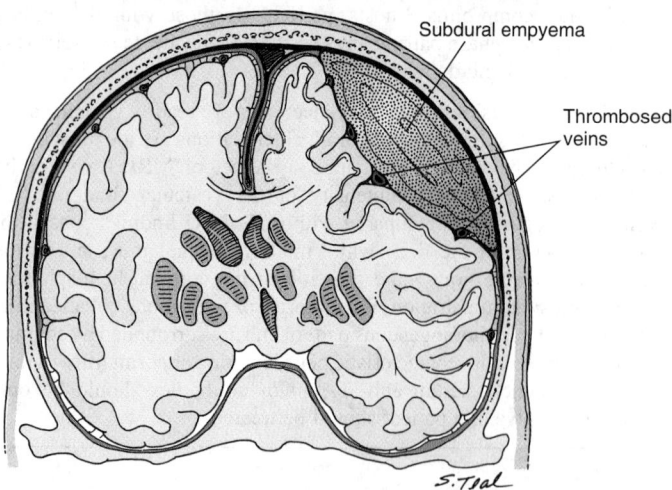

FIGURE 360-5 Subdural empyema is a collection of pus between the dura and arachnoid membranes.

organisms of sinusitis-associated SDE. Staphylococci and gram-negative bacilli are often the etiologic organisms when SDE follows neurosurgical procedures or head trauma. Up to one-third of cases are culture-negative, possibly reflecting difficulty in obtaining adequate anaerobic cultures.

PATHOPHYSIOLOGY   Sinusitis-associated SDE develops as a result of either retrograde spread of infection from septic thrombophlebitis of the mucosal veins draining the sinuses or contiguous spread of infection to the brain from osteomyelitis in the posterior wall of the frontal or other sinuses. SDE may also develop from direct introduction of bacteria into the subdural space as a complication of a neurosurgical procedure. The evolution of SDE can be extremely rapid because the subdural space is a large compartment that offers few mechanical barriers to the spread of infection. In patients with sinusitis-associated SDE, suppuration typically begins in the upper and anterior portions of one cerebral hemisphere and then extends posteriorly. SDE is often associated with other intracranial infections including epidural empyema (40%), cortical thrombophlebitis (35%), and intracranial abscess or cerebritis (>25%). Cortical venous infarction produces necrosis of underlying cerebral cortex and subcortical white matter, with focal neurologic deficits and seizures (see below).

CLINICAL PRESENTATION   A patient with SDE typically presents with fever and a progressively worsening headache. The diagnosis of SDE should always be suspected in a patient with known sinusitis who presents with new CNS signs or symptoms. Patients with underlying sinusitis frequently have symptoms related to this infection. As the infection progresses, focal neurologic deficits, seizures, nuchal rigidity, and signs of increased ICP commonly occur. Headache is the most common complaint at the time of presentation; initially it is localized to the side of the subdural infection but then becomes more severe and generalized. Contralateral hemiparesis or hemiplegia is the most common focal neurologic deficit and can occur from the direct effects of the SDE on the cortex or as a consequence of venous infarction. Seizures begin as partial motor seizures that then become secondarily generalized. Seizures may be due to the direct irritative effect of the SDE on the underlying cortex or result from cortical venous infarction (see above). In untreated SDE, the increasing mass effect and increase in ICP cause progressive deterioration in consciousness, leading ultimately to coma.

DIAGNOSIS   MRI (Fig. 360-6) is superior to CT in identifying SDE and any associated intracranial infections. The administration of gadolinium greatly improves diagnosis by enhancing the rim of the empyema and allowing the empyema to be clearly delineated from the underlying brain parenchyma. Cranial MRI is also extremely valuable in identifying sinusitis, other focal CNS infections, cortical venous infarction, cerebral edema, and cerebritis. CT may show a crescent-shaped hypodense lesion over one or both hemispheres or in the interhemispheric fissure. Frequently the degree of mass effect, exemplified by midline shift, ventricular compression, and sulcal effacement, is far out of proportion to the mass of the SDE.

CSF examination should be avoided in patients with known or suspected SDE as it adds no useful information and is associated with the risk of cerebral herniation.

DIFFERENTIAL DIAGNOSIS   The differential diagnosis of the combination of headache, fever, focal neurologic signs, and seizure activity that progresses rapidly to an altered level of consciousness includes subdural hematoma, bacterial meningitis, viral encephalitis, brain abscess, superior sagittal sinus thrombosis, and acute disseminated encephalomyelitis. The presence of nuchal rigidity is unusual with brain abscess or epidural empyema and should suggest the possibility of SDE when associated with significant focal neurologic signs and fever. Patients with bacterial meningitis also have nuchal rigidity but do not typically have focal deficits of the severity seen with SDE.

℞ TREATMENT

SDE is a medical emergency. Emergent neurosurgical evacuation of the empyema, either through burr-hole drainage or craniotomy, is the definitive step in the management of this infection. Empirical antimicrobial therapy should include a combination of a third-generation cephalosporin (e.g., cefotaxime or ceftriaxone), vancomycin, and metronidazole (see Table 360-2 for dosages). Parenteral antibiotic therapy should be continued for a minimum of 4 weeks. Specific diagnosis of the etiologic organisms is made based on Gram's stain and culture of fluid obtained via either burr holes or craniotomy; the initial empirical antibiotic coverage can be modified accordingly.

PROGNOSIS   Prognosis is influenced by the level of consciousness of the patient at the time of hospital presentation, the size of the empyema, and the speed with which therapy is instituted. Long-term neurologic sequelae, which include seizures and hemiparesis, occur in up to 50% of cases.

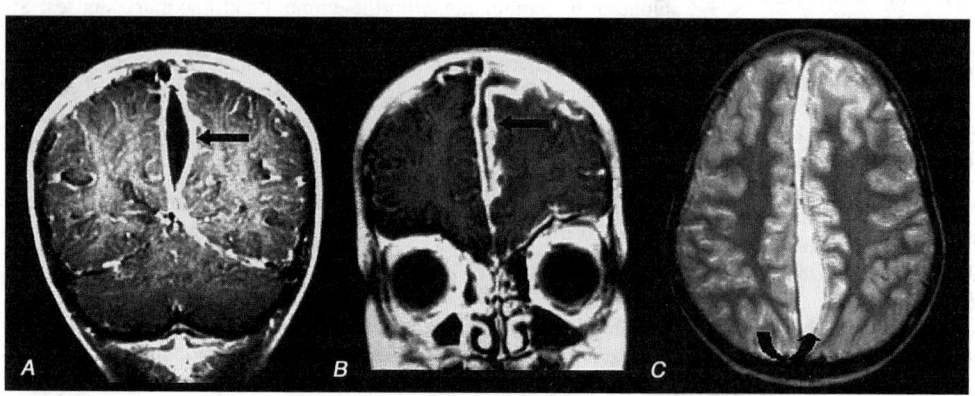

FIGURE 360-6 Subdural empyema. There is marked enhancement of the dura and leptomeninges (A, B, straight arrows) along the left medial hemisphere. The pus is hypointense on T1-weighted images (A, B), but markedly hyperintense on the proton density–weighted (C, curved arrow) image. (Courtesy of Joseph Lurito, MD.)

EPIDURAL ABSCESS

Cranial epidural abscess is a suppurative infection occurring in the potential space between the inner skull table and dura (Fig. 360-7).

ETIOLOGY AND PATHOPHYSIOLOGY Epidural abscess is less common than either brain abscess or SDE and accounts for <2% of focal suppurative CNS infections. A cranial epidural abscess develops as a complication of a craniotomy or compound skull fracture or as a result of spread of infection from the frontal sinuses, middle ear, mastoid, or orbit. An epidural abscess may develop contiguous to an area of osteomyelitis, when craniotomy is complicated by infection of the wound or bone flap, or as a result of direct infection of the epidural space. Infection in the frontal sinus, middle ear, mastoid, or orbit can reach the epidural space through retrograde spread of infection from septic thrombophlebitis in the emissary veins that drain these areas or by way of direct spread of infection through areas of osteomyelitis. Unlike the subdural space, the epidural space is really a potential rather than an actual compartment. The dura is normally tightly adherent to the inner skull table, and infection must dissect the dura away from the skull table as it spreads. As a result, epidural abscesses are often smaller than SDEs. Cranial epidural abscesses, unlike brain abscesses, only rarely result from hematogenous spread of infection from extracranial primary sites. The bacteriology of a cranial epidural abscess is similar to that of SDE (see above). The etiologic organisms of an epidural abscess that arises from frontal sinusitis, middle ear infections, or mastoiditis are usually streptococci or anaerobic organisms. Staphylococci or gram-negative organisms are the usual cause of an epidural abscess that develops as a complication of craniotomy or compound skull fracture.

CLINICAL PRESENTATION Patients present with fever (60%), headache (40%), nuchal rigidity (35%), seizures (10%), and focal deficits (5%). Periorbital edema and Potts puffy tumor, reflecting underlying associated frontal bone osteomyelitis, are present in ~40%. In patients with a recent neurosurgical procedure, wound infection is invariably present, but other symptoms may be subtle and can include altered mental status (45%), fever (35%), and headache (20%). The diagnosis should also be considered when fever and headache follow recent head trauma or occur in the setting of frontal sinusitis, mastoiditis, or otitis media.

DIAGNOSIS Cranial MRI is the procedure of choice to demonstrate a cranial epidural abscess. The sensitivity of CT is limited by the presence of signal artifacts arising from the bone of the inner skull table. The CT appearance of an epidural empyema is that of a lens or crescent-shaped hypodense extraaxial lesion. On MRI, an epidural empyema appears as a lentiform or crescent-shaped fluid collection that is hyperintense compared to CSF on T2-weighted images. On T1-weighted images, the fluid collection has a signal intensity that is intermediate between that of brain tissue and CSF. Following the administration of gadolinium, a significant enhancement of the dura is seen on T1-weighted images. In distinction to subdural empyema, signs of mass effect or other parenchymal abnormalities are uncommon.

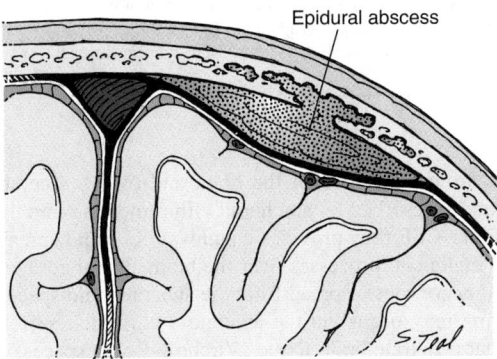

FIGURE 360-7 Cranial epidural abscess is a collection of pus between the dura and the inner table of the skull.

℞ TREATMENT

Immediate neurosurgical drainage is indicated. Empirical antimicrobial therapy, pending the results of Gram's stain and culture of the purulent material obtained at surgery, should include a combination of a third-generation cephalosporin, nafcillin or vancomycin, and metronidazole (Table 360-2). Ceftazidime should be substituted for ceftriaxone or cefotaxime in neurosurgical patients. Meropenem and vancomycin also provide effective empirical therapy in postneurosurgical cases. When the organism has been identified, antimicrobial therapy can be modified accordingly. Antibiotics should be continued for at least 3 weeks after surgical drainage.

PROGNOSIS Mortality is <5% in modern series, and full recovery is the rule in most survivors.

SUPPURATIVE THROMBOPHLEBITIS

DEFINITION Suppurative intracranial thrombophlebitis is septic venous thrombosis of cortical veins and sinuses. This may occur as a complication of bacterial meningitis; SDE; epidural abscess; or infection in the skin of the face, paranasal sinuses, middle ear, or mastoid.

ANATOMY AND PATHOPHYSIOLOGY The cerebral veins and venous sinuses have no valves; therefore, blood within them can flow in either direction. The superior sagittal sinus is the largest of the venous sinuses (Fig. 360-8). It receives blood from the frontal, parietal, and occipital superior cerebral veins and the diploic veins, which communicate with the meningeal veins. Bacterial meningitis is a common predisposing condition for septic thrombosis of the superior sagittal sinus. The diploic veins, which drain into the superior sagittal sinus, provide a route for the spread of infection from the meninges, especially in cases where there is purulent exudate near areas of the superior sagittal sinus. Infection can also spread to the superior sagittal sinus from nearby SDE or epidural abscess. Dehydration from vomiting, hypercoagulable states, and immunologic abnormalities, including the presence of circulating antiphospholipid antibodies, also contribute to cerebral venous sinus thrombosis. Thrombosis may extend from one sinus to another, and often at autopsy thrombi of different histologic ages can be detected in several sinuses. Thrombosis of the superior sagittal sinus is often associated with thrombosis of superior cortical veins and small parenchymal hemorrhages.

The superior sagittal sinus drains into the transverse sinuses (Fig. 360-8). The transverse sinuses also receive venous drainage from small veins from both the middle ear and mastoid cells. The transverse sinus becomes the sigmoid sinus before draining into the internal jugular vein. Septic transverse/sigmoid sinus thrombosis can be a complica-

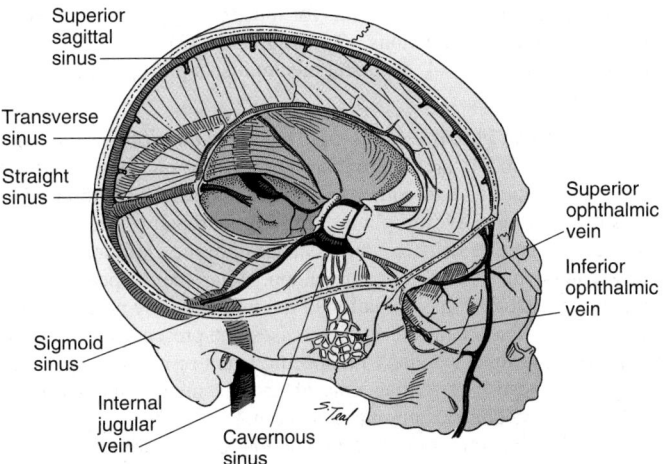

FIGURE 360-8 Anatomy of the cerebral venous sinuses.

tion of acute and chronic otitis media or mastoiditis. Infection spreads from the mastoid air cells to the transverse sinus via the emissary veins or by direct invasion. The cavernous sinuses are inferior to the superior sagittal sinus at the base of the skull. The cavernous sinuses receive blood from the facial veins via the superior and inferior ophthalmic veins. Bacteria in the facial veins enter the cavernous sinus via these veins. Bacteria in the sphenoid and ethmoid sinuses can spread to the cavernous sinuses via the small emissary veins. The sphenoid and ethmoid sinuses are the most common sites of primary infection resulting in septic cavernous sinus thrombosis.

CLINICAL MANIFESTATIONS *Septic thrombosis of the superior sagittal sinus* presents with headache, fever, nausea and vomiting, confusion, and focal or generalized seizures. There may be a rapid development of stupor and coma. Weakness of the lower extremities with bilateral Babinski signs or hemiparesis is often present. When superior sagittal sinus thrombosis occurs as a complication of bacterial meningitis, nuchal rigidity and Kernig's and Brudzinski's signs may be present.

The oculomotor nerve, the trochlear nerve, the abducens nerve, the ophthalmic and maxillary branches of the trigeminal nerve, and the internal carotid artery all pass through the cavernous sinus (Fig. 355-3). The symptoms of *septic cavernous sinus thrombosis* are fever, headache, frontal and retroorbital pain, and diplopia. The classic signs are ptosis, proptosis, chemosis, and extraocular dysmotility due to deficits of cranial nerves III, IV, and VI; hyperesthesia of the ophthalmic and maxillary divisions of the fifth cranial nerve and a decreased corneal reflex may be detected. There may be evidence of dilated, tortuous retinal veins and papilledema.

Headache and earache are the most frequent symptoms of *transverse sinus thrombosis*. A transverse sinus thrombosis may also present with otitis media, sixth nerve palsy, and retroorbital or facial pain (*Gradinego's syndrome*). Sigmoid sinus and internal jugular vein thrombosis may present with neck pain.

DIAGNOSIS The diagnosis of septic venous sinus thrombosis is suggested by an absent flow void within the affected venous sinus on MRI and confirmed by magnetic resonance venography or the venous phase of cerebral angiography. The diagnosis of thrombophlebitis of intracerebral and meningeal veins is suggested by the presence of intracerebral hemorrhage but requires cerebral angiography for definitive diagnosis.

℞ TREATMENT

Septic venous sinus thrombosis is usually treated with antibiotics and hydration. The choice of antimicrobial therapy is based on the bacteria responsible for the predisposing or associated condition. Optimal duration of therapy is unknown, but antibiotics are usually continued for 6 weeks or until there is radiographic evidence of resolution of thrombosis. Anticoagulation with dose-adjusted heparin has been reported to be beneficial in patients with aseptic venous sinus thrombosis; it is also used in the treatment of septic venous sinus thrombosis complicating bacterial meningitis in patients who are worsening despite antimicrobial therapy and intravenous fluids. The presence of a small intracerebral hemorrhage from septic thrombophlebitis is not an absolute contraindication to heparin therapy. Successful management of aseptic venous sinus thrombosis has been reported with urokinase therapy and with a combination of intrathrombus recombinant tissue plasminogen activator (rtPA) and intravenous heparin, but the efficacy of these therapies in septic venous sinus thrombosis is unknown.

FURTHER READING

DE GANS J, VAN DE BEEK D: Dexamethasone in adults with bacterial meningitis. N Engl J Med 347:1549, 2002

DWORKIN MS: A review of progressive multifocal leukoencephalopathy in persons with and without AIDS. Curr Clin Top Infect Dis 22:181, 2002

LU CH et al: Bacterial brain abscess: Microbiological features, epidemiological trends and therapeutic outcomes. Q J Med 95:501, 2002

ROOS KL: Acute bacterial meningitis. Semin Neurol 20:293, 2000

ROSENSTEIN NE et al: Meningococcal disease. N Engl J Med 344:1378, 2001

SOLOMON T et al: West Nile encephalitis, BMJ 326:865, 2003

361 CHRONIC AND RECURRENT MENINGITIS
Walter J. Koroshetz, Morton N. Swartz

Chronic inflammation of the meninges (pia, arachnoid, and dura) can produce profound neurologic disability and may be fatal if not successfully treated. The condition is most commonly diagnosed when a characteristic neurologic syndrome exists for >4 weeks and is associated with a persistent inflammatory response in the cerebrospinal fluid (CSF) (white blood cell count >5/μL). The causes are varied, and appropriate treatment depends on identification of the etiology. Five categories of disease account for most cases of chronic meningitis: (1) meningeal infections, (2) malignancy, (3) noninfectious inflammatory disorders, (4) chemical meningitis, and (5) parameningeal infections.

CLINICAL PATHOPHYSIOLOGY Neurologic manifestations of chronic meningitis (Table 361-1) are determined by the anatomic location of the inflammation and its consequences. Persistent headache with or without stiff neck, and hydrocephalus, cranial neuropathies, radiculopathies, and cognitive or personality changes are the cardinal features. These can occur alone or in combination. When they appear in combination, widespread dissemination of the inflammatory process along CSF pathways has occurred. In some cases, the presence of an underlying systemic illness points to a specific agent or class of agents as the probable cause. The diagnosis of chronic meningitis is usually made when the clinical presentation prompts the astute physician to examine the CSF for signs of inflammation. CSF is produced by the choroid plexus of the cerebral ventricles, exits through narrow foramina into the subarachnoid space surrounding the brain and spinal cord,

TABLE 361-1 Symptoms and Signs of Chronic Meningitis

Symptom	Sign
Chronic headache	+/− Papilledema
Neck or back pain	Brudzinski's or Kernig's sign of meningeal irritation
Change in personality	Altered mental status—drowsiness, inattention, disorientation, memory loss, frontal release signs (grasp, suck, snout), perseveration
Facial weakness	Peripheral seventh CN palsy
Double vision	Palsy of CNs III, IV, VI
Visual loss	Papilledema, optic atrophy
Hearing loss	Eighth CN palsy
Arm or leg weakness	Myelopathy or radiculopathy
Numbness in arms or legs	Myelopathy or radiculopathy
Sphincter dysfunction	Myelopathy or radiculopathy
	Frontal lobe dysfunction
Clumsiness	Ataxia

Note: CN, cranial nerve.

circulates around the base of the brain and over the cerebral hemispheres, and is resorbed by arachnoid villi projecting into the superior sagittal sinus. CSF flow provides a pathway for rapid spread of infectious and malignant processes over the brain, spinal cord, and cranial and spinal nerve roots. Spread from the subarachnoid space into brain parenchyma may occur via the arachnoid cuffs that surround blood vessels that penetrate brain tissue (Virchow-Robin spaces).

Intracranial Meningitis Nociceptive fibers of the meninges (Chap. 14) are stimulated by the inflammatory process, resulting in headache or neck or back pain. Obstruction of CSF pathways at foramina or arachnoid villi may produce *hydrocephalus* and symptoms of raised intracranial pressure (ICP), including headache, vomiting, apathy or drowsiness, gait instability, papilledema, visual loss, impaired upgaze, or palsy of the sixth cranial nerve (CN) (Chap. 258). Cognitive and behavioral changes during the course of chronic meningitis may also result from vascular damage, which may similarly produce seizures, stroke, or myelopathy. Inflammatory deposits seeded via the CSF circulation are often prominent around the brainstem and cranial nerves and along the undersurface of the frontal and temporal lobes. Such cases, termed *basal meningitis*, often present as multiple cranial neuropathies, with visual loss (CN II), facial weakness (CN VII), hearing loss (CN VIII), diplopia (CNs III, IV, and VI), sensory or motor abnormalities of the oropharynx (CNs IX, X, and XII), decreased olfaction (CN I), or facial sensory loss and masseter weakness (CN V).

Spinal Meningitis Injury may occur to motor and sensory roots as they traverse the subarachnoid space and penetrate the meninges. These cases present as multiple radiculopathies with combinations of radicular pain, sensory loss, motor weakness, and sphincter dysfunction. Meningeal inflammation can encircle the cord, resulting in myelopathy. Patients with slowly progressive involvement of multiple cranial nerves and/or spinal nerve roots are likely to have chronic meningitis. Electrophysiologic testing (electromyography, nerve conduction studies, and evoked response testing) may be helpful in determining whether there is involvement of cranial and spinal nerve roots.

Systemic Manifestations In some patients, evidence of systemic disease provides clues to the underlying cause of chronic meningitis. A careful history and physical examination are essential before embarking on a diagnostic workup, which may be costly, prolonged, and associated with risk from invasive procedures. A complete history of travel, sexual practice, and exposure to infectious agents should be sought. Infectious causes are often associated with fever, malaise, anorexia, and signs of localized or disseminated infection outside the nervous system. Infectious causes are of major concern in the immunosuppressed patient, especially in patients with AIDS, in whom chronic meningitis may present without headache or fever. Noninfectious inflammatory disorders often produce systemic manifestations, but meningitis may be the initial manifestation. Carcinomatous meningitis may or may not be accompanied by clinical evidence of the primary neoplasm.

APPROACH TO THE PATIENT

The occurrence of chronic headache, hydrocephalus, cranial neuropathy, radiculopathy, and/or cognitive decline in a patient should prompt consideration of a lumbar puncture for evidence of meningeal inflammation. On occasion the diagnosis is made when an imaging study [computed tomography (CT) or magnetic resonance imaging (MRI)] shows contrast enhancement of the meninges, always abnormal with the exception of dural enhancement after lumbar puncture, neurosurgical procedures, or spontaneous CSF leakage. Once chronic meningitis is confirmed by CSF examination, effort is focused on identifying the cause (Tables 361-2 and 361-3) by (1) further analysis of the CSF, (2) diagnosis of an underlying systemic infection or noninfectious inflammatory condition, or (3) pathologic examination of meningeal biopsy specimens.

Two clinical forms of chronic meningitis exist. In the first, the symptoms are chronic and persistent, whereas in the second there are recurrent, discrete episodes of illness. In the latter group, all symptoms, signs, and CSF parameters of meningeal inflammation resolve completely between episodes without specific therapy. In such patients, the likely etiologies include infection with herpes simplex virus (HSV) type 2; chemical meningitis due to leakage into CSF of contents from an epidermoid tumor, craniopharyngioma, or cholesteatoma; primary inflammatory conditions, including Vogt-Koyanagi-Harada syndrome, Behçet's syndrome (Chap. 307), Mollaret's meningitis, and systemic lupus erythematosus (SLE; Chap. 300); and drug hypersensitivity with repeated administration of the offending agent.

The epidemiologic history is of considerable importance and may provide direction for selection of laboratory studies. Pertinent features include a history of tuberculosis or exposure to a likely case; past travel to areas endemic for fungal infections (the San Joaquin Valley in California and southwestern states for coccidioidomycosis, midwestern states for histoplasmosis, southeastern states for blastomycosis); travel to the Mediterranean region or ingestion of imported unpasteurized dairy products (*Brucella*); time spent in areas endemic for Lyme disease (e.g., Connecticut, New York, Massachusetts); exposure to sexually transmitted disease (syphilis); exposure of an immunocompromised host to pigeons and their droppings (*Cryptococcus*); gardening (*Sporothrix schenkii*); ingestion of poorly cooked meat or contact with a household cat (*Toxoplasma gondii*); residence in Thailand or Japan (*Gnathostoma spinigerum*) or the South Pacific (*Angiostrongylus cantonensis*); rural residence and raccoon exposure (*Baylisascaris procyonis*); and residence in Latin America, the Philippines, or Southeast Asia when eosinophilic meningitis is present (*Taenia solium*).

The presence of focal cerebral signs in a patient with chronic meningitis suggests the possibility of a brain abscess or other parameningeal infection; identification of a potential source of infection (chronic draining ear, sinusitis, right-to-left cardiac or pulmonary shunt, chronic pleuropulmonary infection) supports this diagnosis. In some cases, diagnosis may be established by recognition and biopsy of unusual skin lesions (Behçet's syndrome, cryptococcosis, blastomycosis, SLE, Lyme disease, intravenous drug use, sporotrichosis, trypanosomiasis) or enlarged lymph nodes (lymphoma, tuberculosis, sarcoid, infection with HIV, secondary syphilis, or Whipple's disease). A careful ophthalmologic examination may reveal uveitis [Vogt-Koyanagi-Harada syndrome, sarcoid, or central nervous system (CNS) lymphoma], keratoconjunctivitis sicca (Sjögren's syndrome), or iridocyclitis (Behçet's syndrome) and is essential to assess visual loss from hydrocephalus. Aphthous oral lesions, genital ulcers, and hypopyon suggest Behçet's syndrome. Hepatosplenomegaly suggests lymphoma, sarcoid, tuberculosis, or brucellosis. Herpetic lesions in the genital area or on the thighs suggest HSV-2 infection. A breast nodule, a suspicious pigmented skin lesion, focal bone pain, or an abdominal mass directs attention to possible carcinomatous meningitis.

Imaging Once the clinical syndrome is recognized as a potential manifestation of chronic meningitis, proper analysis of the CSF is essential. However, if the possibility of raised ICP exists, a brain imaging study should be performed before lumbar puncture. If ICP is elevated because of a mass lesion, brain swelling, or a block in ventricular CSF outflow (obstructive hydrocephalus), then lumbar puncture carries the potential risk of brain herniation. Obstructive hydrocephalus usually requires direct ventricular drainage of CSF. In patients with open CSF flow pathways, elevated ICP can occur due to impaired resorption of CSF by arachnoid villi. In such patients, lumbar puncture is usually safe, but repetitive or continuous lumbar drainage may be necessary to prevent relatively sudden death from raised ICP. In some patients, especially with cryptococcal meningitis, life-threatening levels of ICP can occur without visible hydrocephalus on brain imaging.

Contrast-enhanced MRI or CT studies of the brain and spinal cord can identify meningeal enhancement, parameningeal infections (including brain abscess), encasement of the spinal cord (malignancy or inflammation and infection), or nodular deposits on the meninges or nerve roots (malignancy or sarcoidosis) (Fig. 361-1). Imaging studies are also useful to localize areas of meningeal disease prior to meningeal biopsy.

Cerebral angiography may be indicated in patients with chronic meningitis and stroke to identify cerebral arteritis (granulomatous angiitis, other inflammatory or infectious causes).

TABLE 361-2 *Infectious Causes of Chronic Meningitis*

Causative Agent	CSF Formula	Helpful Diagnostic Tests	Risk Factors and Systemic Manifestations
COMMON BACTERIAL CAUSES			
Partially treated suppurative meningitis	Mononuclear or mixed mononuclear-polymorphonuclear cells	CSF culture and Gram stain	History consistent with acute bacterial meningitis and incomplete treatment
Parameningeal infection	Mononuclear or mixed polymorphonuclear-mononuclear cells	Contrast-enhanced CT or MRI to detect parenchymal, subdural, epidural, or sinus infection	Otitis media, pleuropulmonary infection, right-to-left cardiopulmonary shunt for brain abscess; focal neurologic signs; neck, back, ear, or sinus tenderness
Mycobacterium tuberculosis	Mononuclear cells except polymorphonuclear cells in early infection (commonly <500 WBC/μL); low CSF glucose, high protein	Tuberculin skin test may be negative; AFB culture of CSF (sputum, urine, gastric contents if indicated); tuberculostearic acid detection in CSF; identify tubercle bacillus on acid-fast stain of CSF or protein pellicle; PCR	Exposure history; previous tuberculous illness; immunosuppressed or AIDS; young children; fever, meningismus, night sweats, miliary TB on X-ray or liver biopsy; stroke due to arteritis
Lyme disease (Bannwarth's syndrome) *Borrelia burgdorferi*	Mononuclear cells; elevated protein	Serum Lyme antibody titer; Western blot confirmation; (patients with syphilis may have false-positive Lyme titer)	History of tick bite or appropriate exposure history; erythema chronicum migrans skin rash; arthritis, radiculopathy, Bell's palsy, meningoencephalitis–multiple sclerosis-like syndrome
Syphilis (secondary, tertiary) *Treponema pallidum*	Mononuclear cells; elevated protein	CSF VDRL; serum VDRL (or RPR); fluorescent treponemal antibody-absorbed (FTA) or MHA-TP; serum VDRL may be negative in tertiary syphilis	Appropriate exposure history; HIV seropositive individuals at increased risk of aggressive infection; "dementia"; cerebral infarction due to endarteritis
UNCOMMON BACTERIAL CAUSES			
Actinomyces	Polymorphonuclear cells	Anaerobic culture	Parameningeal abscess or sinus tract (oral or dental focus); pneumonitis
Nocardia	Polymorphonuclear; occasionally mononuclear cells; often low glucose	Isolation may require weeks; weakly acid fast	Associated brain abscess may be present
Brucella	Mononuclear cells (rarely polymorphonuclear); elevated protein; often low glucose	CSF antibody detection; serum antibody detection	Intake of unpasteurized dairy products; exposure to goats, sheep, cows; fever, arthralgia, myalgia, vertebral osteomyelitis
Whipple's disease *Tropherema whippelii*	Mononuclear cells	Biopsy of small bowel or lymph node; CSF PCR for *T. whippelii*; brain and meningeal biopsy (with PAS stain and EM examination)	Diarrhea, weight loss, arthralgias, fever; dementia, ataxia, paresis, ophthalmoplegia, oculomasticatory myoclonus
RARE BACTERIAL CAUSES			
Leptospirosis (occasionally if left untreated may last 3–4 weeks)			
FUNGAL CAUSES			
Cryptococcus neoformans	Mononuclear cells; count not elevated in some patients with AIDS	India ink or fungal wet mount of CSF (budding yeast); blood and urine cultures; antigen detection in CSF	AIDS and immune suppression; pigeon exposure; skin and other organ involvement due to disseminated infection
Coccidioides immitis	Mononuclear cells (sometimes 10–20% eosinophils); often low glucose	Antibody detection in CSF and serum	Exposure history—southwestern US; increased virulence in dark-skinned races
Candida sp.	Polymorphonuclear or mononuclear	Fungal stain and culture of CSF	IV drug abuse; post surgery; prolonged intravenous therapy; disseminated candidiasis
Histoplasma capsulatum	Mononuclear cells; low glucose	Fungal stain and culture of large volumes of CSF; antigen detection in CSF, serum, and urine; antibody detection in serum, CSF	Exposure history—Ohio and central Mississippi River Valley; AIDS; mucosal lesions
Blastomyces dermatitidis	Mononuclear cells	Fungal stain and culture of CSF; biopsy and culture of skin, lung lesions; antibody detection in serum	Midwestern and Southeastern USA; usually systemic infection; abscesses, draining sinus, ulcers
Aspergillus sp.	Mononuclear or polymorphonuclear	CSF culture	Sinusitis; granulocytopenia or immunosuppression
Sporothrix schenckii	Mononuclear cells	Antibody detection in CSF and serum; CSF culture	Traumatic inoculation; IV drug use; ulcerated skin lesion
RARE FUNGAL CAUSES			
Xylohypha (formerly *Cladosporium*) *trichoides* and other dark-walled (demateaceous) fungi such as *Curvularia*, *Drechslera*; *Mucor*, *Pseudoallescheria boydii*			

(continued)

TABLE 361-2— (Continued)

Causative Agent	CSF Formula	Helpful Diagnostic Tests	Risk Factors and Systemic Manifestations
PROTOZOAL CAUSES			
Toxoplasma gondii	Mononuclear cells	Biopsy or response to empirical therapy in clinically appropriate context (including presence of antibody in serum)	Usually with intracerebral abscesses common in HIV seropositive patients
Trypanosomiasis *Trypanosoma gambiense* *T. rhodesiense*	Mononuclear cells, elevated protein	Elevated CSF IgM; identification of trypanosomes in CSF and blood smear	Endemic in Africa; chancre, lymphadenopathy; prominent sleep disorder
RARE PROTOZOAL CAUSES			
Acanthamoeba sp. causing granulomatous amebic encephalitis and meningoencephalitis in immunocompromised and debilitated individuals			
HELMINTHIC CAUSES			
Cysticercosis (infection with cysts of *Taenia solium*)	Mononuclear cells; may have eosinophils; glucose level may be low	Indirect hemagglutination assay in CSF; ELISA immunoblotting in serum	Usually with multiple cysts in basal meninges and hydrocephalus; cerebral cysts, muscle calcification
Gnathostoma spinigerum	Eosinophils, mononuclear cells	Peripheral eosinophilia	History of eating raw fish; common in Thailand and Japan; subarachnoid hemorrhage; painful radiculopathy
Angiostrongylus cantonensis	Eosinophils, mononuclear cells	Recovery of worms from CSF	History of eating raw shellfish; common in tropical Pacific regions; often benign
Baylisascaris procyonis (raccoon ascarid)	Eosinophils, mononuclear cells		Infection follows accidental ingestion of *B. procyonis* eggs from raccoon feces; fatal meningoencephalitis
RARE HELMINTHIC CAUSES			
Trichinella spiralis (trichinosis); *Echinococcus* cysts; *Schistosoma* sp. The former may produce a lymphocytic pleocytosis whereas the latter two may produce an eosinophilic response in CSF associated with cerebral cysts (*Echinococcus*) or granulomatous lesions of brain or spinal cord			
VIRAL CAUSES			
Mumps	Mononuclear cells	Antibody in serum	No prior mumps or immunization; may produce meningoencephalitis; may persist for 3–4 weeks
Lymphocytic choriomeningitis	Mononuclear cells	Antibody in serum	Contact with rodents or their excreta; may persist for 3–4 weeks
Echovirus	Mononuclear cells; may have low glucose	Virus isolation from CSF	Congenital hypogammaglobulinemia; history of recurrent meningitis
HIV (acute retroviral syndrome)	Mononuclear cells	p24 antigen in serum and CSF; high level of HIV viremia	HIV risk factors; rash, fever, lymphadenopathy; lymphopenia in peripheral blood; syndrome may persist long enough to be considered as "chronic meningitis"; or chronic meningitis may develop in later stages (AIDS) due to HIV
Herpes simplex (HSV)	Mononuclear cells	PCR for HSV DNA; CSF antibody	Recurrent meningitis due to HSV-2 (rarely HSV-1) often associated with genital recurrences

Abbreviations: AFB, acid-fast bacillus; CSF, cerebrospinal fluid; CT, computed tomography; ELISA, enzyme-linked immunosorbent assay; EM, electron microscopy; FTA, fluorescent treponemal antibody absorption test; MHA-TP, microhemagglutination assay-*T. pallidum*; MRI, magnetic resonance imaging; PAS, periodic acid–Schiff; PCR, polymerase chain reaction; RPR, rapid plasma reagin test; TB, tuberculosis; VDRL, Venereal Disease Research Laboratories test.

Cerebrospinal Fluid Analysis The CSF pressure should be measured and samples sent for bacterial culture, cell count and differential, Gram's stain, and measurement of glucose and protein. In cases without a known cause, CSF should be sent for the Venereal Disease Research Laboratories (VDRL) test, acid-fast bacillus (AFB) stain and culture, wet mount for fungus and parasites, India ink preparation and culture, culture for fastidious bacteria and fungi, assays for cryptococcal antigen and oligoclonal immunoglobulin bands, and cytology. Other specific CSF or blood tests and cultures (Tables 361-2 and 361-3) should be ordered as indicated on the basis of the history, physical examination, or preliminary CSF results (i.e., eosinophilic, mononuclear, or polymorphonuclear meningitis). Rapid diagnosis may be facilitated by serologic tests and polymerase chain reaction (PCR) testing to identify DNA sequences in the CSF that are specific for the suspected pathogen.

In most categories of chronic (not recurrent) meningitis, mononuclear cells predominate in the CSF. When neutrophils predominate after 3 weeks of illness, the principal considerations are *Nocardia asteroides*, *Actinomyces israelii*, *Brucella*, *Mycobacterium tuberculosis* (5 to 10% of early cases only), various fungi (*Blastomyces dermatitidis*, *Candida albicans*, *Histoplasma capsulatum*, *Aspergillus* species, *Pseudallescheria boydii*, *Cladophialophora bantiana*), and noninfectious causes (SLE, exogenous chemical meningitis). When eosinophils predominate or are present in limited numbers in a primarily mononuclear cell response in the CSF, the differential diagnosis includes parasitic diseases (*A. cantonensis*, *G. spinigerum*, *B. procyonis*, or *Toxocara canis* infection, cysticercosis, schistosomiasis, echinococcal disease, *T. gondii* infection), fungal infections (6 to 20% eosinophils along with a predominantly lymphocyte pleocytosis, particularly with coccidioidal meningitis), neoplastic disease (lymphoma, leukemia, metastatic carcinoma), or other inflammatory processes (sarcoidosis, hypereosinophilic syndrome).

It is often necessary to broaden the number of diagnostic tests if the initial workup does not reveal the cause. In addition, repeated samples of large volumes of CSF may be required to diagnose certain infectious and malignant causes of chronic meningitis. For instance, lymphomatous or carcinomatous meningitis may be di-

TABLE 361-3 *Noninfectious Causes of Chronic Meningitis*

Causative Agents	CSF Formula	Helpful Diagnostic Tests	Risk Factors and Systemic Manifestations
Malignancy	Mononuclear cells, elevated protein, low glucose	Repeated cytologic examination of large volumes of CSF; CSF exam by polarizing microscopy; clonal lymphocyte markers; deposits on nerve roots or meninges seen on myelogram or contrast-enhanced MRI; meningeal biopsy	Metastatic cancer of breast, lung, stomach, or pancreas; melanoma, lymphoma, leukemia; meningeal gliomatosis; meningeal sarcoma; cerebral dysgerminoma; meningeal melanoma or B cell lymphoma
Chemical compounds (may cause recurrent meningitis)	Mononuclear or PMNs, low glucose, elevated protein; xanthochromia from subarachnoid hemorrhage in week prior to presentation with "meningitis"	Contrast-enhanced CT scan or MRI Cerebral angiogram to detect aneurysm	History of recent injection into the subarachnoid space; history of sudden onset of headache; recent resection of acoustic neuroma or craniopharyngioma; epidermoid tumor of brain or spine, sometimes with dermoid sinus tract; pituitary apoplexy
Primary inflammation CNS sarcoidosis	Mononuclear cells; elevated protein; often low glucose	Serum and CSF angiotensin-converting enzyme levels; biopsy of extraneural affected tissues or brain lesion/meningeal biopsy	CN palsy, especially of CN VII; hypothalamic dysfunction, especially diabetes insipidus; abnormal chest radiograph; peripheral neuropathy or myopathy
Vogt-Koyanagi-Harada syndrome (recurrent meningitis)	Mononuclear cells		Recurrent meningoencephalitis with uveitis, retinal detachment, alopecia, lightening of eyebrows and lashes, dysacousia, cataracts, glaucoma
Isolated granulomatous angiitis of the nervous system	Mononuclear cells, elevated protein	Angiography or meningeal biopsy	Subacute dementia; multiple cerebral infarctions; recent zoster ophthalmicus
Systemic lupus erythematosus	Mononuclear or PMNs	Anti-DNA antibody, antinuclear antibodies	Encephalopathy; seizures; stroke; transverse myelopathy; rash; arthritis
Behçet's syndrome (recurrent meningitis)	Mononuclear or PMNs, elevated protein		Oral and genital aphthous ulcers; iridocyclitis; retinal hemorrhages; pathergic lesions at site of skin puncture
Chronic benign lymphocytic meningitis	Mononuclear cells		Recovery in 2–6 months, diagnosis by exclusion
Mollaret's meningitis (recurrent meningitis)	Large endothelial cells and PMNs in first hours, followed by mononuclear cells	PCR for herpes; MRI/CT to rule out epidermoid tumor or dural cyst	Recurrent meningitis; exclude HSV-2; rare cases due to HSV-1; occasional case associated with dural cyst
Drug hypersensitivity	PMNs; occasionally mononuclear cells or eosinophils		Exposure to ibuprofen, sulfonamides, isoniazid, tolmetin, ciprofloxacin, phenazopyridine; improvement after discontinuation of drug; recurrent episodes with recurrent exposure
Wegener's granulomatosis	Mononuclear cells	Chest and sinus radiographs; urinalysis; ANCA antibodies in serum	Associated sinus, pulmonary, or renal lesions; CN palsies; skin lesions; peripheral neuropathy

Other: multiple sclerosis, Sjögren's syndrome, neonatal onset multisystemic inflammatory disease (NOMID), and rarer forms of vasculitis (e.g., Cogan's syndrome)

Abbreviations: ANCA, anti-neutrophil cytoplasmic antibodies; CN, cranial nerve; CSF, cerebrospinal fluid; CT, computed tomography; HSV, herpes simplex virus; MRI, magnetic resonance imaging; PCR, polymerase chain reaction; PMNs, polymorphonuclear cells.

agnosed by examination of sections cut from a cell block formed by spinning down the sediment from a large volume of CSF. The diagnosis of fungal meningitis may require large volumes of CSF for culture of sediment. If standard lumbar puncture is unrewarding, a cervical cisternal tap to sample CSF near to the basal meninges may be fruitful.

Laboratory Investigation In addition to the CSF examination, an attempt should be made to uncover pertinent underlying illnesses. Tuberculin skin test, chest radiograph, urine analysis and culture, blood count and differential, renal and liver function tests, alkaline phosphatase, sedimentation rate, antinuclear antibody, anti-Ro and anti-La antibody, and serum angiotensin-converting enzyme level are often indicated. Liver or bone marrow biopsy may be diagnostic in some cases of miliary tuberculosis, disseminated fungal infection, sarcoidosis, or metastatic malignancy. Abnormalities discovered on chest radiograph or chest CT can be pursued by bronchoscopy or transthoracic needle biopsy.

Meningeal Biopsy A diagnostic meningeal biopsy should be strongly considered in patients who are severely disabled, who need chronic ventricular decompression, or whose illness is progressing rapidly. The activities of the surgeon, pathologist, microbiologist, and cytologist should be coordinated so that a large enough sample is obtained and the appropriate cultures and histologic and molecular studies, including electron microscopic and PCR studies, are performed. The diagnostic yield of meningeal biopsy can be increased by targeting regions that enhance with contrast on MRI or CT. With current microsurgical techniques, most areas of the basal meninges can be accessed for biopsy via a limited craniotomy. In a series from the Mayo Clinic reported by Cheng et al., MRI demonstrated meningeal enhancement in 47% of patients undergoing meningeal biopsy. Biopsy of an enhancing region was diagnostic in 80% of cases; biopsy of nonenhancing regions was diagnostic in only 9%; sarcoid (31%) and metastatic adenocarcinoma (25%) were the most common conditions identified.

Approach to the Enigmatic Case In approximately one-third of cases, the diagnosis is not known despite careful evaluation of CSF and potential extraneural sites of disease. A number of the organisms that cause chronic meningitis may take weeks to be identified by cultures. In enigmatic cases several options are available, determined by the extent of the clinical deficits and rate of progression. It is prudent to wait until cultures are finalized if the patient is asymptomatic or symptoms are mild and not progressive. Unfortunately, in many cases progressive neurologic deterioration occurs, and rapid treatment is required. Ventricular-peritoneal shunts may be placed to relieve hydrocephalus, but the risk of disseminating the undiagnosed inflammatory process into the abdomen must be considered.

Empirical Treatment Diagnosis of the causative agent is essential because effective therapies exist for many etiologies of chronic meningitis; if the condition is left untreated, however, progressive damage to the CNS and cranial nerves and roots is likely to occur. Occasionally, empirical therapy must be initiated when all attempts at diagnosis fail. In general, empirical therapy in the United States consists of antimycobacterial agents, amphotericin for fungal infection, or glucocorticoids for noninfectious inflammatory causes. It is important to direct empirical therapy of lymphocytic meningitis at tuberculosis, particularly if the condition is associated with hypoglycorrhachia and sixth and other CN palsies, since untreated disease is fatal in 4 to 8 weeks. In a series from the Mayo Clinic, the most useful empirical therapy was administration of glucocorticoids rather than antituberculous therapy. Carcinomatous or lymphomatous meningitis may be difficult to diagnose initially, but the diagnosis becomes evident with time.

THE IMMUNOSUPPRESSED PATIENT Chronic meningitis is not uncommon in the course of HIV infection. Pleocytosis and mild meningeal signs often occur at the onset of HIV infection, and occasionally low-grade meningitis persists. Toxoplasmosis commonly presents as intracranial abscesses and may also be associated with meningitis. Other important causes of chronic meningitis in AIDS include infection with *Crypto-coccus*, *Nocardia*, *Candida*, or other fungi; syphilis; and lymphoma

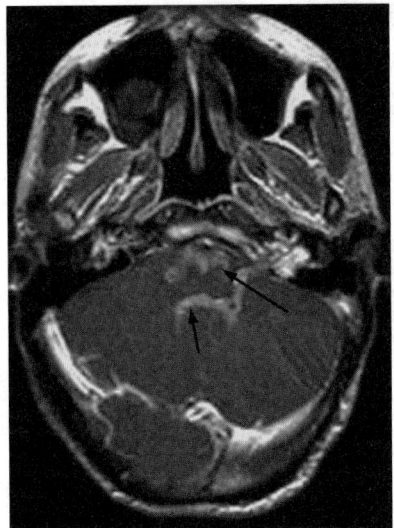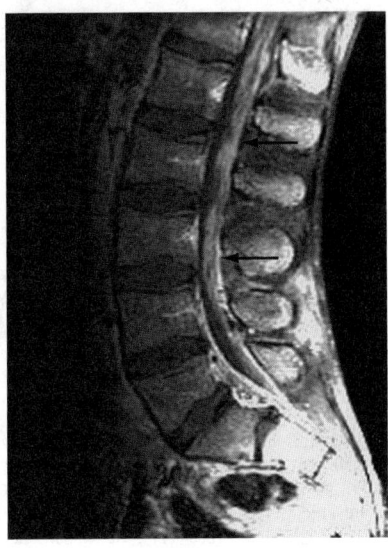

FIGURE 361-1 Primary central nervous system lymphoma. A 24-year-old man, immunosuppressed due to intestinal lymphangiectasia, developed multiple cranial neuropathies. CSF findings consisted of 100 lymphocytes/μL and a protein of 250 mg/dL; cytology and cultures were negative. Gadolinium-enhanced T1 MRI revealed diffuse, multifocal meningeal enhancement surrounding the brainstem (*A*), spinal cord and cauda equina (*B*).

(Fig. 361-1). Toxoplasmosis, cryptococcosis, nocardiosis, and other fungal infections are important etiologic considerations in individuals with immunodeficiency states other than AIDS, including those due to immunosuppressive medications. Because of the increased risk of chronic meningitis and the attenuation of clinical signs of meningeal irritation in immunosuppressed individuals, CSF examination should be performed for any persistent headache or unexplained change in mental state.

FURTHER READING

LAN SH et al: Cerebral infarction in chronic meningitis: A comparison of tuberculous meningitis and cryptococcal meningitis. Q J Med. 94:247, 2001

LILIANG PC et al: Use of ventriculoperitoneal shunts to treat uncontrollable intracranial hypertension in patients who have cryptococcal meningitis without hydrocephalus. Clin Infect Dis. 34:E64, 2002

SMITH JE, AKSAMIT AJ: Outcome of chronic idiopathic meningitis. Mayo Clinic Proc 69:548, 1994

THWAITS G et al: Tuberculous meningitis. J Neurol Neurosurg Psychiatry 68: 289, 2000

---

362 | PRION DISEASES
Stanley B. Prusiner, Bruce Miller

Prions are infectious proteins that cause degeneration of the central nervous system (CNS). Prion diseases are disorders of protein conformation, the most common of which in humans is called Creutzfeldt-Jakob disease (CJD). CJD typically presents with dementia and myoclonus, is relentlessly progressive, and generally causes death within a year of onset. Most CJD patients are between 50 and 75 years of age; however, patients as young as 17 years and as old as 83 years have been recorded.

In mammals, prions reproduce by binding to the normal, cellular isoform of the *prion protein* (PrP^C) and stimulating conversion of PrP^C into the disease-causing isoform (PrP^Sc). PrP^C is rich in α-helix and has little β-structure, while PrP^Sc has less α-helix and a high amount of β-structure (Fig. 362-1). This α-to-β structural transition in the prion protein (PrP) is the fundamental event underlying prion diseases (Table 362-1).

Four new concepts have emerged from studies of prions: (1) Prions are the only known infectious pathogens that are devoid of nucleic acid; all other infectious agents possess genomes composed of either RNA or DNA that direct the synthesis of their progeny. (2) Prion diseases may be manifest as infectious, genetic, and sporadic disorders; no other group of illnesses with a single etiology presents with such a wide spectrum of clinical manifestations. (3) Prion diseases result from the accumulation of PrP^Sc, the conformation of which differs substantially from that of its precursor PrP^C. (4) PrP^Sc can exist in a variety of different conformations, each of which seems to specify a particular disease phenotype. How a specific conformation of a PrP^Sc molecule is imparted to PrP^C during prion replication to produce nascent PrP^Sc with the same conformation is unknown. Additionally, it is

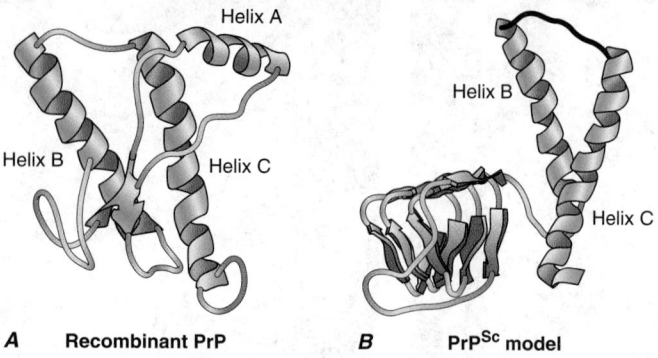

FIGURE 362-1 Structures of prion proteins. *A.* NMR structure of Syrian hamster recombinant (rec) PrP(90–231). Presumably, the structure of the α-helical form of recPrP(90–231) resembles that of PrP^C^. recPrP(90–231) is viewed from the interface where PrP^Sc^ is thought to bind to PrP^C^. Shown are: α-helices A (residues 144–157), B (172–193), and C (200–227). Flat ribbons depict β-strands S1 (129–131) and S2 (161–163). *(Reprinted with permission from H Lui et al: Biochemistry 38:5362, 1999.)* *B.* Theoretical structural model of PrP^Sc^. The 90–160 region has been modeled onto a β-helical architecture while the COOH terminal helices B and C are preserved as in PrP^C^. *(Image prepared by C. Govaerts.)*

unclear what factors determine where in the CNS a particular PrP^Sc^ molecule will be deposited.

SPECTRUM OF PRION DISEASES   The sporadic form of CJD is the most common prion disorder in humans. Sporadic CJD (sCJD) accounts for ~85% of all cases of human prion disease, while inherited prion diseases account for 10 to 15% of all cases (Table 362-2). Familial CJD (fCJD), Gerstmann-Sträussler-Scheinker (GSS) disease, and fatal familial insomnia (FFI) are all dominantly inherited prion diseases that are caused by mutations in the PrP gene.

Although infectious prion diseases account for <1% of all cases and infection does not seem to play an important role in the natural history of these illnesses, the transmissibility of prions is an important biologic feature. *Kuru* of the Fore people of New Guinea is thought to have resulted from the consumption of brains from dead relatives during ritualistic cannibalism. With the cessation of ritualistic cannibalism in the late 1950s, kuru has nearly disappeared with the exception of a few recent patients exhibiting incubation periods of >40 years. Iatrogenic CJD (iCJD) seems to be the result of the accidental inoculation of patients with prions. Variant CJD (vCJD) in teenagers

TABLE 362-1   *Glossary of Prion Terminology*

Prion	*Pro*teinaceous *in*fectious particle that lacks nucleic acid. Prions are composed largely, if not entirely, of PrP^Sc^ molecules. They can cause scrapie in animals and related neurodegenerative diseases of humans such as Creutzfeldt-Jakob disease (CJD).
PrP^Sc^	Disease-causing isoform of the prion protein. This protein is the only identifiable macromolecule in purified preparations of scrapie prions.
PrP^C^	Cellular isoform of the prion protein. PrP^C^ is the precursor of PrP^Sc^.
PrP 27-30	A fragment of PrP^Sc^, generated by truncation of the NH₂-terminus by limited digestion with proteinase K. PrP 27-30 retains prion infectivity and polymerizes into amyloid.
PRNP	PrP gene located on human chromosome 20.
Prion rod	An aggregate of prions composed largely of PrP 27-30 molecules. Created by detergent extraction and limited proteolysis of PrP^Sc^. Morphologically and histochemically indistinguishable from many amyloids.
PrP amyloid	Amyloid containing PrP in the brains of animals or humans with prion disease; often accumulates as plaques.

TABLE 362-2   *The Prion Diseases*

Disease	Host	Mechanism of Pathogenesis
Human		
Kuru	Fore people	Infection through ritualistic cannibalism
iCJD	Humans	Infection from prion-contaminated hGH, dura mater grafts, etc.
vCJD	Humans	Infection from bovine prions
fCJD	Humans	Germ-line mutations in *PRNP*
GSS	Humans	Germ-line mutations in *PRNP*
FFI	Humans	Germ-line mutation in *PRNP* (D178N, M129)
sCJD	Humans	Somatic mutation or spontaneous conversion of PrP^C^ into PrP^Sc^?
sFI	Humans	Somatic mutation or spontaneous conversion of PrP^C^ into PrP^Sc^?
Animal		
Scrapie	Sheep	Infection in genetically susceptible sheep
BSE	Cattle	Infection with prion-contaminated MBM
TME	Mink	Infection with prions from sheep or cattle
CWD	Mule deer, elk	Unknown
FSE	Cats	Infection with prion-contaminated beef
Exotic ungulate encephalopathy	Greater kudu, nyala, or oryx	Infection with prion-contaminated MBM

Abbreviations: BSE, bovine spongiform encephalopathy; CJD, Creutzfeldt-Jakob disease; fCJD, familial Creutzfeldt-Jakob disease; iCJD, iatrogenic Creutzfeldt-Jakob disease; sCJD, sporadic Creutzfeldt-Jakob disease; vCJD, variant Creutzfeldt-Jakob disease; CWD, chronic wasting disease; FFI, fatal familial insomnia; sFI, sporadic fatal insomnia; FSE, feline spongiform encephalopathy; GSS, Gerstmann-Sträussler-Scheinker disease; hGH, human growth hormone; MBM, meat and bone meal; TME, transmissible mink encephalopathy.

and young adults in Europe is the result of exposure to tainted beef from cattle with bovine spongiform encepalopathy (BSE).

Six diseases of animals are caused by prions (Table 362-2). Scrapie of sheep and goats is the prototypic prion disease. Mink encephalopathy, BSE, feline spongiform encephalopathy, and exotic ungulate encephalopathy are all thought to occur after the consumption of prion-infected foodstuffs. The BSE epidemic emerged in Britain in the late 1980s and was shown to be due to industrial cannibalism. Whether BSE began as a sporadic case of BSE in a cow or started with scrapie in sheep is unknown. The origin of chronic wasting disease (CWD), a prion disease endemic in deer and elk in regions of North America, is uncertain.

EPIDEMIOLOGY   CJD is found throughout the world. The incidence of sCJD is approximately one case per million population. Although many geographic clusters of CJD have been reported, each has been shown to segregate with a PrP gene mutation. Attempts to identify common exposure to some etiologic agent have been unsuccessful for both the sporadic and familial cases. Ingestion of scrapie-infected sheep or goat meat as a cause of CJD in humans has not been demonstrated by epidemiologic studies, although speculation about this potential route of inoculation continues. Of particular interest are deer hunters who develop CJD, because up to 90% of culled deer in some game herds have been shown to harbor CWD prions. Studies with Syrian hamsters demonstrate that oral infection with prions can occur, but the process is inefficient compared to intracerebral inoculation.

PATHOGENESIS   The human prion diseases were initially classified as neurodegenerative disorders of unknown etiology on the basis of pathologic changes being confined to the CNS. With the transmission of kuru and CJD to apes, investigators began to view these diseases as infectious CNS illnesses caused by slow viruses. Even though the familial nature of a subset of CJD cases was well described, the significance of this observation became more obscure with the transmission of CJD to animals. Eventually, the meaning of heritable CJD became clear with the discovery of mutations in the *PrP* gene of these patients. The prion concept explains how a disease can manifest as a heritable as well as an infectious illness. Moreover, the hallmark of all prion diseases, whether sporadic, dominantly inherited, or acquired by infection, is that they involve the aberrant metabolism of PrP.

A major feature that distinguishes prions from viruses is the finding that both PrP isoforms are encoded by a chromosomal gene. In humans, the *PrP* gene is designated *PRNP* and is located on the short arm of chromosome 20. Limited proteolysis of PrPSc produces a smaller, protease-resistant molecule of ~142 amino acids designated PrP 27-30; PrPC is completely hydrolyzed under the same conditions (Fig. 362-2). In the presence of detergent, PrP 27-30 polymerizes into amyloid. Prion rods formed by limited proteolysis and detergent extraction are indistinguishable from the filaments that aggregate to form PrP amyloid plaques in the CNS. Both the rods and the PrP amyloid filaments found in brain tissue exhibit similar ultrastructural morphology and green-gold birefringence after staining with Congo red dye.

Prion Strains The existence of prion strains raised the question of how heritable biologic information can be enciphered in a molecule other than nucleic acid. Various strains of prions have been defined by incubation times and the distribution of neuronal vacuolation. Subsequently, the patterns of PrPSc deposition were found to correlate with vacuolation profiles, and these patterns were also used in their characterization.

Persuasive evidence that strain-specific information is enciphered in the tertiary structure of PrPSc comes from transmission of two different inherited human prion diseases to mice expressing a chimeric human-mouse PrP transgene. In FFI, the protease-resistant fragment of PrPSc after deglycosylation has a molecular mass of 19 kDa, whereas in fCJD and most sporadic prion diseases, it is 21 kDa (Table 362-3). This difference in molecular mass was shown to be due to different sites of proteolytic cleavage at the NH₂ termini of the two human PrPSc molecules, reflecting different tertiary structures. These distinct conformations were not unexpected because the amino acid sequences of the PrPs differ.

Extracts from the brains of patients with FFI transmitted disease into mice expressing a chimeric human-mouse PrP transgene and induced formation of the 19-kDa PrPSc, whereas brain extracts from fCJD and sCJD patients produced the 21-kDa PrPSc in mice expressing the same transgene. On second passage, these differences were maintained, demonstrating that chimeric PrPSc can exist in two different conformations based on the sizes of the protease-resistant fragments, even though the amino acid sequence of PrPSc is invariant.

This analysis was extended when patients with sporadic fatal insomnia (sFI) were identified. Although they did not carry a *PRNP* gene mutation, the patients demonstrated a clinical and pathologic phenotype that was indistinguishable from that of patients with FFI. Furthermore, 19-kDa PrPSc was found in their brains, and on passage of prion disease to mice expressing a chimeric human-mouse PrP transgene, 19-kDa PrPSc was also found. These findings indicate that the disease phenotype is dictated by the conformation of PrPSc and not the amino acid sequence. PrPSc acts as a template for the conversion of PrPC into nascent PrPSc. On the passage of prions into mice expressing a chimeric hamster-mouse PrP transgene, a change in the conformation of PrPSc was accompanied by the emergence of a new strain of prions.

Species Barrier Studies on the role of the primary and tertiary structures of PrP in the transmission of prion disease have given new insights into the pathogenesis of these maladies. The amino acid sequence of PrP encodes the species of the prion, and the prion derives its PrPSc sequence from the last mammal in which it was passaged. While the primary structure of PrP is likely to be the most important or even sole determinant of the tertiary structure of PrPC, PrPSc seems to function as a template in determining the tertiary structure of nascent PrPSc mol-

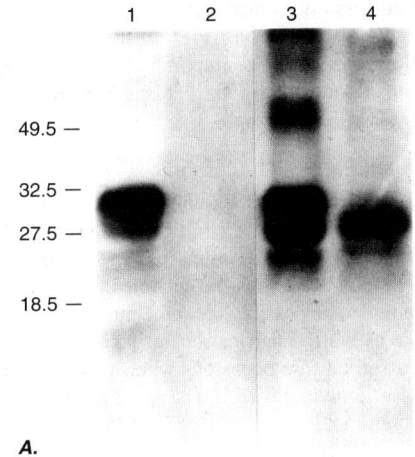

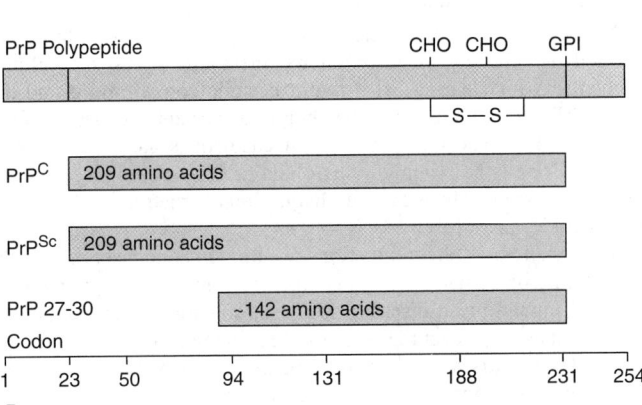

FIGURE 362-2 Prion protein isoforms. *A.* Western immunoblot of brain homogenates from uninfected (lanes 1 and 2) and prion-infected (lanes 3 and 4) Syrian hamsters. Samples in lanes 2 and 4 were digested with proteinase K. PrPC in lanes 2 and 4 was completely hydrolyzed under these conditions, whereas in PrPSc (lane 4), ~67 amino acids were digested from the NH₂-terminus to generate PrP 27–30. The blot was developed with anti-PrP polyclonal rabbit antiserum. Molecular size markers (*left*) are in kilodaltons. *B.* Bar diagram of Syrian hamster PrP, which consists of 254 amino acids. After processing of the NH₂ and COOH termini, both PrPC and PrPSc consist of 209 residues. After limited proteolysis, the NH₂ terminus of PrPSc is truncated to form PrP 27–30 composed of ~142 amino acids. [*Reprinted from Les Prix Nobel T. Frängsmyr (ed), Stockholm, Norstedts Tryckeri, 1998, pp 268–323, with permission.*]

ecules as they are formed from PrPC. In turn, prion diversity appears to be enciphered in the conformation of PrPSc and thus, prion strains seem to represent different conformers of PrPSc.

In general, transmission of prion disease from one species to another is inefficient, in that not all intracerebrally inoculated animals develop disease, and those that fall ill do so only after long incubation times that can approach the natural life span of the animal. This "spe-

TABLE 362-3 *Distinct Prion Strains Generated in Humans with Inherited Prion Diseases and Transmitted to Transgenic Mice*[a]

Inoculum	Host Species	Host PrP Genotype	Incubation Time [days ± SEM] (n/n₀)	PrPSc (kDa)
None	Human	FFI(D178N, M129)		19
FFI	Mouse	Tg(MHu2M)	206 ± 7 (7/7)	19
FFI → Tg(MHu2M)	Mouse	Tg(MHu2M)	136 ± 1 (6/6)	19
None	Human	fCJD(E200K)		21
fCJD	Mouse	Tg(MHu2M)	170 ± 2 (10/10)	21
fCJD → Tg(MHu2M)	Mouse	Tg(MHu2M)	167 ± 3 (15/15)	21

[a] Tg(MHu2M) mice express a chimeric mouse-human PrP gene.

Note: Clinicopathologic phenotype is determined by the conformation of PrPSc in accord with the results of the transmission of human prions from patients with FFI to transgenic mice. FFI, fatal familial insomnia; fCJD, familial Creutzfeldt-Jakob disease.

cies barrier" to transmission is correlated with the degree of similarity between the amino acid sequence of PrP^C in the inoculated host and of PrP^{Sc} in the prion inoculum. The importance of sequence similarity between the host and donor PrP argues that PrP^C directly interacts with PrP^{Sc} in the prion conversion process.

SPORADIC AND INHERITED PRION DISEASES

Several different scenarios might explain the initiation of sporadic prion disease: (1) A somatic mutation may be the cause and thus follow a path similar to that for germ-line mutations in inherited disease. In this situation, the mutant PrP^{Sc} must be capable of targeting wild-type PrP^C, a process known to be possible for some mutations but less likely for others. (2) The activation barrier separating wild-type PrP^C from PrP^{Sc} could be crossed on rare occasions when viewed in the context of a population. Most individuals would be spared, while presentations in the elderly with an incidence of ~1 per million would be seen. (3) PrP^{Sc} may be present at very low levels in some normal cells, where it performs some important, as yet unknown, function. The level of PrP^{Sc} in such cells is hypothesized to be sufficiently low as to be not detected by bioassay. In some altered metabolic states, the cellular mechanisms for clearing PrP^{Sc} might become compromised and the rate of PrP^{Sc} formation would then begin to exceed the capacity of the cell to clear it. The third possible mechanism is attractive since it suggests PrP^{Sc} is not simply a misfolded protein, as proposed for the first and second mechanisms, but that it is an alternatively folded molecule with a function.

More than 30 different mutations resulting in nonconservative substitutions in the human *PRNP* gene have been found to segregate with inherited human prion diseases. Missense mutations and expansions in the octapeptide repeat region of the gene are responsible for familial forms of prion disease. Five different mutations of the *PRNP* gene have been linked genetically to heritable prion disease.

Although phenotypes may vary dramatically within families, specific phenotypes tend to be observed with certain mutations. A clinical phenotype indistinguishable from typical sCJD is usually seen with substitutions at codons 180, 183, 200, 208, 210, and 232. Substitutions at codons 102, 105, 117, 198, and 217 are associated with the GSS variant of prion disease. The normal human PrP sequence contains five repeats of an eight-amino-acid sequence. Insertions from two to nine extra octarepeats frequently cause variable phenotypes ranging from a condition indistinguishable from sCJD to a slowly progressive dementing illness of many years' duration. A mutation at codon 178 resulting in substitution of asparagine for aspartic acid produces FFI if a methionine is encoded at the polymorphic 129 residue on the same allele. Typical CJD is seen if a valine is encoded at position 129 of the same allele.

Human *PRNP* Gene Polymorphisms   Polymorphisms influence the susceptibility to sporadic, inherited, and infectious forms of prion disease. The methionine/valine polymorphism at position 129 not only modulates the age of onset of some inherited prion diseases but can also determine the clinical phenotype. The finding that homozygosity at codon 129 predisposes to sCJD supports a model of prion production that favors PrP interactions between homologous proteins.

Substitution of the basic residue lysine at position 218 in mouse PrP produced dominant-negative inhibition of prion replication in transgenic mice. This same lysine at position 219 in human PrP has been found in 12% of the Japanese population, and this group appears to be resistant to prion disease. Dominant-negative inhibition of prion replication was also found with substitution of the basic residue arginine at position 171; sheep with arginine are resistant to scrapie prions but are susceptible to BSE prions that were inoculated intracerebrally.

INFECTIOUS PRION DISEASES

IATROGENIC CJD   Accidental transmission of CJD to humans appears to have occurred with corneal transplantation, contaminated electroencephalogram (EEG) electrode implantation, and surgical procedures. Corneas from donors with inapparent CJD have been transplanted to apparently healthy recipients who developed CJD after prolonged incubation periods. The same improperly decontaminated EEG electrodes that caused CJD in two young patients with intractable epilepsy caused CJD in a chimpanzee 18 months after their experimental implantation.

Surgical procedures may have resulted in accidental inoculation of patients with prions during their operations, presumably because some instrument or apparatus in the operating theater became contaminated when a CJD patient underwent surgery. Although the epidemiology of these studies is highly suggestive, no proof for such episodes exists.

Dura Mater Grafts   More than 120 cases of CJD after implantation of dura mater grafts have been recorded. All of the grafts were thought to have been acquired from a single manufacturer whose preparative procedures were inadequate to inactivate human prions. One case of CJD occurred after repair of an eardrum perforation with a pericardium graft.

Human Growth Hormone and Pituitary Gonadotropin Therapy   The possibility of transmission of CJD from contaminated human growth hormone (hGH) preparations derived from human pituitaries has been raised by the occurrence of fatal cerebellar disorders with dementia in >120 patients ranging in age from 10 to 41 years. These patients received injections of hGH every 2 to 4 days for 4 to 12 years. If it is assumed that these patients developed CJD from injections of prion-contaminated hGH preparations, the possible incubation periods range from 4 to 30 years. Even though several investigations argue for the efficacy of inactivating prions in hGH fractions prepared from human pituitaries with 6 *M* urea, it seems doubtful that such protocols will be used for purifying hGH because recombinant hGH is available. Four cases of CJD have occurred in women receiving human pituitary gonadotropin.

VARIANT CJD   The restricted geographic occurrence and chronology of vCJD raised the possibility that BSE prions have been transmitted to humans through the consumption of tainted beef. More than 140 cases of vCJD have occurred, with >90% of these in Britain. Because the number of vCJD cases is still small, it not possible to decide if we are at the beginning of a prion disease epidemic in Europe, similar to those seen for BSE and kuru, or if the number of vCJD cases will remain small. What is certain is that prion-tainted meat should be prevented from entering the human food supply.

The most compelling evidence that vCJD is caused by BSE prions was obtained from experiments in mice expressing the bovine PrP transgene. Both BSE and vCJD prions were efficiently transmitted to these transgenic mice and with similar incubation periods. In contrast to sCJD prions, vCJD prions did not transmit disease efficiently to mice expressing a chimeric human-mouse PrP transgene. Earlier studies with nontransgenic mice suggested that vCJD and BSE might be derived from the same source because both inocula transmitted disease with similar but very long incubation periods.

Attempts to determine the origin of BSE and vCJD prions have relied on passaging studies in mice, some of which are described above, as well as studies of the conformation and glycosylation of PrP^{Sc}. One scenario suggests that a particular conformation of bovine PrP^{Sc} was selected for heat resistance during the rendering process and was then reselected multiple times as cattle infected by ingesting prion-contaminated meat and bone meal (MBM) were slaughtered and their offal rendered into more MBM.

NEUROPATHOLOGY   Frequently, the brains of patients with CJD have no recognizable abnormalities on gross examination. Patients who survive for several years have variable degrees of cerebral atrophy.

On light microscopy, the pathologic hallmarks of CJD are spongiform degeneration and astrocytic gliosis. The lack of an inflammatory response in CJD and other prion diseases is an important pathologic feature of these degenerative disorders. Spongiform degeneration is characterized by many 1- to 5-μm vacuoles in the neuropil between nerve cell bodies. Generally, the spongiform changes occur in the cerebral cortex, putamen, caudate nucleus, thalamus, and molecular layer of the cerebellum. Astrocytic gliosis is a constant but nonspecific feature of prion diseases. Widespread proliferation of fibrous astrocytes is found throughout the gray matter of brains infected with CJD prions. Astrocytic processes filled with glial filaments form extensive networks.

Amyloid plaques have been found in ~10% of CJD cases. Purified CJD prions from humans and animals exhibit the ultrastructural and histochemical characteristics of amyloid when treated with detergents during limited proteolysis. In first passage from some human Japanese CJD cases, amyloid plaques have been found in mouse brains. These plaques stain with antisera raised against PrP.

The amyloid plaques of GSS disease are morphologically distinct from those seen in kuru or scrapie. GSS plaques consist of a central dense core of amyloid surrounded by smaller globules of amyloid. Ultrastructurally, they consist of a radiating fibrillar network of amyloid fibrils, with scant or no neuritic degeneration. The plaques can be distributed throughout the brain but are most frequently found in the cerebellum. They are often located adjacent to blood vessels. Congophilic angiopathy has been noted in some cases of GSS disease.

In vCJD, a characteristic feature is the presence of "florid plaques." These are composed of a central core of PrP amyloid, surrounded by vacuoles in a pattern suggesting petals on a flower.

CLINICAL FEATURES Nonspecific prodromal symptoms occur in about a third of patients with CJD and may include fatigue, sleep disturbance, weight loss, headache, malaise, and ill-defined pain. Most patients with CJD present with deficits in higher cortical function. These deficits almost always progress over weeks or months to a state of profound dementia characterized by memory loss, impaired judgment, and a decline in virtually all aspects of intellectual function. A few patients present with either visual impairment or cerebellar gait and coordination deficits. Frequently, the cerebellar deficits are rapidly followed by progressive dementia. Visual problems often begin with blurred vision and diminished acuity, rapidly followed by dementia.

Other symptoms and signs include extrapyramidal dysfunction manifested as rigidity, masklike facies, or choreoathetoid movements; pyramidal signs (usually mild); seizures (usually major motor) and, less commonly, hypesthesia; supranuclear gaze palsy; optic atrophy; and vegetative signs such as changes in weight, temperature, sweating, or menstruation.

Myoclonus Most patients (~90%) with CJD exhibit myoclonus that appears at various times throughout the illness. Unlike other involuntary movements, myoclonus persists during sleep. Startle myoclonus elicited by loud sounds or bright lights is frequent. It is important to stress that myoclonus is neither specific nor confined to CJD. Dementia with myoclonus can also be due to Alzheimer's disease (AD) (Chap. 350), to cryptococcal encephalitis (Chap. 186), or to the myoclonic epilepsy disorder Unverricht-Lundborg disease (Chap. 348).

Clinical Course In documented cases of accidental transmission of CJD to humans, an incubation period of 1.5 to 2.0 years preceded the development of clinical disease. In other cases, incubation periods of up to 30 years have been suggested. Most patients with CJD live 6 to 12 months after the onset of clinical signs and symptoms, whereas some live for up to 5 years.

DIAGNOSIS The constellation of dementia, myoclonus, and periodic electrical bursts in an afebrile 60-year-old patient generally indicates CJD. Clinical abnormalities in CJD are confined to the CNS. Fever, elevated sedimentation rate, leukocytosis in blood, or a pleocytosis in cerebrospinal fluid (CSF) should alert the physician to another etiology to explain the patient's CNS dysfunction.

Variations in the typical course appear in inherited and transmitted forms of the disease. fCJD has an earlier mean age of onset than sCJD. In GSS disease, ataxia is usually a prominent and presenting feature, with dementia occurring late in the disease course. GSS disease typi-

cally presents earlier than CJD (mean age, 43 years) and is typically more slowly progressive than CJD; death usually occurs within 5 years of onset. FFI is characterized by insomnia and dysautonomia; dementia occurs only in the terminal phase of the illness. Rare sporadic cases have been identified. vCJD has an unusual clinical course, with a prominent psychiatric prodrome that may include visual hallucinations and early ataxia, while frank dementia is usually a late sign of vCJD.

DIFFERENTIAL DIAGNOSIS Many conditions may mimic CJD superficially. AD is occasionally accompanied by myoclonus but is usually distinguished by its protracted course and lack of motor and visual dysfunction.

Intracranial vasculitides (Chap. 306) may produce nearly all of the symptoms and signs associated with CJD, sometimes without systemic abnormalities. Myoclonus is exceptional with cerebral vasculitis, but focal seizures may confuse the picture; furthermore, myoclonus is often absent in the early stages of CJD. Stepwise change in deficits, prominent headache, abnormal CSF, and focal magnetic resonance imaging (MRI) or angiographic abnormalities all favor vasculitis.

Neurosyphilis (Chap. 153) may present with dementia and myoclonus that progresses in a relatively rapid fashion but is easily distinguished from CJD by CSF findings, as is cryptococcal meningoencephalitis. A diffuse intracranial tumor (gliomatosis cerebri; Chap. 358) may occasionally be confused with CJD. In rare cases of CNS neoplasia, neuroimaging studies are normal and there are no signs of increased intracranial pressure; however, CSF protein is usually elevated. Adult onset leukodystrophies (ceroid lipofuscinosis; Chap. 350) and myoclonic epilepsy with Lafora bodies (Chap. 348) may be responsible for dementia, myoclonus, and ataxia; but the less acute courses and prominent seizures distinguish them from CJD. A number of diseases that may simulate CJD are easily distinguished by the clinical setting in which they occur. These diseases include anoxic encephalopathy, subacute sclerosing panencephalitis, progressive rubella panencephalitis, herpes simplex encephalitis (in immunoincompetent hosts), dialysis dementia, uremia, and hepatic encephalopathy. When CJD begins atypically, it may for a short time resemble other disorders such as Parkinson's disease, progressive supranuclear palsy (Chap. 351), or progressive multifocal leukoencephalopathy (Chap. 360).

Certain drug intoxications, particularly lithium and bismuth, may produce encephalopathy and myoclonus. The rare condition known as Hashimoto's encephalopathy, which presents with a subacute progressive encephalopathy and myoclonus with periodic triphasic complexes on the EEG, should be excluded in every case of suspected CJD. It is diagnosed by the finding of high titers of antithyroglobulin or antithyroid perioxidase (antimicrosomal) antibodies in the blood, and improves with glucocorticoid therapy. Unlike CJD, fluctuations in severity typically occur in Hashimoto's encephalopathy.

The AIDS dementia complex (Chap. 173) may occasionally imitate CJD in onset, early course, physical signs, computed tomography (CT) findings, and lack of abnormalities on routine CSF studies. The few such patients without manifestations of systemic immunodeficiency (<10%) should be questioned about risk factors and should have serum antibodies to HIV determined.

LABORATORY TESTS The only specific diagnostic tests for CJD and other human prion diseases measure PrP^{Sc}. The most widely used method involves limited proteolysis that generates PrP 27-30, which is detected by immunoassay after denaturation. The conformation-dependent immunoassay (CDI) is based on immunoreactive epitopes that are exposed in PrP^C but buried in PrP^{Sc}. The CDI is extremely sensitive and quantitative and is likely to find wide application in both the post- and antemortem detection of prions. In humans, the diagnosis of CJD can be established by brain biopsy if PrP^{Sc} is detected. If no attempt is made to measure PrP^{Sc}, but the constellation of pathologic changes frequently found in CJD is seen in a brain biopsy, then the diagnosis is reasonably secure (see "Neuropathology," above). Because PrP^{Sc} is not uniformly distributed throughout the CNS, the apparent absence of PrP^{Sc} in a limited sample such as a biopsy does not rule out prion disease. At autopsy, sufficient brain samples should be taken for both PrP^{Sc} immunoassay, preferably by the CDI, and immunohistochemistry of tissue sections.

Whether an antemortem test can be developed using the CDI to detect protease-sensitive forms of PrP^{Sc} in blood is uncertain. Another possibility is such a test based on PrP^{Sc} formation in muscle. PrP^{Sc} accumulation seems to be restricted to the hindlimb muscles in mice but is more widespread in hamsters. Whether muscles in humans and livestock can be identified in which PrP^{Sc} accumulates consistently remains to be established.

To establish the diagnosis of either sCJD or familial prion disease, sequencing the *PRNP* gene must be performed. Finding the wild-type *PRNP* gene sequence permits the diagnosis of sCJD if there is no history to suggest exposure to an exogenous source of prions. The identification of a mutation in the *PRNP* gene sequence that encodes a nonconservative amino acid substitution argues for familial prion disease.

CT may be normal or show cortical atrophy. The MRI scan may show a subtle increased intensity in the basal ganglia with T2- or diffusion-weighted imaging, but this finding is neither sensitive nor specific enough to make a diagnosis.

CSF is nearly always normal but may show minimal protein elevation. Although the stress protein 14-3-3 is elevated in the CSF of some patients with CJD, similar elevations of 14-3-3 are found in patients with herpes simplex virus encephalitis, multi-infarct dementia, and stroke. In AD, 14-3-3 is generally not elevated. In the serum of some patients with CJD, the S-100 protein is elevated, but as with 14-3-3, this elevation is not specific.

The EEG is often useful in the diagnosis of CJD. During the early phase of CJD, the EEG is usually normal or shows only scattered theta activity. In most advanced cases, repetitive, high-voltage, triphasic, and polyphasic sharp discharges are seen, but in many cases their presence is transient. The presence of these stereotyped periodic bursts of <200 ms duration, occurring every 1 to 2 s, makes the diagnosis of CJD very likely. These discharges are frequently but not always symmetric; there may be a one-sided predominance in amplitude. As CJD progresses, normal background rhythms become fragmentary and slower.

CARE OF CJD PATIENTS   Although CJD should not be considered either a contagious or communicable disease, it is transmissible. The risk of accidental inoculation by aerosols is very small; nonetheless, procedures producing aerosols should be performed in certified biosafety cabinets. Biosafety level 2 practices, containment equipment, and facilities are recommended by the Centers for Disease Control and Prevention and the National Institutes of Health. The primary problem in caring for patients with CJD is the inadvertent infection of health care workers by needle and stab wounds. The transmission of prions through the air has never been documented. Electroencephalographic and electromyographic needles should not be reused after studies on patients with CJD have been performed.

There is no reason for pathologists or morgue dieners to resist performing autopsies on patients whose clinical diagnosis was CJD. Standard microbiologic practices outlined here, along with specific recommendations for decontamination, seem to be adequate precautions for the care of patients with CJD and the handling of infected specimens.

DECONTAMINATION OF CJD PRIONS   Prions are extremely resistant to common inactivation procedures, and there is some disagreement about the optimal conditions for sterilization. Some investigators recommend treating CJD-contaminated materials once with 1 *N* NaOH at room temperature, but we believe this procedure may be inadequate for sterilization. Autoclaving at 132°C for 5 h or treatment with 2 *N* NaOH for several hours is recommended for sterilization of prions. The term "sterilization" implies complete destruction of prions; any residual infectivity can be hazardous.

PREVENTION AND THERAPEUTICS   There is no known effective therapy for preventing or treating CJD. The finding that phenothiazines and acridines inhibit PrP^{Sc} formation in cultured cells led to clinical studies of quinacrine in CJD patients. Although quinacrine seems to slow the rate of decline in some CJD patients, no cure of the disease has been observed. In mice, the results of quinacrine treatment are mixed: Some investigators report treatment is ineffective, while others find that quinacrine prolongs the lives of prion-infected mice compared to untreated animals.

Like the acridines, anti-PrP antibodies have been shown to eliminate PrP^{Sc} from cultured cells. Additionally, such antibodies in mice either administered by injection or produced from a transgene have been shown to prevent prion disease when prions are introduced by a peripheral route, such as intraperitoneal inoculation. Unfortunately, the antibodies were ineffective in mice inoculated intracerebrally with prions. Several drugs delay the onset of disease in animals inoculated intracerebrally with prions if the drugs are given around the time of the inoculation.

Structure-based drug design predicated on dominant-negative inhibition of prion formation has produced several promising compounds. Modified quinacrine compounds that are more potent than the parent drug have been found. Whether improving the efficacy of such small molecules will provide general methods for developing novel therapeutics for other neurodegenerative disorders, including AD and Parkinson's disease, as well as amyotrophic lateral sclerosis (ALS), remains to be established.

Financial Disclosure: SBP has a financial interest in InPro Biotechnology, Inc.

FURTHER READING

Bosque PJ et al: Prions in skeletal muscle. Proc Natl Acad Sci USA 99:3812, 2002

May BCH et al: Potent inhibition of scrapie prion replication in cultured cells by bis-acridines. Proc Natl Acad Sci USA 100:3416, 2003

Prusiner SB (ed): *Prion Biology and Diseases*, 2nd ed. Cold Spring Harbor, New York, Cold Spring Harbor Laboratory Press, 2004

Will RG et al: Diagnosis of new variant Creutzfeldt-Jakob disease. Ann Neurol 47:575, 2000

Section 3   Nerve and Muscle Disorders

363 | APPROACH TO THE PATIENT WITH PERIPHERAL NEUROPATHY
Arthur K. Asbury

Peripheral neuropathy is a general term indicating peripheral nerve disorders of any cause; the manifestations of neuropathy may be so diverse that it is difficult for the physician to know where to begin and how to proceed.

The clinical and electrodiagnostic (EDX) approach to evaluation

and management of a neuropathic disorder is summarized in Fig. 363-1. The EDX approach consists of electrophysiologic examination of nerve and muscle, including nerve conduction studies and electromyography. It is part of the evaluation of any neuropathy and is considered to be an extension of the neurologic examination. Using this

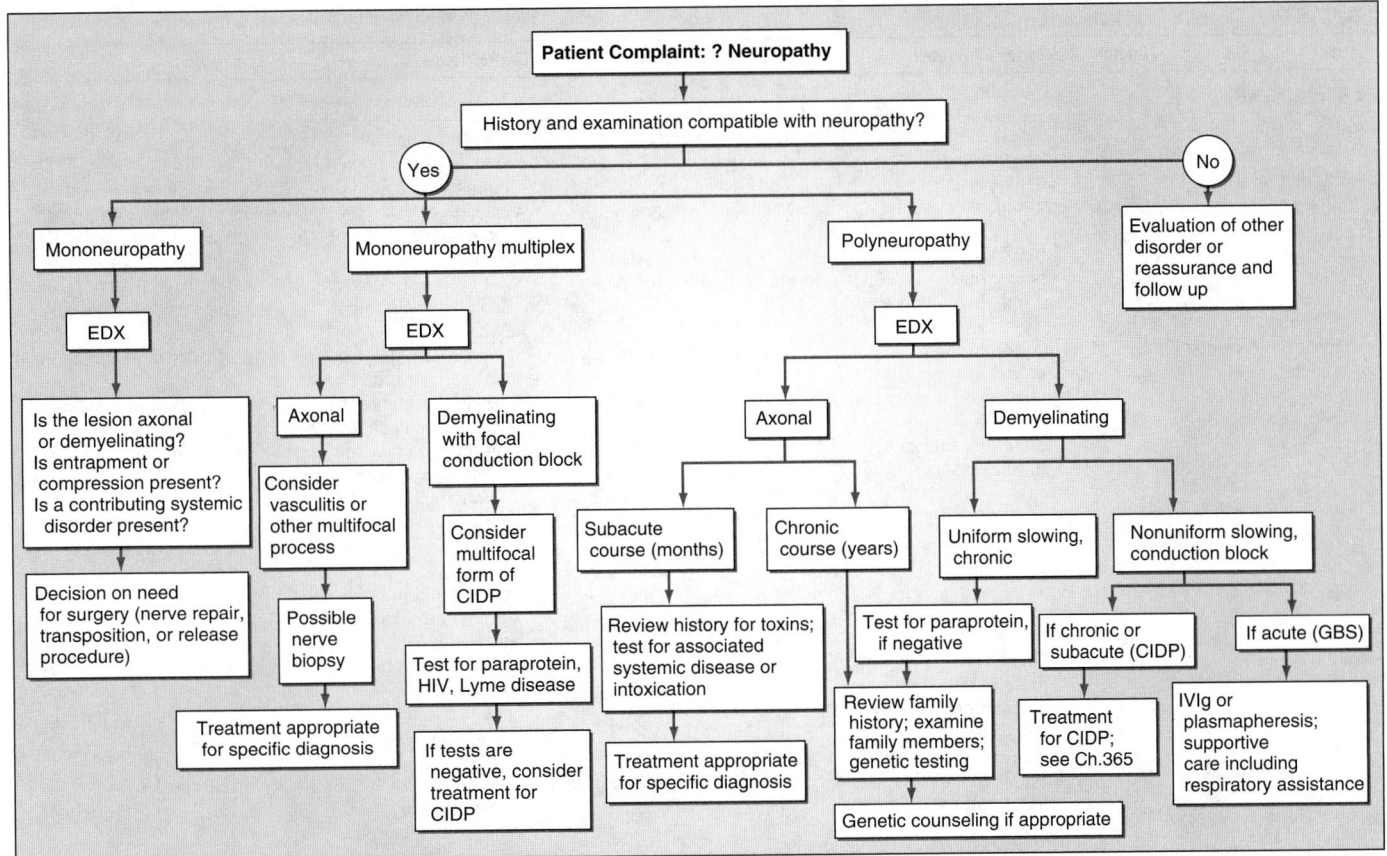

FIGURE 363-1 Approach to the evaluation of peripheral neuropathies. CIDP, chronic inflammatory demyelinating polyradiculoneuropathy; EDX, electrodiagnostic studies; GBS, Guillain-Barré syndrome; IVIg, intravenous immunoglobulin. For management and treatment considerations, see relevant sections of this chapter or of the two succeeding chapters on immune-mediated and on genetically determined neuropathies.

scheme (Fig. 363-1), the examiner determines for each patient the tempo, distribution, and severity of the neuropathy and makes a judgment as to whether the problem represents a mononeuropathy, a mononeuropathy multiplex, or a polyneuropathy. Often this distinction is obvious. With the sum of clinical and EDX information in hand, the differential diagnostic possibilities and treatment options are usually narrowed to a manageable number.

MONONEUROPATHY *Mononeuropathy* refers to focal involvement of a single nerve trunk and therefore implies a local cause. Direct trauma, compression, and entrapment are the usual causes. Ulnar neuropathies, due to lesions either at the ulnar groove or in the cubital tunnel, and median neuropathy due to compression in the carpal tunnel constitute the great majority of mononeuropathies encountered in clinical practice. These are described below, and other common mononeuropathies are listed in Table 363-1. EDX examination is part of the evaluation of mononeuropathies, mainly to judge the nature of the focal lesion (demyelinating or axonal degeneration) and, in severe mononeuropathies, to determine whether any nerve fibers remain in continuity.

In the absence of a history of trauma to the nerve trunk, factors favoring conservative management of a mononeuropathy include sudden onset, no motor deficit, few or no sensory findings (even though pain and sensory symptoms may be present), and no evidence of axonal degeneration by EDX criteria. Factors favoring active measures including surgical intervention are chronicity and worsening neurologic deficit on examination, particularly if motor and EDX evidence suggests that the lesion has produced a degree of wallerian degeneration.

Ulnar Neuropathy Complete ulnar paralysis results in a characteristic claw-hand deformity owing to wasting and weakness of many of the small hand muscles and hyperextension of the fingers at the metacarpophalangeal joints and flexion at the interphalangeal joints. The flex-

ion deformity is most pronounced in the fourth and fifth fingers. Sensory loss occurs over the fifth finger, the ulnar aspect of the fourth finger, and the ulnar border of the palm. The superficial location of the nerve at the elbow makes it a common site of pressure palsy. The ulnar nerve may also become entrapped just distal to the elbow in the cubital tunnel formed by the aponeurotic arch linking the two heads of the flexor carpi ulnaris. Also, prolonged pressure on the base of the palm, as occurs with use of hand tools or bicycle riding, may result in damage to the deep palmar branch of the ulnar nerve, causing weakness of the small hand muscles but no sensory loss (Table 363-1). Management of ulnar neuropathy depends on the timing, site, and severity of the responsible focal lesion. Entrapment of the ulnar nerve within the cubital tunnel may be released surgically, whereas ulnar nerve damage in the condylar groove is managed either conservatively, using padding to protect the nerve, or surgically by an anterior nerve transposition procedure.

Carpal Tunnel Syndrome The median nerve in the carpal tunnel lies in close quarters with nine tendons. Entrapment of the nerve at the wrist (*carpal tunnel syndrome*) is usually due to excessive use of the wrist but on occasion may be secondary to tenosynovitis with arthritis or local infiltration, e.g., by a thickening of connective tissue as in acromegaly or by deposit of amyloid or by one of the mucopolysaccharidoses. Other systemic diseases associated with carpal tunnel syndrome are hypothyroidism, rheumatoid arthritis, and diabetes mellitus, but underlying diseases account for only a small fraction of all cases. The main symptoms of carpal tunnel syndrome are nocturnal paresthesias of thumb, index, and middle fingers. With worsening, numbness occurs in that distribution and is demonstrable by pin examination. Eventually weakness and atrophy of the abductor pollicis brevis (thenar eminence) become evident. The principal treatment of carpal tunnel syndrome is surgical section of the carpal ligament to relieve entrapment.

TABLE 363-1 *Common Mononeuropathies*

Nerve	Origin[a]	Muscles Innervated	Usual Site of Lesion	Clinical Features	Comments
UPPER EXTREMITY					
Suprascapular	C5, C6	Supraspinatus Infraspinatus	Suprascapular notch of scapula	Weakness of lateral rotation of the humerus	No sensory deficit
Long thoracic	C5–C7	Serratus anterior	Variable	Winging of scapula	No sensory deficit
Axillary	C5, C6	Deltoid, teres minor	Near shoulder joint	Weakness of shoulder abduction; atrophy of shoulder	Sensory deficit similar to C5 dorsal root lesion (See Figs. 22-2 and 22-3)
Radial	C5–T1	Triceps, brachioradialis, wrist, finger, and thumb extensors	Spiral groove of humerus	Wrist drop most obvious, also finger and thumb extensors paralyzed	Saturday night palsy (acute compression) is frequent cause
Posterior interosseous branch	C7, C8	Finger and thumb extensors	Edge of supinator muscle below elbow	Finger drop; wrist relatively spared	No sensory deficit
Ulnar	C8, T1	Ulnar flexor of the wrist, long flexors of 4th and 5th digits, and most intrinsic hand muscles	Ulnar groove at the elbow	Weakness of finger adduction and abduction and thumb adduction (see text); interosseous atrophy, claw-hand	May be acute or insidious; sensory symptoms/signs are distinctive (Figs. 22-2 22-3); see also text
			Cubital tunnel	Same as above	Often pain over medial proximal forearm (cubital tunnel)
			Medial base of palm	Intrinsic hand muscles only, interosseous atrophy	No sensory deficit
Median	C6–T1	Abductor pollicis brevis; more proximal muscles include forearm pronator, long finger and thumb flexors	Carpal tunnel	Characteristic sensory symptoms and deficit and inability to make a circle with thumb and index finger	Sensory deficit as per Figs. 22-2 and 22-3 (see text); known as carpal tunnel syndrome
Anterior interosseous branch	C7–T1	Long flexors of thumb and index and middle fingers	Anterior interosseus branch below the elbow	Weakness of pinch; pain in volar forearm	No sensory deficit
LOWER EXTREMITY					
Femoral	L2–L4	Iliopsoas (hip flexor) and quadriceps femoris (knee extensor)	Proximal to inguinal ligament	Knee buckling; absent knee jerk; weak anterior thigh muscles with atrophy	Association with diabetes mellitus; sensory disturbance as per Fig. 22-2
Lateral femoral cutaneous branch	L2, L3	None	Inguinal ligament	Dysesthetic hyperpathia of lateral thigh	Known as meralgia paresthetica
Obturator	L3, L4	Thigh adductors	Intrapelvic or at pubis	Weakness of hip adduction	Sensory deficit on medial thigh
Sciatic	L4–S3	Hamstring muscles, hip abductor, and all muscles below the knee	Near sciatic notch	Severe lower leg and hamstring weakness; flail foot; severe disability	Uncommon except from war wounds; sometimes after a misdirected injection
Posterior tibial	L5–S2	Calf muscles (proximally), toe flexors, and other intrinsic foot muscles	Tarsal tunnel, near medial malleolus	Pain and numbness of sole, weak toe flexors	Known as tarsal tunnel syndrome (see text)
Peroneal	L4–S1	Dorsiflexors of toes and foot, evertors of foot	At neck of fibula	Foot drop and weakness of foot eversion	Sensory deficit is similar in distribution to L5, S1 sensory roots

[a] Spinal segments.

Tarsal Tunnel Syndrome   The distal tibial nerve, along with several tendons and the posterior tibial artery, lies in the tarsal tunnel just posterior to the medial malleolus. Because of its superficial site, the distal tibial nerve is subject to compression or to direct trauma. Causes include sprain or fracture of the ankle, ill-fitting footwear, posttraumatic fibrosis, cysts or ganglia adjacent to the nerve, arthritis, and tenosynovitis. Characteristic symptoms are pain in the ankle and the sole of the foot with paresthesias, particularly while walking. On examination, the tibial nerve trunk in the tarsal tunnel is usually tender to palpation, sensory deficit should be demonstrable on the sole of the foot, and weakness of the toe plantar-flexor muscles may be noted. EDX examination and also nerve block using local anesthetic are useful in establishing the diagnosis. Definitive treatment is extensive surgical decompression of the tibial nerve in the tarsal tunnel. Tarsal tunnel syndrome, in terms of its pathophysiology and management, is similar to carpal tunnel syndrome but is much less common (Table 363-1).

Cranial Mononeuropathy   Mononeuropathy affecting individual cranial nerves is a large subject and is dealt with separately in Chap. 355.

POLYNEUROPATHY   The prototypical picture of polyneuropathy occurs with acquired toxic or metabolic neuropathic states. The first symptoms tend to be sensory and consist of tingling, prickling, burning, or bandlike dysesthesias in the balls of the feet or tips of the toes, or in a general distribution over the soles (Chap. 22). Symptoms and findings are usually symmetric and graded distally and often precede objective motor or sensory signs.

With progression, dysesthesias spread up the lower legs. Pansensory loss is usually found over both feet, ankle jerks are lost, and weakness of dorsiflexion of the toes, best demonstrated in the great toe, is present. In some instances, the process begins with weakness in the feet, without preceding sensory symptoms. As worsening occurs, sensory loss moves centripetally in a graded "stocking" fashion, and the patient may complain that the feet have a numb or "wooden" feeling or may say "I feel as though I'm walking on stumps." Patients have difficulty walking on their heels during examination, and their feet may slap while walking. Later, the knee jerk reflex disappears and foot drop becomes more apparent. By the time sensory disturbance has reached the upper shin, dysesthesias are usually noticed in the tips of the fingers. The degree of spontaneous pain varies but is often considerable. Light stimuli to hypesthetic areas, once perceived, may be experienced as extremely uncomfortable (*hyperpathia*). Unsteadiness of gait may be out of proportion to muscle weakness because of proprioceptive loss.

Worsening is more severe in the legs than in the arms and proceeds in a centripetal, symmetrically graded manner with pansensory loss, areflexia, and muscle atrophy; motor weakness is usually greater in the extensor muscles than in corresponding flexor groups. When the sensory disturbance reaches the elbows and mid-thighs, a tent-shaped area of hypesthesia may often be demonstrated on the lower abdomen. This area will grow broader, and its apex will extend rostrally toward the sternum as the neuropathy worsens. By this time, patients generally cannot stand or walk or hold objects in their hands.

Overall, nerve fibers are affected according to axon length, without regard to root or nerve trunk distribution—hence the aptness of the term *stocking-glove* to describe the pattern of sensory deficit. In general, the motor deficit is also graded, distal, and symmetric.

Although *polyneuropathy* connotes a widespread symmetric process, usually distal and graded, polyneuropathies are quite diverse because of the variability of tempo, severity, mix of sensory and motor features, and presence or absence of positive symptoms. For instance, a patient with a subacute, severely dysesthetic sensory polyneuropathy and alopecia who is in the early phases of thallium intoxication bears little similarity to the patient with a 40-year history of insidiously progressive clumsiness of gait whose findings are foot drop, lower leg atrophy, pes cavus, and minimal asymptomatic distal sensory deficit, all due to a hereditary polyneuropathy (Chap. 364). These two patients fall at opposite ends of the spectrum of polyneuropathy.

The classification of peripheral neuropathies has become increasingly complex as the capacity to discriminate new subgroups and identify new associations with toxins and systemic disorders improves. The important features of each major grouping of polyneuropathies are summarized in Table 363-2, and key aspects of specific polyneuropathies are given in Tables 363-3 to Table 363-6.

MONONEUROPATHY MULTIPLEX (MULTIFOCAL NEUROPATHY) *Mononeuropathy multiplex* refers to simultaneous or sequential involvement of individual noncontiguous nerve trunks, either partially or completely, evolving over days to years. Since the disease process underlying mononeuropathy multiplex affects peripheral nerves in a multifocal and random fashion, progression of the disease favors the neurologic deficit becoming less patchy and multifocal and more confluent and symmetric. As a result, some patients present with what appears to be a distal symmetric neuropathy. Attention to the pattern of early symptoms is therefore important in making the judgment that a particular neuropathy is indeed a mononeuropathy multiplex and not a polyneuropathy.

ASSESSMENT AND DIAGNOSIS OF POLYNEUROPATHY AND MONONEUROPATHY MULTIPLEX Clues to the diagnosis of these neuropathies often lie in unnoticed or forgotten events occurring weeks or months prior to the onset of symptoms. Inquiry should be made about recent viral illnesses; other systemic symptoms; institution of new medications; exposures to solvents, pesticides, or heavy metals; the occurrence of similar symptoms in family members or co-workers; habits concerning alcohol; and the presence of preexisting medical disorders. Patients should be asked if they would feel well if free of their neuropathic symptoms; answers will suggest the presence or absence of an underlying systemic illness.

How did symptoms first appear? Even with distal polyneuropathies, symptoms may appear in the sole of one foot a few days or a week before the other, but usually the patient will describe a distal graded disturbance that moves evenly and symmetrically in centripetal fashion. Symptoms that first appear in the distribution of individual digital nerves, involving only half of a digit at a time, and then gradually spread and coalesce suggest a multifocal process (mononeuropathy multiplex), as might occur with a systemic vasculitis or cryoglobulinemia.

The evolution of neuropathy ranges from rapid worsening over a few days to an indolent process lasting decades. Polyneuropathies that progress slowly, over >5 years, are most likely to be genetically determined, particularly if the major manifestations are distal atrophy and weakness with few or no positive sensory symptoms. Diabetic polyneuropathy and paraproteinemic neuropathies also progress insidiously over 5 to 10 years. Axonal degenerations of toxic or metabolic origin tend to evolve over several weeks to a year or more, and the rate of progression of demyelinating neuropathies is highly variable, ranging from a few days in Guillain-Barré syndrome (GBS; Chap. 365) to many years in others.

Major fluctuations in the course of neuropathy raise two possibilities: (1) relapsing forms of neuropathy and (2) repeated toxic exposures. Slow fluctuation in symptoms taking place over weeks or months (reflecting changes in the activity of neuropathy) should not be confused with day-to-day variation or diurnal undulation of symptoms. The latter are common to all neuropathic disorders. An example is carpal tunnel syndrome, in which dysesthesias may be prominent at night but absent during the day.

Palpation of the nerve trunk to detect enlargement is a frequently forgotten part of the neurologic examination. In mononeuropathy or mononeuropathy multiplex, the entire course of the nerve trunk in question should be explored manually for focal thickening, for the presence of neurofibroma, point tenderness, or Tinel's phenomenon (generation of a tingling sensation in the sensory territory of the nerve

TABLE 363-2	Major Types of Polyneuropathy		
Type of Polyneuropathy	Evolution	Causes	Comments
Axonal			
Acute	Days to weeks	Porphyria	See Table 363-3; also Chap. 337
		Massive intoxications (arsenic; inhalants)	See Table 363-4
		Guillain-Barré syndrome—axonal form	See Chap. 365
Subacute	Weeks to months	Mostly toxic or metabolic polyneuropathies; see Tables 363-3 and 363-4	Treatment involves eliminating the toxins or treating the associated systemic disorder
Chronic	Months to years	<5 years, consider toxic/metabolic causes; >5 years, consider hereditary basis, also diabetic and dysproteinemic causes	See Tables 363-3 and 363-4; also Chap. 364 on hereditary neuropathy
Demyelinating			
Acute	Days to weeks	Almost all are the common form of Guillain-Barré syndrome; see Chap. 365	Rare possibilities include diphtheritic polyneuritis or buckthorn berry intoxication
Subacute	Weeks to months	Mostly relapsing form of CIDP (see Chap. 365)	Rarely, toxins mentioned above plus aurothioglucose and taxol (see Table 363-3)
Chronic	Months to years	Many possibilities including hereditary; inflammatory-autoimmune; dysproteinemias; other metabolic and toxic neuropathies	See Chaps. 364 and 365; also Tables 363-3 and 363-4

Note: CIDP, chronic inflammatory demyelinating polyneuropathy.

TABLE 363-3 Polyneuropathy Associated with Systemic Diseases

Systemic Disease (Occurrence)	Axonal[a]			Demyelinating[a]			Sensory vs. Motor[b]	Autonomic[a]	Comment
	Acute	Subacute	Chronic	Acute	Subacute	Chronic			
Diabetes mellitus (common)	−	±	+	−	±	+	S, SM, rarely M	± to +	See Table 363-5
Uremia (sometimes)	±	+	+	−	−	−	SM	±	Controllable with proper dialysis; curable with successful renal transplant
Porphyria (3 types) (rare)	+	±	−	−	−	−	M or SM	± to +	May be proximal > distal and may have atypical proximal sensory deficits
Hypoglycemia (rare)	±	+	±	−	−	−	M	−	Usually with insulinoma; arms often > legs
Vitamin deficiency, excluding B$_{12}$ (sometimes)	−	+	+	−	−	−	SM	±	Involves thiamine, pyridoxine, folate, pantothenic acid, and probably others
Vitamin B$_{12}$ deficiency (sometimes)	−	±	+	−	−	−	S	−	Neuropathy overshadowed by myelopathy
Critical illness (sepsis) (common)	−	+	±	−	−	−	M > S	−	Sepsis patients severely ill
Chronic liver disease (sometimes)	−	−	−	−	−	+	S or SM	−	Usually mild or subclinical
Primary biliary cirrhosis (rare)	−	±	+	−	−	−	S	−	Intraneural xanthomas; dysesthesias
Primary systemic amyloidosis (rare)	−	±	+	−	−	−	SM	+	Also in amyloidosis with myeloma or macroglobulinemia
Hypothyroidism (rare)	−	−	−	−	±	+	S	−	May respond to thyroid replacement
Chronic obstructive lung disease (rare)	−	±	+	−	−	−	S or SM	−	Severe pulmonary insufficiency
Acromegaly (rare)	−	−	+	−	−	−	S	−	Carpal tunnel syndrome also frequent
Malabsorption (sprue, celiac disease) (sometimes)	−	±	+	−	−	−	S or SM	±	Basis for neuropathy unclear; deficiency?
Carcinoma (sensory) (rare)	−	+	+	−	−	−	Pure S	−	Due to ganglionitis, mostly small cell lung or breast carcinoma; paraneoplastic
Carcinoma (sensorimotor) (sometimes)	−	+	+	−	−	−	SM	±	Sensorimotor axonal neuropathy; mostly with lung cancer
Carcinoma (late) (common)	−	+	+	−	−	−	S > M	±	Mild, probably related to weight loss and wasting
Carcinoma (demyelinating) (sometimes)	−	−	−	+	+	±	SM	−	Acute or relapsing demyelinating neuropathy
HIV infection (sometimes)	−	±	+	−	−	−	S ≫ M	−	Late stages of AIDS; other neuropathies occur; see text
Lyme disease (sometimes)	−	±	+	−	−	−	S > M	−	Variable picture; see text
Lymphoma, including Hodgkin's (sometimes)	−	+	+	+	+	±	See above	±	Same as with carcinomatous types
Polycythemia vera (rare)	−	±	+	−	−	−	S	−	Also CNS manifestations; often shooting pains in limbs
Multiple myeloma, lytic type (sometimes)	−	±	+	−	−	−	S, M, or SM	±	Symptomatic neuropathy uncommon; subclinical neuropathy frequent
Multiple myeloma, osteosclerotic[c] (sometimes)	−	−	±	−	±	+	SM	−	May show severe slowing of nerve conduction velocity
MGUS[d] (sometimes):									
IgA	−	±	+	−	−	−	SM	−	IgM$_\kappa$ mainly; may bind to myelin-associated glycoprotein (MAG) or other glycoconjugates
IgG	−	±	+	−	−	−	SM	−	
IgM	−	−	−	−	±	+	SM or S	−	
Cryoglobulinemia (rare)	−	±	+	−	−	−	SM	−	May be mononeuropathy multiplex in presentation

[a] +, Usually; ±, sometimes; −, rare, if ever.
[b] S, sensory; M, motor; SM, sensorimotor.
[c] Some cases associated with POEMS syndrome (*polyneuropathy, organomegaly, endocrinopathy, M proteins, and skin changes; see Chap. 330).
[d] Monoclonal gammopathy of undetermined significance.

TABLE 363-4 Polyneuropathy Associated with Drugs and Environmental Toxins

	Axonal[a]			Demyelinating[a]			Sensory vs. Motor[b]	Autonomic[a]	CNS[a]	Comment
	Acute	Subacute	Chronic	Acute	Subacute	Chronic				
DRUGS[c]										
Amiodarone (antiarrhythmic)	−	−	+	−	−	+	SM	−	−	Dose-dependent neuropathy, reversible by decreasing dose
Aurothioglucose (antirheumatic)	±	±	−	+	+	−	SM	−	−	Idiosyncratic reaction; ? immune-mediated
Cisplatin (antineoplastic)	−	+	+	−	−	−	S	−	−	Severe sensory neuropathy, also ototoxicity; dose-related
Dapsone (dermatologic agent, e.g., for leprosy)	−	±	+	−	−	−	M	−	−	Dose-related pure motor neuropathy
Disulfiram (antialcoholism agent)	±	+	+	−	−	−	SM	−	±	Usually occurs after months of treatment
Hydralazine (antihypertensive)	−	±	+	−	−	−	S > M	−	−	A pyridoxine antagonist
Isoniazid	−	±	+	−	−	−	SM	±	−	A pyridoxine antagonist; neurotoxic in slow acetylators
Metronidazole (antiprotozoal)	−	−	±	−	−	−	S or SM	−	+	Dose-related central-peripheral distal axonopathy
Misonidazole (radiosensitizer)	−	±	+	−	−	−	S or SM	−	+	Neurotoxicity is the limiting factor
Nitrofurantoin (urinary antiseptic)	−	±	+	−	−	−	SM	−	−	Generally total dose-related; renal failure enhances toxicity
Nucleoside analogues (ddC, ddI, d4T) (antiretroviral agents)	±	+	+	−	−	−	S ≫ M	−	?	Dose-related; painful
Phenytoin (anticonvulsant)	−	−	+	−	−	−	S > M	−	−	After 20–30 years of phenytoin use
Pyridoxine (vitamin)	−	±	+	−	−	−	S	−	−	Occurs with large intake (>300 mg/d)
Statins (HMG CoA reductase inhibitors)	−	±	+	−	−	−	S > M	−	−	Cases reported for most statins
Suramin (antineoplastic)	+	+	−	+	+	−	M > S	−	−	Related to serum levels 350 μg/mL or above
Taxol (antineoplastic)	±	+	±	±	+	±	S > M	−	−	Dose-related
Vincristine (antineoplastic)	−	+	+	−	−	−	S > M	−	−	Sensory symptoms common, hands > feet; motor signs ominous; should stop treatment
TOXINS[c]										
Acrylamide (flocculant; grouting agent)	−	±	+	−	−	−	S > M	±	+	Large-fiber neuropathy; sensory ataxia
Arsenic (herbicide; insecticide)	±	+	+	−	−	−	SM	±	±	Skin changes, Mees' lines in nails; painful; systemic effects
Diphtheria toxin	−	−	−	+	+	−	SM	−	−	Clinically very rare; can be confused with GBS
γ-Diketone hexacarbons (solvents)	−	±	+	−	−	+	SM	±	+	Neurofilamentous swelling of axons; these solvents now in restricted use
Inorganic lead	−	−	+	−	−	−	M > S or M	−	±	Selective motor neuropathy with prominent wrist drop
Organophosphates	−	±	+	−	−	−	SM	−	+	Brain and spinal cord also affected, the latter irreversibly
Thallium (rat poison)	−	+	+	−	−	−	SM	−	+	Also alopecia, Mees' lines in nails; painful

[a] +, Usually; ±, sometimes; −, rare, if ever.

[b] S, sensory; M, motor; SM, sensorimotor.

[c] The following drugs and environmental toxins are also neurotoxic, mainly to the peripheral nervous system:

Drugs: Allopurinol, amitriptyline, chloramphenicol, colchicine, ethambutol, flecainide, indomethacin, lithium, nitrous oxide, perhexiline maleate, podophyllin, sodium cyanate, thalidomide, L-tryptophan.

Environmental toxins: Allyl chloride, buckthorn berry, carbon disulfide, diglycols (either ethylene or propylene), dimethylaminoproprionitrile (DMAPN), ethylene oxide, metallic mercury, methyl bromide, polychlorinated biphenyls, styrene, trichlorethylene, vacor.

Note: CNS, central nervous system; GBS, Guillain-Barré syndrome.

TABLE 363-5 *Classification of Diabetic Neuropathies*

Symmetric
1. Distal, primarily sensory polyneuropathy
   a. Mainly large fibers affected
   b. Mixed[a]
   c. Mainly small fibers affected[a]
2. Autonomic neuropathy
3. Chronically evolving proximal motor neuropathy[a,b]

Asymmetric
1. Acute or subacute proximal motor neuropathy[a,b]
2. Cranial mononeuropathy[b]
3. Truncal neuropathy[a,b]
4. Entrapment neuropathy in the limbs

[a] Often painful.
[b] Recovery, partial or complete, is likely.

by tapping along the course of the nerve trunk); and for pain elicited by stretching of the nerve trunk. In leprous neuritis, fusiform thickening of nerve trunks is frequent, and beading of nerve trunks may be encountered in amyloid polyneuropathy. In genetically determined hypertrophic neuropathies, uniform thickening of all nerve trunks may occur, often to the diameter of one's little finger.

Most neuropathies involve nerve fibers of all sizes, but damage is sometimes restricted either to large or to small fibers. In a polyneuropathy affecting mainly small fibers, diminished pinprick and temperature sensation, often with painful, burning dysesthesias, will predominate, along with autonomic dysfunction, but with relative sparing of motor power, balance, and tendon jerks. Some cases of amyloid and distal diabetic polyneuropathies fall into this category. In contrast, large-fiber polyneuropathy is characterized by areflexia, sensory ataxia, relatively minor cutaneous sensory deficit (even though distal dysesthesias are common), and variable degrees of motor dysfunction, sometimes severe.

For patients with polyneuropathy or mononeuropathy multiplex, standard tests should include a complete blood count and measurement of erythrocyte sedimentation rate, urinalysis, chest x-ray or chest computed tomography (CT) scan, postprandial blood glucose determination, and serum protein electrophoresis. Further tests are dictated by the combined results of the history and the physical and EDX examination (Fig. 363-1).

Electrodiagnosis EDX studies are an essential part of the evaluation of neuropathies and also of myopathies and neuromuscular junction disorders. Such studies indeed are critical in helping to distinguish between these three categories of disease. The EDX examination ordinarily comprises electromyography (EMG) and nerve conduction studies (NCSs). EMG involves recording for electrical potentials from a needle electrode in muscle both at rest and during voluntary contraction of the muscle. Resulting electromyographic patterns are displayed on an oscilloscope screen for analysis. EMG is generally most useful for distinguishing between and among myopathic and neuropathic disorders. Myopathic disorders are marked by small, short-duration, polyphasic muscle action potentials recruited in excessive numbers for a given degree of voluntary muscle contraction. Other patterns characteristic of specific muscle abnormalities can also be observed, such as myotonia (high-frequency discharges that wax or wane).

By contrast, EMG findings in neuropathic disorders are those of muscle denervation. Specifically, denervation features a decrease in the number of motor units[1] activated by maximal effort to contract muscle but an increase in the rate of firing of those remaining motor

units. In long-standing muscle denervation (months or years), motor unit potentials become large and polyphasic. This occurs as a result of collateral reinnervation of nearby denervated muscle fibers by axonal sprouts from surviving motor axons. In brief, when motor axons die back, their muscle fiber domains are taken over by intact neighboring axons. Other EMG features that favor denervation include fibrillations (random, unregulated firing of individual denervated muscle fibers), fasciculations (random, spontaneous firing of motor units, which in chronic states can be markedly enlarged and polyphasic), positive sharp waves, and complex repetitive discharges (Fig. 363-2).

NCSs are carried out by stimulating motor or sensory nerves electrically at two or more sites and recording from either the muscle innervated, for motor nerves (Fig. 363-3), or from yet another site on the stimulated nerve trunk, for sensory nerves. From the data recorded, the velocity of conduction and other informative characteristics of the recorded waveforms can be determined. When a disorder of the neuromuscular junction is suspected, other more specialized techniques are used, including muscle response to repetitive stimulation of nerve and single-fiber EMG. Detailed discussion of the full range of EDX techniques and their application, use, and interpretation may be found in several recent monographs listed in the references.

It is generally not possible to distinguish between axonal and demyelinating disorders by clinical examination alone; here EDX analysis is particularly useful. EDX features of demyelination are slowing of nerve conduction velocity (NCV), dispersion of evoked compound action potentials, conduction block (major decrease in amplitude of muscle compound action potentials on proximal stimulation of the nerve, as compared to distal stimulation), and marked prolongation of distal latencies. In contrast, axonal neuropathies are characterized by a reduction in amplitude of evoked compound action potentials with relative preservation of NCV. The distinction between a primarily demyelinating neuropathy and an axonal neuropathy is crucial because of the differing approaches to diagnosis and management.

EDX studies also help to determine the presence or absence of a sensory involvement when that is not clear by clinical examination alone. It provides information about the distribution of subclinical findings, thus sharpening the diagnostic focus. Other issues that may be clarified by the electrodiagnostician include:

1. The distinction between disorders primary to nerve or to muscle (neuropathy versus myopathy)
2. The distinction between root or plexus involvement and more distal nerve trunk involvement
3. The distinction between generalized polyneuropathic processes and widespread multifocal nerve trunk involvement
4. The distinction between upper and lower motor neuron weakness
5. The distinction, in a given generalized polyneuropathic process, between primary demyelinating neuropathy and primary axonal degeneration
6. The assessment, in both primary axonal and demyelinating neuropathies, of features bearing on the nature, activity, and likely prognosis of the neuropathy, particularly the extent of primary or secondary axonal degeneration
7. The assessment, in mononeuropathies, of the site of the lesion and its major effect on nerve fibers, especially the distinction between demyelinating conduction block and wallerian degeneration
8. The characterization of disorders of the neuromuscular junction
9. The identification, often in muscle of normal bulk and strength, of important features such as chronic partial denervation, fasciculations, and myotonia
10. The analysis of cramp, and its distinction from physiologic contracture

If in a particular instance of progressive polyneuropathy of subacute or chronic evolution the EDX findings are those of an axonopathy, a long list of metabolic states and exogenous toxins comes under consideration (Tables 363-3 and 363-4). If the course is protracted over several years, it raises the likelihood of a hereditary neu-

---

[1] A motor unit is, by definition, an anterior horn cell, its axon, and the motor end plates and muscle fibers it innervates. The number of muscle fibers in a normal motor unit varies widely, from as few as 20 in an extraocular muscle to over 1500 in a large leg muscle (Chap. 21, Fig. 21-2).

TABLE 363-6 *Sensory Neuropathies*

| Cause or Association | Course | Nerve Fiber Size Affected | | Neuronopathy | Comment |
		Small	Large		
TOXINS/DRUGS					
Cisplatin (antineoplastic)	Sub/Chr	+	++	+	Dose-related
Pyridoxine (vitamin, in megadose amounts)	Sub/Chr	+	++	+/−	Dose-related
Taxol (antineoplastic)	Acu/Sub	++	+	−	NGF may be protective
SYSTEMIC DISEASES					
Paraneoplastic	Sub	+	++	++	Most SCLC and breast
Sjögren's syndrome	Sub/Chr	+/−	+	++	Variable presentation
Dysproteinemia (mainly IgM$_\kappa$)	Chr	+	++	−	Demyelinating; may bind to MAG and other myelin glycoproteins
IDIOPATHIC					
Acute sensory neuronopathy	Acu	+/−	++	++	Poor recovery; persistent deficit
Chronic ataxic neuropathy	Chr	+/−	++	Prob.	Gradual progression
HEREDITARY					
Many varieties (see Chap. 364)	Chr	Variable		Some	Progressive

Abbreviations: ++, most; +, some; ±, occasionally; Prob, probable; Acu, acute; Sub, subacute; Chr, chronic; NGF, nerve growth factor; MAG, myelin-associated glycoprotein; SCLC, small-cell lung carcinoma.

ropathy (Chap. 364); family members must be examined and additional attention given to the family history. If the EDX findings indicate primary demyelination of nerve, the approach is entirely different. The possibilities then include acquired demyelinating neuropathy, thought to be immunologically mediated (Chap. 365), and genetically determined demyelinating neuropathies, many of which are marked by uniform and drastic slowing of nerve conduction velocities (Chap. 364).

If the clinical features indicate mononeuropathy multiplex, the EDX question is whether the process is primarily axonal or demyelinating. Almost one-third of all adults with the clinical syndrome of mononeuropathy multiplex have a clear-cut picture of a demyelinating disorder, often with foci of persistent conduction block on EDX examination. Multifocal demyelinating neuropathy may represent part of the spectrum of chronic inflammatory demyelinating polyneuropathy (CIDP) or, if multifocal and only motor, would fit into the related category of multifocal motor neuropathy. →*For further discussion of the management of multifocal motor neuropathy, see Chap. 365.*

The remaining two-thirds of patients with mononeuropathy multiplex have a picture of patchy axonal involvement by EDX examination. Although ischemia should be suspected as the basis of neuropathy in these patients, only about one-half can be shown to have

disease of the vasa nervorum, usually vasculitis. Management of those with proven vasculitis of vasa nervorum is often the same as treatment for systemic vasculitis (Chaps. 306 and 365). If the cause of mononeuropathy multiplex remains undiagnosed even on follow-up, management should be conservative. In many patients the disease will stabilize or reverse, at least partially.

Mononeuropathy multiplex syndrome may also be seen as a manifestation of leprosy, sarcoidosis, certain types of amyloidosis, hypereosinophilia syndrome, cryoglobulinemia, neuroAIDS, and multifocal types of diabetic neuropathy.

Nerve Biopsy The sural nerve at the ankle is the preferred site for cutaneous nerve biopsy. There are few indications to employ this invasive technique. The main one is in asymmetric and multifocal neu-

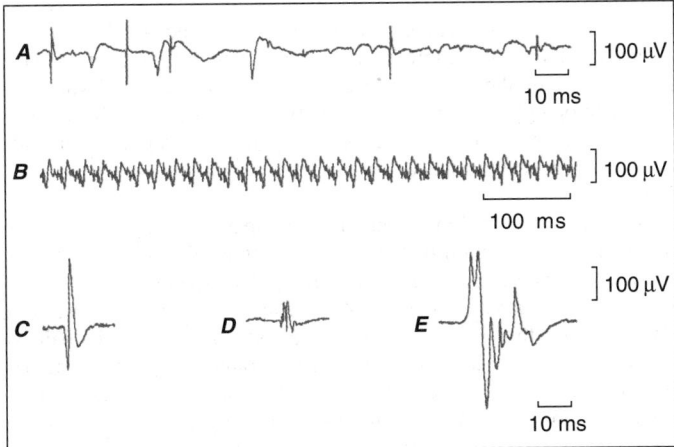

FIGURE 363-2 Activity recorded during EMG. *A.* Spontaneous fibrillation potentials and positive sharp waves. *B.* Complex repetitive discharges recorded in partially denervated muscle at rest. *C.* Normal triphasic motor unit action potential. *D.* Small, short-duration, polyphasic motor unit action potential such as is commonly encountered in myopathic disorders. *E.* Long-duration polyphasic motor unit action potential such as may be seen in neuropathic disorders. (*Courtesy of Prof M.J. Aminoff.*)

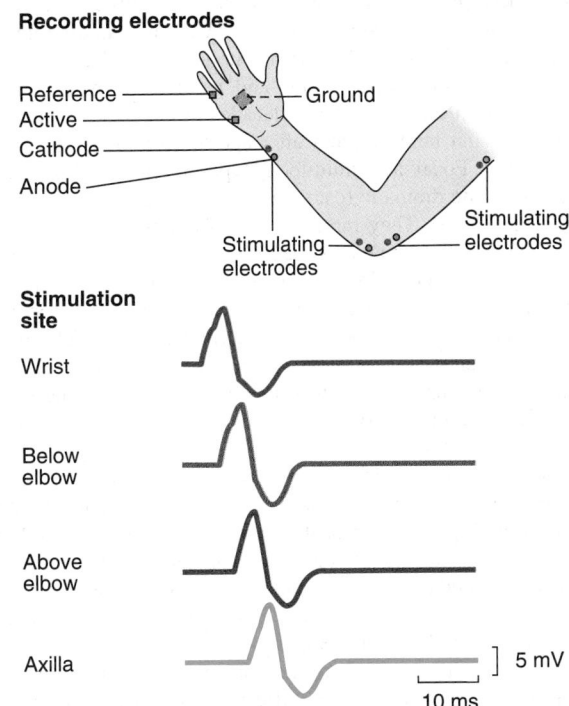

FIGURE 363-3 Arrangement for motor conduction studies of the ulnar nerve. Responses are recorded with a surface electrode from the abductor digiti minimi muscle to supramaximal stimulation of the nerve at different sites and are shown in the lower panel. (*From MJ Aminoff: Electromyography in Clinical Practice: Electrodiagnostic Aspects of Neuromuscular Disease, 3d ed. New York, Churchill Livingstone, 1998.*)

ropathic disorders producing a clinical picture of mononeuropathy multiplex, the basis of which is still unclear after other laboratory investigations are complete. Diagnostic considerations include vasculitis, multifocal demyelinating neuropathies, amyloidosis, leprosy, and occasionally sarcoidosis. Nerve biopsy is also helpful when one or more cutaneous nerves are palpably enlarged. Another clinical application is in establishing the diagnosis in some genetically determined childhood disorders such as metachromatic leukodystrophy, Krabbe's disease, giant axonal neuropathy, and infantile neuroaxonal dystrophy. In all of these recessively inherited diseases, both the central nervous system and the peripheral nervous system are affected.

There is a tendency to carry out sural nerve biopsy in distal symmetric polyneuropathies of subacute or chronic evolution. This practice is discouraged because its yield is low and not worth the risk of wound infection, poor healing, or persistent pain. Nerve biopsy in this situation may be useful as part of an approved research protocol when the biopsy will provide crucial information not otherwise obtainable.

SPECIAL CATEGORIES OF NEUROPATHY   Some neuropathies require individual description because of their importance or distinctiveness.

Diabetic Neuropathies   The neuropathies of diabetes mellitus are classified in Table 363-5. A limitation of this classification is that most patients do not fit neatly into any single category but instead have overlapping clinical features of several. For instance, many diabetic patients with distal, primarily sensory polyneuropathy can also be shown to have autonomic dysfunction, usually in the form of vasomotor disturbance in the limbs and abnormalities of sweating. Similarly, patients who develop a proximal motor syndrome often have dysautonomic features (including sexual impotence in males) and some degree of distal sensory polyneuropathy. To compound matters, such patients appear at risk of developing a cranial mononeuropathy. Pain is a frequent feature of diabetic neuropathies (Table 363-5) but is variable in incidence and degree.

Neuropathies occur in the setting of long-standing hyperglycemia, the principal manifestation of the group of metabolic disorders comprising diabetes mellitus. By far the most common neuropathies related to diabetes mellitus are the diffuse sensory and autonomic types (categories 1 and 2 under "Symmetric" in Table 363-5). Sensory and autonomic polyneuropathy, chronic and indolent in evolution, may first be noticed in the third to fifth decades in patients with juvenile-onset diabetes but tend to occur after age 50 in patients with adult-onset diabetes. Focal and multifocal types of neuropathy are less common but quite dramatic (categories 1, 2, and 3 under "Asymmetric" in Table 363-5). They rarely occur before the age of 45 and are usually subacute or acute in onset. Cranial mononeuropathies are mainly isolated sixth or third nerve palsies. The latter spares the pupil in three-fourths of cases, and some local pain or headache occurs in one-half. Truncal (thoracoabdominal) neuropathy is painful, involves one or more intercostal or lumbar nerves unilaterally, and frequently coexists with asymmetric proximal motor neuropathy in the legs. In asymmetric proximal motor neuropathy (diabetic amyotrophy), the most evident features are weakened muscles innervated by the femoral and obturator nerves (quadriceps femoris, iliopsoas, adductor magnus) and ipsilateral loss of the knee jerk reflex. Sensory deficit is minor, but pain in the hip and anterior thigh may be prominent. In all these multifocal and focal neuropathies, the pain usually subsides within weeks to a year, and function is usually partly or completely recovered. The same is true for symmetric proximal motor neuropathy (category 3 under "Symmetric" in Table 363-5).

Focal and multifocal diabetic neuropathies are considered to be ischemic in origin; ischemia may also underlie symmetric polyneuropathies, which are also thought to involve an abnormality of nerve metabolism.

Management of diabetic neuropathies is directed toward optimal glycemic control and symptomatic pain suppression. In the long-term Diabetes Control and Complications Trial, patients who controlled their diabetes meticulously showed significantly less neuropathy. The role of aldose reductase inhibitors in preventing or reversing diabetic complications, including neuropathy, remains unclear. Entrapment neuropathies are frequently amenable to surgical decompression.

Neuropathies with HIV Infection   Neuropathies are common in infection with HIV, but different types of neuropathy are seen according to the stage of the disease. GBS or CIDP (Chap. 365) are the neuropathies likely to occur following conversion to seropositivity and during the asymptomatic phase of HIV infection. Treatment is the same as for HIV-negative patients. In later, symptomatic stages, mononeuritis multiplex, axonal in nature, can occur; the course is typically subacute or chronic. In some cases, vasculitis of the vasa nervorum has been demonstrated.

A common neuropathy is a distal, symmetric, mainly sensory polyneuropathy, which evolves slowly in the late symptomatic stages of HIV infection and frequently coexists with symptomatic encephalopathy and myelopathy (Table 363-3; Chap. 173). The incidence of late-stage neurologic disorders, including sensory polyneuropathy, appears to be diminishing for HIV-positive individuals on effective highly active antiretroviral therapy (HAART) programs. Sensory polyneuropathy of late-stage HIV infection must be distinguished from toxic polyneuropathy that may result from the use of nucleoside analogue treatment (Table 363-4). At times, nucleoside analogues may precipitate a rapidly evolving, severe polyneuropathy with concurrent lactic acidemia. Clinically the neuropathy can be mistaken for GBS. Also in the late stages, a severe, destructive, subacute, asymmetric polyradiculopathy involving the cauda equina may be seen; it is caused by infection of the nerve roots with cytomegalovirus. Ganciclovir, started early, can arrest the disorder.

Neuropathies with Lyme Disease   A focal or multifocal radiculoneuropathy may occur weeks, months, or even years after primary infection by the tick-borne spirochete *Borrelia burgdorferi*. Although usually sensory and either dysesthetic or painful, the neuropathy is variable in distribution, affecting cranial nerves and spinal roots or nerves in a patchy, asymmetric fashion. Neuropathy is often chronic and persistent; cerebrospinal fluid pleocytosis is the rule. In many, improvement occurs spontaneously, but the course is shortened by treatment with antibiotics, usually intravenous ceftriaxone (Chap. 157).

Herpes Zoster   This is a sensory neuritis due to infection with varicella-zoster virus (VZV) and is characterized by acute inflammation of one or more dorsal root ganglia. Lancinating pain and hyperalgesia over the skin surface supplied by the affected roots occur for 3 to 4 days, followed by the appearance in the same segment of a herpetic eruption characterized by painful raised blisters on reddened bases. Pain usually subsides in a few weeks. If the inflammatory process spreads to involve related motor roots, segmental motor weakness and wasting appear. Paralysis of the oculomotor nerves may occur in conjunction with involvement of the ophthalmic division of the trigeminal ganglion (ophthalmoplegic zoster). Facial paralysis may occur with involvement of the geniculate ganglion and herpetic eruption on the ipsilateral tympanic membrane or external ear canal (Ramsay Hunt syndrome).

In a small proportion of patients, neuropathic pain persists in the dermatomal distribution of the affected ganglia. This pain, known as *postherpetic neuralgia*, is intense, burning, hyperpathic, and unrelenting; it often dominates the lives of those affected. Advancing age is a risk factor for this outcome. In some patients, blunting of the pain to tolerable levels is achieved by use of anticonvulsants such as carbamazepine or gabapentin or a tricyclic antidepressant such as desipramine or norpramin. Recent investigations suggest that postherpetic neuralgia reflects active persistent VZV infection of the ganglion, and that it may respond to intravenous antiviral treatment (Chap. 164).

Leprous Neuritis   This is a major worldwide cause of neuropathy. *Mycobacterium leprae* organisms readily invade Schwann cells in cutaneous nerve twigs, particularly those associated with unmyelinated nerve fibers. *M. leprae* thrives best in the coolest tissues in the body.

Two major forms of leprous neuritis are recognized, tuberculoid and lepromatous, which actually represent the ends of a spectrum of disease, the middle of which is called borderline (dimorphous) leprosy (patchy and multifocal involvement of skin and nerve). The treatment of a given case depends on where it falls in this spectrum (Chap. 151). Tuberculoid (high-resistance) leprosy consists of a single patch of hypesthetic or anesthetic skin in any location. The skin patch is frequently thickened, reddened, or hypopigmented. Few or no *M. leprae* bacilli may be demonstrated. If a superficially placed nerve trunk, typically a cutaneous nerve, courses just beneath the area of affected skin, it may be engulfed in the inflammatory reaction, resulting in an associated mononeuropathy. Such a nerve may be palpably enlarged and beaded. Lepromatous (low-resistance) leprosy is marked by immunologic tolerance; numerous bacilli; and widespread skin thickening, cutaneous anesthesia, and anhidrosis, which spare only the warmest parts of the body, notably the axilla, the groin, and beneath the scalp hair. Motor signs (focal weakness and atrophy) result from damage to mixed nerves lying close to the skin, particularly the median, ulnar, peroneal, and facial nerves.

SPECIAL NEUROPATHIC PRESENTATIONS Some disorders selectively affect the peripheral nervous system, limiting dysfunction to specific systems or sites, such as motor nerves, brachial plexus, or the autonomic nervous system.

Autonomic Neuropathy The autonomic nervous system regulates the visceral organs and vegetative functions (Chap. 354). Many pharmacologic agents modify specific autonomic functions, but autonomic neuropathy (dysautonomia) with structural changes in pre- and postganglionic neurons can also occur. Usually autonomic neuropathy is a manifestation of a more generalized polyneuropathy, as in diabetic neuropathy, GBS, and alcoholic polyneuropathy, but occasionally syndromes of pure pandysautonomia are encountered. Symptoms of dysautonomia are mainly negative (i.e., loss of function) and include postural hypotension with faintness or syncope, anhidrosis, hypothermia, bladder atony, obstipation, dry mouth and dry eyes from failure of salivary and lacrimal glands to secrete, blurring of vision from lack of pupillary and ciliary regulation, and sexual impotence in males. Positive phenomena (hyperfunction) may also occur and include episodic hypertension, diarrhea, hyperhidrosis, and either tachycardia or bradycardia. Management is symptomatic and also directed at the underlying cause, if it can be identified.

Pure Motor Neuropathy Disorders affecting any level of the motor unit—anterior horn cell, motor axon, or neuromuscular junction—can result in a purely lower motor syndrome without sensory disturbance. Distinguishing anterior horn cell disorders (motor neuronopathies) from motor axonopathies may be difficult clinically because they share manifestations (weakness, muscle denervation atrophy, hypo- or areflexia, fasciculations). EDX examination may also fail to localize the primary site of the lesion (neuropathic versus neuronopathic) unless the lesion is demyelinating in nature, in which case it is by definition neuropathic.

Examples of motor neuronopathies include the lower-motor form of amyotrophic lateral sclerosis, poliomyelitis, hereditary spinal muscular atrophies, and adult variant of hexosaminidase A deficiency (Chap. 353). Motor neuropathies may be seen with lead or dapsone intoxication, occasionally with porphyria, and also with multifocal motor neuropathy. The latter is a chronic asymmetric disorder of midlife associated with persistent conduction block on EDX examination, and often high titers of antiganglioside antibodies (particularly anti-GM_1) (Chap. 365). Neuromuscular junction disorders (e.g., Lambert-Eaton myasthenic syndrome, tick bite paralysis, other types of toxic neuromuscular blockade) are purely motor and can be recognized and localized electrodiagnostically (Chap. 366). Some motor-sensory polyneuropathies have predominant motor symptoms and signs, such as hereditary motor-sensory neuropathies, GBS, and CIDP, but the subclinical sensory component is readily demonstrated electrodiagnostically or by quantitative sensory testing.

Pure Sensory Neuropathy Clinical presentations involving primary sensation only (Table 363-6; Chap. 22) are common. Manifestations may (1) reflect mainly large afferent fiber involvement with deficits of vibratory and proprioceptive sense, areflexia, and sensory ataxia with or without tingling dysesthesias; (2) reflect mainly small afferent fiber involvement with numbness and cutaneous hypesthesia to pin-prick and temperature stimuli, often with painful, burning dysesthesias; or (3) be pansensory, with both large- and small-fiber manifestations. The pattern of distribution, although variable, is often distal and symmetric, particularly for large-fiber neuropathies.

The most severe and widespread of these pure sensory syndromes exhibit poor or no recovery, suggesting irreversible lesions of nerve cell bodies in dorsal root and trigeminal ganglia. These are referred to as *sensory neuronopathies*. With sensory neurotoxins, moderate doses lead to potentially reversible neuropathy, but high doses appear to cause irreversible neuronopathy.

Plexopathy This term refers to disorders of either the brachial or the lumbosacral plexus. Lesions of the brachial plexus are characterized by motor and sensory signs different from those expected in either mononeuropathies of the upper limb or polyneuropathies. The usual causes are direct trauma to the plexus, idiopathic brachial neuritis (also called *neuralgic amyotrophy*; Chap. 15), cervical rib or band, infiltration by malignant tumor, or prior radiation therapy. When the upper parts of the brachial plexus, arising from cervical roots 5 through 7, are affected, weakness and atrophy of shoulder girdle and upper arm muscles occur. Injuries to the lower brachial plexus, arising from the eighth cervical and first thoracic roots, produce distal arm weakness, atrophy, and focal sensory deficit in the forearm and hand. In general, idiopathic brachial neuritis, irradiation with >60 Gy (6000 rad), and particular types of trauma (arm jerked downward) result in damage to the upper portions of the brachial plexus. In contrast, infiltration by malignant tumor, cervical rib or band, and certain other types of trauma (arm jerked upward) cause damage to the lower brachial plexus. Lumbosacral plexopathies are less common; they may be due to trauma, including intraoperative damage, retroperitoneal hemorrhage, idiopathic plexitis, or malignant tumor infiltration or may occur in association with long-standing diabetes mellitus.

Cold Effects Cold exerts direct deleterious effects on peripheral nerve, independent of ischemia. Cold injury to nerve occurs after prolonged exposure, usually of a limb, to moderately low temperatures, as with immersion of the feet in seawater; actual freezing of tissue is not required. Axonal degeneration of myelinated fibers is the pathologic expression of cold injury. Frequently, limbs affected by cold injury to nerve show sensory deficit and dysesthesias, cutaneous vasomotor instability, pain, and marked sensitivity to minimal cold exposure, which may persist for years. The pathophysiology of these phenomena is uncertain.

Trophic Changes The array of observable changes in completely denervated muscle, bone, and skin, including hair and nails, is well known, if incompletely understood. It is unclear what portion of the changes is due purely to denervation versus what is due to disuse, immobility, lack of weight bearing, and particularly recurrent, unnoticed, painless trauma. Considerable evidence favors the view that ulceration of skin, poor healing, tissue resorption, neurogenic arthropathy, and mutilation are the result of repeated unheeded injury to insensitive parts. This sequence of events is avoidable with proper attention to and care of the insensitive parts by both patient and physician.

RECOVERY FROM NEUROPATHY In contrast to axons in the central nervous system, peripheral nerve fibers have an excellent ability to regenerate under proper circumstances. The process of regeneration following axonal degeneration may take from 2 months to more than a year, depending on the severity of the neuropathy and the length of regeneration required. Regeneration can take place when the cause of the neuropathy has been eliminated, such as removal from contact with a neurotoxic substance or correction of an abnormal metabolic state. A deficit secondary to demyelination may recover rapidly, since intact axons may remyelinate in just a few weeks. For example, a patient with GBS, in whom demyelination but no secondary axonal degeneration has occurred, may recover to normal strength from bedfastness and paralysis of arms and legs in as little as 3 to 4 weeks.

PERIPHERAL NERVE TUMORS These tumors are mostly benign and can arise on any nerve trunk or twig. Although peripheral nerve tumors can occur anywhere in the body, including the spinal roots and cauda equina, many are subcutaneous in location and present as a soft swelling, sometimes with a purplish discoloration of the skin. Two major categories of peripheral nerve tumors are recognized: neurilemmoma (schwannoma) and neurofibroma. Neurilemmomas are usually solitary and grow in the nerve sheath, rendering the tumor relatively easy to dissect free. In contrast, neurofibromas tend to be multiple, grow in the endoneurial substance, which renders them difficult to dissect, may undergo malignant changes, and are the hallmark of von Recklinghausen's neurofibromatosis (NF1) (Chap. 358).

FURTHER READING

ASBURY AK, THOMAS PK: *Peripheral Nerve Disorders*, 2d ed. Oxford, Butterworth-Heinemann, 1995

BROWN WF et al (eds): *Neuromuscular Function and Disease: Basic, Clinical and Electrodiagnostic Aspects.* Philadelphia, Saunders, 2002

DYCK PJ, THOMAS PK (eds): *Diabetic Neuropathy*, 2d ed, Philadelphia, Saunders, 1999

———, ——— (eds): *Peripheral Neuropathy*, 4d ed. Philadelphia, Saunders, 2004

KATIRJI B et al (eds): *Neuromuscular Disorders in Clinical Practice.* Boston, Butterworth-Heinemann, 2002

LLEWELYN JG: The diabetic neuropathies: Types, diagnosis and management. J Neurol, Neurosurg Psychiatry 74(Suppl 2):15, 2003

MENDELL JR, SAHENK Z: Painful sensory neuropathy. N Engl J Med 348: 1243, 2003

SHAPIRO BE, PRESTON DC: Entrapment and compressive neuropathies. Med Clin North Am 87:663, 2003

STEWART JD: *Focal Peripheral Neuropathies*, 3d ed. Philadelphia, Lippincott Williams & Wilkins, 1999

WILLISON HJ, WINER JB: Clinical evaluation and investigation of neuropathy. J Neurol, Neurosurg Psychiatry 74(Suppl 2):3, 8, 2003

364 | CHARCOT-MARIE-TOOTH DISEASE AND OTHER INHERITED NEUROPATHIES
Phillip F. Chance, Thomas D. Bird

CHARCOT-MARIE-TOOTH DISEASE

GENERAL CLINICAL FEATURES Charcot-Marie-Tooth (CMT) neuropathy comprises a heterogeneous group of inherited peripheral nerve diseases (Table 364-1). Transmission is most frequently autosomal dominant but may also be autosomal recessive or X-linked. An estimated 1 in 2500 persons has a form of CMT, making it one of the most frequently encountered inherited neurologic syndromes.

The neuropathy of CMT affects both motor and sensory nerves. Typical features consist of distal muscle weakness and atrophy, impaired sensation, and absent or hypoactive deep tendon reflexes. Common signs and symptoms are related to muscle weakness, initially involving the feet and legs and later progressing to the hands and forearms. A history of an abnormal high-stepped (steppage) gait with frequent tripping and falling is frequently elicited. Complaints related to foot deformity (pes cavus, or high-arched feet) result from atrophy of intrinsic muscles of the feet. Despite the involvement of sensory nerves in CMT, complaints of limb pain or sensory disturbances are unusual.

Onset is most often during the first or second decade of life, although presentation in mid-adult life is not unusual. The variation in clinical presentation is exceptionally wide, ranging from individuals whose only clinical finding is pes cavus and minimal or no distal muscle weakness to those with severe distal atrophy and marked hand and foot deformity. However, it is unusual for patients with CMT to lose ambulation. There are no therapies that can prevent the onset or delay progression of disability associated with CMT. Patients frequently benefit from physical therapy, use of ankle-foot orthoses (AFOs) to alleviate foot drop, and, in some cases, surgical procedures to the foot. Surgery should be undertaken only when pain or difficulty walking due to severe foot deformity cannot be managed by more conservative means.

CLASSIFICATION BY PHENOTYPE A widely accepted classification system distinguishes demyelinating forms of CMT (also designated as CMT type 1, or CMT1) from those due to axonal degeneration (CMT type 2, or CMT2). Individuals with CMT1 have electrophysiologic findings of reduced motor and sensory nerve conduction velocities (NCVs; typically <38 to 40 m/s) and pathologic findings of hypertrophic demyelinating neuropathy ("onion bulbs"). By contrast, in CMT2 there is relative preservation of the myelin sheath and these individuals have normal or near-normal NCVs. CMT3 refers to Déjerine-Sottas disease

TABLE 364-1 *Forms of Charcot-Marie-Tooth Disease (Hereditary Motor and Sensory Neuropathy) and Related Disorders*

	Locus	Gene	Mechanism
CHARCOT-MARIE-TOOTH TYPE 1			
(HMSNI)			
CMT1A	17p11.2-p12	*PMP22*	AD
CMT1B	1q22-q23	*P₀*	AD
CMT1C	16p12-p13	*SIMPLE*	AD
CMT1D	10q21-q22	*EGR2*	AD/AR
CMTX	Xq13.1	*CX32*	X-linked
CMT4A	8q13-q21	*GDAP1*	AR
CMT4B1	11q22	*MTMR2*	AR
CMT4B2	11p15	*SBF2*	AR
CMT4D (HMSN-Lom)	8q24	*NDRG1*	AR
CMT4F	19q13	*PRX*	AR
CHARCOT-MARIE-TOOTH TYPE 2			
(HMSNII)			
CMT2A	1p35-p36	*KIF1B*	AD
CMT2B	3q13-q22	*RAB7*	AD
CMT2C	12q23-q24	*Unknown*	AD
CMT2D	7p14	*GARS*	AD
CMT2E	8p21	*NEF-L*	AD
CMT2B1	11q21	*LMNA*	AR
DÉJERINE-SOTTAS			
(HMSNIII)			
DSS	17p11.2-p12	*PMP22*	AD
	1q22-p23	*P₀*	AD
	10q21-q22	*EGR2*	AD/AR
	19q13	*PRX*	AD
CONGENITAL HYPOMYELINATION			
CHN	1q22-23	*P₀*	AD
	10q21-q22	*EGR2*	AR/AD
HEREDITARY NEUROPATHY WITH PRESSURE PALSIES			
HNPP	17p11.2-p12	*PMP22*	AD

Abbreviations: PMP22, peripheral myelin protein 22; P_0, myelin protein zero; *SIMPLE*, small integral membrane protein of late endosome; *Cx32*, connexin32; *EGR2* (Krox-20) early growth response 2 gene; *GDAP1*, ganglioside-induced differentiation-associated protein-1; *MTMR2*, myotubularin-related protein-2; *SBF2*, SET binding factor 2; *NDRG1*, N-myc downstream regulated gene1; *PRX*, periaxin; *KIF1B*, kinesin family member 1B; *RAB7*, Ras-associated protein 7; *GARS*, Glycyl-tRNA synthetase; *NEFL*, neurofilament, light polypeptide; *LMNA*, lamin A.

(DSD; see below), CMT4 to autosomal recessive forms of CMT, and CMTX to X-linked varieties.

An alternative classification system designates these disorders as hereditary motor and sensory neuropathies (HMSN); HMSNI refers to CMT1, HMSNII to CMT2, HMSNIII to DSD, and HMSNIV to Refsum disease (see below).

GENETIC CONSIDERATIONS **CMT Neuropathy Type 1A (CMT1A)** Approximately three-quarters of pedigrees with autosomal dominant CMT1 demonstrate linkage to chromosome 17p11.2-12 (CMT1A) and are associated with a tandem 1.5-megabase (Mb) DNA duplication. The duplication is usually inherited as a stable Mendelian trait; however, it may also arise as a de novo event. The de novo duplication is responsible for many sporadic cases of CMT1 and may also account for some cases previously thought to occur on the basis of an autosomal recessive mode of inheritance. When present as a de novo event, the duplication results more commonly from an error in spermatogenesis; however, ~10% of de novo cases have been found to result from an error in oogenesis.

The critical gene for CMT1A is peripheral myelin protein-22 (*PMP22*), which is expressed in Schwann cells. The *PMP22* gene encodes a 160-amino-acid protein localized to the compact portion of peripheral nerve myelin; it contains four putative transmembrane domains and is highly conserved in evolution. The level of expression of *PMP22* is crucial for proper myelination of peripheral nerves. The neuropathy in patients with the duplication results from the presence of three copies of *PMP22* leading to increased expression at this locus. In rare cases, patients homozygous for the CMT1A duplication have been identified, and in some cases these individuals exhibit a more severe phenotype than their heterozygous siblings or parents. As discussed below, monosomic underexpression of *PMP22* results in hereditary neuropathy with liability to pressure palsies (HNPP).

Rare CMT1 pedigrees that are linked to chromosome 17p11.2-p12, yet lack the duplication, may harbor missense mutations within the *PMP22* gene.

DNA testing for CMT1A (including the duplication and sequencing to detect point mutations in *PMP22*) is available and now an accepted part of the evaluation of patients with suspected hereditary neuropathies (see below).

CMT Neuropathy Type 1B (CMT1B) CMT1B is less common than CMT1A; it results from mutations in the human myelin protein zero gene (*MPZ*,

or P_0), which maps to chromosome 1q22-q23. P_0 is the major structural protein component of peripheral nervous system myelin (quantitatively 50% by weight) and represents ~10% of total Schwann cell mRNA. P_0 is a member of the immunoglobulin gene superfamily of cell adhesive molecules and localizes to the compact portion of peripheral nerve myelin. P_0 protein consists of 248 amino acids and contains an intracellular and a glycosylated extracellular domain with a single transmembrane segment. Many different point mutations in the P_0 gene have been found in patients with CMT1B, and these mutations predominantly map to the extracellular domain of its gene product.

At the clinical level it is not possible to differentiate patients with CMT1A from those with CMT1B. Molecular genetic testing is available.

Déjerine-Sottas Disease (CMT3) Patients who never ambulate (or lose the ability to ambulate in infancy or childhood) are sometimes diagnosed as DSD (also called HMSNIII) or congenital hypomyelinating neuropathy (CHN). These disorders are severe, infantile- or childhood-onset, hypertrophic demyelinating polyneuropathies. NCVs are substantially slowed (typically 10 m/s), and elevations in the cerebrospinal fluid (CSF) protein level are typically present. The clinical features of DSD and CHN overlap those of severe CMT1, and for this reason the continued clinical separation of CMT1 and DSD/CHN is perhaps unwarranted. Many cases of DSD or CHN appear to be sporadic, occurring in the absence of a family history of neuropathy.

Molecular genetic studies indicate that DSD and CHN may be associated with point mutations in the P_0 or the *PMP22* genes, although pedigrees have been described that lack mutations in either the P_0, *PMP22*, or *Cx32* gene (see below). Most DSD mutations identified to date appear to function as dominant genetic traits.

Hereditary Neuropathy with Liability to Pressure Palsies HNPP (also called *tomaculous neuropathy*) is an autosomal dominant disorder that produces an episodic, recurrent demyelinating neuropathy. HNPP typically develops during adolescence and may cause attacks of numbness, muscular weakness, and atrophy. Peroneal palsies, carpal tunnel syndrome, and other entrapment neuropathies are manifestations of HNPP. Motor and sensory NCVs are mildly reduced in affected patients as well as in asymptomatic gene carriers. Pathologic changes observed in HNPP include segmental demyelination and tomaculous, or sausage-like, formations in peripheral nerves. Due to overlap of clinical features between HNPP and CMT1, some HNPP patients may be misdiagnosed as having CMT1. Approximately 10% of patients with HNPP present with a brachial neuropathy, which is typically painless. Rare patients with HNPP have been found by magnetic resonance imaging (MRI) to have central nervous system (CNS) demyelination.

The HNPP locus maps to chromosome 17p11.2-p12 and is associated with a 1.5-Mb deletion. The duplicated CMT1A chromosome (described earlier) and the deleted HNPP chromosome are the reciprocal products of unequal crossing-over during meiosis. In the case of HNPP, loss of a copy of the *PMP22* gene and underexpression of this critical myelin gene lead to demyelination. Most HNPP patients have the associated chromosome 17 deletion; however, rare patients with HNPP have been found to have point mutations in the *PMP22* gene. Molecular genetic testing is clinically available.

Treatment for HNPP is largely supportive. Surgical decompression of nerves has been proposed but is controversial. There is some evidence that surgical repair of carpal tunnel syndrome in HNPP is of little benefit and that transposition of the ulnar nerve at the elbow may produce poor results because the nerves are especially sensitive to manipulation and minor trauma.

CMT Neuropathy Type 2 CMT2 is less common than CMT1 and, in general, has a later age of onset, produces less involvement of the intrinsic muscles of the hands, and lacks palpably enlarged nerves. Extensive demyelination with "onion bulb" formation is not present in CMT2. Motor NCVs are normal or only slightly reduced in affected persons. The CMT2A locus maps to chromosome 1p35-p36, and in one pedigree a mutation in KIF1B, an axonal motor protein, was found. Limb ulceration is a notable feature of CMT2B. CMT2B maps to chromosome 3q13-q22 and results from mutations in the *RAB7* gene, a member of the Rab family of ras-related GTPases that function in intracellular membrane trafficking. Further genetic heterogeneity within CMT2 is evidenced by the identification of kindreds with the features of axonal neuropathy, weakness of the diaphragm, and vocal cord paralysis. Such pedigrees carry the designation of CMT2C, which has been mapped to chromosome 12q23-q24. Yet another form of CMT2, designated CMT2D, maps to chromosome 7p14 and results from mutations in the glycyl tRNA synthetase gene (*GARS*). In a large Russian pedigree having an autosomal dominant axonopathy, a CMT2 gene was mapped to chromosome 8p21 (and designated CMT2E), and a mutation was found in the neurofilament-light (*NEFL*) gene.

Additionally, certain P_0 or connexin32 (*Cx32*, see below) mutations have been found to be the underlying genetic defect in a subset of patients with CMT1 or CMTX who were initially thought to have CMT2 because of only mild slowing of NCVs. With these exceptions, DNA testing is not widely available for any form of CMT2.

X-linked CMT Neuropathy The clinical features of X-linked CMT disease (CMTX) include demyelinating neuropathy, absence of male-to-male transmission, and an earlier age of onset and faster rate of progression in males. NCVs vary widely in CMTX from nearly normal to moderately slowed. CMTX accounts for ~10% of all patients thought to have a form of demyelinating CMT (i.e., CMT1). CMTX should be suspected when the commonly associated chromosome 17 duplication is not present and there is no history of father-to-son transmission of the neuropathy.

The gene for CMTX maps to chromosome Xq13-q21 and results from point mutations in the *Cx32* gene. *Cx32* encodes a major component of gap junctions and is structurally similar to PMP22, as both of these proteins contain four putative transmembrane domains in similar orientation. Unlike PMP22 and P_0, which are present in compact myelin, Cx32 is located at uncompacted folds of Schwann cell cytoplasm around the nodes of Ranvier and at Schmidt-Lanterman incisures. This localization suggests a role for gap junctions composed of Cx32 in providing a pathway for the transfer of ions and nutrients around and across the myelin sheath of peripheral nerves. Mutations in the Cx32 protein have been suggested to alter its cellular localization and its trafficking and interfere with cell-to-cell communication. Over 200 different mutations in the *Cx32* gene have been described in patients with CMTX, and the distribution pattern of these mutations suggests that all parts of the Cx32 protein are functionally important. DNA testing is available.

Rare Forms of CMT Mutations in the putative zinc finger domain of the early growth response 2 gene (*EGR2*, or *Krox-20*) or in the small integral membrane protein of the lyzosome/late endosome (*SIMPLE*) gene have been found in CMT1 families that were found to be negative for the CMT1A duplication, as well as for mutations in *PMP22*, P_0, or *Cx32*. EGR2 mutations have also been reported in CHN. EGR2 acts as a direct transactivator of myelination genes in differentiating Schwann cells. SIMPLE has been proposed to play a role in myelin protein degradation and turnover. Mutations have also been found in periaxin (*PRX*), an important structural myelin protein, in demyelinating forms of neuropathy clinically diagnosed as CMT1 or DSD. DNA testing is available for EGR2 and PRX.

Rare families with autosomal recessive motor and sensory neuropathy have been reported, particularly Tunisian families with parental consanguinity. Both demyelinating and axonal types of neuropathy have been described and given the designation CMT4. One form of autosomal recessive demyelinating neuropathy, CMT4A, has been mapped to chromosome 8q13-q21 and is associated with mutations in the ganglioside-induced differentiation-associated protein (GDAP1). CMT4B is characterized by focally folded myelin sheaths and maps

to chromosome 11q23. CMT4B is caused by mutations in the myotubularin-related protein-2 (*MTMR2*), which is thought to be a transcriptional regulator. Additional loci for other rare forms of CMT4 have been found, and in some cases causal genes are known (Table 364-1).

Genetic Evaluation of CMT and HNPP An approach for evaluating a patient suspected of having an inherited peripheral neuropathy is presented in Fig. 364-1. If the proband has evidence for CMT1, determination of NCVs is a useful screening tool for parents and other at-risk family members. The *CMT1* gene is penetrant in early life, and correct disease status can probably be determined by age 5 by screening with NCVs. However, if a proband's nerve conduction is normal or only mildly prolonged, the diagnosis may be CMT2. In this case the screening examination will need to focus on determination of motor unit amplitudes and other electrical signs of denervation. Rare patients have been found to have point mutations in either P_0 or *Cx32*, resulting in very mild demyelination and misclassification as CMT2.

Most CMT1 and CMT2 pedigrees have autosomal dominant inheritance. In pedigrees lacking male-to-male transmission and whenever males are more severely affected than females and have an earlier onset, CMTX should be suspected. Determination of autosomal dominant versus X-linked CMT is important as the genetic counseling for these two modes of inheritance is different. For any form of autosomal dominant CMT, the likelihood of an affected parent (of either sex) having an affected child is 50% for each pregnancy, regardless of the sex of the child. For CMTX, all daughters of an affected father will inherit the gene, and none of the sons will be affected. For a woman with CMTX, there is a 50% likelihood that her children will be affected regardless of their sex.

Sporadic cases in males can be especially difficult to evaluate, as the neuropathy could be nongenetic or the pattern of inheritance could be autosomal dominant, X-linked, or even autosomal recessive. Sporadic cases may also represent de novo duplications (CMT1A) or de novo deletions (HNPP). False paternity is another explanation for apparent sporadic CMT or HNPP.

Molecular genetic testing is currently available for the DNA duplication (or deletion) associated with CMT1A or HNPP and for point mutations in the *PMP22*, P_0, *EGR2*, *PRX*, and *Cx32* genes associated with other forms of CMT1 and CMTX.

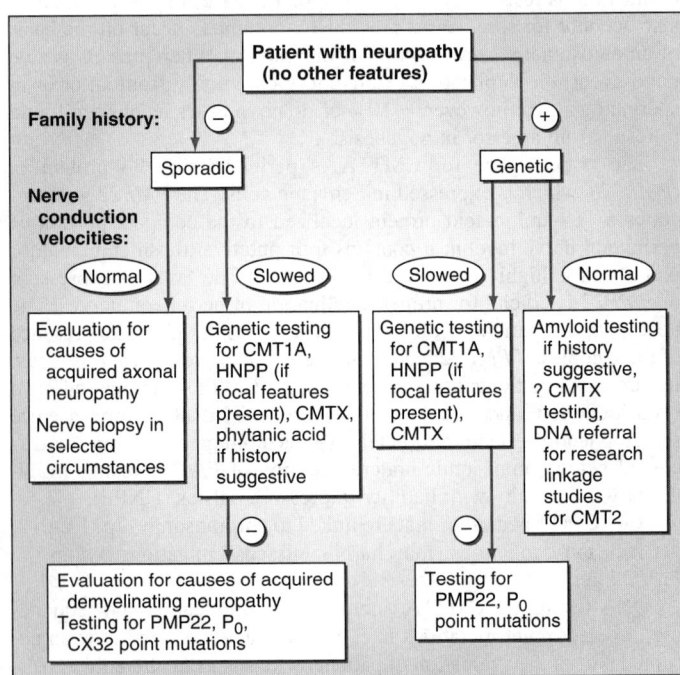

FIGURE 364-1 Evaluation of patients suspected of having an inherited peripheral neuropathy. CMT, Charcot-Marie-Tooth; HNPP, hereditary neuropathy with liability to pressure palsies. (*Modified from Lynch and Chance.*)

CHEMOTHERAPY IN PATIENTS WITH CMT Chemotherapeutic agents known to affect peripheral nerves should be used with great caution in patients with inherited neuropathies, and in the case of vincristine, total avoidance is strongly advised. A number of reports have documented the serious consequences of vincristine treatment administered in standard oncologic dosages in patients with CMT, including CMT1A and CMT2. The complications ranged from the precipitation of severe neuropathies in clinically asymptomatic at-risk individuals, induction of marked worsening in previously symptomatic patients, and even death due to respiratory collapse.

OTHER INHERITED NEUROPATHIES

HEREDITARY SENSORY NEUROPATHIES Hereditary sensory neuropathies (HSNs) are a heterogeneous group of disorders affecting sensory neurons. The most common form of HSN, HSN type I, is an autosomal degenerative disorder of sensory and motor neurons. Phenotypically, distal sensory loss, distal muscle wasting and weakness, and variable neural deafness are observed. The disease involves progressive loss of dorsal root ganglion cells and axons in peripheral nerves. Age of onset is the second decade of life or later. The HSN-I locus maps to chromosome 9q22.1-q22.3 and results from mutations in the serine palmityl transferase (*SPTLC1*) gene. Because of the presence of muscular weakness in some patients with HSN, this disorder may be clinically confused with CMT.

FAMILIAL AMYLOID NEUROPATHY Familial amyloid polyneuropathy (FAP) is an autosomal dominant disorder that classically presents as progressive sensory peripheral neuropathy, with early involvement of the autonomic nervous system and an associated cardiomyopathy. Postmortem studies have shown extensive amyloid deposition in multiple organs throughout the body. Transthyretin (TTR) is the most common constituent amyloid fibril protein deposited in FAP. Several different point mutations in the *TTR* gene have been described in TTR-related FAP, and DNA testing for these mutations is clinically available. →*Amyloidosis is discussed in Chap. 310.*

REFSUM DISEASE This autosomal recessive disorder is characterized by a progressive sensorimotor demyelinating polyneuropathy, associated with cerebellar ataxia and retinitis pigmentosa. Neural deafness, cardiomyopathy, cataracts, and icthyosis are additional features. Onset is in late childhood or early adulthood. Patients often complain of night blindness as the earliest symptom. The CSF protein is typically elevated. Diagnosis is made by demonstration of elevated levels of phytanic acid (a 20-carbon branched-chain fatty acid) in the serum and urine. The disorder appears to be due to a deficiency of a peroxysomal enzyme, phytanic acid oxidase, responsible for alpha oxidation of phytanic acid. Therapy, consisting of avoidance of dietary sources of phytanic acid and plasmapheresis in some cases, is partially effective.

FURTHER READING

BENNETT CL, CHANCE PF: Molecular pathogenesis of hereditary motor, sensory and autonomic neuropathies. Curr Opin Neuro 14:621, 2001

CHANCE PF, SHAPIRO BE: Charcot-Marie-Tooth disease and related disorders, in B Katirji et al (eds): *Neuromuscular Disorders in Clinical Practice.* Philadelphia, Butterworth-Heinemann, pp 513–525, 2002

KAMHOLZ J et al: Charcot-Marie-Tooth disease type 1: Molecular pathogenesis to gene therapy. Brain 123:222, 2000

LYNCH D, CHANCE PF: Inherited peripheral neuropathies. Neurologist 3:277, 1997

MEULEMAN JR, CHANCE PF: Hereditary pressure palsy, in *Neurological Therapeutics: Principles and Practice*, J Noseworthy (ed). London, Martin Dunitz, 2003

SCHERER SS et al: Peripheral neuropathies, in *The Molecular and Genetic Basis of Neurological Disease*, RN Rosenberg et al (eds). Oxford, Butterworth-Heinemann, pp 435–453, 2003

365 GUILLAIN-BARRÉ SYNDROME AND OTHER IMMUNE-MEDIATED NEUROPATHIES
Stephen L. Hauser, Arthur K. Asbury

GUILLAIN-BARRÉ SYNDROME

Guillain-Barré syndrome (GBS) is an acute, frequently severe, and fulminant polyradiculoneuropathy that is autoimmune in nature. It occurs year-round at a rate of about one case per million per month, or ~3500 cases per year in the United States and Canada. Males and females are equally at risk, and in western countries adults are more frequently affected than children.

Clinical Manifestations GBS manifests as rapidly evolving areflexic motor paralysis with or without sensory disturbance. The usual pattern is an ascending paralysis that may be first noticed as rubbery legs. Weakness typically evolves over hours to a few days and is frequently accompanied by tingling dysesthesias in the extremities. The legs are usually more affected than the arms, and facial diparesis is present in 50% of affected individuals. The lower cranial nerves are also frequently involved, causing bulbar weakness and difficulty with handling secretions and maintaining an airway. Most patients require hospitalization, and almost 30% require ventilatory assistance at some time during the illness. Fever and constitutional symptoms are absent at the onset, and, if present, cast doubt on the diagnosis. Deep tendon reflexes usually disappear within the first few days of onset. Cutaneous sensory deficits, e.g., loss of pain and temperature sensation, are usually relatively mild, but functions subserved by large sensory fibers, such as deep tendon reflexes and proprioception, are more severely affected. Bladder dysfunction may occur in severe cases but is usually transient. If bladder dysfunction is a prominent feature and comes early in the course, possibilities other than GBS should be considered, particularly spinal cord disease. Once clinical worsening stops and the patient reaches a plateau, further progression is unlikely.

In severe cases of GBS requiring critical care management, autonomic involvement is common. Usual features are loss of vasomotor control with wide fluctuation in blood pressure, postural hypotension, and cardiac dysrhythmias. These features require close monitoring and management and can be fatal. Pain is another common feature of GBS; several types are encountered. Most common is deep aching pain in weakened muscles, which patients liken to having overexercised the previous day. Other pains in GBS include back pain involving the entire spine and sometimes dysesthetic pain in the extremities as a manifestation of sensory nerve fiber involvement. These pains are self-limited and should be treated with standard analgesics.

Several subtypes of GBS are now recognized, as determined primarily by electrodiagnostic and pathologic distinctions (Table 365-1). A range of limited or regional GBS syndromes may be encountered, although uncommonly. These include (1) the Miller Fisher syndrome (Table 365-1 and see "Immunopathogenesis," below); (2) pure sensory forms; (3) ophthalmoplegia with anti-GQ1b antibodies (see "Immunopathogenesis," below) as part of severe motor-sensory GBS; (4) GBS with severe bulbar and facial paralysis, sometimes associated with antecedent cytomegalovirus (CMV) infection and anti-GM2 antibodies; and (5) acute pandysautonomia.

Antecedent Events Some 75% of cases of GBS are preceded 1 to 3 weeks by an acute infectious process, usually respiratory or gastrointestinal. Culture and seroepidemiologic techniques show that 20 to 30% of all cases occurring in North America, Europe, and Australia are preceded by infection or reinfection with *Campylobacter jejuni*. A similar proportion is preceded by a human herpes virus infection, often CMV or Epstein-Barr virus. Other viruses and also *Mycoplasma pneu-*

TABLE 365-1 Subtypes of Guillain-Barré Syndrome (GBS)

Subtype	Features	Electrodiagnosis	Pathology
Acute inflammatory demyelinating polyneuropathy (AIDP)	Adults affected more than children; 90% of cases in western world; recovery rapid; anti-GM1 antibodies (<50%)	Demyelinating	First attack on Schwann cell surface; widespread myelin damage, macrophage activation, and lymphocytic infiltration; variable secondary axonal damage
Acute motor axonal neuropathy (AMAN)	Children and young adults; prevalent in China and Mexico; may be seasonal; recovery rapid; anti-GD1a antibodies	Axonal	First attack at motor nodes of Ranvier; macrophage activation, few lymphocytes, frequent periaxonal macrophages; extent of axonal damage highly variable
Acute motor sensory axonal neuropathy (AMSAN)	Mostly adults; uncommon; recovery slow, often incomplete; closely related to AMAN	Axonal	Same as AMAN, but also affects sensory nerves and roots; axonal damage usually severe
M. Fisher syndrome (MFS)	Adults and children; uncommon; ophthalmoplegia, ataxia, and areflexia; anti-GQ1b antibodies (90%)	Demyelinating	Few cases examined; resembles AIDP

moniae have been identified as agents involved in antecedent infections. Recent immunization has also been associated with GBS. The swine influenza vaccine, administered widely in the United States in 1976, is the most notable example; influenza vaccines in use from 1992 to 1994, however, resulted in only one additional case of GBS per million persons vaccinated. Older type rabies vaccine, prepared in nervous system tissue, is implicated as a trigger of GBS in developing countries where it is still used; the mechanism is presumably immunization against neural antigens. GBS also occurs more frequently than can be attributed to chance alone in patients with lymphoma, including Hodgkin's disease (Chap. 97), in HIV-seropositive individuals (Chap. 173), and in patients with systemic lupus erythematosus (Chap. 300).

Immunopathogenesis Several lines of evidence support an autoimmune basis for acute inflammatory demyelinating polyneuropathy (AIDP), the most common and best studied type of GBS; the concept extends to all of the subtypes of GBS (Table 365-1).

It is likely that both cellular and humoral immune mechanisms contribute to tissue damage in AIDP. T cell activation is suggested by the finding that elevated levels of cytokines and cytokine receptors are present in serum [interleukin (IL) 2, soluble IL-2 receptor] and in cerebrospinal fluid (CSF) (IL-6, tumor necrosis factor α, interferon-γ). AIDP is also closely analogous to an experimental T cell–mediated immunopathy designated *experimental allergic neuritis* (EAN); EAN is induced in laboratory animals by immune sensitization against protein fragments derived from peripheral nerve proteins, and in particular against the P2 protein. Based on analogy to EAN, it was initially thought that AIDP was likely to be primarily a T cell–mediated disorder; however, abundant data now suggest that autoantibodies directed against nonprotein determinants may be central to many cases.

Circumstantial evidence suggests that all GBS results from immune responses to nonself antigens (infectious agents, vaccines) that misdirect to host nerve tissue through a resemblance-of-epitope (molecular mimicry) mechanism (Fig. 365-1) (Chap. 299). The neural targets are likely to be glycoconjugates, specifically gangliosides (Table 365-2; Fig. 365-2). Gangliosides are complex glycosphingolipids that contain one or more sialic acid residues; various gangliosides participate in cell-cell interactions (including those between axons and glia), modulation of receptors, and regulation of growth. They are typically exposed on the plasma membrane of cells, rendering them susceptible to an antibody-mediated attack. Gangliosides and other glycoconjugates are present in large quantity in human nervous tissues and in key sites, such as nodes of Ranvier. Antiganglioside antibodies, most fre-

quently to GM1, are common in GBS (20 to 50% of cases), particularly in those preceded by *C. jejuni* infection. Furthermore, isolates of *C. jejuni* from stool cultures of patients with GBS have surface glycolipid structures that antigenically cross react with gangliosides, including GM1, concentrated in human nerves. Another line of evidence is derived from experience in Europe with parenteral use of purified bovine brain gangliosides for treatment of various neuropathic disorders. Between 5 and 15 days after injection some recipients developed acute motor axonal GBS with high titers of anti-GM1 antibodies that recognized epitopes at nodes of Ranvier and motor endplates.

Particularly noteworthy is the Miller Fisher syndrome (MFS), which presents as rapidly evolving ataxia and areflexia of limbs without weakness, and ophthalmoplegia often with pupillary paralysis. The MFS variant accounts for ~5% of all GBS cases. Anti-GQ1b IgG antibodies are found in >90% of patients with MFS (Tables 365-1 and 365-2; Fig. 365-2), and titers of IgG are highest early in the course. Anti-GQ1b antibodies are not found in other forms of GBS unless there is extraocular motor nerve involvement. Extraocular motor nerves are enriched in GQ1b gangli-

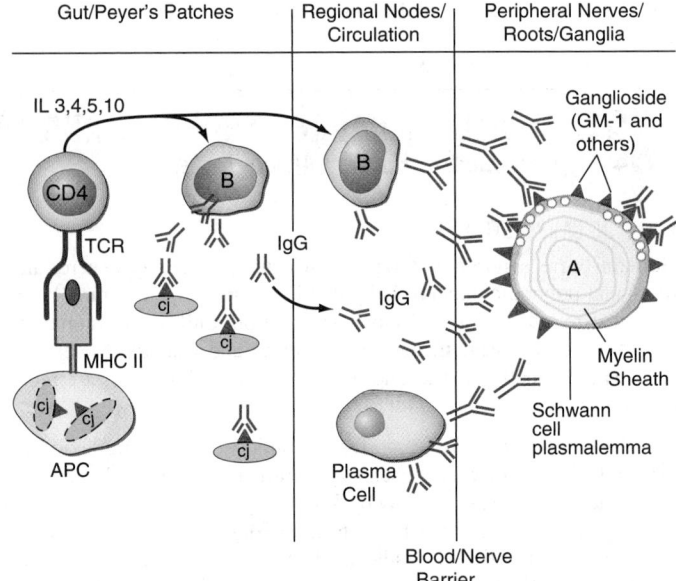

FIGURE 365-1 Postulated immunopathogenesis of GBS associated with *C. jejuni* infection. B cells recognize glycoconjugates on *C. jejuni* (Cj) (triangles) that cross-react with ganglioside present on Schwann cell surface and subjacent peripheral nerve myelin. Some B cells, activated via a T cell–independent mechanism, secrete primarily IgM (not shown). Other B cells (upper left side) are activated via a partially T cell–dependent route and secrete primarily IgG; T cell help is provided by CD4 cells activated locally by fragments of Cj proteins that are presented on the surface of antigen-presenting cells (APC). A critical event in the development of GBS is the escape of activated B cells from Peyers patches into regional lymph nodes. Activated T cells probably also function to assist in opening of the blood-nerve barrier, facilitating penetration of pathogenic autoantibodies. The earliest changes in myelin (right) consist of edema between myelin lamellae and vesicular disruption (shown as circular blebs) of the outermost myelin layers. These effects are associated with activation of the C5b-C9 membrane attack complex and probably mediated by calcium entry; it is possible that the macrophage cytokine tumor necrosis factor (TNF) also participates in myelin damage. B, B cell; MHC II, class II major histocompatibility complex molecule; TCR, T cell receptor; A, axon.

TABLE 365-2 *Principal Anti-Glycolipid Antibodies Implicated in Immune Neuropathies*

Clinical Presentation	Antibody Target	Usual Isotype
ACUTE IMMUNE NEUROPATHIES (GUILLAIN BARRÉ SYNDROMES)		
Acute inflammatory demyelinating polyneuropathy (AIDP)	No clear patterns GM1 most common	IgG (polyclonal)
Acute motor axonal neuropathy (AMAN)	GD1a, GM1, GM1b, Ga1NAc–GD1a (<50% for any)	IgG (polyclonal)
Miller Fisher Syndrome (MFS)	GQ1b (>90%)	IgG (polyclonal)
Acute pharyngeal cervicobrachial neuropathy (APCBN)	GT1a (? Most)	IgG (polyclonal)
CHRONIC IMMUNE NEUROPATHIES		
Chronic inflammatory demyelinating polyneuropathy CIDP (75%)	Po in some	No clear pattern
CIDPa (MGUS associated) (25%)	Neural binding sites	IgG, IgA (monoclonal)
Chronic sensory > motor neuropathy	SPGP, SGLPG (on MAG) (50%)	IgM (monoclonal)
	Uncertain (50%)	IgM (monoclonal)
Multifocal motor neuropathy (MMN)	GM1, Ga1NAc–GD1a, others (25–50%)	IgM (polyclonal, monoclonal)
Chronic sensory atoxic neuropathy	GD1b, GQ1b and other b-series gangliosides	IgM (monoclonal)

Note: MGUS, monoclonal gammopathy of undertermined significance; MAG, myelin-associated glycoprotein.
Source: Modified from HJ Willison, N Yuki: Brain 125:2591, 2002.

osides in comparison to limb nerves. Further, a monoclonal anti-GQ1b antibody raised against *C. jejuni* isolated from a patient with MFS blocked neuromuscular transmission experimentally.

Taken together, these observations provide strong but still inconclusive evidence that autoantibodies play an important pathogenic role in GBS. Although anti-ganglioside antibodies have been studied most intensively, other antigenic targets may also be important. One recent report identified IgG antibodies against Schwann cells and neurons (nerve growth cone region) in some GBS cases. Proof that these antibodies are pathogenic requires that they be capable of mediating disease following direct passive transfer to naïve hosts; this has not yet been demonstrated, although a case of apparent maternal-fetal transplacental transfer of GBS has been described.

Pathophysiology In the demyelinating forms of GBS, the basis for flaccid paralysis and sensory disturbance is conduction block. This finding, demonstrable electrophysiologically, implies that the axonal connections remain intact. Hence, recovery can take place rapidly as remyelination occurs. In severe cases of demyelinating GBS, secondary axonal degeneration usually occurs; its extent can be estimated electrophysiologically. More secondary axonal degeneration correlates with a slower rate of recovery and a greater degree of residual disability. When a primary axonal pattern is encountered electrophysiologically, the implication is that axons have degenerated and become disconnected from their targets, specifically the neuromuscular junctions, and must therefore regenerate for recovery to take place. In motor axonal cases in which recovery is rapid, the lesion is thought to be localized to preterminal motor branches, allowing regeneration and reinnervation to take place quickly.

Laboratory Features CSF findings are distinctive, consisting of an elevated CSF protein level [1 to 10 g/L (100 to 1000 mg/dL)] without accompanying pleocytosis. The CSF is often normal when symptoms have been present for ≤48 h; by the end of the first week the level of protein is usually elevated. A transient increase in the CSF white cell

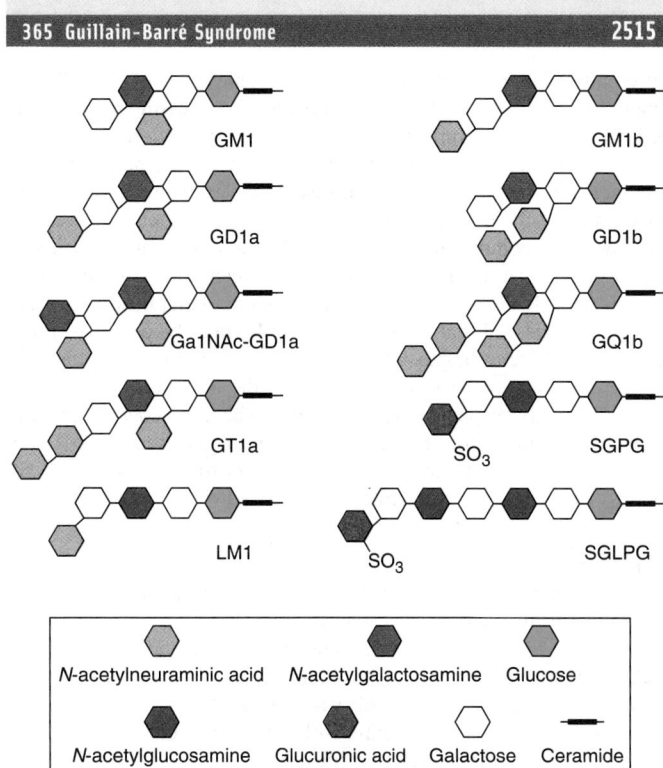

FIGURE 365-2 Glycolipids implicated as antigens in immune-mediated neuropathies. (*Modified from HJ Willison, N Yuki: Brain 125:2591, 2002.*)

count (10 to 100/μL) occurs on occasion in otherwise typical GBS; however, a sustained CSF pleocytosis suggests an alternative diagnosis (viral myelitis) or a concurrent diagnosis (unrecognized HIV infection; Chap. 173). Electrodiagnostic features are mild or absent in the early stages of GBS and lag behind the clinical evolution. In cases with demyelination (Table 365-1), prolonged distal latencies, conduction velocity slowing, evidence of conduction block, and temporal dispersion of compound action potential are the usual features. In cases with primary axonal pathology, the principal electrodiagnostic finding is reduced amplitude of compound action potentials without conduction slowing or prolongation of distal latencies.

Diagnosis GBS is a descriptive entity. The diagnosis is made by recognizing the pattern of rapidly evolving paralysis with areflexia, absence of fever or other systemic symptoms, and characteristic antecedent events (Table 365-3). Other disorders that may enter into the

TABLE 365-3 *Diagnostic Criteria for Guillain-Barré Syndrome*

REQUIRED

1. Progressive weakness of 2 or more limbs due to neuropathy[a]
2. Areflexia
3. Disease course <4 weeks
4. Exclusion of other causes [e.g., vasculitis (polyarteritis nodosa, systemic lupus erythematosus, Churg-Strauss syndrome), toxins (organophosphates, lead), botulism, diphtheria, porphyria, localized spinal cord or cauda equina syndrome]

SUPPORTIVE

1. Relatively symmetric weakness
2. Mild sensory involvement
3. Facial nerve or other cranial nerve involvement
4. Absence of fever
5. Typical CSF profile (acellular, increase in protein level)
6. Electrophysiologic evidence of demyelination

[a] Excluding M. Fisher and other variant syndromes.
Source: Modified from AK Asbury, DR Cornblath: Ann Neurol 27:S21, 1990.

differential diagnosis include acute myelopathies (especially with prolonged back pain and sphincter disturbances); botulism (pupillary reactivity lost early); diphtheria (early oropharyngeal disturbances); Lyme polyradiculitis and other tick-borne paralyses; porphyria (abdominal pain, seizures, psychosis); vasculitic neuropathy (check erythrocyte sedimentation rate, described below); poliomyelitis (fever and meningismus common); CMV polyradiculitis (in immunocompromised patients); critical illness neuropathy; neuromuscular disorders such as myasthenia gravis; or poisonings with organophosphates, thallium, or arsenic. Laboratory tests are helpful primarily to exclude mimics of GBS. Electrodiagnostic features may be minimal, and the CSF protein level may not rise until the end of the first week. If the diagnosis is strongly suspected, treatment should be initiated without waiting for evolution of the characteristic electrodiagnostic and CSF findings to occur. GBS patients with risk factors for HIV or with CSF pleocytosis should have a serologic test for HIV.

℞ TREATMENT

In the vast majority of patients with GBS, treatment should be initiated as soon after diagnosis as possible. Each day counts; ~2 weeks after the first motor symptoms, immunotherapy is no longer effective. Either high-dose intravenous immune globulin (IVIg) or plasmapheresis can be initiated, as they are equally effective (Table 365-4). A combination of the two therapies is not significantly better than either alone. IVIg is often the initial therapy chosen because of its ease of administration and good safety record. IVIg is administered as five daily infusions for a total dose of 2 g/kg body weight. There is some evidence that GBS autoantibodies are neutralized by anti-idiotypic antibodies present in IVIg preparations, perhaps accounting for the therapeutic effect. A course of plasmapheresis, consisting of ~40 to 50 mL/kg plasma exchange (PE) four times over a week, is usually employed. In patients who are treated early in the course of GBS and improve, relapse may occur in the second or third week. Brief retreatment with the original therapy is usually effective. Glucocorticoids have not been found to be effective in GBS. Occasional patients with very mild forms of GBS, especially those who appear to have already reached a plateau when initially seen, may be managed conservatively without IVIg or plasma exchange.

In the worsening phase of GBS, most patients require monitoring in a critical care setting, with particular attention to vital capacity, cardiovascular status, and chest physiotherapy. As noted, ~30% of patients with GBS require ventilatory assistance, sometimes for prolonged periods of time (several weeks or longer). Frequent turning and assiduous skin care are important, as are daily range-of-motion exercises to avoid joint contractures, and daily reassurance as to the generally good outlook for recovery.

Prognosis and Recovery Approximately 85% of patients with GBS achieve a full functional recovery within several months to a year, although minor findings on examination (such as areflexia) may persist. The mortality rate is <5% in optimal settings; death usually results from secondary pulmonary complications. The outlook is worst in patients with severe proximal motor and sensory axonal damage. Such axonal damage may be either primary or secondary in nature (see "Pathophysiology," above), but in either case successful regeneration cannot occur. Other factors that worsen the outlook for recovery are advanced age, a fulminant or severe attack, and a delay in the onset of treatment. Between 5 to 10% of patients with typical GBS have one or more late relapses; such cases are then classsified as chronic inflammatory demyelinating polyneuropathy (CIDP).

CHRONIC INFLAMMATORY DEMYELINATING POLYNEUROPATHY

CIDP is distinguished from GBS by its chronic course. In other respects, this neuropathy shares many features with GBS, including elevated CSF protein levels and the electrodiagnostic findings of acquired demyelination. Most cases occur in adults, and males are affected slightly more often than females. The incidence of CIDP is lower than that of GBS, but due to the protracted course the prevalence is greater.

Clinical Manifestations Onset is usually gradual, sometimes subacute; in a few, the initial attack is indistinguishable from that of GBS. Symptoms are both motor and sensory in most cases. Weakness of the limbs is usually symmetric but can be strikingly asymmetric. There is considerable variability from case to case. Some patients experience a

TABLE 365-4 *Major Clinical Trials of Treatment for Guillain-Barré Syndrome (GBS)*

Trial/Site	Reference	No. Patients (N)/ Follow Up (FU)/ Trial Arms	End Points	Results/p Value	Comment
GBS Study Group; USA/Canada (18 centers)	Neurology 35:1096, 1985	N = 245 FU = 6 months PE vs. none	1. % improved 1 grade at 4 weeks 2. Days to improve 1 grade 3. Days to reach grade 2	1. 59% (PE) vs. 39% (none) $p <. 001$ 2. 19 days (PE) vs. 40 days (none) $p < .001$ 3. 53 days (PE) vs. 85 days (none) $p < .001$	First major trial showing efficacy— prior smaller trials showed conflicting results
French Coop. Group on PE in GBS; France/Switzerland (28 centers)	Ann Neurol 22:753, 1987; Ann Neurol 32:94, 1992	N = 220 FU = 1 year PE vs. none; Albumin vs. FFP in PE arm	1. Days to walk with assistance 2. Days to positive Δ score 3. Albumin vs. FFP	1. 30 days (PE) vs. 44 days (none) $p < .01$ 2. 4 days (PE) vs. 12 days (none) $p < .001$ 3. No significant difference	At 1 year, full strength recovery in 71% (PE) vs. 52% (none); $p = .007$
Dutch GB Study Group; The Netherlands (15 centers)	N Engl J Med 326: 1123, 1992	N = 150 FU = 6 months IVIg vs. PE	1. % improved 1 grade at 4 weeks 2. Days to reach grade 2	1. 53% (IVIg) vs. 34% (PE) $p = .024$ 2. 55 days (IVIg) vs. 70 days (PE) $p = .07$	Patient assignment inadvertently favored IVIg group
Plasma Exchange/ Sandoglobulin GBS Trial (38 centers in 11 countries)	Lancet 349:225, 1997	N = 329 FU = 48 weeks IVIg vs. PE vs. both (3 arms)	1. % improved 1 grade at 4 weeks 2. Secondary end points: days to reach grade 2; days to off-respirator; disability at 48 weeks	No significant difference between the 3 groups for any end points	Nonsignificant trends favoring combined therapy

Abbreviations: PE, plasma exchange; IVIg, high dose intravenous immunoglobulin; FFP, fresh-frozen plasma.
Note: All studies except the French Coop. Group used the London grade scale: 0, healthy; 1, minor symptoms/signs; 2, walk 5 m unassisted; 3, walk 5 m with assistance; 4, bed/chairbound; 5, requiring assisted respiration; 6, dead.

chronic progressive course, whereas others, usually younger patients, have a relapsing and remitting course. Some have only motor findings, and a small proportion present with a relatively pure syndrome of sensory ataxia. Tremor occurs in ~10% and may become more prominent during periods of subacute worsening or improvement. A small proportion have cranial nerve findings, including external ophthalmoplegia. CIDP tends to ameliorate over time with treatment; the result is that many years after onset nearly 75% of patients have reasonable functional status. Death from CIDP is uncommon.

Diagnosis The diagnosis rests on characteristic clinical, CSF, and electrophysiologic findings. The CSF is usually acellular with an elevated protein level, sometimes several times normal. Electrodiagnostically, variable degrees of conduction slowing, prolonged distal latencies, temporal dispersion of compound action potentials, and conduction block are the principal features. In particular, the presence of conduction block is a certain sign of an acquired demyelinating process. Evidence of axonal loss, presumably secondary to demyelination, is present in >50% of patients. Serum protein electrophoresis with immunofixation is indicated to search for monoclonal gammopathy and associated conditions (see "Monoclonal Gammopathy of Undetermined Significance," below). In all patients with presumptive CIDP, it is also reasonable to exclude collagen vascular disease (especially systemic lupus erythematosus), chronic hepatitis, HIV infection, and diabetes mellitus.

Pathogenesis Although there is evidence of immune activation in CIDP, the precise mechanisms of pathogenesis are unknown. Biopsy typically reveals little inflammation and onion-bulb changes (imbricated layers of attenuated Schwann cell processes surrounding an axon) that result from recurrent demyelination and remyelination. The response to therapy suggests that CIDP is immune-mediated; interestingly, CIDP responds to glucocorticoids (see below), whereas GBS does not. Passive transfer of demyelination into experimental animals was recently accomplished using IgG purified from the serum of some patients with CIDP, lending support for a humoral autoimmune pathogenesis. Although the target antigen or antigens in CIDP have not yet been identified, one recent study implicated the myelin protein Po as a potential autoantigen in some patients. Approximately 25% of patients with clinical features of CIDP also have a monoclonal gammopathy of undetermined significance (MGUS). Cases associated with monoclonal IgA or IgG usually respond to treatment as favorably as cases without a monoclonal gammopathy. Patients with IgM monoclonal gammopathy tend to have more sensory findings, a more protracted course, and may have a less satisfactory response to treatment, although this is an area of controversy.

℞ TREATMENT

Most authorities initiate treatment for CIDP when progression is rapid or walking is compromised. If the disorder is mild, management can be expectant, awaiting spontaneous remission. Controlled studies have shown that high-dose IVIg, PE, and glucocorticoids are all more effective than placebo. Initial therapy is usually either IVIg or PE, which appear to be equally effective. IVIg is administered as 0.4 g/kg body weight daily for 5 days; most patients require periodic re-treatment at ~6-week intervals. PE is initiated at two to three treatments per week for 6 weeks; periodic re-treatment may also be required. Treatment with oral glucocorticoids is another option (60 to 80 mg prednisone daily for 1 to 2 months, followed by a gradual dose reduction of 10 mg per month as tolerated), but long-term adverse effects including bone demineralization, gastrointestinal bleeding, and cushingoid changes are problematic. Approximately one-half of patients with CIDP fail to respond adequately to the initial therapy chosen; a different treatment should then be tried. Patients who fail therapy with IVIg, PE, and glucocorticoids may benefit from treatment with immunosuppressive agents such as azathioprine, methotrexate, cyclosporine, and cyclophosphamide, either alone or as adjunctive therapy. Use of these therapies requires periodic reassessment of their risks and benefits.

MULTIFOCAL MOTOR NEUROPATHY

Multifocal motor neuropathy (MMN) is a distinctive but uncommon neuropathy that presents as a slowly progressive motor weakness and atrophy evolving over years in the distribution of selected nerve trunks, associated with sites of persistent focal motor conduction block in the same nerve trunks. Sensory fibers are relatively spared. The arms are affected more frequently than the legs, and >75% of all patients are male. Some cases have been confused with lower motor neuron forms of amyotrophic lateral sclerosis (Chap. 353). Approximately 50% of patients present with high titers of polyclonal IgM antibody to the ganglioside GM1. It is uncertain how this finding relates to the discrete foci of persistent motor conduction block, but high concentrations of GM1 gangliosides are normal constituents of nodes of Ranvier in peripheral nerve fibers. Pathology reveals demyelination and mild inflammatory changes at the sites of conduction block.

Most patients with MMN respond to high-dose IVIg (dosages as for CIDP, above) and some refractory patients have responded to cyclophosphamide. Glucocorticoids and PE are not effective.

NEUROPATHIES WITH MONOCLONAL GAMMOPATHY

MULTIPLE MYELOMA Clinically overt polyneuropathy occurs in ~5% of patients with the commonly encountered type of multiple myeloma, which exhibits either lytic or diffuse osteoporotic bone lesions. These neuropathies are sensorimotor, are usually mild but may be severe, and generally do not reverse with successful suppression of the myeloma. In most cases, electrodiagnostic and pathologic features are consistent with a process of axonal degeneration.

In contrast, myeloma with osteosclerotic features, although representing only 3% of all myelomas, is associated with polyneuropathy in one-half of cases. These neuropathies, which may also occur with solitary plasmacytoma, are distinct because they (1) are usually demyelinating in nature; (2) often respond to radiation therapy or removal of the primary lesion; (3) are associated with different monoclonal proteins and light chains (almost always lambda as opposed to primarily kappa in the lytic type of multiple myeloma); and (4) may occur in association with other systemic findings including thickening of the skin, hyperpigmentation, hypertrichosis, organomegaly, endocrinopathy, anasarca, and clubbing of fingers. These are features of the POEMS syndrome (*p*olyneuropathy, *o*rganomegaly, *e*ndocrinopathy, *M* protein, and *s*kin changes). The pathogenesis of this uncommon syndrome and the explanation for its association with lambda light chains are unknown. Treatment of the neuropathy is best directed at the osteosclerotic myeloma using surgery, radiotherapy, or chemotherapy, as indicated.

Neuropathies are also encountered in other systemic conditions with gammopathy including Waldenström's macroglobulinemia, primary systemic amyloidosis, and cryoglobulinemic states (mixed essential cryoglobulinemia, some cases of hepatitis C).

MONOCLONAL GAMMOPATHY OF UNDETERMINED SIGNIFICANCE Chronic polyneuropathies occurring in association with MGUS are usually associated with the immunoglobulin isotypes IgG, IgA, and IgM. From a clinical standpoint, many of these patients are indistinguishable from patients with CIDP without monoclonal gammopathy (see "Chronic Inflammatory Demyelinating Polyneuropathy," above), and their response to immunosuppressive agents is also similar. An exception is the syndrome of IgM kappa monoclonal gammopathy associated with an indolent, longstanding, sometimes static sensory neuropathy, frequently with tremor and sensory ataxia. Most patients are male and over age 50. In the majority, the monoclonal IgM immunoglobulin binds to a normal peripheral nerve constituent, myelin-associated glycoprotein (MAG), found in the paranodal regions of Schwann cells. Binding appears to be specific for a polysaccharide epitope that is also found in other normal peripheral nerve myelin glycoproteins, P0 and PMP22, and also in other normal nerve-related glycosphingolipids (Fig. 365-1). In the MAG-positive cases, IgM paraprotein is incorporated into the myelin sheaths of affected patients and widens the spacing of the myelin lamellae, thus producing a distinctive ultrastructural pattern. Demyelination and remyelination are the hallmarks of the lesions. The chronic demyelinating neuropathy appears to result from a destabilization of myelin metabolism rather than activation of an immune response. Therapy with chlorambucil or cyclophosphamide often results in improvement of the neuropathy associated with a prolonged reduction in the levels in the circulating paraprotein; chronic use of these alkylating agents is associated with significant risks (Chap. 70). In a small proportion of patients, MGUS will in time evolve into frankly malignant conditions, such as multiple myeloma (Chap. 98) or lymphoma (Chap. 97).

VASCULITIC NEUROPATHY

Peripheral nerve involvement is common in polyarteritis nodosa (PAN), appearing in half of all cases clinically and in 100% of cases at postmortem studies (Chap. 306). The most common pattern is multifocal (asymmetric) motor-sensory neuropathy (mononeuropathy multiplex) due to ischemic lesions of nerve trunks and roots; however, some cases of vasculitic neuropathy present as a distal, symmetric motor-sensory neuropathy. Symptoms of neuropathy are a common presenting complaint in patients with PAN. The electrodiagnostic findings are those of an axonal process. Small- to medium-sized arteries of the vasa nervorum, particularly the epineural vessels, are affected in PAN, resulting in a widespread ischemic neuropathy. A high frequency of neuropathy is also present in allergic angiitis and granulomatosis (Churg-Strauss syndrome).

Systemic vasculitis should always be considered when a subacute or chronically evolving mononeuropathy multiplex occurs in conjunction with constitutional symptoms (fever, anorexia, weight loss, loss of energy, malaise, and nonspecific pains). Diagnosis of suspected vasculitic neuropathy is made by a combined nerve and muscle biopsy, with serial section or skip-serial techniques (Chap. 363).

Approximately one-third of biopsy-proven cases of vasculitic neuropathy are "nonsystemic" in that the vasculitis appears to affect only peripheral nerve. Constitutional symptoms are absent, and the course is more indolent than that of PAN. The erythrocyte sedimentation rate may be elevated, but other tests for systemic disease are negative. Nevertheless, clinically silent involvement of other organs is likely, and vasculitis is frequently found in muscle biopsied at the same time as nerve.

Vasculitic neuropathy may also be seen as part of the vasculitis syndrome occurring in the course of other connective tissue disorders. The most frequent is rheumatoid arthritis, but ischemic neuropathy due to involvement of vasa nervorum may also occur in mixed cryoglobulinemia, Sjögren's syndrome, Wegener's granulomatosis, hypersensitivity angiitis (Chap. 306), and progressive systemic sclerosis (Chap. 303). Management of these neuropathies, including the "nonsystemic" vasculitic neuropathy, consists of treatment of the underlying condition as well as the aggressive use of glucocorticoids and other immunosuppressant drugs, usually cyclophosphamide.

ANTI-HU PARANEOPLASTIC NEUROPATHY

This uncommon immune-mediated disorder manifests as a sensory neuronopathy, i.e., selective damage to dorsal root ganglia. The onset is often asymmetric with dysesthesias and sensory loss in the limbs that soon progress to affect all limbs, the torso, and face. Marked sensory ataxia, pseudoathetosis, and inability to walk, stand, or even sit unsupported are frequent features and are secondary to the extensive deafferentation. Subacute sensory neuronopathy is often idiopathic, but ~25% of cases are paraneoplastic, primarily related to lung cancer, and most of those are small-cell lung cancer (SCLC) (Chap. 87). The target antigens are a family of RNA binding proteins (HuD, HuC, and Hel-N1) that in normal tissues are only expressed by neurons. The same proteins are usually expressed by SCLC, triggering in some patients an immune response characterized by antibodies and cytotoxic T cells that cross-react with the Hu proteins of the dorsal root ganglion neurons, resulting in immune-mediated neuronal destruction. An encephalomyelitis may accompany the sensory neuronopathy and presumably has the same pathogenesis. Neurologic symptoms usually precede, by 1 year on average, the identification of SCLC. The sensory neuronopathy runs its course in a few weeks or months and stabilizes, leaving the patient disabled. Most cases are unresponsive to treatment with glucocorticoids, IVIg, PE, or immunosuppressant drugs.

FURTHER READING

Gong Y et al: Localization of major gangliosides in the PNS: Implications for immune neuropathies. Brain 125:2491, 2002

Hughes RAC et al: Practice parameter: Immunotherapy for Guillain-Barré syndrome. Report of the Quality Standards Subcommittee of the American Academy of Neurology. Neurology 61:736, 2003

Olney RK et al: Consensus criteria for the diagnosis of multifocal motor neuropathy. Muscle Nerve 27:117, 2003

Willison HJ, Yuki N: Peripheral neuropathies and anti-glycolipid antibodies. Brain 125:2591, 2002

366 MYASTHENIA GRAVIS AND OTHER DISEASES OF THE NEUROMUSCULAR JUNCTION
Daniel B. Drachman

Myasthenia gravis (MG) is a neuromuscular disorder characterized by weakness and fatigability of skeletal muscles. The underlying defect is a decrease in the number of available acetylcholine receptors (AChRs) at neuromuscular junctions due to an antibody-mediated autoimmune attack. Treatment now available for MG is highly effective, although a specific cure has remained elusive.

PATHOPHYSIOLOGY   In the neuromuscular junction (Fig. 366-1), acetylcholine (ACh) is synthesized in the motor nerve terminal and stored in vesicles (quanta). When an action potential travels down a motor nerve and reaches the nerve terminal, ACh from 150 to 200 vesicles is released and combines with AChRs that are densely packed at the peaks of postsynaptic folds. The structure of the AChR has been fully elucidated; it consists of five subunits (2α, 1β, 1δ, and 1γ or ϵ) arranged around a central pore. When ACh combines with the binding sites on the AChR, the channel in the AChR opens, permitting the rapid entry of cations, chiefly sodium, which produces depolarization at the end-plate region of the muscle fiber. If the depolarization is sufficiently large, it initiates an action potential that is propagated

along the muscle fiber, triggering muscle contraction. This process is rapidly terminated by hydrolysis of ACh by acetylcholinesterase (AChE), which is present within the synaptic folds, and by diffusion of ACh away from the receptor.

In MG, the fundamental defect is a decrease in the number of available AChRs at the postsynaptic muscle membrane. In addition, the postsynaptic folds are flattened, or "simplified." These changes result in decreased efficiency of neuromuscular transmission. Therefore, although ACh is released normally, it produces small end-plate potentials that may fail to trigger muscle action potentials. Failure of transmission at many neuromuscular junctions results in weakness of muscle contraction.

The amount of ACh released per impulse normally declines on repeated activity (termed *presynaptic rundown*). In the myasthenic patient, the decreased efficiency of neuromuscular transmission combined with the normal rundown results in the activation of fewer and fewer muscle fibers by successive nerve impulses and hence increasing weakness, or *myasthenic fatigue*. This mechanism also accounts for the decremental response to repetitive nerve stimulation seen on electrodiagnostic testing.

The neuromuscular abnormalities in MG are brought about by an autoimmune response mediated by specific anti-AChR antibodies. The anti-AChR antibodies reduce the number of available AChRs at neuromuscular junctions by three distinct mechanisms: (1) accelerated turnover of AChRs by a mechanism involving crosslinking and rapid endocytosis of the receptors; (2) blockade of the active site of the AChR, i.e., the site that normally binds ACh; and (3) damage to the postsynaptic muscle membrane by the antibody in collaboration with complement. The pathogenic antibodies are IgG and are T cell dependent. Thus, immunotherapeutic strategies directed against T cells are effective in this antibody-mediated disease.

How the autoimmune response is initiated and maintained in MG is not completely understood. However, the thymus appears to play a role in this process. The thymus is abnormal in ~75% of patients with MG; in about 65% the thymus is "hyperplastic," with the presence of active germinal centers detected histologically, though the hyperplastic thymus is not necessarily enlarged. An additional 10% of patients have thymic tumors (thymomas). Muscle-like cells within the thymus (myoid cells), which bear AChRs on their surface, may serve as a source of autoantigen and trigger the autoimmune reaction within the thymus gland.

CLINICAL FEATURES MG is not rare, having a prevalence of at least 1 in 7500. It affects individuals in all age groups, but peaks of incidence occur in women in their twenties and thirties and in men in their fifties and sixties. Overall, women are affected more frequently than men, in a ratio of ~3:2. The cardinal features are *weakness* and *fatigability* of muscles. The weakness increases during repeated use (fatigue) and may improve following rest or sleep. The course of MG is often variable. Exacerbations and remissions may occur, particularly during the first few years after the onset of the disease. Remissions are rarely complete or permanent. Unrelated infections or systemic disorders often lead to increased myasthenic weakness and may precipitate "crisis" (see below).

The distribution of muscle weakness often has a characteristic pattern. The cranial muscles, particularly the lids and extraocular muscles, are often involved early in the course of MG, and diplopia and ptosis are common initial complaints. Facial weakness produces a "snarling" expression when the patient attempts to smile. Weakness in chewing is most noticeable after prolonged effort, as in chewing meat. Speech may have a nasal timbre caused by weakness of the palate or a dysarthric "mushy" quality due to tongue weakness. Difficulty in swallowing may occur as a result of weakness of the palate, tongue, or pharynx, giving rise to nasal regurgitation or aspiration of liquids or food. In ~85% of patients, the weakness becomes generalized, affecting the limb muscles as well. The limb weakness in MG is often proximal and may be asymmetric. Despite the muscle weakness, deep tendon reflexes are preserved. If weakness of respiration becomes so severe as to require respiratory assistance, the patient is said to be in *crisis*.

DIAGNOSIS AND EVALUATION (Table 366-1) The diagnosis is suspected on the basis of weakness and fatigability in the typical distribution described above, without loss of reflexes or impairment of sensation or other neurologic function. The suspected diagnosis should always be confirmed definitively before treatment is undertaken; this is essential because (1) other treatable conditions may closely resemble MG, and (2) the treatment of MG may involve surgery and the prolonged use of drugs with adverse side effects.

Anticholinesterase Test Drugs that inhibit the enzyme AChE allow ACh to interact repeatedly with the limited number of AChRs, producing

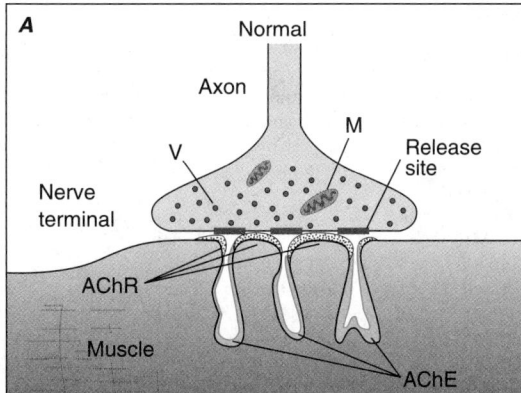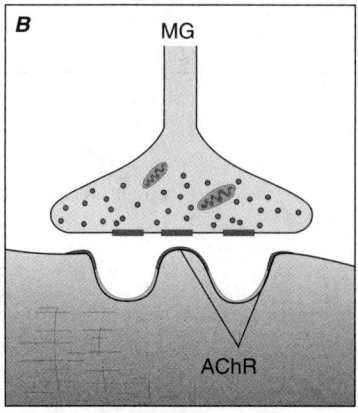

FIGURE 366-1 Diagrams of (*A*) normal and (*B*) myasthenic neuromuscular junctions. V, vesicles; M, mitochondria; AChE, acetylcholinesterase. See text for description of normal neuromuscular transmission. The MG junction shows a normal nerve terminal; a reduced number of AChRs (stippling); flattened, simplified postsynaptic folds; and a widened synaptic space.

improvement in the strength of myasthenic muscles. Edrophonium is used most commonly for diagnostic testing because of the rapid onset (30 s) and short duration (about 5 min) of its effect. An objective endpoint must be selected to evaluate the effect of edrophonium. The examiner should focus on one or more unequivocally weak muscle groups and evaluate their strength objectively. For example, weakness of extraocular muscles, impairment of speech, or the length of time that the patient can maintain the arms in forward abduction may be useful measures. An initial dose of 2 mg of edrophonium is given intravenously. If definite improvement occurs, the test is considered positive and is terminated. If there is no change, the patient is given an additional 8 mg intravenously. The dose is administered in two parts because some patients react to edrophonium with unpleasant side effects such as nausea, diarrhea, salivation, fasciculations, and rarely with severe symptoms of syncope or bradycardia. Atropine (0.6 mg) should be drawn up in a syringe, ready for intravenous administration if these symptoms become troublesome.

False-positive tests occur in occasional patients with other neurologic disorders, such as amyotrophic lateral sclerosis, and in placebo-reactors. False-negative or equivocal tests may also occur. In some cases it is helpful to use a longer-acting drug such as neostigmine (15 mg given orally), since this permits more time for detailed evaluation

TABLE 366-1 *Diagnosis of Myasthenia Gravis (MG)*

History
  Diplopia, ptosis, weakness
  Weakness in characteristic distribution
  Fluctuation and fatigue: worse with repeated activity, improved by rest
  Effects of previous treatments
Physical examination
  Ptosis, diplopia
  Motor power survey: quantitative testing of muscle strength
  Forward arm abduction time (5 min)
  Vital capacity
  Absence of other neurologic signs
Laboratory testing
  Anti-AChR radioimmunoassay: ~85% positive in generalized MG; 50% in ocular MG; definite diagnosis if positive; negative result does not exclude MG. ~40% of AChR antibody-negative patients with generalized MG have anti-MuSK antibodies.
  Edrophonium chloride (Tensilon) 2 mg + 8 mg IV; highly probable diagnosis if unequivocally positive
  Repetitive nerve stimulation; decrement of >15% at 3 Hz: highly probable
  Single-fiber electromyography: blocking and jitter, with normal fiber density; confirmatory, but not specific
  For ocular or cranial MG: exclude intracranial lesions by CT or MRI

Note: AChR, acetylcholine receptor; CT, computed tomography; MRI, magnetic resonance imaging; MuSK, muscle specific tyrosine kinase.
Source: From DB Drachman: N Engl J Med 330:1797, 1994.

TABLE 366-2 *The Congenital Myasthenic Syndromes*

Type	Clinical Features	Electrophysiology	Genetics	End-Plate Effects	Treatment
Slow channel	Most common; weak forearm extensors; onset 2d to 3d decade; variable severity	Repetitive muscle response on nerve stimulation; prolonged channel opening and MEPP duration	Autosomal dominant; α, β, ϵ AChR mutations	Excitotoxic end-plate myopathy; decreased AChRs; postsynaptic damage	Quinidine: decreases end-plate damage; made worse by anti-AChE
Low-affinity fast channel	Onset early; moderately severe; ptosis, EOM involvement; weakness and fatigue	Brief and infrequent channel openings; opposite of slow channel syndrome	Autosomal recessive; may be heteroallelic	Normal end-plate structure	3,4-DAP; anti-AChE
Severe AChR deficiencies	Early onset; variable severity; fatigue; typical MG features	Decremental response to repetitive nerve stimulation; decreased MEPP amplitudes	Autosomal recessive; ϵ mutations most common; many different mutations	Increased length of end plates; variable synaptic folds	Anti-AChE; ?3,4-DAP
AChE deficiency	Early onset; variable severity; scoliosis; may have normal EOM, absent pupillary responses	Decremental response to repetitive nerve stimulation	Mutant gene for AChE's collagen anchor	Small nerve terminals; degenerated junctional folds	Worse with anti-AChE drugs

Abbreviations: AChR, acetylcholine receptor; AChE, acetylcholinesterase; EOM, extraocular muscles; MEPP, miniature end-plate potentials; 3,4-DAP, 3-4-Diaminopyridine.

of strength. In virtually all instances, it is desirable to carry out further testing to establish the diagnosis of MG definitively.

Electrodiagnostic Testing Repetitive nerve stimulation often provides helpful diagnostic evidence of MG. Anti-AChE medication is stopped 6 to 24 h before testing. It is best to test weak muscles or proximal muscle groups. Electric shocks are delivered at a rate of two or three per second to the appropriate nerves, and action potentials are recorded from the muscles. In normal individuals, the amplitude of the evoked muscle action potentials does not change at these rates of stimulation. However, in myasthenic patients there is a rapid reduction in the amplitude of the evoked responses of >10 to 15%. As a further test, a single dose of edrophonium may be given to prevent or diminish this decremental reaction.

Antiacetylcholine Receptor Antibody As noted above, anti-AChR antibodies are detectable in the serum of ~85% of all myasthenic patients but in only about 50% of patients with weakness confined to the ocular muscles. The presence of anti-AChR antibodies is virtually diagnostic of MG, but a negative test does not exclude the disease. The measured level of anti-AChR antibody does not correspond well with the severity of MG in different patients. However, in an individual patient, a treatment-induced fall in the antibody level often correlates with clinical improvement. Recently, antibodies to muscle-specific kinase (MuSK) have been found to be present in about 40% of AChR antibody-negative patients with generalized MG, and their presence is a useful diagnostic test in these patients. MuSK antibodies are not present in AChR antibody-positive patients or in patients with MG limited to ocular muscles. The role of these antibodies in the pathogenesis of MG is as yet uncertain. However, MuSK is known to participate in clustering of AChRs at neuromuscular junctions during development.

Inherited Myasthenic Syndromes The congenital myasthenic syndromes (CMS) comprise a heterogeneous group of disorders of the neuromuscular junction that are not autoimmune but rather are due to genetic mutations in which virtually any component of the neuromuscular

junction may be affected. Alterations in function of the presynaptic nerve terminal or in the various subunits of the AChR or AChE have been identified in the various forms of CMS. These disorders share many of the clinical features of autoimmune MG, including weakness and fatigability of skeletal muscles, in some cases involving extraocular muscles (EOMs), lids, and proximal muscles, similar to the distribution in autoimmune MG. CMS should be suspected when symptoms of myasthenia have begun in infancy or childhood and AChR antibody tests are consistently negative. Features of four of the most common forms of CMS are summarized in Table 366-2. Although clinical features and electrodiagnostic and pharmacologic tests may suggest the correct diagnosis, sophisticated electrophysiologic and molecular analysis are required for precise elucidation of the defect; this may lead to helpful treatment as well as genetic counseling. In the forms that involve the AChR, a wide variety of mutations have been identified in each of the subunits, but the ϵ subunit is affected in ~75% of these cases. In most of the recessively inherited forms of CMS, the mutations are heteroallelic; that is, different mutations affecting each of the two alleles are present.

Differential Diagnosis Other conditions that cause weakness of the cranial and/or somatic musculature include the nonautoimmune CMS discussed above, drug-induced myasthenia, Lambert-Eaton myasthenic syndrome (LEMS), neurasthenia, hyperthyroidism, botulism, intracranial mass lesions, and progressive external ophthalmoplegia. Treatment with penicillamine (used for scleroderma or rheumatoid arthritis) may result in true MG, but the weakness is usually mild, and recovery occurs within weeks or months after discontinuing its use. Aminoglycoside antibiotics or procainamide can cause exacerbation of weakness in myasthenic patients; very large doses can cause neuromuscular weakness in normal individuals.

LEMS is a presynaptic disorder of the neuromuscular junction that can cause weakness similar to that of MG. The proximal muscles of the lower limbs are most commonly affected, but other muscles may be involved as well. Cranial nerve findings, including ptosis of the eyelids and diplopia, occur in up to 70% of patients and resemble features of MG. However, the two conditions are readily distinguished, since patients with LEMS have depressed or absent reflexes, show autonomic changes such as dry mouth and impotence, and show incremental rather than decremental responses on repetitive nerve stimulation. LEMS is caused by autoantibodies directed against P/Q type calcium channels at the motor nerve terminals, which can be detected in ~85% of LEMS patients by radioimmunoassay. These autoantibodies result in impaired release of ACh from nerve terminals. A majority of patients with this syndrome have an associated malignancy, most commonly small-cell carcinoma of the lung, which is thought to trigger the autoimmune response. The diagnosis of LEMS may signal the presence of the tumor long before it would otherwise be detected, permitting early removal. Treatment of the neuromuscular disorder involves plasmapheresis and immunosuppression, as for MG. 3,4 Diaminopyridine (3,4-DAP) and pyridostigmine may be symptomatically

TABLE 366-3 *Disorders Associated with Myasthenia Gravis and Recommended Laboratory Tests*

Associated disorders
  Disorders of the thymus: thymoma, hyperplasia
  Other autoimmune disorders: Hashimoto's thyroiditis, Graves' disease, rheumatoid arthritis, lupus erythematosus, skin disorders, family history of autoimmune disorder
  Disorders or circumstances that may exacerbate myasthenia gravis: hyperthyroidism or hypothyroidism, occult infection, medical treatment for other conditions (aminoglycoside antibiotics, quinine, antiarrhythmic agents)
  Disorders that may interfere with therapy: tuberculosis, diabetes, peptic ulcer, gastrointestinal bleeding, renal disease, hypertension, asthma, osteoporosis, obesity
Recommended laboratory tests or procedures
  CT or MRI of mediastinum
  Tests for lupus erythematosus, antinuclear antibody, rheumatoid factor, antithyroid antibodies
  Thyroid-function tests
  PPD skin test
  Chest radiography
  Fasting blood glucose measurement
  Pulmonary-function tests
  Bone densitometry in older patients

Note: CT, computed tomography; MRI, magnetic resonance imaging; PPD, purified protein derivative.
Source: From RT Johnson, JW Griffin (eds): *Current Therapy in Neurologic Disease*, 4th ed. St. Louis, Mosby Year Book, 1993, p 379.

helpful in LEMS. 3,4-DAP acts by blocking potassium channels, which results in prolonged depolarization of the motor nerve terminals and thereby enhances ACh release. Pyridostigmine prolongs the action of ACh, allowing repeated interactions with AChRs.

Neurasthenia is the historic term for a myasthenia-like fatigue syndrome without an organic basis. These patients may present with subjective symptoms of weakness and fatigue, but muscle testing usually reveals the "jerky release" or "give-away weakness" characteristic of nonorganic disorders; the complaint of fatigue in these patients means tiredness or apathy rather than decreasing muscle power on repeated effort. Hyperthyroidism is readily diagnosed or excluded by tests of thyroid function, which should be carried out routinely in patients with suspected MG. Abnormalities of thyroid function (hyper- or hypothyroidism) may increase myasthenic weakness. Botulism can cause myasthenic-like weakness, but the pupils are often dilated, and repetitive nerve stimulation gives an incremental response. Diplopia that mimics the symptoms of MG may occasionally be due to an intracranial mass lesion that compresses nerves to the EOMs (e.g., sphenoid ridge meningioma), but magnetic resonance imaging (MRI) of the head and orbits usually reveals the lesion.

Progressive external ophthalmoplegia is a rare condition resulting in weakness of the EOMs, which may be accompanied by weakness of the proximal muscles of the limbs and other systemic features. Most patients with this condition have mitochondrial disorders that can be detected on muscle biopsy (Chap. 368).

Search for Associated Conditions (Table 366-3)   Myasthenic patients have an increased incidence of several associated disorders. Thymic abnormalities occur in ~75% of patients, as noted above. Neoplastic change (thymoma) may produce enlargement of the thymus, which is detected by computed tomography (CT) or MRI scanning of the anterior mediastinum. A thymic shadow on CT scan may normally be present through young adulthood, but enlargement of the thymus in a patient >40 years old is highly suspicious of thymoma. Hyperthyroidism occurs in 3 to 8% of patients and may aggravate the myasthenic weakness. Tests of thyroid function should be obtained. Because of the association of MG with other autoimmune disorders, blood tests for rheumatoid factor and antinuclear antibodies should be carried out in all patients. Chronic infection of any kind can exacerbate MG and should be sought carefully. Finally, measurements of ventilatory function are valuable because of the frequency and seriousness of respiratory impairment in myasthenic patients.

Because of the side effects of glucocorticoids and other immunosuppressive agents used in the treatment of MG, a thorough medical investigation should be undertaken, searching specifically for evidence of chronic or latent infection (such as tuberculosis or hepatitis), hypertension, diabetes, renal impairment, and glaucoma.

℞ TREATMENT

(Fig. 366-2) The prognosis has improved strikingly as a result of advances in treatment; virtually all myasthenic patients can be returned to full productive lives with proper therapy. The most useful treatments for MG include anticholinesterase medications, immunosuppressive agents, thymectomy, and plasmapheresis or intravenous immunoglobulin (IVIg).

Anticholinesterase Medications   Anticholinesterase medication produces at least partial improvement in most myasthenic patients, although improvement is complete in only a few. There is no substantial difference in efficacy among the various anticholinesterase drugs; oral pyridostigmine is the one most widely used in the United States. As a rule, the beneficial action of oral pyridostigmine begins within 15 to 30 min and lasts for 3 to 4 h, but individual responses vary. Treatment is begun with a moderate dose, e.g., 60 mg three to five times daily. The frequency and amount of the dose should be tailored to the patient's individual requirements throughout the day. For example, pa-

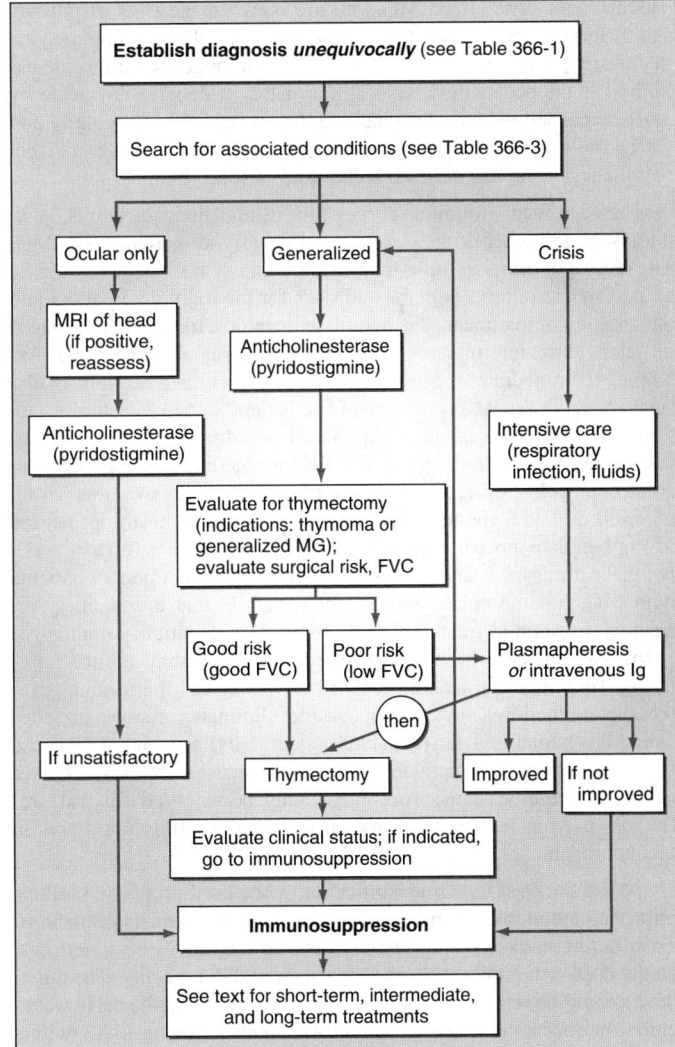

FIGURE 366-2   Algorithm for the management of myasthenia gravis. MRI, magnetic resonance imaging; FVC, forced vital capacity.

tients with weakness in chewing and swallowing may benefit by taking the medication before meals so that peak strength coincides with mealtime. Long-acting pyridostigmine may occasionally be useful to get the patient through the night but should never be used for daytime medication because of variable absorption. The maximum useful dose of pyridostigmine rarely exceeds 120 mg every 3 to 6 h during daytime. Overdosage with anticholinesterase medication may cause increased weakness and other side effects. In some patients, muscarinic side effects of the anticholinesterase medication (diarrhea, abdominal cramps, salivation, nausea) may limit the dose tolerated. Atropine/diphenoxylate or loperamide is useful for the treatment of GI symptoms.

Thymectomy   Two separate issues should be distinguished: (1) surgical removal of thymoma, and (2) thymectomy as a treatment for MG. Surgical removal of a thymoma is necessary because of the possibility of local tumor spread, although most thymomas are benign. In the absence of a tumor, the available evidence suggests that up to 85% of patients experience improvement after thymectomy; of these, ~35% achieve drug-free remission. However, the improvement is typically delayed for months to years. The advantage of thymectomy is that it offers the possibility of long-term benefit, in some cases diminishing or eliminating the need for continuing medical treatment. In view of these potential benefits and of the negligible risk in skilled hands, thymectomy has gained widespread acceptance in the treatment of MG. It is the consensus that thymectomy should be carried out in all patients with generalized MG who are between the ages of puberty and at least 55 years. Whether thymectomy should be recommended in children, in adults >55 years of age, and in patients with weakness limited to the ocular muscles is still a matter of debate. Thymectomy must be carried out in a hospital where it is performed regularly and where the staff is experienced in the pre- and postoperative management, anesthesia, and surgical techniques of total thymectomy.

Immunosuppression   Immunosuppression using glucocorticoids, azathioprine, and other drugs is effective in nearly all patients with MG. The choice of drugs or other immunomodulatory treatments should be guided by the relative benefits and risks for the individual patient and the urgency of treatment. It is helpful to develop a treatment plan based on short-term, intermediate-term, and long-term objectives. For example, if immediate improvement is essential either because of the severity of weakness or because of the patient's need to return to activity as soon as possible, IVIg should be administered or plasmapheresis should be undertaken. For the intermediate term, glucocorticoids and cyclosporine generally produce clinical improvement within a period of 1 to 3 months. The beneficial effects of azathioprine and mycophenolate mofetil usually begin after many months (up to a year), but these drugs have advantages for the long-term treatment of patients with MG. For the occasional patient with MG that is genuinely refractory to optimal treatment with conventional immunosuppressive agents, a course of high-dose cyclophosphamide may induce long-lasting (possibly permanent) benefit by "rebooting" the immune system. At high doses, cyclophosphamide eliminates mature lymphocytes, but hematopoietic precursors (stem cells) are spared, because they express the enzyme aldehyde dehydrogenase, which hydrolyzes cyclophosphamide. This procedure should be reserved for truly refractory patients and administered only in a facility fully familiar with this approach.

GLUCOCORTICOID THERAPY   Glucocorticoids, when used properly, produce improvement in myasthenic weakness in the great majority of patients. To minimize adverse side effects, prednisone should be given in a single dose rather than in divided doses throughout the day. The initial dose should be relatively low (15 to 25 mg/d) to avoid the early weakening that occurs in about one-third of patients treated initially with a high-dose regimen. The dose is increased stepwise, as tolerated by the patient (usually by 5 mg/d at 2- to 3-day intervals), until there is marked clinical improvement or a dose of 50 to 60 mg/d is reached.

This dose is maintained for 1 to 3 months and then is gradually modified to an alternate-day regimen over the course of an additional 1 to 3 months; the goal is to reduce the dose on the "off day" to zero or to a minimal level. Generally, patients begin to improve within a few weeks after reaching the maximum dose, and improvement continues to progress for months or years. The prednisone dosage may gradually be reduced, but usually months or years may be needed to determine the minimum effective dose, and close monitoring is required. Few patients are able to do without immunosuppressive agents entirely. Patients on long-term glucocorticoid therapy must be followed carefully to prevent or treat adverse side effects. The most common errors in glucocorticoid treatment of myasthenic patients include (1) insufficient persistence—improvement may be delayed and gradual; (2) too early, too rapid, or excessive tapering of dosage; and (3) lack of attention to prevention and treatment of side effects. →*The management of patients treated with glucocorticoids is discussed in Chap. 321.*

OTHER IMMUNOSUPPRESSIVE DRUGS   Azathioprine, cyclosporine, mycophenolate mofetil, or occasionally cyclophosphamide is effective in many patients, either alone or in combination with glucocorticoid therapy. Azathioprine has been the most widely used of these drugs because of its relative safety in most patients and long track record. Its therapeutic effect may add to that of glucocorticoids and/or allow the glucocorticoid dose to be reduced. However, up to 10% of patients are unable to tolerate azathioprine because of idiosyncratic reactions consisting of flulike symptoms of fever and malaise, bone marrow depression, or abnormalities of liver function. An initial dose of 50 mg/d should be used to test for adverse side effects. If this dose is tolerated, it is increased gradually until the white blood count falls to ~3000 to 4000/μL. In patients who are receiving glucocorticoids concurrently, leukocytosis precludes the use of this measure. A reduction of the lymphocyte count to <1000/μL and/or an increase of the mean corpuscular volume of red blood cells may be used as indications of adequacy of azathioprine dosage. The typical dosage range is 2 to 3 mg/kg total body weight. The beneficial effect of azathioprine takes at least 3 to 6 months to begin and even longer to peak. In patients taking azathioprine, allopurinol should never be used to treat hyperuricemia, because the two drugs share a common degradation pathway; the result may be severe bone marrow depression due to increased effects of the azathioprine.

Cyclosporine is approximately as effective as azathioprine and is being used increasingly in the management of MG. Its beneficial effect appears more rapidly than that of azathioprine. It may be used alone but is usually used as an adjunct to glucocorticoids to permit reduction of the glucocorticoid dose. The usual dose of cyclosporine is 4 to 5 mg/kg per day, given in two equally divided doses (to minimize side effects). Side effects of cyclosporine include hypertension and nephrotoxicity, which must be closely monitored. "Trough" blood levels of cyclosporine are measured 12 h after the evening dose. The therapeutic range, as measured by radioimmunoassay, is 150 to 200 ng/L.

Mycophenolate mofetil is also useful in the treatment of MG. A dose of 1 g to 1.5 g bid is recommended. Its mechanism of action involves inhibition of purine synthesis by the de novo pathway. Since lymphocytes lack the alternative salvage pathway that is present in all other cells, mycophenolate inhibits proliferation of lymphocytes but not proliferation of other cells. It does not kill or eliminate preexisting autoreactive lymphocytes, and therefore clinical improvement may be delayed for many months to a year, until the preexisting autoreactive lymphocytes die spontaneously. The advantage of mycophenolate lies in its relative lack of adverse side effects, with only occasional production of diarrhea and rare development of leukopenia. This drug may become the choice for long-term treatment of myasthenic patients. Unfortunately, the present cost of mycophenolate may be prohibitively high.

Cyclophosphamide is reserved for occasional patients refractory to the other drugs (see above for discussion of high-dose cyclophosphamide treatment).

Myasthenia Gravis Worksheet

History				
General	Normal	Good	Fair	Poor
Diplopia	None	Rare	Occasional	Constant
Ptosis	None	Rare	Occasional	Constant
Arms	Normal	Slightly limited	Some ADL impairment	Definitely limited
Legs	Normal	Walks/runs fatigues	Can walk limited distances	Minimal walking
Speech	Normal	Dysarthric	Severely dysarthric	Unintelligible
Voice	Normal	Fades	Impaired	Severely impaired
Chew	Normal	Fatigue on normal foods	Fatigue on soft foods	Feeding tube
Swallow	Normal	Normal foods	Soft foods only	Feeding tube
Respiration	Normal	Dyspnea on unusual effort	Dyspnea on any effort	Dyspnea at rest

Examination

BP _____ Pulse _____ Wt _____   Arm abduction time R_____ L_____
Edema _____   Deltoids   R_____ L_____
Vital capacity_____   Biceps   R_____ L_____
Cataracts? R _____ L _____   Triceps   R_____ L_____
EOMS _____   Grip   R_____ L_____
Ptosis time _____   Iliopsoas   R_____ L_____
Face _____   Quadriceps   R_____ L_____
                                           Hamstrings   R_____ L_____
                                           Other   R_____ L_____

FIGURE 366-3   *Abbreviated interval assessment form for use in evaluating treatment for myasthenia gravis.*

Plasmapheresis and Intravenous Immunoglobulin   Plasmapheresis has been used therapeutically in MG. Plasma, which contains the pathogenic antibodies, is mechanically separated from the blood cells, which are returned to the patient. A course of five exchanges (3 to 4 L per exchange) is generally administered over a 2-week period. Plasmapheresis produces a short-term reduction in anti-AChR antibodies, with clinical improvement in many patients. It is useful as a temporary expedient in seriously affected patients or to improve the patient's condition prior to surgery (e.g., thymectomy).

The indications for the use of IVIg are the same as those for plasma exchange: to produce rapid improvement to help the patient through a difficult period of myasthenic weakness or prior to surgery. This treatment has the advantages of not requiring special equipment or large-bore venous access. The usual dose is 2 g/kg, which is typically administered over 5 days (400 mg/kg per day). If tolerated, the course of IVIg can be shortened to administer the entire dose over a 3-day period. Improvement occurs in about 70% of patients, beginning during treatment, or within 4 to 5 days thereafter, and continuing for weeks to months. The mechanism of action of IVIg is not known; the treatment has no consistent effect on the measurable amount of circulating AChR antibody. Adverse reactions are generally not serious but include headache, fluid overload, and rarely aseptic meningitis or renal shutdown. IVIg should rarely be used as a long-term treatment in place of rationally managed immunosuppressive therapy. Unfortunately, there is a growing tendency for physicians unfamiliar with immunosuppressive treatments to rely on repeated IVIg infusions, which are inconvenient, usually produce only intermittent benefit, and are costly. The intermediate and long-term treatment of myasthenic patients requires other methods of therapy outlined earlier in this chapter.

Management of Myasthenic Crisis   Myasthenic crisis is defined as an exacerbation of weakness sufficient to endanger life; it usually consists of respiratory failure caused by diaphragmatic and intercostal muscle weakness. Crisis rarely occurs in properly managed patients. Treatment should be carried out in an intensive care unit staffed with physicians experienced in the management of MG, respiratory insufficiency, infectious disease, and fluid and electrolyte therapy. The possibility that the deterioration could be due to excessive anticholinesterase medication ("cholinergic crisis") is best excluded by temporarily stopping anticholinesterase drugs. The most common cause of crisis is intercurrent infection. This should be treated immediately, because the mechanical and immunologic defenses of the patient can be assumed to be compromised. The myasthenic patient with fever and early infection should be treated like other immunocompromised patients. Early and effective antibiotic therapy, respiratory assistance, and pulmonary physiotherapy are essentials of the treatment program. As discussed above, plasmapheresis or IVIg is frequently helpful in hastening recovery.

PATIENT ASSESSMENT   In order to evaluate the effectiveness of treatment as well as drug-induced side effects, it is important to assess the patient's clinical status at baseline and on repeated interval examinations in a systematic manner. Because of the variability of symptoms of MG, the interval history as well as findings on examination must be taken into account. The most useful clinical tests include forward arm abduction time (up to a full 5 min), forced vital capacity, range of eye movements, and time to development of ptosis on upward gaze. Manual muscle testing or, preferably, quantitative dynamometry of limb muscles, especially proximal muscles, is also important. An interval form can provide a succinct summary of the patient's status and a guide to treatment results; an abbreviated form is shown in Fig. 366-3. A progressive reduction in the patient's AChR antibody level also provides clinically valuable confirmation of the effectiveness of treatment; conversely, a rise in AChR antibody levels during tapering of immunosuppressive medication may predict clinical exacerbation. For reliable quantitative measurement of AChR antibody levels, it is best to compare antibody levels from prior frozen serum aliquots with current serum samples in simultaneously run assays.

FURTHER READING

DRACHMAN DB et al: Treatment of refractory myasthenia gravis: "Rebooting" with high dose cyclophosphamide. Ann Neurol 53:29, 2003

KAMINSKI HJ: *Myasthenia Gravis and Related Disorders.* Totowa, NJ, Humana Press, 2003

KUPERSMITH MJ et al: Development of generalized disease at 2 years in patients with ocular myasthenia gravis. Arch Neurol 60:243, 2003

LINDSTROM JM: Acetylcholine receptors and myasthenia. Muscle Nerve 23:453, 2000

Skeletal muscle diseases, or myopathies, are disorders with structural changes or functional impairment of muscle. These conditions can be differentiated from other diseases of the motor unit (e.g., lower motor neuron or neuromuscular junction pathologies) by characteristic clinical and laboratory findings. →*Myasthenia gravis and related disorders are discussed in Chap. 366; musclar dystrophies and inherited, metabolic, and toxic myopathies in Chap. 368; inflammatory muscle diseases and inclusion body myositis in Chap. 369.*

CLINICAL FEATURES ■ **Muscle Weakness** Symptoms of muscle weakness can be either intermittent or persistent. Disorders causing *intermittent weakness* (Fig. 367-1) include myasthenia gravis, periodic paralyses (hypokalemic, hyperkalemic, and paramyotonia congenita), and metabolic energy deficiencies of glycolysis (especially myophosphorylase deficiency) and fatty acid utilization (carnitine palmitoyltransferase deficiency). The states of energy deficiency cause activity-related muscle breakdown accompanied by myoglobinuria, appearing as light-brown- to dark-brown-colored urine. Most muscle disorders cause *persistent weakness* (Fig. 367-2). In the majority of these, including most types of muscular dystrophy, polymyositis, and dermatomyositis, the proximal muscles are weaker than the distal, and the facial muscles are spared, a pattern referred to as *limb-girdle*. The differential diagnosis is more restricted for other patterns of weakness. Facial weakness (difficulty with eye closure and impaired smile) and scapular winging (Fig. 367-3) are characteristic of facioscapulohumeral dystrophy. Facial and distal limb weakness associated with hand grip myotonia is virtually diagnostic of myotonic dystrophy. When other cranial nerve muscles are weak, causing ptosis and extraocular muscle weakness without diplopia, the most important disorders to consider include oculopharyngeal muscular dystrophy, mitochondrial myopathies, or myotubular myopathy. A pathognomonic pattern exclusive to inclusion body myositis includes loss of strength in both proximal and distal muscles, hand grip weakness, and wasting of quadriceps muscles. Less frequently, but important diagnostically, is the presence of a dropped head syndrome indicative of selective neck extensor muscle weakness. The most common neuromuscular diseases causing this pattern of weakness include myasthenia gravis, polymyositis, and amyotrophic lateral sclerosis. A final pattern, recognized because of preferential distal extremity weakness, is typical of a unique category of muscular dystrophy, the distal myopathies (Chap. 368).

It is important to examine functional capabilities to help disclose certain patterns of weakness (Table 367-1). The Gowers' sign (Fig. 367-4) is particularly useful. Observing the gait of an individual may disclose a lordotic posture caused by combined trunk and hip weakness, frequently exaggerated by toe walking (Fig. 367-5). A waddling gait is caused by the inability of weak hip muscles to prevent hip drop or hip dip. Hyperextension of the knee (genu recurvatum or back-kneeing) is characteristic of quadriceps muscle weakness; and a steppage gait, due to footdrop, accompanies distal weakness.

Any disorder causing muscle weakness may be accompanied by *fatigue*, referring to an inability to maintain or sustain a force (pathologic fatigability). This condition must be differentiated from asthenia, a type of fatigue caused by excess tiredness or lack of energy. Associated symptoms may help differentiate asthenia and pathologic fatigability. Asthenia is often accompanied by a tendency to avoid physical activities, complaints of daytime sleepiness, necessity for frequent naps, and difficulty concentrating on activities such as reading. There may be feelings of overwhelming stress and depression. Thus, asthenia is not a myopathy. In contrast, pathologic fatigability occurs in disorders of neuromuscular transmission and in disorders altering energy production, including defects in glycolysis, lipid metabolism, or mitochondrial energy production. Pathologic fatigability also occurs in chronic myopathies because of difficulty accomplishing a task with less muscle. Pathologic fatigability is accompanied by abnormal clinical or laboratory findings. Fatigue without those supportive features almost never indicates a primary muscle disease.

Muscle Pain (Myalgias), Cramps, and Stiffness Muscle pain can be associated with cramps, spasms, contractures, and stiff or rigid muscles (Chap. 21). In distinction, true myalgia (muscle aching), which can be localized or generalized, may be accompanied by weakness, tenderness to palpation, or swelling. Certain drugs cause true myalgia (Table 367-2).

There are two painful muscle conditions of particular importance, neither of which is associated with muscle weakness. *Fibromyalgia* is a common, yet poorly understood type of myofascial pain syndrome.

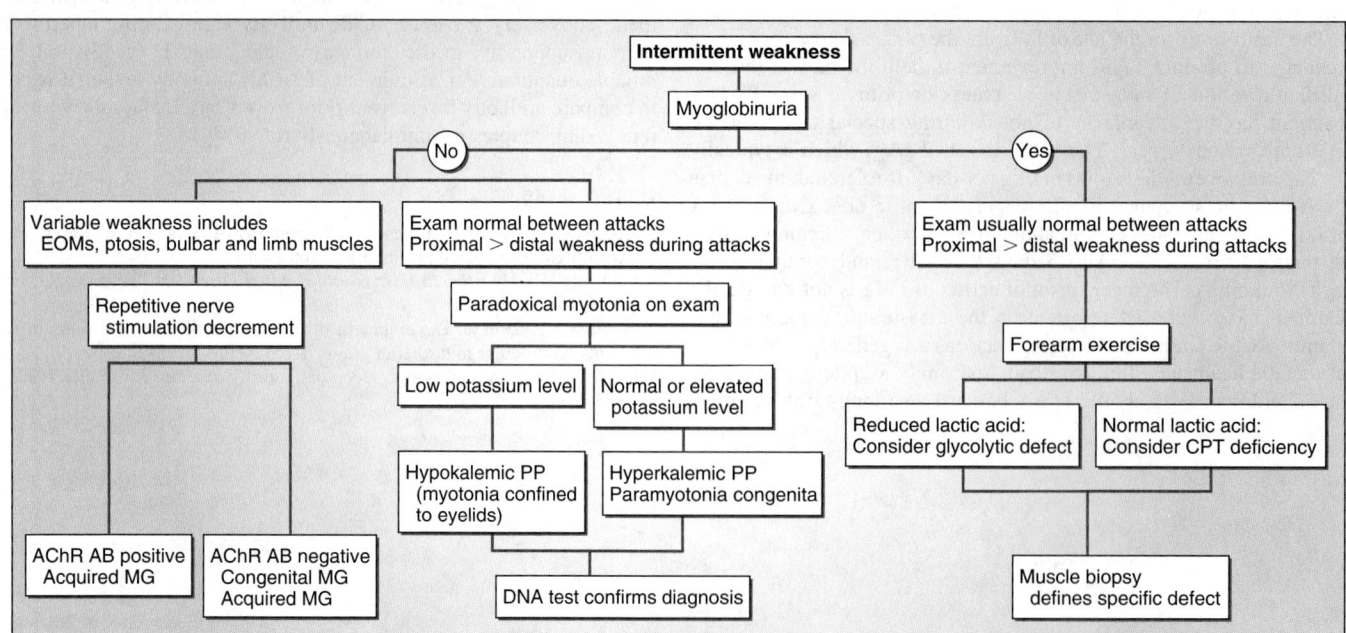

FIGURE 367-1 Diagnostic evaluation of intermittent weakness. EOMs, extraocular muscles; AChR AB, acetylcholine receptor antibody; PP, periodic paralysis; CPT, carnitine palmitoyltransferase; MG, myasthenia gravis.

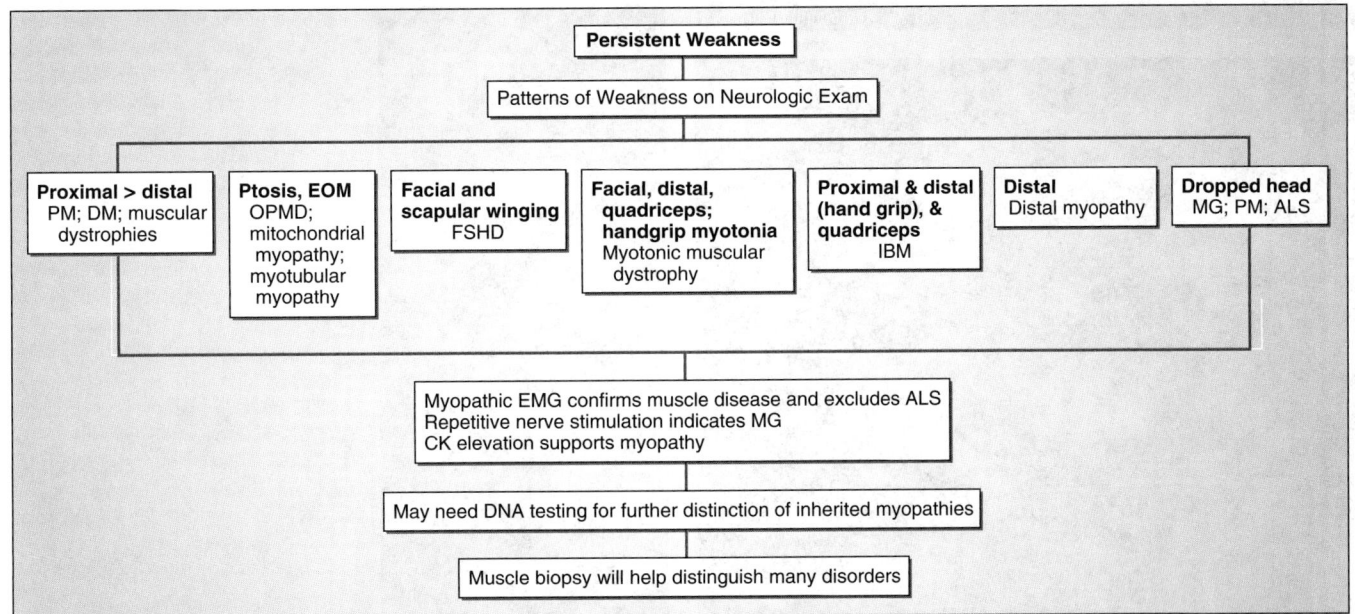

FIGURE 367-2 Diagnostic evaluation of persistent weakness. Examination reveals one of seven patterns of weakness. The pattern of weakness in combination with the laboratory evaluation leads to a diagnosis. EOM, extraocular muscle; OPMD, oculophar-yngeal muscular dystrophy; FSHD, facioscapulohumeral muscular dystrophy; IBM, inclusion body myositis; DM, dermatomyositis; PM, polymyositis; MG, myasthenia gravis; ALS, amyotrophic lateral sclerosis; CK, creatine kinase.

Patients complain of severe muscle pain and tenderness and have specific painful trigger points, sleep disturbances, and easy fatigability. Serum creatine kinase (CK) and erythrocyte sedimentation rate (ESR) are normal (Chap. 315). *Polymyalgia rheumatica* occurs mainly in patients >50 years and is characterized by stiffness and pain in the shoulders, lower back, hips, and thighs (Chap. 306). The ESR is elevated, while serum CK, electromyography (EMG), and muscle biopsy are normal. Temporal arteritis, an inflammatory disorder of medium- and large-sized arteries, usually involving one or more branches of the carotid artery, may accompany polymyalgia rheumatica. Vision is threatened due to ischemic optic neuritis. Glucocorticoids can relieve the myalgias and protect against visual loss.

Localized muscle pain is most often traumatic. A common cause of sudden abrupt-onset pain is a ruptured tendon, which leaves the muscle belly appearing rounded and shorter in appearance compared to the normal side. The biceps brachii and Achilles tendons are particularly vulnerable to rupture. Infection or neoplastic infiltration of the muscle is a rare cause of localized muscle pain.

A *muscle cramp* or *spasm* is a painful, involuntary, localized, muscle contraction with a visible or palpable hardening of the muscle. Cramps are abrupt in onset, short in duration, and may cause abnormal posturing of the joint. The EMG shows firing of motor units, reflecting an origin from spontaneous neural discharge. Muscle cramps often occur in neurogenic disorders, especially motor neuron disease (Chap. 353), radiculopathies, and polyneuropathies (Chap. 363), but are not a feature of most primary muscle diseases. Duchenne muscular dystrophy (Chap. 368) is an exception since calf muscle complaints are a common complaint. Muscle cramps are also common during pregnancy.

A *muscle contracture* is different from a muscle cramp. In both conditions, the muscle becomes hard, but a contracture is associated with energy failure in glycolytic disorders. The muscle is unable to relax after an active muscle contraction. The EMG shows electrical silence. Confusion is created because contracture also refers to a muscle that cannot be passively stretched to its proper length (fixed contracture) because of fibrosis. In some muscle disorders, especially Emery-Dreifuss muscular dystrophy and Bethlem myopathy (Chap.

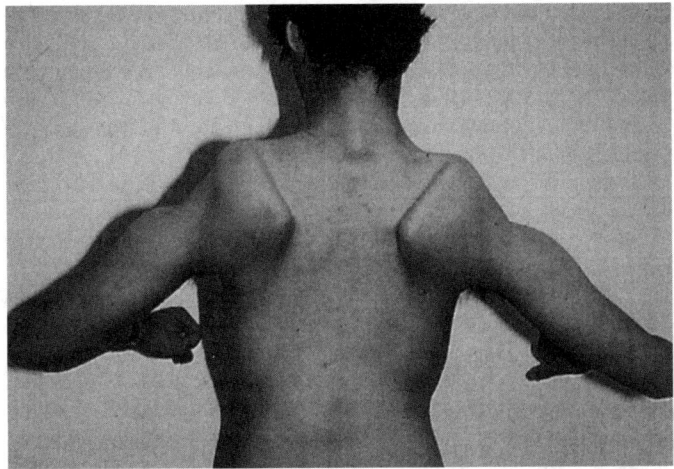

FIGURE 367-3 Facioscapulohumeral dystrophy with prominent scapular winging.

TABLE 367-1 *Observations on Examination That Disclose Muscle Weakness*

Functional Impairment	Muscle Weakness
Inability to forcibly close eyes	Upper facial muscles
Impaired pucker	Lower facial muscles
Inability to raise head from prone position	Neck extensor muscles
Inability to raise head from supine position	Neck flexor muscles
Inability to raise arms above head	Proximal arm muscles (may be only scapular stabilizing muscles)
Inability to walk without hyperextending knee (backkneeing or genu recurvatum)	Knee extensor muscles
Inability to walk with heels touching the floor (toe walking)	Shortening of the Achilles tendon
Inability to lift foot while walking (steppage gait or footdrop)	Anterior compartment of leg
Inability to walk without a waddling gait	Hip muscles
Inability to get up from the floor without climbing up the extremities (Gowers' sign)	Hip muscles
Inability to get up from a chair without using arms	Hip muscles

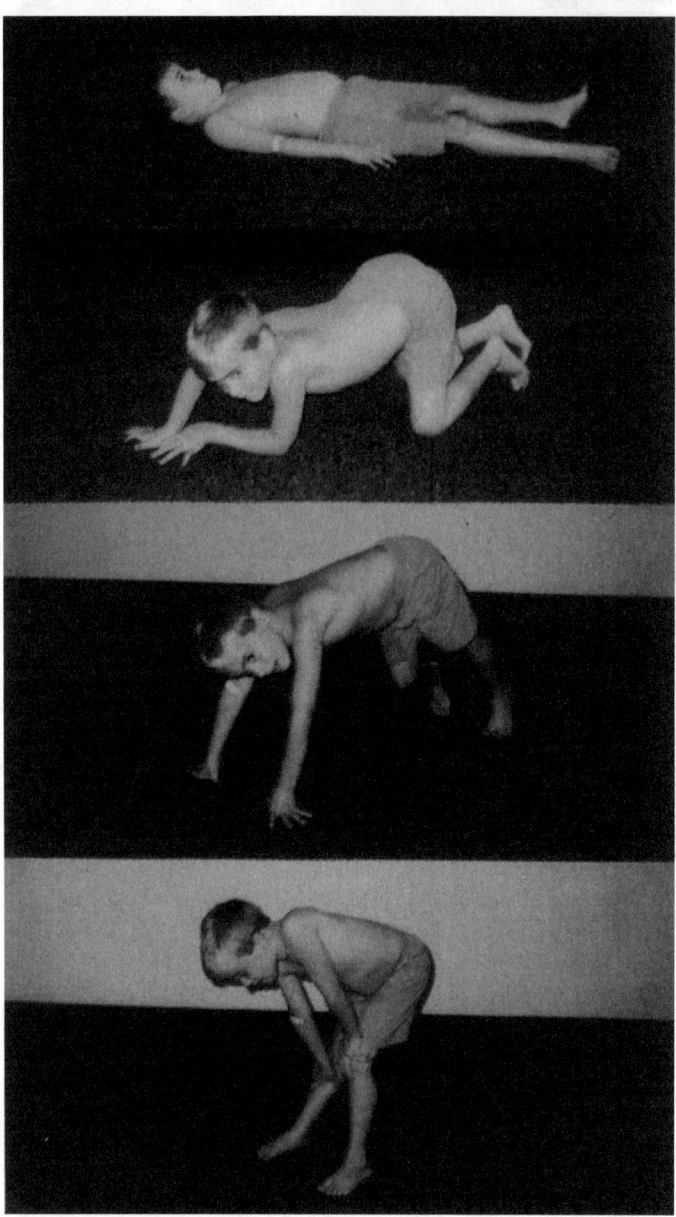

FIGURE 367-4 Gowers' sign showing a patient using arms to climb up the legs in attempting to get up from the floor.

368), fixed contractures occur early and represent distinctive features of the disease.

Muscle stiffness can refer to different phenomena. Some patients with inflammation of joints and periarticular surfaces feel stiff. This condition is different from the disorders of hyperexcitable motor nerves causing stiff or rigid muscles (Chap. 21). In *stiff-person syndrome* spontaneous discharges of the motor neurons of the spinal cord cause involuntary muscle contractions mainly involving the axial (trunk) and proximal lower extremity muscles. The gait becomes stiff and labored, with hyperlordosis of the lumbar spine. Superimposed episodic muscle spasms are precipitated by sudden movements, unexpected noises, and emotional upset. The muscles relax during sleep. Serum antiglutamic acid decarboxylase antibodies are present in approximately two-thirds of cases. In *neuromyotonia* (*Isaac's syndrome*) there is hyperexcitability of the peripheral nerves manifesting as continuous muscle fiber activity. *Myokymia* (continuous undulations of muscle) and impaired muscle relaxation are the result. Muscles of the leg are stiff, and the constant contractions of the muscle cause increased sweating of the extremities. This peripheral nerve hyperexcit-

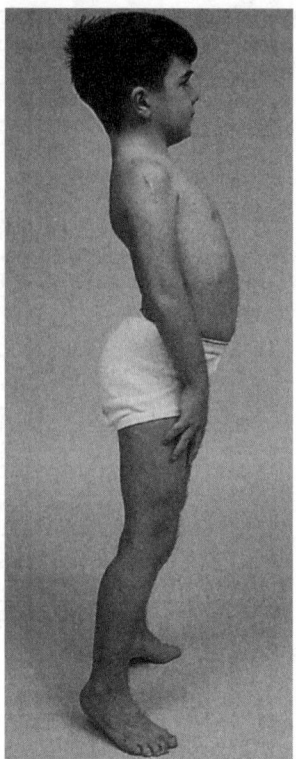

FIGURE 367-5 Lordotic posture, exaggerated by standing on toes, associated with trunk and hip weakness.

ability is antibody-mediated, targeted against voltage-gated potassium channels. The site of origin of the spontaneous nerve discharges is principally in the distal portion of the motor nerves.

Myotonia is a condition of prolonged muscle contraction followed by slow muscle relaxation. It always follows muscle activation, usually voluntary, but may be elicited by mechanical stimulation (percussion myotonia) of the muscle. Myotonia typically causes difficulty in releasing objects after a firm grasp. In myotonic muscular dystrophy, weakness accompanies myotonia. Myotonia also occurs with *myotonia congenita* (a chloride channel disorder), but in this condition muscle weakness is not prominent. *Paramyotonia congenita* (a sodium channel disorder more closely aligned with hyperkalemic periodic paralysis) is named for a paradoxical phenomenon whereby the prolonged muscle contraction, with features virtually indistinguishable from myotonia, is exacerbated by repeated muscle contractions (Chap. 368). In hypokalemic periodic paralysis, myotonia of the eyelids may be present but limb muscles are usually spared.

Muscle Enlargement and Atrophy In most myopathies muscle tissue is replaced by fat and connective tissue, but the size of the muscle is usually not affected. However, in Duchenne and Becker muscular dystrophies, enlarged calf muscles are typical. In the patients with these forms of dystrophy, the enlargement represents true muscle hypertrophy; hence the term "pseudohypertrophy" should be avoided when referring to these patients. The calf muscles remain very strong even late in the course of these disorders. Muscle enlargement can also result from infiltration by sarcoid granulomas, amyloid deposits, bacterial and parasitic infections, and focal myositis.

TABLE 367-2 *Drugs That Cause True Myalgia*

Statins[a]	Emetine
Gemfibrozil	Labetalol
Vincristine	Nifedipine
Zidovudine	D-Penicillamine
Cyclosporine	L-Tryptophan
Gold	Epsilon aminocaproic acid
Danazol	Heroin
Cimetidine	Cocaine
	Methadone

[a] 3-Hydroxy-3-methylglutaryl coenzyme A reductase inhibitors.

LABORATORY EVALUATION   A limited battery of tests can be used to evaluate a suspected myopathy. Nearly all patients require serum enzyme level measurements and electrodiagnostic studies as screening tools to differentiate muscle disorders from other motor unit diseases. The other tests described—DNA studies, the forearm exercise test, and muscle biopsy—are used to diagnose specific types of myopathies.

Serum Enzymes   CK is the preferred muscle enzyme to measure in the evaluation of myopathies. Damage to muscle causes the CK to leak from the muscle fiber to the serum. The MM isoenzyme predominates in skeletal muscle, while CK-MB is the marker for cardiac muscle. Serum CK can be elevated in normal individuals without provocation, presumably on a genetic basis or after strenuous activity, minor trauma (including the EMG needle), a prolonged muscle cramp, or a generalized seizure. Aspartate aminotransferase (AST), alanine aminotransferase (ALT), and lactic dehydrogenase (LDH) are enzymes sharing an origin in both muscle and liver. Problems arise when the levels of these enzymes are found to be elevated in a routine screening battery, leading to the erroneous assumption that liver disease is present when in fact muscle could be the cause. An elevated gamma-glutamyl transferase (GGT) helps to establish a liver origin since this enzyme is not found in muscle. Aldolase is often thought to be a muscle-specific enzyme but is also present in liver.

Electrodiagnostic Studies   EMG, repetitive nerve stimulation, and nerve conduction studies (Chap. 363) are essential methods for evaluation of the patient with suspected muscle disease. In combination they provide the information necessary to differentiate myopathies from neuropathies and neuromuscular junction diseases. Certain features of the EMG will point to an acquired, inflammatory muscle disorder (e.g., irritability on needle placement) versus a long-standing myopathic disorder (lack of irritability) that is more suggestive of a dystrophic process. Both inflammatory and noninflammatory myopathies share findings characterized by excessively recruited (too many) compound muscle action potentials for the degree of effort expended. This degree of recruitment is necessary to compensate for loss of muscle fibers related to the underlying process. The EMG can also be invaluable in helping to choose an appropriately affected muscle to sample for biopsy. The EMG can be used to fully characterize suspected involuntary activity seen during the examination, such as myokymia and myotonia.

DNA Analysis   Advances in molecular diagnosis have evolved over the past decade and now serve as important tools for diagnosis. Certain muscle disorders can be definitively diagnosed by DNA analysis; these are fully discussed in Chap. 368. Nevertheless, important limitations need to be mentioned in seeking a molecular diagnosis. For example, in some disorders, such as Duchenne and Becker dystrophies, two-thirds of patients have deletion- or duplication-mutations that are easy to detect, while the remainder have point mutations that are much more difficult to find. For patients without identifiable gene defects, the muscle biopsy remains the main diagnostic tool.

Forearm Exercise Test   In myopathies with intermittent symptoms, and especially those associated with myoglobinuria, there may be a defect in glycolysis. Many variations of the forearm exercise test exist. For safety, the test should not be performed under ischemic conditions to avoid an unnecessary insult to the muscle, causing rhabdomyolysis. The test is performed by placing a small indwelling catheter into an antecubital vein. A baseline blood sample is obtained for lactic acid and ammonia. The forearm muscles are exercised by asking the patient to vigorously squeeze a sphygmomanometer bulb for 1 min. Blood is then obtained at intervals of 1, 2, 4, 6, and 10 min for comparison with the baseline sample. Normal controls must be established for each laboratory. A three- to fourfold rise of lactic acid is typical. The simultaneous measurement of ammonia serves as a control, since it should also rise with exercise. In patients with myophosphorylase deficiency or other glycolytic defects (Chap. 368), the lactic acid rise will be absent or below normal, while the rise in ammonia will reach control values. If there is lack of effort, neither lactic acid nor ammonia will rise. Patients with selective failure to increase ammonia may have myoadenylate deaminase deficiency. This condition has been reported to be a cause of myoglobinuria, but deficiency of this enzyme in asymptomatic individuals makes interpretation controversial.

Muscle Biopsy   Muscle biopsy analysis is an important step in establishing the final diagnosis of suspected myopathy. The microscopic evaluation uses a combination of techniques—histochemistry, immunocytochemistry with a battery of antibodies, and electron microscopy. Not all techniques need to be used on every case. A specific diagnosis can be established in many disorders. A combination of stains to identify mononuclear cells (polymyositis), complement (dermatomyositis), and amyloid (inclusion body myositis) helps to distinguish the inflammatory myopathies. Mitochondrial and metabolic (e.g., myophosphorylase and acid maltase deficiencies) myopathies demonstrate distinctive histochemical and electron-microscopic profiles. A battery of antibodies is available for the identification of missing components of the dystrophin-glycoprotein complex and related proteins to help diagnose specific types of muscular dystrophies. In addition, the congenital myopathies have distinctive histologic features essential for diagnosis.

FURTHER READING

DAUBE JR: Myokymia and neuromyotonia. Muscle Nerve 24:1711, 2001

GRIGGS RC et al: Evaluation of the patient with myopathy, in *Evaluation and Treatment of Myopathies*, RC Griggs et al (eds). Philadelphia, FA Davis, 1995, pp 17–77

MEINCK HM, THOMPSON PD: Stiff man syndrome and related conditions. Mov Disord 17:853, 2002

THOMPSON PD et al: Statin-associated myopathy. JAMA 289:1681, 2003

VERNINO S, LENNON VA: Ion channel and striational antibodies define a continuum of autoimmune neuromuscular hyperexcitability. Muscle Nerve 26:70, 2002

368   MUSCULAR DYSTROPHIES AND OTHER MUSCLE DISEASES
Robert H. Brown, Jr., Jerry R. Mendell

The muscle disorders discussed in this chapter include diseases that cause acute, subacute, and chronic muscle weakness. Some cause pain in addition to or instead of weakness. →*Dermatomyositis and polymyositis are discussed in Chap. 369.*

HEREDITARY MYOPATHIES

Muscular dystrophy refers to a group of hereditary progressive diseases each with unique phenotypic and genetic features (Table 368-1).

DUCHENNE MUSCULAR DYSTROPHY   This X-linked recessive disorder, sometimes also called *pseudohypertrophic muscular dystrophy*, has an incidence of ~30 per 100,000 live-born males.

Clinical Features   Duchenne dystrophy is present at birth, but the disorder usually becomes apparent between ages 3 and 5. The boys fall frequently and have difficulty keeping up with friends when playing. Running, jumping, and hopping are invariably abnormal. By age 5, muscle weakness is obvious by muscle testing. On getting up from the floor, the patient uses his hands to climb up himself [Gowers' maneu-

TABLE 368-1 *Progressive Muscular Dystrophies*

Type	Inheritance	Defective Gene/Protein	Onset Age	Clinical Features	Other Organ Systems Involved
Duchenne	XR	Dystrophin	Before 5 years	Progressive weakness of girdle muscles Unable to walk after age 12 Progressive kyphoscoliosis Respiratory failure in 2d or 3d decade	Cardiomyopathy Mental impairment
Becker	XR	Dystrophin	Early childhood to adult	Progressive weakness of girdle muscles Able to walk after age 15 Respiratory failure may develop by 4th decade	Cardiomyopathy
Limb-girdle	AD/AR	Several (Tables 368-2, 368-3)	Early childhood to early adult	Slow progressive weakness of shoulder and hip girdle muscles	± Cardiomyopathy
Emery-Dreifuss	XR/AD	Emerin/Lamins A/C	Childhood to adult	Elbow contractures, humeral and peroneal weakness	Cardiomyopathy
Congenital	AR	Several	At birth or within first few months	Hypotonia, contractures, delayed milestones Progression to respiratory failure in some; static course in others	CNS abnormalities (hypomyelination, malformation) Eye abnormalities
Myotonic[a] (DM1, DM2)	AD	DM1: Expansion CTG repeat DM2: Expansion CCTG repeat	Usually 2d decade May be infancy if mother affected (DM1 only)	Slowly progressive weakness of face, shoulder girdle, and foot dorsiflexion Preferential proximal weakness in DM2	Cardiac conduction defects Mental impairment Cataracts Frontal baldness Gonadal atrophy Deafness Coats' (eye) disease
Facioscapulohumeral	AD	Deletion, distal 4q	Before age 20	Slowly progressive weakness of face, shoulder girdle, and foot dorsiflexion	
Oculopharyngeal	AD	Expansion, poly-A RNA binding protein	5th to 6th decade	Slowly progressive weakness of extraocular, pharyngeal, and limb muscles	—

[a] Two forms of myotonic dystrophy, DM1 and DM2, have been identified. Many features overlap (see text).
Abbreviations: XR, X-linked recessive; AD, autosomal dominant; AR, autosomal recessive; CNS, central nervous system.

ver (Fig. 367-4)]. Contractures of the heel cords and iliotibial bands become apparent by age 6, when toe walking is associated with a lordotic posture. Loss of muscle strength is progressive, with predilection for proximal limb muscles and the neck flexors; leg involvement is more severe than arm involvement. Between ages 8 and 10 walking may require the use of braces; joint contractures and limitations of hip flexion, knee, elbow, and wrist extension are made worse by prolonged sitting. By age 12, most patients are wheelchair dependent. Contractures become fixed, and a progressive scoliosis often develops that may be associated with pain. The chest deformity with scoliosis impairs pulmonary function, which is already diminished by muscle weakness. By age 16 to 18, patients are predisposed to serious, sometimes fatal pulmonary infections. Other causes of death include aspiration of food and acute gastric dilation.

A cardiac cause of death is uncommon despite the presence of a cardiomyopathy in almost all patients. Congestive heart failure seldom occurs except with severe stress such as pneumonia. Cardiac arrhythmias are rare. The typical electrocardiogram (ECG) shows an increase net RS in lead V_1; deep, narrow Q waves in the precordial leads; and tall right precordial R waves in V_1. Intellectual impairment in Duchenne dystrophy is common; the average intelligence quotient (IQ) is approximately one standard deviation below the mean. Impairment of intellectual function appears to be nonprogressive and affects verbal ability more than performance.

Laboratory Features Serum creatine kinase (CK) levels are invariably elevated to between 20 and 100 times normal. The levels are abnormal at birth but decline late in the disease because of inactivity and loss

of muscle mass. Electromyography (EMG) demonstrates features typical of myopathy. The muscle biopsy shows muscle fibers of varying size as well as small groups of necrotic and regenerating fibers. Connective tissue and fat replace lost muscle fibers. A definitive diagnosis of Duchenne dystrophy can be established on the basis of dystrophin deficiency in a biopsy of muscle tissue or mutation analysis on peripheral blood leukocytes as discussed below.

GENETIC CONSIDERATIONS Duchenne dystrophy is caused by a mutation of the gene that encodes dystrophin, a 427-kDa protein localized to the inner surface of the sarcolemma of the muscle fiber. The dystrophin gene is >2000 kb in size and thus is one of the largest identified human genes. It is localized to the short arm of the X chromosome at Xp21. The most common gene mutation is a deletion. The size varies but does not correlate with disease severity. Deletions are not uniformly distributed over the gene but rather are most common near the beginning (5' end) and middle of the gene. Less often, Duchenne dystrophy is caused by a gene duplication or point mutation. Identification of a specific mutation allows for an unequivocal diagnosis, makes possible accurate testing of potential carriers, and is useful for prenatal diagnosis.

A diagnosis of Duchenne dystrophy can also be made by western blot analysis of muscle biopsy specimens, revealing abnormalities on the quantity and molecular weight of dystrophin protein. In addition, immunocytochemical staining of muscle with dystrophin antibodies can be used to demonstrate absence or deficiency of dystrophin localizing to the sarcolemmal membrane. Carriers of the disease may demonstrate a mosaic pattern, but dystrophin analysis of muscle biopsy specimens for carrier detection is not reliable.

Pathogenesis Dystrophin is part of a large complex of sarcolemmal proteins and glycoproteins (Fig. 368-1). Dystrophin binds to F-actin at its amino terminus and to β-dystroglycan at the carboxyl terminus. β-Dystroglycan complexes to α-dystroglycan, which binds to laminin in the extracellular matrix (ECM). Laminin has a heterotrimeric molecular structure arranged in the shape of a cross with one heavy chain and two light chains, β1 and γ1. The laminin heavy chain of skeletal muscle is designated laminin α2. Collagen proteins IV and VI are also found in the ECM. Like β-dystroglycan, the transmembrane sarcoglycan proteins also bind to dystrophin; these five proteins (designated α- through ε-sarcoglycan) complex tightly with each other. More recently, other membrane proteins implicated in muscular dystrophy have been found to be loosely affiliated with constituents of the dystrophin complex. These include caveolin-3, α7 integrin, and collagen VI.

The dystrophin-glycoprotein complex appears to confer stability to the sarcolemma, although the function of each individual component of the complex is incompletely understood. Deficiency of one member of the complex may cause abnormalities in other components. For example, a primary deficiency of dystrophin (Duchenne dystrophy) may lead to secondary loss of the sarcoglycans and dystroglycan. The primary loss of a single sarcoglycan (see "Limb-Girdle Muscular Dystrophy," below) results in a secondary loss of other sarcoglycans in the membrane without uniformly affecting dystrophin. In either instance, disruption of the dystrophin-glycoprotein complexes weakens the sarcolemma, causing membrane tears and a cascade of events leading to muscle fiber necrosis. This sequence of events occurs repeatedly during the life of a patient with muscular dystrophy.

℞ TREATMENT

Glucocorticoids, administered as prednisone in a dose of 0.75 mg/kg per day, significantly slow progression of Duchenne dystrophy for up to 3 years. Some patients cannot tolerate glucocorticoid therapy; weight gain in particular represents a significant deterrent for some boys.

BECKER MUSCULAR DYSTROPHY This less severe form of X-linked recessive muscular dystrophy results from allelic defects of the same gene

responsible for Duchenne dystrophy. Becker muscular dystrophy is approximately 10 times less frequent than Duchenne, with an incidence of about 3 per 100,000 live-born males.

Clinical Features The pattern of muscle wasting in Becker muscular dystrophy closely resembles that seen in Duchenne. Proximal muscles, especially of the lower extremities, are prominently involved. As the disease progresses, weakness becomes more generalized. Significant facial muscle weakness is not a feature. Hypertrophy of muscles, particularly in the calves, is an early and prominent finding.

Most patients with Becker dystrophy first experience difficulties between ages 5 and 15 years, although onset in the third or fourth decade or even later can occur. By definition, patients with Becker dystrophy walk beyond age 15, while patients with Duchenne dystrophy are typically in a wheelchair by the age of 12. Patients with Becker dystrophy have a reduced life expectancy, but most survive into the fourth or fifth decade.

Mental retardation may occur in Becker dystrophy, but it is not as common as in Duchenne. Cardiac involvement occurs in Becker dystrophy and may result in heart failure.

Laboratory Features Serum CK levels, results of EMG, and muscle biopsy findings closely resemble those in Duchenne dystrophy. The diagnosis of Becker muscular dystrophy requires western blot analysis of muscle biopsy samples demonstrating a reduced amount or abnormal size of dystrophin. Mutation analysis of DNA from peripheral blood leukocytes reveals deletions or duplications of the dystrophin gene in 65% of patients with Becker dystrophy, approximately the same percentage as in Duchenne dystrophy. In both Becker and Duchenne dystrophies, the size of the DNA deletion does not predict clinical severity; however, in ~95% of patients with Becker dystrophy, the DNA deletion does not alter the translational reading frame of messenger RNA. These "in-frame" mutations allow for production of some dystrophin, which accounts for the presence of altered rather than absent dystrophin on western blot analysis.

℞ TREATMENT

The use of glucocorticoids has not been adequately studied in Becker dystrophy.

LIMB-GIRDLE MUSCULAR DYSTROPHY The syndrome of limb-girdle muscular dystrophy (LGMD) represents more than one disorder. Both males and females are affected, with onset ranging from late in the first decade to the fourth decade. The LGMDs typically manifest with progressive weakness of pelvic and shoulder girdle musculature. Respiratory insufficiency from weakness of the diaphragm may occur, as may cardiomyopathy. Unlike Duchenne dystrophy, intellectual function is unaffected.

A systematic classification of LGMD is based on autosomal dominant (LGMD1) and autosomal recessive (LGMD2) inheritance. Superimposed on the backbone of LGMD1 and LGMD2, the classification employs a sequential alphabetical lettering system (LGMD1A, LGMD2A, etc.). Disorders receive letters in the order in which they are found to have chromosomal linkage. This results in an ever-expanding list of conditions. Presently there are 5 autosomal dominant and 10 autosomal recessive disorders, summarized in Tables 368-2 and 368-3. None of the conditions is as common as the dystrophinopathies; however, prevalence data for the LGMDs have not been systematically gathered for any large heterogeneous population. In referral-based clinical populations, the sarcoglycan deficiencies (LGMD2C, 2D, 2E, 2F) and dysferlinopathies (LGMD2B) have emerged as the most common disorders. Some small group analyses predict that calpain-3 deficiency (LGMD2A) and Fukutin-related protein (FKRP) deficiency (LGMD2I) may rival others for prevalence.

EMERY-DREIFUSS MUSCULAR DYSTROPHY There are two genetically distinct forms of Emery-Dreifuss muscular dystrophy (EDMD). One is

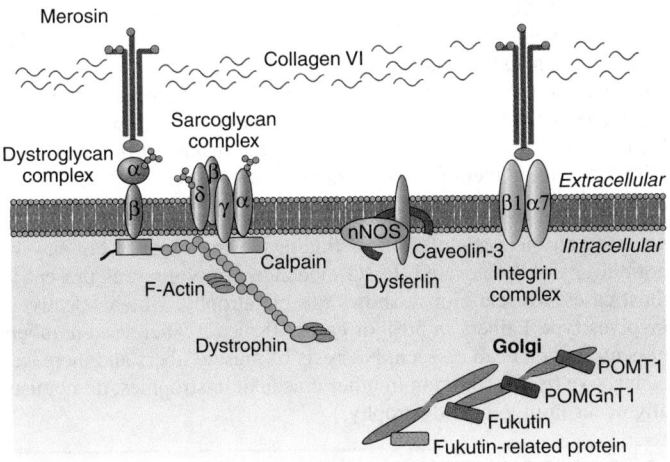

FIGURE 368-1 Selected muscular dystrophy–associated proteins in the cell membrane and Golgi complex. Dystrophin localizes to the cytoplasmic face of the muscle cell membrane. It complexes with two transmembrane protein complexes, the dystroglycans and the sarcoglycans. The dystroglycans bind to the extracellular matrix protein merosin, which is also complexed with α1 and α7 integrins (Tables 368-1, 368-2, 368-3). Dysferlin complexes with caveolin-3 (which binds to neuronal nitric oxide synthase, or nNOS) but not with the dystrophin-associated proteins or the integrins. In each of four congenital dystrophies, there is loss of function of different Golgi-associated proteins: POMT1, POMGnT1, Fukutin, and Fukutin-related protein.

TABLE 368-2 *Autosomal Dominant Limb-Girdle Muscular Dystrophies (LGMDs)*

Disease	Clinical Features	Laboratory Features	Locus or Gene
LGMD1A	Onset 3d to 4th decade Muscle weakness affects distal limb muscles, vocal cords, and pharyngeal muscles	Serum CK 2 × normal EMG mixed myopathy/neuropathy NCS normal	Myotilin
LGMD1B	Onset 1st or 2d decade Proximal lower limb weakness and cardiomyopathy with conduction defects Some cases indistinguishable from Emery-Dreifuss muscular dystrophy with joint contractures	Serum CK 3–5 × normal NCS normal EMG myopathic	Lamin A/C
LGMD1C	Onset in early childhood Proximal weakness Gowers' sign, calf hypertrophy Exercise-related muscle cramps	Serum CK 4–25 × normal NCS normal EMG myopathic	Caveolin-3
LGMD1D	Onset 3d to 5th decade Proximal muscle weakness Cardiomyopathy and arrhythmias	Serum CK 2–4 × normal NCS normal EMG myopathic	Linked to chromosome 7q Gene unidentified
LGMD1E	Childhood onset Proximal muscle weakness	Serum CK usually normal NCS normal EMG myopathic	Linked to chromosome 6q23 Gene unidentified

Abbreviations: CK, creatine kinase; NCS, nerve conduction studies; EMG, electromyography.

inherited as an X-linked disorder, while the other is autosomal dominant. The latter is classified under the rubric of LGMD1B, but clinically the conditions are closely related.

Clinical Features Prominent contractures can be recognized in early childhood and teenage years, often preceding muscle weakness. The contractures persist throughout the course of the disease and are present at the elbows and neck. Muscle weakness affects humeral and peroneal muscles at first and later spreads to a limb-girdle distribution. The cardiomyopathy is potentially life threatening and may result in sudden death. A spectrum of atrial rhythm and conduction defects includes atrial fibrillation and paralysis and atrioventricular heart block. Some patients have a dilated cardiomyopathy. Female carriers of the X-linked variant may have cardiac manifestations that become clinically significant.

Laboratory Features Serum CK may be elevated two-to tenfold. EMG is myopathic. Muscle biopsy shows nonspecific dystrophic features. ECGs demonstrate atrial and atrioventricular rhythm disturbances.

GENETIC CONSIDERATIONS X-linked EDMD arises from defects in the emerin gene encoding a nuclear envelope protein. The autosomal dominant disease is caused by mutations of the *LMNA* gene on chromosome 1q21.2 encoding the lamin proteins A and C. These proteins are alternatively spliced products of the *LMNA* gene that are essential components of the filamentous network underlying the inner nuclear membrane. Loss of structural integrity of the nuclear envelope from defects in emerin or lamin A/C accounts for overlapping phenotypes.

Rx TREATMENT

Supportive care should be offered for neuromuscular disability, including ambulatory aids, if necessary. Stretching of contractures is difficult. Management of cardiomyopathy and arrhythmias can save lives.

MYOTONIC DYSTROPHY Myotonic dystrophy is also known as *dystrophia myotonica* (DM). The condition is composed of at least two clinical disorders with overlapping phenotypes and distinct molecular genetic defects: myotonic dystrophy type 1 (DM1), the classic disease originally described by Steinert, and myotonic dystrophy type 2 (DM2), also called *proximal myotonic myopathy* (PROMM).

Clinical Features The clinical expression of myotonic dystrophy varies widely and involves many systems other than muscle. Affected patients have a typical "hatchet-faced" appearance due to temporalis, masseter, and facial muscle atrophy and weakness. Frontal baldness is characteristic of men with the disease. Neck muscles, including flexors and sternocleidomastoids, and distal limb muscles are involved early. Weakness of wrist extensors, finger extensors, and intrinsic hand muscles impairs function. Ankle dorsiflexor weakness may cause footdrop. Proximal muscles remain stronger throughout the course, although preferential atrophy and weakness of quadriceps muscles occur in many patients. Palatal, pharyngeal, and tongue involvement produce a dysarthric speech, nasal voice, and swallowing problems. Some patients have diaphragm and intercostal muscle weakness, resulting in respiratory insufficiency.

Myotonia, which usually appears by age 5, is demonstrable by percussion of the thenar eminence, the tongue, and wrist extensor muscles. Myotonia causes a slow relaxation of hand grip after a forced voluntary closure. Advanced muscle wasting makes myotonia more difficult to detect.

Cardiac disturbances occur commonly in patients with DM1. ECG abnormalities include first-degree heart block and more extensive conduction system involvement. Complete heart block and sudden death can occur. Congestive heart failure occurs infrequently but may result from cor pulmonale secondary to respiratory failure. Mitral valve prolapse also occurs commonly. Other associated features include intellectual impairment, hypersomnia, posterior subcapsular cataracts, gonadal atrophy, insulin resistance, and decreased esophageal and colonic motility.

Congenital myotonic dystrophy is a more severe form of DM1 and occurs in ~25% of infants of affected mothers. It is characterized by severe facial and bulbar weakness, transient neonatal respiratory insufficiency, and mental retardation.

DM2, or PROMM, has a distinct pattern of muscle weakness affecting mainly proximal muscles. Other features of the disease overlap with DM1, including cataracts, testicular atrophy, insulin resistance, constipation, hypersomnia, and cognitive defects. Cardiac conduction defects occur but are less common, and the hatchet face and frontal baldness are less consistent features. A very striking difference is the failure to clearly identify a congenital form of DM2.

Laboratory Features The diagnosis of myotonic dystrophy can usually be made on the basis of clinical findings. Serum CK levels may be normal or mildly elevated. EMG evidence of myotonia is present in most cases. Muscle biopsy shows muscle atrophy, which selectively involves type 1 fibers in 50% of cases. Typically, increased numbers of central nuclei can be seen. Necrosis of muscle fibers and increased connective tissue, common in other muscular dystrophies, do not usually occur in myotonic dystrophy.

GENETIC CONSIDERATIONS DM1 and DM2 are both autosomal dominant disorders. New mutations do not appear to contribute to the pool of affected individuals. DM1 is transmitted by an intronic mutation consisting of an unstable expansion of a CTG trinucleotide repeat in a serine-threonine protein kinase gene (named *DMPK*) on chromosome 19q13.3. An increase in the severity of the disease phenotype in successive generations (genetic anticipation) is accompanied by an increase in the number of trinucleotide repeats. A similar type of mutation has been identified in fragile X syndrome (Chap. 56). The unstable triplet repeat in myotonic dystrophy can be used for prenatal diagnosis. Congenital disease occurs almost exclusively in infants born to affected mothers; it is possible that sperm with greatly expanded triplet repeats do not function well.

DM2 has been linked to chromosome 3q13.3-q24. At this locus, a DNA expansion mutation consists of a CCTG repeat in intron 1 of the *ZNF9* gene. The gene is believed to encode an RNA binding protein expressed in many different tissues, including skeletal and cardiac muscle.

How the DNA expansions in DM1 and DM2 impair function of muscle and other cells is not well understood. They may alter expression of an adjacent protein kinase gene (DM1), inactivate an important RNA binding protein (DM2), or influence other neighboring genes. In both DM1 and DM2, the mutant RNA appears to form intranuclear inclusions composed of aberrant RNA.

℞ TREATMENT

The myotonia in myotonic dystrophy rarely warrants treatment. Phenytoin is the preferred agent for the occasional patient who requires an antimyotonia drug; other agents, particularly quinine and procainamide, may worsen cardiac conduction. Cardiac pacemaker insertion should be considered for patients with unexplained syncope or advanced conduction system abnormalities with evidence of second-degree heart block, or trifascicular conduction disturbances with marked prolongation of the PR interval. Molded ankle-foot orthoses help prevent footdrop in patients with distal lower extremity weakness.

FACIOSCAPULOHUMERAL (FSH) MUSCULAR DYSTROPHY
This form of muscular dystrophy has a prevalence of ~1 in 20,000. It is distinct from a similar disorder known as scapuloperoneal dystrophy.

Clinical Features The condition typically has an onset in childhood or young adulthood. In most cases, facial weakness is the initial manifestation, appearing as an inability to smile, whistle, or fully close the eyes. Weakness of the shoulder girdles, rather than the facial muscles, usually brings the patient to medical attention. Loss of scapular stabilizer muscles makes arm elevation difficult. Scapular winging (Fig. 367-3) becomes apparent with attempts at abduction and forward movement of the arms. Biceps and triceps muscles may be severely affected, with relative sparing of the deltoid muscles. Weakness is invariably worse for wrist extension than for wrist flexion, and weakness of the anterior compartment muscles of the legs may lead to footdrop.

In most patients, the weakness remains restricted to facial, upper extremity, and distal lower extremity muscles. In 20% of patients, weakness progresses to involve the pelvic girdle muscles, and severe functional impairment and possible wheelchair dependency result.

Characteristically, patients with FSH dystrophy do not have involvement of other organ systems, although labile hypertension is common, and there is an increased incidence of nerve deafness. *Coats' disease*, a disorder consisting of telangiectasia, exudation, and retinal detachment, also occurs.

TABLE 368-3 Autosomal Recessive Limb-Girdle Muscular Dystrophies (LGMDs)

Disease	Clinical Features	Laboratory Features	Locus or Gene
LGMD2A	Onset 1st or 2d decade Tight heel cords Contractures at elbows, wrists, and fingers; rigid spine in some Proximal and distal weakness	Serum CK 3–15 × normal NCS normal EMG myopathic	Calpain-3
LGMD2B	Onset 2d or 3d decade Proximal muscle weakness at onset, later distal (calf) muscles affected Miyoshi myopathy is variant of LGMD2B with calf muscles affected at onset	Serum CK 3–100 × normal NCS normal EMG myopathic Inflammation on muscle biopsy may simulate polymyositis	Dysferlin
LGMD2C–F	Onset in childhood to teenage yrs Clinical condition similar to Duchenne and Becker muscular dystrophies Cardiomyopathy uncommon Cognitive function normal	Serum CK 5–100 × normal NCS normal EMG myopathic	γ, α, β, δ sarcoglycans
LGMD2G	Onset age 10 to 15 Proximal and distal muscle weakness	Serum CK 3–17 × normal NCS normal EMG myopathic	Telethonin
LGMD2H	Onset 1st to 3d decade Proximal muscle weakness	Serum CK 2–25 × normal NCS normal EMG myopathic	TRIM32 gene
LGMD2I	Onset 1st to 3d decade Clinical condition similar to Duchenne or Becker dystrophies Cardiomyopathy (some not all) Cognitive function normal	Serum CK 10–30 × normal NCS normal EMG myopathic	Fukutin-related protein
LGMD2J[a]	Onset 1st to 3d decade Proximal lower limb weakness Mild distal weakness Progressive weakness causes loss of ambulation	Serum CK 1.5–2 × normal NCS normal EMG myopathic	Titin

[a] Tibial muscular dystrophy is a form of titin deficiency with only distal muscle weakness (see Table 368-4).
Abbreviations: CK, creatine kinase; NCS, nerve conduction studies; EMG, electromyography.

Laboratory Features The serum CK level may be normal or mildly elevated. EMG usually indicates a myopathic pattern. The muscle biopsy shows nonspecific features of a myopathy. A prominent inflammatory infiltrate, which is often multifocal in distribution, is present in some biopsy samples. The cause or significance of this finding is unknown.

GENETIC CONSIDERATIONS An autosomal dominant inheritance pattern with almost complete penetrance has been established, but each family member should be examined for the presence of the disease, since ~30% of those affected are unaware of involvement. FSH dystrophy is caused by deletions of tandem 3.3-kb repeats at 4q35. The deletion reduces the number of repeats to a fragment of <35 kb in most patients. This mutation results in an overexpression of upstream genes and a loss of DNA binding of a multiprotein complex mediating transcriptional repression of 4q35 genes. The mutation permits carrier detection and prenatal diagnosis. Most sporadic cases represent new mutations.

℞ TREATMENT

No specific treatment is available; ankle-foot orthoses are helpful for footdrop. Scapular stabilization procedures improve scapular winging but may not improve function.

OCULOPHARYNGEAL DYSTROPHY
This form of muscular dystrophy represents one of several disorders characterized by progressive external ophthalmoplegia, which consists of slowly progressive ptosis and limitation of eye movements with sparing of pupillary reactions for light and accommodation. Patients usually do not complain of diplopia, in contrast to patients having conditions with a more acute onset of ocular muscle weakness (e.g., myasthenia gravis).

TABLE 368-4 *Distal Myopathies*

Disease	Clinical Features	Laboratory Features	Locus/Gene
Welander distal myopathy	Onset in fifth decade Weakness begins in hands Slow progression with spread to distal lower extremities Lifespan normal	Serum CK 2–3 × normal EMG myopathic NCS normal Muscle biopsy shows dystrophic features	AD inheritance Linked to chromosome 2p13
Tibial Muscular dystrophy (Markesbery/Griggs/Udd)	Onset 4th to 8th decade Distal lower extremity weakness (tibial distribution) Upper extremities usually normal Lifespan normal	Serum CK 2–4 × normal EMG myopathic NCS normal Muscle biopsy shows dystrophic features Titin absent in M-line of muscle	AD inheritance Titin
Nonanka distal myopathy (distal myopathy with rimmed vacuoles)	Onset 2d to 3d decade Lower extremity distal weakness Mild distal upper limb weakness may be present early Progression to other muscles sparing quadriceps Ambulation may be lost in 10–15 years	Serum CK 3–10 × normal EMG myopathic NCS normal Dystrophic features on muscle biopsy plus rimmed vacuoles 15–19-nm filaments within vacuoles	AR Allelic to hereditary inclusion body myopathy GNE gene: UDP-*N*-acetylglucosamine 2-epimerase/*N*-acetylmannosamine kinase
Miyoshi myopathy	Onset 2d to 3d decade Lower extremity weakness in posterior compartment muscles Progression leads to weakness in other muscle groups Ambulation lost after 10–15 years in about one-third of cases	Serum CK 20–100 × normal EMG myopathic NCS normal Muscle biopsy shows nonspecific dystrophic features	AR Allelic to LGMD2B (see Table 368-3). Dysferlin

Abbreviations: CK, creatine kinase; AD, autosomal dominant; AR, autosomal recessive; EMG, electromyography; NCS, nerve conduction studies.

Clinical Features   Oculopharyngeal muscular dystrophy has a late onset; it usually presents with ptosis and/or dysphagia in the fourth to sixth decade. The extraocular muscle impairment is less prominent in the early phase but may be severe later. The swallowing problem may become debilitating and result in pooling of secretions and repeated episodes of aspiration. Mild weakness of the neck and extremities also occurs.

Laboratory Features   The serum CK level may be two to three times normal. Myopathic EMG findings are typical. On biopsy, muscle fibers are found to contain vacuoles, which by electron microscopy are shown to contain membranous whorls, accumulation of glycogen, and other nonspecific debris related to lysosomes. A distinct feature of oculopharyngeal dystrophy is the presence of tubular filaments, 8.5 nm in diameter, in muscle cell nuclei.

GENETIC CONSIDERATIONS   Oculopharyngeal dystrophy has an autosomal dominant inheritance pattern with complete penetrance. The incidence is high in French-Canadians and in Spanish-American families of the southwestern United States. Large kindreds of Italian and of eastern European Jewish descent have been reported. The molecular defect in oculopharyngeal muscular dystrophy is a subtle expansion of a modest polyanine repeat tract in a poly-RNA binding protein (PABP2) in muscle.

℞ TREATMENT

Dysphagia can cause inanition, making oculopharyngeal muscular dystrophy a potentially life-threatening disease. Cricopharyngeal myotomy may improve swallowing, although it does not prevent aspiration. Eyelid crutches can improve vision in patients in whom ptosis

obstructs vision; candidates for ptosis surgery must be carefully selected—those with severe facial weakness are not suitable.

DISTAL MYOPATHIES   A group of muscle diseases, the distal myopathies, are notable for their preferential distal distribution of muscle weakness in contrast to most muscle conditions associated with proximal weakness. The major distal myopathies are summarized in Table 368-4.

Clinical Features   Two of the conditions, *Welander distal myopathy* and *tibial muscular dystrophy*, are late-onset disorders, usually manifesting after age 40. *Nonanka distal myopathy* and *Miyoshi myopathy* are distinguished by their early onset in the late teens or twenties. Only Welander disease begins in the hands; all others start in the lower limbs. Miyoshi myopathy is unique in that gastrocnemius muscles are preferentially affected at onset. A clinical feature that makes all of these disorders confusing is that proximal muscles can be affected as the disorders progress (less so for Welander disease than others), perhaps diminishing the entire concept of the distal myopathy. In contrast to many genetic muscle diseases, the distal myopathies are for the most part limited to skeletal muscle.

Laboratory Features   Serum CK is particularly helpful in diagnosing Miyoshi myopathy since it is very elevated. In the other conditions serum CK is only slightly increased. EMGs are myopathic. Muscle biopsy shows nonspecific dystrophic features. In Nonanka distal myopathy rimmed vacuoles, which contain 15- to 19-nm filaments, are common findings. Immune staining for gene product can be helpful in demonstrating titin abnormalities in tibial muscular dystrophy and reduced dysferlin in Miyoshi myopathy.

GENETIC CONSIDERATIONS   Welander and tibial muscular dystrophy are inherited as autosomal dominant disorders, while Nonanka and Miyoshi myopathies are autosomal recessive conditions. The affected genes and their gene products are listed in Table 368-4. The gene for Welander disease awaits identification.

℞ TREATMENT

Occupational therapy is offered for loss of hand function; ankle-foot orthoses can support distal lower limb muscles.

CONGENITAL MYOPATHIES

These rare disorders are distinguished from muscular dystrophies by the presence of specific histochemical and structural abnormalities in muscle. Although primarily disorders of infancy or childhood, three forms that may present in adulthood are described here: central core disease, nemaline (rod) myopathy, and centronuclear (myotubular) myopathy. Other types, such as minicore myopathy (multi-minicore disease), fingerprint body myopathy, and sarcotubular myopathy, are not discussed.

CENTRAL CORE DISEASE   Patients with central core disease may have decreased fetal movements and breech presentation. Hypotonia and delay in motor milestones, particularly in walking, are common. Later in childhood, patients develop problems with stair climbing, running, and getting up from the floor. On examination, there is mild facial, neck-flexor, and proximal-extremity muscle weakness. Legs are more affected than arms. Skeletal abnormalities include congenital hip dislocation, scoliosis, and pes cavus; clubbed feet also occur. Most cases are nonprogressive, but exceptions are well documented. Susceptibility to malignant hyperthermia must be considered as a potential risk factor for patients with central core disease.

The serum CK level is usually normal. Needle EMG demonstrates a myopathic pattern. Muscle biopsy shows fibers with single or multiple central or eccentric discrete zones (*cores*) devoid of oxidative enzymes. Cores occur preferentially in type 1 fibers and represent poorly aligned sarcomeres associated with Z disk streaming.

Autosomal dominant inheritance is characteristic; sporadic cases also occur. The disease is caused by point mutations of the ryanodine receptor gene on chromosome 19q, encoding the calcium-release channel of the sarcoplasmic reticulum of skeletal muscle; mutations of this gene also account for some cases of inherited malignant hyperthermia (Chap. 17). Malignant hyperthermia is an allelic condition; C-terminal mutations of the *RYR1* gene predispose to this complication.

Specific treatment is not required, but establishing a diagnosis of central core disease is extremely important, because these patients have a known predisposition to malignant hyperthermia during anesthesia.

NEMALINE MYOPATHY The term *nemaline* refers to the distinctive presence in muscle fibers of rods or threadlike structures (Greek *nema*, "thread"). Nemaline myopathy is clinically heterogeneous. A severe neonatal form presents with hypotonia and feeding and respiratory difficulties, leading to early death. Nemaline myopathy usually presents in infancy or childhood with delayed motor milestones. The course is nonprogressive or slowly progressive. The physical appearance is striking because of the long, narrow facies, high-arched palate, and open-mouthed appearance due to a prognathous jaw. Other skeletal abnormalities include pectus excavatum, kyphoscoliosis, pes cavus, and clubfoot deformities. Facial and generalized muscle weakness, including respiratory muscle weakness, is common. An adult-onset disorder with progressive proximal weakness may be seen. Myocardial involvement is occasionally present in both the childhood and adult-onset forms. The serum CK level is usually normal or slightly elevated. The EMG demonstrates a myopathic pattern. Muscle biopsy shows clusters of small rods (nemaline bodies), which occur preferentially, but not exclusively, in type 1 muscle fibers. The muscle often shows type 1 muscle fiber predominance. Rods originate from the Z disk material of the muscle fiber.

Five genes have been associated with nemaline myopathy. All code for thin filament–associated proteins, suggesting disturbed assembly or interplay of these structures as a pivotal mechanism. Mutations of the nebulin (*NEB*) gene account for most cases, including both severe neonatal and early childhood forms, inherited as autosomal recessive disorders. Neonatal and childhood cases, inherited as predominantly autosomal dominant disorders, are caused by mutations of the skeletal muscle α-actinin (*ACTA1*) gene. In milder forms of the disease with autosomal dominant inheritance, mutations have been identified in both the slow α-tropomyosin (*TPM3*) and β-tropomyosin (*TPM2*) genes accounting for <3% of cases. Muscle troponin T (*TNNT1*) gene mutations appear to be limited to the Amish population in North America. No specific treatment is available.

MYOTUBULAR (CENTRONUCLEAR) MYOPATHY Three distinct variants of centronuclear myopathy occur. A neonatal form, also known as *myotubular myopathy*, presents with severe hypotonia and weakness at birth. The late infancy–early childhood form presents with delayed motor milestones. Later, difficulty with running and stair climbing becomes apparent. A marfanoid, slender body habitus, long narrow face, and high-arched palate are typical. Scoliosis and clubbed feet may be present. Most patients exhibit progressive weakness, some requiring wheelchairs. Progressive external ophthalmoplegia with ptosis and

varying degrees of extraocular muscle impairment are characteristic of both the neonatal and the late-infantile forms. A third variant, the late childhood–adult form, has an onset in the second or third decade. Patients have full extraocular muscle movements and rarely exhibit ptosis. There is mild, nonprogressive limb weakness and no associated skeletal abnormalities.

Normal or slightly elevated CK levels occur in each of the forms. EMG studies often give distinctive results, showing positive sharp waves and fibrillation potentials, complex and repetitive discharges, and rarely myotonic discharges. Muscle biopsy specimens in longitudinal section demonstrate rows of central nuclei, often surrounded by a halo. In transverse sections, central nuclei are found in 25 to 80% of muscle fibers.

A gene for the neonatal form of centronuclear myopathy has been localized to Xq28; this gene encodes myotubularin, a protein tyrosine phosphatase. Missense, frameshift, and splice-site mutations predict loss of myotubularin function in affected individuals. Carrier identification and prenatal diagnosis are possible. The inheritance pattern for the late infancy–early childhood disorder is probably autosomal recessive, and for the late childhood–adult form is probably autosomal dominant. No specific treatment is available.

DISORDERS OF MUSCLE ENERGY METABOLISM

There are two principal sources of energy for skeletal muscle—fatty acids and glucose. Abnormalities in either glucose or lipid utilization can be associated with distinct clinical presentations that can range from an acute, painful syndrome with rhabdomyolysis and myoglobinuria to a chronic, progressive muscle weakness simulating muscular dystrophy.

GLYCOGEN STORAGE AND GLYCOLYTIC DEFECTS ■ **Disorders of Glycogen Storage Causing Progressive Weakness** ■ *ACID MALTASE DEFICIENCY* Three clinical forms of acid maltase deficiency (*type II glycogenosis*) can be distinguished. The infantile form is the most common, with onset of symptoms in the first 3 months of life. Infants develop severe muscle weakness, cardiomegaly, hepatomegaly, and respiratory insufficiency. Glycogen accumulation in motor neurons of the spinal cord and brainstem contributes to muscle weakness. Death usually occurs by 1 year of age. In the childhood form, the picture resembles muscular dystrophy. Delayed motor milestones result from proximal limb muscle weakness and involvement of respiratory muscles. The heart may be involved, but the liver and brain are unaffected. The adult form begins in the third or fourth decade. Respiratory failure and diaphragmatic weakness are often initial manifestations, heralding progressive proximal muscle weakness. The heart and liver are not involved.

In all forms of acid maltase deficiency, the serum CK level is 2 to 10 times normal. EMG examination demonstrates a myopathic pattern, but other features are especially distinctive, including myotonic discharges, trains of fibrillation and positive waves, and complex repetitive discharges. EMG discharges are very prominent in the lumbosacral paraspinal muscles. The muscle biopsy shows vacuoles containing glycogen and the lysosomal enzyme acid phosphatase. Electron microscopy reveals membrane-bound and free tissue glycogen. Definitive diagnosis is established by enzyme determination in muscle.

Acid maltase deficiency is inherited as an autosomal recessive disorder caused by mutations of the acid maltase gene. Recombinant human α-glucosidase infused intravenously is well tolerated. Clinical benefits in the infantile disease include reduced heart size, improved muscle tone, and longer life.

OTHER GLYCOGEN STORAGE DISEASES WITH PROGRESSIVE WEAKNESS In *debranching enzyme deficiency* (*type III glycogenosis*), a slowly progressive form of muscle weakness can develop after puberty. Rarely, myoglobinuria may be seen. Patients are usually diagnosed in infancy, however, because of hypotonia and delayed motor milestones, hepatomegaly, growth retardation, and hypoglycemia. *Branching enzyme* deficiency (*type IV glycogenosis*) is a rare and fatal glycogen storage disease characterized by failure to thrive and hepatomegaly. Hypotonia and muscle wasting may be present, but the skeletal muscle manifestations are minor compared to liver failure.

Disorders of Glycolysis Causing Exercise Intolerance Five glycolytic defects are associated with recurrent myoglobinuria: *myophosphorylase deficiency (type V glycogenosis), phosphofructokinase deficiency (type VII glycogenosis), phosphoglycerate kinase deficiency (type IX glycogenosis), phosphoglycerate mutase deficiency (type X glycogenosis),* and *lactate dehydrogenase deficiency (glycogenosis type XI).* Myophosphorylase deficiency, also known as *McArdle's disease*, is by far the most common of the glycolytic defects associated with exercise intolerance. These five glycolytic defects result in a common failure to support energy production at the initiation of exercise, although the exact site of energy failure remains controversial.

Clinical muscle manifestations in these five conditions usually begin in adolescence. Symptoms are precipitated by brief bursts of high-intensity exercise, such as running or lifting heavy objects. A history of myalgia and muscle stiffness usually precedes the intensely painful muscle contractures, which may be followed by myoglobinuria. Acute renal failure accompanies significant pigmenturia. Exercise tolerance can be enhanced by a slow induction phase (warm-up) or brief periods of rest, allowing for the start of the "second-wind" phenomenon (switching to utilization of fatty acids).

Certain features help distinguish some enzyme defects. Varying degrees of hemolytic anemia accompany deficiencies of both phosphofructokinase (mild) and phosphoglycerate kinase (severe). In phosphoglycerate kinase deficiency, the usual clinical presentation is a seizure disorder associated with mental retardation; exercise intolerance is an infrequent manifestation.

In all of these conditions, the serum CK levels fluctuate widely and may be elevated even during symptom-free periods. CK levels >100 times normal are expected, accompanying myoglobinuria. All patients with suspected glycolytic defects leading to exercise intolerance should undergo a forearm exercise test (Chap. 367). An impaired rise in venous lactate is highly indicative of a glycolytic defect. In lactate dehydrogenase deficiency, venous levels of lactate do not increase, but pyruvate rises to normal. A definitive diagnosis of glycolytic disease is made by muscle biopsy.

Myophosphorylase deficiency, phosphofructokinase deficiency, and phosphoglycerate mutase deficiency are inherited as autosomal recessive disorders. Phosphoglycerate kinase deficiency is X-linked recessive. Mutations can be found in the respective genes encoding the abnormal proteins in each of these disorders.

Training may enhance the second-wind phenomenon, but attempts to raise blood glucose or to modify these disorders through diet have not proved beneficial.

LIPID AS AN ENERGY SOURCE AND ASSOCIATED DEFECTS Lipid is an important muscle energy source during rest and during prolonged, submaximal exercise. Fatty acids are derived from circulating very low density lipoprotein (VLDL) in the blood or from triglycerides stored in muscle fibers. Oxidation of fatty acids occurs in the mitochondria. To enter the mitochondria, a fatty acid must first be converted to an "activated fatty acid," acyl-CoA. The acyl-CoA must be linked with carnitine by the enzyme carnitine palmitoyltransferase (CPT) I for transport into the mitochondria. CPT I is present on the inner side of the outer mitochondrial membrane. Carnitine is removed by CPT II, an enzyme attached to the inside of the inner mitochondrial membrane, allowing transport of acyl-CoA into the mitochondrial matrix for β-oxidation.

Carnitine Palmitoyltransferase Deficiency CPT II deficiency is the most common recognizable cause of recurrent myoglobinuria, more common than the glycolytic defects. Onset is usually in the teenage years or early twenties. Muscle pain and myoglobinuria occur after prolonged exercise. Strength is normal between attacks. Fasting predisposes to the development of symptoms. In contrast to disorders caused by defects in glycolysis, in which muscle cramps follow short, intense bursts of exercise, the muscle pain in CPT II deficiency does not occur until the limits of utilization have been exceeded and muscle breakdown has already begun. Episodes of rhabdomyolysis may produce severe weakness. In young children and newborns, CPT II deficiency can present with a very severe clinical picture including hypoketotic hypoglycemia, cardiomyopathy, liver failure, and sudden death.

Serum CK levels and EMG findings are both usually normal between episodes. A normal rise of venous lactate during forearm exercise distinguishes this condition from glycolytic defects, especially myophosphorylase deficiency. Muscle biopsy does not show lipid accumulation and is usually normal between attacks. The diagnosis requires direct measurement of muscle CPT.

CPT II deficiency is much more common in men than women (5:1); nevertheless, all evidence indicates autosomal recessive inheritance. A mutation in the gene for CPT II (chromosome 1p36) causes the disease in some individuals. It has been suggested that frequent meals and a low-fat, high-carbohydrate diet can prolong exercise tolerance. Others suggest substituting medium-chain triglycerides in the diet. Neither approach has proved beneficial.

Myoadenylate Deaminase Deficiency The muscle enzyme myoadenylate deaminase converts adenosine 5'-monophosphate (5'-AMP) to inosine monophosphate (IMP) with liberation of ammonia. Myoadenylate deaminase may play a role in regulating adenosine triphosphate (ATP) levels in muscles. Most individuals with myoadenylate deaminase deficiency have no symptoms. There have been a few reports of patients with this disorder who have exercise-exacerbated myalgia and myoglobinuria. Many questions have been raised about the clinical effects of myoadenylate deaminase deficiency, and, specifically, its relationship to exertional myalgia and fatigability, but there is no consensus.

MITOCHONDRIAL MYOPATHIES

In 1972, Olson and colleagues recognized that muscle fibers with significant numbers of abnormal mitochondria could be highlighted with the modified trichrome stain; the term *ragged red fibers* was coined. By electron microscopy, the mitochondria in ragged red fibers are enlarged and often bizarrely shaped and have crystalline inclusions. Since that seminal observation, the understanding of these disorders of muscle and other tissues has expanded (Chap. 56).

Mitochondria play a key role in energy production. Oxidation of the major nutrients derived from carbohydrate, fat, and protein leads to the generation of reducing equivalents. The latter are transported through the respiratory chain in the process known as *oxidative phosphorylation*. The energy generated by the oxidation-reduction reactions of the respiratory chain is stored in an electrochemical gradient coupled to ATP synthesis.

A novel feature of mitochondria is their genetic composition. Each mitochondrion possesses a DNA genome that is distinct from that of the nuclear DNA. Human mitochondrial DNA (mtDNA) consists of a double-strand, circular molecule comprising 16,569 base pairs. It codes for 22 transfer RNAs, 2 ribosomal RNAs, and 13 polypeptides of the respiratory chain enzymes. The genetics of mitochondrial diseases differ from the genetics of chromosomal disorders. The DNA of mitochondria is directly inherited from the cytoplasm of the gametes, mainly from the oocyte. The sperm contributes very little of its mitochondria to the offspring at the time of fertilization. Thus, mitochondrial genes are derived almost exclusively from the mother, accounting for maternal inheritance of some mitochondrial disorders.

Patients with mitochondrial disorders have clinical manifestations that fall into three groups: chronic progressive external ophthalmoplegia (CPEO), skeletal muscle–central nervous system syndromes, and pure myopathy simulating muscular dystrophy.

PROGRESSIVE EXTERNAL OPHTHALMOPLEGIA SYNDROMES WITH RAGGED RED FIBERS The single most common sign of a mitochondrial myopathy is CPEO, occurring in >50% of all mitochondrial myopathies. Varying degrees of ptosis and weakness of extraocular muscles are seen, usually in the absence of diplopia, a point of distinction from disorders with fluctuating eye weakness (e.g., myasthenia gravis).

368 Muscular Dystrophies and Other Muscle Diseases   **2535**

KEARNS-SAYRE SYNDROME (KSS) KSS is a widespread multiorgan system disorder with a defined triad of clinical findings: onset before age 20, CPEO, and pigmentary retinopathy plus one or more of the following features: complete heart block, cerebrospinal fluid protein > 1.0 g/L (100 mg/dL), or cerebellar ataxia. Some patients with CPEO and ragged red fibers may not fulfill all of the criteria for KSS. The cardiac disease includes syncopal attacks and cardiac arrest related to the abnormalities in the cardiac conduction system: prolonged intraventricular conduction time, bundle branch block, and complete atrioventricular block. Death attributed to heart block occurs in about 20% of the patients. Varying degrees of progressive limb muscle weakness and easy fatigability affect activities of daily living. Endocrine abnormalities are common including gonadal dysfunction in both sexes with delayed puberty, short stature, and infertility. Diabetes mellitus is a cardinal sign of mitochondrial disorders and is estimated to occur in 13% of KSS patients. Other less common endocrine disorders include thyroid disease, hyperaldosteronism, Addison's disease, and hypoparathyroidism. Both mental retardation and dementia are common accompaniments to this disorder. Serum CK levels are normal or slightly elevated. Serum lactate and pyruvate levels may be elevated. EMG is myopathic. Nerve conduction studies may be abnormal related to an associated neuropathy. Muscle biopsies reveal ragged red fibers, highlighted in oxidative enzyme stains, many showing defects in cytochrome oxidase. By electron microscopy increased numbers of mitochondria often appear enlarged with paracrystalline inclusions.

KSS is a sporadic disorder. The disease is caused by single mtDNA deletions presumed to arise spontaneously in the ovum or zygote. The most common deletion, occurring in about one-third of patients, removes 4977 bp of contiguous mtDNA. Monitoring for cardiac conduction defects is critical. Prophylactic pacemaker implantation is indicated when electrocardiograms demonstrate a bifascicular block. In KSS no benefit has been shown for supplementary therapies, including multivitamins or coenzyme Q10. Of all the proposed options, exercise might be the most applicable but must be approached cautiously because of defects in the cardiac conduction system.

AUTOSOMAL DOMINANT PROGRESSIVE EXTERNAL OPHTHALMOPLEGIA This condition is caused by nuclear DNA mutations affecting mtDNA copy number and integrity and is thus inherited in a Mendelian fashion. Onset is usually after puberty. Fatigue, exercise intolerance, and complaints of muscle weakness are typical. Some patients notice swallowing problems. The neurologic examination confirms the ptosis and ophthalmoplegia, usually asymmetric in distribution. A sensorineural hearing loss may be encountered. Mild facial, neck flexor, and proximal weakness are typical. Rarely, respiratory muscles may be progressively affected and may be the direct cause of death. Serum CK is normal or mildly elevated. The resting lactates are normal or slightly elevated but may rise excessively after exercise. Spinal fluid protein is normal. The EMG is myopathic, and nerve conduction studies are usually normal. Ragged red fibers are prominently displayed in the muscle biopsy. Southern blots of muscle reveal a normal mtDNA band at 16.6 kb and several additional mtDNA deletion bands with genomes varying from 0.5 to 10 kb.

This autosomal dominant form of CPEO has been linked to loci on three chromosomes: 4q35, 10q24, and 15q22-26. In the chromosome 4q–related form of disease, mutations of the gene encoding the heart and skeletal muscle–specific isoform of the adenine nucleotide translocator 1 (*ANT1*) gene are found. This highly abundant mitochondrial protein forms a homodimeric inner mitochondrial channel through which ADP enters and ATP leaves the mitochondrial matrix. In the chromosome 10q–related disorder, mutations of the gene *C10orf2* are found. Its gene product, *twinkle*, co-localizes with the mtDNA and is named for its punctate, starlike staining properties. The function of twinkle is presumed to be critical for lifetime maintenance of mitochondrial integrity. In the cases mapped to chromosome 15q,

a mutation affects the gene encoding mtDNA polymerase (*POLG*), an enzyme important in mtDNA replication.

Exercise may improve function but will depend on patients' ability to participate.

AUTOSOMAL RECESSIVE CARDIOMYOPATHY AND OPHTHALMOPLEGIA (ARCO) ARCO is a rare mitochondrial disorder clinically important because of an associated life-threatening cardiomyopathy. CPEO is the initial manifestation, occurring between ages 8 and 10. Exercise intolerance and fatigue follow the early symptoms, accompanied by palpitations and chest pain. Examination reveals extraocular muscle weakness, ptosis, facial weakness, reduced muscle bulk, and limb weakness, greater in proximal muscles. A dilated cardiomyopathy is typical, and some patients have conduction system involvement. Death from congestive heart failure occurs as early as age 13. Serum lactate is normal at rest but increases with mild exercise. Serum CK is increased by two- to fourfold. EMG is normal or myopathic. Muscle biopsy demonstrates typical ragged red fibers. Multiple mtDNA deletions are seen on Southern blots of muscle. Echocardiograms show reduced ejection fraction. Conduction block is seen on electrocardiograms. The disease is inherited as an autosomal recessive disorder. The gene has not been identified. Heart failure may require orthotopic cardiac transplantation. Cardiac pacemakers are appropriate for patients with heart block.

mtDNA SKELETAL MUSCLE–CENTRAL NERVOUS SYSTEM SYNDROMES ■ Myoclonic Epilepsy with Ragged Red Fibers (MERRF) The onset of MERRF is variable, ranging from late childhood to middle adult life. Characteristic features include myoclonic epilepsy, cerebellar ataxia, and progressive muscle weakness. The seizure disorder is an integral part of the disease and may be the initial symptom. Cerebellar ataxia precedes or accompanies epilepsy. It is slowly progressive, affects both trunk and limbs, and impairs gait and extremity functions. The third major feature of the disease is muscle weakness in a limb-girdle distribution. Other more variable features include dementia, peripheral neuropathy, optic atrophy, hearing loss, and diabetes mellitus.

Serum CK levels are normal or slightly increased. The serum lactate may be elevated. EMG is myopathic, and in some patients nerve conduction studies show the neuropathy. The electroencephalogram is abnormal, corroborating clinical findings of epilepsy. Typical ragged red fibers are seen on muscle biopsy. MERRF is caused by maternally inherited point mutations of mitochondrial transfer RNA (tRNA) genes. The most common mutation found in 80% of MERRF patients is an A to G substitution at nucleotide 8344 of tRNA lysine (A8344G tRNA^{lys}). Other tRNA^{lys} mutations include base-pair substitutions T8356C and G8363A. Only supportive treatment is possible, with special attention to epilepsy.

MITOCHONDRIAL MYOPATHY, ENCEPHALOPATHY, LACTIC ACIDOSIS, AND STROKE-LIKE EPISODES (MELAS) MELAS is the most common mitochondrial encephalomyopathy. The term *stroke-like* is appropriate because the cerebral lesions do not conform to a strictly vascular distribution. The onset in the majority of patients is before age 20. Seizures, usually partial motor or generalized, are common and may represent the first clearly recognizable sign of disease. The cerebral insults that resemble strokes cause hemiparesis, hemianopia, and cortical blindness. A presumptive stroke occurring before age 40 should place this mitochondrial encephalomyopathy high in the differential diagnosis. Associated conditions include hearing loss, diabetes mellitus, hypothalamic pituitary dysfunction causing growth hormone deficiency, hypothyroidism, and absence of secondary sexual characteristics. In its full expression MELAS leads to dementia, a bedridden state, and a fatal outcome. Serum lactic acid is typically elevated. The spinal fluid protein is also increased but is usually ≤1.0 g/L (100 mg/dL). Muscle biopsies show ragged red fibers. Neuroimaging demonstrates basal ganglia calcification in a high percentage of cases. Focal lesions that mimic infarction are present predominantly in the occipital and parietal lobes. Strict vascular territories are not respected, and cerebral angiography fails to demonstrate lesions of the major cerebral blood vessels.

MELAS is caused by maternally inherited point mutations of mitochondrial tRNA genes. Most of the tRNA mutations are lethal, accounting for the paucity of multigeneration families with this syndrome. The A3243G point mutation in tRNA$^{Leu(UUR)}$ is the most common, occurring in ~80% of MELAS cases. About 10% of MELAS patients have other mutations of the tRNA$^{Leu(UUR)}$ gene including 3252G, 3256T, 3271C, and 3291C. Other tRNA gene mutations have also been reported in MELAS including G583A tRNA^{Phe}, G1642A tRNA^{Val}, G4332A tRNA^{Glu}, and T8316C tRNA^{Lys}. Mutations have also been reported in mtDNA polypeptide-coding genes. Two mutations were found in the ND5 subunit of complex I of the respiratory chain. A missense mutation has been reported at mtDNA position 9957 in the gene for subunit III of cytochrome C oxidase. No specific treatment is available. Supportive treatment is essential for the stroke-like episodes, seizures, and endocrinopathies.

PURE MYOPATHY SYNDROMES   Muscle weakness and fatigue can be the predominant manifestations of mtDNA mutations. When the condition affects exclusively muscle (pure myopathy), the disorder becomes difficult to recognize.

Mitochondrial DNA Depletion Myopathy   This disorder, clinically indistinguishable from muscular dystrophy, usually presents in the neonatal period with weakness, hypotonia, and delayed motor milestones. Some cases are rapidly fatal, with death before age 2. A milder form affects patients at a slightly later age. These patients have slowly evolving proximal muscle weakness simulating Duchenne muscular dystrophy. In some, seizures and cardiomyopathy may be present. Serum CK can reach levels of 20 to 30 times normal. Resting lactates vary from normal to mildly elevated. The EMG is myopathic, and ragged red fibers are seen on muscle biopsy. The mtDNA depletion syndrome is inherited as an autosomal recessive condition. Mutations have been identified in the *TK2* gene on chromosome 16q22 encoding thymidine kinase-2. The affected gene controls the supply of deoxyribonucleotides used for the synthesis of mtDNA. No specific treatment is available. Supportive care follows the approaches outlined for muscular dystrophy.

DISORDERS OF MUSCLE MEMBRANE EXCITABILITY

Muscle membrane excitability is affected in a group of disorders referred to as *channelopathies*. The heart may also be involved, resulting in life-threatening complications (Table 368-5).

CALCIUM CHANNEL DISORDERS OF MUSCLE ■ Hypokalemic Periodic Paralysis (HypoKPP)   Onset occurs at adolescence. Men are more often affected because of decreased penetrance in women. Episodic weakness with onset after age 25 is almost never due to periodic paralyses with the exception of thyrotoxic periodic paralysis (see below). Attacks are often provoked by meals high in carbohydrates or sodium and may accompany rest following prolonged exercise. Weakness usually af-

fects proximal limb muscles more than distal. Ocular and bulbar muscles are less likely to be affected. Respiratory muscles are usually spared but when they are involved, the condition may prove fatal. Weakness may take as long as 24 h to resolve. Life-threatening cardiac arrhythmias related to hypokalemia may occur during attacks. Myotonia, if present, is confined to the eyelids. As a late complication, patients commonly develop severe, disabling proximal lower extremity weakness.

Attacks of thyrotoxic periodic paralysis resemble those of primary hypoKPP. Despite a higher incidence of thyrotoxicosis in women, men, particularly those of Asian descent, are more likely to manifest this complication. Attacks abate with treatment of the underlying thyroid condition.

A low serum potassium level during an attack, excluding secondary causes, establishes the diagnosis. Interattack muscle biopsies show the presence of single or multiple centrally placed vacuoles. Provocative tests with glucose and insulin to establish a diagnosis are usually not necessary and are potentially hazardous. HypoKPP is inherited as an autosomal dominant disorder with incomplete penetrance. Mutations in the voltage-sensitive, skeletal muscle calcium channel (Fig. 368-2) cause the disease.

The acute paralysis improves after the administration of potassium. Muscle strength and electrocardiogram should be monitored. Oral KCl (0.2 to 0.4 mmol/kg) should be given every 30 min. Only rarely is intravenous therapy necessary (e.g., swallowing problems or vomiting present). Administration of potassium in glucose or saline, which may further lower potassium, should be avoided. Mannitol is the preferred vehicle for administration of intravenous potassium. The long-term goal of therapy is to avoid attacks. This may reduce late-onset, fixed weakness. Patients should be made aware of the importance of a low-carbohydrate, low-sodium diet and consequences of intense exercise. Prophylactic administration of acetozolamide (125 to 1000 mg/d in divided doses) reduces or may abolish attacks. Paradoxically the potassium is lowered, but this is offset by the beneficial effect of metabolic acidosis. If attacks persist on acetozolamide, oral KCl should be added. Some patients require treatment with triamterine (25 to 100 mg/d) or spironolactone (25 to 100 mg/d).

SODIUM CHANNEL DISORDERS OF MUSCLE ■ Hyperkalemic Periodic Paralysis (HyperKPP)   The term *hyperkalemic* is misleading since patients are often normokalemic during attacks. The fact that attacks are precipitated by potassium administration best defines the disease. The onset is in the first decade. Attacks are brief and mild, usually lasting 30 min to 4 h. Weakness affects proximal muscles, sparing bulbar muscles. Attacks are precipitated by rest following exercise and fasting. In a variant of this disorder, the predominant symptom is myotonia without weakness (*potassium-aggravated myotonia*). The symptoms are aggravated by cold, and myotonia makes the muscles stiff and painful. This disorder can be confused with paramyotonia and myotonia congenita (described below).

Potassium may be slightly elevated but may also be normal during

TABLE 368-5   *Clinical Features of Periodic Paralysis and Nondystrophic Myotonias*

Feature	Calcium Channel Hypokalemic PP	Sodium Channel Hyperkalemic PP	Paramyotonia Congenita	Potassium Channel Anderson's Syndrome[b]
Mode of inheritance	AD	AD	AD	AD
Age of onset	Adolescence	Early childhood	Early childhood	Early childhood
Myotonia[a]	No	Yes	Yes	No
Episodic weakness	Yes	Yes	Yes	Yes
Frequency of attacks of weakness	Daily to yearly	May be 2–3/d	With cold, usually rare	Daily to yearly
Duration of attacks of weakness	2–12 h	From 1–2 h to >1 day	2–24 h	2–24 h
Serum K$^+$ level during attacks of weakness	Decreased	Increased or normal	Usually normal	Variable
Effect of K$^+$ loading	No change	Increased myotonia, then weakness	Increased myotonia	No change
Effect of muscle cooling	No change	Increased myotonia	Increased myotonia, then weakness	No change
Fixed weakness	Yes	Yes	Yes	Yes

[a] May be paradoxical in paramyotonia congenita.
[b] Dysmorphic features and cardiac arrhythmias are distinguishing features (see text).

Abbreviations: AD, autosomal dominant; AR, autosomal recessive; PP, periodic paralysis.

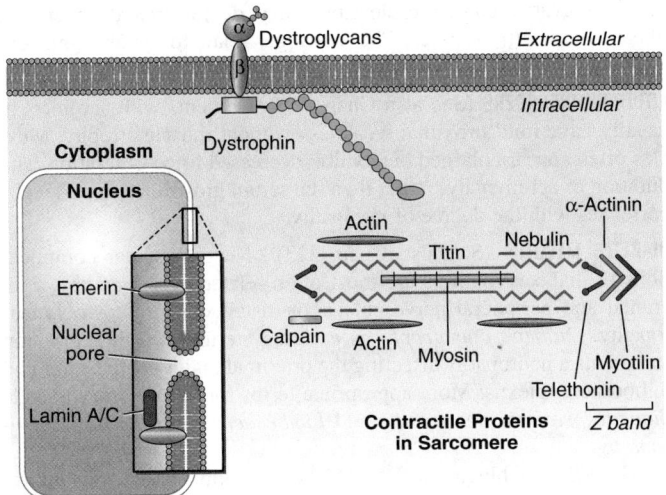

FIGURE 368-2 Selected muscular dystrophy–associated proteins in the nuclear membrane and sarcomere. As shown in the exploded view, emerin and laminin A/C are constitutents of the inner nuclear membrane. Several dystrophy-associated proteins are represented in the sarcomere including titin, nebulin, calpain, telethonin, actinin, and myotilin. The position of the dystrophin-dystroglycan complex is also illustrated.

an attack. The EMG will often demonstrate myotonia during and between attacks. The muscle biopsy shows vacuoles that are smaller, less numerous, and more peripheral compared to the hypokalemic form. Provocative tests by administration of potassium can induce weakness but are usually not necessary to establish the diagnosis. HyperKPP and potassium-aggravated myotonia are inherited as autosomal dominant disorders. Mutations of the voltage-gated sodium channel SCN4A (Fig. 368-3) cause these conditions. For patients with frequent attacks acetozolamide (125 to 100 mg/d) is helpful.

Paramyotonia Congenita In paramyotonia congenita (PC) the attacks of weakness are cold-induced or occur spontaneously and are mild. Myotonia is a prominent feature but worsens with muscle activity (paradoxical myotonia). This is in contrast to classic myotonia in which exercise alleviates the condition. Attacks of weakness are seldom severe enough to require emergency room treatment. Over time patients develop interattack weakness as they do in other forms of periodic paralysis. PC is usually associated with normokalemia or hyperkalemia. Other features are similar to those of hyperKPP. PC is inherited as an autosomal dominant condition; voltage-gated sodium channel mutations (Fig. 368-3) are responsible. Patients with PC seldom seek treatment during attacks. Oral administration of glucose or other carbohydrates hastens recovery. Since interattack weakness may develop after repeated episodes, prophylactic treatment is usually indicated. Thiazide diuretics (e.g., chlorothiazide 250 to 1000 mg/d) and mexiletine (slowly increase dose from 450 mg/d) are reported to be helpful. Patients should be advised to increase carbohydrates in their diet.

POTASSIUM CHANNEL DISORDERS ▪ Andersen's Syndrome This rare disease is characterized by episodic weakness, cardiac arrhythmias, and dysmorphic features (short stature, scoliosis, clinodactyly, hypertelorism, small or prominent low set ears, micrognathia, and broad forehead). The cardiac arrhythmias are potentially serious and life threatening. They include long QT, ventricular ectopy, bidirectional ventricular arrhythmias, and tachycardia. For many years the classification of this disorder was uncertain because episodes of weakness are associated with elevated, normal, or reduced levels of potassium during an attack. In addition, the potassium levels differ among kindreds but are consistent within a family. Inheritance is autosomal dominant, with incomplete penetrance and variable expressivity. The disease is caused by mutations of the inwardly rectifying potassium channel (*kir*) gene. The treatment is similar to that for other forms of periodic paralysis and must include cardiac monitoring. The episodes of weakness may differ between patients because of potassium variability. Acetozolamide will decrease the attack frequency and severity.

CHLORIDE CHANNEL DISORDERS Two forms of this disorder, autosomal dominant (*Thomsen's disease*) and autosomal recessive (*Becker's disease*) are related to the same gene abnormality. Symptoms are noted in infancy and early childhood. The severity lessens in the third to fourth decade. Myotonia is worsened by cold and improved by activity. The gait may appear slow and labored at first but improves with walking. In Thomsen's disease muscle strength is normal, but in Becker's, which is usually more severe, there may be muscle weakness. Muscle hypertrophy is usually present. Myotonia is prominently displayed by EMG recordings. Serum CK is normal or mildly elevated. The muscle biopsy shows hypertrophied fibers. The disease is inherited as dominant or recessive and is caused by mutations of the chloride channel gene (Fig. 368-3). Many patients will not require treatment and learn that the symptoms improve with activity. Medications that can be used to decrease myotonia include quinine, phenytoin, and mexilitene.

ENDOCRINE AND METABOLIC MYOPATHIES

Many endocrine disorders cause weakness. Muscle fatigue is more common than true weakness. The cause of weakness in these disorders is not well defined. It is not even clear that weakness results from

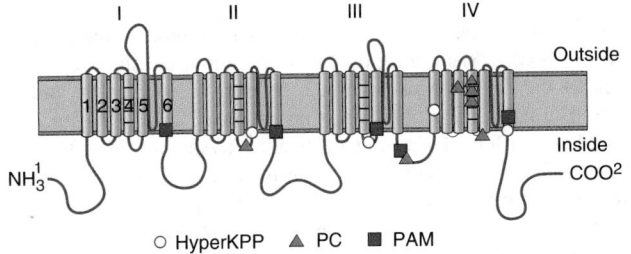

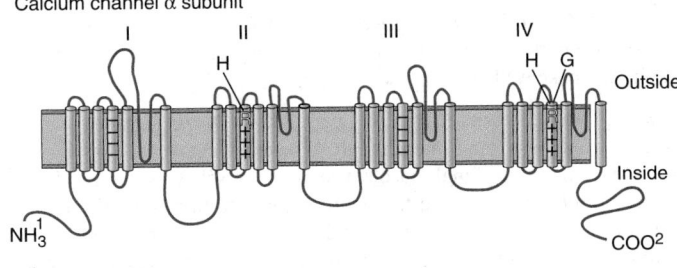

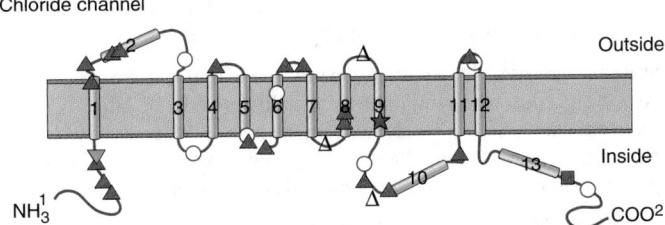

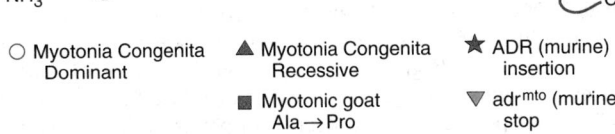

FIGURE 368-3 The sodium and calcium channels are depicted here as containing four homologous domains, each with six membrane-spanning segments. The fourth segment of each domain bears positive charges and acts as the "voltage sensor" for the channel. The association of the four domains is thought to form a pore through which ions pass. Sodium channel mutations are shown along with the phenotype that they confer. HyperKPP, hyperkalemic periodic paralysis; PC, paramyotonia congenita; PAM, potassium-aggravated myotonia. See text for details.

The chloride channel is envisioned to have ten membrane-spanning domains. The positions of mutations causing dominantly and recessively inherited myotonia congenita are indicated, along with mutations that cause this disease in mice and goats.

disease of muscle as opposed to another part of the motor unit, since the serum CK level is often normal (except in hypothyroidism) and the muscle histology is characterized by atrophy rather than destruction of muscle fibers. Nearly all endocrine myopathies respond to treatment.

THYROID DISORDERS (See also Chap. 320)   Abnormalities of thyroid function can cause a wide array of muscle disorders. These conditions relate to the important role of thyroid hormones in regulating the metabolism of carbohydrates and lipids as well as the rate of protein synthesis and enzyme production. Thyroid hormones also stimulate calorigenesis in muscle, increase muscle demand for vitamins, and enhance muscle sensitivity to circulating catecholamines.

Hypothyroidism   Patients with hypothyroidism have frequent muscle complaints, and proximal muscle weakness occurs in about one-third of them. Muscle cramps, pain, and stiffness are common. Features of slow muscle contraction and relaxation occur in 25% of patients, and the relaxation phase of muscle stretch reflexes is characteristically prolonged. The serum CK level is often elevated (up to 10 times normal), even when there is minimal clinical evidence of muscle disease. *Hoffman's syndrome* results in prominent muscle enlargement and weakness with muscle stiffness. The cause of muscle enlargement has not been determined, and muscle biopsy shows no distinctive morphologic abnormalities.

Hyperthyroidism   Patients who are thyrotoxic commonly have proximal muscle weakness and atrophy on examination, but they rarely complain of the deficit. Muscle stretch reflexes are preserved and often brisk. Bulbar, respiratory, and even esophageal muscles may occasionally be affected, causing dysphagia, dysphonia, and aspiration. When bulbar involvement occurs, it is usually accompanied by chronic proximal limb weakness, but occasionally it presents in the absence of generalized thyrotoxic myopathy. Other neuromuscular disorders occur in association with hyperthyroidism, including hypokalemic, myasthenia gravis, and a progressive ocular myopathy associated with proptosis (*Graves' ophthalmopathy*). Serum CK levels are not elevated in thyrotoxic myopathy. The muscle histology usually shows only atrophy of muscle fibers.

PARATHYROID DISORDERS (See also Chap. 332)   ■   **Hyperparathyroidism** Muscle weakness is an integral part of primary and secondary hyperparathyroidism. Proximal muscle weakness, muscle wasting, and brisk muscle stretch reflexes are the main features of this endocrinopathy. Serum CK levels are usually normal or slightly elevated. Serum calcium and phosphorus levels show no correlation with the clinical neuromuscular manifestations. Muscle biopsies show only varying degrees of atrophy without muscle fiber degeneration.

Hypoparathyroidism   An overt myopathy due to hypocalcemia rarely occurs. Neuromuscular symptoms are usually related to localized or generalized tetany. Serum CK levels may be increased secondary to muscle damage from sustained tetany. Hyporeflexia or areflexia is usually present and contrasts with the hyperreflexia in hyperparathyroidism.

ADRENAL DISORDERS (See also Chap. 321)   Conditions associated with glucocorticoid excess cause a myopathy; in fact, steroid myopathy is the most commonly diagnosed endocrine muscle disease. Glucocorticoid excess, either endogenous or exogenous (see "Toxic Myopathies," below), produces various degrees of proximal limb weakness. Muscle wasting may be striking. A cushingoid appearance usually accompanies clinical signs of myopathy. Histologic sections demonstrate muscle fiber atrophy rather than degeneration or necrosis of muscle fibers. Adrenal insufficiency commonly causes muscle fatigue. The degree of weakness may be difficult to asses but is typically mild. In primary hyperaldosteronism (*Conn's syndrome*), neuromuscular complications are due to potassium depletion. The clinical picture is one of persistent muscle weakness. Long-standing hyperaldosteronism may lead to proximal limb weakness and wasting. Serum CK levels may be elevated, and a muscle biopsy may demonstrate degenerating fibers, some with vacuoles. These changes relate to hypokalemia and are not a direct effect of aldosterone on skeletal muscle.

PITUITARY DISORDERS (See also Chap. 318)   Patients with acromegaly usually have mild proximal weakness without muscle atrophy. Muscles often appear enlarged but exhibit decreased force generation. The duration of acromegaly, rather than the serum growth hormone levels, correlates with the degree of myopathy.

DIABETES MELLITUS (See also Chap. 323)   Neuromuscular complications of diabetes mellitus are most often related to neuropathy, with cranial and peripheral nerve palsies or distal sensorimotor polyneuropathy. *Diabetic amyotrophy* is a clumsy term since the condition represents a neuropathy affecting the proximal major nerve trunks and lumbosacral plexus. More appropriate terms for this disorder include *diabetic proximal neuropathy* and *lumbosacral radiculoplexus neuropathy.*

The only notable myopathy of diabetes mellitus is ischemic infarction of thigh muscles. This condition occurs in patients with poorly controlled diabetes and presents with abrupt onset of pain, tenderness, and edema of one thigh. The area of muscle infarction is hard and indurated. The muscles most often affected include the vastus lateralis, thigh adductors, and biceps femoris. Computed tomography or magnetic resonance imaging can demonstrate focal abnormalities in the affected muscle. Diagnosis by imaging is preferable to muscle biopsy, if possible.

VITAMIN DEFICIENCY   Vitamin D deficiency (Chap. 61) due to either decreased intake, decreased absorption, or impaired vitamin D metabolism (as occurs in renal disease) may lead to chronic muscle weakness. Pain reflects the underlying bone disease (*osteomalacia*). Vitamin E deficiency may result from malabsorption. Clinical manifestations include ataxic neuropathy due to loss of proprioception and myopathy with proximal weakness. Progressive external ophthalmoplegia is a distinctive finding. It has not been established that deficiency of other vitamins causes a myopathy.

MYOPATHIES OF SYSTEMIC ILLNESS

Systemic illnesses such as chronic respiratory, cardiac, or hepatic failure are frequently associated with severe muscle wasting and complaints of weakness. Fatigue is usually a more significant problem than weakness, which is typically mild.

Myopathy may be a manifestation of chronic renal failure, independent of the better known uremic polyneuropathy. Abnormalities of calcium and phosphorus homeostasis and bone metabolism in chronic renal failure result from a reduction in 1,25-dihydroxyvitamin D, leading to decreased intestinal absorption of calcium. Hypocalcemia, further accentuated by hyperphosphatemia due to decreased renal phosphate clearance, leads to secondary hyperparathyroidism. Renal osteodystrophy results from the compensatory hyperparathyroidism, which leads to osteomalacia from reduced calcium availability and to osteitis fibrosa from the parathyroid hormone excess. The clinical picture of the myopathy of chronic renal failure is identical to that of primary hyperparathyroidism and osteomalacia. There is proximal limb weakness with bone pain.

Gangrenous calcification represents a separate, rare, and sometimes fatal complication of chronic renal failure. In this condition, widespread arterial calcification occurs and results in ischemia. Extensive skin necrosis may occur, along with painful myopathy and even myoglobinuria.

TOXIC MYOPATHIES

Toxic myopathies are relatively uncommon in clinical practice with the exception of those caused by the cholesterol-lowering agents and glucocorticoids. Others impact practice to a lesser degree but are important to consider in specific situations. Table 368-6 provides a comprehensive list of toxic myopathies with their distinguishing features.

MYOPATHY FROM LIPID-LOWERING AGENTS   All classes of lipid-lowering agents have been implicated in muscle toxicity including fibrates (clo-

TABLE 368-6 Toxic Myopathies

Drugs	Major Toxic Reaction

Lipid-lowering agents
  Fibric acid derivatives
  HMG-CoA reductase
    inhibitors
  Niacin (nicotinic acid)
	Drugs belonging to all three of the major classes of lipid-lowering agents can produce a spectrum of toxicity: asymptomatic serum creatine kinase elevation, myalgias, exercised-induced pain, rhabdomyolysis, and myoglobinuria.

Glucocorticoids	Acute, high-dose glucocorticoid treatment can cause acute quadriplegic myopathy. These high doses of steroids are often combined with nondepolarizing neuromuscular blocking agents but the weakness can occur without their use. Chronic steroid administration produces predominantly proximal weakness.

Nondepolarizing
  neuromuscular blocking
  agents
	Acute quadriplegic myopathy can occur with or without concomitant glucocorticoids.

Zidovudine	Mitochondrial myopathy with ragged red fibers.

Drugs of abuse
  Alcohol
  Amphetamines
  Cocaine
  Heroin
  Phencyclidine
  Meperidine
	All drugs in this group can lead to widespread muscle breakdown, rhabdomyolysis, and myoglobinuria. Local injections cause muscle necrosis, skin induration, and limb contractures.

Autoimmune toxic
  myopathy
  D-Penicillamine
	Use of this drug may cause polymyositis and myasthenia gravis.

Amphophilic cationic
  drugs
  Amiodarone
  Chloroquine
  Hydroxychloroquine
	All amphophilic drugs have the potential to produce painless, proximal weakness associated with autophagic vacuoles in the muscle biopsy.

Antimicrotubular drugs Colchicine	This drug produces painless, proximal weakness especially in the setting of renal failure. Muscle biopsy shows autophagic vacuoles.

fibrate, gemfibrozil), HMG-COA reductase inhibitors (referred to as *statins*), and niacin (nicotinic acid). Myalgia, malaise, and muscle tenderness are the most common manifestations. Muscle pain may be related to exercise. Patients may exhibit proximal weakness. Varying degrees of muscle necrosis are seen, and in severe reactions there are rhabdomyolysis and myoglobinuria. Patients improve with drug cessation. Concomitant use of statins with fibrates and cyclosporine is more likely to cause adverse reactions than use of one agent alone. Elevated serum CK is an important indication of toxicity. Muscle weakness is accompanied by a myopathic EMG, and muscle necrosis is observed by muscle biopsy. Myopathic reactions are indications for stopping the drug.

GLUCOCORTICOID-REALTED MYOPATHIES Glucocorticoid myopathy occurs with chronic treatment or as "acute quadriplegic" myopathy secondary to high-dose, intravenous glucocorticoids. Chronic administration produces proximal weakness accompanied by cushingoid manifestations, which can be quite debilitating; the chronic use of prednisone at a daily dose of ≥30 mg/d is most often associated with toxicity. Patients taking fluorinated glucocorticoids (triamcinolone, betamethasone, dexamethasone) appear to be at especially high risk for myopathy. Patients receiving high-dose, intravenous glucocorticoids for status asthmaticus, chronic obstructive pulmonary disease or other indications may develop severe generalized weakness. Involvement of the diaphragm and intercostal muscles causes respiratory failure and requires ventilatory support. In this setting, the use of glucocorticoids in combination with nondepolarizing neuromuscular blocking agents to further decrease airway resistance is particularly likely to lead to this complication. In chronic steroid myopathy the serum CK is usually normal. Serum potassium may be low. The muscle biopsy in chronic

cases shows preferential type 2 muscle fiber atrophy; this is not reflected in the EMG, which is usually normal. In acute cases with quadraplegic myopathy the muscle biopsy is abnormal, showing a distinctive loss of thick filaments by electron microscopy. By light microscopy there is focal loss of ATPase staining in central or paracentral areas of the muscle fiber. Calpain stains show diffusely reactive atrophic fibers. Withdrawal of glucocorticoids will improve the chronic myopathy. In acute quadriplegic myopathy, recovery is slow. Patients require supportive care and rehabilitation.

MYOPATHY OF NONDEPOLARIZING NEUROMUSCULAR BLOCKING AGENTS Patients may receive nondepolarizing neuromuscular blocking agents because of life-threatening airway resistance. Acute quadriplegic myopathy may result, with or without glucocorticoid use. The clinical features are identical to acute quadriplegic myopathy secondary to glucocorticoids.

DRUG-INDUCED MITOCHONDRIAL MYOPATHY Zidovudine, used in the treatment of HIV infection, is a thymidine analogue that inhibits viral replication by interrupting reverse transcriptase. Myopathy is a well-established complication of this agent. Patients present with myalgias, muscle weakness, and atrophy affecting the thigh and calf muscles. The complication occurs in about 17% of patients treated with doses of 1200 mg/d for 6 months. The introduction of protease inhibitors for treatment of HIV infection has led to lower doses of zidovudine therapy and a decreased incidence of myopathy. Serum CK is elevated and EMG is myopathic. Muscle biopsy shows ragged red fibers with minimal inflammation; the lack of inflammation serves to distinguish zidovudine toxicity from HIV-related myopathy. If the myopathy is thought to be drug related the medication should be stopped or the dosage reduced.

DRUGS OF ABUSE AND RELATED MYOPATHIES Myotoxicity is a potential consequence of addiction to alcohol and illicit drugs. Ethanol is one of the most commonly abused substances with potential to damage muscle. Other potential toxins include cocaine, heroin, and amphetamines. The most deleterious reactions occur from overdosing leading to coma and seizures, causing rhabdomyolysis, myoglobinuria, and renal failure. Direct toxicity can occur from cocaine, heroin, and amphetamines causing muscle breakdown and varying degrees of weakness. The effects of alcohol are more controversial. Direct muscle damage is less certain, since toxicity usually occurs in the setting of poor nutrition and possible contributing factors such as hypokalemia and hypophosphatemia. Alcoholics are also prone to neuropathy and a variety of central nervous system disorders (Chap. 372).

Focal myopathies from self-administration of meperidine, heroin, and pentazocine can cause pain, swelling, muscle necrosis, and hemorrhage. The cause is multifactorial: needle trauma, direct toxicity of the drug or vehicle, and infection. When severe, there may be overlying skin induration and contractures with replacement of muscle by connective tissue. Elevated serum CK and myopathic EMG are characteristic of these reactions. The muscle biopsy shows widespread or focal areas of necrosis. In conditions leading to rhabdomyolysis, patients need adequate hydration to reduce serum myoglobin and protect renal function. In all of these conditions, counseling is essential to limit drug abuse.

DRUG-INDUCED AUTOIMMUNE MYOPATHIES The most consistent drug-related inflammatory or antibody-mediated myopathy is caused by D-penicillamine. This drug chelates copper and is used in the treatment of Wilson's disease. It is also used to treat other disorders including scleroderma, rheumatoid arthritis, and primary biliary cirrhosis. Adverse events include drug-induced polymyositis indistinguishable from the spontaneous disease. The incidence of this inflammatory muscle disease is about 1%. Myasthenia gravis is also induced by D-penicillamine, with a higher incidence estimated at 7%. These disorders resolve with drug withdrawal, although immunosuppressive therapy may be warranted in severe cases.

Scattered reports of other drugs causing an inflammatory myopathy are rare and include a heterogeneous group of agents: cimetidine, phenytoin, procainamide, and propylthiouracil. In most cases, a cause-and-effect relationship is uncertain. A complication of interest was related to L-tryptophan. In 1989 an epidemic of eosinophilia-myalgia syndrome (EMS) in the United States was caused by a contaminant in the product from one manufacturer. The product was withdrawn, and incidence of EMS diminished abruptly following this action.

OTHER DRUG-INDUCED MYOPATHIES Certain drugs produce painless, largely proximal, muscle weakness. These drugs include the amphophilic cationic drugs (amiodarone, chloroquine, hydroxychloroquine) and antimicrotubular drugs (colchicine). Muscle biopsy can be useful in the identification of toxicity since autophagic vacuoles are prominent pathologic features of these toxins.

FURTHER READING

FAN X, ROULEAU GA: Progress in understanding the pathogenesis of oculopharyngeal muscular dystrophy. Can J Neurol Sci 30:8, 2003

FINSTERER J, STOLLBERGER C: The heart in human dystrophinopathies. Cardiology 99:1, 2003

KULLMANN DM, HANNA MG: Neurological disorders caused by inherited ion-channel mutations. Lancet Neurol 1:157, 2002

WIESER T et al: Carnitine palmitoyltransferase II deficiency: Molecular and biochemical analysis of 32 patients. Neurology 60:1351, 2003

369 POLYMYOSITIS, DERMATOMYOSITIS, AND INCLUSION BODY MYOSITIS
Marinos C. Dalakas

The inflammatory myopathies represent the largest group of acquired and potentially treatable causes of skeletal muscle weakness. They are classified into three major groups: polymyositis (PM), dermatomyositis (DM), and inclusion body myositis (IBM).

CLINICAL FEATURES The prevalence of the inflammatory myopathies is estimated at 1 in 100,000. PM as a stand-alone entity is a rare disease affecting adults. DM affects both children and adults, and women more often than men. IBM is three times more frequent in men than in women, more common in Caucasians than blacks, and is most likely to affect persons >50 years of age.

These disorders present as progressive and often symmetric muscle weakness. Patients usually report increasing difficulty with everyday tasks requiring the use of proximal muscles, such as getting up from a chair, climbing steps, stepping onto a curb, lifting objects, or combing hair. Fine-motor movements that depend on the strength of distal muscles, such as buttoning a shirt, sewing, knitting, or writing, are affected only late in the course of PM and DM, but fairly early in IBM. Falling is common in IBM because of early involvement of the quadriceps muscle with buckling of the knees. Ocular muscles are spared, even in advanced, untreated cases; if these muscles are affected, the diagnosis of inflammatory myopathy should be questioned. Facial muscles are unaffected in PM and DM, but mild facial muscle weakness is common in patients with IBM. In all forms of inflammatory myopathy, pharyngeal and neck-flexor muscles are often involved, causing dysphagia or difficulty in holding up the head (*head drop*). In advanced and rarely in acute cases, respiratory muscles may also be affected. Severe weakness, if untreated, is almost always associated with muscle wasting. Sensation remains normal. The tendon reflexes are preserved but may be absent in severely weakened or atrophied muscles, especially in IBM where atrophy of the quadriceps and the distal muscles is common. Myalgia and muscle tenderness may occur in a small number of patients, usually early in the disease, and particularly in DM associated with connective tissue disorders. Weakness in PM and DM progresses subacutely over a period of weeks or months and rarely acutely; by contrast, IBM progresses very slowly, over years, simulating a late-life muscular dystrophy (Chap. 368) or slowly progressive motor neuron disorder (Chap. 353).

SPECIFIC FEATURES (Table 369-1) ■ **Polymyositis** The actual onset of PM is often not easily determined, and patients typically delay seeking medical advice for several months. This is in contrast to DM, in which the rash facilitates early recognition (see below). PM mimics many other myopathies and is a diagnosis of exclusion. It is a subacute inflammatory myopathy affecting adults, and rarely children, who *do not have* any of the following: rash, involvement of the extraocular and facial muscles, family history of a neuromuscular disease, history of exposure to myotoxic drugs or toxins, endocrinopathy, neurogenic disease, muscular dystrophy, biochemical muscle disorder (deficiency

TABLE 369-1 *Features Associated with Inflammatory Myopathies*

Characteristic	Polymyositis	Dermatomyositis	Inclusion Body Myositis
Age at onset	>18 yr	Adulthood and childhood	>50 yr
Familial association	No	No	Yes, in some cases
Extramuscular manifestations	Yes	Yes	Yes
Associated conditions			
Connective tissue diseases	Yes[a]	Scleroderma and mixed connective tissue disease (overlap syndromes)	Yes, in up to 20% of cases[a]
Systemic autoimmune diseases[b]	Frequent	Infrequent	Infrequent
Malignancy	No	Yes, in up to 15% of cases	No
Viruses	Yes[c]	Unproven	Yes[c]
Drugs[d]	Yes	Yes, rarely	No
Parasites and bacteria[e]	Yes	No	No

[a] Systemic lupus erythematosus, rheumatoid arthritis, Sjögren's syndrome, systemic sclerosis, mixed connective tissue disease.
[b] Crohn's disease, vasculitis, sarcoidosis, primary biliary cirrhosis, adult celiac disease, chronic graft-versus-host disease, discoid lupus, ankylosing spondylitis, Behçet's syndrome, myasthenia gravis, acne fulminans, dermatitis herpetiformis, psoriasis, Hashimoto's disease, granulomatous diseases, agammaglobulinemia, monoclonal gammopathy, hypereosinophilic syndrome, Lyme disease, Kawasaki disease, autoimmune thrombocytopenia, hypergammaglobulinemic purpura, hereditary complement deficiency, IgA deficiency.
[c] HIV (human immunodeficiency virus) and HTLV-I (human T cell lymphotropic virus type I).
[d] Drugs include penicillamine (dermatomyositis and polymyositis), zidovudine (polymyositis), and contaminated tryptophan (dermatomyositis-like illness). Other myotoxic drugs may cause myopathy but not an inflammatory myopathy (see text for details).
[e] Parasites (protozoa, cestodes, nematodes), tropical and bacterial myositis (pyomyositis).

of a muscle enzyme), or IBM as excluded by muscle biopsy analysis (see below). As an isolated entity, PM is a rare (and overdiagnosed) disorder; more commonly, PM occurs in association with a systemic autoimmune or connective tissue disease, or with a known viral or bacterial infection. Drugs, especially D-penicillamine or zidovudine (AZT), may also produce an inflammatory myopathy similar to PM.

Dermatomyositis DM is a distinctive entity identified by a characteristic rash accompanying, or more often preceding, muscle weakness. The rash may consist of a blue-purple discoloration on the upper eyelids with edema (heliotrope rash; see Fig. 49-3), a flat red rash on the face and upper trunk, and erythema of the knuckles with a raised violaceous scaly eruption (*Gottron rash*; see Fig. 49-4). The erythematous rash can also occur on other body surfaces, including the knees, elbows, malleoli, neck and anterior chest (often in a *V sign*), or back and shoulders (*shawl sign*), and may worsen after sun exposure. In some patients the rash is pruritic, especially on the scalp, chest, and back. Dilated capillary loops at the base of the fingernails are also characteristic. The cuticles may be irregular, thickened, and distorted, and the lateral and palmar areas of the fingers may become rough and cracked, with irregular, "dirty" horizontal lines, resembling *mechanic's hands*. The weakness can be mild, moderate, or severe enough to lead to quadraparesis. At times, the muscle strength appears normal, hence the term *dermatomyositis sine myositis*. When muscle biopsy is performed in such cases, however, significant perivascular and perimysial inflammation is seen.

DM usually occurs alone but may overlap with scleroderma and mixed connective tissue disease. Fasciitis and thickening of the skin, similar to that seen in chronic cases of DM, have occurred in patients with the *eosinophilia-myalgia syndrome* associated with the ingestion of contaminated L-tryptophan.

Inclusion Body Myositis

In patients ≥50 years of age, IBM is the most common of the inflammatory myopathies. It is often misdiagnosed as PM and suspected only later when a patient with presumed PM does not respond to therapy. Weakness and atrophy of the distal muscles, especially foot extensors and deep finger flexors, occur in almost all cases of IBM and may be a clue to early diagnosis. Some patients present with falls because their knees collapse due to early quadriceps weakness. Others present with weakness in the small muscles of the hands, especially finger flexors, and complain of inability to hold objects such as golf clubs or perform tasks such as turning keys or tying knots. On occasion, the weakness and accompanying atrophy can be asymmetric and selectively involve the quadriceps, iliopsoas, triceps, biceps, and finger flexors, resembling a lower motor neuron disease. Dysphagia is common, occurring in up to 60% of IBM patients, and may lead to episodes of choking. Sensory examination is generally normal; some patients have mildly diminished vibratory sensation at the ankles that presumably is age-related. The pattern of distal weakness, which superficially resembles motor neuron or peripheral nerve disease, results from the myopathic process affecting distal muscles selectively. Disease progression is slow but steady, and most patients require an assistive device such as cane, walker, or wheelchair within several years of onset.

In at least 20% of cases, IBM is associated with systemic autoimmune or connective tissue diseases. Familial aggregation of typical IBM may occur; such cases have been designated as *familial inflammatory IBM*. This disorder is distinct from *hereditary inclusion body myopathy* (h-IBM), which describes a heterogeneous group of recessive, and less frequently dominant, inherited syndromes; the h-IBMs are noninflammatory myopathies. A subset of h-IBM that spares the quadriceps muscles has emerged as a distinct entity. This disorder, originally described in Iranian Jews and now seen in many ethnic groups, is linked to chromosome 9p1 and results from mutations in the UDP-*N*-acetylglucosamine 2-epimerase/*N*-acetylmannosamine kinase (*GNE*) gene.

ASSOCIATED CLINICAL FINDINGS ■ Extramuscular Manifestations

These may be present to a varying degree in patients with PM or DM, including:

1. *Systemic symptoms*, such as fever, malaise, weight loss, arthralgia, and Raynaud's phenomenon, especially when inflammatory myopathy is associated with a connective tissue disorder.
2. *Joint contractures*, mostly in DM and especially in children.
3. *Dysphagia and gastrointestinal symptoms*, due to involvement of oropharyngeal striated muscles and upper esophagus, especially in DM and IBM.
4. *Cardiac disturbances*, including atrioventricular conduction defects, tachyarrhythmias, dilated cardiomyopathy, and a low ejection fraction. Congestive heart failure and myocarditis may also occur, either from the disease itself or from hypertension associated with long-term use of glucocorticoids.
5. *Pulmonary dysfunction*, due to weakness of the thoracic muscles, interstitial lung disease, or drug-induced pneumonitis (e.g., from methotrexate), which may cause dyspnea, nonproductive cough, and aspiration pneumonia. Interstitial lung disease may precede myopathy or occur early in the disease and develops in up to 10% of patients with PM or DM, most of whom have antibodies to t-RNA synthetases, as described below.
6. *Subcutaneous calcifications*, in DM, sometimes extruding on the skin and causing ulcerations and infections.

Association with Malignancies Although all the inflammatory myopathies can have a chance association with malignant lesions, especially in older age groups, the incidence of malignant conditions appears to be specifically increased only in patients with DM and not in PM or IBM. The most common tumors associated with DM are ovarian cancer, breast cancer, melanoma, colon cancer, and non-Hodgkin lymphoma. The extent of the search that should be conducted for an occult neoplasm in adults with DM depends on the clinical circumstances. Tumors in these patients are usually uncovered by abnormal findings in the medical history and physical examination and not through an extensive blind search. The weight of evidence argues against performing expensive, invasive, and nondirected tumor searches. A complete annual physical examination with pelvic, breast (mammogram, if indicated), and rectal examinations (with colonoscopy according to age and family history); urinalysis; complete blood count; blood chemistry tests; and a chest film should suffice in most cases. In Asians, nasopharyngeal cancer is common, and a careful examination of ears, nose, and throat is indicated.

Overlap Syndromes These describe the association of inflammatory myopathies with connective tissue diseases. A well-characterized overlap syndrome occurs in patients with DM who also have manifestations of systemic sclerosis or mixed connective tissue disease, such as sclerotic thickening of the dermis, contractures, esophageal hypomotility, microangiopathy, and calcium deposits (Table 369-1). By contrast, signs of rheumatoid arthritis, systemic lupus erythematosus, or Sjögren's syndrome are very rare in patients with DM. Patients with the overlap syndrome of DM and systemic sclerosis may have a specific antinuclear antibody, the anti-PM/Scl, directed against a nucleolar-protein complex.

PATHOGENESIS An autoimmune etiology of the inflammatory myopathies is indirectly supported by an association with other autoimmune or connective tissue diseases; the presence of various autoantibodies; an association with specific major histocompatibility complex (MHC) genes; demonstration of T cell–mediated myocytotoxicity or complement-mediated microangiopathy; and a response to immunotherapy.

Autoantibodies and Immunogenetics Various autoantibodies against nuclear antigens (antinuclear antibodies) and cytoplasmic antigens are found in up to 20% of patients with inflammatory myopathies. The antibodies to cytoplasmic antigens are directed against ribonucleoproteins involved in protein synthesis (anti-synthetases) or translational transport (anti-signal-recognition particles). The antibody directed against the histidyl-transfer RNA synthetase, called *anti-Jo-1*, accounts for 75% of all the anti-synthetases and is clinically useful because up to 80% of patients with anti-Jo-1 antibodies have interstitial lung disease. Some patients with the anti-Jo-1 antibody also have Raynaud's phenomenon, nonerosive arthritis, and the MHC molecules DR3 and DRw52. DR3 (molecular designation DRB1*0301, DQB1*0201) occurs in up to 75% of patients with PM and IBM, whereas in juvenile DM there is an increased frequency of DQA1*0501 (Chap. 296).

Immunopathologic Mechanisms In DM, humoral immune mechanisms are implicated, resulting in a microangiopathy and muscle ischemia (Fig. 369-1). Endomysial inflammatory infiltrates are composed of B cells located in proximity to CD4 T cells and macrophages; there is a relative absence of lymphocytic invasion of nonnecrotic muscle fibers. Activation of the complement C5b-9 membranolytic attack complex is thought to be a critical early event that triggers release of proinflam-

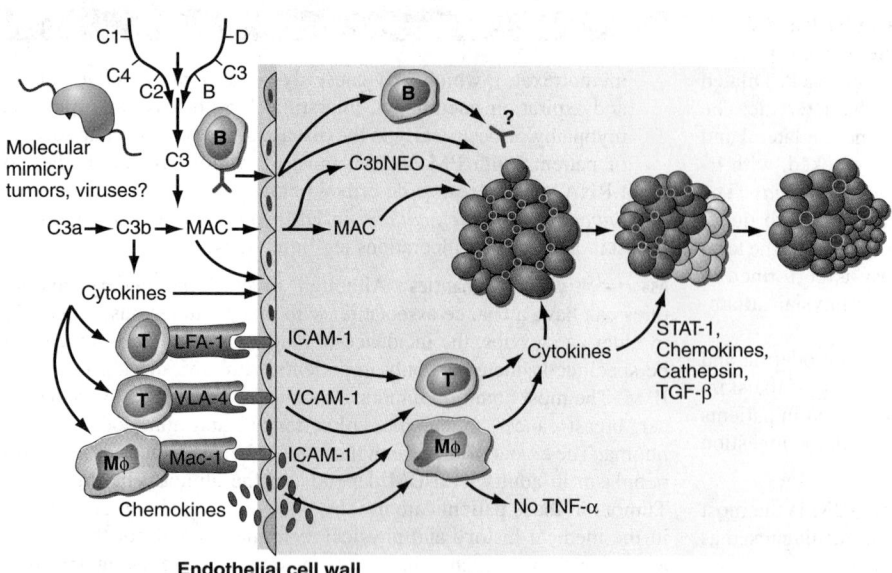

FIGURE 369-1 Immunopathogenesis of dermatomyositis. Autoantibodies (Y) possibly against endothelial cells, induce activation of complement and formation of C3 via the classic or alternative pathway. Activated C3 leads to formation of C3b, C3bNEO, and membrane attack complexes (MAC), which are deposited in and around the endothelial cell wall of the endomysial capillaries. Deposition of MAC leads to destruction of capillaries, ischemia, or microinfarcts most prominent in the periphery of the fascicles, and perifascicular atrophy. B cells, CD4 T cells, and macrophages (Mφ) traffic from the circulation to the muscle. Endothelial expression of vascular cell adhesion molecule (VCAM) and intercellular adhesion molecule (ICAM) is induced by cytokines released by the mononuclear cells. Integrins, specifically very late activation antigen (VLA)-4 and leukocyte function-associated antigen (LFA)-1, bind VCAM and ICAM and promote T cell and macrophage infiltration of muscle through the endothelial cell wall.

matory cytokines and chemokines, induces expression of vascular cell adhesion molecule (VCAM) 1 and intracellular adhesion molecule (ICAM) 1 on endothelial cells, and facilitates migration of activated lymphoid cells to the perimysial and endomysial spaces. Necrosis of the endothelial cells, reduced numbers of endomysial capillaries, ischemia, and muscle-fiber destruction resembling microinfarcts occur. The remaining capillaries often have dilated lumens in response to the ischemic process. Larger intramuscular blood vessels may also be affected in the same pattern. Residual perifascicular atrophy reflects the endofascicular hypoperfusion that is prominent in the periphery of the muscle fascicles.

By contrast, in PM and IBM a mechanism of T cell–mediated cytotoxicity is likely. CD8 T cells, along with macrophages, initially surround and eventually invade and destroy healthy, nonnecrotic muscle fibers that aberrantly express class I MHC molecules. MHC-I expression, absent from the sarcolemma of normal muscle fibers, is probably induced by cytokines secreted by activated T cells and macrophages. The CD8/MHC-I complex is characteristic of PM and IBM; its detection has now become necessary to confirm the histologic diagnosis of PM, as discussed later. The cytotoxic CD8 T cells contain perforin and granzyme granules directed towards the surface of the muscle fibers and capable of inducing myonecrosis. Analysis of T cell receptor molecules expressed by the infiltrating CD8 cells have revealed clonal expansion and conserved sequences in the antigen-binding region, both suggesting an antigen-driven T cell response. Whether the putative antigens are endogenous (e.g., muscle) or exogenous (e.g., viral) sequences is unknown. Viruses have not been identified within the muscle fibers. Key molecules involved in T cell–mediated cytotoxicity are depicted in Fig. 369-2.

The Role of Nonimmune Factors in IBM   In IBM, the presence of vacuoles (almost always in fibers not invaded by T cells) together with β-amyloid deposits within the vacuolated muscle fibers and abnormal mitochondria with cytochrome oxidase–negative fibers suggest that, in addition to the autoimmune component, there is also a degenerative process. Similar to Alzheimer's disease, the amyloid deposits in IBM are immunoreactive against amyloid precursor protein (APP), chymotrypsin, apolipoprotein E, and phosphorylated tau, but it is unclear whether these deposits are directly pathogenic or represent secondary

phenomena. The same is true for the mitochondrial abnormalities, which may also be secondary to the effects of aging or a bystander effect of upregulated cytokines.

Association with Viral Infections and the Role of Retroviruses   Several viruses, including coxsackieviruses, influenza, paramyxoviruses, mumps, cytomegalovirus, and Epstein-Barr virus, have been indirectly associated with myositis. For the coxsackieviruses, an autoimmune myositis triggered by molecular mimicry has been proposed because of structural homology between histidyl-transfer RNA synthetase that is the target of the Jo-1 antibody (see above) and genomic RNA of an animal picornavirus, the encephalomyocarditis virus. Sensitive polymerase chain reaction (PCR) studies, however, have repeatedly failed to confirm the presence of such viruses in muscle biopsies.

The best evidence of a viral connection in PM and IBM is with the retroviruses. Some individuals infected with HIV or with human T cell lymphotropic virus I (HTLV-1) develop PM or IBM; a similar disorder has been described in nonhuman primates infected with the simian immunodeficiency virus. The inflammatory myopathy may occur as the initial manifestation of a retroviral infection, or myositis may develop later in the disease course. Retroviral antigens have been detected only in occasional endomysial macrophages and not within the muscle fibers themselves, suggesting that persistent infection and viral replication within the muscle do not occur. Histologic findings are identical to retroviral-negative PM or IBM. This disorder should be distinguished from a toxic myopathy related to long-term therapy with AZT, characterized by fatigue, myalgia, mild muscle weakness, and mild elevation of creatine kinase (CK). AZT-induced myopathy, which generally improves when the drug is discontinued, is a mitochondrial disorder characterized histologically by "ragged-red" fibers. AZT inhibits γ-DNA polymerase, an enzyme found solely in the mitochondrial matrix.

DIFFERENTIAL DIAGNOSIS   The clinical picture of the typical skin rash and proximal or diffuse muscle weakness has few causes other than DM. However, proximal muscle weakness without skin involvement can be due to many conditions other than PM or IBM.

Subacute or Chronic Progressive Muscle Weakness   This may be due to denervating conditions such as the spinal muscular atrophies or amyotrophic lateral sclerosis (Chap. 353). In addition to the muscle weakness, upper motor neuron signs in the latter and signs of denervation detected by electromyography (EMG) aid in the diagnosis. The muscular dystrophies (Chap. 368) may be additional considerations; however, these disorders usually develop over years rather than weeks or months and rarely present after the age of 30. It may be difficult, even with a muscle biopsy, to distinguish chronic PM from a rapidly advancing muscular dystrophy. This is particularly true of facioscapulohumeral muscular dystrophy, dysferlin myopathy, and the dystrophinopathies where inflammatory cell infiltration is often found early in the disease. Such doubtful cases should always be given an adequate trial of glucocorticoid therapy and be screened for the respective genetic defect. Search for the MHC/CD8 lesion by immunocytochemistry is helpful to identify cases of PM as mentioned above. Some metabolic myopathies, including glycogen storage disease due to myophosphorylase or acid maltase deficiency, lipid storage myopathies due to carnitine deficiency, and mitochondrial diseases, produce weakness that is often associated with other characteristic clinical signs; diagnosis rests upon histochemical and biochemical studies of the muscle biopsy. The endocrine myopathies such as those due to hypercorticosteroidism, hyper- and hypothyroidism, and hyper- and hypoparathyroidism require the appropriate laboratory investigations for diagnosis. Muscle wasting in patients with an underlying neoplasm may be due to disuse, cachexia, or rarely to a paraneoplastic neuromyopathy (Chap. 87).

Diseases of the neuromuscular junction, including myasthenia gravis or the Lambert-Eaton myasthenic syndrome, cause fatiguing weakness that also affects the eye and cranial muscles (Chap. 366). Repetitive nerve stimulation and single-fiber EMG studies aid in diagnosis.

Acute Muscle Weakness This may be caused by an acute neuropathy such as Guillain-Barré syndrome (Chap. 365), transverse myelitis (Chap. 356), a neurotoxin (Chap. 368), or a viral infection such as poliomyelitis or West Nile virus (Chap. 360). When acute weakness is associated with painful muscle cramps, rhabdomyolysis, and myoglobinuria, it may be due to metabolic disorders including a glycogen storage disease such as myophosphorylase deficiency or carnitine palmityltransferase deficiency (Chap. 368). Acute viral infections may cause a similar syndrome. Several animal parasites, such as protozoa (*toxoplasma, trypanosoma*), cestodes (*cysticerci*), and nematodes (*trichinae*), may produce a focal or diffuse inflammatory myopathy known as *parasitic polymyositis. Staphylococcus aureus, Yersinia, Streptococcus*, or other anaerobic bacteria may produce a suppurative myositis, known as *tropical polymyositis*, or *pyomyositis*. Pyomyositis, previously rare in the west, is now occasionally seen in AIDS patients. Other bacteria, such as *Borrelia burgdorferi* (Lyme disease) and *Legionella pneumophila* (Legionnaire's disease) may infrequently cause myositis.

Patients with periodic paralysis develop episodes of recurrent painless acute muscle weakness, always beginning in childhood. Chronic alcoholics may develop painful myopathy with myoglobinuria after a bout of heavy drinking or present with a painless, acute hypokalemic myopathy, which is completely reversible with replacement therapy; other times they show an asymptomatic elevation of serum CK and myoglobin. Acute muscle weakness with myoglobinuria may occur with prolonged severe hypokalemia or with hypophosphatemia and hypomagnesemia, often seen in chronic alcoholics and in patients on nasogastric suction receiving parenteral hyperalimentation.

Macrophagic Myofasciitis This distinctive inflammatory muscle disorder presents as diffuse myalgias, fatigue, and mild muscle weakness. Muscle biopsy reveals pronounced infiltration of the connective tissue around the muscle by sheets of periodic acid–Schiff-positive macrophages and occasional CD8 T cells. The CK or erythrocyte sedimentation rate is variably elevated. Most patients respond to glucocorticoid therapy, and the overall prognosis seems favorable. Histologic involvement is focal and limited to sites of previous vaccinations, which may have been administered months or years earlier. This disorder, which to date has not been observed outside of France, has been linked to an aluminum-containing substrate used in vaccine preparation.

Drug-Induced Myopathies D-Penicillamine and procainamide may produce a true myositis resembling PM, and a DM-like illness had been associated with the contaminated preparations of L-tryptophan. As noted above, AZT causes a mitochondrial myopathy. Other drugs may elicit a toxic noninflammatory myopathy that is histologically different from DM, PM, or IBM. These include the cholesterol-lowering agents such as clofibrate, lovastatin, simvastatin, or provastatin, especially

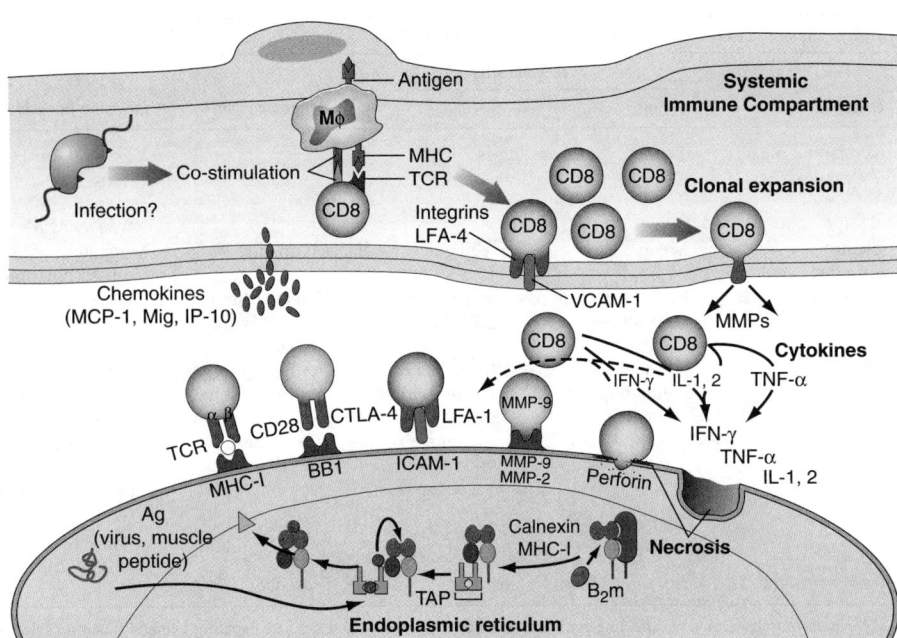

FIGURE 369-2 Cell-mediated mechanisms of muscle damage in polymyositis (PM) and inclusion body myositis (IBM). Antigen-specific CD8 cells are expanded in the periphery, cross the endothelial barrier, and bind directly to muscle fibers via T cell receptor (TCR) molecules that recognize aberrantly expressed MHC-I. Engagement of co-stimulatory molecules (BB1 and ICOSL) with their ligands (CD28, CTLA-4, and ICOS) along with ICAM-1/LFA-1, stabilize the CD8–muscle fiber interaction. Metalloproteinases (MMP) facilitate the migration of T cells and their attachment to the muscle surface. Muscle fiber necrosis occurs via perforin granules released by the autoaggressive T cells. A direct myocytotoxic effect exerted by the cytokines interferon (IFN)γ, interleukin (IL)1, or tumor necrosis factor (TNF) α may also play a role. Death of the muscle fiber is mediated by necrosis. MHC class I molecules consist of a heavy chain and a light chain [B$_2$ microglobulin (B$_2$M)] complexed with an antigenic peptide that is transported into the endoplasmic reticulum by TAP proteins (Chap. 296).

when combined with cyclosporine or gemfibrozil. Rhabdomyolysis and myoglobinuria have been rarely associated with amphotericin B, ϵ-aminocaproic acid, fenfluramine, heroin, and phencyclidine. The use of amiodarone, chloroquine, colchicine, carbimazole, emetine, etretinate, ipecac syrup, chronic laxative or licorice use resulting in hypokalemia, and glucocorticoids or growth hormone administration have also been associated with myopathic muscle weakness. Some neuromuscular blocking agents such as pancuronium, in combination with glucocorticoids, may cause the acute critical illness myopathy. A careful drug history is essential for diagnosis of these drug-induced myopathies, which do not require immunosuppressive therapy.

Pain on Movement and Muscle Tenderness A number of conditions including *polymyalgia rheumatica* (Chap. 306) and arthritic disorders of adjacent joints may enter into the differential diagnosis of inflammatory myopathy, even though they do not cause myositis. The muscle biopsy is either normal or discloses type II muscle fiber atrophy. Patients with *fibrositis* and *fibromyalgia* (Chap. 315) complain of focal or diffuse muscle tenderness, fatigue, and aching, which is sometimes poorly differentiated from joint pain. In other patients there may be suggestive signs of a collagen vascular disorder, such as an increased erythrocyte sedimentation rate, antinuclear antibody, or rheumatoid factor. Occasionally, there is slight but transient elevation of the serum CK. The muscle biopsy is usually normal and the prognosis favorable. Many such patients show some response to nonsteroidal anti-inflammatory agents, though most continue to have indolent complaints. *Chronic fatigue syndrome*, which may follow a viral infection, can present with debilitating fatigue, fever, sore throat, painful lymphadenopathy, myalgia, arthralgia, sleep disorder, and headache (Chap. 370). These patients do not have muscle weakness, and the muscle biopsy is normal.

DIAGNOSIS The clinically suspected diagnosis of PM, DM, or IBM is confirmed by examining the serum muscle enzymes, EMG findings, and muscle biopsy (Table 369-2).

The most sensitive enzyme is CK, which in active disease can be

TABLE 369-2 *Criteria for Diagnosis of Inflammatory Myopathies*

Criterion	Polymyositis Definite	Polymyositis Probable	Dermatomyositis	Inclusion Body Myositis
Myopathic muscle weakness[a]	Yes	Yes	Yes[b]	Yes; slow onset, early involvement of distal muscles, frequent falls
Electromyographic findings	Myopathic	Myopathic	Myopathic	Myopathic with mixed potentials
Muscle enzymes	Elevated (up to 50-fold)	Elevated (up to 50-fold)	Elevated (up to 50-fold) or normal	Elevated (up to 10-fold) or normal
Muscle biopsy findings[c]	"Primary" inflammation with the CD8/MHC-I complex and no vacuoles	Ubiquitous MCH-I expression but minimal inflammation and no vacuoles[d]	Perifascicular, perimysial, or perivascular infiltrates, perifascicular atrophy	Primary inflammation with CD8/MHC-I complex; vacuolated fibers with β-amyloid deposits; cytochrome oxygenase–negative fibers; signs of chronic myopathy[e]
Rash or calcinosis	Absent	Absent	Present[f]	Absent

[a] Myopathic muscle weakness, affecting proximal muscles more than distal ones and sparing eye and facial muscles, is characterized by a subacute onset (weeks to months) and rapid progression in patients who have no family history of neuromuscular disease, no endocrinopathy, no exposure to myotoxic drugs or toxins, and no biochemical muscle disease (excluded on the basis of muscle-biopsy findings).

[b] In some cases with the typical rash, the muscle strength is seemingly normal (dermatomyositis sine myositis); these patients often have new onset of easy fatigue and reduced endurance. Careful muscle testing may reveal mild muscle weakness.

[c] See text for details.

[d] An adequate trial of prednisone or other immunosuppressive drugs is warranted in probable cases. If, in retrospect, the disease is unresponsive to therapy, another muscle biopsy should be considered to exclude other diseases or possible evolution in inclusion body myositis.

[e] If the muscle biopsy does not contain vacuolated fibers but shows chronic myopathy with hypertrophic fibers, primary inflammation with the CD8/MHC-I complex and cytochrome oxygenase–negative fibers, the diagnosis is probable inclusion body myositis.

[f] If rash is absent but muscle biopsy findings are characteristic of dermatomyositis, the diagnosis is probable DM.

perplasia with tubuloreticular profiles, fibrin thrombi, and obliteration of capillaries. The muscle fibers undergo necrosis, degeneration, and phagocytosis, often in groups involving a portion of a muscle fasciculus in a wedgelike shape or at the periphery of the fascicle, due to microinfarcts within the muscle. This results in perifascicular atrophy, characterized by 2 to 10 layers of atrophic fibers at the periphery of the fascicles. The presence of perifascicular atrophy is diagnostic of DM, *even in the absence of inflammation.*

In IBM, there is endomysial inflammation with T cells invading MHC-I-expressing nonvacuolated muscle fibers; basophilic granular deposits distributed around the edge of slitlike vacuoles (rimmed vacuoles); loss of fibers, replaced by fat and connective tissue, hypertrophic fibers, and angulated or round fibers; eosinophilic cytoplasmic inclusions; abnormal mitochondria characterized by the presence of ragged-red fibers or cytochrome oxidase–negative fibers; amyloid deposits within or next to the vacuoles; and filamentous inclusions seen by electron microscopy in the vicinity of the rimmed vacuoles.

℞ TREATMENT

The goal of therapy is to improve muscle strength, thereby improving function in activities of daily living, and ameliorate the extramuscular manifestations (rash, dysphagia, dyspnea, fever). When strength improves, the serum CK falls concurrently; however, the reverse is not always true. Unfortunately, there is a common tendency to "chase" or treat the CK level instead of the muscle weakness, a practice that has led to prolonged and unnecessary use of immunosuppressive drugs and erroneous assessment of their efficacy. It is prudent to discontinue these drugs if, after an adequate trial, there is no objective improvement in muscle strength whether or not CK levels are reduced. Agents used in the treatment of PM and DM include:

1. *Glucocorticoids.* Oral prednisone is the initial treatment of choice; the effectiveness and side effects of this therapy determine the future need for stronger immunosuppressive drugs. High-dose prednisone, at least 1 mg/kg per day, is initiated as early in the disease as possible. After 3 to 4 weeks, prednisone is tapered slowly over a period of 10 weeks to 1 mg/kg every other day. If there is evidence of efficacy and no serious side effects, the dosage is then further reduced by 5 or 10 mg every 3 to 4 weeks until the lowest possible dose that controls the disease is reached. The efficacy of prednisone is determined by an objective increase in muscle strength and activities of daily living, which almost always occur by the third month of therapy. A feeling of increased energy or a reduction of the CK level without a concomitant increase in muscle strength is not a reliable sign of improvement. If prednisone provides no objective benefit after ~3 months of high-dose therapy, the disease is probably unresponsive to the drug and tapering should be accelerated while the next-in-line immunosuppressive drug is started. Although controlled trials have not been performed, almost all patients with true PM or DM respond to glucocorticoids to *some degree and for some period of time*; in general, DM responds better than PM.

The long-term use of prednisone may cause increased weakness associated with a normal or unchanged CK level; this effect is referred to as *steroid myopathy.* In a patient who previously responded to high

elevated as much as 50-fold. Although the CK level usually parallels disease activity, it can be normal in some patients with active IBM or DM, especially when associated with a connective tissue disease. The CK is always elevated in patients with active PM. Along with the CK, the serum glutamic-oxaloacetic and glutamate pyruvate transaminases, lactate dehydrogenase, and aldolase may be elevated.

Needle EMG shows myopathic potentials characterized by short-duration, low-amplitude polyphasic units on voluntary activation and increased spontaneous activity with fibrillations, complex repetitive discharges, and positive sharp waves. Mixed potentials (polyphasic units of short and long duration) indicating a chronic process and muscle fiber regeneration are often present in IBM. These EMG findings are not diagnostic of an inflammatory myopathy but are useful to identify the presence of active or chronic myopathy and to exclude neurogenic disorders.

Magnetic resonance imaging is not routinely used for the diagnosis of PM, DM, or IBM. However, it may guide the location of the muscle biopsy in certain clinical settings.

Muscle biopsy is the definitive test for establishing the diagnosis of inflammatory myopathy and for excluding other neuromuscular diseases. Inflammation is the histologic hallmark for these diseases; however, additional features are characteristic of each subtype.

In PM the inflammation is *primary*, a term used to indicate that T cell infiltrates, located primarily within the muscle fascicles (endomysially), surround individual, healthy muscle fibers and result in phagocytosis and necrosis. The MHC-I molecule is ubiquitously expressed on the sarcolemma, even in fibers not invaded by CD8+ cells. The CD8/MHC-I lesion is now fundamental for confirming or establishing the diagnosis and to exclude disorders with secondary, nonspecific, inflammation. When the disease is chronic, connective tissue is increased and may react positively with alkaline phosphatase.

In DM the endomysial inflammation is predominantly perivascular or in the interfascicular septae and around, rather than within, the muscle fascicles. The intramuscular blood vessels show endothelial hy-

doses of prednisone, the development of new weakness may be related to steroid myopathy or to disease activity that either will respond to a higher dose of glucocorticoids or has become glucocorticoid-resistant. In uncertain cases, the prednisone dosage can be adjusted arbitrarily: the cause of the weakness is usually evident in 2 to 8 weeks.

2. *Other immunosuppressive drugs.* Approximately 75% of patients ultimately require additional treatment. This occurs when a patient fails to respond adequately to glucocorticoids after a 3-month trial, the patient becomes glucocorticoid-resistant, glucocorticoid-related side effects appear, attempts to lower the prednisone dose repeatedly result in a new relapse, or rapidly progressive disease with evolving severe weakness and respiratory failure develops.

The following drugs are commonly used: (1) *Azathioprine* is well tolerated, has few side effects, and appears to be as effective for long-term therapy as other drugs. The dose is up to 3 mg/kg daily. (2) *Methotrexate* has a faster onset of action than azathioprine. It is given orally starting at 7.5 mg weekly for the first 3 weeks (2.5 mg every 12 h for 3 doses), with gradual dose escalation by 2.5 mg per week to a total of 25 mg weekly. A rare side effect is methotrexate pneumonitis, which can be difficult to distinguish from the interstitial lung disease of the primary myopathy associated with Jo-1 antibodies (described above). (3) *Cyclophosphamide* (0.5 to 1 g IV monthly for 6 months) has limited success and significant toxicity. (4) *Chlorambucil* has variable results. (5) *Cyclosporine* has inconsistent and mild benefit. (6) *Mycophenolate mofetil* has recently shown some effectiveness.

3. *Immunomodulation.* In a controlled trial of patients with refractory DM, intravenous immunoglobulin (IVIg) improved not only strength and rash but also the underlying immunopathology. The benefit is often short-lived ($\leq$8 weeks); repeated infusions every 6 to 8 weeks are generally required to maintain improvement. A dose of 2 g/kg divided over 2 to 5 days per course is recommended. Uncontrolled observations suggest that IVIg may also be beneficial for patients with PM. Neither plasmapheresis nor leukapheresis appears to be effective in PM and DM.

The following sequential empirical approach to the treatment of PM and DM is suggested: *Step 1*: high-dose prednisone; *step 2*: azathioprine or methotrexate; *step 3*: IVIg; *step 4*: a trial, with guarded optimism, of one of the following agents, chosen according to the patient's age, degree of disability, tolerance, experience with the drug, and the patient's general health: cyclosporine, chlorambucil, cyclophosphamide, mycophenolate. Patients with interstitial lung disease may benefit from aggressive treatment with cyclophosphamide.

A patient with presumed PM who has not responded to any form of immunotherapy most likely has IBM or another disease, usually a metabolic myopathy, a muscular dystrophy, a drug-induced myopathy, or an endocrinopathy. In these cases, a repeat muscle biopsy and a renewed search for another cause of the myopathy is indicated.

Calcinosis, a manifestation of DM, is difficult to treat; however, new calcium deposits may be prevented if the primary disease responds to the available therapies. Diphosphonates, aluminum hydrox-

ide, probenecid, colchicine, low doses of warfarin, calcium blockers, and surgical excision have all been tried without success.

IBM is generally resistant to immunosuppressive therapies. Prednisone together with azathioprine or methotrexate is often tried for a few months in newly diagnosed patients, although results are generally disappointing. Because occasional patients may feel subjectively weaker after these drugs are discontinued, some clinicians prefer to maintain some patients on low-dose, every-other-day prednisone or weekly methotrexate in an effort to halt disease progression, even though there is no objective evidence or controlled study to support this practice. In two controlled studies of IVIg in IBM, minimal benefit in up to 30% of patients was found; the strength gains, however, were not of sufficient magnitude to justify its routine use. Another trial of IVIg combined with prednisone was ineffective. Nonetheless, many experts believe that a 2- to 3-month trial with IVIg may be reasonable for selected patients with IBM who experience rapid progression of muscle weakness or choking episodes due to worsening dysphagia.

PROGNOSIS The 5-year survival rate for treated patients with PM and DM is ~95% and the 10-year survival 84%; death is usually due to pulmonary, cardiac, or other systemic complications. Patients severely affected at presentation or treated after long delays, those with severe dysphagia or respiratory difficulties, older patients, and those with associated cancer have a worse prognosis. DM responds more favorably to therapy than PM and thus has a better prognosis. Most patients improve with therapy, and many make a full functional recovery, which is often sustained with maintenance therapy. Up to 30% may be left with some residual muscle weakness. Relapses may occur at any time.

IBM has the least favorable prognosis of the inflammatory myopathies. Most patients will require the use of an assistive device such as a cane, walker, or wheelchair within 5 to 10 years of onset. In general, the older the age of onset in IBM, the more rapidly progressive is the course.

FURTHER READING

ASKANAS V, ENGEL WK: Inclusion body myopathies: Different etiologies, possibly similar pathogenic mechanisms. Curr Opin Neurol 15:525, 2002

DALAKAS MC: The molecular and cellular pathology of inflammatory muscle diseases. Curr Opin Pharmacol 1:300, 2001

———: Understanding the immunopathogenesis of inclusion body myositis: Present and future prospects. Rev Neurol 158:948, 2002

———, HOHLFELD R: Polymyositis and dermatomyositis. Lancet. 362:971, 2003

HILTON-JONES D: Inflammatory myopathies. Curr Opin Neurol 14:591, 2001

MARIE I et al: Polymyositis and dermatomyositis: Short term and long term outcome and predictive factors of prognosis. J Rheumatol 28:2230, 2001

MASTAGLIA FL: Inflammatory myopathies: Clinical, diagnostic and therapeutic aspects. Muscle Nerve 27:407, 2003

SONTHEIMER RD: Dermatomyositis: An overview of recent progress with emphasis on dermatologic aspects. Dermatol Clin 20:387, 2002

Section 4 Chronic Fatigue Syndrome

370 | CHRONIC FATIGUE SYNDROME
Stephen E. Straus

DEFINITION *Chronic fatigue syndrome* (CFS) is the current name for a disorder characterized by debilitating fatigue and several associated physical, constitutional, and neuropsychological complaints (Table 370-1). This syndrome is not new; in the past, patients diagnosed with conditions such as the vapors, neurasthenia, effort syndrome, chronic brucellosis, epidemic neuromyasthenia, myalgic encephalomyelitis, hypoglycemia, multiple chemical sensitivity syndrome, chronic can-

didiasis, chronic mononucleosis, chronic Epstein-Barr virus infection, and postviral fatigue syndrome may have had what is now called CFS. A subset of ill veterans of military campaigns suffer from CFS. The U.S. Centers for Disease Control and Prevention (CDC) has developed diagnostic criteria for CFS based upon symptoms and the exclusion of other illnesses (Table 370-2).

EPIDEMIOLOGY Patients with CFS are twice as likely to be women as men and are generally 25 to 45 years old, although cases in childhood and in later life have been described.

Cases are recognized in many developed countries. Most arise spo-

TABLE 370-1 *Specific Symptoms Reported by Patients with Chronic Fatigue Syndrome*

Symptom	Percentage
Fatigue	100
Difficulty concentrating	90
Headache	90
Sore throat	85
Tender lymph nodes	80
Muscle aches	80
Joint aches	75
Feverishness	75
Difficulty sleeping	70
Psychiatric problems	65
Allergies	55
Abdominal cramps	40
Weight loss	20
Rash	10
Rapid pulse	10
Weight gain	5
Chest pain	5
Night sweats	5

Source: From SE Straus: J Infect Diseases 157:405, 1988; with permission.

radically, but many clusters have also been reported. Famous outbreaks of CFS occurred in Los Angeles County Hospital in 1934; in Akureyri, Iceland, in 1948; in the Royal Free Hospital, London, in 1955; and in Incline Village, Nevada, in 1985. While these clustered cases suggest a common environmental or infectious cause, none has been identified.

Estimates of the prevalence of CFS have depended on the case definition used and the method of study. Chronic fatigue itself is a common symptom, occurring in as many as 20% of patients attending general medical clinics; CFS is far less common. Community-based studies find that 100 to 300 individuals per 100,000 population in the United States meet the current CDC case definition.

PATHOGENESIS The diverse names for the syndrome reflect the many and controversial hypotheses about its etiology. Several common themes underlie attempts to understand the disorder: It is often postinfectious, it is associated with immunologic disturbances, and it is commonly accompanied or even preceded by neuropsychological complaints, somatic preoccupation, and/or depression.

Many studies in the 1980s and 1990s attempted to link CFS to infection with Epstein-Barr virus, a retrovirus, or an enterovirus. In many patients with chronic fatigue, titers of antibodies to several viruses are elevated. Reports that viral antigens and nucleic acids could be specifically identified in patients with CFS have not been confirmed. One study from the United Kingdom failed to detect any association between acute infections and subsequent prolonged fatigue. Another study found that chronic fatigue did not develop after typical upper respiratory infections but did in some individuals after infectious mononucleosis. Thus, while antecedent viral infections are associated with CFS, a direct viral pathogenesis is unproven and unlikely.

Changes in numerous immune parameters of uncertain functional significance have been reported in CFS. Modest elevations in titers of antinuclear antibodies, reductions in immunoglobulin subclasses, deficiencies in mitogen-driven lymphocyte proliferation, reductions in natural killer cell activity, disturbances in cytokine production, and shifts in lymphocyte subsets have been described. None of the immune findings appears in all patients, nor do any correlate with the severity of CFS. Careful comparison of affected and unaffected monozygotic twins showed no substantive immunologic differences. In theory, symptoms of CFS could result from excessive production of a cytokine, such as interleukin 1, that induces asthenia and other flulike symptoms; however, compelling data in support of this long-held hypothesis are lacking.

In some studies, patients with CFS manifest unusual sensitivity to

sustained upright tilting, resulting in hypotension and syncope, so as to suggest a form of dysautonomia.

Disturbances in the hypothalamic-pituitary-adrenal function have been identified in several controlled studies of CFS, with some evidence for normalization in patients whose fatigue abates. These neuroendocrine abnormalities could contribute to the impaired energy and depressed mood of patients.

Mild to moderate depression is present in half to two-thirds of patients. Much of this depression may be reactive, but its prevalence exceeds that seen in other chronic medical illnesses. Some propose that CFS is fundamentally a psychiatric disorder and that the various neuroendocrine and immune disturbances arise secondarily.

MANIFESTATIONS Typically, CFS arises suddenly in a previously active individual. An otherwise unremarkable flulike illness or some other acute stress leaves unbearable exhaustion in its wake. Other symptoms, such as headache, sore throat, tender lymph nodes, muscle and joint aches, and frequent feverishness, lead to the belief that an infection persists, and medical attention is sought. Over several weeks, despite reassurances that nothing serious is wrong, the symptoms persist and other features of the syndrome become evident—disturbed sleep, difficulty in concentration, and depression (Table 370-1).

Depending on the dominant symptoms and the beliefs of the patient, additional consultations may be sought from allergists, rheumatologists, infectious disease specialists, psychiatrists, ecologic therapists, homeopaths, or other professionals, frequently with unsatisfactory results. Once the pattern of illness is established, the symptoms may fluctuate somewhat. Many patients report that diverse complaints are linked—that during periods of greatest fatigue they perceive the most pain and difficulty with concentration. Patients also commonly assert that excessive physical or emotional stress may exacerbate their symptoms.

Most patients remain capable of meeting family, work, or community obligations despite their symptoms; discretionary activities are abandoned first. Some feel unable to engage in any gainful employment. A minority of individuals require help with the activities of daily living.

Ultimately, isolation, frustration, and pathetic resignation can mark the protracted course of illness. Patients may become angry at physicians for failing to acknowledge or resolve their plight. Fortunately, CFS does not appear to progress. On the contrary, many patients experience gradual improvement, and a minority recover fully.

DIAGNOSIS A thorough history, physical examination, and judicious use of laboratory tests are required to exclude other causes of the patient's symptoms. Prominent abnormalities argue strongly in favor of alternative diagnoses. No laboratory test, however, can diagnose this condition or measure its severity. In most cases, elaborate, expensive workups are not helpful. Early claims that magnetic resonance imaging or single photon emission computed tomography can identify

TABLE 370-2 *CDC Criteria for Diagnosis of Chronic Fatigue Syndrome*

A case of chronic fatigue syndrome is defined by the presence of:
1. Clinically evaluated, unexplained, persistent or relapsing fatigue that is of new or definite onset; is not the result of ongoing exertion; is not alleviated by rest; and results in substantial reduction of previous levels of occupational, educational, social, or personal activities; and
2. Four or more of the following symptoms that persist or recur during six or more consecutive months of illness and that do not predate the fatigue:
   - Self-reported impairment in short-term memory or concentration
   - Sore throat
   - Tender cervical or axillary nodes
   - Muscle pain
   - Multijoint pain without redness or swelling
   - Headaches of a new pattern or severity
   - Unrefreshing sleep
   - Postexertional malaise lasting $\geq$24 h

Note: CDC, U.S. Centers for Disease Control and Prevention.
Source: Adapted from K Fukuda et al: Ann Intern Med 121:953, 1994; with permission.

abnormalities in the brain of CFS patients have not withstood further study. The dilemma for patient and clinician alike is that CFS has no pathognomonic features and remains a constellation of symptoms and a diagnosis of exclusion. Often the patient presents with features that also meet criteria for other subjective disorders such as fibromyalgia and irritable bowel syndrome.

℞ TREATMENT

After other illnesses have been excluded, there are several points to address in the long-term care of a patient with chronic fatigue.

The patient should be informed about the illness and what is known of its pathogenesis; its potential impact on the physical, psychological, and social dimensions of life; and its prognosis. Patients are relieved when their complaints are taken seriously. Periodic reassessment is appropriate to identify a possible underlying process that is late in declaring itself and to address intercurrent symptoms that should not be simply dismissed as yet another subjective complaint.

Many symptoms of CFS respond to treatment. Non-steroidal anti-inflammatory drugs alleviate headache, diffuse pain, and feverishness. Allergic rhinitis and sinusitis are common; antihistamines or decongestants may be helpful. Although the patient may be averse to psychiatric diagnoses, depression and anxiety are often prominent and should be treated. Expert psychiatric assessment is sometimes advisable. Nonsedating antidepressants improve mood and disordered sleep and may attenuate the fatigue. Even modest improvements in symptoms can make an important difference in the patient's degree of self-sufficiency and ability to appreciate life's pleasures.

Practical advice should be given regarding life-style. Sleep disturbances are common; consumption of heavy meals with alcohol and caffeine at night can make sleep even more elusive, compounding fatigue. Total rest leads to further deconditioning and the self-image of being an invalid, whereas overexertion may worsen exhaustion and lead to total avoidance of exercise. A moderate, carefully graded regimen should be encouraged and has been proven to relieve symptoms and enhance exercise tolerance.

Controlled therapeutic trials have established that acyclovir, fludrocortisone, and intravenous immunoglobulin, among others, are of little or no value in CFS. Low doses of hydrocortisone provide modest benefit, but they may lead to adrenal suppression. Countless anecdotes circulate regarding other traditional and nontraditional therapies. It is important to guide patients away from those therapeutic modalities that are toxic, expensive, or unreasonable.

The physician should promote the patient's efforts to recover. Controlled trials in the United Kingdom, in Australia, and in the Netherlands showed cognitive-behavioral therapy to be helpful. This approach aims to dispel misguided beliefs and fears about CFS that can contribute to inactivity and despair. For CFS, as for many other conditions, a comprehensive approach to physical, psychological, and social aspects of well-being is in order.

FURTHER READING

ALFARI N, BUCHWALD D: Chronic fatigue syndrome: A review. Am J Psychiat 160:221, 2003

WHITING P et al: Interventions for the treatment and management of chronic fatigue syndrome: A systematic review. JAMA 286:1360, 2001

Section 5   Psychiatric Disorders

371 | MENTAL DISORDERS
Victor I. Reus

Mental disorders are common in medical practice and may present either as a primary disorder or as a comorbid condition. The prevalence of mental or substance use disorders in the United States is 18.5%, resulting in an annual cost of $148 billion dollars, only slightly less than the costs of cardiovascular diseases. Only 15% of these individuals are currently receiving treatment.

The revised 4th edition for use by primary care physicians of the *Diagnostic and Statistical Manual* (DSM-IV-PC) provides a useful synopsis of mental disorders most likely to be seen in primary care practice. The current system of classification is multiaxial and includes the presence or absence of a major mental disorder (axis I), any underlying personality disorder (axis II), general medical condition (axis III), psychosocial and environmental problems (axis IV), and overall rating of general psychosocial functioning (axis V).

Changes in health care delivery underscore the need for primary care physicians to assume responsibility for the initial diagnosis and treatment of the most common mental disorders. Prompt diagnosis is essential to ensure that patients have access to appropriate medical services and to maximize the clinical outcome. Validated patient-based questionnaires have been developed that systematically probe for signs and symptoms associated with the most prevalent psychiatric diagnoses and guide the clinician into targeted assessment. Prime MD (and a self-report form, the PHQ) and the Symptom-Driven Diagnostic System for Primary Care (SDDS-PC) are inventories that require only 10 min to complete and link patient responses to the formal diagnostic criteria of anxiety, mood, somatoform, and eating disorders and to alcohol abuse or dependence.

A physician who refers patients to a psychiatrist should know not only when doing so is appropriate but also how to refer, since societal misconceptions and the stigma of mental illness impede the process. Primary care physicians should base referrals to a psychiatrist on the presence of signs and symptoms of a mental disorder and not simply on the absence of a physical explanation for a patient's complaint. The physician should discuss with the patient the reasons for requesting the referral or consultation and provide reassurance that he or she will continue to provide medical care and work collaboratively with the mental health professional. Consultation with a psychiatrist or transfer of care is appropriate when physicians encounter evidence of psychotic symptoms, mania, severe depression, or anxiety; symptoms of post-traumatic stress disorder (PTSD); suicidal or homicidal preoccupation; or a failure to respond to first-order treatment.→*Eating disorders are discussed in Chap. 65.*

ANXIETY DISORDERS

Anxiety disorders, the most prevalent psychiatric illnesses in the general community, are present in 15 to 20% of medical clinic patients. Anxiety, defined as a subjective sense of unease, dread, or foreboding, can indicate a primary psychiatric condition or can be a component of, or reaction to, a primary medical disease. The primary anxiety disorders are classified according to their duration and course and the existence and nature of precipitants.

When evaluating the anxious patient, the clinician must first determine whether the anxiety antedates or postdates a medical illness or is due to a medication side effect. Approximately one-third of patients presenting with anxiety have a medical etiology for their psychiatric symptoms, but an anxiety disorder can also present with somatic symptoms in the absence of a diagnosable medical condition.

PANIC DISORDER ■ Clinical Manifestations   Panic disorder is defined by the presence of recurrent and unpredictable panic attacks, which are distinct episodes of intense fear and discomfort associated with a variety of physical symptoms, including palpitations, sweating, trembling, shortness of breath, chest pain, dizziness, and a fear of impend-

A discrete period of intense fear or discomfort, in which four or more of the following symptoms developed abruptly and reached a peak within 10 min:

1. Palpitations, pounding heart, or accelerated heart rate
2. Sweating
3. Trembling or shaking
4. Sensations of shortness of breath or smothering
5. Feeling of choking
6. Chest pain or discomfort
7. Nausea or abdominal distress
8. Feeling dizzy, unsteady, lightheaded, or faint
9. Derealization (feelings of unreality) or depersonalization (being detached from oneself)
10. Fear of losing control or going crazy
11. Fear of dying
12. Paresthesias (numbness or tingling sensations)
13. Chills or hot flushes

Source: Diagnostic and Statistical Manual of Mental Disorders, 4th ed.

ing doom or death (Table 371-1). Paresthesias, gastrointestinal distress, and feelings of unreality are also common. Diagnostic criteria also require at least 1 month of concern or worry about the attacks or a change in behavior related to them. The lifetime prevalence of panic disorder is 1 to 3%. Panic attacks have a sudden onset, developing within 10 min and usually resolving over the course of an hour, and they occur in an unexpected fashion. The frequency and severity of panic attacks vary, ranging from once a week to clusters of attacks separated by months of well-being. The first attack is usually outside the home, and onset is typically in late adolescence to early adulthood. In some individuals, anticipatory anxiety develops over time and results in a generalized fear and a progressive avoidance of places or situations in which a panic attack might recur. *Agoraphobia*, which occurs commonly in patients with panic disorder, is an acquired irrational fear of being in places where one might feel trapped or unable to escape (Table 371-2). Typically, it leads the patient into a progressive restriction in lifestyle and, in a literal sense, in geography. Frequently, patients are embarrassed that they are housebound and dependent on the company of others to go out into the world and do not volunteer this information; thus physicians will fail to recognize the syndrome if direct questioning is not pursued.

Differential Diagnosis　A diagnosis of panic disorder is made after a medical etiology for the panic attacks has been ruled out. A variety of cardiovascular, respiratory, endocrine, and neurologic conditions can present with anxiety as the chief complaint. Patients with true panic disorder will often focus on one specific feature to the exclusion of

1. Anxiety about being in places or situations from which escape might be difficult (or embarrassing) or in which help may not be available in the event of having an unexpected or situationally predisposed panic attack or panic-like symptoms. Agoraphobic fears typically involve characteristic clusters of situations that include being outside the home alone; being in a crowd or standing in a line; being on a bridge; and traveling in a bus, train, or automobile.
2. The situations are avoided (e.g., travel is restricted) or else are endured with marked distress or with anxiety about having a panic attack or panic-like symptoms, or require the presence of a companion.
3. The anxiety or phobic avoidance is not better accounted for by another mental disorder, such as social phobia (e.g., avoidance limited to social situations because of fear of embarrassment), specific phobia (e.g., avoidance limited to a single situation like elevators), obsessive-compulsive disorder (e.g., avoidance of dirt in someone with an obsession about contamination), posttraumatic stress disorder (e.g., avoidance of stimuli associated with a severe stressor), or separation anxiety disorder (e.g., avoidance of leaving home or relatives).

Source: Diagnostic and Statistical Manual of Mental Disorders, 4th ed.

others. For example, 20% of patients who present with syncope as a primary medical complaint have a primary diagnosis of a mood, anxiety, or substance-abuse disorder, the most common being panic disorder. The differential diagnosis of panic disorder is complicated by a high rate of comorbidity with other psychiatric conditions, especially alcohol and benzodiazepine abuse, which patients initially use in an attempt at self-medication. Some 75% of panic disorder patients will also satisfy criteria for major depression at some point in their illness.

When the history is nonspecific, physical examination and focused laboratory testing must be used to rule out anxiety states resulting from medical disorders such as pheochromocytoma, thyrotoxicosis, or hypoglycemia. Electrocardiogram (ECG) and echocardiogram may detect some cardiovascular conditions associated with panic, such as paroxysmal atrial tachycardia and mitral valve prolapse. In two studies, panic disorder was the primary diagnosis in 43% of patients with chest pain who had normal coronary angiograms and was present in 9% of all outpatients referred for cardiac evaluation. Panic disorder has also been diagnosed in many patients referred for pulmonary function testing or with symptoms of irritable bowel syndrome.

Etiology and Pathophysiology　The etiology of panic disorder is unknown but appears to involve a genetic predisposition, altered autonomic responsivity, and social learning. Panic disorder shows familial aggregation; the disorder is concordant in 30 to 45% of monozygotic twins, and genome-wide screens have identified suggestive risk loci on 1q, 7p15, 10q, 11p, and 13q. Acute panic attacks appear to be associated with increased noradrenergic discharges in the locus coeruleus. Intravenous infusion of sodium lactate evokes an attack in two-thirds of panic disorder patients, as do the α_2-adrenergic antagonist yohimbine, cholecystokinin tetrapeptide (CCK-4), and carbon dioxide inhalation. It is hypothesized that each of these stimuli activates a pathway involving noradrenergic neurons in the locus coeruleus and serotonergic neurons in the dorsal raphe. Agents that block serotonin reuptake can prevent attacks. It is theorized that panic-disorder patients have a heightened sensitivity to somatic symptoms, which triggers increasing arousal, setting off the panic attack. Accordingly, therapeutic intervention involves altering the patient's cognitive interpretation of anxiety-producing experiences as well as preventing the attack itself.

℞ TREATMENT

Achievable goals of treatment are to decrease the frequency of panic attacks and to reduce their intensity. The cornerstone of drug therapy is antidepressant medication (Tables 371-3, 371-4, and 371-5). The tricyclic antidepressants (TCAs) imipramine and clomipramine benefit 75 to 90% of panic disorder patients. Low doses (e.g., 10 to 25 mg/d) are given initially to avoid transient increased anxiety associated with heightened monoamine levels. Selective serotonin reuptake inhibitors (SSRIs) are equally effective and do not have the adverse effects of TCAs. SSRIs should be started at one-third to one-half of their usual antidepressant dose (e.g., 5 to 10 mg fluoxetine, 25 to 50 mg sertraline, 10 mg paroxetine). Monoamine oxidase inhibitors (MAOIs) are also effective and may specifically benefit patients who have comorbid features of atypical depression (i.e., hypersomnia and weight gain). Insomnia, orthostatic hypotension, and the need to maintain a low-tyramine diet (avoidance of cheese and wine) have limited their use, however. Antidepressants typically take 2 to 6 weeks to become effective, and doses may need to be adjusted based upon the clinical response.

Because of anticipatory anxiety and the need for immediate relief of panic symptoms, benzodiazepines are useful early in the course of treatment and sporadically thereafter (Table 371-6). For example, alprazolam, starting at 0.5 mg qid and increasing to 4 mg/d in divided doses, is effective, but patients must be monitored closely, as some develop dependence and begin to escalate the dose of this medication. Clonazepam, at a final maintenance dose of 2 to 4 mg/d, is also helpful; its longer half-life permits twice-daily dosing, and patients appear less likely to develop dependence on this agent.

Early psychotherapeutic intervention and education aimed at symptom control enhances the effectiveness of drug treatment. Patients can be taught breathing techniques, can be educated about physiologic changes that occur with panic, and can learn to expose themselves voluntarily to precipitating events in a treatment program spanning 12 to 15 sessions. Homework assignments and monitored compliance are important components of successful treatment. Once patients have achieved a satisfactory response, drug treatment should be maintained for 1 to 2 years to prevent relapse. Controlled trials indicate a success rate of 75 to 85%, although the likelihood of complete remission is somewhat lower.

GENERALIZED ANXIETY DISORDER ■ Clinical Manifestations Patients with generalized anxiety disorder (GAD) have persistent, excessive, and/or unrealistic worry associated with muscle tension, impaired concentration, autonomic arousal, feeling "on edge" or restless, and insomnia (Table 371-7). Onset is usually before age 20, and a history of childhood fears and social inhibition may be present. The lifetime prevalence of GAD is 5 to 6%; the risk is higher in first-degree relatives of patients with the diagnosis. Interestingly, family studies indicate that GAD and panic disorder segregate independently. Over 80% of patients with GAD also suffer from major depression, dysthymia, or social phobia. Comorbid substance abuse is common in these patients, particularly alcohol and/or sedative/hypnotic abuse. Patients with GAD worry excessively over minor matters, with life-disrupting effects; unlike in panic disorder, complaints of shortness of breath, palpitations, and tachycardia are relatively rare.

Etiology and Pathophysiology Experimental work suggests that anxiogenic agents share in common the property of altering the binding of benzodiazepines to the γ-aminobutyric acid (GABA)$_A$ receptor/chloride ion channel complex. Benzodiazepines are thought to bind two separate GABA$_A$ receptor sites: type I, which has a broad neuroanatomic distribution, and type II, which is concentrated in the hippocampus, striatum, and neocortex. The antianxiety effects of the various benzodiazepines and side effects such as sedation and memory impairment are influenced by their relative binding to type I and type II receptor sites. Serotonin [5-hydroxytryptamine (5HT)] also appears to have a role in anxiety, and buspirone, a partial 5HT$_{1A}$ receptor agonist, and certain 5HT$_{2A}$ and 5HT$_{2C}$ receptor antagonists (e.g., nefazodone) may have beneficial effects.

TABLE 371-3 Antidepressants

Name	Usual Daily Dose, mg	Side Effects	Comments
SSRIs			
Fluoxetine (Prozac)	10–80	Headache; nausea and other GI effects; jitteriness; insomnia; sexual dysfunction; can affect plasma levels of other meds (except sertraline); akathisia rare	Once daily dosing, usually in A.M.; fluoxetine has very long half-life; must not be combined with MAOIs
Sertraline (Zoloft)	50–200		
Paroxetine (Paxil)	20–60		
Fluvoxamine (Luvox)	100–300		
Citalopram (Celexa)	20–60		
Escitalopram (Lexapro)	10–30		
TCAs			
Amitriptyline (Elavil)	150–300	Anticholinergic (dry mouth, tachycardia, constipation, urinary retention, blurred vision); sweating; tremor; postural hypotension; cardiac conduction delay; sedation; weight gain	Once daily dosing, usually qhs; blood levels of most TCAs available; can be lethal in O.D. (lethal dose = 2 g); nortriptyline best tolerated, especially by elderly
Nortriptyline (Pamelor)	50–200		
Imipramine (Tofranil)	150–300		
Desipramine (Norpramin)	150–300		
Doxepin (Sinequan)	150–300		
Clomipramine (Anafranil)	150–300		
Mixed norepinephrine/ serotonin reuptake inhibitors			
Venlafaxine (Effexor)	75–375	Nausea; dizziness; dry mouth; headaches; increased blood pressure; anxiety and insomnia	Bid-tid dosing (extended release available); lower potential for drug interactions than SSRIs; contraindicated with MAOIs
Mirtazapine (Remeron)	15–45	Somnolence; weight gain; neutropenia rare	Once daily dosing
Mixed-action drugs			
Bupropion (Wellbutrin)	250–450	Jitteriness; flushing; seizures in at-risk patients; anorexia; tachycardia; psychosis	Tid dosing, but sustained release also available; fewer sexual side effects than SSRIs or TCAs; may be useful for adult ADD
Trazodone (Desyrel)	200–600	Sedation; dry mouth; ventricular irritability; postural hypotension; priapism rare	Useful in low doses for sleep because of sedating effects with no anticholinergic side effects
Nefazodone (Serzone)	300–600	Sedation; headache; dry mouth; nausea; constipation	Once daily dosing; no effect on REM sleep unlike other antidepressants
Amoxapine (Asendin)	200–600	Sexual dysfunction	Lethality in overdose; EPS possible
MAOIs			
Phenelzine (Nardil)	45–90	Insomnia; hypotension; anorgasmia; weight gain; hypertensive crisis; tyramine cheese reaction; lethal reactions with SSRIs; serious reactions with narcotics	May be more effective in patients with atypical features or treatment-refractory depression
Tranylcypromine (Parnate)	20–50		
Isocarboxazid (Marplan)	20–60		

Note: ADD, attention deficit disorder; MAOI, monoamine oxidase inhibitor; REM, rapid eye movement; SSRI, selective serotonin reuptake inhibitor; TCA, tricyclic antidepressant; EPS, extrapyramidal symptoms.

℞ TREATMENT

A combination of pharmacologic and psychotherapeutic interventions is most effective in GAD, but complete symptomatic relief is rare. A short course of a benzodiazepine is usually indicated, preferably lorazepam, oxazepam, or temazepam. (The first two of these agents are metabolized via conjugation rather than oxidation and thus do not accumulate if hepatic function is altered.) Administration should be initiated at the lowest dose possible and prescribed on an as-needed basis as symptoms warrant. Benzodiazepines differ in their milligram per kilogram potency, half-life, lipid solubility, metabolic pathways, and presence of active metabolites. Agents that are absorbed rapidly and are lipid soluble, such as diazepam, have a rapid onset of action and a higher abuse potential. Benzodiazepines should generally not be prescribed for >4 to 6 weeks because of the development of tolerance and the risk of abuse and dependence. It is important to warn patients that concomitant use of alcohol or other sedating drugs may be neurotoxic and impair their ability to function. An optimistic approach that encourages the patient to clarify environmental precipitants, anticipate his or her reactions, and plan effective response strategies is an essential element of therapy.

Adverse effects of benzodiazepines generally parallel their relative half-lives. Longer-acting agents, such as diazepam, chlordiazepoxide, flurazepam, and clonazepam, tend to accumulate active metabolites,

TABLE 371-4 *Management of Antidepressant Side Effects*

Symptoms	Comments and Management Strategies
Gastrointestinal	
Nausea, loss of appetite	Usually short-lived and dose-related; consider temporary dose reduction or administration with food and antacids
Diarrhea	Famotidine, 20–40 mg/d
Constipation	Wait for tolerance; try diet change, stool softener, exercise; avoid laxatives
Sexual dysfunction	Consider dose reduction; drug holiday
Anorgasmia/impotence; impaired ejaculation	Bethanechol, 10–20 mg, 2 h before activity, or cyproheptadine, 4–8 mg 2 h before activity, or bupropion, 100 mg bid or amantadine, 100 mg bid/tid
Orthostasis	Tolerance unlikely; increase fluid intake, use calf exercises/support hose; fludrocortisone, 0.025 mg/d
Anticholinergic	Wait for tolerance
Dry mouth, eyes	Maintain good oral hygiene; use artificial tears, sugar-free gum
Tremor/jitteriness	Antiparkinsonian drugs not effective; use dose reduction/slow increase; lorazepam, 0.5 mg bid, or propranolol, 10–20 mg bid
Insomnia	Schedule all doses for the morning; trazodone, 50–100 mg qhs
Sedation	Caffeine; schedule all dosing for bedtime; bupropion, 75–100 mg in afternoon
Headache	Evaluate diet, stress, other drugs; try dose reduction; amitriptyline, 50 mg/d
Weight gain	Decrease carbohydrates; exercise; consider fluoxetine
Loss of therapeutic benefit over time	Related to tolerance? Increase dose or drug holiday; add amantadine, 100 mg bid, buspirone, 10 mg tid, or pindolol, 2.5 mg bid

with resultant sedation, impairment of cognition, and poor psychomotor performance. Shorter-acting compounds, such as alprazolam and oxazepam, can produce daytime anxiety, early morning insomnia, and, with discontinuation, rebound anxiety and insomnia. Although patients develop tolerance to the sedative effects of benzodiazepines, they are less likely to habituate to the adverse psychomotor effects. Withdrawal from the longer half-life benzodiazepines can be accomplished through gradual, stepwise dose reduction (by 10% every 1 to 2 weeks) over 6 to 12 weeks. It is usually more difficult to taper patients off shorter-acting benzodiazepines. Physicians may need to switch the patient to a benzodiazepine with a longer half-life or use an adjunctive medication, such as a beta blocker or carbamazepine, before attempting to discontinue the benzodiazepine. Withdrawal reactions vary in severity and duration; they can include depression, anxiety, delirium, lethargy, diaphoresis, tinnitus, autonomic arousal, adventitious movements, and, rarely, seizures.

Buspirone is a nonbenzodiazepine anxiolytic agent. It is nonsedating, does not produce tolerance or dependence, does not interact with benzodiazepine receptors or alcohol, and has no abuse or disinhibition potential. However, it requires several weeks to take effect and requires thrice-daily dosing. Patients who were previously responsive to a benzodiazepine are unlikely to rate buspirone as equally effective, but patients with head injury or dementia who have symptoms of anxiety and/or agitation may do well with this agent.

Administration of benzodiazepines to geriatric patients requires special care. Such patients have increased drug absorption; decreased hepatic metabolism, protein binding, and renal excretion; and an increased volume of distribution. These factors, together with the likely presence of comorbid medical illnesses and medication, dramatically increase the likelihood of toxicity. Iatrogenic psychomotor impairment can result in falls and fractures, confusional states, or motor vehicle accidents. If used, agents in this class should be started at the lowest possible dose, and effects should be monitored closely. Benzodiazepines are contraindicated during pregnancy and breast-feeding.

Anticonvulsants with GABAergic properties may also be effective against anxiety. Gabapentin, oxcarbazepine, tiagabine, pregabalin, and divalproex have all shown some degree of benefit in a variety of anxiety-related syndromes. Agents that selectively target $GABA_A$ receptor subtypes are currently under development; and it is hoped that these will lack the sedating, memory-impairing, and addicting properties of benzodiazepines.

PHOBIC DISORDERS ■ **Clinical Manifestations** The cardinal feature of phobic disorders is a marked and persistent fear of objects or situations, exposure to which results in an immediate anxiety reaction. The patient avoids the phobic stimulus, and this avoidance usually impairs occupational or social functioning. Panic attacks may be triggered by the phobic stimulus or may occur spontaneously. Unlike patients with other anxiety disorders, individuals with phobias usually experience anxiety only in specific situations. Common phobias include fear of closed spaces (claustrophobia), fear of blood, and fear of flying. Social phobia is distinguished by a specific fear of social or performance situations in which the individual is exposed to unfamiliar individuals or to possible examination and evaluation by others. Examples include having to converse at a party, use public restrooms, and meet strangers. In each case, the affected individual is aware that the experienced fear is excessive and unreasonable given the circumstance. The specific content of a phobia may vary across gender, ethnic, and cultural boundaries.

Phobic disorders are common, affecting ~10% of the population. Full criteria for diagnosis are usually satisfied first in early adulthood, but behavioral avoidance of unfamiliar people, situations, or objects dating from early childhood is common.

In one study of female twins, concordance rates for agoraphobia, social phobia, and animal phobia were found to be 23% for monozygotic twins and 15% for dizygotic twins. A twin study of fear conditioning, a model for the acquisition of phobias, demonstrated a heritability of 35 to 45%, and a genome-wide linkage scan has identified a risk locus on chromosome 14 in a region previously implicated in a mouse model of fear. Animal studies of fear conditioning have indicated that processing of the fear stimulus occurs through the lateral nucleus of the amygdala, extending through the central nucleus and projecting to the periaqueductal gray region, lateral hypothalamus, and paraventricular hypothalamus.

TABLE 371-5 *Possible Drug Interactions with Selective Serotonin Reuptake Inhibitors*

Agent	Effect
Monoamine oxidase inhibitors	Serotonin syndrome—absolute contraindication
Serotonergic agonists, e.g., tryptophan, fenfluramine	Potential serotonin syndrome
Drugs that are metabolized by P450 isoenzymes: tricyclics, other SSRIs, antipsychotics, beta blockers, codeine, terfenadine, astemizole, triazolobenzodiazepines, calcium channel blockers	Delayed metabolism resulting in increased blood levels and potential toxicity—possible fatality secondary to QT prolongation with terfenadine or astemizole
Drugs that are bound tightly to plasma proteins, e.g., warfarin	Increased bleeding secondary to displacement
Drugs that inhibit the metabolism of SSRIs by P450 isoenzymes, e.g., quinidine	Increased SSRI side effects

Note: SSRI, selective serotonin reuptake inhibitor.

℞ **TREATMENT**

Beta blockers (e.g., propranolol, 20 to 40 mg orally 2 h before the event) are particularly effective in the treatment of "performance anxiety" (but not general social phobia) and appear to work by blocking the peripheral manifestations of anxiety, such as perspiration, tachycardia, palpitations, and tremor. MAOIs alleviate social phobia independently of their antidepressant activity, and SSRIs appear to be effective also. Benzodiazepines can be helpful in reducing fearful avoidance, but the chronic nature of phobic disorders limits their usefulness.

Behaviorally focused psychotherapy is an important component of treatment, as relapse rates are high when medication is used as the sole treatment. Cognitive-behavioral strategies are based upon the finding that distorted perceptions and interpretations of fear-producing stimuli play a major role in perpetuation of phobias. Individual and group therapy sessions teach the patient to identify specific negative thoughts associated with the anxiety-producing situation and help to reduce the patient's fear of loss of control. In desensitization therapy, hierarchies of feared situations are constructed and the patient is encouraged to pursue and master gradual exposure to the anxiety-producing stimuli.

Patients with social phobia, in particular, have a high rate of comorbid alcohol abuse, as well as of other psychiatric conditions (e.g., eating disorders), necessitating the need for parallel management of each disorder if anxiety reduction is to be achieved.

TABLE 371-6 Anxiolytics

Name	Equivalent PO dose, mg	Onset of Action	Half-life, h	Comments
Benzodiazepines				
Diazepam (Valium)	5	Fast	20–70	Active metabolites; quite sedating
Flurazepam (Dalmane)	15	Fast	30–100	Flurazepam is a pro-drug; metabolites are active; quite sedating
Triazolam (Halcion)	0.25	Intermediate	1.5–5	No active metabolites; can induce confusion and delirium, especially in elderly
Lorazepam (Ativan)	1	Intermediate	10–20	No active metabolites; direct hepatic glucuronide conjugation; quite sedating
Alprazolam (Xanax)	0.5	Intermediate	12–15	Active metabolites; not too sedating; may have specific antidepressant and antipanic activity; tolerance and dependence develop easily
Chlordiazepoxide (Librium)	10	Intermediate	5–30	Active metabolites; moderately sedating
Oxazepam (Serax)	15	Slow	5–15	No active metabolites; direct glucuronide conjugation; not too sedating
Temazepam (Restoril)	15	Slow	9–12	No active metabolites; moderately sedating
Clonazepam (Klonopin)	0.5	Slow	18–50	No active metabolites; moderately sedating
Non-benzodiazepines				
Buspirone (BuSpar)	7.5	2 weeks	2–3	Active metabolites; tid dosing—usual daily dose 10–20 mg tid; nonsedating; no additive effects with alcohol; useful for agitation in demented or brain-injured patients

STRESS DISORDERS ■ Clinical Manifestations Patients may develop anxiety after exposure to extreme traumatic events such as the threat of personal death or injury or the death of a loved one. The reaction may occur shortly after the trauma (*acute stress disorder*) or be delayed and subject to recurrence (PTSD) (Table 371-8). In both syndromes, individuals experience associated symptoms of detachment and loss of emotional responsivity. The patient may feel depersonalized and unable to recall specific aspects of the trauma, though typically it is reexperienced through intrusions in thought, dreams, or flashbacks, particularly when cues of the original event are present. Patients often actively avoid stimuli that precipitate recollections of the trauma and demonstrate a resulting increase in vigilance, arousal, and startle response. Patients with stress disorders are at risk for the development of other disorders related to anxiety, mood, and substance abuse (especially alcohol). Between 5 and 10% of Americans will at some time in their life satisfy criteria for PTSD, with women more likely to be affected than men.

Risk factors for the development of PTSD include a past psychiatric history and personality characteristics of high neuroticism and extroversion. Twin studies show a substantial influence of genetics on all symptoms associated with PTSD, with less evidence for environment effect.

Etiology and Pathophysiology It is hypothesized that in PTSD there are excessive release of norepinephrine from the locus coeruleus in response to stress and increased noradrenergic activity at projection sites in the hippocampus and amygdala. These changes theoretically facilitate the encoding of fear-based memories. Greater sympathetic responses to cues associated with the traumatic event occur in PTSD, although pituitary adrenal responses are blunted.

℞ **TREATMENT**

Acute stress reactions are usually self-limited, and treatment typically involves the short-term use of benzodiazepines and supportive/expressive psychotherapy. The chronic and recurrent nature of PTSD, however, requires a more complex approach employing drug and behavioral treatments. PTSD is highly correlated with peritraumatic dissociative symptoms and the development of an acute stress disorder

at the time of the trauma. TCAs such as imipramine and amitriptyline, the MAOI phenelzine, and the SSRIs (fluoxetine, sertraline, citalopram, paroxetine) can all reduce anxiety, symptoms of intrusion, and avoidance behaviors, as can prazosin, an α_1 antagonist. Trazodone, a sedating antidepressant, is frequently used at night to help with insomnia (50 to 150 mg qhs). Carbamazepine, valproic acid, or alprazolam have also independently produced improvement in uncontrolled trials. Psychotherapeutic strategies for PTSD help the patient overcome avoidance behaviors and demoralization and master fear of recurrence

TABLE 371-7 Diagnostic Criteria for Generalized Anxiety Disorder

A. Excessive anxiety and worry (apprehensive expectation), occurring more days than not for at least 6 months, about a number of events or activities (such as work or school performance).

B. The person finds it difficult to control the worry.

C. The anxiety and worry are associated with three (or more) of the following six symptoms (with at least some symptoms present for more days than not for the past 6 months): (1) restlessness or feeling keyed up or on edge; (2) being easily fatigued; (3) difficulty concentrating or mind going blank; (4) irritability; (5) muscle tension; (6) sleep disturbance (difficulty falling or staying asleep, or restless unsatisfying sleep).

D. The focus of the anxiety and worry is not confined to features of an Axis I disorder, e.g., the anxiety or worry is not about having a panic attack (as in panic disorder), being embarrassed in public (as in social phobia), being contaminated (as in obsessive-compulsive disorder), being away from home or close relatives (as in separation anxiety disorder), gaining weight (as in anorexia nervosa), having multiple physical complaints (as in somatization disorder), or having a serious illness (as in hypochondriasis), and the anxiety and worry do not occur exclusively during posttraumatic stress disorder.

E. The anxiety, worry, or physical symptoms cause clinically significant distress or impairment in social, occupational, or other important areas of functioning.

F. The disturbance is not due to the direct physiologic effects of a substance (e.g., a drug of abuse, a medication) or a general medical condition (e.g., hyperthyroidism) and does not occur exclusively during a mood disorder, a psychotic disorder, or a pervasive developmental disorder.

Source: Diagnostic and Statistical Manual of Mental Disorders, 4th ed.

TABLE 371-8 *Diagnostic Criteria for Posttraumatic Stress Disorder*

A. The person has been exposed to a traumatic event in which both of the following were present:
  1. The person experienced, witnessed, or was confronted with an event or events that involved actual or threatened death or serious injury, or a threat to the physical integrity of self or others.
  2. The person's response involved intense fear, helplessness, or horror.
B. The traumatic event is persistently reexperienced in one (or more) of the following ways:
  1. Recurrent and intrusive distressing recollections of the event, including images, thoughts, or perceptions.
  2. Recurrent distressing dreams of the event.
  3. Acting or feeling as if the traumatic event were recurring (includes a sense of reliving the experience, illusions, hallucinations, and dissociative flashback episodes, including those that occur on awakening or when intoxicated).
  4. Intense psychological distress at exposure to internal or external cues that symbolize or resemble an aspect of the traumatic event.
  5. Physiologic reactivity on exposure to internal or external cues that symbolize or resemble an aspect of the traumatic event.
C. Persistent avoidance of stimuli associated with the trauma and numbing of general responsiveness (not present before the trauma), as indicated by three or more of the following:
  1. Efforts to avoid thoughts, feelings, or conversations associated with the trauma
  2. Efforts to avoid activities, places, or people that arouse recollections of the trauma
  3. Inability to recall an important aspect of the trauma
  4. Markedly diminished interest or participation in significant activities
  5. Feeling of detachment or estrangement from others
  6. Restricted range of affect (e.g., unable to have loving feelings)
  7. Sense of a foreshortened future (e.g., does not expect to have a career, marriage, children, or a normal life span)
D. Persistent symptoms of increased arousal (not present before the trauma), as indicated by two (or more) of the following:
  1. Difficulty falling or staying asleep
  2. Irritability or outbursts of anger
  3. Difficulty concentrating
  4. Hypervigilance
  5. Exaggerated startle response
E. Duration of the disturbance (symptoms in criteria B, C, and D) is more than 1 month
F. The disturbance causes clinically significant distress or impairment in social, occupational, or other important areas of functioning.

Source: *Diagnostic and Statistical Manual of Mental Disorders*, 4th ed.

of the trauma; therapies that encourage the patient to dismantle avoidance behaviors through stepwise focusing on the experience of the traumatic event are the most effective.

OBSESSIVE-COMPULSIVE DISORDER ■ **Clinical Manifestations** Obsessive-compulsive disorder (OCD) is characterized by obsessive thoughts and compulsive behaviors that impair everyday functioning. Fears of contamination and germs are common, as are handwashing, counting behaviors, and having to check and recheck such actions as whether a door is locked. The degree to which the disorder is disruptive for the individual varies, but in all cases obsessive-compulsive activities take up >1 h/d and are undertaken to relieve the anxiety triggered by the core fear. Patients often conceal their symptoms, usually because they are embarrassed by the content of their thoughts or the nature of their actions. Physicians must ask specific questions regarding recurrent thoughts and behaviors, particularly if physical clues such as chafed and reddened hands or patchy hair loss (from repetitive hair pulling, or trichotillomania) are present. Comorbid conditions are common, the most frequent being depression, other anxiety disorders, eating disorders, and tics. OCD has a lifetime prevalence of 2 to 3% worldwide. Onset is usually gradual, beginning in early adulthood, but childhood onset is not rare. The disorder usually has a waxing and waning course,

but some cases may show a steady deterioration in psychosocial functioning.

Etiology and Pathophysiology A genetic contribution to OCD is suggested by twin studies. Family studies show an aggregation with Tourette's disorder. OCD is also more common in males and in first-born children.

The anatomy of obsessive-compulsive behavior is thought to involve the orbital frontal cortex, caudate nucleus, and globus pallidus. The caudate nucleus appears to be involved in the acquisition and maintenance of habit and skill learning, and interventions that are successful in reducing obsessive-compulsive behaviors also decrease metabolic activity measured in the caudate.

℞ TREATMENT

Clomipramine, fluoxetine, and fluvoxamine are approved for the treatment of OCD. Clomipramine is a TCA that is often tolerated poorly owing to anticholinergic and sedative side effects at the doses required to treat the illness (150 to 250 mg/d). Its efficacy in OCD is unrelated to its antidepressant activity. Fluoxetine (40 to 60 mg/d) and fluvoxamine (100 to 300 mg/d) are as effective as clomipramine and have a more benign side-effect profile. Only 50 to 60% of patients with OCD show adequate improvement with pharmacotherapy alone. In treatment-resistant cases, augmentation with other serotonergic agents, such as buspirone, or with a neuroleptic or benzodiazepine may be beneficial. When a therapeutic response is achieved, long-duration maintenance therapy is usually indicated.

For many individuals, particularly those with time-consuming compulsions, behavior therapy will result in as much improvement as that afforded by medication. Effective techniques include the gradual increase in exposure to stressful situations, maintenance of a diary to clarify stressors, and homework assignments that substitute new activities for compulsive behaviors.

MOOD DISORDERS

Mood disorders are characterized by a disturbance in the regulation of mood, behavior, and affect. Mood disorders are subdivided into (1) depressive disorders, (2) bipolar disorders, and (3) depression in association with medical illness or alcohol and substance abuse (Chaps. 372, 373, and 374). Depressive disorders are differentiated from bipolar disorders by the absence of a manic or hypomanic episode. The relationship between pure depressive syndromes and bipolar disorders is not well understood; depression is more frequent in families of bipolar individuals, but the reverse is not true. In the Global Burden of Disease Study conducted by the World Health Organization, unipolar major depression ranked fourth among all diseases in terms of disability-adjusted life years and was projected to rank second by year 2020. In the United States, lost productivity directly related to depression has been estimated at $44 billion per year.

DEPRESSION IN ASSOCIATION WITH MEDICAL ILLNESS Depression occurring in the context of medical illness is difficult to evaluate. Depressive symptomatology may reflect the psychological stress of coping with the disease, may be caused by the disease process itself or by the medications used to treat it, or may simply coexist in time with the medical diagnosis.

Virtually every class of *medication* includes some agent that can induce depression. Antihypertensive drugs, anticholesterolemic agents, and antiarrhythmic agents are common triggers of depressive symptoms. Among the antihypertensive agents, β-adrenergic blockers and, to a lesser extent, calcium channel blockers are the most likely to cause depressed mood. Iatrogenic depression should also be considered in patients receiving glucocorticoids, antimicrobials, systemic analgesics, antiparkinsonian medications, and anticonvulsants. To decide whether a causal relationship exists between pharmacologic therapy and a patient's change in mood, it may sometimes be necessary to undertake an empirical trial of an alternative medication.

Between 20 and 30% of cardiac patients manifest a depressive disorder; an even higher percentage experience depressive symptomatology when self-reporting scales are used. Depressive symptoms following unstable angina, myocardial infarction, or heart transplant impair rehabilitation and are associated with higher rates of mortality and medical morbidity. Depressed patients often show decreased variability in heart rate (an index of reduced parasympathetic nervous system activity), and this has been proposed as one mechanism by which depression may predispose individuals to ventricular arrhythmia and increased morbidity. Depression also appears to increase the risk of developing coronary heart disease; increased serotonin-induced platelet aggregation has been implicated as a possible cause. TCAs are contraindicated in patients with bundle branch block, and TCA-induced tachycardia is an additional concern in patients with congestive heart failure. SSRIs appear not to induce ECG changes or adverse cardiac events and thus are reasonable first-line drugs for patients at risk for TCA-related complications. SSRIs may interfere with hepatic metabolism of anticoagulants, however, causing increased anticoagulation.

In patients with cancer, the mean prevalence of depression is 25%, but depression occurs in 40 to 50% of patients with cancers of the pancreas or oropharynx. Extreme cachexia, common with some cancers, may be misinterpreted as part of the symptom complex of depression; the higher prevalence of depression in patients with pancreatic cancer nevertheless persists when compared to those with advanced gastric cancer. Initiation of antidepressant medication in cancer patients has been shown to improve quality of life as well as mood. Psychotherapeutic approaches, particularly group therapy, may have some effect on short-term depression, anxiety, and pain symptoms and, speculatively, on recurrence rates and long-term survival.

Depression occurs frequently in patients with *neurologic disorders*, particularly cerebrovascular disorders, Parkinson's disease, dementia, multiple sclerosis, and traumatic brain injury. One in five patients with left-hemisphere stroke involving the dorsal lateral frontal cortex experiences major depression. Late-onset depression in otherwise cognitively normal individuals increases the risk of a subsequent diagnosis of Alzheimer's disease. Both TCA and SSRI agents are effective against these depressions, as are stimulant compounds and, in some patients, MAOIs.

The reported prevalence of depression in patients with *diabetes mellitus* varies from 8 to 27%, with the severity of the mood state correlating with the level of hyperglycemia and the presence of diabetic complications. Treatment of depression may be complicated by effects of antidepressive agents on glycemic control. MAOIs can induce hypoglycemia and weight gain. TCAs can produce hyperglycemia and carbohydrate craving. SSRIs, like MAOIs, may reduce fasting plasma glucose, but they are easier to use and may also improve dietary and medication compliance.

Hypothyroidism is frequently associated with features of depression, most commonly depressed mood and memory impairment. Hyperthyroid states may also present in a similar fashion, usually in geriatric populations. Improvement in mood usually follows normalization of thyroid function, but adjunctive antidepressant medication is sometimes required. Patients with subclinical hypothyroidism can also experience symptoms of depression and cognitive difficulty that respond to thyroid replacement.

The lifetime prevalence of depression in HIV-positive individuals has been estimated at 22 to 45%. The relationship between depression and disease progression is multifactorial and likely to involve psychological and social factors, alterations in immune function, and central nervous system disease. Chronic hepatitis C infection is also associated with depression, which may worsen with interferon-α treatment.

Some chronic disorders of uncertain etiology, such as chronic fatigue syndrome (Chap. 370) and fibromyalgia (Chap. 315), are strongly associated with depression and anxiety and may partially benefit from antidepressant treatment, usually at lower than normal dosing.

DEPRESSIVE DISORDERS ■ Clinical Manifestations *Major depression* is defined as depressed mood on a daily basis for a minimum duration of 2 weeks (Table 371-9). An episode may be characterized by sadness, indifference, apathy, or irritability and is usually associated with: changes in sleep patterns, appetite, and weight; motor agitation or retardation; fatigue; impaired concentration and decision-making; feelings of shame or guilt; and thoughts of death or dying. Patients with depression have a profound loss of pleasure in all enjoyable activities, exhibit early morning awakening, feel that the dysphoric mood state is qualitatively different from sadness, and often notice a diurnal variation in mood (worse in morning hours).

Approximately 15% of the population experiences a major depressive episode at some point in life, and 6 to 8% of all outpatients in primary care settings satisfy diagnostic criteria for the disorder. Depression is often undiagnosed, and, even more frequently, it is treated inadequately. If a physician suspects the presence of a major depressive episode, the initial task is to determine whether it represents unipolar or bipolar depression or is one of the 10 to 15% of cases that are secondary to general medical illness or substance abuse. Physicians should also assess the risk of suicide by direct questioning, as patients are often reluctant to verbalize such thoughts without prompting. If specific plans are uncovered or if significant risk factors exist (e.g., a past history of suicide attempts, profound hopelessness, concurrent medical illness, substance abuse, or social isolation), the patient must be referred to a mental health specialist for immediate care. The physician should specifically probe each of these areas in an empathic and hopeful manner, being sensitive to denial and possible minimization of distress. The presence of anxiety, panic, or agitation significantly increases near-term suicidal risk. Approximately 4 to 5% of all de-

---

TABLE 371-9 *Criteria for Major Depressive Episode*

A. Five (or more) of the following symptoms have been present during the same 2-week period and represent a change from previous functioning; at least one of the symptoms is either (1) depressed mood or (2) loss of interest or pleasure. **Note:** Do not include symptoms that are clearly due to a general medical condition, or mood-incongruent delusions or hallucinations.
  1. Depressed mood most of the day, nearly every day, as indicated by either subjective report (e.g., feels sad or empty) or observation made by others (e.g., appears tearful)
  2. Markedly diminished interest or pleasure in all, or almost all, activities most of the day, nearly every day (as indicated by either subjective account or observation made by others)
  3. Significant weight loss when not dieting or weight gain (e.g., a change of >5% of body weight in a month), or decrease or increase in appetite nearly every day
  4. Insomnia or hypersomnia nearly every day
  5. Psychomotor agitation or retardation nearly every day (observable by others, not merely subjective feelings of restlessness or being slowed down)
  6. Fatigue or loss of energy nearly every day
  7. Feelings of worthlessness or excessive or inappropriate guilt (which may be delusional) nearly every day (not merely self-reproach or guilt about being sick)
  8. Diminished ability to think or concentrate, or indecisiveness, nearly every day (either by subjective account or as observed by others)
  9. Recurrent thoughts of death (not just fear of dying), recurrent suicidal ideation without a specific plan, or a suicide attempt or a specific plan for committing suicide
B. The symptoms do not meet criteria for a mixed episode
C. The symptoms cause clinically significant distress or impairment in social, occupational, or other important areas of functioning
D. The symptoms are not due to the direct physiologic effects of a substance (e.g., a drug of abuse, a medication) or a general medical condition (e.g., hypothyroidism)
E. The symptoms are not better accounted for by bereavement; i.e., after the loss of a loved one, the symptoms persist for >2 months or are characterized by marked functional impairment, morbid preoccupation with worthlessness, suicidal ideation, psychotic symptoms, or psychomotor retardation

Source: *Diagnostic and Statistical Manual of Mental Disorders*, 4th ed.

pressed patients will commit suicide; most will have sought help from a physician within 1 month of their death.

In some depressed patients, the mood disorder does not appear to be episodic and is not clearly associated with either psychosocial dysfunction or change from the individual's usual experience in life. *Dysthymic disorder* consists of a pattern of chronic (at least 2 years), ongoing, mild depressive symptoms that are less severe and less disabling than those found in major depression; the two conditions are sometimes difficult to separate, however, and can occur together ("double depression"). Many patients who exhibit a profile of pessimism, disinterest, and low self-esteem respond to antidepressant treatment. Dysthymic disorder exists in ~5% of primary care patients. The term *minor depression* is used for individuals who experience at least two depressive symptoms for 2 weeks, but who do not meet the full criteria for major depression. Despite its name, minor depression is associated with significant morbidity and disability and also responds to pharmacologic treatment.

Depression is approximately twice as common in women as in men, and the incidence increases with age in both sexes. Twin studies indicate that the liability to major depression in adult women is largely genetic in origin. Negative life events can precipitate and contribute to depression, but genetic factors influence the sensitivity of individuals to these stressful events. In most cases, both biologic and psychosocial factors are involved in the precipitation and unfolding of depressive episodes. The most potent stressors appear to involve death of a relative, assault, or severe marital or relationship problems.

Unipolar depressive disorders usually begin in early adulthood and recur episodically over the course of a lifetime. The best predictor of future risk is the number of past episodes; 50 to 60% of patients who have a first episode have at least one or two recurrences. Some patients experience multiple episodes that become more severe and frequent over time. The duration of an untreated episode varies greatly, ranging from a few months to ≥1 year. The pattern of recurrence and clinical progression in a developing episode are also variable. Within an individual, the nature of attacks (e.g., specific presenting symptoms, frequency and duration of episodes) may be similar over time. In a minority of patients, a severe depressive episode may progress to a psychotic state; in elderly patients, depressive symptoms may be associated with cognitive deficits mimicking dementia ("pseudodementia"). A seasonal pattern of depression, called *seasonal affective disorder*, may manifest with onset and remission of episodes at predictable times of the year. This disorder is more common in women, whose symptoms are anergy, fatigue, weight gain, hypersomnia, and episodic carbohydrate craving. The prevalence increases with distance from the equator, and improvement may occur by altering light exposure.

Etiology and Pathophysiology   Although evidence for genetic transmission of unipolar depression is not as strong as in bipolar disorder, monozygotic twins have a higher concordance rate (46%) than dizygotic siblings (20%), with little evidence for any effect of a shared family environment. A recent study indicated that a functional polymorphism in the serotonin transporter (*5-HTT*) gene may interact with stressful life events to markedly increase risk of depression and suicide. Positron emission tomography (PET) studies show decreased metabolic activity in the caudate nuclei and frontal lobes in depressed patients that returns to normal with recovery. Single-photon emission computed tomography (SPECT) studies show comparable changes in blood flow.

Postmortem examination of brains of suicide victims indicate altered noradrenergic activity, including increased binding to α_1-, α_2-, and β-adrenergic receptors in the cerebral cortex and decreased numbers of noradrenergic neurons in the locus coeruleus. Involvement of the serotonin system is suggested by findings of reduced plasma tryptophan levels, a decreased cerebrospinal fluid level of 5-hydroxyindolacetic acid (the principal metabolite of serotonin in brain), and de-

creased platelet serotonergic transporter binding. An increase in brain serotonin receptors in suicide victims and decreased expression of the cyclic AMP response element-binding (CREB) protein are also reported. Depletion of blood tryptophan, the amino acid precursor of serotonin, rapidly reverses the antidepressant benefit in depressed patients who have been successfully treated. However, a decrement in mood after tryptophan reduction is considerably less robust in untreated patients, indicating that, if presynaptic serotonergic dysfunction occurs in depression, it likely plays a contributing rather than a causal role.

Neuroendocrine abnormalities that reflect the neurovegetative signs and symptoms of depression include (1) increased cortisol and corticotropin-releasing hormone (CRH) secretion, (2) an increase in adrenal size, (3) a decreased inhibitory response of glucocorticoids to dexamethasone, and (4) a blunted response of thyroid-stimulating hormone (TSH) level to infusion of thyroid-releasing hormone (TRH). Antidepressant treatment leads to normalization of these pituitary-adrenal abnormalities. Major depression is also associated with an upregulation of proinflammatory cytokines, which normalizes with antidepressant treatment.

Diurnal variations in symptom severity and alterations in circadian rhythmicity of a number of neurochemical and neurohumoral factors suggest that biologic differences may be secondary to a primary defect in regulation of biologic rhythms. Patients with major depression show consistent findings of a decrease in rapid eye movement (REM) sleep onset (REM latency), an increase in REM density, and, in some subjects, a decrease in stage IV delta slow-wave sleep.

Although antidepressant drugs inhibit neurotransmitter uptake within hours, their therapeutic effects typically emerge over several weeks, implicating adaptive changes in second messenger systems and transcription factors as possible mechanisms of action. Antidepressant drugs have been shown to regulate neural plasticity and cell survival by increasing the expression of brain-derived neurotrophic factor (BDNF) through upregulation of the CREB protein and to alter stress responsivity through an increase in glucocorticoid receptor transcription. Secondary effects on activation of the mitogen-activated protein (MAP) kinase and phosphoinositol-3 kinase/AKT pathways and increased expression of the antiapoptotic protein, Bcl-2, are also thought to be critical to antidepressant actions.

℞ TREATMENT

Treatment planning requires coordination of short-term symptom remission with longer term maintenance strategies designed to prevent recurrence. The most effective intervention for achieving remission and preventing relapse is medication, but combined treatment, incorporating psychotherapy to help the patient cope with decreased self-esteem and demoralization, improves outcome (Fig. 371-1). About 40% of primary care patients with depression drop out of treatment and discontinue medication if symptomatic improvement is not noted within a month, unless additional support is provided. Outcome improves with (1) increased intensity and frequency of visits during the first 4 to 6 weeks of treatment, (2) supplemental educational materials, and (3) psychiatric consultation as indicated. Despite the widespread use of SSRIs, there is no convincing evidence that this class of antidepressant is more efficacious than TCAs. Between 60 and 70% of depressed patients respond to any drug chosen, if it is given in a sufficient dose for 6 to 8 weeks. There is no ideal antidepressant; no current compound combines rapid onset of action, moderate half-life, a meaningful relationship between dose and blood level, a low side-effect profile, minimal interaction with other drugs, and safety in overdose. A rational approach to selecting which antidepressant to use involves matching the patient's preference and medical history with the metabolic and side effect profile of the drug (Tables 371-4 and 371-5). A previous response, or a family history of a positive response, to a specific antidepressant would suggest that that drug be tried first. Before initiating antidepressant therapy, the physician should evaluate the possible contribution of comorbid illnesses and consider their spe-

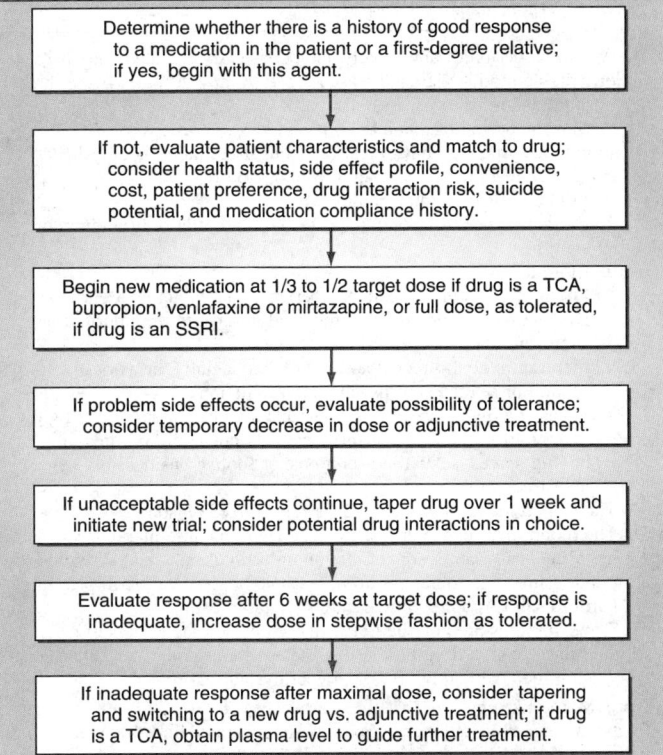

```
┌─────────────────────────────────────────────┐
│  Determine whether there is a history of good response │
│  to a medication in the patient or a first-degree relative; │
│  if yes, begin with this agent. │
└─────────────────────────────────────────────┘
                      │
┌─────────────────────────────────────────────┐
│  If not, evaluate patient characteristics and match to drug; │
│  consider health status, side effect profile, convenience, │
│  cost, patient preference, drug interaction risk, suicide │
│  potential, and medication compliance history. │
└─────────────────────────────────────────────┘
                      │
┌─────────────────────────────────────────────┐
│  Begin new medication at 1/3 to 1/2 target dose if drug is a TCA, │
│  bupropion, venlafaxine or mirtazapine, or full dose, as tolerated, │
│  if drug is an SSRI. │
└─────────────────────────────────────────────┘
                      │
┌─────────────────────────────────────────────┐
│  If problem side effects occur, evaluate possibility of tolerance; │
│  consider temporary decrease in dose or adjunctive treatment. │
└─────────────────────────────────────────────┘
                      │
┌─────────────────────────────────────────────┐
│  If unacceptable side effects continue, taper drug over 1 week and │
│  initiate new trial; consider potential drug interactions in choice. │
└─────────────────────────────────────────────┘
                      │
┌─────────────────────────────────────────────┐
│  Evaluate response after 6 weeks at target dose; if response is │
│  inadequate, increase dose in stepwise fashion as tolerated. │
└─────────────────────────────────────────────┘
                      │
┌─────────────────────────────────────────────┐
│  If inadequate response after maximal dose, consider tapering │
│  and switching to a new drug vs. adjunctive treatment; if drug │
│  is a TCA, obtain plasma level to guide further treatment. │
└─────────────────────────────────────────────┘
```

FIGURE 371-1   A guideline for the medical management of major depressive disorder. SSRI, selective serotonin reuptake inhibitor; TCA, tricyclic antidepressant.

cific treatment. In individuals with suicidal ideation, particular attention should be paid to choosing a drug with low toxicity if taken in overdose. The SSRIs and other newer antidepressant drugs are distinctly safer in this regard; nevertheless, the advantages of TCAs have not been completely superseded. The existence of generic equivalents make TCAs relatively cheap, and for several tricyclics, particularly nortriptyline, imipramine, and desipramine, well-defined relationships among dose, plasma level, and therapeutic response exist. The steady-state plasma level achieved for a given drug dose can vary more than tenfold between individuals. Plasma levels may help in interpreting apparent resistance to treatment and/or unexpected drug toxicity. The principal side effects of TCAs are antihistamine (sedation) and anticholinergic (constipation, dry mouth, urinary hesitancy, blurred vision). Cardiac toxicity due to conduction block or arrhythmias can also occur but is uncommon at therapeutic levels. TCAs are probably contraindicated in patients with serious cardiovascular risk factors. Overdoses of tricyclic agents can be lethal, with desipramine carrying the greatest risk. It is judicious to prescribe only a 10-day supply when suicide is a risk. Most patients require a daily dose of 150 to 200 mg of imipramine or amitriptyline or its equivalent to achieve a therapeutic blood level of 150 to 300 ng/mL and a satisfactory remission; some patients show a partial effect at lower doses. Geriatric patients may require a low starting dose and slow escalation. Ethnic differences in drug metabolism are significant; Hispanic, Asian, and African-American patients generally require lower doses than Caucasians to achieve a comparable blood level.

Second-generation antidepressants include amoxapine, maprotiline, trazodone, and bupropion. Amoxapine is a dibenzoxazepine derivative that blocks norepinephrine and serotonin reuptake and has a metabolite that shows a degree of dopamine blockade. Long-term use of this drug carries a risk of tardive dyskinesia. Maprotiline is a potent noradrenergic reuptake blocker that has little anticholinergic effect but may produce seizures. Bupropion is a novel antidepressant whose mechanism of action is thought to involve enhancement of noradrenergic function. It has no anticholinergic, sedating, or orthostatic side effects and has a low incidence of sexual side effects. It may, however, be associated with stimulant-like side effects, may lower seizure

threshold, and has an exceptionally short half-life, requiring frequent dosing. An extended-release preparation is available.

SSRIs such as fluoxetine, sertraline, paroxetine, citalopram, and escitalopram cause a lower frequency of anticholinergic, sedating, and cardiovascular side effects but a possibly greater incidence of gastrointestinal complaints, sleep impairment, and sexual dysfunction than do TCAs. Akathisia, involving an inner sense of restlessness and anxiety in addition to increased motor activity, may also be more common, particularly during the first week of treatment. A concern is the risk of "serotonin syndrome," thought to result from hyperstimulation of brainstem $5HT_{1A}$ receptors and characterized by myoclonus, agitation, abdominal cramping, hyperpyrexia, hypertension, and potentially death. Serotonergic agonists taken in combination should be monitored closely for this reason. Considerations such as half-life, compliance, toxicity, and drug-drug interactions may guide the choice of a particular SSRI. Fluoxetine and its principal active metabolite, norfluoxetine, for example, have a combined half-life of almost 7 days, resulting in a delay of 5 weeks before steady-state levels are achieved and a similar delay for complete drug excretion once its use is discontinued. All the SSRIs may impair sexual function, resulting in diminished libido, impotence, or difficulty in achieving orgasm. Sexual dysfunction frequently results in noncompliance and should be asked about specifically. Sexual dysfunction can sometimes be ameliorated by lowering the dose, by instituting weekend drug holidays (two or three times a month), or by treatment with amantadine (100 mg tid), bethanechol (25 mg tid) buspirone (10 mg tid), or bupropion (100–150 mg/d). Paroxetine appears to be more anticholinergic than either fluoxetine or sertraline, and sertraline carries a lower risk of producing an adverse drug interaction than the other two. Rare side effects of SSRIs include angina due to vasospasm and prolongation of the prothrombin time. Escitalopram is the most specific of currently available SSRIs and appears to have no specific inhibitory effects on the P450 system.

Venlafaxine, like imipramine, blocks the reuptake of both norepinephrine and serotonin, but it produces relatively little in the way of traditional tricyclic side effects. Unlike the SSRIs, it has a relatively linear dose-response curve. Patients should be monitored for a possible increase in diastolic blood pressure, and multiple daily dosing is required because of the drug's short half-life. An extended-release form is available and has a somewhat lower incidence of gastrointestinal side effects. Nefazadone is a selective $5HT_2$ receptor antagonist that also inhibits the presynaptic reuptake of serotonin and norepinephrine. Its side effects are similar to those of the SSRIs, and twice-daily dosing produces a steady state within 4 to 5 days. The drug is related structurally to trazodone, which is currently used more for its sedative than its antidepressant properties. Nefazadone appears to produce a lower incidence of sexual side effects than do the SSRIs. Mirtazapine is a tetracyclic antidepressant that has a unique spectrum of activity. It increases noradrenergic and serotonergic neurotransmission through a blockade of central α_2-adrenergic receptors and postsynaptic $5HT_2$ and $5HT_3$ receptors. It is also strongly antihistaminic and, as such, may produce sedation.

With the exception of citalopram and escitalopram, each of the SSRIs, as well as nefazadone, may inhibit one or more cytochrome P450 enzymes. Depending on the specific isoenzyme involved, the metabolism of a number of concomitantly administered medications can be dramatically affected. Fluoxetine and paroxetine, for example, by inhibiting 2D6, can cause dramatic increases in the blood level of type 1C antiarrhythmics, while sertraline and nefazadone, by acting on 3A4, may alter blood levels of terfenadine, carbamazepine, and astemizole. Many of these compounds have a narrow therapeutic window and can cause iatrogenic ventricular arrhythmias at toxic levels; thus, the possibility of an adverse drug interaction should always be considered.

The MAOIs are highly effective, particularly in atypical depression, but the risk of hypertensive crisis following intake of tyramine-containing food or sympathomimetic drugs makes them inappropriate as first-line agents. Common side effects include orthostatic hypotension, weight gain, insomnia, and sexual dysfunction. MAOIs should not be used concomitantly with SSRIs, because of the risk of serotonin syndrome, or with TCAs, because of possible hyperadrenergic effects.

Electroconvulsive therapy is at least as effective as medication, but its use is reserved for treatment-resistant cases and delusional depressions. Transcranial magnetic stimulation (TMS) is an investigational treatment of depression that has been shown to have efficacy in several controlled trials; it is uncertain whether the observed benefits were clinically meaningful, however. Vagus nerve stimulation (VNS) appeared to be effective in treatment-resistant depression in an initial open study, only to fail in a controlled trial.

Regardless of the treatment undertaken, the response should be evaluated after ~2 months. Three-quarters of patients show improvement by this time, but if remission is inadequate the patient should be questioned about compliance and an increase in medication dose should be considered if side effects are not troublesome. If this approach is unsuccessful, referral to a mental health specialist is advised. Strategies for treatment then include selection of an alternative drug, combinations of antidepressants, and/or adjunctive treatment with other classes of drugs, including lithium, thyroid hormone, and dopamine agonists. Patients whose response to an SSRI wanes over time may benefit from the addition of buspirone (10 mg tid) or pindolol (2.5 mg tid) or small amounts of a TCA such as desipramine (25 mg bid or tid). Once significant remission is achieved, drug treatment should be continued for at least 6 to 9 months to prevent relapse. In patients who have had two or more episodes of depression, indefinite maintenance treatment should be considered.

It is essential to educate patients both about depression and the benefits and side effects of medications they are receiving. Advice about stress reduction and cautions that alcohol may exacerbate depressive symptoms and impair drug response are helpful. Patients should be given time to describe their experience, their outlook, and the impact of the depression on them and their families. Occasional empathic silence may be as helpful for the treatment alliance as verbal reassurance. Controlled trials have shown that cognitive-behavioral and interpersonal therapies are effective in improving psychological and social adjustment and that a combined treatment approach is more successful than medication alone for many patients.

BIPOLAR DISORDER ■ Clinical Manifestations Bipolar disorder is characterized by unpredictable swings in mood from mania (or hypomania) to depression. Some patients suffer only from recurrent attacks of *mania*, which in its pure form is associated with increased psychomotor activity; excessive social extroversion; decreased need for sleep; impulsivity and impairment in judgment; and expansive, grandiose, and sometimes irritable mood (Table 371-10). In severe mania, patients may experience delusions and paranoid thinking indistinguishable from schizophrenia. Half of patients with bipolar disorder present with a mixture of psychomotor agitation and activation with dysphoria, anxiety, and irritability. It may be difficult to distinguish *mixed mania* from *agitated depression*. In some bipolar patients (*bipolar II disorder*), the full criteria for mania are lacking, and the requisite recurrent depressions are separated by periods of mild activation and increased energy (hypomania). In *cyclothymic disorder*, there are numerous hypomanic periods, usually of relatively short duration, alternating with clusters of depressive symptoms that fail, either in severity or duration, to meet the criteria of major depression. The mood fluctuations are chronic and should be present for at least 2 years before the diagnosis is made.

Manic episodes typically emerge over a period of days to weeks, but onset within hours is possible, usually in the early morning hours. An untreated episode of either depression or mania can be as short as several weeks or last as long as 8 to 12 months, and rare patients have an unremitting chronic course. The term *rapid cycling* is used for pa-

TABLE 371-10   Criteria for a Manic Episode

A. A distinct period of abnormally and persistently elevated, expansive, or irritable mood, lasting at least 1 week (or any duration if hospitalization is necessary)

B. During the period of mood disturbance, three (or more) of the following symptoms have persisted (four if the mood is only irritable) and have been present to a significant degree:
1. Inflated self-esteem or grandiosity
2. Decreased need for sleep (e.g., feels rested after only 3 hours of sleep)
3. More talkative than usual or pressure to keep talking
4. Flight of ideas or subjective experience that thoughts are racing
5. Distractibility (i.e., attention too easily drawn to unimportant or irrelevant external stimuli)
6. Increase in goal-directed activity (either socially, at work or school, or sexually) or psychomotor agitation
7. Excessive involvement in pleasurable activities that have a high potential for painful consequences (e.g., engaging in unrestrained buying sprees, sexual indiscretions, or foolish business investments)

C. The symptoms do not meet criteria for a mixed episode.

D. The mood disturbance is sufficiently severe to cause marked impairment in occupational functioning or in usual social activities or relationships with others, or to necessitate hospitalization to prevent harm to self or others, or there are psychotic features.

E. The symptoms are not due to the direct physiologic effects of a substance (e.g., a drug of abuse, a medication, or other treatment) or a general medical condition (e.g., hyperthyroidism).

Note: Manic-like episodes that are clearly caused by somatic antidepressant treatment (e.g., medication, electroconvulsive therapy, light therapy) should not count toward a diagnosis of bipolar I disorder.

Source: *Diagnostic and Statistical Manual of Mental Disorders*, 4th ed.

tients who have four or more episodes of either depression or mania in a given year. This pattern occurs in 15% of all patients, almost all of whom are women. In some cases, rapid cycling is linked to an underlying thyroid dysfunction and, in others, it is iatrogenically triggered by prolonged antidepressant treatment. Approximately half of patients have sustained difficulties in work performance and psychosocial functioning.

Bipolar disorder is common, affecting ~1% of the population in the United States. Onset is typically between 20 and 30 years of age, but many individuals report premorbid symptoms in late childhood or early adolescence. The prevalence is similar for men and women; women are likely to have more depressive and men more manic episodes over a lifetime.

Differential Diagnosis The differential diagnosis of mania includes toxic effects of stimulant or sympathomimetic drugs as well as secondary mania induced by hyperthyroidism, AIDS, or neurologic disorders, such as Huntington's or Wilson's disease, or cerebrovascular accidents. Comorbidity with alcohol and substance abuse is common, either because of poor judgment and increased impulsivity or because of an attempt to self-treat the underlying mood symptoms and sleep disturbances.

Etiology and Pathophysiology Evidence for a genetic predisposition to bipolar disorder is significant. The concordance rate for monozygotic twin pairs approaches 80%, and segregation analyses are consistent with autosomal dominant transmission. Multiple genes are likely to be involved, with strongest evidence for loci on chromosomes 18p, 18q, 4p, 4q, 5q, 8p, and 21q.

The pathophysiologic mechanisms underlying the profound and recurrent mood swings of bipolar disorder remain unknown. Neuroimaging studies have documented alterations in amygdala volume as well as increases in white matter hyperintensities. Cellular models of changes in membrane Na^+- and K^+-activated ATPase and proposals of disordered signal transduction mechanisms involving the phosphoinositol system and GTP-binding proteins have received the most attention. Neurophysiologic studies suggest that patients with bipolar disorder have altered circadian rhythmicity. Lithium may exert its therapeutic benefit through a resynchronization of intrinsic rhythms keyed to the light/dark cycle (Chap. 24).

Rx TREATMENT (Table 371-11)

Lithium carbonate is the mainstay of treatment in bipolar disorder, although sodium valproate and olanzapine are equally effective in acute mania, as is lamotrigine in the depressed phase. The response rate to lithium carbonate is 70 to 80% in acute mania, with beneficial effects appearing in 1 to 2 weeks. Lithium also has a prophylactic effect in prevention of recurrent mania and, to a lesser extent, in the prevention of recurrent depression. A simple cation, lithium is rapidly absorbed from the gastrointestinal tract and remains unbound to plasma or tissue proteins. Some 95% of a given dose is excreted unchanged through the kidneys within 24 h.

Serious side effects from lithium administration are rare, but minor complaints such as gastrointestinal discomfort, nausea, diarrhea, polyuria, weight gain, skin eruptions, alopecia, and edema are common. Over time, urine-concentrating ability may be decreased, but significant nephrotoxicity does not usually occur. Lithium exerts an antithyroid effect by interfering with the synthesis and release of thyroid hormones. More serious side effects include tremor, poor concentration and memory, ataxia, dysarthria, and incoordination. There is suggestive, but not conclusive, evidence that lithium is teratogenic, inducing cardiac malformations in the first trimester.

In the treatment of acute mania, lithium is initiated at 300 mg bid or tid, and the dose is then increased by 300 mg every 2 to 3 days to achieve blood levels of 0.8 to 1.2 meq/L. Because the therapeutic effect of lithium may not appear until after 7 to 10 days of treatment, adjunctive usage of lorazepam (1 to 2 mg every 4 h) or clonazepam (0.5 to 1 mg every 4 h) may be beneficial to control agitation. Antipsychotics are indicated in patients with severe agitation who respond only partially to benzodiazepines. Patients using lithium should be monitored closely, since the blood levels required to achieve a therapeutic benefit are close to those associated with toxicity.

Valproic acid is an alternative in patients who cannot tolerate lithium or respond poorly to it. Valproic acid may be better than lithium for patients who experience rapid cycling (i.e., more than four episodes a year) or who present with a mixed or dysphoric mania. Tremor and weight gain are the most common side effects; hepatotoxicity and pancreatitis are rare toxicities.

Carbamazepine and oxcarbazepine, although not formally approved by the U.S. Food and Drug Administration (FDA) for bipolar disorder, have clinical efficacy in the treatment of acute mania. Preliminary evidence also suggests that other anticonvulsant agents such as levtiracetam, zonisamide, and topiramate may possess some therapeutic benefit.

The recurrent nature of bipolar mood disorder necessitates maintenance treatment. A sustained blood lithium level of at least 0.8 mEq/L is important for optimal prophylaxis and has been shown to reduce risk of suicide, a finding not yet apparent for other mood stabilizers. Compliance is frequently an issue and often requires enlistment and education of concerned family members. Efforts to identify and modify psychosocial factors that may trigger episodes are important, as is an emphasis on lifestyle regularity. Antidepressant medications are sometimes required for the treatment of severe breakthrough depressions, but their use should generally be avoided during maintenance treatment because of the risk of precipitating mania or accelerating the cycle frequency. Loss of efficacy over time may be observed with any of the mood-stabilizing agents. In such situations, an alternative agent or combination therapy is usually helpful.

Consensus guidelines for the treatment of acute mania and bipolar depression are described in Table 371-12.

SOMATOFORM DISORDERS

CLINICAL MANIFESTATIONS Patients with multiple somatic complaints that cannot be explained by a known medical condition or by the effects of alcohol or of recreational or prescription drugs are com-

TABLE 371-11 *Clinical Pharmacology of Mood Stabilizers*

Agent and Dosing	Side Effects and Other Effects
Lithium Starting dose: 300 mg bid or tid Therapeutic blood level: 0.8–1.2 meq/L	*Common side effects:* Nausea/anorexia/diarrhea, fine tremor, thirst, polyuria, fatigue, weight gain, acne, folliculitis, neutrophilia, hypothyroidism Blood level is increased by thiazides, tetracyclines, and NSAIDs Blood level is decreased by bronchodilators, verapamil, and carbonic anhydrase inhibitors *Rare side effects:* Neurotoxicity, renal toxicity, hypercalcemia, ECG changes
Valproic acid Starting dose: 250 mg tid Therapeutic blood level: 50–125 μg/mL	*Common side effects:* Nausea/anorexia, weight gain, sedation, tremor, rash, alopecia Inhibits hepatic metabolism of other medications *Rare side effects:* Pancreatitis, hepatotoxicity, Stevens-Johnson syndrome
Carbamazepine/oxcarbazepine Starting dose: 200 mg bid for carbamazepine, 150 bid for oxcarbazepine Therapeutic blood level: 4–12 μg/mL for carbamazepine	*Common side effects:* Nausea/anorexia, sedation, rash, dizziness/ataxia Carbamazepine, but not oxcarbazepine, induces hepatic metabolism of other medications *Rare side effects:* Hyponatremia, agranulocytosis, Stevens-Johnson syndrome
Lamotrigine Starting dose: 25 mg/d	*Common side effects:* Rash, dizziness, headache, tremor, sedation, nausea *Rare side effect:* Stevens-Johnson syndrome

Note: NSAID, nonsteroidal anti-inflammatory drug; ECG, electrocardiogram.

monly seen in primary care practice; one survey indicates a prevalence of such complaints of 5%. In *somatization disorder*, the patient presents with multiple physical complaints referable to different organ systems (Table 371-13). Onset is usually before age 30, and the disorder is persistent. Formal diagnostic criteria require the recording of at least four pain, two gastrointestinal, one sexual, and one pseudoneurologic symptom. Patients with somatization disorder often present with dramatic complaints, but the complaints are inconsistent. Symptoms of comorbid anxiety and mood disorder are common and may be the result of drug interactions due to regimens initiated independently by different physicians. Patients with somatization disorder may be impulsive and demanding and frequently qualify for a formal comorbid

TABLE 371-12 *Consensus Guidelines on the Drug Treatment of Acute Mania and Bipolar Depression*

Condition	Preferred Agents
Euphoric mania	Lithium
Mixed/dysphoric mania	Valproic acid
Mania with psychosis	Valproic acid with olanzapine, conventional antipsychotic, or risperidone
Hypomania	Lithium, lamotrigine, or valproic acid alone
Severe depression with psychosis	Venlafaxine, bupropion, or paroxetine *plus* lithium *plus* olanzapine, *or* risperidone; consider ECT
Severe depression without psychosis	Bupropion, paroxetine, sertraline, venlafaxine, *or* citalopram *plus* lithium
Mild to moderate depression	Lithium *or* lamotrigine alone; add bupropion if needed

Note: ECT, electroconvulsive therapy.
Source: From GS Sachs et al: Postgrad Med April, 2000.

TABLE 371-13 *Diagnostic Criteria for Somatization Disorder*

A. A history of many physical complaints beginning before age 30 years that occur over a period of several years and result in treatment being sought or significant impairment in social, occupational, or other important areas of functioning.

B. Each of the following criteria must have been met, with individual symptoms occurring at any time during the course of the disturbance:
 1. *Four pain symptoms:* a history of pain related to at least four different sites or functions (e.g., head, abdomen, back, joints, extremities, chest, rectum, during menstruation, during sexual intercourse, or during urination)
 2. *Two gastrointestinal symptoms:* a history of at least two gastrointestinal symptoms other than pain (e.g., nausea, bloating, vomiting other than during pregnancy, diarrhea, or intolerance of several different foods)
 3. *One sexual symptom:* a history of at least one sexual or reproductive symptom other than pain (e.g., sexual indifference, erectile or ejaculatory dysfunction, irregular menses, excessive menstrual bleeding, vomiting throughout pregnancy)
 4. *One pseudoneurologic symptom:* a history of at least one symptom or deficit suggesting a neurologic condition not limited to pain (conversion symptoms such as impaired coordination or balance, paralysis or localized weakness, difficulty swallowing or lump in throat, aphonia, urinary retention, hallucinations, loss of touch or pain sensation, double vision, blindness, deafness, seizures; dissociative symptoms such as amnesia; or loss of consciousness other than fainting)

C. Either of the following:
 1. After appropriate investigation, each of the symptoms in criterion B cannot be fully explained by a known general medical condition or the direct effects of a substance (e.g., a drug of abuse, a medication)
 2. When there is a related general medical condition, the physical complaints or resulting social or occupational impairment are in excess of what would be expected from the history, physical examination, or laboratory findings

D. The symptoms are not intentionally produced or feigned (as in factitious disorder or malingering).

Source: Diagnostic and Statistical Manual of Mental Disorders, 4th ed.

psychiatric diagnosis. In *conversion disorder*, the symptoms focus on deficits that involve motor or sensory function and on psychological factors that initiate or exacerbate the medical presentation. Like somatization disorder, the deficit is not intentionally produced or simulated, as is the case in factitious disorder (malingering). In *hypochondriasis*, the essential feature is a belief of serious medical illness that persists despite reassurance and appropriate medical evaluation. As with somatization disorder, patients with hypochondriasis have a history of poor relationships with physicians stemming from their sense that they have been evaluated and treated inappropriately or inadequately. Hypochondriasis can be disabling in intensity and is persistent, with waxing and waning symptomatology.

In *factitious illnesses*, the patient consciously and voluntarily produces physical symptoms of illness. The term *Munchausen's syndrome* is reserved for individuals with particularly dramatic, chronic, or severe factitious illness. In true factitious illness, the sick role itself is gratifying. A variety of signs, symptoms, and diseases have been either simulated or caused by factitious behavior, the most common including chronic diarrhea, fever of unknown origin, intestinal bleeding or hematuria, seizures, and hypoglycemia. Factitious disorder is usually not diagnosed until 5 to 10 years after its onset, and it can produce significant social and medical costs. In *malingering*, the fabrication derives from a desire for some external reward, such as a narcotic medication or disability reimbursement.

℞ **TREATMENT**

Patients with somatization disorders are frequently subjected to multiple diagnostic testing and exploratory surgeries in an attempt to find their "real" illness. Such an approach is doomed to failure and does not address the core issue. Successful treatment is best achieved through behavior modification, in which access to the physician is tightly regulated and adjusted to provide a sustained and predictable level of support that is less clearly contingent on the patient's level of presenting distress. Visits can be brief and should not be associated with a need for a diagnostic or treatment action. Although the literature is limited, some patients with somatization disorder may benefit from antidepressant treatment. Fluoxetine and MAOIs have both been found to be useful in reducing obsessive ruminations, dysphoria, and anxious preoccupation in patients with multiple somatic complaints.

The treatment of factitious disorder is complicated in that any attempt to confront the patient usually only creates a sense of humiliation and causes the patient to abandon treatment from that caregiver. A better strategy is to introduce psychological causation as one of a number of possible explanations and to include factitious illness as an option in the differential diagnoses that are discussed. Without directly linking psychotherapeutic intervention to the diagnosis, the patient can be offered a face-saving means by which the pathologic relationship with the health care system can be examined and alternative approaches to life stressors developed.

PERSONALITY DISORDERS

CLINICAL MANIFESTATIONS Personality disorders are characteristic patterns of thinking, feeling, and interpersonal behavior that are relatively inflexible and cause significant functional impairment or subjective distress for the individual. The observed behaviors are not secondary to another mental disorder, nor are they precipitated by substance abuse or a general medical condition. This distinction is often difficult to make in clinical practice, as personality change may be the first sign of serious neurologic, endocrine, or other medical illness. Patients with frontal lobe tumors, for example, can present with changes in motivation and personality while the results of the neurologic examination remain within normal limits. Individuals with personality disorders are often regarded as "difficult patients" in clinical medical practice because they are seen as excessively demanding and/or unwilling to follow recommended treatment plans. Although DSM-IV portrays personality disorders as qualitatively distinct categories, there is an alternative perspective that personality characteristics vary as a continuum between normal functioning and formal mental disorder.

Personality disorders have been grouped into three overlapping clusters. *Cluster A* includes paranoid, schizoid, and schizotypal personality disorders. It includes individuals who are odd and eccentric and who maintain an emotional distance from others. Individuals have a restricted emotional range and remain socially isolated. Patients with schizotypal personality disorder frequently have unusual perceptual experiences and express magical beliefs about the external world. The essential feature of paranoid personality disorder is a pervasive mistrust and suspiciousness of others to an extent that is unjustified by available evidence. *Cluster B* disorders include antisocial, borderline, histrionic, and narcissistic types and describe individuals whose behavior is impulsive, excessively emotional, and erratic. *Cluster C* incorporates avoidant, dependent, and obsessive-compulsive personality types; enduring traits are anxiety and fear. The boundaries between cluster types are to some extent artificial, and many patients who meet criteria for one personality disorder also meet criteria for aspects of another. The risk of a comorbid major mental disorder is increased in patients who qualify for a diagnosis of personality disorder.

℞ **TREATMENT**

Dialectical behavior therapy (DBT) is a cognitive-behavioral approach that focuses on behavioral change while providing acceptance, compassion, and validation of the patient. Several randomized trials have demonstrated the efficacy of DBT in the treatment of personality disorders. Antidepressant medications and low-dose antipsychotic drugs have some efficacy in cluster A personality disorders, while anticonvulsant mood-stabilizing agents and MAOIs may be considered for patients with cluster B diagnoses who show marked mood reactivity, behavioral dyscontrol, and/or rejection hypersensitivity. Anxious or fearful cluster C patients often respond to medications used for axis I anxiety disorders (see above). It is important that the physician and the patient have reasonable expectations vis-à-vis the possible benefit of any medication used and its side effects. Improvement may be subtle and observable only over time.

SCHIZOPHRENIA

CLINICAL MANIFESTATIONS Schizophrenia is a heterogeneous syndrome characterized by perturbations of language, perception, thinking, social activity, affect, and volition. There are no pathognomonic features. The syndrome commonly begins in late adolescence, has an insidious (and less commonly acute) onset, and, classically, a poor outcome, progressing from social withdrawal and perceptual distortions to a state of chronic delusions and hallucinations. Patients may present with positive symptoms (such as conceptual disorganization, delusions, or hallucinations) or negative symptoms (loss of function, anhedonia, decreased emotional expression, impaired concentration, and diminished social engagement) and must have at least two of these for a 1-month period and continuous signs for at least 6 months to meet formal diagnostic criteria. "Negative" symptoms predominate in one-third of the schizophrenic population and are associated with a poor long-term outcome and a poor response to drug treatment. However, marked variability in the course and individual character of symptoms is typical.

The four main subtypes of schizophrenia are catatonic, paranoid, disorganized, and residual. Many individuals have symptoms of more than one type. *Catatonic-type* describes patients whose clinical presentation is dominated by profound changes in motor activity, negativism, and echolalia or echopraxia. *Paranoid-type* describes patients who have a prominent preoccupation with a specific delusional system and who otherwise do not qualify as having *disorganized-type* disease, in which disorganized speech and behavior are accompanied by a superficial or silly affect. In *residual-type* disease, negative symptomatology exists in the absence of delusions, hallucinations, or motor disturbance. The term *schizophreniform disorder* describes patients who meet the symptom requirements but not the duration requirements for schizophrenia, and *schizoaffective disorder* is used for those who manifest symptoms of schizophrenia and independent periods of mood disturbance. Prognosis depends not on symptom severity but on the response to antipsychotic medication. A permanent remission without recurrence does occasionally occur. About 10% of schizophrenic patients commit suicide.

Schizophrenia is present in 0.85% of individuals worldwide, with a lifetime prevalence of ~1 to 1.5%. An estimated 300,000 episodes of acute schizophrenia occur annually in the United States, resulting in direct and indirect costs estimated at >$33 billion.

DIFFERENTIAL DIAGNOSIS The diagnosis is principally one of exclusion, requiring the absence of significant associated mood symptoms, any relevant medical condition, and substance abuse. Drug reactions that cause hallucinations, paranoia, confusion, or bizarre behavior may be dose-related or idiosyncratic; β-adrenergic blockers, clonidine, cycloserine, quinacrine, and procaine derivatives are the most common prescription medications associated with these symptoms. Drug causes should be ruled out in any case of newly emergent psychosis. The general neurologic examination in patients with schizophrenia is usually normal, but motor rigidity, tremor, and dyskinesias are noted in one-quarter of untreated patients.

EPIDEMIOLOGY AND PATHOPHYSIOLOGY Epidemiologic surveys identify several risk factors for schizophrenia including genetic susceptibility, early developmental insults, winter birth, and increasing parental age. Genetic factors are involved in at least a subset of individuals who develop schizophrenia. Schizophrenia is observed in ~6.6% of all first-degree relatives of an affected proband. If both parents are affected, the risk for offspring is 40%. The concordance rate for monozygotic twins is 50%, compared to 10% for dizygotic twins. Schizophrenia-prone families are also at risk for other psychiatric disorders,

including schizoaffective disorder and *schizotypal* and *schizoid personality disorders*, the latter terms designating individuals who show a lifetime pattern of social and interpersonal deficits characterized by an inability to form close interpersonal relationships, eccentric behavior, and mild perceptual distortions.

Despite evidence for a genetic causation, the results of molecular genetic linkage studies in schizophrenia are inconclusive. Major gene effects appear unlikely. Possible susceptibility genes include: neuroregulin-1 at chromosome 8p21; dysbindin at 6p22.3, proline dehydrogenase at 22q11, and G72 at 13q34. Several of these may be involved in glutamatergic regulation, increasing interest in N-methyl-D-aspartate (NMDA)-mediated glutamate signaling as a possible therapeutic target for treatment. One group has reported risk variants in the $\alpha 7$ nicotinic acetycholine receptor subunit gene and linked it to a specific auditory processing deficit.

Schizophrenia is also associated with gestational and perinatal complications, including Rh factor incompatibility, fetal hypoxia, prenatal exposure to influenza during the second trimester, and prenatal nutritional deficiency. Studies of monozygotic twins discordant for schizophrenia have reported neuroanatomic differences between affected and unaffected siblings, supporting a "two-strike" etiology involving both genetic susceptibility and an environmental insult. The latter might involve localized hypoxia during critical stages of brain development.

A number of structural and functional abnormalities have been identified in schizophrenia, including (1) cortical atrophy and ventricular enlargement; (2) specific volume losses in the amygdala, hippocampus, right prefrontal cortex, fusiform gyrus, and thalamus; (3) progressive reduction in cortical volume over time; (4) reduced metabolism in the thalamus and prefrontal cortex; (5) abnormalities of the planum temporale; and (6) changes in the size, orientation, and density of cells in the hippocampus and prefrontal cortex, and decreased numbers of cortical interneurons. These observations have suggested that schizophrenia may result from a disturbance in a cortical striatal–thalamic circuit resulting in abnormalities in sensory filtering and attention.

Schizophrenic individuals are highly distractible and demonstrate deficits in perceptual-motor speed, ability to shift attention, and filtering out of background stimuli. Event-related evoked potential studies of schizophrenia have defined a specific reduction in P300 amplitude to a novel stimulus, which implicates an impairment in cognitive processing. Impaired information processing is also found in unaffected family members.

The *dopamine hypothesis* of schizophrenia is based on the discovery that agents that diminish dopaminergic activity also reduce the acute symptoms and signs of psychosis, specifically agitation, anxiety, and hallucinations. Amelioration of delusions and social withdrawal is less dramatic. Thus far, however, evidence for increased dopaminergic activity in schizophrenia is indirect, although decreased D_2 receptor occupancy by dopamine has recently been shown in drug-naïve patients. An increase in the activity of nigrostriatal and mesolimbic systems and a decrease in mesocortical tracts innervating the prefrontal cortex is hypothesized, although it is likely that other neurotransmitters, including serotonin, acetylcholine, glutamate, and GABA, also contribute to the pathophysiology of the illness. Possible involvement of excitatory amino acids is based on the genetic data cited above and finding that NMDA receptor antagonists and channel blockers, such as phencyclidine (PCP) and ketamine, produce characteristic signs of schizophrenia in normal individuals; cycloserine, an NMDA receptor agonist, can decrease the negative symptoms of psychosis.

 TREATMENT

Antipsychotic agents (Table 371-14) are the cornerstone of acute and maintenance treatment of schizophrenia, and are effective in the treatment of hallucinations, delusions, and thought disorders, regardless of

TABLE 371-14 Antipsychotic Agents

Name	Usual PO Daily Dose, mg	Side Effects	Sedation	Comments
TYPICAL ANTIPSYCHOTICS				
Low-potency				
Chlorpromazine (Thorazine)	100–600	Anticholinergic effects; orthostasis; photosensitivity; cholestasis; QT prolongation	+ + +	EPSEs usually not prominent; can cause anticholinergic delirium in elderly patients
Thioridazine (Mellaril)	100–600			
Mid-potency				
Trifluoperazine (Stelazine)	2–15	Fewer anticholinergic side effects; fewer EPSEs than with higher potency agents	+ +	Well tolerated by most patients
Perphenazine (Trilafon)	4–32		+ +	
Loxapine (Loxitane)	20–250	Frequent EPSEs	+ +	
Molindone (Moban)	50–225	Frequent EPSEs	0	Little weight gain
High potency		No anticholinergic side effects; EPSEs often prominent		Often prescribed in doses that are too high; long-acting injectable forms of haloperidol and fluphenazine available
Haloperidol (Haldol)	0.5–10		0/+	
Fluphenazine (Prolixin)	1–10	Frequent EPSEs	0/+	
Thiothixene (Navane)	2–20	Frequent EPSEs	0/+	
NOVEL ANTIPSYCHOTICS				
Clozapine (Clozaril)	200–600	Agranulocytosis (1%); weight gain; seizures; drooling; hyperthermia	+ +	Requires weekly WBC
Risperidone (Risperdal)	2–6	Orthostasis	+	Requires slow titration; EPSEs observed with doses >6 mg qd
Olanzapine (Zyprexa)	10–20	Weight gain	+ +	Mild prolactin elevation
Quetiapine (Seroquel)	350–700	Sedation; weight gain; anxiety	+ + +	Bid dosing
Ziprasidone (Geodon)	40–60	Orthostatic hypotension	+/+ +	Mimimal weight gain; increases QT interval
Aripiprazole (Abilify)	10–30	Nausea, anxiety, insomnia	0/+	Mixed agonist/antagonist

Note: EPSEs, extrapyramidal side effects; WBC, white blood count.

etiology. The mechanism of action involves, at least in part, blockade of dopamine receptors in the limbic system and basal ganglia; the clinical potencies of traditional antipsychotic drugs parallel their affinities for the D_2 receptor, and even the newer "atypical" agents exert some degree of D_2 receptor blockade. All neuroleptics induce expression of the immediate-early gene c-*fos* in the nucleus accumbens, a dopaminergic site connecting prefrontal and limbic cortices. The clinical efficacy of newer atypical neuroleptics, however, may involve D_1, D_3, and D_4 receptor blockade, α_1- and α_2-noradrenergic activity, and/or altering the relationship between $5HT_2$ and D_2 receptor activity, as well as faster dissociation of D_2 binding.

Conventional neuroleptics differ in their potency and side-effect profile. Older agents, such as chlorpromazine and thioridazine, are more sedating and anticholinergic and more likely to cause orthostatic hypotension, while higher potency antipsychotics, such as haloperidol, perphenazine, and thiothixene, are more likely to induce extrapyramidal side effects. The model atypical antipsychotic agent is *clozapine*, a dibenzodiazepine that has a greater potency in blocking the $5HT_2$ than the D_2 receptor and a much higher affinity for the D_4 than the D_2 receptor. Its principal disadvantage is a risk of blood dyscrasias. Unlike other antipsychotics, clozapine does not cause a rise in prolactin level. Approximately 30% of patients have a better response to these agents than to traditional neuroleptics, suggesting that they will increasingly displace the older-generation drugs. Clozapine appears to be the most effective member of this class and has demonstrated superiority to other atypical agents in preventing suicide; however, its side-effect profile makes it most appropriate for treatment-resistant cases. *Risperidone*, a benzisoxazole derivative, is more potent at $5HT_2$ than D_2 receptor sites, like clozapine, but it also exerts significant α_2 antagonism, a property that may contribute to its perceived ability to improve mood and increase motor activity. Risperidone is not as effective as clozapine in treatment-resistant cases but does not carry a risk of blood dyscrasias. *Olanzapine* is similar neurochemically to clozapine but has a significant risk of inducing weight gain. *Quetiapine* is distinct in having a weak D_2 effect but potent α_1 and histamine blockade. Ziprasidone causes minimal weight gain and is unlikely to increase prolactin, but may increase QT prolongation. Aripiprazole also has little risk of weight gain or prolactin increase but may increase anxiety, nausea, and insomnia as a result of its partial agonist properties.

Conventional antipsychotic agents are effective in 70% of patients presenting with a first episode. Improvement may be observed within hours or days, but full remission usually requires 6 to 8 weeks. The choice of agent depends principally on the side-effect profile and cost of treatment or on a past personal or family history of a favorable response to the drug in question. Atypical agents appear to be more effective in treating negative symptoms and improving cognitive function. An equivalent treatment response can usually be achieved with relatively low doses of any drug selected, i.e., 4 to 6 mg/d of haloperidol, 10 to 15 mg of olanzapine, or 4 to 6 mg/d of risperidone. Doses in this range result in >80% D_2 receptor blockade, and there is little evidence that higher doses increase either the rapidity or degree of response. Maintenance treatment requires careful attention to the possibility of relapse and monitoring for the development of a movement disorder. Intermittent drug treatment is less effective than regular dosing, but gradual dose reduction is likely to improve social functioning in many schizophrenic patients who have been maintained at high doses. If medications are completely discontinued, however, the relapse rate is 60% within 6 months. Long-acting injectable preparations are considered when noncompliance with oral therapy leads to relapses. In treatment-resistant patients, a transition to clozapine usually results in rapid improvement, but a prolonged delay in response in some cases necessitates a 6- to 9-month trial for maximal benefit to occur.

Antipsychotic medications can cause a broad range of side effects, including lethargy, weight gain, postural hypotension, constipation, and dry mouth. Extrapyramidal symptoms such as dystonia, akathisia, and akinesia are also frequent with traditional agents and may contribute to poor compliance if not specifically addressed. Anticholinergic and parkinsonian symptoms respond well to trihexyphenidyl, 2 mg bid, or benztropine mesylate, 1 to 2 mg bid. Akathisia may respond to beta blockers. In rare cases, more serious and occasionally life-threatening side effects may emerge, including ventricular arrhythmias, gastrointestinal obstruction, retinal pigmentation, obstructive jaundice, and neuroleptic malignant syndrome (characterized by hyperthermia, autonomic dysfunction, muscular rigidity, and elevated creatine phosphokinase levels). The most serious adverse effects of clozapine are agranulocytosis, which has an incidence of 1%, and induction of seizures, which has an incidence of 10%. Weekly white blood cell counts are required, particularly during the first 3 months of treatment.

The risk of type 2 diabetes mellitus appears to be increased in schizophrenia, and atypical agents as a group produce greater adverse effects on glucose regulation, independent of effects on obesity, than traditional agents. Clozapine, olanzapine, and quetiapine seem more likely to cause hyperglycemia, weight gain, and hypertriglyceridemia than other atypical antipsychotic drugs. Close monitoring of plasma glucose and lipid levels are indicated with the use of these agents.

A serious side effect of long-term use of the classic antipsychotic agents is *tardive dyskinesia*, characterized by repetitive, involuntary, and potentially irreversible movements of the tongue and lips (bucco-linguo-masticatory triad), and, in approximately half of cases, choreoathetosis (Chap. 21). Tardive dyskinesia has an incidence of 2 to 4% per year of exposure, and a prevalence of 20% in chronically treated patients. The prevalence increases with age, total dose, and duration of drug administration. The risk associated with the newer atypical agents appears to be much lower. The cause may involve formation of free radicals and perhaps mitochondrial energy failure. Vitamin E may reduce abnormal involuntary movements if given early in the syndrome.

Drug treatment of schizophrenia is by itself insufficient. Educational efforts directed toward families and relevant community resources have proved to be necessary to maintain stability and optimize outcome. A treatment model involving a multidisciplinary case-management team that seeks out and closely follows the patient in the community has proved particularly effective.

ASSESSMENT AND EVALUATION OF VIOLENCE

Primary care physicians may encounter situations in which family, domestic, or societal violence is discovered or suspected. Such an awareness can carry legal and moral obligations; many state laws mandate reporting of child, spousal, and elder abuse. Physicians are frequently the first point of contact for both victim and abuser. Between 1 and 2 million older Americans and 1.5 million U.S. children are thought to experience some form of physical maltreatment each year. Spousal abuse is thought to be even more prevalent. One survey of internal medicine practices found that 5.5% of all female patients had experienced domestic violence in the previous year, and that these individuals were more likely to suffer from depression, anxiety, somatization disorder, and substance abuse and to have attempted suicide. When domestic violence is suspected, direct but nonjudgmental questioning should be pursued with each party separately—"Do you feel safe at home?" and "If there's a disagreement or a conflict between the two of you, how is it worked out?" Individuals who are abused may have signs of obvious or suspected physical injury; in addition, abused individuals frequently express low self-esteem, vague somatic symptomatology, social isolation, and a passive feeling of loss of control. Although it is essential to treat these elements in the victim, the first obligation is to ensure that the perpetrator has taken responsibility for preventing any further violence. Substance abuse and/or dependence and serious mental illness in the abuser may contribute to the risk of harm and require direct intervention. Depending on the situation, law enforcement agencies, community resources such as support groups and shelters, and individual and family counseling can be appropriate components of a treatment plan. A safety plan should be formulated with the victim, in addition to providing information about

abuse, its likelihood of recurrence, and its tendency to increase in severity and frequency. Antianxiety and antidepressant medications may sometimes be useful in treating the acute symptoms, but only if independent evidence for an appropriate psychiatric diagnosis exists. Antidepressants are generally not indicated when the diagnosis is linked to the social situation, such as an adjustment disorder with depressed mood. The most important element in treatment is the development of a supportive doctor-patient relationship that avoids further blame of the victim. In certain circumstances, a significant potential for societal violence may be discovered. Sympathetic, but direct, questioning about potential violent impulses, access to weapons, recreational drug use, and specific homicidal ideation is necessary and is sometimes therapeutic in its own right. The existence and possible contribution of such medical conditions as delirium and/or intoxication should be evaluated. Available disposition options for potentially violent patients include police custody, psychiatric hospitalization, and referral to home care, with involvement of family, friends, and caregivers. In deciding which treatment option is most appropriate, clinicians should endeavor to establish an empathic interaction with the patient, while avoiding interventions or stimuli that might precipitate or increase the risk of violent behavior.

MENTAL HEALTH PROBLEMS IN THE HOMELESS

There is a high prevalence of mental disorders and substance abuse among homeless and impoverished people. The total number of homeless individuals in the United States is estimated at 2 to 3 million, one-third of whom qualify as having a serious mental disorder. Poor hygiene and nutrition, substance abuse, psychiatric illness, physical trauma, and exposure to the elements combine to make the provision of medical care challenging. Only a minority of these individuals receive formal mental health care; the main points of contact are outpatient medical clinics and emergency departments. Primary care settings represent a critical site in which housing needs, treatment of substance dependence, and evaluation and treatment of psychiatric illness can most efficiently take place. Successful intervention is dependent on breaking down traditional administrative barriers to health care and recognizing the physical constraints and emotional costs imposed by homelessness. Simplifying health care instructions and follow-up, allowing frequent visits, and dispensing medications in limited amounts that require ongoing contact are possible techniques for establishing a successful therapeutic relationship.

FURTHER READING

ABLON JS, JONES EEJ: Validity of controlled clinical trials of psychotherapy: Findings from the NIMH treatment of depression collaborative research program. Am J Psychiatry 159:775, 2002

COYLE JT, DUMAN RS: Finding the intracellular signaling pathways affected by mood disorder treatments. Neuron 38:157, 2003

FISCHHOFF B, WESSELY S: Managing patients with inexplicable health problems. BMJ 326:595, 2003

KESSLER RC et al: The epidemiology of major depressive disorder: Results from the National Comorbidity Survey Replication (NCSR). JAMA 289: 3095, 2003

WATHEN CN, MACMILLAN HL: Interventions for violence against women: Scientific review. JAMA 289:589, 2003

372 | ALCOHOL AND ALCOHOLISM
Marc A. Schuckit

Alcohol, a drug, is consumed at some time by up to 80% of the population. At low doses alcohol can have some beneficial effects such as decreased rates of myocardial infarction, stroke, gallstones, and possibly vascular or Alzheimer's dementias, but the consumption of more than two standard drinks per day increases the risk for health problems in many organ systems. Heavy repetitive drinking, as is seen in alcohol abuse and dependence, cuts short the life span by an estimated decade in both genders, all cultural groups, and all socioeconomic strata. Even low doses of alcohol have a significant effect on many organ systems, adversely affecting most preexisting disease states and altering the effectiveness or blood levels of most over-the-counter and prescribed medications.

PHARMACOLOGY AND NUTRITIONAL IMPACT OF ETHANOL Ethanol is a weakly charged molecule that moves easily through cell membranes, rapidly equilibrating between blood and tissues. The level of alcohol in the blood is expressed as milligrams or grams of ethanol per deciliter (e.g., 100 mg/dL or 0.10 g/dL); a level of 0.02 to 0.03 results from the ingestion of one to two typical drinks. In round figures, 340 mL (12 oz) of beer, 115 mL (4 oz) of nonfortified wine, and 43 mL (1.5 oz) (a shot) of 80-proof beverage each contain ~10 to 15 g of ethanol; 0.5 L (1 pint) of 86-proof beverage contains ~160 g (about 16 standard drinks), and 1 L of wine contains ~80 g of ethanol. Congeners found in alcoholic beverages, including low-molecular-weight alcohols (e.g., methanol and butanol), aldehydes, esters, histamine, phenols, tannins, iron, lead, and cobalt, may contribute to the adverse health consequences associated with heavy drinking.

Ethanol is a central nervous system (CNS) depressant that decreases neuronal activity, although some behavioral stimulation is observed at low blood levels. This drug has cross-tolerance with other depressants, including benzodiazepines and barbiturates, and all produce similar behavioral alterations. Alcohol is absorbed from mucous membranes of the mouth and esophagus (in small amounts), from the stomach and large bowel (in modest amounts), and from the proximal portion of the small intestine (the major site). The rate of absorption is increased by rapid gastric emptying; by the absence of proteins, fats, or carbohydrates (which interfere with absorption); by the absence of congeners; by dilution to a modest percentage of ethanol (maximum at about 20% by volume); and by carbonation (e.g., champagne).

Between 2% (at low blood alcohol concentrations) and 10% (at high blood alcohol concentrations) of ethanol is excreted directly through the lungs, urine, or sweat, but the greater part is metabolized to acetaldehyde, primarily in the liver. The most important pathway occurs in the cell cytosol where alcohol dehydrogenase (ADH) produces acetaldehyde, which is then rapidly destroyed by aldehyde dehydrogenase (ALDH) in the cytosol and mitochondria (Fig. 372-1). A second pathway in the microsomes of the smooth endoplasmic reticulum (the microsomal ethanol-oxidizing system, or MEOS), is responsible for ≥10% of ethanol oxidation at high blood alcohol concentrations.

While alcohol supplies calories (a drink contains ~300 kJ, or 70 to 100 kcal), these are devoid of nutrients such as minerals, proteins, and vitamins. Alcohol can also interfere with absorption of vitamins in the small intestine and decreases their storage in the liver with effects on folate (folacin or folic acid), pyridoxine (B_6), thiamine (B_1), nicotinic acid (niacin, B_3), and vitamin A.

An ethanol load in a fasting, healthy individual is likely to produce transient hypoglycemia within 6 to 36 h, secondary to the acute actions of ethanol on gluconeogenesis. This can result in glucose intolerance

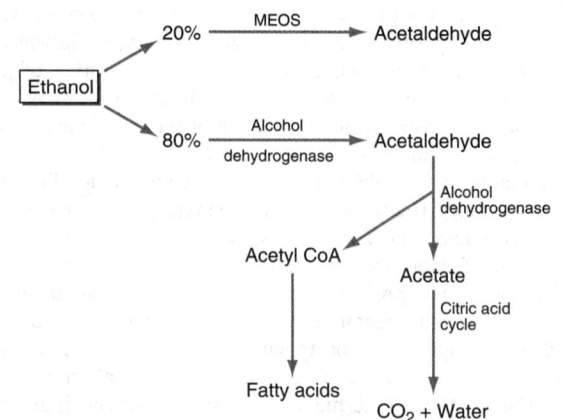

FIGURE 372-1 The metabolism of alcohol.

until the alcoholic has abstained for 2 to 4 weeks. Alcohol ketoacidosis, probably reflecting a decrease in fatty acid oxidation coupled with poor diet or recurrent vomiting, should not be misdiagnosed as diabetic ketosis. With the former, patients show an increase in serum ketones along with a mild increase in glucose but a large anion gap, a mild to moderate increase in serum lactate, and a β-hydroxybutyrate/lactate ratio of between 2:1 and 9:1 (with normal being 1:1).

BEHAVIORAL EFFECTS, TOLERANCE, AND DEPENDENCE The effects of any drug depend on the dose, the rate of increase in plasma, the concomitant presence of other drugs, and the past experience with the agent. With alcohol, an additional factor is whether blood alcohol levels are rising or falling; the effects are more intense during the former period.

Even though "legal intoxication" requires a blood alcohol concentration of at least 80 to 100 mg/dL, behavioral, psychomotor, and cognitive changes are seen at levels as low as 20 to 30 mg/dL (i.e., after one to two drinks) (Table 372-1). Deep but disturbed sleep can be seen at twice the legal intoxication level, and death can occur with levels between 300 and 400 mg/dL. Beverage alcohol is probably responsible for more overdose deaths than any other drug.

The intoxicating effects of alcohol appear to be due to actions at a number of neurotransmitter receptors and transporters. Alcohol enhances γ-aminobutyric acid A ($GABA_A$) receptors and inhibits *N*-methyl-D-aspartate (NMDA) receptors. In vitro studies suggest that additional effects involve inhibition of adenosine uptake and a translocation of the cyclic AMP–dependent protein kinase catalytic subunit from the cytoplasm to the nucleus. Neurons adapt quickly to these actions, and thus different effects may be present during chronic administration and withdrawal.

At least three types of compensatory changes develop after repeated exposure to the drug, producing tolerance of higher ethanol levels. First, after 1 to 2 weeks of daily drinking, *metabolic or pharmacokinetic tolerance* can be seen, with a 30% increase in the rate of hepatic

TABLE 372-1 *Effects of Blood Alcohol Levels in the Absence of Tolerance*

Blood Level, mg/dL	Usual Effect
20	Decreased inhibitions, a slight feeling of intoxication
80	Decrease in complex cognitive functions and motor performance
200	Obvious slurred speech, motor incoordination, irritability, and poor judgment
300	Light coma and depressed vital signs
400	Death

ethanol metabolism. This alteration disappears almost as rapidly as it develops. Second, *cellular or pharmacodynamic tolerance* develops through neurochemical changes that may also contribute to physical dependence. Third, individuals can learn to adapt their behavior so that they can function better than expected under drug influence (*behavioral tolerance*).

The cellular changes caused by chronic ethanol exposure may not resolve for several weeks or longer following cessation of drinking. In the interim, the neurons require ethanol to function optimally, and the individual can be said to be physically dependent. This is distinct from psychological dependence, a concept indicating that the person is psychologically uncomfortable without the drug.

THE EFFECTS OF ETHANOL ON ORGAN SYSTEMS

Although one to two drinks per day in an otherwise healthy and non-pregnant individual can have some beneficial effects, at higher doses alcohol is toxic to most organ systems. Knowledge about the deleterious effects of alcohol helps the physician to identify alcoholic patients and provides information that can be used to help motivate them to abstain. The information offered here generally applies across ages and genders, with common sense differences (e.g., older persons carry higher health risks). It is important to remember that the typical white- or blue-collar alcoholic functions at a fairly high level for years, and that not everyone develops each problem.

CENTRAL NERVOUS SYSTEM Approximately 35% of drinkers may experience a *blackout*, an episode of temporary anterograde amnesia, in which the person forgets all or part of what occurred during a drinking evening. Another common problem, one seen after as few as several drinks, is that alcohol causes alterations between sleep stages and a deficiency in rapid eye movement and deep sleep with resulting prominent and sometimes disturbing dreams later in the night. Finally, alcohol relaxes muscles in the pharynx, which can cause snoring and exacerbate sleep apnea, with symptoms of the latter in 75% of alcoholic men over age 60. As a consequence of alcohol-related impairment in judgment and coordination, at least half of patients with physical trauma have evidence of substance-related impairment, a finding reflecting the fact that 40% of drinkers in the United States have at some time driven while intoxicated.

The effect of alcohol on the nervous system is even more pronounced among alcohol-dependent individuals. Chronic high doses cause *peripheral neuropathy* in 5 to 15% of alcoholics: patients experience bilateral limb numbness, tingling, and paresthesias, all of which are more pronounced distally. *Wernicke's syndrome* (ophthalmoparesis, ataxia, and encephalopathy) and *Korsakoff's syndrome* are seen in <10% of alcoholics as the result of thiamine deficiency, especially in persons with transketolase deficiency (Chap. 258). Approximately 1% of alcoholics develop *cerebellar degeneration*, a syndrome of progressive unsteady stance and gait often accompanied by mild nystagmus; neuroimaging studies reveal atrophy of the cerebellar vermis.

Alcoholics can manifest severe *cognitive problems* including impairment in recent and remote memory for weeks to months after an alcoholic binge. Increased size of the brain ventricles and cerebral sulci are seen in ≥50% of chronic alcoholics, but these changes are often reversible, returning toward normal within a year or so of abstinence. There is no single alcoholic dementia syndrome; rather, this label is used to describe patients who have apparently irreversible cognitive changes (possibly from diverse causes) and chronic alcoholism.

Finally, almost every psychiatric syndrome can be seen temporarily during heavy drinking or subsequent withdrawal. These include intense *sadness* lasting for days to weeks in the midst of heavy drinking in 40% of alcoholics, which is classified as an alcohol-induced mood disorder; temporary severe *anxiety* in 10 to 30% of alcoholics, often beginning during alcohol withdrawal, which can persist for many months after cessation of drinking (alcohol-induced anxiety disorder); and auditory *hallucinations* and/or paranoid delusions in a clear sensorium (*alcohol-induced psychotic disorder*) seen temporarily in 1 to

10% of alcoholics. Treatment of all forms of alcohol-induced psychopathology includes abstinence and supportive care, with the likelihood of full recovery within several days to 4 weeks. A history of alcohol intake is an important consideration in any patient with one of these psychiatric symptoms.

THE GASTROINTESTINAL SYSTEM ▪ Esophagus and Stomach Acute alcohol intake can result in inflammation of the esophagus and stomach, causing epigastric distress and gastrointestinal bleeding. Chronic heavy drinking, if associated with violent vomiting, can produce a Mallory-Weiss lesion, a longitudinal tear in the mucosa at the gastroesophageal junction.

Pancreas and Liver The incidence of acute pancreatitis (~25 per 1000 per year) is almost threefold higher than in the general population, accounting for an estimated 10% or more of the cases of this disorder (Chap. 294). Alcohol impairs gluconeogenesis in the liver with a resulting fall in the amount of glucose produced from glycogen; lactate production increases; and there is a decreased oxidation of fatty acids with an increase in fat accumulation in liver cells. In the healthy individual these changes are reversible, but with repeated exposure to ethanol, more severe changes can occur, including fatty accumulation, alcohol-induced hepatitis, perivenular sclerosis, and cirrhosis, with the latter observed in an estimated 15 to 20% of alcoholics (Chap. 288).

CANCER Drinking as few as 1.5 drinks per day increases a woman's risk of breast cancer 1.4-fold. For both genders, four drinks per day increases the risk for oral and esophageal cancers approximately threefold and rectal cancers by a factor of 1.5; seven to eight or more drinks per day enhances the risks for many cancers by a factor of five.

HEMATOPOIETIC SYSTEM Ethanol causes an increase in red blood cell size [mean corpuscular volume, (MCV)], which reflects the effects on stem cells. If heavy drinking is accompanied by folic acid deficiency, there can also be hypersegmented neutrophils, reticulocytopenia, and a hyperplastic bone marrow; if malnutrition is present, sideroblastic changes can be observed. Chronic heavy drinking can decrease production of most white blood cells, decrease granulocyte mobility and adherence, and impair the delayed-hypersensitivity response to new antigens (with a possible false-negative tuberculin skin test). Finally, many alcoholics have mild thrombocytopenia, which usually resolves within a week of abstinence unless there is hepatic cirrhosis or congestive splenomegaly.

CARDIOVASCULAR SYSTEM Acutely, ethanol decreases myocardial contractility and causes peripheral vasodilation, with a resulting mild decrease in blood pressure and a compensatory increase in cardiac output. Exercise-induced increases in cardiac oxygen consumption are higher after alcohol intake. These acute effects have little clinical significance for the average healthy drinker but can be problematic in men and women with cardiac disease.

The consumption of three or more drinks per day results in a dose-dependent increase in blood pressure, which returns to normal within weeks of abstinence. Heavy drinking is an important contributor to mild to moderate hypertension. Chronic heavy drinking can cause cardiomyopathy, with symptoms ranging from unexplained arrhythmias in the presence of left ventricular impairment to heart failure with dilation of all four heart chambers and hypocontractility of heart muscle. Perhaps one-third of cases of cardiomyopathy are alcohol-induced. Mural thrombi can form in the left atrium or ventricle, while heart enlargement >25% can cause mitral regurgitation. Atrial or ventricular arrhythmias, especially paroxysmal tachycardia, can also occur after a drinking binge in individuals showing no other evidence of heart disease—a syndrome known as the "holiday heart."

Chronic intake of modest doses of alcohol can have some beneficial effects. A maximum of one to two drinks per day may decrease the risk for cardiovascular death, perhaps through an increase in high-density lipoprotein (HDL) cholesterol or changes in clotting mechanisms. In one large national study, cardiovascular mortality was reduced by 30 to 40% among individuals reporting one or more drinks daily compared to nondrinkers, with overall mortality lowest among those consuming approximately one drink per day. Recent data have also corroborated the decreased risk for ischemic, but not hemorrhagic, stroke associated with regular light drinking.

GENITOURINARY SYSTEM CHANGES, SEXUAL FUNCTIONING, AND FETAL DEVELOP-MENT Acutely, modest ethanol doses (e.g., blood alcohol concentrations of $\leq$100 mg/dL) can both increase sexual drive and decrease erectile capacity in men. Even in the absence of liver impairment, a significant minority of chronic alcoholic men may show irreversible testicular atrophy with concomitant shrinkage of the seminiferous tubules, decreases in ejaculate volume, and a lower sperm count (Chap. 325).

The repeated ingestion of high doses of ethanol by women can result in amenorrhea, a decrease in ovarian size, absence of corpora lutea with associated infertility, and spontaneous abortions. Heavy drinking during pregnancy results in the rapid placental transfer of both ethanol and acetaldehyde, which may have serious consequences for fetal development. The *fetal alcohol syndrome* can include any of the following: facial changes with epicanthal eye folds, poorly formed concha, and small teeth with faulty enamel; cardiac atrial or ventricular septal defects; an aberrant palmar crease and limitation in joint movement; and microcephaly with mental retardation. The amount of ethanol and/or time of vulnerability during pregnancy have not been defined, making it advisable for pregnant women to abstain completely.

OTHER EFFECTS OF ETHANOL Between one-half and two-thirds of alcoholics have skeletal muscle weakness caused by acute *alcoholic myopathy*, a condition that improves but which might not disappear with abstinence. Effects of repeated heavy drinking on the *skeletal system* include alterations in calcium metabolism, lower bone density, and less growth in the epiphyses, with an increased risk for fractures and osteonecrosis of the femoral head. *Hormonal changes* include an increase in cortisol levels, which can remain elevated during heavy drinking; inhibition of vasopressin secretion at rising blood alcohol concentrations and the opposite effect at falling blood alcohol concentrations (with the final result that most alcoholics are likely to be slightly overhydrated); a modest and reversible decrease in serum thyroxine (T_4); and a more marked decrease in serum triiodothyronine (T_3).

ALCOHOLISM (ALCOHOL ABUSE OR DEPENDENCE)

Because many drinkers occasionally imbibe to excess, temporary alcohol-related pathology is common in nonalcoholics, especially those in the late teens to the late twenties. When repeated problems in multiple life areas develop, the person is likely to meet criteria for alcohol abuse or dependence.

DEFINITIONS AND EPIDEMIOLOGY *Alcohol dependence* is defined in the Fourth Diagnostic and Statistical Manual (DSM-IV) of the American Psychiatric Association as repeated alcohol-related difficulties in at least three of seven areas of functioning that cluster together over any 12-month period. A special emphasis is placed on tolerance and/or withdrawal, a condition referred to as "dependence with a physiological component," which is associated with a more severe clinical course. Dependence occurs in both men and women and in individuals from all socioeconomic strata and of all racial backgrounds. The diagnosis predicts a course of recurrent problems with the use of alcohol and the consequent shortening of the life span by a decade or more. In the absence of alcohol dependence, an individual can be given a diagnosis of *alcohol abuse* if he or she demonstrates repetitive problems with alcohol in any one of four life areas that include social, interpersonal, legal, and occupational problems, or repeated use in hazardous situations such as driving.

The lifetime risk for alcohol dependence in most western countries is about 10 to 15% for men and 5 to 8% for women. When alcohol

abuse is also considered, the rates are even higher. The typical alcoholic is a blue- or white-collar worker or homemaker and not the stereotypical homeless individual.

GENETICS OF ALCOHOLISM *Alcoholism* is a complex genetically influenced disorder; genes explain about 60% of the risk. The importance of genetic influences is supported by a higher risk in the identical versus fraternal twin of an alcoholic and a fourfold increased risk in children of alcoholics even if adopted at birth and raised without knowledge of their biologic parents.

A variety of independent genetically influenced characteristics likely combine to explain the contribution of hereditary factors. For alcoholism and other substance dependencies, some families appear to carry an enhanced risk through high levels of impulsivity, as can be seen in the antisocial personality disorder. In other families the risk is associated with vulnerability for several independent psychiatric disorders such as schizophrenia and manic-depressive disease. A diminished alcoholism risk is seen in approximately half of Asian men and women; this is due to an inactive form of the enzyme ALDH, which results in higher levels of acetaldehyde following alcohol ingestion. A significant proportion of the vulnerability for alcoholism appears to relate to genes that affect the intensity of the response to alcohol. Most studies have shown that 40% of some subgroups at high risk for future alcoholism (e.g., offspring of alcoholics) require higher blood alcohol concentrations to produce the effects seen at lower blood levels in most other people. This relatively low response to alcohol predicts the risk for alcohol-related problems over the next decade, including alcohol use disorders.

NATURAL HISTORY For the "average" alcoholic, the age of first drink and first problems (e.g., an alcoholic blackout) are similar to those in the general population. However, by the early to mid-twenties, most men and women moderate their drinking (perhaps learning from minor problems), whereas difficulties for alcoholics are likely to escalate, with the first major life problem from alcohol appearing in the mid-twenties. Once established, the course of alcoholism is likely to be one of exacerbations and remissions. As a rule, there is little difficulty in stopping alcohol use when problems develop, and this step is often followed by days to months of carefully controlled drinking. Unless abstinence is maintained, these periods almost inevitably give way to escalations in alcohol intake and subsequent problems. The course is not hopeless, because between half and two-thirds of alcoholics maintain abstinence for years, and often permanently after treatment. Even without formal treatment or self-help groups there is at least a 20% chance of long-term abstinence. However, should the alcoholic continue to drink, the life span is shortened by an average of 10 years, with the leading causes of death, in decreasing order, the result of heart disease, cancer, accidents, and suicide.

IDENTIFICATION OF THE ALCOHOLIC AND INTERVENTION Physicians even in affluent areas should recognize that ~20% of patients have alcoholism. Therefore, it is important to pay attention to the alcohol-related symptoms and signs as well as laboratory tests that are likely to be abnormal in the context of regular consumption of 6 to 8 or more drinks per day. The two blood tests with between 70% and 80% sensitivity and specificity are γ-glutamyl transferase (GGT) (>30 U) and carbohydrate-deficient transferrin (CDT) (>20 U/L); the combination of the two is likely to be more accurate than either alone. Physicians should consider these tests when screening patients for high levels of alcohol intake. These serologic markers of heavy drinking can also be useful in monitoring abstinence as they are likely to return toward normal within several weeks of the cessation of drinking; thus, increases in values of as little as 10% are likely to indicate a resumption of heavy alcohol intake. Other blood tests that can be useful in identifying individuals consuming six or more standard drinks per day include high normal MCVs (>91 μm^3) and serum uric acid (>416 mol/L, or 7 mg/dL). Physical signs and symptoms that can be useful in identifying alcoholism include mild and fluctuating hypertension (e.g., 140/95), repeated infections such as pneumonia, and otherwise unexplained cardiac arrhythmias. Other disorders suggestive of dependence include cancer of the head and neck, esophagus, or stomach as well as cirrhosis, unexplained hepatitis, pancreatitis, bilateral parotid gland swelling, and peripheral neuropathy.

The clinical diagnosis of alcohol abuse or dependence ultimately rests on the documentation of a pattern of difficulties associated with alcohol use; the definition is not based on the quantity and frequency of alcohol consumption. Thus, in screening it is important to probe for life problems and then attempt to tie in use of alcohol or another substance. Information regarding marital or job problems, legal difficulties, histories of accidents, medical problems, evidence of tolerance, etc., is important. While all physicians should be able to take the time needed to gather such information, some standardized questionnaires can be helpful, including the 10-item Alcohol Use Disorder Screening Test (AUDIT). However, these are only screening tools, and a careful face-to-face interview is still required for a meaningful diagnosis. Shorter questionnaires have limited usefulness.

After alcoholism is identified, the diagnosis must be shared with the patient as part of an intervention. The presenting complaint can be used as an entrée to the alcohol problem. For instance, the patient complaining of insomnia or hypertension could be told that these are clinically important symptoms and that physical findings and laboratory tests indicate that alcohol appears to have contributed to the complaints and is increasing the risk for further medical and psychological problems. The physician should share information about the course of alcoholism and explore possible avenues of addressing the problem. This process has been codified under the names of *brief interventions* and *motivational interviewing*. The former has been shown to be effective in decreasing alcohol use and problems when instituted as two 15-min sessions 1 month apart, along with a telephone follow-up reminder. Motivational interviewing uses the clinician's level of concern and understanding of the need for patients to progress through their own stages of enhanced understanding of their problems to optimize their ability to alter their drinking behaviors.

The process of intervention is rarely accomplished in one session. For the person who refuses to stop drinking at the first intervention, a logical step is to "keep the door open," establishing future meetings so that help is available as problems escalate. In the meantime the family may benefit from counseling or referral to self-help groups such as Al-Anon (the Alcoholics Anonymous group for family members) and Alateen (for teenage children of alcoholics).

THE ALCOHOL WITHDRAWAL SYNDROME Once the brain has been repeatedly exposed to high doses of alcohol, any sudden decrease in intake can produce withdrawal symptoms, many of which are the opposite of those produced by intoxication. Features include tremor of the hands (shakes or jitters); agitation and anxiety; autonomic nervous system overactivity including an increase in pulse, respiratory rate, and body temperature; insomnia, possibly accompanied by bad dreams; and gastrointestinal upset. These withdrawal symptoms generally begin within 5 to 10 h of decreasing ethanol intake, peak in intensity on day 2 or 3, and improve by day 4 or 5. Anxiety, insomnia, and mild levels of autonomic dysfunction may persist to some degree for ≥6 months as a protracted abstinence syndrome, which may contribute to the tendency to return to drinking.

At some point in their lives, between 2 and 5% of alcoholics experience withdrawal seizures, often within 48 h of stopping drinking. These rare events usually involve a single generalized seizure, and electroencephalographic abnormalities generally return to normal within several days.

The term *delirium tremens* (DTs) refers to delirium (mental confusion, agitation, and fluctuating levels of consciousness) associated with a tremor and autonomic overactivity (e.g., marked increases in pulse, blood pressure, and respirations). Fortunately, this serious and potentially life-threatening complication of alcohol withdrawal is seen in <5% of alcohol-dependent individuals, with the result that the chance of DTs during any single withdrawal is <1%. DTs are most likely to develop in patients with concomitant severe medical disorders and can usually be avoided by identifying and treating medical conditions.

TREATMENT

Acute Intoxication The first priority is to be certain that the vital signs are relatively stable without evidence of respiratory depression, cardiac arrhythmia, or potentially dangerous changes in blood pressure. The possibility of intoxication with other drugs should be considered, and a blood or urine sample is indicated to screen for opioids or other CNS depressants such as benzodiazepines or barbiturates. Other medical conditions that must be evaluated include hypoglycemia, hepatic failure, or diabetic ketoacidosis.

Patients who are medically stable should be placed in a quiet environment and asked to lie on their side if fatigued in order to minimize the risk of aspiration. When the behavior indicates an increased likelihood of violence, hospital procedures should be followed, including planning for the possibility of a show of force with an intervention team. In the context of aggressiveness, patients should be clearly reminded in a nonthreatening way that it is the goal of the staff to help them to feel better and to avoid problems. If the aggressive behavior continues, relatively low doses of a short-acting benzodiazepine such as lorazepam (e.g., 1 mg orally) may be used and can be repeated as needed, but care must be taken so that the addition of this second CNS depressant does not destabilize vital signs or worsen confusion. An alternative approach is to use an antipsychotic medication (e.g., 5 mg of haloperidol), but this has the potential danger of lowering the seizure threshold. If aggression escalates, the patient might require a short-term admission to a locked ward, where medications can be used more safely and vital signs more closely monitored.

Withdrawal The first step is to perform a thorough physical examination in all alcoholics who are considering stopping drinking, including a search for evidence of liver failure, gastrointestinal bleeding, cardiac arrhythmia, and glucose or electrolyte imbalance.

The second step in treating withdrawal for even the typical well-nourished alcoholic is to offer adequate nutrition and rest. All patients should be given oral multiple B vitamins, including 50 to 100 mg of thiamine daily for a week or more. Most patients enter withdrawal with normal levels of body water or mild overhydration, and intravenous fluids should be avoided unless there is evidence of significant recent bleeding, vomiting, or diarrhea. Medications can usually be administered orally.

The third step in treatment is to recognize that most withdrawal symptoms are caused by the rapid removal of a CNS depressant. Patients can be weaned by administering any drug of this class and gradually decreasing the levels over 3 to 5 days. While many CNS depressants are effective, benzodiazepines have the highest margin of safety and lowest cost and are, therefore, the preferred class of drugs. Benzodiazepines with short half-lives (Chap. 371) are especially useful for patients with serious liver impairment or evidence of preexisting encephalopathy or brain damage, but result in rapidly changing drug blood levels and must be given every 4 h to avoid abrupt fluctuations in blood levels that may increase the risk for seizures. Therefore, most clinicians use drugs with longer half-lives, such as diazepam or chlordiazepoxide, administering enough drug on day 1 to alleviate most of the symptoms of withdrawal (e.g., the tremor and elevated pulse) and then decreasing the dose by 20% on successive days over a period of 3 to 5 days. The approach is flexible; the dose is increased if signs of withdrawal escalate, and the medication is withheld if the patient is sleeping or shows signs of increasing orthostatic hypotension. The average patient requires 25 to 50 mg of chlordiazepoxide or 10 mg of diazepam given orally every 4 to 6 h on the first day.

Treatment of the patient with DTs can be difficult, and the condition is likely to run a course of 3 to 5 days regardless of the therapy employed. The focus of care is to identify medical problems and correct them and to control behavior and prevent injuries. Many clinicians recommend the use of high doses of a benzodiazepine (as much as 800 mg/d of chlordiazepoxide have been reported), a treatment that will decrease the agitation and raise the seizure threshold but probably does little to improve the confusion. Other clinicians recommend the use of antipsychotic medications, such as haloperidol, 20 mg or more per day, an approach less likely to exacerbate confusion but which may increase the risk of seizures. Antipsychotic drugs have no place in the treatment of mild withdrawal symptoms.

Generalized withdrawal seizures rarely require aggressive pharmacologic intervention beyond that given to the usual patient undergoing withdrawal, i.e., adequate doses of benzodiazepines. There is little evidence that anticonvulsants such as phenytoin are effective in drug-withdrawal seizures, and the risk of seizures has usually passed by the time effective drug levels are reached. The rare patient with status epilepticus must be treated aggressively (Chap. 348).

While alcohol withdrawal is often treated in a hospital, efforts at reducing costs have resulted in the development of outpatient detoxification for relatively mild abstinence syndromes. This is appropriate for patients in good physical condition who demonstrate mild signs of withdrawal despite low blood alcohol concentrations and for those without prior history of DTs or withdrawal seizures. Such individuals still require a careful physical examination, evaluation of blood tests, and vitamin supplementation. Benzodiazepines can be given in a 1- to 2-day supply to be administered to the patient by a spouse or other family member four times a day. Patients are asked to return daily for evaluation of vital signs and to come to the emergency room if signs and symptoms of withdrawal escalate.

Rehabilitation of Alcoholics   After completing alcoholic rehabilitation, 60% or more of alcoholics maintain abstinence for at least a year, and many achieve lifetime abstinence. Considering the lack of evidence for the superiority of any specific treatment type, it is best to keep interventions simple.

Maneuvers in rehabilitation fall into several general categories, which are applied to all patients regardless of age or ethnic group. However, the manner in which the treatments are used should be sensitive to the practices and needs of specific populations. First are attempts to help the alcoholic achieve and maintain a high level of motivation toward abstinence. These include education about alcoholism and instructing family and/or friends to stop protecting the person from the problems caused by alcohol. The second step is to help the patient to readjust to life without alcohol and to reestablish a functional lifestyle through counseling, vocational rehabilitation, and self-help groups such as Alcoholics Anonymous. The third component, called *relapse prevention*, helps the person to identify situations in which a return to drinking is likely, formulate ways of managing these risks, and develop coping strategies that increase the chances of a return to abstinence if a slip occurs.

There is no convincing evidence that inpatient rehabilitation is always more effective than outpatient care. However, more intense interventions work better than less intensive measures, and some alcoholics do not respond to outpatient approaches. The decision to hospitalize or place into residential care can be made if (1) the patient has medical problems that are difficult to treat outside a hospital; (2) depression, confusion, or psychosis interferes with outpatient care; (3) there is a severe life crisis that makes it difficult to work in an outpatient setting; (4) outpatient treatment has failed; or (5) the patient lives far from the treatment center. The best predictors of continued abstinence include evidence of higher levels of life stability (e.g., supportive family and friends) and higher levels of functioning (e.g., job skills, higher levels of education, and absence of crimes unrelated to alcohol).

Whether the treatment begins in an inpatient or an outpatient setting, subsequent outpatient contact should be maintained for a minimum of 6 months and preferably a full year after abstinence is achieved. Counseling with an individual physician or through groups focuses on day-to-day living—emphasizing areas of improved functioning in the absence of alcohol (i.e., why it is a good idea to continue to abstain) and helping the patient to manage free time without alcohol, develop a nondrinking peer group, and handle stresses on the job.

The physician serves an important role in identifying the alcoholic, treating associated medical or psychiatric syndromes, overseeing detoxification, referring the patient to rehabilitation programs, and providing counseling. The physician is also responsible for selecting which (if any) medication might be appropriate during alcoholism rehabilitation. Patients often complain of continuing sleep problems or anxiety when acute withdrawal treatment is over, problems that may be a component of protracted withdrawal. Unfortunately, there is no place for hypnotics or antianxiety drugs in the treatment of most alcoholics after acute withdrawal has been completed. Patients should be reassured that the trouble sleeping is normal after alcohol withdrawal and will improve over the subsequent weeks and months. Patients should follow a rigid bedtime and awakening schedule and avoid any naps or the use of caffeine in the evenings. The sleep pattern will improve rapidly. Anxiety can be addressed by helping the person to gain insight into the temporary nature of the symptoms and to develop strategies to achieve relaxation as well as by using forms of cognitive therapy.

While the mainstay of alcoholic rehabilitation involves counseling, education, and cognitive approaches, several medications might be useful. The first is the opioid-antagonist drug naltrexone, 50 to 150 mg/d, which has been reported in several small-scale, short-term studies to decrease the probability of a return to drinking and to shorten periods of relapse. However, at least one longer-term large-scale trial questioned the superiority of naltrexone to placebo, and more studies are required before the cost-effectiveness of this approach can be established. A second medication, acamprosate (Campral), 2 g/d, has been tested in >5000 patients in Europe, with results that appear similar to those reported for naltrexone. Several long-term trials of naltrexone and acamprosate, used individually and in combination, are in progress, and early results are promising. A third medication, which has historically been used in the treatment of alcoholism, is the ALDH inhibitor disulfiram. In doses of 250 mg/d this drug produces an unpleasant (and potentially dangerous) reaction in the presence of alcohol, a phenomenon related to rapidly rising blood levels of the first metabolite of alcohol, acetaldehyde. However, few adequate controlled trials have demonstrated the superiority of disulfiram over placebo. Disulfiram has many side effects, and the reaction with alcohol can be dangerous, especially for patients with heart disease, stroke, diabetes mellitus, and hypertension. Thus, most clinicians reserve this medication for patients who have a clear history of longer-term abstinence associated with prior use of disulfiram and for those who might take the drug under the supervision of another individual (such as a spouse), especially during discrete periods that they have identified as representing high-risk drinking situations for them (such as the Christmas holiday).

Additional support for alcoholics and their relatives and friends is available through self-help groups such as Alcoholics Anonymous (AA). These groups, which typically consist of recovering alcoholics, offer an effective model of abstinence, provide a sober peer group, and make crisis intervention available when the urge to drink escalates. This can help patients optimize their chances for recovery, especially when incorporated into a more structured treatment milieu.

FURTHER READING

FLEMING MF et al: Brief physician advice for problem drinkers: Long-term efficacy and benefit-cost analysis. Alcohol Clin Exp Res 26:36, 2002

KIEFER F et al: Comparing and combining naltrexone and acamprosate in relapse prevention of alcoholism. Arch Gen Psychiatry 60:92, 2003

SCHUCKIT MA et al: A 5-year prospective evaluation of DSM-IV alcohol dependence with and without a physiological component. Alcohol Clin Exp Res 27:818, 2003

It is difficult to imagine modern medical practice without the use of opioid analgesics. These drugs have been part of health care since 300 B.C. Opium and codeine were isolated in the early nineteenth century, opioid-like substances produced by the body were recognized in the 1970s, and the first endogenous opioid was isolated in 1995. As important as these substances are to modern medicine, opioid drugs have many disadvantages, including overdosage and dependency; close to 1 million individuals in the United States are opioid-dependent. All opioid drugs are capable of producing a heroin-like intoxication, as well as tolerance and withdrawal.

PHARMACOLOGY The prototypic opiates, morphine and codeine (3-methoxymorphine), are derived from the milky juice of the poppy *Papaver somniferum*. The semisynthetic drugs produced from the morphine or thebane molecules include hydromorphone, diacetylmorphine (heroin), and oxycodone. The purely synthetic opioids and their cousins include meperidine, propoxyphene, diphenoxylate, fentanyl, buprenorphine, tramadol, methadone, and pentazocine.

Endogenous opioid peptides (i.e., enkephalins, endorphins, dynorphins, and others) have distinct distributions in the central nervous system (CNS) and appear to be natural ligands for opioid receptors. As summarized in (Table 373-1), the receptors with which opioid peptides interact differentially produce analgesia, respiratory depression, constipation, euphoria, and other actions. Substances capable of antagonizing one or more of these actions include nalorphine, levallorphan, cyclazocine, butorphanol, buprenorphine, and pentazocine, each of which has mixed agonist and antagonist properties, as well as naloxone, nalmefene, and naltrexone, which are pure opiate antagonists. The availability of relatively specific antagonists has helped identify at least three different receptor subtypes, including μ receptors, which influence some of the more classic opioid actions such as pain control, reinforcement, constipation, hormone levels, and respiration; κ receptors, with possible similar functions along with sedation and effects on hormones; and δ receptors, thought to relate mostly to analgesia, mood, reinforcement, and breathing. A fourth possible receptor subtype, sensitive to another endogenous peptide, is sometimes called *nociceptin* or *orphanin* and may influence pain. The major features of tolerance, dependence, and withdrawal are thought to be mediated primarily by μ receptors, and these are affected by all prescription opioids.

The most rapid and pronounced effects of opioids occur following intravenous administration, with only slightly less efficient absorption after smoking or inhaling the vapor ("chasing the dragon"). The least intense effects occur after oral consumption. Most of the metabolism of opioids occurs in the liver, primarily through conjugation with glucuronic acid, and only small amounts are excreted directly in the urine or feces. The plasma half-lives of these drugs range from 2.5 to 3 h for morphine to more than 22 h for methadone and even longer for levomethadyl acetate (LAAM).

TABLE 373-1 Actions of Opioid Receptors

Receptor Type	Actions
Mu (μ) (e.g., morphine)	Analgesia, reinforcement euphoria, cough and appetite suppression, decreased respirations, decreased GI motility, sedation, hormone changes, dopamine and acetylcholine release
Kappa (κ) (e.g., butorphanol)	Decreased dysphoria, decreased GI motility, decreased appetite, decreased respiration, psychotic symptoms, sedation, diuresis, analgesia
Delta (δ) (e.g., etorphine)	Hormone changes, appetite suppression, dopamine release

Note: GI, gastrointestinal.

Street heroin is typically only 5 to 10% pure, mixed with sugars, quinine, powdered milk, phenacetin, caffeine, antipyrine, and strychnine. Unexpected increases in the purity of street drugs can cause unintentional lethal overdoses.

ACUTE AND CHRONIC EFFECTS OF OPIOIDS With the exception of overdose and physical dependence, most opioid effects are rapidly reversible. A major danger, however, comes through the use of contaminated needles by intravenous users, which increases the risk of hepatitis B and C, bacterial endocarditis, and infection with HIV (Chap. 173).

Effects on Organ Systems In addition to euphoria and rewarding effects of opioids due to stimulation of a dopaminergic pathway originating in the midbrain and terminating in the nucleus accumbens, CNS effects of opioid drugs include nausea and vomiting (medulla), decreased pain perception (spinal cord, thalamus, and periaqueductal gray region), and sedation (reticular activating system). The adulterants added to street drugs may contribute to nervous system damage, including peripheral neuropathy, amblyopia, myelopathy, and leukoencephalopathy. Acute opioid administration inhibits release of some hormones from the hypothalamus, including corticotropin-releasing factor (CRF) and luteinizing hormone, with a subsequent reduction in some sex hormones, actions that might contribute to the decreased sex drive and problems in handling stress. Other hormonal changes include a decrease in the release of thyrotropin and increases in prolactin and possibly growth hormone (Chap. 318).

Acute changes in the respiratory system include a CNS-mediated decrease in the cough reflex and respiratory depression, which result from a decreased response of the brainstem to carbon dioxide tension, a component of the drug overdose syndrome described below. At even low drug doses, this effect can be clinically significant for individuals with pulmonary disease. Aspiration pneumonia is an additional risk. The gastrointestinal effects of opioids can include nausea and decreased gut motility with resulting constipation and anorexia. Cardiovascular changes tend to be relatively mild, with no direct opioid effect on heart rhythm or myocardial contractility, but orthostatic hypotension can occur, probably secondary to histamine release and dilation of peripheral vessels. Bacterial endocarditis with septic emboli and stroke can occur from contaminated needles.

Opioid Toxicity and Overdosage High doses of opioids can result in a potentially lethal overdose, which may occur in >60% of opioid-dependent persons, especially with the more potent drugs such as fentanyl (80 to 100 times more powerful than morphine). The typical syndrome, which occurs immediately with intravenous overdose, includes shallow and slow respirations, pupillary miosis (with mydriasis once brain anoxia develops), bradycardia, hypothermia, and stupor or coma (Chap. 257). If not treated rapidly, respiratory depression, cardiorespiratory arrest, and death can ensue. Postmortem examination reveals few specific changes except for diffuse cerebral edema. An "allergic-like" reaction to intravenous heroin, perhaps in part related to adulterants, can also occur and is characterized by decreased alertness, frothy pulmonary edema, and an elevation in the blood eosinophil count.

The first step in managing overdose is to support vital signs, using intubation if needed. Definitive treatment is the administration of a narcotic antagonist such as 0.4 mg to 2 mg intravenous or intramuscular naloxone. A response should occur in 1 to 2 min; the dose should be repeated every 2 to 3 min up to 10 mg. Except with buprenorphene overdoses, no response after 10 mg makes an opioid toxic reaction unlikely. It is important to titrate the dose relative to the patient's symptoms to ameliorate the respiratory depression but not provoke a severe withdrawal state; the latter cannot be aggressively treated until overdose-related vital signs are relatively stable. Because the effects of naloxone diminish within 2 to 3 h, the individual must be monitored for at least 24 h after a heroin overdose and 72 h after an overdose of a longer-acting drug such as methadone. For methadone overdose, the substitution of the longer acting naltrexone should be considered. If there is little response to an opioid antagonist, the possibility of a concomitant overdose with a benzodiazepine should be considered and a challenge with intravenous flumazenil, 0.2 mg/min up to a maximum of 3 mg in an hour, might be used.

Treatment of either the typical or the "allergic" type of opioid toxic reaction often requires continued respiratory support (often with oxygen supplementation and positive-pressure breathing for the "allergic" type of overdose), intravenous fluids, pressor agents when needed to support blood pressure, and gastric lavage to remove any remaining drug. Intubation is often required to prevent aspiration in the stuporous or comatose patient. Cardiac arrhythmias and/or seizures may also be part of the opioid toxic reaction, especially with codeine, propoxyphene, or meperidine.

OPIOID ABUSE AND DEPENDENCE ■ Definition and Epidemiology The *Fourth Diagnostic and Statistical Manual* (DSM-IV) of the American Psychiatric Association defines opioid dependence as repeated use of a drug of this class to the point of causing multiple problems. The definition requires evidence of three or more problems in the same year, including tolerance, withdrawal, use of greater amounts of opiates than intended, and use despite consequences. Patients who do not have dependence but demonstrate repeated opioid-related difficulties with the law, impaired ability to meet obligations, use in hazardous situations, or continued use despite problems can be labeled as having abuse.

The use of opioids for intoxication is less prevalent than the use of alcohol, marijuana, and several other drugs. A 2002 national survey of adolescents and young adults reported that 10% of 12th graders (high school seniors) had tried an opioid outside of a doctor's prescription, including almost 2% who had used heroin. Figures for young adults and college students in 2001 were almost 12% and 2%, respectively. In all studies, prevalence rates were only slightly higher in males than females. None of the national surveys offered data regarding the prevalence of dependence, which is estimated as a lifetime risk of about 1%.

Genetics One large study of >3000 male twin pairs reported that there are genetic influences that relate uniquely to heroin dependence and also noted additional genetic factors related to an overall vulnerability toward substance-related problems. The genetic influences operate in the context of additional environmental factors that are likely to relate both to the family of upbringing and the general environment. Genetic factors might influence personality characteristics such as impulsivity and sensation-seeking or susceptibility to develop antisocial personality disorder. Genes relating to the actions of the drug on specific neurochemical systems such as dopamine are also potential candidates for an enhanced vulnerability toward developing opioid dependence.

Natural History While an opioid use disorder can develop in anyone, at least three groups are at increased risk for dependence or misuse. First, a minority of persons with chronic pain syndromes (e.g., back, joint, and muscle disorders) misuse their prescribed drugs. If physical dependence is established, any drop in opioid blood levels can then intensify the pain and promote continued drug intake. Physicians can avoid contributing to physical dependence by helping the patient to accept the goal of moderation rather than disappearance of the pain and to recognize that discomfort may not be completely eliminated (Chap. 11). Analgesic medication should be only one component of treatment and limited to the oral administration of the least potent analgesic that is able to "take the edge off" the pain (e.g., ibuprofen or, if needed, propoxyphene). Behavior-modification techniques, such as muscle relaxation and meditation, and carefully selected exercises should be used as appropriate to help increase function and decrease pain. Finally, nonmedicinal approaches, including electrical transcutaneous neurostimulation for muscle and joint disease, may be useful.

The second group at high risk are physicians, nurses, and pharmacists, primarily because of easy access to opioids. Physicians may begin use to help with sleep or to reduce stress or physical aches and pains, and then escalate doses as tolerance develops. Because of the growing awareness of these problems, programs have been developed to identify and aid substance-impaired physicians, providing peer support and education before problems escalate to the point of licensure revocation. All physicians are advised never to prescribe opioids for themselves or family members.

The third group are those who buy street drugs to get high. While some of these individuals have prior histories of severe antisocial problems, most have a relatively high level of premorbid functioning. The typical person begins using opioids occasionally, often after experimenting with tobacco, then alcohol, then marijuana, and then brain depressants or stimulants. Occasional opiate use, or "chipping," might continue for some time, and some individuals never escalate their intake to the point of developing dependence.

Opioid-dependent individuals are likely to continue to have experience with other drugs. Alcohol may be used to moderate withdrawal problems, to enhance the opioid high, and to serve as a substitute when the opioid is not available, including during methadone and other treatments. Problematic drinking, including alcohol dependence, is seen in about half of opioid-dependent persons. Cocaine appears to be taken for many of the same reasons as alcohol, and is often administered intravenously with the opioid in a mixture known as a "speedball." Another relevant class of drugs is the benzodiazepines, especially among people in methadone maintenance.

Once persistent opioid use is established, severe problems are likely to develop. At least 25% of habitual users die within 10 to 20 years (a mortality rate 15-fold higher than the general population) from suicide, homicide, accidents, or infectious diseases such as tuberculosis, hepatitis, or AIDS. The latter has become an epidemic among injection drug users, with an estimated 60% of these men and women carrying HIV (Chap. 173). Although the majority of opioid-dependent persons experience frequent exacerbations and remissions, it is important to remember that even without treatment ~35% achieve long-term, often permanent, abstinence, especially after the age of 40. As is true with most drugs of abuse, a favorable prognosis is associated with a prior history of marital and employment stability and fewer prior criminal activities unrelated to drugs.

℞ TREATMENT

One key to diagnosis is to discard the erroneous stereotype that opioid-dependent individuals are always unemployed and homeless. Abuse or dependence is possible in any patient who demonstrates symptoms of what might be opioid withdrawal; anyone who has a chronic pain syndrome; physicians, nurses, and pharmacists or others with easy access to opioids; and all patients who repeatedly seek out prescription analgesics. Therefore, before prescribing an opioid analgesic, it is important to gather a complete history that elucidates patterns of life problems and any history of opioid use. If a problem with opioids is suspected, gathering further data from a relative or close friend can be helpful. Additionally, clinicians should search for physical stigmata of misuse (e.g., needle marks) and, when appropriate, screen blood or urine for opioids.

After identifying opioid dependence, the next step is intervention as described for alcoholism in Chap. 372. The need for continuing treatment even after the patient achieves abstinence can be presented, and the availability of help in establishing a drug-free life-style can be emphasized.

Symptoms of Withdrawal Withdrawal symptoms, generally the opposite of the acute effects of the drug, include nausea and diarrhea, coughing, lacrimation, mydriasis, rhinorrhea, profuse sweating, twitching of muscles, and piloerection (or "goose bumps") as well as mild elevations in body temperature, respiratory rate, and blood pressure. In addition, diffuse body pain, insomnia, and yawning occur, along with intense drug craving. Drugs with shorter half-lives, such as morphine or heroin, usually cause symptoms within 8 to 16 h of the last dose; intensity peaks within 36 to 72 h after discontinuation of the drug; and the acute syndrome disappears within 5 to 8 days. A protracted abstinence phase of mild moodiness, autonomic dysfunction, and changes in pain threshold and sleep patterns may persist for ≥6 months and probably contributes to relapse.

Treatment of the Withdrawal Syndrome A thorough physical examination, including an assessment of neurologic function and a search for focal and systemic infections, especially abscesses, is mandatory. Laboratory testing includes assessment of liver function and, in intravenous users, HIV and hepatitis B and C status. Proper nutrition and rest must be initiated as soon as possible.

One treatment of withdrawal requires administration of any opioid (e.g., 10 to 25 mg of methadone bid) on day 1 to decrease symptoms. After several days of a stabilized drug dose, the opioid is then decreased by 10 to 20% of the original day's dose each day. However, detoxification with opioids is proscribed or limited in most states. Thus, pharmacologic treatments often center on relief of symptoms of diarrhea with loperamide, of "sniffles" with decongestants, and pain with nonopioid analgesics (e.g., ibuprofen). Comfort can be enhanced with administration of the α_2-adrenergic agonist clonidine in doses up to 0.3 mg given two to four times a day to decrease sympathetic nervous system overactivity. Blood pressure must be closely monitored. Some clinicians augment this regimen with low to moderate doses of benzodiazepines for 2 to 5 days to decrease agitation. An ultra-rapid detoxification procedure using deep sedation and withdrawal precipitated by naltrexone has been proposed, but has many inherent dangers and little evidence of efficacy.

A special case of opioid withdrawal is seen in the newborn made passively dependent through the mother's drug abuse during pregnancy; withdrawal consists of irritability, crying, a tremor, increased reflexes, increased respiratory rate, diarrhea, vomiting, and sneezing/yawning/hiccuping. Treatment follows the same general steps used in the treatment of the physically dependent adult but using paregoric (0.2 mL orally every 3 to 4 h), methadone (0.1 to 0.5 mg/kg per day), phenobarbital (8 mg/kg per day), or diazepam (1 to 2 mg/kg every 8 h) in decreasing dosages for 10 to 20 days. Dependent infants of mothers on methadone maintenance also benefit by breast feeding while the mother continues to take methadone.

Rehabilitation Despite some differences in demographics, the same general rules for rehabilitation apply to opioid-dependent persons as to alcoholics. The basic strategy includes detoxification and establishment of realistic goals, along with counseling and education to increase motivation toward abstinence. A long-term commitment by the patient to rebuilding a life-style without the substance is essential for preventing relapse.

In most programs, patients are educated about their responsibility for improving their lives, and motivation for abstinence is increased by providing information about the medical and psychological problems that can be expected if dependence continues. Patients and families are encouraged to establish an opioid-free life-style by learning to cope with chronic pain and develop realistic vocational planning (e.g., for pharmacists, physicians, and nurses). The dependent person is also advised to establish a drug-free peer group and to participate in self-help groups such as Narcotics Anonymous. Another important treatment component is relapse prevention aimed at identifying triggers for a return to drugs and developing appropriate coping strategies.

Much of this advice and counseling can be given by the physician or by referring the patients to formal drug programs, including methadone maintenance clinics, programs using narcotic antagonists, and therapeutic communities. Long-term follow-up of treated patients indicates that approximately one-third are completely drug free, and 60% no longer use opioids.

OPIOID MAINTENANCE Maintenance programs with methadone and the longer-acting LAAM should be used only in combination with education and counseling. The goal is to provide a substitute drug that is legally accessible, safer, can be taken orally, and has a long half-life

so that it can be taken once a day. This can help persons who have repeatedly failed in drug-free programs to improve functioning within the family and job, to decrease legal problems, and to improve health. Individuals who stay in methadone maintenance are likely to show improvement in antisocial behavior and employment status.

Methadone is a long-acting opioid optimally dosed at 80 to 120 mg/d (a goal met through slow, careful increases over time). This level is optimally effective in blocking heroin-induced euphoria, decreasing craving, and maintaining abstinence from illegal oipoids. Over three-quarters of patients in well-supervised methadone clinics are likely to remain heroin-free for ≥6 months. Methadone is administered as an oral liquid given once a day at the program, with weekend doses taken at home. The longer-acting analogues, such as LAAM, can be given in doses up to 80 mg two or three times a week. After a period of maintenance (usually 6 months to ≥1 year), the clinician can work to slowly decrease the dose by about 5% per week.

An additional medication that has been used for maintenance treatment involves the μ opioid agonist and κ antagonist buprenorphine. Administered either as a sublingual liquid or tablet, doses of 8 to 12 mg per day (up to 32 mg in some patients) are usually given between 3 and 7 days per week. This drug has several advantages including low overdose danger, easier detoxification than is seen with methadone, and a probable ceiling effect in which higher doses do not increase euphoria. While many studies report equal effectiveness of buprenorphine and methadone, others suggest higher dropout rates or concomitant drug use with buprenorphine. As with all opioids, there is still a danger of misuse.

In the past, the British have used heroin maintenance with goals and guidelines similar to those of current methadone programs. There is no evidence that heroin maintenance has any advantages over methadone maintenance, but the heroin approach increases the risk that the drug will be sold on the streets.

OPIOID ANTAGONISTS The opiate antagonists (e.g., naltrexone) compete with heroin and other opioids at receptors, reducing the effects of the opioid agonists. Administered over long periods with the intention of blocking the opioid "high," these drugs can be useful as part of an overall treatment approach that includes counseling and support. Naltrexone doses of 50 mg/d antagonize 15 mg of heroin for 24 h, and the possibly more effective higher doses (125 to 150 mg) block the effects of 25 mg of intravenous heroin for up to 3 days. To avoid precipitating a withdrawal syndrome, patients must be free of opioids for a minimum of 5 days before beginning treatment with naltrexone and should first be challenged with 0.4 or 0.8 mg of the shorter-acting agent naloxone to be certain they can tolerate the long-acting antagonist. A test dose of 10 mg of naltrexone is then given, which can produce withdrawal symptoms in 0.5 to 2 h. If none appear, the patient can begin with the usual dose of 40 to 150 mg three times per week.

DRUG-FREE PROGRAMS Most opioid-dependent individuals enter treatment programs based primarily on the cognitive behavioral approaches of enhancing commitment to abstinence, helping individuals to rebuild their lives without substances, and preventing relapse. Whether carried out in inpatient or outpatient settings, patients do not receive medications.

A variation of this approach can be used for persons who are having problems maintaining a drug-free state. Here, the basic elements of treatment are incorporated into long-term (often a year or more) residence in a therapeutic community. The person begins with almost full immersion in the environment in which other individuals at various stages of recovery become the primary support group, offering advice and a drug-free atmosphere in which the opioid-dependent person progresses through ever-increasing levels of independence, including assuming a job outside the therapeutic atmosphere.

As is true for treatments of all substance-use disorders, it is likely that counseling, behavioral treatments, and relatively simple approaches to psychotherapy add significantly to a positive outcome.

Most programs focus on teaching participants to cope with stress, enhancing their understanding of personality attributes, teaching better cognitive styles, and, through the process of relapse prevention, addressing issues that might contribute to increased craving, easy access to drugs, or periods of decreased motivation. A combination of these therapies with the approaches described above appears to give the best results.

Finally, it is important to discuss prevention. Except for the terminally ill, physicians should carefully monitor opioid drug use in their patients, keeping doses as low as is practical and administering them over as short a period as the level of pain would warrant in the average person. Physicians must be vigilant regarding their own risk for opioid abuse and dependence, never prescribing these drugs for themselves. For the nonmedical intravenous drug–dependent person, all possible efforts must be made to prevent AIDS, hepatitis, bacterial endocarditis, and other consequences of contaminated needles both through methadone maintenance and by considering needle-exchange programs.

FURTHER READING

DEVRIES TJ, SHIPPENBERG TS: Neural systems underlying opiate addiction. J Neurosci 22:3321, 2002

JOHNSTON LD et al: *Monitoring the Future: National Results on Adolescent Drug Use: Overview of Key Findings*, 2002. Bethesda, MD, National Institute on Drug Abuse, 2003. NIH Publication No. 03-5374.

MATTICK RP et al: Buprenorphine versus methadone maintenance therapy: A randomized double-blind trial with 405 opioid-dependent patients. Addiction 98:441, 2003

SCHUCKIT MA et al: *Drug and Alcohol Abuse: A Clinical Guide to Diagnosis and Treatment*, 5th ed. New York, Plenum, 2000

374 COCAINE AND OTHER COMMONLY ABUSED DRUGS
Jack H. Mendelson, Nancy K. Mello

Cocaine and other psychostimulant drug abuse remains a major public health problem in the United States and throughout the world; its prevalence appears to be increasing in some metropolitan areas for both college students and adults ages 19 to 40. Drug abuse by women continues to parallel abuse of cocaine and other psychostimulant drugs by men; psychostimulant abuse among youth in the United States is a special concern.

The initiation and persistence of drug abuse are determined by a complex interaction of the pharmacologic properties and relative availability of each drug, the personality and expectations of the user, and the environmental context in which the drug is used. Polydrug abuse, the concurrent use of several drugs with different pharmacologic effects, is increasingly common among individuals from all socioeconomic strata. Particularly dangerous forms of polydrug abuse, such as the combined use of heroin and cocaine intravenously, remain a major problem in hospital emergency room settings. Drug abusers may attempt to attenuate one drug effect with another, as when heroin or alcohol is used to modulate the cocaine high. Sometimes one drug is used to enhance the effects of another, as with benzodiazepines and methadone, or cocaine plus heroin in methadone-maintained patients.

Chronic cocaine and psychostimulant abuse may cause a number of adverse health consequences, ranging from pulmonary disease to reproductive dysfunction. Preexisting disorders such as hypertension and cardiac disease may be exacerbated by drug abuse, and the combined use of two or more drugs may accentuate medical complications associated with abuse of one of them.

Drug abuse increases the risk of exposure to HIV. Cocaine and psychostimulant abuse contribute to the risk for HIV infection in part by suppression of immune function. In addition, concurrent use of cocaine and opiates (the "speedball") is frequently associated with needle-sharing by intravenous drug users. Intravenous drug abusers continue to represent the largest single group of persons with HIV infection in several major metropolitan areas in the United States as well as in urban areas in Scotland, Italy, Spain, Thailand, and China.

COCAINE Cocaine is a stimulant and local anesthetic with potent vasoconstrictor properties. The leaves of the *coca* plant (*Erythroxylon coca*) contain ~0.5 to 1% cocaine. The drug produces physiologic and behavioral effects when administered orally, intranasally, intravenously, or via inhalation following pyrolysis (smoking). Cocaine increases synaptic concentrations of the monamine neurotransmitters dopamine, norepinephrine, and serotonin by binding to transporter proteins in presynaptic neurons and blocking reuptake. The reinforcing effects of cocaine appear to be related to effects on dopaminergic neurons in the mesolimbic system.

Prevalence of Use Cocaine is widely available throughout the United States, and cocaine abuse occurs in virtually all social and economic strata of society. The prevalence of cocaine abuse in the general population has been accompanied by an increase in cocaine abuse by heroin-dependent persons, including those in methadone maintenance programs. Intravenous cocaine is often used concurrently with intravenous heroin. This combination purportedly attenuates the postcocaine "crash" and substitutes a cocaine "high" for the heroin "high" blocked by methadone.

Acute and Chronic Intoxication There has been an increase in both intravenous administration and inhalation of pyrolyzed cocaine via smoking. Following intranasal administration, changes in mood and sensation are perceived within 3 to 5 min, and peak effects occur at l0 to 20 min. The effects rarely last more than 1 h. Inhalation of pyrolyzed materials includes inhaling crack/cocaine or smoking coca paste, a product made by extracting cocaine preparations with flammable solvents, and cocaine free-base smoking. Free-base cocaine, including the free base prepared with sodium bicarbonate (crack), has become increasingly popular because of the relative high potency of the compound and its rapid onset of action (8 to 10 s following smoking).

Cocaine produces a brief, dose-related stimulation and enhancement of mood and an increase in cardiac rate and blood pressure. Body temperature usually increases following cocaine administration, and high doses of cocaine may induce lethal pyrexia or hypertension. Because cocaine inhibits reuptake of catecholamines at adrenergic nerve endings, the drug potentiates sympathetic nervous system activity. Cocaine has a short plasma half-life of ~45 to 60 min. Cocaine is metabolized by plasma esterases, and cocaine metabolites are excreted in urine. The very short duration of the euphorigenic effects of cocaine observed in chronic abusers is probably due to both acute and chronic tolerance. Frequent self-administration of the drug (two to three times per hour) is often reported by chronic cocaine abusers. Alcohol is used to modulate both the cocaine high and the dysphoria associated with the abrupt disappearance of cocaine's effects. A metabolite of cocaine, cocaethylene, has been detected in blood and urine of persons who concurrently abuse alcohol and cocaine. Cocaethylene induces changes in cardiovascular function similar to those of cocaine alone, and the pathophysiologic consequences of alcohol abuse plus cocaine abuse may be additive when both are used together.

The prevalent assumption that cocaine inhalation or intravenous administration is relatively safe is contradicted by reports of death from respiratory depression, cardiac arrhythmias, and convulsions associated with cocaine use. In addition to generalized seizures, neurologic complications may include headache, ischemic or hemorrhagic stroke, or subarachnoid hemorrhage. Disorders of cerebral blood flow and perfusion in cocaine-dependent persons have been detected with magnetic resonance spectroscopy (MRS) studies. Severe pulmonary disease may develop in individuals who inhale crack cocaine; this effect is attributed both to the direct effects of cocaine and to residual contaminants in the smoked material. Hepatic necrosis has been reported to occur following crack cocaine use.

Although men and women who abuse cocaine may report that the drug enhances libidinal drive, chronic cocaine use causes significant loss of libido and adversely affects reproductive function. Impotence and gynecomastia have been observed in male cocaine abusers, and these abnormalities often persist for long periods following cessation of drug use. Women who abuse cocaine have reported major derangements in menstrual cycle function including galactorrhea, amenorrhea, and infertility. Chronic cocaine abuse may cause persistent hyperprolactinemia as a consequence of disordered dopaminergic inhibition of prolactin secretion by the anterior pituitary. Cocaine abuse by pregnant women, particularly the smoking of crack, has been associated with both an increased risk of congenital malformations in the fetus and perinatal cardiovascular and cerebrovascular disease in the mother. However, cocaine abuse per se is probably not the sole cause of these perinatal disorders, since many problems associated with maternal cocaine abuse, including poor nutrition and health care status as well as polydrug abuse, also contribute to risk for perinatal disease.

Protracted cocaine abuse may cause paranoid ideation and visual and auditory hallucinations, a state that resembles alcoholic hallucinosis. Psychological dependence on cocaine, indicated by inability to abstain from frequent compulsive use, has also been reported. Although the occurrence of withdrawal syndromes involving psychomotor agitation and autonomic hyperactivity remains controversial, severe depression ("crashing") following cocaine intoxication may accompany drug withdrawal.

℞ TREATMENT

Treatment of cocaine overdose is a medical emergency that is usually best managed in an intensive care unit. Cocaine toxicity produces a hyperadrenergic state characterized by hypertension, tachycardia, tonic-clonic seizures, dyspnea, and ventricular arrhythmias. Intravenous diazepam in doses up to 0.5 mg/kg administered over an 8-h period has been shown to be effective for control of seizures. Ventricular arrhythmias have been managed successfully by administration of 0.5 to 1.0 mg of propranolol intravenously. Since many instances of cocaine-related mortality have been associated with concurrent use of other illicit drugs (particularly heroin), the physician must be prepared to institute effective emergency treatment for multiple drug toxicities.

Treatment of chronic cocaine abuse requires combined efforts of primary care physicians, psychiatrists, and psychosocial care providers. Early abstinence from cocaine use is often complicated by symptoms of depression and guilt, insomnia, and anorexia, which may be as severe as those observed in major affective disorders. Individual and group psychotherapy, family therapy, and peer group assistance programs are often useful for inducing prolonged remission from drug use. A number of medications used for the treatment of various medical and psychiatric disorders have been administered to reduce the duration and severity of cocaine abuse and dependence. However, no available medication is both safe and highly effective for either cocaine detoxification or maintenance of abstinence. Some psychotherapeutic interventions may be effective; however, no specific form of psychotherapy or behavioral modification is uniquely beneficial.

MARIJUANA AND CANNABIS COMPOUNDS *Cannabis sativa* contains >400 compounds in addition to the psychoactive substance, delta-9-tetrahydrocannabinol (THC). Marijuana cigarettes are prepared from the leaves and flowering tops of the plant, and a typical marijuana cigarette contains 0.5 to 1 g of plant material. Although the usual THC concentration varies between 10 and 40 mg, concentrations >100 mg per cigarette have been detected. Hashish is prepared from concentrated resin of *C. sativa* and contains a THC concentration of between 8 to 12% percent by weight. "Hash oil," a lipid-soluble plant extract, may

contain a THC concentration of 25 to 60% percent and may be added to marijuana or hashish to enhance its THC concentration. Smoking is the most common mode of marijuana or hashish use. During pyrolysis, >150 compounds in addition to THC are released in the smoke. Although most of these compounds do not have psychoactive properties, they do have potential physiologic effects.

THC is quickly absorbed from the lungs into blood and is then rapidly sequestered in tissues. It is metabolized primarily in the liver, where it is converted to 11-hydroxy-THC, a psychoactive compound, and >20 other metabolites. Many THC metabolites are excreted through the feces at a rate of clearance that is relatively slow in comparison to that of most other psychoactive drugs.

Specific cannabinoid receptors (CB_1 and CB_2) have been identified in the central nervous system, including the spinal cord, and in the peripheral nervous system. High densities of these receptors have been found in the cerebral cortex, basal ganglia, and hippocampus. B lymphocytes also appear to have cannabinoid receptors. A naturally occurring THC-like ligand has been identified in the nervous system, where it is widely distributed.

Prevalence of Use Marijuana is the most commonly used illegal drug in the United States. Use is particularly prevalent among adolescents; studies suggest that ~37% of high school students in the United States have used marijuana. Marijuana is relatively inexpensive and is often considered to be less hazardous than other controlled drugs and substances. Very potent forms of marijuana (sinsemilla) are now available in many communities, and concurrent use of marijuana with crack/cocaine and phencyclidine is increasing. Marijuana abuse by individuals from all social strata has been increasing.

Acute and Chronic Intoxication Acute intoxication from marijuana and cannabis compounds is related to both the dose of THC and the route of administration. THC is absorbed more rapidly from marijuana smoking than from orally ingested cannabis compounds. Acute marijuana intoxication usually consists of a subjective perception of relaxation and mild euphoria resembling mild to moderate alcohol intoxication. This condition is usually accompanied by some impairment in thinking, concentration, and perceptual and psychomotor function. Higher doses of cannabis may produce behavioral effects analogous to severe alcohol intoxication. Although the effects of acute marijuana intoxication are relatively benign in normal users, the drug can precipitate severe emotional disorders in individuals who have antecedent psychotic or neurotic problems. As with other psychoactive compounds, both set (user's expectations) and setting (environmental context) are important determinants of the type and severity of behavioral intoxication.

As with abuse of cocaine, opioids, and alcohol, chronic marijuana abusers may lose interest in common socially desirable goals and steadily devote more time to drug acquisition and use. However, THC does not cause a specific and unique "amotivational syndrome." The range of symptoms sometimes attributed to marijuana use is difficult to distinguish from mild to moderate depression and the maturational dysfunctions often associated with protracted adolescence. Chronic marijuana use has also been reported to increase the risk of psychotic symptoms in individuals with a past history of schizophrenia. Persons who initiate marijuana smoking before the age of 17 may subsequently develop severe cognitive and neuropsychological disorders, and may be at higher risk for later polydrug and alcohol abuse problems.

Physical Effects Conjunctival injection and tachycardia are the most frequent immediate physical concomitants of smoking marijuana. Tolerance for marijuana-induced tachycardia develops rapidly among regular users. However, marijuana smoking may precipitate angina in persons with a history of coronary insufficiency. Exercise-induced angina may be increased after marijuana use to a greater extent than after tobacco cigarette smoking. Patients with cardiac disease should be strongly advised not to smoke marijuana or use cannabis compounds.

Significant decrements in pulmonary vital capacity have been found in regular daily marijuana smokers. Because marijuana smoking typically involves deep inhalation and prolonged retention of marijuana smoke, marijuana smokers may develop chronic bronchial irritation. Impairment of single-breath carbon monoxide diffusion capacity (DL_{CO}) is greater in persons who smoke both marijuana and tobacco than in tobacco smokers.

Although marijuana has also been associated with adverse effects on a number of other systems, many of these studies await replication and confirmation. A reported correlation between chronic marijuana use and decreased testosterone levels in males has not been confirmed. Decreased sperm count and sperm motility and morphologic abnormalities of spermatozoa following marijuana use have also been reported. Prospective studies demonstrated a correlation between impaired fetal growth and development and heavy marijuana use during pregnancy. Marijuana has also been implicated in derangements of the immune system; in chromosomal abnormalities; and in inhibition of DNA, RNA, and protein synthesis; however, these findings have not been confirmed or related to any specific physiologic effect in humans.

Tolerance and Physical Dependence   Habitual marijuana users rapidly develop tolerance to the psychoactive effects of marijuana and often smoke more frequently and try to secure more potent cannabis compounds. Tolerance for the physiologic effects of marijuana develops at different rates; e.g., tolerance develops rapidly for marijuana-induced tachycardia but more slowly for marijuana-induced conjunctival injection. Tolerance to both behavioral and physiologic effects of marijuana decreases rapidly upon cessation of marijuana use.

Withdrawal signs and symptoms have been reported in chronic cannabis users, with the severity of symptoms related to dosage and duration of use. These include tremor, nystagmus, sweating, nausea, vomiting, diarrhea, irritability, anorexia, and sleep disturbances. Withdrawal signs and symptoms observed in chronic marijuana users are usually relatively mild in comparison to those observed in heavy opiate or alcohol users and rarely require medical or pharmacologic intervention. More severe and protracted abstinence syndromes may occur after sustained use of high-potency cannabis compounds.

Therapeutic Use   Marijuana, administered as cigarettes or as a synthetic oral cannabinoid (dronabinol), has been proposed to have a number of properties that may be clinically useful in some situations. These include antiemetic effects in chemotherapy recipients, appetite-promoting effects in AIDS, reduction of intraocular pressure in glaucoma, and reduction of spasticity in multiple sclerosis and other neurologic disorders. With the possible exception of AIDS-related cachexia, none of these attributes of marijuana compounds is clearly superior to other readily available therapies.

METHAMPHETAMINE   The abuse of methamphetamine, also referred to as "meth," "speed," "crank," "chalk," "ice," "glass," or "crystal," has been declining in many metropolitan areas and communities throughout the United States. This decrease is attributed in part to drug seizures and the closures of clandestine laboratories that produce methamphetamine illegally. Prevention programs focusing upon methamphetamine abuse have also increased.

Most persons who abuse methamphetamine self-administer the drug orally, although there have been reports of methamphetamine administration by inhalation and intravenous injection. Individuals who abuse or become dependent upon methamphetamine state that use of this drug induces feelings of euphoria and decreases fatigue associated with difficult life situations. Adverse physiologic effects observed as a consequence of methamphetamine abuse include headache, difficulty concentrating, diminished appetite, abdominal pain, vomiting or diarrhea, disordered sleep, paranoid or aggressive behavior, and psychosis. Severe, life-threatening toxicity may present as hypertension, cardiac arrythmia or failure, subarachnoid hemorrhage, ischemic stroke, intracerebral hemorrhage, convulsions, or coma. Methamphetamines increase the release of monoamine neurotransmitters (dopamine, norepinephrine, and serotonin) from presynaptic neurons. It is thought that the euphoric and reinforcing effects of this class of drugs are mediated through dopamine and the mesolimbic system, whereas the cardiovascular effects are related to norepinephrine. MRS studies suggest that chronic abuse may injure the frontal areas and basal ganglia of the brain.

Therapy of acute methamphetamine overdose is largely symptomatic. Ammonium chloride may be useful to acidify the urine and enhance clearance of the drug. Hypertension may respond to sodium nitroprusside or α-adrenergic antagonists. Sedatives may reduce agitation and other signs of central nervous system hyperactivity. Treatment of chronic methamphetamine dependence may be accomplished in either an inpatient or outpatient setting using strategies similar to those described above for cocaine abuse.

MDMA (3,4-methylenedioxymethamphetamine), or *Ecstasy*, is a derivative of methamphetamine. Ecstasy is usually taken orally but may be injected or inhaled. In addition to amphetamine-like effects, MDMA can induce hyperthermia and vivid hallucinations and other perceptual distortions.

During the past decade, an eighteenfold increase in MDMA-related emergency room incidents has been reported in the United States. Recent studies have revealed that MDMA induces both brain dopaminergic and serotonergic neurotoxicity. Thus, use of recreational use of MDMA by young persons may significantly increase the risk for subsequent occurrence of severe neuropsychiatric disorders.

LYSERGIC ACID DIETHYLAMIDE (LSD)   The discovery of the psychedelic effects of LSD in 1947 led to an epidemic of LSD abuse during the 1960s. Imposition of stringent constraints on the manufacture and distribution of LSD (classified as a Schedule I substance by the U.S. Food and Drug Administration), as well as public recognition that psychedelic experiences induced by LSD were a health hazard, have resulted in a reduction in LSD abuse. The drug still retains some popularity among adolescents and young adults, however, and there are indications that LSD use among young persons has been increasing in some communities in the United States.

LSD is a very potent drug; oral doses as low as 20 μg may induce profound psychological and physiologic effects. Tachycardia, hypertension, pupillary dilation, tremor, and hyperpyrexia occur within minutes following oral administration of 0.5 to 2 μg/kg. A variety of bizarre and often conflicting perceptual and mood changes, including visual illusions, synesthesias, and extreme lability of mood, usually occur within 30 min after LSD intake. These effects of LSD may persist for 12 to 18 h, even though the half-life of the drug is only 3 h.

Tolerance develops rapidly for LSD-induced changes in psychological function when the drug is used one or more times per day for >4 days. Abrupt abstinence following continued use does not produce withdrawal signs or symptoms. There have been no clinical reports of death caused by the direct effects of LSD.

The most frequent acute medical emergency associated with LSD use is panic episode (the "bad trip"), which may persist up to 24 h. Management of this problem is best accomplished by supportive reassurance ("talking down") and, if necessary, administration of small doses of anxiolytic drugs. Adverse consequences of chronic LSD use include enhanced risk for schizophreniform psychosis and derangements in memory function, problem solving, and abstract thinking. Treatment of these disorders is best carried out in specialized psychiatric facilities.

PHENCYCLIDINE   Phencyclidine (PCP), a cyclohexylamine derivative, is widely used in veterinary medicine to briefly immobilize large animals and is sometimes described as a dissociative anesthetic. PCP binds to ionotropic *n*-methyl-*d*-aspartate (NMDA) receptors in the nervous system, blocking ion current through these channels. PCP is easily synthesized; its abusers are primarily young people and polydrug users. It is used orally, by smoking, or by intravenous injection. It is also used as an adulterant in THC, LSD, amphetamine, or cocaine. The most common street preparation, *angel dust*, is a white granular powder that contains 50 to 100% percent of the drug. Low doses (5 mg) produce agitation, excitement, impaired motor coordination, dysarthria, and analgesia. Users may have horizontal or vertical nystagmus, flushing, diaphoresis, and hyperacusis. Behavioral changes include distortions of body image, disorganization of thinking, and feelings of estrangement. Higher doses of PCP (5 to 10 mg) may produce profuse salivation, vomiting, myoclonus, fever, stupor, or coma. PCP doses of ≥ 10 mg cause convulsions, opisthotonus, and decerebrate posturing, which may be followed by prolonged coma.

The diagnosis of PCP overdose is difficult because the patient's initial symptoms may suggest an acute schizophrenic reaction. Confirmation of PCP use is possible by determination of PCP levels in serum or urine. PCP assays are available at most toxicologic centers. PCP remains in urine for 1 to 5 days following high-dose intake.

PCP overdose requires life-support measures, including treatment of coma, convulsions, and respiratory depression in an intensive care unit. There is no specific antidote or antagonist for PCP. PCP excretion from the body can be enhanced by gastric lavage and acidification of urine. Death from PCP overdose may occur as a consequence of some combination of pharyngeal hypersecretion, hyperthermia, respiratory depression, severe hypertension, seizures, hypertensive encephalopathy, and intracerebral hemorrhage.

Acute psychosis associated with PCP use should be considered a psychiatric emergency since patients may be at high risk for suicide or extreme violence toward others. Phenothiazines should not be used for treatment because these drugs potentiate PCP's anticholinergic effects. Haloperidol (5 mg intramuscularly) has been administered on an hourly basis to induce suppression of psychotic behavior. PCP, like LSD and mescaline, produces vasospasm of cerebral arteries at relatively low doses. Chronic PCP use has been shown to induce insomnia, anorexia, severe social and behavioral changes, and, in some cases, chronic schizophrenia.

POLYDRUG ABUSE Although drug abusers often report a preference for a particular drug, such as alcohol or opiates, the concurrent use of other drugs is common. Multiple drug use often involves substances that may have different pharmacologic effects from the preferred drug. Concurrent use of such dissimilar compounds as stimulants and opiates or stimulants and alcohol is not unusual. The diversity of reported drug use combinations suggests that achieving some perceptible change in state, rather than any particular direction of change (stimulation or sedation), may be the primary reinforcer in polydrug use and abuse. There is also evidence that intoxication with alcohol or opiates is associated with increased tobacco smoking. There is relatively little systematic information available about multiple drug abuse interactions.

However, the combined use of cocaine, heroin, and alcohol increases the risk for toxic effects and adverse medical consequences over risks associated with use of a single drug. One determinant of polydrug use patterns is the relative availability and cost of the drugs. There are many examples of situationally determined drug use patterns. For example, alcohol abuse, with its attendant medical complications, is one of the most serious problems encountered in former heroin addicts participating in methadone maintenance programs.

The physician must recognize that perpetuation of polydrug abuse and drug dependence is not necessarily a symptom of an underlying emotional disorder. Neither alleviation of anxiety nor reduction of depression accounts for initiation and perpetuation of polydrug abuse. Severe depression and anxiety are as frequently the consequences of polydrug abuse as they are the antecedents. There is also evidence that some of the most adverse consequences of drug use may be reinforcing and contribute to the continuation of polydrug abuse.

℞ TREATMENT

Adequate treatment of polydrug abuse, as well as other forms of drug abuse, requires innovative programs of intervention. The first step in successful treatment is detoxification, a process that may be difficult because of the abuse of several drugs with different pharmacologic actions (e.g., alcohol, opiates, and cocaine). Since patients may not recall or may deny simultaneous multiple drug use, diagnostic evaluation should always include urinalysis for qualitative detection of psychoactive substances and their metabolites. Treatment of polydrug abuse often requires hospitalization or inpatient residential care during detoxification and the initial phase of drug abstinence. When possible, specialized facilities for the care and treatment of chemically dependent persons should be used. Outpatient detoxification of polydrug abuse patients is likely to be ineffective and may be dangerous.

Polydrug abuse is a chronic disorder with an unpredictable pattern of remission and recrudescence. Definitive "cures" rarely occur. The physician should continue to assist polydrug abuse patients throughout the cyclic oscillations of this complex behavior disorder, recognizing that resumption of drug use is the rule rather than the exception.

FURTHER READING

CAMI J, FARRE M: Drug addiction. N Engl J Med 349:975, 2003
LYNSKEY MT et al: Escalation of drug use in early-onset cannabis users vs co-twin controls. JAMA 289:427, 2003
WEBER JE et al: Validation of a brief observation period for patients with cocaine-associated chest pain. N Engl J Med 348:510, 2003

375 | NICOTINE ADDICTION
David M. Burns

The use of tobacco leaf to create and satisfy nicotine addiction was introduced to Columbus by Native Americans and spread rapidly to Europe. The use of tobacco as cigarettes, however, is predominantly a twentieth century phenomenon, as is the epidemic of disease caused by this form of tobacco.

Nicotine is the principal constituent of tobacco responsible for its addictive character. Addicted smokers regulate their nicotine intake and blood levels by adjusting the frequency and intensity of their tobacco use both to obtain the desired psychoactive effects and avoid withdrawal.

Unburned cured tobacco contains nicotine, carcinogens, and other toxins capable of causing gum disease and oral cancer. When tobacco is burned, the resultant smoke contains, in addition to nicotine, carbon monoxide and 4000 other compounds that result from volatilization, pyrolysis, and pyrosynthesis of tobacco and various chemical additives

used in making different tobacco products. The smoke is composed of a fine aerosol, with a particle size distribution predominantly in the range to deposit in the airways and alveolar surfaces of the lungs, and a vapor phase. The bulk of the toxicity and carcinogenicity of the smoke resides in the aerosolized particulate phase, which contains a large number of toxic constituents and carcinogenic compounds. The aggregate of particulate matter, after subtracting nicotine and moisture, is referred to as tar. The vapor phase contains carbon monoxide, respiratory irritants, and ciliotoxins as well as many of the volatile compounds responsible for the distinctive smell of cigarette smoke.

The alkaline pH of smoke from blends of tobacco utilized for pipes and cigars allows sufficient absorption of nicotine across the oral mucosa to satisfy the smoker's need for this drug. Therefore, smokers of pipes and cigars tend not to inhale the smoke into the lung, confining the toxic and carcinogenic exposure (and the increased rates of disease) largely to the upper airway for most users of these products. The acidic pH of smoke generated by the tobacco used in cigarettes dramatically reduces absorption of nicotine in the mouth, necessitating inhalation of the smoke into the larger surface of the lungs in order to absorb quantities of nicotine sufficient to satisfy the smoker's addiction. The shift to using tobacco as cigarettes, with resultant increased deposition of smoke in the lung, has created the epidemic of heart disease, lung disease, and lung cancer that dominates the current disease manifestations of tobacco use.

GENETIC CONSIDERATIONS Several genes have been associated with nicotine addiction. Some reduce the clearance of nicotine, and others have been associated with an increased likelihood of becoming dependent on tobacco and other drugs as well as a higher incidence of depression. It is unlikely that genetic factors are the principal determinants of addiction. Rates of smoking initiation among males, and corresponding rates of nicotine addiction, have dropped by almost 50% since the mid-1950s, suggesting that factors other than genetics are important. It is more likely that genetic susceptibility influences the probability that experimentation with tobacco as an adolescent will lead to addiction as an adult.

DISEASE MANIFESTATIONS OF CIGARETTE SMOKING

Over 400,000 individuals die prematurely each year in the United States from cigarette use; this represents approximately one out of every five deaths in the United States. Approximately 40% of cigarette smokers will die prematurely due to cigarette smoking unless they are able to quit.

The major diseases caused by cigarette smoking are listed in Table 375-1. The incidence of smoking-related diseases is proportionately greater in younger than in older smokers, particularly for coronary artery disease and stroke. At older ages, the background rate of disease in nonsmokers increases, diminishing the fractional contribution of smoking and the relative risk; however, absolute excess rates of disease mortality found in smokers compared to nonsmokers increase with increasing age. The organ damage caused by smoking and the number of smokers who die from smoking are both greater among the elderly, as one would expect from a process of cumulative injury.

CARDIOVASCULAR DISEASES Cigarette smokers are more likely than nonsmokers to develop large-vessel atherosclerosis as well as small-vessel disease. Approximately 90% of peripheral vascular disease in the nondiabetic population can be attributed to cigarette smoking, as can ~50% of aortic aneurysms. In contrast, 20 to 30% of coronary artery disease and ~10% of occlusive cerebrovascular disease are caused by cigarette smoking. There is a multiplicative interaction between cig-

arette smoking and other cardiac risk factors such that the increment in risk produced by smoking among individuals with hypertension or elevated serum lipids is substantially greater than the increment in risk produced by smoking for individuals without these risk factors.

In addition to its role in promoting atherosclerosis, cigarette smoking also increases the likelihood of myocardial infarction and sudden cardiac death by promoting platelet aggregation and vascular occlusion. Reversal of these effects may explain the rapid benefit of smoking cessation for a new coronary event demonstrable among those who have survived a first myocardial infarction. This effect may also explain the substantially higher rates of graft occlusion among continuing smokers following vascular bypass surgery for cardiac or peripheral vascular disease, as well as the high failure rate of angioplasty procedures among continuing smokers.

Cessation of cigarette smoking reduces the risk of a second coronary event within 6 to 12 months; rates of first myocardial infarction or death from coronary heart disease also decline within the first few years following cessation. After 15 years of cessation, the risk of a new myocardial infarction or death from coronary heart disease in former smokers is similar to that for those who have never smoked.

CANCER Tobacco smoking causes cancer of the lung, oral cavity, naso-, oro-, and hypopharynx, nasal cavity and paranasal sinuses, larynx, esophagus, stomach, pancreas, liver, kidney (body and pelvis), ureter, urinary bladder, and uterine cervix and also causes myeloid leukemia. There is evidence suggesting that cigarette smoking may play a role in increasing the risk of colorectal and possibly breast cancer. There does not appear to be a causal link between cigarette smoking and cancer of the endometrium, and there is a lower risk of uterine cancer among postmenopausal women who smoke. The risks of cancer increase with the increasing number of cigarettes smoked per day and with increasing duration of smoking, and there are synergistic interactions between cigarette smoking and alcohol use for cancer of the oral cavity, esophagus, and possibly lung. Several occupational exposures also synergistically increase lung cancer risk among cigarette smokers, most notably occupational asbestos and radon exposure.

Cessation of cigarette smoking reduces the risk of developing cancer relative to continuing smoking, but even 20 years after cessation there is a modest persistent increased risk of developing lung cancer.

RESPIRATORY DISEASE Cigarette smoking is responsible for 90% of chronic obstructive pulmonary disease. Within 1 to 2 years of beginning to smoke regularly, many young smokers will develop inflammatory changes in their small airways, although lung function measures of these changes do not predict development of chronic airflow obstruction. After 20 years of smoking, pathophysiologic changes in the lungs develop and progress proportional to smoking intensity and duration. Chronic mucous hyperplasia of the larger airways results in a chronic productive cough in as many as 80% of smokers over age 60. Chronic inflammation and narrowing of the small airways and/or enzymatic digestion of alveolar walls resulting in pulmonary emphysema can result in reduced expiratory airflow sufficient to produce clinical symptoms of respiratory limitation in ~15% of smokers.

Changes in the small airways of young smokers will reverse after 1 to 2 years of cessation. There may also be a small increase in measures of expiratory airflow among individuals who have developed chronic airflow obstruction, but the major change following cessation is a slowing of the rate of decline in lung function with advancing age rather than a return of lung function toward normal.

PREGNANCY Cigarette smoking is associated with several maternal complications of pregnancy: premature rupture of membranes, abruptio placentae, and placenta previa; there is also a small increase in the risk of spontaneous abortion among smokers. Infants of smoking mothers are more likely to experience preterm delivery, have a higher perinatal mortality, are small for their gestational age, have higher rates of infant respiratory distress syndrome, are more likely to die of sudden infant death syndrome, and appear to have a developmental lag for at least the first several years of life.

TABLE 375-1 *Relative Risks for Current Smokers of Cigarettes*

Disease or Condition	Current Smokers Males	Current Smokers Females
Coronary heart disease		
Age 35–64	2.8	3.1
Age ≥65	1.5	1.6
Cerebrovascular lesions		
Age 35–64	3.3	4
Age ≥65	1.6	1.5
Aortic aneurysm	6.2	7.1
Chronic airways obstruction	10.6	13.1
Cancer		
Lip, oral cavity, pharynx	10.9	5.1
Esophagus	6.8	7.8
Stomach	2	1.4
Pancreas	2.3	2.3
Larynx	14.6	13
Lung	23.3	12.7
Cervix		1.6
Kidney	2.7	1.3
Bladder, other urinary organs	3.3	2.2
Sudden Infant Death syndrome		2.3
Infant respiratory distress syndrome		1.3
Low birth weight at delivery		1.8

OTHER CONDITIONS Smoking delays healing of peptic ulcers; increases the risk of osteoporosis, senile cataracts, and macular degeneration; and results in premature menopause, wrinkling of the skin, gallstones and cholecystitis in women, and male impotence.

ENVIRONMENTAL TOBACCO SMOKE Long-term exposure to environmental tobacco smoke increases the risk of lung cancer and coronary artery disease among nonsmokers. It also increases the incidence of respiratory infections, chronic otitis media, and asthma in children as well as causing exacerbation of asthma in children.

PHARMACOLOGIC INTERACTIONS

Cigarette smoking may interact with a variety of other drugs (Table 375-2). Cigarette smoking induces the cytochrome P450 system, which may alter the metabolic clearance of drugs such as theophylline. This may result in inadequate serum levels in smokers as outpatients when the dosage is established in the hospital under nonsmoking conditions. Correspondingly, serum levels may rise when smokers are hospitalized and not allowed to smoke. Smokers may also have higher first-pass clearance for drugs such as lidocaine, and the stimulant effects of nicotine may reduce the effect of benzodiazepines or beta blockers.

OTHER FORMS OF TOBACCO USE

Other major forms of tobacco use are moist snuff deposited between the cheek and gum, chewing tobacco, pipes and cigars, and recently bidi (tobacco wrapped in tendu or temburni leaf and commonly used in India) and clove cigarettes. Oral tobacco use leads to gum disease and can result in oral cancer. All forms of burned tobacco generate toxic and carcinogenic smoke similar to that of cigarette smoke. The differences in disease consequences of use relate to frequency of use and depth of inhalation. The risk of upper airway cancers is similar among cigarette and cigar smokers, while those who have smoked only cigars have a much lower risk of lung cancer, heart disease, and chronic obstructive pulmonary disease. However, cigarette smokers who switch to pipes or cigars do tend to inhale the smoke, increasing their risk; and it is likely that comparable inhalation and frequency of exposure to tobacco smoke from any of these forms of tobacco use will lead to comparable disease outcomes.

A resurgence of cigar and bidi use among adolescents of both genders has raised concerns that these older forms of tobacco use are once again causing a public health problem.

TABLE 375-2 *Interactions of Smoking and Prescription Drugs*

Drug	Interaction
Benzodiazepines	Less sedation
Beta blockers	Reduced lowering of heart rate and blood pressure
Caffeine	Faster metabolic clearance
Chlorpromazine	Decreased serum concentrations[a]
Clomipramine	Decreased serum concentrations[a]
Clozapine	Decreased serum concentrations[a]
Dextropropoxyphene	Less analgesia
Oral estrogens	Increased hepatic clearance
Flecainide	Increased first-pass clearance
Fluphenazine	Decreased serum concentrations[a]
Fluvoxamine	Decreased serum concentrations[a]
Haloperidol	Decreased serum concentrations[a]
Heparin	Faster clearance
Imipramine	Decreased serum concentrations[a]
Insulin	Delayed absorption due to skin vasoconstriction
Lidocaine	Increased first-pass clearance
Mexiletine	Increased first-pass clearance
Olanzapine	Faster clearance
Pentazocine	Less analgesia, possibly increased clearance
Propranolol	Increased first-pass clearance
Tacrine	Faster metabolic clearance
Theophylline	Faster metabolic clearance
Thiothixene	Faster metabolic clearance
Trazodone	Decreased serum concentrations[a]

[a] Clinical implication uncertain.

LOWER TAR AND NICOTINE CIGARETTES

Filtered cigarettes with lower machine-measured yields of tar and nicotine have been recommended as offering lower disease risks. However, these cigarettes commonly use ventilation holes in the filters and other engineering designs to artificially lower the machine measurements. Smokers, however, can compensate and preserve their intake of nicotine (and tar) by changing the manner in which they puff on the cigarette or the number of cigarettes smoked per day. There is no meaningful disease-reduction benefit for smokers who switch to lower-yield cigarettes, and smokers should be discouraged from thinking of low-yield cigarettes as an alternative to cessation.

CESSATION

The process of stopping smoking is often a cyclical one, with the smoker sometimes making multiple attempts to quit and failing before finally being successful. Approximately 70 to 80% of smokers would like to quit smoking, approximately one-third of current smokers attempt to quit each year, and 90% of these unassisted attempts fail. Clinician-based smoking interventions should encourage smokers to try to quit and to use different forms of cessation assistance with each new cessation attempt rather than focusing exclusively on immediate cessation at the time of the first visit.

Physician advice to quit smoking, particularly around an acute illness, is a powerful trigger for cessation attempts, with up to half of patients who are advised to quit making a cessation effort. Other triggers include the cost of cigarettes, media campaigns, and changes in rules to restrict smoking in the workplace.

PHYSICIAN INTERVENTION (Table 375-3)

All patients should be asked whether they smoke, their past experience with quitting, and whether they are currently interested in quitting. Those who are not interested in quitting should be encouraged and motivated to quit; provided a clear, strong, and personalized physician message that smoking is an important health concern; and offered assistance if they become interested in quitting in the future. There is a relationship between the amount of assistance a patient is willing to

TABLE 375-3 *Clinical Practice Guidelines*

Physician actions
Ask: Systematically identify all tobacco users at every visit
Advise: Strongly urge all smokers to quit
Identify smokers willing to quit
Assist the patient in quitting
Arrange follow-up contact

Pharmacologic interventions—first-line therapies
Nicotine gum (1.5)
Nicotine 24-h patch: 21-mg patch for 4 weeks, 14-mg patch for 2 weeks, and 7-mg patch for 2 weeks (1.9)
Nicotine nasal inhaler: one spray to each nostril 1–2 times/h for 3–6 months (2.7)
Nicotine oral inhaler: 6–16 puffs per day for up to 6 months (2.5)
Bupropion: 150 mg/d PO for 3 days followed by 150 mg bid for 7–12 weeks (2.1)

Pharmacologic interventions—second-line therapies
Clonidine: Initial dose 0.1 mg bid PO, or 0.1-mg transdermal patch, increasing to 0.15–0.75 mg/d PO or 0.2-mg patch for 3–10 weeks (2.1)
Nortriptyline: Initial dose 25 mg/d PO, increasing to 75–100 mg/d for 12 weeks (3.2)

Other interventions
Physician or other medical personnel counseling, 10 minutes (1.3)
Intensive smoking cessation program[a] (2.3)
Clinic-based smoking status identification system (3.1)
Counseling by nonclinicians and social support by family and friends
Telephone counseling (1.2)

Note: Numerical value in parentheses is the multiple for cessation success compared to no intervention.

[a] At least four to seven sessions of 20- to 30-min duration, lasting at least 2 weeks, preferably 8 weeks.

accept and the success of the cessation attempt. A quit date should be negotiated, usually not the day of the visit but within the next few weeks, and a follow-up contact by office staff around the time of the quit date should be provided.

There are a variety of nicotine-replacement products, including over-the-counter nicotine patch and gum, as well as nicotine nasal and oral inhalers available by prescription. Recently, antidepressants such as bupropion have also been shown to be effective; some evidence supports the combined use of nicotine-replacement therapy and antidepressants. Nicotine-replacement therapy is provided in different dosages. Clonidine or nortriptyline may be useful for patients who have failed on first-line pharmacologic treatment, or who are unable to use other therapies. Antidepressants are more effective in those with a history of depression symptoms.

Current recommendations are to offer pharmacologic treatment, usually with nicotine replacement therapy and bupropion, to all who will accept it and to provide counseling and other support as a part of the cessation attempt. Cessation advice alone by a physician or his or her staff is likely to increase success compared with no intervention; a more comprehensive approach with advice, pharmacologic assistance, and counseling can increase cessation success by almost threefold.

In order for physicians to incorporate cessation assistance into their practice successfully, it is essential to change the infrastructure in which the physician practices. The following are simple changes: (1) including questions on smoking and interest in cessation on patient-intake questionnaires, (2) asking patients whether they smoke as part of the initial vital sign measurements made by office staff, (3) listing smoking as a problem in the medical record, and (4) automating follow-up contact with the patient on the quit date. These changes are essential to institutionalizing smoking intervention within the practice setting; without this institutionalization, the best intentions of physicians to intervene with their patients who smoke are often lost in the time crush of a busy practice.

PREVENTION

Approximately 90% of individuals who will become cigarette smokers initiate the behavior during adolescence. Factors that promote adolescent initiation are parental or older generation cigarette smoking, tobacco advertising and promotional activities, the availability of cigarettes, and the social acceptability of smoking. The need for an enhanced self-image and to imitate adult behavior is greatest for those adolescents who have the least external validation of their self-worth, which may explain in part the enormous differences in adolescent smoking prevalence by socioeconomic and school performance strata.

Prevention of smoking initiation must begin early, preferably in the elementary school years. Physicians who treat adolescents should be sensitive to the prevalence of this problem. Physicians should ask all adolescents whether they have experimented with tobacco or currently use tobacco, reinforce the facts that most adolescents and adults do not smoke, and explain that all forms of tobacco are both addictive and harmful.

FURTHER READING

INTERNATIONAL AGENCY FOR RESEARCH ON CANCER: *Tobacco Smoke and Involuntary Smoking*. IARC Monographs on the Evaluation of Carcinogenic Risks to Humans. Lyon, France, vol 83, 2003

US DEPARTMENT OF HEALTH AND HUMAN SERVICES: *The Health Consequences of Tobacco Use: A Report of the Surgeon General*. National Center for Chronic Disease Prevention and Health Promotion, Office on Smoking and Health, 2003

———: *Treating Tobacco Use and Dependence*. Clinical Practice Guideline, Public Health Service, DHHS, 2000

376 HEAVY METAL POISONING
Howard Hu

Metals pose a significant threat to health through occupational as well as environmental exposures. One indication of their importance relative to other potential hazards is their ranking by the U.S. Agency for Toxic Substances and Disease Registry, which lists all hazards present in toxic waste sites according to their prevalence and the severity of their toxicity. The first, second, third, and sixth hazards on the list are heavy metals: lead, mercury, arsenic, and cadmium, respectively. Specific information pertaining to each of these metals, including sources and metabolism, toxic effects produced, diagnosis, and the appropriate treatment for poisoning, is summarized in Table 376-1.

Metals are inhaled primarily as dusts and fumes (the latter defined as tiny particles generated by combustion). Metal poisoning can also result from exposure to vapors (e.g., mercury vapor in creating dental amalgams). When metals are ingested in contaminated food or drink or by hand-to-mouth activity (implicated especially in children), their gastrointestinal absorption varies greatly with the specific chemical form of the metal and the nutritional status of the host. Once a metal is absorbed, blood is the main medium for its transport, with the precise kinetics dependent on diffusibility, protein binding, rates of biotransformation, availability of intracellular ligands, and other factors. Some organs (e.g., bone, liver, and kidney) sequester metals in relatively high concentrations for years. Most metals are excreted through renal clearance and gastrointestinal excretion; some proportion is also excreted through salivation, perspiration, exhalation, lactation, skin exfoliation, and loss of hair and nails. The intrinsic stability of metals

TABLE 376-1 *Heavy Metals*

Metal	Main Sources	Metabolism	Toxicity	Diagnosis	Treatment
Arsenic	Smelting and microelectronics industries; wood preservatives, pesticides, herbicides, fungicides; contaminant of deep-water wells; folk remedies; and coal; incineration of these products	Organic arsenic (arsenobentaine, arsenocholine) is ingested in seafood and fish, but is nontoxic; inorganic arsenic is readily absorbed (lung and GI); sequesters in liver, spleen, kidneys, lungs, and GI tract; residues persist in skin, hair, and nails; biomethylation results in detoxification, but this process saturates.	Acute arsenic poisoning results in necrosis of intestinal mucosa with hemorrhagic gastroenteritis, fluid loss, hypotension, delayed cardiomyopathy, acute tubular necrosis, and hemolysis. Chronic arsenic exposure causes diabetes, vasospasm, peripheral vascular insufficiency and gangrene, peripheral neuropathy, and cancer of skin, lung, liver (angiosarcoma), bladder, kidney. Lethal dose: 120–200 mg (adults); 2 mg/kg (children).	Nausea, vomiting, diarrhea, abdominal pain, delirium, coma, seizures; garlicky odor on breath; hyperkeratosis, hyperpigmentation, exfoliative dermatitis, and Mees' lines (transverse white striae of the fingernails); sensory and motor polyneuritis, distal weakness. Radiopaque sign on abdominal x-ray; ECG–QRS broadening, QT prolongation, ST depression, T-wave flattening; 24-h urinary arsenic >67 μmol/d or 50 μg/d; (no seafood × 24 h); if recent exposure, serum arsenic >0.9 μmol/L (7 μg/dL). High arsenic in hair or nails.	If acute ingestion, ipecac to induce vomiting, gastric lavage, activated charcoal with a cathartic. Supportive care in ICU. Dimercaprol 3–5 mg/kg IM q4h × 2 days; q6h × 1 day, then q12h × 10 days; alternative: oral succimer.
Cadmium	Metal-plating, pigment, smelting, battery, and plastics industries; tobacco; incineration of these products; ingestion of food that concentrates cadmium (grains, cereals).	Absorbed through ingestion or inhalation; bound by metallothionein, filtered at the glomerulus, but reabsorbed by proximal tubules (thus, poorly excreted). Biological ½ life: 10–30 y. Binds cellular sulfhydryl groups, competes with zinc, calcium for binding sites. Concentrates in liver and kidneys.	Acute cadmium inhalation causes pneumonitis after 4–24 h; acute ingestion causes gastroenteritis. Chronic exposure causes anosmia, yellowing of teeth, emphysema, minor LFT elevations, microcytic hypochromic anemia unresponsive to iron therapy, proteinuria, increased urinary β_2-microglobulin, calciuria, leading to chronic renal failure, osteomalacia, and fractures.	With inhalation: pleuritic chest pain, dyspnea, cyanosis, fever, tachycardia, nausea, noncardiogenic pulmonary edema. With ingestion: nausea, vomiting, cramps, diarrhea. Bone pain, fractures with osteomalacia. If recent exposure, serum cadmium >500 nmol/L (5 μg/dL). Urinary cadmium >100 nmol/L (10 μg/g creatinine) and/or urinary β_2-microglobulin >750 μg/g creatinine (but urinary β_2-microglobulin also increased in other renal diseases such as pyelonephritis).	There is no effective treatment for cadmium poisoning (chelation not useful; dimercaprol can exacerbate nephrotoxicity). Avoidance of further exposure, supportive therapy, vitamin D for osteomalacia.

(continued)

TABLE 376-1 Heavy Metals—(Continued)

Metal	Main Sources	Metabolism	Toxicity	Diagnosis	Treatment
Lead	Manufacturing of auto batteries, lead crystal, ceramics, fishing weights, etc.; demolition or sanding of lead-painted houses, bridges; stained glass making, plumbing, soldering; environmental exposure to paint chips, house dust (in home built <1975), firing ranges (from bullet dust), food or water from improperly glazed ceramics, lead pipes; contaminated herbal remedies, candies; exposure to the combustion of leaded fuels.	Absorbed through ingestion or inhalation; organic lead (e.g., tetraethyl lead) absorbed dermally. In blood, 95–99% sequestered in RBCs—thus, must measure lead in whole blood (not serum). Distributed widely in soft tissue, with ½ life ~30 days; 15% of dose sequestered in bone with ½ life of >20 years. Excreted mostly in urine, but also appears in other fluids including breast milk. Interferes with mitochondrial oxidative phosphorylation, ATPases, calcium-dependent messengers; enhances oxidation and cell apoptosis.	Acute exposure with blood lead levels (BPb) of > 60–80 μg/dL can cause impaired neurotransmission and neuronal cell death (with central and peripheral nervous system effects); impaired hematopoiesis and renal tubular dysfunction. At higher levels of exposure (e.g., BPb > 80–120 μg/dL), acute encephalopathy with convulsions, coma, and death may occur. Subclinical exposures in children (BPb 25–60 μg/dL) are associated with anemia; mental retardation; and deficits in language, motor function, balance, hearing, behavior, and school performance. Impairment of IQ appears to occur at even lower levels of exposure with no measurable threshold above the limit of detection in most assays of 1 μg/dL. In adults, chronic subclinical exposures (BPb > 40 μg/dL) are associated with an increased risk of anemia, demyelinating peripheral neuropathy (mainly motor), impairments of reaction time, hypertension, ECG conduction delays, interstitial nephritis and chronic renal failure, diminished sperm counts, spontaneous abortions.	Abdominal pain, irritability, lethargy, anorexia, anemia, Fanconi's syndrome, pyuria, azotemia in children with blood lead level (BPb) >80 μg/dL; may also see epiphyseal plate "lead lines" on long bone x-rays. Convulsions, coma at BPb > 120 μg/dL. Noticeable neurodevelopmental delays at BPb of 40–80 μg/dL; may also see symptoms associated with higher BPb levels. In the U.S., screening of all children when they begin to crawl (~6 months) is recommended by the CDC; source identification and intervention is begun if the BPb > 10 μg/dL. In adults, acute exposure causes similar symptoms as in children as well as headaches, arthralgias, myalgias, depression, impaired short-term memory, loss of libido. Physical exam may reveal a "lead line" at the gingiva-tooth border, pallor, wrist drop, and cognitive dysfunction (e.g., declines on the mini-mental status exam); lab tests may reveal a normocytic, normochromic anemia, basophilic stippling, an elevated blood protoporphyrin level (free erythrocyte or zinc), and motor delays on nerve conduction. In the U.S., OSHA requires regular testing of lead-exposed workers with removal if BPb > 40 μg/dL.	Identification and correction of exposure sources is critical. In some U.S. states, screening and reporting to local health boards of children with BPb > 10 μg/dL and workers with BPb > 40 μg/dL is required. In the highly exposed individual with symptoms, chelation is recommended with oral DMSA (succimer); if acutely toxic, hospitalization and IV or IM chelation with edentate calcium disodium (CaEDTA) may be required, with the addition of dimercaprol to prevent worsening of encephalopathy. It is uncertain whether children with asymptomatic lead exposure (e.g., BPb 20–40 μg/dL) benefit from chelation. Correction of dietary deficiencies in iron, calcium, magnesium, and zinc will lower lead absorption and may also improve toxicity. Vitamin C is a weak but natural chelating agent.

(continued)

facilitates tracing and measurement in biologic material, although the clinical significance of the levels measured is not always clear.

Some metals, such as copper and selenium, are essential to normal metabolic function as trace elements (Chap. 61) but are toxic at high levels of exposure. Others, such as lead and mercury, are xenobiotic and theoretically are capable of exerting toxic effects at any level of exposure. Indeed, much research is currently focused on the contribution of low-level xenobiotic metal exposure to chronic diseases and to subtle changes in health that may have significant public health consequences. Research has also begun to determine how genetic factors may modify the impact of metals on health and thereby account, at least in part, for individual susceptibility to metal effects.

The most important component of treatment for metal toxicity is the termination of exposure. *Chelating agents* are used to bind metals into stable cyclic compounds with relatively low toxicity and to enhance their excretion. The principal chelating agents are dimercaprol (British Anti-Lewisite, BAL), edetate (EDTA), succimer (DMSA, dimercaptosuccinic acid), and penicillamine; their specific use depends on the metal involved and the clinical circumstances. Activated charcoal does not bind metals and thus is of limited usefulness in cases of acute metal ingestion.

In addition to the information provided in Table 376-1, several other aspects of exposure, toxicity, or management are worthy of discussion with respect to the four most hazardous toxicants (arsenic, cadmium, lead, and mercury). *Arsenic* exposure from natural contamination of shallow tube wells inserted for drinking water is a huge environmental problem for millions of residents in parts of Bangladesh and Western India. Contamination was formerly considered only a

TABLE 376-1—(Continued)

Metal	Main Sources	Metabolism	Toxicity	Diagnosis	Treatment
Mercury	Metallic, mercurous, and mercuric mercury ($Hg°$, Hg^+, Hg^{2+}) exposures occur in some chemical, metal-processing, electrical-equipment, automotive industries; they are also in thermometers, dental amalgams, batteries. Mercury is dispersed by waste incineration. Environmental bacteria convert inorganic to organic mercury, which then bioconcentrates up the aquatic food chain to contaminate tuna, swordfish, and other pelagic fish.	Elemental mercury ($Hg°$) is not well absorbed; however, it will volatilize into highly absorbable vapor. Inorganic mercury is absorbed through the gut and skin. Organic mercury is well absorbed through inhalation and ingestion. Elemental and organic mercury cross the blood-brain barrier and placenta. Mercury is excreted in urine and feces and has a ½ life in blood of ~60 days; however, deposits will remain in the kidney and brain for years. Exposure to mercury stimulates the kidney to produce metallothionein, which provides some detoxification benefit. Mercury binds sulfhydryl groups and interferes with a wide variety of critical enzymatic processes.	Acute inhalation of $Hg°$ vapor causes pneumonitis and noncardiogenic pulmonary edema leading to death, CNS symptoms, and polyneuropathy. Chronic high exposure causes CNS toxicity (mercurial *erethism*; see diagnosis); lower exposures impair renal function, motor speed, memory, coordination. Acute ingestion of inorganic mercury causes gastroenteritis, the nephritic syndrome, or acute renal failure, hypertension, tachycardia, and cardiovascular collapse, with death at a dose of 10–42 mg/kg. Ingestion of organic mercury causes gastroenteritis, arrhythmias, and lesions in the basal ganglia, gray matter, and cerebellum at doses >1.7 mg/kg. High exposure during pregnancy causes derangement of fetal neuronal migration resulting in severe mental retardation. Mild exposures during pregnancy (from fish consumption) are associated with declines in neurobehavioral performance in offspring. Dimethylmercury, a compound only found in research labs, is "supertoxic"—a few drops of exposure via skin absorption or inhaled vapor can cause severe cerebellar degeneration and death.	Chronic exposure to metallic mercury vapor produces a characteristic intention tremor and mercurial *erethism*: excitability, memory loss, insomnia, timidity, and delirium ("mad as a hatter"). On neurobehavioral tests: decreased motor speed, visual scanning, verbal and visual memory, visuomotor coordination. Children exposed to mercury in any form may develop *acrodynia* ("pink disease"): flushing, itching, swelling, tachycardia, hypertension, excessive salivation or perspiration, irritability, weakness, morbilliform rashes, desquamation of palms and soles. Toxicity from elemental or inorganic mercury exposure begins when blood levels >180 nmol/L (3.6 μg/dL) and urine levels >0.7 μmol/L (15 μg/dL). Exposures that ended years ago may result in a >20-μg increase in 24-h urine after a 2-g dose of succimer. Organic mercury exposure is best measured by levels in blood (if recent) or hair (if chronic); CNS toxicity in children may derive from fetal exposures associated with maternal hair Hg > 30 nmol/g (6 μg/g).	Treat acute ingestion of mercuric salts with induced emesis or gastric lavage and polythiol resins (to bind mercury in the GI tract). Chelate with dimercaprol (up to 24 mg/kg per day IM in divided doses), DMSA (succimer), or penicillamine, with 5-day courses separated by several days of rest. If renal failure occurs, treat with peritoneal dialysis, hemodialysis, or extracorporeal regional complexing hemodialysis and succimer. Chronic inorganic mercury poisoning is best treated with *N*-acetyl penicillamine.

Note: GI, gastrointestinal; ECG, electrocardiogram; ICU, intensive care unit; LFT, liver function tests; RBC, red blood cell; IQ, intelligence quotient; CDC, Centers for Disease Control and Prevention; OSHA, Occupational Safety and Health Administration; CNS, central nervous system.

problem with deep wells; however, the geology of this region allows most residents only a few alternatives for potable drinking water. Serious *cadmium* poisoning from the contamination of food and water by mining effluents in Japan contributed to the 1946 outbreak of "itai-itai" ("ouch-ouch") disease, so named because of cadmium-induced bone toxicity that led to painful bone fractures. Modest exposures from environmental contamination near a smelter in Belgium were recently associated with a lower bone density, a higher incidence of fractures, and a faster decline in height in both men and women, effects that may be related to cadmium's calciuric effect on the kidney. Such research is creating concern that cadmium exposure may be contributing significantly to morbidity and mortality from osteoporosis in the general population.

Advances in our understanding of *lead* toxicity have recently benefited by the development of K-x-ray fluorescence (KXRF) instruments for making safe in vivo measurements of lead levels in bone (which, in turn, reflect cumulative exposure over many years, as opposed to blood lead levels, which mostly reflect recent exposure). High bone lead levels measured by KXRF have been linked to increased risk of hypertension in both men and women from an urban population. In addition, high maternal bone lead levels were found to predict lower birth weight, head circumference, birth length, and neurodevelopmental performance in offspring by age 2. The toxicity of low-level organic *mercury* exposure (as manifested by neurobehavioral performance) is of increasing concern based on studies of the offspring of mothers who ingested mercury-contaminated fish. However, current evidence has not supported the recent contention that ethyl mercury, used as a preservative in multiuse vaccines administered in early childhood, has played a significant role in causing neurodevelopmental problems such as autism.

Finally, a few additional metals deserve brief mention but are not covered in Table 376-1 because of the relative rarity of their being clinically encountered, or the uncertainty regarding their potential toxicities. *Aluminum* contributes to the encephalopathy in patients with severe renal disease who are undergoing dialysis (Chap. 332). High levels of aluminum are found in the neurofibrillary tangles in the cerebral cortex and hippocampus of patients with Alzheimer disease as well as in the drinking water and soil of areas with an unusually high incidence of Alzheimer disease. The experimental and epidemiologic evidence for the aluminum–Alzheimer's disease link is so far relatively weak, however, and it cannot be concluded that aluminum is a causal agent or a contributing factor in neurodegenerative disease. Hexavalent *chromium* is corrosive and sensitizing. Workers in the chromate and chrome pigment production industries have consistently had a greater risk of lung cancer. The introduction of *cobalt* chloride as a fortifier in beer led to outbreaks of fatal cardiomyopathy among heavy consumers. Occupational exposure (e.g., of miners, dry-battery manufacturers, and arc welders) to *manganese* can cause a Parkinsonian syndrome within 1 to 2 years, including gait disorders; postural instability; a masked, expressionless face; tremor; and psychiatric symptoms. With the introduction of methylcyclopentadienyl manganese tricarbonyl (MMT) as a gasoline additive, there is concern for the toxic potential of environmental manganese exposure. *Nickel* exposure induces an allergic response, and inhalation of nickel compounds with low aqueous solubility (e.g., nickel subsulfide and nickel oxide) in occupational settings is associated with an increased risk of lung cancer. Overexposure to *selenium* may cause local irritation of the respiratory system and eyes, gastrointestinal irritation, liver inflam-

mation, loss of hair, depigmentation, and peripheral nerve damage. Workers exposed to certain organic forms of *tin* (particularly trimethyl and triethyl derivatives) have developed psychomotor disturbances, including tremor, convulsions, hallucinations, and psychotic behavior.

Thallium, which is a component of some insecticides, metal alloys, and fireworks, is absorbed through the skin as well as by ingestion and inhalation. Severe poisoning follows a single ingested dose of >1 g or >8 mg/kg. Nausea and vomiting, abdominal pain, and hematemesis precede confusion, psychosis, organic brain syndrome, and coma. Thallium is radiopaque. Induced emesis or gastric lavage is indicated within 4 to 6 h of acute ingestion; Prussian blue prevents absorption and is given orally at 250 mg/kg in divided doses. Unlike other types of metal poisoning, thallium poisoning may be less severe when activated charcoal is used to interrupt its enterohepatic circulation. Other measures include forced diuresis, treatment with potassium chloride (which promotes renal excretion of thallium), and peritoneal dialysis.

FURTHER READING

ALFVÉN T et al: Low-level cadmium exposure and osteoporosis. J Bone Miner Res 15:1579, 2000

CENTENO JA et al: Pathology related to chronic arsenic exposure. Environ Health Perspect 110(Suppl 5):883, 2002

GRANDJEAN P et al: Neurotoxic risk caused by stable and variable exposure to methylmercury from seafood. Ambul Pediatr 3:18, 2003

MISRA UK: Thallium poisoning: Emphasis on early diagnosis and response to haemodialysis. Postgrad Med J 79:103, 2003

ROGAN WJ et al: The effect of chelation therapy with succimer on neuropsychological development in children exposed to lead. N Engl J Med 344:1421, 2001

377 POISONING AND DRUG OVERDOSAGE
Christopher H. Linden, Michael J. Burns

Poisoning refers to the development of dose-related adverse effects following exposure to chemicals, drugs, or other xenobiotics. To paraphrase Paracelsus, the dose makes the poison. In excessive amounts, substances that are usually innocuous, such as oxygen and water, can cause poisoning. Conversely, in small doses, substances commonly regarded as poisons, such as arsenic and cyanide, can be consumed without ill effect. There is, however, substantial individual variability in the response to, and disposition of, a given dose. Some of this variability is genetic, and some is acquired on the basis of enzyme induction or inhibition, or because of tolerance. Poisoning may be local (e.g., skin, eyes, or lungs) or systemic depending on the chemical and physical properties of the poison, its mechanism of action, and the route of exposure. The severity and reversibility of poisoning also depend on the functional reserve of the individual or target organ, which is influenced by age and preexisting disease.

EPIDEMIOLOGY About 5 million poison exposures occur in the United States each year. Most are acute, accidental, involve a single agent, occur in the home, result in minor or no toxicity, and involve children under 6 years of age. Pharmaceuticals are involved in 47% of exposures and 84% of serious or fatal poisonings. Accidental exposures can result from the improper use of chemicals at work or play; product mislabeling; label misreading; mistaken identification of unlabeled chemicals; uninformed self-medication; and dosing errors by nurses, parents, pharmacists, physicians, and the elderly. Excluding the recreational use of ethanol, attempted suicide is the most common reason for intentional exposure. Unintended poisonings may result from the intentional use of drugs for psychotropic effects (abuse) or excessive self-dosing (misuse).

About 5% of exposures require hospitalization. They account for 5 to 10% of all ambulance transports, emergency room visits, and

intensive care unit admissions. Up to 30% of psychiatric admissions are prompted by attempted suicide via overdosage. Overall, the mortality rate is low: 0.4% of all exposures. It is much higher (1 to 2%) in hospitalized patients with nonaccidental (suicidal) overdose, who account for the majority of serious poisonings. Acetaminophen is the pharmaceutical agent most often implicated in fatal poisoning. Overall, carbon monoxide is the leading cause of death from poisoning, but this is not reflected in hospital or poison center statistics because patients with such poisoning are typically dead when discovered and are referred directly to medical examiners.

DIAGNOSIS Although poisoning can mimic other illnesses, the correct diagnosis can usually be established by the history, physical examination, routine and toxicologic laboratory evaluations, and characteristic clinical course. The *history* should include the time, route, duration, and circumstances (location, surrounding events, and intent) of exposure; the name and amount of each drug, chemical, or ingredient involved; the time of onset, nature, and severity of symptoms; the time and type of first aid measures provided; and the medical and psychiatric history.

In many cases the victim is confused, comatose, unaware of an exposure, or unable or unwilling to admit to one. Suspicious circumstances include unexplained illness in a previously healthy person; a history of psychiatric problems (particularly depression); recent changes in health, economic status, or social relationships; and onset of illness while working with chemicals or after ingesting food, drink (especially ethanol), or medications. Patients who become ill soon after arriving from a foreign country or being arrested for criminal activity should be suspected of "body packing" or "body stuffing" (ingesting or concealing illicit drugs in a body cavity). Relevant history may be available from family, friends, paramedics, police, pharmacists, physicians, and employers, who should be questioned regarding the patient's habits, hobbies, behavior changes, available medications, and antecedent events. A search of clothes, belongings, and place of discovery may reveal a suicide note or a container of drugs or chemicals. The imprint code on pills and the label on chemical products may be used to identify the ingredients and potential toxicity of a suspected poison by consulting a reference text, a computerized database, the manufacturer, or a regional poison information center.

The *physical examination* should focus initially on the vital signs, cardiopulmonary system, and neurologic status. The neurologic examination should include documentation of neuromuscular abnormalities such as dyskinesia, dystonia, fasciculations, myoclonus, rigidity, tremors. The patient should also be examined for evidence of trauma and underlying illnesses. Focal neurologic findings are uncommon in poisoning, and their presence should prompt evaluation for a structural central nervous system (CNS) lesion. Examination of the eyes (for nystagmus, pupil size and reactivity), abdomen (for bowel activity and bladder size), and skin (for burns, bullae, color, warmth, moisture, pressure sores, and puncture marks) may reveal findings of diagnostic value. When the history is unclear, all orifices should be examined for the presence of chemical burns and drug packets. The odor of breath or vomitus and the color of nails, skin, or urine may provide diagnostic clues.

The diagnosis of poisoning in cases of unknown etiology primarily relies on pattern recognition. The first step is to assess the pulse, blood pressure, respiratory rate, temperature, and neurologic status and characterize the overall physiologic state as stimulated, depressed, discordant, or normal (Table 377-1). The next step is to consider the underlying causes of the observed physiologic state and attempt to identify a pathophysiologic pattern or toxic syndrome (*toxidrome*) based on further analysis of the vital signs and neurologic status, other physical findings, and the results of ancillary diagnostic tests. Assessing the severity of physiologic derangements (Table 377-2) is useful

in this regard and also for assessing the clinical course and response to treatment. The final step is to attempt to identify the particular agent involved by looking for unique or relatively poison-specific physical or ancillary test abnormalities. This approach is summarized below.

Increased pulse, blood pressure, respiratory rate, temperature, and neuromuscular activity characterize the stimulant toxidromes: sympathetic, anticholinergic, and hallucinogen poisoning and drug withdrawal (Table 377-1). Other features are noted in Table 377-2. Mydriasis, a characteristic feature of all stimulant toxidromes, is most marked in anticholinergic poisoning. This toxidrome is distinguished by the presence of hot, dry, flushed skin; decreased bowel sounds; and urinary retention (Table 377-3). Other stimulant toxidromes increase sympathetic activity and cause diaphoresis, pallor, and increased bowel activity with varying degrees of nausea, vomiting, abnormal distress, and occasionally diarrhea. The absolute and relative degree of vital sign changes and neuromuscular hyperactivity can help distinguish among stimulant toxidromes. Since sympathetics stimulate the peripheral nervous system more directly than do hallucinogens or drug withdrawal, markedly increased vital signs and organ ischemia suggest sympathetic poisoning. Findings helpful in suggesting the particular drug or class causing physiologic stimulation include reflex bradycardia from selective α-adrenergic stimulants (e.g., decongestants), hypotension from selective β-adrenergic stimulants (e.g., asthma therapeutics), limb ischemia from ergot alkaloids, nystagmus from phencyclidine and ketamine (the only physiologic stimulants that cause this finding), and delayed cardiac conduction from high doses

TABLE 377-1 *Differential Diagnosis of Poisoning Based on Physiologic State*

Stimulated	Depressed	Discordant	Normal
Sympathetics	Sympatholytics	Asphyxiants	Nontoxic exposure
Sympathomimetics	α_1-Adrenergic antagonists	Cytochrome oxidase inhibitors	Psychogenic illness
Ergot alkaloids	α_2-Adrenergic agonists	Inert gases	Toxic time-bombs
Methylxanthines	ACE inhibitors	Irritant gases	Slow absorption
Monoamine oxidase inhibitors	Angiotensin receptor blockers	Methemoglobin inducers	Anticholinergics
Thyroid hormones	Antipsychotics	Oxidative phosphorylation inhibitors	Carbamazepine
Anticholinergics	β-adrenergic blockers	AGMA inducers	Concretion formers
Antihistamines	Calcium channel blockers	Alcohol (ketoacidosis)	Dilantin Kapseals
Antiparkinsonian agents	Cardiac glycosides	Ethylene glycol	Drug packets
Antipsychotics	Cyclic antidepressants	Iron	Enteric-coated pills
Antispasmodics	Cholinergics	Methanol	Lomotil
Belladonna alkaloids	Acetylcholinesterase inhibitors	Salicylate	Opioids
Cyclic antidepressants	Muscarinic agonists	Toluene	Salicylates
Muscle relaxants	Nicotinic agonists	CNS syndromes	Sustained-release pills
Mushrooms and plants	Opioids	Extrapyramidal reactions	Slow distribution
Hallucinogens	Analgesics	Hydrocarbon inhalation	Cardiac glycosides
Cannabinoids (marijuana)	GI antispasmodics	Isoniazid	Lithium
LSD and analogues	Heroin	Lithium	Metals
Mescaline and analogues	Sedative-hypnotics	Neuroleptic malignant syndrome	Salicylate
Mushrooms	Alcohols	Serotonin syndrome	Toxic metabolite
Phencyclidine and analogues	Anticonvulsants	Strychnine	Acetaminophen
Withdrawal syndromes	Barbiturates	Membrane-active agents	Carbon tetrachloride
Barbiturates	Benzodiazepines	Amantidine	Cyanogenic glycosides
Benzodiazepines	GABA precursors	Antiarrhythmics	Ethylene glycol
Ethanol	Muscle relaxants	Antihistamines	Methanol
Opioids	Other agents	Antipsychotics	Methemoglobin inducers
Sedative-hypnotics		Carbamazepine	Mushroom toxins
Sympatholytics		Cyclic antidepressants	Organophosphate insecticides
		Local anesthetics	Paraquat
		Opioids (some)	Metabolism disruptors
		Orphenadrine	Antineoplastic agents
		Quinoline antimalarials	Antiviral agents
			Colchicine
			Hypoglycemic agents
			Immunosuppressive agents
			MAO inhibitors
			Metals
			Salicylate
			Warfarins

Note: ACE, angiotensin-converting enzyme; AGMA, anion-gap metabolic alkalosis; GI, gastrointestinal; CNS, central nervous system; LSD, lysergic acid diethylamide; GABA, γ-aminobutyric acid; MAO; monoamine oxidase.

TABLE 377-2 *Severity of Physiologic Stimulation and Depression in Poisoning and Drug Withdrawal*

PHYSIOLOGIC STIMULATION

Grade 1	Anxious, irritable, tremulous; vital signs normal; diaphoresis, flushing or pallor, mydriasis, and hyperreflexia may be present
Grade 2	Agitated; may have confusion or hallucinations but is able to converse and follow commands; vital signs mildly to moderately increased
Grade 3	Delirious; unintelligible speech, uncontrollable motor hyperactivity; moderately to markedly increased vital signs; tachyarrhythmias possible
Grade 4	Coma, seizures, cardiovascular collapse

PHYSIOLOGIC DEPRESSION

Grade 1	Awake, lethargic, or sleeping but arousable by voice or tactile stimulation; able to converse and follow commands; may be confused
Grade 2	Responds to pain but not voice; can vocalize but not converse; spontaneous motor activity present; brainstem reflexes intact
Grade 3	Unresponsive to pain; spontaneous motor activity absent; brainstem reflexes depressed; motor tone, respirations, and temperature decreased
Grade 4	Unresponsive to pain; flaccid paralysis; brainstem reflexes and respirations absent; cardiovascular vital signs decreased

of cocaine and some anticholinergic agents (e.g., antihistamines, cyclic antidepressants, and antipsychotics). Seizures suggest a sympathetic etiology, an anticholinergic agent with membrane-active properties (e.g., cyclic antidepressants, orphenadrine, phenothiazines), or a withdrawal syndrome. Other manifestations of grade 4 physiologic stimulation (Table 377-2) are likely only in sympathetic poisoning.

Decreased pulse, blood pressure, respiratory rate, temperature, and neuromuscular activity are indicative of physiologic depression caused by "functional" sympatholytics (agents that decrease cardiac function and vascular tone as well as symthathetic activity), cholinergic (muscarinic and nicotinic) agents, opioids, and sedative-hypnotic [γ-aminobutyric acid (GABA)-ergic] agents (Tables 377-1 and 377-2). Miosis is also common and most pronounced in opioid and cholinergic poisoning. The latter is distinguished from other depressant toxidromes by the presence of muscarinic and nicotinic signs and symptoms (Table 377-3). Pronounced cardiovascular depression in the absence of significant CNS depression suggests a direct or peripherally acting sympatholytic. In contrast, in opioid and sedative-hypnotic poisoning, vital sign changes are secondary to depression of CNS cardiovascular and respiratory centers (or consequent hypoxemia) and significant abnormalities in these parameters do not occur until there is a marked decrease in the level of consciousness (grade 3 or 4 physiologic depression, Table 377-2). Other clues that suggest the cause of physiologic depression include cardiac arrhythmias and conduction disturbances (due to antiarrhythmics, β-adrenergic antagonists, calcium-channel blockers, digitalis glycosides, propoxyphene, and cyclic antidepressants), mydriasis (due to tricyclic antidepressants, some antiarrhythmics, meperidine, and Lomotil), nystagmus (due to sedative-hypnotics), and seizures (due to cholinergic agents, propoxyphene, cyclic antidepressants).

Discordant or mixed vital sign and neuromuscular abnormalities are characteristic of poisoning by asphyxiants, CNS syndromes, membrane-active agents, and anion-gap metabolic acidosis (AGMA) inducers (Table 377-1). In these conditions, manifestations of physiologic stimulation and physiologic depression occur together or at different times during the clinical course. For example, membrane-active agents can cause simultaneous coma, seizures, hypotension, and tachyarrhythmias. Alternatively, vital signs may be normal but the patient has altered mental status or is obviously sick or clearly symptomatic. Early, pro-

nounced vital sign and mental status changes suggest asphyxiant or membrane-active agent poisoning; the lack of such abnormalities suggests an AGMA inducer, and marked neuromuscular dysfunction without significant vital sign abnormalities suggests a CNS syndrome. As noted below, AGMA inducer poisoning can be distinguished from other causes of AGMA by the serum lactate concentration.

A normal physiologic status and physical examination may be due to a nontoxic exposure, psychogenic illness, or poisoning by "toxic time-bombs," agents that are slowly absorbed, slowly distributed to their sites of action, require metabolic activation, or disrupt metabolic processes (Table 377-1). Diagnosing a nontoxic exposure requires that the identity of the exposure agent be known or that a toxic time-bomb exposure has been excluded and that the time since exposure exceeds the longest known or predicted interval between exposure and peak toxicity. Psychogenic illness (fear of being poisoned, mass hysteria) may also occur after a nontoxic exposure and should be considered when symptoms are inconsistent with the exposure history. Anxiety reactions resulting from a nontoxic exposure can cause mild physiologic stimulation (Table 377-2) and be indistinguishable from toxicologic causes (Table 377-1) without ancillary testing or a suitable period of observation.

Laboratory assessment may be helpful in the differential diagnosis (Fig. 377-1). An increased AGMA is characteristic of advanced methanol, ethylene glycol, and salicylate intoxication but can occur with other agents (Table 377-1) and in any poisoning that results in hepatic, renal, or respiratory failure; seizures; or shock. The serum lactate concentration is low (less than the anion gap) in the former and high (nearly equal to the anion gap) in the latter. An abnormally low anion gap can be due to elevated blood levels of bromide, calcium, iodine, lithium, magnesium, or nitrate. An increased osmolal gap—a difference between the serum osmolality (measured by freezing point depression) and that calculated from the serum sodium, glucose, and blood urea nitrogen of >10 mmol/L—suggests the presence of a low-

TABLE 377-3 *Fundamentals of Poisoning Management*

SUPPORTIVE CARE

Airway protection	Treatment of seizures
Oxygenation/ventilation	Correction of temperature abnormalities
Treatment of arrhythmias	Correction of metabolic derangements
Hemodynamic support	Prevention of secondary complications

PREVENTION OF FURTHER POISON ABSORPTION

Gastrointestinal decontamination	Decontamination of other sites
Syrup of ipecac–induced emesis	Eye decontamination
Gastric lavage	Skin decontamination
Activated charcoal	Body cavity evacuation
Whole-bowel irrigation	
Catharsis	
Dilution	
Endoscopic/surgical removal	

ENHANCEMENT OF POISON ELIMINATION

Multiple-dose activated charcoal	Extracorporeal removal
Forced diuresis	Peritoneal dialysis
Alteration of urinary pH	Hemodialysis
Chelation	Hemoperfusion
	Hemofiltration
	Plasmapheresis
	Exchange transfusion
	Hyperbaric oxygenation

ADMINISTRATION OF ANTIDOTES

Neutralization by antibodies	Metabolic antagonism
Neutralization by chemical binding	Physiologic antagonism

PREVENTION OF REEXPOSURE

Adult education	Notification of regulatory agencies
Child-proofing	Psychiatric referral

molecular-weight solute such as acetone, an alcohol (benzyl, ethanol, isopropanol, methanol), a glycol (diethylene, ethylene, propylene), ether (ethyl, glycol), or an "unmeasured" cation (calcium, magnesium) or sugar (glycerol, mannitol, sorbitol). Ketosis suggests acetone, isopropyl alcohol, or salicylate poisoning. Hypoglycemia may be due to poisoning with β-adrenergic blockers, ethanol, insulin, oral hypoglycemic agents, quinine, and salicylates, whereas hyperglycemia can occur in poisoning with acetone, β-adrenergic agonist, caffeine, calcium channel blockers, iron, theophylline, or Vacor. Hypokalemia can be caused by barium, β-adrenergic agonists, caffeine, diuretics, theophylline, or toluene; hyperkalemia suggests poisoning with an α-adrenergic agonist, a β-adrenergic blocker, cardiac glycosides, or fluoride. Hypocalcemia may be seen in ethylene glycol, fluoride, and oxalate poisoning.

The *electrocardiogram* (ECG) can sometimes be useful for diagnostic purposes. Bradycardia and atrioventricular block may occur in patients poisoned by α-adrenergic agonists, antiarrhythmic agents, beta blockers, calcium channel blockers, cholinergic agents (carbamate and organophosphate insecticides), cardiac glycosides, lithium, magnesium, or tricyclic antidepressants. QRS- and QT-interval prolongation may be caused by hyperkalemia and by membrane-active drugs (Table 377-1). Ventricular tachyarrhythmias may be seen in poisoning with cardiac glycosides, fluorides, membrane-active drugs, methylxanthines, sympathomimetics, and agents that cause hyperkalemia or potentiate the effects of endogenous catecholamines (e.g., chloral hydrate, aliphatic and halogenated hydrocarbons).

Radiologic studies may also be useful. Pulmonary edema (adult respiratory distress syndrome, or ARDS) can be caused by poisoning with carbon monoxide, cyanide, an opioid, paraquat, phencyclidine, a sedative-hypnotic, or salicylate; by inhalation of irritant gases, fumes, or vapors (acids and alkali, ammonia, aldehydes, chlorine, hydrogen sulfide, isocyanates, metal oxides, mercury, phosgene, polymers); or by prolonged anoxia, hyperthermia, or shock. Aspiration pneumonia is common in patients with coma, seizures, and petroleum distillate ingestion. The presence of radiopaque densities on abdominal x-rays suggests the ingestion of calcium salts, chloral hydrate, chlorinated hydrocarbons, heavy metals, illicit drug packets, iodinated compounds, potassium salts, psychotherapeutic agents, lithium, phenothiazines, enteric-coated tablets, or salicylates.

Toxicologic analysis of urine and blood (and occasionally of gastric contents and chemical samples) can sometimes confirm or rule out suspected poisoning. Interpretation of laboratory data requires knowledge of the tests used for screening and confirmation (thin-layer, gas-liquid, or high-performance liquid chromatography; colorimetric and fluorometric assays; enzyme-multiplied, fluorescence polarization, and radioimmunoassays; gas chromatography; mass spectrometry), their sensitivity (limit of detection) and specificity, the preferred biologic specimen for analysis, and the optimal time of specimen sampling. Personal communication with the laboratory is essential. A negative result may mean the substance is not detectable by the test used or that its concentration is too low for detection at the time of sampling. In the latter case, repeating the test at a later time may yield a positive result.

Although rapid screening tests for a limited number of drugs of abuse are available, comprehensive screening tests require 2 to 6 h for completion, and immediate management must often be based on the history, physical examination, and routine ancillary tests. In addition, when the patient is asymptomatic, or when the clinical picture is consistent with the reported history, qualitative screening is neither clinically useful nor cost-effective. It is of greatest value in patients with severe or unexplained toxicity such as coma, seizures, cardiovascular instability, metabolic or respiratory acidosis, and non-sinus cardiac rhythms. Quantitative analysis is useful for poisoning with acetaminophen (Chap.

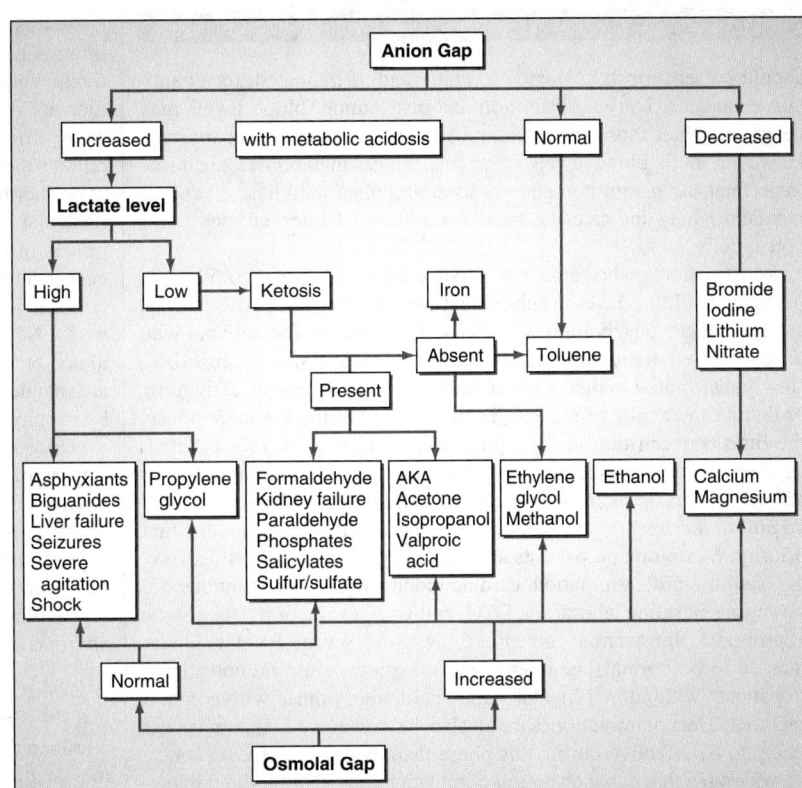

FIGURE 377-1 Differential diagnosis of poisoning based on the results of routine laboratory tests. AKA, alcoholic ketoacidosis; biguanides, metformin, phenformin.

286), acetone, alcohols (including ethylene glycol), antiarrhythmics, anticonvulsants, barbiturates, digoxin, heavy metals, lithium, paraquat, salicylate, and theophylline, as well as for carboxyhemoglobin and methemoglobin. Results can often be available within an hour.

The *response to antidotes* may be useful for diagnostic purposes. Resolution of altered mental status and abnormal vital signs within minutes of intravenous administration of dextrose, naloxone, or flumazenil is virtually diagnostic of hypoglycemia, narcotic poisoning, and benzodiazepine intoxication, respectively. The prompt reversal of dystonic (extrapyramidal) signs and symptoms following an intravenous dose of benztropine or diphenhydramine confirms a drug etiology. Although the reversal of both central and peripheral manifestations of anticholinergic poisoning by physostigmine is diagnostic of this condition, physostigmine may cause arousal in patients with CNS depression of any etiology.

Rx TREATMENT

General Principles Treatment goals include support of vital signs, prevention of further poison absorption, enhancement of poison elimination, administration of specific antidotes, and prevention of reexposure (Table 377-3). Specific treatment depends on the identity of the poison, the route and amount of exposure, the time of presentation relative to the time of exposure, and the severity of poisoning. Knowledge of the offending agents' pharmacokinetics and pharmacodynamics is essential.

During the *pretoxic phase*, prior to the onset of poisoning, decontamination is the highest priority, and treatment is based solely on the history. The maximum potential toxicity based on the greatest possible exposure should be assumed. Since decontamination is more effective when accomplished soon after exposure, the initial history and physical examination should be focused and brief. It is also advisable to establish intravenous access and initiate cardiac monitoring, particularly in patients with potentially serious ingestions or unclear histories.

When an accurate history is not obtainable and a poison causing delayed toxicity or irreversible damage is suspected, blood and urine should be sent for toxicologic screening and, if indicated, for quantitative analysis. During absorption and distribution, blood levels may be greater than those in tissue and may not correlate with toxicity. However, high blood levels of agents whose metabolites are more toxic than the parent compound (acetaminophen, ethylene glycol, or methanol) may indicate the need for additional interventions (antidotes, dialysis).

Most patients who remain or become asymptomatic 4 to 6 h after ingestion will not develop subsequent toxicity and can be discharged safely. Longer observation will likely be necessary for patients who have ingested toxic time-bombs, agents that are slowly absorbed, slowly distributed to their sites of action, require metabolic activation, or disrupt metabolic processes (Table 377-1). During the *toxic phase*, the time between the onset of poisoning and the peak effects, management is based primarily on clinical and laboratory findings. *Effects after an overdose begin sooner, peak later, and last longer than they do after a therapeutic dose.* Resuscitation and stabilization are the first priority. Symptomatic patients should have an intravenous line, oxygen saturation determination, cardiac monitoring, and continuous observation. Baseline laboratory, ECG, and x-ray evaluation may also be appropriate. Intravenous glucose (unless the serum level is documented to be normal), naloxone, and thiamine should be considered in patients with altered mental status, particularly those with coma or seizures. Decontamination should also be considered, but it is less likely to be effective during this phase than during the pretoxic one.

Measures that enhance poison elimination may shorten the duration of toxicity and lessen its severity. However, they are not without risk, which must be weighed against the potential benefit. Diagnostic certainty (usually via laboratory confirmation) is generally a prerequisite. Intestinal dialysis with repetitive doses of activated charcoal is usually safe and can enhance the elimination of many poisons. Diuresis, urinary alkalinization, and chelation therapy enhance the elimination of a relatively small number of poisons, and their use is associated with potential complications. Extracorporeal elimination methods are effective for many poisons, but their expense and risk make their use reasonable only in patients who would otherwise have an unfavorable outcome.

During the *resolution phase* of poisoning, supportive care and monitoring should continue until clinical, laboratory, and ECG abnormalities have resolved. Since chemicals are eliminated sooner from the blood than from tissues, blood levels are usually lower than tissue levels during this phase and again may not correlate with toxicity. This is particularly true when extracorporeal elimination procedures are used. Redistribution from tissues may cause a rebound increase in the blood level after termination of these procedures. When a metabolite is responsible for toxic effects, continued treatment might be necessary in the absence of clinical toxicity.

Supportive Care The goal of supportive therapy is to maintain physiologic homeostasis until detoxification is accomplished and to prevent and treat secondary complications such as aspiration, bedsores, cerebral and pulmonary edema, pneumonia, rhabdomyolysis, renal failure, sepsis, thromboembolic disease, coagulopathy, and generalized organ dysfunction due to hypoxia or shock.

Admission to an intensive care unit is indicated for the following: patients with severe poisoning (coma, respiratory depression, hypotension, cardiac conduction abnormalities, cardiac arrhythmias, hypothermia or hyperthermia, seizures); those needing close monitoring, antidotes, or enhanced elimination therapy; those showing progressive clinical deterioration; and those with significant underlying medical problems. Patients with mild to moderate toxicity can be managed on a general medical service, intermediate care unit, or emergency department observation area, depending on the anticipated duration and level of monitoring needed (intermittent clinical observation versus continuous clinical, cardiac, and respiratory monitoring). Patients who have attempted suicide require continuous observation and measures to prevent self-injury until they are no longer suicidal.

RESPIRATORY CARE Endotracheal intubation for protection against the aspiration of gastrointestinal contents is of paramount importance in patients with CNS depression or seizures as this complication can increase morbidity and mortality. Mechanical ventilation may be necessary for patients with respiratory depression or hypoxia and to facilitate therapeutic sedation or paralysis in order to prevent or treat hyperthermia, acidosis, and rhabdomyolysis associated with neuromuscular hyperactivity. Since clinical assessment of respiratory function is often inaccurate, the need for oxygenation and ventilation is best determined by oximetry or arterial blood gas analysis. The gag reflex is not a reliable indicator of the need for intubation. A patient with CNS depression may maintain airway patency while being stimulated but not if left alone. Those who cannot respond to voice or who are unable to sit and drink fluids without assistance are best managed by prophylactic intubation.

Drug-induced pulmonary edema is usually noncardiac rather than cardiac in origin although profound CNS depression and cardiac conduction abnormalities suggest the latter. Measurement of pulmonary artery pressure may be necessary to establish the cause and direct appropriate therapy. Extracorporeal measures (membrane oxygenation, venoarterial perfusion, cardiopulmonary bypass), partial liquid (perfluorocarbon) ventilation, and hyperbaric oxygen therapy may be appropriate for severe but reversible respiratory failure.

CARDIOVASCULAR THERAPY Maintenance of normal tissue perfusion is critical for complete recovery to occur once the offending agent has been eliminated. If hypotension is unresponsive to volume expansion, treatment with norepinephrine, epinephrine, or high-dose dopamine may be necessary. Intraaortic balloon pump counterpulsation and venoarterial or cardiopulmonary perfusion techniques should be considered for severe but reversible cardiac failure. Bradyarrhythmias associated with hypotension generally should be treated as described in Chap. 213. Glucagon, calcium, and high-dose insulin with dextrose may be effective in both beta blocker and calcium channel blocker poisoning. Antibody therapy may be indicated for cardiac glycoside poisoning.

Supraventricular tachycardia associated with hypertension and CNS excitation is almost always due to agents that cause generalized physiologic excitation (Table 377-1). Most cases are mild or moderate in severity and require only observation or nonspecific sedation with a benzodiazepine. In severe cases or those associated with hemodynamic instability, chest pain, or ECG evidence of ischemia, specific therapy is indicated. When the etiology is sympathetic hyperactivity, treatment with a combined alpha and beta blocker (labetalol), a calcium channel blocker (verapamil or diltiazem), or a combination of a beta blocker and a vasodilator (esmolol and nitroprusside) is preferred. Treatment with an α-adrenergic antagonist (phentolamine) alone may sometimes be appropriate. If the cause is anticholinergic poisoning, physostigmine is the treatment of choice. Supraventricular tachycardia without hypertension is generally secondary to vasodilation or hypovolemia and responds to fluid administration.

Lidocaine and phenytoin are generally safe for ventricular tachyarrhythmias of any etiology. Beta blockers can be hazardous if the arrhythmia is due to sympathetic hyperactivity. For ventricular tachyarrhythmias due to tricyclic antidepressants and probably other membrane-active agents (Table 377-1), class IA, IC, and III antiarrhythmic agents are contraindicated (because of similar electrophysiologic effects), but sodium bicarbonate may be helpful. Magnesium sulfate and overdrive pacing (by isoproterenol or a pacemaker) may be useful in patients with torsades de pointes and prolonged QT intervals. Magnesium and anti-digoxin antibodies should be considered in patients with severe cardiac glycoside poisoning. Invasive (esophageal or intracardiac) ECG recording may be necessary to determine the origin (ventricular or supraventricular) of wide-complex tachycardias (Chap. 214). If the patient is hemodynamically stable, however, it is reasonable to simply observe them rather than to administer another potentially proarrhythmic agent. Arrhythmias may be resistant to drug therapy until underlying acid-base, electrolyte, oxygenation, and temperature derangements are corrected.

CENTRAL NERVOUS SYSTEM THERAPIES Neuromuscular hyperactivity and seizures can lead to hyperthermia, lactic acidosis, and rhabdomyolysis, with their attendant complications, and should be treated aggressively. Seizures caused by excessive stimulation of catecholamine receptors (sympathomimetic or hallucinogen poisoning and drug withdrawal), or decreased activity of GABA (isoniazid poisoning) or glycine (strychnine poisoning) receptors are best treated with agents that enhance GABA activity such as benzodiazepine or barbiturates. Since benzodiazepines and barbiturates act by slightly different mechanisms (the former increases the frequency and the latter increases the duration of chloride channel opening in response to GABA), therapy with both may be effective when neither is effective alone. Seizures caused by isoniazid, which inhibits the synthesis of GABA, may require high doses of pyridoxine (which facilitates the synthesis of GABA). Those resulting from membrane destabilization (beta blocker or cyclic antidepressant poisoning) may require a membrane-active anticonvulsant such as phenytoin as well as GABA enhancers. For poisons with central dopaminergic effects (phencyclidine), a dopamine receptor antagonist, such as haloperidol, may be useful. In anticholinergic and cyanide poisoning, specific antidotal therapy may be necessary. The treatment of seizures secondary to cerebral ischemia or edema, or to metabolic abnormalities should include correction of the underlying cause. Neuromuscular paralysis is indicated in refractory cases. Electroencephalographic monitoring and continuing treatment of seizures are necessary to prevent permanent neurologic damage.

OTHER MEASURES Temperature extremes, metabolic abnormalities, hepatic and renal dysfunction, and secondary complications should be treated by standard therapies.

Prevention of Poison Absorption ■ *GASTROINTESTINAL DECONTAMINATION* Whether or not to perform gastrointestinal decontamination, and which procedure to use, depends on the time since ingestion; the existing and predicted toxicity of the ingestant; the availability, efficacy, and contraindications of the procedure; and the nature, severity, and risk of complications. The efficacy of activated charcoal, gastric lavage, and syrup of ipecac decreases with time, and there are insufficient data to support or exclude a beneficial effect when they are used more than 1 h after ingestion. The average time from ingestion to presentation for treatment is >1 h for children and >3 h for adults. Most patients will recover from poisoning uneventfully with good supportive care alone, but complications of gastrointestinal decontamination, particularly aspiration, can prolong this process. Hence, gastrointestinal decontamination should be performed selectively, not routinely, in the management of overdose patients. It is clearly unnecessary when predicted toxicity is minimal or the time of expected maximal toxicity has passed without significant effect.

Activated charcoal has comparable or greater efficacy, fewer contraindications and complications, is less aversive and invasive than ipecac or gastric lavage, and thus is the preferred method of gastrointestinal decontamination in most situations. Activated charcoal suspension (in water) is given orally via a cup, straw, or small-bore nasogastric tube. The recommended dose is 1 g/kg body weight. Palatability may be increased by adding a sweetener (sorbitol) or a flavoring agent (cherry, chocolate, or cola syrup) to the suspension. Charcoal adsorbs ingested poisons within the gut lumen, allowing the charcoal-toxin complex to be evacuated with stool. The complex can also be removed from the stomach by induced emesis or lavage. In vitro, charcoal adsorbs ≥90% of most substances when given in an amount equal to 10 times the weight of the substance. Charged (ionized) chemicals such as mineral acids, alkalis, and highly dissociated salts of cyanide, fluoride, iron, lithium, and other inorganic compounds are not well adsorbed by charcoal. In animal and human volunteer studies, charcoal decreases the absorption of ingestants by an average of 73% when given within 5 min of ingestant administration, 51% when given at 30 min, and 36% at 60 min. Side effects of charcoal include nausea, vomiting, and diarrhea or constipation. Charcoal may also prevent the absorption of orally administered therapeutic agents.

Complications include mechanical obstruction of the airway, aspiration, vomiting, and bowel obstruction and infarction caused by inspissated charcoal. Charcoal is not recommended for patients who have ingested corrosives because it obscures endoscopy.

Gastric lavage is performed by sequentially administering and aspirating about 5 mL fluid per kilogram of body weight through a no. 40 French orogastric tube (no. 28 French tube for children). Except for infants, where normal saline is recommended, tap water is acceptable. The patient should be placed in Trendelenburg and left lateral decubitus positions to prevent aspiration (even if an endotracheal tube is in place). Lavage decreases ingestant absorption by an average of 52% if performed within 5 min of ingestion administration, 26% if performed at 30 min, and 16% if performed at 60 min. Its efficacy is similar to that of ipecac. Significant amounts of ingested drug are recovered in ~10% of patients. Aspiration is a common complication (occurring in up to 10% of patients), especially when lavage is perfomed improperly. Serious complications (esophageal and gastric perforation, tube misplacement in the trachea) occur in ~1% of patients. For this reason, the physician should personally insert the lavage tube and confirm its placement, and the patient must be cooperative or adequately restrained (with pharmacologic sedation if necessary) during the procedure. Gastric lavage is contraindicated in corrosive or petroleum distillate ingestions because of the respective risks of gastroesophageal perforation and aspiration pneumonitis. It is also contraindicated in those with a compromised unprotected airway and those at risk for hemorrhage or perforation due to esophageal or gastric pathology or recent surgery.

Syrup of ipecac can be used for the home management of patients with accidental ingestions, reliable histories, and mild predicted toxicity. It may delay the administration and decrease the effectiveness of activated charcoal, oral antidotes, and whole-bowel irrigation and is rarely appropriate for patients treated at a health care facility. It is administered orally in a dose of 30 mL for adults, 15 mL for children, and 10 mL for small infants. Clear liquids should also be given. Ipecac irritates the stomach and stimulates the central chemoreceptor trigger zone. Vomiting usually occurs about 20 min after administration. The dose may be repeated if vomiting does not occur. In animal and human volunteer studies, ipecac decreases ingestant absorption by an average of 60% if given within 5 min of ingestant administration, 32% if given at 30 min, and 30% if given at 60 min. Side effects include lethargy in children (12%) and protracted vomiting (8 to 17%). Chronic ipecac use (by patients with anorexia nervosa or bulimia) may cause electrolyte and fluid abnormalities, cardiac toxicity, and myopathy. Except for aspiration, serious complications (e.g., gastric or esophageal tears and perforations) are rare. Ipecac is contraindicated in patients with recent gastrointestinal surgery, CNS depression, or seizures, and in those who have ingested corrosives or rapidly acting CNS poisons (camphor, cyanide, tricyclic antidepressants, propoxyphene, strychnine).

Whole-bowel irrigation is performed by administering a bowel-cleansing solution containing electrolytes and polyethylene glycol (Golytely, Colyte) orally or by gastric tube at a rate of 2.0 L/h (0.5 L/h in children) until rectal effluent is clear. The patient must be in a sitting position. Although data are limited, whole-bowel irrigation appears to be as effective as other decontamination procedures. It is most appropriate for those who have ingested foreign bodies, packets of illicit drugs, slow-release or enteric-coated medications, and agents that are poorly adsorbed by charcoal (e.g., heavy metals). It is contraindicated in patients with bowel obstruction, ileus, hemodynamic instability, and compromised unprotected airways.

Cathartics are salts (disodium phosphate, magnesium citrate and sulfate, sodium sulfate) or saccharides (mannitol, sorbitol) that promote the rectal evacuation of gastrointestinal contents. The most effective cathartic is sorbitol in a dose of 1 to 2 g/kg of body weight. Alone, cathartics do not prevent ingestant absorption and should not be used as a method of gut decontamination. Their primary use is to prevent constipation following charcoal administration. Abdominal cramps, nausea, and occasional vomiting are side effects. Complications of repeated dosing include hypermagnesemia (from magnesium salts) and excessive diarrhea. Cathartics are contraindicated in patients who have ingested corrosives and in those with preexisting diarrhea. Magnesium-containing cathartics should not be used in patients with renal failure.

Dilution (i.e., drinking 5 mL/kg of body weight of water or another clear liquid) is recommended only after the ingestion of corrosives (acids, alkali). It may increase the dissolution rate (and hence absorption) of capsules, tablets, and other solid ingestants and should *not* be used in these circumstances.

Endoscopic or surgical removal of poisons may be useful in rare situations, such as ingestion of a potentially toxic foreign body that fails to transit the gastrointestinal tract, a potentially lethal amount of a heavy metal (arsenic, iron, mercury, thallium), or agents that have coalesced into gastric concretions or bezoars (barbiturates, glutethimide, heavy metals, lithium, meprobamate, salicylates, sustained-release preparations). Patients who become toxic from cocaine due to its leakage from ingested drug packets require immediate surgical intervention.

DECONTAMINATION OF OTHER SITES Immediate, copious flushing with water, saline, or another available clear, drinkable liquid is the initial treatment for topical exposures (exceptions include alkali metals, calcium oxide, phosphorus). Saline is preferred for eye irrigation. A triple wash (water, soap, water) may be best for dermal decontamination. Inhalational exposures should be treated initially with fresh air or oxygen. The removal of liquids from body cavities such as the vagina or rectum is best accomplished by irrigation. Solids (drug packets, pills) should be removed manually, preferably under direct visualization.

Enhancement of Poison Elimination Although the elimination of most poisons can be accelerated by therapeutic interventions, the pharmacokinetic efficacy (removal of drug at a rate greater than that accomplished by intrinsic elimination) and clinical benefit (shortened duration of toxicity or improved outcome) of such interventions are often more theoretical than proven. Hence, the decision to use such measures should be based on the actual or predicted toxicity and the potential efficacy, cost, and risks of therapy.

MULTIPLE-DOSE ACTIVATED CHARCOAL Repetitive oral dosing with charcoal can enhance the elimination of previously absorbed substances by binding them within the gut as they are excreted in the bile, secreted by gastrointestinal cells, or passively diffuse into the gut lumen (reverse absorption or enterocapillary exsorption). Doses of 0.5 to 1 g/kg body weight every 2 to 4 h, adjusted downward to avoid regurgitation in patients with decreased gastrointestinal motility, are generally recommended. Experimentally, this treatment enhances the elimination of nearly all substances tested. Pharmacokinetic efficacy approaches that of hemodialysis for some agents (e.g., phenobarbital, theophylline). Multiple-dose therapy is not effective in accelerating elimination of chlorpropamide, tobramycin, or agents that adsorb poorly to charcoal. Complications include intestinal obstruction, pseudoobstruction, and nonocclusive intestinal infarction in patients with decreased gut motility.

FORCED DIURESIS AND ALTERATION OF URINARY pH Diuresis and ion trapping via alteration of urine pH may prevent the renal reabsorption of poisons that undergo excretion by glomerular filtration and active tubular secretion. Since membranes are more permeable to nonionized molecules than to their ionized counterparts, acidic (low-pK_a) poisons are ionized and trapped in alkaline urine, whereas basic ones become ionized and trapped in acid urine. Saline diuresis can enhance the renal excretion of alcohols, bromide, calcium, chromium, fluoride, isoniazid, lithium, meprobamate, potassium, and thallium. Alkaline diuresis (producing a urine pH $\geq$ 7.5 and a urine output of 3 to 6 mL/kg body weight per hour by adding sodium bicarbonate to an intravenous solution) enhances the excretion of chlorphenoxyacetic acid herbicides, chlorpropamide, diflunisal, fluoride, methotrexate, phenobarbital, sulfonamides, and sa-

licylates. Contraindications include congestive heart failure, renal failure, and cerebral edema. Acid-base, fluid, and electrolyte parameters should be monitored carefully. While acid diuresis can enhance the excretion of amphetamines, chloroquine, cocaine, local anesthetics, phencyclidine, quinidine, quinine, strychnine, sympathomimetics, tricyclic antidepressants, and tocainide, such therapy is not recommended because of potential cardiovascular and renal (myoglobinuric renal failure) complications and lack of clinical efficacy.

EXTRACORPOREAL REMOVAL Peritoneal dialysis, hemodialysis, charcoal or resin hemoperfusion, hemofiltration, plasmapheresis, and exchange transfusion are capable of removing any toxin from the bloodstream. Agents most amenable to enhanced elimination by dialysis have low molecular mass (<500 Da), high water solubility, low protein binding, small volumes of distribution (<1 L/kg body weight), prolonged elimination (long half-life), and high dialysis clearance relative to total-body clearance. Molecular weight, water solubility, or protein binding do not limit the efficacy of the other forms of extracorporeal removal.

Dialysis should be considered in cases of severe poisoning due to acetone, atenolol, barbiturates, bromide, chloral hydrate, ethanol, ethylene glycol, isopropyl alcohol, lithium, methanol, procainamide, theophylline, salicylates, sotalol, and possibly heavy metals. Although hemoperfusion may be more effective in removing some of these poisons, it does not correct associated acid-base and electrolyte abnormalities. Hemoperfusion should be considered in cases of severe poisoning due to caffeine, carbamazepine, carbon tetrachloride, chloramphenicol, dapsone, disopyramide, hypnotic-sedatives (barbiturates, ethchlorvynol, glutethimide, meprobamate, methaqualone), methotrexate, mushrooms (amatoxin-containing), paraquat, phenytoin, procainamide, theophylline, and valproate. Both techniques require central venous access and systemic anticoagulation and often result in transient hypotension. Hemoperfusion may also cause hemolysis, hypocalcemia, and thrombocytopenia. Peritoneal dialysis and exchange transfusion are less effective but may be used when other procedures are either not available, contraindicated, or technically difficult (e.g., in infants). Exchange transfusion may be indicated in the treatment of severe arsine- or sodium chlorate–induced hemolysis, methemoglobinemia, and sulfhemoglobinemia. Although hemofiltration can enhance elimination of aminoglycosides, vancomycin, and metal-chelate complexes, the roles of hemofiltration and plasmapheresis in the treatment of poisoning are not yet defined.

Candidates for extracorporeal removal therapies include patients with severe toxicity who deteriorate despite aggressive supportive therapy; those with potentially prolonged, irreversible, or fatal toxicity; those with dangerous blood levels of toxins; those who lack the capacity for self-detoxification because of liver or renal failure; and those with a serious underlying illness or complication that will adversely affect recovery.

OTHER TECHNIQUES The elimination of heavy metals can be enhanced by chelation, and the removal of carbon monoxide can be increased by hyperbaric oxygenation.

Administration of Antidotes Antidotes counteract the effects of poisons by neutralizing them (e.g., antibody-antigen reactions, chelation, chemical binding) or by antagonizing their physiologic effects (e.g., activation of opposing nervous system activity, provision of competitive metabolic or receptor substrate). Poisons or conditions with specific antidotes include acetaminophen, anticholinergic agents, anticoagulants, benzodiazepines, beta blockers, calcium channel blockers, carbon monoxide, cardiac glycosides, cholinergic agents, cyanide, drug-induced dystonic reactions, ethylene glycol, fluoride, heavy metals, hydrogen sulfide, hypoglycemic agents, isoniazid, membrane-active agents, methemoglobinemia, opioids, sympathomimetics, Vacor, and a variety of envenomations. Antidotes can significantly reduce morbidity and mortality, but most are potentially toxic. Since their safe use requires correct identification of a specific poisoning or syndrome, details of antidotal therapy are discussed with the conditions for which they are indicated (Table 377-4).

Physiologic Condition, Causes	Examples	Mechanism of Action	Clinical Features	Specific Treatments
STIMULATED				
Sympathetics (see also Chap. 374) Sympathomimetics	α_1-Adrenergic agonists (decongestants): phenylephrine, phenylpropanolamine β_2-Adrenergic agonists (bronchodilators): albuterol, terbutaline Nonspecific adrenergic agonists: amphetamines, cocaine, ephedrine	Stimulation of central and peripheral sympathetic receptors directly or indirectly (by promoting the release or inhibiting the reuptake of norepinephrine and sometimes dopamine)	Physiologic stimulation (Table 377-2); reflex bradycardia can occur with selective α_1 agonists; β agonists can cause hypotension and hypokalemia.	Phentolamine, a nonselective α_1-adrenergic receptor antagonist, for severe hypertension due to α_1-adrenergic agonists; propranolol, a nonselective β blocker, for hypotension and tachycardia due to β_2 agonists; labetalol, a β blocker with α-blocking activity, or phentolamine with esmolol, metoprolol, or other cardioselective β blocker for hypertension with tachycardia due to nonselective agents (β blockers, if used alone, can exacerbate hypertension and vasospasm due to unopposed α stimulation).
Ergot alkaloids	Ergotamine, methysergide, bromocriptine, pergolide	Stimulation and inhibition of serotonergic and α-adrenergic receptors; stimulation of dopamine receptors	Physiologic stimulation (Table 377-2); formication; vasospasm with limb (isolated or generalized), myocardial, and cerebral ischemia progressing to gangrene or infarction; hypotension, bradycardia, and involuntary movements can also occur.	Nitroprusside or nitroglycerine for severe vasospasm; prazocin (an α_1 blocker), captopril, nifedipine, and cyproheptidene (a serotonin receptor antagonist) for mild to moderate limb ischemia; dopamine receptor antagonists (antipsychotics) for hallucinations and movement disorders
Methylxanthines	Caffeine, theophylline	Inhibition of adenosine synthesis and adenosine receptor antagonism; stimulation of epinephrine and norepinephrine release; inhibition of phosphodiesterase resulting in increased intracellular cyclic adenosine and quanosine monophosphate	Physiologic stimulation (Table 377-2); pronounced gastrointestinal symptoms and β agonist effects (see above). Toxicity occurs at lower drug levels in chronic poisoning than in acute poisoning.	Propranolol, a nonselective β blocker, for tachycardia with hypotension; any β blocker for supraventricular or ventricular tachycardia without hypotension; elimination enhanced by multiple-dose charcoal, hemoperfusion, and hemodialysis; indications for hemoperfusion or hemodialysis include unstable vital signs, seizures, and a theophylline level of 80 to 100 $\mu g/mL$ after acute overdose and 40 to 60 $\mu g/mL$ with chronic exposure.
Monoamine oxidase inhibitors	Phenelzine, tranylcypromine, selegiline	Inhibition of monoamine oxidase resulting in impaired metabolism of endogenous catecholamines and exogenous sympathomimetic agents	Delayed or slowly progressive physiologic stimulation (Table 377-2); terminal hypotension and bradycardia in severe cases.	Short-acting agents (e.g., nitroprusside, esmolol) for severe hypertension and tachycardia; direct-acting sympathomimetics (e.g., norepinephrine, epinephrine) for hypotension and bradycardia
Anticholinergics Antihistamines	Diphenhydramine, doxylamine, pyrilamine	Inhibition of central and postganglionic parasympathetic muscarinic cholinergic receptors. At high doses, amantidine, diphenhydramine, orphenadrine, phenothiazines, and tricyclic antidepressants have additional nonanticholinergic activity (see below).	Physiologic stimulation (Table 377-2); dry skin and mucous membranes, decreased bowel sounds, flushing, and urinary retention; myoclonus and picking activity. Central effects may occur without significant autonomic dysfunction.	Physostigmine, an acetylcholinesterase inhibitor (see below) for delirium, hallucinations, and neuromuscular hyperactivity. Contraindications include nonanticholinergic cardiovascular toxicity (e.g., cardiac conduction abnormalities, hypotension, and ventricular arrhythmias).
Antiparkinsonian agents	Amantidine, trihexiphenydyl			
Antipsychotics	Chlorpromazine, olanzapine, quetiapine, thioridazine			
Antispasmotics	Clinidium, dicyclomine			
Belladonna alkaloids	Atropine, hyoscyamine, scopolamine			
Cyclic antidepressants	Amitriptyline, doxepin, imipramine			
Muscle relaxants	Cyclobenzaprine, orphenadrine			
Mushrooms and plants	*Amanita muscaria* and *A. pantherina*, henbane, jimson weed, nightshade			

(continued)

Physiologic Condition, Causes	Examples	Mechanism of Action	Clinical Features	Specific Treatments
DEPRESSED				
Sympatholytics α₂-Adrenergic agonists	Clonidine, guanabenz, tetra-hydrozoline and other imidazoline decongestants, tizanidine and other imidazoline muscle relaxants	Stimulation of α₂-adrenergic receptors leading to inhibition of CNS sympathetic outflow; activity at nonadrenergic imidazoline binding sites also contributes to CNS effects.	Physiologic depression (Table 377-2), miosis. Transient initial hypertension may be seen.	Dopamine and norepinephrine for hypotension. Atropine for symptomatic bradycardia. Naloxone for CNS depression (inconsistently effective).
Antipsychotics	Chlorpromazine, clozapine, haloperidol, risperidone, thioridazine	Inhibition of α-adrenergic, dopaminergic, histaminergic, muscarinic, and serotonergic receptors. Some agents also inhibit sodium, potassium, and calcium channels.	Physiologic depression (Table 377-2), miosis, anticholinergic effects (see above), extrapyramidal reactions (see below), tachycardia. Cardiac conduction delays (increased PR, QRS, JT, and QT intervals) with ventricular tachydysrhythmias, including torsades de pointes, can sometimes develop.	Sodium bicarbonate and lidocaine for ventricular tachydysrhythmias associated with QRS prolongation. Magnesium, isoproterenol, and overdrive pacing for torsades de pointes. Avoid class IA, IC, and III antiarrhythmics.
β-Adrenergic blockers	Cardioselective (β₁) blockers: atenolol, esmolol, metoprolol Nonselective (β₁ and β₂) blockers: nadolol, propranolol, timolol Partial β agonists: acebutolol, pindolol α₁ Antagonists: carvedilol, labetalol Membrane-active agents: acebutolol, propranolol, sotalol	Inhibition of β-adrenergic receptors (class II antiarrhythmic effect). Some agents have activity at additional receptors or have membrane effects (see below).	Physiologic depression (Table 377-2), atrioventricular block, hypoglycemia, hyperkalemia, seizures. Partial agonists can cause hypertension and tachycardia. Sotalol can cause increased QT interval and ventricular tachydysrhythmias. Onset may be delayed after sotalol and sustained-release formulation overdose.	Glucagon and calcium for hypotension and symptomatic bradycardia. Atropine, isoproterenol, amrinone, dopamine, dobutamine, epinephrine, and norepinephrine may sometimes be effective. High-dose insulin (with glucose and potassium to maintain euglycemia and normokalemia), electrical pacing, and mechanical cardiovascular support for refractory cases.
Calcium channel blockers	Diltiazem, nifedipine and other dihydropyridine derivatives, verapamil	Inhibition of slow (type L) cardiovascular calcium channels (class IV antiarrhythmic effect).	Physiologic depression (Table 377-2), atrioventricular block, organ ischemia and infarction, hyperglycemia, seizures. Hypotension is usually due to decreased vascular resistance rather than to decreased cardiac output. Onset may be delayed for ≥12 h after overdose of sustained-release formulations.	Calcium and glucagon for hypotension and symptomatic bradycardia. Dopamine, epinephrine, norepinephrine, atropine, and isoproterenol are less often effective but can be used adjunctively. Amrinone, high-dose insulin (with glucose and potassium to maintain euglycemia and normokalemia), electrical pacing, and mechanical cardiovascular support for refractory cases.
Cardiac glycosides	Digoxin, endogenous cardioactive steroids, foxglove and other plants, toad skin secretions (*Bufonidae* sp.)	Inhibition of cardiac Na⁺, K⁺-ATPase membrane pump.	Physiologic depression (Table 377-2); gastrointestinal, psychiatric, and visual symptoms; atrioventricular block with or without concomitant supraventricular tachyarrhythmia; ventricular tachyarrhythmias. Hyperkalemia in acute poisoning. Toxicity occurs at lower drug levels in chronic poisoning than in acute poisoning.	Digoxin-specific antibody fragments for hemodyamically compromising dysrhythmias, Mobitz II or third-degree atrioventricular block, hyperkalemia (>5.5 meq/L; in acute poisoning only). Temporizing measures include atropine, dopamine, epinephrine, phenytoin, and external cardiac pacing for bradydysrhythmias and magnesium, lidocaine, phenytoin, and bretylium for ventricular tachydysrhythmias. Internal cardiac pacing and cardioversion can increase ventricular irritability and should be reserved for refractory cases.

(continued)

TABLE 377-4—*(Continued)*

Physiologic Condition, Causes	Examples	Mechanism of Action	Clinical Features	Specific Treatments
Cyclic antidepressants	Amitriptyline, doxepin, imipramine	Inhibition of α-adrenergic dopaminergic, GABA-ergic, histaminergic, muscarinic, and serotonergic receptors; inhibition of sodium channels (see membrane-active agents); inhibition of norepinephrine and serotonin reuptake.	Physiologic depression (Table 377-2), seizures, tachycardia, cardiac conduction delays (increased PR, QRS, JT, and QT intervals; terminal QRS right axis deviation) with aberrancy and ventricular tachydysrhythmias. Anticholinergic toxidrome (see above).	Hypertonic sodium bicarbonate (or hypertonic saline) and lidocaine for ventricular tachydysrhythmias associated with QRS prolongation. Use of phenytoin is controversial. Avoid class IA, IC, and III antiarrhythmics.
Cholinergics				
Acetylcholinesterase inhibitors	Carbamate insecticides (aldicarb, carbaryl, propoxur) and medicinals (neostigmine, physostigmine, tacrine); nerve gases (sarin, soman, tabun, VX) organophosphate insecticides (diazinon, chlopyriphos, malathion)	Inhibition of acetylcholinesterase leading to increased synaptic acetylcholine at muscarinic and nicotinic cholinergic receptor sites	Physiologic depression (Table 377-2). Muscarinic signs and symptoms: seizures, excessive secretions (lacrimation, salivation, bronchorrhea and wheezing, diaphoresis), and increased bowel and bladder activity with nausea, vomiting, diarrhea, abdominal cramps, and incontinence of feces and urine. Nicotinic signs and symptoms: hypertension, tachycardia, muscle cramps, fasciculations, weakness, and paralysis. Death is usually due to respiratory failure. Cholinesterase activity in plasma and red cells <50% of normal in acetylcholinesterase inhibitor poisoning.	Atropine for muscarinic signs and symptoms. Pralidoxime (2-PAM), a cholinesterase reactivator, for nicotinic signs and symptoms due to organophosphates, nerve gases, or an unknown anticholinesterase.
Muscarinic agonists	Bethanecol, mushrooms (*Boletus*, *Clitocybe*, *Inocybe* sp.), pilocarpine	Stimulation of CNS and postganglionic parasympathetic cholinergic (muscarinic) receptors		
Nicotinic agonists	Lobeline, nicotine (tobacco)	Stimulation of preganglionic sympathetic and parasympathetic and striated muscle (neuromuscular junction) cholinergic (nicotine) receptors		
Sedative-hypnotics (see also Chap. 387)				
Anticonvulsants	Carbamazepine, ethosuximide, felbamate, gabapentin, lamotrigine, levetiracetam, oxcarbazepine, phenytoin, tiagabine, topiramate, valproate, zonisamide	Potentiation of the inhibitory effects of GABA by binding to the neuronal GABA-A chloride channel receptor complex and increasing the frequency or duration of chloride channel opening in response to GABA stimulation. Baclofen and, to some extent, GHB act at the GABA-B rector complex; meprobamate, its metabolite carisoprodol, felbamate, and orphenadrine antagonize N-methyl-D-aspartate (NDMA) excitatory receptors; ethosuximide, valproate, and zonisamide decrease conduction through T-type calcium channels; valproate decreases GABA degradation, and tiagabine blocks GABA reuptake; carbamazepine, lamotrigine, oxcarbazepine, phenytoin, topiramate, valproate, and zonisamide slow the rate of recovery of inactivated sodium channels. Some agents also have α₂ agonist, anticholinergic, and sodium channel blocking activity (see above and below).	Physiologic depression (Table 377-2), nystagmus. Delayed absorption can occur with carbamazepine, phenytoin, and valproate. Myoclonus, seizures, hypertension, and tachyarrhythmias can occur with baclofen, carbamazepine, and orphenadrine. Tachyarrhythmias can also occur with chloral hydrate. AGMA, hypernatremia, hyperosmolality, hyperammonemia, chemical hepatitis, and hypoglycemia can be seen in valproate poisoning. Carbamazepine and oxcarbazepine may produce hyponatremia from SIADH. Some agents can cause anticholinergic and sodium channel (membrane) blocking effects (see above and below).	Flumazenil for benzodiazepine and zolpidem poisoning. Benzodiazepines and barbiturates for seizures. Elimination of phenobarbital and possibly other long-acting agents enhanced by multiple-dose charcoal. Hemodialysis and hemoperfusion may be indicated for severe poisoning by some agents (see "Extracorporeal Removal," in text). See above and below for treatment of anticholinergic and sodium channel (membrane) blocking effects.
Barbiturates	Short-acting: butabarbital, pentobarbital, secobarbital. Long-acting: phenobarbital, primadone			
Benzodiazepines	Ultrashort-acting: estazolam, midazolam, temazepam, triazolam. Short-acting: alprazolam, flunitrazepam, lorazepam, oxazepam. Long-acting: chlordiazepoxide, clonazepam, diazepam, flurazepam. Pharmacologically related agents: zaleplon, zolpidem			
GABA precursors	γ-Hydroxybutyrate (sodium oxybate; GHB), γ-butyrolactone (GBL), 1,4-butanediol.			
Muscle relaxants	Baclofen, carisoprodol, cyclobenzaprine, etomidate, metaxalone, methocarbamol, orphenadrine, propafol, tizanidine and other imidazoline muscle relaxants.			

(continued)

Physiologic Condition, Causes	Examples	Mechanism of Action	Clinical Features	Specific Treatments
Other agents	Chloral hydrate, ethclorvynol, glutethimide, meprobamate, methaqualone, methyprylon			
DISCORDANT				
Asphyxiants				
Cytochrome oxidase inhibitors	Carbon monoxide, cyanide, hydrogen sulfide	Inhibition of mitochrondrial cytochrome oxidase, thereby blocking electron transport and oxidative metabolism. Carbon monoxide also binds to hemoglobin and myoglobin and prevents oxygen binding, transport, and tissue uptake (binding to hemoglobin shifts the oxygen dissociation curve to the left).	Signs and symptoms of hypoxia with initial physiologic stimulation and subsequent depression (Table 377-2); lactic acidosis; normal P_{O_2} and calculated oxygen saturation but decreased oxygen saturation by co-oximetry (that measured by pulse oximetry is falsely elevated but is less than normal and less than the calculated value). Headache and nausea are common with carbon monoxide. Sudden collapse may occur with cyanide and hydrogen sulfide exposure. A bitter almond breath odor may be noted with cyanide ingestion, and hydrogen sulfide smells like rotten eggs.	High-dose oxygen. Inhaled amyl nitrite and IV sodium nitrite and sodium thiosulfate (Lilly cyanide antidote kit) for coma, metabolic acidosis, and cardiovascular dysfunction in cyanide poisoning. Amyl and sodium nitrite (without thiosulfate) for similar toxicity in hydrogen sulfide poisoning. Hyperbaric oxygen for moderate to severe carbon monoxide poisoning and for cyanide or hydrogen sulfide poisoning unresponsive to other measures.
Methemoglobin inducers	Aniline derivatives, dapsone, local anesthetics, nitrates, nitrites, nitrogen oxides, nitro- and nitrosohydrocarbons, phenazopyridine, primaquine-type antimalarials, sulfonamides.	Oxidation of hemoglobin iron from ferrous (Fe^{2+}) to ferric (Fe^{3+}) state prevents oxygen binding, transport, and tissue uptake (methemoglobinemia shifts oxygen dissociation curve to the left). Oxidation of hemoglobin protein causes hemoglobin precipitation and hemolytic anemia (manifest as Heinz bodies and "bite cells" on peripheral blood smear).	Signs and symptoms of hypoxia with initial physiologic stimulation and subsequent depression (Table 377-2), gray-brown cyanosis unresponsive to oxygen at methemoglobin fractions > 15 to 20%, headache, lactic acidosis (at methemoglobin fractions > 45%), normal P_{O_2} and calculated oxygen saturation but decreased oxygen saturation and increased methehemoglobin fraction by co-oximetry (oxygen saturation by pulse oximetry may be falsely increased or decreased but is less than normal and less than the calculated value).	High-dose oxygen. Intravenous methylene blue for methemoglobin fraction > 30%, symptomatic hypoxia, or ischemia (contraindicated in G6PD deficiency). Exchange transfusion and hyperbaric oxygen for severe or refractory cases.
AGMA inducers	Ethylene glycol	Ethylene glycol causes CNS depression and increased serum osmolality. Metabolites (primarily glycolic acid) cause AGMA, CNS depression, and renal failure. Precipitation of oxalic acid metabolite as calcium salt in tissues and urine results in hypocalcemia, tissue edema, and crystalluria.	Initial ethanol-like intoxication, nausea, vomiting, increased osmolar gap, calcium oxalate crystalluria. Delayed AGMA, back pain, renal failure. Coma, seizures, hypotension, ARDS in severe cases.	Gastric aspiration for recent ingestions. Sodium bicarbonate to correct acidemia. Thiamine, folinic acid, magnesium, and high-dose pyridoxine to facilitate metabolism. Ethanol or fomepizole for AGMA, crytalluria or renal dysfunction, ethylene glycol level > 3 mmol/L (20 mg/dL), and for ethanol-like intoxication or increased osmolal gap if level not readily obtainable. Hemodialysis for persistent AGMA, lack of clinical improvement, and renal dysfunction. Hemodialysis also useful for enhancing ethylene glycol elimination and shortening duration of treatment when ethylene glycol level > 8 mmol/L (50 mg/dL).

(continued)

TABLE 377-4— (Continued)

Physiologic Condition, Causes	Examples	Mechanism of Action	Clinical Features	Specific Treatments
	Iron	Hydration of ferric (Fe^{3+}) ion generates H^+. Non-transferrin-bound iron catalyzes formation of free radicals that cause mitochondrial injury, lipid peroxidation, increased capillary permeability, vasodilation, and organ toxicity.	Initial nausea, vomiting, abdominal pain, diarrhea. AGMA, cardiovascular and CNS depression, hepatitis, coagulopathy, and seizures in severe cases. Radiopaque iron tablets may be seen on abdominal x-ray.	Whole-bowel irrigation for large ingestions. Endoscopy and gastrostomy if clinical toxicity and large number of tablets still visible on x-ray. IV hydration. Sodium bicarbonate for acidemia. IV deferoxamine for systemic toxicity, iron level > 90 μmol/L (500 μg/dL).
	Methanol	Methanol causes ethanol-like CNS depression and increased serum osmolality. Formic acid metabolite causes AGMA and retinal toxicity.	Initial ethanol-like intoxication, nausea, vomiting, increased osmolar gap. Delayed AGMA, visual (clouding, spots, blindness) and retinal (edema, hyperemia) abnormalities. Coma, seizures, cardiovascular depression in severe cases. Possible pancreatitis.	Gastric aspiration for recent ingestions. Sodium bicarbonate to correct acidemia. High-dose folinic acid or folate to facilitate metabolism. Ethanol or fomepizole for AGMA, visual symptoms, methanol level > 6 mmol/L (20 mg/dL), and for ethanol-like intoxication or increased osmolal gap if level not readily obtainable. Hemodialysis for persistent AGMA, lack of clinical improvement, and renal dysfunction. Hemodialysis also useful for enhancing methanol elimination and shortening duration of treatment when methanol level > 15 mmol/L (50 mg/dL).
	Salicylate	Increased sensitivity of CNS respiratory center to changes in P_{O_2} and P_{CO_2} stimulates respiration. Uncoupling of oxidative phosphorylation, inhibition of Kreb's cycle enzymes, and stimulation of carbohydrate and lipid metabolism generate unmeasured endogenous anions and cause AGMA.	Initial nausea, vomiting, hyperventilation, alkalemia, alkaluria. Subsequent alkalemia with both respiratory alkalosis and AGMA, and paradoxical aciduria. Late acidemia with CNS and respiratory depression. Cerebral and pulmonary edema in severe cases. Hypoglycemia, hypocalcemia, hypokalemia, and seizures can occur.	IV hydration and supplemental glucose. Sodium bicarbonate to correct acidemia. Alkaline diuresis for systemic toxicity. Hemodialysis for coma, cerebral edema, seizures, pulmonary edema, renal failure, progressive acid-base disturbances or clinical toxicity, salicylate level > 7 mmol/L (100 mg/dL) following acute overdose.
CNS syndromes Extrapyramidal reactions Isoniazid	Antipsychotics (see above), some cyclic antidepressants and antihistamines.	Decreased CNS dopaminergic activity with relative excess of cholinergic activity. Interference with activation and supply of pyridoxal-5-phosphate, a cofactor for glutamic acid decarboxylase, which converts glutamic acid to GABA, results in decreased levels of this inhibitory CNS neurotransmitter; complexation with and depletion of pyridoxine itself; inhibition of nicotine-adenine dinucleotide dependent lactate and hydroxybutyrate dehydrogenases resulting in substrate accumulation.	Akathisia, dystonia, parkinsonism Nausea, vomiting, agitation, confusion; coma, respiratory depression, seizures, lactic and ketoacidosis in severe cases.	Oral or parenteral anticholinergic agent such as benztropine or diphenhydramine. High-dose intravenous pyridoxine (vitamin B_6) for agitation, confusion, coma, and seizures. Diazepam or barbiturates for seizures.

(continued)

Physiologic Condition, Causes	Examples	Mechanism of Action	Clinical Features	Specific Treatments
Lithium		Interference with cell membrane ion transport, adenylate cyclase and Na$^+$, K$^+$-ATPase activity, and neurotransmitter release.	Nausea, vomiting, diarrhea, ataxia, choreoathetosis, encephalopathy, hyperreflexia, myoclonus, nystagmus, nephrogenic diabetes insipidus, falsely elevated serum chloride with low anion gap, tachycardia. Coma, seizures, arrhythmias, hyperthermia, and prolonged or permanent encephalopathy and movement disorders in severe cases. Delayed onset after acute overdose, particularly with delayed-release formations. Toxicity occurs at lower drug levels in chronic poisoning than in acute poisoning.	Whole-bowel irrigation for large ingestions. Consider endoscopic removal if high and rising drug level with progressive clinical toxicity. IV hydration. Hemodialysis for coma, seizures, severe, progressive, or persistent encephalopathy or neuromuscular dysfunction, peak lithium level > 8 meq/L (mmol/L) following acute overdose.
Serotonin syndrome	Amphetamines, cocaine, dextromethorphan, meperidine, MAO inhibitors, selective serotonin (5HT) reuptake inhibitors, tricyclic antidepressants, tramadol, triptans, tryptophan.	Promotion of serotonin release, inhibition of serotonin reuptake, or direct stimulation of CNS and peripheral serotonin receptors (primarily 5HT-1a and 5HT-2), alone or in combination.	Altered mental status (agitation, confusion, mutism, coma, seizures), neuromuscular hyperactivity (hyperreflexia, myoclonus, rigidity, tremors), and autonomic dysfunction (abdominal pain, diarrhea, diaphoresis, fever, flushing, labile hypertension, mydriasis, tearing, salivation, tachycardia). Complications include hyperthermia, lactic acidosis, rhabdomyolysis, and multisystem organ failure.	Serotonin receptor antagonist such as cyproheptadine or chlorpromazine.
Membrane-active agents	Amantidine, antiarrhythmics (class 1 and III agents; some β blockers), antipsychotics (see above), antihistamines (particularly diphenhydramine), carbamazepine, local anesthetics (including cocaine), opioids (meperidine, propoxyphene), orphenadrine, quinoline antimalarials (chloroquine, hydroxychloroquine, quinine), cyclic antidepressants (see above).	Blockade of fast sodium membrane channels prolongs phase 0 (depolarization) of the cardiac action potential, which prolong the QRS duration and promotes reentrant (monomorphic) ventricular tachycardia. Class Ia, Ic, and III antiarrhythmics also block potassium channels during phases 2 and 3 (repolarization) of the action potential, prolonging the JT interval and promoting early after-depolarizations and polymorphic (torsades de pointes) ventricular tachycardia. Similar effects on neuronal membrane channels cause CNS dysfunction. Some agents also block α-adrenergic and cholinergic receptors or have opioid effects (see above and Chap. 373).	QRS and JT prolongation (or both) with hypotension, ventricular tachyarrhythmias, CNS depression, seizures. Anticholinergic effects with amantadine, antihistamines, carbamazepine, disopyramide, antipsychotics, and cyclic antidepressants (see above). Opioid effects with meperidine and propoxyphene (see Chap. 373). Cinchonism (hearing loss, tinnitus, nausea, vomiting, vertigo, ataxia, headache, flushing, diaphoresis) and blindness with quinoline antimalarials.	Hypertonic sodium bicarbonate (or hypertonic saline) for cardiac conduction delays and monomorphic ventricular tachycardia. Lidocaine for monomorphic ventricular tachycardia (except when due to class Ib antiarrhythmics). Magnesium, isoproterenol, and overdrive pacing for polymorphic ventricular tachycardia. Physostigmine for anticholinergic effects (see above.) Naloxone for opioid effects (see Chap. 373). Extracorporeal removal for some agents (see text).

Note: AGMA, anion-gap metabolic acidosis; ARDS, adult respiratory distress syndrome; CNS, central nervous system; GABA, γ-aminobutyric acid; G6PD, glucose-6-phosphate dehydrogenase; MAO, monoamine oxidase; SIADH, syndrome of inappropriate antidiuretic hormone.

Prevention of Reexposure Poisoning is a preventable illness. Unfortunately, some adults and children are poison-prone, and recurrences are common. Adults with accidental exposures should be instructed regarding the safe use of medications and chemicals (according to labeling instructions). Confused patients may need assistance with the administration of their medications. Errors in dosing by health care providers may require educational efforts. Patients should be advised to avoid circumstances that result in chemical exposure or poisoning.

Appropriate agencies and health departments should be notified in cases of environmental or workplace exposure. The best approach with young children and patients with intentional overdose is to limit their access to poisons. In households where children live or visit, alcoholic beverages, medications, household products (automotive, cleaning, fuel, pet-care, toiletry products), nonedible plants, and vitamins should be kept out of reach or in locked or child-proof cabinets. Depressed or psychotic patients should receive psychiatric assessment, disposition, and follow-up. They should be given prescriptions for a limited supply of drugs and with a limited number of refills and be monitored for compliance and response to therapy.

SPECIFIC TOXIC SYNDROMES AND POISONINGS Table 377-4 summarizes the pathophysiology, clinical features, and treatment of toxidromes and poisonings that are common, produce life-threatening toxicity, or require unique therapeutic interventions. In all cases, treatment should include attending to the general principles discussed above, particularly supportive care. Details regarding specific therapies can be found in the references cited here and at *harrisononline.com.* Poisonings not covered in this chapter are discussed in the referenced texts.→*Alcohol, cocaine, hallucinogen, and opioid poisoning and alcohol and opioid withdrawal are discussed in Chaps. 372 to 375; acetaminophen poisoning is discussed in Chap. 286; the neuroleptic malignant syndrome is discussed in Chap. 351; and heavy metal poisoning is discussed in Chap. 376.*

FURTHER READING

AMERICAN ACADEMY OF CLINICAL TOXICOLOGY/EUROPEAN ASSOCIATION OF POISONS CENTERS AND CLINICAL TOXICOLOGISTS: Position Statements on Gastrointestinal Decontamination: Introduction; Ipecac syrup; Gastric lavage; Single-dose activated charcoal; Cathartics; Whole bowel irrigation. Clin Toxicol 35:695, 699, 711, 721, 743, 753, 1997
———: Multi-dose activated charcoal. Clin Toxicol 37:731, 1999
BOSSE GM, MATYUNAS NJ: Delayed toxidromes. J Emerg Med 17:679, 1999
HARDMAN JG et al (eds): *Goodman and Gilman's The Pharmacologic Basis of Therapeutics*, 10th ed. New York, McGraw-Hill, 2001
KLAASSEN CD (ed): *Casarett and Doull's Toxicology: The Basic Science of Poisons*, 6th ed. New York, McGraw-Hill, 2001
LITOVITZ TL et al: 2001 Annual Report of the American Association of Poison Control Centers Toxic Exposure Surveillance System. Am J Emerg Med 20:391, 2002

378 DISORDERS CAUSED BY REPTILE BITES AND MARINE ANIMAL EXPOSURES
Paul S. Auerbach, Robert L. Norris

This chapter outlines general principles for the evaluation and management of victims of venom poisoning or intoxication by certain reptiles and marine creatures and presents a clinical approach to these emergencies. Because the incidence of serious bites and stings is relatively low in developed nations, there remains a paucity of relevant clinical research and literature, and therapeutic decision-making is often based on anecdotal information.

VENOMOUS SNAKEBITE

EPIDEMIOLOGY The venomous snakes of the world are grouped into the families Viperidae (subfamily Viperinae: the Old World vipers; subfamily Crotalinae: the New World and Asian pit vipers), Elapidae (including the cobras, coral snakes, and all Australian venomous snakes), Hydrophiidae (the sea snakes), Atractaspididae (the burrowing asps), and Colubridae (a large group, of which the majority are nonvenomous and only a few species are dangerously toxic to humans). Bite rates are highest in temperate and tropical regions where people subsist by manual agriculture. Global estimates suggest that 30,000 to 40,000 persons die each year from venomous snakebite, but this range is likely an underestimate because of incomplete reporting.

SNAKE ANATOMY/IDENTIFICATION The typical snake-venom apparatus consists of bilateral venom glands—one on each side of the head, below and behind the eye—connected by ducts to hollow, anterior maxillary teeth. In viperids (vipers and pit vipers), these teeth are long mobile fangs that retract against the roof of the mouth when the animal is at rest. In elapids and sea snakes, the fangs are less enlarged and are relatively fixed in an erect position. Venomous snakes can bite without injecting venom. Approximately 20% of pit viper bites and an even higher percentage of bites inflicted by some other snake families (e.g., up to 75% for sea snakes) are "dry."

Differentiation of venomous from nonvenomous snake species can be difficult. Viperids are characterized by somewhat triangular heads (a feature shared with many harmless snakes); elliptical pupils (also seen in some nonvenomous snakes, such as boas and pythons); enlarged maxillary fangs; subcaudal scalation that involves a single scale running the full width of the ventral surface of the tail for several rows just distal to the anal plate (as opposed to two scales in each subcaudal row for most nonvenomous snakes and elapids); and, in the case of pit vipers, the heat-sensing pits (foveal organs), for which they are named, located slightly inferior and anterior to the eyes on each side. Color pattern is notoriously misleading in identifying most venomous

snakes except for the coral snakes, whose other body characteristics are similar to those of harmless colubrids. The American coral snakes can be identified by red, yellow (or white), and black bands completely encircling the body; a few species have red and black bands only. North of Mexico City, the immediate contiguity of red and yellow bands is fairly reliable for distinguishing a coral snake from its many harmless mimics. Further south, differentiation by color pattern is more problematic.

In many areas of the world, such as Australia, enzyme-linked immunoassay (ELISA) kits are available to aid in determining the specific snake species involved in a bite. These kits identify venom in the victim's blood, urine, or wound aspirate. No such kit is commercially available in the United States, however.

VENOMS AND CLINICAL MANIFESTATIONS Snake venoms are complex mixtures of enzymes, low-molecular-weight polypeptides, glycoproteins, and metal ions. Among the deleterious components are hemorrhagins that promote vascular leaking and cause both local and systemic bleeding. Various proteolytic enzymes cause local tissue necrosis, affect the coagulation pathway at various steps, and impair organ function. Myocardial depressant factors reduce cardiac output, and neurotoxins act either pre- or postsynaptically to inhibit peripheral nerve impulses. Most snake venoms have multisystem effects in their victims.

℞ TREATMENT

Field Management Initial (prehospital) measures should focus on rapidly delivering the victim to definitive medical care while keeping him/her as inactive as possible to limit systemic spread of venom. Any other measures employed should at least do no further harm to the victim.

Although mechanical suction has been recommended in the field management of venomous snakebite for many years, there is now literature that demonstrates that this intervention is of little, if any, benefit. The amount of venom extracted from the depot site by devices purported to serve this purpose is minuscule. In addition, there is now preliminary evidence that extended use of such a device (i.e., for longer than 30 min) may actually be detrimental to local tissues.

Despite some evidence that venom can be localized to the bite site by lymph-occlusive constriction bands or by an encompassing wrap combined with splinting (pressure-immobilization), the clinical benefit of these techniques has never been demonstrated. There is concern that severely restricting venom to the bite site may, in fact, worsen local tissue necrosis. If the victim is >1 h from medical care, a constriction band or pressure-immobilization may be considered, but with the realization that one may be sacrificing tissue in order to reduce systemic toxicity. At no time should a totally occlusive arterial tourniquet be employed. Also to be avoided are incising or cooling the bite site, giving the victim an alcoholic beverage, or applying electric shocks. The bitten extremity should be splinted if possible and kept at approximately heart level.

For elapid or sea snake bites, the Australian pressure-immobilization technique, in which the entire bitten extremity is wrapped with an elastic or crepe bandage and then splinted, is highly effective. The bandage is applied with the same snugness used for a sprained ankle. This technique greatly restricts absorption and circulation of these venoms, which tend to cause more limited local tissue effects than viperid venoms.

Hospital Management   In the hospital, the victim should be closely monitored (vital signs, cardiac rhythm, and oxygen saturation) while a history is quickly obtained and a rapid but thorough physical examination is performed. The level of swelling in a bitten extremity should be marked and limb circumferences measured in several locations every 15 min until swelling has stabilized. Large-bore intravenous access in unaffected extremities should be established. Early hypotension is due to pooling of blood in the pulmonary and splanchnic vascular beds. Hours later, hemolysis and loss of intravascular volume into soft tissues may play important roles. Fluid resuscitation with normal saline or Ringer's lactate should be initiated for clinical shock. If the blood pressure response is inadequate after administration of crystalloid (20 to 40 mL/kg of body weight), then a trial of 5% albumin (10 to 20 mL/kg) is in order. If tissue perfusion fails to respond to volume resuscitation and antivenom infusion (see below), vasopressors (e.g., dopamine) should be administered. Invasive hemodynamic monitoring (central venous and/or pulmonary arterial pressures) can be helpful in such cases, although obtaining access is riskier if coagulopathy is present.

Blood should be drawn for laboratory evaluation as soon as possible. Blood typing and cross-matching procedures can be affected over time by circulating venom. Also important are a complete blood count (to evaluate the degree of hemorrhage or hemolysis and effects on platelet count), studies of renal and hepatic function, coagulation studies (to identify signs of consumptive coagulopathy), and testing of urine for blood or myoglobin. In severe cases or in the face of significant comorbidity, arterial blood gas studies, electrocardiography, and chest radiography are indicated.

Attempts to locate a source of appropriate antivenom should begin early in all cases of known venomous snakebite, regardless of symptoms. In the event that signs and symptoms progress rapidly, any delay in the administration of antivenom is dangerous. Antivenoms rarely offer cross-protection against snake species other than those used in their production unless the species are closely related. An example of good cross-protection is that of Australian tiger snake (*Notechis scutatus*) antivenom for sea snake bites (see below). The package insert accompanying a particular antivenom should be consulted for information regarding the spectrum of coverage. In the United States, assistance in finding antivenom can be obtained 24 hours a day from the University of Arizona Poison and Drug Information Center (telephone: 520-626-6016).

Progressive or severe local findings (e.g., soft tissue swelling, ecchymosis, petechiae) or manifestations of systemic toxicity (signs and symptoms or laboratory abnormalities) are indications for the administration of intravenous antivenom in cases of viperid venom poisoning. Victims of bites by elapid snakes, such as coral snakes, should be treated with an appropriate antivenom if the snake has been positively identified. In these cases, local findings are often minimal, the onset of systemic symptoms may be delayed for many hours, and progression may be difficult to halt once manifestations begin. The package insert for the appropriate antivenom should be consulted regarding the method of administration and the optimal dose. Dosing for viperid bites is guided by the severity of the bite (see Table 378-1).

Some manufacturers recommend a skin-testing procedure for potential allergy. Use of any heterologous serum product carries a risk of anaphylactic, anaphylactoid, and delayed-hypersensitivity reactions. Skin testing does not, however, reliably predict which patients will have an allergic reaction to antivenom. The newest available antivenom in the United States (CroFab, Table 378-2) is an ovine antivenom produced by techniques that yield purified Fab antibodies. This product reduces the risk of allergic sequelae, and the manufacturer does not recommend a skin test prior to its use. Table 378-2 compares the two antivenoms available for the treatment of pit viper bites in the United States: Antivenin (Crotalidae) Polyvalent (ACP) and CroFab.

If the risk of allergic reaction is deemed significant (as when a less pure antivenom is being used), the patient should receive pretreatment with appropriate loading doses of intravenous antihistamines (e.g., diphenhydramine, 1 mg/kg to a maximum of 100 mg; and cimetidine, 5 to 10 mg/kg to a maximum of 300 mg). Modest expansion of the patient's intravascular volume with crystalloids may also be beneficial in this regard. Such pretreatment is not necessary when a highly purified Fab antivenom, such as CroFab, is used. Epinephrine should always be immediately available, and the antivenom dose to be administered should be diluted in an appropriate volume of crystalloid. The antivenom should be started slowly, with the physician at the bedside to intervene in the event of an acute reaction. The rate of infusion can be increased gradually in the absence of allergic phenomena until the total starting dose has been administered (over a total period of 1 to 2 h). Further antivenom may be necessary if the patient's clinical condition fails to stabilize or worsens. After stabilization, additional doses of CroFab are recommended because this preparation contains smaller-molecular-weight Fab fragments and is more rapidly cleared from the body than ACP. Laboratory values should be rechecked hourly, particularly if abnormal, until stability is apparent.

TABLE 378-1 *Sample Grading Scale for Use in Viperid Venom Poisoning*

Severity	Local Findings	Systemic Findings		Laboratory Studies
Nonenvenomation (dry bite)	None or puncture wounds only	None	*and*	Normal
Mild	Puncture wounds Pain Soft tissue swelling confined to the bite site	None	*and*	Normal
Moderate	Swelling extending beyond the local bite site	Mild (e.g., nausea, vomiting, muscle fasciculations, paresthesias)	*or*	Mildly abnormal (e.g., mildly abnormal platelet count or fibrinogen, or elevated fibrin split products)
Severe	Generally severe pain and swelling (may be minimal swelling in deep intramuscular or intravenous poisoning)	More severe (respiratory distress, hypotension/shock, evidence of bleeding, etc.)	*or*	Very abnormal

The management of a life-threatening envenomation in a victim with an apparent allergy to antivenom requires significant expertise. Consultation with a poison specialist, an intensive care specialist, and/or an allergist is recommended. Often antivenom can still be administered in these situations under closely controlled conditions and with intensive premedication (e.g., with epinephrine, antihistamines, and glucocorticoids). Preferably, a less immunogenic product (e.g., one composed of Fab fragments) should be used.

Care of the bite wound should include application of a dry sterile dressing and splinting of the extremity with padding between the digits. Once the administration of an indicated antivenom has been initiated, the extremity should be elevated above heart level to relieve edema. Tetanus immunization should be updated as appropriate. Prophylactic antibiotics are unnecessary, as the incidence of secondary infection following venomous snakebite is quite low.

If swelling in the bitten extremity raises concern that subfascial muscle edema may be impeding tissue perfusion (muscle-compartment syndrome), intracompartmental pressures should be checked by any minimally invasive technique (e.g., a wick catheter). If pressures are elevated and remain so despite additional antivenom administration and elevation of the extremity, surgical consultation for possible fasciotomy should be obtained. This complication, fortunately, is rare after snakebites.

Whether or not antivenom is given, any patient with signs of venom poisoning should be observed in the hospital for at least 24 h. A patient with an apparently "dry" bite should be watched for at least 8 h before discharge, as significant toxicity occasionally develops after a delay of several hours. The onset of systemic symptoms is commonly delayed for a number of hours after bites by several of the elapids (including coral snakes) and sea snakes. Patients bitten by these reptiles should be observed in the hospital for 24 h. Any patient requiring antivenom treatment should be admitted to an intensive care setting.

Follow-up care should include referral for physical therapy when needed to return the patient to an optimal level of functioning. In addition, victims of viperid bite should be reevaluated for evidence of recurrent coagulopathy ~48 h after discharge and as needed thereafter. These patients should be warned to avoid any routine surgery for the first few weeks, as occult coagulopathy can recur up to 2 weeks after a viperid bite.

MORBIDITY AND MORTALITY The overall mortality rates for venomous snakebite are low in areas of the world with rapid access to medical care and appropriate antivenom. In the United States, for example, the mortality rate is <1% for victims who receive antivenom. Eastern and western diamondback rattlesnakes (*Crotalus adamanteus* and *C. atrox*, respectively) are responsible for most snakebite deaths in the United States. Snakes responsible for large numbers of deaths in other regions of the world include the cobras (*Naja* spp.) of Asia and Africa, the carpet and saw-scaled vipers (*Echis* spp.) of the Middle East and Africa, Russell's viper (*Daboia russelli*) of the Middle East and Asia, the large African vipers (*Bitis* spp.), and the lancehead pit vipers (*Bothrops* spp.) of Central and South America.

TABLE 378-2 *Comparison of Antivenoms Available for Treatment of Pit Viper Bites in the United States*

	Antivenin (Crotalidae) Polyvalent[a]	CroFab[b]
Available since	1954	2000
Origin	Equine	Ovine
Snakes used in manufacture	*Crotalus adamanteus*	*C. adamanteus*
	C. atrox	*C. atrox*
	C. durissus terrificus	*C. scutulatus*
	Bothrops atrox	*Agkistrodon piscivorus*
Snakes covered	All North, Central, and South American and some Asian pit vipers	All North American pit vipers (and possibly some Latin American pit vipers)
Contains	IgG, equine albumin	Fab fragments
Skin testing recommended by manufacturer	Yes	No
Pretreatment with antihistamines recommended	Yes	No
Dosing		
Dry bite	None	None
Mild	0–5 vials	4–6 vials[c]
Moderately severe	10 vials	4–6 vials[c]
Severe	15–20 vials	6 vials
Repeat dosing	As needed	Repeat starting dose if patient fails to stabilize; after stabilization, 2 vials q6h for 3 more doses
Volume of diluent	1000 mL (reduce for children or in congestive heart failure)	250 mL
Administer over	2 h	1 h
Incidence of anaphylactic/-oid reaction	23–56% (some severe; some deaths)	14% (all relatively mild to date)
Incidence of delayed serum sickness	18–86% (higher with high doses)	16% (more recently, 3% with refinement of manufacturing process)

[a] Wyeth-Ayerst Laboratories, Philadelphia. There are indications that the manufacturer may soon discontinue production of this antivenom.
[b] Savage Laboratories, Melville, NY.
[c] Use of CroFab for a mild to moderate bite should be based on signs of progression of toxicity.

The incidence of morbidity—defined as permanent functional loss in a bitten extremity—is difficult to estimate but is clearly substantial. Such loss may be due to muscle, nerve, or vascular injury or to scar contracture. In the United States, such loss tends to be much more common and severe after rattlesnake bites than after bites by copperheads or water moccasins.

LIZARD BITES

Bites from the two species of venomous lizards (the gila monster, *Heloderma suspectum*, of the southwestern United States and the Mexican beaded lizard, *H. horridum*) are infrequent and usually follow attempts to capture or handle these creatures. Local findings include soft tissue trauma, significant pain, surrounding local edema, and occasionally local cyanosis and ecchymosis. Broken teeth may be embedded in the wounds. The venoms of these lizards are very similar and contain L-amino acid oxidase, phospholipases, hyaluronidase, and kallikreins. Systemic effects may include hypotension, weakness, dizziness, and diaphoresis.

Prehospital care measures for these bites should follow the guidelines listed above for viperid bites. If the biting lizard is still attached to the victim, its jaws may need to be manually pried apart for removal.

The sparseness of data on the pathophysiologic effects of helodermatid venom precludes specific recommendations regarding laboratory evaluation, but routine studies (complete blood count, coagulation studies, electrolyte analysis, blood typing and cross-matching, urinalysis, and electrocardiography) are prudent in anything other than a trivial bite. Wounds should be cleansed thoroughly and irrigated when possible. Tetanus immunization should be updated as indicated. Soft tissue radiography of the bite site and sterile probing under local anesthesia may identify retained teeth. The extremity should be splinted and elevated, but antibiotic treatment is not usually required. Systemic care is supportive (e.g., crystalloid infusion for hypotension). No antivenom exists. Pain due to local venom effects and mechanical trauma can be treated with opiates and regional nerve blocks. The mortality rate is extremely low.

MARINE ENVENOMATIONS

Management of venom poisoning by marine creatures is similar to that of venomous snakebite in that much of the treatment administered is supportive in nature. Prompt and appropriate field therapy may contribute to a successful clinical outcome. A few specific marine antivenoms can be used when appropriate.

INVERTEBRATES *Hydroids, fire coral, jellyfish, Portuguese man-of-war,* and *sea anemones* possess specialized stinging cells called *cnidocytes,* in which reside intracytoplasmic stinging organelles called *cnidae* (including nematocysts). The venoms from these organisms are mixtures of proteins, carbohydrates, and other components. The clinical syndrome following envenomation by any of these species is similar but of variable severity. Victims usually report immediate prickling or burning, pruritus, paresthesias, and painful throbbing with radiation. The skin becomes reddened, darkened, edematous, and/or blistered. A legion of neurologic, cardiovascular, respiratory, rheumatologic, gastrointestinal, renal, and ocular symptoms have been described. Victims in unstable condition with hypotension or respiratory distress should be treated supportively. Anaphylaxis sometimes develops. During stabilization, the skin should be immediately decontaminated with a generous application of vinegar (5% acetic acid), which inactivates nematocysts. Rubbing alcohol (40 to 70% isopropyl alcohol), baking soda (sodium bicarbonate), papain (unseasoned meat tenderizer), fresh lemon or lime juice, or household ammonia may be effective, depending on the species of stinging creature. For the sting of the venomous *box-jellyfish* (*Chironex fleckeri*; Fig. 378-1), vinegar should be used. Perfume, aftershave lotion, and high-proof ethanol are less efficacious and may be detrimental. Shaving the skin helps remove remaining nematocysts. Freshwater irrigation and rubbing lead to further stinging by adherent nematocysts and should be avoided. After decontamination, application of anesthetic ointments (lidocaine, benzocaine), antihistamine creams (diphenhydramine), or steroid lotions (hydrocortisone) may be helpful. Persistent pain after decontamination may be treated with morphine or meperidine. Muscle spasms may respond to 10% calcium gluconate (5 to 10 mL) or diazepam (2 to 5 mg, titrated upwards as necessary) given intravenously. An ovine-derived antivenom is available from Commonwealth Serum Laboratories (see section on antivenom sources, below) for stings from the box-jellyfish found in Australian and Indo-Pacific waters. At the time of this writing, this antivenom has not yet been used to treat envenomation by the box-shaped jellyfish, which may be of the genus *Chiropsalmus,* recently found in Florida waters. Safe Sea, a "jellyfish-safe sun block" (www.nidaria.com) that is applied to the skin before entering the water, inactivates the recognition and discharge mechanisms of nematocysts and has been tested successfully against a number of marine stingers.

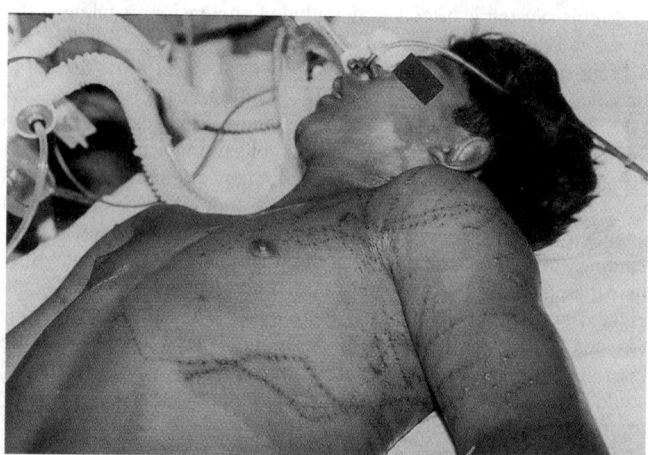

FIGURE 378-1   Skin lesions caused by *Chironex fleckeri* sting. (*Courtesy of Dr. V. Pranava Murthy.*)

Touching a *sea sponge* may result in dermatitis. If contact occurs, the skin should be gently dried and adhesive tape used to remove embedded spicules. Vinegar should be applied immediately and then for 10 to 30 min three or four times a day. Rubbing alcohol may be used if vinegar is unavailable. After spicule removal and skin decontamination, a steroid or antihistamine cream may be applied to the skin. Severe vesiculation should be treated with a 2-week course of systemic glucocorticoids.

Annelid worms (bristleworms) possess rows of soft, cactus-like spines capable of inflicting painful stings. Contact results in symptoms similar to those of nematocyst envenomation. Without treatment, pain usually subsides over several hours, but inflammation may persist for up to a week. Victims should resist the urge to scratch, since scratching may fracture retrievable spines. Visible bristles should be removed with forceps and adhesive tape or a commercial facial peel; alternatively, a thin layer of rubber cement can be used to entrap the spines. Use of vinegar, rubbing alcohol, or dilute ammonia or a brief application of unseasoned meat tenderizer (papain) may provide additional relief. Local inflammation should be treated with topical or systemic glucocorticoids.

Sea urchins possess either hollow, venom-filled, calcified spines or triple-jawed, globiferous pedicellariae with venom glands. Their venom contains several toxic components, including steroid glycosides, hemolysins, proteases, serotonin, and cholinergic substances. Contact with either venom apparatus produces immediate and intensely painful stings. The affected part should be immersed immediately in hot water (see below). Accessible embedded spines should be removed but may break off and remain lodged in the victim. Residual dye from the surface of a spine remaining after the spine's removal may mimic a retained spine but is otherwise of no consequence. Soft tissue radiography or magnetic resonance imaging (MRI) can confirm the presence of retained spines; this finding may warrant referral for attempted surgical removal if the spines are located near vital structures (e.g., joints, neurovascular bundles). Retained spines may cause the formation of granulomas that are amenable to excision or to intralesional injection with triamcinolone hexacetonide (5 mg/mL).

Cone shells are predatory, carnivorous mollusks. The most dangerous of these creatures are found in the Indian and Pacific oceans. A neurotoxic venom comprising multiple peptides is delivered through harpoon-like darts propelled from an extensible proboscis. Clinically, the sting is like that of a bee. The victim may report wound, perioral, and generalized paresthesias. Bulbar dysfunction and systemic muscular paralysis indicate severe envenomation. The sting of the geographer cone (*Conus geographus*) can cause cerebral edema, coma, and death due to respiratory or cardiac failure. Immediately after envenomation, a circumferential pressure-immobilization dressing 15 cm wide should be applied over a gauze pad measuring approximately $7 \times 7 \times 2$ cm that has been placed directly over the sting. The dressing should be applied at venous-lymphatic pressure with the preservation of distal arterial pulses. Once the victim has been transported to the nearest medical facility, the bandage can be released. Provision should be made for cardiovascular and respiratory support.

Serious envenomations and deaths have followed bites of the *Australian blue-ringed octopuses* (*Octopus maculosus* and *O. lunulata*). Although these animals rarely exceed 20 cm in length, their venom contains a potent neurotoxin (maculotoxin) that inhibits peripheral nerve transmission by blocking sodium conductance. Oral and facial numbness develop within several minutes of a serious envenomation and rapidly progress to total flaccid paralysis, including failure of respiratory muscles. If respirations are assisted, the victim may remain awake although completely paralyzed. Since there is no antidote, treatment is supportive. Immediately after envenomation, attempts should be made to limit the dispersion of venom by application of a pressure-immobilization or venous-lymphatic pressure dressing. Hot-water immersion and cryotherapy are ineffective. Artificial respiration should be provided. Even with serious envenomations, significant recovery often takes place within 4 to 10 h. Sequelae are uncommon unless related to hypoxia.

VERTEBRATES A number of marine vertebrates, including stingrays, scorpionfish, catfish, surgeonfish, and weeverfish, can envenomate humans. The management of most of these stings is similar.

A *stingray* injury is both an envenomation and a traumatic wound. The venom, which contains serotonin, 5′-nucleotidase, and phosphodiesterase, causes immediate and intense pain that may last up to 48 h. The wound often becomes ischemic in appearance and heals poorly, with adjacent soft tissue swelling and prolonged disability. Systemic effects include weakness, diaphoresis, nausea, vomiting, diarrhea, dysrhythmias, syncope, hypotension, muscle cramps, fasciculations, paralysis, and (in rare cases) death.

The designation *scorpionfish* encompasses members of the family Scorpaenidae and includes not only scorpionfish but also lionfish and stonefish. A complex venom with neuromuscular toxicity is delivered through 12 or 13 dorsal, 2 pelvic, and 3 anal spines. Pectoral spines do not contain venom. The severity of envenomation depends on the species of fish, the number of stings, and the amount of venom released. In general, the sting of a stonefish is regarded as the most serious (severe to life-threatening); that of the scorpionfish is of intermediate seriousness; and that of the lionfish is the least serious. Like that of a stingray, the sting of a scorpionfish is immediately and intensely painful. Pain from a stonefish envenomation may last for days. The systemic manifestations of scorpionfish stings are similar to those of stingray envenomations but may be more pronounced, particularly in the case of a stonefish sting. The rare deaths following stonefish envenomation usually occur within 6 to 8 h.

Two species of marine *catfish*—*Plotosus lineatus* (the oriental catfish) and *Galeichthys felis* (the common sea catfish)—as well as several species of freshwater catfish are capable of stinging humans. Venom is delivered through a single dorsal spine and two pectoral spines. Clinically, a catfish sting is comparable to that of a stingray, although marine catfish envenomations are generally more severe than those of their freshwater counterparts. *Surgeonfish* (doctorfish, tang), *weeverfish*, *ratfish*, and *horned venomous sharks* have also been implicated in human envenomations.

℞ TREATMENT

The stings of all these marine vertebrates are treated in a similar fashion. Except for stonefish and serious scorpionfish envenomations (see below), no antivenom is available. The affected part should be immersed immediately in nonscalding hot water (113°F/45°C) for 30 to 90 min or until there is significant relief of pain. This measure may inactivate heat-labile components of the venoms. Recurrent pain may respond to repeated hot-water treatment. Cryotherapy is contraindicated. Opiates will help alleviate the pain, as will local wound infiltration or regional nerve block with 1% lidocaine, 0.5% bupivacaine, and sodium bicarbonate mixed in a 5:5:1 ratio. After soaking and anesthetic administration, the wound must be explored and debrided. Radiography (in particular, MRI) may be helpful in the identification and location of foreign bodies. After exploration and debridement, the wound should be vigorously irrigated with warm sterile water, saline, or 1% povidone-iodine in solution. Bleeding can usually be controlled by sustained local pressure for 10 to 15 min. In general, wounds should be left open to heal by secondary intention or be treated by delayed primary closure. Tetanus immunization should be updated. Antibiotic treatment should be considered for serious wounds and for envenomation in immunocompromised hosts. The initial antibiotics should cover *Staphylococcus* and *Streptococcus* spp. If the victim is immunocompromised or an infection develops, antibiotic coverage should be broadened to include *Vibrio* spp.

APPROACH TO THE PATIENT

It is not uncommon for a physician to encounter a patient who has been envenomated by a marine creature that cannot be positively identified at the scene of the envenomation. Therefore, it is useful to be familiar with the local marine fauna and to recognize patterns of injury.

A large puncture wound or jagged laceration, particularly on the lower extremity, that is more painful than one would expect from the size and configuration of the wound is likely a stingray envenomation. Smaller punctures, as described above, represent the activity of a sea urchin or starfish. Stony corals cause rough abrasions and, in rare instances, lacerations or puncture wounds.

Coelenterate (marine invertebrate) stings sometimes create diagnostic skin patterns. A diffuse urticarial rash on exposed skin is often indicative of exposure to fragmented hydroids or larval anemones. A linear, whiplike print pattern appears where a jellyfish tentacle has contacted the skin. In the case of the dreaded box-jellyfish (Fig. 378-1), a cross-hatched, sometimes frosted appearance followed by the development of a dark purple coloration within a few hours of the sting heralds skin necrosis. An encounter with fire coral causes immediate pain and a swollen red skin irritation in the pattern of contact, similar to but more severe than the imprint left by exposure to an intact feather hydroid. Seabather's eruption, caused by thimble jellyfishes and larval anemones, may produce a diffuse rash that consists of clusters of erythematous macules or raised papules, accompanied by intense itching (Fig. 378-2). Toxic sponges (exposure to which usually occurs during handling) create a burning and painful red rash on exposed skin, which may blister and later desquamate. Virtually all marine stingers invoke the sequelae of inflammation, so that local erythema, swelling, and adenopathy are fairly nonspecific.

SOURCES OF ANTIVENOMS AND OTHER ASSISTANCE An antivenom for stonefish (and severe scorpionfish) envenomation, made in Australia by the Commonwealth Serum Laboratories (CSL; 45 Poplar Road, Parkville, Victoria, Australia 3052; www.csl.com.au; 61-3-389-1911; fax: 61-3-389-1434), is available in the United States through the pharmacies of Sharp Cabrillo Hospital Emergency Department, San Diego, CA, at (619) 221-3429, and Community Hospital of Monterey Peninsula (CHOMP) Emergency Department, Monterey, CA, at (408) 625-4900.

Polyvalent sea snake antivenom is available from CSL or CHOMP. If sea snake antivenom is unavailable, tiger snake (*N. scutatus*) antivenom should be used.

Divers Alert Network, a nonprofit organization designed to assist in the care of injured divers, may also help with the treatment of marine

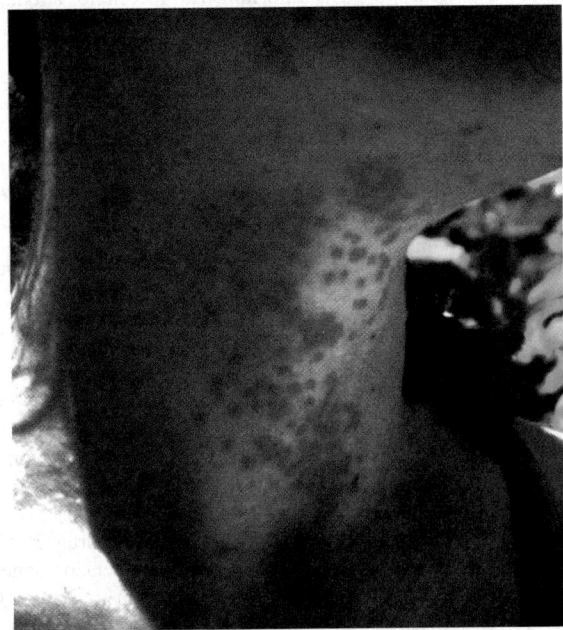

FIGURE 378-2 Erythematous, papular rash typical of seabather's eruption caused by thimble jellyfish and larval anemones. (*Courtesy of Dr. Paul Auerbach.*)

injuries. The network can be reached on the Internet at www.diversalertnetwork.org or by telephone 24 hours a day at (919) 684-8111.

MARINE POISONINGS

CIGUATERA Ciguatera poisoning is the most common nonbacterial food poisoning associated with fish in the United States; most cases occur in Florida and Hawaii. The poisoning involves almost exclusively tropical and semitropical marine coral reef fish. Of reported cases, 75% (except in Hawaii) involve the barracuda, snapper, jack, or grouper. The ciguatera syndrome is associated with at least five polyether sodium channel activator toxins that originate in photosynthetic dinoflagellates (such as *Gambierdiscus toxicus*) and accumulate in the food chain. These toxins are unaffected by freeze-drying, heat, cold, and gastric acid. None of the toxins affects the odor, color, or taste of fish.

The onset of symptoms may come within 15 to 30 min of ingestion and typically takes place within 2 to 6 h. Symptoms then increase in severity over the ensuing 4 to 6 h. Most victims develop symptoms within 12 h of ingestion, and virtually all are afflicted within 24 h. The more than 150 symptoms reported include abdominal pain, nausea, vomiting, diarrhea, chills, paresthesias, pruritus, tongue and throat numbness or burning, sensation of "carbonation" during swallowing, odontalgia or dental dysesthesias, dysphagia, dysuria, dyspnea, weakness, fatigue, tremor, fasciculations, athetosis, meningismus, aphonia, ataxia, vertigo, pain and weakness in the lower extremities, visual blurring, transient blindness, hyporeflexia, seizures, nasal congestion and dryness, conjunctivitis, maculopapular rash, skin vesiculations, dermatographism, sialorrhea, diaphoresis, headache, arthralgias, myalgias, insomnia, bradycardia, hypotension, central respiratory failure, and coma. Death is rare.

Diarrhea, vomiting, and abdominal pain usually develop 3 to 6 h after ingestion of a ciguatoxic fish. Symptoms may persist for 48 h and then generally resolve (even without treatment). A pathognomonic symptom is the reversal of hot and cold tactile perception, which develops in some persons after 3 to 5 days and may last for months. Tachycardia and hypertension have been described, in some cases after potentially severe transient bradycardia and hypotension. More severe reactions tend to occur in persons previously stricken with the disease. Persons who have ingested parrotfish (scaritoxin) may suffer from classic ciguatera poisoning as well as a "second-phase" syndrome (after 5 to 10 days' delay) of disequilibrium with locomotor ataxia, dysmetria, and resting or kinetic tremor. This affliction may persist for 2 to 6 weeks.

The differential diagnosis of ciguatera includes paralytic shellfish poisoning, eosinophilic meningitis, type E botulism, organophosphate insecticide poisoning, tetrodotoxin poisoning, and psychogenic hyperventilation. At present, the diagnosis of ciguatera poisoning is made on clinical grounds because no routinely used laboratory test detects ciguatoxin in human blood. A ciguatoxin enzyme immunoassay or radioimmunoassay may be used to test small portions of the suspected fish, but even these tests may not detect the very small amount of toxin (0.1 ppb) necessary to render fish flesh toxic.

℞ TREATMENT

Therapy is supportive and based on symptoms. Although not of proven efficacy, a slurry of activated charcoal (100 g) in sorbitol may be of limited value if given within 3 h after ingestion. Nausea and vomiting may be controlled with an antiemetic, such as prochlorperazine (2.5 to 5 mg intravenously). Hypotension may require the administration of intravenous crystalloid and, in rare cases, a pressor drug. Bradyarrhythmias that lead to cardiac insufficiency and hypotension generally respond well to atropine (0.5 mg intravenously, up to 2 mg). Cool showers or the administration of hydroxyzine (25 mg orally every 6 to 8 h) may relieve pruritus. Amitriptyline (25 mg orally twice a day)

reportedly ameliorates pruritus and dysesthesias. In three cases unresponsive to amitriptyline, tocainide appeared to be efficacious. Nifedipine has been used to treat headache. Intravenous infusion of mannitol may be beneficial in moderate or severe cases, particularly for the relief of distressing neurologic or cardiovascular symptoms, although the efficacy of this therapy has recently been challenged. The infusion is rendered initially as 1 g/kg per day over 45 to 60 min during the acute phase (days 1 to 5). If symptoms improve, a second dose may be given within 3 to 4 h and repeated on the following day. The mechanism of the benefit against ciguatera intoxication is perhaps hyperosmotic water-drawing action, which reverses ciguatoxin-induced Schwann cell edema. Mannitol may also act in some fashion as a "hydroxyl scavenger."

During recovery from ciguatera poisoning, the victim should exclude the following from the diet: fish (fresh or preserved), fish sauces, shellfish, shellfish sauces, alcoholic beverages, and nuts and nut oils. Consumption of fish in ciguatera-endemic regions should be avoided. All oversized fish of any predacious reef species should be suspected of harboring ciguatoxin. Neither moray eels nor the viscera of tropical marine fish should ever be eaten.

PARALYTIC SHELLFISH POISONING Paralytic shellfish poisoning is induced by the ingestion of any of a variety of feral or aquacultured filter-feeding organisms, including clams, oysters, scallops, mussels, chitons, limpets, starfish, and sand crabs. The origin of their toxicity is the chemical toxin they accumulate and concentrate by feeding on various planktonic dinoflagellates and protozoan organisms. The unicellular phytoplanktonic organisms form the foundation of the food chain, and in warm summer months these organisms "bloom" in nutrient-rich coastal temperate and semitropical waters. A number of dinoflagellates produce a variety of toxins. These planktonic species can release massive amounts of toxic metabolites into the water and cause enormous mortality in bird and marine populations. The paralytic shellfish toxins are water-soluble as well as heat- and acid-stable; they cannot be destroyed by ordinary cooking. The best-characterized and most frequently identified paralytic shellfish toxin is saxitoxin, which takes its name from the Alaska butter clam *Saxidomus giganteus*. A toxin concentration of >75 μg/100 g of foodstuff is considered hazardous to humans. In the 1972 New England "red tide," the concentration of saxitoxin in blue mussels exceeded 9000 μg/100 g of foodstuff. Saxitoxin appears to block sodium conductance, inhibiting neuromuscular transmission at the axonal and muscle membrane levels.

Within minutes to a few hours after ingestion of contaminated shellfish, there is the onset of intraoral and perioral paresthesias, notably of the lips, tongue, and gums, that progress rapidly to involve the neck and distal extremities. The tingling or burning sensation later changes to numbness. Other symptoms rapidly develop and include lightheadedness, disequilibrium, incoordination, weakness, hyperreflexia, incoherence, dysarthria, sialorrhea, dysphagia, thirst, diarrhea, abdominal pain, nausea, vomiting, nystagmus, dysmetria, headache, diaphoresis, loss of vision, chest pain, and tachycardia. Flaccid paralysis and respiratory insufficiency may follow 2 to 12 h after ingestion. In the absence of hypoxia, the victim often remains alert but paralyzed.

℞ TREATMENT

Treatment is supportive and based on symptoms. Since airway loss may be rapid, induced emesis should not be attempted. If the victim comes to medical attention within the first few hours after poison ingestion, the stomach should be emptied by gastric lavage and then irrigated with 2 L (in 200-mL aliquots) of a solution of 2% sodium bicarbonate; this intervention has not been proved to be of benefit but is based on the notion that gastric acidity may enhance the potency of saxitoxin. The administration of activated charcoal (50 to 100 g) and a cathartic (sorbitol, 20 to 50 g) makes empirical sense since these shellfish toxins are believed to bind well to charcoal. Some authors advise against administration of magnesium-based solutions, such as certain cathartics, cautioning that hypermagnesemia may contribute to suppression of nerve conduction.

The most serious problem is respiratory paralysis. The victim should be closely observed in a hospital for at least 24 h for respiratory distress. With prompt recognition of ventilatory failure, endotracheal intubation and assisted ventilation prevent anoxic myocardial and brain injury.

TETRODOTOXIN FISH POISONING Tetrodotoxin is a neurotoxin that has been isolated from four different animal phyla, including puffer fish and the blue-ringed octopus. Humans ingest tetrodotoxin by eating puffer fish (toadfish, globefish, swellfish, porcupine fish) in the form of the delicacy fugu. Ingestion is intended to induce pleasurable sensations of oral tingling. The toxin is found throughout the fish, with high concentrations in the liver, viscera, gonads, and skin. It is stable to extremes of temperature. Tetrodotoxin interferes with central and peripheral neuromuscular transmission in humans via blocking effects on axonal transmission mediated by sodium conductance. In addition, the toxin causes peripheral vasodilation and hypotension, exerting these effects in a dose-dependent fashion.

Symptoms typically develop within 30 min of ingestion but may be delayed by up to 4 h. Death has occurred within 17 min of ingestion. Paresthesias of the lips and tongue are followed by sialorrhea, sweating, headache, weakness, lethargy, ataxia, incoordination, tremor, paralysis, cyanosis, aphonia, dysphagia, seizures, dyspnea, bronchorrhea, bronchospasm, respiratory failure, coma, and hypotension. Gastroenteric symptoms are often severe and include nausea, vomiting, diarrhea, and abdominal pain. Cardiac arrhythmias may precede complete respiratory failure and cardiovascular collapse.

TREATMENT

Therapy is supportive and based on symptoms, with aggressive early airway management. Alpha adrenergic agonists are recommended in addition to intravenous fluids to combat hypotension. Anticholinesterase agents have been used with mixed success.

DOMOIC ACID INTOXICATION In late 1987 in eastern Canada, an outbreak of gastrointestinal and neurologic symptoms (amnestic shellfish poisoning) was documented in persons who had consumed mussels found to be contaminated with domoic acid. In 1991, an epidemic of domoic acid poisoning in the state of Washington was attributed to the consumption of razor clams. A heat-stable neuroexcitatory amino acid whose biochemical analogs are kainic acid and glutamic acid, domoic acid binds to the kainate type of glutamate receptor with three times the affinity of kainic acid and is 20 times as powerful a toxin. Shellfish can be tested for domoic acid by mouse bioassay and high-performance liquid chromatography. The regulatory limit for domoic acid in shellfish is 20 parts per million.

The abnormalities noted within 24 h of ingesting contaminated mussels (*Mytilus edulis*) include arousal, confusion, disorientation, and memory loss. The median time of onset is 5.5 h. Other prominent symptoms include severe headache, nausea, vomiting, diarrhea, abdominal cramps, hiccoughs, arrhythmias, hypotension, seizures, ophthalmoplegia, hemiparesis, mutism, grimacing, agitation, emotional lability, coma, copious bronchial secretions, and pulmonary edema. Histologic study of brain tissue taken at autopsy has shown neuronal necrosis or cell loss and astrocytosis, most prominently in the hippocampus and the amygdaloid nucleus—findings similar to those in animals poisoned with kainic acid. Several months after the primary intoxication, victims still display chronic residual memory deficits and motor neuronopathy or axonopathy. Nonneurologic illness does not persist.

TREATMENT

Therapy is supportive and based on symptoms. Since kainic acid neuropathology seems to be nearly entirely seizure mediated, an emphasis

should be placed on anticonvulsive therapy, for which diazepam appears to be as effective as any other drug.

SCOMBROID Scombroid (mackerel-like) fish include the albacore, bluefin, and yellowfin tuna; mackerel; saury; needlefish; wahoo; skipjack; and bonito. Nonscombroid fish that produce scombroid poisoning include the dolphinfish (Hawaiian mahimahi, *Coryphaena hippurus*), kahawai, sardine, black marlin, pilchard, anchovy, herring, amberjack, and Australian ocean salmon. In the northeastern and mid-Atlantic United States, bluefish (*Pomatomus saltatrix*) has been linked to scombroid poisoning. Because greater numbers of nonscombroid fish are being recognized as scombrotoxic, the syndrome may more appropriately be called *pseudoallergic fish poisoning*.

Under conditions of inadequate preservation or refrigeration, the musculature of these dark- or red-fleshed fish undergoes bacterial decomposition, which includes the decarboxylation of the amino acid L-histidine to histamine, histamine phosphate, and histamine hydrochloride. Histamine levels of 20 to 50 mg/100 g are noted in toxic fish, with levels in excess of 400 mg/100 g on occasion. The toxin is heat stable and is not destroyed by domestic or commercial cooking. Affected fish typically have a sharply metallic or peppery taste; however, they may be normal in appearance, color, and flavor. Not all persons who eat a contaminated fish necessarily become ill, perhaps because of uneven distribution of decay within the fish.

Symptoms develop within 15 to 90 min of ingestion and include flushing (sharply demarcated; exacerbated by ultraviolet exposure; particularly pronounced on the face, neck, and upper trunk), a sensation of warmth without elevated core temperature, conjunctival hyperemia, pruritus, urticaria, angioneurotic edema, bronchospasm, nausea, vomiting, diarrhea, epigastric pain, abdominal cramps, dysphagia, headache, thirst, pharyngitis, burning of the gingiva, palpitations, tachycardia, dizziness, and hypotension. Without treatment, the symptoms generally resolve within 8 to 12 h. The reaction may be more severe in a person who is concurrently ingesting isoniazid because of blockade of gastrointestinal tract histaminase.

TREATMENT

Therapy is directed at reversing the histamine effect with antihistamines, either H-1 or H-2. If bronchospasm is severe, an inhaled bronchodilator—or in rare, extremely severe circumstances, injected epinephrine—may be used. Glucocorticoids are of no proven benefit. Protracted nausea and vomiting, which may empty the stomach of toxin, may be controlled with a specific antiemetic, such as prochlorperazine. The persistent headache of scombroid poisoning may respond to cimetidine or a similar antihistamine if standard analgesics are not effective.

Pfiesteria In the summer of 1997, reports of adverse reactions after casual exposure to Maryland waters infested with the fish-killing dinoflagellate *Pfiesteria piscicida* prompted the Centers for Disease Control and Prevention (CDC) to undertake multistate surveillance and to establish a case definition. The route of exposure is either direct contact with the water or inhalation of aerosols. As defined by the CDC, the human disease syndrome associated with *Pfiesteria* is characterized by either of two groups of signs and symptoms: (1) memory loss, forgetfulness, or confusion *or* acute skin burning on direct contact with infested water; or (2) at least three of the following: headache, rash (flat red sores), eye irritation, upper respiratory irritation, muscle cramps, and gastrointestinal symptoms. The skin lesions—red edematous papules on the extremities and trunk—resolve within a few days to a week after exposure. Since the initial reports, cases have followed either casual exposure to infested water or laboratory work with *Pfiesteria* (which is currently conducted in biohazard III facilities).

Research on *Pfiesteria* has been complicated by a variety of factors, including the lack of a test for detection of its toxins, which have yet to be purified, and the organism's complex life cycle, which includes at least two dozen stages. In nature, the proximity of a school of fish elicits *Pfiesteria*'s transformation into a flagellated zoospore that releases at least two toxins: a water-soluble, neuroactive toxin that kills fish within minutes and a fat-soluble toxin that causes epidermal delamination. Polluted environments appear to favor *Pfiesteria*.

Diagnosis is difficult because the specific toxins have not yet been identified and there is no biomarker for exposure. Detection systems using polymerase chain reaction and fluorescent markers are being developed for rapid identification of the dinoflagellate. Neurocognitive deficits appear to improve significantly within 3 to 6 months after cessation of exposure. No deaths have been reported, and most victims improve without treatment. For the treatment of persistent *Pfiesteria*-associated syndromes, one teaspoon of milk of magnesia each day followed by one scoop of cholestyramine in 8 ounces of water 4 times a day for 2 weeks has been used successfully as an empiric remedy in a limited number of cases.

FURTHER READING

AUERBACH PS (ed): *Wilderness Medicine*, 4th ed. St. Louis, Mosby, 2001

BUSH SP, HARDY DL: Immediate removal of Extractor is recommended. Ann Emerg Med 38:607, 2001

——— et al: Effects of a negative pressure venom extraction device (Extractor) on local tissue injury after artificial rattlesnake envenomation in a porcine model. Acad Emerg Med 7:495, 2000

DART RC et al: A randomized multicenter trial of Crotalinae polyvalent immune Fab (ovine) antivenom for the treatment for crotaline snakebite in the United States. Arch Intern Med 161:2030, 2001

GOLD BS et al: Bites of venomous snakes. N Engl J Med 347:347, 2002

MEIER J, WHITE J (eds): *Handbook of Clinical Toxicology of Animal Venoms and Poisons.* Boca Raton, FL, CRC Press, 1996, pp 89–176

MEYER WP et al: First clinical experiences with a new ovine Fab *Echis ocellatus* snake bite antivenom in Nigeria: Randomized comparative trial with Institute Pasteur Serum (Ipser) Africa antivenom. Am J Trop Med Hyg 56:291, 1997

PEARN J: Neurology of ciguatera. J Neurol Neurosurg Psychiatry 70:4, 2001

379 ECTOPARASITE INFESTATIONS AND ARTHROPOD BITES AND STINGS

James H. Maguire, Richard J. Pollack, Andrew Spielman

Ectoparasites are arthropods or helminths that infest the skin of other animals, from which they derive sustenance. They may penetrate beneath the surface of the host or attach superficially by their mouthparts. These organisms damage their hosts by inflicting direct injury, by eliciting a hypersensitivity reaction, or by inoculating toxins or pathogens. The main medically important ectoparasites are arachnids (including mites and ticks), insects (including lice, fleas, and flies), pentastomes (tongue worms), and leeches. Arthropods may also harm humans through brief encounters in which they take a blood meal or attempt to defend themselves by biting, stinging, or exuding venoms. Various arachnids (spiders, scorpions), insects (including bees, hornets, wasps, ants, flies, bugs, caterpillars, and beetles), millipedes, and centipedes produce ill effects in this manner, as do certain ectoparasites of animals, including ticks, biting mites, and fleas (discussed in this chapter as biting arthropods). More people in the United States die each year as a consequence of arthropod stings than from the bites of poisonous snakes.

ECTOPARASITE INFESTATIONS

SCABIES The human itch mite, *Sarcoptes scabiei*, which infests some 300 million persons each year, is one of the most common causes of itching dermatoses throughout the world. Gravid female mites, measuring 0.3 to 0.4 mm in length, burrow superficially beneath the stratum corneum for a month, depositing two or three eggs a day. Nymphs that hatch from these eggs mature in ~2 weeks through a series of molts and then emerge as adults to the surface of the skin, where they mate and subsequently reinvade the skin of the same or another host. Transfer of newly fertilized female mites from person to person occurs by intimate contact with an infested person and is facilitated by crowding, uncleanliness, and contact with multiple sexual partners. Medical practitioners are at particular risk of infestation. Transmission via sharing of contaminated bedding or clothing is infrequent because these mites die within a day or so in the absence of host contact, depending upon ambient conditions. In the United States, scabies may account for 2 to 5% of visits to dermatologists; involved particularly often are children, immigrants from developing countries, and close household contacts. Outbreaks occur in nursing homes, mental institutions, and hospitals.

The itching and rash associated with scabies derive from a sensitization reaction directed against the excreta that the mite deposits in its burrow (Fig. 379-1). For this reason, an initial infestation remains asymptomatic for 4 to 6 weeks, and a reinfestation produces a hyper-sensitivity reaction without delay. Scratching generally destroys the burrowing mite, but symptoms remain even in its absence. Burrows become surrounded by infiltrates of eosinophils, lymphocytes, and histiocytes, and a generalized hypersensitivity rash later develops in remote sites. By destroying these pathogens, immunity and associated scratching limit most infestations to <15 mites per person. Hyperinfestation with thousands of mites, a condition known as *crusted scabies* or *Norwegian scabies*, may result from glucocorticoid use, immunodeficiency diseases (including AIDS and infection with human T-lymphotropic virus type I), and neurologic and psychiatric illnesses that interfere with itching and scratching.

Patients with scabies report intense itching that worsens at night and after a hot shower. Typical burrows may be difficult to find because they are few in number and may be obscured by excoriations. Burrows appear as dark wavy lines in the epidermis, measure 3 to 15 mm, and end in a small pearly bleb that contains the female mite. Such lesions generally develop on the volar wrists, between the fingers, on the elbows, and on the penis. Small papules and vesicles, often accompanied by eczematous plaques, pustules, or nodules, are symmetrically distributed in these sites and in skin folds under the breasts and around the navel, axillae, belt line, buttocks, upper thighs, and scro-

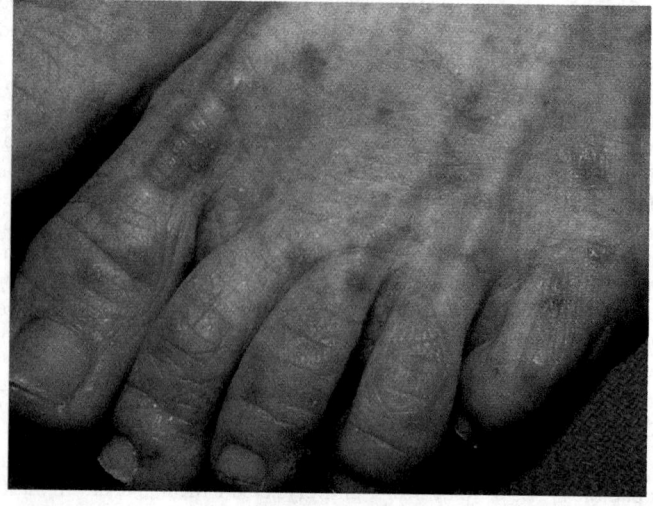

FIGURE 379-1   Scabies showing typical erythematous papules and few linear burrows.

tum. Except in infants, the face, scalp, neck, palms, and soles are spared. Burrows and other typical lesions may be sparse in persons who wash frequently, and topical glucocorticoid treatment and bacterial superinfection may alter the appearance of the rash. Atypical presentations of scabies include bullous lesions, which resemble those of bullous pemphigoid, and vesicular lesions, which resemble those of dermatitis herpetiformis. Superinfection with nephritogenic strains of streptococci has led to acute glomerulonephritis. Crusted scabies resembles psoriasis in its typical widespread erythema, thick keratotic crusts, scaling, and dystrophic nails. Characteristic burrows are not seen in crusted scabies, and patients usually do not itch, although their infestations are highly contagious and have been responsible for outbreaks of classic scabies in hospitals. Bacteremia occurs frequently in AIDS patients with crusted scabies and prominent fissures. Persons with massive infestations occasionally present with diffuse pruritus and generalized papules or with minimal or no cutaneous signs.

A diagnosis of scabies should be considered in patients with pruritus and symmetric polymorphic skin lesions in characteristic locations, particularly if there is a history of household contact with a case. Burrows should be sought and unroofed with a sterile needle or scalpel blade, and the scrapings should be examined microscopically for the mite, its eggs, and its fecal pellets. A drop of mineral oil facilitates removal of the sample. Biopsies or scrapings of papulovesicular lesions may also be diagnostic. In the absence of identifiable mites or mite products, the diagnosis is based on clinical presentation and history. Diverse kinds of dermatitis due to other causes are frequently misdiagnosed as scabies. The possibility of other sexually transmitted diseases should be excluded in adults with scabies.

℞ TREATMENT

For the treatment of scabies, 5% permethrin cream is less toxic than the once commonly used 1% lindane preparations and is effective against lindane-tolerant infestations. Both scabicides are applied thinly but thoroughly behind the ears and from the neck down after bathing and are removed 8 h later with soap and water. Lindane is absorbed through the skin, and its overuse has led to seizures and aplastic anemia. It should not be applied to pregnant women or infants. Alternatives include topical crotamiton cream, benzyl benzoate, and sulfur ointments. Successful treatment of crusted scabies requires the application first of a keratolytic agent such as 6% salicylic acid (to improve the penetration of scabicides) and then of scabicides to the scalp, face, and ears (with care to avoid the eyes). Repeated treatments or the sequential use of several agents may be necessary. A single oral dose of ivermectin (200 μg/kg) effectively treats scabies in otherwise-healthy persons. Patients with crusted scabies may require two or more doses of ivermectin. Although ivermectin may become the agent of choice for treating crusted scabies, it has not yet received approval by the U.S. Food and Drug Administration (FDA) for any form of scabies. Its use should be reserved for persons who fail to respond to topical scabicides, the elderly, persons with generalized eczema, and other persons who may not tolerate topical therapy.

Although effectively treated scabies infestations become noninfectious within a day, itching and rash due to hypersensitivity frequently persist for weeks or months. Unnecessary re-treatment of the affected patients may provoke contact dermatitis. Antihistamines, salicylates, and calamine lotion relieve itching during treatment, and topical glucocorticoids are useful for the pruritus that lingers after effective treatment. An oral antibiotic may be necessary for bacterial superinfections that fail to resolve with antiscabietic therapy. Relapses of scabies may be due to infestations of the scalp when topical therapy is applied only from the neck down. To prevent reinfestations, bedding and clothing should be washed in hot water and dried in a heated dryer, and close contacts, even if asymptomatic, should be treated simultaneously.

OTHER MITE INFESTATIONS Demodectic mites infest the facial skin of virtually all people. The term *follicle mite* is applied both to *Demodex folliculorum*, which resides in hair follicles, and to *D. brevis*, which resides in sebaceous glands. These wormlike mites can be as long as 0.4 mm. They appear not to cause symptoms in humans, although they may be numerous in the skin of individuals with rosacea. Demodectic mange may be severely debilitating in certain domestic animals.

House dust mites of the genus *Dermatophagoides* infest houses throughout the world, living on furniture and rugs and feeding on shed human dander. Exposure to their allergens in the domestic environment causes asthma, rhinitis, conjunctivitis, and eczema in allergic individuals. Management includes immunotherapy with mite extracts and a variety of environmental interventions (e.g., frequent cleaning of floors and upholstered furniture, removal or acaricidal treatment of rugs in bedrooms) to reduce mite density. Although use of a high-efficiency particulate air (HEPA)–filtered vacuum may help remove mites and their food source, it may also exacerbate exposure by propelling mite allergens into the air.

PEDICULOSIS (LOUSE INFESTATION) Nymphs and adults of all three kinds of human louse feed at least once a day, and they ingest human blood exclusively. Head lice (*Pediculus capitis*) infest mainly the hair of the scalp, body lice (*P. humanus*) the clothing, and crab or pubic lice (*Pthirus pubis*) mainly the hair of the pubis. The saliva of lice produces an intensely irritating maculopapular or urticarial rash in sensitized persons. Females of head and pubic lice cement their eggs firmly to hair and body lice mainly to clothing. A nymph hatches after ~10 days of development. The empty egg (nit) may remain affixed for months or longer after the louse has hatched.

Head lice infest ~1% of elementary school–aged children in the United States and are transmitted mainly by direct person-to-person contact. The role of fomites (shared headgear and grooming implements) as a transmission vehicle seems of negligible importance. In the United States, black children are less frequently infested than other children. Excoriations of pruritic lesions on the scalp, neck, and shoulders infrequently lead to oozing, crusting, matting of hair, bacterial infections, and regional lymphadenopathy. Head lice removed from a person generally succumb to desiccation and starvation within a day. Head lice seem unimportant as natural vectors for pathogenic agents.

Body lice remain on clothing except when feeding and generally succumb within a day or two if separated from the human host. These lice mainly infest disaster victims or indigent people who are in close contact with other infested individuals and who change their clothes only infrequently. Transmission by direct contact or by sharing of clothing and bedding is enhanced under crowded conditions. The tendency of the body louse to leave febrile persons or corpses as they become cold may facilitate the transmission of louse-borne typhus, louse-borne relapsing fever, and trench fever (Chap. 158). Trench fever and endocarditis due to *Bartonella quintana* have emerged as diseases of homeless persons living in large cities of the United States and Europe. Pruritic lesions are particularly common around the neckline. Chronic infestations result in a postinflammatory hyperpigmentation and thickening of skin known as *vagabonds' disease*.

The crab or pubic louse is transmitted mainly by sexual contact but can infest eyelashes, axillary hair, and hair in other sites as well as pubic hair. Children with pubic lice generally acquire their infestations from parents rather than via sexual transmission. Polymerase chain reaction analysis of the blood meal of lice may permit identification of host DNA in cases of child abuse or rape. Intensely pruritic lesions and 2- to 3-mm blue macules (maculae ceruleae) develop at the site of bites. Blepharitis commonly accompanies infestations of the eyelashes.

Pediculosis may be suspected upon the detection of nits on hairs or in clothing. Confirmation, however, should await demonstration of a live louse. The dorsoventrally flattened adult louse measures 2 to 4 mm in length and has three pairs of legs ending in claws that enable it to grasp hair shafts or clothing. The oval nits of lice are ~0.8 mm long.

℞ TREATMENT

Generally, treatment is warranted only if live lice are discovered. The presence of nits alone does not form the basis for an active infestation.

Although some lice and their eggs may be removed mechanically by means of a fine-toothed louse or 'nit' comb, this practice often fails to eliminate infestations. Treatment of newly identified active infestations generally relies upon a 10-min application of nonprescription formulations containing 1% permethrin or pyrethrins, with a second application 10 days later. Lice persisting after this treatment may be resistant to pyrethroids. Such chronic infestations may be treated for 8 to 12 h with a prescription formulation of 0.5% malathion. Lindane seems less effective and may pose greater risk, particularly when misused.

Dead or hatched nits, which remain attached to hair sheaths and become translucent or opalescent, may falsely suggest an active infection. Although children infested by head lice are frequently isolated or excluded from school, this practice seems unjustified. Resistance of head lice to permethrin, malathion, and lindane has been reported. Ivermectin may be useful in cases of resistance to both malathion and permethrin but has not been approved for this purpose by the FDA.

Body lice can be eliminated by bathing and by applying topical pediculicides from head to foot. Clothes and bedding are effectively deloused by heat sterilization in a dryer at 65°C for 30 min or by fumigation. Emergency mass delousing of people and clothing may be warranted during periods of civil strife and after natural disasters to reduce the risk of pathogen transmission by body lice. Pubic lice infestations are treated with topical pediculicides except for eyelid infestations (*pthiriasis palpebrum*), which respond to a coating of petrolatum applied for 3 to 4 days or 1% yellow oxide of mercury ointment applied four times daily for 2 weeks.

TUNGIASIS   *Tunga penetrans*, like other fleas, is a wingless, laterally flattened insect measuring 2 to 4 mm in length that feeds on blood. Also known as the chigoe flea, sand flea, or jigger, it occurs in tropical regions of Africa and the Americas. Adults live in sandy soil and burrow under the skin between toes, under nails, or on the soles of bare feet. The fleas engorge on blood and grow from pinpoint to pea size over a 2-week period. The lesions that they produce resemble a white pustule with a central black depression and may be pruritic or painful. Occasional complications include tetanus, bacterial infections, and autoamputation of toes. Tungiasis is treated by removal of the intact flea with a sterile needle or scalpel, tetanus vaccination, and topical application of antibiotics.

MYIASIS   *Myiasis* refers to infestations by maggots, mainly due to the larvae produced by metallic-colored screw-worm flies or botflies. Maggots invade living or necrotic tissue or body cavities and produce different clinical syndromes, depending on the species of fly.

Furuncular Myiasis   In forested parts of Central and South America, larvae of *Dermatobia hominis* (the human botfly) produce boil-like subcutaneous nodules 2 to 3 cm in diameter. The adult female captures a mosquito or other bloodsucking insect and deposits her eggs on its abdomen. When the carrier insect attacks a human or bovine host several days later, the warmth and moisture of the host's surface stimulate these eggs to hatch. The larvae promptly penetrate intact skin. After 6 to 12 weeks, the larvae mature and drop to the ground, where they pupate. The African tumbu fly, *Cordylobia anthropophaga*, produces similar lesions. Dozens of eggs are deposited on sand or drying laundry that is contaminated with urine or sweat. Larvae hatch on contact with the body, penetrate the skin, and produce boils from which they emerge 8 or 9 days later. In North America, larvae of the genus *Cuterebra* (botflies of rabbits and rodents) are an unusual cause of myiasis in persons exposed to eggs in grass or brush. A diagnosis of furuncular myiasis is suggested by uncomfortable lesions with a central breathing pore that emits bubbles when submerged in water. There is often a sensation of movement under the skin that may lead to severe emotional distress. Botfly larvae can be induced to emerge if the air pore is coated with petrolatum or another occlusive substance. Removal of *Dermatobia* larvae is facilitated by injection of a local anesthetic into the surrounding tissue, but surgical excision is often necessary because upward-pointing spines hold the larva firmly in place.

Creeping Dermal Myiasis   Maggots of the horse botfly, *Gasterophilus intestinalis*, do not mature after penetrating human skin but migrate for weeks in the epidermis. The resulting pruritic and serpiginous eruption resembles cutaneous larva migrans caused by *Ancylostoma braziliense*. Horseback riders become infested when eggs deposited on the flank of the horse hatch against their bare legs. The black spines of the larvae can be identified after mineral oil is smeared over the lesion. Larvae are removed with a needle. The larvae of the cattle botfly (*Hypoderma* species) invade more deeply and produce boil-like swellings.

Wound and Body-Cavity Myiasis   Certain flies are attracted to blood and pus, and their newly hatched larvae enter wounds or diseased skin. Larvae of species such as *Lucilia (Phaenicia) sericata*, the green-bottle fly, remain superficial and confined to necrotic tissue and continue to be applied on a limited basis to debride purulent wounds. Other species, including the screw-worms (*Chrysomyia bezziana* in Asia and Africa and *Cochliomyia hominivorax* in Latin America) and the flesh fly (*Wohlfahrtia vigil* in northern North America), invade more deeply into viable tissue and produce large suppurating lesions. Larvae that infest wounds also may infest body cavities such as the mouth, nose, ears, sinuses, anus, vagina, and lower urinary tract, particularly in unconscious or otherwise debilitated patients. The consequences range from harmless colonization to destruction of the nose, meningitis, and deafness. Treatment involves removal of maggots and debridement of tissue.

Other Forms of Myiasis   The maggots responsible for furuncular and wound myiasis may also cause ophthalmomyiasis. Sequelae include nodules in the eyelid, retinal detachment, and destruction of the globe. In addition, the adult sheep botfly, *Oestrus ovis*, may deposit larvae in the eyes of persons tending sheep and goats, and the larvae may produce a conjunctival infestation and acute conjunctivitis. True intestinal myiasis occurs when eggs or larvae of the drone fly (*Eristalis tenax*) are ingested with contaminated food, mature in the gut, and cause enteritis. Most instances in which maggots are found in human feces are the result of larviposition by flesh flies on recently passed stools.

PENTASTOMIASIS   Pentastomids, or tongue worms, are parasites with characteristics of both helminths and arthropods and generally are classified in a separate phylum. The wormlike adults inhabit the respiratory passages of reptiles and carnivorous mammals. Human infestation by *Linguatula serrata* is common in the Middle East and occurs in the Sudan following ingestion of encysted larval stages in raw liver or lymph nodes of sheep and goats, the intermediate hosts. The larvae migrate to the nasopharynx and produce an acute self-limiting syndrome known as *halzoun* (*Marrara* in the Sudan), which is characterized by pain and itching of the throat and ears, coughing, hoarseness, dysphagia, and dyspnea. Severe edema may cause obstruction and necessitate tracheostomy, and ocular invasion has been described. Diagnostic larvae measuring 5 to 10 mm in length are found in the copious nasal discharge or vomitus. Human beings become infected with *Armillifer armillatus* by ingesting eggs in contaminated food or drink or after handling the definitive host, the African python. Larvae encyst in various organs but rarely cause symptoms unless they compress vital structures or perforate an organ during migration. Cysts occasionally require surgical removal as they enlarge during molting, but they are usually encountered as an incidental finding at autopsy. There are reports of the cutaneous larva migrans syndrome due to other pentastomes (*Reighardia* and *Sebekia* species) in Southeast Asia and Central America.

LEECH INFESTATIONS   Medically important leeches are annelid worms that attach to their hosts by means of chitinous cutting jaws and draw blood through muscular suckers. The medicinal leech, *Hirudo medicinalis*, is still used occasionally to reduce venous congestion in surgical flaps or replanted body parts. This practice has been complicated by wound infections, myonecrosis, and sepsis due to *Aeromonas hydrophila*, which colonizes the gullets of commercially available leeches.

Ubiquitous aquatic leeches that parasitize fish, frogs, and turtles readily attach to the skin of humans and avidly suck blood. More notorious are the land leeches (*Haemadipsa*) that live in moist vegetation of tropical rain forests. Attachment is usually painless. Hirudinin, a powerful anticoagulant secreted by the leech, causes continued bleeding after the leech has detached. Healing of the wound is slow, and bacterial infections are not uncommon. Several species of aquatic leeches in Africa, Asia, and southern Europe can enter through the mouth, nose, and genitourinary tract and attach to mucosal surfaces at sites as deep as the esophagus and trachea. Bleeding may be intense. Externally attached leeches are removed by steady gentle traction. Removal is hastened by application of alcohol, salt, vinegar, or a flame to the leech. Internally attached leeches may detach on exposure to gargled saline or may be removed by forceps.

DELUSIONAL INFESTATIONS   The groundless conviction that one is infested with arthropods or other parasites is an extremely difficult disorder to treat and unfortunately is not rare. Patients report infestations of their skin, clothing, or homes and describe sensations of something moving in or on their skin. Excoriations often accompany complaints of pruritus or insect bites. Patients bring in as evidence of infestation specimens that are identified microscopically as plant-feeding or peridomestic arthropods, pieces of skin, vegetable matter, or inanimate objects. In suspected cases, it is imperative to rule out true infestations and neuropathies, environmental irritants such as fragments of fiberglass, and other causes of tingling or prickling sensations. Pharmacotherapy with pimozide, which blocks dopamine receptors, has been more helpful than psychotherapy in treating this disorder.

ARTHROPOD BITES AND STINGS

SPIDER BITES   Of the more than 30,000 recognized species of spider, only about 100 defend themselves aggressively and have fangs sufficiently long to penetrate human skin. The venom that spiders use to immobilize and digest their prey can cause necrosis of skin and systemic toxicity. While the bites of most spiders are painful but not harmful, envenomations of the brown or fiddle spiders (*Loxosceles* species), widow spiders (*Latrodectus* species), and other species may be life-threatening. Identification of the offending spider should be attempted, since specific treatments exist for bites of widow and brown recluse spiders and since injuries attributed to spiders are frequently due to other causes.

Recluse Spider Bites and Necrotic Arachnidism   Severe necrosis of skin and subcutaneous tissue follows envenomation by *Loxosceles reclusa*, the brown recluse spider, and by at least four other species of *Loxosceles*, mainly in the southern and midwestern United States. Other spiders that produce necrotic ulceration include the hobo spider (*Tegenaria agrestis*) in the Pacific Northwest, the sac spiders (*Chiracanthium* species) throughout the United States and abroad, the South American brown spider *Loxosceles laeta* in Central and South America, and other *Loxosceles* species in Africa and the Middle East. All these spiders measure 7 to 15 mm in body length and 2 to 4 cm in leg span. Recluse spiders are brown and have a dark violin-shaped spot on their dorsal surface; hobo spiders are brown with gray markings; and sac spiders may be pale yellow, green, or brown.

These spiders are not aggressive toward human beings and bite only if threatened or pressed against the skin. They hide under rocks and logs or in caves and animal burrows, and they emerge at night to hunt other spiders and insects. They invade homes, particularly in the fall, and seek dark and undisturbed hiding spots in closets, in folds of clothing, or under furniture and rubbish in storage rooms, garages, and attics. Bites often occur while the victim is dressing and are sustained primarily to the arms, neck, and lower abdomen.

The clear viscous venoms of these spiders contain an esterase, alkaline phosphatase, protease, and other enzymes that produce tissue necrosis and hemolysis. Sphingomyelinase B, the most important dermonecrotic factor, binds cell membranes and promotes chemotaxis of neutrophils, leading to vascular thrombosis and an Arthus-like reaction. Initially, the bite is painless or produces a stinging sensation.

Within the next few hours, the site becomes painful and pruritic, with central induration surrounded by a pale zone of ischemia and a zone of erythema. In most cases, the lesion resolves without treatment over 2 to 3 days. In severe cases, the erythema spreads, and the center of the lesion becomes hemorrhagic and necrotic with an overlying bulla. A black eschar forms and sloughs several weeks later, leaving an ulcer that may be ≥25 cm in diameter and eventually a depressed scar. Healing usually takes place within 3 to 6 months but may take as long as 3 years if adipose tissue is involved. Local complications include injury to nerves and secondary infection. Fever, chills, weakness, headache, nausea, vomiting, myalgia, arthralgia, maculopapular rash, and leukocytosis may develop within 72 h of the bite. In rare instances, acute complications such as hemolytic anemia, hemoglobinuria, and renal failure are fatal.

℞ TREATMENT

Initial management includes local cleansing, application of sterile dressings and cold compresses, and elevation and loose immobilization of the affected limb. Analgesics, antihistamines, antibiotics, and tetanus prophylaxis should be administered if indicated. Within the first 48 to 72 h, the administration of dapsone, a leukocyte inhibitor, may halt the progression of lesions that are becoming necrotic. Dapsone is given in oral doses of 50 to 100 mg twice daily after glucose-6-phosphate dehydrogenase deficiency has been ruled out. The efficacy of locally or systemically administered glucocorticoids has not been demonstrated, and a potentially useful *Loxosceles*-specific antivenin has not been approved for use in the United States. Debridement and later skin grafting may be necessary after signs of acute inflammation have subsided, but immediate surgical excision of the wound is detrimental. Patients should be monitored closely for signs of hemolysis, renal failure, and other systemic complications.

Widow Spider Bites   The bite of the female widow spider is notorious for the effect of its potent neurotoxin. *Latrodectus mactans*, the black widow, has been found in every state of the United States except Alaska and is most abundant in the Southeast. It measures up to 1 cm in body length and 5 cm in leg span, is shiny black, and has a red hourglass marking on the ventral abdomen. Other dangerous North American *Latrodectus* species include *L. geometricus* (the brown widow), *L. bishopi* (the red widow), *L. variolus*, and *L. hesperus*, and there are related species in other temperate and subtropical parts of the world.

Widow spiders spin their webs under stones, logs, plants, or rock piles or in dark spaces in barns, garages, and outhouses. Bites are most common in the summer and early autumn and occur when the web is disturbed or when the spider is trapped or provoked. The buttocks or genitals are sites of bites incurred by humans while sitting in an outdoor privy. The initial bite goes unnoticed or is perceived as a sharp pinprick. Two small red marks, mild erythema, and edema develop at the fang entrance site. The oily yellow venom that is injected does not produce local necrosis, and some persons experience no other symptoms. However, α-latrotoxin, the most active component of the venom, binds irreversibly to nerves and causes release and eventual depletion of acetylcholine, norepinephrine, and other neurotransmitters from presynaptic terminals. Within 30 to 60 min, painful cramps spread from the bite site to large muscles of the extremities and the trunk. Extreme rigidity of the abdominal muscles and excruciating pain may suggest peritonitis, but the abdomen is not tender on palpation. Other features include salivation, diaphoresis, vomiting, hypertension, tachycardia, labored breathing, anxiety, headache, weakness, fasciculations, paresthesia, hyperreflexia, urinary retention, uterine contractions, and premature labor. Rhabdomyolysis and renal failure have been reported, and respiratory arrest, cerebral hemorrhage, or cardiac failure may end fatally, especially in very young, elderly, or debilitated persons. The pain begins to subside during the first 12 h but may recur during several days or weeks before resolving spontaneously.

℞ TREATMENT

Treatment consists of local cleansing, application of ice packs, and tetanus prophylaxis. Hypertension that does not respond to analgesics and antispasmodics, such as benzodiazepines or methocarbamol, requires specific antihypertensive medication. Intravenous administration of one or two vials of a widely available equine antivenin rapidly relieves pain and can be life-saving. Because of the risk of anaphylaxis and serum sickness, antivenin should be reserved for severe cases involving respiratory arrest, uncontrollable hypertension, seizures, or pregnancy.

Envenomations by Tarantulas and Other Spiders   Tarantulas are long-lived hairy spiders of which 30 species are found in the United States, mainly in the Southwest. The tarantulas that have become popular household pets are usually imported species with bright colors and a leg span of up to 25 cm. Tarantulas bite only when threatened and cause no more harm than a bee sting, but the venom occasionally provokes deep pain and swelling. Several species are covered with urticating hairs that are brushed off in the thousands when a threatened spider rubs its hind legs across its dorsal abdomen. These hairs penetrate human skin and produce pruritic papules that last for weeks. Failure to wear gloves or to wash the hands after handling the Chilean Rose tarantula, the most popular pet spider, has resulted in transfer of hairs to the eye and devastating ocular inflammation. Treatment of bites includes local washing and elevation of the bitten area, tetanus prophylaxis, and analgesic administration. Antihistamines and topical or systemic glucocorticoids are given for exposure to urticating hairs.

Atrax robustus, the Sydney funnel-web spider of Australia, and *Phoneutria* species, the South American banana spiders, are among the most dangerous spiders in the world because of their aggressive behavior and potent neurotoxins. Envenomation by *A. robustus* causes a rapidly progressive neuromotor syndrome that can be fatal within 2 h. The bite of the banana spiders causes severe local pain followed by profound systemic symptoms and respiratory paralysis that can lead to death within 2 to 6 h. Specific antivenins for envenomation by each of these spiders are available. *Lycosa* species (wolf spiders) are found throughout the world and may produce painful bites and transient local inflammation.

SCORPION STINGS   Scorpions are crablike arachnids that feed on ground-dwelling arthropods and small lizards, which they grasp with a pair of frontal pinchers and paralyze by injecting venom from a stinger on the tip of the tail. Painful but relatively harmless scorpion stings need to be distinguished from the potentially lethal envenomations that are produced by about 30 of the ~1000 known species and cause more than 5000 deaths worldwide each year. Scorpions feed at night and remain hidden during the day in crevices or burrows or under wood, loose bark, or rocks on the ground. They seek cool spots under buildings and often enter houses, where they get into shoes, clothing, or bedding or enter bathtubs and sinks in search of water. Scorpions sting human beings only when disturbed.

Scorpions of the United States   Of the 40 or so scorpion species in the United States, only the bark scorpion (*Centruroides sculpturatus* or *C. exilicauda*) produces a venom that can be lethal. Stings of the other species, such as the common striped scorpion *C. vittatus* and the large *Hadrurus arizonensis*, cause immediate sharp local pain followed by edema, ecchymosis, and a burning sensation. Symptoms typically resolve within a few hours, and skin does not slough. Allergic reactions to the venom sometimes develop.

The deadly *C. sculpturatus* of the southwestern United States and northern Mexico measures ~7 cm in length and is yellow-brown in color. Its venom contains neurotoxins that cause sodium channels to remain open and neurons to fire repetitively. In contrast to the stings of nonlethal species, *C. sculpturatus* envenomations are usually associated with little swelling, but prominent pain, paresthesia, and hy-

peresthesia can be accentuated by tapping on the affected area (the tap test). These symptoms soon spread to other locations; dysfunction of cranial nerves and hyperexcitability of skeletal muscles develop within hours. Patients present with restlessness, blurred vision, abnormal eye movements, profuse salivation, lacrimation, rhinorrhea, slurred speech, difficulty in handling secretions, diaphoresis, nausea, and vomiting. Muscle twitching, jerking, and shaking may be mistaken for a seizure. Complications include tachycardia, arrhythmias, hypertension, hyperthermia, rhabdomyolysis, and acidosis. Symptoms progress to maximal severity in ~5 h and subside within a day or two, although pain and paresthesia can last for weeks. Fatal respiratory arrest is most common among young children and the elderly.

Other Dangerous Scorpions   Envenomations by *Leiurus quinquestriatus* in the Middle East and North Africa, by *Mesobuthus tamulus* in India, by *Androctonus* species along the Mediterranean littoral and in North Africa and the Middle East, and by *Tityus serrulatus* in Brazil cause massive release of endogenous catecholamines with hypertensive crises, arrhythmias, pulmonary edema, and myocardial damage. Acute pancreatitis occurs with stings of *Tityus trinitatis* in Trinidad, and central nervous toxicity complicates stings of *Parabuthus* and *Buthotus* scorpions of South Africa. Tissue necrosis and hemolysis may follow stings of the Iranian *Hemiscorpius lepturus*.

℞ TREATMENT

Identification of the offending scorpion aids in planning therapy. Stings of nonlethal species require at most ice packs, analgesics, or antihistamines. Because most victims of dangerous envenomations (such as those produced by *C. sculpturatus*) experience only local discomfort, they can be managed at home with instructions to return to the emergency department if signs of cranial-nerve or neuromuscular dysfunction develop. Aggressive supportive care and judicious use of antivenin can reduce or eliminate deaths from more severe envenomations. Keeping the patient calm and applying pressure dressings and cold packs to the sting site decrease the absorption of venom. A continuous intravenous infusion of midazolam controls the agitation, flailing, and involuntary muscle movements produced by scorpion stings. Close monitoring during treatment with this drug and other sedatives or narcotics is necessary for persons with neuromuscular symptoms because of the risk of respiratory arrest. Hypertension and pulmonary edema respond to nifedipine, nitroprusside, hydralazine, or prazosin, and bradyarrhythmias can be controlled with atropine.

Commercially prepared antivenins are available in several countries for some of the most dangerous species. A caprine *C. sculpturatus* antivenin (not yet FDA approved) is available as an investigational drug from Arizona State University for use only in Arizona. Because of the risk of anaphylaxis or serum sickness following administration of goat serum, use of the antivenin is controversial. Intravenous administration of antivenin rapidly reverses cranial-nerve dysfunction and muscular symptoms but does not affect pain and paresthesia. The benefit of scorpion antivenin has not been established in controlled trials.

Prevention   In scorpion-infested areas, shoes, clothing, bedding, and towels should be shaken and inspected before being used. Removal of wood, stones, and debris from yards and campsites eliminates hiding places for scorpions, and household spraying of insecticides can deplete their source of food.

CHIGGERS AND OTHER BITING MITES   Chiggers are the larvae of trombiculid (harvest) mites that normally feed on mice in grassy or brush-covered sites in the tropics and subtropics and (less frequently) in temperate areas during warm months. They wait for hosts on low vegetation and attach themselves to passing animals or to people. The larva then pierces the skin of its host and deposits a tubelike structure in the dermis through which it imbibes lymph and tissue juices. This highly antigenic "stylostome" serves as the focus of an exceptionally pruritic papular, papulovesicular, or papulourticarial lesion that may be 2 cm in diameter and that develops within hours of attachment in persons previously sensitized to mite antigen. Feeding mites appear as tiny red vesicles in hair follicles. Scratching invariably destroys the body of a mite attached to a person. These lesions generally vesiculate and develop a hemorrhagic base. Itching and burning last for weeks. The rash is most common on the ankles or near tight-fitting clothes that obstruct the mites' movements. Chiggers are the vectors of scrub typhus in tropical and subtropical parts of Asia. Repellents are useful for preventing chigger bites.

Certain mesostigmatid mites that infest the nests of mice or birds feed on human beings when their usual hosts have been displaced. Intense episodes of itching dermatitis in humans, for example, may follow the removal of trash that has accumulated in a human residence or the departure of pigeons that have been nesting on a window air-conditioner. Other mites that infest grain, straw, cheese, or other animal products occasionally produce similar episodes. Persons who have close contact with dogs—and, to a lesser extent, cats—may develop a self-limited pruritic papulovesicular rash from bites of cheyletiellid mites that cause a mangelike condition in these animals. Mouse mites are the vectors of rickettsialpox in cities of the northeastern United States. Fowl and chicken mites transmit the viruses of St. Louis encephalitis and western equine encephalitis. Although sanitary measures effectively prevent rickettsialpox, removal of accumulated refuse may result in a transient period of elevated risk. Insecticidal applications applied to infested areas can eliminate mites before or while hosts and their nests are removed.

Diagnosis of mite-induced dermatitides (including those caused by chiggers) relies heavily on a history of exposure to the source of the mite, since the tiny mite may escape notice or may fall off or be scratched off the lesions. Antihistamines or topical steroids effectively reduce mite-induced pruritus.

HYMENOPTERA STINGS   Insects that sting to defend their colonies or subdue their prey belong to the order Hymenoptera, which includes apids (bees and bumblebees), vespids (wasps, hornets, and yellow jackets), and ants. Their venoms contain a wide array of amines, peptides, and enzymes that are responsible for local and systemic reactions. Although the toxic effect of multiple stings can be fatal, nearly all of the 100 or more deaths due to hymenopteran stings in the United States each year are the result of allergic reactions.

Bee and Wasp Stings   Honeybees lose their stinging apparatus and the attached venom sac in the act of stinging and subsequently die, while other bees, ants, and vespids can sting numerous times in succession. The familiar honeybees (*Apis mellifera*) and bumblebees (*Bombus* and other genera) generally attack only when a colony is disturbed. The extremely aggressive Africanized honeybees, however, respond to minimal intrusions rapidly and in large numbers. Since their introduction into Brazil in 1957, these "killer bees" have spread through South and Central America to the southern and western United States. The common vespids in the United States include the yellow jackets, notable for the yellow and black bands on their abdomens; the bald-faced hornet, with a black body and a white face; the European hornet, measuring 2.5 to 3.5 cm in length; and the paper wasps, which have variously colored elongate bodies. Vespids sting in defense of their nests, which they often build near human dwellings and suspend from eaves or shubbery, plaster onto walls, or burrow into wood or soil. All vespids feed on sugary substances and decaying meat, and certain of the yellow jackets are annoyingly abundant at recreation sites and around garbage, particularly in the late summer and fall.

Venom is produced in glands at the posterior end of the abdomen and is expelled rapidly by contraction of muscles of the venom sac, which has a capacity of up to 0.1 mL in large insects. The venoms of different species of hymenopterans are biochemically and immunologically distinct. Direct toxic effects are mediated by mixtures of low-molecular-weight compounds such as serotonin, histamine, and acetylcholine and several kinins. Polypeptide toxins in honeybee venom include mellitin, which damages cell membranes; mast cell–degranulating protein, which causes histamine release; apamin, a neurotoxin; and adolapin, which has anti-inflammatory action. Enzymes in venom include hyaluronidase, which allows the spread of other venom components, and phospholipases, which may be among the major venom allergens. There appears to be little cross-sensitization between honeybee and wasp venoms.

Uncomplicated stings cause immediate pain, a wheal-and-flare reaction, and local edema and swelling that subside in a few hours. Stings from accidentally swallowed insects may induce life-threatening edema of the upper airways. Multiple stings can lead to vomiting, diarrhea, generalized edema, dyspnea, hypotension, and collapse. Rhabdomyolysis and intravascular hemolysis may cause renal failure. Death from the direct effects of venom has followed 300 to 500 honeybee stings.

Large local reactions that spread ≥10 cm around the sting site over 24 to 48 h are not uncommon. These reactions may resemble cellulitis but are caused by hypersensitivity rather than secondary infection. Such reactions tend to recur on subsequent exposure but are seldom accompanied by anaphylaxis and are not prevented by venom immunotherapy.

An estimated 0.4 to 4.0% of the U.S. population exhibits clinical immediate-type hypersensitivity to insect stings, and 15% may have asymptomatic sensitization manifested by positive skin tests. Persons who experience severe allergic reactions are likely to have similar reactions after subsequent stings; occasionally, adults who have had mild reactions later experience serious reactions. Mild anaphylactic reactions from insect stings, as from other causes, consist of nausea, abdominal cramping, generalized urticaria, flushing, and angioedema. Serious reactions, including upper airway edema, bronchospasm, hypotension, and shock, may be rapidly fatal. Severe reactions usually begin within 10 min of the sting and only rarely develop after 5 h. Unusual complications, including serum sickness, vasculitis, neuritis, and encephalitis, develop several days or weeks after a sting.

℞ TREATMENT

Stingers from honeybees embedded in the skin should be removed as promptly as possible, using any method available, to limit the quantity of venom delivered. Previous suggestions—that the stinger be scraped or brushed off with a blade or a fingernail but not removed with forceps—simply delay removal and exacerbate the consequences. The site should be cleansed and disinfected and ice packs applied to slow the spread of venom. Elevation of the affected site and administration of analgesics, oral antihistamines, and topical calamine lotion relieve symptoms; application of meat tenderizer containing papain is of no proven value. Large local reactions may require a short course of oral therapy with glucocorticoids. Patients with numerous stings should be monitored for 24 h for evidence of renal failure or coagulopathy.

Anaphylaxis is treated with subcutaneous injection of 0.3 to 0.5 mL of epinephrine hydrochloride in a 1:1000 dilution; treatment is repeated every 20 to 30 min if necessary. Intravenous epinephrine (2 to 5 mL of a 1:10,000 solution administered by slow push) is indicated for profound shock. A tourniquet may slow the spread of venom. Parenteral antihistamines, fluid resuscitation, bronchodilators, oxygen, intubation, and vasopressors may be required. Patients should be observed for 24 h for recurrent anaphylaxis.

PREVENTION   Persons with a history of allergy to insect stings should carry a sting kit with a preloaded syringe containing epinephrine for self-administration in case of a sting. These patients should seek medical attention immediately after using the kit. To avoid stings when outdoors, individuals can wear shoes and protective clothing and avoid attracting insects with sweet foods, bright-colored clothes, perfumes, or cosmetics.

VENOM IMMUNOTHERAPY   Repeated injections of purified venom produce a blocking IgG antibody response to venom and reduce the incidence of recurrent anaphylaxis from between 50 and 60% to <5%. Honeybee, wasp, yellow jacket, and mixed vespid venoms are commercially available for desensitization and for skin testing. Adults with a history of anaphylaxis should undergo desensitization. Results of skin tests and venom-specific radioallergosorbent tests aid in the selection of patients for immunotherapy and guide the design of such treatment. The risk of a systemic reaction to a sting is ~5 to 10% after discontinuation of a ≥5-year course of immunotherapy.

Stings of Fire Ants and Other Ants   All ants that are large enough can injure human beings, and some can secrete repugnant substances when handled. Stinging fire ants are an important medical problem in the United States. The imported fire ants *Solenopsis richteri* and *S. invicta* were introduced from South America into Alabama in 1918 and now infest urban and rural areas of southern states from Texas to North Carolina, with colonies in California, New Mexico, Arizona, and Virginia. They excavate open fields and yards to build tall mounds that can harbor 200,000 worker ants. Slight disturbances of the mounds have provoked massive outpourings of ants and as many as 10,000 stings on a single person. Each year fire ants sting up to 60% of the inhabitants of some cities. Waterborne ants bite on contact during times of flooding. Elderly and immobile persons are at high risk for attacks when fire ants invade dwellings.

Red-brown or brown-black fire ants attach to human skin with powerful mandibles and rotate their bodies around their heads while repeatedly injecting venom with posteriorly situated stingers. The alkaloid venom consists of cytotoxic and hemolytic piperidines and several proteins with enzymatic activity. The initial wheal-and-flare reaction, burning, and itching resolve in ~30 min, and a sterile pustule develops within 24 h. The pustule ulcerates over the next 48 h and then heals a week or 10 days later unless it becomes secondarily infected. Large areas of erythema and edema lasting several days are not uncommon and in extreme cases may compress nerves and blood vessels. Anaphylaxis occurs in ~1 to 2% of persons, and seizures and mononeuritis have been reported. Stings are treated with ice packs, topical glucocorticoids, and oral antihistamines. Covering pustules with bandages and antibiotic ointment may prevent bacterial infection. Epinephrine and supportive measures are indicated for anaphylactic reactions. Whole-body extracts are available for skin testing and immunotherapy, which appears to lower the rate of anaphylactic reactions.

The western United States is home to harvester ants (*Pogonomyrmex* species) as well as to less aggressive fire ants not yet displaced by the introduced species. The painful local reaction following harvester ant stings often extends to lymph nodes and may be accompanied by anaphylaxis. Large Australian bulldog ants and the aggressive South American *Paranopera* ants deliver extremely painful stings and may cause systemic symptoms. Velvet ants that inhabit sandy beaches in the United States and sting the bare feet of bathers are actually wingless female wasps of the genus *Dasymutilla*.

TICK BITES AND TICK PARALYSIS   In the United States, hard ticks (Ixodidae) have increased in abundance since the mid-1900s to become common carriers of vector-borne disease agents. Deer ticks of the genus *Ixodes* transmit the pathogens of Lyme disease, babesiosis, and human anaplasmosis. Other ticks, such as *Dermacentor variabilis* (the dog tick), *D. andersoni* (the wood tick), and *Amblyomma americanum* (the Lone Star tick), are vectors of tularemia, Rocky Mountain spotted fever, Colorado tick fever, human monocytotropic ehrlichiosis, and ehrlichiosis ewingii. Outside the United States, hard ticks transmit pathogenic rickettsiae and arboviruses as well. Soft ticks (Argasidae) of the genus *Ornithodoros* transmit tick-borne relapsing fever (Chap. 156). Except in parts of Africa, soft ticks rarely attack human beings, and relapsing fever occurs only sporadically in the United States. Hard ticks differ from soft ticks by virtue of a dorsal scutum or plate and their preference for wooded, brushy, or weedy habitats. Soft ticks, which are nonscutate and leathery, are generally found in animal burrows and bird nests.

Ticks attach and feed painlessly; blood is their only food. Their secretions, however, produce local reactions, a febrile illness, or paralysis. Soft ticks attach for <1 h and produce erythematous macular lesions up to 2 to 3 cm in diameter. Some species in Africa, the western United States, and Mexico produce painful hemorrhagic lesions. At the site of hard-tick bites, small areas of induration with surrounding erythema and occasionally necrotic ulcers develop. Chronic nodules, or "tick granulomas," reach several centimeters in diameter and may require surgical excision. Tick-induced fever, associated with headache, nausea, and malaise, usually resolves within 24 to 36 h after the tick is removed. Tick paralysis is an ascending flaccid paralysis believed to be caused by a toxin in tick saliva that causes neuromuscular block and decreased nerve conduction. Throughout the world, this rare complication has followed the bites of more than 40 kinds of tick—most commonly, dog and wood ticks in the United States. Children, especially girls with long hair, are most often affected. Weakness begins in the lower extremities 5 to 6 days after the tick's attachment and ascends symmetrically over several days to result in complete paralysis of the extremities and cranial nerves. Deep tendon reflexes are diminished or lacking altogether, but sensory examination and findings on lumbar puncture are typically normal. Removal of the tick generally results in improvement within a few hours and usually in complete recovery after several days. Failure to remove the tick may lead to dysarthria, dysphagia, and ultimately death from aspiration or respiratory paralysis. Diagnosis depends on finding the tick, which often is hidden beneath hair and which, when engorged, may resemble a pedunculated nevus.

An antiserum to the saliva of *Ixodes holocyclus*, the usual cause of tick paralysis in Australia, effectively reverses paralysis caused by these ticks. Ticks should be removed by firm traction with a forceps placed near their point of attachment. The site of attachment should be disinfected (e.g., with tincture of iodine). Mouthparts remaining in the skin may cause persistent irritation or lead to secondary infection. Removal of ticks during the first 48 h of attachment nearly always prevents transmission of the agents of Lyme disease, babesiosis, and erhlichiosis. Gentle handling (to avoid rupture of ticks) and use of gloves may avert accidental contamination with tick fluids containing pathogens. Protective measures against ticks include avoidance of brushy vegetation, removal of ticks from pet dogs and cats, use of protective clothing sprayed with 0.5% permethrin, and application of a repellent containing *N,N*-diethyl-*m*-toluamide (DEET). The cuffs of trousers should be tucked inside the socks. Rather than awaiting results of tick testing or patient seroconversion to Lyme disease, bites thought to be associated with deer ticks may be treated presumptively with a short course of oral antibiotics.

OTHER ARTHROPOD BITES AND ENVENOMATIONS   ■   **Dipteran (Fly and Mosquito) Bites**   In the process of feeding on vertebrate blood, adults of certain fly species inflict painful bites, produce local allergic reactions, or transmit pathogenic agents. Unlike insect stings, insect bites rarely cause anaphylaxis. Mosquitoes are ubiquitous pests and are the vectors of malaria, filariasis, yellow fever, dengue, and viral encephalitides. Female mosquitoes require a blood meal to produce eggs and an environment of standing water in which to deposit them. Their bite typically produces a wheal and later a pruritic papule. A similar reaction follows the bite of tiny but aggressive midges known as "no-see-ums" in the United States, which attack in swarms during warm months, or of other *Culicoides* species that transmit "nonpathogenic" filariae in tropical climates. Nodular lesions at the site of midge bites may last for months. The bite of the small humpbacked blackflies in the genus *Simulium* leaves a bleeding laceration and painful and pruritic sores that are slow to heal; regional lymphadenopathy, fever, or anaphylaxis occasionally ensues. Blackflies are common summertime nuisances in the United States and Canada and are vectors of onchocerciasis in Africa and Latin America. The widely distributed tabanids, including deerflies (*Chrysops* species) and horseflies (*Tabanus* species), are stout flies measuring 10 to 25 mm in length that attack during the day and produce large and painful bleeding punctures. Deerflies transmit loiasis in African equatorial rain forests and tularemia in the United

States and elsewhere. Tsetse flies of the genus *Glossina* transmit African trypanosomiasis in sub-Saharan Africa. Tiny phlebotomine sandflies are the vectors of leishmaniasis, bartonellosis (Carrión's disease), sandfly fever, and other arboviral infections in warm climates. *Stomoxys calcitrans*, the stable fly, which resembles a large housefly, is a fierce biter of human beings and domestic animals and a major pest in seacoast areas. Houseflies do not bite.

℞ TREATMENT

Treatment of fly bites is symptom-based. Topical application of antipruritic agents, glucocorticoids, or antiseptic lotions may relieve the itching and pain. Allergic reactions may require oral antihistamines. Antibiotics may be necessary for large bite wounds that become secondarily infected. Personal protection measures against biting flies include avoidance of infested areas, application of a DEET-containing repellent to exposed skin, and use of protective clothing and bed nets treated with permethrin. Higher concentrations of DEET provide longer-lasting protection, and 10 to 35% DEET provides adequate protection under most conditions. Repellents used on children should contain ≤10% DEET to avoid absorption of toxic levels that may provoke encephalopathy and seizures. Permethrin applied to clothing maintains its potency for at least 2 weeks, even with laundering.

Flea Bites Common human-biting fleas include the dog and cat fleas (*Ctenocephalides* species) and the rat flea (*Xenopsylla cheopis*), which inhabit the nests and resting sites of their hosts. Larval fleas feed on pellets of dried host blood that the adult fleas eject from their rectums while feeding. The high-jumping adults attack human beings or other available warm-bodied animals when the usual host abandons or is driven from its nest. The human flea (*Pulex irritans*) infests human bedding and furniture but mainly in relatively humid buildings that lack central heating. Sensitized persons develop erythematous pruritic papules, urticaria, and occasionally vesicles and bacterial superinfection at the site of the bite. Treatment consists of antihistamines and antipruritics.

Fleas transmit plague, murine typhus, a typhus-like illness due to *Rickettsia felis*, the rat and dog tapeworms, and *Bartonella henselae*. Flea infestations are eliminated by frequent cleaning of the nesting sites and bedding of the host or judicious dusting or spraying of insecticides such as pyrethrin, DDT, or malathion. Flea infestations in the home may abate if pets are treated with veterinary antiparasitic agents and insect growth regulators.

Hemipteran (True Bug) Bites Several true bugs of the family Reduviidae inflict bites that produce allergic reactions and are sometimes painful. The cone-nose bugs, so called because of their elongated heads, include the assassin and wheel bugs, which feed on other insects and bite human beings only in self-defense, and the kissing bugs, which routinely feed on vertebrate blood. Assassin and wheel bugs inhabit many parts of the world, including the United States, where they are notorious for their painful bites. The bites of the nocturnally feeding kissing bugs are painless and occur commonly in groups on the face and other exposed parts of the body. Reactions to such bites depend on prior sensitization and include tender and pruritic papules, vesicular or bullous lesions, giant urticaria, fever, lymphadenopathy, and anaphylaxis. *Triatoma infestans* and other species of kissing bug are the vectors of *Trypanosoma cruzi* in South and Central America and Mexico (causing Chagas' disease), but transmission of *T. cruzi* to humans by bugs indigenous to the United States is exceedingly rare. Bug bites are treated with topical antipruritics or oral antihistamines. Persons with anaphylactic reactions to reduviid bites should keep an epinephrine kit available. The cosmopolitan bedbug (*Cimex* species) hides in crevices in mattresses, bed frames, and other furniture and under loose wallpaper. Bedbugs are increasingly a nuisance in homes, dormitories, and even luxury hotels. The bugs hide during the day and take their blood meal at night. The bedbug's bite is painless, but sensitized persons develop erythema, itching, and wheals around a central hemorrhagic punctum. Bedbugs are not known to transmit pathogens.

Centipede Bites and Millipede Dermatitis The fangs of centipedes of the genus *Scolopendra* can penetrate human skin and deliver a venom that produces intense burning pain, swelling, erythema, and lymphangitis. Dizziness, nausea, and anxiety are occasionally described, and rhabdomyolysis and renal failure have been reported. Treatment includes washing of the site, application of cold dressings, oral analgesic administration or local lidocaine infiltration, and tetanus prophylaxis. Species of *Scolopendra*, measuring up to 25 cm, occur widely in the southern United States and other areas with warm climates worldwide. The smaller house centipede *Scutigera coleoptrata*, which is common throughout the United States, is harmless.

Millipedes, unlike centipedes, do not bite but rather secrete and in some cases eject defensive fluids that burn and discolor human skin. Affected skin turns brown overnight and may blister and exfoliate. Secretions in the eye cause intense pain and inflammation that may lead to corneal ulceration and blindness. Management includes irrigation with copious amounts of water or saline, use of analgesics, and local care of denuded skin. Millipedes are found throughout the world in leaf litter and under rocks.

Caterpillar Stings and Dermatitis The surface of caterpillars of several moth species is covered with hairs or spines that produce mechanical irritation and may contain or be coated with venom. Contact with these caterpillars causes an immediate burning sensation followed by local swelling and erythema and occasionally by regional lymphadenopathy, nausea, vomiting, and headache; shock, seizures, and coagulopathy are rare complications. In the United States, stings are most often caused by caterpillars of the io, puss, saddleback, and brown-tail moths. Contact with even detached hairs of other caterpillars, such as gypsy moth larvae (*Lymantria dispar*), can later produce a pruritic urticarial or papular rash. Spines may be deposited on tree trunks and drying laundry or may be airborne and cause irritation of the eyes and upper airways. Treatment of caterpillar stings consists of repeated application of adhesive or cellophane tape to remove the hairs, which can then be identified microscopically. Local ice packs, topical steroids, and oral antihistamines relieve symptoms.

Beetle Vesication When disturbed, blister beetles extrude cantharidin, a low-molecular-weight toxin that produces thin-walled blisters measuring up to 5 cm in diameter 2 to 5 h after contact with the beetle. The blisters are not painful or pruritic unless broken, and they resolve without treatment in a week to 10 days. Nephritis may follow unusually heavy cantharidin exposure. In the southern United States, blister beetles of several *Epicauta* species are abundant in the summer months. Contact occurs when people sit on the ground, work in the garden, or deliberately handle the beetles. In other countries, different species of beetle produce different vesicants. No treatment is necessary, although ruptured blisters should be kept clean and bandaged until healing is complete.

FURTHER READING

ARLIAN LG: Arthropod allergens and human health. Annu Rev Entomol 47: 395, 2002

AUERBACH PS (ed): *Wilderness Medicine*, 4th ed. St. Louis, Mosby, 2001

BURGESS IF: Human lice and their control. Annu Rev Entomol 49:457, 2004

FRADIN MS: Mosquitoes and mosquito repellents: A clinician's guide. Ann Intern Med 128:931, 1998

GODDARD J: *Physician's Guide to Arthropods of Medical Importance*, 4th ed. Boca Raton, FL, CRC Press, 2002

ISBISTER GK et al: Antivenom treatment in arachnidism. J Toxicol Clin Toxicol 41:291, 2003

MULLEN G, DURDEN L: *Medical and Veterinary Entomology*. Amsterdam, Academic Press, 2002

PETERS W: *A Colour Atlas of Arthropods in Clinical Medicine*. London, Wolfe, 1992

SAFDAR N et al: Autochthonous furuncular myiasis in the United States: Case report and literature review. Clin Infect Dis 36:e73, 2003

WONG HC: Importance of proper identification of stinging insects. Ann Intern Med 132:418, 2000

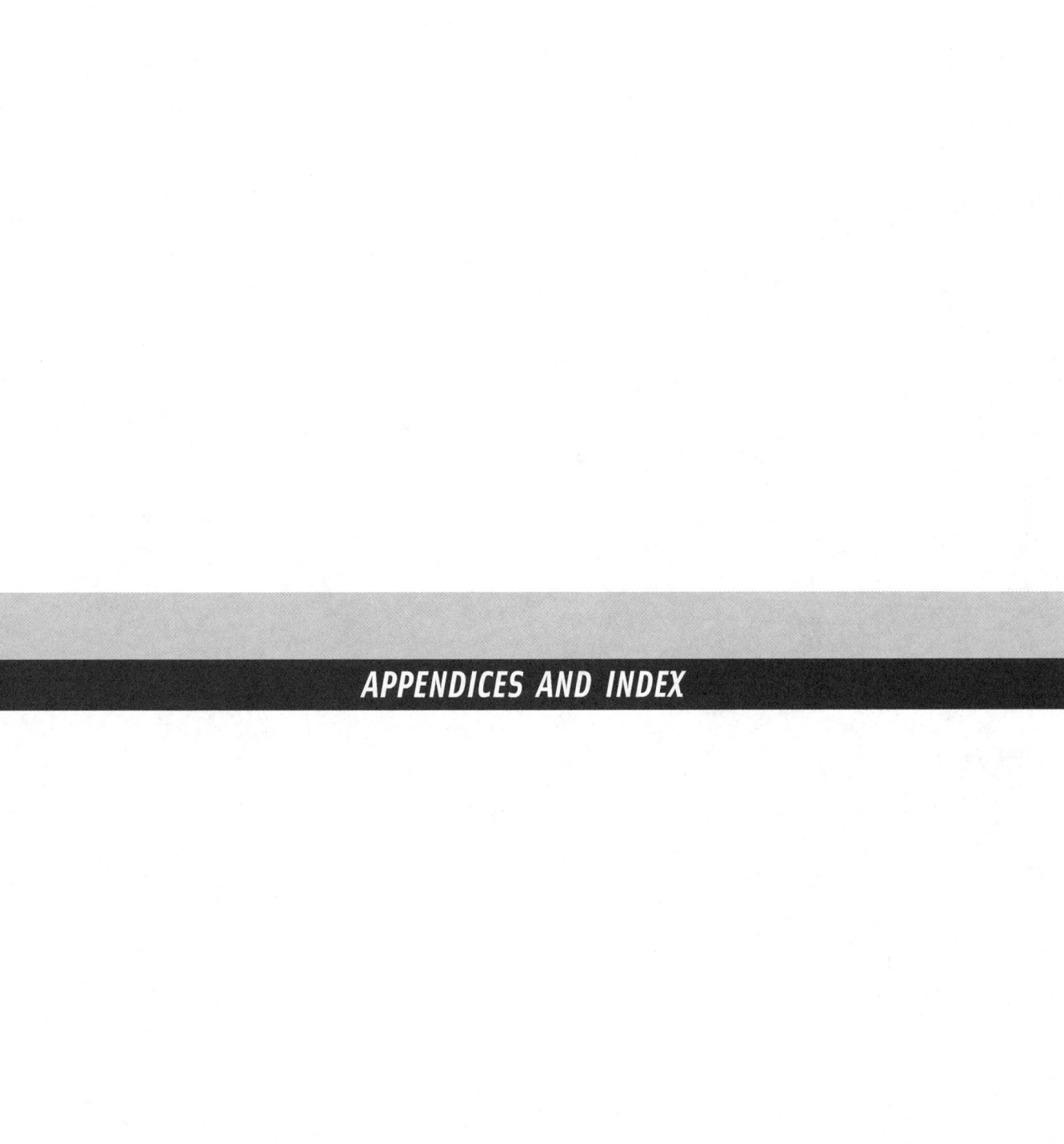

APPENDICES AND INDEX

APPENDICES

APPENDICES: LABORATORY VALUES OF CLINICAL IMPORTANCE
Alexander Kratz, Patrick M. Sluss, James L. Januzzi, Jr., Kent B. Lewandrowski

INTRODUCTORY COMMENTS

The following are tables of reference values for laboratory tests, special analytes, and special function tests. A variety of factors can influence reference values. Such variables include the population studied, laboratory methods and instrumentation, and even the type of container used for the collection of the specimen. Values supplied in this Appendix reflect typical reference ranges in adults. Pediatric reference ranges may vary significantly from adult values. The reference or "normal" ranges given in this appendix may therefore not be appropriate for all laboratories, and these values should only be used as general guidelines. Whenever possible, reference values provided by the laboratory performing the testing should be utilized in the interpretation of laboratory data.

In preparing the Appendix, the authors have taken into account the fact that the system of international units (SI, système international

d'unités) is used in most countries and in some medical journals. However, clinical laboratories may continue to report values in conventional units. Therefore, both systems are provided in the Appendix. The dual system is also used in the text except for (1) those instances in which the numbers remain the same but only the terminology is changed (mmol/L for meq/L or IU/L for mIU/mL), when only the SI units are given; and (2) most pressure measurements (e.g., blood and cerebrospinal fluid pressures), when the traditional units (mmHg, mmH_2O) are used. In all other instances in the text, the SI unit is followed by the conventional unit in parentheses.

Conversion from one system to another can be made as follows:

$$mmol/L = \frac{mg/dL \times 10}{atomic\ weight\ (or\ molecular\ weight)}$$

$$mg/dL = \frac{mmol/L \times atomic\ weight\ (or\ molecular\ weight)}{10}$$

A | REFERENCE VALUES FOR LABORATORY TESTS

TABLE A-1 *Hematology and Coagulation*

Analyte	Specimen	SI Units	Conventional Units
Activated clotting time	WB	70–180 seconds	70–180 seconds
Activated protein C resistance (Factor V Leiden)	P	Not applicable	Ratio > 2.1
Alpha₂ antiplasmin	P	0.80–1.30	80–130%
Antiphospholipid antibody panel			
PTT-LA (lupus anticoagulant screen)	P	Negative	Negative
Platelet neutralization procedure	P	Negative	Negative
Dilute viper venom screen	P	Negative	Negative
Anticardiolipin antibody	S		
IgG		0–15 arbitrary units	0–15 GPL
IgM		0–15 arbitrary units	0–15 MPL
Antithrombin III	P		
Antigenic		220–390 mg/L	22–39 mg/dL
Functional		0.8–1.30 U/L	80–130%
Anti-Xa assay (Heparin assay)	P		
Unfractionated heparin		0.3–0.7 kIU/L	0.3–0.7 IU/mL
Low-molecular-weight heparin		0.5–1.0 kIU/L	0.5–1.0 IU/mL
Danaparoid (Orgaran)		0.5–0.8 kIU/L	0.5–0.8 IU/mL
Bleeding time (adult)		2–9.5 min	2–9.5 min
Bone Marrow: see Table B-3			
Carboxyhemoglobin	WB		
Nonsmoker		0–0.023	0–2.3%
Smoker		0.021–0.042	2.1–4.2%
Clot retraction	WB	0.50–1.00/2 h	50–100%/2 h
Cryofibrinogen	P	Negative	Negative
D-Dimer	P	<0.5 mg/L	<0.5 µg/mL
Differential blood count	WB		
Neutrophils		0.40–0.70	40–70%
Bands		0.0–0.10	0–10%
Lymphocytes		0.22–0.44	22–44%
Monocytes		0.04–0.11	4–11%
Eosinophils		0.0–0.8	0–8%
Basophils		0.0–0.03	0–3%
Erythrocyte count	WB		
Adult males		4.50–5.90 × 10¹²/L	4.50–5.90 × 10⁶/mm³
Adult females		4.00–5.20 × 10¹²/L	4.00–5.20 × 10⁶/mm³
Erythrocyte lifespan	WB		
Normal survival		120 days	120 days
Chromium labeled, half life (t₁/₂)		25–35 days	25–35 days
Erythrocyte sedimentation rate	WB		
Females		1–25 mm/h	1–25 mm/h
Males		0–17 mm/h	0–17 mm/h

(continued)

Analyte	Specimen	SI Units	Conventional Units
Factor II, prothrombin	P	0.60–1.40	60–140%
Factor V	P	0.60–1.40	60–140%
Factor VII	P	0.60–1.40	60–140%
Factor VIII	P	0.50–2.00	50–200%
Factor IX	P	0.60–1.40	60–140%
Factor X	P	0.60–1.40	60–140%
Factor XI	P	0.60–1.40	60–140%
Factor XII	P	0.60–1.40	60–140%
Factor XIII screen	P	Not applicable	No deficiency detected
Factor inhibitor assay	P	<0.5 Bethesda Units	<0.5 Bethesda Units
Ferritin	S		
Male		30–300 μg/L	30–300 ng/mL
Female		10–200 μg/L	10–200 ng/mL
Fibrin(ogen) degradation products	P	<2.5 mg/L	<2.5 μg/mL
Fibrinogen	P	1.50–4.00 g/L	150–400 mg/dL
Folate (folic acid)	S, P		
Normal		7.0–39.7 nmol/L	3.1–17.5 ng/mL
Borderline deficient		5.0–6.8 nmol/L	2.2–3.0 ng/mL
Deficient		<5.0 nmol/L	<2.2 ng/mL
Excess		>39.7 nmol/L	>17.5 ng/mL
Glucose-6-phosphate dehydrogenase (erythrocyte)	WB	Not applicable	No gross deficiency
Ham's test (acid serum)	WB	Negative	Negative
Haptoglobin	S	0.16–1.99 g/L	16–199 mg/dL
Hematocrit	WB		
Adult males		0.41–0.53	41.0–53.0
Adult females		0.36–0.46	36.0–46.0
Hemoglobin			
Plasma	P	0.01–0.05 g/L	1–5 mg/dL
Whole blood:	WB		
Adult males		8.4–10.9 mmol/L	13.5–17.5 g/dL
Adult females		7.4–9.9 mmol/L	12.0–16.0 g/dL
Hemoglobin electrophoresis	WB		
Hemoglobin A		0.95–0.98	95–98%
Hemoglobin A_2		0.015–0.035	1.5–3.5%
Hemoglobin F		0–0.02	0–2.0%
Hemoglobins other than A, A_2, or F		Absent	Absent
Heparin-induced thrombocytopenia antibody	P	Negative	Negative
Homocysteine	P	0–12 μmol/L	0–12 μmol/L
Iron	S	5.4–28.7 μmol/L	30–160 μg/dL
Iron binding capacity	S	40.8–76.7 μmol/L	228–428 μg/dL
Leukocytes			
Alkaline phosphatase (LAP)	WB	Not applicable	13–133/100 neutrophils
Count (WBC)	WB	4.5–11 × 10^9/L	4.5–11.0 × 10^3/mm^3
Mean corpuscular hemoglobin (MCH)	WB	26.0–34.0 pg/cell	26.0–34.0 pg/cell
Mean corpuscular hemoglobin concentration (MCHC)	WB	310–370 g/L	31.0–37.0 g/dL
Mean corpuscular volume (MCV)	WB		
Male (adult)		78–100 fl	78–100 μm^3
Female (adult)		78–102 fl	78–102 μm^3
Methemoglobin	WB		Up to 1% of total hemoglobin
Osmotic fragility of erythrocytes	WB	Not applicable	Increased hemolysis as compared to normal control
Partial thromboplastin time, activated	P	22.1–35.1 s	22.1–35.1 s
Plasminogen	P		
Antigen		84–140 mg/L	8.4–14.0 mg/dL
Functional		0.80–1.30	80–130%
Plasminogen activator inhibitor 1	P	4–43 μg/L	4–43 ng/mL
Platelet aggregation	PRP		>65% aggregation in response to adenosine diphosphate, epinephrine, collagen, ristocetin, and arachidonic acid
Platelet count	WB	150–350 × 10^9/L	150–350 × 10^3/mm^3
Platelet, mean volume	WB	6.4–11 fl	6.4–11.0 μm^3
Prekallikrein assay	P	0.60–1.40	60–140%
Prekallikrein screen	P		No deficiency detected
Protein C	P		
Total antigen		0.70–1.40	70–140%
Functional		0.70–1.40	70–140%
Protein S	P		
Total antigen		0.70–1.40	70–140%
Functional		0.70–1.40	70–140%
Free antigen		0.70–1.40	70–140%
Prothrombin gene mutation G20210A	WB	Not applicable	Not present
Prothrombin time	P	11.1–13.1 s	11.1–13.1 s
Protoporphyrin, free erythrocyte	WB	0.28–0.64 μmol/L of red blood cells	16–36 μg/dL of red blood cells
Red cell distribution width	WB	0.115–0.145	11.5–14.5%

(continued)

Analyte	Specimen	SI Units	Conventional Units
Reptilase time	P	16–24 s	16–24 s
Reticulocyte count	WB	0.005–0.025 red cells	0.5–2.5% red cells
Reticulocyte hemoglobin content	WB	>26 pg/cell	>26 pg/cell
Ristocetin confactor (Functional von Willebrand factor)	P		
Blood group O		0.75 mean of normal	75% mean of normal
Blood group A		1.05 mean of normal	105% mean of normal
Blood group B		1.15 mean of normal	115% mean of normal
Blood group AB		1.25 mean of normal	125% mean of normal
Schilling test, orally administered vitamin B_{12} excreted in urine	U	Not applicable	7–40%
Sickle cell test	WB	Negative	Negative
Sucrose hemolysis	WB	<0.1	<10% hemolysis
Thrombin time	P	16–24 s	16–24 s
Total eosinophils	WB	70–140 × 10⁶/L	70–440/mm³
Transferrin receptor	S, P	9.6–29.6 nmol/L	9.6–29.6 nmol/L
Viscosity			
Plasma	P	1.7–2.1	1.7–2.1
Serum	S	1.4–1.8	1.4–1.8
Vitamin B_{12}	S, P		
Normal		185 pmol/L	>250 pg/mL
Borderline		92–185 pmol/L	125–250 pg/mL
Deficient		<92 pmol/L	<125 pg/mL
von Willebrand factor (vWF) antigen (factor VIII:R antigen)	P		
vWF multimers	P	Normal distribution	Normal distribution
White blood cells: see *Leukocytes*			

Note: P, plasma; PRP, platelet-rich plasma; S, serum; U, urine; WB, whole blood

TABLE A-2 *Immunology*

Analyte	Specimen	SI Units	Conventional Units
Autoantibodies			
Anti-adrenal antibody	S	Not applicable	Negative at 1:10 dilution
Anti–double stranded (native) DNA	S	Not applicable	Negative at 1:10 dilution
Anti-glomerular basement membrane antibodies	S		
Qualitative		Negative	Negative
Quantitative		<5 kU/L	<5 U/mL
Anti-granulocyte antibody	S	Not applicable	Negative
Anti-Jo-1 antibody	S	Not applicable	Negative
Anti-La antibody	S	Not applicable	Negative
Anti-mitochondrial antibody	S	Not applicable	Negative
Antineutrophil cytoplasmic autoantibodies, cytoplasmic (C-ANCA)	S		
Qualitative		Negative	Negative
Quantitative (Antibodies to proteinase 3)		<2.8 kU/L	<2.8 U/mL
Antineutrophil cytoplasmic autoantibodies, perinuclear (P-ANCA)	S		
Qualitative		Negative	Negative
Quantitative (Antibodies to myeloperoxidase)		<1.4 kU/L	<1.4 U/mL
Antinuclear antibody	S	Not applicable	Negative at 1:40
Anti-parietal cell antibody	S	Not applicable	Negative at 1:20
Anti-Ro antibody	S	Not applicable	Negative
Anti-platelet antibody	S	Not applicable	Negative
Anti-RNP antibody	S	Not applicable	Negative
Anti-Scl 70 antibody	S	Not applicable	Negative
Anti-Smith antibody	S	Not applicable	Negative
Anti–smooth muscle antibody	S	Not applicable	Negative at 1:20
Anti-thyroglobulin	S	Not applicable	Negative
Anti-thyroid antibody	S	<0.3 kIU/L	<0.3 IU/mL
Bence Jones protein, serum	S	Not applicable	None detected
Bence Jones protein, urine, qualitative	U	Not applicable	None detected in 50× concentrated urine
Bence Jones Protein, urine, quantitative	U		
κ		<0.03 g/L	<2.5 mg/dL
λ		<0.05 g/L	<5.0 mg/dL
β_2-Microglobulin			
	S	<2.7 mg/L	<0.27 mg/dL
	U	<120 μg/d	<120 μg/d

(continued)

Analyte	Specimen	SI Units	Conventional Units
C-reactive protein	S		
Routine		0.08–3.1 mg/L	0.08–3.1 mg/L
High sensitivity		0.02–8.0 mg/L	0.02–8.0 mg/L
C1-esterase-inhibitor protein	S		
Antigenic		0.12–0.25 g/L	12.4–24.5 mg/dL
Functional		Present	Present
Complement			
C3 (adults)	S	0.86–1.84 g/L	86–184 mg/dL
C4 (adults)	S	0.20–0.58 g/L	20–58 mg/dL
Total complement, EIA (adult)	S	63–145 kU/L	63–145 U/mL
Factor B	S	0.17–0.42 g/L	17–42 mg/dL
Cryoproteins	S	Not applicable	None detected
Immunofixation	S	Not applicable	None detected
Immunoglobulin, quantitation (adult)			
IgA	S	0.60–3.09 g/L	60–309 mg/dL
IgD	S	0–140 mg/L	0–14 mg/dL
IgE	S	24–430 μg/L	10–179 IU/mL
IgG	S	6.14–12.95 g/L	614–1295 mg/dL
IgG_1	S	2.7–17.4 g/L	270–1740 mg/dL
IgG_2	S	0.3–6.3 g/L	30–630 mg/dL
IgG_3	S	0.13–3.2 g/L	13–320 mg/dL
IgG_4	S	0.11–6.2 g/L	11–620 mg/dL
IgM	S	0.53–3.34 g/L	53–334 mg/dL
Joint fluid crystal	JF	Not applicable	No crystals seen
Joint fluid mucin	JF	Not applicable	Only type I mucin present
LE cell test	WB	Negative	Negative
Rheumatoid factor	S, JF	<30 kIU/L	<30.0 IU/mL
Serum protein electrophoresis	S	Not applicable	Normal pattern

Note: JF, joint fluid; P, plasma; S, serum; U, urine; WB, whole blood

TABLE A-3 *Clinical Chemistry*

Constituent	Specimen	SI Units	Conventional Units
Acetoacetate	P	<100 μmol/L	<1 mg/dL
Albumin	S	35–55 g/L	3.5–5.5 g/dL
Aldolase	S	0–100 nkat/L	0–6 U/L
α_1 antitrypsin	S	0.8–2.1 g/L	85–213 mg/dL
Alpha fetoprotein (adult)	S	<15 μg/L	<15 ng/mL
Aminotransferases	S		
Aspartate (AST, SGOT)		0–0.58 μkat/L	0–35 U/L
Alanine (ALT, SGPT)		0–0.58 μkat/L	0–35 U/L
Ammonia, as NH_3	P	6–47 μmol/L	10–80 μg/dL
Amylase	S	0.8–3.2 μkat/L	60–180 U/L
Angiotensin-converting enzyme (ACE)	S	<670 nkat/L	<40 U/L
Anion gap	S	7–16 mmol/L	7–16 mmol/L
Apolipoprotein A-1	S	1.2–2.4 g/L	119–240 mg/dL
Apolipoprotein B	S	0.52–1.63 g/L	52–163 mg/dL
Apo B/Apo A-1 ratio		0.35–0.98	0.35–0.98
Arterial blood gases			
$[HCO_3^-]$		21–28 mmol/L	21–30 meq/L
P_{CO_2}		4.7–5.9 kPa	35–45 mmHg
pH		7.38–7.44	
P_{O_2}		11–13 kPa	80–100 mmHg
β-Hydroxybutyrate	P	<300 μmol/L	<3 mg/dL
β-2-microglobulin	S	1.2–2.8 mg/L	1.2–2.8 mg/L
	U	≤200 μg/L	≤200 μg/L
Bilirubin	S		
Total		5.1–17 μmol/L	0.3–1.0 mg/dL
Direct		1.7–5.1 μmol/L	0.1–0.3 mg/dL
Indirect		3.4–12 μmol/L	0.2–0.7 mg/dL
Brain type natriuetic peptide (BNP)	P	Age and gender specific: <167 ng/L	Age and gender specific: <167 ng/mL
Calcium, ionized	WB	1.1–1.4 mmol/L	4.5–5.6 mg/dL
Calcium	S	2.2–2.6 mmol/L	9–10.5 mg/dL
CA-15-3	S	0–30 kU/L	0–30 U/mL
CA 19-9	S	0–37 kU/L	0–37 U/mL
CA 27-29	S	0–32 kU/L	0–32 U/mL
CA 125	S	0–35 kU/L	0–35 U/mL
Calcitonin	S		
Male		3–26 ng/L	3–26 pg/mL
Female		2–17 ng/L	2–17 pg/mL

(continued)

Constituent	Specimen	SI Units	Conventional Units
Carbon dioxide content (TCO$_2$)	P (sea level)	21–30 mmol/L	21–30 meq/L
Carbon dioxide tension (P$_{CO_2}$)	Arterial blood (sea level)	4.7–5.9 kPa	35–45 mmHg
Carbon monoxide content	WB	Symptoms with 20% saturation of hemoglobin	
Carcinoembryonic antigen (CEA)	S	0.0–3.4 ug/L	0.0–3.4 ng/mL
Ceruloplasmin	S	270–37 mg/L	27–37 ng/dL
Cholinesterase	S	5–12 kU/L	5–12 U/mL
Chloride	S	98–106 mmol/L	98–106 meq/L
Cholesterol: see Table A-7			
Coproporphyrins (types I and III)	U	150–460 μmol/d	100–300 μg/d
C-peptide	S	0.17–0.66 nmol/L	0.5–2.0 ng/mL
Creatine kinase (CK) (total)	S		
Females		0.67–2.50 μkat/L	40–150 U/L
Males		1.00–6.67 μkat/L	60–400 U/L
Creatine kinase-MB	S	0–7 μg/L	0–7 ng/mL
Creatine kinase relative index (ng/mL per total CK U/L) × 100	S	Method dependent	Method dependent
Creatinine	S	<133 μmol/L	<1.5 mg/dL
Erythropoietin	S	5–36 U/L	
Fatty acids, free (nonesterified)	P	0.28–0.89 mmol/L	<8–25 mg/dL
Ferritin	S		
Female		10–200 μg/L	10–200 ng/mL
Male		15–400 μg/L	15–400 ng/mL
Fibrinogen and fibrinogen split products: see Hematology and Coagulation			
Gamma glutamyltransferase	S	1–94 U/L	1–94 U/L
Glucose (fasting)	P		
Normal		4.2–6.4 mmol/L	75–115 mg/dL
Diabetes mellitus		>7.0 mmol/L	>125 mg/dL
Glucose, 2 h postprandial	P	<6.7 mmol/L	<120 mg/dL
Hemoglobin A$_{1c}$	WB	0.038–0.064 Hb fraction	3.8–6.4%
Homocysteine	P	4–12 μmol/L	4–12 μmol/L
Hydroxyproline	U, 24 hour	0–10 μmol/L	0–1.3 mg/d
Iron	S	9–27 μmol/L	50–150 μg/dL
Iron-binding capacity	S	45–66 μmol/L	250–370 μg/dL
Iron-binding capacity saturation	S	0.2–0.45	20–45%
Ketone (acetone)	S, U	Negative	Negative
Lactate dehydrogenase	S	1.7–3.2 μkat/L	100–190 U/L
Lactate	P, venous	0.6–1.7 mmol/L	5–15 mg/dL
Lactate dehydrogenase isoenzymes	S		
Fraction 1 (of total)		0.14–0.25	14–26%
Fraction 2		0.29–0.39	29–39%
Fraction 3		0.20–0.25	20–26%
Fraction 4		0.08–0.16	8–16%
Fraction 5		0.06–0.16	6–16%
Lipase	S	0–2.66 μkat/L	0–160 U/L
Lipids: see Table A-7			
Lipids, triglyceride: see Triglycerides			
Lipoprotein: see Table A-7			
Lipoprotein (a)	S	0–300 mg/L	0–30 mg/dL
Magnesium	S	0.8–1.2 mmol/L	1.8–3 mg/dL
Microalbumin urine			
24-h urine	U	<0.2 g/L or <0.031 g/24 h	<20 mg/L or <31 mg/24 h
Spot AM urine		<0.03 g albumin/g creatinine	<0.03 mg albumin/mg creatinine
Myoglobin	S		
Male		19–92 μg/L	
Female		12–76 μg/L	
5 Nucleotidase	S	0.02–0.18 ukat/L	0–11 U/L
N-telopeptide (cross linked), NTx	U	3–65 nmol/mmol creatinine	3–65 nmol/mmol creatinine
Osmolality			
	P	285–295 mmol/kg serum water	285–295 mosmol/kg serum water
	U	300–900 mmol/kg	300–900 mosmol/kg
Osteocalcin	S	3.1–14 ug/mL	3.1–14 ng/mL
Oxygen content	WB, arterial (sea level)		17–21 vol%
	WB, venous arm (sea level)		10 to 16 vol%
Oxygen percent saturation (sea level)			
	WB, arterial	0.97 mol/mol	97%
	WB, venous, arm	0.60–0.85 mol/mol	60–85%
Oxygen tension (P$_{O_2}$)	WB	11–13 kPa	80–100 mmHg
pH	WB	7.38–7.44	
Parathyroid hormone–related peptide	S	<1.3 pmol/L	<1.3 pmol/L
Phosphatase, acid	S	0.90 nkat/L	0–5.5 U/L
Phosphatase, alkaline	S	0.5–2.0 nkat/L	30–120 U/L

(continued)

TABLE A-3 *Clinical Chemistry—(Continued)*

Constituent	Specimen	SI Units	Conventional Units
Phosphorus, inorganic	S	1.0–1.4 mmol/L	3–4.5 mg/dL
Porphobilinogen	U	None	None
Potassium	S	3.5–5.0 mmol/L	3.5–5.0 meq/L
Prealbumin	S	195–358 mg/L	19.5–35.8 mg/dL
Prostate-specific antigen (PSA)	S		
Female		<0.5 μg/L	<0.5 ng/mL
Male			
<40 years		0.0–2.0 μg/L	0.0–2.0 ng/mL
>40 years		0.0–4.0 μg/L	0.0–4.0 ng/mL
PSA, free, in males 45–75 years, with PSA values between 4 and 20 μg/mL		>0.25 associated with benign prostatic hyperplasia (BPH)	>25% associated with BPH
Protein, total	S	55–80 g/L	5.5–8.0 g/dL
Protein fractions:	S		
Albumin		35–55 g/L	3.5–5.5 g/dL (50–60%)
Globulin		20–35 g/L	2.0–3.5 g/dL (40–50%)
Alpha$_1$		2–4 g/L	0.2–0.4 g/dL (4.2–7.2%)
Alpha$_2$		5–9 g/L	0.5–0.9 g/dL (6.8–12%)
Beta		6–11 g/L	0.6–1.1 g/dL (9.3–15%)
Gamma		7–17 g/L	0.7–1.7 g/dL (13–23%)
Pyruvate	P, venous	60–170 μmol/L	0.5–1.5 mg/dL
Sodium	S	136–145 mmol/L	136–145 meq/L
Transferrin	S	2.3–3.9 g/L	230–390 mg/dL
Triglycerides	S	<1.8 mmol/L	<160 mg/dL
Troponin I	S	0–0.4 μg/L	0–0.4 ng/mL
Troponin T	S	0–0.1 μg/L	0–0.1 ng/mL
Urea nitrogen	S	3.6–7.1 mmol/L	10–20 mg/dL
Uric acid	S		
Males		150–480 μmol/L	2.5–8.0 mg/dL
Females		90–360 μmol/L	1.5–6.0 mg/dL
Urobilinogen	U	1.7–5.9 μmol/d	1–3.5 mg/d
Vasoactive intestinal polypeptide	P	<75 ng/L	<75 pg/mL

Note: P, plasma; S, serum; U, urine; WB, blood

TABLE A-4 *Metabolic and Endocrine Tests*

Analyte	Specimen	SI Units	Conventional Units
Adrenocorticotropin (ACTH)	P	1.3–16.7 pmol/L	6.0–76.0 pg/mL
Aldosterone (adult)			
Supine, normal sodium diet	S, P	55–250 pmol/L	2–9 ng/dL
Upright, normal sodium diet	S, P		2- to 5-fold increase over supine value
Supine, low-sodium diet	S, P		2- to 5-fold increase over normal sodium diet level
Random, low-sodium diet	U	6.38–58.25 nmol/d	2.3–21.0 μg/24 h
Androstenedione (adult)	S	1.75–8.73 nmol/L	50–250 ng/dL
C peptide (adult)	S, P	0.17–0.66 nmol/L	0.5–2.0 ng/mL
Cortisol			
Fasting, 8 AM–Noon	S	138–690 nmol/L	5–25 μg/dL
Noon–8 PM		138–414 nmol/L	5–15 μg/dL
8 PM–8 AM		0–276 nmol/L	0–10 μg/dL
Cortisol, free	U	55–193 nmol/24 h	20–70 μg/24 h
C-peptide (insulin)	S	0.26–0.62 nmol/L	0.78–1.89 ng/mL
Dehydroepiandrosterone (DHEA) (adult)			
Male	S	6.24–41.6 nmol/L	180–1250 ng/dL
Female		4.5–34.0 nmol/L	130–980 ng/dL
DHEA sulfate	S		
Male (adult)		100–6190 μg/L	10–619 μg/dL
Female (adult, premenopausal)		120–5350 μg/L	12–535 μg/dL
Female (adult, postmenopausal)		300–2600 μg/L	30–260 μg/dL
Deoxycorticosterone (DOC) (adult)	S	61–576 nmol/L	2–19 ng/dL
11-Deoxycortisol (adult) (compound S) (8:00 AM)	S	0.34–4.56 nmol/L	12–158 ng/dL
Dihydrotestosterone			
Male	S, P	1.03–2.92 nmol/L	30–85 ng/dL
Female		0.14–0.76 nmol/L	4–22 ng/dL
Dopamine	P	<475 pmol/L	<87 pg/mL
Dopamine	U	425–2610 nmol/d	65–400 g/d
Epinepherine	P		
Supine (30 min)		<273 pmol/L	<50 pg/mL
Sitting		<328 pmol/L	<60 pg/mL
Standing (30 min)		<4914 pmol/L	<900 pg/mL

(continued)

Analyte	Specimen	SI Units	Conventional Units
Epinephrine	U	0–109 nmol/d	0–20 μg/d
Estradiol	S, P		
Female			
Menstruating			
Follicular phase		184–532 pmol/L	<20–145 pg/mL
Mid-cycle peak		411–1626 pmol/L	112–443 pg/mL
Luteal phase		184–885 pmol/L	<20–241 pg/mL
Postmenopausal		217 pmol/L	<59 pg/mL
Male		184 pmol/L	<20 pg/mL
Estrone	S, P		
Female			
Menstruating			
Follicular phase		55–555 pmol/L	1.5–15 pg/mL
Luteal phase		55–740 pmol/L	1.5–20 pg/mL
Postmenopausal		55–204 pmol/L	1.5–5.5 pg/mL
Male		55–240 pmol/L	1.5–6.5 pg/mL
Follicle-stimulating hormone (FSH)	S, P		
Female			
Menstruating			
Follicular phase		3.0–20.0 IU/L	3.0–20.0 U/L
Ovulatory phase		9.0–26.0 IU/L	9.0–26.0 U/L
Luteal phase		1.0–12.0 IU/L	1.0–12.0 U/L
Postmenopausal		18.0–153.0 IU/L	18.0–153.0 U/L
Male		1.0–12.0 IU/L	1.0–12.0 U/L
Fructosamine	S	1.61–2.68 mmol/L	1.61–2.68 mmol/L
Gastrin	S	<100 ng/L	<100 pg/mL
Glucagon	P	20–100 ng/L	20–100 pg/mL
Growth hormone (resting)	S	0.5–17.0 μg/L	0.5–17.0 ng/mL
Human chorionic gonadotropin (HCG) (nonpregnant)	S	<5 IU/L	<5 mIU/mL
17-Hydroxyprogesterone (adult)	S		
Male		0.15 nmol/L	5–250 ng/dL
Female			
Follicular phase		0.6–3.0 nmol/L	20–100 ng/dL
Midcycle peak		3–7.5 nmol/L	100–250 ng/dL
Luteal phase		3–15 nmol/L	100–500 ng/dL
Postmenopausal		≤2.1 nmol/L	≤70 ng/dL
5-Hydroindoleacetic Acid [5-HIAA]	U	10.5–36.6 μmol/d	2–7 mg/d
Insulin	S, P	14.35–143.5 pmol/L	2–20 μU/mL
17 Ketosteroids	U	10–42 μmol/d	3–12 mg/d
Luteinizing hormone (LH)	S, P		
Female			
Menstruating			
Follicular phase		2.0–15.0 U/L	2.0–15.0 U/L
Ovulatory phase		22.0–105.0 U/L	22.0–105.0 U/L
Luteal phase		0.6–19.0 U/L	0.6–19.0 U/L
Postmenopausal		16.0–64.0 U/L	16.0–64.0 U/L
Male		2.0–12.0 U/L	2.0–12.0 U/L
Metanephrine	P	Method dependent	Method dependent
Metanephrine	U	0.03–0.69 mmol/mol creatinine	0.05–1.20 μg/mg creatinine
Norepinephrine	U	89–473 nmol/d	15–80 μg/d
Norepinephrine	P		
Supine (30 min)		650–2423 pmol/L	<110–410 pg/mL
Sitting		709–4019 pmol/L	120–680 pg/mL
Standing (30 min)		739–4137 pmol/L	125–700 pg/mL
Parathyroid hormone (PTH)	S	10–60 ng/L	10–60 pg/mL
Pregnanetriol	U	Age and sex dependent	Age and sex dependent
Progesterone	S, P		
Female			
Follicular		<3.18 nmol/L	<1.0 ng/mL
Midluteal		9.54–63.6 nmol/L	3–20 ng/mL
Male		<3.18 nmol/L	<1.0 ng/mL
Prolactin	S		
Female		0–20 μg/L	1.9–25.9 ng/mL
Male		0–15 μg/L	1.6–23.0 ng/mL
Renin (adult, normal sodium diet)	P		
Supine		0.08–0.83 ng/(L-s)	0.3–3.0 ng/(mL/h)
Upright		0.28–2.5 ng/(L-s)	1–9.0 ng/(mL/h)
Serotonin	WB	0.28–1.14 μmol/L	50–200 ng/mL
Serotonin	Platelet	0.7–2.8 amol/platelet	125–500 ng/10^9 platelets
Sex hormone binding globulin (adult)	S		
Male			13–71 nmol/L
Female			18–114 nmol/L
Somatostatin	P	<25 ng/L	<25 pg/mL

(continued)

Analyte	Specimen	SI Units	Conventional Units
Somatomedin-C (IGF-1) (adult)	S		
16–24 years		182–780 μg/L	182–780 ng/mL
25–39 years		114–492 μg/L	114–492 ng/mL
40–54 years		90–360 μg/L	90–360 ng/mL
>54 years		71–290 μg/L	71–290 ng/mL
Testosterone, total, morning sample	S		
Female		0.21–2.98 nmol/L	6–86 ng/dL
Male		9.36–37.10 nmol/L	270–1070 ng/dL
Testosterone, unbound, morning sample			
Female, adult	S	6.9–107.5 pmol/L	0.2–3.1 pg/mL
Male, adult		416–1386 pmol/L	12.0–40.0 pg/mL
Thyroglobulin	S	0–60 μg/L	0–60 ng/mL
Thyroid binding globulin	S	206–309 μg/L	16–24 μg/dL
Thyroid hormone binding index (THBI or T3RU)	S	0.83–1.17 mol ratio	0.83–1.17
(Free) thyroxine index	S	4.2–13	4.2–13
Thyroid stimulating hormone	S	0.5–4.7 mU/L	0.5–4.7 μU/mL
Thyroxine, total (T4)	S	58–140 nmol/L	4.5–10.9 μg/dL
Triiodothyronine, total (T3)	S	0.92–2.78 nmol/L	60–181 ng/dL
Thyroxine, free (fT4)	S	10.3–35 pmol/L	0.8–2.7 ng/dL
Triiodothyronine, free (fT3)	S	0.22–6.78 pmol/L	1.4–4.4 pg/mL
Vanillylmandelic Acid (VMA)	U, 24 h	7.6–37.9 μmol/d	0.15–1.2 mg/d
Vasoactive intestinal polypeptide (VIP)	P	<75 ng/L	<75 pg/mL

Note: P, plasma; S, serum; U, urine; WB, whole blood

TABLE A-5 *Toxicology and Therapeutic Drug Monitoring*

Drug	Therapeutic Range		Toxic Level	
	Conventional Units	SI Units	Conventional Units	SI Units
Acetaminophen	10–30 μg/mL	66–199 μmol/L	>200 μg/mL	>1324 μmol/L
Amikacin				
Peak	25–35 μg/mL	43–60 μmol/L	>35 μg/mL	>60 μmol/L
Trough	4–8 μg/mL	6.8–13.7 μmol/L	>10 μg/mL	>17 μmol/L
Amitriptyline	120–250 ng/mL	433–903 nmol/L	>500 ng/mL	>1805 nmol/L
Amphetamine	20–30 ng/mL	148–222 nmol/L	>200 ng/mL	>1480 nmol/L
Antiepileptic drugs: see Table 348–8				
Barbiturates, most short-acting			>20 mg/L	>88 μmol/L
Bromide			>1250 μg/mL	>15.6 mmol/L
Carbamazepine	6–12 μg/mL	26–51 μmol/L	>15 μg/mL	>63 μmol/L
Chlordiazepoxide	700–1000 ng/mL	2.34–3.34 μmol/L	>5000 ng/mL	>16.7 μmol/L
Clonazepam	15–60 ng/mL	48–190 nmol/L	>80 ng/mL	>254 nmol/L
Clozapine	200–350 ng/mL	0.6–1 μmol/L		
Cocaine			>1000 ng/mL	>3300 nmol/L
Cyclosporine	Depends on timing after dose and transplant type with ranges of 100–400 ng/mL	Depends on timing after dose and transplant type with ranges of 83–333 nmol/L	Varies with time after dose and transplant type	Varies with time after dose and transplant type
Desipramine	75–300 ng/mL	281–1125 nmol/L	>400 ng/mL	>1500 nmol/L
Diazepam	100–1000 ng/mL	0.35–351 μmol/L	>5000 ng/mL	>17.55 μmol/L
Digoxin	0.8–2.0 ng/mL	1.0–2.6 nmol/L	>2.5 ng/mL	>3.2 μmol/L
Doxepin	30–150 ng/mL	107–537 nmol/L	>500 ng/mL	>1790 nmol/L
Ethanol			>300 mg/dL	>65 mmol/L
Behavioral changes	>20 mg/dL	>4.3 mmol/L		
Clinical intoxication	>100 mg/dL	>1 g/L		
Ethosuximide	40–100 μg/mL	283–708 μmol/L	>150 μg/mL	>1062 μmol/L
Flecainide	0.2–1.0 μg/mL	0.5–2.4 μmol/L	>1.0 μg/mL	>2.4 μmol/L
Gentamicin				
Peak	8–10 μg/mL	16.7–20.9 μmol/L	>10 μg/mL	>21 μmol/L
Trough	<2–4 μg/mL	<4.2–8.4 μmol/L	>4 μg/mL	>8.4 μmol/L
Ibuprofen	10–50 μg/mL	49–243 μmol/L	100–700 μg/mL	485–3395 μmol/L
Imipramine	125–250 ng/mL	446–893 nmol/L	>500 ng/mL	>1784 nmol/L
Lidocaine	1.5–6.0 μg/mL	6.4–26 μmol/L		26–34.2 μmol/L
CNS or Cardiovascular depression			6–8 μg/mL	
Seizures, obtundation, decreased cardiac output			>8 μg/mL	>34.2 μmol/L
Lithium	0.6–1.2 meq/L	0.6–1.2 nmol/L	>2 meq/L	>2 mmol/L
Methadone	100–400 ng/mL	0.32–1.29 μmol/L	>2000 ng/mL	>6.46 μmol/L
Methotrexate	Variable	Variable		
Low dose (1–2 weeks)			>9.1 ng/mL	>20 nmol/L
High dose (48 h)			>227 ng/mL	>0.5 μmol/L

(continued)

TABLE A-5—(Continued)

Drug	Therapeutic Range Conventional Units	SI Units	Toxic Level Conventional Units	SI Units
Morphine	10–80 ng/mL	35–280 μmol/L	>200 ng/mL	>700 nmol/L
Nitroprusside (as thiocyanate)	6–29 μg/mL	103–499 μmol/L		
Nortriptyline	50–170 ng/mL	190–646 nmol/L	>500 ng/mL	>1.9 μmol/L
Phenobarbital	10–40 μg/mL	43–170 μmol/L		
Slowness, ataxia, nystagmus			35–80 μg/mL	151–345 μmol/L
Coma with reflexes			65–117 μg/mL	280–504 μmol/L
Coma without reflexes			>100 μg/mL	>430 μmol/L
Phenytoin	10–20 μg/mL	40–79 μmol/L	>20 μg/mL	>79 μmol/L
Procainamide	4–10 μg/mL	17–42 μmol/L	>10–12 μg/mL	>42–51 μmol/L
Quinidine	2–5 μg/mL	6–15 μmol/L	>6 μg/mL	>18 μmol/L
Salicylates	150–300 μg/mL	1086–2172 μmol/L	>300 μg/mL	>2172 μmol/L
Theophylline	8–20 μg/mL	44–111 μmol/L	>20 μg/mL	>110 μmol/L
Thiocyanate				
After nitroprusside infusion	6–29 μg/mL	103–499 μmol/L		
Nonsmoker	1–4 μg/mL	17–69 μmol/L	>120 μg/mL	>2064 μmol/L
Smoker	3–12 μg/mL	52–206 μmol/L		
Tobramycin				
Peak	8–10 μg/mL	17–21 μmol/L	>10 μg/mL	>21 μmol/L
Trough	<4 μg/mL	<9 μmol/L	>4 μg/mL	>9 μmol/L
Valproic acid	50–150 μg/mL	347–1040 μmol/L	>150 μg/mL	>1040 μmol/L
Vancomycin				
Peak	18–26 μg/mL	12–18 μmol/L	>80–100 μg/mL	>55–69 μmol/L
Trough	5–10 μg/mL	3–7 μmol/L		

TABLE A-6 Vitamins and Selected Trace Minerals

Specimen	Analyte	SI Units	Conventional Units
Aluminum	S	<0.2 μmol/L	<5.41 μg/L
	U, random	5–30 μg/L	0.19–1.11 μmol/L
Arsenic			
	WB	0.03–0.31 μmol/L	2–23 μg/L
	U, 24 h	0.07–0.67 μmol/d	5–50 μg/d
Coenzyme Q10 (ubiquinone)	P	0.5–1.5 mg/L	0.5–1.5 μg/mL
Carotenoids	S	0.9–5.6 μmol/L	50–300 μg/dL
Copper			
	S	11–22 μmol/L	70–140 μg/dL
	U, 24 h	0.047–0.55 μmol/d	3–35 μg/d
Folic acid	RC	340–1020 nmol/L cells	150–450 ng/mL cells
Folic acid	S	7–36 nmol/L cells	3–16 ng/mL cells
Lead (adult)	S	<0.5–1 μmol/L	<10–20 μg/dL
Mercury			
	WB	3.0–294 nmol/L	0.6–59 μg/L
	U, 24 h	<99.8 nmol/L	<20 μg/L
Vitamin A	S	0.7–3.5 μmol/L	20–100 μg/dL
Vitamin B_1 (thiamine)	S	0–75 nmol/L	0–2 μg/dL
Vitamin B_2 (riboflavin)	S	106–638 nmol/L	4–24 μg/dL
Vitamin B_6	P	20–121 nmol/L	5–30 ng/mL
Vitamin B_{12}	S	148–590 pmol/L	200–800 pg/mL
Vitamin C (ascorbic acid)	S	23–57 μmol/L	0.4–1.0 mg/dL
Vitamin D_3, 1,25-dihydroxy	S	60–108 pmol/L	25–45 pg/mL
Vitamin D_3, 25-hydroxy (some labs report as a desirable level rather than a normal range)	P		
Summer		37.4–200 nmol/L	15–80 ng/mL
Winter		34.9–105 nmol/L	14–42 ng/mL
Vitamin E	S	12–42 μmol/L	5–18 μg/mL
Vitamin K	S	0.29–2.64 nmol/L	0.13–1.19 ng/mL
Zinc	S	11.5–18.5 μmol/L	75–120 μg/dL

Note: P, plasma; RC, red cells; S, serum; U, urine; WB, whole blood

TABLE A-7 Classification of LDL, Total, and HDL Cholesterol

LDL cholesterol	
<100	Optimal
100–129	Near or above normal
130–159	Borderline high
160–189	High
≥190	Very high
Total cholesterol	
<200	Desirable
200–239	Borderline high
≥240	High
HDL cholesterol	
<40	Low
≥60	High

Note: HDL, high-density lipoprotein; LDL, low-density lipoprotein
Source: Executive summary of the third report of the national cholesterol education program (NCEP) expert panel on detection, evaluation, and treatment of high blood cholesterol in adults (adult treatment panel III): JAMA 285:2486, 2001.

TABLE B-1 *Cerebrospinal Fluid[a]*

Constituent	SI Units	Conventional Units
Glucose	2.22–3.89 mmol/L	40–70 mg/dL
Lactate	1–2 mmol/L	10–20 mg/dL
Total protein		
Lumbar	0.15–0.5 g/L	15–50 mg/dL
Cisternal	0.15–0.25 g/L	15–25 mg/dL
Ventricular	0.06–0.15 g/L	6–15 mg/dL
Albumin	0.066–0.442 g/L	6.6–44.2 mg/dL
IgG	0.009–0.057 g/L	0.9–5.7 mg/dL
IgG index[b]	0.29–0.59	
Oligoclonal bands (OGB)	<2 bands not present in matched serum sample	
Ammonia	15–47 μmol/L	25–80 μg/dL
CSF pressure		50–180 mmH$_2$O
CSF volume (adult)	~150 mL	
Red blood cells	0	0
Leukocytes		
Total	0–5 mononuclear cells per mm^3	
Differential		
Lymphocytes	60–70%	
Monocytes	30–50%	
Neutrophils	None	

[a] Since cerebrospinal fluid concentrations are equilibrium values, measurements of the same parameters in blood plasma obtained at the same time are recommended. However, there is a time lag in attainment of equilibrium, and cerebrospinal levels of plasma constituents that can fluctuate rapidly (such as plasma glucose) may not achieve stable values until after a significant lag phase.

[b] IgG index = CSF IgG(mg/dL) × serum albumin(g/dL)/Serum IgG(g/dL) × CSF albumin(mg/dL)

TABLE B-2 *Urine Analysis*

	SI Units	Conventional Units
Acidity, titratable	20–40 mmol/d	20–40 meq/d
Ammonia	30–50 mmol/d	30–50 meq/d
Amylase		4–400 U/L
Amylase/creatinine clearance ratio [(Cl$_{am}$/Cl$_{cr}$) × 100]	1–5	1–5
Calcium (10 meq/d or 200 mg/d dietary calcium)	<7.5 mmol/d	<300 mg/d
Creatine, as creatinine		
Female	<760 μmol/d	<100 mg/d
Male	<380 μmol/d	<50 mg/d
Creatinine	8.8–14 mmol/d	1.0–1.6 g/d
Eosinophils	<100 eosinophils/mL	<100 eosinophils/mL
Glucose, true (oxidase method)	0.3–1.7 mmol/d	50–300 mg/d
5-Hydroxyindoleacetic acid (5-HIAA)	10–47 μmol/d	2–9 mg/d
"Microalbumin"	<0.02 g/L	<20 mg/L
Oxalate	228–684 μmol/d	20–60 mg/d
pH	5.0–9.0	5.0–9.0
Phosphate (phosphorus) (varies with intake)	12.9–42.0 mmol/d	400–1300 mg/d
Potassium (varies with intake)	25–100 mmol/d	25–100 meq/d
Protein	<0.15 g/d	<150 mg/d
Sediment		
Bacteria	Negative	
Bladder cells	Negative	
Broad casts	Negative	
Crystals	Negative	
Epithelial cell casts	Negative	
Granular casts	Negative	
Hyaline casts	0–5/low power field	
Red blood cell casts	Negative	
Red blood cells	0–2/high power field	
Squamous cells	Negative	
Tubular cells	Negative	
Waxy casts	Negative	
White blood cells	0–2/high power field	
White cell casts	Negative	
Sodium (varies with intake)	100–260 mmol/d	100–260 meq/d
Specific gravity	1.001–1.035	
Urea nitrogen	214–607 mmol/d	6–17 g/d
Uric acid (normal diet)	1.49–4.76 mmol/d	250–800 mg/d

TABLE B-3 *Differential Nucleated Cell Counts of Bone Marrow Aspirates*

	Mean, %	Range, %	95% Confidence Intervals, %
Myeloid (total)	56.7		
Neutrophilic series (total)	53.6	49.2–65.0	33.6–73.6
Myeloblast	0.9	0.2–1.5	0.1–1.7
Promyelocyte	3.3	2.1–4.1	1.9–4.7
Myelocyte	12.7	8.2–15.7	8.5–16.9
Metamyelocyte	15.9	9.6–24.6	7.1–24.7
Band	12.4	9.5–15.3	9.4–15.4
Segmented	7.4	6.0–12.0	3.8–11.0
Eosinophilic series	3.1	1.2–5.3	1.1–5.2
Basophilic and mast cells	0.1	0–0.2	—
Erythroid (total)	25.6	18.4–33.8	15.0–36.2
Pronormoblasts	0.6	0.2–1.3	0.1–1.1
Basophilic normoblasts	1.4	0.5–2.4	0.4–2.4
Polychromatophilic normoblasts	21.6	17.9–29.2	13.1–30.1
Orthochromatic normoblasts	2.0	0.4–4.6	0.3–3.7
Lymphocytes	16.2	11.1–23.2	8.6–23.8
Plasma cells	1.3	0.4–3.9	0–3.5
Monocytes	0.3	0–0.8	0–0.6
Megakaryocytes	0.1	0–0.4	—
Reticulum cells	0.3	0–0.9	0–0.8
M:E ratio	2.3	1.5–3.3	1.1–3.5

Note: Data are from 12 healthy men.
Source: From SL Perkins: Normal blood and bone marrow values in humans, in GR Lee et al (eds): *Wintrobe's Clinical Hematology*, 10th ed, Philadelphia, Williams and Wilkins, 1999, pp 2738–2748, with permission.

TABLE B-4 *Stool Analysis*

	SI Units	Conventional Units
Bulk		
Wet weight	<197.5 (115 ± 41) g/d	<197.5 (115 ± 41) g/d
Dry weight	<66.4 (34 ± 15) g/d	<66.4 (34 ± 15) g/d
α_1 Antitrypsin	0.98 (±0.17) mg/g dry weight	0.98 (±0.17) mg/g dry weight
Coproporphyrin	600–1500 nmol/d	400–1000 μg/d
Fat		
Adult		<7 g/d
Adult on fat-free diet		<4 g/d
Fatty acid		
Free	0.01–0.10	1–10% of dry matter
Combined as soap	0.005–0.12	0.5–12% of dry matter
Nitrogen	<1.7 (1.4 ± 0.2) g/d	<1.7 (1.4 ± 0.2) g/d
Protein content	Minimal	Minimal
Urobilinogen	68–470 μmol/d	40–280 mg/d
Water	~0.65	~65%

TABLE C-1 *Renal Function Tests*

	SI Units	Conventional Units
Clearances (corrected to 1.72 m² body surface area)		
Measures of glomerular filtration rate (GFR)		
Inulin clearance (Cl)		
Males (mean ± 1 SD)	2.1 ± 0.4 mL/s	124 ± 25.8 mL/min
Females (mean ± 1 SD)	2.0 ± 0.2 mL/s	119 ± 12.8 mL/min
Endogenous creatinine clearance	1.5–2.2 mL/s	91–130 mL/min
Urea	1.0–1.7 mL/s	60–100 mL/min
Measures of effective renal plasma flow and tubular function		
p-Aminohippuric acid clearance (Cl_{PAH})		
Males (mean ± 1 SD)	10.9 ± 2.7 mL/s	654 ± 163 mL/min
Females (mean ± 1 SD)	9.9 ± 1.7 mL/s	594 ± 102 mL/min
Concentration and dilution test		
Specific gravity of urine		
After 12-h fluid restriction	>1.025	>1.025
After 12-h deliberate water intake	≤1.003	≤1.003
Protein excretion, urine	<0.15 g/d	<150 mg/d
Specific gravity, maximal range	1.002–1.028	1.002–1.028
Tubular reabsorption, phosphorus	0.79–0.94 of filtered load	79–94% of filtered load

TABLE C-2 *Gastrointestinal Tests*

Test	SI Units	Conventional Units
Absorption tests		
D-Xylose: after overnight fast, 25 g xylose given in oral aqueous solution		
Urine, collected for following 5 h	33–53 mmol (or >20% of ingested dose	5–8 g (or >20% of ingested dose)
Serum, 1 h after dose	1.7–2.7 mmol/L	25–40 mg/dL
Vitamin A: a fasting blood specimen is obtained and 200,000 units of vitamin A in oil is given orally	Serum level should rise to twice fasting level in 3–5 h	Serum level should rise to twice fasting level in 3–5 h
Bentiromide test (pancreatic function): 500 mg bentiromide (chymex) orally; p-aminobenzoic acid (PABA) measured		
Plasma		>3.6 (±1.1) µg/mL at 90 min
Urine	>50% recovered in 6 h	>50% recovered in 6 h
Gastric juice		
Volume		
24 h	2–3 L	2–3 L
Nocturnal	600–700 mL	600–700 mL
Basal, fasting	30–70 mL/h	30–70 mL/h
Reaction		
pH	1.6–1.8	1.6–1.8
Titratable acidity of fasting juice	4–9 µmol/s	15–35 meq/h
Acid output		
Basal		
Females (mean ± 1 SD)	0.6 ± 0.5 µmol/s	2.0 ± 1.8 meq/h
Males (mean ± 1 SD)	0.8 ± 0.6 µmol/s	3.0 ± 2.0 meq/h
Maximal (after SC histamine acid phosphate, 0.004 mg/kg body weight, and preceded by 50 mg promethazine, or after betazole, 1.7 mg/kg body weight, or pentagastrin, 6 µg/kg body weight)		
Females (mean ± 1 SD)	4.4 ± 1.4 µmol/s	16 ± 5 meq/h
Males (mean ± 1 SD)	6.4 ± 1.4 µmol/s	23 ± 5 meq/h
Basal acid output/maximal acid output ratio	≤0.6	≤0.6
Gastrin, serum	40–200 µg/L	40–200 pg/mL
Secretin test (pancreatic exocrine function): 1 unit/kg body weight, IV		
Volume (pancreatic juice) in 80 min	>2.0 mL/kg	>2.0 mL/kg
Bicarbonate concentration	>80 mmol/L	>80 meq/L
Bicarbonate output in 30 min	>10 mmol	>10 meq

TABLE C-3 *Circulatory Function Tests*

Test	SI Units (Range)	Conventional Units (Range)
Arteriovenous oxygen difference	30–50 mL/L	30–50 mL/L
Cardiac output (Fick)	2.5–3.6 L/m² of body surface area per minute	2.5–3.6 L/m² of body surface area per minute
Contractility indices		
Max. left ventricular *dp/dt (dp/dt)*/DP when DP = 5.3 kPa (40 mmHg)	220 kPa/s (176–250 kPa/s) (37.6 ± 12.2)/s	1650 mmHg/s (1320–1880 mmHg/s) (37.6 ± 12.2)/s
Mean normalized systolic ejection rate (angiography)	3.32 ± 0.84 end-diastolic volumes per second	3.32 ± 0.84 end-diastolic volumes per second
Mean velocity of circumferential fiber shortening (angiography)	1.83 ± 0.56 circumferences per second	1.83 ± 0.56 circumferences per second
Ejection fraction; stroke volume/end diastolic volume (SV/EDV)	0.67 ± 0.08 (0.55–0.78)	0.67 ± 0.08 (0.55–0.78)
End-diastolic volume	70 ± 20.0 mL/m² (60–88 mL/m²)	70 ± 20.0 mL/m² (60–88 mL/m²)
End-systolic volume	25 ± 5.0 mL/m² (20–33 mL/m²)	25 ± 5.0 mL/m² (20–33 mL/m²)
Left ventricular work		
Stroke work index	50 ± 20.0 (g·m)/m² (30–110)	50 ± 20.0 (g·m)/m² (30–110)
Left ventricular minute work index	1.8–6.6 [(kg·m)m²]/min	1.8–6.6 [(kg·m)m²]/min
Oxygen consumption index	110–150 mL	110–150 mL
Maximum oxygen uptake	35 mL/min (20–60 mL/min)	35 mL/min (20–60 mL/min)
Pulmonary vascular resistance	2–12 (kPa·s)/L	20–130 (dyn·s)/cm⁵
Systemic vascular resistance	77–150 (kPa·s)/L	770–1600 (dyn·s)/cm⁵

Note: DP, diastolic pressure
Source: E Braunwald et al, *Heart Disease,* 6th ed. Philadelphia, Saunders, 2001, with permission

---

TABLE C-4 *Summary of Values Useful in Pulmonary Physiology*

	Symbol	Man Age 40, 75 kg, 175 cm Tall	Woman Age 40, 60 kg, 160 cm Tall
PULMONARY MECHANICS			
Spirometry—volume-time curves			
Forced vital capacity	FVC	4.8 L	3.3 L
Forced expiratory volume in 1 s	FEV_1	3.8 L	2.8 L
FEV_1/FVC	FEV_1%	76%	77%
Maximal midexpiratory flow	MMF (FEF 25–27)	4.8 L/s	3.6 L/s
Maximal expiratory flow rate	MEFR (FEF 200–1200)	9.4 L/s	6.1 L/s
Spirometry—flow-volume curves			
Maximal expiratory flow at 50% of expired vital capacity	V_{max} 50 (FEF 50%)	6.1 L/s	4.6 L/s
Maximal expiratory flow at 75% of expired vital capacity	V_{max} 75 (FEF 75%)	3.1 L/s	2.5 L/s
Resistance to airflow			
Pulmonary resistance	RL/(R_L)	<3.0 (cmH₂O/s)/L	
Airway resistance	Raw	<2.5 (cmH₂O/s)/L	
Specific conductance	SGaw	>0.13 cmH₂O/s	
Pulmonary compliance			
Static recoil pressure at total lung capacity	Pst TLC	25 ± 5 cmH₂O	
Compliance of lungs (static)	CL	0.2 L cmH₂O	
Compliance of lungs and thorax	C(L + T)	0.1 L cmH₂O	
Dynamic compliance of 20 breaths per minute	C dyn 20	0.25 ± 0.05 L/cmH₂O	
Maximal static respiratory pressures:			
Maximal inspiratory pressure	MIP	>90 cmH₂O	>50 cmH₂O
Maximal expiratory pressure	MEP	>150 cmH₂O	>120 cmH₂O
LUNG VOLUMES			
Total lung capacity	TLC	6.4 L	4.9 L
Functional residual capacity	FRC	2.2 L	2.6 L
Residual volume	RV	1.5 L	1.2 L
Inspiratory capacity	IC	4.8 L	3.7 L
Expiratory reserve volume	ERV	3.2 L	2.3 L
Vital capacity	VC	1.7 L	1.4 L
GAS EXCHANGE (SEA LEVEL)			
Arterial O₂ tension	Pa_{O_2}	12.7 ± 0.7 kPa (95 ± 5 mmHg)	
Arterial CO₂ tension	Pa_{CO_2}	5.3 ± 0.3 kPa (40 ± 2 mmHg)	
Arterial O₂ saturation	Sa_{O_2}	0.97 ± 0.02 (97 ± 2%)	
Arterial blood pH	pH	7.40 ± 0.02	
Arterial bicarbonate	HCO_3^-	24 + 2 meq/L	
Base excess	BE	0 ± 2 meq/L	
Diffusing capacity for carbon monoxide (single breath)	DL_{CO}	0.42 mLCO/s per mmHg (25 mL CO/min per mmHg)	
Dead space volume	V_D	2 mL/kg body wt	
Physiologic dead space; dead space-tidal volume ratio	V_D/V_T		
Rest		≤35% V_T	
Exercise		≤20% V_T	
Alveolar-arterial difference for O₂	$P(A - a)_{O_2}$	≤2.7 kPa ≤20 kPa (≤20 mmHg)	

TABLE C-5 *Normal Values of Doppler Echocardiographic Measurements in Adults*

	Range	Mean
RVD (cm), measured at the base in apical 4-chamber view	2.6 to 4.3	3.5 ± 0.4
LVID (cm), measured in the parasternal long axis view	3.6 to 5.4	4.7 ± 0.4
Posterior LV wall thickness (cm)	0.6 to 1.1	0.9 ± 0.4
IVS wall thickness (cm)	0.6 to 1.1	0.9 ± 0.4
Left atrial dimension (cm), anteroposterior dimension	2.3 to 3.8	3.0 ± 0.3
Aortic root dimension (cm)	2.0 to 3.5	2.4 ± 0.4
Aortic cusps separation (cm)	1.5 to 2.6	1.9 ± 0.4
Percentage of fractional shortening	34 to 44%	36%
Mitral flow (m/s)	0.6 to 1.3	0.9
Tricuspid flow (m/s)	0.3 to 0.7	0.5
Pulmonary artery (m/s)	0.6 to 0.9	0.75
Aorta (m/s)	1.0 to 1.7	1.35

Note: IVS, interventricular septum; LV, left ventricle; LVID, left ventircular internal dimension; RVD, right ventricular dimension

Source: From A Weyman: *Principles and Practice of Echocardiography,* 2d ed, Philadelphia, Lea & Febiger, with permission.

D | MISCELLANEOUS

TABLE D-1 *Body Fluids and Other Mass Data*

	Reference Range	
	SI Units	Conventional Units
Ascitic fluid: see Chap . . .		
Body fluid		
Total volume (lean) of body weight	50% (in obese) to 70%	
Intracellular	0.3–0.4 of body weight	
Extracellular	0.2–0.3 of body weight	
Blood		
Total volume		
Males	69 mL per kg body weight	
Females	65 mL per kg body weight	
Plasma volume		
Males	39 mL per kg body weight	
Females	40 mL per kg body weight	
Red blood cell volume		
Males	30 mL per kg body weight	1.15–1.21 L/m² of body surface area
Females	25 mL per kg body weight	0.95–1.00 L/m² of body surface area
Body Mass Index	18.5–24.9 kg/m²	18.5–24.9 kg/m²

TABLE D-2 *Radiation-Derived Units*

Quantity	Old Unit	SI Unit	Name for SI Unit (and Abbreviation)	Conversion
Activity	curie (Ci)	Disintegrations per second (dps)	becquerel (Bq)	1 Ci = 3.7×10^{10} Bq 1 mCi = 37 mBq 1 μCi = 0.037 MBq or 37 GBq 1 Bq = 2.703×10^{-11} Ci
Absorbed dose	rad	joule per kilogram (J/kg)	gray (Gy)	1 Gy = 100 rad 1 rad = 0.01 Gy 1 mrad = 10^{-3} cGy
Exposure	roentgen (R)	coulomb per kilogram (C/kg)	—	1 C/kg = 3876 R 1 R = 2.58×10^{-4} C/kg 1 mR = 258 pC/kg
Dose equivalent	rem	joule per kilogram (J/kg)	sievert (Sv)	1 Sv = 100 rem 1 rem = 0.01 Sv 1 mrem = 10 μSv

INDEX

Bold number indicates the start of the main discussion of the topic; numbers with "f" and "t" refer to figure and table pages.

Topical Contents